D0071842

Nursing

A Concept-Based Approach to Learning

VOLUME 1

North Carolina Concept-Based Learning Editorial Board

Pearson

Boston Columbus Indianapolis New York San Francisco Upper Saddle River
Amsterdam Cape Town Dubai London Madrid Milan Munich Paris Montreal Toronto
Delhi Mexico City Sao Paulo Sydney Hong Kong Seoul Singapore Taipei Tokyo

Library of Congress Cataloging-in-Publication Data
Nursing : A Concept-Based Approach to Learning / North Carolina Concept-Based Learning Editorial Board.
p. ; cm.
Includes bibliographical references and index.
ISBN-13: 978-0-13-507806-8 (v.1)
ISBN-10: 0-13-507806-7 (v.1)
ISBN-13: 978-0-13-510351-7 (v. 2)
ISBN-10: 0-13-510351-7 (v.2)
1. Nursing--Textbooks. I. North Carolina Concept-Based Learning Editorial Board.
[DNLM: 1. Nursing. 2. Nursing Care. WY 100 N9726 2011]
RT40.N87 2011
610.73--dc22

2009047837

Publisher: Julie Levin Alexander
Assistant to Publisher: Regina Bruno
Editor-in-Chief: Maura Connor
Assistant to the Editor-in-Chief: Deirdre MacKnight
Executive Acquisitions Editor: Kim Mortimer
Assistant to the Executive Acquisitions Editor: Marion Gottlieb
Editorial Assistant: Luz Costa
Assistant Editor: Sarah Wrocklage
Development Editor: Laura Horowitz, Hearthside Publishing Services
Director of Marketing: David Gesell
Marketing Specialist: Michael Sirinides
Managing Editor, Production: Patrick Walsh
Production Editor: GEX Publishing Services
Production Liaison: Anne Garcia
Media Project Manager: Rachel Collett
Manufacturing Manager: Ilene Sanford
Senior Art Director: Maria Guglielmo-Walsh
Interior Design: GEX Publishing Services
Cover Design: Mary Siener
Manager, Rights and Permissions: Zina Arabia
Manager, Visual Research: Beth Brenzel
Manager, Cover Visual Research & Permissions: Karen Sanatar
Image Permission Coordinator: Vickie Menanteaux
Composition: GEX Publishing Services
Printer/Binder: Courier Kendallville
Cover Printer: Lehigh-Phoenix Color/Hagerstown

Notice: Care has been taken to confirm the accuracy of information presented in this book. The authors, editors, and the publisher, however, cannot accept any responsibility for errors or omissions or for consequences from application of the information in this book and make no warranty, express or implied, with respect to its contents.

The authors and publisher have exerted every effort to ensure that drug selections and dosages set forth in this text are in accord with current recommendations and practice at time of publication. However, in view of ongoing research, changes in government regulations, and the constant flow of information relating to drug therapy and reactions, the reader is urged to check the package inserts of all drugs for any change in indications or dosage and for added warning and precautions. This is particularly important when the recommended agent is a new and/or infrequently employed drug.

Copyright © 2011 by Pearson Education, Inc., Upper Saddle River, New Jersey 07458. All rights reserved. Printed in the United States of America. This publication is protected by Copyright and permission should be obtained from the publisher prior to any prohibited reproduction, storage in a retrieval system, or transmission in any form or by any means, electronic, mechanical, photocopying, recording, or likewise. For information regarding permission(s), write to: Rights and Permissions Department.

Pearson® is a registered trademark of Pearson plc.

10 9 8 7 6 5 4 3

PEARSON

www.pearsonhighered.com

Volume 1:
ISBN-13: 978-0-13-507806-8
ISBN-10: 0-13-507806-7
Volume 2:
ISBN-13: 978-0-13-510351-7
ISBN-10: 0-13-510351-7

CONTRIBUTORS

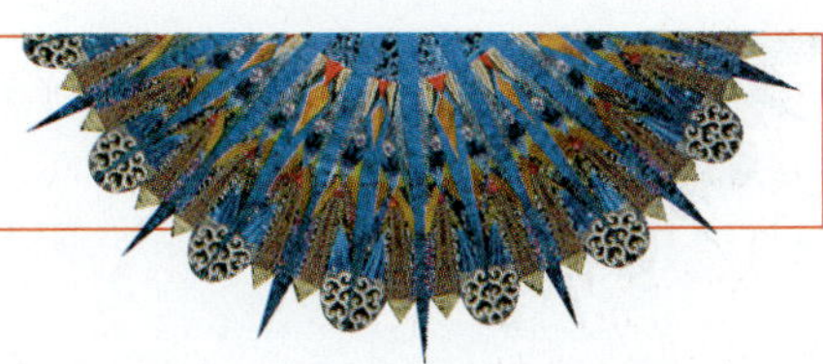

ADVISORY BOARD

Charlotte Blackwell, RN, BSN, MSEd
Wake Technical Community College

Carol Hardin Boles, RN, MSN
Surry Community College

Colleen Burgess, RN, MSN, APRN, BC, EdD
Healthcare Development, Community Outreach and Research
Catawba Valley Community College

Delia Frederick, RN, MSNEd
Southwestern Community College

Robin Harris, RN, BSN, MSEd
College of the Albemarle

Barbara Knopp, RN, MSN
Manager – Education,
North Carolina Board of Nursing

Katherine K. Phillips, RN, MSN
Guilford Technical Community College

Linda Smith, RN, MSN
Johnston Community College

Renee Taylor, RN, BSN
Robeson Community College

Kathy Williford, MSN, RN
NEWH Nursing Consortium

Linda Wright, MSN, RN
Western Piedmont Community College

CONCEPT CONTRIBUTORS

Catherine Borysewicz, MSN, RN, BC, CNE
Carolinas College of Health Sciences

Colleen Burgess, RN, MSN, APRN, BC, EdD
Catawba Valley Community College

Barbara Callahan RN, NCC, BSN, MEd
Lenoir Community College

Sheryl Cornelius, MSN, RN
Mitchell Community College

Rachelle Denney, RN, BSN, MSNC ECU 9/10
Fayetteville Technical Community College

Cathy L. H. Franklin-Griffin, RN, PhD
Surry Community College

Delia Frederick, RN, MSNEd
Southwestern Community College

Martha Freeze, MSN, ACNSBC
Rowan Cabarrus Community College

Barbara Knopp, RN, MSN
Manager – Education
North Carolina Board of Nursing

June Martin, RN, MSN
Forsyth Technical Community College

Debra S. McKinney, MSN, MBA/HCM, RN
University of Phoenix Online

Camille Reese, EdD, MSN, RNC
Mitchell Community College

Marilyn Springle, RN, MSN, FNPBC
Carteret Community College

Linda Wright, MSN, RN
Western Piedmont Community College

EDITORIAL CONSULTANTS

Bruce Goldfarb, BS
Writer

Laura S. Horowitz, BA
Editor
Hearthside Publishing Services

Adelaide R. McCulloch, BA
Editor

Debra S. McKinney, MSN, MBA/HCM, RN
Writer/Consultant

Nancy Peterson, BA
Editor

Kim Wyatt, BSN, MFA
Writer

FOREWORD

During the years of 2006–2008, the Associate Degree Nursing faculty in 55 community colleges were involved in a Curriculum Improvement Project, a collaborative restructuring and revision of the Nursing Education curricula. The outcomes of the Curriculum Improvement Project included a multi-institutional effort that led to the adaptation and implementation of one Nursing Curriculum Standard, which met the standards of all the accrediting agencies and reflected the advances in nursing and health care practices.

Nurse educators across North Carolina investigated issues concerning the large volume of content included in their curricula. The educators agreed that the curriculum was experiencing content overload. After much research and consultation, the statewide team decided that a paradigm shift from a content-laden curriculum to a more conceptual approach to curriculum development and teaching was appropriate.

Much time and research was devoted to identifying and defining the specific concepts to be included in the statewide concept-based curriculum. Best examples of each concept, exemplars, were identified using research data derived from the *Healthy People 2010* report, the Institute of Medicine, the Centers for Disease Control and Prevention, the Joint Commission, the National Institute of Mental Health, the National Institute of Health, the NCLEX Test Plan, Quality & Safety Education for Nurses (QSEN), etc. Using data from these organizations, the statewide team identified exemplars that had high incidence and prevalence throughout the life span, across the health–illness continuum, and in various environmental settings.

The concepts were arranged into the classifications of Individual, Nursing, and Health Care Domains, and the exemplars were assigned to the most appropriate concepts. The statewide project representatives assigned the identified concepts and exemplars to specific courses. In each of the concept-based nursing courses, concepts are presented across the life span, the health–illness continuum, and environmental settings.

Providing a concept-based curriculum is only a single component of the complete curriculum restructuring process needed in order to implement conceptual learning. By shifting from teacher-centered instructional methods to facilitating learner-centered activities, the students emerge from an active, learner-centered environment able to identify the relationship among exemplars and concepts. Using exemplars to facilitate a deeper understanding of a concept facilitates abstract thinking, promotes schema construction, and allows the learner to transfer knowledge to various situations. Once a student is able to understand the connection between and among concepts, then, and only then, can conceptual learning and deep understanding occur.

Many nurse educators from North Carolina made important contributions to the concept-based curriculum. Sincere appreciation is extended to all my professional colleagues throughout the community college system, who have supported the efforts of this work. As project director, I gratefully acknowledge the tireless, unselfish efforts of the Curriculum Improvement Project Steering Committee members: Carol Boles, Colleen Burgess, Linda Smith, Kathy Williford, and Linda Wright. Sincere appreciation is extended to Barbara Knopp, Manager—Education for the North Carolina Board of Nursing, for her support of the project. Dr. Jean Giddens provided invaluable advice and consultation with the Curriculum Improvement Project Team, and I will always be grateful for her significant contributions.

The standardization of the Nursing curriculum at 55 colleges in North Carolina was a collaborative effort of many educators. The search for conceptually written texts and resources was important to the educators as they envisioned the implementation of the new conceptual curriculum and the student-centered learning activities. It is with great optimism that this conceptually written text will meet the needs of nurse educators and nursing students, not only in North Carolina, but across the United States as other states are developing concept-based, standardized curricula.

—Charlotte E. Blackwell

PREFACE

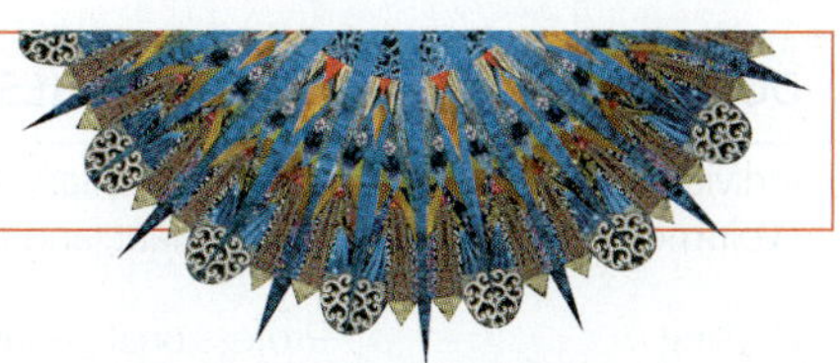

WELCOME!

Congratulations on your decision to enter the profession of nursing! While it will require much hard work, there is nothing more satisfying than making a positive difference in another person's life.

This textbook supports a brand new curriculum, which is the result of collaboration between the North Carolina Curriculum Improvement Project and Pearson Health Science, one of the nation's leaders in medical and educational publishing. Before beginning your journey in nursing, you'll want to know more about this textbook, which has been specially designed to meet the challenges facing nurses in the twenty-first century.

Nursing: A Concept-Based Approach to Learning represents the cutting edge in nursing education. North Carolina has designed the first concept-based nursing curriculum intended for use over the course of a Nursing program.

This curriculum offers a combination of traditional (text) and nontraditional (virtual) learning experiences. The textbooks to be used in the concept-based approach include the two volumes of concepts and a skills manual. The virtual learning opportunities include a computerized nursing kit with practical questions linking concepts together, case studies, and links to websites to further your learning. Individual schools also have the option to access Pearson's *The Neighborhood*, which is the brainchild of Dr. Jean Giddens. *The Neighborhood* is a virtual, web-based learning platform that presents a neighborhood of individuals from various professions and socioeconomic backgrounds with a variety of health alterations and concerns.

The goal of this textbook is to meet your needs and to help you learn and apply the knowledge you acquire to actual client care. This curriculum is dynamic and will be constantly revised to maintain evidenced-based practice. Those of you using the 1st edition have the unique opportunity to guide future editions. Students and professors working with this curriculum will have the opportunity to provide direct feedback to the NC Advisory Board and to Pearson Health Science. This feedback will help improve future versions of the curriculum and will be incorporated into the 2nd edition of this book—almost as soon as the first edition hits North Carolina classrooms. This is because both the NC advisory board and Pearson recognize that the curriculum and your textbooks must meet the changing needs of those using them.

Why Concept-Based Learning?

This curriculum began with a directive from the North Carolina community college presidents to design and implement a new curriculum for nursing programs. Nursing faculty from around the state, led by Charlotte Blackwell, RN, MSN, formed the North Carolina Curriculum Improvement Project (NCCIP). Together, project members examined a variety of resources, including:

- *Educational Rules for Nursing Programs*, 2007, which mandates conceptual teaching, improved utilization of technology, simulation, and evidence-based practice.
- The work of Dr. Jean Giddens, Associate Professor, the College of Nursing, University of New Mexico Health Science Center, an esteemed national nursing curriculum expert and the founder of concept-based learning in nursing.

Through extensive research, the NCCIP team realized the great benefit to students and faculty of a concept-based learning model. A concept-based curriculum sorts information into categories according to common characteristics and provides only the information and skills necessary for students to learn and apply the information when providing client care. For example, in one cohesive section, or exemplar, asthma is discussed within the oxygenation concept. In the exemplar you'll find information essential to providing culturally competent care to individuals with asthma across the life span: Pathophysiology, etiology, clinical manifestations, developmental and cultural considerations, and collaboration are all addressed. Older models addressed asthma separately in adult medical surgical classes, pediatric classes, and then again when studying geriatrics and obstetrics. Bringing all of the information together in one specific exemplar allows students to fully grasp the impact of asthma on a client in any stage of life and meet the nursing care needs of each unique individual.

How Is the Curriculum Organized?

After study and consultation with regional focus groups across the state, the NCCIP team decided on a shift in approach from the old medical model that emphasized the disease to a nursing approach that focused on active, collaborative learning. Through a workshop conducted by Dr. Giddens for nursing faculty from across the state, the team identified content for the new curriculum. Following agreement on the essential concepts, the team identified typical exemplars (the most

DOMAIN	COMPETENCIES
Individual (Volume 1 of text)	Developmentally appropriate client-centered care, collaboration, cultural competence, evidence-based practice, assessment, and communication
Nursing (Volume 2 of text)	Professional behavior, assessment, communication, clinical decision making, and other National League for Nursing Accreditation Committee (NLNAC) competencies for graduates of associate degree programs
Health Care (Volume 2 of text)	Quality improvement, evidence-based practice, informatics, and other elements essential to nursing within the health care system

important topics within the concept to focus on) that would facilitate the learning process for students. These were sorted into three domains of learning: individual, nursing, and health care. Each of these domains contains specific competencies and core elements that provide a comprehensive organizing framework for the curriculum.

Within each domain, the curriculum presents information that is critical to the practice of nursing. Each domain is divided into concepts, and each concept further organizes information into essential exemplars. Within the individual domain, the concept model delineates human systems of functioning, first describing the normal process of each system and then presenting common alterations from normal that are related to the system. These alterations are referred to as *exemplars*. For example, in the concept of oxygenation, the normal process of ventilation and gas exchange is presented, followed by five frequently seen alterations, or exemplars: asthma, acute respiratory distress syndrome, chronic obstructive pulmonary disease, respiratory syncytial virus/bronchiolitis, and sudden infant death syndrome. The information is provided in such a way that students will be able to apply information learned to other alterations in oxygenation in addition to those presented in the curriculum.

Further, the individual domain presents each concept with the underlying premise that no one concept functions without input from various other concepts. As such, this model provides opportunities for students to link concepts and their interactions together. For example, how does oxygenation link to the concept of perfusion? If I provide you with oxygen but your heart isn't beating to circulate the oxygen to the cells of the body, am I meeting your body's oxygen needs?

What Else Does This Curriculum Offer?

Nursing: A Concept-Based Approach to Learning offers a number of special features to help students acquire and use the information presented. These include the following:

- Assessment
- Alterations and Treatments
- Alternative Therapies
- Assessment Interview
- Care Settings
- Client Teaching
- Clinical Manifestations and Therapies
- Developmental Considerations
- Evidence-Based Practice
- Focus on Diversity and Culture
- Medications
- Multisystem Effects
- Nursing Care Plan
- Practice Alert.

Each of these features is further explained in the "User's Guide" section of Volumes 1 and 2 of this text.

The curriculum addresses traditional therapies and treatments as well as newer and alternative therapies. It provides information about diagnostic testing, assessment interviews, case studies and discussion questions, as well as critical thinking questions to promote linkage of concepts, helping students understand that no concept operates independently from other concepts.

SUPPLEMENTS

The following supplements are available for students and instructors.

Supplements for Instructors

INSTRUCTOR'S MANUAL AND RESOURCE GUIDE Each chapter in the Instructor's Manual is thoroughly integrated with the corresponding chapter in *Nursing: A Concept-Based Approach to Learning*, with detailed outlines and suggestions for classroom activities. The Instructor's Manual is available online on MyNursingKit.

TEST BANK Test Item Files with NCLEX®-style questions and complete rationales for correct and incorrect answers mapped to learning outcomes. *Available in TestGen and MS Word.*

Supplements for Students

NURSING: A CONCEPT-BASED APPROACH TO LEARNING SKILLS MANUAL With over 49 concepts, this skills book will ensure skills education is seamlessly integrated into the curriculum.

MYNURSINGKIT MyNursingKit is an online supplement that offers students book-specific learning objectives and practice tests as well as video clips and activities to aid student learning and comprehension.

MyNursingKit also provides instructors with easy and convenient access to important teaching resources, including detailed concepts for lecture and test banks.

Why the Inclusion of Virtual Learning Opportunities?

Nurses and clients alike are using technology more and more to gain access to information. In August 2009, the federal government announced $1.2 billion in grants to help hospitals transition medical records to electronic media. Today's nurses cannot function without advanced technological skills. In recognition of that, the NCCIP board and Pearson are designing new virtual learning opportunities to prepare students for the challenges they will face in the workplace.

Features to Help You Use This Book Successfully

Nursing students face challenges in their education—managing demands on their time, applying research findings, evaluating components of evidence-based practice, and developing their critical-thinking skills. Thus instructors and students alike value the in-text learning aids that we include in our textbooks to meet the challenges of nursing in today's world. We developed a textbook that is easy to learn from and easy to use as a professional reference. The following guide will help you use the text's features and resources to succeed in the classroom, in the clinical setting, on the NCLEX-RN® examination, and in nursing practice.

Each Concept begins with an **overview** of normal presentation and **exemplars** to help students navigate through the concept content.

The **Key Terms** and **Learning Outcomes** at the beginning of each concept highlight important terminology and provide an introductory overview of what will be covered in the concept.

Each Concept begins with an **"About"** section to give students a foundational introduction to the concept.

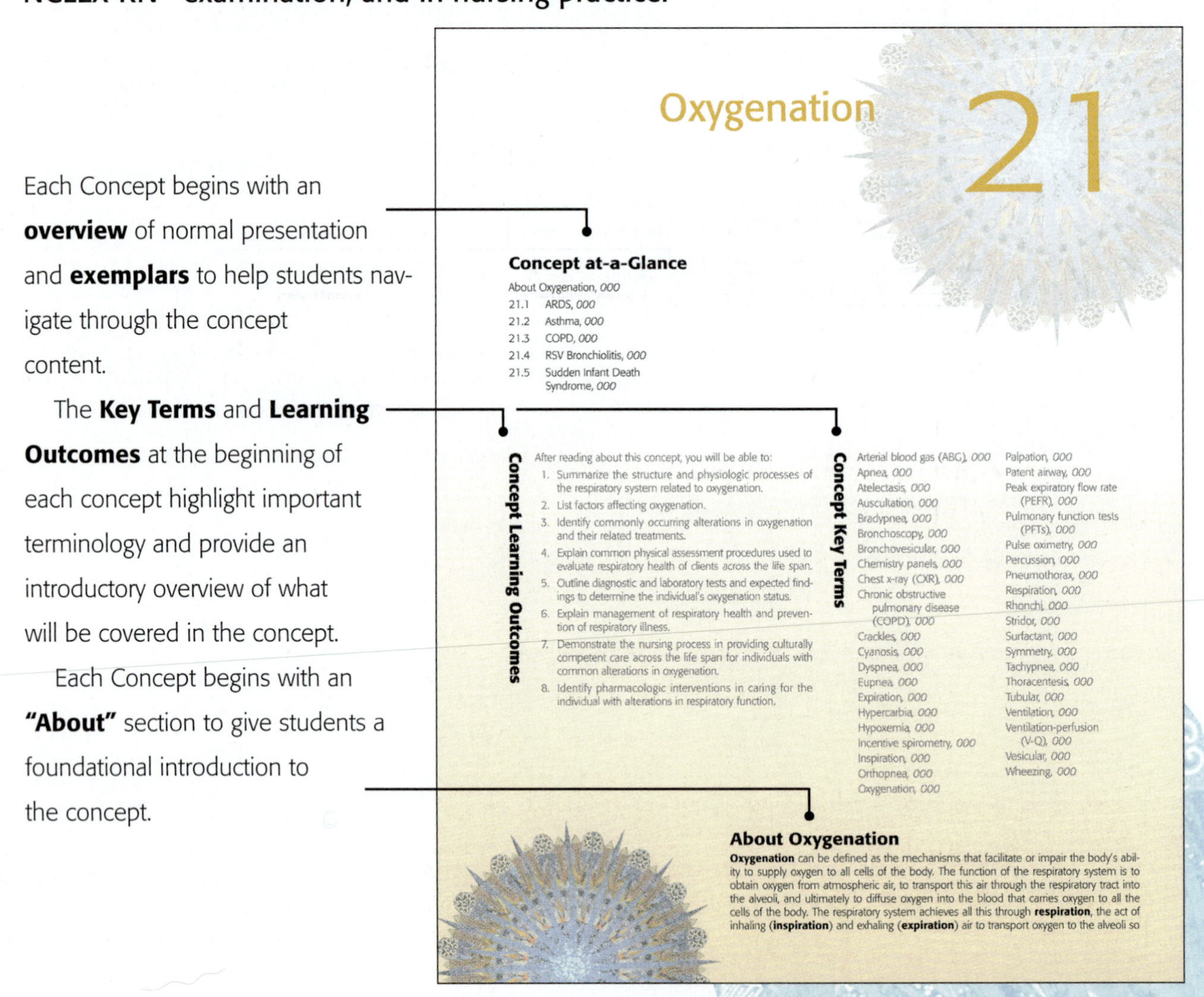

Oxygenation 21

Concept at-a-Glance

About Oxygenation, *000*
21.1 ARDS, *000*
21.2 Asthma, *000*
21.3 COPD, *000*
21.4 RSV Bronchiolitis, *000*
21.5 Sudden Infant Death Syndrome, *000*

Concept Learning Outcomes

After reading about this concept, you will be able to:

1. Summarize the structure and physiologic processes of the respiratory system related to oxygenation.
2. List factors affecting oxygenation.
3. Identify commonly occurring alterations in oxygenation and their related treatments.
4. Explain common physical assessment procedures used to evaluate respiratory health of clients across the life span.
5. Outline diagnostic and laboratory tests and expected findings to determine the individual's oxygenation status.
6. Explain management of respiratory health and prevention of respiratory illness.
7. Demonstrate the nursing process in providing culturally competent care across the life span for individuals with common alterations in oxygenation.
8. Identify pharmacologic interventions in caring for the individual with alterations in respiratory function.

Concept Key Terms

Arterial blood gas (ABG), *000*
Apnea, *000*
Atelectasis, *000*
Auscultation, *000*
Bradypnea, *000*
Bronchoscopy, *000*
Bronchovesicular, *000*
Chemistry panels, *000*
Chest x-ray (CXR), *000*
Chronic obstructive pulmonary disease (COPD), *000*
Crackles, *000*
Cyanosis, *000*
Dyspnea, *000*
Eupnea, *000*
Expiration, *000*
Hypercarbia, *000*
Hypoxemia, *000*
Incentive spirometry, *000*
Inspiration, *000*
Orthopnea, *000*
Oxygenation, *000*
Palpation, *000*
Patent airway, *000*
Peak expiratory flow rate (PEFR), *000*
Pulmonary function tests (PFTs), *000*
Pulse oximetry, *000*
Percussion, *000*
Pneumothorax, *000*
Respiration, *000*
Rhonchi, *000*
Stridor, *000*
Surfactant, *000*
Symmetry, *000*
Tachypnea, *000*
Thoracentesis, *000*
Tubular, *000*
Ventilation, *000*
Ventilation-perfusion (V-Q), *000*
Vesicular, *000*
Wheezing, *000*

About Oxygenation

Oxygenation can be defined as the mechanisms that facilitate or impair the body's ability to supply oxygen to all cells of the body. The function of the respiratory system is to obtain oxygen from atmospheric air, to transport this air through the respiratory tract into the alveoli, and ultimately to diffuse oxygen into the blood that carries oxygen to all the cells of the body. The respiratory system achieves all this through **respiration**, the act of inhaling (**inspiration**) and exhaling (**expiration**) air to transport oxygen to the alveoli so

The concept overview provides the **normal presentation** of the concept, review of anatomy & physiology, assessment & diagnostic tests, alterations from normal, generic nursing care interventions, developmental considerations, and general collaborative care. Each concept overview provides a comprehensive introduction to the concept for the beginning student.

in the alveoli sacs. These passageways for air dilate and contract. The trachea and larger bronchi are supported by C-shaped cartilage rings, as well as by smooth muscle. The smaller bronchioles are supported by smooth muscles only. Bronchioles deliver air to the alveoli. These air passageways dilate and contract as the autonomic nervous system regulates the smooth muscles supporting them. The movement of air within the bronchial tree creates a mixture of sounds of air flowing through a tube and the breeziness of the open alveolar lung fields. This is termed **bronchovesicular** sound.

The lungs are also described in terms of their lobes. The lobes lie obliquely in the thoracic cavity. The right lung has three lobes; the left lung has two lobes. The inferior lobes are the largest. Most of the inferior lobes lie in the posterior thoracic cavity. Each lung has a pleural lining to aid respiration and separate it from the other lung. The pleural lining has two layers, and a minute amount of fluid between the layers allows the structures to glide across one another during respiration.

The final portion of the lower respiratory system is the air sacs. The outcroppings of the air sacs are called alveoli. The alveoli are the portion of the lungs that fulfill the function of

NORMAL PRESENTATION

Adequate oxygenation of the body depends on a healthy, intact respiratory system. The respiratory system obtains oxygen from atmospheric air and transports it into the alveoli, where oxygen diffuses into a capillary and is carried by the blood to all the cells of the body. The respiratory system also passes carbon dioxide from the body.

The upper respiratory system is the inlet for air into the body. The nose is the typical inlet. The nose is midline on the face, with the same color as facial skin. The nose is divided into two nares that are moist, pink, mucosa-lined passageways. The purpose of the nares is to warm, humidify, and filter air as it is breathed into the nose. The upper respiratory tract has two protective mechanisms to prevent foreign matter from entering the lower respiratory tract: sneezing and cilia. Foreign matter that enters the nose irritates the nasal passages and induces sneezing. Sneezing is a reflexive action that clears the upper airway. This reflexive action is active even in the neonatal period. Cilia are microscopic fine hairs within the posterior portion of the nares that

DEVELOPMENTAL CONSIDERATIONS Respiratory Development

INFANTS

- Respiratory rates are highest and most variable in newborns. The respiratory rate of a neonate is 40 to 80 breaths per minute.
- Infant respiratory rates average about 30 breaths per minute.
- Because of the structure of the ribcage infants rely almost exclusively on diaphragmatic movement for breathing. This is seen as abdominal breathing, as the abdomen rises and falls with each breath.

CHILDREN

- The respiratory rate gradually decreases, averaging around 25 breaths per minute in the preschooler and reaching the adult rate of 12 to 18 breaths per minute by late adolescence.
- During infancy and childhood, upper respiratory infections are common but usually not serious. Infants and preschoolers also are at risk for airway obstruction by foreign objects, such as coins and small toys. Cystic fibrosis, a chronic disease usually identified in early childhood, is a congenital disorder that affects the lungs, causing them to become congested with thick, tenacious (sticky) mucus. Asthma is another chronic disease often identified in childhood. The airways of the asthmatic child react to stimuli such as allergens, exercise, or cold air by constricting, becoming edematous, and producing excessive mucus. Airflow is impaired, and the child may wheeze as air moves through narrowed air passages.

OLDER ADULTS

- Older adults are at increased risk for acute respiratory diseases such as pneumonia and chronic diseases such as emphysema and chronic bronchitis. COPD may affect older adults, particularly after years of exposure to cigarette smoke or industrial pollutants.
- Pneumonia may not present with the usual symptom of a fever, but may present with atypical symptoms, such as confusion, weakness, loss of appetite, and increased heart rate and respiration.

Nursing interventions should be directed toward achieving optimal respiratory effort and gas exchange:

- Always encourage wellness and prevention of disease by reinforcing the need for good nutrition, exercise, and immunizations, such as for influenza and pneumonia.
- Increase fluid intake, if not contraindicated by other problems such as cardiac or renal impairment.
- Encourage proper positioning and frequent changing of position to allow for better lung expansion and air and fluid movement.
- Teach the client to use breathing techniques for better air exchange.
- Pace activities to conserve energy.
- Encourage the client to eat more frequent, smaller meals to decrease gastric distention, which can cause pressure on the diaphragm.
- Teach the client to avoid extreme hot or cold temperatures that will further tax the respiratory system.
- Teach actions and side effects of drugs, inhalers, and treatments.

Source: Berman, A., Snyder, S. J., Kozier, B., *fundamentals of nursing: Concepts, process,* Upper Saddle River, NJ: Pearson Education.

Developmental Considerations boxes provide caring interventions throughout the life span for groups such as infants, children, adolescents, the elderly, and pregnant women.

For the concepts in the Individual Domain, there is a presentation of **physical assessment** techniques that includes both normal and abnormal findings to help students differentiate between the two.

Oxygenation Assessment

Technique/Normal Findings	Abnormal Findings
Nasal assessment	
Inspect the nose symmetry. Inspect the nasal cavity using a flashlight. The septum should fall midline and intact. The mucosa of the nares is pink and moist without drainage. Both nares should be patent. (see Figure 21–5 ■)	■ Asymmetry indicates trauma or surgery. ■ Redness and/or swelling is observed. ■ Deviated septum narrows or occludes one naris. ■ Foreign bodies may be found in the nares, especially of infants, toddlers, and preschoolers. ■ Purulent drainage occurs. ■ Watery nasal drainage occurs. ■ Pale turbinates are seen.
Thoracic assessment	
Measure respiratory rate:	■ Bradypnea ■ Tachypnea ■ Apnea
Assess quality of breathing: Determine regularity in timing I:E ratio is 1:2. Assess depth of inspiration. Observe effort to breath.	■ Shortness of breath ■ Dyspnea ■ Orthopnea
Inspection of thoracic cavity	
Anteroposterior diameter is half the transverse diameter. *Normal ratio is 1:2.* (see Figures 21–6 ■ and 21–7 ■)	■ Anteroposterior equals transverse thoracic diameter measurements, called a barrel chest.
Inspection of the muscles of breathing	
The chest walls gently rise and fall with each breath. The muscles in the neck are relaxed. The trachea is midline. The intercostal muscles raise the chest upward and outward with inhalation, then calmly relax with exhalation.	■ Retraction of the intercostals occurs. ■ Sternocleidomastoid muscles of the neck contract. ■ Posturing occurs.
...f the thoracic wall for symmetry	
...nds is observed with ...he chest wall. The tra-	■ Asymmetry of movement occurs. ■ Decreased expansion occurs. ■ The trachea shifts from midline.
... to the respiratory system	
...nation of the cell	Cyanosis is a blue tinge to the skin in fair individuals and gray coloration of the skin in darker pigmented individuals.
...inger and are normally ...il bed to the finger.	Clubbed nail beds have an angle of 180° or greater, depending on the duration of time an individual has had hypoxemia.

Assessment Interview Oxygenation

CURRENT RESPIRATORY PROBLEMS

- Have you noticed any changes in your breathing pattern (e.g., shortness of breath, difficulty in breathing, need to be in upright position to breathe, or rapid and shallow breathing)?
- If so, which of your activities might cause these symptoms to occur?
- How many pillows do you use to sleep at night?

HISTORY OF RESPIRATORY DISEASE

- Have you had colds, allergies, asthma, tuberculosis, bronchitis, pneumonia, or emphysema?
- How frequently have these occurred? How long did they last? And how were they treated?
- Have you been exposed to any pollutants?

LIFESTYLE

- Do you smoke? If so, how much? If not, did you smoke previously, and when did you stop?
- Does any member of your family smoke?
- Is there cigarette smoke or other pollutants (e.g., fumes, dust, coal, asbestos) in your workplace?
- Do you drink alcohol? If so, how many drinks (mixed drinks, glasses of wine, or beers) do you usually have per day or per week?
- Describe your exercise patterns. How often do you exercise and for how long?

PRESENCE OF COUGH

- How often and how much do you cough?
- Is it productive, that is, accompanied by sputum, or nonproductive, that is, dry?
- Does the cough occur during certain activity or at certain times of the day?

DESCRIPTION OF SPUTUM

- When is the sputum produced?
- What is the amount, color, thickness, and odor of the sputum?
- Is it ever tinged with blood?

PRESENCE OF CHEST PAIN

- How does going outside in the heat or the cold affect you?
- Do you experience any pain with breathing or activity?
- Where is the pain located?
- Describe the pain. How does it feel?
- Does it occur when you breathe in or out?
- How long does it last, and how does it affect your breathing?
- Do you experience any other symptoms when the pain occurs (e.g., nausea, shortness of breath or difficulty breathing, lightheadedness, palpitations)?
- What activities precede your pain?
- What do you do to relieve the pain?

Assessment Interviews provide students with sample questions to ask during an assessment, thus helping students to prepare for working with clients.

CLINICAL MANIFESTATIONS AND THERAPIES Eye Injuries

CONDITION AND ETIOLOGY	CLINICAL MANIFESTATIONS	CLINICAL THERAPIES
Corneal abrasion	■ Intense pain and redness ■ Photophobia ■ Tearing	■ Superficial corneal abrasions are diagnosed by touching a sterile fluorescein strip to lower conjunctiva; dye remains where corneal epithelial cells are disrupted. ■ Most corneal abrasions heal spontaneously. Antibiotic ointment may be prescribed and eyes patched in some clients.
Burns (Alkaline burns readily penetrate the cornea and are more serious than acid burns.)	■ Pain and/or complaints of "blindness" or vision loss ■ Swollen eyelids ■ Red, edematous conjunctiva ■ Cloudy or hazy conjunctiva ■ Possible presence of ulcerations	■ For chemical burns, eyes are irrigated, preferably with normal saline. ■ Pupils are dilated to reduce pain and prevent adhesions; after irrigation is complete, eyes are patched and antibiotics are prescribed. ■ Topical anesthetic is applied.
Penetrating and perforating injuries	■ Pain ■ Partial or complete vision loss ■ Possible bleeding or extrusion of eye contents	■ *Note: If foreign object is embedded in or sticking out of eye, do not remove. Immobilize object and protect eye until ophthalmologist arrives. Manage pain.* ■ Irrigation ■ Removal of object using a sterile cotton-tipped applicator or a sterile needle or other equipment ■ Application of antibiotic ointment after removal ■ Application of eye patch ■ Surgery
Blunt trauma	■ Pain and redness ■ Ecchymosis ■ Subconjunctival hemorrhage ■ Hyphema ■ Possible diplopia, enophthalmos ■ Personnel should be aware that retinal hemorrhage is a common presentation of the type of child abuse called shaken-baby syndrome.	■ Client is placed in semi-Fowler's position. ■ Eye is protected with eye shield; also, unaffected eye is patched to minimize eye movement. ■ A carbonic anhydrase inhibitor may be prescribed.
Subconjunctival hemorrhage (caused by coughing, mild trauma, or increased physical activity)	■ Reddened area in conjunctiva	■ Usually heals spontaneously; client should see ophthalmologist if most of sclera is covered or if condition does not clear up in 1–2 weeks.
Periorbital ecchymosis	■ Black eye or bruising of the skin around the eye	■ Ice is applied to eye area (both eyes) for 5–15 minutes every hour for the first 1–2 days after injury (even if only one eye is affected, both eyes may discolor); then warm compresses are applied beginning the second day after injury.
Foreign body on conjunctiva	■ Intense pain or feeling of something in the eye	■ Client must not rub eye; material on surface of eye is removed by closing upper lid over lower lid, irrigating or everting upper lid, visualizing material, and removing it with a slightly damp handkerchief; eye is patched and client transported to emergency department if foreign body cannot be removed.
Detached retina	■ Floaters: irregular dark lines or spots in the field of vision ■ Flashes of light ■ Blurred vision ■ Progressive deterioration of vision ■ Sensation of a curtain or veil being drawn across the field of vision ■ If macula is involved, loss of central vision	■ Prompt treatment to preserve vision ■ Proper positioning ■ Cryotherapy ■ Laser photoco ■ Scleral buckling ■ Laser therapy

Clinical Manifestations and Therapies

The basic clinical manifestations and therapies for the alterations are presented in easy-to-read tables.

Alterations and Treatments

Once the students understand the normal presentation of the concept, the chapter describes the commonly seen alterations from normal and possible treatments. This provides students with a general overview of the exemplars that follow.

ALTERATIONS AND TREATMENTS **Respiratory System**

Alteration	Description	Treatment
Chronic obstructive pulmonary disease (COPD)	COPD is a preventable, treatable disease of compromised airflow within the respiratory system. COPD is a progressive disorder that alters the structures of the respiratory system over time. Inflammation of the mucous membranes of the bronchial tubes occurs as well as loss of elasticity in lung parenchyma.	■ Smoking cessation ■ Avoidance of secondhand smoke ■ Administration of bronchodilators ■ Administration of corticosteroids ■ Use of breathing exercises ■ Respiratory therapy consult ■ Administration of pulmonary function tests ■ Spirometry ■ Complete blood count (CBC), chemistries, and arterial blood gases ■ Taking sputum specimen ■ Administration of oxygen ■ Physical therapy consult ■ Nutritional consult
Asthma	Asthma is a chronic inflammatory disease of the airways. Asthma presents with coughing, wheezing, shortness of breath, chest tightness, and sputum production. Asthma is defined in relation to severity and control as well as to impairments and risk.	■ Smoking cessation ■ Avoidance of secondhand smoke ■ Avoidance of aggravating factors ■ Respiratory therapy consult ■ Measuring daily peak expiratory flow rate ■ Administration of maintenance bronchodilators ■ Administration of maintenance corticosteroids ■ Exercise planning by physical therapy ■ Administration of short-acting bronchodilators for exercise ■ Measuring CBC, chemistry panels, and arterial blood gases ■ Taking a sputum specimen
Respiratory syncytial virus (RSV)	RSV is a highly contagious lower respiratory infection that affects nearly 100% of children younger than 2 years of age. Repeated infections of RSV occur throughout the life span, though subsequent infections tend to be milder.	■ Smoking cessation by caregivers ■ Avoidance of secondhand smoke ■ Separating sick individuals from well individuals ■ Observation of breathing pattern including, rate, rhythm, and quality ■ Teaching the parents or caregiver how to observe breathing patterns ■ Maintaining adequate fluid volume and calories ■ Oral and nasal suctioning ■ Possible use of bronchodilators and corticosteroids
Sudden infant death syndrome (SIDS)	SIDS is the leading cause of death of infants beyond the neonatal period. SIDS occurs most often between the first and the fourth months of life, but may occur up to 1 year of age. The cause of SIDS is not known. Infants who appear healthy are found dead by parents or caregivers. Preventive measures have reduced the incidence of SIDS in developed countries, including the United States.	■ Placing infant on his or her back to sleep ■ Smoking cessation by caregivers ■ Avoidance of secondhand smoke ■ Ensuring a totally smoke-free environment ■ Co-sleeper or same-room sleeping of infant and parents ■ Avoiding bed sharing ■ Maintaining adult-comfort room temperature ■ Breastfeeding ■ Using a pacifier
Acute respiratory distress syndrome (ARDS)	ARDS is a disorder with rapid onset of progressive malfunction of the lungs' ability to take in oxygen. Extensive lung tissue inflammation and small blood vessel injury occurs, followed by malfunction of other organs.	■ Measuring CBC, chemistry panels, and arterial blood gases ■ Taking sputum specimen ■ Administration of oxygen ■ Providing ventilator support ■ Administration of hemodynamic intravenous drugs

After students understand the possible alterations from normal in the Individual Domain concepts, the **Medications** box summarizes pharmacologic management commonly used for those alterations along with related nursing responsibilities.

MEDICATIONS **Pharmacologic Interventions: Glaucoma**

Drug Classifications	Mechanism of Action	Commonly Prescribed Drugs	Nursing Considerations
Antiglaucoma Drugs			
■ Prostaglandins	Drugs for glaucoma work by one of two mechanisms: increasing the outflow of aqueous humor at the canal of Schlemm or decreasing the formation of aqueous humor at the ciliary body. Many agents for glaucoma act by affecting the autonomic nervous system	■ bimatoprost (Lumigan) ■ latanoprost (Xalatan) ■ travoprost (Travatan) ■ unoprostone isopropyl (Rescula)	■ Assess and note eye color, presence of inflammation, exudates, or pain. ■ Note vital signs and most recent liver function test results because these may be altered by the drug.
■ Beta-adrenergic blockers		■ betaxolol (Betoptic) ■ carteolol (Ocupress) ■ levobunolol (Betagan) ■ metipranolol (OptiPranolol) ■ timolol (Betimol, Timoptic, and others)	■ Assess the client for allergies or contraindications to beta-blocker therapy, including asthma, chronic obstructive pulmonary disease (COPD), heart block, and heart failure. ■ Maintain pressure over the lacrimal sac after administration to prevent systemic absorption. ■ Assess for side effects such as bradycardia, hypotension, and depression. ■ Teach about the drug, its dose, administration, and desired and side effects.
■ Alpha$_2$-adrenergic agonists		■ apraclonidine (Iopidine) ■ brimonidine tartrate (Alphagan)	■ Assess the client for contraindications and adverse reactions to adrenergic agonists, including acute angle-closure glaucoma, hypertension, cardiac dysrhythmias, and coronary heart disease. ■ Assess for central nervous system side effects of anxiety, nervousness, and muscle tremors. If these side effects are severe, notify the physician. ■ Assess for a hypersensitivity reaction, including itching, lid edema, and discharge from the eyes. Notify the physician if you notice these signs.
■ Carbonic anhydrase inhibitors		■ acetazolamide (Diamox) ■ brinzolamide (Azopt) ■ methazolamide (Neptazane)	■ Assess for allergies or other contraindications to the use of carbonic anhydrase inhibitors, including known allergy to sulfa, or severe renal or hepatic disease. ■ Monitor for increased drug interactions of amphetamines, procainamide, quinidine, tricyclic antidepressants, and ephedrine

1.1 CONFUSION

KEY TERMS
Confusion, *15*
Delirium, *15*

BASIS FOR SELECTION OF EXEMPLAR
Standards of Nursing Practice
NCLEX

LEARNING OUTCOMES

1. Describe the pathophysiology, etiology, and clinical manifestations of confusion.
2. Identify risk factors associated with confusion.
3. Illustrate the nursing process in providing culturally competent and caring interventions across the life span for individuals with confusion.
4. Formulate priority nursing diagnoses appropriate for an individual with confusion.
5. Create a plan of caring interventions for an individual with confusion.
6. Employ evidence-based caring interventions (or prevention) for an individual with confusion.
7. Assess expected outcomes for an individual with confusion.
8. Discuss therapies used in the collaborative care of an individual with confusion.

OVERVIEW

Confusion is an alteration in cognition that makes it difficult to think clearly, focus attention, or make decisions. It may come on suddenly or gradually, depending on the cause. It can be a one-time event, recurrent, or a constant state of mind. The most important thing to understand about confusion is that it is frequently a symptom and not a diagnosis. Any number of things can cause confusion, including hypoxia, poor perfusion, medications, and disease. The onset of confusion requires thorough assessment to determine the causative agent and improve client outcomes.

Delirium is an acute disorder of cognition that affects functional independence. Confusion, a loss of orientation and memory, can occur in clients of all ages, but it is most commonly seen in older people. The terms *acute confusion* and delirium are used interchangeably by most health professionals, with nurses favoring the use of acute confusion and physicians the term delirium (McCurren & Cronin, 2003, p. 319). Confusion often presents with subtle symptoms, but an attempt should be made to differentiate between acute confusion (delirium) and chronic confusion (dementia) (Table 1–7).

PATHOPHYSIOLOGY AND ETIOLOGY

Delirium often has an abrupt onset; it can be reversed by treating its cause. This contrasts with dementia, often called chronic confusion, which has symptoms that are gradual and irreversible (e.g., Alzheimer's disease). Clients who are confused often know something is wrong and want help. It is important to pay special attention to sudden changes in mood or personality, as these may be signs of delirium related to recent changes in medication, onset of undetected illness, or exacerbation of chronic illness.

Age-related cognitive decline, resulting from slower information processing, mild memory impairment, and decreases in brain volume secondary to loss of some neurons place older clients at increased risk for confusion when they face additional stressors of illness, loss, or change in environment. Depression or other emotional problems can also act as stressors, increasing the likelihood of delirium. It is important to remember that delirium is usually caused by a treatable physical or mental health illness and, when treated typically results in full recovery. Delirium is associated with increased mortality, increased hospital costs, and long-term cognitive and functional impairment (Tullmann, Mion, Fletcher, & Foreman, 2008).

Etiology

Delirium occurs in 6% to 30% of the general hospital population and 7% to 52% of postsurgical clients (Edwards, 2003, p. 347). Delirium in the intensive care unit (ICU) setting is a common problem and has been described as sundown syndrome, ICU psychosis, and ICU syndrome. Delirium or acute confusional state, superimposed on Alzheimer's disease, was found in 8 of 20 older adults with documented dementia (Fick & Foreman, 2000). It is estimated that anywhere from 14% to 80% of all older persons hospitalized for the treatment of an acute physical illness experience an episode of delirium (Foreman, Wakefield, Culp, & Milisen, 2001). Unfortunately, delirium is unrecognized or misdiagnosed by both the physician and the nurse in up to two-thirds of cases (Hanley, 2004, p. 218).

It is not uncommon to think of older adults as the only people who become confused, but this is incorrect. Confusion can occur at any stage of the developmental process and may be caused by alcohol intoxication, low blood sugar, head trauma, fluid and/or

After providing the student with an introduction to the concept, a series of **exemplars** describe alterations from the normal presentation.

The exemplars are set up as discreet modules within the concept so that students can refer to them easily and work through the related learning activities. Each exemplar begins with its own set of Key Terms, Learning Outcomes, and Evidence-Based Selection Criteria for its use as an exemplar within that concept.

At the end of each exemplar module, the student can work through **Review** activities that help the student relate to other concepts, apply critical thinking, analyze case studies, and more. There is also a cross-referenced link to the **Companion Skills Manual**, which contains all the step-by-step skills for students to practice in the lab.

REVIEW Confusion

RELATE: LINK THE CONCEPTS

Linking the concepts of Accountability, Advocacy, Ethics, and Safety with the concept of Cognition:

1. What special responsibilities is the nurse accountable for when caring for a client who is confused?
2. How does the nurse advocate for the confused client?
3. The nurse is caring for a client who is confused and displaying trouble with decision making. If the client declines a treatment essential to obtaining a positive outcome for the client, considering the client's bill of rights, what is the nurse's ethical obligation?
4. What interventions are important for the nurse to initiate in order to maintain safety for the confused client?

READY: GO TO COMPANION SKILLS MANUAL

1. Applying body mechanics
2. Assisting the client with ambulation
3. Assessing appearance and mental status
4. Assessing the neurologic system
5. Bathing an adult client
6. Administering medication
7. Evaluating client safety

REFLECT: CASE STUDY

Clifford is a 64-year-old male who has been married to his wife, Pam, for 40 years. Their only child, 24-year-old Gary, has Down syndrome and lives with them. Clifford is a middle manager for a small manufacturing company where he has worked over the last 20 years.

Overall, Clifford is in good health, although he has recently been undergoing conservative treatment for benign prostate hypertrophy. He has a history of depression. He had a brief episode during college, for which he did not seek treatment. He had another episode shortly after Gary was born, and at the encouragement of his wife, he sought treatment, which consisted of counseling and antidepressant agents. He quit taking the medications after about 6 months and decided he would just learn to deal with depression on his own. Although he has had mild episodes of depression over the years since that time, Clifford has been unwilling to seek

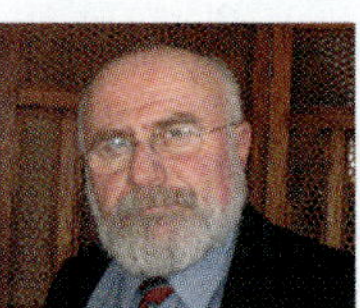
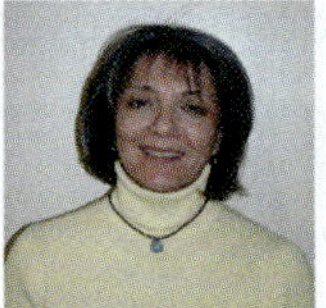
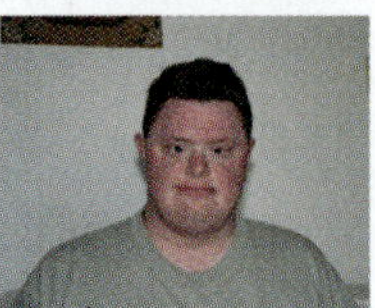

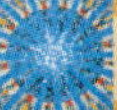

CLIENT TEACHING Fetal Alcohol Syndrome

Fetal alcohol syndrome (FAS) is a preventable cause of mental retardation. About 10% of women consume alcohol while pregnant, and 2% engage in frequent or binge drinking (Suellentrop, Morrow, Williams, D'Angels, 2006). This indicates that all women must receive clear messages about the dangers of drinking while pregnant. Teach all pregnant women that total abstention from alcohol for the entire length of pregnancy is the only completely effective method of preventing FAS. Include this in teaching to all adolescent girls, so they are aware of how alcohol can harm their infant if they become pregnant. Emphasize that the most dangerous time may be early in pregnancy before women commonly know they are pregnant.

Additional boxed features help students make linkages to other concepts, such as **Client Teaching, Focus on Diversity and Culture, Alternative Therapies,** and others.

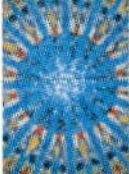

EVIDENCE-BASED PRACTICE Parental Presence During Procedures

Increasingly, parents are permitted to be present during medical procedures performed on their children. Previous resistance to parental presence has been based on the fear that parents would delay or interfere with the procedure, distract or increase the anxiety of the health professionals performing the procedure, or experience heightened anxiety of their own. Studies have investigated parental presence in various situations involving medical procedures such as anesthesia induction, intravenous (IV) starts, and resuscitation (Meyers, Eichhorn, & Guzzetta, 1998; Munro & D'Errico, 2000; Powers & Rubenstein, 1999). In most cases, parents are less anxious if they are able to be present when their child has a procedure, and the ability of health professionals to perform procedures is not affected (Lewandowski & Tesler, 2003; Sacchetti, Paston, & Carraccio, 2005).

The textbook highlights **Evidence-Based Practice** throughout to provide students with the research-based rationales for their nursing care interventions.

PRACTICE ALERT

To determine the impact of the child with mental retardation on the family, the nurse asks parents to describe (1) family activities that include the child, (2) strategies that parents and siblings use to deal with community attitudes about the child, and, (3) in the case of a child with other disabilities, methods of managing the child's care and planning for future care needs.

Practice Alerts integrated into the exemplars teach students about clinical implications that will help them be successful in their clinical experiences.

NURSING CARE PLAN **A Client With Glaucoma and Cataracts**

Lila Rainey is an 80-year-old widow who lives alone in the house she and her late husband built 50 years ago. She has worn glasses for nearsightedness since she was a young girl; she now wears bifocals to correct her near vision as well. She was diagnosed 4 years ago with chronic open-angle glaucoma, for which she takes timolol maleate (Timoptic) 0.5%. Recently she has noticed difficulty reading and watching television despite a new lens prescription. She has stopped driving at night because the glare of oncoming headlights makes it difficult for her to see. Mrs. Rainey's ophthalmologist has told her that she has cataracts but that they do not need to come out until they bother her. Although her glaucoma is still controlled with timolol maleate 0.5%, one drop in each eye twice a day, her intraocular pressure measurements have been gradually increasing. Mrs. Rainey has taken 325 mg of aspirin daily since a transient ischemic attack 8 years ago. She is being admitted to the outpatient surgery unit for cataract removal and intraocular lens implant in her right eye.

ASSESSMENT

Mrs. Rainey is admitted to the eye surgery unit by Susan Schafer, RN. In her assessment, Ms. Schafer finds Mrs. Rainey to be alert and oriented, although apprehensive about her upcoming surgery. Assessment findings include P 86, R 18, BP 134/72 . Mrs. Rainey's neurologic, respiratory, cardiovascular, and abdominal assessments are essentially normal. Her pupils are round and equal and react briskly to light and accommodation. Her conjunctivae are pink; sclera and corneas, clear. Using the ophthalmoscope, Ms. Schafer notes that the red reflex in Mrs. Rainey's right eye is diminished. Ophthalmic examination shows visual acuity of 20/150 OD (right eye) and 20/50 OS (left eye) with corrective lenses. Her intraocular pressures are 21 mmHg OD and 17 mmHg OS. On fundoscopic exam, no disease of the blood vessels, retina, macula, or disc is found. Ms. Schafer reviews the operative procedure with Mrs. Rainey, answering her questions and telling her what to expect after surgery. Following preoperative protocols, Mrs. Rainey is prepared and transported to surgery.

DIAGNOSIS

- Disturbed Sensory Perception: Visual related to myopia and lens extraction
- Anxiety related to anticipated surgery
- Deficient Knowledge related to lack of information regarding postoperative care
- Impaired Home Maintenance related to activity restrictions and impaired vision

PLANNING

Goals of nursing care may include:

- Regain sufficient visual acuity to maintain activities of daily living, including reading and watching television for enjoyment.
- Demonstrate a reduced level of anxiety.
- Demonstrate the procedure for instilling eyedrops post-operatively.
- Demonstrate knowledge of the home care she will require after surgery, signs of complications, and actions to take if complications occur.
- Use appropriate resources to assist with home maintenance until vision stabilizes and activity restrictions are lifted.

IMPLEMENTATION

- Provide a safe environment, placing the call light and personal care items within easy reach.
- Encourage Mrs. Rainey to express her fears about surgery and its potential effect on vision.
- Explain all procedures related to surgery and recovery.
- Instruct Mrs. Rainey to avoid shutting the eyelids tightly, sneezing, coughing, laughing, bending over, lifting, or straining to have a bowel movement. Teach her to wear glasses during the day and an eye shield at night to prevent injury to the surgical site.
- Explain and demonstrate the procedure for administering eyedrops.
- Provide verbal and written instructions about postoperative care, including a schedule of follow-up examinations, potential complications, and actions to take in response.
- Refer Mrs. Rainey to a discharge planner or social worker to help establish a plan for home maintenance.

EVALUATION

Mrs. Rainey is discharged the morning after her surgery. She is visibly relieved when the eye patch is removed because her vision in the operated eye is better than before surgery, even without her glasses. She is able to relate the recommended activity restrictions. Mrs. Rainey administers her own eyedrops before discharge and relates an understanding of the prescribed postoperative care and safety precautions. Mrs. Rainey's daughter plans to visit her mother two or three times a week to help with laundry and vacuuming until Mrs. Rainey can resume all of her household activities. Mrs. Rainey says that she won't "be so scared when I need my other eye done." She understands the chronic nature of her glaucoma and says that her vision is too important for her to neglect her timolol drops and routine eye exams.

For applicable exemplars, students learn to apply the **Nursing Process** and use **Nursing Care Plans**.

NURSING PROCESS

The goal of nursing care is to reduce the incidence of delirium in the client at risk and prevent complications in the delirious client. Routine screening for delirium should be part of the comprehensive plan of care for the older adult or the client at risk. Delirium can be prevented by recognizing high-risk clients and implementing a standardized protocol (Tullmann et al., 2008).

Assessment

Older persons do not develop dementia overnight, so any sudden change in mental status needs to be aggressively evaluated. Delirium must be ruled out because cognitive impairment caused by delirium may be reversible. The development of delirium may indicate decreased reserve capacity of the brain and signal an increased risk for dementia (Alexopoulos, Silver, Kahn, Frances, & Carpenter, 2004). To rate delirium and distinguish delirium from other types of cognitive impairment, the Hartford Institute for Geriatric Nursing *Try This* Assessment Series recommends use of the Confusion Assessment Method (CAM) (Inouye et al., 1990) (Box 1–3). The CAM includes two parts: Part 1 is an assessment instrument that screens for overall cognitive impairment; Part 2 includes only those four features that distinguish delirium. The

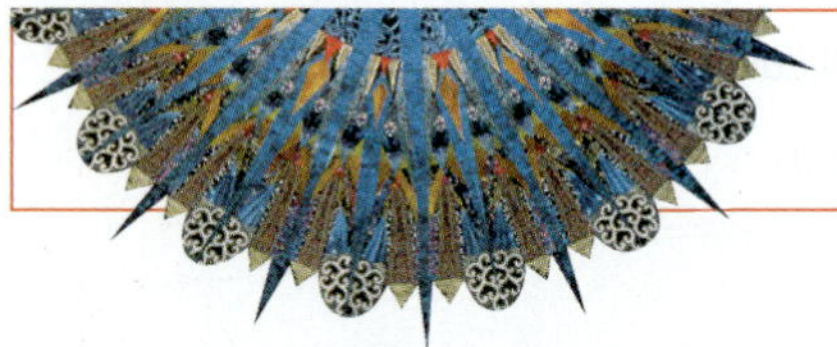

ACKNOWLEDGMENTS

The North Carolina Concept-Based Learning Editorial Board would like to thank the following people for their contributions to this project.

NORTH CAROLINA

The following groups and individuals working for organizations within North Carolina were instrumental in creating this product:

- The North Carolina Community College System (NCCCS)
- The North Carolina Board of Nursing
- The 52 ADN CIP representatives, along with Dr. Jean Giddens.

PEARSON

The following staff from Pearson, our publisher, guided this project from conception through final production:

- Julie Alexander, publisher; Maura Connor, editor-in-chief; Kim Mortimer, executive acquisitions editor; Marion Gottlieb, assistant to the editor-in-chief; and Stephanie Klein, director of development, conceived of this project and provided the vision, staff, and budget to make it happen.
- Deb McKinney and Addy McCulloch gathered all of the content and put it in a consistent, readable format.
- Hearthside Publishing Services and GEX Publishing Services turned our thoughts and manuscript into a beautiful book.

SOURCE BOOKS

The following authors from Pearson generously allowed us to re-purpose their work for this project:

- Priscilla LeMone and Karen Burke, *Medical-Surgical Nursing: Critical Thinking in Client Care,* Fourth Edition
- Audrey Berman, Shirlee J. Snyder, Barbara Kozier, and Glenora Erb, *Kozier & Erb's Fundamentals of Nursing: Concepts, Process, and Practice,* Eighth Edition
- Jane W. Ball and Ruth C. Bindler, *Pediatric Nursing: Caring for Children,* Fourth Edition; and *Child Health Nursing,* Second Edition, along with Kay J. Cowen
- Patricia A. Tabloski, *Gerontological Nursing,* Second Edition
- Linda Eby and Nancy J. Brown, *Mental Health Nursing Care,* Second Edition
- Patricia A. Wieland Ladewig, Marcia L. London, and Michele R. Davidson, *Contemporary Maternal-Newborn Nursing Care,* Seventh Edition
- Donita D'Amico and Colleen Barbarito, *Health & Physical Assessment in Nursing*
- Karen Lee Fontaine, *Mental Health Nursing,* Sixth Edition
- Michael Patrick Adams, Leland Norman Holland, Jr., and Paula Manuel Bostwick, *Pharmacology for Nurses: A Pathophysiologic Approach,* Second Edition
- Kathleen Koerning Blais, Janice S. Hayes, Barbara Kozier, and Glenora Erb, *Professional Nursing Practice: Concepts and Perspectives,* Fifth Edition
- Mary Jo Clark, *Community Health Nursing: Advocacy for Population Health,* Fifth Edition
- Carol Ren Kneisl and Eileen Trigoboff, *Contemporary Psychiatric-Mental Health Nursing,* Second Edition

REVIEWERS

The following nurse educators reviewed the concept and exemplar manuscripts. Their feedback was invaluable:

- Susan S. Barnes, RN, MSN, Guilford Technical Community College
- Charlotte Blackwell, RN, BSN, MSEd, Wake Technical Community College
- Catherine Borysewicz, MSN, RN, BC, CNE, Carolinas College of Health Sciences
- Colleen Burgess, RN, MSN, APRN, BC, EdD, Catawba Valley Community College
- Barbara Callahan, RN, NCC, BSN, MEd, Lenoir Community College
- Teresa Carnevale, RN, MSN, Lenoir-Rhyne University
- Sarah J. Clark, RN, MSN, CCRN, BC, Davidson County Community College
- Faye S. Cook, MSN, RN, Western Piedmont Community College
- Amy G. Crittendon, RN, MSN, CEN, Guilford Technical Community College
- Joyce Estes, RN, MSN, Catawba Community College
- Rhonda Evans, RN, BSN, MSN, Central Carolina Community College
- Amy L. Feaster, RN, MSN, Johnston Community College
- Susan M. Fowler, RN, BSN, MHS, Tri-County Community College
- Delia Frederick, RN, MSNEd, Southwestern Community College
- Gail A. Garren, MSN, RN, University of Phoenix
- Elizabeth Gwyn, MSN, Nurse Educator, Surry Community College
- Robin D. Harris, RN, BSN, MSEd, College of The Albemarle
- Barbara Knopp, RN, MSN, Manager – Education, North Carolina Board of Nursing
- Sarah J. Kulinski, RN. BSN, MA, MSN, Lenoir-Rhyne University, School of Nursing
- June Martin, RN, MSN, Forsyth Technical Community College
- LuAnn Martin, RN, MSN, EdS, Catawba Valley Community College

- Tara McMillan-Queen, AA, BSN, MN, ANP, GNP/RN, APRN, BC, Mercy School of Nursing
- Alisa Montgomery, RN, MSN, CNE, Piedmont Community College
- Tina Ntuen, RN, MSN, Guilford Technical Community College
- Amy Putnam, RN, MSN, Haywood Community College
- Camille N. Reese, EdD, MSN, RN, CNE, Mitchell Community College
- Lori-Ann Sarmiento, RN, MSN, Guilford Technical Community College
- Missy Smiley, RN, BSN, MSN, Wayne Community College
- Jennifer Sugg, RN, BSN, MSN, CCRN, Wayne Community College
- Allison Sutphin, RN, MSN, Cape Fear Community College
- Marie Thomas, RN, PhD, Forsyth Technical Community College
- Kathryn Thornton Tinkelenberg, RN, PhD, School of Nursing, Lenoir-Rhyne University

—Editorial Board

TO THE INSTRUCTOR

The education of professional nurses presents exciting opportunities for faculty and student learning. With the continual outburst of health care information and new technologies, faculty and students may feel they have entered a daily marathon without their best sneakers or a map of the route to help them reach the finish line. Tried and true teaching methods now seem antiquated as faculty compete for students' attention with a variety of new and engaging sources of information and entertainment. Add to this the overwhelming discovery of new knowledge in what has been known as the "information age" has resulted in nursing students feeling overwhelmed by the quantity of knowledge and skills they must gain in order to become practicing nurses.

Faced with these challenges, the 52 presidents in the North Carolina Community College System (NCCCS) appointed a team of nursing education experts to form the Associate Degree in Nursing Curriculum Improvement Project (CIP). The mission of the CIP was to develop a nursing curriculum to address contemporary nursing and workforce issues and to update the proverbial "paper map trail" into a "GPS system" to guide the future of nursing education within the community college system. Quickly the CIP embraced the idea of developing a concept-based nursing curriculum that utilizes today's multi-dimensional matrix of information, technology, communication, high fidelity simulation, and interactive virtual reality.

Recent education initiatives by the North Carolina Board of Nursing also reflect national initiatives and leadership. The Board of Nursing requires nurse educators in North Carolina to address current national trends, mandating conceptual teaching and improved utilization of technology, simulation, and the implementation of evidence-based practice in nursing. (*Education Rules for Nursing Programs, 2007*). An additional directive from the NCCCS was to design a curriculum that was learner-centered and allowed for the ready transfer of student credit from one college to another.

A final force behind the push for change came from North Carolina nursing workforce representatives and The Institute of Medicine's (2003) Task Force Workforce Committee. Both committees warned health educators that, due to the explosion of information and society's demand for technology, accountability, and responsibility, learning needs to be shifted to the learner.

The development of a new concept-based curriculum provides the impetus for educators to transition away from past, antiquated methods of faculty-centered teaching and passive learning and toward active, focused, participative, and collaborative teaching and learning. It offers the opportunity to equip nursing faculty and students with the knowledge and skills necessary to help them reach the finish line together—with the ultimate goal of increasing the competency and ability of nurses to serve the individuals seeking health care in the community.

THE PROCESS

In response to these multiple demands, the CIP Chair, Charlotte Blackwell, RN, MSN, in collaboration with the CIP Steering Committee and the 52 CIP representatives forged ahead to construct what is now known as the NC Concept-Based Nursing Curriculum. The CIP members set out to design a concept-based curriculum under the direction and consultation of Dr. Jean Giddens, an associate professor at the University of New Mexico Health Sciences Center, College of Nursing. Dr. Giddens is an esteemed national nursing curriculum expert and the original author and creator of concept-based learning in nursing education.

In addition, the CIP members consulted and worked collaboratively with Barbara Knopp, Manager—Education, from the North Carolina Board of Nursing Education, and Dr. Sharon Tanner, the National League for Nursing Accreditation Commission (NLNAC) consultant. The CIP members collected data about nursing, health care, and best practices at the national and state health levels. CIP members also conducted meetings and interviews with workforce representatives to elicit feedback about nursing and issues related to entry into practice for graduate nurses.

Faculty collected information from a variety of sources, including but not limited to: the NLNAC competencies for Graduates of Associate Degree Nursing Programs; The Institute of Medicine publications; The PEW Commission; The Joint Commission public health reports; The Institute for Healthcare Improvement; *Healthy People 2010*; Chronic Disease Management IOM Centers for Disease Control; National Center for Health Statistics; Quality & Safety Education for Nurses; and the National Institute of Mental Health. These are just a few of the resources to which faculty turned to inform their decision-making for this project.

As the curriculum began to take shape, a unique opportunity was presented to the CIP Advisory Board. Attuned to national health care initiatives, representatives from Pearson Health Science volunteered their assistance and technology, providing access to their national publishing experts to facilitate the educational transition of this innovative curriculum. Together, CIP and Pearson representatives formed an advisory board for the publication of the NC Concept-Based Curriculum. The practical task of this board was to collaborate and navigate the complex information matrix, and to design, organize, and present the new curriculum in a meaningful manner for students and faculty.

As part of the exploration of concept-based learning, Dr. Giddens presented *The Neighborhood* to the CIP representatives and later to the ADN Council Members. Organized around concepts, *The Neighborhood* presents a variety of families from various professions and socioeconomic backgrounds who interact with their local health care system in a series of stories, which are essentially detailed case studies. Dr. Giddens' labor of love and degree of commitment to the profession of nursing were evident in the presentations. Audiences of nurse educators were enthralled and excited about the learning opportunities presented with this cognitive, experiential, and affective learning pedagogy.

Demonstrating commitment to the CIP project, Pearson representatives negotiated with Jean Giddens to launch *The Neighborhood* along with the new curriculum to enhance concept-based learning activities. *The Neighborhood* is now a virtual, web-based learning platform that gives students and faculty access to its compelling cast of characters with their various health alterations and concerns. This new learning platform adds an invaluable dimension to the construction of knowledge and creates meaning for students and faculty through a combination of cognitive, emotional, spiritual, and developmental stages for the acquisition of knowledge in the art and science of nursing.

THE FOUNDATION FOR THE NEW CURRICULUM

A basic understanding of the development of nursing education standards, curriculum, regulation, legislation and official mechanisms inherent in the process of curriculum development is necessary for both the student and faculty. Only those processes inherent in the development of this curriculum are presented here. The process of the development of the CIP is described within the context of national and state health care trends, the IOM, The National Academy of Science, The National League for Nursing (NLN), and the North Carolina Board of Nursing (NCBON). The National Academy of Science is a non-profit collaboration of scholars engaged in scientific research to advance science and technology for the general welfare of society. By congressional charter, the Institutes of Medicine act under the National Academy of Sciences to identify issues of medical care, research and education (IOM, 2003). The mission of the NLN is to advance quality nursing education and prepare the workforce within an ever-changing health care environment. This curriculum was developed and guided by the NLNAC core competencies for graduates of associate degree nurses.

National Initiatives

The IOM report *Crossing the Quality Chasm: A New Health System for the 21st Century* (2001) called for an interdisciplinary group of health care providers to be convened to reform health care education. As a result of this report, in 2002 a summit of professionals from health disciplines and occupations was assembled. The focus of this summit was to incorporate core competencies into health education. The five core competencies identified through these efforts are patient-centered care, interdisciplinary teams, evidence-based practice, quality improvement, and informatics.

In addition to the IOM reports, as early as the year 2000, the NLN published the *Educational Competencies for Graduates of Associate Degree Nursing Programs.* This document outlines consistent expectations of nursing programs. It challenges nurse educators in nursing programs to facilitate student learning though more effective simulation, virtual learning, and clinical and classroom design, as well as to develop a research base for teaching and learning. Other challenges addressed in this report include advanced technology, increased acuity levels, decreased length of stay, managed care, diverse and multifaceted client population, and diverse settings. The report outlines eight core competencies for graduates of nursing programs: professional behaviors, communication, assessment, clinical decision making, caring interventions, teaching and learning, collaboration, and managing care. (NLN, 2000)

State Initiatives

In response to the IOM reports, the NC Institute of Medicine convened a task force on the NC Nursing Workforce in 2003. The Institute partnered with the North Carolina Area Health Education Centers, the North Carolina Center for Nursing, the North Carolina Hospital Association, and the North Carolina Nurses Association to address issues related to the nursing workforce in North Carolina. They analyzed the current and projected future demand for nursing professionals and paraprofessionals in the NC healthcare industry.

The task force focused on nursing faculty recruitment and retention, nursing education programs, transitions from school to work, and the nursing work environment. In addition, the task force identified that North Carolina needed to address retaining nurses in their jobs and the profession. The task force members agreed that *"all categories* of nursing education programs need to produce more graduates, reduce attrition, and maintain current high pass rates on the NCLEX-RN® exam…" Further suggestions included the development of a Comprehensive Articulation Agreement to improve transfer rates of nursing students from ADN to BSN programs.

The task force also identified nursing workforce goals including producing an adequate number of nurses to meet the state's needs, creating opportunities for nurses to advance education credentials, and elevating the overall level of education of the North Carolina workforce. Recent graduates, employers and supervisors expressed a need for transitional work experiences, such as clinical internships, for newly graduated nurses.

Concurrently, within the state of NC, the Associate Degree Nursing Deans/Directors expressed concerns that nursing courses were not easily transferable among all the community colleges and that some course descriptions did not reflect current nursing practice. The North Carolina Board of Nursing was in the process of revising the education rules for nursing education programs. The Board of Nursing mandated integration of the previously mentioned NC IOM "five practice competencies." At that point the Deans/Directors recommended that Wake Technical Community College in Raleigh, NC, request a grant to fund the Curriculum Improvement Project.

DESIGNING THE NEW CURRICULUM

The CIP grant was awarded to Wake Technical Community College. The Curriculum Improvement Project began with what Ralph Tyler in his classic text in 1949, *Basic Principles of Curriculum and Instruction,* suggested as imperative to curriculum development: a contemporary and current review of the literature. The CIP team's review included the documents previously mentioned, as well as other literature regarding nursing education and practice, education, and conceptual models. Tyler also emphasized (1969) the importance of developing curriculum that is relevant to the learner. The Project Director met with representatives of the North Carolina Board of Nursing to ensure that the curriculum would reflect current nursing practice. The CIP committee members reviewed the results of the state and national workforce initiative in nursing. The CIP Committee and Project Director formed Regional Workforce Focus Groups to identify industry, education, and learner needs.

Upon completion of the first review of current literature and direction from the North Carolina Board of Nursing Education Consultant, the CIP Project Director selected a concept- based model for designing the new curriculum. This concept-based model would incorporate the NLN's *Educational Competencies for Graduates of Associate Degree Nursing Programs.* Next, the CIP team hired a curriculum consultant with expertise in concept-based learning, Dr. Jean Giddens.

The committee embraced a theory of active learning and began with what Tyler (1969) refers to as "constructing." Concept-based learning is rooted in constructivist theory.

Constructivist Theory and Collaborative Learning

Constructivist educational theory is tied to cognitive psychology. This approach emphasizes learners actively constructing their own knowledge and meaning. Constructivism is the product of the work of numerous scholars, such as Jean Piaget, Jerome Bruner, Ernest van Glaserfeld, and Lev Vygotsky. Constructivism, which acknowledges that learning occurs in communities and groups, is the foundation of the collaborative learning movement.

Collaborative learning is at the core of any concept-based curriculum. Collaborative learning is also strongly based in constructivist theory. Learning is about making connections: Neuroscientists have discovered that the brain develops circuitry and grows as a result of experience and learning. Neurologists and cognitive scientists agree that humans build their minds by "constructing" mental structures and "hands-on" concrete application that connects and organizes information.

Andragogy

With this innovative curriculum design, a shift from pedagogy to andragogy is imperative. Knowles (2005) defines andragogy as "the art and science of helping adults learn." Basic assumptions of this theory include the following:

- Belief in the learner's ability to learn
- Learner control over objectives, strategies and evaluation
- Helping students learn for themselves.

Andragogy assumes that the adult learner is qualitatively different from the child or adolescent learner, and educators need to understand those differences. Key differences are (1) the adult learner is self-directing; (2) the adult learner brings a different quality and greater volume of experience; (3) the adult learner approaches the learning activity on a need-to-know basis related to tasks associated with adult roles; (4) the adult learner is problem- and task-centered; and (5) the adult learner's motivations are internal and include self-esteem, recognition, and a better quality of life.

The Whole-Part-Whole (WPW) Learning Model by Knowles (2005) also informed the concept-based curriculum. Whole-Part-Whole learning is a three-stage process. In the first stage, a framework or landscape of learning provides context for and is connected to the learner. In this curriculum, the first stage—or Whole—is the concept. The second stage—the Part—introduces the students to skills, techniques, and processes that constitute new learning. In the NC concept-based curriculum, this stage will be achieved through learning the exemplars of each concept and the skills and techniques provided through the skills manual and clinical experiences. The last stage—the second Whole—links individual parts to allow the learner to comprehend the complete content. The second Whole involves piecing and organizing traces, active learning, repetition, and learning from simple to complex. This will be achieved through the examination of case studies and individual and group student learning projects. The learner must master each part of the framework in order to achieve learning goals.

THE DOMAINS, CONCEPTS, AND EXEMPLARS

The CIP representatives from the community colleges attended a workshop presented by Dr. Giddens and identified content that was considered a "must" for the new curriculum. Dr. Giddens held an additional workshop with the Concept Group Committee to sift through the comprehensive list of imperatives discussed in the previous workshop, and to review, categorize, and complete them. Upon agreement of the essential curriculum concepts, the group members developed typical exemplars for each concept to facilitate learning. CIP committee members also solicited feedback from faculty at their colleges about the prospective curriculum design and content. Their list of selected concepts and exemplars was presented to the CIP Steering Committee.

Upon receipt of the concepts and exemplars, the CIP Steering Committee sorted the concepts and categorized them under the domains of nursing to organize and frame the massive amount of information. As a result, three domains emerged: the individual domain, the nursing domain, and the health care domain, all of which operate within the broader context of environment (See Figure 1). Each of the domains contains specific competencies and core elements essential for nurses entering the work force.

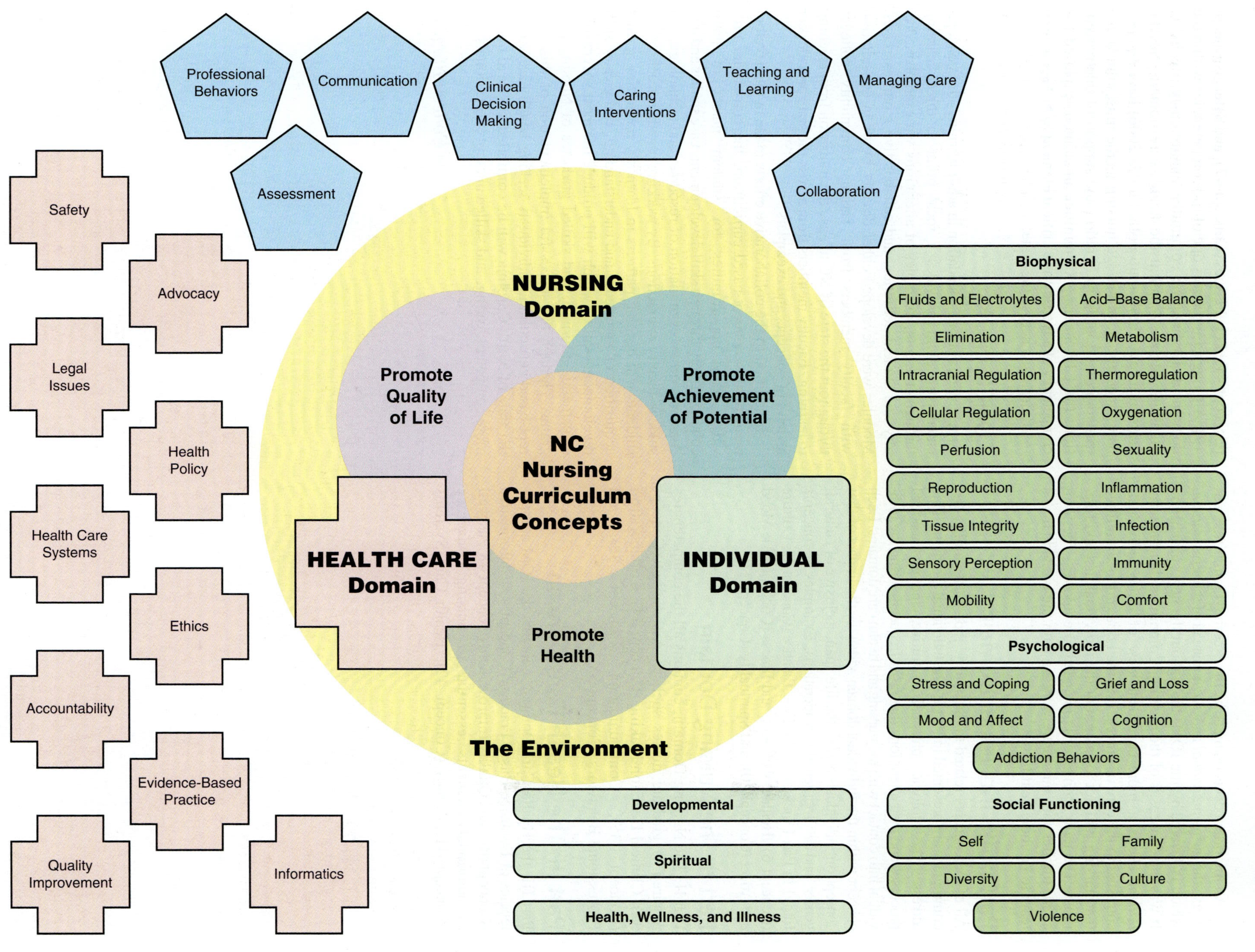
Professional Behaviors
Communication
Clinical Decision Making
Caring Interventions
Teaching and Learning
Managing Care
Assessment
Collaboration
Safety
Advocacy
Legal Issues
Health Policy
Health Care Systems
Ethics
Accountability
Evidence-Based Practice
Quality Improvement
Informatics
NURSING Domain
Promote Quality of Life
Promote Achievement of Potential
NC Nursing Curriculum Concepts
HEALTH CARE Domain
INDIVIDUAL Domain
Promote Health
The Environment
Developmental
Spiritual
Health, Wellness, and Illness
Biophysical
Fluids and Electrolytes
Acid–Base Balance
Elimination
Metabolism
Intracranial Regulation
Thermoregulation
Cellular Regulation
Oxygenation
Perfusion
Sexuality
Reproduction
Inflammation
Tissue Integrity
Infection
Sensory Perception
Immunity
Mobility
Comfort
Psychological
Stress and Coping
Grief and Loss
Mood and Affect
Cognition
Addiction Behaviors
Social Functioning
Self
Family
Diversity
Culture
Violence

An important decision made by the Steering Committee was to use the terms *individual* and *client* instead of the term *patient,* which is favored by the IOM, throughout the new curriculum. It was the consensus of the Steering Committee that the term *patient* elicits a more dependent view of those individuals entrusted to the care of nurses. It is the hope of the committee that nursing will not lose sight of the individual first and foremost. The term *individual* is intended to empower. The term *client* implies that nurses are working with the individual as a team to promote health.

Part I: The Individual Domain

All of the concepts related to the holistic individual, family, and community are presented in Part I: The Individual Domain. This addresses the biologic, physical, cognitive, and psychosocial processes and their alterations that most frequently bring the individual into contact with the nursing and health care domains. Each concept within the individual domain addresses the impact of that concept on individuals across the life span, inclusive of cultural, gender, and developmental considerations. Examples of concepts found in Part I include Acid–Base Balance (Concept 1); Culture (Concept 6); Health, Wellness, and Illness (Concept 13), Mood and Affect (Concept 20), and Spirituality (Concept 27).

Part II: The Nursing Domain

Part II, The Nursing Domain, contains all the competencies required of graduate nurses such as Assessment (Concept 32), Clinical Decision Making (Concept 34), Collaboration (Concept 35), Communication (Concept 36), and Professional Behaviors (Concept 38).

Part III: The Health Care Domain

Part III, the Health Care Domain, contains the IOM competencies of Evidence-Based Practice (Concept 43), Informatics (Concept 46), and Quality Improvement (Concept 48), as well as additional elements essential to nursing: Advocacy (Concept 41), Ethics (Concept 42), Health Care Systems (Concept 44), Legal Issues (Concept 47), and Safety (Concept 49). Although advocacy is one of the competencies within the domain of nursing, the committee unanimously decided to highlight advocacy within the health care domain. Several years in a row, the Gallup polls (2005, 2006) have reported that Americans acknowledge nursing as the most ethical and trusted profession. In recognition and support of this perception, the CIP Steering Committee unanimously placed the competency of advocacy as a critical element to be highlighted in all curricula across the state.

CONCLUSION

Armed with a strong foundation in adult learning, this concept-based curriculum provides a focal point to direct learning through concepts, examples of alterations via exemplars, faculty and student activities, and collaborative group exercises. Modules were developed either directly by or in consultation with faculty members from various community colleges throughout the state of NC to ease the transition from teaching to learning. Faculty members from across the state provide peer reviews of concepts and exemplars.

In addition to the collaborative efforts made in the development of this concept-based curriculum, the curriculum provides many opportunities for student nurses to learn collaboratively through skill development, case studies and discussions, group examination of resources and technology, and student–faculty interactions. By working together, teachers and students will become partners in learning, promoting greater acquisition of knowledge and understanding, and greater skill development—all of which will produce the most successful, empathetic, informed, and skilled graduates of Nursing programs. Through the successful implementation of this concept-based curriculum, individuals seeking health care across the state of North Carolina will be comforted and cared for by more competent, caring, and skilled nursing professionals.

—Colleen Burgess

CONTENTS

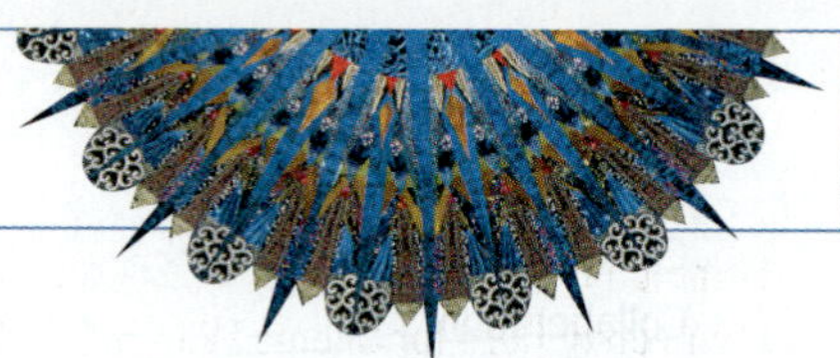

SPECIAL FEATURES

ASSESSMENT

ALTERATIONS AND TREATMENTS

ALTERNATIVE THERAPIES

ASSESSMENT INTERVIEW

CARE SETTINGS

CLIENT TEACHING

CLINICAL MANIFESTATIONS AND THERAPIES

DEVELOPMENTAL CONSIDERATIONS

EVIDENCE-BASED PRACTICE

FAMILY TEACHING

FOCUS ON DIVERSITY AND CULTURE

IMMUNIZATIONS

MEDICATIONS

MULTISYSTEM EFFECTS

NURSING CARE PLAN

The Individual Domain

PART 1

Part I contains the concepts related to the holistic individual, family, and community. The individual domain addresses the biologic, physical, cognitive, and psychosocial processes and their alterations that most frequently bring the individual into contact with the nursing and health care domains. Each concept within the individual domain addresses the impact of that concept on individuals across the life span, inclusive of cultural, gender, and developmental considerations.

Acid–Base Balance 1

Concept at-a-Glance

Concept Learning Outcomes

After reading about this concept, you will be able to:

1. Summarize the structure and physiological processes of the acid–base regulatory systems related to acid–base balance.
2. List factors affecting acid–base balance.
3. Identify commonly occurring alterations in acid–base balance and their related treatments.
4. Explain common physical assessment procedures used to examine acid–base health of clients across the life span.
5. Outline diagnostic and laboratory tests to determine the individual's acid–base status.
6. Explain management of acid–base balance and prevention of imbalances.
7. Demonstrate the nursing process in providing culturally competent and caring interventions across the life span for individuals with common alterations in acid–base balance.
8. Identify pharmacological interventions in caring for the individual with alterations in acid–base balance.

Concept Key Terms

Acidosis, *4*
Acids, *3*
Alkalis, *3*
Alkalosis, *4*
Arterial blood gases (ABGs), *5*
Base excess (BE), *5*
Bases, *3*
Buffers, *4*
Hypercapnia, *5*
Hypocapnia, *5*
Hypoxemia, *5*
$PaCO_2$, *5*
PaO_2, *5*
pH, *3*
Serum bicarbonate, *5*
Volatile acid, *4*

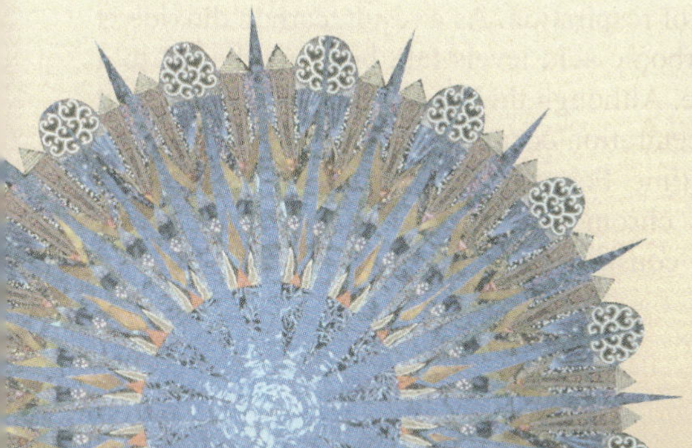

About Acid–Base Balance

Acid–base balance is critical to homeostasis and optimal cellular function. To maintain acid–base balance, the hydrogen ion (H^+) concentration of body fluids must be kept within a relatively narrow range. Hydrogen ions determine the relative acidity of body fluids. **Acids** release hydrogen ions in solution; **bases** (or **alkalis**) accept hydrogen ions in solution. The hydrogen ion concentration of a solution is measured as its **pH**. The relationship between hydrogen ion concentration and pH is inverse: As hydrogen ion concentration increases, the pH falls, and the solution becomes more acidic; as hydrogen ion concentration falls, the pH rises, and the solution becomes more alkaline or basic. The normal pH of body fluids is slightly basic, ranging from 7.35–7.45. (A pH of 7 is neutral.) Normal pH indicates acid–base balance.

Acid–base imbalance can result from any one of several underlying causes and can be an important clue in diagnosing illness or disease. Failure to restore acid–base balance can lead to impairment of organs and critical bodily functions. The body's tolerance for alterations in acid–base levels is very narrow and if pH drops below 7.00 or above 7.6 for even a short time it can quickly result in death. •

REGULATION OF ACID–BASE BALANCE

Metabolic processes in the body continuously produce acids, which fall into two categories: volatile and nonvolatile acids. A **volatile acid** can be eliminated from the body as a gas. Carbonic acid (H_2CO_3) is the only volatile acid produced in the body. It dissociates (separates) into carbon dioxide (CO_2) and water (H_2O); the carbon dioxide is then eliminated through the lungs. All other acids produced in the body are *nonvolatile acids* that must be metabolized or excreted in fluid. Examples include lactic acid (resulting from cellular destruction), hydrochloric acid (found in stomach secretions), phosphoric acid (from the oxidation of phospholipids and phosphoproteins), and sulfuric acid (formed from oxidation of sulfur containing amino acids). Most acids and bases in the body are weak; that is, they neither release nor accept a significant amount of hydrogen ions.

Despite the body's continuous acid production, three systems work together to maintain pH within a normal range: buffer systems, the respiratory system, and the renal system.

Buffer Systems

Buffers are substances that prevent major changes in pH by releasing hydrogen ions. When excess acid is present in body fluid, buffers bind with hydrogen ions to minimize the change in pH. If body fluids become too basic or alkaline, buffers release hydrogen ions, restoring the pH. Although buffers act within a fraction of a second, their capacity to maintain pH is limited. The body's major buffer systems are the bicarbonate–carbonic acid buffer system, the phosphate buffer system, and protein buffers.

The bicarbonate–carbonic acid buffer system can be illustrated by the following equation:

$$CO_2 + H_2O \leftrightarrow H_2CO_3 \leftrightarrow H^+ + HCO_3^-$$

The normal serum bicarbonate level is 24 mEq/L, whereas that of carbonic acid is 1.2 mEq/L. Thus, the ratio of bicarbonate (HCO_3^-) to carbonic acid (H_2CO_3) is 20:1. Although the amounts of bicarbonate and carbonic acid in the body vary to a certain extent, as long as this ratio is maintained, the pH remains within the 7.35–7.45 range (Figure 1–1 ■).

Bicarbonate (HCO_3^-) is a weak base; when an acid is added to the system, the hydrogen ion in the acid combines with bicarbonate and the pH changes only slightly. Carbonic acid (H_2CO_3) is a weak acid produced when carbon dioxide dissolves in water. When a base is added to the system, it combines with carbonic acid and the pH remains within the normal range.

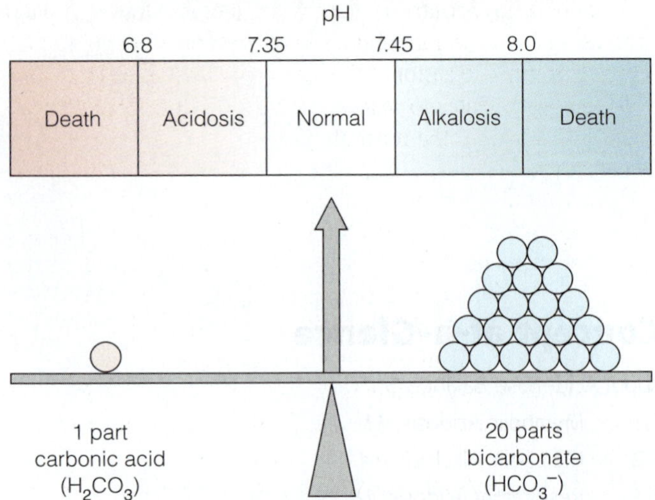

Figure 1–1 ■ The normal ratio of bicarbonate to carbonic acid is 20:1. As long as this ratio is maintained, the pH remains within the normal range of 7.35–7.45.

Adding a strong acid to extracellular fluid (ECF) depletes bicarbonate, changing the 20:1 ratio and causing the pH to drop below 7.35. This is known as **acidosis**. Adding a strong base depletes carbonic acid as it combines with the base, again disrupting the 20:1 ratio. The pH rises above 7.45, a condition known as **alkalosis**.

Inorganic phosphates also serve as extracellular buffers, although their roles are not as important as the bicarbonate–carbonic acid buffer system. Phosphates are, however, important intracellular buffers, helping to maintain a stable pH within the cells. Intracellular and plasma proteins also serve as buffers. Plasma proteins contribute to buffering of ECFs. Proteins in intracellular fluid provide extensive buffering for organic acids produced by cellular metabolism. In red blood cells, hemoglobin acts as a buffer for hydrogen ion when carbonic acid dissociates.

Respiratory System

The respiratory system (and the brain's respiratory center) regulates carbonic acid by eliminating or retaining carbon dioxide. Carbon dioxide is a potential acid; when combined with water, it forms carbonic acid (see previous equation), a volatile acid. Acute increases in carbon dioxide or hydrogen ions in the blood stimulate the brain's respiratory center, increasing both the rate and depth of respiration. As a result, carbon dioxide is eliminated and carbonic acid levels fall, bringing the pH to a more normal range. Although this compensation for increased hydrogen ion concentration occurs within minutes, it becomes less effective over time. For example, clients with chronic lung disease (such as chronic obstructive pulmonary disease, COPD) may have consistently high carbon dioxide levels in their blood.

Alkalosis, by contrast, depresses the respiratory center, decreasing both the rate and depth of respiration and causing carbon dioxide retention. The retained carbon dioxide then combines with water to restore carbonic acid levels and bring the pH back within the normal range.

Renal System

The renal system is responsible for the long-term regulation of acid–base balance. The kidneys normally eliminate excess nonvolatile acids produced during metabolism. The kidneys also regulate bicarbonate levels in ECF by regenerating or reabsorbing bicarbonate ions in the renal tubules. Although the kidneys respond more slowly to changes in pH (over hours to days), they can generate bicarbonate and selectively excrete or retain hydrogen ions as needed. In acidosis, when excess hydrogen ion is present and the pH falls, the kidneys excrete hydrogen ions and retain bicarbonate. In alkalosis, the kidneys retain hydrogen ions and excrete bicarbonate to restore acid–base balance.

NORMAL PRESENTATION

The **$PaCO_2$** measures the pressure exerted by dissolved carbon dioxide in the blood and reflects the respiratory component of acid–base regulation and balance because it is regulated by the lungs. The normal value is 35–45 mmHg. A $PaCO_2$ of less than 35 mmHg is known as **hypocapnia**; a $PaCO_2$ greater than 45 mmHg is known as **hypercapnia**.

PRACTICE ALERT

The abbreviations $PaCO_2$ and PaO_2 are used interchangeably with PCO_2 and PO_2. The *P* stands for partial pressure: the pressure exerted by the gas dissolved in the blood. The *a* indicates that the sample is arterial blood. Because these measurements are rarely done on venous or capillary blood, the *a* is often deleted from the abbreviation.

The **PaO_2** is a measure of the pressure exerted by oxygen that is dissolved in the plasma. Only about 3% of oxygen in the blood is transported in solution; most is combined with hemoglobin. However, it is the dissolved oxygen that is available to the cells for metabolism. As dissolved oxygen diffuses out of plasma into the tissues, more is released from hemoglobin. The normal value for PaO_2 is 80–100 mmHg. A PaO_2 of less than 80 mmHg is indicative of **hypoxemia**. The PaO_2 is valuable for evaluating respiratory function, but it is not used as a primary measurement in determining acid–base status.

The **serum bicarbonate** (HCO_3^-) reflects the renal regulation of acid–base balance. The normal HCO_3^- value is 22–26 mEq/L.

The **base excess (BE)** is a calculated value also known as *buffer base capacity.* The BE measures substances that can accept or combine with hydrogen ions. It reflects the degree of acid–base imbalance by indicating the status of the body's total buffering capacity. It represents the amount of acid or base that must be added to a blood sample to achieve a pH of 7.4. This is essentially a measure of increased or decreased bicarbonate. The normal value for BE for arterial blood is –3.0–+3.0.

Acid–base balance is assessed primarily by measuring **arterial blood gases (ABGs)**. Arterial blood is most often used because it reflects acid–base balance throughout the entire body better than venous or capillary blood that has dispersed oxygen into the tissues and collected carbon dioxide. However, capillary or venous blood gases are occassionally ordered when frequent ABGs have resulted in damage to normal arterial gas sampling sites. Arterial blood also provides information about the effectiveness of the lungs in oxygenating blood. See Appendix B for information on normal and abnormal values and on how to evaluate ABG measurements.

ALTERATIONS

Acid–base imbalances fall into two major categories: acidosis and alkalosis. As noted previously, acidosis occurs when the hydrogen ion concentration increases above normal (pH below 7.35). Alkalosis occurs when the hydrogen ion concentration falls below normal (pH above 7.45).

Acid–base imbalances are further classified as *metabolic* or *respiratory* disorders. In metabolic disorders, the primary change is in the concentration of bicarbonate. In *metabolic acidosis*, the amount of bicarbonate is decreased in relation to the amount of acid in the body (Figure 1–2A ■). It can develop as a result of abnormal bicarbonate losses or as a result of excess nonvolatile acids in the body. The pH falls below 7.35, and the bicarbonate concentration is less than 22 mEq/L. *Metabolic alkalosis*, by contrast, occurs when there is an excess of bicarbonate in relation to the amount of hydrogen ion (Figure 1–2B). The pH is above 7.45, and the bicarbonate concentration is greater than 26 mEq/L.

In respiratory disorders, the primary change is in the concentration of carbonic acid. *Respiratory acidosis* occurs when carbon dioxide is retained, increasing the amount of carbonic acid in the body (Figure 1–3A ■). As a result, the pH falls to less than 7.35, and the $PaCO_2$ is greater than 45 mmHg. When too much carbon dioxide is lost, carbonic acid levels fall and *respiratory alkalosis* develops (Figure 1–3B). The pH rises to above 7.45, and the $PaCO_2$ is less than 35 mmHg. It is important to remember that any condition that causes hypoventilation may result in respiratory acidosis and hypoxemia, while any condition that causes hyperventilation often results in respiratory alkalosis.

Acid–base disorders are further defined as *primary* (simple) and *mixed.* Primary disorders usually are due to one cause. For example, respiratory failure often causes respiratory acidosis due to retained carbon dioxide; renal failure usually causes metabolic acidosis due to retained hydrogen ion and impaired bicarbonate production. Table 1–1 summarizes primary acid–base imbalances with common causes of each. Mixed disorders occur from combinations of respiratory and metabolic disturbances. For example, a client in cardiac arrest develops a mixed respiratory and metabolic acidosis due to lack of ventilation (and retained CO_2) and hypoxia of body tissues that leads to anaerobic metabolism and acid by-products (excess nonvolatile acids).

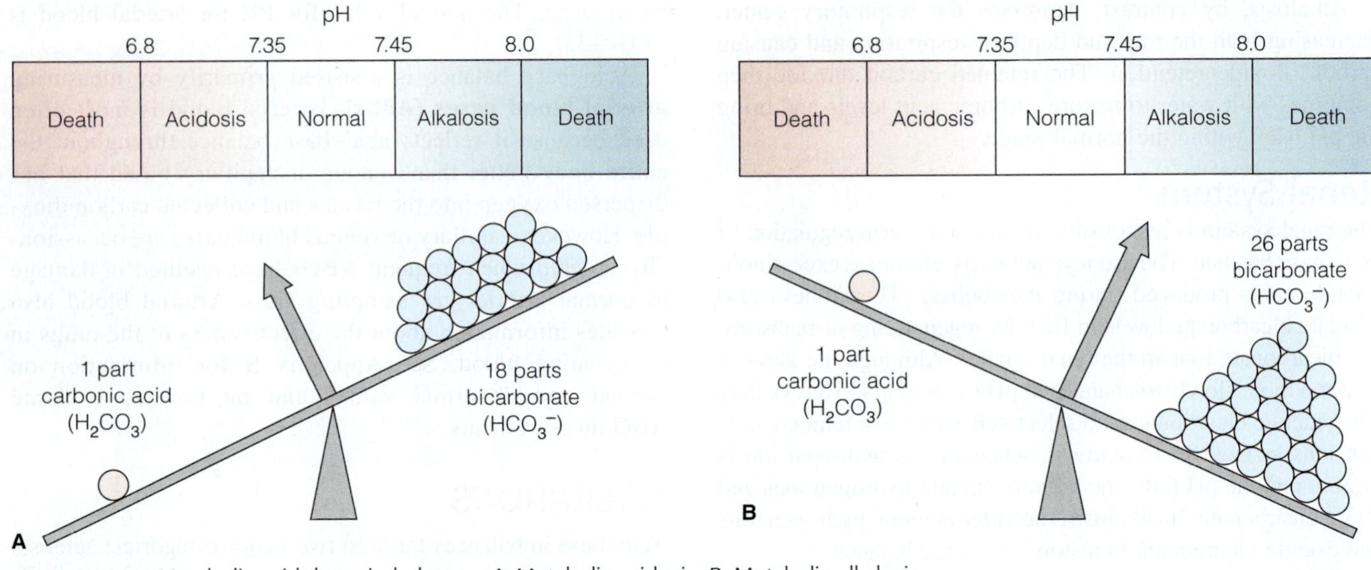

Figure 1–2 ■ Metabolic acid–base imbalances. *A,* Metabolic acidosis. *B,* Metabolic alkalosis.

ALTERATIONS AND TREATMENTS Acid–Base Imbalances

Alteration	Description	Treatments
Respiratory Acidosis	Respiratory acidosis is caused by an excess of dissolved carbon dioxide, or carbonic acid; it can be acute or chronic. *Laboratory findings:* Arterial blood pH less than 7.35 $PaCO_2$ above 45 mmHg HCO_3^- normal or slightly elevated in acute; above 26 mEq/L in chronic	■ Frequently assess respiratory status and lung sounds. ■ Monitor airway and ventilation; assist with insertion of artificial airway and prepare for mechanical ventilation as necessary. ■ Administer pulmonary therapy measures such as inhalation therapy, percussion and postural drainage, bronchodilators, and antibiotics as ordered. ■ Monitor fluid intake and output, vital signs, and ABGs. ■ Administer narcotic antagonists as indicated. ■ Maintain adequate hydration (2–3 L of fluid per day unless contraindicated by other health conditions).
Respiratory Alkalosis	Respiratory alkalosis is caused by hyperventilation, leading to a carbon dioxide deficit. *Laboratory findings (in uncompensated respiratory alkalosis):* Arterial blood pH above 7.45 $PaCO_2$ less than 35 mmHg	■ Monitor vital signs and ABGs. ■ Teach client to breathe more slowly. ■ Reduce stimuli in environment and speak in calm quiet voice.
Metabolic Acidosis	Metabolic acidosis (bicarbonate deficit) may be caused by excess acid in the body or loss of bicarbonate from the body. *Laboratory findings:* Arterial blood pH below 7.35 Serum bicarbonate less than 22 mEq/L $PaCO_2$ less than 38 mmHg with respiratory compensation	■ Monitor ABG values, intake and output, and level of consciousness (LOC). ■ Administer IV sodium bicarbonate carefully as ordered. ■ Treat underlying problem as ordered.
Metabolic Alkalosis	Metabolic alkalosis (bicarbonate excess) may be caused by loss of acid or excess bicarbonate in the body. *Laboratory findings:* Arterial blood pH above 7.45 Serum bicarbonate greater than 26 mEq/L $PaCO_2$ higher than 45 mmHg with respiratory compensation	■ Monitor intake and output closely. ■ Monitor vital signs, especially respirations, and LOC. ■ Administer ordered IV fluids carefully. ■ Treat underlying problem.

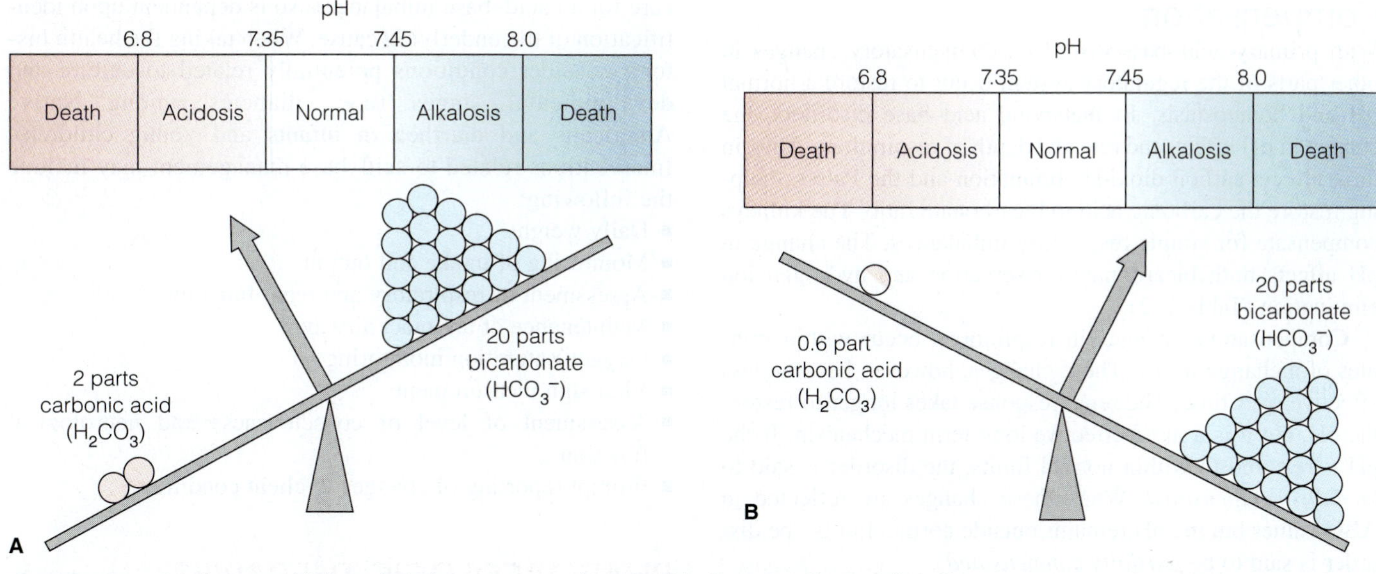

Figure 1–3 ■ Respiratory acid–base imbalances. *A,* Respiratory acidosis. *B,* Respiratory alkalosis.

TABLE 1–1 Common Causes of Primary Acid–Base Imbalances

IMBALANCE	COMMON CAUSES
Metabolic acidosis pH < 7.35 $HCO_3^- < 22$ mEq/L Critical values pH < 7.20 $HCO_3^- < 10$ mEq/L	↑ Acid production ■ Lactic acidosis ■ Ketoacidosis related to diabetes, starvation, or alcoholism ■ Salicylate toxicity ↓ Acid excretion ■ Renal failure ↑ Bicarbonate loss ■ Diarrhea, ileostomy drainage, intestinal fistula ■ Biliary or pancreatic fistulas ↑ Chloride ■ Sodium chloride IV solutions ■ Renal tubular acidosis ■ Carbonic anhydrase inhibitors
Metabolic alkalosis pH > 7.45 $HCO_3^- > 26$ mEq/L Critical values pH > 7.60 $HCO_3^- > 40$ mEq/L	↑ Acid loss or excretion ■ Vomiting, gastric suction ■ Hypokalemia ↑ Bicarbonate ■ Alkali ingestion (bicarbonate of soda) ■ Excess bicarbonate administration
Respiratory acidosis pH < 7.35 $PaCO_2 > 45$ mmHg Critical values pH < 7.2 $PaCO_2 > 77$ mmHg	Acute respiratory acidosis ■ Acute respiratory conditions (pulmonary edema, pneumonia, acute asthma) ■ Opiate overdose ■ Foreign body aspiration ■ Chest trauma Chronic respiratory acidosis ■ Chronic respiratory conditions (COPD, cystic fibrosis) ■ Multiple sclerosis, other neuromuscular diseases ■ Stroke
Respiratory alkalosis pH > 7.45 $PaCO_2 < 35$ mmHg Critical values pH > 7.60 $PaCO_2 < 20$ mmHg	■ Anxiety-induced hyperventilation (e.g., anxiety) ■ Fever ■ Early salicylate intoxication ■ Hyperventilation with mechanical ventilator

Compensation

With primary acid–base disorders, compensatory changes in other parts of the regulatory system occur to restore a normal pH and homeostasis. In metabolic acid–base disorders, the change in pH affects the rate and depth of respirations. This, in turn, affects carbon dioxide elimination and the $PaCO_2$, helping restore the carbonic acid to bicarbonate ratio. The kidneys compensate for simple respiratory imbalances. The change in pH affects both bicarbonate conservation and hydrogen ion elimination (Table 1–2).

Compensatory changes in respirations occur within minutes of a change in pH. These changes, however, become less effective over time. The renal response takes longer to restore the pH, but it is a more effective long-term mechanism. If the pH is restored to within normal limits, the disorder is said to be *fully compensated.* When these changes are reflected in ABG values but the pH remains outside normal limits, the disorder is said to be *partially compensated*.

DIAGNOSTIC TESTS

ABGs are performed to evaluate the client's acid–base balance and oxygenation. Blood gases may be drawn by laboratory technicians, respiratory therapy personnel, or nurses with specialized skills. Because a high-pressure artery is used to obtain blood, it is important to apply pressure to the puncture site for 5 minutes (10–15 minutes if the client is receiving anticoagulant therapy) after the procedure to reduce the risk of bleeding or bruising. When analyzing ABG results, it is important to use a systematic approach. First evaluate each individual measurement; then analyze the interrelationships to determine the client's acid–base status (Box 1–1).

CARING INTERVENTIONS

The goal of treatment is to restore or maintain normal body balance. Treatment of acid–base imbalance depends on identification and treatment of the underlying cause; collaborative care for an acid–base imbalance also is dependent upon identification of the underlying cause. When taking the health history, consider conditions potentially related to culture and developmental stages (e.g., diabetes among Native Americans and diarrhea in infants and young children). Interventions related to acid–base management may include the following:

- Daily weight
- Monitoring of intake and output
- Assessment of respiratory and renal function
- Maintenance of an intact airway
- Oxygen saturation monitoring
- Vital sign measurement
- Assessment of level of consciousness and neurological function
- Prompt reporting of changes in client condition.

PHARMACOLOGIC THERAPIES

Specific pharmacologic therapies are available to treat acidosis and alkalosis. ABG levels must be carefully monitored to prevent overtreatment causing pH to alter in the opposite direction, changing alkalosis to acidosis or acidosis to alkalosis.

Pharmacotherapy of Acidosis

In clients with acidosis, the therapeutic goal is to reverse the effects of excess acids in the blood and return the client to normal pH levels as quickly as possible. The pharmacologic treatment of choice for acute acidosis is administration of sodium bicarbonate infusions, provided that the bicarbonate level is low. Bicarbonate ion acts quickly as a base to neutralize acids in the blood and other body fluids. Carefully monitor the client's ABGs during infusions and watch for signs of alkalosis because this drug can "overcorrect" the acidosis, causing blood pH to turn alkaline. Symptoms of alkalosis include irritability, confusion, cyanosis, slow respirations, irregular pulse, and muscle weakness. If these symptoms occur, withhold the medication and notify the health care provider.

TABLE 1–2 **Compensation for Simple Acid–Base Imbalances**

PRIMARY DISORDER	CAUSE	COMPENSATION	EFFECT ON ABGS
Metabolic acidosis	Excess nonvolatile acids; bicarbonate deficiency	Rate and depth of respirations increase, eliminating additional CO_2.	↓ pH ↓ HCO_3^- ↓ $PaCO_2$
Metabolic alkalosis	Bicarbonate excess	Rate and depth of respirations decrease, retaining CO_2.	↑ pH ↑ HCO_3^- ↑ $PaCO_2$
Respiratory acidosis	Retained CO_2 and excess carbonic acid	Kidneys conserve bicarbonate to restore carbonic acid:bicarbonate ratio of 1:20.	↓ pH ↑ $PaCO_2$ ↑ HCO_3^-
Respiratory alkalosis	Loss of CO_2 and deficient carbonic acid	Kidneys excrete bicarbonate and conserve H^+ to restore carbonic acid:bicarbonate ratio.	↑ pH ↓ $PaCO_2$ ↓ HCO_3^-

Box 1–1 **Interpreting ABGs**

1. Look at the pH.
   - pH < 7.35 = acidosis
   - pH > 7.45 = alkalosis
2. Look at the $PaCO_2$.
   - $PaCO_2 < 35$ mmHg = hypocapnia; more carbon dioxide is being exhaled than normal.
   - $PaCO_2 > 45$ mmHg = hypercapnia; carbon dioxide is being retained.
3. Evaluate the pH–$PaCO_2$ relationship for a possible respiratory problem.
   - If the pH is < 7.35 (acidosis) and the $PaCO_2$ is > 45 mmHg (hypercapnia), retained carbon dioxide is causing increased H^+ concentration and *respiratory acidosis*.
   - If the pH is > 7.45 (alkalosis) and the $PaCO_2$ is < 35 mmHg (hypocapnia), low carbon dioxide levels and decreased H^+ concentration are causing *respiratory alkalosis*.
4. Look at the bicarbonate.
   - If the HCO_3^- is < 22 mEq/L, bicarbonate levels are lower than normal.
   - If the HCO_3^- is > 26 mEq/L, bicarbonate levels are higher than normal.
5. Evaluate the pH, HCO_3^-, and BE for a possible metabolic problem.
   - If the pH is < 7.35 (acidosis), the HCO_3^- is < 22 mEq/L, and the BE is < -3 mEq/L, then low bicarbonate levels and high H^+ concentrations are causing *metabolic acidosis*.
   - If the pH is > 7.45 (alkalosis), the HCO_3^- is > 26 mEq/L, and the BE is $> +3$ mEq/L, then high bicarbonate levels are causing *metabolic alkalosis*.
6. Look for compensation.
   - *Renal compensation*
     a. In respiratory acidosis (pH < 7.35, $PaCO_2 > 45$ mmHg), the kidneys retain HCO_3^- to buffer the excess acid; so the HCO_3^- is > 26 mEq/L.
     b. In respiratory alkalosis (pH > 7.45, $PaCO_2 < 35$ mmHg), the kidneys excrete HO_3^- to minimize the alkalosis; so the HCO_3^- is < 22 mEq/L.
   - *Respiratory compensation*
     a. In metabolic acidosis (pH < 7.35, $HCO_3^- < 22$ mEq/L), the rate and depth of respirations increase, increasing carbon dioxide elimination; so the $PaCO_2$ is < 35 mmHg.
     b. In metabolic alkalosis (pH > 7.45, $HCO_3^- > 26$ mEq/L), respirations slow and carbon dioxide is retained; so the $PaCO_2$ is > 45 mmHg.
7. Evaluate oxygenation.
   - $PaO_2 < 80$ mmHg = hypoxemia; possible hypoventilation
   - $PaO_2 > 100$ mmHg = hyperventilation

The nurse's role in sodium bicarbonate therapy involves carefully monitoring a client's condition and providing education to the client and family about the prescribed treatment. Sodium bicarbonate is given to neutralize acidotic states; so first analyze the ABG reports of pH, carbon dioxide levels (PCO_2), bicarbonate levels ($HCO^-{}_3$), and oxygenation status (PO_2 and O_2 saturation). Assess the client for symptoms associated with acidosis, such as sleepiness, coma, disorientation, dizziness, headache, seizures, and hypoventilation. Also assess the client for causative factors that could produce acidosis, such as diabetes mellitus, shock, and diarrhea. Acidosis is frequently corrected when the underlying disease condition is successfully managed.

Several contraindications and precautions are related to the administration of sodium bicarbonate. Because of the sodium content of this drug, it should be used judiciously in clients with cardiac disease and renal impairment.

Sodium bicarbonate may also be used to alkalinize the urine and speed the excretion of acidic substances. This process is useful in treating overdoses of certain acidic medications such as aspirin and phenobarbital and is useful as adjunctive therapy for certain chemotherapeutic drugs such as methotrexate. Sodium bicarbonate is also used in chronic renal failure to neutralize the metabolic acidosis that occurs when the kidneys cannot excrete hydrogen ion. When IV sodium bicarbonate is given, it causes the urine to become more alkaline. Less acid is reabsorbed in the renal tubules, so more acid and acidic medicine is excreted. This process is known as *ion trapping*. Monitor the client's acid–base status closely and report symptoms of imbalance. Provide care directed toward supporting critical body functions such as cardiovascular, respiratory, and neurological status that may be impaired secondary to the drug overdose.

Sodium bicarbonate (baking soda) is used as a home remedy to neutralize gastric acid, relieving heartburn, and sour stomach. Although occasional use is acceptable, nurses should be aware that clients may misinterpret cardiac symptoms as heartburn and may overuse sodium bicarbonate, leading to systemic alkalosis.

Client education as it relates to sodium bicarbonate should include the goals of therapy, the reasons for obtaining baseline data such as vital signs and electrolyte levels, and possible drug side effects.

CLIENT TEACHING **Sodium Bicarbonate**

Include the following points when teaching clients and their families about sodium bicarbonate:

- Immediately contact the primary health care provider if gastric discomfort continues or is accompanied by chest pain, dyspnea, or diaphoresis.
- Use nonsodium antacids to prevent the absorption of excess sodium or bicarbonate into the systemic circulation.
- Do not use any antacid, including sodium bicarbonate, for longer than 2 weeks without consulting your health care provider.

Pharmacotherapy of Alkalosis

Mild cases of alkalosis can be corrected by administering sodium chloride concurrently with potassium chloride. This combination increases the renal excretion of bicarbonate ion, which indirectly increases the acidity of the blood. More severe alkalosis can be treated with infusions of an acidic drug such as ammonium chloride. The nurse's role in ammonium chloride therapy involves carefully monitoring a client's condition and providing education to clients and their families about the prescribed treatment.

To determine whether ammonium chloride is warranted, assess the pH in ABG reports prior to administration. The major treatment for both metabolic alkalosis and respiratory alkalosis is to attempt to correct first the underlying disease condition creating the imbalance. The administration of ammonium chloride is used in clinical practice only when the alkalosis is so severe that the pH must be restored quickly to prevent life-threatening consequences. This drug is contraindicated in the presence of liver disease because its acidifying action depends on proper liver functioning to convert ammonium ions to urea.

During the IV infusion of ammonium chloride, continually assess for metabolic acidosis and ammonium toxicity. Symptoms of toxic levels of ammonium include pallor, sweating, irregular breathing, retching, bradycardia, twitching, and convulsions. If the client exhibits any of these symptoms, immediately stop the infusion and contact the health care provider.

Also closely monitor the client's renal status because excretion of ammonium chloride depends on normal kidney function. Monitor intake and output ratios, body weight, electrolyte status, and renal function studies for any sign of renal impairment.

In addition, closely monitor the IV infusion site because ammonium chloride is extremely irritating to veins and may cause severe inflammation. Infuse the drug slowly, no more than 5 mL/minute, to prevent ammonia toxicity.

Like sodium bicarbonate, ammonium chloride is used as an ionic trapping agent in the treatment of drug overdoses. Ammonium chloride acidifies urine, which increases the excretion of alkaline substances such as amphetamines, phencyclidine (PCP/angel dust), and other basic substances. Overdoses of alkaline substances can greatly compromise the client's cardiovascular, respiratory, and neurological status. The nursing role for this type of client is directed toward monitoring the client's acid–base status and supporting critical body functions.

Client education as it relates to ammonium chloride should include the goals of therapy, the reasons for obtaining baseline data such as vital signs and the existence of underlying renal disorders, and possible drug side effects.

CLIENT TEACHING **Ammonium Chloride**

Include the following points when teaching clients and families about ammonium chloride:

- Report pain at IV site.
- If medication is taken orally, report diminished appetite, nausea, vomiting, and thirst.
- If medication is given parenterally, report rash, headache, bradycardia, drowsiness, confusion, depression, and excitement alternating with coma.
- Take ammonium chloride tablets for no longer than 6 days.
- Report severe GI upset, fever, chills, and changes in urine or stool color.
- Take medication after meals or use enteric-coated tablets to decrease GI upset; swallow tablets whole.

MEDICATIONS **Acid–Base Imbalance**

Classification	Mechanism of action	Common drugs	Nursing considerations
Electrolyte/Alkaline Agent	Sodium bicarbonate is a drug of choice for correcting metabolic acidosis when bicarbonate is low on ABGs. After dissociation, the bicarbonate ion directly raises the pH of body fluids. Sodium bicarbonate may be given orally if acidosis is mild or intravenously in cases of acute disease. IV concentrations range from 4.2% to 8.4%. Although sodium bicarbonate also neutralizes gastric acid, it is rarely used to treat peptic ulcers due to its tendency to cause uncomfortable gastric distension. After absorption, sodium bicarbonate makes the urine more basic, which aids in the renal excretion of acidic drugs such as barbiturates and salicylates. The oral preparation of sodium bicarbonate is known as *baking soda.*	sodium bicarbonate	■ Give oral sodium bicarbonate 2–3 hours before or after meals and other medications. ■ Do not add oral preparation to calcium-containing solutions. ■ Monitor for symptoms of alkalosis. ■ Note that sodium bicarbonate is contraindicated in clients with hypertension, renal impairment, peptic ulcers, excessive chloride loss due to GI suctioning, diarrhea, or vomiting.
Acidic Agent	Severe metabolic alkalosis may be reversed by the administration of acidic agents such as ammonium chloride. During the hepatic conversion of ammonium chloride to urea, chloride and hydrogen are formed and the pH of body fluids decreases.	ammonium chloride	■ Infuse ammonium chloride slowly to minimize the potential for producing acidosis. ■ Observe for signs of central nervous system depression, which is characteristic of acidosis. ■ Do not administer to clients with serious hepatic or renal impairment or with respiratory acidosis.

1.1 METABOLIC ACIDOSIS

KEY TERMS

Kussmaul's respirations, *12*
Metabolic acidosis, *1*

BASIS FOR SELECTION OF EXEMPLAR

Selected by NC Concept-Based Learning Editorial Board

LEARNING OUTCOMES

After reading about this exemplar, you will be able to:

1. Describe the pathophysiology, etiology, clinical manifestations, and direct and indirect causes of metabolic acidosis.
2. Identify risk factors associated with metabolic acidosis.
3. Illustrate the nursing process in providing culturally competent care across the life span for individuals with metabolic acidosis.
4. Formulate priority nursing diagnoses appropriate for an individual with metabolic acidosis.
5. Create a plan of care for individuals with metabolic acidosis and their family members.
6. Assess expected outcomes for an individual with metabolic acidosis.
7. Discuss therapies used in the collaborative care of an individual with metabolic acidosis.
8. Employ evidence-based caring interventions for an individual with metabolic acidosis.

OVERVIEW

Metabolic acidosis (bicarbonate deficit) is characterized by a low pH (< 7.35) and a low bicarbonate (< 22 mEq/L). It may be caused by excess acid in the body or loss of bicarbonate from the body. When metabolic acidosis develops, the respiratory system attempts to return the pH to normal by increasing the rate and depth of respirations. Carbon dioxide elimination increases, and the $PaCO_2$ falls (< 35 mmHg).

PATHOPHYSIOLOGY AND ETIOLOGY

Three basic mechanisms that can cause metabolic acidosis are as follows:

1. Accumulation of metabolic acids
2. Excess loss of bicarbonate
3. An increase in chloride levels.

An accumulation of metabolic acids can result from excess acid production or impaired renal elimination of metabolic acids. Lactic acidosis develops due to tissue hypoxia and a shift to anaerobic metabolism by the cells. Lactate and hydrogen ions are produced, forming lactic acid. Both oxygen and glucose are necessary for normal cell metabolism. When intracellular glucose is inadequate due to starvation or a lack of insulin to move it into cells, the body breaks down fatty tissue to meet its metabolic needs. In this process, fatty acids are released and converted to ketones; ketoacidosis results. Aspirin (acetylsalicylic acid) breaks down into salicylic acid in the body. Substances such as aspirin, methanol (wood alcohol), and ethylene (contained in antifreeze and solvents) cause a toxic increase in body acids by either breaking down into acid products (salicylic acid) or stimulating metabolic acid production (Porth, 2005). Renal failure impairs the body's ability to excrete excess hydrogen ions and form bicarbonate.

Excess metabolic acids increase the hydrogen ion concentration of body fluids. The excess acid is buffered by bicarbonate, leading to what is known as a high anion gap acidosis.

The pancreas secretes bicarbonate-rich fluid into the small intestine. Intestinal suction, severe diarrhea, ileostomy drainage, or fistulas can lead to excess losses of bicarbonate. Hyperchloremic acidosis can develop when excess chloride solutions (such as NaCl or ammonium chloride) are infused, causing a rise in chloride concentrations. It also may be related to renal disease or administration of carbonic anhydrate inhibitor diuretics. The anion gap remains normal in metabolic acidosis due to bicarbonate loss or excess chloride.

Acidosis depresses cell membrane excitability, affecting neuromuscular function. It also increases the amount of free calcium in ECF by interfering with protein binding. Severe acidosis (pH of 7.0 or less) depresses myocardial contractility, leading to decreased cardiac output. If kidney function is normal, acid excretion and ammonia production increase to eliminate excess hydrogen ions.

Acid–base imbalances also affect electrolyte balance. In acidosis, potassium is retained as the kidney excretes excess hydrogen ion. Excess hydrogen ions also enter the cells, displacing potassium from the intracellular space to maintain the balance of cations and anions within the cells. The effect of both processes is to increase serum potassium levels. Also in acidosis, calcium is released from its bonds with plasma proteins, increasing the amount of ionized (free) calcium in the blood. Magnesium levels may fall in acidosis.

Risk Factors

Metabolic acidosis is rarely a primary disorder; it usually develops during the course of another disease, as follows:

- *Acute lactic acidosis* usually results from tissue hypoxia due to shock or cardiac arrest.
- Clients with type 1 diabetes mellitus are at risk for developing *diabetic ketoacidosis*. (See Concept 18, Metabolism, for more information about diabetes and its complications.)
- *Acute* or *chronic renal failure* impairs the excretion of metabolic acids. (See Concept 11, Fluids and Electrolytes, for more information about renal failure.)
- Diarrhea, intestinal suction, or abdominal fistulas increase the risk for excess *bicarbonate loss*. (See Concept 9, Elimination, for more information related to elimination.)

Other common causes of metabolic acidosis are listed in Table 1–1 on page 5.

CLINICAL MANIFESTATIONS

Metabolic acidosis affects the function of many body systems. Its general manifestations include weakness and fatigue, headache, and general malaise. Gastrointestinal function is affected, causing diminished appetite, nausea, vomiting, and abdominal pain. The level of consciousness may decline, leading to stupor and coma. Cardiac dysrhythmias develop, and cardiac arrest may occur. The skin is often warm and flushed. Skeletal problems may develop in chronic acidosis, as calcium and phosphate are released from the bones. Manifestations of compensatory mechanisms are seen. The respirations are deep and rapid, known as **Kussmaul's respirations**. The client may complain of shortness of breath, or dyspnea.

COLLABORATION

Metabolic acidosis normally results from another primary disorder. Therefore, the focus is on treating the primary disorder, reducing the effects of acidosis on cardiac function, and ensuring adequate oxygenation. Diagnostic tests will include ABGs, serum electrolytes, and tests as indicated by the underlying primary disorder.

Pharmacologic Therapies

To reduce the effects of acidosis on cardiac function, an alkalinizing solution such as bicarbonate may be given if the pH is less than 7.2. Sodium bicarbonate is the most commonly used alkalinizing solution; others include lactate, citrate, and acetate solutions (which are metabolized to bicarbonate). Alkalinizing solutions are given intravenously for severe acute metabolic acidosis. In chronic metabolic acidosis, the oral route is used.

Carefully monitor the client treated with bicarbonate. Rapid correction of the acidosis may lead to metabolic alkalosis and hypokalemia. Hypernatremia and hyperosmolality may develop as well, leading to water retention and fluid overload.

PRACTICE ALERT

As metabolic acidosis is corrected, potassium shifts back into the intracellular space. This can lead to hypokalemia and cardiac dysrhythmias. Carefully monitor serum potassium levels during treatment.

Treatment for diabetic ketoacidosis includes intravenous insulin and fluid replacement. Alcoholic ketoacidosis is treated with saline solutions and glucose. Treatment for lactic acidosis from decreased tissue perfusion (e.g., shock, cardiac arrest) focuses on correcting the underlying problem and improving tissue perfusion. Clients with chronic renal failure and mild or moderate metabolic acidosis may or may not require treatment, depending on the pH and bicarbonate levels. When metabolic acidosis is due to diarrhea, treatment includes correcting the underlying cause and providing fluid and electrolyte replacement.

NURSING PROCESS

Nurses frequently provide care for clients with metabolic acidosis, although the focus of care is usually the underlying disorder (e.g., diabetes mellitus, renal failure) rather than the acidosis itself. For this reason, it is vital for the nurse to be aware of the effects of acidosis and its implications for nursing care.

To promote health in clients at risk for metabolic acidosis, discuss management of the underlying disease process (e.g., type 1 diabetes, renal failure) to help them prevent complications such as diabetic ketoacidosis and metabolic acidosis. Because early manifestations of metabolic acidosis (e.g., fatigue, general malaise, diminished appetite, nausea, abdominal pain) resemble those of common viral disorders such as influenza, stress the importance of promptly seeking treatment if these symptoms develop.

CLINICAL MANIFESTATIONS AND THERAPIES Metabolic Acidosis

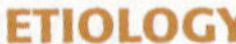

ETIOLOGY	CLINICAL MANIFESTATIONS	CLINICAL THERAPIES
Conditions that increase nonvolatile acids in the blood (e.g., renal impairment, diabetes mellitus, starvation) Conditions that decrease bicarbonate (e.g., prolonged diarrhea) Excessive infusion of chlori1de-containing IV fluids (e.g., NaCl) Excessive ingestion of acids such as salicylates Cardiac arrest	■ Diminished appetite ■ Nausea and vomiting ■ Abdominal pain ■ Weakness ■ Fatigue ■ Headache ■ General malaise ■ Decreasing LOCs ■ Dysrhythmias ■ Bradycardia ■ Warm, flushed skin ■ Skeletal problems ■ Hyperventilation (Kussmaul's respirations) ■ Dyspnea	■ Monitor ABG values, intake and output, and LOC. ■ Position client to facilitate chest expansion. ■ Provide oral care for dry mouth. ■ Administer IV sodium bicarbonate carefully if ordered. ■ Treat underlying problem as ordered.

Assessment

Assessment data related to metabolic acidosis include the following:

- *Health history.* Current manifestations, including diminished appetite, nausea, vomiting, abdominal discomfort, fatigue, lethargy, or other symptoms; duration of symptoms and any precipitating factors such as diarrhea and ingestion of a toxin such as aspirin, methanol, or ethylene; chronic diseases such as diabetes or renal failure, cirrhosis of the liver, or endocrine disorders; current medications
- *Physical assessment.* Mental status and LOC; vital signs including respiratory rate and depth; apical and peripheral pulses; skin color and temperature; abdominal contour and distention; bowel sounds; urine output.

Diagnosis

Nursing management of clients with metabolic acidosis often focuses on the primary disorder (e.g., diabetic ketoacidosis, renal failure); however, the acidosis itself has effects that must be attended to when care is provided. Possible nursing diagnoses for the client with metabolic acidosis may include the following:

- Decreased Cardiac Output
- Risk for Excess Fluid Volume
- Risk for Injury.

Plan

Planning for the client with metabolic acidosis involves identification and treatment of the underlying cause and restoration and maintenance of acid–base balance. Nursing care also includes measures to treat the underlying disorder, such as diabetic ketoacidosis. (Refer to other concepts for a discussion of interventions specific to the underlying disorder.) Potential goals for the client with metabolic acidosis may include the following:

- Client will describe and demonstrate preventive measures related to chronic disease process.
- pH will remain within normal range.
- Disease process causing acid–base imbalance will be controlled to reduce acid production or alkaline loss.
- Client will maintain vital signs within normal range for age and condition.
- Client will maintain baseline cardiac rhythm.
- Client will maintain or regain normal serum electrolyte levels.

Implementation

Metabolic acidosis affects cardiac output by decreasing myocardial contractility, slowing the heart rate, and increasing the risk for dysrhythmias. The accompanying hyperkalemia increases the risk for decreased cardiac output as well. (See Concept 11 for discussion about hyperkalemia.)

Decreased Cardiac Output

- Monitor vital signs, including peripheral pulses and capillary refill. Hypotension, diminished pulse strength, and slowed capillary refill may indicate decreased cardiac output and impaired tissue perfusion. Poor tissue perfusion can increase the risk for lactic acidosis.
- Monitor the ECG pattern for dysrhythmias and changes characteristic of hyperkalemia. Notify the physician of changes. Progressive ECG changes such as widening of the QRS complex indicate an increasing risk of dysrhythmias and cardiac arrest. Dysrhythmias further decrease cardiac output, possibly intensifying the degree of acidosis.
- Monitor laboratory values, including ABGs, serum electrolytes, and renal function studies (serum creatinine and BUN). Frequent monitoring of laboratory values allows evaluation of the effectiveness of treatment as well as early identification of potential problems.

PRACTICE ALERT

Administering bicarbonate to correct acidosis increases the risk for hypernatremia, hyperosmolality, and fluid volume excess.

Risk for Excess Fluid Volume

- Monitor and maintain fluid replacement as ordered. Monitor serum sodium levels and osmolality. Bicarbonate administration can cause hypernatremia and hyperosmolality, leading to water retention.
- Monitor heart and lung sounds, central venous pressure (CVP), and respiratory status. Increasing dyspnea, adventitious lung sounds, a third heart sound (S_3) due to the volume of blood flow through the heart, and high CVP readings are indicative of hypervolemia and should be reported to the care provider.
- Assess for edema, particularly in the back, sacral, and periorbital areas. Initially, edema affects dependent tissues—the back and sacrum in clients who are bedridden. Periorbital edema indicates more generalized edema.
- Assess urine output hourly. Maintain accurate intake and output records. Note urine output less than 30 mL/hour or a positive fluid balance on 24-hour total intake and output calculations. Heart failure and inadequate renal perfusion may lead to decreased urine output.
- Obtain daily weights using consistent conditions. Daily weights are an accurate indicator of fluid balance.
- Administer prescribed diuretics as ordered, monitoring the client's response to therapy. Loop or high-ceiling diuretics such as furosemide can lead to further electrolyte imbalances, especially hypokalemia. This is a significant risk like that seen during correction of metabolic acidosis.

Risk for Injury

Mental status and brain function are affected by acidosis, increasing the risk for injury. The nurse working with clients who exhibit altered mental status related to acidosis should:

- Monitor neurological function, including mental status, LOC, and muscle strength. As the pH falls, mental functioning declines, leading to confusion, stupor, and a decreasing LOC.
- Institute safety precautions as necessary: Keep the bed in its lowest position with side rails raised. These measures help protect the client from injury resulting from confusion or disorientation.
- Keep clocks, calendars, and familiar objects at bedside. Orient to time, place, and circumstances as needed. Allow

significant others to remain with the client as much as possible. An unfamiliar environment and altered thought processes can further increase the risk for injury. Significant others provide a sense of security and reduce anxiety.

Discharge planning and teaching focus on the underlying cause of the imbalance. The client who has developed ketoacidosis as a result of diabetes mellitus, starvation, or alcoholism needs interventions and teaching to prevent future episodes of acidosis. Diet, medication management, and alcohol dependency treatment are vital teaching areas. When metabolic acidosis is related to renal failure, the client should be referred for management of the renal failure itself. Clients who have experienced diarrhea or excess ileostomy drainage leading to bicarbonate loss need information about appropriate diarrhea treatment strategies and need to know when to call their primary care provider.

Evaluation

Expected outcomes of nursing care relate to prevention of acidosis and restoration of normal body balance during disease processes. During the recovery period, pH levels and vital signs should be frequently monitored and the client's condition reassessed in order to revise care plans as necessary. Expected outcomes include the following:

- Client maintains pH within normal range.
- Client's vital signs remain within normal range based on age and condition.
- Client maintains adequate oxygenation of tissues.
- Client is able to describe or demonstrate measures to control disease process to prevent future complications of pH imbalance.

REVIEW Metabolic Acidosis

RELATE: LINK THE CONCEPTS

The ambulance arrives with a client who presents with Kussmaul's respirations and a history of diabetes mellitus.

Linking the exemplar of Metabolic Acidosis with the concept of Metabolism:

1. Based on the client's history, what impact does the nurse expect to find on acid–base balance?
2. When the nurse is assessing this client, what symptoms of diabetic ketoacidosis would be directly related to alterations in pH?

Linking the exemplar of Metabolic Acidosis with the concept of Safety:

3. What precautions would the nurse implement for the client with metabolic acidosis to prevent potential injury?
4. The client with metabolic acidosis becomes confused and disoriented. What nursing care will the nurse provide to this client to maintain safety?

READY: GO TO THE COMPANION SKILLS MANUAL

- Monitoring intake and output
- Oxygen saturation using a pulse oximeter
- Assessing respirations
- Administering medication
- Administering IV fluids
- Measuring weights

REFER: GO TO MYNURSINGKIT

REFLECT: CASE STUDY

Norma James, a 65-year-old widow who lives alone, has a long history of type 2 diabetes mellitus, atrial fibrillation, and hypertension. Her medications include the following:

- Glucotrol 10 mg twice a day
- Captopril 50 mg twice a day
- Digoxin 125 mcg once a day
- Coumadin 5 mg once a day

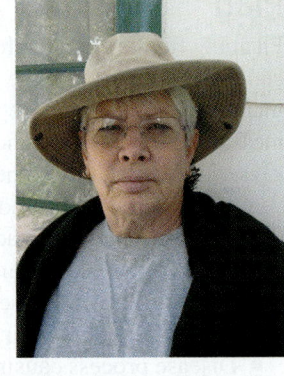

1. What risk factors does this client have for development of metabolic acidosis?
2. What teaching would you perform with this client to reduce the risk of metabolic acidosis when she is seen in the neighborhood clinic for regular check-ups?
3. For what signs and symptoms would you assess Ms. James to rule out possible metabolic acidosis?

1.2 METABOLIC ALKALOSIS

KEY TERM

Metabolic alkalosis, *14*

BASIS FOR SELECTION OF EXEMPLAR

Selected by NC Concept-Based Learning Editorial Board

LEARNING OUTCOMES

After reading about this exemplar, you will be able to:

1. Describe the pathophysiology, etiology, clinical manifestations, and direct and indirect causes of metabolic alkalosis.
2. Identify the risk factors associated with metabolic alkalosis.
3. Illustrate the nursing process in providing culturally competent care across the life span for individuals with metabolic alkalosis.
4. Formulate priority nursing diagnoses appropriate for an individual with metabolic alkalosis.
5. Create a plan of care for individuals with metabolic alkalosis and their family members.
6. Assess expected outcomes for an individual with metabolic alkalosis.
7. Discuss therapies used in the collaborative care of an individual with metabolic alkalosis.
8. Employ evidence-based caring interventions for an individual with metabolic alkalosis.

OVERVIEW

Metabolic alkalosis (bicarbonate excess) is characterized by a high pH (> 7.45) and a high bicarbonate (> 26 mEq/L). It may be caused by loss of acid or excess bicarbonate in the body. When metabolic alkalosis develops, the respiratory system attempts to return the pH to normal by slowing the respiratory rate. Carbon dioxide is retained, and the $PaCO_2$ increases (> 45 mmHg).

PATHOPHYSIOLOGY AND ETIOLOGY

Hydrogen ions may be lost through the kidneys or via gastric secretions or because of a shift of H^+ into the cells. Metabolic alkalosis due to loss of hydrogen ions usually occurs because of vomiting or gastric suction. Gastric secretions are highly acidic (pH 1–3). When these are lost through vomiting or gastric suction, the alkalinity of body fluids increases. This increased alkalinity results from the loss of acid and from selective retention of bicarbonate by the kidneys as chloride is depleted. (Chloride is the major anion in ECF; when it is lost, bicarbonate is retained as a replacement anion.)

Increased renal excretion of hydrogen ions can be prompted by hypokalemia as the kidneys try to conserve potassium, excreting hydrogen ion instead. Hypokalemia contributes to metabolic alkalosis in another way as well. When potassium shifts out of cells to maintain extracellular potassium levels, hydrogen ions shift into the cells to maintain the balance between cations and anions within the cells.

Excess bicarbonate usually occurs as a result of ingesting antacids that contain bicarbonate (such as soda bicarbonate or Alka-Seltzer) or overzealously administering bicarbonate to treat metabolic acidosis. Common causes of metabolic alkalosis are summarized in Table 1–1.

In alkalosis, more calcium combines with serum proteins, reducing the amount of ionized (physiologically active) calcium in the blood. This accounts for many of the common manifestations of metabolic alkalosis. Alkalosis also affects potassium balance: Hypokalemia not only can cause metabolic alkalosis (see above), but also can result from metabolic alkalosis. Hydrogen ions shift out of the intracellular space to help restore the pH, prompting more potassium to enter the cells and depleting ECF potassium. The high pH depresses the respiratory system as the body retains carbon dioxide to restore the carbonic acid to bicarbonate ratio.

Risk Factors

As is the case with other acid–base imbalances, metabolic alkalosis rarely occurs as a primary disorder. Risk factors include hospitalization, hypokalemia, and treatment with alkalinizing solutions (e.g., bicarbonate).

CLINICAL MANIFESTATIONS

Manifestations of metabolic alkalosis occur as a result of decreased calcium ionization and are similar to those of hypocalcemia. They include numbness and tingling around the mouth, fingers, and toes; dizziness; Trousseau's sign; and muscle spasm. As the respiratory system compensates for metabolic alkalosis, respirations are depressed and respiratory failure with hypoxemia and respiratory acidosis may develop.

COLLABORATION

Metabolic alkalosis typically arises as a consequence of an underlying primary disorder. The plan of care and therapeutic regimen will be aimed at controlling alkalosis while treating the underlying cause.

Pharmacologic Therapies

Treatment of metabolic alkalosis includes restoring normal fluid volume and administering potassium chloride and sodium chloride solution. The potassium restores serum and intracellular potassium levels, allowing the kidneys to conserve hydrogen ions more effectively. Chloride promotes renal excretion of bicarbonate. Sodium chloride solutions restore fluid volume deficits that can contribute to metabolic alkalosis. In severe alkalosis, an acidifying solution such as dilute hydrochloric acid or ammonium chloride may be administered. In addition, drugs may be used to treat the underlying cause of the alkalosis.

CLINICAL MANIFESTATIONS AND THERAPIES **Metabolic Alkalosis**

ETIOLOGY	CLINICAL MANIFESTATIONS	CLINICAL THERAPIES
Excessive acid losses due to vomiting or gastric suction Excessive use of potassium-losing diuretics Excessive adrenal corticoid hormones due to ■ Cushing's syndrome. ■ Hyperaldosteronism. ■ Excessive bicarbonate intake from antacids. ■ Parenteral $NaHCO_3$.	■ Confusion ■ Decreasing level of consciousness ■ Hyperreflexia ■ Tetany ■ Dysrhythmias ■ Hypotension ■ Seizures ■ Respiratory failure	■ Monitor intake and output closely. ■ Monitor vital signs, especially respirations and LOC. ■ Administer ordered IV fluids carefully. ■ Administer oxygen as ordered. ■ Treat underlying problem.

Laboratory and Diagnostic Tests

The following laboratory and diagnostic tests may be ordered:

- *ABGs* show a pH greater than 7.45 and bicarbonate level greater than 26 mEq/L. With compensatory hypoventilation, carbon dioxide is retained and the $PaCO_2$ is greater than 45 mmHg.
- *Serum electrolytes* often demonstrate decreased serum potassium (< 3.5 mEq/L) and decreased chloride (< 95 mEq/L) levels. The serum bicarbonate level is high. Although the total serum calcium may be normal, the ionized fraction of calcium is low.
- *Urine pH* may be low (pH 1–3) if metabolic acidosis is caused by hypokalemia. The kidneys selectively retain potassium and excrete hydrogen ion to restore ECF potassium levels. Urinary chloride levels may be normal or greater than 250 mEq/24 hours.
- The *ECG pattern* shows changes similar to those seen with hypokalemia. (See Concept 11, Fluids and Electrolytes, for more information related to symptoms of hypokalemia.) These changes may be due to hypokalemia or to the alkalosis.

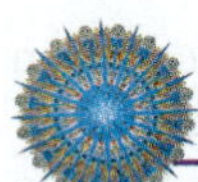

NURSING PROCESS

Health promotion activities focus on teaching clients the risks of using sodium bicarbonate as an antacid to relieve heartburn or gastric distress. Stress the availability of other effective antacid preparations and the need to seek medical evaluation for persistent gastric symptoms.

In the hospital setting, carefully monitor laboratory values for clients at risk for developing metabolic alkalosis, particularly clients undergoing continuous gastric suction.

Assessment

Focused assessment data related to metabolic alkalosis include the following:

- *Health history.* Current manifestations such as numbness and tingling, muscle spasms, dizziness, or other symptoms; duration of symptoms and any precipitating factors such as bicarbonate ingestion, vomiting, diuretic therapy, or endocrine disorders; current medications
- *Physical assessment.* Vital signs, including apical pulse and rate and depth of respirations; muscle strength; deep tendon reflexes
- *Diagnostic tests.* ABGs, serum electrolytes.

Diagnosis

As with metabolic acidosis, nursing care of the client with metabolic alkalosis often focuses on intervening for client responses to the primary problem rather than the alkalosis itself. However, the risk for impaired gas exchange is a priority problem, especially with severe metabolic alkalosis. Possible nursing diagnoses for the client with metabolic alkalosis may include the following:

- Risk for Impaired Gas Exchange
- Deficient Fluid Volume
- Risk for Injury
- Knowledge Deficit.

Plan

Planning for the client with metabolic alkalosis depends on identification and treatment of the underlying cause. Restoring and maintaining normal acid–base balance is the desired outcome. Nursing care also includes measures to treat the underlying disorder, such as hypokalemia. (Refer to other concepts for a discussion of interventions specific to the underlying disorder.) Appropriate outcomes include resolution of the underlying cause and that the client will:

- Return to oxygen saturation level of 95% or greater.
- Return to normal or near normal fluid and electrolyte volumes.

Implementation

Nursing care of the client with metabolic alkalosis is focused on controlling pH while treating the underlying causative disorder and preventing complications.

Impaired Gas Exchange

Respiratory compensation for metabolic alkalosis depresses the respiratory rate and reduces the depth of breathing to promote carbon dioxide retention. As a result, the client is at risk for impaired gas exchange, especially in the presence of underlying lung disease.

- Monitor respiratory rate, depth, and effort. Monitor oxygen saturation continuously, reporting an oxygen saturation level of less than 95% (or as ordered). The depressed respiratory drive associated with metabolic alkalosis can lead to hypoxemia and impaired oxygenation of tissues. Oxygen saturation levels of less than 90% indicate significant oxygenation problems.
- Assess skin color; note and report cyanosis around the mouth. Central cyanosis, seen around the mouth and oral mucous membranes, indicates significant hypoxia.
- Monitor mental status and LOC. Report decreasing LOC or behavior changes such as restlessness, agitation, or confusion. Changes in mental status or behavior may be early signs of hypoxia.
- Place in semi-Fowler's or Fowler's position as tolerated. Elevating the head of the bed facilitates alveolar ventilation and gas exchange.
- Schedule nursing care activities to allow rest periods. The client who is hypoxemic has limited energy reserves, necessitating frequent rest and limited activities.
- Administer oxygen as ordered or as necessary to maintain oxygen saturation levels. Supplemental oxygen can help maintain blood and tissue oxygenation despite depressed respirations.

Deficient Fluid Volume

Clients with metabolic alkalosis often have an accompanying fluid volume deficit.

- Assess intake and output accurately, monitoring fluid balance. In acute situations, hourly intake and output may be indicated. Urine output of less than 30 mL/hour indicates inadequate tissue perfusion, inadequate renal perfusion, and an increased risk for acute renal failure.
- Assess vital signs, CVP, and peripheral pulse volume at least every 4 hours. Hypotension; tachycardia; low CVP; and weak, easily obliterated peripheral pulses indicate hypovolemia.
- Weigh daily under standard conditions (time of day, clothing, and scale). Rapid weight changes accurately reflect fluid balance.
- Administer intravenous fluids as prescribed using an electronic infusion pump. If rapid fluid replacement is ordered, monitor for the following indicators of fluid overload: dyspnea, tachypnea, tachycardia, increased CVP, jugular vein distension, and edema. Rapid fluid replacement may lead to hypervolemia, resulting in pulmonary edema and cardiac failure, particularly in clients with compromised cardiac and renal function.
- Monitor serum electrolytes, osmolality, and ABG values. Rehydration and administration of potassium chloride will affect both acid–base and fluid and electrolyte balance. Careful monitoring is important to identify changes.

Care in the Community

When preparing the client with metabolic alkalosis for discharge, consider the cause of the alkalosis and any underlying factors. For example, provide teaching to the client and family about the following:

- Using appropriate antacids for heartburn and gastric distress
- Using potassium supplements as ordered or eating high-potassium foods to avoid hypokalemia if taking a potassium-wasting diuretic or if aldosterone production is impaired
- Contacting the primary care provider if uncontrolled or extended vomiting develops.

Evaluation

Expected outcomes of nursing care relate to restoration of normal body balance. Revisions in the care plan may need to be made if the client does not respond to some aspect of the plan. Nurses may need to follow up with clients released from hospital care to determine whether clients are continuing to follow instructions for self-monitoring and self-care. Possible outcomes for the client with metabolic alkalosis include the following:

- Client relates antacids that are acceptable for use and will reduce risk of reoccurrence of metabolic alkalosis.
- Client describes proper self-administration procedure for oral potassium supplements.
- Client describes when to notify provider related to changes in daily weight.
- Client's arterial pH returns to normal range.
- Client's serum electrolyte values are within normal range.

REVIEW Metabolic Alkalosis

RELATE: LINK THE CONCEPTS

Linking the exemplar of Metabolic Alkalosis with the concept of Fluids and Electrolytes:

1. What pathophysiological process is involved with metabolic alkalosis that leads to a decrease in mental function?
2. What changes in serum electrolyte levels could indicate a risk for metabolic alkalosis?

Linking the exemplar of Metabolic Alkalosis with the concept of Tissue Integrity:

3. What impact might the client with full thickness burns over 50% of the body experience in regard to acid–base balance?
4. What caring interventions might be implemented (independently by the nurse or collaboratively by the health care team) to prevent metabolic alkalosis?

READY: GO TO THE COMPANION SKILLS MANUAL

- Oxygen saturation: pulse oximetry
- Administering medication
- Preparing client for chest physiotherapy
- Monitoring intake and output
- Measuring weights
- Establishing intravenous infusions

REFER: GO TO MYNURSINGKIT

REFLECT: CASE STUDY

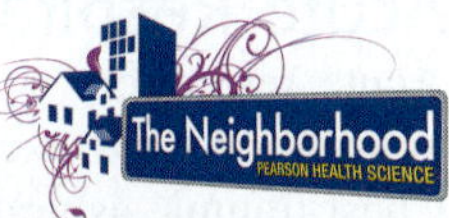

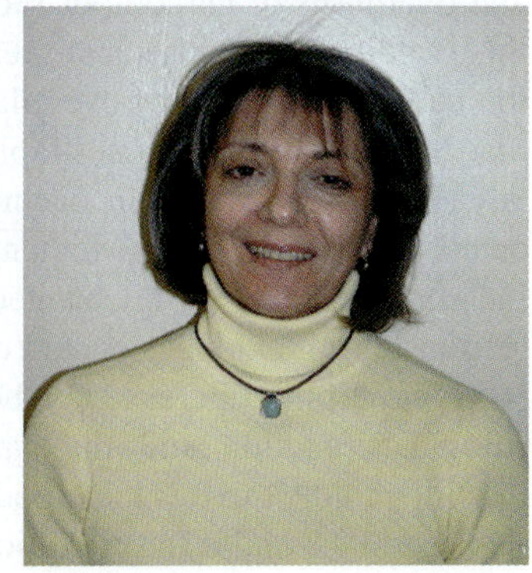

Pam Allen is a 65-year-old female receiving postoperative care after a colectomy. When she wakes up in recovery, she is nauseated and experiences a tremendous amount of pain. She is alarmed by all of the tubes, including intravenous therapy, oxygen, a Foley catheter, and a nasogstric tube. She is told that she had a large cancerous tumor in her lower colon and upper rectum and that the doctors were unable to remove all of it because the tumor had adhered to the side walls of her lower abdominal cavity.

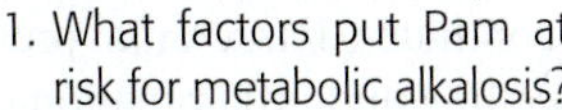

1. What factors put Pam at risk for metabolic alkalosis?
2. What are the priority nursing diagnoses?

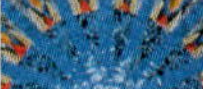

1.3 RESPIRATORY ACIDOSIS

KEY TERMS

Hypercapnia, *18*
Hypoxemia, *18*
Respiratory Acidosis, *18*
Ventilation, *18*

BASIS FOR SELECTION OF EXEMPLAR

Selected by NC Concept-Based Learning Editorial Board

LEARNING OUTCOMES

After reading about this exemplar, you will be able to:

1. Describe the pathophysiology, etiology, clinical manifestations, and direct and indirect causes of respiratory acidosis.
2. Identify risk factors associated with respiratory acidosis.
3. Illustrate the nursing process in providing culturally competent care across the life span for individuals with respiratory acidosis.
4. Formulate priority nursing diagnoses appropriate for an individual with respiratory acidosis.
5. Create a plan of care for individuals with respiratory acidosis and their family members.
6. Assess expected outcomes for an individual with respiratory acidosis.
7. Discuss therapies used in the collaborative care of an individual with respiratory acidosis.
8. Employ evidence-based caring interventions for an individual with respiratory acidosis.

OVERVIEW

Respiratory acidosis is caused by an excess of dissolved carbon dioxide, or carbonic acid. It is characterized by a pH less than 7.35 and a $PaCO_2$ greater than 45 mmHg. Respiratory acidosis may be acute or chronic. In chronic respiratory acidosis, the bicarbonate is higher than 26 mEq/L as the kidneys compensate by retaining bicarbonate.

PATHOPHYSIOLOGY AND ETIOLOGY

Both acute and chronic respiratory acidosis result from carbon dioxide retention caused by alveolar hypoventilation. **Hypoxemia** (decreased oxygen) frequently accompanies respiratory acidosis.

Acute Respiratory Acidosis

Acute respiratory acidosis occurs due to a sudden failure of **ventilation** (the exchange of oxygen and carbon dioxide). Chest trauma, aspiration of a foreign body, acute pneumonia, and overdoses of narcotic or sedative medications can lead to this condition. Because acute respiratory acidosis occurs with the sudden onset of hypoventilation—for example, with cardiac arrest—the $PaCO_2$ rises rapidly and the pH falls markedly. A pH of 7 or lower can occur within minutes, resulting in death if not corrected (Metheny, 2000). Initially, the serum bicarbonate level is unchanged because the compensatory response of the kidneys occurs over hours to days.

Hypercapnia (increased carbon dioxide levels) affects neurological function and the cardiovascular system. Carbon dioxide rapidly crosses the blood–brain barrier. Cerebral blood vessels dilate, and if the condition continues, intracranial pressure increases and *papilledema* (swelling and inflammation of the optic nerve where it enters the retina) develops (Porth, 2005). Peripheral vasodilation also occurs, and the pulse rate increases to maintain cardiac output.

Chronic Respiratory Acidosis

Chronic respiratory acidosis is associated with chronic respiratory or neuromuscular conditions such as COPD, asthma, cystic fibrosis, and multiple sclerosis. These conditions affect alveolar ventilation because of airway obstruction, structural changes in the lung, and limited chest wall expansion. Most clients with chronic respiratory acidosis have COPD with chronic bronchitis and emphysema. In chronic respiratory acidosis, the $PaCO_2$ increases over time and remains elevated. The kidneys retain bicarbonate, increasing bicarbonate levels, and the pH often remains close to the normal range because of adequate metabolic compensation.

The acute effects of hypercapnia may not develop when carbon dioxide levels rise gradually, allowing compensatory changes to occur. When carbon dioxide levels are chronically elevated, the respiratory center becomes less sensitive to the gas as a stimulant of the respiratory drive. The PaO_2 provides the primary stimulus for respirations. Clients with chronic respiratory acidosis are at risk for developing *carbon dioxide narcosis* (with manifestations of acute respiratory acidosis) if the respiratory center is suppressed by administering excess supplemental oxygen. Manifestations include confusions, tremors and convulsions; coma can occur if blood levels of CO_2 reach 70 mmHg or higher.

PRACTICE ALERT

Carefully monitor neurological and respiratory status in clients with chronic respiratory acidosis who are receiving oxygen therapy. Immediately report a decreasing LOC or depressed respirations.

Risk Factors

Acute or chronic lung disease (e.g., pneumonia, COPD) or trauma is the primary risk factor for respiratory acidosis. Other conditions that depress or interfere with ventilation, such as excess narcotic analgesics, airway obstruction, and neuromuscular disease, also are risk factors for respiratory acidosis. Selected causes of respiratory acidosis are listed in Table 1–1.

CLINICAL MANIFESTATIONS

The manifestations of acute and chronic respiratory acidosis differ. In acute respiratory acidosis, the rapid rise in $PaCO_2$ levels causes manifestations of hypercapnia. Cerebral vasodilation causes manifestations such as headache, blurred vision, irritability, and mental cloudiness. If the condition continues, the LOC progressively decreases. Rapid and dramatic changes in ABGs can lead to unconsciousness and ventricular fibrillation, a potentially lethal cardiac dysrhythmia. The skin of the client with acute respiratory acidosis may be warm and flushed, and the pulse rate is elevated.

The manifestations of chronic respiratory acidosis include weakness and a dull headache. Sleep disturbances, daytime sleepiness, impaired memory, and personality changes also may be manifestations of chronic respiratory acidosis Clients with acute respiratory failure require treatment in the emergency department or intensive care unit. The focus is on restoring adequate ventilation and gas exchange.

Acute respiratory acidosis is often the result of inadequate breathing patterns resulting in retained carbon dioxide and inadequate intake of oxygen. Hypoxemia often accompanies hypercapnia as a result, requiring administration of supplemental oxygen. The administration of oxygen to the client with chronic hypercapnia, such as the client with COPD, must be delivered with caution in order to avoid removing the respiratory drive in those who breathe as a result of minor hypoxia. See the exemplar on COPD in Concept 21, Oxygenation, for more information about the administration of oxygen to those with chronic hypercapnia.

COLLABORATION

Care of the client experiencing respiratory acidosis involves the efforts of the entire health care team. A respiratory therapist may providing breathing treatments and related therapies as ordered. Consultation with the pharmacist and the client's primary care provider prevents administration of medications that may be contraindicated. Clients who are using accessory muscles to breathe may require increased caloric intake and the participation of a dietician.

Diagnostic Tests

The following diagnostic tests may be ordered:

- *ABGs* show a pH of less than 7.35 and a $PaCO_2$ of more than 45 mmHg. In acute respiratory acidosis, the bicarbonate level is initially within normal range but increases to greater than 26 mEq/L if the condition persists. In chronic respiratory acidosis, both the $PaCO_2$ and the HCO_3^- may be significantly elevated.
- *Serum electrolytes* may show hypochloremia (chloride level < 98 mEq/L) in chronic respiratory acidosis.
- *Pulmonary function tests* may be done to determine whether chronic lung disease is the cause of the respiratory acidosis. However, these studies are not done during the acute period.

Additional diagnostic tests may be done to identify the underlying cause of the respiratory acidosis. Chest x-ray and sputum studies (cytology and culture) may be ordered to identify an acute or chronic lung disorder. If drug overdose is suspected, serum levels of the drug may be obtained.

CLINICAL MANIFESTATIONS AND THERAPIES Respiratory Acidosis

ETIOLOGY	CLINICAL MANIFESTATIONS	CLINICAL THERAPIES
Acute lung conditions that impair alveolar gas exchange (e.g., pneumonia, acute pulmonary edema, aspiration of foreign body, near-drowning) Chronic lung disease (e.g., asthma, cystic fibrosis, emphysema) Overdose of narcotics or sedatives that depress respiratory rate and depth Brain injury that affects the respiratory center Airway obstruction Mechanical injury	Acute Respiratory Acidosis ■ Headache ■ Warm, flushed skin ■ Elevated pulse ■ Blurred vision ■ Irritability, altered mental status ■ Decreasing LOC ■ Cardiac arrest Chronic Respiratory Acidosis ■ Weakness ■ Dull headache ■ Sleep disturbances with daytime sleepiness ■ Impaired memory ■ Personality changes	■ Frequently assess respiratory status and lung sounds. ■ Evaluate mental status; document and report changes in alertness. ■ Place in semi-Fowler's to Fowler's position as tolerated. ■ Encourage the client with chronic respiratory acidosis to use pursed-lip breathing. ■ Monitor airway and ventilation; insert artificial airway and prepare for mechanical ventilation as necessary. ■ Administer pulmonary therapy measures such as inhalation therapy, percussion and postural drainage, bronchodilators, and antibiotics as ordered. ■ Monitor fluid intake and output, vital signs, and ABGs. ■ Administer narcotic antagonists as indicated. ■ Maintain adequate hydration (2–3 L of fluid per day).

Pharmacologic Therapies

Bronchodilator drugs may be administered to open the airways and antibiotics prescribed to treat respiratory infections. If excess narcotics or anesthetic has caused acute respiratory acidosis, narcotic antagonists such as naloxone may be given to reverse the effects.

Respiratory Support

Treatment of respiratory acidosis, either acute or chronic, focuses on improving alveolar ventilation and gas exchange. Clients with severe respiratory acidosis and hypoxemia may require intubation and mechanical ventilation. The $PaCO_2$ level is lowered slowly to avoid complications such as cardiac dysrhythmias and decreased cerebral perfusion. In clients with chronic respiratory acidosis, oxygen is administered cautiously to avoid carbon dioxide narcosis.

Pulmonary hygiene measures such as deep breathing and coughing exercises, breathing treatments, and percussion and drainage may be instituted. Adequate hydration is important to promote removal of respiratory secretions.

NURSING PROCESS

Nursing care of clients with respiratory acidosis is focused on improving breathing pattern and maintaining a patent airway. Because of the link between smoking and chronic pulmonary diseases, nursing care may include teaching clients how to make healthier lifestyle choices.

Assessment

- *Health history.* Current manifestations (including headache, irritability, and lethargy), difficulty thinking, blurred vision, and other symptoms; duration of symptoms and any precipitating factors such as drug use or respiratory infection; chronic diseases such as cystic fibrosis or COPD; current medications
- *Physical examination.* Mental status and LOC; vital signs; skin color and temperature; rate and depth of respirations, pulmonary excursion, and lung sounds

Diagnosis

Restoring effective alveolar ventilation and gas exchange is the priority of interdisciplinary and nursing care for clients with respiratory acidosis. Possible nursing diagnoses for the client with respiratory acidosis may include the following:

- Impaired Gas Exchange
- Ineffective Airway Clearance
- Anxiety
- Risk for Injury.

Plan

Planning for the client with respiratory acidosis involves both restoration of acid–base balance and appropriate treatment for any underlying disease or cause. Expected outcomes include resolution of the underlying illness and the fact that the client:

- Maintains adequate fluid intake
- Maintains oxygenation saturation greater than 90%
- Maintains normal $PaCO_2$ level
- Maintains pH balance.

Implementation

Frequently assess respiratory status, including rate, depth, effort, and oxygen saturation levels. Decreasing respiratory rate and effort along with decreasing oxygen saturation levels may signal worsening respiratory failure and respiratory acidosis.

PRACTICE ALERT

Frequently assess LOC. A decline in LOC may indicate increasing hypercapnia and the need for increasing ventilatory support (such as intubation and mechanical ventilation).

Impaired Gas Exchange

- Promptly evaluate and report ABG results to the physician and respiratory therapist. Rapid changes in carbon dioxide or oxygen levels may necessitate modification of the treatment plan to prevent complications of overcorrection of respiratory acidosis.
- Place in semi-Fowler's to Fowler's position as tolerated. Elevating the head of the bed promotes lung expansion and gas exchange.
- Administer oxygen as ordered. Carefully monitor response. Reduce the oxygen flow rate or percentage and immediately report increasing somnolence. Supplemental oxygen can suppress the respiratory drive in clients with chronic respiratory acidosis.

Ineffective Airway Clearance

- Frequently auscultate breath sounds (whether on or off a mechanical ventilator). Increasing adventitious sounds or decreasing breath sounds (faint or absent) may indicate worsening airway clearance due to obstruction or fatigue.
- Encourage the client with chronic respiratory acidosis to use pursed-lipped breathing. Pursed-lipped breathing helps maintain open airways throughout exhalation, promoting carbon dioxide elimination. See Box 21–5 on page 1235 in the oxygenation concept for detailed instructions on pursed-lipped breathing.
- Frequently reposition and encourage ambulation as tolerated. Repositioning, sitting at the bedside, and ambulation promote airway clearance and lung expansion.
- Encourage fluid intake of up to 3,000 mL per day as tolerated or allowed. Fluids help liquefy secretions and hydrate respiratory mucous membranes, promoting airway clearance.
- Administer medications such as inhaled bronchodilators as ordered. Inhaled bronchodilators help relieve bronchial spasm, dilating airways.
- Provide percussion, vibration, and postural drainage as ordered. Pulmonary hygiene measures such as these help loosen respiratory secretions so the client can cough them out of their airways.

Anxiety

Anxiety is a common result of both hypoxia and hypercapnia triggered by the neuron's insufficient oxygen supply. Clients with respiratory disorders commonly experience anxiety that

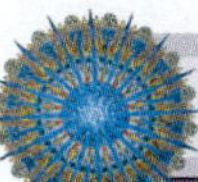

NURSING CARE PLAN **A Client With Acute Respiratory Acidosis**

ASSESSMENT

Marlene Hitz, age 76, is eating lunch with her friends when she suddenly begins to choke and is unable to breathe. After several minutes of trying, an attendant at the senior center successfully dislodges some meat caught in Ms. Hitz's throat, using the Heimlich maneuver. Ms. Hitz is taken by ambulance to the emergency department for follow-up because she was apneic for 3–4 minutes, her respirations are shallow, and she is disoriented. Ms. Hitz is placed in an observation room. Oxygen is started at 4 L/minute per nasal cannula. David Love, the nurse admitting Ms. Hitz, makes the following assessments: T 98.2, P 102, R 36 and shallow, BP 146/92. Skin is warm and dry. Alert but restless and not oriented to time or place, Ms. Hitz responds slowly to questions. Stat ABGs are drawn, a chest x-ray is done, and D5 ½ NS is started intravenously at 50 mL/hour. The chest x-ray shows no abnormality. ABG results are pH 7.30 (normal: 7.35–7.45), $PaCO_2$ 48 mmHg (normal: 35–45 mmHg), PaO_2 92 mmHg (normal: 80–100 mmHg), and HCO_3^- 24 mEq/L (normal: 22–26 mEq/L).

DIAGNOSES

- Impaired Gas Exchange related to temporary airway obstruction
- Anxiety related to emergency hospital admission
- Risk for Injury related to confusion

PLANNING

The desired outcomes for the plan of care specify that Ms Hitz will:

- Regain normal gas exchange and ABG values.
- Be oriented to time, place, and person.
- Regain baseline mental status.
- Remain free of injury.

IMPLEMENTATION

- Monitor ABGs, to be redrawn in 2 hours.
- Monitor vital signs and respiratory status (including oxygen saturation) every 15 minutes for the first hour, then every hour.
- Assess color of skin, nail beds, and oral mucous membranes every hour.
- Assess mental status and orientation every hour.
- Monitor anxiety level as evidenced by restlessness and agitation.
- Maintain a calm, quiet environment.
- Provide reorientation and explain all activities.
- Keep side rails in place and place call bell within reach.

EVALUATION

Ms. Hitz remains in the emergency department for 6 hours. Her ABGs are still abnormal, and David Love now notes the presence of respiratory crackles and wheezes. She is less anxious and responds appropriately when asked who and where she is. Because she has not regained normal gas exchange, Ms. Hitz is admitted to the hospital for continued observation and treatment.

CRITICAL THINKING

1. Why was Ms. Hitz exhibiting confusion? Explain the rationale for your answer, including pathophysiology that contributed to confusion.
2. Had Ms. Hitz not responded adequately to oxygen administration, what would the collaborative team have initiated as the next step in improving her condition?
3. Why might Ms. Hitz have developed respiratory crackles and wheezing, assuming that this was not a pretrauma concern?

is eliminated by improved ventilation and oxygenation. The nurse can help the client reduce anxiety levels through the following interventions:

- Remain with the client and monitor for changes in condition.
- Explain procedures and treatments using short, simple sentences. Providing clearly understood information reduces fear of the unknown.
- Reduce environmental stimuli, and use a calm, reassuring manner. These measures help reduce anxiety.
- Allow supportive family members to remain with the client as much as possible to provide further reassurance.

Risk for Injury

Clients with respiratory acidosis may experience blurred vision and altered level of consciousness, putting them at risk for injuries. Nurses working with these clients should:

- Assess LOC, orientation, and strength frequently.
- Place call bells within reach.
- Encourage client to remain in bed and reduce activity to improve gas exchange and reduce oxygen demands.
- Administer supplemental oxygen as needed to prevent cellular hypoxia and tissue damage.

Care in the Community

Planning and teaching for home care focuses on the problem that caused the respiratory acidosis.

- Teach the client and family about preventive measures and equipment that may be used in the home. The client who developed acute respiratory acidosis as a result of acute pneumonia or chest trauma may require only teaching to prevent future problems.
- If acute respiratory acidosis occurred secondarily to a narcotic overdose, determine whether the drug was prescribed for pain or whether it was an illicit street drug. Provide teaching to the client who requires narcotic medication on

a continuing basis. Refer the client using illicit drugs to a substance abuse counselor, treatment center, or Narcotics Anonymous as appropriate; refer the family to support groups as well.

- For clients with chronic lung disease and their families, discuss ways to avoid future episodes of acute respiratory failure. Encourage the client to receive immunized against pneumococcal pneumonia and influenza. Discuss ways to avoid acute respiratory infections, such as good hand washing, crowd avoidance, and cough etiquette, with the client and family.
- Provide instructions regarding measures to take when respiratory status is further compromised. The client and family should be alert that symptoms such as headache accompanied by blurred vision or weakness, irritability and confusion, or sleep disturbances and memory impairments warrant immediate medical attention. Shortness of breath or activity intolerance can often be the earliest symptoms of worsening respiratory status. Wheezing, grunting, use of accessory muscles, and cyanosis are often late signs.

Evaluation

Nursing care is evaluated based on client's progress in meeting goals, and the plan of care is revised as necessary based on outcomes. Expected outcomes of nursing care for a client with respiratory acidosis include the following:

- Client maintains patent airway.
- Client maintains appropriate breathing patterns to meet oxygen demands.
- Client remains conscious and does not display anxiety indicating potential hypoxia.
- ABG reflects pH and $PaCO_2$ within acceptable range for client.

REVIEW Respiratory Acidosis

RELATE: LINK THE CONCEPTS

Linking the exemplar of Respiratory Acidosis with the concept of Perfusion:

1. Describe the pathophysiological process that leads from cardiac arrest to respiratory acidosis.
2. Describe how pulmonary embolism might impact the client's pH.

Linking the exemplar of Respiratory Acidosis with the concept of Mobility:

3. Regarding the care of an older adult with a hip fracture that was repaired in surgery earlier today, how might the client's reduced mobility increase the risk of respiratory acidosis?
4. What independent and collaborative nursing interventions might be initiated to prevent respiratory acidosis in this client?

READY: GO TO COMPANION SKILLS MANUAL

- Administering oxygen by cannula, face mask, or oxygen tent
- Oxygen saturation: pulse oximetry
- Administering medication
- Preparing client for chest physiotherapy
- Monitoring intake and output
- Measuring weights
- Assessing the appearance and mental status

REFER: GO TO MYNURSINGKIT

REFLECT: CASE STUDY

The Neighborhood
PEARSON HEALTH SCIENCE

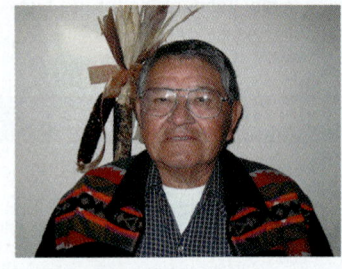

Jimmy Bley is a retired 78-year-old Native American man with moderate emphysema and hearing loss. He spends most of his time surfing the Internet and playing games on the computer. He has smoked a pack of cigarettes a day for 40 years. Mr. Bley has had a persistent, productive cough for a few weeks, but he continues to smoke. Mr. Bley wakes up suddenly in the middle of the night and is unable to catch his breath. He tries to use his inhaler, but this does not seem to help. Mr. Bley is admitted to the intensive care unit with a diagnosis of pneumonia and acute respiratory failure. His initial ABG results are pH 7.31, PaO_2 – 64 $PaCO_2$ – 54 HCO_3 – 31.

1. Why would Mr. Bley's bicarbonate level be elevated at this time?
2. Based on ABG results, how would you assess his acid-base status?
3. What nursing interventions will you implement to promote gas exchange for Mr. Bley?

1.4 RESPIRATORY ALKALOSIS

KEY TERMS

Hyperventilation, *23*
Respiratory alkalosis, *23*

BASIS FOR SELECTION OF EXEMPLAR

Selected by NC Concept-Based Learning Editorial Board

LEARNING OUTCOMES

After reading about this exemplar, you will be able to:

1. Describe the pathophysiology, etiology, clinical manifestations, and direct and indirect causes of respiratory alkalosis.
2. Identify risk factors associated with respiratory alkalosis.
3. Illustrate the nursing process in providing culturally competent care across the life span for individuals with respiratory alkalosis.
4. Formulate priority nursing diagnoses appropriate for an individual with respiratory alkalosis.
5. Create a plan of care for individuals with respiratory alkalosis that includes family members.
6. Assess expected outcomes for an individual with respiratory alkalosis.
7. Discuss therapies used in the collaborative care of an individual with respiratory alkalosis.
8. Employ evidence-based caring interventions for an individual with respiratory alkalosis.

OVERVIEW

Respiratory alkalosis is characterized by a pH greater than 7.45 and a $PaCO_2$ of less than 35 mmHg. It is always caused by **hyperventilation** (unusually fast respiration, or overbreathing), leading to a carbon dioxide deficit.

PATHOPHYSIOLOGY AND ETIOLOGY

In acute respiratory alkalosis, the pH rises rapidly as the $PaCO_2$ falls. Because the kidneys are unable to adapt rapidly to the change in pH, the bicarbonate level remains within normal limits. Anxiety-based hyperventilation is the most common cause of acute respiratory alkalosis. Other physiological causes of hyperventilation include high fever, hypoxia, gram-negative bacteremia, and thyrotoxicosis (excessive amounts of thyroid hormones). Early salicylate intoxication (aspirin overdose), encephalitis, and high progesterone levels in pregnancy directly stimulate the respiratory center, potentially leading to hyperventilation and respiratory alkalosis. Hyperventilation also can occur during anesthesia and mechanical ventilation if the rate and tidal volume (depth) of ventilations is excessive.

If hyperventilation continues, the kidneys compensate by eliminating bicarbonate to restore the bicarbonate to carbonic acid ratio. The bicarbonate level is lower than normal in chronic respiratory alkalosis, and the pH may be close to the normal range.

Alkalosis increases binding of extracellular calcium to albumin, reducing ionized calcium levels. As a result, neuromuscular excitability increases and manifestations similar to hypocalcemia develop. Low carbon dioxide levels in the blood cause vasoconstriction of cerebral vessels, increasing the neurological manifestations of the disorder.

Risk Factors

Anxiety with hyperventilation is the most common cause of respiratory alkalosis; therefore, anxiety disorders increase the risk for this acid–base imbalance. In the client who is critically ill, mechanical ventilation is a risk factor for respiratory alkalosis if breaths per minute or peak pressures are set too high for the client's needs.

CLINICAL MANIFESTATIONS

The manifestations of respiratory alkalosis include lightheadedness, a feeling of panic and difficulty concentrating, circumoral and distal extremity paresthesias (numbness or tingling), tremors, and positive Chvostek's sign (a type of facial spasm, usually indicative of hypocalcemia) and Trousseau's sign (a spasm of the hand and forearm). The client also may experience tinnitus, a sensation of chest tightness, and palpitations (cardiac dysrhythmias). Seizures and loss of consciousness may occur.

ABGs generally show a pH greater than 7.45 and a $PaCO_2$ of less than 35 mmHg. In chronic hyperventilation, there is a compensatory decrease in serum bicarbonate to less than 22 mEq/L, and the pH may be near normal.

COLLABORATION

Management of respiratory alkalosis focuses on correcting the imbalance and treating the underlying cause. It is important to create a calm, quiet, low-stimulation environment to reduce the client's anxiety or panic. ABGs must be ordered prior to administration of medications or oxygen therapy.

Pharmacologic Therapies

A sedative or antianxiety agent may be necessary to relieve anxiety and restore a normal breathing pattern. Additional drugs to correct underlying problems other than anxiety-induced hyperventilation may be ordered.

Respiratory Therapies

Historically, use of paper bags has been a recommended treatment for hyperventilation. While use of paper bags will help to raise carbon dioxide levels in clients with true hyperventilation syndrome, it can also cause hypoxia. Other diseases can mimic hyperventilation (such as myocardial infarction) and use of a paper bag will induce hypoxia causing further cellular damage

CLINICAL MANIFESTATIONS AND THERAPIES **Respiratory Alkalosis**

ETIOLOGY	CLINICAL MANIFESTATIONS	CLINICAL THERAPIES
Hyperventilation due to: ■ Extreme anxiety ■ Elevated body temperature ■ Overventilation with a mechanical ventilator ■ Hypoxia ■ Salicylate overdose ■ Brain stem injury ■ Fever ■ Increased basal metabolic rate	Dizziness Numbness and tingling around mouth, hands, and feet Palpitations Dyspnea Chest tightness Anxiety/panic Tremors Tetany Seizures, loss of consciousness	■ Monitor vital signs, LOC, and ABGs. ■ Encourage client to breathe more slowly; teach breathing and stress reduction techniques. ■ Administer sedative or antianxiety agent as ordered. ■ Monitor ventilator settings. ■ Administer oxygen as ordered. ■ Maintain fluid status.

(Brouhard, 2008). Elevated carbon dioxide levels have been found to trigger panic attacks which can further exacerbate hyperventilation. The best treatment for suspected hyperventilation is to teach breathing exercises, encouraging the client to take slow, regular breaths.

This allows more effective breathing with resulting increases in $PaCO_2$ levels, reducing the pH. If hyperventilation is the result of panic or stress, talking in a calm, low volume can help the client self-calm. Reduced stimuli in the environment will also contribute to slow, regular breathing.

If excessive ventilation by a mechanical ventilator is the cause of respiratory alkalosis, ventilator settings need to be adjusted to reduce the respiratory rate, peek expiratory pressure, and tidal volume. When hypoxia is the underlying cause of hyperventilation, administer oxygen as ordered.

NURSING PROCESS

Nursing care is focused on reducing anxiety through manipulation of the environment to reduce stimuli and to create a sense of peace. This restful environment will help the client breathe more slowly and effectively.

Assessment

- *Health history.* Assess for past history of anxiety disorders and the triggering event for the onset of hyperventilation. Assess for mental health disorders, coping mechanisms, and support systems available to the client.
- *Physical examination.* Assess breath sounds, neurological function, respiratory and cardiac status, and any changes in LOC.

Developmental Considerations

When children threaten to hold their breath to get their way, parents may fear that serious damage will result. However, if the child effectively holds his or her breath long enough, he or she will lose consciousness, the respiratory center will take over involuntary control of respirations, and the child will begin to breathe normally. Usually, the child will take a breath long before fainting. The same is true of the client who is hyperventilating secondary to anxiety because it will cause a light-headed feeling related to insufficient carbon dioxide, causing the client to faint, at which point breathing will return to normal and carbon dioxide will be retained with a return to homeostasis.

Identify clients at risk in the hospital (e.g., clients on mechanical ventilation or clients who have a fever or infection) and monitor assessment data and ABGs to identify early manifestations of hyperventilation and respiratory alkalosis.

Diagnosis

Possible nursing diagnoses for the client with respiratory alkalosis may include the following:

- Ineffective Breathing Pattern
- Anxiety
- Risk for Injury.

Plan

Planning for the client with respiratory alkalosis involves identification and treatment of the underlying cause and restoration of acid–base balance. Appropriate outcomes include resolution of the underlying cause and that the client will:

- Manifest normal respiratory rate and rhythm.
- Maintain safety.
- Maintain appropriate fluid status.

Implementation

The usual cause of hyperventilation and respiratory alkalosis is psychologic, although physiological disorders also can lead to hyperventilation. It is important not only to address the hyperventilation but also to identify the underlying cause.

- Assess respiratory rate, depth, and ease. Monitor vital signs (including temperature) and skin color. Assessment data can help identify the underlying cause, such as a fever or hypoxia.

DEVELOPMENTAL CONSIDERATIONS **Techniques for Reducing Anxiety in Children With Paresthesias**

INFANTS

- Using calming touch
- Using quiet voice
- Swaddling
- Holding quietly

TODDLERS OR PRESCHOOLERS

- Giving a stuffed toy to hug
- Singing familiar, quiet nursery songs
- Acknowledging the child's feelings
- Holding calmly

YOUNG SCHOOL-AGE CHILDREN

- Talking quietly about a happy event
- Telling a familiar story
- Reading a familiar book together
- Explaining that the tingling will go away
- Using simple guided imagery
- Listening supportively

OLDER SCHOOL-AGE CHILDREN OR ADOLESCENTS

- Explaining the reasons for the tingling and explaining that it will go away
- Using guided imagery
- Playing familiar music
- Asking what the child does when anxious or "scared"
- Talking about coping strategies

- Obtain subjective assessment data such as circumstances leading up to the current situation, current health and recent illnesses or medication use, and current manifestations. Subjective data provide clues to the cause and circumstances of the hyperventilation response.
- Reassure the client that he or she is not experiencing a heart attack and that symptoms will resolve when breathing returns to normal. Manifestations of hyperventilation and respiratory alkalosis such as dyspnea, chest tightness or pain, and palpitations can mimic those of a heart attack.
- Instruct the client to maintain eye contact and breathe with you to slow the respiratory rate. These measures help make the client aware of respirations and provide a sense of support and control (Ackley & Ladwig, 2006). Be aware that some clients may be uncomfortable making eye contact for cultural reasons.
- Protect the client from injury. If hyperventilation continues to the point at which the client loses consciousness, respirations will return to normal, as will acid–base balance.
- If the client has experienced repeated episodes of hyperventilation or has a chronic anxiety disorder, refer for counseling. Counseling can help the client develop alternative strategies for dealing with anxiety.

Planning and teaching for home care is directed toward the underlying cause of hyperventilation. If anxiety precipitated the episode, discuss anxiety and stress management strategies with the client. Teach the client how to identify a hyperventilation reaction, provide self-care, and when to seek medical intervention.

Evaluation

Care is evaluated based on the client's ability to meet goals set during the planning stage and the outcomes achieved. Nursing care is reformulated as needed if outcomes are not met. Expected outcomes for the client with respiratory alkalosis include the following:

- Client experiences no subsequent episodes of hyperventilation.
- Client describes strategies for coping with anxiety in the future.
- Family displays ability to contribute to calming client during times of anxiety.
- Client and/or family participates in support groups that will help the client cope with anxiety disorder.

REVIEW Respiratory Alkalosis

RELATE: LINK THE CONCEPTS

Linking the exemplar of Respiratory Alkalosis with the concept of Oxygenation:

1. Why would oxygenation often be a concern when dealing with a client with respiratory alkalosis?
2. For the mechanically ventilated client, what ventilator settings would need to be adjusted if the ABG returned demonstrating respiratory alkalosis?

Linking the exemplar of Respiratory Alkalosis with the concept of Safety:

3. What specific concerns would the nurse have regarding safety for a client with respiratory alkalosis?
4. What safety precautions might the nurse employ to prevent injury to the client with respiratory alkalosis related to hyperventilation caused by anxiety?

READY: GO TO COMPANION SKILLS MANUAL

- Administering medication
- Oxygen saturation: pulse oximetry
- Assessing the appearance and mental status
- Assessing respirations

REFER: GO TO MYNURSINGKIT

REFLECT: CASE STUDY

Tanner Moss is a healthy 13-year-old male who just had surgery for injuries sustained in a bicycle accident. When you enter the room, he is agitated, clutching at his sheets, and states, "I can't breathe!" Respiratory rate is 48 per minute, and pulse rate is 118 per minute.

1. What is your priority nursing intervention?
2. What would you expect ABGs to reveal if drawn at this time?
3. Considering Tanner's developmental stage, how would you help manage his anxiety?

EXPLORE PEARSON mynursingkit™

MyNursingKit is your one stop for online chapter review materials and resources. Prepare for success with additional NCLEX®-style practice questions, interactive assignments and activities, web links, animations and videos, and more!

Register your access code from the front of your book at **www.mynursingkit.com.**

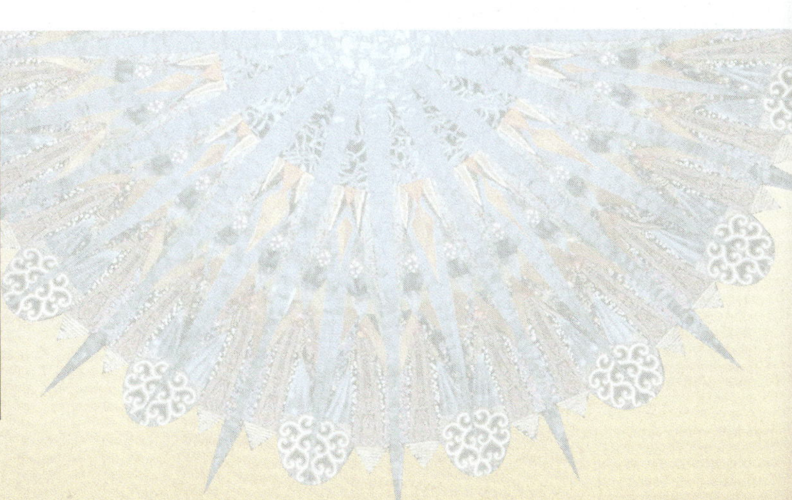

REFERENCES

Ackley, B. J., & Ladwig, G. B. (2006). *Nursing diagnosis handbook: A guide to planning care* (7th ed.). St. Louis, MO: Mosby.

Brouhard, R. (2008). Can I treat hyperventilation syndrome by breathing into a paper bag? Retrieved August 10, 2009, from http://firstaid.about.com/od/shortnessofbreat1/f/07_paper_bags.htm

Metheny, N. M. (2000). *Fluid and electrolyte balance: Nursing considerations* (4th ed.). Philadelphia: Lippincott.

Porth, C. M., & Matfin, G. (2008). *Pathophysiology: Concepts of altered health states* (8th ed.). Philadelphia: Lippincott.

Addiction Behavior

2

Concept at-a-Glance

Concept Learning Outcomes

After reading about this concept, you will be able to:

1. Summarize the physiological and psychological processes that contribute to addiction behaviors.
2. List factors affecting addiction behavior.
3. Identify commonly occurring addiction behaviors and their related treatments.
4. Explain common physical assessment procedures used to assess clients with addiction behaviors across the life span.
5. Outline diagnostic and laboratory tests to determine the individual's addiction status.
6. Explain management of addiction behaviors and their etiologies.
7. Demonstrate the nursing process in providing culturally competent and caring interventions across the life span for individuals with addiction behavior.
8. Identify pharmacological interventions used when caring for individuals with addiction behaviors.

Concept Key Terms

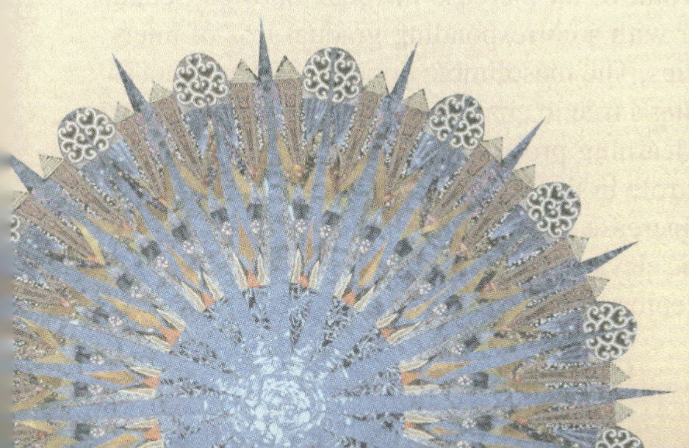

About Addiction Behavior

Addiction is defined as a psychologic or physical need for a substance (such as alcohol) or process (such as gambling) to the extent that the individual will risk negative consequences in an attempt to meet the need. **Addiction behaviors** (also referred to as *addictive behaviors)* are defined as compulsive, problematic patterns of action resulting in psychologic and/or physiologic dependence. •

In our society, many people use substances recreationally to modify mood or behavior. There are, however, wide sociocultural variations in the acceptability of chemical use. Alcohol, caffeine, and tobacco are legal drugs, but the social acceptability of using them varies. Narcotics, sedatives, stimulants, and hallucinogens are often used illegally, and the general population considers recreational use to be socially unacceptable. An individual may abuse any of these substances to the point of becoming addicted and unable to stop, despite dangerous, often life-threatening consequences.

There are other forms of addiction, often referred to as **process addictions**, which include workaholism, gambling, shopping, cutting, pornography, spending and indebtedness, computers, eating disorders, and sexual addictions. Process addictions involve compulsive behaviors that serve to reduce anxiety. Some believe that these behaviors are more closely linked to an obsessive-compulsive disorder, while others see them as addictions resulting from reward deficiency syndrome. Individuals with **reward deficiency syndrome** have a decreased ability to experience pleasure, which drives the person to seek external forms of gratification through the use of substances, pathologic gambling, or other high-risk behaviors. Individuals with reward deficiency syndrome may become addicted to engaging in dangerous activities where there is a possibility of death. BASE jumpers are an example. The acronym BASE stands for "Buildings, Antennas, Spans (or bridges), and Earth (or cliffs)," from which adherents leap. As they jump, their bodies start producing neurotransmitters, which provide the high to which they are addicted.

No specific addictive personality type exists; however, many addicts have several characteristics in common. Addictive behavior associated with alcoholism and other substances is characterized by compulsive preoccupation with obtaining the substance, loss of control over consumption, development of tolerance, dependence, and impaired social and occupational functioning (Weiss & Porrino, 2002). A wide variety of addictive behaviors exist, including but not limited to the following:

- The tendency for addicts to indulge in impulsive risk-taking behaviors
- A low tolerance for frustration and pain
- The tendency of addicts to rebel against social norms and engage in various antisocial and risky behaviors such as stealing, being promiscuous, driving while intoxicated (DWI), and committing violence against others
- The tendency of substance abusers toward anxiety, anger, and low self-esteem, all of which contribute to the likelihood of assaultive behaviors (discussed in more detail in Concept 31, Violence; Exemplar 31.2, Assault and Homicide).

Substance abuse often arises from anxieties. Many people have a desire for social acceptance and initiate drug use to "fit in" with a peer group. Some people may need drugs or alcohol to feel less inhibited while interacting with others.

The term **pseudoaddiction** has been applied to clients who display drug-seeking behaviors but differ from addicts in that they have true underlying pain for which they are seeking relief. These behaviors generally stop when adequate pain control is achieved.

NORMAL PRESENTATION

Addiction needs to be differentiated from dependence. **Dependence** is a physiologic need for a substance that the client cannot control, which results in withdrawal symptoms if the substance (most often a chemical) is withheld. Dependence to a substance also results in the user developing a physiologic **tolerance** for the substance, requiring use of greater quantities to achieve the same effect. Addiction includes the physiologic process of dependence, but also includes a psychologic need that causes addicts to seek out the substance to which they are addicted—at any cost. Addicts may neglect their children, their work, or other responsibilities to meet the need they have for their addiction.

Many different models explain addiction. The biopsychosocial model theorized by psychiatrist George L. Engel has been generally accepted as the most comprehensive theory for the process of addiction. This model links biologic, psychologic, and social factors as contributing to the development of addiction.

A link has been found between addiction and impulse control, although it is not fully understood. Addiction is strongly linked to the dopaminergic system of the brain's reward system. The speed with which someone becomes addicted depends on the substance, the frequency of use, the means of ingestion, the intensity of the high the person obtains, and the person's genetic and psychologic susceptibility. Adequate proof exists that addiction is, at least in part, genetically moderated.

The disease model of addiction holds that addiction is a disease that results from a neurochemical and/or behavioral process. Treatment is aimed at the idea of changing behaviors and supporting positive responses.

The pleasure model, proposed by Nils Bejerot, sees addiction as an emotional fixation acquired through learning that is aimed at obtaining pleasure and avoiding discomfort. If the pleasure that results is sufficiently strong, it induces repetition and overcomes the person's natural drive, resulting in addiction. This model is the basis of zero tolerance for drugs as a prevention strategy.

The cultural model holds that cultural influences play a strong role in the development of and tolerance for an addiction. According to this model, cultures that do not permit use of a substance are likely to have a lower incidence of addiction to that substance. The increase in the prevalence of gambling addiction resulting from loosening of legislation regarding casinos is believed to strengthen the position of those promoting this model.

The neurobiological research into addiction postulates that addiction is the result of an increase in focus on a particular addictive behavior with a corresponding gradual loss of interest in other activities. The mesolimbic dopaminergic system is suspected of playing a role in changing motivation of behavior through a reward learning process. This system is believed to play an important role in the seeking out of rewarding stimuli with a resulting increase in dopamine when the stimulus is received. A chronic elevation of dopamine results in a decrease in dopamine receptors known as **downregulation**, which results in a postsynaptic change in cell permeability. Furthermore, there are areas in the brain that define something as pleasant. When these areas are stimulated as a result of addiction, the substance or behavior takes on an increased level of need. The end result of this process is **anhedonia**, the inability to feel pleasure, causing addicts to look for new ways of reaching the highs they seek.

ALTERATIONS

Addiction can take many different forms, some of which will be discussed later in this concept. Addiction to nicotine, which is considered by some to be one of the most highly addictive substances, may lead to multiple health problems. Some of these include cancers of the lungs, bladder, and colon; heart disease; premature aging; and hypertension. Substance abuse is increasing in the United States and impacts the drug user, the user's family, and society as a whole. Substance abuse in the United States is so common that very few people are unaffected by it.

- One out of four Americans between the ages of 26 and 34 has used cocaine at some time.
- Approximately 5.5% of 19- to 22-year-olds surveyed had used Ecstasy (MDMA) the previous year.
- Two-and-a-half percent of the world's population have used marijuana.
- Six hundred thousand people are estimated to be addicted to heroin (Drug Rehabs.org, 2002).

These statistics only scratch the surface of the number of people dealing with addiction. These figures in combination with figures related to process addictions demonstrate the need for nurses to understand, recognize, and be able to screen clients for past and present addictions and behaviors.

Other alterations related to addiction that are not covered as a part of this concept include but are not limited to the following:

- Anorexia nervosa and bulimia
- Cutting
- Exercise addiction
- Gambling
- Plastic surgery
- Sexual addiction
- Tattoo and piercing addictions.

The Language of Addiction and Recovery

The process of addiction and recovery has its own vocabulary. These terms are used by professionals from all aspects of health care who work with substance-abusing clients and their families. Many of these terms are appropriate regardless of the substance or process being abused. See Table 2–1 for a list of some of these terms and their definitions.

Effects of Addiction on Families

Substance abuse is a family problem. It alters both family problems and behaviors of individual family members. The most devastating effects on a family occur when the abuser is

ALTERATIONS AND TREATMENTS Addictions

Alteration	Description	Treatment
Nicotine addiction	Addiction to nicotine can result from smoking tobacco in the form of cigarettes, cigars, or pipes as well as from chewing tobacco.	■ Medications: Nicotine gum, Chantix, nicotine nasal spray ■ Behavior therapy ■ Support groups
Alcohol addiction	Chronic use of alcohol can lead to addiction resulting in delirium tremens (DTs) if alcohol is not received.	■ Medications: Antabuse ■ Behavioral therapy ■ Support groups ■ 12-step program (e.g., Alcoholics Anonymous [AA]) ■ Detoxification ■ Milieu therapy ■ Family therapy
Substance addiction	Substance addiction may include abuse of heroin, cocaine, marijuana, crack, narcotics, barbiturates, inhalants, or any chemical substance that leads to addiction.	■ Behavior therapy ■ Support groups ■ Detoxification ■ Pharmacologic therapy, which may be required to minimize complications from withdrawal ■ Removal of peers providing substance ■ Milieu therapy ■ 12-step programs ■ Family therapy
Process addictions (sex, gambling, shopping, work)	Process addictions are those behaviors compulsively performed to reduce anxiety; they are considered by some to be a form of obsessive-compulsive disorder.	■ Psychotherapy ■ Behavior therapy ■ Milieu therapy ■ Support groups ■ Family therapy

TABLE 2–1 **Terminology Associated With Substance Abuse**

TERM	DEFINITION
Abstinence	Voluntarily going without drugs or alcohol
Codependence	A cluster of maladaptive behaviors exhibited by significant others of a substance-abusing individual that serves to enable and protect the abuse at the expense of living a full and satisfying life
Co-occurring disorders	Concurrent diagnosis of a substance use disorder and a psychiatric disorder; one disorder can precede and cause the other, such as the relationship between alcoholism and depression
Cross-tolerance	Tolerance to one drug conferring tolerance to another drug
Delirium tremens (DTs)	A medical emergency usually occurring 3–5 days following alcohol withdrawal and lasting 2–3 days; characterized by paranoia, disorientation, delusions, visual hallucinations, elevated vital signs, vomiting, diarrhea, and diaphoresis; also known as alcohol withdrawal delirium
Detoxification	The process of helping an addicted individual safely through withdrawal; commonly referred to as detox
Dual diagnosis	The coexistence of substance abuse/dependence and a psychiatric disorder in one individual (used interchangeably with dual disorder and co-occurring disorders)
Kindling	Brain sensitization to events such as stress, trauma, and the effects of substance use
Korsakoff's psychosis	Secondary dementia caused by thiamine (B_1) deficiency that may be associated with chronic alcoholism; characterized by progressive cognitive deterioration, confabulation, peripheral neuropathy, and myopathy
Physical dependence	A state in which withdrawal syndrome will occur if drug use is discontinued
Polysubstance abuse	The simultaneous use of many substances
Psychologic dependence	An intensive, subjective need for a particular psychoactive drug
Sobriety	The state of habitual refrain from using alcohol or drugs
Tolerance	A state in which a particular dose elicits a smaller response than it formerly did; with increased tolerance, the individual needs higher and higher doses to obtain the desired response
Withdrawal syndrome	A constellation of signs and symptoms that occurs in physically dependent individuals when they discontinue drug use

a parent. Power struggles between abusing and nonabusing partners destroy couples and contribute to a dysfunctional family system. Family relationships begin to deteriorate, and family members become trapped in a cycle of shame, anger, confusion, and guilt. In some families, substance abuse is a contributing factor to emotional neglect and physical or sexual abuse. Often the addict abandons family members and old friends for new relationships in the drug subculture. In other cases, chemically dependent people become more isolated as alcohol or drugs become the main focus of their lives. Some of them are successful in keeping their substance abuse hidden from their colleagues and most of their significant relationships.

Ineffective communication patterns contribute to anxiety and anger. In an attempt to create the illusion of normality, substance abuse is never discussed within or outside the family system. This refusal to acknowledge the existence of a problem contributes to family denial. To avoid embarrassment, family members make excuses to outsiders for the user's behavior. A nonabusing partner may remain in a relationship because of emotional dependency, money, family cohesion, religious compliance, or outward respectability. Other nonabusing partners may threaten to or may actually leave the abuser. At this point, the abuser promises never to drink or use again, the family is reunited, the promise is usually broken, and the family becomes locked into a dysfunctional pattern.

CODEPENDENCY Codependency is a relationship in which a non–substance-abusing partner remains with a substance-abusing partner. The relationship is dysfunctional—the nonabusing partner is hyperresponsible, and the abusing partner is irresponsible. Codependents operate out of fear, resentment, helplessness, and hopelessness. They are obsessively driven to control the user's behavior and to solve the problems the user created. When this is not effective, codependents become exhausted and depressed, but are unable to stop the "helping" behaviors. They often suffer from low self-esteem and fear of abandonment. Codependents are *caretakers,* and this caretaking activity may be a compensation for feelings of inadequacy. Women may be more vulnerable to codependent behavior because they have been socialized to be responsible for the family and often believe they are expected to remain loyal to their partner at all costs. As professionals, nurses must be careful not to blame women for the user's behavior (Martsolf, Sedlak, & Doheny, 2000; Stafford, 2001).

Codependents often engage in **enabling behavior**, which is any action a person takes that consciously or unconsciously facilitates substance dependence. Enabling behaviors (e.g., making excuses for the partner with the employer and lying to others about the abuse) protect the substance abuser from the natural consequences of the problem. Enabling is a response to addiction, not a cause of addiction. The purpose of enabling is the family's instinctual desire to stay together. It is a process of compensating for the dysfunction in one family member and avoiding the issues that threaten the breakup of the family.

Codependent behaviors can continue long after the abusing spouse stops using, the nonabusing spouse ends the marriage, or the children grow up and leave the household. Spouses and children of substance-dependent individuals need healing and treatment as much as—or more than—the addicted family member. A number of support networks and groups, including Adult Children of Alcoholics and Al-Anon, exist to help family members free themselves of addiction behaviors.

THE EFFECTS OF ADDICTION BEHAVIORS ON CHILDREN

The information in this section is based on studies of children of alcoholics (COAs). More research has been done on that group than on children of drug-addicted parents, but the information is generally true for children whose parents are addicted to both street and prescription drugs, partially because many of the addiction behaviors exist regardless of the substance being abused.

It is estimated that one of every eight Americans is a child of an alcoholic parent. Children who grow up in homes where one parent or both parents are alcoholics or drug addicts often suffer the effects their entire lives. Dysfunctional family roles develop around the impact of alcoholism. Despite mysterious events, nonsense language, and threats of impending doom, everyone in the family acts as if the situation were perfectly normal.

Children of alcoholics often believe that they are the cause of the addiction, sometimes because the parent convinces the child that if it were not for what the child did, the parent would not be acting that way. When the alcoholic parent has a tendency toward anger or physical abuse, the children live with fear on an almost daily basis.

Parents preoccupied with alcohol or drugs may jeopardize their children's health and safety. They may use the household budget for drugs. They may disappear for hours or days. They may neglect to cook and clean and to bathe the children and get them to school. Their ability to be emotionally and physically available to their children may be compromised. Their parental judgment is often impaired, and in some cases, children are exposed to criminal activity.

Very early in life, COAs learn to "keep the secret" and not talk about the problem, even with the family. They are taught not to talk about their own feelings, needs, and wants; some learn not to feel at all. Eventually, they repress all feelings and become numb to both pain and joy. The children become objects whose reason for existence is to please the alcoholic parent and to serve that parent's needs. COAs are expected to be in control of their behavior and feelings at all times. They are expected to be perfect and never make mistakes. However, within the family system, no child can ever be perfect "enough." Consistency is necessary for building trust, and alcoholic parents are very unpredictable. Children learn not to expect reliability in relationships. They learn very early that if you do not trust another person, you will not be disappointed.

Children of alcoholics tend to develop one of four patterns of behavior. The *hero,* often the oldest child, becomes the competent caretaker and works on making the family function. The *scapegoat* acts out at home, in school, and in the community. This child takes the focus off the alcoholic parent by getting into trouble and becoming the focus of conflict in the family. The behavior also may be a way to draw attention to the family in an unconscious attempt to seek help. The *lost child* tries to avoid conflict and pain by withdrawing physically and emotionally. The *mascot,* often the youngest child, tries to ease family tension with comic relief used to mask his or her sadness.

In dysfunctional families, designated roles keep the family balanced. Each role is a way to handle the distress and shame of having an alcoholic parent. Every family member has a sense of some control, even though the roles do not change the family system's dysfunction.

Adult COAs grow up denying the stresses of their dysfunctional families. Denial becomes a frequent defense mechanism that only makes situations worse as they proceed through life. The sense of total obligation to the alcoholic parent makes it extremely difficult for adult children to criticize the addicted parent.

Adult COAs grow up without mature adult role models and without the experience of healthy family dynamics. They expect all relationships to be based on power, violence, deceit, and misinformation. They often have difficulty expressing emotion and receiving expressions of feelings. Some grow up to repeat the family pattern by becoming addicted themselves or marrying an addicted person.

Adult COAs often feel a need to change others or to control the environment for the good of others. They typically deny powerlessness and try to solve all problems alone. They blame themselves for not being able to achieve what no one can achieve. Obsessions are common forms of defense, such as constant worrying, preoccupations with work or other activities that bring about good feelings, and compulsive achievement. The obsessive pattern covers the feelings of helplessness and blocks the feelings of anxiety, inadequacy, and fear of abandonment.

ASSESSMENT

The nursing history plays an important role in determining potential addictive behavior. Clients may feel shame, contempt, or embarrassment upon revealing their addiction. In addition, fear of legal reprisal may cause the client to be reluctant to share information if the addiction is to an illegal substance. A trusting nurse–client relationship, along with the nurse's ethical obligation to maintain confidentiality, may help the client share information more freely. By involving family members when gathering assessment data, nurses may uncover addictions the client is hiding. Nurses must help clients understand the importance of disclosure to protect them from potential treatment complications, such as administration of a narcotic to someone with a narcotic addiction. All too often clients admit addiction very late in the cycle of abuse, after permanent damage has already occurred. The nurse's responsibility is to recognize clues while complications are still preventable.

Physical assessment findings are dependent on the nature of the addiction. Clients with an addiction to self-inflicted wounding, called *cutting*, may have many unexplained lacerations, often located in areas that are covered by clothing. Clients addicted to narcotics may demonstrate symptoms described in Exemplar 2.4. When performing a physical assessment, nurses must be alert for symptoms that are abnormal or not within expected boundaries and assess client explanations for inconsistencies. Unless the client comes to the provider under the influence or is referred by an employer, the physical examination may provide the first indications that an addiction is involved.

Clients also may need to be assessed regarding the extent of crisis they are facing in their lives as the result of their addiction behaviors, particularly if a crisis event or behavior motivates them to seek health care. Box 2–1 demonstrates a general crisis assessment that can be used with any client facing crisis and is of particular use for the client whose crisis is the result of addiction behavior.

DIAGNOSTIC TESTS

Diagnostic tests required for clients with addiction will be ordered based on the type of addiction they display. Specific diagnostic tests will be ordered for each type of addiction and may include:

- Serum drug levels
- Toxicology testing
- Chest x-ray for inhaled substances
- Organ biopsies related to damage caused by substance
- Urine, saliva, and serum testing for substance metabolites
- Hair testing to determine substance use within a period of 90 days.

CARING INTERVENTIONS

Nurses may use a number of caring interventions with clients who are addicted or who exhibit addiction behaviors. **Recovery** is generally defined as a state of voluntary sobriety in which the individual maintains personal health and functions normally within society. The goal of all interventions is to move

Box 2–1 Crisis Assessment Related to Substance Abuse

INDIVIDUAL ASSESSMENT

1. What is the most significant stress/problem occurring in your life right now?
2. Has this problem increased the frequency of substance use? (Quantify change in frequency or amount of substance used)
3. Is your addiction behavior causing or contributing to the problem?
4. Who is the problem, or your addiction behavior, impacting? You? Your family? Your employer? The community?
5. How long has this been a problem?
6. Is this a temporary or permanent problem?
7. What does this problem mean to you?
8. What are the factors that cause this problem to continue?
9. Would the problem resolve if you stopped abusing the substance?
10. Have you had similar stresses/problems in the past?
11. What other stresses do you have in your life?
12. How are you managing your usual life roles (partner, parent, homemaker, worker, student, etc.)?
13. In what way has your life changed as a result of this problem?
14. Are you feeling as though you want to harm yourself or others?
15. Describe how you have managed problems in the past.
16. What have you done to try to solve the problem so far?
17. What happened when you tried this?
18. Describe possible resources (e.g., family, friends, employer, teacher; financial, spiritual).
19. Are you interested in abstaining from substance abuse? Are you considering a rehabilitation program?
20. What are your expectations and hopes concerning this problem?
21. What is the most you hope for when this problem is resolved?
22. What is the least you will settle for to resolve this problem?
23. What part of the overall problem is most important to deal with first?

FAMILY ASSESSMENT

1. How do you perceive the current problem and the client's addiction behavior?
2. In what way has the problem and the client's addiction behavior affected your roles in the family?
3. How has your lifestyle changed since this problem began?
4. Describe communication within the family before this current problem.
5. Describe communication within the family since the problem began.
6. How does the family typically manage problems?
7. What has the family done to try and solve the problem so far?
8. What has the family done to try to stop the addiction behavior?
9. What happened when you tried this?
10. How well do you believe the family is coping at this time?
11. Describe possible resources (e.g., extended family, friends; financial).
12. What are your expectations and hopes concerning this problem and the client's addiction behavior?
13. Which part of the overall problem is most important to deal with first?
14. Can the problem be resolved without resolution of the addiction behavior?

COMMUNITY ASSESSMENT

1. What are the special demands of the client's community?
2. What are the living conditions of the neighborhood?
3. Are recreational centers available?
4. Are affordable child care services available?
5. Is there a community mental health center?
6. What support groups are available in the community?
7. Is there a rehabilitation center to help the client resolve addiction behavior issues?
8. What are the possible funding resources?

the client toward treatment and recovery. Nurses must remember that no single intervention is sufficient to ensure recovery, which requires substantial work on the part of the addict. All interventions, even pharmacologic therapies, have one thing in common: They begin with successful communication.

Communication

When nurses care for the client with an addiction, whether it is a substance or a process addiction, establishing a beneficial relationship involves the use of therapeutic communication, which places the client at the center of all communication. This is critical for two reasons: (1) Many clients with addictions have poor communication skills and rely on their addictive behaviors to avoid communications with others, and (2) clients with addictions are experienced at hiding their addictions and avoiding the addiction as the topic of discussion. Although the concept of therapeutic communication is discussed in detail in Exemplar 36.4, it is important here to discuss aspects of communication that greatly benefit the addicted client and family members.

Many clients with addictions or addictive behaviors need assistance with verbal and nonverbal communication. It is important that nurses discuss facial expressions, eye contact, posture, gestures, and interpersonal distance. They should keep in mind that nonverbal communication is culturally determined and teach within those cultural expectations. They can give examples of how being aware of nonverbal communication helps build relationships. Finally, nurses should ask clients to demonstrate a thought or feeling without using words, such as happiness, anger, or frustration. The goal is to increase clients' awareness of their nonverbal communication and that of others.

Conversation is another social skill. Nurses should discuss volume, tone, and rate of speech and model taking turns in speaking and not interrupting. They should have clients practice skills such as initiating conversations, asking questions, making appropriate self-disclosures, and ending conversations gracefully. Assertiveness training is appropriate for clients who are either passive or aggressive in their style of relating to others. Assertive people are able to say no to unreasonable demands and to activities in which they do not want to participate. They are able to express positive and negative feelings in an appropriate manner and accept constructive criticism and praise from other people. Assertiveness may be inappropriate in some cultures, especially those in which children and teens are not allowed to disagree with parents or those in which women are expected to be obedient and submissive to men.

Family Intervention

When addictive behavior reaches a crisis stage, the family and loved ones of an addict may choose to confront the addicted person with the impact of the addict's behavior on others. The objective is to get the addict to agree to seek treatment immediately. This confrontation is called an **intervention**. One goal is to prevent the addict from denying the problem and force the person to face the negative aspects of the behavior. In an intervention, each person in the group tells the addict the negative consequences the addict faces because of the addiction and asks the addict to seek treatment. The family often plans the intervention in advance, usually in consultation with an addiction professional. Typically, the intervention is designed to catch the addict by surprise, but it may take place in a counselor's office, with the addict invited to attend.

The desired result of the intervention is that the addict begins to recognize the impact of the addiction and addiction behaviors on the people who love and support him or her and becomes motivated to seek treatment. When invited to attend a meeting under a counselor's supervision, the addict may be less likely to feel angry or ambushed than when confronted by a surprise intervention. Regardless of the timing of the intervention, the family should make preparations in advance for the addict to enter rehabilitation immediately after the meeting, if the person agrees to seek help. Waiting hours or days can result in a change of mind as the addict's withdrawal or addiction symptoms escalate.

Crisis Intervention

There are many definitions of crisis, most of which concur that a *crisis* is a turning point in a person's life—a point at which the usual resources and coping skills are no longer effective. Two symbols in the Chinese language communicate the meaning of crisis: the symbol for *danger* and the symbol for *opportunity*. This text views a crisis as both a danger and an opportunity.

Throughout life, people experience events to which they must respond. Many of these events are expected life changes that are anticipated at particular ages—graduation, employment, marriage or partnership, and parenthood. Depending on individual circumstances, these expected life changes may evoke crisis states referred to as *maturational crises*. Because of individual differences, not all people choose or have the opportunity to experience all of the expected life changes. Unexpected life changes—such as divorce, serious illness, or death—may result in *situational crises*. It is only when the expected or unexpected event is perceived subjectively as a threat to need fulfillment, safety, or a meaningful existence that the person enters a maturational or situational crisis state.

The addict's poor life management skills frequently result in declining quality of life until a crisis level is reached that causes the person to reexamine his or her choices and consider the need for change. It is during these crisis situations when addicts are most likely to be motivated to seek help to treat their addiction and turn their lives around. The inability to maintain emotional equilibrium is an important feature of a crisis. The state of disequilibrium usually lasts 4–6 weeks. Typically, the high level of anxiety during this short period forces the individual to do one of the following:

- Adapt and return to the previous level of addiction
- Develop more constructive coping skills and seek help for the addiction
- Decompensate to a lower level of functioning.

During this time, people are most receptive to professional intervention. A thorough assessment of support and previous coping behaviors includes an evaluation of the client's self-destructive feelings and behavior. If there is considerable threat to client safety, inpatient intervention may be necessary. Box 2–1 describes crisis assessment from individual, family, and community perspectives. While this assessment can be used for any type of crisis, it is particularly useful in dealing with addictive behavior that has led the client to a crisis situation.

The primary goal of **crisis intervention** is to assist the client in resolving the immediate problem and regaining emotional equilibrium. The minimum goal of intervention is to help clients adapt and return to the pre-crisis level of functioning. The maximum goal is to help clients develop more constructive coping skills and move on to a higher level of functioning without the use of addictive behavior. Assisting the client in crisis resolution may lead to better use of coping mechanisms when dealing with future stressful life events.

The role of nurses in crisis intervention is one of active participation in solving the problem. It is important for nurses to understand that they do *not* take over and make decisions for clients unless clients are suicidal or homicidal.

The nurse's primary focus in crisis intervention is to assist the client in developing skills that enable the client to adapt to or move beyond the crisis state. These skills include behavioral, affective, spiritual, cognitive, and psychosocial skills. The relative importance of these skills varies with each person and each crisis. Most likely, the skills are used in various combinations, with the effectiveness of specific skills depending on the specific event.

Nurses help clients identify alternative ways of resolving the crisis and predict probable consequences for each alternative. This requires the client to gain **behavior skills**, behaviors that help the client resolve problems without resorting to drinking or using. Seeking information is the first step or behavior in a healthy process of problem solving. The next step is choosing an alternative and taking concrete action. The final step is evaluating the consequences and, if necessary, finding solutions again. During the crisis state, the client is more receptive to trying a variety of coping behaviors to decrease anxiety. Nurses must remember to continually reinforce the client's strengths by reviewing the crisis event, the coping effectiveness, and the newly learned methods of problem solving so that the client obtains a reasonable balance. Nurses also provide clients the opportunity to vent their feelings by talking, crying, and even screaming. This allows for emotional discharge of anger, despair, and frustration, a coping skill with which many addicts are unfamiliar. The ability to identify and discuss one's feelings is an adaptive skill. It allows the client to tolerate ambiguity and maintain some hope, behaviors that are very helpful during a crisis period.

Spiritual skills help the individual find meaning in and understand the personal significance of an unexpected event. Finding meaning is an ongoing issue during and after the crisis period. The result of the search depends on the individual's spirituality or philosophy of life. Some people find meaning by focusing on causes beyond themselves. Others believe in divine purpose, in which they find a great source of consolation.

Cognitive skills are thought processes that help the individual cope temporarily and provide long-term resolution of the crisis. Denial is a defense mechanism common to addicted clients and their family members. Denial may be effective temporarily in stabilizing a difficult or volatile situation, but it offers no long-term solutions to the issue causing the crisis (namely, the addiction). A more effective cognitive skill is the ability to redefine the unexpected event. In this instance, the person accepts the basic reality of the event but reshapes the situation into something favorable. For example, the individual might focus on the potential positive outcomes of healthy behaviors or decisions or compare herself or himself with those less fortunate. The goal of adaptive cognitive skills is to maintain a satisfactory self-image and a sense of competence and mastery.

Psychosocial skills enable a person in crisis to maintain relationships with family and friends throughout and after the crisis period. An essential psychosocial skill for addicts to learn is to accept comfort and support offered by others. Family and friends may be sources of information that will enable the person to make wise decisions. Not to be overlooked are community resources such as hotlines, mental health centers, support groups, and self-help groups.

In addition to behavioral, affective, spiritual, cognitive, and psychosocial skills, other factors influence the outcome of unexpected events. Demographic and personal factors influence how a person defines and resolves crises. These factors include age, gender, ethnicity, economic resources, spiritual resources, and past experiences. Factors specific to the event also influence the outcome. Tasks and coping skills vary among biologic, psychologic, environmental, and social crisis events. The more control a person has over these factors, the more adaptive that individual is likely to be. Successful resolution of crisis leads to growth and an increased ability to cope in the future. Failure to resolve the issues contributes to decreased adaptation and potential problems in the future.

Behavioral Therapy

In **behavioral therapy**, clients learn techniques to modify or change their addictive behaviors. Behavioral therapy is based on the principle that all behavior has specific consequences. Behavior is changed by conditioning—a process of reinforcement, punishment, and extinction.

Consequences that lead to an increase in a particular behavior are referred to as **reinforcement**. *Positive reinforcement* provides a reward for the desired behavior, such as the pleasant sensation, or high, that comes from the use of a substance. *Negative reinforcement* removes a negative stimulus to increase the chances that the desired behavior will occur. An example of negative reinforcement is when the family of an addict refuses to support the behavior that results from use of the substance. Consequences that lead to a decrease in undesirable behavior are referred to as **punishment**. *Positive punishment* is the addition of a negative consequence if the undesirable behavior occurs; for example, the addict who drives under the influence is jailed or fined. *Negative punishment* is the removal of a positive reward if the undesirable behavior occurs; for example, the addict who does not show up for work loses his or her job. **Extinction** refers to the progressive weakening of an undesirable behavior through repeated nonreinforcement of the behavior. For example, family members may choose to ignore negative attention-seeking behaviors such as statements like "you're just trying to control my life." If the addict begins to see that these types of angry, provoking statements no longer elicit a response, he or she will (hopefully) be forced to find more appropriate ways to seek attention.

Most behavioral therapists believe that reinforcement is more desirable than punishment. There is no doubt that punishment is effective and sometimes necessary when the behavior is dangerous. But behavior changed through reinforcement is a more desirable clinical outcome than behavior changed through punishment. **Contingency contracts** may be an effective reinforcement process. These contracts operate by "if-then" rules. If the client performs a targeted response, such as abstinence from the addictive behavior (gambling, drug use, cutting, etc.), then the client receives desired reinforcers. Contingency contracts are only as effective as the rewards chosen (e.g., food treats, activities, or privileges). What one person considers a reward, another person may not. When a client is first learning the targeted behavior, rewards are given immediately, along with verbal praise and specific feedback. An example is "Good job. You admitted you have a problem. Here is the reward we talked about."

Token economies are formalized programs of contingency contracts. They are established for all members of a group and are often used with groups of addicts in treatment programs. There are three parts to token economies, as follows:

1. Identifying behaviors that everyone in the group is expected to demonstrate
2. Specifying token rewards for doing those behaviors (e.g., if you face the problems you caused your family as a result of your addiction, you will receive 10 tokens); inappropriate behaviors are also identified for which tokens may be lost
3. Establishing rules for redeeming tokens: what types of activities or privileges may be swapped for tokens, how many tokens each one costs, and when and where tokens are swapped.

Behavioral therapy is well suited to treating addiction behavior because the client must alter familiar coping mechanisms and find means of reducing anxiety other than resorting to the source of the addiction. Nurses are in an ideal position to evaluate client response to treatment. Because they spend a great deal of time with clients, nurses can see developing patterns of behavioral change.

Milieu Therapy

The successful recovery environment involves creating a surrounding for the addict that will support behavior changes, teach new coping measures, and help the client move from addiction to an addiction-free life. This is often referred to as **milieu therapy**. In its earliest conception, *milieu* described a scientifically planned community. Research efforts focused on defining the types of environments that would be most therapeutic for the client facing addiction.

The work of Cummings and Cummings (1962) suggested that the environment (milieu) itself might be a strong force in bringing about changes in client behavior. Kraft (1966) defined the idea of milieu more precisely as a therapeutic community in which the entire social structure of the unit or residence is designed to be part of the helping process. Kraft's idea of a therapeutic community emphasized the social and interpersonal interactions that become the therapeutic tools influencing change in client behavior. This view differed somewhat from the pure idea of milieu therapy, in which the emphasis was on "manipulation" of the environment to effect therapeutic change.

Hildegard Peplau (1952), the mother of psychiatric nursing theory, described the roles of the nurse in the therapeutic milieu. Peplau also described the *therapeutic use of self,* that is, using one's personhood to provide psychiatric nursing care. Within the nurse–client relationship, nurses use their personalities, beliefs, values, feelings, cognitions, and perceptions as they implement holistic nursing practice.

Milieu therapy has certain basic goals, whether the setting is a group home, a community center, a day program, or an inpatient unit. These goals include an emphasis on:

- Clients as responsible people
- Group and social interaction
- Client rights to choose and participate in a variety of treatments
- Informality of relationships with health care professionals.

Milieu therapy also includes clear communication, a safe environment, an activity schedule with therapeutic goals, and a support network. The overall goal behind all of these components is to support the changes in the client's behavior necessary to free the client from addiction. Within this environment, the nurse plays a pivotol role by modeling and teaching desirable behaviors. Often, the nurse is the member of the client's psychiatric team who spends the most time with, and around, the client. The nurse's observations of, and interactions with, the client provide information and opportunities critical to understanding the client's addiction behavior and to helping the client determine a successful path to recovery.

Group Therapy

Therapeutic groups provide support to the members as they work through their problems. **Group therapy** is a beneficial experience in which the group members help each other with psychologic, cognitive, behavioral, and spiritual dysfunctions through a process of change, aided by a professional group therapist.

Groups can be held in an inpatient unit, an outpatient clinic, a community mental health center, or a variety of other settings. Ballinger and Yalom (1995) identified mechanisms of change within a group and called them *curative factors* of group therapy. These factors provide a rationale for a variety of group interventions. Table 2–2 describes the curative factors.

Ballinger and Yalom (1995) also identified two concepts basic to group therapy: the group as a social microcosm and the here-and-now concept. The term **social microcosm** refers to the concept that group members eventually behave in the therapy group the same way they behave with families and friends. The group becomes a living example of how each member relates to others outside the group. The therapist's task is to help members recognize dysfunctional ways of relating to others. As group members interact with one another and

TABLE 2–2 **Curative Factors of Group Therapy**

FACTOR	DESCRIPTION
Instillation of hope	As clients observe other members further along in the therapeutic process, they begin to feel a sense of hope for themselves.
Universality	Through interaction with other group members, clients realize they are not alone in their problems or pain.
Imparting of information	Teaching and suggestions usually come from the group leader but may also be generated by the group members.
Altruism	Through the group process, clients recognize that they have something to give to the other group members.
Corrective recapitulation of the primary family group	Many clients have a history of dysfunctional family relationships. The therapy group is often like a family, and clients can learn more functional patterns of communication, interaction, and behavior.
Development of socializing techniques	Development of social skills takes place in groups. Group members give feedback about maladaptive social behavior. Clients learn more appropriate ways of socializing with others.
Imitative behavior	Clients often model their behavior after the leader or other group members. This trial process enables them to discover what behaviors work well for them as individuals.
Interpersonal learning	Through the group process, clients learn the positive benefits of good interpersonal relationships. Emotional healing takes place through this process.
Existential factors	The group provides opportunities for clients to explore the meaning of their life and their place in the world.
Catharsis	Clients learn how to express their own feelings in a goal-directed way, speak openly about what is bothering them, and express strong feelings about other members in a responsible way.
Group cohesiveness	Cohesiveness occurs when members feel a sense of belonging.

Source: Adapted with permission from Ballinger, B., & Yalom, I. D. (1995). *The theory and practice of group psychotherapy* (4th ed.). New York: Basic Books. Reprinted by permission of BASIC Books a member of Perseus Books Group.

discuss this process, individuals engage in self-reflection, leading to affective, behavioral, cognitive, and spiritual changes. The **here-and-now concept** refers to the present moment of group experience. Although the past and the future have some importance, changes can be made only in the present. People who get stuck in the past ruminate over what was and what might have been. Others spend a great deal of time worrying about the future. The therapist's task is to keep the focus in the present by discussing what happens and why it happens.

Nurses function as group therapists in many different settings, establishing the type of group that is appropriate for the desired outcomes. A single nurse may lead groups, or two cotherapists may share leadership. Initially, the members are strangers, and the leader, as the unifying force, helps the members relate to one another. Some of the important tasks of the group leader include (Ballinger & Yalom, 1995):

- Encouraging members to remain in the group.
- Helping the group develop a sense of cohesiveness.
- Establishing a code of behavior and norms with the group.

Throughout the therapeutic process, the nurse leader assumes two basic roles (Ballinger & Yalom, 1995):

1. *Technical expert:* Using a variety of nondirective or directive approaches, the leader moves the group in a desirable direction. The leader may give explicit directions for conduct or imply suggestions.
2. *Model-setting participant:* The leader shapes behavior by the example set by his or her own personal behavior within the group. The leader molds the group in a health-oriented direction by encouraging adaptive behavior. Through encouraging frank expression of feelings, the leader sets a model in which responsibility and restraint temper honesty with concern for others' feelings and defenses. By modeling the leader's responses, the group members work toward improving interpersonal skills.

Group therapy can be effective with children and adolescents who may be the addict or the children of an addict. In working with young children, the size of the group is usually limited to five. Age and attention span determine the duration of the group session. Group therapy with children is usually activity-oriented and may include daily goal setting, art projects, music or movement therapy, or play therapy.

Because adolescents can reason and talk about their behavior, thoughts, and feelings, group therapy with adolescents is a verbal process rather than an activity process used with children. Peers are very important in teenagers' lives, providing support, feedback, and information. As a result, group therapy with adolescents is often more productive than individual sessions.

There is often a parallel group for the parents of children and adolescents so that the entire family can receive treatment simultaneously. Such a group enables the parents to support each other, learn growth and developmental stages, gain an awareness of their contribution to family dynamics, increase parenting skills, and explore their own needs and problems.

SUPPORT GROUPS Nurses frequently refer clients and their families to support groups, which are very important for mental health clients. In this type of group, members share their thoughts and feelings and help one another examine issues and concerns. The characteristics of support groups include the following:

- Clients define their own needs.
- Members have equal power.
- Groups may or may not be autonomous from mental health professionals.
- Attendance is voluntary.
- Groups may be responsive to a special population (e.g., a bilingual population); those with eating disorders; or those defined by racial, gender, or sexual identity.

Support groups function to educate community members; to help family and friends support the individual; and to act as a crisis support, a source of referrals, and an advocate to help people get their needs met through the health care system. Because people with addictions typically have a very restricted social network, often comprising others with similar addictions, it is important to help clients form a healthier base of support. This helps prevent recidivism into the addictive behavior they are seeking to resolve. As a result, the interpersonal contact of support groups is vitally important. These groups contribute to an increased self-esteem, a sense of identity, increased dignity, and improved self-responsibility.

12-STEP PROGRAMS In the United States, an estimated 3.5 million people attend 12-step programs annually. Twelve-step programs are support groups that offer a spiritual plan for recovery. The first one, Alcoholics Anonymous (AA), originated in Akron, Ohio, in 1935. The first edition of the "Big Book" was published in 1939 and continues today as the principal guideline for AA. Today, worldwide AA membership is estimated at 2 million people scattered across 100 countries. Other 12-step programs emerged in the 1950s and 1960s, including Al-Anon, Narcotics Anonymous (NA), Cocaine Anonymous, Adult Children of Alcoholics, Emotions Anonymous, Gamblers Anonymous, Overeaters Anonymous, and Sex Addicts Anonymous.

The 12-step program consists of prescribed beliefs, values, and behaviors. The sequential plan for recovery is stated in 12 steps, as described in Box 2–2. Step work is considered to be a lifelong process and is usually accomplished with the aid of a sponsor. Twelve-step fellowship includes the activities of the organization, such as helping others, building relationships among members, and sharing joys and hardships.

The only requirement for membership is the sincere desire to change the target behavior. Any interested person can attend open meetings. Closed meetings are reserved for members only. Some 12-step groups cater to demographic subsets such as women, men, adolescents, gays and lesbians, and nurses. There are four common meeting formats:

1. *Open discussion:* Individuals are asked to share thoughts and feelings regarding a general topic introduced at the beginning of the meeting.
2. *Speaker meetings:* One to three members talk for the entire meeting, usually about what life was like before membership, what happened to facilitate membership, and what life is like now as the result of membership.
3. *Big Book or 12-by-12 meetings:* Often called step meetings, the primary focus is on the meaning and practice of the 12 steps.
4. *Birthday meetings:* Once a month, members recognize specified periods of continuous abstinence. They recognize 30-, 60-, and 90-day intervals, as well as 6-, 9-, and 12-month birthdays. Thereafter, birthdays are celebrated annually.

Box 2–2 **The 12 Steps of Alcoholics Anonymous**

WE

1. Admitted we were powerless over alcohol, that our lives had become unmanageable.
2. Came to believe that a Power greater than ourselves could restore us to sanity.
3. Made a decision to turn our will and our lives over to the care of God as we understood Him.
4. Made a searching and fearless moral inventory of ourselves.
5. Admitted to God, to ourselves, and to another human being the exact nature of our wrongs.
6. Were entirely ready to have God remove all these defects of character.
7. Humbly asked Him to remove our shortcomings.
8. Made a list of all persons we had harmed and became willing to make amends to them all.
9. Made direct amends to such people wherever possible, except when to do so would injure them or others.
10. Continued to take personal inventory and when we were wrong promptly admitted it.
11. Sought through prayer and meditation to improve our conscious contact with God as we understood Him, praying only for knowledge of His will for us and the power to carry that out.
12. Having had a spiritual awakening as the result of these steps, we tried to carry this message to alcoholics and to practice these principles in all our affairs.

Source: The Twelve Steps are reprinted with permission of Alcoholics Anonymous World Services, Inc. (A.A.W.S.). Permission to reprint the Twelve Steps does not mean that A.A.W.S. has reviewed or approves the contents of this publication, or that A.A.W.S. necessarily agrees with the views expressed herein. A.A. is a program of recovery from alcoholism only—use of the Twelve Steps in connection with programs and activities which are patterned after A.A., but which address other problems, or in any other non-A.A. context, does not imply otherwise.

Family Therapy

Family therapy is a specialized area of study, and becoming a family therapist requires extensive preparation. In **family therapy**, the family system is treated as a unit and the focus is on family dynamics. The goals are to help families cope, improve their communication and interpersonal skills, establish boundaries, and moderate family cohesion and flexibility. Families strive to maintain balance and harmony. When an addicted member causes the balance to shift, families must use their internal and external resources to adapt. Competent families seem to adapt more efficiently than dysfunctional families.

Change is so frightening or alien to some families that they invest their energies in maintaining the status quo, regardless of how painful that may be. The result is that they seem more interested in enabling the addiction of one of its members than in supporting changes that will improve health.

One of the problems with family therapy is that the Euro-American middle-class heterosexual family ideal has been used as the yardstick for determining "normal family function." This traditional stance has ignored families from other cultures, social classes, and family structures—all of whom may have very different values. Currently, family therapists are committing to not "pathologize" that which is different. Using multicultural theory, they take a more investigative approach and help family members define their unique culture and values.

Family therapy is recommended when the nurse or family determines that the family system is impaired because of the presence of a psychosocial problem or addiction in one or more family members. Schools, courts, and health care providers may identify impairment of family functioning. For family therapy to be successful, all family members must believe that they are part of the problem-solving and decision-making processes and that their personal welfare is always considered. Some advanced practice nurses provide home-based family therapy. This allows the nurse-therapist to observe the family in the natural setting of the home. Comfort with their environment encourages family members to participate. In addition, the therapist becomes a guest; thus, a measure of control remains within the family. Direct observation illuminates family dynamics rather quickly and can effectively guide nursing interventions (Falloon, 2002).

Family therapists help family members look at a number of issues. They assess the family hierarchy, which defines power relationships among the members. They identify subsystems—groups of people within the family who join together to perform various functions—such as the parental or sibling subsystem. Therapists identify and discuss boundaries, which define the degree of emotional closeness among family members and subsystems.

The overall goals of family therapy are to:

- Teach parents better parenting and nurturing skills.
- Reinstate generational boundaries in the family hierarchy.
- Improve family communication.
- Teach the family how to problem solve.

Although most nurses are not family therapists, this is not to say that nurses in the mental health care system do not intervene with families. Nurses in both inpatient and outpatient settings are likely to have a great deal of contact with their clients' families. Family members interact with nurses in a variety of situations, most of which are informal. When nurses work informally with families, they assess for a number of factors, including:

- Relationships between individual members of the family
- Roles that various members of the family assume
- Family communication patterns
- Achievement of the family's developmental tasks
- Normal coping strategies that the family uses
- Past and current efforts to cope with addiction
- Family support systems
- Sociocultural norms and values of the family
- Personal goals for each family member.

Disagreements and conflicts in family relationships are normal. The problem in families with an addictive member is not that they disagree, but that they do not know how to resolve their differences. Families dealing with a member's addiction often become so involved in dysfunctional behavior that they start to see this behavior as normal. Teaching families general principles for resolving conflict is a helpful nursing intervention. Box 2–3 lists eight steps for resolving family disagreements.

PHARMACOLOGIC THERAPIES

Pharmacologic therapies are available to treat and prevent symptoms of withdrawal and to treat overdose. Treating symptoms of withdrawal may involve reducing physiologic cravings for the drug of choice, but it may also involve reducing anxiety to prevent the client from feeding the addiction or to prevent dangerous symptoms associated with sudden withdrawal from powerful substances such as sedatives and hypnotics. A number of pharmacologic therapies are available. Many of these, however, have multiple drug interactions and should be used with caution. For example, disulfiram should never be used during pregnancy and should be used with caution in clients taking phentyoin. See the Medications feature on page 37.

Box 2–3 **Eight Steps Used to Resolve Family Disagreements**

1. *Stay calm.* When people are calm, they think more clearly. People have difficulty remaining calm when they call each other names, become sarcastic, or drag up past injustices. Do not try to solve problems when members are angry.
2. *Express commitment to the relationship.* Arguments often leave people feeling like enemies rather than members of a caring family unit. It is important to defuse that by saying, "I love you. Let's work together to solve this problem."
3. *Identify areas of agreement or success.* Teach people to look for similarities in their viewpoints or to find positive characteristics in the other person. Family members often get stuck on arguing about one small point and overlook the fact that they agree on many other points.
4. *Identify the specific problem.* It is difficult to resolve problems when arguments keep escalating with the addition of more problems.
5. *Express the desired outcome.* Family members should clearly state what they want to happen so that everybody is clear about each other's goals.
6. *Listen carefully to the other person's concerns.* Each person needs to hear what the other person is saying. If necessary, have family members repeat the essence of what they heard to show that they understand. Problems cannot be solved if individuals are planning what they are going to say next, rather than listening carefully to what someone is saying to them.
7. *Seek solutions that benefit the relationship.* Teach family members to brainstorm possible solutions and to look for ways to compromise and meet everyone's needs.
8. *Assess the outcome.* Teach family members to analyze the solution before it is implemented. Does everyone feel respected and heard? Is everyone at least partially satisfied with the solution? If so, the conflict has probably been resolved successfully.

MEDICATIONS Addictions

Classification	Mechanism of action	Common drugs	Nursing considerations
Opioid antagonists	Used to treat a narcotic overdose, these drugs block narcotic receptor sites and quickly reverse the effect of the narcotic if administered via IV therapy.	naloxone	Monitor client condition, including respiratory rate, and anticipate the need for pain management as narcotic effects are reversed.
Acetaldehyde dehydrogenase inhibitor	Inhibits the enzyme that metabolizes alcohol, causing the client to become violently ill if alcohol is consumed while taking this medication. Symptoms include shortness of breath, headache, nausea, and vomiting.	disulfiram	Teach client to avoid all alcohol, including that found in substances such as mouthwash, liquid medications, and food. Use of this medication requires a client who is highly motivated. Assess client's motivational level to quit drinking.
Antiseizure	Raises the threshold of cerebral excitation, reducing the likelihood and severity of seizure activity that can occur as the result of withdrawal from substances such as sedatives and hypnotics.	■ phenytoin ■ carbamazepine ■ valproic acid	Implement seizure precautions to maintain client safety. If a seizure occurs, place a pillow under the client's head and time the seizure, noting client behavior during and after the event.
Nicotine replacement therapy (NRT)	Supplies the body with nicotine to support smoking cessation therapy.	■ nicotine patch ■ nicotine gum ■ nicotine lozenge ■ nicotine nasal spray ■ nicotine inhaler	Client support is an important element of smoking cessation, and clients benefit from behavior modification teaching in addition to pharmacotherapy.
Antidepressant	Some antidepressants have been shown to reduce the craving for nicotine and support smoking cessation programs. Can also be administered to reduce depression occurring as the result of substance withdrawal.	bupropion hydrochloride	Monitor and question clients about thoughts of suicide. Assess for drug side effects, including drowsiness, insomnia, and blurred vision. Teach client about self-administration of medications and symptoms to report.
Nicotine acetylcholine receptor agonist		varenicline	Assess for nicotine withdrawal symptoms such as depression, agitation, and exacerbation of preexisting mental health disorders. Suicide and suicidal ideation have been associated with use of varenicline. Assess clients for thoughts of suicide or changes in mood and affect.

2.1 ALCOHOL ABUSE

KEY TERMS

Alcohol dependence, *40*
Alcohol poisoning, *44*
Alcohol withdrawal delirium, *43*
Alcohol withdrawal syndrome, *43*
Alcoholic dementia, *43*
Alcoholism, *40*
Binge drinking, *40*
Blackouts, *43*
Confabulation, *43*
Korsakoff's psychosis, *43*
Polysubstance abuse, *45*
Wernicke's encephalopathy, *43*

BASIS FOR SELECTION OF EXEMPLAR

Healthy People 2010

LEARNING OUTCOMES

After reading about this exemplar, you will be able to:

1. Describe the pathophysiology, psychopathology, etiology, clinical manifestations, and direct and indirect causes of alcohol abuse.
2. Identify risk factors associated with alcohol abuse.
3. Illustrate the nursing process in providing culturally competent care across the life span for individuals who abuse alcohol.
4. Formulate priority nursing diagnoses appropriate for an individual who abuses alcohol.
5. Create a plan of care for individuals who abuse alcohol and for their family members.
6. Assess expected outcomes for an individual who abuses alcohol.
7. Discuss therapies used in the collaborative care of an individual who abuses alcohol.
8. Employ evidence-based caring interventions for an individual who abuses alcohol.

OVERVIEW

Alcohol is the most commonly used and abused substance in the United States. In 1992, the Joint Committee of the National Council on Alcoholism and Drug Dependence and the American Society of Addiction Medicine defined **alcoholism** as a "primary, chronic disease with genetic, psychosocial, and environmental factors influencing its development and manifestations" (Morse and Flavin, 1992). It is characterized by the behaviors discussed in the About section of this concept: inability to control the primary addictive behavior (drinking), fixation with the drug and continued use of it regardless of consequences, and impaired thought processes.

Alcohol includes liquor, beer, and wine. While much of society sees the use of nicotine and drugs as inappropriate, use of alcohol is still socially acceptable and often encouraged. Alcohol is frequently offered at weddings and other family events, beer is the favorite drink at sports venues across the country, and many grocery stores and restaurants now offer weekly or monthly wine tastings. The availability of alcohol may be the primary reason it is so widely abused. The economic costs of alcohol abuse in the United States were $184.6 billion in 1998, with an anticipated increase of 3.8% per year (NIAAA, 2002). It is estimated that nearly 25% of all people admitted to a general hospital have alcohol problems.

The *pattern of dependence* on alcohol varies from person to person. Some people have a regular daily intake of large amounts of alcohol. Others restrict their use to heavy drinking on weekends or days off from work, often drinking copious amounts in a single session, a type of alcoholism known as **binge drinking**. Some people abstain for long periods of time and then begin their drinking patterns again. At times, people with alcohol dependence can drink with control; at other times, they cannot control the drinking behavior. As the course of alcoholism continues, addiction behaviors appear with increasing frequency. These may include starting the day off with a drink, sneaking drinks throughout the day, gulping alcoholic drinks, shifting from one alcoholic beverage to another, and hiding bottles at work and at home. The alcoholic may give up hobbies and other interests in order to have more time to drink (Liska, 2004).

Alcoholics are separated into two groups. Those with type 1 alcoholism have a later onset, a more psychologic than physical dependence, and guilt related to their alcohol use. Those with type 2 alcoholism demonstrate problems with alcohol at an early age, compulsively seek alcohol, and are socially disruptive when drinking (Chai et al., 2005).

PATHOPHYSIOLOGY AND ETIOLOGY

Alcohol is a central nervous system (CNS) depressant; as such, it acts on neurotransmitters in the brain (e.g., gamma-aminobutyric acid [GABA]). GABA, the most prevalent inhibitory neurotransmitter in the brain, has a major role in decreasing neuronal excitability. Alcohol creates an additive effect with GABA, further inhibiting arousal and depressing the autonomic nervous system. Alcohol decreases glutamate activity, a major excitatory neurotransmitter. This may explain why cross-tolerance effects occur when alcohol and other CNS depressants are used in combination (Varcarolis, 2002). When taken together, alcohol and other CNS depressants (e.g., benzodiazepines and barbiturates) can lead to respiratory depression and death.

Alcohol is absorbed in the mouth, stomach, and digestive tract. The liver metabolizes approximately 95% of the ingested alcohol; the rest is excreted via the skin, kidney, and lungs. Generally, an individual can break down approximately 1 ounce of whiskey every 90 minutes. Factors such as body mass, food intake, and liver function can affect the rate of alcohol absorption.

Dual diagnosis and *dual disorder* are older terms used to describe individuals with co-occurring disorders. One disorder can be an indication of another, such as the relationship between alcoholism and depression. Alcohol dependence and major depression commonly occur together. Research suggests that both illnesses pose a significant risk for development of the other disorder within 1 year's time (Gilman & Abraham, 2001). A depressed person may use self-medication in the form of alcohol to treat the depression, or the alcoholic person may become depressed.

Etiology

Alcoholism (also referred to as **alcohol dependence**) is a major health problem, one that is responsible for 100,000 deaths annually in the United States. Two thirds of the nation's adult population consumes alcohol regularly. An estimated 14 million Americans (approximately 1 in every 13 adults) abuse alcohol or are alcoholics (National Institute on Alcohol Abuse and Alcoholism, 2004). It is estimated that 25–40% of all clients in U.S. general hospital beds (excluding obstetrics and intensive care) are being treated for complications of alcohol-related problems, including trauma, chronic disease, and organ damage (Center on Addiction and Substance Abuse, 1994).

Although the legal drinking age in all 50 states is 21, many underage people obtain and use alcohol. Of the 14 million adults who abused alcohol in 2003, 95% started drinking alcohol before age 21 (SAMHSA, 2004). During 2004, an estimated 142,701 alcohol-related emergency department (ED) visits were made by patients aged 12–20 (OAS, 2006). The rate of underage drinking remains consistently high (about the same in 2004, 2003, and 2002). Approximately 10.8 million people aged 12–20 reported drinking alcohol in the past month (28.7% of this age group). Of these, nearly 7.4 million were binge drinkers and 2.4 million were heavy drinkers. Among people aged 12–20 in 2004, past-month alcohol use rates were lowest among Asians and highest among whites. The highest prevalence of binge and heavy drinking in 2004 was for young adults aged 18–25. The peak rate of both measures occurred at age 21. Thirty-two and a half million people aged 12 and older in 2004 drove under the influence of alcohol at least once in the past year. Table 2–3 lists the top 10 drugs most frequently found in combination with alcohol in ED visits of patients aged 12–20 in 2004.

TABLE 2–3 **Top 10 Combination Drugs Found in Alcohol-Related Emergency Department Visits**

	DRUG	VISITS	PERCENT OF VISITS
	Total alcohol with other drugs	*45,282*	*100%*
1.	Marijuana	22,244	49%
2.	Cocaine	10,066	22%
3.	Stimulants (amphetamine/methamphetamine)	3,805	8%
4.	Alprazolam	3,057	7%
5.	Drug unknown	1,835	3%
6.	Ibuprofen	1,585	3%
7.	Acetaminophen	1,524	3%
8.	Methylenedioxymethamphetamine (MDMA)	1,502	3%
9.	Acetaminophen-hydrocodone	1,436	3%
10.	Heroin	1,323	3%

Source: Office of Applied Studies, SAMHSA, Drug Abuse Warning Network, 2004.

Risk Factors

Genetic factors include an apparent hereditary factor that affects alcohol use and dependence. The discovery in 1990 that the DRD2 A1 allele gene appeared to be associated with alcoholism has led to a growing body of genetic research into substance abuse disorders (Stuart & Laraia, 2005).

Biologic factors were first identified by Jellinek in his disease concept of alcoholism. He hypothesized that addiction to alcohol may have a biochemical basis and identified specific phases of the disease (Jellinek, 1946). Expanding on Jellinek's early work, researchers have implicated low levels of dopamine and serotonin in the development of alcohol dependence (Czermak et al., 2004; Guardia et al., 2000; Nellissery et al., 2003).

Sociocultural factors such as ethnic differences in the way alcohol is metabolized may explain why some individuals choose not to drink. It is hypothesized that the Asian population has a deficiency of aldehyde dehydrogenase (ADH), the chemical in the brain that breaks down alcohol acetaldehyde (Cook et al., 2005). A buildup of acetaldehyde in the brain causes toxic symptoms characterized by vomiting, flushing, and tachycardia. Compared to other ethnic groups, Asian Americans report the lowest prevalence of family history of alcoholism (Ebberhart, Luczak, Avenecy, & Wall, 2003). Caucasians, Hispanics, and African Americans, on the other hand, have sufficient ADH for metabolizing alcohol and report higher alcoholism rates (Bersamin, Paschall, & Flewelling, 2005). Religious background also may correlate with the likelihood that a person will abuse alcohol. Among major religions, people of Jewish faith have the lowest rate of alcoholism, while Roman Catholics have the highest rate.

CLINICAL MANIFESTATIONS

When used in moderation, certain types of alcohol can have positive physiologic effects by decreasing coronary artery disease and protecting against stroke. However, when consumed in excess, alcohol can severely diminish one's ability to function and can ultimately lead to life-threatening conditions. Chronic use of alcohol can cause severe neurologic and psychiatric disorders. Severe damage to the liver occurs with chronic alcohol abuse, and that damage can progress from fatty liver to other liver diseases such as hepatitis and cirrhosis. Chronic alcoholism is the major cause of fatal cirrhosis. Chronic abuse of alcohol also can cause damaging effects to many other systems. These effects include myocardial disease, erosive gastritis, acute and chronic pancreatitis, sexual dysfunction, and an increased risk of breast cancer.

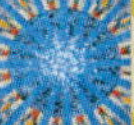

DEVELOPMENTAL CONSIDERATIONS **Alcoholic Fathers and Their Sons**

Genetic research has determined that children of alcoholics (COAs) are at higher risk for developing substance use problems (Conner et al., 2005). This is primarily true with male relatives. One type of alcoholism seen mostly in the sons of alcoholic fathers is associated with an early onset, an inability to abstain, and an antisocial personality (Stuart & Laraia, 2005). Results of one study revealed that adolescent sons of alcoholics with the D(2) dopamine receptor gene (DRD2 A1 allele) tried and got intoxicated on alcohol more often than boys without this genetic marker. In addition, sons of alcoholics tried more and used more substances overall. Boys with the allele developed a more serious tobacco habit and experienced a marijuana high at an earlier age than boys without the allele (Conner et al., 2005).

CRITICAL THINKING IN CLIENT CARE

1. Why is it important to ask your clients if they have a family history of substance abuse?
2. What questions should you ask when assessing for increased risk of substance abuse?
3. Does having a positive family history of substance abuse indicate that a person will develop a substance abuse problem? Why or why not?

CLINICAL MANIFESTATIONS AND THERAPIES **Alcohol Abuse**

ETIOLOGY	CLINICAL MANIFESTATIONS	CLINICAL THERAPIES
DTs as a result of sudden withdrawal of alcohol	■ Confusion ■ Disorientation ■ Agitation ■ Severe autonomic instability ■ Perceptual disturbances ■ Hallucinations—primarily visual but may be tactile ■ Tremors of extremities ■ Anxiety, panic, and paranoia	■ Prescribe benzodiazepines. ■ Reduce stimuli, but keep well lit to minimize visual misinterpretations. ■ If present, treat with antiseizure medications.
Cirrhosis of the liver resulting from damage done by chronic alcoholism	■ Spider angiomata ■ Palmar erythema ■ Muehrcke's nails, Terry's nails, or clubbing ■ Hypertrophic osteoarthropathy ■ Dupuytren's contracture ■ Gynecomastia ■ Hypogonadism ■ Hepatomegaly ■ Ascites ■ Splenomegaly ■ Jaundice ■ Asterixis ■ Weakness, fatigue, anorexia, weight loss	■ Explain that cirrhosis cannot be reversed, but abstaining from alcohol can delay or prevent further damage. ■ Emphasize abstaining from alcohol. ■ Stop any medications that are potentially damaging to the liver, such as acetaminophen. ■ Consider abdominocentesis to reduce ascites. ■ Monitor ammonia levels. ■ Prevent complications such as esophageal varices, hepatic encephalopathy, and hepatorenal syndrome. ■ Monitor for delayed coagulation times and apply pressure to punctures for 10 minutes.
Assaultive behaviors	■ Sexual assault in adolescent and young adult is commonly related to alcohol use. ■ Because of the release of inhibitions, control of emotions such as anger are reduced. ■ Access to weapons increases the risk of assaultive behavior becoming homicide. ■ Spousal or child abuse has strong link to alcohol ingestion.	■ Promote sobriety. ■ Encourage management classes. ■ Provide crisis intervention for family members who have been assaulted. ■ Provide follow-up counseling to reduce posttraumatic stress response.
Esophageal varices, which may result from portal hypertension due to cirrhosis	■ Hematemesis ranging from mild to severe ■ Heartburn ■ Black or tarry stools ■ Decreased urination secondary to hypotension ■ Lightheadedness ■ Shock ■ Weight loss ■ Weakness, fatigue, jaundice ■ Pruritus of hands and feet ■ Edema of lower extremity ■ Mental confusion	■ Encourage abstinence from alcohol. ■ Perform emergency surgery to stop bleeding involving removal of part of the esophagus or cauterization of varicosities. ■ Perform therapeutic endoscopy. ■ Monitor intake and output. ■ Take vital signs frequently during bleeding episodes to monitor for shock. ■ Administer fluids via IV therapy. ■ Administer beta blockers if necessary to reduce incidence of bleeding.
Gastritis	■ Esophageal reflux ■ Decreased appetite ■ Recurrent diarrhea	■ Provide foods that will not exacerbate GI symptoms while meeting nutritional requirements. ■ Teach client to remain upright for 3–4 hours following meals, eat small frequent meals, and avoid gas producing foods. ■ Antidiarrheals, antacids, and H^2 blockers may be appropriate medications to reduce symptoms.
Wernicke's encephalopathy	■ Ataxia ■ Abnormal eye movements ■ Mental confusion ■ Short term memory loss	■ Provide for client safety. ■ Place clocks and calendars to reduce mental confusion. ■ Assess cognition and document findings. ■ Administer IV or IM thiamine. ■ Avoid glucose administration until after thiamine administration. ■ Hydrate client.

Malnutrition is another serious complication of chronic alcoholism; thiamine (B_1) deficiency in particular can result in neurologic impairments. Thiamine depletion is thought to cause the Wernicke-Korsakoff syndrome observed in chronic alcoholics (Stuart & Laraia, 2005). Severe cognitive impairment is a principal feature of Wernicke's encephalopathy and Korsakoff's psychosis. **Wernicke's encephalopathy** is characterized by ataxia (lack of coordination), abnormal eye movements, and confusion. About 80% of people with Wernicke's encephalopathy also develop **Korsakoff's psychosis**, characterized by intact intellectual functioning but an inability to retrieve events from long-term memory or retain new information. **Confabulation**, making up information to fill in memory blanks, develops in a person's attempt to protect self-esteem when confronted with memory loss. Although Wernicke's and Korsakoff's are sometimes considered to be two distinct disorders, they are actually different phases of the same disease, commonly called Wernicke-Korsakoff syndrome. Wernicke's encephalopathy indicates the acute stage of the illness, and Korsakoff's psychosis indicates the chronic stage.

Although alcohol is a CNS depressant, it actually disrupts sleep, thus altering the sleep cycle, decreasing the quality of sleep, intensifying obstructive sleep apnea, and reducing total sleeping time. Heavy drinkers have a higher mortality rate, and many fatalities occur from alcohol-related accidents. Blood alcohol levels (BALs) are highly predictive of CNS effects. Euphoria, reduced inhibitions, impaired judgment, and increased confidence are seen at 0.05% (Kneisl, Wilson, & Trigoboff, 2004). Toxic levels in excess of 0.5% can cause coma, respiratory depression, peripheral collapse, and death (Kneisl et al., 2004). In the United States, the legal level of intoxication is 0.08%.

Chronic consumption of alcohol produces tolerance and creates cross-tolerance to general anesthetics, barbiturates, benzodiazepines, and other CNS depressants. If alcohol is withdrawn abruptly, the brain becomes overly excited because previously inhibited receptors are no longer inhibited (Bayard, McIntyre, Hill, & Woodside, 2004). This hyperexcitability manifests clinically as anxiety, tachycardia, hypertension, diaphoresis, nausea, vomiting, tremors, sleeplessness, and irritability. Severe manifestations of alcohol withdrawal include seizures, convulsions, and DTs. Episodes of DTs have a mortality rate of 1–5% (Kasser, Geller, Howell, & Wartenberg, 2004).

Multisystem Effects

Alcohol is a chemical irritant that has a direct toxic effect on many organ systems, as described in Table 2–4.

Blackouts, a fairly early sign of alcoholism, are a form of amnesia about events that occurred during the drinking period. The alcoholic may carry out conversations and elaborate activities with no loss of consciousness but have no memory of those activities the next day. This may be explained by the toxic effects of alcohol on glutamate transmission necessary for memory storage. A more advanced CNS problem is Wernicke-Korsakoff syndrome, described previously. **Alcoholic dementia** is characterized by impaired abstract thinking and judgment, personality changes, and impaired memory. This is often seen in chronically heavy drinkers (Stern & Sacheim, 2004).

Withdrawal

Alcohol withdrawal syndrome typically begins about 6–8 hours after the alcoholic's last drink. Early symptoms include irritability, anxiety, insomnia, tremors, sweating, and mild tachycardia. In rare cases, the person may experience grand mal seizures or intermittent visual, tactile, or auditory hallucinations. Symptoms of withdrawal usually peak during the second day of abstinence and are likely to show significant improvement by the fourth or fifth day. For individuals who repeatedly withdraw from alcohol, symptoms become worse each time (Reoux & Ries, 2001).

Alcohol withdrawal delirium, sometimes referred to as delirium tremens (DTs), usually occurs on days 2 and 3 but

TABLE 2–4 **Physiologic Complications From Alcohol Dependence**

BODY SYSTEMS	TOXIC EFFECTS
Gastrointestinal (GI)	Esophageal reflux, esophagitis, esophageal varices, gastritis, decreased appetite, malabsorption, recurrent diarrhea, acute or chronic pancreatitis (75% of cases related to alcohol abuse)
Liver	Hepatomegaly, fatty liver, alcoholic hepatitis, cirrhosis, cancer Elevated gamma-glutamyl transpeptidase (GGT) results
Cardiovascular	Hypertension, cardiomyopathy, arrhythmias, increased risk for stroke, coronary artery disease, sudden cardiac death
Respiratory	Pneumonia, bronchitis, tuberculosis
Hematologic	Bone marrow depression, anemia, leukopenia, blood clotting abnormalities
Neurologic	Seizures, peripheral neuropathy, optic neuropathy, Wernicke's encephalopathy, Korsakoff syndrome, alcoholic dementia, impaired cognitive function, labile moods, sleep disturbances
Endocrine	Hyperglycemia, decreased thyroid function
Reproductive	Erectile problems, decreased testosterone, decreased sex drive, menstrual irregularities
Nutritional	Thiamine deficiency, folic acid deficiency, vitamin A deficiency, magnesium deficiency, zinc deficiency

Source: American Psychological Association. (2000). *Diagnostic and statistical manual of mental disorders* (4th ed., Text Revision). Washington, DC: Author; Dunphy, L. M., & Winland-Brown, J. E. (2001). *The art and science of advanced practice nursing.* Philadelphia: Davis; and Naegle, M. A., & D'Avanzo, C. E. (2001). *Addictions and substance abuse: Strategies for advanced practice nursing.* Upper Saddle River, NJ: Prentice Hall.

may appear as late as 14 days after the last drink. The person experiences confusion, disorientation, hallucinations, tachycardia, hypertension or hypotension, extreme tremors, agitation, diaphoresis, and fever. Death may result from cardiovascular collapse or hyperthermia. With improved diagnosis and medical treatment, the mortality rate has dropped from 20% to 1% (American Psychiatric Association, 2000).

Overdose

Signs of alcohol intoxication include nausea, vomiting, lack of coordination, slurred speech, staggering, disorientation, irritability, short attention span, loud and frequent talking, poor judgment, lack of inhibition, labile emotions, and (for some) violent behavior. Alcohol intoxication may result in accidents or falls that cause contusions, sprains, and fractures and facial or head trauma. High BALs may result in unconsciousness, coma, respiratory depression, and death.

Alcohol poisoning is a toxic condition that results from excessive consumption of large amounts of alcohol in a very short period of time. Advanced states of intoxication and alcohol poisoning are critical situations in the emergency department and necessitate careful triage and monitoring to prevent death or permanent disability. Table 2–5 lists symptoms associated with certain BALs.

COLLABORATION

When caring for a client who abuses alcohol, the nurse must work as a collaborative member of a team that may include physicians, psychologists, counselors, nutritionists, and assistive personnel who share the collaborative goal of helping the client achieve sobriety. The treatment team also may include a sponsor. A sponsor is a successfully recovering alcoholic, usually with several years of sobriety, who provides peer counseling and support, often taking the client to 12-step meetings.

Diagnostic Tests

The simplest method of detecting blood alcohol content is by using a breathalyzer. BALs are the main biologic measures for assessment purposes. Knowledge of the symptoms associated with a range of BALs is helpful in ascertaining level of intoxication, level of tolerance, and whether the person accurately reported recent drinking. At 0.10% (after 5–6 drinks in 1–2 hours), voluntary motor action becomes clumsy and reaction time is impaired. The degree of impairment varies with gender, weight, and food ingestion. Small women who drink alcohol on an empty stomach achieve intoxication more quickly than large males who have eaten a full meal. At 0.20% (after 10–12 drinks in 2–4 hours), function of the motor area in the brain is depressed, causing staggering and ataxia (Kneisl et al., 2004). A level above 0.10% without associated behavioral symptoms indicates the presence of tolerance. High tolerance is a sign of physical dependence.

Assessing for withdrawal symptoms is important when the BAL is high. Medications given for treatment of withdrawal from alcohol are usually not started until the BAL is below a set norm (usually below 0.10%) unless withdrawal symptoms become severe. Measurement of BAL may be repeated several times, several hours apart, to determine the body's metabolism of alcohol and at a time it is safe to give the client medication to minimize the withdrawal symptoms.

Treatment of Withdrawal

All CNS depressants, including alcohol, benzodiazepines, and barbiturates, have a potentially dangerous progression of withdrawal. Alcohol and the entire class of CNS depressants share the same withdrawal syndrome. Treatment of severe withdrawal during detoxification is mostly symptomatic through acetaminophen, vitamins, and medications to minimize discomfort.

In managing alcohol withdrawal, the goal is to minimize adverse outcomes such as patient discomfort, seizures, delirium, and mortality and to avoid the adverse effects of withdrawal medications, such as excess sedation (Kasser et al., 2004). Close monitoring is essential to ensure protection of the patient. Critical care monitoring may be indicated to manage alcohol withdrawal delirium, particularly when very high doses of benzodiazepines are needed or when there are significant concurrent medical conditions. Medications such as benzodiazepines are used to minimize the discomfort associated with alcohol withdrawal and to prevent serious adverse effects, particularly seizures (Ntais, Pakos, Kyzas, & Ioannidis, 2005). A symptom-triggered approach to the administration of benzodiazepines during alcohol withdrawal results in less total medication use and requires a shorter duration of treatment (Bayard et al., 2004). The

TABLE 2–5 **Blood Alcohol Levels and Symptoms**

BLOOD ALCOHOL LEVEL (PERCENTAGE OF ALCOHOL IN BLOOD)	BEHAVIOR
0.05	Changes in mood and normal behavior; loosening of judgment and restraint; carefree feelings
0.08–0.10	Clumsy voluntary motor action; legal level of intoxication
0.20	Staggering caused by depression of brain motor area; short-temperedness; shouting; weeping
0.30	Confusion; stupor
0.40	Coma
0.50	Death (usually due to medullar respiratory blocking effects)

Clinical Institute Withdrawal Assessment for Alcohol (CIWA-Ar) is currently recommended to manage the symptoms of acute alcohol withdrawal (McKay, Koranda, & Axen, 2004). In a symptom-triggered regimen, medication is given only when the CIWA-Ar score is higher than 8 points (Bayard et al., 2004).

Two unique medications used to treat alcoholism are disulfiram (Antabuse) and naltrexone (ReVia, Depade). Disulfiram is a form of aversion therapy that prevents the breakdown of alcohol, causing physical illness (intense vomiting) if taken while drinking alcohol. All forms of alcohol, including over-the-counter cough and cold preparations, must be avoided. Naltrexone can help reduce the craving for alcohol by blocking the pathways to the brain that trigger a feeling of pleasure when alcohol and other narcotics are used. Because naltrexone blocks opiate receptors, clients should avoid taking any narcotics, such as codeine, morphine, or heroin, while on naltrexone. Clients also should discontinue all narcotics 7–10 days before starting on naltrexone. It also is recommended that clients wear a medical alert bracelet stating that they are on naltrexone, in case of emergency medical treatment. It is important that clients taking disulfiram or naltrexone also participate in psychosocial treatments such as AA meetings, individual counseling, or group therapy because the desire to "take a break" from treatment can overcome the client's motivation to continue taking the medication. AA meetings and therapy provide supportive support and reinforce clients' efforts to continue treatment. Peer connections made through AA can be especially motivating.

Complementary and Alternative Medicine

Electroencephalograph (EEG) biofeedback, also called *neurotherapy,* has been found to provide some benefit in the treatment of alcoholism (Fontaine, 2005). Many alcoholics and other addicts also have found yoga to be helpful in the recovery process. Both neurotherapy and yoga may provide calming effects on the centers of the brain involved in anxiety and impulse control. Yoga involves maintaining control over one's body and using deep breathing techniques and is frequently hailed as an effective stress reliever.

NURSING PROCESS

Nurses may interact with clients experiencing alcohol abuse or dependence in a variety of settings. The most common setting is an alcohol abuse treatment program where clients are hospitalized for an average of 10–15 days for detoxification and inpatient therapy. These clients may be voluntarily admitted, but many are court-ordered to undergo treatment after charges of DWI or alcohol-related child abuse.

Clients with alcohol abuse or dependence have impaired senses and increased risk-taking behaviors, which can lead to injuries from falls and accidents requiring medical attention. Therefore, hospital EDs as well as medical and surgical units are places where nurses encounter these clients. Occupational nurses and community health nurses also interact with alcohol-abusing clients in employee assistance programs and community health departments. Urgent care centers, pain clinics, and ambulatory care centers are other settings in which clients with alcohol abuse disorders frequently appear for minor health problems associated with chronic disorders related to alcohol abuse or dependence.

In caring for a client who is intoxicated, the focus of nursing care is to maintain the client's safety until the alcohol in the client's system is metabolized. While under the influence of alcohol, the client is not considered mentally competent to make decisions and may not sign a consent form or agree to treatment until his or her BAL decreases to normal limits as defined by state law.

Nursing care of the client with alcohol abuse or dependence is challenging and requires a nonjudgmental atmosphere promoting trust and respect. Efforts at promoting health are aimed at preventing alcohol use among children and adolescents and reducing the risks among adults. Adolescence is the most common phase for the first experience with drugs (Stuart & Laraia, 2005), partly due to the vulnerability of teenagers, who can be quick to succumb to peer pressure. Healthy lifestyles, parental support, stress management, good nutrition, and information about ways to steer clear of peer pressure are important topics for the nurse to provide in school programs.

Nurses have a responsibility to educate their clients about the physiologic effects of alcohol on the body, as well as about ways to manage stress and anxiety. Nurses must encourage and support periods of abstinence while assisting clients to make major changes in lifestyles, habits, relationships, and coping methods.

Assessment

A thorough history of the client's past alcohol use is important to ascertain the possibility of tolerance, physical dependence, or withdrawal syndrome. The following questions are helpful in eliciting a pattern of substance use behavior:

- How many substances has the client used simultaneously (**polysubstance abuse**: the simultaneous use of many substances) in the past?
- How often, how much, and when did the client first use alcohol?
- Is there a history of blackouts, delirium, or seizures?
- Is there a history of withdrawal syndrome, overdoses, and complications from previous alcohol use?
- Has the client ever been treated in an alcohol abuse clinic?
- Has the client ever been arrested for DUI or charged with any criminal offense while using alcohol?
- Is there a family history of alcohol use?

The client's medical history is another important area for assessment and should include the existence of any concomitant physical or mental condition (e.g., HIV, hepatitis, cirrhosis, esophageal varices, pancreatitis, gastritis, Wernicke-Korsakoff syndrome, depression, schizophrenia, anxiety, or personality disorder). Information about prescribed and over-the-counter medications as well as any allergies or sensitivity to drugs is vital. A brief overview of the client's current mental status also is significant.

- Is there a history of abuse (physical or sexual) or family violence?
- Has the client ever tried to commit suicide?
- Is the client currently having suicidal or homicidal ideation?

Information about the client's level of stress and other psychosocial concerns can help in assessing problems with alcohol use, as follows:

- Has the client's alcohol use affected his or her ability to hold a job?
- Has the client's alcohol use affected relationships with spouse, family, friends, or coworkers?
- How does the client usually cope with stress?
- Does the client have a support system that helps in time of need?
- How does the client spend his or her leisure time?

Several screening tools such as the Michigan Alcohol Screening Test (MAST) (Pokorny, Miller, & Kaplan, 1972) and the Brief Drug Abuse Screening Test (B-DAST) (Skinner, 1982) may help the nurse determine the degree of severity of alcohol abuse or dependence. The following screening tools provide a nonjudgmental, brief, and easy method for ascertaining patterns of substance abuse behaviors:

- *Michigan Alcohol Screening Test (MAST) Brief Version* is a 10-question self-administered questionnaire that takes 10–15 minutes to complete. An answer of yes to 3 or more questions indicates a potentially dangerous pattern of alcohol abuse.
- *The CAGE questionnaire* (Ewing, 1984), is more useful when the client may not recognize that he or she has an alcohol problem or is uncomfortable acknowledging it. This questionnaire is designed to be a self-report of drinking behavior, or it may be administered by a professional. One affirmative response raises concern and indicates the need for further discussion and follow-up. Two or more yes answers signify a problem with alcohol that may require treatment.

C Have you ever felt that you should **c**ut down on your drinking?
A Have people **a**nnoyed you by criticizing your drinking?
G Have you ever felt bad or **g**uilty about your drinking?
E Have you ever taken a drink in the morning as an "**e**ye-opener"?

A nonthreatening question such as "How much alcohol do you drink?" is preferable to the judgmental question "You don't drink too much alcohol, do you?" Open-ended questions that elicit more than a simple yes or no answer help to determine the direction of future counseling. The professional should use therapeutic communication techniques to establish trust prior to the assessment process.

Nurses working in medical-surgical units, psychiatric units, and special alcohol abuse units routinely care for patients experiencing acute alcohol withdrawal. Several assessment tools are available to determine the severity of withdrawal symptoms and indicate the need for pharmacologic treatment to manage withdrawal symptoms. An example of a withdrawal assessment tool is the revised Clinical Institute Withdrawal Assessment for Alcohol—Revised (CIWA-Ar) (Sullivan, Sykora, Schneiderman, Naranjo, & Sellers, 1989) (Figure 2–1 ■). This assessment is used widely in clinical and research settings for initial assessment and ongoing monitoring of alcohol withdrawal signs and symptoms.

The CIWA-Ar scale is a validated 10-item assessment tool that can be used to monitor and medicate patients going through alcohol withdrawal. The CIWA-Ar assesses for several alcohol withdrawal symptoms (e.g., high blood pressure, rapid pulse and respirations, tremors, insomnia, irritability, sweating, and convulsions) and results in a score that is used to direct the administration of benzodiazepines or other drugs to relieve associated symptoms of withdrawal and to prevent seizures. A score of 8 points or fewer corresponds to mild withdrawal symptoms. Scores of 9–15 points indicate moderate withdrawal, whereas a score of 15 or greater denotes severe withdrawal and an increased risk of DTs and seizures.

Diagnosis

Nursing diagnoses are individualized to specific client needs. Primary diagnoses may include:

- Risk for Injury
- Risk for Violence
- Ineffective Denial
- Ineffective Coping
- Imbalanced Nutrition: Less Than Body Requirements
- Chronic or Situational Low Self-Esteem
- Deficient Knowledge
- Disturbed Sensory Perception
- Disturbed Thought Processes.

Plan

Goals for client care depend on client needs. The client who denies a problem with alcohol will have far different needs than the client experiencing withdrawal, participating in an alcohol abuse program, or facing serious complications from years of abuse. Possible goals may include the following:

- Client will admit alcohol is controlling his or her life.
- Client will agree to enter an alcohol treatment facility.
- Client will experience no complications (or no further complications) as a result of alcohol abuse or alcohol withdrawal.
- Client will obtain optimal nutritional status.
- Client will remain sober.
- Client will participate in support groups such as AA after discharge from treatment facility.

Implementation

Caring interventions are based on the client's need, diagnoses chosen, and goals set for care. The following interventions are organized by nursing diagnosis.

Risk for Injury and Risk for Violence

- Assess the client's level of disorientation to determine specific risks to safety. Knowledge of the client's level of cognitive functioning is essential to the development of an appropriate plan of care.

Clinical Institute Withdrawal Assessment of Alcohol Scale, Revised (CIWA-Ar)

Patient:_______________________________ **Date:** __________________ **Time:** ________________ (24 hour clock, midnight = 00:00)

Pulse or heart rate, taken for one minute:__________________________ **Blood pressure:**_______

NAUSEA AND VOMITING -- Ask "Do you feel sick to your stomach? Have you vomited?" Observation.
0 no nausea and no vomiting
1 mild nausea with no vomiting
2
3
4 intermittent nausea with dry heaves
5
6
7 constant nausea, frequent dry heaves and vomiting

TREMOR -- Arms extended and fingers spread apart. Observation.
0 no tremor
1 not visible, but can be felt fingertip to fingertip
2
3
4 moderate, with patient's arms extended
5
6
7 severe, even with arms not extended

PAROXYSMAL SWEATS -- Observation.
0 no sweat visible
1 barely perceptible sweating, palms moist
2
3
4 beads of sweat obvious on forehead
5
6
7 drenching sweats

ANXIETY -- Ask "Do you feel nervous?" Observation.
0 no anxiety, at ease
1 mild anxious
2
3
4 moderately anxious, or guarded, so anxiety is inferred
5
6
7 equivalent to acute panic states as seen in severe delirium or acute schizophrenic reactions

AGITATION -- Observation.
0 normal activity
1 somewhat more than normal activity
2
3
4 moderately fidgety and restless
5
6
7 paces back and forth during most of the interview, or constantly thrashes about

TACTILE DISTURBANCES -- Ask "Have you any itching, pins and needles sensations, any burning, any numbness, or do you feel bugs crawling on or under your skin?" Observation.
0 none
1 very mild itching, pins and needles, burning or numbness
2 mild itching, pins and needles, burning or numbness
3 moderate itching, pins and needles, burning or numbness
4 moderately severe hallucinations
5 severe hallucinations
6 extremely severe hallucinations
7 continuous hallucinations

AUDITORY DISTURBANCES -- Ask "Are you more aware of sounds around you? Are they harsh? Do they frighten you? Are you hearing anything that is disturbing to you? Are you hearing things you know are not there?" Observation.
0 not present
1 very mild harshness or ability to frighten
2 mild harshness or ability to frighten
3 moderate harshness or ability to frighten
4 moderately severe hallucinations
5 severe hallucinations
6 extremely severe hallucinations
7 continuous hallucinations

VISUAL DISTURBANCES -- Ask "Does the light appear to be too bright? Is its color different? Does it hurt your eyes? Are you seeing anything that is disturbing to you? Are you seeing things you know are not there?" Observation.
0 not present
1 very mild sensitivity
2 mild sensitivity
3 moderate sensitivity
4 moderately severe hallucinations
5 severe hallucinations
6 extremely severe hallucinations
7 continuous hallucinations

HEADACHE, FULLNESS IN HEAD -- Ask "Does your head feel different? Does it feel like there is a band around your head?" Do not rate for dizziness or lightheadedness. Otherwise, rate severity.
0 not present
1 very mild
2 mild
3 moderate
4 moderately severe
5 severe
6 very severe
7 extremely severe

ORIENTATION AND CLOUDING OF SENSORIUM -- Ask "What day is this? Where are you? Who am I?"
0 oriented and can do serial additions
1 cannot do serial additions or is uncertain about date
2 disoriented for date by no more than 2 calendar days
3 disoriented for date by more than 2 calendar days
4 disoriented for place/or person

Total **CIWA-Ar** Score ______
Rater's Initials ______
Maximum Possible Score 67

The ***CIWA-Ar*** *is not* copyrighted and may be reproduced freely. This assessment for monitoring withdrawal symptoms requires approximately 5 minutes to administer. The maximum score is 67 (see instrument). Patients scoring less than 10 do not usually need additional medication for withdrawal.

Sullivan, J.T.; Sykora, K.; Schneiderman, J.; Naranjo, C.A.; and Sellers, E.M. Assessment of alcohol withdrawal: The revised Clinical Institute Withdrawal Assessment for Alcohol scale (**CIWA-Ar**). *British Journal of Addiction* 84:1353-1357, 1989.

Figure 2–1 ■ Assessment tool for alcohol withdrawal.

- Obtain a drug history as well as urine and blood samples for laboratory analysis of substance content. Subjective history often is not accurate, and knowledge regarding substance use is important for accurate assessment.
- Place the client in a quiet private room to decrease excessive stimuli, but do not leave the client alone if excessive hyperactivity or suicidal ideation is present. Excessive stimuli can increase the client's agitation.
- Frequently orient the client to reality and the environment, ensuring that potentially harmful objects are stored outside the client's access. The client may harm self or others if disoriented and confused.
- Monitor vital signs every 15 minutes until stable. Assess blood alcohol level and assess for signs of intoxication or withdrawal. The most reliable information about withdrawal symptoms comes from BAL and vital signs; they provide information about the need for medication during detoxification.

Ineffective Denial

- Be genuine, honest, and respectful of the client. Keep all promises and convey an attitude of acceptance. The development of a nonjudgmental, therapeutic nurse–client relationship is essential to gain the client's trust.
- Identify maladaptive behaviors or situations that have occurred in the client's life and discuss how the use of alcohol may have been a contributing factor. The first step in combating denial is for the client to recognize the relationship between alcohol use and personal problems.
- Do not accept the use of defense mechanisms such as rationalization or projection as the client attempts to blame others or make excuses for his or her behavior. Use confrontation with care to avoid placing the client on the defensive. Confrontation interferes with the client's ability to use denial.
- Encourage client participation in therapeutic group activities such as AA meetings with other people who are experiencing or have experienced similar problems. Clients often are more accepting of peer feedback than feedback from authority figures.

Ineffective Coping

- Establish a trusting relationship. Trust is essential to the nurse–client relationship.
- Set limits on manipulative behavior and maintain consistency in responses. The alcoholic client is unable to set limits and must begin to accept responsibility without being manipulative.
- Encourage the client to verbalize feelings, fears, or anxieties. Use attentive listening and validate the client's feelings with observations or statements that acknowledge these feelings. Verbalization of feelings helps the client develop insight into behaviors and long-standing problems.
- Explore methods of dealing with stressful situations other than resorting to alcohol use. Provide encouragement for changing to a healthier lifestyle. Teach healthy coping mechanisms (e.g., physical exercise, progressive muscle relaxation, deep breathing exercises, meditation, and imagery). The client needs to know how to adapt to stress without resorting to alcohol use.

Imbalanced Nutrition: Less Than Body Requirements

- Administer vitamins and dietary supplements as ordered by the physician. Vitamin B_1 is necessary to prevent complications from chronic alcoholism (e.g., Wernicke's syndrome).
- Monitor lab work (e.g., total albumin, complete blood count, urinalysis, electrolytes, and liver enzymes) and report significant changes to the physician. Objective laboratory tests provide necessary information to determine the extent of malnourishment.
- Collaborate with a dietitian to determine the number of calories needed to provide adequate nutrition and a realistic weight. Document intake, output, and calorie count. Weigh the client daily if condition warrants. Weight loss or gain is important assessment information for inclusion in the plan of care.
- Teach the importance of adequate nutrition by explaining the Food Guide Pyramid and relating the physical effects of malnutrition on body systems. The client may have inadequate knowledge of proper nutritional habits.

Chronic Low or Situational Low Self-Esteem

- Spend time with the client and convey an attitude of acceptance. Encourage the client to accept responsibility for his or her behaviors and feelings. An attitude of acceptance enhances self-worth.
- Encourage the client to focus on strengths and accomplishments rather than weaknesses and failures. Minimize attention to negative ruminations.
- Encourage participation in therapeutic group activities. Offer recognition and positive feedback for actual achievements. Success and recognition increase self-esteem.
- Teach assertiveness techniques and effective communication techniques such as the use of "I feel" rather than "You make me feel" statements. Previous patterns of communication may have been aggressive and accusatory, causing barriers to interpersonal relationships.

Deficient Knowledge

- Assess the client's level of knowledge and readiness to learn the effects of alcohol on the body. Baseline assessment is required to develop appropriate teaching material.
- Develop a teaching plan that includes measurable objectives. Include significant others if possible. Lifestyle changes often affect all family members.
- Begin teaching with simple concepts and progress to more complex issues. Use interactive teaching strategies and written materials appropriate to the client's educational level. Include information on physiologic effects of alcohol, the propensity for physical and psychologic dependence, and risks to the fetus if the client is pregnant. Active participation and handouts enhance retention of important concepts.

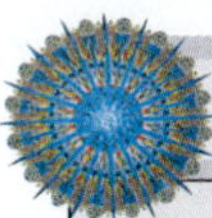

NURSING CARE PLAN **A Client Experiencing Withdrawal From Alcohol**

George Russell, age 58, fell at home and broke his arm. His wife took him to the emergency department where an open reduction internal fixation of his right wrist was performed under general anesthetic in the operating room. He was admitted to the postoperative unit for observation following surgery because he required large amounts of anesthesia during the procedure.

Mr. Russell has a ruddy complexion and looks older than his stated age. He discloses that he was laid off from his factory job 2 years ago and has been working odd jobs until last week, when he was hired by a local assembly plant. His father was a recovering alcoholic, and his 30-year-old son has been treated for alcohol abuse in the past. Mr. Russell states that he knows alcoholism runs in the family, but he believes that he has his drinking under control. However, he cannot remember the events that led up to his fall and how he might have broken his arm.

ASSESSMENT

During the nursing assessment, Mr. Russell is hesitant to provide information and refuses to make eye contact. Prior to his operation, a BAL was drawn because the ER nurse detected alcohol on his breath. His BAL was 0.40%, which is 5 times the legal limit for intoxication. His vital signs are within the upper limits of normal, but he is confused and disoriented with slurred speech and a slight tremor of the hands. He is 6 feet tall and weighs 140 pounds. His total albumin is 2.9 mg, and he has elevated liver enzymes. His wife states that he rarely eats the meals she prepares because he is usually drinking and has no appetite for food.

DIAGNOSES

- Ineffective Individual Coping related to possible hereditary factor and personal vulnerability
- Risk for Injury related to aggressive behavior, unsteady gait, and impaired motor responses
- Ineffective Denial related to inability to recognize maladaptive behaviors caused by substance use
- Imbalanced Nutrition: Less Than Body Requirements related to anorexia manifested by decreased weight and low serum protein levels

PLANNING

- Client will express his true feelings associated with using alcohol as a method of coping with stressful situations.
- Client will identify three adaptive coping mechanisms he can use as alternatives to alcohol in response to stress.
- Client will verbalize the negative effects of alcohol and agree to seek professional help with his drinking.
- Client will be free of injury as evidenced by steady gait and absence of subsequent falls.
- Client will gain 1 pound (0.45 kilogram) per week without evidence of increased fluid retention. Serum albumin levels will return to normal range.

IMPLEMENTATION

- Establish a trusting relationship with the client and spend time with him discussing his feelings, fears, and anxieties.
- Consult with a physician regarding a schedule for medications during detoxification and observe the client for signs of withdrawal syndrome.
- Explain the effects of alcohol abuse on the body and emphasize that prognosis is closely associated with abstinence.
- Teach a relaxation technique that the client believes is useful.
- Provide community resource information about self-help groups and, if the client is receptive, a list of meeting times and phone numbers.
- Consult with a dietitian to determine the number of calories needed to provide adequate nutrition and a realistic weight. Document intake, output, and calorie count.
- Consult with a physician to begin vitamin B_1 (thiamine) and dietary supplements.

EVALUATION

Mr. Russell is discharged from the postoperative unit without complications. He successfully undergoes detoxification and contacts the Employee Assistance Program at his new place of employment. He is on medical leave while his arm completely heals and now attends AA meetings 5 days a week. He reports that he enjoys taking long walks with his wife in the warm weather and that his appetite has returned. He has gained 10 pounds in the past 6 weeks and feels better physically than he has in many years.

CRITICAL THINKING

1. Explain why, during the initial nursing assessment, it would be important to ask questions about Mr. Russell's medication history and his use of other medications.
2. Mr. Russell asks you to explain the risks of taking disulfiram (Antabuse). What should you tell him?
3. Develop a care plan for Mr. Russell for the nursing diagnosis of imbalanced nutrition: less than body requirements. Why is this care plan necessary?

Disturbed Sensory Perceptions

- Observe the client for withdrawal symptoms. Monitor vital signs. Provide adequate nutrition and hydration. Take seizure precautions. These actions provide supportive physical care during detoxification.
- Assess the client's level of orientation frequently. Orient and reassure the client of safety in the presence of hallucinations, delusions, or illusions. The client may be frightened.
- Explain all interventions before approaching the client. Avoid loud noises and talk softly to the client. Decrease external stimuli by dimming lights. Excessive stimuli increase agitation.
- Administer medications according to the detoxification schedule. Benzodiazepines help minimize the discomfort of withdrawal symptoms.

Disturbed Thought Processes

- Give positive reinforcement when thinking and behavior are appropriate or when the client recognizes that delusions are not based in reality. Alcohol can interfere with the client's perception of reality.
- Use simple step-by-step instructions and face-to-face interaction when communicating with the client. The client may be confused or disoriented.
- Express reasonable doubt if the client relays suspicious or paranoid beliefs. Reinforce accurate perception of people or situations. It is important to communicate that you do not share the false belief as reality.
- Do not argue with the client experiencing delusions or hallucinations. Convey acceptance that the client believes a situation to be true but that you do not see or hear what is not there. Arguing with the client or denying the belief serves no useful purpose because delusions are not eliminated.
- Talk to the client about real events and real people. Respond to feelings and reassure the client about being safe from harm. Discussions that focus on the delusions may aggravate the condition. Verbalization of feelings in a nonthreatening environment may help the client develop insight.

The community provides many options for treating alcohol abuse, including a mixture of individual, group, and family therapy. Medical detoxification can occur in hospitals, psychiatric units, special alcohol abuse units, clinics, and outpatient settings. Less restrictive environments include residential rehabilitation programs, halfway houses, and partial hospitalization programs. These programs provide structured environments for the recovering alcohol abuser while the individual maintains a viable presence in the community. In addition, clients can obtain vocational counseling, become involved in self-help groups such as AA, and receive health education.

PRACTICE ALERT

Clients are at highest risk for relapse within the first few months of stopping use of alcohol. An acronym that can assist the client in recognizing behaviors that lead to relapse is **HALT: h**ungry, **a**ngry, **l**onely, and **t**ired. Nurses should emphasize the importance of a balanced diet, adequate sleep, healthy recreation activities, and a caring support system to prevent relapse.

Evaluation

The client is evaluated on the ability to meet goals set during the planning stage of the nursing process. Potential expected outcomes include the following:

- Client controls anxiety to a tolerable level.
- Client displays new coping mechanisms and reduces or eliminates the use of withdrawal.
- Client experiences no complications or new complications as a result of alcohol use or withdrawal.
- Client accepts responsibility for how his or her behavior impacts the family unit.

HEALTH CARE

Legal Issues

The nurse, working in an ED, admits a client accompanied by a police officer who requests that a serum BAL be drawn and tested for use in a court case related to the client's drinking while intoxicated. What are the client's legal rights, and what legal obligations does the nurse have regarding this client's rights of privacy?

Safety

The nurse is caring for a client who was brought to the ED with a BAL of 0.32%. The client is somnolent, is speaking in incomplete sentences that are garbled and difficult to understand, and has a laceration on his forehead. He is admitted to the acute care facility for observation. How will you assess this client's neurologic status to determine whether there is an alteration in level of consciousness reflecting a brain injury or alcohol intoxication?

REVIEW Alcohol Abuse

RELATE: LINK THE CONCEPTS

Linking the exemplar of Alcohol Abuse with the concept of Comfort:

1. Why might the client who has detoxified from alcohol have trouble sleeping?
2. What nursing care might you provide to improve the client's ability to sleep?

Linking the exemplar of Alcohol Abuse with the concept of Infection:

3. What pathophysiology would increase the risk for infection in the client who chronically abuses alcohol?
4. What nursing care would you provide this client to reduce the risk of infection?

REFER: GO TO MYNURSINGKIT

REFLECT: CASE STUDY

Candy Collins, a 46-year-old wife and mother of two, comes to her physician's office seeking help for alcohol abuse. She says her husband has threatened to leave her and take her children with him if she doesn't stop. The nurse determines that Candy drinks at least 5 or 6 alcoholic beverages daily, usually starting after dinner, although sometimes she begins drinking after the children leave for school. The nurse learns Candy's behavior began 5 years ago, shortly after her youngest child began preschool. She denies having blackouts, although she reports occasionally waking in the morning with no memory of the night before.

1. What other data would you want to collect from Candy related to her abuse of alcohol?
2. What treatment would you anticipate as appropriate for this client?
3. What teaching would you provide both Candy and her husband?

2.2 NICOTINE ABUSE

KEY TERMS

Nicotine, *51*

Nicotine replacement therapy (NRT), *53*

BASIS FOR SELECTION OF EXEMPLAR

Institute of Medicine

Healthy People 2010

LEARNING OUTCOMES

After reading about this exemplar, you will be able to:

1. Describe the pathophysiology, etiology, clinical manifestations, and direct and indirect causes of nicotine addiction.
2. Identify risk factors associated with nicotine addiction.
3. Illustrate the nursing process in providing culturally competent care across the life span for individuals with nicotine addiction.
4. Formulate priority nursing diagnoses appropriate for an individual with nicotine addiction.
5. Create a plan of care for individuals with nicotine addiction and their family members.
6. Assess expected outcomes for an individual with nicotine addiction.
7. Discuss therapies used in the collaborative care of an individual with nicotine addiction.
8. Employ evidence-based caring interventions for an individual with nicotine addiction.

OVERVIEW

Cigarette smoking is the single most preventable cause of disease and death in the United States. It is estimated that 443,000 deaths each year are attributable to cigarette smoking (CDC, 2009). This estimate does not include clients exposed to secondhand smoke or clients who consume nicotine by using chewing tobacco. The history of smoking can be dated to as early as 5000 BC and is recorded in many historical records. Nicotine use was considered not only socially acceptable, but also desirable until the dangers became evident in the late 1950s–1960s. Since that time, the U.S. government, health care providers, and anyone invested in promoting healthy lifestyles has worked to make nicotine use socially unacceptable and to help adolescents make better choices than their parents and grandparents did.

Nicotine, a highly addictive chemical found in tobacco, enters the body via the lungs (cigarettes, pipes, and cigars) and oral mucous membranes (chewing tobacco as well as smoking). While smoking is legal, it has become increasingly socially unacceptable, as evidence of the danger of both smoking and breathing in others' secondhand smoke has been demonstrated. Burning of tobacco releases the active substances in the plant, making it available for absorption via the lungs into the bloodstream.

Commercial tobacco contains over 4,000 chemicals, including nicotine, arsenic, and hydrogen cyanide (Table 2–6). Cancer-causing agents in commercial tobacco include nitrosamines, crysenes, cadmium, benzopyrene, polonium 210, nickel, diberiz acidine, urethane, and toluidine. As a result of the combination of chemicals entering the bloodstream, smoking has profound effects on virtually every organ system, ranging from hypertension due to vasoconstriction to suppression of the immune system.

PATHOPHYSIOLOGY AND ETIOLOGY

In low doses, nicotine stimulates nicotinic receptors in the brain to release dopamine (a precursor to norepinephrine) and epinephrine, causing vasoconstriction. This increases the heart rate, blood pressure, and peripheral vascular resistance, increasing the heart's workload. GI effects include an increase in gastric acid secretion, an increase in the tone and motility of GI smooth muscle, nausea, and increased risk of vomiting.

Initially, nicotine increases respiration, mental alertness, and cognitive ability, but eventually it depresses those responses (Kneisl et al., 2004). Moderate doses of nicotine can cause tremors. With high doses, such as acute poisoning from nicotine-containing insecticides, convulsions and death can occur.

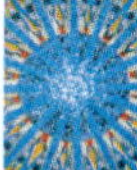

FOCUS ON DIVERSITY AND CULTURE

Smoking

Smoking is acceptable in a number of cultures. For example, in some cultures it is used as part of a ritual to communicate peace, spirituality, and communication. Formal Native American ceremonies, for example, often involve the use of a peace pipe, or calumet. Despite the known health risks of tobacco use, the nurse may need to respect the client's cultural view of smoking as an important ritual.

TABLE 2–6 Common Chemicals Found in Tobacco and Their Effect

CHEMICAL	EFFECT
Benzene	Is a carcinogen associated with leukemia
Formaldehyde	Causes cancer, respiratory, skin, and GI problems
Ammonia	Frees nicotine, turning it into a gas to be absorbed through the lungs or oral mucosa into the bloodstream
Acetone	Simple ketone found in nail polish remover, can be irritating to the tissues and is a CNS depressant
Tar	Is deposited in the lungs from cigarette smoke, reducing elasticity of the alveoli and slowing air exchange
Nicotine	Is one of the most addictive substances known to humans
Carbon monoxide	Is a poisonous gas that is rapidly fatal

Smokers can develop tolerance to nausea and dizziness, which may be experienced with initial use of nicotine, but not to the cardiovascular effects. Furthermore, because of the vasoconstriction, tissue oxygenation can be impaired in areas where vessels are already narrowed by atherosclerosis.

Smokers often have more difficulty falling asleep than nonsmokers do because nicotine acts as a stimulant. Smokers are usually easily aroused and often describe themselves as light sleepers. By refraining from smoking after the evening meal, the person usually sleeps better; moreover, many former smokers report that their sleeping patterns improve once they stop smoking.

Nicotine dependence results from chronic use. Withdrawal symptoms include craving, nervousness, restlessness, irritability, impatience, increased hostility, insomnia, impaired concentration, increased appetite, and weight gain. Gradual reduction in nicotine use seems to prolong suffering. Chronic health problems from smoking have been well established in the form of cancer, heart disease, emphysema, hypertension, and death (Kneisl et al., 2004).

Quitting smoking is thought to be difficult because of the release of dopamine caused by nicotine, which reinforces the addictive craving for more. The highly addictive nature of nicotine plays a factor as well. In 2006, the Massachusetts Department of Health reported that cigarette brands had increased their nicotine content by an average of 10% since 1998. There is evidence that a higher nicotine content in cigarettes could make it much harder for smokers to quit (Brown, 2008, August 31).

Etiology

Smoking is the most common form of recreational drug use, practiced by more than 1 billion people in the majority of human societies. Smoking is now the number one cause of preventable death and disease for both women and men. According to a recent report by the U.S. Surgeon General, who conducted a study on women only, far more women are dying of lung cancer than of breast cancer and around 165,000 women died prematurely from smoking-related diseases such as cancer, stroke, and heart disease (U.S. Department of Health and Human Services, 2005). Pregnant women also face unique health concerns from smoking, including low birth weight and increased risk of premature labor.

Secondhand smoke presents a number of dangers, particularly to children of smokers. According to the Centers for Disease Control and Prevention (CDC):

- Infant children of mothers who smoke are more likely to die from SIDS than children born to nonsmoking mothers.
- Exposure to secondhand smoke causes asthmatic children to have more frequent and severe attacks.
- Children exposed to secondhand smoke are at increased risk for respiratory symptoms and otitis media.
- Mothers who smoke and mothers who are exposed to secondhand smoke are more likely to have lower-birth-weight babies (Centers for Disease Control, 2007).

Risk Factors

Some of the most common factors that influence people to smoke are emotions, social pressure, alcohol use, lack of education, and age. People of lower socioeconomic status are more likely to smoke than those of higher socioeconomic status, partially because smoking is more socially acceptable in groups with fewer resources. Furthermore, quitting smoking is less successful in lower socioeconomic groups because they lack high-quality health education, lack support for quitting, and are exposed to smoking more often.

The leading risk related to smoking is heart disease. Smoking also increases the risk for many other diseases and disorders, including lung, stomach, pancreas, colon, kidney, and bladder cancers; chronic obstructive pulmonary disease (COPD); hypertension; stroke; macular degeneration; cataracts; peripheral vascular disease; Graves' disease; infertility; earlier menopause; dysmenorrhea; impotence; osteoporosis; and degenerative disc disease. Other less serious consequences of smoking include discolored teeth and fingernails, premature aging and wrinkling, bad breath, reduced sense of smell and taste, strong smell of smoke clinging to hair and clothing, and gum disease. Smoking during pregnancy has been associated with preterm labor, spontaneous abortion, low-birth-weight infants, sudden infant death syndrome (SIDS), and learning disorders (Albrecht et al. 2004; Anderson, Johnson, & Batal, 2005).

CLINICAL MANIFESTATIONS

Clinical manifestations of nicotine use are usually nonexistent in the early stages of use and are seen only when a complication such as COPD, cancer, or heart disease occurs. People who smoke for many years often have deep voices secondary to trauma to the vocal cords from the heat of the smoke and the chronic cough they often develop. See Exemplar 3.6, Lung Cancer, in Concept 3, Cellular Regulation, for manifestations of cancers associated with nicotine use; Exemplar 21.3, Chronic Obstructive Pulmonary Disease, in Concept 21, Oxygenation,

CLINICAL MANIFESTATIONS AND THERAPIES **Nicotine Abuse**

ETIOLOGY	CLINICAL MANIFESTATION	CLINICAL THERAPIES
Carcinogens are in commercial cigarettes, cigars, and pipes.	■ Lung cancer ■ Stomach cancer ■ Bladder cancer ■ Oral cancers ■ Laryngeal cancers	■ Chemotherapy ■ Radiation therapy ■ Supportive care ■ Pain management
Smoke, chemicals, and heat from smoke irritate and damage tissues in the respiratory system.	■ Chronic cough ■ COPD ■ Increased mucous production ■ Chronic hypercapnia	■ Bronchodilators ■ Expectorants ■ Oxygen therapy ■ Coughing and deep breathing ■ Positioning ■ Smoking cessation
Damaging effects of secondhand smoke puts those around the smoker at risk.	■ Children at increased risk for upper respiratory tract infections, otitis media ■ Everyone exposed to smoke at risk for cancer secondary to exposure to carcinogens	■ Stop smoking ■ Avoid exposing others to smoke, especially in confined areas with poor ventilation
External exposure to smoke affects cellular regeneration.	■ Wrinkles in the skin ■ Premature aging ■ Yellowing of fingernails and fingers	■ Stop smoking ■ Smoke in well-ventilated area and hold cigarette or cigar so smoke does not pass over fingers
Smell of smoke is prevalent.	■ Reduced sense of smell ■ Hair, skin, and clothing smelling of smoke	■ Stopping smoking is best ■ Smoke in well-ventilated area
Nicotine and other chemicals make smoking very addictive.	■ High level of recidivism when attempting to quit smoking	Provide multiple layers of support when a client chooses to quit, including: ■ Nicotine replacement ■ Pharmacologic therapy ■ Group and individual support ■ Motivational strategies.

for the impact of smoking on lung function; and Exemplars 22.3 and 22.10 in Concept 22, Perfusion, for information related to heart disease and peripheral vascular disease.

COLLABORATION

As with any addiction, the treatment process is a collaborative one. Nicotine addicts benefit from the support of family and friends, especially during times when they would usually be smoking or using tobacco. Although pharmacologic therapies are available over the counter, it is important for the client to discuss treatment with health care providers to minimize symptoms of withdrawal and prevent interactions with prescribed medications. Some clients may seek complementary therapies and support groups to help them quit smoking.

Nicotine Replacement Therapy (NRT)

Nicotine replacement therapy (NRT) helps relieve some of the physiologic effects of withdrawal, including cravings, for clients trying to quit smoking or using tobacco. NRT transdermal patches and gums are available over the counter; nicotine inhalers and nasal sprays are available by prescription only. Use of these nicotine substitution products is not without complications. They do not treat underlying psychologic needs or address addictive behaviors associated with tobacco use. They also come with contraindications and warnings. Nurses should provide information about warnings and contraindications to clients considering NRT. Nurses also should encourage clients to use nicotine therapy in combination with a smoking cessation program that will help them address the psychologic issues related to nicotine abuse.

Smoking Cessation Programs

Smoking cessation programs provide peer support, group therapy, and behavior therapy modifications that can help clients who smoke to quit smoking. The websites of the U.S. Surgeon General, the CDC, the American Heart Association, and the American Lung Association all provide information about smoking cessation programs and other means of quitting smoking.

Complementary Therapies

A number of complementary therapies have been advocated as tools for quitting smoking, hypnotherapy and acupuncture among them. Generally speaking, any therapy that helps reduce client anxiety levels, such as yoga and massage, will lower the likelihood that the client will want to use nicotine to alleviate anxiety.

HYPNOTHERAPY There is conflicting evidence about the success of hypnotherapy as a smoking cessation tool. As with any type of therapy, the qualifications and experience of the therapist have an effect on the success of the therapy. To increase the likelihood of success, nurses should encourage clients who are considering hypnotherapy also to participate in more traditional cessation programs.

NURSING PROCESS

Nurses may interact with clients addicted to nicotine in a variety of settings ranging from acute care to outpatient centers. Nurses often note the smell of smoke on a nicotine user and can implement a plan of care aimed at helping the client make healthier lifestyle choices. Because of the high rate of smoking among clients with mental health disorders, psychiatric facilities are a common place to meet nicotine-addicted clients. It is not uncommon for clients to have addictions to multiple substances, and nurses should assess for other substance abuse problems. A nonjudgmental approach is important when caring for clients addicted to nicotine. Health promotion efforts are directed toward education about making healthy life choices and strategies to support the client in abstaining from nicotine. Through school programs, it is important that nurses provide adolescents with ways to avoid peer pressure, thereby preventing nicotine use.

Assessment

When assessing clients who use nicotine, it is important to assess for amount and frequency of use; length of time nicotine has been used; and the presence of any symptoms indicating possible complications such as a chronic cough, shortness of breath, hypertension, chest pain, or unexpected symptoms. A comprehensive approach to the assessment of substance use is essential to ensure adequate and appropriate intervention. Three important areas to assess are a history of the client's past substance use, medical and psychiatric history, and the presence of psychosocial concerns. Ask questions in a nonthreatening, matter-of-fact manner, phrased so as not to imply wrongdoing (Henderson-Martin, 2000). Open-ended questions that elicit more than a simple yes or no answer help to determine the direction of future counseling (Box 2–4). Part of every assessment of nicotine abusers should be to determine their willingness and motivation to consider abstinence.

The client's medical history is another important area for assessment and should include the existence of any concomitant physical or mental condition. Ask about prescribed and over-the-counter medications as well as any allergies or sensitivity to drugs. A brief overview of the client's current mental status also is significant. Questions to ask may include the following:

- How often do you feel said or depressed?
- Do you have any other family members who use nicotine or other drugs? If so, how much or how often?
- Have you ever thought about hurting yourself? Someone else?

Box 2–4 Examples of Open-Ended Questions for Assessment

- On average, how long have you used nicotine-containing products?
- On a typical day, how many cigarettes (cigars or pipes) do you smoke (or how much tobacco do you chew)?
- When did you last smoke or use tobacco?
- What kinds of problems has nicotine use caused for you and your family, friends, finances, and health? How much money do you think you spend on smoking or tobacco use?
- Tell me about any attempts you've made to quit using nicotine. How long did you quit? What made you return to nicotine use?
- How do you feel about the idea of being nicotine-free? Do you want help to quit now?

Psychosocial Issues

Information about the client's level of stress and other psychosocial concerns can help in the assessment of substance use problems.

- Has the client's nicotine use affected his or her ability to hold or find a job?
- Has the client's nicotine use affected relationships with spouse, family, friends, or coworkers?
- How does the client usually cope with stress?
- Does the client have a support system that helps in time of need?
- How does the client spend leisure time?

Diagnosis

Every client is unique, and the choice of the nursing diagnosis will depend on the type of complications the client may be experiencing as a result of nicotine use. The needs of a client being treated for lung cancer or heart disease after years of smoking will differ from the needs of the adolescent client who may not yet be experiencing adverse effects from the newly begun habit. Possible nursing diagnoses include the following:

- Risk for Injury
- Ineffective Denial
- Ineffective Coping
- Ineffective Airway Clearance
- Anxiety.

Plan

When designing the plan of care, the nurse must put the client's needs, and no other expectations, at the forefront of the plan. If the client has no motivation to make healthier life choices, the nurse must respect the choices the client makes. Goals for client care may include the following:

- Client will verbalize the negative effects, both short-term and cumulative, associated with smoking.
- Client will voice strategies for support with quitting if/when the client is ready to stop smoking.
- Client will identify three activities that can aid in avoiding nicotine use.
- Client will not experience complications as a result of nicotine use.

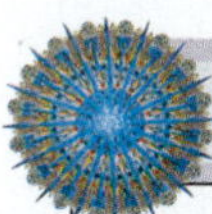

NURSING CARE PLAN **A Client Abusing Nicotine**

Ronald Kohler, age 32, began smoking when he was a junior in high school. His parents tried to discourage his smoking, but they never actually forbade it in their home because both of them smoked and believed it would be hypocritical to hold him to different standards than they practiced. Mr. Kohler says now he wishes his parents had told him all of the negatives and enforced a strict no-smoking rule because, he says, "It would have been easier not to start than it is to quit." Recently, during an annual health exam required by his employer, the physician pointed out early pulmonary changes associated with emphysema. Mr. Kohler denies any symptoms other than a productive cough in the morning upon awakening. Mr. Kohler lives with his wife and two daughters, aged 8 and 5 years of age. His wife strictly forbids smoking in the house and wishes her children did not see their father smoking for fear that they will eventually smoke as adults because of the poor role model he portrays.

ASSESSMENT

During the nursing assessment, Mr. Kohler's vital signs are T_O 37°C (98.6°F), P 80, R 16, BP 138/86. Breath sounds are clear and equal except for mild crackles in the lowest part of the lung bases. He has an intermittent moist, often productive cough, and his oxygen saturation is 91%. Peak flow readings are 480 mL, but he has no baseline for comparison purposes. When questioned, he reports that he has smoked 1 pack of filtered low-tar cigarettes a day on most days but when under stress, he may smoke as much as 2½; packs (or 50 cigarettes) per day. He has tried quitting twice, but both times he lasted less than 24 hours before smoking again. He says he knows he should quit for his girls, his wife would be much happier if he didn't smell like cigarettes when he got close to her, and it would be better for his health, but he reports he is just not interested in quitting because he enjoys the habit and finds that it calms him during times of stress.

DIAGNOSES

- Risk for Injury related to damage to his cardiorespiratory system from cigarette smoke
- Ineffective Denial related to inability to recognize maladaptive behaviors related to smoking

PLANNING

- Client will express his true feelings associated with using nicotine as a method of coping with stressful situations.
- Client will identify three adaptive coping mechanisms he can use as alternatives to nicotine use in response to stress.
- Client will verbalize the negative effects of smoking and agree to consider smoking cessation.
- Client will be free of injury as evidenced by normal cardiorespiratory function on assessment.

IMPLEMENTATION

- Establish a trusting relationship with the client and spend time with him discussing his feelings, fears, and anxieties.
- Explain the effects of nicotine abuse on the body and emphasize that good prognosis is closely associated with abstinence.
- Teach a relaxation technique that the client believes he can use instead of nicotine during times of stress.
- Provide community resource information about self-help groups and, if client is receptive, a list of meeting times and phone numbers.
- Consult with a physician regarding possible use of Chantix (varenicline) if the client chooses that method of smoking cessation.

EVALUATION

Mr. Kohler opts not to quit smoking at this visit but returns in 3 months and is diagnosed with left lower lobe pneumonia and relates that his oldest daughter told him, "Dad, if you loved us, you'd quit smoking because you'd want to be around to walk us down the aisle and meet your grandchildren." He says it made him think about how silly lighting a "stick on fire" was in comparison to that, and he would like to discuss quitting at this visit.

CRITICAL THINKING

1. Explain why it would be important during the initial nursing assessment to include questions about Mr. Kohler's medication history and his use of other medications.
2. Mr. Kohler asks you to explain the risks of taking Chantix (varenicline). What do you tell him?
3. Based on his first visit to the center, develop a care plan for Mr. Kohler for the nursing diagnosis of ineffective denial. Why is this care plan necessary?

Implementation

The nurse's role regarding smoking is to (1) serve as a role model by not smoking; (2) provide educational information regarding the dangers of smoking; (3) help make smoking socially unacceptable (e.g., by posting no-smoking signs in client lounges and offices); and (4) suggest resources such as hypnosis, lifestyle training, and behavior modification to clients who want to stop smoking. Nurses also can promote health related to tobacco by being aware of marketing efforts that target young adults (Ling & Glantz, 2002). The tobacco industry has developed very effective campaigns to encourage smoking among young adults by advertising and sponsoring entertainment events. Nurses can help young adults recognize and resist these marketing efforts.

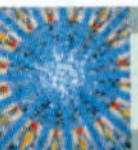

EVIDENCE-BASED PRACTICE Adolescents and Their Control of Tobacco Use

Studies show that in 2003, approximately 3.6 million U.S. children between 12 and 17 years of age (14.4% of that population) used tobacco products. This use increases in older adolescents and young adults, with individuals aged 18–25 years having the highest rate of tobacco use (48.8%) of all Americans (Substance Abuse and Mental Health Services Administration, 2004). In its 2003 study of youth risk behaviors, the CDC found that 27.5% of all adolescents currently use tobacco (Grunbaum et al., 2004). Smoking cigarettes is the most common type of tobacco use. Johnson, Kalaw, Lovato, Baillie, & Chambers (2004) used a grounded theory approach to study how adolescents perceived their smoking, how it fit into a "typical" adolescent framework of experimenting and establishing independence, and how adolescents attempted to control their amount of cigarette use. The researchers found that adolescents go through a process of determining whether smoking is a problem, "crossing the line" to unacceptable tobacco use, using strategies to regain control once the "line" has been crossed, and then "reconstructing" the line at the original usage (e.g., no smoking or very limited cigarette use) or at a higher level of use.

Most adolescents expressed a desire to maintain control of their smoking and not become "addicted." They used strategies such as not buying cigarettes, rationing smokes, limiting the situations in which they would smoke, cutting out "unnecessary" cigarettes, delaying smoking, and "half-butting" (taking a few puffs and saving the butt for later) to limit their use. They also replaced smoking with other activities to gain control, for example, substituting chewing gum, getting help from friends or family to limit or stop their use, using transitions such as moving to a new school to get a "fresh start," and making efforts to quit completely.

The authors conclude that the way adolescents manage their cigarette use, including their active efforts to maintain control over it, may be part of the typical adolescent process of establishing independence and that adolescents do not intend or desire to become addicted to nicotine. Many adolescents who limited smoking went on to quit completely.

Implications

A "harm reduction" approach in which smokers are encouraged to limit their cigarette use validates the adolescent's propensity to establish self-control and may be more effective than a conventional smoking cessation program alone when working with adolescent smokers.

Note: From Johnson, J. L., Kalaw, C., Lovato, C. Y., Baillie, L., & Chambers, N. A. (2004). "Crossing the line: adolescents' experiences of controlling their tobacco use." *Qualitative Health Research, 14*(9), 1276 -1291; Grunbaum, J. A., Kann, L., Kinchen, S., Ross, J., Hawkings, J., Lowry, R., et al. (May 21, 2004). "Youth risk behavior surveillance –United States, 2003." *MMWR Surveillance Summaries, 53 (No. SS-2)*, 1-96; and Substance Abuse and Mental Health Services Administration. (2004). "Results from the 2003 National Survey on Drug Use and Health: National Findings." *Office of Applied Studies, NSDUH Series H-25, DHHS Publication No. SMA 04-3964*. Rockville, MD.

Evaluation

Clients are evaluated based on the goals created during the planning stage. Expected outcomes may include the following:

- Client describes feelings regarding nicotine use, abstinence, and methods of coping without the use of nicotine.
- Client verbalizes negative effects on his or her own life and the lives of loved ones as a result of nicotine use.
- Client is free of injury or complications resulting from nicotine use.
- Client describes strategies that will be or can be useful when beginning a program to quit smoking.

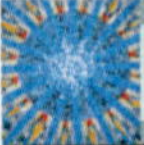

EVIDENCE-BASED PRACTICE Smoking Cessation in Hospitalized Patients

Despite the well-publicized deleterious health effects posed by cigarette smoking and the legally restricted access to cigarettes, smoking remains a persistent problem. Smoking has been banned in stores, malls, hospitals, office buildings, and even restaurants in some jurisdictions. Admission to the hospital provides an excellent opportunity for nurses to assist patients to quit smoking. Patients in hospitals may find it easier to quit in an environment where smoking is restricted or prohibited. In addition, individuals may be more open to cessation efforts when faced with the risks associated with surgery. In a review of the literature, researchers found that high-intensity behavioral interventions that include at least 1 month of follow-up contact were effective in helping hospitalized patients quit smoking (Rigotti, Munafo, Murphy, & Stead, 2005). Health care professionals, especially nurses, can be very instrumental in smoking cessation efforts.

Another literature review provided evidence that nursing interventions for smoking cessation have potential benefits (Rice & Stead, 2005). NRT also increases quit rates with or without additional counseling (Rice & Stead, 2005; Silagy, Lancaster, Stead, & Fowler, 2005). NRT aims to reduce withdrawal from tobacco products by replacing nicotine in the blood. All forms of NRT, available as chewing gum, skin patches, nose spray, inhalers, and tablets, increase the likelihood that a person will succeed in quitting smoking (Silagy et al., 2005). Effective nursing strategies include asking patients about their tobacco use, counseling those who want to quit, reinforcing cessation efforts, and providing early follow-up with those who quit smoking. This evidence points to the important role nurses play in encouraging their clients to quit smoking and the need for nurses to incorporate smoking cessation interventions as part of their standard practice.

Critical Thinking in Client Care

1. You are caring for a 55-year-old man recently hospitalized for acute angina who asks you the best way to stop smoking. What do you do?
2. Do you think nurses and other health care professionals should quit smoking? Why or why not?
3. You are caring for a 12-year-old girl who tells you that she smokes cigarettes occasionally and believes it makes her more popular with her older friends. She admits that she knows that smoking is supposed to be bad for you, but she doesn't see the harm in smoking a few cigarettes every day. How do you respond?

REVIEW Nicotine Abuse

RELATE: LINK THE CONCEPTS

Linking the exemplar of Nicotine Abuse with the concept of Oxygenation:

1. Describe the pathophysiology of the respiratory system and the ability of the alveoli to oxygenate the tissues when a client smokes.
2. While caring for a client who is known to have smoked for more than 30 years, how would you amend your nursing plan of care as related to oxygenation?

Linking the exemplar of Nicotine Abuse with the concept of Grief and Loss:

3. The nurse is caring for a client with terminal lung cancer and is talking with the family. The client's daughter says, "If Dad wanted to stay around and be with us, he wouldn't have made the choice to smoke." How would you respond to this statement and help the family members deal with their anger over the client's lifestyle choices?
4. Why might a client with acute COPD who continues to smoke be denied a lung transplant? How can you help this client (and family) deal with the grief and loss they experience as a result of this decision?

REFER: GO TO MYNURSINGKIT

REFLECT: CASE STUDY

Mr. W., a 50-year-old professional man, has pneumonia and is currently being treated with antibiotics. He smokes two packs of cigarettes a day. Since this bout of pneumonia, he voices concern about his smoking and wonders if he should try to quit again. He states, "I've tried everything and nothing works. The longest I last is about 1 month." He admits to being 30 pounds overweight and states that his wife and he have started walking 30 minutes every evening. His wife also has started making low-fat meals. He is concerned that if he quits smoking, he will gain more weight.

1. What information or knowledge is important for the nurse to remember when assisting a client to advance to the next stage of change?
2. Each contact between a nurse and a client is an opportunity for health promotion. Based on the knowledge or key concepts listed above, what question(s) would you ask Mr. W.?
3. In which state of change is Mr. W. relating to his cigarette smoking? What strategies could you, the nurse, consider?

2.3 PRENATAL SUBSTANCE EXPOSURE

KEY TERMS

Club drugs, *60*
Cocaine, *59*
Crack, *59*
Heroin, *60*
Placenta previa, *60*
Teratogen, *57*

BASIS FOR SELECTION OF EXEMPLAR

Healthy People 2010

LEARNING OUTCOMES

After reading about this exemplar, you will be able to:

1. Describe the pathophysiology, etiology, clinical manifestations, and direct and indirect effects of prenatal substance use on both the mother and the fetus.
2. Identify risk factors associated with prenatal substance use.
3. Illustrate the nursing process in providing culturally competent care across the life span for individuals who abuse substances during pregnancy.
4. Formulate priority nursing diagnoses appropriate for an individual who abuses substances during pregnancy and for her newborn.
5. Create a plan of care for women who abuse substances during pregnancy, their newborns, and their family members.
6. Assess expected outcomes for both the mother who abuses substances during pregnancy and her fetus.
7. Discuss therapies used in the collaborative care of an individual who abuses substances during pregnancy.
8. Employ evidence-based caring interventions for an individual who abuses substance while pregnant.

OVERVIEW

During pregnancy, the fetus is exposed to most of what the mother consumes, uses, or inhales. Any chemical that has the potential to harm the fetus is known as a **teratogen** and can include pesticides, viruses, and medications. If the mother uses or abuses substances, the fetus can experience life-changing alterations ranging from developmental delays to death. Drugs that are commonly misused include tobacco, alcohol, cocaine, marijuana, amphetamines, barbiturates, hallucinogens, club drugs, heroin, and other narcotics. Polysubstance use, which involves multiple substances such as alcohol, tobacco, and illicit drugs, is fairly common and contributes to the risks that a pregnant woman faces.

Drug use during pregnancy, particularly in the first trimester, may adversely affect the health of the woman and the growth and development of the fetus. Unfortunately, prenatal drug use may be the most frequently missed diagnosis in all of maternity care. Physicians and nurses may fail to ask women about drug and alcohol use because of their own lack of knowledge, discomfort, or biases. Often substance-abusing women wait until late in pregnancy to seek health care. Moreover, the substance-abusing woman who seeks early prenatal care may not voluntarily reveal her addiction. Caregivers should ask direct, nonjudgmental questions and be alert for a history or physical signs that suggest substance abuse.

Providing effective prenatal care to chemically dependent women presents many challenges for clinicians. However, pregnancy represents a period in most women's lives when they recognize the need for and are receptive to caring interventions

Table 2–7 identifies common addictive drugs and their effects on the fetus or newborn.

TABLE 2–7 **Possible Effects of Selected Drugs of Abuse/Addiction on Fetus and Newborn**

MATERNAL DRUG	EFFECT ON FETUS/NEWBORN
Depressants	
Alcohol	Mental retardation, microcephaly, midfacial hypoplasia, cardiac anomalies, intrauterine growth restriction (IUGR), potential teratogenic effects, fetal alcohol syndrome (FAS), fetal alcohol effects (FAE)
Narcotics	
Heroin	Withdrawal symptoms, convulsions, IUGR, tremors, irritability, sneezing, vomiting, fever, diarrhea, and abnormal respiratory function
Methadone	Fetal distress, meconium aspiration; with abrupt termination of the drug, severe withdrawal symptoms, preterm labor, rapid labor, abruption Withdrawal symptoms
Barbiturates	
Phenobarbital	Withdrawal symptoms
	Fetal growth restriction
"T's and Blues" (combination of the following)	
Talwin (narcotic)	Safe for use in pregnancy; depresses respiration if taken close to time of birth
Amytal (barbiturate)	See barbiturates
Tranquilizers	
Phenothiazine derivatives	Withdrawal, extrapyramidal dysfunction, delayed respiratory onset, hyperbilirubinemia, hypotonia or hyperactivity, decreased platelet count
Diazepam (Valium)	Hypotonia, hypothermia, low Apgar score, respiratory depression, poor sucking reflex, possible cleft lip
Antianxiety Drugs	
Lithium	Congenital anomalies
Stimulants	
Amphetamines	
Amphetamine sulfate (Benzedrine)	Generalized arthritis, learning disabilities, poor motor coordination, transposition of the great vessels, cleft palate
Dextroamphetamine sulfate (Dexedrine)	Congenital heart defects, biliary atresia, limb reduction defects
Cocaine	Cerebral infarctions, microcephaly, learning disabilities, poor state organization, decreased interactive behavior, CNS anomalies, cardiac anomalies, genitourinary anomalies, sudden infant death syndrome (SIDS)
Nicotine (half to one pack cigarettes/day)	Increased rate of spontaneous abortion, increased incidence of placental abruption, SGA, small head circumference, decreased length, SIDS, attention-deficit/hyperactivity disorder (ADHD) in school-age children
Psychotropics	
PCP ("angel dust")	Withdrawal symptoms
	Newborn behavioral and developmental abnormalities
LSD	Chromosomal breakage
Marijuana	IUGR

PATHOPHYSIOLOGY AND ETIOLOGY

The substance used, the amount of chemical consumed, and the period of gestation when the fetus is exposed all play an important role in determining the effects on the fetus. The greatest potential for gross abnormalities in the fetus occurs during the first trimester of pregnancy, when fetal organs are first developing. The classic period of teratogenesis in a woman with a 28-day cycle extends from day 31 after the last menstrual period (17 days after fertilization) to day 71 (54 days after fertilization) (Niebyl & Simpson, 2007). Many factors influence teratogenic effects, including the specific type of teratogen and the dose, the stage of embryonic development, and the genetic sensitivity of the mother and fetus. Understanding the risks and providing care for the pregnant woman who abuses substances require an understanding of the effects of the chemical in the body.

Substances Commonly Abused During Pregnancy

Client teaching ideally begins before pregnancy with any woman of childbearing age. When assessing the woman, nurses should determine if any substances are currently used that could potentially harm the fetus. If the client admits to substance use, the nurse can focus care on providng strategies to help her make healthier choices with the long-term goal of healthier children.

CAFFEINE Current research reveals no evidence that moderate caffeine intake has teratogenic effects in humans, nor is it linked to intrauterine growth restriction (IUGR), low birth weight, or preterm birth. However, high caffeine intake may be linked to an increased risk of miscarriage (Weng, Odouli, & Li, 2008). In addition, an increased risk of lower birth weight has been found in infants of mothers who consume at least 600 mg of caffeine daily (Bracken, Triche, Belanger, Hellenbrand, & Leaderer, 2003). (The average cup of brewed coffee has 100 mg, a 12 oz can of cola has about 50 mg, and a cup of tea has about 50 mg.) Until more definitive data are available, nurses should advise women about common sources of caffeine, including coffee, tea, colas, and chocolate, and suggest that they limit their caffeine intake to about 300 mg/day (Niebyl & Simpson, 2007).

ALCOHOL Alcohol is a CNS depressant and a potent teratogen. Birth defects related to fetal alcohol exposure can occur in the first 3–8 weeks of gestation, often before the woman even knows she is pregnant. Alcohol use among pregnant women tends to decrease by trimester.

The effects of alcohol on the fetus may result in a group of signs known as fetal alcohol spectrum disorders, also referred to as fetal alcohol syndrome. The spectrum of disorders has characteristic physical and mental abnormalities that vary in severity and combination. Characterized by growth retardation, facial anomalies, and CNS dysfunction of varying severity, fetal alcohol syndrome is the most common preventable cause of mental retardation in the United States. Pregnant women who have more than three drinks per week have an increased risk for miscarriage, while those who have five or more drinks per week increase their risk for intrauterine death by 2 to 3 times that of women who are nondrinkers (Wisner, et al., 2007). There is no definitive answer to how much alcohol a woman can safely consume during pregnancy. Consequently, the expectant woman should avoid alcohol completely. Even low levels of alcohol cannot be recommended (FDA, 2005).

Chronic abuse of alcohol can undermine maternal health by causing malnutrition (especially folic acid and thiamine deficiencies), bone marrow suppression, increased incidence of infections, and liver disease. As a result of alcohol dependence, a woman may have withdrawal seizures in the intrapartal period as early as 12–48 hours after she stops drinking. DTs may occur in the postpartal period, and the newborn may suffer withdrawal syndrome. The nursing staff in the maternal newborn unit must be aware of the manifestations of alcohol abuse so they can prepare for the client's special needs. The care regimen includes sedation to decrease irritability and tremors, seizure precautions, intravenous (IV) fluid therapy for hydration, and preparation for an addicted newborn. Although high doses of sedatives and analgesics may be necessary for the woman, caution is advised because these medications can cause fetal depression.

Breastfeeding generally is not contraindicated if the mother drinks alcohol, although alcohol is excreted in breast milk. Excessive alcohol consumption may intoxicate the infant and inhibit the maternal letdown reflex. Discharge planning for the alcohol-addicted mother and newborn needs to be coordinated with the social services department of the hospital.

COCAINE AND CRACK **Cocaine** is a powerful stimulant of natural origin that acts at the nerve terminals to prevent the reuptake of dopamine and norepinephrine, which in turn results in vasoconstriction, tachycardia, and hypertension. Placental vasoconstriction decreases blood flow to the fetus. The onset of cocaine effects occurs rapidly, but the euphoria lasts only about 30 minutes. Euphoria and excitement are usually followed by irritability, depression, pessimism, fatigue, and a strong desire for more cocaine. This pattern often leads the user to take repeated doses to sustain the effect. Cocaine metabolites may be present in the urine of a pregnant woman for as long as 4–7 days after use.

Cocaine can be taken by IV injection or by snorting the powdered form. **Crack**, a form of freebase cocaine that is made up of baking soda, water, and cocaine mixed into a paste and microwaved to form a rock, can be smoked. Smoking crack leads to a quicker, more intense high because the drug is absorbed through the large surface area of the lungs.

A woman who uses cocaine during pregnancy is at increased risk for acute myocardial infarction, cardiac arrhythmias, ruptured ascending aorta, seizures, cerebrovascular accidents, hyperthermia, bowel ischemia, and sudden death (Cunningham et al., 2005). Cocaine use during pregnancy has been related to abruptio placentae, a partial or total premature separation of a normally implanted placenta. Cocaine use also has been associated with preterm birth, low birth weight, neonatal irritability, and neonatal depression (Schempf, 2007) as well as SIDS and developmental delays as a toddler (King, 2003). Several congenital anomalies in the newborn also have been linked to maternal cocaine use, including, for example, genitourinary anomalies, congenital heart defects, limb reduction defects, and CNS anomalies (Cunningham et al., 2005).

Exposure of the fetus to cocaine in utero increases the risk of IUGR, small head circumference, cerebral infarctions, shorter body length, altered brain development, malformations of the genitourinary tract, and lower Apgar scores. Newborns exposed to cocaine in utero may have neurobehavioral disturbances, marked irritability, an exaggerated startle reflex, labile emotions, and an increased risk of SIDS. Most children who were exposed to cocaine in utero have normal intelligence. In some cases, cocaine-exposed children have subtle behavioral and learning problems; however, a good home environment seems to help reduce those effects (March of Dimes, 2008).

Cocaine crosses into breast milk and may cause symptoms in the breastfeeding infant, including extreme irritability, vomiting, diarrhea, dilated pupils, and apnea. Thus, women who continue to use cocaine after childbirth should avoid nursing.

MARIJUANA Perhaps not surprisingly, marijuana is the most widely used illicit drug among women, both pregnant and nonpregnant (SAMHSA, 2007). The prevalence of marijuana use in society raises many concerns about its effect on the fetus. Research on marijuana use in pregnancy is difficult, however, because it is an illegal drug. Unreliability of reporting, lack of a representative population, inability to determine strength or composition of the marijuana used (including the presence of herbicides), and concurrent use of other drugs are major factors complicating research efforts. To date, there is no strong evidence that marijuana has teratogenic effects on the fetus (Schempf, 2007), although following birth, some infants who were regularly exposed to marijuana in utero appear to have withdrawal symptoms, including trembling and excessive crying (March of Dimes, 2008).

PHENCYCLIDINE (PCP) PCP is a popular hallucinogen that can be smoked, taken orally, or injected intravenously. The drug causes confusion, delirium, and hallucinations with possible feelings of euphoria. The greatest risk for the pregnant woman is overdose or psychotic response. Signs of overdose include hypertension, hyperthermia, diaphoresis, and possible coma, which may jeopardize fetal well-being.

MDMA (ECSTASY) MDMA, better known as Ecstasy, is the most commonly used drug among the many **club drugs**, so called because they have become popular among adolescents and young adults who frequent dance clubs and "raves." Other club drugs include flunitrazepam (Rohypnol), gamma hydroxybutyrate (GHB), and ketamine hydrochloride. PCP and LSD are sometimes classified as club drugs as well.

MDMA is the third most widely used illicit drug in the United States after marijuana and amphetamines. MDMA is taken by mouth, usually as a tablet. It produces euphoria and feelings of empathy for others. It has been widely perceived as a "safe" drug because of a relatively low incidence of adverse reactions. However, adverse responses are very unpredictable and their incidence is growing as MDMA use becomes more commonplace (Gamma, Jerome, Liechti, & Sumnall, 2005). Deaths have also occurred among users. Little is known about the effects of MDMA on pregnancy. Preliminary research using rats suggests that prenatal use of MDMA may be associated with long-term impaired memory and learning in the child. However, the impact of the timing of Ecstasy use by the pregnant woman during fetal brain development may be a critical issue (Koprich et al., 2003).

HEROIN **Heroin** is an illicit CNS depressant narcotic that alters perception and produces euphoria. It is an addictive drug that is generally administered intravenously. Pregnancy in women who use heroin is considered a high risk because of the increased incidence of poor nutrition, iron deficiency anemia, and preeclampsia. Women addicted to heroin also have a higher incidence of sexually transmitted infections because many rely on prostitution to support their drug habit.

The fetus of a heroin-addicted woman is at increased risk for IUGR, meconium aspiration, and hypoxia. The newborn frequently shows signs of heroin addiction such as restlessness; a shrill, high-pitched cry; irritability; fist sucking; vomiting; and seizures. Signs of withdrawal usually appear within 72 hours and may last for several days.

The newborn may exhibit poor consolability for 3 months or more. These behaviors may interfere with successful maternal attachment and increase the risk for parenting problems or abuse in an already high-risk mother.

METHADONE Methadone is the most commonly used therapy for women who are dependent on opioids such as heroin. Methadone blocks withdrawal symptoms and reduces or eliminates the craving for narcotics. Dosage should be individualized at the lowest possible therapeutic level. Methadone crosses the placenta, but the effects on the newborn are inconsistent and do not seem to indicate as much of a dose-related effect on the newborn as previously believed (Jansson, DiPietro, & Elko, 2005). The therapeutic goal is to use methadone to help the mother recover from illicit drug abuse to optimize her health and that of her baby.

TOBACCO In the United States, smoking tobacco during pregnancy is one of the most significant, modifiable causes of poor pregnancy outcomes. Smoking tobacco during pregnancy has a strong association with low-birth-weight infants. In addition, mothers who smoke have an increased risk of preterm birth, premature rupture of the membranes, fetal demise, **placenta previa** (abnormal implantation of the placenta in the lower uterine segment), abruptio placentae, premature rupture of membranes, and preterm birth (Hartmann et al., 2007). Pregnant women who smoke also may participate in other unhealthy behaviors (e.g., alcohol use), further increasing their risk for low-birth-weight infants (Okah, Cai, & Hoff, 2005). Research also links maternal smoking, both during and after pregnancy, with an increased risk of SIDS. Parents who smoke also expose their young children to other risks of secondhand smoke, including middle ear infections, acute and chronic respiratory tract illnesses, and behavioral and learning disabilities (Albrecht et al., 2004).

The specific mechanism of smoking's effect on the fetus is not known. However, the ingredients in cigarette smoke, such as carbon monoxide, nicotine, lead, and cotinine, are toxic to the fetus and decrease the availability of oxygen to maternal and fetal tissues (Cunningham et al, 2005).

In response to public health education campaigns in the United States, smoking during pregnancy has decreased significantly. In fact, approximately 46% of women who smoke quit during pregnancy. Unfortunately, 60–80% of women who quit smoking during their pregnancy resume smoking within a year after childbirth (ACOG, 2005). This finding suggests that although women are aware of the potential impact of smoking on the fetus, they may be less knowledgeable about the effects of passive smoke on the baby.

Any decrease in smoking during pregnancy most likely improves fetal outcome, and researchers continue to explore approaches designed to help women quit smoking. Pregnancy may be a difficult time for a woman to stop smoking, but the nurse should encourage the pregnant woman to reduce the number of cigarettes she smokes daily if she cannot be persuaded to quit entirely. The perceived need to protect her unborn child may increase her motivation.

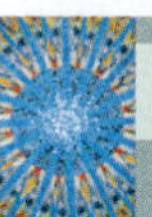

EVIDENCE-BASED PRACTICE **Psychosocial Interventions to Reduce Prenatal Illicit Drug Use**

Clinical Question

What nonpharmacologic interventions are effective in reducing illicit drug use during the prenatal period?

The Evidence

The use of illicit drugs during pregnancy has potentially serious consequences for the mother and her baby. Women who use drugs during the prenatal period are more likely to have low-birth-weight and preterm babies. The effect of nonpharmacologic interventions on outcomes was evaluated through a systematic review conducted by the Cochrane group. Outcomes of interest were attendance and retention in drug treatment, drug abstinence, and neonatal condition. Evidence was gathered from the Cochrane Drug and Alcohol Group register, the Cochrane Central Register of Trials, and three nursing/medical databases. Nine trials involving 546 women were included in this review. Two types of treatments were evaluated—contingency management and motivational interviewing. Conclusions drawn from multiple trials and held to the rigorous standards of the Cochrane Review represent the strongest evidence for practice.

What Is Effective?

The most motivating element was the mother's concern for her baby. Informing the mother about possible fetal and neonatal effects and encouraging entry into drug treatment were most effective. Contingency management was also effective in retaining mothers in treatment programs and in supporting abstinence. Contingency management uses positive, supportive reinforcement for continuation of desired behaviors. These reinforcements are generally concrete and have monetary value. Examples of reinforcements were awarding monetary vouchers or gift cards and giving work and a salary only when the client abstained from drug use. Motivational interviewing, the use of a directive counseling style aimed at changing behavior, was not found to be effective. These studies found that motivational interviewing over three to six sessions may actually lead to poorer retention in treatment.

What Is Inconclusive?

The majority of subjects were African American, single, never married, and unemployed. It is unclear whether these findings can be generalized to other population groups. Only two of the studies included nicotine as a targeted drug, so it is unclear whether these strategies will work for smoking cessation as well. Even when mothers remained abstinent and in treatment, no effect on neonatal outcomes was discovered. More study is needed to determine the specific effects of maternal drug treatment on newborns.

Best Practice

Inform mothers about the effects of their illicit drug use on fetal development and neonatal health. Emphasize to mothers that drug treatment during pregnancy can help them avoid these consequences. You can feel confident using concrete reinforcement to help the mother remain in treatment and abstain from illicit drug use. Directive counseling, on the other hand, is ineffective and may actually decrease the mother's motivation to stay in treatment.

References

Terplan, M., & Lui, S. (2008). Psychosocial interventions for pregnant women in outpatient illicit drug treatment programs compared to other interventions. *Cochrane Database of Systematic Reviews,* Issue 2.

Etiology

In general, the rate of illicit drug use among pregnant women is significantly less than the rate among nonpregnant women. Specifically, approximately 4% of pregnant women aged 15–44 report having used an illicit drug in the past month as compared with 10% of nonpregnant women (SAMHSA, 2007). However, illicit drug usage varies significantly by race and by age, with higher rates among women aged 18–25 than among women aged 26–44. Rates are highest among American Indians and Alaskan Natives (13.7%) and lowest among Asians (3.6%). Rates are 9.8% among blacks, 8.5% among whites, and 6.9% among Hispanics (SAMHSA, 2007).

The incidence of alcohol abuse is highest among women aged 20–40; alcoholism also is seen in teenagers. Among pregnant women aged 15–44, 11.8% used alcohol in a given month. This rate is significantly lower than the rate for nonpregnant women of that same age (53%) (SAMHSA, 2007).

Risk Factors

The Whatcom County Health Department (in the state of Washington) cites 17 identified risk factors for substance abuse, which are outlined in Box 2–5. While these risk factors for substance abuse apply to all clients, they can be of particular assistance to the nurse in trying to evaluate a pregnant woman's risk for substance abuse.

To provide information for caregivers and clients, the U.S. Food and Drug Administration (FDA) has developed the following classification system for all medications administered during pregnancy. This system can be used to help determine the risk of prenatal substance exposure from use of legal medications whether they are abused or prescribed by a physician.

- *Category A:* Controlled studies in women have demonstrated no associated fetal risk. Few drugs fall into this category.
- *Category B:* Animal studies show no risk. There have been no controlled studies in women in particular, but controlled human studies have failed to demonstrate a risk. The penicillins fall into this category.
- *Category C:* Either (1) no adequate animal or human studies are available or (2) animal studies show teratogenic effects but no controlled studies in women are available. Many drugs fall into this category. The lack of information makes this problematic for caregivers. Epinephrine, beta blockers, and zidovudine (a drug used to decrease perinatal transmission of HIV) fall into this category.

Box 2–5 Risk Factors for Substance Abuse

COMMUNITY

1. Availability of drugs
2. Community laws and norms favorable toward drug use
3. Transitions and mobility
4. Low neighborhood attachment and community disorganization
5. Extreme economic deprivation

FAMILY

6. Family history of the problem behavior
7. Family management problems
8. Family conflict
9. Favorable parental attitudes and involvement in the problem behavior

INDIVIDUAL/PEER

10. Alienation and rebelliousness
11. Friends who engage in the problem behavior
12. Favorable attitudes toward the problem behavior
13. Early initiation of the problem behavior
14. Constitutional factors

SCHOOL

15. Early and persistent antisocial behavior
16. Academic failure beginning in late elementary school
17. Lack of commitment to school

Source: The Whatcom County Health Department. Retrieved July 15, 2009, from http://www.co.whatcom.wa.us/health/human/substance_abuse/riskfactors.jsp

CLINICAL MANIFESTATIONS AND THERAPIES **Prenatal Substance Exposure**

ETIOLOGY	CLINICAL MANIFESTATION	CLINICAL THERAPIES
Cocaine abuse	■ Placental abruption ■ Fetal demise ■ Cardiovascular effects—increased heart rate, vasoconstriction, hypertension, myocardial infarction, arrhythmias, cardiomyopathy ■ CNS effects—euphoria, increased energy, excitement, loss of appetite, feeling of increased physical and mental strength, dilated pupils, nausea, vomiting, headache, vertigo, emotional instability, muscle jerks, hallucinations, cocaine psychosis ■ Nasal and sinus diseases if cocaine is snorted	Substance withdrawal using: ■ Behavioral therapy. ■ Recovery environment. ■ Group supportive therapy. ■ Detoxification.
Alcohol abuse	■ Increased risk of miscarriage and stillbirth ■ Low-birth-weight infant ■ Increased risk of learning, speech, attention span, and language disorders in the child born to a mother who abuses alcohol ■ Fetal alcohol syndrome	Substance withdrawal using: ■ Behavioral therapy. ■ Recovery environment. ■ Group supportive therapy. ■ Detoxification. ■ Medication therapy, which generally is not recommended during pregnancy.
Nicotine abuse	■ Miscarriage ■ Placental abruption ■ Premature rupture of membranes ■ Premature birth ■ Low-birth-weight infants ■ Increased risk that child born to a smoker will smoke later in life ■ Premature aging of placenta ■ Arterial spasm, including arteries to placenta ■ Polycythemia in the fetus, leading to possible fetal demise	Substance withdrawal using: ■ Behavioral therapy. ■ Recovery environment. ■ Group supportive therapy. ■ Medication therapy in the form of nicotine replacement with gradual weaning of support.
Narcotic abuse (opioids)	■ Fetal co-addiction ■ Increased risk of premature birth, low-birth-weight infant, newborn respiratory distress, newborn hypoglycemia, and fetal death ■ Respiratory depression in pregnant woman, possibly leading to hypoxia or death ■ Increased risk for infection secondary to use of dirty injection equipment	Substance withdrawal using: ■ Behavioral therapy. ■ Recovery environment. ■ Group supportive therapy. ■ Detoxification. ■ Medication therapy—most commonly methadone

- *Category D:* Evidence of human fetal risk exists, but the benefits of the drug in certain situations are thought to outweigh the risks. Examples of drugs in this category include tetracycline, vincristine, lithium, and hydrochlorothiazide.
- *Category X:* The demonstrated fetal risks clearly outweigh any possible benefit. Examples of drugs in this category include isotretinoin (Accutane), an acne medication, which can cause multiple CNS, facial, and cardiovascular anomalies.

COLLABORATION

Care of the pregnant woman who is a substance abuser is most effective when the woman agrees to try to quit abusing and seeks both prenatal and addiction treatment early in her pregnancy. With the mother's permission, nurses, doctors, and therapists can share information to collaborate in supporting the mother during all phases of treatment.

Complementary Therapies

Yoga classes for women who are pregnant are available in most communities. Yoga can help reduce anxiety and stress, which can decrease a substance abuser's need to use in order to relieve anxiety. Pregnant mothers who want to try yoga should take a class specifically designed for pregnant women from a yoga practitioner who has been trained to work with pregnant women, as some poses are contraindicated during pregnancy.

NURSING PROCESS

The nurse plays an important role in caring for the pregnant woman with a substance abuse problem. Compared to any other health care provider, nurses spend more time with the client; as a result, they are more likely to notice the often subtle signs of substance abuse. It is important that the nurse follow the nursing process, using its cyclical nature for ongoing assessment and care.

Assessment

The substance user is difficult to identify prenatally. Because many drugs are illegal, women may be reluctant to volunteer information about their drug use. The nurse who is familiar with the woman may recognize subtle signs of drug use, including mood swings and appetite changes, and withdrawal symptoms such as depression, irritability, nausea, lack of motivation, and psychomotor changes. As the number of women of childbearing age using substances increases, health care providers must be alert to early signs of use. It is often difficult for a nurse or physician to face the fact that a client is using an illegal substance, but ongoing alertness and an open, nonjudgmental approach are important for early detection. Care must be taken to ask open-ended questions in a nonjudgmental manner. For example, "How much alcohol do you drink per day?" is more helpful than "You don't drink alcohol, do you?" which leads the pregnant woman to believe that it would be inappropriate to admit to alcohol consumption.

Urine screening is valuable, but because cocaine is metabolized rapidly, the drug screen is negative within 24–48 hours after cocaine use. Thus, many expectant mothers who use cocaine probably are not identified.

PRACTICE ALERT

Keep in mind that almost 1 out of 10 women in the United States, regardless of socioeconomic status or ethnic background, is currently abusing a substance. If you consider that possibility with every woman, you will ask the important questions about drug use and be alert for signs of substance abuse.

Because of the prevalence of substance abuse in society today, nurses and other care providers should screen all pregnant women for substance abuse during the health history. Several simple screening tools are available. In addition, the nurse needs to be alert for clues in the woman's history or appearance that suggest substance abuse (Box 2–6).

If abuse is suspected, the nurse needs to ask direct questions, beginning with less threatening questions about use of tobacco, caffeine, and over-the-counter medications. The nurse can then progress to questions about alcohol consumption and finally to questions focusing on past and current use of illicit drugs. The nurse who uses a matter-of-fact and nonjudgmental approach is more likely to elicit honest responses.

Nursing assessment of the woman with a known substance abuse problem focuses on the woman's general health status, with specific attention paid to nutritional status, susceptibility to infections, and evaluation of all body systems. The nurse also assesses the woman's understanding of the impact of substance abuse on herself and her pregnancy.

Box 2–6 Possible Signs of Substance Abuse

HISTORY

- History of vague or unusual medical complaints
- Family history of alcoholism or other addiction
- History of childhood physical, sexual, or emotional abuse
- History of cirrhosis, pancreatitis, hepatitis, gastritis, sexually transmitted infections, or unusual infections such as cellulitis or endocarditis
- History of high-risk sexual behavior
- Psychiatric history of treatment and/or hospitalization

PHYSICAL SIGNS

- Dilated or constricted pupils
- Inflamed nasal mucosa
- Evidence of needle "track marks" or abscesses
- Poor nutritional status
- Slurred speech or staggering gait
- Odor of alcohol on breath

BEHAVIORAL SIGNS

- Memory lapses, mood swings, hallucinations
- Pattern of frequently missed appointments
- Frequent accidents, falls
- Signs of depression, agitation, euphoria
- Suicidal gestures

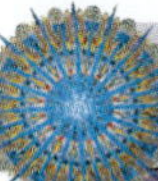

NURSING CARE PLAN A Client Abusing Substances While Pregnant

ASSESSMENT

Kathy Sanderson is a 27-year-old woman who is visiting her gynecologist. She reports a positive home pregnancy test and has come to the doctor's office for confirmation and prenatal care if the provider confirms pregnancy. Ms. Sanderson is in a long-term committed relationship and works full-time as a grammar school teacher. She denies use of alcohol, illegal substances, or any medications. The admitting nurse assesses her and notes dilated pupils, mildly increased temperature, increased heart rate and blood pressure, and extreme talkativeness with rapid speech. Ms. Sanderson has rhinorrhea but denies having a cold, saying she thinks it might be allergies. The nurse suspects possible cocaine use and shares assessment data with the provider, who orders a urine toxicology screen. The provider explains the need for a urine specimen and seeks consent, which the client provides. The results indicate that cocaine, cannabis (marijuana), and alcohol metabolites are present in the urine. When the results are shared with Ms. Sanderson, she begins to cry and admits she drinks occasionally, uses cocaine several times a week, and attended a party last night where marijuana was smoked but denies using it herself. She says that she was afraid to tell the nurse about her drug use because she would be fired from her job if her principal found out.

Physical examination indicates the following:

Height: 172 cm (5'8")
Weight: 57 kg (125 lb)
Temperature: 37.2°C (99°F)
Pulse rate: 102 BPM
Respirations: 22/minute
Blood pressure: 142/90 mmHg
Urine toxicology positive for cannabis, cocaine, and alcohol
Hemoglobin: 10.8
Hematocrit: 33.8%

DIAGNOSIS

Knowledge Deficit related to impact of cocaine and alcohol on the growing fetus and her own health status.

PLANNING

Client will exhibit substance abuse control as evidenced by extensively describing the following:

- Own risk for substance misuse
- Adverse health effects of substance use
- Signs of dependence during substance withdrawal
- Benefits of eliminating substance use.

Client will exhibit knowledge of pregnancy evidenced by extensive description of the following:

- Importance of prenatal care
- Warning signs of pregnancy complications
- Major fetal development milestones.

IMPLEMENTATION

- Establish a therapeutic relationship with Ms. Sanderson.
- Encourage Ms. Sanderson to take control of her own behavior.
- Assist Ms. Sanderson in identifying use of denial as a substitute for confronting the problem.
- Discuss with Ms. Sanderson the impact of substance abuse on her pregnancy and general health.
- Identify constructive goals with Ms. Sanderson to provide alternatives to the use of substances to reduce stress.
- Determine whether codependent or abusive relationships exist within the family.
- Determine Ms. Sanderson's learning needs.
- Appraise Ms. Sanderson's educational level.
- Select appropriate teaching methods and strategies.

EVALUATION

The goals related to knowledge deficit were met. At the prenatal visit, Ms. Sanderson admitted she had a cocaine addiction and agreed to begin rehabilitation therapy immediately. Through counseling, she was able to face her denial and recognize the people in her life who contributed to the problem, as well as those who could help her maintain her resolution to quit using cocaine. After completing an inpatient recovery program, she began attending a 12-step program for ongoing support. She received ongoing prenatal care through the rehabilitation and recovery phase and delivered a healthy, normal baby free of cocaine addiction at 39 weeks' gestation. She continues to attend group support sessions and has not relapsed since the baby was born.

CRITICAL THINKING

1. If the nurse had not noted the subtle assessment findings pointing to cocaine use, how might Ms. Sanderson's outcome have differed?
2. Could the provider have tested Ms. Sanderson's urine for toxicology if Ms. Sanderson had denied permission for the test? Why or why not?
3. While the nurse is working with her, Ms. Sanderson becomes very angry and says, "You don't understand. You've never had to go through this." How might the nurse respond?
4. If Ms. Sanderson had decided not to attend drug rehabilitation and delivered the baby while using cocaine, what follow-up care might the nurse have recommended for this new family?
5. Does the nurse have a responsibility to report Ms. Sanderson's drug use to the school system where she works? Explain your answer.

Diagnosis

Nursing diagnoses that may apply to a woman at risk because of substance abuse include the following:

- Imbalanced Nutrition: Less Than Body Requirements related to inadequate food intake secondary to substance abuse
- Risk for Infection related to use of inadequately cleaned syringes and needles secondary to IV drug use
- Risk for Ineffective Health Maintenance related to a lack of information about the impact of substance abuse on the fetus.

Plan

Prevention of substance abuse during pregnancy is the ideal nursing goal and is best accomplished through education. Unfortunately, many women who abuse substances do not receive regular health care and may not seek care until they are far along in pregnancy. Other goals for client care may include the following:

- Client immediately reduces number of cigarettes smoked to ____ and develops plan to quit smoking within 2 weeks.
- Client attends counseling sessions and/or drug treatment program within 48 hours.
- Client explains effects of substance being abused on fetal health.

Implementation

All women need to be counseled about the effects of alcohol in pregnancy. If heavy consumption is involved, the nurse can refer the pregnant woman to an alcoholic treatment program immediately. Counselors in these programs need to be made aware of a woman's pregnancy before drug therapy is suggested because certain drugs may be harmful to the developing fetus. For example, the drug disulfiram (Antabuse), often used in conjunction with alcohol treatment, is suspected to be a teratogenic agent. If the woman's behavior indicates possible substance abuse problems, the nurse can provide ongoing support and counseling and refer the woman to appropriate professionals.

The nurse's role in providing prenatal care for the woman who abuses substances focuses on ongoing assessment and client teaching. The nurse can provide information about the relationship between substance abuse and existing health problems and the implications for the woman's unborn child. By establishing a relationship of trust and support, the nurse may gain the woman's cooperation. The knowledgeable nurse can discuss possible strategies to help the woman quit (addiction treatment programs, 12-step programs, individual counseling) and suggest a referral for more in-depth assessment by a specialist. Relapse rates are high, even for motivated women, but the nurse's continued support and encouragement are important factors in helping women stop abusing substances.

Preparation for labor and birth should be part of prenatal planning. Fear, tension, or discomfort may be relieved through nonnarcotic psychologic support and careful explanation of the labor process. If pain medication is necessary, it should not be withheld; the notion that it will contribute to further addiction is mistaken. Preferred methods of pain relief include the use of psychoprophylaxis and regional blocks such as epidurals or local anesthetics such as pudendal block and local infiltration. Immediate intensive care should be available for the newborn, who is often depressed, small for gestational age (SGA), and premature.

Evaluation

The ongoing and cyclic nature of the nursing process is especially evident in the prenatal setting. Throughout the course of pregnancy, however, certain criteria can be used to determine the quality of care provided. In essence, nursing care has been effective when the following occur:

- The woman avoids substances and situations that pose a risk to her well-being or that of her child.
- The woman seeks regular prenatal care.
- The woman describes the impact of her substance abuse on herself and her unborn child.
- The woman gives birth to a healthy infant.
- The woman agrees to accept a referral to social services (or another appropriate community agency) for follow-up care after discharge.

REVIEW Prenatal Substance Exposure

RELATE: LINK THE CONCEPTS

Linking the exemplar of Prenatal Substance Exposure with the concept of Development:

1. Explain why the goal of substance use and pregnancy is focused primarily on stopping substance abuse before the woman becomes pregnant.
2. What developmental complications could develop from substance abuse if the woman detoxifies from the substance immediately after the first prenatal visit?

Linking the exemplar of Prenatal Substance Exposure with the concept of Perfusion:

3. What substances reduce perfusion to the neonate? What long-term effects are they likely to have on the growing fetus?

READY: GO TO COMPANION SKILLS MANUAL

REFER: GO TO MYNURSINGKIT

REFLECT: CASE STUDY

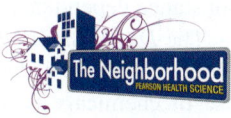

Jessica Riley is an 18-year-old single mother of a 1-year-old son, Ryan. She lives in a small one-bedroom apartment with her boyfriend Casey, who is not Ryan's father. She has had no contact with Ryan's father since before Ryan was born. Jessica works full time as a waitress at a restaurant and struggles financially. She is very grateful for Casey's income because she doesn't know how she would make it financially without him. Jessica dropped out of community college when she learned she was pregnant again. She goes to the community clinic for prenatal care. She likes seeing the nurse midwife because she makes Jessica feel comfortable. At the 24-week visit, Jessica tells the midwife that she tried to stop smoking but hasn't been successful. She tells the midwife that she has stopped drinking alcohol, although she still drinks an occasional beer when Casey insists on having someone to drink with. At her 28-week visit, she reports a problem with constipation. The nurse midwife asks what types of fluids she consumes, and Jessica says that she drinks mostly Coke. The midwife suggests that Jessica decrease the number of soft drinks she consumes and increase her fluid and fiber intake. During the visit, Jessica learns from the ultrasound that the baby is a girl. It never dawns on Jessica to tell the midwife that Casey is smoking marijuana because she doesn't know that it has any impact on her or the baby.

1. What impact will Casey's marijuana use have on Jessica and the fetus?
2. Why would the nurse midwife tell Jessica to reduce her intake of soft drinks?
3. What effect will smoking cigarettes and an occasional beer (1–2 per week) have on the fetus?
4. If you were the nurse caring for Jessica, how would you help her make healthier choices to improve the outcome of her pregnancy?

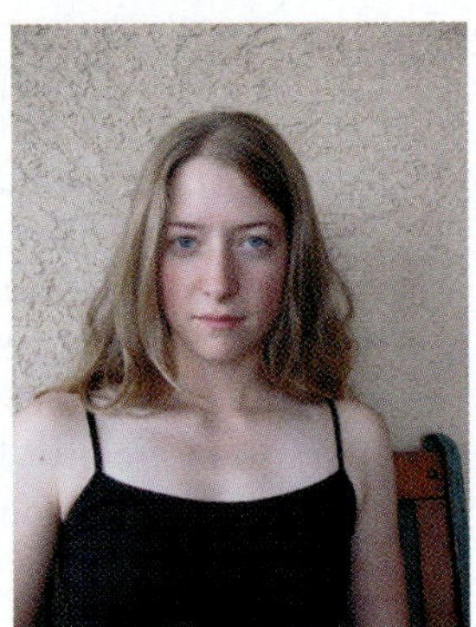

2.4 SUBSTANCE ABUSE

KEY TERMS

Amphetamine, *72*
Caffeine, *71*
Cannabis sativa, *71*
Central nervous system (CNS) depressants, *71*
Co-occurring disorders, *67*
Hallucinogens, *73*
Inhalants, *74*
Kindling, *67*
Opiates, *73*
Psychostimulants, *71*
Substance abuse, *66*
Substance dependence, *66*

BASIS FOR SELECTION OF EXEMPLAR
Healthy People 2010

LEARNING OUTCOMES

After reading about this exemplar, you will be able to:

1. Describe the pathophysiology, etiology, clinical manifestations, and direct and indirect causes of substance abuse.
2. Identify risk factors associated with substance abuse.
3. Illustrate the nursing process in providing culturally competent care across the life span for individuals with substance abuse disorders.
4. Formulate priority nursing diagnoses appropriate for an individual with a substance abuse disorder.
5. Create a plan of care for individuals with a substance abuse disorder and for their family members.
6. Assess expected outcomes for an individual with a substance abuse disorder.
7. Discuss therapies used in the collaborative care of an individual with a substance abuse disorder.
8. Employ evidence-based caring interventions for an individual with a substance abuse disorder.

OVERVIEW

Substance abuse refers to the use of any chemical in a fashion inconsistent with medical or culturally defined social norms despite physical, psychologic, or social adverse effects. Anxiety and depressive disorders frequently occur with substance abuse, and more than 90% of people who commit suicide have a depressive or substance abuse disorder (National Institute of Mental Health, 2004). According to the *Results from the 2004 National Survey on Drug Use and Health: National Findings* (SAMHSA, 2005), 9.4% of the American population aged 12 and older (22.5 million Americans) reported problems with substance dependence or abuse in 2004.

The *Diagnostic and Statistical Manual of Mental Disorders* (4th ed., Text Revision) (DSM-IV-TR) classifies the pathologic use of chemicals as psychoactive substance-related disorders. The words *substance* and *chemical* are used interchangeably. Substance abuse also is defined as recurrent use that results in a failure to manage work, school, or home roles; use in hazardous situations such as driving a car; or use resulting in substance-related legal problems or related interpersonal problems. This diagnosis can be used only for someone who has never been diagnosed as dependent.

Substance dependence occurs when the client can no longer control use of the substance, continues to use despite adverse effects, and experiences withdrawal symptoms without continued use of the substance. Substance-dependent individuals experience tolerance, requiring increasing quantities of the substance to meet the same level of need. People who are dependent on drugs may spend a great deal of time obtaining drugs and limit their usual social, occupational, or recreational activities because of the substance use. As addiction continues, the need for the drug is so powerful that it drives the addict to neglect his or her children, his or her responsibilities, and the law in an effort to obtain drugs (Hyman, 2005). This exemplar focuses on substance dependence, which is the more severe form of the substance-related disorders. See Box 2–7 for the *DSM-IV-TR* diagnostic criteria for substance abuse and substance dependence.

Substance withdrawal symptoms are physiologic, behavioral, cognitive, and affective symptoms that occur after reduction or discontinuance of a drug that has been used heavily over a long period of time. When experiencing withdrawal, most individuals

Box 2–7 *DSM-IV-TR:* Diagnostic Criteria for Substance Abuse Versus Substance Dependence

DIAGNOSTIC CRITERIA FOR SUBSTANCE ABUSE

A. A maladaptive pattern of substance use leading to clinically significant impairment or distress, as manifested by one (or more) of the following, occurring within a 12-month period:
   1. Recurrent substance use resulting in a failure to fulfill major role obligations at work, school, or home
   2. Recurrent substance use in situations in which it is physically hazardous
   3. Recurrent substance-related legal problems
   4. Continued substance use despite having persistent or recurrent social or interpersonal problems caused or exacerbated by the effects of the substance

B. The symptoms have never met the criteria for substance dependence for this class of substance.

DIAGNOSTIC CRITERIA FOR SUBSTANCE DEPENDENCE

A. A maladaptive pattern of substance use leading to clinically significant impairment or distress, as manifested by three (or more) of the following, occurring at any time in the same 12-month period:
   1. Tolerance
   2. Withdrawal
   3. The substance is often taken in larger amounts or over a longer period than was intended.
   4. There is a persistent desire or unsuccessful efforts to cut down or control substance use.
   5. A great deal of time is spent in activities necessary to obtain the substance.
   6. Important social, occupational, or recreational activities are given up or reduced.
   7. The substance use is continued despite knowledge of having a persistent or recurrent physical or psychological problem that is likely to have been caused or exacerbated by the substance.

Source: Reprinted with permission from the American Psychiatric Association. (2000). *Diagnostic and statistical manual of mental disorders* (4th ed., Text Revision) (pp. 197–199). Washington, DC: Author.

find themselves craving the drug, which they know would relieve the withdrawal symptoms. Withdrawal symptoms are specific for each drug (American Psychiatric Association, 2000). Withdrawal is an uncomfortable state lasting several days and, depending on the amount of drugs consumed, may put the client in medical danger. Tolerance is a cumulative state in which a particular dose of the chemical elicits a smaller response than before. With increased tolerance, the individual needs higher and higher doses to obtain the desired effect. When a person is physically addicted to the drug and stops taking it, withdrawal symptoms can occur within hours.

Chemical dependence is a complex, chronic progressive disease that can be fatal if left untreated. While it is true that a disease is not defined as a deficiency of willpower, chemical dependence is composed of several biochemical processes that are subject to voluntary control. In addition, there are psychologic, sociologic, and spiritual aspects to chemical dependence.

A number of types of psychoactive substances are associated with chemical dependence. The days of the so-called pure drug addict or alcoholic are gone. Most people who are chemically dependent are engaged in polysubstance abuse. They may use amphetamines or cocaine to get high and alcohol, diazepam (Valium), or marijuana to come down off the high. Some addicts use sedatives to sleep and amphetamines to wake up. Whatever the pattern, clients must be treated for all secondary, as well as primary, addictions.

While alcohol and nicotine are often abused, they are covered in separate exemplars in this concept. For the purpose of this exemplar, the term *substance abuse* refers specifically to drugs, both legal and illegal, that lead to addiction and dependence.

PATHOPHYSIOLOGY AND ETIOLOGY

The human tendency to seek pleasure and avoid stress and pain is partially responsible for substance abuse. Although far from definite, evidence implicates the endogenous opioid system in the development and maintenance of addictive behaviors. Currently, available data suggest that ethanol increases opioid neurotransmission and that this activation is part of the mechanism responsible for its reinforcing effect (Oswald & Wand, 2004). Although most studies have focused on the role of dopamine D(1) and D(2) receptors in sustaining the addictive danger of drugs, recent studies also have shown that the dopamine D(3) receptor is involved in drug-seeking behavior (Heidbreder et al., 2004). The reinforcing properties of drugs can create a pleasurable experience and reduce the intensity of unpleasant experiences.

The craving that a person has for a particular substance also may be heightened by a phenomenon known as the kindling effect. **Kindling** refers to long-term changes in brain neurotransmission that occur after repeated detoxifications (Bayard et al., 2004). Recurrent detoxifications increase neuron sensitivity and are thought to intensify obsessive thoughts or cravings for a substance. Eventually, the brain responds spontaneously in a dysfunctional manner even when the substance is no longer being used (Stuart & Laraia, 2005). This phenomenon may explain why subsequent episodes of withdrawal from a substance tend to get progressively worse.

Although there is no greater prevalence of psychiatric illness in substance abusers than in the general population, co-occurring disorders are often present. The term **co-occurring disorders** refers to the coexistence of substance abuse or dependence and a psychiatric disorder in one individual. One study describing the prevalence and characteristics of co-occurring serious mental illness (SMI) and substance abuse or dependence found that the most common co-occurring disorders in adult mental health clients were (1) alcohol and/or cannabis abuse with psychoses and heroin and/or (2) alcohol abuse or dependence with depression (Virgo, Bennett, Higgins, Bennett, & Thomas, 2001). Compared with other SMI clients, those who were dually diagnosed were younger, more often male, in less stable accommodations, more likely to be unemployed, and more likely to have more than one psychiatric diagnosis and personality disorder. They also tended to have more crises and to pose greater risk to themselves and others (Virgo et al., 2001).

Etiology

Substance use disorders in the United States cost over $414 billion a year, including the costs of treatment, related health problems, absenteeism, lost productivity, drug-related crime and incarceration, and education and prevention. Illicit drugs are related to 16,000 annual deaths. Studies indicate that alcohol and drugs are a factor in 50% of motor vehicle fatalities and 50% of all violent deaths from any cause. Between 40% and 60% of people seeking treatment are ordered to do so by the court system. The relapse rate for those who have been in treatment is 90% in the first year, with most relapses occurring after 3 months of treatment (Murphy-Parker & Martinez, 2005; Nader & Czoty, 2005; Wright, 2003).

The illicit nature of drug use makes it nearly impossible to retrieve accurate information on the number of drug abusers in the United States. As many as 46–50% of all Americans 12 years of age and older have tried an illegal drug at least once during their life.

It is estimated that drug addiction is a problem for 9–20% of the U.S. population. The prevalence rate for alcohol or drug addiction in the medical population is 25–50%; it is 50–75% in individuals with mental disorders (Miller & Adams, 2005).

In the 1960s, hallucinogens and amphetamines were the most commonly used illegal drugs. In the 1970s, heroin, marijuana, and sedatives were the most popular drugs. The 1980s was the decade of cocaine. Judging by the increase in cocaine-related visits to hospital EDs, hard-core cocaine abuse continues to be a problem in the United States. Eight million Americans use cocaine regularly, with 2.2 million considered dependent. Heroin has become a more popular drug with adolescents and young adults due to the change from injecting it to smoking it. Unfortunately, users mistakenly believe that smoking heroin is not addictive.

Illicit use of prescription drugs is on the rise, especially among adolescents who mistakenly believe that these drugs are safer than illegal drugs. The rapidly escalating abuse of amphetamines, especially Ecstasy, is a significant problem at dance clubs and dance parties known as "raves." Young people take these "love drugs" for increased energy and sexual desire (Compton & Volkow, 2006; O'Malley, 2005).

In the 1800s, alcohol, opiates, cocaine, and marijuana were part of many medications used to treat a variety of illnesses. The addictive potential of these chemicals was not known at the time. Those at highest risk for addiction were physicians, physicians' wives, housewives, and nurses. It is believed that for every male addict, there were three female addicts. By the early 1900s, the process of addiction became clear, but it was believed to be moral failing rather than a disease that could be treated. Addiction was criminalized with passage of the Harrison Narcotic Act of 1914, Prohibition, the Marijuana Tax Act of 1937, the Narcotic Control Act of 1956, the Controlled Substance Act of 1970, and creation of the Drug Enforcement Administration in 1973.

Impaired Nurses

In the early twentieth century, nurses were identified as being at high risk for addiction due to high workloads and high stress levels. There were, however, no treatment options at the time. In the 1960s, nurses and physicians were identified as being at higher risk for narcotic addiction. Little was done about the problem of addiction, and most instances were ignored. When nurses were identified as being addicted or abusing substances, they were either fired or reported to state boards of nursing and disciplined by censure or suspension or by having their professional license revoked. In the 1970s, research on impaired nursing practice began to appear, and in 1982, the American Nurses Association (ANA) passed a resolution entitled "Action on Alcohol and Drug Misuse and Psychological Dysfunctions among Nurses." The hope was to shift the focus from punishment to rehabilitation. In 2002, the ANA adopted an updated resolution entitled "The Profession's Response to the Problems of Addictions and Psychiatric Disorders in Nursing," calling attention again to impaired nursing practice, stressing the need for peer assistance programs (Heise, 2003).

Health care providers are as susceptible as anyone else to developing substance abuse. By the very nature of their roles, dentists, pharmacists, physicians, and nurses are in frequent contact with drugs and are at high risk for substance abuse problems. One study exploring family history of alcohol and drug use in health care professionals found that nurses reported a higher prevalence of alcoholism in their families than did dentists and physicians (Kenna & Wood, 2005). However, no significant differences were found in health care professionals' drinking levels. As a rule, nurses experience many pressures in the workplace and have easy access to drugs. Trinkoff and colleagues (2000) found that nurses reported higher substance use if they had easy access to prescription drugs, increased role strain, and close social connections with substance abusers. Two factors, stronger religious practices and treatment for depressive symptoms, were associated with reduced substance abuse.

Substance abuse and dependence can lead to impaired professional practice; therefore, nurses must act responsibly when coworkers display signs of substance abuse. Health care professionals have a higher risk for opiate abuse than other professionals due to the high accessibility of opiates in their line of work (Trinkoff, Zhou, Storr, & Soeken, 2000). If nurses are showing signs of a substance abuse problem, to help them, their colleagues can find information about impaired nurse programs through state boards of nursing. Warning signs of impaired nurses in the workplace are listed in Table 2–8.

When nurses have an addiction, shame and guilt are magnified. After all, nurses are healers and nurturers. They are not expected to have their own problems, certainly not an addiction that could lead them to take drugs from clients or be less than 100% in control when they are at work.

Early studies suggested that nurses are at higher risk for addiction than the general population. More recent studies contradict these findings and state that most likely, nurses are

TABLE 2–8 **Warning Signs of Impaired Nurses in the Workplace**

AT-RISK SITUATIONS	OBSERVABLE WARNING SIGNS
Easy access to prescription drugs	Inaccurate narcotic counts or frequent missing drugs Client complaints of ineffective pain control, denial of having received pain meds Excessive "wasting" of drugs Likelihood of volunteering to give medications to clients Frequent trips to the bathroom
Role strain	Frequent tardiness or absenteeism, especially before and after scheduled days off Haphazard, shoddy charting Judgment errors in client care Unorganized, erratic behavior; unkempt appearance
Depression	Irritability, unable to focus or concentrate Abrupt mood swings Isolating self, taking long breaks Apathetic, depressed, lethargic Unexplained absences from assigned unit
Signs of alcohol or drug use	Smell of alcohol on breath Excessive use of perfumes, mouthwash, or mints Slurred speech, flushed face, reddened eyes, unsteady gait Long sleeves worn in hot weather to cover up arms
Signs of withdrawal	Tremors, restlessness, sweating Watery eyes, runny nose, stomachaches

not at higher risk for substance abuse (Snow & Hughes, 2003). Nurses now have access to peer assistance and statewide programs to seek treatment and save their licenses. Nurses with substance abuse problems are required to stop practicing and enter a 12-step treatment program for monitoring. Those who abuse substances are banned from client care or administration of narcotics for 1 year (Fletcher, 2004; West, 2002).

Risk Factors

Various risk factors help explain why one person becomes addicted while another does not. Genetic, biologic, psychologic, and sociocultural factors shed light on how a person may abuse or become dependent on a substance.

- *Genetic factors* include an apparent hereditary factor. Evidence supports the D(2) dopamine receptor gene (DRD2 A1 allele) as a genetic marker in adolescent males with increased risk for developing substance use problems (Conner et al., 2005).
- *Biologic factors* were first identified by Jellinek in his disease model of alcoholism. Dopamine and dopamine receptor sites are intricately involved in the complex workings between the nervous system and abusive substances. Any drug's ability to have an impact on the biochemical mechanism of the brain must be able to do so at a receptor site or at a number of receptor sites (Figure 2–2 ■). Most abused substances mimic or block the brain's most important neurotransmitters at their respective receptor sites. For example, heroin and other opiates mimic natural opiate-like neurotransmitters such as endorphin, enkephalin, and dynorphin. In contrast, cocaine and other stimulants block the reuptake of dopamine, serotonin, and norepinephrine (Stuart & Laraia, 2005).
- *Psychologic factors* of substance abuse are examined in psychoanalytic, behavioral, and family system theories. Psychoanalytic theorists view substance abuse as a fixation at the oral stage of development, whereas behavioral theorists see addiction as a learned maladaptive behavior. Family

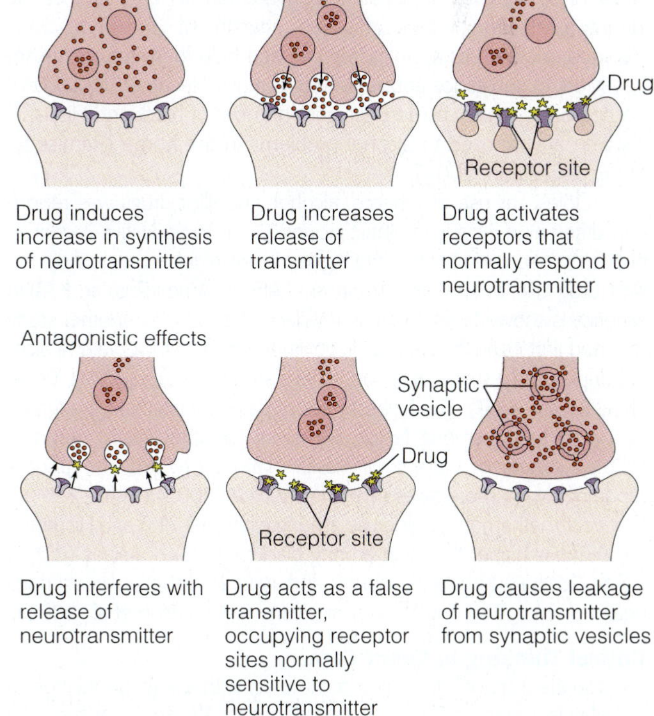

Figure 2–2 ■ Action of abused substances at brain receptor sites.

system theory focuses on the pattern of family relationships throughout several generations. No addictive personality type has been identified; however, several common factors seem to exist among alcoholics and drug users. Many substance abusers have experienced sexual or physical abuse in their childhood and, as a result, have low self-esteem and difficulty expressing emotions. A link also exists between substance abuse and psychiatric disorders such as depression, anxiety, and antisocial and dependent personalities. The habit of using a substance becomes a form of self-medication to cope with day-to-day problems and develops into an addiction over time.

- *Sociocultural factors* often influence individuals' decisions as to when, what, and how they use substances. The way drugs are processed, the degree of acceptance or rejection of drug use, and the finances available to pay for a substance influence what substance is used, how much is used, and what peer pressure the person will face in his or her culture as the abuse becomes evident. Sociocultural factors are especially important influences among teenagers (Box 2–8).

Many factors place a person at risk for substance use, abuse, and dependence. No single cause can explain why one individual develops a pattern of drug use and another person does not. Thorough assessment of these factors is necessary to understand the whole person and to plan appropriate interventions.

Box 2–8 **Substance Dependence Risk Factors in Teenagers**

- Peer pressure, group norms; prosubstance use
- A greater here-and-now orientation than adults; drugs provide immediate gratification
- Rebellion against authority
- Alienation from traditional social and religious values; drugs viewed as a way to individuate and disconnect
- Stressful situations such as a dysfunctional family
- Insecurity and low self-esteem: powerful triggers for compensatory substance abuse

CLINICAL MANIFESTATIONS

Clinical manifestations, and their severity, are dependent on amount, frequency, and specific combination of substances used. Combining two CNS depressants, for example, will produce far more significant manifestations than the use of only one CNS depressant. Some symptoms can be alarming or even fatal. For example, long-term crack use can result in sensory hallucinations, and even the first use of cocaine can result in death for people with never diagnosed cardiac disorders. Specific manifestations are linked to substances in the following section.

FOCUS ON DIVERSITY AND CULTURE **Ethnic Identity and Drug Use**

Ethnic identity plays a unique role in drug use behavior. Patterns of substance use are influenced by cultural norms and practices in addition to other environmental and biologic factors. Adolescents in particular are influenced by ethnic and cultural practices. Positive ethnic identity (i.e., strong ethnic affiliation, attachment, and pride) may "protect" adolescents against drug use and help them form resistant behaviors to substance abuse (Marsiglia, Kulis, Hecht, & Sills, 2004). Compared to white children, a higher number of black and Hispanic children are exposed to alcohol problems in the home (Ramisetty-Mikler & Caetano, 2004).

Adolescent use of tobacco, alcohol, and illicit drugs was reportedly different in racial and ethnic groups. On average, Native American high school seniors revealed the highest levels of tobacco, alcohol, and illicit drug use, while Latin Americans, African Americans, and Asian Americans showed less drug use (Wallace et al., 2002). Another study reported that Asian American college students had a lower rate of alcohol dependence than Caucasian college students (Luczak, Wall, Cook, Shea, & Carr, 2004). The highest rates of past-year methamphetamine use were found among Native Hawaiians or other Pacific Islanders (2.2%), American Indians or Alaska Natives (1.7%), and people reporting two or more races (1.9%) (SAMHSA, 2005) (Figure 2–3 ■). Past-year methamphetamine use among whites (0.7%) and Hispanics (0.5%) was higher than that among blacks (0.1%) or Asians (0.2%) (OAS, 2005a). Substance abuse and type 2 diabetes are serious health problems among Native Americans (Leonardson et al., 2005).

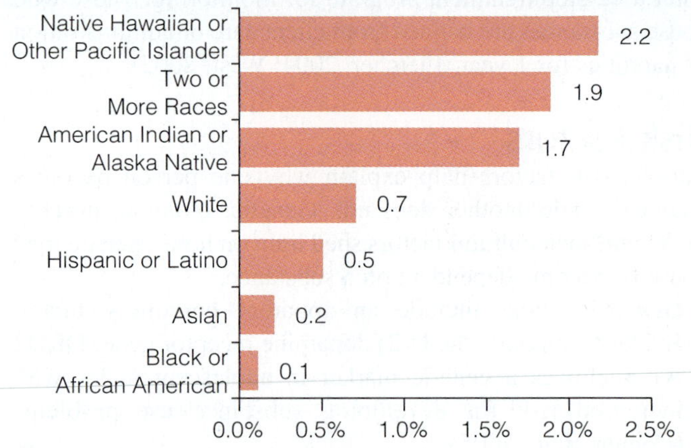

Figure 2–3 ■ Methamphetamine use by race/ethnicity: 2002, 2003, and 2004.

Source: SAMHSA, 2002, 2003, and 2004 NSDUH.

Critical Thinking in Client Care

1. You are a school nurse in a community with a large population of Native Americans, Latin Americans, and African Americans. An increasing problem with alcohol use and binge drinking among the high school students has become evident. The school superintendent asks you for ideas to address this problem. How do you respond?
2. You are caring for a 23-year-old Asian American female brought to the ED by her boyfriend who tells you they were at a college party where she had alcohol for the first time. She is weak, her face is flushed, and she is vomiting violently. What do you do?

Caffeine

Caffeine is a stimulant that increases the heart rate and acts as a diuretic. Although commonly consumed daily in soft drinks, coffee, tea, chocolate, and some pain relievers, an excessive amount of caffeine can cause negative physiologic effects, especially cardiac-related risks. Approximately 300 mg per day is safe for most people, but over 600 mg is considered excessive and is not recommended (Kneisl et al., 2004). Individuals with a history of cardiac disease should be advised to cut down or eliminate caffeine intake altogether. Caffeine, if consumed in large quantities, also can cause higher total cholesterol levels and insomnia.

Many people in today's society recognize the adverse effects of too much caffeine in their system and voluntarily cut down by drinking decaffeinated beverages. A caffeine-addicted person who abruptly withdraws from caffeine will most likely experience headaches and irritability. A rising number of adolescents are developing caffeine dependence by consuming sizable quantities of soft drinks and coffee. In a study investigating caffeine dependence in teenagers, researchers found that 15 out of 36 subjects reported tolerance to caffeine, described withdrawal symptoms after cessation of caffeine intake, reported unsuccessful attempts to control use, and endorsed use despite knowledge of physical or psychologic problems associated with caffeine (Bernstein, Carroll, Thuras, Cosgrove, & Roth, 2002). These results are significant due to the vast number of teens who consume caffeinated beverages.

Cannabis

Cannabis sativa is the source of marijuana. The greatest psychoactive substances are in the flowering tops of the cannabis plant. Marijuana (also know as grass, weed, pot, dope, joint, and reefer) and hashish are the most common derivatives. The psychoactive component of marijuana is an oily chemical known as delta-9-tetrahydrocannabinol (THC). THC activates specific cannabinoid receptors in the brain. Evidence suggests that marijuana may act like opioids and cocaine in producing a pleasurable sensation, probably by causing release of endogenous opioids and then dopamine (Kneisl et al., 2004). Marijuana use can trigger psychosis in schizophrenic clients, and according to recent research, cannabis use may be a risk factor in developing future psychotic symptoms (Ferdinand et al., 2005).

Physiologic effects of cannabis are dose-related and can cause an increase in heart rate and bronchodilation in short-term use. Chronic long-term use can lead to airway constriction, bronchitis, sinusitis, asthma, and increased risk for respiratory cancer (Watson, Benson, & Joy, 2000). The reproductive system also is affected by marijuana use; it causes decreased spermatogenesis and testosterone levels in males and suppresses follicle-stimulating, luteinizing, and prolactin hormones in females, making breastfeeding impossible for new mothers. Birth defects also may be associated with cannabis use. Marijuana crosses the placental barrier and is spread to fetal tissues. Subjective effects of marijuana include euphoria, sedation, and hallucinations. In addition, chronic use of marijuana can result in amotivational behaviors such as apathy, dullness, poor grooming, reduced interest in achievement, and disinterest. At extremely high doses, tolerance and physical dependence result.

Central Nervous System (CNS) Depressants

Central nervous system (CNS) depressants including barbiturates, benzodiazepines, paraldehyde, meprobamate, and chloral hydrate also are subject to abuse. Cross-dependence exists among all CNS depressants, and cross-tolerance can develop to alcohol and general anesthetics. Chronic users of barbiturates require progressively higher doses to achieve subjective effects as tolerance develops, but they develop little tolerance to respiratory depression. The depressant effects related to barbiturates are dose-dependent and range from mild sedation to sleep to coma to death. With larger doses over time and a combination of alcohol and barbiturates, the risk of death increases greatly.

The risk of accidental overdose and death resulting from barbiturates has resulted in decreased use, yet barbiturates are still clinically useful in treating seizure disorders and alcohol withdrawal. Benzodiazepines have replaced barbiturates as the drugs of choice for anxiety-related disorders. Benzodiazepines alone are safer than barbiturates because an overdose of oral benzodiazepines rarely results in death. However, when taken together, CNS depressants (for example, alcohol and benzodiazepines) can result in death.

Psychostimulants

Psychostimulants such as cocaine and amphetamines have a high potential for abuse. Euphoria is the main subjective effect associated with cocaine and amphetamines, leading to addiction. Powdered cocaine has been "snorted" (inhaled through the nostrils) for thousands of years, but a more dangerous method used today is called freebasing. Cocaine base (free-based cocaine, or "crack") is heat-stable and is usually "cooked" in a baking soda solution and smoked (freebasing). Cocaine hydrochloride is diluted or cut before sale, and the pure form ("rocks") is administered intranasally (snorted) or injected intravenously. "Skin popping" is a subcutaneous method that many substance abusers are using to administer drugs, perhaps leading to the formation of abscesses under the skin. A mild overdose of cocaine produces agitation, dizziness, tremor, and blurred vision. A severe overdose produces anxiety, hyperpyrexia, convulsions, ventricular dysrhythmias, severe hypertension, and hemorrhagic stroke with possible angina or myocardial infarction.

The use of cocaine during pregnancy is especially problematic because the drug crosses the placenta and enters the fetal bloodstream. Spontaneous abortion, premature delivery, IUGR, congenital abnormalities, and fetal addiction can result.

Long-term intranasal use of cocaine can cause atrophy of the nasal mucosa, necrosis and perforation of the nasal septum, and lung damage. The growing practice of crack cocaine injection requires serious attention because this new drug use is associated with increased rates of high-risk behaviors. Recent research indicates that injection drug users exhibited significantly higher rates of risky health behaviors. High-risk sexual behaviors were especially prevalent among female crack cocaine injectors. Higher self-reported rates of adverse health outcomes such as sexually transmitted infections, hepatitis C, and abscesses among crack injectors were found, although no differences in rates of HIV infection were self-reported (Buchanan et al., 2006).

Amphetamine is a powerful stimulant that poses a severe health risk to society due to its devastating physical and neurologic consequences, including amphetamine-induced mental disorders. Methamphetamine is illegally manufactured, distributed, and abused and is currently the most widespread amphetamine used in the United States (OAS, 2005a). Methamphetamine is a powerful stimulant drug commonly referred to as *speed; crystal; crank; go;* and, most recently, *ice,* a smokable form of methamphetamine. The manufacture of methamphetamine is a relatively simple process that can be carried out by individuals without special knowledge or expertise in chemistry. Methamphetamine is often taken in combination with other drugs such as cocaine and marijuana and, like heroin and cocaine, can be inhaled, injected, ingested, and smoked.

In 2004, an estimated 1.4 million people aged 12 and older (0.6% of the population) had used methamphetamine in the past year and 600,000 people (0.2% of the population) had used methamphetamine in the past month (OAS, 2005a). The highest rate of methamphetamine use in the past year was found among young adults between the ages of 18 and 25 (1.6%). Methamphetamine use among males (0.7%) was slightly higher than for females (0.5%) (Figure 2–4 ■).

It appears that methamphetamine is an "equal opportunity" drug for addiction without regard to gender, age, race, or sexual preferences. However, the highest percentage rates of methamphetamine use were found among Native Hawaiians or other Pacific Islanders (2.2%), people reporting two or more races (1.9%), and American Indians or Alaska Natives (1.7%) (OAS, 2005a). The lowest rates of methamphetamine use were among whites (0.7%), Hispanics (0.5%), Asians (0.2%), and African Americans (0.1%).

Methamphetamine use has been linked with HIV infection and high rates of sexually transmitted infections in homosexual, heterosexual, and bisexual men and women all over the United States (AIDS Alert, 2005; Brown et al., 2005; Semple, Grant, & Patterson, 2004; Shoptaw et al., 2005). Heterosexual men and women displayed severe to moderate depressive symptoms due to perceived stigma associated with methamphetamine use, emphasizing the importance of identifying and treating depression in this population (Semple et al., 2005). An interesting finding from the 2004 *National Survey on Drug Use and Health* (NSDUH) was that the western half of the United States reported the highest levels of methamphetamine use from 2002 through 2004 (OAS, 2005a). Twelve states including Nevada (2.2%), Wyoming (1.5%), and Montana (1.5%) ranked highest for past-year methamphetamine use. Connecticut (less than 0.1%), New York (0.12%), and North Carolina (0.12%) were among the states with the lowest rates (Figure 2–5 ■).

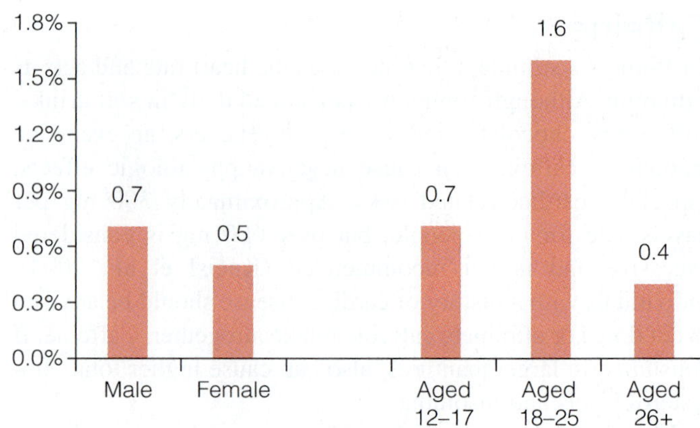

Figure 2–4 ■ Methamphetamine use by gender and age: 2002, 2003, and 2004.

Source: SAMHSA, 2002, 2003, and 2004 NSDUH.

Amphetamines cause arousal and an elevation of mood with a sense of increased strength, mental capacity, self-confidence, and a decreased need for food and sleep. Methamphetamine users in treatment have reported physical symptoms associated with the use of methamphetamine, including weight loss, tachycardia, tachypnea, hyperthermia, insomnia, and muscular tremors (OAS, 2005a). The behavioral and psychiatric symptoms reported most often include violent behavior, repetitive activity, memory loss, paranoia, delusions of reference, auditory hallucinations, and confusion or fright. A psychotic state with hallucinations and paranoia is common with long-term use, requiring treatment similar to other psychotic disorders. The cardiovascular effects of amphetamines are comparable to those of cocaine, including vasoconstriction, tachycardia, hypertension, angina, and dysrhythmias. Tolerance to mood elevation, appetite suppression, and cardiovascular effects develops with amphetamines; however, dependence is more psychologic than physical.

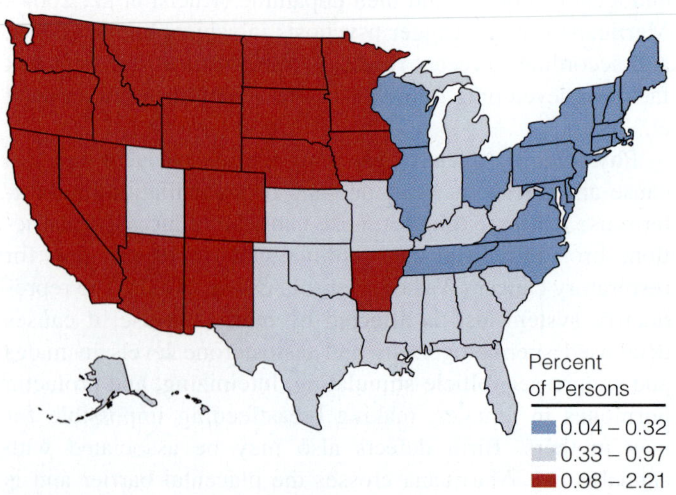

Figure 2–5 ■ Methamphetamine use by state: 2002, 2003, and 2004.

Source: SAMHSA, 2002, 2003, and 2004 NSDUH.

Withdrawal from amphetamines produces dysphoria and craving with fatigue, prolonged sleep, excessive eating, and depression. Although a large number of people cope with amphetamine dependence worldwide, limited evidence exists for effective treatment (Srisurapanont, Jarusuraisin, & Kittirattanapalboon, 2005). In a systematic review of treatment measures for amphetamine dependence and abuse, antidepressants provided little benefit concerning amphetamine use. Both biologic and psychosocial treatments should be further investigated (Srisurapanont et al., 2005). Brief cognitive-behavioral therapy (CBT) was reported to improve methamphetamine users' attempts to resist the urge to use methamphetamine in stressful interpersonal situations (Yen, Wu, Yen, & Ko, 2004). A culturally tailored CBT program was more effective than standard CBT in reducing methamphetamine use and high-risk sexual behaviors (Shoptaw et al., 2005).

Opiates

Opiates such as morphine, meperidine, codeine, hydrocodone, and oxycodone are narcotic analgesics. Some common brand names include Vicodin, Percocet, OxyContin, and Darvon. Narcotic analgesics are a type of pain reliever derived from natural or synthetic opiates. A small percentage of individuals are originally exposed to opiates in the context of prescription pain management; however, most people use opiates under social or illicit circumstances.

The problem of abuse of and addiction to prescribed narcotics resurfaced as a major issue for the United States in the early 2000s and has worsened during the past few years (Compton & Volkow, 2006). In 2004, the number of new nonmedical users of OxyContin was 615,000, with an average age at first use of 24.5 years (SAMHSA, 2005). Figure 2–6 ■ shows a steady increase in the number of initiates from 1995, when OxyContin was first available, through 2003. This increase in opiate abuse seems to reflect, in part, changes in medication prescribing practices, changes in drug formulations, and fairly easy access via the Internet. Although the use of narcotic analgesics for acute pain management looks benign, long-term use has been associated with significant rates of abuse or addiction. OxyContin is a controlled-released form of oxycodone prescribed for the management of moderate to severe pain. OxyContin diversion and abuse has become a major problem in certain areas of the United States, particularly rural areas and Appalachia (Hays, 2004).

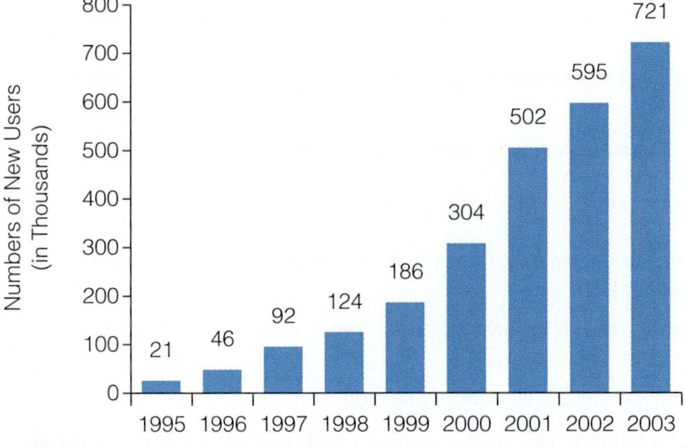

Figure 2–6 ■ Annual numbers of new nonmedical users of OxyContin, 1995–2003.

Source: SAMHSA, 2002, 2003, and 2004 NSDUH.

A retrospective review of 534 medical records revealed that 27% of patients admitted and discharged from an addiction detoxification unit were dependent on prescription opiate medications (Miller & Greenfeld, 2004). The most frequently mentioned medication was Vicodin (hydrocodone) followed by OxyContin (oxycodone). According to data collected by the Drug Abuse Warning Network (DAWN), drug abuse–related ED visits involving narcotic analgesics increased 153% in the nation, from 42,857 visits in 1995 to 108,320 ED visits in 2002 (SAMHSA, 2004). The greatest increases during this period occurred for oxycodone (512%), methadone (176%), hydrocodone (159%), and morphine (116%). Illicit or nonmedical use of OxyContin has been widely cited in recent media reports; however, nonmedical use was found in only 0.4% of the population in 2001 and rarely led to the abuse of other drugs (Sees, Di Marino, Ruediger, Sweeney, & Shiffman, 2005).

Heroin is an opiate that has been abused for many centuries and is usually administered intravenously. It induces a "rush" or "kick" that lasts less than a minute, followed by a sense of euphoria lasting several hours. Tolerance develops to the euphoria, respiratory depression, and nausea, but not to constipation and miosis. Physical dependence occurs with long-term use of opiates. Initial withdrawal symptoms such as drug craving, lacrimation (tear production), rhinorrhea, yawning, and diaphoresis usually take 10 days to run their course. The second phase of opiate withdrawal lasts for months with insomnia, irritability, fatigue, and potential GI hyperactivity and premature ejaculation as problems.

Methadone is a synthetic opiate used to treat chronic pain and addiction to other opiates. Methadone does not hinder one's ability to function productively, as other narcotics do, and it is a viable support for withdrawal (Stuart & Laraia, 2005).

Hallucinogens

Hallucinogens are also called *psychedelics* and include PCP, 3,4-MDMA, D-lysergic acid diethylamide (LSD), mescaline, dimethyltryptamine (DMT), and psilocin. Psychedelics bring on the same types of thoughts, perceptions, and feelings that occur in dreams. PCP (also called *angel dust* and *peace pill*) was developed in the 1950s as an anesthetic similar to ketamine, but due to its severe side effects, its development for human use was discontinued. PCP is known for inducing violent behavior and negative physical reactions such as seizures, coma, and death (OAS, 2005c). The most common route of administration is smoking tobacco, marijuana, or herbal cigarettes laced with PCP powder or the liquid form of PCP.

MDMA, commonly known as Ecstasy, was very popular in the 1980s as a recreational "club drug" associated with dance clubs and "raves" and has reappeared in recent years as a date or rape drug. According to 2003 NSDUH data, approximately 2.1 million people aged 12 and older (0.9%) used Ecstasy during the previous year; however, its use has declined from 3.2 million users in 2002 (SAMHSA, 2005). The rate of past-year Ecstasy use was significantly greater among 18- to 25-year-olds (3.7%) than among 12- to 17-year-olds (1.3%) or people aged 26 and older (0.3%) (SAMHSA, 2005). Parties where other drugs such as marijuana and alcohol are present may lead to easier access or availability of Ecstasy, thereby increasing the chances for first-time Ecstasy use. One study suggests that cannabis use is a powerful risk factor for subsequent first onset of Ecstasy use (Zimmerman et al., 2005). Another study reported approximately 20% of youths aged 16–23 admitted to using one or more of the following drugs: methamphetamine, Ecstasy, LSD, ketamine, GHB, and flunitrazepam (Rohypnol) (Wu, Schlenger, & Gavin, 2006). Females were more likely than males to report using multiple club drugs. Staying in school and getting married were associated with decreased odds of club drug use. On the other hand, criminal behaviors and recent alcohol abuse or dependence increased use of club drugs.

LSD was first used to simulate psychosis. It affects serotonin receptors at multiple sites in the brain and spinal cord. LSD is usually taken orally but can be injected or smoked, as in tobacco- or marijuana-laced cigarettes. The individual's response to a trip, the experience of being high on LSD, cannot be predicted. Psychologic effects (e.g., seeing bursts of radiant colors and seeing objects that appear to breathe) and flashbacks are common. Serotonin imbalance is thought to affect impulse control and may be responsible for uninhibited sexual responses in women who have been given the drug without their knowledge. Other hallucinogens are similar to LSD but have a different potency and course of action. Because physical dependence to hallucinogens does not appear to occur, withdrawal symptoms are not present.

Inhalants

Inhalants are categorized into three types: anesthetics, volatile nitrites, and organic solvents. Nitrous oxide (laughing gas) and ether are the most abused anesthetics. Amyl nitrite, butyl nitrite, and isobutyl nitrite are volatile nitrites used especially by homosexual males to induce venodilation and anal sphincter relaxation. Amyl nitrite is manufactured for medical use, but butyl and isobutyl nitrites are sold for recreational use. Other names for butyl and isobutyl nitrites are *climax, rush,* and *locker room*. Street names for amyl nitrite are *poppers* and *snappers*. Brain damage or sudden death can occur the first, tenth, or hundredth time an individual uses an inhalant, resulting in "sudden sniffing death." This danger makes the use of inhalants more hazardous than some other substances. Street names for other substances can be found in Table 2–9.

Another danger is the wide assortment of organic solvents that are available to and inhaled by young children. Organic solvents are ingested by three different methods: bagging, huffing, and sniffing. *Bagging* involves pouring the solvent in a plastic bag and inhaling the vapor. *Huffing* refers to pouring the solvent on a rag and inhaling. *Sniffing* refers to inhaling the solvent directly from the container. Common organic solvents are toluene, gasoline, lighter fluid, paint thinner, nail polish remover, benzene, acetone, chloroform, and model airplane glue. The effects from inhaling organic solvents are similar to those of alcohol. Prolonged use can lead to multiple toxicities and an increased risk for abusing other substances. Children who used inhalants before the age of 14 were twice as likely to initiate opiate use compared to those who had never tried opiates (Storr, Westergaard, & Anthony, 2005). There are no antidotes for these inhalants; therefore, management of overdose is supportive.

Withdrawal symptoms from opiates and stimulants can be very unpleasant but are generally not life-threatening.

TABLE 2–9 **Common Street Names for Abused Substances**

SUBSTANCE	STREET NAME
Alcohol	Booze, brew, spirits, juice, hooch
Amphetamines	Bennies, crystal, crystal meth, crank, dexies, diet pills, dolls, eye-openers, ice, lid poppers, pep pills, purple hearts, speed, uppers
Barbiturates	Barbs, beans, black beauties, blue angels, candy, downers, goof balls, ludes, nebbies, reds, sleepers, tranks, yellow jackets, yellows
Benzodiazepines	Bennies, blues, rainbows, reds, sopors, yellows
Cocaine	Bernice, bernies, big C, blow, Charlie, coke, dust, girl, heaven, jay, lady, nose candy, nose powder, snow, sugar, white lady Crack: Conan, freebase, rock, toke, white cloud, white tornado
Hallucinogens	Acid, big D, blotter, blue heaven, cap D, deeda, flash, L, mellow yellows, microdots, paper acid, sugar, ticket, yello, Ecstasy
Heroin, morphine	H, horse, harry, boy, M, Miss Emma, scag, "shit," smack, stuff, white junk, white stuff
Marijuana	Acapulco gold, Aunt Mary, broccoli, dope, grass, grunt, hay, hemp, herb, J, joint, joy stick, killer weed, Mary Jane, pot, ragweed, reefer, smoke, weed, "shit"
Opiates	Meperidine (Demerol), hydrocodone (Vicodin), Percocet, oxycodone (OxyContin), and Darvon

TABLE 2–10 **Drugs Used in the Treatment of Substance Withdrawal/Abuse**

DRUG	DOSE	PURPOSE
Benzodiazepines		
1. Chlordiazepoxide (Librium)	15–100 mg	Diminishes anxiety and has anticonvulsant qualities to provide safe withdrawal. May be ordered q4h or prn to manage adverse effects from withdrawal; then dose is tapered to zero.
2. Diazepam (Valium)	4–40 mg	
3. Oxazepam (Serax)	30–120 mg	
4. Lorazepam (Ativan)	2–6 mg	
Vitamins		
1. Thiamine (vitamin B1)	100 mg/day	Prevents Wernicke's encephalopathy
2. Folic acid	1 mg/day	Corrects vitamin deficiency caused by heavy long-term alcohol abuse
3. Multivitamins	1 tab/cap daily	
Anticonvulsants		
1. Phenobarbital	30–320 mg	Controls seizures and acts as a sedative
2. Magnesium sulfate	1 g q6h	Reduces postwithdrawal seizures
Abstinence Medications		
1. Disulfiram (Antabuse)	250 mg/day	Prevents breakdown of alcohol
2. Naltrexone (ReVia)	50 mg/day	Diminishes cravings for alcohol and opioids
3. Acamprosate (Campral)	666 mg BID	Decreases alcohol craving
4. Methadone	40 mg/day	Blocks craving for heroin
Antidepressants		
1. Fluoxetine (Prozac)	20–80 mg/day	Enhances and stabilizes mood and diminishes anxiety
2. Sertraline (Zoloft)	50–200 mg/day	

The client experiencing an acute phase of cocaine withdrawal may become suicidal. Common drugs used in the treatment of substance abuse and withdrawal are presented in Table 2–10.

COLLABORATION

Effective treatment of substance abuse and dependence results from the efforts of an interdisciplinary team specializing in the treatment of psychiatric and substance abuse disorders. Therapies may include detoxification, aversion therapy to maintain abstinence, group and/or individual psychotherapy, psychotropic medications, cognitive-behavioral strategies, family counseling, and self-help groups. Clients suffering from substance abuse can be treated in either an inpatient or outpatient setting. A substance overdose is a life-threatening condition that requires emergency hospitalization to stabilize the client medically before any of the interventions mentioned are implemented. Several diagnostic tests can provide valuable information about the client's physical condition and set the course for treatment.

Diagnostic Testing

The body fluids most often tested for drug content are blood and urine, although saliva, perspiration, and even hair may be tested. More invasive procedures such as serum drug levels are useful in the ED and other hospital settings to treat drug overdoses or complications. Urine drug screening (UDS), which is noninvasive, is the preferred method for detecting substances in the body. Companies often require a UDS of prospective employees before hiring them. In addition, professional and college athletes are now required to submit to random drug testing. Results of UDS are also used in the court system to determine drug use in relation to criminal activity. The length of time that drugs can be found in blood and urine varies according to dosage and metabolic properties of the drug. All traces of the drug may disappear within 24 hours or may still be detectable 30 days later. THC, the psychoactive substance found in marijuana, is stored in fatty tissues (especially the brain and reproductive system) and can be detected in the body for up to 6 weeks (Kneisl et al., 2004).

Emergency Care for Overdose

The care of a client who has overdosed on any substance is a serious medical emergency. Respiratory depression may require mechanical ventilation. The client may become severely sedated and difficult to arouse. Every effort must be made to keep the client awake; however, stupor and coma often results. A seizure is another serious complication that requires emergency treatment. If the overdose was intentional, the client must be monitored constantly for further signs of suicidal ideation. An actively suicidal client must never be left alone. Signs of overdose and withdrawal from major substances are summarized in Table 2–11 along with recommended treatments.

TABLE 2–11 Signs and Treatment of Overdose and Withdrawal

DRUG	OVERDOSE		WITHDRAWAL	
	SIGNS	TREATMENT	SIGNS	TREATMENT
CNS Depressants Alcohol Barbiturates Benzodiazepines	Cardiovascular or respiratory depression or arrest (mostly with barbiturates) Coma Shock Convulsions Death	*If awake:* Keep awake. Induce vomiting. Use activated charcoal to absorb drug. VS q 15 minutes. *Coma:* Clear airway, intubate IV fluids. Perform gastric lavage. Take seizure precautions. Administer hemodialysis or peritoneal dialysis if ordered. Assess VS as ordered. Assess for shock and cardiac arrest.	Nausea and vomiting Tachycardia Diaphoresis Anxiety or agitation Tremors Marked insomnia Grand mal seizures Delirium (after 5–15 years of heavy use)	Carefully titrated detoxification with similar drug NOTE: Abrupt withdrawal can lead to death.
Stimulants Cocaine/crack Amphetamines	Respiratory distress Ataxia Hyperpyrexia Convulsions Coma Stroke Myocardial infarction Death	Antipsychotics Management for: 1. Hyperpyrexia. 2. Convulsions. 3. Respiratory distress. 4. Cardiovascular shock. 5. Acidic urine (ammonium chloride for amphetamine).	Fatigue Depression Agitation Apathy Anxiety Sleepiness Disorientation Lethargy Craving	Antidepressants (desipramine) Dopamine agonist Bromocriptine
Opiates Heroin Meperidine Morphine Methadone	Pupil dilation due to anoxia Respiratory depression arrest Coma Shock Convulsions Death	Narcotic antagonist (Narcan) quickly reverses CNS depression	Yawning, insomnia Irritability Rhinorrhea Panic Diaphoresis Cramps Nausea and vomiting Muscle aches Chills and fever Lacrimation Diarrhea	Methadone tapering Clonidine-naltrexone detoxification Buprenorphine substitution
Hallucinogens LSD	Psychosis Brain damage Death	Ensure low stimuli with minimal light, sound, activity. Have one person "talk down client," reassure. Speak slowly and clearly. Administer diazepam or chloral hydrate for anxiety as ordered.	No pattern of withdrawal	
PCP	Possible hypertensive crisis Respiratory arrest Hyperthermia Seizures	Acidify urine to help excrete drug (cranberry juice, ascorbic acid); in acute stage: ammonium chloride. Minimize stimuli. Do *not* attempt to talk down; speak slowly in low voice. Administer diazepam or Haldol as ordered.		
Inhalants	Intoxication	Support affected systems	No pattern of withdrawal	

TABLE 2–11 Signs and Treatment of Overdose and Withdrawal (continued)

DRUG	OVERDOSE		WITHDRAWAL	
	SIGNS	TREATMENT	SIGNS	TREATMENT
Volatile Solvents such as butane, paint thinner, airplane glue, and nail polish remover	1. Excitation 2. Drowsiness 3. Disinhibition 4. Staggering 5. Lightheadedness 6. Agitation Side effects: 1. Damage to nervous system 2. Death			
Nitrites	Enhanced sexual pleasure	Neurologic symptoms may respond to vitamin B_{12} and folate.		
Anesthetics such as nitrous oxide	Giggling, laughter Euphoria	Chronic users may experience polyneuropathy and myelopathy.		

NURSING PROCESS

Nurses may interact with clients experiencing substance abuse or substance dependence in a variety of settings. The most common setting is an alcohol and drug abuse treatment program where clients are hospitalized for 20–30 days for detoxification and inpatient therapy. These clients may be voluntarily admitted or ordered by the court to undergo treatment. Clients with substance abuse or dependence have impaired senses and risk-taking behaviors that lead to injuries from falls and accidents requiring medical attention. Therefore, hospital emergency departments as well as medical and surgical units are places where nurses frequently encounter these clients. Occupational nurses and community health nurses also interact with substance-abusing clients in employee assistance programs and community health departments. Urgent care centers, pain clinics, and ambulatory care centers are other settings in which clients with substance abuse disorders frequently appear for minor health problems associated with chronic disorders related to substance abuse or dependence.

Nursing care of the client with substance abuse or dependence is challenging and requires a nonjudgmental atmosphere promoting trust and respect. Nurses should provide adults with information on healthy coping mechanisms and relaxation and stress reduction techniques to decrease the risks of substance abuse. Nurses have a responsibility to educate their clients about the physiologic effects of substances on the body. Nurses must encourage and support periods of abstinence while assisting clients to make major changes in lifestyles, habits, relationships, and coping methods. See the Developmental Considerations box on page 76 for a discussion of older clients with substance abuse problems.

Health promotion efforts are aimed at preventing drug use among children and adolescents and reducing the risks among adults. Adolescence is the most common phase for the first experience with drugs (Stuart & Laraia, 2005); therefore, teenagers are a vulnerable population, often succumbing to peer pressure. Healthy lifestyles, parental support, stress management, good nutrition, and information about ways to steer clear of peer pressure are important topics for the nurse to provide in school programs.

Assessment

A comprehensive approach to the assessment of substance use is essential to ensure adequate and appropriate intervention. Therapeutic communication techniques should be used to establish trust prior to the assessment process.

It is important that the nurse asses the client for history of substance use and medical and psychiatric disorders as well as for the presence of psychosocial concerns. Open-ended questions that elicit more than a simple yes or no answer are more effective in eliciting truthful information and may help determine the direction of future counseling. Examples of open-ended questions are provided in Box 2–9.

Box 2–9 Examples of Open-Ended Questions for Assessment of Substance Abuse

- On average, how many days per week do you use drugs?
- On a typical day when you use drugs, how much do you use?
- What is the greatest number of drugs you have used at any one time during the past month?
- What drug(s) did you take before coming to the hospital or clinic?
- How long have you been using the substances?
- How often and how much do you usually use?
- What problems has substance use caused for you and your family, friends, finances, and health?

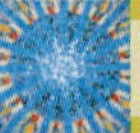

DEVELOPMENTAL CONSIDERATIONS Substance Abuse in the Older Adult

OLDER ADULTS

- Substance abuse in older adults is likely to increase as baby boomers reach retirement age. The number of older adults in need of substance abuse treatment is estimated to increase from 1.7 million in 2001 to 4.4 million in 2020 (Gfroerer, Penne, Pemberton, & Folsom, 2003).
- People of any age can have substance abuse problems, but the consequences in older adults may be more critical. Falls and accidents can rob older adults of their independence, and substance abuse increases the risk of falls by affecting alertness, judgment, coordination, and reaction time.
- Older adults (especially older women) are more likely than younger people to use prescription or over-the-counter medicines, which can be harmful when mixed with alcohol and/or illicit drugs (Lantz, 2005; Simoni-Wastila & Strickler, 2004). Alcohol and drug abuse also can make certain medical problems hard to diagnose, for example, by dulling a pain sensation that might warn of a heart attack.
- Substance abuse and dependence are less likely to be recognized in older adults. A substance abuse problem in an older adult can be difficult to detect because many of the symptoms of abuse (e.g., insomnia, depression, loss of memory, anxiety, musculoskeletal pain) may be confused with conditions commonly seen in older clients (Lantz, 2005). This results in treating the symptoms of abuse rather than diagnosing and treating the abuse itself.
- Older adults who are alcoholics are at greater risk for numerous physical problems and premature death. Alcohol interacts negatively with the natural aging process to increase risks for injuries, hypertension, cardiac dysrhythmias, cancers, GI problems, cognitive deficits, bone loss, and emotional challenges (most notably depression) (Stevenson, 2005).
- Because depression and alcohol abuse are the most frequently found disorders in completed suicides, nurses should routinely screen older adults for substance abuse and mental disorders.

History of Past Substance Use

A thorough history of the client's past substance use is important in order to ascertain the possibility of tolerance, physical dependence, or withdrawal syndrome. The following questions are helpful in eliciting a pattern of substance use behavior:

- How many substances has the client used simultaneously in the past?
- How often, how much, and when did the client first use the substance(s)?
- Is there a history of blackouts, delirium, or seizures?
- Is there a history of withdrawal syndrome, overdoses, and complications from previous substance use?
- Has the client ever been treated in a drug abuse clinic?
- Has the client ever been arrested for driving under the influence or charged with any criminal offense while using drugs?
- Is there a family history of drug use?

Medical and Psychiatric History

The client's medical history is another important area for assessment and should include the existence of any concomitant physical or mental condition (e.g., HIV, hepatitis, cirrhosis, esophageal varices, pancreatitis, gastritis, Wernicke-Korsakoff syndrome, depression, schizophrenia, anxiety, or personality disorder). The nurse should ask about prescribed and over-the-counter medications as well as any allergies or sensitivity to drugs. A brief overview of the client's current mental status is also significant.

- Is there a history of abuse (physical or sexual) or family violence?
- How often does the client experience feelings of sadness or depression?
- What does the client do to relieve feelings of sadness or depression?
- Has the client ever tried to commit suicide?
- Is the client currently having suicidal or homicidal ideation?

Psychosocial Issues

Information about the client's level of stress and other psychosocial concerns can help in the assessment of substance use problems.

- Has the client's substance use affected his or her ability to hold a job?
- Has the client's substance use affected relationships with spouse, family, friends, or coworkers?
- How does the client usually cope with stress?
- Does the client have a support system that helps in time of need?
- How does the client spend his or her leisure time?

Screening Tools

Screening tools such as the B-DAST (Skinner, 1982) may help the nurse determine the degree of severity of substance abuse or dependence. Screening tools provide a nonjudgmental, brief, and easy method to ascertain patterns of substance abuse behaviors. The B-DAST is a yes/no self-administered questionnaire that is useful in identifying people who may be addicted to drugs other than alcohol. A positive response to one or more questions suggests significant drug abuse problems and warrants further evaluation. Because people do not always answer self-report tools truthfully, all clients who screen positive for drug addiction should be evaluated according to other diagnostic criteria.

Nurses working with clients who may experience opiate withdrawal find the Clinical Opiate Withdrawal Scale (COWS) useful for assessing symptoms (Wesson & Ling, 2003). The COWS rates 11 common signs or symptoms of opiate withdrawal. The summed total score of the 11 items can be used to assess the intensity of opiate withdrawal and determine the extent of a patient's physical dependence on opioids. A score of less than 12 on the COWS indicates mild or no opiate withdrawal symptoms, whereas a score of 13 or more indicates moderate to severe withdrawal symptoms.

NURSING CARE PLAN **A Client With Substance Abuse**

ASSESSMENT

Donna Smith is brought to the ED by her husband. She is agitated and can't stand still. Her husband tells the nurse that she has been getting high on crack cocaine on a regular basis. When she didn't come home last night, he called their cell phone company to activate her GPS and found her outside a motel on the highway. He took her home, where she began shouting, yelling, and throwing things and talking about the "men in the trees" who are after her. The nurse conducting the assessment determines that they have two children, ages 11 and 15, living at home.

The nurse collects the following data during assessment:

99.4 ax – 114-20 168/92

Pupils constricted and equally responsive to light

Client is muttering to herself in mosty unintelligible sentences, with phrases such as "men in trees", "gonna get me", and "don't worry" understood among gibberish words. Client says she hears voices and points out things that are not there—apparently having both visual and auditory hallucinations.

Peripheral pulses are 3+ and bounding, sinus tachycardia noted on ECG with frequent premature ventricular contractions, hyperreactive reflexes.

Client is admitted to monitored unit (telemetry) for observation until cardiac and neurological systems are stable.

DIAGNOSES

- Risk for Injury
- Altered Tissue Perfusion
- Interrupted Family Processes
- Ineffective Coping

PLANNING

Goals of care include the following:

- Experience no adverse cardiac event
- Orient to time and place
- ECG will return to normal sinus rhythm
- Neurologic assessment will return to pre-substance use baseline
- Agree to psychosocial intervention to assist in substance avoidance.

IMPLEMENTATION

- Monitor cardiorespiratory function.
- Assess orientation and maintain safety while hallucinating.
- Maintain low stimulation environment until effects of drug subside.
- Maintain hydration to promote excretion of drug from system.
- Obtain complete history of substance use when client's cognitive function returns.
- Administer sedatives and antiarrhythmics as required per orders
- Refer Mr. Smith to a support program for spouses and children.
- Refer to substance abuse program to assist in abstinence once drugs have been cleared from system if client is willing to participate.

EVALUATION

Evaluation of client response may be based on the following expected outcomes:

- Client experiences no cardiac event as the result of cocaine use.
- Client's cognition returns to prior baseline.
- Client admits to having a problem and agrees to seek treatment.

CRITICAL THINKING

1. While the client is experiencing both auditory and visual hallucinations how will the nurse respond if the client insists there is something in the room that is not seen by the nurse?
2. What actions will the nurse implement to maintain the client's safety?
3. After detoxification the client regains normal cognitive function and informs the nurse she is leaving the facility because she wants to "get high again." What is the nurse's legal obligation to this client?

Diagnosis

Nursing diagnoses for clients with substance abuse problems are highly individualized depending on the substance abused, the length of time the client has abused the chemical, and the sources of support available to the client. Common diagnoses used in the care of these clients include the following:

- Risk for Injury
- Risk for Violence
- Ineffective Denial
- Ineffective Coping
- Imbalanced Nutrition: Less Than Body Requirements
- Chronic or Situational Low Self-Esteem
- Deficient Knowledge
- Disturbed Sensory Perceptions
- Disturbed Thought Processes.

Plan

When planning care for the substance-abusing client, it is important to keep goals and expectations reasonable. Substance abuse recovery takes many months and often requires several attempts before abstinence is obtained and maintained. As a result, setting both short- and long-term goals for the client is often most effective.

Short-term goals may include the following:

- Client will admit having a substance abuse problem and having lost control of his or her life as a result.
- Client will seek help to stop using the substance.
- Client will suffer no complications as a result of drug withdrawal symptoms.
- Client will enter a drug rehabilitation program to change the behavior.

Long-term goals may include the following:

- Client will explore the impact of the substance addiction on family, job, and friends.
- Client will describe and recognize his or her denial in avoiding the problems related to substance abuse.
- Client will change his or her thinking and behavior as a result of understanding the negative consequences of substance abuse.
- Client will regularly attend a support group to maintain sobriety from substance use.
- Client will remain free of substance and maintain sobriety.

Implementation

Implications for nursing care in acute and home care settings are combined in this discussion.

Risk for Injury and Risk for Violence

- Assess the client's level of disorientation to determine specific risks to the safety of the client, family members, and others.
- Obtain a drug history as well as urine and blood samples for laboratory analysis of substance content. A client may not admit to using drugs at all or may admit to using only one drug recreationally, when in truth, the client is using one or more drugs regularly. Urine and blood samples provide accurate, objective information.
- Place the client in a quiet private room to decrease excessive stimuli and related agitation, but do not leave the client alone if excessive hyperactivity or suicidal ideation is present.
- If the client is disoriented, frequently orient the client to reality and the environment, ensuring that potentially harmful objects are stored outside the client's access. The client may harm self or others if disoriented and confused.
- Monitor vital signs every 15 minutes until stable. If treatment is dependent on blood or urine levels of a specific drug, reevaluate as instructed by the treating physician.

Ineffective Denial

- Be genuine, honest, and respectful of the client. Keep all promises and convey an attitude of acceptance of the client. The development of a nonjudgmental, therapeutic nurse–client relationship is essential for gaining the client's trust.
- Identify maladaptive behaviors or situations that have occurred in the client's life and discuss how the use of substances may have been a contributing factor. The first step in combating denial is for the client to recognize the relationship between substance use and personal problems.
- Do not accept the use of defense mechanisms such as rationalization or projection as the client attempts to blame others or make excuses for his or her behavior. Use confrontation with caring to avoid placing the client on the defensive. Confrontation interferes with the client's ability to use denial.
- Encourage client participation in therapeutic group activities such as NA meetings. Peer feedback is often more accepted than feedback from authority figures.

Ineffective Coping

- Set limits on manipulative behavior and maintain consistency in responses. Addicted clients are often unable to set limits and must begin to accept responsibility without being manipulative.
- Encourage the client to verbalize feelings, fears, or anxieties. Use attentive listening and validate the client's feelings with observations or statements that acknowledge the feelings. Addicts are inexperienced at verbalizing and sharing feelings and anxieties.
- Explore methods of dealing with stressful situations other than resorting to substance use. Provide encouragement for changing to a healthier lifestyle. Teach healthy coping mechanisms (e.g., physical exercise, progressive muscle relaxation, deep breathing exercises, meditation, and imagery) that will help the client adapt to stress without resorting to drug use.

Imbalanced Nutrition: Less Than Body Requirements

- Administer vitamins and dietary supplements as ordered by the physician.
- Monitor lab work (e.g., total albumin, complete blood count, urinalysis, electrolytes, and liver enzymes) and report significant changes to the physician. Objective laboratory tests provide necessary information to determine the extent of malnourishment.
- Collaborate with a dietitian to determine the number of calories needed to provide adequate nutrition and a realistic weight. Document intake, output, and calorie count. Weigh the client daily if condition warrants. Weight loss or gain impacts development of the care plan.
- Teach the physical effects of malnutrition on body systems. Provide information about adequate nutrition using the Food Guide Pyramid. The client may have inadequate knowledge of proper nutritional habits.

Chronic Low or Situational Low Self-Esteem

- Spend time with the client and convey an attitude of acceptance. Encourage the client to accept responsibility for his or her behaviors and feelings. An attitude of acceptance enhances self-worth.
- Encourage the client to focus on strengths and accomplishments rather than weaknesses and failures. Minimize attention to negative ruminations.
- Encourage participation in therapeutic group activities. Offer recognition and positive feedback for actual achievements. Success and recognition increase self-esteem.
- Teach assertiveness techniques and effective communication techniques such as the use of "I feel" rather than "You

make me feel" statements. Previous patterns of communication may have been aggressive and accusatory, causing barriers to interpersonal relationships.

Deficient Knowledge

- Assess the client's level of knowledge and readiness to learn the effects of drugs and alcohol on the body. Baseline assessment is required to develop appropriate teaching material.
- Develop a teaching plan that includes measurable objectives. Include short-term goals so that the client sees some level of success at an early stage. Include significant others if possible. Lifestyle changes often affect all family members.
- Begin with simple concepts and progress to more complex issues. Use interactive teaching strategies and written materials appropriate to the client's educational level. Include information on physiologic effects of substances, the propensity for physical and psychologic dependence, and risks to the fetus if the client is pregnant. Active participation and handouts enhance retention of important concepts.

Disturbed Sensory Perceptions

- Observe the client for withdrawal symptoms. Monitor vital signs. Provide adequate nutrition and hydration. These actions provide supportive physical care during detoxification.
- Assess the client's level of orientation frequently. Orient and reassure the client of safety in presence of hallucinations, delusions, or illusions.
- Explain all interventions before approaching the client. Avoid loud noises and talk softly to the client. Decrease external stimuli by dimming lights. Excessive stimuli increase agitation.
- Administer medications according to the detoxification schedule. Benzodiazepines may help minimize the discomfort of withdrawal symptoms.

Disturbed Thought Processes

- Provide positive reinforcement when thinking and behavior are appropriate or when the client recognizes that delusions are not based in reality. Drugs and alcohol can interfere with the client's perception of reality.
- Use simple step-by-step instructions and face-to-face interaction when communicating with the client. The client may be confused or disoriented.
- Express reasonable doubt if the client relays suspicious or paranoid beliefs. Reinforce accurate perception of people or situations. It is important to communicate that you do not share the false beliefs as reality.
- Do not argue with the client experiencing delusions or hallucinations. Convey acceptance that the client believes a situation to be true but that you do not see or hear what is not there. Arguing with the client or denying the belief serves no useful purpose because delusions are not eliminated.
- Talk to the client about real events and real people. Respond to feelings and reassure the client that he or she is safe from harm. Discussions that focus on the delusions may aggravate the condition. Verbalization of feelings in a nonthreatening environment may help the client develop insight.

The community provides many options for treating substance abuse, including a mixture of individual, group, and family therapy. Medical detoxification can occur in hospitals, psychiatric units, special substance abuse units, methadone clinics, and outpatient settings. Less restrictive environments include residential rehabilitation programs, halfway houses, and partial hospitalization programs. These programs provide structured environments for the recovering substance abuser while the client maintains a viable presence in the community. In addition, clients can obtain vocational counseling, become involved in self-help groups such as AA or AN, and receive drug and health education.

PRACTICE ALERT

Clients are at highest risk for relapse within the first few months after stopping the abused substance. An acronym that can assist the client in recognizing behaviors that lead to relapse is **HALT:** **h**ungry, **a**ngry, **l**onely, and **t**ired. Nurses should emphasize the importance of a balanced diet, adequate sleep, healthy recreation activities, and a caring support system to prevent relapse.

Evaluation

The client is evaluated based on the ability to meet goals designed during the planning phase of nursing care. Potential positive outcomes may include the following:

- Client suffers no complications from withdrawing from substance.
- Client admits a problem with substance abuse and seeks help.
- Client enters substance abuse program.
- Client can describe choices made that contributed to substance abuse.
- Client attends daily support group meetings after leaving rehabilitation facility.
- Client remains substance-free for (insert time period—days, weeks, months—depending on progress and time sober).

CLIENT TEACHING Substance Abuse

Teach the client and family the following:

- The negative effects of substance abuse, including physical and psychologic complications of substance abuse.
- The signs of relapse and the importance of after-care programs and self-help groups to prevent relapse.
- Information about specific medications that help reduce cravings and maintain abstinence, including the potential side effects, possible drug interactions, and any special precautions to be taken (e.g., avoiding over-the-counter medications such as cough syrup that may contain alcohol)
- Ways to manage stress, including techniques such as progressive muscle relaxation, abdominal breathing techniques, imagery, meditation, and effective coping skills.

In addition, suggest the following resources:

- AA, NA, and other self-help groups
- Employee assistance programs
- Individual, group, and/or family counseling
- Community rehabilitation programs
- National Alliance for the Mentally Ill.

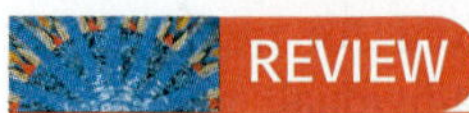

Substance Abuse

RELATE: LINK THE CONCEPTS

Linking the exemplar of Substance Abuse with the concept of Safety:

1. The nurse had surgery a few days ago and is taking a narcotic analgesic to control pain. Is it safe for the nurse to work assigned shifts while taking this medication? Why or why not?
2. You suspect that a coworker whom you admire for his experience and knowledge may be using an illegal drug. What is your best action to maintain client safety? How would you handle this issue?

Linking the exemplar of Substance Abuse with the concept of Violence:

3. How does the abuse of substances affect the risk for violence committed by the client or by others?
4. When working in a substance abuse treatment facility, how can you, as the nurse, protect yourself from acts of violence?

REFER: GO TO MYNURSINGKIT

REFLECT: CASE STUDY

Casey Holmes is a physically fit 23-year-old male who had a troubled youth. His parents divorced when he was very young, and he bounced back and forth between parents—both of whom remarried. Growing up, he often saw his father hit his stepmother when angry. As an adolescent, Casey became involved with a gang and was arrested a few times for petty crimes, such as shoplifting and vandalism. He never finished high school and moved out on his own at the age of 18. Since that time, he has held a number of odd jobs and has made an effort to stay out of trouble.

Casey lives with his pregnant girlfriend Jessica Riley and her son Ryan. He does not particularly like Ryan and thinks Jessica spoils him. He is very proud of the fact that Jessica is pregnant with his baby. He is controlling of Jessica and does not want anybody else looking at her. On most days after work and into the evening, Casey drinks beer and smokes dope with his buddies. He is irritated that Jessica does not party with him as much as she did when they first met. Casey also uses other drugs when he can afford to buy them.

1. What are the priority nursing diagnoses for Casey?
2. What are the implications of his substance abuse on the family?
3. Casey accompanies Jessica to the clinic for one of her prenatal visits. The nurse is aware of Casey's drug use, which Jessica admitted on a prior visit. What should the nurse say to Casey during this visit regarding the impact of his behavior on Jessica and the baby?

PEARSON

EXPLORE mynursingkit™

MyNursingKit is your one stop for online chapter review materials and resources. Prepare for success with additional NCLEX®-style practice questions, interactive assignments and activities, web links, animations and videos, and more!

Register your access code from the front of your book at **www.mynursingkit.com**.

REFERENCES

AIDS Alert. (2005). Studies show link between meth use and HIV infections: Resurgence of STDs tied to drug's use. *AIDS Alert, 20*(9), 97, 99–101.

Albrecht, S. A., Maloni, J. A., Thomas, K. K., Jones, R., Halleran, J., & Osborne, J. (2004). Smoking cessation for pregnant women who smoke: Scientific basis for practice: AWHONN's SUCCESS Project. *Journal of Obstetric, Gynecologic, and Neonatal Nursing, 33*(3), 298–305.

American College of Obstetricians and Gynecologists (ACOG). (2005). *Smoking cessation during pregnancy* (Committee Opinion No. 316). Washington, DC: Author.

American Psychiatric Association (2000). *Diagnostic and statistical manual of mental disorders* (4th ed., Text Revision). Washington, DC: Author.

Anderson, M. E., Johnson, D. C., & Batal, H. A. (2005). Sudden infant death syndrome and prenatal maternal smoking: Rising attributed risk in the back to sleep era. *BMC Medicine, 3*(1), 4.

Baer, J. S., Sampson, P. D., Barr, H. M., Connor, P. D., & Streissquth, A. P. (2003). A 21-year longitudinal analysis of the effects of prenatal alcohol exposure on young adult drinking. *Archives of General Psychiatry, 60*(4), 377–385.

Ballinger, B., & Yalom, I. D. (1995). *The theory and practice of group psychotherapy* (4th ed.). New York: Basic Books.

Bayard, M., McIntyre, J., Hill, K., & Woodside J. (2004). Alcohol withdrawal syndrome. *American Family Physician, 69*(6), 1443–1450.

Bernstein, G. A., Carroll, M. E., Thuras, P. D., Cosgrove, K. P., & Roth, M. E. (2002). Caffeine dependence in teenagers. *Drug and Alcohol Dependence, 55*(1), 1–6.

Bersamin, M., Paschall, M. F., & Flewelling, R. L. (2005). Ethnic differences in relationships between risk factors and adolescent binge drinking: A national study. *Prevention Science, 6*(2), 127–137.

Bracken, M. B., Triche, E. W., Belanger, K., Hellenbrand, K., & Leaderer, B. P. (2003). Association of maternal caffeine consumption with decrements in fetal growth. *American Journal of Epidemiology, 157*(5), 456–466.

Brown, A. H., Domier, C. P., & Rawson, R. A. (2005). Stimulants, sex, and gender. *Sexual Addiction & Compulsivity, 12*(2–3), 169–180.

Brown, D. (2008, August 31). Nicotine up sharply in many cigarettes. *The Washington Post.* Retrieved August 13, 2009, from http://www.washingtonpost.com/wp-dyn/content/article/2006/08/30/AR2006083001418.html

Buchanan, D., Tooze, J. A., Shaw, S., Kinzly, M., Heimer, R., & Singer, M. (2006). Demographic, HIV risk behavior, and health status characteristics of "crack" cocaine injectors compared to other injection drug users in three New England cities. *Drug and Alcohol Dependence, 81*(3), 221–229.

Center on Addiction and Substance Abuse. (1994). *The cost of substance abuse to America's health care system.* Retrieved August 1, 2009, from http://www.marininstitute.org/alcohol_policy/health_care_costs.htm

Centers for Disease Control. (2009). Smoking and tobacco use. Retrieved September 7, 2009, from http://www.cdc.gov/tobacco/

Centers for Disease Control, Office of Smoking and Health. (2007). Children and second hand smoke exposure. Retrieved August 5, 2009, from http://www.cdc.gov/Features/ChildrenAndSmoke/

Chai, Y. G., Oh, D. Y., Chung, E. K., Kim, G. S., Kim, L., Lee, Y. S., et al. (2005). Alcohol and aldehyde dehydrogenase polymorphisms in men with type I and type II alcoholism. *American Journal of Psychiatry, 162*(5), 1003–1005.

Compton, W. M., & Volkow, N. D. (2006). Major increases in opioid analgesic abuse in the United States: Concerns and strategies. *Drug and Alcohol Dependence, 81*(2), 103–107.

Conner, B. T., Noble, E. P., Berman, S. M., Ozkaragoz, T., Ritchie, T., Antolin, T., et al. (2005). DRD2 genotypes and substance use in adolescent children of alcoholics. *Drug and Alcohol Dependence, 79*(3), 379–387.

Cook, T. A., Luczak, S. E., Shea, S. H., Ehlers, C. L., Carr, L. G., & Wall, T. L. (2005). Associations of ALDH2 and ADH1B genotypes with response to alcohol in Asian Americans. *Journal of Studies on Alcohol, 66*(2), 196–204.

Cummings, J., & Cummings, E. (1962). *Ego and milieu.* New York: Atherton Press.

Cunningham, F. G., Leveno, K. J., Bloom, S. L., Hauth, J. C., Gilstrap III, L. C., & Wenstrom, K. D. (2005). *Williams obstetrics* (22nd ed.). New York: McGraw-Hill.

Czermak, C., Lehofer, M., Wagner, E. M., Prietl, B., Lemonis, L., Rohrhofer, A., et al. (2004). Reduced dopamine D_4 receptor mRNA expression in lymphocytes of long-term abstinent alcohol and heroin addicts. *Addiction, 99*(2), 251–257.

DHHS Publication No. SMA 07-4293. Schempf, A. H. (2007). Illicit drug use and neonatal outcomes: A critical review. *Obstetrical & Gynecological Survey, 62*(11), 749–757. U.S. Surgeon General. (21). *U.S. Surgeon General Releases Advisory on Alcohol Use in Pregnancy*. Retrieved March 20, 2008, from http://www.hhs.gov/surgeongeneral/pressreleases/sg02222005.html

Dochterman, J. M., & Bulechek, G. M. (Eds.). (2004). *Nursing interventions classification (NIC)* (4th ed.). St. Louis, MO: Mosby.

Drug Rehabs.org. (2002). *Drug statistics*. Retrieved July 8, 2009, from http://www.drug-rehabs.org/drug-statistics.php#marijuana

Ebberhart, N. C., Luczak, S. E., Avenecy, N., & Wall, T. L. (2003). Family history of alcohol dependence in Asian Americans. *Journal of Psychoactive Drugs, 35*(3), 375–377.

Ewing, J. A. (1984). Detecting alcoholism: The CAGE questionnaire. *Journal of the American Medical Association, 252*(14), 1905–1907.

Falloon, I. R. H. (2002). Cognitive–behavioral family and educational interventions for schizophrenic disorders. In S. G. Hofmann & M. C. Tompson (Eds.), *Treating chronic and severe mental disorders.* New York: Guilford Press.

Ferdinand, R. F., Sondeijker, F., van der Ende, J., Selten, J., Huizink, A., & Verhulst, F. C. (2005). Cannabis use predicts future psychotic symptoms, and vice versa. *Addiction, 100*(5), 612–618.

Fletcher, C. E. (2004). Experience with peer assistance for impaired nurses in Michigan. *Journal of Nursing Scholarship, 36*(1), 92–93.

Fontaine, K. L. (2005). *Complementary and alternative therapies for nursing practice.* Upper Saddle River, NJ: Pearson Education, Inc.

Food and Drug Administration (FDA). (2005). Alcohol warning for pregnant women. *FDA Consumer, 39*(3), 4.

Gamma, A., Jerome, L., Liechti, M. E., & Sumnall, H. R. (2005). Is ecstasy perceived to be safe? A critical survey. *Drug & Alcohol Dependence, 77*(2), 185–193.

Gfroerer, J., Penne, M., Pemberton, M., & Folsom, R. (2003). Substance abuse treatment need among older adults in 2020: The impact of the aging baby-boom cohort. *Drug and Alcohol Dependence, 69*(2), 127–135.

Gilman, S. E., & Abraham, H. D. (2001). A longitudinal study of the order of onset of alcohol dependence and major depression. *Drug & Alcohol Dependence, 63*(3), 277–286.

Grunbaum, J. A., Kann, L., Kinchen, S., Ross, J., Hawkings, J., Lowry, R., et al. (2004, May 21). Youth risk behavior surveillance—United States, 2003. *MMWR Surveillance Summaries, 53* (No. SS-2), 1–96.

Guardia, J., Catafau, A. M., Battle, F., Martin, J. C., Segura, L., Gonzalvo, B., et al. (2000). Striatal dopaminergic D_2 receptor density measured by [1231] iodobenzamide SPECT in the prediction of treatment outcome of alcohol-dependent patients. *American Journal of Psychiatry, 157*, 127–129.

Hartmann, K. E., Wechter, M. E., Payne, P., Salisbury, K., Jackson, R. D., & Melvin, C. L. (2007). Best practice smoking cessation and resource needs of prenatal care providers. *Obstetrics & Gynecology, 110*(4), 765–770.

Hays, L. R. (2004). A profile of OxyContin addiction. *Journal of Addictive Diseases, 23*(4), 1–9.

Heidbreder, C. A., Andreoli, M., Marcon, C., Thanos, P. K., Ashby, C. R., & Gardner, E. L. (2004). Role of dopamine D3 receptors in the addictive properties of ethanol. *Drugs of Today, 40*(4), 355–365.

Heise, B. (2003). The historical context of addiction in the nursing profession: 1850–1982. *Journal of Addictions Nursing, 14*, 117–124.

Henderson-Martin, B. (2000). No more surprises: Screening patients for alcohol abuse. *American Journal of Nursing, 100*(9), 26–32.

Hyman, S. E. (2005). Addiction: A disease of learning and memory. *American Journal of Psychiatry, 162*(8), 1414–1422.

Jansson, L. M., Dipietro, J., & Elko, A. (2005). Fetal response to maternal methadone administration. *American Journal of Obstetrics & Gynecology, 193*(3 Pt 1), 611–617.

Jellinek, E. (1946). *Phases in the drinking history of alcoholics*. New Haven, CT: Hillhouse Press.

Johnson, J. L., Kalaw, C., Lovato, C. Y., Baillie, L., & Chambers, N. A. (2004). Crossing the line: Adolescents' experiences of controlling their tobacco use. *Qualitative Health Research, 14*(9), 1276–1291.

Kasser, C., Geller, A., Howell, E., & Wartenberg, A. (2004). *Detoxification: Principles and protocols*. Chevy Chase, MD: American Society of Addiction Medicine.

Kenna, G. A., & Wood, M. D. (2005). Family history of alcohol and drug use in healthcare professionals. *Journal of Substance Use, 10*(4), 225–238.

King, D. E. (2003). Statistics: Cocaine use and infant development. *International Journal of Childbirth Education, 18*(2), 15.

Kneisl, C. R., Wilson, H. S., & Trigoboff, E. (2004). *Contemporary psychiatric–mental health nursing*. Upper Saddle River, NJ: Pearson-Prentice Hall.

Koprich, J. S., Chen, E. R., Kanaan, N. M., Campbell, N. C., Kordower, J. H., & Lipton, J. W. (2003). Prenatal 3,4-methylenedioxymethamphetamine (ecstasy) alters exploratory behavior, reduces monoamine metabolism, and increases forebrain tyrosine hydroxylase fiber density of juvenile rats. *Neurotoxicology and Teratology, 25*(5), 509–517.

Kraft, A. (1966). The therapeutic community. In S. Arieti (Ed.), *American handbook of psychiatry* (Vol. 2). New York: Basic Books.

Lantz, M. S. (2005). Prescription drug and alcohol abuse in an older woman. *Clinical Geriatrics, 12*(1), 39–43.

Leonardson, G. R., Kemper, E., Ness, F. K., Koplin, B. A., Daniels, M. C., & Leonardson, G. A. (2005). Validity and reliability of the audit and CAGE-AID in Northern Plains American Indians. *Psychological Reports, 97*(1), 161–166.

Lettieri, D. J., Sayers, M., & Pearson, H. W. (1980). *Theories on drug abuse: Selected contemporary perspectives.* Rockville, MD: Department of Health and Human Services.

Ling, P. M., & Glantz, S. A. (2002). Why and how the tobacco industry sells cigarettes to young adults: Evidence from industry documents. *American Journal of Public Health, 92*, 908–916.

Liska, K. (2004). *Drugs and the human body* (7th ed.). Upper Saddle River, NJ: Prentice Hall.

Lu, P. K., Lu, G. P., Lu, D. P., & Lu, W. I. (2004). Managing acute withdrawal syndrome on patients with heroin and morphine addiction by acupuncture therapy. *Acupuncture & Electro-therapeutics Research, 29*(3–4), 187–195.

Luczak, S. E., Wall, T. L., Cook, T. A., Shea, S. H., & Carr, L. G. (2004). ALDH2 status and conduct disorder mediate the relationship between ethnicity and alcohol dependence in Chinese, Korean, and White American college students. *Journal of Abnormal Psychology, 113*(2), 271–278.

__________. (2006). Pregnancy after 35. Retrieved January 16, 2006, from www.marchofdimes.com/printableArticles/14332_1155.asp

March of Dimes (2008). Quick reference: Fact sheets: Illicit drug use during pregnancy. Retrieved from www.marchofdimes.com/printableArticles/14332_1169.asp, September 9, 2009.

Marsiglia, F. F., Kulis, S., Hecht, M. L., & Sills, S. (2004). Ethnicity and ethnic identity as predictors of drug norms and drug use among preadolescents in the U.S. Southwest. *Substance Use & Misuse, 39*(7), 1061–1094.

Martsolf, D. S., Sedlak, C. A., & Doheny, M. O. (2000). Codependency and related health variables. *Archives of Psychiatric Nursing, 14*(3), 150–158.

McKay, A., Koranda, A., & Axen, D. (2004). Using a symptom-triggered approach to manage patients in acute alcohol withdrawal. *Med-Surg Nursing, 13*(1), 15–21.

Miller, N. S., & Greenfeld, A. (2004). Patient characteristics and risk factors for development of dependence on hydrocodone and oxycodone. *American Journal of Therapeutics, 11*(1), 26–32.

Miller, N. S., & Adams, J. (2005). Alcohol and drug disorders. In J. M. Silver, T. W. McAllister, & S. C. Yudofsky (Eds.), *Textbook of traumatic brain injury* (pp. 509–529). Washington, DC: American Psychiatric Press.

Moorhead, S., Johnson, M., & Maas, M. (Eds.). (2004). *Nursing outcomes classification (NOC): Iowa outcomes project* (3rd ed.). St. Louis, MO: Mosby.

Morse, R. M., & Flavin, D. K. (1992). The definition of alcoholism. *Journal of the American Medical Association, 268*(8), 1012–1014. Retrieved August 10, 2009, from http://jama.amaassn.org/cgi/content/abstract/268/8/1012?maxtoshow=&HITS=10&hits=10&RESULTFORMAT=&fulltext=alcoholism&searchid=1&FIRSTINDEX=0&resourcetype=HWCIT

Murphy-Parker, D., & Martinez, R. J. (2005). Nursing students' personal experiences involving alcohol problems. *Archives of Psychiatric Nursing, 19*(3), 150–158.

Nader, M. A., & Czoty, P. W. (2005). PET imaging of dopamine D2 receptors in monkey models of cocaine abuse. *American Journal of Psychiatry, 162*(8), 1473–1482.

National Institute of Mental Health. (2004). *The numbers count: Mental disorders in America* (NIH Publication No. 01-4584). Bethesda, MD: Author. Retrieved February 9, 2005, from http://www.nimh.nih.gov/publicat/numbers.cfm

National Institute on Alcohol Abuse and Alcoholism. (2000). *Updating estimates of the economic costs of alcohol abuse in the United States*. Retrieved August 1, 2009, from http://pubs.niaaa.nih.gov/publications/economic-2000/#introduction

__________. (2004). *Alcoholism: Getting the facts* (NIH Publication No. 96-4153). Bethesda, MD: Author. Retrieved February, 9, 2005, from http://www.niaaa.nih.gov/publications/booklet.htm

Nellissery, M., Feinn, R. S., Covault, J., Gelernter, J., Anton, R. F., Pettinati, H., et al. (2003). Alleles of a functional serotonin transporter promoter polymorphism are associated with major depression in alcoholics. *Alcoholism: Clinical and Experimental Research, 27*(9), 1402–1408.

Niebyl, J. R., & Simpson, J. L. (2007). Drugs and environmental agents in pregnancy and lactation: Embryology, teratology, epidemiology. In S. G. Gabbe, J. R. Niebyl, & J. L. Simpson (Eds.), *Obstetrics: Normal and problem pregnancies* (5th ed.). New York: Churchill-Livingstone.

Nolen-Hoeksema, S. (2004). Gender differences in risk factors and consequences for alcohol use and problems. *Clinical Psychology Review, 24*(8), 981–1010.

North American Nursing Diagnosis Association. (2003). *Nursing diagnoses: Definitions and classification 2003–2004.* Philadelphia: Author.

Ntais, C., Pakos, E., Kyzas, P., & Ioannidis, J. P. (2005). Benzodiazepines for alcohol withdrawal. *The Cochrane Database of Systematic Reviews,* Issue 4, The Cochrane Collaboration. New York: John Wiley & Sons.

Office of Applied Studies (OAS). (2004). Narcotic analgesics, 2002 update. *The Drug Abuse Warning Network (DAWN) Report*, September, 2004. Rockville, MD: Substance Abuse Mental Health Services Administration.

__________. (2005a). Methamphetamine use, abuse, and dependence: 2002, 2003, and 2004. *The NSUDH Report,* September 16, 2005. Rockville, MD: Substance Abuse and Mental Health Services Administration.

__________. (2005b). Substance use among past year Ecstasy users. *The NSUDH Report,* April 29, 2005. Rockville, MD: Substance Abuse and Mental Health Services Administration.

__________. (2005c). Trends in admissions for PCP: 1993–2003. *The NSUDH Report,* October 28, 2005. Rockville, MD: Substance Abuse and Mental Health Services Administration.

__________. (2006). Emergency department visits involving underage drinking. *The Drug Abuse Warning Network (DAWN) Report,* Issue 1. Rockville, MD: Substance Abuse Mental Health Services Administration.

Okah, F. A., Cai, J., & Hoff, G. L. (2005). Term-gestation low birth weight and health compromising behaviors during pregnancy. *Obstetrics and Gynecology, 105*(3), 543–550.

O'Malley, P. (2005). Ecstasy for intimacy: Potentially fatal choices for adolescents and young adults. *Clinical Nurse Specialist, 19*(2), 63–64.

Oswald, L. M., & Wand, G. S. (2004). Opioids and alcoholism. *Physiology & Behavior, 81*(2), 339–358.

Peplau, H. (1952). *Interpersonal relations in nursing.* New York: Putman.

Rice, V. H., & Stead, L. F. (2005). Nursing interventions for smoking cessation. *The Cochrane Database of Systematic Reviews*, Issue 4, The Cochrane Collaboration. New York: John Wiley & Sons.

Pokorny, A. D., Miller, B. A., & Kaplan, H. B. (1972). The brief MAST: A shortened version of the Michigan Alcohol Screening Test. *American Journal of Psychiatry, 129,* 342–345.

Ramisetty-Mikler, S., & Caetano, R. (2004). Ethnic differences in the estimates of children exposed to alcohol problems and alcohol dependence in the United States. *Journal of Studies on Alcohol, 65*(5), 593–599.

Reneman, L., Booij, J., de Bruin, K., Reitsma, J. B., de Wolff, F. A., Gunning, W. B., et al. (2001). Effects of dose, sex, and long-term abstention from use on toxic effects of MDMA (Ecstasy) on brain serotonin neurons. *Lancet, 358*(9296), 1864–1869.

Reoux, J. P., & Ries, R. (2001). Searching for new detoxification strategies. Retrieved September 10, 2006, from www.eurekalert.org/pub_releases/2001-09/ace-sfn091001.php

Rigotti, N. A., Munafo, M. R., Murphy, M. F. G., & Stead, L. F. (2005). Interventions for smoking cessation in hospitalized patients. *The Cochrane Database of Systematic Reviews*, Issue 4, The Cochrane Collaboration. New York: John Wiley & Sons.

Schempf, A. H. (2007). Illicit drug use and neonatal outcomes: A critical review. *Obstetrical & Gynecological Survey, 62*(11), 749–757. U.S. Surgeon General. (21). *U.S. Surgeon General Releases Advisory on Alcohol Use in Pregnancy*. Retrieved March 20, 2008, from http://www.hhs.gov/surgeongeneral/pressreleases/sg02222005.html

Sees, K. L., Di Marino, M. E., Ruediger, N. K., Sweeney, C. T., & Shiffman, S. (2005). Non-medical use of OxyContin tablets in the United States. *Journal of Pain & Palliative Care Pharmacotherapy, 19*(2), 13–23.

Semple, S. J., Grant, I., & Patterson, T. L. (2004). Female methamphetamine users: Social characteristics and sexual risk behavior. *Women & Health, 40*(3), 35–50.

Semple, S. J., Patterson, T. L., & Rant, I. (2005). Methamphetamine use and depressive symptoms among heterosexual men and women. *Journal of Substance Use, 10*(1), 31–47.

Shoptaw, S., Reback, C. J., Peck, J. A., Yang, X., Rotheram-Fuller, E., Larkins, S., et al. (2005). Behavioral treatment approaches for methamphetamine dependence and HIV-related sexual risk behaviors among urban gay and bisexual men. *Drug and Alcohol Dependence, 78*(2), 125–134.

Silagy, C., Lancaster, T., Stead, M., & Fowler, G. (2005). Nicotine replacement therapy for smoking cessation. *The Cochrane Database of Systematic Reviews*, Issue 4, The Cochrane Collaboration. New York: John Wiley & Sons.

Simoni-Wastila, L., & Strickler, G. (2004). Risk factors associated with problem use of prescription drugs. *American Journal of Public Health, 94*(2), 266–268.

Siqueira, L., Diab, M., Bodian, C., & Rolnitzky, L. (2001). The relationship of stress and coping methods to adolescent use. *Substance Abuse, 22*(3), 157–166.

Skinner, H. A. (1982). *Drug Abuse Screening Test (DAST)* (p. 363). Langford Lance, England: Elsevier Science Ltd.

Snow, D., & Hughes, T. (2003). Prevalence of alcohol and other drug use and abuse among nurses. *Journal of Addictions Nursing, 14*, 165–167.

Srisurapanont, M., Jarusuraisin, N., & Kittirattanapalboon, P. (2005). Treatment for amphetamine dependence and abuse. *The Cochrane Database of Systematic Reviews*, Issue 4, The Cochrane Collaboration. New York: John Wiley and Sons.

Stafford, L. L. (2001). Is codependency a meaningful concept? *Issues in Mental Health Nursing, 22,* 273–286.

Stern, Y., & Sacheim, H. A. (2004). Neuropsychiatric aspects of memory and amnesia. In S. C. Yudofsky & R. E. Hales (Eds.), *Essentials of neuropsychiatry and clinical neurosciences* (pp. 201–238). Washington, DC: American Psychiatric Publishing.

Stevenson, J. S. (2005). Alcohol use, misuse, abuse, and dependence in later adulthood. *Annual Review of Nursing Research, 23*, 245–280.

Storr, C. L., Westergaard, R., & Anthony, J. C. (2005). Early onset inhalant use and risk for opiate initiation by young adulthood. *Drug and Alcohol Dependence, 78*(3), 253–261.

Stuart, G. W., & Laraia, M. T. (2005). *Stuart & Sundeen's principles and practice of psychiatric nursing* (8th ed.). St. Louis, MO: Mosby.

Substance Abuse and Mental Health Services Administration (SAMHSA). (2003). *Results from the 2002 National Survey on Drug Use and Health: National Findings* (Office of Applied Studies, NSUDH Series H-22, DHHS Publication No. SMA 03-3836). Rockville, MD: Author.

__________. (2004). *Results from the 2003 National Survey on Drug Use and Health: National Findings* (Office of Applied Studies, NSDUH Series H-25, DHHS Publication No. SMA 04-3964). Rockville, MD: Author.

__________. (2005). *Results from the 2004 National Survey on Drug Use and Health: National Findings* (Office of Applied Studies, NSDUH Series H-28, DHHS Publication No. SMA 05-4062). Rockville, MD: Author.

__________. (2007). *Results from the 2006 National Survey on Drug Use and Health: National Findings.* Rockville MD: Office of Applied Studies (NSDUH Series H-32,

__________. (2004). *Results from the 2003 national survey on drug use and health: National findings (Office of Applied Studies, NSDUH Series H-25,* DHHS Publications No. SMA 04-3964). Rockville, MD. U.S. Department of Health and Human Services, Substance Abuse and Mental Health Services Administration, Office of Applied Studies.

Sullivan, J. T., Sykora, K., Schneiderman, J., Naranjo, C. A., & Sellers, E. M. (1989). Assessment of alcohol withdrawal: The revised Clinical Institute Withdrawal Assessment for Alcohol scale (CIWA-Ar). *British Journal of Addictions, 84*, 1353–1357.

Trinkoff, A. M., Zhou, Q., Storr, C. L., & Soeken, K. L. (2000). Workplace access, negative proscriptions, job strain, and substance use in registered nurses. *Nursing Research, 49*(2), 83–90.

U.S. Department of Health and Human Services. (2005). *At a glance: Women and smoking: A report of the surgeon general–2001*. Rockville, MD: Centers for Disease Control and Prevention, National Center for Chronic Disease Prevention and Health Promotion, Office on Smoking and Health. Retrieved February 9, 2005, from http://www.cdc.gov/tobacco/sgr/sgr_forwomen/ataglance.htm

Varcarolis, E. (2002). *Foundations of psychiatric mental health nursing: A clinical approach* (4th ed.). Philadelphia: W.B. Saunders.

Virgo, N., Bennett, G., Higgins, D., Bennett, L., & Thomas, P. (2001). The prevalence and characteristics of co-occurring serious mental illness (SMI) and substance abuse or dependence in the patients of Adult Mental Health and Addictions Services in eastern Dorset. *Journal of Mental Health, 10*(2), 175–188.

Wallace, J. M., Bachman, J. G., O'Malley, P. M., Johnston, L. D., Schulenberg, J. E., & Cooper, S. M. (2002). Tobacco, alcohol, and illicit drug use: Racial and ethnic differences among U.S. high school seniors. *Public Health Reports, 117*(Suppl. 1), S67–S75.

Watson, S. J., Benson, J. A., & Joy, J. E. (2000). Marijuana and medicine: Assessing the science base: A summary of the 1999 Institute of Medicine Report. *Archives of General Psychiatry, 57*(4), 547–552.

Weiss, F., & Porrino, L. J. (2002). Behavioral neurobiology of alcohol addiction: Recent advances and challenges. *Journal of Neuroscience, 22*(9), 3332–3337.

Weng, X., Odouli, R., & Li, D-K. (2008). Maternal caffeine consumption during pregnancy and the risk of miscarriage: A prospective cohort study. *American Journal of Obstetrics & Gynecology, 198,* 279.e1–279.e8.

Wesson, D. R., & Ling, W. (2003). The clinical opiate withdrawal scale (COWS). *Journal of Psychoactive Drugs, 35*(2), 253–259.

West, M. M. (2002). Early risk indicators of substance abuse among nurses. *Journal of Nursing Scholarship, 34*(2), 187–193.

Wisner, K. L., Sit, D. K. Y., Reynolds, S. K., Altemus, M., Bogen, D. L., Sunder, K. R., et al. (2007). Psychiatric disorders. In S. G. Gabbe, J. R. Niebyl, & J. L. Simpson (Eds.), *Obstetrics: Normal and problem pregnancies* (5th ed.). Philadelphia: Churchill Livingstone.

Wu, L. T., Schlenger, W. E., & Gavin, D. M. (2006). Concurrent use of methamphetamine, MDMA, LSD, ketamine, GHB, and flunitrazepam among American youths. *Drug and Alcohol Dependence, 84*(1), 102–113.

Yen, C., Wu, H., Yen, J., & Ko, C. (2004). Effects of brief cognitive-behavioral interventions on confidence to resist the urges to use heroin and methamphetamine in relapse-related situations. *Journal of Nervous and Mental Disease, 192*(11), 788–791.

Zimmerman, P., Wittchen, H., Waszak, F., Nocon, A., Hofler, M., & Lieb, R. (2005). Pathways into Ecstasy use: The role of prior cannabis use and Ecstasy availability. *Drug and Alcohol Dependence, 79*(3), 331–341.

Cellular Regulation 3

Concept at-a-Glance

Concept Learning Outcomes

After reading about this concept, you will be able to:

1. Summarize the structure and physiologic processes of the cell related to cellular regulation.
2. List factors affecting cellular regulation.
3. Identify commonly occurring alterations in cellular regulation and their related treatments.
4. Explain common physical assessment procedures used to examine cellular health of clients across the life span.
5. Outline diagnostic and laboratory tests used to determine the individual's cellular regulation status.
6. Explain management of cellular regulation and prevention of illnesses caused by alterations in cellular function.
7. Demonstrate the nursing process in providing culturally competent and caring interventions across the life span for individuals with common alterations in cellular regulation.
8. Identify pharmacologic interventions in caring for the individual with alterations in cellular function.

Concept Key Terms

Anaplasia, *88*
Autosomes, *87*
Cell cycle, *88*
Chromosomes, *87*
Differentiation, *88*
Deoxyribonucleic acid (DNA), *86*
Dysplasia, *88*
Homologous chromosomes, *87*
Hyperplasia, *88*
Meiosis, *88*
Metaplasia, *88*
Mitosis, *88*
Ribonucleic acid (RNA), *86*
Sex chromosomes, *87*
Somatic cells, *88*

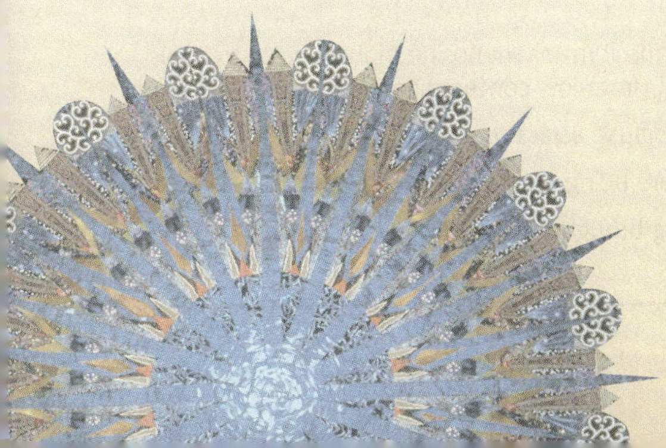

About Cellular Regulation

The cell is the basic unit of life and the working unit of all living systems. Although life starts as a single cell, the developed human body is made up of trillions of cells. There are many different types of specialized cells that function differently depending on their location. For example, pancreatic cells have a very different function than nerve cells. All cells share common features, such as a nucleus containing 46 chromosomes and organelles such as mitochondria.

Cell reproduction, proliferation, and growth are regulated by the body. Alterations in cellular regulation can have devastating consequences for body tissues and functions. ●

NORMAL PRESENTATION

Practically all of the approximately 7.5 trillion cells in the human body are microscopic in size. Although often called building blocks, cells are not brick-shaped objects. They can be flat, round, threadlike, or irregularly shaped. Cells in our bodies can vary greatly in size, shape, and function, but they all share certain common features. Any change in or disturbance to one or more of these common features can result in abnormal cell development or replication. In order to understand alterations in cellular function, it is critical that nurses understand common characteristics of cells.

Cell Membrane

Every cell, regardless of its shape or function, must have a cell membrane in order to maintain its integrity and survive. The membrane is a defined boundary that possesses a definite shape and holds the cell contents together. The cell membrane acts as a protective covering and is responsible for allowing materials in and out of the cell.

The cell membrane, however, allows only certain things in or out of the cell. Because the membrane determines what may pass through, it is a selectively permeable (or semipermeable) membrane. There are several ways substances can be transported across the cell membrane (Table 3–1).

The cell membrane also has identification markers to show that it comes from a specific individual. If a foreign cell shows up (e.g., in a transplanted organ), the body signals an attack on that cell or group of cells.

Cytoplasm

Inside the cell is a watery soup of proteins, nucleic acids, gasses, salts, and other substances that are essential for life. This internal environment of the cell, known as the cytoplasm, must be maintained in balance in order for the cell to survive.

Nucleus and Nucleolus

The nucleus is sometimes described as the brain of the cell. Within the nucleus is the biologic "software" that regulates and directs the activities of the organelles in the cell. The nucleus of a cell is surrounded by a double-walled nuclear membrane. Although this membrane is composed of two layers, it has large pores that allow certain materials to pass in and out.

Chromatin is tightly wound into bundles called chromosomes and is the material found in the nucleus that contains **deoxyribonucleic acid (DNA)**. Coded into DNA are instructions that determine the individual's inherited characteristics, such as hair and eye color, as well as the production of every protein needed by the body. These instructions are called *genes*.

The nucleolus, a spherical body made up of dense fibers is found within the cell nucleus. Its major function is to synthesize the **ribonucleic acid (RNA)** that forms ribosomes.

Centrosomes are tubular structures usually found in pairs in the nucleus. They contain centrioles, which are involved in cell division.

Ribosomes

Ribosomes are organelles found on the endoplasmic reticulum or floating around in the cytoplasm. Ribosomes are made of RNA and assist in the production of enzymes and other proteins needed for cell repair and reproduction.

Endoplasmic Reticulum

The endoplasmic reticulum is a series of channels set up in the cytoplasm; these channels are formed from folded membranes. The endoplasmic reticulum has two distinct forms. The rough endoplasmic reticulum, which has a sandpaperlike appearance due to the ribosomes on its surface, is responsible for the synthesis of protein. Once the protein is synthesized, it is sent to the Golgi apparatus for processing. The smooth endoplasmic

TABLE 3–1 Methods of Cellular Transportation

CELLULAR TRANSPORTATION METHODS	DESCRIPTION
Passive transportation (no energy required)	
Diffusion	Movement of a substance from an area of high concentration to an area of low concentration
Facilitated diffusion	Movement of a substance that is assisted via a "revolving door" in the direction it was already traveling, from an area of high concentration to an area of low concentration
Osmosis	Movement of water across a membrane from areas that have a low concentration of a solute to areas that have a higher concentration until the concentration is the same on both sides of the membrane
Filtration	Application of pressure to force water and dissolved materials across a membrane
Active transport (energy required)	
Active transport pumps	A method that requires additional energy (in the form of adenosine triphosphate) to move substances against the concentration gradient (from low concentration to high concentration)
Endocytosis	Ingestion of substances that are too large to diffuse across the cell membrane
Phagocytosis	Form of endocytosis in which solid particles are being brought into the cell via vesicles
Pinocytosis	Form of endocytosis in which liquid is being brought into the cell via vesicles
Exocytosis	Transportation of material outside of the cell

reticulum has no ribosomes on its surface, making it appear smooth. This endoplasmic reticulum synthesizes lipids (fats) and steroids.

Mitochondria

Mitochondria are tiny, bean-shaped organelles that act as the cell's power plant, providing up to 95% of the body's energy needs for cellular repair, movement, and reproduction. Special enzymes in the mitochondria help to take in oxygen and turn it into energy.

Golgi Apparatus

The Golgi apparatus looks like a bunch of flattened, membranous sacs. Once a protein is received from the endoplasmic reticulum, a portion of the Golgi apparatus envelops the protein, which is pinched off and moved to the cell membrane to be released or secreted. Cells of organs with a high level of secretion or storage, such as the digestive system, contain a larger Golgi apparatus. Salivary glands and pancreatic glands, for example, are made of cells containing a large Golgi apparatus.

Lysosomes

Lysosomes are vesicles containing powerful enzymes that clean up intercellular debris and other waste. They also aid in maintaining health by destroying unwanted bacteria through the process of phagocytosis (process by which microorganisms and cellular debris are engulfed and destroyed).

DNA and Genes

New developments in research seek to provide treatment to the individual client based on genetic components specific to the client's cellular makeup and disease characteristics. While knowledge of the cell, DNA, cell division, chromosomes, and genes has always been important for nurses, it is becoming more essential as the nursing profession begins to deliver a genetic standard of care to the adult client (Figure 3–1 ■).

All human cells except mature red blood cells contain a complete set of DNA molecules. DNA molecules consist of long sequences of nucleotides, or bases, represented by the letters A, G, T, and C. The order of these bases gives the exact instructions for the functioning of that particular cell. Writing the correct order of the bases using A, G, T, and C represents the sequence of the bases in DNA. All of the DNA in a human cell is referred to as the human genome, or the complete set of inheritance for an individual. The human genome includes the DNA in the cell nucleus as well as the DNA in the mitochondria. Each person's genome is unique. Identical (monozygotic) twins are the exception, because they develop from only one fertilized ovum and share identical DNA (Guttmacher & Collins, 2002).

The cell nucleus contains about 6 feet of DNA that is tightly wound and packaged into 23 pairs of **chromosomes** (threadlike strand of DNA in the cell that carries the genes), making a complete set of 46 chromosomes. The structure and number of chromosomes can be shown by a karyotype, or picture, of an individual's chromosomes. There are two copies of each chromosome. One copy, or half of the complete set of these 46 chromosomes, is inherited from the mother, and the other copy, or the

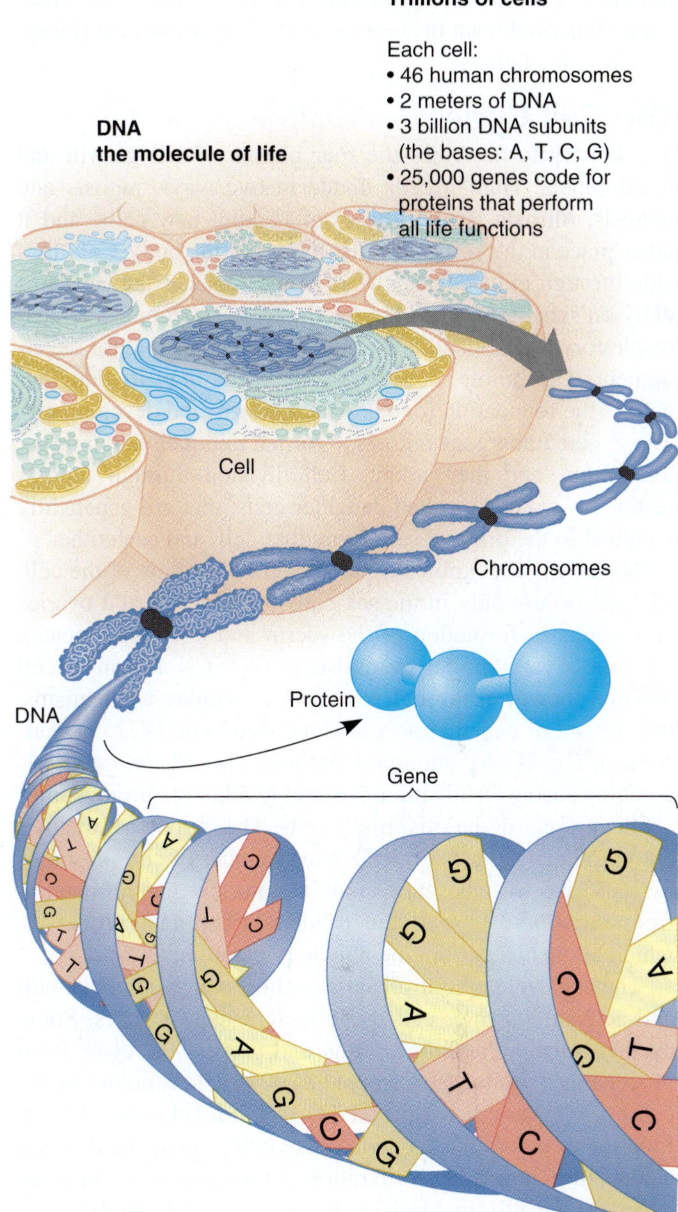
Trillions of cells
Each cell:
• 46 human chromosomes
• 2 meters of DNA
• 3 billion DNA subunits (the bases: A, T, C, G)
• 25,000 genes code for proteins that perform all life functions
DNA
the molecule of life
Cell
Chromosomes
Protein
DNA
Gene

Figure 3–1 ■ Each cell nucleus throughout the body contains the genes, DNA, and chromosomes that make up the majority of an individual's genome. The remaining portion of the human genome is in the mitochondria.

other half of the 46 chromosomes, is inherited from the father. For example, an individual will have two of chromosome 1 (one inherited from the mother and one inherited from the father). These two copies or pairs of inherited chromosomes are called **homologous chromosomes**.

Chromosomes are numbered according to size, with chromosome 1 being the largest and chromosome 22 being the smallest. The first 22 pairs of chromosomes, known as **autosomes**, are alike in males and females. The 23rd pair, the **sex chromosomes**, determines an individual's gender. A female has two copies of the X chromosomes (one copy inherited from each parent), and a male has one X chromosome (inherited from his mother) and a Y chromosome (inherited from his father).

The Cell Cycle

The **cell cycle** describes the four phases of cell growth and development. Human cells divide in two ways, mitosis and meiosis. **Mitosis** is the process of making new cells, and it takes place in the **somatic cells** (tissue) of the body. Cell division through mitosis heals wounds and replaces the cells lost daily on skin surfaces and in the lining of gastrointestinal and respiratory tracts. In addition, mitosis is responsible for development. The mitotic activity of the zygote and its daughter cells is the foundation for a human's growth and development. The zygote undergoes mitosis to form a multicellular embryo, then fetus, and then infant. Cell division through mitosis results in two cells, called daughter cells, that are genetically identical to the original cell, or mother cell, and each other.

Meiosis is also known as the reduction division of the cell. Meiosis occurs only in the sex cells of the testes and ovaries and results in formation of the sperm and oocyte (gametes). Meiosis is very similar to mitosis in that it is a form of cell division; however, through a series of complex mechanisms, the amount of genetic material is reduced in half (23 chromosomes). This is very important, because when the two sex cells combine during fertilization, the total number of chromosomes (46) is present in the offspring's cells. The purpose of meiosis is to produce gametes, to reduce the number of chromosomes by half, and to make new combinations of genetic material from crossing-over and independent assortment processes, which allow diversity in the human population.

The cell cycle is controlled by cyclins, which combine with and activate enzymes called cyclin-dependent kinases. Some cyclins cause a "braking" action and prevent the cycle from proceeding (Dunlop & Campbell, 2000). Checkpoints in the cell cycle ensure that it proceeds in the correct order. A malfunction of any of these regulators of cell growth and division can result in the rapid proliferation of immature cells. In some cases, these cells are considered cancerous (malignant).

Differentiation is a normal process occurring over many cell cycles that allows cells to specialize in certain tasks. For example, some epithelial cells lining the lungs develop into tall columnar cells with cilia. These columnar cells sweep potentially dangerous debris out of the lungs. When adverse conditions occur in body tissues during differentiation, protective adaptations can produce alterations in cells. Some of these alterations are helpful, but in other cases, the cells mutate beyond usefulness and become liabilities (Porth, 2005).

ALTERATIONS

There are a number of potentially unproductive cellular alterations that occur during cell differentiation. These include the following:

- **Hyperplasia** is an increase in the number or density of normal cells. Hyperplasia occurs in response to stress, increased metabolic demands, or elevated levels of hormones. Examples include the hyperplasia of myocardial cells in response to a prolonged increase in the body's demand for oxygen and hyperplasia of uterine cells in response to rising levels of estrogen during pregnancy. Hyperplastic cells are under normal DNA control.
- **Metaplasia** is a change in the normal pattern of differentiation such that dividing cells differentiate into cell types not normally found at that location in the body. The metaplastic cell is normal for its particular type, but it is not in its normal location. Some metaplastic cells are less functional than the cells they replace. Metaplasia is a protective response to adverse conditions, often the result of inflammation. Metaplastic cells are under normal DNA control and are reversible when the stressor or other disruptive condition ceases. An example of metaplasia often occurs in the lungs of smokers when normal columnar ciliated epithelium may be replaced by a squamous stratified epithelium known as squamous metaplasia (Majno & Joris, 2004).
- **Dysplasia** represents a loss of DNA control over differentiation occurring in response to adverse conditions. Dysplastic cells show abnormal variation in size, shape, and appearance and a disturbance in their usual arrangement. Examples of dysplasia include changes in the cervix in response to continued irritation, such as from the human papillomavirus, or leukoplakia on oral mucous membranes in response to chronic irritation from smoking.
- **Anaplasia** is the regression of a cell to an immature or undifferentiated cell type. Anaplastic cell division is no longer under DNA control. Anaplasia usually occurs when a damaging or transforming event takes place inside the dividing, still undifferentiated cell, leading to loss of useful function. Anaplasia may occur in response to overwhelmingly destructive conditions inside the cell or in surrounding tissue (Porth, 2005). It is often associated with malignancies and is one of the criteria used to grade the aggressiveness of the cancer cell.

Although hyperplasia, metaplasia, and dysplasia often reverse after the irritating factor is eliminated, they can lead to malignancy under certain conditions. This is especially true of dysplasia, which represents a loss of DNA control. Anaplasia is not reversible, but the degree of anaplasia determines the potential risk for cancer.

Any one of these differences in cellular regulation have the potential to become cancerous or cause any one of many disorders that can compromise client health. The most common of these are cancer, anemia, sickle cell disorder, leukemia, and polycythemia (see the Alterations and Treatments table and the exemplars that follow). Others you may see, such as endometriosis and HIV, are discussed in other concepts.

Special Issues in Childhood Cancer

This concept discusses treatments and interventions for several types of cancer. Regardless of the type of cancer, there are a number of issues common to the pediatric population. These include oncologic emergencies and psychosocial and developmental considerations related to the illness, its treatment, and issues related to recovery and survival.

ALTERATIONS AND TREATMENTS Cellular Regulation

Alteration	Description	Treatment
Cancer: Breast Lung Colon Ovarian Testicular Prostate	Can be benign or metastatic, depending on location and ability to spread to other areas of the body Cancer cells, especially metastatic cancer, tend to reproduce much faster, to be highly vascular, and to require increased nutritional support to flourish.	■ Chemotherapy ■ Radiation therapy ■ Surgical resection ■ Complementary and alternative therapies such as: ■ Herbs and supplements ■ Massage therapy ■ Guided imagery
Anemia: Iron deficiency Aplastic Hemolytic	Anemias result from insufficient intake or use of chemicals required to produce new red blood cells (RBCs). The result is an inadequate RBC count, causing symptoms related to inadequate oxygen-carrying capability.	■ Aimed at increasing intake of the missing nutrient or chemical required to promote RBC production ■ May include administration of medications to stimulate RBC production in the bone marrow (e.g., epoetin alpha) ■ Blood transfusions
Leukemia	A form of cancer causing excessive and rapid formation of immature white blood cells (WBCs) that do not function as more mature WBCs would.	■ Chemotherapy ■ Radiation therapy ■ Bone marrow transplant ■ Complementary and alternative therapies such as: ■ Herbs and supplements ■ Massage therapy ■ Guided imagery
Sickle cell disorder	RBCs are formed in a sickle shape, increasing risk for clumping in small capillaries and resulting in reduced blood flow to the tissues.	■ Chemotherapy ■ Hydration ■ Pain management ■ Blood transfusions
Polycythemia	Excess production of RBCs results in very viscous blood, increasing risk for cerebrovascular accident, venous stasis, and clotting disorders.	■ Encourage clients to donate blood ■ Smoking cessation ■ Maintain hydration ■ Phlebotomy

ONCOLOGIC EMERGENCIES Oncologic emergencies may result from the cancer itself or as a side effect of treatment. They can be organized into three groups: metabolic, hematologic, and those involving space-occupying lesions. Overall, the most common oncologic emergencies are tumor lysis syndrome, septic shock, brain herniation, spinal cord compression, and superior vena cava compression from a superior mediastinal mass.

Metabolic Emergencies Metabolic emergencies result from the lysis (dissolving or decomposing) of tumor cells, a process called *tumor lysis syndrome*. This cell destruction releases high levels of uric acid, potassium, calcium, and phosphates into the blood, resulting in hyperuricemia, hyperphosphatemia, hypercalcemia, and hyperkalemia. Low levels of sodium result, potentially leading to metabolic acidosis, cardiac arrythmias, and/or renal failure. Tumor lysis syndrome is seen most commonly in children with non-Hodgkin lymphoma (especially the subtype Burkitt lymphoma) and acute lymphocytic leukemia, cancers with high growth rates or large volume (Alavi, Arzanian, Abbasian, et al., 2006; Cantril & Haylock, 2004; Rheingold & Lange, 2006; Spinazze & Schrijvers, 2006).

A second type of metabolic emergency is septic shock. During periods of immune suppression the child is vulnerable to overwhelming infection, resulting in circulatory failure, hypothermia or hyperthermia, tachypnea, mental changes, inadequate tissue perfusion, and hypotension. Septic shock can be fatal (see Concept 15, Exemplar 15.6 for a full description of septicemia and septic shock), but early and aggressive therapy improves outcomes (Haut, 2005).

A third type of metabolic emergency occurs when large amounts of bone are destroyed by treatment, resulting in hypercalcemia (elevated calcium in the serum). Hypercalcemia is most common in children with acute lymphocytic leukemia and rhabdomyosarcoma. Treatment includes hydration and adequate intake of phosphate by oral supplement (Spinazze & Schrijvers, 2006).

Hematologic Emergencies Hematologic emergencies result from bone marrow suppression or infiltration of brain and respiratory tissue with high numbers of leukemic blast cells (hyperleukocytosis). Bone marrow suppression results in anemia and *thrombocytopenia* (decreased platelets) with resultant coagulation disturbance and hemorrhage. Disseminated intravascular coagulation (DIC) occurs in some children and is a life-threatening complication. Gastrointestinal and central nervous system bleeding (strokes) are common. Disruption of normal WBC production and resulting hyperleukocytosis can lead to obstruction of small blood vessels throughout the body.

Treatment involves infusion of packed red blood cells for anemia; and platelet transfusion, vitamin K, and fresh frozen plasma for thrombocytopenia and hemorrhage. Hyperleukocytosis is treated by hydration, bicarbonate infusion, diuresis, allopurinol or urate oxidase, respiratory support, and plasmapheresis if needed (Haut, 2005; Rheingold & Lange, 2006).

Space-Occupying Lesions Extensive tumor growth may result in spinal cord compression, increased intracranial pressure, brain herniation, seizures, massive hepatomegaly, gastrointestinal obstruction, cardiac and respiratory complications, and superior vena cava syndrome (obstruction of the superior vena cava by tumor). These emergencies are often caused by neuroblastoma, medulloblastoma, astrocytoma, Hodgkin disease, or lymphoma. After biopsy of the mass, treatment involves radiation therapy, chemotherapy, and corticosteroids.

PSYCHOSOCIAL NEEDS The diagnosis of cancer is devastating for families. They cannot believe that their vibrant, young child or adolescent has a potentially life-threatening disease. Families are in a state of crisis when the diagnosis is made, with the first response one of shock. At the same time that they are in a state of shock about the diagnosis, parents must gather resources to support the child, make treatment decisions, and adjust family life to integrate the needs of the child with cancer. Some families need to travel a great distance for the child's treatments, and others may have financial constraints that make healthcare costs a major concern. For nearly everyone, parental work schedules and arrangements for other children must be adjusted. Both father and mother should be included in plans of care; extended family members may also be important (Brody & Simmons, 2007). Most cancer treatment will last for a minimum of several months and may last several years, necessitating nearly constant adaptation by the child and family.

The child with cancer reacts to the diagnosis based on age.

- Infants and toddlers are unaware of the severity of the disease and deal with issues such as pain and separation from parents.
- Preschoolers are beginning to understand illness. However, they may think they caused their illness, and often are confused about why the parent cannot make the illness go away.
- School-age children can understand a diagnosis of cancer and benefit from opportunities to talk about the experience.
- Adolescents find contact with others who have gone through their experience reassuring and supportive.

Nearly all children are hospitalized after diagnosis. Care should include close proximity to parents, involvement in self-care appropriate for age, positive relationships with staff, and emotional care (Bjork, Nordstrom, & Hallstrom, 2006). Programs such as group therapy sessions, computer programs about cancer and treatment, and school reintegration can assist youth who are adjusting to cancer.

There has been some controversy about whether children with cancer have higher depression rates than other children. Measurements of depression in children who are getting treatments that influence physical comfort are often not reliable. Anxiety about the disease or treatment may be interpreted as depression, and medications for cancer treatment may influence mood or affect (Kersun & Elia, 2007). Careful assessment of all children with cancer and communication with families to compare the child's present mood to that prior to treatment is important.

CANCER SURVIVAL Children with cancer have a variety of common psychological and physiologic problems, regardless of their specific type of cancer. They and their families are dealing with a complex illness that influences their lives for years. The impact of this experience extends into all areas of function. Over the past 20–30 years, treatment for childhood cancers has been increasingly successful. About 1 in 1,000 young adults is a survivor of childhood cancer, and by 2010 it is expected that 1 in 250 adults will be a cancer survivor (Florin & Hinkle, 2005). The success of new modalities and treatment combinations has, however, created special healthcare needs for many survivors.

Surgery can have many results. Body organs may be removed and manipulated, leading to adhesions, intestinal obstruction, visual impairment, neurological disruption, and sterility. Removal of the spleen can lead to serious infections. Amputation necessitates the need for prosthetic devices and physical rehabilitation.

Radiation has several long-term effects. It can impair the growth of bones and teeth, leading to conditions such as scoliosis, leg length discrepancy, osteoporosis, or poor dental health. Chronic pain can result from skeletal toxicity (Kaste, 2008). Hypothyroidism can be observed in those who have had head and neck radiation (Skinner, Hamish, Wallace, et al., 2006). Cardiotoxicity and pulmonary toxicity can result from mediastinal radiation, while delayed puberty and sterility can result from radiation effects to the cranium and spinal regions. Impaired neurocognitive performance may occur as long-term effects of treatment, especially with higher doses of radiation. Some studies have found lower behavioral and social competence in treated children, and higher rates of posttraumatic stress syndrome (Rourke, Hobbie, Schwartz, et al., 2006).

Secondary cancers, most commonly solid tumors, occur in some survivors. Secondary cancers are also called second malignant neoplasm (SMN), and are those that occur subsequent to the primary cancer and treatment but are of a different histologic type. Cancers of the thyroid, CNS, breast, and skin are examples of secondary neoplasms. Most of these cancers can be effectively treated, emphasizing the need for thorough and frequent monitoring of the treated cancer client (Haddy, Mosher, Dinndorf, et al., 2004). Other chronic conditions, such as heart failure, congestive heart failure, and cognitive dysfunction, are more common in cancer survivors who are adults than in the general population (Twombly, 2007). Reproductive health can pose problems as the survivor reaches young adulthood and wishes to have children.

Chemotherapy can cause a wide variety of effects, both during its administration and for years afterward. Cardiomyopathy can occur with some drugs, especially the anthracyclines. Temporary and/or permanent pulmonary toxicity and renal complications can develop. Neurological effects of some drugs can lead to hearing loss (e.g., cisplatin and ifosfamide), cataracts, and paraplegia (e.g., intrathecal methotrexate for leukemia). Learning disabilities and change in intelligence quotient (IQ) occur in some children. Infertility may result (Nelson & Meeske, 2005). Although radiation is responsible for most secondary tumors, some chemotherapy drugs have also been implicated.

The diagnosis and stress of treatment, along with the risk of recurrence, are significant stressors for the child with cancer. Families may find it difficult to obtain full insurance coverage for the child who has had a prior cancer. Employment can be a potential problem for cancer survivors if employers have concerns about the earlier cancer diagnosis. Most people with cancer report fear of recurrence of the disease, which is a stressor. Depression, suicidal thoughts, and concerns about appearance have been found by some researchers to be more common in survivors of childhood cancer, whereas other researchers have found rates of depression to be similar among those treated for cancer and those in the population at large (Zebrack, Zevon, Turk, et al., 2006). Anxiety, attention deficit, and antisocial behaviors were found to be more common in survivors of leukemia, CNS tumors, or neuroblastoma (Schultz, Ness, Whitton, et al., 2007).

Conversely, hopefulness and the sense of having an added purpose in life can be positive outcomes for many cancer survivors. Some meet with others who have a recent diagnosis, and both children and their families sometimes work on fund-raising events that financially support cancer research. The highest risk for long-term psychological distress in adult survivors of childhood cancer occurs in those with poor health status, low income, low education, and unemployment. Encouraging children with cancer to meet educational goals will maximize their psychological adaptation (Zebrack et al., 2006).

A consensus group of experts identified barriers to optimal care for cancer survivors, including:

- Lack of knowledge about survivorship by healthcare professionals
- Lack of knowledge about risks and care recommendations by the cancer survivor
- Lack of awareness about cancer survivorship by the general public
- Paucity of research on survivorship.

Therefore, additional education of healthcare professionals and the public, as well as research into survivor issues, are recommended (Houldin, Curtiss, & Haylock, 2006; Soliman & Agresta, 2008).

PHYSICAL ASSESSMENT

The assessment of the client with alterations in cellular regulation is highly dependent on where the alteration occurs and the organ systems involved. For example, when the alteration involves cells directly related to the transport of oxygen, an important assessment includes oxygenation and breathing patterns.

Ongoing assessment of all clients with alterations in cellular regulation includes assessment of stress and coping abilities and psychosocial supports. This includes assessing the parents' and caregivers' stress levels and coping abilities and how they are accessing support groups, financial resources, and spiritual and other supports.

Assessment of the client with cancer also includes assessment of the client's nutrition and hydration status. Please refer to Exemplar 3.3, Cancer, for a discussion of nutrition and hydration assessment.

Nurses should assess all clients for early warning signs of cancer and teach clients those signs to watch for and report because early intervention to treat cancer improves outcomes. The early warning signs include change in bowel or bladder habits, a sore that does not heal, unusual bleeding or discharge, thickening or lump in the breast or elsewhere, indigestion or difficulty swallowing, obvious change in wart or mole, or a nagging cough or hoarseness (American Cancer Society, 2006).

Several important areas of client teaching address complementary health practices. They are:

1. Have client, especially children, increase intake of fruits and vegetables. Most people do not eat enough of these foods, and increased intake is associated with lower rates of many cancers. Aim for a minimum of five servings daily.
2. Protect skin with sunscreen. Early excessive exposure to sun, and having had one or repeated severe sunburns during childhood, increase chances of skin cancers developing in adulthood. Clients who work outdoors, athletes, coaches, and others who spend time outside regularly should use sunscreen daily, regardless of the climate in which they live.
3. Discourage smoking among all clients, including children, and make sure that children are not exposed to environmental tobacco smoke. This will decrease the future chance of developing lung cancer.
4. Have homes tested for radon. Be alert for exposure to any potential hazardous substances in the home or on clients' clothes if they work in industries with chemicals or other harmful substances.
5. When there is a history of cancer in the family, particularly if a type associated with familial incidence such as some breast or ovarian cancers, encourage the family to learn more about the cancer and teach children to receive regular surveillance as they enter young adulthood.
6. Inform adolescent and adult clients in all families about screening such as the Papanicolaou test, breast self-examination, and testicular examination that can lead to early detection.

Developmental Assessment of Children

Assessment of the child's physical and neurological development helps in determining the progress made during treatment and provides a baseline for evaluating the long-term effects of treatment. Developmental assessment of children should be performed regularly during treatment for cancer, at times when the child feels well so that the results are accurate. Children under 6 years of age who have cancer should receive regular developmental assessment with a standardized tool such as the Denver II Developmental Screening Test (see Concept 7,

Development). Recommend referral to a neuropsychologist for testing early in treatment and if changes in developmental performance are noted. Observe developmental milestones at each contact with the child and refer for further assessment if regression is observed. Performance in school and social activities with friends provides important information about expected developmental milestones in older children.

DIAGNOSTIC TESTS

Clients with disorders of cellular regulation may need diagnostic tests or procedures to assist in decision-making and treatment. Useful tests may include the following:

- Biopsy
- Bone marrow aspiration
- Computed tomography or computed axial tomography
- Magnetic resonance imaging
- Positron-emission tomography
- Radiograph (x-ray)
- Scans
- Ultrasound
- Complete blood count (CBC)
- Red blood indices
- Serum chemistry panel
- Tumor markers
- Urinalysis
- Lumbar puncture.

CARING INTERVENTIONS

For the client with alterations in cellular regulation, nursing interventions focus on reducing complications and maintaining optimal homeostasis. Interventions common to clients with cellular alterations include those directed at nutrition, activity, breathing, fatigue, and comfort. Nurses also provide interventions and client teaching to help clients manage side effects and provide clients and their families with psychosocial support. These interventions are critical to the client's successful recovery.

Clients with alterations in cellular function may commonly display activity intolerance, which can result in reduced activity, risk for injury, and alterations in skin integrity. Assessing activity tolerance, promoting safety, and helping the client remain as active as possible all play a role in the client's eventual outcome. Clients frequently report fatigue, and nurses can promote an adequate balance of rest, sleep, and activity in order to maintain homeostasis.

Nurses will provide appropriate pain management interventions, both pharmacologic and nonpharmacologic, to clients experiencing discomfort as the result of rapid cellular reproduction (cancer) placing pressure on healthy cells or alterations in cellular function that may result in inadequate oxygenation of tissues (anemias). Pain control may require client teaching to help the client overcome fear of addiction and dependence to narcotics if the need for pharmacologic pain management is anticipated to be long-term.

Nutrition and Hydration

Cells cannot function properly if the body is not provided with all of the essential nutrients. Assessment of nutritional status and promotion of good nutrition plays an important role in supporting the client's recovery as well as reducing the likelihood of cellular alterations.

The high metabolic rate of cancer growth depletes the client's nutritional stores so that many clients are cachectic at the time of diagnosis. In addition, the catabolic effect of chemotherapy and radiation on normal cells necessitates additional cellular replacement. Nurses working with clients being treated for cancer promote healthy nutritional status by performing ongoing assessments, providing client teaching, and initiating interventions to improve nutrition and hydration. Client teaching is directed at a well-rounded diet, including all of the macro- and micronutrients, is an important caring intervention.

The client needs increased nutritional intake at a time when nausea and vomiting are occurring as drug side effects, and when decreased activity and general health status result in diminished appetite. This often leads to extreme concern on the part of parents and caregivers, who may focus excessive attention on the client's intake.

The goals of nutrition therapy during treatment for cancer are to prevent or reverse any nutritional deficiencies, preserve the client's lean body mass, minimize any side effects that influence nutritional state, allow for the growth needs of pediatric clients, and improve overall quality of life (Eldridge, 2004). Administer antiemetic drugs to lessen nausea from chemotherapy. Offer frequent, small meals. It may be helpful to offer the client's favorite foods at times when nausea and vomiting are decreased. Ask the family members what treatments they use to decrease the client's nausea and vomiting and inform them of techniques that may enhance intake. Perform 24-hour dietary recalls to assess the client's intake, and evaluate height and weight regularly. Special nutritional products may be given orally, nasogastric or nasoduodenal tube feedings may be given, or total parenteral nutrition may be necessary. When the client's nutritional status is deteriorating or parenteral nutrition is used, perform weekly studies of serum electrolytes, liver chemistry, glucose, and triglycerides. Partner with both the oncologist and the dietitian to plan interventions appropriate for meeting the needs of individual clients.

Hydration management can be challenging, as the client may not be thirsty but is excreting large numbers of cell fragments and other substances as a result of treatment. Children in particular are at risk for dehydration due to a higher concentration of fluid within the body, Offer frequent, small amounts of fluid. Include frozen ice pops or other fluid-containing foods such as Jell-O, fruit, or soups. Caution should be taken to avoid citrus fruits because acidic foods can exacerbate complications of chemotherapy such as stomatitis. Measure intake and output. To ensure adequate excretion, a number of chemotherapy drugs are given with intravenous fluids. It is important to administer fluids as ordered and to ensure that the recommended urinary output excretion rate is maintained after drug administration.

Manage Treatment Side Effects

All cancer treatments affect some normal body cells as well as cancer cells, causing a wide variety of side effects. Nurses must know all side effects of specific drugs administered and monitor for them. Realize that some side effects are late and may be seen after therapy is completed and provide information about this to clients and their caregivers. Emphasize the importance of all follow-up visits scheduled in the future for monitoring of late effects.

A frequent occurrence is *myelosuppression* or suppression of blood cell production in the bone marrow. Be alert for signs of a decreased white blood cell count, such as infections. *Neutropenia* is present when the absolute neutrophil count (ANC) is less than 500 cells/mm^3 or if between 500 and 1,000 cells/mm^3 when chemotherapy is being given and falling levels are anticipated. At these levels, clients will be given a broad-spectrum antibiotic; granulocyte colony-stimulating factor (G-CSF) may be given. Take the client's temperature, isolate the client from others with infections, and perform serum laboratory studies as ordered.

Protect the client from bruises and be alert for hemorrhage or signs of bleeding such as petechiae, nosebleeds, dark colored or bloody stools, and presence of blood in vomit and urine; these are all effects of thrombocytopenia or decreased platelets. The client may need to receive infusions of platelets if thrombocytopenia is severe. When thrombocytopenia occurs, minimize needle sticks and other intrusive procedures. Be ready to deal with nosebleeds and watch for bleeding gums. Report any bleeding episodes to the oncology specialist. Be sure parents and caregivers know that the client should avoid contact sports or other rough activities and that any healthcare provider, such as a dentist, should be informed of the client's treatment and condition. Infusions to increase platelets are sometimes administered.

Provide Psychosocial Support

A diagnosis of cancer brings with it many emotions for the family. Initially family members experience shock and anger. They need basic information about the disease and the purpose of the tests that will be performed. Instructions often need to be repeated as clients and family members may not process information the first time it is presented due to their increased stress levels. For pediatric clients, assist the parents to plan how and when to tell the child the diagnosis. What the child needs to know is based on his or her developmental level and understanding.

After progressing from the initial state of shock about the diagnosis, the family needs to learn more about the disease, including the pathophysiology, treatment, and expected outcome or the prognosis. Clarify the family's understanding of these areas and be ready to answer questions. Provide both verbal explanations and written material. Clients and family members may talk with friends, purchase books, or search the Internet for information. Find out where they are getting information and provide additional resources when appropriate. Correct misconceptions and misinformation.

The family needs many strategies to deal with the challenge of long-term treatment for cancer. As the client experiences remissions and exacerbations or complications, the family feels alternately hopeful and discouraged. Help the family to identify support systems, and intervene as needed to enhance these systems. Facilitate contact with extended family members who might be of help, faith-based or spiritual connections, social service agencies, and other resources such as Internet and parent and caregiver support groups. Assist clients and caregivers who are concerned about job obligations and financial concerns.

CONSIDERATIONS FOR THE PEDIATRIC CLIENT AND FAMILY

Support for the child with cancer and his or her family includes considering the impact on siblings. They may alternately resent and feel guilty for the sibling's illness. They may not understand the treatments or disease. School progress may be slowed and teachers may not be aware of the sibling's stress. See Evidence-Based Practice: Cancer and Stress.

The child undergoing treatment for cancer needs support appropriate to his or her developmental stage and cognitive level (Figure 3–2 ■). (See Concept 7 for developmental levels and effective support strategies for children of different ages.) Younger children primarily need support during painful procedures and separation from parents. Older children need intervention strategies to assist in working through feelings related to treatments (Figure 3–3 ■). A major developmental task of adolescence is to attain independence and control, but cancer often interferes with adolescents' ability to achieve this task. Therefore, plan nursing strategies that empower adolescents as much as possible. This might include asking them whether

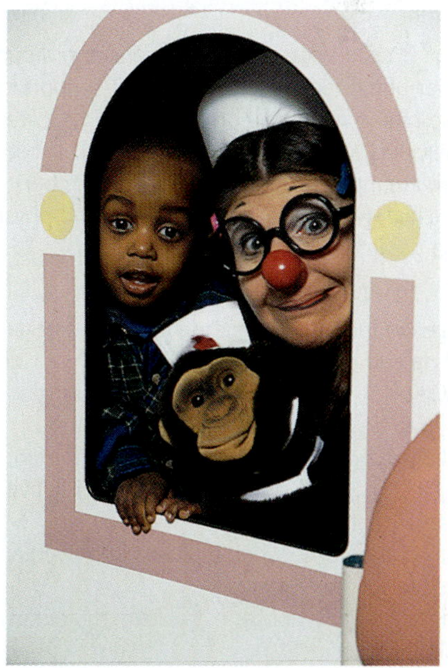

Figure 3–2 ■ Clowns from the Big Apple Clown Care Unit can help to ease the stress of hospitalization for seriously ill children and their families. Here, a clown doctor and her puppet distract a toddler who is waiting for his clinic appointment.

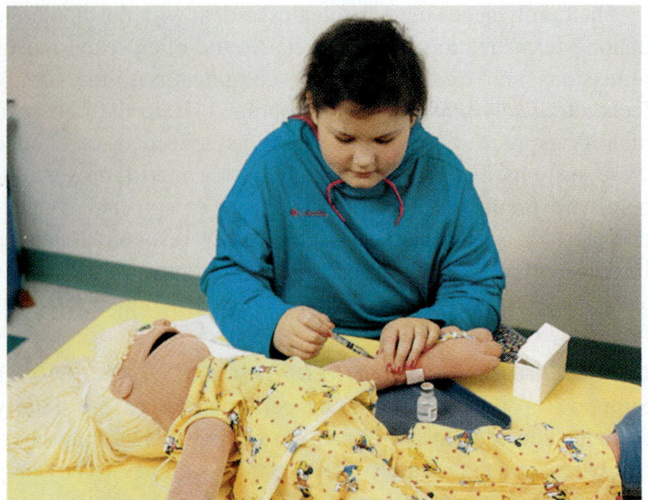

Figure 3–3 ■ A child in a pediatric oncology clinic giving injections to a doll. This type of play therapy helps children deal with fear, thus lowering their stress level.

they prefer morning or afternoon appointments, being placed on a teen unit where they can receive treatments with other teens, and encouraging parents to allow them choices about issues at home.

Talk with the child's teachers before the return to school after treatment to explain the child's condition and assist with plans to prepare the other children. Role-play with the child how to tell friends about any changes in appearance. A nurse or child life specialist could attend the class of a young child to explain what the child is experiencing. Arrange for tutors if necessary to assist the child with schoolwork during hospitalization and home care. Explore the option of summer camp for children with cancer. The Make-a-Wish Foundation strives to make dreams come true for ill children by sponsoring them for a desired activity or outing. Refer the child to this foundation if appropriate.

PHARMACOLOGIC THERAPIES

Pharmacologic therapies play an important role in treating alterations in cellular regulation. Administration of chemotherapy often requires the nurse to obtain advanced training because of the potential for injury to the administering nurse if extreme caution is not exercised. Special gloves are worn that provide greater protection should the medication spill or splash during administration.

Alterations in cellular function are many. This concept and its exemplars provide essential information about the nature of the alterations, risk factors, clinical manifestations, and interventions and treatment options. The exemplars that follow discuss priorities for nursing care and those nursing interventions necessary to assist clients with healing and recovery.

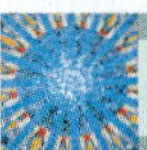

EVIDENCE-BASED PRACTICE **Cancer and Stress**

Problem

The family of a child with cancer experiences profound stress, and each member of the family needs time and support to adjust to the new roles he or she must take on in the family. However, the needs of family members are often overlooked as the ill child becomes the center of treatment and attention. Family members often provide care for the child, which can be emotionally and physically draining, and can also deplete family financial resources.

Evidence

Major changes in the family were identified by a research study that interviewed family members when a child was diagnosed with leukemia (McGrath, Paton, & Huff, 2005). They included:

- Relocation to be closer to the treatment center
- Interruption of normal activities of daily life for family members
- Placing life "on hold" and deferring usual activities, such as classes and vacations
- Readjustment to home when the child improved and the family resumed usual living patterns
- Concerns related to school and employment for family members
- Financial difficulties.

In another study, parents in 86 families that had a child with cancer focused on the needs of the 159 well siblings in those families. About 50% of the parents stated that they anticipated that the well siblings would manifest some problems because of the diagnosis of cancer. Parents frequently observed depression or withdrawal among the siblings, and believed that they had received inadequate information about how to support and help the siblings. Difficulty in scheduling times for the sibling to come to the treatment center and learn more about the cancer treatment was noted. A weekend intervention program for siblings was instituted to offer activities and counseling designed to support siblings. The peer support of meeting with others was helpful to the children (Ballard, 2004).

Implications

Being a family member when a child has cancer is stressful. Both parents and siblings express a need for information about the ill child's condition and treatment. Nurses should provide information at each health encounter and frequently ask what questions the family members have. Ask about siblings and include them in visits when possible. Plan peer support group sessions for the siblings so they can discuss their experiences and feelings with other siblings. In addition to information, support is vital. Ask who the parents and siblings have told about the ill child. Who can they turn to when they want to talk? Who can the parents call upon for help at home? Who can the siblings invite to school performances and other events if the parents are unable to attend?

Critical Thinking Application

Consider the opening scenario that describes Sam, who has leukemia, and his family. *What information do his parents need? How can you best support his older siblings?*

MEDICATIONS **Cellular Regulation**

Drug Groups	Mechanism of Action	Generic Name	Nursing Considerations
Chemotherapy			
Alkylating agents	Form bonds or linkages with DNA, changing the shape and preventing nucleic acids from dividing	chlorambucil, cyclophosphamide, ifosfamide, carmustine, altretamine, busulfan	■ Assess vital signs, CBC, renal and liver function. ■ Monitor for signs of bone marrow depression. ■ May need to hold drug if RBC, WBC, or platelet count decreases. ■ Hydrate before administering. ■ Monitor for and treat nausea. ■ Teach client to avoid foods high in purine and citric acid. ■ Assess skin integrity.
Antimetabolites	Compete for binding sites of nutrients and metabolites needed for cancer growth	methotrexate, pemetrexed, azacitidine, cladribine	■ Monitor for bone marrow suppression. ■ Monitor intake and output and weight. ■ Assess for infection. ■ Most antimetabolites are contraindicated during pregnancy. ■ Closely monitor clients with poor nutritional status, peptic ulcer disease, or ulcerative colitis. ■ Assess for and treat nausea and vomiting. ■ Teach good oral hygiene.
Antitumor antibiotics	More cytotoxic than other antibiotics, their use is usually restricted to a specific type of tumor. They bind to DNA and affect function similar to alkylating agents.	doxorubicin, bleomycin, mitomycin, valrubicin	■ Carefully monitor client's condition. ■ Monitor for bone marrow and cardiac toxicity. ■ Obtain baseline electrocardiogram. ■ Treat side effects such as diarrhea, alopecia, fatigue, nausea, and vomiting.
Hormones and hormone agonists	Useful for treating hormone-dependent cancers, such as breast and testicular cancers, by blocking receptor sites on the cancer cell	dexamethasone, diethylstilbestrol, abarelix, flutamide, histrelin, leuprolide, tamoxifen	■ Contraindicated during pregnancy and lactation. ■ Explain that treatment is most often palliative versus curative. ■ Prepare client for possible development of cross-gender, secondary sex characteristics. ■ Monitor for and reduce risk of infection.
Natural products	Isolated from plants, this group, called miotic inhibitors, affects cell division	vincristine, docetaxel, paclitaxel, etoposide, topotecan hydrochloride	■ Assess baseline vital signs, CBC, and health. ■ Monitor increased risk of allergic reaction ■ Treat side effects, including alopecia.
Biologic response modifiers and miscellaneous anticancer drugs	Stimulate the body's immune system to eliminate the tumor. Less toxic than other antineoplastics.	asparaginase, bexarotene, bortezomib, hydroxyurea, alemtuzumab, trastuzumab	■ Assess for bone marrow depression, pancreatitis, anemia. ■ Reduce risk of infection. ■ Assess fluid status, health, and CBC.
Antianemic			
Iron supplements	Dietary nutrient essential for production of hemoglobin	ferrous fumarate, ferrous gluconate, ferrous sulfate, iron dextran	■ Monitor for gastrointestinal side effects, including constipation, nausea, heartburn, aggravation of peptic ulcer or ulcerative colitis. ■ Teach client that stools will darken. ■ Encourage fluid and fiber intake. ■ Teach client about foods high in iron. ■ If administered parenterally, can stain skin and should be given by Z-track method. ■ If taken in liquid form, avoid contact with teeth.
Folic acid	Dietary nutrient essential for rapidly dividing cells	Folic acid	■ Teach clients about foods high in folic acid.
Vitamin B_{12}	Dietary nutrient essential for rapidly dividing cells	cyanocobalamin	■ Monitor for diarrhea.

3.1 ANEMIA

KEY TERMS

BASIS FOR SELECTION OF EXEMPLAR

American Academy of Pediatrics
American College of Obstetrics and Gynecology
Centers for Disease Control and Prevention
Most common condition
US Preventative Services

LEARNING OUTCOMES

After reading about this exemplar, you will be able to:

1. Describe the pathophysiology, etiology, clinical manifestations, and direct and indirect causes of anemia.
2. Identify risk factors associated with anemia.
3. Illustrate the nursing process in providing culturally competent care across the life span for individuals with anemia.
4. Formulate priority nursing diagnoses appropriate for an individual with anemia.
5. Create a plan of care for individuals with anemia and their family members.
6. Assess expected outcomes for an individual with anemia.
7. Discuss therapies used in the collaborative care of an individual with anemia.
8. Employ evidence-based caring interventions for an individual with anemia.

OVERVIEW

Anemia is an abnormally low number of circulating red blood cells (RBCs), low hemoglobin concentration, or both. Anemia is a common finding in clients, especially women, and may be completely asymptomatic. Routine testing of the RBC count is generally the first indication of anemia unless it becomes severe enough to cause symptoms.

Anemia usually is caused by decreased numbers of circulating RBCs. This decrease may result from blood loss, inadequate RBC production, or increased RBC destruction. Insufficient or defective hemoglobin within RBCs contributes to anemia as well. Insufficient quantities of iron limit hemoglobin production, in turn affecting the production of RBCs.

PATHOPHYSIOLOGY AND ETIOLOGY

A number of different pathologic mechanisms can lead to anemia (Box 3–1). Because RBCs are needed to carry oxygen throughout the body, every type of anemia, regardless of the cause, reduces the oxygen-carrying capacity of the blood. Therefore, anemia results in less oxygen reaching cells and tissues (tissue hypoxia).

When anemia develops gradually and the RBC reduction is moderate, the body's compensatory mechanisms may prevent or mask the appearance of symptoms except during those times when the oxygen needs of the body increase because of exercise or infection. Symptoms develop as RBCs and hemoglobin levels are further reduced. Pallor of the skin, mucous membranes, conjunctiva, and nail beds develops as a result of blood redistribution to vital organs and lack of hemoglobin (Figure 3–4 ■). As tissue oxygenation decreases, the heart and respiratory rates rise in an attempt to increase cardiac output and tissue perfusion. Tissue hypoxia may cause angina, fatigue, dyspnea on exertion, and night cramps. It also stimulates erythropoietin release; in turn, increased erythropoietin activity stimulates RBC production in the bone marrow and may lead to bone pain. Cerebral hypoxia can lead to headache, dizziness, and dim vision. Heart failure may develop in severe anemia.

Box 3–1 **Pathophysiologic Mechanisms of Anemia**

DECREASED RED BLOOD CELL PRODUCTION

- Altered hemoglobin synthesis:
  a. Iron deficiency
  b. Thalassemia
  c. Chronic inflammation
- Altered DNA synthesis:
  a. Vitamin B_{12} malabsorption or deficiency
  b. Folic acid malabsorption or deficiency
- Bone marrow failure:
  a. Aplastic anemia (stem cell dysfunction)
  b. Red cell aplasia
  c. Myeloproliferative leukemias
  d. Cancer metastasis, lymphoma
  e. Chronic infection or inflammation, physical and emotional fatigue

INCREASED RED BLOOD CELL LOSS OR DESTRUCTION

- Acute or chronic blood loss:
  a. Hemorrhage or trauma
  b. Chronic gastrointestinal bleeding, menorrhagia
- Increased hemolysis:
  a. Hereditary cell membrane disorders
  b. Defective hemoglobin—sickle cell anemia or trait
  c. Pyruvate kinase or glucose-6-phosphate dehydrogenase deficiency affecting glycolysis or cell oxidation
  d. Immune mechanisms and disorders (e.g., blood reaction, hypersensitivity responses, and autoimmune disorders)
  e. Splenomegaly and hypersplenism
  f. Infection
  g. Erythrocyte trauma (e.g., caused by cardiopulmonary bypass, hemolytic uremic syndrome)

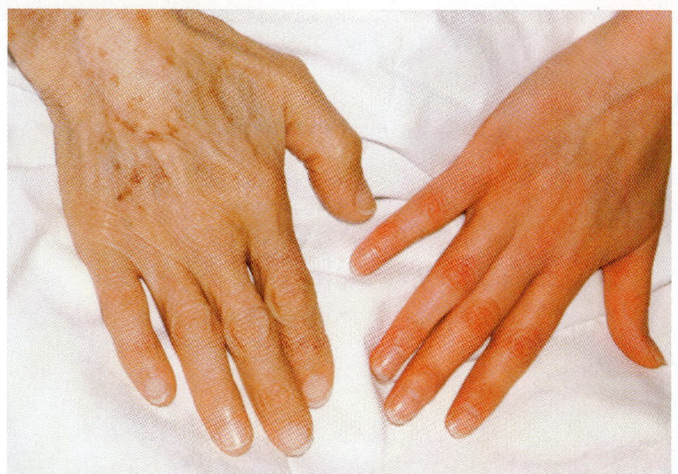

Figure 3–4 ■ The skin of the client with anemia appears pale beside that of a person with a normal hemoglobin and hematocrit.

Source: Westminister Hospital, Photo Researchers, Inc.

With rapid blood loss, blood volume is decreased, as is the oxygen-carrying capacity of the blood. Initial manifestations include tachycardia and tachypnea; the skin may be pale, cool, and clammy as peripheral vessels constrict to maintain blood flow to the heart and brain. With significant blood loss, signs of circulatory shock may occur, including hypotension, tachycardia, decreased level of consciousness, and oliguria. With chronic bleeding, fluid shifts from the interstitial spaces into the vessels, maintaining blood volume. Blood viscosity is reduced, which may result in a systolic heart murmur.

Etiology

Iron deficiency anemia is the most common form of anemia. Excessive iron loss as a result of chronic bleeding is the usual cause of iron deficiency anemia in adults. Menstrual blood loss is the most common cause in adult females. Iron deficiency anemia also may result from inadequate dietary iron intake (<1 mg/day), malabsorption syndromes, or the increased iron requirements associated with pregnancy and lactation. Box 3–2 summarizes common causes of iron deficiency anemia.

Box 3–2 **Causes of Iron Deficiency Anemia**

- Dietary deficiencies:
  - a. Vegetarian diet
  - b. Inadequate protein intake
- Decreased absorption:
  - a. Partial or total gastrectomy
  - b. Chronic diarrhea
  - c. Malabsorption syndromes
- Increased metabolic requirements:
  - a. Pregnancy
  - b. Lactation
- Blood loss:
  - a. Gastrointestinal bleeding (especially caused by ulcers or chronic aspirin use)
  - b. Menstrual losses
- Chronic hemoglobinuria

Iron deficiency anemia is particularly common in older adults and in women of child-bearing age. Iron deficiency anemia can result from chronic, occult (hidden) blood loss caused by slowly bleeding peptic ulcers, gastrointestinal inflammation, hemorrhoids, and cancer. Depending on its severity, anemia may affect all major organ systems.

Iron deficiency anemia is the most common nutritional deficiency in children. It affects 3% of children younger than 2 years, 6–18% of toddlers, 9–11% of adolescent girls, and less than 1% of adolescent boys (Carley, 2003; White, 2005). Pica (consumption of or cravings for nonfood items) is also associated with iron deficiency anemia in pediatric clients. Lead poisoning is associated with anemia and may worsen in those with anemia because lead absorption increases in the anemic state.

Risk Factors

Clients who do not eat a well-balanced diet rich in fresh fruits and vegetables are at increased risk for those anemias caused by nutrient deficiency, including iron deficiency anemia. During child-bearing years, women lose blood during menstruation. Inadequate intake of iron can result in reduced production of RBCs, increasing the risk of this type of anemia.

CLINICAL MANIFESTATIONS

Anemia is categorized by cause: blood loss, nutritional, hemolytic, and bone marrow suppression (aplastic). A neonatal anemia also is recognized. Each type has its own specific pathophysiology and manifestations.

Blood Loss Anemia

When anemia results from acute or chronic bleeding, RBCs and other blood components (e.g., iron) are lost from the body. With acute blood loss, circulating volume decreases. As a result, cardiac output falls. Compensatory mechanisms are activated to maintain cardiac output: The heart rate increases, and peripheral blood vessels constrict. Vessels in the liver, a blood storage organ, also constrict, increasing circulating volume. Fluid shifts from the interstitial spaces into the vascular compartment to maintain blood volume, diluting the cellular components of the blood and reducing its viscosity. If hemorrhage continues, compensatory mechanisms become less effective, increasing the risk for shock and circulatory failure.

In acute blood loss, circulating RBCs are of normal size and shape (normocytic). Early in the hemorrhage, the red blood cell count, hemoglobin, and hematocrit may be normal; as fluid shifts from the interstitial space into the vascular space to maintain circulating volume, however, the RBC count, hemoglobin, and hematocrit fall. If sufficient iron is available, the number of circulating RBCs and hemoglobin levels return to normal within 3–4 weeks after the bleeding episode. Chronic blood loss, on the other hand, depletes iron stores as RBC production attempts to maintain the RBC supply. The resulting RBCs are small (microcytic) and pale (hypochromic).

MULTISYSTEM EFFECTS OF **Anemia**

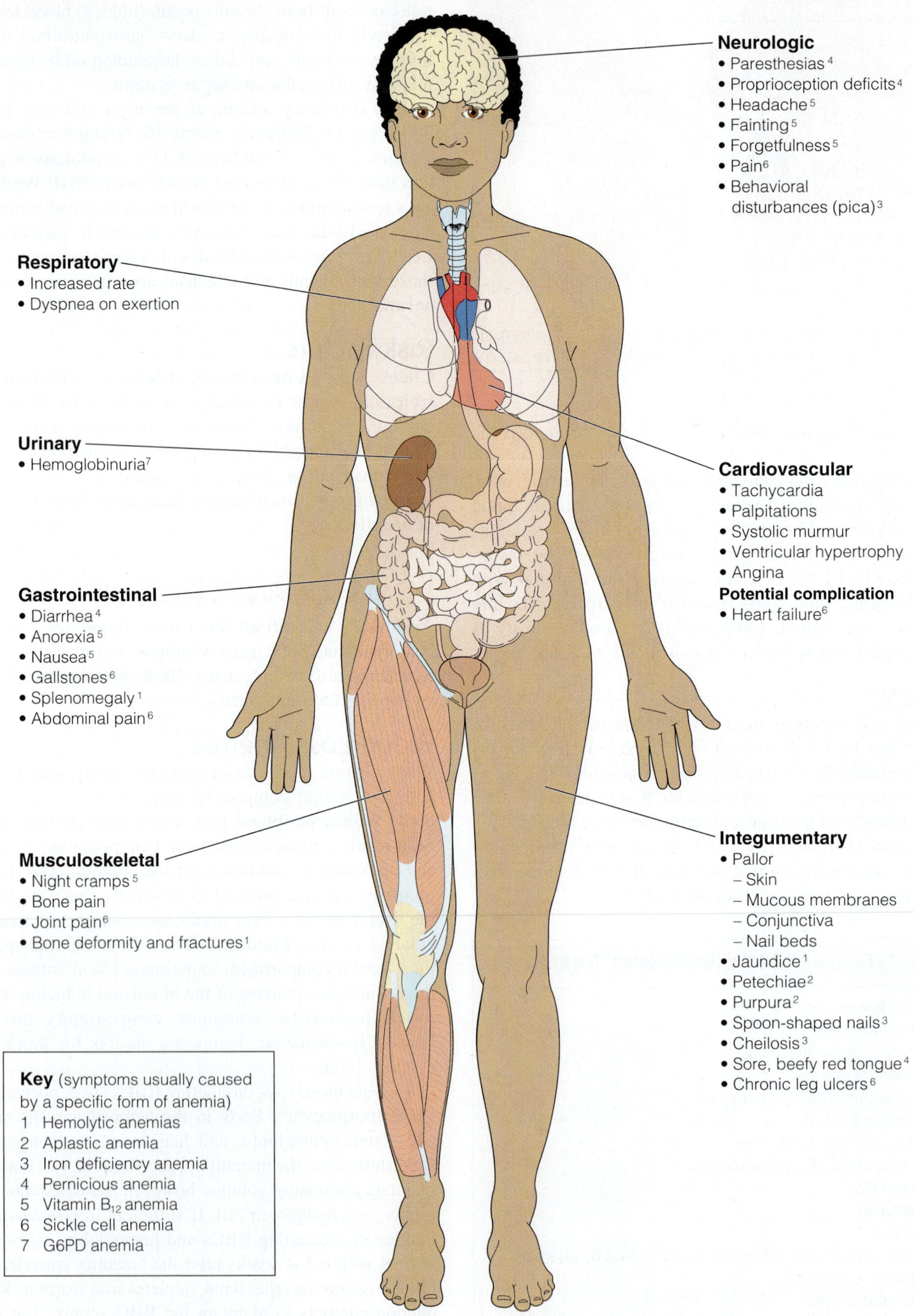

Neurologic
• Paresthesias 4
• Proprioception deficits 4
• Headache 5
• Fainting 5
• Forgetfulness 5
• Pain 6
• Behavioral disturbances (pica) 3
Respiratory
• Increased rate
• Dyspnea on exertion
Urinary
• Hemoglobinuria 7
Cardiovascular
• Tachycardia
• Palpitations
• Systolic murmur
• Ventricular hypertrophy
• Angina
Potential complication
• Heart failure 6
Gastrointestinal
• Diarrhea 4
• Anorexia 5
• Nausea 5
• Gallstones 6
• Splenomegaly 1
• Abdominal pain 6
Integumentary
• Pallor
– Skin
– Mucous membranes
– Conjunctiva
– Nail beds
• Jaundice 1
• Petechiae 2
• Purpura 2
• Spoon-shaped nails 3
• Cheilosis 3
• Sore, beefy red tongue 4
• Chronic leg ulcers 6
Musculoskeletal
• Night cramps 5
• Bone pain
• Joint pain 6
• Bone deformity and fractures 1
Key (symptoms usually caused by a specific form of anemia)
1 Hemolytic anemias
2 Aplastic anemia
3 Iron deficiency anemia
4 Pernicious anemia
5 Vitamin B12 anemia
6 Sickle cell anemia
7 G6PD anemia

Nutritional Anemias

A number of different nutrients are required for normal RBC development (erythropoiesis). Iron is a key nutrient necessary for hemoglobin synthesis. In addition, adequate supplies of protein (and its building blocks, amino acids), vitamins, and other minerals are required. The B vitamins, particularly B_{12} (cobalamin) and folate, play a key role in RBC development. Vitamins C and E also are necessary.

Nutritional anemias result from nutrient deficits that affect RBC formation or hemoglobin synthesis. The nutrient deficit may be caused by inadequate diet, malabsorption of the nutrient, or increased need for the nutrient. The most common types of nutritional anemias are iron deficiency anemia, vitamin B_{12} deficiency anemia, and folic acid deficiency anemia. Vitamin B_{12} and folic acid anemias are sometimes called megaloblastic anemias, because enlarged, nucleated RBCs (megaloblasts) are seen in these anemias.

IRON DEFICIENCY ANEMIA **Iron deficiency anemia** develops when the supply of iron is inadequate for optimal RBC formation (see Box 3–2). The body cannot synthesize hemoglobin without iron. Normally, the body efficiently recycles and stores iron, reusing much of the iron contained in RBCs that are removed from circulation because of age or damage. However, small amounts of iron are continually lost in the feces; therefore, adequate iron intake is necessary for normal hemoglobin synthesis and RBC production.

Iron deficiency anemia results in fewer numbers of RBCs, microcytic and hypochromic RBCs as well as malformed RBCs (poikilocytosis) (Figure 3–5 ■). Chronic iron deficiency may lead to brittle, spoon-shaped nails; cheilosis (cracks at the corners of the mouth); a smooth, sore tongue; and pica.

VITAMIN B_{12} DEFICIENCY ANEMIA Vitamin B_{12} is necessary for DNA synthesis and is found almost exclusively in foods derived from animals. Vitamin B_{12} deficiency occurs when inadequate vitamin B_{12} is consumed or, more commonly, when it is poorly absorbed from the gastrointestinal tract. Deficiency of this vitamin impairs cell division and maturation of the cell nucleus, especially in rapidly proliferating RBCs. As a result, macrocytic (large), misshapen (oval rather than concave) RBCs with thin membranes are produced. Great numbers of these large, immature RBCs enter the circulation. These cells are fragile, incapable of carrying adequate amounts of oxygen, and have a shortened life span.

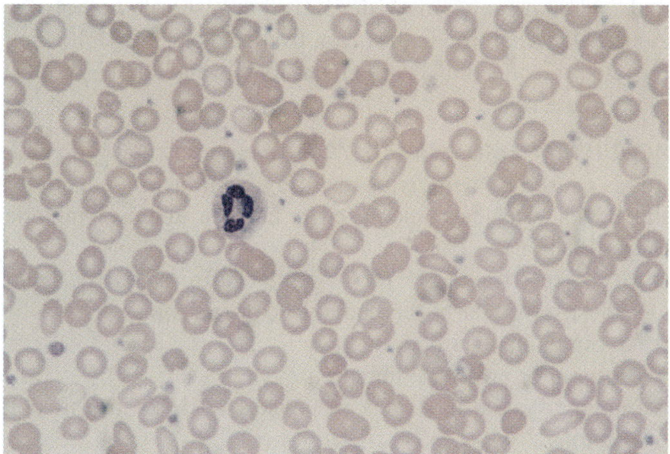

Figure 3–5 ■ A blood smear showing RBCs characteristically seen in iron deficiency anemia. Note the pale color of the RBCs (hypochromic). Many of the cells also are smaller than normal (microcytic) and misshapen, reducing their oxygen-carrying capacity.

Source: Dr. E. Walker, Photo Researchers, Inc.

Failure to absorb dietary vitamin B_{12} is called **pernicious anemia**. It develops from lack of intrinsic factor, a substance secreted by the gastric mucosa. Intrinsic factor binds with vitamin B_{12} and travels with it to the ileum, where the vitamin is absorbed. In the absence of intrinsic factor, vitamin B_{12} cannot be absorbed into the body.

Vitamin B_{12} deficiency may also result from other malabsorption disorders and dietary factors. Resection of the stomach or ileum, loss of pancreatic secretions, and chronic gastritis can affect vitamin B_{12} absorption. Dietary deficiencies of vitamin B_{12} are rare, usually occurring only among strict vegetarians.

Manifestations of vitamin B_{12} deficiency anemia develop gradually, as body stores of the vitamin are depleted. Pallor or slight jaundice and weakness develop. In pernicious anemia, a smooth, sore, beefy red tongue and diarrhea may occur. Because vitamin B_{12} is important for neurologic function, paresthesias (altered sensations, such as numbness or tingling) in the extremities and problems with proprioception (the sense of one's position in space) develop. These manifestations may progress to difficulty maintaining balance as a result of spinal cord damage. Central nervous system manifestations of relatively short duration ($\leq$ 6 months) are reversible with treatment but may be permanent if treatment is delayed (Tierney, McPhee, & Papadakis, 2005).

FOLIC ACID DEFICIENCY ANEMIA Like vitamin B_{12}, folic acid is required for DNA synthesis and normal maturation of RBCs. Folic acid deficiency anemia is characterized by fragile, megaloblastic (large and immature) cells. Folic acid is found in green leafy vegetables, fruits, cereals, and meats, and it is absorbed from the intestines.

Folic acid deficiency anemia as a result of inadequate intake is more common among people who are chronically undernourished. This includes older adults, those with alcoholism, and those addicted to drugs. Those with alcoholism are especially at risk because alcohol suppresses folate metabolism, which forms folic acid. Because increased folic acid requirements also may lead to anemia, pregnant women are at greater risk for anemia due to increased intake of folic acid to promote fetal development. Infants and teenagers can develop temporary folic acid deficiencies during periods of rapid growth. Impaired folic acid absorption and metabolism can cause folic acid deficiency anemia. Malabsorption disorders, such as celiac sprue (a hereditary gastrointestinal disorder characterized by inability to metabolize amino acids found in gluten), and certain medications, such as methotrexate and some chemotherapeutic agents, may be implicated. Causes of folic acid deficiency anemia are summarized in Box 3–3.

The manifestations of folic acid deficiency anemia develop gradually, as folic acid stores are depleted. Signs and symptoms may include pallor, progressive weakness and fatigue,

Box 3–3 Causes of Folic Acid Deficiency Anemia

- Inadequate dietary intake

At risk:

a. Older adults
b. Clients with alcoholism
c. Clients receiving total parenteral nutrition

- Increased metabolic requirements

At risk:

a. Pregnant women
b. Infants and teenagers
c. Clients undergoing hemodialysis
d. Clients with forms of hemolytic anemia

- Folic acid malabsorption and impaired metabolism
  a. Celiac sprue
  b. Chemotherapeutic agents, folate antagonists (methotrexate, pentamidine), or anticonvulsants
  c. Alcoholism

shortness of breath, and heart palpitations. Manifestations similar to those associated with vitamin B_{12} anemia, such as glossitis, cheilosis, and diarrhea, are common. No neurologic symptoms occur with folic acid deficiency anemia, helping differentiate it from vitamin B_{12} deficiency anemia. These two nutritional anemias do, however, sometimes coexist.

Maternal folic acid deficiency is strongly associated with neural tube defects, such as meningomyelocele. The neural tube develops early in the process of fetal development, often before pregnancy is recognized.

Hemolytic Anemias

Hemolytic anemias are characterized by premature destruction (lysis) of RBCs. When RBCs break down, iron and other by-products of their destruction remain in the plasma. RBC lysis (hemolysis) may occur within the circulatory system or as a result of phagocytosis by WBCs, such as circulating monocytes and macrophages in the spleen. In response to hemolysis, the hematopoietic activity of bone marrow increases, leading to increased reticulocytes (immature RBCs) in circulating blood. Most types of hemolytic anemia are characterized by normocytic and normochromic RBCs.

There are many different causes of hemolytic anemias (Box 3–4). The cause may be intrinsic, arising from disorders within the RBC itself, or extrinsic, originating outside the RBC. Intrinsic disorders include cell membrane defects, defects in hemoglobin structure and function, and inherited enzyme deficiencies. Extrinsic causes of hemolytic anemia include drugs, bacterial and other toxins, and trauma. This section discusses thalassemia, acquired hemolytic anemia, and glucose-6-phosphate dehydrogenase anemia. (For details regarding sickle cell anemia, see Exemplar 3.8, Sickle Cell Disorder.)

Box 3–4 Causes of Hemolytic Anemia

INTRINSIC

- Red blood cell membrane defects
- Hemoglobin structure defects (e.g., sickle cell anemia, thalassemia)
- Inherited enzyme defects (e.g., glucose-6-phosphate dehydrogenase deficiency)

EXTRINSIC

- Drugs, chemicals
- Toxins and venoms
- Bacterial and other infections
- Trauma, burns
- Mechanical damage (prosthetic heart valves)

THALASSEMIA **Thalassemia** refers to inherited disorders of hemoglobin synthesis in which either the alpha or beta chains of the hemoglobin molecule are missing or defective. This leads to deficient hemoglobin production and fragile hypochromic, microcytic RBCs called target cells because of their distinctive bull's-eye appearance.

Thalassemia usually affects certain populations. People of Mediterranean descent (southern Italy and Greece) are more likely to have beta-defect thalassemia (often called Cooley's anemia or Mediterranean anemia). People of Asian ancestry, especially from Thailand, the Philippines, and China, more often have alpha-defect thalassemia. Africans and African Americans may have both alpha- and beta-defect thalassemia.

Children with thalassemia major rarely reach adulthood, although repeated blood transfusions may extend their life span (McCance & Huether, 2006). People with thalassemia minor often are asymptomatic.

Manifestations include mild to moderate anemia, mild splenomegaly, bronze skin coloring, and bone marrow hyperplasia. The major form of the disease causes severe anemia, heart failure, and liver and spleen enlargement from increased red cell destruction. Fractures of the long bones, ribs, and vertebrae may result from bone marrow expansion and thinning as a result of increased hematopoiesis. Jaundice, hepatomegaly, and splenomegaly may develop because of hemolysis. Accumulation of iron in the heart, liver, and pancreas following repeated transfusions for treatment may eventually cause failure of these organs.

ACQUIRED HEMOLYTIC ANEMIA Acquired hemolytic anemia is caused by hemolysis resulting from factors outside of the RBCs. Causes of acquired hemolytic anemias include the following:

- Mechanical trauma to RBCs produced by prosthetic heart valves, severe burns, hemodialysis, or radiation
- Autoimmune disorders
- Bacterial or protozoal infection
- Immune-system-mediated responses, such as transfusion reactions
- Drugs, toxins, chemical agents, or venoms.

The manifestations of acquired hemolytic anemia depend on the extent of hemolysis and the body's ability to replace destroyed red blood cells. The anemia itself often is mild to moderate as erythropoiesis increases to replace the destroyed RBCs. The spleen enlarges as it removes damaged or destroyed RBCs. If the breakdown of heme units exceeds the liver's ability to conjugate and excrete bilirubin, jaundice develops. When the condition is severe, bone marrow expands, and bones may be deformed or may develop pathologic fractures. The severity of generalized manifestations of anemia (e.g., tachycardia and pallor) depends on the degree of anemia and deficiency of tissue oxygenation.

GLUCOSE-6-PHOSPHATE DEHYDROGENASE ANEMIA Glucose-6-phosphate dehydrogenase (G6PD) anemia is caused by a hereditary defect in RBC metabolism. It is relatively common in people of African and Mediterranean descent. The defective gene is located on the X chromosome and therefore affects more males than females. There are many variations of this genetic defect.

Glucose-6-phosphate dehydrogenase is an enzyme that catalyzes glycolysis, the process in which an RBC derives cellular energy. A defect in G6PD action causes direct oxidation of hemoglobin, damaging the RBC. Hemolysis usually occurs only when the affected person is exposed to stressors (e.g., drugs such as aspirin, sulfonamides, or vitamin K derivatives) that increase the metabolic demands on RBCs. The G6PD deficiency impairs the necessary compensatory increase in glucose metabolism and causes cellular damage. Damaged RBCs are destroyed over a period of 7–12 days.

When the client is exposed to a stressor that triggers G6PD anemia, symptoms develop within several days. These may include pallor, jaundice, hemoglobinuria (hemoglobin in the urine), and an elevated reticulocyte count. As new RBCs develop, counts return to normal.

Aplastic Anemia

In **aplastic anemia**, the bone marrow fails to produce all three types of blood cells, leading to pancytopenia, a deficiency in both red and white blood cells. Normal bone marrow is replaced by fat. Fortunately, aplastic anemia is rare.

A rare form of aplastic anemia, fanconi anemia, is caused by defects of DNA repair . For approximately 50% of acquired aplastic anemias, however, the underlying cause is unknown (idiopathic aplastic anemia). Other cases follow stem cell damage caused by exposure to radiation or certain chemical substances, such as benzene, arsenic, nitrogen mustard, certain antibiotics (especially chloramphenicol), and chemotherapeutic drugs (McCance & Huether, 2006). Aplastic anemia also may occur with viral infections, such as mononucleosis, hepatitis C, and HIV disease (Porth, 2005).

In aplastic anemia, the number of stem cells in the bone marrow is significantly reduced. The stem cell pool may be less than 1% of normal when the disease is recognized. Anemia develops as the bone marrow fails to replace RBCs that have reached the end of their life span. Remaining RBCs may be normochromic and normocytic, or they may be large, with increased mean corpuscular volume.

Manifestations of aplastic anemia vary with the severity of the pancytopenia. Its onset usually is insidious, but it may be sudden. Manifestations include fatigue, pallor, progressive weakness, exertional dyspnea, headache, and ultimately, tachycardia and heart failure. Platelet deficiency leads to bleeding problems; bleeding gums, excessive bruising, and nosebleeds may be the initial symptoms. A deficiency of WBCs increases the risk of infection, causing manifestations such as sore throat and fever.

Neonatal Anemia

Neonatal anemia may be caused by blood loss, hemolysis/erythrocyte destruction, and impaired RBC production (Aher, Malwatkar, & Kadam, 2008; Rosenberg, 2007). Blood loss (hypovolemia) occurs in utero from placental bleeding (placenta previa or abruptio placentae). Intrapartal blood loss may be fetomaternal, fetofetal, or the result of umbilical cord bleeding. Birth trauma to abdominal organs (adrenal hemorrhage) or the cranium (subgaleal bleed) may produce significant blood loss, and cerebral bleeding may occur because of hypoxia.

Excessive hemolysis of RBCs is usually a result of blood group incompatibilities, but it may be caused by infections. The most common cause of impaired RBC production is a genetically transmitted deficiency in G6PD.

Physiologic anemia of infancy occurs as a result of the normal, gradual drop in hemoglobin for the first 6–12 weeks of life. When the amount of hemoglobin decreases in term infants, the bone marrow begins production of RBCs again, and the anemia disappears.

COLLABORATION

Ensuring adequate tissue oxygenation is the priority of care in treating anemia. Specific therapy is determined by the underlying cause of the disorder. Anemia that results from nutritional deficiencies are addressed through dietary counseling. Some cases of anemia may be treated with drugs. In severe cases, the client with anemia may need a blood transfusion. Table 3–2 outlines interdisciplinary care measures for selected types of anemia. Members of the interdisciplinary health care team may include pharmacists and nutritionists or dieticians in addition to nurses, physicians, and other health care professionals.

Diagnostic Tests

The diagnosis of anemia is established on the basis of laboratory studies. A diet history and analysis can provide information related to food intake. Tests that may be ordered include the following:

- CBC
- Hemoglobin and hematocrit
- Hemoglobin electrophoresis
- Serum iron
- Serum ferritin
- Iron-binding capacity
- Microscopic analysis
- Schilling test
- Bone marrow examination
- Quantitative assay of G6PD.

TABLE 3–2 Interdisciplinary Care Focus for Major Anemias

TYPE OF ANEMIA	INTERDISCIPLINARY CARE
Iron deficiency anemia	■ Increased dietary intake of iron-rich foods ■ Oral or parenteral iron supplements
Vitamin B_{12} deficiency	■ Increased dietary intake of foods containing vitamin B_{12} (e.g., meats, eggs, and dairy products) ■ Oral or parenteral vitamin B_{12} supplements ■ Parenteral vitamin B_{12} for deficiency caused by malabsorption or lack of intrinsic factor
Folic acid deficiency	■ Increased dietary intake of foods rich in folic acid (folate) ■ Oral folic acid supplements ■ Folic acid supplements recommended for women who are pregnant or may become pregnant in order to prevent neural tube defects
Sickle cell anemia	■ Treatment is primarily supportive ■ Hydroxyurea, 10–30 mg · kg^{-1} · day^{-1} ■ Sickle cell crisis: a. Rest b. Oxygen therapy to maintain SaO_2 c. Narcotic analgesia d. Vigorous hydration e. Treatment of precipitating factors ■ Acute chest syndrome: a. Careful hydration; hemodynamic monitoring b. Oxygen therapy c. Transfusion ■ Folic acid supplements ■ Blood transfusions during surgery or pregnancy as necessary ■ Genetic counseling recommended
Thalassemia	■ Regular blood transfusions ■ Folic acid supplements ■ Possible splenectomy ■ Genetic counseling
Aplastic anemia	■ Withdrawal of the causative agent, if known ■ Blood transfusions ■ Bone marrow transplant as indicated

Pharmacologic Therapies

Medications used to treat anemia depend on the underlying cause. Drugs used to treat anemia include the following:

- Ferrous sulfate or other sources of iron
- Folic acid
- Vitamin B_{12}.

Iron replacement therapy is ordered for iron deficiency anemia. Supplemental iron may be given orally or parenterally. Intravenous (IV) administration of iron is becoming more common, particularly in clients with an acute deficiency or an anemia associated with chronic gastrointestinal blood loss, chronic renal failure, and other chronic conditions that increase the need for blood cell production (e.g., cancers). The risk of anaphylaxis is a major concern with IV iron dextran. Other parenteral iron solutions, including IV sodium ferric gluconate (Ferrlecit) and iron sucrose (Venofer), carry a much lower risk of adverse and allergic reactions (Kasper et al., 2005).

Parenteral vitamin B_{12} is given when malabsorption or lack of intrinsic factor leads to vitamin B_{12} deficiency anemia. Folic acid is ordered for women of child-bearing age, pregnant women, and clients with folic acid deficiency or sickle cell anemia to meet the increased demands of the bone marrow. Hydroxyurea, a drug that promotes fetal hemoglobin production, may be prescribed for clients with sickle cell anemia, particularly those with frequent crises or severe disease. Resulting increased levels of fetal hemoglobin interfere with the sickling process and reduce the incidence of painful crises (Kasper et al., 2005).

Erythropoietin may be ordered for clients with low erythropoietin levels (e.g., clients with chronic renal failure) and for people who have anemia associated with other chronic diseases. Erythropoietin is given subcutaneously, and it may be given as often as three times a week in chronic renal failure. Because erythropoietin stimulates RBC production, adequate iron must be present. Clients receiving erythropoietin may require regular IV iron therapy as well (Kasper et al., 2005).

Immunosuppressive therapy with antithymocyte globulin, corticosteroids, and cyclosporine may be used to treat aplastic anemia. Androgens may stimulate blood cell production in some clients with aplastic anemia.

Nutrition

Dietary modifications are recommended for nutritional deficiency anemias, such as iron deficiency anemia, vitamin B_{12} deficiency anemia, or folic acid deficiency anemia. Box 3–5 identifies good sources of dietary iron, vitamin B_{12}, and folic acid.

Blood Transfusion

Blood transfusions may be indicated to treat anemias resulting from major blood loss, such as from trauma or major surgery, and severe anemia regardless of cause. In acute hemorrhage, whole blood may be given to replace both blood cells and volume. A unit of packed RBCs may be given when anemia is severe and the client demonstrates cardiovascular instability or compromise.

Complementary Therapies

Complementary health care practitioners may recommend specific plant enzymes to treat nutritional anemias. Plant enzymes are believed to aid digestion of proteins, fats, and carbohydrates, facilitating absorption of their nutrients. Therapy is determined by the specific type of anemia. Plant enzymes should not be used alone to treat anemia, and it is important to check for possible interactions with prescribed medications before starting therapy.

Box 3–5 **Dietary Sources of Iron, Folic Acid, and Vitamin B_{12}**

IRON

Iron in the diet comes from two sources. The first, heme iron, makes up about one-half of the iron from animal sources. The second, nonheme iron, includes the remaining iron from animal sources and all the iron from plants, legumes, and nuts. Heme iron promotes absorption of nonheme iron from other foods when both forms are consumed at the same time. Absorption of nonheme iron is enhanced by vitamin C and is inhibited by tea and coffee.

SOURCES OF HEME IRON

- Beef
- Chicken
- Egg yolk
- Clams, oysters
- Pork loin
- Turkey
- Veal

SOURCES OF NONHEME IRON

- Bran flakes
- Brown rice
- Whole-grain breads
- Dried beans
- Dried fruits
- Greens
- Oatmeal

SOURCES OF FOLIC ACID

- Green leafy vegetables
- Broccoli
- Organ meats
- Eggs
- Wheat germ
- Asparagus
- Milk
- Yeast
- Kidney beans

SOURCES OF VITAMIN B_{12}

- Liver
- Fresh shrimp and oysters
- Eggs
- Milk
- Kidney
- Meats (muscle)
- Cheese

NURSING PROCESS

Nursing care includes screening clients at risk for anemia in order to promote early intervention to prevent complications. Client teaching is directed toward self-care and will often include dietary counseling.

Assessment

Assessment data to collect for clients with suspected anemia include the following:

- *Health history.* Complaints of shortness of breath with activity, fatigue, weakness, dizziness or fainting, palpitations; history of previous anemia, bleeding episodes; menstrual history (if appropriate); medications; chronic diseases; usual diet and patterns of alcohol intake or cigarette smoking
- *Physical examination.* General appearance, skin color; vital signs, including temperature; heart and lung sounds; peripheral pulses, capillary refill; abdominal tenderness; obvious bleeding or bruising.

Diagnosis

Anemia affects circulating oxygen levels and tissue oxygenation. Priority nursing diagnoses include the following:

- Activity Intolerance
- Altered Oral Mucous Membranes
- Self-Care Deficits
- Risk for Decreased Cardiac Output.

Plan

Treatment goals may include the following:

- The client makes appropriate dietary choices to increase iron intake.
- The client demonstrates appropriate self-administration of supplements.
- The client's RBC count (or hemoglobin) improves.

Implementation

Nursing implementation for the client with anemia is directed toward minimizing the impact of the symptoms while promoting resolution of the condition. Client preferences, culture, and specific symptoms must all be considered before implementing care.

Activity Intolerance

Anemia causes weakness and shortness of breath on exertion. These symptoms are the result of decreased circulating oxygen levels secondary to low hemoglobin levels. Weakness, fatigue, and/or vertigo may occur even during activities of daily living (ADLs), including those associated with self-care, home life, job performance, and social roles.

- Help identify ways to conserve energy when performing necessary or desired activities. Modifying the approach to a particular activity may reduce cardiorespiratory symptoms and activity-related fatigue. Alternative ways of performing tasks (e.g., sitting when performing hygiene care and kitchen tasks) may reduce oxygen demands. In some cases, assistance from others is necessary to conserve energy and reduce symptoms.

- Help the client and family establish priorities for tasks and activities. Because family members may need to assume responsibility for additional tasks, the plan's success depends on mutually established goals.
- Assist to develop a schedule of alternating periods of activity and rest throughout the day. Rest periods decrease oxygen needs, reducing strain on the heart and lungs and allowing restoration of homeostasis before further activities.
- Encourage 8 to 10 hours of sleep at night. Rest decreases oxygen demands and increases available energy for morning activities.
- Monitor vital signs before and after activity. Vital signs provide a measure of activity tolerance. Increased heart and respiratory rates or a change in blood pressure may indicate intolerance of the activity.
- Discontinue activity if any of the following occurs:
  a. Chest pain, breathlessness, or vertigo
  b. Palpitations or tachycardia that does not return to normal within 4 minutes of resting
  c. Bradycardia
  d. Tachypnea or dyspnea
  e. Decreased systolic blood pressure.

  These changes may signify cardiac decompensation resulting from insufficient oxygenation. The intensity, duration, or frequency of the activity needs to be reduced.
- Instruct the client not to smoke. Smoking causes vasoconstriction and increases carbon monoxide levels in the blood, interfering with tissue oxygenation.

Impaired Oral Mucous Membrane

Glossitis, inflammation of the tongue which may cause the tongue and lips to turn red, and cheilosis (fissures or cracks at the corners of the mouth) may occur with nutritional deficiencies of iron, folate, and vitamin B_{12}.

- Monitor the condition of the lips and tongue daily. Glossitis and cheilosis increase the risk for bleeding and infection and may require medical treatment. Pain and discomfort may interfere with oral intake, further worsening the nutritional deficiency.
- Use a mouthwash of saline, saltwater, or half-strength peroxide and water to rinse the mouth every 2–4 hours. Avoid alcohol-based mouthwashes. This cleanses and soothes oral mucous membranes. Alcohol-based mouthwashes further irritate and dry oral tissues.
- Provide frequent oral hygiene (after each meal and at bedtime) with a soft bristle toothbrush or sponge. Removing food debris from painful fissures promotes comfort. A soft toothbrush reduces irritation or bleeding of oral mucosa. Keeping the oral cavity clean also reduces the risk of infection.
- Apply a petroleum-based lubricating jelly or ointment to the lips after oral care. Lubricating ointment helps to retain moisture, facilitate healing, and protect the lips from other drying agents.
- Instruct the client to avoid hot, spicy, or acidic foods. Such foods may further irritate and dry mucous membranes.
- Encourage soft, cool, bland foods. Foods that are soothing to the mucous membranes promote comfort and help maintain adequate food and fluid intake. Minimizing oral pain may also promote compliance with oral care routines.
- Encourage the client to eat four to six small meals with high protein and vitamin content each day. Small, frequent meals may be better tolerated, increasing intake. Nutrient-rich meals promote healing of the mucous membranes.

Risk for Decreased Cardiac Output

Cardiac output may be affected by acute bleeding and volume loss or by heart failure resulting from severe anemia. Impaired tissue oxygenation leads to an increased respiratory rate and dyspnea.

- Monitor vital signs, breath sounds, and apical pulse. Increased cardiac workload can affect the blood pressure, heart, and respiratory rates. Increased blood flow can lead to heart murmur or abnormal heart sounds, such as S_3 or S_4. Tachypnea and dyspnea may affect the depth of respirations, alveolar ventilation, and blood and tissue oxygenation.
- Assess the client for pallor, cyanosis, and dependent edema. Blood is shunted to the vital organs, causing vasoconstriction of skin vessels. This, in addition to lower levels of hemoglobin, causes pallor. Cyanosis, especially of the lips and nail beds, indicates inadequate oxygenation of blood. Dependent edema occurs in response to right ventricular failure.
- Closely monitor the client for manifestations of anaphylaxis (e.g., urticaria, erythema or flushing, edema, wheezing, dyspnea, nausea and vomiting, and anxiety) when administering parenteral iron preparations, particularly

CLIENT TEACHING Home Care for the Client With Anemia

When preparing the client and family for home care, include the following topics:

- Nutritional strategies to address deficiencies
- Prescribed medications, vitamins, or mineral supplements and their appropriate use, intended effect, possible adverse effects, and interactions with food or other medications
- Energy conservation strategies
- Other recommended treatment measures and follow-up
- Inheritance patterns of the disorder
- Symptoms of crisis and manifestations to report to the physician if the anemia is genetically transmitted, such as sickle cell anemia.

In addition, provide referrals for counseling to facilitate decisions about pregnancy as indicated. Refer for nutritional assistance and teaching, home health care, or assistance with self-care and home maintenance activities as needed. Older adults with nutritional anemias may benefit from community services such as senior meals or Meals on Wheels.

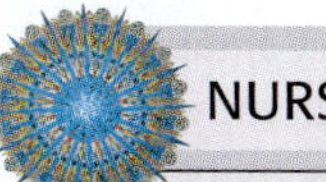

NURSING CARE PLAN A Client With Folic Acid Deficiency Anemia

Sheri Matthews is a 76-year-old widow who lives alone. She tells Lisa Apana, RN, the nurse in her care provider's office, that she liked to cook when her husband was alive, but preparing an entire meal just for herself seems senseless. She relates that her typical day's menu includes coffee for breakfast; a bologna sandwich and coffee for lunch; and a hot dog or two, a few cookies, and a glass of milk for dinner.

ASSESSMENT	DIAGNOSES	PLANNING
Mrs. Matthews's nursing history includes a 20-lb (9-kg) weight loss since her husband died 8 months ago. She states that she sometimes has heart palpitations and always feels weak. Physical assessment show the following: temperature 98.8°F (37.1°C), pulse 110 bpm, respirations 22/min, and BP 90/52 mmHg. Her skin is warm, pale, and dry. Diagnostic tests indicate folic acid deficiency anemia. Mrs. Matthews is started on an oral folic acid supplement and instructed about foods containing folic acid.	■ Activity Intolerance related to weakness secondary to decreased tissue oxygenation ■ Imbalanced Nutrition: Less Than Body Requirements related to lack of motivation to cook and understanding of nutritional needs, as manifested by weight loss of 20 lb and folic acid deficiency ■ Deficient Knowledge related to lack of information about a well-balanced diet and foods containing folic acid	■ The client will verbalize the importance of taking folic acid supplements and eating a balanced diet. ■ The client will gain at least 1 lb (0.45 kg) per week. ■ The client will return to her previous level of physical energy. ■ The client will consume a balanced diet, including foods containing folic acid.

IMPLEMENTATION

- Discuss foods required for a well-balanced diet as well as dietary sources of folic acid.
- Develop a dietary plan with Mrs. Matthews that includes food preferences and foods that are easy and quick to prepare.
- Discuss the importance of taking the folic acid supplement. Advise Mrs. Matthews to continue taking it even after she begins to feel better.
- Help Mrs. Matthews develop a schedule of activities that provides adequate rest and energy for cooking.

EVALUATION

Mrs. Matthews gained 1 lb (0.45 kg) during the first week of treatment. She has met with a nutritionist and has a better understanding of nutritional needs. She states that she can prepare hot meals when she schedules a rest period before and after lunch. Ms. Apana has provided written and verbal information about the folic acid supplement and diet. Mrs. Matthews verbalizes understanding, stating, "I will continue to take the folic acid until the doctor tells me to stop. I'm beginning to enjoy cooking again, now that I have a reason to cook!" Ms. Apana contacts the local senior services representative to determine if Mrs. Matthews is able to participate in the local Meals on Wheels program.

CRITICAL THINKING

1. What is the pathophysiologic basis for Mrs. Matthews's abnormal vital signs during her initial assessment?
2. Design a week's menu that includes foods high in folic acid.
3. Why was Mrs. Matthews placed on a folic acid supplement in addition to dietary modifications?
4. Why is the older adult at increased risk for developing folic acid deficiency anemia? Consider physiologic, economic, and social factors.

iron dextran. If observed, immediately notify the physician, and prepare to administer prescribed drugs, such as diphenhydramine (Benadryl) or epinephrine, as ordered. Institute cardiopulmonary resuscitation measures as necessary. Anaphylaxis, a systemic type I hypersensitivity (allergic) reaction, is a risk when administering parenteral iron preparations, iron dextran in particular. Anaphylaxis can lead to severe cardiopulmonary compromise, necessitating emergency measures to preserve life.

PRACTICE ALERT

Report signs of decreased cardiac output to the physician. Severe anemia can lead to heart failure, necessitating additional treatment.

Self-Care Deficit

Energy expenditures for activities of daily living (ADLs) may cause oxygen demands to exceed supply in the client with severe anemia. This can greatly impair the client's ability to maintain self-care. As a result, clients may need assistance with ADLS in order to maintain self-care and self-esteem as well as reduce cardiac workload.

- Assist the client with ADLs, such as bathing, grooming, and eating, as needed. Assistance decreases energy expenditures and tissue requirements for oxygen, reducing cardiac workload.
- Discuss the importance of rest periods before such activities as dressing. Rest reduces oxygen demand and cardiac workload. The person who is able to perform self-care in ADLs maintains independence, self-esteem, and morale.

Evaluation

Expected outcomes of nursing care include the following:

- The client's laboratory results manifest a normal RBC level.
- The client and/or family verbalizes understanding of the treatment regimen.
- The client consumes the recommended dietary intake.
- The client is free of side effects of oral iron therapy.
- The client is active and able to maintain normal activity levels.
- The pediatric client achieves appropriate growth and development milestones.

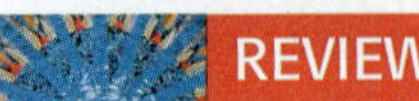

REVIEW Anemia

RELATE: LINK THE CONCEPTS

Linking the exemplar of Anemia with the concept of Development:

1. What effects will anemia have on the development of the school-age child?
2. A young woman is in her fifth month of pregnancy and develops severe anemia. What independent nursing interventions might you initiate to resolve this problem?

Linking the exemplar of Anemia with the concept of Family:

3. What nursing diagnoses does the nurse create for the mother of three who has anemia?
4. What affect will anemia have on family processes?

READY: GO TO COMPANION SKILLS MANUAL

- Monitoring intake and output
- Establishing intravenous infusions
- Assessing the skin
- Assessing the nails
- Assessing an apical pulse
- Assessing respirations
- Assessing blood pressure
- Assessing pulse oximeter
- Assessing the heart rate
- Assessing the respiratory rate

REFER: GO TO MYNURSINGKIT

REFLECT: CASE STUDY

Jessica Riley, 17 years old, is six months pregnant with her first child. The father of the baby has ended their relationship. Jessica tried living with her mother but they fought constantly. Jessica moves into her own apartment. She is working as a waitress to try to support herself and has plans to attend cosmetology school.

1. What preventative interventions would you plan for Jessica to reduce the risk of anemia?
2. How could the development of anemia impact Jessica and her fetus?
3. What nutrition counseling would you provide Jessica to reduce the risk of anemia?

3.2 BREAST CANCER

KEY TERMS

Breast cancer, *106*
Cachexia, *108*
Lumpectomy, *110*
Lymphedema, *110*
Metastasis, *106*
Modified radical mastectomy, *110*
Radical mastectomy, *110*
Segmental mastectomy, *110*
Simple mastectomy, *110*
Staging, *107*

BASIS FOR SELECTION OF EXEMPLAR

Centers for Disease Control and Prevention
Healthy People 2010
Institute of Medicine

LEARNING OUTCOMES

After reading about this exemplar, you will be able to:

1. Describe the pathophysiology, etiology, clinical manifestations, and direct and indirect causes of breast cancer.
2. Identify risk factors associated with breast cancer.
3. Illustrate the nursing process in providing culturally competent care across the life span for individuals with breast cancer.
4. Formulate priority nursing diagnoses appropriate for an individual with breast cancer.
5. Create a plan of care for individuals with breast cancer and their family members.
6. Assess expected outcomes for an individual with breast cancer.
7. Discuss therapies used in the collaborative care of an individual with breast cancer.
8. Employ evidence-based caring interventions for an individual with breast cancer.

OVERVIEW

Breast cancer is the unregulated growth of abnormal cells in breast tissue. It is the most commonly occurring cancer in women and is the second-leading cause of death in women in the United States. The American Cancer Society (ACS) (2006a) estimates that in this country, more than 212,000 women are diagnosed with breast cancer each year, and that approximately 41,000 women die from it annually.

PATHOPHYSIOLOGY AND ETIOLOGY

Cancer of the breast begins as a single, transformed cell and is often hormone dependent. These cancers are classified as noninvasive (in situ) or invasive, depending on the penetration of the tumor into surrounding tissue. Breast cancer may remain a noninvasive disease or an invasive disease without **metastasis** (spreading to other organs), for long periods of time.

Breast cancer may be categorized as carcinoma of the mammary ducts, carcinoma of mammary lobules, or sarcoma of the breast. Most breast cancers are adenocarcinomas and appear to arise in the terminal section of the breast ductal tissue. There are many histologic types of breast cancer, and only examples are described here. The most common type is infiltrating ductal carcinoma. Two atypical types of breast cancer are inflammatory carcinoma and Paget's disease. Inflammatory carcinoma of the breast, a systemic disease, is the most malignant form of breast cancer. Edema with dimpling of the skin that results in the skin looking like the peel of an orange (peau d'orange) is usually present. Paget's disease is a rare type of breast cancer involving infiltration of the nipple epithelium.

Breast cancer can metastasize to other sites through the bloodstream or lymphatic system. The common sites of metastasis of breast cancer are bone, brain, lung, liver, skin, and lymph nodes. **Staging** is a system of classifying cancer according to the size of the tumor, involvement of lymph nodes, and the presence or absence of distant metastasis (Table 3–3). The staging of the breast cancer provides important information for making decisions about treatment options and is also used as a basis for prognosis.

TABLE 3–3 **Staging of Breast Cancer**

STAGE	TUMOR	NODE	METASTASIS
0	Tis—Carcinoma in situ or Paget's disease of the nipple	N0—No regional lymph node metastasis	M0—No evidence of distant metastasis
I	T1—Tumor no larger than 2 cm	N0	M0
IIA	T0—No evidence of primary tumor	N1—Metastasis to movable ipsilateral	M0
	T1	axillary nodes	
	T2—Tumor no larger than 5 cm	N0	M0
IIB	T2	N1	M0
	T3—Tumor larger than 5 cm	N0	M0
IIIA	T0	N2—Metastasis to ipsilateral fixed	M0
	T1	axillary nodes	
	T2		
	T3	N1	M0
		N2	M0
IIIB	T4—Tumor of any size with direct extension to chest wall or skin	Any N	M0
	Any T	N3—Metastasis to ipsilateral internal mammary lymph nodes	M0
IV	Any T	N0 and N1	M1—Distant metastasis

Etiology

Possible causes of breast cancer include environmental, hormonal, reproductive, and hereditary factors. Two breast cancer susceptibility genes have been identified: *BRCA1* on chromosome 17 and *BRCA2* on chromosome 13. These genes may be responsible for the approximately 10% of women with hereditary breast cancer, with genetic mutations causing up to 80% of breast cancer in women younger than 50 years. A woman with identified mutations in *BRCA1*, which is known to be involved in tumor suppression, has a lifetime risk of 56–85% for breast cancer and also has an increased risk for ovarian cancer (Porth, 2005). Mutations of a tumor suppressor gene are also linked to increased risk for breast cancer.

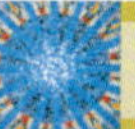

DEVELOPMENTAL CONSIDERATIONS **Older Women With Breast Cancer**

- Although the incidence of breast cancer is increasing among premenopausal women, it is still primarily a disease of older women. However, the needs of older women with breast cancer have been inadequately addressed in the professional literature and popular media.
- Women between the ages of 50 and 65 are the group most likely to benefit from annual screening mammography, yet many women in this age group have never had a mammogram. Failure of physicians to refer older women for mammography is the reason most frequently cited for this statistic; nurse practitioners and female physicians are more likely to refer women for mammography. In addition, promotional campaigns for mammography send a confusing message by showing images of women in their 20s and 30s, for whom mammography is largely ineffective, rather than women in older age groups who are more likely to benefit from mammography.
- For too long, mastectomy was perceived as the only treatment option open to most older women with breast cancer, even those with early-stage disease. Slowly, that perception is changing as breast-conservation treatment gains greater acceptance. The choice of surgical treatment, particularly for older women, is highly individual. Many older women wish to preserve their breasts.
- Although older women with breast cancer may experience coexisting chronic illnesses and impaired physical function, research suggests that they show lower levels of emotional distress compared with younger women. Obviously, the need for services such as personal care, shopping, housekeeping, and transportation increases as the ages of both the woman and the caregiver increase.

Risk Factors

Of the various kinds of risk factors for breast cancer, some can be changed and some cannot. Those that cannot be changed (ACS, 2006a) are the following:

- *Age and gender.* Women are 100 times more likely to have breast cancer than men, and this risk increases with age.
- *Genetic risk factors.* As previously described.
- *Family history of breast cancer.* This includes relatives from either the maternal or paternal side of the family. Having a first-degree relative (mother, sister, or daughter) with breast cancer approximately doubles a person's risk, and having two first-degree relatives increases it fivefold. Having a male family member with breast cancer also poses an increased risk.
- *Personal history of breast cancer.* A woman with cancer in one breast has a three- to fivefold increase in risk for developing a new cancer in the other breast or in a different part of the same breast.
- *Previous breast biopsy.* If earlier breast biopsy specimens were diagnosed as proliferative, then breast disease without atypical hyperplasia increases risk by 1.5- to 2-fold. A previous biopsy result of atypical hyperplasia increases risk by four- to fivefold.
- *Previous chest irradiation.* Radiation of the chest as a child or young woman for other cancer (e.g., Hodgkin's disease) significantly increases the risk.
- *Menstrual history.* Women who begin menstruating before the age of 12 or who have menopause after the age of 50 are at a slightly higher risk.

Lifestyle factors that are associated with risk for breast cancer include using oral contraceptives, not having children or having them after the age of 30, using hormone replacement therapy for more than 5 years, not breast-feeding, drinking alcohol (especially two to five drinks daily), obesity, high-fat diets, physical inactivity, and (possibly) environmental pollution. Breast-feeding, moderate or vigorous physical activity, and maintaining a healthy body weight lower a person's risk for breast cancer.

FOCUS ON DIVERSITY AND CULTURE
Breast Cancer Incidence and Mortality in Women

- Breast cancer is more prevalent in African American women up to the age of 40.
- Breast cancer is more prevalent in white women older than 40 years.
- Asian, Hispanic, and Native American women have a lower risk of developing breast cancer.
- African American women are more likely to die from the cancer because they are often diagnosed at an advanced stage.

CLINICAL MANIFESTATIONS

The manifestations of breast cancer may include a nontender lump in the breast (most often in the upper outer quadrant, the area with the most glandular tissue), abnormal nipple discharge, a rash around the nipple area, nipple retraction, dimpling of the skin, or a change in the position of the nipple (Box 3–6). There may also be nipple pain, scaliness, ulceration, skin irritation, or discharge. Breast cancer is usually painless, but some women report a burning or stinging sensation. Many women with breast cancer have no manifestations, and their tumors are detected by

CLINICAL MANIFESTATIONS AND THERAPIES **Breast Cancer**

ETIOLOGY	CLINICAL MANIFESTATION	CLINICAL THERAPIES
Lymphedema (accumulation of fluid in the soft tissues of the arm) may occur following radical mastectomy secondary to removal of axillary lymph nodes.	Swelling of the arm and hand on the side of the mastectomy May be acute, temporary, and mild if occurring immediately postoperative; acute and painful if occurring 4–6 weeks postoperative; or more commonly, chronic and painless if occurring 18–24 months after surgery	■ Exercise ■ Customized compression sleeve ■ Arm pump ■ Diet and weight control ■ Elevation of the arm ■ Prevention of infection ■ Avoidance of invasive procedures on affected arm
Cachexia is physical wasting from weight loss and loss of muscle mass from rapid growth and reproduction of cancer cells and their need for increased nutrients.	Weight loss, fatigue, weakness, loss of strength, activity intolerance, and constipation are a few of the possible manifestations	■ Nutritional counseling ■ Increased caloric intake ■ Periods of rest and activity ■ Monitoring weight ■ Monitoring intake and output
Memory loss and difficulty concentrating may follow treatment with chemotherapy (sometimes referred to as chemo-brain).	Memory loss, difficulty focusing on tasks, changes in mood and affect, as well as fatigue Generally lasts for 1–2 years after completing treatment	■ Warning clients in advance of possible occurrence, because it can be very frightening to clients ■ Recommendation of memory aids (e.g., making notes) ■ Providing emotional support to clients

Box 3–6 Manifestations of Breast Cancer

- Breast mass or thickening
- Unusual lump in the underarm or above the collarbone
- Persistent skin rash near the nipple area
- Flaking or eruption near the nipple
- Dimpling, pulling, or retraction in an area of the breast
- Nipple discharge
- Change in nipple position
- Burning, stinging, or pricking sensation

mammography, which is discussed in detail in Appendix B. However, most breast cancers are found by the women themselves during breast self-examination (BSE) or a shower, or by their partners during sexual activity.

COLLABORATION

Diagnosis of breast cancer begins with detection of the tumor through mammography, clinical examination, or breast self-examination (Box 3–7). Any palpable mass requires evaluation. Once the diagnosis is made, a number of treatment options are available. The choice of treatment depends on several factors, such as the stage of the cancer, the age of the woman, and the woman's preferences.

Box 3–7 Instructions for Breast Self-Examination

- Lie down on your back, and place your right arm behind your head. (BSE should be done while lying down, because this position spreads breast tissue evenly over the chest wall, making it easier to feel all the breast tissue.)
- Use the finger pads of the middle fingers on your left hand to feel for lumps in the right breast. Use overlapping, dime-sized, circular motions of the finger pads to feel the breast tissue.
- Use three different levels of pressure to feel all the breast tissue. Light pressure is needed to feel the tissue closest to the skin, medium pressure to feel a little deeper, and firm pressure to feel the tissue closest to the chest and ribs. A firm ridge in the lower curve of each breast is normal. Use each pressure level to feel the breast tissue before moving on to the next spot.
- Move around the breast in an up-and-down pattern, starting at an imaginary line drawn straight down your side from the underarm and moving across the breast to the middle of the chest bone (sternum, breastbone). Be sure to check the entire breast area before going down until you feel only ribs and up to the neck or collar bone.
- Repeat the exam on your left breast, using the finger pads of your right hand.
- Stand in front of the mirror with your hands pressing firmly down on your hips. Look at your breasts for any changes in size, shape, contour, or dimpling.
- Examine your underarm while sitting or standing and with your arm only slightly raised.
- If you find any changes, see your health care provider as soon as possible.

Diagnostic Tests

Early detection of breast cancer is possible with clinical breast examination and mammography. Both types of screening are valuable, but mammography can buy a client precious time. Tumors may be present as many as 8–10 years before they can be detected by palpation, and mammography can detect a tumor up to 2 years before it reaches palpable size.

Although controversy exists about the ability of screening mammography to improve mortality rates for women under the age of 50, the ACS recommends annual mammograms beginning at age 40 and clinical breast examination at least every 3 years for women in their 20s and 30s.

Other diagnostic tests include a percutaneous needle biopsy (to define a cystic mass or fibrocystic changes and provide specimens for cytologic examination) and a breast biopsy once a suspicious lump is identified. In aspiration biopsy or fine-needle aspiration biopsy, a needle is used to remove cells or fluid from the breast lesion (Figure 3–6 ■). In many facilities, fine-needle aspiration biopsies are performed using a stereotactic biopsy device; mammography and a computer are used to guide the needle.

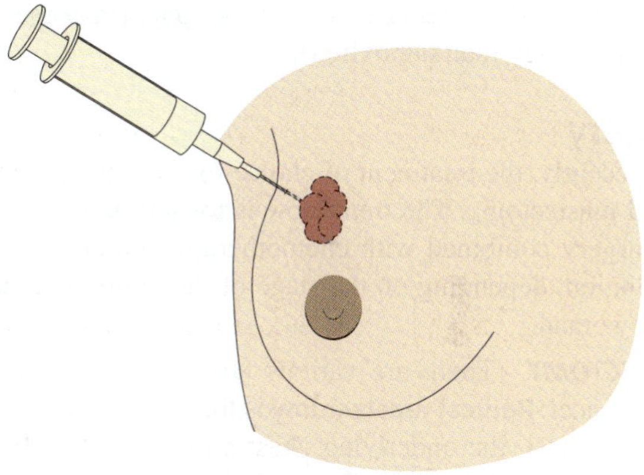

A Aspiration biopsy

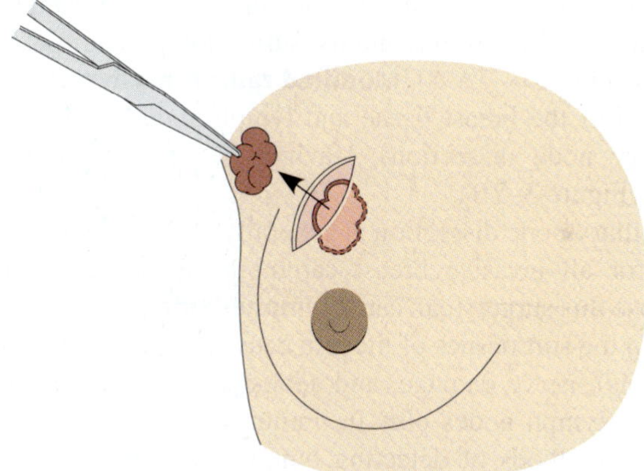

B Excisional biopsy

Figure 3–6 ■ Types of breast biopsy. *A*, In an aspiration biopsy, a needle is used to aspirate fluid or tissue from the breast. *B*, In an excisional biopsy, tissue from the breast lesion is removed surgically.

Pharmacologic Therapies

Tamoxifen citrate (Nolvadex) is an oral medication that interferes with estrogen activity. It is used to treat advanced breast cancer, as an adjuvant for early-stage breast cancer, and as a preventive treatment in women at high risk for developing breast cancer.

Immunotherapy with trastuzumab (Herceptin) is used to stop the growth of breast tumors that express the HER2/neu receptor (which binds an epidermal growth factor that contributes to cancer cell growth) on their cell surface. This drug is a recombinant DNA-derived monoclonal antibody that binds to the receptor, inhibiting tumor cell proliferation.

Chemotherapy has become the standard of care for the majority of breast cancer cases with axillary node involvement. In late metastatic disease, chemotherapy becomes the primary treatment to prolong the woman's life. Adjuvant (additional) systemic therapy following primary treatment for early-stage breast cancer refers to the administration of chemotherapy and other pharmacologic agents. This type of therapy has been widely studied; its use reduces both the rate of recurrence and the rate of death from breast cancer. For example, the drug bevacizumab, when combined with chemotherapy to treat metastatic breast cancer, has extended cancer-free survival; letrozole (an aromatase inhibitor) has reduced the risk of recurrence after surgery (in some cases more effectively than tamoxifen).

Surgery

Until recently, the treatment of choice for breast cancer was a radical mastectomy. The trend now is toward more conservative surgery combined with chemotherapy, hormone therapy, or radiation, depending on the stage of the tumor and the age of the woman.

MASTECTOMY There are various types of mastectomy for breast cancer. **Radical mastectomy** is the removal of the entire affected breast, the underlying chest muscles, and the lymph nodes under the arms. **Simple mastectomy** is the removal of the complete breast only. **Segmental mastectomy** (also referred to as breast conservation surgery or lumpectomy) is the removal of the tumor and the surrounding margin of breast tissues (Figure 3–7A ■). **Modified radical mastectomy** is the removal of the breast tissue and lymph nodes under the arm (axillary node dissection), leaving the chest wall muscles intact (Figure 3–7B).

Axillary node dissection is generally performed during surgery for all invasive breast carcinoma to stage the tumor. Because this surgery can cause **lymphedema** (accumulation of fluid in the soft tissues of the arm caused by removal of lymph channels), nerve damage, and adhesions, and because of the role the lymph nodes play in immune system function, nonsurgical methods of detecting lymph node involvement now are being used. Sentinel node biopsy before a node dissection is conducted by injecting a radioactive substance or dye into the region of the tumor. The dye is carried to the first (sentinel) lymph node to receive lymph from the tumor is therefore be the node most likely to contain cancer cells (if the cancer has metastasized). If the sentinel node is positive, more nodes are removed. If the sentinel node is negative, further node evaluation is usually not indicated.

LUMPECTOMY Breast conservation surgery (**lumpectomy**) may be defined as excision of the primary tumor and adjacent breast tissue followed by radiation therapy. Many women are candidates for this procedure; however, some women, such as those who have multicentric breast neoplasms and those who have large tumors in relation to their breast size, are unsuitable candidates. Selection of women for this procedure is guided by the need for local control of the lesion, cosmetic results, and personal preference.

BREAST RECONSTRUCTION After a mastectomy, some women may choose to have their breast reconstructed. They report that surgical reconstruction of the breast simplifies their

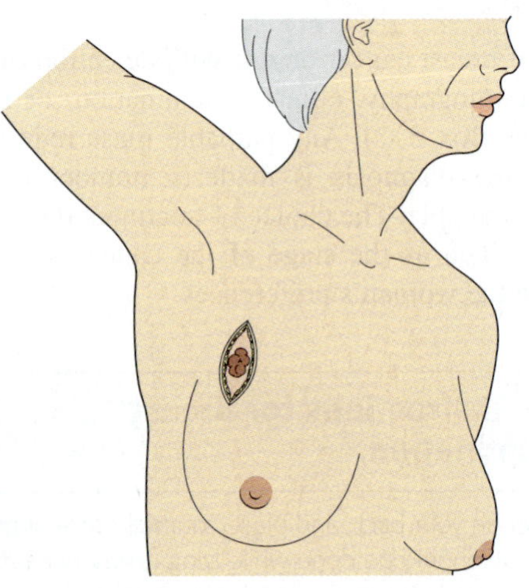

A Lumpectomy

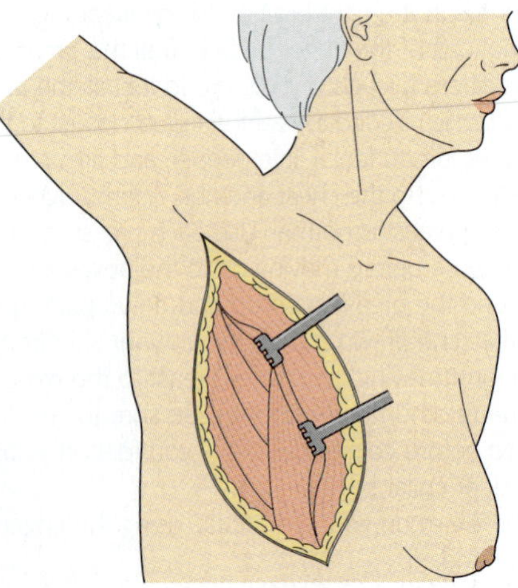

B Modified radical mastectomy

Figure 3–7 ■ Types of mastectomy. *A*, In a lumpectomy, only the tumor and a small margin of surrounding tissue are removed. *B*, In a modified radical mastectomy, all breast tissue and the underarm lymph nodes are removed, but the underlying muscles remain.

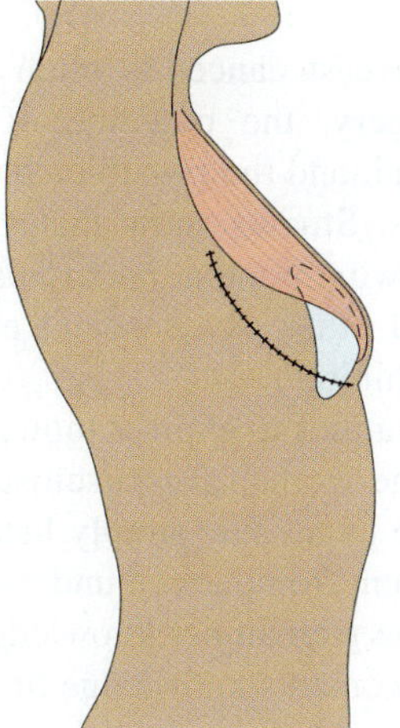

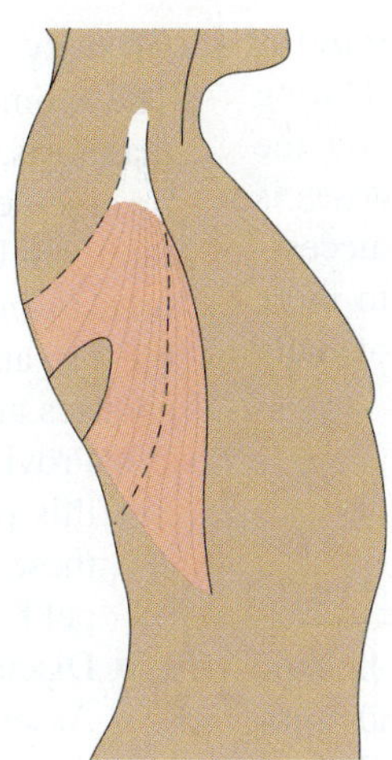

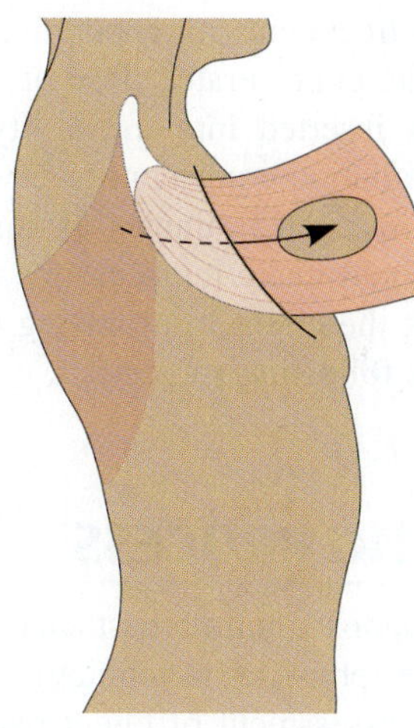

A Implant **B** Latissimus dorsi musculocutaneous flap

Figure 3–8 ■ Types of breast reconstruction surgeries. *A*, A breast implant is inserted under the pectoris muscle. *B*, Autogenous procedurestransfera flap of skin, muscle, and fat from the donor site on the woman's body to the mastectomy site. The most frequently used donor muscle sites are the latissimus dorsi and the rectus abdominis (the TRAM flap).

lives and restores a sense of body integrity. Other women choose to use a removable breast prosthesis, and some women are comfortable without reconstruction or a prosthesis.

Breast reconstruction may be performed at the time of the mastectomy or at any time thereafter, depending on the woman's preference. A number of procedures may be used for the breast reconstruction (Figure 3–8 ■). These include placement of a submuscular implant, use of a tissue expander followed by an implant, transposition of muscle and blood supply from the abdomen or back, or (most often) using the transverse rectus abdominis myocutaneous free-tissue flap.

Radiation Therapy

Radiation therapy typically follows breast cancer surgery to destroy any remaining cancer cells that could cause recurrence or metastasis. If a tumor is unusually large, radiation may be used to shrink the tumor before surgery. Radiation therapy is most commonly used in combination with lumpectomy for early-stage (stage I or II) breast cancer. Palliative radiation therapy is also used to treat chest wall recurrences and some bone metastases to help control pain and prevent fractures. Radiation therapy is administered by means of an external beam or tissue implants.

EVIDENCE-BASED PRACTICE Improving Diagnosis and Treatment of African American Women With Breast Cancer

Clinical Question

Despite efforts to improve both the diagnosis and treatment of women with breast cancer, African American women die more often from breast cancer than any other group. It is believed that this statistic is the result of African American women's advanced stage of disease at diagnosis, primarily because of a delay in seeking treatment.

Evidence

Bradley (2005) conducted a study to examine the variables affecting delay in seeking treatment including the possibility that worry about manifestations of breast cancer in African American women might cause these women to delay seeking treatment. The research found that, although delay in some women does exist, one cannot assume that all African American women delay seeking treatment. The researcher recommended that the relationship between worry and delaying treatment for breast cancer in African American women be further studied.

Best Practice

Nurses must examine multiple factors when considering what may or may not influence African American women to delay seeking diagnosis and treatment for breast cancer. These factors include biologic characteristics and intra- and intercultural differences and similarities as well as perceptions and health beliefs. It is important that nurses do not assume that a delay in seeking care exists, but rather make assessments and design interventions based on consideration of both individual and group cultural differences.

Critical Thinking

1. What barriers to breast cancer screening in women of all races can you identify? Do you think these barriers differ based on culture, race, or socioeconomic level? Why, or why not?
2. Are there barriers to breast cancer screening that might be unique to African American women? To Hispanic women? To Asian American women?
3. What type of questions would you include in a health assessment to identify women who may be worried about breast cancer but have not sought diagnosis?

A new radiation treatment (intraoperative radiotherapy) is provided by a single, concentrated dose of radiation. During surgery, a probe is inserted into the cavity created by the lumpectomy, and radiation equivalent to 6 weeks of doses is emitted for approximately 25 minutes. If this proves successful, the treatment could make lumpectomy available to more women and prevent the client from having 6 weeks of daily radiation treatments following surgery.

NURSING PROCESS

Clients diagnosed with breast cancer require holistic care which addresses physical, psychologic, social, and spiritual needs. Careful assessment of client response to therapy will improve the care planning process.

Assessment

Collect the following data through the health history and physical examination:

- *Health history.* Family history of breast cancer, breast changes, nipple discharge, use of hormone replacement therapy, personal history of breast cancer, previous diagnostic tests and treatment for cancer, menstrual history, pregnancies, alcohol intake, physical activity, dietary history
- *Physical assessment.* Height and weight, breasts, lymph glands.

Further focused assessments are described in the Implementation section that follows.

Diagnosis

Although each woman has individual needs, nursing diagnoses before surgery are concerned with the following:

- Anxiety
- Decisional Conflict
- Grief
- Risk for Infection
- Risk for Injury
- Disturbed Body Image over the loss of a breast.

Plan

Goals for treatment may include the following:

- The client will express feelings regarding diagnosis, treatment, and prognosis.
- The client will not experience infection.
- The client will make informed treatment decisions.
- The family and significant others will provide appropriate support for client.

Implementation

Although each woman has individual needs, nursing diagnoses before surgery are concerned with anxiety, decisional conflict, grief, risk for infection, risk for injury, and disturbed body image over the loss of a breast.

Anxiety

The woman with breast cancer is often anxious about the diagnosis, the surgery, the outcome of surgery if nodal involvement is found, and the possible changes in sexual and family relationships. Studies show that young women with breast cancer, a growing population, are particularly vulnerable for anxiety and other psychosocial effects, as are their spouses and their children.

- Provide opportunities to express thoughts and feelings. In this process, the woman can disclose her fears. During these times, the nurse may simply listen, educate, or dispel fears that stem from lack of understanding.
- Discuss with the woman her knowledge of breast cancer. Assessing the woman's knowledge of breast cancer helps the nurse plan more effective teaching.
- Encourage discussion relating to immediate concerns about resuming her life at home and the changes she must make. Anticipatory guidance can help plan for and cope with changes in her life and relationships.
- Explain the surgical procedure, including information about preoperative medications, anesthesia, and recovery. Knowing what to expect helps decrease anxiety.
- Explain that it is normal to have decreased sensation in the surgical area. Severed or damaged nerves reduce sensation.

Decisional Conflict

The woman with breast cancer must make life-changing decisions about treatment within a relatively brief and highly stressful time. Her age, menopausal status, and the stage of cancer are only some of the factors that affect her decisions. Culture, values, lifestyle, socioeconomic status, and self-esteem also are involved.

- Provide an opportunity for the woman to ask questions; answer questions as simply and directly as possible. Pay attention to body language. Make, but do not force, eye contact. During this time, the woman can process information and make informed decisions.
- Focus on immediate concerns, and provide up-to-date, written material for the woman to review. Written material provides easy reference to information not processed immediately because of anxiety and stress.
- Listen to the woman in a nonjudgmental manner during her decision-making process. Nonjudgmental, empathic listening helps the woman process information and make informed decisions. Only she knows the context of her life.
- If the woman wishes, provide opportunities for her to meet with other women who have had breast cancer surgery. Not all women are ready to meet others in their situation, but opening the door to this resource is appropriate. The woman may choose to talk with these women after the surgery.
- Facilitate a team approach with the surgeon, anesthesiologist, oncologist, plastic surgeon, and other health professionals. Being the woman's advocate during this time of anxiety and decision making reduces the stress of coordinating multiple health care provider schedules.

Grief

Breast surgery, even lumpectomy, alters the appearance of the breast. This loss is expressed through grief. The nurse provides supportive care for the client who is grieving the loss of her breast.

- Listen attentively to expressions of grief, and watch for nonverbal cues (e.g., failure to make eye contact, crying, and silence). Not all women will express grief clearly; sometimes unspoken grief is the most painful. Grief is relieved only when expressed in a nonthreatening environment.
- Allow time to interact, and do not rush interactions. Taking time to be with the woman communicates caring.
- Explain that it is normal to have periods of depression, anger, and denial after breast surgery. All these feelings are appropriate expressions of grief.
- If the woman wishes to do so, involve the partner in helping the woman cope with her loss. Remember that the partner may also be grieving. Not all women want to share their grief, and not all partners are interested and supportive.

Risk for Infection

Like any surgical client, the woman who has breast surgery is at risk for infection. Removal of lymph nodes and the presence of a draining wound increase the risk.

- Assess the surgical dressings for bleeding, drainage, color, and odor every 4 hours for 24 hours, and document your findings. Circle any visible bleeding and drainage on the dressing as a baseline for subsequent assessment. Excessive bleeding or drainage signals postoperative complications that may require emergency attention.
- Observe the incision and IV sites for pain, redness, swelling, and drainage. Assess the drainage system for patency and adequate suction; note the color and amount of drainage. Careful observation for any signs of infection is essential, because the woman's immune system is compromised. IV catheters should be placed on the uninvolved side only.
- Change dressings and IV tubing using aseptic technique. Moist dressings and IV tubing provide sites for bacterial growth. Routine dressing and IV tubing changes using aseptic technique reduce the risk for infection.
- Encourage a protein-rich diet. Discuss the woman's nutritional status with the dietitian, and request a consultation for the woman. Adequate nutrition promotes healing and boosts the immune system.
- Teach the woman how to care for the drainage system, if present (i.e., clean the site, empty the device, and record the amount, color, and type of drainage). The woman is often discharged before removal of the drainage system and dressings and needs teaching to provide self-care.
- At discharge, teach the woman to watch for and report to her health care provider the manifestations of infection: fever, redness or hardness at the surgical site, or purulent drainage. Any of these manifestations should be reported to the physician/surgeon. Knowing the signs and symptoms of infection prepares the woman to seek prompt treatment if infection occurs.
- Explain that the woman may experience scaling, flaking, dryness, itching, rash, or dry desquamation of the skin, particularly after radiation therapy. Impaired skin integrity increases the risk of infection.
- Tell the woman to avoid deodorants and talcum powder on the affected side until the incision is completely healed. These substances may irritate the skin and impede healing.

Risk for Injury

Removal of the lymph nodes puts the woman at risk for injury and long-term complications, such as lymphedema and infection.

- When obtaining blood pressure and starting IVs, use the nonsurgical side. Compression of the arm on the surgical side may cause lymphedema.

CLIENT TEACHING **Breast Cancer**

- Controversy exists about the health effects of silicone. While there is no conclusive evidence that silicone implants induce cancer or autoimmune disease, they are associated with hardening and pain caused by contracture of the capsule around the implant. The implant may rupture, releasing silicone gel, or infection may occur. Saline-filled breast implants may be an alternative.
- Reconstruction can be done immediately after a mastectomy or at any time later on. Some surgeons believe that delayed reconstruction offers better cosmetic results.
- Reconstructive surgery can create a natural-looking breast that makes clothes fit better. Since it has no nerve endings, however, the reconstructed breast has no feeling or sensations.
- If a simple mastectomy is done, an implant approximately the same size as the other breast is placed under the pectoral muscle on the operative side. This creates a breast mound that closely resembles the natural breast in shape and softness. If the implant is placed over the pectoral muscle, a high degree of firmness may occur.
- With a simple mastectomy or modified radical mastectomy, a tissue expander may be used to replace the breast. The tissue expander is placed under the pectoral muscle and gradually expanded with saline injections every 2–3 weeks to stretch the overlying skin and create a pocket. After a period of time, usually 1–2 months, the tissue expander is exchanged for a saline implant.
- With more extensive surgery, such as radical mastectomy, a flap of skin, fat, or muscle is transferred from a donor site to the operative area. A new nipple may be created by using tissue from the opposite nipple or from the inner thigh.
- Reconstructive surgery may require multiple surgeries, including all the risks associated with anesthesia. As the complexity of the procedures increases, so does the risk of complications, such as infection.
- To decrease the risk of a fibrous capsule forming around the implant, it is important to perform breast massage as instructed.

NURSING CARE PLAN **A Woman With Breast Cancer**

Rachel Clemments is a 42-year-old mother of two: Sarah, age 12, and Jennifer, age 18. Because of a family history of breast cancer, she has been closely monitored (annual mammograms and clinical breast examination, monthly BSE, a needle aspiration biopsy with negative findings) for 4 years before her diagnosis. Mrs. Clemments discovers a lump in her left breast during her monthly BSE. An incisional biopsy reveals invasive lobular carcinoma in the left breast. Mrs. Clemments is debating whether to have reconstructive breast surgery. One of her greatest concerns is how her illness will affect her ability to support and care for her daughters. The breast cancer diagnosis seems part of the family legacy. She wonders, "When will it happen to Jennifer? To Sarah?"

ASSESSMENT

During the history, Laura Nelson, RN, the nurse admitting Mrs. Clemments, learns that her mother, two of her aunts, and one sister had been diagnosed with breast cancer. Her mother and one of the aunts died before age 45. Physical assessment findings include temperature 98.5°F (37.0°C), BP 110/62 mmHg, pulse 65 bpm, and respirations 14/min. Her weight is 120 lb (54 kg); she is 66 inches (168 cm) tall. Modified radical mastectomy is performed. Histologic examination shows a 3-cm tumor; axillary node dissection shows that 4 of 16 lymph nodes are positive.

DIAGNOSES

- Risk for Infection related to surgical incision
- Acute Pain related to surgery
- Disturbed Body Image related to loss of breast
- Decisional Conflict About Treatment related to concerns about risks and benefits
- Fear related to disease process/prognosis

PLANNING

- The client will remain free of infection.
- The client will experience minimal pain or discomfort during her recovery.
- The client will maintain a positive body image, regardless of her decision about reconstruction.
- The client will evaluate the treatment options in relation to personal values and decide on a course of action.
- The client will identify the sources of her fear and demonstrate behaviors that may reduce fears.

IMPLEMENTATION

- Teach the client about handwashing and wound care.
- Assess her pain tolerance, and administer analgesics as prescribed.
- Teach her to use caution when moving the arm on the operated side, to avoid lifting heavy objects, and to wear gloves when gardening.
- Encourage her to discuss her thoughts and feelings about her body changes.
- Suggest that she talk with a Reach to Recovery volunteer about her thoughts and feelings.
- Assess her interest in spiritual/religious support, and refer if appropriate.
- Discuss the use of a temporary prosthesis and, later, the fitting of a permanent prosthesis (6–8 weeks after surgery), the need to be fitted by an experienced person, and insurance reimbursement for the prosthesis.
- Discuss the possibility of attending a breast cancer support group where she can draw on the experiences of other women who have undergone mastectomy, chemotherapy, or radiation.
- Encourage her to verbalize her fears about her own prognosis and about her daughters' future risks for breast cancer; assess the need/interest for referral to psychologic counseling.

EVALUATION

At discharge, Mrs. Clemments has no signs of physical complications and is looking forward to being at home with her daughters as temporary caregivers. Mrs. Clemments met with a Reach to Recovery volunteer who brought her a temporary prosthesis and booklets about postmastectomy exercises, chemotherapy, and breast reconstruction. The volunteer also referred her to a local cancer support group. Mrs. Clemments has talked about her concerns related to breast reconstruction. "I want to avoid anything that would increase the risk of complications. The possibility of recurrence and my fear for my daughters' future health are more than enough to worry about."

CRITICAL THINKING

1. What role could genetic counseling play in helping Mrs. Clemments and her daughters better understand the daughters' risks for breast cancer?
2. Describe the types of mastectomies and their implications for nursing care.
3. What medications might help minimize the side effects of chemotherapy?
4. Develop a plan of care for Mrs. Clemments for the nursing diagnosis disturbed sleep pattern.

the elbow. Elevating the arm permits drainage, prevents swelling, and promotes circulation.

- Encourage range-of-motion exercises in the affected arm. Exercise helps develop collateral drainage.
- Explain that lymphedema massage and an elastic compression bandage may help control the swelling after the woman has recovered from surgery. It is important that women know about the resources available after recovery.

Disturbed Body Image

Breast surgery can change the woman's body image. The surgical changes may be compounded by weight gain and other side effects of chemotherapy or hormone therapy. Self-esteem also affects adjustment to a changed body image.

- Assess how the woman views her body. Discuss with the woman what image of herself she had before surgery. Self-image is related to self-esteem. Discuss whether her self-image has changed.
- Explain that redness and swelling in the scar will fade with time. Knowledge that the scar will fade may give the woman a more realistic view of the changes.
- Include the partner and family if possible when discussing the plan of care and ADLs. Request consultation with a psychologist or other professional if the woman is interested. Discussion with the partner and family can facilitate the woman's emotional healing process.
- Offer pamphlets and suggest books and videos that might increase knowledge about what lies ahead. Knowing what to expect can help the woman cope.
- Encourage the woman to look at her incision when she feels ready; often, the reality is not as frightening as what the woman had imagined. Explain that it is normal to be afraid to look. Reassurance that her behavior is normal decreases anxiety.
- If the woman is interested in breast reconstruction, provide written material and encourage her to talk with a plastic surgeon and with women who have had reconstruction. It is important for the woman to be fully knowledgeable about available options to make an informed decision.

PRACTICE ALERT

Offer referral to support groups with women experiencing similar problems. Some women may prefer one-on-one counseling.

Evaluation

Clients are evaluated for expected outcomes based on specific client needs and care planning. Potential outcomes may include the following:

- The client experiences no complications resulting from treatment.
- Side effects from medications are minimized.
- Pain is managed to allow the client to rest and perform essential ADLs.

REVIEW Breast Cancer

RELATE: LINK THE CONCEPTS

Linking the exemplar of Breast Cancer with the concept of Advocacy:

1. How might the nurse advocate for the prevention of breast cancer or its early detection?
2. What role can the nurse play in advocating to make men more aware of the role they can play in breast cancer prevention and early detection?

Linking the exemplar Breast Cancer with the concept of Sexuality:

3. The client, preparing for a radical mastectomy, says, "My husband says if I only have one breast I am only ½ a woman." How can you help this woman adapt to the perceived change in her femininity?
4. Is the impact on a client's sexuality completely reversed if she has plastic surgery to repair the appearance of the breast? Is plastic surgery always an option? Explain your answer.

READY: GO TO COMPANION SKILLS MANUAL

- Monitoring intake and output
- Establishing intravenous infusions
- Maintaining intravenous infusions
- Changing gown for a client with IV
- Performing surgical and antisepsis
- Preparing the client for surgery
- Preparing for a dressing change using individual supplies
- Changing a sterile dressing
- Assessing the skin
- Assessing the client in pain
- Assessing the breasts and axillae

REFER: GO TO MYNURSINGKIT

REFLECT: CASE STUDY

Judy Franklin, 22 years old, has just graduated from college and is about to start a job as a graphic arts designer in a large marketing company. Judy is also planning her wedding to George six months from now. She found a lump in her left breast during self-exam and has come to the doctor for an initial consultation. During the assessment, the nurse learns Judy has not told her fiancée about her findings. Judy will not make eye contact with the nurse and appears distracted during the interview.

1. What nursing diagnoses would be appropriate for Judy?
2. How might you assist Judy to inform her fiancé if the lump is determined to be a malignant tumor?
3. What support interventions would you initiate to help Judy as she waits for the results of diagnostic testing to determine the cause of the lump?

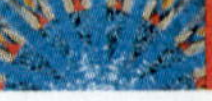

3.3 CANCER

KEY TERMS

BASIS FOR SELECTION OF EXEMPLAR

Centers for Disease Control and Prevention
Healthy People 2010
Institute of Medicine

LEARNING OUTCOMES

After reading about this exemplar, you will be able to:

1. Describe the pathophysiology, etiology, clinical manifestations, and direct and indirect causes of cancer.
2. Identify risk factors associated with cancer.
3. Illustrate the nursing process in providing culturally competent care across the life span for individuals with cancer.
4. Formulate priority nursing diagnoses appropriate for an individual with cancer.
5. Create a plan of care for individuals with cancer and their family members.
6. Assess expected outcomes for an individual with cancer.
7. Discuss therapies used in the collaborative care of an individual with cancer.
8. Employ evidence-based caring interventions for an individual with cancer.

OVERVIEW

Cancer refers to a group of complex diseases whose manifestations depend on which body system is affected and the type of cells involved. It is marked by uncontrolled growth and the spread of abnormal cells. Cancer can affect people of any age, gender, ethnicity, or geographic region. Although the incidence and mortality rates of cancer have continued to decline since 1990, it remains one of the most feared diseases. Even the suggestion of a cancer diagnosis often evokes feelings of hopelessness and helplessness.

Cancer results when normal cells mutate into abnormal, deviant cells that then perpetuate within the body. Cancer can affect any body tissue. Nursing care of the client with cancer is holistic and comprehensive, focusing on cancer not as one disease but as a constellation of many diseases. The nurse recognizes that cancer is a disruptive and life-threatening process that affects the whole person and any significant others. Nursing interventions are based on the understanding that cancer is a chronic disease with acute episodes, that the client is often treated in the home, and that the client is usually treated with a combination of therapeutic modalities. Equally important, the nurse recognizes that caring for the client with cancer involves prevention, early detection, treatment, supportive care, long-term follow-up, and, for some clients, end-of-life care (Oncology Nursing Society, 2006).

Oncology is the study of cancer. The term is derived from the Greek word *oncoma* ("bulk"). Oncologists specialize in caring for clients with cancer; they may be medical doctors, surgeons, radiologists, immunologists, or researchers. The oncology nurse has received specialized training in cancer care and treatment and is an important and significant member of the oncology team. Oncology nurses have special skills in assisting the client and family with the psychosocial issues associated with cancer and terminal illness. Collaboration among health care professionals (e.g., surgeons, oncologists, nurses, social workers) ensures the most effective care and treatment for the client with cancer.

FOCUS ON DIVERSITY AND CULTURE Risk and Incidence of Cancer

- The incidence and mortality rates for all types of cancer are 35–39% lower in Hispanics.
- The incidence of cervical, stomach, and liver cancer is almost twice as high in Hispanics.
- African Americans are more likely to develop cancer than any other ethnic or racial group in the United States.
- African Americans have the highest incidence and mortality for colorectal and lung cancers.
- The incidence of breast cancer is approximately 13% lower in African American women than in white women, but the mortality rate is approximately 28% higher.
- African American men are at least 50% more likely to develop prostate cancer than men of any other ethnic or racial group.
- Cancer incidence and mortality are lower in Native American men and women than in any other ethnic or racial group.

PATHOPHYSIOLOGY AND ETIOLOGY

A **neoplasm** is a mass of new tissue (a collection of cells) that grows independently of its surrounding structures and has no physiologic purpose. The term neoplasm is often used interchangeably with *tumor* (from the Latin word meaning "swelling") Neoplasms are said to be autonomous because of the following:

- They grow at a rate uncoordinated with the needs of the body.
- They share some of the properties of the parent cells but with altered size and shape.
- They do not benefit the host and, in some cases, are actively harmful.

Neoplasms are not completely autonomous, however, because they require a blood supply with nutrients and oxygen to sustain their growth. Neoplasms typically are classified as benign or malignant based on their potential to damage the body and their growth characteristics.

A neoplasm may be classified as benign or malignant. **Benign** means that a growth does not endanger life or health; it tends to not recur after treatment. **Malignant** means that if not treated, a growth will recur, continue to grow, and spread to other sites in the body, ending in death.

Benign Neoplasms

Benign neoplasms are localized growths. They form a solid mass, have well-defined borders, and are frequently encapsulated. Benign neoplasms tend to respond to the body's homeostatic controls. Thus, they often stop growing when they reach the boundaries of another tissue (a process called contact inhibition). They grow slowly and often remain stable in size. Because they are usually encapsulated, benign neoplasms often are easily removed and tend not to recur.

Although typically harmless, benign neoplasms can be destructive if they crowd surrounding tissue and obstruct the function of organs. For example, a benign meningioma (from the meninges of the brain and spinal cord) can cause severely increased intracranial pressure, which progressively impairs the person's cerebral function. Unless the meningioma can be successfully removed, the steadily rising intracranial pressure will eventually lead to coma and death.

Malignant Neoplasms

In contrast to benign neoplasms, malignant neoplasms grow aggressively and do not respond to the body's homeostatic controls. Malignant neoplasms are not cohesive, and they present with an irregular shape. Instead of slowly crowding other tissues aside, malignant neoplasms cut through surrounding tissues, causing bleeding, inflammation, and necrosis (tissue death) as they grow. This invasive quality of malignant neoplasms is reflected in the origin of the word cancer (from the Greek *karkinos*, meaning "crab") Health care professionals are referring to a malignant neoplasm when they use the term cancer.

Malignant cells from the primary tumor may travel through the blood or lymph to invade other tissues and organs of the body and form a secondary tumor. The spreading of malignant neoplasms to other areas of the body—perhaps their most destructive trait—is called **metastasis**. Malignant neoplasms can recur after surgical removal of the primary and secondary tumors and after other treatments. Table 3–4 compares benign and malignant neoplasms.

Malignant neoplasms vary in their degree of differentiation from the parent tissue. Highly differentiated cancer cells try to mimic the specialized function of the parent tissue, but undifferentiated cancers, consisting of immature cells, have almost no resemblance to the parent tissue and so perform no useful function. To make matters worse, undifferentiated cancers rob the body of its energy and nutrition as they grow. Undifferentiated anaplastic cells have little structural or functional relationship to the parent cells and are the basis of many malignant neoplasms. The degree of differentiation of anaplastic cells is a consideration in the classification and staging of neoplasms.

CHARACTERISTICS OF MALIGNANT CELLS Malignant neoplasms may be identified by the following predictable cellular characteristics:

- *Loss of regulation of the rate of mitosis.* This results in rapid cell division and growth of the neoplasm.
- *Loss of specialization and differentiation.* Malignant cells do not perform typical cellular functions. Many produce hormones and enzymes similar to those of the parent tissue, but usually in excessive amounts, possibly revealing their presence.
- *Loss of contact inhibition.* Malignant cells do not respect other cellular boundaries. They easily invade and destroy other tissues.
- *Progressive acquisition of a cancerous phenotype.* Cellular mutation seems to be a sequential process involving successive generations of cells, with each generation becoming more deviant than the previous one. Additionally, malignant cells seem to be "immortal"—that is, they do not stop growing and die, as do normal cells, which have a genetically determined life span.
- *Irreversibility.* The transformation into a malignant cell is irreversible. Rarely does a malignant neoplasm revert to a benign state.

TABLE 3–4 **Comparison of Benign and Malignant Neoplasms**

BENIGN	MALIGNANT
Local	Invasive
Cohesive	Noncohesive
Well-defined borders	Does not stop at tissue border
Pushes other tissues out of the way	Invades and destroys surrounding tissues
Slow growth	Rapid growth
Encapsulated	Metastasizes to distant sites
Easily removed	Not always easy to remove
Does not recur	Can recur

- *Altered cell structure.* Cytologic examination of malignant cells reveals distinct differences in the cell nucleus and cytoplasm as well as an overall cell shape that differs from that of normal cells of the particular tissue type.
- *Simplified metabolic activities.* The work of malignant cells is simpler than that of normal cells; they show an increased synthesis of substances needed for cell division, and they have no need to create proteins for the specialized functions of the tissues they invade.
- *Transplantability.* Malignant cells often break away from the primary tissue site and travel to other locations in the body, where they establish new growths.
- *Ability to promote their own survival.* Malignant cells may create ectopic sites to produce the hormones they need for their growth. By their very presence and their ability to initiate vascular permeability, malignant cells promote the development of nonneoplastic stroma, a connective tissue framework consisting of collagen and other components, which then supports the neoplasm. They may also create their own blood supply. Through a process called angiogenesis, tumor cells secrete a polypeptide angiogenic growth factor that stimulates blood vessels from surrounding normal tissue to grow into the tumor. Finally, malignant cells divert nutrition from the host to meet their own needs, by diffusion when the tumor is less than 1 mm and by means of the newly formed blood vessels thereafter. If unchecked, malignant cells eventually destroy their host Box 3–8.

TUMOR INVASION AND METASTASIS The ability of cancer cells to overtake adjacent tissues (**invasion**) and travel to distant organs (metastasis) is considered their most ominous characteristic. This quality makes treatment a considerable challenge (Hawkins, 2001).

Invasion Aggressive tumors possess several qualities that facilitate invasion:

- *Ability to cause pressure atrophy.* The pressure of a growing tumor can cause atrophy and necrosis of adjacent tissues. The malignancy then moves into the vacated space.
- *Ability to disrupt the basement membrane of normal cells.* Many cancer cells can bind to elements of the basement membrane and secrete enzymes that degrade that physical barrier, thus facilitating their movement into normal tissues, lymph, and blood circulation.

Box 3–8 Characteristics of Malignant Cells

- Loss of regulation of mitotic rate
- Loss of cell specialization
- Loss of contact inhibition
- Progressive acquisition of the cancerous phenotype and immortality
- Irreversibility of cancerous phenotype to greater aggressiveness
- Altered cell structure: differences in cell nucleus and cytoplasm
- Simplified metabolic activity
- Transplantability (metastasis)
- Ability to promote own survival

- *Motility.* Because malignant cells are less tightly bound to each other than normal cells (reduced adhesiveness), they easily separate from the neoplasm and move into surrounding body fluids and tissues.
- *Response to chemical signals from adjacent tissues.* **Chemotaxis** (the movement of cells in response to a chemical stimulus) draws the tumor cells into the normal tissues, possibly as a result of the degrading of the basement membranes of the normal cells. This breakdown of normal cellular membranes releases the chemical stimulus physiologically designed to draw normal phagocytic cells to clean up the debris. Malignant cells are also known to respond chemotactically to the end product of cellular metabolism. Some cancer cells even produce a substance called autocrine motility factor, which calls other malignant cells to a normal tissue. The first invading cells produce this substance, which then actively draws other malignant cells from the primary tumor into the invaded normal tissue.

Metastasis The factors that favor invasion also contribute to the process of metastasis. Metastasis can occur by means of one or more mechanisms, including embolism in the blood or lymph or spread by way of body cavities.

A blood- or lymph-borne metastasis allows a new tumor to be established in a distant organ. Figure 3–9 ■ shows metastasis through the bloodstream. A tumor's ability to metastasize in this manner requires the following steps:

1. Intravasation of malignant cells through blood or lymphatic vessel walls and into the circulation
2. Survival of the malignant cells in the blood (to survive, the cells must escape the notice of the body's immune surveillance; only about 1 in 1,000 cells does so)
3. Extravasation from the circulation and implantation in a new tissue.

The tumor cells tend to clump together, forming an embolus, and continue growing until their size prevents further travel in the vessel or lymph channel. The growing neoplastic mass then uses its invasive abilities (secreting enzymes and motility factor) to move into the nearest organ.

Approximately 60% of metastatic lesions tend to occur in a schema reflecting the pattern of blood or lymph circulation. Some malignant cells, however, defy a bloodborne pattern and actually target specific organs to which they prefer to metastasize. For example, lung cancer frequently metastasizes to the adrenal glands, and breast cancer frequently metastasizes to bone.

Malignant cells that gain access to the lymph channels may travel to a preferred organ and then move into it the same way they emigrate through blood vessels. Alternatively, the malignant cells may become trapped in the lymph node and continue to grow. Eventually, the malignant cells replace the node's tissues. At this point, emboli from the cancerous node disseminate to other nodes, creating a cascade reaction. The malignant cascade causes widespread transfer of the tumor to uncharacteristic sites.

A malignant tumor may break through the walls of the organ in which it is primarily housed, in the process shedding cells into the nearby body cavity. The cells then are free to

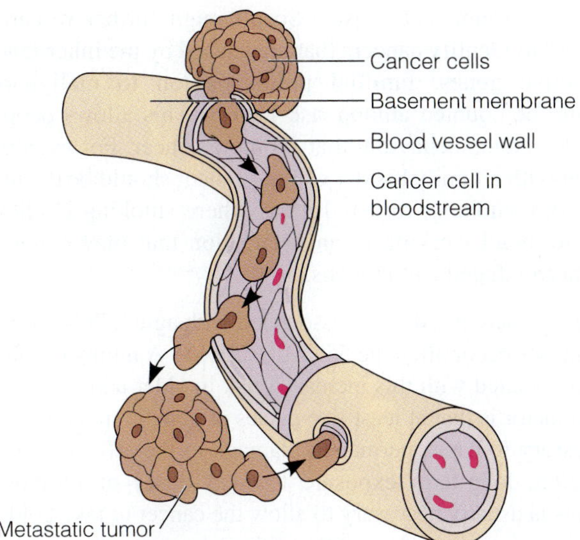

Figure 3–9 ■ Metastasis through the bloodstream. Cancer cells secrete enzymes and a motility factor that disrupt the basement membrane in the blood vessel. In this way, the cancer cells gain access to the circulation. Once in the blood, only about 1 cell in 1000 escapes immune detection, but that can be enough. Undetected cells move out of the blood, again secreting enzymes and cutting through the vessel wall into new tissue. The tissue selected for establishing a new tumor may be downstream from the original tumor, or a chemical attraction may cause the malignant cells to target a specific site. Once in the new site, the malignant multiply and establish a metastatic tumor.

establish new tumors in a distant area of that cavity. For example, malignant cells from a colon cancer may be seeded into the peritoneal cavity, establishing a new tumor in the mesenteric epithelium.

Metastatic lesions are differentiated from primary neoplasms by cell morphology: Metastatic cells do not resemble the tissue in which they reside. The most common sites of metastasis are the lymph nodes, liver, lungs, bones, and brain.

For metastasis to occur, the cancerous cells must avoid detection by the immune system. Thus, impairment of the immune system is a major factor in the establishment of metastatic lesions. Cells may escape detection in several different ways:

- Aggressive cancer cells may compile a large mass (>1 cm) so rapidly that the immune system is unable to overcome the tumor before it takes hold in a new tissue.
- For tumor cells to be recognized as foreign by the immune system, they must display on their surface a special antigen called *tumor-associated antigen* (TAA). TAA marks tumor cells for destruction by the lymphocytes. Some oncogenic viruses depress the expression of TAA on infected cells. Also, some tumors in advanced stages of growth no longer display TAA. Thus, such tumor cells escape detection as they travel through the blood or lymph.
- If the person's immune response is weakened or altered, then a metastatic tumor may take hold with little opposition.

An estimated 50–60% of all cancers have already metastasized by the time the primary tumor is identified. This may account for the current 50% death rate, and it certainly supports the need for client education to facilitate early diagnosis. The time it takes for metastasis to occur is extremely variable and often difficult to predict. Some cancers, such as basal cell carcinomas, do not metastasize. The aggressiveness and location of the tumor, and the state of the person's immune system, determine whether and how rapidly metastasis takes place.

Theories of Carcinogenesis

Theories of **carcinogenesis** (the production or origin of cancer) include the involvement of cellular mutation, oncogenes, and tumor suppressor genes. Central to these theories are two important concepts about the etiology of cancer. First, damaged DNA, whether inherited or from external sources, sets up the necessary initial step for cancer to occur. Second, impairment of the human immune system, from whatever cause, lessens its ability to destroy abnormal cells.

CELLULAR MUTATION The theory of cellular mutation suggests that **carcinogens** (cancer causing substances) cause mutations in cellular DNA. It is believed that the carcinogenic process has three stages: (1) initiation, (2) promotion, and (3) progression. The initiation stage involves permanent damage in the cellular DNA as a result of exposure to a carcinogen (e.g., radiation or chemicals) that was not repaired or that had a defective repair. Promotion may last for years and includes conditions, such as smoking or alcohol use, that act repeatedly on the already affected cells. In the progression stage, further inherited changes acquired during the cell replication develop into a cancer.

ONCOGENES **Oncogenes** are genes that promote cell proliferation and are capable of triggering cancerous characteristics. Oncogenes can be classified according to their overall function. Several oncogenes and their relationship to human cancers have been identified. For example, *BRCA1* and *BRCA2* are associated with breast cancer (Surbone, 2001).

A decrease in the body's immune surveillance may allow the expression of oncogenes; this can occur during times of stress or in response to certain carcinogens. For example, clients with AIDS, who have a decreased number of helper T lymphocytes, have a greater incidence of certain cancers, including non-Hodgkin's lymphoma and Kaposi's sarcoma (Donahue, Wernz, & Cooper, 2000).

TUMOR SUPPRESSOR GENES Tumor suppressor genes normally suppress oncogenes. They can become inactive by deletion or mutation. Inherited cancers have been associated with tumor suppressor genes. An example is p53, a suppressor gene that has been associated with sarcoma and cancer of the breast and brain.

Etiology

A number of agents are known to cause cancer, or at least are strongly linked to certain kinds of cancers. These carcinogens are both external (e.g., chemicals, radiation, and viruses) and internal (e.g., hormones, immune conditions, and inherited mutations). Causal factors may act together or in sequence to initiate or promote carcinogenesis. Ten or more years often pass between exposures or mutations and detectable cancer.

Carcinogens can be categorized in two groups: Genotoxic carcinogens, which directly alter DNA and cause mutations, and promoter substances, which cause other adverse biologic effects, such as cytotoxicity, hormonal imbalances, altered immunity, or chronic tissue damage. Promoter substances do not cause cancer in the absence of previous cell damage (initiation), and they often require high-level and long-term contact with the altered cells.

Although everyone comes into contact with a vast number of substances that are considered carcinogenic, not everyone develops cancer. Other factors, such as genetic predisposition, impairment of the immune response, and repeated exposure to the carcinogen, are necessary for a cancer to develop.

Several viruses have been associated with the development of cancer. These viruses damage cells and induce hyperplastic cell growth. Viral infection may play a role in cell mutation that can progress to malignant cells. Most people are able to suppress this progression (Spitalnick & diSant'Angnese, 2001). Box 3–9 identifies these viruses and the cancers with which they are associated.

In addition, viruses play a significant role in weakening immunologic defenses against neoplasms. For example, human immunodeficiency virus (HIV), which infects helper T lymphocytes and monocytes, impairs the person's protection against certain cancers, such as lymphoma and Kaposi's sarcoma.

Risk Factors

Risk factors make an individual or a population vulnerable to a specific disease or other unhealthy outcome. Risk factors can be divided into those that are controllable and those that are not controllable. Knowledge and assessment of risk factors are especially important in counseling clients and families about measures to prevent cancer.

HEREDITY It is estimated that 5–10% of cancers may have a hereditary component. The familial pattern of some breast and colon cancers has been well documented. Lung, ovarian, and prostate cancers have also shown some familial relationships. The Human Genome Project has identified new cancer-linked genes (Futreal et al., 2001). For most cancers, however, research has yet to distinguish true genetic transfer from environmental causes. So although further research is needed to identify cancers that are caused by the inheritance of defective genes, familial predisposition to malignancies should be counted among risk factors. This allows people at risk to reduce behaviors that promote cancer. For example, a client with a family history of lung cancer should be counseled to avoid smoking, to avoid areas where smoking is allowed, and to avoid working in an occupation that may expose the client to inhaled carcinogens.

AGE Cancer is a disease associated with aging; 76% of cancer diagnoses occur after age 55 (ACS, 2006a). A number of factors are associated with this increased risk in older adults. One possible factor is that at least five cycles of genetic mutations seem necessary to cause permanent damage to the afflicted cells. In addition, long-term exposure to high doses of promotional agents is usually necessary to allow the cancer to take hold. The immune response also alters with aging; its actions become more generalized and less specific (Blaylock, 1998). Another problem is that free radicals (molecules resulting from the body's metabolic and oxidative processes) tend to accumulate in the cells over time, causing damage and mutation.

Hormonal changes that occur with aging can be associated with cancer. Postmenopausal women receiving exogenous estrogen have an increased risk for breast and uterine cancers. Older men are at risk for prostate cancer, possibly as a result of the breakdown of testosterone into carcinogenic forms.

Severe and/or cumulative losses also are implicated in promoting cancer. These losses, which are common to older adults, include the death of a spouse or friends, loss of position and status in society, and a decline in physical abilities (Rossi, 2004). These repeated stressors are related to changes in the immune system that may lead to the development of cancer.

GENDER Gender is a risk factor for certain types of cancer. Breast cancer is the most frequently diagnosed cancer in women; prostate cancer is the most frequently diagnosed cancer in men. The incidence of bladder cancer is about four times higher in men than in women, whereas thyroid cancer occurs more commonly among women (ACS, 2006a).

Box 3–9 **Cancers Associated With Different Viruses**

HERPES SIMPLEX VIRUS TYPES I AND II (HSV-1 AND HSV-2)
- Carcinoma of the lip
- Cervical carcinoma
- Kaposi's sarcoma

HUMAN CYTOMEGALOVIRUS (HCMV)
- Kaposi's sarcoma
- Prostate cancer

EPSTEIN-BARR VIRUS (EBV)
- Burkitt's lymphoma

HUMAN HERPESVIRUS-6 (HHV-6)
- Lymphoma

HEPATITIS B VIRUS (HBV)
- Primary hepatocellular cancer

PAPILLOMAVIRUS
- Malignant melanoma
- Cervical, penile, and laryngeal cancers

HUMAN T-LYMPHOTROPIC VIRUSES (HTLV)
- Adult T-cell leukemia and lymphoma
- T-cell variant of hairy-cell leukemia
- Kaposi's sarcoma

POVERTY The poor are at higher risk for cancer than the population in general. Inadequate access to health care, especially preventive screening and counseling, may be a major factor. Although other factors that may be involved, such as diet and stress, usually come under the category of controllable risks, these risks are frequently uncontrollable in this population.

STRESS Continuous unmanaged stress that keeps hormones such as epinephrine and cortisol at high levels can result in systematic "fatigue" and impaired immunologic surveillance. When the body attempts to adapt to physiologic and psychologic stressors, it goes through a series of stages called the general adaptation syndrome (Rossi, 2004; Selye, 1984). First, the "alarm reaction" occurs, in which adrenal hormones increase, allowing the body to cope with the stressor. Eventually, the body reaches the "stage of resistance," in which the stress hormones are significantly reduced, indicating that adaptation has occurred. If the physiologic adaptation is supported by appropriate coping strategies, the stressor is considered managed, and body systems return to prealarm functioning. However, if adaptation continues and the stress hormones remain elevated, the "stage of exhaustion" sets in. This stage will maintain life, but at great expense to body systems, resulting in general wear-and-tear and depression of the immune system (Rossi, 2004; Selye, 1984).

The role of personality in the causation of cancer is controversial. People with cancer-prone personalities are assumed to be people who have unhealthy coping behaviors for life stressors (Katz & Epstein, 2005). Cancer-prone people are identified as those who tend to others' needs to the exclusion of their own and who rarely ask for help or support, even in personal crises. These people tend to be emotionally—and sometimes even physically—isolated and have a great deal of buried, unexpressed anger. It is thought that this kind of behavior pattern harms the immune system over time, promoting vulnerability to cancer.

Depression is also considered a major risk factor, especially depression that is chronic or related to multiple or major losses. It is thought that depression and hopelessness tend to shut down the energizing chemicals in the body and depress immune responses (Kaye, Morton, Bowcutt, & Maupin, 2000).

DIET Some foods are considered genotoxic, such as the nitrosamines and nitrous indoles found in preserved meats and pickled, salted foods. Other foods, such as high-fat, low-fiber foods—the mainstay of many American diets—promote colon, breast, and sex hormone–dependent tumors. When fish and meat are excessively fried or broiled, potent carcinogenic compounds can form that may cause tumors in the mammary glands, colon, liver, pancreas, and bladder. Also, repeatedly using fat to fry foods at high temperatures produces high levels of polycyclic hydrocarbons, which increase the risk for cancer considerably. Although many people profess to have changed their dietary habits, one only has to observe the large number of people who still frequently lunch on cheeseburgers and french fries (and who teach their children to do the same) to realize that much more educational and motivational work is needed in this area. Other food-related substances believed to increase cancer risk include sodium saccharine, red food dyes, and both regular and decaffeinated coffee.

OCCUPATION Occupational risk might be considered either controllable or uncontrollable. For many people, both education and ability limit their choice of occupation; moreover, during times of high unemployment, changing one's occupation because it poses risk factors may not be a viable option. Federal standards are designed to protect workers from hazardous substances, but many believe that these standards are not strict enough, and that inspections are not frequent enough, to prevent violations.

Specific risks vary according to the occupation. For example, those who work outdoors, such as farmers and construction workers, are exposed to solar radiation. Health care workers, such as x-ray technicians and biomedical researchers, are exposed to ionizing radiation and carcinogenic substances. Exposure to asbestos is a problem for people who work in old buildings with asbestos insulation in the walls.

INFECTION Because a number of viruses have been linked to some cancers, avoiding those specific infections will decrease risk. Although some infections may be unavoidable—Epstein-Barr, for example—others, such as genital herpes and papillomavirus-induced genital warts, can often be avoided by following safer sex practices (e.g., the use of condoms).

TOBACCO USE Lung cancer is considered highly preventable because of its relationship to smoking. The genotoxic carcinogenic substances in tobacco are considered weak; therefore, stopping smoking can reverse the damage it causes. However, many other substances in tobacco are highly promotional, so the larger the dose and the longer the use, the higher the risk for developing cancer. Research has shown a significantly lower risk for death from lung cancer among former smokers compared to current smokers. Smokers who quit before middle age avoid more than 90% of the risk of lung cancer that can be attributed to tobacco (Peto et al., 2000).

Tobacco is also related to other forms of cancer. Smokers face an increased risk for oropharyngeal, esophageal, laryngeal, gastric, pancreatic, and bladder cancers. Pipe and cigar smokers are especially susceptible to oropharyngeal and laryngeal cancers. Oral and esophageal cancers are more common among those who chew tobacco or use snuff. Smokers who have a genetic decrease in alpha$_1$-antitrypsin (an enzyme that protects lung tissue) that results in emphysema face an even higher risk for cancer than smokers without this defect.

Additional research has documented the deleterious effects of secondhand tobacco smoke (Dietrich et al., 2002). Tobacco-specific nitrosamines were recovered in the urine of children living with smokers. It is now accepted that nonsmokers exposed to tobacco smoke over long periods of time, whether in the workplace or in the home, have an increased risk for lung or bladder cancers.

ALCOHOL USE Alcohol promotes cancer by enhancing the contact between carcinogens, such as those in tobacco, and the stem cells that line the oral cavity, larynx, and esophagus

(Porth, 2005). People who both smoke and drink a considerable amount of alcohol daily have an increased risk for oral, esophageal, and laryngeal cancers.

RECREATIONAL DRUG USE Recreational drug use often promotes an unhealthy lifestyle that increases a person's general risk for cancer; for example, drug users often do not maintain adequate nutrition. Furthermore, recreational drugs are implicated as promoters because of their suppressive effect on the immune system. Although it has not been directly implicated in cancer development, marijuana has been demonstrated to cause chromosomal damage that over time also may result in cancer-causing DNA damage and genetic mutations (Khalsa, Genser, Francis, & Martin, 2002). Marijuana smoke is also much more injurious to lung tissue than tobacco smoke (Khalsa et al., 2002).

OBESITY Excessive body fat has been linked to an increased risk for hormone-dependent cancers. Because sex hormones are synthesized from fat, people who are obese often have excessive amounts of the hormones that feed hormone-dependent malignancies of the breast, bowel, ovary, endometrium, and prostate.

SUN EXPOSURE As the protective ozone layer thins, more of the sun's damaging ultraviolet radiation reaches the earth. As a consequence, the rate of skin cancers has increased. Sun-related skin cancers are now considered a problem for all people, regardless of skin color, but people of northern European extraction with very fair skin, blue or green eyes, and light-colored hair are most vulnerable. Older adults with decreased pigment, even those with darker skin, are also more at risk.

CLINICAL MANIFESTATIONS

Much of the nursing care for clients with cancer is related to the generalized effects of cancer on the body and to the side effects of the treatments used to remove or destroy the cancer. Although pathophysiologic effects of the cancer vary with the type and location of the cancer, the effects detailed in this section are common among many types of cancer.

Disruption of Function

Physiologic functioning can be upset by obstruction or pressure. For example, a large tumor in the bowel can stop intestinal motility, resulting in a bowel obstruction. Prostatic tumors can obstruct the bladder neck or urethra, resulting in urine retention. Intracranial pressure can be dangerously increased by a glioma.

Obstruction or pressure can cause anoxia and necrosis of surrounding tissues, which in turn cause a loss of function of the involved organ or tissue. For example, a kidney tumor may progress to renal failure. Pressure against the superior vena cava from an adjacent lung tumor or tumor-infiltrated lymph nodes can interrupt the blood flow to the heart.

In the liver, either a primary hepatocellular cancer or metastatic lesion can have several significant effects:

- In liver parenchymal tissue, it can impair the multiple life-sustaining functions of the liver, such as carbohydrate metabolism, synthesis of plasma proteins, detoxification, and immunologic functions. These functional impairments result in severe nutritional, hormonal, hematologic, and immunologic problems.
- Because more than 1 L of blood per minute passes through the liver via the portal vein, obstruction to this flow by a tumor can cause portal hypertension. This results in backup of fluid and increased pressure in the splanchnic circulation. The end result is ascites (third-spaced fluid in the peritoneal cavity) and varices (friable, overdistended blood vessels) of the esophageal, gastric, mesenteric, and hemorrhoidal vessels.

Hematologic Alterations

Hematologic alterations can impair the normal function of blood cells. For example, in leukemia, a malignant proliferative disease of the hematopoietic (blood cell–producing) system, the immature leukocytes cannot perform the normal protective phagocytic functions, and immunity is compromised. Additionally, the excessive numbers of immature leukocytes in the bone marrow diminish erythrocyte and thrombocyte (platelet) production, resulting in secondary anemia and clotting disorders (Scigliano, Vlachos, Najfeld, & Shank, 2001).

Other examples of hematologic alteration include the following:

- Gastrointestinal tumors disrupt the absorption of vitamin B_{12} and iron.
- Growing tumors need purines and folate and have a unique ability to accumulate and store these substances. Thus, the tumor deprives the bone marrow of these substances, which are needed for erythropoiesis (RBC production).
- Renal cell carcinoma produces its own erythropoietin hormone, which causes an excessively large number of RBCs to be produced and dumped into the bloodstream. The resulting polycythemia causes viscous blood, which impairs circulation, plugs small capillaries, and promotes thrombus formation.

Infection

If the tumor invades and connects two incompatible organs, such as the bowel and the bladder, and thus creates a fistula, infection becomes a serious problem. As they destroy viable tissue and thus their own source of nutrition, tumors may become necrotic; septicemia may result. Some tumors are less efficient in creating capillaries; as a consequence, the center of the tumor may become necrotic and infected. When a tumor grows near the surface of the body, it may erode through to the surface, thus breaking down the natural defenses of intact skin and mucous membranes and providing a site for the entry of microorganisms. Any malignant involvement of the organs or tissues of immunity—such as the liver, bone marrow, Peyer's patches in the small intestine, spleen, or lymph nodes—can seriously impair the immune response, allowing infections to develop in vulnerable tissues.

Hemorrhage

Tumor erosion through blood vessels can cause extensive bleeding, giving rise to severe anemia. Hemorrhage can be serious enough to cause life-threatening hypovolemic shock.

Anorexia-Cachexia Syndrome

A characteristic feature of cancer is the wasted appearance of its victims, called **cachexia**. In many cases, unexplained rapid weight loss is the first symptom that brings the client to a health care provider. This can result from a variety of problems associated with cancer, such as pain, infection, depression, or the side effects of chemotherapy and radiation. Usually, however, the emaciation, malnutrition, and loss of energy are attributed to the anorexia-cachexia syndrome.

This syndrome is specific to cancer because of the effect of cancer cells on the host's metabolism. The neoplastic cells divert nutrition to their own use while causing changes that reduce the client's appetite. Early in the disease, glucose metabolism is altered, causing an increase in serum glucose levels. Through the process of negative feedback, anorexia (loss of appetite) results. In addition, the tumor secretes substances that decrease appetite by altering taste and smell and by producing early satiety. Pain, infection, and depression also contribute to anorexia. Some types of cancers cause specific food aversions, such as to red meat, coffee, or chocolate.

Avaricious cancer cells support their growth through widespread catabolism of the body's tissue and muscle proteins. This catabolism, coupled with inadequate nutrient intake, results in the typical cachexia. Normally, a starvation state reduces the body's basal metabolic rate. However, in many people with cancer, the metabolic rate is increased, probably because of the hyperactive metabolic and reproductive activities of the malignant cells. One theory suggests that cytokinins the body produces in response to the tumor are responsible for both early satiety and cachexia. One specific cytokine, called tumor necrosis factor alpha or cachectin, is believed to enhance the increased metabolic consumption of nutrients. Cancers of the gastrointestinal system further promote anorexia-cachexia by decreasing absorption and use of nutrients; the side effects of some treatment modalities enhance this effect. Figure 3–10 ■ shows the characteristic appearance of a cachectic person.

Paraneoplastic Syndromes

Paraneoplastic syndromes are symptoms that result from chemicals secreted by the tumor and the immune system's response. They may be early warning signs of cancer or indicate complications or return of a malignancy. The most frequent paraneoplastic syndromes are endocrine, occurring when cancers set up ectopic sites of hormone production (Haapoja, 2000). Consider the following examples:

- Breast, ovarian, and renal cancers may set up ectopic parathyroid hormone sites, causing severe hypercalcemia.
- Oat cell and other lung cancers may produce ectopic secretions of insulin (causing hypoglycemia), parathyroid hormone, antidiuretic hormone (causing excessive fluid retention, hypertension, and peripheral edema), and adrenocorticotropic hormone.

Other paraneoplastic syndromes include hematologic abnormalities, such as anemia, thrombocytopenia, and coagulation abnormalities; nephrotic syndrome; cutaneous syndromes; and neurologic syndromes, such as distant tumors that produce increased intracranial pressure (Haapoja, 2000).

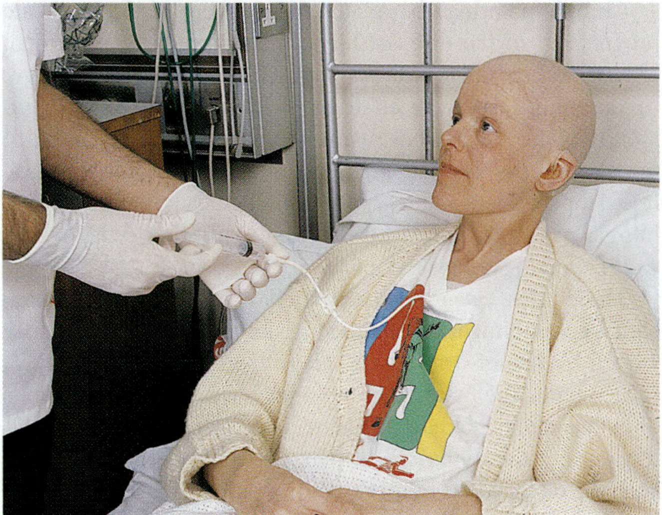

Figure 3–10 ■ Cachectic person. Cancer robs its host of nutrients and increases body catabolism of fat and muscle to meet its metabolic needs.

Source: Simon Fraser/SPL/Photo Researchers, Inc.

Pain

Pain is ranked as one of the most serious concerns of clients, families, and oncology health care professionals. Because pain management for people with cancer has a reputation as being ineffective, the anticipation of pain may engender fear in even the most stoic people. Most persons fear pain and suffering even more than possible death, although pain management strategies have improved tremendously. The findings from a 10-year study of more than 2,000 clients in a palliative care program are encouraging. Following the World Health Organization guidelines for cancer pain relief, 88% of clients reported good to satisfactory pain relief (Zech, Grond, Lynch, Hertel, & Lehmann, 1995). The devastating statistics provided by research in pain have resulted in great improvement in pain management strategies.

TYPES OF CANCER PAIN Cancer pain can be divided into two main categories, acute and chronic, with subgroupings. These classifications serve to indicate appropriate therapeutic approaches. Acute pain has a well-defined pattern of onset, exhibits common signs and symptoms, and is often identified with hyperactivity of the autonomic system. Chronic pain, which lasts more than 6 months, frequently lacks the objective manifestations of acute pain, primarily because the autonomic nervous system adapts to this chronic stress. Unfortunately, chronic pain often results in personality changes, alterations in functional abilities, and lifestyle disruptions that can seriously affect compliance with treatment and the quality of life.

Most clients with cancer who cite acute pain as the primary symptom that led to the diagnosis tend to associate pain with the introduction to their disease. If these clients experience pain during the illness or after therapy, they often perceive the pain as the introduction to another cancer or as a recurrence of the original cancer. Other clients report experiencing pain as a component of cancer therapy. These clients often are able to endure the pain in anticipation of a successful outcome of treatment.

Chronic pain may be related to treatment or may indicate progression of the disease. Identifying the pain as treatment related rather than tumor related is extremely important, because it has a definite effect on the client's psychologic outlook. For the client whose pain is caused by advancement of the disease, psychologic factors play an even more important role. Hopelessness and fear of impending death intensify physiologic pain and contribute to overall suffering (which goes well beyond just physical pain).

Three other categories used to classify clients with cancer pain are worth mentioning: clients with preexisting pain, those with a history of drug abuse, and dying clients with cancer-related pain. The first two groups may have altered perceptions of pain and may not have the anticipated response to pain medication. For the dying client, pain is strongly associated with both the client's and family's confrontation of issues of hopelessness and death. Confronting these issues can intensify the perception of pain.

CAUSES OF CANCER PAIN Direct tumor involvement is the primary cause of the pain experienced by people with cancer. This includes metastatic bone disease, nerve compression, and involvement of visceral organs. The pain from tumor involvement is believed to be mechanical, resulting from stretching of tissues and compression. Chemicals from ischemia or tumor metabolites and toxins that activate and sensitize nociceptors and mechanoreceptors are also responsible for tumor pain.

Side effects or toxic effects of cancer therapies (e.g., surgery, radiation, and chemotherapy) may also cause cancer pain. These are usually the result of traumatized tissue; one example is the oropharyngeal ulcerations that occur with some types of chemotherapy. However, these therapies may also be used to manage pain, such as radiation to decrease pain associated with bone metastasis.

Physical Stress

When the immune system discovers a neoplasm, it tries to destroy it using the resources of the body. The body mounts an all-out assault on the foreign invader, calling on many resources:

- Chemical mediators
- Hormones and enzymes
- Blood cells
- Antibodies
- Proteins
- Inflammatory and immune responses.

These protective responses also mobilize fluid, electrolytes, and nutritional systems. This massive effort requires tremendous energy. (See Concept 11, Fluids and Electrolytes, for specific information on these systems.) If the neoplasm is small enough (i.e., microscopic), the immune system can destroy it, and a tumor will never manifest. A neoplasm of 1 cm is large enough to overwhelm most immune systems; however, the body will continue trying to fight until it reaches the stage of exhaustion and is no longer capable (Selye, 1984). Thus, many clients with cancer present with fatigue, weight loss, anemia, dehydration, and altered blood chemistries (e.g., decreases in electrolytes).

CLINICAL MANIFESTATIONS AND THERAPIES **Cancer**

ETIOLOGY	CLINICAL MANIFESTATION	CLINICAL THERAPIES
Direct tumor involvement with the tissues often results in pain.	Pain often severe in nature and described as any type, depending on the tissue involved	■ Pain management usually requires narcotic analgesics with escalating dosages as tolerance develops
Anorexia-cachexia syndrome often results from rapid growth and reproduction of cancer cells and their need for increased nutrients.	Muscle wasting, weight loss, emaciated appearance, with resulting weakness and fatigue	■ Nutritional counseling ■ Increase caloric intake ■ Reduction in activity level ■ Vitamin and mineral supplementation ■ Dietary supplements, such as liquid formulas, may help provide extra calories between meals
Risk for infection may increase as a result of bone marrow suppression secondary to both the tumor growth and treatments.	Fever, malaise, fatigue with minor infections ranging to septicemia with systemic infection	■ Teach infection-prevention techniques, including hand hygiene, cough etiquette, and crowd avoidance ■ Antimicrobial medications to treat existing infections ■ Monitor and maintain hydration
Paraneoplastic syndrome often results from tumor growth that usually involves the endocrine system but may also involve the kidney, skin, neurologic, or other systems.	Manifestations depend on the system involved. Increased hormone production from ectopic tumor sites will produce symptoms similar to those seen in hypersecretion of hormone.	■ Surgery to remove tumor ■ Palliative treatment of symptoms until tumor reduction therapies diminish impact of tumor ■ Supportive treatment

Psychologic Stress

People confronted with the diagnosis of cancer exhibit a variety of psychologic and emotional responses. Some people see cancer as a death sentence and experience overwhelming grief, often giving up. Others may feel guilt, considering the cancer a punishment for past behaviors, such as smoking, unhealthy eating habits, or delaying diagnosis or treatment. The client may experience anger, especially if the person believes that he or she had been practicing a healthful lifestyle; beneath that anger may reside feelings of powerlessness. Fear is common: fear of the outcome of the illness, fear of the effects of treatment, fear of pain, and fear of death. Some people feel isolated because of the stigma of cancer and old beliefs about contagion. Body image concerns and sexual dysfunction may be present but often unexpressed, especially if the cancer is of the breast or sexual organs or causes visible body changes.

COLLABORATION

A team approach is essential to the care of clients diagnosed with cancer. The possibility for cure is much greater if a cancer is treated in its early stages, when the tumor is small and localized to a single area. Once the cancer has spread to distant sites, cure is much more difficult; thus, it is important to diagnose the disease as early as possible. In an attempt to remove every cancer cell, three treatment approaches are utilized: surgery, radiation therapy, and drug therapy. The nurse's role as a member of the interdisciplinary health care team is discussed in the Nursing Process section that follows.

Diagnostic Tests and Classification

Several procedures are used to diagnose cancer. X-ray imaging, computed tomography (CT), ultrasonography, and magnetic resonance imaging (MRI) can locate abnormal tissues or tumors. However, only microscopic histologic examination of the tissue reveals the type of cell and its structural difference from the parent tissue. Tissue samples are acquired through biopsy, shed cells (e.g., Papanicolaou smear), or collections of secretions (e.g., sputum). Lymph nodes are also biopsied to determine whether metastasis has begun. Simple screening procedures can be used to pick up substances secreted by the tumor, such as the prostate-specific antigen (PSA) blood test now being used to identify early prostatic cancers. Increases in enzymes or hormones released by normal tissues when they are damaged can also contribute to the diagnosis. Increased alkaline phosphatase noted in bone metastases and osteosarcoma is one example of an enzyme increase associated with cancer. Recent research also has identified tumor markers, which are used for early diagnosis, tracking responses to therapy, and devising immunologic treatments.

Some investigators studying chemical mediators of the immune system have noted that communication seems to occur between the chemical mediators and the emotional centers of the brain. A person who states "I feel I have cancer" should be listened to, and the complaint investigated thoroughly.

To help standardize diagnosis and treatment protocols, an elaborate identification system has been developed. This consists of naming the tumor (classification) and describing its aggressiveness (grading) and spread within or beyond the tissue of origin (staging).

Tumors are classified and named by the tissue or cell of origin. Tumor nomenclature often incorporates the Latin stem identifying the tissue from which the tumor arises. For example, a carcinoma arises from epithelial tissue; adjectives are added to further specify the location. A glandular malignancy arising from epithelial tissue is classified as an adenocarcinoma. A tumor arising from supportive tissues is called a sarcoma; the specific type of tissue is added as a prefix. For example, a cancer of fibrous connective tissue is called fibrosarcoma, and a smooth muscle cancer is a leiomyosarcoma. A tumor from seminal or germ tissue is called a seminoma. Table 3–5 compares the nomenclature of benign and malignant neoplasms.

Other names for tumors incorporate the name of the discoverer of that particular cancer, such as Burkitt's lymphoma or Hodgkin's disease. Hematopoietic malignancies (also known as liquid tumors) are usually named by the type of immature blood cell that predominates. For example, myelocytic leukemia is named for the immature form of the granulocyte that is predominant in this malignancy.

GRADING AND STAGING **Grading** evaluates the amount of differentiation (level of functional maturity) of the cell and estimates the rate of growth based on the mitotic rate. Cells that are the most differentiated—that is, cells that are most like the parent tissue and therefore the least malignant—are classified as grade 1 and are associated with a better prognosis. Grade 4 is reserved for the least differentiated and most aggressively malignant cells. Because of the differences inherent in tumor appearance and biologic behavior, grading criteria may vary with different locations and types of tumors.

Staging is used to classify solid tumors and refers to the relative size of the tumor and extent of the disease. The TNM staging system is internationally recognized: The T stands for the relative tumor size, depth of invasion, and surface spread; N indicates the presence and extent of lymph node involvement; and M denotes the presence or absence of distant metastases. Table 3–6 shows the basic outline of the TNM system; however, other systems are also used to differentiate types and locations of tumors (e.g., melanomas, cervical cancer, and Hodgkin's disease).

CYTOLOGIC EXAMINATION For the malignant tissues to be identified by name, grade, and stage, they must first be subjected to histologic and cytologic examination by light or electron microscopy. Specimens are collected by three basic methods:

1. *Exfoliation from an epithelial surface.* Examples include scraping cells from the cervix (Pap smear) or bronchial washings.
2. *Aspiration of fluid from body cavities or blood.* Examples include WBCs for evaluation of hematopoietic cancers, pleural fluid, and cerebrospinal fluid.
3. *Needle aspiration of solid tumors.* This could include the breast, lung, or prostate.

TABLE 3–5 **Nomenclature for Benign and Malignant Neoplasms**

	TISSUE OF ORIGIN	BENIGN	MALIGNANT
Ectoderm/endoderm	Epithelium	Papilloma	Carcinoma
	Gland	Adenoma	Adenocarcinoma
	Liver cells	Hepatocellular adenoma	Hepatocellular carcinoma
	Neuroglia	Glioma	Glioma
	Melanocytes	Melanoma	Malignant melanoma
	Basal cells		Basal cell carcinoma
	Germ cells	Tetroma	Seminoma
Mesoderm	Connective tissue		
	Adipose tissue	Lipoma	Liposarcoma
	Fibrous tissue	Fibroma	Fibrosarcoma
	Bone tissue	Osteoma	Osteosarcoma
	Cartilage	Chondroma	Chondrosarcoma
	Muscle		
	Smooth muscle	Leiomyoma	Leiomyosarcoma
	Striated muscle	Rhabdomyoma	Rhabdomyosarcoma
	Neural tissue		
	Nerve cells	Ganglioneuroma	Neuroblastoma
	Endothelial tissues		
	Blood vessels	Hemangioma	Angiosarcoma
			Kaposi's sarcoma
	Meninges	Meningioma	Malignant meningioma
Hematopoietic tissues	Granulocytes	Granulocytosis	Leukemia
	Plasma cells		Multiple myeloma
	Lymphocytes		Lymphomas

Cytologic examination is also carried out on specimens from biopsied tissues or tumors and on collected body secretions, such as sputum or urine.

After collection, specimens are spread on a glass slide, fixed, and stained if necessary. The morphologic features of the cells are examined, with special attention to the nucleus and cytoplasm. Other special pathologic procedures can be carried out on the specimen, but they must be ordered ahead of time if special preparations of the specimen are necessary.

TUMOR MARKERS A **tumor marker** is a protein molecule detectable in serum or other body fluids. This marker is used as a biochemical indicator for the presence of a malignancy. Small amounts of tumor marker proteins are found in normal body tissues or benign tumors and are not specific for malignancy. However, high levels are suspicious and mandate follow-up diagnostic studies.

Tumor marker tests are currently in the developmental and investigational phase and are most useful for monitoring the

TABLE 3–6 **The TNM Staging System**

	STAGE	MANIFESTATIONS
Tumor	T0	No evidence of primary tumor
	TIS	Tumor in situ
	T1, T2, T3, T4	Ascending degrees of tumor size and involvement
Nodes	N0	No abnormal regional nodes
	N1a, N2a	Regional nodes—no metastasis
	N1b, N2b, N3b	Regional lymph nodes— metastasis suspected
	Nx	Regional nodes cannot be assessed clinically
Metastasis	M0	No evidence of distant metastasis
	M1, M2, M3	Ascending degrees of metastatic involvement of the host, including distant nodes

client's response to therapy and for detecting residual disease. However, one marker, PSA, has received a great deal of media attention as a detector of prostate cancer. As a result, many health care practitioners recommend screening for it in men over age 40, much as Pap smears and mammograms are recommended for women.

Tumor markers fall into two general categories: those derived from the tumor itself and those associated with host (immune) response to the tumor. Examples of tumor markers include the following:

- *Antigens.* These are present in fetal tissue but normally are suppressed after birth. Thus, their presence in large amounts may reflect an anaplastic process in tumor cells. Alpha-fetoprotein and carcinoembryonic antigen (CEA) are oncofetal antigens.
- *Hormones.* Hormones are, of course, present in human blood and tissues in considerable amounts, but very high levels not related to other conditions may signify the presence of a hormone-secreting malignancy. Some common hormones seen as tumor markers include human chorionic gonadotropin, antidiuretic hormone, parathyroid hormone, calcitonin, and catecholamines.
- *Proteins.* These narrow down the type of tissue that may be malignant, although they can also be increased in hyperplastic disorders. Examples of tissue-specific proteins include serum immunoglobin and beta$_2$-microglobulin.
- *Enzymes.* Rapid, excessive growth of a tissue may cause some of the enzymes and isoenzymes normally present in that particular tissue to spill into the bloodstream. Elevated levels can point to either hyperplasia of the tissue or cancer. Prostatic acid phosphatase and neuron-specific enolase are examples. Table 3–7 compares selected tumor-derived markers with their presence in neoplasms and other conditions.

ONCOLOGIC IMAGING Because physical assessment usually cannot detect cancer until the tumor has reached a size that poses a major risk for metastasis, radiologic examination is extremely important in early diagnosis. This diagnostic process may involve routine x-ray imaging (usually for screening only), CT, MRI, ultrasonography, nuclear imaging, angiography, and positron-emission tomography.

X-Ray Imaging Considered the least expensive and least invasive diagnostic procedure, film screen imaging (standard x-ray imaging) is the method of choice for screening such body areas as the breast (mammography), lung, and bone to identify changes in tissue density that may indicate malignancies. X-ray studies are limited in that they do not easily distinguish among calcifications, benign cystic growths, and true malignancies. However, as a screening tool, x-ray imaging can usually reassure the client if findings are negative or encourage follow-up studies if findings are suspicious. X-ray imaging is still the method of choice for lung cancer. Unfortunately, it does not usually reveal tumors until they have reached about 1 cm in size, which is late in their development.

Computed Tomography Computed tomography has greatly advanced the effectiveness of traditional x-ray methods. By applying computers and mathematics to diagnostic imaging, CT allows the visualization of cross-sections of the anatomy. Because CT scans reveal subtle differences in tissue densities, they provide much greater accuracy in tumor diagnosis. This procedure, although more expensive than x-ray imaging, is useful in screening for some cancers such as renal cell and most gastrointestinal tumors. CT scans are especially useful to evaluate possible lymph node involvement.

Magnetic Resonance Imaging Like CT, MRI involves computerized mathematical technology. The client is placed within a strong magnetic field, pulsed radio waves are directed at the client, and transmitted signals based on tissue characteristics are analyzed by a computer. Related diagnostic imaging procedures—positron-emission tomography and single-photon-emission computed tomography—create visible images by measuring electrical impulses from different

TABLE 3–7 **Tumor-Derived Markers Associated With Specific Neoplasms**

	TUMOR MARKER	ASSOCIATED NEOPLASM
Oncofetal antigens	Carcinoembryonic antigen (CEA)	Adenocarcinomas of colon, lung, breast, ovary, stomach, pancreas
	Alpha-fetoprotein (AFP)	Hepatocellular carcinoma, gonadal germ cell tumors (seminoma)
Hormones	Human chorionic gonadotropin (HCG)	Gonadal germ cell tumors
	Calcitonin	Medullary cancer of thyroid
	Catecholamines/metabolites	Pheochromocytoma
Isoenzymes	Prostatic acid phosphatase (PAP)	Adenocarcinoma of prostate
	Neuron-specific enolase (NSE)	Small-cell lung carcinoma, neuroblastoma
Specific proteins	Prostate-specific antigen (PSA)	Adenocarcinoma of prostate
	Immunoglobin	Multiple myeloma
	CA 125	Epithelial ovarian cancer
	CA 19-9	Adenocarcinoma of pancreas, colon
	CA 15-3	Breast cancer

Source: Adapted from Pfeifer, J. D., & Wick, M. R. (1995). The pathologic evaluation of neoplastic disease. In A. I. Holleb, D. J. Fink, & G. P. Murphy (Eds.), *American Cancer Society textbook of clinical oncology* (pp. 75–95). Atlanta: American Cancer Society.

body structures. Although MRI is relatively expensive, it is the diagnostic tool of choice for both screening and follow-up of cranial as well as head and neck tumors.

Because they must be placed inside the diagnostic imaging machine, some clients become claustrophobic during the MRI procedure. This experience has been likened to being encased in a small tube. In addition, some machines make loud thumping sounds that can be frightening if the client is not informed beforehand that this is normal.

Ultrasonography Ultrasonography is relatively safe and noninvasive. It measures sound waves as they bounce off various body structures, giving an image of normal anatomy as well as revealing abnormalities that indicate tumors. Ultrasonography has been adapted for diagnosing some specific tumors. For example, transrectal ultrasonography has provided excellent imaging of early prostate cancers and is used to guide needle biopsy. Ultrasound imaging is also more useful for detecting masses in the denser breast tissue of young women.

Nuclear Imaging Nuclear imaging involves the use of a special scintillation scanner in conjunction with the ingestion or injection of specific radioactive isotopes. This is an invasive, but usually safe, diagnostic method for identifying tumors in various body tissues. For the client with a newly diagnosed cancer, the procedure is often used to check for possible bone or other organ metastases. This evaluation helps the health care provider determine appropriate treatment.

The principle underlying the technology is that certain isotopes have an affinity for specific tissues; for example, radioactive iodine (I-131) has an affinity for the thyroid gland. Malignancies in these tissues sequester an abnormally large amount of the isotope, which then can be traced and measured by the scintillation scanner. This procedure is considered safe, because the amount of isotope used is small enough not to damage normal cells.

Usually, the procedure is only minimally distressing for clients. Drinking the isotope solution is not pleasant but is tolerable; some anxious clients may have difficulty lying still during the scan. Antianxiety medication may help. Some clients may experience nausea from drinking the isotope and require antiemetic drugs to complete the procedure. Client preparation may include complete restriction of fluids and food by mouth or allowing only clear fluids after midnight.

Angiography An expensive and invasive procedure, angiography is used infrequently for tumor diagnosis. Angiography is performed when the precise location of the tumor cannot be identified or the tumor's extent needs to be visualized before surgery.

The procedure involves injecting a radiopaque dye into a major blood vessel proximal to the organ or tissue to be examined. The movement of the dye through the vasculature of the organ or tissue is then traced by means of fluoroscopy or serial x-ray films. In some cases, small catheters are threaded through the vein under fluoroscopy to ensure the specific placement of the dye. Blockage to the flow of the dye indicates the tumor's location. Dye may also be used to identify blood vessels supplying a tumor, allowing the surgeon to know where to safely ligate vessels.

Angiography requires preparation similar to that for minor surgery. This includes ensuring that the client takes in only fluids on the day of the examination, performing skin preparation at the insertion site, and administering sedative drugs before the procedure. Clients should be informed that injection of the dye used to enhance imaging may cause a hot, flushing sensation or nausea and vomiting. Although angiography is usually done on an outpatient basis, the client will be kept in a short-stay unit for several hours and monitored for such complications as bleeding at the catheter insertion site.

DIRECT VISUALIZATION Procedures for direct visualization are invasive but do not require the use of radiography. Examples include the following:

- Sigmoidoscopy (viewing the sigmoid colon with a fiber-optic flexible sigmoidoscope)
- Cystoscopy (viewing the urethra and bladder)
- Endoscopy (viewing the upper gastrointestinal tract)
- Bronchoscopy (inspecting the tracheobronchial tree).

These methods allow visual identification of the organs within the limits of the scope and usually permit biopsy of suspicious lesions or masses. Flexible fiber-optic scopes may be more useful, because they allow deeper penetration than traditional scopes. These procedures all require some client preparation, cause moderate to considerable discomfort, and may require sedation or even anesthesia, as in the case of bronchoscopy. Some procedures, such as sigmoidoscopy and cystoscopy, may be performed in the physician's office and therefore cost less, making them more accessible screening procedures.

Client preparation includes a thorough bowel cleansing before the sigmoidoscopy and cystoscopy; the client may ingest only liquids the morning of the procedure. Because anesthesia may be required, clients undergoing bronchoscopy and endoscopy may be instructed to have nothing by mouth from midnight until the procedure.

A more radical method of direct visualization for suspected malignancies is exploratory surgery with biopsy. In this method, the client undergoes the usual preoperative preparation for the type of surgery anticipated. When the tumor is exposed, a sample of tissue (biopsy) is sent to the pathology laboratory for a "frozen-section" histologic examination. This can be done rapidly, while the client remains on the operating table under anesthesia. If the initial report is negative, the benign mass is usually removed to prevent further symptoms. If the report is positive for cancer, the tumor and, often, the adjacent lymph nodes are resected, along with any other suspicious tissue. The tumor, nodes, and any other specimens are sent to the pathology laboratory for more in-depth analysis. The client then receives the usual postoperative care.

LABORATORY TESTS Most laboratory tests of blood, urine, and other body fluids are used to rule out nutritional disorders and other noncancerous conditions that may be causing the client's symptoms. For example, a CBC helps screen for such problems as anemia, infection, and impaired immunity. Blood chemistries can point out nutritional disturbances and electrolyte imbalances. However, in conjunction with other diagnostic studies, some laboratory tests can be quite useful either in screening for other pathologic conditions or for validating the cancer diagnosis (Kee, 2002). These tests include evaluating levels of enzymes such as alanine aminotransferase, aspartate aminotransferase, and lactic dehydrogenase for liver metastases. Special protein tumor markers, such as PSA for prostate cancer and CEA for colon cancer, are also used. Table 3–8 identifies some useful laboratory tests, their normal values, and their possible indications.

TABLE 3–8 **Laboratory Tests Used for Cancer Diagnosis**

TEST	REFERENCE VALUE	ABNORMALITY INDICATED
Acid phosphatase (ACP)	0.0–0.8 unit/L	Elevated in prostate, breast, and bone cancer and in multiple myeloma
Adrenocorticotropic hormone (ACTH)	8–80 pg/mL	Decreased in adrenal cancer; elevated in pituitary cancer or with tumor that secretes ACTH (bronchiogenic cancer)
Alanine aminotransferase (ALT)	5–35 unit/mL (Frankel)	Moderate elevation in liver cancer
Albumin	3.5–5.0 g/dL	Decreased in malnutrition, metastatic liver cancer
Alkaline phosphatase (ALP)	20–90 unit/L	Elevated in cancer of liver, bone, breast, and prostate, in leukemia, and in multiple myeloma
Alpha-fetoprotein (AFP)	Male and nonpregnant female: < 15 ng/mL	Elevated in germ cell tumors (e.g., seminoma), testicular cancer
Aspartate aminotransferase (AST)	5–40 unit/mL (Frankel)	Elevated in liver cancer
Bilirubin	Total: 0.1–1.2 mg/dL Direct: 0.0–0.3 mg/dL	Elevated in liver and gallbladder cancer
Bleeding time	Ivy method: 3–7 minutes	Prolonged in leukemia and metastatic liver cancer
Blood urea nitrogen (BUN)	5–25 mg/dL	Decreased in malnutrition; increased in renal cancer
Calcitonin	Male: < 40 pg/mL Female: < 20 pg/mL	Elevated to > 500 pg/mL in thyroid medullary cancer, breast cancer, and lung cancer
Calcium (Ca)	4.5–5.5 mEq/L 9.0–11.0 mg/dL	Elevated in bone cancer and ectopic parathyroid hormone production (paraplastic syndrome)
Carcinoembryonic antigen (CEA)	Nonsmokers: 2.5 ng/mL Smokers: 5 ng/mL Neoplasms: > 12 ng/mL	Elevated with gastrointestinal cancers, lung, breast, bladder, kidney, cervical, leukemias Used to evaluate effectiveness of cancer treatment
Chloride (Cl)	95–105 mEq/L	Decreased in vomiting, diarrhea, syndrome of inappropriate antidiuretic hormone (SIADH)
C-reactive protein	> 1:2 titer is positive	Elevated in metastatic cancer and Burkitt's lymphoma
Creatinine	0.5–1.5 mg/dL	Decreased in malnutrition; elevated in most cancers
Dexamethasone suppression test	> 50% reduction in plasma cortisol	Nonsuppression in adrenal cancer and ACTH-producing tumors, severe stress
Estradiol, serum	Female: 20–300 pg/mL Menopausal female: < 20 pg/mL Male: 15–50 pg/mL	Elevated in estrogen-producing tumors and testicular tumors
Fibrinogen	200–400 mg/dL	Decreased in leukemia and as a side effect of chemotherapy
Gamma-glutamyltransferase (GGT)	Male: 10–80 IU/L Female: 5–25 IU/L	Elevated in cancer of liver, pancreas, prostate, breast, kidney, lung, and brain
Fasting blood sugar	70–110 mg/dL	Decreased in malnutrition, cancer of stomach, liver, and lung
Haptoglobin	20–240 mg/dL	Elevated in Hodgkin's disease and cancer of lung, large intestine, stomach, breast, and liver
Hematocrit (Hct)	Male: 40–54% Female: 36–46%	Decreased in anemia, leukemia, Hodgkin's disease, lymphosarcoma, multiple myeloma, and malnutrition and as a side effect of chemotherapy
Hemoglobin (Hgb)	Male: 13.5–18 g/dL Female: 12–16 g/dL 1:3 ratio of Hgb:Hct	Decreased in anemia, many cancers, Hodgkin's disease, leukemia, and malnutrition and as a side effect of chemotherapy

(continued)

TABLE 3–8 Laboratory Tests Used for Cancer Diagnosis (continued)

TEST	REFERENCE VALUE	ABNORMALITY INDICATED
Human chorionic gonadotropin (HCG)	Nonpregnant female: < 0.01 IU/L	Elevated in choriocarcinoma
Insulin	5–25 microunit/mL	Elevated in insulinoma (islet cell tumor) and insulin-secreting cancers (e.g., lung cancer)
Lactic dehydrogenase (LDH)	100–190 IU/L	Elevated in liver, brain, kidney, muscle cancers, acute leukemia, anemia
Occult blood	Negative	Positive in gastric and colon cancers
Serum osmolality	280–300 mOsm/kg H_2O	Decreased in SIADH
Urine osmolality	50–1200 mOsm/kg H_2O	Increased in SIADH
Parathyroid hormone (PTH)	400–900 pg/mL	Increased in PTH-secreting tumors
Platelet (thrombocyte) count	150,000–400,000/mm^3	Decreased in bone, gastric, and brain cancer, in leukemia, and as a side effect of chemotherapy
Potassium (K)	3.5–5.0 mEq/L	Decreased in vomiting and diarrhea and in malnutrition
Prostatic-specific antigen (PSA)	0–4 ng/mL	Elevated from 10 to > 120 ng/mL in prostate cancer
Total protein	6.0–8.0 g/dL	Decreased in malnutrition, gastrointestinal cancer, Hodgkin's disease; elevated in vomiting, diarrhea, multiple myeloma
Red blood cells (RBCs)	Male: 4.6–6.0 million/mm^3 Female: 4.0–5.0 million/mm^3	Decreased in anemia, leukemia, infection, multiple myeloma
Sodium (Na)	135–145 mEq/L	Decreased in SIADH, vomiting; elevated in dehydration
Uric acid	Male: 3.5–8.0 mg/dL Female: 2.8–6.8 mg/dL	Increased in leukemia, metastatic cancer, multiple myeloma, Burkitt's lymphoma, after vigorous chemotherapy
White blood cells (WBCs)		
Total leukocytes	4,500–10,000/mm^3	Elevated in acute infection, leukemias, tissue necrosis; decreased as a side effect of chemotherapy
Neutrophils	50–70%	Elevated in bacterial infection and Hodgkin's disease; decreased in leukemia and malnutrition and as a side effect of chemotherapy
Eosinophils	1–3%	Elevated in cancer of bone, ovary, testes, and brain
Basophils	0.4–1.0%	Elevated in leukemia and healing stage of infection
Monocytes	4–6%	Elevated in infection, monocytic leukemia, and cancer; decreased in lymphocytic leukemia and as a side effect of chemotherapy
Lymphocytes	25–35%	Elevated in lymphocytic leukemia, Hodgkin's disease, multiple myeloma, viral infections, and chronic infections; decreased in malnutrition, cancer, and other leukemias and as a side effect of chemotherapy

Note. All values refer to serum values unless otherwise indicated. Values are approximate; check the reference standards specified by your own agency's laboratory.

Surgery

Surgery is performed to remove a tumor that is localized or when the tumor is pressing on nerves, the airways, or other vital tissues. Surgery lowers the number of cancer cells in the body so that radiation therapy and pharmacotherapy can be more successful. Surgery is not an option for tumors of blood cells or when it would not be expected to extend a client's life span or improve the quality of life.

Pharmacologic Therapies

Pharmacotherapy of cancer may be referred to as **chemotherapy** or antineoplastic drug therapy. Chemotherapy has three general purposes: cure, palliation, or prophylaxis. Because drugs are transported through the blood, they have the potential to reach cancer cells in virtually any location. Certain drugs are able to cross the blood–brain barrier to reach brain tumors. Others are instilled directly into body cavities, such as the urinary bladder, to bring the highest dose possible to the cancer cells without producing systemic side effects.

A simple method of classifying this complex group of drugs includes the following six categories:

1. Alkylating agents
   - Nitrogen mustards
   - Nitrosoureas
2. Antimetabolites
   - Folic acid antagonists
   - Pyrimidine analogs
   - Purine analogs
3. Antitumor antibiotics
4. Natural products
   - Vinca alkaloids
   - Taxanes

- Topoisomerase inhibitors
- Camptothecins

5. Hormone and hormone antagonists
   - Glucocorticoids
   - Androgens and androgen antagonists
   - Estrogens and estrogen antagonists
   - Progestins
6. Biologic response modifiers and immune therapies.

Radiation Therapy

Radiation therapy is an effective way to kill tumor cells through nonsurgical means; approximately 50% of clients with cancer receive radiation therapy as part of their treatment. Radiation therapy is most successful for cancers that are localized, when high doses of ionizing radiation can be aimed directly at the tumor and confined to this area. Radiation treatments may follow surgery to kill any cancer cells left behind following the operation. Radiation is sometimes given as **palliation** (relief of symptoms to improve comfort without expectation of curative effects) for inoperable cancers to shrink the size of a tumor that may be pressing on vital organs and to relieve pain, difficulty breathing, or difficulty swallowing.

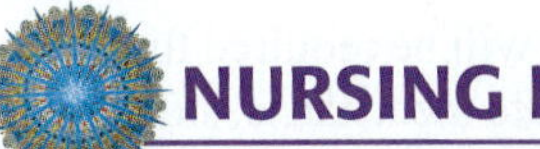

NURSING PROCESS

Nursing care is vitally important to the client's recovery. The client, family, and loved ones are often very frightened by the diagnosis of cancer and require emotional as well as physical support. It is not unusual for clients to become very sick during treatment as a result of complications or if the neoplasm does not respond to treatment. Nursing care focuses on teaching clients about self-care to avoid complications and minimize side effects of treatment as well as on providing emotional, spiritual, and psychologic support.

Assessment

Assessment of the client suspected of having cancer begins with a focused assessment of the organ system involved but then broadens to include a full assessment to determine sites of

Assessment Interview Cancer

The following are appropriate questions to ask the client during the initial interview and at subsequent assessments:

- "What brought you in to see the doctor?" Asking this question allows clients to tell their story in their own way, which may elicit more information than asking specific questions. The answer should elicit not only data about the signs and symptoms but also fears or concerns. If the cancer was discovered during a routine physical examination or checkup, the client may have some difficulty accepting the disease, especially if there were no symptoms. For clients who offer insufficient information in response to this open-ended question, more specific questions may be necessary, such as "Did you have pain or any specific physical problems that caused you to seek health care?"
- "Do you have any other medical conditions or problems that are troubling you at this time?" It may be necessary to ask about specific diseases to help the client focus. For example, "Do you have high blood pressure?" or "Are you having any problems with your lungs?" Information gained from these questions can help you anticipate problems and formulate potential nursing diagnoses related to other diseases that may interact with the cancer.
- "What kinds of physical problems are you having at this time? Do you have pain? Are you nauseated? Have you lost a great deal of weight? Are you so tired you have difficulty carrying on your daily activities? Are you feeling blue or discouraged because of your illness?" For each positive response, ask follow-up questions to narrow down or define the exact nature of the problem. Again, these data help identify what nursing diagnoses should be included in the care plan.
- "What options has your physician suggested for treating your cancer?" The answer will indicate clients' knowledge about their treatment and, possibly, their communication with the physician. Often, under the stress of a cancer diagnosis, clients do not hear or understand what the doctor is saying and are afraid to ask questions. Lack of knowledge indicates a need to collaborate with the physician to explain the information to the client so that the client can absorb and understand it. If the client has a good understanding of the treatment plan, discussing how he or she feels about it can be useful in exposing fears, concerns, and emotional responses.
- "What do you expect to happen as a result of this treatment?" The answer may reveal unrealistic expectations or lack of understanding of consequences of the treatment.
- "What effect is the disease and/or treatment having on your ability to carry on with your usual daily activities?" Additional questions may also be needed to pinpoint the types of limitations. The response to this question should provide information regarding the client's functional status. This information can also be used to identify the need to collaborate with professionals from other disciplines. For example, if the client is the sole financial support of the family and is unable to work, a social worker may be able to help with resources; if the client is extremely weak, referral to a physical therapist may help with energy conservation strategies and strengthening exercises.
- "Who is available to help you at home and run errands for you? Who can provide transportation for you to get to your appointments or treatments? Who can you rely on to be a good listener when you're sad or just to be a comfortable companion? Is there someone you would like to make health care decisions for you if there is a time when you are unable to make them for yourself?" It often seems that the person with cancer is the one who takes care of everyone else; asking for help may be difficult for this person. This information can identify how much support and help the client has access to. The last question introduces the concept of advanced directives and durable power of attorney regarding health care (see Concept 47, Legal Issues).
- "How do you manage your stress or your feelings of discomfort? What helps you feel better? Do you think these measures work well for you?" The responses to these questions provide information about the client's coping strategies and may identify maladaptive strategies, such as alcohol or drug use. Lack of appropriate coping methods can interfere with the client's response to treatment and decrease overall quality of life.

Other assessment questions may be useful at different stages of the client's illness. For example, if the client is not expected to survive the cancer, it is important to ask whether the client has made decisions about last wishes (e.g., for a funeral and burial), whether these have been discussed with significant others, and whether the client has made out a will.

possible metastasis. For example, the client presenting with a lump in the breast will have a focused assessment looking for changes in the breast that may indicate the cause of the lump. However, once the client is diagnosed with metastatic breast cancer, a more thorough assessment will be required that looks for any abnormality that could indicate metastatsis, side effects of treatment, or complications of therapy.

Nurses face a major challenge in educating clients about preventive measures and lifestyle changes to reduce the risk of cancer. At the same time, clients with cancer must be reassured that they are not responsible for having acquired cancer.

Once a cancer diagnosis is established, nurses help clients recover and support them during the rehabilitation phase. In cases of terminal cancer, nurses provide comfort and facilitate positive growth for the client and significant others.

Focused Interview

During this initial phase of the nursing process, collect the following significant data about the client:

- History of the client's disease, including the signs and symptoms that led the client to seek health care
- Other concurrent diseases, such as diabetes
- Current physical or psychologic problems resulting from the cancer, such as pain or depression
- Understanding of the treatment plan
- Expectations of the treatment plan
- Functional limitations due to illness or treatment (Box 14–11)
- Effect of the disease on current lifestyle, including eating and drinking habits
- Reliable support systems or caretakers for the client
- Coping strategies and how well they are working.

Physical Assessment

When screening for cancer, nurses should keep in mind the American Cancer Society's guidelines for early detection (Box 3–10).

As soon as the client is admitted to the health care service or agency, conduct a complete physical assessment to establish a baseline against which to evaluate changes. It is especially important to document the nutritional status of the client using anthropomorphic measurements (i.e., frame size, height, weight, body fat, and muscle mass), and to evaluate laboratory results and note any specific signs and symptoms. Table 3–9 compares the manifestations of good nutrition with those of malnutrition.

It is also important to assess the client's hydration status, especially if the client is not taking oral food and fluids well or is having bouts of vomiting. Box 3–11 lists specific assessments for hydration status. Other recommended assessments are discussed in the Implementation section that follows.

Diagnosis

Specific nursing diagnoses for the client with cancer include the following:

- Anxiety
- Disturbed Body Image
- Anticipatory Grieving
- Risk for Infection
- Risk for Injury
- Imbalanced Nutrition: Less Than Body Requirements
- Impaired Tissue Integrity.

Plan

Nursing goals focus on supporting the whole person and managing specific problems, such as pain, poor nutrition, dehydration, fatigue, adverse emotional responses, altered individual and family coping, and the side effects of medical treatment. Nursing goals may include the following:

- The client will maintain weight within normal range based on height and body type.
- The client will remain hydrated, as evidenced by assessment of skin turgor and mucous membranes.

Box 3–10 **Cancer Screening Guidelines for Asymptomatic People**

COLORECTAL CANCER (MALES AND FEMALES)

- Fecal occult blood test or fecal immunochemical test annually beginning at age 50.
- Flexible sigmoidoscopy every 5 years beginning at age 50.
- Colonoscopy every 10 years.
- Double contrast barium enema every 5 years.

BREAST CANCER (FEMALES)

- Monthly breast self-examination beginning at age 20.
- Clinical breast examination every 3 years from age 20 to 40 and then annually beginning at age 40.
- Mammogram annually beginning at age 40.

CERVICAL AND UTERINE CANCER (FEMALES)

- Papanicolaou (Pap) smear 3 years after beginning vaginal intercourse or by age 21; annually or every 2 years using liquid-based Pap. (After age 30, if a woman has had three or more consecutive satisfactory annual examinations, the Pap test may be performed less frequently at the discretion of her primary care provider.)
- Pap smears may be stopped at age 70 if no abnormal results in the past 10 years.
- Pap smears may be stopped following total hysterectomy.

PROSTATE CANCER (MALES)

- Prostate-specific antigen (PSA) and digital rectal examination annually beginning at age 50 for men who have at least a 10-year life expectancy and for younger men who are at high risk.

HEALTH COUNSELING AND CANCER CHECKUP (MALES AND FEMALES)

- Examination for cancers of the thyroid, testicles, ovaries, lymph nodes, oral region, and skin every 3 years over age 20 and annually over age 40.

Source: From Smith, R. A., Cokkinides, V., & Eyre, H. J. (2006). American Cancer Society recommendations for the early detection of cancer, 2006. *CA: A Cancer Journal for Clinicians, 56*, 11–25.

TABLE 3–9 Signs of Nutritional Status

SYSTEM	GOOD NUTRITION	POOR NUTRITION
General	Alert, energetic, good endurance, psychologically stable	Withdrawn, apathetic, easily fatigued, irritable
	Weight within range for height, age, body size	Over- or underweight
Integumentary	Skin glowing, good turgor, smooth, free of lesions	Skin dull, pasty, scaly-dry, bruises, multiple lesions
	Hair shiny, lustrous, minimal loss	Hair brittle, dull, falls out easily
Head, eyes, ears, nose, and throat	Eyes bright, clear, no fatigue circles	Eyes dull, conjunctiva pale, discoloration under eyes
	Oral mucous membranes pink-red and moist	Oral mucous membranes pale
	Gums pink, firm	Gums red, spongy, and bleed easily
	Tongue pink, moderately smooth, no swelling	Tongue bright to dark red, swollen
Abdomen	Abdomen flat, firm	Abdomen flaccid or distended (ascites)
Musculoskeletal	Firm, well-developed muscles	Flaccid muscles, wasted appearance
	Good posture	Stooped posture
	No skeletal changes	Skeletal malformations
Neurologic	Good attention span, good concentration, astute thought processes	Inattentive, easily distracted, impaired thought processes
	Good reflexes	Paresthesias, reflexes diminished or hyperactive

- The client and family will vocalize feelings related to cancer diagnosis and seek support from others to improve coping.
- The client will relate potential side effects of chosen therapies and list strategies for minimizing or coping with symptoms.

Implementation

Caring interventions for the client with cancer could potentially include any skill or intervention depending on the type and location of the cancer cells. In addition to physical care, clients diagnosed with cancer have acute psychosocial needs that must be addressed in order to promote recovery. The interventions are dependent on the nursing diagnosis; the list provided here is only a sample of the more common client needs.

Anxiety

Early in the disease continuum—for example, during diagnosis and treatment—threats to or changes in health status, physical comfort, role functioning, or even socioeconomic status can cause anxiety. Later, anxiety may result from the anticipation of pain, disfigurement, or the threat of death. In particular, clients whose coping skills have been poor in the past (e.g., in managing anger) may find themselves at a loss to manage this current crisis. The client may manifest overt signs of anxiety: trembling, restlessness, irritability, hyperactivity, stimulation of the sympathetic nervous system (e.g., increased blood pressure, pulse, respiration, excessive perspiration, and pallor), withdrawal, worried facial expressions, and poor eye contact. The client may report insomnia and feelings of tension and apprehension or express concerns regarding perceived changes brought about by the disease and fear of future events.

- Carefully assess the client's level of anxiety (moderate anxiety, severe anxiety, or panic) and the reality of the threats represented in the client's current situation. The level of anxiety and the reality of the perceived threat influence the type of intervention that is appropriate for the client. A client in panic may need medical intervention with appropriate medications, whereas those with moderate or severe anxiety are often managed by the nurse through counseling and teaching new coping skills.
- Establish a therapeutic relationship by conveying warmth and empathy and by listening nonjudgmentally. A client who feels safe in the relationship with the nurse more easily expresses feelings and thoughts. The client will be able to trust the nurse and perhaps be willing to try new behaviors as suggested. The amount of time this relationship may take to develop depends on the client's current emotional and mental state and on the stage of the disease process.
- Encourage the client to acknowledge and express feelings, no matter how inappropriate they may seem to the client. Just by expressing their feelings, clients often can significantly diminish anxiety. Expressing feelings also allows the client to direct energy toward healing and thus has a positive therapeutic effect. Moreover, by acknowledging feelings, especially those the client considers

Box 3–11 Factors to Consider in Assessing Hydration Status

- Intake and output
- Rapid weight changes
- Skin turgor and moisture
- Venous filling
- Vital sign changes
- Tongue furrows and moisture
- Eyeball softness
- Lung sounds
- Laboratory values

unacceptable, the client can lay the groundwork for new coping behaviors.

- Review the coping strategies the client has used in the past, and build on past successful behaviors, introducing new strategies as appropriate. Explain why inappropriate strategies, such as repressing anger or turning to alcohol, are not helpful. The client will be more willing to make changes that build on what has already worked in the past. The client will also be more willing to reject inappropriate strategies if he or she is given a persuasive reason why they have not had the desired effect in managing previous crises.
- Identify resources in the community, such as crisis hotlines and support groups, that can help the client manage anxiety-producing situations. The client may not have support systems available, or the client's significant others may be having their own difficulties in dealing with the cancer diagnosis. Programs such as "I Can Cope," sponsored by the ACS in most communities, provide education, counseling, and support in a group setting with other cancer clients.
- Provide specific information for the client about the disease, its treatment, and what may be expected, especially for those clients with obvious misinformation. Knowing what is to come gives the client a sense of control and enables the client to make decisions. Also, knowing that every effort will be made to keep the client as free of pain as possible can do a great deal to relieve anxiety.
- Provide a safe, calm, and quiet environment for the client in panic. Remain with the client, and administer antianxiety medications as ordered. Staying with the client and displaying calmness and confidence can protect the client from injury and prevent further panic. If the panic does not subside with the nurse's presence and support, referral to the physician for medication management may be necessary.
- Use crisis intervention theory (discussed in Concept 28, Stress and Coping) to promote growth in the client and significant others, regardless of the outcome of the disease. During a major crisis, people can, with assistance, transform the experience from one that causes defeat and despair to one that enhances personal and spiritual growth. If you are not skilled in this area, a referral to an appropriate mental health professional may be helpful to the client and family.

Disturbed Body Image

Cancer and cancer treatments frequently result in major physiologic and psychologic changes in body image. Loss of a body part (e.g., amputation, prostatectomy, or mastectomy), skin changes and hair loss from chemotherapy or radiation therapy, disfigurement of body part (e.g., lymphedema in the affected upper and lower extremities), or creation of unnatural openings on the body for elimination (e.g., colostomy or ileostomy) may have a major effect on the person's self-image. The gaunt, wasted appearance of the client with cachexia or of the draining, malodorous lesions that result when cancer breaks through the skin are other significant etiologies of body image disturbance. This may also give rise to fear of rejection, which plays a major role in sexual dysfunction. In addition to all of the other afflictions the cancer brings about, the client may undergo major changes in appearance and function. The client may exhibit a visible physical alteration of some portion of the body, verbalize negative feelings about the body and/or fear of rejection by others, refuse to look at the affected site, and depersonalize the body change or lost part (e.g., by calling the colostomy "that thing").

- Discuss the meaning of the loss or change with the client. Doing so helps the nurse discover the best approach for this particular client and involves the client more actively in interventions. A small, seemingly trivial loss may have a big impact, especially when viewed in light of the other changes that are occurring in the client's life. Likewise, a major loss may not be as important as the nurse might imagine. To ensure more appropriate and individualized care, evaluate each situation in terms of the reactions of the specific client.
- Observe and evaluate the client's interaction with significant others. People who are important to the client may unintentionally reinforce negative feelings about body image; on the other hand, the client may perceive rejection where none exists.
- Allow denial, but do not participate in the denial; for example, if a client does not want to look at the wound, the nurse may say, "I am going to change the dressing to your breast incision now." During the initial stage of shock at the loss of a body part, denial is a protective mechanism and should not be challenged, nor should it be promoted. A matter-of-fact approach and an empathetic

CLIENT TEACHING **Parents of Children With Cancer**

It is a gross understatement to say that the diagnosis and treatment of a child with cancer causes great anxiety for the parents. Client teaching can help alleviate some of the anxiety parents experience by providing information about key aspects of treatment. Depending on the stage and type of treatment, the following suggestions may be helpful for parents:

- Children in radiation and chemotherapy are fatigued. Provide extra rest periods with shorter activity periods between them.
- Have an overnight bag ready in case the child develops a complication and needs to be taken to stay in the hospital for a few days. Several hospital stays of a few days are normal during treatment.
- When concerned about a symptom in the child, ask the care provider. Parents are often key in identifying problems early.
- Children have poor appetites at times so nutritional intake is needed when they are hungry.
- Remember that children are still at the normal developmental age. Treat them as a reflection of their ages, not as if they are older or younger.
- Try to maintain contact with the child's peer group and family members.
- Seek information from other parents and resources on cancer care.
- Time away for relaxation is important so that parental energy remains high and they are better able to deal with the child's therapy.

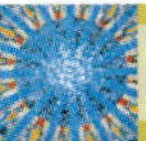

DEVELOPMENTAL CONSIDERATIONS Children With Cancer and Hair Loss

For many parents, especially those with daughters who have cancer, the loss of the child's hair during treatment can be devastating. Ask the parents and the child what this issue is like for them. Prepare them for the fact that hair loss can be rapid or slow. Find out how they plan to cope. Some children want their hair cut very short so its loss will not be as traumatic. Offer resources for wigs, hats, or other ideas. Put them in touch with children who have lost hair and with those who have regrown theirs.

Talk with the child's teachers before the return to school after treatment. Explain the child's condition and assist with plans to prepare the other children. Role-play with the child how to tell friends about any changes in appearance. A nurse or child life specialist could attend the class of a young child to explain what the client is experiencing.

Provide client teaching about the need for the child with hair loss to cover the head, wear sunscreen when outside, and avoid the sun as much as possible to minimize chance of burn to the head, which is prone to burning due to lack of prior sun exposure.

attitude will go far to facilitate the eventual acceptance of the change.

- Assist the client and significant others to cope with the changes in appearance:
  a. Provide a supportive environment.
  b. Encourage the client and significant others to express feelings about the situation.
  c. Give matter-of-fact responses to questions and concerns.
  d. Identify new coping strategies to resolve feelings.
  e. Enlist family and friends in reaffirming the client's worth.

A supportive, safe environment in which feelings are respected and new coping strategies can be tried promotes acceptance, as does reaffirming that the client's worth is not diminished by any physical changes.

- Teach the client or significant others to participate in the care of the afflicted body area. Support and validate their efforts. Active involvement in providing care, such as changing a dressing or emptying a colostomy bag, empowers the client and/or significant others. This intimate involvement also desensitizes feelings about disfigurement and promotes acceptance. Involving significant others reduces the risk of their rejecting the client and can promote closeness. Positive reinforcement from the nurse encourages them to continue these behaviors.
- Teach strategies for minimizing physical changes, such as providing skin care during radiation therapy and dressing to enhance appearance and minimize the change in the body part. Early intervention can limit the negative side effects of treatment and actually promote recovery. Involving the client provides an additional way for the client to be in control of a difficult situation.
- Teach ways to reduce the alopecia that results from chemotherapy and to enhance appearance until the hair grows back:
  a. Discuss the pattern and timing of hair loss. This allows the client to cope with changes and incorporate them into daily activities.
  b. Encourage wearing cheerful, brightly colored head coverings; assist in color coordinating them with usual clothing. Attractive head coverings protect the bald head while allowing the client to feel stylish and well dressed.
  c. Refer to a good wig shop before hair loss is experienced. Hair color and texture can be matched to minimize obvious changes in appearance.
  d. Refer to support programs such as "Look Good … Feel Better," which is sponsored by the ACS and the Cosmetic, Toilet, and Fragrance Association Foundation. A support group can diminish feelings of isolation and provide practical tips for managing problems. For a list of community resources available to clients with cancer, refer to a local phone book.
  e. Reassure that hair will grow back after chemotherapy is discontinued, but also inform that the color and texture of the new hair may be different. Hair loss has been identified as the most distressing symptom by many clients (Ferrell, 2000; Williams, Wood, & Cunningham-Warburton, 1999). Interventions to reduce that loss can have a significant impact on body image concerns. Moreover, knowing what to expect may decrease anxiety and distress.

Anticipatory Grieving

Anticipatory grieving is a response to loss that has not yet occurred. Overall, only 50% of people with cancer fully recover, and certain types of cancer have a much higher death rate. Thus, the client with cancer is often confronted with facing death and making preparations for it. This can be a healthy response that allows the client and family to work through the dying process and achieve growth in the final stage of life. Perceived changes in body image and lifestyle also can prompt anticipatory grieving. The client or significant others may show sorrow, anger, depression, or withdrawal, expressing distress at the potential loss or verbalizing concern about unfinished life business.

- Use the therapeutic communication skills of active listening, silence, and nonverbal support to provide an open environment for the client and significant others to discuss their feelings realistically and to express anger or other negative feelings appropriately. This helps the client and family to get in touch with feelings and confront the possibility of the loss or death.
- Answer questions about illness and prognosis honestly, but always encourage hope. This allows for realistic appraisal of the situation and planning, and it also helps combat feelings of hopelessness and depression.
- Encourage the client who is dying to make funeral and burial plans ahead of time and to be sure the will is in order. Make sure the necessary phone numbers can be

easily located. This gives a sense of control and relieves family members of these concerns at a time when the client is most in need of their support and when they themselves are extremely stressed.

- Encourage the client to continue taking part in activities he or she enjoys, including maintaining employment as long as possible. This gives a sense of continuity of life even in the face of severe losses.

Risk for Infection

Malnutrition, impaired skin and mucous membrane integrity, tumor necrosis, and suppression of WBCs from chemotherapy or radiation therapy may contribute to the risk for infection. Anorexia resulting from nausea and other side effects of treatment, as well as the increased nutritional needs of the cancer cells, deprives the body of nutrients needed for healing, while impaired integrity of skin and mucous membranes (a result of chemotherapy and/or radiation therapy) compromise the first lines of defense against microbial invasion. Cells in the center of large or not very vascular tumors may die from malnutrition, eventually eroding through tissues to increase the risk of sepsis. Bone marrow depression resulting from the effects of certain types of cancers and from chemotherapy undermine the body's ability to respond to infection. The client may exhibit the classic signs of infection: lassitude, fever, anorexia, pain in the affected area, and physical evidence of infection, such as a purulent, draining lesion or wound. If the bone marrow is compromised, the usual signs and symptoms of infection may be absent or reduced.

- Monitor vital signs. Fever and sympathetic nervous system responses, such as increased pulse and respiration, are usual early signs of infection. However, clients with severe immunosuppression may be unable to mount a fever; therefore, the absence of fever cannot rule out infection.
- Monitor WBC counts frequently, especially if the client is receiving chemotherapy known to cause bone marrow suppression. This allows the nurse to notify the physician at the first sign of diminishing WBC counts so that corrective action can be taken.
- Teach the client to avoid crowds, small children, and people with infections when his or her WBC count is at nadir (lowest point during chemotherapy) and to practice scrupulous personal hygiene. During periods of leukopenia, clients may lose immunity to their own natural flora. Careful attention to hygiene reduces the risk of infection. Crowds, which promote contact with a greater variety of infectious agents, and friends with minor infections can be very dangerous for those who are immunosuppressed. Small children should be avoided, because they often have microbes to which most people are usually immune but that the client may not be able to resist.
- Protect skin and mucous membranes from injury. Teach appropriate skin care measures, such as good hygiene, use of a moisturizing lotion to prevent dryness and cracking, frequent changes of position for the bed-bound, and immediate attention to skin breaks or lesions. Ensuring intact skin strengthens the first line of defense against infection.
- Encourage the client to consume a diet high in protein, minerals, and vitamins, especially vitamin C. Improving nutrition decreases the risk of infection. Vitamin C has been shown to help prevent certain types of infection, such as colds.

Risk for Injury

In addition to infection, cancer can pose a risk for injury from, for example, obstruction by a large tumor or one located in a limited body space (e.g., in the brain, bowel, or bronchial airways). If the cancer is one that creates ectopic sites of hormones, elevated levels of hormones that are not under the control of the pituitary gland can injure the client in a variety of ways. Signs of obstruction depend on the organ involved: Bowel obstruction presents with pain, distention, and cessation of bowel activities; obstruction in the brain gives signs of increased intracranial pressure or personality/behavioral change; bronchial obstruction manifests as respiratory distress, cyanosis, and altered arterial blood gases. Ectopic production of parathyroid hormone manifests as high serum calcium levels as well as signs of hypercalcemia; ectopic production of antidiuretic hormone causes fluid retention and manifests as hypertension and peripheral and pulmonary edema.

- Assess frequently for signs and symptoms indicating problems with organ obstruction. Early detection of major problems allows the nurse to seek medical help before the problem evolves into a physiologic crisis.
- Teach the client to differentiate minor problems from those of a serious nature. Encourage the client to consult with the nurse or physician if in doubt or to call 911 if the he or she becomes very ill. Box 3–12 provides guidelines to help clients identify serious problems. Having guidelines for when to call the doctor provides an anxiety-reducing safety net for the client and family and promotes early detection of complications.
- Monitor laboratory values that may indicate the presence of ectopic functioning and report abnormal findings to physicians immediately. Table 3–10 provides laboratory indicators of ectopic functions. Refer to Concepts 1, 11, and 18 for specific signs and symptoms of alterations in acid–base, electrolytes, and endocrine function. Early detection promotes early medical intervention and prevents serious consequences from the ectopic secretion.

Imbalanced Nutrition: Less Than Body Requirements

The anorexia-cachexia syndrome (described earlier in this exemplar) is a common cause of malnutrition in clients with cancer. Metabolism increases in response to increased cancer cell production, while the cancer's parasitic activity reduces the nutrients available to the body. Loss of appetite, food aversion, nausea and vomiting, and painful oral lesions from chemotherapy or radiation may contribute to impaired nutrition. Tumors of the gastrointestinal tract that affect absorption also contribute to the problem. Manifestations include wasted appearance, considerable weight loss over a relatively short period of time, anthropometric measurements below 85% of standard for fat and muscle tissue,

Box 3–12 When to Call for Help

Instruct the client or family member to call the nurse or physician if any of the following signs or symptoms occur:

- Oral temperature greater than 101.5°F (38.6°C)
- Severe headache
- Significant increase in pain at the usual site, especially if the pain is not relieved by the medication regimen; or severe pain at a new site
- Difficulty breathing
- New bleeding from any site, such as rectal or vaginal bleeding
- Confusion, irritability, or restlessness
- Withdrawal, greatly decreased activity level, or frequent crying
- Verbalizations of deep sadness or a desire to end life
- Changes in body functioning, such as the inability to void or severe diarrhea or constipation
- Changes in eating patterns, such as refusal to eat, extreme hunger, or a significant increase in nausea and vomiting
- Appearance of edema in the extremities or significant increase in edema already present.

Instruct the client or family member to call 911 if the client:

- is having much difficulty breathing or if the lips or face has a bluish tinge.
- becomes unconscious or has a convulsion.
- exhibits unmanageable behavior, such as being physically abusive, hurting self, or engaging in uncontrollable activity.

decreases in serum proteins, and negative responses to antigen testing.

- Assess current eating patterns, including usual likes and dislikes, and identify factors that impair food intake. This allows for a more individualized plan based on needs and preferences.
- Evaluate degree of malnutrition:
  a. Check laboratory values for total serum protein, serum albumin and globins, total lymphocyte count, serum transferrin, hemoglobin, and hematocrit. These values represent the laboratory values that are most likely to decrease with malnutrition.
  b. Calculate nitrogen balance and creatinine-height index. Calculate skeletal muscle mass, and compare findings to normal ranges. Urinary creatinine is an index of lean body mass and decreases in malnutrition. Lean muscle mass is catabolized for energy in clients with cancer.
  c. Take anthropometric measurements, and compare them to standards: height, weight, elbow breadth, arm circumference, triceps skinfold thickness, and arm muscle mass. This estimates the degree of wasting; findings below 85% of standard are considered malnutrition.

TABLE 3–10 Laboratory Indicators of Ectopic Functioning

HORMONE	SPECIFIC LABORATORY TEST
Antidiuretic hormone (ADH)	Serum and urine osmolality
Adrenocorticotropic hormone (ACTH)	Plasma ACTH, ACTH suppression test, ACTH stimulation test, urine catecholamines
Calcitonin	Serum calcitonin
Insulin	Serum glucose, glucose tolerance test
Parathyroid hormone (PTH)	Serum PTH Serum calcium
Thyroxine (T_4)	Serum thyroid-stimulating hormone (TSH), triiodothyronine, T_4

- Teach the principles of maintaining good nutrition by using the Food Guide Pyramid and adapting the diet to medical restrictions and current preferences. This tailors the food plan to the client's needs and thereby promotes compliance.
- Manage problems that interfere with eating:
  a. Encourage eating whatever is appealing, and consider adding nutritional supplements, such as Ensure Plus or Isocal, to the diet. It is better to eat something, even if it is not nutritionally balanced.
  b. Eat small, frequent meals. These are more easily digested and absorbed and usually better tolerated by the client with anorexia.
  c. Encourage the client to try icy-cold foods (e.g., ice cream) or those that are more highly seasoned if food has no taste. Chemotherapy and radiation therapy may harm taste buds and prevent distinguishing the taste of foods. Strong seasonings and coldness make food more enjoyable to the client with diminished taste. However, spicy foods are not recommended for clients with stomatitis.
  d. Encourage cold and bland, semisoft and liquid foods for clients with painful oropharyngeal ulcers; use an anesthetic, alcohol-free mouthwash before eating. These foods are less irritating to sensitive mucous membranes; deadening the pain can make chewing and swallowing easier.
  e. Manage nausea and vomiting by administering antiemetic drugs (around-the-clock medication may be an effective preventive measure). Encourage the client to eat small, frequent, low-fat meals with dry foods (e.g., crackers and toast), to avoid liquids with meals, and to sit upright for an hour after meals. Remove emesis basins, and encourage oral hygiene before eating. Dry, low-fat foods are more readily tolerated when nauseated. Removing vomiting cues, such as odor and supplies associated with vomiting, can reduce nausea.
- Teach the client to supplement meals with nutritional supplements, such as Ensure Plus or Isocal, and to take multivitamin and mineral tablets with meals. Suggest increasing calories by adding ice cream or frozen yogurt to the liquid supplement or commercial protein-carbohydrate powders to milk or fruit juice. Because the food intake is usually

less than that needed to maintain or gain weight, these supplements can add calories in a manner often tolerated.

- Teach the client to keep a food diary to document daily intake. If the client can see how little is being consumed, he or she may eat more. A food diary also helps the nurse keep a calorie count and alert the physician if more drastic nutritional measures, such as a feeding tube or parenteral nutrition, need to be instituted.
- Teach the client to administer parenteral nutrition via a central line or other venous access device (VAD). Teach safety measures and care of the VAD, and explain how the pump delivering the solution works. Provide an emergency phone number for help with administration problems. The client with chronic or terminal cancer requiring parenteral nutrition is usually managed at home, so information on how to manage the entire process may be needed.

Impaired Tissue Integrity

The most common impairment of tissue integrity occurs in the oral-pharyngeal-esophageal mucous membranes. It is secondary to the effects of some chemotherapeutic drugs and radiation treatment to the head and neck. The oral-pharyngeal-esophageal tissues are lined with cells that have a high mitotic turnover rate and are therefore vulnerable to many chemotherapeutic drugs. Leukemias, bone marrow transplants, and herpes viral infections are other etiologic factors in the disruption of oral-pharyngeal-esophageal tissue. Box 3–13 lists manifestations of this problem.

- Carefully assess and evaluate the type of tissue impairment present. Identify possible sources, such as chemotherapy or radiation therapy to head and neck. This allows the nurse to implement corrective measures appropriate to the type of problem.
- Implement and teach measures for preventing oropharyngeal infection:
  a. Observe for systemic signs of infection. Be suspicious of any fever that has no apparent cause. This facilitates early identification of an infection before it spreads.
  b. Encourage cleaning teeth gently and using a nonalcohol mouthwash several times a day. This can be done after waking up in the morning, after any oral intake, and before bedtime. Soak dentures nightly in hydrogen peroxide and floss gently with waxed floss after meals and bedtime; this measure may be contraindicated for people with leukemia or thrombocytopenia. Disrupted mucous membranes allow the normal oral bacterial flora into the systemic circulation, which can result in sepsis in those who are immunocompromised. Reducing the oral flora by frequent hygiene decreases the risk of infection.
  c. Culture any oral lesions, and report the problem to the physician. Herpes lesions may not follow a typical pattern in clients who are immunosuppressed. Identifying the cause of the infection, whether viral, fungal, or bacterial, allows the physician to prescribe the appropriate treatment.
- Implement and teach measures for reducing trauma to delicate tissues:
  a. Counteract dry mouth with lubricating and moisturizing agents, such as Gatorade, sugarless gum, and Blistex. This protects mucous membranes from infection and trauma.
  b. Avoid putting sharp instruments in the mouth. Use smooth plastic spoons and forks for eating, especially with a bleeding disorder. Dental work should be done by dental oncologists.
  c. Brush teeth with a very soft toothbrush, and obtain a new toothbrush monthly. If gums are friable and bleeding, clean teeth with a soft cloth or toothpaste over finger. Chlorhexidine mouthwash (Peridex) may be used. This protects gums from trauma and decreases risk of hemorrhage.
- Administer specific medications as ordered to control infection and/or pain:
  a. Acyclovir is often used to treat viral infections.
  b. Systemic antibiotics are used to treat bacterial infections.
  c. Nystatin or clotrimazole solution for "swish and swallow" or lozenges that dissolve slowly in the mouth are used for fungal infections.
  d. Use viscous Xylocaine or various combination mouthwashes before meals and as needed. These agents reduce pain and inflammation. Review the contents of each mouthwash and assist in client teaching to prevent hypersensitivity reactions to ingredients (e.g., to lidocaine).

Box 3–13 Manifestations of Impaired Tissue Integrity

- Small ulcers occur on the tongue and mucous membranes in the mouth and throat.
- Herpes simplex type 1 lesions or vesicles evolve into ulcerations.
- Fungal infections, such as thrush (resulting from *Candida* infections), are manifested by a white, yellow, or tan coating with dry, red, fissured tissue underneath.
- Red, swollen, friable gums bleed with minimal or no trauma.
- **Xerostomia** is excessive dryness of the mucous membranes (caused by chemotherapy or radiation).

Evaluation

When evaluating the client's response to therapy, it is important to remember that while hopeful outcomes would always include client recovery and absence of complications, this is not realistic for all people diagnosed with cancer. In some cases, outcomes may include the client's acceptance of and preparedness for death. Other expected outcomes may include the following:

- The client reports pain level of 3 or less, allowing for adequate rest and performance of ADLs.
- The client reports reduction in side effects of treatment regimen.
- The client experiences no unexpected complications of the disease process or treatment.
- The client demonstrates appropriate dietary choices to increase caloric intake.

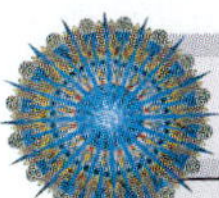

NURSING CARE PLAN **A Client With Cancer**

James Casey, aged 72, is of northern European heritage. He has been receiving medical care for chronic obstructive pulmonary disease, chronic bronchitis, status postmyocardial infarction, and type 1 diabetes mellitus for over 15 years. He reports that he lost his wife from lung cancer 5 years ago and still "misses her terribly." He describes his bad habits as smoking 2 packs of cigarettes a day for 52 years (104 packs/year), one to two 6-packs of beer a week, one "bourbon and water" a night, and "a lot of sugar-free junk food, like french fries." He assures the nurse that he quit smoking 2 years ago when he could no longer walk a block without considerable shortness of breath, and just quit drinking alcohol a few weeks ago at his physician's insistence.

About a year ago, Mr. Casey had a basal cell carcinoma removed from his right ear. Six months ago, cancerous tumors were discovered in his bladder, and he underwent two 6-week chemotherapy courses. His latest report indicates that the tumors have grown back and that no further chemotherapy would be useful. The urologist had considered surgery but believed that Mr. Casey's other medical problems would compromise his chances of survival. Mr. Casey decides to let the disease run its course and to be managed at home through hospice care. Because he lives alone in a modest home, he asks his daughter, Mary, and her family to move in with him to provide care and support during his final months. The daughter accepts, saying she is glad to be able to spend this time with her father; she has been informed of the physical and emotional stress this will entail.

ASSESSMENT

Glynis Jackson, RN, the hospice nurse assigned as case manager for Mr. Casey, completes a health history and physical examination during her first two visits, 1 day apart, in his home. She gathers this information over 2 days to conserve his strength and allow more time for Mr. Casey and his daughter to talk about their concerns.

During the physical assessment, Glynis notes that Mr. Casey is pale, with pink mucous membranes, and thin, with a wasted appearance and a strained, worried facial expression. He complains of severe back pain no longer adequately relieved by Percodan and Vicodin alternating every 2–4 hours. His blood pressure is 90/50 mmHg, right arm in the reclining position with no significant orthostatic change; his apical pulse is 102 bpm, regular and strong; respirations are 24/minute and unlabored; breath sounds are clear but diminished in the bases; oral temperature is 96.8°F.

A tunneled Groshong catheter as a VAD is present in the right anterior chest. There is no drainage, redness, or swelling at the site. The catheter was placed last week when the client was being evaluated at the anesthesiologist's office for pain management, but no medication is running via the VAD. Mary reports that his urinary output is adequate. Approximately 200 mL of yellow, cloudy, nonmalodorous urine is present in the urinal at the bedside from his last voiding.

Mr. Casey states that he spends most of his time either in bed or sitting up in a chair in his room. He reports that he has no energy any more and is unable to walk to the bathroom unassisted, dress himself, or take care of his own personal hygiene. Glynis rates Mr. Casey's functional level at ECOG level 4: capable of only limited self-care, confined to bed or chair 50% or more of waking hours (Karnofsky 10–20). He tells the nurse that his daughter "is working day and night to help me and is looking awfully tired."

Mary reports that Mr. Casey is eating very poorly: He usually eats a small bowl of oatmeal with milk for breakfast and vegetable soup and crackers for lunch, but he tells her that he is too tired for dinner and wants only fruit juice. Mr. Casey tells the nurse that he has no appetite and eats just to please Mary. He does drink at least three to four glasses of water a day plus juice. His fingerstick blood sugars remain within normal range.

His current weight is 120 pounds at 67 inches tall, down from 180 pounds a year ago. He has lost about 30 pounds over the last 2 months.

Available laboratory values from his visit with the doctor show the following: total protein, 4.1 g/dL (normal range, 6.0–8.0 g/dL); albumin, 2.2 g/dL (normal range, 3.5–5.0 g/dL); hemoglobin, 10.2 g/dL (normal range, 13.5–18.0 g/dL); hematocrit, 30.5% (normal range, 40.0–54.0%); blood urea nitrogen: 30 mg/dL (normal range, 5–25 mg/dL, slightly higher in older people); and creatinine, 2.2 mg/dL (normal range: 0.5–1.5 mg/dL).

DIAGNOSES

- Imbalanced Nutrition: Less Than Body Requirements related to anorexia and fatigue
- Risk for Caregiver Role Strain related to severity of Mary's father's illness and lack of help from other family members
- Chronic Pain related to progression of disease process
- Impaired Physical Mobility related to pain, fatigue, and beginning neuromuscular impairment
- Risk for Impaired Skin Integrity related to impaired physical mobility and malnourished state

PLANNING

Goals for care include the following:

- The client will increase oral intake and show improvement in serum protein values.
- The daughter will be able to maintain supportive caretaking activities as long as Mr. Casey needs them.
- The client will have minimal pain for the rest of his life.
- The client will be able to continue his current activity level.
- The client will maintain intact skin.

(continued)

NURSING CARE PLAN **A Client With Cancer** *continued*

IMPLEMENTATION

- Ask about favorite foods, and ask Mary to offer a small portion of one of these foods each day.
- Encourage drinking up to four cans of liquid nutritional supplement with fiber a day, sipping them throughout the day.
- Talk with the physician about prescribing a medication to help stimulate the appetite.
- Plan to have a home health aide come to the home, give him a shower or bed bath daily, and assist his daughter with some of the household chores.
- Talk with Mary about having her adult son and daughter relieve her of the housework and stay with Mr. Casey so that she can get out of the house occasionally. Offer to talk with them if she is uncomfortable doing so.
- Request a volunteer to spend up to 4 hours a day, twice a week with Mr. Casey so that Mary can attend to outside activities and chores.
- Talk with the anesthesiologist, and work out a pain control program, using the VAD and a PCA (patient-controlled analgesia) infusion pump with a continuous morphine infusion.
- Call the infusion therapist to set up the equipment and supplies (including the medication) for the morphine infusion.
- Teach how to use the pump and about the side effects of the morphine infusion, including those that require a call to the nurse for assistance. Teach which untoward effects should be reported.
- Request a physical therapy consultation to evaluate current level of functioning and determine how to maintain current level.
- Instruct Mary to allow ample rest periods for Mr. Casey between activities.
- Order a hospital bed with electronic controls to be delivered to the house.
- Order a special foam pad for bed and chair and a bedside commode from the medical supply house.
- Instruct Mary and the home health aide to inspect skin daily, give good skin care with emollient lotion after bathing, and report any beginning lesions immediately to the nurse.

EVALUATION

Mr. Casey did increase his oral intake a little, sometimes eating the special treats his daughter prepared and drinking one or two cans of liquid nutritional supplement a day. However, his weight did not increase; it stayed at approximately 120 pounds until his death 2 weeks later. His daughter was very grateful for the extra help from the home health aide and the volunteer, though she could not bring herself to ask her son and daughter for help and did not want the nurse to do so. She did become more rested and reported that "Dad and I had some wonderful 3:00 a.m. talks when he couldn't sleep."

Mr. Casey was started on 20 mg of morphine per hour with boluses of 10 mg four times a day, for breakthrough pain. This medication relieved his pain quite well; after 2 days, he was alert enough most of the time to carry on a normal conversation and still walk to the bathroom with help up until 2 days before he died.

The hospital bed simplified Mr. Casey's care and made it much easier for him to rest comfortably and change position. His skin remained intact and in good condition.

Mary reported that Mr. Casey died peacefully in his sleep, about 2 weeks after care was started. She said spending the last weeks of his life together was a healing experience for both of them.

CRITICAL THINKING

1. What other tests could be done to evaluate Mr. Casey's nutritional status?
2. Mr. Casey had severe back pain. What were the possible pathophysiologic reasons for his pain?
3. One of the specified interventions was to consult the physician regarding medication to increase Mr. Casey's appetite. What medications might fulfill that function? What side effects might they have that would contraindicate these medications for Mr. Casey?
4. If Mr. Casey had developed signs and symptoms of sepsis, what manifestations would you expect to see? As the nurse making the home visits, what would be your nursing actions, and in what order of priority?

REVIEW Cancer

RELATE: LINK THE CONCEPTS

Linking the exemplar of Cancer with the concept of Evidence-Based Practice:

1. Why is evidence-based practice of particular importance when caring for clients diagnosed with cancer?
2. What impact on client care could result if the nurse fails to maintain an evidenced based practice?

Linking the exemplar of Cancer with the concept of Health Care Systems:

3. Suggest rationale for why reducing cancer-causing lifestyle choices as suggested by *Healthy People 2010* is so important to reducing costs within the health care system.
4. How large an impact does cancer diagnoses have on the health care system?

READY: GO TO COMPANION SKILLS MANUAL

- Establishing intravenous infusions
- Infusing IV fluids through a central line
- Managing central lines
- Changing a central line dressing
- Assessing vital signs
- Preparing the client for surgery
- Preparing the surgical site
- Preparing for a dressing change using individual supplies
- Changing a sterile dressing
- Assessing the skin
- Assessing the hair
- Assessing the client in pain
- Using the narcotic control system
- Managing pain with a PCA pump

REFER: GO TO MYNURSINGKIT

REFLECT: CASE STUDY

Mandy Leno, 63 years old, has lived with bipolar disorder since young adulthood. She has recently been diagnosed with pancreatic cancer. Ms Leno resides in an inpatient psychiatric unit, where she returns after her diagnosis. She is currently pacing up and down the hall stating that she has big plans for conquering this cancer. She is refusing her medications and does not want to sign the surgical permit to remove the tumor, which may include a pancreectomy. She has been sleeping little and has deep circles under her eyes. She has eaten very little in the last few days. Her urine output is low, she is disheveled, and her clothes are dirty. Mandy is divorced and has no other family nearby. She has a daughter who lives across the country and has three small children.

1. What are the priorities of care for Mandy?
2. Should Mandy's daughter be contacted? Explain your answer.
3. How can you help Mandy to move past her denial and accept the diagnosis in order to plan for treatment?

3.4 COLORECTAL CANCER

KEY TERMS

Colon cancer, *141*
Colorectal cancer, *141*
Colostomy, *144*
Fulguration, *143*
Polyps, *141*

BASIS FOR SELECTION OF EXEMPLAR

Centers for Disease Control and Prevention
Healthy People 2010
Institute of Medicine

LEARNING OUTCOMES

After reading about this exemplar, you will be able to:

1. Describe the pathophysiology, etiology, clinical manifestations, and direct and indirect causes of colorectal cancer.
2. Identify risk factors associated with colorectal cancer.
3. Illustrate the nursing process in providing culturally competent care across the life span for individuals with colorectal cancer.
4. Formulate priority nursing diagnoses appropriate for an individual with colon cancer.
5. Create a plan of care for individuals with colorectal cancer and their family members.
6. Assess expected outcomes for an individual with colorectal cancer.
7. Discuss therapies used in the collaborative care of an individual with colorectal cancer.
8. Employ evidence-based caring interventions for an individual with colorectal cancer.

OVERVIEW

Colon cancer is cancer of the third segment of the large bowel and may or may not include the anus. **Colorectal cancer** involves both the colon and the rectum. While the terms are often used interchangeably, they are different in regards to whether the rectum is involved.

Regular colonoscopies can greatly reduce the risk for colorectal cancer by allowing removal of polyps before they become malignant tumors that invade the bowel and metastasize to other areas of the body. The nurse's role focuses on promoting the need for regular screening as well as reporting the early warning signs of the disease in order to reduce occurrence and improve outcomes.

PATHOPHYSIOLOGY AND ETIOLOGY

Nearly all colorectal cancers are adenocarcinomas that begin as adenomatous **polyps** (small vascular growths on the surface of any mucous membrane, referring in this exemplar to growths on the internal surface of the bowel). Most tumors develop in the rectum and sigmoid colon, although any portion of the colon may be affected (Figure 3–11 ■).

The tumor typically grows undetected, producing few manifestations. By the time manifestations occur, the disease may have spread into deeper layers of the bowel tissue and adjacent organs. Colorectal cancer spreads by direct extension to involve the entire bowel circumference, the submucosa, and outer bowel wall layers. Neighboring structures, such as the liver, greater curvature of the stomach, duodenum, small intestine, pancreas, spleen, genitourinary tract, and abdominal wall, also may be involved by direct extension.

Metastasis to regional lymph nodes is the most common form of tumor spread. This is not always an orderly process; distal nodes may contain cancer cells while regional nodes remain normal. Cancerous cells from the primary tumor may

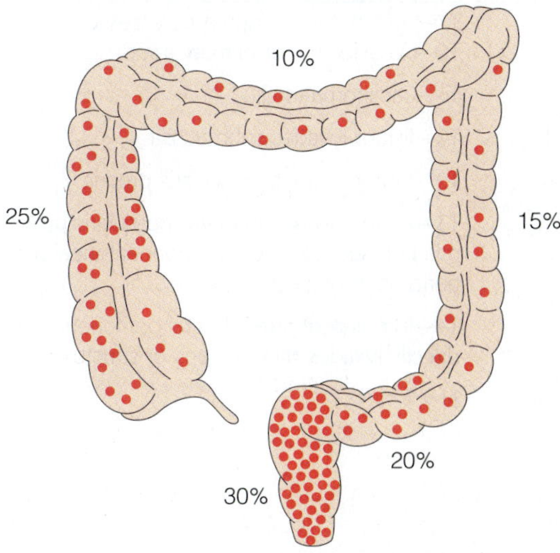

Figure 3–11 ■ The distribution and frequency of cancer of the colon and rectum.

also spread by way of the lymphatic system or circulatory system to secondary sites, such as the liver, lungs, brain, bones, and kidneys. In addition, "seeding" of the tumor to other areas of the peritoneal cavity can occur when the tumor extends through the serosa or during surgical resection.

Current staging methods primarily use the TNM system, as outlined in Table 3–11.

Etiology

Colorectal cancer (cancer of the colon or rectum) is the third most common cancer diagnosed in the United States. In 2005, approximately 145,290 new cases of colorectal cancer were diagnosed in the United States, with approximately 56,290 deaths (28,540 men and 27,750 women) estimated to have resulted from colorectal cancer during that same year (ACS, 2006a).

Earlier diagnosis and improved treatment have improved the survival rate for colorectal cancer. Its incidence, which is nearly equal among men and women, has been declining in the United States for the past 15 years. Colorectal cancer occurs most frequently after age 50. The incidence continues to rise with increasing age. With early diagnosis and treatment, the 5-year survival rate for colorectal cancer is 90%; however, only 39% of colorectal cancers are diagnosed at this early stage.

Risk Factors

A number of risk factors for colorectal cancer have been identified (Box 3–14). Genetic factors are strongly linked to the risk for colorectal cancer. Up to 20% of people who develop colorectal cancer have a family history of the disease (ACS, 2005c). Persons with familial adenomatous polyposis inevitably will develop colon cancer unless the colon is removed. Hereditary nonpolyposis colorectal cancer (also known as Lynch syndrome) is an autosomal dominant disorder that significantly increases the risk for developing colorectal and other cancers. Tumors associated with Lynch syndrome often affect the ascending colon and tend to occur at an earlier age. Inflammatory bowel diseases also increase the risk of colorectal cancer.

Diet plays a role in the development of colorectal cancer. The disease is prevalent in economically prosperous countries where people consume diets high in calories, meat proteins, and fats. This dietary pattern, common in the United States, is thought to increase the population of anaerobic bacteria in the gut. These anaerobes convert bile acids into carcinogens. Diets high in fruits and vegetables, folic acid, and calcium appear to reduce the risk of colorectal cancer. Cereal fiber, once thought to reduce colorectal cancer risk, now does not appear to play a role either way in its development. Other factors that may reduce the risk of colorectal cancer include regular exercise, taking a daily multivitamin, and the use of aspirin and other nonsteroidal anti-inflammatory drugs.

Box 3–14 **Risk Factors for Colorectal Cancer**

- Age older than 50 years
- Polyps of the colon and/or rectum
- Family history of colorectal cancer
- Inflammatory bowel disease
- Exposure to radiation
- Diet: high animal fat and kilocalorie intake

CLINICAL MANIFESTATIONS

Bowel cancer often produces no manifestations until it is advanced. Because it grows slowly, 5–15 years of growth may occur before manifestations develop. The manifestations depend on its location, type and extent, and complications.

TABLE 3–11 **The TNM Staging System for Colorectal Cancer**

STAGE	PRIMARY TUMOR (T)	REGIONAL LYMPH NODES (N)	DISTANT METASTASIS (M)
	TX—Primary tumor cannot be assessed T0—No evidence of primary tumor	NX—Regional lymph node cannot be assessed	MX—Presence of distant metastasis cannot be assessed
Stage 0	Tis—Carcinoma in situ	N0—No regional lymph node metastasis	M0—No distant metastasis
Stage I	T1—Tumor invades submucosa		
	T2—Tumor invades muscularis propria		
Stage II	T3—Tumor invades through muscularis propria into subserosa or into nonperitonealized pericolic or perirectal tissues		
	T4—Tumor perforates visceral peritoneum or directly invades other organs or structures		
Stage III	Any T	N1—Metastasis in one to three pericolic or perirectal lymph nodes	
		N2—Metastasis in four or more pericolic or perirectal lymph nodes	
		N3—Metastasis in any lymph node along course of a major named vascular trunk	
Stage IV	Any T	Any N	M1—Distant metastasis

CLINICAL MANIFESTATIONS AND THERAPIES **Colorectal Cancer**

ETIOLOGY	CLINICAL MANIFESTATION	CLINICAL THERAPIES
Rectal bleeding may occur as the cancer cells invade or irritate the bowel mucosa.	Dark color to stool, blood may or may not be visible without guaiac testing, classic alteration in smell of stools with frank blood, anemia, decreasing hemaglobin and hematocrit, decreased RBC, often asymptomatic unless guaiac tested	■ Surgical removal of tumor and involved segment of bowel ■ Blood transfusions and hydration if blood loss is significant
Change in bowel habits as cancer cells grow	Stools may be pencil thin as the bowel lumen diminishes; diarrhea or constipation	■ Surgical resection of involved bowel ■ Antidiarrheals may be indicated if diarrhea results ■ Monitor for signs of complete obstruction of bowel, including emesis, acute abdominal pain, or abdominal distention, accompanied by absence of stool for several days

Rectal bleeding is often the initial manifestation that prompts clients to seek medical care. Other common early manifestations include a change in bowel habits, either diarrhea or constipation. Pain, anorexia, and weight loss are characteristic in advanced disease. A palpable abdominal or rectal mass may be present. Occasionally, the client presents with anemia from occult bleeding.

COLLABORATION

The client with a diagnosis of colorectal cancer needs a collaborative approach often requiring intervention from surgeons, nurses specializing in care of ostomies, dietary counselors, radiation therapists, as well as the nurse providing primary care. A holistic approach to the client's care improves both client outcomes and chances for survival.

Screening

The ACS (2005c) recommends one of the following testing schedules for early detection of colorectal cancer, beginning at age 50. These options are acceptable choices for average-risk adults:

- Yearly fecal occult blood test or fecal immunochemical test. (For fecal occult blood test, the take-home, multiple-sample method should be used.)
- Flexible sigmoidoscopy every 5 years
- Double-contrast barium enema every 5 years
- Colonoscopy every 10 years.

Diagnostic Tests

Diagnostic and laboratory tests are used for screening, diagnosis, and monitoring purposes. Diagnostic tests include a sigmoidoscopy or colonoscopy as the primary means used to detect and visualize tumors. While flexible sigmoidoscopy can detect 50–65% of colorectal cancers, many clinicians recommend colonoscopy. Tissue for biopsy is obtained at the time of endoscopy to confirm cancerous tissue and evaluate cell differentiation. Current staging methods primarily use the TNM system, as outlined previously in Table 3–11. Radiologic examinations may include a chest x-ray to detect tumor metastasis to the lung, and CT, MRI, or ultrasonic examination may be used to assess tumor depth and involvement of other organs by direct extension or metastasis.

Laboratory tests include a fecal occult blood (by guaiac or hemoccult testing) to detect blood in the feces, a CBC to detect anemia resulting from chronic blood loss and tumor growth, and a CEA level, which is a tumor marker that can be detected in the blood of clients with colorectal cancer. CEA levels are used to estimate prognosis, monitor treatment, and detect cancer recurrence.

Surgery

Surgical resection of the tumor, adjacent colon, and regional lymph nodes is the treatment of choice for colorectal cancer. Options for surgical treatment vary from destruction of the tumor by laser photocoagulation performed during endoscopy to abdominoperineal resection with permanent colostomy. When possible, the anal sphincter is preserved and colostomy avoided.

Other surgical treatment options for small, localized tumors include local excision and fulguration. These procedures also may be performed during endoscopy, eliminating the need for abdominal surgery. Local excision may be used to remove a disk of rectum containing a tumor in clients with a small, well-differentiated, mobile polypoid lesion. **Fulguration**, also known as electrocoagulation, is a procedure used to reduce the size of some large tumors for clients who are poor surgical risks. Fulguration requires general anesthesia and may need to be repeated at intervals.

Most clients with colorectal cancer undergo surgical resection of the colon with anastomosis of the remaining bowel as a curative procedure. The distribution of regional lymph nodes determines the extent of resection, because these may contain metastatic lesions. Most tumors of the ascending, transverse, descending, and sigmoid colon can be resected.

Tumors of the rectum usually are treated with an abdominoperineal resection in which the sigmoid colon, rectum, and anus are removed through both abdominal and perineal incisions. A permanent sigmoid colostomy is performed to provide for elimination of feces.

COLOSTOMY Surgical resection of the bowel may be accompanied by a colostomy for diversion of fecal contents. A **colostomy** is an ostomy made in the colon. It may be created if the bowel is obstructed by the tumor, as a temporary measure to promote healing of anastomoses, or as a permanent means of fecal evacuation when the distal colon and rectum are removed. Colostomies take the name of the portion of the colon from which they are formed: ascending colostomy, transverse colostomy, descending colostomy, and sigmoid colostomy (Figure 3–12 ■).

A sigmoid colostomy is the most common permanent colostomy, particularly for cancer of the rectum. It is usually created during an abdominoperineal resection. This procedure involves removal of the sigmoid colon, rectum, and anus through abdominal and perineal incisions. The anal canal is closed, and a stoma is formed from the proximal sigmoid colon. The stoma usually is located on the lower left quadrant of the abdomen.

When a double-barrel colostomy is performed, two separate stomas are created (Figure 3–13 ■). The distal colon is not removed, but bypassed. The proximal stoma, which is functional, diverts feces to the abdominal wall. The distal stoma, also called the mucous fistula, expels mucus from the distal colon. It may be pouched or dressed with a 4 × 4 gauge dressing. A double-barrel colostomy may be created for cases of trauma, tumor, or inflammation, and it may be temporary or permanent.

An emergency procedure used to relieve an intestinal obstruction or perforation is called a transverse loop colostomy. During this procedure, a loop of the transverse colon is brought out from the abdominal wall and suspended over a plastic rod or bridge, which prevents the loop from slipping back into the abdominal cavity. The loop stoma may be opened at the time of surgery or a few days later at the client's bedside. The bridge may be removed in 1–2 weeks. Transverse loop colostomies are typically temporary.

In a Hartmann procedure, a common temporary colostomy procedure, the distal portion of the colon is left in place and is oversewn for closure. A temporary colostomy may be done to allow bowel rest or healing, such as following tumor resection or inflammation of the bowel. It also may be created following traumatic injury to the colon, such as a gunshot wound. Anastomosis of the severed portions of the colon is delayed, because bacterial colonization of the colon would prevent proper healing of the anastomosis. Approximately 3–6 months following a temporary colostomy, the colostomy is closed, and the colon is reconnected. Clients with temporary colostomies require the same care as clients with permanent colostomies.

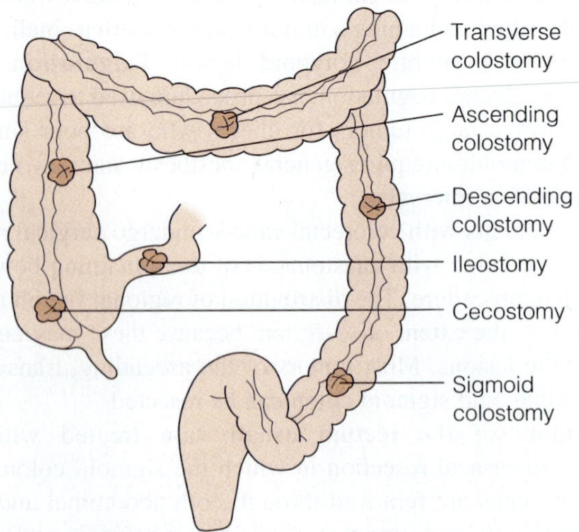

Figure 3–12 ■ Various ostomy levels and sites.

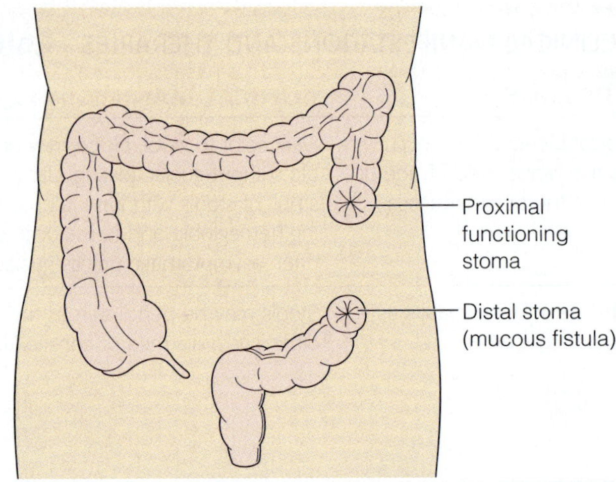

Figure 3–13 ■ A double-barrel colostomy. The proximal stoma is the functioning stoma; the distal stoma expels mucus from the distal colon.

LASER PHOTOCOAGULATION Laser photocoagulation uses a very small, intense beam of light to generate heat in tissues toward which it is directed. The heat generated by the laser beam can be used to destroy small tumors. It is also used for palliative surgery of advanced tumors to remove obstruction. Laser photocoagulation can be performed endoscopically and is useful for clients who cannot tolerate major surgery.

Radiation Therapy

Although radiation therapy is not used as a primary treatment for colon cancer, it is used with surgical resection for treating rectal tumors. Small rectal cancers may be treated with intracavitary, external, or implantation radiation. Rectal cancer has a high rate of regional recurrence following complete surgical resection, particularly when the tumor has invaded tissues outside the bowel wall or regional lymph nodes. Pre- or postoperative radiation therapy reduces the recurrence of pelvic tumors, although the effect of radiation therapy on long-term survival is less clear. Radiation therapy also is used preoperatively to shrink large rectal tumors enough to permit surgical removal of the tumor.

Chemotherapy

Chemotherapeutic agents, such as IV fluorouracil (5-FU) and folinic acid (leucovorin), are also used postoperatively as adjunctive therapy for colorectal cancer. When combined with radiation therapy, chemotherapy reduces the rate of tumor recurrence and prolongs survival for clients with stage II and stage III rectal tumors. The benefit for clients with colon cancer is less clear, but chemotherapy may be used to reduce its spread to the liver and prevent recurrence. Irinotecan (CPT-11) or oxaliplatin also may be used in chemotherapy regimens for colorectal cancer.

NURSING PROCESS

In planning and implementing care, consider both physical care needs and emotional response to the diagnosis. Because colorectal cancer is often advanced at the time of diagnosis, the prognosis, even with treatment, may be poor. Denial and anger are common. Extensive abdominal surgery and a colostomy may be necessary, and the effects of chemotherapy and radiation therapy can leave the client fatigued and discouraged.

Assessment

Collect the following data through the health history and physical examination:

- *Health history.* Usual bowel patterns and any recent changes; weight loss, fatigue, decreased activity tolerance; presence of blood in the stool; pain with defecation, abdominal discomfort, perineal pain; usual diet; family history of colorectal cancer, other specific risk factors, such as inflammatory bowel disease or colon polyps
- *Physical examination.* General appearance; weight; abdominal shape, contour; bowel sounds, abdominal tenderness; stool hemoccult or guaiac.

Diagnosis

Nursing diagnoses for the client with colorectal cancer are individualized to each client's needs and may include:

- Acute Pain
- Imbalanced Nutrition: Less Than Body Requirements
- Anticipatory Grieving
- Risk for Sexual Dysfunction.

Plan

The goals for client outcome are determined by the client's condition, prognosis, amount of tissue involved, and staging of the tumor. Suggested goals may include the following:

- The client will not experience complications related to altered elimination pattern.
- The client will demonstrate proper ostomy care and management.
- The client will verbalize feelings related to diagnosis and prognosis.
- The family and/or significant others will provide adequate emotional and physical support for the client upon discharge.
- The client will make an informed choice related to treatment options.

Implementation

Nursing care includes providing emotional support, teaching, and direct care before and after diagnostic procedures and surgery as well as during adjunctive treatments. Risk for sexual dysfunction should be addressed as a nursing diagnosis if a colostomy has been created.

Acute Pain

The client with colorectal cancer may experience pain related to preparatory procedures, diagnostic examinations, and surgery. Following an abdominoperineal resection, "phantom" rectal pain related to the severing of nerves during the wide excision of the rectum may develop. Finally, the primary tumor itself and, potentially, metastatic tumors may impinge on nerves and other organs, causing pain.

In the early postoperative period, an epidural infusion or client-controlled analgesia often is used to manage pain. Client-controlled analgesia, routine administration of ordered analgesics, or a continuous analgesia delivery system also may be used for pain management when the tumor is far enough advanced to preclude surgical resection. A detailed discussion of pain medications can be found in Exemplar 5.1, Acute and Chronic Pain.

- Monitor for adequate pain relief. Use subjective and objective information, including the location, intensity, and character of the pain, as well as nonverbal signs, such as grimacing, muscle tension, apparent dozing, changes in pulse or blood pressure, and rapid, shallow respirations. The client may assume that pain is to be expected or tolerated or may fear becoming addicted to analgesic medications. Careful questioning and assessment can provide accurate information about pain status, allowing better control of discomfort.
- Ask the client to rate pain using a scale of 0–10. Document the level of pain. Pain is a subjective experience. Clients perceive and respond to pain differently. Religion and ethnic background may affect the response to pain.
- Monitor analgesic effectiveness 30 minutes after administration. Monitor for pain relief and adverse effects. The method of delivery, dosage, or medication itself may need to be adjusted to provide adequate pain relief.
- Assess the incision for inflammation or swelling; assess drainage catheters and tubes for patency. Poorly controlled pain or pain that changes may be related to organ distention from an obstructed nasogastric tube, urinary catheter, or wound drain. It also may indicate an infection.
- Assess the abdomen for distention, tenderness, and bowel sounds. Intra-abdominal bleeding, peritonitis, or paralytic ileus can cause pain that may be confused with incisional pain.
- Administer analgesia before an activity or procedure. Adequate pain relief reduces muscle tension, allowing more comfortable participation in activities.
- Assist with adjunctive comfort measures, such as positioning, diversional activities, management of environmental stimuli, guided imagery, and teaching relaxation techniques. These measures enhance the effects of analgesia by reducing muscle tension.
- Splint incision with a pillow, and teach the client how to self-splint when coughing and deep breathing to prevent respiratory complications related to fear of pain.

Imbalanced Nutrition: Less Than Body Requirements

Bowel preparation for diagnostic procedures, surgery, radiation therapy, and chemotherapy place the client with colorectal cancer at risk for nutritional deficiencies. Fluid and electrolyte replacement is provided following surgery, along with possible total parenteral nutrition. Adequate kilocalorie and nutrient intake are necessary for healing after surgery. Additionally, if the tumor is advanced, metabolic needs may be increased and the appetite decreased.

- Assess nutritional status, using data such as height and weight, skinfold measurements, body mass index, and laboratory data, including serum albumin level. Refer to a dietitian or nutritionist for dietary management. The client who is malnourished before beginning aggressive cancer treatment requires more vigorous nutrition management to promote healing.
- Assess readiness for resumption of oral intake after surgery or procedures using data such as statements of hunger, presence of bowel sounds, passage of flatus, and minimal abdominal distention. Manipulation of the bowel interrupts peristalsis of the gastrointestinal tract. It is important to ensure that peristalsis has resumed before oral intake begins.
- Monitor and document food and fluid intake. Documentation helps identify the adequacy of kilocalories and other nutrient intake.
- Weigh the client daily. Weight fluctuation may indicate adequate or inadequate dietary intake.
- Maintain total parenteral nutrition and central IV lines as ordered. Parenteral nutrition prevents tissue catabolism and promotes healing when food intake is disrupted for more than 2–3 days.
- When oral intake resumes, help the client develop a meal plan that incorporates food preferences and considers the client's schedule and environment. Consideration of likes, dislikes, and circumstances in meal planning promotes adequate intake.

Anticipatory Grieving

When a bowel resection is performed for colorectal cancer, the client needs to adjust to the loss of a major body part as well as to the diagnosis of cancer. Even when the prognosis for recovery is good, many people perceive cancer as fatal. Supporting the client and family during the initial stages of grieving can improve physical recovery as well as psychologic coping and eventual adaptation.

- Work to develop a trusting relationship with the client and family. This increases the nurse's effectiveness in helping them work through the grieving process.
- Listen actively, encouraging the client and family to express their fears and concerns. Assist to identify strengths, past experiences, and support systems:
  a. Demonstrate respect for cultural, spiritual, and religious values and beliefs; encourage use of these resources to cope with losses.
  b. Encourage discussion of the potential impact of loss on individual family members, family structure, and family function. Assist family members to share concerns with one another.
  c. Refer to cancer support groups, social services, or counseling as appropriate.

These resources can be used throughout the grieving process.

Risk for Sexual Dysfunction

Colorectal cancer and ostomy surgery increase the risk for sexual dysfunction, defined as a change in sexual function so that it becomes unsatisfying, unrewarding, or inadequate (NANDA International, 2005). Physical factors that can lead to sexual dysfunction include disruption of nerves and blood vessels that supply the genitals, radiation therapy, chemotherapy, and other medications prescribed after surgery.

Psychologically, a client with an ostomy experiences an altered body image and may develop low self-esteem. The client may feel undesirable and fear rejection. He or she may be concerned about odors or pouch leakage during sexual activity. This emotional stress can also contribute to sexual dysfunction.

- Provide opportunities for the client and family to express feelings about the cancer diagnosis, ostomy, and effects of other treatments. Encouraging verbalization provides an opportunity to validate that feelings of anger and depression are normal responses to the diagnosis and change in body function.
- Provide consistent colostomy care. An accepting attitude and consistent care that provides a secure appliance and controls odor and leakage instill a sense of confidence in the client.
- Encourage expression of sexual concerns. Provide privacy and caregivers who have established trust with the client and family and are comfortable with discussions about sexual concerns. Sexuality is a very private concern to most people. The client and family are not likely to express their concerns openly unless trust has been established.
- Reassure the client and significant other that the effect of physical illness and prescribed interventions on sexuality usually is temporary. The client and partner may misinterpret an initial decrease in libido as evidence that sexual activity will not be possible or resume following recovery.
- Refer the client and partner to social services or a family counselor for further interventions. Clients are often discharged from acute care settings well before concerns about sexual activity surface. Ongoing counseling provides a continuing resource.
- Arrange for a visit from a member of the United Ostomy Association. People who are living and coping with an ostomy can provide information and support, helping the client with a new ostomy overcome feelings of isolation and rejection.

Evaluation

Client outcome is evaluated based on goals of care. Potential expected outcomes may include the following:

- The client will maintain adequate nutritional status.
- The client will maintain adequate hydration.
- The client will report pain level of 3 or less and be able to rest and perform essential daily ADLs.
- The client will explain treatment options and receive support from family in choices related to treatment.

NURSING CARE PLAN **A Client With Colorectal Cancer**

William Cunningham is a 65-year-old retired railroad employee, husband, and father of three grown children. For the past 3 months, Mr. Cunningham has noticed small amounts of blood and occasional mucous in his stools. He has a sensation of pressure in the rectum, and he notices that his stools are smaller in diameter, about the size of pencil. After palpating a mass on digital examination of the rectum, the physician orders a colonoscopy. A large sessile lesion is found in the rectum and biopsied. The pathology report shows the lesion to be adenocarcinoma. Mr. Cunningham is scheduled for an abdominoperineal resection and sigmoid colostomy.

ASSESSMENT	DIAGNOSES	PLANNING
Madonna Hart, RN, completes the admission assessment. Mr. Cunningham states that his bowel habits have recently changed, but he denies pain or other symptoms. Physical assessment findings include temperature 98.4°F (36.9°C), pulse 82 bpm, respirations 18/min, and BP 118/78 mm Hg. He is 70 inches (178 cm) tall and weighs 185 lb (84 kg). Laboratory findings are normal except for the previous pathology report of adenocarcinoma of rectal lesion. Mr. Cunningham states, "I really don't want a colostomy, but if that is what it takes to get rid of this, I'm ready to get it over with."	■ Acute Pain related to surgical intervention ■ Risk for Impaired Skin Integrity (peristomal) related to fecal drainage and pouch adhesive ■ Risk for Constipation/Diarrhea related to effects of surgery on bowel function ■ Disturbed Body Image related to colostomy ■ Risk for Sexual Dysfunction related to wide rectal incision, radiation therapy, and colostomy	■ The client will report pain within an acceptable range that allows ease of movement and ambulation. ■ The client will perform colostomy care using correct technique. ■ The client will demonstrate willingness to discuss changes in sexual function. ■ The client will wear clothing to enhance physical and emotional self-esteem.

IMPLEMENTATION

- Provide analgesia as ordered, evaluating its effectiveness.
- Discuss foods that cause odor and gas.
- Teach colostomy care.
- Maintain consistent nursing personnel assignment to facilitate trust.
- Refer to the local United Ostomy Association.
- Provide a list of local medical supply companies for ostomy supplies.
- Provide for privacy when teaching and discussing concerns about ostomy.

EVALUATION

On discharge, Mr. Cunningham is able to empty and rinse out his colostomy pouch. He is changing the pouch and caring for surrounding skin appropriately. Ms. Hart has given him verbal and written instructions on colostomy care. He verbalizes understanding of phantom rectal pain and the importance of avoiding rectal suppositories. He expresses an understanding of the need to avoid heavy lifting and the importance of follow-up care. Ms. Hart has referred Mr. Cunningham to a home health agency in his community for further questions and follow-up care.

CRITICAL THINKING

1. What is the cause of phantom rectal pain?
2. Why is it important to discuss dietary concerns with a client with a colostomy, especially odor- and gas-forming foods?
3. Outline a plan to teach Mr. Cunningham how to irrigate a colostomy.
4. Develop a care plan for Mr. Cunningham for the nursing diagnosis disturbed body image.

REVIEW Colorectal Cancer

RELATE: LINK THE CONCEPTS

Linking the exemplar of Colorectal Cancer with the concept of Elimination:

1. What alterations in bowel elimination increase the client's risk for colorectal cancer?
2. What preventive teaching can you provide the client with altered bowel elimination to reduce the risk of colorectal cancer?

Linking the exemplar of Colorectal Cancer with the concept of Self:

3. How might a client's self-concept be altered as the result of treatment for colorectal cancer resulting in a colostomy?
4. You are caring for a client with end-stage colorectal cancer who appears emaciated, is cachectic, and has lost most of her hair as a result of treatment. She refuses visitors because she doesn't want friends and loved ones to see her looking like this. What nursing interventions can you implement to help her cope with her altered body-image and self-concept while promoting socialization?

READY: GO TO COMPANION SKILLS MANUAL

- Instructing a client for a colonostomy irrigation
- Monitoring intake and output
- Assessing vital signs
- Preparing the surgical site
- Preparing the client for surgery
- Preparing for a dressing change using individual supplies
- Changing a sterile dressing

- Assessing the abdomen
- Assessing the anus
- Assessing the client in pain
- Using the narcotic control system
- Managing pain with a PCA pump

REFER: GO TO MYNURSINGKIT

REFLECT: CASE STUDY

Pamela is a 65-year-old female who has been married to Clifford for 40 years. Their only child, 24-year-old Gary, has Down syndrome and lives with them. In the past, Pamela worked as an administrative assistant in a law firm. After Gary was born, Pam gave up her career to care for Gary.

Pam frequently experiences constipation, and treats this with over-the-counter agents. She considers the constipation more of an annoyance than anything else. The only medical condition she has ever had requiring treatment was endometrial cancer at age 50. The cancer was diagnosed at a very early stage, and she underwent a total hysterectomy and bilateral salpingo-oophorectomy. Because there was no evidence of lymph node involvement, she was considered cured and has been cancer-free ever since. Her last examination was 14 months ago.

One day Pam experiences diarrhea with an odd reddish-brown color and odor. The next day she returns to experiencing little relief from the constipation that has plagued her. She has been straining to have a bowel movement and notes that her stools are thinner than usual. A few weeks later, while still experiencing constipation and odd-shaped stools, she begins to feel a sense of fullness in her recutm and pelvic area, even after defecation. The appearance of reddish-brown in her stools has been more regular. She has often been feeling tired lately. On Friday afternoon, she finally makes a decision to call for an appointment with her physician about the symptoms. She is told to come to the office on the following Monday morning. She has a feeling of dread and becomes worried that something serious may be wrong.

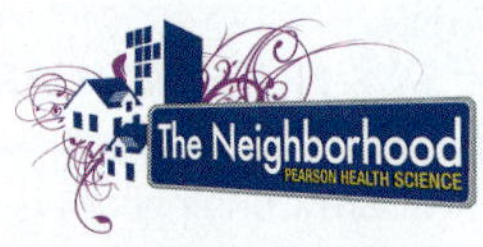

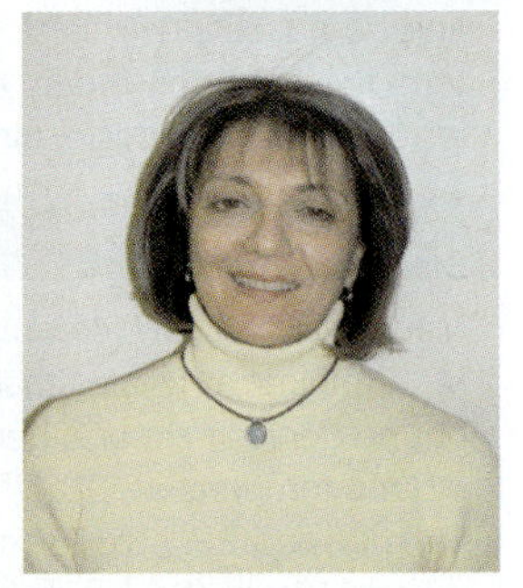

1. What specific symptoms described by Ms. Allen would cause you to suspect colorectal cancer?
2. What diagnostic test would you anticipate will be performed in the doctor's office on her first visit?
3. Develop a plan of care for Ms. Allen addressing both her physical and psychosocial needs.

3.5 LEUKEMIA

KEY TERMS

Acute lymphocytic leukemia (ALL), *150*
Acute myeloid leukemia (AML), *149*
Allogeneic bone marrow transplant, *155*
Autologous bone marrow transplant, *155*
Bone marrow transplant (BMT), *154*
Chronic lymphocytic leukemia (CLL), *151*
Chronic myeloid leukemia (CML), *149*
Leukemia, *148*
Philadelphia chromosome, *149*
Remission, *153*
Stem cell transplant (SCT), *155*

BASIS FOR SELECTION OF EXEMPLAR

Centers for Disease Control and Prevention
Healthy People 2010
Institute of Medicine

LEARNING OUTCOMES

After reading about this exemplar, you will be able to:

1. Describe the pathophysiology, etiology, clinical manifestations, and direct and indirect causes of leukemia.
2. Identify risk factors associated with leukemia.
3. Illustrate the nursing process in providing culturally competent care across the life span for individuals with leukemia.
4. Formulate priority nursing diagnoses appropriate for an individual with leukemia.
5. Create a plan of care for individuals with leukemia and their family members.
6. Assess expected outcomes for an individual with leukemia.
7. Discuss therapies used in the collaborative care of an individual with leukemia.
8. Employ evidence-based caring interventions for an individual with leukemia.

OVERVIEW

Leukemia (literally, "white blood") is a group of chronic malignant disorders of WBCs and WBC precursors. In leukemia, the usual ratio of RBCs to WBCs is reversed. Leukemias are characterized by replacement of bone marrow by malignant immature WBCs, abnormal immature circulating WBCs, and infiltration of these cells into the liver, spleen, and lymph nodes throughout the body.

PATHOPHYSIOLOGY AND ETIOLOGY

Leukemias are classified by their acuity and by the predominant cell type involved. The *acute* leukemias are characterized by an acute onset, rapid disease progression, and immature or undifferentiated blast cells. *Chronic* leukemias, on the other hand, have a gradual onset, prolonged course, and abnormal mature-appearing cells. Lymphocytic (or lymphoblastic) leukemias involve immature lymphocytes and their precursor cells in the bone marrow. Lymphocytic leukemias infiltrate the spleen, lymph nodes, central nervous system, and other tissues. Myeloid (also called myelogenous, myelocytic, or myeloblastic) leukemias involve myeloid stem cells in the bone marrow, interfering with the maturation of all types of blood cells, including granulocytes, RBCs, and thrombocytes (Porth, 2005). Acute lymphoblastic leukemia is the most common type of leukemia in children (Figure 3–14 ■). In adults, acute myeloid leukemia and chronic lymphocytic leukemia

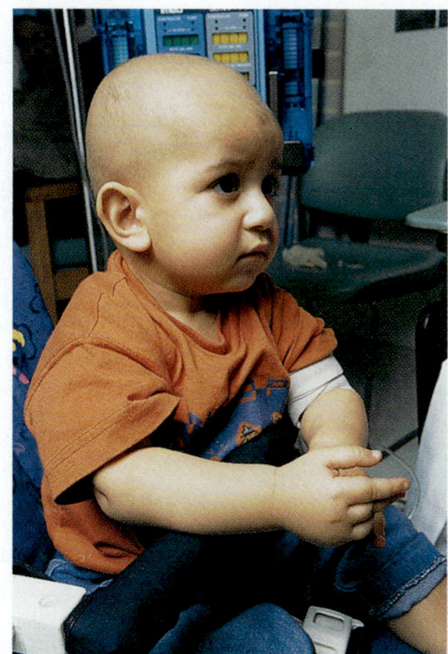

Figure 3–14 ■ Acute lymphoblastic leukemia is the most common type of leukemia in children and the most common cancer affecting children under 5 years of age.

are the most common types (McCance & Huether, 2006). In summary, the general types of leukemia are:

- Acute lymphocytic (lymphoblastic) leukemia
- Chronic lymphocytic leukemia
- Acute myeloid (myeloblastic) leukemia
- Chronic myeloid (myelogenous) leukemia.

The major types of leukemia are summarized in Table 3–12. However, this general system of classifying leukemias does not differentiate subtypes of acute leukemias. The French-American-British (FAB) system for classifying acute leukemias further differentiates acute leukemias by the predominant cell involved and the degree of cell differentiation (Table 3–13).

Acute Myeloid Leukemia

Acute myeloid leukemia (AML) is characterized by uncontrolled proliferation of myeloblasts (the precursors of granulocytes) and hyperplasia of the bone marrow and spleen (Figure 3–15 ■). AML accounts for 80% of acute leukemia cases in adults (Copstead & Banasik, 2005). Treatment induces complete remission in 66% of clients, although only about 30–40% achieve cure or long-term remission (Porth, 2005).

The manifestations of AML result from neutropenia and thrombocytopenia. Decreased neutrophils lead to recurrent severe infections, such as pneumonia, septicemia, abscesses, and mucous membrane ulceration. The manifestations of thrombocytopenia include petechiae, (red or purple spot that looks like a spider caused by a broken capillary), purpura (small areas of subcutaneous bleeding), ecchymoses (bruising), epistaxis (nosebleeds), hematomas, hematuria, and gastrointestinal bleeding. Bone infarctions or subperiosteal infiltrates of leukemic cells may cause bone pain. Anemia is a late manifestation, causing fatigue, headaches, pallor, and dyspnea on exertion. Death usually results from infection or hemorrhage.

Bone marrow aspiration shows a proliferation of immature WBCs. The CBC shows thrombocytopenia and normocytic, normochromic anemia.

Chronic Myeloid Leukemia

Chronic myeloid leukemia (CML) is characterized by abnormal proliferation of all bone marrow elements. This type of leukemia constitutes approximately 15% of adult leukemias. It affects men more frequently than women. The onset of CML typically is between the ages of 30 and 50, although it is seen in children and adolescents as well (Copstead & Banasik, 2005; Porth 2005).

Usually, CML is associated with a chromosome abnormality called the **Philadelphia chromosome**, a balanced translocation of chromosome 22 to chromosome 9 (Figure 3–16 ■). The

TABLE 3–12 **Major Types of Leukemia**

CLASSIFICATION	CHARACTERISTICS	MANIFESTATIONS	TREATMENT
Acute lymphoblastic leukemia (ALL)	Primarily affects children and young adults; leukemic cells may infiltrate the central nervous system	Recurrent infections; bleeding; pallor, bone pain, weight loss, sore throat, fatigue, night sweats, weakness	Chemotherapy; bone marrow transplant (BMT), or stem cell transplant (SCT)
Chronic lymphocytic leukemia (CLL)	Primarily affects older adults; insidious onset and slow, chronic course	Fatigue; exercise intolerance; lymphadenopathy and splenomegaly; recurrent infections, pallor, edema, thrombophlebitis	Often requires no treatment; chemotherapy; BMT
Acute myeloid leukemia (AML)	Common in older adults, may affect children and young adults. Strongly associated with toxins, genetic disorders, and treatment of other cancers	Fatigue, weakness, fever; anemia; headache; bone and joint pain; abnormal bleeding and bruising; recurrent infection; lymphadenopathy, splenomegaly, and hepatomegaly	Chemotherapy; SCT
Chronic myeloid leukemia (CML)	Primarily affects adults; early course slow and stable, progressing to aggressive phase in 3–4 years	*Early:* weakness, fatigue, dyspnea on exertion; possible splenomegaly *Later:* fever, weight loss, night sweats	Interferon alpha; chemotherapy with imatinib mesylate (Gleevec), SCT

TABLE 3–13 French-American-British (FAB) Classification of Acute Leukemia

TYPE	CLASS	PREDOMINANT CELLS	PROGNOSIS
Acute lymphocytic leukemia	L_1	Immature lymphoblasts	> 90% remission rate in children
	L_2	Mature lymphoblasts	Relapse common after 2 or more years of remission
Acute myeloid leukemia	M_0	Undifferentiated cells	Poor
	M_1	Immature myeloblasts	Good; complete response in $\geq$ 65%
	M_2	Mature myeloblasts	Good for 2 or more years of remission
	M_3	Promyelocytes	Good in adults
	M_4	Myelocytes and monocytes	Poorest in adults
	M_5	Poorly or well-differentiated monocytes	Poor
	M_6	Predominant erythroblasts	Variable
	M_7	Megakaryocytes	

fusion gene produced by this translocation, known as *bcr/abl*, is an oncogene capable of initiating a malignancy. Very large doses of ionizing radiation also may induce CML in some clients (Kasper et al., 2005).

People with CML are often asymptomatic in the early stages; in fact, CML is often diagnosed when a routine blood test reveals abnormal cell counts. Anemia causes weakness, fatigue, and dyspnea on exertion. The spleen often is enlarged, causing abdominal discomfort. Within 3–4 years, disease progresses to a more aggressive phase. Rapid cell proliferation and hypermetabolism cause fatigue, weight loss, sweating, and heat intolerance. The spleen enlarges, leading to a sensation of abdominal fullness and discomfort. Platelet function is affected in this stage, leading to bleeding and increased bruising. Finally, the disease evolves to acute leukemia, with blast cell proliferation. This stage, known as the terminal blast crisis phase, is characterized by significant constitutional manifestations, splenomegaly, and infiltration of leukemic cells into the skin, lymph nodes, bones, and central nervous system (Porth, 2005). Survival following the onset of this final stage averages only 2 to 4 months.

Figure 3–15 ■ A blood smear from the bone marrow of a client with acute myeloid leukemia. Note the abnormally large number of myelocyte WBCs (stained purple) among the small RBCs.

Source: Dr. Gopal Murti, Photo Researchers, Inc.

Acute Lymphocytic Leukemia

Acute lymphocytic leukemia (ALL) is the most common type of leukemia in children and young adults. In adults, ALL is rarely seen until late middle age, and then its incidence increases with aging. Genetic factors may play a role in its development, particularly the *bcr/abl* translocation also implicated in CML (Copstead & Banasik, 2005).

Most (80%) cases of ALL result from malignant transformation of B cells, with the remaining 20% arising from T cells. The malignant cells resemble immature lymphocytes (lymphoblasts); however, they do not mature or function effectively

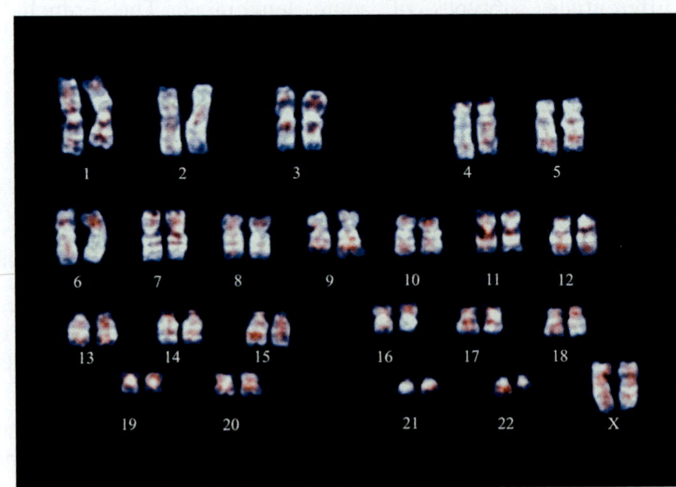

Figure 3–16 ■ The Philadelphia chromosome. Note the chromosomes of pairs 9 and 22. In each instance, the left-hand chromosome of the pair is normal, whereas an exchange of material between chromosomes has made the right-hand chromosome 9 larger and the right-hand chromosome 22 smaller. In stem cells within the bone marrow, the chromosome 22 defect leads to chronic myeloid leukemia.

Source: Addenbrooks Hospital, Photo Researchers, Inc.

to maintain immunity. These lymphoblasts accumulate in the bone marrow, lymph nodes, and spleen as well as in circulating blood. Some types of lymphoma are thought to represent a later stage of the same disease.

The onset of ALL is usually rapid. Lymphoblasts proliferating in bone marrow and peripheral tissues crowd the growth of normal cells (Figure 3–17 ■). Normal hematopoiesis is suppressed, leading to thrombocytopenia, leukopenia, and anemia. Manifestations of infections, bleeding, and anemia develop. Bone pain resulting from rapid generation of marrow elements, lymphadenopathy, and liver enlargement are also common. Infiltration of the central nervous system causes headaches, visual disturbances, vomiting, and seizures.

The CBC shows an elevated WBC count with increased lymphocytes on the differential. The RBC and platelet counts are decreased. Bone marrow studies reveal a hypercellular marrow with growth of lymphoblasts. Combination chemotherapy produces complete remission in 80–90% of adults with ALL.

Chronic Lymphocytic Leukemia

Chronic lymphocytic leukemia (CLL) is characterized by proliferation and accumulation of small, abnormal, mature lymphocytes in the bone marrow, peripheral blood, and body tissues. The abnormal cells are usually B lymphocytes that are unable to produce adequate antibodies to maintain normal immune function. Only approximately 5% of CLL cases involve T cells (Copstead & Banasik, 2005). CLL occurs more commonly in adults, especially older adults (median age, 65 years). CLL is the least common type of the major leukemias.

Chronic lymphocytic leukemia has a slow onset and is often diagnosed during a routine physical examination. If symptoms are present, they usually include vague complaints of weakness or malaise. Possible clinical findings include anemia, infection, and enlarged lymph nodes, spleen, and liver. As in other leukemias, bone marrow hyperplasia is present. Erythrocyte and platelet counts are reduced. Leukocyte counts may be either elevated or reduced, but abnormal cells are always present. In CLL, years may elapse before treatment is required. Survival of this disease averages approximately 7 years.

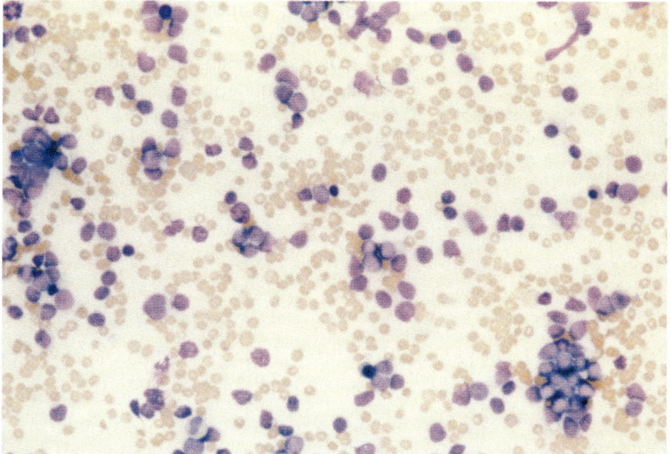

Figure 3–17 ■ A blood smear from the bone marrow of a client with acute lymphocytic leukemia. Note the abnormally large number of lymphocytes (stained purple) crowding the bone marrow. As a result, normal production of RBCs, functional WBCs, and platelets is suppressed.

Source: Dr. Gopal Murti, Photo Researchers, Inc.

Etiology

Although leukemia is often thought of as a childhood disease, it is diagnosed 10 times more often in adults than in children. An estimated 34,810 new cases of leukemia occur annually; slightly more than half are acute leukemia and less than half are chronic leukemia. The ACS (2006a) has estimated that in 2005, approximately 22,570 people died of leukemia. The highest incidence of leukemia is found in the United States, Canada, Sweden, and New Zealand (McCance & Huether, 2006).

The causes of leukemia are not well understood. Some investigators theorize that exposure to infectious agents can predispose people to leukemia. Genetic factors are also believed to play a role in some types of the disease. For instance, children with chromosomal defects, such as Down syndrome, neurofibromatosis type I, Bloom syndrome, and Shwachman syndrome, have an increased incidence of ALL, and chromosomal abnormalities are present in most clients with ALL (Bennett & Konrokji, 2005). Children with immunodeficiency states, such as ataxia-telangiectasia, congenital hypogammaglobulinemia, and Wiskott-Aldrich syndrome, have an increased risk of ALL. Certain racial and ethnic groups have poorer outcomes from leukemia.

Ionizing radiation when in utero and chemical agents such as treatment of an earlier cancer with chemotherapy (alkylating agents and topoisomerase II inhibitors) are thought to play some role in the development of acute nonlymphocytic leukemia. In addition, several chromosomal and genetic abnormalities are associated with acute nonlymphocytic leukemia. For example, trisomy 8 is associated with all subtypes of the disease (Jaff et al., 2006). Leukemia occurs when the stem cells in the bone marrow produce immature WBCs that cannot function normally. These cells proliferate rapidly by cloning instead of through normal mitosis, causing the bone marrow to fill with abnormal WBCs. The abnormal cells then spill out into the circulatory system, where they steadily replace the normally functioning WBCs. As this occurs, the protective lymphocytic functions, such as cellular and humeral immunity, are reduced, leaving the body vulnerable to infections.

The malignant WBCs rapidly fill the bone marrow, replacing stem cells that produce erythrocytes (RBCs) and other blood products, such as platelets, thereby decreasing the amount of these products in circulation. The stem cells are replaced by leukemic clones, eventually resulting in anemia. Clients with leukemia commonly experience abnormal bleeding because of the reduced platelet amounts.

Risk Factors

While the cause of most leukemias is unknown, certain risk factors have been identified. Men are affected more frequently than women. People with certain genetic disorders (e.g., Down syndrome) have a higher incidence of leukemia. Environmental

MULTISYSTEM EFFECTS OF **Leukemia**

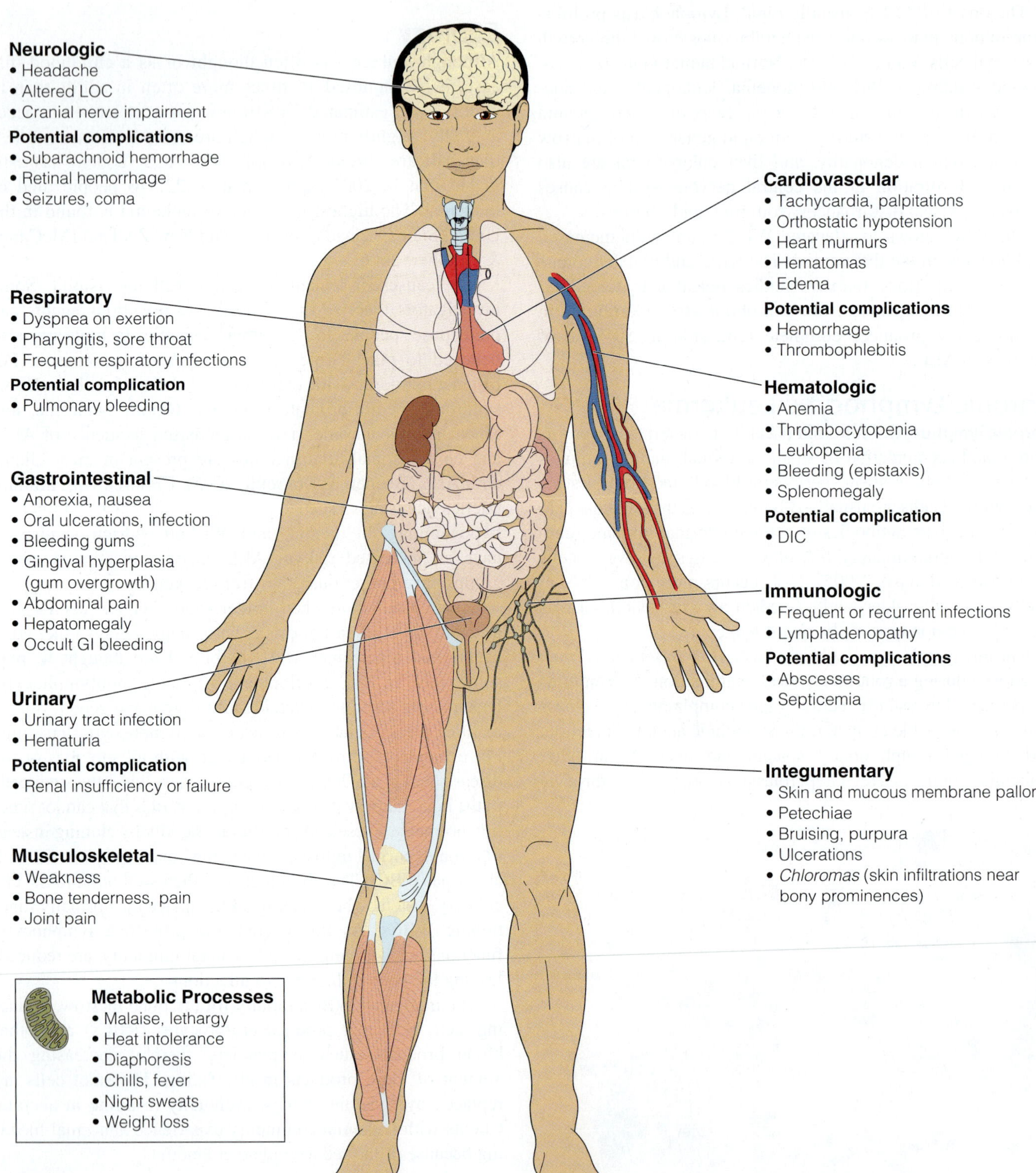
Neurologic
• Headache
• Altered LOC
• Cranial nerve impairment
Potential complications
• Subarachnoid hemorrhage
• Retinal hemorrhage
• Seizures, coma
Respiratory
• Dyspnea on exertion
• Pharyngitis, sore throat
• Frequent respiratory infections
Potential complication
• Pulmonary bleeding
Gastrointestinal
• Anorexia, nausea
• Oral ulcerations, infection
• Bleeding gums
• Gingival hyperplasia (gum overgrowth)
• Abdominal pain
• Hepatomegaly
• Occult GI bleeding
Urinary
• Urinary tract infection
• Hematuria
Potential complication
• Renal insufficiency or failure
Musculoskeletal
• Weakness
• Bone tenderness, pain
• Joint pain
Metabolic Processes
• Malaise, lethargy
• Heat intolerance
• Diaphoresis
• Chills, fever
• Night sweats
• Weight loss
Cardiovascular
• Tachycardia, palpitations
• Orthostatic hypotension
• Heart murmurs
• Hematomas
• Edema
Potential complications
• Hemorrhage
• Thrombophlebitis
Hematologic
• Anemia
• Thrombocytopenia
• Leukopenia
• Bleeding (epistaxis)
• Splenomegaly
Potential complication
• DIC
Immunologic
• Frequent or recurrent infections
• Lymphadenopathy
Potential complications
• Abscesses
• Septicemia
Integumentary
• Skin and mucous membrane pallor
• Petechiae
• Bruising, purpura
• Ulcerations
• *Chloromas* (skin infiltrations near bony prominences)

risk factors play a role as well. Risk factors for myeloid leukemia include cigarette smoking and chemicals such as benzene (present in cigarette smoke and gasoline). Exposure to ionizing radiation increases the risk for several types of leukemia. Clients who have undergone treatment for cancer have an increased risk. The human T-cell leukemia/lymphoma virus-1, a retrovirus, is known to cause certain leukemias and lymphomas (ACS, 2006a).

CLINICAL MANIFESTATIONS

The general manifestations of leukemia (regardless of type) result from anemia, infection, and bleeding. These include pallor, fatigue, tachycardia, malaise, lethargy, and dyspnea on exertion. Infection may cause fever, night sweats, oral ulcerations, and frequent or recurrent respiratory, urinary, integumentary, or other infections. Increased bleeding as a result of thrombocytopenia leads to bruising, petechiae, bleeding gums, and bleeding within specific organs and tissues.

Other manifestations result from leukemic cell infiltration, increased metabolism, and increased leukocyte destruction. Infiltration of the liver, spleen, lymph nodes, and bone marrow causes pain and tissue swelling in the involved areas. Meningeal infiltration may cause manifestations of increased intracranial pressure, such as headache, altered level of consciousness, cranial nerve impairment, nausea, and vomiting. Infiltration of the kidneys may affect renal function, with decreased urine output and increased blood urea nitrogen and creatinine. Increased metabolism causes heat intolerance, weight loss, dyspnea on exertion, and tachycardia. Destruction of large numbers of WBCs releases substantial amounts of uric acid into the circulation; uric acid crystals may obstruct renal tubules, causing renal insufficiency.

COLLABORATION

Treatment for leukemia focuses on achieving remission or cure and relieving symptoms. The methods of treatment may include chemotherapy, radiation therapy, and bone marrow or stem cell transplantation. Cure is more often achieved in children with acute leukemia than in adults, although long-term **remission** (a disease-free period with no signs or symptoms) often can be achieved. The nurse's role as a member of the interdisciplinary health care team is outlined in the Nursing Process that follows this section.

Diagnostic Tests

The following diagnostic tests are ordered when leukemia is suspected:

- *Complete blood count (CBC) with differential* is done to evaluate cell counts, hemoglobin and hematocrit levels, and the number, distribution, and morphology (size and shape) of WBCs.
- *Platelets* are measured to identify possible thrombocytopenia secondary to the leukemia and the risk of bleeding.
- *Bone marrow examination* provides information about cells within the marrow, the type of erythropoiesis, and the maturity of erythropoietic and leukopoietic cells.

Table 3–14 outlines usual diagnostic test results in the various forms of leukemia.

Chemotherapy

Single-agent or combination chemotherapy is the treatment of choice for most types of leukemia, with the goal of eradicating leukemic cells and producing remission. Table 3–15 outlines typical chemotherapeutic regimens for different types of leukemia. Combination chemotherapy reduces drug resistance and toxicity and interrupts cell growth at various stages of the cell cycle, producing a complementary effect of the drugs used.

CLINICAL MANIFESTATIONS AND THERAPIES Leukemia

ETIOLOGY	CLINICAL MANIFESTATION	CLINICAL THERAPIES
Anemia may result because when the bone marrow is so busy producing WBCs, inadequate numbers of RBCs are produced.	Pallor, fatigue, tachycardia, malaise, lethargy, and dyspnea on exertion	■ Improve nutritional status ■ Stimulate RBC production with medications (e.g., epoetin) ■ Blood transfusions ■ Promote rest ■ Monitor vital signs, CBC
Infection risk increases because of immature WBCs that are ineffective in responding to pathogens.	Fever, night sweats, oral ulcerations, and frequent or recurrent respiratory, urinary, integumentary, or other infections	■ Teach infection prevention strategies (e.g., hand hygiene, cough etiquette, crowd avoidance) ■ Teach symptoms to report ■ Antimicrobials as indicated to treat infections ■ Monitor vital signs, CBC
Bleeding may result from reduced coagulation factors, increased fibrinolytic activity and accelerated intravascular coagulation.	Petechia, bruising, bleeding from gums, hematuria, hematemesis, rectal bleeding	■ Monitor coagulation studies ■ Client teaching to reduce injury risk ■ Administration of platelets, clotting factors, ■ Blood replacement if bleeding occurs

TABLE 3–14 **Diagnostic Findings by Type of Leukemia**

TEST	ACUTE MYELOID LEUKEMIA	CHRONIC MYELOID LEUKEMIA	ACUTE LYMPHOCYTIC LEUKEMIA	CHRONIC LYMPHOCYTIC LEUKEMIA
RBC count	Low	Low	Low	Low
Hemoglobin	Low	Low	Low	Low
Hematocrit	Low	Low	Low	Low
Platelet count	Very low	High early, low late	Low	Low
WBC count	Varies	Increased	Varies	Increased
Myeloblasts	Present			
Neutrophils	Decreased	Increased	Decreased	Normal
Lymphocytes		Normal		Increased
Monocytes		Normal/low		
Blasts	Present	Present (crisis)	Present	
Bone marrow	Hypercellular		Hypercellular	
Myeloblasts	Present			
Lymphoblasts			Present	
Lymphocytes				Present

Chemotherapy for leukemia generally is divided into the induction phase and postremission therapy. During induction, drug doses are high to eradicate leukemic cells from the bone marrow. Often, however, these high doses also damage stem cells and interfere with production of normal blood cells. Circulating mature blood cells are not affected, because they are no longer dividing. The degree of bone marrow suppression is influenced by a number of factors, including age, nutritional status, concurrent chronic diseases (e.g., impaired liver or renal function), the drug and drug dose, and previous treatment.

Colony-stimulating factors (CSFs), also called hematopoietic growth factors, often are administered to "rescue" the bone marrow following induction chemotherapy. CSFs are cytokines that regulate the growth and differentiation of blood cells. Factors that support neutrophil maturation, granulocyte-macrophage CSF (GM-CSF) and granulocyte CSF (G-CSF) are commonly used. Bone pain is a common side effect of therapy with these agents. Clients also may experience fevers, chills, anorexia, muscle aches, and lethargy (Kasper et al., 2005).

Once remission has been achieved, postremission chemotherapy is continued to eradicate any additional leukemic cells, prevent relapse, and prolong survival. A single chemotherapeutic agent, combination therapy, or bone marrow transplant may be used for postremission treatment.

Radiation Therapy

Radiation therapy damages cellular DNA. While the cell continues to function, it cannot divide and multiply. Cells that divide rapidly, such as bone marrow and cancer cells (radiosensitive cells), respond quickly to radiation therapy. Although normal cells are affected, they are better able to recover from the damage caused by the radiation compared with cancer cells.

Bone Marrow Transplant

Bone marrow transplant (BMT) is the treatment of choice for some types of leukemia (see Table 3–12). BMT often is used in conjunction with or following chemotherapy or radiation. There are two major categories of BMT: In allogeneic BMT, the bone marrow of a healthy donor is infused into the client

TABLE 3–15 **Chemotherapeutic Regimens Used to Treat Leukemia**

TYPE OF LEUKEMIA	CHEMOTHERAPEUTIC REGIMEN
Acute myeloid leukemia	■ Cytarabine (Cytoxan, an alkylating agent), *with* daunorubicin (Cerubidine, an antitumor antibiotic) *or* idarubicin (Idamycin, an antitumor antibiotic) ■ All-*trans* retinoic acid (ATRA) added for clients with promyelocytic leukemia
Chronic myeloid leukemia	■ Imatinib mesylate (Gleevec), a *bcr/abl* tyrosine kinase (enzyme) inhibitor ■ Hydroxyurea (a DNA inhibitor) *or* homoharringtonine (HHT, a plant alkaloid) if imatinib is not tolerated
Acute lymphocytic leukemia	■ Daunorubicin (Cerubidine, an antitumor antibiotic) *with* vincristine (Oncovin, a plant alkaloid) *with* prednisone *with* asparaginase (Elspar)
Chronic lymphocytic leukemia	■ Fludarabine (Fludara, an antimetabolite) *or* chlorambucil (Chloromycetin, an antitumor antibiotic) ■ Cyclophosphamide (Cytoxan, an alkylating agent), vincristine, and prednisone ■ Cyclophosphamide, doxorubicin (Adriamycin, an antitumor antibiotic), vincristine, and prednisone

with the illness; in autologous BMT, the client is infused with his or her own bone marrow.

ALLOGENEIC BONE MARROW TRANSPLANT **Allogeneic bone marrow transplant** uses bone marrow cells from a donor (often from a sibling with closely matched tissue antigens; closely matched unrelated donors also may be used). Before allogeneic BMT, high doses of chemotherapy and/or total body irradiation are used to destroy leukemic cells in the bone marrow. The donor's bone marrow is aspirated (Figure 3–18 ■) and infused through a central venous line into the recipient. Before BMT and reestablishment of bone marrow function, the client is critically ill and at significant risk for infection and bleeding as a result of the depletion of WBCs and platelets.

AUTOLOGOUS BONE MARROW TRANSPLANT **Autologous bone marrow transplant** uses the client's own bone marrow to restore bone marrow function after chemotherapy or radiation; this procedure is often called bone marrow rescue. In autologous BMT, approximately 1 L of bone marrow is aspirated (usually from the iliac crests) during a period of disease remission. The bone marrow is then frozen and stored for use after treatment. If relapse occurs, lethal doses of chemotherapy or radiation are given to destroy the immune system and malignant cells and to prepare space in the bone marrow for new cells. The filtered bone marrow is then thawed and infused intravenously through a central line. The infused marrow cells slowly become a part of the client's bone marrow, the neutrophil count increases, and normal hematopoiesis takes place.

As in allogeneic BMT, the client is critically ill during the period of bone marrow destruction and immunosuppression. The client is hospitalized in a private room for 6–8 weeks or more. Potential complications include malnutrition, infection, and bleeding.

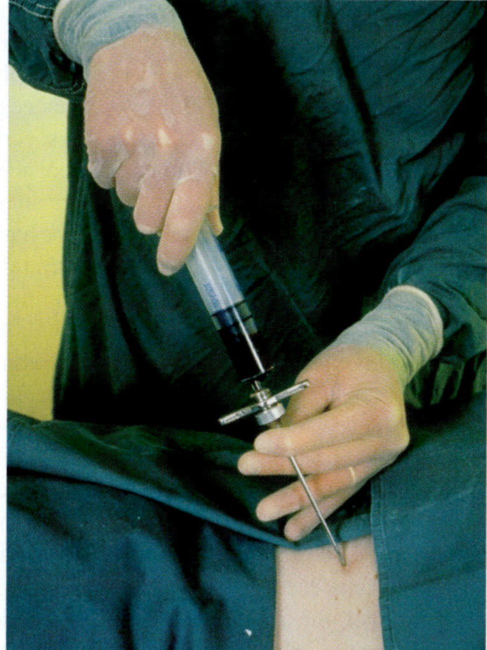

Figure 3–18 ■ Allogeneic bone marrow transplant. Bone marrow from the donor is aspirated, then filtered and infused into the recipient.

Source: Simon Fraser, Photo Researcher, Inc.

Stem Cell Transplant

Allogeneic **stem cell transplant (SCT)** is an alternative to BMT. SCT results in complete and sustained replacement of the recipient's blood cell lines (WBCs, RBCs, and platelets) with cells derived from the donor stem cells. Before SCT, the recipient undergoes treatment similar to that before BMT. The risks for infection and other complications, as well as graft-versus-host disease, are similar as well.

Donors must have tissue that is closely matched with that of the recipient. Before harvesting, hematopoietic growth factors, including G-CSF and GM-CSF, are administered to the donor for 4–5 days. This increases the concentration of stem cells in peripheral blood, allowing it to be used for the transplant instead of bone marrow. Peripheral blood is removed, and WBCs are separated from the plasma, then administered via a large central venous catheter. Large concentrations of stem cells also are present in umbilical cord blood. This may be stored and used in some cases (Kasper et al., 2005).

Graft-Versus-Host Disease

Allogeneic BMT or SCT may precipitate graft-versus-host disease (GVHD), which develops in up to 60% of all clients receiving an allogeneic BMT or SCT (Kasper et al., 2005). In GVHD, immune cells of the donated bone marrow identify the recipient's body tissue as foreign. Consequently, T lymphocytes in the donated marrow attack the liver, skin, and gastrointestinal tract, causing skin rashes progressing to desquamation (loss of skin), diarrhea, gastrointestinal bleeding, and liver damage. Acute GVHD develops within days or weeks of the transplant and is usually marked by a pruritic, maculopapular rash that begins on the palms and soles of the feet and may extend over the entire body. Vaso-occlusive disease of the liver affects up to 25% of allogeneic BMT recipients, with jaundice and elevated liver function tests (Porth, 2005). Chronic GVHD develops later ($\geq$ 100 days after the transplant) and affects 20–50% of clients who survive 6 months or more following allogeneic BMT or SCT (Kasper et al., 2005). It may follow acute GVHD or develop in clients with no previous symptoms. GVHD is treated with antibiotics and steroids; immunosuppressant drugs, such as thalidomide and immunotoxin (XomaZyme), may be used if necessary.

Biologic Therapy

Cytokines, such as interferons and interleukins, are biologic agents that may be used to treat some leukemias. These agents modify the body's response to cancer cells; in some cases, they are cytotoxic as well. Interferons are a complex group of messenger proteins normally produced in response to antigens such as viruses. They have multiple effects, including moderating immune function and inhibiting abnormal cell proliferation and growth. Interferon alpha may be used to treat some leukemias, particularly CML. Side effects commonly associated with interferon therapy include flulike symptoms, persistent fatigue and lethargy, weight loss, and muscle and joint pain.

Complementary Therapies

Although many complementary and alternative medicine therapies have been purported to treat cancer in general, at this time none have been shown to have sustained benefit in treating leukemia. Clinical trials have demonstrated the efficacy of both coping skills training (relaxation and imagery) and hypnosis to significantly reduce oral discomfort associated with leukemia and its treatment (Spencer & Jacobs, 2003).

NURSING PROCESS

When caring for the client with leukemia, the nurse considers the chronic and life-threatening nature of the disease as well as the effects of treatment in planning care.

Assessment

Focused assessment data related to leukemia include the following:

- *Health history.* Complaints of fatigue, weakness, dyspnea on exertion, frequent infections, sore throat, night sweats, bleeding gums, or nose bleeds; recent weight loss; exposure to ionizing radiation (multiple x-rays, residence near a site of radiation or atomic testing) or chemicals (occupational); previous treatment for cancer; history of an immune disorder
- *Physical examination.* Skin and mucous membranes for bruising, purpura, petechiae, ulcers or lesions; pallor; vital signs, including orthostatic vitals; heart and lung sounds; abdominal examination; stool for occult blood.

Diagnosis

Nursing diagnoses for the client with leukemia include the following:

- Risk for Infection
- Imbalanced Nutrition: Less Than Body Requirements
- Impaired Oral Mucous Membrane
- Ineffective Protection (Bleeding)
- Anticipatory Grieving.

FOCUS ON DIVERSITY AND CULTURE
Leukemia Treatment

African American, Hispanic, and Native American clients have statistically poorer outcomes from leukemia treatment than do white and Asian clients. Although the genetic characteristics of certain types of blast cells are associated with the client's response to treatment, these blast cell characteristics are not known to be associated with certain racial groups. Therefore, it is unclear whether the client groups that do not respond as well to treatment have particular genetic characteristics, do not obtain treatment as soon and therefore have more complications of disease, enroll less often in clinical trials, or simply have less access to care at oncology centers. More research is needed to describe and then eliminate the racial and ethnic disparity in leukemia outcomes (Carroll, 2003).

Plan

Goals for client care include the following:

- The client and family members/significant others describe strategies to reduce risk of infection.
- The client remains infection free.
- The pediatric client meets developmental milestones.
- The client expresses feelings related to diagnosis.
- The client meets nutritional needs to maintain growth and/or weight.
- The client reports symptoms of complications in a timely manner.

Implementation

Nurses play a key role in the long-term multidisciplinary treatment of clients with leukemia. The impact of a diagnosis of leukemia and the long-term nature of treatment can severely stress the coping abilities of both the client and the family. Ongoing psychosocial assessment and emotional support are essential. Referral to support groups and social services may be beneficial. Assist the family in exploration of alternative therapies, such as relaxation, imagery, and nutritional support. Be alert for any interactions that could occur between alternative therapies and the medical regimen.

Many clients are treated in an oncology clinic, staying in the hospital only on the day of IV drug administration, and receive oral medications at home. The time at the hospital is used to assess how the family is managing issues such as nutrition, sleep, medication administration, and obtaining psychosocial support. Careful teaching for the family is needed to ensure safe drug administration and identification of issues requiring further care.

Drug side effects may necessitate infusion of platelets or packed RBCs. Special attention to renal function is needed when the client receives cyclophosphamide. Gross hematuria is a side effect of this drug. Hydration with IV fluids to attain a specific gravity of less than 1.010 prevents or reduces the severity of hematuria. It also prepares the kidneys to manage products of tumor cell breakdown. To achieve this desired specific gravity, the client receives IV fluids at 1.5 times maintenance volume for at least 6–8 hours before and at least 1.5 hours after administration of the drug. Other chemotherapeutic drugs have different infusion times, while some do not require hydration before infusion. Check drug references carefully for recommendations with each drug. Evaluate the infusion site before and frequently during infusion. Although extravasation is not as common with central lines used in cancer treatment as in peripheral lines, it still can occur. Many chemotherapeutic agents are extremely toxic to tissues. In addition, lysis of the cancer cells can produce toxic side effects. Careful monitoring of intake and output is required to record the IV fluids, assess kidney functioning, and monitor excretion of by-products from destroyed tumor cells. Monitor specific gravity every 8 hours as well as before and during administration of the drug and when the IV fluids are reduced to maintenance volume levels. Daily weight measurements are important to assist in planning adequate hydration during chemotherapy as well as to measure nutritional status.

Bone marrow suppression necessitates transmission-based precautions. Instruct parents in the prevention of infection, and use nursing care measures to prevent infection as well. Perform careful handwashing; take temperature frequently; give mouth care with antibacterial mouthwashes; and inspect the skin, mouth, rectal area, and central line site for any signs of infection.

Risk for Infection

Changes in WBC function impair the immune and inflammatory responses in the client with leukemia, increasing the risk for infection. WBCs may be immature and ineffective or, in some cases, deficient. Chemotherapy or radiation therapy further depresses bone marrow function and increases the risk for infection.

- Promptly report manifestations of infection: fever, chills, throat pain, cough, chest pain, burning on urination, purulent drainage, and itching and burning in vaginal or rectal areas. Prompt reporting allows timely intervention to prevent overwhelming infection and sepsis.
- Institute infection protection measures:
  a. Maintain protective isolation as indicated.
  b. Ensure meticulous handwashing among all people in contact with the client.
  c. Assist as needed with appropriate hygiene measures.
  d. Restrict visitors with colds, flu, or infections.
  e. Provide oral hygiene after every meal.
  f. Avoid invasive procedures when possible, including injections, IV catheters, catheterizations, and rectal and vaginal procedures. When necessary, use strict aseptic technique for all invasive procedures and monitor carefully for infection.

These precautions minimize exposure to bacterial, viral, and fungal pathogens. Infection is the major cause of death in clients with leukemia. Mucous membranes are especially susceptible to breakdown and infection as a result of tissue damage from chemotherapy or radiation.

- Monitor vital signs, including temperature and oxygen saturation, every 4 hours. Report temperature spikes with chilling, tachypnea, tachycardia, restlessness, change in PaO_2, and hypotension. The inflammatory response may be impaired in leukemia, masking signs of infection until sepsis develops, indicated by manifestations such as those above.
- Monitor neutrophil levels (measured in cubic millimeters) for relative risk for infection: no risk, 2,000–2,500/mm^3; minimal risk, 1,000–2,000/mm^3; moderate risk, 500–1,000/mm^3; severe risk, < 500/mm^3. Neutrophils are the first line of defense against infection. As levels decrease, the risk for infection increases.
- Explain infection precautions and restrictions and their rationale; explain that these measures are usually temporary. Client and family understanding increases compliance and lowers the risk of infection.

Imbalanced Nutrition: Less Than Body Requirements

The client with leukemia may have difficulty meeting nutritional needs because of increased metabolism, fatigue, loss of appetite from radiation, nausea and vomiting from chemotherapy, or painful oral mucous membranes that make chewing and swallowing difficult and/or painful.

- Weigh regularly, and evaluate weight loss over time to determine degree of malnutrition. A weight loss of 10–20% may indicate malnutrition. A minimum intake of nutrients is necessary for health and tissue repair; cancer increases metabolic needs over this basal requirement. Weight loss occurs when metabolic requirements are not met. Both the disease process and its treatment can interfere with nutrient intake.
- Address causative or contributing factors to inadequate food and fluid intake:
  a. Provide mouth care before and after meals; use a soft toothbrush or sponges as necessary.
  b. Provide liquids with different textures and tastes.
  c. Increase liquid intake with meals.
  d. Reduce intake of milk and milk products, which makes mucus more tenacious.
  e. Assist to a sitting position for eating.
  f. Ensure that the environment is clean and odor free.
  g. Provide medications for pain or nausea 30 minutes before meals, if prescribed.
  h. Provide rest periods before meals.
  i. Offer small, frequent meals, including low-fat, high-kilocalorie foods, throughout the day.
  j. Provide commercial supplements, such as Ensure.
  k. Avoid painful or unpleasant procedures immediately before or after meals.
  l. Suggest measures to improve food tolerance, such as eating dry foods when arising, consuming salty foods if allowed, and avoiding very sweet, rich, or greasy foods.

Anorexia, nausea and vomiting, diarrhea, stomatitis, taste changes, and dysphagia often make eating difficult during cancer treatment when good nutrition is most important. Maintaining nutritional status decreases morbidity and mortality by preventing weight loss, improving the response to treatment, minimizing adverse effects, and improving quality of life. Small, frequent meals, especially high-protein, high-kilocalorie foods, are often better tolerated.

Impaired Oral Mucous Membrane

Stomatitis (inflammation and ulceration of the oral mucous membrane) is common in clients with leukemia. Chemotherapy can further impair the integrity of constantly dividing oral tissues.

- Inspect the buccal region, gums, sublingual area, and the throat daily for swelling or lesions. Ask about oral pain or burning. Breakdown of the oral mucous membrane increases the risk of infection and bleeding, causes pain and discomfort with eating and swallowing, and may cause swelling that interferes with the airway.
- Culture any oral lesions. Herpes simplex virus and *Candida* (yeast) are more common in clients with neutropenia. Herpes lesions are usually red, raised, fluid-filled blisters; Candida causes a white coating and patches of white plaque.
- Assist with mouth care and oral rinses with saline or a solution of hydrogen peroxide and water (1:1 or 1:3 hydrogen peroxide and water) every 2–4 hours. Apply petroleum jelly to the lips to prevent dryness and cracking. These measures help prevent infection and increase comfort.

- Encourage use of soft-bristle toothbrush or sponge to clean teeth and gums. Toothbrushes with hard bristles may abrade inflamed mucosa, causing bleeding and increasing the risk of infection.
- Administer medications as ordered to treat infection or relieve pain. Topical antifungal agents such as nystatin may be prescribed to treat *Candida* infections. Topical anesthetics such as lidocaine may be prescribed to relieve comfort and facilitate good oral care.
- Instruct the client to avoid alcohol-based mouthwashes, citrus fruit juices, spicy foods, very hot or very cold foods, alcohol, and crusty foods. Suggest bland, cool foods and cool liquids at least every 2 hours. Avoiding mucosa-traumatizing foods and liquids increases comfort; bland, cool foods and liquids cause the least pain. Intake of adequate fluids is necessary to prevent dehydration.

Ineffective Protection

Bleeding is the second most common cause of leukemia deaths. As platelet counts decrease, the risk of bleeding increases. Tumor lysis syndrome also is a risk in clients with leukemia who are undergoing their initial treatment with chemotherapy. Tumor lysis syndrome develops when a large number of malignant cells are destroyed by treatment with chemotherapy or radiation. The resultant by-products of cell lysis can overwhelm the body's ability to effectively eliminate them, leading to hyperkalemia, hyperphosphatemia with secondary hypocalcemia, and hyperuricemia (Cantril & Haylock, 2004).

- Assess vital signs every 4 hours and body systems every shift for bleeding:
  a. Skin and mucous membranes for petechiae, ecchymoses, and purpura
  b. Gums, nasal membranes, and conjunctiva for bleeding
  c. Vomitus, stool, and urine for visible or occult blood
  d. Vaginal bleeding
  e. Prolonged bleeding from puncture sites
  f. Neurologic changes, such as headache, visual changes, altered mentation, decreased level of consciousness, seizures
  g. Abdomen for complaints of epigastric pain, diminished bowel sounds, increasing abdominal girth, rigidity or guarding

Early identification of bleeding helps prevent significant blood loss and potential shock. Internal hemorrhage may lead to tachycardia, hypotension, pallor, and diaphoresis. Bleeding into the lungs may cause dyspnea; bleeding into the abdomen causes increased girth, pain, and guarding. Intracranial bleeding affects mental status and level of consciousness.

- Avoid invasive procedures, such as rectal temperatures and suppositories, vaginal douches and suppositories, tampons, urinary catheterization, and parenteral injections, if possible. Invasive diagnostic procedures, such as biopsy or lumbar puncture, should not be done if the platelet count is less than 50,000. Invasive procedures can cause tissue trauma and bleeding. Procedures that use large-bore needles should be delayed until the platelet count is increased.
- Apply pressure to injection sites for 3–5 minutes and to arterial punctures for 15–20 minutes. Pressure prevents prolonged bleeding by prompting hemostasis and clot formation.
- Instruct the client to avoid forceful blowing or picking the nose, forceful coughing or sneezing, and straining to have a bowel movement. These activities can damage mucous membranes, increasing the risk for bleeding.
- Monitor and promptly report abnormal blood levels of electrolytes, uric acid, urea nitrogen, and creatinine or

EVIDENCE-BASED PRACTICE Clients With Acute Leukemia and Lymphoma

Clinical Question

Clients with acute leukemia and malignant lymphoma experience a number of distressing manifestations of their disease, including malaise and fatigue, fever, night sweats, infections, and possible hemorrhage. Treatments such as radiation therapy and chemotherapy often have numerous adverse effects as well, including anorexia and nausea, stomatitis, lethargy, malaise, and fatigue.

Evidence

Clients in remission from acute leukemia or malignant lymphoma were surveyed regarding physical problems, their view of help they received and who was of most help during treatment, and the impact of the disease and treatment on their current life (Persson, Hallberg, & Ohlsson, 1997; Persson & Hallberg, 2004). Clients identified energy loss and nutritional problems as being most troublesome during disease treatment. In general, clients with more physical problems were less satisfied with the nursing care they received, suggesting that nurses were less effective in meeting the needs of the sickest clients. Clients continued to experience reduced psychologic and sexual energy as well as a significant need for intimate help and counseling during remission. While family relationships improved, work and finances were negatively impacted by their disease.

Best Practice

Nurses need to actively focus their care on the physical problems experienced during treatment, especially energy loss and nutritional problems. Overwhelming fatigue interferes with the client's ability to provide self-care, but its effects may not be readily apparent to nurses. The long-term effects of reduced psychologic and sexual energy, as well as continued susceptibility to infections, indicate a need for continued follow-up care, teaching, and possibly referral to counseling services.

Critical Thinking

1. Explain the physiologic responses to malignancies and cancer treatments that cause fatigue, malaise, and nutritional problems.
2. Clients undergoing treatment for leukemia, malignant lymphoma, and other cancers may have few outward manifestations of their disease or responses to treatment. Discuss how this apparent well-being may affect the nurses' perception of care needs.
3. How may continued problems of fatigue and lack of psychologic and sexual energy affect family relations?
4. Develop a nursing care plan for a client with acute leukemia to address the nursing diagnosis ineffective sexuality patterns related to fatigue and lack of energy.

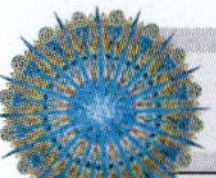

NURSING CARE PLAN **A Client With Acute Myelocytic Leukemia**

Catherine Cole is a 37-year-old secretary who lives with her husband, Ray, and teenage daughter, Amy, in an apartment in a large metropolitan area. Approximately 2 months ago, Mrs. Cole began to tire easily and experience night sweats several times a week. She also noted that she was pale, bruised easily, and was having heavier menstrual periods. Blood tests ordered by her primary care provider are abnormal. She is admitted for a bone marrow biopsy.

ASSESSMENT

Mary Losapio, RN, obtains a nursing history and physical assessment for Mrs. Cole. Mrs. Cole tells her, "I'm so tired, and I have these bruises all over me. I'm so afraid of the results of the bone marrow examination. I don't know what we will do if I have cancer." Mrs. Cole clutches her husband's hand and then begins to cry. Physical assessment data include the following: height, 64 inches (156 cm); weight, 106 lb (48.1 kg); and temperature 100°F, pulse 102 bpm, respirations 22/min, and BP 130/82 mm Hg. Numerous petechiae are scattered over the trunk and arms; ecchymoses are noted on lower right arm and right calf. Oral mucosa is red, with several small ulcerations in buccal areas.

Blood count shows reduced RBCs, hemoglobin, and hematocrit levels. The WBC count is high, with myeloblasts seen on differential. The platelet count is very low. A tentative diagnosis of acute myelogenous leukemia is made.

DIAGNOSES

- Risk for Infection related to altered WBC production and immune function
- Ineffective Protection related to reduced platelet count and risk for bleeding
- Impaired Oral Mucous Membrane secondary to anemia and reduced platelets
- Fatigue related to anemia
- Anxiety related to fear of leukemia diagnosis

PLANNING

- The client will remain free of infection.
- The client will experience no significant bleeding.
- The client will have intact oral mucous membranes.
- The client will manage self-care activities despite fatigue.
- The client will verbalize decreased anxiety.

IMPLEMENTATION

- Place in a private room.
- Limit visitors to immediate family for the present.
- Instruct all staff, the family, and the client to carefully wash hands. Post a sign over the washbasin in the room as a reminder.
- Record vital signs every 4 hours.
- Avoid invasive procedures unless absolutely necessary.
- Monitor for bleeding every 4 hours, including skin, oral mucosa, abdominal assessment, body fluids, and menstrual pad count.
- Instruct to perform oral hygiene every 2 to 4 hours, using a soft-bristle toothbrush.
- Ask the dietitian to work with Mrs. Cole to identify preferred foods. Instruct to avoid foods that may damage oral mucosa, such as very hot, very cold, or highly acidic or spicy foods.
- Provide for periods of rest alternating with activity.
- Teach about the bone marrow biopsy. Allow time for questions and to verbalize fears.
- Refer to the oncology nurse specialist for further teaching and support.

EVALUATION

The bone marrow biopsy confirms the diagnosis of acute myelogenous leukemia. Mrs. Cole is very upset, but she calms as the physician and the oncology nurse discuss treatment plans and the possibility of remission. She decides to have outpatient chemotherapy. During her hospital stay, Mrs. Cole remained free of infection or further bleeding. She tells Ms. Losapio that her mouth feels better, although it is still painful. During routine assessment, Mrs. Cole remarks, "You know, I was so scared when I came here, but I think I am a little less so now. Sometimes not knowing what is wrong is worse than knowing."

CRITICAL THINKING

1. Describe how alterations in WBCs can increase a person's susceptibility to infection.
2. List sources of potential infection for the client who is hospitalized.
3. What is the rationale for having the client do her own oral and physical hygiene?
4. Outline a teaching plan for this client and her family for home care to prevent infection.
5. Develop a care plan for Mrs. Cole for the nursing diagnosis activity intolerance.

manifestations of tumor lysis syndrome. Significant alterations in electrolyte levels can lead to complications, such as cardiac dysrhythmias, muscle weakness or tetany, paresthesias, and mental status changes. Excess uric acid can compromise renal function, and lead to metabolic acidosis and gout.

- Maintain adequate hydration, and administer prescribed medications, such as allopurinol and diuretics, as ordered. Hydration is vital to maintain renal function and promote elimination of tumor lysis by-products. Allopurinol reduces the risk of uric acid crystallization in the kidneys and other tissues (Cantril & Haylock, 2004).

Anticipatory Grieving

The diagnosis of a potentially life-threatening cancer causes actual or perceived losses, such as loss of function, independence, normal appearance, friends, self-esteem, and self. Grieving is the emotional response to those losses. The adaptive process of mourning a loss and resolving grief is called grief work; grief work cannot begin until a loss is acknowledged.

- Discuss the roles of the client and family and the ways in which they managed stressful situations in the past. Assess coping strategies and their effectiveness. Help identify sources of strength and support. Discuss changing roles resulting from the leukemia diagnosis and its effect on spiritual, social, and economic status and usual lifestyle. Evaluate cultural or ethnic factors that affect grief reactions. Grieving is a normal response to a real or potential loss that begins at the time of diagnosis. The timing, duration, and intensity of grief and responses to grief may differ among family members. Share information on diagnosis, role change, and physical loss among all family members to build the foundation for mutual understanding and trust.
- Use therapeutic communication skills to facilitate open discussion of losses and provide permission to grieve. Encouraging discussion of the meaning of the loss helps decrease some of the anxiety associated with the loss. This in turn allows the client and family to examine the current situation and compare it with past situations that they have coped with successfully.
- Provide information about agencies that may help in resolving grief, and make referrals as indicated. Consider self-help groups, cancer support groups, and bereavement groups. Participating in support groups with others who are anticipating or experiencing a similar loss can decrease feelings of isolation.

Evaluation

Expected outcomes for nursing care of the client with leukemia include the following:

- The client is adequately hydrated to allow elimination of drugs and cell components.
- The client maintains normal urinary output.
- The client remains free from infection.
- The client's blood values are maintained within normal limits.
- The client demonstrates adequate knowledge related to the disease process and treatment regimens.

REVIEW Leukemia

RELATE: LINK THE CONCEPTS

Linking the exemplar of Leukemia with the concept of Comfort:

1. When caring for a client diagnosed with leukemia, what nursing diagnoses would you implement to address comfort?
2. What interventions would be appropriate for the client receiving chemotherapy who reports fatigue and difficulty meeting self-care needs?

Linking the exemplar of Leukemia with the concept of Culture:

3. How will you meet the cultural needs of the client who recently moved from Mexico, does not speak English, and has been diagnosed with leukemia?
4. What assessment data will you collect to prioritize nursing diagnoses for a client from India diagnosed with leukemia?

READY: GO TO COMPANION SKILLS MANUAL

- Assessing vital signs
- Assessing appearance and mental status
- Assessing the abdomen
- Hand hygiene
- Latex precautions

REFER: GO TO MYNURSINGKIT

REFLECT: CASE STUDY

Johnny is 4 years old and was brought to the clinic by his mother who reports that she can't put her finger on what's wrong but he has not looked well lately. He is pale, has dark circles under his eyes, bruising on his arms and legs, and his mother states that he does not seem to have any energy lately. Johnny tells you that he is very tired all the time.

1. What is your priority when assessing Johnny during this visit?
2. What client teaching will you provide to maintain Johnny's safety?
3. What interventions will you initiate to support Johnny and his family through a new diagnosis of leukemia?

3.6 LUNG CANCER

KEY TERMS

Brachytherapy, *165*
Bronchogenic carcinomas, *161*
Hemoptysis, *163*
Small-cell carcinomas, *161*
Non-small-cell carcinomas, *161*

BASIS FOR SELECTION OF EXEMPLAR

Centers for Disease Control and Prevention
Healthy People 2010
Institute of Medicine

LEARNING OUTCOMES

After reading about this exemplar, you will be able to:

1. Describe the pathophysiology, etiology, clinical manifestations, and direct and indirect causes of lung cancer.
2. Identify risk factors associated with lung cancer.
3. Illustrate the nursing process in providing culturally competent care across the life span for individuals with lung cancer.
4. Formulate priority nursing diagnoses appropriate for an individual with lung cancer.
5. Create a plan of care for individuals with lung cancer and their family members.
6. Assess expected outcomes for an individual with lung cancer.
7. Discuss therapies used in the collaborative care of an individual with lung cancer.
8. Employ evidence-based caring interventions for an individual with lung cancer.

OVERVIEW

Lung cancer is the leading cause of cancer deaths among all racial groups in the United States, accounting for 31% of all cancer deaths in men and 27% of all cancer deaths in women. In 2005, more than 168,000 people died from lung cancer in the United States; an estimated 184,800 new cases were diagnosed in that same year (ACS, 2006a). It is a major health problem with a grim prognosis: Most people with lung cancer die within 1 year of the initial diagnosis.

PATHOPHYSIOLOGY AND ETIOLOGY

The vast majority of primary lung lesions are **bronchogenic carcinomas** (tumors of the airway epithelium). These tumors are further differentiated by cell type: small-cell carcinoma, adenocarcinoma, squamous cell carcinoma, and large-cell carcinoma. For clinical purposes, the latter three cell types frequently are classified together as non-small-cell carcinomas. **Small-cell carcinomas**, which account for approximately 25% of lung cancers, grow rapidly and spread early. These tumors have paraneoplastic properties; that is, they produce manifestations at sites that are not directly affected by the tumor. Small-cell lung carcinomas can synthesize bioactive products and hormones, such as adrenocorticotropic hormones, antidiuretic hormone, a parathormone-like hormone, and gastrin-releasing peptide. **Non-small-cell carcinomas** account for approximately 75% of lung cancers. Each cell type differs in its incidence, presentation, and manner of spread. Table 3–16 outlines the incidence and unique characteristics of each cell type.

TABLE 3–16 **Comparison of Lung Cancer Cell Types**

CELL TYPE AND PREVALENCE	PRESENTATION AND ASSOCIATED MANIFESTATIONS	SPREAD
Small-cell (oat cell) carcinoma: 20–25% of all lung cancers	Central lesion with hilar mass common, early mediastinal involvement, no cavitation; syndrome of inappropriate antidiuretic hormone (SIADH), Cushing syndrome, thrombophlebitis	Aggressive tumor; > 40% of clients have distant metastasis at time of presentation
Adenocarcinoma: 20–40% of all lung cancers	Peripheral mass involving bronchi; few local symptoms; hypertrophic pulmonary osteoarthropathy	Early metastasis to central nervous system, skeleton, and adrenal glands
Squamous cell carcinoma: 30–32% of all lung cancers	Central lesion located in large bronchi; client presents with cough, dyspnea, atelectasis, and wheezing; hypercalcemia common	Spreads by local invasion
Large-cell carcinoma: 10–15% of all lung cancers	Usually peripheral lesion that is larger than associated with adenocarcinoma and tends to cavitate; gynecomastia, thrombophlebitis	Early metastasis

MULTISYSTEM EFFECTS OF **Lung Cancer**

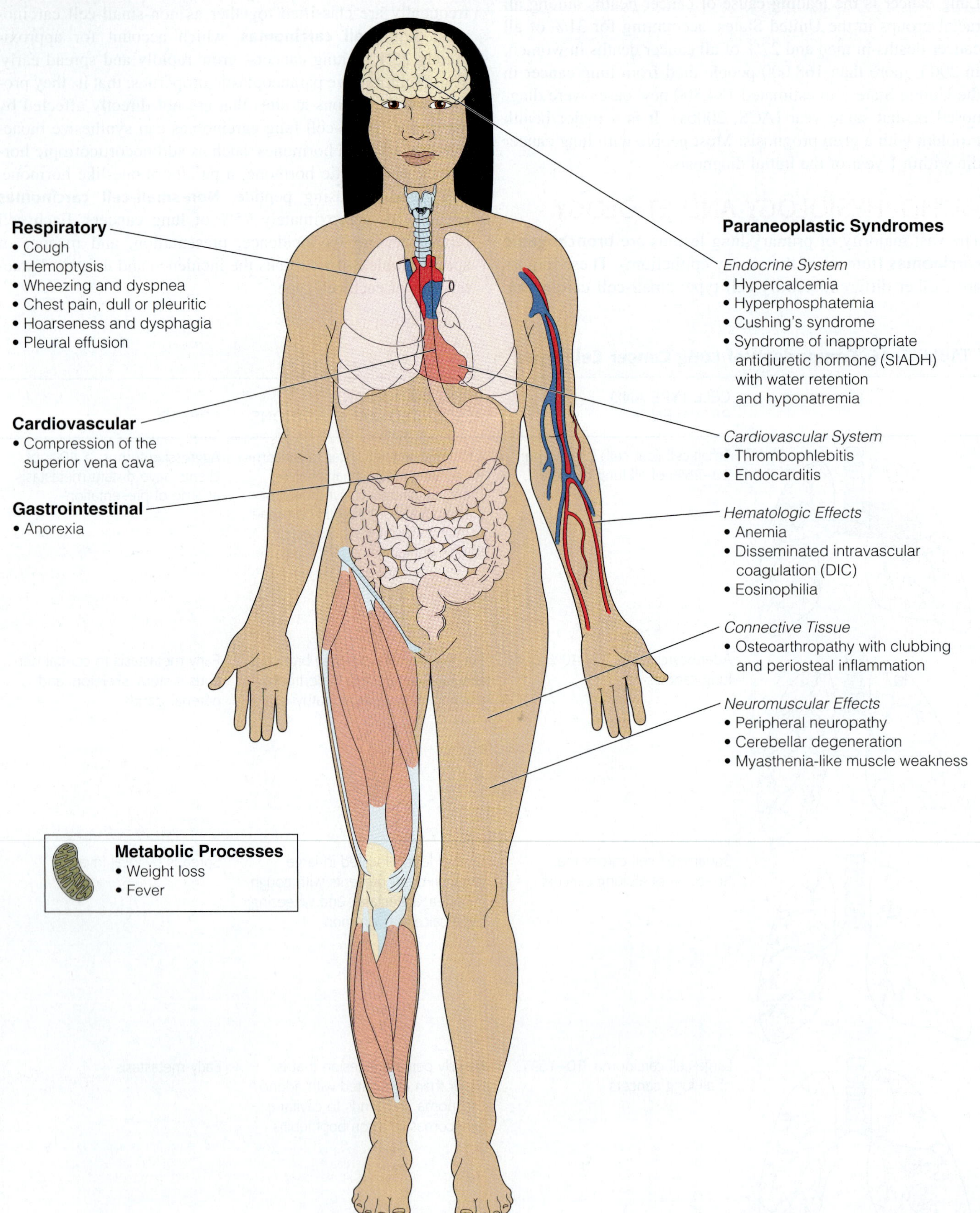

Respiratory
• Cough
• Hemoptysis
• Wheezing and dyspnea
• Chest pain, dull or pleuritic
• Hoarseness and dysphagia
• Pleural effusion
Cardiovascular
• Compression of the superior vena cava
Gastrointestinal
• Anorexia
Metabolic Processes
• Weight loss
• Fever
Paraneoplastic Syndromes
Endocrine System
• Hypercalcemia
• Hyperphosphatemia
• Cushing's syndrome
• Syndrome of inappropriate antidiuretic hormone (SIADH) with water retention and hyponatremia
Cardiovascular System
• Thrombophlebitis
• Endocarditis
Hematologic Effects
• Anemia
• Disseminated intravascular coagulation (DIC)
• Eosinophilia
Connective Tissue
• Osteoarthropathy with clubbing and periosteal inflammation
Neuromuscular Effects
• Peripheral neuropathy
• Cerebellar degeneration
• Myasthenia-like muscle weakness

Bronchogenic cancer, regardless of cell type, tends to be aggressive, locally invasive, and have widespread metastatic lesions. Tumors begin as mucosal lesions that grow to form masses that obstruct the bronchi or invade adjacent lung tissue. All types frequently spread via the lymph system to nodes and other organs, such as the brain, bones, and liver.

Etiology

Lung cancer develops as damaged bronchial epithelial cells mutate over time to become neoplastic. The genetic abnormality commonly seen is on chromosome 3, with loss of genetic material. Alterations of tumor suppressor genes also are seen in some types of lung cancer.

Risk Factors

The incidence of lung cancer varies from state to state and among nations. The incidence increases with age, occurring most commonly in clients over age 50. Family clusters of lung cancer suggest a genetic predisposition; however, exposure to tobacco smoke may be necessary for expression of the trait. Cigarette smoke, which contains 43 known chemical carcinogens and cancer promoters, is clearly the most significant cause of lung cancer (ACS, 2006a). More than 80% of lung cancer cases are related to smoking, and the disease is 10 times more common in those who smoke than in those who do not. There is a dose–response relationship between smoking and lung cancer; the more the person smokes and the longer the person smokes, the greater the risk. Even former smokers who have abstained for a number of years have a higher risk for developing lung cancer compared with those who have never smoked. Exposure to ionizing radiation and inhaled irritants, asbestos in particular, is also recognized as a risk factor for lung cancer (Porth, 2005). Exposure to radon, a radioactive gas, also is identified as a lung cancer risk factor (ACS, 2006a). Radon forms as radium, an element present in the earth's crust, disintegrates. Radon tends to accumulate in closed spaces where air circulation is poor, such as caves, mines, and energy-efficient houses.

CLINICAL MANIFESTATIONS

The manifestations of lung cancer are related to the location and spread of the tumor. Clients may present with symptoms related to the primary tumor, manifestations of metastatic disease, or with systemic symptoms. Initial symptoms often are attributed to smoking or chronic bronchitis. Chronic cough is common, as is hemoptysis. Wheezing and shortness of breath occur as a result of airway obstruction. Dull, aching chest pain occurs as the tumor spreads to the mediastinum; pleuritic pain occurs when the pleura is invaded. Hoarseness and/or dysphagia indicate pressure of the tumor on the trachea or esophagus.

Systemic and paraneoplastic manifestations of lung cancer include weight loss, anorexia, fatigue, and weakness; bone pain, tenderness, and swelling; clubbing of the fingers and toes; and various endocrine, neuromuscular, cardiovascular, and hematologic symptoms. See the Multisystem Effects feature for more details.

Confusion, impaired gait and balance, headache, and personality changes may indicate brain metastasis. Bone metastases cause bone pain, pathologic fractures, and possible spinal cord compression, as well as thrombocytopenia and anemia if bone marrow is invaded. When the liver is affected, symptoms of liver dysfunction and biliary obstruction, including jaundice, anorexia, and upper right quadrant pain, are evident.

Lung cancer has both local and systemic effects. Local effects include cough, excess mucous production, shortness of breath or dyspnea, **hemoptysis** (bloody sputum), and chest pain. Systemic effects may include fever, anorexia and malaise, cyanosis, and other manifestations of impaired gas exchange.

COLLABORATION

Because lung cancer typically is advanced when diagnosed and the prognosis generally is poor, prevention of the disease must be a primary goal for all health care providers. With 80% of lung cancers related to cigarette smoking, reducing tobacco

CLINICAL MANIFESTATIONS AND THERAPIES **Lung Cancer**

ETIOLOGY	CLINICAL MANIFESTATION	CLINICAL THERAPIES
Hypoxia	Shortness of breath, chest pain, reduced oxygen saturation, tachypnea, chronic cough, dyspnea, cyanosis	■ Administer oxygen ■ Reduce activity level ■ Position in Fowler's or tripod position
Paraneoplastic syndrome resulting from growth and metastasis of the tumor	Weight loss, anorexia, fatigue, and weakness; bone pain, tenderness, and swelling; clubbing of the fingers and toes; and various endocrine, neuromuscular, cardiovascular, and hematologic symptoms	■ Surgical removal of tumor ■ Chemotherapy or radiation therapy to reduce metastasis and tumor size ■ Palliative treatment to reduce symptoms ■ Pain management as indicated
Metastasis to brain	Confusion, impaired gait and balance, headache, and personality changes	■ Maintain familiar items in room to promote orientation ■ Protect from falls and risk for injury ■ Explain impact of brain metastasis to family in order to prepare them for personality changes

use can have a significant impact on the death rate from lung cancer—a far greater impact than advances in treatment.

Establishing an accurate diagnosis is the first step in treating lung cancer. Treatment decisions are based on the tumor location, the type of cancer cell, the staging of the tumor, and the client's ability to tolerate treatment. Lung cancer is staged by the tumor size, location, degree of invasion of the primary tumor, and the presence of metastatic disease. Lung cancer staging is summarized in Table 3–17. Surgery is the treatment of choice for most forms of lung cancer.

Diagnostic Tests

Diagnostic tests are based on location and size of the tumor along with client condition. Once lung cancer is diagnosed, additional tests may be ordered to rule out possible metastatis. Common diagnostic tests include:

- *Chest x-ray* usually provides the first evidence of lung cancer. It is particularly reliable as a diagnostic tool when compared with a previous chest x-ray. In high-risk populations, the chest x-ray may be used as a screening tool for lung cancer.
- *Sputum specimen* is sent for cytologic examination to establish the diagnosis of lung cancer. The sputum sample is collected on arising in the morning. If malignant cells are found in the sputum, more expensive and invasive examinations may be unnecessary. However, a sputum sample that is negative for malignant cells does not rule out lung cancer; it may simply indicate that the tumor is not shedding cells into mucous secretions.
- *Bronchoscopy* is frequently done to visualize and obtain a biopsy specimen from the tumor. When a tumor mass or suspicious tissue is identified visually, a cable-activated instrument is used to obtain a tissue specimen. If the tumor cannot be seen, the airways may be flushed with a saline solution (bronchial washing) to obtain cells for cytologic examination.
- *Computed tomography (CT)* is used to evaluate and localize tumors, particularly tumors in the lung parenchyma and pleura. It also is done before needle biopsy to localize the tumor. In addition, CT scanning can detect distant tumor metastasis and evaluate tumor response to treatment.
- *Cytologic examination and biopsy* involve cells or tissue obtained by aspirating fluid from a pleural effusion, percutaneous needle biopsy, and lymph node biopsy. These procedures may be done in an outpatient or a surgical setting.
- *CBC, liver function studies, and serum electrolytes* including calcium are obtained to evaluate for evidence of metastatic disease or paraneoplastic syndromes.
- *Tuberculin test* is performed to rule out tuberculosis as the cause of symptoms and abnormalities seen on chest x-ray.
- *Pulmonary function tests and arterial blood gas* may be performed before the initiation of treatment if the client has manifestations of respiratory insufficiency (e.g., dyspnea, activity intolerance, and low oxygen saturation levels).

These tests are described in greater detail in Appendix B.

Pharmacologic Therapies

Combination chemotherapy (often combined with radiation therapy and/or surgery) is the treatment of choice for small-cell lung cancer because of its rapid growth, dissemination, and sensitivity to cytotoxic drugs. Used in combination, chemotherapeutic drugs allow tumor cells to be attacked at different parts of the cell cycle and in different ways, increasing the effectiveness of therapy. Fifty percent of clients with tumors at early stages achieve complete tumor remission with combination chemotherapy. When a complete tumor response is achieved in the first few cycles of chemotherapy, the chances for long-term survival are much greater.

Combination chemotherapy also is used as an adjunct to surgery or radiation therapy for other types of lung cancer. It may be used to reduce the size of advanced local tumors

TABLE 3–17 The TNM Staging System for Lung Cancer

	PRIMARY TUMOR (T)	REGIONAL LYMPH NODES (N)	DISTANT METASTASIS (M)
	T0—No evidence of primary tumor		
Stage 0	TX—Malignant cells in bronchopulmonary secretions, but no tumor visualized		MX—Presence of distant metastasis cannot be assessed
Stage I	T1S—Carcinoma in situ	N0—No regional lymph node metastasis	M0—No distant metastasis
	T1—Tumor of ≤ 3 cm in diameter, with no evidence of invasion		
Stage II	T2—Tumor of > 3 cm in diameter, or invades visceral pleura, or has associated atelectasis or pneumonitis	N1—Metastasis or direct extension to peribronchial or ipsilateral hilar nodes	
Stage III	T3—Tumor with direct extension into an adjacent structure, or any tumor with associated pleural effusion or atelectasis or pneumonitis of entire lung	N2—Metastasis to ipsilateral mediastinal or subcarinal nodes	
Stage IV	T4—Tumor that invades mediastinum or involves the heart, great vessels, trachea, esophagus, vertebral body, or carina; presence of malignant pleural effusion	N3—Metastasis to contralateral mediastinal, scalene, or supraclavicular nodes	M1—Distant metastasis present

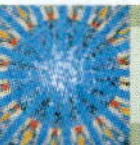

ALTERNATIVE THERAPIES **Lung Cancer**

Research indicates that a significant number of clients diagnosed with lung cancer use complementary and alternative medicine (CAM). In one study of clients with lung cancer in eight European nations, 23.6% used CAM therapies (Molassiotis et al., 2006). The CAM remedies used included herbal medicines, medicinal teas, homeopathy, animal extracts, and spiritual therapies. While these therapies may be safe when used alone, the potential for interactions with conventional medical treatment must be considered. Inquire of clients about their use of complementary and alternative therapies, and inform members of the health care team when such therapies are being used.

before surgery and to lengthen survival when distant metastases are present.

Bronchodilators may be prescribed to reduce airway obstruction. Analgesics and pain management strategies are vital when the cancer is advanced. See Concept 5, Comfort, for more information about postoperative and cancer pain management.

Surgery

Surgery offers the only real chance for a cure in clients with non-small-cell lung cancer. Unfortunately, most tumors are inoperable or only partially resectable at the time of diagnosis. The 5-year survival rate following curative surgery in clients with resectable tumors is approximately 30%, with most clients succumbing to metastatic disease within 5 years (Kasper et al., 2005). The type of surgery performed depends on the location and size of the tumor as well as on the client's pulmonary and general health. The goal of surgery is to remove all involved tissue while preserving as much functional lung as possible. Table 3–18 outlines various surgical procedures used to treat lung cancer.

Radiation Therapy

Radiation therapy is used alone or in combination with surgery or chemotherapy for lung cancer. The goal of treatment may be either cure or symptom relief (palliative). Before surgery, radiation therapy is used to "debulk" tumors. When cancer has spread by direct extension to other thoracic structures and surgery is not feasible, radiation therapy may be the treatment of choice. It also may be used to relieve manifestations such as cough, hemoptysis, pain resulting from bone metastasis, and dyspnea from bronchial obstruction. Complications of lung cancer, such as superior vena cava syndrome, may be treated with radiation. Radiation therapy may be delivered by external beam to the primary tumor site or by intraluminal radiation, or **brachytherapy** with insertion of a radioactive source inside the body near the tumor for more direct effects.

NURSING PROCESS

The client with lung cancer is facing invasive treatments with undesirable side effects, possibly surgery, and typically a poor prognosis for long-term survival. Nursing care needs are diverse, related to respiratory status, the cancer itself and possible metastases, and the treatment plan.

Assessment

Nursing assessment related to lung cancer focuses on identifying risk factors for the disease, early manifestations of lung cancer, and respiratory function in the client undergoing

TABLE 3–18 **Types of Surgery for Lung Cancer**

PROCEDURE	DESCRIPTION	USED FOR
Laser bronchoscopy	Bronchoscopy-guided laser used to resect tumor	Tumors localized in a main bronchus
Mediastinoscopy	Visualization of the mediastinum using an endoscope passed through a suprasternal incision	Evaluation and biopsy of a mediastinal tumor and lymph nodes
Thoracotomy	Incision into the chest wall	Access the lung and thoracic cavity for surgery
Wedge resection	Removal of a small section (wedge) of peripheral lung tissue	Small, peripheral lung tumors
Segmental resection	Removal of an individual bronchovascular segment of a lobe	Peripheral lung tumor with no evidence of extension to the chest wall or metastasis
Sleeve resection (bronchoplastic reconstruction)	Resection of a section of a major bronchus with reconstruction of remaining normal bronchus	Small lesion of a major bronchus
Lobectomy	Removal of a single lung lobe	Tumors confined to a single lobe
Pneumonectomy	Removal of an entire lung	Tumor widespread throughout the lung, involving the main bronchus, or fixed to the hilum

treatment. Collect the following data through the health history and physical examination:

- *Health history.* Current symptoms, including chronic cough, shortness of breath, blood-tinged sputum; systemic manifestations such as recent weight loss, fatigue, anorexia, bone pain; smoking history; occupational exposure to carcinogens; chronic diseases such as chronic obstructive pulmonary disease
- *Physical examination.* Assess respiratory function including respiratory rate, depth, breath sounds, and chest excursion. Oxygenation is assessed using pulse oximetry, arterial blood gas results, and pulmonary function studies.

Diagnosis

Priority nursing diagnoses related to respiratory function include the following:

- Ineffective Breathing Pattern
- Activity Intolerance
- Pain
- Anticipatory Grieving.

Plan

Goals of care may include the following:

- The client expresses feelings related to diagnosis and/or terminal condition.
- The client makes informed decision related to treatment options.
- The client maintains adequate oxygenation.
- The client reports pain at acceptable level to allow for rest.

Implementation

Nurses take a holistic approach to providing care, meeting both the physical and psychosocial needs of the client. Airway and breathing are always the greatest priority. The client who is hypoxic will be anxious, so reducing anxiety is a priority intervention for that client.

Ineffective Breathing Pattern

Breathing pattern and ventilation may be affected by the tumor itself or by treatment of the tumor. Thoracic surgery increases the risk caused by the incision and disruption of the muscles of respiration. Maintaining effective lung ventilation is particularly important postoperatively to reexpand remaining lung tissue and prevent surgical complications.

- Assess and document respiratory rate, depth, and lung sounds at least every 4 hours; evaluate more frequently in the immediate postoperative period or as indicated by condition. Early detection of signs of respiratory compromise or adventitious lung sounds is vital for effective intervention.
- Frequently assess and document pain level (using a standard pain scale); provide analgesics as needed. Pain and attempting to avoid chest movement to prevent additional pain can lead to rapid, shallow respirations and ineffective ventilation.
- Elevate the head of the bed to 60°. Elevating the head of the bed reduces pressure on the diaphragm and permits optimal lung expansion.
- Assist the client to turn, cough, and deep breathe and use incentive spirometry. Help splint the chest with a pillow or blanket when coughing. These measures promote airway clearance.
- Suction airway as needed. Suctioning may be required to remove secretions that the client is unable to cough up and expectorate.
- Provide chest physiotherapy with percussion and postural drainage as needed or ordered. Percussion and postural drainage help maintain airway patency and effective respirations.
- If mechanical ventilation is instituted, work with respiratory therapy and use analgesia or sedation as needed to synchronize respirations with the ventilator. Coordination of the client's respiratory effort with ventilator-delivered breaths is important for fully effective mechanical ventilation.
- Provide reassurance and emotional support. These measures help relieve anxiety and promote an effective breathing pattern.

Activity Intolerance

Both resectional lung surgery and inoperable lung cancer reduce the amount of functional lung tissue and surface area for gas diffusion. This can lead to activity intolerance if the oxygen supply is insufficient to meet the body's oxygen demand.

- Plan rest periods between activities and procedures. Rest periods reduce oxygen demands and fatigue.
- Assist the postoperative client to increase activities gradually. Increasing activity levels gradually improves exercise tolerance.
- Teach measures to conserve energy while performing ADLs, such as sitting while showering and dressing and wearing slip-on shoes. These energy-conserving measures reduce oxygen demand and allow the client to remain independent as long as possible.
- Keep frequently used objects within easy reach. This helps conserve energy.
- Administer oxygen as prescribed. Teach the client and family about home oxygen use if appropriate. Supplemental oxygen can help improve activity and exercise tolerance.
- Encourage maintenance of physical activity to tolerance. Maintaining activity levels to the degree possible improves physical and emotional well-being.
- Allow family members to provide assistance as needed. This helps the client conserve energy and allows the family to retain a sense of usefulness.

Pain

Pain is a priority problem in the postoperative period and in the terminal stages of cancer. Poorly managed pain prolongs recovery from surgery. In the client with terminal cancer, chronic and acute pain must be managed effectively to allow a peaceful death.

- Assess and document pain using a standardized pain scale and objective data. Pain is a subjective experience, best evaluated by the client. Changes in vital signs, guarded movement, or unwillingness to move may indicate unreported pain.

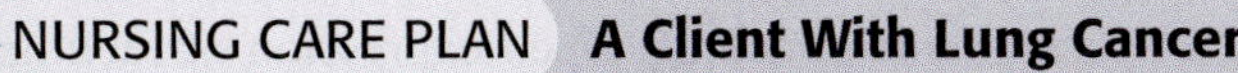

NURSING CARE PLAN A Client With Lung Cancer

After coughing up bloody sputum one morning, James Mueller, a 68-year-old retired mill worker, sees his physician. A chest x-ray shows a suspicious density in the central portion of his right lung. Mr. Mueller is admitted to the hospital the following Monday for diagnostic tests.

ASSESSMENT

Anita Sarros, RN, admits Mr. Mueller to the oncology unit and obtains a nursing history. Mr. Mueller is married and has three grown children. He worked in a local paper mill for 35 years before retiring at age 62. He describes himself as "pretty healthy," except for a chronic smoker's cough. He started smoking as a young man in the army. He has a 50-year smoking history, having smoked a pack a day for 50 years, since age 18. Mr. Mueller says he briefly quit smoking following a small heart attack 3 years ago but started again after 4 months. On further questioning, Mr. Mueller says his cough has been productive for the past few months, especially in the morning, and that he is shorter of breath than usual with activity.

Mr. Mueller's examination data include BP 162/86 mmHg, pulse 78 bpm and regular, respirations 20/min, and temperature 98.4°F (36.9°C). His color is good, and his skin is warm and dry. Inspiratory and expiratory wheezes are noted in right chest, but good breath sounds are heard throughout. No other abnormal findings are noted on examination. The physician orders early morning sputum specimens times 3 days for cytologic examination and schedules a CT scan of the chest the morning after admission.

Mr. Mueller's CBC shows mild anemia, but remaining routine laboratory tests are essentially normal. Sputum cytology is positive for small-cell bronchogenic cancer. The CT scan shows a central mass approximately 4 cm in diameter with involved mediastinal and subclavicular lymph nodes. A small mass is also noted on the lumbar spine. After conferring with his physician and an oncologist, Mr. Mueller decides to undergo a trial course of chemotherapy.

DIAGNOSES

- Ineffective Airway Clearance related to tumor mass
- Risk for Imbalanced Nutrition: Less Than Body Requirements related to effects of chemotherapy
- Risk for Compromised Family Coping related to new diagnosis of lung cancer
- Deficient Knowledge about lung cancer and aids to smoking cessation

PLANNING

- The client will maintain a patent airway.
- The client will maintain current weight.
- The client will express feelings and concerns about the effect of cancer on the family unit.
- The client will participate in care.
- The client will contact appropriate support groups.
- The client will verbalize an understanding of the disease, its treatment, and prognosis.
- The client will develop a plan to stop smoking.

IMPLEMENTATION

- Teach coughing, deep breathing, and hydration measures to facilitate airway clearance.
- Discuss symptoms to report to the physician: increased dyspnea or hemoptysis, severe stridor or wheezing, and chest pain.
- Discuss measures to relieve nausea associated with chemotherapy, including premedication with a prescribed antiemetic.
- Have dietitian consult with Mr. and Mrs. Mueller to develop a diet plan for maintaining ideal weight.
- Discuss possible effects of lung cancer with Mr. and Mrs. Mueller.
- Encourage Mr. and Mrs. Mueller to call a family conference to discuss the disease with their children and grandchildren.
- Evaluate family members' knowledge and understanding of lung cancer, correcting misinformation and teaching as needed.
- Have an American Cancer Society volunteer contact the family.
- Refer to local cancer support group.
- Refer to home health department for follow-up and further teaching.
- Work with Mr. Mueller to develop a plan to stop smoking.
- Ask the physician for a prescription for nicotine patches or gum for Mr. Mueller.

EVALUATION

Mr. Mueller had his first chemotherapy treatment in the hospital and was discharged 4 days after admission. After 3 months of chemotherapy, his tumor shows little regression, and a liver scan reveals further metastasis. He and his wife decide to stop chemotherapy, a decision with which the children reluctantly agree. Mr. and Mrs. Mueller are referred to hospice services. With the help of hospice nurses and volunteers, Mr. Mueller is able to remain at home. His pain is managed initially with oral MS Contin, a sustained-release form of morphine sulfate, and later with an intravenous morphine infusion. Mr. Mueller dies at home with his family at his side 9 months after his diagnosis of lung cancer.

CRITICAL THINKING

1. The oncologist prescribed a chemotherapy regimen of cyclophosphamide, doxorubicin, and vincristine. Describe how each of these drugs works against cancer cells, and discuss the rationale for using this combination.
2. Develop a care plan to deal with the specific side effects for the above treatment regimen.
3. Mr. Mueller had small-cell (oat cell) cancer. How would his presentation and treatment differ if the diagnosis had been non-small-cell adenocarcinoma, stage T2N2M0?

- Provide analgesics as needed to maintain comfort. Postoperative recovery and restoration of function is facilitated by adequate pain management.
- For cancer pain, maintain an around-the-clock medication schedule using narcotic, nonsteroidal anti-inflammatory drugs, and other medications as ordered. Addiction is not a concern in the client with terminal cancer; providing adequate pain relief that does not allow "breakthrough" pain is important.
- Provide or assist with comfort measures, such as massage, positioning, distraction, and relaxation techniques. These techniques promote relaxation and enhance pain relief.
- Assist the client and family to plan and engage in activities that distract from pain, such as reading, watching television, and engaging in social interactions. Distraction helps the client focus away from the pain.
- Spend as much time with the client as possible; allow family members to remain with the client. Physical presence of the nurse and family provides emotional support for the client.

Pain management is discussed further in Exemplar 5.1, Acute and Chronic Pain. Care for the client and the end-of-life is discussed in Exemplar 5.2. A discussion of "presencing" can be found in Concept 27, Spirituality.

Anticipatory Grieving

Because lung cancer often is advanced when diagnosed, the client faces the very real prospect of dying from the disease. Grieving for the anticipated loss of life is a normal response as the client and family begin to adapt to the diagnosis. Nursing care goals are to promote expression of feelings and thoughts about the loss and to help the client and family initiate grief work, make decisions, and use appropriate resources and coping mechanisms to deal with the loss.

- Spend time with the client and family. Time is necessary to develop a trusting, therapeutic relationship.
- Answer questions honestly; do not deny the probable outcome of the disease. Honesty reinforces reality and provides a sense of control over decisions to be made.
- Encourage the client and family to express their feelings, fears, and concerns. Open expression of feelings helps promote understanding and acceptance.
- Assist with understanding the grieving process and acceptance of feelings as normal. Feelings of guilt, anger, or depression may cause the client to withdraw from others. Explanation of the grieving process enhances understanding and ability to cope.
- Help identify strengths and coping measures that have been used effectively in the past. Provide positive reinforcement for effective coping behavior. Past effective coping measures can help the client and family deal with the present situation and regain a sense of control.
- Help the client and family make decisions regarding treatment and care. This also is important to give the client and family a sense of control.
- Encourage use of other support systems, such as spiritual and social groups. Refer the client and family to support groups, social support services, and hospice care as indicated. Provide ACS literature and information as appropriate. These support systems provide emotional support and help the client and family cope with the diagnosis.
- Discuss advance directives, such as do-not-resuscitate orders, and powers of attorney for health care with the client and family. These documents give the client and family a sense of control over medical care provided if the client is no longer able to express his or her own wishes.

Evaluation

Client response to care is evaluated based on goals of care. Expected outcomes may include the following:

- The client chooses treatment option best for his or her needs.
- The client maintains adequate nutritional and hydration status.
- The client achieves pain control within acceptable limits.

REVIEW Lung Cancer

RELATE: LINK THE CONCEPTS

Linking the exemplar of Lung Cancer with the concept of Acid–base Balance:

1. What effect might lung cancer have on the client's acid–base balance?
2. What client teaching will you provide to assist with normalizing acid–base balance?

Linking the exemplar of Lung Cancer with the concept of Infection:

3. What priority client teaching can the nurse provide to reduce the risk of infection in the client diagnosed with lung cancer?
4. When caring for the client with lung cancer, what interventions will you initiate to reduce the risk of infection?

READY: GO TO COMPANION SKILLS MANUAL

- Assessing respirations
- Assessing the client in pain
- Using an incentive spirometer
- Administering oxygen by cannula, face mask, or face tent
- Using an oxygen cylinder
- Inserting an oropharyngeal airway
- Inserting a nasopharyngeal airway
- Oropharangyal, nasopharyngeal, or nasotracheal suctioning
- Caring for the client on a mechanical ventilator

REFER: GO TO MYNURSINGKIT

REFLECT: CASE STUDY

Michael, 66 years old, has abused alcohol for many years and has smoked two packs of cigarettes a day since age 19. He has been diagnosed with lung cancer. Michael is divorced and has two children who are grown and live out of town. Michael lives alone in an apartment and has a girlfriend who also smokes and abuses alcohol. The physician in charge of Michael's care has told Michael that he will need a lobectomy of the left lung, radiation therapy, and chemotherapy. Michael thanks the doctor and tells him he will get back to him. The nurse remains with Michael after is the doctor leaves the room and overhears him whisper under his breath "Fat chance I'm going to do all that. I'd rather die in peace."

1. How would you respond to this statement?
2. What is the priority nursing diagnosis for Michael?
3. What interventions can you initiate to help Michael make the best health care and lifestyle decisions?
4. What will your personal feelings and thought be if you are caring for Michael and he decides not to pursue treatment? How might this bias impact your approach to caring for Michael?

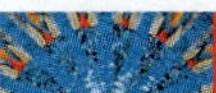

3.7 PROSTATE CANCER

KEY TERMS

Androgens, *169*
Orchiectomy, *172*
Prostatectomy, *170*

BASIS FOR SELECTION OF EXEMPLAR

Centers for Disease Control and Prevention
Healthy People 2010
Institute of Medicine

LEARNING OUTCOMES

After reading about this exemplar, you will be able to:

1. Describe the pathophysiology, etiology, clinical manifestations, and direct and indirect causes of prostate cancer.
2. Identify risk factors associated with prostate cancer.
3. Illustrate the nursing process in providing culturally competent care across the life span for individuals with prostate cancer.
4. Formulate priority nursing diagnoses appropriate for an individual with prostate cancer.
5. Create a plan of care for individuals with prostate cancer and their family members.
6. Assess expected outcomes for an individual with prostate cancer.
7. Discuss therapies used in the collaborative care of an individual with prostate cancer.
8. Employ evidence-based caring interventions for an individual with prostate cancer.

OVERVIEW

Abnormal growth of prostate tissue may be related to benign prostatic hypertrophy (covered in more detail in Concept 9, Elimination), or it may be an indication of prostate cancer. The diagnosis of prostate cancer is very frightening for most men, who fear death, disfigurement, and loss of sexual function.

When diagnosed early, prostate cancer is curable. When the cancer is confined to the prostate at diagnosis, the 5-year survival rate is 100%. Even when the cancer has spread regionally, approximately 95% of clients are alive after 5 years. More than 75% of prostate cancer diagnoses are made at one of these stages (ACS, 2009).

Many men are found to have prostate cancer on autopsy. Usually, the cancer has produced no manifestations or complications, and these men may have died with no knowledge of the developing disease.

PATHOPHYSIOLOGY AND ETIOLOGY

The prostate gland consists primarily of glandular epithelial cells. The exact etiology of prostate cancer is unknown, although **androgens** (hormones synthesized in the testes, ovaries, and adrenal cortex that promote expression of male sex characteristics) are believed to have a role in its development. Almost all primary prostate cancers are adenocarcinomas, and they develop in the peripheral zones of the prostate gland. This location increases the risk of local spread to the prostatic capsule. Despite its proximity to the rectum, metastasis to the bowel is uncommon, because a tough sheet of tissue, Denonvilliers' fascia, acts as an effective physical barrier.

As the tumor enlarges, it may compress the urethra, obstructing urinary flow. The tumor may metastasize and involve the seminal vesicles or bladder by direct extension. Metastasis by lymph and venous channels is common.

Etiology

Cancer of the prostate is the most common type of cancer and the second-leading cause of death among men in North America (American Cancer Society, 2006). It is primarily a disease of older men, increasing in incidence with age, with the majority of cases diagnosed in men older than 65 years. It is estimated that each year, more than 234,000 men will be diagnosed with prostate cancer and approximately 27,000 will die from the disease (American Cancer Society, 2006). Prostate cancer is a major health problem for older men, but the death rate is decreasing as a result of advances in diagnosis and treatment.

Risk Factors

The greatest risk factor for prostate cancer is age. Prostate cancer affects one out of every eight men over the age of 60, and it is more common in older men than bladder cancer (ACS, 2005b). In addition to age, race is a significant risk factor for prostate cancer. Other risk factors being investigated include the following:

- Genetic and hereditary factors, with increased risk in men who have a family history of the disease
- Having a vasectomy, which is believed to increase the levels of circulating free testosterone
- Dietary factors, including a diet high in animal fat and excessive supplemental vitamin A.

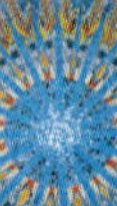

FOCUS ON DIVERSITY AND CULTURE

Risk and Incidence of Prostate Cancer

- African Americans have the highest incidence of prostate cancer in the United States and the world, with rates more than twice as high as those of whites.
- African Americans are more likely to be diagnosed later and to die of prostate cancer, with a mortality rate more than double that of other racial and ethnic groups.
- Asians and Native Americans have the lowest incidence of prostate cancer.

CLINICAL MANIFESTATIONS

Men with early-stage prostate cancer are often asymptomatic. Pain from metastasis to bones is often the initial manifestation noted. Urinary manifestations depend on the size and location of the tumor and on the stage of the malignancy; they are often much like manifestations of benign prostatic hypertrophy: urgency, frequency, hesitancy, dysuria, and nocturia. The man may also notice hematuria or blood in the ejaculate (Porth, 2005). Manifestations of prostate cancer are summarized in Box 3–15.

COLLABORATION

Care of the man with prostate cancer focuses on diagnosis, elimination or containment of the cancer, and prevention or treatment of complications. There are currently no clinical strategies to prevent the development of prostate cancer. Therefore, early detection remains the major emphasis for control of this disease.

The treatment of prostate cancer is complex and depends on the grade and stage of the cancer as well as on the age, general health, and preference of the client. In some cases, for example, when the client with a slow-growing tumor is older or has a limited life expectancy, *watchful waiting* is the treatment of choice. Treatments for prostate cancer include surgery, radiation therapy, and hormone manipulation.

Box 3–14 Manifestations of Prostate Cancer

GENITOURINARY
- Dysuria
- Frequency of urination
- Reduction in urinary stream
- Nocturia
- Hematuria
- Abnormal prostate on digital rectal examination

MUSCULOSKELETAL
- Bone or joint pain
- Migratory bone pain
- Back pain

NEUROLOGIC
- Nerve pain
- Bilateral lower extremity weakness
- Bowel or bladder dysfunction
- Muscle spasms

SYSTEMIC
- Weight loss
- Fatigue

Diagnostic Tests

Although an increasing number of clients are now diagnosed with asymptomatic prostate cancer, many clients with prostate cancer have either locally advanced cancer or distant metastasis at the time of diagnosis. The definitive diagnosis can be made only by biopsy; however, other tests may suggest the presence of prostate cancer.

A *digital rectal examination (DRE)* will find the prostate gland nodular and fixed in the client with prostate cancer. Levels of *prostate-specific antigen (PSA)* are used to diagnose and stage prostate cancer and to monitor response to treatment. Levels depend on age, and there is no specific normal or abnormal level. An increase over time is more significant than one reading. The PSA test is used with a DRE to help detect prostate cancer in men age 50 or older, and it is also used to monitor effects of treatment. Many physicians are using the following ranges (National Cancer Institute, 2004):

- 0–2.5 ng/mL is low.
- 2.6–10 ng/mL is slightly to moderately elevated.
- 10–19.9 ng/mL is moderately elevated.
- 20 ng/mL or more is significantly elevated.

Transrectal ultrasonography may be used when the DRE is abnormal or if the PSA is elevated. In this test, a small probe is inserted in the rectum. The probe gives off sound waves that make a picture of the prostate on a video screen. Guided by this picture, the physician inserts a narrow needle through the rectal wall into the prostate gland, and the needle removes a sample of tissue for examination. Other tests that may be ordered include a urinalysis or cystoscopy. Bone scan, MRI, or CT may be performed to determine the presence of tumor metastasis.

Grade and stage help determine prognosis and guide treatment decisions. Grade (cancer cell differentiation) is determined by the pathologist. Prostate cancer is staged with a variety of tests. Table 3–19 outlines treatment options according to the stage of the cancer.

Surgery

Surgery for prostate cancer generally involves **prostatectomy**, or removal of the prostate. For very early disease in older men, cure may be achieved with a simple prostatectomy (e.g., TURP). Types of prostatectomies include the following:

- *Radical prostatectomy* involves removal of the prostate, prostate capsule, seminal vesicles, and a portion of the bladder neck. Many clients experience varying degrees of urinary incontinence and erectile dysfunction (ED) (Table 3–20). A fairly new treatment is laparoscopic radical prostatectomy, in which small incisions are made in the abdomen and a laparoscope is inserted and used to remove the prostate. Some surgeons do this from an area other than the operating room by using a robotic interface. Nursing research reporting client satisfaction with a discharge program following a

TABLE 3–19 Prostate Cancer Staging and Treatment

STAGE	DESCRIPTION	TREATMENT
I	Confined to prostate, nonpalpable, focal involvement; well differentiated	■ Observation and follow-up ■ Interstitial or external-beam radiation therapy ■ Prostatectomy
II	Confined to prostate, palpable, involves one or both lobes; poorly differentiated	■ Careful observation in selected clients ■ Prostatectomy ■ Interstitial or external-beam radiation therapy ■ Ultrasound-guided percutaneous cryosurgery
III	Extension of the tumor outside the prostate capsule, possible seminal vesicle involvement	■ External-beam radiation therapy ■ Interstitial radiation ■ Radical prostatectomy ■ Adjunctive hormone therapy ■ Palliative surgery (transurethral prostatectomy or TURP – removal of the prostate through the urethra)
IV	Extension of the tumor into surrounding tissues; lymph node involvement or distant metastasis	■ Hormone therapy ■ External-beam radiation therapy ■ Palliative treatment with radiation therapy and/or TURP ■ Radical prostatectomy with orchiectomy ■ Chemotherapy

radical prostatectomy is discussed in the Evidence-Based Practice feature that follows.

- *Retropubic prostatectomy* may be performed because it allows adequate control of bleeding, visualization of the prostate bed and bladder neck, and access to pelvic lymph nodes.
- *Perineal prostatectomy* is often preferred for older men or those who are poor surgical risks. This approach requires less time, and involves less bleeding.
- *Suprapubic prostatectomy* is rarely used, usually when problems with the bladder are expected. Control of bleeding is more difficult because the surgical approach is through the bladder.

TABLE 3–20 Potential Complications Related to Radical Prostatectomy and Radiation Therapy

RADICAL PROSTATECTOMY	RADIATION THERAPY
Erectile dysfunction	Erectile dysfunction[a]
Urethral stricture	Urethral stricture
Fistula/rectal injury	Rectal/anal stricture[a]
Urinary incontinence	Cystitis
Surgical/anesthetic risk	Diarrhea
	Proctitis
	Rectal ulcer
	Bowel obstruction[a]
	Urinary incontinence

[a]Delayed complications; may appear months or years after completion of therapy.

For clients with stage III, locally advanced (beyond the prostatic capsule) cancer, surgery is controversial because of the likelihood of hidden lymph node metastasis and relapse. TURP is not performed as curative therapy, but it may be used to relieve urinary obstruction for men with advanced disease (stage III or IV).

Surgical intervention is now available for men with urinary sphincter insufficiency, which is the major cause of incontinence after prostatectomy. An artificial urinary sphincter is surgically implanted (Figure 3–19 ■). To be eligible, the man must be able to manipulate the pump placed in the scrotum and have adequate cognitive function to know when a problem with the appliance occurs.

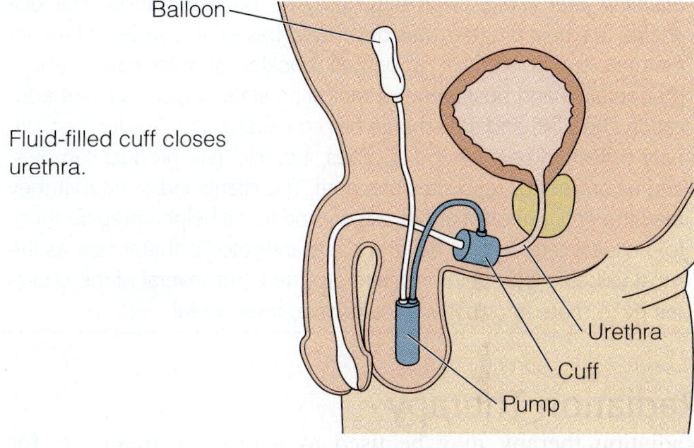

Fluid-filled cuff closes urethra.

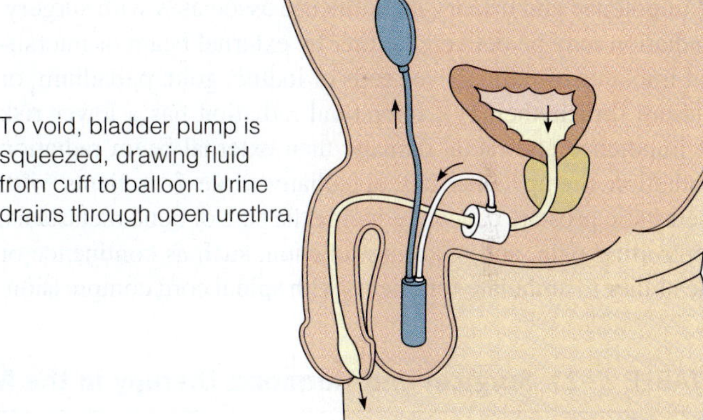

To void, bladder pump is squeezed, drawing fluid from cuff to balloon. Urine drains through open urethra.

After voiding, fluid drains back to cuff, closing urethra.

Figure 3–19 ■ Method of operation of an artificial urinary sphincter.

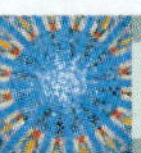

EVIDENCE-BASED PRACTICE Improving Discharge Teaching After Prostatectomy

Clinical Question

The period immediately after hospital discharge for a radical prostatectomy is often a difficult time for men and their families as they cope with the emotional and physical demands of cancer surgery. Deficient knowledge about how long it will take to recover and how to provide care at home can have a major effect on healthy recovery from surgery. Nurses recognize the need to provide discharge teaching before the client leaves the hospital, but this need is often not a part of actual practice.

Evidence

Davison et al. (2004) evaluated a revised program for discharge teaching after a radical prostatectomy for prostate cancer. The discharge teaching program was developed based on a review of the literature. It consisted of a printed booklet of information about preoperative and postoperative radical prostate surgery, a client education checklist, and a discharge bag containing a urinary leg bag, urinary collection bag, wound supplies, incontinence product samples, and a community resources brochure. The clients indicated that they read the entire booklet about surgery and that it helped prepare them for hospital care. Almost half the clients indicated catheter care as the most valuable type of information provided, but several of the clients felt even more information would have been useful.

Best Practice

This type of information is extremely important as the number of clients having radical prostatectomy increases and hospital stays continue to be shortened. Nurses need to provide the type and amount of information required by clients for self-care at home.

Critical Thinking

1. You are caring for a 75-year-old man who has had a radical prostatectomy for prostate cancer. His wife tells you they have always had an active sex life and she hopes this surgery will not change that. What would you say to her?
2. Why would the nursing diagnosis risk for infection be appropriate for a man providing self-care at home following a radical prostatectomy? What type of interventions would you suggest during discharge teaching to reduce this risk?
3. If you were developing a list of community resources for men following prostate surgery, what would you include? How would your list vary for the following situations?
   - A 64-year-old man with a wife and four married children who all live nearby
   - A 77-year-old man who lives alone and has no family
   - A 90-year-old man who will go to an assisted living facility after discharge from the hospital

Radiation Therapy

Radiation therapy may be used as a primary treatment for prostate cancer which reduces the risk of long-term problems of impotence and urinary incontinence associated with surgery. Radiation may be delivered either by external beam or interstitial implants of radioactive seeds of iodine, gold, palladium, or iridium (brachytherapy). Interstitial radiation has a lower risk of impotence and rectal damage than external-beam radiation Radiation therapy also has a palliative role for clients with metastatic prostate cancer, reducing the size of bone metastasis, controlling pain, and restoring function, such as continence or the ability to ambulate for clients with spinal cord compression.

Pharmacologic Therapies

Androgen deprivation therapy is used to treat advanced prostate cancer. Many cells in the growing tumor are androgen dependent and either cease to grow or die if deprived of androgens. Unfortunately, other cancer cells thrive without androgen and are unaffected by therapy to reduce circulating androgens. Therefore, the effects of hormone manipulations vary from complete but temporary regression of the tumor to no response at all.

Strategies to induce androgen deprivation vary from **orchiectomy** (surgical removal of one or both testicles) to oral administration of hormonal agents. Table 3–21 compares surgical and hormone therapies and the advantages and disadvantages of

TABLE 3–21 Surgical and Hormone Therapy in the Management of Advanced Prostate Cancer

TREATMENT	ADVANTAGES	DISADVANTAGES
Orchiectomy	Inexpensive Immediate effect; men report diminished pain from metastasis in the recovery room	Body image problems resulting from loss of testicles
Estrogen compounds (diethylstilbestrol)	Inexpensive Effects reversible	Increased risk of cardiovascular problems More likely to cause gynecomastia, hypertrophy of breast tissue
Luteinizing hormone-releasing hormone agonist (LHRH) (leuprolide)	Effects reversible No cardiovascular risk Monthly administration	Very expensive Subcutaneous injection route Slow onset: up to 4 weeks
Steroidal antiandrogens (megestrol [Megace])	Effects reversible No cardiovascular risk Inexpensive	May not drop testosterone levels sufficiently Weight gain
Nonsteroidal antiandrogens (flutamide; often used in conjunction with LHRH)	Does not alter circulating androgens Blocks some side effects of LHRH May be effective if other methods fail	Very expensive

Note. All hormonal manipulations have the potential disadvantage of loss of libido, erectile dysfunction, hot flashes, and gynecomastia.

each. In addition, new drugs are being developed that block the effects of male hormones, and research is being conducted to demonstrate what mix of hormones is best and at what time in the perioperative period they are most effective.

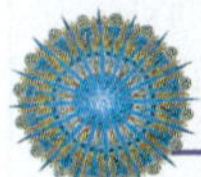

NURSING PROCESS

Nurses plan and provide interventions to help prevent prostate cancer and to facilitate a return to functional health status once prostate cancer is diagnosed. Nurses are in a unique position to increase public awareness about early detection of prostate cancer. Every encounter with men and their families—in clinics, hospital units, or in the home—is an opportunity to provide information about early detection and to identify needs. Several studies have shown a positive correlation between increased awareness of and participation in prostate cancer screening procedures. The ACS has free pamphlets about early detection of prostate cancer, which are useful in educating the public.

One risk factor that can be easily changed is diet. Men should know that they can lower their risk of prostate cancer by eating less red meat and fat. They should include fruits and vegetables as recommended in the new food pyramid; tomatoes, pink grapefruit, and watermelon are high in lycopenes that help prevent damage to DNA and may help lower prostate cancer risk. Other substances that may help lower the risk are vitamin E and selenium.

All men should be given information about the limitations and benefits of testing for early detection and of treatment so they can make an informed decision. The ACS (2005a) recommends that the PSA test and DRE should be offered each year, beginning at age 50, to all men with a life expectancy of at least 10 years. Men at high risk (men of African descent and those with a first-degree relative diagnosed at a younger age) should begin testing at age 45.

Assessment

Collect the following data through the health history and physical examination:

- *Health history.* Risk factors, urinary elimination patterns and manifestations, hematuria, pain
- *Physical assessment.* Digital rectal examination to assess prostate size, symmetry, firmness, and nodules, assess for bladder distention, urinary flow, and urine retention.

Note that a DRE is an advanced nursing assessment.

Diagnosis

Nursing diagnoses for a client with prostate cancer include the following:

- Impaired Urinary Elimination
- Sexual Dysfunction
- Pain.

Plan

Goals of nursing care may include the following:

- The client receives adequate pain management to control pain within tolerable levels.
- The client verbalizes concerns about or symptoms of sexual dysfunction without discomfort.
- The client lists strategies for reducing and coping with urinary incontinence.
- The client maintains adequate urinary output.

Implementation

Nursing care must be provided with sensitivity because clients are often worried about loss of virility, sexual function, and masculinity, and they may be reluctant to discuss these concerns with the nurse. Holistic care must be provided to meet the client's physical, psychosocial, and spiritual needs.

Urinary Incontinence

Urinary incontinence is a disturbing complication following treatment for prostate cancer. Both radical prostatectomy and external-beam radiation therapy can cause incontinence, ranging from a drop or two when the client lifts a heavy object (stress incontinence) to no control at all. Older men may experience involuntary passage of urine soon after a strong sense of urgency to void (urge incontinence). Total and unpredictable loss of urine is classified as total incontinence. The man's reaction to incontinence may be severe even if the incontinence is not great. Many men have significant anxiety at the prospect of an incontinent episode in public, because they feel shame and often guilt about the loss of control.

- Assess the degree of incontinence and its effects on lifestyle. The nurse needs to determine previous urinary patterns and the type of incontinence currently being experienced to plan appropriate interventions.
- Teach Kegel exercises to help restore continence. Pelvic muscle or Kegel exercises can often either eliminate or improve stress incontinence.
- Teach methods to control dampness and odor from stress incontinence:
  a. Do not attempt to prevent accidental voiding by restricting fluids. Not only will the man continue to have incontinent episodes, but his urine will become concentrated, exacerbating the problem with odor.
  b. Manage occasional episodes (one to three small-volume accidents per day) with absorbent pads worn inside the underwear and changed as needed. Most pads are made with a polymer gel that controls odor. Appropriate measures help promote good hygiene, decrease anxiety, and increase comfort.
- Refer to physical therapy or a continence specialist for additional measures to promote continence. Special exercises, restricting some types of fluids, and other measures (e.g., bladder training) can help the client deal with incontinence.
- Explore options such as an external collection device (external catheter or Texas catheter) for the man with total incontinence. This device may improve the man's self-esteem and allow resumption of social activities.
- Encourage verbalizing feelings about the impact of incontinence on quality of life. The degree of incontinence does not necessarily correlate with the perceived level of suffering. Listening to these concerns with sensitivity can help the man work through these feelings and may allow him to move toward a healthy adaptation to his disability.

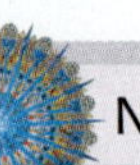

NURSING CARE PLAN A Client With Prostate Cancer

William Turner, a 71-year-old African American, lives with his wife in a small retirement community in Florida. His wife had a stroke 2 years ago, and Mr. Turner does all the cooking and housework. He has been in good health for most of his life, having only "a small touch" of osteoarthritis in his knees and hands. He has noticed a gradual onset of urinary urgency and frequency over the past 2 years but has never had incontinence. During a routine checkup, the nurse practitioner at the local health clinic performs a digital rectal examination and palpates a hard nodule on the surface of Mr. Turner's prostate. After his PSA is found to be elevated, he is referred to a urologist, who diagnoses prostate cancer. Mr. Turner chooses to have surgery, and a radical retropubic prostatectomy and lymph node dissection are performed. The lymph nodes are negative for metastasis. Following surgery, his recovery is uncomplicated. However, the nurse caring for Mr. Turner is concerned about his ability to care for his indwelling catheter because of his arthritis and his wife's physical disabilities from the stroke. The nurse makes a referral to a home health agency to ensure Mr. Turner can manage his care at home. An initial home health assessment is scheduled for the day after Mr. Turner is discharged from the hospital.

ASSESSMENT	DIAGNOSES	PLANNING
The home health nurse notes that the house is clean and neat. Mr. Turner is dressed but still wearing his night urinary drainage bag, although it is 1300. Mr. Turner tells the nurse that his main problem is going to get groceries, because he is embarrassed to be seen with the drainage bag. He says he has not been able to remove the drainage bag and attach the leg bag because of his arthritis. Physical assessment findings include the pelvic incision to be healing without signs of infection. There is no tenderness in his calves, chest pain, or shortness of breath. The urine is yellow, without odor. Mr. Turner does state that he sees no need for the pelvic exercises since he is no longer in the hospital. He also expresses the belief that he is cured of cancer and questions the need for follow-up care.	■ Risk for Stress Urinary Incontinence related to surgical procedure ■ Ineffective Health Maintenance related to inability to care for the urinary drainage system, not understanding need for postoperative exercises, and questions about follow-up care	■ The client will regain urinary continence after catheter removal. ■ The client will change the urinary drainage bag with the appropriate assistance. ■ The client will verbalize the rationale for performing postoperative exercise. ■ The client will verbalize the need for continued follow-up care.

IMPLEMENTATION

- Discuss the possibility of stress incontinence after the catheter is removed.
- Reinforce the need for Kegel exercises while the catheter is still in place.
- Explore Mr. Turner's support system to identify people who could assist him with catheter care, and arrange a teaching session with them.
- Teach Mr. Turner the importance of follow-up care, relating the care to the history of the disease.

EVALUATION

Good friends from Mr. Turner's church have assisted him with care of his drainage bag and have reminded him to do his Kegel exercises several times a day while the catheter is in place. When the catheter is removed, Mr. Turner has only a small amount of urine leakage after voiding. He understands that it may take several weeks for this to resolve. Efforts to help him understand the need for continued medical care are less successful. Mr. Turner continues to state that he is cured, his wife needs him, and he sees no need to go back to the doctor.

CRITICAL THINKING

1. Outline a teaching plan for Mr. Turner for the risk for altered skin integrity related to urinary incontinence.
2. As a result of Mr. Turner's refusal to have ongoing medical care, he might be labeled as noncompliant. Would you make this nursing diagnosis? Why, or why not?
3. If you were the home health nurse making a home visit and found that Mr. Turner had no urinary drainage for 16 hours, what assessments would you make? How would you handle this problem?

Sexual Dysfunction

Surgical treatment for prostate cancer may cause erectile dysfunction and changes in ejaculatory function. Hormone therapy for advanced prostate cancer lowers libido and may also cause erectile dysfunction. The diagnosis of cancer and the body image changes caused by hormone therapy may lower self-esteem, which in turn can diminish sexual desire and willingness to interact sexually with a partner. Most older men are sexually active and fully capable of sustaining an erection. They are likely to fear the effect of treatment on their sexual health. They may allow this concern to guide their decision about the course of treatment, or they may refuse all therapy because of this fear. Reactions vary greatly, and the nurse must maintain a nonjudgmental approach to education and support.

- Assess the man's pretreatment sexual function. Knowledge of previous sexual function is necessary to plan appropriate interventions.
- Teach the man about the actual or potential effects of therapy on sexual function. The incidence of erectile dysfunction varies with different therapies for prostate cancer.
- Provide an opportunity for the man and his partner to discuss implications of and concerns about the diagnosis and

treatment of sexual function. The treatments for prostate cancer often affect the physiology of erection. The man and his partner need support and counseling during the period of adjustment.

- Discuss medical and surgical treatments for erectile dysfunction. Many men are as devastated by the loss of erectile function as they are by the diagnosis of cancer. Information about achieving erection and maintaining sexual intimacy is essential to quality of life.
- Refer for sexual counseling as appropriate. The man and his partner may require therapy beyond that provided by nurses.

Pain

There are many causes of pain in men with advanced prostate cancer. It is not unusual for a client to have three or four distinct pains simultaneously, all from different sources. The most common cause of pain is metastasis to the spinal column, usually the thoracic spine. Other sources of pain include fractures, lymphedema of the lower extremities, and muscle spasms. Because most men with prostate cancer are over the age of 65, many also have pain associated with preexisting conditions, such as osteoarthritis, unrelated to the cancer.

- Assess the intensity, location, and quality of the pain. A cardinal rule of successful pain management is the importance of reducing or eliminating the cause of pain. Appropriate interventions are based on a careful assessment of the client's pain.
- Provide optimal pain relief with prescribed analgesics. It is important the man and his family understand that pain medications should be used on a regular basis to maintain comfort and should not be delayed until pain is severe.
- Teach the man and his family noninvasive methods of pain control. Various modalities can be successful in alleviating pain or reducing its perception, thus enhancing the comfort of the client.

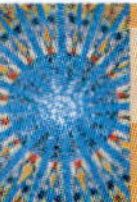

CLIENT TEACHING Home Care for the Client With Prostate Cancer

Depending on the type of treatment, the following topics should be addressed in preparing the client and his family for home care:

- For the man having a surgical procedure: manifestations of infection and excessive bleeding, catheter care, wound care pain management
- For the man receiving radiation therapy:
  a. Danger of radiation damage to others (sleep in a room alone for a week; avoid close contact with pregnant women, infants, and children)
  b. Condom use during sexual contact (ejaculate may be discolored, distressing sexual partner)
- The importance of keeping appointments with health care providers and having yearly PSA and rectal examinations
- If appropriate, community services, such as support groups, home health nurses, and hospice
- Helpful resources:
  a. American Cancer Society (http://www.cancer.org)
  b. American Urological Association (http://www.auanet.org)
  c. National Cancer Institute (http://www.cancer.gov)

Evaluation

Expected outcomes to evaluate client care are based on goals set during the planning stage and may include the following:

- The client rates and reports pain before it becomes intolerable.
- The client discusses sexual function without anxiety or discomfort.
- The client lists strategies for managing urinary incontinence.
- The client maintains adequate urine output without complications related to altered urinary elimination.

REVIEW Prostate Cancer

RELATE: LINK THE CONCEPTS

Linking the exemplar of Prostate Cancer with the concept of Urinary Elimination:

1. What effect might prostate cancer have on the client's ability to urinate if he chooses to treat the cancer by medical, rather than surgical, therapies?
2. How can you promote adequate urinary elimination for this client?

Linking the exemplar of Prostate Cancer with the concept of Tissue Integrity:

3. What nursing interventions can promote tissue integrity in the client who recently had surgical removal of the prostate?
4. Write a teaching plan for the client preparing for discharge to home following prostatectomy.

READY: GO TO COMPANION SKILLS MANUAL

- Performing urinary catheterization
- Performing catheter care and removal
- Assessing the male genitals and inguinal area
- Assessing the client in pain
- Preparing the client for surgery

REFER: GO TO MYNURSINGKIT

REFLECT: CASE STUDY

Maury Blarden is a 45-year-old client who has been diagnosed with prostate cancer. He is married and has a 3-year-old daughter. Maury and his wife own their own company renovating and decorating homes. Maury and Karen have been told that surgery is necessary, along with radiation and chemotherapy. Maury tells the nurse that he and his wife are trying to have another child, hopefully, a boy. He is not sure that he can take the time away from the business for surgery and therapy. The couple has minimal health care coverage and is concerned about the costs of care because they barely make enough to get by.

1. What expected outcomes would be appropriate for this client?
2. Karen asks you, while Maury is out of the room, if the procedure will result in impotence. How will you respond to this question?
3. Will Maury and Karen be able to have children if he decides to undergo surgery? Explain your answer.

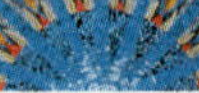

3.8 SICKLE CELL DISORDER

KEY TERMS

Alloimmunization, *179*
Hemoglobinopathy, *176*
Hemosiderosis, *179*
Priapism, *177*
Sickle cell anemia, *176*
Sickle cell crisis, *177*
Sickle cell disorder, *176*
Sickle cell trait, *177*
Sickling, *176*
Vasoocclusive crisis, *178*

BASIS FOR SELECTION OF EXEMPLAR

Centers for Disease Control and Prevention
Healthy People 2010
World Health Organization

LEARNING OUTCOMES

After reading about this exemplar, you will be able to:

1. Describe the pathophysiology, etiology, clinical manifestations, and direct and indirect causes of sickle cell disorder.
2. Identify risk factors associated with sickle cell disorder.
3. Illustrate the nursing process in providing culturally competent care across the life span for individuals with sickle cell disorder.
4. Formulate priority nursing diagnoses appropriate for an individual with sickle cell disorder.
5. Create a plan of care for individuals with sickle cell disorder and their family members.
6. Assess expected outcomes for an individual with sickle cell disorder.
7. Discuss therapies used in the collaborative care of an individual with sickle cell disorder.
8. Employ evidence-based caring interventions for an individual with sickle cell disorder.

OVERVIEW

Sickle cell disorder is a hereditary **hemoglobinopathy**, a type of disorder characterized by replacement of normal hemoglobin with abnormal hemoglobin S (Hgb S) in RBCs. **Sickle cell anemia**, a chronic hemolytic anemia, is the most common type of sickle cell disorder (Table 3–22).

PATHOPHYSIOLOGY AND ETIOLOGY

When the percentage of hemaglobin replaced by Hgb S increases it is called **sickling**. During episodes of sickling, RBCs become abnormally crescent shaped referred to as hemaglobin S or Hgb S. This causes occlusion of small blood vessels, ischemia, and damage to affected organs. Repeated episodes of sickling and unsickling weaken RBC cell membranes. The weakened RBCs are hemolyzed and removed. Consequently, the normal life span of RBCs is greatly reduced in sickle cell disorder, increasing the demand for RBC production. Sickle cell anemia can significantly shorten life span, with most deaths resulting from infection (McCance & Huether, 2006).

The abnormally shaped red blood cell is unable to circulate freely through the blood vessels and become stuck in small vessels, particularly capillaries. These S shaped red blood cells form an occlusion into the smaller vessel much like a traffic jam on a busy highway with the end result of ischemia because the tissues cannot receive the oxygen and nutrients they need nor eliminate the waste products of cellular metabolism. Repeated or prolonged ischemia resulting from sickle cell induced occlusions cause damage to the tissues in organs throughout the body becoming scarred and resulting in impaired function. For example, children with sickle cell disorder can suffer from splenic sequestration when blood is trapped in the spleen, a life-threatening complication. Many children must undergo splenectomy in early childhood, leading to severely compromised immunity. Infection rate is subsequently high because of impaired immunity, and bacterial

TABLE 3–22 SICKLE CELL DISORDERS

SICKLE CELL DISORDER	DESCRIPTION
Sickle cell trait	Most common form of sickle cell disease in the United States Heterozygous condition (child has one sickle cell hemoglobin gene and one normal hemoglobin gene) Child is carrier of sickle cell anemia and rarely has symptoms of the disease
Sickle cell anemia	Homozygous condition (child has two sickle hemoglobin genes) Child is subject to sickle cell crises
Sickle cell syndromes	*Sickle cell–hemoglobin C disease* Second most frequent form of sickle cell disease in African Americans Different from sickle cell anemia only in that the sickle cell assumes a C-shape instead of an S-shape
Rare combination of conditions	*Sickle cell–beta-thalassemia disease* Combination of sickle cell trait and thalassemia trait most often seen in people of Mediterranean descent

FOCUS ON DIVERSITY AND CULTURE Sickle Cell Disorder

Sickle cell disorder tends to affect people whose origins are in equatorial countries, particularly those in central Africa, the Near East, the Mediterranean region, and parts of India. Hispanics from the Caribbean and Central and South America also may have the hemoglobin S (Hgb S) gene. This gene may have originated to protect against lethal forms of malaria, an endemic disease in many equatorial regions.

Sickle cell disorder affects approximately 72,000 people in the United States. In African Americans, sickle cell disorder occurs in 1 out of every 600 births. People from Central and South America, Cuba, Saudi Arabia, India, and Mediterranean countries such as Turkey, Greece, and Italy also may be at risk; sickle cell disorder occurs in 1 of every 1,000 to 1,400 Hispanic American births.

infections are the leading cause of death in young children with sickle cell disorder.

Stroke is a significant risk to children with sickle cell anemia and can lead to developmental delay, mental retardation, and other neurologic outcomes (National Heart, Lung, and Blood Institute, 2002). Other complications of sickle cell disease can include acute chest syndrome with pulmonary hypertension, pulmonary infiltrate, and infection; aplastic crisis or temporary cessation of bone marrow blood cell production; **priapism** (persistent, painful erection of the penis); and gallstone formation (Wilson, Krishnamurti, & Kamat, 2003). Sickling may be triggered by fever and emotional or physical stress. **Sickle cell crisis** is the term used to describe periods when the percentage of hgb S increases resulting in the appearance of symptoms, often marked by acute pain resulting from ischemia Precipitating factors for sickle cell crisis include increased blood viscosity, such as from low fluid intake or fever, and hypoxia or low oxygen tension. Potential causes of hypoxia or low oxygen tension include high altitudes, poorly pressurized airplanes, hypoventilation, vasoconstriction when cold, or an emotionally stressful event. Any condition that increases the body's need for oxygen or alters the transport of oxygen, such as infection, trauma, or dehydration, may result in sickle cell crisis.

Sickled cells can resume a normal shape when rehydrated and reoxygenated. The membrane of these cells becomes more fragile, however, and cell life is shortened to 10–20 days rather than the usual 120 days. In response, bone marrow spaces enlarge to produce more RBCs. Continuous formation and destruction of the child's RBCs contributes to the severe hemolytic anemia that is characteristic of sickle cell anemia (Tanyi, 2003).

Etiology

The disorder is transmitted as an autosomal recessive genetic defect. If both parents have the trait, then with each pregnancy the risk of having a child with the disease is 25%. The HbS gene changes the structure of the beta chain of the hemoglobin molecule. When hypoxemia develops and HbS is deoxygenated, it crystallizes into rodlike structures. Clusters of these rods form long chains that deform the erythrocyte into a crescent or sickle shape (Figure 3–20 ■). The sickled cells tend to clump together and obstruct capillary blood flow, causing ischemia and possible infarction of surrounding tissue.

Risk Factors

The disease is most common among people of African descent. In the United States, 7–13% of African Americans carry the defective gene, having inherited it from one parent (McCance & Huether, 2006); these individuals have **sickle cell trait**. Approximately 40% of their hemoglobin is HbS (Porth, 2005). They are likely to remain asymptomatic unless stressed by severe hypoxia. Less than 1% of African Americans are homozygous for the disorder; that is, less than 1% have inherited a defective gene from both parents. These individuals *have sickle cell disease*; nearly all their hemoglobin is HbS (Porth, 2005). They also are at risk for sickle cell crisis. Those with sickle cell trait as well as those with sickle cell disease are diagnosed with sickle cell disorder. When sickling occurs and symptoms appear the client is diagnosed with sickle cell anemia.

Conditions likely to trigger sickling include hypoxia, low environmental or body temperature, excessive exercise, anesthesia, dehydration, infections, or acidosis. Precipitating factors that contribute to sickle cell crisis are summarized in Box 3–16.

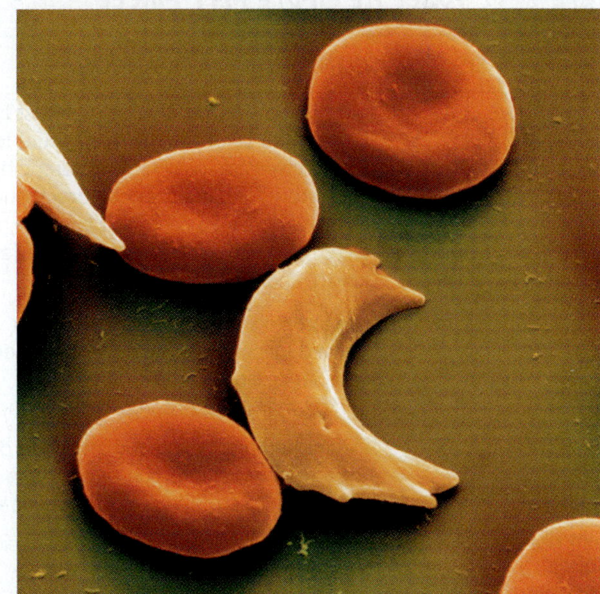

Figure 3–20 ■ Blood smear containing normal red blood cells and sickle cells.

Source: Oliver Meckes and Nicole Ottawa, Photo Researchers, Inc.

Box 3–16 Precipitating Factors Contributing to Sickle Cell Crisis

- Fever
- Dehydration
- Altitude
- Extremes in temperature
- Vomiting
- Emotional distress
- Fatigue
- Alcohol consumption
- Pregnancy
- Elevated hemoglobin levels
- Elevated reticulocyte counts
- Excessive exercise or physical activity
- Acidosis

CLINICAL MANIFESTATIONS

The acute and chronic manifestations of sickle cell anemia arise from episodes of RBC sickling. Sickling causes general manifestations of hemolytic anemia, including pallor, fatigue, jaundice, and irritability. Extensive sickling can precipitate a crisis as a result of occluded circulation, impaired erythropoiesis, or sequestration of large amounts of blood in the liver or spleen (Table 3–23).

A **vasoocclusive** or thrombotic **crisis** occurs when sickling develops in the microcirculation. Obstruction of blood flow by sickled cells that cannot pass through the vessel triggers vasospasm that halts all blood flow. Lack of blood flow leads to tissue ischemia and infarction. Vaso-occlusive crises are painful and last an average of 4–6 days. A simple example of vasoocclusion is the occlusion of blood and resulting pain that one feels when one wraps a rubber band around one's finger too tightly. Infarction of small vessels in the extremities causes painful swelling of the hands and feet; large joints also may be affected. Priapism may develop as well. Abdominal pain may signal infarction of abdominal organs and structures. Infarction also may affect bone marrow or lead to aseptic necrosis of affected bones resulting in pain from avascular necrosis of the bone marrow and is typically experienced in the back, abdomen, chest, and joints. Stroke may result from cerebral vessel occlusion (McCance & Huether, 2006). Skin ulcers may develop as the result of occluded vessels supplying the dermis.

Repeated infarcts associated with sickling can affect the structure and function of nearly every organ system. People with sickle cell disease may develop an enlarged spleen and liver, renal insufficiency, gallstones, and other manifestations of organ dysfunction. Acute chest syndrome, a symptom complex that includes fever, chest pain, an increasing WBC count, and pulmonary infiltrates, may develop, as well as other pulmonary complications, such as pneumonia, pulmonary infarction, and pulmonary embolism (Porth, 2005).

Affected children are usually asymptomatic until 4 to 6 months of age because sickling is inhibited by high levels of fetal hemoglobin. The most common reason for hospitalization of the child with sickle cell anemia is acute painful episodes (Beyer & Simmons, 2004). Children with sickle cell anemia can also experience chest tightness and shortness of breath, which are diagnostic for acute chest syndrome and medical crisis.

Pain intensity and duration vary depending on the individual and the location. Pain may be transient in a localized area, such as the wrist, to severe, generalized pain that lasts for several

TABLE 3–23 TYPES OF SICKLE CELL CRISES

TYPE OF CRISIS	CLINICAL MANIFESTATIONS
Vaso-occlusive crises (thrombotic)	Most common type of crisis; may last for days or weeks. Precipitated by dehydration, exposure to cold, acidosis, or localized hypoxemia. Caused by stasis of blood with clumping of cells in the microcirculation, ischemia, and infarction. Thrombosis and infarction of local tissue may occur if the crisis is not reversed. Cerebral occlusion can result in stroke, manifested by paralysis and/or other central nervous system complications. Extremely painful; symptoms include fever, tissue engorgement, painful swelling of joints in hands and feet, priapism, and severe abdominal pain.
Splenic sequestration	Life-threatening crisis; death can occur within hours. Caused by pooling of blood in the spleen; because the spleen can hold much of the body's blood supply, cardiovascular collapse can result. Clinical manifestations include profound anemia, hypovolemia, and shock.
Aplastic crises	Diminished production and increased destruction of red blood cells. Triggered by viral infection or depletion of folic acid. Signs include profound anemia, pallor, and fatigue.
Acute chest syndrome	Common cause of hospitalization for sickle cell disease. Most common from 2–4 years of age. Pulmonary infiltrate of abnormal blood cells leads to lower respiratory tract symptoms. Clinical manifestations include fever, cough, chest and back pain, dyspnea, and hypoxemia. Pulmonary infection, infarct, and fat embolism may occur and can lead to pulmonary failure and death.

Data from: Bryant (2005) and Wilson et al. (2003).

days or weeks and may require hospitalization. The pain is often severe enough to require opioid analgesics and the use of a client-controlled analgesic pump. Children with sickle cell trait rarely have sickle cell crises. However, because they have some abnormal hemoglobin, they may develop symptoms of the disease under conditions of abnormally low oxygen, such as flying in an unpressurized airplane over 7,000 feet or during anesthesia. The most common symptoms experienced by those with sickle cell trait are splenic infarction and hematuria. However, most persons who carry the trait never have symptoms, even with low oxygen concentrations.

The shortened RBC life span and compromised erythropoiesis can lead to profound aplastic anemia in sickle cell disease. Sequestration crises are marked by pooling of large amounts of blood in the liver and spleen. This sickle cell crisis only occurs in children but is thought to be the cause of sickle cell disease-related deaths in early childhood (Porth, 2005).

COLLABORATION

Optimal care for the client with sickle cell anemia involves the coordinated efforts by members of a health care team. Neonatal screening, early intervention, prophylactic antibiotics, and parent education have allowed children with sickle cell disease to live into adulthood. A nurse with a specialty in genetics, or a genetics counselor, may be involved in sickle cell gene testing and counseling to identify and inform carriers and children who have the disease.

Diagnostic Tests

The initial diagnosis of sickle cell anemia in newborns is often made by testing cord blood using hemoglobin electrophoresis. The sickle-turbidity test (Sickledex) may be used for quick screening purposes in children older than 6 months, once the fetal hemoglobin levels have fallen. Hemoglobin electrophoresis is performed to verify positive Sickledex test results. Newborn screening of infants for hemoglobinopathies occurs in most states. It is recommended that all newborns be screened, because sickle cell disease can occur in several groups in addition to African Americans, such as those of Mediterranean, South American, Arabian, and East Indian descent (Kral et al., 2006). A child's heritage cannot be predicted from appearance or name alone.

Serum analysis of blood reveals the degree of anemia, with hemoglobin of 6–10 g/dL characteristic of severe syndromes (Segal, Hirsh, & Feig, 2002). Reticulocyte values are elevated, demonstrating the marrow activity that attempts to replace destroyed and nonfunctional red cells. These values are monitored regularly to measure the response of the bone marrow and state of the anemia.

> **PRACTICE ALERT**
>
> Neither hot nor cold compresses should be used for pain management in the child with sickle cell anemia. Ischemic tissue is fragile and has reduced sensation, increasing the risk of burn injury from hot compresses while cold compresses promote sickling.

Pain Control, Hydration, and Oxygenation

Parenteral analgesics, such as morphine, are generally administered around the clock or via client-controlled analgesia. Pain medications should not be ordered on an "as needed" basis, because this increases the child's anxiety and delays medication administration. Oral and IV fluid replacement also promotes pain relief, since dehydration is often a cause of crisis. Fluids reduce the viscosity of the blood, so adequate hydration is essential. Oxygen is usually administered to provide comfort and decrease the incidence of pulmonary complications.

Prevention and Treatment of Infection

Children who are functionally asplenic or have had a splenectomy have a resultant decreased capability to fight infection. For this reason, infection is a serious condition requiring immediate attention. Daily prophylactic penicillin VK, 125 mg twice daily, is recommended for children from 2 months to 3 years of age. From 3 to 5 years of age, the recommended dosage is doubled to 250 mg twice daily. Amoxicillin or injections of Bicillin every 3 weeks can be substituted. If the child is allergic to penicillin, erythromycin ethyl succinate, 20 mg/kg divided into two doses, can be used for prophylaxis (Wilson et al., 2003).

When an infection is suspected, cultures (blood, urine, and throat) are obtained to identify the source of infection and the offending organism. Aggressive antibiotic therapy is implemented immediately.

It is recommended that the pneumococcal vaccine (PCV 7 for infants and toddlers or 23-valent for children older than 2 years) be administered to all infants and children with sickle cell disease (National Heart, Lung, and Blood Institute, 2002). The *Haemophilus influenzae* type b (Hib) vaccine series should be started at 2 months of age and continued at recommended ages to prevent infection with Hib, which was once the most common cause of epiglottitis, a life-threatening disorder. Other vaccines, such as the influenza and meningococcal vaccines, may also be administered.

Transfusion of Red Blood Cells

Another therapeutic measure is transfusion of RBCs. The benefits of transfusions include improved blood and tissue oxygenation, a reduction in sickling, and a temporary suppression of the production of RBCs containing HbS (Ogedegbe, 2002). Several types of blood transfusion are used.

A complication associated with frequent transfusions is an overload of iron in the body. The iron is stored in tissues and organs (**hemosiderosis**) because the body has no way of excreting it. For this reason, an iron-chelating drug, such as deferoxamine, may be given with vitamin C to promote iron excretion. Another complication of multiple transfusions is the development of alloimmunization to red cell and platelet antigens (Ogedegbe, 2002). **Alloimmunization** occurs when the child's immune system reacts against antigens on the donated tissues (e.g., blood and stem cells).

Additionally, chronic transfusions have proven to be an effective treatment of stroke complications related to sickle

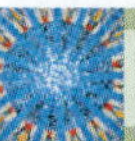

ALTERNATIVE THERAPIES Sickle Cell Anemia and Pain

Management of pain for children with sickle cell disease is a major challenge for both health care providers and families. A nursing study that determined effectiveness of pain control and types of comfort measures used by families provides information that can be applied in caring for children with sickle cell disease in the hospital and at home (Beyer & Simmons, 2004). The mothers in this study described a combination of traditional medicine and complementary approaches. They emphasized the importance of keeping the child healthy, in order to avoid crisis. Avoiding overheating or chilling were listed as important factors. Regular medical checkups, adequate hydration, and immunizations were considered important. Being alert to early signs of pain was also crucial. Families used pharmacologic treatment as well as complementary therapies, such as applying heat by baths and hot towels to decrease pain and increase relaxation; touching, holding, and massaging the extremities or chest and back; praying together; and using distraction and diversionary activities, such as playing games and taking drives. Nurses can learn from and apply these approaches with families. Ask them what they do to identify pain early and alleviate it. Add to the list of interventions the family members can try and then partner with them to evaluate results. Continue to emphasize medical care while integrating the other comfort measures the family and child find helpful into nursing care plans.

cell disease. In children who have had strokes from the disease, periodic transfusions (approximately every 3–4 weeks) can reduce the incidence of future strokes (National Heart, Lung, and Blood Institute, 2002). If administered early in the crisis, blood transfusions may relieve the ischemia caused by vaso-occlusion in major organs and body parts, such as the spleen, lung, kidney, brain, and penis. Exchange transfusion is preferred in order to reduce the potential of fluid volume excess.

Other Therapies

Treatment with hydroxyurea has been helpful in adults and is now being used more frequently in children. This cytotoxic medication decreases production of abnormal blood cells and leads to a lesser amount of pain being experienced. Additionally, hydroxyurea increases fetal hemoglobin production and red cell mean corpuscular volume (Ogedegbe, 2002). Side effects of hydroxyurea include bone marrow suppression, headaches, dizziness, nausea, and vomiting.

Hematopoietic stem cell transplantation may be considered. However, a recurrence of the disease is demonstrated in approximately 10% of recipients.

NURSING PROCESS

Once a child is diagnosed with sickle cell disorder, a comprehensive physical assessment is essential because any body system can be affected. The nurse focuses on providing care to the client as well as teaching both the client and family how to reduce sickling, provide home care, and symptoms to report to the provider immediately.

Assessment

In children who are known to have sickle cell anemia, obtain a detailed history from the parents or child about past crises, precipitating events, medical treatment, and home management. Measure the child's height and weight accurately, and compare them with past measurements (failure to thrive is common). Ask about chronic or acute pain that the child is experiencing. Pain may occur in nearly any body part but most commonly manifests as headache, extremity pain, or abdominal discomfort. Use a pain scale and identify pain perception in each body part where pain exists. Assess the pain management protocols the family has used and what has been most successful.

The ill child with sickle cell disease should receive a careful multisystem assessment. Fever, neurologic changes (e.g., decreased alertness or behavioral changes), and respiratory symptoms are emergency conditions that necessitate prompt treatment. When the child is in crisis, assess pain, and note the presence of any signs of inflammation or infection. Carefully monitor the child for signs of shock (hypotension, changes in level of consciousness, dizziness or lightheadedness, increased capillary refill time).

Sickle cell disease is a chronic illness that interferes with ADLs. Disturbed self-concept and body image, guilt about disturbing the family routines, depression, and isolation can occur. Assess of the child's developmental status with a concentration on friends, family support, and self-concept.

The family of a child with sickle cell disease requires ongoing, thorough psychosocial assessment. If the child is newly diagnosed with the disorder, the family will need assistance to deal with feelings related to the disease's serious, life-threatening nature. Assess parents' understanding of the disease transmission, and ask whether genetic counseling has been obtained. Determine whether the family has adequate health care coverage to pay for the child's medical expenses. Ask older children about their knowledge of the disease, and explore their feelings related to the management of a chronic condition. When siblings or other family members are carriers, they should receive periodic counseling during the life span so that they understand the implications for dating, marriage, and having children.

Diagnosis

Several nursing diagnoses may apply to the child with sickle cell anemia:

- Risk for Impaired Tissue Perfusion (Cerebral)
- Acute Pain

- Caregiver Role Strain
- Risk for Infection
- Interrupted Family Processes
- Delayed Growth and Development
- Impaired Physical Mobility.

Plan

Goals of nursing care include the following:

- The client will experience reducing complications as the result of sickling.
- The caregiver will provide support and assistance as needed.
- The client will meet growth and development needs.
- The client will optimize physical mobility as tolerated.

Implementation

Nursing management for the client in crisis focuses on increasing tissue perfusion, promoting hydration, controlling pain, preventing infection, ensuring adequate nutrition, preventing complications, and providing emotional support to the child and family.

Risk for Impaired Tissue Perfusion

Administer blood transfusions and oxygen as ordered. Because children receive treatment every 3 weeks, nurses commonly start and maintain the lines and infusions used. To prevent hemolysis, the IV fluid used before and after a blood transfusion must be saline rather than D_5W. In small children, the blood is usually infused without saline, because they cannot manage the extra volume.

Monitor for transfusion reactions. Encourage the child to rest. Work with the child and family to avoid emotional stress, and plan with the family for the trips to the health care facility. Any activities that increase cellular metabolism also result in tissue hypoxia, so the family needs assistance to plan the child's daily activities. Schedule caregiving activities and play during hospitalizations and clinic visits to allow for optimal rest.

Acute Pain

Administer prescribed analgesics around the clock during crises. If client-controlled analgesia is used, be sure that the constant infusions run as ordered and that the parent or child understands the use of bolus infusions when needed. Reposition the infant and young child carefully, supporting joints and extremities on pillows or special mattresses. Assist the child to assume a comfortable position. Avoid putting stress on painful joints or other body parts. Pain management is important for comfort, healing, and for promoting physical mobility.

Risk for Infection

Infection makes the child more susceptible to a crisis, and the crisis in turn increases susceptibility to infection. Teach the parents how to administer antibiotics for prophylaxis or treatment of infection. Be sure they have the finances and other resources to obtain and give daily antibiotics. Because infections can be particularly virulent and can cause death in these children, parents should be instructed to obtain immediate care when the child is ill. Encourage the use of the pneumococcal vaccine for all infants and children with the disease. The Hib vaccine series should be started at 2 months of age and continued at recommended ages to prevent another common source of infection.

Delayed Growth and Development

Emphasize the importance of adequate nutrition and hydration to promote growth. Encourage the child to eat a high-protein, high-calorie diet. Emphasize the importance of folic acid and

---

CLIENT TEACHING The Child With Sickle Cell Disorder

- Provide parents with information about sickle cell disease and the child's treatment. Even parents of a child previously diagnosed with the disorder may benefit from information about the disease process and its management. Explain the basic effect of tissue hypoxia and the effects of sickling on circulation.
- Teach parents to look for signs of dehydration, such as dry mucous membranes, weight loss, and sunken fontanelles in infants. Give specific instructions about how many ounces of liquid the child needs to drink each day. Emphasize that increased fluid intake is needed to replace the fluids lost from overheating or exposure to hot weather.
- Make sure both the child and family understand the triggers and precipitating factors for sickle cell crises. Encourage them to avoid situations that cause crises. Instruct the child and parents about signs and symptoms of crises that should be reported to their health care provider.
- Provide the family with careful instructions about infusion therapy. When regular blood infusions are used, the resulting iron overload is damaging to body organs. Children treated with transfusions need infusion of deferoxamine (Desferal) for iron overload. The medication is usually given by subcutaneous or IV routes over 8–10 hours. Prompt recognition of side effects and careful management of the lengthy infusion process are important. The child needs to be monitored for skin reactions and allergic responses. Have parents demonstrate the infusion technique and state what to do in case of reactions. Pain management is needed during infusion as the site may be tender and uncomfortable.
- Instruct parents that it is important to inform all treating physicians and dentists of the child's medical condition. Special precautions are necessary when the child undergoes surgery of any kind, because hypoxia resulting from anesthesia is a major surgical risk. The child should also wear a medical identification tag or bracelet.
- Family members need ongoing support to deal with the stress of having a child with a chronic condition. Provide resources, respite care for parents, and information as needed for siblings.
- Encourage older children with sickle cell anemia to participate in activities with other children between crises but to avoid strenuous physical exertion and contact sports. Play and social interactions that promote learning and development are important.

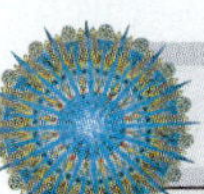

NURSING CARE PLAN **A Client With Sickle Cell Anemia**

Mark Gotham is 10 years old. He was diagnosed with sickle cell anemia shortly after birth. Both his mother and father carry the trait, but neither has the disease. Mark started fifth grade at a new school last week and was worried the kids would make fun of him because of the way he looks. Instead of going to lunch with the other kids, he stayed in the classroom so no one would see how he limps when he walks. He became dehydrated and started to feel severe pain in his right leg. His mother brought him to the emergency room.

ASSESSMENT	DIAGNOSES	PLANNING
Mark is crying in pain and holding his right upper thigh. His vital signs are as follows: 98.4°F (36.9°C), P 128, R 24, BP 138/84. Popliteal, dorsalis pedis, and posterior tibial pulses are palpable in both legs.	■ Ineffective Tissue Perfusion (all systems) related to affinity of hemoglobin for oxygen ■ Risk for Deficient Fluid Volume related to inadequate fluid intake and dehydration ■ Chronic Pain related to chronic physical disability and clustering of sickled cells ■ Risk for Infection related to chronic disease and splenic malfunction ■ Deficient Knowledge (child and parents) related to lack of exposure about cause and treatment of sickle cell anemia	■ The child will show few signs and symptoms of tissue hypoxia. ■ The child will maintain or be restored to adequate hydration. ■ The child will verbalize that pain is controlled. ■ The child will not develop infection. ■ The child and family will verbalize understanding of risk factors for sickle cell crises and how to minimize them.

IMPLEMENTATION

- Instruct the child to avoid physical exertion, emotional stress, low-oxygen environments (e.g., airplanes and high altitudes), and known sources of infection.
- Administer blood transfusions as ordered.
- Perform several caregiving activities together when possible.
- Give oxygen as ordered.
- Administer and teach the family to administer prophylactic transfusions for the child who has had a cerebrovascular accident.
- Calculate the child's daily fluid requirements. Monitor the child's usual fluid consumption and make necessary adjustments. Encourage the child to take fluids. Observe for signs of dehydration.
- Record intake and output.
- Instruct the family to report fever, vomiting, diarrhea, or other signs of fluid imbalance immediately.
- Administer analgesics, such as morphine or hydromorphone (Dilaudid), as ordered. Continuous IV infusion is used for the duration of a painful crisis.
- Position carefully.
- Ask family what pain relief measures are helpful, and integrate them into care for the child.
- Ensure adequate nutrition by providing a high-calorie, high-protein diet. Ensure that the child's immunizations are up-to-date. Report any signs of infection to the physician immediately.
- Isolate the child from possible sources of infection. Instruct parents about signs of infection, and encourage them to seek prompt health care.
- Review the basics of sickle cell disease. Teach the child and family about signs and symptoms of crises.
- Arrange for genetic counseling and testing for sickle cell trait for family members if desired.

EVALUATION

- The child has no shortness of breath and shows no signs of hypoxia.
- The child does not suffer a cerebrovascular accident.
- The child shows signs of adequate hydration.
- The child is pain free, or pain control is significantly improved.
- The child is free of infection.
- The child and parent can verbalize precipitating events of crises.

CRITICAL THINKING

1. What factors in Mark's history may have precipitated sickling?
2. When you admit Mark to the emergency room, what is your priority of care? Explain your answer.
3. What teaching will you provide to reduce the risk of future recurrence of sickling?

vitamin C supplements as prescribed. Perform regular growth measurements, and if slow growth is apparent, perform 24-hour diet recalls and other nutritional assessments.

The child with sickle cell anemia is adversely affected by dehydration. Calculate the child's fluid maintenance requirements (minimum daily fluid intake), and monitor the child's oral fluid intake. Administer IV fluids as ordered. Adjust oral intake as necessary to keep the child well hydrated. Teach clients and parents how to monitor intake and output, and provide client teaching regarding fluid management

PRACTICE ALERT

A priority of nursing care for the client with sickle cell is the prevention of complications of crises. Observe the child for signs of increasing anemia and shock (mental status change, pallor, vital sign changes). Maintain ongoing monitoring of the child's neurologic status for evidence of altered cerebral function. Assess for an enlarged spleen by gentle palpation. Administer blood transfusions and watch the child for any adverse reaction. Assess growth and developmental milestones.

Caregiver Role Strain

Sickle cell anemia is a chronic disease that is accompanied by life-threatening episodic crises. Family members often need support to help them deal with their feelings about the diagnosis and its implications. Explore resources in the home and community to see if parents will be able to administer medications and fluids and to provide adequate nutrition. Assess their knowledge of signs of infection and of sickle cell crisis and when to seek medical care for the child. Refer the parents for genetic counseling, particularly if they plan to have more children. Encourage adolescents and young adults in the family to receive genetic counseling and testing as well. Referrals to support groups and contact with others with the disease can be helpful.

Collaborate with family members, and provide them with ongoing support to deal with the stress of having a child with a chronic condition. Provide resources, including information about respite care for parents and information as needed for siblings. Sickle cell disease and some other hematologic disorders of childhood require that parents provide ongoing monitoring and care for their children with these chronic conditions. Refer parents to support groups such as the National Association of Sickle Cell Disease for further information.

Evaluation

Expected outcomes of nursing care for the child with sickle cell anemia include the following:

- The child expresses that pain is successfully managed to a state of comfort.
- The child demonstrates adequate hydration to prevent cell sickling.
- The child displays no side effects of disease in the respiratory system, central nervous system, and body organs.
- The child has normal immune status and freedom from infection.
- Family and health care personnel promptly recognize and treat complications of the disease.
- The child meets normal growth and developmental milestones.
- Parents and other family members are referred for and receive information to manage and understand the disease.
- The family demonstrates adequate knowledge of the disease and treatment regimens.

REVIEW Sickle Cell Disorder

RELATE: LINK THE CONCEPTS

Linking the exemplar of Sickle Cell Disorder with the concept of Oxygenation:

1. You admit a child in sickle cell crisis. How will you assess oxygenation?
2. How will you promote oxygenation for the client in sickle cell crisis?

Linking the exemplar of Sickle Cell Disorder with the concept of Infection:

3. What teaching priorities will you provide the parents of a young child who has sickle cell disease to reduce the risk of infection?
4. What interventions will you implement during hospitalization for the 9-year-old admitted in sickle cell crisis to reduce the risk of infection?

READY: GO TO COMPANION SKILLS MANUAL

- Assessing the client in pain
- Assessing vital signs
- Managing pain with a PCA pump
- Administering blood transfusions
- Administering oxygen by cannula, face mask, or face tent

REFER: GO TO MYNURSINGKIT

REFLECT: CASE STUDY

Wendell Kozier is a 7-year-old boy with sickle cell anemia. Wendell has been held back in school as the result of his many absences secondary to sickle cell crisis and is now in kindergarten. Wendell is very bright, articulate, and inquisitive. He tells the nurse he wants to play hockey when he grows up. Wendell's dad is African American and his mom is Caucasian and African American. Wendell is in the doctor's office today for a check-up and immunizations. He was discharged from the hospital following sickle cell crisis one month ago.

1. What nursing diagnoses are appropriate for Wendell?
2. How will you respond to Wendell's desire to play hockey? What will you teach his parents about sports and sickle cell crisis?
3. What teaching will you provide to Wendell and his family to help reduce the frequency of sickle cell crisis?

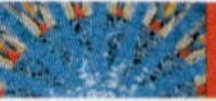

3.9 SKIN CANCER

KEY TERMS

Actinic keratosis, *186*
Basal cell cancer, *185*
Keratotic basal cell carcinoma, *186*
Melanomas, *184*
Microstaging, *188*
Morpheaform basal cell carcinoma, *186*
Nevi, *184*
Nodular basal cell carcinoma, *186*
Pigmented basal cell carcinoma, *186*
Squamous cell cancer, *186*
Superficial basal cell carcinoma, *186*

BASIS FOR SELECTION OF EXEMPLAR

Centers for Disease Control and Prevention
Healthy People 2010
Institute of Medicine

LEARNING OUTCOMES

After reading about this exemplar, you will be able to:

1. Describe the pathophysiology, etiology, clinical manifestations, and direct and indirect causes of skin cancer.
2. Identify risk factors associated with skin cancer.
3. Illustrate the nursing process in providing culturally competent care across the life span for individuals with skin cancer.
4. Formulate priority nursing diagnoses appropriate for an individual with skin cancer.
5. Create a plan of care for individuals with skin cancer and their family members.
6. Assess expected outcomes for an individual with skin cancer.
7. Discuss therapies used in the collaborative care of an individual with skin cancer.
8. Employ evidence-based caring interventions for an individual with skin cancer.

OVERVIEW

The skin, despite its ability to protect the internal body from external damage, is a fragile organ and is subject to damage from ultraviolet (UV) radiation and chemicals. Over time, this damage results in alterations in cellular structure and function, and malignancies of the skin occur.

The skin is a common site for malignant lesions. Many of these lesions are found on skin surfaces that have undergone long-term exposure to the sun or the environment. Malignant skin tumors (**melanomas**) are the most common of all cancers. The nonmelanoma skin cancers are basal cell cancer and squamous cell cancer.

PATHOPHYSIOLOGY AND ETIOLOGY

Skin cancer can be classified as melanoma or nonmelanoma in type. Each classification will be considered independently.

Melanoma

Malignant melanomas arise from melanocytes, cells located at or near the basal layer (the deepest epidermal layer). These cells produce melanin, the dark skin pigment. Melanin is made in granules and transferred to keratinocytes (primary cell of the epidermis), where it accumulates on the superficial side of each keratinocyte and forms a shield of pigment over the nucleus as protection against UV rays. Malignant melanomas can develop wherever there is pigment, but about one-third of them originate in existing **nevi** (moles).

Almost all malignant melanomas are more than 6 mm in diameter, are asymmetric, and initially develop within the epidermis over a long period. While they are still confined to the epidermis, the lesions (called malignant melanoma in situ) are flat and relatively benign. However, when they penetrate the dermis, they mingle with blood and lymph vessels and are capable of metastasizing. At this latter stage, the tumors develop a raised or nodular appearance and often have smaller nodules, called satellite lesions, around the periphery.

The prognosis for survival among people diagnosed with malignant melanoma is determined by several variables, including tumor thickness, ulceration, metastasis, site, age, and gender. Younger clients and women have a somewhat better chance of survival. Tumors on the hands, feet, and scalp have a poorer prognosis; tumors of the feet and scalp are less visible and may not be diagnosed until they grow into the dermis.

PRECURSOR LESIONS The three specific precursor lesions for the development of malignant melanoma are congenital nevi, dysplastic nevi, and lentigo maligna. A precursor lesion is also called a premalignant lesion, a name that indicates that the lesion's risk of becoming malignant is greater than normal.

Congenital Nevi Congenital nevi are present at birth. Some lesions are small; others are large enough to cover an entire body area. Their color can range from brown to black. They are often slightly raised, with an irregular surface and a fairly regular border.

Dysplastic Nevi Dysplastic nevi are also called atypical moles. Although dysplastic nevi are not present at birth, they appear as normal nevi during childhood and become dysplastic (having abnormal development) after puberty. A client with classic dysplastic nevi has more than 100 nevi, at least one of which is larger than 8 mm in diameter and at least one of which has the characteristics of malignant melanoma (asymmetry, irregular border, color variegation, and a diameter of > 6 mm). A familial tendency to dysplastic nevi increases the risk for development of malignant melanoma. However, it is not known whether people with dysplastic nevi and no family history of melanoma face a higher risk for melanoma.

Dysplastic nevi most often appear on the face, trunk, and arms but also are seen on the scalp, female breast, groin, and buttocks. The pigmentation of the nevi is irregular, with mixtures of tan, brown, black, red, and pink. An area of lighter pigmentation is surrounded by a papular area of deeper pigmentation (described as a "fried egg appearance"). The borders of the nevi are irregular.

Lentigo Maligna Lentigo maligna, also called Hutchinson's freckle, is a tan or black patch on the skin that looks like a freckle. It grows slowly, becoming mottled, dark, thick, and nodular. It is usually seen on one side of the face of an older adult who has had a large amount of sun exposure.

CLASSIFICATIONS OF MALIGNANT MELANOMAS Malignant melanomas are classified into different types. The major types are superficial spreading melanoma, lentigo maligna melanoma, nodular melanoma, and acral lentiginous melanoma.

Each of these tumors is characterized by a radial and/or vertical growth phase. During the initial radial phase, which may last from 1–25 years (depending on the type), the melanoma grows parallel to the skin surface. During this phase, the tumor rarely metastasizes and is often curable by surgical excision. However, during the vertical growth phase, atypical melanocytes rapidly penetrate into the dermis and subcutaneous tissue, greatly increasing the risk for metastasis and death.

Superficial Spreading Melanoma Superficial spreading melanoma is the most common type, comprising approximately 70% of all melanomas (Porth, 2005). The lesions are usually flat and scaly or crusty and are approximately 2 cm in diameter. They often arise from a preexisting nevus. This type of melanoma is found on the trunk and back of men and on the legs of women. Superficial spreading melanomas occur more often in women than in men. The median age of occurrence is the 50s.

The radial growth phase lasts from 1–5 or more years. When the lesion enters the vertical growth phase, it grows rapidly, and its color changes from a mixture of tan, brown, and black to a characteristic red, white, and blue. The lesion also develops irregular borders and often has raised nodules and ulcerations (Figure 3–21 ■).

Lentigo Maligna Melanoma Lentigo maligna melanoma often arises from the precursor lesion, lentigo maligna. The lesions are large and tan, with different shades of brown. This type of melanoma makes up 4–10% of malignant melanomas and is the least serious form (Porth, 2005). It occurs on skin that has had long-term sun exposure, such as the face, neck, and sometimes, the dorsal surface of the hands and lower extremities. Lentigo maligna melanoma affects women more than men. It is typically diagnosed in people in their 60s and 70s.

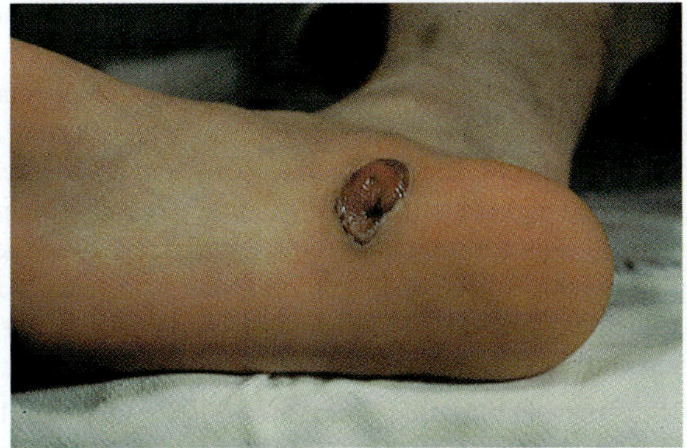

Figure 3–21 ■ Malignant melanoma is a serious skin cancer that arises from melanocytes.

Source: L. Solomon/Custom Medical Stock Photography.

Lentigo maligna melanoma is characterized by a proliferation of atypical melanocytes parallel to the basal layer of the epidermis. The radial growth phase may last from 10 to 25 years, with the lesion growing to as large as 10 cm. The lesion becomes malignant as soon as the melanocytes invade the dermis. In the vertical growth phase, raised nodules may appear on the surface of the lesion. The lesion tends to acquire a freckled or mottled appearance.

Nodular Melanoma Nodular melanoma lesions are raised, dome-shaped, blue-black or red nodules on areas of the head, neck, and trunk that may or may not have been exposed to the sun. The lesions may look like a blood blister, or they may ulcerate and bleed. The lesions arise from unaffected skin rather than from a preexisting lesion. This type makes up 15–30% of malignant melanomas and is often diagnosed in people in their 50s (Porth, 2005).

Nodular melanoma has only a vertical growth phase, but it grows aggressively during that phase. However, the absence of a radial growth phase makes this type of melanoma more difficult to diagnose before it metastasizes.

Acral Lentiginous Melanoma Acral lentiginous melanoma, also called mucocutaneous melanoma, is less common in people with fair skin and more common in people with dark skin. The lesions progress from tan, brown, or black flat lesions to elevated nodules and are approximately 3 cm in diameter. The radial phase lasts from 2 to 5 years. The nodules are found on the palms of the hands, the soles of the feet, the mucous membranes, and the nail beds. Acral lentiginous melanoma affects men and women equally and is most often diagnosed in people in their 50s and 60s.

Nonmelanoma Skin Cancer

Basal cell cancer and squamous cell cancer arise from epithelial tissue but have different pathophysiologies, classifications, and manifestations.

BASAL CELL CANCER **Basal cell cancer** is an epithelial tumor believed to originate either from the basal layer of the epidermis or from cells in the surrounding dermal structures. These tumors are characterized by an impaired ability of the basal cells of the epidermis to mature into keratinocytes, with mitotic division beyond the basal layer. This results in a bulky neoplasm that grows by direct extension and destroys surrounding tissue, including healthy skin, nerves, blood vessels, lymphatic tissue, cartilage, and bone. Basal cell cancer is the most common but least aggressive type of skin cancer, rarely metastasizing.

Basal cell cancers tend to recur. Tumors greater than 2 cm in diameter have a high recurrence rate. Predisposing factors for metastasis are the size of the tumor and the client's resistance to treatment with surgery or chemotherapy. Although they rarely metastasize, untreated basal cell cancers invade surrounding tissue and may destroy body parts, such as the nose or eyelid.

Basal cell cancer is classified into different types: nodular, superficial, pigmented, morpheaform, and keratotic. These types are described below and are summarized in Table 3–24.

Nodular basal cell cancer, the most common type of basal cell cancer, most often appears on the face, neck, and head. The tumor is made up of masses of cells that resemble epidermal basal cells and grow in a bulky, nodular form from lack of keratinization. In early stages, the tumor is a papule that looks like a smooth pimple. It is often pruritic and continues to grow at a steady rate, doubling in size every 6–12 months. As the tumor grows, the epidermis thins but remains intact. The skin over the tumor is shiny, and either pearly white, pink, or flesh colored. Telangiectasis (red, purple, or blue discoloration under the skin caused by abnormal dilation of a vessel) may be visible over the area of the tumor. As the tumor continues to increase in size, the center or periphery may ulcerate, and the tumor develops well-circumscribed borders. It bleeds easily from mild injury.

Superficial basal cell cancer, found most often on the trunk and extremities, is the second most common type of basal cell cancer. This tumor is a proliferating tissue that attaches to the undersurface of the epithelium. The tumor is a flat papule or plaque, often erythematous, with well-defined borders. The tumor may ulcerate and be covered with crusts or shallow erosions (Figure 3–22 ■).

Pigmented basal cell cancer, found on the head, neck, and face, is less common. This tumor concentrates melanin pigment in the center of the basal cancer cells, giving it a dark brown, blue, or black appearance. The border of the tumor is shiny and well defined.

Morpheaform basal cell cancer, the rarest form of basal cell cancer, usually develops on the head and neck. The tumor forms finger-like projections that extend in any direction along dermal tissue planes. The tumor resembles a flat ivory or flesh-colored scar. This form is more likely to extend into and destroy adjacent tissue, especially muscle, nerve, and bone. It is often more difficult to diagnose because of its appearance.

TABLE 3–24 Types and Characteristics of Basal Cell Cancers

TYPE	COMMON LOCATION	MANIFESTATION
Nodular	Face, neck, head	Small, firm papule; pearly, white, pink, or flesh colored; telangiectasis; enlarges; may ulcerate
Superficial	Trunk, extremities	Papules or plaque that is flat, erythematous, or scaling; pink color; well-defined borders; may have shallow erosions and surface crusting
Pigmented	Head, neck, face	Dark brown, blue, or black color; border is shiny and well defined
Morpheaform	Head, neck	Looks like a flat scar; ivory or flesh colored
Keratotic	Ear	Small, firm papule; pearly, white, pink, or flesh colored; may ulcerate.

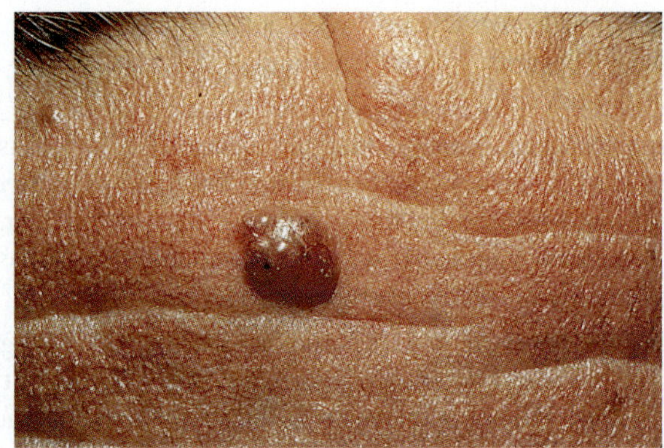

Figure 3–22 ■ A superficial basal cell cancer is characterized by erythema, ulcerations, and well-defined borders.

Source: From American Academy of Dermotolgy. Reprinted with permission. All rights reserved.

Keratotic basal cell cancer (basosquamous) is found on the preauricular and postauricular groove. It contains both basal cells and squamoid-appearing cells that keratinize. Its appearance is much like that of nodular basal cell cancer. This type of basal cell cancer tends to recur locally and also is the type most likely to metastasize.

SQUAMOUS CELL CANCER **Squamous cell cancer** is a malignant tumor of the squamous epithelium of the skin or mucous membranes. It occurs most often on areas of skin exposed to UV rays and weather, such as the forehead, helix of the ear, top of the nose, lower lip, and back of the hands. Squamous cell cancer may also arise on skin that has been burned or has chronic inflammation. This is a much more aggressive cancer than basal cell cancer, with a faster growth rate and a much greater potential for metastasis if untreated.

The tumors arise when the keratinizing cells of the squamous epithelium proliferate, producing a growth that eventually fills the epidermis and invades the dermal tissue planes. Keratinization of some cells is present, and the formation of keratin "pearls" is common. The keratin formation diminishes as the tumor grows. As the tumor grows, the tumor cells increase in number and rate of mitosis, forming odd shapes.

Squamous cell cancer begins as a small, firm, red nodule. The tumor may be crusted with keratin products. As it grows, it may ulcerate, bleed, and become painful. As the tumor extends into the surrounding tissue and becomes a nodule, the area around the nodule becomes indurated (hardened) (Figure 3–23 ■).

Recurrent squamous cell cancer can be invasive, increasing the risk of metastasis. Invasive squamous cell cancer may arise from preexisting skin lesions, such as scars and actinic keratosis, and extend into the dermis (called intraepidermal squamous cell cancer). This form appears as a slightly raised erythematous plaque with well-defined borders. Metastasis occurs most often via the lymphatics. The degree of risk for metastasis depends on the size and depth of penetration of the tumor.

Actinic Keratosis **Actinic keratosis**, also called senile or solar keratosis, is an epidermal skin lesion directly related to chronic sun exposure and photodamage. Actinic keratosis may progress to squamous cell carcinoma. Less than 1% of early

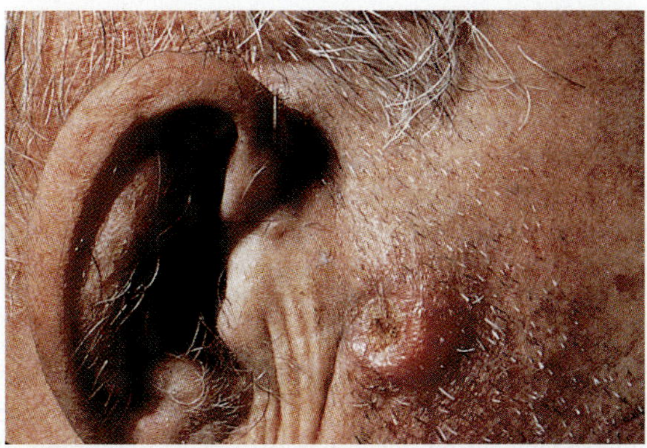

Figure 3–23 ■ As a squamous cell cancer grows, it tends to invade surrounding tissue. It also ulcerates, may bleed, and is painful.

Source: From American Academy of Dermotolgy. Reprinted with permission. All rights reserved.

lesions become malignant, but many of those that persist progress to malignancy (Porth, 2005). Because of this tendency, the lesions are classified as premalignant.

Actinic keratosis lesions are erythematous, rough macules a few millimeters in diameter. They are often shiny but may be scaly; if the scales are removed, the underlying skin bleeds. They occur in multiple patches, primarily on the face, dorsa of the hands, the forearms, and sometimes, on the upper trunk (Figure 3–24 ■). Enlargement or ulceration of the lesions suggests transformation to malignancy.

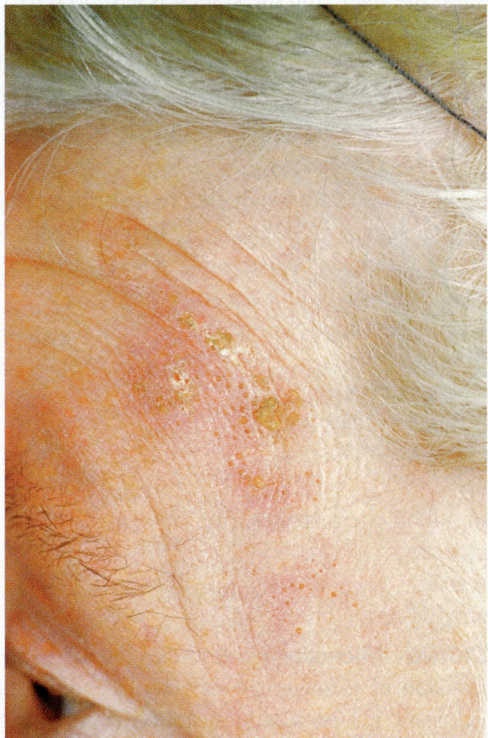

Figure 3–24 ■ The effects of long-term sun exposure are illustrated in this epidermal skin lesion, call actinic keratosis.

Source: Medical-On-Line, Ltd.

Etiology

One of the leading causes of skin cancer is exposure to the sun. Research has indicated that tanning beds are among the most dangerous form of UV exposure, and it has been suggested they should be banned because of the high risk of skin cancer that results from their use (Roberts, Hornung, & Polk, 2009). Other factors contributing to etiology includes age, skin type, skin color, and genetic predisposition.

Risk Factors

Risk factors vary according to type of lesion. Melanoma, nonmelanoma, and actinic keratosis each have specific considerations related to risk.

MELANOMA SKIN CANCER Although the exact cause of melanoma is unknown, certain risk factors are associated with the disease. The risk factors for melanoma are listed in Box 3–17.

Behaviors and skin characteristics that increase the risk for pediatric melanoma include light-colored eyes, freckling, fair skin, blond or red hair, family history of melanoma, blistering sunburns before 12 years of age, frequent sun exposure without the use of sunscreen, melanocytic nevi, and immunosuppression (Strouse, Fears, Tucker, & Wayne, 2005).

NONMELANOMA SKIN CANCER Multiple etiologic factors are involved in the development of nonmelanoma skin cancer, including environmental factors and host factors. Unknown factors may also play a role.

Environmental Factors The environmental factors implicated in the nonmelanoma skin cancers are UV radiation, pollutants, chemicals, ionizing radiation, viruses, and physical trauma.

Ultraviolet radiation from the sun is believed to be the cause of most nonmelanoma skin cancers. Sunlight contains both short-length rays (UVB) and long-length rays (UVA). UVB rays are absorbed by the top layer of skin and cause sunburn. UVA rays penetrate deeper into the skin layers, causing tissue damage. Both types of rays are believed to cause DNA alterations and also suppress T-cell and B-cell immunity. The amount of UV radiation reaching the earth is increasing, most likely from depletion of the ozone layer surrounding the

Box 3–17 **Risk Factors for Melanoma Skin Cancer**

- A high number of moles, or large moles
- Fair skin, freckling, blond hair, or blue eyes
- Close relative with the disease
- Men with gene changes from a family history of breast or ovarian cancer
- Treatment with medications that suppress the immune system
- Too much exposure to UV radiation from sunlight, tanning lamps, or tanning booths
- Age older than 50 years
- Xeroderma pigmentosus, a rare, inherited disease in which people are less able to repair damage caused by sunlight
- Past history of melanoma

planet. The U.S. Environmental Protection Agency predicts that for every 1% decrease in the ozone layer, a corresponding 1–3% increase in cases of nonmelanoma skin cancer per year will occur.

Geographic, environmental, and lifestyle factors affect the amount of exposure to the sun and the risk for nonmelanoma skin cancer. People who live in latitudes close to the equator and those who live at higher altitudes receive greater UV radiation exposure. The amount of clothing worn, the time of day, and the amount of time in the sun also determine the amount of exposure. Exposure to UV radiation in tanning booths has also been implicated in the development of nonmelanoma skin cancer.

Certain chemicals have long been associated with nonmelanoma skin cancer. Polycyclic aromatic hydrocarbons, found in mixtures of coal, tar, asphalt, soot, and mineral oils, have been linked with skin cancers. Psoralens, used in conjunction with UVA for treatment of psoriasis and cutaneous T-cell lymphoma, increase the risk of squamous cell cancer.

Other factors associated with nonmelanoma skin cancer are the use of ionizing radiation, viruses, and physical trauma. X-ray therapy for tinea capitis and the use of radium to treat other malignancies are risk factors. Human papillomavirus is implicated in the development of squamous cell cancer, as is damage to the skin from burns.

Host Factors Certain host factors increase the risk for nonmelanoma skin cancer. These include skin pigmentation as well as the presence of premalignant lesions.

Skin pigmentation is an important factor in the development of nonmelanoma skin cancer. The amount of melanin pigment produced by the melanocytes determines a person's skin color. The more melanin, the more the skin is protected from the damage produced by UV rays. Thus, African Americans, Asian Americans, and people of Mediterranean descent have a much lower incidence of nonmelanoma skin cancer than do people who have fair complexions and tend to freckle or sunburn easily, such as people of Irish, Scandinavian, or English ancestry.

Although most people have numerous pigmented lesions on their body, almost all of these are normal. However, a major risk factor in the development of nonmelanoma skin cancer is a change in an existing lesion or the presence of a premalignant lesion, such as actinic keratosis. Organ transplant recipients who undergo immunosuppression to prevent rejection are also at risk for the development of squamous cell cancer.

ACTINIC KERATOSIS The prevalence of actinic keratosis is highest in people with light-colored skin. These lesions are rare in people with dark skin.

CLINICAL MANIFESTATIONS

The clinical manifestations of each type of skin cancer differ. It is often possible to determine the likelihood of a specific classification based on appearance, although further testing is generally done to confirm the diagnosis. Table 3–25 summarizes the clinical manifestations of skin cancers.

COLLABORATION

Care of the client with skin cancer requires a collaborative team of health care providers in order to promote early detection and prompt intervention and to improve client outcomes. Numerous treatment options may be offered, and the nurse's role is to help the client make an informed decision about the treatment option that is best for his or her needs and circumstances.

Nonmelanoma

Treatment of nonmelanoma skin cancer focuses on removal of all malignant tissue using such methods as surgery, curettage and electrodesiccation, cryotherapy, or radiotherapy. These modalities offer a greater than 90% cure rate. After the malignant tissue is removed, the client should have regular examinations for recurrence.

Melanoma

The management of the client with malignant melanoma begins with identification, diagnosis, and tumor staging. If treatable, the tumor is removed through surgical excision. Malignant melanoma is also treated with chemotherapy, immunotherapy, and radiation therapy. Other therapies used with success include biologic therapies with interleukin-2 and interferon and therapeutic vaccines containing melanoma antigens.

IDENTIFICATION Malignant melanoma is most often found on the trunk of men and on the lower extremities of women. Nevertheless, it is important for the client to have a complete physical examination and total skin assessment. In addition to a visual examination of all skin surfaces, palpation of regional lymph nodes, the liver, and the spleen is essential to assess for metastasis when a melanoma is suspected or found.

A change in the color or size of a nevus is reported in 70% of people diagnosed with a malignant melanoma. The ABCD rule is used to assess suspicious lesions (Box 3–18).

DIAGNOSTIC TESTS In addition to biopsy of any suspicious lesion, diagnostic tests are conducted to determine whether the tumor has metastasized. Because malignant melanoma may metastasize to any organ or tissue of the body, a variety of tests may be conducted, including the following:

- Microscopic examination
- Biopsy
- Tests for metastasis
  - a. Liver function tests
  - b. CT of the liver
  - c. CBC
  - d. Serum blood chemistry profile
  - e. Chest x-ray
  - f. Bone scan
  - g. CT or MRI of the brain.

MICROSTAGING **Microstaging** describes the assessment of the level of invasion of a malignant melanoma and the maximum tumor thickness. In the Clark system of microstaging, the vertical growth of the lesion is measured from the epidermis to the subcutaneous tissue to determine the level of invasion (Figure 3–25 ■). However, variations in individual skin thicknesses and different anatomic sites can affect the accuracy of

TABLE 3–25 Clinical Manifestations of Skin Cancers

SKIN CANCER	CLINICAL MANIFESTATIONS
Melanoma	
Congenital nevi, precursor to melanoma	■ Range in color from brown to black ■ Often slightly raised, with an irregular surface and fairly regular border ■ Can range in size from small to covering entire body
Dysplastic nevi, precursor to melanoma	■ Have irregular pigmentation with mixtures of tan, brown, black, red, and pink ■ May have an area of lighter pigmentation surrounded by a popular area of deeper pigmentation ■ Irregular borders ■ Often appear on the face, trunk, and arms but can be seen on the scalp, female breast, groin, buttocks
Lentigo maligna, precursor to melanoma	■ Tan or black patch on the skin that looks like a freckle ■ Grows slowly, becoming mottled, dark, thick, and nodular ■ Usually seen on one side of the face in an older adult who has had a large amount of sun exposure
Malignant melanoma	■ Asymmetrical, with an irregular border ■ Color variegation ■ Diameter $>$ 6 mm (the size of a pencil eraser)
Nonmelanomas	
Basal cell	
Nodular basal cell carcinoma	■ Papule that looks like a smooth pimple that grows at a steady rate ■ Skin over the tumor that is shiny and may be pearly white, pink, or flesh-colored ■ Chance of visible telangiectasis ■ Tumor that may ulcerate at the center or periphery and bleed easily from mild injury
Superficial basal cell carcinoma	■ Appears as a flat papule or plaque, often erythematous, with well-defined borders ■ Tumor that may ulcerate and be covered with crusts or shallow erosions ■ Most common on the trunk and extremities
Pigmented basal cell carcinoma	■ Dark brown, blue, or black, with a shiny surface and well-defined borders ■ Typically found on the head, face, and neck
Morpheaform basal cell carcinoma	■ Resembles a flat ivory or flesh-colored scar that forms finger-like projections that extend along dermal tissue planes ■ Usually develops on the head and neck
Keratotic basal cell carcinoma	■ Appears similar to nodular basal cell carcinoma
Squamous cell cancer	■ Begins as a small, firm, red nodule that may be crusted with keratin products ■ Tumors that ulcerate, bleed, and become painful as they grow ■ Causes the area around the nodule to harden as the tumor extends into the surrounding tissue and becomes a nodule ■ Most common on areas of skin exposed to ultraviolet rays and weather, such as the forehead, helix of the ear, top of the nose, lower lip, and back of the hands
Other types of lesions	
Actinic keratosis	■ Erythematous, rough macules a few millimeters in diameter ■ Often shiny but may be scaly; if the scales are removed, the underlying skin bleeds ■ Occur in multiple patches, primarily on the face, dorsa of the hands, the forearms, and sometimes, on the upper trunk ■ Enlargement or ulceration of the lesions that suggests transformation to malignancy

Box 3–18 The ABCD Rule

Using the ABCD rule to assess for melanoma:
A = asymmetry (one half of the nevus does not match the other half)
B = border irregularity (edges are ragged, blurred, or notched)
C = color variation or dark black color
D = diameter greater than 6 mm (size of a pencil eraser)

the measurement. In the Breslow system, an adaptation of the Clark system of assessment, the vertical thickness is measured from the granular level of the epidermis to the deepest level of tumor invasion. This determination is important, because as the thickness of the melanoma increases, survival rate decreases.

After the thickness and depth of the tumor are determined, a clinical stage is assigned. The traditional three-stage system is still used, although it does not include tumor thickness. The

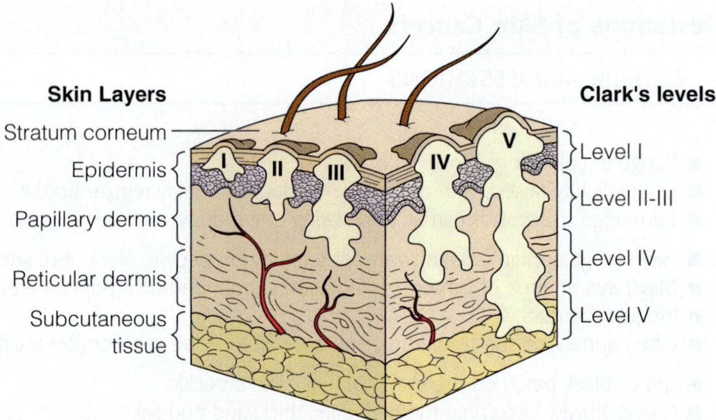

Figure 3–25 ■ Clarks' levels for staging measure the invasion of a melanoma from the epidermis to the subcutaneous tissue.

American Joint Committee on Cancer has adopted a four-stage system that includes tumor thickness, level of invasion, lymph node involvement, and evidence of metastasis.

TREATMENTS Surgical excision is the preferred treatment for malignant melanoma. Other methods of treatment are chemotherapy, immunotherapy, and radiation therapy.

Surgery If a biopsy identifies the lesion as a melanoma, a wide excision is performed that includes the full thickness of the skin and subcutaneous tissue. Because the risk of local recurrence for thin melanomas (those < 0.76 mm) is quite low, margins of 0.5–1.0 cm of normal skin are excised around the tumor. Thick tumors require a 1- to 3-cm margin excision because they are at risk for local recurrence or satellite lesions.

Regional lymph nodes are the most common sites for metastasis of malignant melanoma. Standard surgical treatment for clinically suspicious lymph node involvement includes excision of the primary lesions as well as surgical dissection of the involved lymph nodes. Elective lymph node dissection (ELND) in the treatment of localized malignant melanoma remains controversial. Advocates of ELND believe that the procedure benefits clients with intermediate-thickness tumors, because approximately 20% of people whose lymph nodes were clinically negative at diagnosis show some metastasis on removal of the nodes. Those opposed to ELND believe the risks associated with the procedure are too high for the 80% of people who have no evidence of metastasis after removal of the nodes.

Surgery also is indicated for palliative management of isolated metastasis. Removal of metastatic tumors in the brain, liver, lung, gastrointestinal tract, or subcutaneous tissue may relieve symptoms and prolong life.

Immunotherapy Immunotherapy is a relatively new treatment modality for malignant melanoma. The role of the immunologic response initially was recognized because of the numerous spontaneous remissions seen in clients with melanoma—a higher occurrence than with any other adult tumor. In addition, researchers have recently identified tumor-specific antigen-antibodies in clients with melanoma. This also has stimulated an interest in immunotherapeutic interventions for the treatment of malignant melanoma.

Agents such as interferons, interleukins, monoclonal antibodies, bacille Calmette-Guérin, levamisole, transfer factors, and tumor vaccines have been used to treat melanoma, with varying response rates. The effectiveness of these agents, used either alone, in combination with chemotherapy, or in combination with each other, is under investigation.

Radiation Therapy Melanoma responds to higher-dose radiation, especially if the tumor is small. Response rates to radiation therapy depend on the site of the tumor, the thickness of the tumor, the type of melanoma, and the client's general health but may range from 0 to 71%. Radiation frequently is used for palliation of symptoms resulting from metastasis to the brain, bone, lymph nodes, gastrointestinal tract, skin, or subcutaneous tissue. Liver and lung metastases are not treated with radiation therapy, because a loss of organ function may result.

Emerging Treatments Melanoma skin cancer research is ongoing and directed toward more specific methods of diagnosis and treatment. Examples of emerging treatments include the following:

- *Gene therapy:* Clinical trials are in progress to test the effectiveness of adding certain genes to the malignant cells.
- *Melanoma DNA research:* Knowledge of how UV light harms DNA is increasing, providing support for referral to genetic counseling for people with a strong family history of melanoma.
- *Immune therapy:* Vaccines are being developed to make an individual immune to his or her melanoma cells, or to train the person's immune cells to fight the cancer.
- *Staging:* Very sensitive new tests can better detect the spread of melanoma to lymph nodes and can possibly better identify people who could be helped by a treatment such as immunotherapy after surgery.

NURSING PROCESS

Nursing care of clients diagnosed with any form of skin cancer requires careful assessment and documentation of lesions, monitoring for any change in appearance, and support of the client's physical and emotional needs. Fear of death, altered body image, and painful treatments often result from the diagnosis, and the nurse needs to provide holistic care that addresses both the physical and emotional needs of the client.

Assessment

Clients with skin cancer should undergo a skin assessment. Specific health history questions and assessments for skin cancer are outlined in Box 3–19.

Diagnosis

Although many different nursing diagnoses may be appropriate for the client with a malignant melanoma, common responses are the following:

- Impaired Skin Integrity
- Hopelessness
- Anxiety.

Plan

Planning care for the client diagnosed with skin cancer is highly individualized, depending on where the cells are located, the presence of metastasis, and the age of the client. Suggested goals for care may include the following:

- The client reports need to examine all skin lesions for changes or unusual appearance.
- The client avoids sun exposure and does not use tanning beds.
- The client expresses feelings related to diagnosis of skin cancer.
- The client describes different treatment options available and the pros and cons of each in order to make an informed decision about treatment.

Implementation

In addition to providing client care, nurses play an important role in promoting awareness of skin cancer prevention. Teaching the need for sun protection and avoidance of tanning beds is an important role for the nurse advocate.

Impaired Skin Integrity

Malignant melanomas not only destroy skin layers but also invade body structures. Certain types of melanomas may ulcerate before diagnosis, and treatment typically involves some type of surgical biopsy and excision. Any open lesion or incision increases the risk for secondary infection.

- Monitor for manifestations of infection, such as fever, tachycardia, malaise, incisional erythema, swelling, pain, or drainage that increases or becomes purulent. Intact skin is the first line of defense against infection; impaired skin integrity increases the risk for infection. If infection is present, the client may have both systemic and local manifestations.
- Keep the incision line clean and dry by changing dressings as necessary. Moisture increases the risk of infection.
- Follow principles of medical and surgical asepsis when caring for the client's incision. Teach family members and visitors the importance of careful handwashing. Maintain standard precautions if drainage is present. Careful handwashing is essential in preventing the spread of infection.

Box 3–19 **Nursing Assessment for Skin Cancer**

INTERVIEW QUESTIONS

- Have any members of your family ever been treated for skin cancer?
- Have you had a skin cancer removed from any part of your body?
- Have you noticed any change in the size, shape, or color of a mole, wart, birthmark, or scar?
- Do you have any moles, warts, birthmarks, or scars that itch, are painful, have crusting, or bleed?
- In what parts of the country or world have you lived?
- Have you ever been badly sunburned?
- Do you visit tanning salons?
- Are you exposed to any hazardous chemicals in your job?
- Have you been taught how to examine your skin? If so, how do you do this examination? How often?

PHYSICAL ASSESSMENT

1. Ask the client to remove all clothing and put on an examination gown. Ensure good light; natural, bright light is best for inspection of lesions. The client may sit, stand, or lie down.
2. Inspect and palpate the skin. Stretching the skin tightly during assessment facilitates assessment of nodular and scaly lesions and lesions in the dermis. Assess for the following:
   a. Obvious lesions
   b. Visible swellings
   c. Alterations in normal contour and borders of nevi
   d. Enlarged lymph glands
   e. Skin or mucosal discolorations
   f. Areas of ulceration, scaling, crusting, or erosion.
3. The order of assessment is as follows:
   a. Head and neck: entire scalp, eyelids, external ear, auditory canals, external surface of the nose, internal surface of the nose, the oral cavity, facial skin, the facial glands (parotid, submaxillary, sublingual)
   b. Thyroid and neck, including lymph glands
   c. Chest and abdomen, with special attention under pendulous breasts, in skin folds, and in areas covered with hair
   d. Back and buttocks, with special attention to the area between the buttocks
   e. Extremities, with special attention to the axillae, nail beds, webs between the fingers and toes, and soles of the feet
   f. External genitals, with special attention to skin folds, mucous membranes, and areas covered with hair.
4. Measure and record a description of all skin lesions on an anatomic chart. Take photographs (if possible) of any suspicious lesion, and include them in the client's record for future reference.

Aseptic techniques are necessary when caring for any surgical incision to prevent infection.

- Encourage and maintain adequate caloric and protein intake in the diet. Suggest a consultation with the dietitian if the client does not want to eat. Adequate kilocalories and protein are necessary for proper healing. The client with cancer has increased metabolic needs; if these needs are not met, nutritional problems that impair healing may result.

Hopelessness

Hopelessness is an emotional state in which a person feels there is no possibility that life will improve. Clients who experience hopelessness are often withdrawn, passive, and apathetic.

The diagnosis of malignant melanoma threatens the quality and quantity of life as the client faces the possibility or reality of metastasis; the possibility that the cancer may recur and cause death; and alterations in self-concept, roles, and relationships. Inspiring hope in clients during this health crisis is a legitimate nursing action.

- Provide an environment that encourages the client to identify and express feelings, concerns, and goals:
  a. Use active listening, ask open-ended questions, and reflect on the client's statements.
  b. Acknowledge and respect feelings of apathy and/or anger as expressions of distress.
  c. Convey an empathetic understanding of fears and concerns.
  d. Provide opportunities to express positive emotions, such as hope, faith, a sense of purpose, and the will to live.
  e. Explore the client's perceptions, and modify or clarify them if necessary by providing information and correcting misconceptions.
  f. Encourage the client to identify support systems and sources of strength and coping in the past.

Verbalizing feelings, concerns, and goals allows others to validate or correct them, promotes a therapeutic nurse–client relationship, and fosters feelings of self-worth. Expressing positive emotions and calling on support systems and sources of strength that were effective in coping with past crises help the person resolve the crisis and develop hope.

- Encourage active participation in self-care as well as in mutual decision making and goal setting. Meeting self-care needs and making decisions about care increase personal confidence in one's capacity for coping.
- Encourage a focus not only on the present but also on the future: Review past occasions for hope, discuss the client's personal meaning of hope, establish and evaluate short-term goals with the client and family, and encourage them to express hope for the future. The nurse mobilizes the client's resources to strengthen motivation, hope, and the will to live.

Anxiety

The intensity of anxiety, aroused by a perceived threat, depends on the severity of the present situation and on the client's ability to handle the threat. Anxiety is one of the most common psychosocial responses in clients with cancer. Anxiety increases at the time of diagnosis and remains a constant emotion throughout the course of treatment, regardless of treatment type or setting. Interventions center on helping the client recognize the manifestations of anxiety, determining whether the client wishes to do anything about the anxiety, and facilitating coping strategies.

- Provide reassurance and comfort:
  a. Set aside time to sit quietly with the client.
  b. Speak slowly and calmly.
  c. Convey empathetic understanding by touch and supporting present coping mechanisms, such as crying and talking.
  d. Do not make demands or expect the client to make decisions.

Coping behaviors differ from situation to situation and from person to person. Anxiety at moderate to severe levels narrows perceptions and the ability to function.

- Decrease sensory stimuli by using short, simple sentences; focusing on the here and now; and providing concise information. Higher levels of anxiety result in a focus on the present, inability to concentrate, and difficulty in understanding verbal communications.
- Provide interventions that decrease anxiety levels and increase coping:
  a. Provide accurate information about the illness, treatment, and expected length of recovery.
  b. Encourage discussion of expected physical changes and ways to minimize disfigurement through cosmetics and clothing.
  c. Include family members in teaching sessions.
  d. Encourage participation in care.

Although the prognosis and treatment of melanoma depend on various factors, the prognosis of complete cure is decreased with metastasis. Surgical incisions include excision with wide margins, which may cause disfigurement. Active participation

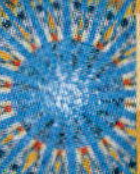

CLIENT TEACHING The Client With Malignant Melanoma

Health education for the client and family experiencing the diagnosis and treatment of malignant melanoma involves self-care and ongoing self-monitoring. Education for the client and family is specific to the type of treatment. In addition to wound care, clients who have had a lymph node dissection need instructions on how to protect against bleeding, trauma, and infection. Address the following topics:

- The importance of regular medical checkups every 3 months for the first 2 years, every 6 months for the next 5 years, and yearly thereafter
- How proper self-care combined with regular medical care can help the client lead a fairly normal life
- If assistance for home care is necessary, referrals to a community health agency or a home care agency, as well as referral to a local cancer support group if desired. Other resources in this area include the following:
  a. The American Cancer Society (http://www.cancer.org)
  b. The Skin Cancer Foundation (http://www.skincancer.org)

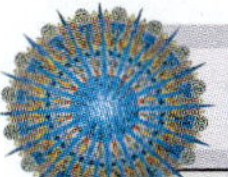

NURSING CARE PLAN A Client With Malignant Melanoma

Geoff Sanders, aged 69, is retired from the U.S. Postal Service. He has always been an avid participant in outdoor sports. When he was younger, he played baseball and tennis, and for the last 10 years, he has played golf at least twice a week. He now lives in Connecticut, but as a younger man, he lived in Florida for almost 15 years. Mr. Sanders has a variety of warts and moles and rarely pays attention to them. However, after taking a shower one day he noticed that a mole on his left lower leg looked bigger and darker. Mr. Sanders had just seen a public announcement on television about the dangers of changes in moles, and he immediately called his primary HMO physician for an appointment at the dermatology clinic.

ASSESSMENT

On arriving at the clinic, Mr. Sanders is interviewed and examined by Tom Hall, a clinical nurse specialist. Following the assessment, Tom documents the following information.

Mr. Sanders has a family history of skin cancer; his father had several squamous cell cancers removed from his face. Mr. Sanders has numerous nevi on his body; the one causing concern is located on the medial anterior left leg, 2 inches below the patella. Mr. Sanders states that the mole has been present for years but that he noticed just yesterday that it has become larger and darker. On further questioning, he states that the mole itches sometimes but has never hurt or bled. Mr. Sanders lived in Florida for 15 years and now experiences a sunburn early each summer before he tans. The sunburn involves the lower legs because Mr. Sanders wears shorts during his twice-weekly golf game.

A complete skin assessment reveals various freckles, warts, and nevi. With the exception of the nevus that prompted Mr. Sanders to come to the clinic, all lesions appear normal. The nevus in question is raised, 3 cm in diameter, with irregular borders and a nodular surface. It is variegated in color, with various shades of brown. The skin surrounding the nevus is slightly erythematous. Inguinal lymph nodes are not enlarged or painful. Tom Hall takes a photograph of the lesion with Mr. Sanders's permission.

Following the assessment, Mr. Sanders discusses the lesion with a surgeon, who recommends excision. They discuss the possibility of skin cancer and the importance of early detection and treatment. Mr. Sanders is scheduled for a biopsy of the nevus under a local anesthetic the following morning. Following the biopsy, histologic examination reveals lentigo maligna melanoma. Staging of the tumor reveals that it is a melanoma in situ, with no metastasis to regional lymph nodes. Mr. Sanders undergoes a wide excision of the lesion the following afternoon.

DIAGNOSES

- Impaired Skin Integrity related to excision of melanoma from the left lower leg
- Risk for Infection related to surgical wound on left lower leg
- Acute Pain related to wide excision of melanoma on left lower leg
- Anxiety related to diagnosis of skin cancer

PLANNING

- The client will demonstrate complete healing of the incision without manifestations of infection.
- The client will verbalize relief of pain by the time the incision is healed.
- The client will verbalize fears and concerns about his diagnosis.

IMPLEMENTATION

- Make the first dressing change, but ensure that Mr. Sanders can safely change the dressing himself before discharge the day after surgery.
- On discharge, provide adequate dressings and tape for the first home dressing change; include in the discharge instructions necessary information about where to buy supplies and how many dressing supplies will be needed.
- Review and provide written instruction for prescribed systemic antibiotic and pain medication.
- Provide written instructions for dressing change, manifestations of infection, and phone number of clinic; stress importance of calling if any abnormal symptoms occur.
- Teach how to protect the incision from bumps and to protect the site from irritants.
- Discuss diagnosis, positive outlook for treatment of melanoma in situ, and the client's concerns.
- Stress importance of lifelong regular health care evaluations to identify any recurrence or metastasis.

EVALUATION

Mr. Sanders returned to the dermatology clinic 1 week after his surgical incision. His incision is well approximated and shows no signs of infection. He is taking his antibiotic four times a day as prescribed and reports that his need for pain medications is decreasing. During his clinic visit the following week, Tom Hall removes the sutures and assesses the wound as healed. Mr. Sanders completed his antibiotics and no longer requires pain medications. He says he is still "scared to death" about having cancer, but he has decided to join a local cancer support group. He also says he had gotten a list of skin safety rules from the American Cancer Society and will be sure to cover up and use sunscreens when he plays golf. Mr. Sanders makes an appointment for follow-up care in 3 months.

(continued)

NURSING CARE PLAN A Client With Malignant Melanoma *continued*

CRITICAL THINKING

1. Consider reasons why people who notice a change in a skin lesion put off seeking health care. What can nurses do to effect change?
2. Design a teaching plan for young adults for preventing skin cancers.
3. What would you say to Mr. Sanders if he called the clinic and said that the antibiotics were making him sick and he didn't think he needed them anyway?
4. Design a nursing care plan for Mr. Sanders for the diagnosis powerlessness.

in care gives the client some control over the future and is often an effective means of coping with anxiety.

Evaluation

Nursing care is evaluated based on the client's progress in meeting goals of care. Possible expected outcomes used to evaluate care include the following:

- The client makes informed decision regarding treatment options.
- The client avoids sun exposure and use of tanning bed.
- The client copes with alterations in body image in a constructive way.

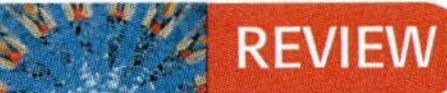

REVIEW Skin Cancer

RELATE: LINK THE CONCEPTS

Linking the exemplar of Skin Cancer with the concept of Development:

1. What teaching points will you include when teaching a group of teens about skin cancer prevention?
2. How will you respond to an adolescent girl who tells you she has to use the tanning bed or she looks too pale and ugly?

Linking the exemplar of Skin Cancer with the concept of Advocacy:

3. How can you, as a student nurse, advocate for clients to reduce the rate of skin cancer as the result of tanning bed usage?
4. What is the role of the nurse advocate in reducing the rate of skin cancer diagnosis?

READY: GO TO COMPANION SKILLS MANUAL

- Assessing the skin
- Assessing the client in pain
- Preparing the client for surgery
- Preparing the surgery site
- Performing surgical and antisepsis

REFER: GO TO MYNURSINGKIT

REFLECT: CASE STUDY

Roe Jefferson is a nurse on vacation in Hampton Bays, Long Island. Roe has worked in pediatrics for 4 years now and really enjoys her work with parents and children. As she walks along the beach, she sees families with kids swimming and sunning themselves. She notices there are no umbrellas and, when not in the water, the children are not wearing hats and shirts. Several families have infants in car seats sitting in the sun.

1. What interventions would you implement to advocate for the children on the beach if you were Roe?
2. What is the teaching priority for families regarding the use of sunscreen?
3. What safety strategies would you teach families when they plan a day at the beach?

EXPLORE PEARSON mynursingkit™

MyNursingKit is your one stop for online chapter review materials and resources. Prepare for success with additional NCLEX®-style practice questions, interactive assignments and activities, web links, animations and videos, and more!

Register your access code from the front of your book at **www.mynursingkit.com**.

REFERENCES

Aher, S., Malwatkar, K., & Kadam, S. (2008). Neonatal anemia. *Seminars in Fetal & Neonatal Medicine, 13*, 239–247.

American Cancer Society. (2005). *What are the risk factors for colorectal cancer?* Retrieved October 28, 2009, from http://www.cancer.org/docroot/CRI/content/CRI_2_4_2X_What_are_the_risk_factors_for_colon_and_rectum_cancer.asp?rnav=cri

American Cancer Society. (2006). *Cancer Facts & Figures 2006.* Atlanta: American Cancer Society.

American Cancer Society (ACS). (2009). Prostate cancer. Retrieved October 24, 2009, from http://www.cancer.org/docroot/CRI/CRI_2_3x.asp?dt=36

Bennett, J. M., & Konrokji, R. S. (2005). The myelodysplastic syndromes: Diagnosis, molecular biology and risk assessment. *Hematology, 10*(Suppl 1), 258–269.

Beyer, J. E., & Simmons, L. E. (2004). Home treatment of pain for children and adolescents with sickle cell disease. *Pain Management Nursing, 5*, 126–135

Blaylock, R. L. (1998). Neurodegeneration and aging of the central nervous system: Prevention and treatment by phytochemicals and metabolic nutrients. *Integrative Medicine, 1*(3), 117–133, 135–141.

Bradley, P. (2005). The delay and worry experience of African American women with breast cancer. *Oncology Nursing Forum, 32*(2), 243–249.

Bryant, R. (2005). Asthma in the pediatric sickle cell patient with acute chest syndrome. *Journal of Pediatric Health Care, 19*, 157–162.

Cantril, C. A., & Haylock, P. J. (2004). Tumor lysis syndrome. *American Journal of Nursing, 104*(4), 49–52.

Carley, A. (2003). Anemia: When is it iron deficiency? *Pediatric Nursing, 29*, 128–133.

Carroll, W. L. (2003). Race and outcome in childhood acute lymphoblastic leukemia. *Journal of the American Medical Association, 290*, 2061–2062.

Copstead, L. C., & Banasik, J. L. (2005). *Pathophysiology* (3rd ed.). St. Louis, MO: Elsevier/Saunders.

Davison, B. J., Moore, K., MacMillan, H., Bisaillon, A., & Wiens, K. (2004). Patient evaluation of a discharge program following a radical prostatectomy. *Urology Nursing, 24*(6), 483–489.

Dietrich, M., Block, G., Norkus, E. P., Hudes, M., Traber, M. G., Cross, C. E., et al. (2002). Smoking and exposure to environmental tobacco smoke decrease some plasma antioxidants and increase gamma-tocopherol in vivo after adjustment for dietary antioxidant intakes. *American Journal of Clinical Nutrition, 77*(1), 160–166.

Donahue, B. R., Wernz, J. C., & Cooper, J. S. (2000). HIV-associated malignancies. In J. D. Roseblatt, P. Okunieff, & J. V. Sitzmann (Eds.), *Clinical oncology: A multidisciplinary approach for physicians and students* (8th ed., pp. 199–207). Philadelphia: W. B. Saunders.

Dunlop, R. J., & Campbell, C. W. (2000). Cytokines and advanced cancer. *Journal of Pain & Symptom Management, 20*(3), 214–232.

Ferrell, B. (2000). Article captures the essence and meaning of alopecia. *Oncology Nursing Forum, 27*, 17.

Futreal, P. A., Kasprzyk, A., Birney, E., Mullikin, J. C., Wooster, R., & Stratton, M. R. (2001). Cancer and genomics. *Nature, 409*(6822), 850–852.

Guttmacher, A. E., & Collins, F. (2002). Genomic medicine: A primer. *New England Journal of Medicine, 347*, 1512–1527.

Haapoja, I. (2000). Paraneoplastic syndromes. In C. H. Yarbro, M. H. Frogge, M. Goodman, & S. L. Groenwald (Eds.), *Cancer nursing: Principles and practice* (5th ed., pp. 792–812). Boston: Jones & Bartlett.

Hawkins, R. (2001). Mastering the intricate maze of metastasis. *Oncology Nursing Forum, 28*(6), 959–965.

Jaff, N., Chelghoum, Y., Elhamri, M., Tigaud, I., Michallet, M., & Thomas, X. (2006). Trisomy 8 as sole anomaly or with other clonal aberrations in acute myeloid leukemia: Impact on clinical presentation and outcome. *Leukemia Research, 31*, 67–73.

Kasper, D. L., Braunwald, E., Fauci, A. S., Hauser, S. L., Longo, D. L., & Jameson, J. L. (Eds.). (2005). *Harrison's principles of internal medicine* (16th ed.). New York: McGraw-Hill.

Katz, L. S., & Epstein, S. (2005). The relation of cancer-prone personality to exceptional recovery from cancer: A preliminary study. *Advances in Mind-Body Medicine, 21*(3/4), 6–20.

Kaye, J., Morton, J., Bowcutt, M., & Maupin, D. (2000). Stress, depression, and psychoneuroimmunology. *Journal of Neuroscience Nursing, 32*, 93–100.

Kee, J. L. (2002). *Laboratory and diagnostic tests with nursing implications* (6th ed.). Upper Saddle River, NJ: Prentice Hall Health.

Khalsa, J. H., Genser, S., Francis, H., & Martin, B. (2002). Clinical consequences of marijuana. *Journal of Clinical Pharmacology, 42*(11 Supplement), 7S–10S.

Kral, M. C., Brown, R. T., Connelly, M., Cure, J. K., Besenski, N., Jackson, S. M., & Abboud, M. R. (2006). Radiographic predictors of neurocognitive functioning in pediatric sickle cell disease. *Journal of Child Neurology, 21*, 37–44.

McCance, K. L., & Huether, S. E. (2006). *Pathophysiology: The biologic basis for disease in adults & children* (4th ed.). St. Louis, MO: Mosby.

Majno, G., & Joris, I. (2004). *Cells, tissues, and disease: Principles of general pathology* (2nd ed.). New York: Oxford University Press.

Molassiotis, A., Panteli, V., Patiraki, E., Ozden, G., Platin, N., Madsen, E., et al. (2006). Complementary and alternative medicine use in lung cancer patients in eight European countries. *Complementary Therapies in Clinical Practice, 12*(1), 34–39.

NANDA International. (2005). *Nursing diagnoses: Definitions & classification 2005–2006.* Philadelphia: NANDA International.

National Cancer Institute. (2004). The prostate-specific antigen (PSA) test: Questions and answers. Retrieved from http://cis.nci.nih.gov/fact/5_29.htm

National Heart, Lung, and Blood Institute. (2002). *The management of sickle cell disease.* Retrieved June 1, 2004, from http://www.nhlbi.nih.gov/health/prof/blood/sickle/sc_mngt.pdf

Ogedegbe, H. O. (2002). Sickle cell disease: An overview. *Laboratory Medicine, 7*, 515–543.

Oncology Nursing Society. (2006). *Oncology Nursing Society position paper on quality cancer care.* Retrieved May 11, 2006, from http://www.ons.org/publications/positions/QualityCancerCare.shtml

Persson, L., & Hallberg, I. R. (2004). Lived experience of survivors of leukemia or malignant lymphoma. *Cancer Nursing, 27*(4), 303–313

Persson, L., Hallberg, I. R., & Ohlsson, O. (1997). Survivors of acute leukemia and highly malignant lymphoma—retrospective views of daily life problems during treatment and when in remission. *Journal of Advanced Nursing, 25*(1), 68–78

Peto, R., Darby, S., Deo, H., Silcocks, P., Whitley, E., & Doll, R. (2000). Smoking, smoking cessation, and lung cancer in the UK since 1950: Combination of national statistics with two case-control studies. *BMJ, 321*(7257), 323–329.

Porth, C. (2005). *Pathophysiology: Concepts of altered health states* (7th ed.). Philadelphia: Lippincott.

Roberts, D., Hornung, C., & Polk Jr., H. (2009, July). Another duel in the sun: Weighing the balances between sun protection, tanning beds, and malignant melanoma. *Clinical Pediatrics, 48*(6), 614–622. Retrieved August 21, 2009, from Academic Search Complete database.

Rosenberg, A. A. (2007). The neonate. In S. G. Gabbe, J. R. Niebyl, & J. L. Simpson (Eds.), *Obstetrics: Normal and problem pregnancies* (5th ed., pp. 523–565). Philadelphia, PA: Churchill Livingstone/Elsevier.

Rossi, E. L. (2004). Stress-induced alternative gene splicing in mind-body medicine. *Advances in Mind-Body Medicine, 20*(2), 12–19.

Scigliano, E., Vlachos, A., Najfeld, V., & Shank, B. (2001). The leukemias. In P. Rubin (Ed.), *Clinical oncology: A multidisciplinary approach for physicians and students* (pp. 565–614). Philadelphia: W. B. Saunders.

Segal, G. B., Hirsh, M. G., & Feig, S. A. (2002). Managing anemia in pediatric office practice: Part 1. *Pediatrics in Review, 23*, 75–83.

Selye, H. (1984). *The stress of life* (2nd ed. rev.). New York: McGraw-Hill.

Spencer, J. W., & Jacobs, J. J. (2003). *Complementary and alternative medicine: An evidence-based approach* (2nd ed.). St. Louis, MO: Mosby

Spitalnick, P. F., & diSant'Agnese, P. A. (2001). The pathology of cancer. In P. Rubin (Ed.), *Clinical oncology: A multidisciplinary approach for physicians and students* (pp. 47–61). Philadelphia: W. B. Saunders.

Strouse, J. J., Fears, T. R., Tucker, M. A., & Wayne, A. S. (2005). Pediatric melanoma: Risk factor and survival analysis of the surveillance, epidemiology, and end results database. *Journal of Clinical Oncology, 23*, 4735–4741.

Surbone, A. (2001). Ethical implications of genetic testing for breast cancer susceptibility. *Critical Reviews in Oncology-Hematology, 40*(2), 149–157.

Tanyi, R. A. (2003). Sickle cell disease: Health promotion and maintenance and the role of primary care nurse practitioners. *Journal of the American Academy of Nursing Practitioners, 15*, 389–397.

Tierney, L. M., Jr., McPhee, S. J., & Papadakis, M. A. (Eds.). (2005). *Current medical diagnosis & treatment* (44th ed.). New York: McGraw-Hill.

White K. E. (2005). Anemia is a poor predictor of iron deficiency among toddlers in the United States: For heme the bell tolls. *Pediatrics, 115*, 315–320.

Williams, J., Wood, C., & Cunningham-Warburton, P. (1999). A narrative study of chemotherapy-induced alopecia. *Oncology Nursing Forum, 26*, 1463–1468.

Wilson, R. E., Krishnamurti, L., & Kamat, D. (2003). Management of sickle cell disease in primary care. *Clinical Pediatrics, 42*, 753–761.

Zech, D., Grond, S., Lynch, J., Hertel, D., & Lehmann, K. (1995). Validation of World Health Organization Guidelines for cancer pain relief: A 10-year prospective study. *Pain, 63*, 65–76.

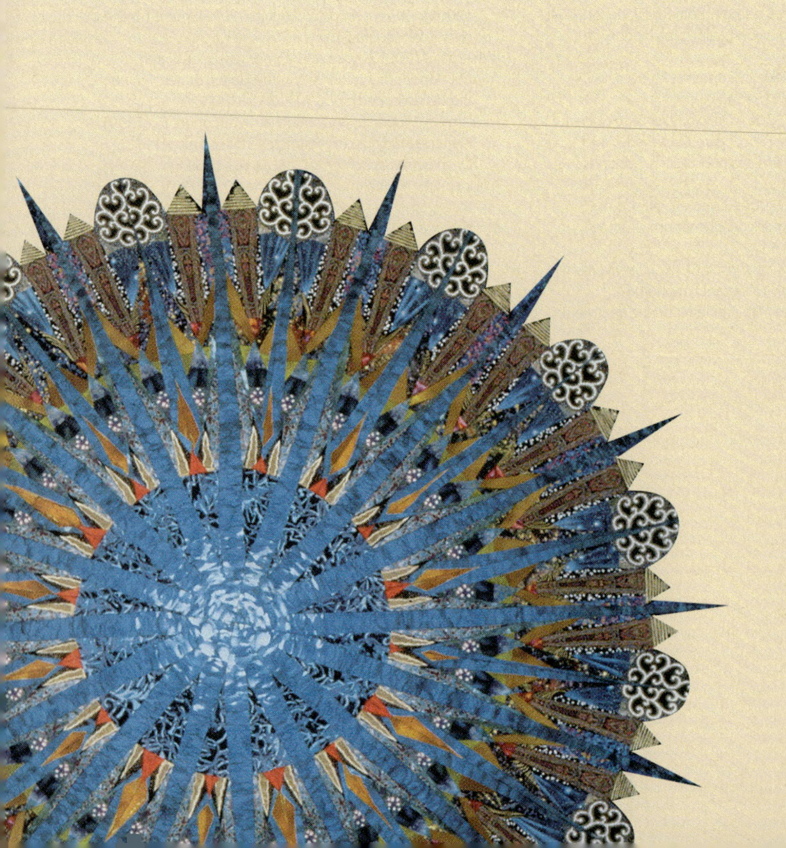

Cognition

4

Concept at-a-Glance

Concept Learning Outcomes

After reading about this concept, you will be able to:

1. Summarize the structure and physiologic processes of the neurological system related to cognition.
2. List factors affecting cognition.
3. Identify common alterations in cognition and their related treatments.
4. Explain common physical assessment procedures used to evaluate the cognitive status of clients across the life span.
5. Outline diagnostic and laboratory tests to determine causes of alteration in the individual's cognitive status.
6. Explain management of altered cognition and prevention of cognitive dysfunction.
7. Demonstrate the nursing process in providing culturally competent care across the life span for individuals with common alterations in cognition.
8. Identify pharmacologic interventions in caring for the individual with alterations in cognitive function.

Concept Key Terms

Adaptive functioning, *201*
Akathisia, *207*
Anomia, *207*
Aphasia, *207*
Ataxia, *207*
Carphologia, *207*
Cognition, *197*
Constructional difficulty, *207*
Cognitive development, *198*
Dementia, *206*
Developmental disability, *201*
Down syndrome, *201*
Dysphagia, *207*
Echolalia, *207*
Fetal alcohol syndrome, *202*
Floccillation, *207*
Fragile X syndrome, *202*
Functional assessments, *202*
Learning disabilities, *200*
Long-term memory, *199*
Mental retardation, *201*
Paraphasia, *207*
Perception, *199*
Recent memory, *199*
Sensory memory, *199*
Short-term memory, *199*

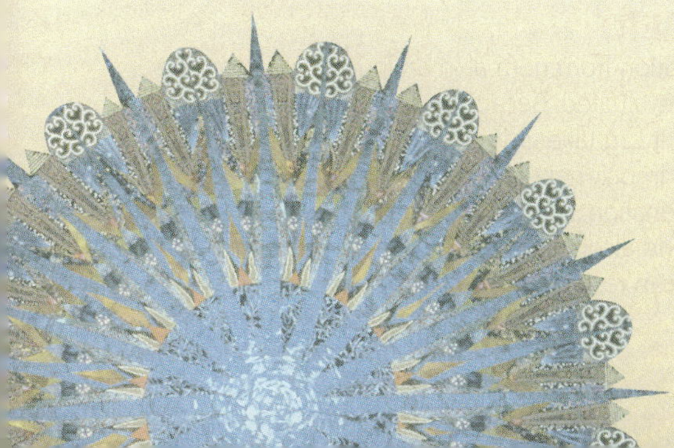

About Cognition

Cognition is a complicated process by which an individual learns, stores, retrieves, and uses information. Cognitive processing supports reasoning, problem solving, remembering, interpreting, and communicating. The nervous system is responsible for control of cognitive function and both voluntary and involuntary activities.

Joan is a 58-year-old registered nurse working in a busy urban emergency department. Sometimes Joan has to think to remember a term she has used frequently throughout her nursing career, and she jokes that she's having a "senior moment." She tells stories and laughs about not being able to find her keys, searching for her eyeglasses only to find they are propped up on her head, or calling her children by the wrong name. Though she may joke about her memory and growing older, Joan is an excellent nurse who has a great deal of experience and acts as a resource for new staff members in the emergency department. Joan's situation raises two very important questions: Is cognitive loss an inevitable result of the aging process or is it an indication of a disease process that requires further diagnostic testing? Do all older people lose cognitive function? ●

NORMAL PRESENTATION

The ability to think and learn makes us human. It enables us to be rational, to make good judgments, to interpret the world around us, and to learn new skills. **Cognitive development** refers to the manner in which people learn to think, reason, and use language. It involves a person's intelligence, perceptual ability, and ability to process information. Cognitive development represents a progression of mental abilities from illogical to logical thinking, from simple to complex problem solving, and from concrete thinking to understanding abstract concepts. It is important to note that sensory alterations can cause changes in cognitive functioning (Wahl & Heyl, 2003).

Cognitive Theories

All developmental theories are simply that—theories. A theory is developed to explain a collection of observations or facts and to predict future occurrences. As such, no one theory can explain all of reality, and all theories have some strengths and some weaknesses.

The most widely known cognitive theorist is Jean Piaget. His theory of cognitive development has contributed to other theories, such as Kohlberg's theory of moral development and Fowler's theory of the development of faith. According to Piaget (1966), based on his observations and work with children, cognitive development is an orderly, sequential process in which a variety of new experiences (stimuli) are needed before intellectual abilities can develop. He believed that age and maturational ability largely influence the child's view of the world. Given nurturing experiences, the child's ability to think matures naturally (Ginsberg & Opper, 1988; Piaget, 1972). Piaget's cognitive developmental process is divided into four major phases: the sensorimotor phase, the preoperational phase, the concrete operational phase, and the formal operational phase. These phases are explained in detail in the Development concept.

Although Piaget's theory of cognitive development provides a useful framework for examining and understanding the thought process of young children, like all theories it is not perfect. He developed the theory mainly by observation of his own three children. It may lack some applicability in cross-cultural contexts, and it does not explain the importance of social contexts in learning. Two other important cognitive theories expand the work of Piaget and may provide assistance for nurses:

1. Lev Vygotsky (1896–1934) agreed with Piaget's theory of a child's cognition. However, he believed that children are embedded in social contexts that influence learning. With guidance and assistance from parents and others, children learn tasks that are impossible for them to master alone. Vygotsky also viewed the social structure of language as essential to development of thought (Santrock, 2005; Vygotsky, 1962).
2. Information processing is another theory of cognitive development that views attention and memory as the most important parts of learning, rather than the structures Piaget described. Infants tend to habituate or become bored with the same stimuli and therefore are more attentive to, and learn from, new stimuli that are introduced to them. Long-term and short-term memory both are important to learning. The older child actively engages in strategies to assist with memorization, thereby playing an active part in learning (Meltzoff & Gopnick, 1997; Santrock, 2005).

Nursing Practices

Cognitive theory is essential to pediatric nursing. The nurse must understand a client's thought processes in order to design stimulating activities and meaningful, appropriate teaching plans. Health teaching is tailored to the understanding of cognitive stages. For example, a nurse can expect a toddler to be egocentric and literal; therefore, explanations to the toddler should focus on the needs of the toddler rather than on the needs of others. A child's concept of time suggests how far in advance the nurse should prepare that child for procedures. Similarly, the nurse's decision to offer manipulative toys, read stories, draw pictures, or give the child reading material to explain health care measures depends on the child's cognitive stage of development. A teenager can be expected to use rational thinking and to reason; therefore, when explaining the need for a medication to a teen, a nurse can outline the consequences of taking and not taking the medication, enabling the adolescent client to make a rational decision. Nurses must remember, however, that the range of normal cognitive development is broad, despite the age ranges attributed to each level. When teaching adults, nurses may become aware that some adults are more comfortable than others with concrete thought and some are slower to acquire and apply new information.

PRACTICE ALERT

Any change or deviation from normal in an individual's cognitive function should be evaluated. Because a number of factors can influence cognition, it can take time to determine the reason behind a change or impairment in cognitive function. Stress, grief, impairment of oxygenation, head injury, obstructive sleep apnea, stroke, embolism, and alcohol and drug abuse are just some of the conditions that can result in impaired cognitive ability.

Cognitive Abilities and Aging

Piaget's phases of cognitive development end with the formal operations phase. However, considerable research on cognitive abilities and aging is already beginning to provide insight into changes in cognition experienced by older adults, both as part of the normal aging process and through alterations that sometimes develop as people age. The brain loses mass with aging. In addition, blood flow to the brain decreases, the meninges thicken, and brain metabolism slows. Little is known about the effect of these physical changes on the cognitive functioning of the older adult. Lifelong mental activity, particularly verbal activity, helps the older adult retain a high level of cognitive function and maintain long-term memory.

Intellectual capacity includes perception, cognitive agility, memory, and learning. Declines in any of these abilities can affect cognition.

PERCEPTION **Perception**, or the ability to interpret the environment, depends on the acuteness of the senses. If the aging person's senses are impaired, the ability to perceive the environment and react appropriately is diminished. Changes in the nervous system may also affect perceptual capacity.

COGNITIVE ABILITY In older adults, changes in cognitive abilities are more often a difference in speed than in ability. Overall, the older adult maintains intelligence, problem solving, judgment, creativity, and other well-practiced cognitive skills. Intellectual loss generally reflects a disease process (e.g., atherosclerosis) that causes the blood vessels to narrow and diminishes perfusion of nutrients to the brain. Most older adults do not experience cognitive impairments; only 15% of older men and 11% of older women manifest moderate or severe memory impairment (FIFAS, 2004). Cognitive impairment that interferes with normal life is not considered part of normal aging. A decline in intellectual abilities that interferes with social or occupational functions should always be regarded as abnormal. Family members should be advised to seek prompt medical evaluation.

MEMORY Memory is also a component of intellectual capacity and involves the following steps:

1. Momentary perception of stimuli from the environment, referred to as **sensory memory**.
2. Storage in **short-term memory** (information held in the brain for immediate use or what one has in mind at a given moment). An example of this type of memory is when an individual calls directory assistance for a telephone number and remembers the number only for the brief time needed to dial the number. Short-term memory also deals with the recent past few minutes to a few hours, which is often referred to as **recent memory**.
3. Encoding, in which the information leaves short-term memory and enters **long-term memory**, the repository for information stored for periods longer than 72 hours and usually weeks and years. Memories of childhood friends, teachers, and events are stored in long-term memory. Older people who remember the flowers in their wedding bouquet or the names of the boys on their dance card are drawing from long-term memory.

In older adults, retrieval of information from long-term memory can be slower, especially if the information is not frequently used. Most age-related differences, however, occur in short-term memory. Older adults tend to forget the recent past. This forgetfulness can be improved by using memory aids, making notes or lists, and placing objects in consistent locations.

LEARNING Older people need additional time for learning, largely because of problems in retrieving information. Motivation is also important. Older adults have more difficulty in learning information they do not consider meaningful; therefore, the nurse should be particularly careful to discover what is meaningful to the older adult before attempting client education.

Cognitive Function in Older Adults

Normal, healthy aging is not characterized by cognitive and mental disorders (U.S. Department of Health and Human Services, 2001). Some cognitive abilities may decline with age, some may improve, and some stay relatively stable. These changes are highly variable from one person to another as a person ages and may even vary within a person over time. Most older people will not have significant memory impairment, but many may experience slight problems with word finding and remembering names. Usually, these problems are mild and the older person can compensate for them. Levels of educational attainment within the older population have increased significantly and are projected to continue to increase over the next decade. Higher education levels are linked to better health outcomes and a higher standard of living in retirement. However, even though older people share similar generational experiences, there may be considerable diversity among them. Life experiences, health status, race, culture, sexual orientation, and a variety of other factors can make an older person who did not finish high school think and act more like a college professor and vice versa.

Normally, an older person's mental health and cognition remain relatively stable. For those functions that do change, the change is usually not severe enough to cause significant impairment in daily life or social ability. Severe changes and sudden loss of cognitive function are usually symptoms of a physical or mental illness, such as Alzheimer's disease, stroke, or serious depression. The following are some general cognitive changes that are considered normal age-related changes (American Psychological Association, 2008):

- Information-processing speed declines with age, resulting in a slower learning rate and greater need for repetition of information.
- The ability to divide attention between two tasks shows age-related decline.
- The ability to switch attention rapidly from one auditory input to another shows age-related decline (visual input switching ability does not change significantly with age).
- The ability to maintain sustained attention or perform vigilance tasks appears to decline with age.
- The ability to filter out irrelevant information appears to decline with age.

- Short-term or primary memory remains relatively stable.
- Long-term or secondary memory exhibits more substantial age-related changes, with a greater decline for recall than for recognition. (Cueing improves performance of long-term memory.)
- Most aspects of language are well preserved, such as use of language sounds and meaningful combinations of words. Vocabulary improves with age. However, word finding, naming ability, and rapid word list generation decline with age.
- Visuospatial task ability such as drawing and construction ability declines with age.
- Abstraction and mental flexibility show some age-related decline.
- Accumulation of practical experience, or wisdom, continues until the very end of life.

PRACTICE ALERT

Normal healthy older persons who forget where they put the keys can be assured there is no significant memory problem, but if they forget what a key is for or how to use it, they should be referred for further evaluation and treatment.

Decline of intellectual function is generally greater in older people who develop disease and disability than in those who remain healthy. Many impairments in cognitive capacity, mood, and performance that formerly were attributed to "normal aging" are now known to be associated with psychiatric illness or physical disease. Significant changes in mood, cognitive ability, and personality should never be dismissed as normal aging, but always aggressively assessed and referred for treatment.

Late adulthood is no longer seen as a period of growth cessation and arrested cognitive development, but rather a period of continued growth with the opportunity for development of unique capacities (Ebersole, Hess, & Lugfen, 2004). Education, pulmonary health, general health, and activity levels all influence cognitive activity in later life. Older adults often have a positive outlook and seek challenges and activities that maintain their well-being. Since most changes of aging are gradual, the older person adjusts to the changes over time. Methods for coping with age-associated cognitive changes follow:

- Making lists, posting appointments on calendars, and writing "notes to self"
- Using memory training and memory enhancement techniques (for instance, when meeting a new person for the first time, trying to link his or her name to a common object or easily remembered item)
- Playing computer games that emphasize eye–hand coordination and memory of shapes, colors, and objects
- Keeping the mind challenged and mentally active (reading daily, completing a crossword puzzle, playing bridge, etc.)
- Using assistive devices such as pill boxes and preprogrammed telephones, and reliance on habits such as parking in the same place in the mall parking lot to reduce chances of forgetting vital information
- Seeking support and encouragement from others
- Staying positive and hopeful for the future, including laughing at oneself when appropriate. ("You won't believe what I did today. I showed up for my doctor's appointment with one brown and one black shoe! Oh well, at least I'm not a slave to fashion!")

A nurse who is beginning to notice changes in an older client's cognitive activity can suggest and encourage use of these methods and other coping techniques to assist the client in adjusting to the changes and maintaining a positive outlook.

Older adults must be able to monitor their cognitive abilities and adapt to changes in their memory skills to function safely in their everyday lives. Some people with severe cognitive deficits may continue to engage in behaviors that are unsafe for them, such as driving, cooking, and trying to live independently. Others with good memories may live in continual fear that they are developing Alzheimer's disease whenever they forget a name or an appointment.

It is difficult to predict whether an older person who has mild problems with memory will develop more severe memory loss. Some older people try to hide or cover up memory problems because they fear restrictions on their freedoms and living situation. Memory changes may result from a variety of causes, including Alzheimer's disease, depression, underlying psychiatric illness, physical illness, medications, vitamin deficiencies, and sensory impairments. Any alteration or concern over cognitive abilities should be assessed to identify reversible causes of memory loss and institute appropriate safety measures in a supportive environment.

ALTERATIONS

Pediatric Cognitive Disorders

A wide array of cognitive conditions occur in childhood. Some are mild and not diagnosed until a child has difficulty in school, while others may be associated with physical signs that are visible at birth.

LEARNING DISABILITIES **Learning disabilities** involve neurological conditions in which the brain cannot receive or process information in the normal manner. They are common in young children, affecting approximately 8–10% of school children. Often the impairment is in only one or two types of learning, making diagnosis difficult. Common types of learning disorders are listed and described in Box 4–1. Children may have difficulty in processing visual information that is manifested in reading, writing, and mathematics performance. Others may have more difficulty with oral information, leading to problems in language development and reading (Kelly & Aylward, 2005; National Center for Learning Disabilities, 2004).

The causes of learning disorders are complex. Sometimes they are related to low birth weight or problems during the perinatal period. Children suspected of having a disability should be evaluated and diagnosed by a learning specialist such as a psychologist with specialty training. A series of cognitive and developmental tests are most commonly used. Brain scanning with magnetic resonance imaging (MRI) is

Box 4–1 Learning Disorders

DISORDER	CLINICAL MANIFESTATIONS
Dyslexia	Difficulty with writing, reading, spelling
Dyscalculia	Difficulty with mathematics and computation
Dysgraphia	Difficulty with writing, spelling, and composition
Dyspraxia	Difficulty with manual dexterity and coordination

showing promise for providing diagnostic clues, but is not yet commonly used or available in most communities. Some disabilities may have a genetic component, since their occurrence is more common when other family members are affected. Treatments generally involve teaching children how to compensate for the difficulties by using capabilities that are intact. Some children will require accommodations, such as having all material presented in class provided to them in writing, or being given extra time to complete tests. Children with learning disabilities should have individualized education plans (IEPs) established with realistic goals for school performance. These plans are normally developed collaboratively by the classroom teacher, a learning specialist, and the child's parents.

Nursing Management

Nurses play a major role in identifying children with learning disabilities. In fact, the pediatrician's office is frequently the first place a parent will take a child if the parent suspects something is wrong with the child's development. Nurses may also encounter families during health promotion visits or in other settings when parents relay concerns about the child's behavior at home or in day care or about the child's performance or difficulty in some aspect of school. The nurse should ask whether there is a family history of learning problems, and evaluate the child's history for prematurity, low birth weight, head injury, seizure activity, and other chronic health conditions. The nurse assesses the child for the following developmental milestones, which can indicate a learning disability:

- Inability to phrase sentences together by 2.5 years of age
- Inability to use speech that is understandable at least 50% of the time by age 3 years
- Inability to tie shoes, button clothes, hop, or cut with scissors by kindergarten
- Inability to sit for a short story by 3–5 years (Kelly & Aylward, 2005).

A number of screening tools exist to help nurses and other professionals screen children for suspected learning disabilities in order to determine whether a referral is necessary.

A nurse who suspects a child may have a learning disability should refer the family to the school or other testing resource. The nurse should partner with the family to plan for the child's learning needs. This includes helping the family to work closely with the child, providing a setting at home to maximize potential for learning, building healthy self-esteem in the child, and assisting the family in working with the school to establish annual goals for the child. A multidisciplinary team, including teachers, therapists, and the family, commonly works within the school to plan for the child's learning needs (Lambros & Leslie, 2005). In some states, a special agency or network exists for diagnosing children younger than kindergarten age, and a nurse or primary care provider can refer a family for diagnostic procedures before a child enters school. Because most children with learning disabilities can learn to perform well in their areas of strength and compensate for areas of difficulty, early intervention is key to their success and to building a positive self-image regarding their abilities.

MENTAL RETARDATION **Mental retardation** is defined as significant limitation in intellectual functioning and adaptive behavior. It is manifested in differences in conceptual, social, and practical life skills and begins before the age of 18 years (American Association of Mental Retardation, 2004). Later events that lead to limitations in function are referred to as brain injury. Intellectual functioning is generally characterized by an IQ below 70–75 and significant impairment in **adaptive functioning** (the ability of an individual to meet the standards expected for his or her cultural group). The individual with mental retardation has adaptive deficits in at least two areas, such as communication, self-care, home living, social/interpersonal skills, use of community resources, self-direction, functional academic skills, work, leisure, health, or safety. A low IQ score by itself does not necessarily correlate with impairment in adaptive skills. The child should be evaluated within the contexts of the individual's cultural and community environments. The IQ score and the level of adaptive skills together determine the severity of mental retardation.

Mental retardation is one type of developmental disability. A **developmental disability** is any of a variety of chronic conditions that are characterized by mental and/or physical impairment. Other examples are pervasive developmental disorder, cerebral palsy, and sensory loss. A developmental disability begins by the age of 21 years and lasts throughout life (Bhasin, Brocksen, Avchen, & Braun, 2006). Early detection, diagnosis, and treatment can greatly increase the chances of a successful and productive life for an individual with a developmental disability.

Mental retardation occurs in 12 per 1,000 children, a decrease from 15.5 per 1,000 one decade ago (Bhasin et al., 2006). The causes of mental retardation can be grouped into three general categories: prenatal errors in the development of the central nervous system (CNS), prenatal or postnatal changes in the biologic environment of the person, and external forces leading to CNS damage. In each instance, the precipitating factor causes a change in the form, function, and adaptation of the CNS. Table 4–1 provides examples of common causes of mental retardation for each category.

Three common conditions associated with mental retardation from the prenatal category are Down syndrome, fragile X syndrome, and fetal alcohol syndrome. In the United States, about 1 in 1,000 infants, or 5,500 infants each year, are born with **Down syndrome** (Centers for Disease Control and Prevention,

TABLE 4–1 Common Conditions Associated With Mental Retardation

PRENATAL CONDITIONS	BIOLOGIC ENVIRONMENT	EXTERNAL FORCES
Down syndrome	Inborn errors of metabolism (e.g., phenylketonuria, hypothyroidism)	Traumatic brain injury (e.g., accident)
Fragile X syndrome		Poison ingestion (acute or chronic)
Fetal alcohol syndrome		Hypoxia/anoxic insult
Maternal infection (e.g., rubella, cytomegalovirus)		Infection (e.g., meningitis)
		Environmental deprivation

2006). The condition is caused by an extra chromosome; the child has 47 rather than 46 chromosomes. The most common chromosome affected is 21, so that the child often has trisomy 21, or three copies instead of two of chromosome 21. In addition to mental retardation and physical signs, the child with Down syndrome is at higher risk of developing other conditions such as cardiac defects, hearing loss, strabismus, gastrointestinal problems, orthodontic conditions, thyroid disease, dermatologic conditions, and leukemia (Van Cleve, Cannon, & Cohen, 2006).

Fragile X syndrome is caused by a single recessive gene abnormality on the X chromosome. The faulty gene creates a deficiency in the FMR1 protein that leads to brain changes. The condition is often associated with other conditions such as attention deficit/hyperactivity disorder (ADHD), anxiety, and autism (Hagerman, 2006).

Fetal alcohol syndrome (FAS) is caused by the effect of ethyl alcohol on the developing fetus. The term *fetal alcohol spectrum disorder* (FASD) describes the wide range of effects from the condition, which can range from FAS to a milder condition called fetal alcohol effects (FAE) (Caley, Shipkey, Winkelman et al., 2006). Alcohol ingestion by the pregnant woman can influence the development of many body organs, and its effects can range from mild to severe. In spite of the warnings regarding use of alcohol during pregnancy, alcohol use remains a leading cause of mental retardation, affecting 2 in 1,000 births in the United States, or 8,000 to 12,000 infants annually (Troshinksy, 2004).

Fetal alcohol syndrome is more common in groups with a higher intake of alcohol. The rate in Native American and Alaskan Native communities is 10 times the rate in the general population (Troshinksy, 2004). Because some Native American tribes have a high rate of alcoholism, the federal government has joined with them to lower that risk among this ethnic group. On some reservations, such as the Yakama Nation in Washington State, alcoholic beverages are not sold and educational programs are in place to discourage use of alcohol among pregnant women.

Phenylketonuria and hypothyroidism are two common biochemical causes of mental retardation. Other causes are traumatic brain injury and infections of the CNS.

Clinical Manifestations Mild mental retardation was originally described as an IQ between 50 and 70, with moderate retardation between 35 and 50, severe retardation between 20 and 35, and profound retardation below 20. Although an IQ below 70 is considered indicative of retardation, the functional assessment of the child is now considered a more accurate identification of children's performance and needs. **Functional assessments** can include diagnostic testing, but they primarily involve detailed observations of the behavior, responses, and abilities a child uses in both the home and school settings. In other words, these assessments look at how a child functions on a daily basis in his or her environment. Children who are mentally retarded manifest delays in all areas of development, including motor movement, language, and adaptive behavior. They usually achieve developmental milestones more slowly than the average child. These developmental delays may be the first indication to parents and care providers of the child's condition.

Mental retardation is sometimes accompanied by sensory impairment, speech problems, motor and orthopedic disabilities, and seizure disorders. Of children with mental retardation, 10–30% manifest at least one such disorder. Table 4–2 lists several physical characteristics associated with Down syndrome, fragile X syndrome, and fetal alcohol syndrome.

Diagnostic Tests Mental retardation is diagnosed and initial treatment is planned in a multistep process that involves a multidisciplinary team that includes the parents. This team usually includes a developmental specialist, physician, geneticist, nurse, teacher, language therapist, and rehabilitation specialists. See Box 4–2 for a description of the *DSM-IV-TR* for mental retardation.

The team will begin by conducting a comprehensive history and evaluation of the child's physical characteristics, developmental level, and intellectual and adaptive functioning. Laboratory tests such as chromosome analysis, blood enzyme levels, and lead levels or cranial imaging may be ordered to provide additional information. A three-generation family history is generally performed (Moeschler, Shevell, & American Academy of Pediatrics, 2006).

Developmental screening using a test such as the Denver II can help to identify children who may be at risk of developmental delay. A neurologic examination may indicate asymmetry of movement or strength, irritability or lethargy, or abnormal pitch to an infant's cry. Because mental retardation may be accompanied by physical abnormalities, it is important

TABLE 4–2 Characteristics of Three Common Conditions Associated With Mental Retardation

DOWN SYNDROME (See Figure 4–1 ■)	FRAGILE X SYNDROME	FETAL ALCOHOL SYNDROME (See Figure 4–2 ■)
Small head (microcephaly)	Long face	Flat midface
Flattened forehead	Prominent jaw	Low nasal bridge
Wide, short neck	Large ears	Long philtrum with narrow upper lip
Epicanthal eye folds	Frequent otitis media	Short upturned nose
White spots on eye iris (Brushfield spots)	Large testicles	Poor coordination
Congenital cataracts	Epicanthal eye folds	Failure to thrive
Flat nose	Strabismus	Skeletal and joint abnormalities
Small, low-set ears	High-arched palate	Hearing loss
Protruding tongue	Scoliosis	
Short broad hands	Pliable joints	
Simian line on palm		
Wide space between first and second toes		
Hearing loss		
Increased incidence of diabetes, congenital heart defect, and leukemia		
Hypotonia		

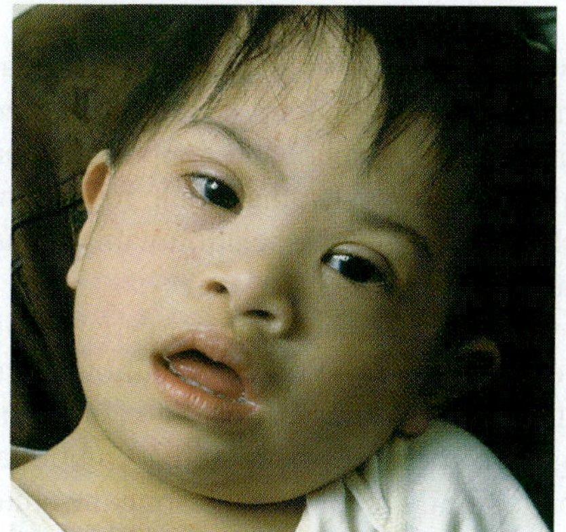

Figure 4–1 ■ A child with Down syndrome.

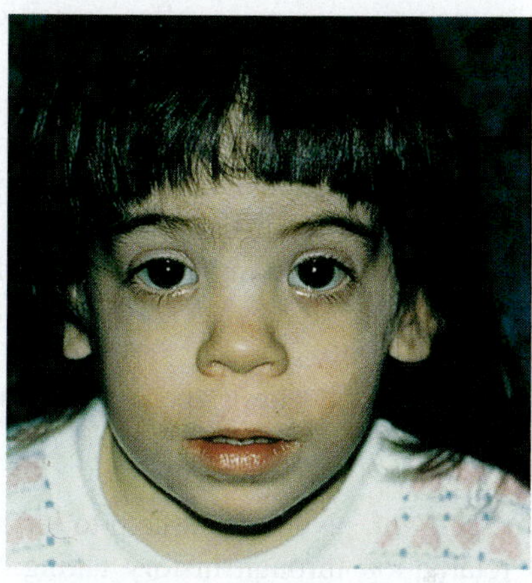

Figure 4–2 ■ A child with fetal alcohol syndrome.

Courtesy of Dr. Sterling Clarren, Seattle, WA, and Vancouver, BC. From Clarren, S. F. H. Smith, D.W. (1978). The fetal alcohol syndrome. New England Journal of Medicine, 298, 1063–1067.

to observe the child for facial symmetry, distance between the eyes, level of the ears, hair growth, and palmar creases. These abnormalities may be cues to other health problems.

Clinical Therapy Based on the results of the evaluation, the multidisciplinary team will plan the support needed to maximize the child's potential for development. Management focuses on early intervention to improve the degree of adaptive functioning. Simultaneous treatment of associated physical, emotional, and behavioral problems is provided. Depending on the child's condition, special education programs and physical or occupational therapy may be necessary. At all stages, the multidisciplinary team obtains the permission of, discusses test results with, and makes recommendations to the parent. Parents' understanding of and participation in this process are critical to the success of any treatment plan, and the parents' permission is required for any treatment to be provided.

Box 4–2 *DSM-IV-TR* Diagnostic Criteria for Mental Retardation

A. Significantly subaverage intellectual functioning: an IQ of approximately 70 or below on an individually administered IQ test (for infants, a clinical judgment of significantly subaverage intellectual functioning).

B. Concurrent deficits or impairments in present adaptive functioning (i.e., the person's effectiveness in meeting the standards expected for his or her age by his or her cultural group) in at least two of the following areas: communication, self-care, home living, social/interpersonal skills, use of community resources, self-direction, functional academic skills, work, leisure, health, and safety.

C. The onset is before age 18 years.

Source: Reprinted with permission from the *Diagnostic and Statistical Manual of Mental Disorders*, Text Revision, Fourth Edition, (Copyright © 2000). American Psychiatric Association.

PRACTICE ALERT

Prematurity and low birth weight place the child at risk of displaying below-normal cognitive development. Premature and low-birth-weight infants need frequent, thorough neurologic and developmental examinations, particularly in the first 2 years of life. Premature infants are expected to reach developmental milestones at approximately the same age as infants born at normal gestational age. For example, an infant born 2 months prematurely should be evaluated on milestones of an infant 2 months younger than the infant's current chronological age. The infant gradually catches up and reaches the chronological age milestones by about 2 years of age. Nurses should encourage parents to keep health promotion appointments and be sure the child receives developmental screening at each visit.

The child may require supportive care and assistance with activities of daily living (ADLs). The plans for intervention change as the child grows and family situations evolve. Some classes and community agencies offer transitional classes when children who are mentally retarded reach adolescence and young adulthood. These services help teach self-care skills that may enable some youth to live in group homes or other community settings. Families can receive help in planning for the child's future as parents look toward retirement. Information is provided on living options, health insurance, work opportunities, and other needs. Agencies that provide these services can also offer respite services for parents and other family members who have spent much time with the child for many years.

Nursing Management Nurses can help to identify children with mental retardation through history taking, observation, and developmental screening during early childhood. The history should provide information about the mental and adaptive functioning of birth parents and other family members, as mental retardation can have a genetic component. The pregnancy and birth history can provide important information relating to the mother's alcohol and drug use during pregnancy. Nurses should be alert for a history of difficult pregnancy and problems during delivery.

When genetic conditions in the family predispose family members to mental retardation, careful assessment of the child is needed. Children from deprived environments or those at risk from environmental hazards, such as lead poisoning, are more likely to manifest mental retardation.

Many children with mental retardation are not diagnosed with the condition until they reach school age, particularly if the condition is mild or moderate. Early intervention, however, can help to enhance the child's functioning later. During home visits or clinic appointments, in child care centers, and during hospitalization, nurses should be alert for signs of developmental delays, multiple (more than three) physical anomalies associated with a specific condition, or neurologic alterations. Developmental assessment should be part of each health care visit.

Once the diagnosis of mental retardation has been made, the nurse assesses the adaptive functioning of the child and family. A functional assessment of the child should be performed, including toileting, dressing, and feeding skills. The child's language, sensory, and psychomotor functioning are assessed, as well as the home and community for safety hazards. The nurse observes how the family is managing with the child. The availability of services, such as support groups for parents and special education opportunities for children, is assessed. The coping skills of family members are evaluated.

Several nursing diagnoses may be appropriate for the child with mental retardation, depending on the degree, cause, and outcome of the condition. Diagnoses that relate to impairments in adaptive functioning and family impact include the following:

- Delayed Growth and Development related to neonatal disease or condition
- Imbalanced Nutrition; Less Than Body Requirements related to inability to ingest sufficient food
- Self-Care Deficit (dressing, toileting, bathing) related to developmental disability
- Impaired Verbal Communication related to developmental disability
- Risk for Injury related to lack of understanding of environmental hazards
- Compromised Family Coping related to the child's developmental variations.

Prevention is important for some types of mental retardation. All pregnant women or those who are trying to become pregnant should stop ingestion of alcohol and nonprescription drugs. Encourage regular prenatal visits; these help to prevent premature births, which have a higher association with mental retardation than birth at term.

Nearly all children with mental retardation are cared for in the community; however, they may have conditions that require periodic hospitalization or frequent health care visits. When needed, nursing care focuses on providing emotional support and information to family members, assisting the child with adaptive functioning, and fostering parental management of the child's activities. When possible, the nurse uses preventive teaching to lower the risk of mental retardation.

Family members need empathy and support both at the time of diagnosis and in the ensuing years. Following initial diagnoses, parents may enter an acute or chronic state of grief over the loss of the perfect child. The nurse should encourage them to verbalize their feelings. Introducing them to parents of other mentally retarded children may provide assistance and support as they learn how to manage the child's needs. The availability of respite care to provide parents with a break from caretaking is discussed. Other family members may also be experiencing grief or guilt and should be given an opportunity to talk about their feelings.

Parents need honest information and answers to their questions about the child's condition. The nurse should reinforce information provided by genetic counselors and other health care professionals. Parents need help accessing information about community resources designed to assist children with mental retardation. Such resources include the Zero to Three Project, special education preschools and schools, county health services, and respite care. The nurse refers parents to Internet sources and helps them to interpret information received and analyze its strengths and limitations. The nurse should ask parents if they

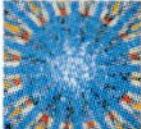

CLIENT TEACHING Fetal Alcohol Syndrome

Fetal alcohol syndrome (FAS) is a preventable cause of mental retardation. About 10% of women consume alcohol while pregnant, and 2% engage in frequent or binge drinking (Suellentrop, Morrow, Williams, D'Angels, 2006). This indicates that all women must receive clear messages about the dangers of drinking while pregnant. Teach all pregnant women that total abstention from alcohol for the entire length of pregnancy is the only completely effective method of preventing FAS. Include this in teaching to all adolescent girls, so they are aware of how alcohol can harm their infant if they become pregnant. Emphasize that the most dangerous time may be early in pregnancy before women commonly know they are pregnant.

have questions about individualized education plans (IEPs), and review federal and state laws and services that might be helpful to the family, including the following:

- Administration on Developmental Disabilities (ADD) is the U.S. organization that ensures that the Developmental Disabilities Act goals are met. The agency implements the Developmental Disabilities and Bill of Rights Act of 2000 and seeks to enhance life through training activities, educating the community, eliminating barriers, and influencing policy (Administration for Children and Families, 2004).
- State councils on developmental disabilities (SCDDs) are present in each state to increase integration of children with developmental disabilities.
- Public Law (PL) 94–142 of 1975 mandates that all children, even those with handicaps, be provided with public education and related services (Box 4–3).
- PL 99–457 of 1986 expanded the services of PL 94–142 to include children from birth to 5 years who need special education. Its focus is the importance of fostering development and enhancing the capacity of families to meet the needs of children.
- PL 101–336 of 1990 is known as the American Disabilities Act (ADA). It prohibits discrimination and ensures equal opportunity for persons with disabilities in employment, state and local government services, public accommodations, commercial facilities, and transportation.
- Individuals with Disabilities Education Act Amendments (IDEA) of 1997 strengthened the academic expectations and accountability for children with disabilities.

Box 4–3 Education for All Handicapped Children Act

The Education for All Handicapped Children Act, P.L. 94–142, provides free appropriate public education to all handicapped children between 2 and 21 years of age. Amendments to this act in 1986 (P.L. 99–457) encouraged states to provide early intervention services for infants and toddlers with developmental delay by providing federal funding. This act and its amendments also include language specifically designed to protect the rights of parent and child and to ensure parent participation in the educational process.

PRACTICE ALERT

To determine the impact of the child with mental retardation on the family, the nurse asks parents to describe (1) family activities that include the child, (2) strategies that parents and siblings use to deal with community attitudes about the child, and, (3) in the case of a child with other disabilities, methods of managing the child's care and planning for future care needs.

Children with mental retardation require close supervision because they may lack an understanding of common hazards. The nurse ensures safety in the hospital environment. The nurse assists parents in providing safety at home and school and teaching their child such necessary skills as pedestrian safety. Both physical and emotional safety should be considered. This type of child may be overly trusting of others and can be at risk for physical or sexual abuse.

Parents should be encouraged in efforts to maximize the child's areas of strength and identify needs related to adaptive behaviors. The nurse refers parents to resources to assist in the areas of adaptive functioning in which the child has impairment, such as communication, self-care activities, or social skills. During hospitalization, the nurse can support parents' efforts to maintain the child's skills in toileting, dressing, and self-care by planning interventions to use the skills being taught at home.

The child with mental retardation needs ongoing care throughout childhood, and adaptation of interventions as development occurs and the family's needs evolve. Parents often act as case managers for the child's care. The nurse can assist parents as necessary to acquire the skills required to coordinate the child's plan of care. The child's needs should be evaluated regularly and the parents asked to assist with the treatment plan as necessary. The nurse assists with plans for education and services such as physical or speech therapy. Most children with mental retardation have an IEP designed to meet their specific learning needs. Parents, nurses, and other professionals such as teachers and language therapists are part of the team that establishes this plan. All team members work together to promote optimal development and socialization. As the child reaches adolescence, education is directed toward a vocation, issues of sexuality, and the goal of independent living, when appropriate.

Specific guidelines for care are available for the child with Down syndrome. These guidelines suggest times for evaluation of hearing, growth, cardiac function, and other areas designed for early identification and treatment of associated disorders (Van Cleve & Cohen, 2006). There are specific growth grids for children with Down syndrome, and specific topics to suggest for anticipatory guidance during health care visits.

The expected outcomes of nursing care depend on the child's needs and developmental level. Early in the diagnostic phase, desired outcomes may involve the family's understanding of the diagnosis and the child's special needs. Later outcomes may focus on the child's communication and self-help skills. Outcomes related to cognitive performance and adaptive skills may be developed during childhood.

PRACTICE ALERT

Children with learning disabilities or mental retardation are at greater risk of abuse than their typically developing peers. They may also have more difficulty verbalizing or explaining the abuse. The reasons for this risk are many, including the increased emotional and economic stress these children place, unintentionally of course, on their parents. Nurses working with children with these special needs should be alert for any evidence of abuse, but should also be aware that some disabilities can cause injuries that mimic abuse. After careful assessment, a nurse who suspects a child has been abused should immediately report her suspicions to the local child protective services agency.

Dementia

Dementia is a progressive loss of cognitive function. It is critical that dementia be differentiated from delirium, an acute and reversible syndrome. Both may be characterized by changes in memory, judgment, language, mathematic calculation, abstract reasoning, and problem-solving ability.

Dementia affects multiple cortical functions. Impairments of cognitive function are usually accompanied by deterioration in emotional control, social behavior, and motivation. People with dementia lose their ability to solve problems and may experience personality changes including agitation and hallucinations. All forms of dementia result from death of neurons and/or the loss of communication among the cells. Although the exact cause is not always known, many forms of dementia are characterized by abnormal structures in the brain called inclusions. While a genetic component clearly exists in the development of some kinds of dementia, there may be no known family history of the condition in an individual who develops dementia.

It is estimated that as many as 6.8 million people in the United States have dementia, and at least 1.8 million of those are severely affected. Studies of some communities have found that almost half of all people age 85 and older have some form of dementia. However, despite increased incidence in older people, dementia is not a normal part of aging (National Institute of Neurological Disorders and Stroke, 2005b).

Many diseases and conditions may cause dementia, including Alzheimer's disease, vascular dementia, Huntington's disease, Creutzfeldt-Jakob disease, metabolic disorders, poisoning and anoxia, and medications. Table 4–3 provides an overview of its most common causes. Doctors do not diagnose dementia unless two or more brain functions (such as memory, language skills, perception, reasoning, or judgment) are significantly impaired without loss of consciousness. The most common type of dementia is Alzheimer's disease (AD).

Even though the actual cause of all dementias may not be known, risk factors for developing one or more kinds of dementia have been identified. These include advancing age, a family history of a disease that causes dementia, smoking and alcohol use, atherosclerosis, high cholesterol and plasma homocysteine levels, diabetes, mild cognitive impairment, and Down syndrome.

People often experience other conditions that may mimic dementia. These include the following:

- Age-related cognitive decline, resulting from slower information processing and mild memory impairment. With aging, the brain often decreases in volume and some neurons are lost. These changes are normal and are not considered a part of dementia.
- Mild cognitive impairment, which may progress to dementia, but is not severe enough to be initially diagnosed as such.
- Depression or other emotional problems that cause people to be passive, slow, confused, or forgetful.
- Delirium, characterized by confusion, rapidly altering mental states, disorientation, and possible personality changes. Delirium is usually caused by a treatable physical or mental health illness and, when treated, results in a full recovery.

Dementia can be difficult to diagnose in its early stages, primarily because an individual experiencing dementia may not notice these slight gradual changes until they become more pronounced or he or she may deny experiencing any changes. This can present challenges for family members: An older person with early dementia may blame others for hiding or stealing his or her

TABLE 4–3 **Common Causes of Dementia**

NAME	CAUSE AND PRIMARY PATHOPHYSIOLOGY
Alzheimer's disease (the most common cause of dementia in people age 65 and older)	Cause is unknown; characterized by two abnormalities in the brain: amyloid plaques and neurofibrillary tangles.
Vascular dementia (the second most common cause of dementia)	Caused by brain damage from cerebrovascular and cardiovascular problems (usually strokes). May also be caused by cerebral blood vessel damage from genetic disorders, endocarditis, myeloid angiopathy, vasculitis, and profound hypotension.
Lewy body dementia	Cause is usually unknown, although familial cases have been reported. Cells die, and remaining cells in the substantia nigra contain abnormal structures called Lewy bodies.
Frontotemporal dementia	Nerve cells, especially in the frontal and temporal lobes, degenerate. In many people, abnormal tau protein accumulates in neurofibrillary tangles.

TABLE 4–4 Common Deficits Associated With Dementia

DEFICIT	CLINICAL MANIFESTATIONS
Akathisia	Inability to keep still; feeling of restlessness
Anomia	Difficulty naming persons or objects; no impairment of comprehension
Aphasia/paraphasia	Impairment of comprehension and expression of language (both verbal and written)
Ataxia	Poor muscle control during voluntary movement, poor balance
Carphologia/floccillation	Involuntary, repeated picking at bedding and clothing
Constructional difficulty	Difficulty assembling blocks, drawing or copying three-dimensional figures
Dysphagia	Difficult or painful swallowing
Echolalia	Involuntary repetition of words or sentences just spoken by another person

belongings when, in reality, he or she has simply misplaced them. These delusions can be hurtful to family and friends who are attempting to assist the older person and may result in increased social isolation and conflict within the family.

An individual with dementia may experience one or more of several cognitive deficits. These can be mild, as in the case of anomia, or more pronounced, as with paraphasia. Some of these deficits are listed in Table 4–4.

Other alterations related to cognition that are not addressed as part of this concept include, but are not limited to, mental illness.

PHYSICAL ASSESSMENT

A physical assessment should be conducted at each office visit or health care interaction to determine any potential changes in the cognitive state of an older person. Nurses should conduct a cognitive assessment using tools such as those listed in Table 4–5. One of the most frequently used is the Mini-Mental State Exam (MMSE), a short, 30-question test used to assess the extent of cognitive impairment. The MMSE can be used to assess for changes in cognitive function over time. Frequently used as a screening tool for Alzheimer's disease, the MMSE assesses cognitive function in a number of areas, including language, mathematics, memory, and motor skills.

Nurses should also be alert for any need to assess for depression in the older individual, particularly one who has recently experienced a dramatic life change. Typical changes that can result in depression include moving out of a lifelong home to a new environment and the loss of a spouse or family member. The Geriatric Depression Scale (GDS) is a screening instrument used in many clinical settings to assess depression in older people. The GDS is a 30-item (long version) or 15-item (short version) instrument with questions that can be answered "yes" or "no." An older person can complete the GDS alone by circling the correct answer, or have it read to him or her. When tested in various groups of older people, the GDS was found to distinguish successfully between depressed and nondepressed older people (Yesavage et al., 1983). The GDS can be used for screening physically healthy or ill individuals and those with cognitive impairment (Hartford Institute for Geriatric Nursing, 2008). Older people scoring above 10 should be referred for further assessment. The Cornell Depression Scale (CDS) can be used to screen for depression in older adults with severe cognitive impairments (MMSE below 15).

The Senses and Cognition

Clients who are out of contact with reality may display illusional, delusional, and hallucinatory speech and behaviors, such as talking to themselves (auditory hallucinations); reacting to objects, noises, or other people in strange ways (illusions); or discussing false beliefs (delusions). Direct questioning may increase the client's anxiety and escalate the abnormal behavior or cause confusion. The nurse should use direct questioning only when the client appears to be in control and in touch with reality.

TABLE 4–5 Tools for Assessment of Mental Status

TOOL	ASSESSMENT
Mini-Mental State Examination (MMSE)	Cognitive status—conducted via interview
Addenbrooke's Cognitive Examination	Detects early dementia
Confusion Assessment Method (CAM)	Tests for delirium
Telephone Interview Telephone Interview for Cognitive Status (TICS)for Cognitive Status (TICS)	Similar to MMSE, cognitive function assessed via telephone interview
Cornell Scale for Depression in Dementia	Assessment of behavioral problems
Dementia Symptoms Scale	Assessment of behavioral problems
Psychogeriatric Dependency Rating Scale	Assessment of behavioral problems
Hopkins Competency Assessment Test	Assessment of ability to make decisions about health care
General Health Questionnaire	Assessment of emotional disturbance in those with normal cognitive ability
Hamilton Depression Rating Scale	Assessment of depression in clients with impaired cognition
Short Portable Mental Status Questionnaire (SPMSQ)	Assessment of organic brain deficit

Cognitive Assessment

Techniques and Normal Findings | **Abnormal Findings Special Considerations**

Mental Status

The nurse assesses the mental status of the client when meeting the client for the first time. This process begins with taking the health history and continues with each client contact.

A variety of tools are available to conduct mental status assessment. These tools are described in Table 4–5.

1. Instruct the client.

- Explain to the client that you will be conducting a variety of tests. Tell the client that you will provide instructions before beginning each examination. Explain that moving about and changing position during the examination will be required. Provide reassurance that the tests will not cause discomfort; however, the client must inform you of problems if they arise during any part of the assessment. Identify the types of equipment you will use and describe the purpose in relation to neurologic function. Tell the client that you will begin the assessment with some general questions about the present and past. Then you will ask the client to respond to number and word questions.

2. Position the client.

- The client should be sitting on the examination table wearing an examination gown (see Figure 4–3 ■).

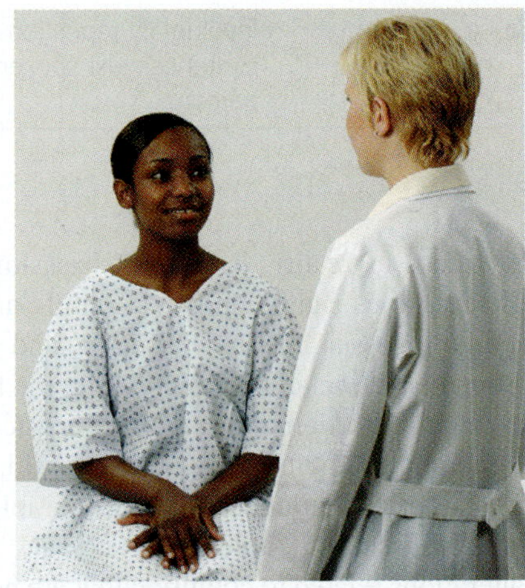

Figure 4–3 ■ Positioning the client.

3. Observe the client.

- Look at the client and note hygiene, grooming, posture, body language, facial expressions, speech, and ability to follow directions.

Changes could be indicative of depression, schizophrenia, organic brain syndrome, or obsessive-compulsive disorder.

4. Note the client's speech and language abilities.

- Throughout the assessment, note the client's rate of speech, ability to pronounce words, tone of voice, loudness or softness (volume) of voice, and ability to speak smoothly and clearly.
- Assess the client's choice of words, ability to respond to questions, and ease with which a response is made.

Changes in speech could reflect anxiety, Parkinson's disease, depression, or various forms of aphasia.

5. Assess the client's sensorium.

- Determine the client's orientation to date, time, place, and reason for being here. Grade the level of alertness on a scale from full alertness to coma.

Neurologic disease can produce a sliding or changing degree of alertness. Change in the level of consciousness may be related to cortical or brain stem disease. A stroke, seizure, or hypoglycemia could also contribute to a change in the level of consciousness.

Cognitive Assessment (continued)

Techniques and Normal Findings | **Abnormal Findings Special Considerations**

6. Assess the client's memory.

- Ask for the client's date of birth, Social Security number, names and ages of any children or grandchildren, educational history with dates and events, work history with dates, and job descriptions. Ask questions for which the response can be verified.

Loss of long-term memory may indicate cerebral cortex damage, which occurs in Alzheimer's disease.

7. Assess the client's ability to calculate problems.

- Start with a simple problem, such as 4 + 3, 8 ÷ 2, and 15 − 4.
- Progress to more difficult problems, such as (10 × 4) − 8, or ask the client to start with 100 and subtract 7 (100 − 7 = 93, 93 − 7 = 86, 86 − 7 = 79, and so on).
- Remember to use problems that are appropriate for the developmental, educational, and intellectual level of the client.
  - Asking the client to calculate change from one dollar for the purchase of items costing 25, 39, and 89 cents is a quick test of calculation.

Inability to calculate simple problems may indicate the presence of organic brain disease, or it may simply indicate lack of exposure to mathematical concepts, nervousness, or an incomplete understanding of the examiner's language. In an otherwise unremarkable assessment, a poor response to calculations should not be considered an abnormal finding.

8. Assess the client's ability to think abstractly.

- Ask the client to identify similarities and differences between two objects or topics, such as wood and coal, king and president, orange and apple, and pear and celery. Quote a proverb and ask the client to explain its meaning. For example:
  - "A stitch in time saves nine."
  - "The empty barrel makes the most noise."
  - "Don't put all your eggs in one basket."
- Be aware that age and culture influence the ability to explain American proverbs and slang terms.

Responses made by the client may reflect lack of education, mental retardation, or dementia. Clients with personality disorders such as schizophrenia or depression may make bizarre responses.

9. Assess the client's mood and emotional state.

- Observe the client's body language, facial expressions, and communication technique. The facial expression and tone of voice should be congruent with the content and context of the communication.
- Ask if the client generally feels this way or if he or she has experienced a change and if so over what period of time.
- Ask the client if it is possible to identify an event or incident that fostered the change in mood or emotional state.
- The client's mood and emotions should reflect the current situation or response to events that trigger mood change or call for an emotional response (e.g., a change in health status, a loss, or a stressful event).

Lack of congruence of facial expression and tone of voice with the content and context of communication may occur with neurologic problems, emotional disturbance, or a psychogenic disorder such as schizophrenia or depression.

Lack of emotional response, lack of change in facial expression, and flat voice tones can indicate problems with mood or emotional responses. Other abnormal findings in relation to mood and emotional state include anxiety, depression, fear, anger, overconfidence, ambivalence, euphoria, impatience, and irritability. Mood disorders are associated with bipolar disorder, anxiety disorders, and major depression.

10. Assess perceptions and thought processes.

- Listen to the client's statements. Statements should be logical and relevant. The client should complete his or her thoughts.
- Determining the client's awareness of reality assesses perception.

Disturbed thought processes can indicate neurologic dysfunction or mental disorder.

Disturbances in sense of reality can include hallucination and illusion. These are associated with mental disturbances as seen in schizophrenia.

11. Assess the client's ability to make judgments.

- Determine if the client is able to evaluate situations and to decide upon a realistic course of action. For example, ask the client about future plans related to employment.
- The plans should reflect the reality of the client's health, psychological stability, and family situation and obligations. The client's responses should reflect an ability to think abstractly.

Impaired judgment can occur in emotional disturbances, schizophrenia, and neurologic dysfunction.

Assessment Interview Cognition

The following questions are helpful in gathering additional information. The nurse should preface these questions by explaining to the client that some of them may seem silly or unimportant, but they are helpful in assessing memory.

- What is your name?
- How old are you?
- Where were you born?
- Where are you right now?
- What day of the week is it? What is the date?
  Questions 1 through 5 determine whether the client is oriented to person, place, and time.
- What would you take with you if a fire broke out?
  This tests the client's ability to make a judgment.
- Count backward from 10 to 1.
  This question tests cognitive function.
- What did you have for breakfast?
  This question tests recent memory.
- Who were the last two presidents?
  This tests remote memory.
- Describe what the following statement means: People who live in glass houses shouldn't throw stones.
  This question tests the client's ability to do abstract or symbolic thinking.
- Are you having any problems thinking? If so, describe what happens.
  The client may not be able to answer this question if a thought disorder is present. Clients with bipolar disorders and who are manic describe their thoughts as "racing."
- Do you have trouble making decisions? Describe what happens when you have to make a decision.
  The inability to make decisions may indicate depression or low self-esteem.
- Do you ever hear voices, see objects, or experience other sensations that don't make sense? If so, describe your experiences.
  The client who is out of touch with reality may experience auditory, visual, gustatory, somatic, and olfactory hallucinations (hearing, seeing, tasting, feeling, and smelling stimuli that are not real). Discussing hallucinatory experiences in detail may reinforce them for the client; therefore, it is important not to dwell on these symptoms with the client.
- If you hear voices, do they tell you what you must do?
  The nurse asks this question to determine if the client is experiencing command hallucinations. These are dangerous hallucinations that may lead the client to self-destructive behavior or to harm others.
- Do you ever misinterpret objects, sounds, or smells? If so, please describe.
  Clients who are very anxious or out of contact with reality may experience illusions (misinterpretation of environmental stimuli).

It is important to assess the content of a client's hallucinations and delusions in order to provide for the client's safety and the safety of others. Command hallucinations tell clients to carry out acts against themselves or others that are usually harmful. These command hallucinations may be part of an elaborate delusional system in which clients feel persecuted or in danger. In some cases, clients are disturbed by these thoughts and share them with others. In other situations, clients keep their thoughts to themselves, and these thoughts do not become apparent until they commit some violent act. A client who demonstrates these symptoms should be referred to a psychiatric/mental health nurse or clinical specialist who has the skill and expertise needed to uncover hallucinatory and delusional thinking without exacerbating the symptoms.

PHARMACOLOGIC THERAPIES

Pharmacologic treatment and research of chemicals to treat cognitive disorders are primarily aimed at reducing the effect of Alzheimer's disease, which is discussed in the Confusion exemplar. Though acetylcholinesterase inhibitors have been the mainstay in the treatment of Alzheimer's dementia, several other agents are being investigated for their possible benefit in delaying the progression of Alzheimer's, including anti-inflammatory agents, cyclooxygenase 2 (COX-2) inhibitors, estrogen, ginkgo biloba, and antioxidants. Agitation accompanying delusions, dementia, and delirium may be treated with antipsychotic agents, such as risperidone (Risperdal) and olanzapine (Zyprexa). Conventional antipsychotics such as haloperidol (Haldol) are occasionally prescribed, although extrapyramidal side effects often limit their use. Anxiety and depression, which may occur less frequently than agitation with delusions, dementia, and delirium, may be treated with anxiolytics, including buspirone (BuSpar) or some of the benzodiazepines, to control unease and apprehension. Mood stabilizers such as sertraline (Zoloft), citalopram (Celexa), or fluoxetine (Prozac) are given when major depression interferes with daily activities. Although Alzheimer's is the most common cause of dementia, there are other causes as well. A physician working with a client who exhibits dementia will likely conduct a number of tests to rule out other causes, and prescribe other or additional medications as necessary to address other or additional conditions that may cause dementia. One example is excess calcium, which has been found to cause lesions and narrow blood vessels in the brain. A physician may prescribe a calcium channel blocker in addition to acetylcholinesterase inhibitors for a client with dementia.

4.1 ALZHEIMER'S DISEASE

KEY TERMS

Affect, *211*
Agraphia, *215*
Alzheimer's disease *211*
Amyloid plaques, *212*
Apraxia, *215*
Astereognosis, *215*
Neurofibrillary tangles, *212*
Sundowning, *215*
Tau, *212*

BASIS FOR SELECTION OF EXEMPLAR

National Institute of Mental Health
National Center for Health Statistics
Healthy People 2010
Centers for Disease Control and Prevention

LEARNING OUTCOMES

After reading about this exemplar, you will be able to:

1. Describe the pathophysiology, etiology, clinical manifestations, and direct and indirect causes of Alzheimer's disease.
2. Identify risk factors associated with Alzheimer's disease.
3. Illustrate the nursing process in providing culturally competent care across the life span for individuals with Alzheimer's disease.
4. Formulate priority nursing diagnoses appropriate for an individual with Alzheimer's disease.
5. Create a plan of care for individuals with Alzheimer's disease and their family members.
6. Assess expected outcomes for an individual with Alzheimer's disease.
7. Discuss therapies used in the collaborative care of an individual with Alzheimer's disease.
8. Employ evidence-based caring interventions for an individual with Alzheimer's disease.

OVERVIEW

Dementia is a progressive loss of cognitive function characterized by changes in memory, judgment, language, mathematic calculation, abstract reasoning, and problem-solving ability. The client's **affect**, which is an outward manifestation of what a person is feeling, is often affected as cognition becomes significantly impacted. It is important to differentiate between *dementia* (chronic, irreversible) and *delirium* (acute, usually reversible), which is characterized by a reduced ability to focus and maintain attention with altered perception (Table 4–6).

The most common cause of dementia is **Alzheimer's disease** (AD), although there are many other types. AD is named after Dr. Alois Alzheimer, who first described the disease in a 55-year-old woman in 1906. As many as 5.3 million people in the United States have AD, costing health insurance entities and businesses as much as $148 billion in direct and indirect costs (Alzheimer's Association, 2009). Although AD is more common in people over age 65, its onset may occur as early as middle adulthood. Clients with AD live about 8–10 years following diagnosis, although some live as long as 20 years. The cause of death is often aspiration pneumonia because of the loss of the ability to swallow late in the disease (NINDS, 2005i).

It is estimated that about 1 million people with AD are cared for in the home. The burden of care is frequently on women—wives and daughters—who are themselves aging. AD is devastating for the families and caregivers of its victims. Caregivers often experience physical and emotional exhaustion while they render continuous care. Caregiving is complicated when the client no longer recognizes family members or close friends. The nurse's responsibility is to provide supportive nursing care, accurate information, and referral assistance as needed. It is important for the nurse to do an ongoing assessment of both the client and caregiver because changes will occur as the client's condition deteriorates.

Many long-term care facilities offer specialized units for clients with AD, especially those in advanced stages of the disease. The gerontological nurses working in Alzheimer's units have specialized knowledge and help family members understand and cope with the disease process affecting their loved one.

PATHOPHYSIOLOGY AND ETIOLOGY

Memory loss is usually the first sign of AD. Memory deficits are initially subtle; family members and friends may not suspect a problem until the disease progresses and manifestations become more noticeable. Family members and clients with AD also may deny the manifestations and hide deficits until the person exhibits unsafe or extremely unusual behavior. Progression of the disease varies, but the course is one of deteriorating cognition and judgment with eventual physical decline and total inability to perform activities of daily living

TABLE 4–6 **Dementia and Delirium Compared**

	DEMENTIA	DELIRIUM
Onset	Onset of impairment generally slow and insidious	Onset usually sudden; acute development of impairment of orientation, memory, cognitive function, judgment, and affect
Essential feature	Not based on disordered consciousness; however, delirium, stupor, and coma may occur	Clouded state of consciousness
Etiology	Generally caused by irreversible alteration of brain function	Caused by temporary, reversible, diffuse disturbances of brain function
Course	No diurnal fluctuations. Clinical course usually progresses over months or years, ending in death.	Short, diurnal fluctuations in symptoms. Clinical course is usually brief, although it may last for months. Untreated, prolonged delirium may cause permanent brain destruction and lead to dementia.
History	Onset: insidious Duration: months to years Course: consistent deterioration with occasional lucid moments	Onset: sudden Duration: hours to days Course: fluctuating arousal
Motor signs	None (until late) Speech is usually normal in early stages, but word-finding difficulties progress.	Postural tremor, restless, hyperactive, or sluggish Slurred speech, reflecting disorganized thinking
Mental status	Attention generally normal in early stages; inattention progresses	Fluctuations in attention
Memory	Memory impairment; recent memory affected before remote	Impaired by poor attention
Language	Aphasia in later stages	Normal or mild misnaming of objects
Perception	Hallucinations not prominent, although cognitive impairment may lead to paranoid delusions	Visual, auditory, and/or tactile hallucinations
Pronounced mood/affect	Disinterested and/or disinhibited	Fear and suspiciousness may be prominent; anxiety, depression, anger, irritability, or euphoria may occur.
Review of systems	Extraneural organ systems usually involved	History of systemic illness or toxic exposure
EEG	Normal or mildly slow	Pronounced diffuse slowing of fast cycles relates to state of arousal.

(ADLs). As the client's abilities to perform tasks decrease, the caregiver's burdens increase until eventually the caregiver must perform the most basic ADLs for the client.

Pathophysiological changes associated with AD are degenerative and result in gross atrophy of the cerebral cortex. As the disease destroys brain cells, two types of abnormalities occur: neurofibrillary tangles and amyloid plaques.

Neurofibrillary tangles are thick, insoluble clots of protein inside the damaged brain cells or neurons. They result when **tau**, a kind of protein in the neurons, becomes distorted and twisted. Tau normally holds together the microtubules, which guide nutrients and molecules to the end of the axon. In AD, tau changes and twists into pairs of filaments, which then join to form tangles. Because tau no longer maintains the transport system, communication between neurons is lost. Death of neurons may follow, contributing to the development of dementia.

When groups of nerve cells (especially the terminal axons) degenerate and clump around an amyloid core in the spaces between the neurons of the brain, they form **amyloid plaques**. These plaques consist primarily of insoluble deposits of beta-amyloid, a protein fragment from a larger protein called amyloid precursor protein (APP), mixed with other neurons and nonnerve cells. The enzyme beta-secretase appears to play a key role in increasing the buildup of amyloid plaques. The plaques, which develop first in areas used for memory and cognition, disrupt transmission of nerve impulses. It is not yet known whether plaque formation causes AD or is a by-product of the AD process.

Galanin is a neuropeptide thought to play a role in the pathophysiology of AD. Galanin rescues neurons that are in distress by slowing down the cells and eventually immobilizing them so that repairs can be made. The destruction of cells in AD leads to twice the normal level of galanin as the condition worsens. Excess galanin inhibits access to memory, especially visual memory, which may explain why people with AD easily become lost in their own neighborhoods because they

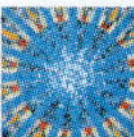

FOCUS ON DIVERSITY AND CULTURE Caring for Family Members With Alzheimer's Disease

Cultural variations play a large role in determining where older adults diagnosed with Alzheimer's disease will receive care. In Japan and China, family commitment to older adults is strong and family members prefer to care for their aging parents and relatives in the home, avoiding institutionalization in favor of shared responsibilities among children, grandchildren, and extended family members. Those from European cultures may attempt home care but often consider long-term care facilities when the needs of the older adult exceed the ability of the family to provide safe care. Families from Latino cultures place great value on family, including extended family, and care decisions are often made as a group with preference given to providing care of the older adult diagnosed with AD in the home, although institutionalization is considered if required to maintain safety of both the client and family.

cannot remember landmarks. Drug antagonists to galanin do not cross the blood–brain barrier and must be injected directly into the brain. Researchers are trying to develop oral antagonists because of their potential to slow the progression of this disease (Counts et al., 2006).

The death of neurons in AD follows a specific pattern. The first nerves to die are in the limbic system, the center for emotion and memory. The limbic system interprets emotional responses from the cerebral cortex, and the hippocampus, a part of the limbic system, is involved in memory storage. Destruction of the hippocampus results in loss of recent memory. Remote memory loss occurs more slowly, possibly because the memories are stored in more than one location in the brain. AD often brings on depression related to limbic system damage, as well as damage to the locus ceruleus, which modulates mood and stress response. The destruction of neurons spreads toward the surface of the brain, killing nerve cells in the cerebral cortex. Various symptoms appear as the destruction spreads throughout the four lobes. See Table 4–7 for symptoms related to central nervous system (CNS) destruction.

Blood flow to the affected areas of the brain decreases. Computed tomography (CT) scans may show brain atrophy, widened cortical sulci, and enlarged cerebral ventricles. AD is characterized by atrophy of the cortical area of the brain and loss of neurons, especially in the parietal and temporal lobes. With significant atrophy and loss of brain tissue, the ventricles enlarge (a form of hydrocephalus) (Porth, 2005). As AD progresses, more areas of the brain are affected, with manifestations correlating to those areas. For example, neuronal and neurotransmitter losses in the parietal lobe result in problems with perception and interpretation of environmental stimuli; and deficits in the frontal lobe cause changes in personality and emotional lability (exaggerated changes in mood).

Several structural and chemical changes in the brain occur with AD, especially in the hippocampus and the frontal and temporal lobes of the cerebral cortex. As AD destroys neurons in the hippocampus and related structures, short-term memory fails and the ability to perform easy and familiar tasks declines. The effect of AD on neurons in the cerebral cortex is loss of language skills and judgment. Emotional outbursts and behavior changes (such as tendency to wander and agitation) begin to occur and become more frequent as the disease progresses. Eventually, other areas of the brain are affected; all affected areas begin to atrophy, and the person becomes totally helpless and unresponsive.

Etiology

Alzheimer's disease is the most common degenerative neurologic disorder and the most common cause of cognitive impairment in older adults (Porth, 2005). It accounts for approximately two thirds of cases of dementia in the United States, affecting adults in middle to late life. AD accounts for 60–70% of late-onset dementia and affects about 4.8 million Americans. The current annual costs are approximately $200 billion in the United States, $3.9 billion in Canada, and $87 billion in Europe. AD strikes 1 of 12 people older than 65, 1 of 3 people older than 80, and almost 1 of 2 people older than 85. Onset usually occurs late in life, but

TABLE 4–7 CNS Pathways of Destruction

AREA	FUNCTION	SYMPTOMS
Limbic system	Memory, interpretation of emotion	Problems with recent and later remote memory; depression; apathy; unstable affect
Hippocampus	Memory storage	Decreased ability to learn; memory loss
Frontal lobe	Cognition, planning; motor aspects of speech; control of movement; control of outbursts; insight into own behavior	Problems with planning activities; inability to carry out skilled, purposeful movement; catastrophic reactions and emotional outbursts; delusions; inability to walk, talk, swallow
Parietal lobe	Sensory speech and ability to recognize written words; proprioception; ability to recognize objects and their function	Inability to recognize familiar places, people, and purpose of common household objects; expressive aphasia; agraphia; agnosia; hallucinations; seizures; falls
Temporal lobe	Memory, judgment, learning; ability to understand spoken words	Receptive aphasia; problems with memory and learning new concepts or activities
Occipital lobe	Ability to understand written words	Inability to read with comprehension; hallucinations

in rare cases, the disorder appears at age 40 or 50. Slightly more women than men are affected, even when controlling for a longer life span (Wimo, Winblad, Shah, Chin, Zhang, & McRae, 2004).

Two types of AD exist: familial AD (FAD), which follows an inheritance pattern, and sporadic AD, which has no obvious inheritance pattern. Approximately 15–20% of AD cases are inherited. Because FAD often begins at a much younger age than AD, it also is referred to as early-onset AD. Early-onset AD occurs in people aged 30–65; late onset AD occurs in people aged 65 and older. Early-onset AD is relatively rare and often progresses more rapidly than late-onset AD.

GENETICS The cause of AD is unknown, but is likely a combination of aging and genetic and environmental factors. Research continues in an effort to understand the biochemical events responsible for the destruction of brain cells. Research currently is focused on the role of chromosomes 1, 14, 19, and 21 and the APP gene. APP is the precursor of beta-amyloid protein, which accumulates into plaques in AD.

People with Down syndrome, which is caused by an extra copy of chromosome 21 that includes the APP gene, are at high risk for lesions in the brain similar to those seen in AD. It is estimated that 75% of people with Down syndrome older than 60 have dementia, with neurobiological changes postmortem that are indistinguishable from those of AD (Krasuski, Alexander, Horwitz, Rapoport, & Schapiro, 2002).

Consensus is against genetic testing for AD. Tests are promising but lack the sensitivity and specificity for routine use. All of the possible genetic mutations also are unknown, which limits the predictability of genetic testing. If testing is available in the future, it will be necessary to protect against genetic discrimination by employers and insurers.

Risk Factors

As a person ages, the risk of developing AD increases. With numbers of older adults increasing, the incidence of AD is predicted to increase as well. The risk factors for AD are older age, family history, and female gender.

One environmental risk factor for AD is traumatic head injury. People who have experienced severe head injuries have a significant increase in the deposition of amyloid protein in the brain. The injury may decrease the functional reserves of the brain. It also is possible that damage to the blood–brain barrier allows entry of toxic products or somehow makes the brain more susceptible to the effects of aging (Lucas, Rothwell, & Gibson, 2006).

Protective Factors

Cigarette smoking may be a protective factor in both early- and late-onset AD. Smoking facilitates nicotinic receptor function and appears to delay signs and symptoms of AD.

The better educated people are, the less likely they are to experience dementia. It is believed that mental stimulation actually builds many more synapses between neurons, which allow individuals to better withstand the damages of disease. The same process is true for physical exercise. Drinking up to three glasses of wine daily is associated with a lower risk for AD. Intake of liquor or beer does not seem to provide protection (Larson et al., 2006; Ngandu et al., 2006).

CLINICAL MANIFESTATIONS

Warning signs for AD include the following:

- Memory loss that affects job skills
- Difficulty performing familiar tasks
- Problems with language
- Disorientation to time and place
- Poor or decreased judgment
- Problems with abstract thinking
- Likelihood of misplacing things
- Changes in mood or behavior
- Changes in personality
- Loss of initiative.

Recognizing early manifestations is important because early diagnosis can maximize quality of life and allow the affected person to plan for the future.

Mild cognitive impairment is often described as memory loss without dementia. In some cases, it may be a transitional state between normal aging and AD. In other cases, the cognitive impairment never worsens. If possible, it is important to distinguish between the two situations, as pharmacologic therapies exist that make it possible to delay the progression of AD (Modrego, Fayed, & Pina, 2005; Rose, 2005).

See Table 4–8 for a comparison of normal aging and Alzheimer's disease.

The average course of AD is 5–10 years, but the range may be 2–20 years. People who have early-onset AD often

TABLE 4–8 **Changes in Normal Aging and Changes in Alzheimer's Disease Compared**

NORMAL AGING	ALZHEIMER'S DISEASE
Recent memory more impaired than remote memory	Recent and remote memory profoundly affected
Difficulty in recalling names of people and places	Inability to recall names of people and places
Decreased concentration	Inability to concentrate
Writing things down is helpful in stimulating memory.	Inability to write; nothing stimulates memory
Changes do not interfere with daily functioning.	Changes cause an inability to function at work, in a social relationship, and at home.
Insight into forgetful behavior is preserved.	With progression, the person has no insight into changes that have occurred.

deteriorate more rapidly. The progression is divided roughly into three stages:

- **Stage 1 (Mild)** typically lasts 2–4 years, during which time the person is alert and sociable but forgetfulness begins to interfere with daily living. A client typically appears physically healthy and alert, and cognitive deficits may go undetected by the client unless thorough and periodic evaluations are performed. Family members may notice changes before the client does. Clients in stage 1 may seem restless, forgetful, or uncoordinated; they may lack spontaneity; and they may be disoriented as to time and date, although for some, this may come later. They display short-term memory loss and mild cognitive deficits that they attempt to cover up, and some problems occur with depth perception. In addition to lapses in memory, family members may notice subtle changes in personality or problems in doing simple calculations. AD clients and families may consciously or unconsciously compensate for cognitive deficits by adjusting schedules and routines.
- **Stage 2 (Moderate)** is often the longest stage of the disease, lasting 2–12 years. Memory deficits are more apparent, and the client is less able to behave spontaneously. Clients may wander and get lost, even in their own homes. Although progression of manifestations continues and orientation to place and time deteriorates, AD clients may still have periods of mental lucidity and engage in time-oriented conversations. Generally, however, clients become more confused and lose their sense of time, leading to changes in sleeping patterns, agitation, and stress. They have changes in personality, visuospatial deficits, impaired motor skills, and impaired judgment. They may demonstrate repetitive behavior and eat ravenously. AD clients are less able to make even simple decisions and to adapt to environmental changes and are often unable to carry out ADLs. **Sundowning** is another behavioral change that is characterized by increased agitation, time disorientation, and wandering behaviors during afternoon and evening hours; it is accelerated on overcast days. There is a deterioration of intellect, logic, behavior, and daily functioning. Diagnosis most often occurs during this stage. Day care or assisted home care may be necessary to ensure safety.
- **Stage 3 (Severe)** may last 1–2 years or longer and brings increasing dependence, with inability to communicate, loss of urinary and fecal continence, and progressive loss of cognitive abilities. People at this stage can no longer do basic self-care activities and usually require 24-hour care. They are extremely confused and lose most of their long-term memory. Communication skills are usually absent, and the client is frequently mute. Cognitive abilities and motor skills are grossly decreased or absent. Common complications include pneumonia, dehydration, malnutrition, falls, depression, delusions, seizures, and paranoid reactions. AD clients in this stage are indifferent to food and lose weight. They are unable to recognize family, friends, and even themselves. The average life expectancy is 1–2 years from the onset of stage 3, although the individual may live as long as 10 years. Most people with AD are institutionalized during this final stage of the disease. Death frequently occurs from pneumonia secondary to aspiration.

Language deficits are common in stage 2. They include *paraphasia* (using the wrong word), *echolalia* (repetition of words or phrases), and *scanning speech,* in which the client appears to search for words. Eventually, as the person moves into stage 3, total aphasia (absence of speech) may occur. Frustration and depression are common among AD clients as the full extent and implications of the deficits become obvious.

The AD client slowly loses the ability to perform simple tasks required for hygiene or eating because sequencing of tasks is lost. For example, the client may open a can of soup but not remember to pour it into a pan to heat it. Instead, the client might place the can directly on the burner and leave the heat on high even after a smoke alarm sounds. The AD client may falsely interpret the smoke alarm as a ringing telephone, a tornado warning siren, or an ambulance siren. Thus, safety is a high priority for the client in stage 2.

Sensorimotor deficits in stage 2 include **apraxia**, the inability to perform purposeful movements and use objects correctly; **astereognosis**, the inability to identify objects by touch; and **agraphia**, the inability to write properly. Problems related to malnutrition and decreased fluid intake, such as anemia and constipation, may be evident. Sleep pattern disturbances also are common and are related to the loss of time orientation, sundowning phenomenon, and depression.

Up to 50% of people with AD experience a comorbid depression, which increases the level of disability and hastens death. See Table 4–9 for a comparison of depression and dementia. It is imperative that depression from irreversible dementia be recognized and differentiated. Only through recognition can appropriate treatment measures be initiated (Zubenko et al., 2003).

It is critical that all other disease processes be identified and treated before a person is diagnosed with AD. Hamdy, Turnball, and Edwards (1994) developed the following differential diagnosis tool based on the word *dementia*:

D **Drugs and Alcohol.** Older adults often purchase over-the-counter medications, have many medications prescribed, and sometimes borrow medication from friends.

E **Eyes and Ears.** People who cannot hear or see well often appear confused.

M **Metabolic and Endocrine Diseases.** Disruptions such as electrolyte imbalance, hypothyroidism, and uncontrolled diabetes may mimic dementia.

E **Emotional Disorders.** Mood and schizophrenic disorders may be mistaken for AD.

N **Nutritional Deficiencies.** These may mimic dementia.

T **Tumors and Trauma.** Disorders of the CNS may be confused with AD.

I **Infection.** Infections of the urinary tract and pneumonia in older adults may lead to confusion. Clients might not have an elevated temperature.

A **Arteriosclerosis.** A decreased blood flow to the brain, brain attacks, and multi-infarct dementia often mimic AD.

TABLE 4–9 Depression and Dementia Compared

DEPRESSION	DEMENTIA
Relatively rapid onset	Insidious onset
Symptoms progress rapidly	Symptoms progress slowly
Able to recall recent events	Has difficulty recalling recent events
Has long-term memory	As disease progresses, loses long-term memory
"Don't know" answers are common	Uses confabulation rather than admitting "don't know"
Attention span normal	Impaired attention span
Affect is depressed	Affect is shallow and labile
Oriented to person, time, and place	Unable to recognize familiar people and places; becomes lost in familiar environments; disoriented as to time
Apathetic in relationship to ADLs	Struggles to perform ADLs and is frustrated as a result

Like any client with a chronic or progressive disease, AD clients can have good and bad days at any stage. A client in stage 1 or 2 may be more motivated and happier when visiting with family, which may cause the client to exhibit fewer symptoms during the visit. This in turn may cause family members who do not see the client often to believe that the client is not doing as poorly as others have described. A difficult or challenging event such as client hospitalization following a fall or caregiver illness and substitution may cause a temporary decline in client functioning.

As clients progress from stage 2 to stage 3, they often experience increased agitation, sometimes to the point of exhibiting aggression against caregivers. Nurses working with these clients should assess caregiver safety at each health care interaction if the AD client is being cared for in the home.

CLINICAL MANIFESTATIONS AND THERAPIES Alzheimer's Disease

ETIOLOGY	CLINICAL MANIFESTATIONS	CLINICAL THERAPIES
Stage 1	■ Short-term memory loss ■ Mild cognitive deficits that may go unnoticed ■ Problems with depth perception ■ Problems with simple mathematical calculations	■ Pharmacologic therapies include cholinesterase inhibitors, angiotensin-converting enzyme inhibitors ■ Behavioral modifications such as making lists, adapting schedules and routines, verbal reminders
Stage 2	■ Orientation to time and place deteriorates ■ Impaired motor skills ■ Impaired judgment ■ Increased appetite ■ Increased anger and frustration ■ Decrease in daily functioning ■ Communication challenges—repeating sentences, having difficulty getting words out	■ Continuation of pharmacologic therapies and behavior modifications ■ Assistance with daily living as indicated by manifestations and progression of disease ■ Safety measures, such as rails in bathrooms to protect from falls and alarms or buzzers on doors to alert family members of wandering
Stage 3	■ Inability to perform ADLs ■ Increasing lack of response to stimuli ■ Indifference towards food ■ Extreme confusion ■ Loss of cognitive abilities and long-term memory Later: ■ Absent or grossly affected motor skills ■ Loss of gag reflex, ability to swallow	■ Liquid nutrition or feeding tubes as warranted by manifestations ■ frequent repositioning ■ 24-hour nursing care is required.

COLLABORATION

The most effective approach to Alzheimer's disease occurs with the coordinated efforts of the multidisciplinary team. AD clients beginning to lose language skills may benefit from speech therapy. Speech therapists may be able to slow down the aphasic process and restore partial swallowing function. Dieticians and nutritionists can examine a client's drug regimen and dietary behaviors and make suggestions for meal planning based on client preferences that may improve client energy levels and decrease symptoms, especially side effects of medications (e.g., constipation).

Physical therapists can maintain or increase range of motion, improve muscle tone, improve coordination, and increase endurance for exercise. Occupational therapists can provide additional sensory stimulation and self-care training programs. Social workers can provide individual or group therapy for families of people with AD; moreover, they can help with community resources or institutional placement. Pastoral counselors can help clients and families meet religious and spiritual needs.

Pharmacologic Therapies

No known treatment can stop or reverse the mental deterioration of Alzheimer's disease. The goals of medication are to improve ability or slow decline in cognition and ADLs with minimal side effects. Current medications either inhibit cholinesterase or regulate glutamic acid, an excitatory amino acid. Other drugs may be used to manage symptoms such as anxiety, depression, or agitation. Researchers are looking for ways to increase the amount of acetylcholine (ACh) in the brain. Because it is digested in the gastrointestinal tract, ACh cannot be taken orally. Three medications approved by the U.S. Food and Drug Administration (FDA) increase the availability of ACh in the synapses by inhibiting the enzyme cholinesterase responsible for the breakdown of ACh. These medications are donepezil (Aricept), rivastigmine (Exelon), and galantamine (Reminyl). Galantamine is a cholinesterase inhibitor that also includes nicotinic receptor–modulating activity.

Cholinesterase inhibitors do not cure AD, but may slow the progression of the disorder. In some cases, this is almost as good as a cure. Because AD usually strikes late in life, delaying its onset by a year would decrease the incidence (for those near the end of life) and delay nursing home placement in many cases. Cholinesterase inhibitors are not effective for those with advanced AD. The side effects are usually transient, occurring at the onset of treatment, and include nausea, diarrhea, sweating, bradycardia, and insomnia. Taking the medication after breakfast may decrease side effects.

Preliminary research suggests that angiotensin-converting enzyme inhibitors also may slow the progression of AD (Ohrui et al., 2004). Memantine (Namenda) has been approved for the treatment of moderate to severe AD. This new drug targets the excitatory amino acids such as glu. Excess glu is associated with the death of neuronal nerve cells found in neurodegenerative disorders. The drug appears to correct the glu imbalance by acting as a receptor antagonist (Laustsen & Wimmett, 2005).

Because concomitant depression may increase functional disability, antidepressant medications are prescribed for people with depressive symptoms. Antipsychotic medications may decrease agitation, aggression, paranoid thinking, and poor impulse control. In 2005, the FDA issued a public health advisory regarding increased risk of death associated with the use of all second-generation antipsychotics in older adults with dementia. Clinicians must decide when the benefits of antipsychotics outweigh the potential harm.

Selegiline (El-depryl), a selective monoamine oxidase B inhibitor approved for motor dysfunction of Parkinson disease, may delay functional decline but does not improve cognitive performance. Citalopram (Celexa), a selective serotonin receptor inhibitor antidepressant, is helpful for behavioral disturbances and psychotic symptoms (DeDeyn et al., 2005).

Medication should not be overused to sedate and calm clients. For those clients experiencing sleep problems, the use of hypnotics is contraindicated because the medication does not improve sleep patterns and often increases confusion and sedation during awake periods. Medications used for agitation and aggression include trazodone (Desyrel), buspirone (BuSpar), carbamazepine (Tegretol), and valproate (Depakote).

Very early pilot studies suggest that intravenous immunoglobulin (IVIg) may slightly reverse the disease process in AD (Hayden, 2007). IVIg is a combination of many antibiotics that is already used for some autoimmune diseases. It is thought that antiamyloid antibodies in IVIg attach to beta-amyloid and remove it from the brain.

Alternative Therapies

ANTIOXIDANTS Antioxidants are a group of vitamins, minerals, enzymes, and herbs that help protect the body from naturally occurring free radicals. As the body goes through its normal processes and oxygen is used to provide cellular fuel, some of the oxygen molecules lose one of their two electrons. When they do, the formerly stable oxygen molecules become dangerous free radicals that try to stabilize themselves by stealing another electron from stable molecules, thus damaging them and creating more free radicals. An excess of free radicals is, in part, responsible for the effects of aging and is implicated in degenerative conditions such as AD (Fontaine, 2005).

As people age, they produce fewer antioxidants and may benefit from dietary antioxidants such as vitamin C, vitamin E, carotenoids, the mineral selenium, and the hormone melatonin. Herbs with antioxidant properties include bilberry, ginkgo, grape seed extract, green tea, and flavonoids. Fruits and vegetables are the primary sources for antioxidants, although they also are available in the form of supplements. At the top of the list in providing antioxidants are fruits and vegetables with the deepest colors, such as prunes, raisins, blueberries, blackberries, raspberries, garlic, kale, cranberries, strawberries, spinach, broccoli, and beets (Berman & Brodaty, 2004).

MEDICATIONS For Older Adults With Alzheimer's Disease

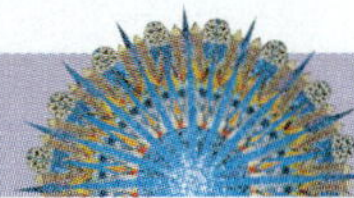

An often underutilized source of collaboration in caring for the client with AD is the pharmacist. Pharmacists can help families and caregivers by looking at the entire regimen of drugs and supplements a client is taking and suggesting ways they can be made more efficient based on the pharmacist's knowledge of the drugs and their interactions. The pharmacist may suggest an antidepressant be taken in the morning rather than at bedtime or suggest a certain medicine be taken with food or not be taken at the same time with a different medicine. Even small changes such as these can make a difference for a client and family.

Commonly Used Medications for Older Persons With Alzheimer's Disease

Drug Class	Name	Dose Range (mg)/Frequency*	Comments
Selected Antidepressant Medications			
Selective serotonin reuptake inhibitors	Fluoxetine (Prozac) Paroxetine (Paxil) Sertraline (Zoloft) Citalopram (Celexa) Escitalopram (Lexapro)	10–40 mg/day 10–40 mg/day 50–200 mg/day 20–30 mg/day 10 mg/day	With older adults, any new medication should be initiated at a lower dose and a longer time period should be allowed before increasing the dosage. Medications that are highly protein bound may be problematic and medications with anticholinergic properties should be avoided. Other considerations include onset of action and indications for treatment of both depression and generalized anxiety syndrome.
Other	Mirtazapine (Remeron) Trazodone (Desyrel) Venlafaxine (Effexor) Duloxetine (Cymbalta)	15–45 mg/day 25–50 mg/bid-tid 75–225 mg/day 20–60 mg/daily	Trazodone and mirtazapine may be useful in older persons who suffer from insomnia.
Selected Drugs Used in Treatment of Delusions and Hallucinations			
Typical neuroleptics	Haloperidol (Haldol)	0.5–2 mg/daily	Do not give a drug with a long half-life for an intermittent symptom of short duration.
Atypical neuroleptics	Risperidone (Risperdal) Olanzapine (Zyprexa) Quetiapine (Seroquel)	0.25–1.5 mg/daily 2.5–10 mg/daily 25–100 mg/bid-tid	
Selected Medications to Treat Anxiety			
Several Antidepressants Are Also Useful for Anxiety: Duloxatine (Cymbalta), Venlafaxine (Effexor XR), Escitalopram (Lexapro), and Paroxetine (Paxil)			
Benzodiazepines	Lorazepam (Ativan) Alprazolam (Xanax) Oxazepam (Serax) Clonazepam (Klonopin)	0.5–1 mg/bid-tid 0.25–0.5 mg/tid 10–20 mg/tid-qid 0.25–0.5 mg/bid	Side effects are sedation, impaired motor coordination, akathesia, risk of falls, memory loss, respiratory or central nervous system depression, and paradoxical reaction. Must be tapered slowly. Azaspirone
Buspirone (BuSpar)	5–20 mg/tid		Side effects are headache, nausea, drowsiness, and lightheadedness.

* bid = twice a day, tid = three times a day, qid = four times a day, qam = every morning, qhs = every evening

Note: All of these medications contain a black box warning for use in older adults and the risks and benefits of treatment need to be discussed with families.

OMEGA-3 FATTY ACIDS Omega-3 fatty acids, especially the component DHA (docosahexaenoic acid), are essential for optimal functioning of neuronal synapses in the brain. Good sources of omega-3 fatty acids are fish oil, including salmon, mackerel, herring, sardines, and cod liver oil. Eating too many omega-6 vegetable fats such as corn oil and other processed oils makes the neuronal membranes rigid and can destroy DHA. Low levels of DHA are a risk factor for low mental performance and AD.

PHOSPHATIDYL SERINE Phosphatidyl serine is a component of the nerve cell membrane that helps keep nerve cell membranes flexible. A dose of 300 mg/day for 1 month followed by

100 mg/day thereafter often improves memory. Phosphatidyl serine from cow brains is rich in DHA and increases levels of dopamine (DA) and norepinephrine (NE). As a supplement, it may be combined with ginkgo (Brown & Gerbarg, 2000).

MELATONIN Insomnia is a frequent problem among people with AD. Melatonin, a hormone secreted by the pineal gland, plays a critical role in the regulation of the day–night cycle. As people age, they produce less melatonin, and for those with AD, the disturbance is even more pronounced. Studies have shown that melatonin is effective in inducing sleep and has no notable side effects. Slow-release melatonin often improves the sleep pattern in people with AD.

DEHYDROEPIANDROSTERONE Dehydroepiandrosterone (DHEA) is a corticosteroid produced primarily in the adrenal glands. In addition to serving as a precursor to testosterone and estrogen, DHEA may be involved in regulating a person's mood and sense of well-being. The method of action is unclear, but it may stimulate gamma-aminobutyric acid (GABA) receptors or increase 5-HT levels. Because little is known about long-term risks, DHEA is probably best used under medical supervision. The usual dose is up to 90 mg/day.

SAMe SAMe (S-adenosylmethionine), a compound made by every cell in the body, helps produce DA, 5-HT, and NE. In addition, SAMe (pronounced sam-ee) improves cell membrane flexibility. Low levels of SAMe have been found in people with AD. SAMe should be used with caution in people who have a history of cardiac arrhythmia.

LECITHIN Lecithin is a major component of cell membranes. Nerve cells and the protective membranes surrounding the brain are composed largely of lecithin. High doses of lecithin may be helpful for people with AD. Most lecithin is derived from soybeans, but recently, egg lecithin has become popular.

MUSIC THERAPY Neurohormone and neurotransmitter levels may change because of music therapy. One study of people with AD found that 30–40 minutes of music therapy in the morning 5 days a week for 4 weeks resulted in significant increases in serum melatonin concentration. Levels continued to rise even after the music therapy had been discontinued for 6 weeks. Some clinical effects were clients' ability to sing and learn new songs, an increased ability to follow rhythmic patterns, an ability to anticipate endings of phrases and songs, an improved ability to follow changes in tempo, and increased social interaction with peers and therapists (Kumar, Tims, & Gruess, 1999).

TOUCH THERAPY Management of agitation is one goal of alternative practices. Massage therapy relaxes and calms people with AD. One study evaluated the effect of therapeutic touch (TT) on 10 individuals with AD. A significant decrease in vocalization and pacing or walking was observed over time with the treatment of TT (Woods & Dimond, 2002).

ANIMAL-ASSISTED THERAPY A nursing study investigated the use of fish aquariums in dementia-specific inpatient units. Residents exposed to the aquarium experienced an increase in nutritional intake and significant weight gain (Edwards & Beck, 2002).

NURSING PROCESS

There is no cure for AD; the main objective of care is to provide an environment that matches the client's functional abilities. Nurses, physicians, physical therapists, and social workers collaborate with the client's family to provide the least restrictive environment in which the client can function safely.

Clients with AD often require intensive, supportive nursing interventions directed at the physical and psychosocial responses to illness. Equally important, the nurse can facilitate the long-term support of these clients by providing teaching and referrals to follow-up care in the community.

Assessment

The nursing assessment is comprised of the health history and physical examination. Further focused assessments are described with nursing interventions later in this exemplar.

- *Health history.* Family member/caregiver support, living arrangements, ability to carry out ADLs, drug use, work history (e.g., exposure to metals), previous history of multiple strokes, brain injury or brain infection, family history of dementia, sleep pattern, changes in cognition and memory, ability to communicate, changes in behavior
- *Physical assessment.* Height/weight, orientation, abstract reasoning, mental status

Nurses should also be alert for these signs:

- Symptoms of depression
- Risk factors for suicide
- Changes in cognitive function
- Medications that increase risk of falls
- Signs of physical abuse or neglect
- Alterations in skin integrity (at greatest risk during stage 3)
- Tooth decay, gingivitis, loose teeth
- Dietary pattern
- Any problems with bowel or urinary elimination
- Activity/exercise and sleep/rest patterns
- Family and social activities and interests.

Mental status examinations such as those described in the Cognitive Assessment feature in this concept (page 208) are frequently used in assessing clients at risk for or suspected of AD. One of the most frequently used is the Mini-Mental State Exam, which can help assess the level of cognitive impairment as well as the progression of impairment over time. This tool looks at several areas of cognitive functioning, including orientation, short-term memory, and language. More information can be found at the publisher's website, www.minimental.com.

The health history and physical assessment may indicate the need for laboratory testing or a CT scan or magnetic resonance imaging (MRI) to rule out other disorders that may mimic AD, such as dementia as a side effect of medication or a B-vitamin deficiency.

Diagnosis

Appropriate nursing diagnoses may be dependent on the stage of AD. The suggested nursing diagnoses are as follows:

- Impaired Memory is an appropriate nursing diagnosis in stage 1 AD.
- Chronic Confusion may be appropriate late in stage 1 and throughout stage 2 of AD.

Diagnoses appropriate at all stages of AD include the following:

- Risk for Injury
- Anxiety
- Hopelessness
- Caregiver Role Strain.

Plan

As seen with nursing diagnoses, the choice of outcome will be dictated by the stage of the illness, the cognitive dysfunction, and the number of family members participating in caring for the client. Suggested outcomes include the following:

- Client will remain free of injury.
- Client will navigate home environment with modifications as needed.
- Client will participate in grooming and hygiene activities with prompting and supervision.
- Client will obtain a minimum of 7 uninterrupted hours of sleep a night.
- Client will utilize memory aids such as alarm clocks (may be an appropriate outcome for stage 1 clients).

Planning for the AD client also may include appropriate outcomes for primary caregivers, including participation in activities that provide stress relief for the caregiver as well as appropriate nutrition, sufficient sleep, and (as necessary) additional community supports such as home health.

Implementation

During the early stage of AD, nursing care focuses on helping the client make minor adaptations to the environment. As the client becomes progressively unable to manage self-care tasks, more adaptations are required. Equally important, the caregiver needs much support—both physical and psychosocial—as the client becomes increasingly dependent.

Early diagnosis allows for inclusion of the client in making decisions and plans for the future. The client's participation helps prevent the struggle that families face to make decisions about care in the later stages when these issues cannot be discussed with the client. People with dementia should be given an opportunity to establish advance directives. As early as practicable, they should select a health care proxy or medical power of attorney to carry out their wishes (Rempusheski & Hurley, 2000). Educated decision making should be established and maintained throughout the progressive course, with the roles changing from the early stage when older adults can represent themselves to later stages when their proxy presents their wishes. With a better understanding of the progression of the disease, families should be encouraged to be realistic about the demands of caregiving and avoid making promises such as "I'll never put you in a nursing home" that may not be realistic in the long run.

Progression of dementia does not occur uniformly in all individuals. Health teaching should be geared to the older adult's current stage and the anticipated issues. As the disease progresses, the role of the caregiver becomes more active to compensate for the older adult's cognitive losses and the development of behavioral symptoms. Families will need support from their professional caregivers as they make and live through some of the most difficult decisions of their lives—selecting life-prolonging treatments that may increase discomfort or choosing care that will provide comfort but may be seen as hastening death. Palliative care is often the only choice, as more aggressive measures will not alter the course of the disease and only result in prolonged discomfort for the client. Nurses can help guide older adults and their families as they face some of these difficult end-of-life choices.

Impaired Memory

In the early stage, techniques to help with memory loss should be included in teaching for both the client and caregiver.

- Suggest complementary therapies such as meditation, massage, or exercise. These activities can help reduce stress, which can aggravate memory loss.
- Suggest using a calendar, keeping lists of reminders, or asking someone else to provide reminders of appointments and events. Written or verbal reminders are helpful if memory is impaired.
- Recommend using a medication box labeled with days and times. A medication box is a good way to remember to take medications.
- If safety is a concern (such as turning on the stove and forgetting it), suggest using alternatives such as a microwave. Program emergency numbers into the telephone. Ask the client to consider a Lifeline telephone program. These measures can increase safety.
- Suggest using cues such as an alarm on a watch or a pocket computer to trigger actions at designated times. Cues are often helpful when memory loss is a problem.
- Suggest that the client carry a wallet card that identifies names and phone numbers of caregivers and close family or friends. These measures can increase safety in the event of an emergency.

PRACTICE ALERT

Many of the medications that treat AD today help the client maintain cognitive functioning for a longer period of time. If a client forgets to take medications or does not take them at the prescribed intervals, cognitive functioning can be greatly impaired in a very short period of time. While medication boxes can help clients remember to take medications, the client or caregiver must be sufficiently competent to put the appropriate pills in the appropriate boxes for this cue to be successful. The nurse should assess the client's manner of following medication schedules at each health care interaction and the supports the client has for doing so. A phone call to the client's pharmacy can establish whether refills are being sought on a timely basis.

Chronic Confusion

Clients with AD often have memory deficits that make functioning in a nonstructured environment difficult. Many of the nursing interventions for this diagnosis need to be modified over time as the client continues to lose cognitive function.

- Label rooms, drawers, and other items as needed. Visual cues promote the highest possible degree of independence for the client.
- Remove potential hazards (e.g., guns, sharp knives, and potentially harmful liquids or chemicals) from the environment. Ensuring safety is a critical factor in providing care.
- Keep environmental stimuli to a minimum. Decrease noise levels; speak in a calm, low voice; and take an unhurried approach. Minimizing sensory input and maintaining a calm manner may decrease anxiety.
- Begin each interaction by identifying yourself and calling client by name. See Box 4–4 for other communication techniques. These techniques provide information for the client with memory loss.
- Limit questions to those that require a simple yes or no response. Questions need to be appropriate to the client's ability as decision making and verbal skills decline.
- Orient to the environment, person, and time as able; place large, easy-to-read calendars and clocks in the client's line of vision. Make references to the season or day of the week when conversing with the client. Orient the client according to level of ability; orienting to precise time may not be possible in the later stages of AD.
- Provide boundaries by affixing red or yellow tape to the floor. Boundaries help the client stay within safe areas.
- Provide continuity in nursing staff. This not only promotes consistency of care for the client, but also more accurate determination of changes in the client's condition.

Box 4–4 **Communicating With the Client With AD**

- Face the client and talk directly to the client; call the client by name.
- When first approaching the client, identify yourself.
- Use simple sentences and words with few syllables.
- Speak in a calm, low voice.
- Ask one question at a time. Use questions that require only a yes or no response.
- Keep nonverbal communication relaxed and parallel to the verbal communication.
- Avoid giving the impression of being in a hurry; try to have a relaxed approach.
- Observe for anxiety—wringing hands, pacing, darting eye movements—and alter your approach to decrease anxiety.
- Avoid arguing with client. Do not insist on orienting client to reality; the client's point of reference may not be based in reality.
- Give plenty of time for the client with AD to process what you are trying to say; do not expect clients to perform skills beyond their abilities.
- Repeat explanations in simple terms.

- Repeat explanations simply and as needed to decrease anxiety. Loss of short-term memory leads to loss of a point of reference; eventually, AD clients think they are experiencing everything for the first time.

Risk for Injury

DECREASING THE RISK OF FALLS AD clients with chronic confusion are at risk for falls. To help clients and caregivers decrease this risk, the nurse should help clients and caregivers

- assess usual environments for hazards such as throw rugs, electrical cords, and slick floors.
- observe areas of special concern, such as the bathroom, kitchen, and stairs, and modify as needed; for example, provide skidproof surfaces and mark stairs to show depth.
- evaluate muscle strength and gait; consult a physical therapist to plan exercises to increase strength and balance.
- check shoes for fit and support.
- inquire about alcohol use and medications that affect balance or cause mobility problems.
- use night-lights and increase daytime lighting in dark areas such as hallways.
- keep traffic areas free from clutter.

DECREASING THE INJURIES RELATED TO COGNITIVE IMPAIRMENTS Clients and caregivers may need to make additional changes to decrease the risk for injury, not only to the client, but also to family members and caregivers. These changes include addressing both specific safety and more generalized safety issues. Encourage families to do the following:

- Secure items that may be mistakenly ingested, such as cleaning preparations and houseplants.
- Modify potentially unsafe areas such as unenclosed porches.
- Provide double lock systems to outside doors and doors to rooms that are off limits.
- Protect from fire hazards; for example, make matches and cigarettes inaccessible.
- Fence the yard with a locked gate to prevent wandering.
- Modify the controls on the oven and stove.
- Adjust the water heater to a safe temperature.
- Plan a calling system for emergencies; have children call at about the same time every day as a check.
- Ensure that the cognitively impaired family member has no access to objects in the home such as knives and guns.

PRACTICE ALERT

One of the greatest sources of conflict for the AD client and family revolves around the AD client and driving. Many AD clients see their independence as being closely related to their ability to drive. For some clients, their car may be a particular source of pride. Discussions about use of the car may provoke great anger and anxiety in the client. It is not uncommon for families to ask health care professionals for guidance in how to handle this situation. Because of the many other sources of strain in family relationships, family members may be unwilling to "play the heavy" and physically take the car keys away. Nurses can assist family members by reinforcing the need for safety with the client. Nurses can offer the client a self-assessment tool to help the client evaluate the ability to drive or refer the client and family to a senior driver evaluation program. Sometimes an independent evaluation may be sufficient to convince an AD client to stop driving. Another option is for the doctor to write a letter to the local department of motor vehicles, requesting a formal evaluation of the client's driving ability or, in some states, requesting that the client's driving privilege be revoked on medical grounds.

Anxiety

Managing the AD client's behaviors associated with anxiety, restlessness, and confusion is a major challenge confronting nurses and caregivers. Frequently, clients are relatively calm in the morning hours, only to experience increasing periods of agitation in the afternoon and evening hours. The AD client may even awaken from a night's sleep with confusion, fearfulness, or panic attacks.

- Monitor for early behaviors of fatigue and agitation. Early assessment of problems results in prompt intervention to promote rest or to remove the client from the situation causing anxiety.
- Remove from situations that are causing increased anxiety, such as noisy activities involving large groups. High-stimulus situations may increase anxious feelings and agitation.
- Keep daily routine as consistent as possible. Providing a structured day enhances feelings of familiarity and decreases stress.
- Schedule rest periods or quiet times throughout the day. Fatigue contributes to anxiety and lowers the ability to tolerate stress.
- Provide quiet activities in the afternoon or early evening, such as listening to favorite music. Quiet activities may help decrease sundowning.
- If confusion and agitation persist or escalate, assess for physical causes such as decreased oxygenation, infections, fatigue, constipation, and electrolyte imbalance. Physical factors can increase agitation in clients with AD.
- Use TT or gentle hand massage. These activities induce relaxation and have a calming effect.

PRACTICE ALERT

A sudden change in the life of an AD client can have gravely disabling effects for the AD client. Caregiver illness, hospitalization, or death increases anxiety levels and may cause a temporary or permanent progression of the disease. Resulting substitution of caregivers or temporary environmental changes such as going to stay with another family member or being admitted to a nursing home can quickly increase confusion and decrease client function. If possible, transitions to new environments should be carefully planned for the AD client to maximize coping mechanisms and decrease anxiety.

Hopelessness

As the client and family recognize the effects of AD on their lives, they may feel a sense of hopelessness. A diagnosis of AD can be devastating to a family, regardless of the family's coping skills and ability to anticipate problems. The irreversible and increasingly degenerative nature of the disorder tends to diminish hope. Even when feelings of hope are restored to a client or family, they can diminish again as the client progresses through the stages of the disease and as personal and financial resources are used to care for the client.

- Assess the client's and family's response to the diagnosis and understanding of AD; encourage expression of feelings. Understanding the client/family's perspective enables the nurse to dispel myths about AD.
- Provide realistic information about the disorder; provide information at the client/family's level of understanding. Client and family may need to have separate sessions. Factual information provides a foundation for decision making.
- Avoid criticizing or judging expressed feelings. An environment accepting of the expression of real feelings promotes further expressions of feelings and a willingness to discuss other issues.
- Support positive family bonds and enhance communication among family members; promote mutual positive regard. Strong family relationships can provide direction for living and convey a willingness to share the burden.
- Encourage the client to make as many decisions as possible. Self-determination enhances a feeling of control over a situation and may give a sense of hope.
- Encourage client and family to call the nurse or clinic with questions about the disease or medications. Returning these calls in a timely fashion provides support for the client and family that increases the trusting relationship and can give the client and family a sense of hope.
- Encourage the client and family to seek spiritual guidance that previously inspired hope. The client's religious affiliation can serve as an important support system. Religious faith can inspire hope beyond present circumstances.
- Return client and family phone calls in a timely fashion. Understand that families calling for information may be trying to gain reassurance or reinforcement to help calm or provide explanations to the client with AD. Timely information from the nurse has a direct impact on client and family hopelessness, as it helps them feel that someone who knows more about the disease than they do is in their "corner."

Caregiver Role Strain

Most caregivers of clients with AD are spouses or other family members. Because AD is a chronic and eventually debilitating disorder, caregivers often experience extreme stress in caring for their loved one. The caregiving spouse faces not only the responsibility for the client's multiple physical demands, but also economic and psychosocial stressors. Fear of the future,

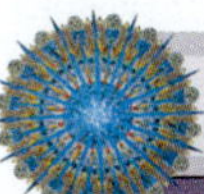

NURSING CARE PLAN A Client With Alzheimer's Disease

ASSESSMENT

Arthur and Ruth Joste, both aged 73, have been married for 47 years; he is a retired history teacher, and she has been a homemaker. They have four children; two live in the same town, and two live out of state. Arthur has noticed that he is having problems remembering friends' names and phone numbers; his wife has been asking him if he is driving in the correct direction when they go shopping.

Mrs. Joste has severe osteoarthritis and is unable to lift heavy objects or perform anything but light housekeeping tasks. For about 18 months, Mrs. Joste has been aware of her husband's progressive cognitive decline, including forgetting current news from last night's newspaper, miscalculating checkbook balances, neglecting his hygiene needs, and confusing their children's and grandchildren's names. The Jostes are referred to a neurologist for evaluation.

Martha Spital, RN, assesses Mr. Joste at the neurologist's office. She notes that he is unable to recall his home address without prompting, to name the correct date (although he does know the day of the week), to subtract serial 7s more than twice, and to recall two of three objects. He is alert to his surroundings. Mrs. Joste states that the problems seem to be getting worse with time and that she has had to "cover up" mistakes for her husband. Mr. Joste seems easily agitated, and his wife reports that his sleep habits are "jumbled"; he has long periods of wakefulness in the nighttime hours.

Following a thorough evaluation and diagnostic testing to rule out other possible disorders, the neurologist tells the couple that Mr. Joste has probable dementia of the Alzheimer's type. Both have feared this diagnosis; they want to know how they can be sure that Mr. Joste has this disease and what they can do to prevent further decline. Both are obviously much saddened, and they verbalize their feelings of being overwhelmed. The Jostes stated that they intend to remain in their home "for as long as we can."

DIAGNOSES

- Chronic Confusion related to deterioration of brain function and dementia
- Self-Care Deficits related to forgetfulness and declining physical abilities
- Risk for Injury related to decreased orientation
- Disturbed Sleep Pattern related to time disorientation
- Caregiver Role Strain (wife) related to need to care for self and husband

PLANNING

Based on Mr. Joste's current condition and the anticipated progression of the disease, reasonable goals include the following:

- Remain free of injury
- Navigate home environment with modifications as needed
- Participate in grooming and hygiene activities with prompting and supervision
- Obtain a minimum of 7 uninterrupted hours of sleep a night
- Have Mrs. Joste participate in a minimum of two out-of-home activities a week.

IMPLEMENTATION

The home health nurse, Erick Montane, RN, makes a home visit to evaluate the environment, assess available support, and determine needs. He meets two of the Jostes' children, Dawn and Jay, who live in the same community and are willing to participate as much as possible in providing care and modifying the home.

Mr. Montane discusses the importance of establishing and maintaining a consistent daily routine. He emphasizes the importance of matching activities to Mr. Joste's mental abilities to avoid frustration and increased agitation. Mr. Montane recommends labeling drawers, such as Mr. Joste's sock drawer, with their contents. Labeling rooms may eventually be necessary.

Because his inability to comprehend and process information distresses and agitates Mr. Joste, Mr. Montane teaches the family to modify their communications to fit Mr. Joste's cognitive ability, such as using simple, direct statements and directions.

Mr. Montane recommends that family members keep background noise to a minimum because this may be a source of confusion.

After assessing the home, Mr. Montane makes the following recommendations about safety:

- Remove throw rugs from hallways and tack down any remaining carpets.
- Secure the kitchen, bathroom, and workshop cabinets as well as the controls on the oven and stove.
- Modify the doors so that negotiating locks requires a two-step system of unlocking, such as with a deadbolt and a key.
- Provide extra lighting in dark areas, especially a night-light in the bathroom.

Mr. Montane explains that Mrs. Joste will need assistance with housekeeping as Mr. Joste continues to decline. Mr. Montane provides referrals to community services, including Meals On Wheels, which can supply a daily meal. He also suggests that the Jostes obtain the services of a home health aide to provide daily hygiene care. Most of the remaining home maintenance needs can be met with the children's help.

For approximately 3 months, Mr. and Mrs. Joste and the two children attend the weekly local support group meetings for AD and related disorders; thereafter, Mrs. Joste attends with her daughter.

(continued)

NURSING CARE PLAN **A Client With Alzheimer's Disease** *continued*

EVALUATION

Six months after the initial home visit and family planning session, Mr. Joste

- has not had a fall, a burn, or another injury.
- has periods of confusion when outside his home, but 90% of the time is oriented to place when at home.
- has attended several support group meetings until 3 months ago. Currently, his wife attends weekly, and a daughter occasionally accompanies her. Mrs. Joste has continued to participate in their church and maintains contact with a few friends. She is finding it harder to leave her husband unattended for even a few minutes.
- is able to clean and dress himself with prompting; he is not able to choose his own clothing. If hygiene articles are "set up" (e.g., if the toothpaste is placed on the toothbrush), he remembers to perform the hygiene activity. The children have been replacing buttons and zippers with Velcro closures on his clothing.
- sleeps an average of 6 hours a night with a 30-minute nap in the afternoon; this pattern is consistent with his previous sleep pattern.
- has seemed to be more easily agitated for the past month. He wanders from room to room, apparently looking for something. These behaviors are worse in the evening and on cloudy days. Mrs. Joste acknowledges her progressive inability to care for her husband.

CRITICAL THINKING

1. Develop a tool to teach safety needs for family members and a client with AD.
2. List five interventions to decrease agitation in cognitively impaired older adults; give three additional examples of activities suited to an older adult with AD who has osteoarthritis.
3. You are caring for a client in stage 2 AD. She is 65 inches (165 cm) tall and weighs 132 lb (59.9 kg); she has lost 3 lb in the past month. The client has difficulty focusing on eating and is easily agitated. Describe your plan for ensuring that she has adequate nutrition.

loss of income, and loss of companionship and a mate—combined with fatigue—make the caregiver vulnerable. Caregivers may become physically and mentally exhausted and socially isolated because of the overwhelming responsibilities of providing total care to the incapacitated family member.

- Teach the caregivers self-care techniques such as taking rest periods and avoiding fatigue. Fatigue adds to stress and potentially leads to poor decision making.
- Have the caregivers list and regularly take part in physical activities they enjoy, such as walking or swimming. Regular physical exercise decreases stress.
- Refer the caregivers to local AD support groups. Suggest books pertinent to the subject. Explicit suggestions in locating support systems and providing specific information promotes coping.
- Refer the caregivers to Meals On Wheels, home health, respite care, and other community services. Community agencies can relieve some of the daily care burdens, thus providing time for other activities. Programs that support caregivers have been shown to delay nursing home placement for the client.
- Ensure that the family knows that hospice care is available during the end stages of AD. Hospice services can support the family during this difficult time.

Community-Based Care

Teaching for clients and families initially centers on explaining the disorder and exploring available support systems. Anticipate the need to reexplain the disorder and its consequences because clients and families may be in shock or denial during the initial period of the disease.

In addition to explaining the anticipated changes with AD, suggest practical solutions to identified problems. It is important to evaluate both the client and caregivers; interventions must be appropriate for the family's situation and resources. Maintaining the least restrictive environment that promotes safety for the client is a major goal of teaching. Using memory cues such as labeling drawers to indicate the specific types of clothing and labeling rooms can help orient the client and foster independence. Consistency in the environment and daily routine is an essential part of care. Emphasizing realistic expectations means adjusting care and communication techniques to the client's level of ability.

Address the following topics for home care of the client and for the caregiver:

- Take advantage of support groups and peer counseling, which are helpful in handling caregiver stress.
- Keep in mind that a person with AD who is confused or agitated is not comfortable and is usually frightened.
- Plan care that matches the person's level of coping, using a consistent routine.
- Provide regular rest periods to decrease the client's stress and fatigue. (These do not increase nighttime wandering.)
- Plan care for the caregiver. Periodic adult day care or respite care during the initial stages, with plans for increasing assistance to meet the client's daily needs as the disease progresses, may be sufficient. Referrals to the appropriate agency for long-term care, including skilled nursing facilities, may be indicated. Family members may need help adjusting to the idea of extended care but may be relieved to relinquish the physical care needs.
- Suggest the following resources:
  a. Alzheimer's Association
  b. Alzheimer's Disease and Related Disorders Association
  c. Alzheimer's Disease Education and Referral Center
  d. National Institute of Neurological Disorders and Stroke.

Evaluation

The client's and family's ability to meet the chosen outcomes is evaluated and the plan of care amended as needed, which will become more important as degeneration continues. The goal of nursing care is to encourage independence, maintain as much cognitive function as possible, and provide support to both the client and caregiver.

HEALTH CARE

Advocacy

The nurse must act as an advocate for clients who are unable to advocate for themselves. The nurse also must advocate for the caregivers who often carry the majority of the burden related to AD as the client becomes increasingly dependent.

Evidence-Based Practice

It is important that the nurse remain informed of changes in nursing care of clients with AD because many new therapies, both pharmacological and nonpharmacological, are being researched. It is hoped that better therapies will slow the progression of AD, and only a well-informed nurse can advocate for the client using the most up-to-date evidence-based practice.

Health Care System

As an increasing number of baby boomers become elderly, the number of clients anticipated to be diagnosed with AD is expected to increase dramatically, placing an increased strain on the health care system.

Legal Issues

The importance of involving the client in planning for the future when first diagnosed with AD cannot be overemphasized. While the client is still competent to plan care, it is important for advanced directives and a medical power of attorney to be determined so that the future can be delivered as the client wishes and the strain of legal decisions can be removed from the caregivers.

Safety

People with AD or other types of dementia experience increasing safety needs as their condition deteriorates. Judgment becomes impaired as the disease progresses, and some environmental modification is needed to help the older adult remain safe.

REVIEW Alzheimer's Disease

RELATE: LINK THE CONCEPTS

Mary O'Boyle, aged 62, has been increasingly forgetful lately. She finds it so embarrassing when she can't remember a dear friend's name or where she put the car keys when she gets home that she tends to try to minimize the concern by saying things such as "Oh well, a senior moment is to be expected every now and then." Her daughter has noticed that she is using the phrase more often and worries that her mother may not be safe living at home alone any longer. She talks her mother into seeing a doctor who performs a number of tests to rule out other causes and eventually diagnoses Mrs. O'Boyle as having stage 1 AD.

Linking the exemplar of Alzheimer's Disease with the concept of Legal Issues:

1. What plans and interventions would the nurse who is caring for this family initiate to meet the legal needs of the client?
2. At what point would Mrs. O'Boyle be considered legally incompetent to make decisions for herself, including medical decisions regarding her treatment plan?

Linking the exemplar of Alzheimer's Disease with the concept of Safety:

3. When performing a home care assessment, what types of things might you look for to indicate whether it is safe for Mrs. O'Boyle to live at home?
4. What recommendations could you make to allow Mrs. O'Boyle to remain in her home and function independently for as long as possible?

READY: GO TO COMPANION SKILLS MANUAL

- Assessing home for safe environment
- Evaluating client's safety
- Evaluating caregiver's safety
- Assessing for elder abuse
- Assessing the neurologic system

REFER: GO TO MYNURSINGKIT

REFLECT: CASE STUDY

You have been working with a client's family for 3 years in an outpatient clinic that treats clients with AD. The client's illness has progressed, and his health has deteriorated, but his family is still able to care for him at home. He lives with his 40-year-old daughter, her husband, and their three children. His wife died 5 years ago. The client is now in stage 2 of the illness. He has experienced progressive memory loss and communication difficulties, and his sundowning and wandering behaviors have gradually increased. His daughter says, "He just seems to make up things when he can't remember." She wants to keep him at home a little longer and is aware that this cannot go on long term.

1. What should you consider as you develop interventions with the daughter to ensure the client's safety at home?
2. The family has asked for help in improving communication with the client. What communication guidelines would you discuss with them?
3. The daughter states that the client wanders from room to room and calls out for his deceased wife. What interventions for wandering would you suggest to the family?
4. The family has asked for help in managing the increased confusion and agitation that occurs later in the day. What measures would you suggest to promote optimal conduct and impulse control?

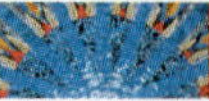

4.2 CONFUSION

KEY TERMS

Confusion, *226*
Delirium, *226*

BASIS FOR SELECTION OF EXEMPLAR

Standards of Nursing Practice
NCLEX-RN®

LEARNING OUTCOMES

After reading about this exemplar, you will be able to:

1. Describe the pathophysiology, etiology, and clinical manifestations of confusion.
2. Identify risk factors associated with confusion.
3. Illustrate the nursing process in providing culturally competent and caring interventions across the life span for individuals with confusion.
4. Formulate priority nursing diagnoses appropriate for an individual who exhibits confusion.
5. Create a plan of caring interventions for an individual who displays confusion.
6. Employ evidence-based caring interventions for an individual displaying confusion.
7. Assess expected outcomes for an individual displaying confusion.
8. Discuss therapies used in the collaborative care of an individual displaying confusion.

OVERVIEW

Confusion is an alteration in cognition that makes it difficult to think clearly, focus attention, or make decisions. It may come on suddenly or gradually, depending on the cause. It can be a one-time event, recurrent, or a constant state of mind. The most important thing to understand about confusion is that it is frequently a symptom and not a diagnosis. Any number of things can cause confusion, including hypoxia, poor perfusion, medications, and disease. The onset of confusion requires thorough assessment to determine the causative agent and improve client outcomes.

Delirium is an acute disorder of cognition that affects functional independence. Confusion, a loss of orientation and memory, can occur in clients of all ages, but it is most commonly seen in older people. The terms *acute confusion* and delirium are used interchangeably by most health professionals, with nurses favoring the use of acute confusion and physicians the term delirium (McCurren & Cronin, 2003, p. 319). Confusion often presents with subtle symptoms, but an attempt should be made to differentiate between acute confusion (delirium) and chronic confusion (dementia) (see Table 4–6).

PATHOPHYSIOLOGY AND ETIOLOGY

Delirium often has an abrupt onset; it can be reversed by treating its cause. This contrasts with dementia, often called chronic confusion, which has symptoms that are gradual and irreversible (e.g., Alzheimer's disease). Clients who are confused often know something is wrong and want help. It is important to pay special attention to sudden changes in mood or personality, as these may be signs of delirium related to recent changes in medication, onset of undetected illness, or exacerbation of chronic illness.

Age-related cognitive decline, resulting from slower information processing, mild memory impairment, and decreases in brain volume secondary to loss of some neurons place older clients at increased risk for confusion when they face additional stressors of illness, loss, or change in environment. Depression or other emotional problems can also act as stressors, increasing the likelihood of delirium. It is important to remember that delirium is usually caused by a treatable physical or mental health illness and, when treated typically results in full recovery. Delirium is associated with increased mortality, increased hospital costs, and long-term cognitive and functional impairment (Tullmann, Mion, Fletcher, & Foreman, 2008).

Etiology

Delirium occurs in 6–30% of the general hospital population and 7–52% of postsurgical clients (Edwards, 2003, p. 347). Delirium in the intensive care unit (ICU) setting is a common problem and has been described as sundown syndrome, ICU psychosis, and ICU syndrome. Delirium or acute confusional state, superimposed on Alzheimer's disease, was found in 8 of 20 older adults with documented dementia (Fick & Foreman, 2000). It is estimated that anywhere from 14–80% of all older persons hospitalized for the treatment of an acute physical illness experience an episode of delirium (Foreman, Wakefield, Culp, & Milisen, 2001). Unfortunately, delirium is unrecognized or misdiagnosed by both the physician and the nurse in up to two-thirds of cases (Hanley, 2004, p. 218).

It is not uncommon to think of older adults as the only people who become confused, but this is incorrect. Confusion can occur at any stage of the developmental process and may be caused by alcohol intoxication, low blood sugar, head trauma, fluid and/or electrolyte imbalances, nutritional deficiencies, hypothermia, hypoxia, medications, sepsis, or sleep deprivation. In older adults, onset of illness may also cause mental confusion.

Risk Factors

Older adults are at risk for delirium, especially when hospitalized, because they often have other chronic medical problems (e.g., chronic obstructive pulmonary disease, hypertension, stroke). Many elders also take numerous medications with anticholinergic, narcotic, or sedative effects that increase the risk for delirium. Undertreating pain can contribute to the risk as well. Many older adults have vision or hearing loss, which makes it easy to misunderstand what they see or hear, further contributing to confusion. All of these risks plus the unfamiliar surroundings and routine of a hospital, possible sleep deprivation, stress, and sensory overload compound the older adult's risk for developing delirium.

CLINICAL MANIFESTATIONS

Manifestations of confusion can range from very subtle symptoms, such as forgetting where one is or what one is doing, to acute loss of cognitive function. Clients may be unable to correctly answer questions related to time, place, person, or thing. They may become agitated, aggressive, fearful, anxious, or withdrawn. Symptoms may come on suddenly, or at specific times of the day. Sundown syndrome is manifested by confusion that occurs after sunset and usually resolves when the sun rises in the morning.

Features of delirium include fluctuations in alertness ranging from stuporous to hypervigilance. Clients are often inattentive, are easily distractible, have difficulty shifting attention from one focus to another, and often have difficulty keeping track of what is being said. They are disoriented to time and place but should not be disoriented to person. Memory testing reveals inability to recall recent events, instructions, names, events, activities, and current news. Thinking is disorganized and speech is often rambling, irrelevant, incoherent, unclear or showing an illogical flow of ideas. Confused clients will switch unpredictably from topic to topic and have difficulty expressing needs or concerns. Speech may be garbled. Severe delirium may include perceptual disturbances such as illusions and visual or auditory hallucinations and misperceptions that lead clients to call a stranger by a relative's name. Psychomotor activity may be hypoactive, hyperactive, or mixed subtypes (Tullmann et al., 2008).

NURSING PROCESS

The goal of nursing care is to reduce the incidence of delirium in the client at risk and prevent complications in the delirious client. Routine screening for delirium should be part of the comprehensive plan of care for the older adult or the client at risk. Delirium can be prevented by recognizing high-risk clients and implementing a standardized protocol (Tullmann et al., 2008).

Assessment

Older persons do not develop dementia overnight, so any sudden change in mental status needs to be aggressively evaluated. Delirium must be ruled out because cognitive impairment caused by delirium may be reversible. The development of delirium may indicate decreased reserve capacity of the brain and signal an increased risk for dementia (Alexopoulos, Silver, Kahn, Frances, & Carpenter, 2004). To rate delirium and distinguish delirium from other types of cognitive impairment, the Hartford Institute for Geriatric Nursing *Try This* Assessment Series recommends use of the Confusion Assessment Method (CAM) (Inouye et al., 1990) (Box 4–5). The CAM includes two parts: Part 1 is an assessment instrument that screens for overall cognitive impairment; Part 2 includes only those four features that distinguish delirium. The tool can be administered in less than 5 minutes. It closely correlates with DSM-IV criteria for delirium. See the Best Practices feature: The Confusion Assessment Method for the Intensive Care Unit (CAM-ICU). When the older client's cognitive status appears to be impaired, the nurse should request the client's permission to include a family member or caregiver in the assessment to supplement and verify the information the patient reports.

Because of the role depression can play in increasing the risk for delirium, it is important to screen the older adult. The GDS and the CDS can be used to screen for depression in older clients as previously described.

The client should be assessed for risk factors including baseline cognitive function, medication history, and environment. The nurse looks for manifestations of pain, metabolic disturbances, dehydration, infection, or impaired mobility that can contribute to the development of confusion. The nurse should assess for evidence of delirium at least every 8 hours (Tullmann et al., 2008).

Diagnosis

Nursing diagnoses are individualized based on client needs and cause of confusion, but may include the following:

- Insomnia
- Disturbed Sleep Patterns
- Self-Care Deficit
- Acute or Chronic Confusion
- Wandering
- Impaired Memory
- Impaired Verbal Communication
- Caregiver Role Strain.

Plan

Nursing care is planned based on client needs and must consider factors such as safety, support systems, and ability to provide self-care. Potential outcomes may include the following:

- Absence of confusion
- Cognitive status returned to baseline
- Discharged to same destination as prehospitalization
- Able to perform activities of daily living.

Implementation

The nurse must provide a therapeutic environment for the confused client. Interventions include fostering orientation by frequently reassuring and reorienting the client through the use of calendars, clocks, caregiver identification, explanation of all activities, and clear communication. Appropriate sensory stimulation is provided by reducing

Box 4–5 The Confusion Assessment Method for the Intensive Care Unit (CAM-ICU)

FEATURES AND DESCRIPTIONS	ABSENT	PRESENT
I. ACUTE ONSET OR FLUCTUATING COURSE*		
A. Is there evidence of an acute change in mental status from the baseline? B. Or, did the (abnormal) behavior fluctuate during the past 24 hours, that is, tend to come and go or increase and decrease in severity as evidenced by fluctuations on the Richmond Agitation Sedation Scale (RASS) or the Glasgow Coma Scale?		
II. INATTENTION†		
Did the patient have difficulty focusing attention as evidenced by a score of less than 8 correct answers on either the visual or auditory components of the Attention Screening Examination (ASE)?		
III. DISORGANIZED THINKING		
Is there evidence of disorganized or incoherent thinking as evidenced by incorrect answers to three or more of the 4 questions and inability to follow the commands? Questions 1. Will a stone float on water? 2. Are there fish in the sea? 3. Does 1 pound weigh more than 2 pounds? 4. Can you use a hammer to pound a nail? Questions and Commands 1. Are you having unclear thinking? 2. Hold up this many fingers. (Examiner holds 2 fingers in front of the patient.) 3. Now do the same thing with the other hand (without holding the 2 fingers in front of the patient). (If the patient is already extubated from the ventilator, determine whether the patient's thinking is disorganized or incoherent, such as rambling or irrelevant conversation, unclear or illogical flow of ideas, or unpredictable switching from subject to subject.)		
IV. ALTERED LEVEL OF CONSCIOUSNESS		
Is the patient's level of consciousness anything other than alert, such as being vigilant or lethargic or in a stupor or coma? Alert: spontaneously fully aware of environment and interacts appropriately Vigilant: hyperalert Lethargic: drowsy but easily aroused, unaware of some elements in the environment or not spontaneously interacting with the interviewer; becomes fully aware and appropriately interactive when prodded minimally Stupor: difficult to arouse, unaware of some or all elements in the environment or not spontaneously interacting with the interviewer; becomes incompletely aware when prodded strongly; can be aroused only by vigorous and repeated stimuli and as soon as the stimulus ceases, stuporous subject lapses back into unresponsive state Coma: unarousable, unaware of all elements in the environment with no spontaneous interaction or awareness of the interviewer so that the interview is impossible even with maximal prodding		
Overall CAM-ICU Assessment (Features 1 and 2 and either Feature 3 or 4):	**Yes____**	**No____**

**The scores included in the 10-point RASS range from a high of 4 (combative) to a low of _5 (deeply comatose and unresponsive). Under the RASS system, patients who were spontaneously alert, calm, and not agitated were scored at 0 (neutral zone). Anxious or agitated patients received a range of scores depending on their level of anxiety: 1 for anxious, 2 for agitated (fighting ventilator), 3 for very agitated (pulling on or removing catheters), or 4 for combative (violent and a danger to staff). The scores _1 to _5 were assigned for patients with varying degrees of sedation based on their ability to maintain eye contact: _1 for more than 10 seconds, _2 for less than 10 seconds, and _3 for eye opening but no eye contact. If physical stimulation was required, then the patients were scored as either_4 for eye opening or movement with physical or painful stimulation or _5 for no response to physical or painful stimulation. The RASS has excellent interrater reliability and intraclass correlation coefficients of 0.95 and 0.97, respectively, and has been validated against visual analog scale and geropsychiatric diagnoses in 2 ICU studies.*

†In completing the visual ASE, the patients were shown 5 simple pictures (previously published) at 3-second intervals and asked to remember them. They were then immediately shown 10 subsequent pictures and asked to nod "yes" or "no" to indicate whether they had or had not just seen each of the pictures. Since 5 pictures had been shown to them already, for which the correct response was to nod "yes," and 5 others were new, for which the correct response was to nod "no," patients scored perfectly if they achieved 10 correct responses. Scoring accounted for either errors of omission (indicating "no" for a previously shown picture) or for errors of commission (indicating "yes" for a picture not previously shown). In completing the auditory ASE, patients were asked to squeeze the rater's hand whenever they heard the letter A during the recitation of a series of 10 letters. The rater then read 10 letters from the following list in a normal tone at a rate of 1 letter per second: S, A, H, E, V, A, A, R, A, T. A scoring method similar to that of the visual ASE was used for the auditory ASE testing.

Source: The Confusion Assessment Method for the Intensive Care Unit (CAM-ICU). Ely, E. W., Inouye, S. K., Bernard, G. R., Gordon, S., Francis, J., May, L., Truman, B., Speroff, T., Gautam, S., Margolin, R., Hart, R. P., & Dittus, R. (2001). Delirium in mechanically ventilated patients: Validity and reliability of the confusion assessment method for the intensive care unit (CAM-ICU). *JAMA, 286*(21), 2703–2710. Table 1, p. 2705. © American Medical Association. All rights reserved.

NURSING CARE PLAN **A Client With Delirium**

ASSESSMENT

Mr. Dalton is a 75-year-old man who has been admitted to the hospital. He fell in his home and suffered a fractured left hip and had an open reduction with internal fixation this morning. When Mr. Dalton first arrived, he was quiet and pleasant but now he is agitated, attempting to get out of bed, yelling, and throwing his sheets on the floor. The nurse attempts to reason with him and reassure him, but he is not responding.

The nurse suspects Mr. Dalton is delirious because his symptoms had an acute onset. Delirium poses a common and serious problem in older patients with hip fracture. Systematic determination of an older person's mental status is of major importance for early recognition and treatment of delirium. The nurse knows that delirium can be caused by any of the following factors:

- Infection
- Medications (antihistamines, anticholinergics, benzodiazepines)
- Anesthesia
- Electrolyte imbalance
- Pain
- Sleep disturbance
- Underlying dementia (diagnosed or undiagnosed).

A complete assessment of each of these factors using standardized assessment instruments is indicated while the older person is protected from injury.

DIAGNOSES

Nursing diagnoses that may be appropriate for Mr. Dalton include the following:

- Acute Confusion
- Previously Altered Thought Processes (if previously diagnosed with cognitive impairment)
- Risk for Imbalanced Fluid Volume (overhydration or dehydration)
- Risk for Injury (due to falls)
- Impaired Verbal Communication
- Impaired Physical Mobility
- Delayed Surgical Recovery
- Acute Pain
- Anxiety
- Fear.

PLANNING

The expected outcomes for the plan of care specify that Mr. Dalton will

- be free from injury.
- begin to exhibit resolution of his symptoms of delirium.
- experience correction of the underlying mechanisms causing his delirium.
- receive consultation, assessment, and treatment from appropriate members of the interdisciplinary team, including physicians, nurses, physical therapists, dietitians, social workers, and others as appropriate to resolve and improve his delirium.

IMPLEMENTATION

The following nursing interventions may be appropriate for Mr. Dalton:

- Establish a therapeutic relationship by being present and using gentle touch and a soft voice for communication.
- Review all current medications.
- Evaluate basic laboratory studies (complete blood count, serum electrolytes, and urinalysis).
- Provide supportive and restorative care.
- Treat behavioral symptoms.
- Correct sensory deficits (place glasses and hearing aids if used by the older person).
- In consultation with the physician, consider further testing as appropriate that may include chest radiology, blood culture, drug levels, serum B12, thyroid function tests, pulse oximetry, electrocardiogram, brain imaging, lumbar puncture, or electroencephalogram.
- Administer medications as ordered by the physician (haloperidol 0.5–2.0 mg or lorazepam 0.5 to 2.0 mg by mouth every 4–6 hours).
- Reassure, educate, and involve family.
- Maintain a quiet and peaceful environment to decrease noise stimuli to the extent possible.

EVALUATION

The nurse will consider the plan a success based on the following criteria:

- Mr. Dalton will return to normal cognitive and physical function.
- He will be free from injury.
- He will cooperate with a rehabilitation program and be discharged to home or a rehabilitation facility (as appropriate).

ETHICAL DILEMMA

Mr. Dalton's daughter requests that he be restrained to prevent falls. She has seen older persons with waist restraints and feels the use of this device will keep her father safe from injury. The nurse wishes to be responsive to the daughter's request, but professional standards indicate that restraints can worsen delirium and injure the older person. The ethical dilemma involves threats to the older person's and surrogate's autonomy versus nonmaleficence or the desire to do no harm. The nurse should educate and inform the daughter regarding the risks of entrapment and strangulation that accompany the use of restraints. Agitation and anxiety can be exacerbated as the older person fights to free himself from the restraints, and larger doses of medication may be needed to reduce symptoms. Physical restraints should be used cautiously (if at all) and only as a last resort. Additionally, a delirious physically restrained older person will need constant observation to prevent injury, entrapment, and strangulation.

(continued)

NURSING CARE PLAN A Client With Delirium *(continued)*

CRITICAL THINKING

1. How would you explain the diagnosis of Alzheimer's disease to a family?
2. What resources are available in your community or professional setting to assist older persons and their families caring for a loved one with dementia?
3. Identify three major changes you would like to see implemented in your clinical agency that would facilitate the care of older persons with dementia.
4. Caring for older persons with cognitive impairments (dementia and delirium) can be stressful for nurses and other health care providers. What types of support services and resources in the clinical setting would assist you to provide the highest quality care to older persons with cognitive impairments?

noise, maintaining adequate lighting, and performing one task at a time. The nurse helps the client to obtain adequate sleep, maximize mobility, and create an environment that contains familiar objects from home. Family and friends should be encouraged to stay at the bedside, and consistency of caregivers is optimum. The nurse should communicate clearly, provide simple explanations, reassure and educate the family, and minimize invasive procedures. Pharmacological interventions for confusion should be the last resort and used only when all other measures have proven ineffective (Tullmannet al., 2008). Box 4–6 lists nursing interventions to help promote a therapeutic environment for the client with acute confusion/delirium.

Evaluation

Clients are evaluated based on ability to meet outcomes; the nursing plan of care is adapted as indicated. In addition to evaluating client outcomes, a decrease in the occurrence of delirium should become a measure of the quality of care delivered by all facilities that care for older adults.

Box 4–6 Promoting a Therapeutic Environment for a Client With Acute Confusion/Delirium

- Wear a readable name tag.
- Address the person by name and introduce yourself frequently: "Good morning, Mr. Richards. I am Betty Brown. I will be your nurse today."
- Identify time and place as indicated: "Today is December 5, and it is 8:00 in the morning."
- Ask the client, "Where are you?" and orient the client to place (e.g., nursing home) if indicated.
- Place a calendar and clock in the client's room. Mark holidays with ribbons, pins, or other means.
- Speak clearly and calmly to the client, allowing time for your words to be processed and for the client to respond.
- Encourage family to visit frequently unless this activity causes the client to become hyperactive.
- Provide clear, concise explanations of each treatment procedure or task.
- Eliminate unnecessary noise.
- Reinforce reality by interpreting unfamiliar sounds, sights, and smells; correct any misconceptions of events or situations.
- Schedule activities (e.g., meals, bath, activity and rest periods, treatments) at the same time each day to provide a sense of security. If possible, assign the same caregivers.
- Provide adequate sleep.
- Keep glasses and hearing aid within reach.
- Ensure adequate pain management.
- Keep familiar items in the client's environment (e.g., photographs), and keep the environment uncluttered. A disorganized, cluttered environment increases confusion.
- Keep room well lit during waking hours.

REVIEW Confusion

RELATE: LINK THE CONCEPTS

Linking the exemplar of Confusion with the concept of Ethics:

1. You overhear an unlicensed assistive personnel (UAP) talking with a confused client while bathing her. The UAP is agreeing with the client's delusions and misperceptions. What is your ethical obligation to this client?
2. A client who is confused is requesting to sign out of the hospital against medical advice and insisting he'll call his lawyer if you don't bring him the form to sign. What is your ethical obligation to this client? How will you respond to this demand?

Linking the exemplar of Confusion with the concept of Assessment:

3. While caring for an older adult who was alert and oriented on admission and suddenly became confused, what assessments would you make to determine possible causes of the change in cognition displayed?

4. While caring for a pediatric client you notice the child has suddenly become confused and is making comments that are inappropriate. What would you assess on this client?

READY: GO TO COMPANION SKILLS MANUAL

- Applying body mechanics
- Assisting the client with ambulation
- Assessing appearance and mental status
- Assessing the neurologic system
- Bathing an adult client
- Administering medication
- Evaluating client's safety

REFLECT: CASE STUDY

Clifford is a 64-year-old male who has been married to his wife, Pam, for 40 years. Their only child, 24-year-old Gary, has Down syndrome and lives with them. Clifford is a middle manager for a small manufacturing company where he has worked over the last 20 years.

Overall, Clifford is in good health, although he has recently been undergoing conservative treatment for benign prostate hypertrophy. He has a history of depression. He had a brief episode during college, for which he did not seek treatment. He had another episode shortly after Gary was born, and at the encouragement of his wife, he sought treatment, which consisted of counseling and antidepressant agents. He quit taking the medications after about 6 months and decided he would just learn to deal with depression on his own. Although he has had mild episodes of depression over the years since that time, Clifford has been unwilling to seek treatment because he fears the social stigma of being labeled medically depressed and is concerned his employer will discover it through his use of the medical benefits. It is Clifford's opinion that his employer would perceive depression as a sign of weakness. Overall, he has done well without the medications.

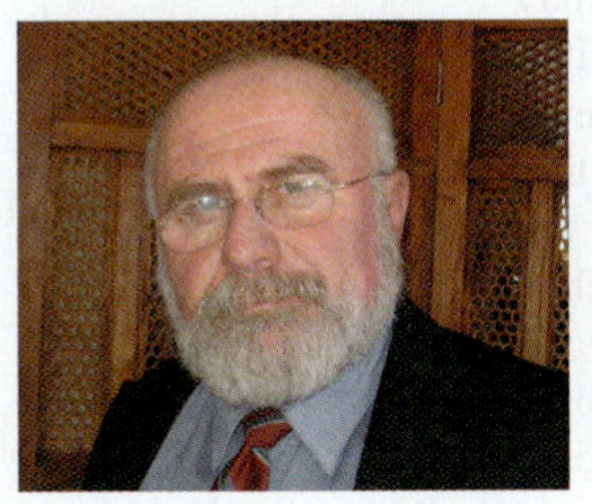

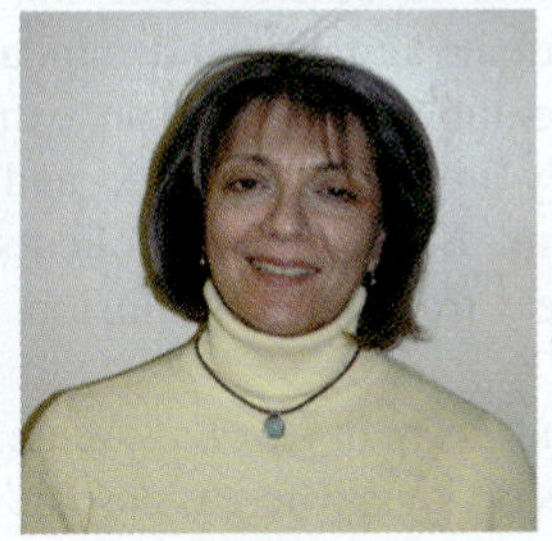

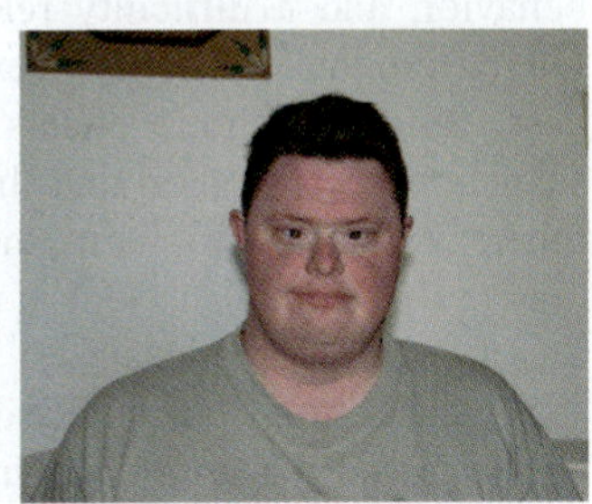

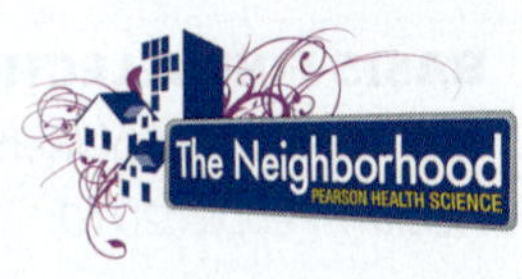

Clifford has been thinking about retiring within the next few years. He and his wife have always planned to do some traveling, but mostly he looks forward to escaping the busy and stressful work environment. Clifford and Gary are involved with activities at his church; they also enjoy a walk each evening after supper. Clifford belongs to a bowling league and is at the bowling alley a couple of evenings a week.

Clifford is admitted to the acute care hospital for a transurethral resection of the prostate (TURP). He has been very anxious about having the procedure because of the risk of impotence. His surgery goes smoothly, and he experiences no complications. In the immediate postoperative period, Clifford has a three-way Foley catheter inserted, with continuous bladder irrigation. He experiences pain and has occasional bladder spasms because of blood clots. The day after surgery, the nurse enters Clifford's room and he asks why the hospital bed was brought to his room and calls the nurse by his wife's name. The nurse assesses Clifford and determines he is confused.

1. What factors may increase the risk of confusion in this client?
2. What interventions would the nurse initiate for Clifford if he were to display confusion?
3. What nursing diagnosis would be appropriate for Clifford if he were to display confusion?
4. What assessment tools would the nurse use to assess Clifford if he were to display confusion?

4.3 SCHIZOPHRENIA

KEY TERMS

Alogia, *237*
Anhedonia, *238*
Attention impairment, *240*
Avolition, *241*
Brief psychotic disorder, *235*
Catatonic excitement, *237*
Catatonic inhibition, *237*
Concrete thinking, *240*
Declarative memory, *240*
Delusions, *232*
Dystonias, *243*
Echopraxia, *237*
Extrapyramidal side effects (EPS), *243*
Hallucinations, *232*
Illusions, *232*
Involuntary admission, *250*
Loose association, *236*
Negative symptoms, *232*
Nicotinic receptors, *211*
Paranoia, *232*
Positive symptoms, *232*
Procedural memory, *240*
Psychiatric (psychosocial) rehabilitation, *244*
Psychosis, *232*
Schizoaffective disorder, *235*
Schizophrenia, *232*
Schizophreniform disorder, *235*
Selective perception, *239*
Sensory overload, *239*
Shared psychotic disorder, *235*
Stigma, *250*
Systematized, *239*
Tardive dyskinesia, *243*
Voluntary admission, *250*

BASIS FOR SELECTION OF EXEMPLAR

National Institute of Mental Health

Healthy People 2010

LEARNING OUTCOMES

After reading about this exemplar, you will be able to:

1. Describe the pathophysiology, etiology, clinical manifestations, and direct and indirect causes of schizophrenia.
2. Identify risk factors associated with schizophrenia.
3. Illustrate the nursing process in providing culturally competent care across the life span for individuals with schizophrenia.
4. Formulate priority nursing diagnoses appropriate for an individual with schizophrenia.
5. Create a plan of care for individuals with schizophrenia and their family members.
6. Assess expected outcomes for an individual with schizophrenia.
7. Discuss therapies used in the collaborative care of an individual with schizophrenia.
8. Employ evidence-based caring interventions for an individual with schizophrenia.

OVERVIEW

Severe mental illness can be incapacitating for the client and intensely frustrating for family members and those who interact with the client on a regular basis. Before the 1950s, clients with acute mental dysfunction were institutionalized, often for their entire lives.

A **psychosis** or psychotic disorder is a mental health condition characterized by **delusions** (firm ideas and beliefs not founded in reality), **hallucinations** (perceptions of seeing, hearing, or feeling something that is not there), **illusions** (distorted perceptions of actual sensory stimuli), disorganized behavior, and a difficulty relating to others. Behavior may range from total inactivity to extreme agitation and combativeness. Some psychotic clients exhibit **paranoia**, an extreme suspicion and delusion that they are being followed and that others are trying to harm them. Because these clients are unable to distinguish what is real from what is illusion, they are often viewed as insane.

Psychoses may be classified as *acute* or *chronic*. Acute psychotic episodes occur over hours or days, whereas chronic psychoses develop over months or years. Sometimes psychosis can be attributed to an identifiable cause such as brain damage, overdoses of certain medications, extreme depression, chronic alcoholism, or drug addiction. Genetic factors are known to play a role in some psychoses. Unfortunately, the vast majority of psychoses have no identifiable cause.

Schizophrenia is the most common psychotic disorder. Many other conditions can cause bizarre behavior, and these should be distinguished from schizophrenia. **Schizophrenia** is a combination of disordered thinking, perceptual disturbances, behavioral abnormalities, affective disruptions, and impaired social competency. This means that the person has difficulty thinking clearly, knowing what is real, managing feelings, making decisions, and relating to others. Typically, the person is fairly normal early in life, experiences subtle changes after puberty, and undergoes severe symptoms in late teens to early adulthood. The early age of onset often shatters the lives of its victims and robs them of the opportunity for a productive adult life.

Schizophrenia is a disorder of the brain and is a devastating and often disabling disorder that affects not only the individual, but also family, friends, and the community as a whole. Although it is referred to as a single disease, it is more accurately described as a spectrum of disorders characterized by a broad range of symptoms, physiological malfunctions, etiologies, and prognoses. Included in the syndrome of schizophrenia are schizoid personality disorder, schizotypal personality disorder, paranoid personality disorder, schizoaffective disorder, schizophreniform disorder, delusional disorder, brief psychotic disorder, shared psychotic disorder, and schizophrenia.

Symptoms of schizophrenia are commonly described as *positive* or *negative.* **Positive symptoms** are excessive or added behaviors that are not normally seen in healthy adults, such as delusions. **Negative symptoms** are the loss of normal function normally seen in mentally healthy adults, such as the ability to care for one's self. Relatives of people who have schizophrenia are often included in the spectrum because they are thought to have a genetic predisposition to schizophrenia but might not necessarily demonstrate full or any clinical manifestations of schizophrenia (Gottesman & Petronis, 2003; Seeman, 2004).

PATHOPHYSIOLOGY AND ETIOLOGY

Neurodevelopment studies demonstrate evidence of abnormal brain development in peopole with schizophrenia. The basic flaw seems to be that certain nerve cells migrate to the wrong areas when the brain is first taking shape, leaving small regions of the brain permanently out of place or miswired. In some cases, the neurons of the cortex may be deficient. From a developmental perspective, it is not known whether these cells form normally and then fail to thrive or whether they are malformed from the beginning.

The question arises that if schizophrenia begins in utero, why does it not manifest for 20 years? Recent studies show that some people with schizophrenia may have early signs that are overlooked or misunderstood. For example, a child might sit up a month later than other children or speak 3 months later than other children of the same age. These signs may indicate a slight maturational lag in brain function that is later associated with schizophrenia. Later in childhood, there may be evidence of lagging development and cognitive perceptual abnormalities.

One factor related to the delay in the appearance of significant symptoms may be formation of the myelin sheath, which does not form on the outside of many brain cells until late adolescence. Between the ages of 16 and 22, there are also progressive changes in cortical interactions, especially between the left prefrontal and temporal regions. This failure of the cortex to reorganize during adolescence may be the final neurodevelopmental failure of schizophrenia.

Neurochemical factors likely involve dopamine (DA), serotonin (5-HT), norepinephrine (NE), glutamate, and gamma-aminobutyric acid (GABA) neurotransmission. At times, neurotransmitters work together (synergistically) to trigger the same biochemical reaction, while at other times, they act as antagonists, with one inhibiting the action of another.

Glu, involved in learning and memory, may be responsible for some of the cognitive symptoms of schizophrenia. Glu is necessary for the breakdown of DA and other transmitters, which affects the efficiency of prefrontal information processing. Glu receptors have a role in regulating the migration and pruning of neurons during brain development and, thus, may play a role in the structural abnormalities that have been seen in schizophrenia. Excessively high levels of NE are associated with positive symptoms, while paranoid symptoms have been related to increased DA activity.

No single neurotransmitter is clearly responsible for schizophrenia. The important concept may be homeostasis, the absolute level of any neurotransmitter being much less important than its relative level with respect to all other transmitters. There also may be an undiscovered neurochemical factor. It will be a long time before this is understood clearly (Keltner, 2005; Yasuno et al., 2004).

On a larger scale, new brain imaging studies have revealed abnormalities of brain structure in schizophrenia. Although no single brain region has been found to be involved in the pathology of schizophrenia, the areas most noted for abnormalities include the prefrontal cortex, temporal lobes, hippocampus, limbic system, thalamus, and ventricles. See Box 4–7 for a list of brain abnormalities in schizophrenia.

The reason the brains of people with schizophrenia may not "look the same" clinically may be a function of individual deviations in brain structure. In some cases, tissue volume is decreased in specific areas; in other cases, cerebral blood flow is disrupted; in some clients, utilization of glucose and oxygen is decreased; and in still more clients, ventricular size is increased. Individuals with childhood-onset schizophrenia demonstrate greater loss of cortical gray matter than those with later development of the disorder. The corpus callosum is defective in some people with schizophrenia. The resulting misconnection of the hemispheres may contribute to the affective symptoms and social isolation (Brambilla et al., 2005; Gogtay et al., 2004; Kim, Ha, & Kwon, 2004).

An example of one deviation is that decreased blood flow to the thalamus may affect the ability of the brain to filter sensory signals, causing a person to be flooded with sensory information. (Refer to Figure 4–4 ■.) Changes in cerebral blood flow suggest abnormalities in the density, size, or configuration of blood vessels in a person with schizophrenia. Structural abnormalities are only the result of some abnormal process and do not provide much information about the process.

For some people with schizophrenia, there is a deficiency of **nicotinic receptors** in the hippocampus, an area of the brain involved with new sensory stimuli and memory formation.

Box 4–7 **Central Nervous System Abnormalities in Schizophrenia**

INCREASED VENTRICULAR SIZE

DECREASED VOLUME
- Temporal lobes
- Hippocampus
- Prefrontal cortex
- Limbic system
- Thalamus

DECREASED CEREBRAL BLOOD FLOW
- Temporal lobes
- Basal ganglia
- Thalamus

DECREASED BLOOD GLUCOSE AND OXYGEN UTILIZATION
- Frontal lobes
- Basal ganglia

DECREASED ACTIVITY
- Prefrontal cortex

DECREASED NICOTINIC RECEPTORS
- Hippocampus

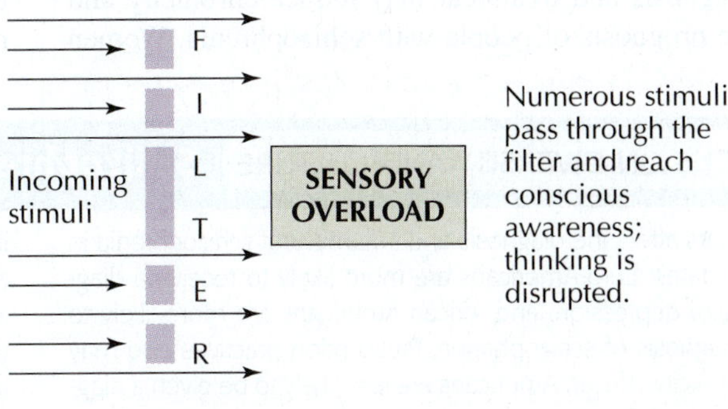

Figure 4–4 ■ Impaired sensory filtering in schizophrenia.

Clients who smoke may be self-medicating with nicotine, which improves their attentiveness and ability to lay down memories. Nicotine may be especially reinforcing because it stimulates DA release in the nucleus accumbens and the prefrontal cortex. DA deficiency and low activity in these regions are linked to the negative symptoms of schizophrenia. Only about 25% of the general U.S. population smokes, compared with 58–92% of people with schizophrenia. Nicotine addiction, therefore, is a serious problem for people with this disorder (Olincy et al., 2006).

Etiology

Schizophrenia is diagnosed in about 1% of the U.S. population. Schizophrenia is recognized worldwide and affects about 1% of the population in different cultures. For unknown reasons, there are small populations with increased incidence, such as second-generation African Caribbean people living in the United Kingdom. The symptoms of schizophrenia tend to be universal, but culture affects how the symptoms are interpreted (Phillips, Yang, Li, & Li, 2004).

The onset and progression of schizophrenia are variable. It is believed that people with an abrupt onset of the illness have a different form of schizophrenia than those whose onset is more insidious. The majority develop the disorder in adolescence or young adulthood, with only 10–15% of cases first diagnosed in people older than 45. Schizophrenia rarely occurs for the first time in old age. Only about 10% of people with diagnosed schizophrenia experience the onset of symptoms after the age of 40 (APA, 2008).

Some symptoms of schizophrenia, such as hallucinations and delusions, appear to decline with age, but symptoms such as apathy and withdrawal may place the older adult at high risk for social isolation and neglect. People with late-onset schizophrenia have more delusions, which are often persecutory and bizarre. They are more likely to exhibit vivid hallucinations but have fewer cognitive disruptions and negative symptoms. It is thought that late-onset schizophrenia may be a less severe form of the disorder (Friedman et al., 2002).

In some cases, the disorder progresses through relapse and remission. In other cases, it takes a long-term, stable course, while in some clients, a long-term, progressively deteriorating course evolves. Much too often, the illness results in lifelong problems coping with everyday living that reflect irreversible neurobiological deficits.

Early diagnosis and treatment may reduce chronicity and improve the prognosis of people with schizophrenia. Women tend to have a later onset of illness, better treatment response, shorter and less frequent relapses, and an overall higher quality of life than their male counterparts (Seeman, 2004).

Individuals with schizophrenia have a 20% shorter life expectancy than the general population. Accidents, suicide, and homicide account for one third of these premature deaths. Two thirds die of coronary heart disease, hypertension, emphysema, or complications of type 2 diabetes mellitus. In part, this is attributable to a lifestyle with poor dietary habits, obesity, high rates of smoking, and the use of alcohol and street drugs. Side effects of antipsychotic medication include weight gain and metabolic syndrome (Ryan, Collins, & Thakore, 2003).

The age of onset for schizoaffective disorder, as with schizophrenia, is typically late adolescence or early adulthood. Schizophrenia is equally common in men and women. Men typically are diagnosed earlier. Women are more likely than men to have their diagnosis switched from schizophrenia to schizoaffective disorder.

The cause of schizophrenia has not been determined, although several theories have been proposed. Many studies support the view of environmental factors and genetic susceptibility as causes. In some individuals, a genetic defect may contribute to abnormal development of the brain or a neurochemical malfunction, whereas in other cases, factors such as nutrition, toxins, or trauma might interact in a genetically vulnerable person, resulting in schizophrenia. In still other cases, the cause may be completely environmental, such as lack of prenatal care, complications at birth, or exposure to maternal viral infections. People with schizophrenia are more likely to have experienced complications at birth, and are more likely to experience an earlier onset and greater severity of the disorder.

Risk Factors

It is well recognized that there is a genetic component in schizophrenia, and 85% of susceptibility to schizophrenia may be genetic. However, the amount of genetic vulnerability is not known because no single gene has been identified as a risk factor for schizophrenia. It is likely that a number of genes are involved and that different genes may be involved in different families. There also may be a different pattern of inheritance in early-onset versus late-onset schizophrenia. It is likely that the early-onset type has a higher genetic load for schizophrenia (Gochman et al., 2004).

A person has an 8% risk for schizophrenia if a sibling has the disorder, a 13% risk if one parent is affected, a 10–15% risk of sharing the disorder with a dizygotic twin, a 40–50%

FOCUS ON DIVERSITY AND CULTURE Schizophrenia

Cultural factors affect the diagnosis and treatment of schizophrenia in the United States. Euro-Americans are more likely to receive a diagnosis of major depression, and African Americans are more likely to receive a diagnosis of schizophrenia. Prescription practices also may vary with ethnicity. African Americans are less likely to be given a diagnosis of comorbid depression than are Euro-Americans, leaving these clinically significant symptoms untreated. African Americans are more likely than Euro-Americans to receive psychotropic medications above recommended levels. In addition, African Americans are more likely to experience tardive dyskinesia than are Euro-Americans (Buchanan, Kreyenbuhl, Zito, & Lehman, 2002; Practice Guideline for the Treatment of Patients with Schizophrenia, 2004; Wonodi, Adami, Cassady, Sherr, Avila, & Thaker, 2004).

risk if both parents are affected, and a 50% risk if a monozygotic twin has schizophrenia. In addition, 21% of first-degree relatives of individuals with schizophrenia have schizotypal personality disorder or other traits in the schizophrenic spectrum (Tamminga, Thaker, & Medoff, 2004). Figure 4–5 ■ illustrates the average risk for development of schizophrenia.

In monozygotic twins, prenatal factors do not always affect each twin to the same extent. Because the hands are formed at the same time cells are migrating to the cerebral cortex during the second trimester of pregnancy, they have been a site for the indirect study of brain development. In studying sets of twins in which one has schizophrenia and the other does not, it was found that the affected twin had a number of small deformities in the hands and greater differences in fingerprints than the sibling. There was also a significant prenatal size difference between the twins during the second trimester. Conditions that could result in brain injury at this stage of development include anemia, anoxia, ischemia, maternal alcohol or drug abuse, toxin exposure, or viral infection (Tarrant & Jones, 2000).

Advanced paternal age may be a risk factor for schizophrenia and the other schizophrenia spectrum disorders. Compared with children of fathers younger than 25 years, the risk doubled for children of fathers in their 40s and tripled in children of men older than 50. The etiology is believed to involve mutations in the sperm (Sipos et al., 2005).

The more protective factors a person has, the less the chance of developing the disorder. Only a few people have such a strong genetic vulnerability that schizophrenia is almost inevitable. The majority of the population has little or no risk for schizophrenia. In between are people who may develop the disorder if stressed enough but who also could survive and not experience schizophrenia if not sufficiently stressed.

CLINICAL MANIFESTATIONS

Each of the disorders along the spectrum of schizophrenia exhibits some differentiation in manifestations. In **schizoaffective disorder**, clients have symptoms that appear to be a mixture of schizophrenia and mood disorders. The person experiences one or more of the following psychotic symptoms: delusions, hallucinations, disorganized speech, disorganized behavior, and negative symptoms. In addition, the person experiences symptoms of mood disorders, which may be major depressive symptoms (e.g., depressed mood, insomnia or hypersomnia, and feelings of worthlessness), manic symptoms (e.g., decreased need for sleep, racing thoughts, inflated self-esteem, and unrestrained behaviors), or mixed symptoms. Schizoaffective disorder is most likely a distinct syndrome resulting from a high genetic liability to mood disorders and schizophrenia. Clients with schizoaffective disorder often have difficulty maintaining job or school functioning, experience problems with self-care, are socially isolated, and often have suicidal ideation. The prognosis of schizoaffective disorder is somewhat better than that for schizophrenia but significantly worse than the prognosis for mood disorders (Siever & Davis, 2004).

In **brief psychotic disorder**, there is a rapid onset of at least one of the following psychotic symptoms: delusions, hallucinations, disorganized speech, or disorganized and strange behavior. The episode lasts at least 1 day but less than 1 month, after which the person returns to the premorbid level of functioning.

The symptoms of **schizophreniform disorder** are the same but last at least 1 month and less than 6 months. One third of people with schizophreniform disorder return to premorbid levels of functioning, whereas two thirds progress to the diagnosis of schizophrenia or schizoaffective disorder.

In **shared psychotic disorder**, a person who is in a close relationship with another person who is delusional comes to share the delusional beliefs. This most commonly occurs between two people but may involve more individuals, such as when children adopt a parent's delusional beliefs (APA, 2000).

The classic subtypes of schizophrenia described in the *Diagnostic and Statistical Manual of Mental Disorders* (4th ed., Text Revision) (*DSM-IV-TR*) (Box 4–8) (undifferentiated, catatonic, paranoid, disorganized, and residual) are difficult to apply and have many symptoms in common. Diagnoses are often changed from one category to another as symptoms fluctuate; thus, the classification is unstable. See the *DSM-IV-TR* Criteria feature for the descriptions of the subtypes of schizophrenia. The classic subtypes have given way to new systems

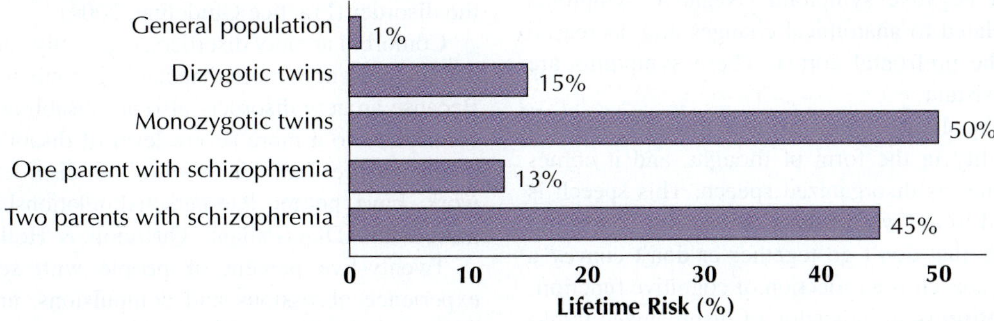

Figure 4–5 ■ Average risk for developing schizophrenia.

Sources: Gottesman, I. I, & Petronis, A. (2003). Schizophrenia genetics obscured by the realities of complex diseases. NAMI Advocate, 1(4), 31–32; Siever, L. J., & Davis, K. L. (2004). The pathophysiology of schizophrenia disorders: Perspectives from the spectrum. *American Journal of Psychiatry, 161*(3), 398–413; Tamminga, C. A., Thaker, G. K., & Medoff, D. R. (2004). Neuropsychiatric aspects of schizophrenia. In S. C. Yudofsky & R. E. Hales (Eds.), *Essentials of neuropsychiatry and clinical neurosciences* (pp. 457–487). Washington, DC: American Psychiatric Publishing.

Box 4–8 ***DSM-IV-TR*** **Diagnostic Criteria for Schizophrenia Subtypes**

PARANOID TYPE

A type of schizophrenia in which the following criteria are met:

a. Preoccupation with one or more delusions or frequent auditory hallucinations.
b. None of the following is prominent: disorganized speech, disorganized or catatonic behavior, or flat or inappropriate affect.

DISORGANIZED TYPE

A type of schizophrenia in which the following criteria are met:

a. All of the following are prominent:
b. The criteria are not met for catatonic type.

CATATONIC TYPE

A type of schizophrenia in which the clinical picture is dominated by at least two of the following:

1. Motoric immobility as evidenced by catalepsy (including waxy flexibility) or stupor
2. Excessive motor activity (that is apparently purposeless and not influenced by external stimuli)
3. Extreme negativism (an apparently motiveless resistance to all instructions or maintenance of a rigid posture against attempts to be moved) or mutism
4. Peculiarities of voluntary movement as evidenced by posturing (voluntary assumption of inappropriate or bizarre postures), stereotyped movements, prominent mannerisms, or prominent grimacing
5. Echolalia or echopraxia.

UNDIFFERENTIATED TYPE

A type of schizophrenia in which symptoms that meet Criterion A are present, but the criteria are not met for the paranoid, disorganized, or catatonic type.

RESIDUAL TYPE

A type of schizophrenia in which the following criteria are met:

a. Absence of prominent delusions, hallucinations, disorganized speech, and grossly disorganized or catatonic behavior.
b. There is continuing evidence of the disturbance, as indicated by the presence of negative symptoms or two or more symptoms listed in Criterion A for schizophrenia, present in an attenuated form (e.g., odd beliefs, unusual perceptual experiences).

Source: Reprinted with permission from the *Diagnostic and Statistical Manual of Mental Disorders*, Fourth Edition, Text Revision, (Copyright 2000). American Psychiatric Association.

of classification. The most widely used system is one of positive symptoms, negative symptoms, and thought disorganization. This arrangement represents symptom types that are probably semi-independent of one another.

Positive symptoms are most likely the result of physiological changes, including increased DA function in the subcortical areas of the brain and decreased glucose utilization in the brain. Women are more likely to exhibit more positive than negative symptoms. Medication is often successful in diminishing positive symptoms. Table 4–10 lists the positive symptoms of schizophrenia.

Negative symptoms of schizophrenia are related to decreased motivation and drive, the inability to express feelings, and the lack of spontaneity and curiosity. Negative symptoms are listed in Table 4–10. Men are more likely to exhibit prominent negative symptoms. Negative symptoms are most likely related to anatomical changes and decreased DA function in the prefrontal cortex. These symptoms are more treatment-resistant.

Schizophrenia is often referred to as a thought disorder, which is abnormality in the form of thought, and it comes across to the listener as disorganized speech. This speech is sometimes referred to as "word salads" because it comes out in strings of words that don't go together or don't convey a meaning. Because speech is a reflection of cognitive functioning, **loose association** is an indication of disorganized thinking. A person has a loose association when verbal ideas shift from one topic to another, there is no apparent relationship between thoughts, and the person speaking is unaware that the topics are unconnected. (Bowie, Tsapelas, Friedman, Parrella, White, & Harvey, 2005).

Comorbid Disorders

It is not uncommon for people with schizophrenia to experience a comorbid disorder. More than 50% of people with schizophrenia have problems with alcohol or drugs at some point during their illness. Many people with schizophrenia use alcohol or drugs to self-medicate and to feel better. More than half are nicotine-dependent. Prompt recognition and treatment of this dual diagnosis problem is essential for effective treatment.

Suicide accounts for the majority of premature deaths among people with schizophrenia. It is estimated that as many as half of this population experience suicidal ideation, make suicide attempts, or both. Ten percent are successful suicides. Risk factors include a young age, a high socioeconomic status background, a high intelligence quotient (IQ) with a high level of pre-illness academic achievement, and a severe course of the disorder (Practice Guideline, 2004).

Comorbid anxiety disorders, especially social anxiety disorder, are present in more than half of people with schizophrenia. Because anxiety disorders also are disabling, the combination contributes to a more severe level of disability and decreased quality of life. Individuals with both disorders are less able to work, have poorer interpersonal relationships, and struggle more with ADLs (Pallanti, Quercioli, & Hollander, 2004).

Twenty-five percent of people with schizophrenia also experience obsessions and compulsions, and of this group, 26% could be diagnosed with obsessive–compulsive disorder. Typically, these clients are preoccupied with the content of their delusions and may ruminate for hours over their upsetting thoughts (Nechmad et al., 2003).

People with late-onset schizophrenia, diagnosed at age 45 or older, appear to be at high risk for AD. In one study, half the

TABLE 4–10 **Symptoms of Schizophrenia**

POSITIVE SYMPTOMS	NEGATIVE SYMPTOMS
Behavioral	
Hyperactivity	Decreased activity level
Bizarre behavior	Limited speech; conversation difficult
	Minimal self-care
Affective	
Inappropriate affect	Blunted or flat affect
Overreactive affect	Anhedonia
Hostility	
Perceptual	
Hallucinations	Inability to understand sensory information
Sensory overload	
Cognitive	
Delusions	Concrete thinking
Disorganized thinking	Attention impairment
Loose associations	Memory deficits
Suspiciousness	Impaired problem solving
	Lack of motivation
Social	
Aloof and stilted interactions	Social withdrawal, isolation
	Poor rapport with others
	Inadequate social and occupational skills

subjects developed dementia between 1 and 5 years following a diagnosis of schizophrenia (Brodaty, Sachdev, Koschera, Monk, & Cullen, 2003).

There are many different presentations of schizophrenia depending on the type, age of onset, and progression. It is unlikely that one client would present with all of the manifestations listed here. All clients must be assessed to determine which of these common manifestations they are experiencing.

Catatonic Manifestations

Catatonia is a frequent psychomotor syndrome in people with schizophrenia. **Catatonic excitement** includes hyperactivity and bizarre behavior and is a positive symptom of the disorder. *Hyperactive behavior* most typically occurs during a period of relapse. Excitement may become so great that it threatens the person's safety or that of others. Behavior may also be unpredictable. Schizophrenia can cause people to engage in bizarre behavior such as repeating rhythmic gestures, doing ritualistic postures, or demonstrating freakish facial or body movements. Some people will imitate other people's movements (**echopraxia**) or words (echolalia) or may senselessly repeat the same word or phrase for hours or days. Another positive characteristic is a decreased awareness of one's own behavior. It is not unusual to hear clients describe their behavior as being under the influence of alien forces or of other people (Kruger, Bagby, Hoffler, & Braunig, 2003).

Catatonic inhibition involves decreased activity level; limited speech; minimal self-care; and, at times, a trancelike state. Catatonic inhibition is a negative symptom of schizophrenia. The decreased activity level includes a reduction of energy, initiative, and spontaneity. There is a loss of natural gracefulness in body movements that results in poor coordination: Activities may be carried out in a robotlike fashion. People with schizophrenia often have limited speech, referred to as **alogia**, which makes it difficult for them to carry on a continuous conversation or to say anything new. They may say very little on their own initiative or in response to questions from others; some individuals with schizophrenia may be mute for several hours to several days. Some clients experience decreased responsiveness and appear to be in a trancelike state.

Another difficulty for individuals and their significant others is a deterioration in appearance and manners. Self-care

CLINICAL MANIFESTATIONS AND THERAPIES Schizophrenia

ETIOLOGY	CLINICAL MANIFESTATIONS	CLINICAL THERAPIES
Control cognition problems resulting from schizophrenia	Positive and negative symptoms	Psychopharmacology ■ Antipsychotic medications ■ Mood stabilizing agents ■ Benzodiazepines
Inability to function successfully in the community	Lack of skills for successful living, learning, and working in the community	Psychiatric rehabilitation
Isolation and withdrawal	Avoidance behaviors, difficulty maintaining relationships	Group therapy
Poor coping skills, inability to self-care and keep a job	Clients assigned to a specific multidisciplinary team that delivers all services when and where the client needs them with the goal of preventing rehospitalization	Assertive community treatment (ACT)
ALTERNATIVE THERAPIES		
Auditory hallucinations	Placement of transcranial magnetic stimulation (TMS) on left temporal lobe may decrease frequency and duration of hallucinations.	TMS
Fatty acid deficiency	Increased fish oil intake in the form of omega-3 fatty acids may reduce positive and negative symptoms and dyskinesia side effects.	Omega-3 fatty acids
Excitation or agitation	Use of aromas, specifically basil, bergamot, chamomile, frankincense, juniper, lavender, lemon balm, and sandalwood, may induce a sense of calm.	Aromatherapy
		Acupuncture

may become minimal; clients may need to be reminded to bathe, shave, brush their teeth, and change their clothes. Because of confusion and distraction, people with schizophrenia may not conform to social norms of dress and behavior.

Only a minority of people with schizophrenia demonstrate violent behavior. Risk factors include male sex; a history of being poor, unskilled, or uneducated; a history of arrests; and a history of violent behavior. Some clients become violent when they act on the basis of their delusions and hallucinations. Comorbid alcohol and drug abuse increases the risk for violent behavior, as does severe akathisia (Practice Guideline, 2004).

Manifestations Related to Affect

Positive affective characteristics include inappropriate affect, overreactive affect, and hostility. *Inappropriate affect* occurs when the person's emotional tone is not related to the immediate circumstances. An *overreactive affect* is appropriate to the situation but out of proportion to it. Negative affective characteristics include blunted or flat affect and anhedonia. A *blunted affect* describes a dulled emotional response to a situation, and a *flat affect* describes the absence of visible cues to the person's feelings. Schizophrenia can make it difficult for people to identify and communicate feelings. Clients with schizophrenia show less emotion, laugh less, and cry less. The nurse should not confuse the inability to *express* emotions with the inability to *experience* emotions. Table 4–11 gives examples of descriptors of affect.

Anhedonia, the inability to experience pleasure, causes many people with schizophrenia to feel emotionally barren. This may lead to eccentric social interaction and social withdrawal. Clients may not take much interest in the things around them, even things they used to find enjoyable. If the world feels "flat as cardboard," clients may not feel it is worth the effort to get out and do things.

People with schizophrenia have a normal ability to experience unpleasant emotions and often experience worries and fears. With little warning, some people with schizophrenia become hostile as anger turns into aggression with the intent to do harm.

Manifestations Related to Perception

Positive perceptual characteristics include hallucinations and sensory overload. Hallucinations are real to the person having them and may be triggered by anxiety or by functional changes in the CNS. The same brain area is activated when clients listen to audible speech as when they experience auditory hallucinations. In other words, the brain reacts as if it is unable to

TABLE 4–11 Descriptors of Affect

AFFECT	EXAMPLE
Appropriate	Juan cries when learning of the death of his father.
Inappropriate	When told it is time to turn off the TV and go to bed, Joe begins to laugh uproariously.
Stable	During a card game, Don smiles and laughs at the appropriate social interchanges.
Labile	During a friendly checkers game, Sean, who has been laughing, suddenly knocks the board off the table in anger. He then begins to laugh and wants to continue the game.
Elevated	Connor bounces around the cafeteria, laughing and singing and telling his classmates how wonderful everything is.
Depressed	Leo sits slumped in a chair with a sad facial expression, teary eyes, and minimal body movement.
Overreactive	Kathy screams and curses when her child spills a glass of milk on the floor.
Blunted	When Tom learns of his full-tuition scholarship, he responds with only a small smile.
Flat	When Juanita's mother tells her that her favorite dog has died, Juanita simply says, "Oh," and gives no indication of an emotional response.

distinguish between its own internally generated speech and actual audible speech.

The most common type of hallucination is an *auditory hallucination*, or the hearing of voices or unusual noises. The voice is often that of God, the devil, a neighbor, or a relative; the voice may say bad or good things; and the voice seems to come from an external source. Auditory hallucinations occur in 50–80% of people with schizophrenia.

The next most common type is a *visual hallucination*, which is usually nearby, clearly defined, and moving. Visual hallucinations are often accompanied by auditory hallucinations.

Tactile, *olfactory*, and *gustatory hallucinations* are uncommon and are more likely to occur in people who are undergoing substance withdrawal or abusing drugs.

Hallucinations may have considerable control over the person's behavior. It is not unusual for people having auditory hallucinations to carry on a conversation with one of the voices. After a period of time, many people realize that if they admit they hear voices, they will be labeled as "sick" or "crazy." To avoid being labeled, people having auditory hallucinations may be very evasive about their hallucinations.

The body's sensory systems receive information from the environment and from the body through stimuli transmitted to the brain. Humans do not, however, consciously perceive much of this sensory information. Sensory information is processed in a series of relay stations in the brain where irrelevant stimuli are inhibited. This allows the brain to filter out unnecessary and distracting information—a process called **selective perception**—and focus on what is important at the given moment. Schizophrenia often disrupts the filtering process, causing **sensory overload**. When there are too many messages arriving at the cerebral cortex at the same time, thinking becomes disorganized and fragmented.

The negative perceptual characteristic in schizophrenia is the inability to understand sensory information. People with schizophrenia sometimes have a hard time making sense of everyday sights, sounds, and feelings. Their perception of what is going on around them may be distorted so that ordinary things are distracting or frightening. They may be overly sensitive to background noises, colors, and shapes.

Humans are highly evolved in face recognition. Survival demands that humans be able to distinguish between friend and foe, between related and unrelated, and between familiar and unfamiliar. People with schizophrenia often fail to recognize a previously seen face, which is likely related to dysfunction in the visual cortex. This may contribute to difficulties in social interactions (Onitsuka et al., 2005).

Alterations in Cognitive Function

Schizophrenia impairs many cognitive functions, such as thought formation, memory, language, attention, and executive functions. This impairment interferes with daily functioning more than any other group of symptoms. Positive cognitive characteristics of schizophrenia are delusions, disorganized thinking, and loose associations.

Delusions are false beliefs that cannot be changed by logical reasoning or evidence. Even though delusions are the product of brain dysfunction, clients attempt to make sense of them in the context of who they are. Thus, people in an underdeveloped country might believe that evil shamans are after them, while in Canada, they may believe that the Royal Canadian Mounted Police are following them. When there is an extensively developed central delusional theme from which conclusions are deduced, the delusions are termed **systematized**. There are a number of delusional types: grandiosity (delusions of grandeur), persecution, control, somatic, religious, erotomanic, ideas of reference, thought broadcasting, thought withdrawal, and thought insertion (Table 4–12). It is believed that delusions represent dysfunctions in the information-processing circuits in and between the hemispheres of the brain. The severity of delusions can be a valuable indicator in monitoring the course of the illness.

TABLE 4–12 Examples of Delusions

DELUSION	EXAMPLE
Grandiosity	"Within 1 month I am going to be a billionaire and own 14 houses and 20 cars. I will be so rich and successful that Bill Gates and Alan Greenspan are going to call me for financial advice."
Persecution	"My neighborhood wants me dead or alive. They think I hold all of their secrets. They have tapped my phone and peek through my windows 24 hours a day."
Control	"My mother put a voodoo curse on me. She can control all of my thoughts and emotions through a remote-control car. I am completely under her spell."
Religious	"God told me that I am his Chosen One. I can perform miracles. I know this is real because my rosary beads revealed this to me."
Erotomanic	"I can have any guy I want. Matt Damon called me last night but I couldn't go out because I already had a date with Tom Cruise."
Sin and guilt	"I can't do anything right. I always mess everything up. I had so many friends from school, but now no one will come and see me because I am a failure."
Somatic	"I have a hammer in my heart. It pounds daggers in it all day long. Don't you hear it? Someday soon it is going to pound so hard that my heart will come flying out of my chest onto the floor."
Ideas of reference	"The headline of the *New York Times* told me that I have been assigned to stop crime. I am issuing a nationwide bulletin telling people to turn in their guns and knives. I take my assignments very seriously."
Thought broadcasting	"I don't have to tell you that. You already know because you can read my mind."
Thought withdrawal	"I'm trying to tell you something, but I keep losing it because someone keeps stealing my thoughts."
Thought insertion	"You think this is me talking, but it really isn't. My husband keeps putting these thoughts in my head."

Grandiosity, also known as *delusions of grandeur*, is an exaggerated sense of importance or self-worth. It is often accompanied by beliefs of magical thinking. An example of grandiosity may be the client who believes they are king or president and expect others to behave accordingly toward them.

People with schizophrenia may experience *delusions of persecution*. They may believe that someone is trying to harm them and, therefore, that any personal failures in life are the fault of these harmful others.

Delusions of control occur when people believe that feelings, impulses, thoughts, or actions are not their own, but are being imposed by some external force. *Religious delusions* involve false beliefs with religious or spiritual themes. People with *erotomanic delusions* believe that a person, usually someone famous and of higher status, is in love with them. Preoccupation with the "fantasy" lover may lead to stalking. Occasionally, the stalker turns violent, not because of hatred of the person, but because the object of their obsession cannot fulfill the romantic delusions.

Somatic delusions occur when people believe something abnormal and dangerous is happening to their bodies that in no way refers to the person with schizophrenia, but is interpreted as related to the person. *Thought broadcasting* occurs when people believe that others can hear their thoughts. *Thought withdrawal* is the belief that others are able to remove thoughts from one's mind. *Thought insertion* is the belief that others are able to put thoughts into one's mind.

As previously discussed, disorganized thinking is another effect of schizophrenia. Adaptation to the environment and effective coping depend not only on learned responses, but also on flexibility of the brain in organizing this incoming information.

The negative cognitive characteristics of schizophrenia are concrete thinking, attention impairment, memory deficits, impaired problem solving, lack of motivation, and lack of insight. These symptoms are most likely related to dysfunctions in the cerebral cortex.

Concrete thinking is characterized by a focus on facts and details and an inability to generalize or think abstractly. If someone were to ask a client what brought him or her to the hospital, the client would likely say, "a car."

Attention impairment interferes with the processing of information and the response to such information. A person with attention impairment has poor concentration and is easily distracted. Disturbances include responding to irrelevant external stimuli and difficulty completing tasks.

Declarative memory is memory related to people and facts, is consciously accessible, and can be verbally expressed. **Procedural memory** does not require conscious awareness and involves the memory of motor skills and procedures. *Memory deficits* in schizophrenia are one of the most severely impaired functions and explain the day-to-day difficulties that people with schizophrenia encounter. The area of declarative memory is primarily affected. The processes of responding emotionally, forming impressions about people, and drawing inferences, as well as many other high-level cognitive functions, are supported by declarative memory. Therefore, a person may display inappropriate behavior or make poor judgments when memory is impaired by schizophrenia (Kim et al., 2004).

Impaired problem solving may occur for a number of reasons. A person may be unaware that a problem exists, have impaired judgment, be unable to think logically, be unable to make a decision, or be unable to plan or follow through with a decision. Because one of the problems with schizophrenia is faulty information processing, a person with schizophrenia needs more time to think and problem-solve.

Lack of motivation, referred to as **avolition**, is the inability to persist in goal-directed activities. Clients may have trouble starting projects or following through with projects once begun. Their inability to persist at work or school activities results in significant employment or academic difficulties. At the extreme, these individuals may have to be reminded to do simple things such as taking a bath or changing clothes.

Poor insight, or lack of awareness of one's own mental illness, is more common in people with schizophrenia than in those with schizoaffective disorder or with major depressive disorder. Between 70% and 90% of clients have little awareness of their illness. Poor insight means that individuals have difficulty identifying their symptoms, which has implications for agreeing with treatment plans, recognizing early signs of relapse, and seeking treatment. Clients often believe that any difficulties they experience result from external causes. Insight often does not improve as the other symptoms improve (Flashman, 2004; Rickelman, 2004).

Effects of Manifestations on Interpersonal Relationships

The primary positive social characteristic of schizophrenia is one of aloof and stilted interactions with others. People with schizophrenia may use outdated or very formal language and may have difficulty carrying on a conversation. The negative social characteristics of schizophrenia are social withdrawal/isolation, poor rapport with others, and inadequate social and occupational skills. Social withdrawal/isolation may result from paranoid delusions, severe difficulty participating in conversations, or an inability to experience feelings of friendship or intimacy.

Inadequate social skills can interfere with the ability to develop rapport with others. These ineffective skills may drive away friends and family members who do not understand the behavior, further increasing the client's sense of isolation. People with schizophrenia may be socially incompetent, in part because they are unable to perceive the subtle cues critical to interpersonal interactions. To be able to understand body cues during an interaction, one must be able to think abstractly. People with schizophrenia understand concrete cues better than abstract cues. For example, although a person with schizophrenia can identify and recall what someone said and did, the person is less able to identify the emotional tone behind the words or comprehend the motivation for the interaction. Occupational skills may be problematic because of cognitive disruptions, behavioral abnormalities, inability to manage feelings, or inadequate social skills.

Most people with schizophrenia experience cycles of relapse and remission. Families who have a loved one with a long-term medical illness such as debilitating heart disease usually receive social support and sympathy. But members of families with a loved one suffering from schizophrenia are often avoided. The expense of long-term therapy, medications, and intermittent hospital stays drains many families. Mental health services are poorly covered in most medical insurance policies.

People with schizophrenia are not indifferent to their emotional and social environments. The emotional climate of the family has been shown to play a role in the rate of relapse of the disorder. Clients who live in families that are highly critical, hostile, and overinvolved (referred to as high expressed emotion [EE]) have a significantly higher relapse rate than those who live in a supportive and caring family system. Families that are highly negative or excessively intrusive to the client can accelerate the time to relapse by causing physiological arousal and increased symptoms. On average, the relapse rate among clients who are not in family therapy is almost 3 times as high as the rate for those in family therapy (Jungbauer, Wittmund, Dietrich, & Angermeyer, 2003).

Age-Specific Characteristics of Schizophrenia

Childhood-onset schizophrenia is diagnosed when the onset of psychotic symptoms occurs before 12 years of age and before the completion of brain maturation. This form of schizophrenia is severe and may have a stronger genetic predisposition than other forms (Sporn et al., 2004). Childhood-onset schizophrenia, also referred to as pediatric schizophrenia, occurs in 1 in 10,000 children. However, the prevalence of schizophrenia increases after puberty and reaches adult levels by late adolescence (Remschmidt & Theisen, 2005).

Most children who develop schizophrenia seem healthy at birth and during the first years of life. Subtle behavioral and cognitive characteristics often precede the first psychotic episode. These signs include higher-than-expected rates of abnormal speech and motor abnormalities such as clumsiness and abnormal movements.

The brain is altered in the disease, with progressively enlarged ventricles and nervous system arousal. Impaired glucose metabolism is often present. Onset is usually slow with increasing intensity over time. Most often the child demonstrates restlessness, poor appetite, and social withdrawal over a period of several weeks to months. Behavioral problems, slowed development, and minor neurological symptoms may occur. In addition, clients experience isolation, decline in IQ over several years, and diminishing school performance. Prior to developing psychotic symptoms, there is a high rate of special education placement and failed grades (Sporn et al., 2004).

Symptoms in children are similar to those seen in adults, although the content of children's hallucinations and delusions comes from their experiences. For example, rather than believing that the FBI is following them, children may believe that a cartoon villain is out to get them.

During adolescence, acute schizophrenia can occur suddenly while the teenager is making plans to leave home to attend college, marry, or work in another area. Onset of symptoms may be triggered by a stressor such as an important loss (death of a significant other, parent, child, or friend).

The majority of older adults with schizophrenia have had the disorder since youth. A number of older adults with early-onset schizophrenia show substantial improvement in symptoms, especially the positive symptoms, over the course of a lifetime.

COLLABORATION

Schizophrenic clients benefit when they are supported by a multidisciplinary team that includes their treating physician, the nurse, counselors, and close family and support people. For example, a homeless client with schizophrenia may receive support from the physician and nurse at a local free clinic, the director or a staff member from the homeless shelter, a counselor or therapist, and a professional at a job placement center. A team comprising these individuals can help the client prioritize goals and can direct treatment and support interventions to assist the client in improving functioning and relationship skills with the goal of finding the client a permanent, stable living situation and a job.

Collaborative treatment is highly individualized because of varying responses to different forms of therapy. While one client may respond well to a specific treatment, other treatments may have no effect at all. All too often the decision regarding the best therapy is based on a trial-and-error method that looks for the best outcome that will provide the client with the greatest independence and freedom from symptoms.

Pharmacologic Therapies

The primary goal of pharmacotherapy for schizophrenic clients is to reduce psychotic symptoms to a level that allows the client to maintain normal functioning, including caring for self and employment. From a pharmacological perspective, therapy has both positive and negative aspects. Although many symptoms of psychosis can be controlled with current drugs, adverse effects are common and often severe.

The antipsychotic agents do not cure schizophrenia, and symptoms remain in remission only as long as the client chooses to take the drug. The relapse rate for clients who discontinue their medication is 60–80%. In terms of efficacy, there is little difference in the various antipsychotic drugs and there is no single drug of choice for schizophrenia. Selection of a specific drug is based on clinician experience, the occurrence of side effects, and the needs of the client. The experience and skills of the physician and mental health nurse are particularly valuable in achieving successful psychiatric pharmacotherapy.

The conventional antipsychotics, sometimes called first-generation or typical antipsychotics, include the phenothiazine and phenothiazine-like agents. The first effective drug used to treat schizophrenia was the low-potency phenothiazine chlorpromazine (Thorazine), approved by the FDA for this use in 1954. Seven phenothiazines are now available to treat mental illness. All seven block the excitement associated with the positive symptoms of schizophrenia, although they differ in their potency and side-effect profiles (Table 4–13). Hallucinations and delusions often begin to diminish within days. Other symptoms, however, may require as long as 7–8 weeks of pharmacotherapy to improve. Because of the high rate of recurrence of psychotic episodes, pharmacotherapy should be considered long-term, often for the life of the client. Phenothiazines are thought to act by preventing DA and serotonin from occupying their receptor sites in certain regions of the brain.

Although phenothiazines revolutionized the treatment of severe mental illness, they exhibit numerous adverse effects that can limit pharmacotherapy. Anticholinergic effects such as dry mouth, postural hypotension, urinary retention, and constipation are common. Ejaculation disorders occur in a high percentage of male clients taking phenothiazines; delay in achieving orgasm (in both men and women) is a common cause for noncompliance. Menstrual disorders are common. Each phenothiazine has a slightly different side-effect spectrum. Unlike many other drugs whose primary action is on the CNS (e.g., amphetamines, barbiturates, anxiolytics, and alcohol), antipsychotic drugs do not cause physical or psychological dependence. They also have a wide safety margin between a therapeutic and lethal dose; deaths due to overdoses of antipsychotic drugs are uncommon.

TABLE 4–13 Adverse Effects of Conventional Antipsychotic Agents

EFFECT	DESCRIPTION
Acute dystonia	Severe spasms, particularly the back muscles, tongue, and facial muscles; twitching movements
Akathisia	Constant pacing with repetitive, compulsive movements
Anticholinergic effects	Dry mouth, tachycardia, blurred vision, constipation
Hypotension	Particularly severe when client moves quickly from a recumbent to an upright position
Neuroleptic malignant syndrome	High fever, confusion, muscle rigidity, and high serum creatine kinase; can be fatal
Parkinsonism	Tremor, muscle rigidity, stooped posture, and shuffling gait
Sedation	Usually diminishes with continued therapy
Sexual dysfunction	Impotence and diminished libido
Tardive dyskinesia	Bizarre tongue and face movements such as lip smacking and wormlike motions of the tongue; puffing of cheeks, uncontrolled chewing movements

Extrapyramidal side effects (EPS) are a particularly serious set of adverse reactions to antipsychotic drugs. EPS include acute dystonia, akathisia, Parkinsonism, and tardive dyskinesia. Acute **dystonias** occur early in the course of pharmacotherapy and involve severe muscle spasms, particularly of the back, neck, tongue, and face. Akathisia, the most common EPS, is an inability to rest or relax. The client paces, has trouble sitting or remaining still, and has difficulty sleeping. Symptoms of phenothiazine-induced Parkinsonism include tremor, muscle rigidity, stooped posture, and a shuffling gait. Long-term use of phenothiazines may lead to **tardive dyskinesia**, which is characterized by unusual tongue and face movements such as lip smacking and wormlike motions of the tongue. Tardive dyskinesia may be reversible if prompt intervention is provided. If EPS are reported early and the drug is withdrawn or the dosage is reduced, the side effects can be reversible. With higher doses given for prolonged periods, the extrapyramidal symptoms may become permanent. The nurse must be vigilant in observing and reporting EPS, as prevention is the best treatment.

With the conventional antipsychotics, it is not always possible to control the disabling symptoms of schizophrenia without producing some degree of EPS. In these clients, drug therapy may be warranted to treat EPS symptoms. Concurrent pharmacotherapy with an anticholinergic drug may prevent some of the extrapyramidal signs. For acute dystonia, benztropine (Cogentin) may be given orally or parenterally. Levodopa (Dopar, Larodopa), common in the treatment of Parkinson's disease, is usually contraindicated for the schizophrenic client because its ability to increase DA function antagonizes the action of the phenothiazines. Beta-adrenergic blockers and benzodiazepines are sometimes given to reduce signs of akathisia.

The efficacy of the nonphenothiazine antipsychotic medications is equal to that of the phenothiazines. Although the incidence of sedation and anticholinergic side effects is less, EPS may be common, particularly in older adults.

The conventional nonphenothiazine antipsychotic class consists of drugs whose chemical structures are dissimilar to the phenothiazines. Introduced shortly after the phenothiazines, initially the nonphenothiazines were expected to produce fewer side effects. Unfortunately, this appears not to be the case. The spectrum of side effects for the nonphenothiazines is identical with that of the phenothiazines, although the degree to which a particular effect occurs depends on the specific drug. In general, the nonphenothiazine agents cause less sedation and fewer anticholinergic side effects than chlorpromazine (Thorazine) but exhibit an equal or even greater incidence of extrapyramidal signs. Concurrent therapy with other CNS depressants must be carefully monitored because of the potential additive effects. Drugs in the nonphenothiazine class have the same therapeutic effects and efficacy as the phenothiazines. They also are believed to act by the same mechanism as the phenothiazines, that is, by blocking postsynaptic D_2 DA receptors. As a class, they offer no significant advantages over the phenothiazines in the treatment of schizophrenia.

Atypical antipsychotics treat both positive and negative symptoms of schizophrenia. They have become drugs of choice for treating psychoses. The approval of clozapine (Clozaril), the first atypical antipsychotic, marked the first major advance in the pharmacotherapy of psychoses since the discovery of chlorpromazine decades earlier. Clozapine and the other drugs in this class are called second-generation, or atypical, because they have a broader spectrum of action than the conventional antipsychotics, controlling both the positive and negative symptoms of schizophrenia. Furthermore, at therapeutic doses, they exhibit their antipsychotic actions without producing the EPS effects of the conventional agents. Some drugs, such as clozapine, are especially useful for clients with whom other drugs have proved unsuccessful.

The mechanism of action of the atypical agents is largely unknown, but they are thought to act by blocking several different receptor types in the brain. Like the phenothiazines, the atypical agents block DA D_2 receptors. However, the atypicals also block serotonin (5-HT) and alpha-adrenergic receptors, which is thought to account for some of the properties of the atypical agents. Because the atypical agents are only loosely bound to D_2 receptors, they produce fewer EPS than the conventional antipsychotics.

Although there are fewer side effects with atypical antipsychotics, adverse effects are still significant and clients must be carefully monitored. While most antipsychotics cause weight gain, the atypical agents are associated with obesity and its risk factors. Risperidone (Risperdal) and some of the other antipsychotic drugs increase prolactin levels, which can lead to menstrual disorders, decreased libido, and osteoporosis in women. In men, high prolactin levels can cause lack of libido and impotence. There also is concern that some atypical agents alter glucose metabolism, which can lead to type 2 diabetes.

Owing to side effects caused by conventional and atypical antipsychotic medications, a new drug class was developed to better meet the needs of clients with psychoses (Bailey, 2003). The new class is called *dopamine system stabilizers* or DA partial agonists. Aripiprazole (Abilify) received FDA approval in November 2002 for the treatment of schizophrenia and schizoaffective disorder. Because aripiprazole controls both the positive and negative symptoms of schizophrenia, it is grouped in Table 4–14 with the atypical antipsychotic drugs. Aripiprazole-treated clients appear to exhibit fewer EPS than clients treated with haloperidol (Haldol). Side effects include headache, nausea/vomiting, fever, constipation, and anxiety.

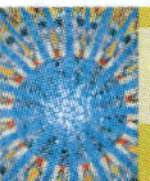

DEVELOPMENTAL CONSIDERATIONS

Older Adults

The use of medications in older clients is problematic at times. These individuals are likely to have other medical illnesses and to be taking multiple medications. Because of their age, older clients are at an increased risk for drug interactions and side effects. Low doses of the second-generation antipsychotics are the drugs of choice.

TABLE 4–14 **Atypical Antipsychotic Drugs**

DRUG	ROUTE AND ADULT DOSE (MAX DOSE WHERE INDICATED)	ADVERSE EFFECTS
aripiprazole (Abilify)	PO; 10–15 mg/day (max: 30 mg/day)	*Tachycardia, transient fever, sedation, dizziness, headache, light-headedness, somnolence, anxiety, nervousness, hostility, insomnia, nausea, vomiting, constipation, parkinsonism, akathisia* <u>Agranulocytosis, neuroleptic malignant syndrome (rare)</u>
clozapine (Clozaril)	PO; start at 25–50 mg/day and titrate to a target dose of 50–450 mg/day in 3 days; may increase further (max: 900 mg/day)	
olanzapine (Zyprexa)	Adult: PO; start with 5–10 mg/day; may increase by 2.5–5 mg every week (range 10–15 mg/day; max: 20 mg/day). Geriatric: PO; start with 5 mg/day	
quetiapine fumarate (Seroquel)	PO; start with 25 mg bid; may increase to a target dose of 300–400 mg/day in divided doses	
risperidone (Risperdal)	PO; 1–6 mg bid; increase by 2 mg daily to an initial target dose of 6 mg/day	
ziprasidone (Geodon)	PO; 20 mg bid (max: 80 mg bid)	

Italics indicate common adverse effects; <u>underlining</u> indicates serious adverse effects.

During the first episode of schizophrenia, the majority of individuals respond quickly to relatively low doses of antipsychotic medication. Later episodes require higher doses, and 5–25% of people with schizophrenia become resistant to the effects of medications. Side effects force other clients to decrease or stop their medication, which is a significant factor in relapse. The determination of which medication to use is often made on the basis of an individual side effect profile, which is determined by medication history. If an individual has a history of EPS, the individual would most likely be prescribed a second-generation antipsychotic. If the person is prone to weight gain and high blood lipid levels, the person would most likely be prescribed a first-generation antipsychotic (Navon & Ozer, 2003).

Psychiatric Rehabilitation

The field of **psychiatric (psychosocial) rehabilitation** grew out of a need to create opportunities for people with persistent psychiatric disability to increase their skill levels. The rehabilitation approach emphasizes the development of skills and support necessary for successful living, learning, and working in the community. This approach creates *collaborative partnerships* with all interested people—clients, families, friends, and mental health providers. It is assumed that the client will be "in charge" of setting goals for where and how to live, work, learn, socialize, and enjoy recreation. Rehabilitation is an ongoing process. It also is different from the traditional approach to long-term clients, which assumes that people with schizophrenia cannot make decisions and will continue to deteriorate in spite of interventions. It is now known that a substantial number of people with schizophrenia adjust well and lead satisfactory lives.

People who have severe and persistent mental illness differ little from the general population. They want work that is meaningful and self-enhancing and the opportunity to socialize with others. Psychiatric rehabilitation is anchored in the values of hope and optimism that people can grow, learn, and make changes in their lives. Other values include promotion of choices, self-determination, and individual responsibility. The essential element of self-help is power. People who are persistently ill need power and control in their relationships with professionals, in their own lives, and in the way resources are allocated. This allows them to take personal responsibility for where they are in their lives and where they are going (Lecomte, Wallace, Perreault, & Caron, 2005).

A nurse who functions as a resource for clients must not only be competent, but also be compassionate and caring. This includes searching for talents and skills in clients even when these traits are obscured by multiple relapses and low self-esteem. The nurse's role is to teach skills, to coach skills as needed in a variety of social and work situations, and to identify supports in the community of choice. In this way, the nurse will promote independent living and successful coping for people with psychiatric disabilities.

Group Therapy

Group therapy is an effective psychosocial treatment method for people with schizophrenia. It helps prevent the withdrawal and social isolation that may occur for people who are persistently ill. For those who live alone, the group may be their primary opportunity to relate to others. The group setting also provides an opportunity to discuss and help one another solve problems in everyday living, with employment difficulties, or with interpersonal conflicts. There are several types of group therapy. Some groups are highly structured, while others may be more spontaneous. Some groups may have a very narrow topic range, such as assertiveness training, while others may have a broader range, such as general problems living in the community. Groups focus on peer support, with an emphasis on development skills and changing behavior. Groups also are used for teaching and social support.

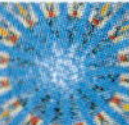

FOCUS ON DIVERSITY AND CULTURE **Culture Views and Treatments of Mental Illness**

Some cultures have very different perspectives on the cause of and treatment for mental illness. The foundation of many of these mental health treatments involves herbs and spiritual healing methods. Native Americans may be treated by the community's traditional "medicine man," who may treat mental symptoms with a sweat lodge and herbs. Hispanics may seek treatment from a folk healer, called a curandero; and they may use herbs such as chamomile, spearmint, and sweet basil for mental conditions. Members of some cultures may use amulets or charms to protect the wearer from evil spirits that are believed to cause mental illness.

Assertive Community Treatment

People who are psychiatrically disabled are often ill-prepared to find and maintain the multiple services needed to function in the community. One approach to helping clients is the assertive community treatment (ACT) program. Clients are assigned to a specific multidisciplinary team that delivers all services when and where the client needs them. The main goal of the program is to prevent rehospitalization by providing comprehensive, integrated community services. The ACT program provides 24-hour coverage, including emergencies. Studies show that ACT reduces time spent in the hospital, improves housing stability, decreases the occurrence of symptoms, and improves quality of life (Marshall & Lockwood, 2000).

Electroconvulsive Therapy

Electroconvulsive therapy (ECT) may be used in combination with second-generation antipsychotics for individuals with schizophrenia or schizoaffective disorder who have not responded to medication alone. Other candidates for ECT are people with unremitting depressive symptoms or severe suicidal ideation and behaviors (Practice Guideline, 2004).

Alternative Therapies

Cultural beliefs, as well as the frustration that often occurs when traditional therapies are not completely effective, have led clients to try therapies involving complementary and alternative medicine (CAM) with a goal of improved quality of life. Some of these CAM therapies have been researched to objectively determine their impact on symptom control, while others may be in the earliest stage of study to determine their usefulness in treating schizophrenia.

TRANSCRANIAL MAGNETIC STIMULATION Transcranial magnetic stimulation (TMS) is the use of a magnetic field that passes through the skull, which causes cells in the cerebral cortex to fire. More studies have been conducted in the use of TMS for depression than for schizophrenia. Initial studies indicate that TMS of the left temporal–parietal area may decrease the frequency and duration of auditory hallucinations and may modulate other symptoms of schizophrenia (Saenger, 2004).

OMEGA-3 FATTY ACIDS Individuals with a deficiency of omega-3 fatty acids will find the addition of fish oil helpful. It may not be that people with schizophrenia have a low intake; rather, they may need more to overcome a metabolic disorder that uses essential fatty acids at a faster rate. Initial studies suggest that omega-3 fatty acids reduce positive and negative symptoms and the side effects of dyskinesia. The recommended dosage is 5 g/day, usually 7 or 8 capsules. The maximum dosage is 15 g/day. Taking the capsules at night with orange juice cuts down on the fishy aftertaste (Emsley, Myburgh, Oosthuizen, & van Rensburg, 2002).

AROMATHERAPY Olfactory receptors are the only sensory pathways that open directly to the brain. Nerve cells relay this information directly to the limbic system, influencing emotions and behavior. Inhaling essential oils through the use of a diffuser or making use of essential oils in massage may be beneficial in inducing a sense of calmness. The following oils are most helpful: basil, bergamot, chamomile, frankincense, juniper, lavender, lemon balm, and sandalwood. Coriander improves memory and mental function.

ACUPUNCTURE The Chinese claim to have successfully treated schizophrenia with acupuncture. Research in Western medical practice is just beginning in this area. A 6-month study in Texas showed a decrease in the duration of hospital stays for individuals treated with acupuncture (Gerber, 2000).

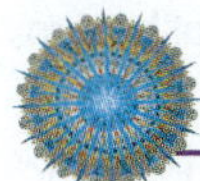

NURSING PROCESS

Assessment

Assessing a client who is suspected of having a psychosis is much different from assessing a client who may have a broken bone or who has an oxygen impairment. The assessment of client health history, family or caregiver reports, and direct observation of performance are essential to assessing client responses to illness and functional status for a client with or suspected of having schizophrenia. Clients are usually able to provide accurate information about their history with psychiatric disability and their current experiences. However, when clients are acutely ill, it may be difficult to obtain information from them directly. This is especially true for those experiencing delusions and hallucinations. Family members, roommates, friends, group-home supervisors, or case managers may be the initial data sources when a client is admitted to an acute care setting.

Health History

Nurses performing an assessment of the client with schizophrenia will ask the client and family members for examples of unusual behavior. Nurses should try to avoid asking leading questions. and should try to elicit detailed information about specific behaviors. Likely behavioral indicators include catatonic behaviors; significant changes in appearance; and, infrequently, violent behaviors. Because schizophrenic clients often experience alterations in perception, the nurse will assess for those through direct observation and through interviews with family members and others with whom the client interacts on a regular basis.

The assessment must include questions about early behaviors, success or failure at school and work, other health conditions and any related treatments, and previous experiences with mental health services and therapies.

Cultural Influences

A nurse must consider a person's cultural and religious backgrounds when assessing individuals from cultures that are different from those of the nurse. In some cultures, experiences labeled as delusional or hallucinatory are expected normal experiences. Differences in styles of expression of feelings may be misunderstood and labeled as pathological when, in fact, they are completely normal for that cultural group (APA, 2000).

Physical

There are several additional physical health indicators for schizophrenia. Abnormalities in the ability to identify smells may be a marker of cerebral dysfunction in schizophrenia. Individuals have difficulty with odor detection, odor identification, and odor recognition memory. Research shows that people with schizophrenia are unable to identify smells that have a pleasing scent, just as they are unable to experience pleasure. The circuitry of the prefrontal brain regions used to assess emotional and olfactory pleasure appears to be dysfunctional (Turetsky, Moberg, Arnold, Doty, & Gur, 2003).

Schizophrenia is characterized by disturbed sleep patterns. This contributes to an impaired ability to process information and a decline in working memory (Keshavan, Cashmere, Miewald, & Yeragani, 2004).

Individuals with schizophrenia are at high risk for polydipsia, a condition in which a person ingests excessive amounts of liquids, as high as 10 L. This can lead to hyponatremia, which may result in death. Symptoms include nausea and vomiting, diarrhea, headaches, delirium, ataxia, stupor, muscle tremors, seizures, and coma. Smoking makes the condition even more serious because nicotine causes release of the antidiuretic hormone, leading to increased water retention (Broome, 2004).

Diagnosis

There are many potential nursing diagnoses for clients with schizophrenia. In synthesizing the assessment data, consider the following:

- How well clients are functioning in daily life
- What their skills and talents are
- How stable their affect is
- How well they are able to communicate
- How well they are getting along with others
- How well they function at work.

Following is a list of the common diagnoses applicable to people with schizophrenia (North American Nursing Diagnosis Association, 2009):

- Risk for Self-Directed Violence related to command hallucinations
- Risk for Other-Directed Violence related to suspiciousness, fear, and command hallucinations
- Disturbed Sensory Perception, Auditory and Visual, related to disruptions in temporal lobe and occipital lobe, causing hallucinations
- Impaired Verbal Communication related to cognitive disruptions
- Impaired Social Interaction related to withdrawal, preoccupation with symptoms, lack of a supportive network, and negative reaction by others to client's social behavior
- Chronic Low Self-Esteem related to feeling different from others; chronic nature of the disorder
- Anxiety related to environmental stimuli; reduced contact with reality
- Fatigue related to hyperactivity
- Noncompliance related to decreasing or stopping prescribed medication
- Self-Care Deficit Bathing/Hygiene related to an inability to remember steps in self-care; low motivation
- Knowledge Deficit related to not understanding disease process
- Imbalanced Nutrition: More Than Body Requirements, related to side effects of antipsychotic medications
- Caregiver Role Strain related to fear of unknown, lack of social support, need to care for family member, and inappropriate behavior on part of client
- Impaired Home Maintenance related to being homeless.

Plan

Based on the assessment data, select outcomes appropriate to the nursing diagnoses. Three broad outcomes are as follows:

1. Reducing or eliminating symptoms
2. Improving quality of life and adaptive functioning, including improving family relationships
3. Enabling recovery by helping clients attain personal life goals.

Once outcomes are established, the nurse and the client mutually identify goals for change. Client goals are specific behavioral measures that the nurse, clients, and significant others identify as realistic and attainable. Following are examples of goals appropriate for people with schizophrenia:

- Communicates clearly
- Completes ADLs appropriately
- Exhibits increased attention span
- Makes appropriate decisions
- Displays affect appropriate to the situation
- Denies hallucinations
- Verbalizes logical thought processes
- Interacts well with others
- Develops occupational skills.

Implementation

Once the nursing diagnoses, outcome criteria, and goals have been identified, the plan of care is developed to assist clients toward a higher level of functioning and an enriched quality of life. Priorities of care for clients with schizophrenia are as follows:

- Prevention of violence towards self or others
- Altered cognition

- Compromised social relationships
- Risk for injury.

Nurses have many opportunities to assist people with schizophrenia in a variety of settings. These contacts may be long-term relationships or may take place during crisis periods. Clients should be cared for in the least restrictive setting that is both safe and effective for treatment. Indications for hospitalization include the client's being a danger to self or others, the client's being unable to care for self and needing constant supervision, or a new onset of a psychotic episode.

For the plan of care to be effective, clients must identify their priority concerns. Change is more likely to happen when clients are invested in the treatment process. Families, significant others, or caregivers should be actively involved in the plan of care and be taught to implement many of the interventions.

A good nurse–client relationship is one of the most effective nursing interventions. With rapport, communication, and trust, the nurse can help clients meet the outcome criteria they have identified. A nurse who listens to clients, accepts them for who they are, and understands their perspective is more likely to empower them and thereby help them achieve their highest level of functioning.

Nicotine Addiction

People with schizophrenia have a very high rate of nicotine dependence and have been a difficult group of individuals to involve in smoking cessation programs, in part because many self-medicate in an effort to improve symptoms. For many clients, the reward center in the brain functions below normal and nicotine stimulates this area. In fact, smoking may be one of the few dependable sources of pleasure for clients. Research has shown that clients know the disadvantages of smoking but believe they are outweighed by the advantages of smoking. Thus, it continues to be a challenge to motivate these individuals to quit smoking. Smoking cessation interventions should include nicotine replacement therapies and behavioral approaches. The desired outcome is that the client quits smoking.

Need for Positive Reinforcement

Clients benefit from regular positive reinforcement. Therefore, it is important that the nurse acknowledge the progress that clients make and celebrate their successes. As they are able to accomplish more ADLs, increase interactions with others, cope with side effects of medication, and live more independently, the nurse's support reinforces their personal gains (Dearing, 2004). The desired outcome is that clients will continue making positive behavioral changes.

Need for Family Education

Schizophrenia often strikes adolescents or young adults, leaving parents confused and frightened. Whether the child is living at or away from home, is employed or unemployed, parents report feeling a never-ending sense of responsibility for the child, which is at times overwhelming. Parents are likely to experience sorrow and grief as they begin to deal with the impact of their child's illness. Knowing that this is likely to occur, nurses can offer anticipatory guidance and interventions.

Parents want information and some level of involvement in their child's treatment plan. The question that health care professionals must answer is how to include the family within the context of client confidentiality. The desired outcomes are that clients and families will do the following:

- Verbalize an accurate understanding of the disorder
- Balance protective behaviors while encouraging independence
- Develop an advance directive
- Utilize effective communication skills
- Implement a problem-solving process to manage family issues
- Negotiate individual roles and responsibilities within the family
- Participate in family therapy.

Before intervening with the family, the nurse should discover answers to the following questions:

- How much does the family know about the illness?
- How do family members react to symptoms?
- Is their reaction helpful or hurtful?
- How does the client respond to the family?
- Does the client understand the distress the family experiences?

Because so many people are afraid of and uninformed about schizophrenia, many families try to hide it from friends and deal with it on their own. The nurse must reach out to these families and offer them support and education. Family education often is conducted in a group setting, which enables families to begin to build a support network. The nurse must help them understand that they are not responsible for their loved one developing schizophrenia and have no reason to feel guilty. They need to learn about the nature of schizophrenia and the variety of available treatment programs. The nurse may ask the client to teach the family what it is like to have schizophrenia. Similarly, the family members can share their observations and experiences.

Families need practical solutions on how to manage on a day-to-day basis. The nurse can assist families in achieving a balance between being protective and encouraging independence. For example, families should try to do things *with* the individuals rather than *for* them so that clients are able to regain their sense of self-confidence. Increased family education often decreases caregiver burden and improves the quality of life for all family members (Czuchta & McCay, 2001). Box 4–9 provides an outline for family education.

Box 4–9 **Family Education**

- Information about the disorder
- Ways to manage symptoms
- Expectations during recovery
- Role of medications
- Ways to handle crises
- Warning signs of suicide
- Early signs of relapse
- Housing and social resources
- Self-help groups

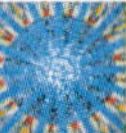

CLIENT TEACHING Effective Communication Styles for Families

Implementing effective communication styles is a way that families can decrease stress and improve family relationships. The nurse should choose a nonthreatening event and model new ways of talking and listening. The nurse can utilize role playing and coach the family in these new skills. The four basic communication skills are as follows (Miklowitz, 2004):

1. Expressing positive feelings. When sharing feelings, family members are coached to use "I" language, such as "I feel pleased when you come out of your bedroom in the morning."
2. Using active listening. Family members are coached to ask clarifying questions of the speaker and to use nonverbal attending behavior such as eye contact and nodding of the head.
3. Making positive requests for change. These requests should be specific and linked to a feeling, such as "I would really like it if you could help with the dishes after supper."
4. Expressing negative feelings. Family members are reminded to use "I" language because "you" language leads to conflict. Rather than saying, "You are so lazy," it would be more effective to say, "I worry about you when it seems so difficult for you to participate in family activities."

Ask the family to pick a time and topic to practice these skills at home. The more family members try the new skills, the more automatic the skills will become. Just as problem-solving skills are taught to individual clients, the problem-solving process is taught to families. A quick review of teaching the problem solving process follows.

- Identify and define the problem.
- List possible solutions.
- List advantages and disadvantages of each solution.
- Choose the best solution or combination of solutions.
- Develop an implementation plan.
- Evaluate the results of the action.

Families may need help in setting expectations and limits on inappropriate behavior. The positive symptoms of schizophrenia can cause a great deal of family stress. That is also true of the negative symptoms, which are often misinterpreted as laziness or uncooperativeness. Families must understand that clients are not trying to be stubborn or difficult, but rather fail to understand the importance of the desired behavior due to lack of insight. Explain that just because clients can verbally describe a problem does not mean that they can act on that knowledge. This information may help family members be more supportive.

Families can encourage their loved ones to stick with the treatment program, take their medications, and avoid alcohol and drugs. It is important to recognize early signs of relapse to prevent acute episodes and rehospitalization. Family members can ask clients with schizophrenia to agree that if any family members notice warning signs of a relapse, it is okay for them to contact the physician so that the medication can be adjusted to stabilize the condition. All threats of suicide should be taken very seriously. Families should have an identified contact person they can call for help. If the situation becomes desperate, the family should call 911.

Clients are encouraged to develop an *advance directive* indicating permission for treatment in the case of future acute episodes. Advance directives assist the family and caregivers who must make decisions for clients when they are unable to make the decision themselves. Health care providers are given important information about the client's preferences for treatment. Family and friends experience less conflict and guilt during times of psychiatric crises.

To prevent or delay relapse, it is critical to intervene with families who have high EE, that is, those who are highly critical, hostile, and overinvolved. Clients who live in high EE situations have much higher relapse rates than those living in low EE environments. The nurse must teach family members to moderate displays of all emotion in an effort to provide a neutral emotional climate. They may need assistance in defining and reshaping appropriate boundaries.

It is within the rights of a family to decide that a member who has an illness must get treatment for it. The family also should establish appropriate rules that must be followed. After an acute episode, the family may disagree over illness management around such issues as medication compliance; work/school activities; sleep–wake routines; or use of tobacco, alcohol, or drugs. Some families may disagree over role responsibilities and financial management. If the client is unwilling to comply with or modify behavior, the family may choose to look for alternative living arrangements.

Clients who are discharged from an acute hospitalization episode with medication as the primary intervention have a 50% rehospitalization rate within 6–9 months. *In contrast, clients discharged with medication who continue family therapy have only a 2–10% rehospitalization rate.* Family therapy moves beyond family education and helps people cope with the disorder of schizophrenia. Families learn how to manage conflict, avoid criticizing one another, decrease overprotective behaviors, and develop appropriate expectations of one another. Often this is best accomplished with the help of a family therapist.

Evaluation

Coping with schizophrenia is a lifelong process for most clients. Recovery rates from the first acute episode of schizophrenia are high, with almost 85% achieving remission. Remission is accomplished when symptoms no longer interfere with life. This is often referred to as the *stable phase*. The majority of clients alternate between acute psychotic episodes and stable phases. The current focus is on preventing relapse by maintaining medication and other treatment options.

About 25% of individuals with schizophrenia are resistant to treatment and experience a "downward spiral" of functioning. They often become dependent on others for food, clothing, and housing. The negative symptoms and cognitive dysfunctions are more severe in this group. Recovery is a longer-term phenomenon than remission and is characterized by few, if any, symptoms and an ability to function well in

NURSING CARE PLAN A Client With Schizophrenia

ASSESSMENT

Jacob Franklin is a 19-year-old college freshman living away from home for the first time. He is attending a college that is 3 hours from where his family lives. He was a good student in high school and decided to enter the electrical engineering program. During his first semester, his grades were poor and he flunked three of his five classes. When he returns home for the holiday school break his mother is shocked by his appearance. His hair is dirty, his clothes look as though he's slept in them for several nights, he is unshaven, and she describes his eyes as "flat and lifeless." His father hears him in his room talking to someone and assumes that he is talking to school friends on his cell phone until his father finds Jacob's cell phone in the kitchen. When he talks with Jacob about Jacob's experiences at school, it quickly becomes clear that Jacob kept to himself, developed no friends, and was very withdrawn.

Jacob's parents suspect that something is seriously wrong with their son and make an appointment with their family doctor.

A neurological history and examination reveals altered ability to identify smells, disturbed sleep patterns, difficulty remembering details, altered information processing, and polydipsia. Jacob's speech is stilted, and he uses very formal language, making it difficult to hold a conversation with him. He displays inadequate problem-solving skills for his age and cannot remember the nurse's name within 3 minutes of being reminded. While Jacob denies auditory or visual hallucinations, despite an empty room, he is observed talking in an animated fashion as though talking with someone. The physician suspects a diagnosis of schizophrenia, which is later confirmed after Jacob visits a psychiatrist.

DIAGNOSES

- Risk for Self-Directed Violence
- Altered Thought Process related to disruptions in cognitive processes such as delusions, loose association, concrete thinking
- Impaired Social Interaction related to withdrawal, preoccupation with symptoms, lack of a supportive network, negative reaction by others to client's social behavior
- Self-care Deficit Bathing/Hygiene related to an inability to remember steps in self-care; low motivation
- Knowledge Deficit related to not understanding disease process

PLANNING

In this early stage of the diagnostic process, nursing care is focused on helping the client and family understand the disease process and treatment options and helping them work through the grief and loss related to the diagnosis. Goals for treatment include the following:

- Client will remain safe from command hallucinations or suicide.
- Client and family will make informed decisions related to treatment options.
- Client will communicate clearly.
- Client will complete ADLs appropriately.
- Client will verbalize logical thought processes.

IMPLEMENTATION

An important priority of care is client safety. Command hallucinations may order Jacob to harm, mutilate, or kill himself or others. Some clients have delusions so intense for so long that suicide seems like the only way to escape the pain of being persecuted or controlled by out side forces. Living with such a complex chronic illness induces feelings of hopelessness and depression, which, in turn, increases suicide risk.

- Teach family the importance of providing supervision for Jacob when he is not hospitalized.
- Explore Jacob's mental state to determine if he has had thoughts of suicide or of harming himself or others.
- Administer medications as ordered to reduce intensity and occurrence of hallucinations.
- With reduction of symptoms, when Jacob is ready to learn, teach him the importance of following medication regimen, self-administration of medication, and symptoms that must be reported immediately.
- Because Jacob is legally an adult and has the right to privacy of medical information, discuss the fact that he must give permission to include his family in care planning and problem solving.
- Do not leave Jacob alone when he is hallucinating.
- Talk slightly louder using short, simple phrases and use Jacob's name.
- Assess for clues that Jacob may be hallucinating, such as:
  - Smiling or laughing inappropriately.
  - Talking to someone whom the nurse cannot see.
  - Showing slowed verbal responses.
- Ask Jacob to describe what is happening. Assess for content of hallucinations. Help him identify needs that may be reflected in the content of the hallucination, such as:
  - Power and control of decisions that affect daily life.
  - Ability to express anger.
  - Self-esteem issues.
- Ask which coping methods Jacob has used to manage hallucinations.
- When symptoms improve, teach Jacob to avoid social stigma by pretending to use the cell phone if he must respond to hallucination.
- Teach Jacob and his family about disease process, treatment options, support groups, and resources.
- Support Jacob and his family as they attempt to cope with the diagnosis.

EVALUATION

Jacob is admitted to a mental health facility specializing in the care of young adults. He is started on low-dose antipsychotic medication and responds quickly. He participates in group therapy, family counseling, and ACT. When he is discharged, he decides, with his family's approval, to live at home and attend a local community college until he is ready to try living independently again.

CRITICAL THINKING

1. What interventions would you initiate or recommend to help Jacob deal with the stigma associated with the diagnosis of schizophrenia?
2. What family teaching would you provide Jacob's family to help them recognize and respond to symptoms Jacob demonstrates?
3. How can nurses advocate in the community for clients with mental health problems?

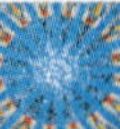

FOCUS ON DIVERSITY AND CULTURE Schizophrenia and Homelessness

Approximately one third of the homeless population has a persistent mental illness such as schizophrenia. The figure rises to 66% when chemical dependence is included in the estimate. In addition, all people, if left homeless for a sufficient period, will develop less effective coping skills and demonstrate some type of mental disorder (Bradford, Gaynes, Kim, Kaufman, & Weinberger, 2005; Philpot, 2005). Perhaps nothing is more upsetting than the sight of an individual who is homeless and clearly experiencing severe psychiatric problems. The image of a disheveled man angrily responding to voices only he can hear is an example of society's failure to address the problems of homelessness and mental illness. Homeless women with persistent mental illness represent one of the most vulnerable segments of society. They frequently face a choice between the dangers of life on the street and the hazards of overcrowded, unsafe, and poorly supervised shelters. Rape and physical battery are a daily risk for these women (Tucker, Wenzel, Straus, Ryan, & Golinelli, 2005).

Homeless people with persistent mental illness are often fearful and distrustful of the mental health system. The community health nurse must be prepared to work with homeless people in nonclinical settings, including on the streets, in shelters, on subways, in bus terminals, and in other public areas. The nurse will need a combination of patience, persistence, and understanding. Depending on the needs and wants of a particular person, providing food, clothing, or simply company can be essential in developing a therapeutic relationship (Dearing, 2004).

the community over a long period of time. Those who recover experience fewer cognitive and social problems during the acute phase of the illness (Andreasen, Carpenter, Kane, Lasser, Marder, & Weinberger, 2005; Scott, Kingdon, & Turkington, 2004).

HEALTH CARE

Advocacy

One of the primary functions of the nurse is to be an advocate for the wishes of the mentally ill client. At times, the nurse may function much the same way as an advance directive. The Patient Self-Determination Act became federal law in 1990. This law states that clients have a right to participate in their own care. In addition, health care professionals are required to inform clients of the right to accept or refuse medical care, including medication. The nurse also advocates for the client with family members and other people the client considers important, helping to foster communication and maintain a positive nurturing relationship.

Health Policy

Mental illness often carries a **stigma** (a collection of negative attitudes and beliefs that lead people to fear, reject, avoid, and discriminate against people with mental illness) with which families and clients may find difficulty coping. The nurse can help eradicate this stigma by attempting to educate the public and to influence public policy changes to provide financing and regulations to care for the mentally ill.

Legal Issues

When hospitalization is required, the client can be admitted voluntarily or involuntarily. **Voluntary admission** occurs when a client, for the purpose of assessment and treatment of a mental disorder, consents to hospitalization and signs a document indicating such fact. If clients choose to leave the hospital, they must give written notice of their intention to leave the facility. The number of hours or days between notice of intention and actual discharge is determined by individual states. This notification period provides the health care team the time needed to complete discharge arrangements or to seek authorization through the court system for further hospitalization.

Commitment, or **involuntary admission**, detains the client in a psychiatric facility without the client's permission. In most states, this occurs because the client is considered a danger to self or others, but a few states have altered their laws by including the criterion of preventing significant physical or mental deterioration. Adults can be held temporarily until a court hearing determines that there is clear and convincing evidence of danger or need for treatment.

Clients with mental health disorders do not lose constitutional, legal, or ethical rights when they receive treatment for a mental disorder. See Box 4–10 for a list of clients' rights.

Safety

The nurse has a role in maintaining a safe and protective environment for the client, family, and health care team. Special precautions are required with violent or potentially violent clients.

Box 4–10 Client Rights

- Right to confidentiality and privacy
- Right to informed consent
- Right to treatment
- Right to refuse treatment
- Right to least restrictive environment
- Right to communicate with others
- Right to freedom from unnecessary restraints and seclusion
- Right to participate in legal matters
- Right to religious freedom
- Right to consensual sexual relationships

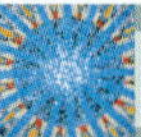

EVIDENCE-BASED PRACTICE Schizophrenia and Physical Activity

Beebe, L. H. (2006). Describing the health parameters of outpatients with schizophrenia. *Applied Nursing Research, 19*, 43–47.

What is the study about?

Examine, among persons living with schizophrenia, physical health parameters and psychiatric symptoms as related to those three types of disease.

How was the study done?

- Quantitative descriptive pilot study of 11 veterans living with schizophrenia (9 men, 2 women) and receiving care from a veteran's outpatient facility in the Southeast.
- Sample included 9 Whites and 2 African Americans.
- Approved by an institutional review board.
- Investigated participant aerobic fitness, body mass index (BMI), body fat, severity of psychopathology, and perceptions of their own health.
- All participants medically approved to participate in a moderate exercise program; none reported a history of cardiovascular, neuromuscular, endocrine, or other disorders that would bar safe participation in the study.
- A trained research assistant unaware of treatment grouping obtained data over an 8-week period.
- All data obtained at same time of day to control for possible circadian variation and medication effects.
- Physical health measured by BMI, body fat percentages, and test of aerobic fitness: the 6-minute walking distance (6MWD).
- BMI calculated using height in meters and weight in kilograms.
- Body fat percentage assessed via three skinfold measures using calipers at three specific body sites.
- In 6MWD, participants walked around a path until signaled to stop; distance was measured to nearest foot.
- Severity of psychopathology measured by Positive and Negative Syndrome Scale (PANSS) and self-reported health perception by Duke Health Profile.

What were the results of the study?

- Subjects walked a distance ranging from 1,114 to 1,912 feet, with an average of 1,407 feet. Healthy men and women walk an average of 1,641 feet. BMIs ranged from 21.83 to 43.09, with an average of 31.58.
- 10 of 11 subjects exceeded the Centers for Disease Control (CDC) threshold for overweight (BMI between 25 and 29.9); 7 fell into the CDC category of obese (BMI>30).
- PANSS showed that the men were less ill on all scales than the women.
- White patients (n=9) had more negative symptoms and African American patients (n=2) more positive symptoms.
- Duke questionnaire revealed that none of the participants saw themselves as having a disability due to their diagnosis of schizophrenia, yet all had a history of inconsistent work patterns and 9 collected disability benefits from Veterans Affairs.
- Most common physical diagnoses were hypertension and peptic ulcer disease; the most commonly prescribed medications were antihypertensives.

What additional questions might I have?

- What results would be found from a larger sample?
- Since this was a pilot study, what follow-up studies might be planned to validate findings?
- How long had the participants been diagnosed with schizophrenia, and did length of diagnosis correlate with poorer physical health outcomes?
- What was the age range of the subjects; did younger patients experience fewer or milder physical health problems?

How can I use this study?

- Nurses caring for persons living with schizophrenia need to promote health by being attuned both to patients' mental and physical health.
- This kind of health promotion will involve addressing not only mental status but also physical fitness, good nutrition, and staying physically well.
- Nurses must monitor the physical health parameters of persons living with schizophrenia and make referrals as needed.
- All patients who receive medical clearance should be encouraged to participate in a physical fitness regimen.

Source: Contributed by Dolores Huffman, PhD, RN, Associate Professor of Nursing, Purdue University Calumet, Hammond, Indiana.

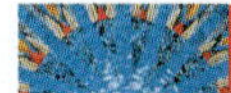

REVIEW Schizophrenia

RELATE: LINK THE CONCEPTS

The client is a 22-year-old man diagnosed with schizophrenia 5 years ago. He was admitted to the hospital when he stopped taking his medications and had an acute exacerbation of positive symptoms. After 2 weeks in the psychiatric facility, his condition has stabilized and he has achieved remission. The nurse caring for him would like to help him quit smoking.

Linking the exemplar of Schizophrenia with the concept of Addiction:

1. What interventions might the nurse initiate, both collaboratively and independently, to lead the client to decide to quit smoking and support him through the process to improve the likelihood of success?
2. Why is the client with schizophrenia at increased risk of addiction?

Linking the exemplar of Schizophrenia with the concept of Development:

3. What developmental milestones might this client be at increased risk of not meeting?
4. How could the nurse foster normal development at various stages in the developmental process in clients diagnosed with schizophrenia?

READY: GO TO COMPANION SKILLS MANUAL

- Assessing the appearance and mental status
- Managing clients in restraints
- Applying wrist or ankle restraint
- Applying a mummy immobilizer
- Maintaining nurse's safety
- Evaluating client's safety

REFER: GO TO MYNURSINGKIT

REFLECT: CASE STUDY

Sara is a 41-year-old woman who was diagnosed with schizophrenia 15 years ago. She has a history of childhood sexual abuse. She has been able to live at home with her husband except for a few brief periods of hospitalization. Lately, her thinking has become more disorganized and her therapist has recommended that she come to the day treatment program. The themes of the interaction below include raping and hurting little children and wanting to return to infancy, a period of time when she felt safe and cared for.

Conversation between Nurse and Sara:

SARA: I killed a man when I was 6 years old, and he was raping and killing little babies. I killed him. Then my friends told me to run, so I ran. I got away with my underpants on. My twin brother died—he committed suicide. [crying]

NURSE: Would you like to talk about this?

SARA: Not right now. I loved my brother. [Sobbing] I really miss him. You know I build houses.

NURSE: You do?

SARA: Yes, I start out 14 feet tall and when I'm done I've shrunk to 14 inches. [Smiles and laughs]

NURSE: You shrink?

SARA: Yes, the aliens come and get me at night and tell me they'll make me safe, and they make me into a baby and take care of me.

NURSE: Do you feel safe as a baby?

SARA: Yes, no one can hurt me then. They protect me. [Smiling]

NURSE: [Silence]

SARA: My husband exhibits me, you know. [Laughs]

NURSE: Can you explain "exhibits"? I don't understand.

SARA: He took movies of us having sex and set me down and showed them to me. He told me I had grown into a beautiful woman. He still loves me, you know, and I still love him even though I slapped him 3,600 times in the head.

NURSE: How did you feel about his exhibiting you?

SARA: It was okay because I really do love him. I was attached to my husband at the waist in the bedroom. [Laughs] [Puts finger to ear and pauses]

NURSE: Are you hearing voices?

SARA: No, I have synthetic eardrums, and I hear a buzz sometimes. Do you know I saved little boys from Alcatraz? I saved them to keep them safe. [Laughs]

NURSE: I didn't know that. What did you save them from?

SARA: I saved them from the men raping them. They were raping and killing all those little boys. The president gave me permission to save as many as I could.

NURSE: Is it a good feeling when you are able to help others?

SARA: I build spaceships at night and escape to bars for smokes, and men buy me whiskey.

CRITICAL THINKING QUESTIONS

1. How would you assess Sara's cognition?
2. What goals might you set for Sara?
3. What interventions would help you achieve those goals, both collaborative and independent?

PEARSON

EXPLORE mynursingkit™

MyNursingKit is your one stop for online chapter review materials and resources. Prepare for success with additional NCLEX®-style practice questions, interactive assignments and activities, web links, animations and videos, and more!

Register your access code from the front of your book at **www.mynursingkit.com**.

REFERENCES

Administration for Children and Families. (2004). About ADD. Retrieved July 15, 2005, from http://www.acf.dhhs.gov/programs/add/about/htm

Agency on Aging. (2004). *Alzheimer's resource room: Professionals and providers*. Retrieved June 11, 2006, from http://www.aoa.gov/ALZ/Public/alzprof/alz_prof.asp

Alexopoulos, G., Silver, J., Kahn, D., Frances, A., & Carpenter, D. (Eds.). (2004). Treatment of agitation in older persons with dementia. Expert Knowledge Systems. Retrieved December 13, 2004, from http://www.psychguides.com

Alzheimer's Association. (2009). Alzheimer's disease fast facts and figures. Retrieved June 21, 2009, from http://www.alz.org/alzheimers_disease_facts_figures.asp

American Association of Mental Retardation. (2004). Definition of mental retardation. Retrieved July 15, 2004, from http://www.aamr.org/Policies/faq_mental_retardation.shtml

American Psychiatric Association. (2000). *Diagnostic and statistical manual of mental disorders* (4th ed., text revision). Washington, DC: Author.

American Psychiatric Association, Committee on Nomenclature and Statistics. (2000). *Diagnostic and statistical manual of mental disorders* (4th ed., text revision) (*DSM-IV-TR*). Washington, DC: Author.

American Psychological Association. (2008). What practitioners should know about working with older adults. Retrieved February 14, 2008, from http://www.apa.org/pi/aging/practitioners/executive.html

Andreasen, N. C., Carpenter, W. T., Kane, J. M., Lasser, R. A., Marder, S. R., & Weinberger, D. R. (2005). Remission in schizophrenia. *American Journal of Psychiatry, 162*(3), 441–449.

Askin-Edgar, S., White, K. E., & Cummings, J. L. (2004). Neuropsychiatric aspects of Alzheimer's disease and other dementing illnesses. In S. C. Yudofsky & R. E. Hales (Eds.), *Essentials of neuropsychiatry and clinical neurosciences* (pp. 421–456). Washington, DC: American Psychiatric Publishing.

Bachmann, S., Schröder, J., Bottmer, C., Torrey, E. F., & Yolken, R. H. (2005). Psychopathology in first-episode schizophrenia and antibodies to boxoplasma gondii. *Psychopathology, 38*(2), 87–90.

Bailey, K. (2003). Aripiprazole: The newest antipsychotic agent for the treatment of schizophrenia. *Psychosocial Nursing and Mental Health Services, 41*(2), 14–18.

Berman, K., & Brodaty, H. (2004). Tocopherol (vitamin E) in Alzheimer's disease and other neurodegenerative disorders. *CNS Drugs, 18*(12), 807–825.

Bhasin, T. K., Brocksen, S., Avchen, R. N., & Braun, K. V. (2006). Prevalence of four developmental disabilities among children aged 8 years—Metropolitan Atlanta developmental disabilities surveillance program, 1996 and 2000. *Morbidity and Mortality Weekly Report, 55,* SS–1, 1–9.

Bowie, C. R., Tsapelas, I., Friedman, J., Parrella, M., White, L., & Harvey, P. D. (2005). The longitudinal course of thought disorder in geriatric patients with chronic schizophrenia. *American Journal of Psychiatry, 162*(4), 793–795.

Bradford, D. W., Gaynes, B. N., Kim, M. M., Kaufman, J. S., & Weinberger, M. (2005). Can shelter-based interventions improve treatment engagement in homeless individuals with psychiatric and/or substance misuse disorders? *Medical Care, 43*(8), 763–768.

Brambilla, P., Cerini, R., Gasparini, A., Versace, A., Andreone, N., Vittorini, E., et al. (2005). Investigation of corpus callosum in schizophrenia with diffusion imaging. *Schizophrenia Research, 79*(2), 201–210.

Brodaty, H., Sachdev, P., Koschera, A., Monk, D., & Cullen, B. (2003). Long-term outcome of late-onset schizophrenia. *British Journal of Psychiatry, 183*(1), 213–219.

Broome, M. E. (2004). Polydipsia screening tool. *Archives of Psychiatric Nursing, 18*(2), 49–59.

Brown, A. S., Begg, M. D., Gravenstein, S., Schaefer, C. A., Wyatt, R. J., Bresnahan, M., et al. (2004). Serologic evidence of prenatal influenza in the etiology of schizophrenia. *Archives of General Psychiatry, 61*(8), 774–780.

Brown, R. P., & Gerbarg, P. L. (2000). Integrative psychopharmacology. In P. R. Muskin (Ed.), *Complementary and alternative medicine and psychiatry* (pp. 1–66). Washington, DC: American Psychiatric Press.

Buchanan, R. W., Kreyenbuhl, J., Zito, J. M., & Lehman, A. (2002). Relationship of the use of adjunctive pharmacological agents to symptoms and level of function in schizophrenia. *American Journal of Psychiatry, 159*(6), 1035–1043.

Burbaeva, G. S., Boksha, I. S., Tereshkina, E. B., Savushkina, O. K., Starodubtseva, L. I., & Turishcheva, M. S. (2005). Glutamate metabolizing enzymes in prefrontal cortex of Alzheimer's disease patients. *Neurochemical Research, 30*(11), 1443–1451.

Caley, L. M., Shipkey, N., Winkelman, T., Dunlap, C., & Rivera, S. (2006). Evidence-based review of nursing interventions to prevent secondary disabilities in fetal alcohol spectrum disorder. *Pediatric Nursing, 32,* 155–162.

Cannon, M., Jones, P. B., & Murray, R. M. (2002). Obstetric complications and schizophrenia: Historical and meta-analytic review. *American Journal of Psychiatry, 159*(7), 1080–1092.

Centers for Disease Control and Prevention. (2004a). Developmental disabilities. Retrieved July 15, 2004, from http://www.cdc.gov.ncbddd.dd.default.htm

Compton, M. T. (2005). Cigarette smoking in individuals with schizophrenia. *Medscape Psychiatry & Mental Health, 8*(2), 1–6.

Corrigan, P. W. (2005). Motivational interviewing of people with schizophrenia. *Medscape Psychiatry & Mental Health, 8*(2), 1–5. www.medscape.com/viewarticle/515818

Counts, S. E., Chen, E. Y., Che, S., Ikonomovie, M. D., Wuu, J., Ginsberg, S. D., et al. (2006). Galanin fiber hypertrophy within the cholinergic nucleus basalis during the progression of Alzheimer's disease. *Dementia and Geriatric Cognitive Disorders, 21*(4), 205–214.

Czuchta, D. M., & McCay, E. (2001). Help-seeking for parents of individuals experiencing a first episode of schizophrenia. *Archives of Psychiatric Nursing, 15*(4), 159–170.

Dearing, K. S. (2004). Getting it, together: How the nurse patient relationship influences treatment compliance for patients with schizophrenia. *Archives of Psychiatric Nursing, 18*(5), 155–163.

DeDeyn, P. P., Katz, I. R., Brodaty, H., Lyons, B., Greenspan, A., & Burns, A. (2005). Management of agitation, aggression and psychosis associated with dementia. *Clinical Neurology and Neurosurgery, 107*(6), 497–508.

Dochterman, J. M., & Bulechek, G. M. (Eds.). (2004). *Nursing interventions classification (NIC)* (4th ed.). St. Louis, MO: Mosby.

Dowling, J. E. (2004). *The great brain debate: Nature or nurture?* Washington, DC: Joseph Henry Press.

Ebersole, P., Hess, P., & Lugfen, A. (2004). *Toward healthy aging: Human needs and nursing response* (6th ed.). St. Louis, MO: Mosby.

Edwards, N. (2003). Differentiating the three D's: Delirium, dementia, and depression. *Medsurg Nursing, 12*(6), 347–357.

Edwards, N. E., & Beck, A. M. (2002). Animal-assisted therapy and nutrition in Alzheimer's disease. *Western Journal of Nursing Research, 24*(6), 697–712.

Emsley, R., Myburgh, C., Oosthuizen, P., & van Rensburg, S. J. (2002). Randomized, placebo-controlled study of ethyl-eicosapentaenoic acid as supplemental treatment in schizophrenia. *American Journal of Psychiatry, 159*(9), 1596–1598.

Federal Interagency Forum on Aging-Related Statistics (FIFAS). (2004). *Older Americans 2004: Key indicators of well-being.* Washington, DC: U.S. Government Printing Office.

Fick, D., & Foreman, M. (2000). Consequences of not recognizing delirium superimposed on dementia in hospitalized elderly individuals. *Gerontology Nursing,* 26(1), 30–40.

Flashman, L. A. (2004). Disorders of insight, self-awareness, and attribution in schizophrenia. In B. D. Beitman & J. Nair (Eds.), *Self-awareness deficits in psychiatric patients* (pp. 129–158). New York: W.W. Norton & Company.

Fontaine, K. L. (2005). *Complementary & alternative therapies for nursing practice* (2nd ed.). Upper Saddle River, NJ: Prentice Hall.

Foreman, M. D., Wakefield, B., Culp, K., & Milisen, K. (2001). Delirium in elderly patients: An overview of the state of the science. *Journal of Gerontological Nursing, 27*(4), 13–20. *Journal of Gerontological Nursing, 26,* 30–40.

Friedman, J. I., Harvey, P. D., McGurk, S. R., White, L., Parrella, M., Raykov, T., et al. (2002). Correlates of change in function status of institutionalized geriatric schizophrenic patients. *American Journal of Psychiatry, 159*(8), 1388–1394.

Galderisi, S., Mau, M., Mucci, A., Cassano, G. B., Invernizzi, G., Rossi, A., et al. (2002). Historical, psychopathological, neurological, and neuropsychological aspects of deficit schizophrenia. *American Journal of Psychiatry, 159*(6), 983–990.

Gerber, R. (2000). *Vibrational medicine for the 21st century.* New York: Eagle Brook.

Ginsberg, H., & Opper, S. (1988). *Piaget's theory of intellectual development* (3rd ed.). Paramus, NJ: Prentice Hall.

Gochman, P. A., Greenstein, D., Sporn, A., Gogtay, N., Nicolson, R., Keller, A., et al. (2004). Childhood onset schizophrenia: Familial neurocognitive measures. *Schizophrenia Research, 71,* 43–47.

Gogtay, N., Sporn, A., Clasen, L. S., Nugent, T. F. III, Greenstein, D., Nicolson, R., et al. (2004). Comparison of progressive cortical gray matter loss in childhood-onset schizophrenia with that in childhood-atypical psychoses. *Archives of General Psychiatry, 61*(1), 17–22.

Gottesman, I. I., & Petronis, A. (2003). Schizophrenia genetics obscured by the realities of complex diseases. *NAMI Advocate, 1*(4), 31–32.

Hagen, B. F., & Mitchell, D. L. (2001). Might within the madness: Solution-focused therapy and thought-disordered clients. *Archives of Psychiatric Nursing, 15*(2), 86–93.

Hagerman, R. J. (2006). Lessons from fragile X regarding neurobiology, autism, and neurodegeneration. *Journal of Developmental and Behavioral Pediatrics, 27,* 63–74.

Hanley, C. (2004). Delirium in the acute care setting. *Medsurg Nursing, 13*(4), 217–225.

Hartford Institute for Geriatric Nursing. (2008). *Best nursing practices in care for older adults.* Try this: The geriatric depression scale. Retrieved February 14, 2008, from http://www.hartfordign.org/trythis/issue04.pdf

Hayden, T. (2007). Antibody may be the body's natural defense against Alzheimer's disease. *Neurology Reviews, 15*(7), 36.

Hummer, M., Malik, P., Gasser, R. W., Hofer, A., Kemmler, G., Naveda, R. C. M., et al. (2005). Osteoporosis in patients with schizophrenia. *American Journal of Psychiatry, 162*(1), 162–167.

Inouye, S., van Dyck, C., Alessi, C., Balkin, S., Siegal, A., & Horwitz, R. (1990). Clarifying confusion: The confusion assessment method. A new method for the detection of delirium. *Annals of Internal Medicine, 113*(12), 941–948.

Jungbauer, J., Wittmund, B., Dietrich, S., & Angermeyer, M. C. (2003). Subjective burden over 2 months in parents of patients with schizophrenia. *Archives of Psychiatric Nursing, 17*(3), 126–134.

Kelly, C., & McCreadie, R. G. (1999). Smoking habits, current symptoms, and premorbid characteristics of schizophrenia patients in Nithsdale, Scotland. *American Journal of Psychiatry, 156*(11), 1751–1757.

Kelly, D. P., & Aylward, G. P. (2005). Identifying school performance problems in the pediatric office. *Pediatric Annals, 34,* 288–298.

Keltner, N. L. (2005). Genomic influences on schizophrenia-related neurotransmitter systems. *Journal of Nursing Scholarship, 37*(4), 322–328.

Keshavan, M. S., Cashmere, J. D., Miewald, J., & Yeragani, V. K. (2004). Decreased nonlinear complexity and chaos during sleep in first episode schizophrenia. *Schizophrenia Research, 71*(2), 263–272.

Keshavan, M. S., Duggal, H. S., Veeragandham, G., McLaughlin, N. M., Montrose, D. M., Haas, G. L., et al. (2005). Personality dimensions in first-episode psychosis. *American Journal of Psychiatry, 162*(1), 102–109.

Kim, M. S., Ha, T. H., & Kwon, J. S. (2004). Neurological abnormalities in schizophrenia and obsessive-compulsive disorder. *Current Opinions in Psychiatry, 17*(3), 215–220.

Krasuski, J. S., Alexander, G. E., Horwitz, B., Rapoport, S. I., & Schapiro, M. B. (2002). Relation of medial temporal lobe volumes to age and memory function in nondemented adults with Down syndrome. *American Journal of Psychiatry, 159*(1), 74–81.

Kruger, S., Bagby, R. M., Hoffler, J., & Braunig, P. (2003). Factor analysis of the catatonia rating scale and catatonic symptom distribution across four diagnostic groups. *Comprehensive Psychiatry, 44*(6), 472–482.

Kumar, A. M., Tims, F., & Gruess, D. G. (1999). Music therapy increases serum melatonin levels in patients with Alzheimer's disease. *Alternative Therapies, 5*(6), 49–57.

Lambros, K. M., & Leslie, L. K. (2005). Management of the child with a learning disorder. *Pediatric Annals, 34,* 275–287.

Larson, E. B., Wang, L., Bowen, J. D., McCormick, W. C., Terri, L., Crane, P., et al. (2006). Exercise is associated with reduced risk for incident dementia among persons 65 years of age and older. *Annals of Internal Medicine, 144*(2), 73–81.

Laustsen, G., & Wimmett, L. (2005). 2004 drug approval highlights: FDA update. *The Nurse Practitioner, 30*(2), 14–29.

Lawson, W. B. (2000). Issues in pharmacotherapy for African Americans. In P. Ruiz (Ed.), *Ethnicity and psychopharmacology* (pp. 37–53). Washington, DC: American Psychiatric Press.

Lucas, S. M., Rothwell, N. J., & Gibson, R. M. (2006). The role of inflammation in CNS injury and disease. *British Journal of Pharmacology, 147*(Suppl. 1), S232–S240.

Lecomte, T., Wallace, C. J., Perreault, M., & Caron, J. (2005). Consumers' goals in psychiatric rehabilitation and their concordance with existing services. *Psychiatric Services, 56*(2), 209–211.

Marshall, M., & Lockwood, A. (2000). Assertive community treatment for people with severe mental illness. *Cochrane Database Systematic Reviews, 2,* CD001089.

McCurren, C., & Cronin, S. N. (2003). Delirium: Elders tell their stories and guide nursing practice. *Medsurg Nursing, 12*(5), 318–323.

McDevitt, J., Wilbur, J., Kogan, J., & Briller, J. (2005). A walking program for outpatients in psychiatric rehabilitation. *Biological Research for Nursing, 7*(2), 87–97.

Meltzoff, A., & Gopnick, A. (1997). *Words, thoughts, and theories.* Cambridge, MA: MIT Press.

Miklowitz, D. J. (2004). Family therapy. In S. L. Johnson & R. L. Leahy (Eds.), *Psychological treatment of bipolar disorder* (pp. 184–202). New York: Guilford Press.

Moberg, P. J., Roalf, D. R., Gur, R. E., & Turetsky, B. I. (2004). Smaller nasal volumes as stigmata of aberrant neurodevelopment in schizophrenia. *American Journal of Psychiatry, 161*(12), 2314–2316.

Modrego, P. J., Fayed, M., & Pina, M. A. (2005). Conversion from mild cognitive impairment to probable Alzheimer's disease predicted by brain magnetic resonance spectroscopy. *American Journal of Psychiatry, 162*(4), 667–675.

Moeschler, J. B., Shevell, M., and the American Academy of Pediatrics Committee on Genetics. (2006). Clinical genetic evaluation of the child with mental retardation or developmental delays. *Pediatrics, 117,* 2304–2316.

Mueser, K. T., Bond, G. R., & Drake, R. E. (2001). Community-based treatment of schizophrenia and other severe mental disorders: Treatment outcomes. *Medscape Mental Health, 6*(1). www.medscape.com/Medscape/psychiatry/journal/2001/v06.n01/

NANDA International. (2005). *NANDA nursing diagnoses: Definitions and classification 2005–2006*. Philadelphia: Author.

NANDA International. (2007). *NANDA nursing diagnoses: Definitions and classification 2007–2008*. Philadelphia: Author.

National Center for Learning Disabilities. (2004). *Learning disability*. Retrieved May 25, 2004, from http://www.ldanatl.org

National Institute of Neurological Disorders and Stroke. (2005a). *Amyotrophic lateral sclerosis fact sheet*. Retrieved from http://www.ninds.nih.gov/disorders/amyotrophiclateralsclerosis/detail_amyotrophiclateralsclerosis_pr.htm

__________. (2005i). *The dementias: Hope through research*. Retrieved from http://www.ninds.nih.gov/disorders/alzheimersdisease/detail/alzheimersdisease_pr.htm

Navon, L., & Ozer, N. (2003). Ordinary logic in unordinary lay theories: A key to understanding proneness to medication nonadherence in schizophrenia. *Archives of Psychiatric Nursing, 17*(3), 108–116.

Nechmad, A., Ratzoni, G., Poyurovsky, M., Meged, S., Avidan, G., Fuchs, C., et al. (2003). Obsessive-compulsive disorder in adolescent schizophrenia patients. *American Journal of Psychiatry, 160*(5), 1002–1004.

Ngandu, T., Helkala, E. L., Soininen, H., Winblad, B., Tuomilehto, J., Nissinen, A., et al. (2006). Alcohol drinking and cognitive functions. *Dementia and Geriatric Cognitive Disorders, 23*(3), 140–149.

North American Nursing Diagnoses Association.(2007). Nursing Diagnoses Definitions and Classification 2005–2006. Philadelphia: Author.

North American Nursing Diagnoses Association.(2009). Nursing Diagnoses Definitions and Classification 2005–2006. Philadelphia: Author.

Ohrui, T., Tomita, N., Sato-Nakagawa, T., Matsui, T., Maruyama, M., Niwa, K., et al. (2004). Effects of brain-penetrating ACE inhibitors on Alzheimer disease progression. *Neurology, 63*(7), 1324–1325.

Olincy, A., Harris, J. G., Johnson, L. L., Pender, V., Kongs, S., Allensworth, D., et al. (2006). Proof-of-concept trial of an alpha7 nicotinic agonist in schizophrenia. *Archives of General Psychiatry, 63*(6), 630–638.

Onitsuka, R., Nestor, P. G., Gurrera, R. J., Shenton, M. E., Kasai, K., Frumin, M., et al. (2005). Association between reduced extraversion and right posterior fusiform gyrus gray matter reduction in chronic schizophrenia. *American Journal of Psychiatry, 162*(3), 599–601.

Pallanti, S., Quercioli, L., & Hollander, E. (2004). Social anxiety in outpatients with schizophrenia. *American Journal of Psychiatry, 161*(1), 53–58.

Phillips, M. R., Yang, G., Li, S., & Li, Y. (2004). Suicide and the unique prevalence pattern of schizophrenia in mainland China. *Lancet, 364*(9439), 1016–1017.

Philpot, T. (2005). From hotel to home. *Nursing Standard, 19*(51), 22–23.

Piaget, J. (1966). *Origins of intelligence in children*. New York: Norton.

Piaget, J. (1972). *The child's conception of the world*. Totowa, NJ: Littlefield, Adams Co.

Porth, C. M. (2005). *Pathophysiology: Concepts of altered health states* (7th ed.). Philadelphia: Lippincott.

Practice Guideline for the Treatment of Patients with Schizophrenia (2nd ed.). (2004). Supplement to the *American Journal of Psychiatry, 161*(2), 1–56.

Rempusheski, V. F., & Hurley, A. C. (2000). Advance directives and dementia. *Journal of Gerontological Nursing, 26*(10), 27–33.

Remschmidt, J., & Theisen, F. M. (2005). Schizophrenia and related disorders in children and adolescents. *Journal of Neural Transmission, 69,* 121–124.

Rickelman, B. L. (2004). Anosognosia in individuals with schizophrenia: Toward recovery of insight. *Issues in Mental Health Nursing, 25*(3), 227–242.

Rose, K. M. (2005). Mild cognitive impairment in Hispanic Americans: An overview of the state of the science. *Archives of Psychiatric Nursing, 19*(5), 205–209.

Ryan, M. C. M., Collins, P., & Thakore, J. H. (2003). Impaired fasting glucose tolerance in first episode, drug-naïve patients with schizophrenia. *American Journal of Psychiatry, 160*(2), 284–289.

Saenger, E. (2004). Treatment-resistant schizophrenia: An expert interview with Ralph Hoffman. *Medscape Psychiatry & Mental Health, 9*(2), 1–4. www.medscape.com/viewarticle/496285

Santrock, J. (2005). *Life-span development* (9th ed.). Boston: McGraw-Hill.

Schutte, D. L., & Holston, E. C. (2006). Chronic dementing conditions, genomics, and new opportunities for nursing interventions. *Journal of Nursing Scholarship, 38*(4), 328–334.

Scott, J., Kingdon, D., & Turkington, D. (2004). Cognitive behavior therapy for schizophrenia. In J. H. Wright (Ed.), *Cognitive-behavior therapy* (pp. 1–24). Washington, DC: American Psychiatric Press.

Seeman, M. V. (2004). Gender differences in the prescribing of antipsychotic drugs. *American Journal of Psychiatry, 161*(8), 1324–1333.

Seshadri, S., Beiser, K. A., Selhub, J., Jacques, P. R., Rosenberg, I. H., D'Agostino, R. B., et al. (2002). Plasma homocysteine as a risk factor for dementia and Alzheimer's disease. *New England Journal of Medicine, 346*(7), 476–483.

Siever, L. J., & Davis, K. L. (2004). The pathophysiology of schizophrenia disorders: Perspectives from the spectrum. *American Journal of Psychiatry, 161*(3), 398–413.

Sipos, A., Rasmussen, F., Harrison, G., Tynelius, P., Lewis, G., Leon, D. A., et al. (2005). Paternal age and schizophrenia: A population based cohort study. *British Medical Journal, 330*(7483), 147–148.

Sporn, A. L., Addington, A. M., Gogtay, N., Ordonez, A. E., Gornick, M., Clasen, L., et al. (2004). Pervasive developmental disorder and childhood-onset schizophrenia. *Biological Psychiatry, 55*(10), 989–994.

St. Clair, D., Xu, M., Wang, P., Yu, Y., Fang, Y., Zhang, F., et al. (2005). Rates of adult schizophrenia following prenatal exposure to the Chinese famine of 1959–1961. *JAMA, 294*(5), 557–562.

Suellentrop, K., Morrow, B., Williams, L., & D'Angels, D. (2006). Monitoring progress toward advising material and infant Healthy People 2010 objectives: 19 states, Pregnancy Risk Assessment Monitoring System (PKAmg) 2000–2003. *Morbidity and Mortality* Weekly Reports, 55 (5509), 1–11.

Tamminga, C. A., Thaker, G. K., & Medoff, D. R. (2004). Neuropsychiatric aspects of schizophrenia. In S. C. Yudofsky & R. E. Hales (Eds.), *Essentials of neuropsychiatry and clinical neurosciences* (pp. 457–487). Washington, DC: American Psychiatric Publishing.

Tarrant, C. J., & Jones, P. B. (2000). Biological markers as precursors to schizophrenia. In J. L. Rapoport (Ed.), *Childhood onset of "adult" psychopathology* (pp. 65–102). Washington, DC: American Psychiatric Press.

Torrey, E. F., & Yolken, R. H. (2003). Toxoplasma gondii and schizophrenia. *Emerging Infectious Diseases, 9*(11), 1375–1380.

Troshinksy, L. (2004). Fetal alcohol syndrome. Closing the gap. *Newsletter of the Office of Minority Health*. U.S. Department of Health and Human Services, Jan–Feb 2004, 4–5.

Tsai, Y. F., & Ku, Y. C. (2005). Self-care symptom management strategies for auditory hallucinations among inpatients with schizophrenia at a veterans' hospital in Taiwan. *Archives of Psychiatric Nursing, 19*(4), 194–199.

Tucker, J. S., Wenzel, S. L., Straus, J. B., Ryan, G. W., & Golinelli, D. (2005). Experiencing interpersonal violence. *Violence Against Women, 11*(10), 1319–1340.

Turetsky, B. I., Moberg, P. J., Arnold, S. E., Doty, R. L., & Gur, R. E. (2003). Low olfactory bulb volume in first-degree relatives of patients with schizophrenia. *American Journal of Psychiatry, 160*(4), 703–708.

Tuszynski, M. H., Thal, L., Pay, M., Salmon, D. P., U, H. S., Bakay, R., et al. (2005). A phase 1 clinical trial of nerve growth factor gene therapy for Alzheimer's disease. *Nature Medicine, 11*(5), 551–555.

Van Cleve, S. N., Cannon, S., & Cohen, W. I. (2006). Part II: Clinical practice guidelines for adolescents and young adults with Down syndrome: 12 to 21 years. *Journal of Pediatric Health Care, 20,* 198–205.

Van Cleve, S. N., & Cohen, W. I. (2006). Part I: Clinical practice guidelines for children with Down syndrome from birth to 12 years. *Journal of Pediatric Health Care, 20,* 47–54.

Vygotsky, L. (1962). *Thought and language*. Cambridge, MA: MIT Press.

Wahl, H., & Heyl, V. (2003). Connection between vision, hearing, and cognitive function. *Generations, 27*(1), 39–47.

Wimo, A., Winblad, B., Shah, S. N., Chin, W., Zhang, R., & McRae, T. (2004). Impact of donepezil treatment for Alzheimer's disease on caregiver time. *Current Medical Research Opinion, 20*(8), 1221–1225.

Wonodi, I., Adami, H. M., Cassady, S. L., Sherr, J. D., Avila, M. T., & Thaker, G. K. (2004). Ethnicity and the course of tardive dyskinesia in outpatients presenting to the motor disorders clinic at the Maryland psychiatric research center. *Journal of Clinical Psychopharmacology, 24*(6), 592–598.

Woods, D. L., & Dimond, M. (2002). The effect of therapeutic touch on agitated behavior and cortisol in persons with Alzheimer's disease. *Biological Research for Nursing, 4*(2), 104–114.

Yasuno, F., Suhara, T., Okubo, Y., Sudo, Y., Inoue, M., Ichimiya, T., et al. (2004). Low dopamine D2 receptor binding in subregions of the thalamus in schizophrenia. *American Journal of Psychiatry, 161*(6), 1016–1022.

Yesavage, J., Brink, T., Rose, T., Lum, O., Huang, V., Adey, M., et al. (1983). Development and validation of a geriatric depression screening scale: A preliminary report. *Journal of Psychiatric Research, 17,* 37–49.

Zubenko, G. S., Zubenko, W. N., McPherson, S., Spoor, E., Marin, D. B., Farlow, M. R., et al. (2003). A collaborative study of the emergence and clinical features of the major depressive syndrome of Alzheimer's disease. *American Journal of Psychiatry, 160*(5), 857–866.

Comfort

5

Concept at-a-Glance

Concept Learning Outcomes

After reading about this concept, you will be able to:

1. Summarize the physiological processes related to comfort.
2. List factors affecting comfort.
3. Identify commonly occurring alterations in comfort and their related treatments.
4. Explain common physical assessment procedures used to assess the comfort of clients across the life span.
5. Outline diagnostic and laboratory tests to determine the individual's comfort status.
6. Demonstrate the nursing process in providing culturally competent and caring interventions across the life span for individuals with common alterations in comfort.
7. Identify pharmacological interventions in caring for the individual with alterations in comfort.

Concept Key Terms

Acute pain, *257*
Cancer pain, *257*
Chronic fatigue syndrome, *258*
Chronic pain, *257*
Comfort, *255*
End-of-life care, *257*
Fatigue, *258*
Fibromyalgia, *258*
Hypersomnia, *258*
Insomnia, *258*
Narcolepsy, *258*
Pain, *256*
Parasomnia, *258*
Sleep apnea, *258*
Sleep hygiene, *260*
Tender points, *258*

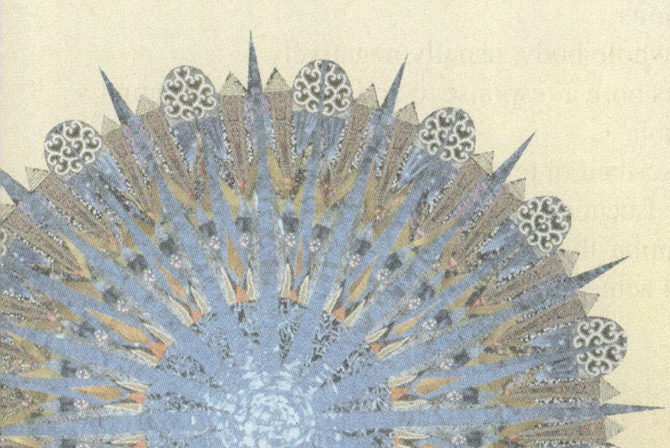

About Comfort

The word **comfort** is defined by Merriam-Webster as (1) "to give strength or hope to" and (2) "to ease the grief or trouble of." Katharine Kolcaba (2003) provides an excellent definition for purposes of student nurses, stating that comfort is "the immediate experience of being strengthened by having needs for relief, ease, and transcendence met in four contexts (physical, psychospiritual, social, and environmental); much more than the absence of pain." In the quoted definition, *ease* relates to a sense of calm or contentment; *relief* is the experience of being and feeling well, or being *comfortable*; and *transcendence* is the state in which one rises above problems or pain.

For the client in crisis, the nurse is the most immediate, recognizable source of comfort. It is the nurse's responsibility to provide comfort in all of the contexts. The nurse achieves this by demonstrating presence and by providing information and explanations, kindness and concern, referrals to resources, and timely and appropriate caring interventions.

There are any number of reasons for the nurse to provide comfort to a client, but the most significant reason is also the simplest: Comfort promotes healing. Comfort counteracts stress, which can impair sleep and nutrition; allows body, mind, and spirit to enter into processes of recovery and rehabilitation; and restores the sense of self and self-esteem.

Taken on a continuum, one might see the "normal" end of comfort as being warm and well fed, on a sofa with a blanket and some close friends, watching a movie. On the extreme opposite end, one would find starvation or torture. Looking at that continuum, one could argue that the state of being comfortable is the state of being most wholly oneself, with a high measure of relief, ease, and transcendence in each of Kolbaca's contexts. •

NORMAL PRESENTATION

The individual experiences a state of comfort when all needs are met in the physical, psychospiritual, social, and environmental contexts. When this happens, the individual experiences feelings of ease, relief, and/or transcendence. Essentially, the individual feels *comfort*able with physical well-being (no pain, sufficient energy, restful sleep), psychospiritual well-being, social circumstances, and/or environmental habitat and events.

Subjectively, the client may express a feeling of contentment and ease. Objectively, the nurse may note vital signs within normal range for the client and an expression of calmness in facial appearance, vocalization, and body language.

Because comfort has a high rate of subjectivity, it is important for the nurse working with a client to understand what is "comfortable" or "normal" for the client. Some clients may have difficulty articulating this or may have such a high tolerance for discomfort that it may be difficult to determine an appropriate baseline. For example, a client with severe persistent asthma may have such a history of poor sleep that waking up three times a night even without symptoms is normal. A woman who has worked for the Peace Corps in Africa for several years may be unperturbed by an extra day's stay in the hospital; she may welcome the rest and relatively quiet environment. However, an Olympic athlete, who is used to getting 8 hours of active exercise each day, might find the extra day of confinement and rest intolerable.

A number of neurological and medical functions and processes are typically associated with comfort. These include pain and the absence of pain; sleep and rest; nutrition and fluids; and sensory perceptions of heat, cold, odor, and noise. This concept will discuss some common alterations in comfort that are frequently encountered by the nurse, as well as the complexities involved in providing comfort to the client at the end of life.

ALTERATIONS

Any number of illnesses and conditions can result in client discomfort. But how is discomfort defined? What aspects of discomfort can the nurse address to help the client return to a state of ease, relief, and transcendence? Pain, fatigue, and anxiety come quickly to mind. Anxiety is addressed in Concept 28, Stress and Coping. In this concept, pain, end-of-life care, fatigue, fibromyalgia, and sleep and rest disorders are discussed.

Pain

The simplest opposite of comfort is pain. The widely agreed-upon definition of **pain** is "an unpleasant sensory and emotional experience associated with actual or potential tissue damage, or described in terms of such damage" (American Pain Society [APS], 2003; Gordon, 2003). Pain is a subjective response to both physical and psychological stressors. All people experience pain at some point during their lives. Although pain usually is experienced as uncomfortable and unwelcome, it also plays a protective role, warning of potentially health-threatening conditions. For this reason, pain is increasingly referred to as the *fifth vital sign*, with recommendations to assess pain with each vital sign assessment. The Joint Commission (JCAHO, 2001) has established pain standards that identify the relief of pain as a client right. These standards also require health care facilities to implement specific procedures for, and provider education on, pain assessment and management.

Each individual pain event is a distinct and personal experience influenced by physiological, psychological, cognitive, sociocultural, and spiritual factors. Pain is the symptom most associated with describing oneself as ill, and it is the most common reason for seeking health care. Although there are many definitions and descriptors of pain, the one most relevant is that pain is "whatever the person experiencing it says it is, and existing whenever the person says it does" (McCaffery, 1979, p. 11). This definition acknowledges the client as the only person who can accurately define and describe his or her own pain and serves as the basis for nursing assessment and care of clients in pain. It also supports the values and beliefs about pain necessary for holistic nursing care, including the following:

- Only the person affected can experience pain; that is, pain has a personal meaning.
- If the client says he or she has pain, the client is in pain. All pain is real.
- Pain has physical, emotional, cognitive, sociocultural, and spiritual dimensions.
- Pain affects the whole body, usually negatively.
- Pain may serve as both a response to and a warning of actual or potential trauma.

Pain may be described in terms of location, duration, intensity, and etiology. Location, intensity, and etiology are discussed in the exemplar that follows. *Duration* establishes the difference between acute and chronic pain.

DURATION When pain lasts only through the expected recovery period, it is described as **acute pain**, whether it has a sudden or slow onset and regardless of the intensity. **Chronic pain**, on the other hand, is prolonged, usually recurring or persisting over 6 months or longer, and interferes with functioning. Acute and chronic pain result in different physiological and behavioral responses, as shown in Table 5–1. Although experts may disagree on whether the cutoff point for chronic pain should be 1, 3, or 6 months after onset or expected healing time, NANDA specifies the accepted nursing diagnosis of *chronic pain* to be mild to severe, constant or recurring, without an anticipated or predictable end, and lasting for longer than 6 months (Ackley & Ladwig, 2006).

The categories differentiating chronic cancer (malignant) pain from chronic nonmalignant pain have also been problematic. **Cancer pain** may result from the direct effects of the disease and its treatment, or it may be unrelated to the disease and its treatment in individuals with cancer. Over the years, other diagnoses have been included in the malignant pain category, such as HIV/AIDS pain or burn pain, which tends to be treated more aggressively than "nonmalignant pain."

End-of-Life Care

End-of-life care refers to the nursing care provided to a client who is dying or who is near death. While many think of end-of-life care in the context of the older adult, a client of any age may experience life-threatening illness requiring end-of-life care. Clients at this stage can no longer care for themselves and rely on nurses, family members, and other caregivers to provide life's most basic necessities.

Dying clients and their families look to their nurse to educate, support, and guide them throughout the dying process. This intimate position allows the nurse to advocate for improved quality of life for the person with serious illness. According to the Hospice and Palliative Nurses Association (HPNA, 2003), "achieving quality of life, especially at the end of life, is contingent upon competent, 'state of the art' professional nursing care" (p. 1). Informed understanding of the client's values, wishes, and goals allows the nurse to attend to the client's physical, emotional, psychosocial, and spiritual needs.

Death is as natural a part of life as is birth. Although birth is embraced with joy and celebration, death is frequently denied and often prolonged for the sake of the living. Nurses have a unique opportunity and an obligation to help clients and their families through the dying process. Viewing death as a natural process—not a medical failure—is of utmost importance. The nurse who helps the client die comfortably and with dignity provides the following benefits of good nursing care:

- Attention to pain and symptom control
- Relief of psychosocial distress
- Coordinated care across settings with high-quality communication between health care providers
- Preparation of the client and family for death
- Clarification and communication of goals of treatment and values
- Support and education during the decision-making process, including the benefits and burdens of treatment.

Source: National Consensus Project [NCP] for Quality Palliative Care, 2004.

Nurses must be confident in their clinical skills when caring for the dying. They must be aware of the ethical, spiritual, and legal issues they may confront while providing end-of-life care.

End-of-life care requires a team approach. Nurses work together with treating physicians, other health care professionals, and family members to ensure the comfort of the dying client. Nurses often provide referrals for services for family members as well as the client. These may include referrals to home health services, social services agencies, and grief and loss counselors. Nurses provide and teach many comforting and health promoting interventions, such as turning the client to relieve pressure, bathing the client who is confined to bed, assisting with toileting, and dressing and feeding the client. Shaving, hair washing, nail care, and oral care all help the client to maintain dignity and feel comfortable during this time. The nurse provides these and teaches family members how to provide them as well.

TABLE 5–1 Comparison of Acute and Chronic Pain

ACUTE PAIN	CHRONIC PAIN
Mild to severe	Mild to severe
Sympathetic nervous system responses:	Parasympathetic nervous system responses:
Increased pulse rate	Vital signs normal
Increased respiratory rate	
Elevated blood pressure	
Diaphoresis	Dry, warm skin
Dilated pupils	Pupils normal or dilated
Related to tissue injury; resolves with healing	Continues beyond healing
Client appears restless and anxious	Client appears depressed and withdrawn
Client reports pain	Client often does not mention pain unless asked
Client exhibits behavior indicative of pain: crying, rubbing area, holding area	Pain behavior often absent

PRACTICE ALERT

Providing simple caring interventions such as shaving a client or washing the client's hair is essential to helping the client maintain dignity and promoting trust with family members. Imagine that a grown daughter flies across country to her dying father's bedside. She walks into his hospital room. She sees that he's clean, his hair is freshly washed, and his face is freshly shaven. Although she knows he cannot see or respond to her, she sees that his glasses and hearing aids are nearby and well cared for. How does this make her view the nurses caring for him? What comfort does this provide for her?

Each dying client, regardless of age, brings special challenges to the nurses providing end-of-life care. Nurses working with these clients must use active listening, be especially observant and sensitive, and provide a calm and reassuring manner at all times.

Fatigue

Fatigue may be a product of insufficient sleep, overexertion, illness, or a side effect of medication. Fatigue is not the same as feeling tired. **Fatigue** is characterized by a lack of energy and motivation that may or may not be accompanied by drowsiness. Common causes of fatigue (Mayo Clinic, 2008) include the following:

- Anemia (including iron deficiency anemia)
- Sleep disorders
- Depression or grief
- Pregnancy
- Respiratory disorders
- Hypothyroidism
- Use of alcohol or drugs.

Fatigue may result from the course of normal events, as in the kind of fatigue experienced by the parents of a new baby. It may also result from a single occurrence of enormous impact. Acute fatigue is often associated with the body's continued biological responses following disaster, such as a hurricane. Acute fatigue normally resolves with rest or with the resolution of the underlying cause, such as an acute infection. Chronic fatigue may not resolve as easily. Chronic fatigue may be experienced as an effect of a long-term illness or as a side effect of the medications required to treat a lengthy illness. Some individuals experience **chronic fatigue syndrome**, a complex disorder in which the client experiences unrelenting fatigue and associated symptoms that cannot be otherwise explained for a period of six months or longer.

Fibromyalgia

An estimated 5 million Americans suffer from **fibromyalgia**, a chronic disorder characterized by widespread musculoskeletal pain, fatigue, and multiple tender points. **Tender points** refers to tenderness that occurs in precise, localized areas, particularly in the neck, spine, shoulders, and hips. People with this syndrome may also experience sleep disturbances, morning stiffness, irritable bowel syndrome, anxiety, and other symptoms. Although the symptoms present as muscle pain, stiffness, and weakness, it is considered by many to be a problem of abnormal central nervous system (CNS) functioning, particularly as it relates to the way nerves process pain.

Sleep and Rest Disorders

Sleep is a basic human need, a universal biological process common to all people. Humans spend about one third of their lives asleep. We require sleep for many reasons: to cope with daily stresses, to prevent fatigue, to conserve energy, to restore the mind and body, and to enjoy life more fully. Sleep enhances daytime functioning. It is vital for not only optimal psychological functioning but also physiological functioning, as the rate of healing of damaged tissue is greatest during sleep (Robinson, Weitzel, & Henderson, 2005, p. 263). Sleep is an important factor in a person's quality of life. Yet a 2006 report from the Institute of Medicine (IOM) states that sleep disorders and sleep deprivation constitute an unmet public health problem. It is estimated that 50 million to 70 million Americans suffer from a chronic disorder of sleep and wakefulness that hinders daily functioning and adversely affects health (IOM, 2006, p. 24). Numerous *Sleep in America* polls by the National Sleep Foundation reflect that Americans, from infants to older adults, need more sleep.

Many members of the general public and health professionals are unaware of the consequences of chronic sleep loss (e.g., increased risk of hypertension, diabetes, obesity, depression, heart attack, and stroke). Almost 20% of all serious car crash injuries are associated with driver sleepiness (IOM, 2006, p. 25). As a result, the IOM report made a number of recommendations, including (a) increasing financial investments in interdisciplinary somnology (the study of sleep) and sleep medicine research training, (b) increasing public awareness by establishing a multimedia public education campaign, (c) increasing education and training of health care professionals in somnology and sleep medicine, (d) developing new technologies for the diagnosis and treatment of sleep disorders, and (e) monitoring the American population's sleep patterns and the prevalence and health outcomes associated with sleep disorders (IOM, 2006).

A knowledge of common sleep disorders can help nurses assess the sleep complaints of their clients and, when appropriate, make a referral to a specialist in sleep disorders medicine. This concept discusses insomnia, hypersomnia, narcolepsy, sleep apnea, insufficient sleep, and **parasomnias**, behaviors that may interfere with sleep and may occur during sleep. **Insomnia** is described as the inability to fall asleep or remain asleep. **Hypersomnia** refers to conditions where the affected individual obtains sufficient sleep at night, but still cannot stay awake during the day. Clients with **narcolepsy** experience sleep attacks or excessive daytime sleepiness. **Sleep apnea** is characterized by frequent short breathing pauses during sleep.

ALTERATIONS AND TREATMENTS Comfort

Alteration	Description	Treatment
Acute pain	Pain of varying severity, location, and etiology that lasts fewer than 6 months. In addition to the pain itself, manifestations include: ■ Nausea and vomiting ■ Restlessness ■ Rapid/shallow respirations ■ Elevated blood pressure.	Pharmacological pain management: ■ Narcotic analgesics ■ Anti-inflammatory ■ Nonnarcotic analgesics ■ Miscellaneous analgesics. Nonpharmacological therapy: ■ Massage ■ Diversional therapies ■ Nerve stimulation.
Chronic pain	Pain of varying severity, location, and etiology that lasts 6 months or more (even if intermittent). In addition to the pain itself, manifestations include: ■ Heart rate and blood pressure below normal ranges ■ Depression ■ Irritability ■ Impaired mobility and/or activity.	Pharmacological pain management: ■ Nonnarcotic analgesics such as NSAIDs ■ Antidepressants may reduce nerve-related pain ■ Anti-inflammatory medications ■ Antispasmodic or muscle relaxants ■ Narcotic analgesics as last resort. Nonpharmacological therapy: ■ Guided imagery ■ Massage ■ Nerve stimulation units ■ Diversional activities (music, involvement in hobbies, aroma therapy) ■ Chiropractic interventions ■ Physical therapy ■ Applications of heat or cold ■ Relaxation techniques ■ Positioning.
End-of-life care	■ Loss of muscle tone ■ Slowing of circulation ■ Change in respirations ■ Sensory impairments	■ Palliative care or more aggressive care as chosen by client and family ■ Comforting caring interventions, e.g., bathing, nail care, turning, and repositioning
Fatigue	■ Restlessness ■ Irritability ■ Drowsiness ■ Depression ■ Anxiety	■ Improved sleep hygiene ■ Counseling ■ Pharmacological and nonpharmacological therapies
Fibromyalgia	■ Widespread pain, especially at tender points ■ Insomnia ■ Chronic fatigue	■ Local heat application ■ Massage ■ Stretching exercises ■ Selective serotonin norepinephrine uptake inhibitors
Sleep-rest disorders	■ Insomnia ■ Hypersomnia ■ Narcolepsy ■ Parasomnias ■ Insufficient sleep ■ Sleep apnea	■ Improved sleep hygiene ■ Pharmacological therapies as appropriate ■ Relaxation techniques, massage, other complementary and alternative medicine (CAM) therapies ■ Continuous positive airway pressure

ASSESSMENT

The nursing history plays an important role in determining the client's level of discomfort. Some clients may not even realize the extent to which the area of discomfort is impacting their lives. Nurses should determine to what extent the client's discomfort is affecting his or her ability to perform activities of daily living. While specific assessments, interviews, and scales are discussed with each exemplar of this concept, the nurse, at a minimum, should assess for the following:

- Length of time the problem has persisted
- Times of day or activities during or following which the problem becomes worse
- Nature and duration of client's sleep; nature of bedtime rituals
- Effect of the client's discomfort on other family members

- Nature of the client's support network
- Client's eating habits, including types of food, portion sizes, and times of day that the client eats.

A thorough physical exam is necessary, in part to rule out any underlying previously undiagnosed illness or disorder that may be causing the client's discomfort. For clients experiencing pain, nurses may palpate painful areas for presence of edema, and location and nature of the pain.

DIAGNOSTIC TESTS

A number of diagnostic tests may be ordered to determine if there is an underlying biological cause of the client's discomfort or to gain more information in addition to the physical assessment. X-rays, for example, may be necessary to determine if a fracture is causing a client pain. A white blood cell count (WBC) may also be ordered if there is indication of infection causing pain, such as an open wound, inflammation, or a fever. For the client verbalizing continuous or chronic fatigue and dyspnea on exertion, diagnostic tests such as hemoglobin and hematocrit (H & H) to check iron levels and oxygen-carrying ability of the red blood cells may be ordered. Reports of poor sleeping patterns may indicate the need for a sleep study.

CARING INTERVENTIONS

Caring interventions depend on the area of discomfort for the client. The first intervention is active listening to assure the client that his or her discomfort is acknowledged. Active listening components are an environment as free from distractions as possible, sitting at eye level with the client, asking open-ended questions (that cannot be answered with just "yes" or "no"), observing facial expressions and body language, and verifying information obtained.

Sleep Hygiene

An important caring intervention that may be implemented for all clients experiencing discomfort, regardless of the etiology of their discomfort, is the promotion of good sleep hygiene. Even for clients experiencing great pain, good sleep hygiene can help improve the quality of their sleep.

Sleep hygiene is a term referring to interventions used to promote sleep. Nurses can promote knowledge of sleep hygiene by teaching about sleep habits, support of bedtime rituals, the provision of a restful environment, specific measures to promote comfort and relaxation, and appropriate use of hypnotic medications. Nurses trying to help clients who need to improve their sleep hygiene should do the following:

- Promote bedtime rituals or presleep routines that are conducive to comfort and relaxation. Altering or eliminating such routines can affect a client's sleep. Common bedtime routines for adults include listening to music, reading, taking a soothing bath, and praying. Appropriate bedtime rituals for children include reading a bedtime story, holding a favorite toy or blanket, kissing everyone goodnight, and praying with other family members.
- Encourage maintenance of a restful environment. All people need a sleeping environment with minimal noise, a comfortable room temperature, appropriate ventilation, and appropriate lighting. A low light source may provide comfort to children or those in a strange environment.
- Promote comfort and relaxation to help the client fall and stay asleep. The following interventions, either provided by the nurse or used by the client, may help improve rest and relaxation:
  - Provide loose-fitting nightwear.
  - Assist clients with hygienic routines.
  - Make sure the bed linen is smooth, clean, and dry.
  - Assist or encourage the client to void before bedtime.
  - Offer to provide a back massage before sleep.
  - Position dependent clients appropriately to aid muscle relaxation, and provide supportive devices to protect pressure areas.
  - Schedule medications, especially diuretics, to prevent nocturnal awakenings.
  - For clients who have pain, administer analgesics 30 minutes before sleep.

For hospitalized clients, sleep problems are often related to the hospital environment or their illness. Assisting the client to sleep in such instances can be challenging to a nurse, often involving scheduling activities, administering analgesics, and providing a supportive environment. Explanations and a supportive relationship are essential for the fearful or anxious client.

Different types of hypnotics may be prescribed depending on the type of sleep problem (e.g., difficulties falling asleep or difficulties maintaining sleep). Drugs with longer half-lives are often prescribed for difficulties maintaining sleep but must be used with caution for older adults.

Bedtime rituals for institutionalized clients may include assisting with a hand and face wash, providing a massage or hot drink, freshening pillows, and providing extra blankets as needed.

Nurses should help clients reduce environmental distractions and provide a room temperature that is satisfactory to the client. Some interventions to reduce environmental distractions in hospitals, especially noise, are listed in Box 5–1.

Nurses working in a hospital, rehabilitation facility, or long-term care facility should try to take into consideration individual circadian rhythms. An early riser may welcome receiving respiratory therapy first thing in the morning but not appreciate a bath and linen change after supper when he or she is tired and ready for sleep.

PHARMACOLOGIC THERAPIES

Potential interventions include pharmacological therapies (medication) and/or nonpharmacological therapies. Nonpharmacological therapies may be alternative (instead of pharmacological therapies) or complementary (in addition to pharmacological and/or other nonpharmacological therapies). Therapies linked to the physical, psychospiritual, environmental, and social domains are outlined in Table 5–2.

Box 5–1 Reducing Environmental Distractions in Hospitals

- Close window curtains if street lights shine through.
- Close curtains between clients in semiprivate and larger rooms.
- Reduce or eliminate overhead lighting; provide a night light at the bedside or in the bathroom.
- Use a flashlight to check drainage bags, etc. without turning on the overhead lights.
- Ensure a clear pathway around the bed to avoid bumping the bed and jarring the client during sleeping hours.
- Close the door of the client's room.
- Adhere to agency policy about times to turn off communal televisions or radios.
- Lower the ring tone of nearby telephones.
- Discontinue use of the paging system after a certain hour (e.g., 2,100 hours) or reduce its volume.
- Keep required staff conversations at low levels; conduct nursing reports or other discussions in a separate area away from client rooms.
- Wear rubber-soled shoes.
- Ensure that all cart wheels are well oiled.
- Perform only essential noisy activities during sleeping hours.

TABLE 5–2 **Therapies Related to Discomfort**

DIMENSION OF DISCOMFORT	THERAPY
Physical: Inflammation/infection/pain	Pharmacological: Anti-inflammatory/antibiotic/antipyretic Nonpharmacological: Herbs; imaging
Psychospiritual	Pharmacological: Antidepressants Nonpharmacological: Spiritual support
Environmental	Pharmacological: Antianxiety/antidepressants Nonpharmacological: Aromatherapy/music therapy/environmental changes
Social	Pharmacological: Antianxiety Nonpharmacological: Psychotherapy; companionship

5.1 ACUTE AND CHRONIC PAIN

KEY TERMS

Acute pain, *262*
Breakthrough pain, *264*
Central pain, *264*
Chronic pain, *263*
Coanalgesic, *274*
Hyperalgesia, *264*
Incident pain, *264*
Nerve block, *278*
Neuralgias, *264*
Neuropathic pain, *262*
Nociceptor, *263*
Pain, *262*
Pain threshold, *271*
Pain tolerance, *271*
Phantom pain, *264*
Physiological pain, *262*
Placebo, *278*
Psychogenic pain, *264*
Referred pain, *263*
Sensitization, *271*
Somatic pain, *263*
Spinal cord stimulation (SCS), *279*
Visceral pain, *263*

BASIS FOR SELECTION OF EXEMPLAR

Fifth vital sign
Standards of Nursing Practice

LEARNING OUTCOMES

After reading about this exemplar, you will be able to:

1. Describe the pathophysiology, etiology, clinical manifestations, and direct and indirect causes of acute and chronic pain.
2. Identify risk factors associated with acute and chronic pain.
3. Illustrate the nursing process in providing culturally competent care across the life span for individuals with acute and chronic pain.
4. Formulate priority nursing diagnoses appropriate for individuals with acute and chronic pain.
5. Create a plan of care for individuals with acute and chronic pain and their family members.
6. Assess expected outcomes for individuals with acute and chronic pain.
7. Discuss therapies used in the collaborative care of individuals with acute and chronic pain.
8. Employ evidence-based caring interventions for individuals with acute and chronic pain.

OVERVIEW

Pain is an unpleasant and highly personal experience that may be imperceptible to others while consuming all parts of the person's life. The widely agreed-upon definition of **pain** is "an unpleasant sensory and emotional experience associated with actual or potential tissue damage, or described in terms of such damage" (American Pain Society [APS], 2003; Gordon, 2003). Three parts of this definition have important implications for nurses. First, pain is a physical *and* emotional experience, not all in the body or all in the mind. Second, it is in response to actual *or* potential tissue damage, so there may not be abnormal lab or radiographic reports despite real pain. Finally, pain is described in terms of such damage. This final component is aligned with McCaffery's often quoted definition of pain: "Pain is whatever the experiencing person says it is, existing whenever he says it does" (McCaffery & Pasero, 1999, p. 17). Given that some clients are reluctant to disclose the presence of pain unless prompted, nurses will not know of the client's pain until they assess for it. Additionally, it is clear that nonverbal clients (e.g., preverbal children, intubated clients, the cognitively impaired) experience pain that demands nursing assessment and treatment even if clients are unable to "describe in terms" the nature of their discomfort. Pain can be described in terms of location, intensity, etiology, and duration. Duration is discussed in the About Comfort section of this concept.

Location

Classifications of pain based on where it is in the body (e.g., headache, backache, chest pain) may be useful in determining the client's underlying problems or needs, or it may be problematic given that most clients don't fit neatly into one of the categories. Location of pain is, however, a very important component to note. For example, if after knee surgery, a client reports moderately severe chest pain, the nurse must act immediately to further evaluate and treat this discomfort. Complicating the categorization of pain by location is the fact that some pains radiate (spread or extend) to other areas (e.g., low back to legs). Pain may be referred (appear to arise in different areas) to other parts of the body. For example, cardiac pain may be felt in the shoulder or left arm, with or without chest pain.

Intensity

To avoid ambiguity, categorizing pain according to intensity (mild, moderate, severe) or the underlying physiology (somatic, visceral, neuropathic) has emerged as a useful way to identify types of pain (Figure 5–1 ■). Serlin, Mendoza, Nakamura, Edwards, and Cleeland (1995) conducted a large-scale international study that confirmed earlier classifications of pain by intensity using a standard 0 (no pain) to 10 (worst possible pain) scale. Linking the rating to health and functioning scores, pain in the 1–3 range is deemed mild pain, a rating of 4–6 is moderate pain, and pain reaching 7–10 is ranked severe pain and is associated with the worst outcomes.

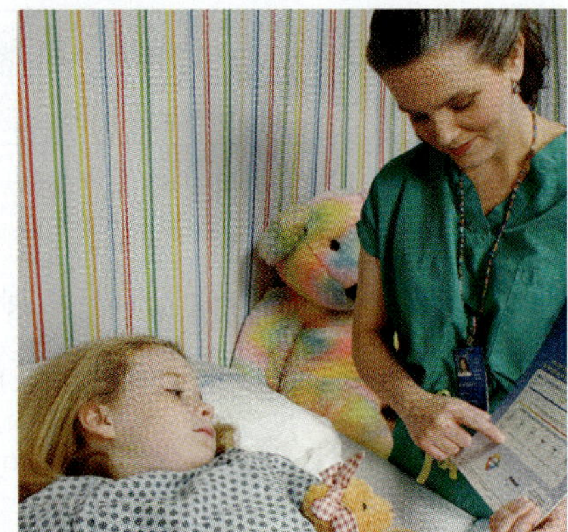

Figure 5–1 ■ The nurse is having the child rate her pain by pointing to the face that most closely matches the way she feels. Note her stuffed animals that provide comfort.

Etiology

Types of pain can be designated by etiology under the broad categories of physiological pain and neuropathic pain. **Physiological pain** is experienced when an intact, properly functioning nervous system sends signals that tissues are damaged, requiring attention and proper care. For example, the pain experienced following a cut or broken bone alerts the person to avoid further damage until it is properly healed. Once stabilized or healed, the pain goes away; thus this pain is transient. There may also be persistent forms of physiological pain. For example, a person who has lost the protective cartilage in joints will have pain when he or she stresses those joints, as the bone-to-bone contact damages tissues. This common form of arthritis produces pain in millions of sufferers, some of whom have intermittent pain, while others have constant pain that persists for years.

Neuropathic pain is experienced by people who have damaged or malfunctioning nerves. The nerves may be abnormal due to illness (e.g., postherpetic neuralgia, diabetic peripheral neuropathy), injury (e.g., phantom limb pain, spinal cord injury pain), or undetermined reasons.

Regardless of the type of pain the client is experiencing, it is the nurse's responsibility to assess for etiology, location, duration, and severity and to help the client determine the best course necessary to alleviate the pain.

TYPES OF PAIN

There are several types of pain, with the most common classifications being *acute* and *chronic* pain. *Breakthrough, central, phantom,* and *psychogenic* pain are also discussed in this exemplar.

Acute Pain

As discussed previously, pain may be described in terms of location, duration, intensity, and etiology. Pain is classified as either acute or chronic. **Acute pain** has a sudden onset, is usually temporary, and is localized. Pain that lasts for less than 6 months and has an identified cause is classified as acute pain. The onset is usually sudden, most often resulting from tissue injury from trauma, surgery, or inflammation. The pain is usually sharp and localized, although it may radiate. The three major types of acute pain are as follows:

- **Somatic pain** arises from nerve receptors originating in the skin or close to the surface of the body. Somatic pain may be either sharp and well localized or dull and diffuse. It is often accompanied by nausea and vomiting.
- **Visceral pain** arises from body organs. Visceral pain is dull and poorly localized because of the low number of **nociceptors**, the nerve receptors for pain. The viscera are sensitive to stretching, inflammation, and ischemia but relatively insensitive to cutting and temperature extremes. Visceral pain is associated with nausea and vomiting, hypotension, and restlessness. It often radiates or is referred. It may be described as cramping, intermittent pain, or colicky pain.
- **Referred pain** is pain that is perceived in an area distant from the site of the stimuli. It commonly occurs with visceral pain, as visceral fibers synapse at the level of the spinal cord, close to fibers innervating other subcutaneous tissue areas of the body (Figure 5–2 ■). Pain in a spinal nerve may be felt over the skin in any body area innervated by sensory neurons that share the same spinal nerve route. Body areas defined by spinal nerve routes are called *dermatomes*.

Acute pain warns of actual or potential injury to tissues. As a stressor, it initiates the fight-or-flight autonomic stress response. Characteristic physical responses include tachycardia, rapid and shallow respirations, increased blood pressure, dilated pupils, sweating, and pallor. The person experiencing the pain responds to this threat with anxiety and fear. This psychological response may further increase the physical responses to acute pain.

Chronic Pain

Chronic pain is prolonged pain, usually lasting longer than 6 months. It is not always associated with an identifiable cause. The heart rate and blood pressure may fall within normal ranges due to physiological adaptation, but hormonal stress responses to pain persist. Chronic pain lowers the pain threshold as a result of the depletion of serotonin and endorphin levels in the neurons; this leads to depression and irritability (Schaffer & Yucha, 2004). Unlike acute pain, chronic pain has a much more complex and poorly understood purpose.

Chronic pain can be subdivided into four categories:

1. *Recurrent acute pain* is characterized by relatively well-defined episodes of pain interspersed with pain-free episodes. Examples of recurrent acute pain include migraine headaches and sickle cell crises.

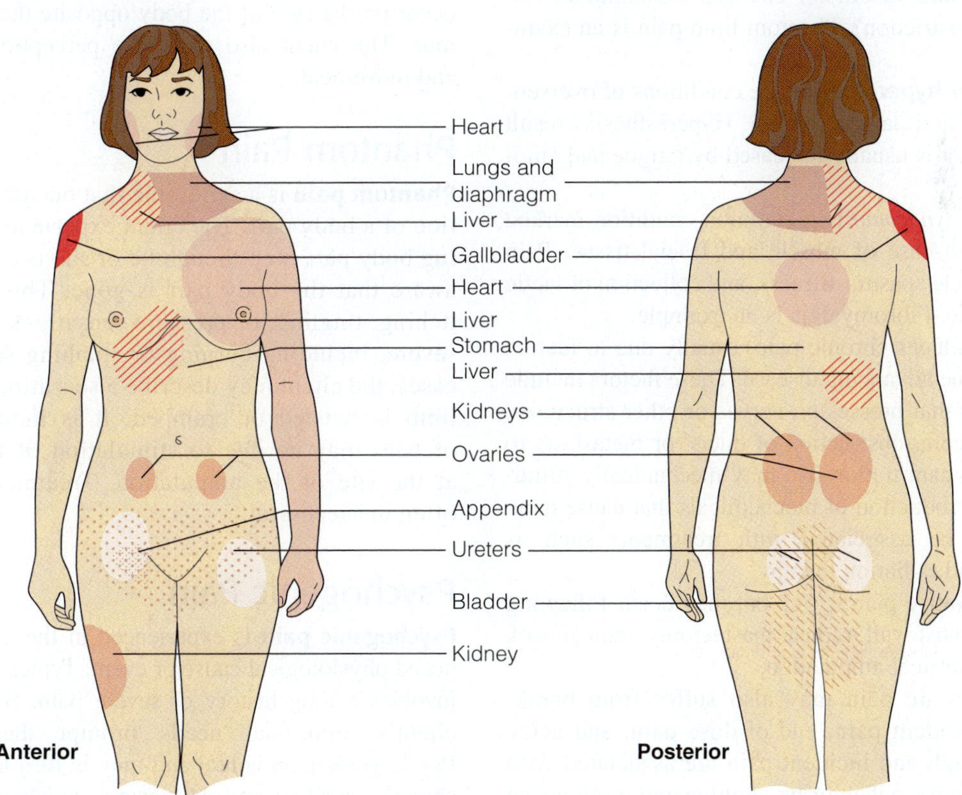

Figure 5–2 ■ Referred pain is the result of the convergence of sensory nerves from certain areas of the body before they enter the brain for interpretation. For example, a toothache may be felt in the ear, pain from inflammation of the diaphragm may be felt in the shoulder, and pain from ischemia of the heart muscle (angina) may be felt in the left arm.

2. *Ongoing time-limited pain* is identified by a defined time period. Some examples are cancer pain, which ends with control of the disease or death, and burn pain, which ends with rehabilitation or death.
3. *Chronic nonmalignant pain* is non-life-threatening pain that nevertheless persists beyond the expected time for healing. Chronic lower back pain falls into this category.
4. *Chronic intractable nonmalignant pain syndrome* is similar to simple chronic nonmalignant pain but is characterized by the person's inability to cope well with the pain and sometimes by physical, social, and/or psychological disability resulting from the pain.

The client with chronic pain often is depressed, withdrawn, immobile, irritable, and/or controlling. Although chronic pain may range from mild to severe and may be continuous or intermittent, the unrelenting presence of the pain often results in the pain itself becoming the pathological process requiring intervention. The most common chronic pain condition is lower back pain. Other common chronic pain conditions include the following (McCance & Huether, 2002):

- **Neuralgias** are painful conditions that result from damage to a peripheral nerve caused by infection or disease. Postherpetic neuralgia (following shingles) is an example.
- *Complex regional pain syndrome* is a neuropathic pain that results from nerve damage. It is characterized by continuous severe, burning pain. These conditions follow peripheral nerve damage and present the symptoms of pain, vasospasm, muscle wasting, and vasomotor changes (vasodilation followed by vasoconstriction). Phantom limb pain is an example (Porth, 2005).
- *Hyperesthesias or* **hyperalgesias** are conditions of oversensitivity to tactile and painful stimuli. Hyperesthesias result in diffuse pain that is usually increased by fatigue and emotional lability.
- *Myofascial pain syndrome* is a common condition marked by injury to or disease of muscle and fascial tissue. Pain results from muscle spasm, stiffness, and collection of lactic acid in the muscle. Fibromyalgia is an example.
- Cancer often produces chronic pain, usually due to factors associated with the advancing disease. These factors include a growing tumor that presses on nerves or other structures, stretching of viscera, obstruction of ducts, or metastasis to bones. The malignant tumor also may mechanically stimulate pain or the production of biochemicals that cause pain. Pain also may be associated with treatments such as chemotherapy and radiation therapy.
- Chronic postoperative pain is rare but may occur following incisions in the chest wall, radical mastectomy, radical neck dissection, and surgical amputation.
- Clients with chronic pain may also suffer from breakthrough pain, incident pain, end-of-dose pain, and acute pain. Breakthrough and incident pain are associated with coughing or activity but may be spontaneous without an identifiable cause. End-of-dose pain refers to an increasing awareness of pain prior to the next scheduled dose of controlled-release analgesia.

Breakthrough Pain

Breakthrough pain is pain that exceeds baseline treated or untreated pain (Svendsen et al., 2005). It is often described as a sudden flare that exceeds the analgesic effect of long-acting pain medications; it is sometimes associated with the ending of an *analgesic*. Whether the pain is *malignant* or nonmalignant in origin, treated or untreated, breakthrough pain is temporary and often debilitating. An increase in the baseline dose of analgesic to prevent breakthrough pain or administration of doses timed in relation to patterns of breakthrough pain may be needed.

Incident pain is a subtype of breakthrough pain. It is predictable pain precipitated by an event or activity such as coughing, changing position, or being touched. Clients at rest sometimes report their pain to the prescriber as very tolerable only to cry out in pain when subsequently attempting to change positions in bed or stand. Clients experience incident pain when the activity or incident begins.

Central Pain

Central pain is related to a lesion in the brain that may spontaneously produce high-frequency bursts of impulses that are perceived as pain. A vascular lesion, tumor, trauma, or inflammation within the brain may cause central pain. Thalamic pain is one of the most common types. Thalamic pain is severe, spontaneous, and often continuous. Hyperesthesia (an abnormal sensitivity to touch, pain, or other sensory stimuli) may occur on the side of the body opposite the lesion in the thalamus. The client also may lose perception of body position and movement.

Phantom Pain

Phantom pain is a syndrome that occurs following amputation of a body part. The client experiences pain in the missing body part even though he or she is completely mentally aware that the body part is gone. This pain may include itching, tingling, or pressure sensations, or it may be more severe, including burning or stabbing sensations. In some cases, the client may describe a sensation that an amputated limb is twisted or cramped. It is thought that this type of pain may be due to stimulation of the severed nerves at the site of the amputation. Treatment is complex and often unsuccessful.

Psychogenic Pain

Psychogenic pain is experienced in the absence of any diagnosed physiological cause or event. Typically psychogenic pain involves a long history of severe pain. It is thought that the client's emotional needs prompt the pain sensations. Psychogenic pain is real and may in turn lead to physiological changes, such as muscle tension, which may produce further pain. This condition may result from interpersonal conflicts, a need for support from others, or a desire to avoid a stressful or traumatic situation. Depression is often present.

PATHOPHYSIOLOGY AND ETIOLOGY

The peripheral nervous system is composed of two types of neurons: sensory and motor. Pain is perceived through the sensory neurons and responded to through the motor neurons. Connections or synapses occur within the spinal cord and again within the central nervous system (CNS), where cognitive analysis of the painful stimulus leads to a response. A highly intense pain may prompt an immediate reflex response that precedes awareness of the pain.

Nociceptors (Figure 5–3 ■) are located at the ends of small afferent neurons and are woven throughout all tissues of the body except the brain. Nociceptors are especially numerous in the skin and muscles. Pain occurs when biological, mechanical, thermal, electrical, or chemical factors stimulate nociceptors (Table 5–3). The intensity and duration of the stimuli determine the sensation. Long-lasting, intense stimulation produces greater pain than brief, mild stimulation.

Nociceptors are stimulated either by persistent mechanical, chemical, or thermal stimuli to the cell or by the local release of biochemicals secondary to cell injury. *Bradykinin*, a polypeptide element of the kinin protein system (McCance & Huether, 2002), appears to be the most abundant and potent pain-producing chemical; other biochemical sources of pain include prostaglandins, histamine, hydrogen ions, and potassium ions. These biochemicals are thought to bind to nociceptors in response to noxious stimuli causing the nociceptors to initiate pain impulses.

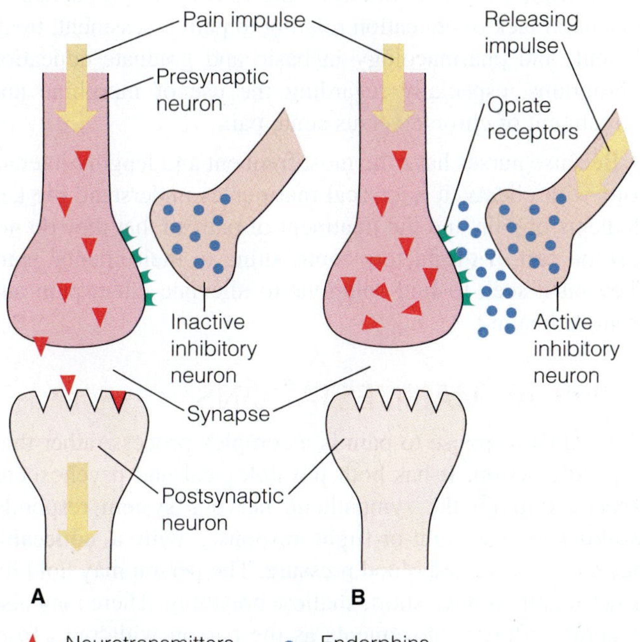

Figure 5–3 ■ *A*, Pain impulse causes presynaptic neuron to release burst of neurotransmitters across synapse. These bind to postsynaptic neuron and propagate impulse. *B*, Inhibitory neuron releases endorphins, which bind to presynaptic opiate receptors. Neurotransmitter release is inhibited, and pain impulse is interrupted.

TABLE 5–3 **Pain Stimuli**

CAUSATIVE FACTOR	EXAMPLE
Microorganisms (e.g., bacteria, viruses)	Meningitis
Inflammation	Sore throat
Impaired blood flow	Angina
Invasive tumor	Colon cancer
Radiation	Therapy for cancer
Heat	Sunburn
Obstruction	Kidney stone
Spasm	Colon cramping
Compression	Carpal tunnel syndrome
Decreased movement	Pain after cast removal
Stretching or straining	Sprained ankle
Fractures	Fractured hip
Swelling	Arthritis
Deposits of foreign tissue	Endometriosis
Chemicals	Skin rash
Electricity	Electrical burn
Conflict, difficulty in life	Psychogenic pain

Pain Theories

Three theories about pain include *specific theory*, *pattern theory*, and *gate theory*.

SPECIFIC THEORY Pain neurons are specific and unique. Sensations go directly to the brain for interpretation. The "pain" message that reaches the brain is equal in intensity to the "pain" message that was transmitted by the nociceptor. Psychological effects on pain perception are not recognized in this theory.

PATTERN THEORY The perception of pain depends on the pattern of the stimulus, thus may be interpreted differently by different individuals. Psychosocial impacts are not recognized in this theory, just differences in perception based on differences in stimuli patterns.

GATE THEORY Pain impulses can be modified at the spinal cord level before they reach the brain. The gate theory (Melzack & Wall, 1965) proposes that "gates" exist at the dorsal horn synapses in the spinal cord. The gates may be open to let pain stimuli through to the brain or may "close" to inhibit transmission of the stimuli to the brain.

Etiology

Epidemiological studies estimate that most people have experienced pain in the last month, and between one third and one half of adults live with some form of chronic pain (APS, 1999; Elliott, Smith, Penny, Smith, & Chambers, 1999), with the prevalence higher among the older populations (Reyes-Gibby, Aday, & Cleeland, 2002). Approximately 25 million

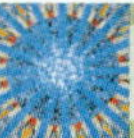

ALTERNATIVE THERAPIES **Pain Control**

The gate control theory helps explain why complementary pain management techniques are effective in helping to control pain. Stimulation of the larger A-delta fibers by ice or nonpainful touch and pressure such as massage causes the substantia gelatinosa in the dorsal horn of the spinal cord to "close the gate" and decrease the transmission of pain impulses to the brain (Huether & Defriez, 2006).

Americans live with persistent pain described as "very severe," causing them to be unable to work or independently perform activities of daily living (APS, 1999). Severe or persistent pain affects all body systems causing potentially serious health problems while increasing the risk of complications, delays in healing, and an accelerated progression of fatal illnesses (Arnstein, 2003). Even if the original cause of the pain heals, the changes in the nervous system resulting from suboptimal pain management can result in the development of incurable chronic pain (Arnstein, 1997; Katz, Jackson, Kavanagh, & Sandler, 1996). Persistent pain also contributes to insomnia, weight gain, constipation, hypertension, deconditioning, chronic stress, and depression (Dodd et al., 2001; Monteiro-Cruz & Mattos-Pimenta, 2001; Wilson, Eriksson, D'Eon, Mikail, & Emery, 2002). These effects interfere with work, recreation, domestic activities, and personal care activities to the point that leads many sufferers to question if life is worth living (Hitchcock, Ferrell, & McCaffery, 1994). Effective pain management is an important aspect of nursing care to promote healing, prevent complications, reduce suffering, and prevent the development of incurable pain states.

Risk Factors

Risks for incurring pain include internal and external environmental factors. Safety features and practices protect against external risks. Healthy life styles protect against internal risks.

Risks for enhanced perception of new pain may include physical effects of previous pain (discomfort) or decreased functional ability; psychosocial effects such as alteration in social relationships or self-esteem; emotional effects such as diminished leisure or depression; spiritual issues such as questioning the meaning of suffering; financial effects such as inability to work and earn money; and/or cultural issues such as belief that minorities, females, and older adults often receive less than optimal pain management.

A number of specific factors contribute to risk for pain. Preoperative anxiety, younger age, and chronic pain are associated with severe postoperative pain. Clients who are vulnerable to stress and have an impaired cortisol response are more susceptible to persistent pain following a motor vehicle accident. Risk factors related to inadequate pain relief for lower back pain include a previous history of lower back pain, lifting weights, lack of exercise, emotional distress, and dissatisfaction with employment (Bruckenthal, 2008).

Risk factors related to inadequate pain relief include barriers from the client and family perspective, as well as barriers from the health care provider perspective. Patricia Berry (2005) lists the barriers to assessment and treatment of pain from the perspective of the client and family:

1. The belief that "good" clients don't complain.
2. Pain is inevitable with aging, so older adults should not complain.
3. Strong medicine only comes in injectable form and do not want "shots."
4. Side effects of pain medicine are worse than the pain itself.
5. Addiction to pain medicine is common (a misconception).
6. "Strong" pain medicine should be used only for very severe pain.
7. Morphine is used only when the individual is dying.

Berry (2005) identifies additional barriers to the successful treatment of client pain from the health care provider's perspective:

- Health care professionals are better judges of pain than the client is.
- Pain is often not seen as important as other indicators in the hospital.
- Only opioids are effective in severe pain.
- Opioids cause respiratory depression.
- Fear of double effect (unintentionally causing harm when trying to do good).
- Confusion over addiction/tolerance/physical dependence.
- General lack of education relating to pain assessment, treatment, and pharmacology in basic and graduate education programs, especially regarding the use of morphine and treatment of chronic versus acute pain.

Because nurses have the most frequent and lengthy interactions with clients, it is critical that nurses understand the key elements of pain and the treatment of pain so that they do not become part of the factors contributing to their clients' pain. They must seek to find solutions to alleviate client pain and promote healing.

CLINICAL MANIFESTATIONS

The body's response to pain is a complex process rather than a specific action. It has both physiological and psychosocial aspects. Initially the sympathetic nervous system responds, resulting in the fight-or-flight response, with a noticeable increase in pulse and blood pressure. The person may hold his or her breath or have short, shallow breathing. There may also be some reflexive movements as the person withdraws from the painful stimuli (Figure 5–4 ■). Over a matter of minutes or hours, the pulse and blood pressure return to baseline despite the persistence of pain. Contrary to the adaptation noted in vital signs, the pain fibers themselves adapt very little and become sensitized in a way that intensifies, prolongs, and/or spreads the pain.

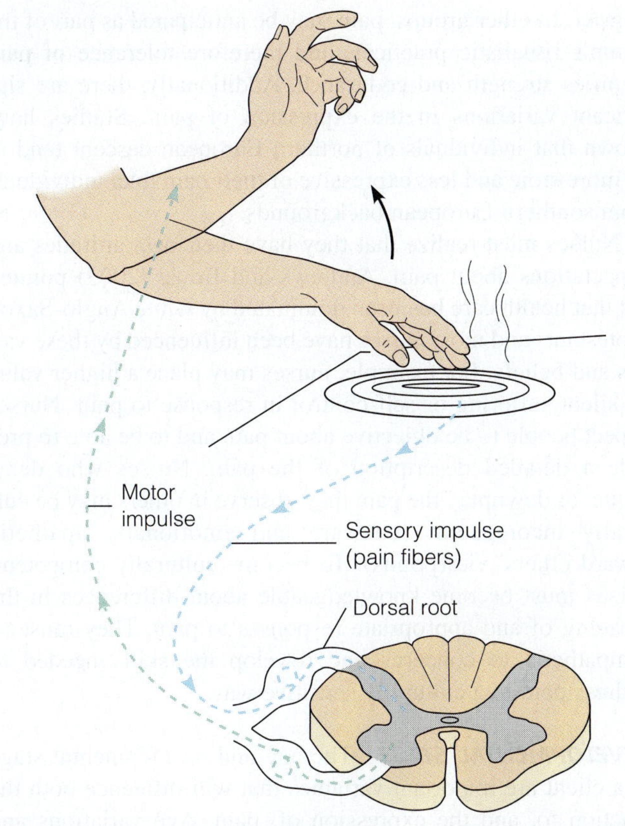

Figure 5–4 ■ Proprioceptive reflex to pain stimulus.

Unrelieved pain has been noted to have a potentially harmful effect on the person's well-being. Pain interferes with sleep, affects appetite, and lowers the quality of life for clients and their family members. A natural response to pain is to stop activity, tense muscles, and withdraw from the pain-provoking activities. This reduced mobility may produce muscle atrophy and painful spasm, putting the person at risk of complications related to immobility and/or cardiopulmonary deconditioning.

Uncontrolled pain impairs immune function, which slows healing and increases susceptibility to infections and dermal ulcers. The short, shallow breathing that accompanies pain produces atelectasis, lowers circulating oxygen levels, and increases cardiac workload. Undertreated pain also increases morbidity and mortality for a wide variety of conditions, including speeding metastasis of cancer and extending cardiac damage during a heart attack (Page, Ben-Eliyahu, Yirmiya, & Liebeskind, 1993; Puntillo & Weiss, 1994). The physical stress and emotional distress of severe or prolonged pain can contribute to the development of a wide variety of physical and emotional disorders.

Persistent, severe pain changes the nervous system in a way that intensifies, spreads, and prolongs the pain, risking the development of incurable chronic pain syndromes. Beginning at 24 hours, persistent unrelieved severe pain changes the structure and function of the nervous system in a way that prolongs and intensifies the pain experience. A windup phenomenon occurs, tipping the balance in the substantia gelatinosa heavily in the

CLINICAL MANIFESTATIONS AND THERAPIES Acute and Chronic Pain

ETIOLOGY	CLINICAL MANIFESTATIONS	CLINICAL THERAPIES
Acute pain	Pain of varying severity, location, and etiology, which lasts less than 6 months. In addition to the pain itself, manifestations include: ■ Nausea and vomiting ■ Restlessness ■ Rapid/shallow respirations ■ Elevated blood pressure.	Pharmacological pain management: ■ Narcotic analgesics ■ Anti-inflammatory agents ■ Nonnarcotic analgesics ■ Miscellaneous analgesics. Nonpharmacological therapy: ■ Massage ■ Diversional therapies ■ Nerve stimulation.
Chronic pain	Pain of varying severity, location, and etiology, which lasts 6 months or more (even if intermittent). In addition to the pain itself, manifestations include: ■ Heart rate and blood pressure below normal ranges ■ Depression ■ Irritability ■ Impaired mobility and/or activity.	Pharmacological pain management: ■ Nonnarcotic analgesics such as NSAIDs ■ Antidepressants may reduce nerve-related pain ■ Anti-inflammatory medications ■ Antispasmodic or muscle relaxants ■ Narcotic analgesics as last resort. Nonpharmacological therapy: ■ Guided imagery ■ Massage ■ Nerve stimulation units ■ Diversional activities (music, involvement in hobbies, aroma therapy) ■ Chiropractic interventions ■ Physical therapy ■ Applications of heat or cold ■ Relaxation techniques ■ Positioning.

direction of excitation, and establishing new nerve growth, including the development of reverberating loops, which further prolong, spread, and intensify the noxious stimuli (Arnstein, 1997). The pain threshold is lowered, and the cells are said to be sensitized. Sensitization of the CNS is reflected by spontaneous neuron firing, reduced thresholds or increased responsiveness to afferent inputs, prolonged after-discharges to repeated stimulation, and expansion of the peripheral receptive field of dorsal horn neurons. A similar process can occur in the peripheral nerves, when sensitized, normally innocuous stimuli (e.g., light touch) may be perceived as painful. Thus, to prevent the development of persistent pain and promote overall health and well-being, the nurse must act to promote optimal and expedient pain control.

Factors That Affect Responses to Pain

Numerous factors can affect a person's perception of, and reaction to, pain. These include the person's ethnic and cultural values, developmental stage, environment and support people, and previous pain experiences, and the meaning of the current pain to the person.

ETHNIC AND CULTURAL VALUES Ethnic background and cultural heritage have long been recognized as factors that influence both a person's reaction to pain and the expression of that pain. Behavior related to pain is a part of the socialization process. For example, individuals in one culture may have learned to be expressive about pain, whereas individuals from another culture may have learned to keep those feelings to themselves and not bother others.

Although there appears to be little variation in pain threshold, cultural background can affect the level of pain that an individual is willing to tolerate. In some Middle Eastern and African cultures, self-infliction of pain is a sign of mourning or grief. In other groups, pain may be anticipated as part of the group's ritualistic practices, and therefore tolerance of pain signifies strength and endurance. Additionally, there are significant variations in the expression of pain. Studies have shown that individuals of northern European descent tend to be more stoic and less expressive of their pain than individuals from southern European backgrounds.

Nurses must realize that they have their own attitudes and expectations about pain. Andrews and Boyle (2003) pointed out that health care has been dominated by white Anglo-Saxon Protestants and most nurses have been influenced by these values and beliefs. For example, nurses may place a higher value on silent suffering or self-control in response to pain. Nurses expect people to be objective about pain and to be able to provide a detailed description of the pain. Nurses who deny, refute, or downplay the pain they observe in others may be culturally incompetent (unaware and emotionally apathetic toward others' viewpoints). To become culturally competent, nurses must become knowledgeable about differences in the meaning of and appropriate responses to pain. They must be sympathetic to concerns and develop the skills needed to address pain in a culturally sensitive way.

DEVELOPMENTAL STAGE The age and developmental stage of a client are important variables that will influence both the reaction to, and the expression of, pain. Age variations and related nursing interventions are presented in Table 5–4.

The field of pain management for infants and children has grown significantly. It is now accepted that anatomical, physiological, and biochemical elements necessary for pain transmission are present in newborns regardless of their gestational age. The American Academy of Pediatrics and the Canadian Paediatric Society (2000) recommend that environmental, nonpharmacological, *and*

FOCUS ON DIVERSITY AND CULTURE Cultural Differences in Responses to Pain

Expressions of pain vary from culture to culture and may vary from person to person within a culture.

AFRICAN AMERICANS

- Some believe pain and suffering is a part of life and is to be endured.
- Some may deny or avoid dealing with the pain till it becomes unbearable.
- Some believe that prayer and laying on of hands will free a person from suffering and pain.

MEXICAN AMERICANS

- May tend to view pain as a part of life and as an indicator of the seriousness of an illness.
- Some believe that enduring pain is a sign of strength.

PUERTO RICANS

- Many tend to be loud and outspoken in their expressions of pain. This is a socially learned way to cope and it is important for the nurse to not judge or disapprove.

ASIAN AMERICANS

- Chinese culture values silence. As a result, some clients may be quiet when in pain because they do not want to cause dishonor to themselves and their family.
- Japanese may have a stoic (minimal verbal and nonverbal expressions) response to pain. They may even refuse pain medication.
- Filipino clients may believe that pain is "God's will." Some older Filipino clients may refuse pain medication.

NATIVE AMERICANS

- In general, Native Americans are quiet, are less expressive verbally and nonverbally, and may tolerate a high level of pain. They tend to not request pain medication and may tolerate pain until they are physically disabled.

ARAB AMERICANS

- Pain responses are considered private and reserved for immediate family, not with health professionals. As a result, this may lead to conflicting perceptions between the family members and the nurse regarding the effectiveness of the client's pain relief.

Source: From *Transcultural Communication in Nursing*, 2nd ed., by C. Munoz & J. Luckmann, 2005, From Clifton Park: Delmar Learning; *Transcultural Concepts in Nursing Care*, 4th ed., by M. M. Andrews & J. S. Boyle, 2003, Philadelphia: Lippincott Williams & Wilkins.

TABLE 5–4 **Age Variations in the Pain Experience**

AGE GROUP	PAIN PERCEPTION AND BEHAVIOR	SELECTED NURSING INTERVENTIONS
Infant	Perceives pain. Responds to pain with increased sensitivity. Older infant tries to avoid pain; for example, turns away and physically resists.	Give a glucose pacifier. Use tactile stimulation. Play music or tapes of a heartbeat.
Toddler and preschooler	Develops the ability to describe pain and its intensity and location. Often responds with crying and anger because child perceives pain as a threat to security. Reasoning with child at this stage is not always successful. May consider pain a punishment. Feels sad. May learn there are gender differences in pain expression. Tends to hold someone accountable for the pain.	Distract the child with toys, books, pictures. Involve the child in blowing bubbles as a way of "blowing away the pain." Appeal to the child's belief in magic by using a "magic" blanket or glove to take away pain. Hold the child to provide comfort. Explore misconceptions about pain.
School-age child	Tries to be brave when facing pain. Rationalizes in an attempt to explain the pain. Is responsive to explanations. Can usually identify the location and describe the pain. With persistent pain, may regress to an earlier stage of development.	Use imagery to turn off "pain switches." Provide a behavioral rehearsal of what to expect and how it will look and feel. Provide support and nurturing.
Adolescent	May be slow to acknowledge pain. Recognizing pain or "giving in" may be considered weakness. Wants to appear brave in front of peers and not report pain.	Provide opportunities to discuss pain. Provide privacy. Present choices for dealing with pain. Encourage music or TV for distraction.
Adult	Behaviors exhibited when experiencing pain may be gender-based behaviors learned as a child. May ignore pain because to admit it is perceived as a sign of weakness or failure. Fear of what pain means may prevent some adults from taking action.	Deal with any misconceptions about pain. Focus on the client's control in dealing with the pain. Allay fears and anxiety when possible.
Older adult	May have multiple conditions presenting with vague symptoms. May perceive pain as part of the aging process. May have decreased sensations or perceptions of the pain. Lethargy, anorexia, and fatigue may be indicators of pain. May withhold complaints of pain because of fear of the treatment, of any lifestyle changes that may be involved, or of becoming dependent. May describe pain differently, that is, as "ache," "hurt," or "discomfort." May consider it unacceptable to admit or show pain.	Thorough history and assessment is essential. Spend time with the client and listen carefully. Clarify misconceptions. Encourage independence whenever possible.

pharmacological interventions be used to prevent, reduce, or eliminate pain in neonates. Physiological indicators may vary in infants, so behavioral observation is recommended for pain assessment (Ball & Bindler, 2003). Children may be less able than an adult to articulate their experience or needs related to pain, which may result in their pain being undertreated. However, children as young as 3 years can accurately report the location and intensity of their pain if it is evaluated properly.

With puberty comes the emergence of some pain syndromes, particularly for women. Unfortunately, women are overrepresented in a large number of painful disorders, including headaches, fibromyalgia, lupus, and menstrual-related disorders. Men are more vulnerable to pain related to their occupational or risk-taking patterns, including burn pain, post-trauma pain, and pain related to HIV/AIDS. A needless disparity is that the very young, the very old, women, and ethnic minorities are undertreated for their pain more frequently than their adult male counterparts.

Studies have shown that chronic pain affects 25–50% of older adults living in the community and 45–80% of those in nursing homes (American Geriatrics Society [AGS], 1998). With the number of older adults in our society increasing dramatically, by 2030, nurses will be caring for older adults in all settings of care in greater numbers.

Older adults constitute the largest group of individuals seeking health care services. The prevalence of pain in the older population is generally higher due to both acute and chronic disease conditions. Pain threshold does not appear to change with aging, although the effect of analgesics may increase due to physiological changes related to drug metabolism and excretion (Stanley, Blair, & Beare, 2005).

ENVIRONMENT AND SUPPORT PEOPLE A strange environment such as a hospital, with its noises, lights, and activity, can compound pain. In addition, the lonely person who is without a support network may perceive pain as severe, whereas the person who has supportive people around may perceive less pain. Some people prefer to withdraw when they are in pain, whereas others prefer the distraction of people and activity around them. Family caregivers can be a significant support for a person in pain. With the increase in outpatient and home care, families are assuming an increased responsibility for the management of pain. Education related to the assessment and management of pain can positively affect the perceived quality of life for both clients and their caregivers (McCaffery & Pasero, 1999).

Expectations of significant others can affect a person's perceptions of and responses to pain. In some situations, for example, girls may be permitted to express pain more openly than boys. Family role can also affect how a person perceives or responds to pain. For instance, a single mother supporting three children may ignore pain because of her need to stay on the job. The presence of support people often changes a client's reaction to pain. For example, toddlers often tolerate pain more readily when supportive parents or nurses are nearby.

PAST PAIN EXPERIENCES Previous pain experiences alter a client's sensitivity to pain. People who have personally experienced pain or who have been exposed to the suffering of someone close are often more threatened by anticipated pain than people without a pain experience. In addition, the success or lack of success of pain relief measures influences a person's expectations for relief and future response to interventions. For example, a person who has tried several nondrug pain relief measures without success may have little hope about the helpfulness of nursing interventions and may demand medication as the only thing that helps the pain.

MEANING OF PAIN Some clients may accept pain more readily than others, depending on the circumstances and the client's interpretation of its significance. A client who associates the pain with a positive outcome may withstand the pain amazingly well. For example, a woman giving birth to a child or an athlete undergoing knee surgery to prolong his career may tolerate pain better because of the benefit associated with it. These clients may view the pain as a temporary inconvenience rather than a potential threat or disruption to daily life.

By contrast, clients with unrelenting chronic pain may suffer more intensely. Chronic pain affects the body, mind, spirit, and social relationships in an undesirable way. Physically, the pain limits functioning and contributes to the disuse or deconditioning alluded to previously. For many, the change in activities of daily living (e.g., eating, sleeping, toileting) also takes a toll. The side effects of the many medications used to try to control the pain also place a heavy burden on the body. Mentally, individuals with chronic pain change their outlook, becoming more pessimistic, often to the point of helplessness and hopelessness. Mood often becomes impaired when pain persists, because the sadness of being unable to do important or enjoyable activities combines with self-doubts and learned helplessness to produce depression. Anxiety, worry, and uncertainty about coping with the pain may escalate emotionally, to the point of panic. Spiritually, pain may be viewed in a variety of ways. It may be perceived as a punishment for wrongdoing, a betrayal by the higher power, a test of fortitude, or a threat to the essence of who the person is. Pain may be a source of spiritual distress, or it may be a source of strength and enlightenment. Socially, pain often strains valued relationships, in part because of the impaired ability to fulfill role expectations.

Myths and Misconceptions About Pain

Myths and misconceptions about pain and its management are common in both health care professionals and clients. Following are some of the most common of these myths:

- *Pain is a result, not a cause.* According to the traditional view of pain, pain is only a symptom of a condition. However, it is now recognized that unrelieved or poorly relieved pain itself sets up further responses, such as immobility, anger, and anxiety; pain may also delay healing and rehabilitation.
- *Chronic pain is really a masked form of depression.* Serotonin plays a chemical role in pain transmission and is also the major modulator of depression. Therefore, pain and depression are chemically related, not mutually exclusive. It is common to find them coexisting.
- *Narcotic medication is too risky to be used to treat chronic pain.* This common misconception often deprives clients of the most effective source of pain relief. It is true that other methods should be tried first; if, however, they prove ineffective, narcotics should be considered as an appropriate alternative.
- *It is best to wait until a client has pain before giving medication.* It is now widely accepted that anticipating pain has a noticeable effect on the amount of pain a client experiences. Offering pain relief before a pain event is well on its way can lessen the pain.
- *Many clients lie about the existence or severity of their pain.* Very few clients lie about their pain.
- *Postoperative pain is best treated with intramuscular injections.* The most commonly used postoperative pain relief for many years was meperidine (Demerol) given intramuscularly. However, meperidine has many adverse effects, such as irritating tissues and producing the CNS stimulant normeperidine. In addition, meperidine is short acting. Most contemporary experts do not recommend its use to manage postoperative pain (Cohen & Schecter, 2005).
- *Pain relief interferes with diagnosis.* There is a prevailing attitude in the emergency department (ED) that pain relief can interfere with diagnosis. Research about treating pain with analgesics in the ED consistently shows no impact on physical assessment findings or diagnosis (Pasero, 2003). Despite a prevailing attitude that pain management is an essential part of good-quality medical care, pain management in the ED is difficult because of the short-term associations with clients, increased vigilance against drug abuse, and the myth that diagnosis is impaired by pain relief.

Children and Pain

As discussed previously, developmental stage plays a role in the responses to and expression of pain. In addition to physiological responses to pain, children may exhibit behaviors as a response to or expression of pain. A knowledge of pain as it relates to children will help the nurse provide appropriate interventions to children in pain.

NEONATAL PATHOPHYSIOLOGY Some question whether neonates have the ability to feel pain like other children. All of the necessary peripheral and CNS anatomical structures and functional ability to process pain are developed early in the fetal life, between the first and second trimesters. Additionally, the hypothalamic-pituitary-adrenal axes are developed, enabling the newborn to release catecholamines and cortisol in response to stress (Hall & Anand 2005). However, there are some differences in the nociceptive processing between infants and adults due to neurophysiological and cognitive immaturity. As a result of these differences, the distance from the site of pain to the newborn's brain is short and the descending neurotransmitters are underdeveloped. This makes the newborn less able to modulate pain impulses (Walden, 2007, p. 361). Therefore, preterm and full-term newborns may be more sensitive to pain stimuli than older infants and children because of the immaturity of the descending control mechanisms that enable older infants and children to reduce the transmission of pain.

Sensitization (an increased reaction to pain over time, or a reduced threshold for reaction to painful stimuli) occurs at the cellular, peripheral, and spinal levels, and increasing evidence suggests that pain sensitization leads to increased skin sensitivity and an increased neural response in infants (von Baeyer, Marche, Rocha, & Salmon, 2004). By 6 months of age, infants have a memory of pain and demonstrate anticipatory fear of pain with immunizations and pin pricks (Hall & Anand, 2005).

PHYSIOLOGICAL CONSEQUENCES OF PAIN Unrelieved pain is stressful and has many undesirable physiological consequences on several body systems. In addition to elevations in vital signs, there is an increased release of catecholamines, glucagon, and corticosteroids. This can result in a catabolic state that can have a serious effect on newborns and young infants with higher metabolic rates and fewer nutritional reserves. Pain in the newborn and infant drains energy resources the infant needs for growth and healing. The autonomic nervous system becomes unstable, reflected in changes in vital signs, oxygen saturation, vagal tone, and palmar sweating (American Academy of Pediatrics, Committee on Fetus and Newborn, 2006).

The child with acute postoperative pain takes shallow breaths and suppresses coughing to avoid more pain. These self-protective actions increase the potential for respiratory complications. Unrelieved pain may delay the return of normal gastric and bowel functions and cause a stress ulcer. Loss of appetite associated with pain decreases nutritional intake and delays the healing process.

Repeated pain experiences in newborns and infants are thought to cause changes in the **pain threshold** (the point at which the pain is perceived), the perception of pain, and **pain tolerance** (duration of time or intensity of pain a child will endure before demonstrating pain responses) throughout life. Because the pain pathways continue to develop during infancy and childhood, the painful experiences may have an impact on the development of the overall pain system. Repeated pain experiences may lead to hyperalgesia (increased response to a pain stimulus because of peripheral sensitization) and a decreased pain threshold, potentially leading to increased physiological and behavior responses to future painful events (Brislin & Rose, 2005).

BEHAVIORAL CONSEQUENCES OF PAIN Children learn about pain through the first experience and develop a pain memory. The pain experience may also cause an infant or child to respond in different ways. Sensitization may cause the child to have a lower tolerance for pain, display more distress, or develop a fear-avoidance behavior. Some children become accustomed to the pain stimulus, such as a child with diabetes who reports lower pain intensity with insulin injections over time. Other children report no change in pain intensity over time to similar painful experiences, or they have no pattern in pain intensity response (von Baeyer et al., 2004).

Infants display increased distress at cues tied to prior painful experiences, such as skin preparation for a heel stick, indicating that they are sensitized to pain and possibly are anticipating pain (von Baeyer et al., 2004). During prolonged periods of pain, newborns become passive, with few movements and little facial expression, appearing to try to conserve energy (American Academy of Pediatrics, 2006). Newborn males who were circumcised without analgesia demonstrated more pain with immunizations than uncircumcised males (Young, 2005). Concerns are increasing that the long-term consequences of pain in newborns include emotional, behavioral, and learning disabilities (American Academy of Pediatrics, 2006). For example, low-birth-weight infants who experienced painful episodes rated medical procedures as more painful at 8–10 years of age than did full-term newborns (Young, 2005).

Children who were untreated with analgesia for a painful procedure reported greater pain levels during a second painful procedure despite being given adequate analgesia, compared to children given adequate analgesia for both procedures who reported less pain during the second painful procedure. This study provided evidence that children who are not treated with analgesia may have a changed reaction to a future painful event (von Baeyer et al., 2004). Fear, anxiety, poor coping abilities, and lack of a support person can increase the child's perception of pain (Verghese & Hannallah, 2005). Younger children demonstrate more distress with pain than older children who are able to use coping strategies (Young, 2005).

BARRIERS TO PAIN MANAGEMENT IN CHILDREN Health care professionals once believed that infants and children feel less pain than adults. Underestimation and undertreatment of infants and children for pain continues today (O'Rourke, 2004). Barriers to effective pain management are related to the knowledge deficits about pain assessment and the fear of addiction when analgesia is prescribed as a routine treatment (Plaisance & Logan, 2006). In addition, pain assessment of infants and young children is more difficult and complex than assessment of adults. For a review of past myths and the contrasting reality, see Table 5–5.

Research has shown that past beliefs about the ability of infants and children to perceive pain were incorrect. Even the smallest infants do feel and remember pain. Effective pain treatment is the right of every infant and child. In 2001, the Joint Commission introduced standards for pain assessment, management, and evaluation of clients of all accredited hospitals (see Box 5–2).

TABLE 5–5 Misconceptions About Pain in Infants and Children

MYTH	REALITY
Neonates and infants are incapable of feeling pain. Children do not feel pain with the same intensity as adults because a child's nervous system is immature.	An infant develops most of the anatomical and functional requirements for pain processing early in fetal life (Walden, 2007, p. 361). Preterm and full-term newborns may be more sensitive to pain stimuli because their immature spinal cord descending pain control mechanisms do not allow them to reduce the transmission of pain as occurs in older children and adults (von Baeyer et al., 2004).
Infants are incapable of expressing pain.	Infants express pain with both behavioral and physiological cues that can be assessed.
Infants and children have no memory of pain.	Preterm infants have been noticed to associate the smell of alcohol with heel sticks and try to pull the foot away to avoid the pain. Infants cry in anticipation of immunizations (Young, 2005).
Parents exaggerate their child's pain.	Parents know their child and are able to identify when the child is in pain.
Children are not in pain if they can be distracted or they are sleeping.	Children use distraction (engaging in a pleasant activity to help focus attention on something other than pain) to cope with pain, but they soon become exhausted when coping with pain and fall asleep.
Repeated experience with pain teaches the child to be more tolerant of pain and cope with it better.	Older children may habituate to some painful stimuli, such as repeated insulin injections. Other children may have an exaggerated response to pain because of pain sensitization (von Baeyer et al., 2004).
Children tolerate discomfort well. They become accustomed to pain after having it for a while.	Children do not tolerate pain any better than adults. Infants may develop pain sensitivity with repeated exposure and have a higher pain reaction (von Baeyer et al., 2004).
Children recover more quickly than adults from painful experiences such as surgery.	Children heal quickly from surgery, but they have the same amount of pain from surgery as an adult.
Children tell you if they are in pain. They do not need medication unless they appear to be in pain.	Children may be too young to express pain or afraid to tell anyone other than a parent about the pain. The child may fear the treatment for pain will be worse than the pain itself.
Children without obvious physical reasons for pain are not likely to feel pain.	The cause of pain cannot always be determined. The feeling of pain is subjective and should be accepted by nurses.
Children run the risk of becoming addicted to pain medication when it is used for pain management.	Addiction is extremely rare when the child is treated for an acute condition (less than 1%) (Plaisance & Logan, 2006).

DEVELOPMENTAL ASPECTS OF PAIN PERCEPTION, MEMORY, AND RESPONSE Although every infant and child perceives pain, their understanding, response to pain, and memory of painful events change as they develop. A number of factors influence the pain perceived by the child, including maturation of the nervous system, the child's developmental stage, and previous pain experiences.

Box 5–2 Joint Commission Pain Management Standards

The Joint Commission standards for the assessment and management of pain in clients in accredited hospitals and other health care organizations were introduced in 2001 and remain in force today. Standard RI.2.160 states that clients have the right to pain management. The health care facility must plan, support, and coordinate activities and resources to ensure that pain is recognized and addressed appropriately and in accordance with the care, treatment, and services provided, including the following:

- Assessing for pain
- Educating all relevant providers about assessing and managing pain
- Educating clients and families, when appropriate, about their roles in managing pain and the potential limitations and side effects of pain treatments.

Source: © Joint Commission Resources: Comprehensive Accreditation Manual for Hospitals (CAMH). Oakbrook Terrace, IL: Joint Commission on Accreditation of Healthcare Organizations, 2007. Reprinted with permission.

The child's memory and response to anticipated pain are also related to developmental stage. As described earlier, newborns and infants develop a memory of pain. Preschool-age children demonstrate pain memory by making efforts to delay a painful procedure. Children also report more pain intensity when recalling a past painful experience than when they rated it at the time of its occurrence (von Baeyer et al., 2004).

A child's responses to acute or chronic pain are also influenced by other factors (Anthony & Schanberg, 2005):

- *Cognitive-behavioral factors*: Understanding of the pain source, cognitive development, expectations of the nature of the pain, coping skills or use of a pain control strategy such as distraction
- *Emotional factors*: Fear, anxiety, frustration, anger, depression, and psychological adjustment
- *Biological factors*: Genetics, disease activity, medications, pain processing
- *Environmental factors*: Parent pain experience, parent coping and adjustment, family relationships, school and social relationships, responses of health care providers

Depending on their developmental stage, children use different coping strategies to deal with their pain (such as escape, postponement or avoidance, diversion, and imagery).

Children may not complain of pain for several reasons:

- Some children believe they need to be brave.
- Preschoolers and adolescents may assume the nurse knows they have pain.
- Other children may be afraid that the injection to relieve pain will hurt more than the pain already does.

Pain and Older Adults

Few studies have examined the relationship between pain perception and aging. Those studies that have enrolled older adults have found that, with the exception of skin sensation, nociception appears not to change with age, although pain tolerance decreases (Gloth, 2001). Certain types of visceral pain may be less severe in the older adult, and that may explain the higher incidence of silent myocardial infarction and the less dramatic presentation of peptic ulcer disease (Moore & Clinch, 2004). The younger adult experiencing myocardial infarction will most often report severe, crushing chest pain, often with radiation down the left arm, sweating, and tremor. However, the older adult may report vague complaints of pain that can be attributed to heartburn or sour stomach, the presence of nausea and vomiting, or unexplained fatigue or falls. Box 5–3 lists the common causes of pain in older adults.

ACUTE PAIN IN OLDER ADULTS Acute pain in the older adult most often results from surgery, medical procedures, or injury (Herr, Bjoro, Steffensmeier, & Rakel, 2006). When acute pain occurs, it is important for the nurse to adequately identify the source of the pain and facilitate treatment of the underlying disease or trauma whenever possible. Conditions that cause acute pain in older adults include exacerbations of degenerative joint disease; flare-ups of chronic conditions such as gout or rheumatoid arthritis; trauma from falls including muscle strain, bone fractures, bumps, and bruises; skin problems such as burns, decubitus ulcers, and skin tears; presence of infection such as urinary tract infection; pleuritic pain in pneumonia and the neuropathic pain of herpes zoster (shingles); constipation; and postoperative pain from surgical intervention.

CHRONIC PAIN IN OLDER ADULTS Chronic pain that continues over a prolonged period of time affects one in five persons aged 65 and older. This persistent pain may be related to musculoskeletal disorders (spinal stenosis, osteoporosis with compression fractures, osteoarthritis, degenerative disk disease, arthritis, and related disorders), cancer, or neuropathic disorders. Other common conditions include back pain, chronic respiratory disorders, and the ischemic pain of vascular disease. All older adults suffering from chronic pain are candidates for pharmacological therapy (Partners Against Pain, 2002).

Approximately 45–80% of nursing home residents, who often have a variety of physical ailments, are estimated to be in substantial pain that is often undertreated (AGS, 2002). Although good coping mechanisms and family support can lower pain levels, depression can exacerbate pain. It is recommended that nurses routinely screen for depression when working with older adults with chronic pain. A comprehensive pain treatment plan is needed to treat the biopsychosocial needs of the older adult. A vicious chronic pain cycle can occur with negative consequences, including decreased socialization, withdrawal from daily life, fatigue, sleep disturbance, irritability, and physical deconditioning, and other signs of stress and depression (Bishop & Morrison, 2007).

COLLABORATION

Effective pain relief results from collaboration among health care providers. Pain clinics are centers staffed by a team of health care professionals who use a multidisciplinary approach to managing chronic pain. Therapies may include traditional pharmacological agents as well as herbs, vitamins, and other dietary supplements; nutritional counseling; psychotherapy; biofeedback; hypnosis; acupuncture; massage; and other treatments. Hospices for dying clients also provide a multifaceted approach to pain management.

Diagnostic Tests

Pain assessment tools are used to evaluate pain in clients; laboratory tests are not routinely used to assess pain. Prolonged, severe pain produces a physiological stress response that includes the chemical release of catecholamines, cortisol, aldosterone, and other corticosteroids. Elevated blood glucose levels also occur (Huether & Defriez, 2006). Existing conditions such as infection, trauma, and anemia or stress also cause the vital sign changes seen with sudden pain. While laboratory and diagnostic tests may be performed to determine cause of pain, there is no testing specific to quantify pain. Pain is subjective and is highly dependent on the client's description in order to diagnose.

Box 5–3 **Conditions Associated With Pain in Older Adults**

- Degenerative joint disease
- Rheumatoid arthritis
- Chronic back pain
- Osteoporosis (with and without spinal fracture)
- Neuropathic pain (with diabetes mellitus and postherpetic neuralgia)
- Gastroesophageal reflux disease
- Peripheral vascular disease
- Poststroke syndromes
- Immobility, contractures
- Headache
- Oral problems and gum disease
- Amputation
- Pressure ulcers
- Angina and other cardiac disease
- Cancer pain and pain from resulting treatment

Source: Thomas, D., Flaherty, J., & Morley, J. (2001). The management of chronic pain in long-term care settings. *Supplement to the Annals of Long-Term Care*, November. Newtown Square, PA: MultiMedia Health Care/Freedom.

Pharmacologic Therapies

Pharmacological pain management involves the use of opioids (narcotics), nonopioids/nonsteroidal anti-inflammatory drugs (NSAIDs), and **coanalgesic** drugs, medications that are not classified as pain medications but may be used in conjunction with them (see Box 5–4). The principles of modern analgesic use are built on a foundation established by the World Health Organization (WHO) three-step approach to treating cancer pain (Figure 5–5 ■). This approach focuses on aligning the proper analgesic with the intensity of pain. This approach has evolved into what is currently termed *rational polypharmacy*, which demands that health care professionals be aware of all ingredients of medications that alleviate pain and use combinations to reduce the need for high doses of any one medication, and to maximize pain control with a minimum of side effects or toxicity. These multidrug strategies, combined with multimodal therapy (use of nondrug approaches like heat/relaxation) "may permit opioid dose reduction and improve patient outcomes" (APS, 2003, p. 34).

World Health Organization (WHO) Three-Step Approach

For clients with mild pain (1–3 on a 0–10 scale), step 1 of the analgesic ladder, nonopioid analgesics (with or without a coanalgesic) is the appropriate starting point. If the client has mild pain that persists or increases despite using full doses of step 1 medications, or if the pain is moderate (4–6 on a 0–10 scale), then a step 2 regimen is appropriate. At the second step, a weak opioid (e.g., codeine, tramadol, pentazocine) or a combination of opioid and nonopioid medicine (e.g., oxycodone with acetaminophen, hydrocodone with ibuprofen) is provided with or without coanalgesic medications. If the client has moderate pain that persists or increases despite using full doses of

Box 5–4 Categories and Examples of Analgesics

NONOPIOID ANALGESICS/NSAIDS

- Acetaminophen (Tylenol, Datril)
- Acetylsalicylic acid (aspirin)
- Choline magnesium trisalicylate (Trilisate)
- Diclofenac sodium (Voltaren)
- Ibuprofen (Motrin, Advil)
- Indomethacin sodium trihydrate (Indocin)
- Naproxen (Naprosyn), naproxen sodium (Anaprox)
- Celecoxib (Celebrex)
- Piroxicam (Feldene)
- Meloxicam (Mobic)

MIXED OR WEAK OPIOID ANALGESICS

- Butorphanol (Stadol)
- Hydrocodone (Lortab, Vicodin)
- Codeine (Tylenol No. 3, Empirin No. 3)
- Tramadol (Ultram, Ultracet)
- Propoxyphene napsylate (Darvon-N, Darvocet-N)

STRONG OPIOID ANALGESICS

- Fentanyl citrate (Sublimaze, transdermal patches)
- Hydromorphone hydrochloride (Dilaudid)
- Meperidine hydrochloride (Demerol)
- Morphine sulfate (morphine)
- Methadone (Dolophiné)

COANALGESICS

- Tricyclic antidepressants (nortriptyline)
- Anticonvulsants (gabapentin)
- Topical local anesthetic (Lidoderm)
- Hydroxyzine (Vistaril)

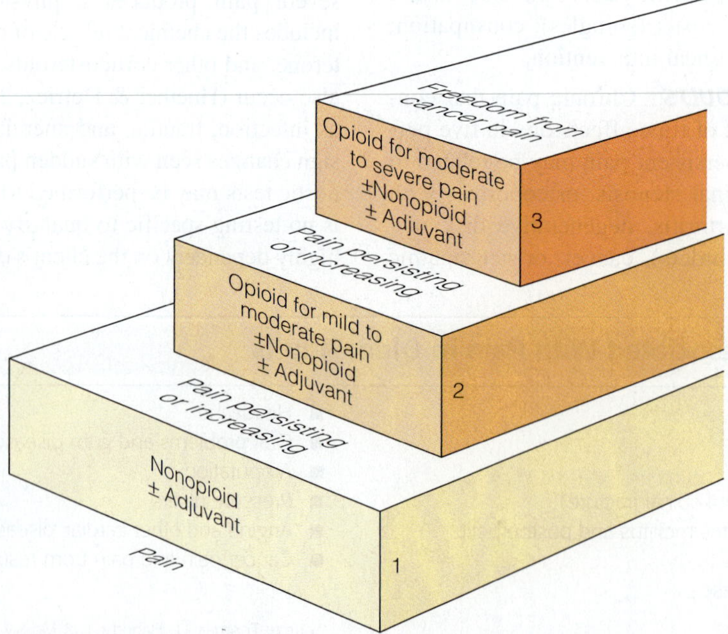

Figure 5–5 ■ The WHO three-step analgesic ladder.

Source: From: Cancer Pain Relief, 2nd ed., by World Health Organization, 1996, Geneva: Author. © World Health Organization (WHO), 2006. All rights reserved.

step 2 medications, or if the pain is severe (7–10 on a 0–10 scale), then a step 3 regimen is medically indicated. At the third step, strong opiates (e.g., morphine, hydromorphone, fentanyl) are administered and titrated in around-the-clock scheduled doses until the pain is relieved or dose-limiting respiratory depression occurs.

PRACTICE ALERT

Combining opioid and nonopioid analgesics is frequently overlooked. Each has different side effects, mechanisms of action, and toxicity profile. Alternating the two or giving them at the same time creates no danger and often produces a synergistic rather than merely additive effect.

Nonopioids/NSAIDs

Nonopioids include acetaminophen and *nonsteroidal anti-inflammatory drugs (NSAIDs)* such as ibuprofen or aspirin. NSAIDs have anti-inflammatory, analgesic, and antipyretic effects, whereas acetaminophen has only analgesic and antipyretic effects. The anti-inflammatory action relieves pain by interfering with the cyclooxygenase (COX) chemical cascade that is activated by damaged tissue. The COX chemical reactions produce prostaglandins and other inflammatory chemicals that cause a firing of nociceptive fibers. The COX-1 specific isoforms are found in platelets, the gastrointestinal (GI) tract, kidneys, and most other tissue, and are believed to be the cause of the well-known side effects of NSAIDs (GI bleed, diminished renal blood flow, inhibited clotting, etc.).

In the 1990s a second isoform (COX-2) was found and believed to be specific only for pain and inflammation. The resulting new "safer" (COX-2 selective) NSAIDs were tested, approved, and widely used. These drugs demonstrated significantly less GI bleeding, but uncommon cardiovascular events and rare skin problems in susceptible individuals prompted the U.S. Food and Drug Administration (FDA) to request a withdrawal of rofecoxib (Vioxx) in 2004 and a few months later to have valdecoxib (Bextra) also withdrawn from the marketplace. On April 6 and 7, 2005, a memorandum and a public health advisory (respectively) were issued from the FDA warning consumers of the increased risk of serious cardiovascular events from the use of NSAIDs, both COX-2 selective and nonselective products. All prescription NSAIDs now must carry the strong "black box" warning of the risks of using these drugs. Even nonprescription NSAIDs (e.g., aspirin, ibuprofen, naproxen) must be labeled to warn consumers of the potential dangers of using those products (FDA, 2005).

PRACTICE ALERT

Many health care professionals underestimate the effectiveness of ordinary aspirin and acetaminophen. The ordinary dose of aspirin or acetaminophen relieves as much pain as 1.5 mg of parenteral morphine, whereas standard doses of mixed analgesics (e.g., Tylenol No. 3 or Percocet) are approximately equivalent to 2.5–5 mg of morphine.

Individual drugs in this category vary little in their analgesic potency but do vary in their anti-inflammatory properties, metabolism, excretion, and side effects. These drugs have a ceiling effect and a narrow therapeutic index. The *ceiling effect* means that once the maximum analgesic benefit is achieved, more drug will not produce more analgesia; however, more toxicity may occur. The *narrow therapeutic index* indicates that there's not much margin for safety between the dose that produces a desired effect and the dose that may produce a toxic, even lethal effect. The most common side effect of nonopioid analgesics is gastrointestinal, such as heartburn or indigestion. These effects can become toxic or lethal when silent GI bleeding occurs. Given the interference with platelet aggregation, a small stomach ulcer can bleed a lot, making it a potentially life-threatening condition. Clients should be taught to take NSAIDs with food and a full glass of water and be routinely monitored by a health care professional if they take these preparations daily for more than a couple of weeks.

Acetaminophen (Tylenol) has a different mechanism of action and side effect/toxicity profile. It does not affect platelet function and rarely causes GI distress, ulcers, or kidney, skin, or cardiovascular problems. It was not included in the public health advisory issued by the U.S. Food and Drug Administration (FDA); however, hepatotoxicity, and possible renal toxicity, does occur with high doses or with long-term use. Generally, 10 g of acetaminophen is considered a lethal dose, with 6 g per day causing measurable liver damage. It is recommended that otherwise young and healthy people limit their acetaminophen consumption to less than 4 g per day, with susceptible individuals (e.g., older adults, people with a history of alcoholism, dehydration, or liver disease) limiting their consumption to 2.4 g per day or fewer. Given that acetaminophen is so well tolerated, it is often a hidden ingredient in over-the-counter (OTC) remedies (e.g., pain, fever, allergy, cough and cold preparations), so clients must be instructed to read the ingredient list of all OTC medicines they take. Table 5–6 provides consumption parameters for medications that contain acetaminophen. Table 5–7 lists common misconceptions about nonopioids.

TABLE 5–6 Consumption Parameters for Common Pain Medications Containing Acetaminophen

Medication	Total Daily Tablet Limit (2.5–4 g Acetaminophen)*
Tylenol No. 3	8–12 tablets
Percocet	8–12 tablets
Lortab	5–8 tablets
Vicodin	5–8 tablets
Tylox	5–8 tablets
Darvocet-N 100	3–6 tablets
Vicodin ES (750 mg)	3–5 tablets

*Clients at risk for toxicity (e.g., older adults, liver disease, alcohol consumption, cardiac disease, pulmonary disease) to consume at low end of the range.

TABLE 5–7 **Misconceptions About Nonopioids**

MISCONCEPTION	CORRECTION
Regular daily use of NSAIDs is much safer than taking opioids.	Side effects from long-term use of NSAIDs are considerably more severe and life threatening than the side effects from daily doses of oral morphine or other opioids. The most common side effect from long-term use of opioids is constipation, whereas NSAIDs can cause gastric ulcers, increased bleeding time, and renal insufficiency. Acetaminophen can cause hepatotoxicity.
A nonopioid should not be given at the same time as an opioid.	It is safe to administer a nonopioid and opioid at the same time. Giving a dose of nonopioid at the same time as a dose of opioid poses no more danger than giving the doses at different times. In fact, many opioids are compounded with a nonopioid (e.g., Percocet [oxycodone and acetaminophen]).
Administering antacids with NSAIDs is an effective method of reducing gastric distress.	Administering antacids with NSAIDs can lessen distress but may be counterproductive. Antacids reduce the absorption and therefore the effectiveness of the NSAID by releasing the drug in the stomach rather than in the small intestine where absorption occurs.
Nonopioids are not useful analgesics for severe pain.	Nonopioids alone are rarely sufficient to relieve severe pain, but they are an important part in the total analgesic plan. One of the basic principles of analgesic therapy is: Whenever pain is severe enough to require an opioid, adding a nonopioid should be considered.
Gastric distress (e.g., abdominal pain) is indicative of NSAID-induced gastric ulceration.	Most clients with gastric lesions have no symptoms until bleeding or perforation occurs.

Source: Reprinted from *Pain: Clinical Manual,* 2nd ed., by M. McCaffery and C. Pasero, 1999, St. Louis, MO: Mosby. Copyright © 1999, Mosby, Inc., with permission from Elsevier.

Opioids

There are three primary types of opioids:

1. *Full agonists.* These pure opioid drugs bind tightly to mu receptor sites, found throughout the body and particularly in the medulla, producing maximum pain inhibition by producing an agonist effect that also depresses respiratory drive. A full *agonist analgesic* includes morphine (e.g., Kadian, MS Contin), oxycodone (e.g., Percocet, OxyContin), and hydromorphone (e.g. Dilaudid, Palladone). There is no ceiling on the level of analgesia from these drugs; their dose can be steadily increased to relieve pain. There is also no maximum daily dose limit unless they are in compound with a nonopioid analgesic drug such as acetaminophen, which has a daily maximum limit of 2,400–4,000 mg.
2. *Mixed agonists-antagonists. Agonist-antagonist analgesic* drugs can act like opioids and relieve pain (agonist effect) when given to a client who has not taken any pure opioids. However, they can block or inactivate other opioid analgesics when given to a client who has been taking pure opioids (antagonist effect). These drugs include dezocine (Dalgan), pentazocine hydrochloride (Talwin), butorphanol tartrate (Stadol), and nalbuphine hydrochloride (Nubain). They block the mu receptor site and activate a kappa receptor site. If a client has been receiving a mu agonist (e.g., morphine, Percocet, or Vicodin for pain) daily for more than a couple of weeks, the administration of a mixed agonist-antagonist may result in an immediate and severe withdrawal reaction. These drugs also have a ceiling effect that limits the dose. They are not recommended for use with terminally ill clients. In the opioid-naïve client with acute pain (e.g., migraine headache), these agents have a favorable effect and low side effect burden.
3. *Partial agonists.* Partial agonists have a ceiling effect in contrast to a full agonist. These drugs, such as buprenorphine (Buprenex), block the mu receptors or are neutral at that receptor but bind at a kappa receptor site. This drug has good analgesic potency and is emerging as an alternative to methadone for opioid maintenance/narcotic treatment programs. The safety and favorable side effect profile make it an increasingly popular choice.

WEAK OR MIXED OPIOID ANALGESICS These analgesics include drugs that are weak opioids (e.g., propoxyphene, codeine, tramadol), mixed agonist-antagonist drugs, or combination opioids with nonopioid (NSAIDs) analgesic compounds. These medicines are generally two to four times more potent that nonopioids alone and carry some of the risks of both drug classes. With a rare exception, these are controlled substances and must be ordered by a physician or nurse practitioner, adhering to applicable federal and state laws. These drugs also have a ceiling effect and a maximum daily dose limit. There are advantages to giving combination drugs, such as lowering the amount of any one medicine needed in a 24-hour period, thus reducing the potential for side effects or toxicity. However, nurses need to be familiar with each medication and be aware of daily dose limits of the ingredients as well as the potential to receive duplicate medications for different clinical indications (e.g., Tylenol in the mixed drug, Tylenol for fever, and Tylenol in the headache preparation).

Among the weak opioids, there is a narrow therapeutic index. Codeine at doses of 30–60 mg produces dose-limiting gastrointestinal distress in many people. Propoxyphene produces a by-product that irritates nerves and muscles, and tramadol lowers seizure threshold. The mixed agonist-antagonist drugs have some properties of naloxone (Narcan), and thus in individuals who have been on opioids for a period of time, these drugs can cause a serious withdrawal reaction. Therefore, mixed agonist-antagonist medications (Talwin, Stadol, Nubain, etc.) may be a first opioid tried, but the client is not switched from another opioid to these preparations.

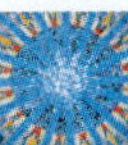

FOCUS ON DIVERSITY AND CULTURE Codeine Use

Codeine gets its analgesic properties with its conversion to morphine by the liver; however, about 10% of Caucasians are unable to convert codeine to morphine because they lack the CYP2D6 enzyme. The Chinese population produces less morphine from codeine than Caucasians due to a genetic polymorphism (Bell, 2006). Children with these genetic differences may have limited or no analgesic response to codeine. This demonstrates why response to pain medications must be carefully monitored.

STRONG OPIOID ANALGESICS Pure agonist opioid analgesics include opium derivatives, such as morphine, hydromorphone, oxycodone, fentanyl, and methadone (APS, 2003). *Opioid* is the pharmacological class of pain relievers, many of which are "scheduled" as a controlled substance (narcotic) due to the potential for misuse. Pure agonist opioids relieve pain primarily by binding to mu receptors in the peripheral and central nervous systems. In addition to pain reduction, changes in mood may make the person feel more comfortable even though the pain persists. As the most potent class of pain relievers, these drugs are indicated for severe pain, or when other medications have failed to control moderately severe or worse pain. Among this class, meperidine (Demerol) has received a lot of attention in recent years as a medication to avoid because of its short half-life, toxic metabolite, and potential to induce seizures with repeated doses.

OPIOID SIDE EFFECTS When administering any analgesic, the nurse must review side effects. Side effects of the opioids typically include respiratory depression, sedation, nausea/vomiting, urinary retention, blurred vision, sexual dysfunction, and constipation. The most concerning adverse effect of opioids is respiratory depression (e.g., 8 per minute or less), which usually occurs early in therapy among opioid-naïve clients; with dose escalation; or in clients with drug–drug or drug–disease interactions. In the event of respiratory depression due to opioid therapy, the client will appear overly sedated, and respirations will be slow and deep with periods of apnea. The nurse needs to assess a client's level of alertness and respiratory rate for baseline data before administering narcotics. See the sedation rating scale in Box 5–5. Often clients will manifest an increase in sedation *before* they manifest a decrease in respiratory rate and depth. Early recognition of an increasing level of sedation or respiratory depression will enable the nurse to implement appropriate measures promptly (e.g., pulse oximetry monitoring, obtaining an order to decrease the opioid dosage). Box 5–6 provides suggested measures to prevent and treat side effects of opioid analgesics.

Box 5–5 Sedation Scale

S = Sleep, easy to arouse
1 = Awake and alert
2 = Slightly drowsy, easily aroused
3 = Frequently drowsy, arousable, drifts off to sleep during conversation
4 = Somnolent, minimal or no response to physical stimulation

Source: Reprinted from *Pain: Clinical Manual,* 2nd ed. (p. 267), by M. McCaffery and C. Pasero, 1999. St. Louis, MO: Mosby. Copyright © 1999, Mosby, Inc., with permission from Elsevier.

PRACTICE ALERT

Constipation is an almost universal adverse effect of opioid use. All clients should receive prophylactic stimulant laxative therapy, unless contraindicated. Stool softeners are not useful alone but are a good choice when combined with a stimulant laxative (e.g, Senokot-S). If those products are ineffective, a regimen of cathartic laxatives (e.g., bisacodyl), followed by more aggressive forms of treatment (e.g., osmotic laxatives, enema, manual disimpaction) may be necessary.

Older adults are particularly sensitive to the analgesic properties of opioids and may require less medication, or medication administered at less frequent intervals, than younger clients. This sensitivity may be related to reduced or delayed excretion of the drug in older adults. As such, the clinical pearl of "start low (25–50% dose reduction) and go (titrate) slow" is often followed in the older population (AGS, 2002).

PRACTICE ALERT

Assessing for sedation and respiratory status is critical during the first 12–24 hours after starting opioid therapy. The most critical period is during the peak effect of the first dose (15 minutes if administered intravenously; first hour after intramuscular, oral, or rectal route). An exception is with opioids administered via the spinal route. Respiratory depression may increase over time with epidural infusions and with intrathecal analgesia; respiratory depression may manifest 24 hours after the spinal injection even after the analgesic effect has worn off. In general, the longer the client receives opioids, the wider the safety margin as the client develops a tolerance to the sedative and respiratory depressive effects of the drug.

Coanalgesics

Coanalgesic agents have properties that may reduce pain alone or in combination with other analgesics, relieve other discomforts, potentiate the effect of pain medications, or reduce the pain medication's side effects. Examples of coanalgesics that relieve pain are antidepressants (support the function of the pain-modulating system), anticonvulsants (stabilize nerve membranes, reducing excitability and spontaneous firing), and local anesthetics (block the transmission of pain signals). Anxiolytics, sedatives, and antispasmodics are examples of medicines that relieve other discomforts; however, they do not alleviate pain and thus should be used in addition to rather than instead of analgesics. Examples of

Box 5–6 Common Opioid Side Effects, Preventive, and Treatment Measures

CONSTIPATION
- Increase fluid intake (e.g., 6–8 glasses daily).
- Increase fiber and bulk-forming agents to the diet (e.g., fresh fruits and vegetables). Increasing exercise is often ineffective in controlling this type of constipation.
- Administer daily stool softeners combined with a mild laxative (e.g., Senokot-S) as a first line of prevention against constipation for clients on opioid maintenance therapy.
- Stimulants (bisacodyl), osmotic laxatives (lactulose, sorbitol, and polyethylene glycol), enemas (tap water and sodium phosphate), and even prokinetic agents (metoclopramide) may be needed for refractory cases of constipation (Kurz & Sessler, 2003).

NAUSEA AND VOMITING
- Inform client that tolerance to this emetic effect generally develops after several days of opiate therapy.
- Provide an antiemetic (antihistamines [e.g., Vistaril, Phenergan], antimuscarinics [e.g., cyclizine, hyoscine], and dopamine receptor antagonists [e.g., Haldol]) as indicated.
- Change the dose or analgesic agent as indicated.

SEDATION
- Inform client that tolerance usually develops over 3–5 days.
- Consider the administration of a stimulant (e.g., Dexedrine or Ritalin) or an alternative route of administration (e.g., epidural) for clients with persistent pain and sedation.
- Observe client for evidence of respiratory depression that may occur with sedation.

RESPIRATORY DEPRESSION
- Administer an opioid antagonist, such as naloxone hydrochloride (Narcan), cautiously by diluting 1 ampule in 10 mL of saline and then administering 1 cc/minute until the respirations are greater than10 breathes per minute. Make provisions for repeat administration, continuous infusion, or a longer-acting version of a reversal agent as the half-life of naloxone is considerably shorter than most opioids being reversed. As a result, as naloxone wears off he symptoms of opioid overdose will return.
- Stop, change, or slow the administration of opioids until respirations are restored.

PRURITUS
- Apply cool packs, lotion, and diversional activity.
- Administer an antihistamine (e.g., diphenhydramine hydrochloride [Benadryl]).
- Inform client that tolerance also develops to pruritus.

URINARY RETENTION
- May need to catheterize client, or change or lower the analgesic dose.
- Administer narcotic antagonist (naloxone hydrochloride [Narcan]) or longer acting reversal agent (methylnaltrexone is pending FDA approval). Extreme caution is urged with the use of Narcan.

medications used to reduce the side effects of analgesics include stimulants, laxatives, and antiemetics.

Coanalgesics appear to be particularly beneficial for the management of neuropathic pain. Tricyclic antidepressant drugs seem to be particularly useful for central neuropathic pain, which often manifests as pain with a burning, unusual, or stinging quality. Anticonvulsant drugs, such as gabapentin seem particularly useful for peripheral neuropathic conditions that often present with a stabbing, shooting, or electrical-shock quality. Local anesthetics such as the Lidoderm patch also alleviate neuropathic as well as other types of pain, and are particularly useful for clients with the skin sensitivity known as allodynia. There is a growing scientific and clinical basis for the use of these medications in relieving pain, especially for persistent pain that is not relieved by the analgesic classes of medication alone.

Administration of Placebos

A **placebo** is "any medication or procedure, including surgery, that produces an effect in a client because of its implicit or explicit intent and not because of its specific physical or chemical properties" (McCaffery & Pasero, 1999). *Placebos* often take the form of sugar pills, saline injections, minuscule doses of drugs, or sham procedures designed to be void of any known therapeutic value. In contrast, the *placebo effect* is a perceptible, measurable, and desirable consequence which exceeds the anticipated biological changes and may occur as a result of interpersonal factors such as the presence of a caring person or a healing intent (Arnstein, 2003). Some professionals try to justify the use of placebos to elicit the desirable placebo effect or in a misguided attempt to determine if the client's pain is "real." The use of placebos, outside the context of an approved research study, is deceptive and represents fraudulent and unethical treatment. The American Society for Pain Management Nursing (2005) and other professional organizations have published position papers that adamantly oppose the use of placebos without consent.

A common myth among health care professionals is that using narcotics for pain treatment poses a real threat of addiction. Actually, when the medications are used as recommended, there is little to no risk of addiction. Rather, if pain is not adequately treated, the client may seek more and more narcotic relief, thus increasing the risk of an adversarial relationship with the provider and a weakening of the trust relationship between client and provider (Trame, 2002) (see Box 5–7).

Nonpharmacological Invasive Therapies

A **nerve block** is a chemical interruption of a nerve pathway, effected by injecting a local anesthetic into the nerve. Nerve blocks are widely used during dental work. The injected drug blocks nerve pathways from the painful tooth, thus stopping the transmission of pain impulses to the brain. Nerve blocks are often used to relieve the pain of whiplash

Box 5–7 Pain Management and Drug Abuse History

Clients addicted to pain relievers often experience inadequate dosing of medications for pain. When providers suspect or learn of drug abuse, they tend to order lower doses than they would for a person of similar size and injury. Despite significant data showing very little addiction as the result of treating pain with adequate analgesia, prescribers still undertreat pain in clients with addictions. Addiction is a neurophysiological disease; when clients with addiction have injuries, they usually need greater doses of pain medication because of the tolerance they have developed from repeated exposure to opioids. Even clients without an addiction may exhibit behaviors suggesting addiction when pain is undertreated (Trame, 2002).

Cook and colleagues (2004) report an experiment to evaluate provider attitudes about prescribing analgesics for those in acute pain with a history of drug abuse. They sent questionnaires to 745 physicians in one county and received 120 responses. Sixty-six of the responders received the case of a seriously burned client with no mention of addiction; 54 responders received the case of an acutely burned client with heroin addiction. The physicians were provided the same selection of analgesics and dosages for both clients in the case studies. The physicians' prescribing practices were significantly different for the two clients; the client with heroin addiction was prescribed significantly more nonopioid analgesics than the nonaddicted client. Furthermore, there was no significant difference in the dosages prescribed for the two clients despite the risk for greater tolerance to opiates by the heroin-addicted client. The authors suggest that prescribers may be uninformed about the pathophysiology of addiction and increased need for analgesia in addiction. They also observe that analgesics may be rationed to addicted persons in an effort to wean them from their addiction. During the acute stress of injury or infection, however, withholding pain medication is an added stressor. The client will benefit from detoxification and recovery management after the acute phase is over. Nurses attempting to advocate for the comfort needs of an addicted client may encounter increased resistance without good explanations. This creates an ethical as well as a professional dilemma.

Providing analgesics for a client with chronic pain who has a history of addiction or ongoing addiction may be even more challenging. Clients may be fearful that their pain will be undertreated or that addiction will return or increase if the pain is treated with opioids (Compton & Athanasos, 2003). It is important to clearly communicate all needed information about medications and accessibility to providers. Dose escalation may be monitored with careful assessment and random urine screens. Treatment for addiction should be included in the care plan to minimize the risk of addiction or relapse.

injury, lower back disorders, bursitis, and cancer. With the intention of quieting "pain generators" (irritable nerves that cause the pain), a combination of a long-acting local anesthetic and a steroid is injected adjacent to the problem nerve (e.g., lumbar epidural steroid injections, joint injections). The local anesthetic should provide relief for several hours, before the effect of the steroid begins a day or two later. Often a series of three injections are scheduled weeks or months apart. Each subsequent injection should result in a longer duration of pain relief. No more than three injections per year are recommended because of the mineral-robbing effect steroids have on bones in the area. For longer-lasting results after a nerve block has worked, more permanent blocks may be attempted. The "permanent" blocks involve damaging nerves with alcohol, phenol, or radio frequency (heat). These nerve-killing procedures are controversial, as nerve fibers often regenerate and the pain returns in a significant proportion of clients.

Pain conduction pathways can be interrupted surgically. Because this disruption is permanent, surgery is performed only as a last resort, generally for intractable pain. Several surgical procedures may be performed. A *cordotomy* obliterates pain. Temperature sensation below the level of the spinothalamic portion of the anterolateral tract is severed. This procedure is usually done for pain in the legs and trunk. *Rhizotomy* interrupts the anterior or posterior nerve root between the ganglion and the cord. Interruption of anterior motor nerve roots stops spasmodic movements that accompany paraplegia. Interruption of posterior sensory nerve roots eliminates pain in areas innervated by that specific nerve root. Rhizotomies are generally performed on cervical nerve roots to alleviate pain of the head and neck from cancer or neuralgia, and increasingly they use radio frequency technologies.

In *neurectomy*, peripheral or cranial nerves are interrupted to alleviate localized pain, such as pain in the lower leg or foot arising from a vascular occlusion. In a *sympathectomy*, pathways of the sympathetic division of the autonomic nervous system are severed. This procedure eliminates vasospasm, improves peripheral blood supply, and thus is effective in treating painful vascular disorders such as Raynaud's disease.

Spinal cord stimulation (SCS) is used with persistent pain that has not been controlled with less invasive therapies. SCS involves the insertion of an electrode (may be a single-channel or multichannel device) adjacent to the spinal cord in the epidural space. The electrode(s) is (are) attached to an impulse-generator (external or implanted) that sends electric impulses to the spinal cord to control pain. The client is awake during the insertion procedure to aid in the optimal placement of the electrodes.

Nonpharmacological Pain Management

Nonpharmacological pain management consists of a variety of physical, cognitive-behavioral, and lifestyle pain management strategies that target the body, mind, spirit, and social interactions (see Table 5–8). Physical modalities include cutaneous stimulation, ice or heat, immobilization or therapeutic exercises, transcutaneous electrical nerve stimulation (TENS), and acupuncture. Mind–body (cognitive–behavioral) interventions include distracting activities, relaxation techniques, imagery, meditation, biofeedback, hypnosis, cognitive–reframing, emotional counseling, and spiritually directed approaches such as therapeutic touch or Reiki. Lifestyle management approaches

TABLE 5–8 Nonpharmacological Interventions for Pain Control

TARGET DOMAIN OF PAIN CONTROL	INTERVENTION
Body	Reducing pain triggers, promoting comfort Massage Applying heat or ice Electric stimulation (TENS) Positioning, bracing (selective immobilization) Acupressure Diet, nutritional supplements Exercise, pacing activities Invasive interventions (e.g., blocks) Sleep hygiene
Mind	Relaxation, imagery Self-hypnosis Pain diary, journal writing Distracting attention Repatterning thinking Attitude adjustment Reducing fear, anxiety, stress Reducing sadness, helplessness Information about pain
Spirit	Prayer, meditation Self-reflection about life and pain Meaningful rituals Energy work (e.g., therapeutic touch, Reiki) Spiritual healing
Social interactions	Functional restoration Improved communication Family therapy Problem solving Vocational training Volunteering Support groups

include symptom monitoring, stress management, exercise, nutrition, pacing activities, disability management, and other approaches needed by many clients with persistent pain that has drastically changed their lives.

Complementary and Alternative Medicine

Clients with chronic pain are turning to complementary and alternative medicine for pain relief with increasing frequency. Although the use of some herbs and supplements may be contraindicated for clients using traditional pharmacological therapies or whose pain stems from disease, a number of other therapies may be safe and effective for those clients seeking additional sources of relief.

MASSAGE Massage is a comfort measure that can aid relaxation, decrease muscle tension, and ease anxiety, in part because the physical contact communicates caring. It can also decrease pain intensity by increasing superficial circulation to the area. Massage can involve the back and neck, hands and arms, or feet. The use of ointments or liniments may provide localized pain relief with joint or muscle pain. Massage is contraindicated in areas of skin breakdown, suspected clots, or infections.

REPATTERNING UNHELPFUL THINKING Some people harbor strong self-doubts, unrealistic expectations (e.g., "I just want someone to make the pain go away"), rumination (e.g., "I keep thinking about my pain and the person who did this to me"), helplessness (e.g., "I can't do anything"), and magnification (e.g., "My life is ruined, I'll never be a good parent because of my pain"). These cognitive patterns have been identified as important contributors to treatment failures, the intensification of pain, disability, and depression (Arnstein, Caudil, Mandle, Norris, & Beasley, 1999; DeGood & Kiernan, 1997). Nurses can help by challenging the truthfulness and helpfulness of these thoughts, and replacing them with realistic and confidence-building ones that are particularly powerful predictors of more effective coping, better clinical outcomes, and improved quality of life (Caudill, 2002).

ACUPUNCTURE To restore the flow of energy, acupuncturists insert sterile, hair-thin needles at points along the meridians. The needles are rotated, twirled, or accompanied by a weak electrical current and are often left in several minutes or longer. Acupuncturists also may apply heat or use finger pressure. Clients feel little, if any, pain. Some people experience sensations of warmth, tingling, heaviness, or a dull ache.

Evidence now indicates that acupuncture reduces pain by triggering the release of endogenous opioids. This may explain why many of the analgesic effects of acupuncture can be partially or completely blocked by the use of opioid antagonists such as naloxone. Acupuncture also stimulates the nervous system to release ACTH, a chemical that aids in fighting inflammation; prostaglandins, which help wounds heal more quickly; and other substances that may promote nerve regeneration.

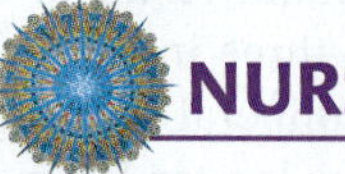

NURSING PROCESS

Assessment

Pain assessments consist of two major components: (1) a pain history to obtain facts from the client and (2) direct observation of behaviors, physical signs of tissue damage, and secondary physiological responses of the client. The goal of assessment is to gain an objective understanding of a subjective experience. Box 5–8 provides one example of a helpful mnemonic to make a complete pain assessment.

Pain History

While taking pain histories, the nurse must provide an opportunity for clients to express in their own words how they view the pain and the situation. This will help the nurse understand what the pain means to each client and how each client copes with it. Remember that each client's pain experience is unique and that the client is the best interpreter of the pain experience. This history should be geared to the specific client. For example, questions asked of an accident victim would be different from those asked of a postoperative client or one suffering from chronic

Box 5–8 Mnemonic for Pain Assessment: COLDERR

Character: describe the sensation (e.g., sharp, aching, burning),
Onset: when it started, how it has changed,
Location: where it hurts (all locations),
Duration: constant versus intermittent in nature,
Exacerbation: factors that make it worse,
Relief: factors that make it better (medications and other factors), and
Radiation: pattern of shooting/spreading/location of pain away from its origin.

Source: Reprinted from "Optimizing Perioperative Pain Management," 2002, by P. M. Arnstein. *AORN Journal, 76*(5): 812–818. Copyright © 2002 with permission of Elsevier.

pain. The initial pain assessment for someone in severe acute pain may consist of only a few questions before intervention occurs. In addition, the nurse may focus on the following:

- Previous pain treatment and effectiveness
- When and what analgesics were last taken
- Other medications being taken
- Allergies to medications.

For the person with chronic pain, the nurse may focus on the client's coping mechanisms, effectiveness of current pain management, and ways in which the pain has affected the client's body, thoughts and feelings, activities, and relationships.

Data that should be obtained in a comprehensive pain history include pain location, intensity, quality, patterns, precipitating factors, alleviating factors, associated symptoms, effect on activities of daily living (ADLs), past pain experiences, meaning of the pain to the person, coping resources, and affective responses. Questions to elicit these data are listed in the Assessment Interview.

Pain Intensity or Rating Scales

The single most important indicator of the existence and intensity of pain is the client's report of pain. In practice, however, McCaffery, Ferrell, and Pasero (2000) found that nurses tend to use less reliable measures for assessing pain. The top factors identified by nurses were culturally influenced (e.g., facial expressions, verbalization, request for relief). In addition, studies have shown that health care providers may underrate or overrate the pain intensity (Bergh & Sjostrom, 1999). Pain intensity scales are easy-to-use and reliable tools for determining the client's pain intensity. Such scales provide consistency for nurses to communicate with the client and other health care providers. To avoid confusion, scales should use a 0–10 range with 0 indicating "no pain" and the highest number indicating the "worst pain possible" for that individual. An 11-point (0–10) rating scale is shown in Figure 5–6 ■. The inclusion of word modifiers on the scale can assist some clients who find it difficult to apply a number level to their pain. For example, after ruling out "0" and "10" (neither no pain nor the worst possible pain), a nurse can ask the client if it is mild (2), mild to moderate (4), moderate to severe (6), or severe (8).

Another way to evaluate the intensity of pain for clients who are unable to use the numeric rating scales is to determine the extent of pain awareness and degree of interference with functioning. For example, 0 = no pain, 2 = awareness of pain only when paying attention to it, 4 = can ignore pain and do things, 6 = can't ignore pain, interferes with functioning, 8 = impairs ability to function or concentrate, and 10 = intense, incapacitating pain. It is believed that the degree to which pain interferes with functioning is a good marker for the severity of pain, especially for those with chronic pain.

Another scale sometimes used to assess pain is the Edmonton Symptom Assessment System, which uses a 0–10 scale ranking not only pain but also symptoms such as fatigue, drowsiness, nausea, depression, anxiety, feelings of wellbeing, shortness of breath, and appetite (Bruera, Kuehn, Miller, Selmser, & Macmillan, 1991).

This scale is particularly useful for the client taking narcotics for chronic pain who may choose to tolerate higher levels of pain to avoid the side effects of chronic opioid use.

Assessment Interview Pain History

- *Location:* Where is your discomfort?
- *Quality:* Tell me what your discomfort feels like.
- *Intensity:* On a scale of 0–10, with "0" representing no pain (substitute the word they use, e.g., no burning) and 10 representing the worst possible pain (e.g., burning sensation), how would you rate the degree of discomfort you are having right now?
- *Pattern*
  a. Time of onset: When did or does the pain start?
  b. Duration: How long have you had the pain, or how long does it usually last?
  c. Constancy: Do you have pain-free periods? When? And for how long?
- *Precipitating factors:* What triggers the pain or makes it worse?
- *Alleviating factors:* What measures or methods have you found helpful in lessening or relieving the pain? What pain medications do you use?
- *Associated symptoms:* Do you have any other symptoms (e.g., nausea, dizziness, blurred vision, shortness of breath) before, during, or after your pain?
- *Effects on ADLs:* How does the pain affect your daily life (e.g., eating, working, sleeping, and social and recreational activities)?
- *Past pain experiences:* Tell me about past pain experiences you have had and what was done to relieve the pain.
- *Meaning of pain:* What does having this pain mean to you? Does it signal something about the future or past? What worries or scares you the most about your pain?
- *Coping resources:* What do you usually do to help you deal with pain?
- *Affective response:* How does the pain make you feel? Anxious? Depressed? Frightened? Tired? Burdened?

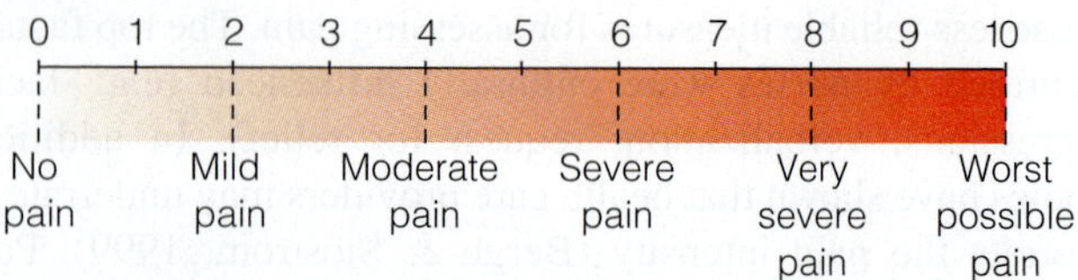

Figure 5–6 ■ An 11-point pain intensity scale with word modifiers.

PRACTICE ALERT

Perception is reality. The client's self-report of pain is what must be used to determine pain intensity. The nurse is obligated to record the pain intensity as reported by the client. By challenging the believability of the client's report, the nurse is undermining the therapeutic relationship and preventing the fulfillment of advocacy and helping people with pain, which is called for in the American Nurses Association (ANA) 2005 Scope and Standards of Practice in Pain Management Nursing.

When noting pain intensity, it is important to determine any related factors that may be affecting the pain. When the intensity changes, the nurse needs to consider the possible cause. For example, the abrupt cessation of acute abdominal pain may indicate a ruptured appendix. Several factors affect the perception of intensity: (a) the amount of distraction, or the client's concentration on another event; (b) the client's state of consciousness; (c) the level of activity; and (d) the client's expectations.

Not all clients can understand or relate to numerical pain intensity scales. These include preverbal children, older adults with impairments in cognition or communication, and people who do not speak English. For these clients the Wong-Baker FACES Rating Scale (Figure 5–7 ■) may be easier to use (Wong, Hockenberry-Eaton, Wilson, Winkelstein, & Schwartz, 2001). The face scale includes a number scale in relation to each expression so that the pain intensity can be documented.

When clients are unable to verbalize their pain for reasons of age, mental capacity, medical interventions, or other factors, nurses need to accurately assess the intensity of each client's pain and the effectiveness of the pain management interventions. For these clients, the nurse must rely on observation of behavior.

For effective use of pain rating scales, clients need not only to understand the use of the scale but also to be educated about how the information will be used to determine changes in their condition and the effectiveness of pain management interventions. Clients should also be asked to indicate what level of comfort is acceptable so that they can perform specific activities (Acello, 2000). To align the client's goals and expectations with reality, it is important to note that acute pain can typically be cut by 50% and chronic pain cut by 25%. To ensure that optimal pain management is achieved, the client works together with professionals toward established goals of pain reduction and functional improvement.

The use of a pain rating scale together with a pain flow sheet (Figure 5–8 ■) has been shown to be effective in improving pain management (McCaffery & Pasero, 1999). Documentation can be completed by the nurse, the client, or a caregiver and used in acute, outpatient, and home care settings.

PRACTICE ALERT

Assessing pain in the neonate can be challenging because he or she cannot report pain. Symptoms of pain in infants may include crying, lethargy, hypertension, hypotension, tachycardia, bradycardia, or apnea. Due to the wide array of symptoms that can indicate pain in the infant, any change in the child's condition should result in the nurse's consideration of a possible relationship to pain. Please refer to the Neonatal Infant Pain Scale in the accompanying Skills Manual to learn more about how to assess the neonate and infant for pain.

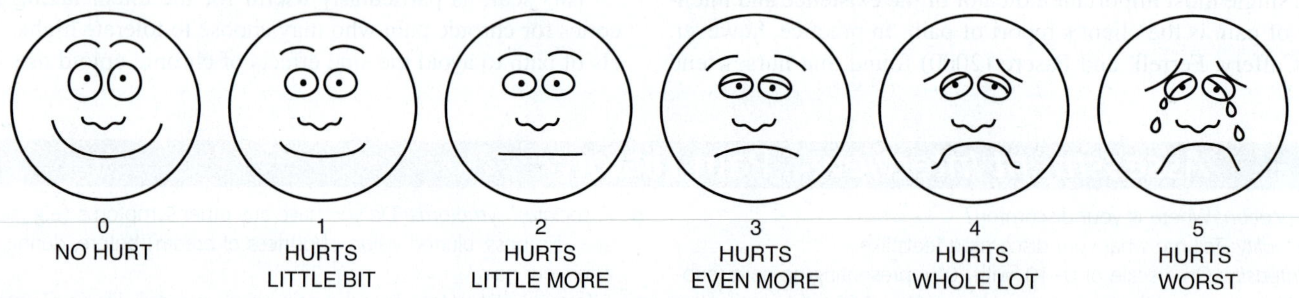

Explain to the person that each face is for a person who feels happy because he has no pain (hurt) or sad because he has some or a lot of pain. Face 0 is very happy because he doesn't hurt at all. Face 1 hurts just a little bit. Face 2 hurts a little more. Face 3 hurts even more. Face 4 hurts a whole lot. Face 5 hurts as much as you can imagine, although you don't have to be crying to feel this bad. Ask the person to choose the face that best describes how he is feeling.

Rating scale is recommended for persons aged 3 years and older.

Brief word instructions: Point to each face using the words to describe the pain intensity. Ask the child to choose the face that best describes own pain and record the appropriate number.

Figure 5–7 ■ The Wong-Baker FACES Rating Scale.

Source: From *Wong's Essentials of Pediatric Nursing*, 6th ed. (p. 1301), by D.L. Wong, M. Hockenberry-Eaton, D. Wilson, M.L. Winkelstein, and P. Schwartz. 2001. St. Louis, MO: Mosby. Copyright by Mosby, Inc. Reprinted with permission.

Sunrise Hospital and Medical Center & Sunrise Children's Hospital
Pain Management Flow Sheet

SR-1420 (6/00)

***Monitoring Guidelines outlined on back of form**

Patient's stated pain level goal:__________

Mode of Administration

A-PO opioid and nonopioid medications
B-PCA Infuser Basal with Patient Control
C-Continuous Infusion
D-Epidural Infuser Continuous Basal Only
E-Epidural Infuser Basal & Patient Control
F-Intermittent IV/IM Injection
G-Transdermal opioids
H-On-QPump
I-Per Rectum

Level of Pain Assessment Scales

Faces Pain Rating Scale

0 ....2..........4..........6..........8..........10

1-10 Pain Scale

0 - - - - - - - - - - - - - - - - 10

No pain or pain relieved — Worst pain imaginable

0-10 Sum Scale

A. Vocal
0 = Positive/ETT
1 = Whimpers
2 = Crying
3 = Screaming

C. Facial
0 = Smiling
1 = Neutral
2 = Frown/grimace
3 = Clenched teeth

B. Body Movement
0 = Moves easily
1 = Neutral shifting
2 = Tense/flailing limbs

D. Touching (localizing)
0 = Notouching
1 = Reaching/patting
2 = Grabbing

Location of Pain:

Right — Left — Left — Right

A = No pain
B-Z = Use letters to mark location of pain on graph

Frequency of Pain:
0 = Occasional **F** = Frequent **C** = Constant

Type of Pain
A = Burning
B = Stabbing
C = Radiating
D = Sharp
E = Shooting
F = Dull
G = Isolated
H = Other

Date																		
Time																		
Initials																		
Mode of Admin																		
Level of Pain																		
Location of Pain																		
Frequency of Pain																		
Type of Pain																		
Arousal Score																		
Non-Pharm. Intervent.																		
Analgesia Order																		
Reason for Order																		
Side Effects																		
Adverse Effects **(Y/N)**																		
Sensory Function **Epidural Only**																		
Motor Function **Epidural Only**																		
Neuro Score **Epidural Only**																		
Catheter Site **Epidural Only**																		
Cath Integrity **Epidural Only**																		
O_2 Saturation																		
Respirations																		
Pulse																		
Blood Pressure																		
See Nursing Notes **(Y/N)**																		

Initials	**Signature**

Patient Identification Label

Arousal Score:
0 = Alert
1 = Medically sedated/ETT
2 = Drowsy
3 = Somnolent
4 = Asleep

Non-Pharmacologic Interventions L
C = Cold
D = Distraction
H = Heat
HO = Holding
I = Imagery
M = Massage
MU = Music
P = Pacifier
PO = Positioning
R = Relaxation
RO = Rocking
S = SecurityObject
T = TensUnit
O = Other

Analgesia Order:
1 = Increase in dosage/rate
2 = Decrease in doseage/rate
3 = Extra bolus
4 = PRN medication for break-through pain
5 = Discontinue

Reason for Analgesia Order:
1 = Unrelieved pain
2 = Decreased arousal/neuroscore
3 = Side effects (Seebelow)
4 = Discontinue therapy/change to oral route
5 = Adverse drug reactions
(Document all adverse drug reactions in Nsg notes and complete an ADR report)

Side Effects: **0** = None
A = Anxiety
C = Confused
Co = Constipation
I = Itching
N = Nausea
R = Respiratory Depression
U = Urinary Rentention
V = Vomiting

Sensory Function **Epidural Only**
0 = Moves all extremities well
1 = Unable to move all extremities well

Motor Function **Epidural Only**
0 = Able to feel tactile pressure
1 = Unable to feel tactile pressure

Neuro Score: **Epidural Only**
0 = No numbness, no weakness
1 = Medically sedated/ETT
2 = Numbness with out weakness
3 = Numbness and weakness

Catheter Site: **Epidural Only**
1 = No redness, drainage, inflammation or swelling
2 = Red, inflamed
3 = Visable clear drainage
4 = Visable purulent drainage
5 = Visable serosanguinous/sanguinous drainage
6 = Swelling

Catheter Integrity Upon Removal: Epidural Only
1 = Catheter tip visually intact
2 = Catheter NOT visually intact-See Nsg Notes

Figure 5–8 ■ Pain Management Flow Sheet.

Source: Courtesy of Aprille Ciaverella, RN, and Lori Townsend, RN, at Sunrise Hospital and Medical Center and Sunrise Children's Hospital, Las Vegas, NV.

Diagnosis

NANDA includes the following diagnostic labels for clients experiencing pain or discomfort:

- Acute Pain
- Chronic Pain.

When writing the diagnostic statement, the nurse should specify the location (e.g., right ankle pain, left frontal headache). Related factors, when known, should also be part of the diagnostic statement and can include both physiological and psychological factors. For example, in addition to the injurious agent, related factors may include deficient knowledge of pain management techniques or fear of drug tolerance or addiction.

Because the presence of pain can affect so many facets of a person's functioning, additional nursing diagnoses may be appropriate for the client experiencing pain, including:

- Hopelessness related to feelings of continual pain
- Anxiety related to past experiences of poor control of pain and to anticipation of pain
- Ineffective Coping related to prolonged continuous back pain, ineffective pain management, and inadequate support systems
- Ineffective Health Maintenance related to chronic pain and fatigue
- Self-Care Deficit (Specify) related to poor control of pain
- Deficient Knowledge (Pain Control Measures) related to lack of exposure to information resources
- Impaired Physical Mobility related to arthritic pain in knee and ankle joints
- Insomnia related to increased pain perception at night.

Plan

The plan for client improvement is developed with the client and may include any of the following goals:

- Client will report reduction in pain to allow for comfort.
- Client will be able to contribute to self-care activities.
- Client will obtain adequate relief from pain to allow for mobility.
- Client will obtain adequate pain relief to allow for sleep.

Implementation

The primary nursing diagnoses for clients in pain are acute pain and chronic pain. The interventions for these diagnoses are combined in this discussion.

- Assess the characteristics of the pain by asking the client to:
  a. Point to the pain location or mark the pain location on a figure drawing. Pain location provides information about the etiology of the pain and the type of pain being experienced.
  b. Rate the intensity of the pain by using a pain scale (1–10, with 10 being the worst pain ever experienced), a visual analog scale (a scale on which pain is marked on a continuum from no pain to severe pain), or with word descriptors. *Use the same scale with each assessment.* The intensity of pain is a subjective experience. The perception of the intensity of pain is affected by the client's degree of concentration or distraction, state of consciousness, and expectations. Some body tissues are more sensitive than others.

PRACTICE ALERT

Do not assume that the older client or the client with a cognitive impairment is not having pain or is unable to identify its intensity.

  c. Describe the quality of the pain, saying, for example, "Describe what your pain feels like." If necessary, provide word descriptors for the client to select. Descriptive terms provide insight into the nature and perception of the pain. In addition, the location and type of pain (for example, acute versus chronic) affect the quality.
  d. Describe the pattern of the pain, including time of onset, duration, persistence, and times without pain. It is also important to ask whether the pain is worse at regular times of the day and whether it has any relationship to activity. The pattern of pain provides clues about cause and location.
  e. Describe any precipitating or relieving factors. Precipitating factors include sleep deficits, anxiety, temperature extremes, excessive noise, anxiety, fear, depression, and activity.
  f. Describe the meaning of the pain, including its effects on lifestyle, self-concept, roles, and relationships. Clients with acute pain may believe the pain is a normal response to injury or that it signals serious illness and death. Pain is a stressor that may affect the ability of the client to cope effectively. The client with chronic pain often has concerns about addiction to pain medication, costs, social interactions, sexual activities, and relationships with significant others.
- Monitor manifestations of pain by taking vital signs; assessing skin temperature and moisture; observing pupils; observing facial expressions, position in bed, guarding of body parts; and noting restlessness. Autonomic responses to pain may result in increased blood pressure, tachycardia, rapid respirations, perspiration, and dilated pupils. Other responses to pain include grimacing, clenching the hands, muscle rigidity, guarding, restlessness, and nausea. The client with chronic pain may have an unexpressive, tired facial appearance.

PRACTICE ALERT

Consider pain the fifth vital sign and assess clients for pain every time you check temperature, pulse, respirations, and blood pressure.

- Communicate belief in the client's pain by verbally acknowledging the presence of the pain, listening carefully to the description of pain, and acting to help the client manage the pain. Because pain is a personal, subjective experience, the nurse must convey belief in the client's pain. By conveying belief in the client's pain, the nurse reduces anxiety and thereby lessens pain. See the Evidence-Based Practice feature on page 285.

- Provide optimal pain relief with prescribed analgesics, determining the preferred route of administration. Provide pain-relieving measures for severe pain on a regular around-the-clock basis or by self-administration (such as with a client-controlled analgesic [PCA] pump). The client is part of the decision-making process and can exert some control over the situation by choosing the administration route. Analgesics are usually most effective when they are administered before pain occurs or becomes severe. Around-the-clock administration has been proven to provide better pain management for both acute and chronic pain. Do not crush or break or allow clients to chew controlled-release oral preparations; a dose meant to be slowly absorbed that is absorbed rapidly may lead to a toxic overdose and death. Capsules containing pellets for controlled-release medications can be opened and sprinkled over soft foods; the pellets should not be crushed, chewed, or dissolved (Vallerand, 2003).
- Evaluate and monitor the effects of analgesics and other pain-relieving measures and teach family members or significant others to be alert for adverse reactions to pain medications. Sedation, constipation, nausea, and dizziness are common side effects. Excessive sedation can progress to significant respiratory depression (Pasero & McCaffery, 2002). Check oxygen saturation q2 at the beginning of opioid therapy and after increasing dosage (Pasero & McCaffery, 2002). Prevent falls that may result from sedation or dizziness. If the client has symptoms of excessive opioid dosage, antidotes are available. Narcan (naloxone) is used for morphine overdose. Use caution to titrate Narcan slowly. Never push an entire dose all at once. Administer only enough Narcan to eliminate adverse effects such as respiratory depression or excessive sedation. If excessive Narcan is administered, the client may experience acute withdrawal and will have no pain relief. It may take considerable time to reestablish a therapeutic comfort level.
- Determine the level of sedation the client with tolerate. For clients with chronic pain or cancer pain who need high doses of opioids, sedation may interfere with quality of life and neither the client nor the family want the client so sedated. Several classes of drugs are being used to counteract sedation. They are usually given in the morning so they will not interfere with sleep throughout the night. Amphetamines, especially methylphenidate (Ritalin), are the most commonly used; modafinil (Provigil) has been used for several years, and donepezil (Aricept), which is used for the symptoms of Alzheimer's disease, reduces sedation and fatigue (Bourdeanu, Loseth, & Funk, 2005).
- Teach the client and family nonpharmacological methods of pain management, such as relaxation, distraction, and cutaneous stimulation. These techniques are especially useful when used in conjunction with pain medications and may also be useful in managing chronic pain.
- Provide comfort measures, such as changing positions, back massage, oral care, skin care, and changing bed linens. Basic comfort measures for personal cleanliness,

EVIDENCE-BASED PRACTICE The Client Experiencing Pain

Pain that is not adequately managed is the focus of regulatory agencies, professional health care organizations, and consumer groups. Despite well-defined guidelines for pain management, there is a gap between guideline standards of care and implementation of care. Observational studies of pain management are valuable because they are time sensitive. Relying on nurses' self-report of pain management introduces bias and loses currency. In the study by Manias et al. (2005), nurses were observed in 2-hour periods of high environmental, client, and nursing activity. Examination of the collected observations by independent analysts revealed six categories of response to clients' pain. The pain was (1) responded to effectively; (2) prioritized as less important than completing medication administration, vital sign assessment, taking telephone calls, or dressing changes; (3) ignored because cues were missed; (4) treated as part of the medication administration regimen and given or withheld according to schedule; (5) prevented through comfort measures, medicating before pain was present or was going to occur as with dressing changes, teaching the importance of early communication about pain; and (6) was only addressed reactively, after the painful experience.

Because pain management is mandatory with regulatory agencies such as The Joint Commission, attention to clients' self-reported pain scores is increasing. It is valuable to have the informative detail this study provides. Communication among nurses, physicians, and clients is key to pain relief. The pharmacology and the nonpharmacology of pain relief need to be taught and reviewed regularly. Environmental distractions and interruptions are associated with less attention to pain management. Few conditions have higher priority for the client than pain relief, but the study revealed that nurses accept pain as a normal component of the postoperative surgery experience. Administrators need to be aware that competing responsibilities impact nurses' ability to provide effective pain management. Those responsibilities include documentation, admitting new clients, and completing discharge teaching and arrangements. Pain management is an important component of professional nursing; nurses should be supported in their efforts to address pain with compassion and efficiency.

Critical Thinking in Client Care

1. Reflect on your own experiences with pain. Will those experiences facilitate or hinder your assessments and interventions for clients in pain?
2. You are caring for a young man who has multiple injuries from a motorcycle accident. He tells you his pain is so bad that "he just wants to die." How would you respond?
3. You are caring for an 80-year-old man with diabetes who has had his left foot amputated for gangrene. He is restless and moaning. Another nurse tells you to give only one-half of the ordered dose of narcotics because "he is old and there is a danger of respiratory depression." What would you do?
4. Why do you think nurses tend to underestimate and undermedicate pain?

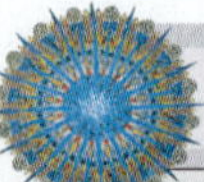

NURSING CARE PLAN **A Client With Chronic Pain**

Susan Akers, aged 37, is currently being seen at an outpatient clinic for chronic nonmalignant pain. She works at a local paper factory. She has a 3-year history of neck and shoulder pain that usually is accompanied by headaches. She believes the pain is related to lifting objects at work, but it is now precipitated by activities of daily living. Susan is absent from work approximately three times a month and states that the absences are due to her pain and headaches. She has been seeking care in the local emergency department on the average of twice monthly for injections for pain. She does not regularly use medications but does take Darvocet-N 100 and Valium as needed (usually two to three times a day). Ms. Akers is divorced and has two children. She states that she has several friends in the area, but her parents and siblings live in another part of the United States.

ASSESSMENT

During the nursing history, Susan rates her pain during an acute episode as a 7 on a 1–10 scale. She states that lifting objects and moving her hands and arms above shoulder level precipitate sharp pain. The pain never really goes away, but it does decrease with upper extremity rest. She says that when she lifts a lot at work she has difficulty sleeping at night. She takes two Darvocet-N 100 tablets every 4 hours when the pain is severe, but does not get complete relief.

DIAGNOSIS

- Chronic Pain related to muscle inflammation

PLANNING

- Client will return for follow-up visits with a journal of activities and pain experiences.
- After 3–5 days on regularly scheduled doses of pain medication, client will report a decrease in the level of pain from 7 to 3 or 4 on a 1–10 scale.
- Client will report a decrease in number of absences from work.
- Client will modify activities at work and at home, especially when pain is intense.

IMPLEMENTATION

- Encourage discussion of pain, and acknowledge belief in Susan's report of pain.
- Consult with a physician for a nonnarcotic analgesic with a minimum of side effects, and instruct in maintaining regular dosing schedules.
- For episodes of acute pain, take narcotic analgesics as soon as the pain begins and every 4 hours while continuing the dosage of nonnarcotic analgesic.
- Teach one relaxation technique that is personally useful.
- Explore distraction techniques such as listening to music, watching comedies, or reading.
- Provide clinic phone number and instruct to call if pain is unrelieved with narcotic and nonnarcotic analgesics.

EVALUATION

Susan returns for scheduled follow-up visits with a completed journal of her activities and associated pain. She reports that taking oral narcotic analgesics has relieved her pain and that within 3 weeks nonnarcotic analgesics brought her pain under control. She also reports that her supervisor has reassigned her to a position that requires no lifting. She now rates her pain at 2 or 3 on a 1–10 scale. She has missed only 1 day of work in the last 3 months and reports that her children and friends have helped with her household tasks when she has requested they do so.

CRITICAL THINKING

1. Describe three factors that support the statement "Pain is a personal experience."
2. Susan asks you how often she should take her pain medications. Do you tell her to (a) take them on a regular basis or (b) wait until she experiences pain? Why?
3. Develop a care plan for Susan for the nursing diagnosis of risk for constipation. Why is this necessary?

skin care, and mobility promote physical and psychosocial well-being, lessening the perception of pain.

- Provide client and family teaching, and make referrals if necessary to assist with coping, financial resources, and home care. The client (and family) with pain requires information about medications, noninvasive techniques for pain management, and sources of assistance with home-based care. The client with acute pain requires information about the expected course of pain resolution.

Community-Based Care

Teaching of the client and family includes:

- Specific drugs to be taken, including the frequency, potential side effects, possible drug interactions, and any special precautions to be taken (such as taking with food or avoiding alcohol)
- How to take or administer the drugs (see Table 5–9)
- The importance of taking pain medications before the pain becomes severe

TABLE 5–9 **Providing Long-Term Analgesia at Home**

ROUTE	DRUG	NURSING IMPLICATIONS
Oral	Oxycodone (OxyContin)	Available in a timed-release formulation for 12-hour dosing and as fast-acting formulations (OxyIR,OxyFAST) for breakthrough pain.
Oral	Morphine (Kadian)	Formulated of timed-release particles in a capsule. If client can't swallow the capsule, may be sprinkled over food or given by nasogastric or gastric tube.
Transdermal	Fentanyl (Duragesic)	Absorbed slowly through the skin; allows 72-hour dose schedule. Up to 14 hours to achieve therapeutic level when discontinued therapeutic effect will decay slowly.
Transdermal	Lidocaine (Lidoderm)	Effective for 12 hours for various neuropathic pains. Monitor clients also taking Class 1 antiarrhythmic drugs for increased effects.
Transmucosal	Fentanyl citrate (Actiq)	A lozenge formulation used to treat breakthrough cancer pain in opioid-tolerant clients.

- An explanation that the risk of addiction to pain medications is very small when they are used for pain relief and management
- The importance of scheduling periods of rest and sleep.

In addition, suggest the following resources:

a. Pain clinics
b. Community support groups
c. American Cancer Society
d. American Pain Society.

Evaluation

The nurse evaluates the effectiveness of pain control measures by assessing the client's pain and questioning the client to determine if adequate pain relief has been obtained. Time for pain relief is highly dependent on route of analgesic administration, type of nonpharmacological intervention, and client's pain level prior to initiation of therapy. Oral medications may take up to an hour to provide relief, while intravenous medications should begin working within minutes. If inadequate relief of pain is obtained, further intervention is required until the client is comfortable.

In addition to evaluating pain relief it is also important to evaluate vital signs, particularly if narcotics have been administered. Respiratory effort and blood pressure should be monitored to avoid complications.

Objective data may validate and/or conflict with subjective data. Vital signs that continue to be out of baseline for client, guarded body position, tensed facial muscles, restlessness, and diaphoresis all indicate presence of pain. The nurse asks more focused evaluation questions, records the information, and amends the nursing plan of care as needed.

REVIEW Acute and Chronic Pain

RELATE: LINK THE CONCEPTS

Linking the exemplar of Acute and Chronic Pain with the concept of Culture:

1. When caring for a client who appears to be in pain, but denies it, how might understanding of the client's culture help you interpret the dichotomy between body language and reported pain?
2. How might interpretations and interventions for pain differ among cultures?

Linking the exemplar of Acute and Chronic Pain with the concept of Stress and Coping:

3. What alterations in stress and coping would you anticipate when a client experiences chronic pain?
4. When caring for a mother with acute pain over the past few weeks, the client relates she has just not had the energy to deal with her children. How is pain impacting this mother's ability to cope with her children's needs?

READY: GO TO COMPANION SKILLS MANUAL

- Applying dry heat measures
- Applying compresses and moist packs
- Applying dry cold measures
- Assessing the client in pain
- Using the narcotic control system

REFER: GO TO MYNURSINGKIT

REFLECT: CASE STUDY

Mr. Wind is an 82-year-old Cherokee Indian man. His history includes anterior-septal MI, brown lung disease, and congestive heart failure. Mr. Wind has painful joints in the morning that make it difficult for him to walk. He comes to the doctor's office for a routine checkup and sees the nurse practitioner. His appointment is at 2:00 p.m. At 2:30 p.m., he is called back to a treatment room where he waits another 20 minutes before the nurse practitioner arrives.

1. How might psychosocial and cultural issues impact the accuracy of a comfort assessment by the nurse practitioner?
2. How can assessment of pain levels demonstrate a worsening physiological condition?
3. What teaching points will the nurse stress to help Mr. Wind manage his chronic joint pain?

5.2 END-OF-LIFE CARE

KEY TERMS

Advance directive, *289*
Closed awareness, *289*
Death anxiety, *299*
Do-not-intubate order, *296*
Do-not-resuscitate order, *290*
Durable power of attorney, *290*
End of life, *288*
Euthanasia, *290*
Health care surrogate, *290*
Hospice care, *291*
Living will, *289*
Mutual presence, *298*
Open awareness, *298*
Palliative care, *291*

LEARNING OUTCOMES

After reading about this exemplar, you will be able to:

1. Describe the pathophysiology, etiology, clinical manifestations, and direct and indirect causes of symptoms seen in clients at the end of life.
2. Illustrate the nursing process in providing culturally competent care across the lifespan for individuals at the end of life.
3. Formulate priority nursing diagnoses appropriate for an individual at the end of life.
4. Create a plan of care for individuals at the end of life and their family members.
5. Assess expected outcomes for clients at the end of life and their family members.
6. Discuss therapies used in the collaborative care of an individual at the end of life.
7. Employ evidence-based caring interventions for an individual at the end of life.

BASIS FOR SELECTION OF EXEMPLAR

Priority Areas for National Action
Transforming Areas for Quality Improvement (IOM)
National Roundtable on Health Care Quality
Standards of Nursing Practice

OVERVIEW

End-of-life (the final weeks of life when death is imminent) nursing care that ensures a peaceful death was mandated by the International Council of Nurses (1997) and further supported by the American Association of Colleges of Nursing (AACN, 1999). The following are selected competencies necessary for nurses to provide high-quality end-of-life care as defined by the AACN (1999):

- Promote the provision of comfort care to the dying as an active, desirable, and important skill and an integral component of nursing care (Figure 5–9 ■).
- Communicate effectively and compassionately with the client, family, and health care team members about end-of-life issues.
- Recognize one's own attitudes, feelings, values, and expectations about death and the individual, cultural, and spiritual diversity existing in those beliefs and customs.
- Demonstrate respect for the client's views and wishes during end-of-life care.
- Use scientifically based standardized tools to assess symptoms (e.g., pain, dyspnea, constipation, anxiety, fatigue, nausea/vomiting, and altered cognition) experienced by clients at the end of life.
- Use data from symptom assessment to plan and intervene in symptom management using state-of-the-art traditional and complementary approaches.
- Assist the client, family, colleagues, and one's self to cope with suffering, grief, loss, and bereavement in end-of-life care.

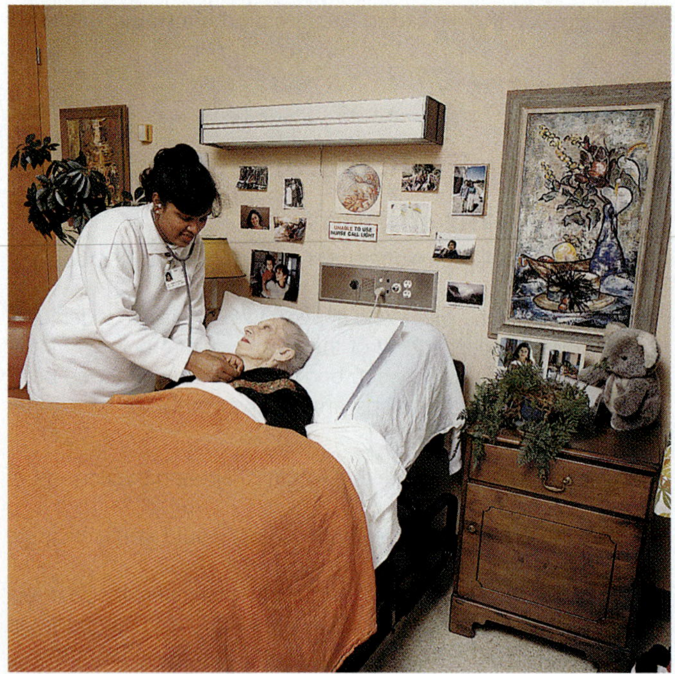

Figure 5–9 ■ The nurse helps the client visualize the hospital room as a safe, comfortable place to be by surrounding the client with familiar pictures and objects.

PATHOPHYSIOLOGY AND ETIOLOGY

The 10 leading causes of death accounting for 80% of all death in the United States in 2008 include, ranked in descending order, heart disease, malignant neoplasms, cerebrovascular disease, chronic lower respiratory disease, accidents, diabetes mellitus, influenza and pneumonia, Alzheimer's disease, renal disease, and septicemia (National Center for Health Statistics, 2008). Often, the exact cause of death is difficult to determine in an older adult. For example, an older adult with Alzheimer's disease may fall, fracture a hip, and die shortly after the injury. The actual cause of the fall, however, may have been a myocardial infarction that was not detected. The death certificate may indicate either a fall or Alzheimer's disease as the cause of death while the true cause was the myocardial infarction.

Etiology

Most Americans, regardless of age, would prefer to die in their own homes rather than institutions. However, about 50% of Americans die in hospitals, 25% in long-term care facilities, 20% at home or the home of a loved one, and 5% in other settings, including inpatient hospices (NCP, 2004). Almost half the population aged 65 and older will spend some time in a long-term care facility prior to death, and many deaths occur shortly after transfer from the long-term care facility to the hospital (Strumpf, Tuch, Stillman, Parrish, & Morrison, 2004). Data from numerous studies demonstrate high degrees of symptom distress in hospitalized clients and long-term care residents, high use of burdensome technologies among the seriously ill, caregiver burden on families, and problems with communication between clients, families, and caregivers about the goals of care and medical decisions that should follow (Last Acts, 2002; NCP, 2004; Quill, 2000; SUPPORT Principal Investigators, 1995).

When a national survey asked how the current health care system does in caring for dying people, only 3% of respondents answered excellent, 8% responded very good, 31% responded good, 33% responded fair, and 25% responded poor (Last Acts, 2002). Most professionals agree that there is much room for improvement in view of these results.

NURSING CONSIDERATIONS FOR END-OF-LIFE CARE

Nurses care for the dying client in CCUs, emergency departments, hospital units, long-term care facilities, and clients' homes. Regardless of the setting, the client's wishes about death should be respected. The Dying Person's Bill of Rights (see Box 5–9) states that each person has "the right to be cared for by caring, sensitive, knowledgeable people who will attempt to understand my needs and will be able to gain some satisfaction in helping me face my death" (Barbus, 1975).

Legal and Ethical Issues

Issues such as those involved in advance directives and living wills, euthanasia, and quality of life are especially important to nurses in upholding the specific care requests of their clients.

ADVANCE DIRECTIVES **Advance directives** are legal documents that allow a person to plan for health care and/or financial affairs in the event of incapacity. They include living wills, health care surrogates (sometimes referred to as a health care proxy or power of attorney), and durable power of attorney.

- **Living will:** A document that provides written directions about life-prolonging procedures to provide instructions when a person can no longer communicate in a life-threatening situation.

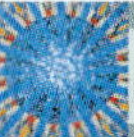

EVIDENCE-BASED PRACTICE **End-of-Life Care**

End-of-life care is emerging as a major concern in the United States. Although many people die in the hospital, little research has been done about deaths in the critical care unit (CCU). Clients are not admitted to the CCU to die, but approximately 20% of critical care clients do not live to be discharged from the hospital. Most deaths in the CCU occur in undesirable situations, for example, when clients do not respond to the advanced technology and decide to forgo further treatment or are comatose or receiving mechanical ventilation. In most instances, clients dying in the CCU are isolated from family members. The purpose of this study (Kirchhoff, Spuhler, Walker, Hutton, Cole, & Clemmer, 2000) was to address the largely unstudied area of CCU nursing care by conducting focus groups of CCU nurses.

Implications for Nursing

Regardless of the setting for end-of-life care, nurses need to ensure that clients are as free from pain as possible and that the comfort and dignity of the client are maintained. In addition, family members should be given time to begin to accept the dying process. This may be facilitated by having the family member provide physical care and lie in bed with the client and by providing time and space for family rituals and saying good-bye. Nurses also need to show the family that they care and are involved. However, nurses face the dilemmas of sometimes having a less optimistic outlook than physicians, of approving or not approving of the use of extraordinary measures to preserve life, and of not wanting to share feelings following a death or share too much.

Critical Thinking in Client Care

1. What environmental differences between a regular hospital unit and a CCU that might make quality end-of-life care more difficult for nurses?
2. The family of a client in the CCU says to you, "Uncle Al is going to die, isn't he?" What would you need to know before responding? How would you respond?
3. A CCU client who previously had been improving suddenly dies. The staff are saddened, and several are in tears. A more experienced nurse says, "Oh, you just have to go on. There's nothing else to do." Do you agree? Why or why not?

Source: Data from Kirchhoff, K., Spuhler, V., Walker, L., Hutton, A., Cole, B., & Clemmer, T. (2000). Intensive care nurses' experiences with end-of-life care. *American Journal of Critical Care, 9*(1), 35–42.

Box 5–9 The Dying Person's Bill of Rights

I have the right to be treated as a living human being until I die.
I have the right to maintain a sense of hopefulness however changing its focus may be.
I have the right to express my feelings and emotions about my approaching death in my own way.
I have the right to participate in decisions concerning my care.
I have the right to expect continuing medical and nursing attention even though cure goals must be changed to comfort goals.
I have the right not to die alone.
I have the right to be free from pain.
I have the right to have my questions answered honestly.
I have the right not to be deceived.
I have the right to have help from and for my family in accepting my death.
I have the right to die in peace and with dignity.
I have the right to retain my individuality and not be judged for my decisions which may be contrary to the beliefs of others.
I have the right to be cared for by caring, sensitive, knowledgeable people who will attempt to understand my needs and will be able to gain some satisfaction in helping me face my death.

Source: From "The Dying Person's Bill of Rights," by A. J. Barbus, 1975, created at the workshop *The Terminally Ill Patient and the Helping Person*, Lansing, MI: South Western Michigan Inservice Education Council.

- **Health care surrogate:** An individual who has been selected to make medical decisions when a person is no longer able to make them for himself or herself.
- **Durable power of attorney:** A document that can delegate the authority to make health, financial, and/or legal decisions on a person's behalf. It must be in writing and must state that the designated person is authorized to make health care decisions. In some states, the client may execute a health care power of attorney and have a separate durable power of attorney that addresses financial and legal decisions.

A living will is a legal document that formally expresses a person's wishes regarding life-sustaining treatment in the event of terminal illness or permanent unconsciousness. It is not a type of durable power of attorney and usually does not designate a substitute decision maker. It is the responsibility of the nurse as client advocate to request and record the client's preference for care and include it in the plan of care. The nurse's documentation helps communicate these preferences to the other members of the health care team.

All facilities that receive Medicare and Medicaid funds are required to provide all clients with written information and counseling about advance directives and the institution's policies governing them. The specific terms of this requirement are found in the Patient Self-Determination Act. A copy of the signed advance directive must be kept in the client's medical record, but clients do not have to sign it in order to be treated. Nurses are the ones in close contact with clients, so they bear much of the responsibility for ensuring the client's wishes in this area are followed. Although advance directives do not ease the pain of seeing clients die, they do help nurses provide clients with the care that the clients have chosen.

DO-NOT-RESUSCITATE ORDERS A **do-not-resuscitate order** (DNR, or "no-code") is written by the physician for the client who has a terminal illness or is near death. This order is usually based on the wishes of the client and family that no cardiopulmonary resuscitation be performed for respiratory or cardiac arrest. A comfort-measures-only order indicates that no further life-sustaining interventions are necessary and that the goal of care is a comfortable, dignified death. Agency protocols should be established that define "comfort care" for consistency in nursing care. Confusing or conflicting DNR orders create dilemmas, because nurses are involved in resuscitation and either begin CPR or ensure that unwanted attempts do not occur. The American Nurses Association (ANA) has made specific recommendations related to a DNR order (Box 5–10). The ANA further recommends that guidelines and policies be developed to help resolve conflicts between clients and their families, between clients and health care professionals, and among health care professionals.

Box 5–10 The ANA Position on Nursing Care and Do-Not-Resuscitate Decisions

- The choices and values of the competent client should always be given highest priority, even when these wishes conflict with those of health care providers and families.
- In the case of the incompetent or never competent client, any existing advance directives or the decisions of surrogate decision makers acting in the client's best interest should be determinative.
- The DNR decision should always be a subject of explicit discussion among the client, the family, any designated surrogate decision maker acting in the client's best interest, and the health care team. The decision should include consideration of the efficacy and desirability of CPR, a balancing of benefits and burdens to clients, and therapeutic goals.
- DNR orders must be clearly documented, reviewed, and updated periodically to reflect changes in the client's condition.
- Nurses have a responsibility to educate clients and their families about various forms of advance directives such as living wills and durable power of attorney.
- If it is the nurse's personal belief that his or her moral integrity is compromised by professional responsibility to carry out a particular DNR order, the nurse should transfer the responsibility for the client's care to another nurse.

Source: From *Task Force on the Nurse's Role in End of Life Decisions* by ANA Board of Directors, 1992.

EUTHANASIA The term **euthanasia** (from the Greek for "painless, easy, gentle, or good death") is now commonly used to signify a killing prompted by some humanitarian motive. There are many arguments for and against euthanasia, and nurses have often found themselves at the center of the debate. As a result, nurses have pushed for the development of appropriate guidelines and procedures for DNR orders. When no such orders exist, the nurse faces a dilemma. Certainly, there are situations in which the nurse's role is clear. For example, it is considered malpractice to participate in "slow codes" (in which the nurse does not hurry to alert the emergency team when a terminally ill client who does not have a DNR order stops breathing).

The natural death laws seek to preserve the notion of voluntary versus involuntary euthanasia. In voluntary euthanasia, the competent adult client or loved one of the client and a physician make the decision to withdraw life support with the knowledge that it will result in the client's death. For example, removal of the use of mechanical ventilation for a client who has a terminal condition at the client's request would be classified as voluntary euthanasia and is legal in most locations. Involuntary euthanasia ("mercy killing") is generally performed by administering a lethal dose of medication that will result in the client's death. Administering a large dose of narcotic to a client diagnosed with amyotrophic lateral sclerosis at the client's urging to avoid degenerative symptoms when the client's condition is too advanced to allow the client to administer the medications to himself would be an example of involuntary euthanasia. It is illegal to perform involuntary euthanasia in most areas of the country with the exception of Oregon, which has passed euthanasia laws. Because care settings offer many complex and technological interventions, it is not likely that the ethical aspects of euthanasia will soon be resolved. However, advance directives do give clients a much more active role in decisions about their own care.

Settings and Services for End-of-Life Care

Settings and services for end-of-life care range from the critical care unit in a hospital to the client's own home. Two methods of providing end-of-life care—palliative care and hospice care—are described in this section.

Palliative Care

In the late 1990s, the World Health Organization defined **palliative care** as an approach that improves the quality of life of clients and their families facing life-threatening illness by preventing, assessing, and treating pain and other physical, psychosocial, and spiritual problems (National Consensus Project for Quality Palliative Care, 2004). Palliative care is a multidisciplinary care strategy designed to relieve the physical, social, emotional, and spiritual suffering in clients and their families by managing symptoms and monitoring all aspects of suffering during the course of the client's illness (Korones, 2007). Nursing interventions that help the client enhance quality of life, reduce pain and suffering, optimize functionality, and promote appropriate goal setting and decision making are integral to the provision of excellent palliative care. Regardless of the stage of the disease or the need for curative therapies, palliative care is appropriate for clients with life-limiting, serious illness.

Palliative care is appropriate for some conditions that may possibly be cured, but treatment failure is also possible, as in cases of advanced or progressive cancer or severe congenital heart defects. Particularly for children, care may be palliative from the time of diagnosis, as in cases of severe forms of osteogenesis imperfecta or certain chromosomal disorders. Other conditions that should be considered for palliative care include muscular dystrophy, severe immune deficiency, cystic fibrosis, and severe respiratory failure (Himelstein, Hilden, Boldt, & Weissman, 2004). Palliative care is especially appropriate when provided to older adults who have the following:

- Acute, serious, life-threatening illness (such as stroke, trauma, major myocardial infarction, and cancer where cure or reversibility may or may not be a realistic goal but the burden of treatment is high).
- Progressive chronic illness (such as end-stage dementia, congestive heart failure, renal or liver failure, and frailty).

Palliative care may take place across all settings including hospitals, outpatient clinics, long-term care facilities, or the home. The client and family are supported during the dying and bereavement process. The care provided emphasizes quality of life and living as full a life as possible up until the moment of death.

HOSPICE CARE The hospice movement began in the United States in the 1970s. Since 1974, over 7 million clients and families have received end-of-life care at home as well as in long-term care settings and hospitals through hospice programs, with escalating use in recent years (NCP, 2004). The work of nurse leaders such as Florence Wald, Dame Cicely Saunders (also a physician), and Jeanne Quint Benoliel highlighted the need for "competent, expert, evidence-based care provided in a way that embodies compassion, respect for dignity, and an appreciation for the whole person and the family" (HPNA, 2003b, p. 1). Another nurse leader, Harriet Goetz, published an approach to care for the dying in 1962 emphasizing therapeutic communication and symptom management techniques to provide comfort. Current standards of comprehensive and compassionate hospice and palliative nursing care are built upon the foundation of the work of these nurse leaders (HPNA, 2003b).

Hospice care can be defined as the support and care for persons in the last phase of an incurable disease so that they may live as fully and comfortably as possible (National Hospice and Palliative Care Organization [NHPCO], 2000). In the early 1980s, Congress added a hospice benefit to the Medicare program that was designed to support dying clients with an expected prognosis of less than 6 months to live if the disease ran its usual course. However, it is often difficult to predict with accuracy how long a client will live, especially when the diagnosis is chronic in nature (renal failure, congestive heart failure, cancer, or progressive dementia). Many hospices are expanding service options so that clients and families can receive palliative care long before the last 6 months of life to meet the needs of clients dying from chronic illnesses (Dembner, 2004).

Clients and families often seek hospice care when two physicians have determined that the client has 6 months or less to live and the dying person and family are agreeable with care and comfort over aggressive medical intervention. Hospice care focuses on the whole person by caring for the body, mind, and spirit. The goal is for the client to live his or her last days as fully and comfortably as possible. To achieve this goal, an interdisciplinary team of physicians, nurses, therapists, home health aids, pharmacists, pastoral counselors, social workers, and trained lay volunteers assist the family and caregivers in providing care. The hospice nurse assumes the role of specialist in the management of pain and control of symptoms and assesses the client's and family's coping mechanisms, available resources to care for the client, the client's wishes, and the support systems in place.

Hospice personnel may work with caregivers and clients in the home, long-term care facilities, other long-term care settings, and hospitals. Hospitals may have affiliated hospices and some home health agencies promote their own home care hospices. Freestanding hospices that provide a homelike atmosphere in which care is provided by trained staff at the facility are also available. Reimbursement for hospice services is provided by Medicare, Medicaid, private health insurance companies, and some health maintenance organizations. Some hospices accept donations for care; others may have access to charitable foundations. All hospices encourage family involvement and promote death with dignity. Because the experience of the dying and death of a loved one deeply affects the family, supportive care is provided to family and caregivers throughout the illness trajectory and for a period after the death has occurred.

There are many misconceptions and myths about hospice care. Table 5–10 illustrates common myths and facts regarding hospice.

Cultural and Religious Considerations in Providing End-of-Life Care

People of many cultural backgrounds reside in the United States. Culture encompasses dimensions such as race, ethnicity, gender, age, abilities/disabilities, sexual orientation, religion and spirituality, and socioeconomic status (Mazanec & Panke, 2006). An ever-changing system, culture is shaped over time as beliefs, values, and lifestyle patterns are passed from generation to generation. Sensitivity and empathy are essential when caring for a dying person from a different culture. Each dying client is a unique individual with cultural preferences that influence the specialized needs of the client, the family, and their caregivers. (See Concept 6 for a thorough discussion of culture.)

Despite efforts to improve access to palliative care to all older adults, improvements are not reaching minority populations (Krakauer, Crenner, & Fox, 2002). The SUPPORT Principal Investigators (1995) reported that fewer resources were expended on African American clients than on Caucasians with similar disease processes; other studies have noted that minority clients are significantly less likely to

TABLE 5–10 **Myths and Facts Regarding Hospice**

MYTH	FACT
Medicare provides only 6 months of hospice care, so enrollment should be delayed as long as possible.	Medicare law does not limit the hospice benefit, but Medicare regulations often discourage a longer length of stay. Clients may enroll when their physician judges their life expectancy to be 6 months or less.
All hospice care is the same.	Hospices vary widely in the services they provide. Visit and observe services before choosing or recommending one for care.
Clients cannot receive curative treatments while on hospice.	Clients must sign a statement choosing hospice care instead of curative therapies to treat their terminal illness. Medicare will still pay for covered benefits for any health problems that are not related to the terminal diagnosis.
Hospice means giving up hope. Hospices help people die.	Hope for comfort and relief of pain is always present. Hospice workers do not hasten death.
Hospice helps only when advice is needed regarding pain medication.	Hospice care is holistic and goes beyond traditional medical care.
You cannot keep your own doctor on hospice.	Most hospices have working relationships with the referring physician.
Hospice is only for cancer clients.	Hospice is available to all clients with a variety of diagnoses, including those with cancer, dementia, and heart and lung diseases.
Hospice is only for the sick family member.	Hospice supports all family members during the illness and supports the family for 1 year after the death.
Hospice is a place, so you must leave home to go there.	Most hospice care is delivered in the home, although inpatient care is available to those with no in-home caregiver or to those whose families are overwhelmed by providing the care.
Hospice is expensive.	In general, hospice costs less than traditional hospital or long-term care.

Source: Adapted from Labyak, 2001. *Home Healthcare Nurse*, 20;3 (March 2002): 148.

receive appropriate pain management. Many minority clients have an underlying mistrust of the health care system (Mazanec & Panke, 2006). It is well documented in the literature that African-American clients often wish for aggressive life-sustaining interventions in the face of terminal disease. These clients may choose feeding tubes and CPR because of fears of being denied health care similar in scope to that of Caucasians.

Religion and spirituality play an important role in forming beliefs and practices that are paramount when death is imminent. Feelings of guilt, remorse, comfort, or peacefulness may all be related to religious beliefs. Religious customs are extremely important to many dying clients, and concerns or fears intensify as death nears. It is important to remember that each client's spiritual reactions to situations are highly individualized, regardless of the client's religious faith. Requests by family or clients to seek spiritual counseling should be met with respect. Many health care facilities have chaplains, clergy, social workers, and others to assist staff. Spiritual care should be individualized and made available to the terminal client.

At times, a religious belief may help the client in determining the type of end-of-life care to request. Nurses must be aware of concerns the client may have and respond therapeutically. The age-old question of why this is happening may take on religious tones or thoughts. Punishment, atonement, God's will, or hope for a miracle may all be discussed or alluded to by the client. Follow the client's lead in discussing spiritual needs and beliefs. Serious illnesses frequently initiate a search for life's meaning and questions may arise regarding the individual's purpose in life. Even the client's emotional response to pain may be influenced by religious or spiritual beliefs.

When discussing religion or spirituality with the client, it is important to assist the client's efforts to seek meaning. Nurses who feel unable to assist clients in discussions of spirituality should make referrals to others on the team with skills and knowledge in this area. Spiritual care interventions that may be chosen by the client to affirm life and hope include renewal of vows, faith readings, guided meditation, receiving sacraments, spiritual life review, and discussion of spiritual pain (ELNEC, 2006).

It is common for a person of Catholic faith to wish to receive the Sacrament of the Sick to give spiritual strength and prepare for death. A religious item such as a rosary or medal may bring comfort. The Jewish believer may want to see a rabbi and participate in prayers. In Judaism, burial is performed as soon as possible and before the Sabbath. Muslims may prefer that a family member be notified as soon as death occurs. It is best to wait for the family member since because Muslims typically observe special washing and shrouding procedures. Muslims also may prefer that the family wash the body. The body is then placed in a position that faces Mecca. If there is no family member to prepare the body, the staff may do so provided that gloves are worn. In Muslim faiths, cremation is not accepted, and burial of the body takes place as quickly as possible.

END-OF-LIFE CARE FOR CHILDREN

Palliative care is provided to children and their families in many of the same circumstances in which it is provided to adults. It is also an option for very preterm neonates and for children with lethal genetic anomalies. Palliative care may occur in the home, hospital, or other facility. Children may require these services for many years. Box 5–11 discusses nursing roles for providing palliative and end-of-life care to children.

About 8,600 children each day could benefit from palliative care that acknowledges their limited life expectancy and severity of illness. Unfortunately, many do not receive it (Rushton, 2005). Some of the most common reasons for seeking a palliative care consultation or conference include the following (Rushton, Reder, Hall, et al., 2006):

- The client has a disease that will limit his or her life span.
- Death could potentially occur within the next 6–12 months.
- A major clinical event has occurred related to the child's condition (e.g., relapse, need for transplant).
- The frequency of clinic visits has changed due to the client's symptoms.
- There is a change or deterioration in the client's response to treatment, pain intensity, energy, functional status, respiratory function, mental status, or quality of life.
- The family and health care team are in conflict over goals of care.

Box 5–11 **Nursing Roles in Improving Pediatric Palliative and End-of-Life Care**

The nurse and other members of the health care team work collaboratively to improve end-of-life care for children and their families through the following actions:

- Plan nursing care for children with life-threatening medical conditions and their families that matches the child's physical, cognitive, emotional, and spiritual level of development.
- Implement family-centered care, ensuring that families are part of the care team and that their beliefs, feelings, and desires are respected.
- Plan and provide compassionate care for children with life-threatening conditions and for their families beginning at the time of diagnosis through death and bereavement.
- Seek information, education, and mentoring to gain proficiency and skill in working effectively with children who are dying and their families.
- Work within the health care facility to promote needed changes that will improve the palliative, end-of-life, and bereavement care for children and their families.
- Participate in research designed to increase health care professionals' understanding of clinical, cultural, organizational, and other practices or perspectives that can improve palliative, end-of-life, and bereavement care for children and their families.

Source: Reprinted with permission from "Working Principles for Pediatric Palliative, End-of-Life and Bereavement Care," from "When Children Die: Improving Palliative and End-of-Life Care for Children and Their Families," Summary, p. 7—Box S.1. © 2003 by the National Academy of Sciences, Courtesy of the National Academies Press, Washington, D.C.

Barriers to providing effective pediatric palliative care can be attitudinal, educational, institutional, regulatory, or financial factors. Examples of barriers include the following:

- Health care professionals inexperienced in palliative care
- Poor reimbursement for the time-intensive nature of care
- Objections to providing palliative care along with curative care
- Difficulty in communicating about the death
- Association of palliative care with giving up or hopelessness
- Fragmentation of medical and psychosocial/spiritual services.

Other significant barriers in the provision of palliative care to children are adult denial that children die and the natural human instinct to attempt to preserve a child's life at any cost (Himelstein, 2005). As a result of any combination of these barriers, children may live for a prolonged time with a life-limiting condition without the palliative care supports and services that could improve quality of life. See the core elements of palliative care in Box 5–12.

Advance Care Planning

Advance care planning for a child's death should include the following (Himelstein et al., 2004):

- Identify the decision makers and make sure all on the health care team are aware.
- Describe the expected changes in the child's functional ability and quality of life as the disease progresses.
- Determine whether the family's and child's goals are curative, comfort, or not known at this time.
- Help the family make decisions about medical interventions that are desired and how intervention decisions should be modified as the child's health status changes (Box 5–13).
- Provide anticipatory guidance about changes to expect when the child is near death and identify who will help the family manage the child's symptoms.

Adolescents should participate in any advance planning discussions. (See the Developmental Considerations feature.) Research has suggested that the adolescent's experience with a serious medical condition rather than age is a better indicator of decision-making capability (Hartman, 2004). The adolescent may express a desire to refuse treatment or request withdrawal of treatment. Open and honest discussion with the adolescent can help parents and the health care team to determine if he or she fully understands the implications of terminating curative therapy. If the intent is to avoid more painful procedures, then the adolescent needs to be informed about options for pain relief. Because of the adolescent's desire for autonomy, information about all choices should be provided, including but not limited to withdrawal of treatment. However, the adolescent may have reached the acceptance stage in the grieving process and is ready for death to occur. Once parents are satisfied that the adolescent has reached a resolution based on facts, it may be easier for the parents to support and respect the adolescent's wishes. The nurse who has established a trusting relationship with the adolescent may be able to help him or her recognize the parents' wishes to continue nurturing and protecting their child.

Box 5–12 **Core Elements of Palliative Care for Children**

- Provides care to children with chronic or life-threatening illnesses, conditions, or injury.
- Services are family centered, with the goals and preferences of the client and family integrated with the support and guidance in decision making by the health care team.
- Palliative care ideally begins at the time of diagnosis of a life-threatening or debilitating condition and continues until the child is cured or dies, into the bereavement period.
- Regular assessments are performed to help clients and families understand changes in condition and how those changes impact care goals and future treatment.
- An interdisciplinary care team provides palliative care, and includes physicians, nurses, psychologists, pharmacists, chaplains, social workers, child life therapists, and other needed health professionals.
- A major focus of care is on the relief of pain and suffering associated with other condition symptoms.
- Effective communication strategies are used to help the child and family develop care goals and make health care decisions.
- The health care team needs to be skilled in the care of the dying child and bereaved family.
- Palliative care should be provided in all health care delivery settings and be accessible to all children in need of services.
- Evaluation of the care processes and outcomes should be performed to promote high-quality care.

Source: Adapted from *National Consensus Project for Quality Palliative Care.* (2004). Clinical practice guidelines for quality palliative care pp. 5–7. Retrieved September 19, 2007, from http://www.nationalconsensusproject.org/guidelines

Box 5–13 **Research: Advance Care Planning**

In a small study, the parents of 17 children with noncancerous chronic progressive conditions were interviewed about their experiences with the process of advance care planning. The advance care plans were followed for 8 of the children. Parents reported that talking about the child's death was difficult, but the process of doing advance planning benefited the children and the family because it ensured the best care for the child by focusing on the child's quality of life and prevented unnecessary suffering (Hammes, Klevan, Kempf, et al.& Williams, 2005).

DEVELOPMENTAL CONSIDERATIONS
Adolescents and Self-Determination

The Patient Self-Determination Act of 1990 (PSDA) supports the rights of persons 18 years of age or older to make decisions about their medical care. Although many adolescents younger than 18 have the cognitive skills necessary for decision making and are involved in decisions concerning their care, the PSDA limits their legal rights. Creative strategies are needed to develop a model of decision-making rights and responsibilities for adolescents that is built on the PSDA and shared with parents who ultimately will be responsible for decisions on care.

Ethical Issues Surrounding a Child's Death

A child's death can be emotionally charged, potentially resulting in misunderstandings and conflicts between families and health care providers. The more common ethical issues that need to be addressed include withdrawal of or withholding treatment, parental treatment refusal, and DNR orders.

WITHDRAWING OR WITHHOLDING TREATMENT The decision to withdraw or withhold life-sustaining treatments from the dying infant or child is extremely difficult and highly emotional for the parents. Some parents misunderstand and believe that withdrawing treatment means discontinuing all care. Some parents feel that discontinuing aggressive treatment is a form of abandonment, and it may lead them to feel as though they contributed to the child's death (Baergen, 2006). The decision to withhold nutrition and hydration is particularly difficult for parents because they often associate the provision of food with nurturing and love. Other treatments, including certain medications, mechanical ventilation, and dialysis, may also be withdrawn if the child's outcome is inevitable death and continuation of the treatment prolongs the dying process or causes more suffering than benefit.

PRACTICE ALERT

Care must be used in how parents are asked to withdraw or forgo therapies. An effective communication strategy is to inform parents that an intervention was initiated to give the child the best chance at recovery, but it has not been effective and is not beneficial for the child. When asking to withhold therapy such as cardiopulmonary resuscitation, it is helpful to indicate that the therapy is not effective in reversing overwhelming illness or brain damage (Levetown, 2005).

The nurse may feel conflicted when parents are unable to discontinue aggressive therapies that the nurse feels are extending the child's suffering. Consultation with the hospital ethics committee can help the nurse clarify issues involved and reduce the emotions associated with the conflict. During the consultation, an unbiased professional collects facts about the child's condition, clarifies the beliefs and values of parents and health professionals, and improves communication while investigating options for compromise (Rushton, 2004). In some cases, the parents may wish to prolong a pain-free dying process until an important family member has had a chance to say good-bye (Jacobs, 2005).

CONFLICTS REGARDING PARENTAL REFUSAL OF TREATMENT Parents and health care providers sometimes disagree over what, if any, medical interventions should be provided when the child is dying. Parents may refuse treatments because of religious convictions or because they wish to avoid prolonging the child's life in order to provide a peaceful death (Institute of Medicine, 2003). Initiating highly technical, but possibly futile, interventions may cause emotional and financial stress that can overwhelm parents.

The health care team may initiate court intervention to appoint a surrogate legal guardian in certain situations when recommended care is refused. Intervention is based on the legal principle that failure to obtain adequate medical care for a child violates state child neglect laws (Institute of Medicine, 2003). The nurse or health care team should also consult with the hospital's ethics committee to help resolve the conflict. The nurse is sometimes in the uncomfortable position of trying to provide care to the infant or child while

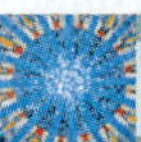

EVIDENCE-BASED PRACTICE Improving the Quality of Pediatric End-of-Life Care in the PICU

Problem

The majority of children who die due to life-limiting conditions die in the hospital setting, often in the pediatric intensive care unit (PICU). Two thirds of deaths in the PICU follow withdrawal of life-sustaining therapies. The parents' perspectives with regard to improving their child's quality of care in this setting are important.

Evidence

A study involving 56 parents of children who had died in the PICU 1–4 years previously focused on their priorities and recommendations for improving quality end-of-life care and communication in the PICU. Six priorities were identified, including honest and complete information, ready access to staff, coordinator of communication and care, emotional expression and support by staff as it conveys caring for the child and family, preservation of the integrity of the parent–child relationship, and faith (Meyer, Ritholz, Burns, & Truog, 2006). Another study was conducted by interviewing 36 parents of children who had died in three hospitals. The interviews addressed what mattered to parents of children with life-threatening conditions. Continuity of care was valued by parents as it resulted in relationships and a sense of their children and themselves being known as individuals. Continuity of care also led to improved communication between the health care providers and parents and to greater confidence of parents in the quality of care their child received (Heller & Solomon, 2005).

Implications

Identifying the specific care valued by parents during this time is important for planning nursing care and multidisciplinary palliative care. Facilitating opportunities for regular communication that include full disclosure of information about the child's condition by a single familiar person may help reduce conflicting information provided by other health care providers and assist with decision making. Additional options of communication such as family conferences, staff-family journals, e-mail, and office hours at the bedside may help improve communication. Planning of care and communication should ensure that family-centered care is integrating values important to the family.

Critical Thinking Application

Consider the special needs of the parents of a newborn with a cardiac congenital anomaly that cannot be corrected by surgery. Identify the most common patterns of communication with family members in the NICU and evaluate their effectiveness in promoting family-centered care and decision making. Suggest two other communication methods that could improve communication with family members and improve the family's perception of care that its newborn receives.

in an adversarial rather than a supportive relationship with the parents. The nurse should demonstrate proper concern and care of the child in these cases and seek support and guidance to work with the family as needed.

DO-NOT-RESUSCITATE ORDERS A physician may ask parents faced with a child's inevitable death as a result of a terminal illness or condition to consider a DNR or **do-not-intubate order (DNI)**, choosing not to resuscitate or take other lifesaving interventions for a child who stops breathing. In some cases the term "allow natural death" may be used. For children with end-stage, irreversible life-limiting conditions, the family and health care providers must decide if a resuscitation attempt would be in the child's best interest. Factors influencing the decision for a DNR or DNI status include allowing the child to die with dignity and the possibility of causing more harm and suffering if resuscitative measures are implemented. Parents require ongoing support as they may feel they are "giving up" on their child. When an adolescent is the client, the adolescent should be involved in discussions and have a role in decision making.

When faced with the decision of requesting a DNR or DNI for its child, the family requires honest information. It is essential that the family understand that the child will continue to receive further care or interventions such as oxygen, suctioning, pain control, and supportive nursing care in the presence of a DNR order. If a child with a DNR order requires anesthesia or surgery, a discussion of the DNR order should occur when obtaining informed consent for the procedure. Parents may choose to temporarily suspend the DNR order or to keep it active during the perioperative period, and their wishes should be respected (Fallat, Deshpande, & Section on Surgery, 2004).

CLINICAL MANIFESTATIONS

Although each person responds differently, certain manifestations are common in the dying process regardless of the pathology causing death. Most manifestations are related to changes in four main areas: loss of muscle tone, slowing of circulation, changes in respirations, and changes in sensory impairments. Manifestations of dying and impending death are discussed in more complete detail in Concept 12, Exemplar 12.2, Death and Dying.

In many cases, the client and family choose palliative care, and the nurse's primary responsibility is to ensure that the client is as comfortable as possible, physically, mentally, emotionally, and spiritually. Box 5–14 lists caring interventions that provide physical comfort to clients nearing death.

COLLABORATION

As discussed previously, a great deal of collaboration is required when caring for the client at the end of life. Nurses have responsibility for notifying both physicians and family members of changes in client symptoms that may signal a need for a change in the care plan, be it simple, such as an order for a change in pain medication, or more complex, such as the need for a decision regarding artificial nutrition and hydration. Regardless of the decisions of the client and family, the nurse has an ethical responsibility to provide comfort to the client during this time.

Clinical Therapies to Prolong Life

The decision to use clinical therapies such as feeding tubes and cardiopulmonary resuscitation at the end of life can be a difficult one for both the client and family members. Nurses

CLINICAL MANIFESTATIONS AND THERAPIES End-of-Life Care

ETIOLOGY	CLINICAL MANIFESTATIONS	CLINICAL THERAPIES
Loss of muscle tone	■ Relaxation of facial muscles ■ Difficulty speaking, swallowing ■ Decreased gastrointestinal activity ■ Retention of feces ■ Decreased sphincter control as evidenced by incontinence ■ Diminished movement	■ Treatment is palliative and aimed at maintaining client comfort and hygiene. ■ Assure ability to swallow without aspirating before offering food and fluids. ■ Provide support for family members grief.
Slowing of circulation	■ Diminished sensation ■ Cyanosis of the extremities ■ Slower and weaker pulse ■ Decreased blood pressure	■ Treatment is palliative to maintain comfort. ■ Provide support for family members grief.
Changes in respiration	■ Rapid, shallow, irregular or abnormally slow respiration ■ Noisy breathing (the "death rattle") ■ Mouth breathing ■ Dry oral mucous membranes	■ Treatment is palliative to maintain comfort. ■ Provide support for family members grief.
Sensory impairments	■ Blurred vision ■ Impaired taste and smell	■ Treatment is palliative to maintain comfort. ■ Provide support for family members grief.

Box 5–14 Providing Comfort for the Client Nearing Death

- Maintain clean skin and bed linens.
- Use a draw sheet to turn the client as often as possible so the client is comfortable.
- Position the client to promote comfort and protect bony areas with padding. Reposition the client and raise the head of the bed if fluids accumulate in the upper airways and back of the throat.
- Use bed pads or insert a Foley catheter (if ordered) for urinary incontinence.
- Use gentle massage to improve circulation and shift edema.
- Provide small, frequent sips of fluids, ice chips, or Popsicles.
- Provide oral care using a soft moist brush or glycerin swab.
- Clean secretions from the eyes and nose.
- Administer ordered pain medications as needed to maintain comfort.
- Administer oxygen as prescribed to relieve dyspnea.

must be able to communicate the nature of these interventions, their purposes, and how they may or may not impact the client's health.

USE OF FEEDING TUBES FOR ARTIFICIAL NUTRITION AND HYDRATION Clients with multiple comorbidities, cognitive deficits, and life-limiting, progressive illness often experience decreased appetite with loss of interest in eating and drinking and subsequent weight loss (HPNA, 2003a). Dysphagia related to advancing dementia or terminal illness may contribute to this issue. As clients near the end of life, most will be unable or will refuse to take food and fluids by mouth (HPNA, 2003a). These changes can cause distress, especially for families and other caregivers, and may lead to questions about artificial nutrition and hydration (ANH).

The decision to institute ANH should take into account possible benefits and risks. ANH traditionally has been assumed to meet several therapeutic goals: prolong life, prevent aspiration pneumonia and "starvation," maintain independence and physical function, improve nutritional status, assist in healing of pressure ulcers, and decrease suffering and discomfort at the end of life (HPNA, 2003a; Lacey, 2005). These goals, however, are not supported in the literature. Studies have shown that long-term care facility residents living with feeding tubes have survival rates similar to those of residents living without, and aspiration rates are higher in clients with feeding tubes (Lacey, 2005). Furthermore, artificial nutrition and nutritional supplements do not enhance frail clients' strength and physical function (ELNEC, 2006; Hallenbeck, 2005; HPNA, 2003a). Also contrary to expectations, most actively dying clients do not experience hunger even if they have inadequate caloric intake. In fact, risks such as increased infection, sensory deprivation, and restraint use have led researchers and palliative care experts to discourage the use of feeding tubes in dying clients and those with advanced dementia. Collaboration with other health care professionals (nutritionists and speech therapists) is indicated to explore alternatives to artificial nutrition techniques.

Adult clients who feel strongly that they do not want tube feedings should inform their health care surrogates and specify this wish in their living wills. Administration of ANH is considered a medical treatment and thus can be accepted or rejected by the client. This right reflects respect for client autonomy. Client teaching regarding the risks involved with the use of feeding tubes may be beneficial for family members who do not understand that withholding nutrition will not result in pain or discomfort to the client.

CARDIOPULMONARY RESUSCITATION Cardiopulmonary resuscitation (CPR) is administered to a person experiencing cardiac or respiratory arrest; simply put, it is the process of restarting the heartbeat and/or breathing after one or both have stopped. This intervention is most successful when it occurs in the hospital, specifically in the ICU. However, when the client is frail, has multiple chronic conditions, and is nearing the end of life, CPR is significantly less effective. Several studies have demonstrated that attempts at resuscitation in long-term care residents are rarely successful (Gordon, 2003). The decision to designate a client with a DNR order is usually made by the client, his or her family, the nurse, physician, and others on the health care team. In most health care facilities, the physician or primary health care provider must write the DNR order in the chart for it to be legal; if no order is written, CPR must be administered by default if the need arises. It can be very upsetting for the nurse to provide CPR to the ill client, who may suffer injury from anoxia, broken ribs, and aspiration.

When the nurse approaches the client and the family for clarification of the client's code status, it is best to discuss the issue as fully and objectively as possible. Facts should be presented with empathy and by conveyance of the idea that the nurse will support whatever reasonable decision is made. This conversation should be part of an ongoing discussion of the client's wishes and goals for end-of-life care. According to the ANA, "the efficacy and desirability of CPR attempts, a balancing of benefits and burdens to the client, and therapeutic goals should be considered" (ANA, 2003a, p. 1). The nurse should emphasize that the decision not to resuscitate is not condemning that person to die. Rather, the nurse is helping the person decide whether medical intervention might reverse the death process and even prohibit a peaceful death. The process of letting go may be painful for both the client and the family.

The Use of Complementary and Alternative Medicine in Palliative Care

A number of complimentary and alternative therapies may provide comfort to the dying client. A study conducted at 15 U.S. hospice organizations and funded in part by the National Center for Complementary and Alternative Medicine found that massage and touch therapy provided significant relief for cancer clients receiving treatment through those hospices. Clients reported significant relief in areas of pain, physical and emotional distress, and quality of life. Greater relief was experienced by the clients who received massage therapy than by those who received touch therapy (Kutner J, Smith M, Corbin S, et al., 2008).

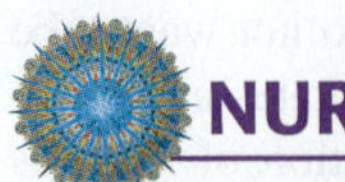

NURSING PROCESS

Assessment

End-of-life assessments involve determining the client's state of awareness about her or his condition; assessing for signs of approaching death; assessing the client's needs for spiritual and emotional comfort; assessing the client's DNR and health care proxy status.

State of Awareness

In cases of terminal illness, the nurse needs to assess the state of awareness shared by the dying person and the family. This affects the nurse's ability to communicate freely with clients and other health care team members and to assist in the grieving process. Three types of awareness that have been described are closed awareness, mutual pretense, and open awareness (Glaser & Strauss, 1965).

In **closed awareness**, the client is not made aware of impending death. The family members may choose this because they do not completely understand why the client is ill or they believe the client will recover. The primary care provider may believe it is best not to communicate a diagnosis or prognosis to the client. Nursing personnel are confronted with an ethical problem in this situation. See Concept 42 for further information on ethical dilemmas.

With **mutual pretense**, the client, family, and health care personnel know that the prognosis is terminal but do not talk about it and make an effort not to raise the subject. Sometimes the client refrains from discussing death to protect the family from distress. The client may also sense discomfort on the part of health care personnel and therefore not bring up the subject. Mutual pretense permits the client a degree of privacy and dignity, but it places a heavy burden on the dying person, who then has no one in whom to confide.

With **open awareness**, the client and others know about the impending death and feel comfortable discussing it, even though it is difficult. This awareness provides the client an opportunity to finalize affairs and even participate in planning funeral arrangements.

Not all people are comfortable with open awareness. Some believe that terminal clients acquire knowledge of their condition even if they are not directly informed. Others believe that clients remain unaware of their condition until the end. It is difficult, however, to distinguish what clients know from what they are willing to accept or acknowledge.

Approaching Death

Nursing care and support for the dying client and family include making an accurate assessment of the physiological signs of approaching death. In addition to signs related to the client's specific disease, certain other physical signs are indicative of impending death. The four main characteristic changes the nurse should assess are as follows:

1. *Loss of Muscle Tone.* Relaxation of the facial muscles (e.g., the client's jaw may sag); difficulty speaking; difficulty swallowing and gradual loss of the gag reflex; decreased activity of the gastrointestinal tract, with subsequent nausea; accumulation of flatus; abdominal distention; retention of feces, especially if narcotics or tranquilizers are being administered; possible urinary and rectal incontinence due to decreased sphincter control; diminished body movement.
2. *Slowing of the Circulation.* Diminished sensation; mottling and cyanosis of the extremities; cold skin, first in the feet and later in the hands, ears, and nose (the client, however, may be warm if he or she has a fever); slower and weaker pulse; decreased blood pressure.
3. *Changes in Respirations.* Rapid, shallow, irregular, or abnormally slow respirations; noisy breathing, referred to as the death rattle, due to mucus collecting in the throat; mouth breathing, dry oral mucous membranes.
4. *Changes in Sensory Impairment.* Blurred vision; impaired senses of taste and smell.

Various consciousness levels may exist just before death. Some clients are alert, whereas others are drowsy, stuporous, or comatose. Hearing is thought to be the last sense lost.

Assessing for Spiritual and Emotional Comfort

The spiritual and emotional comfort of the dying client and family is an essential part of end-of-life care. Whether the client is in a long-term care facility, a hospital, a hospice center, or at home, the client needs to have things around which he or she finds comforting. These may include pictures of family, drawings made by children or grandchildren, religious icons, prayer books, plants, a CD or other music player, books, whatever items are comforting to the client. The nurse should work with the family to determine what will provide emotional and spiritual comfort to the client.

Assessment Interview The Comfort of the Dying Client

Ask the client, or if the client cannot respond, ask the spouse, partner, or significant others:

- What kinds of things did the client like to do before becoming ill?
- What daily routines did the client observe at home before becoming ill?
- What family members are the client closest to? Are there any pictures of those family members which we can place in the room?
- Is there a family member who cannot come to visit with whom the client would like to speak to by phone every day?
- Does the client observe specific prayer times? Is there a family minister or religious leader you would like to have visit?
- Is there a DNR order or health care surrogate?
- Is there anyone you would like us to contact now or when death occurs?

Diagnosis

A variety of nursing diagnoses may be appropriate for the client who is nearing death. These may include:

- Acute or Chronic Pain
- Death Anxiety
- Risk for Caregiver Role Strain
- Compromised Family Coping.

Plan

The nursing plan of care will be written in consultation with the client and support people. Appropriate goals of nursing care often include:

- Maintain client comfort
- Support family members and loved ones as they grieve
- Maintain client hygiene
- Prevent complications such as pressure ulcers or loss of skin integrity
- Support and comfort client to reduce fear and anxiety related to death.

Implementation

The nurse caring for the client at the end of life is responsible for providing a number of caring interventions in accordance with the care plan. While these will always be individualized, it is reasonable for the nurse to expect to address client pain, death anxiety, and compromised family coping during the course of caring for the client.

Acute or Chronic Pain

- Monitor manifestations of pain by taking vital signs; assessing skin temperature and moisture; observing pupils; observing facial expressions, position in bed, guarding of body parts; and noting restlessness. Autonomic responses to pain may result in increased blood pressure, tachycardia, rapid respirations, perspiration, and dilated pupils. Other responses to pain include grimacing, clenching the hands, muscle rigidity, guarding, restlessness, and nausea.
- Use an appropriate assessment instrument (such as those provided in the Exemplar 5.1 or in the skills manual) to assess the client's pain. Use the same assessment consistently.
- Communicate belief in the client's pain by verbally acknowledging the presence of the pain, listening carefully to the description of pain, and acting to help the client manage the pain. Because pain is a personal, subjective experience, the nurse must convey belief in the client's pain. By conveying belief in the client's pain, the nurse reduces anxiety and thereby lessens pain.
- Provide optimal pain relief with prescribed analgesics, determining the preferred route of administration. Provide pain-relieving measures for severe pain on a regular around-the-clock basis or by self-administration, such as with a client-controlled analgesia (PCA) pump. The client should be part of the decision-making process and allowed to exert some control over the situation by choosing the administration route as long as the client remains competent. Analgesics are usually most effective when they are administered before pain occurs or becomes severe.

Death Anxiety

Death anxiety is worry or fear related to death or dying. It may be present in clients who have an acute life-threatening illness, who have a terminal illness, who have experienced the death of a family member or friend, or who have experienced multiple deaths in the same family.

- Explore the client's knowledge of the situation. For example, ask, "What has your doctor told you about your condition?" This informs you of the client's knowledge base about the condition and about his or her ability to make informed decisions.
- Ask the client to identify specific fears about death. This provides data about any unrealistic expectations or misperceptions.
- Determine the client's perceptions of strengths and weaknesses in coping with death. Identifying past strengths can help the client cope with loss, illness, and death.
- Ask the client to identify areas in which the client needs help. This determines whether available resources are adequate.
- Encourage independence and control in decisions about treatment and care. This promotes self-esteem, decreases feelings of powerlessness, and allows the client to retain dignity in dying.
- Facilitate access to culturally appropriate spiritual rituals and practices. This provides spiritual comfort.
- Explain advance directives and assist with them if necessary. Advance directives help ensure that the client's wishes for end-of-life care are carried out.
- Encourage life review and reminiscence. Life review is self-affirming.
- Encourage activities such as listening to music, aromatherapy, massage, or relaxation exercises. These activities decrease anxiety.
- Suggest keeping a journal or leaving a written legacy. A written document provides continuing support to others after death.

Compromised Family Coping

The death of a family member can cause great disruption in a family, particularly the death of a child or the death of a parent who has young children. By providing comfort, information, and referral for the family of a dying client, nurses strengthen the family's ability to cope with the death.

- Dying parents may ask the nurse about leaving memories for their child. Suggestions that the nurse could offer include making videos for the child to watch at special occasions, such as birthdays and high school graduation, or writing letters or birthday cards for the child to read at those times.
- Refer family members to the local hospice provider or another organization that supports dying families. These organizations offer support groups for family members who

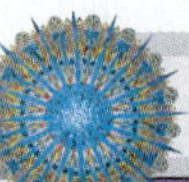

NURSING CARE PLAN The Client at the End of Life

ASSESSMENT

Tom Crandall is a 75-year-old man with advanced Alzheimer's disease. Three weeks ago, he became very agitated and began having difficulty swallowing. He was transferred from his assisted living facility to a hospital with a psychiatric gerontology unit. Once transferred, Mr. Crandall experienced a steady decline in health, and he was transferred to the acute care area of the facility after experiencing a major stroke. He is arousable, but seems unaware of his surroundings. He is currently receiving oxygen via a face mask and enteral nutrition. The treating physician has called his family and asked them to come to the hospital, advising that Mr. Crandall is unlikely to live much longer.

DIAGNOSES

- Risk for Impaired Skin Integrity
- Ineffective Breathing Pattern
- Ineffective Peripheral Tissue Perfusion

PLANNING

The nursing plan of care includes the following goals:

- Maintain client comfort
- Support family grieving process
- Prevent or minimize alteration of skin integrity
- Meet client's hygiene needs.

IMPLEMENTATION

The nurses caring for Mr. Crandall implement the following interventions:

- Reposition Mr. Crandall every 2 hours to prevent pressure ulcers and promote tissue perfusion.
- Administer medications as ordered.
- Bathe client and change linen as needed to maintain client comfort.
- Provide oral care every 2 hours.
- Encourage family to express feelings about client's terminal condition.
- Prepare family for signs and symptoms of impending death.

EVALUATION

Shortly after the family's arrival Mr. Crandall died with family members surrounding him. He died peacefully with a gradual decrease in respirations and heart rate without regaining consciousness. His family members expressed appreciation that they had the opportunity to tell him they loved him one last time.

CRITICAL THINKING

1. When the nurses were checking Mr. Crandall's blood pressure he would cry out as if in pain. How would you direct the nursing staff to respond to this finding?
2. What recommendation or request would you make of the provider regarding Mr. Crandall's tube feedings? Explain your answer.
3. Mr. Crandall's daughter asks if he will be placed on a mechanical ventilator to support his breathing. How would you respond to this question?

have lost a spouse, parents who have lost a child, and therapy services for children who have lost a sibling or parent.

- Assist the primary caregiver of the dying client at home to arrange for respite services. Friends, church members, volunteer organizations, and home health organizations are all sources of assistance for running errands or for sitting with the dying client while the caregiver gets some rests or attends to personal needs.
- Refer the family to resources for financial support as necessary.

Evaluation

Client care is evaluated based on the following expected outcomes:

- Client's comfort is maintained throughout the dying process.
- Client is supported by nursing and/or family presence at time of death.
- Family members are informed and prepared for client's dying process.

REVIEW End-of-Life Care

RELATE: LINK THE CONCEPTS

Linking the exemplar of End-of-Life Care with the concept of Family:

1. What is the priority nursing diagnoses for the family of the client with a terminal illness requiring end of life care?
2. What teaching points would you provide the family of a terminal client regarding end of life care?

Linking the exemplar of End-of-Life Care with the concept of Grief and Loss:

3. How can the nurse support the family's need to prepare for loss of a family member while meeting the client's need for end-of-life care?
4. Describe your plan of care for helping the family of a terminal school-age child provide end-of-life care for the child while meeting its need to grieve.

READY: GO TO COMPANION SKILLS MANUAL

- Meeting the physiologic needs of the dying client
- Performing postmortem care
- Assessing the client in pain
- Administering a tube feeding
- Providing total parental nutrition

REFER: GO TO MYNURSINGKIT

REFLECT: CASE STUDY

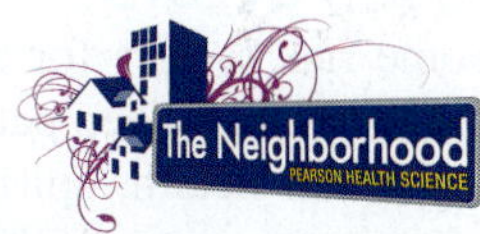

Pam Allen is a middle-aged woman who recently experienced a recurrence of colon cancer. She is dying. Pam and her husband, Clifford, have elected for Pam to stay at home. Her health care team includes a hospice nurse, a social worker, and her treating physician. Friends and church members have been bringing food for the Allen family, and Clifford has discussed his fears about Pam's death with the social worker.

Pam has had very little to eat or drink this week and is rarely urinating. The hospice nurse notices that she has abdominal fullness (ascites) due to the accumulation of fluid in the peritoneal cavity and appears more jaundiced. Her pain continues. She is agitated and has difficulty speaking. At today's visit, the hospice nurse records the following vital signs: 98_R degrees F – 99-30 (shallow) 100/66

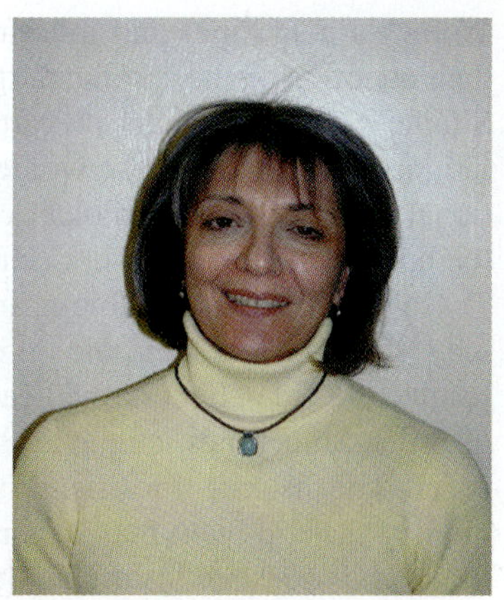

1. What is the priority of care for Pam on this visit?
2. Based on the current assessment, what information would you provide Clifford?
3. Would you consider notifying the physician of current findings? Why or why not?

5.3 FATIGUE

KEY TERMS

Acute fatigue, *301*
Chronic fatigue, *301*
Chronic fatigue syndrome, *302*
Fatigue, *301*

BASIS FOR SELECTION AS EXEMPLAR

Centers for Disease Control and Prevention

LEARNING OUTCOMES

After reading about this exemplar, you will be able to:

1. Describe the pathophysiology, etiology, clinical manifestations, and direct and indirect causes of fatigue.
2. Identify risk factors associated with fatigue.
3. Illustrate the nursing process in providing culturally competent care across the life span for individuals with fatigue.
4. Formulate priority nursing diagnoses appropriate for an individual with fatigue.
5. Create a plan of care for individuals with fatigue and their family members.
6. Assess expected outcomes for an individual with fatigue.
7. Discuss therapies used in the collaborative care of an individual with fatigue.
8. Employ evidence-bases caring interventions for an individual with fatigue.

OVERVIEW

Fatigue is characterized by a lack of energy and motivation that may or may not be accompanied by drowsiness. Fatigue is subjective, in that what causes the feeling of weariness in one individual may not be perceived in the same way by another person. One's perception of fatigue is influenced by culture and by the capacity to carry out expected or required daily activities (ELNEC, 2006).

Think back to a time when you considered yourself to be fatigued. How would you describe it? What cultural impacts informed your perception? What caused the perceived fatigue? How did it impact how your thoughts, actions, interactions with others? What relieved the fatigue? As an advocate for clients, you should strive for self-awareness about the reality of fatigue and its potential impact on quality of life.

PATHOPHYSIOLOGY AND ETIOLOGY

Fatigue is normally a symptom of other conditions and illnesses. It may result from a variety of causes, including the following:

- Chronic illness
- Life-threatening illness or injury
- Sleep disturbances (e.g., insomnia)
- Pain
- Grief or anxiety
- Side effects of medication
- Autoimmune disorders
- Chronic lung disorders.

When one is fatigued, the body's reserves of energy are exhausted on either a short-term or long-term basis. Often the tissues of the body are not receiving the oxygen and nourishment needed to carry on the activities of daily life at the "normal" or expected level. An individual may have fatigue as a result of excessive physical work, such as a construction worker might experience; as a result of mental overload, such as an English teacher grading papers might experience; as a result of profound illness, such as a cancer client may experience; or as a result of a combination of stressors and insufficient sleep, such as a working mother with a sick child might experience.

Acute fatigue can result from a variety of causes. Sleep deprivation, regardless of cause, sensory overload, acute or chronic illness, and acute or chronic pain are just a few of the many etiologies of acute fatigue. Acute fatigue normally resolves on treatment of the underlying cause. For example, nursing students may find themselves experience acute fatigue during exam week. This type of fatigue is normally resolved the first weekend following the conclusion of exams.

Chronic fatigue normally results from an ongoing illness, condition, or situation that may not be resolved quickly.

Women's magazines and morning television frequently focus their attention on the chronic fatigue that working mothers face. Single working mothers in particular are at risk for chronic fatigue. For most of these women, fatigue resolves with additional support, such as an older child being able to help around the house, or a flexible work schedule. (See Box 5–15.)

Clients with chronic illness, and often their family members, may struggle with chronic fatigue. Sometimes this fatigue results as a side effect of medications used to treat the primary disorder. Sometimes fatigue is associated directly with the disorder. This is true for clients with chronic obstructive pulmonary disease, who may experience periods of hypercapnia, in which tissues are insufficiently supplied with oxygen.

Chronic fatigue which is not associated with another primary disorder and which is unresolved by sufficient rest may be the result of chronic fatigue syndrome.

Chronic Fatigue Syndrome

Chronic fatigue syndrome is an unexplained persistent or recurring chronic fatigue that is not alleviated by substantial rest and that greatly impacts the client's levels of activity in all area. To be diagnosed with chronic fatigue syndrome, four or more of the following symptoms must have persisted or recurred for a period of six or more consecutive months:

- Substantial impairment of short-term memory or concentration
- Sore throat
- Multiple-joint pain absent the presence of edema
- Muscle pain
- Tender lymph nodes
- Unrefreshing sleep
- Postactivity malaise lasting more than 24 hours.

Chronic fatigue syndrome may not be diagnosed without ruling out a number of other illnesses for which fatigue is a primary manifestation. These include untreated hypothyroidism, major depressive disorders, eating disorders, sleep apnea, narcolepsy, dementias, and the side effects of medications. Severe obesity also excludes a diagnosis of chronic fatigue syndrome.

Box 5–15 Behaviors and Conditions That Contribute to Women's Fatigue

- *Crash dieting* can result in poor nutrition and contribute to lethargy. Combining a crash diet with water pills or diuretics can result in hypokalemia, even to life-threatening levels.
- *High-fat, low-carb* diets contribute to fatigue. Complex carbohydrates are needed for energy. Whole grains, lean meats and fish, and lots of fruits and vegetables are best.
- *Hypoactive thyroid* can result in fatigue. Women comprise 70% of the population with underactive thyroids.
- *Anxiety* may result in a number of sleepless nights. Women who find themselves worrying to the extent that they cannot fall asleep at night, or that they wake up in the middle of the night and cannot go back to sleep, should seek professional help for their anxiety.

Source: Adapted from P. Leider. (2006). When women's fatigue signals danger. Retrieved August 15, 2009 from http://www.cbsnews.com/stories/2006/01/30/earlyshow/health/main1259346.shtml?tag=contentMain;contentBody

Risk Factors

Some risk factors for acute fatigue include less than optimal lifestyle (poor sleep patterns, poor nutrition, too much activity, emotional health, spiritual health), exposure to extreme elements, surgery, and infection.

Risk factors for chronic fatigue include chronic diseases (such as cancer, congestive heart failure, blood dyscrasias, advanced renal disease, rheumatoid arthritis, HIV/AIDS, coronary artery disease), disability, extensive and long-term medication regimens, radiation therapy, chemotherapy, and delay in addressing symptoms of distress.

Chronic fatigue syndrome may follow a cold, influenza, bronchitis, mononucleosis, or develop gradually without a clear initiating event. Approximately 500,000 people in the United States are affected each year. Since the majority of those affected are well-educated white females from the upper middle socioeconomic stratum, the syndrome was initially called "yuppie flu." It is currently believed that causes may be genetic, environmental, viral, transient trauma, toxins, and/or stress.

CLINICAL MANIFESTATIONS

Clinical manifestations may include changes from baseline vital signs, electrolyte imbalances, pallor, pale conjunctiva, stooped posture and slow gait, decreased cognition, flat to depressed affect, lack of energy, change in muscle tone, and dyspnea upon mild exertion. However, the best indicator is the client's subjective comments of tiredness, weakness, exhaustion, and/or weariness.

COLLABORATION

The simplest fatigues are resolved with sufficient sleep. Fatigues with a more complicated etiology, such as fatigue related to anemia or depression, require a supportive health care team to help the client resolve his or her fatigue. For the client whose fatigue stems from lack of sleep due to depression or anxiety, counseling and behavior therapy may help the client improve coping mechanisms and acquire improved sleep hygiene in order to improve sleep. Other clients may benefit from diagnostic testing to determine if there is an underlying biological etiology that may explain the client's fatigue.

Diagnostic Tests

Diagnostic tests are often ordered to find the underlying cause of fatigue and can include virtually any test. However, typical labs to determine the cause of fatigue fall into the following classifications:

1. Oxygenation status (pulse oximetry; arterial blood gases, pulmonary function studies, chest x-ray, or ventilation-perfusion studies)
2. Oxygen-carrying status (hemoglobin; hematocrit, red blood cell count)
3. Metabolism function (thyroid studies, blood glucose, or catecholamine levels).

CLINICAL MANIFESTATIONS AND THERAPIES Fatigue

ETIOLOGY	CLINICAL MANIFESTATION	CLINICAL THERAPIES
Anemia	■ Mild anemia, typically asymptomatic ■ Moderate anemia exhibiting as fatigue, pale skin and mucous membranes ■ Severe anemia may result in shortness of breath, dizziness, orthostatic hypotension, activity intolerance, hypoxia	Therapies depend on cause of anemia but may include: ■ Hydration ■ Nutrition supplements ■ Decreased activity levels ■ Fall prevention ■ Monitoring of vital signs, hemoglobin, and hematocrit ■ Nutrition counseling.
Anxiety	■ Insomnia ■ Hypersomnia ■ Restlessness ■ Irritability ■ Diminished appetite ■ Activity intolerance ■ Depression, ineffective coping	■ Improved sleep hygiene ■ Pharmacological sleeping aids ■ Relaxation techniques ■ Graded exercise program
Pain	■ Nausea and vomiting ■ Restlessness ■ Elevated blood pressure ■ Irritability ■ Insufficient sleep	■ Treatment of underlying cause of pain ■ Pharmacological pain management ■ CAM therapies, including massage, acupuncture

Pharmacologic Therapies

The pharmacological interventions vary depending on the root cause of the fatigue. For example, a client with marked iron-deficiency anemia may receive erythropoietin. Erythropoietin can increase the hemoglobin level and produce positive effects on energy, activity, and quality of life. However, for the client suffering from depression and sleep deprivation fatigue, a tricyclic antidepressant such as nortriptyline can improve sleep, thus reducing fatigue.

Other pharmacological interventions include stimulants that increase appetite and energy levels; selective serotonin reuptake inhibitors, which improve sleep and decrease anxiety and pain; and pain medications.

Nonpharmacologic Therapies

A variety of nonpharmalogic therapies may benefit the client struggling with fatigue. Nurses should assist the client to determine his or her "best" time of day to engage in activities.

MEDICATIONS Fatigue

Class of Drug	Examples	Mechanism of Action	Comments
Stimulants	Methylphenidate	Stimulate CNS and respiratory centers, increases appetite and energy levels, improves mood, reduces sedation.	Starting dose 1.5–10 mg q am and 12 noon, titrate to effect
Antidepressants		Reduce depressive symptoms associated with fatigue. Can improve sleep. Primary choice for treatment of depression in cancer clients.	
Selective serotonin reuptake inhibitors (SSRIs)	Paroxetine Fluoxetine	Inhibit serotonin reuptake.	Some SSRIs have long half-lives and should be used cautiously in the terminally ill.
Tricyclic antidepressants	Desipramine Nortriptyline	Block reuptake of various neurotransmitters at the neuronal membrane. Can improve sleep.	Starting dose 10–25 mg qhs
Erythropoietin		Increase hemoglobin with effects on energy, activity and overall quality of life while decreasing transfusion requirements.	150 units/kg sq q 3 times a week

Source: Adapted from American Association of Colleges of Nursing and the City of Hope National Medical Center. (2000). Pharmacologic treatments for fatigue, In Module 3: Symptom Management module. *The End-of-Life Nursing Education Consortium (ELNEC) – Core Training Curriculum.* Duarte, CA: Authors. Used with Permission.

If the client is a morning person, for example, the client may benefit from engaging in more challenging activities during the morning, and reserving other periods of the day for more enjoyable activities and rest periods. Graded exercise programs, where the client gradually builds stamina for exercise, may be helpful. Physical therapy and occupational therapy can help the client improve strength and stamina. In addition, the therapists may be helpful in assisting the client to identify activities that he or she enjoys enough to engage in on a regular basis. Improved sleep hygiene, which is discuss in detail in Exemplar 5.5, may also help the client get more and better rest.

Complementary and Alternative Medicine

Complementary and alternative medicine provides a number of techniques that can help clients relax and get more and better rest. Massage, acupuncture, hydrotherapy, aromatherapy, relaxation techniques, and calming herbs can all benefit the client struggling with fatigue. Clients attempting to use herbal remedies need to be aware of possible contraindications. Chamomile tea, for example, is a popular tea to drink at bedtime, but is contraindicated for clients with ragweed allergies. Nurses should ask all clients struggling with fatigue about complementary and nonpharmacological therapies that they are using.

NURSING PROCESS

An important component to treating a client with fatigue is determining the underlying cause. Thorough assessment of the client's symptoms along with measures to promote rest are priority areas of focus.

Assessment

Assessment of the client complaining of fatigue involves a physical examination and health history. As part of the health history, the nurse may ask the following questions:

1. Are you feeling weak, tired, or wiped out?
2. How long does it last?
3. Is there a pattern?
4. How does your fatigue affect your normal activities of daily living? Your relationships with family members?
5. Is there a part of your body that feels more tired than another?
6. What medications are you taking? Have you been taking any medications to help you sleep? If so, do these have any effect?
7. Do you feel anxious or depressed?
8. Do you have difficulty concentrating?
9. Do you have any preexisting conditions?

As part of the physical examination, the nurse will assess the following:

1. *Vital signs:* fever, increased pulse rate, weak pulse are indicators of stress and potential for fatigue.
2. *Client mobility*: nausea and/or dyspnea upon exertion indicate stress and potential for fatigue.
3. *Hydration status:* poor skin turgor and/or lowered blood pressure indicate poor hydration and potential for fatigue.
4. *Muscle strength, symmetry, and endurance:* deficits indicate muscular, skeletal, and/or nervous system challenges and potential for fatigue.

Diagnosis

Diagnoses will be made depending on the cause of the client's fatigue. The client with chronic fatigue syndrome may be experiencing great difficulty with ADLs, to the point that he or she may be at risk in other health areas. Some appropriate diagnoses may be the following:

- Fatigue
- Activity Intolerance
- Ineffective Self Health Management
- Disturbed Sleep Pattern
- Readiness for Enhanced Self Care
- Ineffective Coping.

Plan

An appropriate plan of care, made in collaboration with the client, may include the following goals of care:

- The client will be able to explain the importance of bedtime rituals and good sleep hygiene and create a bedtime routine to promote rest.
- The client will make changes in daily routine for periods of rest.
- The client will experience improvement in duration and quality of sleep.
- The client will optimize ability to perform ADLs.

Implementation

When implementing care to reduce fatigue, it is important to consider the client's cultural and developmental needs regarding sleep rituals. Fatigue is a subjective symptom so careful attention must be given to clients' assessment of how they are feeling.

Ineffective Coping

- Assess the client's social support network and usual methods of coping. This will help both the nurse and the client identify people and mechanisms that can help the client cope more effectively with the disease.
- Support the client's social network. When the nurse expresses confidence and support in the client's social network, the client will feel more confident about asking for support from the network.
- Encourage client involvement in making care decisions. This gives the client a greater sense of self-worth and control over the situation, increasing coping abilities.
- Assist the client in setting both short-term and long-term goals. Short-term goals allow the client to feel a sense of pride in accomplishments made early in the healing process, while long-term goals give the client something greater to work toward.

Evaluation

Evaluations are conducted at intervals from subjective data (how the client feels) and objective data (vital signs back to baseline, activity without dyspnea, nutritional status, normal lab results). The return of capacity in meeting demands of activities of daily living indicates abatement of fatigue.

Note that for chronic fatigue syndrome, although antiviral, antidepressant, and immune modulators have been tried, little effect has been noted. Instead, interventions to control the symptoms are ordered. Such interventions include nonsteroidal anti-inflammatory drugs (NSAIDs) to decrease body aches and fever and nonsedating antihistamines to relieve allergy symptoms. Nonpharmacological interventions include a well-balanced diet (avoiding sugar, caffeine, alcohol, tobacco); nighttime sleep free from interruptions (avoiding daytime naps); family support; massage; imagery; and graded exercise.

REVIEW Fatigue

RELATE: LINK TO CONCEPTS

Linking the exemplar of Fatigue with the concept of Infection:

1. How does infection and/or inflammation put a person at risk for fatigue?
2. Is fatigue more likely to be acute or chronic as the result of infection?

Linking the exemplar of Fatigue with the concept of Oxygenation:

3. How does uncontrolled asthma put a client at risk for fatigue?
4. What strategies could the asthmatic client use to decrease risk for fatigue?

REFER: GO TO MYNURSINGKIT

REFLECT: CASE STUDY

Mr. Joe Harmon is an 82-year-old man of Asian heritage. He is a World War II Army Air Force veteran who suffered a massive anteroseptal myocardial infarction (MI) at the age of 57. His MI was secondary to brown lung disease. Since the age of 57, he has been hospitalized three times for chronic obstructive pulmonary disease (COPD) and for congestive heart failure (CHF). His skin color is ruddy, his conjunctiva is pale pink, he walks with a stooped posture, and he experiences dyspnea after walking 100 feet. He states that he feels "OK, just tired most of the time."

1. When obtaining Mr. Harmon's vital signs what readings would you anticipate?
2. What diagnostic tests do you anticipate might be useful to determine the cause of Mr Harmon's fatigue?
3. What nursing diagnoses would be appropriate for Mr. Harmon's plan of care?
4. Develop a teaching plan to discuss with Mr. Harmon and his wife.

5.4 FIBROMYALGIA

KEY TERM

Fibromyalgia, *305*
Tender points, *305*

BASIS FOR SELECTION OF EXEMPLAR

Chronic Disease Management

LEARNING OUTCOMES

After reading about this exemplar, you will be able to:

1. Describe the pathophysiology, etiology, clinical manifestations, and direct and indirect causes of fibromyalgia.
2. Identify risk factors associated with fibromyalgia.
3. Illustrate the nursing process in providing culturally competent care across the life span for individuals with fibromyalgia.
4. Formulate priority nursing diagnoses appropriate for an individual with fibromyalgia.
5. Create a plan of care for individuals with fibromyalgia and their family members.
6. Assess expected outcomes for an individual with fibromyalgia.
7. Discuss therapies used in the collaborative care of an individual with fibromyalgia.
8. Employ evidenced-based caring interventions for an individual with fibromyalgia.

OVERVIEW

Fibromyalgia is a common rheumatic syndrome characterized by musculoskeletal pain, stiffness, and multiple **tender points**, tenderness that occurs in precise, localized areas, particularly in the neck, spine, shoulders, and hips. Fibromyalgia affects more than 6 million Americans, 90% of them women between 20 and 50 years of age (National Fibromyalgia Research Association, 2004). The cause is unknown, but possible etiologies include sleep disorders, depression, infections, and an altered perception of normal stimuli. Fibromyalgia can be a complication of hypothyroidism, rheumatoid arthritis, or (in men) sleep apnea. It closely resembles chronic fatigue syndrome, except that musculoskeletal pain is predominant in fibromyalgia, whereas fatigue is a more significant feature of chronic fatigue syndrome.

PATHOPHYSIOLOGY AND ETIOLOGY

No inflammatory, structural, or physiological muscle changes have been demonstrated in fibromyalgia. A connection between fibromyalgia and the central nervous sytem is being studied. One possibility is described by the central sensitization theory, which holds that people with fibromyalgia have a lower pain threshold due to increased sensitivity in the brain to pain signals. It is hypothesized that this sensitivity results from an abnormal increase in levels of the neurotransmitters in the brain that signal pain (Mayo Clinic, 2009). The National Institute of Arthritis and Musculoskeletal and Skin Diseases (2005a) is conducting research to better understand why people with fibromyalgia have increased sensitivity to pain, the role of stress hormones in the body, the effect of genetics, and what medications or behavioral treatments are most effective.

Risk Factors

Risk factors for fibromyalgia include being female, being 20–50 years of age, having a family history of fibromyalgia, and having another rheumatic disorder, such as rheumatoid arthritis or system lupus erythematosus. Disturbed sleep patterns are highly associated with fibromyalgia, although it is unclear whether they are a cause of fibromyalgia or a result.

CLINICAL MANIFESTATIONS

A gradual onset of chronic, achy muscle pain is typical, although the onset may be sudden, occasionally following a viral illness. The pain may be localized or involve the entire body. The neck, spine, shoulders, and hips are often affected. Pain is produced by palpating localized tender points (Figure 5–10 ■). Local tightness or muscle spasm may also occur. Systemic manifestations of fibromyalgia include fatigue, sleep disruptions, headaches, morning stiffness, painful menstrual periods, and problems with thinking and memory (called the "fibro fog"). Pain and fatigue are aggravated by exertion.

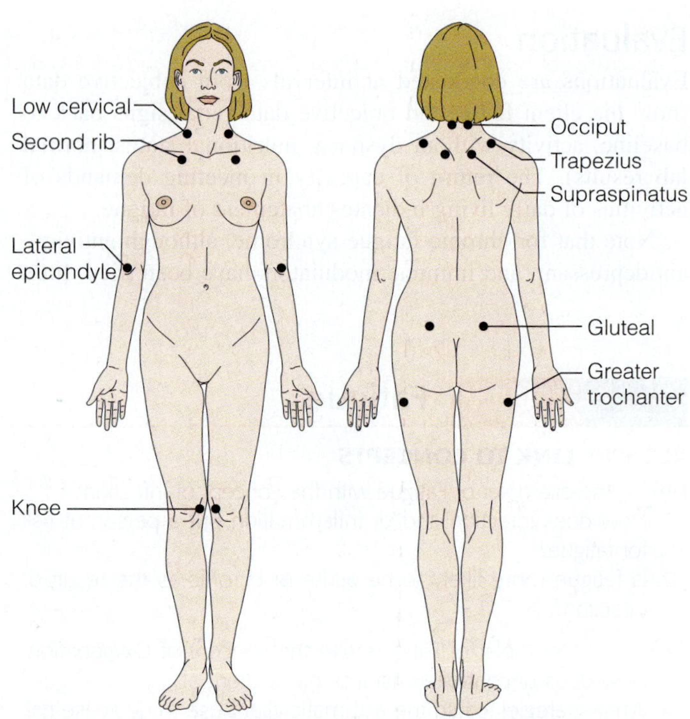

Figure 5–10 ■ Location of "tender points" in fibromyalgia.

COLLABORATION

Fibromyalgia is exceedingly difficult to treat. The client's health care team may try a combination of therapies before finding a treatment regimen that provides relief for the client. Nurses and physicians working with a client with fibromyalgia should not rule out consultations with or referrals to occupational and physical therapists, nutritionists and dieticians, and CAM therapy providers.

Diagnostic Tests

There are no diagnostic tests that can be used to evaluate fibromyalgia. Because of the high correlation of the symptoms of fibromyalgia with rheumatic disorders and chronic fatigue

CLINICAL MANIFESTATIONS AND THERAPIES Fibromyalgia

ETIOLOGY	CLINICAL MANIFESTATIONS	CLINICAL THERAPIES
Pain	■ Widespread pain lasting 3 months or longer ■ Pain at 11 of 18 tender points upon palpation	■ Local heat application ■ Massage ■ Stretching exercises ■ Selective serotonin norepinephrine uptake inhibitors
Sleep disruptions	■ Insomnia ■ Restless leg syndrome	■ Improved sleep hygiene ■ Tricyclic antidepressants
Fatigue	■ Chronic fatigue ■ Acute fatigue exacerbations, often associated with exercise or increased activity	■ Rest ■ Stress reduction techniques

syndrome, those disorders should be ruled out before a diagnosis of fibromyalgia is made. Fibromyalgia also may occur as a complication of hypothyroidism, so thyroid function studies are performed.

Pharmacologic Therapies

There is no single pharmacologic therapy guaranteed to treat fibromyalgia. A number of medications, however, have been shown to be effective. Efficacy may vary greatly among individuals, and a client may have to try more than one before finding a medication that is helpful.

SELECTIVE SEROTONIN REUPTAKE INHIBITORS Selective serotonin reuptake inhibitors (SSRIs) and selective serotonin norepinephrine uptake inhibitors (SSNIs) have been found to be effective in reducing many of the symptoms associated with fibromyalgia. For prolonged therapy, they are much safer than tricyclic antidepressants, which are also popular (Podolecki, Podolecki, & Hrycek, 2009). Milnacipran is an SSNI that inhibits norepinephrine uptake at a greater rate than serotonin uptake. The FDA approved the use of milnacipran in treating fibromyalgia in January 2009. Side effects of SSNIs include nausea, constipation, increased heart rate, hypertension, and dry mouth. Hyponatremia has been associated with taking Milnacipran. SSNIs may be contraindicated for use in clients with depression, as these medications have been associated with a worsening of symptoms (Formulary Journal, 2009).

TRICYCLIC ANTIDEPRESSANTS Tricyclic antidepressants also inhibit the reuptake of serotonin and norepinephrine, and, to a lesser extent, that of dopamine. Amitriptyline, a tricyclic antidepressant, has been shown to promote better sleep and relieve manifestations of fibromyalgia. Side effects include constipation, urinary retention, dry mouth, increased heart rate, nausea, increased appetite, and weight gain, among others.

Complementary and Alternative Medicine

Studies done on a myriad of therapies including light therapy using tanning beds, resistance training, and whole body vibration show such variance in results and historically use such a small number of participants that these cannot be recommended with any degree of confidence. Acupuncture is widely sought as a remedy for all types of pain. Although acupuncture has not been shown to provide pain relief in clients with fibromyalgia, it has been shown to have some effect on fatigue and anxiety level in clients with fibromyalgia (Habib, 2006).

NURSING PROCESS

Pain control is a priority focus of nursing care. Clients require a great deal of support as they seek a diagnosis because fibromyalgia is often diagnosed only after other diagnoses are ruled out. Clients often find it very frustrating to wait for a diagnosis as they undergo one diagnostic test after another.

Assessment

The diagnosis of fibromyalgia is based on the history and physical assessment. The diagnostic criteria developed by the American College of Rheumatology (Box 5–16) are a history of widespread pain for at least 3 months and pain at 11 of the 18 tender points on palpation.

Diagnosis

Nursing diagnoses that may be appropriate for the client with fibromyalgia include:

- Disturbed Sleep Pattern
- Readiness for Enhanced Sleep
- Fatigue
- Activity Intolerance
- Acute Pain.

Box 5–16 **1990 Criteria for the Classification of Fibromyalgia**

1. HISTORY OF WIDESPREAD PAIN

Definition. Pain is considered widespread when all of the following are present: pain in the left side of the body, pain in the right side of the body, pain above the waist, and pain below the waist. In addition, axial skeletal pain (cervical spine or anterior chest or thoracic spine or low back) must be present. In this definition, shoulder and buttock pain is considered as pain for each involved side. "Low back" pain is considered lower segment pain.

2. PAIN IN 11 OF 18 TENDER POINT SITES ON DIGITAL PALPATION

Definition. Pain on digital palpation must be present in at least 11 of the following 18 sites:

Occiput: Bilateral, at the suboccipital muscle insertions.

Low cervical: Bilateral, at the anterior aspects of the intertransverse spaces at C5–C7.

Trapezius: Bilateral, at the midpoint of the upper border.

Supraspinatus: Bilateral, at origins, above the scapula spine near the medial border.

Second rib: Bilateral, at he second costochondral junctions, just lateral to the junctions on upper surfaces.

Lateral epicondyle: Bilateral, 2 cm distal to the epicondyles.

Gluteal: Bilateral, in upper outer quadrants of buttocks in anterior fold of muscle.

Greater trochanter: Bilateral, posterior to the trochanteric prominence.

Knee: Bilateral, at the medial fat pad proximal to the joint line.

- Digital palpation should be performed with an approximate force of 4 kg. For a tender point to be considered "positive" the subject must state that the palpation was painful. "Tender" is not to be considered "painful."
- For classification purposes, clients will be said to have fibromyalgia if both criteria are satisfied. Widespread pain must have been present for at least 3 months. The presence of a second clinical disorder does not exclude the diagnosis of fibromyalgia.

Source: Wolfe, F, Smythe HA, Yunus MB, Bennett RM, Bombardier C, Goldenberg DL, et al. (1990). The American College of Rheumatology 1990 criteria for the classification of fibromyalgia: report of the multicenter criteria committee. *Arthritis Rheum 33*:160–172.

Plan

Goals developed when designing the nursing plan of care may include:

- Pain relief
- Improve activity tolerance
- Balanced periods of exercise and rest
- Promote client self-care through client education.

Implementation

This disorder may resolve spontaneously or become chronic and recurrent. The client with fibromyalgia needs reassurance of the benign nature of the disorder along with validation of its reality.

Activity Intolerance

- Assess current activity level and tolerance of that activity. Assess vital signs. This provides baseline information to plan an activity program and assess response to that activity.
- Encourage the client to establish priorities and include rest periods or naps when scheduling daily activities. This provides a sense of control over activities and helps maintain self-esteem. Scheduled rest periods help restore energy and decrease fatigue.
- Encourage delegation of some responsibilities to family members. Delegation helps maintain the client's involvement and role in family decisions and responsibilities, while conserving energy for those activities identified as high priority by the client.

Fatigue

- Inquire about feelings of malaise (a vague feeling of body weakness or discomfort) and fatigue, particularly fatigue that is not improved with rest.
- Encourage verbalization of feelings about the impact of the disease and fatigue on lifestyle. Discussion of feelings helps the client clarify values and may assist in identifying priorities.
- Encourage enjoyable but quiet activities, such as reading, listening to music, or hobbies. Enjoyable activities help decrease feelings of fatigue. Quiet activities conserve energy while yielding a sense of accomplishment.

Care in the Community

Nursing care for clients with fibromyalgia is supportive and educational, provided in community settings such as clinics and other primary care settings. It is important to validate clients' concerns and reassure them that their symptoms are not "all in the head." This syndrome is recognizable and manageable; its course is not progressive. Teach clients about the disorder, and reassure them that it resolves uneventfully in most instances. Provide verbal and written instructions about the use of heat, exercise, stress-reduction techniques, and prescribed medications to relieve manifestations. In addition, suggest the following resources:

- Fibromyalgia Network
- National Fibromyalgia Research Association
- American College of Rheumatology
- National Institute of Arthritis and Musculoskeletal and Skin Diseases.

Evaluation

Client care is evaluated based on the following suggested expected outcomes:

- Client is able to reduce pain sufficiently to allow for periods of activity and sleep
- Client voices feelings related to chronic condition
- Client obtains adequate follow-up
- Client avoids use of narcotics or addictive substances to avoid substance addiction.

REVIEW Fibromyalgia

RELATE: LINK THE CONCEPTS

Linking the exemplar of Fibromyalgia with the concept of Development:

1. How might the pain of fibromyalgia impact the developmental tasks of the client?
2. What would be your expected findings when performing a developmental assessment of a 32-year-old with fibromyalgia?

Linking the exemplar of Fibromyalgia with the concept of Addiction Behaviors:

3. What factors put the client with fibromyalgia at risk for the development of addiction behaviors?
4. What would you plan for the client with fibromyalgia to assist in the prevention of addiction behaviors?

READY: GO TO COMPANION SKILLS MANUAL

- Assessing the client in pain

REFER: GO TO MYNURSINGKIT

REFLECT: CASE STUDY

Nancy Franklin is a 49-year-old physical therapist with a history of alcoholism. She has not had a drink in 10 years. She was recently in a car accident and sustained whiplash of the shoulders and neck. After 3 months of treatment, Nancy's pain has not improved, so the physician refers Nancy to a specialist who diagnoses her with fibromyalgia. Nancy now has trouble getting out of bed in the morning, sleeps most of the morning, and takes naps in the afternoon. Several of the parents of the children that she treats have complained because she is chronically late or does not show up for appointments at all. Nancy is returning to the fibromyalgia clinic today for a follow-up visit and she is 30 minutes late.

1. What is your priority nursing diagnosis for Nancy?
2. What referral might you recommend for Nancy?
3. What is your plan of care to assist Nancy in coping with the diagnosis of fibromyalgia?

5.5 SLEEP-REST DISORDERS

KEY TERMS

BASIS FOR SELECTION OF EXEMPLAR

Common condition

Centers for Disease Control and Prevention

LEARNING OUTCOMES

After reading about this exemplar, you will be able to:

1. Describe the pathophysiology, etiology, clinical manifestations, and direct and indirect causes of sleep-rest disorders.
2. Identify risk factors associated with sleep-rest disorders.
3. Illustrate the nursing process in providing culturally competent care across the life span for individuals with sleep-rest disorders.
4. Formulate priority nursing diagnoses appropriate for an individual with sleep-rest disorders.
5. Create a plan of care for individuals with sleep-rest disorders and their family members.
6. Assess expected outcomes for an individual with sleep-rest disorders.
7. Discuss therapies used in the collaborative care of an individual with sleep-rest disorders.
8. Employ evidence-based caring interventions for an individual with sleep-rest disorders.

OVERVIEW

A knowledge of common sleep disorders can help nurses assess the sleep complaints of their clients and, when appropriate, make a referral to a specialist in sleep disorders medicine. Although sleep disorders are typically categorized for the purpose of research as dyssomnias, parasomnias, and disorders associated with medical or psychiatric illness, it is usually more appropriate for clinicians to focus on the client's symptoms (e.g., insomnia, excessive sleepiness, and abnormal events) occurring during sleep (parasomnias). For an explanation of the pathophysiology of sleep, please see Concept 13, Health, Wellness, and Illness.

COMMON SLEEP DISORDERS

There are a number of disorders associated with the inability to obtain adequate sleep and rest. While **insomnia** is the term used for the inability to fall asleep or remain asleep, there are a number of conditions that can cause this disorder.

Insomnia

Persons with insomnia awake not feeling rested. Insomnia is the most common sleep complaint in America. Acute insomnia lasts one to several nights and is often caused by personal stressors and/or worry. If the insomnia persists for longer than a month, it is considered chronic insomnia. More often, people experience chronic intermittent insomnia, which means difficulty sleeping for a few nights, followed by a few nights of adequate sleep before the problem returns (National Sleep Foundation, 2005a).

Hypersomnia

Hypersomnia refers to conditions where the affected individual obtains sufficient sleep at night but still cannot stay awake during the day. Hypersomnia can be caused by medical conditions, for example, CNS damage and certain kidney, liver, or metabolic disorders, such as diabetic acidosis and hypothyroidism. Rarely does hypersomnia have a psychological origin.

Narcolepsy

Narcolepsy is a disorder of excessive daytime sleepiness caused by the lack of the chemical hypocretin in the area of the CNS that regulates sleep. Clients with narcolepsy have sleep attacks or excessive daytime sleepiness, and their sleep at night usually begins with a sleep-onset REM period (dreaming sleep occurs within the first 15 minutes of falling asleep). The majority of clients also have cataplexy or the sudden onset of muscle weakness or paralysis in association with strong emotion, sleep paralysis (transient paralysis when falling asleep or waking up), hypnagogic hallucinations (visual, auditory, or tactile hallucinations at sleep onset or when waking up), and/or fragmented nighttime sleep.

For clients with narcolepsy, poor nocturnal sleep is not the cause of their excessive daytime sleepiness; many clients, particularly younger clients, have sound restorative nocturnal sleep but still cannot stay awake during the daytime.

Onset of symptoms tends to occur between ages 15 and 30, with symptom severity usually stabilizing within the first 5 years of onset. CNS stimulants such as methylphenidate (Ritalin) or amphetamines have been used to reduce excessive daytime sleepiness. Antidepressants, both older monoamine oxidase (MAO) inhibitors and the newer serotonergic antidepressants, are usually quite effective for controlling cataplexy. In 1999, the FDA, approved modafinil (Provigil) for control of excessive daytime sleepiness in narcoleptic clients. Although its exact mechanism of action is unknown, it has fewer side effects, and a lower potential for abuse. A second drug, sodium oxybate (Xyrem), approved in 2002 for the treatment of cataplexy, has also been shown to reduce excessive daytime sleepiness in clients with narcolepsy. Because Xyrem is difficult to administer (it is available only as a liquid and taken at bedtime and then again 2.5–4 hours after sleep onset) and its use is tightly controlled by the FDA, only those clients whose symptoms are not controlled by other medications are usually offered Xyrem. Only one pharmacy in the United States is allowed to dispense Xyrem. As a result, clients need to allow adequate time for obtaining their medications from the central pharmacy.

Sleep Apnea

Sleep apnea is characterized by frequent short breathing pauses during sleep. Although all individuals have occasional periods of apnea during sleep, more than five apneic episodes or five breathing pauses longer than 10 seconds/hour is considered abnormal and should be evaluated by a sleep medicine specialist. Symptoms suggestive of sleep apnea include loud snoring, frequent nocturnal awakenings, excessive daytime sleepiness, difficulties falling asleep at night, morning headaches, memory and cognitive problems, and irritability. Although sleep apnea is most frequently diagnosed in men and postmenopausal women, it may occur during childhood.

The periods of apnea, which last from 10 seconds to 2 minutes, occur during REM or NREM sleep. Frequency of episodes ranges from 50 to 600 per night. Because these apneic pauses are usually associated with an arousal, clients frequently report that their sleep is nonrestorative and that they regularly fall asleep when engaging in sedentary activities during the day.

Three common types of sleep apnea are obstructive apnea, central apnea, and mixed apnea. *Obstructive apnea* occurs when the structures of the pharynx or oral cavity block the flow of air. The person continues to try to breathe; that is, the chest and abdominal muscles move. The movements of the diaphragm become stronger and stronger until the obstruction is removed. Enlarged tonsils and adenoids, a deviated nasal septum, nasal polyps, and obesity predispose the client to obstructive apnea. An episode of obstructive sleep apnea usually begins with snoring; thereafter, breathing ceases, followed by marked snorting as breathing resumes. Toward the end of each apneic episode, increased carbon dioxide levels in the blood cause the client to wake.

Central apnea is thought to involve a defect in the respiratory center of the brain. All actions involved in breathing, such as chest movement and airflow, cease. Clients who have brainstem injuries and muscular dystrophy, for example, often have central sleep apnea. At this time, there is no available treatment. *Mixed apnea* is a combination of central apnea and obstructive apnea.

Treatment for sleep apnea is directed at the cause of the apnea. For example, enlarged tonsils may be removed. Other surgical procedures, including laser removal of excess tissue in the pharynx, reduce or eliminate snoring and may be effective in relieving the apnea. In other cases, the use of a nasal **continuous positive airway pressure (CPAP)** device at night is effective in maintaining an open airway. Weight loss may also help decrease the severity of symptoms.

Sleep apnea profoundly affects a person's work or school performance. In addition, prolonged sleep apnea can cause a sharp rise in blood pressure and may lead to cardiac arrest. Over time, apneic episodes can cause cardiac arrhythmias, pulmonary hypertension, and subsequent left-sided heart failure.

PRACTICE ALERT

Partners of clients with sleep apnea may become aware of the problem because they hear snoring that stops during the apneic period and then restarts. Surgical removal of tonsils or other tissue in the pharynx, if it is not the cause of the sleep apnea, can actually worsen the situation by removing the snoring and, thus, the warning that apnea is occurring.

Insufficient Sleep

Healthy individuals who obtain less sleep than they need will experience sleepiness and fatigue during the daytime hours. Depending on the severity and chronicity of this voluntary, albeit unintentional sleep deprivation, individuals may develop attention and concentration deficits, reduced vigilance, distractibility, reduced motivation, fatigue, malaise, and occasionally diplopia and dry mouth. The cause of these symptoms may or may not be attributed to insufficient sleep, since many Americans believe that 6.8 hours of sleep is sufficient to maintain optimal daytime performance. In fact, the sleep times of Americans have decreased dramatically over the past decade, with adults averaging only 6.8 hours of sleep on weekdays and 7.4 hours on weekends. All age groups, not just adults and adolescents, are getting less than the recommended amounts of sleep. Even 4- to 5-year-old children now average less than 9.5 hours of sleep, approximately 1.5 to 2.5 hours less than recommended.

Although the effects of obtaining less than optimal amounts of sleep are generally considered benign, there is growing evidence that insufficient sleep can have significant deleterious effects. Staying awake 19 consecutive hours produces the same impairments in reaction times and cognitive function as a blood alcohol level of 0.05, and staying awake for 24 consecutive hours has the same effects on reaction times and cognitive function as being legally drunk (with a blood alcohol level of 0.1). Nurses who report reduced hours of sleep are more likely to make an error, have difficulty staying awake on duty, and have difficulty staying awake while driving home from work than those who obtained more sleep.

When clients report obtaining more sleep on weekends or days off, it usually indicates that they are not obtaining sufficient sleep. Convincing the client to obtain more sleep may be difficult, but it can result in the resolution of their daytime symptoms.

Parasomnias

A **parasomnia** is behavior that may interfere with sleep and may even occur during sleep. The *International Classification of Sleep Disorders* (American Sleep Disorders Association, 2005) subdivides parasomnias into arousal disorders (e.g., sleepwalking, sleep terrors), sleep–wake transition disorders (e.g., sleeptalking), parasomnias associated with REM sleep (e.g., nightmares), and others (e.g., bruxism). Box 5–17 describes examples of parasomnias.

Box 5–17 **Parasomnias**

- *Bruxism:* Usually occurring during stage II NREM sleep, this clenching and grinding of the teeth can eventually erode dental crowns, cause teeth to come loose, and lead to deterioration of the temporomandibular joint and temporomandibular joint syndrome.
- *Enuresis:* Bed-wetting during sleep can occur in children over 3 years old. More males than females are affected. It often occurs 1 to 2 hours after falling asleep, when rousing from NREM stages III and IV.
- *Periodic limb movements disorder (PLMD):* In this condition, the legs jerk twice or three times per minute during sleep. It is most common among older adults. This kicking motion can wake the client and result in poor sleep. The condition may be treated with medications such as those otherwise used for Parkinson's disease. PLMDs differ from restless leg syndrome (RLS), which occurs whenever the person is at rest, not just at night when sleeping. RLS may occur during pregnancy or be due to other medical problems that can be treated.
- *Sleeptalking:* Talking during sleep occurs during NREM sleep before REM sleep. It rarely presents a problem to the person unless it becomes troublesome to others.
- *Somnambulism:* Somnambulism (sleepwalking) occurs during stages III and IV of NREM sleep. It is episodic and usually occurs 1 to 2 hours after falling asleep. Sleepwalkers tend not to notice dangers (e.g., stairs) and often need to be protected from injury.

Risk Factors

The two main risk factors of insomnia are older age and female gender (IOM, 2006, p. 91). Women suffer sleep loss in connection with hormonal changes (e.g., menstruation, pregnancy, and menopause). The incidence of insomnia increases with age, but it is thought that this is caused by some other medical condition.

Risk factors for obstructive sleep apnea, in addition to male gender, include increasing age and obesity. Large neck circumference (>17 inches in men and >16 inches in women) also is a known risk factor for obstructive sleep apnea (Porth, 2005). Use of alcohol and other CNS depressants may contribute to sleep apnea.

It is difficult to judge the incidence and prevalence of sleep disorders, as many go unreported and diagnosed. Estimates regarding sleep apnea vary widely: The National Heart, Blood, and Lung Institute estimates 12 million Americans have sleep apnea, while the National Sleep Foundation puts that number at closer to 18 million (Reuters, 2009). A study recently published has found that sleep-disordered breathing is associated with higher mortality rates, as much as 46% in men ages 40–70 with severe cases of sleep apnea (Punjabi, Caffo, Goodwin, et al., 2009).

Sleep and the Older Adult

Most older adults require 6–10 hours of sleep nightly. Less than 4 or more than 8 hours of sleep is associated with higher mortality rates than those sleeping 8 hours (Kripke, Garfinkle, Wingard, Klauber, & Marler, 2002). Often, the time it takes to fall asleep serves as a good indicator of whether a person is getting enough sleep. Those who fall asleep almost immediately upon placing their head on the pillow may be sleep deprived. When an older adult's sleep requirements are not met, a sleep deficit accumulates with resulting loss of overall daytime function. When a person regularly loses 1–2 hours of sleep each night, the lack of sleep can accumulate, leading to chronic excessive sleepiness. Lifestyle factors like irregular sleep schedules; use of caffeine, tobacco, and alcohol; excessive time spent in daytime napping; and certain medications can make sleep problems worse. In 2002, driver sleepiness was the principle cause of over 100,000 motor vehicle accidents and about 4% of all fatal crashes (Clinical Advisor, 2007).

Older adults may nap more often during the day, thus further disrupting normal circadian patterns. While one "cat nap" a day of 30 minutes or less in the early afternoon was found not to disrupt the nighttime sleep of older adults, more frequent daytime napping can be disruptive (Doghramji, 2000). If an older adult normally requires 8 hours of sleep in a 24-hour period and 2–3 hours of sleep occur during the daytime hours, the person cannot expect to enjoy 8 hours of uninterrupted sleep at night. The older adult may toss and turn, become frustrated with the inability to sleep, and suffer further disruption in the sleep–wake patterns. For good sleepers, the bed and bedroom are strong cues for drowsiness and sleep; for poor sleepers, these places signal alertness, frustration, and sleeplessness.

Sleep disruption is common in older adults with psychosocial problems. Life stresses when combined with predisposing emotional factors such as depression and anxiety may be related to the onset of sleep problems (Jao & Alessi, 2004). Many studies identify anxiety, stress, and depression as major deterrents to falling and staying asleep in people of all ages. Psychosocial influences that may disrupt sleep include social isolation, caregiving stress and strain, and grief and bereavement (Fragoso & Gill, 2007).

Mental health problems associated with poor sleep include anxiety, depression, and substance abuse disorders (Clinical Advisor, 2007). Sleep problems identified in depressed older adults include difficulty in falling asleep, increased frequency of early morning awakenings, and frequent daytime napping. For some older women, sleep problems begin during menopause. Menopause, the cessation of menstruation resulting from declines in estrogen levels, is associated with a variety of behavioral changes, including hot flashes and mood swings. Hot flashes that occur routinely during sleep can lead to fatigue, irritability, and chronic sleep disruption, establishing a poor sleep pattern that persists into old age for many women (Fragoso & Gill, 2007). Older depressed adults are more likely to report somatic complaints like sleep problems and changes in appetite rather than feeling "sad" or "blue."

Younger people are more likely to acknowledge the connection between sleep disturbances and emotional problems; therefore, the nurse should be aware of this connection.

Various health problems and the medications used to treat them are associated with sleep disruption in older adults. Pulmonary disease, heart disease, arthritis, dementia associated with Alzheimer's disease, and depression may cause sleep disruption. Diseases of the cardiac and respiratory system are often associated with orthopnea and shortness of breath. Persons with heart failure are often asked "the pillow question" as an indicator of the stability and progression of their disease. The nurse should ask, "How many pillows do you sleep with at night? Is this your usual number of pillows?" Older adults with severe heart failure may find it necessary to sleep sitting nearly upright to allow the lungs to clear fluid and breathe, but this position may not offer adequate support for the back and the head during deep sleep (Figure 5–11 ■).

Physical discomfort or pain can be a major deterrent for sleep. Older adults with pain take longer to fall asleep and have an increased number of nighttime awakenings. Pain makes it difficult to achieve a comfortable sleeping position, may cause tension and muscle spasms, and may keep an older adult awake during the night if pain medication wears off (Jao & Alessi, 2004). A common source of pain in older adults is the chronic pain resulting from osteoarthritis. This disease often results in chronic pain of the knee or hip and was reported to disrupt sleep in one third of the respondents of the National Survey of Self-Care and Aging Study (Wilcox, Brenes, Levine, et al., 2000). Further, older adults who experience chronic pain may also limit daytime activities, resulting in physical inactivity, deconditioning or loss of physical strength and function, and further disruption of the sleep–activity cycle. Acutely ill hospitalized clients may also experience pain from surgical incisions, pain from the trauma or injury that was the cause of the hospitalization, or discomfort from intravenous tubing, indwelling urinary catheters, or other instrumentation (Figure 5–12 ■).

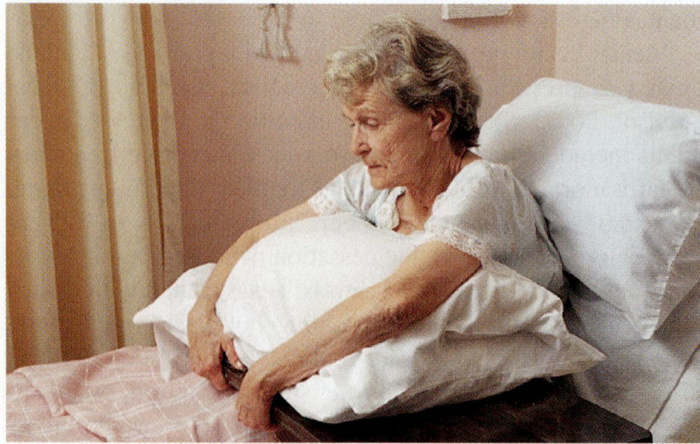

Figure 5–11 ■ Sleep may be difficult for older persons with heart and lung disease.

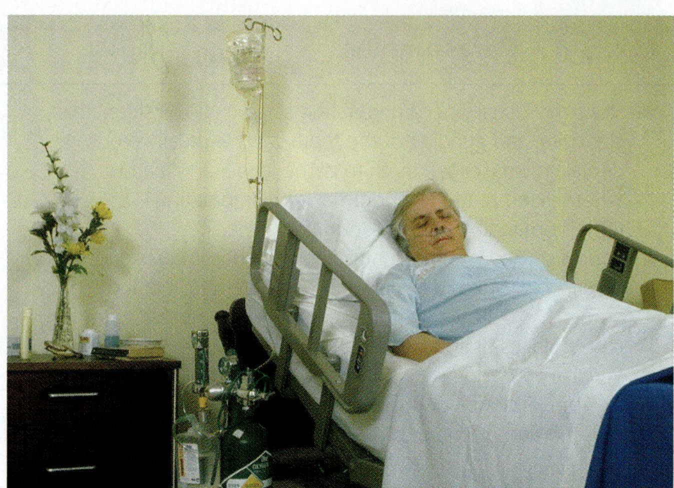

Figure 5–12 ■ Sleep disturbances are common in institutional settings.

Older adults with dementia endure even more sleep disruptions than other older adults do. Sleep disruptions common in dementia such as those with Alzheimer's disease include breakdown of the normal sleep–wake cycle with short periods of fragmented sleep occurring throughout a 24-hour period, reduced stage 3 and REM sleep, and no stage 4 sleep (Jao & Alessi, 2004). Older adults with dementia may suffer other problems as a result of their impairment such as social isolation, boredom, nursing home placement, excessive daytime napping, and periods of agitation or restlessness throughout the evening or night.

CLINICAL MANIFESTATIONS

Manifestations of sleep disorders vary according to the nature of the disorder. Symptoms vary from sleeplessness to excessive sleepiness and fatigue. Symptoms such as irritability, distractibility, and morning headaches also are indicative of sleep disorders. Because lack of sleep is associated with the onset of a number of chronic conditions, the nurse working with a client reporting frequent or chronic difficulty sleeping or staying awake should thoroughly assess the client (CDC, 2009). This will elicit information that may indicate the presence of either a sleep disorder or another developing medical condition.

COLLABORATION

Clients with a suspected sleep disorder may benefit from a collaborative health care team that includes the nurse, the client's primary care physician, a sleep disorder specialist (often a pulmonologist), a counselor, and a CAM therapy provider such as an acupuncturist. Sleep disorders can be very difficult to treat; a holistic approach in which the client's health care providers communicate and collaborate may serve to provide relief for the client in both the short and long term.

CLINICAL MANIFESTATIONS AND THERAPIES **Sleep-Rest Disorders**

ETIOLOGY	CLINICAL MANIFESTATIONS	CLINICAL THERAPIES
Insomnia	■ Inability to fall asleep or remain asleep	■ Improved sleep hygiene ■ Relaxation techniques and CAM therapies ■ Pharmacologic therapy ■ Counseling, if etiology of insomnia is anxiety
Obstructive Sleep Apnea	■ Loud, cyclic snoring ■ Periods of apnea lasting 15–120 seconds during sleep ■ Gasping or choking during sleep ■ Restlessness, thrashing during sleep ■ Daytime fatigue and sleepiness ■ Morning headache ■ Personality changes, depression ■ Intellectual impairment ■ Impotence ■ Hypertension	■ Weight reduction ■ Abstinence from alcohol ■ Nasal CPAP
Narcolepsy	Excessive daytime drowsiness caused by lack of hypocretin; other symptoms include: ■ Sleep attacks ■ Cataplexy ■ Sudden onset muscle weakness ■ Sleep paralysis.	■ Stimulants such as methylphenidates or amphetamines ■ Antidepressants
Insufficient Sleep	■ Fatigue ■ Drowsiness ■ Attention deficits ■ Reduced motivation ■ Increased distractibility	

Diagnostic Studies

Sleep is measured objectively in a sleep disorder laboratory by **polysomnography (PSG)**, a recording of the biophysical changes that a client experiences during sleep. An **electroencephalogram (EEG)** measures and records the brains electrical activity; an *electromyogram (EMG)* records muscle activity; and an *electro-oculogram (EOG)* records eye movements. These tests are recorded simultaneously by placing electrodes on the scalp to record brain waves (EEG), on the outer canthus of each eye to record eye movement (EOG), and on the chin muscles to record the structural electromyogram (EMG). The electrodes transmit electric energy from the cerebral cortex and muscles of the face to pens that record the brain waves and muscle activity on graph paper. Respiratory effort and airflow, electrocardiogram (ECG), leg movements, and oxygen saturation are also monitored. Oxygen saturation is determined by monitoring with a pulse oximeter, a light-sensitive electric cell that attaches to the ear or a finger. Oxygen saturation and ECG assessments are of particular importance if sleep apnea is suspected. Through polysomnography, the client's activity (movements, struggling, noisy respirations) during sleep can be assessed. Such activity of which the client is unaware may be the cause of arousal during sleep.

Pharmacologic Therapies

Sleep medications often prescribed on a as-needed (prn) basis for clients include the sedative-hypnotics, which induce sleep, and antianxiety drugs or tranquilizers, which decrease anxiety and tension. When prn sleep medications are ordered in institutional settings, the nurse is responsible for making decisions with the client about when to administer them. These medications should be administered only with complete knowledge of their actions and effects and only when indicated.

Both nurses and clients need to be aware of the actions, effects, and risks of the specific medication prescribed. Although medications vary in their activity and effects, considerations include the following:

- Sedative-hypnotic medications produce a general CNS depression and an unnatural sleep; REM or NREM sleep is altered to some extent, and daytime drowsiness and a morning hangover effect may occur. Some of the new hypnotics, such as zolpidem (Ambien), do not alter REM sleep or produce rebound insomnia when discontinued. (For an explanation of REM and NREM sleep, please see Concept 13, Health, Wellness, and Illness.)
- Antianxiety medications decrease levels of arousal by facilitating the action of neurons in the CNS that suppress

responsiveness to stimulation. These medications are contraindicated in pregnant women because of their associated risk of congenital anomalies, and in breast-feeding mothers because the medication is excreted in breast milk.

- Sleep medications vary in their onset and duration of action and will impair waking function as long as they are chemically active. Some medication effects can last many hours beyond the time that the client's perception of daytime drowsiness and impaired psychomotor skills have disappeared. Clients need to be cautioned about such effects and about driving or handling machinery while the drug is in their system.
- Sleep medications affect REM sleep more than NREM sleep. Clients need to be informed that one or two nights of increased dreaming (REM rebound) are usual after the drug is discontinued after long-term use.
- Initial doses of medications should be low and increases added gradually, depending on the client's response. Older adults, in particular, are susceptible to side effects because of their metabolic changes; they need to be closely monitored for changes in mental alertness and coordination. Clients need to be instructed to take the smallest effective dose and then only for a few nights or intermittently as required.
- Regular use of any sleep medication can lead to tolerance over time (e.g., 4–6 weeks) and rebound insomnia. In some instances, this may lead clients to increase the dosage. Clients must be cautioned about developing a pattern of drug dependency.
- Abrupt cessation of barbiturate sedative-hypnotics can create withdrawal symptoms such as restlessness, tremors, weakness, insomnia, increased heart rate, seizures, convulsions, and even death. Long-term users need to taper their medications under the supervision of a specialist.

About half of the clients who seek medical intervention for sleep problems are treated with sedative-hypnotics (Vitiello, 1999). Sometimes the prescription of hypnotics can be appropriate. For example, women with chronic difficulties maintaining sleep or nonrestorative sleep associated with menopausal symptoms often benefit by the prescription of 10 mg of zolpidem, a low dose that was documented to be both safe and efficacious in this population. Hypnotics are not appropriate if clients have any symptoms suggestive of sleep-related breathing disorders, or decreased renal and/or hepatic function.

TABLE 5–11 **Selected Sedative-Hypnotic Medications Used for Insomnia**

MEDICATION	HALF-LIFE
Chloral hydrate (Noctec)	7–10 hours
Eszopiclone (Lunesta)	6 hours
Ethchlorvynol (Placidyl)	10–20 hours
Flurazepam (Dalmane)	47–100 hours
Glutethimide (Doriden)	1–12 hours
Lorazepam (Ativan)	10–20 hours
Melatonin	1 hour
Temazepam (Restoril)	9–15 hours
Triazolam (Halcion)	1.5–5.5 hours
Zaleplon (Sonata)	1 hour
Zolpidem (Ambien)	2.6 hours

Table 5–11 ■ presents some of the common medications used for enhancing sleep and the half-life of these medications. The half-life represents how long it takes for half of the medication to be metabolized and eliminated by the body; hence, those with shorter half-lives are less likely to cause residual drowsiness after administration, but may be less effective for the treatment of sleep maintenance insomnia.

Clinical Therapies for Sleep Apnea

Mild to moderate obstructive sleep apnea may be treated by weight reduction, alcohol abstinence, improving nasal patency, and avoiding the supine position for sleep. Although weight reduction often cures the disorder, maintaining optimal weight is difficult. Oral appliances designed to keep the mandible and tongue forward also may be prescribed.

Nasal CPAP (continuous positive airway pressure) is the treatment of choice for obstructive sleep apnea. Positive pressure generated by an air compressor and administered through a tight-fitting nasal mask (Figure 5–13 ■) splints the pharyngeal airway, preventing collapse and obstruction. With proper training, this device is well tolerated by the client. Nasal airways can become dry and irritated with CPAP, so an in-line humidifier or a room humidifier is recommended. A newer device, the **BiPAP** ventilator (bilevel positive airway pressure), delivers higher pressures during inhalation and lower pressures during expiration, providing less resistance to exhaling.

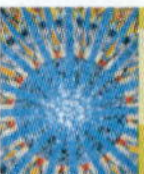

DEVELOPMENTAL CONSIDERATIONS **Clinical Therapies for Children With Obstructive Sleep Apnea**

Adenotonsillectomy is the most common treatment for obstructive sleep apnea syndrome (OSAS), and resolution of the condition occurs in the majority of children. Children at higher risk for respiratory complications in the immediate postoperative period include those with severe OSAS, neuromuscular disorders, morbid obesity, craniofacial abnormalities, and children under age 3 years (Darrow, 2007). In rare cases, an artificial airway is placed (nasopharyngeal or endotracheal tube) to maintain the airway overnight (Darrow, 2007). Polysomnography is usually repeated about 6–8 weeks after surgery to determine if any residual OSAS remains.

Weight loss strategies are implemented for obese children. Continuous positive airway pressure is used for children with surgical contraindications or those with persistent OSAS (craniofacial anomalies, Down syndrome, or neuromuscular disorders) after adenotonsillectomy. CPAP levels are set at the pressure that eliminates apneic episodes, sleep arousals, and hypoxemia. Pressure levels may need to be changed as the child grows. Craniofacial surgery or even tracheostomy may be treatment options in some cases. Oxygen is not usually prescribed as it decreases the ventilatory drive.

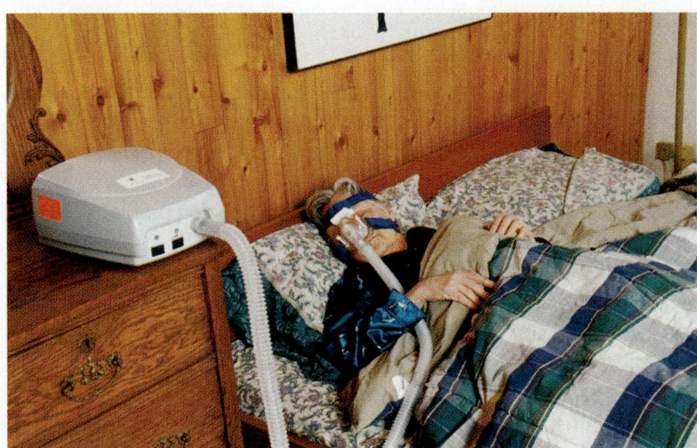

Figure 5–13 ■ A client using a nasal mask and CPAP to treat sleep apnea.

Tonsillectomy and adenoidectomy may relieve upper airway obstruction in some clients. Excision of obstructive tissue from the soft palate, uvula, and posterior lateral pharyngeal wall may be accomplished by *uvulopalatopharyngoplasty (UPPP)*. Although only about 50% of these surgeries are successful in treating sleep apnea, UPPP is useful in selected cases. In severe cases, tracheostomy may also be performed to bypass the area of obstruction.

Complementary and Alternative Therapies

Many older adults use herbal or natural remedies to promote sleep. Melatonin is a hormone produced in the pineal gland and plays a role in the regulation of sleep. Melatonin is sold in many pharmacies and health food stores and is effective for some older adults with sleep disturbances due to decreased levels of melatonin. Doses of 0.5–3 mg have been suggested for sleep. It should be taken approximately 2 hours before bedtime. Melatonin has been found to significantly improve sleep onset in older adults with insomnia; however, it has been found not to affect sleep quality, number of awakenings after sleep onset, total sleep time, or sleep architecture (National Institutes of Health [NIH], 2008a). The most commonly reported side effects include nausea, dizziness, and drowsiness. Melatonin is generally considered safe for short-term use, and no significant drug interactions have been described. Because melatonin has a short half-life (about 40 minutes), a controlled-release formulation is recommended to maintain sleep throughout the entire sleep cycle (Reuben, Herr, Pacala, et al., 2008).

Additional natural remedies include herbal chamomile tea (if the person has no allergies to ragweed or daisies), hops, lemon balm, and valerian (NIH, 2008b). Valerian root has been used since Greek and Roman times. A dose of 400–450 mg of the extract will shorten sleep latency similarly to a short-acting benzodiazepine. The NIH concluded that there is not enough hard evidence to support the effectiveness of valerian in treating insomnia. Common side effects include headache, dizziness, itchiness, and gastrointestinal upset. Older adults taking valerian should be warned that there can be toxic interactions with other medications such as alcohol, sedating drugs, benzodiazepines, and barbiturates. Sometimes a small evening snack such as a glass of milk or a turkey sandwich may promote sleep onset because of the natural tryptophan contained in these foods.

Cognitive–behavioral therapy (CBT), a short-term goal-focused therapy, has been used to improve sleep. CBT interventions include sleep restriction (limiting the time spent in bed), stimulus formation (learning to associate the bed with sleep and rest), biofeedback, and relaxation techniques. CBT has been shown to be effective in improving sleep efficiency and significantly decreasing insomnia symptoms in a majority of older adults studied (Goldsmith, 2007).

GUIDED IMAGERY An integrative therapist can lead the client through guided imagery. Imagining a peaceful scene while in a dark room with lowered stimuli may provide the extra relaxation needed to induce sleep. Drinking a glass of warm milk before and wearing loose comfortable clothing during the imagery can increase the benefits of this nonpharmacological approach to inducing sleep.

NURSING PROCESS

Clients experiencing sleep disorders often report a great deal of frustration and annoyance with sleepless nights. However, more than just an annoyance, risks of injury increase dramatically in tired people. In addition to care of the client's sleeplessness, it is important for nurses to promote injury prevention by teaching strategies to reduce risk such as not driving when tired, using caution with potentially dangerous equipment, and fire prevention if the client smokes.

Assessment

The nurse assesses the client for sleep integrity by interviewing and taking a sleep history. The majority of the data collected at this point is subjective. A partner may provide additional information on the client's sleep habits. Parents are valuable to provide information regarding children's sleep patterns. Sleep assessment scales, such as the Epworth Sleepiness Scale used for older adults, can be helpful in collecting information to inform the care plan. See the Assessment Interview and Epworth Sleepiness Scale provided in this exemplar for more information. Objective data includes vital signs, muscle tone, reflexes, observation of level of consciousness and orientation, and coordination. Pallor, dark circles under the eyes, and irritability may suggest sleep deprivation.

Diagnosis

Obvious nursing diagnoses are insomnia and sleep deprivation. Other diagnoses may vary by client, and include the following:

- Readiness for Enhanced Sleep related to poor sleep hygiene
- Disturbed Sleep Pattern
- Anxiety related to diagnosis of a sleep disorder
- Ineffective Breathing Pattern related to sleep apnea
- Risk for Impaired Gas Exchange related to sleep apnea
- Deficient Knowledge related to sleep hygiene
- Activity Intolerance related to insufficient sleep
- Risk for Injury related to somnambulism
- Fatigue.

Assessment Interview Sleep Disturbances

ADULTS

- How would you describe your sleeping problem? What changes have occurred in your sleeping pattern? How often does this happen?
- How many cups of coffee, tea, or caffeinated beverages do you drink per day? Do you drink alcohol? If so, how much?
- Do you have difficulty falling asleep?
- Do you wake up often during the night? If so, how often?
- Do you wake up earlier in the morning than you would like and have difficulty falling back to sleep?
- How do you feel when you wake up in the morning?
- Do you sleep more than usual? If so, how often do you sleep?
- Do you have periods of overwhelming sleepiness? If so, when does this happen?
- Have you ever suddenly fallen asleep in the middle of a daytime activity? Does anything unusual happen when you laugh or get angry?
- Has anyone ever told you that you snore, walk in your sleep, or stop breathing for a while when sleeping?
- What have you been doing to deal with this sleeping problem? Does it help?
- What do you think might be causing this problem? Do you have any medical condition that might be causing you to sleep more (or less)? Are you receiving medications for an illness that might alter your sleeping pattern? Are you experiencing any stressful or upsetting events or conflicts that may be affecting your sleep?
- How is your sleeping problem affecting you?

OLDER ADULTS: THE EPWORTH SLEEPINESS SCALE (ESS)

How likely are you to doze off or fall asleep in the following situations, in contrast to feeling just tired? This refers to your usual way of life in recent times. Even if you have not done some of these things recently try to work out how they would have affected you. Use the following scale to choose the most appropriate number for each situation:

0 = would *never* doze
1 = *slight* chance of dozing
2 = *moderate* chance of dozing
3 = *high* chance of dozing

SITUATION	CHANCE OF DOZING
Sitting and reading	
Watching television	
Sitting inactive in a public place (e.g., a theater or meeting)	
As a passenger in a car for an hour without a break	
Lying down to rest in the afternoon when circumstances permit	
Sitting and talking to someone	
Sitting quietly after a lunch without alcohol	
In a car, while stopped for a few minutes in the traffic	
TOTAL SCORE	

Score Results

1–6	Congratulations, you are getting enough sleep!
7–8	Your score is average.
9 and up	Very sleepy and should seek medical advice

Source: The Epworth Sleepiness Scale (ESS). M.W. Johns. (1991). A new method for measuring daytime sleepiness: The Epworth sleepiness scale, *Sleep, 14,* 540–545. Permission from the Associated Professional Sleep Societies, LLC, September 2006.

CHILDREN WITH OBSTRUCTIVE SLEEP APNEA SYNDROME

- Does your child snore? If so how often, and how loudly?
- Do you ever see your child struggling to breathe during sleep? Or stop breathing at night or during naps?
- Does your child become restless during sleep or assume unusual sleep positions?
- Does your child wet the bed?
- Does your child exhibit signs of being excessively sleepy or tired during the day? At school?
- Does your child complain of morning headaches?
- Does your child often breathe with the mouth open?
- Is your child having difficulty with schoolwork or relationships?
- Does your child have any signs of hyperactivity or aggressiveness?
- Does your child fall asleep in less than 30 minutes in a motor vehicle?

Source: Adapted from Peeke, K., Hershberger, M., & Marriner, J. (2006). Obstructive sleep apnea syndrome in children. *Pediatric Nursing, 32*(5), 489–494.

Plan

The major goal for clients with sleep disturbances is to maintain (or develop) a sleeping pattern that provides sufficient energy for daily activities. Other goals may relate to enhancing the client's feeling of well-being or improving the quality and quantity of the client's sleep. The nurse plans specific nursing interventions to reach the goal based on the etiology of each nursing diagnosis. Appropriate goals for the client with a sleep disturbance may include the following:

- The client will sleep through the night.
- The client will use relaxation techniques 30–45 minutes prior to bedtime.
- The client will maintain a consistent bedtime.
- The client will use good sleep hygiene.
- The client will reduce or remove environmental distractions from the bedroom.

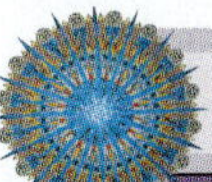

NURSING CARE PLAN **A Client With a Sleep-Rest Disorder**

ASSESSMENT	DIAGNOSIS	PLANNING
Jack Harrison is a 36-year-old police officer assigned to a high-crime police precinct. One week ago he received a surface bullet wound to his arm. Today he arrives at the outpatient clinic to have the wound redressed. While speaking with the nurse, Mr. Harrison mentions that he has recently been promoted to the rank of detective and has assumed new responsibilities. He states that since his promotion, he has experienced increasing difficulty falling asleep and sometimes staying asleep. He expresses concern over the danger of his occupation and his desire to do well in his new position. He complains of waking up feeling tired and irritable. **Physical Examination** Height: 185.4 cm (62") Weight: 85.7 kg (189 lb) Temperature: 37.0°C (98.6°F) Pulse: 80 bpm Respirations: 18/minute Blood pressure: 144/88 mmHg **Diagnostic Data** CBC within normal range, x-ray left arm: evidence of superficial soft tissue injury	Insomnia related to anxiety (as evidenced by difficulty falling and remaining asleep, fatigue, and irritability)	■ Client will sleep through the night. ■ Client will feel refreshed after sleep. ■ Client will not use pharmacological sleep aids.

IMPLEMENTATION

- Determine the client's sleep and activity pattern.
- Encourage Mr. Harrison to establish a bedtime routine to facilitate transition from wakefulness to sleep.
- Encourage him to eliminate stressful situations before bedtime.
- Instruct Mr. Harrison and significant others about factors (e.g., physiological, psychological, lifestyle, frequent work shift changes, excessively long work hours, and other environmental factors) that contribute to sleep pattern disturbances.
- Discuss with Mr. Harrison and his family comfort measures, sleep-promoting techniques, and lifestyle changes that can contribute to optimal sleep.
- Monitor bedtime food and beverage intake for items that facilitate or interfere with sleep.
- Seek to understand Mr. Harrison's perspective of a stressful situation.
- Encourage verbalization of feelings, perceptions, and fears.
- Discuss specific situations or individuals that threaten Mr. Harrison or his family.
- Assist him to use coping responses that have been successful in the past.

EVALUATION

Outcome met. Mr. Harrison acknowledges his insomnia is a somatic expression of his anxiety regarding job promotion and fear of failing. He states that talking with the police department counselor has been helpful. He is practicing relaxation techniques each night and sleeps an average of 7 hours a night. Mr. Harrison expresses a feeling of being rested upon awakening.

CRITICAL THINKING

1. What further information would be helpful to obtain from Mr. Harrison about his sleep problem?
2. What suggestions can you make that may help him develop better sleep habits?
3. What are the most common problems that interfere with clients' ability to sleep?

Implementation

Culturally competent, caring interventions that include the client, family, and indicated members of the interdisciplinary team can help establish or reestablish a restful sleep–wake cycle and an effective sleep pattern for the client.

Disturbed Sleep Pattern

- Assess sleep pattern and existing conditions that may affect sleep, such as depression and pain.
- Explain the disease process, options for treatment, and potential side effects.
- Review the client's medications to determine if medications may be interfering with sleep.
- Teach how to modify lifestyle activities that affect sleep:
  a. Alternate periods of activity with rest; avoid naps close to bedtime.
  b. Incorporate diet modifications, such as limiting caffeine and alcohol intake.
  c. Adapt the environment to aid sleep (e.g., darken the room and decrease noises).

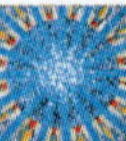

DEVELOPMENTAL CONSIDERATIONS Promoting Sleep in the Older Client

People of any age, but especially older adults, are unable to sleep well if they feel cold. Changes in circulation, metabolism, and body tissue density reduce the older adult's ability to generate and conserve heat. To compound this problem, hospital gowns have short sleeves and are made of thin polyester. Bedsheets also are often made of polyester rather than a warm fabric, such as cotton flannel. The following interventions can be used to keep older adults warm during sleep:

- Before the client goes to bed, warm the bed with prewarmed bath blankets.
- Use 100% cotton flannel sheets or apply thermal blankets between the sheet and bedspread.
- Encourage the client to wear own clothing, such as flannel nightgown or pajamas, socks, leg warmers, long underwear, sleeping cap (if scalp hair is sparse), or sweater, or use extra blankets.

Emotional stress obviously interferes with a person's ability to relax, rest, and sleep, and inability to sleep further aggravates feelings of tension. Sleep rarely occurs until a person is relaxed. Relaxation techniques can be encouraged as part of the nightly routine. Slow, deep breathing for a few minutes followed by slow, rhythmic contraction and relaxation of muscles can alleviate tension and induce calm.

Community-Based Care: Sleep Apnea

Obstructive sleep apnea usually is treated in the home. Nursing care focuses on teaching the client and family about equipment use and strategies to decrease contributing factors such as obesity and alcohol intake. Effective sleep apnea management depends on the client's willingness to participate in care. Provide teaching about the following topics:

- Relationship between obesity and sleep apnea
- Plans, resources, and referrals as needed for weight loss (e.g., programs such as Weight Watchers to provide additional support)
- Relationship of alcohol and sedatives to sleep apnea; referral to an alcohol treatment program or Alcoholics Anonymous as indicated
- How to use CPAP if ordered
- The importance of using CPAP continuously at night
- Measures to reduce airway dryness, including supplemental humidity and an adequate fluid intake to maintain moist mucous membranes.

If a support group for people with sleep apnea syndrome is available in the local area, refer the client and family to the group.

Evaluation

Using data collected during care and the desired outcomes developed during the planning stage as a guide, the nurse judges whether client goals and outcomes have been achieved. Data collection may include (a) observations of the duration of the client's sleep, (b) questions about how the client feels on awakening, or (c) observations of the client's level of alertness during the day.

If the desired outcomes are not achieved, the nurse and client should explore the reasons, which may include answers to the following questions:

- Were etiological factors correctly identified?
- Has the client's physical condition or medication therapy changed?
- Did the client comply with instructions about establishing a regular sleep–wake pattern?
- Did the client avoid ingesting caffeine?
- Did the client participate in stimulating daytime activities to avoid excessive daytime naps?
- Were all possible measures taken to provide a restful environment for the client?
- Were the comfort and relaxation measures effective?

REVIEW Sleep-Rest Disorder

RELATE: LINK THE CONCEPTS

Linking the exemplar of Sleep-Rest Disorder with the concept of Development:

1. How do requirements for sleep vary across developmental stages?
2. What assessment differences might you expect in sleep deprivation across the life span?

Linking the exemplar of Sleep-Rest Disorders with the concept of Sexuality:

3. How might sleep-rest disorders impact the client's sexual relationship with her significant other?
4. What interventions would you initiate for the couple when one of the partners has a sleep-rest disorder?

REFER: GO TO MYNURSINGKIT

- Sleep apnea video
- Diagnosing sleep apnea application
- Client with difficulty falling asleep case study
- Client with sleep disorder care plan activity

REFLECT: CASE STUDY

Jennifer Leno is a 30-year-old nursing student who works 20 hours each week, carries a full-time academic load, and has an 8-year-old child. She begins to drink energy drinks at night to stay awake to study. However, after 2 months of 5 hours of sleep a night and three energy drinks each day, she begins to have problems going to sleep. Her friend Janie offers Jennifer zolpidem (Ambien) to help her relax.

1. What might be causing Jennifer's insomnia?
2. What is zolpidem and is it likely to be effective in treating Jennifer's symptoms?
3. If you were a friend of Jennifer's as well, what would you advice would you give her?

PEARSON

EXPLORE mynursingkit™

MyNursingKit is your one stop for online chapter review materials and resources. Prepare for success with additional NCLEX®-style practice questions, interactive assignments and activities, web links, animations and videos, and more!

Register your access code from the front of your book at **www.mynursingkit.com**.

REFERENCES

Acello, B. (2000). Meeting JCAHO standards for pain control. *Nursing, 30*(3), 52–54.

Ackley, B. J., & Ladwig, G. B. (2006). *Nursing diagnosis handbook* (7th ed.). St. Louis, MO: Mosby Elsevier.

Adams, M.P., & Holland, N. (2005). *Pharmacology for nurses* (2nd ed.). Prentice Hall.

American Academy of Pediatrics, Committee on Fetus and Newborn. (2006). Prevention and management of pain in the neonate: An update. *Pediatrics, 118*(5), 2231–2241.

American Academy of Pediatrics & Canadian Paediatric Society. (2000). Prevention and management of pain and stress in the neonate. *Pediatrics, 105*(2), 454–461.

American Association of Colleges of Nursing (AACN). (1999). *Peaceful death: Recommended competencies and curricular guidelines for end-of-life nursing care.* Washington, DC: Author.

American Geriatrics Society (AGS) Clinical Practice Guidelines. (1998). The management of chronic pain in older persons. *Journal of the American Geriatrics Society, 46*, 635–651.

American Geriatrics Society (AGS). (2002). The management of persistent pain in older persons. *Journal of the American Geriatrics Society, 50* (6 Suppl.), S205–S224.

American Nurses Association. (2003a). *Position statement on nursing care and do-not-resuscitate (DNR) decisions.* Washington, DC: Author.

American Nurses Association. (1992b). *Report from the task force on the nurse's role in end of life decisions.* Kansas City: Author.

American Pain Society (APS). (1999). *Chronic pain in America: Roadblocks to relief.* Retrieved June 22, 2006, from http://www.ampainsoc.org/whatsnew/toc_road.htm

American Pain Society (APS). (2003). *Principles of analgesic use in the treatment of acute pain and cancer pain* (5th ed.). Glenview, IL: Author.

American Sleep Disorders Association. (2005). *The international classification of sleep disorders: Diagnostic and coding manual.* Lawrence, KS: Allen Press.

American Society for Pain Management Nursing. (2005). *Position paper: Use of placebos in pain management.* Retrieved June 22, 2006, from http://aspmn.org/pdfs/Use%20of%20Placebos.pdf

Andrews, M. M., & Boyle, J. S. (2003). *Transcultural concepts in nursing care* (4th ed.). Philadelphia: Lippincott Williams & Wilkins.

Anthony, K. K., & Schanberg, L. E. (2005). Pediatric pain syndromes and management of pain in children and adolescents with rheumatic disease. *Pediatric Clinics of North America, 52*, 611–639.

Arnstein, P. M. (1997). The neuroplastic phenomenon: A physiologic link between chronic pain and learning. *Journal of Neuroscience Nursing, 29*(3), 179–186.

Arnstein, P. M. (2003). Comprehensive assessment and management of chronic pain. *Nursing Clinics of North America, 38*, 403–417.

Arnstein, P., Caudil, M., Mandle, C. L., Norris, A., & Beasley, R. (1999). Self efficacy as a mediator of the relationship between pain intensity, disability and depression in chronic pain patients. *Pain, 80*(3), 483–491.

Baergen, R. (2006). How hopeful is too hopeful? Responding to unreasonably optimistic parents. *Pediatric Nursing, 32*(5), 482–486.

Ball, J. W., & Bindler, R. C. (2003). *Pediatric nursing: Caring for children* (3rd ed.). Upper Saddle River, NJ: Prentice Hall.

Ball, J.W., & Binder, R.M.W. (2007). *Pediatric nursing* (4th ed.). Upper Saddle River, NJ: Pearson Education.

Barbus, A. J. (1975). The Dying Person's Bill of Rights. *American Journal of Nursing, 75*(1), 99.

Bell, E. A. (2006). Is codeine a useful medication in pediatrics? *Infectious Diseases in Children, 19*(7), 12.

Bergh, I., & Sjostrom, B. (1999). A comparative study of nurses' and elderly patients' ratings of pain and pain tolerance. *Journal of Gerontological Nursing, 25*(5), 30–36.

Berman, A.J., Snyder, S., Kozier, B.J., & Erb, G. (2007). *Fundamentals of nursing* (8th ed.). Upper Saddle River, NJ: Pearson Education.

Berry. P.H. (Editor). (2005). *HPNA: Core curriculum for the generalist hospice and palliative nurse.* (2nd ed.). Dubuque, Iowa: Kendall/Hunt Publishing Company.

Bishop, T. F., & Morrison, S. (2007). Geriatric palliative care–part I: Pain and symptom management. *Clinical Geriatrics, 15*(1), 25–32.

Bourdeanu, L., Loseth, D. B., & Funk, M. (2005). Management of opioid-induced sedation in patients with cancer. *Clinical Journal of Oncology Nursing, 9*(6), 705–711.

Brislin, R. P., & Rose, J. B. (2005). Pediatric acute pain management. *Anesthesiology Clinics of North America, 23*, 789–814.

Bruckenthal, P. (2008) Risk factors associated with the onset of persistent pain. Retrieved August 15, 2009 from http://cme.medscape.com/viewarticle/576473

Bruera, E., Kuehn, N., Miller, M., Selmser, P., & Macmillan, K. (1991). The Edmonton Symptom Assessment Scale (ESAS): A simple method for the assessment of palliative care patients. *Journal of Palliative Care, 7*, 6–9.

Caudill, M. A. (2002). *Managing pain before it manages you* (revised ed.). New York: Guilford Press.

Centers for Disease Control. (2009). *Sleep and sleep disorders: a public health challenge.* Retrieved October 17, 2009, from http://www.cdc.gov/sleep/

Clinical Advisor. (2007). *Managing excessive sleepiness.* Highlights from Symposia held at the AANP National Conference and AAPA Annual Conference, *1*(4), Program ID 0709411.

Cohen, M. J., & Schecter, W. P. (2005). Perioperative pain control: A strategy for management. *Surgical Clinics of North America, 85*, 1243–1257.

Compton, P., & Athanasos, P. (2003). Chronic pain, substance abuse and addiction. *Nursing Clinics of North America, 38*, 525–537.

Cook, L., Sefcik, E., & Stetina, P. (2004). Pain management in the addicted population: A case study comparison of prescriptive practice. *Journal of Addictions Nursing, 15*, 11–14.

Darrow, D. H. (2007). Surgery for pediatric sleep apnea. *Otolaryngology Clinics of North America, 40*, 855–875.

DeGood, D. E., & Kiernan, B. D. (1997). Pain related cognitions as predictors of pain treatment outcomes. *Advances in Medical Psychotherapy, 9*, 73–90.

Dembner, A. (2004, September 14). Hospices widen care services. *Boston Globe*, B24.

Dodd, M., Janson, S., Facione, N., Faucett, J., Froelicher, E. S., Humphreys, J., et al. (2001). Advancing the science of symptom management. *Journal of Advanced Nursing, 33*(5), 668–676.

Doghramji, D. (2000). *Sleepless in America: Diagnosing and treating insomnia.* Retrieved February 22, 2008, from http://www.medscape.com/viewprogram/347

Elliott, A. M., Smith, B. H., Penny, K. I., Smith, W. C., & Chambers, W. A. (1999). The epidemiology of chronic pain in the community. *Lancet, 354*, 1248–1252.

End-of-life Nursing Education Consortium (ELNEC). (2000). *Training program.* American Association of Colleges & City of Hope; Clearwater, Florida: The Hospice Institute of the Florida Suncoast.

End of Life Nursing Education Consortium (ELNEC). (2006). Promoting advanced practice nursing in palliative care. Duarte, CA: City of Hope National Medical Center and Washington, DC: American Association of Colleges of Nursing.

Fallat, M. E., Deshpande, J. K., & Section on Surgery, Section on Anesthesia and Pain Medicine, and Committee on Bioethics. (2004). Do-not-resuscitate orders for pediatric patients who require anesthesia and surgery. *Pediatrics, 114*(6), 1686–1692.

FDA: U.S. Food and Drug Administration. (2005). *FDA Public Health Advisory: FDA announces important changes and additional warnings for COX-2 selective and non-selective non-steroidal anti-inflammatory drugs (NSAIDs).* Retrieved June 22, 2006, from http:// www.fda.gov/cder/drug/advisory/COX2.htm

Formulary Journal. (2009). Milnacipran (Savella): Selective norepinephrine and serotonin reuptake inhibitor approved for the management of fibromyalgia. Retrieved August 15, 2009, from http://formularyjournal.modernmedicine.com/formulary/Modern+Medicine+Now/Milnacipran-Savella-Selective-norepinephrine-and-s/ArticleStandard/Article/detail/579380

Fragoso, C., & Gill, T. (2007). Sleep complaints in community-living older persons: A multifactorial geriatric syndrome. *Journal of the American Geriatrics Society, 55*, 1853–1866.

Glaser, B., & Strauss, A. (1965). *Awareness of dying.* Chicago: Aldine.

Gloth, F. (2001). Pain management in older adults: Prevention and treatment. *Journal of the American Geriatrics Society, 49*, 188–199.

Goldsmith, C. (2007, February 26). Insomnia: Sleepless in America. *Nursing Spectrum*, New England Edition, 18–21.

Gordon, M. (2003). CPR in long-term care: Mythical benefits or necessary ritual. *Annals of Long-Term Care, 11*(4), 41–49.

Habib, Lisa. (2006). Acupuncture good for fibromyalgia? Retrieved August 15, 2009, from http://www.webmd.com/news/20060616/acupuncture-good-for-fibromyalgia

Hall, R. W., & Anand, K. J. S. (2005). Short- and long-term impact of neonatal pain and stress: More than an ouchie. *NeoReviews, 6*(2), e69–e74.

Hallenbeck, J. (2005). Fast facts and concepts #11: Tube feed or not tube feed? *End of life Physician Education Resource Center.* Retrieved October 30, 2007, from http://www.eperc.mcw.edu

Hammes, B. J., Klevan, J., Kempf, M., & Williams, M. S. (2005). Pediatric advance care planning. *Journal of Palliative Medicine, 8*(4), 766–773.

Hartman, R. G. (2004). Dying young: Cues from the courts. *Archives of Pediatrics and Adolescent Medicine, 158*, 615–619.

Heller, K. S., & Solomon, M. Z. (2005). Continuity of care and caring: What matters to parents of children with life-threatening conditions. *Journal of Pediatric Nursing, 20*(5), 335–346

Herr, K., Bjoro, K., & Decker, S. (2006). Tools for assessment of pain in nonverbal older adults with dementia: A state-of-the-science review. *Journal of Pain and Symptom Management, 31*(2), 170–192.

Herr, K., Bjoro, K., Steffensmeier, J., & Rakel, B. (2006). *Acute pain management in older adults.* Iowa City, IA: University of Iowa Gerontological Nursing Interventions Research Center, Research Translation and Dissemination Core.

Himelstein, B. P. (2005). Palliative care in pediatrics. *Anesthesiology Clinics of North America, 23*, 837–856.

Himelstein, B. P., Hilden, J. M., Boldt, A. M., & Weissman, D. (2004). Pediatric palliative care. *New England Journal of Medicine, 350*(17), 1752–1762.

Hitchcock, L. S., Ferrell, B. R., & McCaffery, M. (1994). The experience of chronic non-malignant pain. *Journal of Pain and Symptom Management, 9*(5), 312–318.

Hospice and Palliative Nurses Association (HPNA). (2003a). *HPNA position statement: Artificial nutrition and hydration in end-of-life care.* Pittsburg, PA: Author. Retrieved October 25, 2007, from http://www.hpna.org

Hospice and Palliative Nurses Association (HPNA). (2003b). *HPNA position statement: Value of professional nurse in end-of-life care.* Pittsburg, PA: Author. Retrieved August 14, 2007, from http://www.hpna.org

Huether, S. E., & Defriez, C. B. (2006). Pain, temperature regulation, sleep, and sensory function. In K. L. McCance & S. E. Huether (Eds.), *Pathophysiology: The biologic basis for disease in adults and children* (5th ed., pp. 447–462). St. Louis, MO: Mosby–Year Book.

Institute of Medicine (IOM). (2003). Patterns of childhood death in America. In *When children die: Improving palliative and end-of-life care for children and their families* (pp. 41–71). Washington, DC: National Academy Press.

Institute of Medicine (IOM). (2006). *Sleep disorders and sleep deprivation: An unmet public health problem.* Washington, DC: Author.

International Council of Nurses. (1997). *Basic principles of nursing care.* Washington, DC: American Nurses Publishing.

Jacobs, H. H. (2005). Ethics in pediatric end-of-life care: A nursing perspective. *Journal of Pediatric Nursing, 20*(5), 360–369.

Jao, D., & Alessi, C. (2004). Sleep disorders. In C. Landefeld, R. Palmer, M. Johnson, C. Johnston, & W. Lyons (Eds.), *Current geriatric diagnosis and treatment.* New York: Lange Medical Books/McGraw-Hill.

Joint Commission on Accreditation of Healthcare Organizations (JCAHO). (2001). *Joint Commission on Accreditation of Healthcare Organizations pain standards for 2004.* Available from http://www.jcaho.org

Katz, J., Jackson, M., Kavanagh, B. P., & Sandler, A. N. (1996). Acute pain after thoracic surgery predicts long-term post-thoracotomy pain. *Clinical Journal of Pain, 12*, 50–55.

Kirchhoff, K., Spuhler, V., Walker, L., Hutton, A., Cole, B., & Clemmer, T. (2000). Intensive care nurses' experiences with end-of-life care. *American Journal of Critical Care, 9*(1), 35–42.

Kolcaba, K. (2003). *Comfort theory and practice: A vision for holistic health care and research.* New York: Springer Publishing Company.

Korones, D. N. (2007). Pediatric palliative care. *Pediatrics in Review, 28*(8), e46–e56.

Krakauer, E., Crenner, C., & Fox, K. (2002). Barriers to optimum end-of-life care for minority patients. *Journal of the American Geriatrics Society, 50*, 182–190.

Kripke, D., Garfinkle, L., Wingard, D., Klauber, M., & Marler, M. (2002). Mortality associated with sleep duration and insomnia. *Archive of General Psychiatry, 59*, 131–136.

Kurz, A., & Sessler, D. I. (2003). Opioid-induced bowel dysfuntion: Pathophysiology and potential new therapies. *Drugs, 63*(7), 649–671.

Lacey, D. (2005). Tube feeding, antibiotics, and hospitalization of long-term care facility residents with end-stage dementia: Perceptions of key medical decision-makers. *American Journal of Alzheimer's Disease and Other Dementias, 20*(4), 211–219.

Last Acts. (2002). *Means to a better end: A report on dying in America.* Retrieved August 27, 2007, from http://www.lastacts.org

Levetown, M. (2005). Deciding to allow my child to die in the intensive care unit. *Pediatric Critical Care Medicine, 6*(5), 604–605.

Manias, E., Bucknall, T., & Botti, M. (2005). Nursing strategies for managing pain in the postoperative setting. *Pain Management Nursing, 6*(1), 18–29.

Mayo Clinic. (2009). Fibromyalgia: Causes. Retrieved August 15, 2009 from http://www.mayoclinic.com/health/fibromyalgia/DS00079/DSECTION=causes

Mayo Clinic. (2008). Causes of Fatigue. Retrieved October 17, 2009, from http://www.mayoclinic.com/health/fatigue/MY00120/DSECTION=causes

Mazanec, P., & Panke, J. T. (2006). Cultural considerations in palliative care. In B. R. Ferrell & N. Coyle (Eds.), *Textbook of palliative nursing* (pp. 623–633). Oxford, England: Oxford University Press.

McCaffery, M. (1979). *Nursing management of the patient with pain.* Philadelphia: Lippincott.

McCaffery, M., Ferrell, B. R., & Pasero, C. (2000). Nurses' personal opinions about patients' pain and their effect on recorded assessments and titration of opioid doses. *Pain Management Nursing, 1*(3), 79–87.

McCaffery, M., & Pasero, C. (1999). *Pain: Clinical manual* (2nd ed.). St. Louis, MO: Mosby.

McCance, K., & Huether, S. (2002). *Pathophysiology: The biologic basis for disease in adults and children.* (4th ed.). St. Louis, MO: Mosby.

Melzack, R., & Wall, P. D. (1965). Pain mechanisms: A new theory. *Science,150*, 971–979.

Meyer, E. C., Ritholz, M. D., Burns, J. P., & Truog, R. D. (2006). Improving the quality of end-of-life care in the pediatric intensive care unit: Parents' priorities and recommendations. *Pediatrics, 117*(3), 649–657.

Monteiro-Cruz, D. A. L., & Mattos-Pimenta, C. A. (2001). Chronic pain: Nursing diagnosis or syndrome? *Nursing Diagnosis, 12*(4), 117–127.

Moore, A., & Clinch, D. (2004). Underlying mechanism of impaired visceral pain perception in older people. *Journal of the American Geriatrics Society, 52*, 132–136.

National Center for Health Statistics. (2008). *Deaths-leading causes. Fast stats.* Retrieved September 24, 2008, from http://www.cdc.gov/nchs/FASTATS/lcod.htm

National Consensus Project (NCP) for Quality Palliative Care. (2004). *Clinical practice guidelines for quality palliative care,* Retrieved September 19, 2007, from http://www.nationalconsensusproject.org/guidelines

National Hospice and Palliative Care Organization. (2000). *Hospice fact sheet.* Alexandria, VA: Author. Retrieved September 14, 2002, from http://www.nhpco.org

National Institute of Arthritis and Musculoskeletal and Skin Diseases. (2005a). *Fibromyalgia.* Retrieved from http://www.niams.nih.gov/hi/topics/fibromyalgia/ffibro.htm

National Institutes of Health (NIH). (2008a). *Melatonin for sleep disorders.* Retrieved February 22, 2008, from http://ahrq.gov/clinic/epcsums/melatsum.htm

National Institutes of Health (NIH). (2008b). *Valerian.* Retrieved February 22, 2008, from http://ods.od.nih.gov/factsheets/Valerian.asp

National Fibromyalgia Research Association. (2004). *Fibromyalgia syndrome.* Retrieved from http://www.nfra.net/

National Sleep Foundation. (2005a). *Insomnia.* Retrieved June 29, 2006, from http://www.sleepfoundation.org/sleeptionary/index.php?id=19

O'Rourke, D. (2004). The measurement of pain in infants, children and adolescents: From policy to practice. *Physical Therapy, 84*(6), 560–570.

Page, G. G., Ben-Eliyahu, S., Yirmiya, R., & Liebeskind, J. C. (1993). Morphine attenuates surgery-induced enhancement of metastatic colonization in rats. *Pain, 54*(1), 21–28.

Partners Against Pain. (2002). *Senior care: The management of persistent pain in older persons.* Retrieved October 4, 2007, from http://www.partnersagainstpain.com

Pasero, C. (2003). Pain in the emergency department. Withholding pain medication is not justified. *American Journal of Nursing, 103*(7), 73–74.

Pasero, C., & McCaffery, M. (2002). Pain control: Monitoring sedation: It's the key to preventing opioid-induced respiratory depression. *American Journal of Nursing, 102*(2), 67, 69.

Plaisance, L., & Logan, C. (2006). Nursing students' knowledge and attitudes regarding pain. *Pain Management Nursing, 7*(4), 167–175.

Podolecki, T., Podolecki, A., & Hrycek, A. (2009). Fibromyalgia: pathogenic, diagnostic, and therapeutic concerns. *Polish Archives of Internal Medicine, 119*(3), 157–160.

Porth, C. (2005). *Pathophysiology: Concepts of altered health states* (7th ed.). Philadelphia: Lippincott.

Punjabi, N. M., Caffo, B. S., Goodwin, J. L., Gottlieb, D. J., Newman, A. B., O'Connor, G. T., Rapoport, D. M. (2009). Sleep-disordered breathing and mortality: a prospective cohort study. *PLOS Medicine, 6* (8): e1000132.doi:10.1371/journal.pmd.1000132. Retrieved August 18, 2009 from http://www.plosmedicine.org/article/info%3Adoi%2F10.1371%2Fjournal.pmed.1000132

Puntillo, K. A., & Weiss, S. J. (1994). Pain: Its mediators and associated morbidity in critically ill cardiovascular surgical patients. *Nursing Research, 43*, 31–36.

Quill, T. (2000). Perspectives on care at the close of life. Initiating end of life discussions with seriously ill patients: Addressing the "elephant in the room." *Journal of the American Medical Association, 284* (19), 2501–2507.

Reuben, D., Herr, K., Pacala, J., Pollick, B., Potter, J., & Semla, T. (2008). *Geriatrics at your fingertips* (9th ed.). Malden, MA: Blackwell.

Reuters. (2009). Sleep apnea raises death risk 46 percent. Retrieved August 18, 2009 from http://news.yahoo.com/s/nm/20090818/sc_nm/us_sleep_death

Reyes-Gibby, C. C., Aday, L., & Cleeland, C. (2002). Impact of pain on self-rated health in community-dwelling older adults. *Pain, 95*, 75–82.

Robinson, S. B., Weitzel, T., & Henderson, L. (2005). The sh-h-h-h project. Nonpharmacological interventions. *Holistic Nursing Practice, 19*(6), 263–266.

Rushton, C. H. (2004). Ethics and palliative care in pediatrics. *American Journal of Nursing, 104*(4), 54–63.

Rushton, C. H. (2005). A framework for integrated pediatric palliative care: Being with dying. *Journal of Pediatric Nursing, 20*(5), 311–325.

Rushton, C. H., Reder, E., Hall, B., Comello, K., Sellers, D. E., & Hutton, N. (2006). Interdisciplinary interventions to improve pediatric palliative care and reduce health care professional suffering. *Journal of Palliative Medicine, 9*, 922–933.

Schaffer, S. D., & Yucha, C. B. (2004). Relaxation & pain management. *American Journal of Nursing, 104*(8), 75–76, 78–79, 81–82.

Serlin, R. C., Mendoza, T.R., Nakamura, Y., Edwards, K. R., & Cleeland, C. S. (1995). When is cancer pain mild, moderate or severe? Grading pain severity by its interference with function. *Pain, 61*, 277–284.

Stanley, M., Blair, K. A., & Beare, P. G. (2005). *Gerontological nursing: Promoting successful aging with older adults* (3rd ed.). Philadelphia: F. A. Davis.

Strumpf, N. E., Tuch, H., Stillman, D., Parrish, P., & Morrison, N. (2004). Implementing palliative care in the nursing home. Annals of Long-Term Care, 12(11), 35–41.

SUPPORT Principal Investigators. (1995). A controlled trial to improve care for seriously ill hospitalized patients. The study to understand prognoses and preferences for outcomes and risks of treatment. *Journal of the American Medical Association, 274*(20), 1591–1598.

Svendsen, K. B., Andersen, S., Arnason, S., Arnér, S., Breivik, H., Heiskanen, T., et al. (2005). Breakthrough pain in malignant and non-malignant diseases: A review of prevalence, characteristics and mechanisms. *European Journal of Pain 9*, 195–206.

Trame, C. (2002). Pharmacology consult: Just what are we treating—addiction or pain? *Clinical Nurse Specialist, 16*(1), 295–297.

Vallerand, A.H. (2003). The use of long-acting opiods in chronic pain management. *Nursing Clinics of North America, 38*, 435–445.

Verghese, S. T., & Hannallah, R. S. (2005). Postoperative pain management in children. *Anesthesiology Clinics of North America, 23*, 163–184.

Vitiello, M. V. (1999). Effective treatments for age-related sleep disturbances. *Geriatrics, 54*, 47–52.

Von Baeyer, C. L., Marche, T. A., Rocha, E. M., & Salmon, K. (2004). Children's memory for pain: Overview and implications for practice. *Journal of Pain, 5*(5), 241–249.

Walden, M. (2007). Pain in the newborn and infant. In C. Kenner & J. W. Lott, *Comprehensive neonatal nursing: An interdisciplinary approach* (4th ed., pp. 360–371). Philadelphia: Elsevier Saunders.

Wilcox, S., Brenes, G., Levine, D., Sevick, M. A., Shumaker, S. A., & Craven, T. (2000). Factors related to sleep disturbance in older adults experiencing knee pain or knee pain with radiographic evidence of knee osteoarthritis. *Journal of the American Geriatrics Society, 48*, 1241–1251.

Wilson, K. G., Eriksson, M. Y., D'Eon, J. L., Mikail, S. F., & Emery, P. C. (2002). Major depression and insomnia in chronic pain. *Clinical Journal of Pain, 18*(2), 77–83.

Wolfe, F, Smythe HA, Yunus MB, Bennett RM, Bombardier C, Goldenberg DL, et al. (1990). The American College of Rheumatology 1990 criteria for the classification of fibromyalgia: report of the multicenter criteria committee. *Arthritis Rheum 33*:160–172.

Wong, D. L., Hockenberry-Eaton, M., Wilson, D., Winkelstein, M. L., & Schwartz, P. (2001). *Essentials of pediatric nursing* (6th ed.). St. Louis, MO: Mosby.

Young, K. D. (2005). Pediatric procedural pain. *Annals of Emergency Medicine, 45*(2), 160–171.

6 Culture

Concept at-a-Glance

Concept Learning Outcomes

After reading about this concept, you will be able to:

1. Contrast factors that differ between and among cultures.
2. Identify cultural differences in the characteristics and behaviors of individuals.
3. Demonstrate the nursing process in providing culturally competent care across the life span.
4. Describe variations of social behaviors found in different cultures.
5. Discuss how cultural and religious differences and preferences may affect an individual's lifestyle and health care choices.

Concept Key Terms

Acculturation, 322
Assimilation, 322
Culture, 322
Cultural groups, 322
Enculturation, 322
Ethnic groups, 323
Multiculturalism, 323
Race, 323
Religion, 325
Stereotyping, 323
Subculture groups, 323

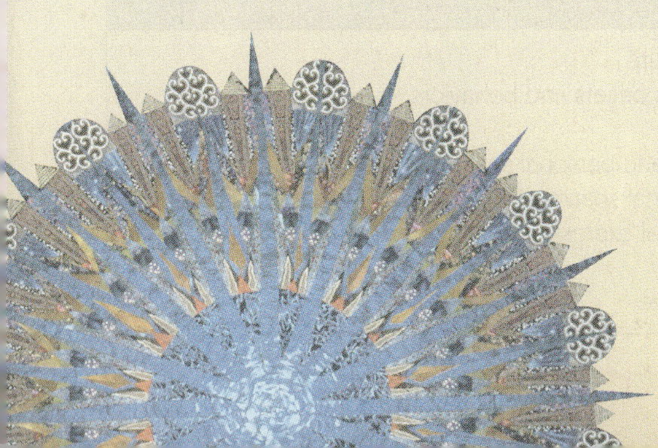

About Culture

A Chinese client is admitted to a hospital but refuses to enter his assigned hospital room—room 444. Although quiet just moments earlier, the client is now very anxious and shouting in his native language as he quickly walks down the hall away from his room. What might have caused this change in the client's behavior?

The answer can be found in the values and beliefs of the client. In the Chinese culture, many people believe the number 4 is a bad omen and must be avoided. The Chinese client could perceive the number 444 as a bad sign for his continued health if he stays in that room. ●

WHAT IS CULTURE?

Social identity includes the cultural practices that differentiate one social group from another. The people within a social group share a common identity. Their social memory gives the cultural group a history of behaviors, rituals, and other social practices as well as religious practices. Social groups have a variety of traditions and practices regarding marriage, family, art, music, religion, science, and leadership. Change may come from within or from outside of the social group, and the group may need to modify its cultural practices so that the culture itself will survive these changes.

Not everyone embraces the idea of working with other cultures. To be successful professionals, nurses must learn to recognize their own cultural biases and how to address them. One important thing nurses should remember in this regard is that a person's ethnic identity does not necessarily communicate anything about his or her cultural values or patterns of behavior. Culture provides identity for its members, but within a single culture or ethnic group, individuals choose how much of their culture they will practice and incorporate in daily life. It is important for health care professionals to consider a client as an individual first and as a member of a culture or ethnic group second.

Aspects of Culture

Culture refers to the patterns of behavior and thinking that people living in social groups learn, develop, and share. A society is a group of people who share a common culture, rules of behavior, and basic social organization. Culture is learned by people living together in a society. As described in the Focus on Diversity and Culture feature that follows, cultural characteristics, such as customs, beliefs, values, language, and socialization patterns, are passed from generation to generation. **Cultural groups** are racial, ethnic, religious, or social groups with specific group behaviors and characteristics that are learned and shared, including language, customs, beliefs, and values.

Box 6–1 How Cultural Behaviors are Learned

Cultural behaviors are learned by

- observing others doing the behavior.
- hearing instructions on how to do the behavior.
- imitating others doing the behavior.
- getting reinforcement for doing the behaviors others do.
- internalizing the behaviors.
- spontaneously doing the behaviors without thinking about it.

Culture is transmitted from one generation to the next through language, material objects, rituals and customs, institutions, and art. Through use of a common language, people learn how to live by the rules governing the society and how to earn money or trade goods or services to meet basic needs, such as food and shelter. Culture can influence everything the members of a society think and do.

ENCULTURATION **Enculturation**, or cultural transmission, is the process of children learning culture from adults. People biologically inherit many physical traits and behavioral instincts; people socially inherit culture. A person must learn culture from other people in a society. Enculturation occurs in families until the children are ready to leave and establish their own households. However, it may continue among family members who live close to each other, celebrate religious holidays together, or otherwise work to maintain the culture within their family. For additional information about how cultural behaviors are learned, see Box 6–1.

All the people in a society keep the characteristics of the culture alive. The culture can be preserved in the art, music, and traditions of the cultural group. Because culture is adaptive, these characteristics may be modified over the years as people use culture to adjust to changes in the world around them. The process of enculturation will adapt to these changes.

Different societies can come together and share or exchange culture as well. People may move from one cultural group to another. **Assimilation** the process of adapting to and integrating characteristics of the dominant culture as one's own. Cultures benefit by exchanging ideas, natural resources, people, and goods. (For information on using assimilation to help clients learn new skills, see the Client Teaching feature.) **Acculturation** is the process of not only adapting to another culture but also accepting the majority group's culture as one's

FOCUS ON DIVERSITY AND CULTURE Cultural Characteristics

- History of origin
- Holiday customs
- Styles of dress
- General world view
- Religious beliefs and practices
- Foods and eating patterns
- Values
- Roles and patterns of relationships
- Leadership structure
- Health and illness beliefs and behaviors
- Social systems
- Concept of time and personal space
- Concept of personal space
- Gestures and facial expressions
- Concept of self
- Common language

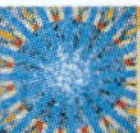

CLIENT TEACHING Using the Assimilation Process

Whatever the client's cultural background, use the assimilation process to help the client learn a new skill that will be needed at home:

- Assess the client's cultural beliefs as they relate to the new skill.
- Introduce a new skill by having the client observe as it is demonstrated.
- Explain each step of using the new skill.
- Have the client perform the new skill while the nurse observes and helps.
- Have the client practice the new skill to improve his or her performance.
- Have the client perform the skill at home without assistance from a nurse.
- When the skill has been assimilated, the client can perform it at home without having to think about how to do it.

own. Language, customs, religious practices, or traditions can be adapted from one culture to another. Because culture is complex, members of a cultural group may engage in many behaviors and habits unconsciously, making them difficult to explain to others.

Sometimes, smaller cultural groups within a larger society maintain their customs and other cultural traits. **Subculture groups** are minority groups characterized by specific norms, beliefs, and values that coexist with a dominant culture. The members of a subculture group may share distinct dress, rituals, or language. Examples of subculture groups are street gangs, mountain folk, and pop-group followers (e.g., "Dead Heads").

MULTICULTURALISM **Multiculturalism** is defined as many subcultures coexisting within a given society in which no one culture dominates. In a multicultural society, human differences are accepted by most people, leading to a desire to overcome racism, sexism, and other forms of discrimination (Multiculturalism Definitions, 2008). Classrooms in these communities are culturally diverse, and students have different levels of socialization and learning styles.

In the United States, one driver of multiculturalism has been immigration. People from nearly every country in the world have come to the United States in search of a new way of life. Many, such as the Hmong people immigrating from Asia, sought freedom from an oppressive government. Others sought religious freedom, and still others freedom from poverty. Each family or group of immigrants brings its own culture with it, adding to what has been called the "melting pot" that is the United States. The ideal of the melting pot is the assimilation of multiple ethnic groups with their cultural practices into an American national identity with national allegiance and values.

Typically, families and groups from the same country will relocate to a specific area or neighborhood, which helps them to maintain their native language, traditions, and ways of worship. These **ethnic groups** have common racial characteristics—for example, nationality, language, values, and customs—and they share a cultural heritage. Examples of ethnic groups are the large Cuban-American population living in and around Miami, Florida; the Lakota Sioux, one of three major ethnic groups that make up the Great Sioux Nation; and the Hmong populations living in western North Carolina.

Immigrant groups often maintain use of their native language in their homes and places of worship for several generations. Children may speak their native language in the home and English at school, and families retain ties to their country of origin and continue native cultural practices. As these families have children and grandchildren, however, customs such as food preparation and eating habits, dress, and celebration of holidays survive, but other cultural traditions become lost as the descendants of the original immigrants assimilate further into American culture. Today, the multiple cultures in the United States may be better described as "a tossed salad"—each group intermingles with other cultures but maintains its own separate identity and cultural heritage. These differences can impact how individuals and families interact with health care providers and other professionals. Nurses working in areas with people of many cultures must be careful to respect each client's culture.

RACE **Race** refers to socially defined populations that have in common genetically transmitted physical characteristics, such as skin color, bone structure, and other genetic traits. Today, the U.S. Bureau of the Census recognizes six categories of race: Native American, African American, Asian American, Native Hawaiians or Other Pacific Islanders, White (European American), and Some Other Race (available to people who do not think they belong in the other race categories). The Census Bureau asks questions to determine Hispanic/Latino status separate from race. This subject is discussed in greater detail in the concept of Diversity.

STEREOTYPING **Stereotyping** refers to generalizing that all individuals in a group are the same. Stereotyping does help to provide a frame of reference regarding people from other cultures, but it also can lead to misunderstandings and miscommunication. One example is the still pervasive tendency that Americans have to group all Asian Americans together despite the many countries that they represent and the fact that many Asian-American families have been U.S. citizens for several generations (for more information on this tendency, see the Asian-Nation website at http://www.asian-nation.org).

Use of stereotypes also can have grave, long-standing effects on the people of a culture or an ethnic group. Nowhere is this more clear than in the effects of segregation in the American South. Segregation and racial prejudices have contributed to a general lack of trust and apprehension among some African Americans in the South related to accepting and following medical recommendations (Betancourt & Ananeh-Firemping, 2004). While less prevalent today, it remains a factor in how

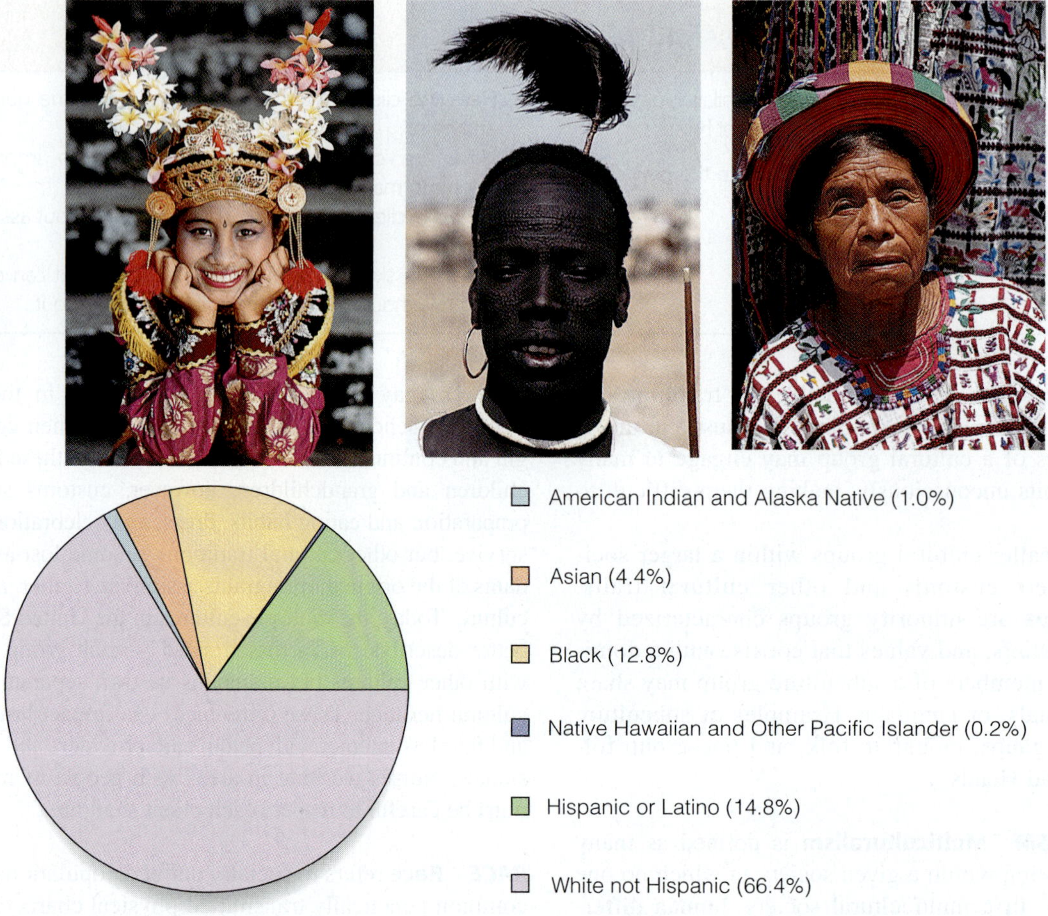

Figure 6–1 ■ Different cultural heritages are parts of the population in America.

Source: Graph from U.S. Bureau of the Census. (2007). State & County QuickFacts. Retrieved from http://quickfacts.census.gov/qfd/states/00000.html; Steve Vidler/SuperStock; Robert Caputo/Stock Boston; Arvind Garg/Getty Images, Inc.–Liaison.

some African Americans view working with health care professionals. Regardless of the reason why a client may be reluctant to follow treatment recommendations, the best way the nurse can address this reluctance is by building a relationship of respect and trust. Often, respectful communication and a sincere desire for the client's health and well-being can overcome any cultural is understandings.

Culture in the United States

According to the U.S. Census (2007) Bureau, the estimated population of United States in 2006 was 299,398,484. In addition to the six races defined by the Census Bureau and the ethnicity known as Hispanic/Latino, there are an uncountable number of cultures, subcultures, and ethnic groups. Some of these are easily defined, but many are not. Children whose parents come from different cultures may not identify with either parent's culture (Figure 6–1 ■).

The culture of the United States is Western, and Western culture often is associated with economic liberalization (free trade), democratization (or representative government), and scientific advancement (technology and gadgets). As a result of large numbers of immigrants arriving from many countries throughout this country's history, the culture of the United States also is multicultural (Figure 6–2 ■). These various cultures are represented by numerous professional, ethnic, religious, recreational, demographic, or social groups with which individuals may identify or to which they may belong (Figure 6–3 ■). Some examples are the National Association for the Advancement of Colored People (NAACP), a civil rights organization; the American Irish Historical Society, a cultural organization; and the National Association of Hispanic Nurses, a professional organization.

Within the United States, the federal government as well as state and local governments have instituted any number of policies supporting this multicultural population. Some of these government multicultural policies (modified from Multiculturalism, 2004) are as follows:

- Acceptance of multiple citizenship
- Support for minority holidays and celebrations
- Support for music and arts from minority cultures
- Acceptance of traditional and religious dress in schools and public places (Figure 6–4 ■)
- Encouragement of minority representation in education, politics, and the workforce.

Government at the federal, state, and local levels supports education. The primary unofficial language is American English, although government agencies frequently offer programs and print publications in other languages. Many religions

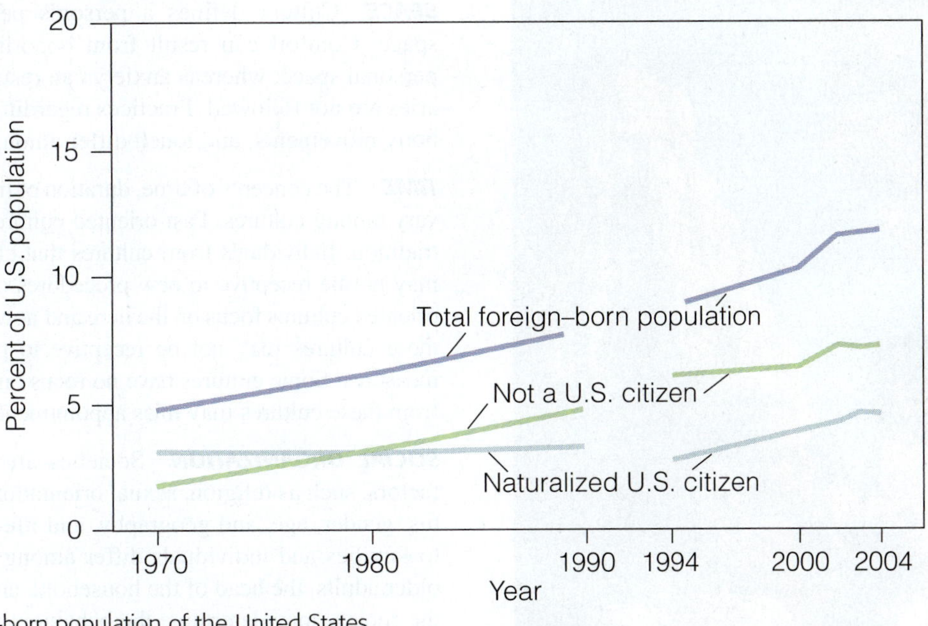

Figure 6–2 ■ Foreign-born population of the United States.

Source: Centers for Disease Control and Prevention. U. S. Census Bureau.

are practiced, including Protestant Christianity, Catholicism, Judaism, Hinduism, Islam, and Buddhism. **Religion** refers to a set of doctrines accepted by a group of people who gather together regularly to worship that offer a means to relate to God or a higher power, nature, and their spiritual being. Religion plays a greater role in some communities than in others: One town may sponsor a living nativity at Christmas, while the next may ban religious spectacles on government property altogether. Family arrangements in the United States are exceedingly diverse, including the nuclear family, single-parent families, childless couples, and blended families.

Influenced by many of the cultures within its borders, American culture includes a few general values and attitudes toward social behaviors (Essortment, 2008):

- Importance placed on punctuality and time sensitivity
- Distaste for pushiness, condescension, and bullying
- Intolerance of line jumping or not waiting one's turn
- Acceptance of casual and formal attire at the same events
- Liberation of women (feminism)
- Acceptance of political discussions (if not specific)
- Appreciation of efficiency at work and in social situations.

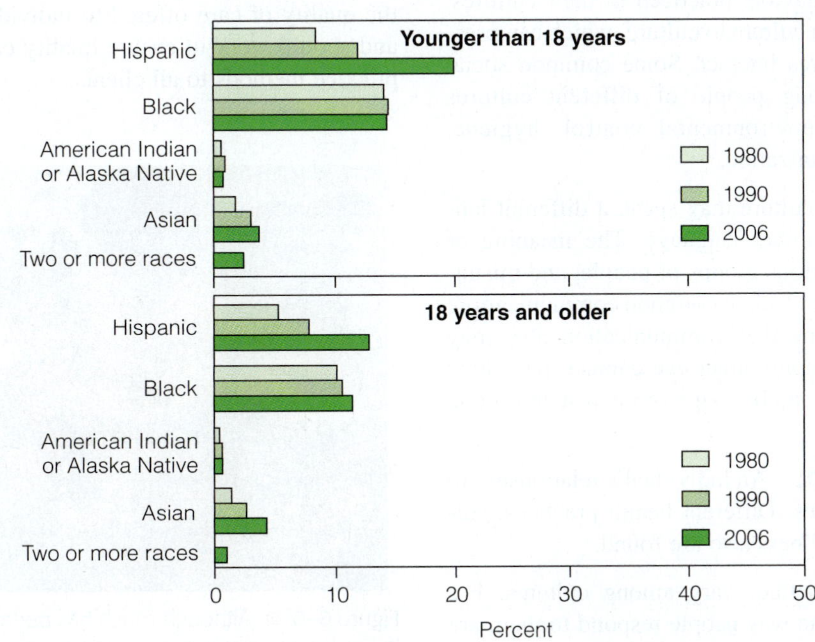

Figure 6–3 ■ Population of the United States by race and ethnicity.

Source: Centers for Disease Control and Prevention, National Center for Health Statistics. (2006). Health, United States, 2006, Figure 3. Data from U.S. Bureau of the Census.

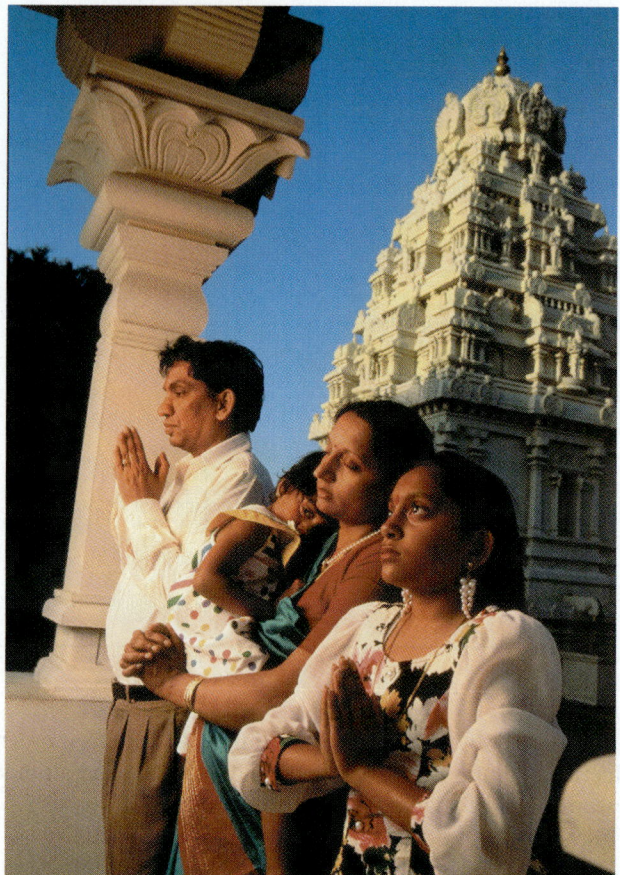

Figure 6–4 ■ Subcultures can maintain heritage and identity through dress, foods eaten, and daily activities.

Source: Steve Liss Photography

CULTURAL DIFFERENCES

Variations in Social Behavior

People learn the social behaviors practiced in their cultures. These behaviors differ from culture to culture, which can present challenges when cultures interact. Some common social behavioral variations among people of different cultures involve communication, environmental control, hygiene, space, time, and social organization.

COMMUNICATION Each culture may speak a different language or a variation of another language. The meaning of words can differ among various groups of people, and misunderstandings may result from lack of common communication.

Misinterpretation of nonverbal communication also may lead to problems. For example, direct eye contact may show disrespect in some cultures and be a sign of interest and active listening in others.

ENVIRONMENTAL CONTROL An individual's relationship to nature varies among cultures. Different health practices, values, and experiences with illness also are found.

HYGIENE Cleanliness practices vary among cultures. For example, body odors and the way people respond to them are different among various societies. Cultural practices determine whether body odors are disguised, ignored, or enhanced.

SPACE Culture defines a person's perception of personal space. Comfort can result from honoring the boundaries of personal space, whereas anxiety can result when these boundaries are not followed. Practices regarding proximity to others, body movements, and touch differ among cultures.

TIME The concepts of time, duration of time, and points in time vary among cultures. Past-oriented cultures, for example, value tradition. Individuals from cultures that closely follow tradition may not be receptive to new procedures or treatments. Present-oriented cultures focus on the here and now, and individuals from these cultures may not be receptive to preventive health care measures. Some cultures have no focus on time, and individuals from these cultures may miss appointments or be late.

SOCIAL ORGANIZATION Societies are influenced by many factors, such as religion, sexual orientation, socioeconomic status, gender, age, and geography, and life-cycle factors relative to families and individuals differ among cultures. The role of older adults, the head of the household, and men and women in the society may determine the behaviors of these individuals.

Disparities in Health Care

In 2002, the Institute of Medicine (IOM) released a report on disparities in the United States regarding the types and quality of health services that racial and ethnic minorities receive. The IOM report explored factors that might contribute to inequities in care and contained recommended policies and practices to eliminate these inequities.

The IOM found significant variation in the rates of medical procedures by race even when income, age, and severity of conditions were comparable. This research indicates that U.S. racial and ethnic minorities are less likely to receive medical care, and when they do, receive lower quality of services (Figures 6–5 ■ and 6–6 ■). Nurses should be alert to practices (formal and informal) in their work environment that impact the quality of care offered to individuals of any ethnic group and should work to ensure quality care and provision of best practice methods to all clients.

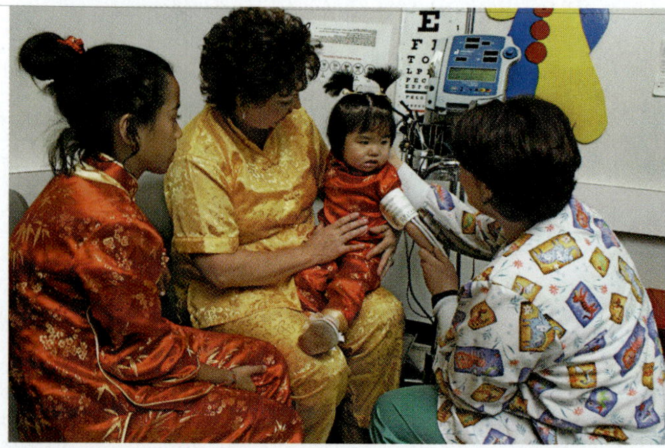

Figure 6–5 ■ Although much has been done to improve the quality of health services received by American cultural and ethnic minorities, these services are still in need of continued reform.

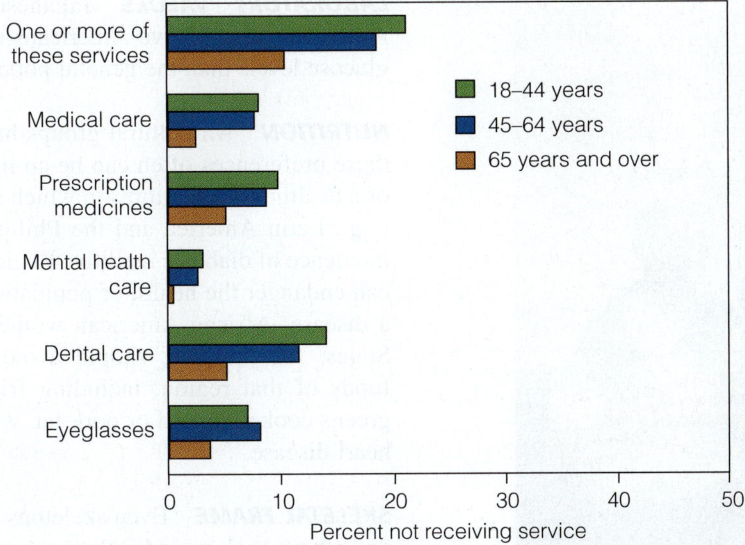

Figure 6–6 ■ Percentage not receiving needed health services because of cost, 2005.

Source: Centers for Disease Control and Prevention, National Center for Health Statistics, Health, United States, 2007, Figure 21. Data from National Health Interview Survey.

The recommendations for reducing these disparities in health care include increasing awareness of them among the public, health care providers, insurance companies, and policy makers. More minority health care providers are needed in underserved communities, and more interpreters are needed in clinics and hospitals to improve the quality of care. The IOM report suggests educating health care professionals to increase their cultural competence with different populations and inform them of how discrimination and racism affect the provision of health care. Including information about health care disparities in the curriculum is one way to educate nurses early in their careers (IOM, 2002).

PHYSICAL ASSESSMENT

Cultural differences can affect the physical assessment in several ways. Biological variations in cultural groups are the simplest and most obvious differences that nurses will deal with in their professional careers. Differences in values, beliefs, and religions can be more challenging, however, and often require nurses to go the extra mile to ask the right questions to obtain very important information regarding a client's health and perceptions of Western medicine.

Differences in Values and Beliefs

The assessment process includes asking questions about mental status and psychological disorders. The beliefs and values of a culture define normal and abnormal behaviors and thinking processes, so the client's culture may view mental status and psychological disorders as having psychological, physical, social, spiritual, or emotional origins. Learning about cultural expectations of behaviors and ways of thinking helps nurses to understand the client's mental status.

Cultures may explain mental problems in different ways. People from some cultures may believe that those with mental problems need to be avoided because of mystical, magical, or evil powers. Some cultures believe mental problems are punishments for sins or wrong deeds done in this life or, as sometimes is the case among Indian and Asian populations that practice Hinduism, a previous life. Culturally sensitive nurses ask questions to determine how family members and others from the client's culture may view someone with a mental illness.

Biological Variations

People differ genetically and physiologically. These biological variations among individuals, families, and races produce differences in susceptibility and response to various diseases among people of different cultures and all walks of life (Figure 6–7 ■).

SUSCEPTIBILITY TO DISEASE Certain ethnic groups or races may tend toward developing specific diseases. African Americans, for example, have a higher incidence of hypertension and sickle cell anemia. Cardiovascular disease is the number-one killer of American women, and African-American women are at greater risk from this disease compared to women from any other ethnic group (Centers for Disease Control and Prevention, 2009). Native Americans have a higher incidence of tuberculosis. Sometimes, however, an individual's susceptibility to disease is not so obvious but may be discerned as a nurse takes a health history, including the health of any parents, grandparents, and siblings.

GROWTH AND DEVELOPMENT Average adult size, growth rate, and shape vary among individuals because of genetic and environmental factors. Nutritional status influences growth as well: Children with inadequate diets may have slowed development.

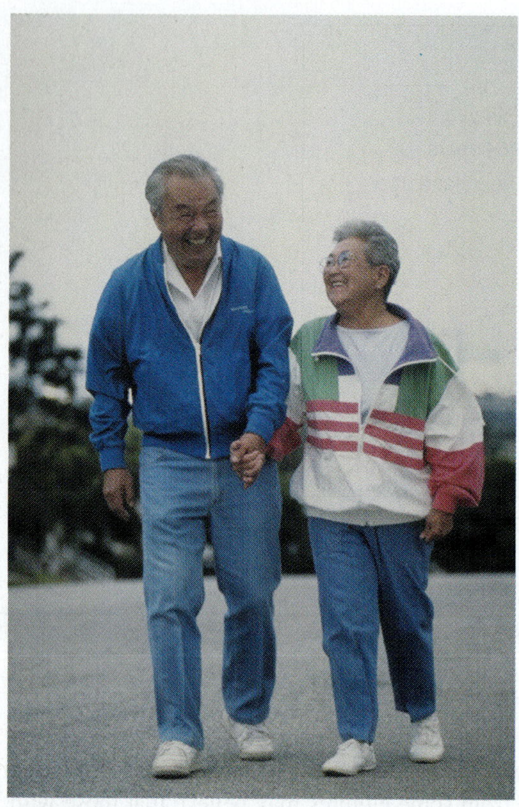

Figure 6–7 ■ Those of different cultures also have biological variations. This couple of Japanese descent are likely to have higher blood glucose levels than the general population.

Source: PhotoEdit Inc.

LABORATORY VALUES Japanese Americans, Hispanic Americans, and Native Americans usually have higher blood glucose levels than the general population.

NUTRITION All cultural groups have food preferences, and these preferences often can be an indicator or even the cause of a health issue. Cultures in which sugar cane is a major crop (e.g., Latin America and the Philippines) have an increased incidence of diabetes mellitus. Regional food preferences also can endanger the health of populations already susceptible to a disease. African-American women in the southern United States, for example, should avoid some of the traditional foods of that region, including fried chicken and fish and greens cooked in lard or pork fat, which increase their risk of heart disease.

SKELETAL FRAME Even skeletons show differences in racial and ethnic backgrounds. Native Americans have an increased incidence of back problems. African-American and white men usually are taller than Asian-American and Mexican-American men. Small-framed white women of European descent are predisposed to osteoporosis.

SKIN COLOR This most obvious difference among individuals has important implications for health care providers. Darker skin tones require closer inspection to observe changes (as when assessing for changes in oxygenation). African Americans and Native Americans have lower incidences of skin cancer because of higher levels of melanin.

6.1 VALUES AND BELIEFS

KEY TERMS

Belief system, *329*
Cultural competence, *331*
Cultural values, *328*
World view, *329*

LEARNING OUTCOMES

After reading about this exemplar, you will be able to:

1. Describe the role of belief systems in the development of culture.
2. Discuss common rules reflecting basic values found in many cultures.
3. Identify ways in which culture influences beliefs and values.
4. Relate the impact of beliefs and values on health care and lifestyle choices.
5. Develop a nursing plan of care reflecting respect for the client's values and beliefs.

OVERVIEW

Culture includes a society's values, beliefs, assumptions, principles, myths, legends, and norms. People use these to help them define meaning, identify acceptable behaviors, choose emotional reactions, and determine appropriate actions in given situations. Values and belief systems are part of a culture, as are family relationships and roles (Figure 6–8 ■). To understand client behaviors better, the nurse must identify which cultures are present demographically in a given area, learn more about those cultures by reading or attending a class about them, and apply that knowledge and experiences in providing client care.

Values reflect an underlying system of beliefs. **Cultural values** describe preferred ways of behaving or thinking that are sustained over time and used to govern a cultural group's actions and decisions. When people live together in a society, cultural values determine the rules they live by each and every day.

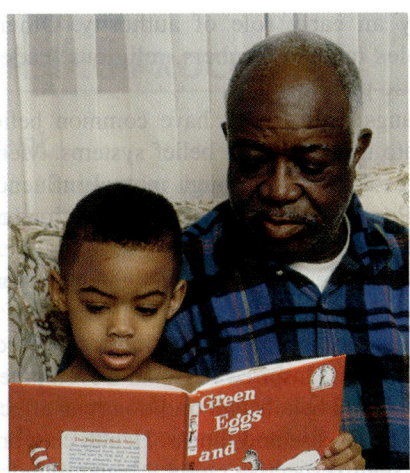

Figure 6–8 ■ Cultural beliefs and practices include family relationships and roles.

These rules may be variously stated, but they basically address the same values. Examples of these rules in Western culture include the following:

- Don't steal from others.
- Respect other people's property.
- Don't hurt others.
- Don't take another's mate.
- Share your food and clothing with those who are in need.
- Speak truthfully based on what you see.
- Respect your elders for their wisdom and experience.
- Respect God or a higher power.
- Respect nature and your environment.

Characteristics of culture include observable behaviors as well as the unseen values that influence those behaviors. Cultural practices have meaning that gives the group its world view and that reflects the social organization of the culture as a whole. The organization of a culture or society includes the following elements:

- A physical element: the geographic area in which the society is located
- An infrastructure element: the framework of the systems and processes that keep the society functioning
- A behavioral element: the way people in the society act and react to each other
- A cultural element: all the values, beliefs, assumptions, and norms that comprise a code of conduct for acceptable behaviors within the society.

Each culture has its own world view or understanding of the world. A **world view** refers to how the people in a culture perceive ideas and attitudes about the world, other people, and life in general.

A culture's world view supports its overall **belief system**, which is developed to explain the mysteries of the universe and of life that each society tries to understand (Figure 6–9 ■). What is the meaning of life? How do individuals know their purpose in life? What is reality? How much can be known about values and beliefs? Some world-view questions concern God or a higher power. Is there a God? How was the universe created? What happens after death? A culture's belief systems influence an individual's decisions and actions in society regarding everything from the preparation of food to rituals of death and burial (for an example, see the Focus on Diversity and Culture feature that follows). Scientific and medical advancements may or may not impact a culture's belief systems.

Beliefs systems differ in every culture. The beliefs of a society are passed from generation to generation by word of mouth. As cultures interact with other cultures and assimilate, some cultural beliefs become lost, some are kept, and others adapt to incorporate parts of other cultures.

Children learn the belief system of their culture from parents and other family members who teach them any number of values and beliefs, including those about what is "right or wrong." Multicultural societies like the that of the United States have a mix of traditional moral basics. The differences may originate from religious beliefs or social conditions. People make decisions about "right or wrong," and as things change, people adapt and the culture evolves.

Belief systems are based on people's experiences of the world. As people's knowledge and understanding grow, their belief systems expand. Knowing why we believe what we believe builds self-awareness and understanding of differences in our own beliefs compared with the beliefs of others.

One way people develop beliefs is by analyzing and critically thinking about causation How does one thing cause another? This is logical thinking and rational problem solving. The skills of evidence-based believing develop as individuals mature and learn. Events are measurable, and facts are supported by scientific studies.

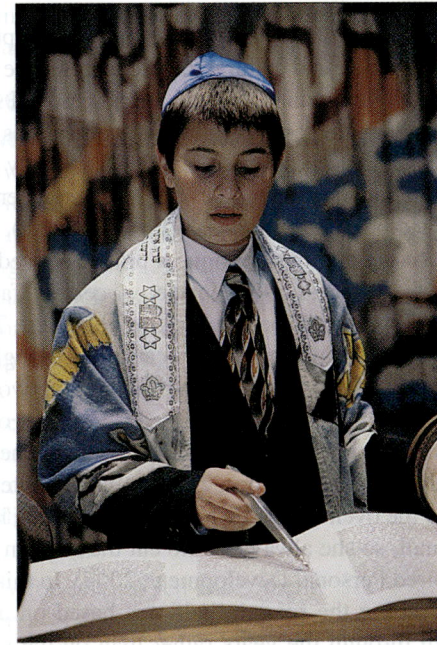

Figure 6–9 ■ Cultures try to understand and give meaning to life through spiritual beliefs, social values, and acceptable behaviors.

FOCUS ON DIVERSITY AND CULTURE How Culturally Sensitive Are You?

To help you identify areas where you can improve when providing nursing care to culturally different people, answer the following questions by checking Yes or No:

____ Yes ____ No I accept values of others even when different from my own.
____ Yes ____ No I accept beliefs of others even when different from my own.
____ Yes ____ No I accept that the male and female roles may vary among different cultures.
____ Yes ____ No I accept that religious practices may influence how a client responds to illness, health problems, and death.
____ Yes ____ No I accept that alternative medicine practices may influence a client's response to illness and health problems.
____ Yes ____ No I accept cultural diversity in my clients.
____ Yes ____ No I attend educational programs to enhance my knowledge and skills in providing care to diverse cultural groups.
____ Yes ____ No I understand that clients who are unable to speak English may be very proficient in their own languages.
____ Yes ____ No I try to have written materials in the client's language available when possible.
____ Yes ____ No I use interpreters when available to improve communication.

If you have more No responses than Yes responses, you may not be as culturally sensitive as you could be. The purpose of this self-assessment is to increase your awareness of areas where you can improve to develop your cultural sensitivity.

The Focus on Diversity and Culture feature above will help you examine your own cultural competence and sensitivity.

In the United States, there are plenty of opportunities to encounter differences resulting from cultural diversity, and these encounters require cultural competence Some demographic areas have experienced culturally varied client populations for decades, and other areas of the country have only recently seen increases in immigrant populations. Health practices, beliefs about illness and disease, decisions to enter health care systems, and responses to health care providers are some of the topics influenced by cultural differences. Understanding these differences and being able to communicate will enhance the nurse's effectiveness in eliminating barriers to providing health care.

Diversity also has increased within the health care professions. In the United States, these professions were once open only to whites, but over time, all the health care professions, including nursing, have opened to students and practitioners from all races and cultures. This increasing diversity among health care professionals is slowly impacting how Western health care is perceived among individuals from other cultures, but there are still gains to be made and barriers to be overcome.

Developing cultural competence is a continuous process. The LEARN model (American Medical Student Association, 2007) is a tool for developing cultural competency. Below is a modification of this model to help the nurse include cultural behaviors in a client's health care:

Listen to the client's perception of the problem.
Explain your perception of the problem and of the treatments ordered by the physician.
Acknowledge and discuss the differences and similarities between these two perceptions.
Review the ordered treatments while remembering the client's cultural parameters.
Negotiate agreement. Assist the client in understanding the medical treatments ordered by the physician, and have the client help to make decisions about those treatments as appropriate (e.g., choosing cultural foods that are permitted on an ordered diet).

Box 6–2 provides a chance to put the LEARN model into practice.

No one becomes culturally aware or culturally sensitive overnight. There is a process by which nursing students (and other individuals) learn cultural confidence, with learning taking place in a fairly predictable sequence:

1. Students begin by developing cultural awareness of how culture shapes beliefs, values, individual power, and social power.
2. Students develop cultural knowledge about the differences, similarities, and inequalities in experience and practice among various societies.

Box 6–2 Critical Thinking Exercise: The LEARN Model

An Arab couple has come to Nurse Smith's clinic because the wife, who is 6 months pregnant, is not feeling well. The husband speaks English well, but the wife's proficiency in English is more limited. Both are dressed in American-style clothes. During the assessment, Nurse Smith determines that the couple has a 9-month-old and a 2-year-old at home. Nurse Smith also learns that the husband is the head of the household, making most of the major decisions for the family, and that the wife has sole responsibility for the family's care and daily living needs. The wife presents with exhaustion and elevated blood pressure. After obtaining a urine specimen, the physician diagnoses toxemia and orders the wife to be on strict bed rest and to return in two weeks. While the husband conveys concern for his wife's health, he is reluctant to have her treatment disrupt the household routine.

1. What NANDA diagnoses might Nurse Smith identify for this family?
2. Using the LEARN model, describe how Nurse Smith could discuss the situation and the doctor's recommendations with both the husband and wife.

NURSING PROCESS

Assessment

During the initial assessment interview with clients and their families, include focused questions to identify cultural behaviors, health beliefs, illness practices, and cultural needs. This information can be used in planning culturally sensitive care. A helping relationship with clients and families involves spending time with them, building trust, and showing a desire to better understand their values and beliefs.

Assessment questions may include the following areas:

- Does the client follow culturally specific traditions? If so, how closely? Where does the client see himself or herself on a heritage continuum ranging from strict devotion to a mix of cultural influences? To what extent has the client been socialized to an American lifestyle?
- Are there specific practices regarding types of foods eaten or not eaten? How are foods prepared? At what times are meals scheduled?
- Are unique customs followed in the home that the client needs to maintain while he or she is away? Are there specific times for these practices?
- What does the family consist of for the client? What members of the family stay in the home with the client? How will family members participate in the client's care?
- Does the client speak and understand the English language? Is another language spoken in the home?

Physical cues can guide a nurse in choosing assessment questions. For example, consider the following:

- *Clothing*. If a client is wearing clothes that are traditional in his or her native land, the nurse may want to ask additional questions to identify cultural practices impacting health care.
- *Adult family members present for the assessment*. This signals an increased possibility for family involvement in decision making related to health care practices
- *Young children present for an assessment of their mother*. This may indicate the family lacks sufficient supports for the mother to come alone, and it may prompt the nurse to ask questions related to self-care and caregiver role strain. This can be true among families regardless of cultural background.

When clients speak languages other than English or are not proficient in English, minimal assessment information from clients can be obtained with the following questions:

- What language do you speak? Do you speak any English?
- How long have you lived here?
- What do you think caused your problem?
- When did it start?
- Why do you think it started when it did?
- What does your sickness do to you?
- How severe is your sickness?
- What do you fear about your sickness?
- What kind of treatment do you think you need?
- Are there any religious practices we need to know about?
- Who is your family?
- Who makes decisions most of the time?
- Who can you go to for help when you need it?

Diagnosis

No NANDA nursing diagnoses exclusively address culture. However, differences in cultural behaviors, beliefs, and values could potentially cause clients many problems. Cultural misunderstandings or miscommunications also may result from different perceptions of health and of the illness diagnosed. The following are examples of NANDA nursing diagnoses that may be appropriate for clients of different cultures (depending on individual situations):

- Powerlessness
- Spiritual Distress
- Risk for Impaired Religiosity
- Disturbed Thought Processes
- Fear
- Decisional Conflict
- Noncompliance
- Anxiety
- Ineffective Health Maintenance
- Ineffective Coping
- Acute Pain
- Impaired Social Interaction.

Plan

Planning culturally appropriate care requires knowledge of the client's values and belief system. Nursing care is best planned in conjunction with the client in order to determine those actions that would best suit the client's needs. Goals may include:

- Client states that plan of care is in keeping with cultural beliefs and values.
- Client participates in the creation of the plan of care.
- Client modifies plan of care to be consistent with cultural beliefs and values.

Implementation

DEVELOPING CULTURAL COMPETENCE Nurses provide care to individuals from many different cultures. To be culturally sensitive, nurses must have cultural information and be able to apply this knowledge to improve the quality of their nursing care. Nurses need to avoid stereotyping and personal bias, which may raise barriers to culturally sensitive behaviors. Nurses need to understand their own world views to appreciate differences in their client's cultural world view.

Cultural competence is the ability to apply the knowledge and skills needed to provide quality care for clients from different cultures. Culture competence has some basic characteristics, including the following:

1. Valuing diversity
2. Capacity for cultural self-assessment
3. Awareness of the different dynamics present when cultures interact
4. Knowledge about different cultures
5. Adaptability in providing nursing care that reflects an understanding of cultural diversity.

FOCUS ON DIVERSITY AND CULTURE How Culturally Sensitive Are You?

To help you identify areas where you can improve when providing nursing care to culturally different people, answer the following questions by checking Yes or No:

____ Yes ____ No I accept values of others even when different from my own.
____ Yes ____ No I accept beliefs of others even when different from my own.
____ Yes ____ No I accept that the male and female roles may vary among different cultures.
____ Yes ____ No I accept that religious practices may influence how a client responds to illness, health problems, and death.
____ Yes ____ No I accept that alternative medicine practices may influence a client's response to illness and health problems.
____ Yes ____ No I accept cultural diversity in my clients.
____ Yes ____ No I attend educational programs to enhance my knowledge and skills in providing care to diverse cultural groups.
____ Yes ____ No I understand that clients who are unable to speak English may be very proficient in their own languages.
____ Yes ____ No I try to have written materials in the client's language available when possible.
____ Yes ____ No I use interpreters when available to improve communication.

If you have more No responses than Yes responses, you may not be as culturally sensitive as you could be. The purpose of this self-assessment is to increase your awareness of areas where you can improve to develop your cultural sensitivity.

The Focus on Diversity and Culture feature above will help you examine your own cultural competence and sensitivity.

In the United States, there are plenty of opportunities to encounter differences resulting from cultural diversity, and these encounters require cultural competence Some demographic areas have experienced culturally varied client populations for decades, and other areas of the country have only recently seen increases in immigrant populations. Health practices, beliefs about illness and disease, decisions to enter health care systems, and responses to health care providers are some of the topics influenced by cultural differences. Understanding these differences and being able to communicate will enhance the nurse's effectiveness in eliminating barriers to providing health care.

Diversity also has increased within the health care professions. In the United States, these professions were once open only to whites, but over time, all the health care professions, including nursing, have opened to students and practitioners from all races and cultures. This increasing diversity among health care professionals is slowly impacting how Western health care is perceived among individuals from other cultures, but there are still gains to be made and barriers to be overcome.

Developing cultural competence is a continuous process. The LEARN model (American Medical Student Association, 2007) is a tool for developing cultural competency. Below is a modification of this model to help the nurse include cultural behaviors in a client's health care:

Listen to the client's perception of the problem.
Explain your perception of the problem and of the treatments ordered by the physician.
Acknowledge and discuss the differences and similarities between these two perceptions.
Review the ordered treatments while remembering the client's cultural parameters.
Negotiate agreement. Assist the client in understanding the medical treatments ordered by the physician, and have the client help to make decisions about those treatments as appropriate (e.g., choosing cultural foods that are permitted on an ordered diet).

Box 6–2 provides a chance to put the LEARN model into practice.

No one becomes culturally aware or culturally sensitive overnight. There is a process by which nursing students (and other individuals) learn cultural confidence, with learning taking place in a fairly predictable sequence:

1. Students begin by developing cultural awareness of how culture shapes beliefs, values, individual power, and social power.
2. Students develop cultural knowledge about the differences, similarities, and inequalities in experience and practice among various societies.

Box 6–2 Critical Thinking Exercise: The LEARN Model

An Arab couple has come to Nurse Smith's clinic because the wife, who is 6 months pregnant, is not feeling well. The husband speaks English well, but the wife's proficiency in English is more limited. Both are dressed in American-style clothes. During the assessment, Nurse Smith determines that the couple has a 9-month-old and a 2-year-old at home. Nurse Smith also learns that the husband is the head of the household, making most of the major decisions for the family, and that the wife has sole responsibility for the family's care and daily living needs. The wife presents with exhaustion and elevated blood pressure. After obtaining a urine specimen, the physician diagnoses toxemia and orders the wife to be on strict bed rest and to return in two weeks. While the husband conveys concern for his wife's health, he is reluctant to have her treatment disrupt the household routine.

1. What NANDA diagnoses might Nurse Smith identify for this family?
2. Using the LEARN model, describe how Nurse Smith could discuss the situation and the doctor's recommendations with both the husband and wife.

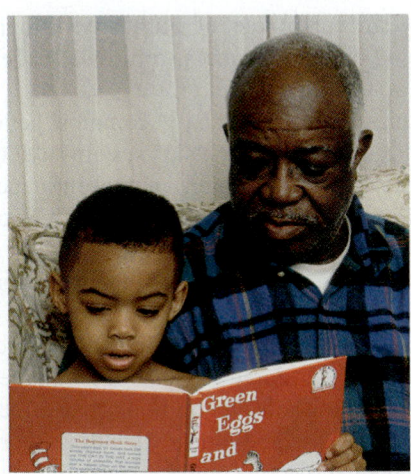

Figure 6–8 ■ Cultural beliefs and practices include family relationships and roles.

These rules may be variously stated, but they basically address the same values. Examples of these rules in Western culture include the following:

- Don't steal from others.
- Respect other people's property.
- Don't hurt others.
- Don't take another's mate.
- Share your food and clothing with those who are in need.
- Speak truthfully based on what you see.
- Respect your elders for their wisdom and experience.
- Respect God or a higher power.
- Respect nature and your environment.

Characteristics of culture include observable behaviors as well as the unseen values that influence those behaviors. Cultural practices have meaning that gives the group its world view and that reflects the social organization of the culture as a whole. The organization of a culture or society includes the following elements:

- A physical element: the geographic area in which the society is located
- An infrastructure element: the framework of the systems and processes that keep the society functioning
- A behavioral element: the way people in the society act and react to each other
- A cultural element: all the values, beliefs, assumptions, and norms that comprise a code of conduct for acceptable behaviors within the society.

Each culture has its own world view or understanding of the world. A **world view** refers to how the people in a culture perceive ideas and attitudes about the world, other people, and life in general.

A culture's world view supports its overall **belief system**, which is developed to explain the mysteries of the universe and of life that each society tries to understand (Figure 6–9 ■). What is the meaning of life? How do individuals know their purpose in life? What is reality? How much can be known about values and beliefs? Some world-view questions concern God or a higher power. Is there a God? How was the universe created? What happens after death? A culture's belief systems influence an individual's decisions and actions in society regarding everything from the preparation of food to rituals of death and burial (for an example, see the Focus on Diversity and Culture feature that follows). Scientific and medical advancements may or may not impact a culture's belief systems.

Beliefs systems differ in every culture. The beliefs of a society are passed from generation to generation by word of mouth. As cultures interact with other cultures and assimilate, some cultural beliefs become lost, some are kept, and others adapt to incorporate parts of other cultures.

Children learn the belief system of their culture from parents and other family members who teach them any number of values and beliefs, including those about what is "right or wrong." Multicultural societies like the that of the United States have a mix of traditional moral basics. The differences may originate from religious beliefs or social conditions. People make decisions about "right or wrong," and as things change, people adapt and the culture evolves.

Belief systems are based on people's experiences of the world. As people's knowledge and understanding grow, their belief systems expand. Knowing why we believe what we believe builds self-awareness and understanding of differences in our own beliefs compared with the beliefs of others.

One way people develop beliefs is by analyzing and critically thinking about causation How does one thing cause another? This is logical thinking and rational problem solving. The skills of evidence-based believing develop as individuals mature and learn. Events are measurable, and facts are supported by scientific studies.

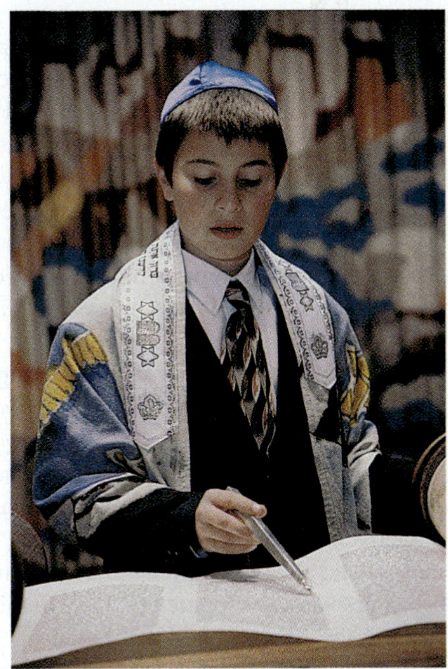

Figure 6–9 ■ Cultures try to understand and give meaning to life through spiritual beliefs, social values, and acceptable behaviors.

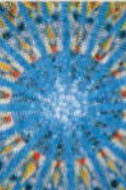

FOCUS ON DIVERSITY AND CULTURE

The Peoplehood Model

An example of cultures having distinct beliefs and practices can be found with Native American tribes. Each tribe has a distinct language, territory, specific ceremonial cycles, and sacred history that tells how it came into existence and incorporates expected interactions with the environment, ceremony guidelines, and expected behaviors with others within the community. Figure 6–10 ■ shows Tom Holm's Peoplehood Model, in which the four factors overlap and interact with each other (Cornsilk and Blythe, 2008).

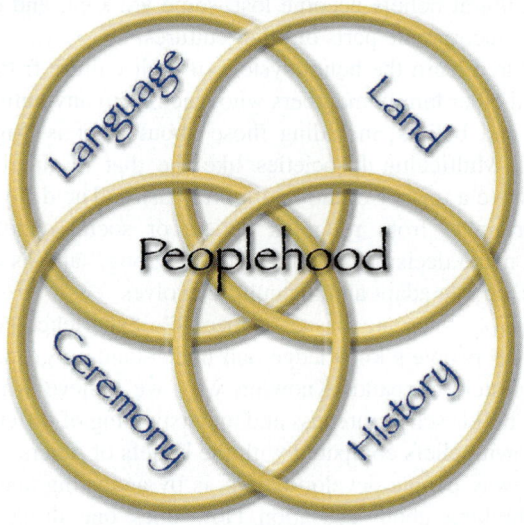

Figure 6–10 ■ The Peoplehood model of Native Americans.

Source: Cornsilk, C., & Blythe, F. (Executive Producers). (2006, November). *Indian country diaries*. Peoplehood. New York and Washington, DC: Public Broadcasting Service. Retrieved from http://www.pbs.org/indiancountry.

Another method of developing beliefs is by adopting traditional beliefs. Family and cultural traditions influence our belief systems through family bias, societal prejudices, and social culture. These beliefs are passed on through generations and often are accepted without questions. What was necessary in an earlier generation may no longer be useful for later generations but still be retained because of tradition (Figure 6–11 ■).

How might generations continue a practice based on tradition rather than necessity? Consider a certain family that always cut roasts in half before cooking the meat. The third-generation daughter said she did it because she thought it made the meat more tender. The second generation woman (the daughter's mother) said she had learned it from her own mom, and she thought it was done to reduce cooking time and save energy. And the first-generation woman (the daughter's grandmother) said the oven she had when she was raising her family was very small, so she always had to cut the roast in half to fit inside (Inspired Personal Development, 2007). In this case, the practice of cutting the roast in half was based on a tradition passed down through the years rather than on the size of the family oven.

Beliefs can be adopted from people who have authority in our lives. In addition to giving us traditional beliefs, parents play an early role of authority. Other people in authority roles include teachers, religious leaders, doctors, or charismatic people.

Clubs, gangs, and groups have common beliefs that are integrated into the members' belief systems. Members adopt the identity of the group through mutual influence of values and beliefs. Personal attitudes become reflections of the group, giving beliefs by association.

Another influence on beliefs is enlightenment or revelation. Enlightenment may come from the experience of "a gut feeling" or from intuition. This inspiration is not predictable and may give us insight (Inspired Personal Development, 2007).

Culturally based beliefs and traditions can affect the course and outcome of disease and illness. Health care providers and clients bring their respective cultural backgrounds and expectations to a medical interview. Their cultural differences can present barriers to necessary care. Some areas in which barriers can arise include the following:

- The importance of family in managing illness and disease
- The belief that illnesses are not always strictly a biological problem
- Cultural assumptions about disease and illness that may influence the presentation of symptoms or the response to treatments
- Failure of clients to see a pattern of repeated illness as a chronic condition rather than their symptoms as unrelated occurrences
- Cultural beliefs that discussing prognosis and risks with clients can influence outcomes or be dangerous.

While cultural beliefs and behaviors change over the years as a cultural group adapts to new ideas and conditions, some individuals may retain traditional behaviors and thinking and continue to follow the beliefs and practices as always. Tension may increase when different health belief systems conflict with each other. The result may be anxiety, anger, or fear. The health care provider's cultural sensitivity may reduce this discomfort by showing a nonjudgmental attitude of respect.

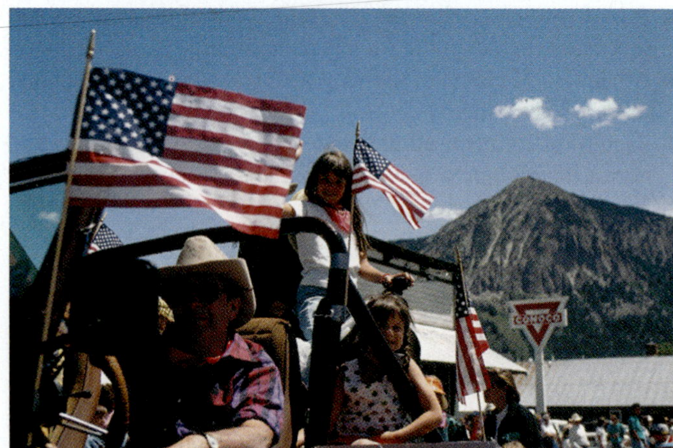

Figure 6–11 ■ Cultural beliefs are passed on through generations as traditions. In this photo, a family from Crested Butte, Colorado, celebrates the 4th of July.

Source: Omni-Photo Communications, Inc.

EVIDENCE-BASED PRACTICE A Model of Ethical Multiculturalism

The Harper Model is an evidenced-based model of ethical multiculturalism (Figure 6–12 ■) developed and presented at the 34th Annual Transcultural Nursing Society Conference (Harper, 2008). This model includes key attributes of cultural competence and the relationship to a continuum of ethical philosophies. Dr. Harper has said, "Cultural competence occurs on a continuum. Even when you believe you are competent, you can always learn more!" (Harper, 2008).

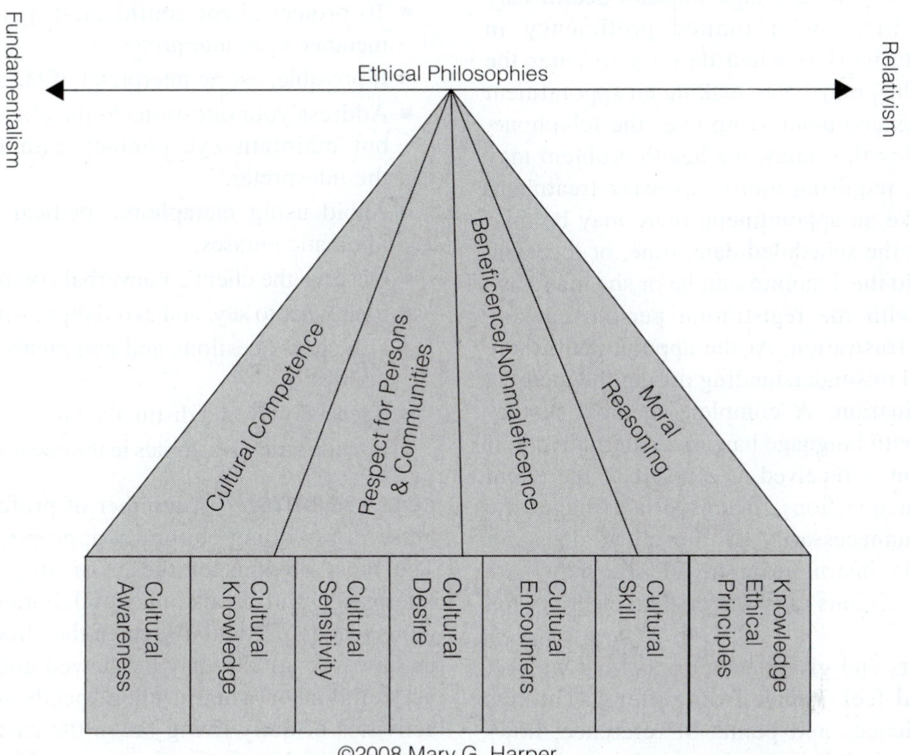

Figure 6–12 ■ This model shows how components of cultural competence are obtained through ethical influences, knowledge, and experience with the culture.

Source: Mary Harper, University of Central Florida. Reprinted with permission.

3. Students develop cultural understanding of problems and issues facing societies and cultures when values, beliefs, and behaviors are compromised by another culture.
4. Students develop cultural sensitivity to the cultural beliefs, values, and behaviors of their clients. This reflects an awareness of their own cultural beliefs, values, and behaviors that may influence their nursing practice.
5. Students develop cultural competence and provide care that respects the cultural values, beliefs, and behaviors of their clients.

Hopefully, at the end of this sequence, nursing students will have developed a model of ethical multiculturalism, as described in the Evidence-Based Practice feature that follows.

MAINTAINING CULTURAL COMPETENCE Maintaining cultural competence is an ongoing process. Nurses continually assess, modify, and evaluate the care provided to culturally diverse clients. Reframing questions can show sensitivity and respect for different cultural beliefs. Active listening can assist nurses in understanding cultural differences. Four significant factors need to be considered:

- Clinical differences among people of different cultures and ethnic groups. For example, African Americans have a higher incidence of hypertension, and some Native-American tribes have a higher incidence of diabetes.
- A need both to have interpreters when languages differ and to understand differences in the meaning of words when communicating with clients who speak various languages.
- Respect for the belief systems of others and the effects of those beliefs on well-being, including when clients use alternative health care practices instead of traditional Western medicine.
- Trust between clients and nurses as part of the helping relationship. Authority figures are not accepted readily in some cultures. Trust both in the nurse and in the care provided need to be established.

Implementation of cultural competence involves many aspects of the nursing process. These aspects include communication, using an interpreter, and collaboration. Institutions such as hospitals also need to develop and implement cultural competence to address the cultural and language needs of an increasingly multicultural client population.

COMMUNICATION The United States is a country of many cultures, and health care professionals need to have a basic understanding of how language impacts health care delivery systems. Clients with limited proficiency in English often run into barriers when they try to enter the health care system. They may delay making an appointment because of difficulties communicating over the telephone, for example, and during this delay, the health problem may become more severe, requiring more expensive treatment. If the client does make an appointment, there may be misunderstandings about the scheduled date, time, or location. If the client makes it to the appointment, he or she may have difficulty speaking with the registration person, causing additional delay and frustration. At the appointment, there may be confusion and misunderstanding during the medical interview and examination. A complete medical history may not be possible with language barriers. Alternatively, if inaccurate information is received as a result of the client misunderstanding the questions, inappropriate diagnostic tests may be done unnecessarily. If the client does not understand take-home instructions, he or she may take inappropriate actions. Clients must understand clearly what is required of them.

The brain interprets and gives meaning to what we see, hear, taste, smell, and feel. People from different cultures have different experiences and points of reference, however, so two people from different cultures who are experiencing the same reality will interpret it in entirely different ways. For example, someone makes the "OK" gesture. How would this be interpreted? What if the person is from a culture in which this gesture is obscene? Or what if the person is from a culture in which this gesture has romantic connotations? Behavior has no meaning unless the observer interprets the behavior and gives it meaning. The mind has been culturally trained, so different cultures will produce different interpretations.

USING AN INTERPRETER Many clients do not speak English, and even if clients do speak English, their speech may be limited or lack proficiency. Any facility receiving federal funding from the U.S. Department of Health and Human Services is required to communicate effectively with clients or risk the loss of that funding (American Medical Student Association, 2007). Having bilingual nurses available is one strategy to address the language barrier. Another strategy is providing access to language banks through electronic or telephone systems nurses can dial up for interpreter services. Unless a client brings an interpreter with her, however, an interpreter may not have any previous knowledge of the client. Nurses can ask a client or family with limited English proficiency if the family works with any area service organizations that provide interpreters. These organizations attempt to provide competent interpreters who build relationships with families over time.

Guidelines for using an interpreter include the following:

- When possible, use an interpreter to translate and provide meaning behind the words.
- To protect client confidentiality, avoid using a family member as an interpreter.
- If possible, use an interpreter of the same sex as the client.
- Address your questions to the client, not the interpreter, but maintain eye contact with both the client and the interpreter.
- Avoid using metaphors, medical jargon, similes, and idiomatic phrases.
- Observe the client's nonverbal communication.
- Plan what to say, and avoid rephrasing or hesitating.
- Use short questions and comments. Ask one question at a time.
- Speak slowly and distinctly, but not loudly.
- Provide written materials in the client's language as available.

COLLABORATION A number of professionals can assist a nurse in providing culturally appropriate care for a family. The most obvious of these, as already discussed, is the interpreter. Nurses also may collaborate with a client's religious leader, particularly when the client wants clarification on how a treatment may be viewed under the laws of his or her religion or when a client needs some assistance with activities of daily living (as in the case of the Arab couple with whom Nurse Smith was working). Churches, synagogues, and mosques can provide support and often services to their members.

Nurses should take a holistic approach to their nursing care and recognize the wholeness of all clients, regardless of their diverse cultural, racial, ethnic, religious, or other background or heritage (Figure 6–13 ■). Accepting clients as they are can give comfort to the families as well as to the clients, which can increase compliance with the treatment regimen. The Client Teaching feature that follows discusses how communication between parents and nurses can help to bring about a collaborative relationship.

HOSPITALS, LANGUAGE, AND CULTURE The Joint Commission (2008) conducted a study called *Hospitals, Language, and Culture: A Snapshot of the Nation* that investigated how 60 hospitals across the United States were addressing cultural and language needs among an increasingly multicultural client population. The Joint Commission found there was no one-size-fits-all solution; the process of becoming more culturally competent was unique to each organization.

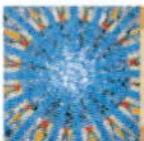

CLIENT TEACHING Communication Between Parents and Nurses

When children enter the health care system, it is usually the parents that provide information about what is wrong with the child, how long a problem has been occurring, what they have tried to do to help the problem, and so on. Taking care of children is a collaborative effort between parents, nurses, and other health care providers. Mutual respect and support are healthy attitudes that will facilitate the child's health care experience.

Parents may need to learn how best to communicate with nurses and other health care professionals. Some suggestions that can be given to parents to support this communication include the following:

- Keep records of all medical treatments, immunizations, major illnesses, routine medications, hospitalizations, diagnostic tests results, and screening results.
- Write down any questions about the care or treatment of childhood conditions, illnesses, developmental progress, behavioral or mental concerns, or preventive measures.
- Become familiar with a child's daily habits of eating, sleeping, playing, learning activities, social interactions, usual schedule each day, emotional expressions, and interactions with pets and other family members.

Some suggestions for nurses to support this communication include the following:

- Provide information to parents, and be available to answer any questions they might have.
- Be honest and real with the parents.
- Respect family dynamics and values, and find opportunities for using them in the care of the child.
- Maintain open communication with parents and other family members.

Based on the data gathered, the Joint Commission identified some issues and offered recommendations for how organizations could develop cultural competence:

- Identify the needs of client populations served in the community, and assess how well current practices are meeting these needs.
- Bring various health care providers in the organization together to gain their perspectives on and experiences with providing care, barriers to working with different cultures, and gaps in the services delivered.
- Initiate a continuous monitoring process for assessment and evaluation of cultural and language needs.
- Improve the services provided to meet the needs of clients using the resources available to the organization.

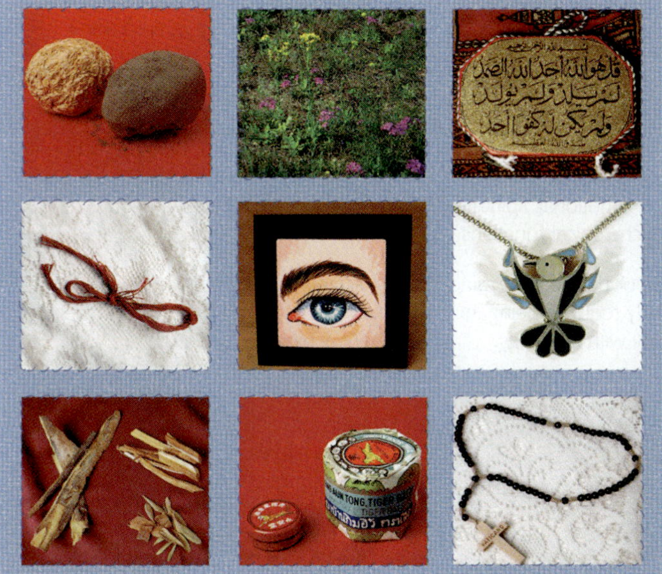

Figure 6–13 ■ Cultures use various symbols and traditions for health beliefs and practices.

The case of a middle-aged Chinese client refusing pain medication following nasal surgery illustrates cultural competence. When asked why he refused, he replied his discomfort was bearable and he could survive without any medication. Later, the nurse found him restless and uncomfortable and again offered pain medication. Again, he refused, explaining that her responsibilities at the hospital were far more important than his comfort, and that he did not want to impose. Only after the nurse firmly insisted that the client's comfort was one of her most important responsibilities did he finally agree to take the medication.

Among Asian people, health is considered a state of spiritual and physical harmony with nature. There is a need for balance between yin and yang. When an imbalance occurs, illness results. Asian clients do not usually complain about pain or physical problems because they are taught self-restraint and the priority of group over individual needs. Another factor that may be involved in this case is that initial refusal of something offered is seen as a gesture of courtesy; this client may have considered it impolite to agree to the pain medication the first time it was offered. The best approach for the nurse is to consider the client's need for pain medication even if the client has not requested or even refuses relief from pain. Then, if the client still refuses, the nurse should respect his or her wishes.

Evaluation

Nursing care is evaluated by comparing client outcomes with goals established for nursing diagnoses that are identified following appropriate assessment. The nursing process includes cultural sensitivity specific to the client. Nurses should consider the impact of the client's beliefs and behaviors on achievement of the goals established. If cultural differences are a factor, the nursing care plan needs to be modified to include cultural influences that support the client in reaching expected outcomes.

The nursing process organizes the nursing care of clients, beginning with assessment and ending with evaluation. Cultural sensitivity can be included in every phase of the nursing process to support both clients and their families. The following cultural issues need to be addressed throughout the nursing process (modified from Russell Consulting, 2005):

- Routines of daily life both in and out of the home
- Customs and practices
- Level of education and training
- Ceremonies, celebrations, and events that clients follow
- How health care decisions are made
- The head of the household's role
- Verbal and nonverbal communication
- Physical environment and boundaries of personal space
- Organizational structure of the home.

ALTERNATIVE HEALTH CARE

Health practices involving exercise, diet, and environment are beneficial to clients. However, some clients may believe in health care practices that fall outside the scope of Western medicine. Acupuncture and yoga are two excellent and increasingly familiar examples (Table 6–1).

Cultural health practices must be respected and not ignored, because they are important to clients. If nontraditional health practices have no negative impact on the client, it may be important for the client to continue using them.

Alternative medical health and mental health treatments are becoming increasingly popular among the general population as well. Many people are adopting alternative healing practices from different cultures, such as Buddhist meditation, Asian acupuncture, Native-American sweat lodges, and Chinese herbal medicines. The importance in the healing process of body, mind, and spirit and of being in harmony with nature are common themes in many cultural healing practices and rituals (Corkindale, 2008).

TABLE 6–1 **Examples of Cultural Health Care Practices**

TYPE OF SYSTEM	VIEW OF ILLNESS	EMPHASIS	VIEW OF HEALTH	INTERVENTIONS
Ayurveda (India)	State of imbalance in body systems	Interdependence of health and quality of societal life	Mental health—good memory, comprehension, intelligence, and reasoning ability Emotional health—evenly balanced emotional state and sense of well-being Physical health—abundant energy and proper functioning of senses, digestion, and elimination	Lifestyle interventions are major preventative and therapeutic approaches.
Traditional Chinese Medicine	Imbalance or interruption in the flow of qi	Mind, body, spirit, and emotions are never separated.	Balance of qi Body's organ systems have physical, emotional, spiritual, and psychological functions.	Herbal medicine, acupuncture, acupressure, massage, heat therapy, qigong, tai chi, and nutritional lifestyle counseling
Native American Healing	Illness begins in the head, and individual must get rid of ideas that predispose to illness. If the mind is negative the body will be drained.	Spirituality and medicine are inseparable.	Balance or harmony of mind and body requires being in harmony with all things.	Medicine women and men act as channels through which Great Power helps others achieve well-being. Health care often is dispensed through a ritual or ceremony with healer entering into a loving and compassionate relationship with client, and they join or merge as process unfolds. Use of sweat lodge, singing, pipe ceremony, sun dance, and vision question
Curanderism (Latin American)	Disease is caused by social, psychological, physical, and spiritual factors that can come from natural or supernatural forces.	Encompasses mind, body, spirit, and soul	Health is achieved by maintaining balance, such as hot and cold or spiritual and physical.	Use of plant remedies, loving touch massage, prayer, channeling of advice from helpful spirits, and heart-to-heart talks in addition to Western medical practices Practice is dependent on local area, with different practices in different areas.

REVIEW Values and Beliefs

RELATE: LINK THE CONCEPTS

You are a nurse working in a children's rehabilitation center. A 6-year-old girl who is recovering from a car accident comes to your center for an extended stay. She speaks a little English. Her family has recently moved here from China, and her parents speak very little English. Although, they are grateful for the help they are receiving, they are very stressed about their daughter's situation.

Linking the exemplar of Values and Beliefs with the concept of Communication:

1. How might the nurse assess this family's values and beliefs in light of the family's inability to speak English?
2. How might involvement of an interpreter to facilitate communication impact the client and her family's values and beliefs? How can you overcome this problem?

Linking the exemplar of Values and Beliefs with the concept of Advocacy:

3. How can you advocate for this client's values and beliefs while she is institutionalized?
4. The client's family wishes to pray at the child's bedside using candles, which are not allowed because of the risk for fire related to oxygen use. How can you advocate for this family while maintaining safety?

REFER: GO TO MYNURSINGKIT

REFLECT: CASE STUDY

Jesus Hernandez is a 5-year-old boy and a client at the pediatric clinic where you are employed. His family are immigrants from Mexico; he speaks a little English. His mother, Senora Hernandez, speaks very little English. Her older daughter, Maria, is 15 and speaks English fairly well. Maria usually acts as interpreter for the family.

Jesus is diagnosed with allergic asthma. His pediatrician prescribes Singulair once a day, to be taken at night; a steroid inhaler to be taken morning and night; and an albuterol inhaler to be used before recess and whenever he is short of breath, but not more than two puffs every 6 hours. The pediatrician also refers Jesus to an allergist for further evaluation.

1. How can you, as the nurse, be sure that his mother understands the medication instructions?
2. How can you be sure she understands his condition and at what point she may need to take him to the emergency room if his breathing deteriorates?
3. What dangers are possible as the result of having Maria interpret and how might you resolve this issue?

EXPLORE PEARSON mynursingkit™

MyNursingKit is your one stop for online chapter review materials and resources. Prepare for success with additional NCLEX®-style practice questions, interactive assignments and activities, web links, animations and videos, and more!

Register your access code from the front of your book at **www.mynursingkit.com**.

REFERENCES

American Academy of Family Physicians. (2007). Cultural competence self-test. Retrieved May 14, 2009, from http://www.aafp.org/fpm/20001000/58cult.html#boxb

American Association of Colleges of Nursing. (2006). *Cultural competency in baccalaureate nursing education*. Retrieved May 14, 2009, from http://www.aacn.nche.edu

American Medical Student Association. (2007). *Cultural competency in medicine*. Retrieved May 14, 2009, from http://www.amsa.org/programs/gpit/cultural.cfm

Berman, A., Snyder, S. J., Kozier, B., & Erb, G. (2008). *Kozier & Erb's fundamentals of nursing: Concepts, process, and practice* (8th ed.). Upper Saddle River, NJ: Pearson Education.

Betancourt, J. R., & Ananeh-Firemping, O. (2004). *Not me! Doctors, decisions and disparities in health care*. Retrieved May 14, 2009, from http://www.medscape.com/viewarticle/480602

Centers for Disease Control and Prevention, U.S. Department of Health and Human Services. (2007). *Health, United States, 2007*. Chartbook on trends in the health of Americans. Retrieved May 14, 2009, from http://www.cdc.gov/nchs/data/hus/hus07.ped#contents

Centers for Disease Control and Prevention, U.S. Department of Health and Human Services. (2009). Women and heart disease fact sheet. Retrieved May 14, 2009, from http://www.cdc.gov/DHDSP/library/fs_women_heart.htm

Collins, S. D. (2006). Is cultural competency required in today's nursing care? *NSNA IMPRINT, Feb/Mar*, 52–54. Retrieved May 14, 2009, from http://www.nsna.org/pubs/imprint/febmar06/impfeb_feat_collins.pdf

Corkindale, D. F. (2008). *Healing traditions in multi-cultural America*. Retrieved May 14, 2009, from http://www.debbiecorkindale.com/multicultural.html

Cornsilk, C., & Blythe, F. (Executive Producers). (2006, November). *Indian country diaries*. Peoplehood. New York and Washington, DC: Public Broadcasting Service. Retrieved from http://www.pbs.org/indiancountry

Craven, R. F., & Hirnle, C. J. (2007). *Fundamentals of nursing human health and function* (5th ed.). Philadelphia: Lippincott Williams & Wilkins.

Cultural Diversity in Nursing. Transcultural Nursing. (2008). *Cultural competence*. Retrieved May 14, 2009, from http://www.culturediversity.org/cultcomp.htm

Culturally sensitive nursing care. (2008). Retrieved May 14, 2009, from http://www.megaessays.com/viewpaper/88079.html

Department of Education, Science, and Training. (2008). *Current models of multicultural education*. Retrieved May 14, 2009, from http://www.dest.gov.au/archive/HIGHERED/nursing?pubs?multi_cultural/5.htm

DiversityRx. (2008). *Why language and culture are important*. Retrieved May 14, 2009, from http://www.diversityrx.org/htmL/ESLANG.htm

essortment. (2008). *American culture for foreigners*. Retrieved May 14, 2009, from http://www.essortment.com/all/americanculture_rtjl.htm

Harper, M. G. (2008). *Evaluation of the antecedents of cultural competence*. University of Central Florida. Retrieved from http://www.tcns.org

Hooker, R. (2008). *World civilizations*. Retrieved May 14, 2009, from http://wsu.edu/~dee/WORLD.HTM

Inspired Personal Development. (2007). *The big 5 that develop your belief system*. Retrieved May 14, 2009, from http://www.inspired-personal-development.com/belief-system.html

Institute of Medicine of the National Academies. (2002). *Unequal treatment: Confronting racial and ethnic disparities in health care*. Washington, DC: National Academy of Sciences.

Jay, G. (2008). *What is multiculturalism*? Milwaukee, WI: University of Wisconsin.

The Joint Commission. (2008). *Hospitals, language, and culture: A snapshot of the nation*. Retrieved May 14, 2009, from http://www.jointcommission.org/PatientSafety/HLC

Management Sciences for Health. (2009). *The provider's guide to quality and culture*. Retrieved from http://erc.msh.org/

Multicultural Nursing Education. (2008). *National review of nursing education*. Retrieved from http://www.dest.gov.au/archive/HIGHERED/nursing/pubs/multi_cultural/5.htm

Multiculturalism. (2004). Retrieved June 3, 2009, from http://www.wikinfo.org/index.php/Multiculturalism

Multiculturalism definition. (2008). Retrieved from http://www.answers.com/topic/multiculturalism

Peace Corps. (2003). *Culture matters: The Peace Corps cross cultural workbook*. Retrieved from http://peacecorps.gov/multimedia/pdf/library/T0087_culturematters.pdf

Persistent Stereotypes About Asian Americans. (2009). Retrieved from http://www.asian-nation.org/

Potter, P. A., & Perry, A. G. (2009). *Fundamentals of nursing* (7th ed.). St. Louis, MO: Mosby.

Rusbult, C. (2007). What is a worldview?—Definition & introduction. Retrieved from http://www.asa3.org/ASA/education/views/index.html

Russell Consulting Cooperation. (2005). Understanding organizational cure. Retrieved from http://www.russellconsultinginc.com/docs/white/culture.html

Society of the United States. (2008). Retrieved from http://en.wikipedia.org/wiki/Society_of_the_United_States

Transcultural Nursing Society. (2008). Retrieved from http://www.tcns.org

U.S. Bureau of the Census. (2007). State & County QuickFacts. Retrieved from http://quickfacts.census.gov/qfd/states/00000.html

Values and Beliefs as Components of Culture: An Introduction (2008). Retrieved from http://www.wsu.edu/gened/learn-modules/top_culture/values-beliefs/values-beliefs-intro.html

What is culture? (2008). Retrieved from http://dictionary.reference.com/browse/culture

Wilkinson, J. M., & Van Leuven, K. (2007). *Fundamentals of nursing theory, concepts & applications*. Philadelphia: F.A. Davis.

Wilson-Stronks, A., Galvez, E., & The Joint Commission (2007). Exploring cultural and linguistic services in the nation's hospitals: A report of findings. Retrieved from http://www.jointcommission.org/PatientSafety

Development 7

Concept at-a-Glance

Concept Learning Outcomes

After reading about this concept, you will be able to:

1. Differentiate between the terms *growth* and *development*.
2. Describe essential principles related to development.
3. List factors that influence development.
4. Describe the stages of development according to various theorists.
5. Compare Peck's and Gould's stages of adult development.
6. Compare Kohlberg's and Gilligan's theories of moral development.
7. Compare Fowler's and Westerhoff's stages of spiritual development.
8. Explain contemporary developmental approaches such as temperament theory, ecologic theory, and the resilience framework.
9. Recognize major developmental milestones for clients at each stage of development.
10. Discuss the importance of developmentally appropriate care in meeting client's needs.

Concept Key Terms

Accommodation, *347*
Adaptation, *347*
Adaptive mechanisms, *343*
Adaptation phase, *350*
Adjustment phase, *350*
Animism, *360*
Assimilation, *347*
Associative play, *360*
Autosomal chromosomes, *340*
Centration, *360*
Cephalocaudal development, *340*
Cognitive development, *347*
Conservation, *360*
Cooperative play, *363*
Defense mechanism, *343*
Development, *340*
Developmental stage, *340*
Developmental task, *345*
Dramatic play, *361*
Ecologic theory, *350*
Ego, *343*
Egocentrism, *360*
Expressive jargon, *359*
Expressive speech, *357*
Fixation, *344*
Growth, *339*
Id, *340*
Libido, *343*
Magical thinking, *360*
Moral, *350*
Moral behavior, *350*
Moral development, *350*
Morality, *350*
Nature, *350*
Nurture, *350*
Object permanence, *360*
Parallel play, *358*
Personality, *343*
Protective factors, *350*
Proximodistal development, *340*
Puberty, *364*
Receptive speech, *357*
Resilience, *350*
Risk factors, *350*
Self-efficacy, *348*
Sex chromosomes, *340*
Solitary play, *356*
Superego, *343*
Temperament, *340*
Transductive reasoning, *360*
Unconscious mind, *343*

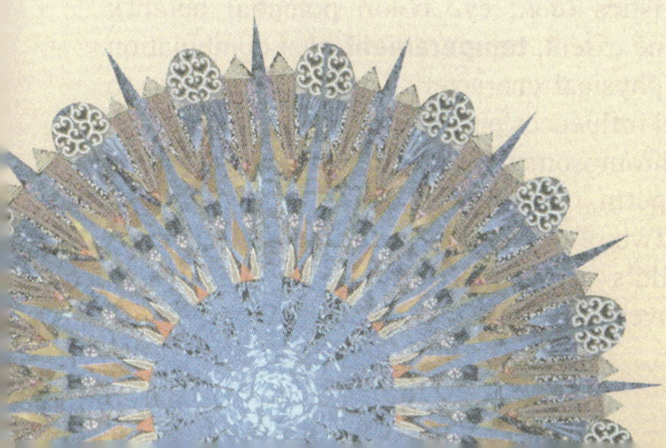

About Development

The terms *growth* and *development* both refer to dynamic processes. Often used interchangeably, these terms have different meanings. **Growth** refers to physical change and increase in size. It can be measured quantitatively. Indicators of growth include height, weight, bone size, and dentition. The pattern of physiologic growth is similar for all people. However, growth rates vary during different stages of growth and development. The growth rate is rapid during the prenatal, neonatal, infancy, and adolescent stages and slows during childhood. Physical growth is minimal during adulthood.

Development is an increase in the complexity of function and skill progression, the capacity and skill of a person to adapt to the environment. Development is the behavioral aspect of growth (e.g., a person develops the ability to walk, to talk, and to run). •

Growth and development are independent, interrelated processes. For example, an infant's muscles, bones, and nervous system must grow to a certain point before the infant is able to sit up or walk. Growth generally takes place during the first 20 years of life; development takes place throughout the life span. The following are principles of growth and development:

- Growth and development are continuous, orderly, sequential processes influenced by maturational, environmental, and genetic factors.
- All humans follow the same pattern of growth and development.
- The sequence of each stage is predictable, although the time of onset, the length of the stage, and the effects of each stage vary with each person.
- Learning can either help or hinder the maturational process, depending on what is learned.
- Each **developmental stage** (level of achievement) has its own characteristics. For example, Piaget suggested that in the sensorimotor stage (birth to 2 years) children learn to coordinate simple motor tasks.
- Growth and development occur in a **cephalocaudal** direction, that is, starting at the head and moving toward the trunk, legs, and feet (Figure 7–1 ■). This pattern is particularly obvious at birth, when the head of the infant is disproportionately large.
- Growth and development occur in a **proximodistal** direction, that is, from the center of the body outward (see Figure 7–1). For example, infants can roll over before they can grasp an object with the thumb and second finger.
- Development proceeds from simple to complex, or from single acts to integrated acts. To accomplish the integrated act of drinking and swallowing from a cup, for example, the child must first learn a series of single acts: eye–hand coordination; grasping; hand–mouth coordination; controlled tipping of the cup; and then mouth, lip, and tongue movements to drink and swallow.
- Development becomes increasingly differentiated. Differentiated development begins with a generalized response and progresses to a specific skilled response. For example, an infant's initial response to a stimulus involves the total body, but a 5-year-old child can respond more specifically with laughter or fear.
- Certain stages of growth and development are more critical than others. It is known, for example, that the first 10–12 weeks after conception are critical. The incidence of congenital anomalies as a result of exposure to certain viruses, chemicals, or drugs is greater during this stage than during others.

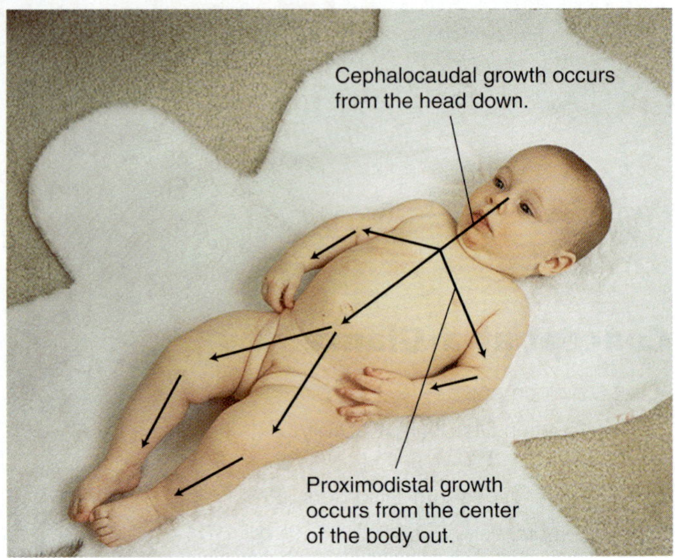
Cephalocaudal growth occurs from the head down.
Proximodistal growth occurs from the center of the body out.

Figure 7–1 ■ In normal cephalocaudal growth, the child gains control of the head and neck before the trunk and limbs. In normal proximodistal growth, the child controls arm movements before hand movements. For example, the child reaches for objects before being able to grasp them. Children gain control of their hands before their fingers; that is, they can hold things with the entire hand before they can pick something up with just their fingers.

- The pace of growth and development is uneven. It is known that growth is greater during infancy than during childhood. Asynchronous development is demonstrated by rapid growth of the head during infancy and the extremities at puberty.
- The rate of a person's growth and development is highly individual; however, the sequence of growth and development is predictable. Stages of growth usually correspond to certain developmental changes (Table 7–1).

FACTORS INFLUENCING DEVELOPMENT

Many factors can influence growth and development. Knowledge of these factors helps the nurse to intervene to promote positive growth and development of the individual. Both genetic and environmental factors contribute to individual differences.

Genetics

The genetic inheritance of an individual is established at conception. It remains unchanged throughout life and determines physical characteristics (e.g., eye color, potential height); gender; and, to some extent, **temperament**, that combination of biological and physical characteristics that is specific to each individual and influences personality and behavior. Each child inherits 23 chromosomes from the mother's egg and 23 from the father's sperm, resulting in a unique individual with 46 chromosomes. Two of these are **sex chromosomes**, which determine the child's gender; the rest, called **autosomal chromosomes**, govern all remaining characteristics. Every

TABLE 7–1 **Stages of Growth and Development**

STAGE	AGE	SIGNIFICANT CHARACTERISTICS	NURSING IMPLICATIONS
Neonatal	Birth to 28 days	Behavior is largely reflexive and develops to more purposeful behavior.	Assist parents to identify and meet unmet needs.
Infancy	1 month to 1 year	Physical growth is rapid.	Control the infant's environment so that physical and psychological needs are met.
Toddlerhood	1 to 3 years	Motor development permits increased physical autonomy. Psychosocial skills increase.	Safety and risk-taking strategies must be balanced to permit growth.
Preschool	3 to 6 years	The preschooler's world is expanding. New experiences and the preschooler's social role are tried during play. Physical growth is slower.	Provide opportunities for play and social activity.
School age	6 to 12 years	Stage includes the preadolescent period (10–12 years). Peer group increasingly influences behavior. Physical growth is slower.	Allow time and energy for the school-age child to pursue hobbies and school activities. Recognize and support child's achievement.
Adolescence	12 to 18 years	Self-concept changes with biological development. Values are tested. Physical growth accelerates. Stress increases.	Assist adolescents to develop coping behaviors. Help adolescents develop strategies for resolving conflicts.
Young adulthood	18 to 40 years	A personal lifestyle develops. Person establishes a relationship with a significant other and a commitment to something.	Accept adult's chosen lifestyle and assist with necessary adjustments relating to health. Recognize the person's commitments. Support change as necessary for health.
Middle adulthood	40 to 65 years	Lifestyle changes due to other changes; for example, children leave home, occupational goals change.	Assist clients to plan for anticipated changes in life, to recognize the risk factors related to health, and to focus on strengths rather than weaknesses.
Older adulthood			
Young-old	65 to 74 years	Adaptation to retirement and changing physical abilities is often necessary. Chronic illness may develop.	Assist clients to keep mentally, physically, and socially active and to maintain peer group interactions.
Middle-old	75 to 84 years	Adaptation to decline in speed of movement, reaction time, and increasing dependence on others may be necessary.	Assist clients to cope with loss (e.g., hearing, sensory abilities and eyesight, death of loved one). Provide necessary safety measures.
Old-old	85 and older	Increasing physical problems may develop.	Assist clients with self-care as required, and with maintaining as much independence as possible.

chromosome carries many genes that determine physical characteristics, intellectual potential, personality type, and other traits. Children are born with the potential for certain features; however, their interaction with the environment influences how and to what extent particular traits are manifested. For example, a child may have the potential for a high level of intellectual performance, but if he or she lives in an environment without access to supports such as education and proper nutrition, that potential may never be reached.

Since chromosomes and genes carry messages that encode for certain characteristics, they also can carry diseases. Children can be affected by chromosomal disorders, such as fragile X or Down syndrome, which involve either altered numbers or altered structure of chromosomes. Although some of these mutations are incompatible with life and result in fetal death, live births can occur with others. Chromosomal disorders may be caused by an array of factors, such as radiation exposure, parental age, or parental disease states; however, sometimes their causes cannot be determined.

Some children inherit genes that lead to diseases such as cystic fibrosis; others may have a mutation that manifests in the disease. A family history of these diseases is usually present, but because genes sometimes mutate, an initial incidence of a genetic disorder may appear with no identifiable history.

Prenatal Influences

Some Asian cultures calculate age from the time of conception. This practice acknowledges the profound influence of the prenatal period.

The mother's nutrition and general state of health play a part in pregnancy outcome. Poor nutrition can lead to low-birth-weight infants and infants with compromised neurologic performance, slow development, or impaired immune status with resultant high disease rates. Low maternal stores of iron can result in anemia in the infant (American Academy of Pediatrics, 2004). Maternal smoking is associated with low-birth-weight infants. Ingestion of alcoholic beverages, including beer and wine, during pregnancy may lead to fetal alcohol syndrome or fetal alcohol effects. Substance abuse by the mother may result in neonatal addiction, convulsions, hyperirritability, poor social responsiveness, and other neurologic disturbances of the infant, as well as changes in neurobehavioral and cognitive function of children (Huizink & Mulder, 2006).

Even prescription or nonprescription drugs may adversely affect the fetus. This was brought to general attention when the drug thalidomide, commonly prescribed in Europe to treat nausea during the 1950s, resulted in the birth of infants with limb abnormalities to women who had taken the drug during pregnancy. Differences in physiology related to gastric emptying, renal clearance, drug distribution, and other factors contribute to variations in pharmacokinetics during pregnancy. Drugs can cause teratogenesis (abnormal development of the fetus) or mutagenesis (permanent changes in the fetus' genetic material) (McCarter-Spaulding, 2005). Certain drugs can cause bleeding, stained teeth, impaired hearing, or other defects in the infant. The U.S. Food and Drug Administration (FDA) has established risk categories for drugs in pregnancy.

Some maternal illnesses are harmful to the developing fetus. One example is rubella (German measles), which is rarely a serious disease for adults but can cause deafness, vision defects, heart defects, and mental retardation in the fetus if it is acquired by a pregnant woman. A fetus can also acquire diseases such as AIDS and HIV infection or hepatitis B from the mother.

Chronic maternal distress or depression can affect the fetus. Excess stress hormones such as cortisone pass through the placenta, and can result in lower birth weight and size. Recent studies indicate that maternal distress during pregnancy can also affect a baby's temperament and neurobehavioral development (Diego, 2006).

Radiation, chemicals, and other environmental hazards may adversely affect a fetus when the mother is exposed to these influences during her pregnancy. The best outcomes for infants occur when mothers eat well; exercise regularly; seek early prenatal care; refrain from use of drugs, alcohol, tobacco, and excessive caffeine; and follow general principles of good health.

Family and Parenting

An environmental factor that is extremely important in the development of children is the profile of family characteristics. The family is an important component in every child's life and plays an essential role in fostering the development of youth. Parenting is a significant concept in families. The effects of parenting interact with a child's individual characteristics to influence risk and protective factors, personality characteristics, and developmental outcomes.

The families into which individuals are born influence them profoundly. Children are supported in different ways and acquire different world views depending on such factors as whether they have one or two parents or stepparents, whether one or both parents work, how many siblings are present, and whether an extended family is close. When working with a child or family, the nurse should take note of variations in family structure such as single parent, homosexual parents, extended family, and stepparents.

Cultural Influences

Another factor that influences development is culture, both through traditional practices and due to genetic variations among some ethnic groups. The traditional customs of the many cultural groups represented in North America influence the development of children in these groups. Nutritional practices of various ethnic groups may influence the rate of growth for infants. In addition, development may be influenced by childrearing practices. For example, the Native American practice of carrying infants on boards often delays walking compared to the norm measured in some developmental tests. Children who are carried by straddling the mother's hips or back for extended periods have a low incidence of developmental hip dysplasia since this keeps their hips in an abducted position. It is important for nurses to take cultural practices into account when performing developmental screening; some tests may not be culturally sensitive and can inaccurately label a child as delayed when the pattern of development is simply different in the group, perhaps due to family's childrearing practices. In these cases there is no lasting delay in any milestone, but variation in acquiring skills may occur.

All cultural groups have rules regarding patterns of social interaction. Schedules of language acquisition are determined by the number of languages spoken and the amount of speech in the home. The particular social roles men and women assume in the culture affect school activities and ultimately career choices. Attitudes toward touching and other methods of encouraging developmental skills vary among cultures.

Genetic traits common in certain ethnic or cultural groups may predispose children to being at the upper or lower ranges of growth and may influence other physical characteristics. Genetic variations also make certain groups more prone to develop certain diseases.

Nutrition

Adequate nutrition is an essential component of growth and development. For example, poorly nourished children are more likely to get infections than are well-nourished children. In addition, poorly nourished children may not attain their full height potential. Inadequate nutrition during pregnancy and the first few years of life may also impact brain development. If the brain is not properly nourished children will fall behind on development. Children who are severely malnourished may have permanent brain damage and may even die.

Environment

A few environmental factors that can influence growth and development are the living conditions of the child (e.g., homelessness), socioeconomic status (e.g., poverty versus financial stability), climate, and community (e.g., providing developmental support versus exposing the child to hazards).

Health

Illness or injury can affect growth and development. Being hospitalized is stressful for a child and can affect the child's coping mechanisms. Prolonged or chronic illness may affect normal developmental processes, including psychosocial development.

GROWTH AND DEVELOPMENT THEORIES

Growth and development are commonly thought of as having five major components: psychosocial, cognitive, moral, spiritual, and biophysical. Researchers have advanced several theories about the various stages and aspects of growth and development, particularly with regard to infant and child development. A discussion of some of the major theories follows.

Psychosocial Theories

Psychosocial development refers to the development of personality. **Personality**, a complex concept that is difficult to define, can be considered as the outward (interpersonal) expression of the inner (intrapersonal) self. It encompasses a person's temperament, feelings, character traits, independence, self-esteem, self-concept, behavior, ability to interact with others, and ability to adapt to life changes.

Many theorists have attempted to account for psychosocial development in humans. These theories often explain the development of a person's personality and the causes of behavior.

FREUD (1856–1939) Sigmund Freud introduced a number of concepts about development that are still used today. The **unconscious mind** is the part of a person's mental life of which he or she is unaware. This concept of the unconscious is one of Freud's major contributions to the field of psychiatry. The **id** resides in the unconscious and, operating on the pleasure principle, seeks immediate pleasure and gratification. The **ego**, the realistic part of the person, balances the gratification demands of the id with the limitations of social and physical circumstances. The methods the ego uses to fulfill the needs of the id in a socially acceptable manner are called defense mechanisms or adaptive mechanisms. **Defense mechanisms**, or **adaptive mechanisms** as they are more commonly called today, are the result of conflicts between the id's impulses and the anxiety created by the conflicts due to social and environmental restrictions. The third aspect of the personality, according to Freud, is the superego. The **superego** contains the conscience and the ego ideal. The conscience consists of society's "do not's," usually resulting from parental and cultural expectations. The ego ideal comprises the standards of perfection toward which the individual strives. Freud also proposed that the underlying motivation to human development is a dynamic, psychic energy, which he called **libido**. According to Freud's theory of psychosexual development, the personality develops in five overlapping stages from birth to adulthood. The libido changes its location of emphasis within the body from one stage to another. Therefore, a particular body area has special significance to a client at a particular stage. The first three stages (oral, anal, and phallic) are called *pregenital stages*. The culminating stage is the *genital stage*. Table 7–2 indicates characteristics for each stage.

Freudian theory asserts that the individual must meet the needs of each developmental stage to move successfully to the next. For example, during the oral stage, nurses can assist an infant's development by making feeding a pleasurable experience. This provides comfort and security for the infant. Freud

TABLE 7–2 **Freud's Five Stages of Development**

STAGE	AGE	CHARACTERISTICS	IMPLICATIONS
Oral	Birth to 1½ years	Mouth is the center of pleasure (major source of gratification and exploration). Security is primary need. Major conflict: weaning.	Feeding produces pleasure and a sense of comfort and safety. Feeding should be pleasurable and provided when required.
Anal	1½ to 3 years	Anus and bladder are the sources of pleasure (sensual satisfaction, self-control). Major conflict: toilet training.	Controlling and expelling feces provide pleasure and sense of control. Toilet training should be a pleasurable experience.
Phallic	4 to 6 years	The child's genitals are the center of pleasure. Masturbation offers pleasure. Other activities can include fantasy, experimentation with peers, and questioning of adults about sexual topics. Major conflict: the Oedipus or Electra complex, which resolves when the child identifies with parent of same sex. (The Oedipus complex refers to the male child's attraction to his mother and hostile attitudes toward his father. The Electra complex refers to the female child's attraction to her father and hostile attitudes toward her mother.)	The child identifies with the parent of the opposite sex and later takes on a love relationship outside the family. Encourage identity.
Latency	6 years to puberty	Energy is directed toward physical and intellectual activities. Sexual impulses tend to be repressed. Relationships between peers of the same sex develop.	Encourage child with physical and intellectual pursuits. Encourage sports and other activities with same-sex peers.
Genital	Puberty and after	Energy is directed toward full sexual maturity and function and development of skills needed to cope with the environment.	Encourage separation from parents, achievement of independence, and decision making.

also emphasized the importance of infant–parent interaction. Therefore, the nurse, as a caregiver, should provide a warm, caring atmosphere for an infant and assist parents to do so when the infant returns to their care.

If the person does not achieve a satisfactory progression at one stage, the personality becomes fixated at that stage. **Fixation** is immobilization or the inability of the personality to proceed to the next stage because of anxiety. For example, making toilet training a positive experience during the anal stage enhances the child's feeling of self-control. If, however, the toilet training was a negative experience, the resulting conflict or stress can delay or prolong progression through that stage or cause a person to regress to a previous stage. Ideally, an individual progresses through each stage with balance between the id, ego, and superego.

ERIKSON (1902–1996) Erik H. Erikson (1963, 1968) adapted and expanded Freud's theory of development to include the entire life span, believing that people continue to develop throughout life. He described eight stages of development (Table 7–3).

Erikson's theory proposes that life is a sequence of developmental stages or levels of achievement. Each stage signals a task that must be accomplished. The resolution of the task can be complete, partial, or unsuccessful. Erikson believed that the more successful an individual is at each developmental stage, the healthier the personality of the individual will be. Failure to complete any developmental stage interferes with the person's ability to progress to the next level. These developmental stages can be viewed as a series of crises. Successful resolution of these crises supports healthy ego development. Failure to resolve the crises damages the ego.

Erikson's eight stages reflect both positive and negative aspects of the critical life periods. The resolution of the conflicts at each stage enables the person to function effectively in society. Each phase has its own developmental task, and the individual must find a balance between, for example, trust and mistrust (Stage 1) or integrity and despair (Stage 8). See Figures 7–2 ■ and 7–3 ■.

When using Erikson's developmental framework, nurses should be aware of indicators of positive and negative resolution of each developmental stage. According to Erikson, the environment is highly influential to development. Nurses can enhance a client's development by being aware of the individual's developmental stage and assisting with the development of coping skills related to stressors experienced at that specific level. Nurses can strengthen a client's positive resolution of a developmental task by providing the individual with appropriate opportunities and encouragement. For example, a 10-year-old child (industry versus inferiority) can be encouraged to be creative, to finish schoolwork, and to learn how to accomplish these tasks within the limitations imposed by health status. An older adult can be encouraged to maintain generativity (care for and connection

TABLE 7–3 **Erikson's Eight Stages of Development**

STAGE	AGE	CENTRAL TASK	INDICATORS OF POSITIVE RESOLUTION	INDICATORS OF NEGATIVE RESOLUTION
Infancy	Birth to 18 months	Trust versus mistrust	Learning to trust others	Mistrust, withdrawal, estrangement
Early childhood	18 months to 3 years	Autonomy versus shame and doubt	Self-control without loss of self-esteem; ability to cooperate and to express oneself	Compulsive self-restraint or compliance; willfulness and defiance
Late childhood	3 to 5 years	Initiative versus guilt	Learning the degree to which assertiveness and purpose influence the environment; beginning ability to evaluate one's own behavior	Lack of self-confidence; pessimism, fear of wrongdoing; overcontrol and overrestriction of own activity
School age	6 to 12 years	Industry versus inferiority	Beginning to create, develop, and manipulate; developing sense of competence and perseverance	Loss of hope, sense of being mediocre; withdrawal from school and peers
Adolescence	12 to 20 years	Identity versus role confusion	Coherent sense of self; plans to actualize one's abilities	Feelings of confusion, indecisiveness, and possible antisocial behavior
Young adulthood	18 to 25 years	Intimacy versus isolation	Intimate relationship with another person; commitment to work and relationships	Impersonal relationships; avoidance of relationship, career, or lifestyle commitments
Adulthood	25 to 65 years	Generativity versus stagnation	Creativity, productivity, concern for others	Self-indulgence, self-concern, lack of interests and commitments
Maturity	65 years to death	Integrity versus despair	Acceptance of worth and uniqueness of one's own life; acceptance of death	Sense of loss, contempt for others

Source: "Figure of Erickson's Stages of Personality Development," from *Childhood and society* by Erik H. Erikson. © 1950, 1963 by W. W. Norton & Company Inc., renewed © 1978, 1991 by Erik H. Erikson. Used by permission of W. W. Norton & Company, Inc.

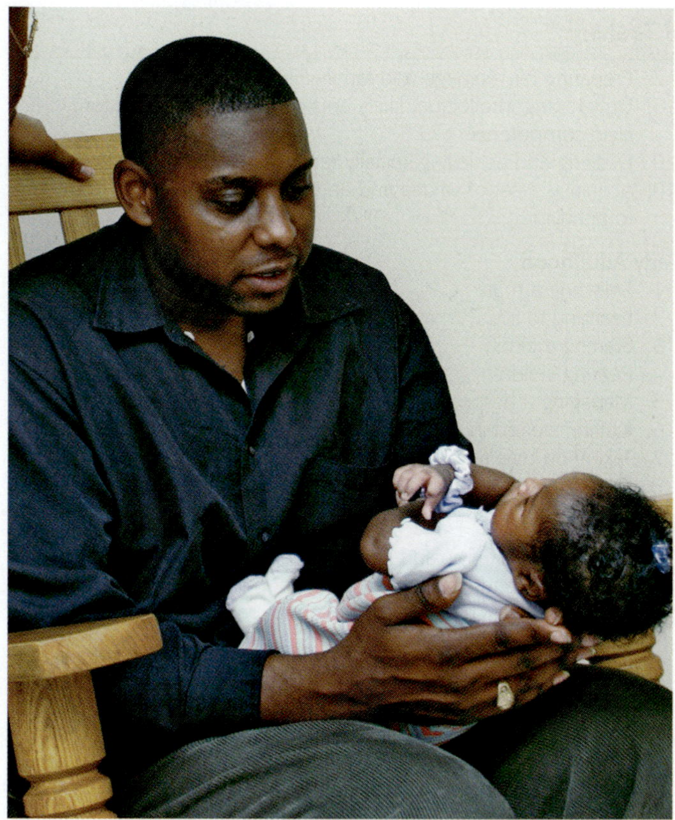

Figure 7–2 ■ Note that the parent and infant faces are in the same plane. This "en face" position enables both to examine the other's face and establish eye contact, fostering attachment between parent and child.

with others) in order to avoid a sense of stagnation, or a feeling of disconnectedness that increases self-absorption and loneliness.

Erikson emphasized that people must change and adapt their behavior to maintain control over their lives. In his view, no stage in personality development can be bypassed, but

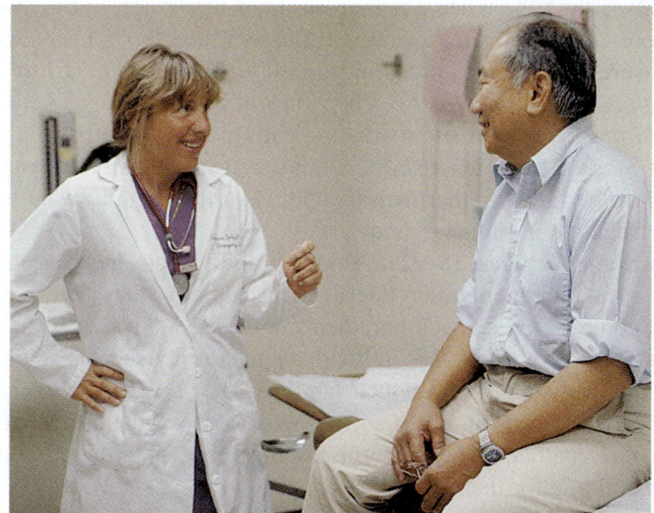

Figure 7–3 ■ Regular assessments can help older adults maintain their health and independence, contributing to achievement of integrity versus despair.

people can become fixated at one stage or regress to a previous stage under anxious or stressful conditions. For example, a middle-aged woman who has never satisfactorily resolved the identity versus role confusion task might regress to an earlier stage when stressed by an illness with which she cannot cope.

HAVIGHURST (1900–1991) Robert Havighurst believed that learning is basic to life and people continue to learn throughout life. He described growth and development as occurring in six stages, each associated with 6–10 tasks to be learned (Table 7–4).

Havighurst promoted the concept of developmental tasks in the 1950s. A **developmental task** is "a task which arises at or about a certain period in the life of an individual, successful achievement of which leads to his happiness and to success with later tasks, while failure leads to unhappiness in the individual, disapproval by society, and difficulty with later tasks" (Havighurst, 1972, p. 2).

Havighurst's developmental tasks provide a framework that the nurse can use to evaluate a person's general accomplishments. However, some nurses find that the broad categories limit its usefulness as a tool in assessing specific accomplishments, particularly those of infancy and childhood. In a multicultural society, the definition of successful completion of tasks may vary with values and belief systems as well (e.g., not all individuals may wish to marry or bear children), making these tasks less relevant for some.

VYGOTSKY (1896–1934) Lev Vygotsky, referred to as a "social constructivist," explored the concept of cognitive development within a social, historical, and cultural context, arguing that adults guide children to learn, and that development depends on the use of language, play, and extensive social interaction. These ideas have been used in treatment of children with learning disorders, autism, mental handicaps, and other disabilities (Edwards, 2002). These ideas also support the benefit of adult social learning opportunities through group interaction and observation. Vygotsky truly supported social learning and reinforcement through work, group discussion, and other means.

PECK (1968–) Theories and models about adult development are relatively recent compared with theories of infant and child development. Research into adult development has been stimulated by a number of factors, including increased longevity and healthier old age. In the past, development was viewed as complete by the time of physical maturity, and aging was considered a decline following maturity. The emphasis was on the negative aspects rather than the positive aspects of aging. However, Robert Peck believes that, although physical capabilities and functions decrease with old age, mental and social capacities tend to increase in the latter part of life.

Peck proposes three developmental tasks during old age, in contrast to Erikson's one (integrity versus despair):

1. **Ego differentiation versus work-role preoccupation.** An adult's identity and feelings of worth are highly dependent on that person's work role. On retirement, people may

TABLE 7–4 Havighurst's Age Periods and Developmental Tasks

Infancy and Early Childhood

1. Learning to walk
2. Learning to take solid foods
3. Learning to talk
4. Learning to control the elimination of body wastes
5. Learning sex differences and sexual modesty
6. Achieving psychologic stability
7. Forming simple concepts of social and physical reality
8. Learning to relate emotionally to parents, siblings, and other people
9. Learning to distinguish right from wrong and developing a conscience

Middle Childhood

1. Learning physical skills necessary for ordinary games
2. Building wholesome attitudes toward oneself as a growing organism
3. Learning to get along with age-mates
4. Learning an appropriate masculine or feminine social role
5. Developing fundamental skills in reading, writing, and calculating
6. Developing concepts necessary for everyday living
7. Developing conscience, morality, and a scale of values
8. Achieving personal independence
9. Developing attitudes toward social groups and institutions

Adolescence

1. Achieving new and more mature relations with age-mates of both sexes
2. Achieving a masculine or feminine social role
3. Accepting one's physique and using the body effectively
4. Achieving emotional independence from parents and other adults
5. Achieving assurance of economic independence
6. Selecting and preparing for an occupation
7. Preparing for marriage and family life
8. Developing intellectual skills and concepts necessary for civic competence
9. Desiring and achieving socially responsible behavior
10. Acquiring a set of values and an ethical system as a guide to behavior

Early Adulthood

1. Selecting a mate
2. Learning to live with a partner
3. Starting a family
4. Rearing children
5. Managing a home
6. Getting started in an occupation
7. Taking on civic responsibility
8. Finding a congenial social group

Middle Age

1. Achieving adult civic and social responsibility
2. Establishing and maintaining an economic standard of living
3. Assisting teenage children to become responsible and happy adults
4. Developing adult leisure-time activities
5. Relating oneself to one's spouse as a person
6. Accepting and adjusting to the physiologic changes of middle age
7. Adjusting to aging parents

Later Maturity

1. Adjusting to decreasing physical strength and health
2. Adjusting to retirement and reduced income
3. Adjusting to death of a spouse
4. Establishing an explicit affiliation with one's age group
5. Meeting social and civil obligations
6. Establishing satisfactory physical living arrangements

Source: Havighurst, R. J. (1972). *Developmental tasks and education.* (3rd ed.). Boston, MA: Allyn and Bacon. Copyright © 1972 Pearson Education. Reprinted by permission of the publisher.

experience feelings of worthlessness unless they derive their sense of identity from a sufficient number of roles that one such role can replace the work role or occupation as a source of self-esteem. For example, a man who likes to garden or golf can obtain ego rewards from those activities, replacing rewards formerly obtained from his occupation.

2. **Body transcendence versus body preoccupation.** This task calls for the individual to adjust to decreasing physical capacities and at the same time maintain feelings of well-being. Preoccupation with declining body functions reduces happiness and satisfaction with life.
3. **Ego transcendence versus ego preoccupation.** Ego transcendence is the acceptance without fear of one's death as inevitable. This acceptance includes being actively involved in one's own future beyond death. Ego preoccupation, by contrast, results in holding onto life and a preoccupation with self-gratification.

GOULD (1935–) Roger Gould is another theorist who has studied adult development. He believes that transformation is a central theme during adulthood: "Adults continue to change over the period of time considered to be adulthood and developmental phases may be found during the adult span of life" (Gould, 1972, p. 33). According to Gould, the 20s is the time when a person assumes new roles, in the 30s role confusion often occurs, in the 40s the person becomes aware of time limitations in relation to accomplishing life's goals, and in the 50s the acceptance of each stage as a natural progression of life marks the path to adult maturity.

- **Stage 1 (ages 16–18).** Individuals consider themselves part of the family rather than individuals; they begin to want to separate from their parents.
- **Stage 2 (ages 18–22).** Although individuals have established autonomy, they feel it is in jeopardy; they feel they could be pulled back into their families.
- **Stage 3 (ages 22–28).** Individuals feel established as adults and autonomous from their families. They see themselves as well-defined but still feel the need to prove themselves to their parents. They see this as the time for growing and building for the future.
- **Stage 4 (ages 29–34).** Marriage and careers are well established. Individuals question what life is all about and wish to be accepted as they are, no longer finding it necessary to prove themselves.

- **Stage 5 (ages 35–43).** This is a period of self-reflection. Individuals question long-held values as well as life itself. They see time as finite, with little time left to shape the lives of adolescent children.
- **Stage 6 (ages 43–50).** Personalities are seen as set. Time is accepted as finite. Individuals are interested in social activities with friends and spouse and desire both sympathy and affection from spouse.
- **Stage 7 (ages 50–60).** This is a period of transformation, with a realization of mortality and a concern for health. There is an increase in warmth and a decrease in negativism. The spouse is seen as a valuable companion (Gould, 1972, pp. 525–527).

JUNG'S THEORY OF INDIVIDUALISM This theory hypothesizes that as a person ages, the shift of focus is away from the external world (extroversion) toward the inner experience (introversion). At this stage of life, the older person will search for answers to many of life's riddles and try to find the essence of the "true self." To age successfully, the older person will accept past accomplishments and failures (Jung, 1960). Older persons subscribing to Jung's theory may spend a lot of time in contemplation and introspection.

DISENGAGEMENT THEORY Introduced by Cummings and Henry in 1961, this controversial theory asserts that the appropriate pattern of behavior in later life is for the older person and society at large to engage in a mutual and reciprocal withdrawal. Thus, when death occurs, neither the older individual nor society is disadvantaged, and social equilibrium is maintained. Mandatory retirement forces some older people to withdraw from work-related roles, accelerating the process of disengagement. In some cultures, older people remain engaged, active, and busy throughout their lives.

CONTINUITY THEORY This theory advances the idea that successful aging involves maintaining or continuing previous values, habits, preferences, family ties, and all other linkages that have formed the basic underlying structure of adult life. Older age is not viewed as a time that should trigger major life readjustment, but rather as just a time to continue being the same person (Havighurst et al., 1963). According to this theory, the pace of activities may be slowed. The older person may drop activities pursued in earlier life that did not bring satisfaction and genuine happiness. For some, relief from constant time pressures and deadlines is one of the benefits of old age.

Piaget's Theory of Cognitive Development

Cognitive development refers to the manner in which people learn to think, reason, and use language. It involves a person's intelligence, perceptual ability, and ability to process information. Cognitive development represents a progression of mental abilities from illogical to logical thinking, from simple to complex problem solving, and from understanding concrete ideas to understanding abstract concepts.

The most widely known cognitive theorist is Jean Piaget. His theory of cognitive development has contributed to other theories, such as Kohlberg's moral development and Fowler's development of faith theories, both discussed in this chapter.

According to Piaget (1966), cognitive development is an orderly, sequential process in which a variety of new experiences (stimuli) must exist before intellectual abilities can develop. Piaget divides cognitive development into five major phases: the sensorimotor phase, the preconceptual phase, the intuitive thought phase, the concrete operations phase, and the formal operations phase. A detailed discussion of these phases, and how the nurse can incorporate his or her knowledge of them into nursing plans and interventions, can be found in the Cognition concept.

A person develops through each of these phases; each phase has its own unique characteristics (Table 7–5). In each phase, the person uses three primary abilities: assimilation, accommodation, and adaptation. **Assimilation** is the process through which humans encounter and react to new situations by using the mechanisms they already possess. In this way, people acquire knowledge and skills as well as insights into the world around them. **Accommodation** is a process of change whereby cognitive processes mature sufficiently to allow the person to solve problems that were unsolvable before. This adjustment is possible chiefly because new knowledge has been assimilated. **Adaptation**, or coping behavior, is the ability to handle the demands made by the environment.

Nurses can use Piaget's theory of cognitive development when developing teaching strategies. For example, a nurse can expect a toddler to be egocentric and literal; therefore, explanations to the toddler should focus on the needs of the toddler rather than on the needs of others. A 13-year-old can be expected to use rational thinking and to reason; therefore, when explaining the need for a medication, a nurse can outline the consequences of taking and not taking the medication, enabling the adolescent to make a rational decision. Nurses must remember, however, that the range of normal cognitive development is broad, despite the ages arbitrarily associated with each level. When teaching adults, nurses may become aware that some adults are more comfortable with concrete thought and are slower to acquire and apply new information than are other adults.

Behaviorism

Behaviorist theory states that learning takes place when an individual's reaction to a stimulus is either positively or negatively reinforced. The more rapid, consistent, and positive the reinforcement, the more likely a behavior is to be learned and retained.

B.F. Skinner believed that organisms learn as they respond to or "operate on" their environment. His research led to the concept of *operant conditioning*, in which he maintained that rewarded or reinforced behavior will be repeated; behavior that is punished will be suppressed. Most of his work was with laboratory animals.

Social Learning Theory

Albert Bandura (1925–), a contemporary psychologist, believes that children learn attitudes, beliefs, customs, and values through their social contacts with adults and other children. Children imitate (or model) the behavior they see; if the behavior is positively reinforced, they tend to repeat it. However, Bandura also believes that people can consciously choose how

TABLE 7–5 **Piaget's Phases of Cognitive Development**

PHASES AND STAGES	AGE	SIGNIFICANT BEHAVIOR
Sensorimotor phase	Birth to 2 years	
Stage 1: Use of reflexes	Birth to 1 month	Most action is reflexive.
Stage 2: Primary circular reaction	1 to 4 months	Perception of events is centered on the body. Objects are extension of self.
Stage 3: Secondary circular reaction	4 to 8 months	The external environment is acknowledged. Changes in the environment are actively made.
Stage 4: Coordination of secondary schemata	8 to 12 months	A goal can be distinguished from a means of attaining it.
Stage 5: Tertiary circular reaction	12 to 18 months	Individual tries and discovers new goals and ways to attain goals. Rituals are important.
Stage 6: Inventions of new means	18 to 24 months	Individual interprets the environment by mental image; uses make-believe and pretend play.
Preconceptual phase	2 to 4 years	Individual uses an egocentric approach to accommodate the demands of an environment. Everything is significant and relates to "me." Individual explores the environment. Language development is rapid. Words are associated with objects.
Intuitive thought phase	4 to 7 years	Egocentric thinking diminishes. Individual thinks of one idea at a time, includes others in the environment. Words express thoughts.
Concrete operations phase	7 to 11 years	Individual solves concrete problems; begins to understand relationships such as size; understands right and left; is cognizant of viewpoints.
Formal operations phase	11 to 15 years	Individual uses rational thinking. Reasoning is deductive and futuristic.

Source: Adapted from Piaget, J. (1966). *The origin of intelligence.* Copyright © 1966 International Universities Press, Inc. Reprinted with permission.

to act, such as deciding to handle problems by talking rather than using violence. The external environment (the behavior of others) and the child's internal processes are both key elements in the behaviors the child manifests (Bandura, 1986, 1997a).

Bandura believes that an important determinant of behavior is **self-efficacy**, or the expectation that someone can produce a desired outcome. For example, if adolescents believe they can avoid use of drugs or alcohol, they are more likely to do so. A child who has confidence in his or her ability to exercise regularly or lose weight has a greater chance of success with these behavior changes. Parents who have confidence in their ability to care adequately for their infants are more likely to do so (Bandura, 1997b).

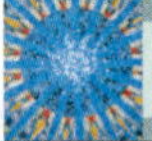

EVIDENCE-BASED PRACTICE **Self-Efficacy**

Clinical Question

Nurses often provide information for parents and children that will encourage them to adopt healthy lifestyles. Providing information may not be enough; many of us know about healthy behaviors but do not consistently apply them. The concept of self-efficacy helps to explain why some people take on healthy behaviors, whereas others do not. People who are convinced they can make a positive change are more likely to do so. A number of research projects test and apply self-efficacy in teaching about health. Two examples follow.

Evidence

A federally funded study sought to measure the effectiveness of a preventive parent training program among low-income families with small children. The weekly sessions involved viewing a videotape and discussing positive and negative parenting skills observed. The researchers compared characteristics of the parents who chose to attend the sessions, including a measure of parental self-efficacy, or belief that they could manage a range of tasks and situations in caring for their young children. Parents with lower self-efficacy scores were significantly more likely to enroll in and attend the parenting training sessions (Garvey, Julion, Fogg, et al., 2006).

Mothers who have a greater degree of self-efficacy about their ability to breastfeed are significantly more likely to begin and to continue breastfeeding. A Breastfeeding Self-Efficacy Scale has been developed to identify both risk and protective factors that influence the self-efficacy of new mothers. Educational level, support from other women, quality of postpartum care, maternal anxiety, and plans made for feeding method all influence the breastfeeding self-efficacy scores of women (Dennis, 2006).

Best Practice

In addition to providing information about health behaviors, nurses need to integrate methods to increase self-efficacy in teaching projects with families. Assessments should be designed to identify self-efficacy of parents and children around health topics of interest. Interventions can then be planned to enhance the self-efficacy of family members.

Critical Thinking

Nurses can apply the concept of self-efficacy in teaching children and families.

1. Plan a teaching project for school-age children to foster healthy eating. Include expected outcomes for the children and interventions.
2. Could your outcome be improved if you focus not just on getting the content across, but also on increasing the belief and confidence that the children will be able to integrate the new behaviors into their lives?
3. What activities could your teaching plan include that would be likely to improve the self-efficacy of these school-age children?

TABLE 7–6 **Nine Parameters of Personality—Chess and Thomas**

PARAMETER	DESCRIPTION	SCORING
Activity level	Degree of motion during eating, playing, sleeping, bathing	High, medium, or low
Rhythmicity	Regularity of schedule maintained for sleep, hunger, elimination	Regular, variable, or irregular
Approach or withdrawal	Response to a new stimulus such as a food, activity, or person	Approachable, variable, or withdrawn
Adaptability	Degree of adaptation to new situations	Adaptive, variable, or nonadaptive
Threshold of responsiveness	Intensity of stimulation needed to elicit a response to sensory input, objects in the environment, or people	High, medium, or low
Intensity of reaction	Degree of response to situations	Positive, variable, or negative
Quality of mood	Predominant mood during daily activity and in response to stimuli	Positive, variable, or negative
Distractibility	Ability of environmental stimuli to interfere with the child's activity	Distractible, variable, or nondistractible
Attention span and persistence	Amount of time devoted to activities (compared with other children of the same age) and the degree of ability to stick with an activity in spite of obstacles	Persistent, variable, or nonpersistent

Source: Data from Chess, S., & Thomas, A. (1996). *Temperament: Theory and practice*. Philadelphia: Brunner/Mazel Publishers.

Temperament Theory

Chess and Thomas (1995, 1996) recognize the innate qualities of personality that each individual brings to the events of daily life. They view the child as an individual who both influences and is influenced by the environment. However, Chess and Thomas focus on one specific aspect of development—the wide spectrum of behaviors possible in children, identifying nine parameters of response to daily events (Table 7–6). Infants generally display clusters of responses, which Chess and Thomas have classified into three major personality types (Box 7–1). Although most children do not demonstrate all behaviors described for a particular type, they usually show a grouping indicative of one personality type (Chess & Thomas, 1995, 1996).

Box 7–1 **Patterns of Temperament—Chess and Thomas**

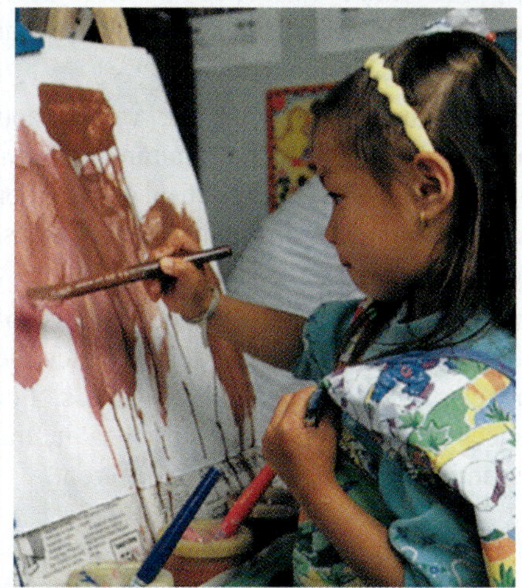

The "easy" child is generally moderate in activity; shows regularity in patterns of eating, sleeping, and elimination; and is usually positive in mood and when subjected to new stimuli. The easy child adapts to new situations and is able to accept rules and work well with others. About 40% of children in the New York Longitudinal Study displayed this personality type.

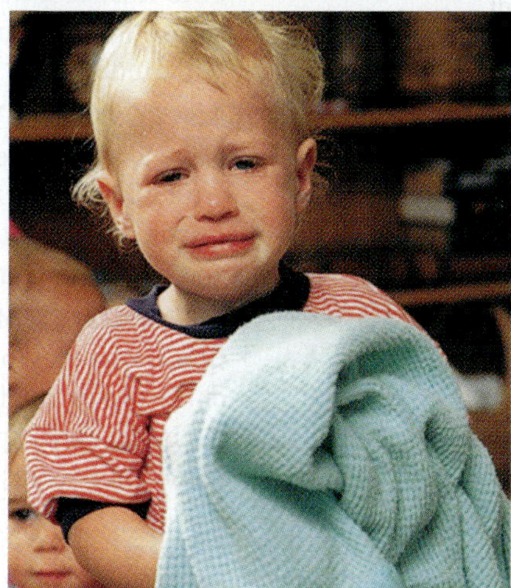

The "difficult" child displays irregular schedules for eating, sleeping, and elimination; adapts slowly to new situations and persons; and displays a predominantly negative mood. Intense reactions to the environment are common. The New York Longitudinal Study found that approximately 10% of children display this personality type.

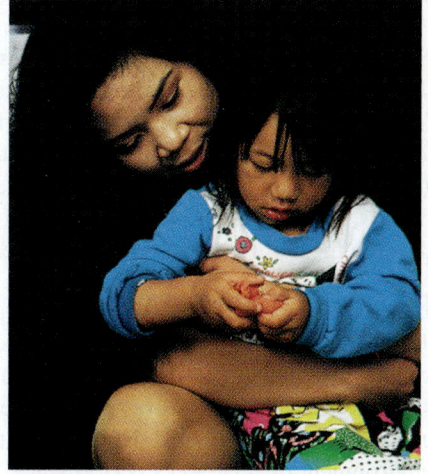

The "slow-to-warm-up" child has reactions of mild intensity and is slow to adapt to new situations. The child displays initial withdrawal followed by gradual, quiet, and slow interactions with the environment. About 15% of children in the New York Longitudinal Study displayed this personality type.

The remaining 35% of children studied showed some characteristics of each personality type.

Source: Ball, J. W., Bindler, R. C, & Cowen, K. J. (2010). *Child health nursing: Partnering with children and families* (2nd ed.). Upper Saddle River, NJ: Pearson Education.

Longitudinal research has demonstrated that personality characteristics displayed during infancy are often consistent with those seen later in life. The ability to predict future characteristics is not possible, however, because of the complex and dynamic interaction of personality traits and environmental reactions.

Resiliency Theory

Why do some children have such different behavioral outcomes from others coming from similar backgrounds? A theory that examines the individual's characteristics as well as the interaction of these characteristics with the environment is the resiliency model. **Resilience** is the ability to function with healthy responses, even when experiencing significant stress and adversity (Stewart, Reid, & Mangham, 1997). In this model, the individual or family members experience a crisis that provides a source of stress, and the family interprets or deals with the crisis based on resources available. Families and individuals have **protective factors** that provide strength and assistance in dealing with crises and **risk factors** that promote or contribute to their challenges. Risk and protective factors can be identified in children, in their families, and in their communities. A typical crisis for a young child might be a transfer to a new child care provider. Protective factors for a child transferring to a new provider could involve past positive experiences with new people and an "easy" temperament. An additional protective factor might be the level of understanding the new child care provider has about the adaptation needs of young children to new experiences. Risk factors for a child experiencing this type of transition might include repeated moves to new care providers, limited close relationships with adults, and a "slow-to-warm-up" temperament.

Once confronted by a crisis, the child and family first experience the **adjustment phase**. This phase is characterized by disorganization and unsuccessful attempts at meeting the crisis. In the **adaptation phase**, the child and family meet the challenge and use resources to deal with the crisis (Malone, 1998). Adaptation may lead to increasing resilience, as the child and family learn about new resources and inner strengths and develop the ability to deal more effectively with future crises.

Ecologic Theory

The relative importance in human development of heredity versus environment—or nature versus nurture—is controversial among theorists. **Nature** refers to the genetic or hereditary capability of an individual. **Nurture** refers to the effects of the environment on a person's performance. Contemporary developmental theories increasingly recognize the interaction of nature and nurture in determining the child's development.

The ecologic theory of development was formulated by Urie Bronfenbrenner to explain the child's unique relationship in all of life's settings, from close to remote (Bronfenbrenner, 1986, 2005; Bronfenbrenner, McClelland, Ceci, Moen, & Wethington, 1996). **Ecologic theory** emphasizes the presence of mutual interactions between the child and these various settings. Neither nature nor nurture is considered more important. Bronfenbrenner believes each child brings a unique set of genes—and specific attributes such as age, gender, health, and other characteristics—to his or her interactions with the environment. The child then interacts in many settings at different levels or systems (Figure 7–4 ■). The five systems of ecologic theory are microsystem, mesosystem, exosystem, macrosystem, and chronosystem.

MICROSYSTEM This level is defined as the daily, consistent, close relationships such as home, child care, school, friends, and neighbors. For the child with a chronic illness requiring regular care, the health care providers may even be part of the microsystem. In the ecologic model, the child influences each of these settings in addition to being influenced by them, with reciprocal interactions.

MESOSYSTEM This level includes relationships of microsystems with one another. For example, two microsystems for most children are the home and the school. The relationships between these microsystems are shown by parents' involvement in their children's school. This involvement, in turn, influences the effects of both the home and school settings on the children.

EXOSYSTEM This level of ecologic theory is composed of those settings that influence the child even though the child is not in close daily contact with the system. Examples are the parents' jobs and the governing board of the local school district. Although the child may not go to the parents' workplaces, he or she can be influenced by policies related to health care, sick leave, inflexible work hours, overtime, travel, or even the mood of the boss (through its impact on the parent). The child's needs may influence a parent to give up a certain job or to work harder to obtain money for the child's education. Likewise, when a local school board votes to ban certain books or to finance a field trip, the child is influenced by these decisions; the child, in turn, can help establish an atmosphere that will guide future school board decisions.

MACROSYSTEM This level includes the beliefs, values, and behaviors expressed in the child's environment. Culture is a powerful influence on the macrosystem, as is the political system. For instance, a democratic system creates different beliefs, values, and even eating practices from those of an anarchic system.

CHRONOSYSTEM This final level brings the perspective of time to the previous settings. The time period during which the child grows up influences views of health and illness. For example, the experiences of children with influenza in the nineteenth versus twentieth centuries were quite different.

Moral Theories

Moral development, a complex process not fully understood, involves learning what one should and should not do. It is more than merely the imprinting of parents' rules and virtues or values on children. The term **moral** means "relating to right and wrong." The terms *morality, moral behavior*, and *moral development* need to be distinguished from each other. **Morality** refers to the requirements necessary for people to live together in society, **moral behavior** is the way a person perceives and responds to those requirements, and **moral development** is the pattern of change in moral behavior with age.

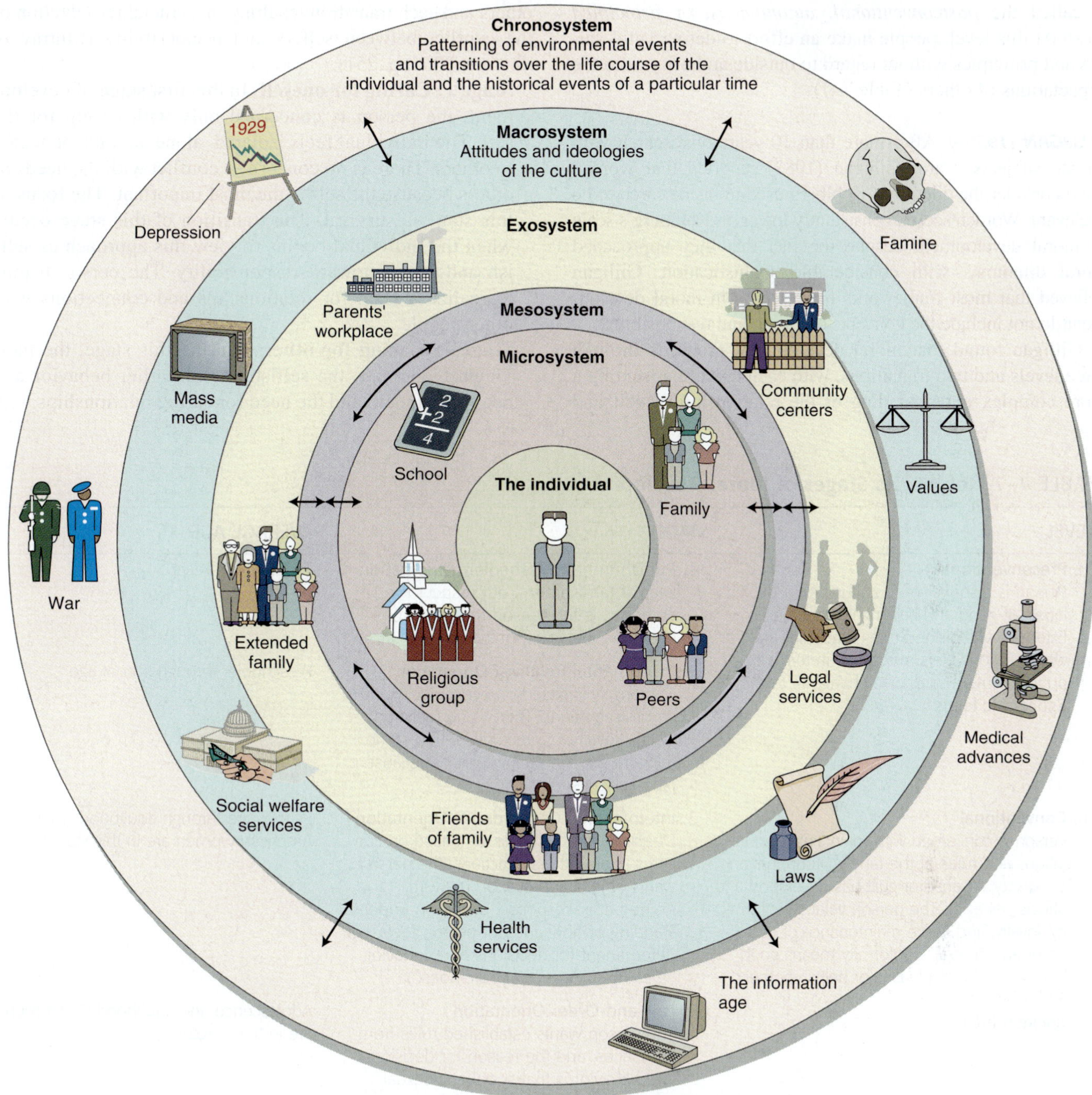

Figure 7–4 ■ Bronfenbrenner's ecologic theory of development views the individual as interacting within five levels or systems.

Source: Redrawn from Santrock, J. W. (2005). *Life span development*. Madison, WI: Brown & Benchmark. Based on Bronfenbrenner's (1979, 1986) works in Contexts of child rearing: Problems and prospects. *American Psychologist, 34*, 844–850; Ecology of the family as a context for human development: Research perspectives. *Developmental Psychology, 22*, 723–742.

KOHLBERG (1927–1987) Lawrence Kohlberg's theory specifically addresses moral development in children and adults (Kohlberg, 1981, 1984). The morality of an individual's decision was not Kohlberg's concern; rather, he focused on the reasons an individual makes a decision. According to Kohlberg, moral development progresses through three levels and six stages. Levels and stages are not always linked to a certain developmental stage, because some people progress to a higher level of moral development than others.

At Kohlberg's first level, called the *premoral* or *preconventional level,* children are responsive to cultural rules and labels of good and bad, right and wrong. However, children interpret these in terms of the consequences of their actions—punishment or reward. At the second level, the *conventional level*, the individual is concerned about maintaining the expectations of the family, group, or nation, and sees this as right. The emphasis at this level is on conformity and loyalty to one's own expectations as well as society's. Level III is called the *postconventional, autonomous*, or *principled level*. At this level, people make an effort to define valid values and principles without regard to outside authority or to the expectations of others (Table 7–7).

GILLIGAN (1936–) After more than 10 years of research with female subjects, Carol Gilligan (1982) reported that women often consider the dilemmas Kohlberg used in his research to be irrelevant. Women scored consistently lower on Kohlberg's scale of moral development despite the fact that they approached moral dilemmas with considerable sophistication. Gilligan believed that most frameworks for research in moral development do not include the concepts of caring and responsibility.

Gilligan found that moral development proceeds through three levels and two transitions, with each level representing a more complex understanding of the relationship of self and others and each transition resulting in a crucial reevaluation of the conflict between selfish and responsibility (Murray & Zentner, 2001, p. 251).

Stage 1: Caring for oneself In this first stage of development, the person is concerned only with caring for the self. The individual feels isolated, alone, and unconnected to others. There is no concern or conflict with the needs of others because the self is the most important. The focus of this stage is survival. The transition of this stage occurs when the individual begins to view this approach as selfish and moves toward responsibility. The person begins to realize a need for relationships and connections with other people.

Stage 2: Caring for others During this stage, the individual recognizes the selfishness of earlier behavior and begins to understand the need for caring relationships with

TABLE 7–7 **Kohlberg's Stages of Moral Development**

LEVEL	STAGE	AVERAGE AGE
I. **Preconventional** Person is responsive to cultural rules of labels of good and bad, right or wrong. Externally established rules determine right or wrong actions. Person reasons in terms of punishment, reward, or exchange of favors. **Egocentric focus**	1. **Punishment and Obedient Orientation** Fear of punishment, not respect for authority, is the reason for decisions, behavior, and conformity.	Toddler to 7 years
	2. **Instrumental Relativist Orientation** Conformity is based on egocentricity and narcissistic needs. There is no feeling of justice, loyalty, or gratitude. "I'll do something if I get something for it or because it pleases you."	Preschooler through school age
II. **Conventional** Person is concerned with maintaining expectations and rules of the family, group, nation, or society. A sense of guilt has developed and affects behavior. The person values conformity, loyalty, and active maintenance of social order and control. Conformity means good behavior or what pleases or helps another and is approved. **Societal focus**	3. **Interpersonal Concordance Orientation** Decisions and behavior are based on concerns about others' reactions; the person wants others' approval or a reward. An empathic response, based on understanding of how another person feels, is a determinant for decisions and behavior. ("I can put myself in your shoes.")	School age through adulthood (Most American women are in this stage.)
	4. **Law-and-Order Orientation** The person wants established rules from authorities, and the reason for decisions and behavior is that social and sexual rules and traditions demand the response. ("I'll do something because it's the law and my duty.")	Adolescence and adulthood (Most men are in this stage.)
III. **Postconventional** The person lives autonomously and defines moral values and principles that are distinct from personal identification with group values. He or she lives according to principles that are universally agreed on and that the person considers appropriate for life. **Universal focus**	5. **Social Contract Legalistic Orientation** The social rules are not the sole basis for decisions and behavior because the person believes a higher moral principle applies, such as equality, justice, or due process.	Middle-aged or older adult Only 20% or fewer of Americans achieve this stage.
	6. **Universal Ethical Principle Orientation** Decisions and behaviors are based on internalized rules, on conscience rather than social laws, and on self-chosen ethical and abstract principles that are universal, comprehensive, and consistent.	Middle-aged or older adult Few people attain or maintain this stage. Examples of this stage are seen in times of crisis or extreme situations.

Source: Murray, R. B., Zentner, J. P., & Yakimo, R. (2009). *Health promotion strategies through the life span* (pp. 32–33). Upper Saddle River, NJ: Pearson Prentice Hall. Adapted with permission.

others. Caring relationships bring with them responsibility. The definition of responsibility includes self-sacrifice, where "good" is considered to be "caring for others." The individual now approaches relationships with a focus on not hurting others. This approach causes the individual to be more responsive and submissive to others' needs, often to the exclusion of meeting one's own needs. A transition from goodness to truth occurs when the individual recognizes that the lack of balance between caring for oneself and caring for others in this approach can cause difficulties with relationships. The woman makes decisions on personal intentions and consequences of actions rather than on how she thinks others will react (Murray & Zentner, 2001, p. 253).

Stage 3: Caring for self and others During this last stage, a person sees the need for a balance between caring for others and caring for the self. The concept of responsibility now includes responsibility for the self and for other people. Care remains the focus on which decisions are based. However, the person recognizes the interconnections between the self and others and realizes that if one's own needs are not met, other people may also suffer.

Gilligan (1982) believes that because women often see morality in the integrity of relationships and caring, the moral problems they encounter are different from those of men. Men tend to consider what is right to be what is just, whereas for women what is right is taking responsibility for others as a self-chosen decision (p. 140). The ethic of justice, or fairness, is based on the idea of equality: Everyone should receive the same treatment. This is the development path usually followed by men and widely accepted by moral theorists. By contrast, the ethic of care is based on the premise of nonviolence: No one should be harmed. This is the path typically followed by women but given little attention in the literature of moral theory.

In discussing the development of maturity, Gilligan (1982) stated that both viewpoints blend "in the realization that just as inequality adversely affects both perspectives in an unequal relationship, so too violence is destructive for everyone involved" (p. 174). The blending of these two perspectives could give rise to a new view of human development and a better understanding of human relations.

Spiritual Theories

The spiritual component of growth and development refers to individuals' understanding of their relationship with the universe and their perceptions about the direction and meaning of life.

FOWLER James Fowler describes the development of faith as a force that gives meaning to a person's life. He uses the term *faith* as a form of knowing, a way of being in relation to "an ultimate environment." To Fowler, "faith is a relational phenomenon; it is an active 'mode-of-being-in-relation' to another or others in which we invest commitment, belief, love, risk and hope" (Fowler & Keen, 1985, p. 18). Fowler's stages in the development of faith are described in Table 7–8.

Fowler's theory and developmental stages were influenced by the work of Piaget, Kohlberg, and Erikson. Fowler believes that the development of faith is an interactive process between the individual and his or her environment (Fowler, Streib, & Keller, 2004). In each of Fowler's stages, new patterns of thought, values, and beliefs are added to those the individual already holds; therefore, the stages must follow in sequence. Faith stages, according to Fowler, are separate from Piaget's cognitive stages: They evolve from a combination of knowledge and values.

WESTERHOFF (1933–) John Westerhoff describes faith as a way of being and behaving that evolves from an experienced faith, guided by parents and others during a person's infancy and childhood, to an owned faith that is internalized in adulthood and serves as a directive for personal action (Table 7–9). For the client who is ill, faith—whether in a higher authority (e.g., God, Allah, Jehovah), in the client's own self, in the health care team, or in a combination of all—provides strength and trust.

TABLE 7–8 **Fowler's Stages of Spiritual Development**

STAGE	AGE	DESCRIPTION
0. Undifferentiated	0 to 3 years	Infant unable to formulate concepts about self or the environment
1. Intuitive-projective	4 to 6 years	A combination of images and beliefs given by trusted others, mixed with the child's own experience and imagination
2. Mythic-literal	7 to 12 years	Private world of fantasy and wonder; symbols referring to something specific; dramatic stories and myths used to communicate spiritual meanings
3. Synthetic-conventional	Adolescent or adult	World and ultimate environment structured by the expectations and judgments of others; interpersonal focus
4. Individuating-reflexive	After 18 years	Constructing one's own explicit system; high degree of self-consciousness
5. Paradoxical-consolidative	After 30 years	Awareness of truth from a variety of viewpoints
6. Universalizing	Maybe never	Becoming an incarnation of the principles of love and justice

Source: Fowler, J., & Keen, S. (1985). *Life maps: Conversations in the journey of faith.* Waco, TX: Word Books; and Hollander, A. (1980). *How to help your child have a spiritual life: A parents' guide to inner development.* New York: A and W Publishers. Adapted with permission.

TABLE 7–9 **Westerhoff's Four Stages of Faith**

STAGE	AGE	BEHAVIOR
Experienced faith	Infancy/early adolescence	Experiences faith through interaction with others who are living a particular faith tradition
Affiliative faith	Late adolescence	Actively participates in activities that characterize a particular faith tradition; experiences awe and wonderment; feels a sense of belonging
Searching faith	Young adulthood	Through a process of questioning and doubting own faith, acquires a cognitive as well as an affective faith
Owned faith	Middle adulthood/old age	Puts faith into personal and social action and is willing to stand up for what the individual believes, even against the nurturing community

Source: Westerhoff, J. *Will our children have faith?* (1976). New York: Seabury Press. Reprinted with permission from the author.

Growth and Development Through the Life Span

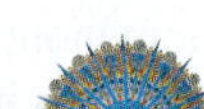

Nurses use information about developmental milestones to assess children, to identify those with delays, and to plan interventions that will foster development. To do so requires a comprehensive understanding of expected physical growth and development, cognitive abilities, and psychosocial characteristics (Fine & Mayer, 2006; Johnson & Marlow, 2006). Potential risks—such as prematurity, international adoption, and presence of health problems—necessitate a more frequent and in-depth assessment of observed milestones. Nurses compare the expected findings with assessment results, making referrals for further evaluation when appropriate, and using the results to plan nursing interventions.

INFANT (BIRTH TO 1 YEAR)

Can you imagine tripling your present weight in a single year? Or becoming proficient in understanding fundamental words in a new language and even speaking a few? These and many more accomplishments take place in the first year of life. Starting as a mainly reflexive creature, the infant can walk and communicate by the year's end. Never again in life is development so swift.

Physical Growth and Development

The first year of life is one of rapid change for the infant. The infant's birth weight usually doubles by about 5 months and triples by the end of the first year. Height increases by approximately 1 foot during this year. Teeth begin to erupt at about 6 months, and by the end of the first year, the infant has six to eight deciduous teeth. Physical growth is closely associated with type and quality of feeding.

Body organs and systems, although not fully mature at 1 year of age, function differently than they did at birth. Kidney and liver maturation helps the 1-year-old excrete drugs or other toxic substances more readily than in the first weeks of life. The changing body proportions mirror changes in developing internal organs (Figure 7–5 ■). Maturation of the nervous system is demonstrated by increased control over body movements, enabling the infant to sit, stand, and walk. Sensory function also increases as the infant begins to discriminate visual images, sounds, and tastes (Table 7–10).

Cognitive Development

The brain continues to increase in complexity during the first year of life. Most of the growth involves maturation of cells, with only a small increase in cell number. This growth of the brain is accompanied by development of its functions. One has only to compare the behavior of an infant shortly after birth with that of a 1-year-old to understand the incredible maturation of brain function. The newborn's eyes widen in response to sound; the 1-year-old turns to the sound and recognizes its significance. The 2-month-old cries and coos; the 1-year-old says a few words and understands

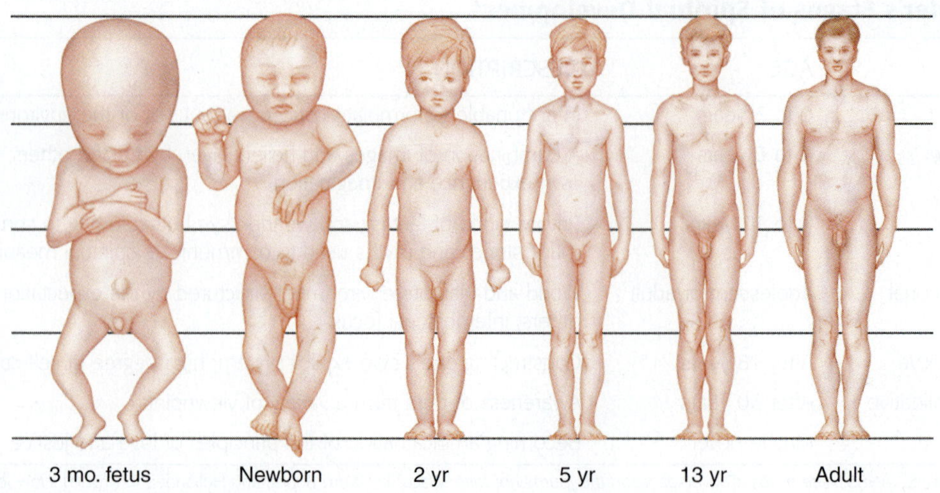

Figure 7–5 ■ Body proportions at various ages.

TABLE 7–10 **Growth and Development Milestones During Infancy**

AGE	PHYSICAL GROWTH	FINE MOTOR ABILITY	GROSS MOTOR ABILITY	SENSORY ABILITY
Birth to 1 month	Gains 5–7 oz (140–200 g)/ week. Grows 1.5 cm (1/2 in.) in first month. Head circumference increases 1.5 cm (1/2 in.)/month.	Holds hand in fist. Draws arms and legs to body when crying.	Inborn reflexes such as startle and rooting are predominant activity. May lift head briefly if prone. Alerts to high-pitched voices. Comforts with touch.	Prefers to look at faces and black-and-white geometric designs. Follows objects in line of vision.
2 to 4 months	Gains 5–7 oz (140–200 g)/ week. Grows 1.5 cm (1/2 in.)/ month. Head circumference increases 1.5 cm (1/2 in.)/month. Posterior fontanel closes. Eats 120 mL/kg/24 h (2 oz/lb/24 h).	Holds rattle when placed in hand. Looks at and plays with own fingers. Brings hands to midline.	Moro reflex fading in strength. Can turn from side to back and then return. Head lag when pulled to sitting position decreases; sits with head held in midline with some bobbing. When prone, holds head and supports weight on forearms.	Follows objects 180 degrees. Turns head to look for voices and sounds.
4 to 6 months	Gains 5–7 oz (140–200 g)/ week. Doubles birth weight 5–6 months. Grows 1.5 cm (1/2 in.)/month. Head circumference increases 1.5 cm (1/2 in.)/month. Teeth may begin erupting by 6 months. Eats 100 mL/kg/24 h (1 1/2 oz/lb/24 h).	Grasps rattles and other objects at will; drops them to pick up another offered object. Mouths objects. Holds feet and pulls to mouth. Holds bottle. Grasps with whole hand (palmar grasp). Manipulates objects.	Holds head steady when sitting. Has no head lag when pulled to sitting. Turns from abdomen to back by 4 months and then back to abdomen by 6 months. When held standing supports much of own weight.	Examines complex visual images. Watches the course of a falling object. Responds readily to sounds.
6 to 8 months	Gains 3–5 oz (85–140 g)/ week. Grows 1 cm (3/8 in.)/month. Growth rate slower than first 6 months.	Bangs objects held in hands. Transfers objects from one hand to the other. Pincer grasp begins at times.	Most inborn reflexes extinguished. Sits alone steadily without support by 8 months. Likes to bounce on legs when held in standing position.	Recognizes own name and responds by looking and smiling. Enjoys small and complex objects at play.
8 to 10 months	Gains 3–5 oz (85–140 g)/ week. Grows 1 cm (3/8 in.)/month.	Picks up small objects. Uses pincer grasp well.	Crawls or pulls whole body along floor by arms. Creeps by using hands and knees to keep trunk off floor. Pulls self to standing and sitting by 10 months. Recovers balance when sitting.	Understands words such as "no" and "cracker." May say one word in addition to "mama" and "dada." Recognizes sound without difficulty.
10 to 12 months	Gains 3–5 oz (85–140 g)/ week. Grows 1 cm (3/8 in.)/month. Head circumference equals chest circumference. Triples birth weight by 1 year.	May hold crayon or pencil and make mark on paper. Places objects into containers through holes.	Stands alone. Walks holding onto furniture. Sits down from standing.	Plays peek-a-boo and patty cake.

many more. The 6-week-old grasps a rattle for the first time; the 1-year-old reaches for toys and begins to feed himself or herself.

The infant's behaviors provide clues about thought processes. Piaget's work outlines the infant's actions in a set of rapidly progressing changes in the first year of life. The infant receives stimulation through sight, sound, and feeling, which the maturing brain interprets. This input from the environment interacts with internal cognitive abilities to enhance cognitive functioning.

Psychosocial Development

The infant relies on interactions with primary care providers to meet needs and then begins to establish a sense of trust in other adults and in children. As trust develops, the infant becomes comfortable in interactions with a widening array of people.

PLAY An 8-month-old infant is sitting on the floor, grasping blocks and banging them on the floor. When a parent walks by, the infant laughs and waves hands and feet wildly (Figure 7–6 ■). The infant plays primarily alone with toys (**solitary play**) but enjoys the presence of adults or other children. Physical capabilities enable the infant to move toward and reach for objects of interest.

Cognitive ability is reflected in manipulation of the blocks to create different sounds. Social interaction enhances play. The presence of a parent or other person increases interest in surroundings and teaches the infant different ways to play.

The play of infants begins in a reflexive manner. When infants move extremities or grasp objects, they experience the foundations of play. They gain pleasure from the feel and sound of these activities, and gradually perform them purposefully. For example, when a parent places a rattle in the hand of a 6-week-old infant, the infant grasps it reflexively. As the hands move randomly, the rattle makes an enjoyable sound. The infant learns to move the rattle to create the sound and then finally to grasp the toy at will to play with it.

The next phase of infant play focuses on manipulative behavior. The infant examines toys closely, looking at them, touching them, and placing them in his or her mouth. The infant learns a great deal about texture, qualities of objects, and all aspects of the surroundings. At the same time, interaction with others becomes an important part of play. The social nature of play is obvious as the infant plays with other children and adults.

Toward the end of the first year, the infant's ability to move in space enlarges the sphere of play. Once infants crawl or walk, they can get to new places, find new toys, discover forgotten objects, or seek out other people for interaction. Play is a reflection of every aspect of development, as well as a method for enhancing learning and maturation (Table 7–11).

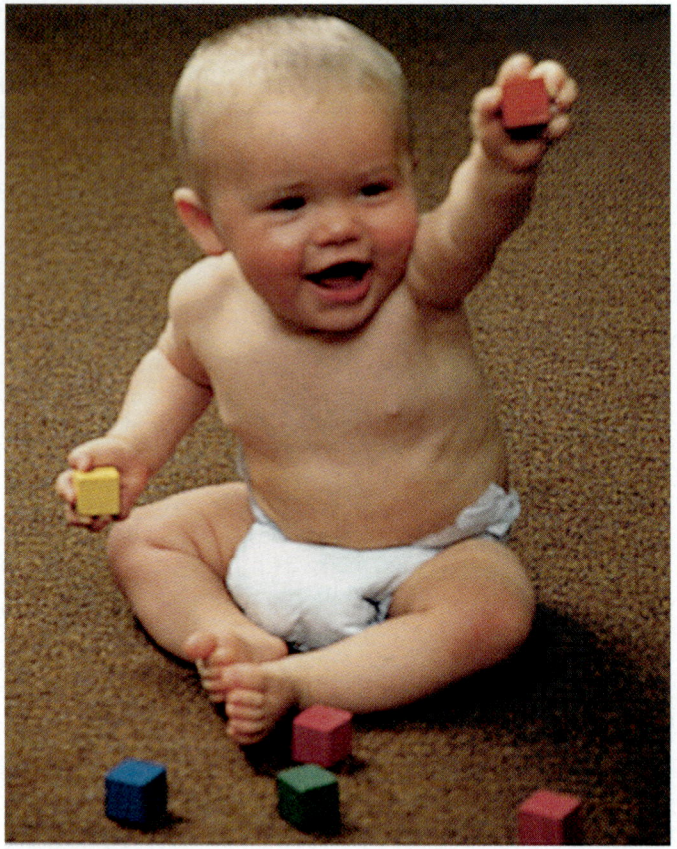

Figure 7–6 ■ Garrett shows us that an 8-month-old child can play with blocks, demonstrating physical, cognitive, and social capabilities.

TABLE 7–11 Psychosocial Development During Infancy

AGE	PLAY AND TOYS	COMMUNICATION
Birth to 3 months	■ Prefers visual stimuli of mobiles, black-and-white patterns, mirrors ■ Responds to auditory stimuli such as music boxes, tape players, soft voices ■ Responds to rocking and cuddling ■ Moves legs and arms while adult sings and talks ■ Likes varying stimuli—different rooms, sounds, visual images	■ Coos ■ Babbles ■ Cries
3 to 6 months	■ Prefers noise-making objects that are easily grasped like rattles ■ Enjoys stuffed animals and soft toys with contrasting colors	■ Vocalizes during play and with familiar people ■ Laughs ■ Cries less ■ Squeals and makes pleasure sounds ■ Babbles multisyllabically (mamamamama)
6 to 9 months	■ Likes teething toys ■ Increasingly desires social interaction with adults and other children ■ Favors soft toys that can be manipulated and mouthed	■ Increases vowel and consonant sounds ■ Links syllables together ■ Uses speechlike rhythm when vocalizing with others
9 to 12 months	■ Enjoys large blocks, toys that pop apart and go back together, nesting cups and other objects ■ Laughs at surprise toys like jack-in-the-box ■ Plays interactive games like peek-a-boo ■ Uses push-and-pull toys	■ Understands "no" and other simple commands ■ Says "dada" and "mama" to identify parents ■ Learns one or two other words ■ Receptive speech surpasses expressive speech

> FOCUS ON DIVERSITY AND CULTURE
> **Reaching Developmental Milestones**
>
> In traditional Native American families, children are allowed to unfold and develop naturally at their own pace. Children wean and toilet train themselves with little interference or pressure from parents. The nurse should be sensitive to the childrearing practices of the family and support them in these culturally accepted practices, rather than imposing Western beliefs on reaching developmental milestones.

PERSONALITY AND TEMPERAMENT Why does one infant frequently awaken at night crying while another sleeps for 8 to 10 hours undisturbed? Why does one infant smile much of the time and react positively to interactions while another is withdrawn around unfamiliar people and frequently frowns and cries? Such differences in responses to the environment are believed to be inborn characteristics of temperament. Infants are born with a tendency to react in certain ways to noise and to interact differently with people. They may display varying degrees of regularity in activities of eating and sleeping, and manifest a capacity for concentrating on tasks for different amounts of time.

The nursing assessment identifies personality characteristics of the infant that the nurse can share with the parents. With this information, the parents can appreciate more fully the uniqueness of their infant and design experiences to meet the infant's needs. Parents can learn to modify the environment to promote adaptation. For example, an infant who does not adapt easily to new situations may cry, withdraw, or develop another way of coping when adjusting to new people or places. Parents might be advised to use one or two babysitters rather than engaging new sitters frequently. If the infant is easily distracted when eating, parents can feed the infant in a quiet setting to encourage a focus on eating. Although the infant's temperament is unchanged, the ability to fit with the environment is enhanced.

COMMUNICATION Even at a few weeks of age, infants communicate and engage in two-way interaction; they express comfort by soft sounds, cuddling, and eye contact. The infant displays discomfort by thrashing the extremities, arching the back, and crying vigorously. From these rudimentary skills, communication ability continues to develop until the infant speaks several words at the end of the first year of life (see Table 7–9). Nonverbal methods continue to be a primary method of communication between parent and child.

Nurses assess communication to identify possible abnormalities or developmental delays. Language ability may be assessed with the Denver II Developmental Test or other specialized language screening tools. Normal infants and toddlers understand (**receptive speech**) more words than they can speak (**expressive speech**). Abnormalities may be caused by a hearing deficit, developmental delay, or lack of verbal stimulation from caretakers. Further assessment may be required to pinpoint the cause of the abnormality.

Nursing interventions focus on providing a stimulating and comforting environment. Parents are encouraged to speak to infants and teach words. Hospital nurses should include the infant's known words when providing care, and provide nonverbal support by hugging and holding. Nurses planning interventions should consider the family's cultural patterns for communications and development.

TODDLER (1 TO 3 YEARS)

Toddlerhood is sometimes called the first adolescence. The child, who months before was merely an infant, from 1–3 years is now displaying independence and negativism. Pride in newfound accomplishments emerges during this time.

Physical Growth and Development

The rate of growth slows during the second year of life. The child requires limited food intake during this time, a change that may cause concern to the parent. The nurse should reassure parents with these concerns that this is a normal occurrence in their child's development. By age 2 years, the birth weight has usually quadrupled and the child is about one-half of the adult height. Body proportions begin to change, with longer legs and a smaller head in proportion to body size than during infancy. The toddler has a pot-bellied appearance and stands with feet apart to provide a wide base of support. By approximately 33 months, eruption of deciduous teeth is complete, with 20 teeth present.

Gross motor activity develops rapidly (Table 7–12) as the toddler progresses from walking to running, kicking, and riding a tricycle. As physical maturation occurs, the toddler develops the ability to control elimination patterns.

TABLE 7–12 **Growth and Development Milestones During Toddlerhood**

AGE	PHYSICAL GROWTH	FINE MOTOR ABILITY	GROSS MOTOR ABILITY	SENSORY ABILITY
1–2 years	■ Gains 8 oz (227 g) or more per month. ■ Grows 3.5–5 in. (9–12 cm) during this year. ■ Anterior fontanel closes.	■ By end of second year, builds a tower of four blocks. ■ Scribbles on paper. ■ Can undress self. ■ Throws a ball.	■ Runs. ■ Walks up and down stairs. ■ Likes push- and pull-toys.	Visual acuity 20/50
2–3 years	■ Gains 1.4–2.3 kg (3–5 lb)/year. ■ Grows 5–6.5 cm (2–2.5 in.)/year.	■ Draws a circle and other rudimentary forms. ■ Learns to pour. ■ Is learning to dress self.	■ Jumps. ■ Kicks ball. ■ Throws ball overhand.	

Cognitive Development

During the toddler years, the child moves from the sensorimotor to the preoperational stage of development. The early use of language awakens in the 1-year-old the ability to think about objects or people when they are absent. Object permanence is well developed.

At about 2 years of age, the increasing use of words as symbols enables the toddler to use preoperational thought. Rudimentary problem solving, creative thought, and an understanding of cause-and-effect relationships are now possible.

Psychosocial Development

The toddler is soundly rooted in a trusting relationship and feels more comfortable in asserting autonomy and separating from primary care providers. It is important for toddlers to begin asserting their autonomy within the context of safe places and relationships that promote their interaction with both adults and other children.

PLAY Many changes in play patterns occur between infancy and toddlerhood. The toddler's motor skills enable him or her to bang pegs into a pounding board with a hammer. The social nature of toddler play is also readily seen. Toddlers find the company of other children pleasurable, even though socially interactive play may not occur. Toddlers tend to play with similar objects side-by-side, occasionally trading toys and words (Figure 7–7 ■). This is called **parallel play**. This playtime with other children assists toddlers to develop social skills. Toddlers engage in play activities they have seen at home, such as pounding with a hammer and talking on the phone. This imitative behavior helps them to learn new actions and skills.

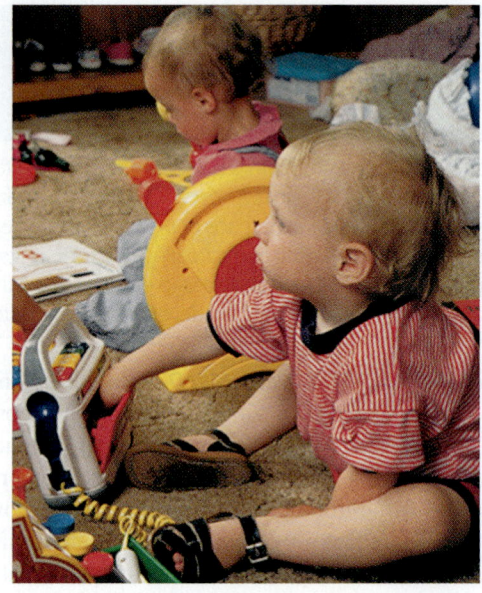

A

B

Figure 7–7 ■ *A*, Two children are displaying typical parallel play, since they enjoy playing near other children, but are not engaging in social interactions with each other. Which cognitive and motor skills are these children developing? *B*, Imitative play such as pushing and pulling a vacuum allows this toddler to develop gross and fine motor skills.

Physical skills are manifested in play as toddlers push and pull objects, climb in and out and up and down, run, ride a Big Wheel, turn the pages of books, and scribble with a pen. Both gross motor and fine motor abilities are enhanced during this age period.

Cognitive understanding enables the toddler to manipulate objects and learn about their qualities. Stacking blocks and placing rings on a building tower teach spatial relationships and other lessons that provide a foundation for future learning. Various kinds of play objects should be provided for the toddler to meet play needs. These play needs can easily be met whether the child is hospitalized or at home (Table 7–13).

PERSONALITY AND TEMPERAMENT The toddler retains most of the temperamental characteristics identified during infancy, but may demonstrate some changes. The normal developmental progression of toddlerhood also plays a part in responses. For example, the infant who previously responded positively to stimuli, such as a new babysitter, may appear more negative in toddlerhood. The increasing independence characteristic of this age is shown by the toddler's use of the word *no*. The parent and child constantly adapt their responses to each other and learn anew how to communicate with each other.

COMMUNICATION Because the individual's capacity for development of language skills is greatest during the toddler period, adults should communicate frequently with children in this age group. This communication is critical not only to the toddler's ability to communicate simple wants and needs, but also to cognitive and language development, as they affect the toddler's future literacy. Toddlers also begin to learn the subtleties of language, as they begin to imitate words and speech intonations, as well as the social interactions and nonverbal gestures that they observe.

At the beginning of toddlerhood, the child may use four to six words in addition to "mama" and "dada." Receptive speech (the ability to understand words) far outpaces expressive

TABLE 7–13 **Psychosocial Development During Toddlerhood**

AGE	PLAY AND TOYS	COMMUNICATION
1–3 years	■ Refines fine motor skills by use of cloth books, large pencil and paper, wooden puzzles. ■ Facilitates imitative behavior by playing kitchen, grocery shopping, toy telephone. ■ Learns gross motor activities by riding Big Wheel tricycle, playing with soft ball and bat, molding water and sand, tossing ball or bean bag. ■ Cognitive skills develop by educational television shows, music, stories, and books.	■ Increasingly enjoys talking. ■ Vocabulary grows expotentially, especially when spoken and read to. ■ Needs to release stress by pounding board, frequent gross motor activities, and occasional temper tantrums. ■ Likes contact with other children and learns interpersonal skills.

speech. By the end of toddlerhood, however, the 3-year-old has a vocabulary of almost 1,000 words and uses short sentences.

Communication occurs in many ways, some of which are nonverbal. Toddler communication includes pointing, pulling an adult over to a room or object, and speaking in **expressive jargon** (using unintelligible words with normal speech intonations as if truly communicating in words). Other communication methods include crying, pounding or stamping feet, displaying a temper tantrum, or other means that illustrate dismay. These powerful communication methods can upset parents, who often need suggestions for handling them. Adults can best assist the toddler by verbalizing the feelings shown by the toddler, by saying things like, "You must be very upset that you cannot have that candy. When you stop crying you can come out of your room." Verbalizing the child's feeling and then ignoring further negative behavior ensures that the parent is not unintentionally reinforcing the inappropriate behavior. While the toddler's search for autonomy and independence creates a need for such behavior, an upset toddler may respond well to holding, rocking, and stroking.

Parents and nurses can promote a toddler's communication by speaking frequently, naming objects, giving single-step directions, explaining procedures in simple terms, expressing feelings that the toddler seems to be displaying, and encouraging speech. The toddler from a bilingual home is at an optimal age to learn two languages. If the parents do not speak English, the toddler will benefit from a child care experience that will expose him or her to English in addition to his or her native language.

The nurse who understands the communication skills of toddlers is able to assess expressive and receptive language and communicate effectively, thereby promoting positive health care experiences for these children. Parents often need ideas of strategies for communication with the young child.

PRESCHOOL CHILD (3 TO 6 YEARS)

The preschool years are a time of new initiative and independence. Most children are in a child care center or school for part of the day, and they learn a great deal from this social contact. Language skills are well developed, and the child is able to understand and speak clearly. Endless projects characterize the world of busy preschoolers. They may work with play dough to form animals, then cut out and paste paper, then draw and color.

Physical Growth and Development

Preschoolers grow slowly and steadily, with most growth taking place in long bones of the arms and legs. The short, chubby toddler gradually gives way to a slender, long-legged preschooler (Table 7–14).

Physical skills continue to develop. The preschooler runs with ease, holds a bat, and throws balls of various types. Writing ability increases, and the preschooler enjoys drawing and learning.

TABLE 7–14 **Growth and Development Milestones During the Preschool Years**

PHYSICAL GROWTH	FINE MOTOR ABILITY	GROSS MOTOR ABILITY	SENSORY ABILITY
Gains 1.5–2/5 kg (3–5 lb)/year. Grows 4–6 cm (1 1/2–2 1/2 in.)/year.	Uses scissors. Draws circle, square, cross. Draws at least a six-part person. Enjoys art projects such as pasting, stringing beads, using clay. Learns to tie shoes at end of preschool years. Buttons clothes. Brushes teeth. Eats three meals, with snacks. Uses spoon, fork, and knife.	Throws a ball overhand. Climbs well. Rides tricycle.	Visual acuity continues to improve. Can focus on and learn letters and numbers.

The preschool period is a good time to encourage good dental habits. Children can begin to brush their own teeth with parental supervision and help in reaching all tooth surfaces. Parents should floss children's teeth, give fluoride as ordered if the water supply is not fluoridated, and schedule the first dental visit so the child can become accustomed to the routine of periodic dental care.

Cognitive Development

The preschooler exhibits characteristics of preoperational thought. Symbols or words are used to represent objects and people, enabling the young child to think about them. This is a milestone in intellectual development; however, the preschooler still has some limitations in thought (Table 7–15).

It is important to understand the preschooler's thought processes in order to plan appropriate teaching for health care and development of health habits.

Psychosocial Development

The preschooler is more independent in establishing relationships with others. The child interacts closely with children and adults as well as being able to plan and carry out activities.

PLAY The preschooler has begun to play in a new way (Figure 7–8 ■). Toddlers simply play side by side with friends, each engaging in his or her own activities; preschoolers interact with others during play. One child cuts out colored paper while his or her friend glues it on paper in a design. This new type of interaction is called **associative play**.

In addition to this social dimension, other aspects of play also differ. The preschooler enjoys large motor activities such as swinging, riding a tricycle, and throwing a ball. Increasing manual dexterity is demonstrated in greater complexity of drawings and manipulation of blocks and modeling. These changes necessitate planning of playtime to include appropriate activities. Preschool programs and child life departments in hospitals help meet this important need.

Materials provided for play can be simple but should guide activities in which the child engages. Because fine motor activities are popular, paper, pens, scissors, glue, and a variety of other such objects should be available. The child can use them to create important images such as pictures of people, hospital beds, or friends. A collection of dolls, furniture, and clothing can be manipulated to represent parents and children, nurses and physicians, teachers, or other significant people.

TABLE 7–15 **Characteristics of Thought Identified by Piaget**

CHARACTERISTIC	DEFINITION	DEVELOPMENT STAGE	NURSING IMPLICATIONS
Object permanence	Ability to understand that when something is out of sight it still exists	Sensorimotor period, especially in coordination of secondary schemes substage from 8–12 months	Before development of object permanence, babies will not look for toys or other objects out of sight; as the concept is developing they are concerned when a parent leaves, since they are not certain the parent will return.
Egocentrism	Ability to see things only from one's own point of view	Preoperational thought	Peers or others who have gone through an experience will not impress the preschooler; teaching should focus on what an experience will be like to the child.
Transductive reasoning	Connecting two events in a cause-effect relationship simply because they occur together in time	Preoperational thought	Ask the child what he or she thinks caused an occurrence; ask how the two events are connected; correct misconceptions to lessen child's guilt.
Centration	Focusing only on one particular aspect of a situation	Preoperational thought	Listen to the child's comments and deal with concerns in order to be able to present new concepts to the child.
Animism	Giving lifelike qualities to nonliving things	Preoperational thought	Ask preschool children to describe how a machine works, or how the trees move. Provide opportunities to learn about machines that may move and make noises (intravenous pumps, magnetic resonance imaging) to decrease fears.
Magical thinking	Believing that events occur because of one's thoughts or actions	Preoperational thought	Ask young children how they became ill, or what caused a parent's or sibling's illness. Correct misconceptions when the child blames self for causing problems by wishing someone ill or having bad behavior.
Conservation	Knowing that matter is not changed when its form is altered	Concrete operational thought	Before conservation of thought is reached, the child may think that gender can be changed when hair is cut, the leg under a cast is broken in separate pieces. Ask perceptions and clarify misconceptions.

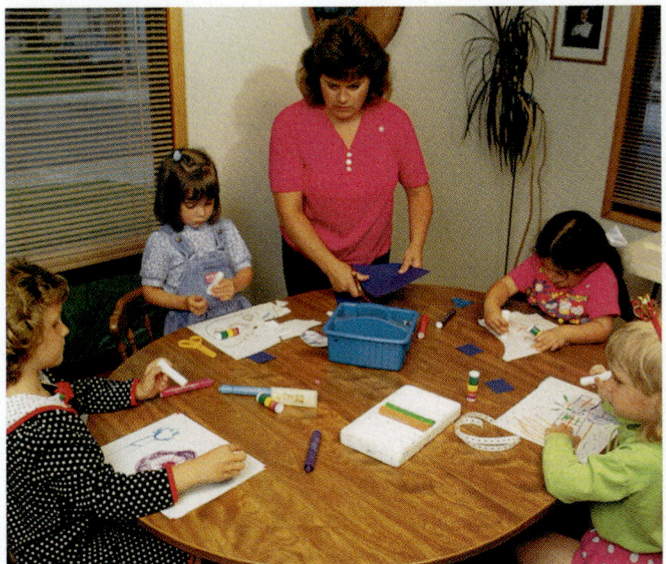

Figure 7–8 ■ Preschoolers have well-developed language, motor, and social skills, and they can work creatively together on an art project, as this group is doing at an in-home child care center.

Because fantasy life is so powerful at this age, the preschooler readily uses props to engage in **dramatic play**, that is, the living out of the drama of human life.

The nurse can use playtime to assess the preschooler's developmental level, knowledge about health care, and emotions related to health care experiences. Observations about objects chosen for play, content of dramatic play, and pictures drawn can provide important assessment data. The nurse can also use play periods to teach the child about health care procedures and offer an outlet for expressing emotions (Table 7–16).

PERSONALITY AND TEMPERAMENT Characteristics of personality observed in infancy tend to persist over time. The preschooler may need assistance as these characteristics are expressed in the new situations of preschool or nursery school. An excessively active child, for example, will need gentle, consistent handling to adjust to the structure of a classroom. Encourage parents to visit preschool programs to choose the one that would best foster growth in their child. Some preschoolers enjoy the structured learning of a program that focuses on cognitive skills, while others are happier and more open to learning in a small group that provides much time for free play. Nurses can help parents to identify their child's personality or temperament characteristics and to find the best environment for growth.

COMMUNICATION Language skills blossom during the preschool years. The vocabulary grows to over 2,000 words, and children speak in complete sentences of several words and use all parts of speech. They practice these newfound language skills by endlessly talking and asking questions.

The sophisticated speech of preschoolers mirrors the development occurring in their minds and helps them to learn about the world around them. However, this speech can be quite deceptive. Although preschoolers use many words, their grasp of meaning is usually literal and may not match that of adults. These literal interpretations have important implications for health care providers. For example, the preschooler who is told she will be "put to sleep" for surgery may think of a pet recently euthanized; the child who is told that a dye will be injected for a diagnostic test may think he is going to die; mention of "a little stick" in the arm can cause images of tree branches rather than of a simple immunization.

Concrete visual aids such as pictures of a child undergoing the same procedure or a book to read together enhance teaching by meeting the child's developmental needs. Handling medical equipment such as intravenous bags and stethoscopes increases interest and helps the child to focus. Teaching may have to be done in several short sessions rather than one long session.

Some general approaches:

- Allow time for the child to integrate explanations.
- Verbalize frequently to the child.
- Use drawings and stories to explain care.
- Use accurate names for bodily functions.
- Allow choices.

The preschooler's social growth and increased communication skills make these years the perfect time to introduce concepts related to problem solving and conflict resolution. Puzzles and manipulative toys help foster early problem-solving skills. Children in this age group can learn to calm themselves by learning how to take deep breaths and count to 3 or 5 when they are upset. Many preschool programs employ special curricula that help teachers and parents assist children in developing essential conflict resolution skills. Using language to resolve conflict is a protective factor that decreases the likelihood of children choosing inappropriate or violent behavior to try to get what they want or bring a distressing interaction to a close.

TABLE 7–16 **Psychosocial Development During Preschool Years**

AGE	PLAY AND TOYS	COMMUNICATION
3–6 years	Associative play is facilitated by simple games, puzzles, nursery rhymes, songs. Dramatic play is fostered by dolls and doll clothes, play houses and hospitals, dress-up clothes, puppets. Stress is relieved by pens, paper, glue, scissors. Cognitive growth is fostered by educational television shows, music, stories and books.	Developed and uses all parts of speech, occasionally incorrectly. Communicates with a widening array of people. Play with other children is a favorite activity. Health professionals can ■ verbalize and explain procedures to children. ■ use drawings and stories to explain care. ■ use accurate names for bodily functions. ■ allow the child to talk, ask questions, and make choices.

SCHOOL-AGE CHILD (6 TO 12 YEARS)

Errol, 10 years old, arrives home from school shortly after 3 p.m. each day. He immediately calls his friends and goes to visit one of them. They are building models of cars and collecting baseball cards. Endless hours are spent on these projects and on discussions of events at school that day.

Nine-year-old Karen practices soccer two afternoons a week and plays in games each weekend. She also is learning to play the flute and spends her free time at home practicing. Although practice time is not her favorite part of music, Karen enjoys the performances and wants to play well in front of her friends and teacher. Her parents now allow her to ride her bike unaccompanied to the store or to a friend's house.

These two school-age children demonstrate common characteristics of their age group. They are in a stage of industry in which it is important to the child to perform useful work. Meaningful activities take on great importance and are usually carried out in the company of peers. A sense of achievement in these activities is important to developing self-esteem and to preventing a sense of inferiority or poor self-worth.

Physical Growth and Development

School age is the last period in which girls and boys are close in size and body proportions. As the long bones continue to grow, leg length increases (see Figure 7–5). Fat gives way to muscle, and the child appears leaner. Jaw proportions change as the first deciduous tooth is lost at 6 years and permanent teeth begin to erupt. Body organs and the immune system mature, resulting in fewer illnesses among school-age children. Medications are less likely to cause serious side effects, because they can be metabolized more easily. The urinary system can adjust to changes in fluid status. Physical skills are also refined as children begin to play sports, and fine motor skills are well developed through school activities (Table 7–17).

Although it is commonly believed that the start of adolescence (age 12 years) heralds a growth spurt, the rapid increases in size commonly occur during school age. Girls may begin a growth spurt as early as 9 or 10 years of age and boys a year or so later (Figure 7–9 ■). Nutritional needs increase dramatically with this spurt.

The loss of the first deciduous teeth and the eruption of permanent teeth usually occur at about age 6 years, or at the beginning of the school-age period. Of the 32 permanent teeth, 22–26 erupt by age 12 years and the remaining molars follow during the teenage years. The school-age child should be closely monitored to ensure that brushing and flossing are adequate, that fluoride is taken if the water supply is not fluoridated, that dental care is obtained to provide for examination of teeth and alignment, and that loose teeth are identified before surgery or other events that may lead to loss of a tooth.

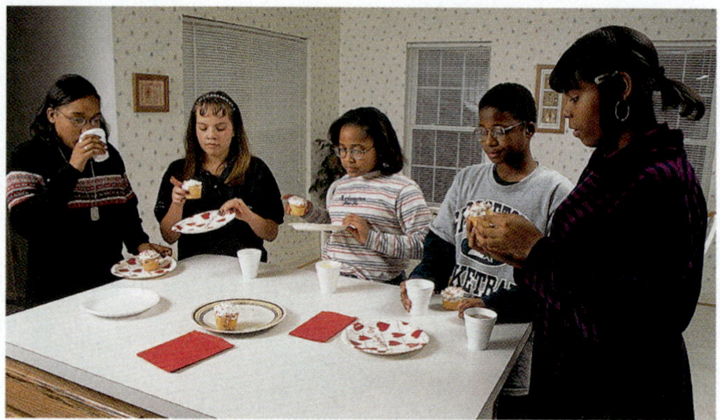

Figure 7–9 ■ Because girls have a growth spurt earlier than boys, girls often are taller than boys of the same age.

Cognitive Development

The child enters the stage of concrete operational thought at about age 7 years. This stage enables school-age children to consider alternative solutions and solve problems. However, school-age children continue to rely on concrete experiences and materials to form their thought content.

During the school-age years, the child learns the concept of conservation (that matter is not changed when its form is altered). At earlier ages, a child believes that when water is poured from a short, wide glass into a tall, thin glass, there is more water in the taller glass. The school-age child recognizes that, although it may look like the taller glass holds more water, the quantity is the same. The concept of conservation is helpful when the nurse explains medical treatments. The school-age child understands that an incision will heal, that a cast will be removed, and that an arm will look the same as before once the intravenous infusion is removed.

Psychosocial Development

The school-age child has many friends and cooperatively interacts with others to accomplish tasks. The child develops a sense of accomplishment from activities and relationships.

PLAY When the preschool teacher tries to organize a game of baseball, both the teacher and the children become frustrated. Not only are the children physically unable to hold a bat and hit a ball, but they seem to have no understanding of the rules

TABLE 7–17 **Growth and Development Milestones During the School-Age Years**

PHYSICAL GROWTH	FINE MOTOR ABILITY	GROSS MOTOR ABILITY	SENSORY ABILITY
Gains 1.4–2.2 kg (3–5 lb)/year.	Plays card and board games.	Roller skates or ice skates.	Is able to concentrate for longer periods.
Grows 4–6 cm (1 1/2–2 1/2 in.)/year.	Enjoys craft projects.	Jumps rope. Rides two-wheeler.	Can read.

TABLE 7–18 **Psychosocial Development During the School-Age Years**

AGE	ACTIVITIES	COMMUNICATION
6–12 years	Gross motor development is fostered by ball sports, skating, dance lessons, water and snow skiing/boarding, biking. A sense of industry is fostered by playing a musical instrument, gathering collections, starting hobbies, playing board and video games. Cognitive growth is facilitated by reading, crafts, word puzzles, schoolwork.	Use of language is mature. Is able to converse and discuss topics for increasing lengths of time. Spends many hours at school and with friends in sports or other activities. Health professionals can ■ assess child's knowledge before teaching. ■ allow the child to select rewards following procedures. ■ teach techniques such as counting or visualization to manage difficult situations. ■ include both parent and child in health care decisions.

of the game and do not want to wait for their turn at bat. By 6 years of age, however, children have acquired the physical ability to hold the bat properly and may occasionally hit the ball. School-age children also understand that everyone has a role—the pitcher, the catcher, the batter, the outfielders. They cooperate with one another to form a team, are eager to learn the rules of the game, and want to ensure that these rules are followed exactly (Table 7–18).

The characteristics of play exhibited by the school-age child include cooperation with others and the ability to play a part in order to contribute to a unified whole. This type of play is called **cooperative play**. The concrete nature of cognitive thought leads to a reliance on rules to provide structure and security. Children have an increasing desire to spend much of their playtime with friends, which demonstrates the social component of play. Play is an extremely important method of learning and living for the school-age child. Active physical play has decreased in recent years as television viewing and playing of computer games have increased, leading to poor nutritional status and high rates of overweight among children.

When a child is hospitalized, the separation from playmates can lead to feelings of sadness and purposelessness. School-age children often feel better when placed in multibed units with other children. Games can be devised even for wheelchair-bound children. Normal, rewarding parts of play should be integrated into care. Friends should be encouraged to visit or call a hospitalized child. Discharge planning for the child who has had a cast or brace applied should address the activities in which the child can participate and those the child must avoid. Nurses should reinforce the importance of playing games with friends to both parents and children.

PERSONALITY AND TEMPERAMENT The enduring aspects of temperament continue to be manifest during the school years. The child classified as "difficult" at an earlier age may now have trouble in the classroom. Nurses may advise parents to provide a quiet setting for homework and to reward the child for concentration. For example, after completing homework, the child may watch a television show. Creative efforts and alternative methods of learning should be valued. Encourage parents to see their children as individuals who may not all learn in the same way. The "slow-to-warm-up" child may need encouragement to try new activities and to share experiences with others, whereas the "easy" child will readily adapt to new schools, people, and experiences.

COMMUNICATION During the school-age years, the child should learn how to correct any lingering pronunciation or grammatical errors. Vocabulary increases, and the child learns about parts of speech in school. school-age children enjoy writing and, while in the hospital, can be encouraged to keep a journal of their experiences as a method of dealing with anxiety. The literal translation of words characteristic of preschoolers is uncommon among school-age children.

Following are some communication strategies helpful with the school-age child:

- Provide concrete examples of pictures or materials to accompany verbal descriptions.
- Assess knowledge before planning the instruction.
- Allow child to select rewards following procedures.
- Teach techniques such as counting or visualization to manage difficult situations.
- Include child in discussions and history with parent.

SEXUALITY Although children become aware of sexual differences between genders during preschool years, they deal much more consciously with sexuality during the school-age years. As children mature physically, they need information about their bodily changes so that they can develop a healthy self-image and an understanding of the relationships between their

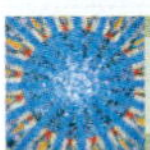

ALTERNATIVE THERAPIES **Music and Art Therapy**

Most children are accustomed to listening to music via earphones or earbuds. They should be encouraged to bring their favorite music to the hospital as a means of stress reduction. It may also reduce the need for sedation during diagnostic tests or uncomfortable procedures (DeLoach Walworth, 2005). Musical instruments and artistic tools such as paints and brushes, markers, and clay are frequently used in hospital and other care settings to help children express fears and anxieties about their illnesses. Just as important, these tools can assist children in sharing their desires and dreams for health and wellness.

bodies and sexuality. Children become interested in sexual issues and are often exposed to erroneous information on television shows, in magazines, or from friends and siblings. Schools and families need to use opportunities to teach school-age children factual information about sex and to foster healthy concepts of self and others. It is advisable to ask occasional questions about sexual issues to learn how much the child knows and to provide correct information when answers demonstrate confusion.

Both friends and the media are common sources of erroneous ideas. Appropriate and inappropriate touch should be discussed, with lists of trusted people who can be approached (teachers, clergy, school counselors, family members, neighbors) to discuss any episodes with which the child feels uncomfortable. Because even these trusted people can be implicated in inappropriate episodes, the nurse should encourage the child to go to more than one person, an important approach if the child is uncomfortable about a relationship with any individual.

ADOLESCENT (12 TO 18 YEARS)

Adolescence is a time of passage signaling the end of childhood and the beginning of adulthood. Although adolescents differ in behaviors and accomplishments, they are all in a period of identity formation. If a healthy identity and sense of self-worth are not developed in this period, role confusion and purposeless struggling will ensue. The adolescents in your care will represent various degrees of identity formation, and each will offer unique challenges.

Physical Growth and Development

The physical changes ending in **puberty**, or sexual maturity, begin near the end of the school-age period. The prepubescent period is marked by a growth spurt at an average age of 10 years for girls and 13 years for boys, although there is considerable variation among children. The increase in height and weight is generally remarkable and is completed in 2–3 years (Table 7–19). The growth spurt in girls is accompanied by an increase in breast size and growth of pubic hair. Menstruation occurs last and signals achievement of puberty. In boys, the growth spurt is accompanied by growth in size of the penis and testes and by growth of pubic hair. Deepening of the voice and growth of facial hair occur later, at the time of puberty.

During adolescence children grow stronger and more muscular and establish characteristic male and female patterns of fat distribution. The apocrine and eccrine glands mature, leading to increased sweating and a distinct odor to perspiration. All body organs are now fully mature, enabling the adolescent to take adult doses of medications.

The adolescent must adapt to a rapidly changing body for several years. These physical changes and hormonal variations offer challenges to identity formation.

Cognitive Development

Adolescence marks the beginning of Piaget's last stage of cognitive development, the stage of formal operational thought. The adolescent no longer depends on concrete experiences as the basis of thought but develops the ability to reason abstractly. Such concepts as justice, truth, beauty, and power can be understood. The adolescent revels in this newfound ability and spends a great deal of time thinking, reading, and talking about abstract concepts.

The ability to think and act independently leads many adolescents to rebel against parental authority. Through these actions, adolescents seek to establish their own identity and values. While this behavior is normal for adolescents, it can create a number of difficulties at home and school as adolescents try to balance their needs to express themselves and the expectations of parents, teachers, and other authority figures.

Psychosocial Development

The adolescent is mature in relationships with others. Establishing a meaningful identity is the key aspect that the teen is working on during relationships and activities.

ACTIVITIES Maturity leads to new activities. Adolescents may drive, ride buses, or bike independently. They are less dependent on parents for transportation and spend more time with friends. Activities include participation in sports and extracurricular school activities, as well as "hanging out" and attending movies or concerts with friends (Table 7–20). The peer group becomes the focus of activities, regardless of the teen's interests. Peers are important in establishing identity and providing meaning. Although same-sex interactions predominate, boy–girl relationships are more common than at earlier stages. Adolescents thus participate in and learn from social interactions fundamental to adult relationships.

PERSONALITY AND TEMPERAMENT Characteristics of temperament manifested during childhood usually remain stable in the teenage years. For instance, the adolescent who was a calm, scheduled infant and child often demonstrates initiative to regulate study times and other routines. Similarly, the adolescent who was an easily stimulated infant may now have a

TABLE 7–19 **Growth and Development Milestones During Adolescence**

PHYSICAL GROWTH	FINE MOTOR ABILITY	GROSS MOTOR ABILITY	SENSORY ABILITY
Variation in age of growth spurt During growth spurt, girls gain 7–25 kg (15–55 lb) and grow 2.5–20 cm (2–8 in.); boys gain approximately 7–29.5 kg (15–65 lb) and grow 11–30 cm (41/2–12 in.).	Skills are well developed.	New sports activities are attempted and muscle development continues. Some lack of coordination is common during growth spurt.	Sensory ability is fully developed.

TABLE 7–20 **Psychosocial Development During Adolescence**

AGE	ACTIVITIES	COMMUNICATION
12–18 years	Sports—ball games, gymnastics, water and snow skiing/boarding, swimming, school sports School activities—drama, yearbook, class office, club participation Quiet activities—Reading, schoolwork, television, computer, video games, music	Increasing communication and time with peer group—movies, dances, driving, eating out, attending sports events Applying abstract thought and analysis in conversations at home and school

messy room, a harried schedule with assignments always completed late, and an interest in many activities. It is also common for an adolescent who was an easy child to become more difficult because of the psychological changes of adolescence and the need to assert independence.

As during the child's earlier ages, the nurse's role may be to inform parents of different personality types and to help them support the teen's uniqueness while providing necessary structure and feedback. Nurses can help parents understand their teen's personality type and work with the adolescent to meet expectations of teachers and others in authority.

COMMUNICATION All parts of speech are used and understood by the adolescent. Colloquialisms and slang are commonly used with the peer group. The adolescent often studies a foreign language in school, having the ability to understand and analyze grammar and sentence structure.

The adolescent increasingly leaves the home base and establishes close ties with peers. These relationships become the basis for identity formation. A period of stress or crisis generally occurs before a strong identity can emerge. The adolescent may try out new roles by learning a new sport or other skills, experimenting with drugs or alcohol, wearing different styles of clothing, or trying other activities. It is important to provide positive role models and a variety of experiences to help the adolescent make wise choices.

The adolescent also has a need to leave the past, to be different, and to change from former patterns to establish a self-identity. Rules that are repeated constantly and dogmatically will probably be broken in the adolescent's quest for self-awareness. This poses difficulties when the adolescent has a health problem that requires ongoing care, such as diabetes or a heart problem. Introducing the adolescent to other teens who manage the same problem appropriately is usually more successful in getting the adolescent to comply with a care plan than telling the adolescent what to do.

Privacy should be ensured during the taking of health histories or interventions with teens. Even if a parent is present for part of a history or examination, the adolescent should be given the opportunity to relay information to or ask questions of the health care provider alone. The adolescent should be given a choice of whether to have a parent present during an examination or while care is provided. Most information shared by an adolescent is confidential. Some states mandate disclosure of certain information to parents such as an adolescent's desire for an abortion. In these cases, the adolescent should be informed of what will be disclosed to the parent.

Setting up teen rooms (recreation rooms for use only by adolescents) or separate adolescent units in hospitals can provide necessary peer support during hospitalization. Most adolescents are not pleased when placed on a unit or in a room with young children. Nurses and care staff should allow adolescents the freedom of choice whenever possible, including preferences for evening or morning bathing, the type of clothes to wear while hospitalized, timing of treatments, and visitation guidelines. Use of contracts with adolescents may increase adherence with health care recommendations. Firmness, gentleness, choices, and respect must be balanced during care of adolescent clients.

Some specific communication strategies that help with the adolescent:

- Provide written and verbal explanations.
- Direct history and explanations to teen alone; then include parent.
- Allow for safe exploration of topics by suggesting that the teen is similar to other teens. ("Many teens with diabetes have questions about.... How about you?")
- Arrange meetings for discussions with other teens.

SEXUALITY With maturation of the body and increased secretion of hormones, the adolescent achieves sexual maturity. This complex process involves growing interactions with members of the opposite sex, an interplay of the forces of society and family, and identity formation. The early adolescent progresses from dances and other social events with members of the opposite sex to the late adolescent who is mature sexually and may have regular sexual encounters. About 47% of all high school students in the United States have had intercourse and 34% are currently sexually active. Only 63% used a condom at their last sexual encounter, putting this age group at high risk of acquiring sexually transmitted infections (Eaton, Kann, Kinchen, et al., 2006).

Teenagers need information about their bodies and emerging sexuality. They should understand the interests and forces they experience. Including sex education in school classes and health care encounters is important. Information on methods to prevent sexually transmitted diseases is given, with most school districts now providing some teaching on HIV. Far more common risks to teens, however, are diseases such as gonorrhea, herpes, and hepatitis. Health histories should include questions on sexual activity, sexually transmitted diseases, and birth control use and understanding. Most hospitals routinely perform pregnancy screening on adolescent girls before elective procedures.

Adolescents will benefit from clear information about sexuality, an opportunity to develop relationships with adolescents in various settings, an open atmosphere at home and school where problems and issues can be discussed, and previous experience in problem solving and decision making. Sexual issues should be among topics that adolescents can discuss openly in a variety of settings. Alternatives and support for their decisions should be available.

Some adolescents identify with a sexual minority group such as lesbian, gay, bisexual, or transgendered. These teens are at particular risk of being stigmatized and harassed by other youth or adults. They are more likely to suffer a variety of problems such as isolation, rejection by significant others, violence, suicide, and sexual risk-taking (Rew, Whittaker, Taylor-Seehafer, & Smith, 2005). Nurses are instrumental in helping these youths by providing information for them and their parents, integrating sexual minority content into sexual education curricula, and providing referrals for health and social care when needed. Nurses must examine their own beliefs and communication styles to provide culturally competent care. They can promote trust and acceptance among youth and in the general school community (Bakker & Cavender, 2003). Additionally, the nurse who encounters a sexually active teenager should remember that he or she may be the very first health care provider with whom the teenager discusses his or her sexuality. The nurse who refrains from asserting his or her own beliefs and who emphasizes open communication and active listening will strengthen the teen's confidence in the health care system and increase the likelihood that the teen will seek help from a health care professional in the future.

ADULT

The adult years commonly are divided into three stages: young adulthood (ages 18–40), middle adulthood (ages 40–65), and older adulthood (over age 65). Although developmental markers are not as clearly delineated in the adult as in the infant or child, specific changes in intellectual, psychosocial, and spiritual development, as well as in physical structures and functions do occur with aging (see Tables 7–3, 7–4, 7–7, 7–8 and Multisystem Effects of Aging on page 367). Applying a variety of developmental theories is important to the holistic care of the adult client as nurses perform assessments, implement care, and teach.

The Young Adult

From ages 18–25, the healthy young adult is at the peak of physical development. All body systems are functioning at maximum efficiency. During the 30s, some normal physiologic changes begin. A comparison of physical status for young adults during their 20s and 30s is shown in Table 7–21.

Many individualized psychosocial stressors may affect the young adult. Choices must be made about education, occupation, relationships, independence, and lifestyle. The young adult without adequate education or job skills may face unemployment, poverty, homelessness, and limited access to health care.

Physical assessment of the young adult includes height and weight, blood pressure, and vision. During the health history, the nurse should ask specific questions about substance use, sexual activity and concerns, exercise, eating habits, menstrual history and patterns, coping mechanisms, any familial chronic illnesses, and family changes.

The Middle Adult

The middle adult, ages 40–65, has physical status and function similar to that of the young adult. However, many changes take place between ages 40 and 65. Table 7–22 lists the physical changes that normally occur in the middle years.

Physical assessment of the middle adult includes all body systems, including blood pressure, vision, and hearing. Monitoring for risks and onset of cancer symptoms is essential. During the health history, the nurse should ask specific questions about food intake and exercise habits, substance abuse, sexual concerns, changes in the reproductive system, coping mechanisms, and family history of chronic illnesses.

TABLE 7–21 **Physical Status and Changes in the Young Adult Years**

ASSESSMENT	STATUS DURING THE 20S	STATUS DURING THE 30S
Skin	Smooth, even temperature	Beginning of wrinkles
Hair	Slightly oily, shiny	Beginning of graying
	Beginning of balding	Balding
Vision	Snellen 20/20	Some loss of visual acuity and accommodation
Musculoskeletal	Strong, coordinated	Some loss of strength and muscle mass
Cardiovascular	Maximum cardiac output	Slight decline in cardiac output
	60–90 beats/min	60–90 beats/min
	Mean BP: 120/80	Mean BP: 120/80
Respiratory	Rate: 12–20	Rate: 12–20
	Full vital capacity	Decline in vital capacity

MULTISYSTEM EFFECTS OF **Aging**

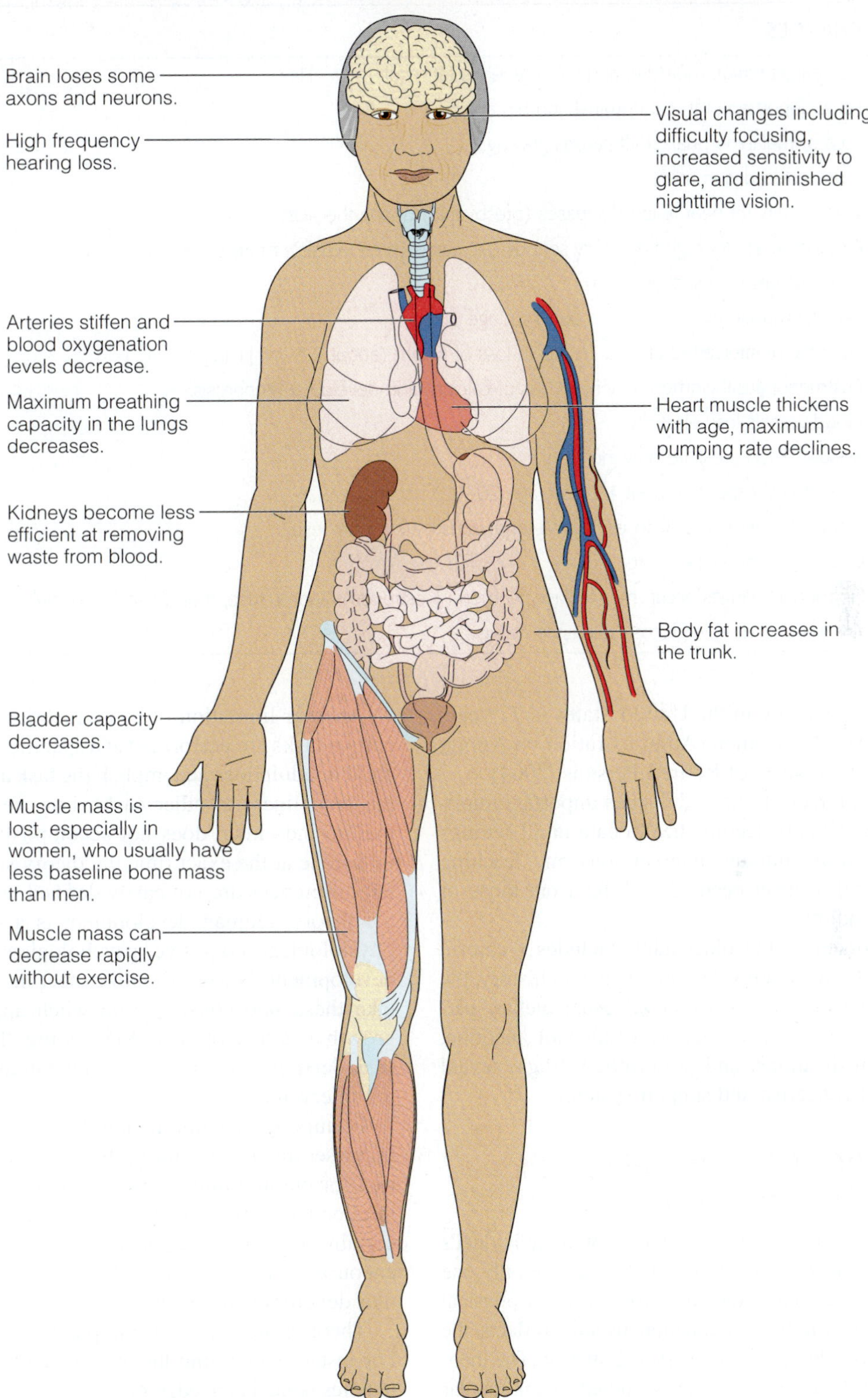

Brain loses some axons and neurons.
High frequency hearing loss.
Visual changes including difficulty focusing, increased sensitivity to glare, and diminished nighttime vision.
Arteries stiffen and blood oxygenation levels decrease.
Maximum breathing capacity in the lungs decreases.
Heart muscle thickens with age, maximum pumping rate declines.
Kidneys become less efficient at removing waste from blood.
Body fat increases in the trunk.
Bladder capacity decreases.
Muscle mass is lost, especially in women, who usually have less baseline bone mass than men.
Muscle mass can decrease rapidly without exercise.

The Older Adult

The older adult period begins at age 65, but it can be further divided into three periods: the young-old (65–74 years), the middle-old (75–84 years), and the old-old (age 85 years and older). With increasing age, a number of normal physiologic changes occur, as listed in Table 7–23.

The older adult population is increasing more rapidly than any other age group. In the last century, the number of adults in the United States living to age 65 or older increased from 3.1 million in 1900 to an estimated 40.2 million in 2010. There will be 71 million older adults by the year 2030, more than twice the number in 2000 (35 million).

TABLE 7–22 **Physical Changes in the Middle Adult Years**

ASSESSMENT	CHANGES
Skin	Decreased turgor, moisture, and subcutaneous fat result in wrinkles.
	Fat is deposited in the abdominal and hip areas.
Hair	Loss of melanin in hair shaft causes graying.
	Hairline recedes in men.
Sensory	Visual acuity for near vision decreases (presbyopia) during the 40s.
	Auditory acuity for high-frequency sounds decreases (presbycusis); more common in men.
	Sense of taste diminishes.
Musculoskeletal	Skeletal muscle mass decreases by about age 60.
	Thinning of intervertebral discs results in loss of height (about 2.5 cm [1 in.]).
	Postmenopausal women may have loss of calcium and develop osteoporosis.
Cardiovascular	Blood vessels lose elasticity.
	Systolic blood pressure may increase.
Respiratory	Loss of vital capacity (about 1 L from age 20–60) occurs.
Gastrointestinal	Large intestine gradually loses muscle tone; constipation may result.
	Gastric secretions are decreased.
Genitourinary	Hormonal changes occur: menopause, women (↓ estrogen); andropause, men (↓ testosterone).
Endocrine	Gradual decrease in glucose tolerance occurs.

The average life expectancy in the United States is 72 years for men and 79 years for women (Administration on Aging, 2003; American Association of Retired Persons, 2004).

The increasing number of older adults has important implications for nursing. Clients needing health care in all settings will be older, requiring nursing interventions and teaching specifically designed to meet needs that differ from those of young and middle adults.

Physical assessment of the older adult includes a careful examination of all body systems. During the health history, the nurse should ask specific questions about usual dietary patterns; elimination; exercise and rest; use of alcohol, nicotine, over-the-counter medications, and prescription drugs; sexual concerns; financial concerns; and support systems.

APPLYING GROWTH AND DEVELOPMENT CONCEPTS TO NURSING PRACTICE

Different theories explain one or more aspects of an individual's growth and development. Typically, theorists examine only one aspect of development, such as the cognitive, moral, or physical aspect. The area chosen for examination usually reflects the researcher's academic discipline and personal interest. The theorists may also limit the population that is studied to a particular part of the life span, such as infancy, childhood, or adulthood.

Although such theories can be useful, they have limitations. First, the theory chosen may explain only one aspect of the growth and development process. Yet a person does not develop in fragmented sections but rather as a whole human being. Thus, the nurse may find it necessary to apply several theories to gain an adequate understanding of the growth and development of a client.

Another limitation of some theories is the suggestion that certain tasks are performed at a specific age. In most cases, the child or adult does accomplish the task at the time specified by the guidelines. In other cases, however, the nurse may find that an individual does not accomplish the task or meet the milestone at the exact time the theory suggests. Such individual differences are not easily defined or categorized by a single theory. Human development is a complex synthesis of physiological, cognitive, psychological, moral, and spiritual development. Nurses should expect individual variations and take these into consideration when applying theories about growth and development. In so doing, they will be better able to understand a client's development and plan effective nursing interventions.

In nursing, developmental theories can be useful in guiding assessment, explaining behavior, and providing a direction for nursing interventions. An understanding of a child's intellectual ability helps a nurse to anticipate and explain certain reactions, responses, and needs. Nurses can then encourage client behavior that is appropriate for that particular developmental stage.

Theories are also useful in planning a nursing intervention. For instance, choosing the appropriate toy for a 3-year-old boy requires some knowledge of the physical and cognitive development of the child, as well as a sensitivity to individual preferences.

In adult care, knowledge about the physical, cognitive, and psychologic aspects of the aging process is a fundamental aspect of administering sensitive nursing care. For example, nurses can use their familiarity with the theories of development to help clients understand and anticipate the psychosocial changes that take place after retirement or the physical limitations that come with aging.

TABLE 7–23 Physical Changes in the Older Adult Years

ASSESSMENT	CHANGES
Skin	■ Decreased turgor and sebaceous gland activity result in dry, wrinkled skin. Melanocytes cluster, causing "age spots" or "liver spots."
Hair and nails	■ Scalp, axillary, and pubic hair thins; nose and ear hair thickens. Women may develop facial hair. ■ Nails grow more slowly; may become thick and brittle.
Sensory	■ Visual field narrows, and depth perception is distorted. ■ Pupils are smaller, reducing night vision. ■ Lenses yellow and become opaque, resulting in distortion of green, blue, and violet tones and increased sensitivity to glare. ■ Production of tears decreases. ■ Sense of smell decreases. ■ Age-related hearing loss progresses, involving middle- and low-frequency sounds. ■ Threshold for pain and touch increases. ■ Alterations in proprioception (sense of physical position) may occur.
Musculoskeletal	■ Loss of overall mass, strength, and movement of muscles occurs; tremors may occur. ■ Loss of bone structure and deterioration of cartilage in joints results in increased risk of fractures and limitation of range of motion.
Cardiovascular	■ Systolic blood pressure rises. ■ Cardiac output decreases. ■ Peripheral resistance increases, and capillary walls thicken.
Respiratory	■ Loss of vital capacity continues as the lungs become less elastic and more rigid. ■ Anteroposterior chest diameter increases; kyphosis occurs. ■ Although blood carbon dioxide levels remain relatively constant, blood oxygen levels decrease by 10–15%.
Gastrointestinal	■ Production of saliva decreases, and declining number of taste buds reduces the number of accurate receptors for salt and sweet. ■ Gag reflex is decreased, and stomach motility and emptying are reduced. ■ Both large and small intestines undergo some atrophy, with decreased peristalsis. ■ The liver decreases in weight and storage capacity; incidence of gallstones increases; pancreatic enzymes decrease.
Genitourinary	■ Kidneys lose mass, and the glomerular filtration rate is reduced (by nearly 50% from young adulthood to old age). ■ Bladder capacity decreases, and the micturition reflex is delayed. Urinary retention is more common. ■ Women may have stress incontinence; men may have an enlarged prostate gland. ■ Reproductive changes in men occur: ▪ Testosterone decreases. ▪ Sperm count decreases. ▪ Testes become smaller. ▪ Length of time to achieve an erection increases; erection is less full. ■ Reproductive changes in women occur: ▪ Estrogen levels decrease. ▪ Breast tissue decreases. ▪ Vagina, uterus, ovaries, and urethra atrophy. ▪ Vaginal lubrication decreases. ▪ Vaginal secretions become alkaline.
Endocrine	■ Pituitary gland loses weight and vascularity. ■ Thyroid gland becomes more fibrous, and plasma T_3 decreases. ■ Pancreas releases insulin more slowly; increased blood glucose levels are common. ■ Adrenal glands produce less cortisol.

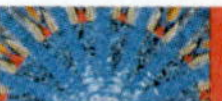

7.1 ATTENTION DEFICIT HYPERACTIVITY DISORDER

KEY TERMS

Attention deficit disorder (ADD), *370*
Attention deficit hyperactivity disorder (ADHD), *370*

BASIS FOR SELECTION OF EXEMPLAR
National Institute of Mental Health

LEARNING OUTCOMES

After reading about this exemplar, you will be able to:

1. Describe the pathophysiology, etiology, clinical manifestations, and direct and indirect causes of ADHD.
2. Identify risk factors associated with ADHD.
3. Illustrate the nursing process in providing culturally competent care across the life span for individuals with ADHD.
4. Formulate priority nursing diagnoses appropriate for an individual with ADHD.
5. Create a plan of care for individuals with ADHD and their family members.
6. Assess expected outcomes for an individual with ADHD.
7. Discuss therapies used in the collaborative care of an individual with ADHD.
8. Employ evidence-based caring interventions for an individual with ADHD.

OVERVIEW

Attention deficit disorder (ADD) is a variation in central nervous system processing characterized by developmentally inappropriate behaviors involving inattention. When hyperactivity and impulsivity accompany inattention, the disorder is called **attention deficit hyperactivity disorder (ADHD)**. The latter is the more common condition that affects from 6–9% of all school-age children (Froehlich, et al.; Wolraich, et al., 2005). Boys are affected almost 4 times more often than girls. Children with ADHD have been shown to be at higher risk for injury due primarily to lack of attention to risk situations (National Center on Birth Defects and Developmental Disabilities, 2004a).

At one time, ADHD was considered strictly a childhood condition, outgrown in adolescence and of little consequence for adults. Research indicates, however, that the disorder persists into adulthood in 30–70% of individuals. Hyperactivity and impulsivity may improve as the child nears adulthood, with inattentiveness appearing as the most persistent characteristic. The adolescent may have difficulty due to the increasing cognitive demands of school (Reiff, 2006). Physical hyperactivity often changes to verbal hyperactivity in adults (Nierenberg et al., 2005). ADHD is a known risk factor among adults for antisocial behavior, substance abuse, involvement in serious accidents, academic underachievement, and low occupational success. In adults, inattention is more persistent than hyperactivity or impulsivity.

Roughly one third of adults with ADHD are not diagnosed until after 18 years of age. Approximately half of adults with ADHD go on to have a child with the disorder, suggesting a genetic component to the disease (American Medical Association, 2004). Overall estimates of ADHD in the U.S. population stand at 5 million, with approximately half of those cases undiagnosed (Federwisch, 2005).

PATHOPHYSIOLOGY AND ETIOLOGY

The pathophysiology of ADD/ADHD is unclear, but some brain characteristics provide clues. There may be a deficit in the catecholamines dopamine and norepinephrine in some children, lowering the threshold for stimuli input. The disorder is marked by a delay in brain maturation in the areas of self-regulation. Increased input from stimuli and decreased self-regulation cause the hallmark inability to inhibit stimuli and motor activity. Some children exhibit additional problems such as aggressive behaviors, learning disabilities, and motor disorders.

Risk Factors

Although a variety of physical and neurologic disorders are associated with ADHD, children with identifiable causes represent a small proportion of this population. There are probably many types of attention deficit that result from several different mechanisms involving interaction of genetic, biologic, and environmental risk factors. Examples of known associations include exposure to high levels of lead in childhood and prenatal exposure to alcohol or tobacco smoke. Other prenatal factors associated with a higher incidence of ADHD include preterm labor, impaired placenta functioning, and impaired oxygenation. Seizures and serious head injury are other potential associations. Genetic factors may be important, as well as family dynamics and environmental characteristics. Although ADHD occurs more commonly within families (25% have a first-degree relative with the disorder), a single gene has not been located and a specific mechanism of genetic transmission is not known. It is believed that a genetic predisposition interacts with the child's environment, so that both factors contribute to the appearance of the condition. Family stress, poverty, and poor nutrition may be contributing factors in some cases. Daily television exposure at ages 1–3 years is associated with attentional problems at 7 years (Christakis, Zimmerman, DiGiuseppe, & McCarty, 2004).

CLINICAL MANIFESTATIONS

Children with ADD and ADHD have problems related to decreased attention span, impulsiveness, and/or increased motor activity (Figure 7–10 ■). Symptoms can range from mild to severe. The child has difficulty completing tasks, fidgets constantly, is frequently loud, and interrupts others. Sleep disturbances are common. Because of these behaviors, the child often has difficulty developing and maintaining social relationships and may be shunned or teased by other children. This only increases the anxiety of the already compromised child, whose behavior is set on a downward-spiraling course (Brown et al., 2005).

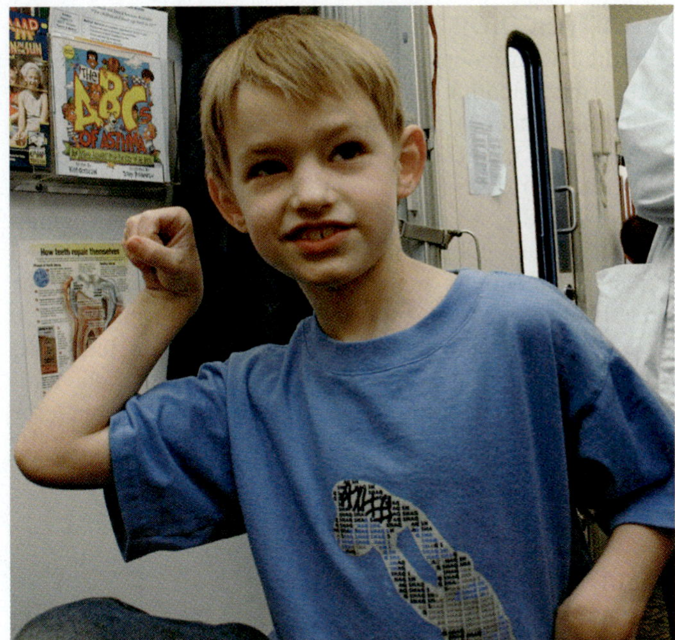

Figure 7–10 ■ This child with ADHD was challenged by a visit to a health care facility for dental care. He found it difficult to remain in the chair for the examination, and once it was over, he rapidly ran from one piece of equipment to another in the facility. He asked what things were for but did not wait for answers. His engaging personality emerged as he posed briefly for a picture. Such behaviors can be exhausting for parents to manage and may create safety hazards in the health care setting.

Typically, girls with ADHD show less aggression and impulsiveness than boys, but far more anxiety, mood swings, social withdrawal, rejection, and cognitive and language problems. Girls tend to be older at the time of diagnosis.

COLLABORATION

The successful diagnosis and treatment of the child or adult with ADHD requires a collaborative effort that may involve any combination of the following: parents, nurses, and physicians; teachers and school personnel or coworkers; mental health specialists and speech and language therapists. Diagnosis begins with a careful history of the child, including family history, birth history, growth and developmental milestones, behaviors such as sleep and eating patterns, progression and patterns in school, social and environmental conditions, and reports from parents and teachers. A physical examination should be performed to rule out neurologic diseases and other health problems. The mental health specialist then tests the child and administers questionnaires to the parent and teacher. It is important to identify other conditions that may mimic ADD/ADHD or exist in conjunction with the disorders. These conditions may include depression, anxiety, learning disorder, conduct disorder, or oppositional defiant disorder (Adesman, 2003).

Specific diagnostic criteria must be applied to all children with the potential diagnosis of ADD or ADHD. Behaviors at home and school or at day care must be evaluated because abnormal patterns in two settings are needed for diagnosis. The diagnosis of ADD can be difficult due to the absence of hyperactivity behaviors. A variety of tests are available for the trained professional to use in establishing the diagnosis (Table 7–24).

TABLE 7–24 **Screening Tests for ADD/ADHD**

TEST	SOURCE
Vanderbilt Parent and Teacher Scales	Wolraich, M. L., Feurer, I. D., Hannah, J. N., et al. (1998). Obtaining systematic teaching reports of disruptive behavior disorders with your DSM-IV. *Journal of Abnormal Child Psychology, 26,* 141–152. Wolraich, M. L., Lambert, W., Doffing M. A., Bickman, L., Simmons, T., & Worley, K. (2003). Psychometric properties of the Vanderbilt ADHD diagnostic parent rating scale in a referred population. *Journal of Pediatric Psychology, 28,* 559–567.
Connors' Parent and Teacher Rating Scales—Revised—Long Form	Olfson, M., Gameroff, J. J., Marcus, S. C., & Jensen, P. S. (2003). National trends in the treatment of attention deficit hyperactivity disorder. *American Journal of Psychiatry, 160,* 1071–1077.
Swanson, Nolan and Pelham Questionnaire II Teacher and Parent Rating Scale (SNAP-IV)	Swanson, J. M. (1992). *School-based assessments and interventions for ADD students.* Irvine, CA: KC Publications.
Disruptive Behavior Disorder Scale	Pelham, W. E., Gnagy, E. M., Greenslade, K. E., & Milich, R. (1992). Teacher ratings of DSM-III-R symptoms for disruptive behavior disorders. *Journal of the American Academy of Child and Adolescent Psychiatry, 31,* 210–218.
ADHD Rating Scale	DuPaul, G. J., & Rapport, M. D. (1993). Does methylphenidate normalize the classroom performance of children with attention deficit disorder? *Journal of American Academy of Child and Adolescent Psychiatry, 32,* 190–198.
Revised Behavior Problem Checklist	Quay, H. C., & Peterson, D. R. (1987). *Manual for the Revised Behavior Problem Checklist.* Coral Gables, FL: University of Miami.
Child Behavior Checklist	Achenback, T. M. (1991). *Manual for the child behavior checklist/4–18 and the 1991 profile.* Burlington: University of Vermont.

Source: Data from Liu, Y. H., & Leslie, L. K. (2003). Diagnosing ADHD: Putting AAP guidelines to the test—and into practice. *Contemporary Pediatrics, 20*(12), 51–73; Brown, R. T. et al. (2005). Treatment of attention-deficit/hyperactivity disorder: Overview of the evidence. *Pediatrics, 115,* 749–757.

Based on the findings, desired outcomes are established for the child's performance and management of the disorder. Treatment is established to meet the desired behavioral outcomes and includes a combination of approaches, such as environmental changes, behavior therapy, and pharmacotherapy (Brown et al., 2005). It is expected that treatment will be long-term.

Children are frequently diagnosed with the disorder soon after they begin school, when demands for attentive behavior increase. See Box 7–2 for *DSM-IV-TR* diagnostic criteria for attention deficit hyperactivity disorder.

Children are usually brought for evaluation when behaviors escalate to the point of interfering with the daily functioning of teachers or parents. When children have learning disabilities or anxiety disorders, the problem is commonly misdiagnosed as ADHD without further evaluation of the child's symptoms. Obtaining an accurate diagnosis by a pediatric mental health specialist is vital (Brown et al., 2005; Wolraich et al., 2005).

Although ADHD was once thought to be a disorder of childhood that gradually improved with age, it is now believed that symptoms continue into adulthood and that careful management in childhood assists in lessening problems of social functioning later in life.

Pharmacologic Therapy

Children with moderate to severe ADD/ADHD are treated with pharmacotherapy (Table 7–25). Methylphenidate (Ritalin, Concerta) is most often prescribed. A skin patch that releases medication over a 9-hour period is now available, facilitating ease of administration (Anderson & Scott, 2006). Usually, a favorable response (a decrease in impulsive behaviors and an increase in the ability to sit still and attend to an activity for at least 15 minutes) is seen in the first 10 days of treatment and frequently with the first few doses. Other medications that may be used include dextroamphetamine (Dexedrine or Adderall), the tricyclic antidepressants desipramine and imipramine, and the antidepressant bupropion (Wellbutrin) (Brown et al., 2005; Wolraich et al., 2005).

Environmental Supports

Children with ADHD often benefit from environmental changes. Decreasing stimulation by turning off the television, keeping the environment quiet, and maintaining an orderly

Box 7–2 *DSM-IV-TR* Diagnostic Criteria for Attention Deficit Hyperactivity Disorder

A. Either 1 or 2:

1. Inattention: Six (or more) of the following symptoms of inattention have persisted for at least 6 months to a degree that is maladaptive and inconsistent with developmental level:
   a. Often fails to give close attention to details or makes careless mistakes in schoolwork, work, and other activities
   b. Often has difficulty sustaining attention in tasks or play activities
   c. Often does not seem to listen when spoken to directly
   d. Often does not follow through on instructions and fails to finish schoolwork, chores, or duties in the workplace (not due to oppositional behavior or failure to understand instructions)
   e. Often has difficulty organizing tasks and activities
   f. Often avoids, dislikes, or is reluctant to engage in tasks that require sustained mental effort (such as schoolwork or homework)
   g. Often loses things necessary for tasks or activities (e.g., toys, school assignments, pencils, books, or tools)
   h. Is often easily distracted by extraneous stimuli
   i. Is often forgetful in daily activities
2. Hyperactivity-impulsivity: Six (or more) of the following symptoms of hyperactivity-impulsivity have persisted for at least 6 months to a degree that is maladaptive and inconsistent with developmental level:

   Hyperactivity

   a. Often fidgets with hands or feet or squirms in seat
   b. Often leaves seat in classroom or in other situations in which remaining seated is expected
   c. Often runs about or climbs excessively in situations in which it is inappropriate (in adolescents or adults, may be limited to subjective feelings of restlessness)
   d. Often has difficulty playing or engaging in leisure activities quietly
   e. Is often "on the go" or acts as if "driven by a motor"
   f. Often talks excessively

   Impulsivity

   g. Often blurts out answers before questions have been completed
   h. Often has difficulty awaiting turn
   i. Often interrupts or intrudes on others (e.g., butts into conversations or games)

B. Some hyperactive-impulsive or inattentive symptoms that caused impairment were present before age 7 years.

C. Some impairment from the symptoms is present in two or more settings (e.g., at school [or work] and at home).

D. There must be clear evidence of clinically significant impairment in social, academic, or occupational functioning.

E. The symptoms do not occur exclusively during the course of a pervasive developmental disorder, schizophrenia, or other psychotic disorder and are not better accounted for by another mental disorder (e.g., mood disorder, anxiety disorder, dissociative disorder, or a personality disorder).

Reprinted with permission from the *Diagnostic and Statistical Manual of Mental Disorders*, Fourth Edition, Text Revision. Copyright © 2000 American Psychiatric Association.

TABLE 7–25 Medications Used to Treat ADHD

MEDICATION	ACTION AND INDICATION	NURSING MANAGEMENT
Methylphenidate	A derivative of piperidine that acts like amphetamine. May work in ADHD treatment by inhibiting reuptake of dopamine and norepinephrine, thereby enhancing catecholamine effects in the nervous system, improving attention span and task performance. Schedule II drug in Schedule of Controlled Substances.	Available as Ritalin, Methylin, Focalin, Concerta, and Metadate in a variety of forms and formula. A skin patch (Daytrana) is now approved for use. The variety of available forms makes it important to read labels carefully and to inform families about proper administration of the child's specific type of drug. The most common side effects are headache, insomnia, and anorexia. Periodic growth measurements and cardiac assessments are needed. Behavior and school performance should be monitored.
Amphetamine salts (amphetamine, dextroamphetamine, lisdexamfetamine)	Synthetic sympathomimetic amine with stimulant effect on central nervous system. Increases release of norepinephrine and dopamine by blocking their reuptake. Schedule II drug in Schedule of Controlled Substances.	Available as Dexedrine, (DextroStat), and Adderall. Read labels and instruct in proper administration. Anorexia, weight loss, insomnia, and headache are common side effects. Monitor vital signs, cardiac status, and growth measurements periodically.
Atomoxetine	This is the first nonstimulant drug for treatment of ADHD. It inhibits norepinephrine reuptake. Decreases hyperactivity and impulsivity of ADHD and may assist with improving mood and decreasing anxiety.	Available in various doses as Strattera. Recommended starting dose for children is 0.5 mg/kg/day. Has been shown to have long-lasting effect of 1 day or longer. Side effects are uncommon and transient, with dyspepsia or vomiting, fatigue, decreased appetite, and dizziness most common. Instruct the child to change position slowly if dizziness occurs; caution teen not to drive until effects of drug are clear. Perform periodic growth measurements. The U.S. Food and Drug Administration (FDA) has warned about uncommon side effects of hepatotoxicity and suicidal ideation.

Source: Data from Smoot, L. C., Boothby, L. A., & Gillett, R. C. (2007). Clinical assessment and treatment of ADHD in children. *International Journal of Clinical Practice 61*, 1730–1773. Pliszka, S. R. (2007). Pharmacologic treatment of attention-deficit hyperactivity disorder. Efficacy, safety and mechanism of action. *Neuropsychological Review 17*, 61–72.

and clutter-free desk or study area without distraction, for example, may help the child to stay focused on the task at hand. Another relatively simple change is appropriate classroom placement, preferably in a small class with a teacher who can provide close supervision and a structured daily routine. Consistent limits and expectations should be set for the child. Children living in chaotic homes and communities may function better if the environment can be simplified. When aggressive behaviors occur, therapeutic approaches such as play and group therapy may be useful.

Behavior Therapy

Behavior therapy involves rewarding the child for desired behaviors and applying consequences for undesirable behaviors. Children may be rewarded by praise or earn points toward a movie or another desired outing for staying seated during meals or quietly listening in a classroom. Cues are established so that a child can subtly be reminded when impulsive or hyperactive behaviors are escalating. All adults who are in close contact with the child, such as parents and teachers, must be informed and involved in the established behavioral program.

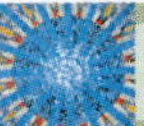

ALTERNATIVE THERAPIES **ADD and ADHD**

There are many claims in the media about what causes ADD and ADHD. Parents may want to try a variety of approaches in addition to or instead of traditional behavioral therapy and medication. Some common complementary therapies include elimination of dietary components such as highly processed foods, sugar, aspartame, or yeast. Other therapies include use of supplements such as iron, magnesium, zinc, and vitamin B_6. Herbs such as pycnogenol, melatonin, echinacea, St. John's wort, and gingko biloba are sometimes used, as are visual and auditory training. Parents do not typically tell health care providers about the use of herbs; 70–75% of parents have not discussed their use during health care visits. The nurse should ask parents about alternative therapies used and investigate what is known about them in order to share this information with parents (Rojas & Chan, 2005).

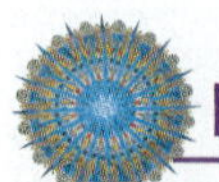

NURSING PROCESS

Assessment

The nurse often encounters the family who is concerned about the child's behavior before a diagnosis has been made. Ask about family and birth history and have the parents describe the child's behaviors. Perform developmental testing and look specifically for attention span and physical activity. Refer the family to their pediatric health care home for further assessment, then to a mental health care specialist who is experienced in diagnosing ADHD.

The nurse may encounter the child with ADHD in the hospital when parents bring the child for treatment of an injury (e.g., fracture) or another problem. Explore in detail the parents' report of the child's attention span. Usually within a few minutes in an unstructured setting or waiting area, the child with ADHD becomes restless and searches for distraction. Gather information about the child's activity level and impulsiveness. Be alert for information that reveals a serious problem, such as hurting animals or other children. Obtain information about distractibility, attention deficit in activities of daily living, characteristic ways of reacting, and the extent of impulsiveness when the child is receiving medication. Find out how the family manages at home and what treatments are being applied.

Diagnosis

Examples of nursing diagnoses that may be appropriate for a child with ADHD include the following:

- Impaired Verbal Communication related to altered perceptions
- Impaired Social Interaction related to chronic episodes of impulsive behavior
- Chronic Low Self-Esteem related to behaviors associated with ADD/ADHD
- Risk for Injury related to high level of impulsiveness and excitability
- Risk for Caregiver Role Strain related to management of the child with unpredictable moods and high energy.

Plan

Prevention can focus on discouraging regular television exposure for young children from 1–3 years and encouraging daily vigorous physical activity for all children.

The nursing care of the hospitalized child with ADD/ADHD focuses on administering medications, managing the child's environment, implementing behavioral management plans, providing emotional support to the child and family, promoting self-esteem, and ensuring ongoing care. Care in the community includes using the same components along with guiding parents to appropriate resources when needed.

Implementation

Children with ADHD present a number of challenges to their parents and teachers. The nurse may need to provide client teaching to both parents and teachers regarding medications and their side effects, the importance of decreasing stimuli and minimizing distractions, and the need for consistency and patience with behavior management plans. Some trial and error may be necessary before the child's treatment team (including parents and teachers) find the combination of therapies that is most effective for the child.

Administer Medications

Stimulant and nonstimulant medications increase the child's attention span and decrease distractibility. Be alert for the common side effects of these medications, including anorexia, insomnia, and tachycardia. Administering medication early in the day helps to alleviate insomnia. Anorexia can be managed by giving medication at mealtimes. Careful periodic monitoring of weight, height, and blood pressure is necessary. Instruct families about the abuse potential of stimulant drugs; they should be locked up and administered only as directed.

Minimize Environmental Distractions

The child may need to be placed in an environment with minimal distractions. Potentially harmful equipment should be kept out of reach. Television and video game time needs to be monitored and limited. Use shades to darken the room during naps or at bedtime and minimize noise. Teach parents to minimize distractions at home during periods when the child needs to concentrate (e.g., when doing schoolwork) (Figure 7–11 ■). Visits to areas such as shopping malls and playgrounds may need to be limited. Plenty of daily exercise and minimal use of television/video games may assist the child in concentrating when needed for schoolwork. When the child is hospitalized, minimizing environmental distractions may mean a room with only one other child.

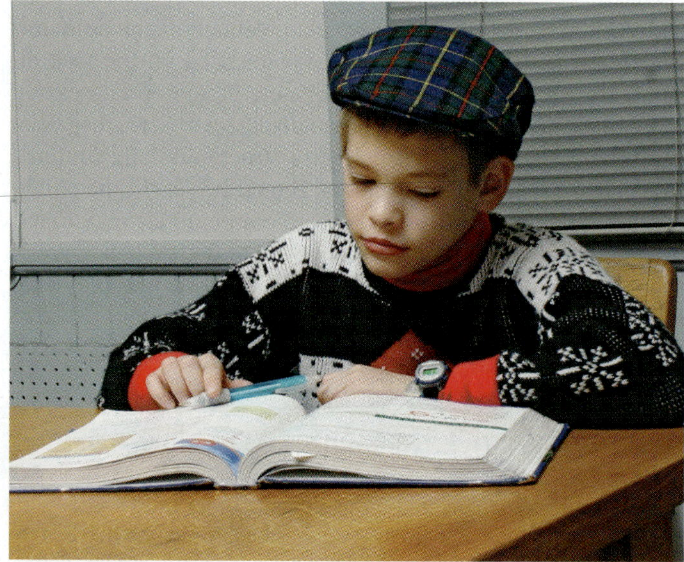

Figure 7–11 ■ Managing the environment to provide quiet places with minimal distractions is often necessary for the child with ADHD. This boy reads and does homework in a room with few pictures, no music, and only the book with homework on the table. He also is assisted by structure, such as a scheduled time for homework, with short breaks to walk around every 10–15 minutes.

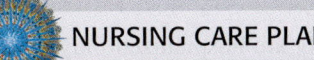

NURSING CARE PLAN A Client With Attention Deficit Disorder

ASSESSMENT

Melanie Taylor, 8 years old, visits her pediatrician's office for a routine check-up. Her mother, Melinda, reports Melanie is not doing well in school and she is a difficult child to raise. Upon further questioning Mrs. Taylor reports her daughter is forgetful, has trouble focusing, and often does not respond to her name being called. She has to repeatedly ask her to perform her chores, get ready for bed, or do her homework. Melanie doesn't sleep well at night, and crawls into her parents' bed most nights. One night Mrs. Taylor awoke to find Melanie watching TV at 2 a.m. in the family room. Melanie's teacher has suggested she be evaluated for possible ADD.

The nurse interviews Melanie who says she doesn't like school because "it's too hard" and the teacher "always tells me to sit still."

Upon reviewing Melanie's medical history the nurse finds the client's growth and development have been normal to date. Mrs. Taylor's pregnancy and delivery were unremarkable

The physical examination is normal although the nurse notes Melanie often requires repetition of instructions such as "Touch your finger to your nose" before she complies. Both Melanie and her mother appear tired and yawn several times during the nurse's time with them.

The provider speaks with Melanie and Mrs. Taylor suggesting the signs and symptoms are highly suspicious of attention deficit disorder (ADD) and provides a referral for the family to meet with a psychologist specializing in the care of clients with this disorder.

The nurse provides Ms. Taylor a Connor's Parent Rating Scale to complete and gives her a copy of the Teacher Rating Scale to give to Melanie's teacher for completion before seeing the counselor, who will evaluate the results.

DIAGNOSES

- Risk for Situational Low Self-Esteem
- Disturbed Sleep Pattern
- Risk for Caregiver Role Strain
- Fatigue

PLANNING

- The client (Melanie) will sleep through the night, remaining in her own bed.
- The client will participate in a therapeutic regimen as recommended by the physician.
- The client's parents and teachers will participate in the therapeutic regimen.
- The client will increase her ability to remain on task by five minute intervals over a period of 6–8 weeks, until she can remain on task for a minimum of 20 minutes at a time.
- The client will keep track of her belongings.
- The client will respond when spoken to the first time.

IMPLEMENTATION

- Explain diagnosis in terms Melanie can understand taking care to help Melanie understand she is not "abnormal" but "unique" in how her brain works.
- Help Ms. Taylor set rules related to sleep that will promote Melanie's sleep hygiene.
- Assist client to understand how her potential diagnosis of ADD impacts her thinking as well as how treatment can help her perform better in school.
- Determine if Melanie of Ms. Taylor have questions related to ADD.
- Suggest strategies for helping Melanie improve her concentration and memory such as lists.
- Teach positive behavioral skills through role play, role modeling, and discussion.
- Convey confidence in client's and mother's ability to handle situation.
- Encourage increased responsibility for self, as appropriate.
- Encourage Melanie to accept new challenges.
- Monitor Melanie's statements of self-worth and frequency of self-negating verbalizations.

EVALUATION

Ms. Taylor and Melanie return at the end of 3 months. Ms. Taylor reports that Melanie is doing better at paying attention both at home and at school, and that she is able to maintain attention for 20 minutes "most of the time." Both of them are sleeping better. Melanie is able to answer the nurse's questions readily and describes things that she does to keep track of her belongings and try to stay on task. Melanie voices pride in her improvement at school.

CRITICAL THINKING

1. Ms. Taylor asks the nurse, privately out of range of Melanie's hearing, if the diagnosis resulted from something she did as a parent or while pregnant. How would you respond?
2. Melanie tells the nurse, "I'm so stupid compared to the other kids in my class. I guess ADD means I'm brain damaged." How would you respond?
3. Is it possible to adequately treat ADD without the use of medications? Explain your answer.

Implement Behavioral Management Plans

Behavior modification programs can help to reduce specific impulsive behaviors. An example is setting up a reward program for the child who has taken medication as ordered or completed a homework assignment. Depending on the child's age, the rewards may be daily as well as weekly or monthly. For example, one completed homework assignment might be rewarded with 30 minutes of basketball or a bike ride and assignments completed for a week might be rewarded with participation in an activity of the child's choice on the weekend.

If punishment is necessary, the behavior should be corrected while simultaneously supporting the child as a person. Punishment is generally withdrawal of a privilege and should follow the offense quickly, as the child may not otherwise connect the punishment with the behavior.

Provide Emotional Support

Children with ADD/ADHD offer a special challenge to parents, teachers, and health care providers. Parents must cope simultaneously with managing the difficult needs and demands of a hard-to-handle child, obtaining appropriate evaluation and treatment, and understanding and accepting the diagnosis, even when the child exhibits different behaviors with different people.

Family support is essential. Educate both the parents and the child about the importance of appropriate expectations and consequences of behaviors. Teach skills that will help as the child grows older: making lists of tasks to accomplish; following routines for eating, sleeping, recreation, and schoolwork; minimizing stimuli in the environment when completing work; and asking teachers and friends to identify when behavior is inappropriate.

When the child is hospitalized for another condition, the time may provide a brief respite from constant care by the parent. The activity, impulsivity, and general high energy of children with ADHD can fatigue parents. When the child is hospitalized, parents may want to spend a few hours each day at home or at a nearby residence for families. Ask them how they manage at home and offer ideas for respite care.

Promote Self-Esteem

Help the child to understand the disorder at an appropriate developmental level and facilitate a trusting relationship with health care providers. Assist the child with social skills through the use of role playing, small group play, and modeling. Promote the child's self-esteem by emphasizing the positive aspects of behavior and treating instances of negative behavior as learning opportunities. Help the child to develop ego strengths (the conscious ability to screen outside stimuli and to control internal demands), which will result in better impulse control and thus increase the child's self-esteem over time. Encourage skills at which the child excels and consider the use of support groups for children in school (Barber, Grubbs, & Cottrell, 2005). Praise the hospitalized child for lying still for a procedure, taking a medication on time, or helping a staff member carry toys around to other children.

Care in the Community

Most children with ADD/ADHD are hospitalized only when they need care for another condition. Parents need support to understand the diagnosis and to learn how to manage the child. Explain what the diagnosis is and what is known about attention deficit disorders. Provide written materials, Internet sites, and an opportunity to ask questions.

Emphasize the importance of a stable environment at home as well as at school. At home, the child may have difficulty staying on task. Parents need to consider the child's age and developmental appropriateness of tasks, give clear and simple instructions, and provide frequent reminders to ensure completion. Routines in the evening can promote good sleep patterns.

The nurse can serve as a liaison to teachers and school personnel or as the case manager for the child. See Box 7–3 for suggestions on how parents and teachers can work together to improve the school experience for a child with ADD/ADHD. An Individualized Education Plan (IEP) may be needed, with clear expected outcomes stated for the child's behaviors. IEPs or periods of instruction free from the distractions of the entire class may enable the child to improve school performance. Parents may have difficulty understanding the need for these approaches because the child often tests at above average intelligence.

Reinforce the importance of providing a structured environment free from unnecessary external stimuli. Make sure that parents understand behavioral approaches that will help the child, the administration of prescribed medications, and the importance of returning for health care visits to monitor for side effects. Medication should be safely locked away at home to keep it away from other children and to prevent illegal use of the controlled substance. An Individualized Health Plan may be needed for medication management at school.

Parents may have heard about ADD/ADHD in the media and may have questions about its cause and management. Providing information about complementary and alternative treatments is a nursing role. The National Institutes of Health sponsors the National Center for Complementary and Alternative Medicine (NCCAM), which is a reliable source for parents and professionals.

As the child grows older, provide explanations about the disorder and information about techniques that will assist in dealing with problems. Emphasize the importance of doing homework or other tasks requiring concentration in a quiet environment

FOCUS ON DIVERSITY AND CULTURE
Mental Health and Stigma

Many families who have a child with ADHD are embarrassed and feel shame because of the diagnosis, especially in certain cultures (e.g., some Asian groups) and in very structured and highly achieving families. When taking histories from family members, be sensitive to the stigma some may feel. In a private setting, ask about the family's feelings regarding a mental health disorder. Is there someone in the family with whom they can talk about the diagnosis? Provide information in a nonjudgmental manner and, if appropriate, provide support from other families with similar experiences.

Box 7–3 School Suggestions for Children With ADD/ADHD

Parents can work with teachers to provide a school environment that fosters attention and learning. Some ideas that may be helpful include the following:

- Have the child sit near the front of the class.
- Plan a reminder that is apparent to the teacher and student but not to other children when the child needs to concentrate on attention. This might be an object placed on the student's desk or a light hand placed on the shoulder or arm.
- Give instructions verbally and in written form and repeat them more than once.
- Provide opportunities to take notes and make lists of assignments and mark off when accomplished. Have a planned time to go through the child's backpack daily to find notices and to ensure that homework is completed and in a uniform location.
- Use computers for making lists and taking notes. The child may need to listen in class, record the teacher, and take notes later from the recording.
- If the child has well-developed fine or gross motor skills, integrate motor movement into learning situations whenever possible.
- Provide quiet places with minimal distraction for examinations. Offer additional time.
- Allow time for organizing clothing, desk, and other areas.
- Go over assignments and tests with the child in person to explain areas that are understood and those that need attention.
- Find the child's areas of excellence and allow for performance in these ways. Some children are talented in dance; others, in art or extemporaneous speech.
- Never call the child names, make fun of behavior or performance, or call the child "hyperactive" in front of other children, teachers, or parents.

Adapted from Call-Schmidt & Maharaj, 2004; Stein & Barren, 2003.

without background noise from a television or radio. Encourage children with ADHD to keep assignment notebooks and use checklists to help them accomplish specific tasks.

Evaluation

Expected outcomes of nursing care for the child with ADD or ADHD include the following:

- The parents and child demonstrate understanding of the disorder.
- The family accurately and safely manages medication administration.
- The child demonstrates an increase in attentiveness and a decrease in hyperactivity, impulsivity, and sleep disturbance.
- The child displays formation of a positive self-image.
- The child manifests formation of healthy social interactions with peers and family.
- The child achieves educational performance to maximum potential.

REVIEW Attention Deficit Hyperactivity Disorder

RELATE: LINK THE CONCEPTS

Linking the exemplar of Attention Deficit Hyperactivity Disorder with the concept of Family:

1. How can the nurse support the family of a child with ADHD?
2. What if the family is a single parent? A grandparent?

Linking the exemplar of Attention Deficit Hyperactivity Disorder with the concept of Safety:

3. What interventions are important for the nurse to initiate to maintain the safety of a client with ADHD?
4. When caring for an adolescent with ADHD how would you teach automobile safety?

REFER: GO TO MYNURSINGKIT

REFLECT: CASE STUDY

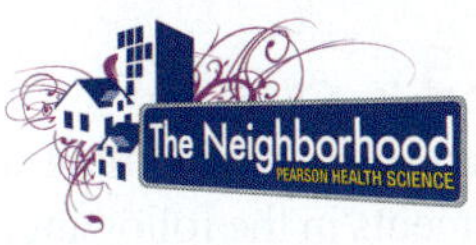

Jason is an active, healthy 11-year-old boy. He is currently in fifth grade at the public elementary school near his home. He lives with his mother Evelyn and his 14-year-old sister Jenna. He has not had much contact with his father. Jason's home life has been somewhat stressful the last year or so because of ongoing fights between his mother and oldest sister Jessica; the conflict resulted in Jessica moving out of the house. Jason gets along well with his mother, but he has typical sibling conflicts with Jenna.

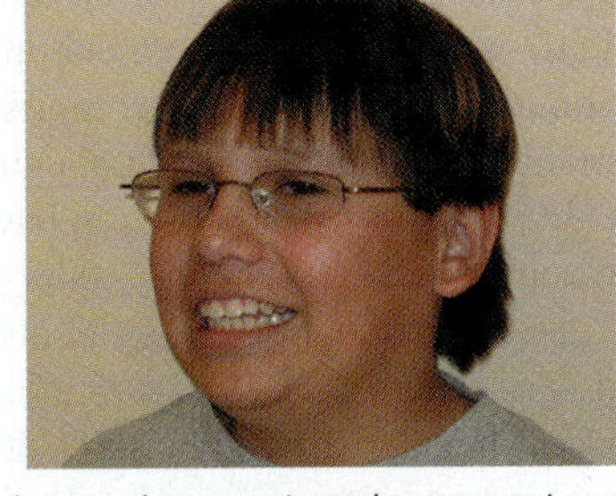

Jason has had problems in school for the last 3 years. Teachers report that he has difficulty staying on task and won't follow directions. Although he made some progress last year with his fourth-grade teacher, his grades have been consistently poor. His mother tries to help him with homework after school or in the evening; these sessions frequently turn into battlegrounds. It takes Jason hours to complete fairly simple assignments, resulting in a great deal of frustration for both Jason and his mother. The fact that he frequently comes home from school with headaches further aggravates the situation.

In addition to problems with academics, Jason has problems with social interactions. His teachers find him to be disruptive in the classroom. During the past year, he has often been sent to the principal's office for misbehaving. He has few friends and is a frequent target of teasing at school. Most of his time at home is spent playing video and computer games and watching TV.

1. What are the priorities of nursing care for Jason?
2. What outcomes would be appropriate for this client?
3. What independent nursing interventions would you initiate for this client?

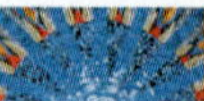

7.2 AUTISM SPECTRUM DISORDERS

KEY TERMS

Autistic spectrum disorders (ASDs), *378*
Echolalia, *379*
Pervasive developmental disorders (PDDs), *378*
Stereotypy, *379*

BASIS FOR SELECTION OF EXEMPLAR

National Institute of Mental Health

LEARNING OUTCOMES

After reading about this exemplar, you will be able to:

1. Describe the pathophysiology, etiology, clinical manifestations, and direct and indirect causes of autism.
2. Identify risk factors associated with autism.
3. Illustrate the nursing process in providing culturally competent care across life span for individuals with autism.
4. Formulate priority nursing diagnoses appropriate for an individual with autism.
5. Create a plan of care for individuals with autism and their family members.
6. Assess expected outcomes for an individual with autism.
7. Discuss therapies used in the collaborative care of an individual with autism.
8. Employ evidence-based caring interventions for an individual with autism.

OVERVIEW

It is estimated that 12–16% of children have a developmental or behavioral disorder. One of the most common sets of disorders is pervasive developmental disorders. **Pervasive developmental disorders (PDDs)** begin in early childhood and are characterized by impaired social interactions and communication, with restricted interests, activities, and behaviors (Centers for Disease Control and Prevention, 2006). The PDDs comprise five disorders:

- Autistic disorder (autism)
- Asperger syndrome
- Rett's disorder
- Childhood disintegrative disorder
- Pervasive developmental disorder not otherwise specified (PDD-NOS).

Three of the disorders are commonly called **autistic spectrum disorders (ASDs)**: autism, Asperger syndrome, and PDD-NOS. About 5.7–6.6 children in 1,000 have an ASD, with about half of the cases comprised of autistic disorder (commonly called autism). Although incidence varies geographically, about 1 in 150 children have autism (Centers for Disease Control and Prevention, 2006; Schieve, Rice, Boyle et al., 2006). This incidence represents an increase from previously described levels. Before 1985, about 0.4–0.5 children in 1,000 were diagnosed with an ASD. It is unclear whether there is a real increase in cases or simply improved techniques in making the diagnosis, as well as an enlarged diagnostic category that includes more children (Johnson, Myers, & the Council on Children with Disabilities, 2007). ASDs are 2–15 times more common in males than in females, with the higher proportion more common in highly functioning Asperger syndrome (Johnson et al., 2007). Peak age at diagnosis is 6–11 years, but symptoms often begin at 18–24 months of age.

Children and adults with ASDs often suffer from impairments of language, cognition, and social skills that make them seem different from others. These clients, however, are no different from anyone else: They seek respect, love, affection, and understanding. They can be funny, happy, sad, confused, scared, or angry. Like anyone else, the client with ASD interacts with the health care system for different reasons and at different times. This exemplar discusses how nurses can meet some of the special needs of clients with autism spectrum disorders and their families.

PATHOPHYSIOLOGY AND ETIOLOGY

The etiology of ASDs is unknown, although they are biologically based with multiple and complex phenotypes as the cause. Researchers are looking into the roles that genetic transmission, immune responses, and neuroanatomy may play in ASDs. Neurotransmitters such as dopamine, serotonin, and opioids also are a focus of research. Brain size (and therefore head circumference) may be enlarged in the young child with the disorder (DiCicco-Bloom et al., 2006). Data on increased head size in ASD and magnetic resonance imaging (MRI) results suggest that the disorder is due to malfunction of the cortex and the connectivity among brain regions (Williams & Minshew, 2007).

Risk Factors

Fetal alcohol syndrome, fragile X syndrome, phenylketonuria, Down syndrome, and tuberous sclerosis are all associated with a higher-than-normal incidence (Johnson et al., 2007) of autism spectrum disorders. Environmental factors likely interact with genetic phenotype in many cases of the condition. Advanced parental age, rubella infection in pregnancy, and teratogens have been associated with ASDs. Despite concern expressed in earlier medical and lay press reports, there has been no demonstrated relationship of measles-mumps-rubella vaccine, nor mercury-containing vaccines with the incidence of ASDs (Richler et al., 2006; D'Souza, Fombonne, & Ward, 2006; Katz, 2006).

CLINICAL MANIFESTATIONS

The essential features typically become apparent by the time a child is 3 years of age. They reflect impairments in the following:

- Social interactions
- Communication
- Ability to adapt to new situations
- Attention span and ability to organize responses to situations (Volkmar, Wiesner, & Westphal, 2006).

Social interactions are always complex and involve perceptions of the other person as well as social behaviors. The autistic child does not learn the common characteristics of these social interchanges. As a result, the child may be unable to converse normally, may fail to initiate conversations, and may fail to understand or observe nonverbal behavior.

Children with autism manifest disturbances in the rate or sequence of development, with onset of abnormal functioning in at least one of the following areas prior to age 3: social interaction, language used in social interactions, and imaginative play.

A primary finding is impairment in social interactions. Autistic children are unable to relate to people or to respond to social and emotional cues. In addition, autistic children engage in **stereotypy**, or rigid and obsessive behavior. Characteristically, these repetitive behaviors in affected children include head banging, twirling in circles, biting themselves, and flapping their hands or arms. Frequently, a child's behavior is self-stimulating or self-destructive. Responses to sensory stimuli are frequently abnormal and include an extreme aversion to touch, loud noises, and bright lights. Emotional lability (rapid, significant mood changes) is common (Figure 7–12 ■).

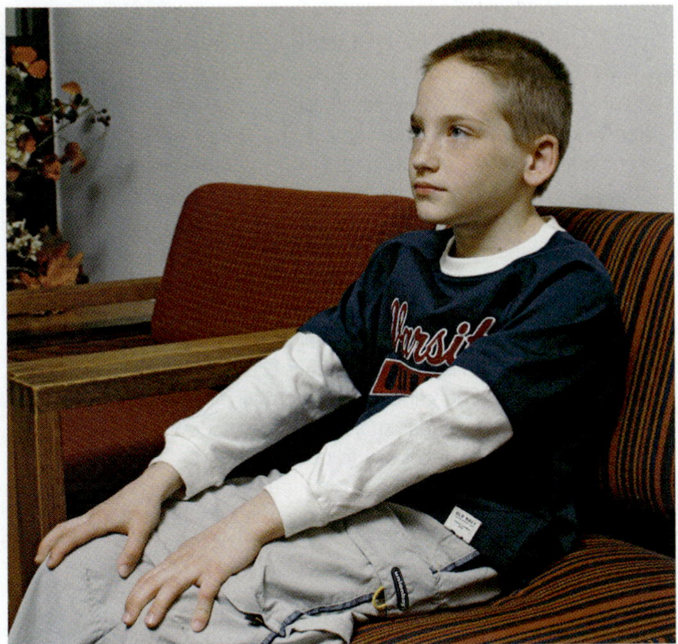

Figure 7–12 ■ This child with autism sits stiffly in the chair and engages in rhythmic rocking behavior. He has a disengaged appearance and does not readily interact with other children or adults who are in his environment.

Communication difficulties or delays in speech and language are common and are often the first symptoms that lead to diagnosis. Absence of babbling and other communication by 1 year, absence of two-word phrases by 2 years, and deterioration of previous language skills are characteristic of autism. Language acquisition develops normally in children with Asperger syndrome. Some children with Asperger syndrome exhibit abnormal verbal and nonverbal communication patterns, such as lack of eye contact. Children and adults with Asperger syndrome can participate fully in conversations, but may show characteristic behaviors such as marked lack of eye contact and lack of emotional reciprocity. They may or may not understand humor and other subtleties of language.

Autistic children may eventually learn to talk—in some cases well—but their speech is likely to show certain abnormalities, such as the following:

- Using *you* in place of *I*
- Engaging in **echolalia** (a compulsive parroting of a word or phrase just spoken by another)
- Repeating questions rather than answering them
- Being fascinated with rhythmic, repetitive songs and verses.

Behaviors of children with autism spectrum disorders show several differences from other children's behaviors. Children

CLINICAL MANIFESTATIONS AND THERAPIES **Autistic Spectrum Disorders (Pervasive Developmental Disorders)**

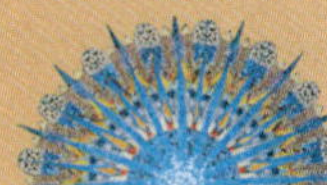

DISORDER	CLINICAL MANIFESTATIONS	CLINICAL THERAPIES
Autistic disorder	Impaired social, communicative, and behavioral development is usually noted in the first year of life.	Early intervention is key to maximal performance. Interventions focus on improving behaviors and communication skills, providing physical and occupational therapy, structuring play interactions with other children, and educating parents about the child's needs.
Asperger syndrome	Impaired social interactions with normal language development for age; pitch, tone, and other speech characteristics may be abnormal. Verbal skills involving spelling and vocabulary are high, with concept formation, language flexibility, and comprehension low.	Social interactions and speech and language therapy for pragmatics are the focus of therapy.
PDD-NOS	Severe social impairment without meeting *DSM* criteria for other types of ASD.	Behavioral therapy focuses on building social and language skills.

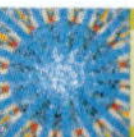

DEVELOPMENTAL CONSIDERATIONS Adults With Autism

Children with ASDs become adults with ASDs; there is no cure. Children who receive timely intervention and whose parents and treatment teams collaborate to find the best treatment for them as individuals have the greatest chance of becoming successfully functioning adults. Adults with ASDS continue to struggle with communication skills, especially understanding nonverbal communication, and socialization. These clients are most successful when they seek employment opportunities and activities that play to their strengths.

Many communities provide job training and supervised work programs for adults with ASDs. Many adults with high functioning autism or Asperger syndrome can function normally in their communities, becoming fully employed and living independently. Others need more support and may choose to continue to live with their parents or to reside in a group living environment that provides additional support. A number of government programs exist to assist these individuals with financial support. Information on these programs is available from the Social Security Administration (National Institute of Mental Health, 2009).

Unfortunately, there is a lack of research on adults with autism, especially the geriatric population. Few clinics exist that specifically treat disabled adults with ASDs, making it challenging for these adults to get the best level of care. Many adults with ASDs who cannot function independently or whose families can no longer provide care for them end up being financially subsidized by the state. With the steady rise in the number of children diagnosed with autism comes a resulting increase in the number of adults with the disorder. The financial impact on state governments is significant and is likely to increase steadily for many years. This is all the more reason that children with ASDs be identified early, so that they may have access to treatments and therapies that give them the best chance to become fully functioning adults.

with ASDs may have a great difficulty dealing with new situations and typically show agitation and withdrawal when routines are changed. Children with ASDs do not commonly explore objects, but have stereotyped behaviors. They may line up objects, play with the same objects over and over, and have certain rituals that must be performed. They often become upset if these normal routines are disrupted. Rituals may involve eating only certain types or colors of foods or eating in specific patterns.

Autistic children may manifest disturbances in the rate or sequence of development. Children with autism may be cognitively impaired, but they can demonstrate a wide range of intellectual ability and functioning. Cognitive impairment may be manifested early in life by slow developmental progression, particularly in social skills. Children with Asperger syndrome are of at least average intelligence, and some are highly gifted. Some children with ASDs are impaired in particular areas of development, while others are above normal. About 25% have macrocephaly, with reduced head size at birth, followed by excessive growth at 1–2 months and 6–14 months (Courchesne, Carper, & Akshoomoff, 2003). However, most children with ASDs have a normal appearance.

COLLABORATION

A number of agencies and resources are available to support the child with an autism spectrum disorder. Many communities have an interdisciplinary task force or team that meets regularly to review services available in their area for children with special needs, including ASDs. Public schools are charged with the responsibility of facilitating and providing services for children with ASDs and other disabilities. Nurses frequently serve on multidisciplinary teams to ensure that medical and mental health needs of these clients are included in supportive plans. Team members for a client with ASD may include any combination of the following: a nurse, a physician, a mental health professional, a classroom teacher, a speech therapist, an occupational or physical therapist, and parents.

Diagnostic Tests

Diagnosis is based on the presence of specific criteria, as described in the American Psychiatric Association's *Diagnostic and Statistical Manual of Mental Disorders*, 4th edition (*DSM-IV-TR*). See Box 7–4 for the autistic disorder, Box 7–5 for Asperger syndrome, and the *DSM-IV* for specific criteria for PDDs. Table 7–26 lists several screening tests that are useful in ASDs. Additional testing is done to rule out other causes of the child's behavior. Tests may include neuroimaging (computed tomography [CT] scan or MRI), lead screening, DNA analysis, and electroencephalogram.

Therapies

Early intervention assists in maximizing the child's potential by improving developmental skills and decreasing severity of symptoms, as well as establishing helpful support for parents (Giarelli, Souders, Pinto-Martin, Bloch, & Levy, 2005;

FOCUS ON DIVERSITY AND CULTURE Hispanics and Autism

Hispanics are diagnosed with autism far less frequently than are members of non-Hispanic groups. This is more likely the result of lack of access to services and lack of Spanish-speaking professionals in the United States than to any biomedical or genetic factor. As with any other culture, early intervention is critical to identifying and providing appropriate therapies and supports to the Hispanic child with autism. Nurses working with Hispanic families who do not have insurance should refer them to the local health department or department of social services to see whether their children qualify for Medicaid or the Child Health Insurance Plan. Nurses working in hospitals or health departments should ask whether families have a medical home and help them find one if they do not. Clinics offering developmental screenings to children should have at least one staff member trained to administer a valid, reliable screening tool that has been developed specifically for use with Spanish-speaking children and is not simply a tool that has been translated into Spanish.

Box 7–4 *DSM-IV-TR* Diagnostic Criteria for Autistic Disorder

A. A total of six or more items from 1, 2, and 3, with at least two from 1, and one each from 2 and 3:
   1. Qualitative impairment in social interaction, as manifested by at least two of the following:
      a. Marked impairment in the use of multiple nonverbal behaviors such as eye-to-eye gaze, facial expression, body posture, and gestures to regulate social interaction
      b. Failure to develop peer relationships appropriate to developmental level
      c. A lack of spontaneous seeking to share enjoyment, interests, or achievements with other people
      d. Lack of social or emotional reciprocity
   2. Qualitative impairments in communication as manifested by at least one of the following:
      a. Delay in, or total lack of, the development of spoken language (not accompanied by an attempt to compensate through alternative modes of communication such as gesture or mime)
      b. In individuals with adequate speech, marked impairment in the ability to initiate or sustain a conversation with others
      c. Stereotyped and repetitive use of language or idiosyncratic language
      d. Lack of varied, spontaneous make-believe play or social imitative play appropriate to developmental level
   3. Restricted repetitive and stereotyped patterns of behavior, interests, and activities, as manifested by at least one of the following:
      a. Encompassing preoccupation with one or more stereotyped and restricted patterns of interest that is abnormal either in intensity or in focus
      b. Apparently inflexible adherence to specific, nonfunctional routines or rituals
      c. Stereotyped and repetitive motor mannerisms (e.g., hand or finger flapping or twisting, or complex whole-body movements)
      d. Persistent preoccupation with parts of objects

B. Delays or abnormal functioning in at least one of the following areas, with onset prior to age 3 years: (1) social interaction, (2) language as used in social communication, or (3) symbolic or imaginative play.

C. The disturbance is not better accounted for by Rett's disorder or childhood disintegrative disorder.

Reprinted with permission from the *Diagnostic and Statistical Manual of Mental Disorders,* Fourth Edition, Text Revision. Copyright © 2000 American Psychiatric Association.

Rogers & Vishmara, 2008). Children are taught how to focus and apply learning. Treatment focuses on behavior management to reward appropriate behaviors, foster positive or adaptive coping skills, and facilitate effective communication. The goals of treatment are to reduce rigidity or stereotypy (repetitive, obsessive, machinelike movements) and other maladaptive behaviors. Often the child must be physically restrained from aggressive or self-destructive behaviors. Some parents choose to use complementary therapies such as vitamin supplements and dimethylglycine. Foods such as sugar, aspartame, milk products, and wheat are sometimes eliminated from the diet.

Box 7–5 *DSM-IV-TR* Diagnosis Criteria: Asperger Disorder

A. The diagnosis of Asperger disorder is made when the following symptoms are present:
   1. Qualitative impairment in social interactions, as manifested by at least two of the following:
      a. Marked impairment in the use of multiple nonverbal behaviors such as eye-to-eye gaze, facial expression, body postures, and gestures to regulate social interaction
      b. Failure to develop peer relationships appropriate to developmental level
      c. A lack of spontaneous seeking to share enjoyment, interests, or achievements with other people
      d. Lack of social or emotional reciprocity
   2. Restrictive and repetitive and stereotyped patterns of behavior, interests, and activities as manifested by at least one of the following:
      a. Encompassing preoccupation with one or more stereotyped and restricted patterns of interest that is abnormal either in intensity or focus
      b. Apparently inflexible adherence to specific, nonfunctional routines or rituals
      c. Stereotyped and repetitive motor mannerisms (e.g., hand or finger flapping or twisting, or complex whole-body movements)
      d. Persistent preoccupation with the parts of objects
   3. The disturbance causes clinically significant impairment in social, occupational, or other important areas of functioning.
   4. There is no clinically significant general delay in language (e.g., single words used by age 2 years, communicative phrases used by age 3 years).
   5. There is no clinically significant delay in cognitive development or in the development of age appropriate self-help skills, adaptive behavior (other than social interaction), and curiosity about the environment in childhood.
   6. Criteria are not met for another specific pervasive developmental disorder or schizophrenia.

Source: Reprinted with permission from the *Diagnostic and Statistical Manual of Mental Disorders,* Fourth Edition, Text Revision. Copyright © 2000 American Psychiatric Association.

TABLE 7–26 **Screening Tests for Autism Spectrum Disorders**

TEST	SOURCE
Clinical Practice Guidelines–Early Intervention Program of the New York State Department of Health	www.health.state.ny.us
Checklist for Autism in Toddlers (CHAT) or Modified Checklist for Autism in Toddlers (MCHAT)	Scambler, D., Rogers, S. J., & Wehner, E. A. (2001). Can the checklist for autism in toddlers differentiate young children with autism from those with developmental delays? *Journal of the American Academy of Child and Adolescent Psychiatry, 40,* 1457–1463.
Autism Diagnostic Interview–Revised	Lord, C., Rutter, M., & LeConteur, A. (1994). Autism Diagnostic Interview–Revised: A revised version of a diagnostic interview for caregivers of individuals with possible pervasive developmental disorder. *Journal of Autism and Developmental Disorders, 24,* 659–685.
Detection of Autism by Infant Sociability Interview (DAISI)	Hopson, R. P. (1993). *Autism and the development of mind.* Hillsdale, NJ: Erlbaum.
Screening Tool for Autism in Two-Year-Olds	Stone, W. L., Coonrod, E., & Osley, O. (2000). Brief report: Screening Tool for Autism in Two-Year-Olds (STAT): Development and preliminary data. *Journal of Autistic and Developmental Disorders, 30,* 607–612.
Autism Behavior Checklist	Gillberg, C., Nordin, V., & Ehlers, S. (1996). Early detection of autism: Diagnostic instruments for clinicians. *European Child and Adolescent Psychiatry, 5*(2), 67–74.
Autism Diagnostic Observation Schedule–Generic (ADOS-G)3p1.5	Lord, C., et al. (2000). The Autism Diagnostic Observation Schedule–Generic: A standard measure of social and communication deficits associated with the spectrum of autism. *Journal of Autism and Developmental Disorders, 30,* 205–233.
Childhood Autism Rating Scale (CARS)	Schopler, E., Reichler, R. J., & Renner, B. R. (1988). *The Childhood Autism Rating Scale (CARS).* Los Angeles: Western Psychological Services.
Developmental Checklist-Early Screen (DBC-ES)	Gray, K. M., Tonge, B. J., Sweeney, D. J. & Einfeld, S. L. (2007). Screening for autism in young children with developmental delay: An evaluation of the Developmental Behaviour Checklist-Early Screen.
Childhood Asperger Syndrome Test (CAST)	Williams, J. et al., (2005). The CAST (Childhood Asperger Syndrome Test): Test accuracy. *Autism, 9,* 45–68.

Medications are used with some children to treat associated disorders, but they are not effective in treatment of autistic syndrome itself. Medications used for associated conditions include stimulants, selective serotonin reuptake inhibitors (SSRIs), and mood stabilizers.

The overall prognosis for children with ASDs to become functioning members of society is guarded. The extent to which adequate adjustment is achieved varies greatly. Successful adjustment is more likely for children with higher IQs, adequate speech, and access to specialized programs.

Alternative Therapies

Some parents who have a child with autism choose to use complementary and alternative medicine (CAM), such as touch therapy or a gluten-free diet, in an attempt to help the child. It is important to note that CAM therapies have not been adequately evaluated; therefore, there is an insufficient research base to support or refute them individually or as a whole.

One approach includes dietary therapy with vitamin A, vitamin C, vitamin B6, magnesium, and omega-3 fatty acids. The use of gluten-free or casein-free diets has gained popularity in recent years. Parents have tried drug therapies that include secretin, a pancreatic gastrointestinal peptide, and Pepcid or other antacids. Some parents believe that detoxification by limiting certain dietary intake or using Epsom salt baths can be helpful (Levy & Hyman, 2003). Others may choose to investigate whether their child may benefit from chelation therapy, a form of detoxification that removes metals such as lead and mercury from the body. Like many alternative therapies for autism, this therapy has been considered controversial by some and embraced by others.

Nurses can help parents evaluate studies on complementary care and encourage parents to initiate only one treatment at a time; the effectiveness of any one treatment cannot be measured properly if it is initiated in conjunction with other therapies. At each health care interaction, the nurse working with a client with ASD should ask about therapies being used and discuss safeguards to avoid any undesired side effects.

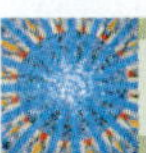

ALTERNATIVE THERAPIES **The GFCF Diet**

Many parents of children with ASDs choose to implement a gluten-free, casein-free (GFCF) diet. This has gained sufficient popularity that there are entire websites and programs devoted to this diet. Essentially, the GFCF diet eliminates the proteins gluten and casein from the client's diet. Gluten is normally found in wheat, barley, and rye. Casein is found in dairy products, including milk, cheese, and eggs. Nurses working with clients considering the GFCF diet should encourage them to consult with a nutritionist or registered dietician who can help them make sure that they plan GFCF meals that will meet their child's nutritional needs.

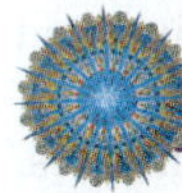

NURSING PROCESS

Assessment

The nurse may encounter the child with ASD when parents seek care for a suspected hearing impairment, speech difficulty, or developmental delay. Early and frequent developmental screening of all children can help in referral for thorough assessment and identification of cases. Parents may report abnormal interaction such as lack of eye contact, disinterest in cuddling, minimal facial responsiveness, and failure to talk. Be alert to observations by the parents that the baby or young child does not look at them or provide other developmental or behavioral cues (Beauchesne & Kelley, 2004). Initial assessment focuses on language development, response to others, and hearing acuity. Become familiar with the following "red flags" of the American Academy of Neurology and Child Neurology Society that require immediate evaluation.

- No babbling or communication gestures by 12 months
- No single word by 16 months
- No spontaneous two words by 24 months
- Loss of language or social skills previously achieved (Johnson et al., 2007)

Ask about birth history, including possible neonatal exposure to drugs or alcohol. Carefully evaluate the child for history of developmental milestones and refer for abnormalities. Perform developmental screening that considers several areas of development, including motor activity, social skills, and language, or refer the family to a professional or community resource that provides such screenings. Recall that the child may have normal performance in one area such as motor skills and delayed development in another area such as language skills. Likewise, language may be normal for age but social interactions may be quite delayed. Include questions about adaptive skills such as toilet training and feeding patterns. Inquire about school performance because some areas may be normal while others are delayed. Observe the child in play situations and evaluate the use of creative and exploratory play versus more repetitive patterns. Perform hearing and vision screening if possible to rule out sensory problems.

When a child with a diagnosis of autistic disorder is hospitalized for a concurrent problem, obtain a history from the parents regarding the child's routines, rituals, and likes and dislikes, as well as ways to promote interaction and cooperation. Autistic children may carry a special toy or object that they play with during times of stress. Ask parents about these objects and their use.

Ask about the child's behaviors and observe them on admission. Obtain a history of acute and chronic illnesses and injuries. Ask about eating patterns and food restrictions. Inquire about CAM in a nonjudgmental and supportive manner.

Diagnosis

Nursing diagnoses must be tailored to fit the individual needs of the child. Diagnoses that may be appropriate for children with autistic syndromes include the following:

- Impaired Verbal Communication
- Impaired Social Interaction related to developmental disability
- Disturbed Thought Processes
- Risk for Injury related to cognitive impairment
- Risk for Caregiver Role Strain related to the chronic demands of child's condition
- Compromised Family Coping.

Plan

Nursing care focuses on stabilizing environmental stimuli, providing supportive care, enhancing communication, maintaining a safe environment, giving the parents anticipatory guidance, and providing emotional support. Appropriate outcomes for a child with ASD may include the following:

- The child will remain free of injury.
- The child will acquire communication strategies that enable communication with others.
- The child will be able to perform self-care to maximum potential.
- The child will demonstrate consistent developmental progress.
- The child will participate in small group activities with family members or peers.
- The child's symptoms will be managed successfully.

Implementation

Working with children with autism spectrum disorder and their families requires patience, sensitivity, and understanding. While some parents may be aggressive about seeking information and resources, others may be too overwhelmed and exhausted by caring for their child to do this. For these parents, the nurse may be the most important, most accessible, and most caring resource available to them. Nurses must take the time to provide client teaching and support and affirm parents' efforts to help their children.

Stabilize Environmental Stimuli

Children with ASDs interpret and respond to the environment differently than other individuals. Sounds that are not distressing to the average person may be interpreted by autistic children as louder, more frightening, and overwhelming. They may respond to different sounds or environment by withdrawing, crying, or using ritualistic behaviors such as arm-flapping, which may or may not be self-injurious.

The child needs to be oriented to new settings such as a classroom or hospital room and may adjust best to a small classroom or a hospital room with only one other child. Encourage parents to bring the child's favorite objects from home. Try to keep these objects in the same places because the child with ASD does not cope well with changes in the environment.

Provide Supportive Care

Developing a trusting relationship with the autistic child is often difficult. Adjust communication techniques and teach to the child's developmental level. Ask parents about the child's usual home routines and maintain these routines as much as possible when the child is out of the home.

Because self-care abilities are often limited, the child may need assistance to meet basic needs. When possible, schedule daily care and routine procedures at consistent times to maintain predictability. Identify rituals for nap time and bedtime and maintain them to promote rest and sleep. Integrate patterns that facilitate intake of nutritious foods at mealtimes. School programs and IEPs can help the child learn self-care skills. Parents are integral parts of the treatment team when the child's learning goals are established in early intervention or school programs. If the child is hospitalized, encourage parents to remain with the child and to participate in daily care planning.

All clients with ASD need emotional support. Children who are developing successfully may face new challenges with the onset of the emotional and hormonal changes of adolescence. As social circles develop in middle and high school, the adolescent with autism may become more painfully aware of being different from other teenagers (Autism Speaks, 2009). The nurse may see this when a parent brings in a child after a scuffle at school or for help with increasing self-destructive behaviors as the child struggles to deal with the many changes. The nurse can provide crucial information about the physical changes adolescents experience and help the parent modify the plan of care to include opportunities for building new skills the child needs to navigate this difficult time.

Enhance Communication

Because children with autism have impaired communication, nursing care focuses on utilizing and improving communication with the child. Speech is used when possible; short, direct sentences are usually best (Galinat, Barcalow, & Krivda, 2005). If the child responds well to visual cues, then pictures, computers, and other visual aids may form an important part of interaction. Some children are able to learn and communicate through sign language.

Children with autism spectrum disorders benefit greatly from speech and language therapy. Encourage parents of these children to maintain close contact with speech therapists. Use of consistent communication techniques at home and at school provides further stability for the child and increases opportunities for successful communication.

Maintain a Safe Environment

Monitor autistic children at all times, including bath time and bedtime. Close supervision ensures that the child does not obtain any harmful objects or engage in dangerous behaviors. For the child who engages in head banging or other abusive behaviors, bicycle helmets and hand mitts can be the least restrictive method for providing safety. They enable the child to participate in activities and engage in a social environment to the degree possible.

Provide Anticipatory Guidance

Many children with autism spectrum disorders will require lifelong supervision and support, especially if the disorder is accompanied by mental retardation. Some children may grow up to lead independent lives, although they will have social limitations with impaired interpersonal relationships. Encourage parents to promote the child's development through behavior modification and specialized educational programs. The overall goal is to provide the child with the guidance, education, and support necessary for optimal functioning.

Care in the Community

Families of autistic children need a great deal of support to cope with the challenges of caring for the autistic child. They experience the challenges of families who have a child with a chronic disorder. Participating in parent support groups and learning how to reframe the condition to view its positive aspects are helpful strategies (Luther, Canham, & Cureton, 2005). Many communities offer training programs for parents, in addition to support groups. Help parents identify resources for child care, such as special toddler programs and preschools.

The child may need specialized transportation services or other social supports. The school-age child will need an IEP. The parent or primary caretaker often has difficulty obtaining respite care and may need assistance to find suitable resources. Siblings of the autistic child may need help explaining the disorder to their friends or teachers. The nurse can be instrumental in assisting these siblings in understanding and explaining autism. Family support programs are available in some states to provide assistance to parents.

Genetic counseling should be offered to the family. Information on immunizations is necessary because parents may have heard about a potential connection between immunization and the disorder. They should be encouraged to have the child immunized on the recommended schedule. Parents may have questions about where to find information on complementary and alternative therapies.

Local support groups for parents of autistic children are available in most areas. Families can also be referred to the Autism Society of America for information.

Evaluation

At each health care interaction, the nurse should discuss with the child's progress with the parents. The nurse should discuss any injuries that have occurred since the previous visit and the steps being taken to prevent recurrence. The nurse should ask parents what type of environments the child is in during the day, paying particular attention to the frequency of transitions and changes in caregivers. For example, a child with ASD who attends school or an early intervention program at a preschool will do well having the same caregiver drop off the child in the morning and pick up the child at the end of the school day.

For children who are enrolled in early intervention programs or who have IEPs at school, the nurse should participate as part of the treatment team when possible. If this is not possible, the nurse should ask the parent how the child's treatment is progressing and continue to encourage open communication between the parents and the treatment team. For children who are taking medication to treat a comorbid disorder such as depression or ADHD, the nurse should, with parent permission, provide the necessary information to the treatment team so that the team is aware of potential side effects.

REVIEW Autism Spectrum Disorders

RELATE: LINK THE CONCEPTS

Linking the exemplar of Autism Spectrum Disorders with the concept of Family:

1. How can the nurse support the family of a child with autism?
2. How might other children in the family be impacted by a sibling with autism?

Linking the exemplar of Autism Spectrum Disorders with the concept of Safety:

3. What interventions are important for the nurse to initiate to maintain the safety of a client with autism?
4. What would be important at school?

REFER: GO TO MY NURSINGKIT

REFLECT: CASE STUDY

Chad, age 4, was recently diagnosed with an autistic disorder. Chad's mother keeps ruminating about her pregnancy, wondering what she did that "caused" Chad's illness. Chad recently became angry and reacted by banging his head against the wall. His parents told the nurse they do not believe that the doctor made the right diagnosis.

1. Based on the case study, what are the priorities of nursing care for Chad?
2. Based on the statement made by Chad's parents, what are his parents experiencing?
3. How might the nurse locate resources to help Chad's parents learn more about having a child with autism? What resources might the nurse find?

7.3 CEREBRAL PALSY

KEY TERMS

Cerebral palsy (CP), *385*

BASIS FOR SELECTION OF EXEMPLAR

Centers for Disease Control and Prevention

LEARNING OUTCOMES

After reading about this exemplar, you will be able to:

1. Describe the pathophysiology, etiology, clinical manifestations, and direct and indirect causes of cerebral palsy.
2. Identify risk factors associated with cerebral palsy.
3. Illustrate the nursing process in providing culturally competent care across the life span for individuals with cerebral palsy.
4. Formulate priority nursing diagnoses appropriate for an individual with cerebral palsy.
5. Create a plan of care for individuals with cerebral palsy and their family members.
6. Assess expected outcomes for an individual with cerebral palsy.
7. Discuss therapies used in the collaborative care of an individual with cerebral palsy.
8. Employ evidence-based caring interventions for an individual with cerebral palsy.

OVERVIEW

Cerebral palsy (CP) is a group of chronic conditions affecting body movement, coordination, and posture that results from a nonprogressive abnormality of the immature brain. CP is often the result of some type of insult to the developing brain of the fetus, neonate, or infant that occurs in the later stages of pregnancy, during birth, or within the first two years after birth. The impact of the disease can range from mild to profound mobility issues; CP may or may not include mental retardation.

Cerebral palsy is a common chronic disorder of childhood, occurring in an estimated 2 to 3 per 1000 births (Nehring, 2004). Four types of motor dysfunction are seen with CP—spastic, dyskinetic, ataxic, and mixed—related to the location of brain insult. Children with severe impairment of mobility and feeding skills have a greater risk of dying during childhood (Liptak & Accardo, 2004).

PATHOPHYSIOLOGY AND ETIOLOGY

The exact insult leading to CP may not be identifiable if it occurs during the prenatal period. After delivery, the cause of the insult is more likely to be identified. Insults may include any combination of hypoxic-ischemic encephalopathy, vascular, metabolic, infectious, toxic, teratogenic, traumatic, or genetic events. The insult alters muscle tone, muscle stretch reflexes, postural reactions, and primitive reflexes and may also result in seizures, mental retardation, and/or hearing problems. The outcome depends on the area of the brain affected, the severity of the event, the duration of the insult, and the child's age at the time of the event.

The exact pathogenesis is multifactorial and not clearly understood. It is believed that damage is done to the motor areas of the brain, impairing the body's ability to control movement and adjust posture appropriately. CP is neither contagious nor inherited and is not progressive. It cannot be cured, but it can be managed.

CP is often identified when children fail to meet expected developmental milestones and diagnostic testing is ordered to pinpoint the reason for the delay. Symptoms and manifestations vary from person to person depending on the exact neurologic impact of the event.

Etiology

Most CP cases are believed to be caused by congenital, hypoxic, ischemic, or infectious intrauterine insults to the central nervous system (CNS) (McKearnan, Kieckhefer, Engel, Jensen, & Labyak, 2004). The risk for CP is increased when intrauterine infection (chorioamnionitis) is documented (Van Eerden & Bernstein, 2003). Injury to the immature periventricular white matter in fetuses and premature infants is thought to be the most common cause of CP (Johnston, Ferriero, Vannucci, & Hagberg, 2005). At one time, hypoxia was considered the primary culprit for CP, but studies revealed that only 4% of children with CP were found to have experienced a known hypoxic event (Speer & Hankins, 2003).

The rate of CP increases with decreasing gestational age; approximately 20% of infants born before 27 weeks' gestational age are diagnosed with CP (Ancel et al., 2006). Birth asphyxia is believed to account for only 9% of CP cases. No reduction of incidence of CP has been noted since the use of electronic fetal heart rate monitoring was implemented (Van Eerden & Bernstein, 2003). In young children, CNS infection and head trauma are the major sources of acquired brain injury and subsequent motor dysfunction.

Risk Factors

Increased risk for CP is found in mothers older than 40 or younger than 20 years of age, fathers who are 20 years of age or younger, and mothers or fathers with African American ethnicity. The risk is highest in first-born children and in children born subsequent to the fourth child. Prematurity, multiple births, low birth weight, blood type incompatibility, neonatal sepsis, and hyperbilirubinemia place the infant at higher risk for development of CP. Multiple risk factors at the same time can further increase the odds of developing CP.

CLINICAL MANIFESTATIONS

Cerebral palsy is characterized by abnormal muscle tone and lack of coordination, with spasticity found in the majority of cases (Table 7–27). Children have a variety of symptoms depending on their age (Figure 7–13 ■). See Table 7–26 for symptoms by type of central nervous system injury. There is wide variability in symptoms depending on the area of the brain involved and the degree of anoxia.

Children with CP usually are delayed in meeting developmental milestones. For example, at 6 months of age, they may

TABLE 7–27 Clinical Characteristics of Cerebral Palsy

CLINICAL CHARACTERISTICS	DEFINITIONS
Hypotonia	Floppiness, increased range of motion of joints, diminished reflex response
Hypertonia	Tense, tight muscles
Rigidity	Uncoordinated, awkward, stiff movements;
Spasticity	scissoring or crossing of the legs; exaggerated reflex reactions
Athetosis	Constant involuntary writhing motions that are more severe distally
Ataxia	Poor muscle control during voluntary movement, poor balance
Hemiplegia	Involvement of one side of the body, with the upper extremities being more dysfunctional than the lower extremities
Diplegia	Involvement of all extremities, but the lower extremities are more affected than the upper, usually spastic
Quadriplegia	Involvement of all extremities with the arms in flexion and legs in extension

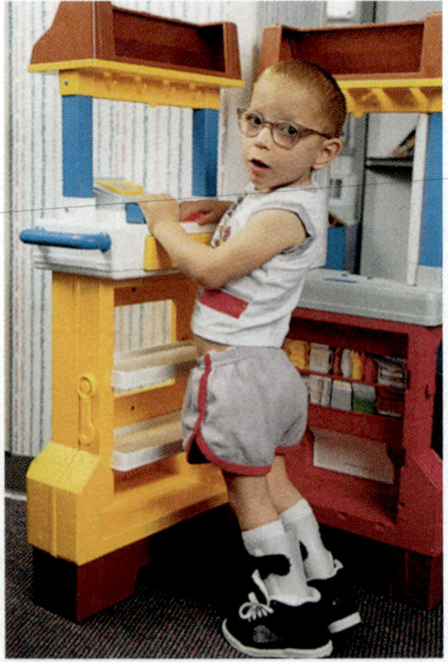

Figure 7–13 ■ A child with cerebral palsy has abnormal muscle tone and lack of coordination.

CLINICAL MANIFESTATIONS AND THERAPIES Cerebral Palsy

CLASSIFICATION AND TYPE OF INSULT	CLINICAL MANIFESTATIONS	CLINICAL THERAPIES
Spastic	Persistent hypertonia, rigidity	■ Physical therapy ■ Muscle relaxants ■ Braces, splints, and orthotics
Cerebral cortex or pyramidal tract injury	Exaggerated deep tendon reflexes	■ In addition to therapies used for spastic CP, surgery may be required to loosen contractures or to repair curvature of the spine.
75% of cases	Persistent primitive reflexes Leads to contractures and abnormal curvature of the spine	
Dyskinetic	Impairment of voluntary muscle control accompanied by appearance of involuntary movements (e.g., tics, chorea)	
Extrapyramidal, basal ganglia injury	Bizarre twisting movements	
10–15% of cases	Tremors, difficulty with fine and purposeful motor movements Exaggerated posturing Rigid muscle tone when awake and normal or decreased muscle tone when asleep Inconsistent muscle tone that may change hour to hour or day to day	
Ataxic Cerebellar (extrapyramidal) injury	Abnormalities of voluntary movement involving balance and position of the trunk and limbs	■ Canes, crutches, walkers, and other orthotics may be needed to promote mobility.
5–10% of cases	Difficulty controlling hand and arm movements when reaching Increased or decreased muscle tone Hypotonia in infancy Muscle instability and wide-based, unsteady gait	
Mixed Injuries to multiple areas	No dominant motor pattern Unique compensatory movements and posture to maintain control over specific neuromotor deficits Combination of characteristics from other types	

have persistent back arching, show little spontaneous movement, and be unable to sit up. They frequently have other problems, including visual defects such as strabismus (abnormal alignment of the eyes or "crossed eyes"), nystagmus (involuntary rapid eye movement), or refractory errors; hearing loss; language delay; speech impediment; or seizures. Feeding may be difficult because of oral motor involvement. Approximately 75% of children with CP have mental retardation or learning disabilities (Liptak & Accardo, 2004).

Collaboration

Care of the client with CP requires a collaborative care team including nurses, physical therapists, occupational therapists, physicians, orthotics, speech therapists, dietitians, and social services. CP is a lifelong condition that requires special consideration, particularly in the growing child who quickly outgrows orthotic devices and must meet changing developmental needs.

Diagnostic Tests

Diagnosis is usually based on clinical findings. CP is difficult to diagnose in the early months of life, as it must be distinguished from other neurologic conditions and signs may be subtle. Suspicious findings include an infant who is small for his or her age or has a history of prematurity; low Apgar score (0–3 at 5 minutes); or inflammatory, traumatic, or anoxic event (Van Eerden & Bernstein, 2003). However, the majority of children who develop CP have normal Apgar scores at birth. Ultrasonography can be used to detect fetal and neonatal abnormalities of the brain, such as intraventricular hemorrhage. Neuromotor tests are used to evaluate the presence of normal movement patterns and absence of primitive reflexes and abnormal tone. Once CP is suspected, CT scans, MRI, and positron emission tomography may be performed.

Clinical Therapy

It is not uncommon for children who are delayed in meeting developmental milestones or have neuromuscular abnormalities at 1 year of age to show gradual improvement in function. Half of the infants suspected to be at risk for CP at 1 year of age are unimpaired neurologically by 2 years of age due to physical maturation (Pelligrino, 2002).

Clinical therapy focuses on helping the child develop to a maximum level of independence. Referrals are made for physical, occupational, and speech therapy, as well as special education to improve motor function and ability. Braces and splints, serial casting, and positioning devices (prone wedges, standers, and sidelyers) are used to promote range of motion, skeletal alignment, stability, and control of involuntary movements. They are also used to prevent contractures. Physical therapy and occupational therapy promote optimal independent functioning.

Surgery

Surgical interventions may be required to improve function by balancing muscle power and stabilizing uncontrollable joints. The Achilles tendon may be lengthened to increase range of motion in the ankle, which allows the heel to touch the floor and thus improves ambulation. The hamstrings may be released to correct knee flexion contractures. Other procedures may be performed to improve hip adduction or correct the foot's natural position. A dorsal rhizotomy may be performed for spastic diplegia to cut the afferent fibers that contribute to spasticity; however, some muscle weakness may result from the procedure (Pelligrino, 2002).

Pharmacologic Therapy

Medications are given to control seizures, to control spasms (skeletal muscle relaxants, baclofen, and benzodiazepines), and to minimize gastrointestinal side effects (cimetidine or ranitidine). Baclofen is administered by intrathecal pump to decrease muscle tone and vasospasms when oral administration is ineffective or causes side effects (Pelligrino, 2002). See Figure 7–14 ■. Botulinum toxin injection into specific muscles is a relatively new therapy used to help control spasticity (Buck, 2003).

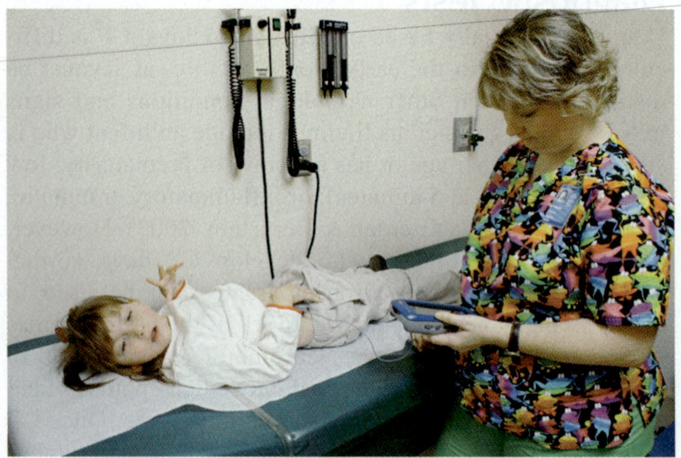

Figure 7–14 ■ This child is having a baclofen pump filled.

Early Intervention Programs

The prognosis for infants and children with CP depends on the level of physical involvement and on the presence of intellectual, visual, or hearing deficits. Early intervention programs can significantly improve performance. Many children with hemiplegia or ataxia show some improvement with maturation and are able to ambulate. Others need assistance with mobility and activities of daily living. They are usually cared for in their homes, although some receive care in long-term care facilities.

NURSING PROCESS

Nursing care focuses on early intervention, prevention of complications, and support of children and families to help them cope with the diagnosis of CP.

Assessment

Be alert for children whose histories indicate an increased risk for CP. Assess all children at each health care visit for developmental delays. Note any orthopedic, visual, auditory, or intellectual deficits. Assess for newborn reflexes, which may persist beyond the normal age in a child with CP. Identify infants who appear to have abnormal muscle tone or abnormal posture (child has an arched back, child becomes stiff when moving against gravity, child's neck or extremities have increased or decreased resistance to passive movement). A child with asymmetric or abnormal crawling using two or three extremities indicates a motor problem. Hand dominance before the preschool years is another sign of a motor problem. Record dietary intake as well as height and weight percentiles for children suspected to have or to be diagnosed with the condition.

PRACTICE ALERT

Evaluate all infants who show symptoms of developmental delays, feeding difficulties caused by poor sucking, or abnormalities of muscle tone. Two simple screening assessments are as follows:

- Place a clean diaper on the 6–12 month old infant's face. The infant without special needs will use two hands to remove it, but the infant with CP will use one hand or will not remove the cloth at all.
- Turn the infant's head to one side. A persistent asymmetric tonic neck reflex (beyond 6 months of age) indicates a pathologic condition. Suspect CP in any infant who has persistent primitive reflexes.

Diagnosis

Nursing diagnoses for the child with CP vary depending on the type of CP, the particular child's symptoms and age, and the family situation. The accompanying Nursing Care Plan includes several diagnoses that may be appropriate. Additional nursing diagnoses may include the following:

- Risk for Constipation related to low intake of fiber and fluids and insufficient physical activity
- Impaired Tissue Integrity related to decreased physical mobility and limited self-care ability

- Impaired Verbal Communication related to hearing and/or speech impairment
- Impaired Home Maintenance related to child's developmental disability and inadequate support system
- Chronic Pain related to spasticity and stretching exercises to prevent contractures
- Delayed Growth and Development related to lack of muscle strength or limited social interaction
- Caregiver Role Strain related to caring for chronically ill child with special needs.

Plan

Because the condition can range from mild to severe and may involve numerous manifestations, care planning must be highly individualized on the basis of specific needs of each individual. It may include the following goals:

- The client will demonstrate appropriate growth and development.
- The client will maintain an appropriate diet to meet nutritional needs.
- The client and family will monitor bony prominences to avoid altered skin integrity.

Implementation

Interventions need to be adapted to the particular child and family. Nursing care focuses on providing adequate nutrition, maintaining skin integrity, promoting physical mobility, promoting safety, promoting growth and development, teaching parents how to care for the child, and providing emotional support.

Provide Adequate Nutrition

Children with CP require high-calorie diets or supplements to the diet because of feeding difficulties associated with spasticity. Many children have difficulty chewing and swallowing. Give the child small amounts of soft foods at a time. Utensils with large, padded handles may be easier for the child to use.

Maintain Skin Integrity

Take special care to protect the bony prominences from skin breakdown. Monitor the skin under splints and braces for redness. If the skin is red, the braces or splints should be removed and not replaced until the redness is gone.

Proper body alignment should be maintained at all times. Support the child with pillows, towels, and bolsters whether the child is in bed or in a chair. Support the head and body of a floppy infant. A child with spasticity may have scissored, extended legs, and a child with athetoid movements may be difficult to carry and transport.

Promote Physical Mobility

Range-of-motion exercises are essential to maintain joint flexibility and to prevent contractures. Consult with the child's physical therapist and help with recommended exercises. Teach parents to position the child to foster flexion rather than extension so that the child can more easily interact with the environment (for example, by bringing objects closer to the face). Consider the use of therapeutic massage or relaxation training to manage pain associated with spasticity and stretching exercises (McKearnan et al., 2004).

Adaptive and assistive technology may be needed to promote mobility and communication. Assistive technology is any item, equipment, or product customized for use to promote the functional capabilities and independence of an individual with disabilities. Examples include computers, adaptive utensils, and customized wheelchairs. Refer parents to the appropriate resources for help obtaining adaptive devices. Encourage parents to bring in the child's adaptive appliances (braces, positioning devices) for use during hospitalization.

Promote Safety

Safety belts should be used for children in strollers and wheelchairs. An adaptive care safety seat may be needed to transport the child safely. A child with chronic seizures should wear a helmet to protect against further injury.

Promote Growth and Development

Remember that many children with CP are physically disabled but not necessarily intellectually disabled. Use terminology appropriate for the child's developmental level. Help the child develop a positive self-image to ensure emotional health and social growth. Adaptive devices may be available to help the child with CP to communicate more independently. Children with a hearing impairment may need a referral to learn American Sign Language or other communication methods. Provide audio and visual activities for the child who is quadriplegic.

Foster Parental Knowledge

Teach parents about the disorder and arrange sessions to teach them about all of the child's special needs. Teach administration, desired effects, and side effects of medications prescribed for seizures. Make sure parents are aware of the need for dental care for children taking anticonvulsants and other medications, as they can impact oral health.

Parents also may need suggestions for amending parenting strategies to promote the child's autonomy and abilities.

Provide Emotional Support

Parents require emotional support to help them cope with the diagnosis. Listen to the parents' concerns and encourage them to express their feelings and ask questions. Explain what they can expect from future treatment. Refer parents to individual and family counseling if appropriate. Work with other health care professionals to help families adjust to this chronic disease.

Evaluation

Clients are evaluated based on their ability to meet goals identified in the plan of care, which may include the following:

- Client's growth is appropriate for age.
- Client meets developmental milestones appropriate for age.
- Client's nutritional status is adequate for age and energy needs.

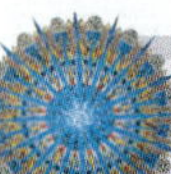

NURSING CARE PLAN A Client With Cerebral Palsy

ASSESSMENT

Justine McBride is a 2-year-old African American child. Her mother was 41 when she delivered Justine, and Justine's father was 45. Justine is the seventh child in the family. Her mother works outside the home as a chemistry teacher at the local high school, and her father is an accountant for a large firm. Justine's mother became concerned that Justine was not walking when she turned 14 months old; all of her other children were walking by 12 months of age. Diagnostic tests were performed, and Justine was diagnosed with spastic CP.

Examination of Justine demonstrates scissoring of the legs when prone, stiff movements of arms and legs, hyperreflexia, and muscular rigidity.

DIAGNOSES

- Impaired Physical Mobility related to decreased muscle strength and control
- Imbalanced Nutrition: Less Than Body Requirements related to difficulty in chewing and swallowing and high metabolic needs
- Ineffective Therapeutic Regimen Management: Family related to excessive demands made on family with child's complex care needs

PLANNING

Goals for Justine's care include the following:

- Justine will reach maximum physical mobility and all developmental milestones.
- Justine will receive adequate visual sensory/perceptual input to maximize developmental outcome.
- Justine will exhibit normal growth patterns for height, weight, and other physical parameters.
- Justine's family will successfully support all of its members.
- Justine will participate in activities to maximize development.

IMPLEMENTATION

Recreation Therapy: *Purposeful use of recreation to promote relaxation and enhancement of social skills.*

- Refer the family to an early intervention program. Encourage contact with other children. If Justine is hospitalized, place her in a room with other children whenever possible.
- Work with Justine's preschool to develop an IEP that encourages interaction with peers and a variety of activities that support development.
- Investigate recreational programs for children with disabilities and share information with the parents.

Family Mobilization: *Utilization of family strengths to influence Justine's health in a positive direction.*

- Allow chances for parents to verbalize the impact of CP on the family. Refer to other parents and support groups.
- Explore community services for rehabilitation, respite care, child care, and other needs and refer family as appropriate.
- During home and office visits, review Justine's achievements and praise the family for care provided.
- Teach the family skills needed to manage Justine's care (e.g., medication administration, muscle stretching, physical rehabilitation, seizure management).
- Teach case management techniques.
- Involve Justine's older siblings in her care. Review with parents the needs of all children in the family.

Nutrition Management: *Assistance with or provision of a balanced dietary intake of foods and fluids.*

- Monitor height and weight and plot on a growth grid. Perform hydration status assessment.
- Teach the family techniques to promote caloric and nutrient intake.
- Position Justine upright for feedings.
- Place foods far back in the mouth to overcome tongue thrust.
- Use soft and blended foods.
- Allow extra time for chewing and swallowing.
- Obtain adaptive handles for utensils and encourage self-feeding skills.
- Apply manual jaw control technique if it helps the child to control jaw movement.
- Perform frequent respiratory assessment. Teach the family to avoid aspiration pneumonia.

Exercise Therapy, Joint Mobility: *Use of active and passive body movement to maintain or restore joint flexibility.*

- Perform development assessment and record age of achievement of milestones (e.g., reaching for objects, sitting).
- Plan activities to use gross and fine motor skills (e.g., holding a pen or eating utensils, reaching for toys and rolling over).
- Allow time for the child to complete activities.
- Perform range-of-motion exercises every 4 hours for the child who is unable to move body parts. Position the child to promote tendon stretching (e.g., foot plantar flexion instead of dorsiflexion, legs extended instead of flexed at knees and hips).
- Arrange for and encourage parents to keep appointments with a rehabilitation therapist.
- Teach the family to maintain appropriate brace wear.

EVALUATION

The client's progress in meeting the goals of care is based on the following expected outcomes:

Joint Movement—Active: *Range of motion of joints with self-initiated movement.*

- Justine reaches maximum physical mobility and all developmental milestones.

Nutritional Status: Nutrient Intake: *Adequacy of nutrients taken into the body.*

- Justine shows normal growth patterns for height, weight, and other physical parameters.

NURSING CARE PLAN A Client With Cerebral Palsy *continued*

Family Functioning: *Ability of the family to meet the needs of its members through developmental transitions.*

- Justine demonstrates appropriate growth and developmental progress. The family successfully supports all of its members.

Play Participation: *Use of activities as needed for enjoyment, entertainment, and development by children.*

- Justine engages in activities to maximize development.

CRITICAL THINKING

1. What support groups exist in your area that could help Justine's family cope with this diagnosis?
2. Why is involvement of the older siblings important?
3. How would you assess Justine's cognitive ability? Is cognition always impacted by CP?

CARE SETTINGS Care of the Child With CP in the Community

Children with CP need continuous support in the community. A case manager, such as the parent or a nurse, is often needed to coordinate care. Parents may need financial assistance to provide for the child's needs and to obtain appliances such as braces, wheelchairs, or adaptive utensils. As they grow, children need new adaptive devices, ongoing developmental assessment and care planning, and, sometimes, surgery. Although the brain lesion does not change, it manifests differently as the child grows. For example, once the child begins to walk, the extensor tone may cause tightening of the Achilles cord. Braces may decrease deformities, but surgery may be needed eventually.

Early intervention programs can help parents meet their child's special needs, by providing physical, occupational, and speech therapy. Early education programs also help meet the child's educational needs. The child often needs an Individual Education Plan (IEP) or an Individual Family Service Plan (for children younger than three years of age) to maximize learning potential. The nurse can be instrumental in helping parents meet the needs of the child with CP in preschools, schools, offices, clinics, and other settings. In addition, the nurse makes referrals, as appropriate, to support groups and organizations such as the United Cerebral Palsy Association and Shriners Hospitals.

An individualized transition plan developed during adolescence assists the family and adolescent with CP to develop plans for adult living. Vocational training options can be explored. The young adult (18–21 years) may be able to move into a group home or live independently if desired.

REVIEW Cerebral Palsy

REVIEW: LINK THE CONCEPTS

Linking the exemplar of Cerebral Palsy with the concept of Comfort:

1. How might you help to promote comfort in a child with CP who is required to wear braces and orthotics to bed at night?
2. If spasticity of muscles cause pain, what nonpharmacologic strategies might you recommend?

Linking the exemplar of Cerebral Palsy to the concept of Cognition:

3. While caring for a child diagnosed with CP who also has mild cognitive impairment, how would you help the child become increasingly autonomous in performing range-of-motion exercises?
4. How might you encourage this child's parents to promote autonomy?

READY: GO TO COMPANION SKILLS MANUAL

- Assisting the client to use crutches
- Assisting the client to use a walker
- Monitoring intake and output
- Applying dry heat measures
- Applying dry cold measures

REFER: GO TO MYNURSINGKIT

REFLECT: CASE STUDY

Frangelica Gonzalez, 12 years old, was born with CP. She began working with physical therapists when she was less than 1 year old and has worn braces on her legs and used crutches to allow her greater mobility for as long as she can remember. Her mother and father have always told her she can overcome any challenge and do anything other children do if she tries hard enough. As a result of her parent's encouragement and support, Frangelica is a member of the school swim team, plays jazz piano, and has a large circle of friends. She has a younger brother who is 9 years old, an older brother who is 15 years old, and an identical twin sister who is healthy and does not have CP.

Lately her parents have noticed that Frangelica is moody, often seeming depressed, and her twin sister told their mother that Frangelica is "tired of being different." Frangelica has been waking in the morning offering various physical complaints as reasons why she can't go to school that day, ranging from a stomachache to a sore foot.

1. Why might Frangelica suddenly be feeling different and trying to find reasons not to go to school?
2. What strategies might you recommend to Frangelica's parents to help her cope with the developmental changes she is experiencing?
3. What strategies might you recommend to Frangelica to explore and cope with her feelings?

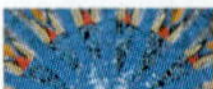

7.4 FAILURE TO THRIVE

KEY TERMS

Failure to thrive (FTT), *392*

BASIS FOR SELECTION OF EXEMPLAR

Centers for Disease Control

Health People 2010

World Health Organization

LEARNING OUTCOMES

After reading about this exemplar, you will be able to:

1. Describe the pathophysiology, etiology, clinical manifestations, and direct and indirect causes of failure to thrive.
2. Identify risk factors associated with failure to thrive.
3. Illustrate the nursing process in providing culturally competent care across the life span for individuals with failure to thrive.
4. Formulate priority nursing diagnoses appropriate for an individual with failure to thrive.
5. Create a plan of care for individuals with failure to thrive and their family members.
6. Assess expected outcomes for an individual with failure to thrive.
7. Discuss therapies used in the collaborative care of an individual with failure to thrive.
8. Employ evidence-based caring interventions for an individual with failure to thrive.

OVERVIEW

Failure to thrive (FTT) describes a syndrome in which an infant falls below the fifth percentile for weight and height on a standard growth chart or is falling in percentiles on a growth chart (Pillitteri, 2003). This disorder accounts for 1–5% of pediatric hospitalizations in children under 1 year of age, and many more children are managed in community settings. From 5–10% of low-birth-weight infants are affected (Behrman, Kliegman, & Jenson, 2004).

PATHOPHYSIOLOGY AND ETIOLOGY

Etiology

The cause of FTT can be organic, as in congenital acquired immune deficiency syndrome (AIDS), inborn errors of metabolism, neurologic disease, and esophageal reflux. However, most cases of FTT are nonorganic in origin. FTT resulting from nonorganic causes is called *feeding disorder of infancy or early childhood.*

Risk Factors

Infants who are deprived of mothering, especially from 3–15 months of age, will not learn to form significant relationships or to trust others. Touch, cuddling, and visual and auditory stimulation are all critical for the infant. Through these mechanisms, the baby comes to know self and the environment. Infants who fail to establish a loving, responsive relationship with a caregiver often fail to develop normally.

Infants and children whose parents or caretakers suffer from depression, substance abuse, mental retardation, or psychosis, or who have a history of abuse are at risk for FTT. Their parents may be socially and emotionally isolated or may lack knowledge of infant nutritional and nurturing needs. A multifactorial and reciprocal interaction pattern may exist whereby the parent does not offer enough food or is not responsive to the infant's hunger cues and, as a result, the infant is irritable, not soothed, and does not give clear cues about hunger. Preterm and small-for-gestational-age babies more commonly have eating disorders (Block & Krebs, 2005).

CLINICAL MANIFESTATIONS

The characteristics of this feeding disorder are persistent failure to eat adequately with no weight gain or with weight loss in a child under 6 years of age. The disorder is not associated with other medical conditions or mental disorders; it is not caused by lack of or unavailability of food (American Psychiatric Association Working Group on Eating Disorders, 2000). Infants with feeding disorders refuse food, may have erratic sleep patterns, are irritable and difficult to soothe, fall well under expected growth patterns, and are often developmentally delayed (Figure 7–15 ■).

Infants with inorganic FTT show delayed development without any physical cause. They are often malnourished and fail to gain weight and grow normally. Behavior may be apathetic, withdrawn, demonstrate poor eye contact, and the child may lack anticipated stranger danger.

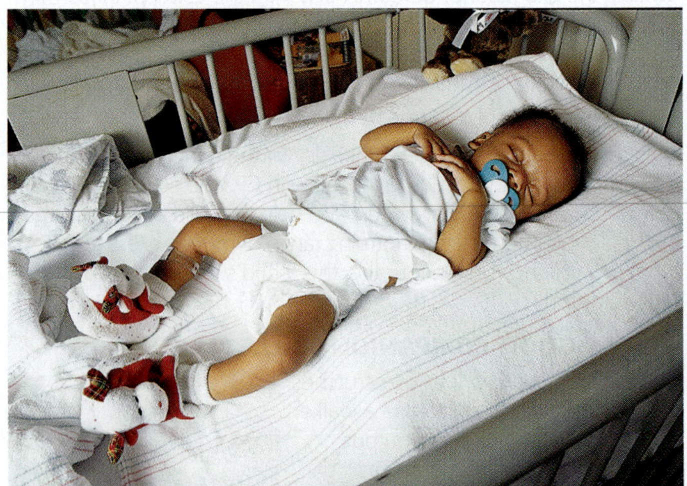

Figure 7–15 ■ Infants with failure to thrive may not look severely malnourished, but they fall well below the expected weight and height norms for their age and population. This infant, who appears to be about 4 months old, is actually 8 months old. He has been hospitalized for examination of his failure to thrive and treatment of the eating disorder.

COLLABORATION

A thorough history and physical examination are needed to rule out any chronic physical illness. The infant or child may be hospitalized so that health care providers can establish a routine for feeding and sleeping. The goals of treatment are to provide adequate caloric and nutritional intake, promote normal growth and development, and assist parents in developing feeding routines and responding to the infant's cues of physical and psychologic hunger.

NURSING PROCESS

Nursing care is directed toward improving the child's nutritional intake with the end result of increasing growth and health of the child. This may be accomplished through parent teaching; observation of child–parent interactions, especially during feeding times; and careful recording of height and weight on growth charts.

Assessment

Assessment of the child is essential for establishing the best intervention plan. Take accurate measurement of weight, height, BMI, and percentiles each time a child interacts with a health care provider to develop an important record of growth patterns over time. This helps to identify the child with an eating disorder. The child's activity level, developmental milestones, and interaction patterns also provide important information. When feeding the child, observe how the child indicates hunger or satiety, the ability of the child to be soothed, and general interaction patterns such as eye contact, touch, and cuddliness.

Ask parents about stressors in their lives that may prevent or interefere with appropriate interaction with the child. Questions about the pregnancy and delivery can elicit information about early disturbances in the child–parent relationship. Ask whether there are other children in the family and whether they have experienced feeding problems. It is important for the nurse to observe the child's and parents' behaviors when the parents feed the child; cues given by each person and interactional modes such as rocking, singing, talking, and body postures are important.

Diagnosis

Nursing diagnoses pertinent for the young child with failure to thrive may include the following:

- Imbalanced Nutrition: Less Than Body Requirements related to inability to ingest proper amounts of food
- Delayed Growth and Development related to inadequate intake
- Risk for Impaired Parenting related to lack of knowledge about nutritional needs
- Fatigue related to malnutrition.

Plan

The goals of the nursing care for the child with failure to thrive may include the following:

- Child will attain adequate growth and normal development.
- The parent–child relationship will improve.
- Parental understanding of the child's nutritional requirements will improve.
- Complications associated with poor nutrition will be prevented.

Implementation

Nursing care centers on performing a thorough history and physical assessment, observing parent–child interactions during feeding times, and providing necessary teaching to enable parents to respond appropriately to their child's needs. The child is often hospitalized initially so that staff members can establish feeding and sleeping patterns and evaluate the child's physical growth. Accurate weights, nutritional assessments, and developmental evaluation should be done to see if the child grows more normally. Additional diagnostic tests may be given to rule out organic causes of the poor growth.

Once a diagnosis of nonorganic FTT is confirmed, parents become involved in feeding the child. Observations of feeding and continued careful physical assessments are needed. Teach parents to record carefully the child's intake at each meal or feeding. Teach parents how to understand and respond to the child's cues of hunger and satiety. Teach them to hold, rock, and touch the infant during feeding and to establish eye contact with infants and older children.

Upon discharge, refer parents to an early childhood intervention agency that can continue monitoring the home situation. Agency staff can observe feeding during a home visit and evaluate stresses and behavior patterns among family members. Frequent growth measurement and development must be ensured so that the child is adequately nourished. Parents may need referral to community resources to help them manage stressful situations and to enhance their parenting skills.

Evaluation

The child's outcomes are largely evaluated based on the following:

- Growth and development of the child improve.
- The parent–child relationship improves.
- The parent voices a specific action plan to improve and maintain appropriate growth of child.
- The child experiences no long-term complications as a result of FTT.

FOCUS ON DIVERSITY AND CULTURE
Growth Measurement

Each child should maintain a height and weight growth pattern similar to the population standard. It may be normal for Asian American children to be below the fifth percentile on growth charts and not have an eating disorder. American children tend to be larger, and growth charts are based on American averages. Suspect an eating disorder when the infant or child falls one standard deviation below the curve and fails to gain weight or loses weight over several months.

REVIEW Failure to Thrive

RELATE: LINK THE CONCEPTS

Linking the exemplar of Failure to Thrive with the concept of Acid–Base Balance:

1. How might excessive protein metabolism as the result of inadequate sources of energy supply from dietary intake impact the client's acid–base balance?
2. How might altered glucose metabolism as a result of inadequate caloric intake impact the client's acid–base balance?

Linking the exemplar of Failure to Thrive with the concept of Elimination:

3. How might inadequate caloric and nutrient intake impact elimination?
4. If caloric and nutrient intake is increased suddenly, how might the client's elimination habits be impacted?

READY: GO TO COMPANION SKILLS MANUAL

- Measuring height
- Measuring weight
- Measuring body mass index
- Administering a tube feeding

REFER: GO TO MYNURSINGKIT

REFLECT: CASE STUDY

Hilary is born 8 weeks prematurely at 32 weeks' gestation to a single adolescent mother. Hilary remains in the neonatal intensive care unit for 10 weeks until she is stable enough to be discharged. Her mother tries to visit at least once a week and is sometimes able to visit more often depending on whether someone can give her a ride to and from the hospital.

Hilary returns for her 6-week check-up and is found to have gained only 2 ounces, increasing her weight from 5 lb 2 oz (2.32 kg) to 5 lb 4 oz (2.38 kg). The provider schedules a follow-up visit for 2 weeks from now, and the nurse explains Hilary's nutritional requirements. Two weeks later, when Hilary returns, she has lost 1 ounce in weight.

1. Does Hilary qualify as having FTT? Explain your answer.
2. Do you suspect an organic or inorganic cause of her failure to gain weight?
3. Develop a nursing plan of care for Hilary.

PEARSON

EXPLORE mynursingkit™

MyNursingKit is your one stop for online chapter review materials and resources. Prepare for success with additional NCLEX®-style practice questions, interactive assignments and activities, web links, animations and videos, and more!

Register your access code from the front of your book at **www.mynursingkit.com**.

REFERENCES

Adesman, A. (2003). A diagnosis of ADHD? Don't overlook the probability of comorbidity! *Contemporary Pediatrics, 20*(12), 91–106.

Administration on Aging, U.S. Department of Health and Human Services. (2003). *Statistics: A profile of older Americans, 2003.* Retrieved May 4, 2009, from http://www.aoa.gov/AoAroot/Aging_Statistics/Profile/2003/4.aspx#figure1

American Academy of Pediatrics. (2004). *Pediatric nutrition handbook* (5th ed.). Elk Grove Village, IL: Author.

American Association of Retired Persons. (2004). *Profile of older Americans, 2004.* Washington, DC: Resource Services Group.

American Medical Association. (2004). *Breaking news: The social and economic impact of ADHD.* Retrieved June 7, 2005, from http://www.ama-assn.org/ama/pub/category/print/12869.html

American Psychiatric Association. (2000). *Diagnostic and statistical manual of mental disorders* (4th ed., text revision). Washington, DC: American Psychiatric Association.

American Psychiatric Association Working Group on Eating Disorders. (2000). Practice guidelines for the treatment of patients with eating disorders. *American Journal of Psychiatry, 157,* 1–39.

Ancel, P. Y., Livinec, F., Larroque, B., Marret, S., Arnaud, C., Pierrat, V., et al. (2006). Cerebral palsy among very preterm children in relation to gestational age and neonatal ultrasound abnormalities: The EPAPAGE cohort study. *Pediatrics, 117*(3), 828–835.

Anderson, V. R., & Scott, L. J. (2006). Methylphenidate transdermal system: In attention-deficit hyperactivity disorder in children. *Drugs, 66,* 1117–1126.

Autism Speaks. (2009). Teens and adults. Retrieved August 15, 2009, from http://www.autismspeaks.org/howtogrow/index.php?WT.svl=Top_Nav

Bakker, L. J., & Cavender, A. (2003). Promoting culturally competent care for gay youth. *Journal of School Nursing, 19,* 65–72.

Bandura, A. (1986). *Social foundations of thought and actions: A social cognitive theory.* Englewood Cliffs, NJ: Prentice Hall.

Bandura, A. (1997a). *Self-efficacy: The exercise of control.* New York: W. H. Freeman.

Bandura, A. (1997b). *Self-efficacy in changing societies.* New York: Cambridge University Press.

Barber, S., Grubbs, L., & Cottrell, B. (2005). Self-perception in children with attention deficit/hyperactivity disorder. *Journal of Pediatric Nursing, 20,* 235–245.

Beauchesne, M. A., & Kelley, B. R. (2004). Evidence to support parental concerns as an early indicator of autism in children. *Pediatric Nursing, 30,* 57–67.

Behrman, R. E., Kliegman, R. M., & Jenson, H. B. (2004). *Nelson textbook of pediatrics* (17th ed.). Philadelphia: Saunders.

Block, R.W., & Krebs, N. F. (2005). Failure to thrive as a manifestation of child neglect. *Pediatrics, 116,* 1234–1237.

Bronfenbrenner, U. (1986). Ecology of the family as a context for human development: Research perspectives. *Developmental Psychology, 22,* 723–742.

Bronfenbrenner, U. (Ed.). (2005). *Making human beings human: Bioecological perspectives on human development.* Thousand Oaks, CA: Sage Publications.

Bronfenbrenner, U., McClelland, P. D., Ceci, S. J., Moen, P., & Wethington, E. (1996). *The state of Americans.* New York: Free Press.

Brown, R. T., Amler, R. W., Freeman, W. S., Perrin, J. M., Stein, M. T., Feldman, H. M., et al. (2005). Treatment of hyperactivity disorder: Overview of the evidence. *Pediatrics, 115,* e749–e757.

Buck, M. L. (2003). Clinical applications for botulinum toxin type A in pediatric patients. *Pediatric Pharmacology, 9*(3), Retrieved April 18, 2003, from http://www .medscape.com/viewarticle/451626

Call-Schmidt, T., & Maharaj, G. (2004). Using nonpharmacological treatments in conjunction with stimulant medications for children with ADHD. *Journal of Pediatric Health Care, 18,* 255–259.

Centers for Disease Control and Prevention. (2006). Improved national prevalence estimates for 18 selected major birth defects—United States, 1999–2001. *Morbidity and Mortality Weekly Report, 54,* 1301–1305.

Chess, S., & Thomas, A. (1995). *Temperament in clinical practice.* New York: Guilford Press.

Chess, S., & Thomas, A. (1996). *Temperament: Theory and practice.* Philadelphia: Brunner/Mazel Publishers.

Chess, S., & Thomas, A. (1999). *Goodness of fit: Clinical applications from infancy through adult life.* Philadelphia: Brunner/Mazel Publishers.

Christakis, D. A., Zimmerman, F. J., DiGiuseppe, D. L., & McCarty, C. A. (2004). Early television exposure and subsequent attentional problems in children. *Pediatrics, 113,* 708–713.

Courchesne, E., Carper, R., & Akshoomoff, N. (2003). Evidence of brain overgrowth in the first year of life in autism. *Journal of the American Medical Association, 290,* 337–344.

Cummings, E., & Henry, W. (1961). *Growing old: The process of disengagement.* New York: Basic Books.

Dennis, C. L. (2006). Identifying predictors of breastfeeding self-efficacy in the immediate postpartum period. *Research in Nursing and Health, 28,* 256–268.

DiCicco-Bloom, E., Lord, C., Zwaigenbaum, L., Courchesne, E., Dager, S. R., Schmitz, C., et al. (2006). The developmental neurobiology of autism spectrum disorder. *Journal of Neuroscience, 26,* 6897–6906.

Diego, M. A., Jones, N. A., Field, T., Hernandez-Reif, M., Schanberg, S., Kuhn, C., et al. (2006). Maternal psychological distress, prenatal cortisol, and fetal weight. *Psychosomatic Medicine, 68,* 747–753.

D'Souza, Y., Fombonne, E., & Ward, B. J. (2006). No evidence of persisting measles virus in peripheral blood mononuclear cells from children with autism spectrum disorder. *Pediatrics 118,* 1664–1675.

Eaton, D. K., Kann, L., Kinchen, S., Ross, J., Hawkins, J., Harris, W. A., et al. (2006). Youth risk behavior surveillance—United States, 2005. *Morbidity and Mortality Weekly Report, 55*(SS05), 1–108.

Edwards, M. E. (2002). Attachment, mastery, and interdependence: A model of parenting processes. *Family Process, 41*(3), 389–404.

Erikson, E. (1963). *Childhood and society.* New York: W.W. Norton.

Erikson, E. (1968). *Identity: Youth and crisis.* New York: W.W. Norton.

Federwisch, A. (2005). Paying attention: Helping families cope with ADHD. *Nurseweek, 18*(21), 10–12.

Fowler, J., & Keen, S. (1985). *Life maps: Conversations in the journey of faith.* Waco, TX: Word Books.

Fowler, J. W., Streib, H., & Keller, B. (2004). *Manual for faith development research* (3rd ed.). Bielefeld, Germany: Research Center for Biographical Studies in Contemporary Religion; Atlanta: Center for Research in Faith and Moral Development, Emory University.

Froehlich, T. E., Lanphear, B. P., Epstein, J. N., Barbaresi, W. J., Katusic, S. K., & Kahn, R. S. (2007). Prevalence, recognition, and treatment of attention-deficit/hyperactivity disorder in a national sample of US children. *Archives of Pediatrics and Adolescent Medicine, 161,* 857–864.

Galinat, K., Barcalow, K., & Krivda, B. (2005). Caring for children with autism in the school setting. *Journal of School Nursing, 21,* 208–217.

Garvey, C., Julion, W., Fogg, L., Kratovil, A., & Gross, D. (2006). Measuring participation in a prevention trial with parents of young children. *Research in Nursing & Health, 29,* 212–222.

Giarelli, E., Souders, M., Pinto-Martin, J., Bloch, J., & Levy, S. E. (2005). Intervention pilot for parents of children with autistic spectrum disorder. *Pediatric Nursing, 31,* 389–399.

Gilligan, C. (1982). *In a different voice: Psychological theory and women's development.* Cambridge, MA: Harvard University Press.

Gould, R. L. (1972). The phases of adult life: A study in developmental psychology. *American Journal of Psychiatry, 129,* 33–43.

Havighurst, R. J. (1972). *Developmental tasks and education* (3rd ed.). Boston: Allyn & Bacon.

Huizink, A. C., & Mulder, E. J. (2006). Maternal smoking, drinking, or cannabis use during pregnancy and neurobehavioral and cognitive functioning in human offspring. *Neuroscience and Biobehavior Review, 30,* 24–41.

Johnson, C. P., Myers, S. M., and the Council on Children with Disabilities (2007). Identification and evaluation of children with autism spectrum disorders. *Pediatrics, 120,* 1183–1215.

Johnston, M.V., Ferrio, D. M., Vannucci, S. J., & Hagberg, H. (2005). Models of cerebral palsy: Which ones are best? *Journal of Child Neurology,* 20(12), 984–987.

Johnston, M. V., & Kinsman, S. (2004c). Microcephaly. In R. E. Behrman, R. M. Kliegman, & H. B. Jepson, *Nelson textbook of pediatrics* (17th ed., pp. 1988–1989). Philadelphia: Saunders.

Katz, S. L. (2006). Has the measles-mumps-rubella vaccine been fully exonerated? *Pediatrics 118,* 1744–1745.

Kohlberg, L. (1981). *Essays on moral development: Vol. 1. The philosophy of moral development.* San Francisco: Harper & Row.

Kohlberg, L. (1984). *Essays on moral development: Vol. 2. The psychology of moral development.* San Francisco: Harper & Row.

Levy, S. E., & Hyman, S. L. (2003). Use of complementary and alternative treatment for children with autistic spectrum disorders is increasing. *Pediatric Annals, 32,* 685–691.

Liptak, G. S., & Accardo, P. J. (2004). Health and social outcomes of children with cerebral palsy. *Journal of Pediatrics, 145*(Suppl.), S36–S41.

Luther, E. H., Canham, D. L., & Cureton, V. Y. (2005). Coping and social support for parents of children with autism. *Journal of School Nursing, 21,* 40–47.

Malone, J. A. (1998). The resiliency model of family stress, adjustment, and adaptation. In B. Vaughan-Cole, M. A. Johnson, J. A. Malone, & B. L. Walker. *Family nursing practice* (pp. 49–60). Philadelphia: W.B. Saunders.

McCarter-Spaulding, D. E. (2005). Medications in pregnancy and lactation. *MCN: American Journal of Maternal/Child Nursing, 30,* 10–17.

McKearnan, K. A., Kieckhefer, G. M., Engel, J. M., Jensen, M. P., & Labyak, S. (2004). Pain in children with cerebral palsy: A review. *Journal of Neuroscience Nursing, 36*(5), 252–259.

Murray, R. B., & Zentner, J. P. (2001). *Health promotion strategies through the life span* (7th ed.). Upper Saddle River, NJ: Prentice Hall.

National Center on Birth Defects and Developmental Disabilities. (2004a). *ADHD: Attention-deficit/hyperactivity disorder.* Retrieved June 16, 2005, from http://www/ cdc.gov/ncbddd/adhd/injury.htm

National Institute of Mental Health. (2009). Adults with autism spectrum disorder. Retrieved July 20, 2009, from http://www.nimh.nih.gov/health/publications/autism/ adults-with-an-autism-spectrum-disorder.shtml

Nehring, W. M. (2004). Cerebral palsy. In P. J. Allen & J. A. Vessey (Eds.), *Primary care of the child with a chronic condition* (4th ed., pp. 327–346). St. Louis, MO: Mosby.

Nierenberg, A. A., Miyahara, S., Spencer, T., Wisniewski, S. R., Otto, M. W., Simon, N., et al. (2005). Clinical and diagnostic implications of lifetime attention-deficit/ hyperactivity disorder comorbidity in adults with bipolar disorder. *Biological Psychiatry, 57*(11), 1467–1473.

Peck, R. (1968). Psychological developments in the second half of life. In B. L. Neugarten (Ed.), *Middle age and aging.* Chicago: University of Chicago Press.

Pelligrino, L. (2002). Cerebral palsy. In M. L. Batshaw (Ed.), Children with disabilities (5th ed., pp. 443–466). Baltimore: Paul H. Brooks Publishing Co.

Piaget, J. (1966). *Origins of intelligence in children.* New York: W.W. Norton.

Pillitteri, A. (2003). *Maternal & child health nursing: Care of the childbearing & childrearing family* (4th ed.). Philadelphia: Lippincott Williams & Wilkins.

Reiff, M. I. (2006). ADHD: A guide to assessment and diagnosis. *Psychiatric Times, 5*(8), 104. Retrieved December 12, 2007, from http://www.psychiatrcitimes .com/topic/ADHD

Rew, L., Whittaker, T. A., Taylor-Seehafer, M. A., & Smith, L. R. (2005). Sexual health risks and protective resources in gay, lesbian, bisexual, and heterosexual homeless youth. *Journal of Specialists in Pediatric Nursing, 10,* 11–19.

Richler, J., Luyster, R., Risi, S., Hsu, W. L. Dawson, G., Bernier, R., et al. (2006). Is there a "regressive phenotype" of autism spectrum disorder associated with the measles-mumps-rubella vaccine? A CPEA Study. *Journal of Autism and Developmental Disorders, 36,* 299–316.

Rogers, S. J., & Vishmara, L. A. (2008). Evidence-based comprehensive treatments for early autism. *Journal of Clinical Child and Adolescent Psychology, 37,* 8–38.

Rojas, N. L., & Chan, E. (2005). Old and new controversies in the alternative treatment of attention-deficit-hyperactivity disorder. *Mental Retardation and Developmental Disability Research Review, 11,* 116–130.

Schieve, L. A., Rice, C., Boyle, C., Visser, S.M., & Blumberg, S. J. (2006). Mental health in the United States: Parental report of diagnosed autism in children ages 4–17 years – United States, 2003–2004. *Morbidity and Mortality Weekly Report, 55,* 481,487.

Speer, M., & Hankins, G. D. (2003). Defining the true pathogenesis and pathophysiology of neonatal encephalopathy and cerebral palsy. *Journal of Perinatology, 23,* 179–180.

Stein, M. A., & Barren, M. (2003). Welcome progress in the diagnosis and treatment of ADHD in adolescence. *Contemporary Pediatrics, 20*(8), 83–107.

Stewart, M., Reid, G., & Mangham, C. (1997). Fostering children's resilience. *Journal of Pediatric Nursing, 12,* 21–31.

Van Eerden, P., & Bernstein, P. S. (2003). Summary of the publication, "Neonatal encephalopathy and cerebral palsy: Defining the pathogenesis and pathophysiology" by the ACOG Task Force on Neonatal Encephalopathy and Cerebral Palsy. *Medscape OB/GYN & Women's Health, 8*(2) Retrieved July 10, 2003, from http://www.medscape.com/viewarticle/457882_

Volkmar, F. R., Wiesner, L. A., & Westphal, A. (2006). Healthcare issues for children on the autism spectrum. *Current Opinions in Psychiatry, 19,* 361–366.

Westerhoff, J. (1976). *Will our children have faith?* New York: Seabury Press.

Williams, D. L., & Minshew, N. J. (2007). Understanding autism and related disorders: What has imaging taught us? *Neuroimaging Clinics of North America, (17),* 495–509.

Witt, C. (2003). Detecting developmental dysplasia of the hip. *Advances in Neonatal Care, 3,* 65–75.

Wolraich, M. L., Wibbelsman, C. J., Brown, T. E., Evans, S. W., Gotlieb, E. M., Knight, J. R., et al. (2005). Attention-deficit/hyperactivity disorder among adolescents: A review of the diagnosis, treatment, and clinical implications. *Pediatrics, 115,* 1734–1746.

8 Diversity

Concept at-a-Glance

BASIS FOR SELECTION OF CONCEPT

Healthy People 2010

Concept Learning Outcomes

After reading about this concept, you will be able to:

1. Define terms used in the study of diversity.
2. List factors that contribute to diversity.
3. Describe the importance of the nurse's self-knowledge regarding prejudgment and bias related to diversity.
4. Contrast the diverse needs of various groups of clients based on race, age, gender, sexual orientation, and membership in a vulnerable population.
5. Create a plan of care for the client that considers the client's needs related to the client's individual diversity.

Concept Key Terms

Ageism, *401*
Bias, *398*
Bisexuals, *400*
Cross-dressing, *400*
Discrimination, *398*
Diversity, *398*
Heterosexism, *401*
Heterosexual, *400*
Homophobia, *400*
Homosexual, *400*
Intersex, *400*
Lesbian, *400*
Prejudice, *398*
Race, *404*
Sexual orientation, *400*
Stereotyping, *398*
Transsexuals, *400*
Vulnerable populations, *403*
Xenophobia, *398*

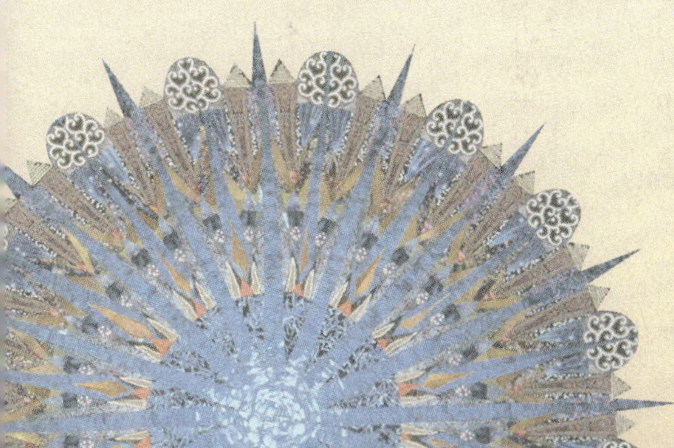

About Diversity

Imagine a large campground with people from various cities and states staying in tents and campers. Everyone has returned to camp to prepare the evening meal when suddenly a bear crashes the picnic and heads for the area where the children are playing. Do you think everyone in the camp would react at the same time and in the same way? Why or why not? What factors would influence people's responses? The key to the answers lies in understanding diversity. Based on a number of characteristics and experiences, some campers may scream, some may freeze, others may run to save the children, while still others may turn and run away. Even if everyone in the camp came from the same cultural background, differences in age, gender, personality, and experience would make many of them react differently under the circumstances. This difference in response is diversity, the unique attributes that combine to make all people one of a kind. •

FACTORS THAT CONTRIBUTE TO DIVERSITY

Nurses must never forget that human beings are different regardless of culture, race, or population sector. **Diversity** refers to the unique variations among and between individuals, variations that are informed by genetics and cultural background, but that are refined by experience and personal choice. Although people from a given culture share certain beliefs, values, and experiences, often there is widespread intragroup diversity. This diversity causes individuals to look at health care, lifestyle choices, and treatment options in different ways. It further impacts how clients will respond to medications, surgical procedures, and client teaching, often in ways that may not be anticipated. Diversity is the reason individualization of nursing care is so important, because unlike the claims of some clothing manufacturers, one size does *not* fit all. To optimize the outcome for each individual when planning and delivering care for a client, the nurse must consider culture, client needs, and diverse client responses.

One of the major goals of *Healthy People 2010* is to eliminate health disparities by gender, race, or ethnicity; education; income; disability; geographic location; and sexual orientation. To achieve that goal, the Health Resources and Services Administration (HRSA) aims to increase the number of underrepresented racial and ethnic groups entering the nursing profession (Public Health Foundation, 2009). Greater diversity among nursing professionals will result in improved understanding of clients from diverse groups (Figure 8–1 ■). However, this diversity can create conflict if others' unique perspectives are not taken into consideration. Stereotyping, prejudice, and discrimination can threaten the delivery of health care services and impact client outcomes. Nurses need to understand and recognize these attitudes in themselves and others in order to reduce their effects on the clients they serve.

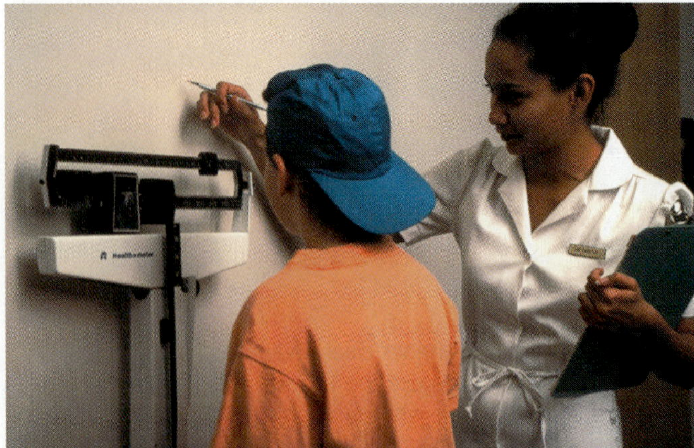

Figure 8–1 ■ Hispanic nurses made up less than 2% of the population of nurses in 2004.

Stereotyping refers to the act of making assumptions that all people in a given group are the same. For example, a nurse may assume that all women are highly verbal or that all older people have numerous health problems. Stereotyping may be based on generalizations founded in research, or it may be based on assumptions unrelated to reality. For example, research indicates that women tend to be more verbal than men, but a specific woman may not be more verbal than men in general. Stereotyping that is unrelated to reality is frequently an outcome of prejudice. Nurses need to realize that not all people of a specific group have the same health beliefs, practices, and values. Therefore, it is essential for nurses to identify a specific client's beliefs, needs, and values rather than assume they are the same as those attributable to the larger group.

Prejudice, or **bias**, is a negative belief or preference that is generalized about a group that leads to "prejudgment." Prejudice occurs because the person making the judgment does not understand the individual or the individual's diverse background or because the person making the judgment generalizes an experience of one individual from a group to all members of that group. A related concept is **xenophobia**—the fear or dislike of people different from oneself. While prejudice often refers to racial differences, it also can refer to negative beliefs about older adults, the homeless, or those from other groups outside the person's realm of understanding. Nurses, in particular, tend to hold prejudices against those who make unhealthy lifestyle choices such as smoking and overeating. Prejudice can lead to **discrimination**, the differential treatment of individuals or groups based on categories such as race, age, weight, gender, or social class, occurs when a person acts on prejudice and denies other people one or more of their fundamental rights (Figure 8–2 ■). Discrimination also occurs when a person acts on prejudice to deny someone from a particular group the same opportunities provided to other groups.

SOURCE OF DIVERSITY

The family, as the basic unit of society, teaches values that impact how individual family members view differences in others outside the family. The family also teaches values regarding the expected role of different members of society. For example, if the man is considered the breadwinner and leader of the family, while the woman is expected to care for the home and family, their children may believe that a woman who acts as breadwinner is overly ambitious or abandoning her family.

The following factors contribute to one's individual diversity:

- Age
- Gender
- Sexual orientation
- Socioeconomics
- Living arrangements
- Race
- Culture
- Education
- Life experiences.

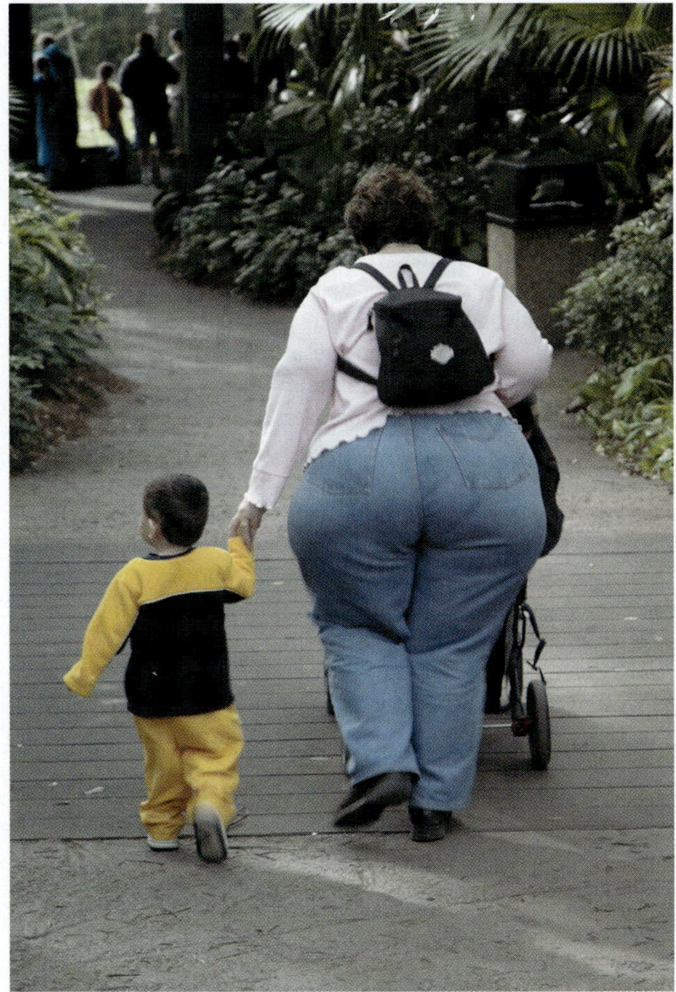

Figure 8–2 ■ Obese people face discrimination from many sources. Nurses should avoid discriminating against obese clients.

Those are just the primary factors that play a role in impacting how people approach life and problem solving. Personality also factors into diversity, with some people being shy, some being outspoken, others being confrontational, while still others being peacekeepers. Culture is discussed in more detail in Concept 6, Culture, and personality differences are explained in Concept 24, Self. This concept examines in greater detail the remaining factors related to diversity and looks at how they impact nursing practice.

GENDER

Differences in men and women vary by culture and in different societies. Some cultures assign specific roles, responsibilities, and positions in both the family and the community (Ostlin, Eckermann, Mishra, Nkowane, & Wallstam, 2007). While Western culture aims to minimize the differences in men and women with the belief that the sexes are equal, nonetheless men and women are more than just biologically different. Depending on the beliefs their families taught, men and women may take "traditional" roles, with the women caring for the home and family while the man earns an income. Increasingly, however, both men and women work outside the home in order to make ends meet. These parents usually share child care or divide the responsibilities in a way that works best for their family. In recent years, more fathers have become stay-at-home dads while the mothers take on the financial responsibilities. This trend has resulted from a combination of the recession that began in 2007–2008, the fact that women are beginning to achieve jobs that pay sufficient wages to enable them to financially support their families, and the increasing social acceptability of women in roles outside the home.

Differences between men and women go beyond anatomy and physiology and cultural or social definitions. Compared to women, men typically are less verbal and more action-oriented, having stronger skills in logic, mathematics, and coordination; women tend to be more skilled in languages, perceiving and responding to others' needs, and the arts. However, these are general tendencies: Even within genders, individual diversity is expected; for example, some women may be highly coordinated, mathematically skilled, and disinterested in the arts. No conclusion about an individual can ever be drawn based on a simple term such as *woman* or *man.*

How the male and female roles are defined greatly influences how men and women manage health, wellness, and illness. This can be demonstrated by viewing the differences in mortality and morbidity between men and women of different cultures as well as their involvement in health prevention and health promotion programs.

The genders also differ in access to and control over resources and decision-making power in the family and community. The extent of these differences is often cultural. Gender and sex, often in interaction with socioeconomic circumstances, influence exposure to health risks, access to health information and services, health outcomes, and the social and economic consequences of ill health. Therefore, it is crucial to recognize the root causes of gender inequities when designing the nursing plan of care. Health promotion and disease prevention and treatment need to address gender differences equally if positive outcomes are to be obtained. For example, millions of women are injured as the result of spousal or significant other abuse, but the magnitude and health consequences of domestic violence against women have often been neglected in both research and policy (Garcia-Moreno, 2002).

When planning and implementing health promotion and disease prevention strategies, nurses should not neglect the importance of gender (Cristofides, 2001; Ostlin, 2002; Roses Periago, 2004). Generally, there seems to be an assumption that interventions will be just as effective for men as for women. Many health promotion programs are gender-blind and are based on research that neither accounted for nor controlled for the sex of the study participants. "Many health promotion strategies aim at reducing risky behaviors, such as smoking, while ignoring the material, social and psychological conditions within which the targeted behaviors are embedded" (Ostlin et al, 2007).

Until the last decade, most new medications were tested only on white men, with no consideration that women or people of other ethnicities respond differently. Only in the mid 1990s did pharmaceutical companies begin to look at the difference between male and female responses. Understanding the differences in responses between genders has led to research on how drugs affect women as well as those from different races and cultural backgrounds. As a result, scientists are finding that some drugs are more effective for women while others are more effective for men. One example is Seldane (terfenadine), which was removed from the market when it was associated with torsades de pointes, a condition that occurs most commonly in women because women have longer Q-T intervals than men.

In addition to the way in which men and women respond to health promotion, they also display different needs with regard to their response to the same diagnosis. For example, the traditional symptom of crushing chest pain as a primary indicator of myocardial infarction has been found to be primarily a male response. Women with myocardial infarction are more likely to experience extreme fatigue that extends to pain in the jaw, back, or shoulder if not treated early in the symptomatology. Biologic differences such as genetics, hormones, and metabolic influences combine to play a part in shaping different symptoms as well as morbidity and mortality rates (Doyal, 2001). Gender differences have been shown in both responses to and perceptions of pain.

Research also indicates a distinct gender difference in approach to seeking health care. Women are more likely to report symptoms early when visiting the health care provider, while men often postpone seeking care until the problem interferes with their daily lives. Further research is needed to determine whether this contributes to the longer life span of women in the United States.

About 1 in every 2,000 babies is born with an **intersex** condition in which there are contradictions among chromosomal gender, gonadal gender, internal organs, and external genital appearance. The gender of such an infant is ambiguous, as the child is born with some parts usually associated with males and some parts usually associated with females. Intersex anatomy may not be apparent at birth. Sometimes it is undetected until puberty, until the person is identified as an infertile adult, or until the person dies and is autopsied. For more information, refer to the Intersex Society of North America website at www.isna.org.

By improving their understanding of how gender differences impact client health, nurses can develop a plan of care that meets the specific and unique health care needs of each client. It is important that nurses not allow their own gender bias or preconceived beliefs to affect their ability to assess and plan appropriate care for the individual client. Health-promoting interventions aimed at inclusion in a safe and supportive environment promote a trusting nurse–client relationship. Nurses should promote an environment in which clients can access essential services that address the differences between men and women in an equitable manner. When planning care, nurses who take into consideration the biologic differences and social vulnerability of men and women are more likely to see positive outcomes for their clients.

SEXUAL ORIENTATION

An individual's attraction to people of the same sex, opposite sex, or both sexes is referred to as **sexual orientation**. Sexual orientation is a continuum ranging from those who have a strong preference for a partner of the same sex to those who strongly prefer someone of the opposite sex. **Homosexual** individuals prefer a partner of the same sex, with the term **lesbian** used to describe women who prefer to develop intimate relationships with other women. **Heterosexual** individuals prefer a partner of the opposite sex to develop an intimate relationship. Individuals who are attracted to people of both genders are referred to as **bisexuals**.

The medical profession considers **transsexuals** to have a condition called *gender dysphoria* (strong and persistent feelings of discomfort with one's assigned gender) or *gender identity disorder.* For the transsexual person, sexual anatomy is not consistent with gender identity. Those who are born physically male but who are emotionally and psychologically female are called male-to-female (MTF) transsexuals. Those who are born female but who are emotionally and psychologically male are called female-to-male (FTM) transsexuals. Most transsexuals report that they have felt gender dysphoria since early childhood. They often suffer for many years and try to hide the situation from family and friends for fear of being considered "crazy." Being transgendered puts women and men at extreme risk of ridicule, humiliation, and prejudice. As self-understanding and acceptance increase, many transsexuals live part- or full-time as members of the other sex. **Cross-dressing** (dressing in the clothing of the other sex) not only makes their outward appearance consistent with their inner identity and gender role, but also makes them more comfortable with themselves. Their sexual orientation may be heterosexual, homosexual, or bisexual.

The origins of sexual orientation still are not well understood. Some biologic theories describe sexual orientation in terms of the genetic composition of the individual. Psychologic theories stress the role of early learning experiences and cognitive processes. Other theories acknowledge the confluence of genetics and the environment in the development of sexual orientation.

Estimates of the percentage of the population with a homosexual orientation vary, although the usual figure is 5–10% of men and 2–4% of women (Mooney, Knox, & Schacht, 2009). Because these individuals grow up acutely aware of the discrimination they face in North America, many do not disclose their sexual orientation; thus, actual figures are not available.

The discrimination that gay and lesbian seniors and their caregivers face in the health care system was identified in a study by Brotman, Ryan, & Cormier (2003). The study found that homosexual clients are reluctant to share their sexual orientation with health care providers based on past experiences with biases and fear of experiencing prejudice. The study challenges nurses to examine their beliefs and overcome their biases. The most common bias is **homophobia** (fear, hatred, or mistrust of gays and lesbians often expressed in overt

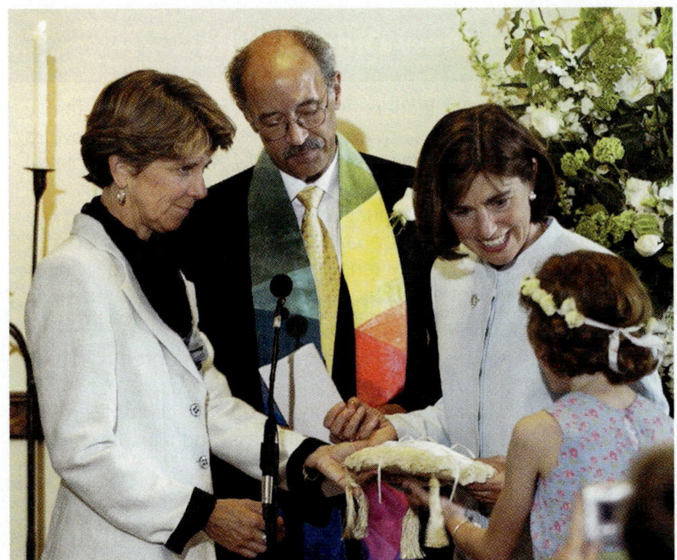

Figure 8–3 ■ Hillary and Julie Goodridge were married in Boston on Monday, May 17, 2004, on the first day of state-sanctioned marriage in the United States. As of 2010, six states sanction gay marriage.

displays of discrimination) or **heterosexism** (view of heterosexuality as the only correct sexual orientation). Often this bias is displayed in subtle and invisible ways that create obstacles to achieving full equality for the homosexual client. Caregivers who provide home care for the homosexual client face unique challenges as the result of laws and health care provider's attitudes.

Laws differ by state on the legality of same-sex marriage, civil unions, and the rights of the homosexual partner to make health care decisions when the client is unable to make independent decisions. It is important that each nurse know the laws in the state in which he or she practices (Figure 8–3 ■).

AGE

American society values youth. The Focus on Culture and Diversity feature describes how different cultures view elders. **Ageism** is a term that describes the deep and profound prejudice in American society against older adults (Meiner & Lueckenotte, 2006). It is a discrimination based solely on age. Unfortunately, this negative attitude toward aging or older adults exists among some health care professionals (Ebersole, Hess, Touhy, & Jett, 2005; Mauk, 2006). This attitude is another reason for nurses to examine their personal beliefs and values toward elders.

Ageism contributes to the development of negative stereotypes about older adults. Stereotypes occur when younger people do not understand or identify with older adults as unique human beings. Instead, they generalize undesirable characteristics (e.g., senile, old-fashioned, unproductive, inflexible) to all older adults. Many negative attitudes about aging are based on myths and incorrect information (Table 8–1). As a result, it is important for nurses to provide accurate information about aging. This has been found to be an effective intervention for reducing negative stereotypes and improving attitudes about aging (Miller, 2004).

Ageism can be subtle and often goes unrecognized by many in the health care industry. The beliefs that all elderly are sickly, lack mental acuity, are less likely to recover from illness, or need help in meeting their daily needs are just a few ways that ageism is displayed. Nurses display ageism when they refer to clients in language that diminishes them (Figure 8–4 ■).

PRACTICE ALERT

Do not address older adults with terms like Honey or Sweetie; it is disrespectful. Instead, use the client's name.

The act of making care decisions with family members instead of involving the client is another act of ageism that often occurs when the client is still competent to make independent decisions.

TABLE 8–1 **Myths and Realities of Aging**

MYTH	REALITY
People consider themselves to be old at 65.	People feel old based on their health and functional ability rather than their chronological age.
In today's society, families no longer care for older people.	In the United States, 80% of the care of older adults is provided by their families.
As people grow older, it is natural for them to want to withdraw from society.	Because older people are unique individuals, each of them responds differently to society.
By age 70, an individual's psychologic growth is complete.	People never lose their capacity for psychologic growth.
In old age, there is an inevitable decline in all intellectual abilities.	A few areas of cognitive ability decline in older adulthood, but other areas show improvement.
Older adults cannot learn complex new skills.	Older adults are capable of learning new things, but the speed with which they process information slows with age.
Older people decrease the level of their sexual activity because they are less able to perform sexually.	If sexual activity in older people declines, it is because of social reasons (e.g., loss of a partner) or risk factors such as diseases and adverse effects from medication.
Most old people are depressed and should be allowed to withdraw from society.	About one third of older people exhibit depressive symptoms; however, depression is a treatable condition at any age.

Note: From C. A. Miller, *Nursing for Wellness in Older Adults,* 4th ed. Copyright © Lippincott, Williams & Wilkins, 2004. Reprinted with permission.

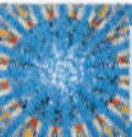

FOCUS ON DIVERSITY AND CULTURE How Different Cultures View Older Adults

CHINESE

- Traditional Chinese values place the family and society over the individual. Many American-born Chinese may not be as traditional as their elders, but they still hold values of respect for older adults and authority.
- The oldest son has obligations toward the family and is expected to respect and care for his parents.
- The tradition of filial piety is the value of total respect for the family, especially the older family members. This respect for older adults was advocated by Confucius, the famous Chinese philosopher; many Chinese and Chinese American families choose to follow these ancient principles.

NATIVE AMERICAN

- Traditionally, older adults are respected for their wisdom, experience, and knowledge.
- Older adults, regardless of tribe, assume significant roles as teachers and caretakers of the young.

VIETNAMESE

- Older adults are given high respect in Vietnamese society. They are considered the carriers of tradition, knowledge, and wisdom. Age is considered an asset, not a liability.
- Elderly grandparents and parents live with the family for support and care.
- Older adults may prepare meals and care for grandchildren if both the husband and wife work.
- Older adults are the leaders and decision-makers in the family and are often sought for advice. When these older adults move to the United States, they can become socially and culturally isolated for many reasons (e.g., lack of English skills, age, and lack of training for work). In contrast, younger family members become more Americanized and may behave in ways their elders do not approve of. This can create tension in families where older adults feel ignored and not respected.

BLACK/AFRICAN AMERICAN

- Older adults are respected, obeyed, and considered a source of wisdom.
- To survive to old age is often considered an accomplishment reflecting personal strength, resourcefulness, and faith.

HISPANIC/LATINO

- Older adults are held in high esteem.
- Old age is viewed as a positive time in one's life.
- Care for older adults is provided by the extended family. Children are expected to care for their elderly parents.

KOREAN

- Traditional Koreans value filial piety and respect for older adults.
- In Korean culture, children are taught to respect their elders whether they are right or wrong.
- Children are expected to take care of their parents in old age.
- Two important family holidays that are celebrated with feasts include the 60th and 70th birthdays.

EDUCATION, ABILITIES, AND LIFE EXPERIENCES

Individual education and ability levels range from the very well-educated professional to illiterate but able adults to adults of low intellectual ability. Nurses must be able to interact with clients having different abilities and educational experiences.

Highly Educated Adults

If the client you were assigned to care for in clinical was a registered nurse, would it alter your approach to providing client care and teaching? What if the client was a physician? Many nurses agree that it would alter their approach to care because they would anticipate that the client knows as much or more than they do. These care decisions are based on a perceived expectation regarding the client's education and experience that can be confirmed only through a thorough assessment. However, even well-educated adults may not possess information about their conditions. Some well-educated adults possess a great deal of information but few coping skills to use upon learning of the diagnosis. Only through assessment can the nurse determine what the client's entry-level knowledge is about the diagnosis and whether the client has the capacity to receive and act on new information. As for any other client, care for a well-educated professional must be individualized.

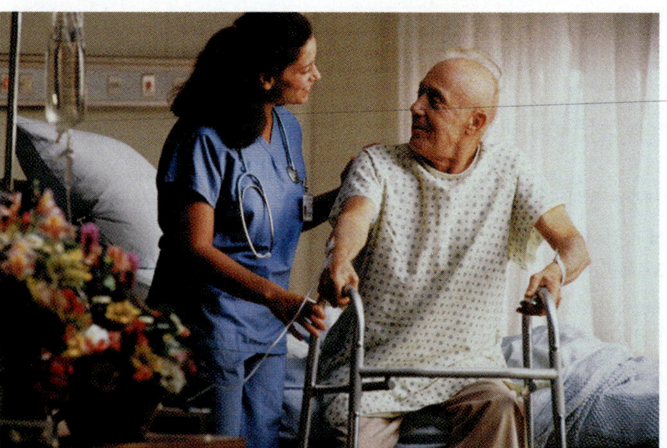

Figure 8–4 ■ Speak directly to elderly clients, addressing them by name.

Low-Literacy Clients

Current research indicates that, in the United States, there is growing illiteracy involving health-related material (Hanzel, 2008). An estimated 90 million citizens may be unable to function adequately in the health care system as a result of this fact alone (Bryan, 2008). Findings indicate a correlation with level of education and the ability to read health-related literature. The inability to read health-related literature also impacts mortality rates (Baker et al, 2008). The Joint Commission on Accreditation of Healthcare Organizations plans to revise hospital accreditation standards to include diversity, language, and health literacy requirements for client care processes to improve education for those with health care information illiteracy (Anonymous, 2009).

When caring for clients, nurses should perform a thorough assessment of the clients' ability to read before providing them with written health care material. Even successful clients with high socioeconomic status may be marginally or functionally illiterate. For that reason, it is important not to draw conclusions about the client's ability to read based solely on lifestyle or achievements in other areas. The topics of health literacy and the ability to work with clients with low literacy levels are discussed in further detail in Concept 13, Health, Wellness, and Illness.

Clients With Intellectual Disabilities

Intellectual disabilities also may be a factor in the care of a diverse population. Over the last 30 years, a range of terms have been used to describe people with intellectual disabilities. *Mental deficiency*, *mental retardation*, *mental handicap*, *developmental disability*, and *learning disability* are examples. Clients with an intellectual disability and their families experience poorer health care compared with the general population. Living with an intellectual disability is often challenged by coexisting complex and chronic conditions such as gastrointestinal and respiratory conditions (Goddard, Davidson, Daly, & Mackey, 2008). It is important that nurses working with these clients develop trusting relationships so they can communicate successfully with the clients as well as with family members and caregivers.

Educational Biases in Nursing

Educational bias also exists in the profession of nursing. This fact is easy to expose by discussing entry-level educational requirements with a group of nurses. Health care facilities often propagate this bias by promoting beliefs that only those nurses with specified levels of education can safely perform techniques, manage staff, or contribute to data collection for research and quality assurance. The word that commonly precedes a statement of bias is *only,* as in "You are only a. . . ." Nurses working with nurses, with other health care professionals, with paraprofessionals, and even with volunteers must try to achieve relationships of respect and trust regardless of educational levels. Doing so benefits nurses and clients alike.

Whether caring for a client with advanced degrees or a client with a known intellectual disability, the nurse must use caution in drawing biased conclusions. A thorough assessment of what the client knows, how the client best learns new information, and what the client's willingness and ability are in contributing to planning care are of utmost importance in delivering high quality care aimed at achieving the best possible outcome and fostering autonomy for the client.

VULNERABLE POPULATIONS

Vulnerable populations are social groups with inadequate access to health care because they lack resources and are exposed to more risk factors. They may be made vulnerable by financial circumstances, place of residence, health, age, functional or developmental status, inability to communicate effectively, presence of chronic or terminal illness or disability, personal characteristics, sexual preferences, and immigration status. All vulnerable populations are less able than others to safeguard their needs and interests adequately. In conceptual terms, the most vulnerable are those households with the fewest choices and the greatest number of limiting factors.

Groups commonly considered members of vulnerable populations include the homeless, foster children who are shuttled from family to family with no real connection, abused women with or without children, and people living in poverty. A primary focus of health care—and *Healthy People 2010*—is to reduce the disparity in access to health care among these groups.

Clients from vulnerable populations are more likely to develop health problems because they have the greatest number of risk factors and the fewest options for managing those risks. They often have limited access to health care and are more dependent on others for helping them meet their health care needs. Those from vulnerable populations are likely to be older, living in poverty, homeless, in abusive relationships, mentally ill, chronically ill, or children. It is not uncommon for those considered vulnerable to belong to more than one of these groups. These individuals face multiple challenges, statistically poorer outcomes and shorter life spans, and higher mortality and morbidity rates due to cumulative or combinations of risk factors. They may be from any culture, ethnicity, age, or gender, although they are more likely to be women than men.

Nurses face many challenges when caring for vulnerable populations. Because of health care disparities, clients from vulnerable populations often present with acute and serious illnesses due to lack of early intervention or preventive care. Their needs are complex and many. Many of them have multiple chronic conditions that can complicate care still further. Assessing the client from a vulnerable population requires the nurse to investigate all systems, determine stressors and coping mechanisms, and help the client identify potential resources.

Flaskerud and Winslow created the Vulnerable Populations Model for Research and Practice, relating resource availability and relative risk to health status (Fkasjerydm et al., 2002). The model focuses on the provision of economic and social resources with the goal of empowering individuals to participate in research and in health prevention, screening, and treatment. The welfare of vulnerable populations is dependent on the nation's willingness to provide the necessary programs to promote health and well-being. Other issues impacting the provision of health care to vulnerable populations include accessibility and transportation. Impoverished children living in very rural communities, for example, may not have access to fluoridated water and may be an hour from the nearest dentist who accepts Medicaid.

The Homeless Client

Among the most vulnerable clients are those who are homeless. In cities, 40% of the homeless population may consist of families with children (U.S. Conference of Mayors, 2005). Homeless clients presents unique and complex challenges because they often live in dangerous, unsanitary conditions; have diets that are severely lacking in nutrients; and have very few resources for coping with illness. They must find shelter and food every day and cannot predict what the next day will bring (Figure 8–5 ■). The homeless have difficulty obtaining, keeping, and storing medications. There is a high incidence of substance abuse and mental illness that limits their ability to provide self-care still further. Another important nursing intervention in addition to providing care to the homeless is the identification of resources to help these clients.

Undocumented Immigrants

It is estimated that some 11.6 million undocumented immigrants live in the United States, and that approximately 8.8 million of them are from other countries in North America with most of them originating from Mexico (Department of Homeland Security). A statewide study found that between 1990–2004, one out of four new residents in the state of North Carolina was an undocumented immigrant. North Carolina ranks 9th in the nation with more than 300,000 (Pew Hispanic Center, 2008) undocumented immigrants.

Undocumented immigrants often do not seek health care until their condition becomes critical. This behavior results from a complex combination of factors. Many are uninsured, do not speak English, and have not yet learned the culture of their new homeland. Many believe that accessing health care will result in legal consequences, up to and including deportation. These factors combine to create fear in the undocumented immigrant client who needs medical attention.

Special health care concerns related to this population include lack of preventative care, inadequate immunization status, and lack of past medical records. Because they enter the country without border screening, risks of diseases such as tuberculosis and HIV are much higher. Many receive their health information from television, the Internet, or family members, which can lead to misinformation and improper treatment.

In most states across the country, health care facilities are not required to ask for proof of citizenship when providing care, nor are they required to report people seeking care who are undocumented. In some states, cost of care may be covered by Medicaid if the client cannot afford to pay.

When providing care to clients who may be or are known to be undocumented immigrants, the nurse has the ethical and moral imperative to deliver the same high quality care delivered to any client. Use of an interpreter will improve the quality of communication if the client does not speak English or does not speak English well enough to understand the information presented. Thorough screening, nursing history, and assessment contribute to determining both current condition as well as risks, preventative care needs, and understanding of self-care upon discharge. Because access to health care for this population is unpredictable, nurses should maximize each opportunity to care for and teach the client.

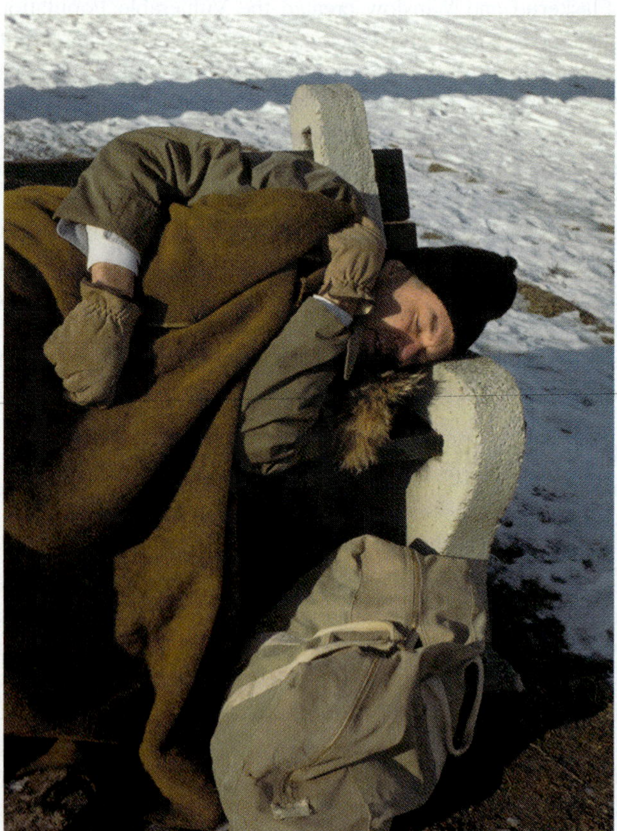

Figure 8–5 ■ This homeless man has spent the night on a park bench in St. Paul, Minnesota.

RACE

Race refers to socially defined populations that have common genetically transmitted characteristics such as skin color and bone structure. Statistics of race in the population can be complicated to interpret and change over time. In 2008, the United States Bureau of the Census reported that over 66% of Americans identify themselves as White and nearly 15% identify themselves as Hispanic or Latino while projecting that by 2050, the Hispanic population will increase to 24% of the total, while white non-Hispanics will decrease to 50% of the total.

While diversity in nursing is improving, nurses are predominantly white and, in percentage, are disproportionate to the demographic profile of the United States. Table 8–2 compares the percentages of American Indian, Asian/Pacific Islander, black non-Hispanic, Hispanic, and White non-Hispanic nurses in 2004 (Public Health Foundation, 2009).

Shared risk factors for certain diseases among individuals of similar racial backgrounds are most likely the result of shared genetics. For example, hypertension is commonly found in African Americans, while rheumatoid arthritis is more common among the European White population. Awareness of racial risk factors is an important component to assessment of the client.

TABLE 8–2 **Percentages of American Indian, Asian/Pacific Islander, Black Non-Hispanic, Hispanic, and White Non-Hispanic Nurses in 2004**

POPULATION	PERCENT
American Indian/Alaska Native	0.4
Asian/Pacific Islander and Other	3.3
Black non-Hispanic	4.6
Hispanic	1.8
White non-Hispanic	88.4
Two or more races	1.5

Source: From "The Registered Nurse Population: Preliminary Findings from the National Sample Survey of Registered Nurses, March 2004," by the U.S. Department of Health and Human Services Health Resources and Service Administration Bureau of Health Professions. Retrieved April 21, 2006, from http://bhpr.hrsa.gov/healthworkforce/reports/rnpopulation/preliminaryfindings.htm

NURSING CARE PLAN **Diversity in Planning Health Care**

ASSESSMENT

Mary Burke is a 26-year-old mother with three children; she and her children are currently homeless. Ms. Burke dropped out of high school when she was 15 years old and pregnant with her first child. She and her boyfriend moved in together and had plans of building a comfortable life for their family, but soon she had three children and her boyfriend was sentenced to 10 years in prison. Two years ago she was diagnosed with type 2 diabetes. Shortly after the diagnosis, she lost her job cleaning rooms at a local hotel because she missed too much time due to illness. She and her children have been intermittently homeless when she can't find a job and doesn't have the money to pay the rent.

In the past 6 months, Ms. Burke has been admitted four times to the acute care facility through the emergency department when she was found unconscious secondary to diabetic ketoacidosis (DKA). Each time she is admitted, her blood glucose levels are too high to register on the glucose meter and return from the lab greater than 600. The nurses caring for her have reviewed self-care instructions repeatedly, and she seems to understand what she is taught. Ms. Burke has been brought to the emergency department again today in DKA, and her children are playing quietly in the waiting area.

Serum blood glucose level 643
Vital signs: 98.2°F, P 118, R 32, BP 97/48
Weight: 110 lb (50 kg) (6 pounds less than when last seen)
Height: 66 in. (167.64 cm)
Difficult to arouse, slurred speech, fruity smell to breath

DIAGNOSES

- Risk-Prone Health Behaviors as evidenced by recurrent DKA
- Decisional Conflict related to meeting family's basic needs versus meeting own health needs
- Ineffective Health Maintenance as evidenced by recurrent DKA
- Noncompliance in Diabetic Management as evidenced by recurrent DKA

PLANNING

Goals for Ms. Burke's care include the following:

- Ms. Burke will take personal actions to promote wellness, recovery, and rehabilitation based on professional advice.
- Ms. Burke will participate in health care decision making in selecting and evaluating health care options to achieve desired outcomes.
- Ms. Burke will identify personal health threats and perform basic care activities to promote health.
- Noncompliance will decrease as demonstrated by adherence to diabetic regimen and plan of care developed in consultation with Ms. Burke.

IMPLEMENTATION

Risk-Prone Behaviors

- Promote behavioral change.
- Provide information and support Ms. Burke to make healthy decisions regarding care.
- Provide reassurance, acceptance, and encouragement.
- Develop and provide instructions and learning experiences to facilitate voluntary adaptation of behavior conducive to health.
- Collaborate with client to identify and prioritize care goals; then develop a plan to achieve goals.

Decisional Conflict

- Assess client's understanding of available choices.
- Evaluate client's level of distress.
- Assess decision-making skills and usual patterns of decision making.
- Determine if differences exist between client's and nurse's view of the client's condition.
- Involve available resources to help improve Ms. Burke's ability to make better choices.

Ineffective Health Maintenance

- Assist in securing and managing finances to meet health care needs.
- Facilitate location and use of appropriate health services.
- Reinforce self-directed changes initiated by Ms. Burke to achieve personally important goals.
- Facilitate improved community support of Ms. Burke.
- Create a teaching program designed to address Ms. Burke's particular needs.

Noncompliance

- Facilitate Ms. Burke's location and use of appropriate health services.
- Promote Ms. Burke's ability to process and comprehend information.
- Collaborate with client to identify and prioritize care goals.
- Assist Ms. Burke to understand diabetic self-care needs.

EVALUATION

After assessing Ms. Burke's perception of barriers to adequate self-care, it was determined that when Ms. Burke was unable to find a job, she and the children would frequently eat at fast-food restaurants and split a hamburger, French fries, and milk shakes. It also was determined that Ms. Burke was unable to store diabetic supplies and glucose monitoring equipment during periods of homelessness. The facility's nutrition counselor and social services were called in. Together the health care team helped Ms. Burke find subsidized housing, provided coupons to be used at the local grocery store for food, and directed her to a neighborhood clinic that would assist in providing monitoring and follow-up care for her condition. Ms. Burke was discharged with a supply of insulin, syringes, a glucose monitor, and several bottles of glucose monitoring sticks. The clinic reports that she regularly attends appointments and has been maintaining improved serum blood sugars and that her children's growth and development also have improved.

(continued)

NURSING CARE PLAN Diversity in Planning Health Care *continued*

CRITICAL THINKING

1. Why was Ms. Burke noncompliant with the medical regimen?
2. If it had not been possible to find permanent shelter for Ms. Burke and her children, how might the nurse have helped her improve compliance with diabetic self-care?
3. How would the outcome have been different if the nurse had viewed the situation as hopeless and failed to intervene?

DIVERSITY AS A CONCEPT IN PROVISION OF HEALTH SERVICES

Nursing must change to meet the needs of an increasingly diverse population that brings lifestyles, beliefs, and health care choices that may differ from those of the nurse actually providing client care. Valuing the diverse needs of the clients from different backgrounds serves to increase client comfort, improve client outcomes, and strengthen the nurse–client relationship. It also increases client involvement in care planning, which improves compliance with the treatment regimen. Clients can reach their full potential only when the nurse creates a care plan that places value on how clients prefer to do things and encourages change in only those patterns that could be harmful (Spector, 2004).

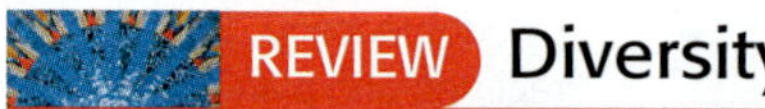

Diversity

RELATE: LINK THE CONCEPTS

Linking the concept of Diversity with the concept of Advocacy:

1. What obligation does the nurse hold to advocate for the client who is a member of a vulnerable population?
2. What obligation does the client have when the nurse works as an advocate for him or her?

Linking the concept of Diversity with the concept of Development:

3. How might a pediatric client's development be impacted if his or her mother is homeless?
4. How might an adolescent's development be impacted by the realization that he or she is homosexual?

REFER: GO TO MYNURSINGKIT

REFLECT: CASE STUDY

Mrs. Rivera, a 79-year-old woman of Mexican heritage, is admitted to a long-term care facility. Neither she nor her immediate family members speak, write, read, or understand English. She has been a life-long member of an orthodox Catholic church and will not allow staff to help her undress and tells a translator she is very modest and does not want the nursing staff to examine her under her clothing. When asked about advanced directives, living wills, or medical power or attorney both the client and the family inform the staff, "That is none of your business."

1. What client teaching will the nurse provide through the use of a medical interpreter?
2. How can the nurse advocate for Mrs. Rivera's diversity requirements while maintaining facility policy and the client's health-care needs?
3. What nursing diagnoses and interventions would be appropriate for Mrs. Rivera's plan of care?

EXPLORE PEARSON **mynursingkit**™

MyNursingKit is your one stop for online chapter review materials and resources. Prepare for success with additional NCLEX®-style practice questions, interactive assignments and activities, web links, animations and videos, and more!

Register your access code from the front of your book at **www.mynursingkit.com.**

REFERENCES

Anonymous. (2009). JCAHO to address diversity, language, health literacy. *Nevada RNformation, Reno, 14*(4), 12.

Baker, D.W., Wolf, M.S., Feinglass, J., & Thompson, J.A. (2008). Health literacy, cognitive abilities, and mortality among elderly persons. *Journal of General Internal Medicine, 23*(6), 723–726. Retrieved from EBSCO database.

Brotman, S., Ryan, B., Collins, S., & Chamberland, L. (2007). Coming out to care: Caregivers of gay and lesbian seniors in Canada. *The Gerontologist, 47*(4), 490–504.

Brotman, S., Ryan, B., & Cormier, R. (2003). The health and social service needs of gay and lesbian elders and their families in Canada. *The Gerontologist, 43,* 192–202.

Brotman, S., Ryan, B., & Meyer, E. (2006). The health and social service needs of gay and lesbian elders: Final report, Montreal, Quebec, Canada: McGill University School of Social Work.

Bryan, C (2008). Provider and policy response to reverse the consequences of low health literacy. *Journal of Health Care Management, 53*(4), 230–241. Retrieved from EBSCO database on 6/11/09.

Cristofides, N. (2001). How to make policies more gender sensitive. In J. Samet & Y. Joon-Young (Eds.), *Women and the tobacco epidemic: Challenges for the 21st century.* World Health Organization, Geneva.

Doyal, L. (2001). Sex, gender, and health: the need for a new approach. *British Medical Journal, 323*(7320), 1061–1064. Retrieved from http://proquest.umi.com.ezproxy.apollolibrary.com/pqdweb?did=92366641&sid=1&Fmt=4&clientId=13118&RQT=309&VName=PQD

Ebersole, P., Hess, P., Touhy, T., & Jett, K. (2005). *Gerontological nursing & healthy aging* (2nd ed.). Philadelphia: Elsevier Mosby.

Fkasjerydm, J. H., Lesser, J., Dixon, E., Anderson, N., Conde, F., Kim, S., et al. (2002). Health disparities among vulnerable popultions: Evolution of knowledge over five decades in nursing research publications. *Nursing Research, 51*(2), 74–85.

Flaskerud, J. H., & Winslow, B. J. (1998). Conceptualizing vulnerable populations health-related research. *Nursing Research, 47*(2), 69–78.

Garcia-Moreno, C. (2002) Violence against women: Consolidating a public health agenda. In G. Sen, A. George, & P. Ostlin (Eds.), *Engendering international health: The challenge of equity.* MIT Press, Cambridge.

Goddard, L., Davidson, P. M., Daly, J., & Mackey, S. (2008). People with an intellectual disability in the discourse of chronic and complex conditions: An invisible group? *Australian Health Review, 32*(3), 405–415.

Hanzel, J. L. (2008). *An assessment of patient health literacy levels.* (Doctoral dissertation, North Dakota State University, 2008). Retrieved from http://proquest.umi.com.ezproxy.apollolibrary.com/pqdweb?did=1633339031&sid=7&Fmt=2&clientId=13118&RQT=309&VName=PQD

Mauk, K. L. (2006). *Gerontological nursing: Competencies for care.* Boston: Jones & Bartlett.

Meiner, S. E., & Lueckenotte, A. (2005). *Gerontological nursing* (3rd ed.). Philadelphia, PA: Mosby.

Miller, C. A. (2004). *Nursing for wellness in older adults: Theory and practice* (4th ed.). Philadelphia: Lippincott Williams & Wilkins.

Mooney, L. A., Knox, D., & Schacht, C. (2009). *Understanding social problems* (6th ed.). Belmont, CA: Wadsworth, Cengage Learning.

Ostlin, P. (2002). Gender perspective on socioeconomic inequalities in health. In J. Mackenbach & M. Bakker (Eds.), *Reducing inequalities in health: A European perspective.* London: Routledge.

Ostlin, P., Eckermann, E., Mishra, U. S., Nkowane, M., & Wallstam, E. (2007). Gender and health promotion: A multisectoral policy approach. *Health Promotion International, 21*(S1), 25–35.

Pew Hispanic Center (2008). *Hispanics and health care in the United States: Access, information, and knowledge* retrieved September 14, 2008, from http://pewhispanic.org/surveys/

Public Health Foundation. (2009). *Council on linkages between academia and public health practices.* Retrieved September 17, 2009, from http://www.phf.org/link/NLMlitsearch2009.pdf

Roses Periago, M., Fescina, R., and Ramón-Pardo, P. (2004). Steps for preventing infectious diseases in women. *Emerging Infectious Diseases, 10,* 1968–1973.

Spector, R. E. (2004). *Cultural diversity in health & illness* (6th ed.). Upper Saddle River, NJ: Prentice Hall.

U.S. Census Bureau. (2008). *U.S. populations projections.* Retrieved September 18, 2009, from http://www.census.gov/population/www/projections/projectionsagesex.html

U.S. Conference Of Mayors. (2005). *Conference of Mayors - Sodexho USA hunger and homelessness survery 2004.* Retrieved September 18, 2009, from http://usmayors.org/usmayornewspaper/documents/01_10_05/hunger.asp

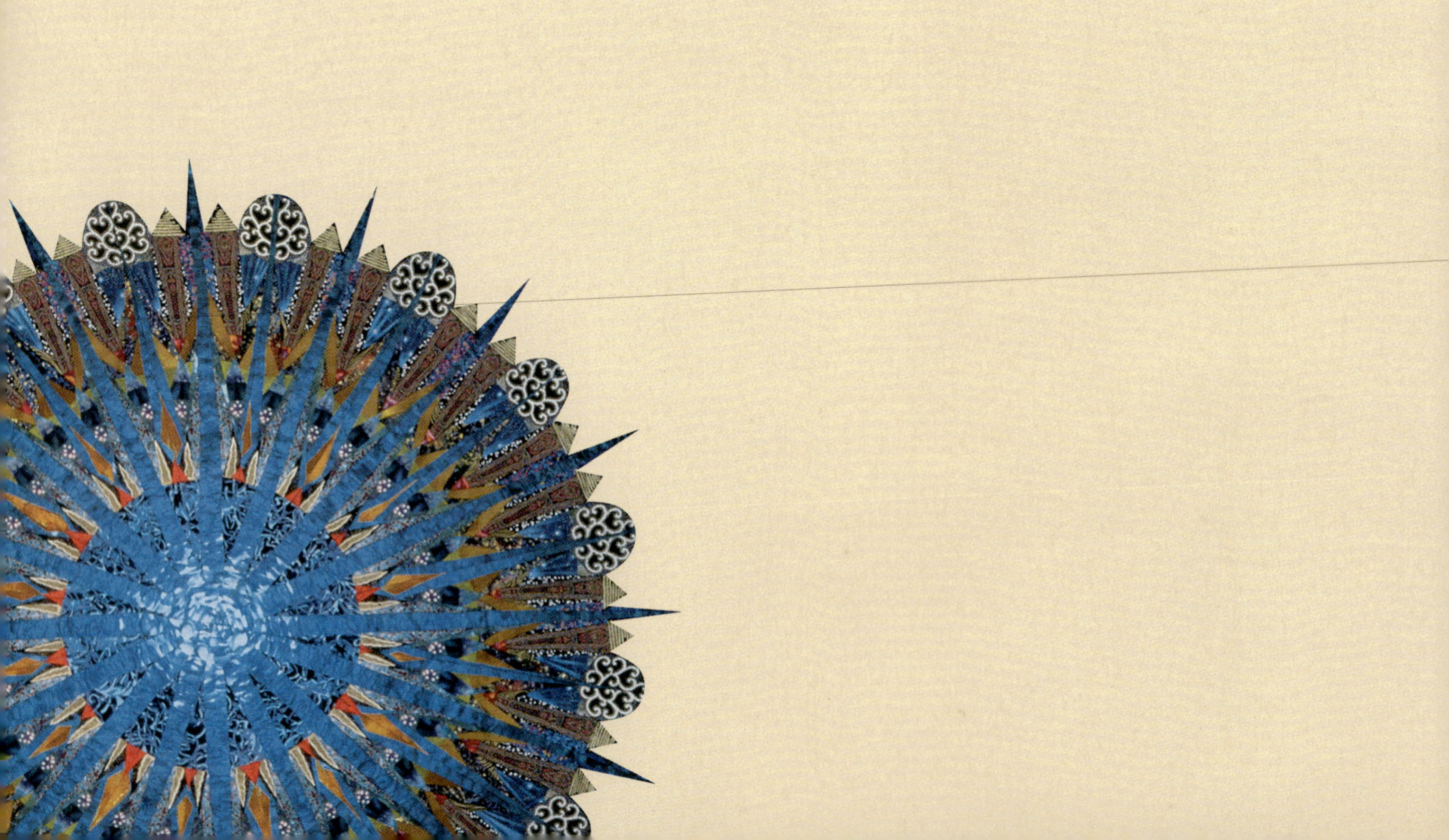

Elimination

9

Concept at-a-Glance

Concept Learning Outcomes

After reading about this concept, you will be able to:

1. Summarize the structure and physiologic processes of the renal and gastrointestinal systems related to elimination.
2. List factors affecting elimination.
3. Identify commonly occurring alterations in elimination and their related treatments.
4. Outline diagnostic and laboratory tests to determine the individual's elimination status.
5. Explain management of urinary and bowel health and prevention of alterations in elimination.
6. Explain management of urinary and bowel health and prevention of urinary and bowel illness.
7. Demonstrate the nursing process in providing culturally competent care across the life span for individuals with common alterations in elimination.
8. Identify pharmacologic interventions in caring for individuals with alterations in urinary and bowel function.

Concept Key Terms

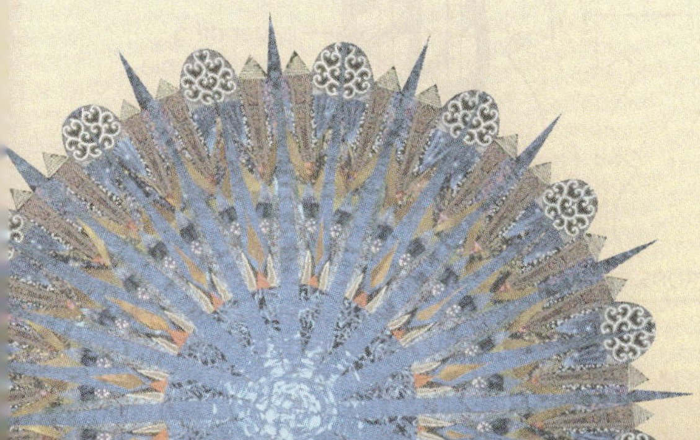

About Elimination

This concept will discuss the process of urinary and gastrointestinal elimination. The term **elimination** refers to the secretion and excretion of body wastes from the kidneys and intestines and any alterations from normal of those processes. Using the nursing process, along with critical thinking and scientific rationales, to make decisions about the care of clients of all ages who are experiencing alterations in elimination, nurses can work with clients to optimize their health and well-being.

Elimination processes are intertwined in the physiology of the human body. Alterations in elimination often indicate alterations from normal in other physiologic areas, side effects from medications, or improper levels of hydration or nutrition. Because nurses frequently are the first health care professionals to determine that a client is experiencing problems with elimination, nurses must be familiar with the different alterations in elimination, their risk factors, and how these alterations affect other physiologic processes. •

Urinary Elimination

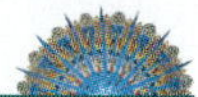

Urinary elimination habits depend on social, cultural, personal, and physical factors. In North America, most people are accustomed to privacy and clean, even decorative, surroundings while they eliminate.

Personal habits regarding urinary elimination are affected by the social propriety of leaving to urinate, the availability of a private and clean facility, and initial training. Elimination is essential to health, and it can be postponed for only so long before the urge becomes too great to control.

NORMAL PRESENTATION

Urinary elimination depends on effective functioning of the upper urinary tract (kidneys and ureters) and the lower urinary tract (urinary bladder, urethra, and pelvic floor). Figure 9–1 ■ shows the anatomic structures of the urinary tract.

Kidneys

The paired kidneys are situated on either side of the spinal column, behind the peritoneal cavity. The right kidney is slightly lower than the left because of the position of the liver. The kidneys are the primary regulators of fluid and acid–base balance in the body. The functional units of the kidneys—the nephrons (Figure 9–2 ■)—filter the blood and remove metabolic wastes. In the average adult, 1,200 mL of blood, or approximately 21% of the cardiac output, passes through the kidneys every minute. Each kidney contains approximately 1 million nephrons. Each nephron has a **glomerulus**, a tuft of capillaries surrounded by the Bowman's capsule. The endothelium of glomerular capillaries is porous, allowing fluid and solutes to move readily across this membrane into the capsule. Plasma proteins and blood cells are too large to cross the membrane normally. Glomerular filtrate, which is made up of water, electrolytes, glucose, amino acids, and metabolic wastes, is similar in composition to plasma.

From the Bowman's capsule, the filtrate moves into the tubule of the nephron. In the proximal convoluted tubule, most of the water and electrolytes are reabsorbed. Solutes, such as glucose, are reabsorbed in the loop of Henle, proximal tubule, and collecting ducts; however, other substances also are secreted into the filtrate, concentrating the urine. In the distal convoluted tubule, additional water and sodium are reabsorbed under the control of hormones such as antidiuretic hormone

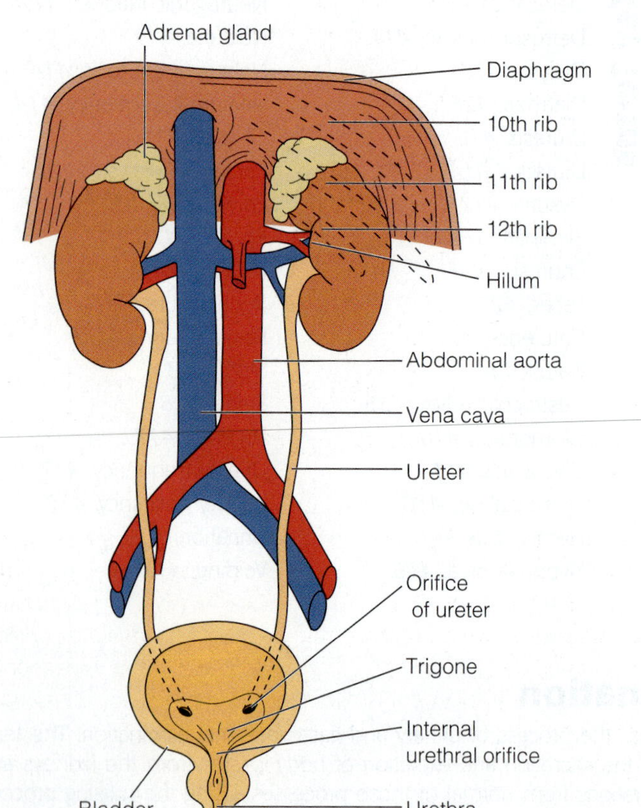

Figure 9–1 ■ Anatomic structures of the urinary tract.

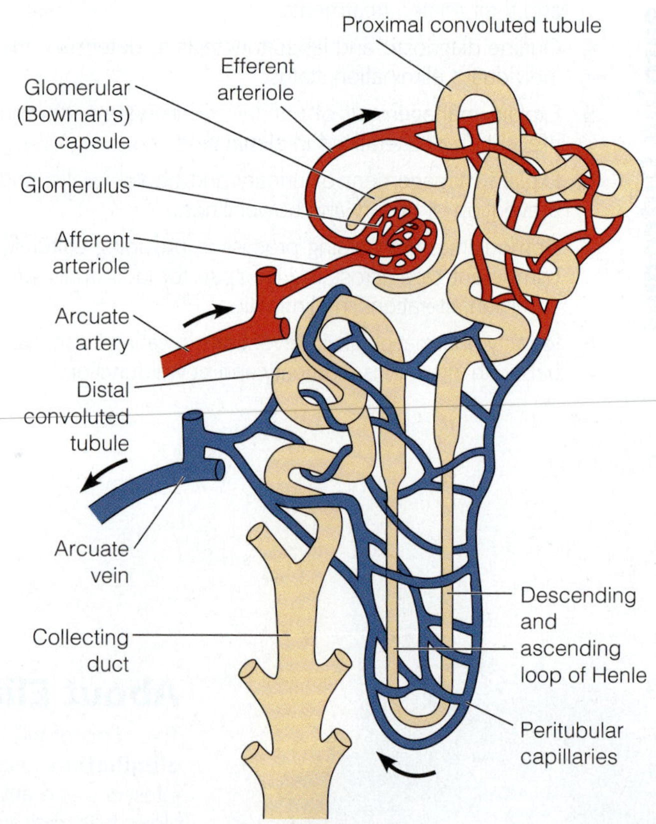

Figure 9–2 ■ Nephrons of the kidneys.

(ADH) and aldosterone. This controlled reabsorption allows fine regulation of fluid and electrolyte balance in the body. When fluid intake is low or the concentration of solutes in the blood is high, ADH is released from the anterior pituitary, more water is reabsorbed in the distal tubule, and less urine is excreted. By contrast, when fluid intake is high or the blood solute concentration is low, ADH is suppressed. Without ADH, the distal tubule becomes impermeable to water, and more urine is excreted. Aldosterone also affects the tubule. When aldosterone is released from the adrenal cortex, sodium and water are reabsorbed in greater quantities, increasing the blood volume and decreasing the urinary output.

Ureters

Once the urine is formed in the kidneys, it moves through the collecting ducts into the calyces of the renal pelvis and, from there, into the ureters. In the adult, the ureters are 25–30 cm (10–12 in.) in length and approximately 1.25 cm (0.5 in.) in diameter. The upper end of each ureter is funnel shaped as it enters the kidney. The lower ends of the ureters enter the bladder at the posterior corners of the floor of the bladder. At the junction between the ureter and the bladder, a flap-like fold of mucous membrane acts as a valve to prevent backflow of urine up the ureters.

Bladder

The urinary bladder (vesicle) is a hollow, muscular organ that serves as a reservoir for urine and as the organ of excretion. When empty, it lies behind the symphysis pubis. In men, the bladder lies in front of the rectum and above the prostate gland; in women, it lies in front of the uterus and vagina (Figures 9–3 ■ and 9–4 ■). The bladder wall is made up of four layers: (a) an inner mucous layer; (b) a connective tissue layer; (c) three layers of smooth muscle fibers, some of which extend lengthwise, some obliquely, and some more or less circularly; and (d) an outer serous layer. The smooth muscle layers are collectively called the **detrusor muscle** The detrusor muscle allows the bladder to expand as it fills with urine and to contract as it releases urine to the outside of the body during voiding (D'Amico & Barbarito, 2007). At the base of the bladder is the trigone, a triangular area marked by the ureter openings at the posterior corners and the opening of the urethra at the anteroinferior corner.

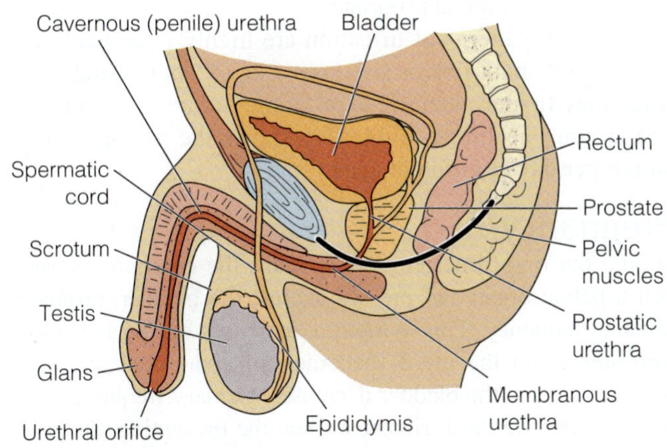

Figure 9–3 ■ Male urogenital system.

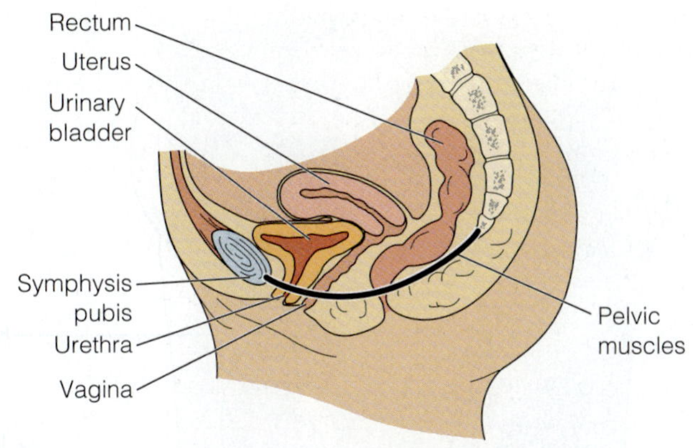

Figure 9–4 ■ Female urogenital system.

The bladder is capable of considerable distention because of rugae (folds) in the mucous membrane lining and because of the elasticity of its walls. When full, the dome of the bladder may extend above the symphysis pubis; in extreme situations, it may extend as high as the umbilicus. Normal bladder capacity is between 300 and 600 mL of urine.

Urethra

The urethra extends from the bladder to the urinary **meatus** (opening). In the adult woman, the urethra lies directly behind the symphysis pubis, anterior to the vagina, and is between 3 and 4 cm (1.5 in.) in length (see Figure 9–4). The urethra serves only as a passageway for the elimination of urine. The urinary meatus is located between the labia minora, in front of the vagina and below the clitoris. The male urethra is approximately 20 cm (8 in.) in length and serves as a passageway for semen, as well as for urine (see Figure 9–3). In men, the meatus is located at the distal end of the penis.

In men and women both, the urethra has a mucous membrane lining that is continuous with the bladder and the ureters. Thus, an infection of the urethra can extend through the urinary tract to the kidneys. Women are particularly prone to urinary tract infections (UTIs) because of their short urethras and the proximity of the urinary meatus to the vagina and anus.

Pelvic Floor

The vagina, urethra, and rectum pass through the pelvic floor, which consists of sheets of muscles and ligaments that support the viscera of the pelvis (see Figures 9–3 and 9–4). The pelvic floor muscles are under voluntary control and are important in controlling urination. Specific sphincter muscles contribute to the continence mechanism (Figure 9–5 ■). These muscles can become weakened by pregnancy and childbirth, chronic constipation, decrease in estrogen (menopause), being overweight, aging, and lack of general fitness. The internal sphincter muscle situated in the proximal urethra and the bladder neck is composed of smooth muscle under involuntary control. It provides active tension

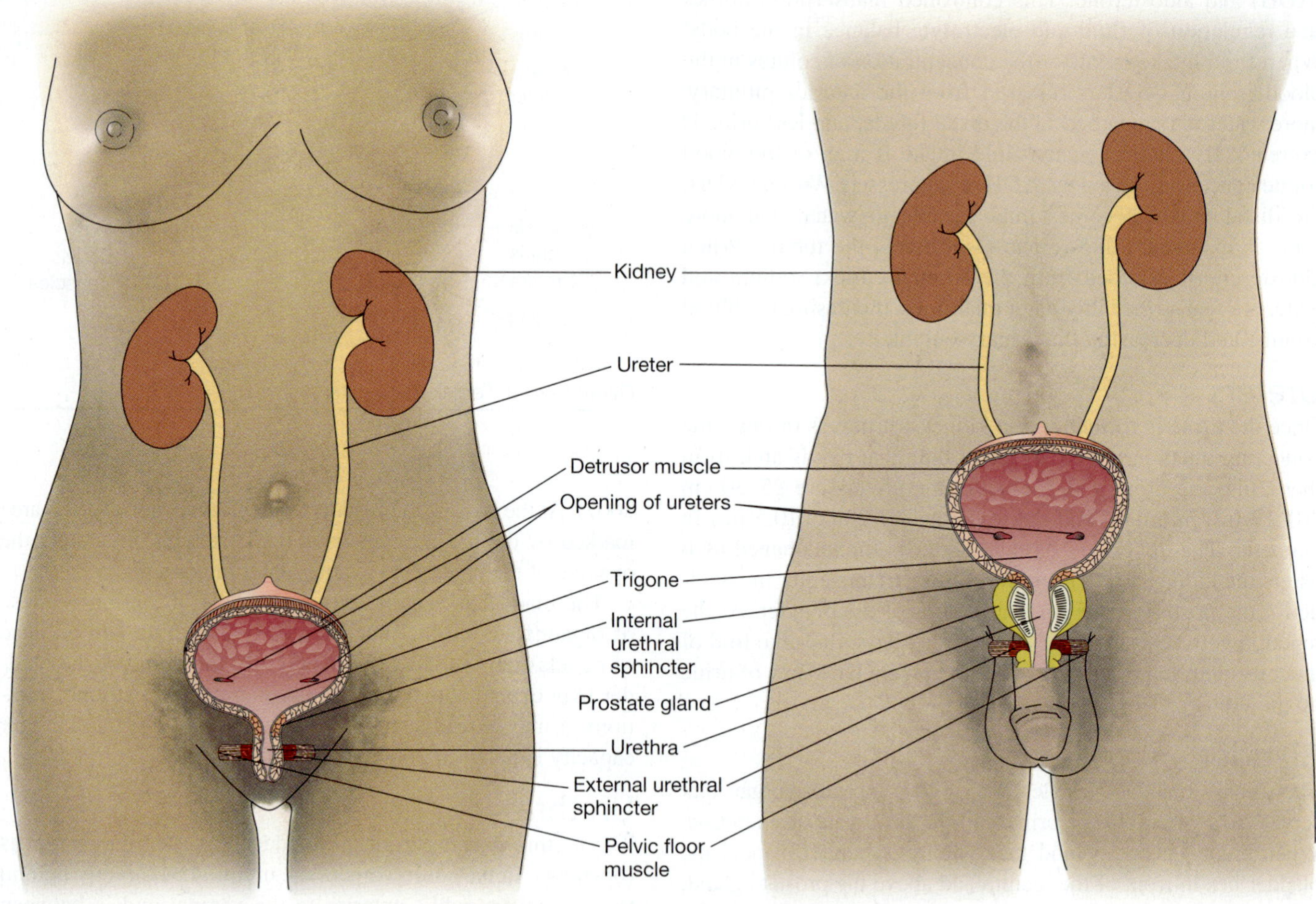

Figure 9–5 ■ Female and male urinary bladders and urethras, showing sphincter muscles.

Source: Custom Medical Stock Photo, Inc.

designed to close the urethral lumen. The external sphincter muscle is composed of skeletal muscle under voluntary control, allowing the individual to choose when urine is eliminated.

Urination

Micturition, **voiding**, and **urination** all refer to the process of emptying urinary bladder. Urine collects in the bladder until pressure stimulates special sensory nerve endings, called stretch receptors, in the bladder wall. This stimulation occurs when the adult bladder contains between 250 and 450 mL of urine. In children, a considerably smaller volume (50–200 mL) stimulates these nerves.

The stretch receptors transmit impulses to the spinal cord—specifically to the voiding reflex center located at the level of the second to fourth sacral vertebrae, causing the internal sphincter to relax and stimulating the urge to void. If the time and place are appropriate for urination, the conscious portion of the brain relaxes the external urethral sphincter muscle, and urination takes place. If the time and place are inappropriate, the micturition reflex usually subsides until the bladder becomes more filled and the reflex is stimulated again.

Voluntary control of urination is possible only if the nerves supplying the bladder and urethra, the neural tracts of the cord and the brain, and the motor area of the cerebrum are all intact. The individual must be able to sense that the bladder is full. Injury to any of these parts of the nervous system—for example, by a cerebral hemorrhage or a spinal cord injury above the level of the sacral region—results in intermittent involuntary emptying of the bladder. Older adults whose cognition is impaired may not be aware of the need to urinate or be able to respond to this urge appropriately.

Although patterns of urination are highly individual, most people void about five or six times a day. People usually void when they first awaken in the morning, before they go to bed, and around mealtimes. Table 9–1 shows the average urinary output per day at different ages.

Pregnancy

During the first trimester of pregnancy, the enlarging uterus is still a pelvic organ and presses against the bladder, producing urinary frequency. This symptom decreases during the second trimester when the uterus becomes an abdominal organ and pressure against the bladder decreases. Urinary frequency reappears during the third trimester when the presenting part of the uterus descends into the pelvis and again presses on the bladder, thus reducing bladder capacity, contributing to hyperemia, and irritating the bladder. The ureters elongate and dilate above the pelvic brim; this is especially the case for the right ureter. The glomerular filtration rate (GFR) rises by as much as 50% beginning in the second trimester, and it remains elevated until birth. To compensate for this increase, renal tubular reabsorption also increases. However, **glycosuria** (excretion of carbohydrates into the urine) sometimes arises during pregnancy because of the kidneys' inability to reabsorb all the glucose filtered by the glomeruli. Glycosuria may be normal or may indicate gestational diabetes, so it always warrants further testing. Presence of protein, blood, or white cells is always considered to be abnormal and should be evaluated.

The postpartum woman has an increased bladder capacity, swelling and bruising of the tissue around the urethra, decreased sensitivity to fluid pressure, and decreased sensation of bladder filling. Consequently, the postpartum woman is at risk for overdistention, incomplete bladder emptying, and buildup of **residual urine** (urine that remains in the bladder after voiding). Women who have had an anesthetic block have inhibited neural functioning of the bladder and are more susceptible to bladder distention, difficulty with voiding, and bladder infections. In addition, immediate postpartum use of oxytocin (to facilitate uterine contractions following expulsion of the placenta) has an antidiuretic effect. After oxytocin is discontinued, the woman will experience rapid bladder filling (Cunningham et al., 2005).

Urinary output increases during the early postpartum period (first 12–24 hours) because of puerperal diuresis. The kidneys must eliminate an estimated 2,000–3,000 mL of extracellular fluid with a normal pregnancy, causing rapid filling of the bladder. As a result, adequate bladder elimination is an immediate concern. Women with preeclampsia, chronic hypertension, or diabetes experience greater fluid retention than other women do, and postpartum diuresis increases accordingly. If urine stasis exists, the chance for a UTI increases because of bacteriuria and the presence of dilated ureters and renal pelves, which persist for approximately 6 weeks after birth. A full bladder also may increase the tendency of the uterus to relax by displacing the uterus and interfering with its contractility, increasing the risk for hemorrhage. In the absence of infection, the dilated ureters and renal pelves return to prepregnant size by the end of the sixth week.

TABLE 9–1 Average Daily Urine Output by Age

AGE	AMOUNT (mL)
1 to 2 days	15–60
3 to 10 days	100–300
10 days to 2 months	250–450
2 months to 1 year	400–500
1 to 3 years	500–600
3 to 5 years	600–700
5 to 8 years	700–1,000
8 to 14 years	800–1,400
14 years through adulthood	1,500
Older adulthood	1,500 or less

Newborns

The GFR of the newborn's kidney is low compared to that of the adult. Because of this physiologic decrease in kidney glomerular filtration, the newborn's kidney is unable to dispose of water rapidly when necessary. Full-term newborns are less able to concentrate urine because the tubules are short and narrow. The limited tubular reabsorption of water and limited excretion of solutes (principally sodium, potassium, chloride, bicarbonate, urea, and phosphate) in the growing newborn also reduce the newborn's ability to concentrate urine, and because the newborn has difficulty concentrating urine, the effect of excessive insensible water loss or restricted fluid intake is unpredictable. The newborn kidney also is limited in dilutional capabilities. These limitations regarding concentration and dilution are important considerations in monitoring fluid therapy to prevent dehydration or overhydration. The newborn attains the ability to concentrate urine fully by 3 months of age.

Many newborns void immediately after birth, and the voiding frequently goes unnoticed. Among healthy newborns, 93% void by 24 hours after birth, and 100% void by 48 hours after birth (Thureen, Deacon, Hernandez, & Hall, 2005). A newborn who has not voided by 48 hours should be assessed for adequacy of fluid intake, bladder distention, restlessness, and symptoms of pain. If any of these signs are observed, the appropriate clinical personnel should be notified.

The initial bladder volume is 6–44 mL of urine. Unless edema is present, normal urinary output often is limited, and voiding is scanty until fluid intake increases. For the first 2 days after birth, the newborn voids from 2 to 6 times daily, with a urine output of 15 mL • kg^{-1} • day^{-1}. The newborn subsequently voids from 5 to 25 times every 24 hours, with a volume of 25 mL • kg^{-1} • day^{-1}.

After the first voiding episode, the newborn's urine frequently is cloudy (because of mucus content) and has a high specific gravity, which decreases as fluid intake increases. Occasionally, pink stains ("brick dust spots") appear on the diaper. These are caused by urates and are innocuous. During early infancy, normal urine is straw colored and almost odorless, although odor can occur when certain drugs are given, metabolic disorders exist, or infection is present.

FACTORS AFFECTING URINARY ELIMINATION

Numerous factors affect the volume and characteristics of the urine produced and the manner in which it is excreted.

Developmental Factors

Factors specific to infants, preschoolers, school-age children, and older adults can affect the elimination of urine.

INFANTS Urine output varies according to fluid intake but gradually increases to between 250 and 500 mL a day during the first year. Infants are born without urinary control and may urinate as often as 25 times a day. Most will develop urinary control between 2 and 5 years of age. Control during the daytime normally precedes control during the nighttime.

PRESCHOOLERS A preschooler is able to take responsibility for independent toileting. Parents must realize that accidents occur; however, the child should never be punished or chastised for a toileting accident. Because children at this age often forget to wash their hands or flush the toilet, they require reminders and appropriate adult modeling. Young children also require instruction in wiping themselves. Girls should be taught to wipe from front to back to prevent contamination of the urinary tract by feces.

SCHOOL-AGE CHILDREN The school-age child's elimination system reaches maturity during this period. The kidneys double in size between 5 and 10 years of age. During this period, the child urinates six to eight times a day.

Enuresis which is defined as the involuntary passing of urine when control should be established (approximately 5 years of age), can be a problem for some school-age children. About 10% of all 6 year olds experience difficulty controlling the bladder.

Nocturnal enuresis, or bed-wetting, is the involuntary passing of urine during sleep. It has many causes but basically occurs because the child fails to awaken when the bladder empties (Nield & Kamat, 2004, p. 409). The incidence of nocturnal enuresis decreases as the child matures, and bed-wetting should not be considered a problem until after 6 years of age. Nocturnal enuresis may be referred to as primary when the child has never achieved nighttime urinary control. Secondary enuresis is that which appears after the child has achieved dryness for a period of 6 consecutive months. Often, it is related to another problem, such as constipation, stress, or illness, and may resolve when the cause is eliminated. Recent research indicates that primary and secondary nocturnal enuresis both may be related to poor daytime voiding habits, and children should be taught to be aware of the sensation of needing to void (Robson, Leung, & Van Howe, 2005).

OLDER ADULTS The excretory function of the kidneys diminishes as people age, but function usually does not diminish significantly below normal levels unless a disease process intervenes. Arteriosclerosis can reduce blood flow, impairing renal function. As a person ages, the number of functioning nephrons decreases to some degree, impairing the kidney's filtering abilities. Conditions that alter normal fluid intake and output, such as influenza or surgery, can compromise the kidney's ability to filter, maintain acid–base balance, and maintain electrolyte balance in older adults, and the amount of time necessary for these processes to return to normal functioning also increases as a person ages. The decrease in kidney function also places older adults at higher risk for toxicity from medications when excretion rates are longer.

The more noticeable changes as a person ages are related to the bladder. Reports of urinary urgency and urinary frequency are common. In men, these changes often are caused by an enlarged prostate gland; in women, they may be caused by weakened muscles supporting the bladder or by weakness of the urethral sphincter. The capacity of the bladder and its ability to empty both diminish as a person ages. This explains the need for older adults to awaken at night to void (**nocturnal frequency**) and the increase in retention of residual urine. The increased retention of residual urine predisposes the older adult to bladder infection. Table 9–2 shows a summary of the developmental changes that affect urinary output.

Psychosocial Factors

For many people, a set of conditions helps stimulate the micturition reflex. These conditions include privacy, normal position, sufficient time, and occasionally, running water. Circumstances that do not allow for the client's accustomed conditions may produce anxiety and muscle tension. When this happens, the person is unable to relax the abdominal and perineal muscles and the external urethral sphincter, and voiding is inhibited. People also may voluntarily suppress urination because of perceived time pressures; for example, nurses often ignore the urge to void until they are able to take a break. This behavior can increase the risk of UTIs.

Fluid and Food Intake

The healthy body maintains a balance between the amount of fluid ingested and the amount of fluid eliminated. When the amount of fluid intake increases, the output normally increases. Certain fluids, such as alcohol, increase fluid output by inhibiting the production of ADH. By contrast, food and fluids that are high in sodium can cause fluid retention so that the body will be able to maintain the normal concentration of electrolytes. Some foods and fluids can change the color of urine: Beets can cause urine to appear red; foods containing carotene can cause yellow discoloration of the urine.

Medications

Many medications, particularly those affecting the autonomic nervous system, interfere with the normal urination process and may cause retention (Box 9–1). **Diuretics** (e.g., chlorothiazide and furosemide) increase urine formation by preventing the reabsorption in the bloodstream of water and electrolytes from the tubules of the kidney. Some medications may alter the color of the urine.

Muscle Tone

Good muscle tone is important to maintain the elasticity and contractility of the detrusor muscle, allowing the bladder to fill adequately and empty completely. Clients who require long-term use of a retention catheter may develop poor bladder muscle tone because continuous drainage of urine prevents the bladder from filling and emptying normally. Pelvic muscle tone also contributes to the ability to store and empty urine.

Pathologic Conditions

Some diseases and conditions can affect the formation and excretion of urine. Diseases of the kidneys may affect the ability of the nephrons to produce urine. Abnormal amounts of protein or

TABLE 9–2 **Changes in Urinary Elimination Through the Life Span**

STAGE	VARIATIONS
Fetuses	The fetal kidney begins to excrete urine between the 11th and 12th weeks of development.
Infants	Ability to concentrate urine is minimal; therefore, urine appears light yellow. Because of neuromuscular immaturity, voluntary urinary control is absent.
Children	Kidney function reaches maturity between the first and second year of life; urine is concentrated effectively and appears a normal amber color. Between 18 and 24 months of age, the child starts to recognize bladder fullness and is able to hold urine beyond the urge to void. At approximately 2.5–3 years of age, the child can perceive bladder fullness, hold urine after the urge to void, and communicate the need to urinate. Full urinary control usually occurs at 4 or 5 years of age; daytime control is usually achieved by 3 years of age. The kidneys grow in proportion to overall body growth.
Adults	The kidneys reach maximum size between 35 and 40 years of age. After 50 years, the kidneys begin to diminish in size and function. Most shrinkage occurs in the cortex of the kidney as individual nephrons are lost.
Older adults	An estimated 30% of nephrons are lost by 80 years of age. Renal blood flow decreases because of vascular changes and a decrease in cardiac output. The ability to concentrate urine declines. Bladder muscle tone diminishes, causing increased frequency of urination and nocturia (voiding two or more times at night). Diminished bladder muscle tone and contractibility may lead to residual urine in the bladder after voiding, increasing the risk of bacterial growth and infection. Urinary incontinence may occur because of mobility problems or neurologic impairments.

blood cells may be present in the urine, or the kidneys may virtually stop producing urine altogether, a condition known as **renal failure**. Heart and circulatory disorders, such as heart failure, shock, or hypertension, can affect blood flow to the kidneys, interfering with urine production. When abnormal amounts of fluid are lost through another route (e.g., vomiting or high fever), the kidneys retain water, and urinary output decreases.

Processes that interfere with the flow of urine from the kidneys to the urethra also affect urinary excretion. A urinary stone (calculus) may obstruct a ureter, blocking urine flow from the kidney to the bladder. Hypertrophy of the prostate gland, a common condition affecting older men, may obstruct the urethra, impairing urination and bladder emptying.

Box 9–1 **Medications That May Cause Urinary Retention**

- Anticholinergic and antispasmodic medications, such as atropine and papaverine
- Antidepressant and antipsychotic agents, such as phenothiazines and monoamine oxidase inhibitors
- Antihistamine preparations, especially those containing pseudoephedrine (e.g., Claritin-D and Sudafed)
- Antihypertensive agents, such as hydralazine (Apresoline) and methyldopate (Aldomet)
- Antiparkinsonism drugs, such as levodopa, trihexyphenidyl (Artane), and benztropine mesylate (Cogentin)
- Beta-adrenergic blockers, such as propranolol (Inderal)
- Opioids, such as hydrocodone (Vicodin)

Surgical and Diagnostic Procedures

Some surgical and diagnostic procedures affect the passage of urine and even the urine itself. The urethra may swell after cystoscopy (endoscopy of the urinary bladder), and surgical procedures on any part of the urinary tract may result in some postoperative bleeding, which can cause the urine to be tinged red or pink for a time.

Spinal anesthetics can affect the passage of urine because they decrease the client's awareness of the need to void. Swelling in the lower abdomen because of surgery on structures adjacent to the urinary tract (e.g., the uterus) also can affect voiding.

AGE-RELATED CHANGES IN THE URINARY SYSTEM

It is difficult to differentiate normal aging of the genitourinary system from changes related to common conditions found in older people. It is prudent, therefore, to keep an open mind when discussing age-related changes.

Renal function begins to decline around 40 years of age but does not create significant issues for an otherwise healthy individual until the ninth decade of life. At that time, decreases in GFR, renal blood flow, maximal urinary concentration, and response to sodium loss are marked. Renal function in an 85-year-old person is approximately 50% of that in a 30-year-old person (Timiras & Leary, 2007). Sclerosis may be found in as many as 40% of the remaining glomeruli, and fibrous changes in the interstitial tissues may be found in older persons without kidney disease (Bailey & Sands, 2003; Wiggins, 2003). Blood flow to the kidney decreases as a result of atrophy in the supplying blood vessels, particularly in the renal cortex. In addition, the proximal tubules decrease in number and length. Compared with a young adult, an older adult usually has a lower creatinine clearance, has urine that is more dilute (lower specific gravity), and typically excretes lower levels of glucose, acid, and potassium. As these changes progress, the serum creatinine level and the blood urea nitrogen (BUN) will increase (Esposito et al., 2007). In addition, the kidneys of older adults excrete more fluid and electrolytes during the night than during the day, and more urine is formed at night, potentially interrupting sleep patterns.

One very important consequence of these changes is impaired excretion of drugs and their metabolites, making older adults extremely susceptible to drug overdose and other adverse effects of medication (even when administered within a normal dose range). This is of particular concern for the older adult with multiple health impairments who requires several types of pharmacologic therapies. Another consequence of age-related changes is an increased probability of hyperkalemia, particularly when potassium-sparing diuretics, angiotensin-converting enzyme inhibitors, nonsteroidal anti-inflammatory drugs, or beta-blockers are used (Timiras & Luxenberg, 2007). The older adult's decreased ability to concentrate urine results in an increased susceptibility to dehydration, a problem that is further complicated by a deficit in the thirst response; therefore, the older person may not feel thirsty even when significantly dehydrated. In addition, an older adult who has concerns about incontinence may choose not to drink for fear of an incontinence accident. These changes also produce a decline in the ability of older adults to respond to a fluid overload by increasing urine production.

Changes in the bladder and urethra also occur with aging. The bladder becomes more fibrous, with a subsequent decrease in capacity and an increase in residual urine (Huether & McCance, 2005). Autonomic regulation of the bladder by the nervous system decreases as a person ages, affecting contraction of both the detrusor muscle and the external sphincter. The detrusor muscle becomes less contractile but also somewhat unstable. This means that the older adult is subject both to the inability to empty the bladder completely and to involuntary contractions of the bladder (Ouslander & Johnson, 2003). Age-related weakening also occurs in the voluntary pelvic floor muscles, which are important in controlling the release of urine from the urethra. These changes make older adults more likely to have difficulty delaying urination and predispose them to urinary incontinence and UTI. However, it is important for the nurse to remember that even though some anatomic and physiologic changes make incontinence more probable with increased age, urinary incontinence is not a normal part of aging.

Older adults tend to have higher basal levels of ADH than younger adults do, and the pituitary responds more vigorously to osmotic stimuli by secreting more ADH than in younger people (Timiras & Leary, 2007). Although ADH is released as a response to hypotension and hypovolemia (low blood volume), its action is blunted in older adults, requiring the release of more hormones to achieve the desired antidiuretic effect. In addition, the aging kidney is less responsive to circulating ADH, producing urine that is poorly concentrated and rich in sodium. This puts the older adult at increased risk of **hyponatremia**, an abnormally low concentration of sodium in the blood that can be magnified with the use of diuretics.

ALTERATIONS

A number of diseases and processes can interfere with the flow of blood to the kidneys or of urine from the kidneys, interfering with the production and elimination of urine.

Altered Urine Production

Polyuria (or **diuresis**) is the production of abnormally large amounts of urine by the kidneys—often several liters more than the client's usual daily output. Polyuria can occur after excessive fluid intake, a condition known as **polydipsia**, or it may be associated with diseases such as diabetes mellitus, diabetes insipidus, and chronic nephritis. Polyuria can cause excessive fluid loss, leading to intense thirst, dehydration, and weight loss.

The terms "anuria" and "oliguria" are used to describe decreased urinary output. **Anuria** refers to an absence of urine production, whereas **oliguria** refers to a low urine output, usually less than 500 mL a day or 30 mL an hour for an adult. Although oliguria may occur as a result of abnormal fluid losses or a lack of fluid intake, it often indicates impaired blood flow to the kidneys or impending renal failure, and it should be reported promptly to the primary care provider. Rapid restoration of renal blood flow and urinary output can prevent renal failure and its complications.

Should the kidneys become unable to function adequately, some mechanism of filtering the blood is necessary to prevent illness and death. This filtering is done through renal **dialysis**, a technique by which fluids and molecules pass through a semipermeable membrane according to the rules of osmosis. The two most common methods of dialysis are hemodialysis and peritoneal dialysis. In **hemodialysis**, the client's blood flows through vascular catheters, passes by the dialysis solution in an external machine, and then returns to the client. In **peritoneal dialysis**, the dialysis solution is instilled into the abdominal cavity through a catheter, allowed to rest there while the fluid and molecules exchange, and then removed through the catheter. Both hemodialysis and peritoneal dialysis must be performed at frequent intervals until the client's kidneys can resume the filtering function.

Altered Urinary Elimination

Despite normal production of urine, a number of factors or conditions can affect its elimination. Urinary frequency, nocturia, urgency, and dysuria often are manifestations of underlying conditions such as a UTI. Enuresis, incontinence, retention, and neurogenic bladder may be either a manifestation of an underlying condition or the primary problem affecting elimination of urine.

Selected factors associated with altered patterns of urinary elimination are identified in Table 9–3.

Urinary frequency is voiding at frequent intervals—that is, more than four to six times a day. An increased intake of fluid causes some increase in the frequency of voiding. Conditions such as UTI, stress, and pregnancy can cause frequent voiding of small quantities (50–100 mL) of urine. Total fluid intake and output may be normal. **Nocturia** (voiding at night) usually is expressed in terms of the number of times the person gets out of bed to void—for example, "nocturia ×4."

Urgency is the sudden strong desire to void. Whether or not a great deal of urine is present in the bladder, the person feels a need to void immediately. Urgency often accompanies psychologic stress and irritation of the trigone and urethra. It also is common in people who have poor external sphincter control and unstable bladder contractions. It is not a normal finding.

Dysuria means voiding that is either painful or difficult. It can accompany a stricture (decrease in diameter) of the urethra, UTI, and injury to the bladder and urethra. Often, clients will say they have to push to void or that burning accompanies or follows voiding. The burning may be described as severe, like a hot poker, or more subdued, like sunburn. **Urinary hesitancy** (a delay and difficulty in initiating voiding) is associated often with dysuria.

Adults and children can experience enuresis. Diurnal (daytime) enuresis may be persistent and pathologic in origin. It affects women and girls more frequently than it does men and boys. The occurrence of enuresis after voluntary bladder control has been acquired successfully should be reported to the primary care provider.

Impaired neurologic function can interfere with the normal mechanisms of urinary elimination, resulting in a **neurogenic bladder**. The client with a neurogenic bladder does not perceive bladder fullness and is unable to control the urinary sphincters. The bladder may become flaccid and distended or spastic, with frequent involuntary urination. For additional details, see the Alterations and Treatments features.

TABLE 9–3 **Selected Factors Associated With Altered Urinary Elimination**

PATTERN	SELECTED ASSOCIATED FACTORS
Polyuria	Ingestion of fluids containing caffeine or alcohol Prescribed diuretic Presence of thirst, dehydration, and weight loss History of diabetes mellitus, diabetes insipidus, or kidney disease
Oliguria, anuria	Decrease in fluid intake Signs of dehydration Presence of hypotension, shock, or heart failure History of kidney disease Signs of renal failure, such as elevated BUN and serum creatinine Edema, hypertension
Frequency or nocturia	Pregnancy Increase in fluid intake UTI
Urgency	Presence of psychologic stress UTI
Dysuria	Urinary tract inflammation, infection, or injury Hesitancy, hematuria, pyuria (pus in the urine), and frequency
Enuresis	Family history of enuresis Difficult access to toilet facilities Home stresses
Incontinence	Bladder inflammation or other disease Difficulties in independent toileting (mobility impairment) Leakage when coughing, laughing, sneezing Cognitive impairment
Retention	Distended bladder on palpation and percussion Associated signs, such as pubic discomfort, restlessness, frequency, and small urine volume Recent anesthesia Recent perineal surgery Presence of perineal swelling Medications prescribed Lack of privacy or other factors inhibiting micturition

ALTERATIONS AND TREATMENTS Urinary Elimination Problems

Alteration	Description	Treatment
Urinary incontinence	Involuntary leakage of urine	■ Kegel exercises ■ Surgery ■ Bladder training
Urinary retention	Incomplete emptying or inability to empty bladder completely	■ Credé maneuver ■ Urinary catheter insertion
Prostatic hypertrophy	Enlargement of the prostate—may be benign or malignant	■ Surgical removal ■ Medications
Cancer of the urinary system	Abnormal cellular growth within the organs of the urinary tract	■ Surgery ■ Chemotherapy ■ Radiation therapy
Kidney stones	Formation of calculi within the calyx of the kidney, causing severe pain when moving through ureters	■ Administration of pain medication ■ Lithotripsy ■ Dietary alteration to reduce risk of recurrence ■ Increased fluid intake
Renal failure	Insufficient or absent kidney function	■ Administration of diuretics if some kidney function remains ■ Dialysis (hemodialysis or peritoneal dialysis) ■ Kidney transplantation
Infection of the urinary system	Pathogens within the sterile urinary system creating infection, which can occur in the bladder, ureter, or kidney	■ Administration of antibiotics if infection is caused by bacterium ■ Increased fluid intake ■ Cranberry juice to increase urine pH

PHYSICAL ASSESSMENT

Physical assessment, a health assessment interview that collects subjective data, and diagnostic tests are used to assess urinary system function. Box 9–2 shows sample documentation for an assessment of urinary system function, and the following Urinary Assessments feature provides additional information. Table 9–4 lists characteristics of normal and abnormal urine, and the following Assessment Interview feature gives further details regarding urinary elimination.

Box 9–2 Sample Documentation

ASSESSMENT OF URINARY SYSTEM FUNCTION

Home visit made to 66-year-old woman with end-stage chronic kidney failure. Skin pale and oral mucous membranes dry. 4+ edema in ankles and feet. Eyelids swollen. Skin tight and shiny over abdomen and bilateral lower extremities. Abdomen distended and tender on light palpation; further palpation deferred. Urinary bladder not palpable. Urine output for past 24 hours is 15 mL.

Urinary Assessment

Technique/Normal Findings	Abnormal Findings
Skin Assessment	
Inspect the skin and mucous membranes, noting color, turgor, and excretions. *The color of skin and mucous membranes should be even and appropriate to the age and race of the client; skin should be dry with no visible excretions.*	■ Pallor of the skin and mucous membranes may indicate kidney disease with resultant anemia. ■ Decreased turgor of the skin may indicate dehydration. ■ Edema (generalized or in the lower extremities) may indicate fluid volume excess. (Changes in skin turgor may indicate renal insufficiency with either excess fluid loss or retention.) ■ An accumulation of uric acid crystals, called uremic frost, may be seen on the skin of the client with late-stage renal failure.
Abdominal Assessment	
Inspect the abdomen, noting size, symmetry, masses or lumps, swelling, distention, glistening, or skin tightness. *The abdomen should be slightly concave, symmetric, without distention or masses.*	■ Enlargements or asymmetry may indicate a hernia or superficial mass. ■ If the urinary bladder is distended, it rises above the symphysis pubis as a rounded mass. ■ Distention, glistening, or skin tightness may be associated with fluid retention. ■ Ascites is an accumulation of fluid in the peritoneal cavity.

Urinary Assessment (continued)

Technique/Normal Findings | **Abnormal Findings**

Urinary Meatus Assessment

This technique is not part of a routine assessment, but it is an important component in clients with health problems of the urinary system.

For the male client: **With the client in a sitting or standing position, compress the tip of the glans penis with your gloved hand to open the urinary meatus (Figure 9–6 ■).**

For the female client: **With the client in the dorsal lithotomy position, spread the labia with your gloved hand to expose the urinary meatus.**

The urinary meatus should be midline and free of redness, lesions, or discharge.

- Increased redness, swelling, or discharge from the urinary meatus may indicate infection or sexually transmitted infection.
- Ulceration of the urinary meatus may indicate a sexually transmitted infection.
- Hypospadias is displacement of the urinary meatus to the ventral surface of the penis.
- Epispadias is displacement of the urinary meatus to the dorsal surface of the penis.

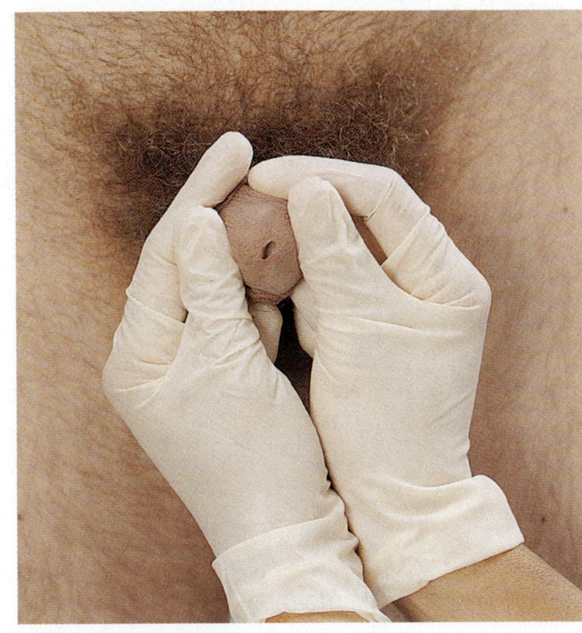

Figure 9–6 ■ Inspecting the urinary meatus of the male.

Kidney Assessment

Auscultate the renal arteries by placing the bell of the stethoscope lightly in the areas of the renal arteries, located in the left and right upper abdominal quadrants. *Bruits are not normally heard over the renal arteries.*

- Systolic bruits ("whooshing" sounds) may indicate renal artery stenosis.

Percuss the kidneys for tenderness or pain. *No tenderness or pain should be elicited.*

- Tenderness and pain on percussion of the costovertebral angle suggest glomerulonephritis or glomerulonephrosis.

Palpate the kidneys. The lower pole of the right kidney may be palpable with deep palpation; the remaining right kidney and the left kidney are normally not palpable. *If palpable, they should be nontender, bilaterally of appropriate size and density, without palpable masses.*

- A mass or lump may indicate a tumor or cyst.
- Tenderness or pain on palpation may suggest an inflammatory process.
- A soft kidney that feels spongy may indicate chronic renal disease.
- Bilaterally enlarged kidneys may suggest polycystic kidney disease.
- Unequal kidney size may indicate hydronephrosis.

Bladder Assessment

Percuss the bladder for tone and position. *The bladder should be midline without dullness.*

- A dull percussion tone over the bladder of a client who has just urinated may indicate urinary retention.

Palpate the bladder (over the symphysis pubis and abdomen) for distention. *The bladder is normally not palpable.*

- A distended bladder may be palpated at any point from the symphysis pubis to the umbilicus and is felt as a firm, rounded organ. It indicates urinary retention.

TABLE 9–4 Characteristics of Normal and Abnormal Urine

CHARACTERISTIC	NORMAL	ABNORMAL	NURSING CONSIDERATIONS
Amount in 24 hours (adult)	1,200–1,500 mL	1,200 mL A large amount over intake	Normally, urinary output is approximately equal to fluid intake. Output of less than 30 mL/hr may indicate decreased blood flow to the kidneys and should be reported immediately.
Color, clarity	Straw, amber Transparent	Dark amber Cloudy Dark orange Red or dark brown Mucous plugs, viscid, thick	Concentrated urine is darker in color. Dilute urine may appear almost clear, or very pale yellow. Some foods and drugs may color urine. Red blood cells in the urine (hematuria) may be evident as pink, bright red, or rusty brown urine. Menstrual bleeding also can color urine but should not be confused with hematuria. White blood cells, bacteria, pus, or contaminants (e.g., prostatic fluid, sperm, vaginal drainage) may cause cloudy urine.
Odor	Faint, aromatic	Offensive	Some foods (e.g., asparagus) cause a musty odor; infected urine can have a fetid odor; urine high in glucose has a sweet odor.
Sterility	No microorganisms present	Microorganisms present	Urine in the bladder is sterile. Urine specimens, however, may be contaminated by bacteria from the perineum during collection.
pH	4.5–8	8<4.5	Freshly voided urine is somewhat acidic. Alkaline urine may indicate a state of alkalosis, a UTI, or a diet high in fruits and vegetables. More acidic urine (low pH) is found in starvation, with diarrhea, or with a diet high in protein foods or cranberries.
Specific gravity	1.010–1.025	1.02<1. 010	Concentrated urine has a higher specific gravity; diluted urine has a lower specific gravity.
Glucose	Not present	Present	Glucose in the urine indicates high blood glucose levels (>180 mg/dL) and may be indicative of undiagnosed or uncontrolled diabetes mellitus.
Ketone bodies (acetone)	Not present	Present	Ketones, the end product of the breakdown of fatty acids, are not normally present in the urine. They may be present in the urine of clients who have uncontrolled diabetes mellitus, who are in a state of starvation, or who have ingested excessive amounts of aspirin.
Blood	Not present	Occult (microscopic) Bright red	Blood may be present in the urine of clients who have a UTI, kidney disease, or bleeding from the urinary tract.

Note: Urine outputs below 30 mL/hr may indicate low blood volume or kidney malfunction. Nurses monitor urine output and should notify the primary provider if urine output averages less than 30 mL/hr over a 4-hour period of time.

DIAGNOSTIC TESTS

The results of diagnostic tests of urinary system function are used to support the diagnosis of a specific disease, to provide information to identify or modify the appropriate medication or therapy used to treat the disease, and to help nurses monitor the client's responses to treatment and nursing care interventions. Diagnostic tests to assess the structures and functions of the urinary system are described in the Diagnostic Tests appendix and summarized in the bulleted list that follows.

- Urine may be tested for characteristics and components through routine analysis, a urine culture, a postvoiding residual urine, and a 24-hour collection for creatinine. Results of these tests include findings to serve as baseline data, to support the diagnosis of various health problems, to evaluate the ability to empty the bladder of urine, and to evaluate renal function. (Table 9–5).
- The ability to empty the bladder of urine may be evaluated by an ultrasonic bladder scan to examine for residual urine; uroflowmetry to measure the volume of urine voided per second; and cystometrography to evaluate bladder capacity, neuromuscular functions of the bladder, urethral pressures, and causes of bladder dysfunction.
- Radiologic examinations include intravenous pyelography (IVP), retrograde pyelography, and renal arteriography or angiography. These examinations are useful in visualizing (via radiographs) the urinary tract to identify abnormal size, shape, and function of the kidneys, kidney pelvis, and ureters, and to detect renal **calculi** (stones), tumors, or cysts.
- A cystoscopy allows direct visualization of the bladder wall and urethra. During this procedure, small stones can be removed, a sample of tissue may be taken for biopsy, and retrograde pyelography may be done. If a contrast dye is instilled in the bladder, then fistulas, tumors, or ruptures can be identified.
- Noninvasive tests include renal ultrasound, computed tomography (CT), magnetic resonance imaging (MRI), and

Assessment Interview Urinary Elimination

The assessment interview conducted by the nurse provides critical information about urinary function. The nurse should be direct but polite, recognizing that discussing urinary function can be embarrassing to many clients. Initially, the nurse should ask the client to describe the frequency of urination and any problems with urination. During the remainder of the interview, the nurse should use the vocabulary the client uses (to ensure understanding). In addition to recording the client's answers, the nurse should record any abnormalities that he or she observes in the client, such as swelling and changes in skin integrity.

VOIDING PATTERN

- How many times do you urinate during a 24-hour period?
- Has this pattern changed recently?
- Do you need to get out of bed to void at night? How often?

DESCRIPTION OF URINE AND ANY CHANGES

- How would you describe your urine in terms of color, clarity (clear, transparent, or cloudy), and odor (faint or strong)?

URINARY ELIMINATION PROBLEMS

What problems have you had or do you now have with passing your urine?

- Passage of small amounts of urine?
- Voiding at intervals that are more frequent?
- Trouble getting to the bathroom in time or feeling an urgent need to void?
- Painful voiding?
- Difficulty starting urine stream?
- Frequent dribbling of urine or a feeling of bladder fullness associated with voiding small amounts of urine?
- Reduced force of stream?
- Accidental leakage of urine? If so, when does this occur (e.g., when coughing, laughing, or sneezing; at night; during the day)?
- Past urinary tract illness, such as infection of the kidney, bladder, or urethra; urinary calculi; surgery of kidney, ureters, or bladder?

FACTORS INFLUENCING URINARY ELIMINATION

- *Medications.* Do you take any medications that could increase urinary output or cause urinary retention? Nurses should note the name and specific dosage of all medications because the individual may not be aware that a medication could influence elimination.
- *Fluid intake.* What amount and kind of fluid do you take each day (e.g., six glasses of water, two cups of coffee, three cola drinks with or without caffeine)?
- *Environmental factors.* Do you have any problems with toileting (mobility, removing clothing, toilet seat too low, facility without grab bar)?
- *Stress.* Are you experiencing any major stress? If so, what are the stressors? Do you think these affect your urinary pattern?
- *Disease.* Have you had or do you have any illnesses that may affect urinary function, such as hypertension, heart disease, neurologic disease, cancer, prostatic enlargement, or diabetes?
- *Diagnostic procedures and surgery.* Have you recently had a cystoscopy or anesthetic?

---

renal scan. These tests are used to identify and evaluate kidney size and structure as well as renal or perirenal masses and obstructions. In addition, a renal scan may be used to evaluate kidney blood flow, perfusion, and urine production.

- A kidney biopsy is done to obtain tissue for use in diagnosing or monitoring kidney disease.

Regardless of the type of diagnostic test, the nurse is responsible for explaining the procedure and any special preparations needed as well as assessing for medication use that may affect the outcome of the tests. It is critical that the nurse ensures the client fully understands the conditions under which the test will be administered and which preparations the

TABLE 9–5 **Normal and Abnormal Findings: Urinalysis**

CHARACTERISTIC OR COMPONENT	NORMAL RESULTS	ABNORMAL FINDING WITH POSSIBLE CAUSE
Color	Light straw to amber yellow	■ Red, dark, smoky color may be the result of blood in the urine (hematuria or menstrual blood). ■ Cloudy urine occurs from infection. ■ Colorless urine indicates very dilute urine, such as in overhydration, kidney disease, alcohol ingestion, or diabetes insipidus. ■ Very dark yellow urine indicates dehydration and/or fever. ■ Red or red brown urine may be caused by sulfisoxazole-phenazopyridine (Azo Gantrisin), phenytoin (Dilantin), cascara, chlorpromazine (Thorazine), docusate calcium and phenolphthalein (Doxidan); and by carrots, rhubarb, and food coloring. ■ Orange urine is caused by fever, urobilin, phenazopyridine (Pyridium), amidopyrine, nitrofurantoin, sulfonamides, carrots, beets, and food coloring. ■ Blue or green urine is caused by Pseudomonas, amitriptyline (Elavil), methylene blue, methocarbamol (Robaxin), and yeast concentrate. ■ Brown or black urine is caused by Lysol poisoning, melanin, bilirubin, methemoglobin, porphyrin, cascara, and injectable iron.
Appearance	Clear	■ Hazy or cloudy urine indicates bacteria, pus, RBCs, WBCs, phosphates, prostatic fluid spermatozoa, or urates. ■ Milky urine is the result of fats or pyuria. ■ Yellow foam results from bilirubin, bile, or severe cirrhosis of the liver. ■ A dark yellow to brownish color is seen with deficient fluid volume.

(continued)

TABLE 9–5 **Normal and Abnormal Findings: Urinalysis** **(continued)**

CHARACTERISTIC OR COMPONENT	NORMAL RESULTS	ABNORMAL FINDING WITH POSSIBLE CAUSE
Odor	Aromatic	■ Ammonia smell increases as urine stands outside the body. ■ Urinary tract infection (UTI) causes a foul or unpleasant odor, depending on the causative organism. ■ Asparagus causes a distinctive odor. ■ Mousy odors result from phenylketonuria. ■ Sweet or fruity odors occur in starvation and diabetic ketoacidosis.
pH	4.5–8.0	■ < 4.5: metabolic acidosis, respiratory acidosis, diet high in meat protein, ammonium chloride and mandelic acid. ■ > 8.0: bacteriuria, UTI, antibiotics (neomycin, kanamycin), sulfonamides, sodium bicarbonate, acetazolamide (Diamox), potassium citrate.
Specific gravity	1.005–1.030	■ < 1.005: diabetes insipidus, overhydration, renal disease, severe potassium deficit.
Protein	2–8 mg/dL	■ > 8 mg/dL: proteinuria, exercise, fever, stress, acute infection, kidney disease, lupus erythematosus, leukemia, multiple myeloma, cardiac disease, toxemia of pregnancy, septicemia, lead, mercury, neomycin, barbiturates, sulfonamides.
Glucose	Negative	■ > 15 mg/dL or +4: diabetes mellitus, stroke, Cushing's syndrome, anesthesia, glucose infusions, severe stress, infections, ascorbic acid, aspirin, cephalosporins, and epinephrine.
Ketones	Negative	■ +1 to +3: ketoacidosis, starvation, high-protein diet.
RBCs	Rare	■ > 2 per low-power field: kidney trauma, kidney diseases, renal calculi, cystitis, excess aspirin, anticoagulants, sulfonamides, menstrual contamination.
WBCs	3–4	■ > 4 per low-power field: UTI, fever, strenuous exercise, kidney diseases.
Casts	Occasional hyaline	■ Fever, kidney diseases, heart failure.

Source: LeMone, P., & Burke, K. (2008). *Medical-surgical nursing: Critical thinking in client care* (4th ed. p. 832). Upper Saddle River, NJ: Pearson Education.

client may need to take in advance (e.g., fasting) for tests to be accurate and successful. The nurse also supports the client during the examination as necessary, documents the procedures as appropriate, and monitors the results of the tests.

Blood levels of two metabolically produced substances, urea and creatinine, are used routinely to evaluate renal function. Both substances normally are eliminated by the kidneys through filtration and tubular secretion. Urea, the end product of protein metabolism, is measured as BUN. Creatinine is produced in relatively constant quantities by the muscles. The **creatinine clearance** test uses 24-hour urine and serum creatinine levels to determine the GFR, a sensitive indicator of renal function. Other tests related to urinary functions include collection of a urine specimen, measurement of specific gravity, and visualization procedures.

CARING INTERVENTIONS

The primary purpose for performing nursing interventions associated with elimination of urine is to maintain the integrity of the urinary system, which eliminates excess fluid and wastes, thereby promoting homeostasis.

Care of the client with altered urinary output is determined by the cause and severity of the problem. Clients with reduced urine output secondary to dehydration will require increased fluid intake. Poor kidney perfusion or function may require the addition of medications such as diuretics. If renal function is severely compromised or nonfunctional, the client may require dialysis (peritoneal or hemodialysis) or kidney transplantation.

Aseptic technique is essential whenever performing procedures that could introduce bacteria into the urinary tract. Washing hands, using sterile gloves, and maintaining a closed urinary collection system decrease the incidence of ascending bladder contamination and subsequent UTI. Maintaining aseptic technique throughout dialysis procedures is necessary to prevent infection in grafts, fistulas, and catheters.

Consult your skills manual for step-by-step descriptions of the following caring interventions related to urinary elimination:

- Measurement of intake and output
- External urine collection systems
- Urinary catheterization
- Bladder irrigation
- Suprapubic catheter care
- Collecting specimens from a closed urinary system
- Urinary diversions
- Hemodialysis.

MEDICATIONS Urinary Elimination

Drug classifications	Mechanism of action	Commonly prescribed drugs	Nursing considerations
Anticholinergic agents	These reduce urgency and frequency by blocking muscarinic receptors in the detrusor muscle of the bladder, thereby inhibiting contractions and increasing storage capacity. They can be useful in relieving symptoms associated with voiding in clients who have neurogenic bladder, reflex neurogenic bladder, or urge urinary incontinence.	Oxybutynin	■ Monitor for constipation, dry mouth, urinary retention, blurred vision, and (in older adults) mental confusion. Symptoms may be dose related. ■ Start with small doses for clients older than 75 years. ■ Oxybutynin is contraindicated in clients with urinary retention, gastrointestinal (GI) motility problems (partial or complete GI obstruction, paralytic ileus), or uncontrolled narrow-angle glaucoma.
Cholinergic agents or parasympathomimetics	These medications stimulate bladder contraction and facilitate voiding.	Bethanechol chloride (Urecholine)	■ Do not administer to clients with GI or urinary tract obstructions, asthma, bradycardia, hypotension, or Parkinson's disease. ■ May increase serum aspartate aminotransferase, amylase, and lipase levels. ■ Effect of medications is antagonized by angel's trumpet, jimson weed, or scopolia. ■ Overdose is treated with atropine sulfate.
Diuretics: loop, thiazide, potassium-sparing, and miscellaneous type	Each type of diuretic works in a specific place within the nephron to increase fluid excretion and prevent fluid reabsorption.		■ Monitor hydration and electrolyte balance. ■ Monitor vital signs, and be alert for signs of hypotension secondary to fluid loss. ■ Monitor serum BUN, creatinine, electrolyte, and other pertinent laboratory values. ■ Clients taking potassium-sparing diuretics should avoid salt substitutes.

PHARMACOLOGIC THERAPIES

Pharmacologic therapy for urinary elimination includes diuretics to increase the production of urine, anticholinergic medications to reduce urinary frequency and treat incontinence related to urgency, and cholinergic medications to stimulate bladder contractions and promote urination, especially in clients with difficulty voiding. See the Medications feature for additional information.

There are four subclassifications of diuretics based on where and how they act in the kidney. Loop diuretics, as the name implies, work in the loop of Henle by blocking reabsorption of sodium and chloride. Thiazide diuretics act on the distal tubule to block sodium reabsorption and increase potassium and water excretion. Potassium-sparing diuretics work in the distal tubule allowing sodium to be excreted while restoring much of the potassium to the body, thereby avoiding the large potassium loss seen with other types of diuretics. Finally, diuretics that cannot be otherwise classified make up a miscellaneous group; this group includes carbonic anhydrase inhibitors and osmotic diuretics.

Bowel Elimination

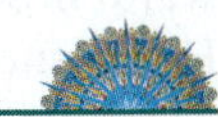

Nurses frequently are consulted or involved in assisting clients with fecal elimination problems. These problems can be embarrassing to clients and can cause considerable discomfort. The elimination of feces is a prominent public topic in North America. For example, laxative advertisements, which describe feelings such as tiredness because of irregularity, keep the subject in the public consciousness. Some older adults are preoccupied with their bowels. People who have had a bowel movement once a day for 75 years can view missing one day as a serious problem.

NORMAL PRESENTATION

The excreted waste products from the bowel are referred to as **feces** or **stool**. Individuals (especially children) may use very different terms for a bowel movement. The nurse may need to try several common words before finding one the client understands.

Defecation is the expulsion of feces from the anus and rectum. It is also called a bowel movement. The frequency of defecation is highly individual, varying from several times a day to two or three times a week. The amount defecated also varies from person to person.

Normal feces are made up of approximately 75% water and 25% solid materials. They are soft but formed. If the feces are propelled very quickly along the large intestine, there is inadequate time for most of the water in the chyme to be reabsorbed, and the feces will be more fluid, containing perhaps 95% water. Normal feces require a normal fluid intake; feces that contain less water may be hard and difficult to expel. Feces normally are brown, chiefly because of the presence of stercobilin and urobilin, which are derived from bilirubin (a red pigment in bile). Another factor that affects fecal color is the action of bacteria, such as *Escherichia coli* or *Staphylococcus* sp., which normally are present in the large intestine. The action of microorganisms on the chyme also is responsible for the odor of feces.

An adult usually forms 7–10 L of **flatus** (gas) in the large intestine every 24 hours. The gases include carbon dioxide, methane, hydrogen, oxygen, and nitrogen. Some are swallowed with food and fluids taken by mouth. Others are formed through the action of bacteria on the chyme in the large intestine. Still other gas diffuses from the blood into the gastrointestinal tract.

Bowel Elimination and Pregnancy

During pregnancy, elevated progesterone levels cause smooth muscle relaxation, resulting in delayed gastric emptying and decreased peristalsis. As a result, the pregnant woman may complain of bloating and constipation. These symptoms are aggravated as the enlarging uterus displaces the stomach upward and the intestines are moved laterally and posteriorly. The cardiac sphincter also relaxes, and heartburn (pyrosis) may occur as a result of **reflux**, a backward flow of acidic secretions into the lower esophagus. Hemorrhoids frequently develop in late pregnancy from constipation and from pressure on vessels below the level of the uterus.

In the postpartum period the bowels tend to be sluggish following birth because of the lingering effects of progesterone, decreased abdominal muscle tone, and bowel evacuation associated with the labor and birth process. A woman who has had an episiotomy, lacerations, or hemorrhoids may tend to delay elimination for fear of increasing her pain or because she believes her stitches will be torn if she bears down. In refusing or delaying the bowel movement, the woman may cause increased constipation and pain when bowel elimination finally occurs.

The woman who has had a cesarean birth may experience some initial discomfort from flatulence, which can be relieved by early ambulation and use of antiflatulent medications. Chamomile or peppermint tea also may be helpful in reducing discomfort from flatulence. It may take a few days for the bowel to regain its tone, especially if general anesthesia was used. The woman who has had a cesarean or a difficult birth may benefit from stool softeners.

FACTORS AFFECTING BOWEL ELIMINATION

Defecation patterns vary at different stages of life. Circumstances of diet, fluid intake and output, activity, psychologic factors, lifestyle, medications and medical procedures, and disease also affect defecation.

Developmental Factors

Newborns and infants, toddlers, children, and older adults are groups within which members have similarities in elimination patterns.

NEWBORNS AND INFANTS Term newborns usually pass meconium within 8–24 hours of life and almost always within 48 hours. **Meconium** is formed in utero from the amniotic fluid and its constituents, intestinal secretions, and shed mucosal cells. It is recognized by its thick, tarry black or dark green appearance. Transitional (thin brown to green) stools consisting of part meconium and part fecal material are passed for the next day or two, and then the stools become entirely fecal. Generally, the stools of a breast-fed newborn are pale yellow (but may be pasty green) and usually are more liquid and more frequent than those of formula-fed newborns, whose stools are paler (Figure 9–7 ■).

Frequency of bowel movement varies but ranges from one every 2 or 3 days to as many as 10 movements daily. Totally breast-fed infants often progress to stools that occur every 5–7 days. Mothers should be counseled that the newborn is not constipated as long as the bowel movement remains soft.

Infants pass stool frequently, often after each feeding. Because the intestine is immature, water is not well absorbed, and the stool is soft, liquid, and frequent. When the intestine matures, bacterial flora increase. After solid foods are introduced, the stool becomes firmer and less frequent.

TODDLERS Some control of defecation starts at between 1.5 and 2 years of age. By this time, children have learned to walk, and their nervous and muscular systems are sufficiently well developed to permit bowel control. A desire to control daytime bowel movements and to use the toilet generally starts when the child becomes aware of the discomfort caused by a soiled diaper and the sensation that indicates the need for a bowel movement. Daytime control typically is attained by 2.5 years of age, after a process of toilet training.

SCHOOL-AGE CHILDREN AND ADOLESCENTS School-age children and adolescents have bowel habits similar to those of adults. Patterns of defecation vary in frequency, quantity, and consistency. Some school-age children may delay defecation because of an activity such as play.

OLDER ADULTS Constipation is the most common bowel management problem in the older adult population (Mauk, 2005). This is caused, in part, by reduced activity levels, inadequate fluid and fiber intake, and muscle weakness. Many older people believe that "regularity" means a bowel movement every day.

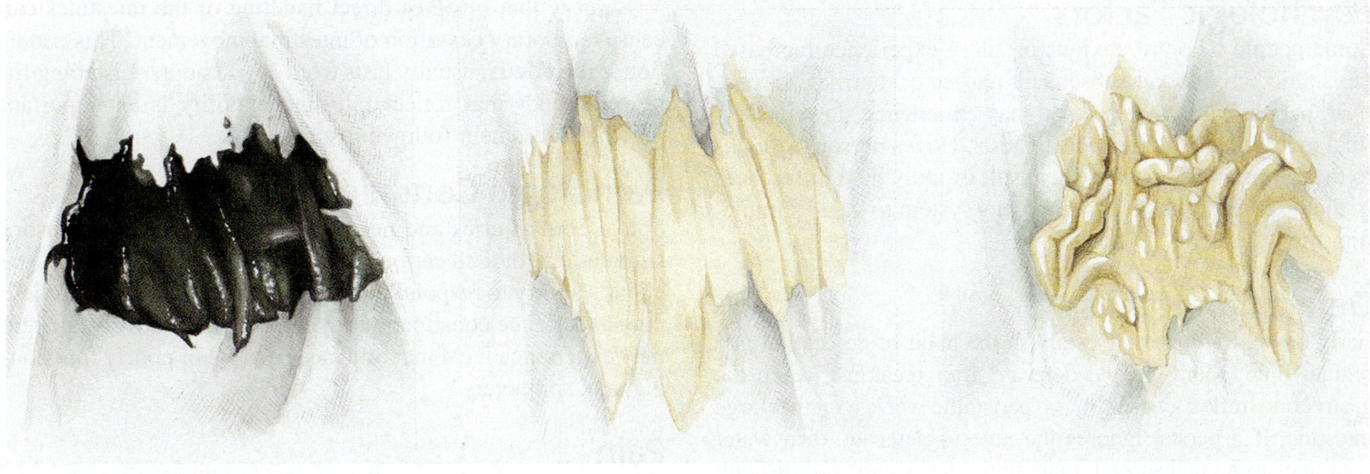

Figure 9–7 ■ Newborn stool samples.

Those who do not meet this criterion often seek over-the-counter preparations to relieve what they believe to be constipation. Older adults should be advised that normal patterns of bowel elimination vary considerably. For some, a normal pattern may be every other day; for others, a normal pattern may be twice a day. Adequate roughage in the diet, adequate exercise, and six to eight glasses of fluid daily are essential preventive measures for constipation. A cup of hot water or tea at a regular time in the morning also is helpful for some. Responding to the **gastrocolic reflex** (increased peristalsis of the colon after food has entered the stomach) is an important consideration as well. For example, toileting is recommended 5–15 min after meals—especially after breakfast, when the gastrocolic reflex is strongest (Hinrichs & Huseboe, 2001, p. 23).

The older adult should be warned that consistent use of laxatives inhibits natural defecation reflexes and is thought to cause, rather than cure, constipation. The habitual user of laxatives eventually requires larger or stronger doses because the effect is progressively reduced with continual use. Laxatives also may interfere with the body's electrolyte balance and reduce the absorption of certain vitamins. The reasons for constipation can range from lifestyle habits (e.g., lack of exercise) to serious malignant disorders (e.g., colorectal cancer). The nurse should evaluate carefully any complaints of constipation. A change in bowel habits over several weeks with or without weight loss, pain, or fever should be referred to a primary care provider for a complete medical evaluation.

Diet

Sufficient bulk (cellulose, fiber) in the diet is necessary to provide fecal volume. Bland diets and low-fiber diets lack bulk and therefore create insufficient residue of waste products to stimulate the reflex for defecation. Low-residue foods, such as rice, eggs, and lean meats, move more slowly through the intestinal tract. Increasing fluid intake with such foods increases their rate of movement.

Certain foods are difficult, or even impossible, for some people to digest. This difficulty can result in digestive upsets and, in some instances, the passage of watery stools. Irregular eating also can impair regular defecation. Individuals who eat at the same times every day usually have a regularly timed, physiologic response to the food intake and a regular pattern of peristaltic activity in the colon.

Spicy foods can produce diarrhea and flatus in some individuals. Excessive sugar also can cause diarrhea. Other foods that may influence bowel elimination include the following:

- Gas-producing foods, such as cabbage, onions, cauliflower, bananas, and apples
- Laxative-producing foods, such as bran, prunes, figs, chocolate, and alcohol
- Constipation-producing foods, such as cheese, pasta, eggs, and lean meat.

Fluid

Healthy fecal elimination usually requires a daily fluid intake of 2,000–3,000 mL, but even when fluid intake is inadequate or output (e.g., urine or vomitus) is excessive, the body continues to reabsorb fluid from the chyme as it passes along the colon. The chyme becomes drier than normal, however, resulting in hard feces. In addition, reduced fluid intake slows the passage of chyme along the intestines, further increasing the reabsorption of fluid from the chyme. If, on the other hand, chyme moves abnormally quickly through the large intestine, there is less time for fluid to be absorbed into the blood, and soft or even watery feces will result.

Activity

Activity stimulates peristalsis, facilitating the movement of chyme along the colon. Weak abdominal and pelvic muscles often are ineffective in increasing the intra-abdominal pressure during defecation or in controlling defecation. Weak muscles can result from lack of exercise, immobility, or impaired neurologic functioning. Clients confined to bed are often constipated.

Psychologic Factors

Some people who are anxious or angry experience increased peristaltic activity and subsequent nausea or diarrhea. In contrast, people who are depressed may experience slowed intestinal motility, resulting in constipation. How a person responds to these emotional states is the result of individual differences in the response of the enteric nervous system to vagal stimulation from the brain.

Defecation Habits

Early bowel training may establish the habit of defecating at a regular time. Many people defecate after breakfast, when the gastrocolic reflex causes mass peristaltic waves in the large intestine. If a person ignores the urge to defecate, then water continues to be reabsorbed, making the feces hard and difficult to expel. When the normal defecation reflexes are inhibited or ignored, these conditioned reflexes tend to be progressively weakened. When habitually ignored, the urge to defecate ultimately is lost. Adults may ignore these reflexes because of the pressures of time or work. Hospitalized clients may suppress the urge because of embarrassment about using a bedpan, because of lack of privacy, or because defecation is too uncomfortable.

Medications

Some drugs have side effects that can interfere with normal elimination. Large doses of certain tranquilizers and repeated administration of morphine or codeine cause constipation by decreasing gastrointestinal activity through their action on the central nervous system. Iron tablets, which have an astringent effect, act more locally on the bowel mucosa to cause constipation. A variety of other drugs cause diarrhea.

Some medications directly affect elimination. **Laxatives** are medications that stimulate bowel activity and assist in fecal elimination. Other medications soften stool, facilitating defecation. Certain medications suppress peristaltic activity and may be used to treat diarrhea.

Medications also affect the appearance of the feces. Any drug that causes gastrointestinal bleeding (e.g., aspirin products) can cause the stool to be red or black. Iron salts cause black stool because of the oxidation of the iron. Antibiotics may cause a gray-green discoloration. Antacids can cause a whitish discoloration or white specks in the stool. Pepto-Bismol, a common over-the-counter drug, causes stools to be black.

Diagnostic Procedures

Before certain diagnostic procedures, such as visualization of the colon (colonoscopy or sigmoidoscopy), the client is restricted from ingesting food or fluid. The client also may be given a cleansing enema before the examination. In these instances, normal defecation usually will not occur until eating resumes.

Anesthesia and Surgical Procedures

General anesthetics cause the normal colonic movements to cease or slow by blocking parasympathetic stimulation to the muscles of the colon. Clients who have regional or spinal anesthesia are less likely to experience this problem.

Surgery that involves direct handling of the intestines can cause temporary cessation of intestinal movement. This condition, called **ileus**, usually lasts from 24–48 hours. Listening for bowel sounds that reflect intestinal motility is an important nursing assessment following surgery.

Pathologic Conditions

Spinal cord injuries and head injuries can reduce the sensory stimulation for defecation. Impaired mobility may limit the client's ability to respond to the urge to defecate, and the client may experience constipation as a result. Alternatively, a client may experience fecal incontinence because of poorly functioning anal sphincters.

Pain

Clients who experience discomfort when defecating (e.g., following hemorrhoid surgery) often suppress the urge to defecate to avoid the pain. These clients can experience constipation as a result. Clients taking narcotic analgesics for pain also may experience constipation as a side effect of the medication.

ALTERATIONS

Four common problems are related to fecal elimination: diarrhea, flatulence, constipation, and bowel incontinence. Constipation and bowel incontinence will be discussed later in this concept. For more details, see the Alterations and Treatments feature.

Diarrhea

Diarrhea refers to the passage of liquid feces and an increased frequency of defecation. The opposite of constipation, it results from rapid movement of fecal contents through the large intestine. Rapid passage of chyme reduces the time available for the large intestine to reabsorb water and electrolytes. Some people pass stool with increased frequency, but diarrhea is not present unless the stool is relatively unformed and excessively liquid. The person with diarrhea finds it difficult or impossible to control the urge to defecate for very long. Often, spasmodic cramps are associated with diarrhea. Bowel sounds usually increase. With persistent diarrhea, irritation of the anal region, extending to the perineum and buttocks, generally results. Fatigue, weakness, malaise, and emaciation are the results of prolonged diarrhea.

Diarrhea is thought to be a protective flushing mechanism when caused by irritants in the intestinal tract. It can create serious fluid and electrolyte losses in the body, however, and these losses can develop within frighteningly short periods of time, particularly in infants, small children, and older adults. Table 9–6 lists some of the major causes of diarrhea and the physiologic responses of the body.

The irritating effects of diarrhea stool increase the risk for skin breakdown. The area around the anal region should be kept clean and dry and be protected with zinc oxide or other ointment. In addition, a fecal collector can be used.

ALTERATIONS AND TREATMENTS Bowel Elimination

Alteration	Description	Treatment
Constipation	Infrequent passage of hard stool	▪ Increase fluid and fiber intake. ▪ Increase activity level. ▪ Administer enema. ▪ May require medications (e.g., laxatives, stool softeners, cathartics). ▪ Evaluate medication profile for gastrointestinal side effects.
Diarrhea	Passage of liquid stools	▪ Increase fluid intake. ▪ Administer antidiarrheal medications. ▪ Assess for cause (medications, diet, bacterial infection).
Bowel incontinence	Inability to control release of feces	▪ Administer bowel training. ▪ Treat with surgery (sphincter repair and fecal diversion or colostomy).
Impaction	Mass or collection of hardened feces in the folds of the rectum	▪ Digital removal may be necessary. ▪ Administer enema as necessary. ▪ Increase fluid and fiber intake to prevent recurrence. ▪ Evaluate medication profile for gastrointestinal side effects. ▪ Improve defecation habits, and reduce constipation.
Bowel cancer	Abnormal growth of cells in the bowel	▪ Take preventive measures, and make an early diagnosis. ▪ Remove surgically. ▪ Administer chemotherapy or radiation therapy.
Obstruction	Blockage in the bowel preventing or reducing the passage of fecal material	▪ Remove blockage surgically.

Flatulence

There are three primary sources of flatus: action of bacteria on the chyme in the large intestine, swallowed air, and gas that diffuses between the bloodstream and the intestine.

Most gases that are swallowed are expelled through the mouth by eructation (belching). Large amounts of gas can accumulate in the stomach, however, resulting in gastric distention. The gases formed in the large intestine are chiefly absorbed through the intestinal capillaries into the circulation. **Flatulence** is the presence of excessive flatus in the intestines and leads to stretching and inflation of the intestines (intestinal distention). Flatulence can occur in the colon from a variety of causes, including foods (e.g., cabbage and onions), abdominal surgery, or narcotics. If the gas is propelled by increased colon activity before it can be absorbed, it may be expelled through the anus. If excessive gas cannot be expelled through the anus, it may be necessary to insert a rectal tube to remove it.

PHYSICAL ASSESSMENT

Assessment of fecal elimination includes taking a nursing history; performing a physical examination of the abdomen, rectum, and anus; and inspecting the feces. The nurse also should review any data obtained from relevant diagnostic tests. For more details, see the Bowel Assessment and Assessment Interview features.

TABLE 9–6 Major Causes of Diarrhea

CAUSE	PHYSIOLOGIC EFFECT
Psychologic stress (e.g., anxiety)	Increased intestinal motility and secretion of mucus
Medications	Inflammation and infection of mucosa caused by overgrowth of pathogenic intestinal microorganisms
Antibiotics	Irritation of intestinal mucosa
Iron	Irritation of intestinal mucosa
Cathartics	Incomplete digestion of food or fluid
Allergy to food, fluid, drugs	Increased intestinal motility and secretion of mucus
Intolerance of food or fluid	Reduced absorption of fluids
Diseases of the colon (e.g., malabsorption syndrome, Crohn's disease)	Inflammation of the mucosa, often leading to ulcer formation

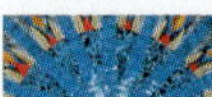

Bowel Assessment

Technique/Normal Findings | **Abnormal Findings**

Abdominal Assessment

Inspect abdominal contour, skin integrity, venous pattern, and aortic pulsation. *Abdomen should be slightly concave with intact skin. There should not be distended veins or obvious aortic pulsations.*

- Generalized abdominal distention may be seen in gas retention or obesity.
- Lower abdominal distention is seen in bladder distention, pregnancy, or ovarian mass.
- General distention and an everted umbilicus are seen with ascites and/or tumors.
- A scaphoid (sunken) abdomen is seen in malnutrition or when fat is replaced with muscle.
- **Striae** (whitish-silver stretch marks) are seen in obesity and during or after pregnancy.
- Spider angiomas may be seen in liver disease.
- Dilated veins are prominent in cirrhosis of the liver, ascites, portal hypertension, or venocaval obstruction.
- Pulsation is increased in aortic aneurysm.

Auscultate all four quadrants of the abdomen with the diaphragm of the stethoscope. Begin in the lower right quadrant, where bowel sounds are almost always present. *Normal bowel sounds (gurgling or clicking) occur every 5–15 seconds. Listen for at least 5 minutes in each of the four quadrants to confirm the absence of bowel sounds.*

- **Borborygmus** (hyperactive high-pitched, tinkling, rushing, or growling bowel sounds) is heard in diarrhea or at the onset of bowel obstruction.
- Bowel sounds may be absent later in bowel obstruction, with an inflamed peritoneum, and/or following surgery of the abdomen.

Auscultate the abdomen for vascular sounds with the bell of the stethoscope. *No sounds (bruits, venous hum, or friction rub) other than bowel sounds should be auscultated.*

- **Bruits** (blowing sound due to restriction of blood flow through vessels) may be heard over constricted arteries. A bruit over the liver may be heard in hepatic carcinoma.
- A venous hum (continuous medium-pitched sound) may be heard over a cirrhotic liver.
- Friction rubs (rough grating sounds) may be heard over an inflamed liver or spleen.

Percuss the abdomen in all four quadrants. *Normally, tympany is heard over the stomach and gas-filled bowels.*

- Dullness is heard when the bowel is displaced with fluid or tumors or filled with a fecal mass.

Palpate the abdomen in all four quadrants. Use a circular motion to move the abdominal wall over underlying structures. Feel for masses and note any tenderness or pain the client may have during this part of the exam. Palpate lightly at first (0.5–0.75 in.), then more deeply (1.5–2 in.) with caution. If a mass is palpated, ask the client to raise head and shoulders. *There should be no abdominal masses or pain on palpation.*

- A mass in the abdomen may become more promiznent when the head and shoulders are raised, as will a ventral abdominal wall hernia. If the mass is no longer palpable, it is deeper in the abdomen.

PRACTICE ALERT

Never use deep palpation in a client who has had a pulsatile abdominal mass, renal transplant, polycystic kidneys, or is at risk for hemorrhage.

- In cases of peritoneal inflammation, palpation causes abdominal pain and involuntary muscle spasms.
- Abnormal masses include aortic aneurysms, neoplastic tumors of the colon or uterus, and a distended bladder or distended bowel due to obstruction.
- A rigid, boardlike abdomen may be palpated when the client has a perforated duodenal ulcer.

Palpate for rebound tenderness. Press the fingers into the abdomen slowly and release the pressure quickly. *Releasing pressure should not cause or increase pain.*

- In peritoneal inflammation, pain occurs when the fingers are withdrawn.
- Right upper quadrant pain occurs with acute cholecystitis.
- Upper middle abdominal pain occurs with acute pancreatitis.
- Right lower quadrant pain at McBurney's point occurs with acute appendicitis.
- Left lower quadrant pain is seen in acute diverticulitis.

Inguinal Area Assessment

Inspect the inguinal area for bulges after asking the client to bear down. *The inguinal area is normally free of bulges.*

- Bulges that appear in the inguinal area when the client bears down may indicate a **hernia** (a defect in the abdominal wall that allows abdominal contents to protrude outward).

Bowel Assessment (continued)

Technique/Normal Findings	Abnormal Findings
Palpate the inguinal area with the gloved hand. Ask the client to shift weight to the left to palpate the right inguinal area and vice versa. Place your right index finger upward into the inguinal area and ask the client to bear down or cough. *Bulging or masses are normally not palpable.*	■ A bulge or mass may indicate a hernia.
Perianal Assessment	
Inspect the perianal area. Wearing gloves, spread the client's buttocks apart. Observe the area, and ask client to bear down as if trying to have a bowel movement. *The perianal area should be intact, without obvious lesions.*	■ Swollen, painful, longitudinal breaks in the anal area may appear in clients with anal fissures. (These are caused by the passing of large, hard stools or by diarrhea.) ■ Dilated anal veins appear with hemorrhoids. ■ A red mass may appear with prolapsed internal hemorrhoids. ■ Doughnut-shaped red tissue at the anal area may appear with a prolapsed rectum.
Palpate the anus and rectum. Lubricate the gloved index finger and ask the client to bear down. Touch the tip of your finger to the client's anal opening. Flex the index finger, and slowly insert it into the anus, pointing the finger toward the umbilicus (Figure 9–8 ■). Rotate the finger in both directions to palpate any lesions or masses. *There should be no masses in the anus or rectum.*	■ Movable, soft masses may be polyps. ■ Hard, firm, irregular embedded masses may indicate carcinoma.

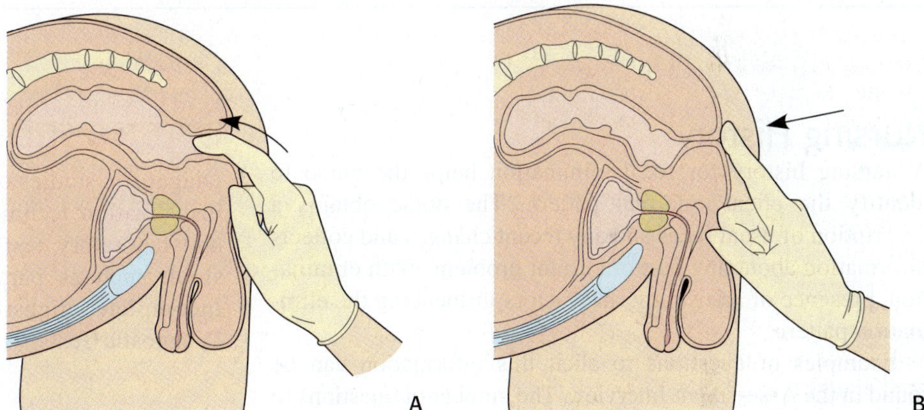

Figure 9–8 ■ Digital examination of the *A*, rectum and *B*, anus.

Technique/Normal Findings	Abnormal Findings
Fecal Assessment	
Inspect the client's feces. After palpating the rectum, withdraw your finger gently. Inspect any feces on the glove. Note color and/or presence of blood. Also use gloved fingers to note consistency. *Stool should be soft with no blood present, either on the stool or as occult blood.*	
Test the feces for occult blood. Use a testing kit such as Occultest or Hemoccult II. *There should be no blood in the feces.*	■ A positive occult blood test requires further testing for colon cancer or gastrointestinal bleeding due to peptic ulcers, ulcerative colitis, or diverticulosis.
Note the odor of the feces. *No distinctly foul odors should be present.*	■ Distinctly foul odors may be noted with stools containing blood or extra fat or in cases of colon cancer.

Assessment Interview Fecal Elimination

DEFECATION PATTERN

- When do you usually have a bowel movement?
- Has this pattern changed recently?

DESCRIPTION OF FECES AND ANY CHANGES

- Have you noticed any changes in the color, texture (hard, soft, watery), shape, or odor of your stool recently?

FECAL ELIMINATION PROBLEMS

- What problems have you had or do you now have with your bowel movements (constipation, diarrhea, excessive flatulence, seepage, or incontinence)?
- When and how often do they occur?
- What do you think causes these problems (food, fluids, exercise, emotions, medications, disease, surgery)?
- What have you tried to solve the problems, and how effective was it?

FACTORS INFLUENCING ELIMINATION

- *Use of elimination aids.* What routines do you follow to maintain your usual defecation pattern? Do you use natural aids such as specific foods or fluids (e.g., a glass of hot lemon juice before breakfast), laxatives, or enemas to maintain elimination?
- *Diet.* What foods do you believe affect defecation? What foods do you typically eat? What foods do you avoid? Do you take meals at regular times?
- *Fluid.* What amount and kind of fluid do you take each day (e.g., six glasses of water, two cups of coffee)?
- *Exercise.* What is your usual daily exercise pattern? (Obtain specifics about exercise rather than asking whether it is sufficient; ideas of what is sufficient vary among individuals.)
- *Medications.* Have you taken any medications that could affect the intestinal tract (e.g., iron or antibiotics)? (Note the name and specific dosage of all medications because the client may not be aware what medications may affect elimination.)
- *Stress.* Are you experiencing any stress? Do you think this affects your defecation pattern? If so, how?

PRESENCE AND MANAGEMENT OF OSTOMY

- What is your usual routine with your colostomy/ileostomy?
- What type of appliance do you wear, and did you bring a spare with you?
- What problems, if any, do you have with it?
- How can the nurses help you manage your colostomy/ileostomy?

Nursing History

A nursing history for fecal elimination helps the nurse to identify the client's normal pattern. The nurse obtains a description of usual feces and any recent changes and collects information about any past or current problems with elimination, presence of an ostomy, and factors influencing the elimination pattern.

Examples of questions to elicit this information can be found in the Assessment Interview. The number of questions to ask is adapted to the individual client, according to the client's responses in the first three categories listed.

When obtaining data about the client's defecation pattern, the nurse needs to understand that the time of defecation and the amount of feces expelled are as individual as the frequency of defecation. Often, the patterns that individuals follow depend largely on early training and convenience.

Physical Examination

Physical examination of the abdomen in relation to fecal elimination problems includes inspection, auscultation, percussion, and palpation with specific reference to the intestinal tract. Auscultation precedes palpation, because palpation can alter peristalsis. Examination of the rectum and anus includes inspection and palpation.

Inspecting the Feces

Observe the client's stool for color, consistency, shape, amount, odor, and presence of abnormal constituents.

DIAGNOSTIC TESTS

Diagnostic studies of the gastrointestinal tract include direct visualization techniques, indirect visualization techniques, and laboratory tests for abnormal constituents within the stool, such as parasites, microorganisms, or products of incomplete digestion. For details, see Appendix B, Diagnostic Tests.

CARING INTERVENTIONS

Medical management of altered bowel elimination is based on the diagnosed problem impacting elimination. Treatment for minor problems may include increasing the amount of fiber and fluid in the diet. Medications such as laxatives, antidiarrheal agents, or stool softeners may be indicated. Clients with more acute problems, such as obstruction, ulceration, perforation, or cancer, may require surgical resection of the bowel with or without creation of an ostomy. Medical management of obstructions may involve gut rest with placement of a nasogastric tube.

PHARMACOLOGIC THERAPIES

Medications for management of bowel elimination may be given to promote bowel movement, to promote absorption of excess fluid in the intestine, or to coalesce gas or reduce the production of gas. For details regarding medications, see the Medications feature.

MEDICATIONS Bowel Elimination

Drug Classifications	Mechanism of Action	Commonly Prescribed Drugs	Nursing Considerations
Laxatives: bulk-forming agents, stool softeners, stimulants, saline or osmotic laxatives, herbal agents, and miscellaneous agents	Promote bowel movement	Psyllium hydrophilic mucilloid, methylcellulose, docusate sodium, senna, mineral oil, and Epsom salts	■ Contraindicated in clients with nausea, cramps, colic, vomiting, or undiagnosed abdominal pain. Also contraindicated in clients after abdominal surgery. ■ Should not be used continuously, because they weaken bowel's natural response to fecal distention. ■ Before administration, assess abdomen for distention, bowel sounds, and bowel patterns. ■ Teach clients preventive measures for constipation to avoid overdependence on laxatives.
Antidiarrheal agents	Slow motility of the intestines or promote absorption of excess fluid in the intestine	Diphenoxylate with atropine, camphorated opium tincture, difenoxin with atropine, loperamide, bismuth salts, and furazolidone	■ Monitor fluid and electrolyte status. ■ Contraindicated in clients with severe dehydration, electrolyte imbalance, liver and renal disorders, and glaucoma. ■ Teach clients to seek medical care if diarrhea does not subside in 2 days, fever develops, or dehydration occurs.
Antiflatulent agents	Coalesce gas bubbles and facilitate passage	Simethicone	■ Teach clients to seek medical care if symptoms persist or recur. ■ Side effects include bloating, constipation, diarrhea, gas, and heartburn.

9.1 BENIGN PROSTATIC HYPERTROPHY

KEY TERMS

Androgen, *432*
Benign prostatic hypertrophy (BPH), *432*
Continuous bladder irrigation (CBI), *439*
Detrusor muscles, *433*
Digital rectal examination (DRE), *436*
Dihydrotestosterone (DHT), *432*
Diverticula, *433*
Hydronephrosis, *433*
Hydroureter, *433*
Hyperplasia, *432*
Hypertrophy, *432*
Prostate specific antigen (PSA), *434*
Prostatitis, *432*
Prostatodynia, *432*
Transurethral incision of the prostate (TUIP), *435*
Transurethral needle ablation (TUNA), *435*
Transurethral resection of the prostate (TURP), *435*
TURP syndrome, *439*
Uroflowmetry, *436*

BASIS FOR SELECTION OF EXEMPLAR

Most common condition
National Institutes of Health

LEARNING OUTCOMES

After reading about this exemplar, you will be able to:

1. Describe the pathophysiology, etiology, clinical manifestations, and direct and indirect causes of benign prostatic hypertrophy.
2. Identify risk factors associated with benign prostatic hypertrophy.
3. Illustrate the nursing process in providing culturally competent care across the life span for individuals with benign prostatic hypertrophy.
4. Formulate priority nursing diagnoses appropriate for an individual with benign prostatic hypertrophy.
5. Create a plan of care for individuals with benign prostatic hypertrophy and their family members.
6. Assess expected outcomes for an individual with benign prostatic hypertrophy.
7. Discuss therapies used in the collaborative care of an individual with benign prostatic hypertrophy.
8. Employ evidenced-based caring interventions for an individual with benign prostatic hypertrophy.

OVERVIEW

Prostatitis is a term used to refer to different types of inflammatory disorders of the prostate gland. **Prostatodynia** is a condition in which the client experiences the symptoms of prostatitis but shows no evidence of inflammation or infection. **Benign prostatic hypertrophy (BPH)**, on the other hand, is an age-related, nonmalignant enlargement of the prostate gland commonly seen in the aging male.

While BPH is discussed casually by health care providers, it can be a cause for great anxiety in the aging man who fears loss of his virility and ability to maintain a satisfying sex life. Radical surgeries, the only treatment choice many years ago, often left men impotent, and the stories from those days still circulate as current fact. Client education and support play an important role in providing nursing care to men diagnosed with BPH.

Benign prostatic hypertrophy is the most common benign neoplasm in men. It is characterized by a nonmalignant enlargement of the prostate gland that decreases the outflow of urine by obstructing the urethra, causing difficult urination. Although BPH typically begins in a mans forties, he may not experience symptoms until much later, depending on how his individual condition progresses. BPH is not considered to be a precursor to prostate cancer.

PATHOPHYSIOLOGY AND ETIOLOGY

The prostate gland borders the urethra near the lower part of the bladder. About the size of a chestnut (2 cm), it is partially palpable through the front wall of the rectum because it lies just anterior to the rectum (Figure 9–9 ■). The prostate is composed of glandular structures that continuously secrete a milky alkaline solution. During sexual intercourse, glandular activity increases and the alkaline secretions flow into the urethra. Because sperm motility is reduced in an acidic environment, these secretions aid sperm transport. In addition, the prostate gland produces about one third of all semen.

The two necessary preconditions for BPH are age 50 and older and the presence of testes. Men who are castrated before puberty do not develop BPH. The androgen that mediates prostatic growth at all ages is **dihydrotestosterone (DHT)**, which is formed in the prostate from testosterone. An **androgen** is a hormone that stimulates the development and maintenance of male sex characteristics. Although androgen levels decrease in aging men, the aging prostate appears to become more sensitive to available DHT. Estrogen, produced in small amounts in men, appears to sensitize the prostate gland to the effects of DHT. Increasing estrogen levels associated with aging or a relative increase in estrogen related to testosterone levels may contribute to prostatic hyperplasia.

Benign prostatic hypertrophy begins as small nodules in the periurethral glands, which are the inner layers of the prostate. The prostate enlarges through formation and growth of nodules (**hyperplasia**) and enlargement of glandular cells (**hypertrophy**). These changes occur over a long period of time. The pathophysiologic effects result from a combination of factors, including urethral resistance to the effects of BPH, intravesical pressure during voiding, detrusor muscle strength, neurologic functioning, and general physical health.

Etiology

Benign prostatic hypertrophy affects 50% of men between the ages of 51 and 60 years and 90% of men over age 80 (National Institute of Diabetes and Digestive and Kidney Diseases, 2001). BPH is classified three ways. Microscopic benign prostatic hypertrophy is diagnosable only by histologic changes. Macroscopic BPH is characterized by palpable enlargement of the gland during rectal examination (Wei, Calhoun, &

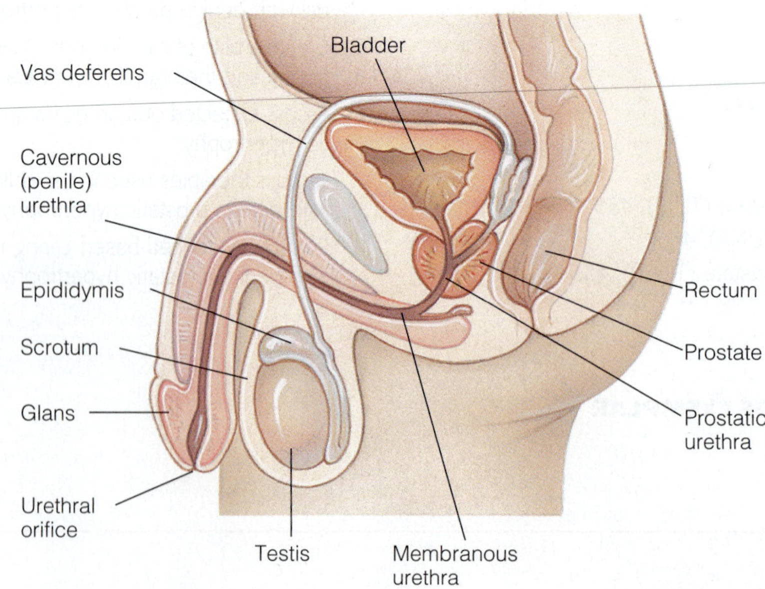

Figure 9–9 ■ Gross anatomy of the male reproductive organs.

Jacobsen, 2007). Clinical benign prostatic hypertrophy refers to observable symptoms related to BPH (Wei et al., 2007). The growth of the prostate is influenced by androgens and occurs mostly in the transitional zone that surrounds the urethra (Letran & Brawer, 1999).

Risk Factors

Although the exact cause of BPH is unknown, risk factors include the following:

- Age
- Family history
- Race (highest in African Americans and lowest in native Japanese)
- Diet high in meat and fats.

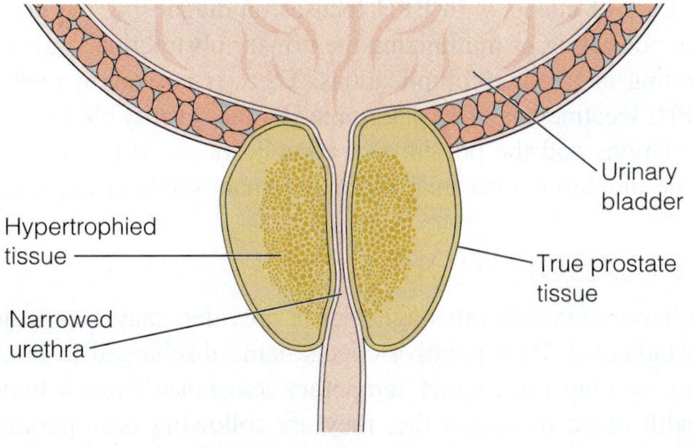

Figure 9–10 ■ Benign prostatic hyperplasia.

CLINICAL MANIFESTATIONS

Although the symptoms of BPH are sometimes referred to as nuisances, they can have a profound effect on daily living. The expanding prostatic tissue compresses the urethra (Figure 9–10 ■) and causes partial or complete obstruction of the outflow of urine from the urinary bladder. Despite the fact that the **detrusor muscles** hypertrophy to compensate for increased resistance to urinary flow, decreased bladder compliance and bladder instability eventually result. These changes manifest as symptoms of obstruction (weak urinary stream, increased time to void, hesitancy, incomplete bladder emptying, and postvoid dribbling) and irritation (frequency, urgency, incontinence, nocturia, dysuria, and bladder pain). Urinary retention may become chronic, resulting in overflow incontinence with an increase in intraabdominal pressure. Clients often report sensations of incomplete bladder emptying. There is little correlation between the size of the prostate gland and the urinary manifestations.

PRACTICE ALERT

Urinary retention in men with BPH can be precipitated by several classes of medications, including those with anticholinergic properties and over-the-counter medications for the common cold, such as decongestants.

Unless the enlarging mass is reduced, multiple complications may occur. As urine is retained in the bladder, increasing bladder distention occurs. **Diverticula** (saclike projections of mucosa through the muscular layer of the colon) on the bladder wall result from the distention. The distention also may obstruct the ureters. Infection, more common in retained urine and in diverticula, may ascend from the bladder to the kidneys. Possible complications include **hydroureter** (distention of the ureter with urine), **hydronephrosis** (accumulation of urine in the renal pelvis as a result of obstructed outflow), and renal insufficiency.

CLINICAL MANIFESTATIONS AND THERAPIES Benign Prostatic Hypertrophy

ETIOLOGY	CLINICAL MANIFESTATIONS	CLINICAL THERAPIES
Pressure on the urethra	■ Frequency ■ Urgency ■ Hesitancy ■ Dribbling after urination ■ Incomplete bladder emptying ■ Dysuria ■ Bladder pain	■ Monitor for potential urinary tract infections (UTIs). ■ May monitor mild cases while more severe cases will require surgical intervention. ■ Monitor prostate-specific antigen to rule out cancer. ■ Assess using International Prostate Symptom Score (IPSS) and treat symptoms. ■ May find pharmacotherapy useful if hyperplastic tissue is androgen-dependent and smooth muscle contraction within the prostate exacerbates urinary obstruction.
Complete or significant blockage of urethra by prostate	■ Inability to void ■ Frequent UTIs ■ Hematuria ■ Bladder stones ■ Renal insufficiency secondary to BPH ■ Difficulty or inability to pass a urinary catheter ■ Bladder distention ■ Bladder pain	■ Surgical removal of the prostate can be performed using a TURP or suprapubic approach. ■ Transurethral microwave thermotherapy uses microwave heat to destroy excess prostate tissue and is less invasive than traditional surgery.

Care of clients with BPH focuses on diagnosing the disorder, correcting or minimizing the urinary obstruction, and preventing or treating complications. There is no way to reverse BPH. Treatment is often determined by the severity of the manifestations and the presence of complications. Mild cases are often monitored over time and may remain stable or improve.

COLLABORATION

Collaboration with other agencies or providers may or may not be indicated. Postoperative clients being discharged to home may or may not require temporary assistance from a home health nurse to ensure that they are following postoperative care procedures. For family members of clients who require a great deal of assistance and who choose to recover at home, referral to an agency that provides caregiver respite or home health services may be helpful. The nurse plays an essential role in assessing the postoperative needs of the client and family and working with them to make sure they are able to manage the recovery process successfully.

Treatment for BPH includes managing urge incontinence and decreasing the other urinary symptoms. Alpha-adrenergic blocking medications such as tamsulosin and doxazosin mesylate may be prescribed. Saw palmetto is an over-the-counter herbal preparation that appears to be effective in improving BPH symptoms and has relatively few side effects (Chow, 2001).

Diagnostic Tests

A man presenting with symptoms of BPH may be offered several diagnostic tests with the dual purpose of identifying BPH and ruling out other causes of the symptoms. These tests include a blood test for **prostate specific antigen (PSA)** (a protein produced in the cells of the prostate gland), a cystoscopy, postvoid residual collection or ultrasound, an intravenous pyelogram, and urodynamic studies (Wei et al., 2007).

Pharmacologic Therapy

Medications such as alpha blockers and 5-alpha reductase inhibitors have dramatically reduced the need for surgery to control the symptoms of BPH. When urinary retention becomes resistant to other treatments or renal insufficiency due to bladder outlet obstruction develops, surgical intervention may be recommended (NKUDIC, 2007b).

Treatment with medications is based on two considerations: The hyperplastic tissue is androgen-dependent, and smooth muscle contraction within the prostate can exacerbate urinary obstruction (Table 9–7). The first consideration is usually addressed by treatment for mild prostate enlargement with finasteride (Proscar) or dutasteride (Avodart), both of which are antiandrogen agents that inhibit the conversion of testosterone to DHT and cause the enlarged prostate to shrink in size. Potential side effects include impotence, decreased libido, and decreased volume of ejaculate. Client and family education includes the information that crushed tablets should not be handled by pregnant women because the drug may be absorbed through the skin and be harmful to a male fetus.

Excessive smooth muscle contraction in BPH may be blocked with alpha-adrenergic antagonists such as terazosin (Hytrin), doxazosin (Cardura), tamsulosin (Flomax), and alfuzosin (Uroxatral). These medications relieve obstruction and increase the flow of urine. They may cause orthostatic hypotension. Client and family teaching includes making position changes slowly to avoid dizziness and accidental falls; taking and recording blood pressure; and checking with the healthcare provider before taking any medication for coughs, colds, or allergies (because these over-the-counter medications may contain an adrenergic agent). Federal research found that using finasteride and doxazosin together is more effective than using each alone to relieve manifestations and prevent the progression of BPH (NKUDIC, 2004).

Certain commonly used medications have been found to worsen symptoms of BPH. Alpha-adrenergic agents, which include decongestants such as pseudoephedrine and phenylephrine, may activate alpha$_1$-adrenergic receptors in the bladder neck, causing restriction of urine flow. Drugs with anticholinergic side effects such as antihistamines, TCAs, and phenothiazines may also adversely affect BPH. Testosterone and other

TABLE 9–7 Agents for Benign Prostatic Hyperplasia

DRUG	ROUTE AND ADULT DOSE (MAXIMUM DOSE WHERE INDICATED)	ADVERSE EFFECTS
Alpha-Adrenergic Blockers		
doxazosin (Cardura)	po; 1–8 mg/day	*Orthostatic hypotension, headache, dizziness*
prazosin (Minipress)	1 mg qid or bid	First-dose phenomenon (severe hypotension and syncope), tachycardia
tamsulosin (Flomax)	po; 0.4 mg 30 min after a meal (max: 0.8 mg/day)	
terazosin (Hytrin)	po; start with 1 mg at bedtime, then 1–5 mg/day (max: 20 mg/day)	
5-Alpha-Reductase Inhibitors		
dutasteride (Avodart)	po; 0.5 mg/day	*Sexual dysfunction, decreased libido, decreased ejaculate volume*
finasteride (Proscar)	po; 5 mg/day	No serious adverse effects

Italics indicate common adverse effects; underlining indicates serious adverse effects.

anabolic steroids may increase prostate enlargement, increasing the physical obstruction of the urethra. Elderly men should avoid drugs that worsen symptoms of BPH.

Surgery

Men who have urinary retention, recurrent urinary tract infection, hematuria, bladder stones, or renal insufficiency secondary to BPH are candidates for surgical intervention. Surgical treatment may be performed by minimally invasive surgery or through transurethral, open, or laser surgery.

MINIMALLY INVASIVE SURGERY Because medications are not effective for all men, a number of procedures have been developed to relieve the manifestations of BPH that are less invasive than traditional surgery. *Transurethral microwave thermotherapy* uses microwaves to heat and destroy excess prostate tissue. During the procedure, a cooling system protects the urinary tract. The procedure takes about an hour and can be performed on an outpatient basis. Although microwave procedures do not cure BPH, they do reduce urinary manifestations. These procedures do not cause impotence or incontinence.

The **transurethral needle ablation (TUNA)** system uses low-level radio frequency through twin needles to burn away a region of the enlarged prostate. Shields protect the urethra. TUNA improves the flow of urine through the urethra. It does not cause impotence or incontinence.

TRANSURETHRAL SURGERY **Transurethral resection of the prostate (TURP)** is the surgical procedure used most often. Obstructing prostate tissue is removed using the wire loop of a resectoscope and electrocautery inserted through the urethra (Figure 9–11 ■). No external incision is necessary. During the procedure, the surgeon uses the resectoscope to remove obstructing tissue one piece at a time. The tissue is flushed into the bladder with fluid and then flushed out at the end of the operation. This surgery has potential risks, however, including postoperative hemorrhage or clot retention, inability to void, and UTI. Other possible complications are incontinence, impotence, and retrograde ejaculation.

In the **transurethral incision of the prostate (TUIP)** procedure, small incisions are made in the smooth muscle where the prostate is attached to the bladder. The gland is split to reduce pressure on the urethra. No tissue is removed, so this procedure is most appropriate for men with smaller prostate glands. TUIP can be done on an outpatient basis, and it has the additional advantage of there being less risk of postoperative retrograde ejaculation than is associated with TURP and other prostatectomy procedures.

OPEN SURGERY When the prostate gland is very large, an open prostatectomy may be used. These procedures are discussed in Concept 3: Cellular Regulation, Exemplar 3.7: Prostate Cancer.

LASER SURGERY In laser surgery, the surgeon uses a cystoscope to pass the YAG laser fiber through the urethra into the prostate and then vaporizes obstructing prostate tissue with several short bursts of energy. Advantages of laser surgery include decreased blood loss and a more rapid recovery

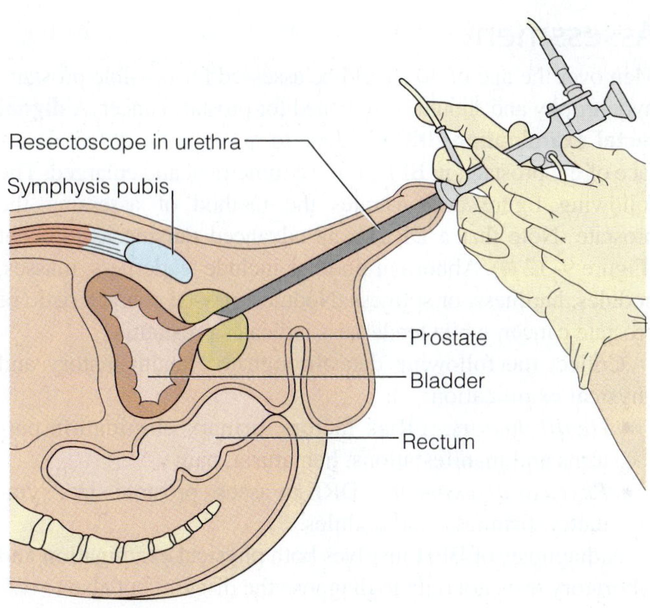

A Transurethral resection of the prostate

Figure 9–11 ■ In a transurethral resection of the prostate, a resectoscope inserted through the urethra is used to remove excess prostate tissue.

time. However, this method may not be as effective for larger prostates.

NEW TREATMENTS Newer treatments for BPH include minimally invasive procedures such as balloon urethroplasty and placement of intraurethral stents to maintain patency of the urethra. Balloon urethroplasty is a simple procedure in which a balloon-tipped catheter is inserted in the narrowed portion of the urethra and inflated. Inflation of the balloon widens the urethra, relieving obstruction. These procedures can be done as outpatient surgery.

Complementary and Alternative Therapies

Phytotherapy is the use of plants or plant extracts for medical treatment. Several plant extracts have been used for years in Europe to treat BPH and are being used more often in the United States. Plants sometimes used as phytotherapy for BPH include saw palmetto berry; the bark of *Pygeum africanum;* the roots of *Echinacea, purpurea*, and *Hypoxis rooperi;* and the leaves of the trembling poplar. The mechanisms of action of these extracts are unknown, but men report they are effective in relieving manifestations (Tierney, McPhee, & Papadakis, 2004).

NURSING PROCESS

The nurse who is caring for a client with BPH must be sensitive to the man's concerns and fears and provide education and support. Therapeutic communication will help the nurse obtain a thorough and complete history and assist the client with discussing sensitive topics.

Assessment

Men over the age of 40 should be assessed for possible prostatic hypertrophy and should be screened for prostate cancer. A **digital rectal examination (DRE)** is done to examine the external surface of the prostate; in BPH, it is asymmetrical and enlarged. The following figure demonstrates the method of assessing the prostate. Note that a DRE is an advanced nursing assessment (Figure 9–12 ■). Abnormal findings include tenderness, masses, nodules, hardness, or softness. Nodules may be characteristic of prostate cancer, while tenderness indicates prostatitis.

Collect the following data through the health history and physical examination:

- *Health history.* Risk factors, urinary elimination patterns and manifestations, hematuria, pain
- *Physical assessment.* DRE to assess prostate size, symmetry, firmness, and nodules.

A diagnosis of BPH involves both physical examination and laboratory tests not only to diagnose the disease, but also to differentiate it from prostate cancer. Examination of the creatinine levels of the blood is conducted to assess for kidney damage.

The client's urine is examined for white blood cells (WBCs), red blood cells (RBCs), and bacteria. Urinary function is assessed by measuring residual urine (amount of urine remaining in the bladder after voiding) with ultrasonography or postvoiding catheterization (more than 100 mL is considered high) and through **uroflowmetry**, which measures urine flow rate (normal is greater than 14 mL/sec). A finding of less than 10 mL/sec indicates obstruction.

Prostate-specific antigen levels are obtained to rule out prostate cancer. PSA is a glycoprotein produced only in the cytoplasm of benign and malignant prostate cells; the serum level corresponds with the volume of both benign and malignant prostate tissue.

In addition to diagnostic tests, the clients own subjective experiences with BPH are included in the diagnosis and treatment. For example, the International Prostate Symptom Score (IPSS) (Box 9–3) uses a scale of 0 (not at all) to 5 (almost always) to collect data about several subjective factors, including feeling as though the bladder did not empty with urinating; needing to urinate within 2 hours after urinating; starting and stopping the stream several times while urinating; and straining to urinate. This questionnaire also asks how many times during the night the man needs to urinate and how the man feels about having the disorder.

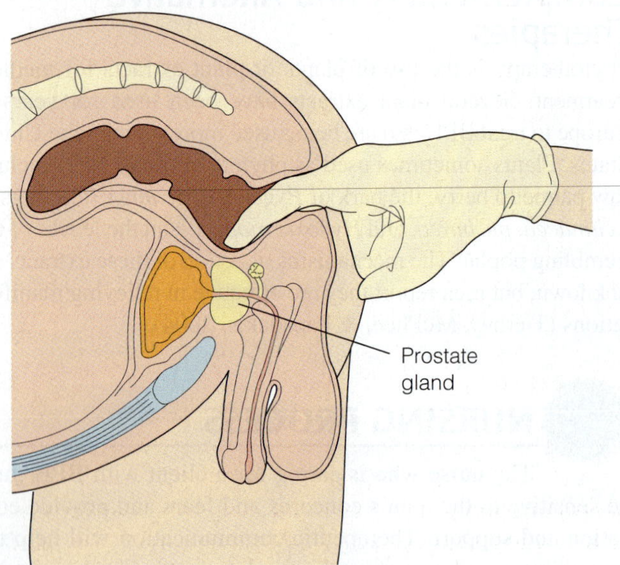

Figure 9–12 ■ Palpating the prostate gland.

Diagnosis

Nursing diagnoses that may be considered for clients with BPH include the following:

- Deficient Knowledge
- Urinary Retention
- Risk for Infection
- Risk for Imbalanced Fluid Volume
- Urinary Incontinence.

Plan

The nursing plan of care should be individualized to meet client needs; every client will require goals specific to his situation. However, commonly created goals may include the client being able to do the following:

- Regain urinary continence after catheter removal
- Verbalize the rationale for performing postoperative exercise
- Verbalize the need for continued follow-up care
- Verbalize warning signs of urinary tract infection
- Verbalize proper administration of prescribed medications and adverse affects that should be reported to provider
- Report pain of 3 or less and obtain adequate pain relief to allow for comfort.

Implementation

Care of the client with BPH will differ based on treatment decisions and need for surgical intervention. In this section, care is divided into preoperative and postoperative care.

Preoperative Care

Tactful but thorough preoperative care, education, and support are critical to the client's subjective view of the surgery as well as to its objective outcomes. The nurse should assess the client's and family's knowledge about the surgery. Most men are unsure of the function of the prostate gland and even the prostate's exact location, although its relationship to sexual and urinary function is at least generally known. This lack of knowledge, coupled with the growing number of treatment options, is confusing to many men. Clients may be confused about the surgical approach because there are several different methods. Client teaching will help reduce client anxiety related to fear of the unknown.

Verify informed consent was signed. Inform the client that he will have a urinary catheter when he returns from surgery and that he may have a drain in his incision, depending on the type of surgery performed. Explain that he also will be wearing sequential pneumatic compression stockings. Bowel preparation with a 2% neomycin enema may be ordered to cleanse the bowel in the event a perineal approach is used.

Box 9–3 International Prostate Symptom Score (IPSS)

To calculate your voiding symptom severity, make a response (by clicking on one response box) for each of the 7 questions below. After responding to all 7 questions, click on "Calculate." Note the total symptom score and read the commentary at bottom.

During the last month or so how often have you.	Not at all	Less than 1 time in 5	Less than 1/2 the time	About 1/2 the time	More than 1/2 the time	Almost always
1. had a sensation of not emptying your bladder completely after urinating?	0 ❍	1 ❍	2 ❍	3 ❍	4 ❍	5 ❍
2. had to urinate again less than two hours after you have urinated?	0 ❍	1 ❍	2 ❍	3 ❍	4 ❍	5 ❍
3. how often have you stopped and started several times when you urinated?	0 ❍	1 ❍	2 ❍	3 ❍	4 ❍	5 ❍
4. found it difficult to postpone urination?	0 ❍	1 ❍	2 ❍	3 ❍	4 ❍	5 ❍
5. had a weak urinary stream?	0 ❍	1 ❍	2 ❍	3 ❍	4 ❍	5 ❍
6. had to push or strain to urinate?	0 ❍	1 ❍	2 ❍	3 ❍	4 ❍	5 ❍
During the last month...	**None**	**1 time**	**2 times**	**3 times**	**4 times**	**5 times or more**
7. how many times did you most typically get up to urinate from the time you went to bed at night until the time you got up in the morning?	0 ❍	1 ❍	2 ❍	3 ❍	4 ❍	5 ❍

Source: http://www.usrf.org/questionnaires/AUA_SymptomScore.html

Understanding of the scope of preoperative activities and postoperative conditions reduces patient anxiety and increases patient cooperation with postoperative care.

Men may be anxious about the outcome of their surgery and its potential long-term effects on their sexuality. The nurse communicates willingness to address any concerns or anxiety by maintaining a professional approach and creating a trusting relationship.

Postoperative Care

Maintain the usual postoperative assessments. Monitor vital signs closely for the first 24 hours and regularly thereafter. The client who has had prostate surgery is at risk for hemorrhage and infection. Changes in vital signs are often the earliest manifestations of these complications. Maintain accurate intake and output records, including amounts of irrigating solution used. Frequently assess patency of any catheters and drains. Monitor color and character of urine. Catheters may become occluded by blood clots or kinks, interfering with urinary drainage and increasing the risk of hemorrhage.

Assess and manage the client's pain, which may include incisional pain, bladder spasms, or abdominal cramps due to intestinal gas. Analgesics and nonsteroidal anti-inflammatory drugs (NSAIDs) are administered on a routine and prn basis to control incisional pain. Bladder spasms may be accompanied by strong urges to void and urine leakage around the catheter. Belladonna and opium (B & O) suppositories may be used to relieve bladder spasms.

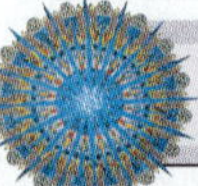

NURSING CARE PLAN **A Man With Benign Prostatic Hypertrophy**

William Turner, a 71-year-old African American, lives with his wife in a small retirement community in Florida. His wife had a stroke 2 years ago, and Mr. Turner does all of the cooking and housework. He has been in good health for most of his life, having only a small touch of osteoarthritis in his knees and hands. He has noticed a gradual onset of urinary urgency and frequency over the past 2 years and has found it increasingly difficult to begin his stream. During a routine check-up, the nurse practitioner at the local health clinic performs a DRE and palpates Mr. Turner's prostate, finding it enlarged. After Mr. Turner's PSA is found to be normal, he is referred to a urologist, who diagnoses BPH. Mr. Turner chooses to have surgery, and a TURP is performed. Following surgery, his recovery is uncomplicated. However, the nurse caring for Mr. Turner is concerned about his ability to care for his indwelling catheter because of his arthritis and his wife's physical disabilities from the stroke. The nurse makes a referral to a home health agency to ensure that Mr. Turner can manage his care at home. An initial home health assessment is scheduled for the day after Mr. Turner is discharged from the hospital.

ASSESSMENT

The home health nurse notes that the house is clean and neat. Mr. Turner is dressed but is still wearing his night urinary drainage bag even though it is 1300. Mr. Turner tells the nurse that his main problem is going to get groceries because he is embarrassed to be seen with the drainage bag. He says that he has not been able to remove the drainage bag and attach the leg bag because of his arthritis. Physical assessment finds no tenderness in his calves, chest pain, or shortness of breath. The urine is yellow, without odor or sedimentation. Mr. Turner does state that he sees no need for the pelvic exercises since he is no longer in the hospital.

DIAGNOSES

- Risk for Stress Urinary Incontinence related to surgical procedure
- Ineffective Health Maintenance related to inability to care for the urinary drainage system, lack of understanding about the need for postoperative exercises, and questions about follow-up care
- Need for continued follow-up care

PLANNING

Planning care is done in collaboration with Mr. Turner to improve outcomes and include the following goals:

- Regain urinary continence after catheter removal.
- Change the urinary drainage bag with the appropriate assistance.
- Verbalize the rationale for performing postoperative exercise.
- Verbalize the need for continued follow-up care.

IMPLEMENTATION

- Discuss the possibility of stress incontinence after the catheter is removed.
- Reinforce the need for Kegel exercises while the catheter is still in place.
- Explore Mr. Turner's support system to identify people who can assist him with catheter care and arrange a teaching session with them.
- Teach Mr. Turner the importance of follow-up care, relating the care to the history of the disease.

EVALUATION

The client's care is evaluated based on the goals of care established during the planning phase. Good friends from Mr. Turner's church have assisted him with care of his drainage bag and have reminded him to do his Kegel exercises several times a day while the catheter is in place. When the catheter is removed, Mr. Turner has only a small amount of leaking of urine after voiding. He understands that it may take several weeks for this to resolve. Efforts to help him understand the need for continued medical care are less successful. Mr. Turner continues to state that he is cured, his wife needs him, and he sees no need to return to the doctor.

CRITICAL THINKING

1. Outline a teaching plan for Mr. Turner for the risk for altered skin integrity related to urinary incontinence.
2. As a result of Mr. Turner's refusal to have ongoing medical care, he might be labeled as noncompliant. Would you make this nursing diagnosis? Why or why not?
3. If you were the home health nurse making a home visit and found that Mr. Turner had no urinary drainage for 16 hours, what assessments would you make? How would you handle this problem?

Maintain antiembolic stockings and pneumatic compression devices as ordered. Assist with leg exercises and ambulation as ordered. These are important preventive measures because the man who has had prostate surgery is at risk for developing thromboemboli. Encourage the client to maintain a liberal fluid intake of 2–3 L a day and explain that increased fluids reduce burning upon urination after catheter removal, as well as the risk of UTI.

For the first 24–48 hours, a client with a transurethral resection of the prostate (TURP) should be monitored for hemorrhage, evidenced by frankly bloody urinary output, presence of large blood clots, decreased urinary output, increased bladder spasms, decreased hemoglobin and hematocrit, tachycardia, and hypotension. Notify the physician if any of these manifestations occur. Postoperative hemorrhage may be arterial or venous and may be precipitated by movement, bladder spasms, or an obstructed urinary drainage system.

Instruct the client with a three-way indwelling catheter with traction to keep his leg straight while the traction is applied. A No. 18–22 Fr three-way catheter with a 30–45 mL balloon usually is inserted following a TURP. The inflated balloon is pulled down into the prostatic fossa, and the catheter tubing is pulled down and taped to the client's leg to apply pressure against the operative site, preventing bleeding.

Pressure on the urethra by the large catheter and on the internal sphincter by the catheter's balloon stimulates the micturition reflex. Explain that the presence of a urinary catheter will cause the sensation of needing to void, but it is important not to strain when trying to void around the catheter or when having a bowel movement. Straining to void or to have a bowel movement may stimulate bladder spasms and increase pain; it also may increase the risk for bleeding. Explain that bladder spasms, experienced as lower abdominal pressure or pain and a desire to urinate, may occur. Ensure that the client understands that this is an expected sensation and that medications can help alleviate this discomfort. Administer pain medications at regular intervals.

Continuous bladder irrigation (CBI) is used to prevent the formation of blood clots, which can obstruct urinary output. If the client has CBI, assess the catheter and the drainage tubing at regular intervals. Maintain the rate of flow of irrigating fluid to keep the output light pink or colorless. Assess the urinary output every 1–2 hours for color, consistency of amount, and presence of blood clots; assess for bladder spasms. Bladder distention resulting from output obstruction increases the risk of bleeding. Irrigating fluids are continuously infused and drained at a rate to keep urine light pink or colorless. Bladder spasms and urine that is frankly bloody, contains many blood clots, or is decreased in amount are indicators of obstruction and bleeding.

Assess for fluid volume excess and hyponatremia, called **TURP syndrome**, which is manifested by hyponatremia, decreased hematocrit, hypertension, bradycardia, nausea, and confusion. If these manifestations occur, notify the physician. TURP syndrome results from the absorption of irrigating fluids during and after surgery. Untreated, it may result in dysrhythmias and/or seizures.

If the client does not have CBI, follow agency procedure and physician orders for irrigating the indwelling catheter (usually when the urine is frankly bloody or has numerous large blood clots or when bladder spasms increase). In most instances, using sterile technique, gently irrigate the catheter with 50 mL of irrigating solution at a time until the obstruction is relieved or the urine is clear. Ensure equal input and output of irrigating fluid. Intermittent irrigation may be used to prevent obstruction of urinary drainage.

Following catheter removal, assess the amount, color, and consistency of urine. Explain that the client may experience burning upon urination, that dribbling after urination is a common experience, and that the urine may contain small blood clots after catheter removal. The CBI and catheter usually are removed in the 24–48 hours following surgery. Urinary control may be improved by teaching the client to start and stop the urine stream several times during each voiding and by having the client practice Kegel exercises. Regaining full control may take up to 1 year.

If the man had a retropubic prostatectomy, assess the abdominal incision for the presence of urine or increased or purulent drainage. Because the bladder is not entered during a retropubic prostatectomy, no urine should be found on the dressing.

If the man had a suprapubic prostatectomy, assess urinary output from both the suprapubic and urethral catheters. The man with a suprapubic prostatectomy often has two separate closed

Box 9–4 Discharge Instructions for Men After Prostate Surgery

ACTIVITY

The healing period lasts from 4 to 8 weeks. Avoid strenuous activity and heavy lifting. Except for short rides, do not drive for 2 weeks. Do take long walks; take stairs slowly and carefully. Continue exercises that you did in the hospital to prevent blood clots in the legs. You can take showers, but avoid tub baths while the catheter is in place.

BLEEDING

Bleeding can occur any time after surgery. It is fairly common after a bowel movement, coughing, or increased exercise. If you notice blood in the urine, increase fluids and rest until the urine is clear. If heavy bleeding plugs the channel, call the care provider immediately. Avoid aspirin and NSAIDs for at least 2 weeks.

BOWEL MOVEMENTS

Keep bowel movements regular and soft to avoid pressure on the prostate area. Drink fruit juices and take mild laxatives or stool softeners as ordered.

DIET

Resume your normal diet. Increase fluids to 10 glasses (8 oz) daily. Avoid alcohol unless otherwise advised by your physician.

SEXUAL INTERCOURSE

To avoid bleeding, do not have sex for 6 weeks after surgery. You may still have erections even with the catheter in place. When you resume sex, ejaculate will flow back into the bladder, so you will express little or no semen.

URINATION

After your catheter is removed, you may experience some burning, stinging, or leakage for several weeks, and you may pass small blood clots occasionally. These symptoms will disappear as the area heals. It is best to use pads to control leakage.

WORK

If work is not strenuous, you may return in 4 weeks; otherwise, wait 6–8 weeks.

PLEASE CALL IMMEDIATELY IF:

- You are unable to urinate.
- Bleeding is not controlled by fluids and rest or bleeding is excessive.
- You have chills and fever or severe abdominal pain.
- Your scrotum becomes swollen and tender.
- You have pain in one calf, chest pain, or difficulty breathing.

drainage systems: one from the suprapubic incision and one from a urethral catheter. Assess the abdominal dressing for urinary drainage and change saturated dressings frequently. Consult with a skin care specialist if urinary dressing results in skin irritations. Following removal of the urethral catheter (usually 2–4 days after surgery), based on physician orders, clamp the suprapubic catheter and encourage the man to void. Assess residual urine by unclamping the suprapubic catheter and measuring urinary output after voiding. If residual urine is 75 mL or less with several voidings, remove the suprapubic catheter.

The man with a perineal prostatectomy should be assessed for perineal drainage and manifestations of infection. Rectal temperatures and enemas are contraindicated because they may precipitate bleeding. Use a T-binder or padded scrotal support to hold the dressing in place. (The location of the dressing makes application difficult.) Following removal of the dressing and perineal sutures, heat lamps or sitz baths may be used to provide heat and promote healing. Teach the man to perform perineal irrigations with sterile normal saline as ordered and as instructed after each bowel movement. Because of the proximity of the incision to the anus, special wound care is necessary to prevent infection.

Depending on a client's choice of treatment, the procedure may be performed on an outpatient basis. The client having a TURP, although hospitalized for the surgery, may be discharged within 2 days after surgery if there are no complications. Home care often involves care of an indwelling urinary catheter.

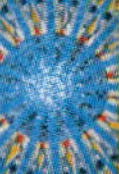

CLIENT TEACHING Caring for Catheters and Drainage Bags

Teaching how to care for the catheter and drainage bag includes the following information:

- Change from the daytime leg drainage bag to a larger night drainage bag. A larger bag suspended from the bed frame at night permits gravity drainage of urine and prevents reflux of urine into the bladder.
- Avoid strapping on the leg bag too tightly, which can decrease venous return and increase risk for thrombophlebitis (swelling of the veins) and embolic complications such as pulmonary emboli.
- Place a soft cloth between the leg bag and thigh to decrease friction and to absorb dampness under the bag, reducing the risk of skin irritation.
- Empty the leg bag every 3–4 hours during waking hours to prevent overfilling.
- Promptly report to the urologist any unexpected changes in urine color, urine consistency, urine odor, hematuria, evidence of frank bleeding, or large blood clots, as well as a lack of or significant decrease in urine output.

Evaluation

A client's individualized plan of care is developed in collaboration with the client and will include outcomes identified with the client's participation. The client's condition is regularly evaluated based on those outcomes. If an outcome is not met, the nurse reviews the plan of care with the client to determine necessary changes. Potential outcomes may include the following:

- Client is continent.
- Client maintains adequate pain control to allow for comfort and performance of ADLs.
- Client is asymptomatic, or symptoms are less severe.
- Client describes symptoms to report to the provider upon occurrence.
- Client lists over-the-counter medications to be avoided.

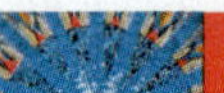

REVIEW Benign Prostatic Hypertrophy

RELATE: LINK THE CONCEPTS

Linking the exemplar of Benign Prostatic Hypertrophy with the concept of Sexuality:

1. How can you talk with an older man about the impact of BPH on his sexuality without making him uncomfortable?
2. How can you assess his concerns, fears, and knowledge regarding the impact of BPH on his sexuality?

Linking the exemplar of Benign Prostatic Hypertrophy with the concept of Infection:

3. What pathophysiology of BPH could increase the risk of UTIs?
4. What nursing interventions can the nurse initiate to reduce the risk of UTIs?

READY: GO TO COMPANION SKILLS MANUAL

- Measuring intake and output
- Using a bladder scanner
- Performing urinary catheritization
- Performing catheter care and removal
- Performing bladder irrigation
- Maintaining continuous bladder irrigation
- Providing suprapubic catheter care
- Obtaining a urine specimen from a closed drainage system
- Assessing the male genitals and inguinal area

REFER: GO TO MYNURSINGKIT

REFLECT: CASE STUDY

Clifford Allen is a 64-year-old male married to his wife Pam for 40 years. They live with their 24-year-old son Gary, who was born with Down syndrome. Mr. Allen is a middle manager for a small manufacturing company where he has worked for the last 20 years. Overall, Mr. Allen is in good health, although he has been undergoing treatment recently for BPH. He has a history of depression for which he does not seek treatment because he fears the social stigma connected to the diagnosis. Mr. Allen has been considering retiring within the next few years so he and his wife can travel, but mostly to escape the stressful work environment. He enjoys bowling and is involved with activities at church. He and his wife walk each evening after supper.

One evening while bowling, he notices that his bladder feels somewhat full. Mr. Allen calls to make an appointment to see his urologist for a follow-up examination. He has been taking finasteride (Proscar) for the last 6 months but does not believe it has been particularly effective. He still has trouble urinating and believes his symptoms are worse than before he started taking the drug. When he sees the urologist 2 weeks later, he reports that he often feels his bladder is full after voiding, he has difficulty starting his stream, and his stream is weak once started. He gets up frequently at night to void. His score on the American Urological Association Symptom Index is 28, up from 18 six months ago. The urologist confirms that the medication has not been effective and schedules further tests, including a uroflowmetry test, a postvoid residual test, a PSA blood test, and a urinalysis. Results from the uroflowmetry and postvoid residual test show a significant obstruction of urinary flow. The PSA is negative, and the urinalysis is consistent with bladder inflammation. A TURP is recommended in the upcoming weeks.

1. To determine his understanding of the procedure, what will the nurse want to ask this client upon admission to the surgical center?
2. What teaching will the nurse prepare regarding postoperative self-care?
3. Design a nursing plan of care for this client postoperatively.

9.2 BLADDER INCONTINENCE AND RETENTION

KEY TERMS

Bladder training, *445*
Habit training, *445*
Hydronephrosis, *445*
Scheduled toileting, *445*
Urinary incontinence, *441*
Urinary retention, *445*

BASIS FOR SELECTION OF EXEMPLAR

Institute of Medicine
Chronic Disease Management

LEARNING OUTCOMES

After learning about this exemplar, you will be able to:

1. Describe the pathophysiology, etiology, clinical manifestations, and direct and indirect causes of bladder incontinence and retention.
2. Identify risk factors associated with bladder incontinence and retention.
3. Illustrate the nursing process in providing culturally competent care across the life span for individuals with bladder incontinence and retention.
4. Formulate priority nursing diagnoses appropriate for an individual with bladder incontinence and retention.
5. Create a plan of care for an individual with bladder incontinence and retention that includes family members and caregivers.
6. Assess expected outcomes for an individual with bladder incontinence and retention.
7. Discuss therapies used in the collaborative care of an individual with bladder incontinence and retention.
8. Employ evidence-based caring interventions (or prevention) for an individual with bladder incontinence and retention.

OVERVIEW

When caring for clients with urinary tract disorders, it is important to consider the client's modesty in voiding, possible difficulty in discussing the genitals, embarrassment about being exposed for examination and testing, and fear of changes in body image or function. These psychosocial issues may interfere with the client's willingness to seek help, discuss treatment, and learn about preventive measures. Nursing interventions for clients with urinary tract disorders are directed toward primary prevention, early detection, and management of the disorder through health teaching and nursing care.

URINARY INCONTINENCE

Urinary incontinence or involuntary urination, is a symptom, not a disease. It is the most common manifestation of impaired bladder control. It can have a significant impact on the client's life, creating physical problems, such as skin breakdown, and it can lead to psychosocial problems, including embarrassment, isolation, and social withdrawal.

Incidence and Prevalence

Approximately 17 million people in the United States have some degree of urinary incontinence (Mason, Newman, & Palmer, 2003). The estimated annual cost of managing urinary incontinence is $10 billion. Although urinary incontinence is especially common among older clients, it is not a normal consequence of aging, and it can be treated. An estimated 30% or more of older women living in the community experience urinary incontinence. In long-term care, foster care, and homebound populations, the incidence is approximately 50% (Mason et al., 2003; Tierney, McPhee, & Papadakis, 2005). Despite these statistics, the actual prevalence of urinary incontinence is nearly impossible to determine. Embarrassment and the availability of products to protect clothing and prevent detection contribute to clients not seeking evaluation and treatment of incontinence.

Etiology and Pathophysiology

Urinary continence requires a bladder that is able to expand and contract and sphincters that can maintain a urethral pressure higher than that of the bladder. Incontinence results when the pressure within the urinary bladder exceeds urethral resistance, allowing urine to escape. Any condition causing higher-than-normal bladder pressures or reduced urethral resistance can potentially result in incontinence. Relaxation of the pelvic musculature, disruption of cerebral and nervous system control, and disturbances of the bladder and its musculature are common contributing factors.

Incontinence may be an acute, self-limited disorder, or it may be chronic. The causes may be congenital or acquired, reversible or irreversible. Congenital disorders associated with incontinence include epispadias (absence of the upper wall of the urethra), and meningomyelocele (a neural tube defect in which a portion of the spinal cord and its surrounding meninges protrude through the vertebral column). Central nervous system or spinal cord trauma, stroke, and chronic neurologic disorders, such as multiple sclerosis and Parkinson's disease, are examples of acquired, irreversible causes of incontinence. Reversible causes include medications (e.g., diuretics and sedatives), prostatic enlargement, vaginal and urethral atrophy, UTI, and fecal impaction. Fecal impaction occurs when a mass of hard, dry stool will not void with a normal bowel movement. Vaginal childbirth also may contribute to urinary incontinence. In addition, acute confusion can cause incontinence that may or may not be reversible, depending on the underlying cause of the confusion.

Incontinence commonly is categorized as stress incontinence, urge incontinence (also known as overactive bladder), overflow incontinence, and functional incontinence. Table 9–8 summarizes each type with its physiologic cause and associated factors. Mixed incontinence (elements of both stress and urge incontinence) is common. Total incontinence is loss of all voluntary control over urination, with urine loss occurring without stimulus and in all positions.

Common causes of incontinence include UTI, urethritis, pregnancy, hypercalcemia, volume overload, delirium, restricted mobility, stool impaction, and psychologic causes (Morantz, 2005, p. 175). Urinary incontinence can be broken into two categories: acute and chronic.

ACUTE INCONTINENCE Many factors can contribute to acute, or reversible, incontinence, including polyuria, exposure to irritants, infection, urinary retention, use of pharmaceuticals, stool impaction or constipation, atrophic urethritis or vaginitis, restricted mobility or dexterity, psychologic conditions, and delirium or acute confused state. Some of these factors are readily reversible, with a decrease in symptoms if not complete resolution of urinary incontinence.

CHRONIC INCONTINENCE There are different types of chronic incontinence, including stress, urge, reflex, retention with overflow, and functional incontinence. Each type of chronic incontinence has a different etiology.

Risk Factors

Women are much more susceptible than men to urinary incontinence. Smokers have a higher risk for urinary incontinence, as do older adults who are housebound or living in nursing homes (see the Developmental Considerations feature that follows). Obesity, diabetes, inactivity, depression, and neurological disorders (e.g., stroke) are all risk factors for urinary incontinence. Individuals who experience two or more UTIs per year also are at higher risk.

Certain medications can cause urinary incontinence. These include medications that affect the adrenergic system, diuretics, and calcium-channel blockers.

Clinical Manifestations

Symptoms of urinary incontinence include the inability to avoid urinating until a bathroom can be found, inability to urinate, increased rate of urination, leakage, uncontrollable

TABLE 9–8 **Types of Urinary Incontinence**

	DESCRIPTION	PATHOPHYSIOLOGY	CONTRIBUTING FACTORS
Stress	Loss of urine associated with increased intraabdominal pressure during sneezing, coughing, lifting; quantity of urine lost usually is small	Relaxation of pelvic musculature and weakness of urethra and surrounding muscles and tissues leads to decreased urethral resistance	■ Multiple pregnancies ■ Decreased estrogen levels ■ Short urethra, change in angle between bladder and urethra ■ Abdominal wall weakness ■ Prostate surgery ■ Increased intra-abdominal pressure caused by tumor, ascites, obesity
Urge	Involuntary loss of urine associated with a strong urge to void	Hypertonic or overactive detrusor muscle leads to increased pressure within bladder and inability to inhibit voiding	■ Neurologic disorders, such as stroke, Parkinson's disease, multiple sclerosis; peripheral nervous system disorders ■ Detrusor muscle overactivity associated with bladder outlet obstruction, aging, or disorders such as diabetes
Overflow	Inability to empty bladder, resulting in overdistention and frequent loss of small amounts of urine	Outlet obstruction or lack of normal detrusor activity leads to overfilling of bladder and increased pressure	■ Spinal cord injuries below S_2 ■ Diabetic neuropathy ■ Prostatic hypertrophy ■ Fecal impaction ■ Drugs, especially those with anticholinergic effect
Functional	Incontinence resulting from physical, environmental, or psychosocial causes	Ability to respond to the need to urinate is impaired	■ Confusion or dementia ■ Physical disability or impaired mobility ■ Therapy or sedation ■ Depression ■ Regression

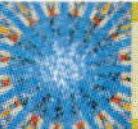

DEVELOPMENTAL CONSIDERATIONS The Institutionalized Older Adult and Self-Care Deficit

Functional incontinence may be the predominant problem in an institutionalized older adult. Limited mobility, impaired vision, dementia, lack of access to facilities and privacy, and tight staffing patterns increase the risk for incontinence in previously continent residents. The primary problem in functional incontinence is an outside factor that interferes with the ability to respond normally to the urge to void. An immobilized client may wet the bed if a call light is not within reach; a client with Alzheimer's disease may perceive the urge to void but be unable to interpret its meaning or respond by seeking a bathroom. For these clients, self-care deficit in toileting is a primary problem.

To assist clients with self-care, the nurse should do the following:

- Assess physical and mental abilities and limitations, usual voiding pattern, and ability to assist with toileting. A thorough assessment allows planned interventions to address specific needs and promote independence.
- Provide assistive devices. such as raised toilet seats, grab bars, a bedside commode, or night lights, as needed to facilitate independence. Fostering independence in toileting bolsters self-concept and maintains a positive body image.
- Plan a toileting schedule based on the client's normal elimination patterns to achieve a urine output of approximately 300 mL with each voiding. Allowing the bladder to fill to a point at which the urge to void is experienced and then emptying it completely helps to maintain normal bladder capacity and bacteriostatic functions.
- Position for ease of voiding—sitting for females, standing for males—and provide privacy. Normal positioning, usual toileting facilities, and privacy all enhance the ability to void on schedule and empty the bladder completely.
- Adjust fluid intake so that the majority of fluids are consumed during times of the day when the client is most able to remain continent. Unless fluids are restricted, maintain a fluid intake of at least 1.5–2.0 L per day. An adequate fluid intake is vital to promote hydration and urinary function. Overly concentrated urine can irritate the bladder, increasing incontinence.
- Assist with clothing that is easily removed (e.g., elastic-waist pants or loose dresses). Velcro and zipper fasteners may be easier to use than snaps and buttons. Clothing that is difficult to remove can increase the risk of incontinence in clients with mobility problems or impaired dexterity.

wetting, and frequent bladder infections. A number of medications and therapies are available to help individuals experiencing urinary incontinence.

MEDICATIONS Both stress and urge incontinence may improve with drug treatment. Drugs that contract the smooth muscles of the bladder neck may reduce episodes of mild stress incontinence. Imipramine (Tofranil), an antidepressent, is an effective preparation. It can make people drowsy, however, so it typically is taken at night. Adverse effects, such as dizziness and irregular heartbeat, and contraindications with a number of other medications may limit its use.

When incontinence is associated with postmenopausal atrophic vaginitis, estrogen therapy may be effective. Options include systemic estrogens and local creams. Clients with urge incontinence may be treated with preparations that increase bladder capacity. The primary drugs used to inhibit detrusor muscle contractions and increase bladder capacity include oxybutynin (Ditropan and the extended-release form, Ditropan XL), an anticholinergic drug, and tolterodine (Detrol and its longer-acting form, Detrol LA), a more specific antimuscarinic agent. These drugs can be taken once or twice a day and have fewer side effects than less-specific anticholinergic drugs. Drugs with anticholinergic effects are contraindicated for the client with acute glaucoma. Urinary retention is a potential side effect that must be considered when these drugs are used.

SURGERY Surgery may be used to treat stress incontinence associated with cystocele or urethrocele and overflow incontinence associated with an enlarged prostate gland. Suspension of the bladder neck (Box 9–5), a technique that brings the angle between the bladder and urethra closer to normal, is

Box 9–5 **Nursing Care of the Client Undergoing Bladder Neck Suspension**

PREOPERATIVE CARE

- Discuss the need to avoid straining and the use of the Valsalva maneuver postoperatively. *Straining and increased abdominal pressure during the Valsalva maneuver may place excessive stress on suture lines and interfere with healing.*
- Suggest measures such as increasing fluid and fiber intake and using a stool softener to prevent postoperative constipation.

POSTOPERATIVE CARE

- Monitor urine output, including quantity, color, and clarity. Expect urine to be pink initially, then to clear gradually. *Bright red urine, excessive vaginal drainage, or incisional bleeding may indicate hemorrhage. Instrumentation of the urinary tract increases the potential for UTI; cloudy urine may be an early sign.*
- Maintain stability and patency of suprapubic and/or urethral catheters. Secure catheters in position. *Maintaining bladder decompression eliminates pressure on suture lines. Preventing movement of or pulling on catheters reduces the risk for resultant pressure on surgical incisions.*
- Carefully monitor urine output after catheter removal. Difficulty voiding is common following catheter removal. *Early intervention to prevent bladder distention is important to prevent pressure on suture lines.*
- If the urethral or suprapubic catheter will remain in place on discharge, teach proper care to the client and family members as needed. *Appropriate self-care and early recognition of problems reduce the risk for significant complications.*

effective in treating stress incontinence associated with urethrocele in 80–95% of clients. A laparoscopic, vaginal, or abdominal approach may be used to perform this surgery.

Prostatectomy, using either the transurethral or suprapubic approach, is indicated for the client who is experiencing overflow incontinence as a result of an enlarged prostate gland and urethral obstruction.

Other surgical procedures of potential benefit in the treatment of incontinence include implantation of an artificial sphincter, formation of a urethral sling to elevate and compress the urethra, augmentation of the bladder with bowel segments to increase bladder capacity, and injection of collagen along the urethra to narrow the urinary passageway and support more normal urethral positioning.

COMPLEMENTARY THERAPIES Biofeedback and relaxation techniques may help to reduce episodes of urinary incontinence. Biofeedback uses electronic monitors to teach conscious control over physiologic responses of which the individual is not normally aware. Developing an awareness of perceptible information allows the client to gain voluntary control over urination. Biofeedback is widely used to manage urinary incontinence.

For more information, see the Evidence-Based Practice feature.

HEALTH PROMOTION Although urinary incontinence rarely has serious physical effects, it frequently has significant psychosocial effects, and it can lead to lowered self-esteem, social isolation, and even institutionalization (Lauver, Gross, Ruff, & Wells, 2004). The nurse should get the word out—informing all clients that urinary incontinence is not a normal consequence of aging and that treatments are available. To reduce the incidence of urinary incontinence, the nurse should teach all women to perform pelvic floor muscle (Kegel) exercises (Box 9–6) to improve perineal muscle tone. Women should be urged to seek advice from their primary care practitioner about using topical or systemic hormone therapy during menopause to maintain perineal tissue integrity. Older men should be advised to have routine prostate examinations to prevent urethral obstruction and overflow incontinence. Pelvic floor muscle exercises also may benefit men who experience urinary incontinence following prostatectomy, but evidence supporting this is limited (Moore & Gray, 2004).

PRACTICE ALERT

Clients who have difficulty emptying the bladder completely should not to stop urine flow while voiding in order to identify the pelvic floor muscles. Repeated interruption of micturition can interfere with complete bladder emptying and increase the risk for UTI.

CLIENT TEACHING Client teaching is essential for clients who experience problems with urinary incontinence and for their family members. The nurse should discuss the following points with clients to help prevent UTI and urinary incontinence:

- Maintain a generous fluid intake (see the Practice Alert feature that follows). Reduce or eliminate fluid intake after the evening meal to reduce nocturia.
- Wear comfortable clothing that is easy to remove for toileting.
- Maintain good hygiene, but do not bathe more often than necessary. Frequent bathing and use of feminine hygiene sprays or douches may dry perineal tissues, increasing the risk of UTI or urinary incontinence.

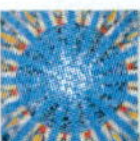

EVIDENCE-BASED PRACTICE **Urinary Incontinence**

An accurate diagnosis of stress urinary incontinence often is made based on clinical data, but motor urge incontinence generally is more difficult to diagnose accurately without urodynamic testing. This presents a difficulty for nurses and nurse practitioners in planning care for clients with incontinence when urologic testing is not feasible or readily available. A model developed by Gray, McClain, Peruggia, Patrie, and Steers (2001) may be useful in addressing this problem in adults whose cognitive abilities are intact. By comparing client data with urodynamic testing results, this team of researchers identified factors predictive of motor urge incontinence. These factors included age, gender, and three key symptoms: diurnal frequency (urinating more often than every 2 hours while awake), nocturia (awakening with the urge to urinate more than once per night if younger than 65 years and twice per night if older than age 65), and urge incontinence (urine loss associated with a strong desire to urinate). The presence of all three symptoms was more than 92% predictive of motor urge incontinence in study participants of all ages (range, 18–89 years; median, 61 years) and both genders.

Implications for Nursing

Asking specific questions about urinary tract symptoms can facilitate accurate identification of the nursing diagnosis *Urge Urinary Incontinence*. Accurate diagnosis is vital to planning and implementing appropriate care measures and to achieving the desired outcome—namely, continence. Successful treatment promotes self-esteem and provides positive reinforcement for continuing planned strategies.

Critical Thinking in Client Care

1. What nursing care measures and client teaching will you provide for the client with stress incontinence that may not be appropriate or necessary for the client with urge incontinence? What nursing care measures and client teaching will you provide for the client with urge incontinence but not stress incontinence?
2. Identify circumstances in which it may not be possible or feasible to have the client undergo urodynamic testing to differentiate stress, urge, or mixed (stress and urge) incontinence.
3. The clients in the study by Gray et al. lived independently in the community with no known or visible cognitive impairment. Can the data in this study be generalized to clients residing in a long-term care facility? Can the results be applied to all types of incontinence? Why, or why not?

Source: Gray, M., McClain, R., Perrugia, M., Patrie, J., & Steers, W. D. (2001). A model for predicting motor urge urinary incontinence. *Nursing Research, 50*(2), 116–122.

Box 9–6 Pelvic Floor Muscle (Kegel) Exercises

- Identify the pelvic muscles with these techniques:
  a. Stop the flow of urine during voiding, and hold for a few seconds (see the Practice Alert feature that follows).
  b. Tighten the muscles at the vaginal entrance around a gloved finger or tampon.
  c. Tighten the muscles around the anus as though resisting defecation.
- Perform exercises by tightening pelvic muscles, holding for 10 seconds, and then relaxing for 10–15 seconds. Continue the sequence (tighten, hold, relax) for 10 repetitions.
- Keep abdominal muscles and breathing relaxed while performing exercises.
- Initially, exercises should be performed twice a day, working up to four times a day.
- Encourage exercising at a specific time each day or in conjunction with another daily activity (e.g., bathing or watching the news). Establish a routine, because these exercises should be continued for life.
- Assistive devices, such as vaginal cones, and biofeedback may be useful for clients who have difficulty identifying appropriate muscle groups.

- Perform pelvic muscle (Kegel) exercises several times a day to increase perineal muscle tone.
- Reduce consumption of caffeine-containing beverages (e.g., coffee, tea, and colas), citrus juices, and artificially sweetened beverages containing NutraSweet.
- Use behavioral techniques to reduce the frequency of incontinence. **Scheduled toileting** is toileting at regular intervals (e.g., every 2–4 hours). **Habit training** is toileting the client on a schedule that corresponds with the normal pattern. **Bladder training** gradually increases the bladder capacity by increasing the intervals between voidings and resisting the urge to void.
- See your primary care provider regularly for a pelvic or prostate examination.
- For women, discuss possible benefits and risks of hormone replacement therapy, physical therapy, or surgery to treat incontinence.
- Report any change in urine color, odor, or clarity or symptoms such as burning, frequency, or urgency to your primary care provider.

PRACTICE ALERT

Limiting total fluid intake to less than 1.5–2.0 L per day is not recommended for clients with urinary incontinence. Inadequate fluid increases urine concentration, leading to bladder wall irritation and possibly increasing problems of urge incontinence.

URINARY RETENTION

When bladder emptying is impaired, urine accumulates and the bladder becomes overdistended, a condition known as **urinary retention**. Overdistention of the bladder causes poor contractility of the detrusor muscle, further impairing urination. If the problem persists, more serious problems, such as **hydronephrosis** (accumulation of urine in the renal pelvis as a result of obstructed outflow) can result. Common causes of urinary retention include prostatic hypertrophy (enlargement), surgery, and some medications.

Clients with urinary retention may experience overflow voiding or incontinence, eliminating from 25–50 mL of urine at frequent intervals. The bladder is firm and distended on palpation and may be displaced to one side of midline.

Etiology and Pathophysiology

Either mechanical obstruction of the bladder outlet or a functional problem can cause urinary retention. Benign prostatic hypertrophy (BPH) is a common cause, with difficulty initiating and maintaining urine flow often being the presenting complaint in men. Acute inflammation associated with infection or trauma of the bladder, urethra, or perineal tissues also may interfere with micturition. Scarring caused by repeated UTIs can lead to urethral stricture and a mechanical obstruction. Bladder calculi also may obstruct the urethral opening from the bladder.

Risk Factors

A number of factors may increase an individual's risk for urinary retention. Surgery, particularly abdominal or pelvic surgery, may disrupt function of the detrusor muscle, leading to retention of urine.

Drugs also may interfere with detrusor muscle function. Anticholinergic medications, such as atropine, glycopyrrolate (Robinul), propantheline bromide (Pro-Banthine), and scopolamine hydrochloride (Transderm-Scop), can lead to acute urinary retention and bladder distention. Many other drug groups have anticholinergic side effects and may cause urinary retention. Among these are antianxiety agents, such as diazepam (Valium); antidepressant and tricyclic drugs, such as imipramine (Tofranil); antiparkinsonian drugs (L-dopa); antipsychotic agents; and some sedative/hypnotic drugs. In addition, antihistamines, which are common in over-the-counter cough, cold, allergy, and sleep-promoting drugs, have anticholinergic effects and may interfere with bladder emptying. Diphenhydramine (Benadryl) is an example of a nonprescription antihistamine.

Voluntary urinary retention (particularly common among nurses!) may lead to overfilling of the bladder and a loss of detrusor muscle tone. Accidents to or infections of the brain or spinal cord can increase a client's risk for urinary retention. Diabetes, stroke, pelvic trauma, multiple sclerosis, and BPH all increase the risk for urinary retention.

Clinical Manifestations

The client with urinary retention is unable to empty the bladder completely and may feel discomfort because of this inability. The client may have difficulty starting urination and may

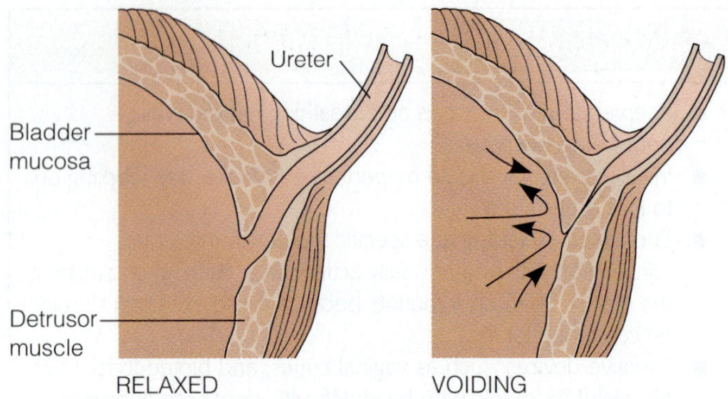

Figure 9–13 ■ A competent vesicoureteral junction.

be able to produce only a weak flow. Overflow voiding or incontinence may occur, with 25–50 mL of urine eliminated at frequent intervals. Assessment reveals a firm, distended bladder that may be displaced to one side of midline. Percussion of the lower abdomen reveals a dull tone, reflective of fluid in the bladder. Urinary retention is confirmed using a bladder scan or by inserting a urinary catheter (if possible) and measuring the urine output. Use of a bladder scan is preferred to reduce the risk of UTI (Teng, Huang, Kuo, & Bih, 2005).

Severe urinary retention with resulting bladder distention impairs the ability of the vesicoureteral junction to prevent backflow of urine into the ureters (Figure 9–13 ■). Reflux of urine from the distended bladder distends the ureters (hydroureter) and kidneys (hydronephrosis). Hydronephrosis impairs renal function, and acute renal failure can result.

MEDICATIONS Cholinergic medications, such as bethanechol chloride (Urecholine), that promote contraction of the detrusor muscle and emptying of the bladder may be used. A medication with no anticholinergic side effects may be substituted when urinary retention is related to drug therapy.

SURGERIES AND PROCEDURES An indwelling urinary catheter or intermittent straight catheterization can prevent urinary retention and overdistention of the bladder. Mechanical obstructions are treated by removing or repairing the obstruction when possible. Resection of the prostate gland may be done for urinary retention related to BPH. Bladder calculi are removed, and measures to prevent their formation are instituted.

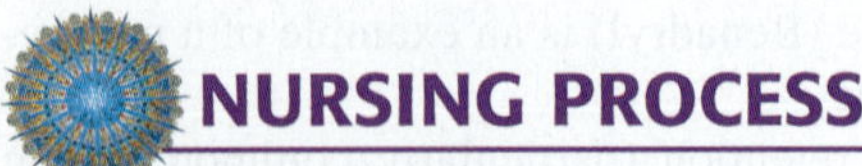

NURSING PROCESS

Assessment

The preliminary assessment and identification of the symptoms of urinary incontinence and retention are truly within the scope of nursing practice. All clients should be asked about their voiding patterns. Clients with mild symptoms may not even realize that they are experiencing a problem. Older adults who are incontinent while in their home or who manage to contain or conceal their incontinence from others do not consider themselves to be incontinent. Therefore, if these older adults are asked whether they are incontinent, they may deny it. However, asking if they lose urine when they don't want to may provide more accurate information (Palmer & Newman, 2006). If incontinence is described, a thorough history and assessment is indicated.

A complete assessment of a client's urinary function includes the following:

- *Health history.* Voiding diary; frequency of urination, amount of urine loss, and activities associated with incontinence; methods used to deal with incontinence; use of Kegel exercises or medications; any chronic diseases, medications, or alternative health therapies, related surgeries, and so on; effects of incontinence or retention on usual activities, including social activities
- *Physical examination.* Physical and mental status, including any physical limitations or impaired cognition; inspection, palpation, and percussion of abdomen for bladder distention; inspection of perineal tissues for redness, irritation, or tissue breakdown; observation for bulging of bladder into vagina when bearing down; assessment of pelvic muscle tone as indicated; assessment hydration status, and examination of urine.

Diagnosis

NANDA International (2007) includes one general diagnostic label for urinary elimination problems: Impaired Urinary Elimination, dysfunctional in urine elimination. other, more specific NANDA nursing diagnoses related to urinary elimination are subcategories of this diagnosis:

- Functional Urinary Incontinence
- Reflex Urinary Incontinence
- Stress Urinary Incontinence
- Total Urinary Incontinence
- Urge Urinary Incontinence
- Overflow Urinary Incontinence
- Urinary Retention.

Box 9–7 lists definitions of NANDA diagnoses related to incontinence. Box 9–8 lists clinical examples of assessment data clusters and related nursing diagnoses, outcomes, and interventions.

Box 9–7 **Definitions of NANDA Incontinence Diagnoses**

- Functional Urinary Incontinence: inability of usually continent person to reach toilet in time to avoid unintentional loss of urine
- Reflex Urinary Incontinence: involuntary loss of urine at somewhat predictable intervals when a specific bladder volume is reached
- Stress Urinary Incontinence: sudden leakage of urine occurring with activities that increase abdominal pressure
- Total Urinary Incontinence: continuous and unpredictable passage of urine
- Urge Urinary Incontinence: involuntary passage of urine occurring soon after a strong sense of urgency to void

Source: Adapted from Moorhead, S., Johnson, M., & Meridean M. (2004). *Nursing outcomes classification (NOC)* (3rd ed.). Copyright © 2004 with permission from Elsevier.

Box 9–8 **Identifying Nursing Diagnoses, Outcomes, and Interventions: Clients With Urinary Elimination Disorders**

Data Cluster: Mrs. Amy Brown, 75, reports accidental loss of urine before she is able to reach the toilet. She is aware of the urge to void but states, "Because of my stroke I sometimes can't get there soon enough."

Nursing diagnosis/ definition	Sample desired outcomes/ definition	Indicators	Selected interventions/ definition	Sample NIC activities
Functional Urinary Incontinence: Inability of usually continent person to reach toilet in time to avoid unintentional loss of urine	Urinary Continence [0502]: *Control of the elimination of urine from the bladder*	Consistently demonstrated: ■ Responds to urge in timely manner ■ Gets to toilet between urge and passage of urine ■ Voids >150 mL each time	Prompted Voiding [0640]: *Promotion of urinary continence through the use of timed verbal toileting reminders and positive social feedback for successful toileting*	■ Determine client awareness of continence status by asking if wet or dry. ■ Prompt up to three times to use toilet or substitute, regardless of continence status. ■ Give positive feedback by praising desired toileting behavior. ■ Document outcomes of toileting session.
Data Cluster: Anthony Cherry, a teenager with a spinal cord injury, has no awareness of bladder filling, the urge to void, or feelings of bladder fullness. He reports loss of urine at fairly regular intervals.				
Reflex Urinary Incontinence: Involuntary loss of urine at somewhat predictable intervals when a specific bladder volume is reached	Urinary Elimination [0503]: *Collection and discharge of urine*	Not compromised: ■ Elimination pattern ■ Complete bladder emptying ■ Urine amount ■ Urine clarity	Urinary Catheterization: Intermittent [0582]: *Regular periodic use of a catheter to empty the bladder*	■ Teach client/family purpose, supplies, method, and rationale of intermittent catheterization. ■ Demonstrate procedure, and have a return demonstration. ■ Determine catheterization schedule based on a comprehensive assessment.
Data Cluster: Tammy Tyndale reports dribbling whenever she laughs, coughs, or sneezes. She is 8 months pregnant.				
Stress Urinary Incontinence: Sudden loss of urine occurring with activities that increase abdominal pressure	Symptom Control [1608]: *Personal actions to minimize perceived adverse changes in physical and emotional functioning*	Consistently demonstrated: ■ Use of preventive measures ■ Use of available resources	Pelvic Muscle Exercise [0560]: *Strengthening and training the levator ani and urogenital muscles through voluntary repetitive contraction to decrease stress, urge, or mixed types of urinary incontinence*	■ Instruct client to tighten, then relax the ring of muscle around urethra and anus, as if trying to prevent urination or bowel movement. ■ Provide positive feedback for doing exercises as prescribed.
Data Cluster: Mrs. Gail Brady reports urinary urgency, difficulty in getting to the bathroom in time, frequency (more often than every 2 hours), and leakage of urine when unable to reach the toilet in time.				
Urge Urinary Incontinence: *Involuntary passage of urine occurring soon after a strong sense of urgency to void*	Tissue Integrity: Skin and Mucous Membranes [1101]: *Structural intactness and normal physiological function of skin and mucous membranes*	Not compromised: ■ Skin integrity	Urinary Bladder Training [0570]: *Improving bladder function for those with urge incontinence by increasing the bladder's ability to hold urine and the client's ability to suppress urination*	■ Keep a continence record for 3 days to establish voiding pattern. ■ Establish interval for toileting, preferably more than 2 hours. ■ Reduce toileting interval by 30 minutes if more than three incontinence episodes in 24 hours. ■ Increase interval by 30 minutes if no incontinence episodes for 3 days until optimal 4-hour interval is reached.

Note: The NOC numbers for desired outcomes and the NIC numbers for nursing interventions are listed in brackets following the appropriate outcome or intervention. Outcomes, indicators, interventions, and activities selected are only a sample of those suggested by NOC and NIC and should be further individualized for each client.

Problems of urinary elimination also may become the etiology for other problems the client experiences. Examples include the following:

- Urinary retention and invasive procedures, such as catheterization or cystoscopic examination, can put a client at risk for infection.
- Incontinence is a risk factor for low self-esteem and social isolation because it is considered to be socially unacceptable and therefore can be physically and emotionally distressing to clients. Often, the client is embarrassed about dribbling or having an accident and may restrict normal activities for this reason.
- Incontinence increases risk for impaired skin integrity. Bed linens and clothes saturated with urine irritate and macerate the skin. Prolonged skin dampness leads to dermatitis (inflammation of the skin) and subsequent formation of dermal ulcers.
- Functional incontinence is a risk factor for self-care deficits in toileting.
- Impaired urinary function associated with a disease process may put a client at risk for deficient or excess fluid volume.
- A client who has a urinary diversion ostomy may develop a disturbed body image.
- Clients who require new self-care skills to manage (e.g., a new urinary diversion ostomy) may be at risk of deficient knowledge regarding management of their care.
- An incontinent client who is being cared for by a family member for extended periods may be at risk for caregiver role strain as well as for deteriorating family relationships as a result of that strain.

Plan

Goals established for a client will depend on the diagnosis and defining characteristics. Examples of overall goals for clients with urinary elimination problems may include the following:

- Maintain or restore a normal voiding pattern.
- Regain normal urine output.
- Prevent associated risks, such as infection, skin breakdown, fluid and electrolyte imbalance, and lowered self-esteem.
- Perform toilet activities independently, with or without assistive devices.
- Contain urine with the appropriate device, catheter, ostomy appliance, or absorbent product.

Appropriate preventive and corrective nursing interventions that relate to these goals must be identified. Specific nursing activities associated with each of these interventions can be selected to meet the client's individual needs. Box 9–7 and the Nursing Care Plan feature at the end of this exemplar show examples of clinical applications of these using NANDA, NIC, and NOC designations.

Planning for Home Care

To provide for continuity of care, the nurse must consider the client's needs for teaching and assistance with care in the home. Discharge planning includes assessment of client and family resources and abilities for self-care, available financial resources, and need for referrals and home health services. The Care Settings feature on urinary elimination outlines an assessment of home care capabilities related to urinary elimination problems and needs. The Client Teaching feature addresses the learning needs of the client and family.

CARE SETTINGS Urinary Elimination

CLIENT AND ENVIRONMENT

- Self-care abilities: Ability to consume adequate fluids, to perceive bladder fullness, to ambulate and get to the toilet, to manipulate clothing for toileting, and to perform hygiene measures after toileting
- Current level of knowledge: Fluid and dietary intake modifications to promote normal patterns of urinary elimination, bladder training methods, and specific techniques to promote voiding care for indwelling catheter or ostomy (if appropriate)
- Assistive devices required: Ambulatory aids such as walker, cane, or wheelchair; safety devices such as grab bars; toileting aids such as raised toilet seat, urinal, commode, or bedpan; presence of a urinary catheter
- Physical layout of the toileting facilities: Presence of mobility aids; toilet at correct height to enable elders to get up after voiding
- Home environment factors that interfere with toileting: Distance to the bathroom from living areas or bedrooms; barriers such as stairways, scatter rugs, clutter, or narrow doorways that interfere with bathroom access; lighting (including night lighting)
- Urinary elimination problems: Type of incontinence and precipitating factors; manifestations of urinary tract infection such as dysuria, frequency, urgency; evidence of prostatic hypertrophy and effect on urination; ability to perform self-catheterization and care for other urinary elimination devices such as indwelling catheter, urinary diversion ostomy, or condom drainage

FAMILY

- Caregiver availability, skills, and responses: Ability and willingness to assume responsibilities for care, including assisting with toileting, intermittent catheterization, indwelling catheter care, urinary drainage devices or ostomy care; ready access to laundry facilities; access to and willingness to use respite or relief caregivers
- Family role changes and coping: Effect on spousal and family roles, sleep/rest patterns, sexuality, and social interactions
- Financial resources: Ability to purchase protective pads and garments, supplies for catheterization or ostomy care

COMMUNITY

- Environment: Access to public restrooms and sanitary facilities
- Current knowledge of and experience with community resources: Medical and assistive equipment and supply companies, home health agencies, local pharmacies, available financial assistance, support and educational organizations

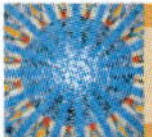

CLIENT TEACHING Urinary Elimination in the Home Setting

FACILITATING URINARY ELIMINATION SELF-CARE

- Teach the client and family to maintain easy access to toilet facilities, including removing scatter rugs and ensuring that halls and doorways are free of clutter.
- Suggest graduated lighting for nighttime voiding: a dim night-light in the bedroom and low-wattage hallway lighting.
- Advise the client and family to install grab bars and elevated toilet seats as needed.
- Provide for instruction in safe transfer techniques. Contact physical therapy to provide training as needed.
- Suggest clothing that is easily removed for toileting, such as elastic waist pants or Velcro closures.

PROMOTING URINARY ELIMINATION

- Instruct the client to respond to the urge to void as soon as possible; avoid voluntary urinary retention.
- Teach the client to empty the bladder completely at each voiding.
- Emphasize the importance of drinking eight to ten 8-ounce glasses of water daily.
- Teach female clients about pelvic muscle exercises to strengthen perineal muscles.
- Inform the client about the relationship between tobacco use and bladder cancer and provide information about smoking cessation programs as indicated.
- Teach the client to promptly report any of the following to the primary care provider: pain or burning on urination, changes in urine color or clarity, malodorous urine, or changes in voiding patterns (e.g., nocturia, frequency, dribbling).

ASEPSIS

- Teach the client to maintain perineal-genital cleanliness, washing with soap and water daily and cleansing the anal and perineal area after defecating.
- Instruct female clients to wipe from front to back (from the urinary meatus toward the anus) after voiding, and to discard toilet paper after each swipe.
- Provide information about products to protect the skin, clothing, and furniture for clients who are incontinent. Emphasize the importance of cleaning and drying the perineal area after incontinence episodes. Instruct in the use of protective skin barrier products as needed.
- Teach clients with an indwelling catheter and their family about care measures such as cleaning the urinary meatus, managing and emptying the collection device, maintaining a closed system, and bladder irrigation or flushing if ordered.
- For clients with a urinary diversion, teach about care of the stoma, drainage devices, and surrounding skin. For continent diversions, teach the client how to catheterize the stoma to drain urine.
- For clients with an indwelling catheter or urinary diversion, emphasize the importance of maintaining a generous fluid intake (2.5–3 quarts daily) and of promptly reporting changes in urinary output, signs of urinary retention such as abdominal pain, and manifestations of urinary tract infection such as malodorous urine, abdominal discomfort, fever, or confusion.

MEDICATIONS

- Emphasize the importance of taking medications as prescribed. Instruct the client to take the full course of antibiotics ordered to treat a urinary tract infection, even though symptoms are relieved.
- Inform the client and family about any expected changes in urine color or odor associated with prescribed medications.
- For clients with urinary retention, emphasize the need to contact the primary care provider before taking any medication (even over-the-counter medications such as antihistamines) that may exacerbate symptoms.
- For clients taking medications that may damage the kidneys (e.g., aminoglycoside antibiotics), stress the importance of maintaining a generous fluid intake while taking the medication.
- Suggest measures to reduce anticipated side effects of prescribed medications, such as increasing intake of potassium-rich foods when taking a potassium-depleting diuretic such as furosemide.

DIETARY ALTERATIONS

- Teach the client about dietary changes to promote urinary function, such as consuming cranberry juice and foods that acidify the urine to reduce the risk of repeated urinary tract infections or forming calcium-based urinary stones.
- Instruct clients with stress or urge incontinence to limit their intake of caffeine, alcohol, citrus juices, and artificial sweeteners because these are bladder irritants that may increase incontinence. Also, teach clients to limit their evening fluid intake to reduce the risk of nighttime incontinence episodes.

MEASURES SPECIFIC TO URINARY PROBLEMS

- Provide instructions for clients with specific urinary problems or treatments such as
  a. timed urine specimens.
  b. urinary incontinence.
  c. urinary retention.
  d. retention catheters.

REFERRALS

- Make appropriate referrals to home health agencies, community agencies, or social services for assistance with resources such as grab bars and raised toilet seats, providing wheelchair access to bathrooms, obtaining toileting aids such as commodes, urinals, or bedpans, and services such as home health aides for assistance with activities of daily living.

COMMUNITY AGENCIES AND OTHER RESOURCES

- Provide information about resources for durable medical equipment such as commodes or raised toilet seats, possible financial assistance, and medical supplies such as drainage bags, incontinence briefs, or protective pads.
- Suggest additional sources of information and help such as the National Council of Independent Living, United Ostomy Association, National Association for Continence, and Simon Foundation for Continence.

Implementation

Independent nursing interventions for clients with urinary incontinence who are returning to their home or a residential facility include (a) a behavior-oriented continence training program that may consist of bladder training, habit training, prompted voiding, pelvic muscle exercises, and positive reinforcement; (b) meticulous skin care; and (c) for male clients, application of an external drainage device (condom-type catheter device). Other interventions include promoting adequate fluid intake, maintaining normal voiding habits, and assisting with toileting; also, see the following Practice Alert feature. Clients must be alert and physically able or have caregivers who can assist with implementing the plan of care so that the plan can be followed.

PRACTICE ALERT

Stress incontinence in women may be successfully treated by insertion (under local anesthesia) of a transvaginal tape sling to support the urethra.

Successful home care for a client will involve a combination of the following strategies:

- *Education*, which involves the client, family and any non-family caregivers, including private nursing providers and respite caregivers.
- *Bladder training*, which requires that the client postpone voiding, resist or inhibit the sensation of urgency, and void according to a timetable rather than according to the urge to void. The goals are to gradually lengthen the intervals between urination to correct the client's frequent urination, to stabilize the bladder, and to diminish urgency. This form of training may be used for clients who have bladder instability and urge incontinence. Delayed voiding provides larger voided volumes and longer intervals between voiding. Initially, voiding may be encouraged every 2–3 hours except during sleep, and then every 4–6 hours. A vital component of bladder training is inhibiting the urge-to-void sensation. To do this, instruct the client to practice deep, slow breathing until the urge diminishes or disappears. This is performed every time the client has a premature urge to void.
- *Habit training*, also referred to as timed voiding or scheduled toileting, which attempts to keep clients dry by having them void at regular intervals. With habit training, no attempt is made to motivate the client to delay voiding if the urge occurs. This approach can be effective in children who are experiencing urinary dysfunction. Biofeedback therapy, in which the child is taught to relax the pelvic floor, also can decrease incidents of wetting (Shei Dei Yang & Cheng Wang, 2005).
- *Prompted voiding,* which supplements habit training by encouraging the client to use the toilet (prompting) and reminding the client when to void.
- *Pelvic muscle exercises*, which includes the following technique: Ask the client to think of the perineal muscles as an elevator. When the client relaxes, the elevator is on the first floor. To perform the exercise, contract the perineal muscles, bringing the elevator to the second, third, and fourth floors. Keep the elevator on the fourth floor for a few seconds, and then gradually relax the area. When the exercise is properly performed, contraction of the muscles of the buttocks and thighs is avoided. Pelvic muscle exercises can be performed anytime, anywhere, sitting or standing—even when voiding. Specific client instructions for performing these exercises are summarized in the Client Teaching feature.

Maintaining Skin Integrity

Skin that is continually moist becomes macerated (softened). Urine that accumulates on the skin is converted to ammonia, which is very irritating to the skin. Because both skin irritation and maceration predispose the client to skin breakdown and ulceration, the incontinent person requires meticulous skin care. To maintain skin integrity, the nurse washes the client's perineal area with mild soap and water or a commercially prepared no-rinse cleanser after episodes of incontinence, rinses it thoroughly if soap and water were used, dries it gently and thoroughly, and provides clean, dry clothing or bed linen. The nurse applies barrier ointments or creams to protect the skin from contact with urine. If it is necessary to pad the client's clothes for protection, the nurse should use products that absorb wetness and leave a dry surface in contact with the skin. Clients returning home or to a care facility should be instructed in techniques for maintaining skin integrity.

Specially designed incontinence draw sheets, which provide significant advantages over standard draw sheets, may be used for incontinent clients confined to bed. These sheets are like a standard draw sheet but are double layered, with a quilted upper nylon or polyester surface and an absorbent viscose rayon layer below. The rayon soaker layer generally has a waterproof backing on its underside. Fluid (i.e., urine) passes through the upper quilted layer and is absorbed and dispersed by the viscose rayon, leaving the quilted surface dry to the touch. This absorbent sheet helps maintain skin integrity; it does not stick to the skin when wet, decreases the risk of bedsores, and reduces odor.

Maintaining Normal Voiding Habits

Prescribed medical therapies often interfere with a client's normal voiding habits. When a client's urinary elimination pattern is adequate, the nurse helps the client adhere to normal voiding habits as much as possible (Box 9–9).

Promoting Urination

Nursing measures to promote urination include placing the client in normal voiding position and providing for privacy. Additional measures include running water, placing the client's hands in warm water, pouring warm water over the perineum, and taking a warm sitz bath.

In acute urinary retention, catheterization may be necessary to relieve bladder distention and prevent hydronephrosis. Use a relatively small catheter (16 French for a man, 14 French for a woman). A coudé-tipped catheter is passed more easily in the older man with an enlarged prostate. Using 2% lidocaine gel (10 mL injected into the male urethra, or 6 mL injected into the female urethra) reduces discomfort during catheterization and the risk of catheter-associated infection, and it promotes pelvic muscle relaxation (Bardsley, 2005). Carefully observe the client as the distended bladder drains. See the following Practice Alert feature for additional information.

Box 9–9 Maintaining Normal Voiding Habits

POSITIONING

- Assist the client to a normal position for voiding: standing for male clients; for female clients, squatting or leaning slightly forward when sitting. These positions enhance movement of urine through the tract by gravity.
- If the client is unable to ambulate to the lavatory, use a bedside commode for females and a urinal for males standing at the bedside.
- If necessary, encourage the client to push over the pubic area with the hands or to lean forward to increase intra-abdominal pressure and external pressure on the bladder.

RELAXATION

- Provide privacy for the client. Many people cannot void in the presence of another person.
- Allow the client sufficient time to void.
- Suggest the client read or listen to music.
- Provide sensory stimuli that may help the client relax. Pour warm water over the perineum of a female or have the client sit in a warm bath to promote muscle relaxation. Applying a hot water bottle to the lower abdomen of both men and women may also foster muscle relaxation.
- Turn on running water within hearing distance of the client to stimulate the voiding reflex and to mask the sound of voiding for people who find this embarrassing.
- Provide ordered analgesics and emotional support to relieve physical and emotional discomfort to decrease muscle tension.

TIMING

- Assist clients who have the urge to void immediately. Delays only increase the difficulty in starting to void, and the desire to void may pass.
- Offer toileting assistance to the client at usual times of voiding, for example, on awakening, before or after meals, and at bedtime.

FOR CLIENTS WHO ARE CONFINED TO BED

- Warm the bedpan. A cold bedpan may prompt contraction of the perineal muscles and inhibit voiding.
- Elevate the head of the client's bed to Fowler's position, place a small pillow or rolled towel at the small of the back to increase physical support and comfort, and have the client flex the hips and knees. This position simulates the normal voiding position as closely as possible.

PRACTICE ALERT

Some clients may experience a vasovagal response, becoming pale, sweaty, and hypotensive if the bladder is rapidly drained. Draining urine in 500-mL increments and clamping the catheter for 5–10 minutes between increments may prevent this response. Hematuria, the presence of blood in the urine, also may occur with rapid bladder decompression. Promptly notify the physician if hematuria develops.

Home care for the client with urinary retention varies depending on the cause. Some clients may be taught intermittent self-catheterization. Nurses should instruct all clients who have experienced urinary retention to avoid over-the-counter drugs that affect micturition, especially those with an anticholinergic effect (allergy and cold medications, many nonprescription sleep aids). Other home care measures include double-voiding (urinate, remain on the toilet for 2–5 min, and then urinate again); scheduled voiding; or when other measures fail, an indwelling catheter. When an indwelling catheter is necessary, teach the client and family to use clean technique when changing from an overnight bag to a leg bag, and to report promptly any signs of UTI to the primary care provider.

Assisting With Toileting

Clients who are weakened by a disease process or impaired physically may require assistance with toileting. The nurse should assist these clients to the bathroom and remain with them if they are at risk for falling. The bathroom should contain an easily accessible call signal to summon help if needed. Clients also must be encouraged to use handrails placed near the toilet. For clients who are unable to use bathroom facilities, provide urinary equipment close to the bedside (e.g., urinal, bedpan, or commode) and the necessary assistance to use them.

Coping With Social Isolation

Urinary incontinence increases the risk for social isolation because of embarrassment, fear of not having ready access to a bathroom, body odor, or other factors. In turn, social isolation can increase problems of incontinence because normal cues and relationships are lost and the need to remain dry becomes less of a concern. To assist clients in the area of social isolation, the nurse should do the following:

- Assess for reasons and extent of social isolation. Verify the degree of social isolation with the client or significant other. Do not assume that social isolation is related only to urinary incontinence. Other problems frequently associated with aging (e.g., a hearing deficit) may be primary or contributing factors.
- Refer the client for urologic examination and incontinence evaluation. Clients who assume that urinary incontinence is a normal part of the aging process may not be aware of treatment options.
- Explore alternative coping strategies with the client, significant other, staff, and other health care team members. Protective pads or shields, good perineal hygiene, scheduled voiding, and clothing that does not interfere with toileting can enhance continence.

Community-Based Care

Because urinary incontinence is a contributing factor to the institutionalization of many older people, client and family teaching can have a significant impact on a client maintaining independence and residence in the community. Address possible causes of incontinence and appropriate treatment measures. Refer for urologic examination if one has not already completed. Discuss fluid intake management, perineal care, and products for clothing protection.

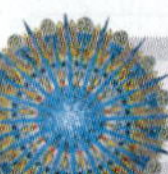

NURSING CARE PLAN A Client With Impaired Urinary Elimination

ASSESSMENT

Mrs. Patrice Ross, 46 years old, is the mother of eight children ranging in age from 10 to 4 years of age with one set of triplets who are now 6 years old. Mrs. Ross visits her health provider, reporting urinary incontinence when she coughs, sneezes, or laughs hard. The admitting nurse learns that Mrs. Ross has been experiencing this since her last child was born 4 years ago. However, Mrs. Ross says that the problem has gotten worse within the past few months and now when she has to void, she feels as though she must hurry to prevent leakage. She reports that when she urinates, she has to bear down to completely empty her bladder, but she denies frequency, burning, hesitancy, or nocturia. When asked about what she has been doing to control the problem, she reports that she has cut back on fluid intake when she knows she must leave her home in order to avoid possible accidents and that she has begun using peri-pads to catch any leakage. Physical examination detects a mild bladder prolapse into the vagina. Mrs. Ross requests help to resolve the problem.

DIAGNOSES

- Stress Urinary Incontinence
- Readiness for Enhanced Fluid Balance
- Risk for Impaired Social Interaction

PLANNING

Demonstrates urinary continence as evidenced by:

- Describing a plan for treating stress incontinence
- Maintaining a voiding frequency of more than q2h.

Knowledge: Treatment regimen [1813] as evidenced by substantial:

- Description of self-care responsibilities for ongoing care
- Description of self-monitoring techniques.

Fluid balance will be achieved, as evidenced by:

- Urine specific gravity
- Serum electrolytes
- Hemaglobin and hematocrit
- Balanced intake and output.

IMPLEMENTATION

- Instruct client to monitor urinary elimination, including consistency, odor, volume, and color.
- Instruct client to drink a minimum of 1500 mL (six 8 oz glasses) of fluids per day.
- Help client select appropriate incontinence garment or pad for short-term management while more definitive treatment is designed.
- Instruct client about which signs and symptoms to report to the health care provider (e.g., burning on urination, hematuria, oliguria).
- Instruct client on use of Kegel exercises to strengthen pelvic muscles.

EVALUATION

Outcomes partially met. Following the appointment, Mrs. Ross reports a reduction in leakage as a result of frequent urination to keep bladder empty and improved control after practicing Kegel exercises regularly several times per day. She discussed with her surgeon possible surgery to repair the bladder prolapse and has opted to delay surgery until she can evaluate the effects of nonsurgical treatment. She has maintained adequate fluid intake and reports that she no longer fears being embarrassed when she goes out with friends. She continues to wear a peri-pad when she leaves the house.

CRITICAL THINKING

1. Considering Mrs. Rosss history and assessment data, what factors contributed to her development of stress incontinence?
2. The primary care provider has suggested possible surgery, but Mrs. Ross has opted to delay this treatment until medical management can be evaluated. How can the nurse respond to Mrs. Rosss decision?
3. What risk factors will the nurse want Mrs. Ross to be aware of as a result of stress incontinence? What teaching will the nurse provide to decrease risk?

Evaluation

Using the overall goals anddesired outcomes identified in the planning stage, the nurse collects data to evaluate the effectiveness of nursing activities. The Nursing Care Plan feature on urinary elimination lists examples of desired outcomes for the identified goals.

If the desired outcomes are not achieved, the nurse should explore the reasons before modifying the care plan. For example, the following are examples of questions that must be considered if the outcome "Remains dry between voidings and at night" is not met:

- What is the client's perception of the problem?
- Does the client understand and comply with the health care instructions provided?
- Is access to toilet facilities a problem?
- Can the client manipulate clothing for toileting? Are there adjustments that can be made to allow easier disrobing?
- Are scheduled toileting times appropriate?
- Is there adequate lighting for nighttime toileting?

- Are mobility aids (e.g., walker, elevated toilet seat, or grab bar) needed? If these aids are currently used, are they appropriate or adequate? If assistance from a family member or caregiver is needed, is that available and appropriate?
- Is the client performing pelvic floor muscle exercises appropriately as scheduled?
- Is the client's fluid intake adequate? Does the timing of fluid intake require adjustment (e.g., restricted after dinner)?
- Is the client restricting caffeine, citrus juice, carbonated beverages, and artificial sweetener intake?
- Is the client taking a diuretic? If so, when is the medication taken? Do the times require adjustment (e.g., taking second dose no later than 4 p.m.)?
- Should continence aids (e.g., a condom catheter or absorbent pads) be considered or used?

REVIEW Bladder: Incontinence and Retention

RELATE: LINK THE CONCEPTS

The nurse admits an 83-year-old client with medical diagnosis of congestive heart failure, chronic renal failure, and diabetes mellitus. While the nursing history is being taken, the client says she takes her diuretic in the morning and then spends the next few hours in the bathroom, because if she goes too far away, she ends up "wetting her pants" and then has to "clean up the mess." She says she gets so thirsty in the afternoon that she drinks several glasses of water but stops drinking fluids after 6 p.m. to avoid "wetting the bed." The client's skin turgor is poor, and assessment reveals possible dehydration.

Linking the exemplar of Bladder: Incontinence and Retention with the concept of Fluids and Electrolytes:

1. What recommendations and client teaching should the nurse provide this client to prevent further dehydration?
2. What lab values should the nurse review to confirm potential dehydration?

While caring for a 41-year-old busy executive of a thriving small business, she informs you she has been experiencing bladder incontinence when she laughs, coughs, or sneezes and that it is causing embarrassment at work. She blames it on having had five children.

Linking the exemplar of Bladder: Incontinence and Retention with the concept of Self:

3. What impact is bladder incontinence having on this client's self image?
4. What recommendations might you make for this client to reduce her feelings of shame and self-consciousness?

READY: GO TO COMPANION SKILLS MANUAL

- Collecting a routine urine specimen
- Performing urinary catheterization
- Performing catheter care and removal
- Performing bladder irrigation
- Providing suprapubic catheter care
- Providing hemodialysis
- Providing ongoing care of hemodialysis
- Terminating hemodialysis

REFER: GO TO MYNURSINGKIT

REFLECT: CASE STUDY

Mr. Justin Gardner is a 26-year-old man who fractured his third thoracic vertebra when he fell while rock climbing. In preparation for transfer to a rehabilitation center, the doctor orders discontinuation of the client's indwelling urinary catheter and PRN straight catheterization to reduce urinary retention.

1. What assessment data will the nurse collect to determine the presence of urinary retention?
2. What signs and symptoms would the nurse recognize as indicative of the need for straight catheterization?
3. What nursing diagnosis would be appropriate for this client?
4. What client teaching will this client require, related to urinary retention, before discharge if he is to provide safe home care for himself?

9.3 BOWEL: INCONTINENCE, CONSTIPATION, AND IMPACTION

KEY TERMS

Constipation, *464*
Encopresis, *467*
Fecal impaction, *468*
Fecal incontinence, *468*
Ulcerative colitis, *465*

BASIS FOR SELECTION OF EXEMPLAR

Institute of Medicine
Chronic Disease Managment
Standards of Nursing Practice

LEARNING OUTCOMES

After learning about this exemplar, you will be able to:

1. Describe the pathophysiology and etiology of incontinence, constipation, and impaction.
2. Identify risk factors associated with incontinence, constipation, and impaction.
3. Illustrate the nursing process in providing culturally competent care across the life span for individuals with incontinence, constipation, and impaction.
4. Formulate priority nursing diagnoses appropriate for an individual with incontinence, constipation, and impaction.
5. Create a plan of care for an individual with incontinence, constipation, and impaction that includes family members and caregivers.
6. Assess expected outcomes for an individual with incontinence, constipation, and impaction.
7. Discuss therapies used in the collaborative care of an individual with incontinence, constipation, and impaction.
8. Employ evidence-based care (or prevention) for an individual with incontinence, constipation, impaction, clinical manifestations, direct and indirect causes.

OVERVIEW

Disorders of intestinal absorption and bowel elimination can affect not only functional elimination status but also other functional health patterns including, but not limited to, health perception and management, nutritional and metabolic, activity and exercise, self-perception and self-concept, and sexuality and reproductive health patterns. Bowel function can be affected by inflammations, infections, tumors, obstructions, or changes in structure.

Clients with intestinal disorders often face extensive diagnostic testing, surgery, and permanent changes in physical appearance and lifestyle. Nursing care is directed toward returning to or maintaining homeostasis, meeting the client's physiologic needs, providing emotional support, and educating the client to adapt to changes in lifestyle.

Few body functions respond as readily to internal and external influences as the process of defecation. Factors affecting the gastrointestinal tract directly, such as food intake and bacterial population, affect the number and consistency of stools. Indirect factors, such as psychologic stress or voluntary postponement of defecation, also affect elimination. It is important to evaluate each client's bowel elimination against his or her own normal pattern.

CONSTIPATION

Constipation may be defined as fewer than three bowel movements per week or difficult passage of stools. This infers either the passage of dry, hard stool or the passage of no stool. It occurs when the movement of feces through the large intestine is slow, allowing time for additional reabsorption of fluid from the large intestine. Difficult evacuation of stool and increased effort or straining of the voluntary muscles of defecation are associated with constipation. The individual also may have a feeling of incomplete stool evacuation after defecation. Careful assessment of a client's habits is necessary before a diagnosis of constipation is made. Box 9–10 lists the frequent defining characteristics of constipation.

Constipation affects older adults more frequently than younger people. Recent studies indicate that approximately 20–35% of people older than 65 years report recurrent constipation and laxative use. Although fecal transit in the large intestine slows with aging, the increased incidence of constipation in older adults is thought to relate more to impaired general health status, increased medication use, and decreased physical activity.

The loss of teeth makes chewing and swallowing food difficult. Ill-fitting, broken, or lost dentures also alter nutritional status. Periodontal disease with subsequent loss of natural teeth is one such factor, because the accompanying inability to chew foods results in a diet of soft, nonfibrous foods. Lack of fresh fruits and vegetables or other sources of bulk or fiber contributes to the pattern of constipation. The older adult may self-limit daily fluid intake, especially water, to decrease frequency of urination, unintentionally increasing the potential for constipation.

Constipation is a common complaint of pregnant women. In pregnancy, mechanical pressure from the growing uterus contributes to displacement of the small intestine and reduces motility. The increased secretion of progesterone further reduces motility because of decreased gastric tone and increased smooth muscle relaxation; thus, the emptying time of the stomach and bowel is prolonged. Hemorrhoids (swollen and inflamed veins in the anus and rectum) frequently develop in late pregnancy from constipation and from pressure on vessels below the level of the uterus, causing the pregnant woman further discomfort.

Box 9–10 Sample Defining Characteristics of Constipation

- Decreased frequency of defecation
- Hard, dry, formed stools
- Straining at stool; painful defecation
- Reports of rectal fullness or pressure or of incomplete bowel evacuation
- Abdominal pain, cramps, or distention
- Diminished appetite, nausea
- Headache

Risk Factors

Many causes and factors contribute to constipation, including the following:

- Insufficient fiber intake
- Insufficient fluid intake
- Insufficient activity or immobility
- Irregular defecation habits
- Change in daily routine
- Lack of privacy
- Chronic use of laxatives or enemas
- Irritable bowel syndrome
- Pelvic floor dysfunction or muscle damage
- Poor motility or slow transit
- Neurologic conditions (e.g., Parkinson's disease), stroke, or paralysis
- Emotional disturbances (e.g., depression or mental confusion)
- Medications (e.g., opioids, iron supplements, antihistamines, antacids, and antidepressants).

Constipation itself can cause health problems for some clients. In children, it often is associated with a UTI. Straining associated with constipation often is accompanied by holding the breath, and this can present serious problems for people with heart disease, brain injuries, or respiratory disease: Holding one's breath while bearing down increases intrathoracic pressure and vagal tone, slowing the pulse rate (LeMone & Burke, 2008).

Pathophysiology

Constipation may be a primary problem or a manifestation of another disease or condition. Acute constipation, a definite change in the bowel elimination pattern, often is caused by an organic process. A change in bowel patterns that persists or becomes more frequent or severe may be caused by a tumor or other partial bowel obstruction. With chronic constipation, functional causes that impair storage, transport, and evacuation mechanisms impede the normal passage of stools.

Psychogenic factors are the most common causes of chronic constipation. These factors include postponing defecation when the urge is felt and the perception of satisfaction with defecation. Clients often use laxatives and enemas to stimulate a bowel movement when constipation is perceived. Overuse of these measures can lead to real intestinal problems which further aggravate the condition. For example, cathartic colon (impaired colonic motility and changes in bowel structure) mimics **ulcerative colitis** (a disease that causes sores in the lining of the rectum and colon) in that the normal pouch-like or saccular appearance of the colon is lost. Melanosis coli is a brownish-black discoloration of the colon mucosa. Both cathartic colon and melanosis coli may be caused by long-term laxative use. Table 9–9 lists selected causes of constipation.

Clinical Manifestations

The manifestations of constipation include having bowel movements less often than the usual pattern, frequent flatus, abdominal discomfort, diminished appetite, straining to have a bowel movement, and the passage of hard, dry stools.

With significant constipation or long-term dependence on laxatives or enemas, fecal impaction may develop. Impaction may also occur after barium administration for radiologic examination. Fecal impaction is felt as a rock-hard or putty-like mass of feces in the rectum. Abdominal cramping and a full sensation in the rectal area may be manifestations of impaction. Watery mucus or foul-smelling liquid stool may be passed around the impaction, causing the client to complain of diarrhea.

Manifestations of constipation that may appear on examination include an abdomen that may appear somewhat distended as well as reduced bowel sounds. If an impaction is present, digital examination of the rectum reveals a palpable, hard or putty-like fecal mass.

Simple or chronic constipation is treated with education (a daily bowel movement is not necessary for health), modification of diet, and exercise routines. If the problem is acute or does not resolve, further diagnostic examination may be ordered. This may include a barium enema to identify bowel structure, tumors, or diverticula. If the problem is acute, a sigmoidoscopy or colonoscopy may be used for evaluation and biopsy. For more information, see Box 9–11.

MEDICATIONS Laxative and cathartic preparations are used to promote stool evacuation. Milder preparations generally are known as laxatives; those known as cathartics have a stronger effect. Most laxatives are appropriate only for short-term use. Cathartics and enemas interfere with normal bowel reflexes and should not be used for simple constipation. Laxatives should never be given if an intestinal obstruction, abdominal pain, fecal impaction, rectal fissures, ulcerated hemorrhoids, Crohn's disease, ulcerative colitis, or chronic inflammatory bowel disease are suspected (Peate, 2003). When the bowel is obstructed, laxatives or cathartics may cause serious mechanical damage and perforate the bowel.

The only laxatives that are appropriate and safe for long-term use are bulking agents, such as psyllium seed, calcium polycarbophil, and methylcellulose. These agents act by increasing the bulk of the feces and drawing water into the bowel to soften it.

Pharmacologic management of severe constipation usually occurs in two stages. The first stage involves softening the stool with medications such as lactulose, and the second stage involves evacuation of stool with a laxative. The evacuation phase is the most difficult for the client and for caregivers who may be managing the constipation of a child or older adult (Clayden & Keshtgar, 2003).

Once a stool softener has been administered, the most effective means to evacuate the stool while causing the least amount of stress and anxiety to the client is considered. Suppositories and enemas can cause fear in children. Polyethylene glycol electrolyte solution (GoLYTELY) can be administered orally or instilled via a nasogastric tube to promote stool evacuation (Biggs & Dery, 2006). More recently, electrolyte-free polyethylene glycol (MiraLAX) has been used effectively (Kinservik & Friedhoff, 2004). Once the stool has been evacuated, a routine stimulant laxative is given to prevent reaccumulation of stool in the bowel. The stimulant laxative of choice usually is Senokot or Bisacodyl (Biggs & Dery, 2006).

TABLE 9–9 **Selected Causes of Constipation**

FACTOR	RELATED CAUSE
Activity	Lack of exercise; bed rest
Dietary	Highly refined, low-fiber foods; inadequate fluid intake
Drugs	Antacids containing aluminum or calcium salts; narcotic analgesics; anticholinergic agents; many antidepressants, tranquilizers, and sedatives; antihypertensive agents, such as ganglionic blockers, calcium-channel blockers, beta-adrenergic blockers, and diuretics; iron salts
Large bowel	Diverticular disease, inflammatory disease, tumor, obstruction; changes in rectal or anal structure or function
Psychogenic	Voluntary suppression of urge; perceived need to defecate on schedule; depression
Systemic	Advanced age; pregnancy; neurologic conditions (e.g., trauma, multiple sclerosis, tumors, cerebrovascular accident, parkinsonism); endocrine and metabolic disorders (e.g., hypothyroidism, hypercalcemia, uremia, porphyria)
Other	Chronic laxative or enema use

Box 9–11 Constipation and the Older Adult

Constipation and perceived constipation are common problems in older adults. Although constipation is not a normal consequence of aging, factors such as slowed peristalsis, lowered activity levels, reduced food and fluid intake, and decreased sensory perception contribute to the higher incidence of constipation seen in older adults. Chronic diseases such as diabetes, mobility problems, and medications also increase the risk of constipation in older adults.

Cultural influences and advertising lead many older adults to believe that a daily bowel movement is important for health. This belief contributes to an increased incidence of perceived constipation in older adults. Because of this perception, the older adult may come to rely on laxatives, suppositories, or enemas to facilitate regular bowel movements. These external aids to defecation can further impair the ability to maintain "normal" bowel habits (a movement of soft stool every 2–3 days).

NUTRITION Foods are recommended for clients experiencing constipation. Vegetable fiber is largely indigestible and cannot be absorbed, so it increases stool bulk. Fiber also helps to draw water into the fecal mass, softening the stool and making defecation easier. Raw fruits and vegetables are good sources of dietary fiber, as is cereal bran. Use two to three teaspoons of unprocessed bran with meals (sprinkled on fruit or cereal), or up to one-quarter cup daily, to supply adequate fiber.

Fluids also are important to maintain bowel motility and soft stools. The client should drink six to eight glasses of fluid per day. It is important to advise the client to increase fluid intake when dietary fiber is initially increased to decrease flatus and help maintain softer stools.

ENEMAS Significant or chronic constipation or fecal impaction may require administration of an enema. As a general rule, enemas should be used only in acute situations and only on a short-term basis. They also may be ordered to prepare the bowel for diagnostic testing or examination.

DEVELOPMENTAL CONSIDERATIONS Constipation is a common complaint in the pediatric population and accounts for approximately 25% of referrals made to pediatric gastroenterologists (Coughlin, 2003). Because defecation patterns vary among children, identification of an abnormal pattern is sometimes difficult. Infants usually have several bowel movements a day. Breast-fed infants may have bowel movements as frequently as every feeding or just one bowel movement every several days. Because of differences in fat digestion and absorption, bottle-fed infants are more prone to hard stools (Coughlin, 2003). For a young child, one bowel movement a day may be normal. As the child grows, however, three to four bowel movements a week may be a normal pattern. Constipation is characterized by "pebble-like, hard stools for a majority of bowel movements for at least 2 weeks, firm stools ≤ 2 times per week for at least 2 weeks, and no evidence of structural, endocrine, or metabolic disease" (Lembo & Camilleri, 2003). Constipation in children can be influenced by a variety of factors. Refer to Table 9–10 for further information.

Constipation during infancy is rare, and most often, it is caused by mismanagement of diet. The transition from formula to cow's milk may cause a transient constipation, because the bowel must adjust to the increased protein content of cow's milk.

Constipation occurs most frequently in toddlers and preschoolers. This increased incidence often is associated with learning to control body functions. Many children do not like the sensations of a bowel movement and may begin withholding stool, which accumulates in and dilates the rectum until the next urge to defecate. The increasingly hard and painful bowel movement reinforces the child's behavior, and a pattern develops (Clayden & Keshtgar, 2003). For information about constipation and stool toileting refusal, see Box 9–12.

TABLE 9–10 Influential Factors In Childhood Constipation

PHYSICAL FACTORS IN INFANCY	PHYSICAL FACTORS IN CHILDREN	PSYCHOLOGICAL FACTORS IN CHILDREN
Familial stool patterns	Hypertrophied rectum	Embarrassment/shame related to soiling resulting from early or coercive toilet training, or lack of privacy
High milk and low fiber intake	Residual stool blockage (fecalith)	
Cow's milk allergy	Overflow fecal soiling around a solid stool	
Hard stools	Poor rectal sensation	Fear of pain from hard stool
Dehydration	Diseases that influence gastrointestinal or neurologic systems (e.g., celiac disease, cerebral palsy)	Being too busy to use the bathroom
Perianal group A streptococcal infection		Parental blame/anger related to soiling and toileting refusal
Medications (e.g., diuretics) and analgesia		
Intestinal or anal conditions (e.g., Hirschsprung disease), cystic fibrosis, anorectal malformations		Teasing and bullying related to incontinence
		Decreased mobility/activity

Source: Adapted from Clayden, G., & Keshtgar, A. S. (2003). Management of childhood constipation. *Postgraduate Medical Journal, 79*, 616–621. Used with permission.

Box 9–12 Bowel Elimination and STR

A recent study was conducted to determine whether constipation and painful bowel elimination occur as a result of or before stool toileting refusal (STR). In this prospective longitudinal study of toilet training, 380 children between the ages of 17 and 19 months were followed (Blum, Taubman, & Nemeth, 2004). Researchers found that when hard or painful bowel movements or painful bowel elimination were associated with STR, the first episode of constipation generally occurred before the STR (Blum et al., 2004). This suggests that constipation is a chronic problem for many children and that it is not being treated effectively. Thus, painful bowel elimination associated with hard bowel movements contribute to, rather than result from, STR (Blum et al., 2004).

Constipation in the school-age child and adolescent usually results in overflow fecal incontinence. Some children with constipation are discovered during their school years after being evaluated for recurrent UTIs or enuresis (Clayden & Keshtgar, 2003).

Constipation may occur as a result of limited time for toileting. Busy school-age children may delay toileting, and adolescents participating in sports or other extracurricular activities may have limited time for toileting. Children also may be hesitant to use an unfamiliar bathroom. Encouragement from parents and relaxation of bathroom privileges at school promote regularity and return of previous bowel patterns within a short time. Children and adolescents may need to get up earlier to have breakfast and time for toileting before going to school.

Constipation may follow surgery, especially in children who are immobilized, such as by traction or a body cast. Stool softeners and a diet high in fiber and fluids are given to prevent and treat constipation.

CLINICAL THERAPY Dietary management is the treatment of choice for constipation that has no underlying pathologic cause. Constipation in young infants usually can be corrected by increasing the amount of fluids or adding 2 ounces of pear or apple juice to daily intake. Increasing physical activity and fluid intake may be effective for some children.

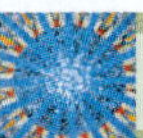

ALTERNATIVE THERAPIES Herbal Laxatives

Herbal laxatives are used by some cultures as complementary therapies. The safety and effectiveness of many of these laxatives have not been established in children. Psyllium, for example, has been approved for use as an ingredient in bulk-forming laxatives, but no studies have evaluated its safety or effectiveness in treating constipation in children. Cascara sagrada and senna are stimulant laxatives that have been approved by the U.S. Food and Drug Administration for use in children older than 2 years to treat constipation. Stimulant laxatives should be used with caution in children, however, because they can lead to dependency as well as to abdominal pain. Senna also has been associated with skin problems in children, including diaper rash and blistering (Gardiner & Kemper, 2005).

Removing constipating foods (e.g., bananas, rice, and cheese) from the child's diet often reduces the constipation. Increasing the child's intake of high-fiber foods (whole-grain breads, raw fruits, and vegetables) and fluids also promotes bowel elimination. A single glycerin suppository or enema may be needed to remove hard stool, followed by dietary and fluid management.

BEHAVIOR MANAGEMENT Behavior modification may prove beneficial to managing constipation. For younger children, providing rewards for overcoming the fear of toilets or for toileting at routinely scheduled times can be effective. Older children also respond to rewards (Clayden & Keshtgar, 2003). These rewards can be simple items, such as an afternoon spent with the parent playing a game. For children with psychological issues, child and family psychotherapy may be necessary. In these cases, the family is referred to a child and family counselor.

ENCOPRESIS

Encopresis is an abnormal elimination pattern characterized by recurrent soiling or passage of stool at inappropriate times by a child who should have achieved bowel continence. Encopresis is reported to occur in 55% of boys and 35% of girls with constipation (Biggs & Dery, 2006). Children with primary encopresis have never achieved bowel control. Children with secondary encopresis have had bowel continence for several months.

Encopresis usually is associated with voluntary or involuntary retention of stool in the lower bowel and rectum. This leads to constipation, dilation of the lower bowel, and incompetence of the inner sphincter. The retention of stool usually is a result of being "too busy"—the child puts off going to the bathroom because activities are occurring and leaving would be an inconvenience. The retention of stool leads to constipation that is untreated and chronic. Loose stool leaks around the hard feces, and the child becomes unaware of a need to eliminate. Soiling may occur during the day or night. Bowel movements are irregular, painful, small, and hard. The child may be ridiculed by peers because of his or her offensive body odor. This rejection leads to withdrawal and behavioral problems, often resulting in altered school performance and attendance. The child continues to hold stool because the passage has become painful. Parents commonly seek health care, believing that the child has diarrhea or constipation.

The underlying constipation that leads to encopresis may be caused by the stress of environmental changes (e.g., birth of a sibling, moving to a new house, attending a new school), issues of anger and control related to bowel training, diet, a full schedule of activities, or a genetic predisposition.

A thorough history, physical examination, and diagnostic studies (possibly including barium enema) are necessary to rule out organic causes and anatomic abnormalities. Examination of mental health and cognitive functioning may be indicated. Information about the child's toilet-training habits and parents' attitudes concerning those habits is obtained. A dietary history, including eating habits and types of foods eaten, often is helpful as well. Physical examination sometimes reveals a nontender mass in the lower abdomen.

Treatment may include behavior modification techniques, dietary changes, use of lubricants to clear the bowel of impacted stool and encourage normal defecation, and psychotherapy. Behavior modification programs that reward and reinforce appropriate toileting habits can be successful. Dietary changes include incorporating high-fiber foods, such as fruits, vegetables, and whole-grain cereals, into the diet. Limiting intake of refined and highly processed foods and dairy products also may be helpful. Drugs, such as mineral oil, bulk-forming laxatives, and stool softeners, are used temporarily to empty the bowel. The child should sit on the toilet for several minutes after the morning and evening meals. It takes several months for the bowel to be retrained to respond to sphincter stimulation. Psychotherapy involving the child and family may be indicated in instances of dysfunctional parent–child relationships.

Nursing Management

Prevention of encopresis is the nursing goal. Nurses should partner with parents to teach toilet-training techniques, emphasizing the child's developmental readiness. Encourage parents to praise the child for successes and to avoid punishment and power struggles. Encourage high-fiber diets and regular times for elimination.

Nursing care centers on educating the child and parents about the disorder and its treatment and on providing emotional support. Explain the treatment plan, including dietary changes and use of laxatives or stool softeners. Reassure the child that he or she has a healthy body and, with treatment, will achieve normal functioning. Nurses should monitor the child for at least 6 months to be certain new patterns become established.

FECAL IMPACTION

Fecal impaction is a mass or collection of hardened feces in the folds of the rectum. Impaction results from prolonged retention and accumulation of fecal material. In severe impactions, the feces accumulate and extend well up into the sigmoid colon and beyond. Fecal impaction can be recognized by the passage of liquid fecal seepage (diarrhea) without normal stool, as the liquid portion of the feces seeps out around the impacted mass. Impaction also can be assessed by digital examination of the rectum, during which the hardened mass often can be palpated.

Along with fecal seepage and constipation, symptoms include rectal pain and a frequent but nonproductive desire to defecate. A generalized feeling of illness results: The client becomes anorexic, the abdomen becomes distended, and nausea and vomiting may occur.

The causes of fecal impaction usually are poor defecation habits and constipation. Barium used in radiologic examinations of the upper and lower gastrointestinal tracts also can be a causative factor. After these examinations, laxatives or enemas usually are taken to ensure removal of the barium.

Digital examination of the impaction through the rectum should be done gently and carefully. Although digital rectal examination is within the scope of nursing practice, some agency policies require a primary care provider's order for digital manipulation and removal of a fecal impaction.

Although fecal impaction generally can be prevented, treatment of impacted feces sometimes is necessary. When fecal impaction is suspected, the client often is given an oil retention enema, a cleansing enema 2–4 hours later, and daily additional cleansing enemas, suppositories, or stool softeners. If these measures fail, manual removal may be necessary.

FECAL INCONTINENCE

Fecal incontinence, also called bowel incontinence, refers to the loss of voluntary ability to control fecal and gaseous discharges through the anal sphincter. It occurs less frequently than urinary incontinence but is no less distressing to the client. The incontinence may occur at specific times, such as after meals, or it may occur irregularly. Two types of bowel incontinence are described: partial and major. Partial incontinence is the inability to control flatus or to prevent minor soiling. Major incontinence is the inability to control feces of normal consistency.

Fecal incontinence generally is associated with impaired functioning of the anal sphincter or its nerve supply, such as in some neuromuscular diseases, spinal cord trauma, and tumors of the external anal sphincter muscle. Multiple factors contribute to fecal incontinence, including both physiologic and psychologic conditions (Box 9–13). Bowel incontinence usually is considered to be a manifestation of a disorder rather than a disorder unto itself. Clients often do not reveal fecal incontinence in discussing health concerns. Little information is available about its incidence and prevalence. Because many of the etiologic factors are more prevalent in the older adult, older clients are more often affected (see Evidence-Based Practice feature).

Box 9–13 **Selected Causes of Fecal Incontinence**

NEUROLOGIC CAUSES

- Spinal cord injury or disease
- Head injury, stroke, or brain tumor
- Degenerative neurologic disease, such as multiple sclerosis, amyotrophic lateral sclerosis, dementia
- Diabetic neuropathy

LOCAL TRAUMA

- Obstetric tears
- Anorectal injury
- Anorectal surgery with sphincter damage

INFLAMMATORY PROCESSES

- Infection
- Radiation

OTHER PHYSIOLOGIC CAUSES

- Diarrhea
- Stool impaction
- Pelvic floor relaxation or loss of sphincter tone
- Tumors

PSYCHOLOGIC CAUSES

- Depression
- Confusion and disorientation

The rate of fecal incontinence among older adults living in the community has been reported to be 4–17%, compared with 2% in the general community population and 20 to 54% in older nursing home residents (Bliss, Fischer, & Savik, 2005, p. 36). Fecal incontinence is an emotionally distressing problem that ultimately can lead to social isolation. Afflicted persons withdraw into their homes or, if in the hospital, the confines of their room to minimize the embarrassment associated with soiling.

Several surgical procedures are used for the treatment of fecal incontinence. These include repair of the sphincter and fecal diversion or colostomy.

Pathophysiology

The most common causes of fecal incontinence are those that interfere with either sensory or motor control of the rectum and anal sphincters. If the external sphincter is paralyzed as a result of spinal cord injury or disease, defecation occurs automatically when the internal sphincter relaxes with the defecation reflex. If sphincter muscles have been damaged or excessive pelvic floor relaxation has occurred, it may not be possible to override the defecation reflex with voluntary control.

Age-related changes in anal sphincter tone and response to rectal distention increase the risk for fecal incontinence in older adults. Resting and maximal anal sphincter pressures are decreased, particularly in older women. In addition, less rectal distension is needed to produce sustained relaxation of the anal sphincter in older women.

Clinical Manifestations

The diagnosis of fecal incontinence includes client history and physical examination of the pelvic floor and anus to evaluate muscle tone and rule out a fecal impaction. Impaired sphincter muscles may be palpable on digital examination. Anorectal manometry or a rectal motility test may be used to evaluate the functional ability of the sphincter muscles. In this test, a small, flexible balloon catheter is introduced into the rectum, and pressures are measured in the rectum and internal and external sphincters. Normally, rectal dilation causes the internal sphincter to relax and the external sphincter to contract. Sigmoidoscopy also may be used to examine the rectum and anal canal.

Management of fecal incontinence is directed toward the identified cause. Medications to relieve diarrhea or constipation may be prescribed. A high-fiber diet, ample fluids, and regular exercise are helpful for many clients. Exercises to improve sphincter and pelvic floor muscle tone (Kegel exercises) may be of long-term benefit. Clients also may benefit from using loperamide before meals and prophylactically before running errands or leaving the house (Tierney et al., 2005). Biofeedback therapy may be used for mentally alert clients with intact sphincter muscles but low muscle tone. With motivation and reinforcement, clients achieve improved sphincter control in response to a stimulus. The goal of biofeedback is to improve sensation, coordination, and strength of the sphincter muscle (Halverson, 2005).

When damage to the sphincter or rectal prolapse (protrusion of rectal mucous membrane through the anus) is the cause of fecal incontinence, surgical repair is the treatment of choice. Surgery also may be indicated when conservative measures have not been effective. Permanent colostomy (the creation of an opening from the large bowel on the abdominal wall) is a last-choice option for some clients, but it can control fecal output when other measures fail.

RISK FOR IMPAIRED SKIN INTEGRITY Good skin care is vital for the client with fecal incontinence. Stool contains enzymes and other irritating substances that promote skin breakdown when they are not promptly removed. This can lead

EVIDENCE-BASED PRACTICE **What Self-Care Practices Do Older Adults Use for Fecal Incontinence?**

Researchers conducted the first systematic investigation of self-care for fecal incontinence (FI) among older adults living in the community. The purpose of the study was to describe the self-care practices used and to examine factors associated with the number of self-care practices and willingness to report FI to a health care practitioner. FI was described as accidental leakage of stool during the past 12 months. A 51-item survey was distributed at four HMO primary care clinics in the Midwest. The clinic staff offered surveys to individuals 65 years or older who lived in the community. More than 1,300 surveys were received, primarily from women.

The results indicated that the most common self-care practices for managing FI were changing diet (e.g., avoiding certain foods); wearing a sanitary panty liner, pad, or brief; and reducing activity or exercise. A significant difference was found in the number and types of self-care practices between men and women. Fifty-two percent of men, compared with 19% of women, did not use any self-care practices to manage FI. Only 43% of the respondents discussed their FI with a health care practitioner, with no significant difference between men and women. More of those who had a health problem or disability that caused FI or who were not sure about the cause of FI consulted with a health professional.

The study has some limitations in that it was based on self-report rather than a more rigorous method, such as observation. Also, the population included older adults who visited HMO clinics, and as a result, generalization for the population at large is limited.

The findings indicate that nurses who care for older adults living in the community must inquire routinely about FI. Discussing FI, and especially new-onset FI, with a client allows the health care practitioner to provide appropriate follow-up to ascertain if the FI is a symptom of a health problem. Some older adults believe that FI is a normal part of aging and therefore may minimize its significance. If the FI is not health related, the nurse needs to assess the self-care practices of the older adult and if those practices are effective. The authors also suggest future research be conducted to investigate the reasons for the differences between men and women regarding self-care practices for FI.

Source: Bliss, D., Fischer, L., & Savik, K. (2005). Managing fecal incontinence: self-care practices of older adults. *Journal of Gerontological Nursing,* Copyright © 2005 SLACK, Inc. Reprinted with permission.

to pressure ulcers, particularly when a neurologic disorder (e.g., spinal cord injury, dementia, or stroke) impairs mobility.

Good skin care includes the following:

- Clean the skin thoroughly with mild soap and water after each bowel movement. Toilet tissue may be more irritating to the skin and less effective in removing fecal material.
- Apply a skin barrier cream or ointment after each bowel movement. These help protect the skin from irritating substances in the feces.
- If incontinence pads or briefs are used, check frequently for soiling and change when feces is noted. Although these help to protect bedding and clothing from soiling, they can contribute to skin breakdown if they are not checked and changed frequently.

COMMUNITY-BASED CARE Managing fecal incontinence is a challenging problem for the client, family, and caregivers. For the client with intact cognition, it can be psychologically devastating. The client may become socially isolated from fear of odor or soiling clothing. The client's self-esteem may suffer from a sense of lost control over body functions and the inability to provide self-care. It is important to stress that incontinence is never normal (i.e., aging alone is not a cause of incontinence) and often is treatable. Encourage the client to seek medical evaluation of the problem.

Topics for client and family education include the following:

- Recommended dietary measures, such as consuming a high-fiber diet and ample fluids to maintain soft, formed stool or maintaining a low-residue diet to reduce the number of stools
- Suggestions for regular exercise to stimulate bowel peristalsis and regular evacuation
- Use of bulk-forming laxatives, such as psyllium seed (Metamucil), to provide stool bulk and reduce the number of small, liquid stools
- Prescribed medications (e.g., loperamide to reduce the number of stools), their appropriate use, and management of adverse effects (e.g., constipation)
- Bowel training program, including techniques for digital anal stimulation, inserting suppositories, or administering enemas as recommended (For digital anal simulation, teach the client to insert a lubricated, gloved finger through the anal sphincter into the rectum 1.5–2 in. while seated on the toilet or commode and then use a circular, side-to-side movement to gently stretch the rectal wall until the internal sphincter relaxes.)
- The importance of good skin care, particularly if neurologic impairment is present
- The potential benefits and associated risks of biofeedback and surgical treatment, if recommended
- Referrals for home care or community health services as indicated.

COLLABORATION

Collaboration for the client with bowel elimination issues frequently will involve a nutritionist who can help support the client making any needed changes in diet or dietary patterns. Nurses also may want to consult with the client's pharmacist, who may be able to provide additional information regarding medications and supplements being taken and any related side effects. Physical therapists may offer important points on exercise within the client's range of motion that can promote bowel health and management. Nurses working with children who have problems with bowel elimination should encourage parents to work with teachers and school dieticians to support the child in improving dietary habits that support healthy bowel elimination.

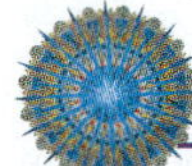

NURSING PROCESS

Assessment

- *Health history.* The nurse and client discuss the extent, onset, and duration of incontinence; identified contributing factors; history of spinal cord or anorectal injury or surgery; chronic diseases, such as diabetes, multiple sclerosis, or other neurologic disorders; medications and use of alternative therapies; nutrition; and hydration patterns.
- *Physical examination.* The nurse palpates and assesses the abdomen for firmness or tenderness as well as for the presence of any mass (retained stool). Bowel sounds should be assessed. If a digital rectal examination is performed, the nurse assesses for the presence of stool in the rectum. The nurse also assesses for hemorrhoids, anal fissures, or other abnormalities of the abdomen or perineum.

Diagnosis

NANDA International (2007) includes the following diagnostic labels for fecal elimination problems:

- Bowel Incontinence
- Constipation
- Risk for Constipation
- Perceived Constipation
- Diarrhea.

Clinical application of selected diagnoses is shown in Box 9–14 and at the end of the exemplar in the Nursing Care Plan.

Fecal elimination problems may affect many other areas of human functioning and, as a consequence, may be the etiology of other NANDA diagnoses. Examples include the following:

- Risk for Impaired Skin Integrity, related to
  a. bowel incontinence
  b. prolonged diarrhea
- Low Self-Esteem, related to
  a. fecal incontinence
  b. need for assistance with toileting
- Disturbed Body Image, related to bowel incontinence
- Deficient Knowledge (Bowel Training), related to lack of previous experience
- Anxiety, related to
  a. lack of control of fecal elimination
  b. response of others to fecal incontinence.

Box 9–14 Clients With Fecal Elimination Problems

Data Cluster: Mary Kuoko has had involuntary leakage of stool. She states her clothing is soiled several times a day, and says she is too embarrassed to go out with her friends because of the fecal odor. Her last bowel movement was more than 3 days ago. Digital examination reveals impaction.

Nursing diagnosis/ definition	Sample desired outcomes/ definition	Indicators	Selected interventions/ definition	Sample NIC activities
Bowel Incontinence: Change in normal bowel habits, characterized by involuntary passage of stool	Bowel Continence [0500]: *Control of passage of stool from the bowel*	Consistently demonstrated ■ Evacuates stool at least every 3 days ■ Responds to urge in a timely manner ■ Describes relationship of food intake to stool consistency	Bowel Management [0430]: *Establishment and maintenance of a regular pattern of bowel elimination* Bowel Incontinence Care [0410]: *Promotion of bowel continence and maintenance of perianal skin integrity*	■ Instruct on foods high in fiber as appropriate. ■ Give warm liquids after meals as appropriate. ■ Initiate a bowel training program as appropriate. ■ Wash perianal area with soap and water, and dry it thoroughly after each stool. ■ Monitor for adequate bowel evacuation. ■ Monitor diet and fluid requirements.

Note: The NOC numbers for desired outcomes and the NIC numbers for nursing interventions are listed in brackets following the appropriate outcome or intervention. The outcomes, indicators, interventions, and activities selected are only a sample of those suggested by NOC and NIC.

Plan

The major goals for clients with fecal elimination problems include the following:

- Maintaining or restoring normal bowel elimination pattern
- Maintaining or regaining normal stool consistency
- Preventing associated risks, such as fluid and electrolyte imbalance, skin breakdown, abdominal distention, and pain.

Implementation

Caring interventions include promoting regular defecation, digital removal of fecal impaction, bowel training programs, and use of a fecal incontinence pouch. The two Client Teaching features also address aspects of fecal elimination and healthy defecation.

Promoting Regular Defecation

The nurse can help clients to achieve regular defecation by attending to (a) the provision of privacy, (b) timing, (c) nutrition and fluids, (d) exercise, and (e) positioning.

PRIVACY Privacy during defecation is extremely important to most people. The nurse should provide as much privacy as possible for such clients but may need to stay with those who are too weak to be left alone. Some clients also prefer to wipe, wash, and dry themselves after defecating. A nurse may need to provide water, a washcloth, and a towel for this purpose.

TIMING A client should be encouraged to defecate when the urge is recognized. To establish regular bowel elimination, the client and nurse can discuss when mass peristalsis normally occurs and provide time for defecation. Many people have well-established routines. Other activities, such as bathing and ambulating, should not interfere with the defecation time.

NUTRITION AND FLUIDS The diet a client needs for regular, normal elimination varies depending on the kind of feces the client currently has, the frequency of defecation, and the types of foods that the client finds assist with normal defecation.

For constipation, increase the daily fluid intake, and instruct the client to drink hot liquids and fruit juices, especially prune juice. Include fiber in the diet—that is, foods such as raw fruit, bran products, and whole-grain cereals and bread.

For flatulence, limit carbonated beverages, the use of drinking straws, and chewing gum—all of which increase the ingestion of air. Gas-forming foods, such as cabbage, beans, onions, and cauliflower, should be avoided as well.

EXERCISE Regular exercise helps clients to develop a regular defecation pattern. A client with weak abdominal and pelvic muscles, which impede normal defecation, may be able to strengthen them with the following isometric exercises:

- In a supine position, the client tightens the abdominal muscles as though pulling them inward, holding them for about 10 seconds and then relaxing them. This should be repeated 5–10 times each session and four times a day, depending on the client's health.
- Again in a supine position, the client can contract the thigh muscles and hold them contracted for about 10 seconds, repeating the exercise 5–10 times each session and four times a day. This helps the client confined to bed gain strength in the thigh muscles, thereby making it easier to use a bedpan.

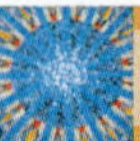

CLIENT TEACHING Fecal Elimination

FACILITATING TOILETING

To facilitate successful client toileting, nurses should do the following:

- Ensure safe and easy access to the toilet. Make sure lighting is appropriate, scatter rugs are removed or securely fastened, and so on.
- Facilitate instruction as needed about transfer techniques.
- Suggest ways that garments can be adjusted to make disrobing easier for toileting (e.g., Velcro closing on clothing).

MONITORING BOWEL ELIMINATION PATTERN

- Nurses should instruct the client, if appropriate, to keep a record of time and frequency of stool passage, any associated pain, and color and consistency of the stool.

DIETARY ALTERATIONS

- Nurses should provide clients with information about required food and fluid alterations to promote defecation or manage diarrhea.

MEDICATIONS

- Medications should be discussed with the client at each health care interaction. Discussions should address problems associated with overuse of laxatives, if appropriate, and the use of alternatives to laxatives, suppositories, and enemas. Nurses also should discuss the addition of a fiber supplement if the client is taking a constipating medication.
- Discuss the addition of a fiber supplement if the client is taking a constipating medication.

MEASURES SPECIFIC TO ELIMINATION PROBLEM

- Nurses should provide instructions associated with specific elimination problems and treatment, including
  a. constipation,
  b. diarrhea, and
  c. ostomy care.

COMMUNITY AGENCIES AND OTHER SOURCES OF HELP

A number of agencies and resources are available to clients who need assistance. Nurses should be informed about what is available in their community and provide the following:

- Appropriate referrals to home care or community care for assistance with resources such as installation of grab bars and raised toilet seats, structural alterations for wheelchair access, homemaker or home health aide services to assist with activities of daily living, and enterostomal therapy nurse for assistance with stoma care and selection of ostomy appliances.
- Information about companies from which durable medical equipment (e.g., raised toilet seats, commodes, bedpans, and urinals) can be purchased, rented, or obtained free of charge and supplies (e.g., incontinence pads or ostomy irrigating supplies and appliances) can be obtained.
- Additional sources of information and help, such as ostomy self-help and support groups or clubs.

POSITIONING Although the squatting position best facilitates defecation, the best position on a toilet seat for most people seems to be leaning forward.

For clients who have difficulty sitting down and getting up from the toilet, an elevated toilet seat can be attached to a regular toilet. Clients then do not have to lower themselves as far onto the seat or lift themselves as far off the seat. Elevated toilet seats can be purchased for use in the home.

An enema is a solution introduced into the rectum and large intestine. The action of an enema is to distend the intestine and, sometimes, to irritate the intestinal mucosa, increasing peristalsis and the excretion of feces and flatus.

Digital Removal of a Fecal Impaction

Digital removal involves breaking up the fecal mass with a finger in the rectum and then removing the mass in portions. Because the bowel mucosa can be injured during this procedure, some agencies restrict and specify the personnel who are permitted to conduct digital disimpaction. Rectal stimulation also is contraindicated for some people because it may cause an excessive vagal response, resulting in cardiac arrhythmia. Before disimpaction is performed, an oil retention enema should be given and held for 30 minutes. After a disimpaction, the nurse can use various interventions to remove any remaining feces, such as a cleansing enema or insertion of a suppository.

Because manual removal of an impaction can be painful, the nurse may use, if the agency permits, 1–2 mL of lidocaine (Xylocaine) gel on a gloved finger inserted into the anal canal as far as the nurse can reach. The lidocaine will anesthetize the anal canal and rectum and should be inserted 5 minutes before the disimpaction.

Digital removal of a fecal impaction is performed as follows:

1. If indicated, obtain assistance from a second person who can comfort the client during the procedure.
2. Ask the client to assume a left-side-lying position with the knees flexed and the back toward the nurse.
3. Place a bed pad under the client's buttocks and a bedpan nearby to receive stool.
4. Drape the client for comfort and to avoid unnecessary exposure of the body.
5. Put on a pair of clean gloves, and liberally lubricate the index finger to be inserted.

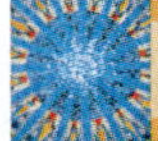

CLIENT TEACHING Healthy Defecation

SOME TEACHING POINTS FOR HEALTHY DEFECATION

- Establish a regular exercise regimen.
- Include high-fiber foods, such as vegetables, fruits, and whole grains, in the diet.
- Maintain fluid intake of 2,000–3,000 mL a day.
- Do not ignore the urge to defecate.
- Allow time to defecate, preferably at the same time each day.
- Avoid over-the-counter medications to treat constipation and diarrhea.

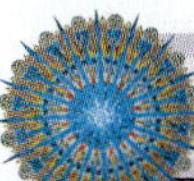

NURSING CARE PLAN Altered Bowel Elimination

ASSESSMENT	DIAGNOSIS	PLANNING
Mrs. Emma Brown is a 78-year-old who has been a widow for 9 months. She lives alone in a low-income housing complex for older adults. Her two children live with their families approximately 150 miles away. She has always enjoyed cooking for her family; however, now that she is alone, she does not cook for herself. As a result, she has developed irregular eating patterns and tends to prepare soup-and-toast meals. She gets little exercise and has had bouts of insomnia since her husband's death. For the past month, Mrs. Brown has been having a problem with constipation. She states that she has a bowel movement about every 3–4 days and that her stools are hard and painful to excrete. Mrs. Brown decides to attend the health fair sponsored by the housing complex and seeks assistance from the county public health nurse. The nurse conducts a physical examination and finds the following: Height: 162 cm (5'4") Weight: 65 kg (143 lb) Temperature: 36.2°C (97.2°F) Pulse: 82 bpm Respirations: 20/min Blood pressure: 128/74 mmHg Active bowel sounds, abdomen slightly distended Diagnostic tests: CBC: Hgb 10.8 Urinalysis negative	Constipation related to low-fiber diet and inactivity (as evidenced by infrequent, hard stools; painful defecation; abdominal distention)	■ Mrs. Brown will make appropriate choices for her menu to increase fiber in her diet based on her food likes and dislikes. ■ Mrs. Brown will increase her activity level as tolerated with any coexisting medical conditions. ■ Mrs. Brown will increase her fluid intake after consulting with her primary provider to determine any contraindications. ■ Mrs. Brown will choose healthy fluids to consume in order to increase intake (i.e., low-sugar fluids if diabetic, low-sodium fluids if fluid retention is an issue). ■ Mrs. Brown will list all medications she is currently taking, including over-the-counter medications and supplements, and recognize their contribution to constipation.

IMPLEMENTATION

- Identify factors (e.g., medications, diet) that may cause or contribute to constipation.
- Encourage increased fluid intake unless contraindicated.
- Evaluate medication profile for side effects, contraindications.
- Teach Mrs. Brown how to keep a food diary.
- Instruct Mrs. Brown on a high-fiber diet as appropriate.
- Instruct Mrs. Brown on the relationship of diet, exercise, and fluid intake to constipation and impaction.

EVALUATION

Outcome not met. Mrs. Brown has kept a food diary and is able to identify the need for more fluid and fiber but has not consistently included fiber in her diet. She has started a walking program with a neighbor, but is able to walk for only 10 minutes at a time twice a week. She states that her last bowel movement was 3 days ago.

CRITICAL THINKING

1. You learn that Mrs. Browns stools have been liquid, have been in very small amounts, and have been occurring at infrequent intervals, generally when she feels the urge to defecate. What additional data is important to obtain from her? What are you screening for?
2. What nursing intervention is most appropriate before making suggestions to correct or prevent the problem Mrs. Brown is experiencing?
3. What suggestions can you give Mrs. Brown about maintaining a regular bowel pattern?
4. Explain why cathartics and laxatives generally are contraindicated for people in Mrs. Browns situation.
5. How would you amend Mrs. Browns plan of care based on her lack of achieving optimal outcomes?

6. Gently insert the index finger into the rectum, and move the finger along the length of the rectum.
7. Loosen and dislodge stool by gently massaging around it. Break up stool by working the finger into the hardened mass, taking care to avoid injury to the mucosa of the rectum.
8. Carefully work stool downward to the end of the rectum and remove it in small pieces. Continue to remove as much fecal material as possible. Periodically assess the client for signs of fatigue, such as facial pallor, diaphoresis, or change in pulse rate. Manual stimulation should be minimal.
9. Following disimpaction, assist the client to clean the anal area and buttocks. Then, assist the client onto a bedpan or commode for a short time, because digital stimulation of the rectum often induces the urge to defecate.

Bowel Training Programs

For clients who have chronic constipation, frequent impactions, or fecal incontinence, bowel training programs may be helpful. The program is based on factors within the client's control and is designed to help the client establish normal defecation. Such matters as food and fluid intake, exercise, and defecation habits are all considered. Before beginning such a program, clients must understand it and want to be involved. The major phases of the program are as follows:

- Determine the client's usual bowel habits and factors that help and hinder normal defecation.
- Design a plan with the client that includes the following:
  a. Fluid intake of approximately 2,500–3,000 mL per day
  b. Increase in fiber in the diet
  c. Intake of hot drinks, especially just before the usual defecation time
  d. Increase in exercise
- Maintain the following daily routine for 2–3 weeks:
  a. To stimulate peristalsis, administer a cathartic suppository (e.g., Dulcolax) 30 minutes before the client's defecation time to stimulate peristalsis.
  b. When the client experiences the urge to defecate, assist the client to the toilet or commode or onto a bedpan. Note the length of time between the insertion of the suppository and the urge to defecate.
  c. Provide the client with privacy for defecation and a time limit (30–40 minutes usually is sufficient).
  d. Teach the client to lean forward at the hips, to apply pressure on the abdomen with the hands, and to bear down for defecation. These measures increase pressure on the colon. Straining should be avoided because it can cause hemorrhoids.
- Provide positive feedback when the client successfully defecates. Refrain from negative feedback if the client fails to defecate.
- Offer encouragement to the client, and convey that patience often is required. Many clients require weeks or months of training to achieve success.

PRACTICE ALERT

Provide room odor control with deodorizer tablets, sprays, or other devices. Controlling odor is important to preserve the client's self-esteem.

Fecal Incontinence Pouch

To collect and contain large volumes of liquid feces, the nurse may place a fecal incontinence collector pouch around the anal area. The purpose of the pouch is to prevent progressive perianal skin irritation and breakdown as well as frequent linen changes necessitated by incontinence. In many agencies, the pouch is replacing the more traditional approach of inserting a large Foley catheter into the client's rectum and inflating the balloon to keep it in place—a practice that may damage the rectal sphincter and rectal mucosa. A rectal catheter also increases peristalsis and incontinence by stimulating sensory nerve fibers in the rectum.

A fecal collector is secured around the anal opening and may or may not be attached to drainage. Pouches are best applied before the perianal skin becomes excoriated. If perianal skin excoriation is present, the nurse either (a) applies a dimethicone-based moisture-barrier cream or alcohol-free barrier film to the skin to protect it from feces until it heals and then applies the pouch or (b) applies a skin barrier or hydrocolloid barrier underneath the pouch to achieve the best possible seal.

Nursing responsibilities for clients with a rectal pouch include (a) regular assessment and documentation of the perianal skin status, (b) changing the bag every 72 hours or sooner if leakage occurs, (c) maintaining the drainage system, and (d) providing explanations and support to the client and support people.

Some clients (e.g., those who are quadriplegic or paraplegic, or after trauma or stroke) may be treated for fecal incontinence by surgical repair of a damaged sphincter or an artificial bowel sphincter. The artificial sphincter consists of three parts: a cuff around the anal canal, a pressure-regulating balloon, and a pump that inflates the cuff. The cuff is inflated to close the sphincter, maintaining continence. To have a bowel movement, the client deflates the cuff. The cuff automatically reinflates in 10 minutes. Management of this device usually is specific to the model being used; contact the manufacturing company for details. Administering enemas and rectal medications may be harmful with this device in place.

Evaluation

The goals established during the planning phase are evaluated according to specific desired outcomes that are also established during that phase. Examples of these were shown previously in Box 9–12. Other examples are shown in the Nursing Care Plan feature for this exemplar.

If the desired outcomes are not achieved, the nurse should explore the reasons. The nurse might consider some or all of the following questions:

- Were the client's fluid intake and diet appropriate?
- Was the client's activity level appropriate?
- Are prescribed medications or other factors affecting the gastrointestinal function?
- Do the client and family understand the provided instructions well enough to comply with the required therapy?
- Were sufficient physical support and emotional support provided?

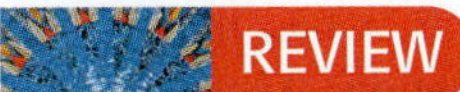

REVIEW Bowel: Incontinence, Constipation, and Impaction

RELATE: LINK THE CONCEPTS

Linking the exemplar of Bowel: Incontinence, Constipation, and Impaction with the concept of Mobility:

1. What impact does the concept of mobility have on elimination?
2. How can the nurse promote normal bowel elimination in the client with altered mobility?

Linking the exemplar of Bowel: Incontinence, Constipation, and Impaction with the concept of Metabolism:

3. When caring for a client with liver disease, what special precautions must the nurse implement related to bowel elimination?
4. When caring for a client diagnosed with hypothyroidism, what nursing implementations can be initiated to reduce the impact of this disorder on bowel elimination?

READY: GO TO COMPANION SKILLS MANUAL

- Removing a fecal impaction
- Developing a regular bowel routine
- Inserting a rectal tube
- Obtaining and testing stool specimen
- Collecting infant stool specimen
- Collecting stool for bacterial culture
- Teaching parents to test for pinworms
- Collecting stool for ova and parasites
- Implementing the Zassi Bowel Management System™
- Administering an enema
- Administering a retention enema
- Applying a fecal ostomy pouch

REFER: GO TO MYNURSINGKIT

REFLECT: CASE STUDY

Mr. Justin Gardner is a 26-year-old man who fractured his third thoracic vertebrae when he fell while rock climbing. The client is incontinent of feces secondary to sensory loss and the inability to feel the need to defecate.

1. Is there anything that can be implemented to return bowel continence to this client? Explain your answer.
2. What skin care precautions will the nurse implement to maintain skin integrity?
3. What nursing diagnosis would be appropriate for this client?
4. What client teaching will this client require, related to bowel continence, before discharge if he is to provide effective home care for himself?

9.4 URINARY CALCULI

KEY TERMS

Calcium oxalate, *466*
Calcium phosphate, *466*
Extracorporeal shock wave lithotripsy (ESWL), *469*
Hydronephrosis, *467*
Lithiasis, *466*
Lithotripsy, *469*
Nephrolithiasis, *466*
Nephrolithotomy, *470*
Nucleation, *466*
Pyelolithotomy, *470*
Renal colic, *467*
Staghorn stones, *466*
Struvite stones, *466*
Ureterolithotomy, *470*
Uric acid stones, *466*
Urinary calculi, *466*
Urolithiasis, *466*

BASIS FOR SELECTION OF EXEMPLAR

Most common condition

LEARNING OUTCOMES

After reading about this exemplar, you will be able to:

1. Describe the pathophysiology, etiology, clinical manifestations, and direct and indirect causes of urinary calculi.
2. Identify risk factors associated with urinary calculi.
3. Illustrate the nursing process in providing culturally competent care across the life span for individuals with urinary calculi.
4. Formulate priority nursing diagnoses appropriate for an individual with urinary calculi.
5. Create a plan of care for individuals with urinary calculi and their family members.
6. Assess expected outcomes for an individual with urinary calculi.
7. Discuss therapies used in the collaborative care of an individual with urinary calculi.
8. Employ evidence-based caring interventions for an individual with urinary calculi.

OVERVIEW

Urinary calculi, often referred to as kidney stones, is a very painful disorder caused by the development of one small crystal or many small crystals. These calculi can lodge anywhere in the urinary tract, risking obstruction and resulting in kidney damage. Clients who experience the pain of renal calculi, caused by the movement of a multifaceted crystal that irritates the lining of the ureter as it scrapes against it, often report it as being the most painful experience of their lives. As a result, pain management is an important consideration when caring for clients with this disorder.

Urinary calculi are the most common cause of upper urinary tract obstruction (Porth, 2005). The term **lithiasis** means "stone formation." When the stones form in the kidney, the condition is known as **nephrolithiasis**; when they form elsewhere in the urinary tract (for example, the bladder), the condition is called **urolithiasis**. Stones may form and obstruct the urinary tract at any point (Figure 9–14 ■). In the United States and other industrialized countries, renal (or kidney) stones are most common.

PATHOPHYSIOLOGY AND ETIOLOGY

Normally, a balance exists in the kidneys between the need to conserve water and the need to eliminate poorly soluble materials such as calcium salts. This balance is affected by factors such as diet, environmental temperature, and activity. Protective inorganic and organic substances in the urine, such as pyrophosphate, citrate, and glycoproteins, normally inhibit stone formation.

Three factors contribute to urolithiasis: supersaturation, **nucleation** (formation of a crystal from a liquid), and lack of inhibitory substances in the urine. When the concentration of an insoluble salt in the urine is very high (i.e., when the urine is supersaturated), crystals may form (nucleation). Usually, these crystals disperse and are eliminated because the bonds holding them together are weak. However, a nucleus of crystals may develop stable bonds to form a stone. More often, crystals form around an organic matrix, or mucoprotein nucleus, to become a stone. The stimulus required to initiate crystallization in supersaturated urine may be minimal. Things as simple as ingesting a meal high in insoluble salt or decreased fluid intake as that which occurs during sleep can allow the concentration to increase to the point where precipitation occurs and stones form and grow. When fluid intake is adequate, no stone growth occurs. The acidity or alkalinity of the urine and the presence or absence of calculus-inhibiting compounds also affects lithiasis.

Most kidney stones (75–80%) are calcium stones, composed of **calcium oxalate** and/or **calcium phosphate**. These stones are generally associated with high concentrations of calcium in the blood or urine. **Uric acid stones** develop when the urine concentration of uric acid is high. They are more common in men and may be associated with gout. Genetic factors contribute to the development of uric acid stones and calcium stones. **Struvite stones** are associated with UTI caused by urease-producing bacteria such as *Proteus.* These stones can grow to become very large, filling the renal pelvis and calyces. They are often called **staghorn stones** because of their shape. Cystine stones, which are rare, are associated with a genetic defect. The types of renal calculi, contributing factors, and recommended dietary modifications are listed in Table 9–11.

Etiology

Most urinary stones form in the renal pelvis and are composed primarily of calcium salts. Urolithiasis affects up to 720,000 people annually in the United States (Tierney,

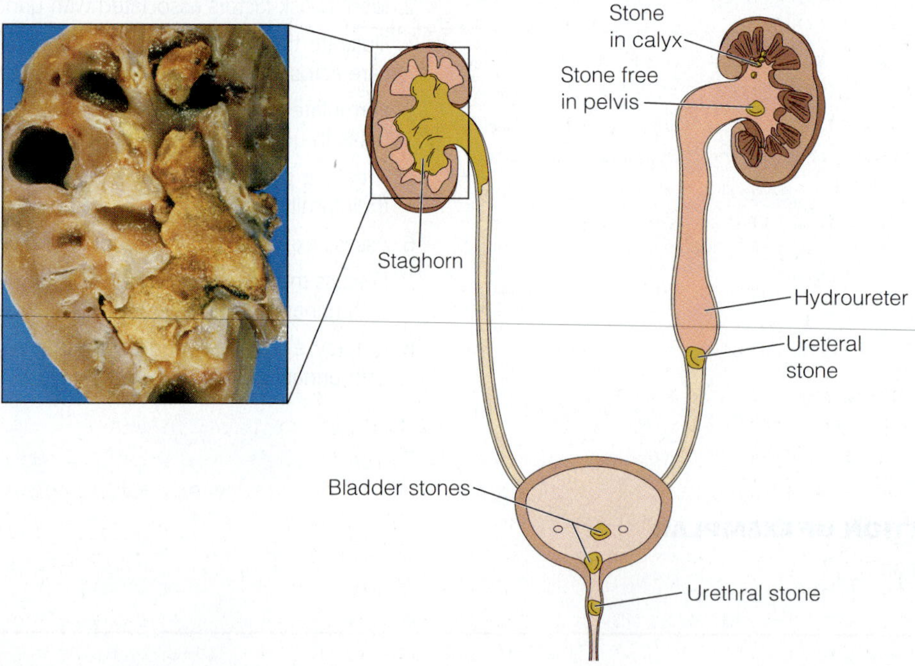

Figure 9–14 ■ Development and location of calculi in the urinary tract.

Source: Dr. E. Walker/Photo Researchers, Inc.

TABLE 9–11 **Risk Factors and Interventions for Renal Calculi**

STONE TYPE AND INCIDENCE	RISK FACTORS	MANAGEMENT
Calcium phosphate and/or oxalate 75–80%	Hypercalciuria and hypercalcemia: Hyperparathyroidism, immobility, bone disease, vitamin D intoxication, multiple myeloma, renal tubular acidosis, prolonged steroid intake, alkaline urine, dehydration, inflammatory bowel disease	Pharmacology: Thiazide, diuretics, phosphates, calcium-binding agents. Dietary: Limit foods high in calcium and oxalate, increase foods that acidify urine Other: Increase hydration, exercise
Struvite 15–20%	UTIs, especially *Proteus* infections	Pharmacology: Antibiotic therapy for UTI Other: Surgical intervention or lithotripsy to remove stone
Uric acid 5–10%	Gout, increased purine intake, acid urine	Pharmacology: Potassium citrate, allopurinol Dietary: Low purine diet Other: Increase hydration
Cystine (uncommon)	Genetic defect, acid urine	Pharmacology: Penicillamine, sodium bicarbonate Dietary: Sodium restriction Other: Increase hydration

McPhee, & Papadakis, 2005). In the United States, the incidence varies by region, with the highest frequency in southern and midwestern states. Males are affected 2 or 3 times more often than females (Porth, 2005). Calculi are more common among whites than blacks. Most people affected are in young or middle adulthood.

Risk Factors

Although the majority of stones are idiopathic (having no demonstrable cause), a number of risk factors have been identified. The greatest risk factor for stone formation is a prior personal or family history of urinary calculi. A genetic predisposition toward the accumulation of certain mineral substances in the urine or a congenital lack of protective factors may explain the familial link. Other identified risk factors include dehydration with resultant increased urine concentration; immobility; and excess dietary intake of calcium, oxalate, or proteins. Gout, hyperparathyroidism, and urinary stasis or repeated infections also contribute to calculus formation. Loss of calcium from the bones (e.g., due to immobility) and dehydration are major risk factors for urinary stones.

CLINICAL MANIFESTATIONS

The symptoms caused by urinary calculi vary with their size and location. (See the following Clinical Manifestations and Therapies box.) Manifestations develop from obstructed urine flow with resulting distention and from tissue trauma caused by passage of the rough-edged crystalline stone.

Calculi affecting the kidney calyces and pelvis may cause few symptoms. If the stone has gradually or partially obstructed urinary flow, dull, aching flank pain may be present, but renal calculi often are silent, without symptoms. Bladder calculi may cause few symptoms other than dull suprapubic pain with exercise or after voiding.

Renal colic, acute, severe flank pain on the affected side, develops when a stone obstructs the ureter, causing ureteral spasm. The pain of renal colic may radiate to the suprapubic region, groin, and external genitals (the scrotum or labia). The severity of the pain often causes a sympathetic response with associated nausea; vomiting; pallor; and cool, clammy skin.

Manifestations of UTI, including chills and fever, frequency, urgency, and dysuria, may accompany urinary calculi at any level. Calculi may cause trauma to the urinary tract, resulting in gross or microscopic hematuria. Gross hematuria is often the only sign of bladder stones.

Complications

Urinary stones may obstruct urine flow at any point of the urinary tract, leading to complications such as hydronephrosis and urinary stasis with subsequent infection. Occurrence of these complications requires alteration to the nursing plan of care.

OBSTRUCTION Stones can obstruct the urinary tract at any point, from the calyces of the kidney to the distal urethra, impeding the outflow of urine. If the obstruction develops slowly, there may be few or no symptoms, whereas sudden obstruction (e.g., blockage of a ureter by a passing stone) may cause severe manifestations. Urinary tract obstruction can ultimately lead to renal failure. The degree of obstruction, its location, and the duration of impaired urine flow determine the effect on renal function.

HYDRONEPHROSIS The kidneys continue to produce urine, causing increased pressure and distention of the urinary tract behind the obstruction. **Hydronephrosis** (accumulation of urine in the renal pelvis as a result of obstructed outflow) and hydroureter (distention of the ureter with urine) are possible results. If the pressure is not relieved, the collecting tubules, proximal tubules, and glomeruli of the kidney are damaged, causing a gradual loss of renal function.

Acute hydronephrosis typically causes colicky pain on the affected side. The pain may radiate into the groin. Chronic

CLINICAL MANIFESTATIONS AND THERAPIES Urinary Calculi

ETIOLOGY	CLINICAL MANIFESTATIONS	CLINICAL THERAPIES
Acute hydronephrosis caused by the development of a sudden obstruction of urine flow	■ Acute, colicky pain; may radiate into groin ■ Hematuria, pyuria ■ Fever ■ Nausea, vomiting, abdominal pain	■ Lithotripsy or surgical removal of the stone ■ IV therapy ■ Thiazide diuretics if stone is caused by excess calcium ■ Dietary modification ■ Monitoring of BUN and creatinine to determine extent of kidney damage ■ Client teaching to reduce risk factors and prevent reoccurrence
Chronic hydronephrosis caused by gradual development of obstruction of urine flow	■ May be asymptomatic until complete obstruction develops ■ Dull, aching flank pain ■ Hematuria, pyuria ■ Fever ■ Palpable flank mass	■ Lithotripsy or surgical removal of the stone ■ Evaluation of kidney function ■ Dietary modification ■ IV therapy ■ Client teaching to reduce risk of reoccurrence
Kidney stones	■ Often asymptomatic ■ Dull, aching flank pain ■ Microscopic hematuria ■ Manifestations of UTI	■ Hydration ■ Thiazide diuretics ■ Monitoring of hemoglobin and hematocrit ■ Limits on foods high in calcium ■ Calcium binding agents
Ureteral stones	■ Renal colic ■ Acute, severe flank pain on affected side ■ Likelihood of pain radiating to suprapubic region, groin, and external genitals ■ Nausea; vomiting; pallor; and cool, clammy skin	■ Hydration ■ Monitoring of hemoglobin and hematocrit ■ Limits on foods high in calcium ■ Calcium binding agents ■ Analgesics for pain (morphine sulfate); NSAIDs (indomethacin) ■ Thiazide diuretics ■ IV fluids
Bladder stones	■ May be asymptomatic ■ Dull suprapubic pain, possibly associated with exercise or voiding ■ Gross or microscopic hematuria ■ Manifestations of UTI	If asymptomatic, often no treatment other than increasing hydration and monitoring for hematuria

hydronephrosis develops slowly and may have few manifestations other than dull, aching back or flank pain. When hydronephrosis is significant, a palpable mass may be felt in the flank region. Hematuria and signs of UTI such as pyuria, fever, and discomfort may occur. Gastrointestinal symptoms such as nausea, vomiting, and abdominal pain may accompany hydronephrosis.

INFECTION The urinary stasis associated with partial or complete obstruction increases the risk of UTI. Upper or lower urinary tract infections may develop.

COLLABORATION

Collaborative care for clients diagnosed with urinary calculi focuses on relieving acute symptoms, destroying or removing stones, and preventing further stone formation. Asymptomatic stones (those not causing pain, infection, or obstruction) are treated conservatively.

Diagnostic Testing

The following laboratory and diagnostic tests may be ordered when urinary calculi are suspected:

- Urinalysis to assess for hematuria and the possible presence of WBCs and crystal fragments. Urine pH is helpful in identifying the type of stone.
- Chemical analysis of any stones passed in the urine determines the type of stone and suggests measures to prevent further stone formation. Retrieving stones or teaching the client to do so is a nursing responsibility. All urine is strained and may be saved. Any visible stones or sediment is sent for analysis.
- Urine calcium, uric acid, and oxalate levels measure the amount of these substances excreted over a 24-hour period and may be assessed to help identify possible causes of lithiasis. Elevated calcium levels occur in hyperparathyroidism, Cushing's syndrome, and osteoporosis, all of which may contribute to lithiasis. Uric acid levels may be elevated in clients with gout and those at risk for forming uric acid calculi. Urine

oxalate excretion may help to differentiate calcium oxalate from calcium phosphate stones.

- Serum calcium, phosphorus, and uric acid levels may be obtained to help identify factors contributing to calculus formation.
- KUB (kidneys, ureters, and bladder) may be used to identify calculi as opacities in the kidneys, ureters, and bladder.
- Renal ultrasonography may be used to detect stones and evaluate the kidneys for possible hydronephrosis.
- Computed tomography (CT) scan of the kidney, with or without contrast medium, may be used to provide a computer-generated photograph that shows calculi, ureteral obstruction, and other renal disorders.
- Intravenous pyelogram (IVP) may be done to visualize the kidneys, ureters, and bladder after injection of a contrast medium. This procedure is of particular importance when KUB, renal ultrasonography, and CT scan fail to demonstrate clear evidence of urinary calculi.
- Cystoscopy is used to visualize and possibly remove calculi from the urinary bladder and distal ureters.

Pharmacologic Therapy

An acute episode of renal colic is treated with analgesia and hydration. A narcotic analgesic such as morphine sulfate is given, often intravenously, to relieve pain and reduce ureteral spasm. Indomethacin, a nonsteroidal anti-inflammatory drug (NSAID), given as a suppository, may reduce the amount of narcotic analgesia required for acute renal colic. Oral or intravenous fluids reduce the risk of further stone formation and promote urine output.

After analysis of the calculus, various medications may be ordered to inhibit or prevent further lithiasis. A thiazide diuretic, frequently prescribed for calcium calculi, acts to reduce urinary calcium excretion and is very effective in preventing further stones. Potassium citrate alkalinizes urine (raises the pH), and is often prescribed to prevent stones that tend to form in acidic urine (uric acid, cystine, and some forms of calcium stones). See Table 9–11 for other preparations related to types of stones. Nursing responsibilities focus on teaching the client about the prescribed medication, its importance in preventing further stone formation, and potential adverse effects.

Surgery

Treatment of existing calculi depends on the location of the stone, extent of obstruction, renal function, presence or absence of UTI, and client's general state of health. In general, the stone is removed if it is causing severe obstruction, infection, unrelieved pain, or serious bleeding (Kasper et al., 2005).

Lithotripsy, using sound or shock waves to crush a stone, is the preferred treatment for urinary calculi. Several techniques may be used. **Extracorporeal shock wave lithotripsy (ESWL)** is a noninvasive technique for fragmenting kidney stones by using shock waves generated outside the body. Acoustic shock waves are aimed under fluoroscopic guidance at the stone (Figure 9–15 ■). These shock waves travel through soft tissue without causing damage, but shatter the stone as its greater density stops their progress. Repeated shock waves pulverize the stone into fragments small enough to be eliminated in the urine.

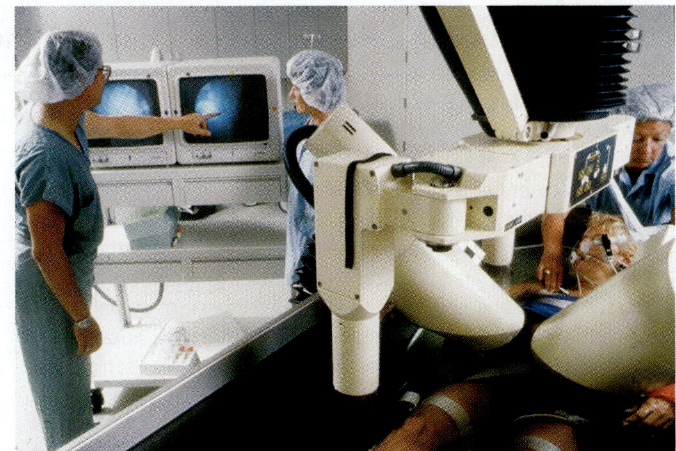

Figure 9–15 ■ Extracorporeal shock wave lithotripsy. Acoustic shock waves generated by the shock wave generator travel through soft tissue to shatter the urinary stone into fragments, which are then eliminated in the urine.

The procedure may require 30 minutes to 2 hours to complete. Generally, intravenous sedation is adequate to maintain comfort during the procedure (Way & Doherty, 2003). See Box 9–15 for nursing care of the client undergoing a lithotripsy procedure.

Lithotripsy also may be performed using a percutaneous ultrasonic or laser technique. Percutaneous ultrasonic lithotripsy uses a nephroscope inserted into the kidney pelvis through a small flank incision (Figure 9–16 ■). The stone is fragmented using a small ultrasonic transducer, and the fragments are removed

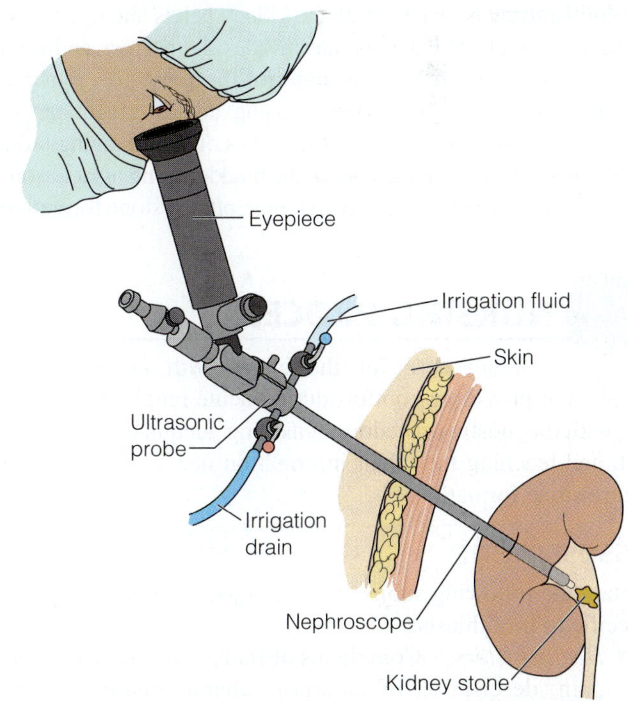

Figure 9–16 ■ Percutaneous ultrasonic lithotripsy. A nephroscope is inserted into the renal pelvis, and ultrasonic waves are used to fragment the stone. Then the fragments are removed through the nephroscope.

Box 9–15 Nursing Care of the Client Having Lithotripsy

PREOPERATIVE CARE

Verify informed consent was signed. Assess knowledge and understanding of the procedure, providing information as needed. Anxiety is reduced and recovery is enhanced and hastened when the client is fully prepared for surgery. Follow directions from the radiology department, physician, or anesthetist for withholding food and fluids and for bowel preparation prior to surgery. Conscious sedation, general anesthesia, or spinal anesthesia may be required depending on the procedure. Fecal material in the bowel may impede fluoroscopic visualization of the kidney and stone.

POSTOPERATIVE CARE

- In the initial period, monitor vital signs frequently. The kidney is highly vascular; therefore, hemorrhage and resulting shock are potential complications of lithotripsy. Bleeding may be internal or retroperitoneal and difficult to detect. Monitor amount, color, and clarity of urine output. Urine is often bright red initially, but bleeding should diminish within 48–72 hours. Cloudy urine may indicate the presence of an infection.
- Maintain placement and patency of urinary catheters. Anchor ureteral catheters or nephrostomy tubes securely. Irrigate gently if ordered. A kinked or plugged catheter may result in hydroureter, hydronephrosis, and kidney damage. Decreased urinary output and flank pain are possible symptoms of obstructed urine flow. Excessive force in irrigation may cause trauma and bleeding.
- Prepare for discharge by teaching care of the indwelling catheter, urine collection device, and incision site (if present). Teach signs and symptoms to report: urine leakage from incision for more than 4 days, symptoms of infection, pain, bright hematuria. Many clients are discharged with dressings and catheters in place. The client and family need necessary information to provide self-care.
- Teach measures to reduce the risk of further lithiasis. Many clients have repeated episodes of lithiasis and renal colic. Prevention of stone formation is important to preserve renal function.

through the nephroscope. Laser lithotripsy is an alternative to ultrasonic lithotripsy. Laser beams are used to disintegrate the stone without damaging soft tissue. A nephroscope or a ureteroscope (passed up the ureter from the bladder during cystoscopy) is used to guide the laser probe into direct contact with the stone. A double J stent may be inserted into the affected ureter to maintain its patency following ESWL or other lithotripsy procedures.

On rare occasions, surgical intervention is necessary to remove a calculus in the renal pelvis or ureter. **Ureterolithotomy** is an incision in the affected ureter to remove a calculus. **Pyelolithotomy** is incision into the kidney pelvis and removal of a stone. A staghorn calculus that invades the calyces and renal parenchyma may require a **nephrolithotomy** for removal. Bladder stones may be removed using an instrument passed through a cystoscope to crush the stones. The remaining stone fragments are then irrigated out of the bladder using an acid solution to counteract the alkalinity that precipitated stone formation.

NURSING PROCESS

Nursing care for the client with urolithiasis is directed at providing comfort during acute renal colic, assisting with diagnostic procedures, ensuring adequate urinary output, and teaching the client information necessary to prevent future stone formation.

Assessment

Obtain the following subjective and objective assessment data specific to urolithiasis:

- *Health history.* Complaints of flank, back, or abdominal pain; description of radiation, characteristics, timing, aggravating or relieving factors; other symptoms such as nausea and vomiting; possible contributing factors such as dehydration; previous or family history of kidney stones; current or previous treatment measures
- *Physical examination.* General appearance, including position, vital signs, skin color, temperature, moisture, turgor; abdominal, flank, or costovertebral tenderness; amount, color, and characteristics of urine (presence of hematuria, bacteria, pyuria, pH).

Assessment guidelines for percussion and palpation of the kidneys are demonstrated in the following Assessment feature. Note that the kidneys of an older client are more difficult to palpate abdominally because the mass of the adrenal cortex decreases with age. The nurse should omit blunt percussion in a frail older person. Instead, palpation of the costovertebral angles and flanks can be used to reveal any pain or tenderness.

Diagnosis

Possible nursing diagnoses for the client with urinary calculi may include the following:

- Acute Pain
- Impaired Urinary Elimination
- Deficient Knowledge
- Anxiety
- Risk for Imbalanced Nutrition
- Risk for Infection.

Plan

Goals appropriate for the client with urinary calculi must be individualized to meet each client's specific needs but may include:

- Requesting analgesics as needed at onset of pain and reporting effective pain relief within 20 minutes of parenteral analgesic administration.
- Maintaining urine output of 2500 mL in each 24-hour period without signs of infection or obstruction.
- Verbalizing understanding of disease process to include dietary changes that may reduce the risk of reoccurrence of calculi formation.
- Demonstrating reduced anxiety by nonverbal gestures and return of vital signs to baseline.

Kidney Assessment

Techniques and Normal Findings | **Abnormal Findings Special Considerations**

General Survey

A quick survey of the client enables the nurse to identify any immediate problem as well as the client's ability to participate in the assessment.

1. Instruct the client.

- Explain that you will be looking, listening, touching, and tapping on parts of the abdomen. Tell the client you will explain each procedure as it occurs. Tell the client to report any discomfort and that you will stop the examination if the procedure is uncomfortable.

2. Position the client.

- Begin the examination with the client in a supine position with the abdomen exposed from the nipple line to the pubis (see Figure 9–17 ■).

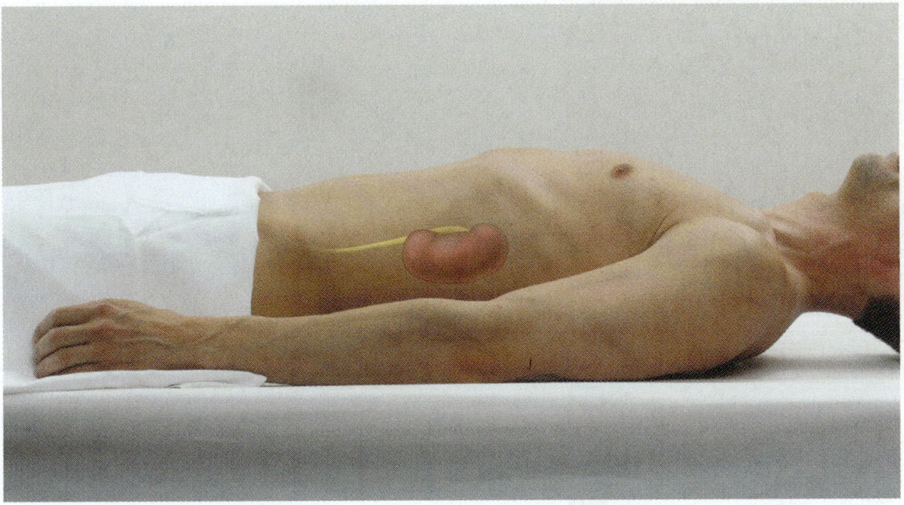

Figure 9–17 ■ Position the client.

3. Assess the general appearance.

- Assess general appearance and inspect the client's skin for color, hydration status, scales, masses, indentations, or scars.
- The client should not show signs of acute distress and should be mentally alert and oriented.

Abnormal findings:

- Clients with kidney disorders frequently look tired and complain of fatigue. If a kidney disorder is suspected, it is important to look for signs of circulatory overload (pulmonary edema) or peripheral edema (puffy face or fingers), or indications of pruritus (scratch marks on the skin).
- Elevated nitrogenous wastes (azotemia) in the blood contribute to mental confusion.

4. Inspect the abdomen for color, contour, symmetry, and distention.

- It may be helpful to stand at the foot of the exam table and inspect the abdomen from there (see Figure 9–18 ■).

Abnormal findings:

- A distended bladder may be visible in the suprapubic area, indicating the need to void and perhaps the inability to do so.

Kidney Assessment

Techniques and Normal Findings | **Abnormal Findings Special Considerations**

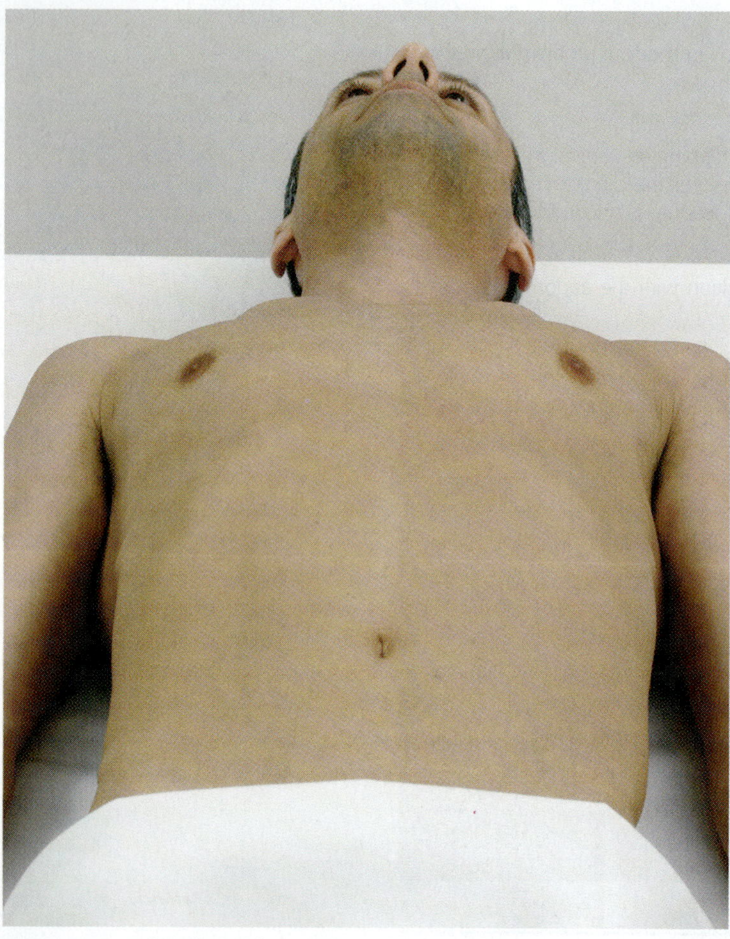

Figure 9–18 ■ Inspecting the abdomen from the foot of the bed.

- Note that visual inspection of the suprapubic area may confirm the presence or absence of a distended bladder.
- Normally, the client's abdomen is not distended, is relatively symmetrical, and is free of bruises, masses, and swellings.

- Many diseases may contribute to abdominal distention. These include renal conditions such as polycystic kidney disease; enlarged kidneys, as seen in acute pyelonephritis; ascites (accumulation of fluid) due to hepatic disease; and displacement of abdominal organs. Pressure from the abdominal contents on the diaphragm may alter the client's breathing pattern.

5. Ausculate the right and left renal arteries to assess circulatory sounds.

- Gently place the bell of the stethoscope over the extended midclavicular line (MCL) on either side of the abdominal aorta, which is located above the level of the umbilicus (see Figure 9–19 ■).

Kidney Assessment

Techniques and Normal Findings | **Abnormal Findings Special Considerations**

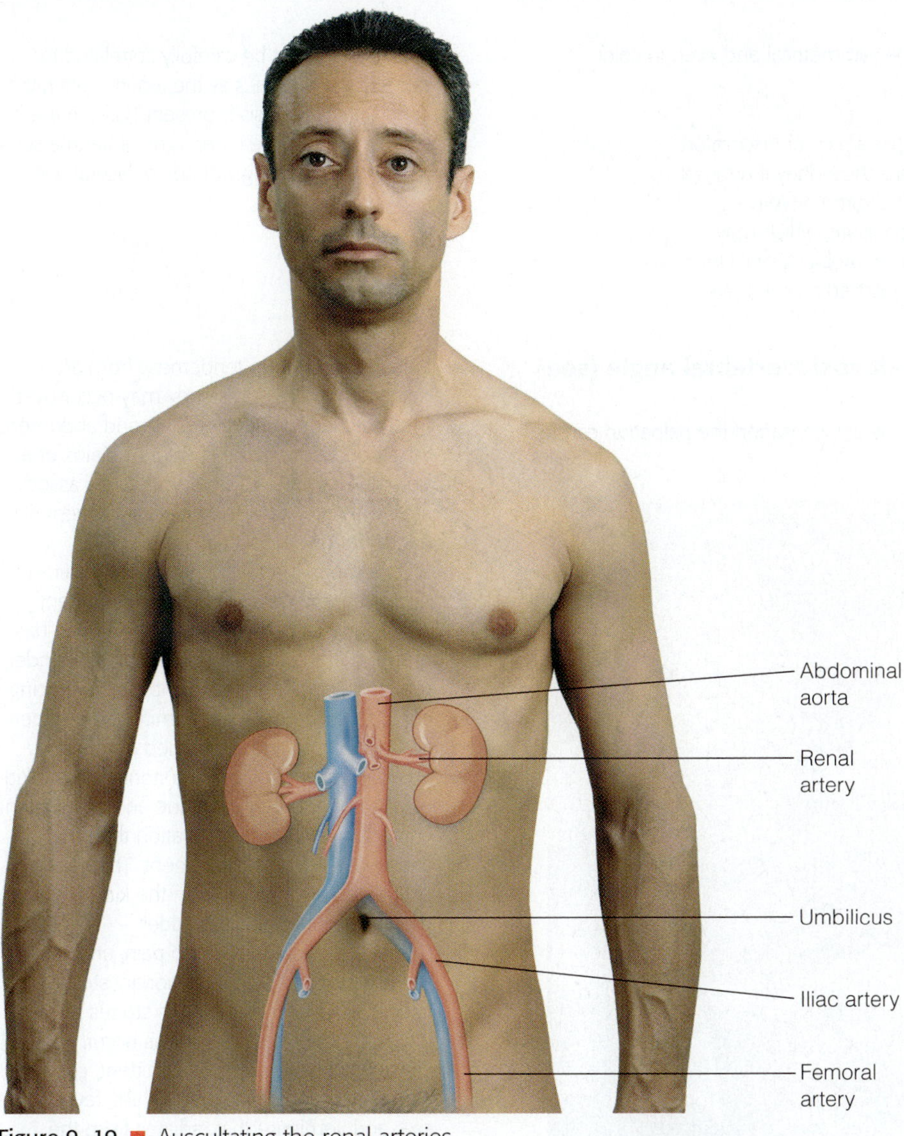

Figure 9–19 ■ Auscultating the renal arteries.

- Be sure to auscultate both the right and left sides, and over the epigastric and umbilical areas.
- In most cases, no sounds are heard; however, an upper abdominal bruit is occasionally heard in young adults and is considered normal. On a thin adult, renal artery pulsation may be auscultated.

THE KIDNEYS AND FLANKS

1. Position the client.

- Place the client in a sitting position facing away from you with the client's back exposed.

2. Inspect the left and right costovertebral angles for color and symmetry.

- The color should be consistent with the rest of the back.

- A protrusion or elevation over a costovertebral angle occurs when the kidney is grossly enlarged or when a mass is present.

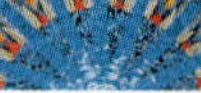

Kidney Assessment

Techniques and Normal Findings | **Abnormal Findings Special Considerations**

3. Inspect the flanks (the side areas between the hips and the ribs) for color and symmetry.

- The costovertebral angles and flanks should be symmetrical and even in color.

PRACTICE ALERT

Do not percuss or palpate the client who reports pain or discomfort in the pelvic region. Do not percuss or palpate the kidney if a tumor of the kidney is suspected, such as a neuroblastoma or Wilms' tumor. Palpation increases intra-abdominal pressure, which may contribute to intraperitoneal spreading of this neuroblastoma. Deep palpation should be performed only by experienced practitioners.

- This finding must be carefully correlated to other diagnostic cues as the assessment proceeds. If ecchymosis is present (Grey Turner's sign), there may be other signs of trauma such as blunt, penetrating wounds or lacerations.

4. Gently palpate the area over the left costovertebral angle (see Figure 9–20 ■).

- Watch the reaction and ask the client to describe any sensation the palpation causes. Normally, the client expresses no discomfort.

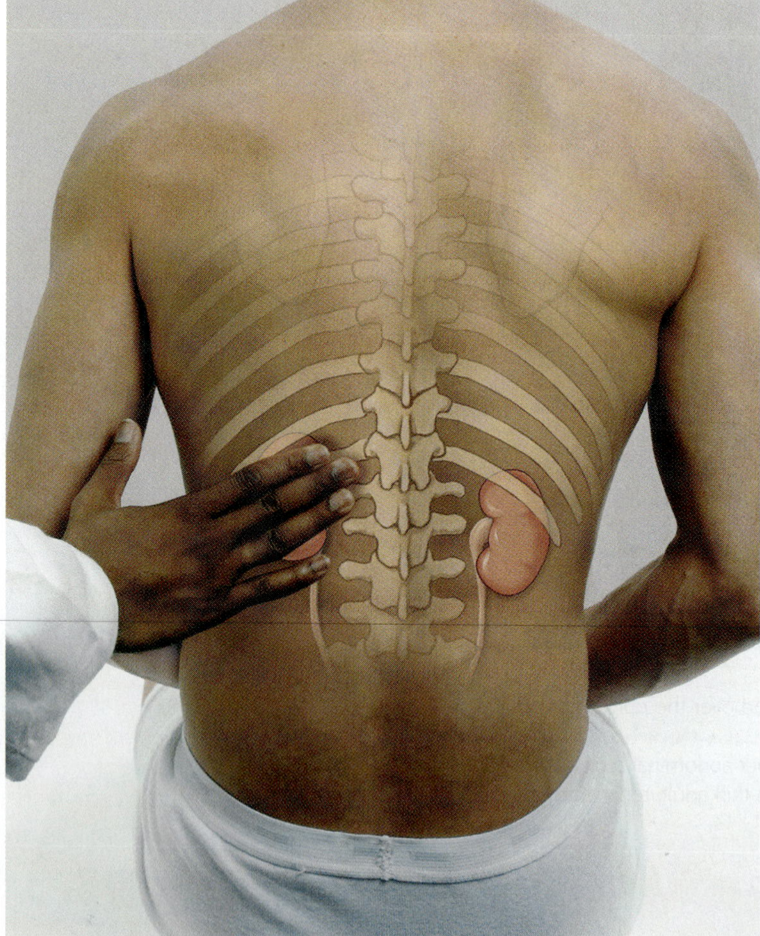

Figure 9–20 ■ Palpating the costovertebral angle.

- Pain, discomfort, or tenderness from an enlarged or diseased kidney may occur over the costovertebral angle, flank, and abdomen. When questioned, the client complains of a dull, steady ache. This type of pain is associated with polycystic formation, pyelonephritis, and other disorders that cause kidney enlargement. In the client with polycystic kidney disease, a sharp, sudden, intermittent pain may mean that a cyst in the kidney has ruptured. If the costovertebral angle is tender, red, and warm, and the client is experiencing chills, fever, nausea, and vomiting, the underlying kidney could be inflamed or infected.
- The pain caused by calculi (stones) in the kidney or upper ureter is unique and different in character, severity, and duration than that caused by kidney enlargement. This pain occurs as calculi travel from the kidney to the ureters and the urinary bladder.
- Some clients experience no pain, and others feel excruciating pain. A stationary stone causes a dull, aching pain. As stones travel down the urinary tract, spasms occur. These spasms produce sharp, intermittent, colicky pain (often accompanied by chills, fever, nausea, and vomiting) that radiates from the flanks to the lower quadrants of the abdomen, and in some cases, the upper thigh and scrotum or labium.
- If the client reports severe pain, hematuria (blood in the urine) or oliguria (diminished volume of urine), and nausea and vomiting, it is important to be alert for hydroureter, a frequent complication that occurs when a renal calculus moves into the ureter. The calculus blocks and dilates the ureter, causing spasms and severe pain. Hydroureter can lead to shock, infection, and impaired renal function. If the nurse suspects hydroureter or obstruction at any point in the urinary tract, medical collaboration must be sought immediately.

Kidney Assessment

Techniques and Normal Findings | **Abnormal Findings Special Considerations**

5. Use blunt or indirect percussion to further assess the kidneys.

- Place your left palm flat over the left costovertebral angle.
- Thump the back of your left hand with the ulnar surface of your right fist, causing a gentle thud over the costovertebral angle (see Figure 9–21 ■).

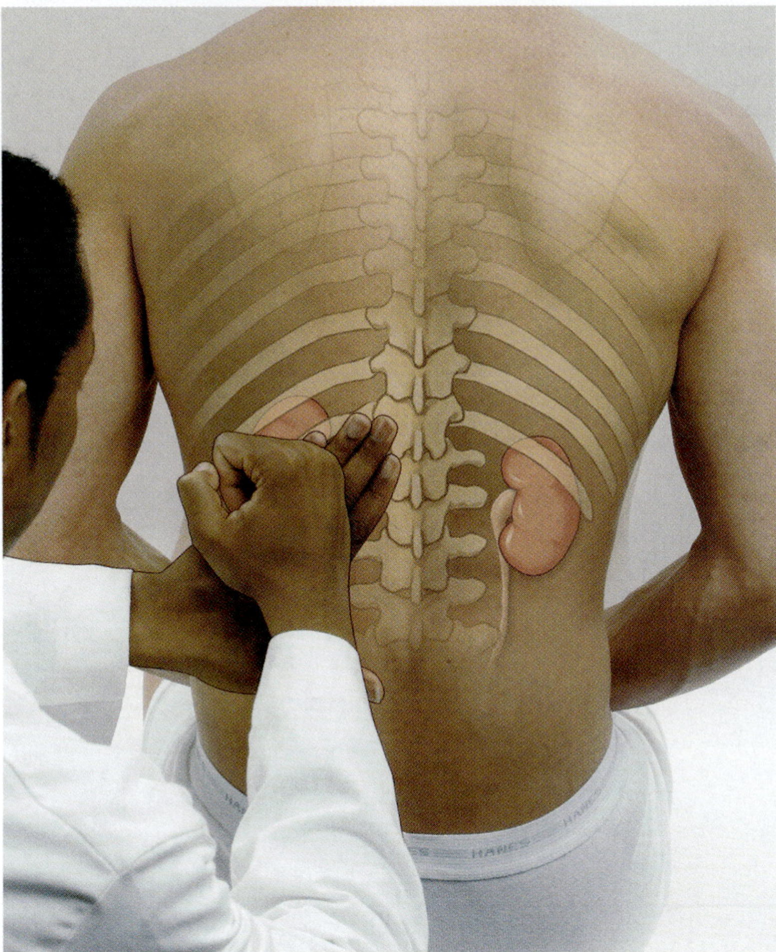

Figure 9–21 ■ Blunt percussion over the left costovertebral angle.

- Repeat the procedure on the right side. Ask the client to describe the sensation as you examine each side.
- The client should feel no pain or tenderness with pressure or percussion.

- Pain or discomfort during and after blunt percussion suggests kidney disease. This finding is correlated with other assessment findings.

THE LEFT KIDNEY

1. Attempt to palpate the lower pole of the left kidney.

- Although it is not usually palpable, attempt to palpate the lower pole of the kidney for size, contour, consistency, and sensation. Note that the rib cage obscures the upper poles.

- When enlargement occurs in the presence of conditions such as neoplasms and polycystic disease, the kidneys may be palpable. Otherwise, they are rarely palpable.

PRACTICE ALERT

Because deep kidney palpation can cause tissue trauma, novice nurses should not attempt either deep palpation or capture of the kidney unless supervised by an experienced nurse or nurse practitioner. Deep kidney palpation should not be done in clients who have had a recent kidney transplant or an abdominal aortic aneurysm.

Kidney Assessment

Techniques and Normal Findings

- Position the client in a supine position. All palpation should be performed from the client's right side.
- While standing on the client's right side, reach over the client and place your left hand between the posterior rib cage and the iliac crest (the left flank).
- Place your right hand on the left upper quadrant of the abdomen lateral and parallel to the left rectus muscle just below the costal margin.
- Instruct the client to take a deep breath. As the client inhales, lift the client's left flank with your left hand and press deeply with your right hand (approximately 4 cm) to attempt to palpate the lower pole of the kidney (see Figure 9–22 ■).

Abnormal Findings Special Considerations

- Care must be taken not to mistake an enlarged spleen for an enlarged left kidney. An enlarged kidney feels smooth and rounded, whereas an enlarged spleen feels sharper, with a more delineated edge.

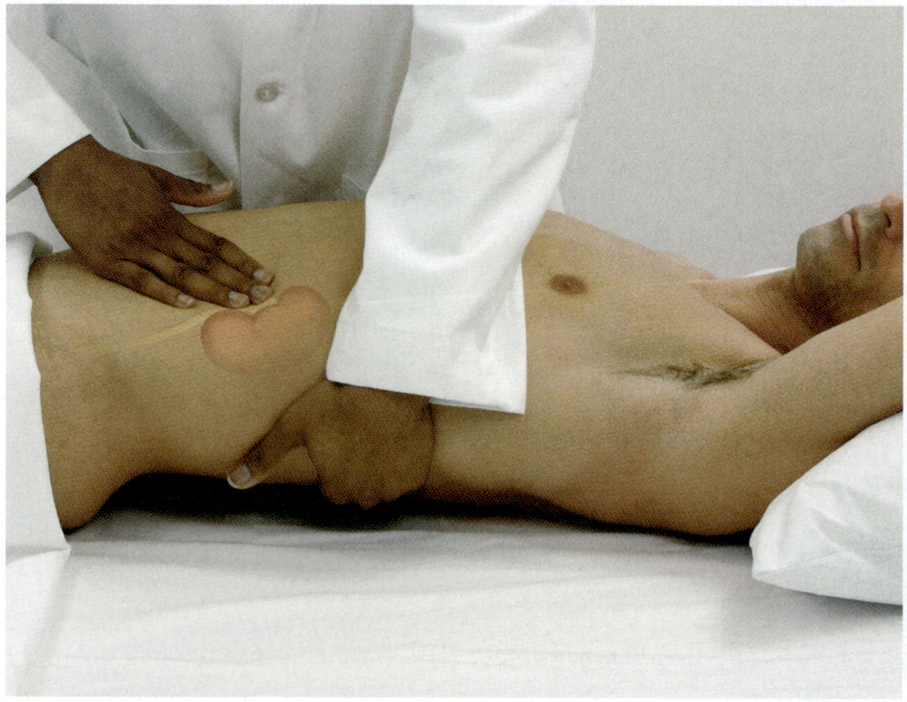

Figure 9–22 ■ Palpating the left kidney.

2. Attempt to capture the left kidney.

- Because of its position deep in the retroperitoneal space, the left kidney is not normally palpable. The capture maneuver may enable you to palpate it. This maneuver is possible because the kidneys descend during inspiration and slide back into their normal position during exhalation.
- Standing on the client's right side, place your left hand under the client's back to elevate the flank as before. Place your right hand on the left upper quadrant of the abdomen lateral and parallel to the left rectus muscle with the fingertips just below the left costal margin. Instruct the client to take a deep breath and hold it. As the client inhales, attempt to capture the kidney between your two hands. Ask the client to exhale slowly and then to briefly hold the breath. At the same time, slowly release the pressure of your fingers.
- As the client exhales, you will feel the captured kidney move back into its previous position. The kidney surface should be rounded, smooth, firm, and nontender.

Abnormal Findings Special Considerations

- An enlarged palpable kidney could be painful for the client. This suggests tumor, cyst, or hydronephrosis.

Kidney Assessment

Techniques and Normal Findings	Abnormal Findings Special Considerations
THE RIGHT KIDNEY	
1. Attempt to palpate the lower pole of the right kidney. ■ Standing on the client's right side, place your left hand under the back parallel to the right twelfth rib (about halfway between the costal margin and iliac crest) with your fingertips reaching for the costovertebral angle. Place your right hand on the right upper quadrant of the abdomen lateral to the right rectus muscle and just below the right costal margin. ■ Instruct the client to take a deep breath. As the client inhales, lift the flank with your left hand and use deep palpation to feel for the lower pole of the kidney.	
2. Attempt to capture the right kidney. ■ Place your left hand under the client's right flank. ■ Place your right hand on the right upper quadrant of the abdomen with the fingertips lateral and parallel to the right rectus muscle just below the right costal margin. ■ Instruct the client to take a deep breath and hold it. As the client inhales, attempt to capture the kidney between your two hands. ■ Ask the client to exhale slowly and then to briefly hold the breath. At the same time, slowly release the pressure of your fingers. ■ As the client exhales you will feel the captured kidney move back into its previous position. The kidney surface should be rounded, smooth, firm, and nontender. ■ The lower pole of the right kidney is palpable in some individuals, especially in thin, relaxed females. If palpable, the lower pole of the kidney has a smooth, firm, uninterrupted surface. ■ During the capture maneuver, some clients describe a nonpainful sensation as the kidney slides between the nurse's fingers back into its normal position.	■ It is important not to mistake an enlarged liver for an enlarged right kidney. An enlarged kidney feels smooth and rounded, whereas an enlarged liver is closer to the midline and has a more distinct border. Polycystic kidney disease or carcinoma should be suspected when there is gross enlargement of the kidney. The kidneys may be two or three times their normal size in clients with polycystic disease.

Implementation

In collaboration with the health care team, the nurse will provide culturally appropriate caring interventions to assure the comfort the client and promote continuing health following discharge. While treating client pain may be the most immediate intervention, client teaching and health promotion help the client maintain urinary health beyond the current need for health care intervention.

Acute Pain

Pain is the primary outward manifestation of urolithiasis, particularly when a stone lodges in a ureter, causing acute obstruction and distention. Invasive and noninvasive procedures to remove or crush stones also may be painful. Clients undergoing surgery also experience incisional pain. The intensity of renal colic pain can cause a vasovagal response with resulting hypotension and syncope. It is important to provide for the client's safety.

- Assess pain using a standard pain scale and its characteristics. Administer analgesia as ordered and monitor its effectiveness. The intensity, type of pain, and its responsiveness to analgesia provide valuable clues as to its cause. Regularly administering prescribed analgesics controls pain more effectively than waiting until pain becomes intolerable. Administering an ordered NSAID on a routine schedule may significantly reduce the need for narcotic analgesia in clients with renal colic.
- Unless contraindicated, encourage fluid intake and ambulation in the client with renal colic. Increased fluids and ambulation increase urinary output, facilitating movement of the calculus through the ureter and decreasing pain.
- Use nonpharmacologic measures such as positioning, moist heat, relaxation techniques, guided imagery, and diversion as adjunctive therapy for pain relief. Adjunctive pain relief measures can enhance the effectiveness of analgesics and other prescribed treatment.
- If surgery has been performed, monitor urinary output, catheters, incision, and wound drainage. Pain may be a symptom of proximal distention due to a blocked catheter. Infection or hematoma at the surgical site can increase pain significantly.

Impaired Urinary Elimination

Obstruction of the urinary tract is the primary problem associated with urolithiasis. A stone that completely obstructs the ureter can lead to hydronephrosis and kidney damage on the affected side. Report symptoms of hydronephrosis, such as dull flank pain or aching and changes in renal function studies (BUN and serum creatinine). Because the other kidney continues to function, urine output may not fall significantly with obstruction of one ureter. A rising BUN and serum creatinine may be early signs of renal failure. Obstruction can ultimately lead to stasis, infection, or irreversible renal damage.

- Monitor amount and character of urine output. If catheterized, measure output hourly. Document any hematuria, dysuria, frequency, urgency, and pyuria. Strain all urine for stones, saving any recovered stones for laboratory analysis. The amount of urine output helps determine possible urinary tract obstruction and adequacy of hydration. Hematuria, gross or microscopic, is often associated with calculi and with procedures used to remove stones, such as cystoscopy or lithotripsy. A change in the amount of hematuria may indicate stone passage or a complication. Dysuria, frequency, urgency, and cloudy urine are symptoms of UTI, often associated with urolithiasis. Antibiotic therapy may be required. Analysis of stones recovered from the urine can direct measures used to prevent further lithiasis.
- Maintain patency and integrity of all catheter systems. Secure catheters well, label as indicated, and use sterile technique for all ordered irrigations or other procedures. A kinked or plugged catheter, particularly a ureteral catheter or nephrostomy tube, may damage the urinary system. Labeling catheters can prevent mistakes such as inappropriate irrigation and clamping. Any catheter increases the risk of infection; aseptic technique in all procedures reduces this risk.

Deficient Knowledge

The client with urolithiasis has multiple learning needs. These include information about the disease and its possible consequences, understanding of any diagnostic or therapeutic procedures performed, and strategies to prevent future lithiasis. The nurse working with a client with urolithiasis should:

- Assess understanding and previous learning. Relating information to previously learned material enhances retention and understanding.
- Present all material in a manner appropriate to knowledge base, developmental and educational levels, and current needs. Learning is an active process that requires the client's participation. Tailoring teaching to the individual increases client involvement and compliance with the care plan.
- Teach about all diagnostic and treatment procedures. Knowing what to expect reduces anxiety, enhances compliance, and hastens recovery.
- If the client will be managed at home or in the community, teach the client to:
  a. Collect and strain all urine, saving any stones.
  b. Report stone passage to the physician and bring in the stone for analysis.
  c. Report to physician any changes in the amount or character of urine output.

When pain can be managed with oral analgesics, urinary stones are managed at home or in the community. The client needs to know how and why to collect the calculus as well as what the indicators of complications are, such as reduced urine output and cloudy or bloody urine.

- Teach measures to prevent further urolithiasis.
  a. Increase fluid intake to 2500–3500 mL per day.
  b. Follow recommended dietary guidelines.
  c. Maintain activity level to prevent urinary stasis and bone resorption (loss).
  d. Take medications as prescribed.

The risk of recurrent lithiasis is approximately 50%; however, this risk can be reduced through measures used to prevent conditions favoring stone formation.

- Teach about the relationship between urinary calculi and UTI, emphasizing preventive measures and the importance of prompt treatment. UTI promotes urolithiasis and thus requires prompt treatment to reduce this risk.

Preparing the Client for Discharge

The client with urinary calculi needs to know how to manage existing stones and what to do to reduce the risk of future stone formation. Discuss the following topics to prepare the client and family for home care:

- Importance of maintaining a fluid intake adequate to produce 2.0–2.5 quarts of urine per day
- Prescribed medications, their management, and potential adverse effects
- Dietary recommendations
- Prevention, recognition, and management of UTI
- Any further diagnostic or treatment measures planned.

Health Promotion

Discuss with all clients the importance of maintaining an adequate fluid intake. Stress the need to increase fluid intake during warm weather and strenuous exercise or physical labor. Discuss the relationship between weight-bearing activity and retention of calcium in the bones. Encourage all clients to remain as physically active as possible to prevent bone resorption and possible hypercalciuria.

Instruct clients with known gout to maintain a generous fluid intake so as to produce at least 2 L of urine every day.

CLIENT TEACHING **Urinary Calculi**

When the client is to be discharged with dressings, a nephrostomy tube, or a catheter, teach the client and family about the following:

- How to change dressings, maintaining aseptic technique
- How to assess the wound and skin for healing and possible complications such as infection or skin breakdown
- How to manage drainage systems and maintain their patency
- How to empty drainage bags and assess urine output
- When to contact the physician and what the recommendations are for follow-up care.

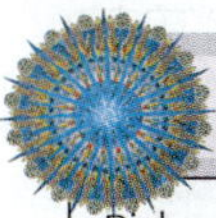

NURSING CARE PLAN **A Client With Urinary Calculi**

Richard Leton, age 44, owns a small business. He is admitted to the medical unit from the emergency department after awakening at 4 a.m. with severe right-sided pain. His CBC is normal, and urinalysis reveals microscopic hematuria but no protein or bacteria. A renal ultrasound shows a 4–5 mm stone partially obstructing the right ureter.

Stephen Phillips, Mr. Leton's admitting nurse, notes that Mr. Leton is pale, diaphoretic, and very anxious. Mr. Leton complains of nausea and asks for an emesis basin. Mr. Leton received 4 mg of intravenous morphine sulfate shortly after admission to the ED, approximately 2.5 hours ago. He denies pain at this time but says, "I'm scared to death that it'll come back—I couldn't even move, it hurt so bad."

ASSESSMENT

Mr. Leton's history reveals no previous episodes of renal calculi. He felt well until the pain awakened him during the night. He admits that he has been working under a deadline to complete a construction project and that he probably has not been drinking enough fluids "considering how hot it's been." Physical assessment findings include T_O 100.4°F (38.0°C) po, P 98, R 24, and BP 160/86. Color is pale to ashen, skin cool and moist. Abdomen firm with moderate tenderness in the right upper outer quadrant. The ED physician orders an IV of 5% dextrose in 1/2 normal saline at 200 mL/h until nausea is relieved, then PO fluids of at least 3000 mL/24 h; morphine sulfate (MS) 2–10 mg IV prn severe pain; indomethacin (Indocin) 50 mg per rectal suppository q8h; promethazine (Phenergan) 25 mg po or per suppository q6h prn nausea; activity to tolerance; and strain all urine, sending recovered stones for analysis.

DIAGNOSES

- Anxiety related to anticipation of recurrent severe pain
- Risk for Imbalanced Nutrition: Less Than Body Requirements related to nausea
- Acute Pain related to partial obstruction of right ureter by calculus
- Impaired Urinary Elimination related to partial obstruction of ureter by calculus
- Deficient Knowledge related to lack of information about disease process, contributing factors, and management

PLANNING

To return to health and achieve expected outcomes, Mr. Leton's goals for care include the following:

- Demonstrate reduced anxiety by relaxed facial expression, vital signs within his normal range, and ability to rest when not disturbed.
- Consume at least 50% of diet and 100% of ordered fluids without nausea or vomiting.
- Request analgesia as needed at onset of pain; report effective pain relief.
- Maintain urine output of 2500 mL/24 h with no signs of infection or obstruction (such as increased pain, dysuria, pyuria, or hematuria).
- Relate an understanding of the process of urolithiasis and contributing factors.
- Verbalize dietary and fluid intake and other measures to reduce risk of future stone formation.

IMPLEMENTATION

The nurse caring for Mr. Leton should:

- Reassure that measures to prevent further episodes of renal colic are being implemented and that medication is available to relieve pain promptly.
- Assess the effectiveness of analgesia and its adverse effects, especially nausea.
- Maintain IV as ordered until oral fluid intake exceeds 200 mL of fluid per hour while awake.
- Measure and strain all urine. Assess urine for color, clarity, and odor.
- Teach about urolithiasis and its risk factors, especially as they relate to Mr. Leton.
- Teach Mr. Leton the importance of maintaining a high fluid intake, especially when working outdoors in hot weather; recommended dietary modifications and their rationale; ordered medications and their effects; ways to identify and prevent UTI; and symptoms that should be reported to the physician.

EVALUATION

Mr. Leton's care is evaluated based on the goals of nursing care. Mr. Leton passed the obstructing stone the evening after admission and is discharged the following day. On discharge, he denies pain or nausea, his urine is clear and pale yellow, and urinalysis is normal. Laboratory analysis shows that the calculus was calcium. Mr. Leton is able to state the importance of continuing a high fluid intake. He verbalizes that he will reduce his intake of calcium-rich foods such as milk and milk products and that he will increase his intake of foods to acidify his urine. He is able to list foods to include in his diet. He states, "You'd better believe I'll follow my diet, drink my water, and make sure I don't get an infection. I hope to never feel pain like that again!"

(continued)

NURSING CARE PLAN A Client With Urinary Calculi *continued*

CRITICAL THINKING

1. What factors contributed to the onset and timing of Mr. Leton's ureteral colic?
2. What is the rationale for administering indomethacin, an NSAID, to a client with ureteral colic?
3. Why did Mr. Phillips include a nursing intervention to assess for a relationship between Mr. Leton's nausea, his pain, and the ordered analgesic agent?

Discuss the risk of lithiasis with clients who have frequent UTIs and teach measures to reduce the incidence of UTI and the risk for lithiasis.

Evaluation

The client is evaluated based on the selected outcomes and nursing diagnoses, and the plan of care is amended depending on the client's response to interventions. While straining of the client's urine may indicate that the stone has passed, it is important to assess the client for possible complications such as infection or kidney damage. Expected outcomes include the following:

- Client reports pain of 3 or less and is comfortable enough to perform ADLs.
- Client remains infection-free.
- Client chooses appropriate diet to prevent recurrence of renal calculi.
- Client demonstrates adequate fluid intake.

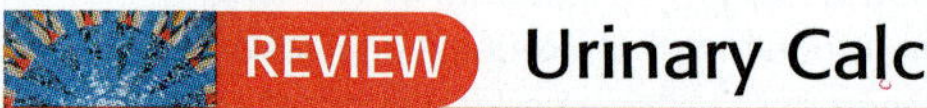

Urinary Calculi

RELATE: LINK THE CONCEPTS

You are caring for a client with urinary calculi who is experiencing severe pain that he ranks as an 11 on the 1–10 scale, with 10 being the worst pain he's ever felt.

Linking the exemplar of Urinary Calculi with concept of Comfort:

1. Describe both pharmacologic and nonpharmacologic strategies you would use to relieve the client's pain.
2. What expected outcomes would you assess as indicating that pain management techniques were successful?

Linking the exemplar of Urinary Calculi with the concept of Culture:

3. How would you respond if the client informed you of a website he looked at last night that recommended increasing magnesium intake to cure kidney stones instead of following the therapy recommended by his provider?
4. The client with urinary calculi has already been seen several times for the same diagnosis. What cultural assessment would you perform to determine if there is a cultural link to the recurrent diagnosis?

READY: GO TO COMPANION SKILLS MANUAL

The following skills related to this concept can be found in your skills book:

- Assessing the abdomen
- Assessing the client in pain
- Collecting a routine urine specimen
- Monitoring intake and output
- Performing urine tests
- Preparing for medication administration
- Using the narcotic control system
- Administering intravenous medications using IV push

REFER: GO TO MYNURSINGKIT

REFLECT: CASE STUDY

Guy Markson, 28, is a business executive with a sedentary lifestyle. His wife says that he is always telling her that he needs to exercise more, but business meetings and job responsibilities seem to get in the way of his plans to work out. Lately, he's been even busier than usual and sometimes forgets to eat lunch or dinner unless he has a business lunch, which is usually red meat and wine.

Mr. Markson called his physician today, reporting excruciating pain under his rib cage on the left side of his back, saying that when his urine looked bloody, he knew he had to do something. The doctor ordered a renal ultrasound, serum laboratory testing (calcium, uric acid, BUN, creatine, phosphorus) and urinalysis to include urine calcium. The doctor instructed Mr. Markson to go to the emergency department, which would coordinate the ordered tests and inform him of the results.

When Mr. Markson arrives at the hospital, the nurse administers morphine sulfate for pain and indomethacin by suppository and initiates IV normal saline at 150 mL/hour. A renal ultrasound is performed, and Mr. Markson receives a diagnosis of a 6 mm stone completely obstructing the left ureter, with resulting acute hydronephrosis. Based on results of diagnostic tests, it is suspected that the stone is a uric acid stone, although further testing will be performed on it when removed. The doctor recommends ESWL as the initial treatment and admits Mr. Markson to the acute care facility.

1. As the nurse admitting this client to the unit, what preparations will you make for the client while awaiting his arrival from the emergency department?
2. What nursing diagnosis would be appropriate for this client?
3. Following successful lithotripsy and confirmation that the stone was composed of uric acid, what discharge teaching will you provide to the client and his wife?

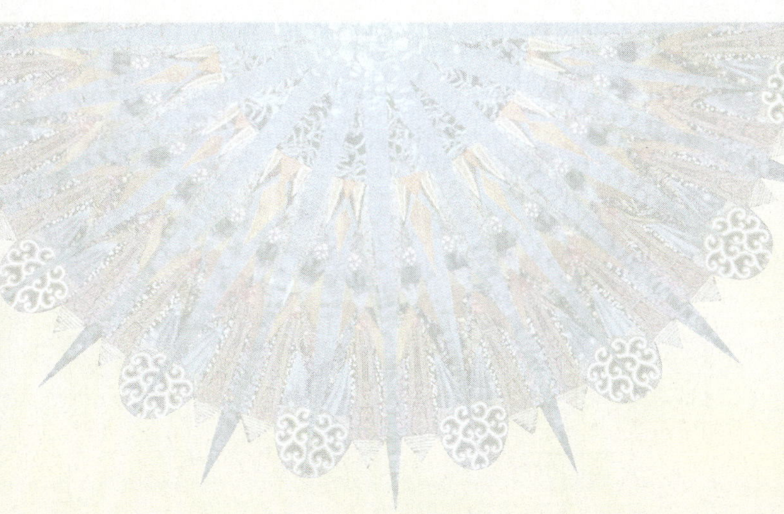

PEARSON

EXPLORE mynursingkit™

MyNursingKit is your one stop for online chapter review materials and resources. Prepare for success with additional NCLEX®-style practice questions, interactive assignments and activities, web links, animations and videos, and more!

Register your access code from the front of your book at **www.mynursingkit.com**.

REFERENCES

Bailey, J. L., & Sands, J. M. (2003). Renal disease. In W. R. Hazzard, J. P. Blass, J. B. Halter, J. G. Ouslander, & M. E. Tinetti (Eds.). *Principles of geriatric medicine and gerontology* (5th ed., pp. 551–568). New York: McGraw-Hill.

Balch, J. F., & Stengler, M. (2004). *Prescription for natural cures: A self-care guide for treating health problems with natural remedies including diet and nutrition, nutritional supplements, bodywork, and more.* Hoboken, NJ: Wiley & Sons.

Ball, J. W., & Bindler, R. C. (2006). *Child health nursing.* Upper Saddle River, NJ: Prentice Hall.

Bardsley, A. (2005). Use of lubricant gels in urinary catheterization. *Nursing Standard, 20*(8), 41–46.

Biggs, W. S., & Dery W. H. (2006). Evaluation and treatment of constipation in infants and children. *American Family Physician, 73*(3), 469–477.

Bliss, D. Z., Fischer, L., & Savik, K. (2005). Managing fecal incontinence: Self-care practices of older adults. *Journal of Gerontological Nursing, 31*(7), 35–44.

Blum, J., Taubman, B., & Nemeth, N. (2004). During toilet training, constipation occurs before stool toileting refusal. *Pediatrics, 113,* 1791–1792.

Cavagnaro, S. M. F. (2005). Infeccion urinaria en la infancia [Urinary infection in infancy]. *Revista Chilena de Infectologia, 222,* 161–168.

Chow, R. D. (2001). Benign prostatic hyperplasia: Patient evaluation and relief of obstructive symptoms. *Geriatrics, 56*(3), 33–38.

Clayden, G., & Keshtgar, A. S. (2003). Management of childhood constipation. *Postgraduate Medical Journal, 79,* 616–621.

Coughlin, E. C. (2003). Assessment and management of pediatric constipation in primary care. *Pediatric Nursing, 29,* 296–302.

Cunningham, F. G., Leveno, K. J., Bloom, S. L., Hauth, J. C., Gilstrap III, L. C., & Wenstrom, K. D. (2005.) *Williams obstetrics* (22nd ed.). New York: McGraw-Hill.

D'Amico, D., & Barbarito, C. (2007). *Health & physical assessment in nursing.* Upper Saddle River, NJ: Pearson Education.

Dochterman, J. M., & Bulechek, G. M. (2004). *Nursing interventions classification (NIC)* (4th ed.). St. Louis, MO: Mosby.

Esposito, C., Plati, A., Mazzullo, T., Fasoli, G., De Mauri, A., Grosjean, D., et al. (2007). Renal function and functional reserve in healthy elderly individuals. *Journal of Nephrology, 20,* 617–625.

Gardiner, P., & Kemper, K. J. (2005). Which herbs and supplements spell relief? *Contemporary Pediatrics, 22*(8), 50–55.

Gray, M. (2004). Clinical practice: Stress urinary incontinence in women. *Journal of the American Academy of Nurse Practitioners, 16*(5), 188–197.

Gray, M., McClain, R., Peruggia, M., Patrie, J., & Steers, W. D. (2001). A model for predicting motor urge urinary incontinence. *Nursing Research, 50*(2), 116–122.

Halverson, A. L. (2005). Nonoperative management of fecal incontinence. *Clinics in Colon and Rectal Surgery, 16*(1), 17–20.

Hinrichs, M., & Huseboe, J. (2001). Research-based protocol: Management of constipation. *Journal of Gerontological Nursing, 27*(2), 17–28.

Hsieh, C. (2005). Treatment of constipation in older adults. *American Family Physician, 72*(11), 2277–2284.

Huether, S., & McCance, K. (2005). *Understanding pathophysiology.* St. Louis, MO: Mosby.

Kasper, D. L., Braunwald, E., Fauci, A. S., Hauser, S. L., Longo, D. L., & Jameson, J. L. (Eds.). (2005). *Harrison's principles of internal medicine* (16th ed.). New York: McGraw-Hill.

Kinservik, M. A., & Friedhoff, M. M. (2004). The efficacy and safety of Polyethylene Glycol 3350 in the treatment of constipation in children. *Pediatric Nursing, 30*(3), 232–237.

Lauver, D. R., Gross, J., Ruff, C., & Wells, T. J. (2004). Patient-centered interventions: Implications for incontinence. *Nursing Research, 53*(6S), S30–S35.

Lembo, A., & Camilleri, M. (2003). Chronic constipation. *The New England Journal of Medicine, 349,* 1360.

Lemone, P., & Burke, K. (2004). *Medical-surgical nursing* (3rd ed.). Upper Saddle River, NJ: Pearson Prentice Hall.

Letran, J. L., & Brawer, M. K. (1999). Disorders of the prostate. In W. R. Hazzard, J. P. Blass, W. H. Ettinger, J. B. Halter, & J. G. Ouslander (Eds.). *Principles of geriatric medicine and gerontology* (4th ed., pp. 809–821). New York: McGraw-Hill.

Madsen, D., Sebolt, T., Cullen, L., Folkedahl, B., Mueller, T., Richardson, C., et al. (2005). Listening to bowel sounds: An evidence-based practice project. *American Journal of Nursing, 105*(12), 40–49.

Mason, D. J., Newman, D. K., & Palmer, M. H. (2003). Changing UI practice. *American Journal of Nursing, 103*(3) Supplement, 2–3.

Mauk, K. L. (2005). Preventing constipation in older adults. *Nursing, 35*(6), 22–23.

Moore, K. N., & Gray, M. (2004). Urinary incontinence in men. *Nursing Research, 53*(6S), S36–S41.

Moorhead, S., Johnson, M., & Maas, M. (2004). *Nursing outcomes classification (NOC)* (3rd ed.). St. Louis, MO: Mosby.

Morantz, C. A. (2005). ACOG guidelines on urinary incontinence in women. *American Family Physician, 72*(1), 175–178.

NANDA International. (2007). NANDA nursing diagnoses: Definitions and classification 2007–2008. Philadelphia: Author.

National Institute of Diabetes and Digestive and Kidney Diseases. (2001). *Kidney and urologic diseases statistics for the United States* (NIH Publication No. 02-3895). Washington, DC: U.S. Department of Health and Human Services.

National Kidney and Urologic Diseases Information Clearinghouse (NKUDIC). (2004). *Prostate enlargement: Benign prostatic hyperplasia.* Retrieved from http://kidney.niddk.nih. gov/kudiseases/pubs/prostateenlargement/index.htm

National Kidney and Urologic Diseases Information Clearinghouse (NKUDIC). (2007b). *Urinary retention.* Retrieved July 1, 2008, from http://kidney.niddk.nih.gov/kudiseases/pubs/UrinaryRetention/index.htm

Nield, L. S., & Kamat, D. (2004). Enuresis: How to evaluate and treat. *Clinical Pediatrics, 43*(5), 409–415.

Ouslander, J. G., & Johnson, T. M. (2003). Incontinence. In W. R. Hazzard, J. P. Blass, J. B. Halter, J. G. Ouslander, & M. E. Tinetti (Eds.). *Principles of geriatric medicine and gerontology* (5th ed., 1571–1586). New York: McGraw-Hill.

Palmer, M. H., & Newman, D. K. (2004). Urinary incontinence in nursing homes: Two studies show the inadequacy of care. *American Journal of Nursing, 104*(11), 57–59.

Palmer, M. H., & Newman, D. K. (2006). Bladder control: Educational needs of older adults. *Journal of Gerontological Nursing, 32*(1), 28–32.

Peate, I., (2003). Nursing role in the management of constipation: Use of laxatives. *British Journal of Nursing, 12*(19), 1130–1136.

Porth, C. M. (2005). *Pathophysiology: Concepts of altered health states* (7th ed.). Philadelphia: Lippincott.

Robson, W. L. M., Leung, A. K. C., & Van Howe, R. (2005). Primary and secondary nocturnal enuresis: Similarities in presentation. *Pediatrics, 115,* 956–959.

Shei Dei Yang, S., & Cheng Wang, C. (2005). Outpatient biofeedback relaxation of the pelvic floor in treating pediatric dysfunctional voiding: A short-course program is effective. *Urologia Internationalis, 74*(2), 118–122.

Sparks, A., Boyer, D., Gambrel, A., Lovet, M., Johnson, J., Richards, T., et al. (2004). The clinical benefits of the bladder scanner: A research synthesis. *Journal of Nursing Care Quality, 19*(3), 188–192.

Teng, C. H., Huang, Y. H., Kuo, B. J., & Bih, L. I. (2005). Application of portable ultrasound scanners in the measurement of post-void residual urine. *Journal of Nursing Research, 13*(3), 216–223.

Thureen, P. J., Deacon, J., Hernandez, J., & Hall, D. M. (2005). *Assessment and care of the well newborn* (2nd ed.). Philadelphia: Saunders.

Tierney, L., McPhee, S., & Papadakis, M. (Eds.). (2004). *Current medical diagnosis & treatment* (43rd ed.). Stamford, CT: Appleton & Lange.

Tierney, L. M., Jr., McPhee, S. J., & Papadakis, M. A. (Eds.). (2005). *Current medical diagnosis & treatment* (44th ed.). New York: McGraw-Hill.

Timiras, M. L., & Leary, J. (2007). The kidney, lower urinary tract, body fluids, and the prostate. In P. S. Timiras (Ed.). *Physiological basis of aging and geriatrics* (4th ed., pp. 297–313). New York: Informa Healthcare.

Timiras, M. L., & Luxenberg, J. S. (2007). Pharmacology and drug management in the elderly. In P. S. Timiras (Ed.). *Physiological basis of aging and geriatrics* (4th ed., pp. 355–361). New York: Informa Healthcare.

Way, L. W., & Doherty, G. M. (2003). *Current surgical diagnosis & treatment* (11th ed.). New York: McGraw-Hill.

Wei, J. T., Calhoun, E., & Jacobsen, S. J. (2007). Benign prostatic hyperplasia. In M. S. Litwin & C. S. Saigal (Eds.). *Urologic diseases in America* (pp. 44–69). (NIH Publication No. 07–5512). Washington, DC: U.S. Government Printing Office.

Wiggins, J. (2003). Changes in renal function. In W. R. Hazzard, J. P. Blass, J. B. Halter, J. G. Ouslander, & M. E. Tinetti (Eds.). *Principles of geriatric medicine and gerontology* (5th ed., pp. 543–549). New York: McGraw-Hill.

Family 10

Concept at-a-Glance

Concept Learning Outcomes

After reading about this concept, you will be able to:

1. Describe the functions of the family and the roles each member fulfills.
2. Outline the elements of the family system.
3. Describe characteristics of different types of families.
4. Identify the components of a family health assessment.
5. Identify four parenting styles and analyze their impact on child personality development.
6. Describe the effect of major family changes on children.

Concept Key Terms

Adolescent family, *486*
Blended family, *487*
Binuclear family, *487*
Boundaries, *494*
Childless family, *486*
Discipline, *492*
Ecomap, *493*
Emotional availability, *496*
Extended family, *485*
Extended kin network family, *485*
Family, *484*
Family-centered care, *484*
Family-centered nursing, *484*
Family cohesion, *495*
Family communication, *493*
Family coping mechanisms, *497*
Family development, *488*
Family flexibility, *496*
Foster family, *486*
Genogram, *493*
Intragenerational family, *487*
Joint custody, *487*
Limit setting, *490*
Nuclear family, *485*
Parenting, *490*
Punishment, *492*
Resiliency, *497*
Single-parent family, *486*
Stepfamily, *486*
Traditional family, *485*
Two-career family, *486*

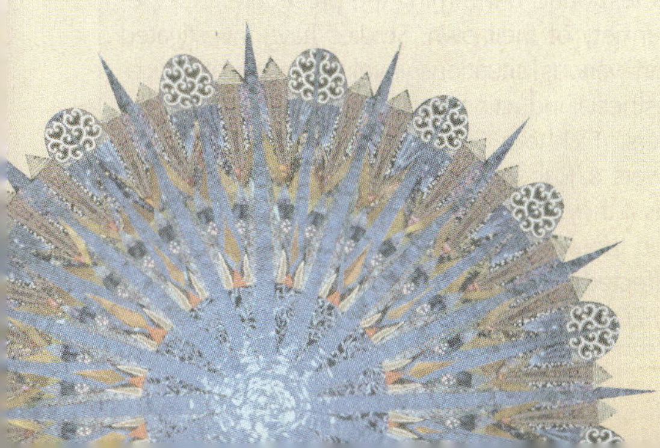

About Family

Do you ever find yourself sounding like your mother or father? Do you find yourself providing first aid for a minor problem at home and realize you are doing what you saw your grandparents do instead of what you learned in class? How big an influence does/did your family have on who you are today? If you suddenly became ill and needed to be admitted to the hospital, would your first call be to your family?

This concept will study the role of the family in development, childrearing, health promotion, and response to alterations in health status. Nurses assess and plan health care for three types of clients: the individual, the family, and the community. The beliefs and values of each person and the support he or she receives come, in large part, from the family and are reinforced by the community. Thus, an understanding of family dynamics and the context of the community assists the nurse in planning care. When a family is the client, the nurse determines the health status of the family and its individual members, the level of family functioning, family interaction patterns, and family strengths and weaknesses. •

NORMAL PRESENTATION

The family is a basic unit of society. It consists of those individuals, male or female, youth or adult, legally or not legally related, genetically or not genetically related, whom the others consider to be their significant persons. The U.S. Bureau of the Census (2006) defines a **family** as individuals who are joined together by marriage, blood, adoption, or residence in the same household. More broadly, however, families are generally characterized by bonds of emotional closeness, sharing, and support. A family may be a self-identified group of two or more persons joined together by sharing resources and emotional closeness. Family members can also include "honorary relatives" of the family, whether or not they are related by blood, marriage, or adoption, or even living in the same household. The family as defined by its members is likely to be dynamic because membership changes over time. In today's world it is even more likely that extended family members will live in different cities, states, or even countries. So, there is no *typical* family.

Within families, members are guided by a common set of values that bind them together. These family values are greatly influenced by external factors including cultural background, social norms, education, environmental influences, and socioeconomic status, as well as beliefs held by peers, coworkers, political and community leaders, and other individuals outside the family unit. Because of the influence of these external factors, a family's values may change considerably over the years.

A family is generally understood to be a safe haven for its members as they learn group values, norms, and acceptable behaviors. However, child abuse and neglect is a significant problem and can occur within any family configuration.

Roles of the family include the following:

- Caring, nurturing, and educating children; teaching children how to get along in the world
- Maintaining the continuity of society by transmitting the family's knowledge, customs and traditions, values, and beliefs to children
- Receiving and giving love
- Preparing children to become productive members of society
- Meeting the needs of its members, including protection and economic support
- Serving as a buffer between its members and environmental and societal demands while advocating or addressing the interests and needs of the individual family members.

Individual family members take on certain social and gender roles and hold a designated status within the family based on the values and beliefs that bind the family together. These values and beliefs may evolve from the family's religious or cultural values and practices, social norms, education, and other influences to which parents were exposed during childhood, adolescence, and early adult years. Parental roles, including childrearing practices and beliefs, are usually learned through a socialization process during childhood and adolescence.

Parents have important roles that involve childrearing and the long-term care of children until they reach adulthood. Depending on their other roles in society, parents work to nurture and rear children, helping them meet role expectations. Parents must also meet the needs of and provide economic support for the family. Children also learn specific roles through a socialization process. Parents set expectations of behavior with discipline and modeling of appropriate behavior.

Ideally, the family is a child's source of strength and support, the major constant in the child's life. Families are intimately involved in their children's physical and psychological well-being, and they play a vital role in the health promotion and health maintenance of their children. By respecting the family's role, strengths, and experiences with the health care system, nurses have an opportunity to develop an effective partnership with the child and family as they make health care decisions that promote the child's health. This partnership between nurses and families is known as **family-centered care**.

In the nursing profession, interest in the family unit and its impact on the health, values, and productivity of individual family members is expressed by **family-centered nursing**, nursing that considers the health of the family as a unit in addition to the health of individual family members.

Functions of the Family

The economic resources the family needs are secured by adult members. The family protects the physical health of its members by providing adequate nutrition and health care services. Family

EVIDENCE-BASED PRACTICE **Parental Presence During Procedures**

Increasingly, parents are permitted to be present during medical procedures performed on their children. Previous resistance to parental presence has been based on the fear that parents would delay or interfere with the procedure, distract or increase the anxiety of the health professionals performing the procedure, or experience heightened anxiety of their own. Studies have investigated parental presence in various situations involving medical procedures such as anesthesia induction, intravenous (IV) starts, and resuscitation (Meyers, Eichhorn, & Guzzetta, 1998; Munro & D'Errico, 2000; Powers & Rubenstein, 1999). In most cases, parents are less anxious if they are able to be present when their child has a procedure, and the ability of health professionals to perform procedures is not affected (Lewandowski & Tesler, 2003; Sacchetti, Paston, & Carraccio, 2005).

nutritional and lifestyle practices directly affect the developing health attitudes and lifestyle practices of the children.

In addition to providing an environment conducive to physical growth and health, the family creates an atmosphere that influences the cognitive and the psychosocial growth of its members. Children and adults in healthy, functional families receive support, understanding, and encouragement as they progress through predictable developmental stages, as they move in or out of the family unit, and as they establish new family units. In families where members are physically and emotionally nurtured, individuals are encouraged to achieve their potential in the family unit. As individual needs are met, family members are able to reach out to others in the family, the community, and the larger society.

Families from different cultures are an integral part of North America's rich heritage. Each family has values and beliefs that are unique to its culture of origin and shape the family's structure, methods of interaction, health care practices, and coping mechanisms. These factors interact to influence the health of families. Families of a particular culture may cluster to form mutual support systems and to preserve their heritage; however, this practice may isolate them from the larger society (Figure 10–1 ■).

Although every family is unique, all families have certain structural and functional features in common. Family structure (family roles and relationships) and family function (interactions among family members and with the community) provide the following:

- *Interdependence:* The behaviors and level of development of individual family members constantly influence and are influenced by the behaviors and level of development of all other members of the family.
- *Maintaining boundaries:* The family creates boundaries that guide its members, providing a distinct and unique family culture. This culture, in turn, provides values.
- *Adapting to change:* The family changes as new members are added, current members leave, and the development of each member progresses.
- *Performing family tasks:* Essential tasks maintain the stability and continuity of the family. These tasks include physical maintenance of the home and the people in the home, the production and socialization of family members, and the maintenance of the psychological well-being of members.

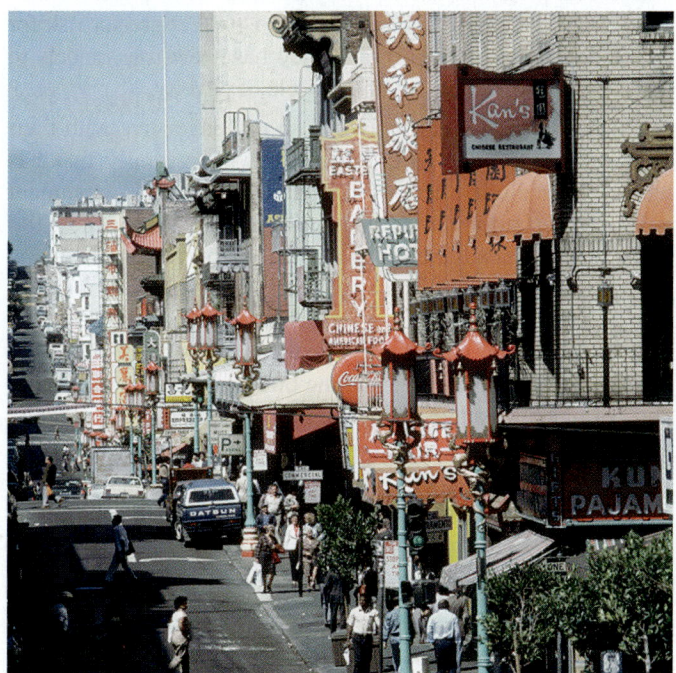

Figure 10–1 ■ Cultural clustering.

Courtesy of Morton Beebe/Corbis.

Types of Families in Today's Society

Families consist of persons (structure) and their responsibilities within the family (roles). Governmental data are grouped by types of *households*: married couples with children, married couples without children, other family households (single-parent families), men living alone, women living alone, and other nonfamily households. Some families live in houses, some in apartments; some live in urban areas, some in rural towns, and some are homeless. Various types of families exist in contemporary American society.

NUCLEAR FAMILY A family structure of parents and their offspring is known as the **nuclear family**. The nuclear family consists of a husband, a wife, and their shared biological children. Although the nuclear family was once the norm in the United States, it is no longer the most common type of family.

EXTENDED FAMILY The relatives of nuclear families, such as grandparents or aunts and uncles, compose the **extended family**. In some families, members of the extended family live with the family. Although members of the extended family may live in different areas, they may be a source of emotional or financial support for the family. An extended family may share household and childrearing responsibilities with parents, siblings, or other relatives. According to the U.S. Bureau of the Census, 4.1 million children live in an extended family with at least one parent and usually a grandparent (U.S. Census Bureau, 2002). Grandparents may raise children because the parents are unable to care for them. Grandparents endure emotional, physical, and financial stresses when taking on the childrearing role of one or more grandchildren.

EXTENDED-KIN NETWORK FAMILY Another example of an extended family is the **extended-kin network family**. This is a specific form of an extended family in which two nuclear families of primary or unmarried kin live in close proximity to each other. The family shares a social support network, chores, goods, and services. This type of family model is common in the Latino community. Multigenerational arrangements of this sort are more common in non-U.S. cultures and workingclass families.

TRADITIONAL FAMILY The **traditional family** is viewed as an autonomous unit in which both parents reside in the home with their children, the mother often assuming the nurturing role and the father providing the necessary economic resources. In today's society both men and women are less bound to traditional role patterns. For example, fathers are more likely to be involved with the household chores, their children, and family life (Figure 10–2 ■). In 2004, the U.S. Bureau of the Census reported 26.5 million fathers in married-couple families, 98,000 of whom were stay-at-home fathers (caring for 336,000 children). This was the first time the number of stay-at-home parents was analyzed in the census. Of all the families with children, the percentage consisting of married couples decreased between 1980 and 1996 and has since remained constant at about 68% (Fields, 2003).

TWO-CAREER FAMILY In **two-career families** (or dual-career families), both partners are employed by choice or by necessity. They may or may not have children. Two-career families have steadily increased since the 1960s because of increased career opportunities for women, a desire to increase the family's standard of living, and economic necessity. Today, two-thirds of all two-parent families are this type. Dual-career families have to address issues related to child care, household chores, and spending time together. The need to find good quality, affordable child care is one of the greatest stresses working parents face.

SINGLE-PARENT FAMILY Of all types of households, about 9% (12 million) are **single-parent families** and the number continues to increase (Fields, 2003). Several reasons for the increasing rate of single-parent families are as follows (Friedman, Bowden, & Jones, 2003):

- High rates of divorce
- Large amount of financial aid available to one-parent families with dependent children
- Loss of stigma associated with unwed motherhood
- Growth in number of births to never-married mothers.

Of these families, 10 million are headed by women and 2 million by men. In 2000, 26.7% of children under 18 years of age lived with a single parent, and almost 1 in 10 children lived with a never-married parent (Lugaila & Overturf, 2004; U.S. Department of Health and Human Services, 2001). There are many reasons for single parenthood, including death of a spouse, separation, divorce, birth of a child to an unmarried woman (whether the pregnancy was planned), or adoption of a child by a single man or woman. The stresses of single parenthood are many: child care concerns, financial concerns, role overload and fatigue from managing daily tasks, and social isolation. Single-parent families often face difficulties because the sole parent may lack social and emotional support, need assistance with childrearing issues, or face financial strain. Single-parent families experience higher rates of poverty, which has important implications for the children (Denham, 2005). Depending on social support and family resources, the single parent may be stressed from working to support the family, maintaining household responsibilities, serving as both mother and father, and attempting to have a personal life. Single mothers are often at risk for poverty due to lack of child support, unequal pay for work performed, work skill deficiencies, and cutbacks in social welfare programs. An important nursing consideration for working with single parents is assessing their strengths and needs in providing care to the child, such as after-school and back-up child care arrangements that enable the parent to fulfill work commitments. Nurses working with a single-parent family should determine if the family has access to all resources available to support growth and development, such as school breakfast and lunch programs that provide nutritional support.

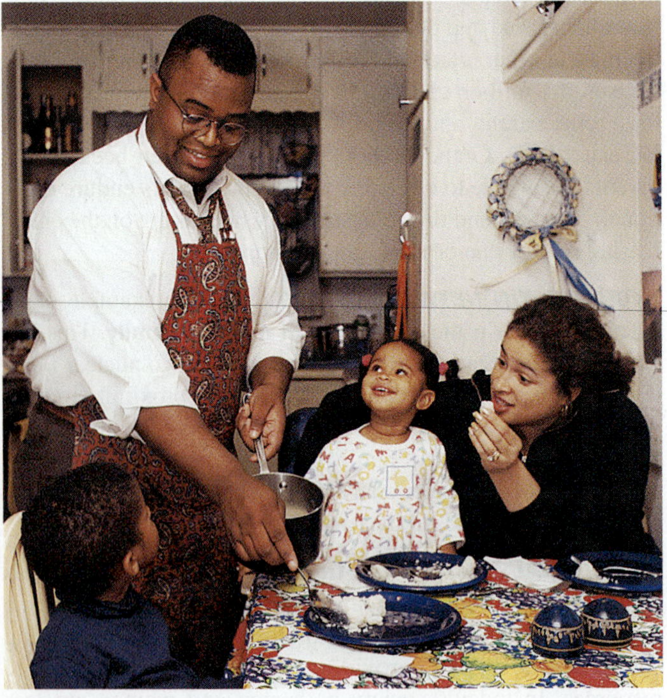

Figure 10–2 ■ Role patterns within traditional families are changing.

ADOLESCENT FAMILY The birth rate among teenagers peaked in 1991 and has decreased progressively since then to 47.7 births per 1,000 women aged 15–19 in 2000 (Alan Guttmacher Institute, 2004). Rates are highest among Black teens, followed by Latina females, and then White women. These young parents are often developmentally, physically, emotionally, and financially ill prepared to undertake the responsibility of parenthood. Adolescent pregnancies frequently interrupt or stop formal education. Children born to adolescents are often at greater risk for health and social problems, and they have few role models to assist them in breaking out of the cycle of poverty.

FOSTER FAMILY Children who can no longer live with their birth parents may require placement with a family that has agreed to include them temporarily. The legal agreement between the **foster family** and the court to care for the child includes the expectations of the foster parents and the financial compensation they will receive. A family (with or without its own children) may house more than one foster child at a time or different children over many years. Hopefully, at some time the fostered child can return to the birth parent(s) or be legally and permanently adopted by other parents.

CHILDLESS FAMILY **Childless families** (also known as child-free families) are a growing trend. In some cases a family is child-free by choice; in other cases, a family is childless because of issues related to infertility or other medical conditions that present risks to the woman or fetus should the woman become pregnant.

STEPFAMILY A **stepfamily** consists of a biologic parent with children and a new spouse who may or may not have children. This family structure has become increasingly common in the

United States because of high rates of divorce and remarriage. These families are also known as remarried, reconstituted, or blended families. There are no official statistics on the number of blended families, but a commonly accepted view is that about one of every three Americans is a member of a stepfamily.

Stepfamily models have both strengths and challenges. Stepfamilies may have fewer financial issues and may offer a child a new support person and role model. Remarriage also provides a new opportunity for a successful relationship for the parents; however, the relationship between stepparents and stepchildren can be strained. Stresses occur as blended families get acquainted with each other, respect differences, and establish new patterns of behavior. These stresses can include discipline issues, adjustment problems, role ambiguity, strain with the other biologic parent, and communication issues. When **blended families** with children form after the divorce or death of a parent, adjustment can be particularly challenged by the normal processes of grief and loss. Important nursing considerations include directing families to resources that may help reduce the potential conflicts associated with different parenting styles, discipline, and manipulative behaviors of children that can develop with the blended family.

PRACTICE ALERT

Children have the best emotional, behavioral, and educational outcomes when they live with two mutually committed parents who collaborate on childrearing and who have adequate social and financial resources (American Academy of Pediatrics Task Force on the Family, 2003).

BINUCLEAR FAMILY A **binuclear family** is a postdivorce family in which the biologic children are members of two nuclear households, both that of the father and that of the mother. The children alternate between the two homes. This is also called coparenting and involves joint custody. In **joint custody**, both parents have equal responsibility and legal rights, regardless of where the children live. The binuclear family model enables both parents to be involved. It is a model for effective communication. It enables both biological parents to be involved in a child's upbringing and provides additional support and role models from extended family members. Special nursing considerations in this family type involve ensuring that health promotion guidance and education for care of the child with an acute or chronic condition are communicated effectively to both biological parents.

INTRAGENERATIONAL FAMILY In some cultures, and as people live longer, more than two generations may live together. Children may continue to live with their parents even after having their own children, or the grandparents may move in with their grown children's families after some years of living apart. In other situations, a generation is skipped or missing; that is, grandparents live with and care for their grandchildren, but the children's parents are not a part of this family. Many life events and choices can lead to this type of family.

HETEROSEXUAL COHABITING FAMILY Cohabiting (or communal) families consist of unrelated individuals or families who live under one roof. This may include never-married individuals as well as divorced or widowed persons. According to the 2000 U.S. Census, approximately 2.9 million children under 18 years of age live with a parent and unmarried partner (Peterson, 2003). Biological children may result from the relationship, or in some cases children of one parent are present and help form a blended cohabitating family. Special concerns exist regarding the increased likelihood of the couple separating—approximately 50% in 5 years versus 20% for married couples (Peterson, 2003). Reasons for cohabiting may be a need for companionship, a desire to achieve a sense of family, testing a relationship or commitment, or sharing expenses and household management. Cohabiting families illustrate the flexibility and creativity of the family unit in adapting to individual challenges and changing societal needs. These families are less stable for the children because of the disruption associated with separation (American Academy of Pediatrics Task Force on the Family, 2003).

An important nursing consideration for children who live in informal cohabiting families is that the nonbiological parent has no legal authority to seek emergency medical care for the child. However, in the case of a true emergency that could result in loss of life or diminished functioning, health professionals are obligated to provide care and obtain consent as soon as possible afterwards. The nonbiological parent also may not have any knowledge of the child's medical history.

GAY AND LESBIAN FAMILIES Gay and lesbian families include those in which two or more people who share a same-sex orientation live together (with or without children), and those in which a gay or lesbian single parent rears a child. Children in these families may be from a previous heterosexual union, or be born to or adopted by one or both member(s) of the same-sex couple. For example, a biological child may be born to one of the partners through artificial insemination or through a surrogate mother. According to the 2000 U.S. Census, 96% of all U.S. counties have at least one gay or lesbian couple with children under 18 years in the household (Urban Institute, 2003). Small studies that have evaluated children reared by gay and lesbian couples found that the children show no significant differences from children reared in other types of families. Lesbian and gay couples function much like heterosexual couples, and children who are adopted or born into the family are highly valued. Children raised in gay and lesbian families may face unique issues in interacting with peers and in revealing their parents' sexual orientation. Homosexual adults form gay and lesbian families based on the same goals of caring and commitment seen in heterosexual relationships. In addition, the structure of gay and lesbian families is as diverse as that of heterosexual families—including stepfamilies and single-parent families. Children raised in these family units develop sex role orientations and behaviors similar to children in the general population. These children have been found to have the same advantages and expectations for health, adjustment, and development as children born into heterosexual families (American Academy of Pediatrics, 2002). Lesbian and gay parents are believed to be as effective as heterosexual couples in providing a supportive and healthy environment for their children (American Psychological Association, 2004).

PRACTICE ALERT

It is important to identify the biological or adoptive parent, or a caregiver's legal documentation proving the right to medical decision making, when obtaining consent for the child's health care.

Children in these families typically have only one biological or adoptive legal parent. The other partner is the coparent and has no legal parental status in the majority of states. Only seven states (California, Connecticut, Massachusetts, New Jersey, New York, Pennsylvania, Vermont) and the District of Columbia have considered legislative actions to ensure the security of children whose parents are gay or lesbian by guaranteeing access to the second parent of joint adoption rights (Urban Institute, 2003). Coparent adoption would help maintain the child's rights to a continuing relationship if the legal parent dies or becomes incapacitated, or if the parents separate. Either parent could then provide consent for health care and make other important decisions on behalf of the child. Financial support of the child also would be more assured if one parent dies or parents separate. Nursing considerations in this type of family involve respect for the relationship between partners and recognition of the nurturing capacity in these families.

Legal issues for same-sex couples are significant and constantly changing. Domestic partner policies extend the same rights and privileges to the partner of a nonmarried employee of the same or opposite gender as would be offered to spouses. California Family Code Section 297–297.5 defines domestic partners as "two adults who have chosen to share one another's lives in an intimate and committed relationship of mutual caring." Numerous state and federal laws have been introduced in the United States to allow or prohibit same-sex marriages or civil unions. It can be a challenge for the nurse to keep current on how such legislation affects health care issues such as insurance coverage and the right to consent for health care.

SINGLE ADULTS LIVING ALONE Individuals who live by themselves represent a significant portion of today's society. Of younger adults 18–34 years of age, about 10% live alone, with little variation between males and females. However, among adults 65 years and older, about 20% of men live alone, whereas about 40% of women live alone (Fields, 2003). Singles include young self-supporting adults who have recently left the nuclear family as well as older adults living alone. Young adults typically move in and out of living situations and may have membership in family, nonfamily household, and living alone categories at different times. Older adults may find themselves single through divorce, separation, or the death of a spouse, but generally remain living alone for the remainder of their lives.

Family Development Frameworks

Family development refers to the dynamics or changes that a family experiences over time, including changes in relationships, communication patterns, roles, and interactions. Although each family is unique, the members go through a set of fairly predictable changes. (See Box 10–1 for a new family dynamic.) For example, Duvall (1977) developed an eight-stage family life cycle that describes the developmental process each family encounters. This model is based on the nuclear family (Table 10–1). The oldest child serves as a marker for the family's developmental stages except in the last two stages, when children are no longer present. Couples with more than one child may find themselves in overlapping stages, with developmental advances occurring simultaneously. Other family development models have been developed to address the stages and developmental tasks facing the unattached young adult, the gay and lesbian family, those who divorce, and those who remarry.

FAMILY FUNCTIONING

Transition to Parenthood

Choosing to become a parent is a major life change for adults. From the time of a child's birth, the parents experience stresses and challenges along with feelings of pride and excitement.

Box 10–1 The "Sandwich Generation"

Adults who care for their own children and one or more of their own parents belong to a group that has come to be known as the "Sandwich Generation." This group of adults faces an incredible amount of stress trying to meet the diverse needs of young children and adolescents as well as aging parents. One of the chief sources of stress for these families is financial insecurity. A family with limited financial resources may face taking the aging parent into their own home or placing an aging parent who is no longer independent into a senior care facility that is below standard. If a family has very young children, taking an aging parent with dementia into the home can present either real or perceived hazards to the young children, increasing the stress level of the entire family. In addition, a member of the sandwich generation often faces additional stress addressing the elder parent's needs while still trying to get his or her own children off to school and to extracurricular activities and maintain his or her own full-time job. End-of-life issues can be a great source of stress and conflict for these families.

A nurse who is assessing an adult who cares for both his or her own children and his or her aging parents may diagnose any one of several conditions including, but not limited to, the following: Ineffective Self Health Management, Sleep Deprivation or Disturbed Sleep Pattern, Risk for Situational Low Self-Esteem, Interrupted Family Processes, and Compromised Family Coping.

CRITICAL THINKING

In small groups, discuss what assessment questions would be appropriate when working with a client who is a member of the "sandwich generation." Discuss what caring interventions might be appropriate, and what outcomes could be developed in collaboration with the client.

TABLE 10–1 **The Eight-Stage Family Life Cycle**

STAGE I	Beginning families	Marriage between partners, identification as partners, establishing goals for future, and interaction and building relationships with kin
STAGE II	Childbearing families	Birth of first child, new role as parents, integrating new family member into existing family
STAGE III	Families with preschool children	Establishing family network, socialization of children, reinforcing independence in children when separating from parents
STAGE IV	Families with school-age children	Facilitating peer relationships while maintaining family dynamics and adjusting to outside influences
STAGE V	Families with teenagers	Increase in children's independence and autonomy; parents' concerns shift to aging parents, careers, and marital relationship
STAGE VI	Families launching young adults	Readjustment of marital relationship; parents and children establish separate identities outside the family unit
STAGE VII	Middle-aged parents	Renewed marital relationship, new outside interests, fewer family responsibilities, new roles as grandparents and as in-laws, increased concern for aging parents, death, and disability of older generation
STAGE VIII	Retirement and old age	End of career, shift to retirement, maintain functioning during the aging process, maintain marital relationship, adjust to potential loss of spouse, friends, and siblings, prepare for eventual death

Source: Adapted from Duvall, Elizabeth M. *Marriage and family development* (5th ed.). Published by Allyn and Bacon, Boston, MA. Copyright © 1977 by Pearson Education. Adapted by permission of the publisher; and Friedman, M. M. (1998). *Family nursing: Research, theory, and practice* (4th ed., p. 113). Reprinted by permission of Pearson Education, Upper Saddle River, NJ.

Mothers and fathers both adjust their lifestyles to give priority to parenting. The baby is dependent for total care 24 hours a day, and this often results in sleep deprivation, irritability, less personal time, and less time for the couple's relationship. In addition, the family with a new baby often experiences a change in financial status.

Several factors influence how well the parents adjust to their new role. Social support provided to the mother, especially by the father, is important for the mother's adjustment. Marital happiness during pregnancy is an important factor for the adjustment of both parents. Infants with significant health conditions or those with difficult temperaments can cause parents extra stress and affect their adjustment to the parenting role.

With the birth of the first child, mothers and fathers both have challenges related to renegotiating their employment to accommodate family and child care time (Box 10–2). Fathers are sometimes additionally challenged to develop closeness with the infant and learn how to care for the infant, especially when they may not have had role models or any previous child care experience. Most parents find that caring for infants and children takes more time than anticipated.

Nurses can help parents through this important transition by listening to the challenges the parents describe during the infant's first health visits. Encourage fathers as well as mothers to attend and participate in health promotion visits with the health care provider. Answer questions and offer ideas to address described problems that the parents may be too tired to solve on their own. Help parents recognize that their frustrations and feelings regarding the challenges of infant care are normal. Encourage both parents to become active in caring for the infant and to gain comfort in that care. Help both parents find activities that they enjoy with regard to infant care that will encourage interaction and bonding with the infant.

Parental Influences on the Child

The qualities of family relationships and behaviors are important aspects of family strengths and functioning. Positive family relationships are characterized by parent–child warmth and supportiveness. Warm parent–child relationships can buffer children from stress and promote positive cognitive and social outcomes. Parents who are warm and place high demands on their children for appropriate behavior have children who tend to be content, self-reliant, self-controlled, and open to learning in school.

Mothers and fathers both contribute to the psychological, emotional, and social health and development of their children. Both parents provide affection, nurturing, and comfort. They teach children life skills and healthy lifestyles. Fathers play an important role in the sexual identity and gender role

Box 10–2 **Medical and Family Leave Act**

Eligible parents of newborns and adopted children are entitled to 12 weeks of unpaid leave during any 12-month period initially authorized under the federal Medical and Family Leave Act of 1993. Vacation or sick leave may be used to pay for time away from work, depending on the employer's leave policies. This act also applies if a child, spouse, or parent of the employee develops a serious health condition. The employee is entitled to return to the previous position or an equivalent position with all the same pay, benefits, and other conditions. The Act carries some additional conditions and requirements, including that employees are only eligible if they have worked for a covered employer for 1,250 hours over the previous 12 months. More information on the Act can be found at www.dol.gov.

Source: Family and Medical Leave, Public Law 103-3, February 5, 1999. 5 U.S.C. 6381–6387; 5 CFR part 630, subpart L. Adapted with permission.

development of both male and female children. Both mothers and fathers promote the social competence, academic achievement, and problem-solving abilities of their children (American Academy of Pediatrics, 2004).

Family Size

The size of the family influences the amount of attention children get. In small families parents often have more time to give attention to the children, encourage achievement, meet family expectations, and support involvement in community activities. Children in larger families are encouraged to be cooperative to support family functioning. The children usually receive less personal attention from the parents and often turn to others in the family for needed support. Family finances may be more limited. Children may adopt a specialized family role to gain recognition, such as the "responsible one," "the clown," or "the black sheep."

Sibling Relationships

Siblings are a child's first peers and often have a lifelong relationship. Siblings, especially those of the same gender or who are close in age, tend to have a closer relationship because they often share many common experiences through childhood and adolescence. In general, the parents have greater influence than siblings on children who are more widely spaced in age. However, the older sibling may be a very strong role model for younger siblings.

Sibling rivalry between children exists at times in all families. Within the family children learn to share, compete, and compromise with siblings. Some siblings take on roles such as protector, problem solver, friend, and supporter for dealing with issues in the family and in the environment. Some siblings learn to work well together to maintain privacy or to form a coalition for negotiating with the parents. An older sibling helps reinforce rules and roles in the family by prompting and inhibiting certain patterns of behavior in the younger siblings. However, one sibling may test the waters by breaking a previously implicit rule to determine what rule flexibility is allowed in the family.

Children develop different personalities because of a need to establish distinct identities for themselves and be seen as unique in the family. It has not been possible to reproduce earlier research findings that birth order was associated with specific personality traits of individual children in a family (Craig & Baucum, 2002). Siblings may share some experiences, but they are often exposed to different environmental experiences that help shape their personalities (Craig & Baucum, 2002). Firstborn children do have some advantages, such as more favorable treatment in the family. They tend to have slightly higher IQs and greater achievement in school and in their careers (Craig & Baucum, 2002). Their intellectual development may be enhanced through experiences of teaching their younger siblings.

PARENTING

The family is an important component in the lives of all children, and it plays an essential role in fostering the development of infants, children, and youth. A significant concept in families is that of parenting. **Parenting** is a leadership role in the family in which children are guided to learn acceptable behaviors, beliefs, morals, and rituals of the family and to become socially responsible, contributing members of society. The manner in which children are parented, in combination with their individual personality traits and characteristics, influences their developmental outcomes.

Parents have responsibility for providing children stability through nurturance, safety, and structure in a family that undergoes frequent changes over time. The child needs to have physical and emotional space to grow and develop. Parents also provide their children with the values, beliefs, rituals, and behaviors learned and transmitted across family generations.

To be successful, parents should implement reasonable, consistent **limit setting** (established rules or guidelines for behavior) on children's autonomy while the children are still learning values and self-control. At the same time, parents need to foster their children's curiosity, initiative, and sense of competence. Parents use different styles to parent their children. Parental warmth and control are two major factors that are important in children's development. Parental warmth refers to the amount of affection and approval displayed. Parental control refers to how restrictive the parents are regarding rules. See Table 10–2 for the characteristics associated with parental warmth and control.

Diana Baumrind (1971), an important contemporary child developmentalist, proposed classifications of parenting styles that are still well accepted today. She identified three main types of parenting styles—(*authoritarian*, *authoritative*, and *permissive*)—and described the influences each style has on children. One additional parenting style, called *indifferent*, exists in some families. While families will generally tend to use one style, they may vary their style for certain situations. See Table 10–3 for characteristics or parenting styles defined by level of warmth and control, and the associated child outcomes.

Authoritarian Parents

Authoritarian parents tend to be punitive and adhere to rigid rules, or to be more dictatorial. Parents who use this style might say, "Because I'm your parent, that's why," "A rule is a rule," or "Just do what I say." While this style sets firm limits, those limits or rules are not negotiable or open to any discussion. Parents expect family beliefs and principles to be accepted without question. Children have no opportunity to participate in the family decision-making process. Children with authoritarian parents do not develop the skills to examine why a certain behavior is desirable or how their actions might influence others.

Authoritative Parents

Authoritative parents use firm control to set limits, but they establish an atmosphere with open discussion or are more democratic. Limits for behavior are clear, consistent, and reasonable, but the children are encouraged to talk about why certain behaviors occurred and how the situations might be handled differently another time. Parents set and stick to established routines, so children have clear expectations of appropriate behavior. Authoritative parents provide explanations about

TABLE 10–2 **Characteristics of Significant Parenting Attributes**

PARENTING ATTRIBUTE	PARENTAL WARMTH	PARENTAL CONTROL
High level	■ Warm, nurturing ■ Expressing affection and smiling at children frequently ■ Limiting criticism, punishment ■ Expressing approval of child	■ Restrictive control of behavior ■ Surveying and enforcing compliance with rules ■ Encouraging children to fulfill their responsibilities ■ Sometimes limiting freedom of expression
Low level	■ Cool, hostile ■ Quick to criticize or punish ■ Ignoring children ■ Rarely expressing affection or approval ■ Sometimes rejecting children	■ Permissive, minimally controlling ■ Making fewer demands ■ Making fewer restrictions on behavior or expression of emotion ■ Permitting freedom in exploring environment

inappropriate behaviors at a child's level of understanding. Children are allowed to express their opinions and objections, and some flexibility is permitted when appropriate. However, parents make it clear that they are the ultimate authority for decisions. Children with authoritative parents develop a sense of social responsibility because they converse about their responsibilities and approaches.

Permissive Parents

Permissive parents show a great deal of warmth, but set few controls or restraints on the children's behavior. Parents are so intent on showing unconditional love that they fail to perform some important parenting functions. Children are allowed to regulate their own behavior. Discipline is inconsistent, and parents may threaten punishment but not follow through. Both extremes result in excessive permissiveness, and the children do not learn socially acceptable limits of behavior. As the parents do not impose any controls on the children, the children end up controlling the parents.

Indifferent Parents

Indifferent parents do not display much interest in their children or in their roles as parents. They do not demonstrate affection or approval of the children, and they do not set lim-

TABLE 10–3 **Parenting Styles by Level of Warmth and Control**

PARENTING STYLE	WARMTH/CONTROL	BEHAVIOR OF PARENTS	CHILD OUTCOMES
Authoritarian	High control Low warmth	■ Highly controlling, issue commands and expect them to be obeyed ■ Little communication with children, avoid lengthy verbal discussions with children ■ Have inflexible rules ■ Permit little independence	■ Have no negotiation skills ■ Have no ability to direct and initiate own activities ■ Frustrated in efforts to achieve autonomy ■ May become fearful, withdrawn, and unassertive ■ Girls often passive and dependent during adolescence ■ Boys often rebellious and aggressive
Authoritative	Moderately high control High warmth	■ Set reasonable limits on behavior ■ Accept and encourage growing autonomy of children ■ Engage in open communication with children ■ Have flexible rules	■ More willingly accept restrictions ■ Tend to be more self-reliant, self-controlled, and socially competent ■ Have higher self-esteem ■ Perform better in school
Permissive	Low control High warmth	■ Have few or no restraints ■ Give unconditional love ■ Communication flows from child to parent ■ Provide much freedom and little guidance ■ Provide no limit setting	■ Often unable to cooperate and negotiate with others ■ May become rebellious, aggressive, or socially inept, self-indulgent, or impulsive ■ May have difficulty being accepted by peers or being accepted and effective in a work setting ■ May be creative, active, and outgoing
Indifferent	Low control Low warmth	■ Provide no limit setting ■ Lack affection for children ■ Focus on stress in own lives ■ May show hostility or neglect	■ Often have the worst outcomes such as destructive impulses and delinquent behavior

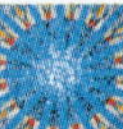

CLIENT TEACHING Guidelines for Promoting Acceptable Behavior in Children

The nurse can assist parents in handling their child's misbehavior by helping them to:

- Set realistic expectations and directions for behavior based on the child's age and understanding; consistently enforce the expected directions and behaviors.
- Focus on promoting appropriate and desirable behaviors in the child.
- Model or suggest appropriate behavior.
- Review expected behavior for special situations, such as a family party, going to the movies, or other social event.
- Help the child distinguish between inside and outside voice and behaviors.
- Praise or reward the child using appropriate behaviors.
- Tell the child about his or her inappropriate behavior as soon as it begins, and offer guidelines for changing behavior or provide a distraction.
- When reprimanding the child, focus on the behavior rather than stating that the child is bad. Explain how the behavior is inappropriate, how it makes you, as the parent, and any other person involved feel. Avoid ridicule or accusation that can take the form of shame or criticism, as these actions can affect the child's self-esteem if repeated often enough.
- Be alert for situations when the child could misbehave, such as when tired or overexcited. Use a distraction to control or calm the child.
- Help children gain self-control with friendly reminders (e.g., count to 3, as soon as the clothes are on the doll, as soon as you finish the game) regarding the timing for transition to the next event of the day, such as bedtime, putting the toys away, or washing hands before dinner.
- Discuss reasons and social rules for expected behaviors when the child is old enough to understand.

its or controls on the children. This may occur because they do not care, or because their lives are so stressed that they have no time or energy left for the children (Craig & Baucum, 2002).

Assessing Parenting Styles

Nurses assess parenting styles by asking families how they handle situations that require limit setting. As previously described, an authoritative style is preferred because of its positive outcomes for child behavior and learning. The nurse in all settings is often in a position to discuss parenting styles and to offer suggestions for managing certain types of child behaviors that are frustrating to the family. Keep in mind that children are all different, and parents often must vary their parenting styles for different children in the family. For example, the child's temperament is often tied to her or his behavioral style. One child may need very clear limits, with discussion and reinforcement, while a sibling may immediately respond to the parents' limit setting without a need for discussion of the situation.

Discipline and Limit Setting

Discipline is a method for teaching children the rules for how to behave in society and what is expected in different circumstances. **Punishment** is the action taken to enforce the rules when the child misbehaves. Parenting styles play an important role in the type of discipline and punishment parents use with children. When clear limits are set and consistently maintained, as with authoritative parenting, punishment may be needed less often. Limit setting and firm control of those limits are important discipline methods that allow children to learn to what extent they can safely and independently operate within the environment. Firm limits also help children feel secure; they are reassured by consistency and the sense of protection the limits are perceived to provide. Punishment helps children learn that misbehavior has consequences, and may affect other individuals. This helps children develop a sense of responsibility for their behavior.

ASSESSMENT OF FAMILY FUNCTIONING

The incidence of family violence has increased in recent years. Statistics are not accurate because many cases remain unreported. Family violence includes abuse between intimate partners, child abuse, and elder abuse, and it may include physical, mental, and verbal abuse as well as neglect. Nurses should be alert to the symptoms of family violence and take appropriate measures to report it and obtain resources for the family. More information about violence can be found in Concept 31, Violence.

Family Assessment

The purpose of family assessment is to determine the level of family functioning, clarify family interaction patterns, identify family strengths and weaknesses, and describe the health status of the family and its individual members. Also important are family living patterns, including communication, childrearing, coping strategies, and health practices. Family assessment gives an overview of the family process and helps the nurse identify areas that need further investigation. Nurses carry out a detailed assessment in specific target areas as they become more acquainted with the family and begin to understand family needs and strengths more fully. The nurse's understanding of a family's structure helps provide insight into the family's support system and needs. In planning interventions, nurses need to focus not only on problems, but also on family strengths and resources as part of the nursing care plan (see Box 10–3).

To obtain an accurate and concise family assessment, the nurse needs to establish a trusting relationship with the parent(s) and the family. Data are best collected in a comfortable, private environment, free from interruptions.

Assessment begins with a complete health history. The nurse focuses first on the family unit and then on the individuals in that family. Taking a health history is one of the most effective ways to identify existing or potential health problems. Using a genogram will aid the nurse in visualizing how

Box 10–3 **Family Assessment Guide**

FAMILY STRUCTURE
- Size and type of family
- Name, age, and gender of family members
- Family relationship of all people residing within the household

FAMILY ROLES AND FUNCTIONS
- Family members working outside the home; type of work and satisfaction with it
- Household roles and responsibilities and how tasks are distributed
- Ways childrearing responsibilities are shared
- Major decision maker and methods of decision making
- Family members' satisfaction with roles, the way tasks are divided, and the way decisions are made

PHYSICAL HEALTH STATUS
- Current physical health status of each member
- Perceptions of own and other family members' health
- Preventive health practices (e.g., status of immunizations, oral hygiene practices, regularity of vision examinations)
- Routine health care; when and why primary care provider was last seen

INTERACTION PATTERNS
- Ways of expressing affection, love, sorrow, anger, and so on
- Most significant family member in person's life
- Openness of communication with all family members

FAMILY VALUES
- Cultural and religious orientations; degree to which cultural and religious practices are followed
- Use of leisure time and whether leisure time is shared with total family unit
- Family's view of education, teachers, and the school system
- Health values: how much emphasis is put on exercise, diet, preventive health care

COPING RESOURCES
- Degree of emotional support offered to one another
- Availability of support persons and affiliations outside the family (e.g., friends, church memberships, mentors)
- Sources of stress
- Methods of handling stressful situations and conflicting goals of family members
- Financial ability to meet current and future needs

all family members are genetically related to each other and grasping how patterns of chronic conditions occur within the family unit. **Genograms** consist of visual representations of gender showing lines of birth descent through the generations (Figure 10–3 ■). The history is followed by physical assessment of family members. If further evaluation is indicated, a referral is made to the appropriate health care professional.

The nurse should also develop an ecomap for family members, individually and as a group, to document the family unit's energy expenditures within the community setting. **Ecomaps** visualize how the family unit interacts with the external community environment, including schools, religious commitments, occupational duties, and recreational pursuits (Figure 10–4 ■). When the focus is on health, the appraisal includes information on lifestyle behaviors and health beliefs. The nurse uses data from the health appraisal to formulate a health profile. The health profile provides the data necessary to determine wellness or establish a nursing diagnosis, and to plan appropriate nursing interventions to promote optimal health through lifestyle modification.

Health Beliefs

To promote health, the nurse must understand the health beliefs of individuals and families. Health beliefs may reflect a lack of information or misinformation about health or disease. They may also include folklore and practices from different cultures. Because of the many advances in medicine and health care during the last few decades, clients may have outdated information about health, illness, treatment, and prevention. The nurse is frequently in a position to give information or correct misconceptions. This function is an important component of the nursing care plan.

Family Communication Patterns

Family communication is measured by focusing on the listening and speaking skills, self-disclosure, and tracking abilities of the family as a group. In high-functioning families each person does the following:

- Listens—is empathetic and attentive
- Speaks—speaks for oneself and does not speak for others
- Self-discloses—shares personal feelings about oneself and others in the family
- Tracks—stays on the topic at hand.

Families who communicate well are better able to adapt and cope. Families who find communication difficult may experience lower levels of expressiveness, vague requests to one another, an inability to comprehend each other's messages, frequent interruption of one another, speaking for others, and high levels of verbalized hostility.

Another aspect of family communication is the family's strategy to resolve conflict. The ability to resolve differences is based on the family's capacity to talk about areas of disagreement and its mutual willingness to negotiate and reach acceptable solutions. Problem-solving skills are critical to smooth family functioning. Without these skills, families seem to use strategies such as confrontation or avoidance, which are ineffective in reducing stress and do not resolve conflict satisfactorily. Children who grow up in families that use appropriate problem-solving skills are more successful at avoiding and resolving conflicts both at home and in school.

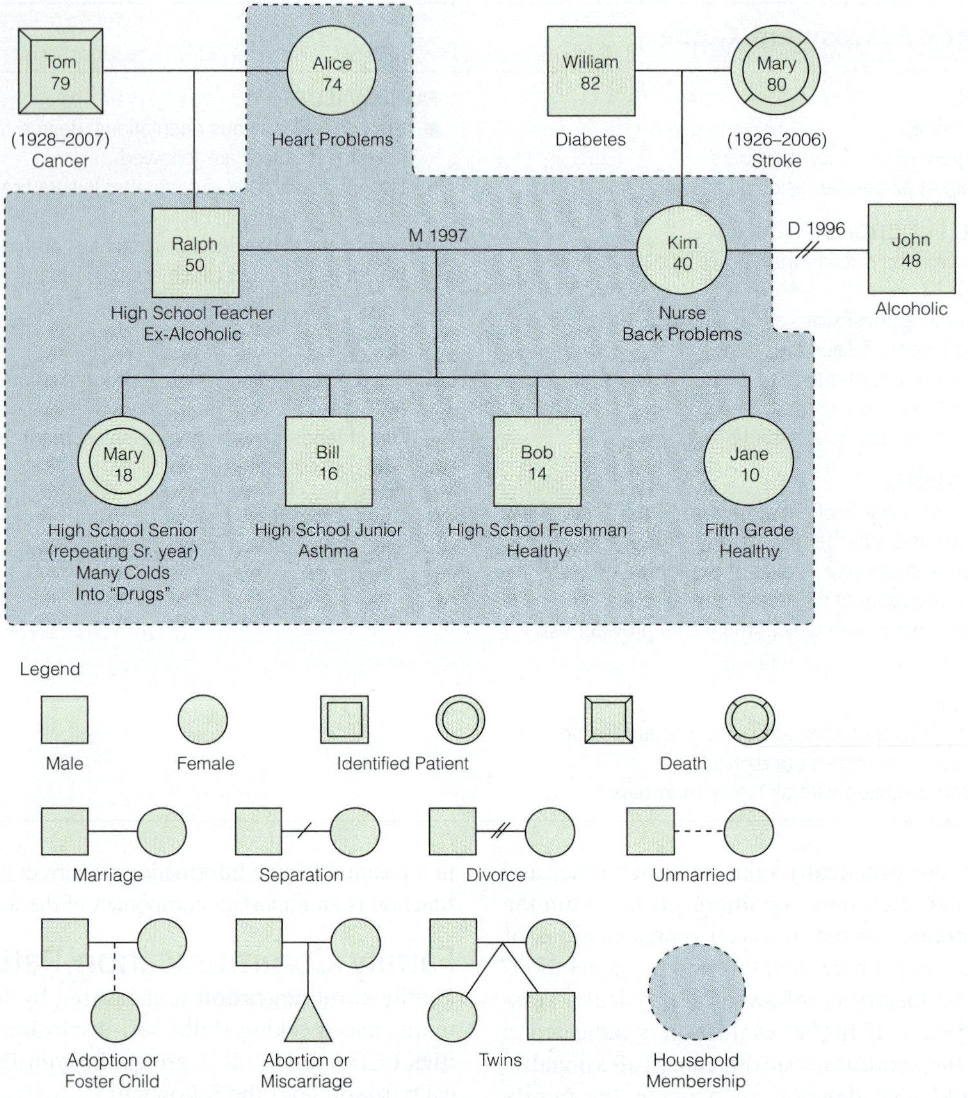

Figure 10–3 ■ Example of a family genogram with accompanying legend (symbols used in genograms).

The effectiveness of family communication determines the family's ability to function as a cooperative, growth-producing unit. Messages are constantly being communicated among family members, both verbally and nonverbally. The information transmitted influences how members work together, fulfill their assigned roles in the family, incorporate family values, and develop skills to function in society. Intrafamily communication plays a significant role in the development of self-esteem, which is necessary for the growth of personality.

Families that communicate effectively transmit messages clearly. Members are free to express their feelings without fear of jeopardizing their standing in the family. Family members support one another and have the ability to listen, empathize, and reach out to one another in times of crisis. When the needs of family members are met, they are more able to reach out to meet the needs of others in society.

When patterns of communication among family members are dysfunctional, messages are often communicated unclearly. Verbal communication may be incongruent with nonverbal messages. Power struggles may be evidenced by hostility, anger, or silence. Members may be cautious in expressing their feelings because they cannot predict how others in the family will respond. When family communication is impaired, the growth of individual members is stunted. Members often turn to other systems to seek personal validation and gratification.

The nurse needs to observe intrafamily communication patterns closely. Nurses should pay special attention to who does the talking for the family, which members are silent, how disagreements are handled, and how well the members listen to one another and encourage the participation of others. Nonverbal communication is important because it gives valuable clues about what people are feeling.

Boundaries

Boundaries are the invisible lines that define the amount and kind of contact allowable among members of the family and between the family and outside systems. Boundaries determine the patterns of how, when, and to whom family members

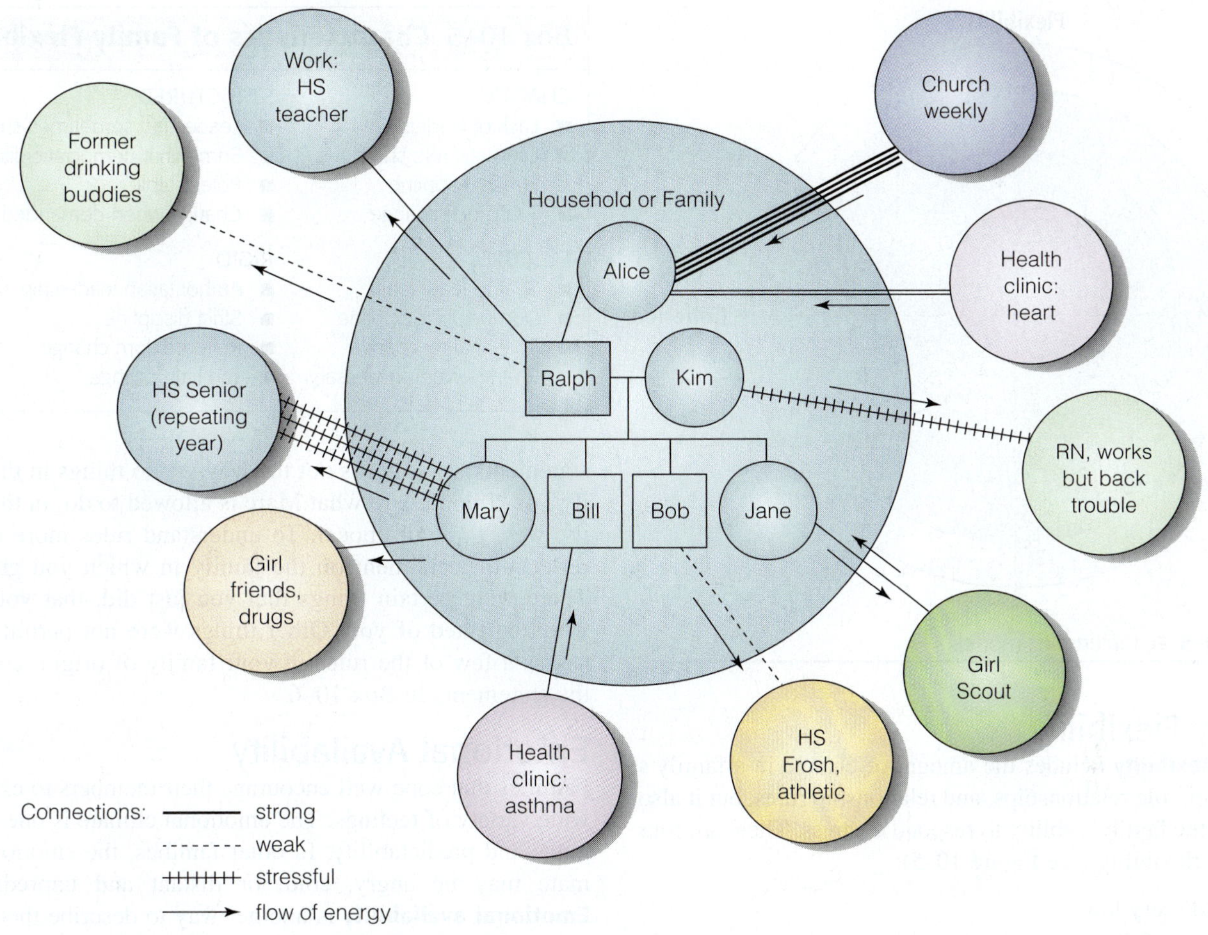

Figure 10–4 ■ Example of a family ecomap. Many more components may be added to the map.

relate. Boundaries define the divisions among the spousal, parental, and sibling subsystems.

- *Clear boundaries:* Firm yet flexible; family members are supported and nurtured but also allowed a certain degree of autonomy.
- *Rigid boundaries:* Family members are isolated from one another and there is little room for negotiation and individual development.
- *Diffuse boundaries:* Everyone is into everyone else's business; there is little distinction between family members and there is too much negotiation, resulting in a loss of autonomy.

In the modern Western nuclear family, competent families have clear hierarchical boundaries between generations in terms of power, authority, and responsibility. Competent adult leadership provides an emotional climate that considers everyone's needs and provides a sense of security. Members spend time apart, as well as time together. Mutual respect is also a boundary issue. Competent families respect and value the individual's opinions and feelings. The family system tolerates individual differences and honors different opinions.

Boundaries are a social construction and, as such, are culturally determined. What appears to be a boundary violation in one culture may be acceptable in another culture. For example, how family members respect privacy in regard to toileting, bathing, changing clothes, and sleeping arrangements varies by culture. Multigenerational boundaries in terms of power and authority vary from culture to culture.

Family Cohesion

Family cohesion is defined as the emotional bonding between family members. There are four levels of cohesion (Figure 10–5 ■):

1. Disengaged (very low)
2. Separated (low to moderate)
3. Connected (moderate to high)
4. Enmeshed (very high).

In Western, developed societies, it is believed that the central ranges of cohesion (separated and connected) contribute to optimal family competency. The extremes (disengaged or enmeshed) are seen as less adaptive. Disengaged families seem almost like a group of strangers who happen to be living together. There is little loyalty or closeness in a disengaged family. Members of enmeshed families cannot develop a separate identity, and each person must yield autonomy to belong to the family. Uniqueness is experienced as distance, and individuality is viewed as alienation and disloyalty (Olson, 1996). See Box 10–4 for characteristics of family cohesion.

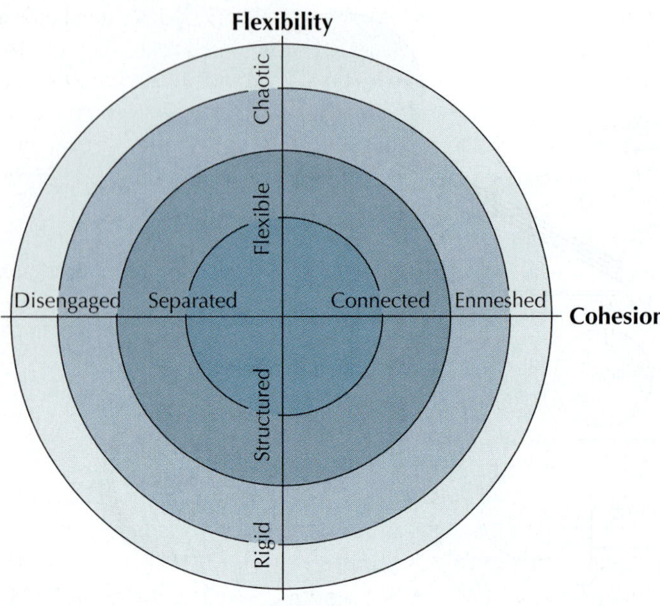

Figure 10–5 ■ Circumplex model.

Family Flexibility

Family flexibility ncludes the amount of change in a family's leadership, role relationships, and relationship rules, but it also refers to the family's ability to respond to stress. There are four levels of flexibility (see Figure 10–5):

1. Rigid (very low)
2. Structured (low to moderate)
3. Flexible (moderate to high)
4. Chaotic (very high).

As with the levels of family cohesion, it is believed that the central ranges (structured and flexible) are more conducive to family adaptation, with the extremes (rigid and chaotic) being less competent (Olson, 1996). See Box 10–5 for characteristics of family flexibility.

Rules determine appropriate roles and relationship patterns within the family. Rules express the family's values, forming a boundary around each family which screens outside information for compatibility with its value system. If the message is not congruent with the family's values, such statements as, "That is not the way we do things in this family," or "I don't care what Marc is allowed to do; in this family, we . . ." will appear. To understand rules more clearly, reflect for a moment on the family in which you grew up. There were certain things that you just did, that you knew were expected of you. Other things were not permitted. To assess a few of the rules in your family of origin, complete the statements in Box 10–6.

Box 10–4 **Characteristics of Family Cohesion**

DISENGAGED
- Little closeness
- Little loyalty
- High independence

SEPARATED
- Low–moderate closeness
- Some loyalty
- Interdependent with more independence than dependence

CONNECTED
- Moderate–high closeness
- High loyalty
- Interdependent with more dependence than independence

ENMESHED
- Very high closeness
- Very high loyalty
- High dependency

Box 10–5 **Characteristics of Family Flexibility**

CHAOTIC
- Lack of leadership
- Dramatic role shifts
- Erratic discipline
- Too much change

FLEXIBLE
- Shared leadership
- Democratic discipline
- Role-sharing change
- Change when necessary

STRUCTURED
- Leadership sometimes shared
- Somewhat democratic discipline
- Roles stable
- Change when demanded

RIGID
- Authoritarian leadership
- Strict discipline
- Roles seldom change
- Too little change

Emotional Availability

Families that cope well encourage their members to express a wide variety of feelings. The emotional climate is one of intimacy and predictability. In other families, the emotional climate may be angry, cold, or distant and unpredictable. **Emotional availability** is another way to describe the quality of parent-child interactions. Areas for assessment include parental sensitivity, structuring, nonintrusiveness, and nonhostility. Parental sensitivity is assessed by how parents pick up on children's emotional signals and how appropriately parents express their own emotions. Parental structuring refers to the ability of parents to support learning and exploration without overwhelming the child's autonomy. Parental nonintrusiveness refers to the parents' availability to the child without being interfering, overprotective, or overwhelming. Nonhostility refers to ways of interacting with the child that are patient and pleasant. When angry, parents express their anger in an appropriately controlled manner (Biringen, 2000).

Box 10–6 **Assessing Rules in Your Family of Origin**

In my family, we were never allowed to . . .
In my family, we were always expected to . . .
In my family, girls were required to . . .
In my family, girls were allowed to . . .
In my family, girls were forbidden to . . .
In my family, boys were required to . . .
In my family, boys were allowed to . . .
In my family, boys were forbidden to . . .
In my family, household responsibilities were determined by . . .
In my family, we handled conflict by . . .
In my family, the most important thing in life for women is . . .
In my family, the most important thing in life for men is . . .

Family Competency

Competency is found in many family arrangements. More important than the form or type of family are the family's relational resources and adaptive abilities. The most distinctive trait of competent families is the ability to manage stress productively. Simply put, adaptive families evolve and shift with changing situations. This is often referred to as **resiliency**. Walsh (1998) describes family resiliency as the "process of coming to terms with all that has happened, reaching new emotional and relational equilibrium with changed circumstances, and becoming more resourceful in facing whatever lies ahead." Life crises and developmental transitions can stimulate family growth and transformation. Resilient families make it through crises such as disability and death with a renewed sense of confidence and purpose.

Family Coping Mechanisms

Family coping mechanisms are the behaviors families use to deal with stress or changes imposed from either within or without the family. Coping mechanisms can be viewed as an active method of problem solving developed to meet life's challenges. The coping mechanisms families and family members develop reflect their individual resourcefulness. Families may use coping patterns rather consistently over time or may change their coping strategies when new demands are made on the family. The success of a family largely depends on how well it copes with the stresses it experiences.

Nurses working with families realize the importance of assessing coping mechanisms as a way of determining how families relate to stress. Also important are the resources available to the family. Internal resources, such as knowledge, skills, effective communication patterns, and a sense of mutuality and purpose within the family, assist in the problem-solving process. In addition, external support systems promote coping and adaptation. These external systems may be extended family, friends, religious affiliations, health care professionals, or social service agencies. The development of social support systems is particularly valuable today because many families, due to stress, mobility, or poverty, are isolated from the resources that would traditionally have helped them cope with stress.

10.1 FAMILY HEALTH PROMOTION

KEY TERMS

Feedback, *498*
Input, *497*
Negative feedback, *498*
Output, *498*
Positive feedback, *498*
Structural-Functional theory, *498*
Subsystem, *497*
Suprasystem, *497*
System, *497*
Systems theory, *497*
Throughput, *498*

Basis for Selection of Exemplar

National Institute of Mental Health (NIMH)
ATI NCLEX-RN® test plan

LEARNING OUTCOMES

After reading about this exemplar, you will be able to:

1. Describe the nurse's role in health promotion for the family.
2. Explain the definitions, functions, and developmental stages and tasks of the family.
3. Identify theoretical frameworks used in family health promotion.
4. Identify common risk factors regarding family health.
5. Assess family functioning using the family competency model.
6. Employ evidence-based practice to develop caring interventions using the nursing process for family health promotion.

OVERVIEW

Applying Theoretical Frameworks to Families

A variety of theoretical frameworks provide the nurse with a holistic overview of health promotion for families across the life span. The major theoretical frameworks nurses use in promoting the health of families are systems theory and structural-functional theory.

SYSTEMS THEORY A **system** is a set of interacting identifiable parts or components. The basic concepts of general systems theory were proposed in the 1950s. One of its major proponents, Ludwig von Bertalanffy (1980), introduced **systems theory** as a universal theory that could be applied to many fields of study. Nurses are increasingly using systems theory to understand not only biologic systems but also systems in families, communities, and nursing and health care. General systems theory provides a way of examining interrelationships and deriving principles.

Systems may be complex and the systems components are often studied as **subsystems**. For family systems, the subsystems would be individuals. Looking back up the hierarchy, the systems above other systems are referred to as **suprasystems**—the family is the suprasystem of the individual. See Figure 10–6 ■ for a hierarchy of the human system.

A system depends on the quality and quantity of its input, throughput, output, and feedback. **Input** consists of information,

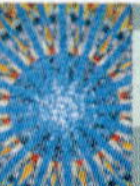

EVIDENCE-BASED PRACTICE Are Adolescent Mothers Able to Promote a Healthy Life for Their Families?

Much of the research on families headed by adolescent mothers has focused on the negative health aspects of these family units. Yet family and community theory suggest that no unit, family, or community will continue to exist with only negative factors. Black and Ford-Gilboe conducted a study with 41 adolescent mothers to test the families' resilience and ability to promote healthy lifestyles. The young mothers were asked to provide verbal responses to items on three questionnaires designed to gather information on the mothers' health-promoting lifestyle practices and demographic background. The results validated the theoretical relationships between increased family resilience and the teenage mother's ability to promote healthy lifestyles for herself and her children.

Implications

Nursing focuses on the complete individual by assessing for both positive and negative health behaviors and risks. In the past, families headed by young single mothers tended to be viewed only in negative terms. By conducting research to examine the positive strengths of these types of family units, nursing is helping to place these families in a more positive light.

Source: Black, C., & Ford-Gilboe, M. (2004). Adolescent mothers: Resilience, family health, work, and health promoting practices. *Journal of Advanced Nursing, 48*, 351–360. Reprinted with permission.

material, or energy that enters the system. After the input is absorbed by the system, it is processed into a form that is useful to the system. This transformation is called **throughput**. For example, food is input to the digestive system; it is digested (throughput) so that it can be used by the body. **Output** from a system is energy, matter, or information the system gives out as a result of its processes. Output from the digestive system includes caloric energy, nutrients, urine, and feces.

Feedback is the mechanism by which some of the output of a system is returned to the system as input. Feedback enables a system to regulate itself by redirecting the system's output back into the system as input, thus forming a feedback loop. This input influences the behavior of the system and its future output. **Negative feedback** inhibits change; **positive feedback** stimulates change.

The biologic system can be subdivided into the neurologic, musculoskeletal, respiratory, circulatory, gastrointestinal, and urinary subsystems, among others. Each subsystem can be subdivided in turn. For example, the urinary system consists of the kidneys, the ureters, and the bladder; the circulatory system consists of the heart and the blood vessels; the neurologic system consists of the brain, the spinal cord, and the nerves. The biologic system can also be subdivided into categories of needs or functional health patterns or activities of daily living, such as nutrition and hydration, sleep/rest, activity/exercise, elimination, and so on.

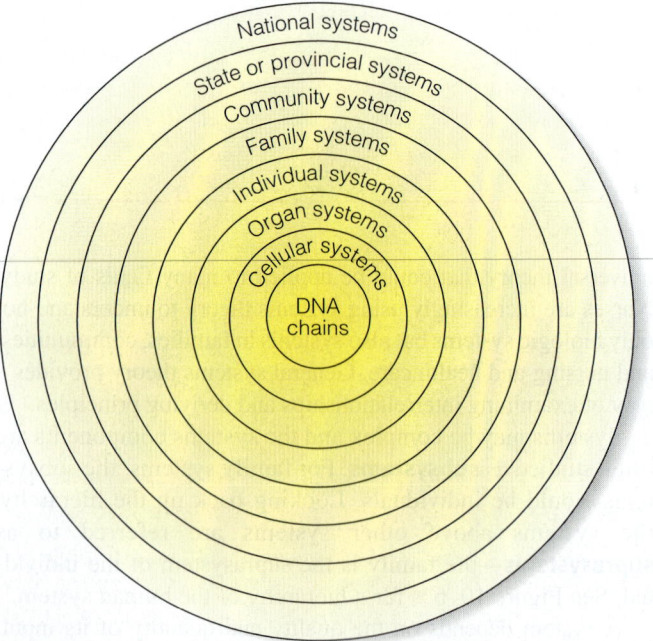

Figure 10–6 ■ A common system hierarchy.

The family unit can also be viewed as a system. Its members are interdependent, working toward specific purposes and goals. Families, as open systems, are continually interacting with and influenced by other systems in the community. Boundaries regulate the input from other systems that interact with the family system; they also regulate output from the family system to the community or to society. Boundaries protect the family from the demands and influences of other systems. Families are likely to welcome input from without, encouraging individual members to adapt beliefs and practices to meet the changing demands of society, seek out health care information, and use community resources.

In understanding the complexity of family systems, consider how family members communicate, how they establish and maintain boundaries, how cohesive and flexible they are, and how emotionally available they are to others in the family. Understanding these interactions will provide a general idea of how well the family is able to adapt and function, both in everyday life and in the face of adversity.

STRUCTURAL-FUNCTIONAL THEORY The **structural-functional theory**, as the name implies, focuses on family structure and function. The structural component of the theory addresses the membership of the family and the relationships among family members. Intrafamily relationships are complex because of the numerous relationships that exist within the family structure—mother–daughter, brother–sister, spouse–partner, and so on. These relationships are constantly evolving as children mature and leave the family nest and as adults age and become more dependent on others to meet their daily needs.

The functional aspect of the theory examines the effects of intrafamily relationships on the family system, as well as their effects on other systems. Some of the main functions of the family include developing a sense of family purpose and affiliation, adding and socializing new members, and providing and distributing care and services to members. A healthy family organizes its members and resources to meet family goals; it functions in harmony, working toward shared goals.

Nurses generally use a combination of theoretical frameworks in promoting the health of individuals and families. For example, the nurse may provide education for the mother of a toddler who is struggling to accomplish the developmental stage of autonomy described by Erikson (1963). Simultaneously, the nurse may guide the same family in its stressful transition period between developmental stages as their older school-age child becomes an adolescent.

Family Developmental Stages and Tasks

The family, like the individual, has developmental stages and tasks. Each stage brings change, requiring adaptation; each new stage also brings family-related risk factors for alterations in health. The nurse must consider the client's needs both at specific developmental stages and within a family with specific developmental tasks. Family developmental stages and developmental tasks are described next; related risk factors and health problems for each stage are listed in Table 10–4.

COUPLE Two people living together (with or without being married) are in a period of establishing themselves as a couple. The developmental tasks of the couple include adjusting to living together as a couple, establishing a mutually satisfying relationship, relating to kin, and deciding whether to have children (in those of child-bearing age).

FAMILY WITH INFANTS AND PRESCHOOLERS The family with infants or preschoolers must adjust to having and supporting the needs of more than two members, with at least one member who is incapable of supporting him- or herself. Other developmental tasks of the family at this stage are developing an attachment between parents and children, adjusting to the economic costs of having more members, coping with energy depletion and lack of privacy, and carrying out activities that enhance growth and development of the children.

FAMILY WITH SCHOOL-AGE CHILDREN The family with school-age children has the developmental tasks of adjusting to the expanded world of children in school and encouraging educational achievement. A further task is promoting joint decision making between children and parents.

FAMILY WITH ADOLESCENTS AND YOUNG ADULTS The developmental tasks of the family with adolescents and young adults focus on transition. While providing a supportive home base and maintaining open communications, parents must balance freedom with responsibility and release adult children as they seek independence.

FAMILY WITH MIDDLE ADULTS The family with middle adults (in which the parents are middle aged and children are no longer at home) has the developmental tasks of maintaining ties with older and younger generations and planning for retirement. If the family consists of just the middle-aged couple, they have the developmental task of reestablishing the relationship and (if necessary) acquiring the role of grandparents.

FAMILY WITH OLDER ADULTS The older adult family has the developmental tasks of adjusting to retirement, adjusting to aging, and coping with the loss of a spouse. If a spouse dies, further tasks include adjusting to living alone or closing the family home.

Risk Factors

RISK FOR HEALTH PROBLEMS Risk assessment helps the nurse identify individuals and groups at higher risk than the general population of developing specific health problems, such as stroke, diabetes, and lung cancer. The vulnerability of family units to health problems may be based on the maturity level of individual family members, heredity or genetic factors, sex or race, sociologic factors, and lifestyle practices.

MATURITY FACTORS Families with members at both ends of the age continuum are at risk of developing health problems. Families entering childbearing and child rearing phases experience many changes in roles, responsibilities, and expectations. The many, often conflicting, demands on the family cause stress and fatigue, either or both of which may impede growth of individual family members and the functioning of the group as a unit. Adolescent mothers, because of their developmental level and lack of knowledge about parenthood, are more likely to develop health problems, as are single-parent families, because of role overload experienced by the head of the household. Many elderly persons feel a lack of purpose and decreased self-esteem. These feelings can reduce their motivation to engage in health-promoting behaviors, such as exercise or community and family involvement.

HEREDITARY FACTORS Persons born into families with a history of certain diseases, such as diabetes or cardiovascular disease, are at greater risk of developing these conditions. A detailed family health history that includes genetically transmitted disorders is crucial to the identification of persons and families at risk. These data are used not only to monitor the health of individual family members, but also to recommend modifications in health practices that potentially reduce the risk, minimize the consequences, or postpone the development of genetically related conditions.

GENDER OR RACE FACTORS Some family units or family members may be at risk of developing a disease by reason of gender or race. Men, for example, are at greater risk of having cardiovascular disease at an earlier age than women, and women are at greater risk of developing osteoporosis, particularly after menopause. Although it is sometimes difficult to separate genetic factors from cultural factors, certain risk factors seem to be related to race. Sickle cell anemia, for example, is a hereditary disease limited to people of African descent, and Tay-Sachs is a neurodegenerative disease that occurs primarily in descendants of eastern European Jews.

SOCIOLOGIC FACTORS Poverty is a major problem that affects not only the family but also the community and society. Poverty is a real concern among the rising number of single-parent families. As the number of these families increases, poverty will affect a larger number of growing children.

TABLE 10–4 **Family-Related Risk Factors for Alterations in Health**

STAGE	RISK FACTORS	HEALTH PROBLEMS
Couple, or family with infants and preschoolers	■ Lack of knowledge about family planning, contraception, and sexual and marital roles ■ Inadequate prenatal care ■ Altered nutrition: inadequate nutrition, overweight, underweight ■ Smoking, alcohol/drug abuse ■ Lack of knowledge about child health and safety ■ Low socioeconomic status ■ First pregnancy before age 16 or after age 35 ■ Rubella, syphilis, gonorrhea, AIDS	■ Premature pregnancy ■ Low-birth-weight infant ■ Birth defects ■ Injury to infant or child ■ Accidents
Family with school-age children	■ Unsafe home environment ■ Working parents with inappropriate or inadequate resources for child care ■ Low socioeconomic status ■ Child abuse or neglect ■ Multiple, closely spaced children ■ Repeated infections, accidents, and hospitalizations ■ Unrecognized and unattended health problems ■ Poor or inappropriate nutrition ■ Toxic substances in the home	■ Behavior problems ■ Speech and vision problems ■ Learning disabilities ■ Communicable diseases ■ Physical abuse ■ Cancer ■ Developmental delay ■ Obesity, underweight
Family with adolescents and young adults	■ Family values of aggressiveness and competition ■ Lifestyle and behavior leading to chronic illness (substance abuse, inadequate diet) ■ Lack of problem-solving skills ■ Conflicts between parent and children	■ Violent death and injury ■ Alcohol/drug abuse ■ Unwanted pregnancy ■ Suicide ■ Sexually transmitted infections ■ Domestic abuse
Family with middle adults	■ High-cholesterol diet ■ Overweight ■ Hypertension ■ Smoking, alcohol abuse ■ Physical inactivity ■ Personality patterns related to stress ■ Exposure to environment: sunlight, radiation, asbestos, or water or air pollution ■ Depression ■ Age	■ Cardiovascular disease (coronary artery disease and cerebrovascular disease) ■ Cancer ■ Accidents ■ Suicide ■ Mental illness
Family with older adults	■ Depression ■ Drug interactions ■ Chronic illness ■ Death of spouse ■ Reduced income ■ Poor nutrition ■ Lack of exercise ■ Past environment and lifestyle	■ Impaired vision and hearing ■ Hypertension ■ Acute illness ■ Chronic illness ■ Infectious diseases (influenza, pneumonia) ■ Injuries from burns and falls ■ Depression ■ Alcohol abuse

When ill, the poor are likely to put off seeking services until the illness reaches an advanced state and requires longer or more complex treatment. Although the health of the people of industrialized nations has improved significantly during the past century, this progress has not benefited all segments of society, particularly the poor.

LIFESTYLE FACTORS Many diseases are preventable, the effects of some diseases can be minimized, or the onset of disease can be delayed through lifestyle modifications. Certain cancers, cardiovascular disease, adult-onset diabetes, and tooth decay are among the lifestyle diseases. The incidence of lung cancer, for example, would be greatly reduced if people stopped smoking. Good nutrition, dental hygiene, and use of fluoride—in the water supply, in toothpaste, as a topical application, or as a supplement—have been shown to reduce dental decay or caries, one of America's most prevalent health problems.

Other important lifestyle considerations are exercise, stress management, and rest. Today, health professionals have the knowledge to prevent or minimize the effects of some of the main causes of disease, disability, and death. The challenge is to disseminate information about prevention and to motivate families to make lifestyle changes before the onset of illness.

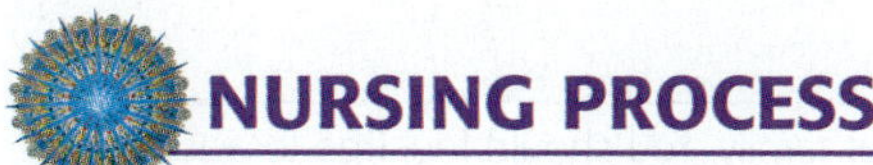

NURSING PROCESS

Assessment

Family Assessment Tools

Family assessment tools can be used to gather additional information about the family's functioning and can place particular focus on family stresses, coping strategies, and family strengths. Information about the way the family functions in nurturing its members, problem solving, and communicating may help identify strategies that are potentially more effective for managing the child's health care. These strategies, such as collaborating with the family in planning for health maintenance and health promotion strategies, enable the nurse to work more effectively with the family.

Family Ecomap

An ecomap illustrates the family's relationships and interactions with the social networks in the community, enabling the nurse and other health care providers to visualize the family's social network. By having family members participate in preparing the ecomap, it is possible to obtain information about how the family perceives or receives social support, as well as the strength of family relationships with significant other persons and organizations. The ecomap provides an opportunity to identify the community resources the family uses and to highlight any potential community resources that may help promote the family's health. See Figure 10–7 ■ for a sample ecomap.

Family APGAR

The Family APGAR is a quick five-item questionnaire that may be used as an initial screening tool for family assessment. The five family concepts measured are family adaptability, partnership, growth, affection, and resolve (Table 10–5). This five-item questionnaire can be administered quickly to family members over 10 years of age. Ask all family members to complete a separate copy of the questionnaire to gain a picture of the family's perspective on family functioning. Be concerned if the majority of responses fall in the "hardly ever" category or if responses vary a lot among family members. This may indicate a family that needs much more support to cope with the demands of daily life and provide insight into health maintenance and health promotion needs.

Home Observation for Measurement of the Environment (HOME)

The HOME Inventory is an assessment tool developed to measure the quality and quantity of stimulation and support available in the home environment (Caldwell & Bradley, 1984). Four age-specific scales are available (birth to 3 years,

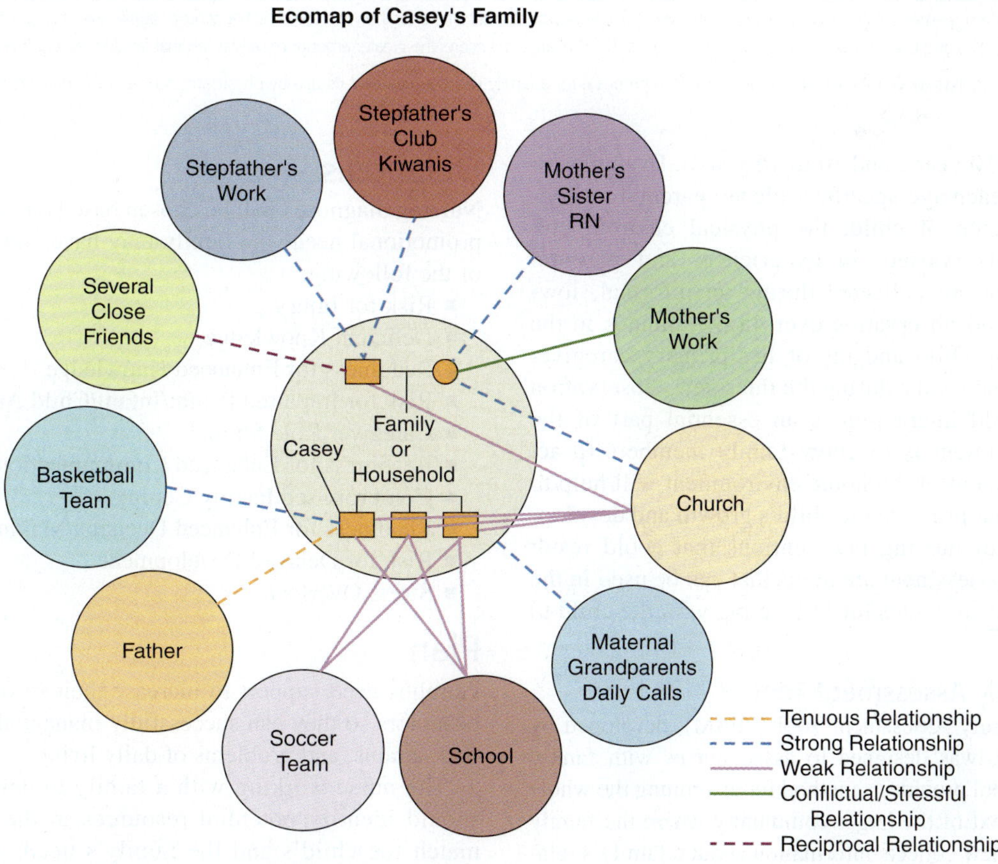

Figure 10–7 ■ An ecomap illustrates the family's relationships and interactions with groups and individuals in the immediate external environment.

TABLE 10–5 The Family APGAR Questionnaire

Directions: The following questions have been designed to help us better understand you and your family. You should feel free to ask questions about any item in the questionnaire. The space for comments should be used when you wish to give additional information or if you wish to discuss how the question is applied to your family. Please try to answer all questions. Family is defined as the individual(s) with whom you usually live. If you live alone, your "family" consists of persons with whom you now have the strongest emotional ties.*

For each question, check only one box.

	ALMOST ALWAYS 2	SOME OF THE TIME 1	HARDLY EVER 0
I am satisfied that I can turn to my family for help when something is troubling me. Comments:______			
I am satisfied with the way my family talks over things with me and shares problems with me. Comments:______			
I am satisfied that my family accepts and supports my wishes to take on new activities or directions. Comments:______			
I am satisfied with the way my family expresses affection and responds to my emotions, such as anger, sorrow, and love. Comments:______			
I am satisfied with the way my family and I share time together. Comments:______			

**Note:* Depending on which member of the family is being interviewed, the interviewer may substitute for the word *family* either *spouse*, *significant other*, *parents*, or *children*. Responses are scored 2, 1, 0 and totaled. The total score ranges from 0 to 10. The larger the score, the greater amount of satisfaction that family member has with family functioning.

Source: Adapted from: Smilkstein, G. (1978). The family APGAR: A proposal for a family function test and its use by physicians. *Journal of Family Practice,* (6), 1231–1239.

3 to 6 years, 6 to 10 years, and 10 to 15 years). Examples of subscales within each age-specific scale are parental responsiveness, acceptance of child, the physical environment, learning materials, variety in experience, and parental involvement. Data are collected during an informal, low-stress interview and observation over 45–90 minutes in the home setting. The child and his or her primary caregiver must be present and awake during the interview. Observation of the parent–child interaction is an essential part of the assessment. The intent is to allow family members to act normally. Assessment of the home environment will help to identify factors that promote the child's growth and development. Examples of nursing interventions that could result from the HOME assessment are items that can be used in the home for toys and strategies for interacting with the child to promote learning.

Friedman Family Assessment Tool

The Friedman Family Assessment Tool (FFAM), developed by Marilyn Friedman, was designed to assist nurses with family assessment. This tool provides a method for examining the whole family in the context of the larger community where the family resides. The interview collects information about a family's relationships, functioning, strengths, and problems. The short form for this assessment tool is provided in Box 10–7.

Diagnosis

Nursing diagnoses will be chosen based on what type of health promotional needs the family may have and may include any of the following:

- Risk for Injury
- Deficient Knowledge
- Readiness for Enhanced Knowledge
- Risk for Impaired Parent/Infant/Child Attachment
- Caregiver Role Strain
- Readiness for Enhanced Communication
- Compromised Family Coping
- Readiness for Enhanced Decision Making
- Risk for Delayed Development
- Stress Overload.

Plan

Families need support to increase their resources and coping behaviors so they can successfully manage the multiple stressors, strains, and problems of daily living.

The nurse working with a family to develop a care plan should identify potential resources in the community that match the child's and the family's needs for support. The nurse will collaborate with the family to discuss those resources and to select the ones that are acceptable to the

Box 10–7 **Friedman Family Assessment Tool**

The following form is shortened for ease in assessing a family. If you are not sure what data should be covered in each of the assessment areas, please refer to the original reference, where more detailed questions/areas are presented.

Before using the following guidelines in completing family assessments, note that not all areas included will be germane for each of the families visited. The guidelines are comprehensive and allow depth when probing is necessary. Do not feel that every subarea needs to be covered when the broad area of inquiry poses no problems to the family or concern to the health worker. Second, by virtue of the interdependence of the family system, opportunities for repetition will arise. The assessor should try not to repeat data, but to refer the reader back to sections where this information has already been described.

IDENTIFYING DATA

1. Family Name
2. Address and Phone
3. Family Composition: The Family Genogram
4. Type of Family Form
5. Cultural (Ethnic) Background
6. Religious Identification
7. Social Class Status
8. Social Class Mobility

DEVELOPMENTAL STAGE AND HISTORY OF FAMILY

9. Family's Present Developmental Stage
10. Extent of Family Developmental Tasks Fulfillment
11. Nuclear Family History
12. History of Family of Origin of Both Parents

ENVIRONMENTAL DATA

13. Characteristics of Home
14. Characteristics of Neighborhood and Larger Community
15. Family's Geographical Mobility
16. Family's Associations and Transactions With Community

FAMILY STRUCTURE

17. Communication Patterns
    - Extent of Functional and Dysfunctional Communication (types of recurring patterns)
    - Extent of Emotional (Affective) Messages and How Expressed
    - Characteristics of Communication Within Family Subsystems
    - Extent of Congruent and Incongruent Messages
    - Types of Dysfunctional Communication Processes Seen in Family
    - Areas of Closed Communication
    - Familial and Contextual Variables Affecting Communication
18. Power Structure
    - Power Outcomes
    - Decision-Making Process
    - Power Bases
    - Variables Affecting Family Power
    - Overall Family System and Subsystem Power (Family Power Continuum Placement)
19. Role Structure
    - Formal Role Structure
    - Informal Role Structure
    - Analysis of Role Models (optional)
    - Variables Affecting Role Structure
20. Family Values
    - Compare the family to American core values or family's reference group values and/or identify important family values and their importance (priority) in family
    - Congruence Between the Family's Values and the Family's Reference Group or Wider Community
    - Disparity in Value Systems
    - Presence of Value Conflicts in Family
    - Effect of the Above Values and Value Conflicts on Health
    - Status of Family

(continued)

Box 10–7 **Friedman Family Assessment Tool** (continued)

FAMILY FUNCTIONS

21. Affective Function
    - Mutual Nurturance, Closeness, and Identification
    - Separateness and Connectedness
    - Family's Need-Response Patterns
22. Socialization Function
    - Family Childrearing Practices
    - Adaptability of Childrearing Practices for Family Form and Family's Situation
    - Who Is (Are) Socializing Agent(s) for Child(ren)?
    - Value of Children in Family
    - Cultural Beliefs That Influence Family's Childrearing Patterns
    - Social Class Influence on Childrearing Patterns
    - Estimation About Whether Family Is at Risk for Childrearing Problems and if so, Indication of High-Risk Factors
    - Adequacy of Home Environment for Children's Needs to Play
23. Health Care Function
    - Family's Health Beliefs, Values, and Behavior
    - Family's Definitions of Health-Illness and Its Level of Knowledge
    - Family's Perceived Health Status and Illness Susceptibility
    - Family's Dietary Practices
    - Adequacy of Family Diet (recommended 3-day food history record)
    - Function of Mealtimes and Attitudes Toward Food and Mealtimes
    - Shopping (and its planning) Practices
    - Person(s) Responsible for Planning, Shopping, and Preparation of Meals
    - Sleep and Rest Habits
    - Physical Activity and Recreation Practices
    - Family's Therapeutic and Recreational Drug, Alcohol, and Tobacco Practices
    - Family's Role in Self-Care Practices
    - Medically Based Preventive Measures (physicals, eye and hearing tests, immunizations, dental care)
    - Complementary and Alternative Therapies
    - Family Health History (both general and specific diseases—environmentally and genetically related)
    - Health Care Services Received
    - Feelings and Perceptions Regarding Health Services
    - Emergency Health Services
    - Source of Payments for Health and Other Services
    - Logistics of Receiving Care

FAMILY STRESS, COPING, AND ADAPTATION

24. Family Stressors, Strengths, and Perceptions
    - Stressors Family is Experiencing
    - Strengths That Counterbalance Stressors
    - Family's Definition of the Situation
25. Family Coping Strategies
    - How the Family Is Reacting to the Stressors
    - Extent of Family's Use of Internal Coping Strategies (past/present)
    - Extent of Family's Use of External Coping Strategies (past/present)
    - Dysfunctional Coping Strategies Used (past/present; extent of use)
26. Family Adaptation
    - Overall Family Adaptation
    - Estimation of Whether Family is in Crisis
27. Tracking Stressors, Coping, and Adaptation Over Time

Source: Friedman, M. M., Bowden, V. R., & Jones, E. G. (2003). *Family nursing: Research, theory, and practice* (5th ed., pp. 593–594). Upper Saddle River, NJ: Prentice Hall. Reprinted with permission.

NURSING CARE PLAN

ASSESSMENT	DIAGNOSES	PLANNING
Ms. Blankenship, a single mother, brings her 2-year-old son in for routine immunizations. After he has received his immunizations, while waiting the required 20 minutes before leaving, Ms. Blankenship reveals that she recently lost her job because her child became ill and she had to miss work. She says that she has found a new job, but that the salary is much lower and she will not be able to afford day care for the child. She is considering taking the job anyway because she would be working nights and the child sleeps through the night. She spoke with a neighbor who has agreed to listen for him in case he awakens.	■ Decisional Conflict ■ Compromised Family Coping ■ Risk for Impaired Parenting	■ Ms. Blankenship will be able to state the risks related to leaving a child home alone. ■ Ms. Blankenship will learn of other resources available to help her care for her child in a safe environment. ■ Ms. Blankenship will discuss available choices she has without risking child's safety.

IMPLEMENTATION

- Assess client's understanding of available choices.
- Provide information about risks associated with leaving child home alone.
- Teach problem-solving and decision-making processes.
- Provide referrals to social services to help meet financial needs.
- Provide decision-making support.

EVALUATION

Ms. Blankenship has an appointment to meet with social services and has decided not to make a decision until she has an opportunity to explore other options. She has enrolled in a once-a-week parenting class that provides on-site child care during each class.

CRITICAL THINKING

1. Is the diagnosis of risk for impaired parenting accurate? Why or why not?
2. Upon calling Ms. Blankenship and making the evaluation, what else can the nurse do to help Ms. Blankenship meet her outcomes?
3. If Ms. Blankenship made the choice to leave the child home alone at night, what would your obligation as a nurse require you to do?

family, to increase the likelihood that the family will follow through with the plan. In some cases it may be necessary to collaborate with a multidisciplinary team, including social workers to help the family obtain assistance to overcome barriers such as transportation, financial, geographic, and any other that interfere with the child's health care. The nurse should make sure the family has a care coordinator, especially when a family member initially seems unable to assume the case management role. The nurse may also assist the family in obtaining resources by such actions as role rehearsal, providing instructions and support when making an initial call, or connecting with another family support person who can help with resource linkage. The nurse will refer families with moderate or severe dysfunction to community resources for social support and counseling as appropriate.

Outcomes are determined based on the needs of the family and may include any of the following:

- Children will achieve developmental milestones in social, self-regulatory behavior or cognitive, language, or gross or fine motor skills.
- Family will display or describe actions to manage stressors that tax family resources.
- Family system will meet the needs of its members during developmental transitions.
- Family members will demonstrate actions to improve the overall health and social competence of family unit.

Implementation

Establishing a therapeutic relationship with the family is an important intervention in and of itself. This relationship should be characterized by empathy and trust, as well as the development of mutually identified goals for the family's needs. To help families develop resiliency, the nurse should focus on family competence and strengths, and acknowledge and validate their emotions. The nurse provides information in a clear, timely, and sensitive manner. Questions are asked to help direct the family's thinking rather than providing them with all of the answers. The nurse works with families by teaching them to identify solutions until they are able to problem solve independently. The family's ethnic and religious background need to be considered in developing intervention recommendations.

Evaluation

Evaluation will be based on the family's progress toward goals and outcomes mutually determined by the family and nurse. The following are indicators that outcomes are being met and progress is being achieved:

- Family members' behaviors collectively demonstrate cohesion, strength, and emotional bonding.
- The family system has the capacity to successfully adapt and function competently after adversity or crisis.

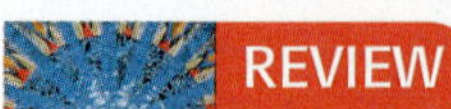

REVIEW Family Health Promotion

RELATE: LINK THE CONCEPTS

Linking the exemplar of Family Health Promotion with the concept of Culture:

1. How does the nurse incorporate the family's cultural beliefs into health promotion teaching?
2. How might the family's cultural beliefs impact their health behaviors?

Linking the exemplar of Family Health Promotion with the concept of Advocacy:

3. How can the nurse advocate for the vulnerable population family in the community?
4. What responsibilities does the nurse have to advocate for families?

REFER: GO TO MYNURSINGKIT

REFLECT: CASE STUDY

The home health nurse has been visiting a 90-year-old woman and her younger sister who live alone in a large farmhouse. The women have been active in caring for each other and their residence. During one of the home visits, they confide that the farm is too much for them, but they admit that they do not want to tell their families because they are afraid that they will be put into a nursing home.

1. What community resources are available to assist the sisters to live independently?
2. How should the family be involved in the decision making?
3. What signs can alert the nurse that the sisters are unable to care for themselves?
4. Should the nurse contact the family without the sisters' knowledge? Why or why not?

10.2 FAMILY RESPONSE TO HEALTH ALTERATIONS

KEY TERMS

Family burden, *507*
Family recovery, *508*
Family support, *509*
Friend support, *509*
Objective family burden, *507*
Professional support, *509*
Spiritual support, *509*
Stigma, *507*
Subjective family burden, *508*

LEARNING OUTCOMES

After reading about this exemplar, you will be able to do the following:

1. Create a nursing care plan utilizing the nursing process to support family functioning when facing health alterations in a family member.
2. List the categories of family strengths that help families develop and cope with stressors.
3. Identify a variety of family support services that might be available in a community.
4. Describe how family type may influence nursing care of the childbearing family.

Basis for Selection of Exemplar

Centers for Disease Control and Prevention (CDC)
The Joint Commission (JCAHO)
Institute for Healthcare Improvement (IHI)

OVERVIEW

Although some clients are totally alone in the world, most have one or more people who are significant in their lives. These significant others may be related or bonded to the client by birth, adoption, marriage, or friendship. Although not always meeting traditional definitions, people (or even pets) significant to the client are the client's family. The nurse includes the family as an integral component of care in all health care settings.

Illness of a family member is a crisis that affects the entire family system. The family is disrupted as members abandon their usual activities and focus their energy on restoring family equilibrium. Roles and responsibilities the ill person previously assumed are delegated to other family members, or those functions remain undone for the duration of the illness. The family experiences anxiety because members are concerned about the sick person and the resolution of the illness. This anxiety is compounded by additional responsibilities when there is less time or motivation to complete the normal tasks of daily living. See Box 10–8 for some factors that determine the impact of illness on the family unit.

The family's ability to deal with the stress of illness depends on the members' coping skills. Families with good communication skills are better able to discuss how they feel about the illness and how it affects family functioning. They

Box 10–8 Factors Determining the Impact of Illness on the Family

- The nature of the ilness, which can range from minor to life threatening
- The duration of the illness
- The residual effects of the illness, ranging from none to permanent disability
- The meaning of the illness to the family and its significance to family systems
- The financial impact of the illness, which is influenced by factors such as insurance and ability of the ill member to return to work
- The effect of the illness on future family functioning (for instance, previous patterns may be restored or new patterns may be established)

can plan for the future and are flexible in adapting these plans as the situation changes. An established social support network provides strength, encouragement, and services to the family during the illness. During health crises, families must realize that turning to others for support is a sign of strength rather than weakness. Nurses can be part of the support system for families, or they can identify other sources of support in the community.

During a crisis, families are often drawn together by a common purpose. In this time of closeness, family members have the opportunity to reaffirm personal and family values and their commitment to one another. Indeed, illness may provide a unique opportunity for family growth.

The Nurse's Role With Families Experiencing Illness

Nurses committed to family-centered care involve both the ailing individual and the family in the nursing process. Through their interaction with families, nurses can give support and information, although the ailing individual needs to give permission regarding what information can be shared with family members. Nurses make sure that not only the individual but also each family member understands the disease, its management, and the effect of these two factors on family functioning.

The Family of the Client With a Chronic Illness

The client with a chronic illness may be hospitalized for diagnosis and treatment when he or she experiences acute exacerbations, but the care of the client is primarily and usually provided at home. Chronic illness in a family member is a major stressor that may cause changes in family structure and function, as well as in how family developmental tasks are performed.

Many different factors affect family responses to chronic illness; family responses in turn affect the client's response to and perception of the illness. Factors influencing response to chronic illness include personal, social, and economic resources; the nature and course of the disease; and demands of the illness as perceived by family members. Clients with chronic illness, and their families, may be at risk for depression. Nursing considerations for a client with a chronic illness include being alert to symptoms of depression, both in the client and in his or her close family members.

PATHOPHYSIOLOGY AND ETIOLOGY

Severe Mental Illness and the Family System

Family members of individuals with mental illness often share in the many losses that accompany the illness. Families are the major source of support and rehabilitation for their loved ones. Of clients discharged from acute care, 65% return to their families. At any given time, 40–50% of the 48 million Americans who are severely and persistently mentally ill live with their families on a regular basis. Even when clients do not live at home, the families are often the only source of support. In the United States, care for the mentally ill has become as much family based as community based. Caring for a mentally ill family member can result in overwhelming emotional and economic stress on the family system (Rose, Mallinson, & Gerson, 2006). In an ideal world, family members would be supportive and effective in dealing with an ill family member. The person with the mental disorder (client) would not act out (or threaten to act out). In reality, family relationships can be conflicted. When clients try to assert their autonomy, families worry about what will happen and become critical or try to control the situation. As families struggle with guilt and fear, clients feel rejected and abandoned. Clients may also experience shame over being mistrusted and monitored.

Family Burden

Families have important needs of their own in response to their loved one's mental illness. Severe and persistent mental illness often puts the family under catastrophic levels of stress. As families respond to the grief and trauma, they need empathy and support from health care professionals.

Family burden is the overall level of distress experienced as a result of the mental illness. The **objective family burden** is related to the actual, identifiable family problems associated with the person's mental illness. One burden the family must manage relates to *symptomatic behaviors*. The family's loved one's deficit behaviors—such as lack of motivation, difficulty in completing tasks, isolation from others, inability to manage money, poor grooming and personal care, and poor eating and sleeping behavior—can be of great concern to families. Intrusive or acting-out behaviors—such as lack of consideration for others, excessive arguing, conflicts with neighbors and friends, damaging material possessions, inappropriate sexual behavior, suicide attempts, substance abuse, and violent outbursts—are very disturbing to family members. These behaviors may be more episodic than the deficit behaviors but may have more severe immediate consequences. This family burden may lead to loss of independence and increased responsibility as families try to cope with day-to-day living. This burden includes disruption in household functioning, restriction of social activities, and financial hardship due to medical bills and the cost of their loved one's economic burden.

Another objective burden related to family problems is caregiving. Families may find that community services are not always available and not always satisfactory. Inadequate funding results in lack of treatment programs and lack of services for families themselves. Families also find themselves negotiating with the legal and criminal justice system. With few long-term psychiatric facilities available, many people who would have previously been cared for in state hospitals now find themselves in jails and prisons. Often, the "crimes" with which they are charged are misdemeanors resulting from their symptoms of mental illness, such as disorderly conduct, trespassing, and drunkenness.

A third objective burden that families must cope with is the burden of **stigma**, which is a collection of negative attitudes and beliefs that lead people to fear, reject, avoid, and discriminate against people with mental illness. In response to stigma, people with mental disorders internalize these attitudes and become ashamed of themselves and their illness. People with mental illness continue to be ostracized from mainstream society. Families may become isolated as they avoid others who misunderstand the illness. When a family member has cancer or heart disease, other people respond with kindness. When a family member has a mental disorder, the response is often avoidance because there is a perception of unpredictability and danger. Thus, stigma severely limits support from extended family and friends. As they and their loved one face multiple discriminations, families may feel isolated and shameful, may lose self-esteem, and may run the risk of self-stigmatization (Rose, Mallinson, & Gerson, 2006; Stengler-Wenzke, Trosbach, Dietrich, & Angermeyer, 2004).

The **subjective family burden** is defined as the psychological distress of the family members in relation to the objective burden. They often experience frustration, anxiety, depression, hopelessness, and helplessness. Families also experience intense feelings of grief and loss. They must mourn for the person they knew before the onset of the illness and the potential loss of hopes, dreams, and expectations. They live with a sense of chronic sorrow for those loved ones who experience periods of remission and relapse. There is also a sense of empathetic pain as they watch their family member become a victim of the illness. Living with and caring for a person with mental illness can have a tremendous impact on the family. Some families cope fairly well, whereas others are easily exhausted and give up (Jungbauer, Wittmund, Dietrich, & Angermeyer, 2003). See Box 10–9 for descriptions of the language of family pain.

Family Recovery

Family response to the mental illness of a family member can vary depending on what stage the family (or members of a family) is in. Family response, formally known as "**family recovery**" to mental illness within the family, has three pronounced stages. A nurse may adjust his or her approach adjust caring interventions for a family depending on the family's stage of recovery.

Box 10–9 The Language of Family Pain

Catastrophe: Watching as your loved one slips away. This is like a horror movie in which the hero/heroine (loved one) is utterly transformed by some unseen, monstrous force.

Torture: The agony of watching a loved one experience relentless pain and suffering without being able to make it stop. The absolute panic when he or she refuses your assistance, rejects your help, resists your protection at the time when it is most needed.

Anguish: The pain of having loved ones turn on those who are trying to help them, attack them angrily, or blame them for their difficulties.

Horror/fear: A dread that the ill person will do something terrible to his- or herself or others.

Nightmare: Rejection, labeling, and ostracism by the mental health system when we are trying to help.

Source: Reprinted with permission from Burland, J. (1999). *NAMI provided education program*. Arlington, VA: National Alliance for the Mentally Ill.

Stage 1 of family recovery involves discovery and denial. Family members are often the first to notice that another member is exhibiting unusual behavior. The family's initial response may range from minimizing (it's not so serious) to denial (it's just a phase). This response is a temporary, rather than maladaptive, reaction to avoid a painful reality. As the family members attempt to explain the changes to others, they may attribute the changes to something more socially acceptable than mental illness. For example, they might tell others that the person is suffering from exhaustion or an endocrine problem, or that stress at school or work is causing the difficulties. Others' prejudice and the family's avoidance of stigma can lead to family isolation and loss of relationships outside the immediate family system.

Stage 2 of family recovery involves recognition and acceptance. As it becomes more evident that a significant problem exists, families begin to search for reasons and solutions by gathering available information. Families start to develop their own image of the disease process and expectations of mental health professionals. Many families also hope for what was in the past and for what might be in the future. It is very sad to lose a close family member to mental illness. Many people do not believe that mental illness is a brain disease. If the disorder begins in childhood, it is easier to think that it is a result of bad parenting because good parenting should be able to fix it. That is like telling parents of a child with leukemia that if they were better parents they could stop those white cells from growing. When a person experiences a mental disorder, expectations and dreams may necessitate alteration. Some clients come through the experience of mental illness able to develop meaningful and productive lives. Others, who do not respond to current treatment strategies, may have to grieve the loss of their hopes and dreams (Tweedell, Forchuk, Jewell, & Steinnagel, 2004).

Stage 3 of family recovery involves coping and competence. This includes the day-to-day efforts necessary to cope with all the changes in the family. When people become persistently and severely mentally ill, they may have difficulty carrying out their family roles and responsibilities. In this case, other family members must assume those roles and come to terms with an altered family lifestyle. Family members develop cognitive, emotional, and behavioral coping strategies to live with their loved one who is experiencing a mental disorder. As they take stock of the challenges, constraints, and resources, they are better able to make the most of their options.

Coping strategies protect the affected family member and maintain the stability of family functioning. These strategies include expressing affection, suggesting alternatives, reducing conflict, seeking social support, and trying to make the best of the family members' experiences by focusing on the positive parts of the relationship with the ill family member.

Rose (1997) describes four family support sources:

- Professional support
- Friend support
- Family support
- Spiritual support.

Professional support may come from any one or a number of professionals in the community who exhibit a nonblaming and respectful attitude toward families, and who provide information on how to respond to symptoms and help in locating community resources, such as housing or vocational training. **Friend support** comes from non-family members, such as close friends and coworkers. Friend support is most valued when the concern is genuine and stigma is minimized. **Family support** often comes in the form of tangible assistance, such as respite care for family members and physical presence in times of crisis. Many families find emotional strength from their religious faith. They find **spiritual support** as they search for meaning through relationships and feeling connected with others. Supportive relationships build and sustain courage, helping families make the best of their difficult lives.

When families learn to cope effectively, the intense focus on the ill family member lightens as other members, moving through the adjustment process, begin to focus on caring for themselves and reconnecting with others outside the family. The family adapts to its changed circumstances and continues to function successfully.

The final stage of family recovery is personal and political advocacy. This stage involves working with the mental health system to obtain treatment. Family members want to be seen as partners in treatment and do not want to be excluded from discussions and treatment recommendations. Ideally, professionals, clients, and families all work together in joint problem solving. At times, the issue of client confidentiality is raised. Family members generally respect confidentiality but do need information about treatments, medications, resources, and ways to cope with certain behaviors.

Some families go on to educate the public about mental illness and lobby for improved public policy and legislation, often through the National Alliance on Mental Illness (NAMI), an organization composed of clients, families, and professionals. NAMI actively lobbies for improved legislation and improved health care benefits at local, state, and federal levels.

FAMILY-CENTERED CARE IN PEDIATRIC NURSING

Family-centered care is a philosophy of health care in which a mutually beneficial partnership develops between families, the nurse, and other health professionals as appropriate. In this way the priorities and needs of the family are addressed when the family seeks health care for the child. Each party respects the knowledge, skills, and experience that the other brings to the health care encounter (Table 10–6). This contrasts family-focused care, in which health professionals provide care from the position of an expert. In family-focused care, the expert health professional directs care, tells the family what to do, and intervenes for the child and family as a unit.

TABLE 10–6 **Elements of Family-Centered Care and Recommendations for Nursing Practice**

ELEMENTS	NURSING PRACTICE RECOMMENDATIONS
Family at the center: Incorporate into policy and practice the recognition that the family is the constant in a child's life, while the service systems and support personnel within those systems fluctuate, and that the illness or injury of a child affects all members of the family system.	■ Establish a therapeutic relationship with the family. ■ Perform a comprehensive family assessment in collaboration with the family, identifying both strengths and needs. ■ Use the family assessment when working with the family to plan, implement, and evaluate care, considering the impact of the child's illness or injury on the entire family, with special attention to the siblings. ■ Provide siblings with information about their sibling's illness/injury at an appropriate developmental level and answer questions honestly. ■ Promote sibling visitation in hospital settings and participation in home care activities. ■ Identify extended family members who should receive information and be included in the educational process.
Family-professional collaboration: Facilitate family professional collaboration at all levels of hospital, home, and community care for the following: ■ Care of an individual child ■ Program development, implementation, evaluation, and evolution ■ Policy formation	■ Develop provider–family relationships that are guided by goals and expectations of both the family and the provider. ■ Ensure that parents are integral and critical collaborators in the decision-making process about their child's care. Involve children and adolescents in the decision-making process as appropriate for their cognitive and emotional development. ■ Assure parents 24-hour access to their children and facilitate their participation in the child's care. ■ Provide parents with the option to stay with their child during procedures and tests, and provide ways for the parent to support the child during the procedure. ■ Provide comfort and hygiene facilities for families who spend long hours at the facility or travel great distances. ■ Promote the family's development of expertise in the special care of their child, fostering family independence and empowerment. ■ Incorporate parents and children into the quality assessment/improvement process. ■ Integrate family members into institutional and community advisory groups and in policy development.

(continued)

TABLE 10–6 **Elements of Family-Centered Care and Recommendations for Nursing Practice (continued)**

ELEMENTS	NURSING PRACTICE RECOMMENDATIONS
Family-professional communication: Exchange complete and unbiased information between families and professionals in a supportive manner at all times.	■ Provide information about the child's problem, prognosis, and needs in a manner that respects the child and family as individuals and promotes two-way dialogue. ■ Encourage the family to share information about the child and the illness/injury so that care planning and decisions are made in the most informed and collaborative manner.
Cultural diversity of families: Incorporate into policy and practice the recognition and honoring of cultural diversity, strengths, and individuality within and across all families, including ethnic, racial, spiritual, social, economic, educational, and geographic diversity.	■ Practice family-centered care in a culturally competent manner with respect and sensitivity for the wide range of families with diverse values and beliefs. ■ Seek to understand the family's beliefs and practices related to race, culture, and ethnicity when developing relationships and collaborating in the child's health care. ■ Seek to understand and respect the family's religious/spiritual beliefs and practices and integrate these into the child's care, as the family desires. ■ Assist the family to address care issues related to socioeconomic status, insurance status, geography, and access to health care. ■ Integrate training programs on diversity, cultural understanding, and culturally competent care into staff development programs.
Coping differences and support: Recognize and respect different methods of coping. Implement comprehensive policies and programs that provide families with the developmental, educational, emotional, spiritual, environmental, and financial supports needed to meet their diverse needs.	■ Assess the strengths and weaknesses of the family's coping strategies and its resiliency factors and characteristics. Identify maladaptive coping mechanisms and assist the family to augment its coping efforts. ■ Assess and support the family's needs and desires for support and assist the family in accessing and accepting assistance from support networks as needed or desired.
Family-centered peer support: Encourage and facilitate family-to-family support and networking.	■ Educate parents about parent-to-parent and family support resources and assist them to access such resources in the institution and community. ■ Provide access to psychoeducational groups that might be useful to parents, siblings, or ill/injured children.
Specialized service and support systems: Ensure that hospital, home, and community service and support systems for children needing specialized health and developmental care and their families are flexible, accessible, and comprehensive in responding to diverse family-identified needs.	■ Provide collaborative, flexible, accessible, comprehensive, and coordinated services to children and their families. ■ Provide comprehensive case management/care coordination for children and families with ongoing care needs. ■ Along with families, take an active role in advocating for the needs of ill and injured children.
Holistic perspective of family-centered care: Appreciate families as families and children as children, recognizing that they possess a wider range of strengths, concerns, emotions, and aspirations beyond their need for specialized health and developmental services and support.	■ Encourage attention to the normal developmental needs and developmental tasks of the entire family unit and individual family members. ■ Encourage and facilitate the development of individual and family identities beyond a focus on illness or injury. ■ Facilitate "normalization" as valued and desired by the family.

Source: Reprinted with permission from Burland, J. (1999). NAMI provider education program. Arlington, VA: National Alliance for the Mentally Ill.

Promoting Family-Centered Care

Collaborating with families in providing health care is essential to promoting the best outcome when caring for children. Families have important knowledge to share about their child, their child's health condition, and how their child responds to various actions and events. They also need access to information that will make it possible for them to fully participate in planning and decision making.

PRACTICE ALERT

Some health care facilities are developing family resource centers to provide consumer information and support. In most cases, the resource center is a consumer-oriented health library with staffing, but peer support services may be coordinated through the center as well (Institute for Family Centered Care, 2004). Families can be supported in accessing useful information that helps them become informed decision makers about their child's care. Resources can often be provided in the preferred language and at appropriate reading level.

FOCUS ON DIVERSITY AND CULTURE
Family-Centered Care

When working to establish a family-centered relationship with families of various ethnic groups, consider the possibility that an extended family may need to be consulted. For example, Native Americans may consult tribal elders (considered part of the extended family) before agreeing to health care for their child. In some Hispanic cultures, major decisions for the child's health care include input from grandparents and other extended family members. It is important for the nurse to learn more about the strengths of the family network to better assist the family in planning the child's care at home (Ochieng, 2003).

Parents often need to assess their strengths in managing their ongoing family and caregiving responsibilities before planning how to add more caregiving responsibilities to their routine. Strategies that the nurse and parents collaboratively develop for the child's care must mesh with the family's cultural and ethnic illness-related behaviors, experiences, and beliefs (Sullivan-Bolyai, Sadler, Knafl et al., 2004). The child's opinions should also be integrated in the strategies for care. In almost all cases, the child leaves the health care setting and the family assumes responsibility for providing needed care in the home. The family caregivers must not feel alienated from a health care system they need for continuing assistance. See Box 10–10 for guidelines for effective collaboration.

Family involvement is also valuable in the development of policies and guidelines for family-centered care in all types of health care settings. A family's experiences while receiving care in the health care setting may reveal valuable insights, perspectives, and realities that could lead to improved quality of care and satisfaction with care. Feedback could be provided on such issues as how comfortable they felt in the setting; their understanding of information provided to them; and the attitudes they sensed from health professionals (Hanson & Randall, 1999). Parents who have been supported in developing leadership skills can be empowered to serve on advisory boards or councils representing the family and community perspectives. Guidelines for working with families as advisors and tools for assessing the family-centered policies in various health care settings are available from the Institute of Family-Centered Care.

Parents can also perform a valuable role in family-to-family support networks by serving as mentors to new families entering the health care system for a new chronic condition. In addition, parents may help raise awareness about specific health care issues, serve as advocates for public policy issues, and assist with fundraising activities.

PRACTICE ALERT

When providing care to children, recall that the family is central to all health care interventions with parents and child as the partners in care. It is important to consider how a health care setting's written policies, procedures, and literature for families refer to families and what attitudes these materials convey. Words like *policies*, *allowed*, and *not permitted* imply that hospital personnel have authority over families in matters concerning their children. Words like *guidelines*, *working together*, and *welcome* communicate an openness and appreciation for families in the care of their children.

Box 10–10 **Guidelines for Effective Collaboration**

Parents have a role in developing an effective collaborative relationship with nurses and other health professionals. Parents often become experts in their child's health condition, and learn to advocate for their child. They also must learn to communicate effectively with the health professionals caring for their child, and in the process develop a trusting relationship.

Tips for parents for improved communication follow (Allshouse & Goldberg, 2003):

- Keep a journal that includes your observations about your child's behavior, eating habits, illness, temperature, or anything else that might be helpful to the health care providers caring for your child.
- Keep a copy of your child's medical records, including test and procedure results.
- Write out questions and do not hesitate to ask for clarification if you don't understand an answer provided.
- Be realistic about what you can expect from your child's nurses and doctors. They cannot solve all your problems or answer all your questions. They also can become frustrated at times by a child's condition or lack of answers to questions. Try to let your health care providers know you appreciate their time and efforts on behalf of your child.

Communication tips for nurses include the following:

- Provide information and honestly discuss issues of concern to both the family and health care providers.
- Engage in creative problem solving and identify options for needed care that conform to the family's values and functioning.
- Demonstrate respect for the family's choices and methods for providing needed care.
- Continue to collaborate with the child and family and be willing to continue problem solving as new issues arise.

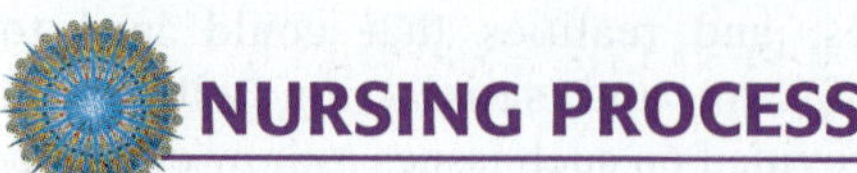

NURSING PROCESS

Assessment

The nurse assesses the family's readiness and ability to provide continued care and supervision at home when warranted. Support for the family is essential. The following information should be considered when performing any family assessment and developing a client's plan of care:

- Cohesiveness and communication patterns within the family
- Family interactions that support self-care
- Number of friends and relatives available
- Family values and beliefs about health and illness
- Cultural and spiritual beliefs
- Developmental level of the client and family.

Family History

The family history is a review of the client's family to determine if any genetic or familial patterns of health or illness might shed light on the client's current health status. For example, if the client has a family history of type 1 diabetes, the nurse will question the client closely about signs of the disease. These signs include increased appetite, frequent urination, and weight loss. The family history begins with a review of the immediate family, parents, siblings, children, grandparents, aunts, uncles, and cousins. The nurse should encourage the client to recall as many generations as possible to develop a complete picture. If the client provides data about a genetic or familial disease, it is helpful to interview older members of the family for additional information. Adopted children, spouses, and other individuals living with the client may not be related by blood; however, their health history should be reviewed because the client's concern may have an environmental basis. For example, illnesses may be associated with secondhand smoke in the spouse or child of a smoker, or illness may be associated with exposure to toxins or fumes carried into the home on the clothing of a spouse or family member. The nurse documents information collected from the client and the family in a family genogram. The family genogram, also known as a pedigree or family tree, is the most effective method of recording the large amount of data gathered from a family's health history.

As nurses, we must focus our attention on the family, both as the context for the individual and as the unit of care. It is important to assess and involve families because they are in a position to be affected by and to influence the course of an individual's problems. The questions we ask influence how we view the family. For example, if we ask only about problems, we are likely to "find" problems in the family. On the other hand, if we also include questions about resourcefulness, we have an increased chance of discovering family competency. Questions shape our experience of and our interactions with clients and families. The following questions are examples for assessing the resourcefulness of the family system:

- What do you hope for in the future?
- How will your life be different when your concerns are no longer problems?
- What strengths, resources, and knowledge do you have to deal with the problems?

Assessment includes gathering information on how partners, parents, and children in the family experience or react to the client's symptoms. Nurses must learn how others are affected by problems and how they have attempted to cope with problems. If we want to know the family, we must listen to its story. The family's story will tell us who the members are and what is meaningful to them. Telling their stories also allows families to make sense of any confusion.

Clients, families, and nurses collaborate to identify the family's strengths, resources, and social support and try to identify problems that might cause stress for any of the family members. Factors in assessing clients and their families include family communication, conflict resolution, boundaries, cohesion, flexibility, emotional availability, leadership patterns, and overall family functionality.

Diagnosis

Data gathered during a family assessment may lead to the following nursing diagnoses:

- Interrupted Family Processes, a change in family relationships
- Readiness for Enhanced Family Coping, effective management of adaptive tasks by family members involved with the client's health challenge, who now exhibits desire and readiness for enhanced health and growth in regard to self and in relation to the client
- Disabled Family Coping, behavior of significant person (family member or other primary person) that disables his or her capacities to effectively address tasks essential to either person's adaptation to the health challenge
- Impaired Parenting, inability of the primary caretaker to create, maintain, or regain an environment that promotes the optimum growth and development of the child
- Impaired Home Maintenance, inability to independently maintain a safe growth-promoting immediate environment
- Caregiver Role Strain, difficulty in performing family caregiver role.

Examples of contributing factors for one selected diagnosis, desired outcomes to evaluate the achievement of client goals, and the effectiveness of nursing interventions are listed in Table 10–7.

Plan

Being sensitive to cultural differences is important in assessment and planning care. Knowing who makes most of the decisions in the family, especially in health care, helps the

TABLE 10–7 **Identifying Nursing Diagnoses, Outcomes, and Interventions: Clients With Disruption in Family Health**

DATA CLUSTER: Mr. and Mrs. G's 6-year-old son has just been diagnosed with acute leukemia. they also have a 9-year-old daughter and a 4-year-old son.

NURSING DIAGNOSIS/ DEFINITION	SAMPLE DESIRED OUTCOMES*: DEFINITION	NOC INDICATORS	SELECTED INTERVENTIONS	SAMPLE NIC ACTIVITIES
Interrupted family processes: Change in family relationships	Family coping [2600]: Family actions to manage stressors that tax family resources	Often demonstrated: ■ Involves family members in decision making ■ Uses stress reduction strategies ■ Arranges for respite care.	Family integrity promotion [7100]: Promotion of family cohesion and unity Normalization promotion [7200]: Assisting parents and other family members of children with chronic illness or disabilities in providing normal life experiences for their children and families	■ Determine family understanding of illness. ■ Tell family members it is safe and acceptable to use typical expressions of affection. ■ Refer for family therapy as indicated. ■ Deemphasize uniqueness of child's condition. ■ Involve siblings in care and activities of child as appropriate.
	Psychosocial adjustment: Life change [1305]: Adaptive psychosocial response of an individual to a significant life change	Sometimes demonstrated: ■ Sets realistic goals ■ Reports of feeling empowered.	Family process maintenance [7130]: Minimization of family process disruption effects	■ Determine typical family processes. ■ Discuss strategies for normalizing family life with family members.

*The NOC# for desired outcomes and the NIC# for nursing interventions are listed in brackets after the appropriate outcome or intervention. Outcomes, indicators, interventions, and activities in this table are only a sample of those suggested by NOC and NIC and should be further individualized for each client.

nurse know to whom to direct questions in order to obtain information and also whom to instruct. The extended family unit is found in many cultures, and different health beliefs and health practices may exist within the family. Older members of the family may continue their traditional practices, whereas younger members may have had more exposure to modern practices. Building a trusting relationship with these families by talking with them about their beliefs and practices is the first step toward planning more effective care.

Nursing needs to focus on assisting the family to plan realistic goals/outcomes and strategies that enhance family functioning, such as improving communication skills, identifying and utilizing support systems, and developing and rehearsing parenting skills. Anticipatory guidance may assist well-functioning families in preparing for predictable developmental transitions that occur in the life of families.

In helping families reintegrate the ill person into the home, nurses use data gathered during family assessment to identify family resources and deficits. By formulating mutually acceptable goals for reintegration, nurses help families cope with the realities of the illness and the changes it may have brought about. Such changes may include new roles and functions of family members or the need to provide continued medical care to the ill or recovering person. Working together, nurses and families can create environments that restore or reorganize family functioning during illness and throughout the recovery process.

Implementation

Nursing interventions are based on the medical diagnoses, nursing diagnoses, and selected goals or outcomes (see Table 10–7).

After carefully planned instruction and practice, families are given an opportunity to demonstrate their ability to provide care under the supportive guidance of the nurse. When the care indicated is beyond the capability of the family, nurses work with families to identify available resources that are socially and financially acceptable.

It is important to remember that standardized teaching plans may not be effective for clients with chronic illness and their families. Rather, these clients and their families should be given the freedom to choose appropriate literature, self-help or support groups, and interactions with others who have the same illness.

Evaluation

In evaluating the success of the family care plan, the nurse assesses for the presence of the indicators identified for the chosen outcomes. If the indicators are present, it is likely that the outcome has been achieved. If the indicators or outcomes are partially or not met, all aspects of the family situation must be reexamined: Have the intervention activities been carried out? Are the indicators and outcomes appropriate? Is the nursing diagnosis proper? Has the medical condition or diagnosis changed?

Recognition of individual and family strengths helps to maintain wellness and also directs behavior in crisis situations. If a plan of care has to be modified to be more effective, these strengths should be identified and utilized.

REVIEW Family Response to Health Alterations

RELATE: LINK THE CONCEPTS

Mrs. Ann Bell, an 82-year-old widow, was diagnosed with Alzheimer's disease several years ago. She lives with her daughter and son-in-law and their two children, aged 16 and 10 years. Mrs. Bell has begun wandering, especially at night, and has started small fires when she attempts to cook and forgets about the pot on the stove. Mrs. Bell's daughter, Laura, accompanies her mother to her physician's appointment today and relates that the stress of caring for her mother, in addition to her other obligations to her family, is becoming increasingly difficult.

Linking the exemplar of Family Response to Health Alterations with the concept of Grief and Loss:

1. How can the nurse help the family to cope with the loss they feel related to Mrs. Bell's cognitive degeneration?
2. How can you help Mrs. Bell's grandchildren identify their feelings of grief and loss and work as a family to deal with these feelings?

Linking the exemplar of Family Response to Health Alterations with the concept of Stress and Coping:

3. What strategies can you suggest to help this family deal with the stress of Mrs. Bell's cognitive degeneration?
4. What referrals can you make to reduce Mrs. Bell's daughter's caregiver role strain?

REFER: GO TO MYNURSINGKIT

REFLECT: CASE STUDY

Casey, a 16-year-old, is recuperating from injuries sustained in a motor vehicle crash in which he was the passenger. He was not wearing a seatbelt and experienced a brain injury after striking the windshield. His cognitive and motor functions are impaired. After a 7-day acute care hospital stay, he was moved to an inpatient rehabilitation hospital, where he has been for the past 5 days. He is much more responsive to stimuli and to family members 12 days after his injury. Physical therapy is provided twice a day to promote range of motion and muscle tone and to prevent contractures. Plans are being made to discharge him home with outpatient rehabilitation care within the next 5 days. A case manager will be assigned to coordinate his health care services.

Casey lives with his mother, two half-brothers (10 and 6 years old), and stepfather. Both his mother and stepfather are employed full time and are trying to determine how to manage care for Casey once he returns home. Casey's father has not been actively involved in his life since the divorce 12 years ago. Casey's grandparents reside in the same town and may provide the family some support.

1. What family supports will Casey need as he continues his rehabilitation for the brain injury?
2. What family assessment information is needed to effectively plan nursing care for this adolescent and his family?
3. Does this family have strengths and coping strategies that will help them adapt to Casey's disability?

Casey's family is coping with his initial survival of a serious brain injury, and facing a long rehabilitation process. The family is just now recognizing that life as they have known it is changing. Casey is totally dependent for care, including bathing, toileting, feeding, and mobilizing. While he is expected to regain self-care abilities, the impact of the injury on his cognitive ability and future functioning is unknown.

Casey's extended family has provided support for the family during the past 12 days, but the level of support in the future weeks will decrease because of other family obligations. Casey's mother has already initiated a leave of absence from work so she can care for him when he returns home; however, this will mean the family has reduced income during that time period. Casey's younger brothers have been able to visit him, and they are very anxious because Casey cannot talk with them. They have been trying to avoid bothering their mother and father during this time, but they are wondering when life will be more normal and they can again participate in their usual afterschool activities.

1. What information about the family strengths, needs, and resilience can be identified from the chapter opening scenario, the ecomap on page 501, and the previous information?
2. What additional information would be helpful to know about family strengths and needs prior to developing a nursing care plan?
3. Based on your assessment of the family and challenges facing them, list at least one nursing diagnosis (additional to those listed on page 502) that addresses issues important in planning nursing care for Casey and his family.
4. Describe the use of family-centered care principles in planning Casey's nursing care in collaboration with the family.
5. What potential parenting issues could this family anticipate for Casey and his brothers?

PEARSON

EXPLORE mynursingkit™

MyNursingKit is your one stop for online chapter review materials and resources. Prepare for success with additional NCLEX®-style practice questions, interactive assignments and activities, web links, animations and videos, and more!

Register your access code from the front of your book at **www.mynursingkit.com**.

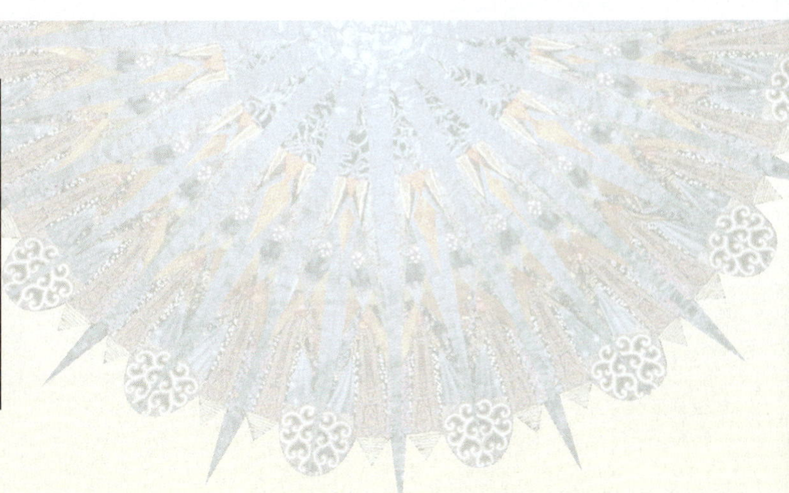

REFERENCES

Alan Guttmacher Institute. (2004). *U.S. teenage pregnancy statistics: Overall trends, trends by race and ethnicity and state-by-state information*. New York: Author.

Allshouse, C., & Goldberg, P. F. (2003). *Working with doctors: A parent's guide to navigating the health system*. Minneapolis, MN: Pacer Center.

American Academy of Pediatrics. (2004). Fathers and pediatricians: Enhancing men's roles in the care and development of their children. *Pediatrics, 113*(5), 1406–1411.

American Academy of Pediatrics Committee on Early Childhood, Adoption, and Dependent Care. (2000). Developmental issues for young children in foster care. *Pediatrics, 106*(5), 1145–1150.

American Academy of Pediatrics Committee on Early Childhood, Adoption, and Dependent Care. (2002). Health care of young children in foster care. *Pediatrics, 109*(3), 536–541.

American Academy of Pediatrics Committee on Hospital Care and the Institute of Family Centered Care. (2003). Family-centered care and the pediatrician's role. *Pediatrics, 112*(3), 691–696.

American Academy of Pediatrics Committee on Psychosocial Aspects of Child and Family Health. (2002). Coparent or second parent adoption by same-sex parents. *Pediatrics, 111*(6), 1541–1571.

American Academy of Pediatrics Task Force on the Family. (2003). Family pediatrics: Report on the Task Force on the Family. *Pediatrics, 111*(6), 1541–1571.

American Nurses Association. (1998). *Culturally competent assessment for family violence*. Washington, DC: American Nurses Publishing.

American Psychological Association. (2004). *Sexual orientation, parents, and children: APA Policy Statement*. Retrieved May 6, 2006, from http://www.apa.org/pi/lgbc/policy/parents.html

Baumrind, D. (1971). Current patterns of parental authority. *Developmental Psychology, 4*, 1–103.

Biringen, Z. (2000). Emotional availability: Conceptualization and research findings. *American Journal of Orthopsychiatry, 70*(1), 104–114.

Black, C., & Ford-Gilboe, M. (2004). Adolescent mothers: Resilience, family health work and health-promoting practices. *Journal of Advanced Nursing, 48*, 351–360.

Byrd, M., & Garwick, A. (2004). A feminist critique of research on interracial family identity: Implications for family health. *Journal of Family Nursing, 10*, 302–320.

Caldwell, B. M., & Bradley, R. H. (1984). *The home observation for measurement of the environment*. Little Rock: University of Arkansas.

Craig, G. J., & Baucum, D. (2002). *Human development* (9th ed.). Upper Saddle River, NJ: Prentice Hall.

Denham, S. A. (2005). Family structure, function, and process. In S. M. H. Hanson, V. Gedaly-Duff, & J. R. Kaakinen, *Family health care nursing* (3rd ed., pp. 119–156). Philadelphia: F. A. Davis.

Doane, G. H., & Varcoe, C. (2004). *Family nursing as relational inquiry*. Philadelphia: Lippincott Williams & Wilkins.

Dochterman, J., & Bulechek, G. B. (Eds.). (2004). *Nursing interventions classification (NIC)* (4th ed.). St. Louis, MO: Mosby.

Duvall, E.M. (1977). *Marriage and family development* (5th ed.). New York: Harper & Row.

Erikson, E. (1963). *Childhood and society* (2nd ed.). New York: W.W. Norton.

Family and Medical Leave, Public Law 103-3, February 5, 1999. 5 U.S.C. 6381–6387; 5 CFR part 630, subpart L. Retrieved July 9, 2004, from http://www.opm.gov/pca/leave/HTMS/fmlafac2.asp

Fields, J. (2003). *America's families and living arrangements: 2003*. Current Population Reports, P20–553. Washington, DC: U.S. Bureau of the Census.

Friedman, M. M., Bowden, V. R., & Jones, E. G. (2003). *Family nursing: Research, theory and practice* (5th ed.). Upper Saddle River, NJ: Prentice Hall.

Hanson, J. L., & Randall, V. F. (1999). Evaluating and improving the practice of family-centered care. *Pediatric Nursing, 25*(4), 445–449.

Institute for Family Centered Care. (2004). Patient and family resource centers. Retrieved May 7, 2009, from http://www.familycenteredcare.org/advance/topics/pafam-resource.html

Jungbauer, J., Wittmund, B., Dietrich, S., & Angermeyer, M. C. (2003). Subjective burden over 12 months in parents of patients with schizophrenia. *Archives of Psychiatric Nursing, 17*(3), 126–134

Lewandowski, L. A., & Tesler, M. D. (Eds.). (2003). *Family-centered care: Putting it into action. The SPN/ANA guide to family-centered care*. Washington, DC: American Nurses Association.

Locsin, R. C. (2003). Culture perspectives. The integration of family health, culture, and nursing: Prescriptions and practices. *Holistic Nursing Practice, 17*(1), 8–10.

Lugaila, T., & Overturf, J. (2004). *Children and the households they live in: 2000. CENSR-14*. Washington, DC: U.S. Bureau of the Census.

McGuinness, T. M., Noonan, P., & Dyer, J. G. (2005). Family history as a tool for psychiatric nurses. *Archives of Psychiatric Nursing, 19*(3), 116–124.

Meyers, T. A., Eichhorn, D. J., & Guzzetta, C. E. (1998). Do family members want to be present during CPR? A retrospective study. *Journal of Emergency Nursing, 24*(5), 400–405.

Moorhead, S., Johnson, M., & Maas, M. (Eds.). (2004). *Nursing outcomes classification (NOC)* (3rd ed.). St. Louis, MO: Mosby.

Munro, H., & D'Errico, C. (2000). Parental involvement in perioperative anesthetic management. *Journal of PeriAnesthesia Nursing, 15*(6), 397–400.

NANDA International. (2007). *NANDA nursing diagnoses: Definitions and classification 2007–2008*. Philadelphia: NANDA.

Ochieng, B. M. N. (2003). Minority ethnic families and family-centered care. *Journal of Child Health Care, 7*(2), 123–132.

Olson, D. H. (1996). Clinical assessment and treatment interventions using the family circumplex model. In F. W. Kaslow (Ed.), *Handbook of relational diagnosis and dysfunctional family patterns* (pp. 59–77). New York: John Wiley & Sons.

Peterson, K. S. (2003, September 18). Unmarried with children: For better or worse? *USA Today*, pp. 1A, 8A.

Powers, K. S., & Rubenstein, J. S. (1999). Family presence during invasive procedures in pediatric intensive care unit: A prospective study. *Archives of Pediatric and Adolescent Medicine, 153*, 955–958.

Rigazio-DiGilio, S. A. (2005). *Community genograms: Using individual, family, and cultural narratives with clients*. New York: Teacher's College Press.

Rose, L. E. (1997). Caring for caregivers: Perceptions of social support. *Journal of Psychosocial Nursing, 35*(2), 17–24.

Rose, L. E., Mallinson, R. K., & Gerson, L. D. (2006). Mastery, burden and areas of concern among family caregivers of mentally ill persons. *Archives of Psychiatric Nursing, 20*(1), 41–51.

Sacchetti, A., Paston, C., & Carraccio, C. (2005). Family members do not disrupt care when present during invasive procedures. *Academic Emergency Medicine, 12*(5), 477–479.

Sgarbossa, D., & Ford-Gilboe, M. (2004). Mother's friendship quality, parental support, quality of life, and family health work in families led by adolescent mothers with preschool children. *Journal of Family Nursing, 10*, 232–261.

Stengler-Wenzke, K., Trosbach, J., Dietrich, S., & Angermeyer, M. C. (2004). Experience of stigmatization of relatives of patients with obsessive compulsive disorder. *Archives of Psychiatric Nursing, 18*(3),88–96.

Sullivan-Bolyai, S., Sadler, L., Knafl, K. A., & Gillis, C. L. (2004). Great expectations: A position description for parents as caregivers: Part II. *Pediatric Nursing, 30*(1), 52–56.

Tweedell, D., Forchuk, C., Jewell, J., & Steinnagel, L. (2004). Families' experience during recovery of nonrecovery from psychosis. *Archives of Psychiatric Nursing, 18*(1), 17–25.

U.S. Census Bureau. (2002). Living arrangements of children under 18 years of age: 1960 to present. Retrieved May 6, 2009, from http://www.census.gov/population/socdemo/hh-fam/cps2002/tabC3-all.pdf

U.S. Census Bureau. (2004). *"Stay-at-home" parents top 5 million*. Washington, DC: Author. Retrieved May 6, 2009, from http://www.census.gov/Press-Release/www/releases/archives/families_households/003118.html

U.S. Census Bureau (2006). *Definition: Household and family*. Retrieved May 6, 2009, from http://www.census.gov/population/www/cps/cpsdef.html

U.S. Conference of Mayors. (2004). *A status report on hunger and homelessness in America's cities: 2004*. Retrieved May 5, 2006, from http://www.usmayors.org/uscm/us_mayor_newspaper/documents/01_10_05/hunger_survey.asp

U.S. Department of Health and Human Services. (2001). Indicators of welfare reform. Annual Report to Congress 2001. Table Birth 4. Washington, DC: Author.

Urban Institute. (2003). *Gay and lesbian families in the Census: Couples with children*. Washington, DC: Author. Retrieved January 28, 2004, from http://www.urban.org

von Bertalanffy, L. (1980). *General system theory* (revised from original 1969). New York: George Braziller.

Wilkerson, S. A., & Loveland-Cherry, C. J. (2004). Johnson's behavioral system model. In J. J. Fitzpatrick & A. L. Whall (Eds.), *Conceptual models of nursing: Analysis and application* (4th ed., pp. 83–103). Upper Saddle River, NJ: Prentice Hall Health.

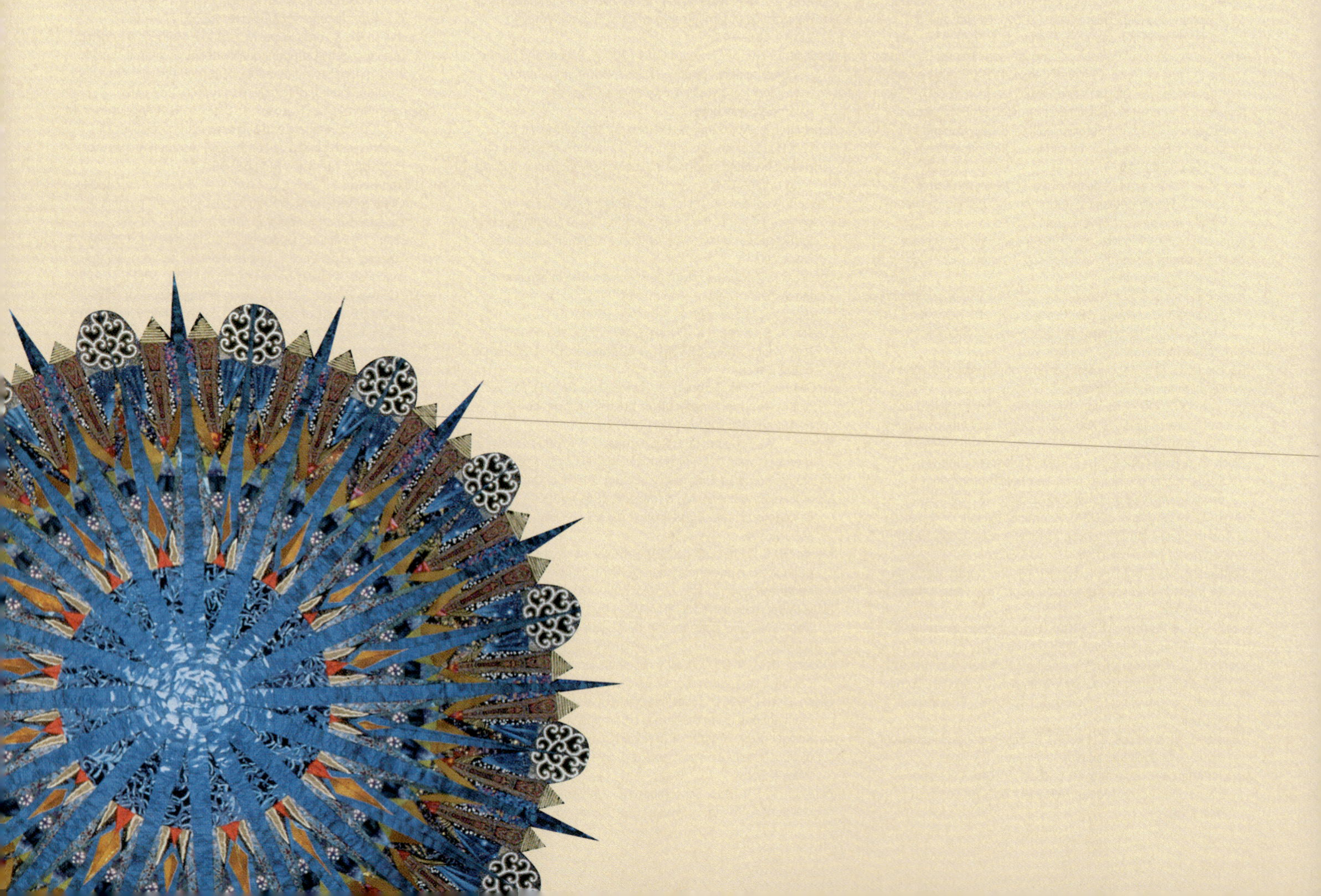

Fluids and Electrolytes

11

Concept at-a-Glance

Concept Learning Outcomes

After reading about this concept, you will be able to:

1. Summarize the structure and physiological processes involved in maintaining fluid and electrolyte balance.
2. Identify factors affecting fluid and electrolyte balance.
3. Identify commonly occurring alterations in fluid and electrolyte balance and their related treatment.
4. Explain common physical assessment procedures use to examine fluid and electrolyte balance in clients across the life span.
5. Outline diagnostic and laboratory tests to determine the individual's fluid and electrolyte status.
6. Explain management of fluid and electrolyte balance and prevention of alterations.
7. Demonstrate the nursing process in providing culturally competent and caring interventions across the life span for individuals with common alterations in fluid and electrolyte balance.
8. Identify pharmacological interventions in caring for the individual with alterations in fluid and electrolyte balance.

Concept Key Terms

Active transport, *521*
Anion, *518*
Body surface area, *526*
Cation, *518*
Colloid, *519*
Colloid osmotic pressure, *520*
Crystalloid, *519*
Dehydration, *521*
Diffusion, *520*
Edema, *529*
Electrolyte, *517*
Extracellular fluid, *578*
Filtration, *521*
Fluid volume deficit, *531*
Fluid volume excess, *531*
Hematocrit, *531*
Hydrostatic pressure, *521*
Hyperkalemia, *532*
Hypernatremia, *532*
Hypertonic, *520*
Hypokalemia, *532*
Hyponatremia, *532*
Hypotonic, *520*
Insensible fluid loss, *522*
Interstitial fluid, *518*
Intracellular fluid, *518*
Intravascular fluid, *518*
Ions, *518*
Isotonic, *520*
Milliequivalent, *518*
Obligatory losses, *523*
Oncotic pressure, *520*
Osmolality, *520*
Osmosis, *519*
Osmotic pressure, *520*
Saline, *520*
Solutes, *518*
Solvent, *520*
Tonicity, *520*
Transcellular fluid, *518*

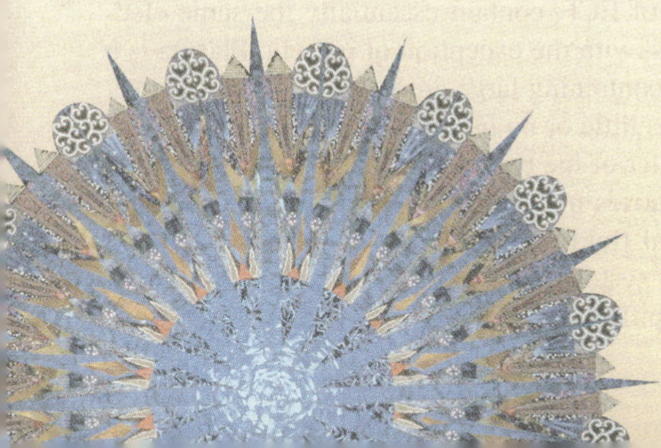

About Fluids and Electrolytes

The body is largely composed of fluid in many forms. Blood, serum, saline, albumin, urine, bile, hormones, cerebrospinal fluid—these are just a few of the fluids required for homeostasis, the delicate balance of fluids and electrolytes that promotes the body's functions.

Within each of these fluids are **electrolytes**, charged ions capable of conducting electricity, in various concentrations and combinations. Learning what fluids contain specific electrolytes can help you identify causes of electrolyte imbalances in clients. This will allow you to specifically design care to restore homeostasis.

Homeostasis depends on multiple physiologic processes. Fluid and electrolyte balance is critical to maintaining good health. Fluid and electrolyte imbalance can result in a variety of conditions, such as dehydration and renal failure, and can also impact both chronic and acute illnesses. In turn, almost every illness has the potential to threaten this crucial balance. Even in daily living, excessive temperatures or vigorous activity can disturb the balance if adequate intake of water and salt is not maintained. Therapeutic measures can also disturb the body's homeostasis unless water and electrolytes are replaced. •

NORMAL PRESENTATION

The proportion of the human body composed of fluid is surprisingly large. Approximately 60% of the average healthy adult's weight is water, the primary body fluid. In good health, this volume remains relatively constant and the person's weight varies by less than 0.2 kg (0.5 lb) in 24 hours, regardless of the amount of fluid ingested.

Water is vital to health and normal cellular function, serving as

- a medium for metabolic reactions within cells;
- transporter for nutrients, waste products, and other substances;
- a lubricant;
- an insulator and shock absorber;
- one means of regulating and maintaining body temperature.

Age, sex, and body fat affect total body water. Infants have the highest proportion of water, accounting for 70–80% of their body weight. The proportion of body water decreases with aging. In people older than 60 years of age, water represents only about 50% of the total body weight. Women also have a lower percentage of body water than men. Women and older adults have reduced body water due to lower muscle mass and a greater percentage of fat tissue. Fat tissue is essentially free of water, whereas lean tissue contains a significant amount of water. Water makes up a greater percentage of a lean person's body weight than that of an obese person.

Distribution and Composition of Body Fluids

The body's fluid is divided into two major compartments, intracellular and extracellular.

Both of these contain oxygen from the lungs, dissolved nutrients from the gastrointestinal tract, excretory products of metabolism such as carbon dioxide, and charged particles called **ions**. The composition of fluids varies from one body compartment to another.

Many salts dissociate in water; that is, they break up into electrically charged ions. The salt sodium chloride breaks up into one ion of sodium (Na^+) and one ion of chloride (Cl^-). These charged particles are called electrolytes because they are capable of conducting electricity. The number of ions that carry a positive charge, called **cations**, and ions that carry a negative charge, called **anions**, should be equal. Examples of cations are sodium (Na^+), potassium (K^+), calcium (Ca^{2+}), and magnesium (Mg^{2+}). Examples of anions are chloride (Cl^-), bicarbonate (HCO_3^-), phosphate (HPO_4^{2-}), and sulfate (SO_4^{2-}).

Electrolytes generally are measured in milliequivalents per liter of water (mEq/L) or milligrams per 100 mL (mg/100 mL). The term **milliequivalent** refers to the chemical combining power of the ion, or the capacity of cations to combine with anions to form molecules. This combining activity is measured in relation to the combining activity of the hydrogen ion (H^+). Thus, 1 mEq of any anion equals 1 mEq of any cation. Clinically, the milliequivalent system is most often used. However, nurses need to be aware that different systems of measurement may be found when interpreting laboratory results. For example, calcium levels frequently are reported in milligrams per deciliter (1 dL = 100 mL) instead of milliequivalents per liter. It also is important to remember that laboratory tests are usually performed using blood plasma, an extracellular fluid. Although these results may reflect what is happening in the ECF, it generally is not possible to directly measure electrolyte concentrations within the cell.

INTRACELLULAR FLUID **Intracellular fluid (ICF)** is found within the cells of the body. It constitutes approximately two-thirds of the total body fluid in adults.

Intracellular fluid is vital to normal cell functioning. It contains **solutes** (substances that dissolve in liquid) such as oxygen, electrolytes, and glucose, and provides a medium in which metabolic processes of the cell take place.

The composition of intracellular fluid differs significantly from that of extracellular fluid. Potassium and magnesium are the primary cations present in ICF, and phosphate and sulfate the major anions. As in extracellular fluid, other electrolytes are present within the cell, but in much smaller concentrations (Figure 11–1 ■).

EXTRACELLULAR FLUID **Extracellular fluid (ECF)** is found outside the cells and accounts for about one-third of total body fluid. It is subdivided into compartments. The two main compartments of ECF are intravascular and interstitial. **Intravascular fluid**, or plasma, accounts for approximately 20% of the ECF and is found within the vascular system. **Interstitial fluid**, accounting for approximately 75% of the ECF, surrounds the cells. The other compartments of ECF are the lymph and transcellular fluids. Examples of **transcellular fluid** are cerebrospinal, pericardial, pancreatic, pleural, intraocular, biliary, peritoneal, and synovial fluids.

In extracellular fluid, the principal electrolytes are sodium, chloride, and bicarbonate. Other electrolytes such as potassium, calcium, and magnesium are also present but in much smaller quantities. Plasma and interstitial fluid, the two primary components of ECF, contain essentially the same electrolytes and solutes, with the exception of protein. Plasma is a protein-rich fluid, containing large amounts of albumin; interstitial fluid contains little or no protein. Although extracellular fluid is in the smaller of the two compartments, it is the transport system that carries nutrients to and waste products from the cells. Interstitial fluid transports wastes from the cells by way of the lymph system as well as directly into the blood plasma through capillaries.

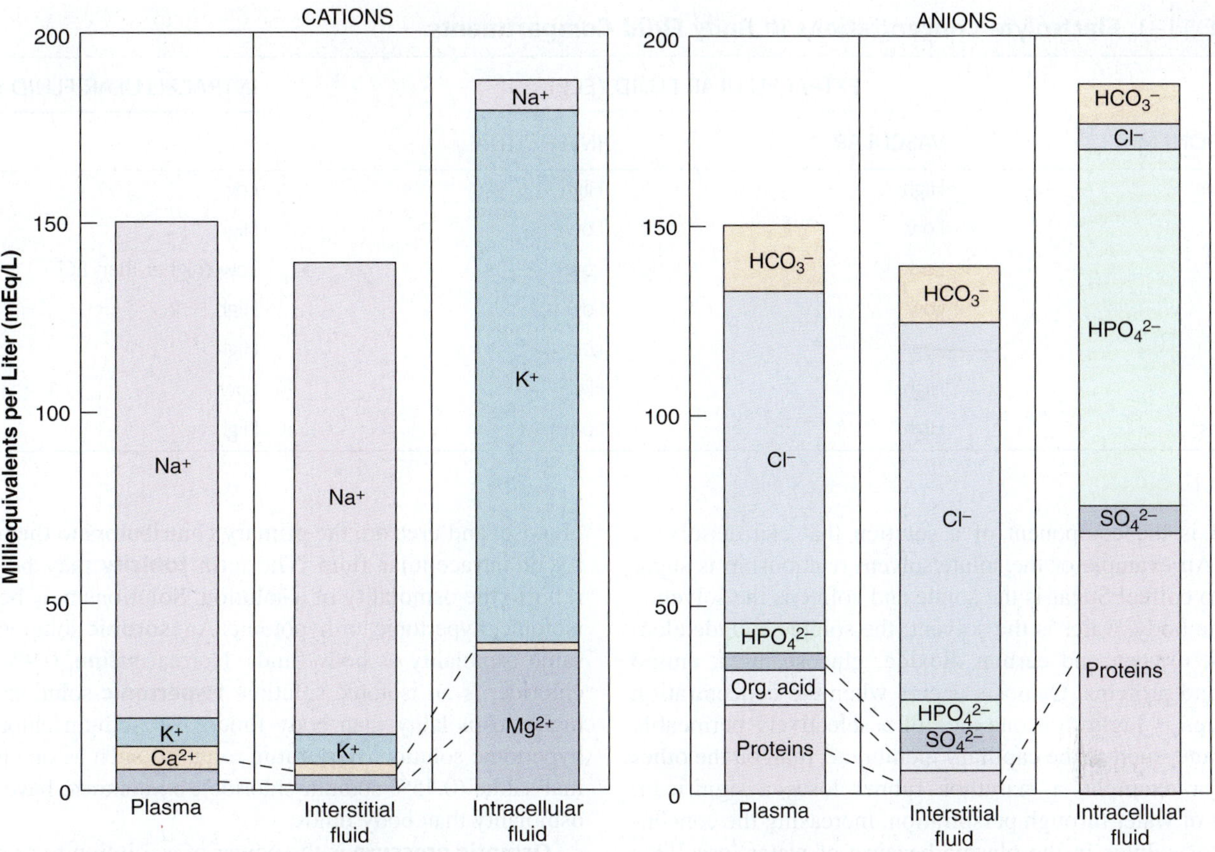

Figure 11–1 ■ Electrolyte composition (cations and anions) of body fluid compartments.

Source: Martini, F, H., Haylard, R. A. (1998). *Fundamentals of anatomy and physiology interactive* (Media Edition) (4th ed.). Reproduced with permission of Pearson Education, Inc., Upper Saddle River, New Jersey.

Maintaining a balance of fluid volumes and electrolyte compositions in the fluid compartments of the body is essential to health. Normal and unusual fluid and electrolyte losses must be replaced if homeostasis is to be maintained (Box 11–1).

Other body fluids such as gastric and intestinal secretions also contain electrolytes. Excessive loss of these fluids from the body (for example, with severe vomiting or diarrhea or when gastric suction removes the gastric secretions) is of particular concern, as fluid and electrolyte imbalances can result. Table 11–1 shows electrolyte concentrations in body fluid compartments.

Box 11–1 Linking Concepts

Fluid and electrolyte imbalance is critical to maintaining homeostasis. Just two examples of the important role that fluids and electrolytes play are given here.

FLUIDS, ELECTROLYTES, AND COGNITION
Imbalance of fluids and electrolytes can severely affect cognition. Moderate to severe dehydration can result in confusion in the healthiest adult. Fluid and electrolyte imbalance can also be a factor in delirium, and best practice dictates that fluid and electrolyte levels be assessed through diagnostic testing when a patient presents with symptoms of delirium.

FLUIDS, ELECTROLYTES, AND PERFUSION
Clients with imbalance in fluid and electrolytes, particularly fluid and sodium, may increase intravascular fluid content resulting in stress on the cardiovascular system. Clients with perfusion disorders are frequently placed on medications that can cause a fluid and/or electrolyte imbalance.

Movement of Body Fluids

The body fluid compartments are separated from one another by cell membranes and the capillary membrane. While these membranes are completely permeable to water, they are considered to be selectively permeable to solutes as substances move across them with varying degrees of ease. Small particles such as ions, oxygen, and carbon dioxide move easily across these membranes, but larger molecules such as glucose and proteins have more difficulty moving between fluid compartments. The methods by which electrolytes and other solutes move are osmosis, diffusion, filtration, and active transport.

OSMOSIS **Osmosis** is the movement of water across cell membranes, from the less concentrated solution to the more concentrated solution (Figure 11–2 ■). In other words, water moves toward the higher concentration of solute in an attempt to equalize the concentrations.

Solutes may be **crystalloids** (salts that dissolve readily into true solutions) or **colloids** (substances such as large protein molecules that do not readily dissolve into true solutions). A

TABLE 11–1 **Electrolyte Concentrations in Body Fluid Compartments**

	EXTRACELLULAR FLUID (ECF)		INTRACELLULAR FLUID (ICF)
COMPONENTS	VASCULAR	INTERSTITIAL	
Na^+	High	High	Low
K^+	Low	Low	High
Ca^{++}	Low	Low	Low (higher than ECF)
Mg^{++}	Low	Low	High
Pi	Low	Low	High
Cl^-	High	High	Low
Proteins	High	Low	High

solvent is the component of a solution that can dissolve a solute. An example of the solute/solvent relationship is sugar added to coffee: Sugar is the solute and coffee is the solvent.

In the body, water is the solvent; the solutes include electrolytes, oxygen and carbon dioxide, glucose, urea, amino acids, and proteins. Osmosis occurs when the concentration of solutes is higher on one side of a selectively permeable membrane, such as the capillary membrane, than on the other side. For example, a marathon runner loses a significant amount of water through perspiration, increasing the concentration of solutes in the plasma because of water loss. This higher solute concentration draws water from the interstitial space and cells into the vascular compartment to equalize the concentration of solutes in all fluid compartments. Osmosis is an important mechanism for maintaining homeostasis and fluid balance.

The concentration of solutes in body fluids is usually expressed as the **osmolality**. Osmolality is determined by the total solute concentration within a fluid compartment and is measured as parts of solute per kilogram of water.

Osmolality is reported as milliosmols per kilogram (mOsm/kg). Sodium is by far the greatest determinant of osmolality, with glucose and urea also contributing. Potassium, glucose, and urea are the primary contributors to the osmolality of intracellular fluid. The term **tonicity** may be used to refer to the osmolality of a solution. Solutions may be termed isotonic, hypertonic, or hypotonic. An **isotonic** solution has the same osmolality as body fluids. Normal **saline**, 0.9% sodium chloride, is an isotonic solution. **Hypertonic** solutions have a higher osmolality than body fluids; 3% sodium chloride is a hypertonic solution. **Hypotonic** solutions such as one-half normal saline (0.45% sodium chloride), by contrast, have a lower osmolality than body fluids.

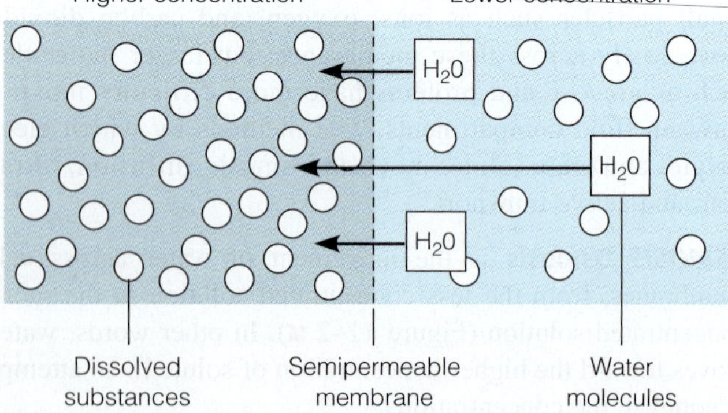

Figure 11–2 ■ Osmosis: Water molecules move from the less concentrated area to the more concentrated area in an attempt to equalize the concentration of solutions on two sides of a membrane.

Osmotic pressure is the power of a solution to draw water across a semipermeable membrane. When two solutions of different solute concentrations are separated by a semipermeable membrane, the solution of higher solute concentration exerts a higher osmotic pressure, drawing water across the membrane to equalize the concentrations of the solutions. For example, infusing a hypertonic intravenous solution such as 3% sodium chloride will draw fluid out of red blood cells (RBCs), causing them to shrink. On the other hand, a hypotonic solution administered intravenously will cause the RBCs to swell as water is drawn into the cells by their higher osmotic pressure. In the body, plasma proteins exert an osmotic draw called **colloid osmotic pressure** or **oncotic pressure**, pulling water from the interstitial space into the vascular compartment. This is an important mechanism in maintaining vascular volume.

DIFFUSION **Diffusion** is the continual intermingling of molecules in liquids, gases, or solids brought about by the random movement of the molecules. For example, two gases become mixed by the constant motion of their molecules. The process of diffusion occurs even when two substances are separated by a thin membrane. In the body, diffusion of water, electrolytes, and other substances occurs through the "split pores" of capillary membranes.

The rate of diffusion of substances varies according to (a) the size of the molecules, (b) the concentration of the solution, and (c) the temperature of the solution. Larger molecules move less quickly than smaller ones because they require more energy to move about. With diffusion, the molecules move from a solution of higher concentration to a

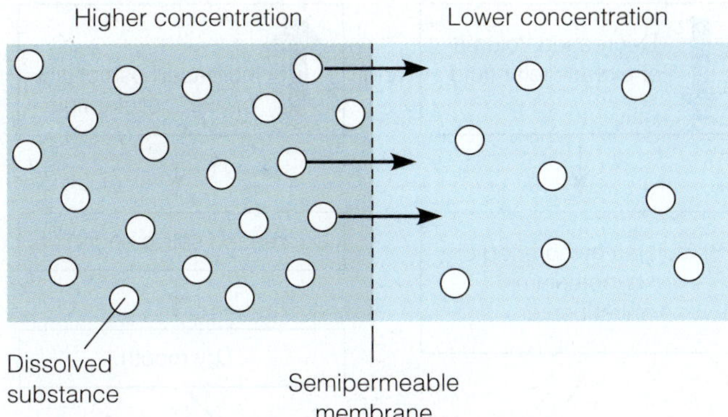

Figure 11–3 ■ Diffusion: The movement of molecules through a semipermeable membrane from an area of higher concentration to an area of lower concentration.

solution of lower concentration (Figure 11–3 ■). Increases in temperature increase the rate of motion of molecules and therefore the rate of diffusion.

FILTRATION **Filtration** is a process whereby fluid and solutes move together across a membrane from one compartment to another. The movement is from an area of higher pressure to one of lower pressure. An example of filtration is the movement of fluid and nutrients from the capillaries of the arterioles to the interstitial fluid around the cells. The pressure in the compartment that results in the movement of the fluid and substances dissolved in fluid out of the compartment is called filtration pressure. **Hydrostatic pressure** is the pressure a fluid exerts within a closed system on the walls of its container. The hydrostatic pressure of blood is the force blood exerts against the vascular walls (e.g., the artery walls). The principle involved in hydrostatic pressure is that fluids move from the area of greater pressure to the area of lesser pressure. Using the example of the blood vessels, the plasma proteins in the blood exert a colloid osmotic or oncotic pressure (see the earlier section on Osmosis) that opposes the hydrostatic pressure and holds the fluid in the vascular compartment to maintain the vascular volume. When the hydrostatic pressure is greater than the osmotic pressure, the fluid filters out of the blood vessels. The filtration pressure in this example is the difference between the hydrostatic pressure and the osmotic pressure (Figure 11–4 ■).

ACTIVE TRANSPORT Substances can move cell membranes from a less concentrated solution to a more concentrated one by **active transport** (Figure 11–5 ■). This process differs from diffusion and osmosis in that metabolic energy is expended. In active transport, a substance combines with a carrier on the outside surface of the cell membrane, and together they move to the inside surface of the cell membrane. Once inside, they separate, and the substance is released to the inside of the cell. Each substance requires a specific carrier, active transport requires enzymes, and energy is expended.

Active transport is particularly important in maintaining the differences in sodium and potassium ion concentrations of ECF and ICF. Under normal conditions, sodium concentrations are higher in the extracellular fluid, and potassium concentrations are higher inside the cells. To maintain these proportions, the active transport mechanism (the sodium-potassium pump) is activated, moving sodium from the cells and potassium into the cells.

Regulating Body Fluids

In a healthy person, the volumes and chemical composition of the fluid compartments stay within narrow, safe limits. Normally, fluid intake and fluid loss are balanced. Illness can upset this balance so that the body has too little or too much fluid. Fluid imbalance can result in a number of illnesses and conditions. The most common example is probably **dehydration**, a condition that occurs when a body does not take in as much water as it loses or lacks sufficient reserves to maintain proper function.

FLUID INTAKE During periods of moderate activity at moderate temperature, the average adult drinks about 1,500 mL per day but needs 2,500 mL per day, an additional 1,000 mL. This added volume is acquired from foods and the oxidation of these foods during metabolic processes. Interestingly, the water content of food is relatively large, contributing about 750 mL per day. The water content of fresh vegetables is approximately 90%, of fresh fruits about 85%, and of lean meats around 60%.

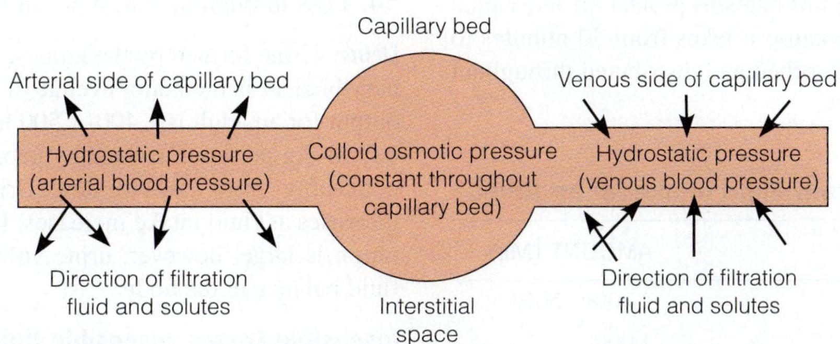

Figure 11–4 ■ Schematic of filtration pressure changes within a capillary bed. On the arterial side, arterial blood pressure exceeds colloid osmotic pressure, so that water and dissolved substances move out of the capillary into the interstitial space. On the venous side, venous blood pressure is less than colloid osmotic pressure, so that water and dissolved substances move into the capillary.

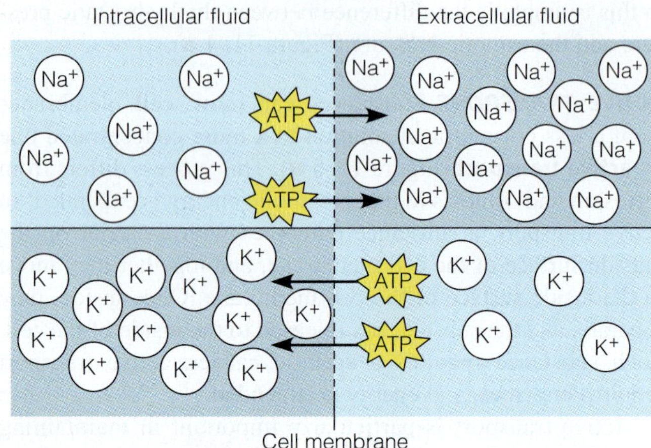

Figure 11–5 ■ An example of active transport. Energy (ATP) is used to move sodium molecules and potassium molecules across a semipermeable membrane against sodium's and potassium's concentration gradients (i.e., from areas of lesser concentration to areas of greater concentration).

Water as a byproduct of food metabolism accounts for most of the remaining fluid volume required. This quantity is approximately 200 mL per day for the average adult (Table 11–2).

The thirst mechanism is the primary regulator of fluid intake. The thirst center is located in the hypothalamus of the brain. A number of stimuli trigger this center, including the osmotic pressure of body fluids, vascular volume, and angiotensin (a hormone released in response to decreased blood flow to the kidneys). For example, a long-distance runner loses significant amounts of water through perspiration and rapid breathing during a race, increasing the concentration of solutes and the osmotic pressure of body fluids. This increased osmotic pressure stimulates the thirst center, causing the runner to experience the sensation of thirst and the desire to drink to replace lost fluids.

Thirst is normally relieved immediately after drinking a small amount of fluid, even before it is absorbed from the gastrointestinal tract. However, this relief is only temporary, and the thirst returns in about 15 minutes. The thirst is again temporarily relieved after the ingested fluid distends the upper gastrointestinal tract. These mechanisms protect the individual from drinking too much, because it takes from 30 minutes to 1 hour for the fluid to be absorbed and distributed throughout the body. See Figure 11–6 ■.

TABLE 11–2 **Average Daily Fluid Intake for an Adult**

SOURCE	AMOUNT (ML)
Oral fluids	1,200–1,500
Water in foods	1,000
Water as by-product of food metabolism	200
Total	2,400–2,700

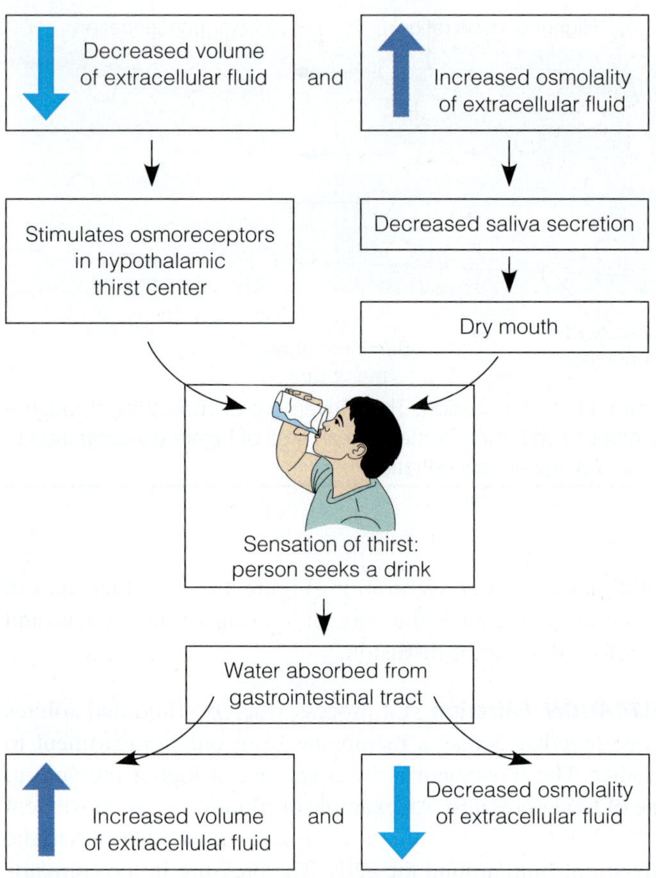

Figure 11–6 ■ Factors stimulating water intake through the thirst mechanism.

FLUID OUTPUT Fluid losses from the body counterbalance the adult's 2,500-mL average daily intake of fluid, as shown in Table 11–3. There are four routes of fluid output:

1. Urine
2. Insensible loss through the skin as perspiration and through the lungs as water vapor in the expired air
3. Noticeable loss through the skin
4. Loss through the intestines in feces.

Urine Urine formed by the kidneys and excreted from the urinary bladder is the major avenue of fluid output. Normal urine output for an adult is 1,400–1,500 mL per 24 hours, or at least 0.5 mL/kg per hour. In healthy people, urine output may vary noticeably from day to day. Urine volume automatically increases as fluid intake increases. If fluid loss through perspiration is large, however, urine volume decreases to maintain fluid balance in the body.

Insensible Losses **Insensible fluid loss** occurs through the skin and lungs. It is called insensible because it is usually not noticeable and cannot be measured. Insensible fluid loss through the skin occurs in two ways. Water is lost through

TABLE 11–3 Average Daily Fluid Output for an Adult

ROUTE	AMOUNT (ML)
Urine	1,400–1,500
Insensible losses	
Lungs	350–400
Skin	350–400
Sweat	100
Feces	100–200
Total	2,300–2,600

diffusion and perspiration (which is noticeable but not measurable). Water losses through diffusion are not noticeable but normally account for 300–400 mL per day. This loss can be significantly increased if the protective layer of the skin is lost due to burns or large abrasions. Perspiration varies depending on factors such as environmental temperature and metabolic activity. Fever and exercise increase metabolic activity and heat production, thereby increasing fluid losses through the skin.

Another type of insensible loss is the water in exhaled air. In an adult, this is normally 300–400 mL per day. When respiratory rate accelerates due to changes such as exercise or an elevated body temperature, this loss can increase.

Feces The chyme that passes from the small intestine into the large intestine contains water and electrolytes. The volume of chyme entering the large intestine in an adult is normally about 1,500 mL per day. Of this amount, all but about 100 mL is reabsorbed in the proximal half of the large intestine.

Certain fluid losses are required to maintain normal body function. These are known as **obligatory losses**. An adult must excrete approximately 500 mL of fluid through the kidneys each day to eliminate metabolic waste products from the body. Losses of water through respirations, through the skin, and in feces are also obligatory losses, necessary for temperature regulation and elimination of waste products. The total of all these losses is approximately 1,300 mL per day.

MAINTAINING HOMEOSTASIS The volume and composition of body fluids are regulated through several homeostatic mechanisms. The body's systems work together to contribute to this regulation. As the kidneys regulate and filter waste, they return electrolytes such as potassium and sodium to the blood for use. The cardiovascular and respiratory systems ensure the body has adequate oxygen to function and use fluids and electrolytes appropriately. The immune system destroys foreign particles and pathogens that can undermine homeostasis. Hormones such as antidiuretic hormone (ADH; also known as arginine vasopressin or AVP), the renin-angiotensin-aldosterone system, and atrial natriuretic factor are involved, as are mechanisms to monitor and maintain vascular volume.

Illness or injury to any one system can negatively impact homeostasis. Some illnesses and diseases, such as cancers, impact homeostasis directly by their very presence in the body. They also impact homeostasis indirectly by the nature of the treatments required to rid the body of the illness itself. Chemotherapy, which can wreak havoc on fluid and electrolyte balance, is a prime example of such a treatment.

Kidneys The kidneys are the primary regulator of body fluids and electrolyte balance. They regulate the volume and osmolality of extracellular fluids by regulating water and electrolyte excretion. The kidneys adjust the reabsorption of water from plasma filtrate and ultimately the amount excreted as urine. Although 135–180 L of plasma per day is normally filtered in an adult, only about 1.5 L of urine is excreted. Electrolyte balance is maintained by selective retention and excretion by the kidneys. The kidneys also play a significant role in acid–base regulation, excreting hydrogen ion (H^+) and retaining bicarbonate.

Antidiuretic Hormone Antidiuretic hormone, which regulates water excretion from the kidney, is synthesized in the anterior portion of the hypothalamus and acts on the collecting ducts of the nephrons. When serum osmolality rises, ADH is produced, causing the collecting ducts to become more permeable to water. This increased permeability allows more water to be reabsorbed into the blood. As more water is reabsorbed, urine output falls and serum osmolality decreases because the water dilutes body fluids. Conversely, if serum osmolality decreases, ADH is suppressed, the collecting ducts become less permeable to water, and urine output increases. Excess water is excreted, and serum osmolality returns to normal. Other factors also affect the production and release of ADH, including blood volume, temperature, pain, stress, and some drugs such as opiates, barbiturates, and nicotine. (See Figure 11–7 ■.)

Renin-Angiotensin-Aldosterone System Specialized receptors in the juxtaglomerular cells of the kidney nephrons respond to changes in renal perfusion. This initiates the renin-angiotensin-aldosterone system. If blood flow or pressure to the kidney decreases, renin is released. Renin causes the conversion of angiotensinogen to angiotensin I, which is then converted to angiotensin II by angiotensin-converting enzyme. Angiotensin II acts directly on the nephrons to promote sodium and water retention. In addition, it stimulates the release of aldosterone from the adrenal cortex. Aldosterone also promotes sodium retention in the distal nephron. The net effect of the renin-angiotensin-aldosterone system is to restore blood volume (and renal perfusion) through sodium and water retention.

Atrial Natriuretic Factor Atrial natriuretic factor (ANF) is a peptide-hormone released from cells in the atrium of the heart in response to excess blood volume and stretching of the atrial walls. Acting on the nephrons, ANF promotes sodium wasting and acts as a potent diuretic, thus reducing vascular volume. ANF also inhibits thirst, reducing fluid intake.

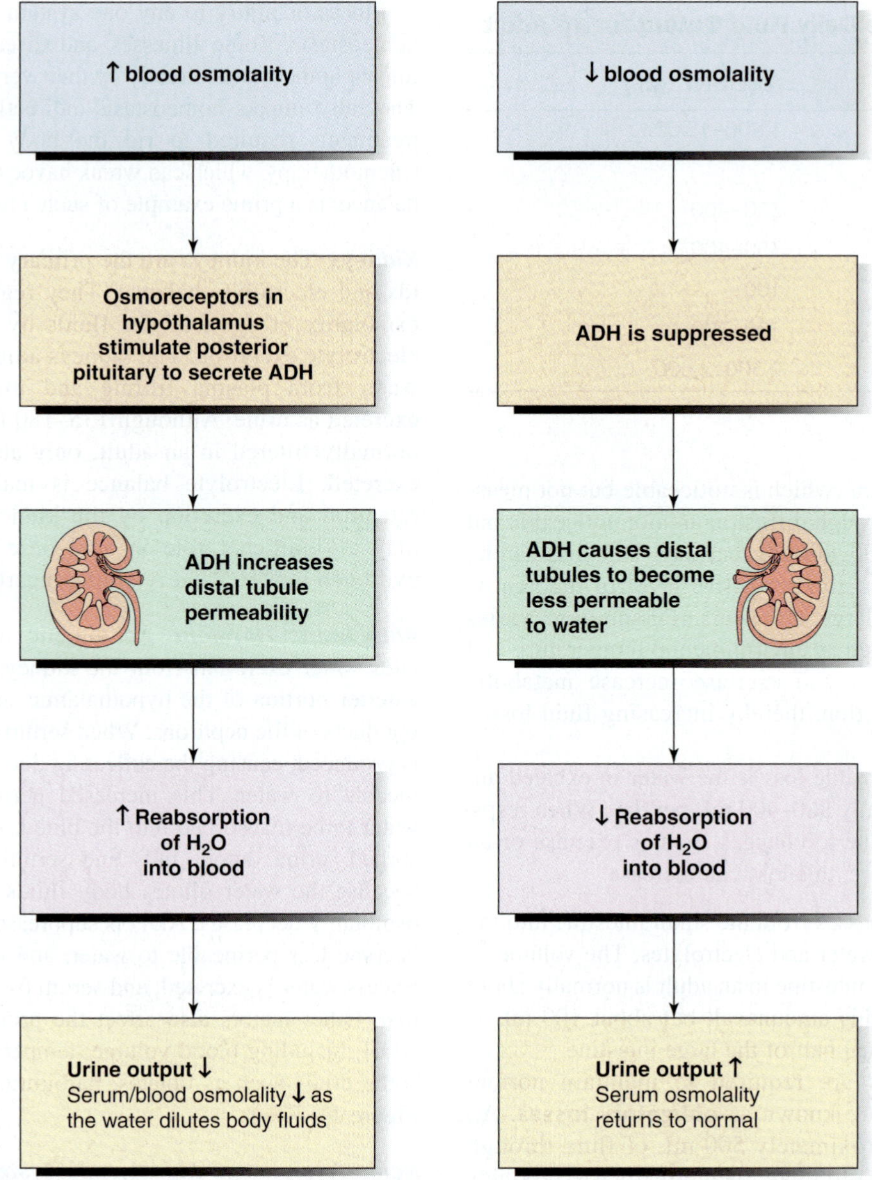

Figure 11–7 ■ Antidiuretic hormone (ADH) regulates water excretion from the kidneys.

Regulating Electrolytes

Electrolytes are present in all body fluids and fluid compartments. Just as maintaining the fluid balance is vital to normal body function, so is maintaining electrolyte balance. Although the concentration of specific electrolytes differs between fluid compartments, a balance of cations (positively charged ions) and anions (negatively charged ions) always exists. Electrolytes are important for the following:

- Maintaining fluid balance
- Contributing to acid–base regulation
- Facilitating enzyme reactions
- Transmitting neuromuscular reactions.

Most electrolytes enter the body through dietary intake and are excreted in the urine. The body does not store some electrolytes, such as sodium and chloride, which must be consumed daily to maintain normal levels. Potassium and calcium, on the other hand, are stored in the cells and bone, respectively. When serum levels drop, ions can shift out of the storage "pool" into the blood to maintain adequate serum levels for normal functioning. The regulatory mechanisms and functions of the major electrolytes are summarized in Table 11–4.

SODIUM (NA^+) Sodium is the most abundant cation in extracellular fluid and a major contributor to serum osmolality. Normal serum sodium levels are 135–145 mEq/L. Sodium functions largely in controlling and regulating water balance. When sodium is reabsorbed from the kidney tubules, chloride and water are reabsorbed with it, thus maintaining ECF volume. Sodium is found in many foods including bacon, ham, processed and canned foods and processed cheeses, and table salt.

POTASSIUM (K^+) Potassium is the major cation in intracellular fluids, with only a small amount found in plasma and interstitial fluid. ICF levels of potassium are usually 125–140 mEq/L,

TABLE 11–4 **Regulation and Functions of Electrolytes**

ELECTROLYTE	REGULATION	FUNCTION
Sodium (Na^+)	■ Renal reabsorption or excretion ■ Aldosterone increases Na^+ reabsorption in collecting duct of nephrons	■ Regulating ECF volume and distribution ■ Maintaining blood volume ■ Transmitting nerve impulses and contracting muscles
Potassium (K^+)	■ Renal excretion and conservation ■ Aldosterone increases K^+ excretion ■ Movement into and out of cells ■ Insulin helps move K^+ into cells; tissue damage and acidosis shift K^+ out of cells into ECF	■ Maintaining ICF osmolality ■ Transmitting nerve and other electrical impulses ■ Regulating cardiac impulse transmission and muscle contraction ■ Skeletal and smooth muscle function ■ Regulating acid–base balance
Calcium (Ca^{2+})	■ Redistribution between bones and ECF ■ Parathyroid hormone and calcitriol increase serum Ca^{2+} levels; calcitonin decreases serum levels	■ Forming bones and teeth ■ Transmitting nerve impulses ■ Regulating muscle contractions ■ Maintaining cardiac pacemaker (automaticity) ■ Blood clotting ■ Activating enzymes such as pancreatic lipase and phospholipase
Magnesium (Mg^{2+})	■ Conservation and excretion by kidneys ■ Intestinal absorption increased by vitamin D and parathyroid hormone	■ Intracellular metabolism ■ Operating sodium–potassium pump ■ Relaxing muscle contractions ■ Transmitting nerve impulses ■ Regulating cardiac function
Chloride (Cl^-)	■ Excreted and reabsorbed along with sodium in the kidneys ■ Aldosterone increases chloride reabsorption with sodium	■ HCl production ■ Regulating ECF balance and vascular volume ■ Regulating acid–base balance ■ Buffer in oxygen–carbon dioxide exchange in RBCs
Phosphate (PO_4^-)	■ Excretion and reabsorption by the kidneys ■ Parathyroid hormone decreases serum levels by increasing renal excretion ■ Reciprocal relationship with calcium: increasing serum calcium levels decrease phosphate levels; decreasing serum calcium increases phosphate	■ Forming bones and teeth ■ Metabolizing carbohydrate, protein, and fat ■ Cellular metabolism; producing ATP and DNA ■ Muscle, nerve, and RBC function ■ Regulating acid–base balance ■ Regulating calcium levels
Bicarbonate (HCO_3^-)	■ Excretion and reabsorption by the kidneys ■ Regeneration by kidneys	■ Major body buffer involved in acid–base regulation

whereas normal serum potassium levels are 3.5–5.0 mEq/L. The ratio of intracellular to extracellular potassium must be maintained for neuromuscular response to stimuli. Potassium is a vital electrolyte for skeletal, cardiac, and smooth muscle activity. It is involved in maintaining acid–base balance as well, and it contributes to intracellular enzyme reactions. Potassium must be ingested daily because the body does not conserve it. Many fruits and vegetables, meat, fish, and other foods contain potassium.

CALCIUM (CA²⁺) The vast majority, 99%, of calcium in the body is in the skeletal system, with a relatively small amount in extracellular fluid. Although this calcium outside the bones and teeth amounts to only about 1% of the total calcium in the body, it is vital in regulating muscle contraction and relaxation, neuromuscular function, and cardiac function. ECF calcium is regulated by a complex interaction of parathyroid hormone calcitonin, and calcitriol, a metabolite of vitamin D. When calcium levels in the ECF fall, parathyroid hormone and calcitriol cause calcium to be released from bones into ECF and increase the absorption of calcium in the intestines, thus raising serum calcium levels. Conversely, calcitonin stimulates the deposition of calcium in bone, reducing the concentration of calcium ions in the blood.

With aging, the intestines absorb calcium less effectively and more calcium is excreted via the kidneys. Calcium shifts out of the bone to replace these ECF losses, increasing the risk of osteoporosis and fractures of the wrists, vertebrae, and hips. Lack of weight-bearing exercise (which helps keep calcium in the bones) and vitamin D deficiency (usually due to inadequate exposure to sunlight) contribute to this risk.

Milk and milk products are the richest sources of calcium, with other foods such as dark green leafy vegetables and canned salmon containing smaller amounts. Many clients benefit from calcium supplements.

Serum calcium levels are often reported in two ways, based on how it circulates in the plasma. Approximately 50% of serum calcium circulates in a free, ionized, or unbound form. The other 50% circulates in the plasma bound to either plasma proteins or other nonprotein ions. The normal total serum calcium levels, which range from 8.5–10.5 mg/dL, represent both bound and unbound calcium. The normal ionized serum calcium, which ranges from 4.0–5.0 mg/dL, represents calcium circulating in the plasma in free, or unbound, form (Hayes, 2004b).

MAGNESIUM (MG²⁺) Magnesium is primarily found in the skeleton and intracellular fluid. It is the second most abundant intracellular cation, with normal serum levels of

1.5–2.5 mEq/L. It is important for intracellular metabolism, particularly in the production and use of adenosine triphosphate (ATP). Magnesium also is necessary for protein and DNA synthesis within the cells. Only about 1% of the body's magnesium is in ECF; here it is involved in regulating neuromuscular and cardiac function. Maintaining and ensuring adequate magnesium levels are an important part of care of clients with cardiac disorders. Cereal grains, nuts, dried fruit, legumes, and green leafy vegetables are good sources of magnesium in the diet, as are dairy products, meat, and fish.

CHLORIDE (CL^-) Chloride is the major anion of ECF, and normal serum levels are 95–108 mEq/L. Chloride functions with sodium to regulate serum osmolality and blood volume. The concentration of chloride in ECF is regulated secondarily to sodium; when sodium is reabsorbed in the kidney, chloride usually follows. Chloride is a major component of gastric juice, as hydrochloric acid (HCl), and is involved in regulating acid–base balance. It also acts as a buffer in the exchange of oxygen and carbon dioxide in RBCs. Chloride is found in the same foods as sodium.

PHOSPHATE PO_{4^-} Phosphate is the major anion of intracellular fluids. It also is found in ECF, bone, skeletal muscle, and nerve tissue. Normal adult serum levels of phospate range from 2.5 to 4.5 mg/dL. Children have much higher phosphate levels than adults, with that of a newborn nearly twice that of an adult. Higher levels of growth hormone and a faster rate of skeletal growth probably account for this difference. Phosphate is involved in many chemical actions of the cell; it is essential for functioning of muscles, nerves, and red blood cells. It is also involved in the metabolism of protein, fat, and carbohydrate. Phosphate is absorbed from the intestine and is found in many foods such as meat, fish, poultry, milk products, and legumes.

BICARBONATE HCO_{3^-} Bicarbonate is present in both intracellular and extracellular fluids. Its primary function is regulating acid–base balance as an essential component of the carbonic acid–bicarbonate buffering system. Extracellular bicarbonate levels are regulated by the kidneys: Bicarbonate is excreted when too much is present; if more is needed, the kidneys both regenerate and reabsorb bicarbonate ions. Unlike other electrolytes that must be consumed in the diet, bicarbonate is produced through metabolic processes in adequate amounts to meet the body's needs.

Factors Affecting Body Fluid and Electrolyte Balance

The ability of the body to adjust fluid and electrolyte balance is influenced by age, gender and body size, environmental temperature, and lifestyle.

AGE ***Pediatric Differences*** Infants and young children differ physiologically from adults in ways that make them vulnerable to fluid and electrolyte imbalances. Infants lose more fluid through the kidneys because immature kidneys are less able to conserve water than adult kidneys. In addition, infants' respirations are more rapid and their **body surface area** (BSA; relationship between height and weight measured in square meters) is proportionately greater than that of adults, increasing insensible fluid losses. This greater percentage of body surface area also puts them at greater risk when burned.

The percentage of body weight that is composed of water also varies with age (Figure 11–8 ■). The percentage is highest at birth (and higher in premature than in full-term infants) and decreases with age (Figure 11–9 ■). Neonates and young infants have a proportionately larger extracellular fluid volume than older children and adults because their brain and skin (both rich in interstitial fluid) constitute a greater proportion of their body weight. Because much of our extracellular fluid is exchanged each day, infants have a high daily fluid requirement with little fluid volume reserve, making them vulnerable to dehydration. As an infant grows, the proportion of water inside the cells increases, the extracellular amount decreases in comparison, and the risk of fluid imbalance begins to decrease.

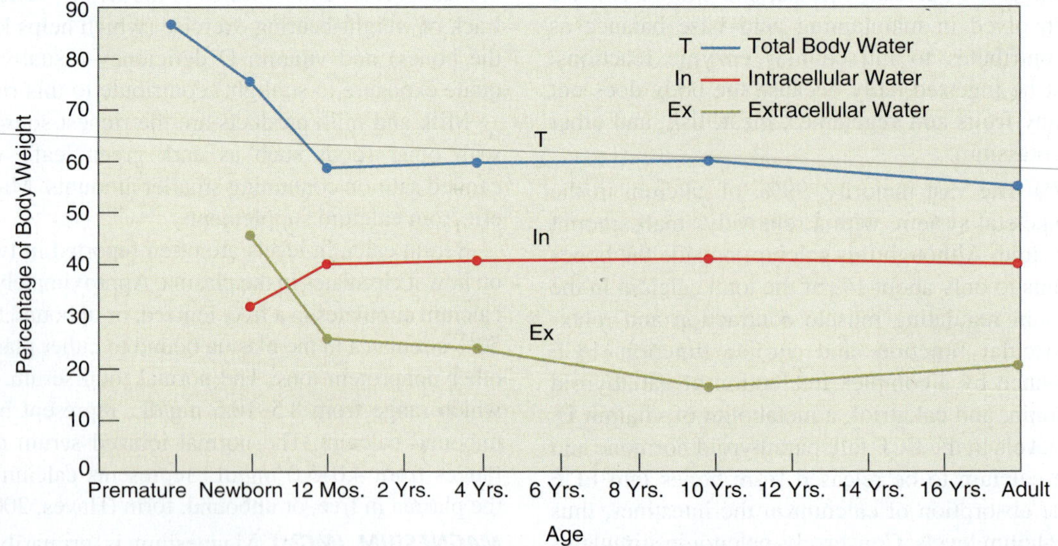

Figure 11–8 ■ The major body fluid compartments at various ages. *Extracellular fluid* is composed mainly of vascular fluid (fluid in blood vessels) and interstitial fluid (fluid between the cells and outside the blood and lymphatic vessels.) *Intracellular fluid* is that within cells.

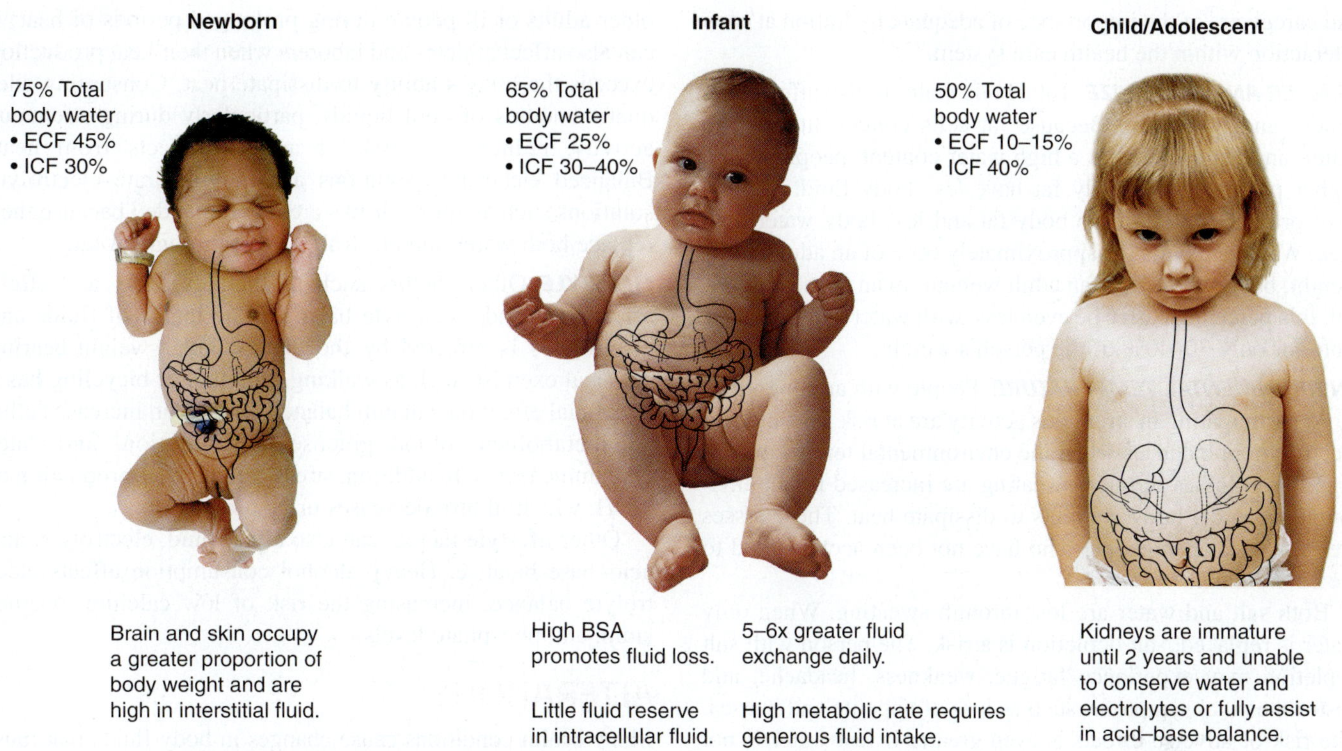
Newborn
75% Total body water
• ECF 45%
• ICF 30%
Brain and skin occupy a greater proportion of body weight and are high in interstitial fluid.
Infant
65% Total body water
• ECF 25%
• ICF 30–40%
High BSA promotes fluid loss.
Little fluid reserve in intracellular fluid.
5–6x greater fluid exchange daily.
High metabolic rate requires generous fluid intake.
Child/Adolescent
50% Total body water
• ECF 10–15%
• ICF 40%
Kidneys are immature until 2 years and unable to conserve water and electrolytes or fully assist in acid–base balance.

Figure 11–9 ■ The newborn and infant have a high percentage of body weight comprised of water, especially extracellular fluid, which is lost from the body easily. Note the small stomach size, which limits ability to rehydrate quickly.

Infants and children under 2 years of age lose a greater proportion of fluid each day than do older children and adults and are thus more dependent on adequate intake. Respiratory illnesses, stomach viruses resulting in vomiting or diarrhea, and burns can all result in fluid or electrolyte imbalance in an infant or young child, increasing the risk for serious complications. A nurse working with parents of a young child presenting with these conditions should take time to explain the importance of monitoring the child's hydration until the child returns to health.

In addition, respiratory and metabolic rates are high during early childhood. These factors lead to greater water loss from the lungs and greater water demand to fuel the body's metabolic processes (Figure 11–10 ■). Because of these factors, the exercising child dehydrates easily and must consume more fluid during physical activity, particularly during hot weather (Committee on Sports Medicine and Fitness, 2000).

When fluid status is compromised, a number of body mechanisms activate to help restore balance. Several of these mechanisms occur in the kidneys. The kidneys conserve water and needed electrolytes while excreting waste products and drug metabolites. In children under 2 years of age, however, the glomeruli, tubules, and nephrons of the kidneys are immature. They are therefore unable to conserve or excrete water and solutes effectively. Because more water is generally excreted, the infant and young child can become dehydrated or develop electrolyte imbalances quickly. Children under 2 years of age also have difficulty regulating electrolytes such as sodium and calcium. Renal response to high solute loads is slower and less developed, with function improving gradually during the first year of life.

Older Adults In elderly people, the normal aging process may affect fluid balance. The thirst response often is blunted. Antidiuretic hormone levels remain normal or may even be elevated, but the nephrons become less able to conserve water in response to ADH. Increased levels of ANF seen in older adults may also contribute to this impaired ability to conserve water. These normal changes of aging increase the risk of dehydration. When combined with the increased likelihood of heart diseases, impaired renal function, and multiple drug regimens, the older adult's risk for fluid and electrolyte imbalance is significant. Nurses should take the opportunity to remind older adults

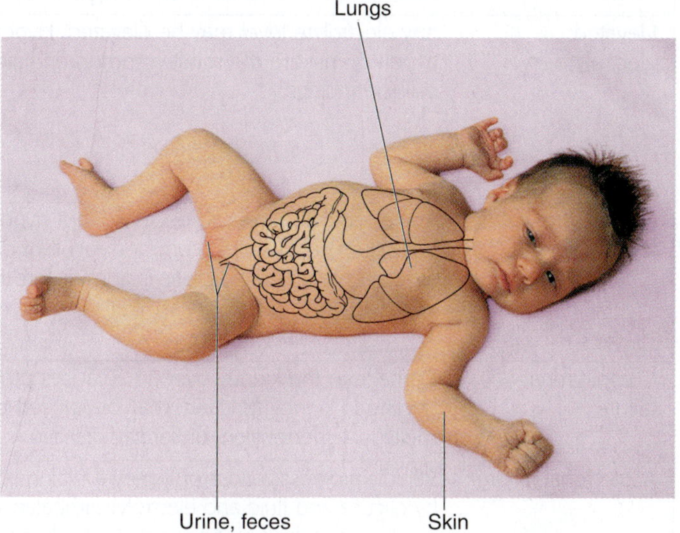
Lungs
Urine, feces
Skin

Figure 11–10 ■ Normal routes of fluid excretion from infants and children.

and caregivers of the importance of adequate hydration at each interaction within the health care system.

GENDER AND BODY SIZE Total body water is also affected by gender and body size. Because fat cells contain little or no water, and lean tissue has a high water content, people with a higher percentage of body fat have less body fluid. Women have proportionately more body fat and less body water than men. Water accounts for approximately 60% of an adult man's weight, but only 52% for an adult woman. In an obese individual, this percentage may be even less, with water being responsible for only 30–40% of the person's weight.

ENVIRONMENTAL TEMPERATURE People with an illness and those participating in strenuous activity are at risk for fluid and electrolyte imbalances when the environmental temperature is high. Fluid losses through sweating are increased in hot environments as the body attempts to dissipate heat. These losses are even greater in people who have not been acclimatized to the environment.

Both salt and water are lost through sweating. When only water is replaced, salt depletion is a risk. The person with salt depletion may experience fatigue, weakness, headache, and gastrointestinal symptoms such as loss of appetite and nausea. The risk of adverse effects is even greater if lost water is not replaced. Body temperature rises, and the person becomes at risk for heat exhaustion or heatstroke. Heatstroke may occur in older adults or ill people during prolonged periods of heat; it can also affect athletes and laborers when their heat production exceeds the body's ability to dissipate heat. Consuming adequate amounts of cool liquids, particularly during strenuous activity, reduces the risk of adverse effects from heat. Balanced electrolyte solutions and carbohydrate–electrolyte solutions such as sports drinks are recommended because they replace both water and electrolytes lost through sweat.

LIFESTYLE Other factors such as diet, exercise, and stress affect fluid and electrolyte balance. The intake of fluids and electrolytes is affected by the diet. Regular weight-bearing physical exercise such as walking, running, or bicycling has a beneficial effect on calcium balance. Stress can increase cellular metabolism, blood glucose concentration, and catecholamine levels. In addition, stress can increase production of ADH, which in turn decreases urine production.

Other lifestyle factors can also affect fluid, electrolyte, and acid–base balance. Heavy alcohol consumption affects electrolyte balance, increasing the risk of low calcium, magnesium, and phosphate levels.

ALTERATIONS

Many health conditions cause changes in body fluids that must be regulated and managed. Sometimes management of fluid status in the home or in a short-term ambulatory facility can prevent

ALTERATIONS AND TREATMENTS Fluids and Electrolytes

Alterations	Description	Treatment
Fluid volume deficit–dehydration	Fluids are lost secondary to diarrhea, vomiting, inability to take in fluids, excessive perspiration, or increased basal metabolic rate due to fever, hyperthyroidism, or medications.	Administer fluids via either the oral or intravenous route and treat the underlying cause.
Fluid volume excess	Too much fluid in the body may be caused by excessive fluid intake (intravenous fluid administration, water intoxication) or inadequate fluid excretion (e.g., kidney failure, poor perfusion to the kidneys secondary to congestive heart failure, low cardiac output, hypertension).	Administer diuretics to increase fluid excretion, reduce fluid intake, and elevate head of bed if dyspnea results from pulmonary edema.
Elevated electrolyte level	Any electrolyte level may be elevated. Hypernatremia and hyperkalemia are the most common and significant extracellular findings.	Limit intake of the elevated electrolyte. Administration of glucose and insulin will lower serum potassium levels by driving potassium from the extracellular space into the intracellular space. Diuretics will increase potassium and sodium loss but will also remove fluid.
Low electrolyte level	Any electrolyte level can decrease, but hypokalemia (low potassium) is the most common result of diuretics unless a potassium sparing diuretic is administered.	Administer electrolyte supplement, monitor serum electrolyte levels, monitor for symptoms associated with electrolyte imbalance. For example, low potassium levels can cause cardiac arrhythmias, and client should be placed on cardiorespiratory monitor.
Chronic renal failure	Damage to the kidney over time causes progressive decline in kidney function; may be caused by diabetes mellitus, hypertension, or cardiac disease.	Initially may be treated with diuretics, progresses to need for dialysis and/or kidney transplant.
Acute renal failure	Rapidly progressive loss of kidney function is characterized by oliguria and fluid and electrolyte imbalances. Can be the result of disturbed blood supply to the kidneys, toxins, or kidney trauma; may be reversible or permanent.	Administer dialysis, monitor fluid and electrolyte balance, transplant kidney, treat the underlying cause.

more serious illness or hospitalization. Examples of conditions that commonly require fluid, electrolyte, or acid–base balance include gastroenteritis, burns, kidney disorders, oral fluid restriction for surgery, anorexia or bulimia, and dehydration and electrolyte imbalances that can result from athletics in hot weather.

PHYSICAL ASSESSMENT

Evaluating clients for fluid and electrolyte status is an important nursing care function. Components of the assessment include (a) the nursing history, (b) physical assessment of the client, (c) clinical measurements, and (d) review of laboratory test results.

Nursing History

The nursing history is particularly important for identifying clients who are at risk for fluid and electrolyte imbalances. The current and past medical history reveals conditions such as chronic cardiac disease or diabetes mellitus that can disrupt normal balances. Medications prescribed to treat acute or chronic conditions (e.g., diuretic therapy for hypertension) also may put the client at risk for altered homeostasis. Functional, developmental, and socioeconomic factors must also be considered in assessing the client's risk. Older people and very young children, clients who must depend on others to meet their needs for food and fluid intake, and people who cannot afford or do not have the means to cook food for a balanced diet (e.g., homeless people) are at greater risk for fluid and electrolyte imbalances.

When obtaining the nursing history, the nurse needs not only to recognize risk factors but also to obtain data about the client's food and fluid intake, fluid output, and the presence of signs or symptoms suggesting altered fluid and electrolyte balance. The Assessment Interview provides examples of questions to elicit information regarding fluid and electrolyte balance.

Physical Assessment

Physical assessment to evaluate a client's fluid and electrolyte status focuses on the skin, the oral cavity and mucous membranes, the eyes, the cardiovascular and respiratory systems, and neurologic and muscular status. Often, the agency will use a standardized form or computer software to help the nurse make sure that certain elements of physical assessment are conducted consistently between visits and from one patient to the next. In addition to these important tools, the nurse should also make note of anything unusual in the client's physical appearance. For example, **edema**, which is swelling caused by excess fluid trapped in bodily tissue, may be readily observed in a client's extremities and recorded during the physical assessment. Data from the physical assessment are used to expand and verify information obtained in the nursing history.

Clinical Measurements

Three simple clinical measurements that the nurse can initiate without a primary care provider's order are daily weights, vital signs, and fluid intake and output.

DAILY WEIGHTS Daily weight measurements provide a relatively accurate assessment of a client's fluid status. Significant changes in weight over a short time (e.g., more than 5 lbs in a week or less) indicate acute fluid changes. Each kilogram (2.2 lbs) of weight gained or lost is equivalent to 1 L of fluid gained or lost. Such fluid gains or losses indicate changes in total body fluid volume rather than in any specific compartment. Rapid losses or gains of 5–8% of total body weight indicate moderate to severe fluid volume deficits or excesses. Regular assessment of weight is particularly important for clients in the community and extended-care facilities who are at risk for fluid imbalance. For these clients, measuring intake and output may be impractical because of lifestyle or problems with incontinence. Regular weight measurement, taken daily, every other day, or weekly, provides valuable information about the client's fluid volume status.

VITAL SIGNS Changes in the vital signs may indicate, or in some cases precede, fluid, electrolyte, and acid–base imbalances. For example, elevated body temperature may be a result of dehydration or a cause of increased body fluid losses.

Tachycardia is an early sign of hypovolemia. Pulse volume will decrease in fluid volume deficit and increase in fluid volume excess. Irregular pulse rates may occur with electrolyte imbalances.

Blood pressure, a sensitive measure to detect blood volume changes, may fall significantly with fluid volume deficit (FVD) and hypovolemia or increase with fluid volume excess (FVE). Postural, or orthostatic, hypotension may also occur with FVD and hypovolemia.

FLUID INTAKE AND OUTPUT The measurement and recording of all fluid intake and output (I & O) during a 24-hour period provides important data about the client's fluid and electrolyte balance.

Most agencies have a form for recording I & O, usually a bedside record on which the nurse lists all items measured and the quantities per shift. Some agencies have another form for recording the specifics of intravenous fluids, such as the type of solution, additives, time started, amounts absorbed, and amounts remaining per shift.

It is important to inform clients, family members, and all caregivers that accurate measurements of the client's fluid intake and output are required. Explain why and emphasize the need to use a bedpan, urinal, commode, or in-toilet collection device (unless a urinary drainage system is in place). Instruct the client not to put toilet tissue into the container with urine. Clients who wish to be involved in recording fluid intake measurements need to be taught how to compute the values and which foods are considered fluids.

To measure fluid intake, the nurse records each fluid item taken (if the client has not already done so) on the I & O form, specifying the time and type of fluid. All of the following fluids need to be recorded:

- Oral fluids
- Ice chips
- Foods that are or tend to become liquid at room temperature
- Tube feedings
- Parenteral fluids
- Intravenous medications
- Catheter or tube irrigants.

Fluid and Electrolyte Assessments

System	Assessment Focus	Technique	Possible Abnormal Findings
Skin	Color, temperature, moisture	Inspection, palpation	Flushed, warm, very dry Moist or diaphoretic Cool and pale
	Turgor	Gently pinch up a fold of skin over sternum or inner aspect of thigh for adults, on the abdomen or medial thigh for children	Poor turgor: Skin remains tented for several seconds instead of immediately returning to normal position
	Edema	Inspect for visible swelling around eyes, in fingers, and in lower extremities	Skin around eyes is puffy, lids appear swollen; rings are tight; shoes leave impressions on feet
		Compress the skin over the dorsum of the foot, around the ankles, over the tibia, in the sacral area	Depression remains (pitting)
Mucous membranes	Color, moisture	Inspection	Mucous membranes dry, dull in appearance; tongue dry and cracked
Eyes	Firmness	Gently palpate eyeball with lid closed	Eyeball feels soft to palpation
Fontanels (infant)	Firmness, level	Inspect and gently palpate anterior fontanel	Fontanel bulging, firm Fontanel sunken, soft
Cardiovascular system	Heart rate	Auscultation, cardiac monitor	Tachycardia, bradycardia; irregular; dysrhythmias
	Peripheral pulses	Palpation	Weak and thready; bounding
	Blood pressure	Auscultation of Korotkoff's sounds	Hypotension
		BP assessment lying and standing	Postural hypotension
	Capillary refill	Palpation	Slowed capillary refill
	Venous filling	Inspection of jugular veins and hand veins	Jugular venous distention; flat jugular veins, poor venous refill
Respiratory system	Respiratory rate and pattern	Inspection	Increased or decreased rate and depth of respirations
	Lung sounds	Auscultation	Crackles or moist rales
Neurologic	Level of consciousness (LOC)	Observation, stimulation	Decreased LOC, lethargy, stupor, or coma
	Orientation, cognition	Questioning	Disoriented, confused; difficulty concentrating
	Motor function	Strength testing	Weakness, decreased motor strength
	Reflexes	Deep-tendon reflex (DTR) testing	Hyperactive or depressed DTRs
	Abnormal reflexes	*Chvostek's sign:* Tap over facial nerve about 2 cm anterior to tragus of ear	Facial muscle twitching including eyelids and lips on side of stimulus
		Trousseau's sign: Inflate a blood pressure cuff on the upper arm to 20 mmHg greater than the systolic pressure, leave in place for 2–5 minutes	Carpal spasm: contraction of hand and fingers on affected side

Assessment Interview Fluid and Electrolyte Balance

CURRENT AND PAST MEDICAL HISTORY

- Are you currently seeing a health care provider for treatment of any chronic diseases such as kidney disease, heart disease, high blood pressure, diabetes insipidus, or thyroid or parathyroid disorders?
- Have you recently experienced any acute conditions such as gastroenteritis, severe trauma, head injury, or surgery? If so, describe them.

MEDICATIONS AND TREATMENTS

- Are you currently taking any medications on a regular basis such as diuretics, steroids, potassium supplements, calcium supplements, hormones, salt substitutes, or antacids?
- Have you recently undergone any treatments such as dialysis, parenteral nutrition, or tube feedings or been on a ventilator? If so, when and why?

FOOD AND FLUID INTAKE

- How much and what type of fluids do you drink each day?
- Describe your diet for a typical day. (The nurse should pay particular attention to the client's intake of protein, whole grains, fruits, vegetables, and foods high in sodium content.)
- Have you made any recent changes in your food or fluid intake, for example, as a result of following a weight-loss program?
- Are you on any type of restricted diet?
- Has your food or fluid intake recently been affected by changes in appetite, nausea, or other factors such as pain or difficulty breathing?

FLUID OUTPUT

- Have you noticed any recent changes in the frequency or amount of urine output?
- Have you recently experienced any problems with vomiting, diarrhea, or constipation? If so, when and for how long?
- Have you noticed any other unusual fluid losses such as excessive sweating?

FLUID AND ELECTROLYTE IMBALANCES

- Have you gained or lost weight in recent weeks?
- Have you recently experienced any symptoms such as excessive thirst, dry skin or mucous membranes, dark or concentrated urine, or low urine output?
- Do you have problems with swelling of your hands, feet, or ankles? Do you ever have difficulty breathing, especially when lying down or at night? How many pillows do you use to sleep?
- Have you recently experienced any of the following symptoms: difficulty concentrating or confusion; dizziness or feeling faint; muscle weakness, twitching, cramping, or spasm; excessive fatigue; abnormal sensations such as numbness, tingling, burning, or prickling; abdominal cramping or distention; heart palpitations?

Source: Berman, A., Snyder, S. J., Kozier, B., & Erb, G. (2008). *Kozier & Erb's fundamentals of nursing: Concepts, process, and practice* (8th ed., p. 1445). Upper Saddle River, NJ: Pearson Education.

To measure fluid output, measure the following fluids (remember to observe appropriate infection control precautions):

- Urinary output
- Vomitus and liquid feces (The amount and type of fluid and the time of output need to be specified.)
- Tube drainage, such as gastric or intestinal drainage
- Wound drainage and draining fistulas.

Fluid intake and output measurements are totaled at intervals pursuant to agency protocol or physician instruction, and the totals are recorded in the client's permanent record.

To determine whether the fluid output is proportional to fluid intake or whether there are any changes in the client's fluid status, the nurse (a) compares the total 24-hour fluid output measurement with the total fluid intake measurement, and (b) compares both to previous measurements. Urinary output is normally equivalent to the amount of fluids ingested; the usual range is 1,500–2,000 mL in 24 hours, or 40–80 mL in 1 hour (0.5 mL/kg per hour). Clients whose output substantially exceeds intake are at risk for **fluid volume deficit**. By contrast, clients whose intake substantially exceeds output are at risk for **fluid volume excess**. In assessing the client's fluid balance, it is important to consider additional factors that may affect intake and output. The client who is extremely diaphoretic or who has rapid, deep respirations has fluid losses that cannot be measured but must be considered in evaluating fluid status.

When there is a significant discrepancy between intake and output or when fluid intake or output is inadequate (for example, a urine output of less than 500 mL in 24 hours or less than 0.5 mL/kg per hour in an adult), this information should be reported to the charge nurse or primary care provider.

DIAGNOSTIC TESTS

Many laboratory studies may be conducted to determine the client's fluid and electrolyte status. Some of the more common tests are discussed here.

Serum Electrolytes

Serum electrolyte levels are often routinely ordered for any client admitted to the hospital as a screening test for electrolyte imbalances. The most commonly ordered serum tests are for sodium, potassium, chloride, magnesium, and bicarbonate ions. Normal values of commonly measured electrolytes are shown in Box 11–2. Some primary care providers use a diagram format (Figure 11–11 ■) for keeping track of the client's electrolytes when documenting in their progress notes.

Complete Blood Count (CBC)

The complete blood count, another basic screening test, includes information about the hematocrit (Hct). The **hematocrit** measures the volume (percentage) of whole blood that is composed of RBCs. Because the hematocrit is a measure of the volume of cells in relation to plasma, it is affected by changes in plasma volume. Thus, the hematocrit increases with severe dehydration and decreases with severe overhydration. Normal hematocrit values are 40–54% (men) and 37–47% (women).

Box 11–2 Normal Electrolyte Values for Adults*

VENOUS BLOOD	
Sodium	135–145 mEq/L
Potassium	3.5–5.0 mEq/L
Chloride	95–108 mEq/L
Calcium (total)	4.5–5.5 mEq/L or 8.5–10.5 mg/dL
(ionized)	56% of total calcium (2.5 mEq/L or 4.0–5.0 mg/dL)
Magnesium	1.5–2.5 mEq/L or 1.6–2.5 mg/dL
Phosphate (phosphorus)	1.8–2.6 mEq/L or 2.5 – 4.5 mg/dL
Serum osmolality	280–300 mOsm/kg water

**Note:* Normal laboratory values vary from agency to agency.

Osmolality

Serum osmolality is a measure of the solute concentration of the blood. The particles included are sodium ions, glucose, and urea (blood urea nitrogen, or BUN). Serum osmolality can be estimated by doubling the serum sodium, because sodium and its associated chloride ions are the major determinants of serum osmolality. Serum osmolality values are used primarily to evaluate fluid balance. Normal values are 280–300 mOsm/kg. An increase in serum osmolality indicates a fluid volume deficit; a decrease reflects a fluid volume excess.

Urine osmolality is a measure of the solute concentration of urine. The particles included are nitrogenous wastes, such as creatinine, urea, and uric acid. Normal values are 500–800 mOsm/kg. An increased urine osmolality indicates a fluid volume deficit; a decreased urine osmolality reflects a fluid volume excess.

Urine Specific Gravity

Specific gravity is an indicator of urine concentration that can be performed quickly and easily by nursing personnel. Normal specific gravity ranges from 1.005–1.030 (usually 1.010–1.025). When the concentration of solutes in the urine is high, the specific gravity rises; in very dilute urine with few solutes, it is abnormally low.

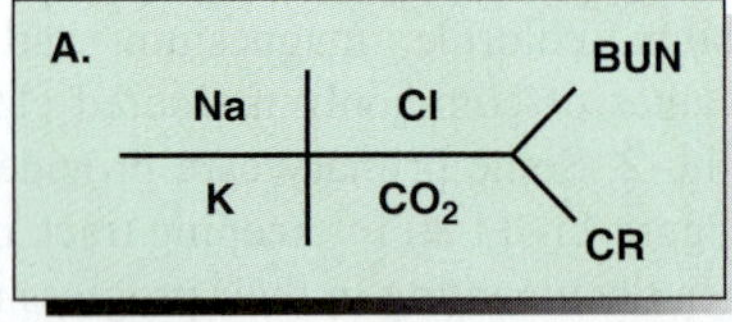

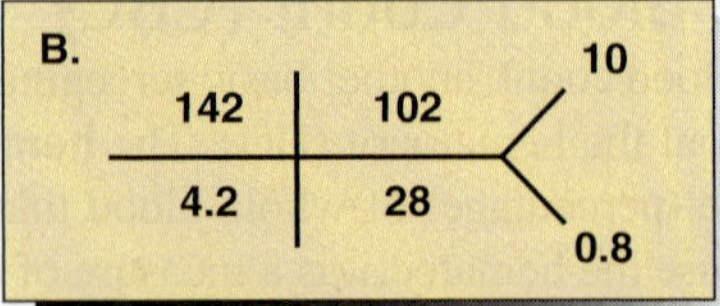

Figure 11–11 ■ *A*, Format for a diagram of serum electrolyte results. *B*, Example that may be seen in a primary care provider's documentation notes.

Urine Sodium and Chloride Excretion

These are indicators of renal perfusion that can provide useful information about a client's fluid status. With hypovolemia, aldosterone is secreted. This will cause reabsorption of sodium and chloride, which results in decreased levels of sodium and chloride, less than 20 mEq/L each (Elgart, 2004).

CARING INTERVENTIONS

Alterations in fluid and electrolytes may occur as a primary event or as a secondary response to a preexisting disease state or a sudden traumatic event. When alterations of fluid and electrolytes exceed the narrow limits consistent with health, the body needs to adjust quickly. The severity of fluid and electrolyte imbalance determines whether treatment will consist of oral replacements or the initiation of intravenous therapy. Intravenous fluids may be ordered for the client with a fluid volume deficit if replacement oral fluids cannot be taken in sufficient quantity. Electrolyte supplements may be used to replace electrolyte deficits. Diuretics may be ordered to reduce fluid volume excess.

Consult your skills manual for step-by-step descriptions of the following caring interventions related to fluids and electrolytes:

- Initiating intravenous therapy
- Intravenous management
- Monitoring fluid balance
- Medication administration
- Blood transfusions.

PHARMACOLOGIC THERAPIES

Pharmacological therapies are aimed at replacing what has been lost or deleting what may be excessive in order to restore a normal balance to the body's fluid and electrolytes. Fluids are replaced in an attempt to put back what is lost so blood loss is replaced with blood transfusions, albumins, or other large-molecule protein solutions (colloid). Fluids lost secondary to excessive diuresis, perspiration, inadequate intake, or insensible water loss are replaced using crystalloids.

Electrolyte correction is highly dependent on the specific electrolyte and whether the body is in deficit or in excess. For example, elevated potassium levels (sometimes referred to as **hyperkalemia**) are ultimately corrected by dialysis, but treatments such as administration of glucose and insulin can help to drive potassium back into the cell where elevated levels will create less risk. A deficit in potassium is known as **hypokalemia**, and is frequently a side-effect of diuretics. Sodium excess, often seen in clients with reduced production of antidiuretic hormone (ADH), may be corrected by administration of ADH. Sodium excess may be referred to as **hypernatremia**, whereas a deficit in sodium is known as **hyponatremia**. Sodium deficiency may be treated with oral supplementation or, if the deficiency is severe or life threatening, intravenous supplementation may be administered.

MEDICATIONS **Fluids and Electrolytes**

Drug Groups	Mechanism of Action	Common Drugs	Nursing Considerations
Electrolyte supplements	Restore electrolyte balance by replacing.	Sodium chloride–sodium supplement Potassium chloride–potassium supplement	■ Monitor serum electrolyte levels, intake and output, vital signs.
Colloids	Proteins, starches, or other large molecules remain in the blood for a long time and act as a volume expander.	Serum albumin, dextran 40	■ Carefully monitor client's condition, laboratory values, and renal function.
Crystalloids	Intravenous solutions that contain electrolytes and other agents that mimic the body's extracellular fluid are used to replace depleted fluid and promote urine output.	5% dextrose and water, normal saline solution, lactated ringer's, 5% dextrose and 1/2 normal saline	■ Monitor client's fluid and electrolyte status.
Diuretics	Promote urine output.	Furosemide, hydrochlorothiazide, aldactone	■ Monitor intake and output, daily weight, serum electrolytes, and hydration status.

11.1 ACUTE RENAL FAILURE

KEY TERMS

Acute renal failure (ARF), *534*
Acute tubular necrosis (ATN), *534*
Anuria, *541*
Arteriovenous (AV) fistula, *545*
Azotemia, *534*
Catabolism, *550*
Continuous renal replacement therapy (CRRT), *543*
Dialysate, *543*
Dialysis, *543*
Diuresis, *538*
Glomerular filtration rate (GFR), *534*
Hematuria, *539*
Hemodialysis, *543*
Hemolysis, *537*
Hyperphosphatemia, *538*
Hypervolemia, *547*
Hypocalcemia, *538*
Hypoperfusion, *534*
Hypovolemia, *535*
Ischemia, *534*
Nephrotoxins, *534*
Oliguria, *534*
Osteodystrophy, *540*
Peritoneal dialysis, *543*
Pitting edema, *538*
Proteinuria, *540*
Renal failure, *534*
Renal insufficiency, *537*
Tetany, *548*
Ultrafiltration, *544*

BASIS FOR SELECTION OF EXEMPLAR

Healthy People 2010

LEARNING OUTCOMES

After reading about this exemplar, you will be able to:

1. Describe the pathophysiology, etiology, clinical manifestations, and direct and indirect causes of acute renal failure.
2. Identify risk factors associated with acute renal failure.
3. Illustrate the nursing process in providing culturally competent care across the life span for individuals with acute renal failure.
4. Formulate priority nursing diagnoses appropriate for an individual with acute renal failure.
5. Create a plan of care for individuals with acute renal failure and their family members.
6. Assess expected outcomes for an individual with acute renal failure.
7. Discuss therapies used in the collaborative care of an individual with acute renal failure.
8. Employ evidence-based caring interventions for an individual with acute renal failure.

OVERVIEW

The kidneys control fluid and electrolyte balance as well as acid–base balance, and they help to control blood pressure, thereby helping to maintain homeostasis. Normally only one functioning kidney is necessary to maintain homeostasis. When both kidneys fail to function properly, fluids accumulate and electrolyte levels are altered, and this affects many systems within the body. Heart rate increases in an attempt to accommodate excess fluid, and muscle function is impacted by electrolyte imbalance. Cerebral edema may occur. Death will result within a few days if appropriate treatment is not initiated.

Renal failure is a condition in which the kidneys are unable to remove accumulated metabolites from the blood, resulting in altered fluid, electrolyte, and acid–base balance. The cause may be a primary kidney disorder, or renal failure may be secondary to a systemic disease or other urologic defects. Renal failure may be either acute or chronic. When acute, renal failure has an abrupt onset and may be reversed with prompt intervention. Chronic renal failure is a silent disease, which progresses slowly and with few symptoms until the kidneys are severely damaged and unable to meet the excretory needs of the body. Both forms of renal failure are characterized by **azotemia** (increased levels of nitrogenous wastes in the blood). In this exemplar, we discuss the acute form of renal failure.

Acute renal failure (ARF) is a rapid decline in renal function with azotemia and fluid and electrolyte imbalances. The most common causes of ARF are **ischemia** (insufficient blood supply) and **nephrotoxins** (substances that damage nerves or nerve tissue). The kidneys are particularly vulnerable to both because of the amount of blood that passes through them. A fall in blood pressure or volume can cause ischemia of kidney tissues. Nephrotoxins in the blood damage renal tissue directly.

PATHOPHYSIOLOGY AND ETIOLOGY

The causes and pathophysiology of ARF are commonly categorized as prerenal, intrinsic, and postrenal. Prerenal ARF is the most common, accounting for approximately 55% of the total. In prerenal ARF, **hypoperfusion** (decreased blood flow) leads to ARF without directly affecting the integrity of kidney tissues. Intrinsic (or intrarenal) ARF, caused by direct damage to functional kidney tissue, is responsible for another 40%. Urinary tract obstruction with resulting kidney damage is the precipitating factor for postrenal ARF, the least common form (~5%). Table 11–5 summarizes the causes of ARF, and Figure 11–12 ■ outlines the pathophysiology of ARF.

PRERENAL ARF Prerenal ARF results from conditions that affect renal blood flow and perfusion. Any disorder that significantly decreases vascular volume, cardiac output, or systemic vascular resistance can affect renal blood flow. Prerenal ARF is common, particularly in trauma, surgical, and critically ill clients.The kidneys normally receive 20 to 25% of the cardiac output to maintain the **glomerular filtration rate (GFR)** (the rate at which fluid is filtered through the kidneys). A drop in renal blood flow to less than 20% of normal causes the GFR to fall. As the filtration of substances by the glomeruli is reduced, less reabsorption of substances in the tubule is required. As a result, kidney cells require less energy and oxygen, and their metabolism slows. Prerenal ARF is rapidly reversed when blood flow is restored, and the renal parenchyma remains undamaged. Unresolved ischemia can lead to tubular cell necrosis and significant nephron damage (Kasper et al., 2005; Porth, 2005). Intrinsic ARF caused by ischemic injury may result.

POSTRENAL ARF Obstructive causes of ARF are classified as postrenal. Any condition that prevents urine excretion can lead to postrenal ARF. Benign prostatic hypertrophy is the most common precipitating factor. Others include renal or urinary tract calculi and tumors. Children may experience **oliguria** (decreased urine output) or normal or increased urine output. Renal failure without oliguria usually indicates a less severe renal injury.

INTRINSIC (INTRARENAL) ARF Intrinsic or intrarenal failure is characterized by acute damage to the renal parenchyma and nephrons. Intrarenal causes include diseases of the kidney itself and acute tubular necrosis, the most common intrarenal cause of ARF.

In acute glomerulonephritis, glomerular inflammation can reduce renal blood flow and cause ARF. Vascular disorders affecting the kidney, such as vasculitis (inflammation of the blood vessels), malignant hypertension, and arterial or venous occlusion, can damage nephrons sufficiently to result in ARF.

ACUTE TUBULAR NECROSIS Nephrons are especially susceptible to injury from ischemia or exposure to nephrotoxins. **Acute tubular necrosis (ATN)** (the destruction of tubular epithelial cells) causes an abrupt and progressive decline of renal function. Prolonged ischemia is the primary cause of ATN. When ischemia and nephrotoxin exposure occur concurrently, the risk

TABLE 11–5 **Causes of Acute Renal Failure**

	CAUSE	EXAMPLES
Prerenal	Hypovolemia	Hemorrhage, dehydration, excess fluid loss from gastrointestinal tract, burns, wounds
	Low cardiac output	Heart failure, cardiogenic shock
	Altered vascular resistance	Sepsis, anaphylaxis, vasoactive drugs
Intrarenal	Glomerular/microvascular injury	Glomerulonephritis, disseminated intravascular coagulation, vasculitis, hypertension, toxemia of pregnancy, hemolytic uremic syndrome
	Acute tubular necrosis	Ischemia resulting from conditions associated with prerenal failure; toxins, such as drugs, heavy metals; hemolysis; rhabdomyolysis (muscle cell breakdown)
	Interstitial nephritis	Acute pyelonephritis, toxins, metabolic imbalances, idiopathic
Postrenal	Ureteral obstruction	Calculi, cancer, external compression
	Urethral obstruction	Prostatic enlargement, calculi, cancer, stricture, blood clot

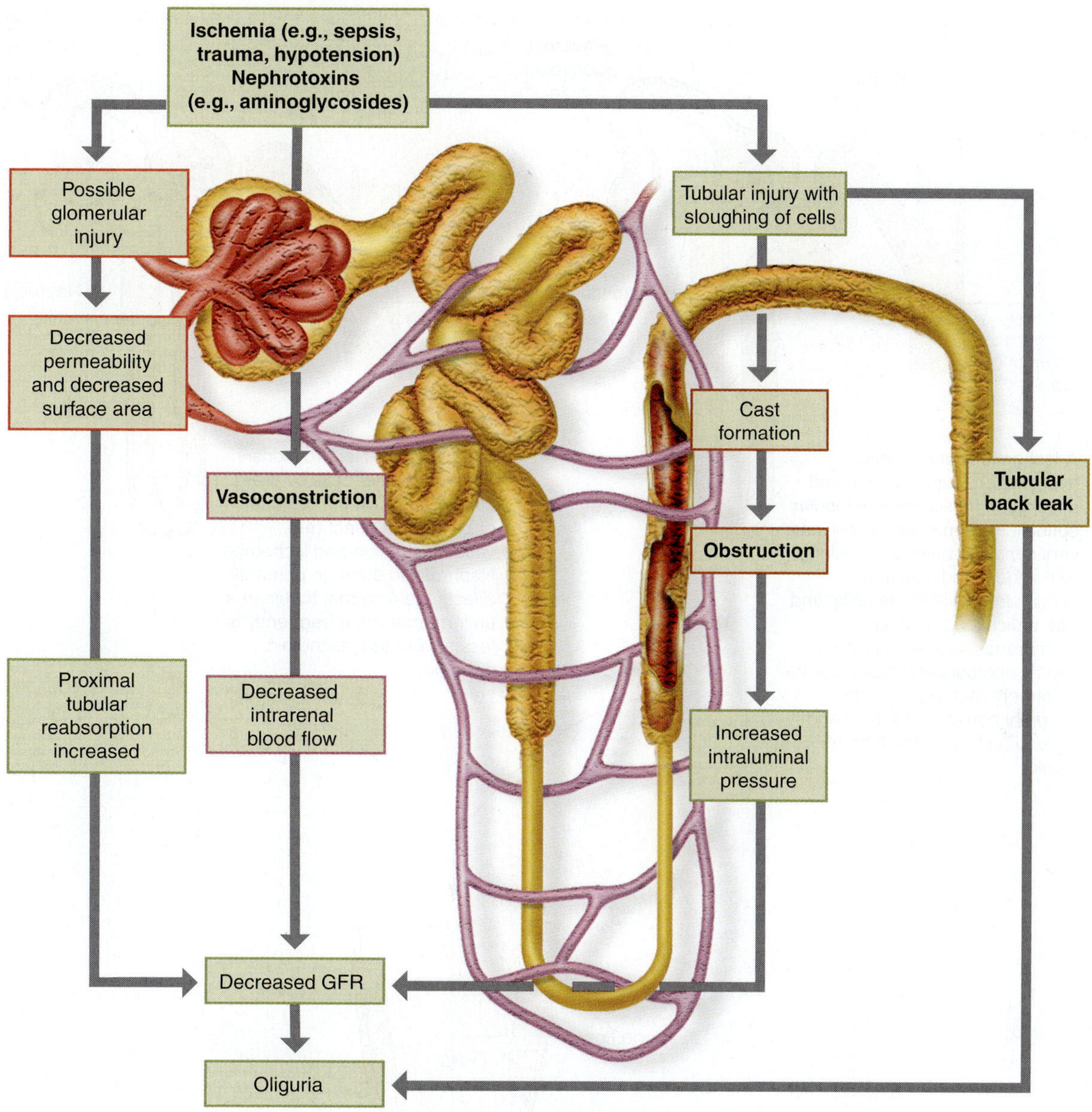

Figure 11–12 ■ The pathophysiology of acute renal failure.

for ATN and tubular dysfunction is especially high. See Figure 11–13 ■ for the pathogenesis of ARF caused by ATN. Risk factors for ischemic ATN include major surgery, severe **hypovolemia** (decreased circulating blood volume), sepsis, trauma, and burns. The impact of ischemia resulting from vasodilation and fluid loss in sepsis, trauma, and burns often is compounded by toxins released by bacteria or from damaged tissue. Injury to the tubule resulting in ATN is the most frequent cause of intrinsic renal failure in children.

Ischemia lasting more than 2 hours causes severe and irreversible damage to kidney tubules, with patchy cellular necrosis and sloughing. The GFR is significantly reduced as a result of ischemia, activation of the renin–angiotensin system, and tubular obstruction by cellular debris, which raises the pressure in the glomerular capsule.

Common nephrotoxins associated with ATN include the aminoglycoside antibiotics and radiologic contrast media. Many other drugs (e.g., nonsteroidal anti-inflammatory drugs and some chemotherapeutic drugs), heavy metals (e.g., mercury and gold), and some common chemicals (e.g., ethylene glycol [antifreeze]) are also potentially toxic to the renal tubule. The risk for ATN is higher when nephrotoxic drugs are given to older clients or to clients with preexisting renal insufficiency, and when used in combination with other nephrotoxins. Dehydration increases the risk by increasing the toxin concentration in nephrons.

Nephrotoxins destroy tubular cells by both direct and indirect effects. As tubular cells are damaged and lost through necrosis and sloughing, the tubule becomes more permeable. This increased permeability results in filtrate reabsorption, further reducing the ability of the nephron to eliminate wastes.

Rhabdomyolysis (muscle cell breakdown) may account for 7–15% of all cases of ARF (Criddle, 2003; Russell, 2005). It is caused by release of excess myoglobin from injured skeletal

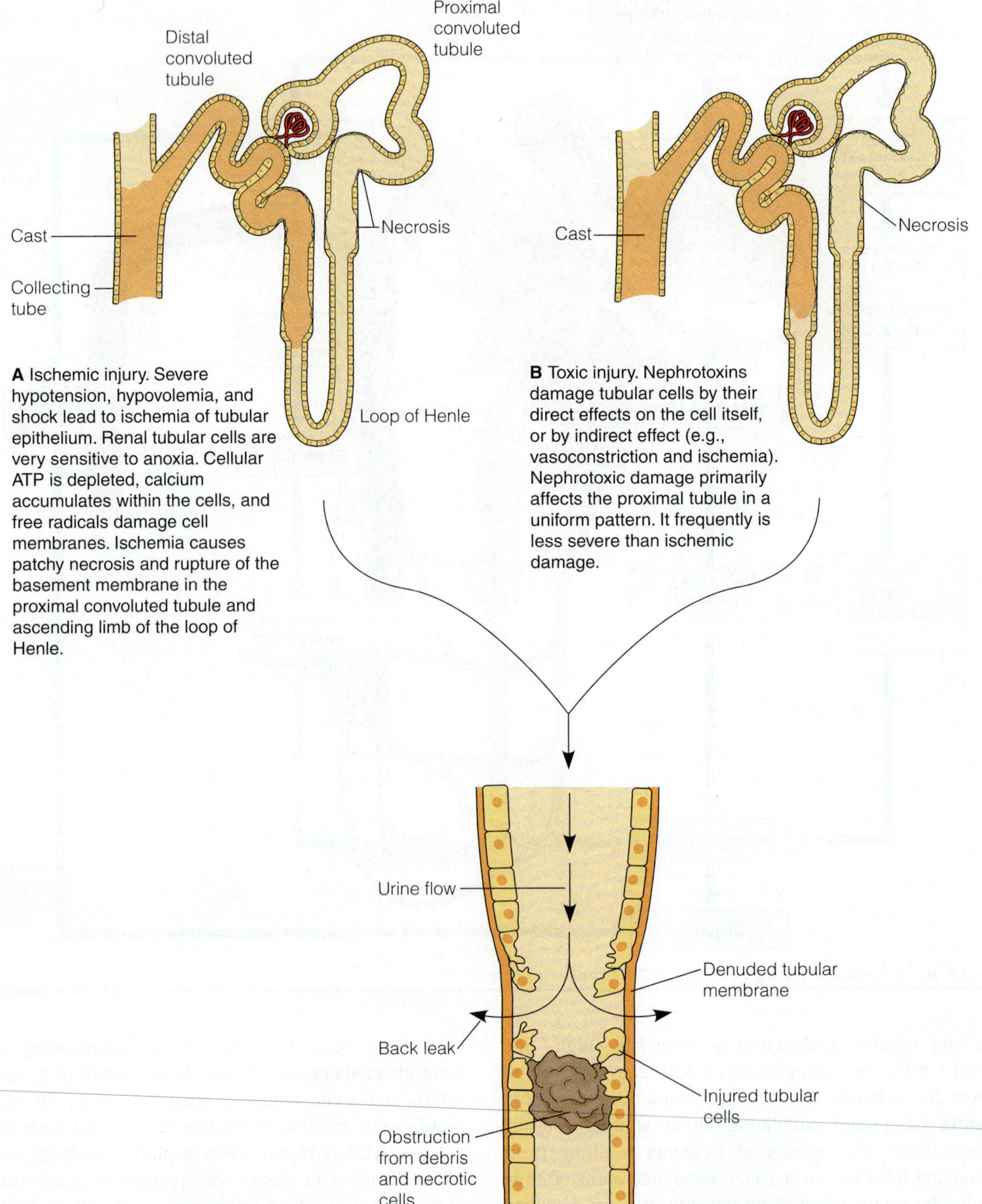

Proximal convoluted tubule
Distal convoluted tubule
Cast
Necrosis
Collecting tube
Cast
Necrosis
A Ischemic injury. Severe hypotension, hypovolemia, and shock lead to ischemia of tubular epithelium. Renal tubular cells are very sensitive to anoxia. Cellular ATP is depleted, calcium accumulates within the cells, and free radicals damage cell membranes. Ischemia causes patchy necrosis and rupture of the basement membrane in the proximal convoluted tubule and ascending limb of the loop of Henle.
Loop of Henle
B Toxic injury. Nephrotoxins damage tubular cells by their direct effects on the cell itself, or by indirect effect (e.g., vasoconstriction and ischemia). Nephrotoxic damage primarily affects the proximal tubule in a uniform pattern. It frequently is less severe than ischemic damage.
Urine flow
Denuded tubular membrane
Back leak
Injured tubular cells
Obstruction from debris and necrotic cells
C Injured tubular cells release intracellular debris, which combines with proteins within the tubules to form casts. These casts, together with sloughed necrotic cells, occlude the tubular lumen, increasing tubular pressure and disrupting the flow of glomerular filtrate. Glomerular filtration slows. The increased pressure pushes filtrate out of the damaged tubule into interstitial tissues (back leak). Renal blood flow and glomerular filtration may be further reduced by intrarenal angiotension II release and vasoconstriction.

Figure 11–13 ■ Acute tubular necrosis (ATN). In ATN, tubular epithelial cells are destroyed by either ischemic or toxic injury.

muscles. Myoglobin is a protein that acts as the oxygen reservoir for muscle fibers, much as hemoglobin does for blood. Muscle trauma, strenuous exercise, hyperthermia or hypothermia, drug overdose, infection, and other factors can precipitate rhabdomyolysis. The myoglobin clogs renal tubules, causing ischemic injury, and contains an iron pigment that directly damages the tubules. **Hemolysis** (red blood cell [RBC] destruction) releases hemoglobin into the circulation, with much the same effect as rhabdomyolysis.

Etiology

Approximately 5% of all hospitalized clients develop ARF; the incidence jumps to as much as 30% in critical and special care units (Kasper et al., 2005). The mortality rate for ARF in seriously ill clients is up to 75%. This high death rate is probably more related to the populations affected by ARF—older clients and the critically ill—than to the disorder itself (Porth, 2005).

ARF occurs in approximately one fifth of older adults (Bailey & Sands, 2003) and may comprise up to 10% of all older adults admitted to acute care settings (Jassal, Fillit, & Oreopoulos, 1998). Prerenal causes are common in older adults and lead to poor perfusion of the kidney. In adults of any age, renal causes may be secondary to chronic diseases, such as hypertension and diabetes mellitus (Table 11–6).

ARF is seen in 2–3% of children cared for in pediatric intensive care units, and up to 8% of infants cared for in neonatal intensive care units (Vogt & Avner, 2007). Potential causes include hemolytic uremic syndrome, acute glomerulonephritis, sepsis, poisoning, hypovolemia, obstructive uropathy, and complication of cardiac surgery. Recently, hematologic-oncologic complications, bone marrow transplantation, and respiratory failure have become more common causes of ARF (Bock, 2005). In some cases, a combination of factors leads to the development of ARF. Children who recover from ARF may have residual kidney damage and compromised renal function.

Risk Factors

Risk factors for ARF include major trauma or surgery, infection, hemorrhage, severe heart failure, severe liver disease, and lower urinary tract obstruction. Drugs and radiologic contrast media that are toxic to the kidney also increase the risk for ARF.

Older adults develop ARF more frequently because of their higher incidence of serious illness, hypotension, major surgeries, diagnostic procedures, and treatment with nephrotoxic drugs. Decrease in kidney function associated with aging also puts older adults at greater risk for kidney failure.

The child with **renal insufficiency** (decrease in the kidneys' ability to conserve sodium and concentrate the urine) is at greater risk for fluid loss with illness. In cases of acute gastrointestinal (GI) illness, these children are at greater risk for dehydration and ARF.

CLINICAL MANIFESTATIONS

The course of ARF caused by acute tubercular necrosis typically includes three phases: initiation, maintenance, and recovery.

Initiation Phase

The initiation phase may last hours to days. It begins with the initiating event (e.g., hemorrhage) and ends when tubular injury occurs. If ARF is recognized and the initiating event is treated effectively during this phase, the prognosis is good. The initiation phase of ARF is often asymptomatic, however, making it difficult to identify ARF before the appearance of the manifestations of the maintenance phase.

Maintenance Phase

The maintenance phase of ARF is characterized by a significant fall in GFR and tubular necrosis. Oliguria may develop, although many clients continue to produce normal or near-normal

TABLE 11–6 Causes of Renal Failure in Older Adults

PRERENAL CAUSES	RENAL CAUSES	POSTRENAL CAUSES
Dehydration	Acute glomerulonephritis	Benign prostatic hyperplasia
Shock	Aminoglycoside antibiotics	Prostate cancer
Vomiting and diarrhea	Sepsis	Bladder cancer
Surgery	Acute pyelonephritis	Calculi
Cardiac failure	Aneurysms	Fecal impaction
Diuretics	Cholesterol embolus	Urethral strictures
Nonsteroidal anti-inflammatory drugs	Allergic response to radiocontrast media	Gynecologic cancers
Angiotensin-converting enzyme inhibitors	Renal hypertension secondary to renal artery stenosis	
Hypotension	Diabetic nephropathy	

Source: Bailey & Sands (2003); Beers & Berkow (2004); Wiggins (2003).

CLINICAL MANIFESTATIONS AND THERAPIES Acute Renal Failure

ETIOLOGY	CLINICAL MANIFESTATION	CLINICAL THERAPIES
Anemia	Fatigue Pallor Dizziness, confusion, lethargy Tachycardia, tachypnea, hypotension	■ Iron supplementation ■ Administration of epoetin ■ Blood transfusion ■ Therapies aimed at treating the underlying cause of ARF
Fluid volume excess	Dependent **pitting edema** (edema that retains indentation caused by pressure) Respiratory crackles Dyspnea, pulmonary edema, hypoxemia Weight gain Tachycardia Jugular vein distention	■ Fluid restriction ■ Sodium-restricted diet ■ Diuretics ■ Dialysis
Hyperkalemia	Ventricular arrhythmias Tall, peaked T waves; widened QRS Cardiac arrest Smooth muscle hyperactivity Nausea and vomiting Abdominal cramping Diarrhea Muscle weakness Paresthesias Flaccid paralysis	■ Removal of all potassium from intravenous solutions ■ Low-potassium diet ■ Administration of glucose and insulin to drive potassium into the cell ■ Potassium-absorbing enema solutions ■ Dialysis

amounts of urine (nonoliguric ARF). Even though urine may be produced, the kidney cannot efficiently eliminate metabolic wastes, water, electrolytes, and acids from the body during the maintenance phase of ARF. Azotemia, fluid retention, electrolyte imbalances, and metabolic acidosis develop. These abnormalities are more severe in the client with oliguria than in the client without oliguria, leading to a poorer prognosis with oliguria.

During the maintenance phase, salt and water retention cause edema, increasing the risk for heart failure and pulmonary edema. Impaired potassium excretion leads to hyperkalemia (increased levels of potassium in the blood). When the serum potassium level is greater than 6.0–6.5 mEq/L, manifestations of its effect on neuromuscular function develop. These include muscle weakness, nausea and diarrhea, electrocardiographic changes, and possible cardiac arrest. Other electrolyte imbalances include **hyperphosphatemia** (increased blood levels of phosphate) and **hypocalcemia** (decreased blood levels of calcium). Metabolic acidosis results from impaired hydrogen ion elimination by the kidneys.

Anemia develops after several days of ARF because of suppressed erythropoietin secretion by the kidneys. Immune function may be impaired, increasing the risk for infection. Other manifestations of the maintenance phase include the following:

- Confusion, disorientation, agitation or lethargy, hyperreflexia, and possible seizures or coma because of azotemia and electrolyte and acid–base imbalances
- Anorexia (loss of appetite), nausea, vomiting, and decreased or absent bowel sounds
- Uremic syndrome (if ARF is prolonged; see the exemplar on chronic renal failure that follows).

Recovery Phase

The recovery phase of ARF is characterized by a process of tubule cell repair and regeneration and gradual return of the GFR to normal or pre-ARF levels. **Diuresis** (excretion of abnormally large quantities of urine) may occur as the nephrons and GFR recover, promoting retained salt, water, and solutes to be excreted. Serum creatinine, blood urea nitrogen (BUN), potassium, and phosphate levels remain high and may continue to rise in spite of increasing urine output. Renal function improves rapidly during the first 5–25 days of the recovery phase and continues to improve for up to 1 year.

Renal failure has different presentations in older and younger adults. In younger adults, marked oliguria is the most dramatic symptom of ARF, but older adults may not display this symptom. Postural hypotension (a decrease in blood pressure when the client sits or stands) is common in clients with prerenal ARF (Bailey & Sands, 2003), and the nurse is in a position to monitor for this finding. BUN and serum creatinine levels increase, and dependent edema may be present (Table 11–7). Ultrasound may demonstrate changes in the size of the kidney, or presence of calculi, in renal and postrenal causes.

TABLE 11–7 Comparison of Signs and Symptoms of Renal Failure in Older Adults

SIGNS AND SYMPTOMS	ACUTE RENAL FAILURE	CHRONIC RENAL FAILURE
Onset	Sudden onset	Gradual onset
Blood pressure	Postural hypotension	Hypertension
Electrolytes	Increased blood urea nitrogen (BUN) and serum creatinine	Increased serum phosphate, calcium, BUN, creatinine, potassium Decreased serum calcium Metabolic acidosis
Edema	Dependent edema	Generalized edema
Well-being	Fatigue and drowsiness	Fatigue and drowsiness
Urine output	Possible decreased urine output	Volume decline over time
Gastrointestinal symptoms	Nausea and vomiting Rapid weight loss	Nausea and vomiting Anorexia Weight loss
Other symptoms	Flank pain	Decreased glomerular filtration rate Anemia Pruritus, uremic "bronzing," and uremic odor Altered mental status

Source: Bailey & Sands (2003); Beers & Berkow (2000); Jassal et al. (1998).

Pediatric manifestations characteristically begin with a healthy child who suddenly becomes ill with nonspecific symptoms that indicate a significant illness or injury. These symptoms may include any combination of the following: nausea, vomiting, lethargy, edema, gross **hematuria** (blood in the urine), oliguria, and hypertension. These manifestations result from electrolyte imbalances (Table 11–8), uremia (excessive amounts of urea in the blood), and fluid overload. The child appears pale and lethargic.

COLLABORATION

Preventing ARF is a goal in caring for all clients, especially those in high-risk groups. Maintaining adequate vascular volume, cardiac output, and blood pressure are vital to preserving kidney perfusion, as is avoiding nephrotoxic drugs whenever possible. When a nephrotoxic drug or substance must be used, the risk of ARF can be reduced by using the minimum effective dose, maintaining hydration, and eliminating other known

TABLE 11–8 Electrolyte Imbalances in Acute and Chronic Renal Failure in Children

ELECTROLYTE IMBALANCE	CAUSE	CLINICAL MANIFESTATIONS
Hyperkalemia (excess potassium in the blood)	Results from inability to adequately excrete potassium derived from diet and catabolized cells. In metabolic acidosis, potassium also moves from intracellular fluid to extracellular fluid.	■ Peaked T waves, widening of QRS waves on electrocardiogram ■ Dysrhythmias: ventricular dysrhythmias, heart block, ventricular fibrillation, cardiac arrest ■ Diarrhea ■ Muscle weakness
Hyponatremia (decreased potassium in the blood)	In the acute oliguric phase, hyponatremia is dilutional, related to the accumulation of fluid in excess of solute.	■ Change in level of consciousness ■ Muscle cramps ■ Anorexia ■ Abdominal reflexes, depressed deep tendon reflexes ■ Cheyne-Stokes respirations ■ Seizures
Hypocalcemia (decreased calcium in the blood)	Phosphate retention (hyperphosphatemia) caused by impaired renal function depresses the serum calcium concentration. Calcium is deposited in injured cells.	■ Muscle tingling ■ Changes in muscle tone ■ Seizures ■ Muscle cramps and twitching
	Hyperkalemia and metabolic acidosis may mask the common clinical manifestations of severe hypocalcemia.	■ Positive Chvostek's sign (contraction of facial muscles after tapping facial nerve just anterior to parotid gland)

nephrotoxins from the medication regimen. When discharging a client with instructions to avoid nephrotoxic drugs, the nurse should encourage the client to contact his or her pharmacist. Adding that information to the client's pharmacy history will help the client to avoid nephrotoxic drugs that may be prescribed in the future.

If a client develops ARF, maintaining the fluid and electrolyte balance is a key goal in managing the condition. Other goals in the treatment of ARF include the following:

1. To identify and correct the underlying cause
2. To prevent additional kidney damage
3. To restore the urine output and kidney function
4. To compensate for renal impairment until kidney function is restored.

The complex nature of renal failure makes an interdisciplinary approach critical. The nurse, nephrologist, and nutritionist are essential members of the care team. Consultation with a nephrologist is important in limiting kidney damage and decreasing mortality (Bailey & Sands, 2003). Consultation with a cardiologist may be necessary, particularly for clients with a preexisting cardiac condition. In the older adult, nutritional support is especially important. Weight loss of up to 1 lb per day is expected in the older adult with ARF. Any attempt to prevent the weight loss may overtax multiple systems and lead to cardiac failure. For example, the use of nutritional supplements that are high in calories may be contraindicated in the older adult with ARF. Allowing weight loss to occur during this acute phase may better protect the long-term health of the older adult. Dehydration in the older adult is a causative factor in ARF; therefore, fluid restrictions should be modest (Jassal et al., 1998).

Diagnostic Tests

Diagnostic tests are used to identify the cause of ARF and monitor its effects on homeostasis. These tests include the following:

- *Urinalysis* often shows the following abnormal findings in ARF:
  a. A fixed specific gravity of 1.010 (equal to the specific gravity of plasma), because the tubules are unable to concentrate the filtrate
  b. **Proteinuria** (excess protein in urine) if glomerular damage is the cause of ARF
  c. The presence of RBCs (caused by glomerular dysfunction), white blood cells (WBCs; related to inflammation), and renal tubular epithelial cells (indicating ATN)
  d. Cell casts, which are protein and cellular debris molded in the shape of the tubular lumen (in ARF, RBCs, WBCs, and renal tubular epithelial casts may be present; brownish-pigmented casts and positive tests for occult blood indicate hemoglobinuria or myoglobinuria)
- *Serum creatinine* and *BUN* are used to evaluate renal function. In ARF, serum creatinine levels increase rapidly, within 24–48 hours of the onset. Creatinine levels generally peak within 5–10 days. Creatinine and BUN levels tend to increase more slowly when urine output is maintained. The onset of recovery is marked by a halt in the rise of the serum creatinine and BUN.
- *Serum electrolytes* are monitored to evaluate the fluid and electrolyte status. The serum potassium rises at a moderate rate and is often used to indicate the need for dialysis. Hyponatremia is common because of the water excess associated with ARF.
- *Arterial blood gas* studies often show a metabolic acidosis caused by the kidneys' inability to adequately eliminate metabolic wastes and hydrogen ions.
- *Complete blood count (CBC)* shows reduced RBCs, moderate anemia, and a low hematocrit. ARF affects erythropoietin secretion and RBC production. Iron and folate absorption may also be impaired, further contributing to anemia.
- *Renal ultrasonography* is used to identify obstructive causes of renal failure and to differentiate ARF from end-stage chronic renal failure. In ARF, the kidneys may be enlarged, whereas in chronic renal failure, they typically appear small and shrunken.
- *Computed tomography* may be done to evaluate kidney size and identify possible obstructions.
- *Intravenous pyelography, retrograde pyelography,* or *antegrade pyelography* may be used to evaluate kidney structure and function. Radiologic contrast media are used with extreme caution because of their potential nephrotoxicity. Retrograde pyelography, in which contrast dye is injected into the ureters, and antegrade pyelography, in which the contrast medium is injected percutaneously into the renal pelvis, are preferred, because they have fewer nephrotoxic effects than intravenous pyelography.
- *Renal biopsy* may be necessary to differentiate between acute and chronic renal failure.
- *Radiographic studies* may be helpful in determining ARF in pediatric clients, because these studies will indicate the size of the kidney. A common cause of ARF in children is **osteodystrophy** (a complex bone disease process of chronic kidney disease in which increased resorption of bone is caused by chronic hyperparathyroidism).

Pharmacologic Therapies

The primary focus in drug management for ARF is to restore and maintain renal perfusion and to eliminate drugs that are nephrotoxic from the treatment regimen. Intravenous fluids and blood volume expanders are given as needed to restore renal perfusion. Dopamine (Intropin), administered in low doses by intravenous infusion, increases renal blood flow. Dopamine is a sympathetic neurotransmitter that improves cardiac output and dilates blood vessels of the mesentery and kidneys when given in low therapeutic doses.

If restoration of renal blood flow does not improve urinary output, a potent loop diuretic, such as furosemide (Lasix), or an osmotic diuretic, such as mannitol, may be given with intravenous fluids. The purpose for giving a potent diuretic is twofold. First, if nephrotoxins are present, the combination of fluids and potent diuretics may, in effect, "wash out" the nephrons, reducing toxin concentration. Second, establishing urine output may prevent oliguria and reduce the degree of azotemia and fluid and electrolyte imbalances. Furosemide also may be used to manage salt and water retention associated with ARF.

MEDICATIONS Acute Renal Failure

Classification	Mechanism of Action	Common Drugs	Nursing Considerations
Loop diuretics	The loop diuretics, named for their primary site of action in the loop of Henle, are high-ceiling diuretics (the response increases with increasing doses). These are highly effective diuretics used in early ARF to reestablish urine flow and convert oliguric renal failure to nonoliguric renal failure. Loop diuretics may be given with intravenous dopamine to promote renal blood flow. In ATN caused by a nephrotoxin, loop diuretics are used to clear the toxin from the nephrons more rapidly. Loop diuretics cause potassium wasting, which is generally not a concern in ARF because renal failure impairs normal potassium elimination.	Bumetanide (Bumex) Ethacrynic acid (Edecrin) Furosemide (Lasix) Torsemide (Demadex)	■ Assess weight and vital signs for baseline data. ■ Monitor intake and output, daily weight (or more frequently as ordered), vital signs, skin turgor, and other indicators of fluid volume status frequently. ■ Assess for orthostatic hypotension; these potent diuretics can lead to hypovolemia. ■ Monitor laboratory results, especially serum electrolyte, glucose, blood urea nitrogen, and creatinine levels. ■ Administer as ordered: a. Furosemide, undiluted at a rate of no more than 20 mg/min b. Ethacrynic acid, 50 mg diluted with 50 mL of normal saline at a rate of no more than 10 mg/min c. Bumetanide, undiluted over at least 1 min or diluted in lactated Ringer's solution, normal saline, or 5% dextrose in water for infusion d. Torsemide, undiluted over at least 2 min. ■ Assess response. Urine output typically increases within 10 min after intravenous administration. ■ Monitor hearing and for complaints such as tinnitus. High doses of loop diuretics increase the risk of ototoxicity, especially with ethacrynic acid. These effects may be reversible if they are detected early and the drug is discontinued. ■ Avoid administering concurrently with other ototoxic agents, such as aminoglycoside antibiotics and cisplatin. ■ Health education for the client and family: a. Unless contraindicated, maintain a fluid intake of 2–3 quarts per day. b. Rise slowly from lying or sitting positions, because a fall in blood pressure may cause light-headedness. c. Take in the morning and, if ordered twice a day, in the late afternoon to avoid sleep disturbance. d. Take with food or milk to prevent gastric distress. e. Nonsteroidal anti-inflammatory drugs interfere with the effectiveness of loop diuretics and should be avoided.
Osmotic diuretics	The osmotic diuretics act by increasing the osmotic draw in the blood and urine. In the blood, the effect is to pull extracellular water into the vascular system, increasing the GFR. These substances are then freely filtered in the glomerulus and increase the osmotic draw of the urine, inhibiting water reabsorption. The effect is to increase urine volume and flow. In addition, osmotic diuretics dilute waste products in the urine, decreasing the risk of renal damage because of excess concentrations.	Mannitol (Osmitrol, Isotel) Urea (Ureaphil)	■ Assess urine output. Osmotic diuretics are used in early renal failure to maintain urine output but are contraindicated in **anuria** (inability of kidneys to produce urine). A test dose may be administered; urine output of 30 mL/hr following the test dose shows an adequate response. ■ Do not give these diuretics to clients who have heart failure or are severely dehydrated. These drugs increase vascular volume and may worsen heart failure. They are not effective unless extracellular volume is adequate. ■ Administer mannitol intravenously, diluting before use if indicated. Check solution for crystallization. Dissolve crystals by warming the solution slightly. Infuse 15–25% mannitol solutions through a filter over 30–90 min. ■ Administer urea intravenously, diluting in 100 mL of 5 or 10% dextrose in water for every 30 g of urea. Administer no faster than 4 mL/min through a filter. ■ Monitor vital signs, breath sounds, and urinary output. ■ Discontinue the drug if signs of heart failure or pulmonary edema develop or if renal function continues to decline. ■ Instruct client and family to report shortness of breath, headache, chest pain, or dizziness immediately.

(continued)

MEDICATIONS **Acute Renal Failure** (continued)

Classification	Mechanism of Action	Common Drugs	Nursing Considerations
Electrolytes and electrolyte modifiers	Calcium chloride or gluconate and sodium bicarbonate are administered intravenously in the initial management of hyperkalemia. Calcium is also administered to correct hypocalcemia and reduce hyperphosphatemia (calcium and phosphate have a reciprocal relationship in the body; as the level of one rises, the level of the other falls). Sodium bicarbonate helps to correct acidosis and move potassium back into the intracellular space. Sodium polystyrene sulfonate is not used to replace an electrolyte but to remove excess potassium from the body by exchanging sodium for potassium in the large intestine.	Calcium chloride Calcium gluconate Sodium bicarbonate Sodium polystyrene sulfonate (Kayexalate)	■ Assess serum electrolyte levels before and during therapy. Report rapid shifts or adverse responses to the physician. ■ Administer as appropriate: a. Intravenous calcium chloride at less than 1 mL/min; intravenous calcium gluconate at 0.5 mL/min. Inject into a large vein through a small-bore needle; avoid infiltration, because extravasation of intravenous solution will cause tissue necrosis. b. Intravenous sodium bicarbonate infusion over 4–8 hr; oral tablets as prescribed. c. Sodium polystyrene sulfonate as an oral solution mixed with sorbitol to prevent constipation, or as a retention enema mixed with warm water. Leave in the bowel for 30–60 min, irrigate using a small tap-water enema. ■ Monitor for adverse reactions, such as dysrhythmias, electrolyte imbalances, and metabolic alkalosis. ■ Health education for the client and family: a. Intravenous calcium may make you light-headed; remain in bed for at least 30 min after administration. b. Chew sodium bicarbonate tablets and follow with 8 oz of water. Do not take with milk. c. Retain the sodium polystyrene sulfonate enema as long as possible.

Aggressive management of hypertension limits renal injury when ARF is associated with disorders such as toxemia and pregnancy-induced hypertension. Angiotensin-converting enzyme inhibitors or other antihypertensive medications are used to control arterial pressures.

All drugs that are either directly nephrotoxic or that may interfere with renal perfusion (e.g., potent vasoconstrictors) are discontinued. Nonsteroidal anti-inflammatory drugs, nephrotoxic antibiotics, and other potentially harmful drugs are avoided throughout the course of ARF.

The client in ARF has an increased risk of GI bleeding, probably related to the stress response and impaired platelet function. Regular doses of antacids, histamine H_2-receptor antagonists (e.g., famotidine or ranitidine), or a proton-pump inhibitor (e.g., omeprazole [Prilosec]) are often ordered to prevent GI hemorrhage.

Hyperkalemia may require active intervention as well as restricted potassium intake. Serum levels greater than 6.5 mEq/L are treated to prevent cardiac effects of hyperkalemia. With significant hyperkalemia, calcium chloride, bicarbonate, and insulin and glucose may be given intravenously to reduce serum potassium levels by moving potassium into the cells. A potassium-binding exchange resin, such as sodium polystyrene sulfonate (Kayexalate, SPS Suspension), may be given orally or by enema. This agent removes potassium from the body by exchanging sodium for potassium, primarily in the large intestine. When given orally, it is often combined with sorbitol to prevent constipation. Rectally, it is instilled as a retention enema, allowed to remain in the bowel for approximately 30–60 minutes, and then irrigated out using a tap-water enema.

Aluminum hydroxide (ALternaGEL, Amphojel, Nephrox), an antacid, is used to control hyperphosphatemia in renal failure. It binds with phosphates in the GI tract, which are then excreted in the feces.

Because many drugs are eliminated from the body by the kidney, drug dosages may need to be adjusted. Doses within the usual range can lead to potentially toxic blood levels, because their elimination is slowed and their half-life prolonged. Nursing implications for medications commonly prescribed for the client with ARF are summarized in the Medications feature.

Fluid Management

Once vascular volume and renal perfusion are restored, fluid intake is usually restricted. The restricted daily fluid intake is calculated by allowing 500 mL for insensible losses (respiration, perspiration, and bowel losses) and adding the amount excreted as urine (or lost in vomitus) during the previous 24 hours. For example, if a client with ARF excretes 325 mL of urine in 24 hours, allow the client a fluid intake (including oral and intravenous fluids) of 825 mL for the next 24 hours. Carefully monitor fluid balance by using accurate weight measurements and the serum sodium as the primary indicators.

Initial emergency treatment of children with fluid depletion focuses on rapid fluid replacement with 20 mL/kg of saline or lactated Ringer's solution given over 5 to 10 minutes and repeated as needed. This ensures renal perfusion and stabilizes blood pressure.

Albumin may also be administered when blood loss is the cause of the client's circulatory depletion. If oliguria persists after restoration of adequate fluid volume, intrinsic renal damage is suspected.

Nutrition

Renal insufficiency and the underlying disease process increase the rate of catabolism and decrease the rate of anabolism (body tissue repair). The client with ARF needs adequate nutrients and calories to prevent catabolism. Proteins are limited to 0.6 g/kg of body weight per day to minimize the degree of azotemia. Dietary proteins should be of high biologic value (rich in essential amino acids). Carbohydrates are increased to maintain adequate calorie intake and provide a protein-sparing effect.

Parenteral nutrition providing amino acids, concentrated carbohydrates, and fats may be instituted when the client cannot consume an adequate diet (e.g., because of nausea, vomiting, or underlying critical illness). The disadvantages of parenteral nutrition in the client with ARF are the high volume of fluid required and the risk for infection through the venous line.

Renal Replacement Therapy

Manifestations of uremia, organ dysfunction caused by accumulated metabolic wastes, severe fluid overload, hyperkalemia, or metabolic acidosis in a client with renal failure, indicate a need to replace renal function. **Dialysis** is the diffusion of solute molecules across a semipermeable membrane from an area of higher solute concentration to one of lower concentration according to the rules of osmosis. It is used to remove excess fluid and metabolic waste products in renal failure. Early use of dialysis can reduce the rate of complications. Dialysis may also be used to rapidly remove nephrotoxins in ATN. While dialysis compensates for lost renal elimination functions, it does not replace lost erythropoietin production. Anemia is a continuing problem for the client receiving dialysis.

In dialysis, blood is separated from a dialysis solution (**dialysate**) by a semipermeable membrane. Either **hemodialysis**, a procedure in which blood flows through vascular catheters, is pumped through the dialyzer unit, and returned to the client, or **peritoneal dialysis**, which uses the peritoneum surrounding the abdominal cavity as the dialyzing membrane, may be used for the client with ARF. **Continuous renal replacement therapy (CRRT)**, in which blood is continuously circulated through a highly porous hemofilter from artery to vein or from vein to vein, is a newer form of dialysis that may be used to treat ARF.

HEMODIALYSIS Hemodialysis uses the principles of diffusion and ultrafiltration to remove electrolytes, waste products, and excess water from the body. Blood is taken from the client via a vascular access and is pumped to the dialyzer (Figure 11–14 ■). The porous membranes of the dialyzer unit allow small molecules (e.g., water, glucose, and electrolytes)

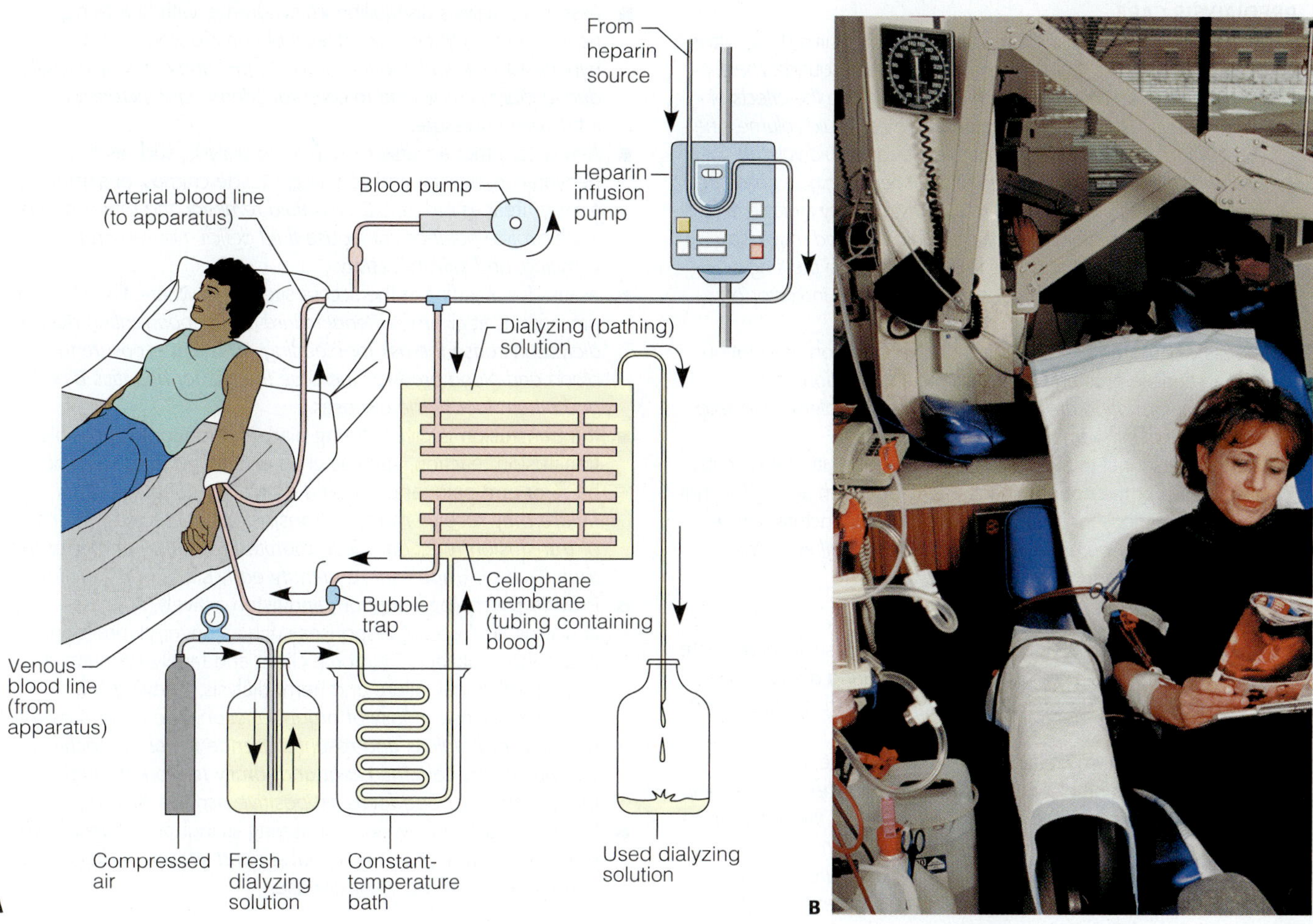

Figure 11–14 ■ *A*, The components of a hemodialysis system. *B*, A woman receiving kidney dialysis.

to pass through but block larger molecules (e.g., serum proteins and blood cells). The dialysate, a solution of approximately the same composition and temperature as normal extracellular fluid, passes along the other side of the membrane. Small solute molecules move freely across the membrane by diffusion. The direction of movement for any substance is determined by the concentrations of that substance in the blood and the dialysate. Electrolytes and waste products (e.g., urea and creatinine) diffuse from the blood into the dialysate. If it is necessary to add something to the blood, such as calcium to replace depleted stores, it can be added to the dialysate to diffuse into the blood. Excess water is removed by creating a hydrostatic pressure of the blood moving through the dialyzer that is higher than that of the dialysate, which flows in the opposite direction. This process is known as **ultrafiltration**.

Initially, clients with ARF typically undergo daily hemodialysis. As their condition improves, clients may change to three to four sessions per week as indicated. Hemodialysis is not used if the client is hemodynamically unstable (e.g., with hypotension or low cardiac output). The following are complications associated with hemodialysis:

- Hypotension, the most frequent complication during hemodialysis, may result from changes in serum osmolality, rapid removal of fluid from the vascular compartment, vasodilation, and other factors.
- Bleeding may result from altered platelet function associated with uremia and the use of heparin during dialysis.
- Infection (local or systemic) may result from WBC damage and immune system suppression. *Staphylococcus aureus* septicemia is commonly associated with contamination of the vascular access site. Clients on chronic hemodialysis have higher rates of hepatitis B, hepatitis C, cytomegalovirus, and HIV infection than the general population.

Box 11–3 describes nursing care for the client undergoing hemodialysis.

CONTINUOUS RENAL REPLACEMENT THERAPY Clients with ARF may be unable to tolerate hemodialysis and rapid fluid removal if their cardiovascular status is unstable (e.g., because of trauma, major surgery, or heart failure). Continuous renal replacement therapy, which allows more gradual fluid and solute removal, often is used for these clients. In CRRT, blood is continuously circulated from an artery to a vein or

Box 11–3 **Nursing Care of the Client Undergoing Dialysis**

PREDIALYSIS CARE

- Assess vital signs, including orthostatic blood pressures (lying, sitting, and standing), apical pulse, respirations, and lung sounds. *These data provide baseline information to help evaluate the effects of hemodialysis. Hypertension may indicate excess fluid volume. The client who is hypotensive may not tolerate rapid fluid volume changes during dialysis. Abnormal heart sounds (e.g., a gallop or murmur) and changes in heart rate or rhythm may indicate excess fluid volume or electrolyte imbalance. Fluid overload may also cause dyspnea, tachypnea, and rales or crackles in the lungs.*
- Record weight. *Weight changes are an effective indicator of fluid volume.*
- Assess vascular access site for a palpable pulsation or vibration and an audible bruit and for inflammation. *Infection and thrombus formation are the most common problems affecting the access site in hemodialysis clients.*
- Alert all personnel to avoid using the extremity with the vascular access site (or the nondominant arm, if long-term access has not been established) for blood pressures or venipuncture. *These procedures may damage vessels and lead to failure of the arteriovenous fistula.*

POSTDIALYSIS CARE

- Assess and document vital signs, weight, and vascular access site condition. *Rapid fluid and solute removal during dialysis may lead to orthostatic hypotension, cardiopulmonary changes, and weight loss.*
- Monitor BUN, serum creatinine, serum electrolyte, and hematocrit levels between dialysis treatments. *These values help to determine the effectiveness of the treatment, the need for fluid and diet restrictions, and the timing of future dialysis sessions. The anemia associated with renal failure does not improve with dialysis, and iron and folate supplements or periodic blood transfusions may be needed.*
- Assess for dialysis disequilibrium syndrome, with headache, nausea and vomiting, altered level of consciousness, and hypertension. *Rapid changes in BUN, pH, and electrolyte levels during dialysis may lead to cerebral edema and increased intracranial pressure.*
- Assess for other adverse responses to dialysis, such as dehydration, nausea and vomiting, muscle cramps, or seizure activity. Treat as ordered. *Excess fluid removal and rapid changes in electrolyte balance can cause fluid deficit, nausea and vomiting, and seizure activity.*
- Assess for bleeding at the access site or elsewhere. Use standard precautions at all times. *Renal failure and heparinization during dialysis increase the risk for bleeding. Frequent exposure to blood and blood products increase the risk for hepatitis B or C and other bloodborne diseases.*
- If a transfusion is given during dialysis, monitor for possible transfusion reaction, such as chills and fever; dyspnea; chest, back, or arm pain; and urticaria or itching. *Clients in renal failure may receive multiple transfusions, increasing the risk of transfusion reaction. Close monitoring during and after the transfusion is important to identify early signs of a reaction.*
- Provide psychologic support, and listen actively. Address concerns, and accept responses such as anger, depression, and noncompliance. Reinforce client and family strengths in coping with renal failure and hemodialysis. *Grieving is a normal response to loss of organ function. The client may feel hopeless or helpless and resent dependence on a machine. The nurse can help the client and family to work through these responses and focus on positive aspects of living.*
- Refer to social services and counseling as indicated. *Clients with renal failure may need additional support services to help them adapt to and live with their disease.*

TABLE 11–9 **Continuous Renal Replacement Therapies**

TYPE	INDICATIONS	DESCRIPTION
Continuous arteriovenous hemofiltration (CAVH)	Remove fluid and some solutes	Arterial blood circulates through a hemofilter, then returns to client through venous line; ultrafiltrate collects in a drainage bag.
Continuous arteriovenous hemodialysis (CAVHD)	Remove fluid and waste products	Arterial blood circulates through a hemofilter surrounded by dialysate, then returns to client through venous line; ultrafiltrate collects in a drainage bag.
Continuous venovenous hemodialysis (CVVHD)	Remove fluid and waste products	Venous blood circulates through a hemofilter surrounded by dialysate, then returns to client through double-lumen venous catheter; ultrafiltrate collects in a drainage bag.

from a vein to a vein through a highly porous hemofilter for a period of 12 hours or more. Excess water and solutes, such as electrolytes, urea, creatinine, uric acid, and glucose, drain into a collection device. Fluid may be replaced with normal saline or a balanced electrolyte solution as needed during CRRT. This slower process helps to maintain hemodynamic stability and avoid complications associated with rapid changes in composition of the extracellular fluid. The most common CRRT techniques are outlined in Table 11–9.

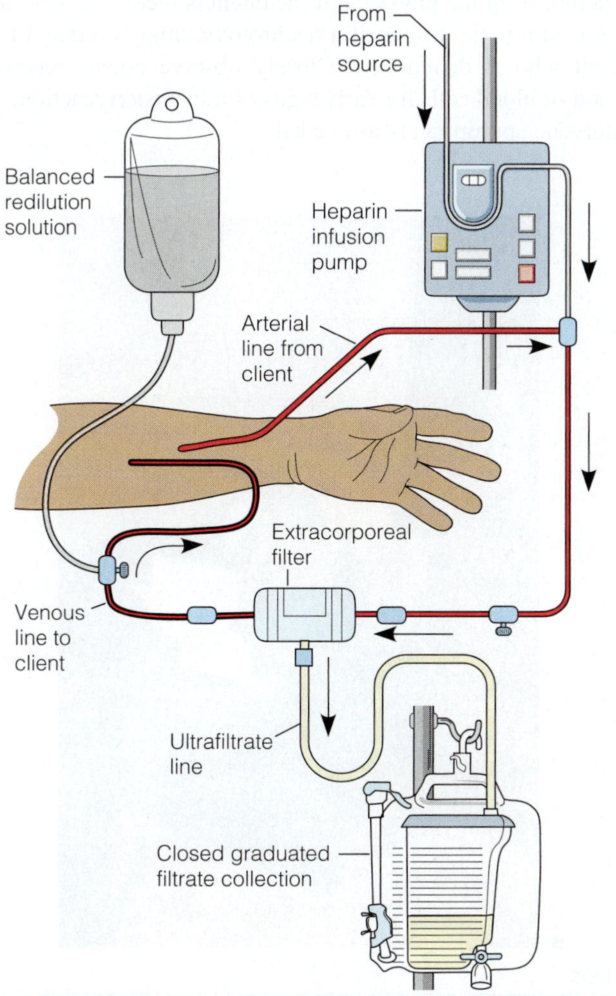

Figure 11–15 ■ Continuous arteriovenous hemofiltration (CAVH).

Typically, CRRT is performed in an intensive care unit or specialized nephrology unit. Both arterial and venous lines are required for some types of CRRT (Figure 11–15 ■); for others, a double-lumen venous catheter is used. Strict aseptic technique is vital in caring for vascular access sites to reduce the risk of infection.

VASCULAR ACCESS FOR HEMODIALYSIS AND CONTINUOUS RENAL REPLACEMENT THERAPY Acute or temporary vascular access for hemodialysis or CRRT usually is gained by inserting a double-lumen catheter into the subclavian, jugular, or femoral vein. The double-lumen catheter has a central partition separating the blood-withdrawal side of the catheter from the return side. Blood is drawn into the catheter through small openings in the proximal portion of the catheter, and it is returned to the circulation through an opening in the distal end of the catheter to avoid withdrawing the blood that has just been dialyzed.

For longer-term vascular access, an **arteriovenous (AV) fistula** (creation of an artificial connection between a vein and an artery) is created (Figure 11–16 ■). In preparation for fistula formation, the nondominant arm is not used for venipuncture or blood pressure measurement during renal failure. The fistula is created by surgical anastomosis of an artery and vein, usually the radial artery and cephalic vein. It takes about a month for the fistula to mature so that it can be used for taking and replacing blood during dialysis. A functional AV fistula has a palpable pulsation and a bruit on auscultation. Avoid venipunctures and blood pressures on the arm with the fistula.

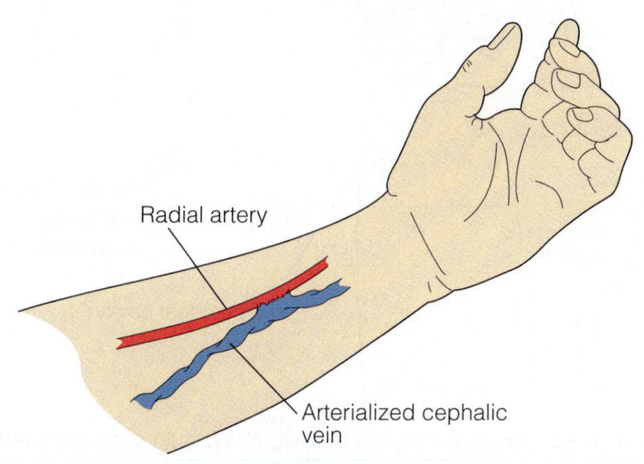

Figure 11–16 ■ An arteriovenous fistula.

In chronic renal failure, an *arteriovenous graft* is most often used for vascular access. The graft, a tube made of Gortex, is surgically implanted and connects the artery and the vein. Blood flows through the graft from the artery to the vein. Occasionally, an *external AV shunt* connecting a peripheral artery with a peripheral vein is used for vascular access. Ideally, an AV fistula or graft is created as soon as the potential need for long-term renal replacement therapies is identified (Dinwiddie, 2004).

The rate of complications and mortality associated with catheter access is higher than with AV fistulas or grafts; however, localized AV fistula, graft, or shunt problems can occur. Infection and clotting or thrombosis are the most common shunt problems. Aneurysms may also develop. Both infection and thrombosis can lead to systemic manifestations, such as septicemia and embolization. These local complications may cause the fistula or graft to fail, necessitating development of a new site. The psychologic impact of AV fistula or graft failure is significant, often causing depression and low self-esteem.

PERITONEAL DIALYSIS In peritoneal dialysis, the highly vascular peritoneal membrane serves as the dialyzing surface (Figure 11–17 ■) Warmed, sterile dialysate is instilled into the peritoneal cavity through a catheter inserted into the peritoneal cavity. Metabolic waste products and excess electrolytes diffuse into the dialysate while it remains in the abdomen. Water movement is controlled using dextrose as an osmotic agent to draw it into the dialysate. The fluid is then drained by gravity out of the peritoneal cavity into a sterile bag. This process of dialysate infusion, dwell time of the solution in the abdomen, and drainage is repeated at prescribed intervals.

Because excess fluid and solutes are removed more gradually in peritoneal dialysis, this type of renal replacement therapy poses less risk for the unstable client; however, this slower rate of metabolite removal can be a disadvantage in clients with ARF. Peritoneal dialysis increases the risk for developing peritonitis, and it is contraindicated for clients who have had recent abdominal surgery, significant lung disease, or peritonitis.

See Box 11–4 for nursing care for the client having peritoneal dialysis.

NURSING PROCESS

ARF often can be prevented by measures that maintain fluid volume and cardiac output and that reduce the risk of exposure to nephrotoxins. Carefully monitor critically ill, postoperative, and other at-risk clients for early signs of hypovolemia (low urine output, altered mental status, and changes in vital signs, skin color, or temperature). Promptly report a fall in urine output to less than 30 mL/hr and other evidence of decreased cardiac output. Maintain intravenous fluids as ordered. Alert the physician if the client is receiving more than one nephrotoxic drug or if a nephrotoxic drug is ordered for a client who is dehydrated. Closely observe clients receiving blood or blood cells for early signs of transfusion reaction, and intervene appropriately as needed.

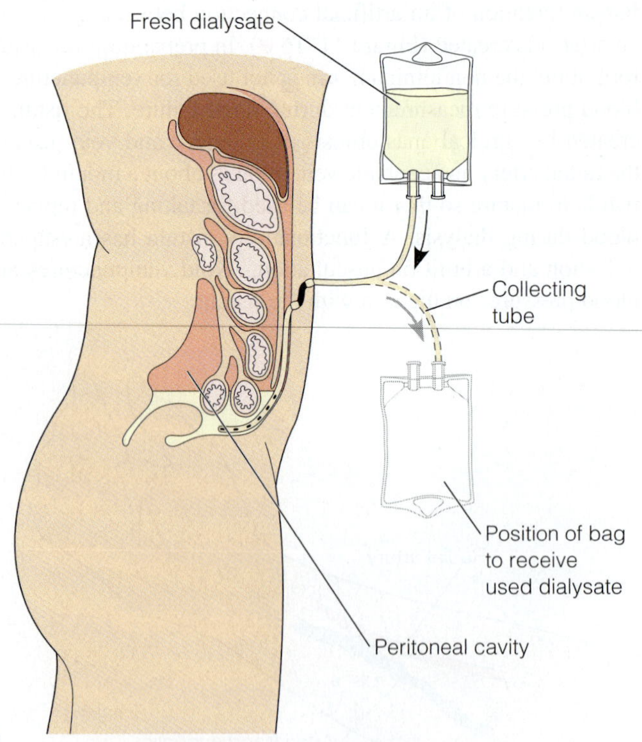

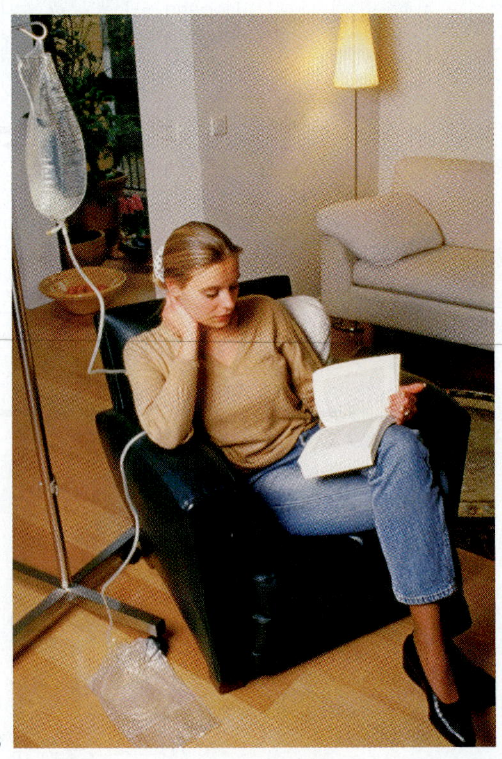

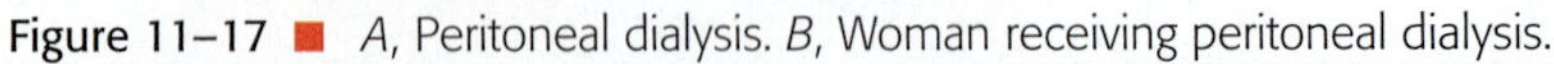
Figure 11–17 ■ *A*, Peritoneal dialysis. *B*, Woman receiving peritoneal dialysis.

Box 11–4 **Nursing Care of the Client Undergoing Peritoneal Dialysis**

PREDIALYSIS CARE

- Document vital signs, including temperature, orthostatic blood pressures (lying, sitting, and standing), apical pulse, respirations, and lung sounds. *These baseline data help to assess fluid volume status and tolerance of the dialysis procedure. Hypertension, abnormal heart or lung sounds, or dyspnea may indicate excess fluid volume. Poor respiratory function may affect the ability to tolerate peritoneal dialysis. Temperature measurement is vital, because infection is the most common complication of peritoneal dialysis.*
- Weigh daily or between dialysis runs as indicated. *Weight is an accurate indicator of fluid volume status.*
- Note blood urea nitrogen (BUN), serum electrolyte, creatinine, pH, and hematocrit levels before peritoneal dialysis and periodically during the procedure. *These values are used to assess the efficacy of treatment.*
- Measure and record abdominal girth. *Increasing abdominal girth may indicate retained dialysate, excess fluid volume, or early peritonitis.*
- Maintain fluid and dietary restrictions as ordered. *Fluid and diet restrictions help to reduce* ***hypervolemia*** *(increased circulating blood volume) and control azotemia.*
- Have the client empty the bladder before catheter insertion. *Emptying the bladder reduces the risk of inadvertent puncture.*
- Warm the prescribed dialysate solution to body temperature (98.6°F or 37°C) using a warm-water bath or heating pad on low setting. *Dialysate is warmed to prevent hypothermia.*
- Explain all procedures and expected sensations. *Knowledge helps to reduce anxiety and elicit cooperation.*

INTRADIALYSIS CARE

- Use strict aseptic technique during the dialysis procedure and when caring for the peritoneal catheter. *Sterile technique reduces the risk for peritonitis.*
- Add prescribed medications to the dialysate. Prime the tubing with solution, and connect it to the peritoneal catheter, taping connections securely and avoiding kinks. *This allows the dialysate to flow freely into the abdominal cavity and prevents leaking or contamination.*
- Instill the dialysate into the abdominal cavity over a period of approximately 10 min. Clamp tubing, and allow the dialysate to remain in the abdomen for the prescribed dwell time. Keep drainage tubing clamped at all times during instillation and dwell time. Dialysate should flow freely into the abdomen if the peritoneal catheter is patent. *Dialysis, the exchange of solutes and water between the blood and dialysate, occurs across the peritoneal membrane during the dwell time.*
- During instillation and dwell time, observe closely for signs of respiratory distress, such as dyspnea, tachypnea, or crackles. Place in Fowler's or semi-Fowler's position, and slow the rate of instillation slightly to relieve respiratory distress if it develops. *Respiratory compromise may result from overly rapid filling or overfilling of the abdomen or from a diaphragmatic defect that allows fluid to enter the thoracic cavity.*
- After prescribed dwell time, open the drainage tubing clamps, and allow the dialysate to drain by gravity into a sterile container. Note the clarity, color, and odor of returned dialysate. *Blood or feces in the dialysate may indicate organ or bowel perforation; cloudy or malodorous dialysate may indicate an infection.*
- Accurately record the amount and type of dialysate instilled (including any added medications), dwell time, and amount and character of the drainage. *When more dialysate drains than has been instilled, excess fluid has been lost (output). If less dialysate is returned than has been instilled, a fluid gain has occurred (intake).*
- Monitor BUN, serum electrolyte, and creatinine levels. *These values are used to assess the effectiveness of dialysis.*
- Troubleshoot for possible problems during dialysis:
  a. Slow dialysate instillation. Increase the height of the container, and reposition the client. Check tubing and catheter for kinks. Check abdominal dressing for wetness, indicating leakage around the catheter.
  b. Excess dwell time.
  c. Poor dialysate drainage. Lower the drainage container, reposition, and check for tubing kinks. Check abdominal dressing.

Slow dialysate flow may be related to a partially obstructed tube or catheter. Prolonged dwell time may lead to water depletion or hyperglycemia. Tubing or catheter obstruction can also interfere with dialysate drainage.

POSTDIALYSIS CARE

- Assess vital signs, including temperature. *Comparison of pre- and postdialysis vital signs helps to identify beneficial and adverse effects of the procedure.*
- Time meals to correspond with dialysis outflow. *Scheduling meals while the abdomen is empty of dialysate enhances intake and reduces nausea.*
- Teach the client and family about the procedure. *The client may elect to use peritoneal dialysis at home to manage end-stage renal disease and prevent uremia.*

Assessment

Both subjective and objective data are useful when assessing the client with ARF. The client's history and physical assessment can provide clues about the initiating event for ARF. Impaired perfusion for as few as 30 minutes may cause significant renal ischemia, so it is crucial to get a thorough history. For pediatric and older clients, assessments should include input from immediate family members or caregivers.

- *Health history.* Complaints of anorexia, nausea, weight gain, or edema; recent exposure to a nephrotoxin, such as an aminoglycoside antibiotic or radiologic procedure using an injected contrast medium; previous transfusion reaction; chronic diseases, such as diabetes, heart failure, or kidney disease
- *Physical examination.* Vital signs, including temperature; urine output (amount, color, clarity, specific gravity, presence of blood cells or protein); weight; skin color; peripheral pulses; presence of edema (periorbital or dependent); lung sounds, heart sounds, and bowel tones

PRACTICE ALERT

The unexpected and acute nature of the child's hospitalization creates anxiety for both parents and the child. Assess for feelings of anger, guilt, or fear associated with the hospitalization. Such feelings are likely if ARF developed as a result of dehydration, a preventable injury, or poisoning. Assess coping mechanisms, family support systems, and level of stress.

Diagnosis

The client with ARF has numerous nursing care needs related both to the renal failure and to the underlying condition that precipitated it. Priority nursing care needs relate to fluid volume alterations, appetite and nutrition, and teaching/learning. Appropriate nursing diagnoses may include any of the following:

- Excess Fluid Volume related to renal dysfunction and sodium retention
- Imbalanced Nutrition: Less Than Body Requirements related to anorexia, nausea, vomiting, and catabolic state
- Ineffective Renal Tissue Perfusion related to hypovolemia, sepsis, or drug toxicity
- Risk for Altered Skin Integrity related to uremia and reduced tissue perfusion
- Risk for Altered Cardiac Perfusion Secondary to hyperkalemia
- Risk for Infection related to invasive procedures and monitoring equipment and diminished immune functioning
- Compromised Family Coping related to sudden hospitalization and uncertain prognosis.

Plan

Nursing care focuses on preventing complications, maintaining fluid balance, administering medications, meeting nutritional needs, preventing infection, and providing emotional support to the client and family. Possible outcomes, created in collaboration with the client and family, include the following:

- The client's weight returns to baseline measurement.
- The client's urine output is greater than 30 mL/hr.
- The client's hemoglobin and hematocrit values are within normal limits.
- The client's serum electrolytes are within normal limits.
- The client's pulse rate, volume, and rhythm return to baseline.

FOCUS ON DIVERSITY AND CULTURE

Religious and Cultural Preferences

The client with ARF may have religious and cultural preferences that affect the condition and its treatment. Food preferences may put the client at risk for fluid or electrolyte imbalance. Religious practices, such as frequent daily prayers and religious policies against transfusions or dialysis, may impact implementation of care.

Implementation

The care of each client will vary based on the cause of ARF and the specific needs of the individual client. Ensuring compliance with the treatment plan is the best way to prevent complications. Careful monitoring of vital signs, intake and output, serum electrolytes, and level of consciousness can alert the nurse to changes that indicate potential complications. Be sensitive to any cultural or religious practices, even if it means scheduling appointments or nursing activities around scheduled prayer times.

- Maintain hourly intake and output records. Accurate intake and output records help to guide therapy, especially fluid restrictions.
- Weigh the client daily or more frequently as ordered. Use standard technique (same scale, clothing, or coverings) to ensure accuracy. Rapid weight changes are an accurate indicator of fluid volume status, particularly in the client with oliguria client.
- Assess vital signs at least every 4 hours. Hypertension, tachycardia, and tachypnea may indicate excess fluid volume.
- Assess breath and heart sounds, neck veins for distention, and back and extremities for edema; report abnormal findings.
- If not contraindicated, place client in semi-Fowler's position to enhance cardiac and respiratory function.
- Report abnormal serum electrolyte values and manifestations of electrolyte imbalance. The client with ARF is at particular risk for the following electrolyte imbalances:
  a. *Hyperkalemia* caused by impaired potassium excretion. Manifestations include irritability, nausea, diarrhea, abdominal cramping, cardiac dysrhythmias, and electrocardiographic changes.
  b. *Hyponatremia* caused by water retention. Manifestations include nausea, vomiting, and headache, with possible central nervous system manifestations of lethargy, confusion, seizures, and coma. If the serum sodium concentration rises and the client's weight falls, insufficient fluids are being administered. If the serum sodium level falls and the client's weight increases, excessive fluids are being administered.
  c. *Hyperphosphatemia* caused by decreased phosphate excretion. Manifestations include hyperreflexia, paresthesias, and possible **tetany** (tonic muscle spasms). ARF impairs electrolyte and water excretion, causing multiple electrolyte imbalances.
- Turn the client frequently, and provide good skin care. Edema decreases tissue perfusion and increases the risk of skin breakdown, especially in the older or debilitated client.
- Restrict fluids as ordered. Provide frequent mouth care, and encourage use of hard candies to decrease thirst. If ice chips are allowed, include the water content (approximately half the total volume) as intake. Fluids are restricted to minimize fluid retention and complications of fluid volume excess.
- Administer medications with meals. Giving oral medications with meals minimizes ingestion of excess fluids.

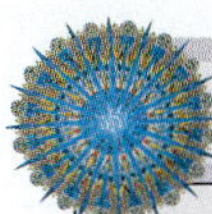

NURSING CARE PLAN A Client With Acute Renal Failure

Judy Devak is driving home late one evening when she loses control of her car trying to avoid hitting a deer in the road. Her car strikes a tree and rolls into a deep ditch beside the road, out of sight of passing cars. The wreck is not discovered until 2 hours later. On arrival at the accident scene, the paramedics find Ms. Devak hypotensive: BP 90/60 mmHg, pulse 120 bpm, and respirations 24/min. She is alert and in severe pain, with a fractured right femur. After immobilizing Ms. Devak's neck and back and extricating her from the car, the paramedics apply a traction splint to her leg and transport her to the local hospital.

ASSESSMENT

Katie Leaper, RN, obtains a nursing history on Ms. Devak's admission to the intensive care unit (ICU). Ms. Devak indicates that she has been healthy, having experienced only minor illnesses and chickenpox as a child. She has never been hospitalized and has no known allergies to medications. Ms. Devak is not currently taking prescription or nonprescription drugs. Physical assessment findings include temperature 97.4°F (36.3°C) oral, pulse 100 bpm, respirations 18/min, and BP 124/68 mmHg. Ms. Devak's skin is pale, cool, and dry, with multiple scrapes, minor abrasions, and bruises on her face and extremities. Nurse Leaper notes a linear bruise on her chest and abdomen from the seat belt. Ms. Devak's lung sounds are clear, heart tones normal, and abdomen tender but soft to palpation. Right leg alignment is maintained with skeletal traction. One unit of whole blood was infused before ICU admission; a second unit is currently infusing. An indwelling urinary catheter and a nasogastric tube are in place.

During the first few hours after admission, Ms. Leaper notes that Ms. Devak's hourly output has dropped from 55 to 45 to 28 mL of clear yellow urine. The physician orders a 500-mL intravenous fluid challenge, STAT urinalysis, BUN, and serum creatinine. The fluid challenge elicits only a slight increase in urine output. Urinalysis results show a specific gravity of 1.010 and the presence of white blood cells, red and white cell casts, and tubular epithelial cells in the sediment. Ms. Devak's BUN is 28 mg/dL; her serum creatinine is 1.5 mg/dL. The physician diagnoses probable ARF and orders a nephrology consultation. In addition, the physician orders aluminum hydroxide, 10 mL every 2 hours per nasogastric tube, and ranitidine, 50 mg intravenously every 8 hours.

DIAGNOSES

- Acute Pain related to injuries sustained in accident
- Anxiety related to being in the ICU
- Risk for Excess Fluid Volume related to impaired renal function
- Impaired Physical Mobility related to skeletal traction
- Ineffective Protection related to injuries and invasive procedures

PLANNING

- Client will report adequate pain control.
- Client will verbalize reduced anxiety.
- Client will maintain stable weight and vital signs within normal range.
- Client will maintain skin integrity.
- Client will use the trapeze appropriately to adjust position in bed while maintaining body alignment.
- Client will remain free of infection, bleeding, or respiratory distress.

IMPLEMENTATION

- Maintain patient-controlled anesthesia.
- Assess frequently for pain control and response to analgesia.
- Encourage expression of thoughts, feelings, and fears about condition and placement in ICU.
- Document vital signs and heart and lung sounds at least every 4 hours.
- Weigh every 12 hours.
- Document hourly intake and output.
- Restrict fluids as ordered, including diluent for all intravenous medications as intake.
- Assist with mouth care every 3–4 hours; allow frequent rinsing of mouth and ice chips as allowed.
- Assist with position changes at least every 2 hours; teach use of the overhead trapeze.
- Monitor frequently for signs of infection, bleeding, or respiratory distress.

EVALUATION

After just over 3 days of oliguria, Ms. Devak's urine output increases. By the end of the fourth day, she is excreting 60–80 mL/hr of urine. Although her BUN, serum creatinine, and potassium levels remain high, they never reach a critical point, and dialysis is not required. She is transferred from the ICU on the fifth day after admission. When Ms. Devak is able to begin eating, she is placed on a low-potassium diet, restricted to 50 g of protein. Her renal function gradually improves. By discharge, results of her renal function studies, including BUN and serum creatinine, are nearly normal. Ms. Devak verbalizes an understanding of the need to avoid nephrotoxins, such as nonsteroidal anti-inflammatory drugs, until allowed by her physician.

CRITICAL THINKING

1. What was the most likely specific precipitating factor for Ms. Devak's ARF? Did anything else contribute to her risk?
2. Why did the physician prescribe aluminum hydroxide and ranitidine? Consider both the ARF and Ms. Devak's placement in the ICU.
3. Ms. Devak is at risk for respiratory distress related to potential fluid volume excess. How does her fractured femur further contribute to risk for respiratory distress?
4. Develop a care plan for Ms. Devak for the nursing diagnosis of deficient diversional activity.

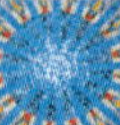

DEVELOPMENTAL CONSIDERATIONS Nutrition and Children With Acute Renal Failure

- Children are at risk for malnutrition because of their high metabolic rate during acute renal failure. Parenteral or enteral feeding may be used initially to minimize protein catabolism.
- The diet is tailored to the individual child's needs for calories, carbohydrates, fats, and amino acids or protein hydrolysates. Depending on the degree of renal failure, sodium, potassium, and phosphorus may be restricted.
- Initiate oral feedings as soon as tolerated.
- A multidisciplinary team review with a nutritionist may be necessary.

Imbalanced Nutrition: Less Than Body Requirements

Anorexia and nausea associated with renal failure often interfere with food intake and nutrition. In addition, the disease process leading to ARF may contribute to increased nutritional needs for healing concurrently with decreased food intake. The nurse working with the client with Imbalanced nutrition: less than body requirements related to ARF should:

- Monitor and record food intake, including the amount and type of food consumed. A detailed intake record helps to guide decisions about nutritional status and necessary supplements.
- Weigh the client daily. Weight changes over time (days to weeks) reflect nutritional status, while rapid weight changes are more reflective of fluid volume status. In ARF, weight may remain stable or increase because of fluid retention even though tissue mass is being lost.
- Arrange for consultation with a dietician. A registered dietician can assist in planning meals within prescribed limitations that consider the client's food preferences, especially if the client follows cultural or religious mandates regarding foods. Diets restricted in protein, salt, and potassium can be unpalatable; intake and appetite improve when preferred foods are included as allowed.
- Engage the client in planning daily menus. Participation in meal planning increases the client's sense of control and autonomy.
- Allow family members to prepare meals within dietary restrictions. Encourage family members to eat with the client. Familiar foods and social interaction encourage eating and increase enjoyment of meals.
- Provide frequent, small meals or between-meal snacks. These measures promote food intake in the client who is fatigued or anorectic.
- Administer antiemetics as ordered, and provide mouth care before meals. Nausea and a metallic taste in the mouth, common manifestations of uremia, can decrease food intake.
- Administer parenteral nutrition as ordered if the client is unable to eat or tolerate enteral nutrition. Preventing or slowing tissue **catabolism** (the breakdown of body proteins) is important for the client with ARF.
- Assess anxiety level and ability to comprehend instruction. Tailor information and presentation to the client's developmental level and physical, mental, and emotional status. The client with ARF may be critically ill or have uremic effects that hinder learning. During the initial stages of ARF, it may be necessary to limit information to immediate concerns, such as treatment of the underlying cause of the kidney failure.
- Assess knowledge and understanding. To enhance understanding and retention, relate the information presented to previous learning.
- Teach client and immediate family about diagnostic tests and therapeutic procedures. Teaching reduces anxiety and improves understanding and cooperation.
- Discuss dietary and fluid restrictions. These measures may be continued after discharge.
- If the client is discharged before the recovery phase of ARF, teach the signs and symptoms of complications, including fluid volume excess or deficit, heart failure, and electrolyte imbalances. Explain to the client that urine output increases as kidney function returns, but that the concentrating ability of the nephrons and electrolyte excretion remain impaired. This impaired function increases the risk of excess fluid loss, possible dehydration, orthostatic hypotension, and electrolyte imbalance.
- Teach client how to monitor weight, blood pressure, and pulse. These are important means of assessing fluid status.
- Instruct client to avoid nephrotoxic drugs and chemicals for up to 1 year following an episode of ARF. During recovery, nephrons are vulnerable to damage by nephrotoxins, such as nonsteroidal anti-inflammatory drugs, some antibiotics, radiologic contrast media, and heavy metals. Because alcohol can increase the nephrotoxicity of some materials, discourage alcohol ingestion.

Evaluation

Evaluation of the client with ARF is based on resolution of symptoms and prevention of complications. Data to be evaluated include weight, cardiac rhythm, vital signs, breath sounds, oxygen saturation, serum electrolyte levels, intake and output, and hemoglobin and hematocrit. The client should be evaluated for response to treatment as well as for understanding of the disease process and self-care requirements. Expected outcomes of nursing care include the following:

- The client's fluid status is balanced with edema-associated weight loss, and electrolyte and acid–base balance is restored.
- The client's nutritional needs are met.
- The client acquires no secondary infections.

REVIEW Acute Renal Failure

RELATE: LINK THE CONCEPTS

Linking the exemplar of Acute Renal Failure with the concept of Elimination:

1. Nurses frequently get so busy they don't take time to go to the bathroom to urinate until it can no longer be postponed. Explain how this behavior increases the risk of ARF.
2. What would you teach a client who reported this behavior to reduce their risk of ARF?

Linking the exemplar of Acute Renal Failure with the concept of Acid–Base Balance:

3. What laboratory results would you review to determine the acid–base balance of the client with ARF?
4. What acid–base finding would you anticipate when caring for a client with ARF?

READY: GO TO COMPANION SKILLS MANUAL

- Administering blood components
- Monitoring intake and output
- Care of the AV fistula or graft
- Assisting with peritoneal dialysis catheter insertion
- Conducting peritoneal dialysis procedures
- Providing hemodialysis procedures
- Providing hemodialysis
- Providing ongoing care of the client receiving hemodialysis
- Terminating dialysis
- Maintaining central venous dial-lumen dialysis catheter
- Performing venipuncture
- Establishing an intravenous infusion
- Using an infusion pump or controller
- Maintaining infusions
- Maintaining intermittent-infusion devices
- Changing the gown of a client with an IV
- Discontinuing infusion devices

REFER: GO TO MY NURSING KIT

REFLECT: CASE STUDY

Missy is a healthy 4-year-old who seems to be in perpetual motion. She came home from preschool today and told her mother she was tired and wanted to take a nap. Her mother immediately sensed there was something wrong, because Missy never volunteers to take a nap. Missy's appetite was diminished at dinner, and although she appeared pale, she went to bed that night without complaint.

The following morning, Missy looks very ill, refuses to get out of bed, and hasn't urinated since 8 p.m. the evening before. Missy's mother brings her to the pediatrician's office, where Missy is diagnosed with ATN. Her pediatrician admits Missy to the local acute care facility. You are the nurse admitting Missy to the pediatric unit.

1. What questions would you ask Missy's mother to determine contributory factors of the development of acute tubular necrosis?
2. What orders would you anticipate from the health care provider to prevent the development of ARF?
3. What independent nursing orders would you develop to provide holistic, family-centered care for Missy?
4. What nursing diagnosis would be appropriate for Missy's plan of care?

11.2 CHRONIC RENAL FAILURE

KEY TERMS

Chronic renal failure (CRF), *552*
End-stage renal disease (ESRD), *552*
Nephrectomy, *560*
Paresthesias, *556*
Uremia, *554*
Uremic fetor, *556*
Uremic frost, *558*

BASIS FOR SELECTION OF EXEMPLAR

Healthy People 2010

LEARNING OUTCOMES

After reading about this exemplar, you will be able to:

1. Describe the pathophysiology, etiology, clinical manifestations, and direct and indirect causes of chronic renal failure.
2. Identify risk factors associated with chronic renal failure.
3. Illustrate the nursing process in providing culturally competent care across the life span for individuals with chronic renal failure.
4. Formulate priority nursing diagnoses appropriate for an individual with chronic renal failure.
5. Create a plan of caring interventions for individuals with chronic renal failure and their family members.
6. Assess expected outcomes for an individual with chronic renal failure.
7. Discuss therapies used in the collaborative care of an individual with chronic renal failure.
8. Employ evidence-based caring interventions for an individual with chronic renal failure.

OVERVIEW

The internal environment of the body normally remains in a relatively constant or homeostatic state. The kidneys help to maintain homeostasis by regulating the composition and volume of extracellular fluid. They excrete excess water and solutes and, when deficits occur, can conserve water and solutes. In addition, the kidneys help to regulate acid–base balance, and they excrete metabolic wastes. Regulation of blood pressure is also a key function of the kidneys.

Both primary kidney disorders (e.g., glomerulonephritis) and systemic diseases (e.g., diabetes mellitus) can affect renal function. In North America, more than 26 million people are affected by kidney diseases (National Kidney Foundation, 2009). Every year, approximately 3.6 of every 1,000 people in the United States develop **end-stage renal disease (ESRD)**, the final phase of **chronic renal failure (CRF)** in which little or no kidney function remains. Chronic renal disease is a major cause of lost work time and wages (U.S. Renal Data System [USRDS], 2008). Ironically, the increased prevalence of chronic renal disease in recent years is partially related to the success of dialysis and transplantation.

Renal function is dependent on an adequate supply of blood. Blood supports renal cell metabolism and is vital to kidney function, the nephron in particular. Only with sufficient blood supply can the kidney regulate fluid, electrolyte, and acid–base balance and serve as a major organ of excretion. Vascular disorders, therefore, can have a significant impact on renal function. Hypertension causes arteriosclerotic lesions in the afferent (leading into) and efferent (going out of) arterioles and the glomerular capillaries. The GFR declines, and tubular function is affected, resulting in proteinuria and microscopic hematuria. Approximately 10% of deaths attributed to hypertension result from renal failure (Kasper et al., 2005).

Although the kidneys usually recover from acute injury, many chronic conditions can lead to progressive renal tissue destruction and loss of function. Nephron units are lost and renal mass decreased, with progressive deterioration of glomerular filtration, tubular secretion, and reabsorption. This process of CRF may progress slowly for many years without being recognized. Eventually, the kidneys are unable to excrete metabolic wastes and to regulate fluid and electrolyte balance adequately—the condition known as ESRD, the final stage of CRF. Because of the increasing prevalence of CRF and ESRD, *Healthy People 2010* selected chronic kidney disease as one of its focus areas (see Box 11–5).

PATHOPHYSIOLOGY AND ETIOLOGY

The pathophysiology of CRF involves a gradual loss of entire nephron units. In the early stages, as nephrons are destroyed, remaining functional nephrons hypertrophy (enlarge as a result of an increase in size of the constituent cells). Glomerular capillary flow and pressure increase in these nephrons, and more solute particles are filtered to compensate for lost renal mass. This increased demand predisposes the remaining nephrons to glomerular sclerosis (scarring), resulting in their eventual destruction. This process of continued loss of nephron function may persist even after the initial disease process has resolved (Kasper et al., 2005). Table 11–10 outlines common pathologic processes leading to nephron destruction and ESRD.

The course of CRF is variable, progressing over a period of months to many years. In the early stage, known as decreased renal reserve, unaffected nephrons compensate for the lost nephrons. The GFR is approximately 50% of normal, and the client is asymptomatic, with normal BUN and serum creatinine levels. As the disea552se progresses and the GFR falls to between 20–50% of normal, azotemia and some manifestations of renal insufficiency may be seen. Any further insult to the kidneys (e.g., infection, dehydration, exposure to nephrotoxins, or urinary tract obstruction) at this stage can further reduce function and precipitate the onset of renal failure or overt uremia. Renal failure is characterized by a GFR of less than 20% of normal. The serum creatinine and BUN levels rise sharply (Figure 11–18 ■), the client becomes oliguric, and manifestations of uremia are seen. Finally, in ESRD, the GFR is less than 5% of normal, and renal replacement therapy is

Box 11–5 *Healthy People 2010*: Chronic and End-Stage Renal Disease (ESRD)

PREVALENCE

- Some 10–12 million people over the age of 12 have chronic renal disease.
- ESRD results from chronic damage to the kidneys over a decade or more.
- Diabetes and hypertension increase the risk for ESRD.
- The number of new cases of ESRD is increasing and correlates to an increase in cases of type 2 diabetes mellitus.
- African Americans are at the highest risk for renal disease.
- American Indians, Native Alaskans, Asians, and Pacific Islanders have higher rates of renal disease than whites.
- Mexicans have a high risk for renal disease related to higher incidence of type 2 diabetes mellitus.

OBJECTIVES

- Decrease the rate of new cases of ESRD.
- Increase the number of dialysis patients on waiting lists for transplant.
- Decrease kidney failure caused by diabetes.

ACTIONS

- Early identification of people at risk
- Control of diabetes and hypertension
- Education related to diet and exercise

TABLE 11–10 **Pathophysiology of Chronic Renal Failure**

CAUSE	EXAMPLES
Diabetic nephropathy	Changes in the glomerular basement membrane, chronic pyelonephritis, and ischemia lead to sclerosis of the glomerulus and gradual destruction of the nephron.
Hypertensive nephrosclerosis	Long-standing hypertension leads to renal arteriosclerosis and ischemia, resulting in glomerular destruction and tubular atrophy.
Chronic glomerulonephritis	Bilateral inflammatory process of the glomeruli leads to ischemia, nephron loss, and shrinkage of the kidney.
Chronic pyelonephritis	Chronic infection commonly associated with an obstructive or neurologic process and vesicoureteral reflux leads to reflux nephropathy (renal scarring, atrophy, and dilated calyces).
Polycystic kidney disease	Multiple bilateral cysts gradually destroy normal renal tissue by compression.
Systemic lupus erythematosus	Basement membrane damage by circulating immune complexes leads to focal, local, or diffuse glomerulonephritis.

necessary to sustain life (Kasper et al., 2005; Porth, 2005). Table 11–11 summarizes the stages of CRF.

Etiology

Renal failure is common and costly. Each year, nearly 354,000 clients with ESRD undergo dialysis, approximately 18,000 have kidney transplants, and another 77,000 are awaiting kidney transplants (National Kidney and Urologic Diseases Information Clearinghouse [NKUDIC], 2009). The annual cost to Medicare alone of treating clients with ESRD is $23 billion (USRDS, 2008). The cost is also measured in lives and lifestyle. The 5-year survival rate for clients undergoing dialysis is 31.9% (NKUDIC, 2004). Although many clients report satisfaction with their quality of life, clients on dialysis are often unable to work, and family structures may disintegrate under the strain of treatment.

The incidence of ESRD is increasing, particularly in older adults. In 2006, more than 110,000 people started treatment for ESRD, compared with 93,000 in 2001 (NKUDIC, 2004, 2009). African Americans have the highest incidence of ESRD, followed by Native Americans, Asians, and European Americans (USRDS, 2005).

Risk Factors

Conditions causing CRF typically involve diffuse, bilateral disease of the kidneys with progressive destruction and scarring of the entire nephron. Diabetes is the leading cause of ESRD in all population groups in the United States. Hypertension closely follows diabetes as a major cause of ESRD; in many clients, these disorders coexist (USRDS, 2005).

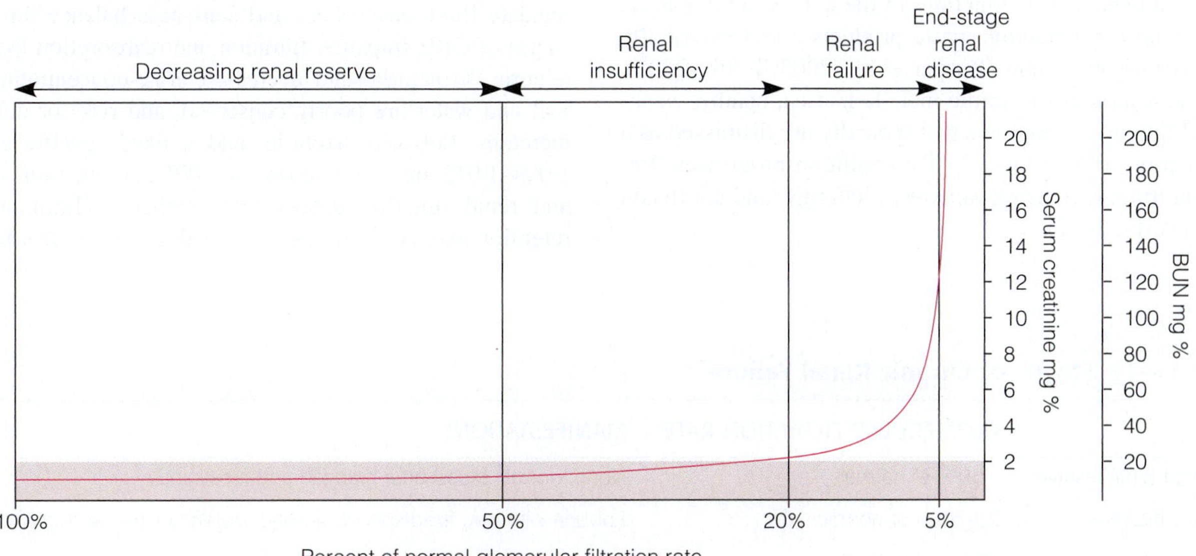

Figure 11–18 ■ The relationship of renal function to blood urea nitrogen and serum creatinine values through the course of chronic renal failure.

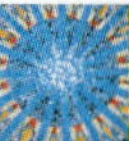

DEVELOPMENTAL CONSIDERATIONS Renal Failure in the Older Adult

Structural and functional changes occur in the aging kidney. Structurally, the number of nephrons decreases. Functionally, the GFR decreases, resulting in decreased renal clearance of drugs. Urine-concentrating ability decreases, and the kidney is less able to conserve sodium. Renal compensation for acid–base imbalances takes longer. Despite these changes, the kidney retains its ability to regulate fluid and electrolyte homeostasis remarkably well unless additional stresses are added. Any additional stressors, such as hypotension, exposure to nephrotoxic drugs, or an inflammatory process like glomerulonephritis, may precipitate renal failure in the older adult.

The manifestations of renal failure often are missed in aging clients (e.g., edema may be attributed to heart failure or high blood pressure to preexisting hypertension). Serum creatinine levels may rise slowly. Because older adults have less muscle mass, they produce less creatinine, a by-product of muscle cell metabolism. Likewise, the blood urea nitrogen may remain within normal limits.

The same measures are used to treat renal failure in older adults as in younger people. Hemodialysis, peritoneal dialysis, and renal transplantation are appropriate if necessary. Treatment options (including conservative treatment or no treatment) and their potential benefits and ramifications should be explained clearly to the client and caregivers.

ASSESSING FOR HOME CARE

A number of factors should be considered in assessing the older adult's ability to manage treatment such as dialysis at home:

- Does the client have reasonable access to a dialysis center or outpatient unit? Is transportation available?
- Would home hemodialysis be appropriate? Is a caregiver available who can be trained to manage dialysis? Does the client's home have appropriate electrical and plumbing fixtures?
- Would continuous ambulatory peritoneal dialysis be appropriate? Does the client have the manual dexterity, will, and cognitive ability to manage dialysis infusions? If not, would intermittent peritoneal dialysis using a dialyzing machine be more appropriate?
- Are family members or other support persons available to assist the client as needed?

RESOURCES FOR HOME CARE

The following resources may be useful for clients with kidney disease:

- American Association of Kidney Patients
  800-749-2257
  813-636-8100
  http://www.aakp.org
- American Kidney Fund
  800-638-8299
  866-300-2900 (Spanish help line)
  http://www.kidneyfund.org
- National Kidney Foundation
  800-622-9010
  http://www.kidney.org

CLINICAL MANIFESTATIONS

CRF often is not identified until its final, uremic stage is reached. **Uremia**, which literally means "urea in the blood," refers to the syndrome or group of symptoms associated with ESRD. In uremia, fluid and electrolyte balance is altered, the regulatory and endocrine functions of the kidney are impaired, and accumulated metabolic waste products affect essentially every other organ system (Kasper et al., 2005; Porth, 2005). Early manifestations of uremia include nausea, apathy, weakness, and fatigue—symptoms that typically are dismissed as a viral infection or influenza. As the condition progresses, frequent vomiting, increasing weakness, lethargy, and confusion develop (Porth, 2005).

For a list of the signs and symptoms of CRF in older adults, see Table 11–7. For a list of electrolyte imbalances in children with CRF, see Table 11–8.

Fluid and Electrolyte Effects

Loss of functional kidney tissue impairs the kidneys' ability to regulate fluid, electrolyte, and acid–base balance. In the early stages of CRF, impaired filtration and reabsorption lead to proteinuria, hematuria, and decreased urine-concentrating ability. Salt and water are poorly conserved, and risk for dehydration increases. Polyuria, nocturia, and a fixed specific gravity of 1.008–1.012 are common (Porth, 2005). As the GFR decreases and renal function deteriorates further, sodium and water retention may occur, necessitating salt and water restrictions.

TABLE 11–11 Stages of Chronic Renal Failure

STAGE	GLOMERULAR FILTRATION RATE	MANIFESTATIONS
Decreased renal reserve	~50% of normal	None; normal blood urea nitrogen and creatinine
Renal insufficiency	20–50% of normal	Polyuria with low, fixed specific gravity; azotemia; anemia; hypertension
Renal failure	<20% of normal	Increasing azotemia; edema; metabolic acidosis; hypercalcemia; possible uremia
End-stage renal disease	<5% of normal	Kidney atrophy and fibrosis; overt uremia

MULTISYSTEM EFFECTS OF **Uremia**

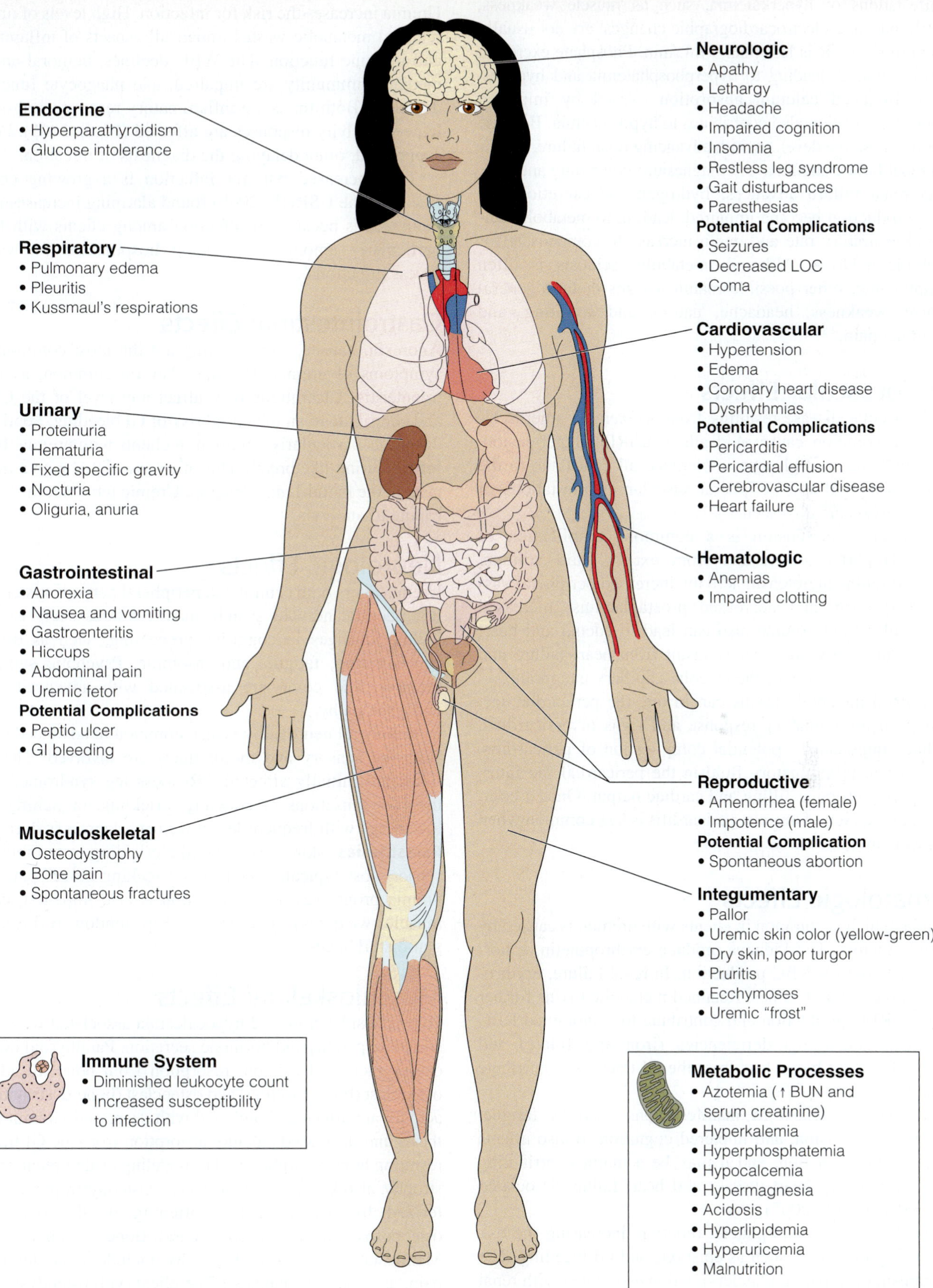
Neurologic
• Apathy
• Lethargy
• Headache
• Impaired cognition
• Insomnia
• Restless leg syndrome
• Gait disturbances
• Paresthesias
Potential Complications
• Seizures
• Decreased LOC
• Coma
Endocrine
• Hyperparathyroidism
• Glucose intolerance
Respiratory
• Pulmonary edema
• Pleuritis
• Kussmaul's respirations
Cardiovascular
• Hypertension
• Edema
• Coronary heart disease
• Dysrhythmias
Potential Complications
• Pericarditis
• Pericardial effusion
• Cerebrovascular disease
• Heart failure
Urinary
• Proteinuria
• Hematuria
• Fixed specific gravity
• Nocturia
• Oliguria, anuria
Hematologic
• Anemias
• Impaired clotting
Gastrointestinal
• Anorexia
• Nausea and vomiting
• Gastroenteritis
• Hiccups
• Abdominal pain
• Uremic fetor
Potential Complications
• Peptic ulcer
• GI bleeding
Reproductive
• Amenorrhea (female)
• Impotence (male)
Potential Complication
• Spontaneous abortion
Musculoskeletal
• Osteodystrophy
• Bone pain
• Spontaneous fractures
Integumentary
• Pallor
• Uremic skin color (yellow-green)
• Dry skin, poor turgor
• Pruritis
• Ecchymoses
• Uremic "frost"
Immune System
• Diminished leukocyte count
• Increased susceptibility to infection
Metabolic Processes
• Azotemia (↑ BUN and serum creatinine)
• Hyperkalemia
• Hyperphosphatemia
• Hypocalcemia
• Hypermagnesia
• Acidosis
• Hyperlipidemia
• Hyperuricemia
• Malnutrition

Hyperkalemia develops as renal failure progresses. Manifestations of hyperkalemia, such as muscle weakness, paresthesias, and electrocardiographic changes, are not usually seen until the GFR is less than 5 mL/min. Phosphate excretion is also impaired, leading to hyperphosphatemia and hypocalcemia. Reduced calcium absorption caused by impaired vitamin D activation also contributes to hypocalcemia. Because hypermagnesemia develops with advancing renal failure, clients with renal failure should avoid magnesium-containing antacids.

As renal failure advances, hydrogen ion excretion and buffer production become impaired, leading to metabolic acidosis. Respiratory rate and depth increase to compensate for metabolic acidosis. Although metabolic acidosis is often asymptomatic, other possible manifestations include general malaise, weakness, headache, nausea and vomiting, and abdominal pain.

Cardiovascular Effects

Cardiovascular disease resulting from accelerated atherosclerosis is a common cause of death in ESRD. Hypertension, hyperlipidemia, and glucose intolerance all contribute to the process. Cerebral and peripheral vascular manifestations of atherosclerosis are also seen.

Systemic hypertension is a common complication of ESRD. Hypertension results from excess fluid volume, increased renin–angiotensin activity, increased peripheral vascular resistance, and decreased prostaglandins. Increased extracellular fluid volume also can lead to edema and heart failure. Pulmonary edema may result from heart failure and increased permeability of the alveolar capillary membrane.

Retained metabolic toxins can irritate the pericardial sac, causing an inflammatory response and signs of pericarditis. Cardiac tamponade, a potential complication of pericarditis, occurs when inflammatory fluid in the pericardial sac interferes with ventricular filling and cardiac output. Once a common complication of uremia, pericarditis is less common when dialysis is initiated early.

Hematologic Effects

Anemia, which is common in clients with uremia, is caused by multiple factors. The kidneys produce erythropoietin, a hormone that controls RBC production. In renal failure, erythropoietin production declines. Retained metabolic toxins further suppress RBC production and contribute to a shortened RBC life span. Nutritional deficiencies (iron and folate) and increased risk for blood loss from the GI tract also contribute to anemia.

Anemia contributes to manifestations such as fatigue, weakness, depression, and impaired cognition. It also affects cardiovascular function, and it may be a major contributing factor to coronary heart disease and heart failure associated with ESRD (Porth, 2005).

Renal failure impairs platelet function, increasing the risk of bleeding disorders, such as epistaxis and GI bleeding. The mechanism of impaired platelet function associated with renal failure is poorly understood.

Immune System Effects

Uremia increases the risk for infection. High levels of urea and retained metabolic wastes impair all aspects of inflammation and immune function. The WBC declines, humoral and cell-mediated immunity are impaired, and phagocyte function is defective. Both the acute inflammatory response and delayed hypersensitivity responses are affected (Porth, 2005). Fever is suppressed, often delaying the diagnosis of infection.

This increased risk for infection is a growing concern. Recently, the USRDS (2008) found alarming increases in hospitalizations because of infection among clients with ESRD, particularly among those being hospitalized for vascular access infections.

Gastrointestinal Effects

Anorexia, nausea, and vomiting are the most common early symptoms of uremia. Hiccups also are common, as is gastroenteritis. Ulcerations may affect any level of the GI tract and contribute to an increased risk of GI bleeding. Peptic ulcer disease is particularly common in clients with uremia. **Uremic fetor** (a urine-like breath odor often associated with a metallic taste in the mouth) may develop. Uremic fetor can further contribute to anorexia.

Neurologic Effects

Uremia alters both central and peripheral nervous system function. Central nervous system manifestations occur early and include changes in cognitive processing, such as difficulty concentrating, fatigue, and insomnia. Psychotic symptoms, seizures, and coma are associated with advanced uremic encephalopathy.

Peripheral neuropathy is also common in advanced uremia. Both the sensory and motor tracts are involved. The lower limbs are initially affected. "Restless leg syndrome," which involves sensations of crawling, prickling, or itching of the lower legs with frequent leg movement, increases during rest. **Paresthesias** (skin sensations like prickling or numbing) and sensory loss typically occur in a "stocking-glove" pattern. As uremia progresses, motor function is also impaired, causing muscle weakness, decreased deep tendon reflexes, and gait disturbances.

Musculoskeletal Effects

Hyperphosphatemia and hypocalcemia associated with uremia stimulate parathyroid hormone secretion. Parathyroid hormone causes increased calcium resorption from bone. In addition, osteoblast (bone-forming) and osteoclast (bone-destroying) cell activity are affected. Combined with decreased vitamin D synthesis and decreased calcium absorption from the GI tract, the resulting bone resorption and remodeling lead to renal osteodystrophy, also known as renal rickets. Osteodystrophy is characterized by osteomalacia (softening of the bones) and osteoporosis (decreased bone mass). Bone cysts may develop. Manifestations of osteodystrophy include bone tenderness, pain, and muscle weakness. The client with osteodystrophy is at increased risk for spontaneous fractures (Porth, 2005).

CLINICAL MANIFESTATIONS AND THERAPIES Chronic Renal Failure

ETIOLOGY	CLINICAL MANIFESTATIONS	CLINICAL THERAPIES
Uremia	Hyperparathyroidism Glucose intolerance Pulmonary edema Pleuritis Kussmaul's inspirations Proteinuria Hematuria Fixed specific gravity Nocturia Oliguria Anorexia, nausea, vomiting, gastroenteritis Hiccups Abdominal pain, peptic ulcer, gastrointestinal bleeding Uremic fetor Osteodystrophy, bone pain, spontaneous fractures Apathy, lethargy, headache, impaired cognition, insomnia, restless leg syndrome, gait disturbance, gait disturbances Hypertension, edema, coronary heart disease or failure Anemias, impaired clotting Pallor, uremic skin color, dry skin, poor skin turgor, pruritus	■ Often when uremia develops, the only option is dialysis. ■ Serum electrolytes, BUN, creatine, arterial blood gas (pH), lipid level monitoring ■ Cardiorespiratory monitoring ■ Accurate intake and output ■ Diuretic administration ■ Fluid restriction ■ Dietary consult may be needed to improve nutrition status.
Anemia	Fatigue Pallor Dizziness, confusion, lethargy Tachycardia, tachypnea, hypotension	■ Iron supplementation ■ Administration of epoetin ■ Blood transfusion ■ Therapies aimed at treating the underlying cause of acute renal failure
Fluid volume excess	Dependent pitting edema Respiratory crackles Dyspnea, pulmonary edema, hypoxemia Weight gain Tachycardia Jugular vein distention	■ Fluid restriction ■ Sodium restricted diet ■ Diuretics ■ Dialysis
Hyperkalemia	Ventricular arrhythmias Tall, peaked T waves; widened QRS Cardiac arrest Smooth muscle hyperactivity Nausea and vomiting Abdominal cramping Diarrhea Muscle weakness Paresthesias Flaccid paralysis	■ Removal of all potassium from intravenous solutions ■ Low-potassium diet ■ Administration of glucose and insulin to drive potassium into the cell ■ Potassium-absorbing enema solutions ■ Dialysis

Endocrine and Metabolic Effects

Accumulated waste products of protein metabolism are a primary factor in the effects and manifestations of uremia. Serum creatinine and BUN levels are significantly elevated. Uric acid levels increase, contributing to an increased risk of gout. Tissues become resistant to the effects of insulin in uremia, leading to glucose intolerance. High blood triglyceride levels and lower-than-normal levels of high-density lipoprotein contribute to the accelerated atherosclerotic process.

CRF affects reproductive function. Pregnancies are rarely carried to term, and menstrual irregularities are common. Reduced testosterone levels, low sperm counts, and impotence affect the male client with ESRD.

Dermatologic Effects

Anemia and retained pigmented metabolites cause pallor and a yellowish hue to the skin in clients with uremia. Dry skin with poor turgor, a result of dehydration and sweat gland atrophy, is common. Bruising and excoriations are common as well. Metabolic wastes not eliminated by the kidneys may deposit in the skin, contributing to itching or pruritus. In advanced uremia, high levels of urea in the sweat may result in **uremic frost** (crystallized deposits of urea on the skin).

COLLABORATION

Early management of CRF focuses on eliminating factors that may further decrease renal function and on measures to slow the progression of the disease to ESRD. Treatment goals for clients in all stages of development include:

- Maintain nutritional status while minimizing the accumulation of toxic waste products and manifestations of uremia.
- Identify and treat complications of CRF.
- Prepare for renal replacement therapies such as dialysis or renal transplant.

Treatment of CRF should be modified for the older adult. The restrictions on fluid intake and dietary protein should be less stringent, because most older adults have already decreased their protein and sodium intakes (Jassal et al., 1998) as well as their fluid intake. Constipation, a concern for many older adults, especially those who curb their own fluid intake, may exacerbate the hyperkalemia that accompanies CRF. Nursing and medical management for regularity are important contributions to the treatment plan. Thinning and dry skin is a common concern for all older adults, and the pruritus of CRF can present a real challenge. Careful skin care by the nurse, including moisturizing the skin, will be much appreciated by the older client.

Diagnostic Tests

Diagnostic tests are used both to identify CRF and to monitor kidney function. A number of tests may be performed to determine the underlying renal disorder. Once the diagnosis is established, renal function is monitored primarily through blood levels of metabolic wastes and electrolytes.

- *Urinalysis* is done to measure urine specific gravity and detect abnormal urine components. In CRF, the specific gravity may be fixed at approximately 1.010, equivalent to that of plasma. This fixed specific gravity is the result of impaired tubular secretion, reabsorption, and urine-concentrating ability. Abnormal proteins, blood cells, and cellular casts may also be noted in the urine.
- *Urine culture* is ordered to identify any urinary tract infection that may hasten the progress of CRF.
- *BUN* and *serum creatinine* are obtained to evaluate kidney function in eliminating nitrogenous waste products. Levels of both are monitored to assess the progress of renal failure. A BUN of 20–50 mg/dL signals mild azotemia; levels greater than 100 mg/dL indicate severe renal impairment. Uremic symptoms are seen when the BUN is around 200 mg/dL or higher. Serum creatinine levels of greater than 4 mg/dL indicate serious renal impairment.
- *Creatinine clearance* evaluates the GFR and renal function. In early CRF (renal insufficiency), the GFR is more than 20% of normal, and the creatinine clearance is 30 mL/min or greater. As the disease progresses and the stage of renal failure is reached, the GFR is reduced to less than 20% of normal and the creatinine clearance to 15–29 mL/min. In ESRD, the GFR is less than 5% of normal, and the creatinine clearance is less than 15 mL/min (Kasper et al., 2005).
- *Serum electrolytes* are monitored throughout the course of CRF. The serum sodium may be within normal limits or low because of water retention. Potassium levels are elevated but usually remain below 6.5 mEq/L. Serum phosphate is elevated, and the calcium level is decreased. Metabolic acidosis is identified by a low pH, low CO_2, and low bicarbonate levels.
- *CBC* reveals moderately severe anemia with a hematocrit of 20–30% and a low hemoglobin. The number of RBCs and platelets is reduced.
- *Renal ultrasonography* is done to evaluate kidney size. In CRF, kidney size decreases as nephrons are destroyed and kidney mass is reduced.
- *Kidney biopsy* may be done to identify the underlying disease process if this is unclear. It is also used to differentiate acute from CRF. Kidney biopsy may be performed in surgery or done percutaneously using needle biopsy.

Pharmacologic Therapies

CRF affects both the pharmacokinetics and pharmacodynamics of drug therapy. Most medications are excreted primarily by the kidney. The half-life and plasma levels of many drugs increase in CRF. Drug absorption may decrease when phosphate-binding agents are administered concurrently. Proteinuria can significantly reduce plasma protein levels, leading to manifestations of toxicity when highly protein-bound drugs are given. In addition, any potentially nephrotoxic agent should be used with extreme caution. Avoid drugs eliminated by the kidney, such as meperidine, metformin (Glucophage), and other oral hypoglycemic agents, (Kasper et al., 2005).

Furosemide or other loop diuretics may be prescribed to reduce extracellular fluid volume and edema. Diuretic therapy also can reduce hypertension and cause potassium wasting, lowering serum potassium levels. Other antihypertensive agents are used to maintain the blood pressure within normal levels, slow the progress of renal failure, and prevent complications of coronary heart disease and cerebral vascular disease. Angiotensin-converting enzyme inhibitors are preferred, although any class of antihypertensive agent may be prescribed.

Other drugs may be used to manage electrolyte imbalances and acidosis. Sodium bicarbonate or calcium carbonate may be used to correct mild acidosis. Oral phosphorus–binding agents, such as calcium carbonate or calcium acetate, are given to lower serum phosphate levels and normalize serum calcium levels. Aluminum hydroxide may be used in acute treatment of hyperphosphatemia. It is limited to short-term use, however, because of complications such as encephalopathy and osteodystrophy associated with long-term administration of aluminum-containing preparations (Tierney et al., 2005). Vitamin D supplements may be given to improve calcium absorption.

If the client's serum potassium rises to dangerously high levels, a combination of bicarbonate, insulin, and glucose may be given intravenously to promote potassium movement into the cells. Sodium polystyrene sulfonate (Kayexalate), a potassium-ion exchange resin, can be given either orally or rectally (as an enema).

Folic acid and iron supplements are given to combat anemia associated with CRF. A multiple vitamin preparation is also often prescribed, because anorexia, nausea, and dietary restrictions may limit nutrient intake.

Nutrition and Fluid Management

As renal function declines, the elimination of water, solutes, and metabolic wastes is impaired. Accumulation of these wastes in the body leads to uremic symptoms. Instituted early in the course of CRF, dietary modifications can slow the progress of nephron destruction, reduce uremic symptoms, and help to prevent complications.

Unlike carbohydrates and fats, the body is unable to store excess proteins. Unused dietary proteins are degraded into urea and other nitrogenous wastes, which are then eliminated by the kidneys. Protein-rich foods also contain inorganic ions, such as hydrogen ion, phosphate, and sulfites, that are eliminated by the kidneys. Research has shown that restricting dietary protein intake slows the progression of CRF and reduces uremic symptoms (Kasper et al., 2005). A daily protein intake of 0.6 g/kg body weight, or approximately 40 g/day for an average male client, provides the amino acids necessary for tissue repair. Proteins should be of high biologic value, rich in the essential amino acids. Carbohydrate intake is increased to maintain energy requirements and provide approximately 35 kcal/kg each day.

Water and sodium intake are regulated to maintain the extracellular fluid volume at normal levels. Water intake of 1–2 L/day is generally recommended to maintain water balance. Sodium is restricted to 2 g/day initially. More stringent water and sodium restrictions may be necessary as renal failure progresses. Instruct the client to monitor his or her weight daily and to report any weight gain in excess of 5 pounds over a 2-day period.

When the GFR falls to less than 10–20 mL/min, potassium and phosphorous intake are also restricted. Potassium intake is limited to less than 60 –70 mEq/day (normal intake is ~100 mEq/day) (Tierney et al., 2005). Caution the client and caregivers to avoid using salt substitutes, which typically contain high levels of potassium chloride. Foods high in phosphorus include eggs, dairy products, and meat.

Renal Replacement Therapies

When pharmacologic and dietary management strategies are no longer effective to maintain fluid and electrolyte balance and prevent uremia, dialysis or kidney transplantation is considered. The most common therapies for ESRD in the United States are hemodialysis performed in a dialysis center, followed by peritoneal dialysis and kidney transplant (NKUDIC, 2009). A number of considerations, including the client's age, concurrent health problems, donor availability, and personal preference, influence the choice of long-term treatment.

A number of considerations affect the choice of long-term treatment. Hemodialysis and peritoneal dialysis each have advantages and disadvantages. Establishing vascular access for hemodialysis may take several months. Planning ahead to develop the access before dialysis is necessary can ease the transition to dialysis. Also, when dialysis treatments will be performed at home, initiating client instruction before the treatments are required can result in more effective learning. If a family member will serve as a dialysis helper, begin training before the onset of uremia.

If transplantation is considered, tissue typing and identification of potential living related donors can be done before the onset of ESRD. To make an informed decision, both the client and the potential donor need to understand the risks, benefits, and options available. If the decision for transplant is made early, dialysis can potentially be avoided.

DIALYSIS The most common therapies for ESRD in the United States are hemodialysis performed in a dialysis center, followed by peritoneal dialysis and kidney transplant (NKUDIC, 2004). Both hemodialysis and peritoneal dialysis can be done in the home, but few clients use home hemodialysis. Of the two, peritoneal dialysis is typically the choice for at-home treatment. Because the morbidity and mortality for each are comparable, factors such as the desire and ability to manage home care, employment, and availability of a dialysis center become the primary factors influencing the choice of hemodialysis or peritoneal dialysis.

Clients on long-term dialysis have a higher risk for complications and death than the general population. Many have other severe diseases along with ESRD. Infection and cardiovascular disease are common causes of illness and death. The 1-year survival rate for clients receiving dialysis is nearly 78%; long-term survival, however, falls to 32% at 5 years and about 9% at 10 years (NKUDIC, 2004).

The decision to initiate dialysis is not easy. Like insulin therapy for the client with diabetes, dialysis manages the symptoms of ESRD but does not cure it. Dialysis is a constant factor of life, requiring thinking and planning ahead at all times. Clients on dialysis may not be able to maintain a job. Families often fall apart with the day-to-day stress. Even with dialysis, the client may have constant flulike symptoms, never feeling truly well. Clients on hemodialysis may see themselves as powerless because of their dependence on others for treatment. On the other hand, home peritoneal dialysis places a continuing burden on the client to maintain treatment. In the end, the client may choose to discontinue treatment, preferring death over continued dialysis.

Hemodialysis and peritoneal dialysis each have advantages and disadvantages. Both can be done in the home, but few clients use home hemodialysis. Of the two, peritoneal dialysis is typically the choice for at-home treatment. Because the morbidity and mortality for each are comparable, issues such as the desire and ability to manage home care, employment, and availability of a dialysis center become the primary factors influencing the choice of hemodialysis or peritoneal dialysis.

Clients on long-term dialysis have a higher risk for complications and death than the general population. Many also have other severe diseases along with ESRD. Infection and cardiovascular disease are common causes of illness and death.

Hemodialysis for ESRD typically is done three times a week for a total of 9–12 hours. The amount of dialysis needed (or dialysis dose) is determined individually by factors such as body size and residual renal function, dietary intake, and concurrent illness. Hypotension and muscle cramps are common complications during hemodialysis treatments. Infection and vascular access problems are common long-term complications of hemodialysis. Cardiovascular disease is the leading cause of death for clients receiving hemodialysis. The death rate from cardiovascular disease is higher among clients receiving hemodialysis than among those receiving peritoneal dialysis or kidney transplant (Kasper et al., 2005). (See the previous exemplar on ARF and Box 11–3 for more information about hemodialysis and related nursing care.)

Peritoneal dialysis is currently used by approximately 10% of people who require long-term dialysis in the United States. In Canada and Europe, 35–45% of clients with ESRD are treated with peritoneal dialysis. In Third World countries, peritoneal dialysis is used to treat the majority of clients with ESRD.

Continuous ambulatory peritoneal dialysis (CAPD) is the most common form of peritoneal dialysis used. Dialysate (2 L) is instilled into the peritoneal cavity, and the catheter is sealed. The client can then continue normal daily activities, emptying the peritoneal cavity and replacing the dialysate every 4–6 hours. No special equipment is needed. A variation of CAPD is continuous cyclic peritoneal dialysis (CCPD), which uses a delivery device during nighttime hours and a continuous dwell during the day. CAPD can be performed anywhere, and CCPD allows for home treatment at night, leaving the client free during the day.

Peritoneal dialysis has several advantages over hemodialysis. Heparinization and vascular complications associated with an AV fistula are avoided. The clearance of metabolic wastes is slower but more continuous, avoiding rapid fluctuations in extracellular fluid composition and associated symptoms. The client on CAPD is often allowed more liberal intake of fluids and nutrients. While glucose absorbed from dialysate can increase blood glucose levels in the client with diabetes, regular insulin can be added to the infusion to manage hyperglycemia. The client on peritoneal dialysis is better able to self-manage the treatment regimen, reducing feelings of helplessness.

The major disadvantages of peritoneal dialysis include less effective elimination of metabolites and increased risk of infection (peritonitis). Peritoneal dialysis may not be effective for large clients with no residual kidney function. Serum triglyceride levels increase with peritoneal dialysis. Finally, the presence of an indwelling peritoneal catheter may cause a body image disturbance. (See *Renal Replacement Therapy* in Exemplar 11.1, Acute Renal Failure, for more information about dialysis and Box 11–4 for more information about nursing care for the client undergoing peritoneal dialysis.)

KIDNEY TRANSPLANT Kidney transplant has become the treatment of choice for many clients with ESRD. Kidneys are the solid organ most commonly transplanted; to date, kidney transplantation is the most successful of transplantation procedures. The first kidney transplant was performed in 1954; the donor and recipient were identical twins. Kidney transplant as a treatment for ESRD is limited primarily by the availability of organs. In 2008, more than 16,000 people received a kidney transplant; however, approximately 80,000 people are currently awaiting a transplant (Organ Procurement and Transplantation Network, 2009).

Kidney transplant improves both survival and quality of life for the client with ESRD. The client on dialysis has a 64.3% probability of surviving after 2 years of dialysis; the transplant recipient has a greater than 90% probability of survival after 2 years. At 5 years, the difference is even greater: 33% for dialysis compared with 80.6% for those who receive a transplant from a deceased donor, and nearly 90% when the donated organ comes from a living donor (NKUDIC, 2009). Quality of life improves dramatically once the client is no longer tethered to a dialysis catheter, machine, or center. Dietary and fluid restrictions are reduced, and the body image is more "whole."

Most transplanted kidneys are obtained from cadavers; however, transplants from living donors are increasing. In 2004, a total of 41.5% of transplanted kidneys, came from living donors, most of whom were related to the recipient (United Network for Organ Sharing [UNOS], 2005). With both cadaver and living donor transplants, a close match between blood and tissue type is desired. Human leukocyte antigens are compared between the donor and recipient; six antigens in common is considered to be a "perfect" match. The success of well-matched living-donor transplants is better than that for cadaver organ transplants, with a 1-year graft survival of 97.6% for living-donor transplants compared to 93.7% for cadaver transplants (NKUDIC, 2004). Close tissue matching probably accounts for the better outcome with living donors. People with normal kidneys who are in good physical health may donate a kidney. Pre-donation counseling is vital: **Nephrectomy** is major surgery, and the donor faces the risk that trauma or disease may affect the remaining kidney in the future. If the transplant fails, the psychologic impact on the donor can be significant. Nursing care of the client having a nephrectomy is summarized in Box 11–6.

Cadaver kidneys are obtained from people who meet the criteria for brain death, are younger than 65 years, and are free of systemic disease, malignancy, or infection, including HIV and hepatitis B or C. Kidneys are removed after brain death has been determined and are preserved by hypothermia or a technique called continuous hypothermic pulsatile perfusion. A kidney preserved by hypothermia must be transplanted within 24 to 48 hours. Continuous hypothermic pulsatile

Box 11–6 **Nursing Care of the Client Having a Nephrectomy**

PREOPERATIVE CARE

- Provide routine preoperative care as outlined in Concept 16, Exemplar 16.1.
- Report abnormal laboratory values to the surgeon. *Bacteriuria, blood coagulation abnormalities, or other significant abnormal values may affect surgery and postoperative care.*
- Discuss operative and postoperative expectations as indicated, including the location of the incision and anticipated tubes, stents, and drains. *Preoperative teaching about postoperative expectations reduces anxiety for the client and family during the early postoperative period.*

POSTOPERATIVE CARE

- Provide routine postoperative care as described in Exemplar 16.1.
- Frequently assess urine color, amount, and character, noting any hematuria, pyuria, or sediment. Promptly report oliguria or anuria, as well as changes in urine color or clarity. *Preserving function of the remaining kidney is critical; frequent assessment allows early intervention for potential problems.*
- Note the placement, status, and drainage from ureteral catheters, stents, nephrostomy tubes, or drains. Label each clearly. Maintain gravity drainage; irrigate only as ordered. *Maintaining drainage tube patency is vital to prevent potential hydronephrosis. Bright bleeding or unexpected drainage may indicate a surgical complication.*
- Support the grieving process and adjustment to the loss of a kidney. *Loss of a major organ leads to a body image change and grief response. When renal cancer is the underlying diagnosis, the client may also grieve the loss of health and potential loss of life.*
- Provide the following home care instructions for the client and family:
  a. The importance of protecting the remaining kidney by preventing UTI, renal calculi, and trauma. *Damage to the remaining kidney by UTI, renal calculi, or trauma can lead to renal failure.*
  b. Maintain a fluid intake of 2,000–2,500 mL per day. *This important measure helps prevent dehydration and maintain good urine flow.*
  c. Gradually increase exercise to tolerance, avoiding heavy lifting for a year after surgery. Participation in contact sports is not recommended to reduce the risk of injury to the remaining kidney. *Lifting is avoided to allow full tissue healing. Trauma to the remaining kidney could seriously jeopardize renal function.*
  d. Care of the incision and any remaining drainage tubes, catheters, or stents. *This routine postoperative instruction is vital to prepare the client for self-care and prevent complications.*
  e. Report signs and symptoms to the physician, including manifestations of UTI (dysuria, frequency, urgency, nocturia, cloudy, malodorous urine) or systemic infection (fever, general malaise, fatigue), redness, swelling, pain, or drainage from the incision or any catheter or drain tube site. *Prompt treatment of postoperative infection is vital to allow continued healing and prevent compromise of the remaining kidney.*

perfusion, however, allows up to 3 days before transplantation. The system used to allocate cadaver kidneys for transplantation is outlined in Box 11–7.

The donor kidney is placed in the lower abdominal cavity of the recipient, and the renal artery, vein, and ureter are anastomosed (Figure 11–19 ■). The renal artery of the donor kidney is connected to the hypogastric artery, and the renal vein is connected to the iliac vein. The ureter is connected to one of the recipient's ureters or directly to the bladder, using a tunnel technique to prevent reflux. Nursing care for the client having a kidney transplant is outlined Box 11–8.

Unless the donor and recipient are identical twins, the grafted organ stimulates an immune response to reject the transplanted organ. Immunosuppressive drugs minimize this response. Azathioprine or mycophenolate mofetil are commonly used, often in combination with prednisone, a corticosteroid. Cyclosporine, a potent immunosuppressive, also may be used. These drugs suppress a portion of the immune system and the inflammatory response, increasing the risk for infections and cancers with long-term therapy.

Glucocorticoids such as prednisone and methylprednisolone are used for maintenance immunosuppression and to treat acute rejection episodes. Side effects of long-term corticosteroid use include impaired wound healing, emotional disturbances, osteoporosis, and cushingoid effects on glucose, protein, and fat metabolism.

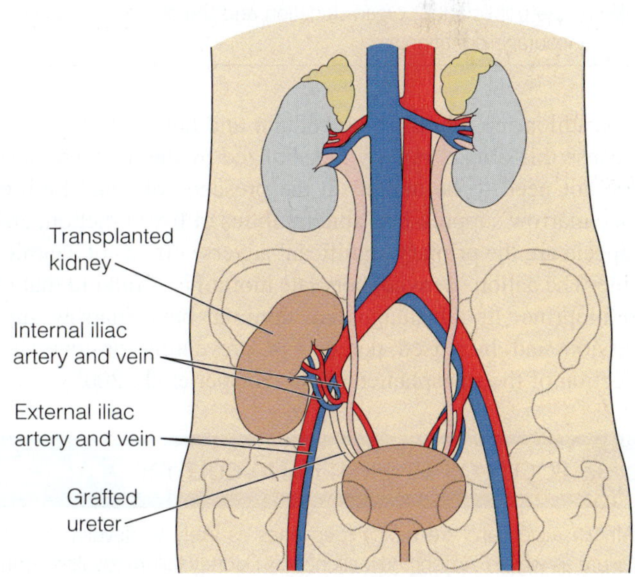

Figure 11–19 ■ Placement of a transplanted kidney in the iliac fossa with anastomosis to the hypogastric artery, iliac vein, and bladder.

Box 11–7 How Cadaver Kidneys Are Allocated for Transplant

The scarcity of organs for transplant raises questions about how cadaver kidneys are allocated—who receives a kidney, and who does not. Past inequities in the allocation process (e.g., more men than women, more whites than people of color, more rich than poor, and more young than old) led to the development of the UNOS in 1986. UNOS has established policies for organ distribution, including kidneys, hearts, livers, and other transplanted organs.

UNOS maintains national, regional, and local lists of clients awaiting transplants. When an organ becomes available, donor information is entered into the UNOS computer. The computer then runs a match program, generating a list of clients ranked by criteria such as blood and tissue type, organ size, and medical urgency of the client. Factors such as time on the waiting list and distance between the donor and the transplant center also are considered. A candidate with a perfect match (six human leukocyte antigens in common) and compatible blood type gets priority for the kidney, regardless of region or geographic area. Otherwise, the list of clients in the local area is checked first, then the regional list of clients awaiting transplant. If no match is found in the region, the organ becomes available to clients nationwide.

The UNOS allocation system, standardized fees, and Medicare coverage for transplantation have done much to ensure equitable access to available kidneys. Still, controversy exists. Clients with resources for travel may register in several different regions for an organ. Up to 10% of clients receiving a transplant in any center may be foreign nationals competing with U.S. citizens for scarce organ resources. A transplant center can accept or reject a candidate for transplant who has lost a kidney because of noncompliance with treatment regimens.

As long as the demand for kidneys exceeds the supply of donor organs, it is likely that controversy will exist regarding their allocation. Nurses can help by identifying potential donors and contacting the transplant coordinator. In addition, nurses can inform the public about organ donation and the allocation system, and encourage donation.

Azathioprine inhibits both cellular and humoral immunity. Because this drug is rapidly metabolized by the liver, the dose may not need to be altered in the presence of renal failure. Bone marrow suppression, abnormalities of liver function, and alopecia are the primary significant adverse effects of azathioprine. The action of mycophenolate mofetil is similar to that of azathioprine. Its advantages are minimal bone marrow suppression and increased potency in preventing or reversing rejection of the transplanted organ (Kasper et al., 2005).

Cyclosporine primarily affects cellular immunity, the helper T cells in particular. Among its many adverse effects, which include hepatotoxicity and hirsutism, nephrotoxicity is a primary concern for the client having a kidney transplant.

Even with immunosuppressive therapy, however, the transplanted kidney can be rejected at any time. Either acute or chronic rejection may develop. Acute rejection develops within months of the transplant. It is caused by a cellular immune response with T-lymphocyte proliferation (Porth, 2005). Few manifestations may be apparent other than a rise in serum creatinine and possible oliguria. Methylprednisolone, a glucocorticoid, and OKT3 monoclonal antibody are used to manage acute rejection episodes. OKT3 can cause severe systemic reactions, including chills, fever, hypotension, headache, and possible pulmonary edema (Kasper et al., 2005). Chronic rejection, which may develop months to years following the transplant, is a major cause of graft loss. Both humoral and cellular immune responses are involved in chronic rejection. It does not respond to increased immunosuppression. The presenting manifestations of chronic rejection—progressive azotemia, proteinuria, and hypertension—are those of progressive renal failure.

Hypertension is a possible complication of kidney transplant, resulting from graft rejection, renal artery stenosis, or renal vasoconstriction. Clients may develop glomerular lesions and manifestations of nephrosis. Hypertension and altered blood lipids (increased low-density lipoprotein and decreased high-density lipoprotein levels) increase the risk of death from myocardial infarction and stroke following transplant (Kasper et al., 2005).

Long-term immunosuppression has adverse effects as well. Infection is a continuing threat. Bacterial and viral infections may develop, as well as fungal infections of the blood, lungs, and central nervous system. Tumors are also common, with carcinoma in situ of the cervix, lymphomas, and skin cancers most prevalent. The risk of congenital anomalies is increased in infants whose mothers have undergone immunosuppressive therapy. Corticosteroid use may lead to bone problems, GI disorders (e.g., peptic ulcer disease), and cataract formation.

Complementary Therapies

Clients with CRF should avoid herbal supplements, which can contain minerals that may be harmful to the kidneys or contraindicated with one or more medications the client might be taking. Nurses should encourage clients and their caregivers to discuss the use of any over-the-counter or complementary therapies with the physician.

FOCUS ON DIVERSITY AND CULTURE African Americans and Kidney Disease

African Americans are nearly four times as likely to develop kidney failure as whites. Among new clients with kidney failure resulting from high blood pressure, more than half are African American. Among new clients with kidney failure resulting from diabetes, more than a third are African American. Considering that African Americans make up approximately 12% of the population of the United States, these figures are significant. Because kidney failure resulting from diabetes or high blood pressure accounts for 70% of new kidney failure cases, nurses working with African American clients who have high blood pressure or diabetes should take the opportunity for client teaching at every health care interaction (National Kidney Disease Education Program, 2005). It is critical for African American clients with high blood pressure or diabetes to understand the risk for renal failure and the importance of following their treatment regimens.

Box 11–8 **Nursing Care of the Client Having a Kidney Transplant**

PREOPERATIVE CARE

- Provide routine preoperative care.
- Assess knowledge and feelings about the procedure, answering questions and clarifying information as needed. Listen to and address concerns about surgery, the source of the donor organ, and possible complications. *Addressing concerns and reducing preoperative anxiety improve postoperative recovery.*
- Continue dialysis as ordered. *Continued renal replacement therapy is necessary to manage fluid and electrolyte balance and prevent uremia before surgery.*
- Administer immunosuppressive drugs as ordered before surgery. *Immunosuppression is initiated before transplantation to prevent immediate graft rejection.*

POSTOPERATIVE CARE

- Provide routine postoperative care.
- Maintain urinary catheter patency and a closed system. *Catheter patency is vital to keep the bladder decompressed and prevent pressure on suture lines. A closed drainage system minimizes the risk for urinary tract infection.*
- Measure urine output every 30–60 minutes initially. *Careful assessment of urine output helps to determine fluid balance and transplant function. Acute tubular necrosis is a common early complication, usually caused by tissue ischemia during the period between removal of the kidney from the donor and transplantation. Oliguria is an early sign.*
- Monitor vital signs and hemodynamic pressures closely. *Diuresis may occur immediately, resulting in hypovolemia, low cardiac output, and impaired perfusion of the transplanted kidney.*
- Maintain fluid replacement, generally calculated to replace urine output over the previous 30 or 60 minutes, milliliter for milliliter. *Fluid replacement is vital to maintain vascular volume and tissue perfusion.*
- Administer diuretics as ordered. *Loop and/or osmotic diuretics, such as furosemide or mannitol, may be used to promote postoperative diuresis.*
- Remove the catheter within 2–3 days or as ordered. Encourage the client to void every 1–2 hours, and assess frequently for signs of urinary retention following catheter removal. *The bladder may have atrophied before surgery, reducing its capacity. Urinary retention places stress on suture lines and increases the risk of infection.*
- Monitor serum electrolytes and renal function tests. *These tests are used to monitor graft function and fluid and electrolyte status. Electrolyte imbalances may develop as the transplanted kidney begins to function and diuresis occurs. Elevated serum creatinine and blood urea nitrogen levels may be early signs of rejection or graft failure.*
- Monitor for possible complications:
  a. *Hemorrhage* from an arterial or venous anastomosis can be either acute or insidious. Indicators include swelling at the operative site, increased abdominal girth, and signs of shock, including changes in vital signs and level of consciousness. *Hemorrhage is a surgical emergency, requiring prompt recognition and treatment to preserve the graft.*
  b. *Ureteral anastomosis failure* causes urine leakage into the peritoneal cavity. It may be marked by decreased urine output with abdominal swelling and tenderness. *Failure of the ureteral anastomosis requires surgical intervention.*
  c. *Renal artery thrombosis* is characterized by an abrupt onset of hypertension and reduced GFR. *Renal artery thrombosis can result in transplant failure.*
  d. *Infection* resulting from immunosuppression is an immediate and continuing risk. The inflammatory response is blunted, and infection may not significantly elevate the temperature. Monitor for signs such as change in level of consciousness, cloudy or malodorous urine, or purulent drainage from the incision. *Prevention and prompt treatment of infections is particularly important in the client with immunosuppression.*
- Include the following in predischarge teaching for the client and family:
  a. Use and effects of prescribed medications, including antihypertensive medications, immunosuppressive agents, prophylactic antibiotics, and others as ordered.
  b. Monitoring of vital signs (including temperature) and weight.
  c. Manifestations of organ rejection, such as swelling and tenderness over the graft site, fever, joint aching, weight gain, and decreased urinary output. Stress the importance of promptly reporting signs and symptoms to the physician.
  d. Ordered or recommended dietary restrictions, such as restricted carbohydrate and sodium intake, and increased protein intake.
  e. Measures to prevent infection, such as avoiding crowds and obviously ill individuals.

The client and family will manage care after discharge and therefore need a thorough understanding of what to expect, how to monitor graft status, and measures to reduce the adverse effects of medications.

- Provide psychologic support, addressing concerns and providing information as needed. *The client knows that transplant success is not guaranteed. In addition, the client has often been managing a chronic disease independently and is used to having a degree of control. Providing information and allowing the client to retain control relieves anxiety and improves recovery.*

NURSING PROCESS

Measures to reduce the risk of CRF focus on preventing kidney disease and appropriately managing diabetes and hypertension. Nurses should promote early and effective treatment of all infections, particularly skin and pharyngeal infections caused by streptococcal bacteria. Discuss measures to reduce the risk for urinary tract infections, and stress the importance of prompt treatment to eradicate the infecting organism. Discuss the relationship between diabetes, hypertension, and kidney disease. Emphasize that maintaining blood glucose levels and blood pressure within the recommended ranges reduces the risk of adverse effects on the kidneys. Ensure that all clients with less-than-optimal renal function are well hydrated, particularly when a nephrotoxic drug is prescribed or anticipated. Finally, encourage the client with ESRD to investigate options for early transplantation to avoid long-term dialysis.

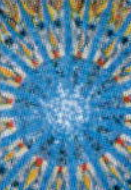

FOCUS ON DIVERSITY AND CULTURE
Jehovah's Witnesses

Some Jehovah's Witnesses are against blood transfusions, but many permit dialysis and organ transplantation if appropriate considerations are made. Organ transplantation for a Jehovah's Witness normally requires removal of all blood from the organ before transplanting it in the Jehovah's Witness. Similarly, dialysis requires banking of the client's own blood to fill the machine if that becomes necessary.

Assessment

Both subjective and objective data are used to assess the client with CRF:

- *Health history.* Complaints of anorexia, nausea, weight gain, or edema; current treatment (if any), including type and frequency of dialysis or previous kidney transplant; chronic diseases, such as diabetes, heart failure, or kidney disease
- *Physical examination.* Mental status; vital signs, including temperature, heart and lung sounds, and peripheral pulses; urine output (if any); weight; skin color, moisture, and condition; presence of edema (periorbital or dependent); bowel tones; and presence and location of an AV fistula, shunt, or graft, or peritoneal catheter.

Diagnosis

Nursing diagnoses for clients with CRF may include the following:

- Ineffective Tissue Perfusion: Renal
- Imbalanced Nutrition: Less Than Body Requirements
- Excess Fluid Volume
- Impaired Skin Integrity
- Risk for Infection
- Disturbed Body Image.

Plan

The plan of care, made in collaboration with the client, may include the following goals:

- The client verbalizes fluid allotment allowed throughout the day.
- The client's weight decreases and approaches baseline level.
- The client breathes comfortably, with clear breath sounds.
- The client remains free of infection.
- The client shares feelings regarding change in body image.

Implementation

Whether the client with ESRD is facing long-term dialysis or renal transplantation, a number of nursing care needs can be identified. This section focuses on nursing care related to impaired renal function, nutritional deficits caused by dietary restrictions and nausea, increased risk for infection, and changes in body image. See the Nursing Care Plan feature that follows for additional potential nursing diagnoses and interventions for the client with CRF.

Ineffective Tissue Perfusion: Renal

Capillaries are an integral part of the nephron. As nephrons are destroyed, kidney perfusion progressively declines. As renal perfusion and nephron function fall, the kidney is less able to maintain fluid and electrolyte balance and to eliminate waste products from the body.

- Monitor intake and output; vital signs, including orthostatic blood pressures; and weight. Weight changes are a more accurate indicator of fluid volume status in the oliguric or anuric client than intake and output measurements.These provide important data to identify changes in fluid volume.
- Restrict fluids as ordered. As renal function declines, the ability to eliminate excess fluid is impaired.
- Monitor respiratory status, including lung sounds, every 4 to 8 hours. Fluid volume overload may lead to heart failure and possible pulmonary edema.
- Monitor BUN, serum creatinine, pH, electrolytes, and CBC. Report significant changes. As renal function declines, progressive azotemia with increasing BUN and serum creatinine appears. Metabolic acidosis develops as the kidney is unable to eliminate hydrogen ions and conserve bicarbonate. Hyponatremia, hyperkalemia, hyperphosphatemia, and hypocalcemia are associated with renal failure. The RBC count, hemoglobin, and hematocrit decline because of deficient erythropoietin to stimulate cell production in the bone marrow. An acute fall in hemoglobin and hematocrit may indicate GI bleeding, a risk in clients with ESRD.
- Report manifestations of electrolyte imbalances, such as cardiac dysrhythmias and other electrocardiographic changes.
- Administer antihypertensive medications as ordered. Hypertension management is an important factor in slowing the progression of CRF.
- Time activities and procedures to allow rest periods. The anemia associated with CRF may cause significant fatigue and activity intolerance.

Imbalanced Nutrition: Less Than Body Requirements

Anorexia, nausea, and vomiting are common manifestations of ESRD and uremia. The metallic taste associated with uremia combined with a diet restricted in protein and sodium will compound loss of appetite. This increases the risk that food intake will be insufficient to meet metabolic needs. Catabolism exacerbates azotemia and uremia, resulting in muscle tremors and possible tetany, and Kussmaul's respirations. Manifestations of electrolyte imbalance may indicate the need for intervention.

- Administer medications to treat electrolyte imbalances as ordered. Carefully monitor for desired and adverse effects. Impaired renal function affects drug elimination and increases the risk for toxic effects. Medications may be prescribed to help maintain electrolyte and acid–base balance and prevent adverse effects of imbalances.
- Monitor food and nutrient intake as well as episodes of vomiting. Careful monitoring helps to determine the adequacy of intake.

- Weigh the client daily before breakfast. This provides the most accurate measurement. Remember that a gain of 2 pounds or more over a 24-hour period is more likely to reflect fluid retention than a gain in body mass.
- Administer antiemetic agents 30–60 minutes before eating. Antiemetics reduce nausea and the risk of vomiting with food intake.
- Assist with mouth care before meals and at bedtime. Mouth care improves taste, stimulates the appetite, and maintains the integrity of oral mucous membranes.
- Serve small meals, and provide between-meal snacks. Small meals are less likely to prompt nausea and help to improve food intake.
- Arrange for a dietary consultation. Provide preferred foods to the extent possible, and involve the client in planning daily menus. Encourage family members to bring food as dietary restrictions allow. Providing preferred foods within restrictions promotes intake.
- Monitor nutritional status by tracking weight; laboratory values, such as serum albumin and BUN; and anthropometric measurements. Indicators of impaired nutrition develop gradually and may be subtle. Careful assessment is important.
- Administer parenteral nutrition as prescribed. Routinely monitor blood glucose levels, and use strict aseptic technique when handling the solution and venous access site. Parenteral nutrition may be necessary to prevent catabolism and increasing azotemia. Hyperglycemia and infection are risks associated with parenteral nutrition. Immune system suppression associated with renal failure further increases the risk for infection.

Risk for Infection

CRF affects the immune system and leukocyte function, increasing susceptibility to infection. Invasive devices required for hemodialysis or peritoneal dialysis add to this risk. The client who has had a kidney transplant remains on immunosuppressive therapy for life, further depressing the immune system and increasing the risk for infection.

- Use standard precautions and good handwashing technique at all times. Handwashing is a primary means of preventing the transfer of organisms. Clients who are on hemodialysis or who have had multiple blood transfusions to treat anemia have an increased risk for hepatitis B, hepatitis C, and HIV infection.
- Monitor temperature and vital signs at least every 4 hours. A low-grade fever or increased pulse rate may indicate an infection in the client who is immunosuppressed.
- Monitor WBC count and differential. Increased WBCs may indicate a bacterial infection; decreased WBCs may indicate viral infection. A shift in the differential showing more immature WBCs (bands) in circulation is another indicator of infection.
- Culture urine, peritoneal dialysis fluid, and other drainage as indicated. Culture is performed to verify the presence of pathogens.
- Monitor clarity of dialysate return. Dialysate should return clear in the client undergoing peritoneal dialysis. Cloudy dialysate may indicate peritonitis, the most common complication of peritoneal dialysis, and should be reported and cultured.
- Provide good respiratory hygiene, including position changes, coughing, and deep breathing. These measures improve clearance of respiratory secretions, reducing the risk for infection.
- Restrict visits from people who are obviously ill. Teach the client and family about the risk for infection and measures to reduce the spread of infection. Because the client's resistance to infection is impaired, extra caution is required to prevent unnecessary exposures.

Disturbed Body Image

Chronic disease and impaired kidney function can affect the client's body image. Hemodialysis requires an AV fistula or shunt, while peritoneal dialysis requires a permanent peritoneal catheter. Although kidney transplant can restore an image of wholeness, a visible scar remains, and the organ may be perceived as "foreign."

- Involve the client in care, including meal planning, dialysis, and catheter, port, or incision care to the extent possible. Involvement improves acceptance and stimulates discussion about the effect of the disease and treatment measures on the client's life (see the Evidenced-Based Practice feature).
- Encourage expression of feelings and concerns, accepting perceptions and feelings without criticism. Self-expression enhances the client's self-worth and acceptance.
- Include the client in decision making, and encourage self-care. Increased autonomy enhances the client's sense of control, independence, and self-worth.
- Support positive gains, but do not support denial. The client may have difficulty accepting the renal failure, but adaptation to the loss is important.
- Help the client to develop and achieve realistic goals. Realistic goals allow the client to see progress.

DEVELOPMENTAL CONSIDERATIONS **The Child With Chronic Renal Failure**

- Physical activity is important to help children maintain optimal health and self-esteem.
- Nurses should encourage children with CRF to participate in developmentally appropriate activities as tolerated.
- Nurses may partner with children to establish routine plans for physical activity as tolerated that will help to promote strong bones.
- Nurses should encourage parents to promote children's participation in age-appropriate activities to minimize the psychologic consequences of coping with a chronic disease.

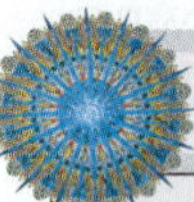

NURSING CARE PLAN **A Client With End-Stage Renal Disease**

Walter Cohen, 45 years old, is the print shop manager at a local community college. He has had a type 1 diabetes mellitus since the age of 20 and was diagnosed with diabetic nephropathy 10 years ago. Despite blood pressure control with antihypertensive medications and frequent blood glucose monitoring with insulin coverage, he developed overt proteinuria 5 years ago and has now progressed to end-stage renal disease. He enters the nephrology unit for temporary hemodialysis to relieve uremic symptoms. While there, a continuous ambulatory peritoneal dialysis (CAPD) catheter will be inserted. Mr. Cohen's desire to continue working is the primary factor in his choice of CAPD over hemodialysis.

ASSESSMENT

Richard Gonzalez, Mr. Cohen's care manager, obtains a nursing assessment. Mr. Cohen states that his diabetes has always been difficult to control. He has had numerous hypoglycemic episodes and has been hospitalized "four or five times" for ketoacidosis. Recently, he has developed symptoms of peripheral neuropathy and increasing retinopathy. He attributed his lack of appetite, nausea, vomiting, and fatigue over the past month to "a touch of the flu." His weight remained stable, so he did not worry about not eating much.

Physical assessment findings include temperature 97.8°F (36.5°C) oral, pulse 96 bpm, respirations 20/min, and BP 178/100 mmHg. His skin is cool and dry, with minor excoriations on forearms and lower legs. His breath odor is fetid. Scattered fine rales are noted in bilateral lung bases, and a soft S_3 gallop is noted at cardiac apex. Bilateral pitting edema of lower extremities to just below the knees is observed; fingers and hands are also edematous. Abdominal assessment is essentially normal, with hypoactive bowel sounds. Urinalysis shows a specific gravity of 1.011, gross proteinuria, and multiple cell casts. CBC results are as follows: red blood cells, 2.9 million/mm^3; hemoglobin, 9.4 g/dL; hematocrit, 28%. Blood chemistry abnormalities include the following: BUN, 198 mg/dL; creatinine, 18.5 mg/dL; sodium, 125 mEq/L; potassium, 5.7 mEq/L; calcium, 7.1 mg/dL; and phosphate, 6.8 mg/dL. A temporary jugular venous catheter will be placed for hemodialysis the next day, followed by peritoneal catheter insertion later in the week.

DIAGNOSES

- Excess Fluid Volume related to failure of kidneys to eliminate excess body fluid
- Imbalanced Nutrition: Less Than Body Requirements related to effects of uremia
- Impaired Skin Integrity of Lower Extremities related to dry skin and itching
- Risk for Infection related to invasive catheters and impaired immune function

PLANNING

- Client will adhere to the prescribed fluid restriction of 750 mL/day.
- Client will demonstrate reduced extracellular fluid volume by weight loss, decreased peripheral edema, clear lung sounds, and normal heart sounds.
- Client will consume and retain 100% of prescribed diet, including snacks.
- Client will demonstrate healing of lower extremity skin lesions.
- Client will remain free of infection.
- Client will demonstrate appropriate peritoneal catheter care and CAPD.

IMPLEMENTATION

- Space fluids, allowing 400 mL from 7 a.m. to 3 p.m., 200 mL from 3 p.m. to 11 p.m., and 100 mL from 11 p.m. to 7 a.m.
- Provide mouth care at least every 4 hours and before every meal.
- Keep sugarless hard candy and ice chips at the bedside; include ice consumed as fluid intake.
- Weigh daily before breakfast; monitor vital signs and heart and lung sounds every 4 hours.
- Document intake and output every 4 hours.
- Arrange dietary consultation for menu planning.
- Administer prescribed antiemetic 1 hour before meals.
- Monitor food intake, noting percentage and types of food consumed.
- Clean lesions on lower extremities every 8 hours and assess healing.
- Teach CAPD procedure and peritoneal catheter care.
- Assist to identify strengths and needs in health regimen management.

EVALUATION

Mr. Cohen was hospitalized for 2 weeks, undergoing four hemodialysis sessions to reduce uremic symptoms. An arteriovenous fistula has been created in his left arm in case he should need hemodialysis in the future. He begins peritoneal dialysis the second week, and by discharge, he is able to manage the catheter care and dialysis runs with the help of his wife. His heart and lung sounds are normal, and he has minimal peripheral edema on discharge. The excoriations on his legs have healed. His temperature is normal, and no evidence of infection is noted. Mr. Cohen remains anorectic and slightly nauseated but is eating most of his prescribed diet and snacks. He has lost 10 pounds with excess fluid removal by dialysis, but his weight remains stable during the second week. Mr. Cohen and his wife have been introduced to another client who has been on CAPD for several years and promises to help them with problem solving.

CRITICAL THINKING

1. How does diabetes mellitus damage the kidneys and lead to end-stage renal disease? Why is this more significant for a client with type 1 diabetes mellitus than for someone with type 2 diabetes mellitus?
2. Why do high levels of urea in the blood often cause changes in cognition and mental status? What manifestations of encephalopathy would you expect to see?
3. How might Mr. Cohen's insulin dosage and diet need to be changed with the institution of peritoneal dialysis? Why?
4. Develop a care plan for the nursing diagnosis disturbed body image.

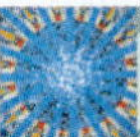

EVIDENCE-BASED PRACTICE The Client on Hemodialysis

Evidence

In a study of clients undergoing hemodialysis for CRF, researchers in Sweden looked at suffering on three levels: related to sickness and treatment, related to care provided, and related to the client's unique life experience and existence (Hagren et al., 2001). The study included 15 clients between ages 50 and 86.

The researchers identified dependence on the hemodialysis machine and dependence on caregivers as the primary sources of suffering in these clients. This dependence and the loss of freedom associated with hemodialysis affected the marital and family relationships and the social lives of the sufferers. Accepting dependence on the hemodialysis machine, being seen as an individual by caregivers, and promoting autonomy relieved clients' suffering.

Implications for Nursing

Treating all clients with end-stage renal disease holistically, respecting their individual and unique characteristics and experiences, is vital to promoting acceptance and autonomy. Listen carefully and respond appropriately to each person's concerns. Discuss the effects of the disease and its treatment on the client's life, marital and family relationships, and socialization. Suggest strategies to maintain independence and provide relief for caregivers. When appropriate, discuss alternatives to hemodialysis for treating end-stage renal disease, such as kidney transplant or peritoneal dialysis. Peritoneal dialysis may be managed independently by the client, reducing dependence on others and time spent in treatment.

Critical Thinking in Client Care

1. Identify assessment tools and data you could use to evaluate degree of suffering in the client receiving long-term hemodialysis.
2. In addition to the above, what interventions can you, as the nurse, implement to promote autonomy and acceptance of hemodialysis in the client with end-stage renal disease?
3. Develop a teaching plan for families and significant others to help them promote acceptance and autonomy in the client undergoing long-term hemodialysis.

- Provide positive reinforcement and feedback. These measures support growth and adaptation.
- Reinforce effective coping strategies. Reinforcement helps the client to develop positive versus negative strategies for coping.
- Facilitate contact with a support group or other community members affected by renal failure. The client benefits by providing and receiving support in a group of people going through similar circumstances.
- Refer for mental health counseling as indicated or desired. Counseling can help the client to develop effective coping and adaptation strategies.

Care in the Community

Teaching for home care includes the following topics:

- Nature of the kidney disease and renal failure, including expected progression and effects
- Monitoring weight, vital signs, and temperature
- Prescribed dietary and fluid restrictions (Involve the client, a dietitian, and the family member usually responsible for cooking. Include strategies to manage nausea and relieve thirst within allowed fluid limits.)
- How to assess and protect a fistula or shunt for hemodialysis (or the extremity to be used if one is anticipated)
- Peritoneal catheter care and the procedure for peritoneal dialysis as indicated (Include a family member or significant other, in case the client is unable to perform the procedure independently at some time.)
- Following kidney transplant, prescribed medications, adverse effects and their management, infection prevention, graft protection, and manifestations of organ rejection.

Refer to a dietitian for diet planning and counseling. If home hemodialysis is planned, refer the designated dialysis helper for formal training. Both the National Kidney Foundation and the American Association of Kidney Patients may be able to provide support and educational materials for the client with ESRD. Local and state chapters of these organizations can provide additional support.

Evaluation

CRF and ESRD are long-term processes that require management by the client. No matter what treatment option the client chooses (hemodialysis, peritoneal dialysis, or renal transplantation), day-to-day management falls to the client and family. When evaluating the client, an important aspect to consider is the client and family's readiness to assume self-care and management.

HEALTH CARE

What impact do lifestyle choices, such as tobacco use, obesity, and alcohol abuse, have on the health care system when considering the increased risk for diseases such as hypertension, renal failure, and cardiac disease?

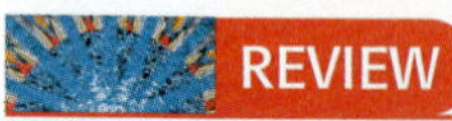

REVIEW Chronic Renal Failure

RELATE: LINK THE CONCEPTS

Linking the exemplar of Chronic Renal Failure with the concept of Perfusion:

1. When providing health promotion education to the community, what information could you provide to improve overall perfusion and, as a result, reduce the risk of kidney damage resulting in CRF?
2. What impact would CRF have on the cardiovascular system of the client? What assessments would indicate the client is experiencing cardiovascular complications?

Linking the exemplar of Chronic Renal Failure with the concept of Development:

3. How does CRF impact a pediatric client's development?
4. What nursing interventions may be helpful in promoting normal development in the pediatric client with CRF?

READY: GO TO COMPANION SKILLS MANUAL

- Administering Continuous Ambulatory Peritoneal Dialysis (CAPD)
- Changing dressings for client receiving CAPD
- Administering blood components
- Monitoring intake and output
- Providing hemodialysis
- Providing ongoing care of the client receiving hemodialysis
- Terminating dialysis
- Maintaining central venous dual-lumen dialysis catheter
- Care of the AV fistula or graft

REFER: GO TO MYNURSINGKIT

REFLECT: CASE STUDY

Joe Jenkins is a 45-year-old African American who has been a long-distance truck driver for the past 20 years. He is admitted to the hospital with complaints of nausea for several weeks, weakness, fatigue, and loss of appetite. He has been feeling very depressed. He has a past medical history of type 1 diabetes mellitus, hypertension, and diabetic nephropathy. On admission, his vital signs are temperature T_O 98.7°F, P 96, R 20, BP 170/110. He has bilateral pitting edema of the lower extremities. His fingers and hands are also edematous. He complains of dry and itching skin. His urine is dark, frothy, and scanty. A specimen is collected for a urinalysis, and blood work is drawn and sent to the laboratory. Urinalysis results show a specific gravity of 1.011, gross hematuria, and 3+ protein. His blood work reveals a BUN of 198 mg/dL and creatinine of 12.5 mg/dL. Based on his past medical history of diabetes, hypertension, and diabetic nephropathy, and on the current findings, a medical diagnosis of CRF is established. Based on Mr. Jenkins' assessment and past medical history, the nursing diagnosis of impaired urinary elimination is identified as the highest priority for planning nursing care.

1. What would be the priority nursing interventions when admitting Mr. Jenkins to the acute care facility?
2. What teaching will this client need considering his prediagnosis lifestyle?
3. What alterations will Mr. Jenkins need to make in his life if daily dialysis is required?

11.3 FLUID AND ELECTROLYTE IMBALANCE

KEY TERMS

Anasarca, *582*
Anorexia, *577*
Ascites, *582*
Dehydration, *569*
Dyspnea, *582*
Fluid volume deficit (FVD), *569*
Fluid volume excess, *579*
Hypercalcemia, *591*
Hyperchloremia, *589*
Hypermagnesemia, *594*
Hypertonic dehydration, *570*
Hypochloremia, *589*
Hypomagnesemia, *593*
Hypophosphatemia, *595*
Hypotonic dehydration, *569*
Iatrogenic, *582*
Isotonic dehydration, *569*
Isotonic fluid volume deficit, *569*
Isotonic imbalances, *569*
Oncotic pressure, *580*
Orthopnea, *582*
Osmolar imbalances, *569*
Polyuria, *582*
Third spacing, *570*

BASIS FOR SELECTION OF EXEMPLAR

Standards of Nursing Practice

LEARNING OUTCOMES

After reading about this exemplar, you will be able to:

1. Describe the pathophysiology, etiology, and clinical manifestations of fluid and electrolyte imbalance.
2. Identify risk factors associated with fluid and electrolyte imbalance.
3. Illustrate the nursing process in providing culturally competent care across the life span for individuals with fluid and electrolyte imbalance.
4. Formulate priority nursing diagnoses appropriate for an individual with fluid and electrolyte imbalance.
5. Create a plan of care for individuals with fluid and electrolyte imbalance and their family members.
6. Assess expected outcomes for an individual with fluid and electrolyte imbalance.
7. Discuss therapies used in the collaborative care of an individual with fluid and electrolyte imbalance.
8. Employ evidence-based caring interventions for an individual with fluid and electrolyte imbalance.

EXEMPLAR OVERVIEW

The human body's balance of fluids and electrolytes is delicate, and this balance is easily disrupted by the simplest of means, such as playing outside on a hot, sunny day. Mild imbalances may be treated quickly and typically resolve without any long-term effects. However, more severe imbalances that are complicated by other disease processes or that last too long can create serious short-term and long-term effects; the chemistry of the body leaves little room for error. Furthermore, the wide-ranging, multisystem impact of imbalance, if overlooked, can have severe and serious, life-threatening consequences.

A number of factors, including illness, trauma, surgery, and medications, can affect the body's ability to maintain fluid and electrolytes. The kidneys play a major role in maintaining fluid and electrolyte balance, and renal disease is a significant cause of imbalance. Clients who are confused or unable to communicate their needs are at risk for inadequate fluid intake. Vomiting, diarrhea, or nasogastric suction can cause significant fluid losses. Tissue trauma, such as burns, causes fluid and electrolytes to be lost from damaged cells. Decreased blood flow to the kidneys as a result of impaired cardiacfunction stimulates the renin–angiotensin–aldosterone system, causing sodium and water retention. Medications such as diuretics or corticosteroids can result in abnormal losses of electrolytes and in fluid loss or retention. Diabetic ketoacidosis, cancer, and head injury may also lead to electrolyte imbalances.

Fluid and electrolyte imbalance is actually a broad term covering a number of disorders. Fluid or any electrolyte may become excessive or deficient, causing an imbalance within the body. To complicate matters still further, electrolytes in combination with other electrolytes or fluid may create imbalance. It is important to understand the need to monitor serum electrolyte values carefully and to consider the possibility of a fluid or electrolyte imbalance when the client presents with a new, unexpected sign or symptom. Fluid and electrolyte imbalances can be classified in terms of fluid volume deficit, fluid volume excess, and electrolyte imbalance.

Fluid imbalances are of two basic types: isotonic and osmolar. **Isotonic imbalances** occur when water and electrolytes are lost or gained in equal proportions so that the osmolality of body fluids remains constant. **Osmolar imbalances** involve the loss or gain of only water so that the osmolality of the serum is altered. Thus, four categories of fluid imbalances may occur:

1. An isotonic loss of water and electrolytes
2. An isotonic gain of water and electrolytes
3. A hyperosmolar loss of water only
4. A hypo-osmolar gain of water only.

These four imbalances are referred to, respectively, as fluid volume deficit, dehydration (hyperosmolar imbalance), fluid volume excess, and overhydration (hypo-osmolar imbalance).

Fluid Volume Deficit and Dehydration

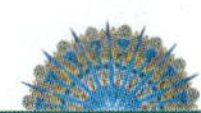

OVERVIEW

Fluid volume deficit (FVD) is a decrease in intravascular, interstitial, and/or intracellular fluid in the body. FVD is a relatively common problem that may exist alone or in combination with other electrolyte or acid–base imbalances. **Dehydration** refers to loss of fluid alone, even though it often is used interchangeably with FVD.

PATHOPHYSIOLOGY AND ETIOLOGY

FVD can develop slowly or rapidly, depending on the type of fluid loss. Loss of extracellular fluid volume can lead to hypovolemia (decreased circulating blood volume). Often, electrolytes are lost along with fluid, resulting in an **isotonic fluid volume deficit**. When both water and electrolytes are lost, the serum sodium level remains normal, although levels of other electrolytes, such as potassium, may fall. Fluid is drawn into the vascular compartment from the interstitial spaces as the body attempts to maintain tissue perfusion. This eventually depletes fluid in the intracellular compartment as well.

Hypovolemia stimulates regulatory mechanisms to maintain circulation. The sympathetic nervous system is stimulated, as is the thirst mechanism. Antidiuretic hormone and aldosterone are released, prompting sodium and water retention by the kidneys. Severe fluid loss can lead to cardiovascular collapse.

Another classification of FVD is by location of the deficiency, whether extracellular or intracellular. Extracellular FVD occurs when there is not enough fluid in the extracellular compartment (vascular and interstitial). Depending on the cause of the deficit, sodium may be at a normal, low, or elevated level. Each level is described as a specific type of dehydration:

- **Isotonic dehydration** *(or isonatremic dehydration):* This occurs when fluid loss is not balanced by intake and the losses of water and sodium are in proportion. The serum sodium is therefore within normal limits even though the circulating blood volume is lowered. Most of the fluid lost is from the extracellular component. This type of dehydration is commonly manifested through such symptoms as vomiting and diarrhea.
- **Hypotonic dehydration** *(or hyponatremic dehydration).* This occurs when fluid loss is characterized by a proportionately greater loss of sodium than of water. Serum sodium is below normal levels. Compensatory fluid shifts occur from the extracellular to intracellular components in an attempt to establish normal proportions, thus leading to even greater extracellular dehydration. Hypotonic dehydration may result from severe and prolonged vomiting and diarrhea, burns, and renal disease. Administering intravenous fluid without electrolytes as treatment for dehydration increases client risk for hypotonic dehydration.

- **Hypertonic dehydration** *(or hypernatremic dehydration).* This occurs when sodium loss is proportionately less than water loss. Serum sodium is above normal levels. Compensatory fluid shifts from the intracellular to extracellular components occur as the body attempts to establish normal proportions. The extracellular component therefore remains fairly normal, delaying the onset of signs and symptoms of dehydration until the condition is quite serious. Neurologic symptoms reflecting intracellular imbalance may occur simultaneously with more common symptoms of dehydration. The condition may result from health problems, such as diabetes insipidus, or administration of intravenous fluid or tube feedings with high electrolyte levels.

The body continuously attempts to compensate for fluid and electrolyte imbalance by shifting fluid and electrolytes from one component to another. Therefore, it is rare for only one type of dehydration to occur; the fluid and electrolyte status and symptoms are constantly changing. Ongoing assessment and management is essential to nursing care.

Third Spacing

Fluid and electrolyte balance is essential to supporting vascular function. A shift of fluid from the vascular space into an area where it is not available to support normal physiologic processes is known as **third spacing**. The trapped fluid represents a volume loss and is unavailable for normal physiologic processes. Fluid may be sequestered in the abdomen or bowel or in other actual or potential body spaces, such as the pleural or peritoneal space. Fluid may also become trapped within soft tissues following trauma or burns.

In many cases, fluid is sequestered in interstitial tissues and is thus unavailable to support cardiovascular function. Surgery triggers adaptive stress responses and the release of stress hormones (adrenocorticotropic hormone, cortisol, and catecholamines). These hormones increase blood glucose levels to provide increased fuel for metabolic processes and lead to vasoconstriction that redistributes blood to vital organs (the heart and brain). Renal blood flow falls, stimulating the renin–angiotensin–aldosterone system. This promotes sodium and water retention to maintain intravascular volume. The blood vessel and tissue damage caused by surgery stimulate the release of inflammatory mediators, such as histamine and prostaglandins. These substances lead to local vasodilation and increased capillary permeability, allowing fluid to accumulate in interstitial tissues.

Assessing the extent of FVD resulting from third spacing is difficult. Because there is no loss or gain of fluid but, rather, a shift in compartments, third spacing may not be reflected by changes in weight or intake-and-output records and may not become apparent until after organ malfunction occurs (Metheny, 2000).

Etiology

FVDs may be the result of excessive fluid losses, insufficient fluid intake, or failure of regulatory mechanisms and fluid shifts within the body. The most common cause of FVD is excessive loss of GI fluids, which can result from vomiting, diarrhea, GI suctioning, intestinal fistulas, or intestinal drainage. Other causes of fluid losses include the following:

- Excessive renal losses of water and sodium from diuretic therapy, renal disorders, or endocrine disorders
- Water and sodium losses during sweating from excessive exercise or increased environmental temperature
- Hemorrhage
- Chronic abuse of laxatives and/or enemas.

Inadequate fluid intake may result from lack of access to fluids, inability to request or to swallow fluids, oral trauma, or altered thirst mechanisms. Excessive exercise during very hot weather without sufficient fluid replacement can lead to fluid and electrolyte imbalance. Athletes and those whose jobs require them to expend enormous amounts of energy in hot climates, such as military personnel and ROTC candidates, are also frequently at risk for fluid imbalance.

Burns of the skin usually involve huge loss of body fluids, including water and electrolytes, particularly sodium. Hypotonic dehydration is the type most commonly seen in the initial period after a burn. Because serum proteins are also lost, body fluid is more likely to leak into interstitial spaces, causing edema and further contributing to the fluid deficit. The kidneys decrease urine production because of their decreased blood flow, which leads to lowered urinary output. While the fluid imbalance of burns is therefore very complicated, the first imbalance encountered is often that of dehydration with accompanying hyponatremia.

For burns, gastroenteritis, and other illnesses, initial dehydration in the first 3 days reflects a high loss of extracellular fluid. Approximately 80% of the fluid loss is extracellular and only approximately 20% is intracellular. Over time the relationship begins to change so that in illnesses lasting longer than 3 days, approximately 60% of fluid loss is extracellular while 40% is intracellular (Johns Hopkins Hospital, 2005). Because the electrolyte composition of extracellular and intracellular fluids differs, electrolyte management needs to be adapted in long-term conditions.

Children are more likely than adults to experience imbalance from exercise. Because children have a larger body surface area, they can gain more heat from the environment when it is hot and lose more when it is cold (Binkley et al., 2002). In addition, the high metabolic rate of children is further increased during exercise so that fluid lost in metabolism is significant. Children may not feel thirsty and so fail to drink even when dehydrated (Committee on Sports Medicine and Fitness, 2000).

A number of conditions may contribute to fluid imbalance in pediatric clients. Radiant heat (phototherapy) used to treat hyperbilirubinemia increases insensible water loss through the skin. The increased respiratory rate of pediatric clients increases insensible water loss from the lungs. Children are at increased risk for fever, which increases the metabolic rate and, therefore, the water demands of metabolism (for each degree of Celsius increase above 37°, 0.42 $mL \cdot kg^{-1} \cdot hr^{-1}$ of additional fluid is needed).

Vomiting and diarrhea are common manifestations of disease in children throughout the world. Each year, up to 5 million children—300–500 of whom live in the United States—die from dehydration related to diarrhea. Each year, some 220,000 U.S. children are hospitalized (9% of pediatric hospitalizations), and approximately 1.5 million receive care on an outpatient basis for dehydration resulting from diarrhea (Dale, 2004; Dennehy, 2005; Nager & Wang, 2002).

Infants may also experience FVD through increased water loss in low-birth-weight infants who are kept under radiant warmers to maintain heat (Figure 11–20 ■). Their high body surface area puts them at risk of dehydration as a result of insensible fluid loss through the skin. Adrenal insufficiency, accumulation of extracellular fluid in a "third space" (e.g., the peritoneal cavity), and overuse of diuretics may also result in FVD in children. Overuse of diuretics is most often seen in adolescents with bulimia.

Older adults have fewer intracellular reserves, contributing to rapid development of dehydration. A blunted thirst perception and altered hormone response also contribute to the development of dehydration in the older adult. Without intervention, mortality from dehydration can exceed 50% in the older adult population (Suhayda & Walton, 2002).

Risk Factors

Older adults are at particular risk for FVD. Dehydration is one of the 10 most common hospital admitting diagnoses for older adults (Suhayda & Walton, 2002). As mentioned, the older adult has fewer intracellular reserves, contributing to rapid development of dehydration. Blunted thirst perception, altered hormone response, and decreased total body water can also predispose the older person to dehydration, especially when additional hydration stressors like fever or exudative wounds occur. The dependent geriatric client who requires assistance with eating may be fed without consideration of making sure adequate fluids are provided. These clients may be reluctant to ask someone to help them take a drink. Food service workers should be encouraged to leave unfinished beverage containers at the bedside within reach of the client. Placing liquids in spillproof containers can also help older debilitated clients to drink adequate amounts of fluids. Dependence on others with lack of free access to fluids, altered thirst, and voluntary fluid restrictions for fear of incontinence or reliance on others for toileting are factors that can contribute to inadequate fluid intake and chronic dehydration (Box 11–9).

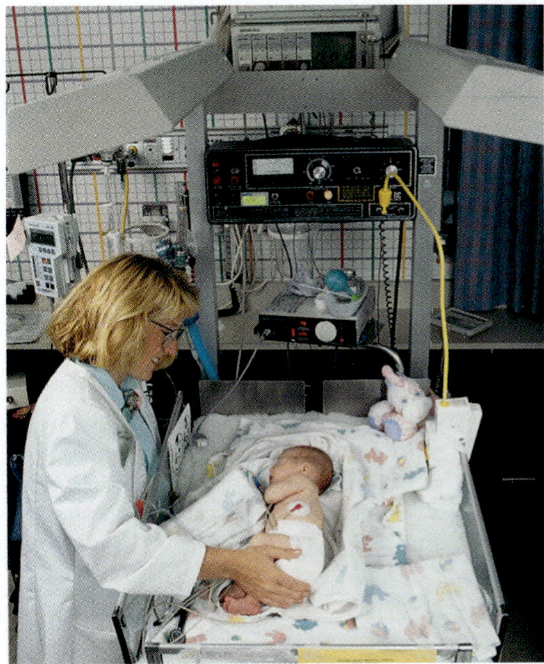

Figure 11–20 ■ Use of an overhead warmer or phototherapy increases insensible fluid excretion through the skin, thus increasing the fluid intake needed.

Pregnancy carries risk for FVD, especially during the first trimester, when vomiting from morning sickness or blood loss during a spontaneous abortion (miscarriage) are most likely to occur. During the first prenatal visit, pregnant women should be taught how to avoid dehydration, the proper fluids to consume, and to avoid caffeine, alcohol, and diet drinks.

The younger and smaller the child, the greater the risk for dehydration. As discussed previously, infants and smaller children have a higher body surface area and experience greater insensible fluid losses. Exposure to common childhood illnesses with symptoms of vomiting, diarrhea, or fever increase the child's risk as well.

CLINICAL MANIFESTATIONS

Symptoms of dehydration relate to the severity or degree of the body water deficit. They result from both the decreased fluid (e.g., diminished turgor and mucous membrane moisture) and the body's response to the fluid deficit (e.g., pulse and blood pressure changes). A water loss of as little as 1 to 2% impairs cognition and physical performance. Loss of 7% of body water can lead to circulatory collapse. With a rapid fluid loss (e.g., hemorrhage or uncontrolled vomiting), manifestations of hypovolemia develop rapidly. When the loss of fluid occurs more gradually, the client's fluid volume may become very low before symptoms develop.

Initial symptoms may be as simple as thirst. As fluid loss increases, however, lethargy, dry mucous membranes, reduced urine output, and weakness develop. Manifestations of acute fluid loss are similar to those associated with hypovolemic shock and include hypotension, tachycardia, tachypnea, decreased or absent urine output, and decreased cardiac output. Coma and death may result if treatment is not initiated.

Because rapid weight loss is a good indicator of FVD, it is critical to weigh clients who are at risk for FVD daily. Each liter of body fluid weighs approximately 1 kg (2.2 lb). The severity of the FVD can be estimated by the percentage of rapid weight loss:

- A loss of 2–5% of total body weight represents mild FVD.
- A loss of 6–9% represents moderate FVD.
- A loss of 10% or greater represents severe FVD.

Box 11–9 Dehydration Risk Factors and Symptoms in the Older Adult

DEHYDRATION RISK FACTORS

Physical changes of aging

- ↓ Total body water
- ↓ Lean body mass
- ↓ Thirst from aging, medication, or disease
- Impaired angiotensin production

Lack of free access to fluids:

- Dependency on others
- Cognitive impairment
- Physical impairment

Voluntary fluid restriction to manage:

- Incontinence
- Nocturia
- Diuretic side effect
- Limited physical movement due to mobility or pain issues

Increased insensitive fluid losses:

- Sweating from fever or climate
- ↑ Respiratory rate
- Vomiting
- Diarrhea
- Polyuria
- Exudative wound or fistula

SYMPTOMS OF DEHYDRATION

Darkened urine
↓ Urine output
Confusion
Lethargy
Headache
Light-headedness
Sunken eyes
Dry mucous membranes
Dry axillae
Long tongue furrows
Postural changes in pulse and blood pressure

Loss of interstitial fluid causes skin turgor (the skin's ability to return to normal shape after being pinched) to diminish. When pinched, the skin of a client with FVD remains elevated. Loss of skin elasticity with aging makes this assessment finding less accurate in older adults. Tongue turgor is not generally affected by age; therefore, assessing the size, dryness, and longitudinal furrows of the tongue may be a more accurate indicator of FVD.

Postural or orthostatic hypotension is a sign of hypovolemia. A drop of more than 15 mmHg in systolic blood pressure when changing from a lying to standing position often indicates loss of intravascular volume. Venous pressure falls as well, causing flat neck veins, even when the client is recumbent. Loss of intravascular fluid causes the hematocrit to increase.

Compensatory mechanisms to conserve water and sodium and maintain circulation account for many of the manifestations

CLINICAL MANIFESTATIONS AND THERAPIES Fluid Volume Deficit and Dehydration

ETIOLOGY	CLINICAL MANIFESTATION	CLINICAL THERAPIES
Decreased cardiac output	Hypotension (may be orthostatic or postural initially) Tachycardia Weak pulse Tachypnea Reduced urine output or very concentrated urine with high specific gravity	■ Administer fluid replacement. ■ Administer isotonic intravenous solutions. ■ Monitor vital signs frequently. ■ Monitor intake and output. ■ Assess serum electrolytes and hematocrit. ■ Conduct urine specific gravity and osmolality. ■ Monitor central venous presssure.
Inadequate fluid supply to the tissues	Dry, cracked skin Dry mucous membranes Hematocrit increases Poor skin turgor Weight loss	■ Administer isotonic or mildly hypotonic solutions. ■ Measure weight daily. ■ Monitor serum electrolytes and serum osmolality. ■ Monitor hemoglobin and hematocrit.
Third spacing	Edema Symptoms of FVD No weight loss	■ Administer hypertonic intravenous fluid.

MULTISYSTEM EFFECTS OF **Fluid Volume Deficit (FVD)**

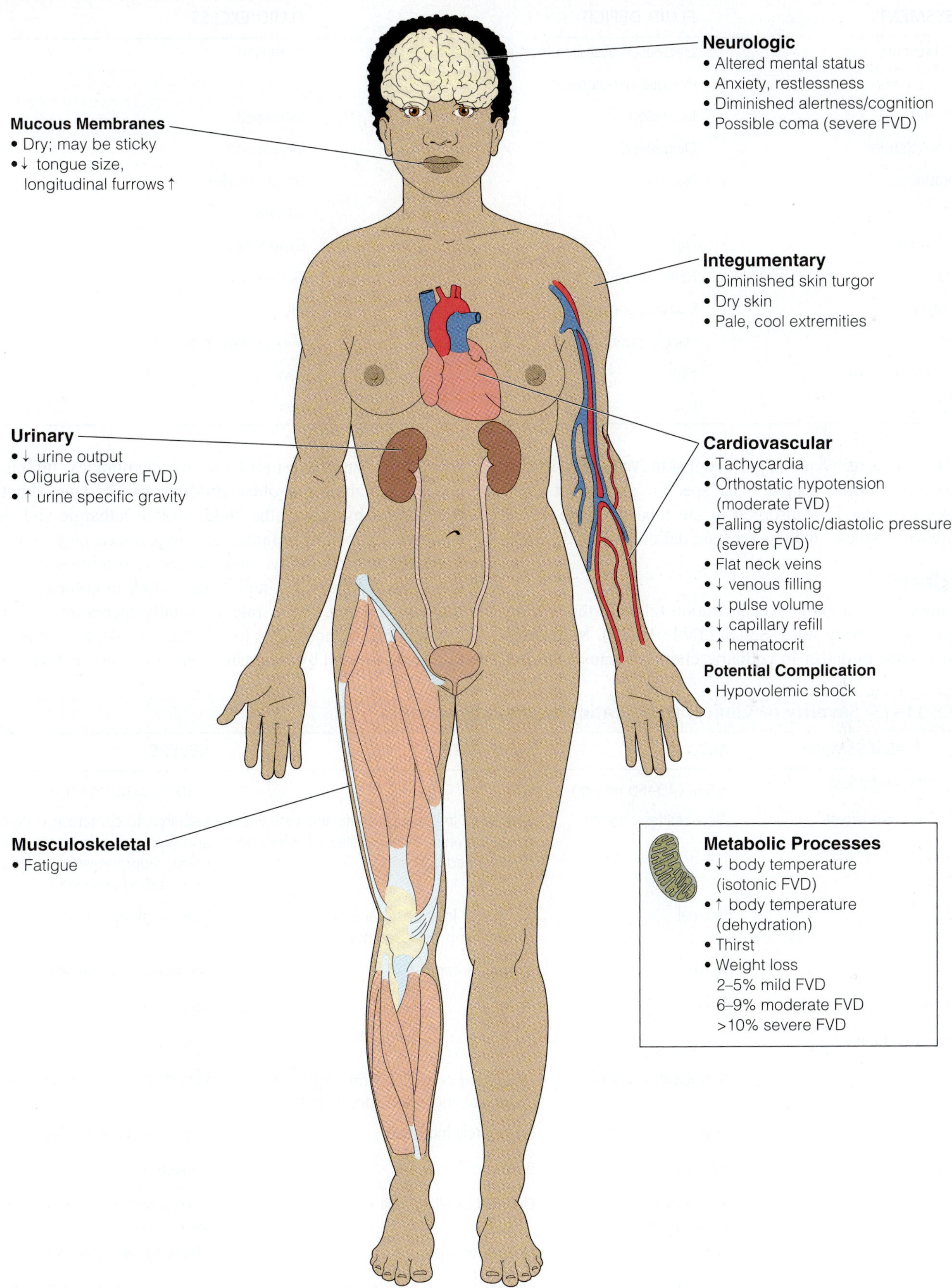

Neurologic
• Altered mental status
• Anxiety, restlessness
• Diminished alertness/cognition
• Possible coma (severe FVD)
Mucous Membranes
• Dry; may be sticky
• ↓ tongue size, longitudinal furrows ↑
Integumentary
• Diminished skin turgor
• Dry skin
• Pale, cool extremities
Urinary
• ↓ urine output
• Oliguria (severe FVD)
• ↑ urine specific gravity
Cardiovascular
• Tachycardia
• Orthostatic hypotension (moderate FVD)
• Falling systolic/diastolic pressure (severe FVD)
• Flat neck veins
• ↓ venous filling
• ↓ pulse volume
• ↓ capillary refill
• ↑ hematocrit
Potential Complication
• Hypovolemic shock
Musculoskeletal
• Fatigue
Metabolic Processes
• ↓ body temperature (isotonic FVD)
• ↑ body temperature (dehydration)
• Thirst
• Weight loss
2–5% mild FVD
6–9% moderate FVD
>10% severe FVD

TABLE 11–12 **Comparison of Assessment Findings in Clients With Fluid Imbalance**

ASSESSMENT	FLUID DEFICIT	FLUID EXCESS
Blood pressure	Decreased systolic blood pressure	Increased
	Postural hypotension	
Heart rate	Increased	Increased
Pulse amplitude	Decreased	Increased
Respirations	Normal	Moist crackles
		Wheezes
Jugular vein	Flat	Distended
Edema	Rare	Dependent
Skin turgor	Loose, poor turgor	Taut
Output	Low, concentrated	May be low or normal
Urine specific gravity	High	Low
Weight	Loss	Gain

of FVD, such as tachycardia, pale, cool skin (vasoconstriction), and decreased urine output. The specific gravity of urine increases as water is reabsorbed in the tubules. Table 11–12 compares assessment findings for fluid deficit and fluid excess.

Children

As mentioned, symptoms of dehydration relate to the severity or degree of the body water deficit (Table 11–13). Mild dehydration is hard to detect in pediatric clients, because children appear alert and have moist mucous membranes. Infants may become irritable, and older children may become thirsty. In moderate dehydration, the child is often lethargic and sleepy. Children, especially infants, may experience periods of restlessness and irritability. Skin turgor is diminished, mucous membranes appear dry, and urine is dark in color and diminished in amount. Pulse rate is usually increased, and blood pressure can be normal or low (Table 11–14). Severe dehydration is manifested by increasing lethargy or nonresponsiveness,

TABLE 11–13 **Severity of Clinical Dehydration in Pediatric Clients**

CLINICAL ASSESSMENT	MILD	MODERATE	SEVERE
% of body weight lost	≤5% (40–50 mL/kg)	6–9% (60–90 mL/kg)	≥10% (≥100 mL/kg)
Level of consciousness	Alert, restless, thirsty	Irritable or lethargic (infants and very young children); alert, thirsty, restless (older children and adolescents)	Lethargic to comatose (infants and young children); often conscious, apprehensive (older children and adolescents)
Blood pressure	Normal	Normal or low; postural hypotension children and adolescents)	Low to undetectable
Pulse	Normal	Normal or rapid	Tachycardia or bradycardia
Skin turgor	Normal	Poor	Very poor
Mucous membranes	Moist	Dry	Parched
Urine	May appear normal	Decreased output (<1 mL $\cdot$ kg^{-1} $\cdot$ hr^{-1}) dark color; increased specific gravity	Very decreased or absent output
Thirst	Slightly increased	Moderately increased	Greatly increased unless lethargic
Fontanelle	Normal	Sunken	Sunken
Extremities	Warm; normal capillary refill	Delayed capillary refill (>2 sec)	Cool, discolored, delayed capillary refill (>3–4 sec)
Respirations	Normal	Normal or rapid	Changing rate and pattern
Deep	Normal	Slightly sunken, decreased tears	Deeply sunken, absent tears

TABLE 11–14 **Clinical Manifestations of Extracellular Fluid Volume Deficit**

ETIOLOGY	CLINICAL MANIFESTATIONS
Decreased fluid volume	Weight loss Sunken fontanel (infant)
Inadequate circulating blood volume to offset the force of gravity when in upright position	Postural blood pressure drop
Dizziness	Decreased intravascular volume
Increased small-vein filling time	Delayed capillary refill time
	Flat neck veins when supine
Inadequate circulation to the brain	Dizziness, syncope
Inadequate circulation to the kidneys	Oliguria
Cardiac reflex response to decreased intravascular volume	Thready, rapid pulse
Decreased interstitial fluid volume	Decreased skin turgor

markedly decreased blood pressure, rapid pulse, poor skin turgor, dry mucous membranes, seizure activity, and markedly decreased or absent urinary output.

Older Adults

Manifestations of FVD may be more difficult to recognize in the older adult. A change in mental status, memory, or attention may be an early sign. Skin turgor is less reliable as an indicator of dehydration, although assessing turgor over the sternum or on the inner aspect of the thigh may be more effective. Dry oral mucous membranes and tongue furrows also are indicative of dehydration. Chronic dehydration may result in dry, itchy skin; dull-appearing, brittle hair; and loss of thirst reflex. Orthostatic, or postural, vital signs may not demonstrate typical changes in the dehydrated older adult. (Bennett, Thomas, & Riegel, 2004) found that chronic dehydration among older adults seeking treatment at emergency departments was often missed in nursing assessments because of the absence of more typical symptoms. Other common signs of dehydration, such as dry oral membranes and upper body weakness, may be better indicators of dehydration in the older adult.

COLLABORATION

The diagnosis of dehydration is best accomplished by clinical observations. A major observation that provides clues about the degree of dehydration is the percentage of weight loss. A synthesis of studies on dehydration showed that abnormal capillary refill time, skin turgor, and abnormal respirations were the most useful clinical signs of dehydration to assist in identifying the disorder (Steiner, DeWalt, & Byerly, 2004).

Diagnostic Tests

The serum electrolyte panel may be helpful in severe and continuing dehydration that is complicated by electrolyte imbalance or acidosis. The test includes serum electrolytes, creatinine, and glucose. Elevated BUN (>17 mg/dL) and low serum bicarbonate (LESTHEN16 mmol/L) are also useful in identifying moderate and severe dehydration (Wathen, MacKenzie, & Bothner, 2004). The results can be used to target the fluid type and amount to best meet the imbalances identified. Urine specific gravity may provide useful information in adults and older children who are dehydrated. However, because of the inability of the child under 2 years of age to concentrate urine effectively, a rising specific gravity may not be seen as definitively in the younger dehydrated child.

Clinical Therapies

Medical management depends on accurate identification of the degree of dehydration. The treatment of extracellular FVD is administration of fluid containing sodium. This may be accomplished by oral rehydration therapy or by intravenous fluids.

ORAL REHYDRATION Oral rehydration is the safest and most effective treatment for FVD in alert clients who are able to take oral fluids. Adults require a minimum of 1,500 mL of fluid per day, or approximately 30 mL/kg body weight (ideal body weight is used to calculate fluid requirements for clients who are obese), for maintenance. Fluids are replaced gradually, particularly in older adults, to prevent rapid rehydration of the cells. In general, fluid deficits are replaced at a rate of approximately 30 to 50% of the deficit per 24 hours.

With mild fluid deficits, in which the loss of electrolytes has been minimal (e.g., moderate exercise in warm weather), fluid replacement may be accomplished with water alone. When the fluid deficit is more severe, and when electrolytes have also been lost (e.g., FVD caused by vomiting and/or diarrhea, strenuous exercise for longer than an hour or two), a carbohydrate/electrolyte solution, such as a sports drink, ginger ale, or a rehydrating solution (e.g., Pedialyte or Rehydralyte), is more appropriate. These solutions provide sodium, potassium, chloride, and calories to help meet metabolic needs.

Oral rehydration therapy has been used for a number of years in developing countries without an accessible supply of intravenous fluids. More recently, the benefits of using this therapy early to prevent severe dehydration and to treat mild and moderate dehydration in children living in developed countries has been recognized. Solutions are available commercially that contain water, carbohydrate (glucose), sodium, potassium, chloride, and lactate. Some clinicians allow lactose-free milk, breast milk, or half-strength milk to be given in addition to oral rehydration therapy solution. A WHO/UNICEF solution was developed for use with cholera and is not generally used for diarrhea treatment in the United States, because its sodium and chloride loads are higher than that of other commercial solutions (Box 11–10).

INTRAVENOUS FLUIDS When the fluid deficit is severe or the client is unable to ingest fluids, the intravenous route is used to administer replacement fluids (Table 11–15). Isotonic electrolyte solutions (0.9% NaCl or Ringer's solution) are used to expand plasma volume in clients who are hypotensive or to

Box 11–10 Oral Rehydration and Maintenance Fluids for Mild and Moderate Dehydration

- Cerealyte
- Equalyte
- Hydralyte
- Infalyte
- Kaolectrolyte
- Lytren
- Nutrilyte
- Pedialyte
- Pediatric Oral Maintenance Solution (ORS)
- Rehydralyte
- Resol
- ReVital
- Ricelyte
- WHO/UNICEF oral rehydration solution

TABLE 11–15 **Commonly Administered Intravenous Fluids**

	FLUID AND TONICITY	USES
Dextrose in water	5% dextrose in water (D_5W)	Replaces water losses
Solutions	Isotonic	Provides free water necessary for cellular rehydration Lowers serum sodium in hypernatremia
	10% dextrose in water ($D_{10}W$)	Provides free water
	Hypertonic	Provides nutrition (supplies 340 kcal/L)
	20% dextrose in water ($D_{20}W$)	Supplies 680 kcal/L
	Hypertonic	May cause diuresis
	50% dextrose in water ($D_{50}W$)	Supplies 1,700 kcal/L
	Hypertonic	Used to correct hypoglycemia
Saline solutions	0.45% sodium chloride	Provides free water to replace hypotonic fluid losses
	Hypotonic	Maintains levels of plasma sodium and chloride
	0.9% sodium chloride	Expands intravascular volume
	Isotonic	Replaces water lost from extracellular fluid
		Used with blood transfusions
		Replaces large sodium losses (as from burns)
	3% sodium chloride	Corrects serious sodium depletion
	Hypertonic	
Combined dextrose and saline solution	5% dextrose and 0.45% sodium chloride	Provides free water
	Isotonic	Provides sodium chloride
		Maintenance fluid of choice if there are no electrolyte imbalances
Multiple electrolyte solutions	Ringer's solution	Expands the intracellular fluid
	Isotonic (electrolyte concentrations of sodium, potassium, chloride, and calcium are similar to plasma levels)	Replaces extracellular fluid losses
	Lactated Ringer's solution	Replaces fluid losses from burns and the lower gastrointestinal tract Fluid of choice for acute blood loss

replace abnormal losses, which are usually isotonic in nature. Normal saline (0.9% NaCl) tends to remain in the vascular compartment, increasing blood volume. When administered rapidly, however, this solution can precipitate acid–base imbalances, so balanced electrolyte solutions, such as lactated Ringer's solution, are preferred to expand plasma volume. Often, Ringer's lactate is administered intravenously followed by or accompanied with dilute saline, such as one-half or one-quarter normal saline. This fluid combination replenishes the extracellular fluid volume and adds solutes to return the body fluid to normal.

Five percent dextrose in water or 0.45% NaCl (one-half normal saline) is given to provide water to treat total body water deficits. D_5W is isotonic (similar in tonicity to the plasma) when administered and thus does not provoke hemolysis of RBCs. The dextrose is metabolized to carbon dioxide and water, leaving free water available for tissue needs. Hypotonic saline solution (0.45% NaCl with or without added electrolytes) or 5% dextrose in 0.45% sodium chloride may be used as maintenance solutions. These solutions provide additional electrolytes (e.g., potassium), a buffer (lactate or acetate) as needed, and water. When dextrose is added, they also provide a minimal number of calories.

A fluid challenge (the rapid administration of a designated amount of intravenous fluid) may be performed to evaluate fluid volume when urine output is low and cardiac or renal function is questionable. A fluid challenge helps to prevent fluid volume overload resulting from intravenous fluid therapy when cardiac or renal function is compromised.

In children under 2 years of age, the glomeruli, tubules, and nephrons of the kidneys are immature. They are thus unable to conserve or excrete water and solutes effectively. Because more water is generally excreted, the infant and young child can become dehydrated or develop electrolyte imbalances quickly. In addition, infants have a weaker transport system for ions and bicarbonate, placing them at greater risk for acidosis and acid–base imbalances. Children under 2 years of age also have difficulty regulating electrolytes, such as sodium and calcium. Renal response to high solute loads is slower and less developed, with function improving gradually during the first year of life. As a result, fluid challenge must be administered with caution in young children.

NURSING PROCESS

Nurses are responsible for identifying clients at risk for FVD, initiating and carrying out measures to prevent and treat FVD, and monitoring the effects of therapy. Health promotion activities focus on teaching clients to prevent FVD. Discuss the importance of maintaining adequate fluid intake, particularly when exercising and during hot weather. Advise clients to use commercial sports drinks to replace both water and electrolytes when exercising during warm weather. Instruct clients to maintain fluid intake when ill, particularly during periods of fever, when diarrhea is a problem.

Assessment

Carefully monitor clients at risk for abnormal fluid losses through routes such as vomiting, diarrhea, nasogastric suction, increased urine output, fever, or wounds. Monitor fluid intake in clients with decreased level of consciousness, disorientation, nausea, **anorexia** (loss of appetite), and physical limitations. Assess hydration by looking at skin for dryness, flakiness, or scaling as well as tenting when skin is pinched up (skin turgor). Check oral mucous membranes for dryness.

Nurses should assess both fluid and nutritional intake in the older adult. Older clients may consciously or unconsciously decrease fluid intake, because they do not feel thirsty when it is appropriate to drink, they fear incontinence or nocturia, or they lack the mobility to have easy access to beverages. Embarrassment also may be a factor for the older client who

EVIDENCE-BASED PRACTICE Clients With Imbalanced Fluid Volume

Nurses caring for clients with a fluid volume imbalance frequently monitor both 24-hour intake and output records and daily weights. These measurements require caregiver time and may provide redundant data.

Nurse managers on three nursing units compared the results of continuous 48-hour intake and output records with daily weights for a total of 73 selected clients on their units. Their findings suggest that even when compliance with recording accurate intake and output is optimal, it is an unreliable measure of actual fluid balance (Wise et al., 2000).

Implications for Nursing

As the United States begins to struggle with health care reforms, hospitals have begun pledging new efforts at cost containment. Added to this struggle is a significant shortage of licensed nurses that continues to be predicted for the first part of this century. Tight resources will require more efficient nursing practices to maintain quality care. This study suggests that for the majority of clients (the exceptions being clients with kidney disease or those on a fluid restriction), accurate daily weight measurements are a better indicator of fluid balance than intake and output records.

Critical Thinking in Client Care

1. What factors can you identify that would affect the accuracy of intake and output records?
2. What measures can you and your institution take to ensure accurate daily weight measurements?
3. Compare intake and output records and daily weights for your assigned clients. Is the balance between intake and output accurately reflected by day-to-day weight changes? If not, what factors can you identify that might account for this discrepancy?

Source: Adapted from Wise, L. C., et al. (2000). Evaluating the reliability and utility of cumulative intake and output. *Journal of Nursing Care Quality*, *14*(3), 37–42.

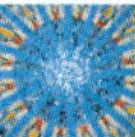

DEVELOPMENTAL CONSIDERATIONS Assessing Older Adults: Fluid Volume Deficit

- Some older adults experience postural hypotension, even when well hydrated.
- Allow the older adult to stand quietly for a full minute before rechecking blood pressure and pulse when measuring orthostatic vital signs.
- Because skin turgor diminishes with age, upper body weakness and dry oral membranes may be more reliable signs of dehydration in the older client.

needs assistance with toileting. Dehydration may lead to confusion, digestion problems, constipation, and bladder infections.

Collect the following assessment data through the health history interview and physical examination:

- *Health history.* Risk factors, such as medications and acute or chronic renal or endocrine disease; precipitating factors, such as hot weather, extensive exercise, lack of access to fluids, and recent illness (especially if accompanied by fever, vomiting, and/or diarrhea); and onset and duration of symptoms
- *Physical assessment.* Weight; vital signs, including orthostatic blood pressure and pulse; peripheral pulses and capillary refill; jugular neck vein distention; skin color, temperature, and turgor; level of consciousness and mentation; urine output. (See the Developmental Considerations feature for physical assessment of the older adult.)

Diagnosis

Appropriate nursing diagnoses may include the following:

- Deficient Fluid Volume
- Ineffective Peripheral Tissue Perfusion related to hypovolemia
- Risk for Injury related to postural hypotension
- Confusion
- Activity Intolerance.

Plan

Appropriate outcomes, planned together with clients and caregivers, may include the following:

- The client will achieve electrolyte and fluid balance.
- The client will drink 1,500 mL of fluid per day.
- The client will relate the need to replace fluids lost during exercise with sports drinks.
- The client will return to normal hydration status and not develop hypovolemic shock.
- The parents will relate strategies for preventing the child from becoming dehydrated.
- The parents will describe appropriate home management of fluid replacement for diarrhea and vomiting.
- The parents will describe when to seek health care if a child's condition worsens.

Implementation

The focus of care for the client with FVD is on managing the effects of the deficit and preventing complications.

- Record intake and output accurately; occasionally, hourly intake and output may be indicated.
- Weigh the client daily with the same scale and in same or similar clothing (young children should be weighed without clothing). Compare to past weights and calculate weight loss.

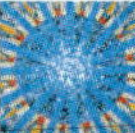

EVIDENCE-BASED PRACTICE Use of Oral Rehydration Therapy

In spite of the recommendation of the American Academy of Pediatrics (Provisional Committee on Quality Improvement, 1996) and other groups to use outpatient oral rehydration therapy (ORT) for mild and moderate dehydration, many health care providers continue to hospitalize these children and administer intravenous therapy (Nager & Wang, 2002). Hospitalization is expensive and disruptive for families, but care providers state that it seems easier than keeping a child in an outpatient setting for several hours to institute ORT.

Several analyses of studies performed with children have demonstrated the success and efficacy of ORT (Fonseca et al., 2004). To study the possibility of decreased treatment time, a study with 96 children from 3–36 months of age randomly assigned the moderately dehydrated children to receive either rapid nasogastric hydration or rapid intravenous (IV) hydration. Both methods were accomplished within 3 hours in an emergency department and were effective in treating children for dehydration. However, the nasogastric rehydration was significantly less expensive. The authors offer the possibility of rapid rehydration as a cost-effective management technique for children who are moderately dehydrated (Nager & Wang, 2002). In another study of 18 moderately dehydrated children with gastroenteritis, half were given ORT, and half were started on intravenous therapy. The length of treatment in the emergency department was significantly lower for the ORT group than for the IV group, and ORT required significantly less staff time. Parents reported greater satisfaction with ORT therapy, and the outcomes for the children were comparable (Atherly-John, Cunningham, & Crain, 2002).

Nurses can support ORT for children with mild or moderate dehydration. Teach parents to keep appropriate fluids at home and to institute the therapy early during vomiting and diarrhea episodes. Monitor children receiving the therapy in outpatient settings, whether by traditional oral therapy or rapid nasogastric hydration.

- Take vital signs, central venous pressure (CVP), and peripheral pulse volume at least every 4 hours.
- Administer and monitor intake of fluids as prescribed.
- Administer intravenous fluid using an electronic infusion pump.
- Monitor laboratory values (electrolytes, BUN, creatinine, osmolality, and urine specific gravity).
- Monitor for changes in level of consciousness and mental status.
- Reposition every 2 hours if client is unable to move independently.
- Initiate safety precautions to avoid falls secondary to dizziness or loss of balance.
- Teach client and family how to reduce orthostatic hypotension:
  a. Move from one position to another in stages; for example, raise the head of the bed before sitting up, and sit for a few minutes before standing.
  b. Avoid prolonged standing.
  c. Rest in a recliner rather than in bed during the day.
  d. Use assistive devices to pick up objects from the floor rather than stooping.
- Teach importance of maintaining adequate fluid intake (at least 1,500 mL/day).
- Teach how to prevent fluid deficit:
  a. Avoid exercising during extreme heat.
  b. Increase fluid intake during hot weather.
  c. If vomiting, take small frequent amounts of ice chips or clear liquids, such as weak tea, flat cola, or ginger ale.
  d. Reduce intake of coffee, tea, and alcohol, which increase urine output and can cause fluid loss (recent studies have called into question the diuretic effects of caffeine).

In mild or moderate dehydration, oral rehydration fluid is the first intervention for pediatric clients (Fonseca, Holdgate, & Craig, 2004; Spandorfer et al., 2005). It is given in frequent small amounts; for example, 1–3 tsps of fluid every 10–15 minutes is a useful guideline for starting oral rehydration. For the first 2–4 hours of treatment, 50 mL of fluid for each kilogram of the child's weight should be the target intake. Instruct parents to continue to administer 1 tsp every 2–3 minutes even if the child vomits, because small amounts of the fluid may still be absorbed. Children are often treated in special sections of emergency departments or outpatient clinics for several hours to begin hydration. Oral or nasogastric tube feedings of oral rehydration are administered while monitoring response.

Sugar facilitates the absorption of sodium in oral rehydration fluids. Teach parents not to give diet beverages for oral rehydration, because they contain no sugar and will not be effectively absorbed. However, if an oral rehydration solution is too concentrated, it can worsen the diarrhea. Juice and cola are highly concentrated and should be diluted to half-strength when given to a child who has diarrhea. Encourage parents to keep an oral rehydration solution in liquid or powder form on hand at all times and to use these solutions rather than juice or soda when the child first develops diarrhea.

Evaluation

Evaluate the client's progress toward meeting the outcomes created in collaboration with the client, and adjust the nursing plan of care as indicated. The more acutely ill client with a severe FVD may require evaluation of his or her condition every few minutes to hourly until progress is made.

Expected outcomes of nursing care for the client with dehydration include the following:

- The client has water and electrolytes that are balanced in intracellular and extracellular compartments as measured by serum electrolytes, hematocrit, and assessment findings.
- The client's urinary output is within normal limits.
- The client's fluid intake is adequate to meet maintenance needs.
- The client's vital signs are within normal limits.

Fluid Volume Excess

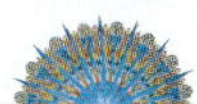

OVERVIEW

Fluid volume excess results when both water and sodium are retained in the body. Fluid volume excess may be caused by fluid overload (excess water and sodium intake) or by impairment of the mechanisms that maintain homeostasis leading to excess intravascular fluid (hypervolemia) and excess interstitial fluid (edema).

PATHOPHYSIOLOGY AND ETIOLOGY

Extracellular fluid volume excess occurs when there is too much fluid in the extracellular compartment (vascular and interstitial). This imbalance may also be called saline excess or extracellular volume overload. If total body sodium content is increased, it causes an increase in total body water. Because the increase in sodium and water is isotonic, the serum sodium and osmolality remain normal, and the excess fluid remains in the extracellular space.

Stress responses activated before, during, and immediately after surgery commonly lead to increased antidiuretic hormone and aldosterone levels, leading to sodium and water retention. In the immediate postoperative period, however, this additional fluid tends to be sequestered in interstitial tissues and unavailable to support cardiovascular and renal function (see earlier discussion of third spacing in this concept). This sequestered fluid is reabsorbed into the circulation within approximately 48–72 hours after surgery. Although it is then normally eliminated through a process of diuresis, clients with heart or kidney failure are at risk for developing fluid overload.

Interstitial Fluid Volume Excess (Edema)

Interstitial fluid volume excess, or edema, is an abnormal increase in the volume of the interstitial fluid. It may be caused by an extracellular fluid volume excess, or it may result from other causes.

Box 11–11 Clinical Conditions that Cause Edema

EDEMA CAUSED BY INCREASED BLOOD HYDROSTATIC PRESSURE

Increased Capillary Blood Flow
- Inflammation
- Local infection

Venous Congestion
- Extracellular fluid volume excess
- Right heart failure
- Venous thrombosis
- External pressure on vein
- Muscle paralysis

EDEMA CAUSED BY DECREASED BLOOD OSMOTIC PRESSURE

Increased Albumin Excretion
- Nephrotic syndrome (albumin leaks into urine)
- Protein-losing enteropathies (excess albumin in feces)

Decreased Albumin Synthesis
- Kwashiorkor (low-protein, high-carbohydrate starvation diet provides too few amino acids for liver to make albumin)
- Liver cirrhosis (diseased liver unable to make enough albumin)

EDEMA CAUSED BY INCREASED INTERSTITIAL FLUID OSMOTIC PRESSURE

Increased Capillary Permeability
- Inflammation
- Toxins
- Hypersensitivity reactions
- Burns

EDEMA CAUSED BY BLOCKED LYMPHATIC DRAINAGE
- Tumors
- Goiter
- Parasites that obstruct lymph nodes
- Surgery that removes lymph nodes

The causes of edema are best understood in the context of normal capillary dynamics. Fluid moves between the vascular and interstitial compartment by the process of filtration. Filtration is the net result of forces that tend to move fluid in opposing directions. The strongest forces will determine the direction of fluid movement.

At the capillary level, two forces (blood hydrostatic pressure and interstitial osmotic pressure) tend to move fluid from the capillaries into the interstitial fluid, while two other forces (blood colloid osmotic pressure and interstitial fluid hydrostatic pressure) tend to move fluid in the opposite direction (from the interstitial fluid into the capillaries). The net result of these forces usually moves fluid from the capillaries into the interstitial compartment at the arterial end of the capillaries and fluid from the interstitial compartment back into the capillaries at the venous end of the capillaries. This process brings oxygen and nutrients to the cells and removes carbon dioxide and other waste products.

Edema occurs if the balance of these four forces is altered so that excess fluid either enters or leaves the interstitial compartment. This may occur through increased blood hydrostatic pressure, decreased blood colloid osmotic pressure, increased interstitial fluid osmotic pressure, or blocked lymphatic drainage. Various clinical conditions are associated with these altered forces (Box 11–11):

1. *Increased blood hydrostatic pressure.* When extracellular fluid volume excess occurs, the increased fluid volume in the vascular compartment congests the veins. The pressure against the sides of the capillary is increased, and more fluid then enters the interstitial compartment.
2. *Decreased blood colloid osmotic pressure.* Much of the osmotic pressure that pulls fluid into the capillaries results from the presence of albumin and other plasma proteins made by the liver. The part of the blood osmotic pressure that is caused by plasma proteins is often called **oncotic pressure**, or blood colloid osmotic pressure. Any condition that decreases plasma proteins will decrease blood colloid osmotic pressure and cause edema. For example, if a clinical condition causes large amounts of albumin to leak into the urine, the liver will not be able to make albumin fast enough to replace it. As a result, the plasma protein level will fall, decreasing the blood osmotic pressure. Without this pulling force to return fluid to the capillaries, edema will occur. This is the cause of the edema that occurs in clients who have nephrotic syndrome. Another cause is prolonged surgical procedures with significant blood loss. Intravenous fluids and blood may be infused during surgery to replace these losses, but plasma proteins are lost and not fully restored by infusion, causing edema in the postoperative period.
3. *Increased interstitial fluid osmotic pressure.* Ordinarily, only a few small proteins enter the interstitial fluid, and the interstitial fluid osmotic pressure is small. If the capillary becomes abnormally permeable to proteins, however, the influx of large amounts of proteins into the interstitial fluid causes a dramatic increase in interstitial fluid osmotic pressure. This increased pulling force keeps an abnormal amount of fluid in the interstitial compartment. This mechanism plays an important part in edema caused by a bee sting or a sprained ankle. It occurs to a greater extent in burns, leading to swelling at the same time that there is a great loss of fluid volume through the burned skin.
4. *Blocked lymphatic drainage.* The lymph vessels normally drain small proteins and excess fluid from the interstitial compartment and return them to the blood vessels. If this process is blocked, fluid accumulates in the interstitial compartment. This may occur when a tumor blocks lymphatic drainage.

CLINICAL MANIFESTATIONS AND THERAPIES Fluid Volume Excess

ETIOLOGY	CLINICAL MANIFESTATION	CLINICAL THERAPIES
Congestive heart failure	Dependent edema Distended neck veins Pulmonary edema Tachycardia Dyspnea Hypoxia Respiratory crackles White or pink foamy sputum Liver enlargement Loss of appetite Nausea Weakness Fatigue Decreased activity tolerance Nocturia Paroxysmal nocturnal dyspnea Ascites Cardiogenic shock	■ Diuretics ■ Fluid restrictions ■ Fowler's or high Fowler's position ■ Oxygen ■ Medications may include cardiac glycosides, angiotensin-converting enzyme inhibitors, phosphodiesterase inhibitors, and β-adrenergic agonists (particularly dobutamine) ■ Monitor lab values: serum electrolytes, brain natriuretic peptide, blood urea nitrogen, creatine, urinalysis, alanine aminotransferase, aspartate aminotransferase, lactate dehydrogenase, bilirubin, total protein, albumin levels, thyroid function tests, and arterial blood gas ■ Chest X-ray ■ Electrocardiography ■ Hemodynamic monitoring ■ Intra-arterial pressure monitoring ■ Central venous pressure monitoring
Liver cirrhosis	Weight loss Weakness Anorexia Disrupted bowel function Portal hypertension Bleeding Ascites Jaundice Neurologic changes Peripheral edema Anemia Esophageal varices	■ Avoid hepatotoxic drugs ■ Diuretics ■ Lactulose and neomycin ■ β-blocker ■ Ferrous sulfate and folic acid ■ Antacid ■ Antianxiety drugs ■ Low-sodium, low-ammonia diet with vitamin and mineral supplements ■ Paracentesis ■ Hemodynamic monitoring
Adrenal tumor	Increased aldosterone production Water and sodium retention Edema Fluid volume excess	■ Removal of the tumor ■ Diuretics ■ Monitoring serum electrolytes, hemoglobin, and hematocrit ■ Cardiorespiratory monitoring ■ Oxygen
Over administration of intravenous fluids	Edema Pulmonary edema Shortness of breath Orthopnea Hypertension Reduced peripheral perfusion	■ Administration of diuretics ■ Elevate the head of the bed ■ Cardiorespiratory and oxygen saturation monitoring ■ Administration of oxygen ■ Daily weights ■ Accurate measurement of intake and output ■ Fluid restriction

Edema causes swelling, which may be localized or generalized. The swelling of tissue may cause pain and restrict motion. Edema that results from extracellular fluid volume excess or right-sided heart failure usually occurs in the dependent portion of the body, often observed in the ankles; in a client who is supine in bed, it is seen in the sacral area or in the scrotal area in men. The skin over an edematous area often appears thin and shiny.

Etiology

Fluid volume excess usually results from conditions that cause retention of both sodium and water. These conditions include heart failure, cirrhosis of the liver, renal failure, adrenal gland disorders, corticosteroid administration, and stress conditions causing the release of antidiuretic hormone and aldosterone. Other causes include an excessive intake of sodium-containing foods, drugs that cause sodium retention, and the administration of excess amounts of sodium-containing intravenous fluids (such as 0.9% NaCl or Ringer's solution). This **iatrogenic** (induced by the effects of treatment) cause of fluid volume excess primarily affects clients with impaired regulatory mechanisms.

Risk Factors

A decrease in cardiovascular reserve or a decrease in cardiac output may result from deconditioning and/or disease or from the natural aging processes. The older adult is at greater risk for fluid volume excess, in part because of natural reductions in kidney function that occur with aging. Additional stressors, such as hypertension, diabetes, or cardiac disease, increase the risk still further.

An increase in fluid volume is anticipated with normal pregnancy, but conditions such as preeclampsia may cause abnormal retention of fluid, resulting in increased stress on the body. Pregnant women with preeclampsia are taught that mild to moderate edema of the lower extremities (dependent edema) is to be anticipated, but edema of the face or hands or severe edema of the lower extremities must be reported to the provider immediately.

The clients with heart disease, kidney dysfunctions, or diabetes with peripheral vascular disease are at increased risk. Any disease that impairs blood flow to the kidney, such as hypertension, can potentially cause fluid volume excess. Any client receiving intravenous therapy is at risk if careful monitoring of infusion rate and type of solution is not carefully monitored.

CLINICAL MANIFESTATIONS

The following manifestations of fluid volume excess relate to both the excess fluid and its effects on circulation:

- The increase in total body water causes weight gain (>5% of body weight) over a short time period.
- Circulatory overload causes manifestations such as:
  a. A full, bounding pulse
  b. Distended neck and peripheral veins (distended neck veins are difficult to assess in infants)
  c. Increased central venous pressure (>11–12 cm of water)
  d. Cough, **dyspnea** (labored or difficult breathing), and **orthopnea** (difficulty breathing when supine)
  e. Moist crackles (rales) in the lungs or, if severe, pulmonary edema (excess fluid in pulmonary interstitial spaces and alveoli)
  f. **Polyuria** (greatly increased urine output)
  g. **Ascites** (excess fluid in the peritoneal cavity)
  h. Peripheral edema or, if severe, **anasarca** (severe, generalized edema).
- Dilution of plasma by excess fluid causes a decreased hematocrit and BUN.
- Possible cerebral edema (excess water in brain tissues) can lead to altered mental status and anxiety.

Heart failure is not only a potential cause of fluid volume excess, it is also a potential complication of the condition if the heart is unable to increase its workload to handle the excess blood volume. Severe fluid overload and heart failure can lead to pulmonary edema, a medical emergency.

COLLABORATION

Managing fluid volume excess focuses on prevention in clients at risk, treating its manifestations, and correcting the underlying cause. Management includes limiting sodium and water intake and administering diuretics. A consultation with a dietician or nutritionist may help the client to make appropriate food choices and provide the staff with a better understanding of client food preferences.

Diagnostic Tests

The following laboratory tests may be ordered:

- *Serum electrolytes* and *serum osmolality* are measured. Serum sodium and osmolality usually remain within normal limits.
- *Serum hematocrit* and *hemoglobin* often are decreased because of plasma dilution from excess extracellular fluid.

Additional tests of renal and liver function (e.g., serum creatinine, BUN, and liver enzymes) may be ordered to help determine the cause of fluid volume excess if it is unclear.

Pharmacologic Therapies

Diuretics are commonly used to treat fluid volume excess. They inhibit sodium and water reabsorption, increasing urine output. The three major classes of diuretics, each of which acts on a different part of the kidney tubule, are as follows:

1. *Loop diuretics,* which act in the ascending loop of Henle.
2. *Thiazide-type diuretics,* which act on the distal convoluted tubule
3. *Potassium-sparing diuretics,* which affect the distal nephron.

Fluid Management

Fluid intake may be restricted in clients who have fluid volume excess. The amount of fluid allowed per day is prescribed by the primary care provider. All fluid intake must be calculated, including fluid consumed at meals and that used to administer medications orally or intravenously. Some foods may be higher in fluid content (e.g., watermelon, oranges, and soups) and must be considered as well. Box 11–12 provides guidelines for clients with a fluid restriction.

Dietary Management

Because sodium retention is a primary cause of fluid volume excess, a sodium-restricted diet often is prescribed. Americans typically consume more than 4 or 5 g of sodium every day; recommended sodium intake is 500 to 2,400 mg/day. The primary dietary sources of sodium are the salt shaker, processed foods, and foods themselves (Box 11–13).

Box 11–12 **Fluid Restriction Guidelines**

- Subtract requisite fluids (e.g., ordered intravenous fluids, fluid used to dilute intravenous medications) from total daily allowance.
- Divide remaining fluid allowance:
  a. Day shift: 50% of total
  b. Evening shift: 25 to 33% of total
  c. Night shift: Remainder
- Explain the fluid restriction to the client and family members.
- Identify preferred fluids and intake pattern of client.
- Place allowed amounts of fluid in small glasses (gives perception of a full glass).
- Offer ice chips (when melted, ice chips are approximately half the frozen volume).
- Provide frequent mouth care.
- Provide sugarless chewing gum (if allowed) to reduce thirst sensation.

A mild sodium restriction can be achieved by instructing the client and primary food preparer in the household to reduce the amount of salt in recipes by half, avoid using the salt shaker during meals, and avoid foods that contain high levels of sodium (either naturally or because of processing). In moderate and severely sodium-restricted diets, salt is avoided altogether, as are all foods containing significant amounts of sodium.

NURSING PROCESS

Nursing care focuses on preventing fluid volume excess in clients at risk and on managing problems resulting from its effects. Health promotion related to fluid volume excess focuses on teaching preventive measures to clients who are at risk (e.g., clients who have heart or kidney failure). Discuss the relationship between sodium intake and water retention. Provide guidelines for a low-sodium diet, and teach clients to carefully read food labels to identify "hidden" sodium, particularly in processed foods. Instruct clients who are at risk to weigh themselves on a regular basis, using the same scale, and to notify their primary care provider if they gain more than 5 pounds in a week or less.

Carefully monitor clients receiving intravenous fluids for signs of hypervolemia. Reduce the flow rate and promptly report manifestations of fluid overload to the physician.

Assessment

Collect assessment data through the health history interview and physical examination:

- *Health history.* Risk factors, such as medications, heart failure, and acute or chronic renal or endocrine disease; precipitating factors, such as a recent illness, change in diet, or change in medications; recent weight gain; complaints of persistent cough, shortness of breath, swelling of feet and ankles, or difficulty sleeping when lying down

Box 11–13 **Foods High in Sodium**

HIGH IN ADDED SODIUM

Processed Meat and Fish
- Bacon
- Sausage
- Luncheon meat and other cold cuts
- Smoked fish

Selected Dairy Products
- Buttermilk
- Cottage cheese
- Cheeses
- Ice cream

Processed Grains
- Graham crackers
- Most dry cereals

Most Canned Goods
- Meats
- Vegetables
- Soups

Snack Foods
- Salted popcorn
- Nuts
- Potato chips/pretzels
- Gelatin desserts

Condiments and Food Additives
- Barbecue sauce
- Saccharin
- Catsup
- Pickles
- Chili sauce
- Soy sauce
- Meat tenderizers
- Salted margarine
- Worcestershire sauce
- Salad dressings

NATURALLY HIGH IN SODIUM
- Brains
- Oysters
- Kidney
- Shrimp
- Clams
- Dried fruit
- Crab
- Spinach
- Lobster
- Carrots

- *Physical assessment.* Daily weight, preferably using the same scale and wearing the same or similar clothing; vital signs; peripheral pulses and capillary refill; jugular neck vein distention; edema; lung sounds (crackles or wheezes), dyspnea, cough, and sputum; urine output; and mental status.

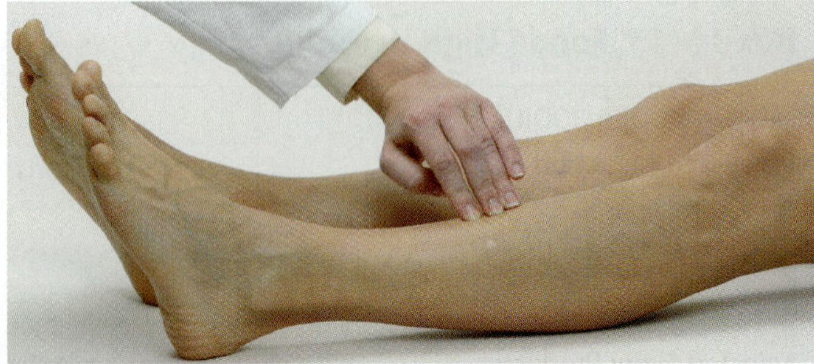

Figure 11–21 ■ Palpating for edema over the tibia.

More specifically, check for edema of the legs by pressing the skin for at least 5 seconds over the tibia, behind the medial malleolus, and over the dorsum of each foot (Figure 11–21 ■). If edema is present, you should grade it on a scale of 1+ mild to 4+ severe (see Figure 11–22 ■). Assess for periorbital edema, swollen puffy eyelids that may result from crying or fluid volume excess. Men may experience scrotal edema, because the scrotum is in the dependent position when sitting.

Measure the child's intake and output, and weigh the diapers of infants. You can tell if a child's weight gain is the result of normal growth or the development of extracellular fluid volume excess by looking at the speed with which the increase develops. Sudden weight gain (e.g., 0.5 kg [1 lb] in 1 day) is caused by the accumulation of fluid. A gain of 0.5 kg overnight is caused by retention of approximately 500 mL of saline.

Assess the character of the pulse, and observe for neck vein distention when the client is sitting (usually visible only in adults and older children). Monitor for signs of pulmonary edema (an indication of severe imbalance) by listening to lung sounds in the dependent lung fields (crackles) and assessing for respiratory distress (rapid respiratory rate, use of accessory muscles of respiration). Observe for edema.

FOCUS ON DIVERSITY AND CULTURE

Sodium Use

To adapt teaching about low-sodium diets to the cultural practices of a family, ask the family members what types of food they usually eat. Help them to choose low-sodium foods from their diets and to avoid high-sodium foods. This approach is more effective than giving the same list of restricted foods to each family.

For example, some Asians use monosodium glutamate to flavor foods. They should be encouraged to add this at the table for family members who can have extra sodium rather than to use it during cooking. Many Hispanic groups use large amounts of cheese that contain significant sodium. Encourage them to look for low-sodium cheese and substitute cottage cheese for other types, because it is lower in sodium. Low-sodium milk is available and is a good option for young children. Canned foods tend to have high sodium, so teach all families to use fresh or frozen produce rather than canned.

The potential for a client (especially a small child) to develop a fluid overload is present whenever an isotonic intravenous solution containing sodium is being administered. Careful assessment of infusion rates is essential to all client care but especially when caring for pediatric clients. Therefore, monitor the infusion rate frequently and carefully, and use a pump when possible to aid in accurate administration.

Diagnosis

Appropriate nursing diagnosis may include the following:

- Excess Fluid Volume
- Risk for Impaired Skin Integrity
- Risk for Impaired Gas Exchange
- Activity Intolerance
- Ineffective Health Maintenance.

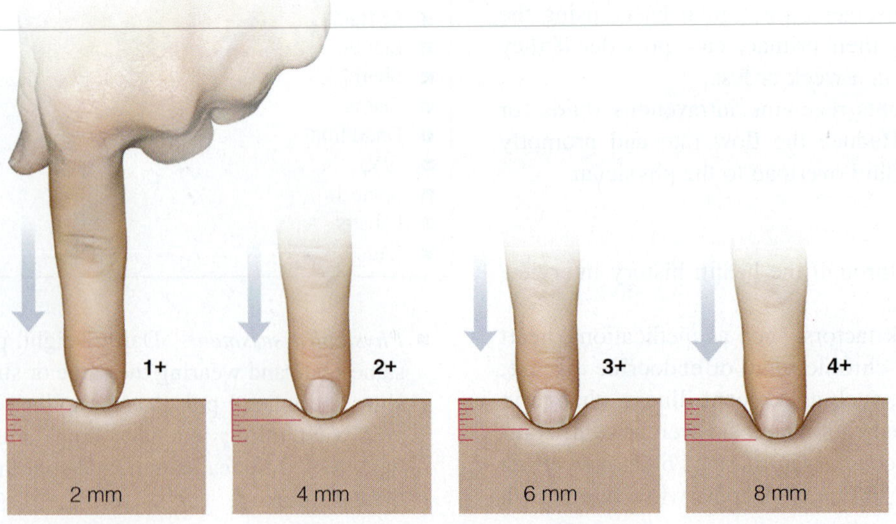

Figure 11–22 ■ Grading pitting edema.

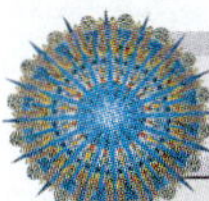

NURSING CARE PLAN **A Client With Fluid Volume Excess**

Dorothy Rainwater is a 45-year-old Native American woman hospitalized with acute renal failure that developed as a result of acute glomerulonephritis. She is expected to recover, but she has very little urine output. Ms. Rainwater is a single mother of two teenage sons. Until her illness, she was active in caring for her family, her career as a high school principal, and community activities.

ASSESSMENT

Ms. Rainwater's nurse notes that she is in the oliguric phase of acute renal failure and that her urine output for the previous 24 hours was 250 mL; this low output has been constant for the past 8 days. Ms. Rainwater gained 1 lb (0.45 kg) in the past 24 hours. Laboratory test results from that morning are as follows: sodium, 155 mEq/L (normal, 135–145 mEq/L); potassium, 5.3 mEq/L (normal, 3.5–5.0 mEq/L); calcium, 7.6 mg/dL (normal, 8.0–10.5 mg/dL), and urine specific gravity, 1.008 (normal, 1.010–1.030). Ms. Rainwater's serum creatinine and blood urea nitrogen are high; however, her arterial blood gases are within normal limits.

The nurse's assessment of Ms. Rainwater yields the following:

- BP 160/92; P 102, with obvious neck vein distention; R 28, with crackles and wheezes; head of bed elevated 30°; and T_O 98.6°F.
- Periorbital and sacral edema present; 3+ pitting bilateral pedal edema; and skin cool, pale, and shiny.
- Alert, oriented, and responds appropriately to questions.
- Client states she is thirsty, slightly nauseated, and extremely tired.

Ms. Rainwater is receiving intravenous furosemide and is on a 24-hour fluid restriction of 500 mL plus the previous day's urine output to manage her fluid volume excess.

DIAGNOSES

- Excess Fluid Volume related to acute renal failure
- Risk for Impaired Skin Integrity related to fluid retention and edema
- Risk for Impaired Gas Exchange related to pulmonary congestion
- Activity Intolerance related to fluid volume excess, fatigue, and weakness

PLANNING

- The client will regain fluid balance, as evidenced by weight loss, decreasing edema, and normal vital signs.
- The client will experience decreased dyspnea.
- The client will maintain intact skin and mucous membranes.
- The client will increase activity levels as prescribed.

IMPLEMENTATION

- Weigh at 6:00 a.m. and 6:00 p.m. daily.
- Assess vital signs and breath sounds every 4 hours.
- Measure intake and output every 4 hours.
- Obtain urine specific gravity every 8 hours.
- Restrict fluids as follows: 350 mL from 7:00 a.m. to 3:00 p.m.; 300 mL from 3:00 p.m. to 11:00 p.m.; and 100 mL from 11:00 p.m. to 7:00 a.m. Client prefers water or apple juice.
- Turn every 2 hours, following schedule posted at the head of bed. Inspect and provide skin care as needed; avoid vigorous massage of pressure areas.
- Provide oral care every 2–4 hours (client can brush her own teeth; caution client not to swallow water); use moistened applicators as desired.
- Elevate head of bed to 30–40°; client prefers to use own pillows.
- Assist to recliner chair at bedside for 20 minutes two or three times a day. Monitor ability to tolerate activity without increasing dyspnea or fatigue.

EVALUATION

At the end of the shift, the nurse evaluates the effectiveness of the plan of care and continues all diagnoses and interventions. Ms. Rainwater gained no weight, and her urinary output during this shift is 170 mL. Her urine specific gravity remains at 1.008. Her vital signs are unchanged, but her crackles and wheezes have decreased slightly. Her skin and mucous membranes are intact. Ms. Rainwater tolerated the bedside chair without dyspnea or fatigue.

CRITICAL THINKING

1. What is the pathophysiologic basis for Ms. Rainwater's increased respiratory rate, blood pressure, and pulse?
2. Explain how elevating the head of the bed 30° facilitates respirations.
3. Suppose Ms. Rainwater says, "I would really like to have all my fluids at once instead of spreading them out." How would you reply, and why?
4. Outline a plan for teaching Ms. Rainwater about diuretics.

CLIENT TEACHING Low-Sodium Diet

- Reducing sodium intake helps the body to excrete excess sodium and water.
- The body needs less than one tenth of a teaspoon of salt per day.
- Approximately one third of sodium intake comes from salt added to foods during cooking and at the table, one fourth to one third comes from processed foods, and the rest comes from food and water naturally high in sodium.
- Sodium compounds are used in foods as preservatives, leavening agents, and flavor enhancers.
- Many nonprescription drugs (e.g., analgesics, cough medicine, laxatives, and antacids), toothpastes, and mouthwashes contain high amounts of sodium.
- Low-sodium salt substitutes are not really sodium free; they may contain half as much sodium as regular salt.
- Use salt substitutes sparingly; larger amounts often taste bitter instead of salty.
- The preference for salt will eventually diminish.
- Salt, monosodium glutamate, baking soda, and baking powder contain substantial amounts of sodium.
- Read labels.
- In place of salt or salt substitutes, use herbs, spices, lemon juice, vinegar, and wine as flavoring when cooking.

Plan

Outcomes are designed in collaboration with the client and may include the following:

- The client regains fluid balance.
- The client has clear lung fields with eupneic breathing.
- The client maintains intact skin.
- The client avoids infection of skin wounds (if present).
- The client shows increased activity tolerance.
- The client makes appropriate food choices to limit sodium.

Implementation

Nursing interventions for the client with fluid volume excess may include the following:

- Weigh the client daily.
- Maintain intake and output records.
- Administer oral fluids carefully.
- Perform oral hygiene at least every 2 hours.
- Teach client and significant others about sodium-restricted diet.
- Administer prescribed diuretics, and monitor response to therapy.
- Report significant changes in serum electrolyte or osmolality.
- Teach client how to safely self-administer diuretics after discharge.
- Reposition client every 2 hours.
- Reduce shearing or friction to skin.
- Provide a low-pressure alternative mattress, foot cradle, heel protectors, and other devices to reduce pressure on tissues.
- Place in Fowler's position if dyspnea or orthopnea is present.
- Monitor oxygen saturation and arterial blood gas results.
- Elevate area of edema (if possible) to encourage fluid reabsorption into extracellular fluid compartment.

Evaluation

Evaluate changes in weight, respirations, and edema to determine the client's response to treatment. To evaluate client understanding of dietary teaching, encourage the client to participate in making appropriate diet choices from the menu. Revise the nursing plan of care as indicated based on client's progress toward meeting outcomes.

Electrolyte Imbalance

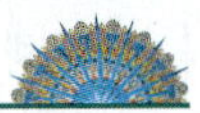

OVERVIEW

All body fluids contain electrolytes in varying concentrations, depending on the type and location of fluid. When a serum electrolyte value is reported from the laboratory, it provides information about the concentration of that electrolyte in the blood. It does not necessarily reflect the concentration of the electrolyte in other body compartments.

Electrolytes are normally gained and lost in relatively equal amounts, so the body remains in balance. However, when a client has an abnormal route of loss, such as vomiting, wound drainage, diuretic administration, or nasogastric suction, electrolyte balance can be disturbed. Monitoring for signs of imbalance is an important part of nursing care for clients at risk.

Signs and symptoms of electrolyte imbalance can be very subtle if the imbalance is minimal. Moderate to severe electrolyte imbalance often produces multisystem effects and can lead to death if not reversed. When caring for a client in the acute care facility, it is important to consider the role of electrolytes in maintaining homeostasis and watch for signs of imbalance. It is often important to assess the client's new symptom in regard to possible electrolyte imbalance.

While electrolytes are taught individually to make it easier to learn about them, it is important to understand the interaction between all electrolytes and fluid. Imbalance rarely occurs with only one electrolyte. For example, if sodium is lost, chloride often accompanies it; fluid volume excess often dilutes other electrolytes, resulting in lower serum levels; and gastric suctioning causing hypokalemia also causes loss of magnesium, sodium, and chloride as well as acid–base imbalance.

Table 11–16 reviews alterations in electrolyte balance. Lists of conditions resulting in specific electrolyte imbalance are not comprehensive but describe only the more common causes.

TABLE 11–16 **Electrolyte Imbalances**

CONDITION	ETIOLOGY	CLINICAL MANIFESTATION	CLINICAL THERAPIES	NURSING CARE
ELECTROLYTE: SODIUM (NA+); NORMAL 135–145 MEQ/L; HIGHEST CONCENTRATION FOUND IN EXTRACELLULAR FLUID.				
Hyponatremia Critical value, <120 mEq/L	■ Diuretics ■ Kidney disease ■ Adrenal insufficiency ■ Vomiting ■ Diarrhea ■ Excessive gastrointestinal (GI) suctioning ■ Irrigating GI tubes with water instead of saline ■ Repeated tap water enemas ■ Excessive sweating ■ Loss of skin surfaces (burns) ■ Water gain from heart failure, renal failure, cirrhosis of the liver of syndrome of inappropriate antidiuretic hormone ■ Excessive administration of hypotonic intravenous (IV) fluid	■ Decrease osmolality. ■ Fluid shifts from extracellular fluid (ECF) to intracellular fluid causing cellular edema Manifestations depend on rapidity of onset and cause. **Na, 120–125 mEq/L** ■ Muscle cramps ■ Weakness ■ Fatigue ■ Anorexia ■ Nausea and vomiting ■ Abdominal cramps ■ Diarrhea **Na, <120 mEq/L** ■ Headache ■ Depression ■ Dulled sensorium ■ Personality changes ■ Irritability ■ Lethargy ■ Hyperreflexia ■ Muscle twitching ■ Tremors **Very low levels** ■ Convulsions ■ Coma ■ Death	**Diagnostic Tests** ■ Serum sodium ■ Serum osmolality ■ 24-hour urine sodium **Medications** ■ Sodium containing fluids administered (normal saline or isotonic Ringer's solution) ■ Loop diuretics if normal or excess ECF volume **Treatments** ■ Treat the underlying cause ■ Increase intake of sodium containing foods ■ Fluid restrictions	**Assessment** ■ Identify clients at risk (athletes or laborers who perspire profusely and drink water in large quantities, people who lack air conditioning in hot weather). ■ Client teaching to drink fluids containing sodium to replace-perspiration. ■ Asses for symptoms. **Diagnosis** ■ (Risk for) Imbalanced Fluid Volume ■ Risk for Ineffective Cerebral Tissue Perfusion **Interventions** ■ Monitor input and output (I&O), daily weight, and calculate fluid balance. ■ Use IV flow device to administer hypertonic saline solutions. ■ Help client understand rationale for and adapt to fluid restrictions if ordered. ■ Monitor electrolytes and serum osmolality. ■ Assess for neurological change. ■ Assess muscle strength and tone and deep tendon reflexes.
Hypernatremia Critical Value, >160 mEq/L	■ Altered thirst or inability to respond to thirst ■ Profuse sweating ■ Diarrhea ■ Diabetes insipidus ■ Oral electrolyte solutions	■ Hyperosmolality of ECF ■ Cellular dehydration ■ Thirst ■ Increased temperature ■ Dry, sticky mucous membranes ■ Restlessness ■ Weakness	Corrected slowly to avoid cerebral edema **Diagnostic Tests** ■ Serum sodium ■ Serum osmolality ■ Water deprivation test	**Assessment** ■ Identify risk factors. ■ Monitor lab results. ■ Duration of symptoms ■ Precipitating factors **Diagnosis** ■ (Risk for) Imbalanced Fluid Volume

(continued)

TABLE 11–16 Electrolyte Imbalances (continued)

CONDITION	ETIOLOGY	CLINICAL MANIFESTATION	CLINICAL THERAPIES	NURSING CARE
	■ Hyperosmolar tube feeding formulas ■ Excess IV fluids ■ Sodium gained in excess of water (excess intake of salt or hypertonic IV solutions) ■ Water lost in excess of sodium (watery diarrhea or increased insensible water loss from fever, burns, or hyperventilation) ■ Fluid volume excess or FVD may accompany	Brain shrinks as cells contract, causing mechanical traction that can lead to bleeding ■ Altered mentation ■ Decreasing level of consciousness ■ Muscle twitching ■ Seizures ■ Coma ■ Death	**Medications** ■ Oral or IV water replacement ■ Hypotonic IV fluids ■ Diuretics to increase sodium excretion	■ Risk for Ineffective Cerebral Tissue Perfusion ■ Risk for Injury **Interventions** ■ Monitor I&O, daily weight, and calculate fluid balance. ■ Monitor neurologic function, including mental status, level of consciousness, and any symptoms. ■ Institute safety precautions as indicated (seizure precautions, bed in low position, side rails up). ■ Reorient if needed and keep familiar objects at bedside. ■ Instruct caregivers of debilitated clients to offer fluids regularly or notify physician if alternate method of fluid delivery is needed. ■ Possible low-sodium diet. ■ Teach proper use of diuretics as indicated.
ELECTROLYTE: CHLORIDE (CL^-); NORMAL, 98–106 MEQ/L; HIGHEST CONCENTRATION FOUND IN EXTRACELLULAR FLUID.				
Hypochloremia	■ Not commonly seen alone but results from another electrolyte or fluid imbalance ■ Loss of body fluid ■ Vomiting, diarrhea, sweating, high fever ■ Drugs such as bicarbonate, corticosteroids, diuretics, and laxatives ■ Metabolic alkalosis	■ Only seen with severe imbalance ■ Low serum chloride ■ Pediatric clients are often small for age ■ Skin tenting ■ Poor peripheral perfusion ■ Confusion, apathy, disorientation, lethargy ■ Seizures, stupor ■ Scaphoid abdomen or distended abdomen	**Diagnostic Tests** ■ Serum electrolytes ■ Arterial blood gas Treatments ■ Increase salt in diet. ■ Add chloride to infusing IV fluids (e.g., KCl) depending on other electrolyte levels. ■ Treat the underlying cause.	**Assessment** ■ Identify clients at risk (long-term gastric suction, bulimia with purging, first trimester of pregnancy with excessive vomiting). ■ Assess muscles, vital signs, respiratory strength, peripheral perfusion. ■ Assess neurologic status. ■ Assess abdomen and bowel sounds. ■ Chart growth in pediatric clients.

TABLE 11–16 **Electrolyte Imbalances** (continued)

CONDITION	ETIOLOGY	CLINICAL MANIFESTATION	CLINICAL THERAPIES	NURSING CARE
	■ Hyponatremia usually lowers chloride levels as well ■ Overconsumption of licorice ■ Hyperaldosteronism	■ Hyperactive bowel sounds ■ Muscle wasting, atrophy, and hypotonia ■ Shallow breathing		**Diagnosis** ■ Risk for Imbalanced Fluid Volume ■ Risk for Injury **Interventions** ■ Monitor lab results. ■ Monitor neurologic status. ■ Teach clients proper diet management. ■ Encourage fluids. ■ Record intake and output.
Hyperchloremia	■ Diarrhea ■ Renal failure ■ Overactive parathyroid glands ■ Comorbid with diabetes or hypernatremia ■ Use of carbonic anhydrase inhibitors, hormonal treatments, and polypharmacy ■ Metabolic acidosis ■ Respiratory alkalosis	■ May be asymptomatic if minor deficiency ■ May lead to poor control of blood glucose in diabetics ■ Kussmaul's respirations ■ Weakness ■ Intense thirst	**Diagnostic Tests** ■ Serum electrolytes ■ Arterial blood gas ■ Hemoglobin and hematocrit ■ Serum or urine osmolality **Medications** ■ Diuretics ■ Increase fluids—oral or IV **Treatments** ■ Treat the underlying cause. ■ Dialysis	**Assessment** ■ Identify clients at risk. ■ Assess blood sugar more frequently on diabetics. ■ Assess lab findings. ■ Assess current medications. ■ Assess respirations and muscle strength. **Diagnosis** ■ (Risk for) Imbalanced Fluid Volume ■ Risk for Ineffective Cerebral Tissue Perfusion **Interventions** ■ Monitor I&O, daily weight, and calculate fluid balance. ■ Initiate safety interventions to prevent falls related to weakness. ■ Encourage oral fluid intake.
ELECTROLYTE: POTASSIUM (K^+); NORMAL, 3.5–5.0 MEQ/L; HIGHEST CONCENTRATION FOUND INSIDE THE CELL.				
Hypokalemia Critical value, <2.5 mEq/L	■ Potassium-wasting diuretics ■ Corticosteroids ■ Amphotericin B ■ Large doses of some antibiotics ■ Hyperaldosteronism ■ Glucosuria ■ Osmotic diuresis ■ Severe vomiting ■ Gastric suction	■ Dysrhythmias ■ Electrocardiogram (ECG) changes (flat or inverted T wave, development of U wave, depressed ST segment) ■ Nausea and vomiting ■ Anorexia ■ Decreased bowel sounds	**Diagnostic Tests** ■ Serum potassium, sodium and calcium ■ Arterial blood gas ■ Renal function tests ■ 12-lead ECG ■ Digitalis level (if indicated) ■ Serum myoglobin ■ Creatine kinase	**Assessment** ■ Identify clients at risk. ■ Assess for symptoms. ■ Continuous cardiac rhythm assessment, especially those below critical levels. ■ Monitor muscle strength and tone and assist with self-care activities as needed. ■ Monitor bowel sounds and assess for abdominal distention.

(continued)

TABLE 11–16 Electrolyte Imbalances (continued)

CONDITION	ETIOLOGY	CLINICAL MANIFESTATION	CLINICAL THERAPIES	NURSING CARE
	■ Loss of intestinal fluids ■ Inadequate intake ■ Alkalosis ■ Rapid tissue repair ■ Clients receiving long-term IV therapy without potassium ■ Presence of excess insulin	■ Ileus ■ Muscle weakness ■ Leg cramps ■ Increased risk for digitalis toxicity ■ Symptoms magnified if serum calcium levels are high ■ Insulin secretion suppressed ■ Reduced ability of kidneys to concentrate urine ■ Rhabdomyolysis may result from extended hypokalemia ■ Symptoms most acute when potassium lost rapidly	**Medications** ■ Potassium acetate (Tri K) ■ Potassium bicarbonate (K^+ Care ET) ■ Potassium citrate (K-Lyte) ■ Potassium chloride (K-Lease, Micro-K, Apo-K) ■ Potassium gluconate (Kaon Elixir, Royonate)	**Diagnosis** ■ Risk for Injury related to muscle weakness ■ Decreased Cardiac Output ■ Ineffective Peripheral Tissue Perfusion ■ Ineffective Health Maintenance related to lack of knowledge about diuretic therapy and potassium supplementation. **Interventions** ■ Monitor serum potassium levels and digitalis levels if indicated. ■ Maintain I&O. ■ Monitor vital signs, including orthostatic vital signs and peripheral pulses. ■ Continuous monitoring of cardiac rhythm. ■ Administer parenteral forms of potassium slowly and well diluted—NEVER given as IV push or rapid bolus, and always run on an electronic infusion device. Assess IV site for infiltration, which can cause serious tissue necrosis. Best if administered through a central line. ■ Teach clients to replace abnormal fluid losses with sports drinks containing sodium and potassium. ■ Provide diet teaching. ■ Teach clients how to take diuretics and potassium supplements properly.
Hyperkalemia Critical value, >6.5 mEq/L	■ Renal failure ■ Potassium-sparing diuretics ■ Excess potassium intake—rare with normal kidney function ■ Adrenal insufficiency	■ Altered cell membrane potential affecting heart, skeletal muscle, and GI tract ■ Tall, peaked T waves, widened QRS ■ Dysrhythmias ■ Cardiac arrest		**Assessment** ■ Identify clients at risk. ■ Continuous monitoring of cardiac rhythm, especially with potassium levels approaching or above critical values.

TABLE 11–16 **Electrolyte Imbalances** **(continued)**

CONDITION	ETIOLOGY	CLINICAL MANIFESTATION	CLINICAL THERAPIES	NURSING CARE
	■ Aged blood transfusions ■ Acidosis (greater with metabolic than respiratory acidosis) ■ Severe tissue trauma ■ Chemotherapy with cellular destruction ■ Starvation ■ Trimethoprim ■ Some nonsteroidal anti-inflammatory drugs **GUARD AGAINST** pseudohyperkalemia caused by hemolyzed blood specimens giving falsely high potassium readings.	■ Smooth muscle hyperactivity ■ Nausea and vomiting ■ Abdominal cramping ■ Diarrhea ■ Muscle weakness ■ Paresthesias ■ Flaccid paralysis	**Diagnostic Tests** ■ Serum electrolytes ■ Arterial blood gas ■ ECG ■ Digitalis level if indicated **Medications** ■ Calcium gluconate ■ Regular insulin and glucose ■ B_2-agonist by nebulizer ■ Sodium bicarbonate to treat acidosis ■ Sodium polystyrene sulfonate (Kayexalate) ■ Diuretics if renal function is normal **Treatments** ■ Dialysis	■ Assess for numbness, tingling, abdominal cramping, GI symptoms. ■ Assess for use of salt substitutes, potassium supplements, chronic disease, renal failure, and current medications. ■ Assess apical pulses, bowel sounds, muscle strength, ECG pattern. **Diagnosis** ■ Risk for Decreased Cardiac Output ■ Activity Intolerance related to skeletal muscle weakness ■ Risk for Ineffective Health Maintenance related to inadequate knowledge of recommended diet (or medications) **Interventions** ■ Monitor I&O, daily weight, serum electrolytes, and cardiac rhythm. ■ Teach clients taking potassium supplements how to take them safely. ■ Assist with self-care activities as needed. ■ Monitor for fluid volume excess.
ELECTROLYTE: CALCIUM (CA_2^+); NORMAL, 8.5–10 MG/DL; HIGHEST CONCENTRATION BOUND TO PHOSPHORUS IN FORM OF THE MINERALS IN BONES AND TEETH, REMAINDER IS FOUND IN EXTRACELLULAR FLUID.				
Hypocalcemia Critical value, <6.0 mg/dL	■ Following parathyroidectomy ■ Malabsorption disorders ■ Alkalosis ■ Inadequate vitamin D ■ Older adults, especially women ■ Lactose intolerance ■ Alcoholism ■ Reduced calcium intake ■ Inactivity promotes calcium loss from bones	■ Tetany ■ Paresthesias ■ Muscle spasms ■ Positive Chvostek's sign **Positive Trousseau's sign** is seen in clients with low calcium; manifested by muscle spasms in the hand and forearm after application of a blood pressure cuff inflated higher than systolic blood pressure and left in place for 3 minutes.	**Diagnostic Tests** ■ Total serum calcium ■ Serum albumin ■ Serum magnesium ■ Serum phosphate ■ Parathyroid hormones ■ ECG ■ Bone density scan **Medications** ■ Oral or IV calcium (calcium chloride or calcium gluconate)	**Assessment** ■ Identify clients at risk (elderly, postmenopausal women, clients with chronic disability and those who cannot perform weight bearing activities). ■ Assess for numbness and tingling around the mouth and hands and feet, abdominal pain, shortness of breath. ■ Assess for acute or chronic disease such as pancreatitis, liver or kidney disease. ■ Assess deep tendon reflexes, Chvostek's sign, Trousseau's sign, respiratory rate and depth, vital signs and apical pulse.

(continued)

TABLE 11–16 **Electrolyte Imbalances** **(continued)**

CONDITION	ETIOLOGY	CLINICAL MANIFESTATION	CLINICAL THERAPIES	NURSING CARE
	■ Drugs can interfere with calcium absorption or promote excretion ■ Decrease in estrogen levels as with menopause ■ Acute pancreatitis ■ Lack of sun exposure ■ Loop diuretics, calcitonin, anticonvulsants, phosphates, and calcitonin ■ Hypomagnesemia ■ Acute renal failure with hyperphosphatemia ■ Massive transfusion of banked blood	■ Laryngospasm ■ Seizures ■ Anxiety, confusion, psychosis ■ Decreased cardiac output ■ Hypotension ■ Dysrhythmias ■ Abdominal cramping ■ Diarrhea ■ Muscle weakness, fatigue ■ Decreased deep tendon reflexes ■ Personality changes ■ Altered mental status ■ Decreasing level of consciousness ■ Abdominal pain ■ Constipation ■ Anorexia, nausea, vomiting ■ Dysrhythmias ■ Hypertension ■ Polyuria, thirst		**Diagnosis** ■ Risk for Injury ■ Risk for Ineffective Cerebral Tissue Perfusion **Interventions** ■ Monitor I&O, daily weight, and calculate fluid balance. ■ Monitor IV site carefully if infusing calcium for venous sclerosis or extravasation. ■ Teach diet high in calcium rich foods. ■ Report changes in respiratory status, neuromuscular irritability and seizure activity. ■ Administer calcium slowly. ■ Maintain quiet environment. ■ Continuous monitoring of ECG during IV calcium administration.
Hypercalcemia Critical value, >13.0 mg/dL	■ Increased reabsorption of calcium from bones ■ Hyperparathyroidism ■ Bone malignancies or tumors ■ Following kidney transplant ■ Chronic renal failure ■ Excess vitamin D ■ Overuse of calcium based antacids ■ Excessive milk ingestion ■ Thiazide diuretics and lithium interfere with calcium excretion	■ Decreased neuromuscular excitability ■ Muscle weakness ■ Depressed deep tendon reflexes ■ Reduced GI motility ■ Strengthened cardiac contractions and decreased heart rate leading to heart blocks ■ Excess sodium and water loss with increased thirst	**Diagnostic Tests** ■ Serum electrolytes with total serum calcium ■ Serum parathyroid hormone ■ Digitalis levels ■ ECG ■ Bone density scans **Medications** ■ IV fluids (isotonic saline) ■ Loop diuretics ■ Calcitonin ■ Bisphosphonates	**Assessment** ■ Identify clients at risk. ■ Assess muscle strength and tone, GI function, mentation, dietary intake of calcium containing foods, vital signs, bowel sounds, deep tendon reflexes. ■ Review diagnostic test results. ■ Assess for signs of digitalis toxicity. ■ Assess vital signs frequently. **Diagnosis** ■ Risk for Injury ■ Risk for Excess Fluid Volume

TABLE 11–16 **Electrolyte Imbalances** **(continued)**

CONDITION	ETIOLOGY	CLINICAL MANIFESTATION	CLINICAL THERAPIES	NURSING CARE
		■ Altered mental status, personality changes, confusion, impaired memory, acute psychosis ■ Hypertension ■ Increased gastric acid secretion leading to peptic ulcer development ■ Pancreatitis from calcium deposits in pancreatic ducts ■ Increased risk of kidney stones ■ Coma ■ Death	■ Sodium phosphate or potassium phosphate ■ Plicamycin (Mithracin) ■ Glucocorticoids (cortisone)	**Interventions** ■ Monitor I&O and calculate fluid balance. ■ Promote motility in clients as soon as possible. ■ Teach benefits of regular weight-bearing activities. ■ Consume fluids that increase acidity of urine to prevent stone formation. ■ Initiate safety precautions if confusion or change in mental status. ■ Promote fluid intake. ■ Use caution when turning, positioning or transferring client. ■ Elevate head of bed.
ELECTROLYTE: MAGNESIUM (MG_2^+); NORMAL, 1.6–2.6 MG/DL; HIGHEST CONCENTRATION FOUND IN EXTRACELLULAR FLUID.				
Hypomagnesemia Critical value, <1 mg/dL	■ Loss of GI fluids (diarrhea, ileostomy, intestinal fistula) ■ Disruption of nutrient absorption in small intestine ■ Chronic alcoholism ■ Protein-calorie malnutrition or starvation ■ Endocrine disorders (diabetic ketoacidosis [DKA]) ■ Loop or thiazide diuretics, aminoglycoside antibiotics, amphotericin B and cyclosporine	■ Increased excitability of neuromusculature with muscle weakness and tremors ■ Hyperreactive reflexes ■ Positive Chvostek's sign ■ Positive Trousseau's sign ■ Paresthesias ■ Seizures, tetany ■ Changes in mental status, mood, and personality ■ Hallucinations and psychoses ■ Increased heart rate	**Diagnostic Tests** ■ Serum electrolytes ■ ECG with prolonged PR, widened QRS, depressed ST, T-wave inversion **Medications** ■ Oral or IV magnesium; may also be given deep intramuscular	**Assessment** ■ Assess for clients at risk (hospitalized clients with protein-calorie malnutrition). ■ Monitor serum electrolyte levels. ■ Assess GI function. ■ Assess cardiac rhythm, rate, and vital signs. ■ Assess deep tendon reflexes frequently. **Diagnosis** ■ Risk for Injury ■ Risk for Ineffective Cerebral Tissue Perfusion ■ Risk for Decreased Cardiac Output

(continued)

TABLE 11–16 **Electrolyte Imbalances** (continued)

CONDITION	ETIOLOGY	CLINICAL MANIFESTATION	CLINICAL THERAPIES	NURSING CARE
	■ Rapid administration of citrated blood ■ Kidney disease ■ Often occurs with low potassium and calcium levels	■ Increased risk of cardiac ventricular dysrhythmias and sudden death ■ Increases risk of digitalis toxicity ■ Vasoconstriction ■ Dysphagia, anorexia, nausea, vomiting, diarrhea ■ Tachycardia, dysrhythmias, hypertension		**Interventions** ■ Monitor I&O, daily weight, and calculate fluid balance. ■ Teach importance of well-balanced diet particularly in people at risk. ■ Maintain quiet dark environment. ■ Initiate continuous cardiorespiratory monitoring. ■ Report and treat dysrhythmias as indicated.
Hypermagnesemia Critical value, > 4.7 mg/dL	■ Renal insufficiency or failure ■ Excess intake of antacids or laxatives ■ Excess magnesium administration ■ Pregnant women treated for preeclampsia	■ Depressed neuromuscular transmission and central nervous system depression ■ Muscle weakness, depressed deep tendon reflexes ■ Lethargy, drowsiness ■ Nausea and vomiting ■ Hypotension, bradycardia, cardiac arrest ■ Flushing, sweating, feeling of warmth ■ Respiratory depression ■ Coma	**Diagnostic Tests** ■ Serum electrolytes **Medications** ■ Withhold all medications containing magnesium (antacids, IV solutions, enema solutions). ■ Administer calcium gluconate to reverse effects of high magnesium level. **Treatment** ■ Dialysis may be instituted to remove excess magnesium. ■ Mechanical ventilation may be needed. ■ Pacemaker to maintain adequate cardiac output	**Assessment** ■ Identify clients at risk. ■ Assess vital signs, cardiac rhythm, respiratory effectiveness, oxygenation. ■ Assess mental status, deep tendon reflexes, muscle strength, GI function. **Diagnosis** ■ Decreased Cardiac Output ■ Risk for Ineffective Breathing Pattern ■ Risk for Injury ■ Risk for Ineffective Health Maintenance **Interventions** ■ Initiate continuous cardiorespiratory monitor. ■ Perform frequent neurological examinations (frequency determined by severity of Mg elevation). ■ Teach client about safe use of magnesium-containing supplements, antacids, laxatives, or enemas.

TABLE 11–16 Electrolyte Imbalances (continued)

CONDITION	ETIOLOGY	CLINICAL MANIFESTATION	CLINICAL THERAPIES	NURSING CARE
ELECTROLYTE: PHOSPHATE (PO_4^-); NORMAL, 2.5–4.5 MG/DL (VARIES WITH AGE); FOUND MOSTLY IN INTRACELLULAR FLUID.				
Hypophosphatemia Critical value, <1 mg/dL	■ Shift of phosphorus into cells ■ IV glucose administration ■ Total parenteral nutrition without phosphorus ■ Aluminum- or magnesium-based antacids ■ Diuretic therapy ■ Alcoholism ■ Decreased GI absorption ■ Increased renal excretion ■ Refeeding syndrome ■ Anabolic steroids ■ Hyperventilation and respiratory alkalosis ■ DKA, stress response, extensive burns	■ Paresthesias ■ Muscle weakness ■ Muscle pain and tenderness ■ Confusion, decreasing level of consciousness ■ Irritability, lack of coordination ■ Seizures, coma ■ Bone pain, osteomalacia ■ Anorexia, dysphagia ■ Decreased bowel sounds ■ Possible acute respiratory failure ■ Hemolytic anemia ■ Increase creatine phosphokinase ■ Acute rhabdomyolysis leading to renal failure ■ Chest muscle weakness interferes with ventilation	**Diagnostic Tests** ■ Serum electrolyte levels **Medications** ■ Oral phosphate supplement ■ IV phosphate if acute deficiency **Treatment** ■ Improved diet	**Assessment** ■ Identify clients at risk (malnourished, alcoholic, receiving IV glucose, on diuretic therapy, taking antacids). ■ Assess neurologic function, level of consciousness, coordination. ■ Assess GI function, swallowing. ■ Assess vital signs, oxygenation. ■ Assess for bone or muscle pain. **Diagnosis** ■ Impaired Physical Mobility ■ Ineffective Breathing Pattern ■ Decreased Cardiac Output ■ Risk for Injury **Interventions** ■ Assist with activities of daily living as needed. ■ Instruct client on proper use of diuretics, antacids. ■ Teach manifestations of hypophosphatemia and when to report signs and symptoms to provider. ■ Teach the importance of a well-balanced diet.
Hyperphosphatemia Critical value, even mild elevations increase risk	■ Renal failure ■ Chemotherapy ■ Muscle tissue trauma ■ Sepsis ■ Severe hypothermia ■ Heat stroke ■ Rapid administration of phosphate containing solutions including phosphate enemas ■ Excess vitamin D intake ■ Disruptions in calcium levels	■ For each 1 mg/dL increase in serum phosphate, the risk of coronary artery calcification increases by 21% (Fore, 2008) ■ Circumoral and peripheral paresthesias ■ Muscle spasms ■ Tetany ■ Soft-tissue calcification	**Diagnostic Tests** ■ Serum phosphate and calcium levels **Medications** ■ Oral calcium containing antacids ■ IV normal saline **Treatment** ■ Treatment of the underlying disease ■ Dialysis	**Assessment** ■ Identify clients at risk. ■ Monitor lab values. ■ Assess for manifestations. **Diagnosis** ■ Risk for Decreased Cardiac Tissue Perfusion ■ Risk for Injury ■ Risk for Ineffective Health Maintenance **Interventions** ■ Monitor I&O, daily weight, and calculate fluid balance.

Source: Mckinney, Ramont, D'Anna, and Webb. (2011). *Bridging to RN: Preparation and Refresher.* Upper Saddle River, NJ: Pearson.

HEALTH CARE

Evidence-Based Practice

Review the literature, and find a research article indicating a recommended best practice related to treatment of fluid and/or electrolyte imbalance.

Safety

Why would safety be of concern to the client with a fluid and/or electrolyte imbalance?

REVIEW Fluid and Electrolyte Imbalance

RELATE: LINK THE CONCEPTS

Linking the exemplar of Fluid and Electrolyte Imbalances with the concept of Cognition:

1. What impact do you anticpate a fluid and electrolyte imbalance may have on an older client's cognition?
2. What expected outcomes are appropriate for the client with confusion and hyperkalemia?

Linking the exemplar of Fluid and Electrolyte Imbalances with the concept of Elimination:

3. You are caring for a client with acute nausea, vomiting, and diarrhea. What impact do you anticpate this having on the client's fluid and electrolyte balance and how can you minimize this impact?
4. What focused assessment is a priority for the client with chronic renal failure who has a potassium level of 5.5?

READY: GO TO COMPANION SKILLS MANUAL

- Monitoring intake and output
- Assessing weight
- Establishing intravenous infusions
- Maintaining intravenous infusions
- Administering an enema

REFER: GO TO MYNURSINGKIT

REFLECT: CASE STUDY

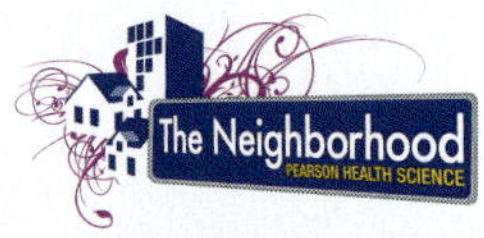

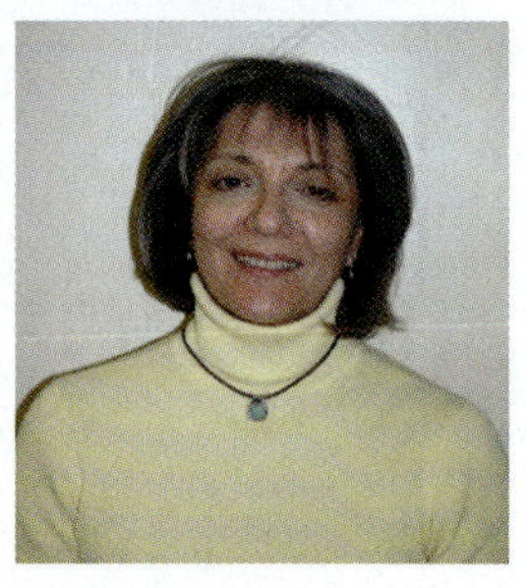

Pamela Allen is a 65-year-old woman who has been married to Clifford for 40 years. Their only child, Gary, has Down syndrome and lives with them. Mrs. Allen stopped working after Gary was born to care for him. She has recently been diagnosed with advanced colorectal cancer and had surgery last month (colectomy and colostomy). Because the tumor extended into the perineum and lymph nodes, she has been advised to start radiation and chemotherapy. She previously underwent treatment for endometrial cancer at age 50 but did not receive chemotherapy or radiation at that time.

1. When caring for Mrs. Allen during administration of chemotherapy, what issues might you anticipate could result in fluid and electrolyte imbalance?
2. If Mrs. Allen experiences dehydration following chemotherapy administration, what suggestions could the nurse recommend to improve fluid status?
3. As a result of chemotherapy and radiation causing bowel irritation, Mrs. Allen develops severe acute diarrhea. What changes would you recommend to Mrs. Allen's fluid intake to maintain adequate fluid balance and normal electrolyte levels?

PEARSON

EXPLORE mynursingkit™

MyNursingKit is your one stop for online chapter review materials and resources. Prepare for success with additional NCLEX®-style practice questions, interactive assignments and activities, web links, animations and videos, and more!

Register your access code from the front of your book at **www.mynursingkit.com**.

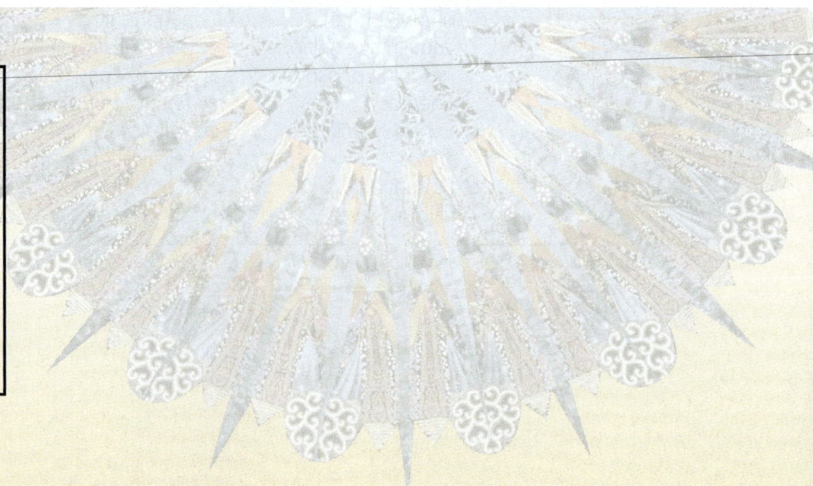

REFERENCES

Atherly-John, Y. C., Cunningham, S. J., & Crain, E. F. (2002). A randomized trial of oral vs intravenous rehydration in a pediatric emergency department. *Archives of Pediatric and Adolescent Medicine, 156,* 1240–1243.

Bailey, J.L., & Sands, J. M. (2003). Renal disease. In W. R. Hazzard, J. P. Blass, J. B. Halter, J.G. Ouslander, & M. E. Tinetti (Eds.), *Principles of geriatric medicine and gerontology* (5th ed., pp. 551–568). New York: McGraw-Hill.

Ball, J. W., & Bindler, R. C. (2008). *Pediatric nursing: Caring for children* (4th ed.). Upper Saddle River, NJ: Pearson, Inc.

Beers, M. H., & Berkow, R. (Eds.). (2004). *The Merck manual of diagnosis and therapy* (17th ed.). Merck & Co., Inc. Internet edition provided by Medical Services, USMEDSA, USHH.

Bennett, J. A., Thomas, V., & Riegel, B. (2004). Unrecognized chronic dehydration in older adults. Examining prevalence rate and risk factors. *Journal of Gerontological Nursing, 30*(1), 22–28.

Binkley, H. M., Beckett, J., Casa, D.J., Kleiner, D. M., & Plummer, P. E. (2002). National Athletic Trainers' Association position statement: Exertional heat illnesses. *Journal of Athletic Training, 37,* 329–343.

Bock, K. R. (2005). Renal replacement therapy in pediatric critical care medicine. *Current Opinion in Pediatrics, 17,* 368–371.

Centers for Disease Control and Prevention. (2002). Guidelines for the prevention of intravascular catheter-related infections. *Morbidity and Mortality Weekly Report, 51*(10), 1–29.

Committee on Sports Medicine and Fitness. (2000). Climatic heat stress and the exercising child and adolescent. *Pediatrics, 106,* 158–159.

Criddle, L. M. (2003). Rhabdomyolysis. Pathophysiology, recognition, and management. *Critical Care Nurse, 23*(6), 14–22, 24–26, 28+.

Dale, J. (2004). Oral rehydration solutions in the management of acute gastroenteritis among children. *Journal of Pediatric Health Care, 18,* 211–212.

Dennehy, P. H. (2005). Acute diarrheal disease in children: Epidemiology, prevention, and treatment. *Infectious Disease Clinics of North America, 19,* 585–602.

Dinwiddie, L. C. (2004). Managing catheter dysfunction for better patient outcomes: A team approach. *Nephrology Nursing Journal, 31*(6), 653–660, 661–662, 671.

Fonseca, B. K., Holdgate, A., & Craig, J. C. (2004). Enteral vs. intravenous rehydration therapy for children with gastroenteritis. *Archives of Pediatrics & Adolescent Medicine, 158,* 483–490.

Food and Drug Administration (FDA). (2004). Bar code label requirements for human drug products and biological products. *Federal Register, 69* (38), 9119–9171.

Fore, K. (2008). High serum phosphate increases vascular calcification. *Medpage Today.* Retrieved March 29, 2009, from http://www.medpagetoday.com/Nephrology/GeneralNephrology/12115

Hadaway, L. C. (2003). Infusing without infecting. *Nursing, 33* (10), 58–64.

Hagren, B., Petterson, I. M., Severinsson, E., Lutzon, K., & Clyne, H. (2001). The haemodialysis machine as a lifeline: Experiences of suffering from end-stage renal disease. *Journal of Advanced Nursing, 34*(2), 196–202.

Jassal, V., Fillit, H., & Oreopoulos, D. G. (1998). Diseases of the aging kidney. In R. Tallis, H. Fillit, & J. C. Brocklehurst (Eds.), *Brocklehurst's textbook of geriatric medicine and gerontology* (5th ed., pp. 949–971). Edinburgh, Scotland: Churchill Livingstone.

Johns Hopkins Hospital. (2005). *The Harriet Lane handbook* (17th ed.). St. Louis: Mosby.

Just the facts: Fluids & electrolytes. (2005). Philadelphia: Lippincott Williams & Wilkins.

Kasper, D.L., Braunwald, E., Fauci, A. S., Hauser, S. L., Longo, D. L., & Jameson, J. L. (Eds.). (2005). *Harrison's principles of internal medicine* (16th ed.). New York: McGraw-Hill.

Metheny, N.M. (2000). *Fluid and electrolyte balance: Nursing considerations* (4th ed.). Philadelphia: Lippincott.

Nager, A. L., & Wang, V. J. (2002). Comparison of nasogastric and intravenous methods of rehydration in pediatric patients with acute dehydration. *Pediatrics, 109,* 566–572.

NANDA International. (2009). *NANDA nursing diagnoses: Definitions and classification 2009–2011.* Philadelphia: Wiley-Blackwell.

National Kidney and Urologic Diseases Information Clearinghouse. (2004). *Kidney and urologic disease statistics for the United States* (NIH Publication No. 04-3895). Retrieved from http://www.niddk.nih.gov/kudiseases/kidney/pubs/kustats

National Kidney and Urologic Diseases Information Clearinghouse. (2009). *Kidney and urologic disease statistics for the United States.*Retrieved July 20, 2009, from http://kidney.niddk.nih.gov/kudiseases/pubs/kustats/index.htm

National Kidney Disease Education Program. (2005). *Kidney disease in African Americans.* Retrieved July 20, 2009, from http://www.nkdep.nih.gov/news/campaign/african_americans.htm

National Kidney Foundation. (2009). Kidney Disease. Retrieved July 14, 2009, from http://www.kidney.org/kidneydisease/

Organ Procurement and Transplantation Network. (2009). Retrieved July 20, 2009, from http://optn.transplant.hrsa.gov/latestData/rptData.asp

Porth, C. M. (2005). *Pathophysiology: Concepts of altered health states* (7th ed.). Philadelphia: Lippincott Williams & Wilkins.

Provisional Committee on Quality Improvement, Subcommittee on Acute Gastroenteritis. (1996). Practice parameter: The management of acute gastroenteritis in young children. *Pediatrics, 97,* 424–436.

Russell, T.R. (2005). Acute renal failure related to rhabdomyolysis: Pathophysiology, diagnosis, and collaborative management. *Nephrology Nursing Journal, 32*(4), 409–417.

Spandorfer, P.R., Alessandrini, E. A., Joffe, M. D., Localio, R., & Shaw, K. N. (2005). Oral versus intravenous rehydration of moderately dehydrated children: A randomized, controlled trial. *Pediatrics, 115*(2), 295–301.

Steiner, M. J., DeWalt, D. A., & Byerly, J.S. (2004). Is this child dehydrated? *JAMA, 291,* 2746–2754.

Suhayda, R., & Walton, J. C. (2002). Preventing and managing dehydration. *MEDSURG Nursing, 11*(6), 267–278.

Tierney, L. M., McPhee, S. J., & Papadakis, M.A. (2005). *Current medical diagnosis and treatment* (44th ed.). New York: Lange Medical Books/McGraw-Hill.

United Network for Organ Sharing: Organ Donation and Transplantation (2005). U.S. Transplantation Data. Retrieved from http://www.unos.org/data/default.asp?display Type=usData

U.S. Renal Data System. (2008). 2006 Annual Data Report: *Atlas of end-stage renal disease in the United States.* Bethesda, MD: National Institutes of Health, National Institute of Diabetes and Digestive and Kidney Diseases.

Vogt, B. A., & Avner, E. D. (2007). Toxic neuropathies: Renal failure. In R. M. Kliegman, R.E. Berman, H.B. Jenson, & B. F. Stanton (Eds.), *Nelson textbook of pediatrics* (18th ed., pp. 2204–2219). Philadelphia: Saunders.

Wathen, J. E., MacKenzie, T., & Bothner, J. P. (2004). Usefulness of the serum electrolyte panel in the management of pediatric dehydration treated with intravenously administered fluids. *Pediatrics, 114,* 1227–1234.

Wiggins, J. (2003). Changes in renal function. In W.R. Hazzard, J. P. Blass, J. B. Halter, J.G. Ouslander, & M. E. Tinetti (Eds.), *Principles of geriatric medicine and gerontology* (5th ed., pp. 543–549). New York: McGraw-Hill.

Wise, L. C., Mersch, J., Racioppi, J., Crosier, J., & Thompson, C. (2000). Evaluating the reliability and utility of cumulative intake and output. *Journal of Nursing Care Quality, 14*(3), 37–42.

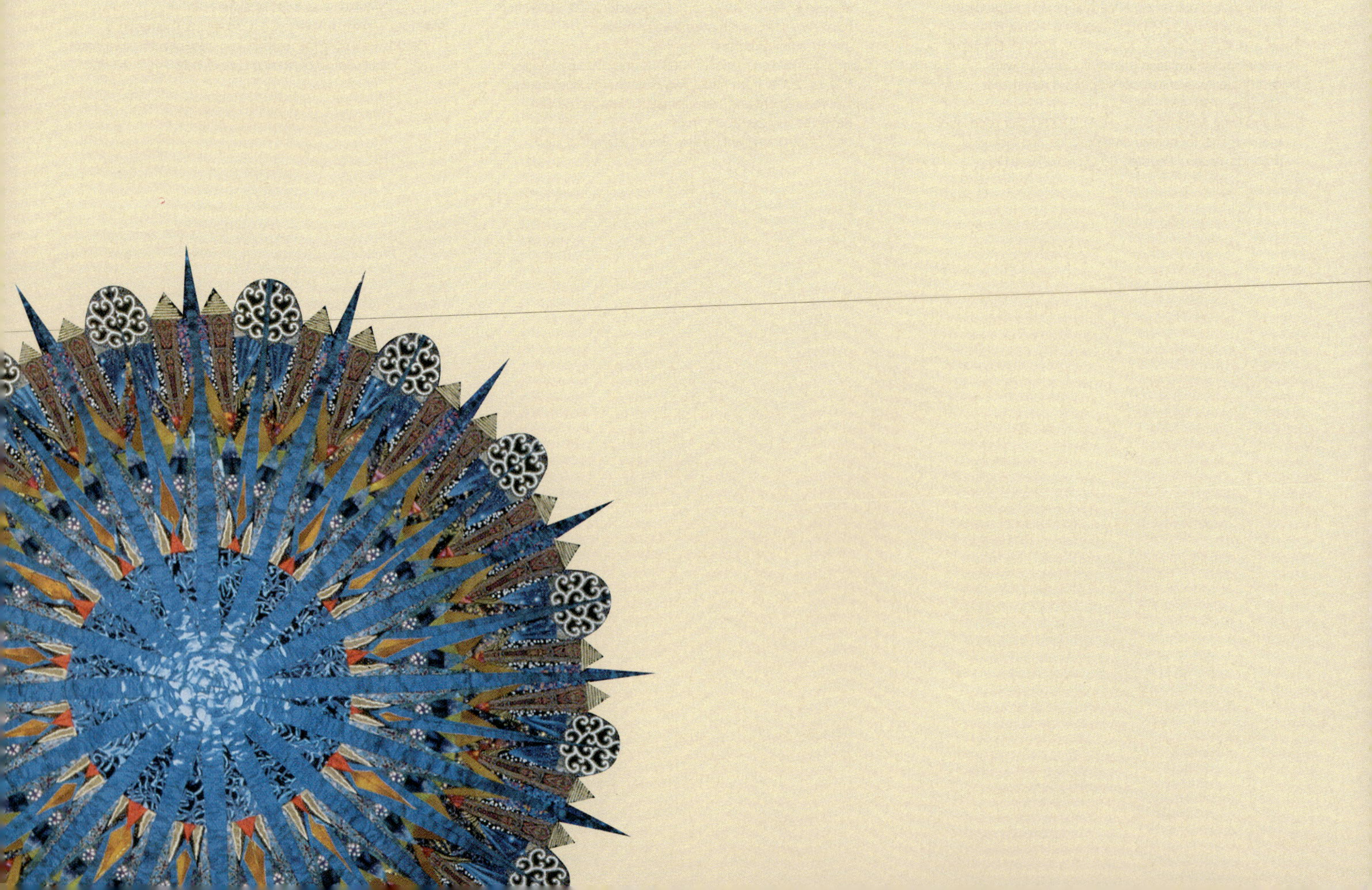

Grief and Loss 12

Concept at-a-Glance

Concept Learning Outcomes

After reading about this concept, you will be able to:

1. Deconstruct situations that could potentially cause feelings of grief or loss.
2. Contrast different cultural responses to, and means of displaying, grief and loss.
3. Examine different theories related to the grieving process.
4. Contrast normal grief responses to those that indicate an alteration in the grieving process.
5. Apply theories of growth and development to the expressions and manifestations of grief.
6. Develop a nursing plan of care for the client working through the grieving process.
7. Develop appropriate nursing diagnoses for the client experiencing grief or loss.
8. Assess expected outcomes for an individual experiencing grief or loss.

Concept Key Terms

Actual loss, *600*
Anticipatory grief, *601*
Anticipatory loss, *600*
Bereavement, *601*
Complicated grief, *601*
Disenfranchised grief, *606*
Grief, *601*
Hospice, *608*
Loss, *600*
Mourning, *601*
Perceived loss, *600*

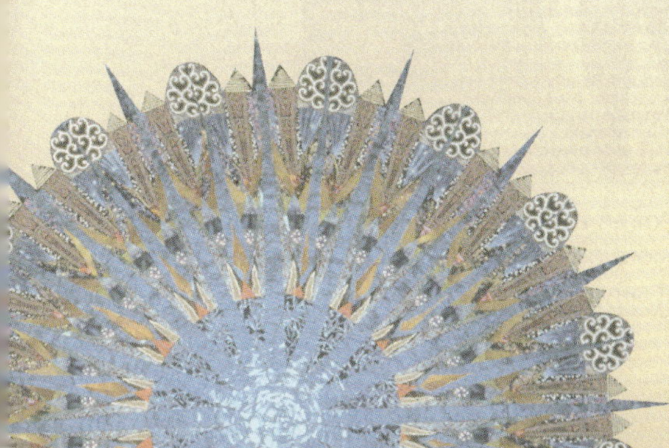

About Grief and Loss

Every individual experiences loss, grief, and death at some time during his or her life. People may suffer the loss of valued relationships through life changes such as relocation; separation; divorce; and the death of a parent, spouse, or friend. People may grieve changing life roles when they watch grown children leave home or when they retire from their lifelong work. The loss of valued material objects through theft or natural disaster also can evoke feelings of grief and loss. When people's lives are affected by civil or national strife, they may grieve the loss of valued ideals such as safety, freedom, and democracy.

In the clinical setting, the nurse encounters clients who may be experiencing grief related to declining health, loss of a body part or ability, terminal illness, or the impending death of self or a significant other. The nurse also may work with clients in community settings who are grieving losses related to personal crisis (e.g., divorce or separation) or disaster (war, earthquakes, terrorism, or hurricanes). Therefore, it is important for the nurse to understand the significance of loss and develop the ability to assist clients as they work through the grieving process.

Nurses may interact with dying clients and their families or caregivers in a variety of settings from a fetal demise (death of an unborn child), to the adolescent victim of an accident, to the elderly client who finally succumbs to a chronic illness. Nurses must recognize the various influences on the dying process—legal, ethical, religious and spiritual, biologic, personal—and be prepared to provide sensitive, skilled, and supportive care to everyone affected. ●

LOSS AND GRIEF

Loss is an actual or potential situation in which something that is valued is altered or no longer available. People can experience the loss of body image, a significant other, a sense of well-being, a job, personal possessions, or beliefs. Illness and hospitalization often produce losses.

Death is a fundamental loss. Although death is inevitable, it can stimulate both the dying individual and his or her survivors to gain greater understanding of themselves and others. Death can be viewed as the dying person's final opportunity to experience life in ways that bring significance and fulfillment. People experiencing loss often search for the meaning of the event, and it is generally accepted that finding meaning is necessary for healing to occur. However, people can be well adjusted without searching for meaning, and even those who find meaning may not see it as an end point, but rather as an ongoing process.

Types and Sources of Loss

There are two general types of loss: actual and perceived. An **actual loss** is one that can be recognized by others. A **perceived loss** is experienced by one person but cannot be verified by others. Psychologic losses are often perceived losses in that they are not directly verifiable. For example, a woman who leaves her employment to care for her children at home may perceive a loss of independence and freedom. Both types of loss can be anticipatory. An **anticipatory loss** is one that is experienced before the loss actually occurs. For example, a woman whose husband is dying may experience actual loss in anticipation of his death.

Loss can be viewed as situational or developmental. The loss of one's job, the death of a child, or the loss of functional ability due to acute illness or injury are *situational losses.* Losses that occur in the process of normal development such as the departure of grown children from the home, retirement from a career, and the death of aged parents are *developmental losses* that can, to some extent, be prepared for and anticipated.

There are several sources of loss: (1) loss of an aspect of oneself—a body part, a physiologic function, or a psychologic attribute; (2) loss of an object external to oneself; (3) separation from an accustomed environment; and (4) loss of a loved or valued person.

ASPECT OF SELF The loss of an aspect of self changes a person's body image even though the loss may not be obvious. A face scarred from a burn or a leg lost to amputation is generally obvious to people (Figure 12–1 ■); loss of part of the stomach or loss of ability to feel emotion may not be as obvious.

Both physical and psychological losses can have an impact on self-image. For example, an older adult in the early stages of Alzheimer's may experience a great blow to his or her self-esteem when he or she is forced to surrender his or her driving privileges a result of the changes that he or she is experiencing in cognitive functioning due to his or her disease. The degree to which these losses affect a person largely depends on the integrity of the person's body image or self-esteem.

EXTERNAL OBJECTS Loss of external objects includes (1) loss of inanimate objects that have importance to the person, such as the loss of money or the burning down of the family's home, and (2) loss of animate (live) objects such as pets, which provide love and companionship.

FAMILIAR ENVIRONMENT Separation from an environment and people in that environment who provide security can result in a sense of loss. The 6-year-old is likely to feel loss when first leaving the home environment to attend school. The university student who moves away from home for the first time also experiences a sense of loss.

LOVED ONES The loss of a loved one or valued person through illness, divorce, separation, or death can be disturbing. In some illnesses (such as Alzheimer's disease), a person may undergo personality changes that make friends and family feel that they have lost that person long before the person dies.

The death of a loved one is a permanent and complete loss. In contemporary American society, people may be uncomfortable talking about death and being around people who are dying. There is a tendency to consider using extraordinary measures to prolong and preserve life.

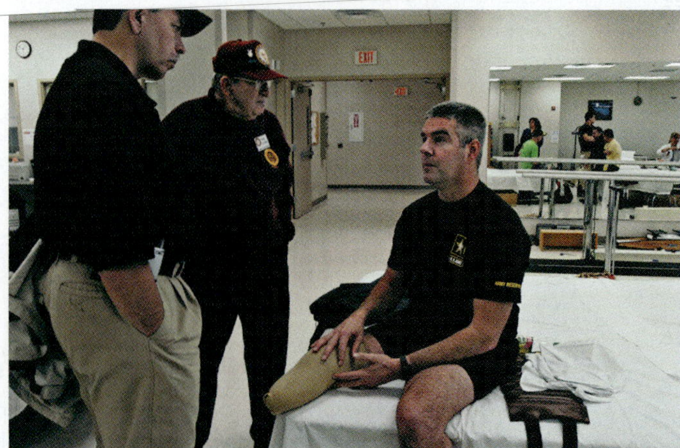

Figure 12–1 ■ Loss of an aspect of self is common in those serving in the military, as loss of an appendage or a functional ability is one of the hazards of serving in combat situations.

Source: Getty Images

Grief, Bereavement, and Mourning

Grief is the total response to the emotional experience related to loss. Grief is manifested in thoughts, feelings, and behaviors associated with overwhelming distress or sorrow. **Bereavement** is the subjective response experienced by the surviving loved ones after the death of a person with whom they have shared a significant relationship. **Mourning** is the behavioral process through which grief is eventually resolved or altered; it is often influenced by culture, spiritual beliefs, and custom (Figure 12–2 ■). Grief and mourning are experienced not only by the person who faces the death of a loved one, but also by the person who suffers other kinds of losses. Grieving is essential for good mental and physical health. It allows the individual to cope with the loss gradually and to accept it as part of reality. Grief is a social process; it is best shared and carried out with the assistance of others.

Working through one's grief is important because bereavement may have potentially devastating effects on health. Symptoms that may accompany grief include anxiety, depression, weight loss, difficulty swallowing, vomiting, fatigue, headaches, dizziness, fainting, blurred vision, skin rashes, excessive sweating, menstrual disturbances, palpitations, chest pain, and dyspnea. The bereaved also may experience alterations in libido; in concentration; and in patterns of eating, sleeping, activity, and communication.

Although bereavement can threaten health, a positive resolution of the grieving process may enrich the individual with new insights, values, challenges, openness, and sensitivity. For some, the pain of loss, although diminished, recurs for the rest of their lives.

TYPES OF GRIEF RESPONSES A normal grief reaction may be abbreviated or anticipatory. *Abbreviated grief* is brief but genuinely felt. This can occur when the lost object is not significantly important to the grieving person or may have been replaced immediately by another equally esteemed object. **Anticipatory grief** is experienced in advance of the event, such as the wife who grieves before her ailing husband dies. A young girl may grieve in advance of an operation that will leave a scar on her body. Because many of the normal symptoms of grief will have been expressed during the anticipation, the reaction when the loss actually occurs is sometimes quite abbreviated.

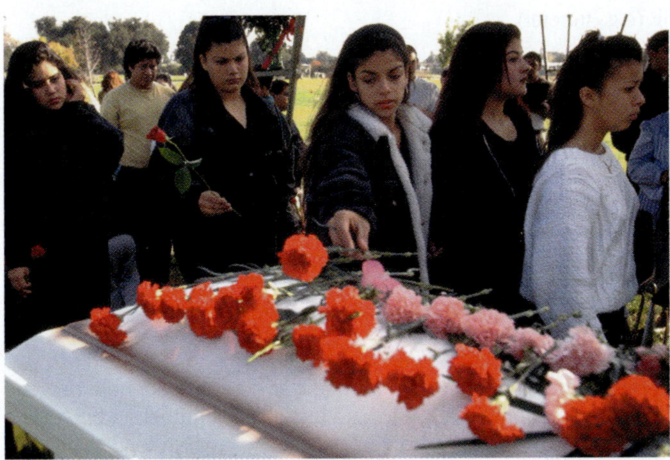

Figure 12–2 ■ Hispanic teenagers lay red carnations on the casket of the victim of a drive-by shooting.

Source: PhotoEdit Inc.

THEORIES RELATED TO GRIEVING Many authors have described stages or phases of grieving. Perhaps the most well-known theory was presented by Kübler-Ross (1969), who described five stages: denial, anger, bargaining, depression, and acceptance (Table 12–1). Engel (1964) identified six stages of grieving: shock and disbelief, developing awareness, restitution, resolving the loss, idealization, and outcome (Table 12–2). Sanders (1998) described five phases of bereavement: shock, awareness, conservation/withdrawal, healing, and renewal (Table 12–3).

Martocchio (1985) described five clusters of grief—shock and disbelief; yearning and protest; anguish, disorganization, and despair; identification in bereavement; and reorganization and restitutio—and maintained that there is no single correct way (or correct timetable) by which a person progresses through the grief process. Whether a person can succeed in integrating the loss and how this is accomplished are related to that person's individual development and personal makeup. In addition, individuals responding to the very same loss cannot be expected to follow the same pattern or schedule in resolving their grief, even while they support each other.

Rando (1991, 1993, 2000) has written extensively on the subject of grief, describing three categories of responses: avoidance, confrontation, and accommodation. Avoidance is similar to Kübler-Ross's phases of denial, anger, and bargaining and to Engel's phase of shock and disbelief. Confrontation is the most upsetting phase for the grieving person facing the loss. Accommodation is the phase in which the person begins to resume more usual activities, feels better, and places the loss in perspective.

MANIFESTATIONS OF GRIEF

Following a loss, the nurse assesses the grieving client or family members to determine the phase or stage of grieving. Physiologically, the body responds to a current or anticipated loss with a stress reaction. The nurse can assess the clinical signs of this response as discussed in Concept 28, Stress and Coping.

Manifestations of grief that are considered normal include verbalization of the loss, crying, sleep disturbance, loss of appetite, and difficulty concentrating. **Complicated grief** may be characterized by extended time of denial, impairment of functioning, depression, severe physiologic symptoms, or suicidal thoughts.

Factors Influencing the Loss and Grief Responses

A number of factors affect a person's response to a loss or death. These include age, significance of the loss, culture, spiritual beliefs, gender, socioeconomic status, support systems, and the cause of the loss or death. Nurses can learn general concepts about how these factors influence the grieving experience, but their makeup and significance vary from individual to individual.

TABLE 12–1 Client Responses and Nursing Implications in Kübler-Ross's Stages of Grieving

STAGE	BEHAVIORAL RESPONSES	NURSING IMPLICATIONS
Denial	Client refuses to believe that loss is happening. Client is not ready to deal with practical problems, such as a prosthesis after the loss of a leg. Client may assume artificial cheerfulness to prolong denial.	Verbally support client but do not reinforce denial. Examine your own behavior to ensure that you do not share in client's denial.
Anger	Client and/or family may direct anger at nurse or staff about matters that normally would not bother them.	Help client understand that anger is a normal response to feelings of loss and powerlessness. Avoid withdrawal or retaliation; do not take anger personally. Deal with needs underlying any angry reaction. Provide structure and continuity to promote feelings of security. Allow clients as much control as possible over their lives.
Bargaining	Client seeks to bargain to avoid loss. May express feelings of guilt or fear of punishment for past sins, real or imagined.	Listen attentively and encourage client to talk to relieve guilt and irrational fear. If appropriate, offer spiritual support.
Depression	Client grieves over what has happened and what cannot be. Client may talk freely (e.g., reviewing past losses such as money or job) or may withdraw.	Allow client to express sadness. Communicate nonverbally by sitting quietly without expecting conversation. Convey caring by touch.
Acceptance	Client comes to terms with loss. Client may have decreased interest in surroundings and support people. Client may want to begin making plans (e.g., will, prosthesis, altered living arrangements).	Help family and friends understand client's decreased need to socialize. Encourage client to participate as much as possible in the treatment program.

TABLE 12–2 Engel's Stages of Grieving

STAGE	BEHAVIORAL RESPONSES
Shock and disbelief	Refuses to accept loss. Has stunned feelings. Accepts the situation intellectually, but denies it emotionally.
Developing awareness	Reality of loss begins to penetrate consciousness. Anger may be directed at agency, nurses, or others.
Restitution	Conducts rituals of mourning (e.g., funeral). Resolves the loss. Attempts to deal with painful void. Still unable to accept new love object to replace lost person or object. May accept more dependent relationship with support person. Thinks over and talks about memories of the lost object.
Idealization	Produces image of lost object that is almost devoid of undesirable features. Represses all negative and hostile feelings toward lost object. May feel guilty and remorseful about past inconsiderate or unkind acts to lost person. Unconsciously internalizes admired qualities of lost object. Reminders of lost object evoke fewer feelings of sadness. Reinvests feelings in others.
Outcome	Behavior is influenced by several factors: importance of lost object as source of support, degree of dependence on relationship, degree of ambivalence toward lost object, number and nature of other relationships, and number and nature of previous grief experiences (which tend to be cumulative).

Note: From Engel, G. L. (1964). Grief and Grieving. *American Journal of Nursing, 64*(9), 93–98. Copyright © Lippincott, Williams & Wilkins. Adapted with permission.

TABLE 12–3 **Sander's Phases of Bereavement**

PHASE	DESCRIPTION	BEHAVIORAL RESPONSES
Shock	Survivors are left with feelings of confusion, unreality, and disbelief that the loss has occurred. They are often unable to process the normal thought sequences. Phase may last from a few minutes to many days.	Disbelief. Confusion. Restlessness. Feelings of unreality. Regression and helplessness. State of alarm. Physical symptoms: dryness of mouth and throat, sighing, weeping, loss of muscular control, uncontrolled trembling, sleep disturbance, and loss of appetite. Psychologic symptoms: preoccupation with thoughts of the deceased and psychologic distancing.
Awareness of loss	Friends and family resume normal activities. The bereaved experience the full significance of their loss.	Separation anxiety. Conflicts. Acting out emotional expectations. Prolonged stress. Physical symptoms: crying and sleep disturbance. Psychologic symptoms: anger, guilt, frustration, shame, oversensitivity, disbelief and denial, dreaming, sense of presence of the deceased, and fear of death.
Conservation/ withdrawal	During this phase, survivors feel a need to be alone to conserve and replenish both physical and emotional energy. The social support available to the bereaved has decreased, and they may experience despair and helplessness.	Physical symptoms: weakness, fatigue, need for more sleep, and a weakened immune system. Psychologic symptoms: withdrawal, obsessional review, grief work, and ultimately a renewal of hope.
Healing: the turning point	During this phase, the bereaved move from distress about living without their loved one to learning to live more independently.	Assuming control. Identity restructuring. Relinquishing roles, such as spouse, child, or parent. Physical symptoms: increased energy, sleep restoration, immune system restoration, and physical healing. Psychologic symptoms: forgiving, forgetting, searching for meaning, and hope.
Renewal	In this phase, survivors move on to a new self-awareness, an acceptance of responsibility for self, and learning to live without the loved one.	Functional stability. Revitalization. Assumption of responsibility for self-care needs. Psychologic symptoms: loneliness, anniversary reactions, and a reaching out to others.

Note: Sanders, C. M. (1998). *Grief: The mourning after: Dealing with adult bereavement* (2nd ed.). New York: John Wiley & Sons. Reprinted with permission.

AGE Age affects a person's understanding of and reaction to loss. With familiarity, people usually increase their understanding and acceptance of life, loss, and death.

People do not usually experience the loss of loved ones at regular intervals. As a result, preparing for these experiences is difficult. Coping with other losses, such as the loss of a pet, the loss of a friend, and the loss of youth or a job, can help people anticipate the more severe loss of death of loved ones by teaching them successful coping strategies.

Childhood Children differ from adults not only in how they understand loss and death, but also in how they are affected by the loss of others. The loss of a parent or another significant person can threaten the child's ability to develop, sometimes resulting in regression. Assisting the child with the grief experience includes helping the child regain the normal continuity and pace of emotional development.

Some adults assume that children do not have the same need as adults to grieve the loss of others. In situations of crisis and loss, children are sometimes pushed aside or protected from the pain. They can feel afraid, abandoned, and lonely. Careful work with bereaved children is especially necessary because experiencing a loss in childhood can have serious effects later in life (Figure 12–3 ■).

Early and Middle Adulthood As people grow, they come to experience loss as part of normal development. By middle age, for example, the loss of a parent through death seems a more normal occurrence compared to the death of a young person. Coping with the death of an aged parent has even been viewed as an essential developmental task of the middle-aged adult.

The middle-aged adult can experience losses other than death. For example, losses resulting from impaired health or body function and losses of various role functions can be

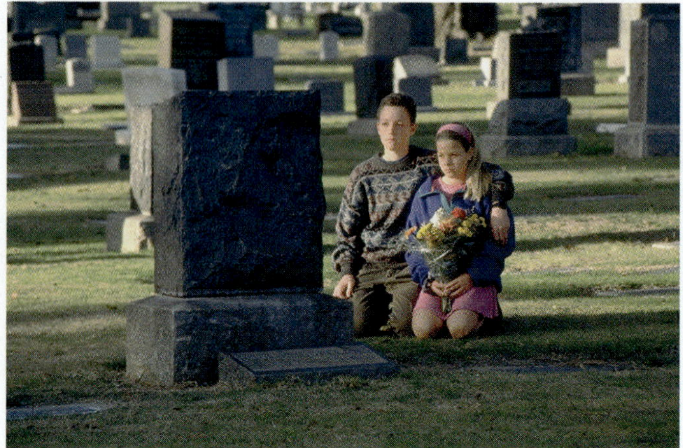

Figure 12–3 ■ Children experience the same emotions of grief as adults do.

difficult to accept. How the middle-aged adult responds to such losses is influenced by previous experiences with loss, the individual's sense of self-esteem and coping mechanisms, and the strength and availability of support.

Late Adulthood Losses experienced by older adults include loss of health, mobility, independence, and work role. Limited income and the need to change one's living accommodations also can lead to feelings of loss and grieving.

For older adults, the loss through death of a longtime mate is profound. Although individuals differ in their ability to deal with such loss, research suggests that health problems for widows and widowers increase following the death of the spouse (Caserta, Lund, & Obray, 2004). Because the majority of deaths occur among elderly people and because the number of elderly people is increasing in North America, nurses need to be alert to the potential problems of older grieving adults.

SIGNIFICANCE OF THE LOSS The significance of a loss depends on the perceptions of the individual experiencing the loss. One person may experience a great sense of loss over a divorce; another may find it only mildly disrupting. The following factors affect the significance of the loss:

- Importance of the lost person, object, or function
- Degree of change required because of the loss
- The person's beliefs and values.

For older adults who have already encountered many losses, an anticipated loss such as their own death may not be viewed as highly negative; they may be apathetic about it instead of reactive. More than fearing death, some fear losing control or becoming a burden.

CULTURE Culture influences an individual's reaction to loss. How grief is expressed is often determined by customs. Unless an extended family structure exists, grief is handled by the nuclear family. The death of a family member in a small nuclear family typically leaves a great void because the same few individuals fill most of the roles. In cultures where several generations and extended family members reside in the same household or within close proximity, the impact of a family member's death may be softened because the roles of the deceased are quickly filled by other relatives.

Some people have adopted the belief that grief is a private matter to be endured internally. Therefore, feelings tend to be repressed and may remain unidentified. People who have been socialized to "be strong" and "make the best of the situation" may not express deep feelings or personal concerns when they experience a serious loss.

Some cultural groups value social support and the expression of loss. In some groups, expressions of grief through wailing, crying, and other outward expressions are acceptable and encouraged. Other groups may frown on this demonstration as a loss of control, favoring a more quiet and stoic expression of grief. In cultural groups where strong kinship ties are maintained, physical and emotional support and assistance are provided by family members.

SPIRITUAL BELIEFS Spiritual beliefs and practices greatly influence an individual's reaction to loss and subsequent behavior. Most religious groups have practices related to dying, which are often important to the dying client and support people. To provide support at a time of death, nurses need to understand the client's beliefs and practices. See the following Focus on Diversity and Culture and Table 12–4 for more information on diverse cultural and spiritual perspectives about death and dying.

GENDER The gender roles into which many people are socialized in the United States and Canada affect their reactions at times of loss. Men are frequently expected to "be strong" and to show very little emotion during grief, whereas it is acceptable for women to show grief by crying. Often when a wife dies, the husband, who is the chief mourner, is expected to repress his own emotions and to comfort sons and daughters in their grieving.

FOCUS ON DIVERSITY AND CULTURE Diverse Perspectives on Death

Cultural differences are important to consider when working with families dealing with the death of a loved one. Examples of differences include the following (Dratler, Burns, & Dratler, 2006):

- African Americans often place great importance on the presence of their families and the expression of emotions. They value shared decision making between the patient and family members. Many African Americans value suffering as a meaningful spiritual experience.
- Asian families often want to protect the terminally ill from knowing about their condition. So decisions are usually made by family members. They often prefer aggressive treatments.
- In some Filipino cultures, words are considered so powerful that talking about the patient's death is believed to make it happen. As a result, they may refuse to discuss any medical options.
- Hispanics generally believe the family should be responsible for making health care decisions. Faith is very important in times of death. They also believe that death is a natural part of life, and the anniversary of a loved one's death is celebrated every year.

TABLE 12–4 **Spiritual Traditions in Mourning and After-Death Rites**

FAITH-BASED OR SPIRITUAL GROUP	POSSIBLE RITUALS	ORGAN DONATION OR AUTOPSY BELIEFS
Native American	Beliefs and practices vary widely. Navajo do not touch the deceased or their belongings. Body must be as whole as possible for the afterlife.	Organ donation and autopsy vary among tribes.
Buddhism	Last-rite chanting takes place at bedside. Cremation is preferred.	Organ donation is considered an act of mercy; autopsy is an individual choice.
Catholicism	Sacrament of the sick is administered. Obligation exists to take ordinary but not extraordinary means to prolong life. Deceased is buried. Novenas (prayers) are said for 9 days.	Autopsy and organ donation are acceptable.
Christian Science	Medical help is not likely to be sought to prolong life. Family decides how body and parts are disposed.	Organ donation is not acceptable.
Hinduism	There are no restrictions regarding the right-to-die issue. Religious prayers are chanted before and after death. Thread is tied around the wrist to signify a blessing; it is not removed. Body is bathed and massaged in oils, dressed in new clothes, and then cremated. Men and women display outward grief.	Autopsy and organ donation are acceptable.
Islam	Attempts to shorten life are prohibited. Deathbed should be turned to face the northeast, and room may be perfumed. Passages from the Quran are read to the dying patient. Body is washed only by a Muslim of the same gender and is wrapped in a white shroud.	Organ donation is acceptable. Autopsy is acceptable only for medical or legal reasons.
Jehovah's Witness	Use of extraordinary means to prolong life is an individual choice. Burial is determined by family preference.	Autopsy is acceptable if required by law. A decision regarding organ donation is made with input from religious leaders.
Judaism	If death is imminent, there is no need to prolong life. Dying patient should not be left alone. Body is ritually washed, and embalming is prohibited. Burial takes place within 24–48 hours; all body parts must be buried together. There is a 7-day mourning period (shiva).	Autopsy is permitted in certain circumstances. Organ donation may be acceptable.
Mennonite	They do not believe that life must be continued at all cost.	Autopsy and organ donation are acceptable.
Mormonism	If death is inevitable, a peaceful and dignified death is preferred. Deceased is buried in temple clothes.	Autopsy is permitted with permission of next of kin; organ donation is an individual choice.
Protestantism	Burial or cremation is an individual decision.	Organ donation and autopsy are individual decisions.
Seventh-Day Adventist	Prolonging life is preferred.	Disposal of body and burial are individual decisions. Autopsy and organ donation are acceptable.

Source: Adapted from Spector, R. E. (2009). *Cultural diversity in health and illness* (7th ed., pp. 139–142). Upper Saddle River, NJ: Prentice Hall Health; Purnell, L. D., & Paulanka, B. J. (2005). *Guide to culturally competent health care.* Philadelphia: F. A. Davis Company.

Gender roles also affect the significance of changes in body image to clients. A man might consider his facial scar to be "macho," but a woman might consider hers ugly. Thus, the woman would be more likely to see the change as a loss.

SOCIOECONOMIC STATUS The socioeconomic status of an individual often affects the support system available at the time of a loss. A pension plan or insurance, for example, can offer a widowed or disabled person a choice of ways to deal with a loss; a person who is confronted with severe loss and economic hardship may not be able to cope with either.

SUPPORT SYSTEM The people closest to the grieving individual are often the first to recognize and provide needed emotional, physical, and functional assistance. However, because many people are uncomfortable or inexperienced in dealing with loss, the usual support people may withdraw from the grieving individual. In addition, support may be available when the loss first occurs, but as the support people return to their usual activities, the grieving person's need for ongoing support may go unmet. Sometimes the grieving individual is unable or unready to accept support when it is offered.

CAUSE OF LOSS OR DEATH Individual and societal views on the cause of a loss or death may significantly influence the grief response. Some diseases, such as cardiovascular disorders, are considered "clean" and engender compassion, whereas others may be viewed as repulsive and less unfortunate. A loss or death that is beyond the control of those involved may be more acceptable than one that is preventable, such as a drunk driving accident. Injuries or deaths occurring during respected activities, such as "in the line of duty," are considered honorable, whereas those occurring during illicit activities may be considered the individual's just rewards.

ALTERATIONS

Disenfranchised grief occurs when a person is unable to acknowledge the loss to other people. Situations in which this occurs often relate to a socially unacceptable loss that cannot be spoken about, such as committing suicide, having an abortion, or giving up a child for adoption. Other examples include losses of relationships that are socially unsanctioned and may not be known to other people (such as homosexuality or extramarital affairs).

Complicated grief exists when the strategies to cope with the loss are maladaptive. Many factors can contribute to complicated grief, including a prior traumatic loss, family or cultural barriers to the emotional expression of grief, sudden death, strained relationships between the survivor and the deceased, and lack of adequate support for the survivor (Egan & Arnold, 2003).

Complicated grief may take several forms. *Unresolved or chronic grief* is extended in length and severity. The same signs are expressed as with normal grief, but the bereaved also may have difficulty expressing the grief, may deny the loss, or may grieve beyond the expected time. With *inhibited grief*, many of the normal symptoms of grief are suppressed and other effects, including somatic, are experienced instead. *Delayed grief* occurs when feelings are purposely or subconsciously suppressed until a much later time. A survivor who appears to be using dangerous activities as a method to lessen the pain of grieving may be experiencing *exaggerated grief*. Complicated grief that continues beyond 2 years after the death is considered *pathological grief*.

Complicated grief after a death may be inferred, based on cultural beliefs, from the following data or observations:

- The client fails to grieve; for example, a husband does not cry at or absents himself from his wife's funeral.
- The client avoids visiting the grave and refuses to participate in memorial services even though these practices are a part of the client's culture.
- The client becomes recurrently symptomatic on the anniversary of a loss or during holidays.
- The client develops persistent guilt and lowered self-esteem.
- Even after a prolonged period, the client continues to search for the lost person. Some may consider suicide to effect reunion.
- A relatively minor event triggers symptoms of grief.
- Even after a period of time, the client is unable to discuss the deceased with composure; for example, the client's voice cracks and quivers and eyes become moist.
- After the normal period of grief, the client experiences physical symptoms similar to those of the person who died.
- The client's relationships with friends and relatives worsen following the death.

Many factors contribute to unresolved grief after a death:

- Ambivalence (intense feelings, both positive and negative) toward the lost person
- A perceived need to be brave and in control; fear of losing control in front of others
- Endurance of multiple losses, such as the loss of an entire family, which the bereaved finds too overwhelming to contemplate
- Extremely high emotional value invested in the dead person; failure to grieve in this instance helps the bereaved avoid the reality of the loss
- Uncertainty about the loss—for example, when a loved one is missing in action
- Lack of support systems.

NURSING PROCESS

While the nursing process is individualized to the client, some aspects of the nursing process are valuable to any client experiencing grief and loss, regardless of the client's age, culture, or background. To tailor the nursing process, the nurse takes into consideration the grieving client's cognitive and developmental level, cultural background, and family and financial support systems.

Assessment

Nursing assessment of the client experiencing a loss includes three major components: (1) nursing history, (2) assessment of personal coping resources (Box 12–1), and (3) physical assessment. During the routine health assessment of every client, the nurse poses questions regarding previous and current losses. The nurse must explore the nature and significance of the loss to the client.

If there is a current or recent loss, greater detail is needed in the assessment. Because clients do not always associate physical ailments with emotional responses such as grief, the nurse may need to probe to identify possible loss-related stresses. If the client reports significant losses, it is important to examine how the client usually copes with loss and what resources are available to assist the client in coping. Data regarding general health status; other personal stressors; cultural and spiritual traditions, rituals, and beliefs related to loss and grieving; and the person's support network are needed to determine a plan of care. (See the following Assessment Interview.) In assessing the client's response to a current loss, the nurse may identify complicated grief best treated by a

Box 12–1 Grieving Assessment: Personal Coping Resources

CLIENT
- *Knowledge:* Client's understanding of the implications of the loss
- *Self-care abilities:* Skill in caring for self based on physical abilities that may have been altered or affected by the loss (for example, if a caregiver died, determine to what extent that person was responsible for assisting the client with ADLs)
- *Current coping:* Stage in the grieving or bereavement process
- *Current manifestations of the grief response:* Adaptive or maladaptive signs and symptoms; cultural or spiritually based behaviors
- *Role expectations:* Client's perception of the need to return to work or family roles

FAMILY
- *Knowledge:* Various family members' perception of the loss
- *Support people's availability and skills:* Sensitivity to the client's emotional and physical needs; ability to provide an accepting environment; ability to provide assistance with ADLs (if needed)
- *Role expectations:* Family perception of client's need to return to work or family roles

COMMUNITY
- *Resources:* Availability and familiarity with possible sources of assistance (e.g., grief support groups, religious or spiritual centers, counseling services, and physical care providers)

health care professional who is an expert in assisting such clients. If the nursing assessment reveals severe physical or psychologic signs and symptoms, the client should be referred to an appropriate care provider.

Communication with grieving clients needs to be relevant to their stage of grief. Whether the client is angry or depressed affects how the client hears messages and how the nurse interprets the client's statements.

Diagnosis

Nursing diagnoses (NANDA International, 2007) relating specifically to grieving include the following:

- *Grieving:* A normal complex process that includes emotional, physical, spiritual, social, and intellectual responses and behaviors by which individuals, families, and communities incorporate an actual, anticipated, or perceived loss into their daily lives.
- *Complicated Grieving:* A disorder that occurs after the death of a significant other in which the experience of distress accompanying bereavement fails to follow normative expectations and manifests in functional impairment. *Risk for Complicated Grieving* replaced *Risk for Dysfunctional Grieving* in 2007, which had been added as a new diagnosis in 2005.

Other nursing diagnoses may include:

- *Interrupted Family Processes:* The loss has such impact on the individual and family that usual effective roles and interactions are negatively affected.
- *Risk-prone Health Behavior:* The client has great difficulty placing the loss in a perspective that is appropriate for his or her other life activities.
- *Risk for Loneliness:* The death of a significant other is related to the loss of relationships with others.

Plan

The client's plan of care is tailored to the nature of the loss and the clients cognitive and developmental level. The plan of care may include family, social, or financial supports.

Assessment Interview Loss and Grieving

PREVIOUS LOSSES
- Have you ever lost someone or something very important to you?
- Have you or your family ever moved to a new home or location?
- What was it like for you when you first started school? Moved away from home? Got a job? Retired?
- Are you physically able to do all of the things you used to do?
- Has anyone important or close to you died?
- Do you think there will be any losses in your life in the near future?

If there has been previous grieving:
- Tell me about (the loss). What was losing __________ like for you?
- Did you have trouble sleeping? Eating? Concentrating?
- What kinds of things did you do to make yourself feel better when something like that happened?
- Did you observe any spiritual or cultural practices when you had a loss like that?
- Whom did you turn to when you were very upset about (the loss)?
- How long did it take you to feel more like yourself again and go back to your usual activities?

If there is a current loss:
- What have you been told about (the loss)? Is there anything else you would like to know or don't understand?
- What changes do you think this (illness, surgery, problem) will cause in your life? What do you think it will be like without (the lost object)?
- Have you ever experienced a loss like this before?
- Can you think of anything good that might come of this?
- What kind of help do you think you will need? Who is going to be helping you with this loss?
- Are there any people or organizations in your community that might be able to help?

CURRENT GRIEVING
- Are you having trouble sleeping? Eating? Concentrating? Breathing?
- Do you have any pain or other new physical problems?
- What are you doing to help yourself deal with this loss?
- Are you taking any drugs or medications to help you cope with this loss?

The overall goals for clients who are grieving the loss of body function or a body part may include the following:

- Client looks at body part
- Client participates in learning self-care related to the change in body function
- Client participates in rehabilitation.

The goals for clients who are grieving the loss of a loved one or thing may include the following:

- Client remembers the deceased loved one without feeling intense pain
- Client redirects emotional energy into own life
- Client demonstrates adjustment to the actual or impending loss.

Implementation

The skills most relevant to situations of loss and grief are listening attentively, using open and closed questioning, paraphrasing, clarifying and reflecting feelings, and summarizing. *Presencing*, the act of just being with the client, is also a helpful skill; presencing is discussed in greater detail in Concept 27, Spirituality. Responses that give advice and evaluation, that interpret and analyze, and that give unwarranted reassurance are less helpful. To ensure effective communication, the nurse must make an accurate assessment of what is appropriate for the client.

In addition to using effective communication skills, the nurse implements a plan to provide client and family teaching and to help the client work through the stages of grief.

Facilitating Grief Work

To assist the client with the grief process, the nurse should do the following:

- Explore and respect the client's and family's ethnic, cultural, religious, and personal values in their expressions of grief.
- Teach the client or family what to expect in the grief process, including that certain thoughts and feelings are normal (acceptable) and that labile emotions, feelings of sadness, guilt, anger, fear, and loneliness, will stabilize or lessen over time. Knowing what to expect may lessen the intensity of some reactions.
- Encourage the client to express and share grief with support people. Sharing feelings reinforces relationships and facilitates the grief process.
- Teach family members to encourage the client's expression of grief and not to push the client to move on or enforce their own expectations of appropriate reactions. If the client is a child, encourage family members to be truthful and to allow the child to participate in mourning rituals and in the grieving activities of others.
- Encourage the client to resume normal activities on a schedule that promotes physical and psychologic health. Some clients may try to return to normal activities too quickly. However, a prolonged delay in return may indicate complicated grieving.

Providing Emotional Support

To provide emotional support to the client or family, nurses should do the following:

- Use silence and personal presence along with techniques of therapeutic communication. These techniques enhance exploration of feelings and let clients know that the nurse acknowledges their feelings.
- Acknowledge the grief of the client's family and significant others. Family members and support people are part of the grieving client's world.
- Offer choices that promote client autonomy. Clients need to have a sense of some control over their own lives at a time when much control may not be possible.
- Provide appropriate information regarding how to access community resources: clergy, support groups, and counseling services.
- Suggest additional sources of information and help, such as
  a. **Hospice** organizations, which provide both physical and psychological care for the dying client and family,
  b. The Grief Recovery Institute,
  c. Partnership for Caring: America's Voice for the Dying,
  d. the American Association of Retired Persons, and
  e. Compassionate Friends (for those who have lost a child).

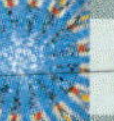

EVIDENCE-BASED PRACTICE Is There a Better Way to Treat Complicated Grief?

This study compared standard treatment for complicated grief interpersonal psychotherapy (IPT) with a new method—complicated grief treatment (CGT). The research was prompted by the fact that complicated grief is a debilitating disorder associated with important negative health consequences but that the results of existing treatments have been disappointing. A total of 83 women and 12 men aged 18–85 recruited from a university-based psychiatric research clinic as well as a satellite clinic in a low-income African American community were randomly assigned to receive IPT (n = 46) or CGT (n = 49). Each participant received 16 sessions over about 19 weeks. IPT focuses on restoring effective interpersonal functioning of the grieving person. CGT has greater emphasis on reviewing the loss, coping with depression, and facing difficult situations. Both treatments produced improvement in complicated grief symptoms. The improvement was statistically significantly better and faster for CGT than for IPT.

Implications

The "gold standard" in research is the randomized clinical trial. This study is reported to be the first of its kind to examine a population of people experiencing complicated grief. Although CGT was more effective than the standard, it still achieved results in only half the participants. Thus, the study provides evidence that one treatment may be more beneficial than another, but more research is needed to identify truly effective treatment for a broad population. The nurse may use these results to recommend that clients experiencing complicated grief may achieve greater resolution of symptoms with CGT if IPT has not been successful.

Note: From "Shear, K., Frank, E., Houck, P. R., & Reynolds, C. F. (2005). Treatment of complicated grief: A randomized controlled trial. *Journal of the American Medical Association, 293,* 2601–2608.

Evaluation

Evaluating the effectiveness of nursing care of the grieving client is difficult because of the long-term nature of the life transition. Criteria for evaluation must be based on goals set by the client and family.

Client goals and related desired outcomes for a grieving client will depend on the characteristics of the loss and the client. If outcomes are not achieved, the nurse needs to explore why the plan was unsuccessful. Such exploration begins with reassessing the client in case the nursing diagnoses were inappropriate. The following are examples of questions guiding the exploration.

- Do the client's grieving behaviors indicate dysfunctional grieving or another nursing diagnosis?
- Is the expected outcome unrealistic for the given time frame?
- Does the client have additional stressors previously not considered that are affecting grief resolution?
- Have nursing orders been implemented consistently, compassionately, and genuinely?

The work of grieving is some of the most difficult emotional work that people do. It can have serious consequences on physical health. Imagine the young child whose mother has died suddenly starting to wet the bed or the octogenarian in an assisted living center who recently lost her husband of 40 years suddenly complaining of unexplained chronic pain. Regardless of the client and the nature of the grief, the nurse is in an excellent position to determine the effects of grieving on the client and to help the client transition through the grieving process.

12.1 CHILDREN'S RESPONSE TO LOSS

KEY TERM

Death anxiety, *613*

BASIS FOR SELECTION OF EXEMPLAR

Standards of Nursing Practice

LEARNING OUTCOMES

After reading about this exemplar, you will be able to:

1. Apply knowledge of development to the pediatric client's understanding of, and response to, grief, loss, and death.
2. Contrast cultural differences in the child's response to and display of grief and loss.
3. Formulate a nursing plan of care for the child grieving common losses experienced in childhood.
4. Develop a nursing plan of care for the family anticipating the loss of the pediatric client.
5. Select appropriate nursing diagnoses for the pediatric client and family coping with loss and grief.
6. Relate appropriate nursing goals for the pediatric client and family coping with loss and grief.
7. Demonstrate appropriate nursing interventions when caring for the pediatric client coping with loss and grief.
8. Assess expected outcomes from which to evaluate the pediatric client's progress through the grieving process.

OVERVIEW

Children, even very young children, experience grief and loss. The nurse caring for the child and family experiencing death, loss, and grief must consider the personal, ethical, legal, spiritual, cultural, and biologic influences on these individuals. This enables the nurse to provide supportive and sensitive care to the child and family and assist them through the grieving process.

Sources of loss for children may include:

- Loss of a loved one (e.g., parent, sibling, grandparent, friend, child care provider, pet)
- Loss of an aspect of oneself, such as a body part or function (e.g., amputation, organ failure, hearing or vision loss)
- Loss of an object (e.g., favorite toy)
- Separation from an accustomed environment (e.g., relocation to new neighborhood or new school).

THE CHILD'S EXPERIENCE WITH DEATH AND LOSS

For children, major losses associated with death include the death of a parent, death of a grandparent, death of a sibling, and death of a friend. Children also experience loss through a myriad of circumstances not related to the death of a person, including parental separation or divorce, loss of a pet, loss of a possession, and relocation. The significance of the loss to the child determines the amount and type of grieving the child experiences. Children differ from adults in their understanding of loss and death but, like adults, they miss the loved one who died. Their understanding and behavioral responses vary according to their developmental level and their previous experience with loss and death (Table 12–5).

Death of a Parent

In the United States, 1 in every 20 children will experience the death of one or both parents (Kirwin & Hamrin, 2005). The death of a parent is an extremely traumatic event for a child, and it has significant impact on the child's self-concept, health, and social and economic circumstances. All children who have lost a parent experience emotional distress, but some internalize their feelings. Internalizing those feelings may lead to insomnia, learning problems, and health issues such as headaches and abdominal pain.

The child's reaction to the death of a parent is greatly influenced by the manner in which the surviving parent reacts to the death and supports the child. When the bereaved parent is grieving the loss of a spouse, parenting responsibilities may be

TABLE 12–5 The Child's Developmental Understanding of Death, Potential Behaviors, and Nursing Considerations

UNDERSTANDING OF DEATH	POTENTIAL BEHAVIORS	NURSING MANAGEMENT
Infant		
Cognitive Stage: Sensorimotor Perceives death as separation and abandonment. Senses disruption in home, tenseness of caregivers, and altered routines. Senses separation.	Resists cuddling or clings more than usual. Protests and shows despair from disruption in caretaking. Has problems feeding. Cries excessively. Sleeps more than usual.	■ Provide a sense of security by being with the infant or child and by holding and hugging him or her. ■ Verbally tell the infant or child you will be there to provide care. ■ Try to return to usual routines. ■ Be tolerant of regressive behaviors.
Toddler		
Cognitive Stage: Preoperational Has no understanding of true concept of death. Is aware someone is missing; separation anxiety. Is unable to distinguish death from temporary separation or abandonment	Regresses to younger stage of development. Is clingy and whiny, cries. Refuses to let surviving parent out of sight, is fearful. Shows distress by biting, hitting, crying. Has problems eating and sleeping. Alternates between grieving behavior and playing behavior. May have more physical illnesses.	■ Encourage parent to hold and cuddle the toddler to help reduce the fear of separation. ■ Follow familiar routines. ■ Be tolerant of regressive behaviors. ■ Talk and answer questions in terms the child will understand.
Preschooler		
Cognitive Stage: Preoperational Believes death is temporary and the dead person will return. May see death as punishment. Believes bad thoughts cause death. Displays magical thinking (believes the dead person can be brought back to life or that he or she is the cause of death). Has beginning experience with death of animals and plants.	Regresses to younger stage of development, has problems with bowel and bladder control, throws tantrums. Uses play activities to cope with strong feelings. Asks when deceased will come back. May fear going to sleep, has nightmares, is afraid of dark. Has crying spells. Seems morbidly fascinated with death. Asks many questions. Complains of abdominal pain.	■ Listen to the child and answer questions honestly. ■ Try to return to usual routines and provide reassurance that you will be with the child. ■ Be understanding and nonjudgmental about regression in developmental tasks. ■ Keep memories alive with pictures and other things that remind the child of the loved one. ■ Participate in rituals such as going to the cemetery, releasing helium balloons, and planting flowers. ■ Provide play activities.
School-Age Child		
Cognitive Stage: Concrete Operations Understands difference between temporary separation and death. By 6–9 years, understands that death is permanent. May have magical thinking about death, such as death is a person like the grim reaper, or think that death is contagious. May have guilt or assume blame for the death. May not realize that death can occur at any age.	Shows regressive behaviors when under stress. Has angry outbursts, disruptive behaviors. Fears being abandoned and fears death of others, worries about surviving family members. May refuse to go to school. Cries, is moody, may become more withdrawn and distant. May try to comfort parents by taking over tasks. May deny sadness by hiding tears and acting more like adults to seem less different than peers Shows decreased concentration for school work. Has psychosomatic complaints—stomachache or headache.	■ Listen to the child and answer questions honestly. ■ Return to usual routines and activities. ■ Keep memories alive through activities such as art, music, a memory book, a quilt, and a garden. ■ Share Internet resources. ■ Use coping support groups. ■ Encourage family to seek faith-based support.
Adolescent		
Cognitive Stage: Formal Operations Is intellectually capable of understanding death. Recognizes that all people and self must die. Has a better grasp of association between illness and death. Is conflicted about sense of invincibility and fear of death. Is able to recognize effect of death on others.	Uses abstract and philosophic reasoning. May seek comfort from friends (girls). Displays mood swings, withdraws from friends. Has problems eating and sleeping. May feel angry or guilty. Displays acting-out or risk-taking behavior, delinquency, suicide attempts, inappropriate sexual behaviors, drug or alcohol use.	■ Be available and foster open communication. ■ Share your own grief and feelings with the adolescent. ■ Keep memories alive with pictures and other things that remind the teen of the loved one. ■ Access counseling and support groups. ■ Share Internet resources. ■ Encourage the child to seek faith-based support.

Source: Data from Hinds, P. S., Oakes, L. L., Hicks, J., & Anghelescu, D. L. (2005). End-of-life care for children and adolescents. *Seminars in Oncologic Nursing, 21*(1), 53–62; Kirwin, K. M., & Havrin, V. (2005). Decreasing the risk of complicated bereavement and future psychiatric disorders in children. *Journal of Child and Adolescent Psychiatric Nursing, 18*(2), 62–78; Auman, M. J. (2007). Bereavement support for children. *Journal of School Nursing, 23*(1), 34–39; and Korones, D. N. (2007). Pediatric palliative care. *Pediatrics in Review, 28*(8), e46–e56.

overwhelming. As with adults, the death of a parent changes the life of the child forever. Children do not quickly bounce back after the death of a parent. Children need continued support, understanding, and counseling over time to prevent negative complications of grief.

Additional losses for the child may occur as the result of a parent's death. The death may bring about relocation or a change in living arrangements. For example, the child may have to live with a noncustodial parent, a grandparent, or another extended family member. The family's financial status may change as a result of the loss of a wage earner. Older children may be expected to assume more responsibility for the home or younger siblings, allowing them less time with peers and recreational activities.

Death of a Grandparent

The death of a grandparent is often the first experience a child has with the death of a significant individual. The child's grandparent may have had a special role in the development of the child's understanding of trust, love, and belonging. With an understanding of a grandparent's death, the child also may come to the realization that his or her parents will die as well.

PRACTICE ALERT

Communicating with children about death is often a difficult task for parents. Because the words used to describe death may vary by culture, nurses should learn the terminology that cultural groups use in their community. Parents and other adults should avoid euphemisms such as "she has gone to sleep" because this may confuse children and hinder their understanding of the finality of death. Parents and health care providers should not be afraid to use the word *death* or *dead* when explaining these concepts to children. After discussing death with children, adults should always provide them with the opportunity to ask questions and express their feelings.

The child's reaction to the loss of a grandparent depends on the significance of the grandparent to the child. In many families and cultures, grandparents are important influences in the child's life. Children may be raised by a grandparent, they may be cared for by a grandparent while the parents work, or they may reside in the same household with the grandparent. Grandparents are often a child's link to his or her heritage through the grandparents' storytelling and sharing of family history. Therefore, the influence of the grandparent on the child may have considerable meaning to the child, and the impact of a grandparent's death may be as significant as the death of a parent.

Death of a Friend

Children may experience the death of a friend due to a chronic condition, an acute illness, or an injury. Because children with chronic and life-threatening conditions are living longer and are better able to attend school and engage in social activities, they are likely to develop close friendships with other children. The childhood friends and schoolmates of chronically ill children should be prepared for the potential death according to their developmental level. When a friend dies suddenly, such as through violence or unintentional injury, there is no time for preparation. Whether the death of a friend was anticipated or sudden, the child experiences the same stages of grief as with other losses. The death of a peer may bring about the first realization that older adults are not the only ones who die. The child's sense of invulnerability may be shaken.

Some schools offer grief support and counseling to provide opportunities for students to express their grief and sadness following the death of a peer. Developing a memorial is often helpful for children. Planting a tree, hanging a plaque, or creating a play area at school in memory of the deceased child helps the child's friends express their grief. (See Table 12–6 for additional resources.)

Other Potentially Significant Losses

For many children, the first significant loss is that of a pet. A pet is often viewed by the child as a source of unconditional love and acceptance. The child typically views a pet as a friend, companion, and member of the family. The child may experience a pet's loss because of death (anticipated or unexpected) or because the pet ran away or was stolen. How the parents and other adults support the child and handle the loss can impact the manner in which the child learns to cope with loss and death later in life.

Parents should offer honest, simple, and developmentally appropriate explanations to help the child understand what happened. Telling a child that because the dog was old and sick, it had to be "put to sleep" may cause anxiety in the 4-year-old about what will happen when he or she sleeps at night. The 8-year-old who is told "God was lonely, so he took Cocoa to live with him" may become concerned about what other possessions God may want.

Suggestions for helping the child cope with the loss of a pet include burying the pet and holding a memorial service, talking about good memories of the pet, planting flowers or a tree in memory of the pet, and creating a scrapbook.

FACTORS INFLUENCING FAMILY RESPONSES TO DEATH AND LOSS

Cultural traditions and practices, spiritual beliefs, and the child's developmental level are central factors that influence a child's and family's response to death and loss. These become even more important when the loss being experienced is the death of the child.

Culture

Recognizing and understanding a family's cultural traditions and practices when it is experiencing the death of a child helps nurses provide individualized care to the dying child and family. Some families, believing that grief is a private matter, may internalize and repress their feelings. Other families may believe that outward demonstrations of

TABLE 12–6 **Books for Children Who Experience the Death of a Family Member or Friend**

BOOK	PUBLISHER	AGE GROUP
A Separate Peace, by John Knowles	New York: MacMillan	12 and up
Blackwater, by Eve Bunting	New York: Harper Collins	12 and up
When a Friend Dies: A Book for Teens About Grieving & Healing, by Marilyn E. Gootman	Minneapolis, MN: Free Spirit Press	12 and up
Bridge to Terabithia, by Katherine Paterson	New York: Harper Collins	10–14
On My Honor, by Marion Dane Bauer	New York: Bantam Doubleday Dell Publishing	8–12
Sunflower Promise, by Kathleen Maresh Hemery	Omaha, NE: Centering Corporation	8–12
Charlotte's Web, by E. B. White	New York: Harper and Row	5–10
Children Also Grieve: Talking About Death and Healing, by Linda Goldman	Philadelphia: Jessica Kingsley	5–10
If Nathan Were Here, by Mary Bahr	Grand Rapids, MI: Eerdmans Books for Young Readers	5–10
Tell Me Papa: Answers to Questions Children Ask About Death and Dying, by Joy Johnson and Dr. Marvin Johnson	Omaha, NE: Centering Corporation	4–10
I Know I Made It Happen: Children and Guilt, by Lynn Blackburn	Omaha, NE: Centering Corporation	4–8
Missing Hannah: Based on a True Story of Sudden Infant Death Syndrome, by Darlene Kane	Bloomington, IN: Author House	4–8

Source: Smith, C. (2005). Death, general: Resource list. Retrieved September 16, 2007, from http://www.nursingconsult.com/das/patient/body/010072/24810.html?preview=t&printing; and National Sudden Infant Death Resource Center. (2006). New additions to the NSIDRC resource library. Retrieved November 10, 2006, from http://www.sidscenter.org. Copyright © 2009 RelayHealth and/or its affiliates. All rights reserved.

grief are acceptable; they may even be encouraged. It is important to note that not all families observe traditional rites and rituals. For more information, see Focus on Diversity and Culture: Diverse Perspectives on Death on page 604.

Faith-Based Beliefs and Spirituality

In providing family-centered care, the nurse should understand that death ceremonies and rituals are based on culture and spiritual beliefs. These are important because they help families prepare for the death and ease the family member's passage to death (Lobar, Youngblut, & Brooten, 2006). Many groups want to keep a vigil to prevent the dying person from being alone; some groups, such as Irish Catholics, maintain a tradition of keeping vigil with the body until the time of burial. Other groups cry loudly and wail as a sign that they care about the dying person.

When dealing with death and dying, faith and spirituality may be a fundamental coping mechanism (Flannelly, Weaver, & Costa, 2004). Faith-based or spiritual leaders may be helpful to families. Most faith groups have specific practices related to death, which may be expressed through prayer, meditation, rituals, worship, music, art, and dance. See Table 12–4 on page 605 for an overview of faith-based traditions in mourning and after-death rites. Faith-based practices also are significant as a means of coping with grief (Figure 12–4 ■). An individual's spiritual beliefs and practices considerably influence his or her reactions to loss and subsequent behavior. It is particularly important that the nurse assess the family's faith or spiritual beliefs when the dying family member is a child.

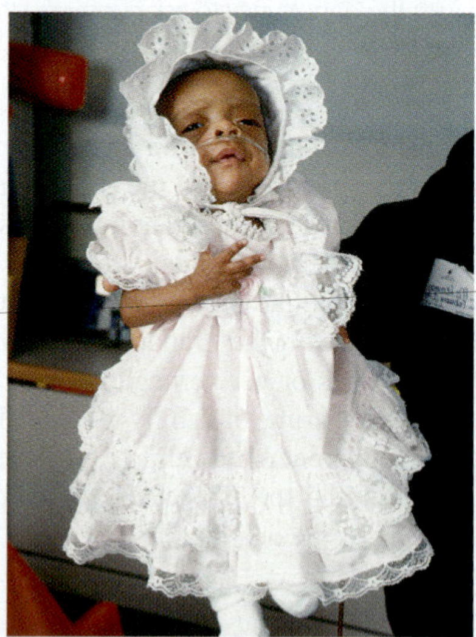

Figure 12–4 ■ Religious rituals such as baptism and the blessing of an ill infant may provide great comfort to the family. When the infant is stable, a traditional baptism may be performed in the home or church with family and friends present. When the infant has a life-threatening illness, baptism may be performed in the hospital by a chaplain or health professional.

Awareness of Dying by Developmental Age

A child's awareness of death develops more rapidly when he or she is experiencing the progression of a disease and related medical treatment. Children with life-threatening illnesses often learn about death and their own illness from exposure to other seriously ill and dying children during hospitalization or clinic visits.

Infants and toddlers are not actually aware of death; they are aware of and react to changes in normal routines and parental nonverbal communication. Toddlers may know that they "feel bad," but they do not understand that their physical symptoms are associated with impending death (Figure 12–5 ■).

Preschool children can see their bodies deteriorate and feel the effects of medications used during disease progression and treatment. Changes in self-concept occur as they perceive these body changes. The preschool child often describes illness in terms of mutilation to the body. The child may realize that he or she is dying because of these physical changes, as well as the reactions of parents and hospital staff.

School-age children also have subtle fears about body integrity and anxieties related to the serious nature of their illness. This greater preoccupation with illness is considered by many professionals as the child's version of **death anxiety**, a feeling of apprehension or fear of death. Children may express death anxiety as a concern with treatments that invade the body or interfere with normal body functions.

Adolescents have a mature understanding of death, but the normal developmental milestones of adolescence add to their challenges in facing a terminal illness. They are struggling to establish their own identity and plans for the future. At a time when body image is extremely important, they may be faced with the possibility of mutilation and disfigurement. Dying adolescents are often isolated from their peers during a period when peers are the most essential social group. Adolescents with terminal illnesses may be angry because they recognize their loss at a time when the whole world is opening up to them.

Adolescents should not be expected to handle feelings the same way adults do. Adolescents often avoid expressing anger, an expected stage of grieving, toward the family by seeking to control and direct these feelings elsewhere. Adolescents often become angry at changes in treatment procedures, lack of explanations, and threats to their independence. As death nears, the adolescent may permit comfort and support and may accept care from warm and loving family members as long as he or she is not treated condescendingly.

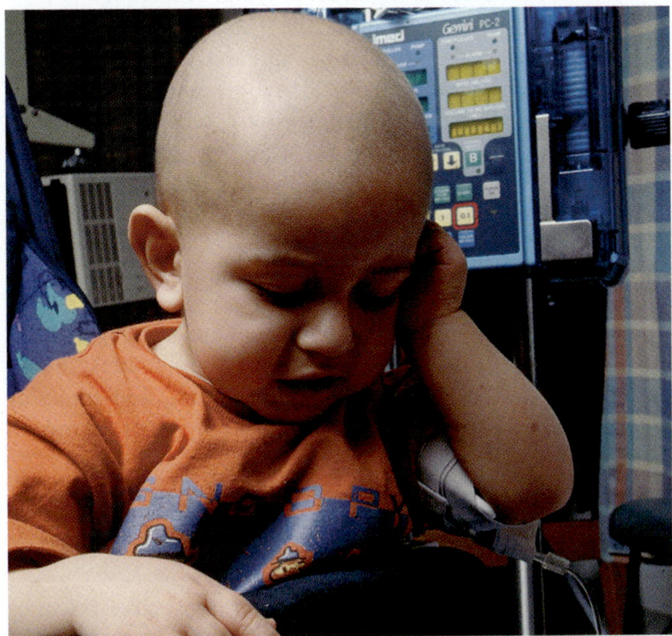

Figure 12–5 ■ The toddler with a life-threatening disorder recognizes that he or she feels bad and that routines are different. His or her anxiety may increase due to the concern and feelings of sadness that his or her parents exhibit.

COLLABORATION

Involvement of family counselors or those who work specifically with children may help the child's and family cope with the loss of a loved one. Family counselors are often used when a child has lost a parent or family member, but they also may by helpful when a child loses a classmate, friend, or teacher. When the loss results from violence, such as school shootings or mass casualty events (e.g., 9/11), grief counselors can help children face the many emotions that develop as well as reduce the impact of post-traumatic stress disorder.

NURSING PROCESS

Whether families are facing a child's illness or the child is to be told about the loss of a loved one, parents often ask the nurse for help in reducing the impact on the child. While parents know their child best, the nurse can provide resources and information to help them break the bad news in a manner consistent with the developmental needs of the child.

Assessment

Nursing assessment of the child's and family's coping with loss includes a psychosocial assessment of all family members, an assessment of cultural and spiritual influences on the child and individual family members, and an assessment of the child's and family's social support system.

Kübler-Ross (1983) noted that children are more fearful of abandonment than death. The terminally ill child is reported to grieve losing function and the future, as well as leaving family members behind in sorrow (Hinds, Schum, Baker, & Wolfe, 2005). The child may feel a "conspiracy of silence" that leads the child to avoid the subject in an attempt to protect the parents from the truth. The child may believe that expressing an awareness of death and related fears will place added emotional burdens on family members. The result is that both parents and child miss the opportunity to share the comfort and love that could make the death more peaceful for all of them. The types of questions children may ask include the following:

- What will death be like? Will I have pain?
- What will happen to me when I die? What happens after I die?
- Will I be punished for the bad things I have done?
- When will I be with [person(s) closest to child] again?
- Will an angel come to take me away? What does heaven look like?
- Will my parents be all right?
- Can you come with me?
- Will you remember me?

Assessment of the family includes assisting family members to express their fears and concerns and to cope with the realization that the child is going to die. Assess the parents' ability to talk with the child about his or her impending death. Conduct an assessment of personal coping skills. To evaluate the individual's ability to cope, ask questions regarding previous and current losses, the nature of the loss, and the significance of the loss. The information that should be discussed in the assessment includes cultural and spiritual traditions, rituals, beliefs related to loss and grieving, other stressors, and social support.

Diagnosis

Examples of nursing diagnoses that apply to the child and family experiencing a loss include the following:

- Fear (child) related to unanswered questions and concerns of abandonment
- Death Anxiety (child) related to own or other's impending death
- Hopelessness related to failure of therapies to prolong life
- Grieving related to imminent death of a loved one
- Disabled Family Coping related to sudden death of a child or family member.

Plan

The nurse may serve as a source of comfort and information for the child experiencing a loss. Goals of care may include the following:

- The child freely expresses feelings and thoughts related to the loss.
- The child is able to explain the loss in developmentally appropriate terms.
- The child will receive spiritual guidance as needed.

Implementation

Nursing care of the dying child and family focuses on ensuring physical comfort, providing client teaching regarding physical processes and methods of comfort, and providing emotional and spiritual support as appropriate.

Spiritual Support

- Assist the child to feel balance and connection with a greater power.
- Assess the family's cultural, religious, or spiritual beliefs and practices.
- Ask the family if it would like to have a spiritual leader notified or present.
- Facilitate the observance of religious, cultural, or spiritual rituals.

For more information regarding providing spiritual support to clients and their families, please see Concept 27, Spirituality.

End-of-Life

Promote physical comfort and psychologic peace in the final phase of life as follows:

- Provide information to the family about the signs and symptoms of approaching death.
- Encourage parents to invite close family members or friends to share the death vigil.
- Provide information about nursing interventions and medications used to keep the client comfortable. Reassure parents that regular assessments of the child's comfort are performed.
- Provide information about comfort measures parents can provide to the child, such as singing, massage, warm blankets, a cool cloth to the head, praying, or reading.
- Educate the parents about the signs and symptoms of death and, if the child is being cared for at home, the actions they should take if the child's condition changes drastically or the child dies.

For more information, see the exemplar about Death and Dying that follows, and the exemplar discussing End-of-Life Care in Concept 5, Comfort.

Evaluation

The child must be allowed to go through the grieving process at his or her own pace. Nurses and family members should periodically assess the child's understanding and thoughts regarding the loss to ensure that the child is not taking on

Assessment Interview Questions to Assess Spiritual Needs of the Child and Family

- Which spiritual rituals and resources have significance to the child and family?
- What is the child's understanding of the spiritual aspects surrounding life and death?
- What cultural influences have significance to the dying child and family, such as the concept of an afterlife and ways to prepare for it?
- What are the cultural practices, rites, and rituals related to the dying child and family?
- Should the child's death occur with the immediate family or with an extended family group?

feelings of guilt or responsibility for the death of another. Expected outcomes to be evaluated include the following:

- The child is able to discuss the loss and use developmentally appropriate terms to explain what it means to him or her.
- The child recognizes personal lack of responsibility for his or her own death or the loss of a loved one.
- The child with a terminal illness is able to talk about personal fears or concerns related to the dying process.

REVIEW Children's Response to Loss

RELATE: LINK THE CONCEPTS

Linking the exemplar Children's Response to Loss with the concept of Immunity:

1. How does the stress of loss impact the functioning of the immune system?
2. What strategies could you promote to support the immune system while a client is experiencing grief and loss?

Linking the exemplar Children's Response to Loss with the concept of Development:

3. While assessing a 4-year-old whose mother died 2 years ago you find the child has some small delays in developmental milestones. Why might this happen?
4. What interventions can you initiate to help this child meet future developmental milestones?

REFER: GO TO MYNURSINGKIT

REFLECT: CASE STUDY

Jason Riley is an active, healthy 11-year-old boy. He is currently in the 5th grade at the public grade school near his home. He lives with his mother Evelyn and his 14-year-old sister Jenna. He has never had much contact with his father. Jason's home life has been somewhat stressful this last year or so because of fighting between his mom and oldest sister Jessica, who moved out and lives in her own apartment with her new baby. Jason gets along well with his mom and oldest sister, but has typical sibling conflicts with his sister Jenna.

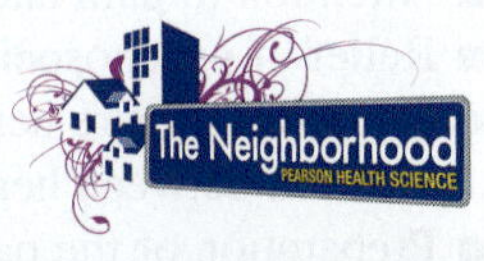

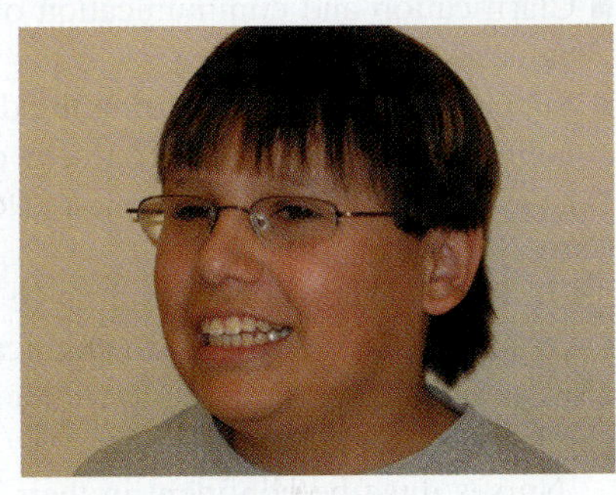

Jason is not doing well in school, academically or socially this year. He tells his sister that he gets teased a lot because he doesn't have a father. His mother has been told by the teachers that he is disruptive in class. Jason and his mom are in the clinic for a well-child check today.

1. Based on Jason's developmental level, what loss might he be grieving?
2. How is Jason's grief impacting his daily life?
3. How might you, the nurse, guide both Jason and his mother to help Jason discuss and cope with his feelings of loss in a more constructive manner?

12.2 DEATH AND DYING

LEARNING OUTCOMES

After reading about this exemplar you will be able to:

1. Describe the physiologic processes and clinical manifestations of impending death.
2. Formulate priority nursing diagnoses appropriate for the terminal client and his or her family members.
3. Create a plan of care for the terminal client that includes family members and loved ones.
4. Identify culturally competent, developmentally appropriate, caring interventions for the dying client and his or her family.
5. Analyze your own beliefs and fears related to death and dying.
6. Formulate strategies for assisting nurses to cope with their feelings of grief and loss related to the death of a client.

BASIS FOR SELECTION OF EXEMPLAR

Standards of Nursing Practice

OVERVIEW

Death, the process of dying, and the client's response to and perception of that process are highly individualized. The client with terminal lung cancer dies in a different manner than the client killed instantly in a motor vehicle accident. The former has time to consider death, and perhaps even to fear it or accept it; the latter is relieved of any feelings and considerations. Similarly, responses of family members to death—whether imminent or sudden, expected or unexpected—vary greatly. To support the range of clients and their families (and their various responses), the nurse needs a solid understanding of the physiologic process of death and dying. Before understanding these processes and working with the dying client, however, each nurse must examine his or her own thoughts and fears about death.

THE NURSE'S RESPONSE TO DEATH AND DYING

Death is as natural a part of life as birth. Although birth is embraced with joy and celebration, death is frequently denied and often prolonged for the sake of the living. Nurses have a unique opportunity and an obligation to help clients and their families through the dying process. Nurses learn to do this by confronting their own feelings about death and seeking guidance and mentorship when confronting death during clinical experiences. While a student, the nurse learns how to acknowledge and accept death as part of life and realizes that the nurse grieves the loss of clients. Viewing death as a natural process—not a medical failure—is of utmost importance. The nurse who helps the client die in comfort and with dignity provides the following benefits of good nursing care:

- Attention to pain and symptom control
- Relief of psychosocial distress
- Coordinated care across settings with high-quality communication between health care providers
- Preparation of the patient and family for death
- Clarification and communication of goals of treatment and values
- Support and education during the decision-making process, including the benefits and burdens of treatment.

Source: National Consensus Project (NCP) for Quality Palliative Care, 2004).

To achieve these goals, the nurse must be well-educated, have appropriate support in the clinical setting, and develop a close collaborative partnership with hospice and palliative care service providers.

Nurses must be confident in their clinical skills when caring for the dying client and be aware of the ethical, spiritual, and legal issues they may confront while providing end-of-life care. Many believe that the first step in the process is confronting their own fears about death and dying. By addressing their fears, nurses are better able to help clients and families when they are confronted with impending death. The nurse may then more objectively recognize and respect the client's and family's values and choices that guide their decisions at the end of life.

Facing one's mortality may help clarify beliefs and values. As death nears, the meaning of hope shifts from striving for a cure to achieving relief from pain and suffering. There is no "right" or "correct" way to die; each person faces death in a unique and individual way. To prepare to work with the dying, nurses may want to consider the questions in Table 12–7. Answering these questions will increase nurses' awareness of their feelings about death and dying so that they are better prepared to comfort and care for others.

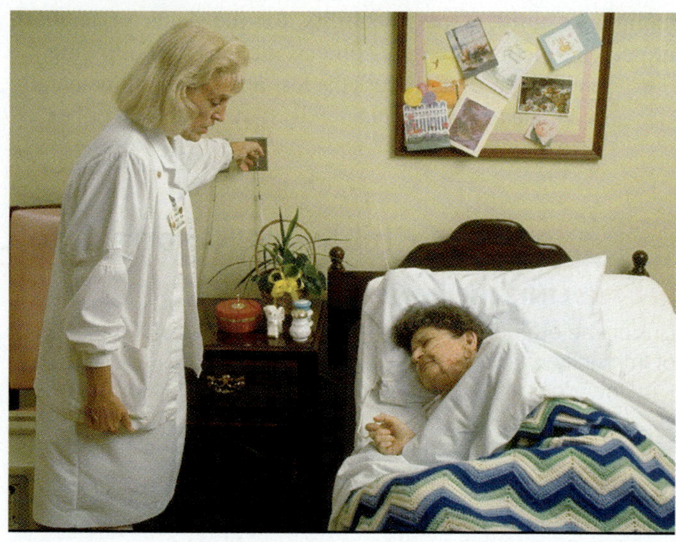

Figure 12–6 ■ Providing compassionate and holistic end-of-life care allows the nurse to apply a wide range of skills.

By coming to terms with their own feelings about death, nurses can better meet the emotional, spiritual, social, and physical needs of their clients. Often it is the caregiver who bonds with the dying client and is present when the last breath is taken. The nurse's presence is a way of expressing compassionate caring. In this way, nurses enter into another person's reality and use all of their skills of compassionate care. This is a humbling and beautiful privilege. It is a celebration of a life lived (Figure 12–6 ■).

Caring for Children Who Die

Children are highly valued by society because of their potential future contributions. Because children are expected to have a normal life span, the death of a child is often viewed as a tragedy. Caring for dying children is especially stressful and demanding for health care professionals. Health professionals caring for a dying child may feel a sense of helplessness, a feeling that they have failed the child, and sadness for the child's shortened life (Beale, Baile, & Aaron, 2005). Nurses involved in long-term relationships with children experience grief when the children die. Some nurses may cope by distancing themselves socially from the dying child and the family to

TABLE 12–7 **Questions and Critical Thinking in Preparation to Care for Dying Patients**

QUESTION FOR CONSIDERATION	CRITICAL THINKING APPLICATION
Have I ever seen a dead body?	Identify and overcome feelings regarding the lifeless body of another.
What are my own views of death?	Recognize feelings that death indicates a failure of the medical model.
Have I experienced the death of a close friend or relative?	By contemplating the death of a loved one, different emotions emerge including feelings of sadness and perhaps relief or joy for a life well lived.
How would I like to be remembered by my family and friends?	The way we hope to be remembered often adds purpose and meaning to our lives.
What age do I think I will be when I die?	Death in old age is often seen as a natural end to a long and productive life.
How do I think I will die?	The fear of death is often accompanied by fear of pain, suffering, and isolation from family and friends. These fears may be greater than the fear of death itself.

maintain composure and a professional demeanor and to protect themselves from the pain of repeated loss.

Caring for the dying child may be especially difficult for nurses with young children of their own. They tend to identify with the child, making it more likely that they will have difficulty dealing with the death in a professional manner. Nurses may not recognize the dying child's anxiety and fears because of their own defenses and feelings of helplessness.

Nurses who work with terminally ill children and their families require special preparation to meet the needs of these clients and, at the same time, to manage their own feelings and stress. Mentorship with experienced hospice nurses, as well as additional educational experiences, may help promote professional nursing care. Nurses who work with dying children and their families must learn to cope effectively with grief and to develop empathy, competence, and confidence in their ability to provide humane and effective nursing care.

Nurses should feel free to express their sorrow and grief for the child and family. Some nurses attend funeral and memorial services when invited by the client's family. Attending these services may help nurses deal with their own grief and promote closure. In addition, the presence of nurses who provided care to the child may offer the family continued support because it displays a way of demonstrating continuing culturally appropriate care for the deceased child and the family. See the following feature regarding families' appreciation of the support that health professionals provide.

Nurses who work in emergency departments caring for children who die suddenly or who work in hospice settings and hospital units caring for terminally ill children need support systems to help balance the stresses of their work. The workplace should provide resources that help nurses handle the stress and overwhelming feelings they experience when working with children who die. Educational seminars on compassion fatigue may help nurses identify coping strategies (Meadors & Lamson, 2008). Support systems may include discussions with peers or debriefing group sessions with mental health professionals that provide an opportunity for nurses to discuss their feelings and concerns (Figure 12–7 ■). Participating in team decisions regarding the dying client's palliative plan of care helps many nurses manage their distress.

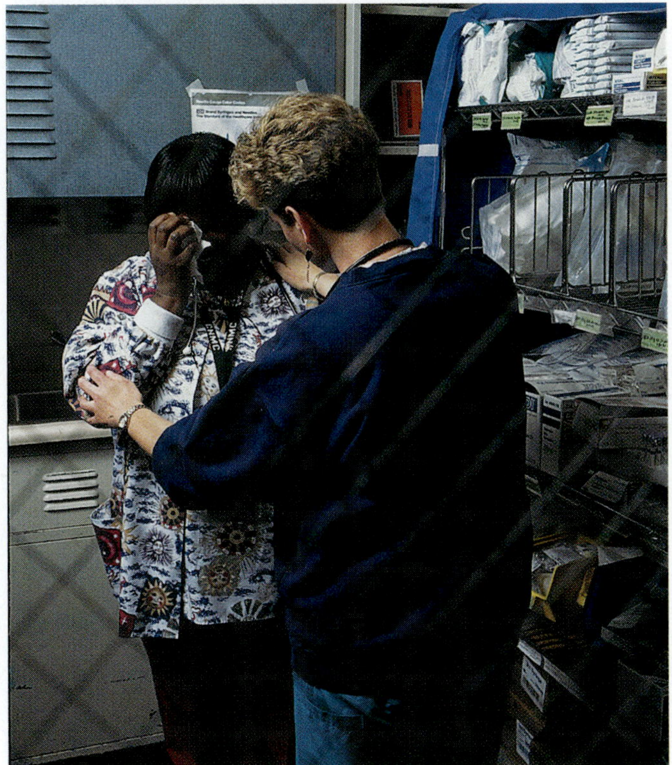

Figure 12–7 ■ Nurses need to express their own grief in a supportive environment after a child's death. Sharing with colleagues the sadness and grief or futility of resuscitation efforts often help nurses continue to provide supportive care to the next family who needs compassionate care.

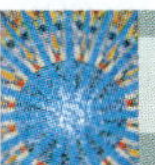

EVIDENCE-BASED PRACTICE **Family Support After Death**

In a small study, 12 parents of children who died in a pediatric intensive care unit (PICU) were interviewed to explore their experiences with staff support after the child's death. Findings revealed that parents placed great importance on the hospital's memorial service. All parents attended the memorial service and found some closure in returning to the hospital setting. Parents also appreciated receiving cards, telephone calls, and visits from staff members and valued their attendance at the child's funeral. Parents expressed disappointment when nurses and physicians did not participate in these activities (Macdonald, Liben, Carnevale, Rennick, & Wolf, 2005).

PHYSIOLOGIC CHANGES IN THE DYING CLIENT

Death is a highly individualized process that may occur rapidly or slowly. Physiologic changes are a part of the dying process. These changes result in any or all of the manifestations listed in Box 12–2 as death nears. The discussion that follows includes treatments and related nursing care. Additional information also may be found in Concept 5, Exemplar 5.2, End-of-Life Care.

Box 12–2 **Manifestations of Impending Death**

- Difficulty talking or swallowing
- Nausea, flatus, abdominal distention
- Urinary and/or bowel incontinence, constipation
- Decreased sensation, taste, and smell
- Weak, slow, and/or irregular pulse
- Decreasing blood pressure
- Decreased, irregular, or Cheyne-Stokes respirations
- Changes in level of consciousness
- Restlessness, agitation
- Coolness, mottling, and cyanosis of the extremities

Pain

Pain is a common problem for clients at the end of life; pain in death is what people often say they fear the most. Pain, a subjective experience, is influenced by the client's emotions, previous experiences with pain, and family and culture. Unfortunately, pain is often undertreated at the end of life (Tierney, McPhee, & Papadakis, 2004) because physicians and nurses fear that addiction or harm will result from the high dose of opioids necessary to control pain at the end of life. However, nearly all pain at the end of life can be managed without causing addiction or hastening death through respiratory depression. It is of utmost importance to keep the client comfortable through general comfort measures (Box 12–3) and through the administration of medications as ordered for pain, neuropathic pain (which is rarely relieved by opioids), seizures, and/or anxiety. The pathophysiology, treatment, and nursing care of clients experiencing pain are discussed in Concept 5, Exemplar 5.1.

> **PRACTICE ALERT**
> There is no maximum allowable dose at a person's end of life for opioids such as morphine sulfate; the dose should be increased to whatever is necessary to relieve pain. Meperidine (Demerol) is not useful for chronic pain because it has a short half-life and a toxic metabolite that can cause irritability and seizures (Tierney et al., 2004).

Dyspnea

Respiratory changes, including dyspnea, are normal as death nears. Dyspnea is a subjective experience, and the client often reports having a feeling of suffocation, shortness of breath, or tightness in the chest. Up to 50% of dying clients have severe dyspnea, especially those with lung tumors (primary or metastatic), restrictive lung disease, or pleural effusion (Tierney et al., 2004). Regardless of the terminal illness or fatal injury, the final cause of death is a lack of oxygen to the brain.

Box 12–3 Providing Comfort for the Client Nearing Death

- Maintain clean skin and bed linens.
- Use a draw sheet to turn the client as often as possible so the client is comfortable.
- Position the client to promote comfort and protect bony areas with padding. Reposition the client and raise the head of the bed if fluids accumulate in the upper airways and back of the throat.
- Use bed pads or insert a Foley catheter (if ordered) for urinary incontinence.
- Use gentle massage to improve circulation and shift edema.
- Provide small, frequent sips of fluids, ice chips, or Popsicles.
- Provide oral care using a soft moist brush or glycerin swab.
- Clean secretions from the eyes and nose.
- Administer ordered pain medications as needed to maintain comfort.
- Administer oxygen as prescribed to relieve dyspnea.

As death nears, respirations often become fast or slow, shallow and labored. The client may have apnea or Cheyne-Stokes respirations (regular periods of deep, rapid breathing followed by no breaths for 5–30 seconds). Fluid may accumulate in the lungs, causing rales and rhonchi, especially in clients who are well hydrated and are having difficulty swallowing or coughing. Although these sounds are not painful for the client, they may be treated with oxygen, opioids (to improve respirations and decrease anxiety), and medications to decrease secretions (atropine, scopolamine, hyoscyamine, or glycopyrrolate). Note that oxygen and suctioning are only temporary measures and (especially with suctioning) may be traumatic for the client. Nursing care to improve respirations includes keeping the head of the bed elevated. Keeping the room cool and providing a breeze from a fan often make the client more comfortable.

> **PRACTICE ALERT**
> Morphine is the medication of choice for palliative treatment of dyspnea. Nebulized morphine may be used. While it is often more effective than morphine given by other routes, it increases the risk of bronchospasm. Nebulized morphine is contraindicated in clients with chronic obstructive pulmonary disease because of the risk of respiratory depression and increasing hypercapnia.

Anorexia, Nausea, and Dehydration

Anorexia and a decrease in food and fluid intake are normal in the dying client. Anorexia may be a protective mechanism; the breakdown of body fats results in ketosis, which leads to a sense of well-being and helps decrease pain. Parenteral or enteral feedings do not improve symptoms or prolong life and may actually cause discomfort. As weakness and difficulty swallowing progress, the gag reflex is decreased and clients are at increased risk for aspiration if oral foods or fluids are given. Client teaching for the family is called for during this time, as some family members may not understand the physiologic changes that make eating difficult or risky. Instead, they may associate the client's lack of appetite or inability to eat as "giving up."

Nausea, with or without vomiting, is a common problem in dying clients. Nausea and vomiting may be caused by reduced gastric emptying, constipation, bowel obstruction, a side effect of morphine, uremia, or hypercalcemia. If the client is conscious and complains of nausea, antiemetics such as prochlorperazine (Compazine) or ondansetron (Zofran) should be administered.

Dehydration is less of a problem than overhydration. Forcing fluids or initiating intravenous fluids for hydration may increase fluid in the lungs, peripheral edema, ascites, and vomiting. Dehydration in the client nearing death primarily causes discomfort from dry mouth and thirst. The client should be given small sips of water, or an atomizer can be used to spray the inside of the mouth. Nurses should provide oral care at least every 2 hours and more often if the client is breathing through the mouth. Glycerin swabs may be used to provide moisture to the lips.

Altered Levels of Consciousness

Neurologic dysfunction results from any or all of the following: decreased cerebral perfusion, hypoxemia, metabolic acidosis, sepsis, an accumulation of toxins from liver and renal failure, the effects of medications, and disease-related factors. These changes may result in a decreased level of consciousness or agitated delirium. Clients with terminal delirium may be confused, restless, or agitated. Moaning, groaning, and grimacing often accompany the agitation and may be misinterpreted as pain. Level of consciousness often decreases to the point where the client cannot be aroused. Although decreased consciousness and agitation are normal states at the end of life, they are distressing to the client's family.

Confusion or agitation may be treated based on its cause (e.g., by relieving pain or dyspnea). Other medications include low doses of neuroleptics, tranquilizers, or antianxiety medications. A client near death often has altered cerebral function, so the nurse must stand near the bedside and speak clearly. Hearing is thought to be the last sense a dying client loses, so the nurse should not whisper or engage in conversation with the family as if the client were not there.

Hypotension

As death nears, cardiac output and intravascular blood volume decrease. As a result, blood pressure gradually decreases and the pulse is often rapid and irregular. The extremities are cooler, and cyanosis is present in nail beds, skin, and lips. The skin on the legs and in dependent areas may become mottled in color. Renal perfusion decreases, and the kidneys cease to function. Urinary output is scanty. The client will have tachycardia, hypotension, cool extremities, and cyanosis with skin mottling.

Support for the Client and Family

As the client's condition deteriorates, the nurse's knowledge of the client and family guides the care provided. It may be necessary to provide opportunities for clients to express personal preferences about where they want to die and about funeral and burial arrangements. If the family thinks this is morbid, the nurse should explain that it helps clients to keep a sense of control as they approach death.

The client needs the opportunity to say good-bye to others. The nurse should encourage and support the client and family as they terminate relationships as a necessary part of the grief process. The nurse acknowledges that termination is painful and, if the client or family prefers, stays with them during this time. Family members are often afraid to be present at the moment of death, yet dying alone is the greatest fear expressed by clients. Nurses should inquire about the cultural and religious preferences of the client and family and provide opportunities for them to visit with faith leaders or practice rituals for dying according to their culture or religion.

DEATH

The manifestations listed in Box 12–4 are seen after death occurs, and they are the basis for pronouncing death. They appear gradually and not in any particular order. Pronouncement of death is legally required by a physician or another health care provider to confirm death. The time of death, with any related data, is documented in the client's chart.

Box 12–4 **Manifestations of Death**

- Absence of respirations, pulse, and heartbeat
- Fixed and dilated pupils; eyes may stay open
- Release of stool and urine
- Waxen color (pallor) as blood settles to dependent areas
- Drop in body temperature
- Lack of reflexes
- Flat encephalogram

The nurse also may fear being present at the moment of the client's death. In fact, Kübler-Ross (1969) noted that the nurse's fear of death frequently interferes with the ability to provide support for the dying client and the family. Thoughts such as "Please, God, don't let him die on my shift" are common, and they express the nurse's emotional turmoil in dealing with the task. Nurses who have worked through their own feelings about death and dying are more at ease in assisting the dying client toward a peaceful death.

After the death, the family is encouraged to acknowledge the pain of loss. The nurse's presence and support as the bereaved express their sorrow, anger, or guilt can help them begin a healthy grieving process. Resolution of grief begins with acceptance of the loss. The nurse can encourage this acceptance by maintaining open, honest dialogue and by providing the family with the opportunity to view, touch, hold, and kiss the person's body. As family members realize the finality of the death, they are often comforted by the presence of the nurse who cared for the client during the final days.

POSTMORTEM CARE

The nurse documents the time of death (required for the death certificate and all official records), notifies the physician, and assists the family (if needed) in the choice of a funeral home. If the client dies at home, death must be pronounced before the body is removed. In some states and in some situations, nurses can pronounce death; for specifics, state practice acts, laws, and agency policy can be consulted. All jewelry is removed and given to the family unless the family asks that it be left on. The body is kept in place until the family is ready and gives permission. If an autopsy is required or requested, the body must be left undisturbed (e.g., no tubes are removed) for transportation to the medical examiner.

Documentation of the death is finished by sending the body to the morgue or funeral home (for a death in the hospital or long-term care setting) and by submitting the completed death certificate and required paperwork to the appropriate state agency for registration.

NURSING PROCESS

Nursing care of the dying client requires great sensitivity. Clients may be fearful or, having accepted their impending death, they may be very serene. Family members may be emotional and often require the nurse's support. Nurses can provide a great deal of support by being present and available to clients as the time of death nears.

Assessment

The nurse caring for the dying client and the family will assess for signs of approaching death; the client's needs for physical, spiritual, and emotional comfort; and the status of any advanced directives.

Assessing for Signs of Approaching Death and Physical Comfort

- Take vital signs every 2 hours or as ordered.
- Include the fifth vital sign, pain, as part of the assessment of vital signs. Nurses are responsible for ensuring that clients are as physically comfortable as possible during this time. If pain medication or other comforting interventions are not providing relief, contact the treating physician to determine if an increase in dosage or alternative medications are appropriate.
- Assess for signs of impending death. Inform client and family members of noticeable changes, such as weak or irregular pulse, changes in respirations, or changes in level of consciousness.

Assessing for Spiritual and Emotional Comfort

The spiritual and emotional comfort of the dying client and family is an essential part of end-of-life care. Whether the client is in a long-term care facility, in a hospital, in a hospice center, or at home, the client needs to have comforting items nearby. These may include pictures of family, drawings made by children or grandchildren, religious icons, prayer books, plants, a CD or another music player, books, whatever items are comforting to the client. The nurse should work with the family to determine what will provide emotional and spiritual comfort to the client.

Diagnosis

A number of diagnoses may be appropriate for the dying client and the family, including the following:

- Anticipatory Grieving
- Death Anxiety
- Acute or Chronic Pain
- Fear
- Risk for Compromised Human Dignity
- Risk for Caregiver Role Strain.

Plan

The nurse, health care team, client, and family members or caregivers as designated by the client will collaborate to develop the plan of care. Appropriate outcomes may include the following:

- The client will maintain human dignity throughout the dying process.
- The client will remain free of pain throughout the dying process.
- The client will participate in the decision-making process as long as he or she is competent to do so.
- The family will receive the emotional support needed throughout the dying process.

Implementation

The nurse working with the dying client and the family is responsible for communicating changes in client health status and providing a wide array of caring interventions at a time when the client and family are most in need of support and consideration.

Risk for Compromised Human Dignity

All terminally ill clients reach a point when they can no longer care for themselves. When this occurs, they are at risk for compromised human dignity; they are completely dependent on others for physical care, emotional support, and mental and spiritual nourishment. This is true even for the comatose client. Nurses are responsible for implementing caring interventions to prevent impairments in skin integrity, prevent and alleviate pain, and maintain client hygiene. Nursing care for the comatose client or the client with a very low level of consciousness or cognition includes:

- Using artificial tears if the client does not blink
- Keeping lights at a low level
- Keeping skin clean and dry
- Covering only with a light blanket
- Using adult incontinence pads or pants for incontinence
- Turning every 2 hours and maintaining joint positions.

Fear

Nurses who regularly assist clients and families to understand changes in their health status and the implications of these changes can alleviate many commonly held fears. Common fears and concerns of the dying include the following:

- Death itself
- Thoughts of a long or painful death
- Thoughts of facing death alone
- Thoughts of dying in a long-term care facility or hospital
- Loss of body control, such as bowel or bladder incontinence
- Inability to make decisions concerning care
- Loss of consciousness
- Financial costs and the thought of becoming a burden to others
- Thoughts of dying before having a chance to put personal affairs in order.

The nurse can assist the older client in addressing some of these fears by ensuring client comfort and support. Often the nurse is present for the client and family and can communicate compassion through caring acts (e.g., adjusting the client's position in bed and fluffing the pillow). Nurses also can help alleviate fears by providing family members the opportunity to observe religious and spiritual rituals with the dying client. Offering to call the family's minister or spiritual leader, providing space and time, and scheduling nursing interventions around specific prayer times can provide a great deal of comfort to clients and families during this time. Additional supportive interventions may include the following:

- Refer clients and families to social services and other agencies that provide financial support.

- Provide bedside activities and distractions to decrease boredom and to limit obsessing about death. Schools, churches, and civic organizations are excellent sources of volunteers who read to clients; play cards or board games with clients; or sit, pray, or simply listen to music with clients.
- Encourage clients who are able to form support groups to discuss fears and ways to alleviate them.
- Ensure clients who are still competent have the opportunity to visit with their lawyer or financial representative so that they can make necessary arrangements regarding wills and advanced directives.

Evaluation

Client care is evaluated based on the comfort level of the client during the dying process and the family's perception of the event. Possible expected outcomes related to the terminal client may include the following:

- Client's wishes prior to death are supported or met, as possible
- Family, loved ones, and client are able to support one another throughout the process
- Client experiences no discomfort during the dying process
- Client reaches the acceptance stage prior to death.

REVIEW Death and Dying

RELATE: LINK THE CONCEPTS

Linking the exemplar of Death and Dying with the concept of Culture:

1. When caring for a client who just died how can you support the family's request to hold a ceremony and prepare the body according to its customs?
2. What priority interventions will you implement for the family visiting the bedside of the client who is dying from lung cancer who are from South America and speak no English?

Linking the exemplar of Death and Dying with the concept of Comfort:

3. What appropriate response will you make to a family member who states that he or she cannot stand to watch his or her father gasp for air and asks you to do something to make him more comfortable?
4. What are your priorities of care for the client dying at home and his or her family?

REFER: GO TO MYNURSINGKIT

REFLECT: CASE STUDY

Julianna Converse, a 38-year-old, has been diagnosed with metastatic breast cancer. She had a radical mastectomy of the left breast one month ago. Diagnostic tests indicate metastasis to the brain and bone. She is currently being treated with chemotherapy and radiation. Julianna is married to Frank and they have 3 children: Paul, age 17; Mary, age 12; and Johnny, age 8. Julianna has recently quit her job as a buyer for a major clothing chain due to her treatments and extreme fatigue. Julianna has been told her chance for survival is very slim and she has accepted her likely death. She is trying to put her affairs in order while she has the energy to do the things that are important to her. She has contacted friends and family to help her plan for the future care of her children. Julianna is in the clinic today for chemotherapy and appears depressed and sad. Her chest is excoriated from the radiation treatments, her hair is brittle and falling out, and she has very little energy.

1. How can you assess your assumption of depression and sadness?
2. What is your priority nursing diagnosis for Julianna?
3. Describe a conversation you might have with Julianna using therapeutic communication to help her express her feelings?
4. What resources could you recommend to Julianna to help her plan for her family's future?

12.3 ELDER'S RESPONSE TO LOSS

KEY TERMS

Ageism, *622*
Disenfranchised grief, *622*

BASIS FOR SELECTION OF EXEMPLAR

Standards of Nursing Practice

LEARNING OUTCOMES

After reading about this exemplar you will be able to:

1. Apply knowledge of development to the older client's understanding of, and response to, grief, loss, and death.
2. Contrast cultural differences in the older client's response to and display of grief and loss.
3. Apply the nursing process to supporting the older client's need to grieve.
4. Develop a nursing plan of care for the older client and family facing the loss of a child.
5. Select appropriate nursing diagnoses for the older client and family coping with loss and grief.
6. Relate appropriate nursing goals for the older client and family coping with loss and grief.
7. Demonstrate appropriate nursing interventions when caring for the older client coping with loss and grief.
8. Assess expected outcomes for an older client's coping with the grieving process.

OVERVIEW

For the older adult, the grieving process is complicated by a number of factors. It is helpful for nurses working with older adults to understand psychologic factors that can impact the older adult's responses to loss.

Mental Health Issues and Older Adults

Undiagnosed and untreated mental disorders such as depression may complicate grieving responses. Older people evidence fewer diagnosable psychiatric disorders than younger people, excluding cognitive impairment. Major population-based surveys find that the overall prevalence of mental disorders for older adults is lower than for any other age group. Only cognitive impairments such as Alzheimer's disease show a definite age-associated increase. Despite the fact that about 20% of older people suffer from mental health problems including anxiety, severe cognitive impairments, and mood disorders, many older adults are denied access to mental health services for a variety of factors. Some of these factors include missed diagnosis of psychologic problems, denial of problems, funding issues, lack of coordination between mental health and aging care providers, shortages of health professionals with expertise in geriatric mental health, and the perceived stigma that many older people attach to having a psychologic problem. The rate of utilization of mental health services is lower in older people than in any other age group, and it is estimated that only half of those older adults with mental health problems receive mental health services (American Association for Geropsychiatry, 2008).

Older adults can evidence a variety of psychologic problems, including almost all of those experienced by younger adults. Some of these problems may be newly onset, the result of late-life stress or neuropathology, and others may be recurrences of psychologic problems experienced in earlier life. As with physical problems, the older adult may experience multiple psychologic symptoms or syndromes that make recognition and diagnosis challenging for the gerontologic nurse and other health care providers. In addition, psychologic problems can result from and coexist with physical problems.

Factors Affecting Loss in Special Populations

Racial and ethnic minorities bear a greater burden from unmet mental health needs. Thus, losses that they suffer have a greater impact on their overall health and productivity, regardless of age. Most minority groups are less likely than whites to use services, and they receive poorer quality mental health care despite having similar rates of mental health problems in the community. Racial and ethnic minorities and older gay men and lesbians are especially at risk. Similar prevalence, combined with lower utilization and poorer quality of care, means that minority communities have a higher proportion of individuals with unmet mental health needs. As a result, disproportionate numbers of minority older adults are not fully benefiting from the opportunities that others have to enjoy growing old. The major barriers these clients face include the cost of care, societal stigma, and fragmentation of services. Additional barriers include health care providers' lack of awareness of cultural issues, bias, inability to speak the older person's language, and the older person's fear and mistrust of treatment (U.S. Surgeon General, 2003). Lack of opportunity increases both the likelihood of loss and the severity of the older adult's response to loss.

The older population is highly heterogeneous and includes a diverse mix of immigrants, refugees, and multigenerational Americans with vastly different histories, languages, spiritual practices, demographic patterns, and cultures. Generations within the same minority family may represent different racial or cultural orientation, religious affiliation and practices, societal values, and attitudes toward the larger society. Minority elders may be considered especially vulnerable and at risk for mental health problems because of **ageism** (negative stereotypes toward elderly adults) and cultural bias.

Older Adults and Change

While all of these factors place older adults at greater risk for more serious diagnoses such as complicated grieving, they do not mean that older adults cannot meet the challenges that come with death and loss. Older adults can prepare for and

FOCUS ON DIVERSITY AND CULTURE Grieving Norms

Every culture has established grieving norms and denies such emotions to people deemed to have insignificant losses. **Disenfranchised grief** results from a loss that cannot be openly acknowledged, socially validated, or publicly mourned. Typically, there are three categories of disenfranchised grief:

- The relationship is not recognized.
- The loss is not recognized.
- The griever is not recognized.

Some people negate the loss of relationships that are not socially sanctioned, such as nontraditional relationships, extramarital affairs, or same-gender relationships. Some believe that relationships that existed primarily in the past do not need to be mourned, such as former friends, past lovers, or former spouses. In the following examples, which family members are at risk for disenfranchised grief?

1. A 70-year-old woman dies in her assisted living facility, leaving behind her homosexual partner of 10 years and her grown children from a heterosexual marriage that ended 25 years ago.
2. An 85-year-old man dies in his home, leaving behind his 40-year-old second wife, their 6-year-old son, and his grown daughters from a previous marriage.

How do the risks for disenfranchised grief change if the couple in the second question are an interracial couple? If the woman who dies in the first question is Jewish and her partner is agnostic?

respond to psychosocial changes by developing and using effective coping strategies they have developed earlier in life. With each day that passes, the opportunity for change, both positive and negative, presents itself. A rich, full life usually encompasses joyous and sad events. Some older people experience many significant losses as they age. The positive coping mechanisms that a person developed and used earlier in life may be inadequate in later life. Thus, depression or another serious mental health problem may result from an inability to cope, and additional services and support may be needed. Although older adults suffer from major depressive disorders less often than younger adults, about 5 million older adults experience depressive symptoms (Hartford Institute for Geriatric Nursing, 2008).

Nurses working with older adults who are experiencing grief and loss must help them find new coping mechanisms to replace those that have become inadequate or inaccessible. For example, imagine a Roman Catholic wife and mother who, after raising her children, found comfort in attending daily Mass at her church. Shortly after her husband dies, she falls and breaks her hip, requiring surgery and 3–4 months of rehabilitation in a skilled nursing facility. She can no longer attend Mass every day. What nursing interventions would help her learn new coping mechanisms for dealing with the loss of her husband and the loss, even though it may be temporary, of her mobility?

BEREAVEMENT

Most older adults experience the loss or death of loved ones, including spouses, family members, and friends. While bereavement is considered a normal reaction to loss and death, pathologic grief occurs in some older adults. Symptoms of complicated grief in older adults are essentially the same as those of younger adults. They include preoccupation with death, excessive guilt, an overwhelming sense of loss and worthlessness, marked psychomotor retardation, and functional impairment. The length of time spent grieving is culturally determined and is a function of the individual's resources and the circumstances of death. In the United States, a 2-year period of grief in the older adult is considered normal; grief persisting longer than 2 years is considered *pathologic*. However, establishing preconceived time frames and judging others according to various theories quickly becomes problematic. In some cultures, bereavement lasts for the lifetime of the survivor. Traditional Greek widows wear black for the rest of their lives (Figure 12–8 ■). The professional standard of care regarding the grieving older person should not be time-related. Rather, it should focus on the prevention of grief-related psychiatric disorders, profound depression, medical illness, and social incapacitation (American Psychological Association, 2008).

Factors that can affect the duration and course of grieving include:

- *Centrality or significance of the loss.* If the person who died occupied a central place in the survivor's life (either physically or emotionally), the loss will be harder to bear. An older person with psychologic attachments to others will receive support and assistance after the loss.
- *Health of the survivor.* An older person with robust mental and physical health will be better able to cope with the loss of a loved one and complete the work of grieving. Unresolved issues from the past, feelings of ambiguity toward the one who died, and unresolved or incomplete coping with previous losses can complicate the grieving process and prolong the time required to grieve. When the survivor is experiencing changes in cognitive function, such as Alzheimer's disease, loss of a spouse can be especially devastating, both physically and mentally. If the spouse was the survivor's primary caregiver, the loss is even greater, and the resulting changes due to the loss of the caregiver may result in rapid deterioration of the survivor's cognitive and physical condition.
- *Survivor's religious or spiritual belief system.* Personal religion or spirituality can be deeply integrated into the older person's perspective and positively influence the grieving process. When an older person believes a loved one has lived a meaningful life and has passed into the care of a higher power, a sense of self-worth and acceptance of the death may occur. However, the gerontologic nurse should be aware that older people who are religious are not necessarily spiritual and vice versa. Some people attend church or temple for the social and recreational opportunities and find very little comfort from the religion when it is needed most. Other older people may have grown away from organized

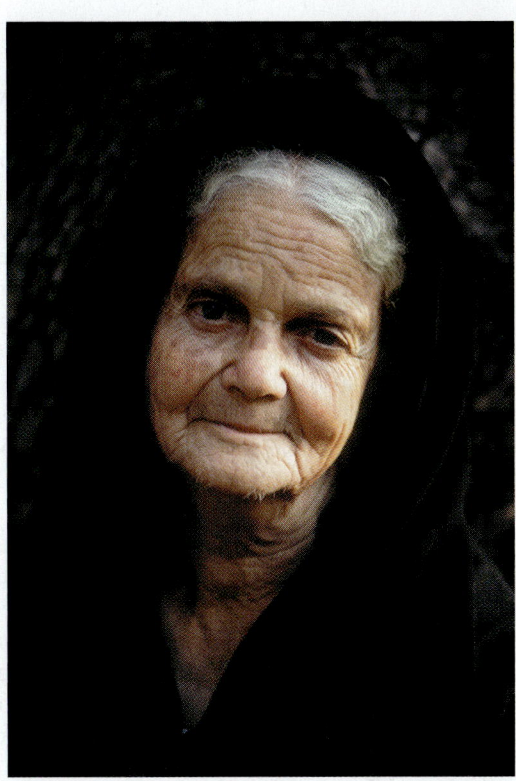

Figure 12–8 ■ This elderly woman from Crete is wearing the traditional black headdress of a widow.

Source: Robert Fried Photography

religion but still possess a deep and abiding faith in God and the meaning of life.

- *History of substance abuse.* Older people who have used drugs or alcohol to cope with unpleasant life events and serious losses in the past may consider using these substances again. Careful monitoring and support of these older adults is warranted.
- *Nature of the death.* Sudden deaths that are a result of trauma, natural disaster, or violent acts may be more difficult to bear, thereby resulting in a prolonged grieving process. These deaths, in addition to the great personal loss the survivor feels, also may trigger more symbolic losses, such as loss of trust, security, and control. These older adults may experience the double psychologic burden of bereavement and post-traumatic stress reaction. Symptoms include feelings of shock, horror, and numbness. Recurrent violent and frightening dreams may disrupt sleep and cause daytime anxiety. These older adults may focus on retelling the horrific events of the death, return to the scene of the crises, overidentify with the deceased, and focus on pictures and objects. The gerontologic nurse can assist older people with their grief, helping them gain mastery and control over the trauma by urging them to seek mental health services and counseling while providing support.

PRACTICE ALERT

Some older adults will grieve the loss of a pet to the same extent as the loss of a family member. The centrality of the loss is the predictor of the depth and duration of grief, not the societal value of the being that has died.

NURSING PROCESS

As the client ages, loss becomes a more frequent occurrence. How the client copes with grief and loss is often related to past experiences. A thorough nursing history can give the nurse a greater understanding of what the current loss means to the client.

Assessment

The nursing assessment of the older adult who is grieving includes the following:

- *Health History.* Assess the nature of the loss, amount of time that has passed since the loved one died, the activities in which the client participated to honor the loss (e.g., attending the funeral), change in sleep patterns, change in appetite or eating habits, and past and current coping mechanisms.
- *Examination of Resources.* What familial, social, and financial support does the client have to help with the grieving process? What restrictions or barriers exist for the client accessing these supports?
- *Physical Examination.* Assess vital signs, including pain; changes in cognitive skills; symptoms of depression; and changes in symptomatology from baseline.

Diagnosis

Appropriate nursing diagnoses for the older adult experiencing loss may be many and will depend on the adult's coping mechanisms, resources, physical health, and perception of the loss. These diagnoses may include the following:

- Grieving
- Risk for Complicated Grieving
- Disturbed Sleep Pattern
- Risk for Spiritual Distress
- Risk for Acute Confusion
- Death Anxiety
- Hopelessness.

Plan

The nurse should create a plan of care in collaboration with the client; family members; and any other significant others who provide emotional, physical, or financial support to the grieving client. Appropriate outcomes may include the following:

- The client will be able to express grief in appropriate ways.
- The client will be able to participate in mourning rituals honoring the deceased.
- The client will maintain (or resume) healthy eating and sleeping patterns.
- The client will resume normal activities following the loss.

Implementation

Care of the grieving older client will be influenced by the client's culture, the meaning of the loss to the client, and the strength of the coping measures used by the client. The responses of individual clients to a loss differ significantly, and nursing care must be individualized.

Hopelessness

As the client recognizes the loss, he or she may feel a sense of hopelessness. The client may not have the coping skills to deal effectively with the loss and its consequences without additional support. The nurse can provide support to the client encountering hopelessness during the grieving process.

- Assess the client's responses to the loss. Encourage expression of feelings.
- Provide information about the grieving process at the client's level of understanding. Factual information helps assure the client that feelings related to grief are normal.
- Avoid criticizing or judging the client's feelings. An environment that is accepting and promotes client self-expression promotes continued expressions of feelings and a willingness to discuss other issues.
- Support positive family bonds and enhance communication among family members; promote mutual positive regard. Strong family relationships can provide direction and motivation for living.
- Encourage the client to make as many decisions as possible. Self-determination enhances a feeling of control over a situation and may give a sense of hope.
- Encourage the client and family to seek spiritual guidance that previously inspired hope. The client's church or faith is a legitimate support system.

Evaluation

In the evaluation of the effectiveness of nursing care of the grieving older adult, it is important to consider what is most important to the client and to allow the client time to work through the grieving process. Potential outcomes that may be used to evaluate care include the following:

- Client grieves appropriately based on personal importance of the event and cultural beliefs
- Client voices feelings related to the loss
- Client copes with the emotions in a healthy manner.

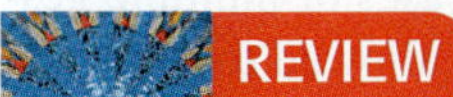

REVIEW Elder's Response to Loss

RELATE: LINK THE CONCEPTS

Linking the exemplar of Elder's Response to Loss with the concept of Mood and Affect:

1. Describe the types of losses the elderly experience and why those losses put them at risk for depression.
2. How will you assist the elderly man who has had to give up his home and move to an assisted living facility to adjust to this change? What other losses do you anticipate this client may be coping with?

Linking the exemplar of Elder's Response to Loss with the concept of Mobility:

3. What are your goals for the elderly client who has lost the use of his or her legs?
4. Create a plan of care for an elderly client who lives alone and is wheelchair bound.

REFER: GO TO MYNURSINGKIT

REFLECT: CASE STUDY

Peter Murphy is an 86-year-old man who has arthritis that is particularly advanced in his lower extremities due to injuries he sustained playing pro football. He has also been diagnosed with congestive heart failure and peripheral vascular disease. His lower extremities are becoming increasingly weak and he has fallen several times. His primary provider is strongly encouraging him to use a wheelchair for safety.

Pete lives in an apartment by himself since his wife died 3 years ago. With help from neighbors he manages to care for himself and his small dog in his second-floor apartment. His neighbor, Mary, does his laundry for him once a week and takes him to the local senior center every morning with her husband. Pete gets his breakfast and lunch at the center and returns home around 4 p.m. Pete is extremely upset about the idea of being confined to a wheelchair because he feels his independence is being threatened. Mary's car is not big enough to take him and a scooter or wheelchair to the senior center where he finds his primary source of support and friendship. Pete is at the clinic today for follow-up care, and his primary provider is encouraging Pete to decide about the type of chair he would like to use.

1. What assessment data would help you determine Pete's risk for depression or, possibly, suicide?
2. How can you help Pete cope with his grief over the need to rely on a wheelchair?
3. What are your priority nursing diagnoses and goals of care for Pete?

12.4 PERINATAL LOSS

KEY TERMS

Disseminated intravascular coagulation (DIC), *626*
Fetal demise, *626*
Intrauterine fetal death (IUFD), *626*
Miscarriage, *626*
Perinatal loss, *626*
Spontaneous abortion, *626*
Stillbirth, *626*

BASIS FOR SELECTION OF EXEMPLAR

Standards of Nursing Practice

LEARNING OUTCOMES

After reading about this concept, you will be able to:

1. Describe the pathophysiology, etiology, clinical manifestations, and causes of perinatal loss.
2. Identify risk factors associated with perinatal loss.
3. Illustrate the nursing process in providing culturally competent care across the life span for individuals and their loved ones experiencing perinatal loss.
4. Formulate priority nursing diagnoses appropriate for individuals and their loved ones experiencing perinatal loss.
5. Create a plan of care for individuals and their loved ones experiencing perinatal loss.
6. Assess expected outcomes for individuals and their loved ones experiencing perinatal loss.
7. Discuss therapies used in the collaborative care of individual experiencing perinatal loss.
8. Employ evidence-based caring interventions for individuals and their loved ones experiencing perinatal loss.

OVERVIEW

Pregnancy is often a time of hope and anticipation of the birth of a healthy new baby. Parents facing the birth of a child with serious health issues, the loss of the neonate, or the possibility of a premature birth grieve the normal healthy baby they had pictured. Parents of infants born prematurely often say that they would like to have another baby just to experience birth the way they expected it to be. Even when the premature baby has no long-term issues and comes home healthy and thriving, parents still talk about feeling cheated because they did not have a "normal" birthing experience and grieve the loss.

Perinatal loss is death of a fetus or infant that occurs between the time of conception and the end of the newborn period 28 days after birth. **Intrauterine fetal death (IUFD)** occurs after 20 weeks gestation and is often referred to as **stillbirth** or **fetal demise**. **Miscarriage** and **spontaneous abortion** are terms used to describe the loss of a fetus prior to 20 weeks' gestation.

PATHOPHYSIOLOGY AND ETIOLOGY

Prolonged retention of the dead fetus may lead to the development of **disseminated intravascular coagulation (DIC)**, also called *consumption coagulopathy*, in the mother. After the release of thromboplastin from the degenerating fetal tissues into the maternal bloodstream, the extrinsic clotting system is activated, triggering the formation of multiple tiny blood clots. Fibrinogen and factors V and VII are subsequently depleted, and the woman begins to display symptoms of DIC. Fibrinogen levels begin a linear descent 3–4 weeks after the death of the fetus and continue to decrease in the absence of appropriate medical intervention.

Besides DIC, other adverse outcomes can occur if the onset of labor and subsequent birth are delayed. Women with prolonged retention of a dead fetus are more prone to infection. A resulting infection can cause endometritis or sepsis. The longer the pregnancy continues, the higher the incidence of maternal infection.

Although immediate induction is routinely performed, there may be situations in which induction is delayed, such as maternal refusal or the presence of a multiple gestation. In these cases, fibrinogen levels are monitored weekly or biweekly to identify and prevent progressive coagulopathy from occurring (Lindsey, 2006). In cases of fetal death in the presence of a multiple gestation, some perinatologists opt to do a single set of coagulation labs, whereas others do no laboratory assessment. DIC rarely occurs in cases of multiple gestations where the remaining fetus(es) are allowed to grow and mature (Lindsey, 2006).

Etiology

Antepartal fetal deaths, although infrequent, account for about half of all perinatal mortality in the United States (Druzin, Smith Jr., Gabbe, & Reed, 2007). The *perinatal mortality rate (PMR)* is defined as late fetal deaths (over 28 gestational weeks) plus the first 6 days of life (National Center for Health Statistics, 2006). It is estimated that 70–90% of stillbirths occur before the onset of labor, with more than 50% occurring between 20 and 28 weeks' gestation (Druzin et al., 2007). The cause may be unknown, or it may result from any of a number of physiologic maladaptations—asphyxia; congenital malformations; and superimposed pregnancy complications including preeclampsia or eclampsia, abruptio placentae, placenta previa, diabetes, renal disease, cord accidents, fetal growth restriction, and alloimmunization. Perinatal loss associated with birth defects may occur as a result of congenital anomalies or may occur if the fetus is exposed to teratogens late in the pregnancy (Blackburn, 2007). Other fetal deaths occur with no apparent cause (Box 12–5).

Perinatal loss in industrialized countries has declined in recent years as early diagnosis of congenital anomalies and advances in genetic testing techniques have increased the use of elective termination. Surprisingly, other reproductive advances have increased the incidence of fetal death. It appears that fetal death occurs more frequently in monochorionic twins. Because most monochorionic twins are conceived naturally, they have a higher incidence of loss. Most twins

Box 12–5 Factors Associated With Perinatal Loss

FETAL FACTORS
- Chromosomal disorders
- Birth defects not chromosomal in nature
- Anencephaly, open neural tube defects, isolated hydrocephalus, congenital heart defects
- Nonimmune hydrops fetalis
- Infections
- Complications of multiple gestations

MATERNAL FACTORS
- Prolonged pregnancy
- Diabetes
- Chronic hypertension
- Preeclampsia/eclampsia
- Advanced maternal age
- Hereditary thrombophilias
- Antiphospholipid syndrome
- Uterine rupture
- Rh disease
- Ascending bacteria from the vagina

PLACENTAL AND OTHER FACTORS
- Placenta previa
- Abruptio placentae
- Cord accident
- Premature rupture of membranes
- Substance abuse
- Unknown factors

conceived via assisted reproductive technology are dichorionic placentation (Sperling et al., 2006). Pregnancies conceived by in vitro fertilization have higher rates of loss and complications (placenta abruption, fetal loss after 24 weeks' gestation, gestational hypertension, placenta previa, and cesarean births) (Shevell et al., 2005). In addition, certain genetic testing procedures such as amniocentesis and chorionic villus sampling (CVS) can actually cause fetal loss.

In developing countries, infection plays a significant role in fetal mortality. Ascending bacterial organisms include *Escherichia coli*, group B streptococci, and *Ureaplasma urealyticum.* These infections can occur before or after the membranes have ruptured, resulting in fetal demise. Viral causes of fetal demise include parvovirus and coxsackievirus. *Toxoplasma gondii*; *Listeria monocytogenes*; and the organisms that cause leptospirosis, Q fever, and Lyme disease also have been identified as causative factors for stillbirth. Untreated syphilis is associated with a high stillbirth rate, as is malaria infection when contracted for the first time by the mother during the pregnancy (Gibbs & Roberts, 2007). These infections carry a much higher morbidity and mortality rate in developing countries.

Identifying the causative factor of fetal loss helps many families progress through the grieving process. Information obtained from a postmortem examination or postmortem studies can provide vital information related to the cause of the fetal death, the possibility for reoccurrence, and closure for the couple. The information also can be used to help with recurrence and future preconceptional counseling, pregnancy management, prenatal diagnostic procedures, and neonatal management (Lindsey, 2006). The types of studies and tests performed depend on the parents' past history, medical history, and preferences for extent of testing. Chromosome studies should be considered if the couple has a history of other second or third trimester losses or if either parent has a suspected balanced translocation or mosaic chromosomal pattern. Fetuses who are dysmorphic, have growth retardation, are hydropic, or have anomalies or other signs of chromosomal abnormalities may be candidates for chromosomal studies (anomalies) (Lindsey, 2006).

If an intra-amniotic infection is the suspected cause, cultures of the placenta and the fetus should be obtained. If specific infections are being considered, both IgM and IgG antibodies should be drawn to determine whether an acute infectious process occurred.

A careful visual inspection for obvious defects or abnormalities should be made of all stillborn infants at the time of birth. The placenta and membranes also should be closely examined and the placenta sent to pathology for further testing. The umbilical cord should be inspected for true knots, a velamentous insertion, lack of Wharton's jelly, or a short cord to determine whether a cord accident was the cause. If a specific cause is suspected, blood tests and x-rays can be performed to verify the suspicions (Lindsey, 2006). An autopsy is the best way to determine the cause of death; however, in the event that the parents decline an autopsy, an MRI also can provide detailed information (Lindsey, 2006).

Most practitioners perform a complete blood count (CBC) and antibody screen upon the mother's admission. Because diabetes is a causative factor, a random or postpartum glucose level can be obtained to rule out this cause. If diabetes is identified, a hemoglobin A1C should be performed. Additional maternal factors also can be evaluated. Additional tests that may be performed are listed in Table 12–8.

Risk Factors

Paternal causes of fetal death also may be examined. One recent study determined that paternal exposure to pesticides resulted in a higher rate of fetal deaths when compared with pregnancies conceived by men who were not exposed to pesticides occupationally (Ronda, Regidor, Garcia & DomÌnguez, 2005).

Certain maternal conditions also can be associated with higher rates of fetal death. Past maternal exposure to some bacterial and viral antigens may produce an autoimmune response that results in fetal death (Silver, 2007). Women with acquired and immune thrombophilia have higher rates of miscarriage and fetal demise than those without hematologic alterations (Michels & Tiu, 2007).

CLINICAL MANIFESTATIONS

Many women first report an absence of fetal activity, although some women fail to recognize this change in fetal activity. Diagnosis of IUFD is confirmed by visualization of the fetal heart with absence of heart action on ultrasound. Some practitioners routinely have a second ultrasound performed or have a second practitioner verify the absence of cardiac activity before making the diagnosis. When a fetal demise occurs, maternal estriol levels fall. Without medical intervention, most women have spontaneous labor within 2 weeks of fetal death. The once common practice of waiting for the onset of labor has largely been abandoned in recent years because the risks of complications increase with delaying the birth. It is

TABLE 12–8 **Tests to Determine the Cause of Fetal Loss**

FETAL TESTING	MATERNAL TESTING
Fetal blood tests and x-rays	Diabetes testing
Autopsy or MRI	CBC with platelet count
Placental studies	Kleihauer-Betke test
Chromosomal studies (if indicated)	Abnormal antibody testing (lupus anticoagulant, anticardiolipin antibodies)
	Thyroid-stimulating hormone (TSH) levels
	Infectious disease testing (rubella, syphilis, malaria, toxoplasmosis, cytomegalovirus)
	Hereditary thrombophilia testing
	Toxicology testing

estimated that 60% of fetal deaths have no known case. In 25% of all fetal deaths, the cause remains unknown even after an autopsy (Lindsey, 2006). The specific cause is more difficult to identify when time since the death is prolonged. Prompt birth increases the ability to identify the cause of death.

In modern practice, most women with a diagnosed fetal demise are given the option of waiting a few days or scheduling an induction procedure immediately. Most women elect for an induction within a day or two of the final diagnosis. One study determined that women who waited more than 24 hours experienced more prolonged anxiety compared with women who underwent induction within 6 hours of diagnosis (Lindsey, 2006). The mode of induction depends on the gestational age of the fetus, the readiness of the cervix, and the previous mode of birth. In women who have had a previous cesarean birth, a repeat cesarean may be performed because the use of Pitocin or prostaglandin agents can increase the risk of a uterine rupture. Women with an unfavorable cervix may be given vaginal prostaglandin agents, misoprostol, or laminaria tents. Women whose gestations are less than 16 weeks may have a laminaria tent inserted into the cervix before a dilatation and extraction procedure. *Laminaria tents* are made from the stems of brown seaweed that are cut, shaped, dried, sterilized, and packaged in specific sizes. Laminaria tents work by drawing water out of the cervical tissue, allowing the cervix to soften and dilate. They are commonly used to dilate the cervix in preterm gestations when induction is warranted. They may be placed before surgical procedures or inductions of labor.

Women less than 28 weeks' gestation are typically given prostaglandin E_2 (PGE_2) 10–20 mg vaginal suppositories every 4–6 hours or oral or vaginal misoprostol 400 mcg every 4–6 hours until spontaneous labor occurs (Lindsey, 2006). Because PGE_2 suppositories can cause severe vomiting and diarrhea, women are commonly pretreated with antiemetic and antidiarrheal preparations to prevent or lessen these unpleasant side effects (Lindsey, 2006). Recent studies have shown that misoprostol is more effective than other regimens, resulting in fewer side effects and shorter times to childbirth (Prairie et al., 2007).

Women who are term and have not had a previous cesarean birth or another uterine scar may undergo an induction of labor. Women with an unfavorable cervix may be given cervical ripening agents such as vaginal prostaglandin agents. Induction with Pitocin can be performed following the same protocol as any other term induction of labor.

GRIEVING THE LOSS

The behaviors that couples exhibit while mourning may be associated with the five stages of grieving described by Kübler-Ross (1969). (See the About section for detailed discussion.) Often the first stage is *denial* of the death of the fetus. Even when the initial health care provider suspects fetal demise, the couple is hoping that a second opinion will be different. Some couples may not be convinced of the death until they see and hold the stillborn infant after birth. The second stage is *anger*, resulting from feelings of loss, loneliness, and perhaps guilt. The anger may be projected at significant others and members of the health care team, or it may be absent when the death is sudden and unexpected. The mother may attempt to identify a specific event that caused the death or may blame herself. *Bargaining*, the third stage, may or may not be present depending on the couple's preparation for the death of the fetus. If the death is unanticipated, the couple may not have time for bargaining. Bargaining is more commonly seen when the death is expected, such as in the case of a known lethal congenital anomaly. It is marked by the couple making mental trade-offs in exchange for the fetus being healthy. In the fourth stage, *depression* is evidenced by preoccupation, weeping, and withdrawal. Changing hormonal levels in the first 24–48 hours after the birth may compound the depression and associated grief. The final stage, *acceptance*, occurs when resolution occurs. This stage is highly individualized and may take months to years to complete.

NURSING PROCESS

Nursing care of the family experiencing a perinatal loss is focused on meeting the mother's physiologic needs as well as supporting the family's grieving process. Men and women tend to grieve differently, so couples may need assistance in interpreting each other's behavior.

Assessment

The mother's communication to the nurse of cessation of fetal movement is frequently the first indication of fetal death. It is followed by a gradual decrease in the signs and symptoms of pregnancy. Fetal heart tones are absent, and fetal movement is no longer palpable. Once fetal demise is established, the nurse assesses the family members' ability to adapt to the loss. Open communication between the mother, her partner, and the members of the health care team contributes to a realistic understanding of the medical condition and its associated treatments. The nurse may discuss prior experiences the family members have had with loss and what they believe their perceived coping abilities were at that time. Identifying the family's social supports and resources is also important.

Perinatal loss also may occur in the intrapartum period as a result of an intrapartum complication such as an unresolved shoulder dystocia, a prolapsed umbilical cord, or abruptio placentae. In such emergency situations, members of the health care team often focus on the physical needs of the mother and an attempt to save the fetus's life. Commonly, the family is not told that a perinatal death has occurred until after the infant is delivered. Thus, the parents are faced with the sudden and completely unanticipated death of their infant. The most common reaction is protest or disbelief. Although the physician or certified nurse-midwife (CNM) informs the family of the death, the nurse continues one-on-one care with the family, providing both physical and emotional support throughout this crucial period. The nurse assists the family members in the grief process and explores their immediate wishes for viewing and holding the deceased child.

Diagnosis

Nursing diagnoses that may apply include the following:

- Anticipatory Grieving related to imminent loss of a child
- Powerlessness related to lack of control in current situational crisis
- Ineffective Denial related to the unexpected death of the fetus
- Compromised Family Coping related to death of a child/unresolved feelings regarding perinatal loss
- Interrupted Family Processes related to fetal demise
- Hopelessness related to sudden, unexpected fetal loss
- Risk for Spiritual Distress related to intense suffering secondary to unexpected fetal loss.

Plan

Goal setting for the family experiencing a prenatal loss may include the following:

- Extended family or support systems are available to help the grieving parents cope with their loss.
- Parents express grief over the loss of the fetus.
- Parents avoid taking undue or unreasonable responsibility for fetal loss.

Implementation

Most facilities have an established protocol to follow in the event of perinatal death. It typically provides a holistic focus for family-centered nursing care. It is often helpful for the nurse to view the stillborn baby before talking to the parents so that the nurse can prepare the parents for what to expect regarding the baby's appearance. The nurse can then point out normal things about the baby. It is important that the entire health care team be notified so multidisciplinary care can be initiated. When fetal death has been confirmed before admission, the entire staff on the unit is informed so it can avoid making inappropriate remarks. Many facilities have a symbol, such as a card with a leaf or a cluster of flowers, that is placed on the mother's door to inform all staff members of the loss.

PRACTICE ALERT

Lack of experience may make the nurse feel awkward in helping the family in pain because of a prenatal loss. A good start and an appropriate statement is "I'm so sorry for your loss. How can I help?"

Preparing the Family for the Birth

Upon arrival at the facility, the couple with a known or suspected fetal demise should be placed in a private room immediately. When possible, the woman should be in the room that is farthest from other laboring women. Care should be taken not to leave the couple in the waiting room with other expectant parents or visitors waiting for news from other women in labor.

Allow the couple to remain together as much as they like. Provide privacy as needed and maintain a supportive environment. Give the couple complete information about what to expect and what will happen. Encourage and answer their questions. At all times, a nurse stays with the couple so they do not feel alone and isolated; however, cues that the couple wants to be alone should be assessed continuously. Some couples may want outside support, such as family members or friends, to be present during the labor. The nurse facilitates the couple's wishes.

When possible, the same nurse should provide care for the couple so a therapeutic relationship is established. As the relationship develops, the nurse provides solace by listening to the couple without offering explanations. The nurse also provides ongoing opportunities for the couple to ask questions. It is not uncommon for the family to ask the same questions repeatedly. This is part of the initial grief process. The nurse should provide clear explanations and straightforward answers. The nurse also arranges for other members of the multidisciplinary team to interact with the family. If a grief counselor is available, the nurse should arrange an initial meeting with the couple. If the family wants to see a spiritual advisor, the nurse offers to contact the hospital chaplain or another cleric. A social worker is commonly involved. The nurse typically coordinates members of the multidisciplinary team so a comprehensive plan of care can be initiated.

The nurse explains details of the plan of care and allows the family members to ask questions and make decisions for their labor and birth preferences. The availability of anesthesia and analgesia should be reviewed. Typically, the woman can have pain medication whenever she prefers. The nurse facilitates the participation of the woman and her partner in the labor and birth process.

In contrast to a typical birth experience, the birth of a stillborn infant marks both the beginning and the end. For that reason, it is imperative that all of the couple's and family's wishes and preferences be respected. During this period, the family may be overwhelmed and may have difficulty making decisions. The nurse needs to assist the couple in exploring their feelings and help them make decisions about who will be present and what rituals will occur during and following the birth. Examples of birth preferences include:

- Using music, dimmed lighting, or other environmental preferences
- Laboring or birthing in a specific position
- Having the infant placed on the mother's chest immediately after birth
- Allowing the father to cut the umbilical cord
- Including other family members or friends at the birth.

Sometimes couples worry that others may view their preferences as "strange" or "wrong." The nurse can reassure the family members that it is their personal experience and that there are no right or wrong feelings or preferences.

The couple may have waves of overwhelming grief, disbelief, or sadness. The nurse needs to encourage the couple to express their grief. It is not uncommon for one partner to attempt to put on a "brave front," thinking that by showing grief, he or she will make the other partner feel worse. It also is not uncommon for partners to have intense feelings that they are unable to share. Encourage partners to express their emotions freely to the extent they are able. Help them understand that each of them may experience different feelings.

Supporting the Family in Viewing the Stillborn Infant

Advocates of seeing the stillborn infant believe that viewing the infant assists in dispelling denial and enables the couple to progress to the next step in the grieving process. If they choose to see their stillborn infant, prepare the couple for what they will see by saying, "She is going to feel cold," "He is going to be blue," or other appropriate statements. If the parents have shared the name they chose for their baby, use that name in discussing the baby (e.g., "Jessie's face is bruised."). Another common practice is to wrap the infant in a blanket or to use a hat to cover a birth defect. This allows the parents to view the infant before they see the birth defect. Most parents eventually remove the covering to inspect the infant; however, applying a covering allows them time to adjust to the appearance.

Some families hold their infant for a short time before returning him or her to the nurse, whereas others want to spend a great deal of time with the infant. The nurse allows the family members to remain with the infant for as long as they choose. Some parents may elect to bathe or dress their stillborn; the nurse supports them in their choice. Some couples may want other family members, friends, or their other children to see the infant. The nurse acts as an advocate to ensure that the family's wishes are respected.

Providing Discharge Care

Most facilities prepare a remembrance box or package for the family to take home. This typically consists of a photograph of the infant or family, a card with the baby's footprints, a crib card, an identification band, a lock of hair, and possibly a blanket or clothing worn by the infant. If the couple declines the package, the hospital often keeps these items for a specific period of time in case the parents change their minds.

After the birth, the couple can be given the option of an early discharge (as early as 6–8 hours after the birth). Facility protocol dictates where mothers are transferred after a perinatal loss. Some hospitals have the women remain on the labor and birthing unit; others give the mother the option of choosing a postpartum room or a room on a medical unit. If the mother is transferred to a postpartum unit, care is given to put her in a room far away from other rooms and the newborn nursery. As stated before, it is imperative that all staff members, as well as student nurses, be notified of the mother's status.

Discharge focuses on the physical considerations and adaptation of the mother. The nurse provides the mother with postpartum directions for follow-up care, written materials, and a phone number for questions. The woman also should be given information about her milk coming in and interventions to follow to decrease the discomfort associated with engorgement.

Additional information should be given on the grief process (Figure 12–9 ■). The nurse can prepare the couple to return home by emphasizing that others may not know what to say and that even loved ones may make inappropriate comments because they do not know how to respond to grief and loss. This helps prepare the couple for other's reactions. If there are siblings, each usually progresses through age-appropriate grieving. Provide the parents with information about normal mourning reactions, both psychologic and physiologic.

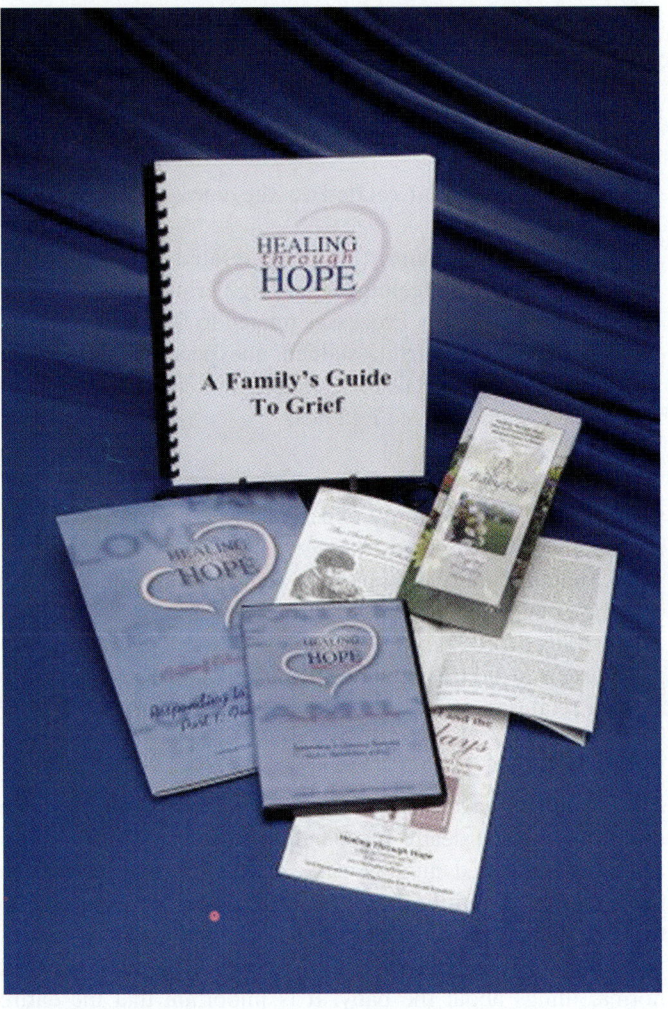

Figure 12–9 ■ Bereavement literature.

Source: Healing through Hope.

When caring for a family suffering from a perinatal loss, understand that the nurse experiences many of the same grief reactions as the parents of a stillborn infant. The nurse should have access to colleagues and family members for counseling and support.

Facilitating the Family's Grief Work

The parents of a stillborn infant suffer a devastating experience that precipitates an intense emotional trauma. During the pregnancy, the couple has already begun the attachment process, which now must be terminated through the grieving process. Thus, facilitating the family's grief work is a critical nursing intervention—one that requires skill, sensitivity, and compassion.

Following discharge, some families may need closure of the intrapartum event to progess with their grief work. A consultation can be scheduled with the practitioner that

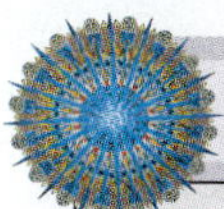

NURSING CARE PLAN For a Family Experiencing Perinatal Loss

Irina Borodina, aged 26, G1P0 at 27 weeks' gestation, arrives with her husband, Anton, at the labor and birthing unit, stating she has been cramping over the last 3 hours and does not feel the baby move. Fetal heart tones are absent. Additional assessments, including an ultrasound, confirm a fetal demise. The physician informs Irina and Anton of the loss, and they decide to undergo an immediate induction. The nurse explains what will occur during labor and what care the body of their deceased child will receive after birth.

During labor, Irina is quiet and she and her husband periodically weep. During the birth, the room is darkened and quiet. Anton asks to see the baby, a male. The nurse explains that the baby is very small, wraps the tiny body in a blanket, and gives it to the father to hold. Irina turns away, crying, and asks the nurse why her baby died. She sobs that she did everything the doctors advised and does not understand what went wrong. "It's not fair!" she says. "Why did God do this to me?" The nurse explains that tests can be performed to help determine why their baby died, but Irina withdraws and does not appear to be listening. She tells the nurse that she is exhausted and asks to be alone with her husband. The nurse removes the body from the room and informs the couple that they can ask to see the baby again if they choose.

When the nurse checks on the couple a few minutes later, they seem calmer. However, when she asks whether they would like to view the baby now, Irina bursts into tears again and shouts at the nurse, "Why can't you just leave us alone?" Her husband quietly suggests that they phone their priest and ask him to bless the baby, but Irina shakes her head despondently. "I prayed so hard all these months, and God took our baby away anyway! Why should I turn to him now?"

ASSESSMENT	DIAGNOSIS	PLANNING
Subjective: Exhaustion, crying, feelings of bewilderment. **Objective:** Hyperventilation during admission, anorexia, pulse 120, respirations 20, restless. Refuses to view baby. Refuses visit from priest. States, "It's not fair!" Blames God for "taking our baby away."	■ Spiritual Distress as evidenced by refusal to view or hold baby, statement of anger at God for taking baby away, and refusal to participate in customary religious practices	■ The clients will participate in seeing and holding the baby, while verbalizing thoughts and feelings associated with the loss. ■ The clients will openly expresses feelings concerning the loss. ■ The clients will verbalize understanding of cause of the baby's death. ■ The client will request to see and hold baby. ■ The clients will accept offer of visit from spiritual advisor.

IMPLEMENTATION

- Provide factual information as soon as it is available about the cause of the fetal demise if known.
- Provide consistency in nursing staff assignments for the client.
- Prepare the baby for viewing.
- Encourage the parents to see, touch, and name the baby.
- Offer remembrances of the baby for the parents to keep.
- Provide an opportunity for religious or spiritual counseling and practices.

EVALUATION

The client communicates feelings of sadness, helplessness, and anger.
The client verbalizes understanding of physiologic etiology of her loss.
The client views, holds, and calls baby by name while saying good-bye.
The client accepts visit from spiritual advisor and verbalizes spiritual comfort.

CRITICAL THINKING

1. How can the nurse promote the grieving process for a couple who has experienced perinatal loss?
2. What types of nursing behaviors might squelch the grieving process?
3. What factors might affect the grief reaction to a perinatal loss?

cared for them during the pregnancy and birth. Families may also want to read the results of tests performed during the intrapartum period and the autopsy report. The couple should be provided with a copy of the medical records and encouraged to ask questions, express their feelings, and ask for clarification.

After a perinatal loss has occurred, nurses and members of the health care team routinely refer families for counseling services. A counselor who specializes in perinatal issues can provide expertise and assist the couple in their grieving. Partners should be allowed to verbalize their fears and concerns about future pregnancies. When appropriate, referrals to genetic counselors, religious support people, and social service agencies should be provided.

Besides referral information, the woman should receive scheduled follow-up phone calls to assess the family's functioning and its progress with grief work. During these follow-up phone calls, pertinent information can be given and additional resources can be identified.

As the grief process ensues, families should be encouraged to implement cultural, religious, or social customs that will assist them in grieving and mourning. The nurse should advise the family members that certain upcoming milestones, such as holidays, future birthdays, baby showers, Mother's Day, Father's Day, and other social events, may trigger their grief. The family can better cope with these events when it is adequately prepared.

Referring the Family to Community Services

Although most facilities have an established protocol for families experiencing perinatal loss, communities are establishing more comprehensive step-by-step intervention programs to assist these families. Community support groups that focus on perinatal loss can provide an important support network and resources. Specialized groups, such as those focused on early pregnancy loss, stillbirth, and perinatal loss associated with specific congenital anomalies, allow families the opportunity to interact with peers who have lost infants under similar circumstances. The nurse provides the group name, contact person (if possible), and phone number. Various books written by mothers who have lost children are available in bookstores and are valuable resources for grieving parents.

Internet technology allows many individuals to share resources and information and to participate in online support groups. Internet resources can be effective for all families and may be the only resources available for families who live in rural, underserved areas.

Specialized community outreach programs are another community resource that can provide assistance to grieving families. One example is an early community intervention program that provides counseling to parents whose fetus has a known lethal congenital anomaly. In perinatal hospice programs, parents are given the opportunity to explore options such as choosing elective termination or waiting for the onset of spontaneous labor or a medically indicated induced labor. For families wanting to continue their pregnancy, the program typically assigns a multidisciplinary team that provides compassionate care, ongoing counseling, referral to support groups, and spiritual guidance (Ramer-Chrastek & Thygesen, 2005).

Caring for the Couple Who Has Experienced Loss in a Previous Pregnancy

Couples who have had a previous perinatal loss typically enter a subsequent pregnancy with conflicting feelings and may experience ambivalence, fear, and anxiety. They often relive their past experience when another pregnancy occurs. Some couples conceive soon after a loss, whereas others wait years. Some couples enter a subsequent pregnancy with grief work largely completed, whereas others are still experiencing unresolved grief.

The nurse caring for a couple who has had a previous loss needs to be kind, compassionate, and patient. Couples need specific information and clear explanations of all prenatal information. Referrals to a genetic counselor should be made when appropriate. Some couples may want to consult with a perinatologist. If unresolved grief issues are present or the family experiences extreme anxiety, counseling may be beneficial.

Interventions to decrease anxiety can help the couple tremendously. At the first visit, an ultrasound can be performed to verify the presence of the fetal heart. In early pregnancy, women may be fearful when first trimester pregnancy symptoms begin to resolve. It may be helpful for these women to make weekly visits for a period of time simply to hear the fetal heartbeat. This intervention may continue to help until the woman begins to feel fetal movement. Throughout the pregnancy, the office or clinic nurse can play a key role by providing reassurance and answering questions the woman may have.

Women with a previous loss typically receive additional antepartum testing throughout the pregnancy. Ultrasounds can provide reassurance and assess fetal growth and development, placental functioning, and cord variations. Nonstress testing and biophysical profiles can be performed weekly after 32 weeks' gestation to ensure fetal well-being. Fetal kick counts should be initiated at 28 weeks and continue until birth. Because placental functioning can decline in postdate pregnancies, women with a previous loss should give birth when their child is due or when the pregnancy is at term—they should not go over their due date.

Many women who have had a previous perinatal loss continue to experience stress and anxiety, even after the birth of a healthy infant (Ramer-Chrastek & Thygesen, 2005). Postpartum and nursery nurses should assess for ongoing stress and anxiety and be prepared to provide additional support to these families.

Evaluation

Anticipated outcomes of nursing care include the following:

- Family members express their feelings about the death of their baby.
- Family members participate in decision making regarding the labor, birth, and immediate postpartum period.
- Family members participate in the decision of whether to see their baby and other decisions about the baby.
- The family has resources available for continued support.
- Family members know what community resources are available and have names and phone numbers if they choose to use them.
- The family is moving into and through the grieving process.

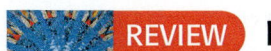

REVIEW Perinatal Loss

RELATE: LINK THE CONCEPTS

Linking the exemplar of Perinatal Loss with the concept of Family:

1. What impact does perinatal loss have on the entire family including father, siblings of the fetus, and grandparents?
2. How can the family members be helped to both support the mother and cope with their own feelings of loss?

Linking the exemplar of Perinatal Loss with the concept of Reproduction:

3. What implications does a perinatal loss have on future pregnancies?
4. How might the needs of this mother differ if she had experienced other perinatal losses and was currently childless?

REFER: GO TO MYNURSINGKIT

REFLECT: CASE STUDY

Betty Jane Walker, 29 years old, is 30 weeks pregnant. She lives with her husband, Rick, and their three children ages 6, 5, and 3. She and her husband describe their marriage as average. He has a history of alcohol abuse but is currently functioning well and owns his own business in the city, commuting via train. Betty is a stay-at-home mom who enjoys reading and playing the piano when she can find the time. Betty is an excellent cook, likes to play bridge, and enjoys golf. She rarely gets time to pursue her hobbies, but does find time to read a few evenings a week. Rick ignores the children for the most part, working all day and burying himself in the newspaper and TV at night. Betty learned last week that the fetus had died and the provider recommended waiting for the normal labor process to begin. Betty visits her provider today because she isn't feeling well.

1. What is the priority nursing diagnosis for Betty?
2. How can you assess Betty's current coping related to the perinatal loss?
3. Betty asks you how to tell her other children about the loss of the baby. What counseling will you provide?
4. How will you respond if Betty tells you that, in some ways, the loss of the fetus is somewhat of a relief?

PEARSON

EXPLORE mynursingkit™

MyNursingKit is your one stop for online chapter review materials and resources. Prepare for success with additional NCLEX®-style practice questions, interactive assignments and activities, web links, animations and videos, and more!

Register your access code from the front of your book at **www.mynursingkit.com**.

REFERENCES

American Association for Geropsychiatry. (2008). Geriatrics and mental health: The facts. Retrieved February 14, 2008, from http://www.aagpgpa.org/prof/facts_mh.asp

American Psychological Association. (2008). What practitioners should know about working with older adults. Retrieved February 14, 2008, from http://www.apa.org/pi/aging/practitioners/executive.html

Beale, E. A., Baile, W. F., & Aaron, J. (2005). Silence is not golden: Communicating with children dying from cancer. *Journal of Clinical Oncology, 23*(15), 3629–3631.

Blackburn, S. T. (2007). *Maternal, fetal, and neonatal physiology: A clinical perspective* (3rd ed.). Philadelphia: Saunders.

Caserta, M. S., Lund, D. A., & Obray, S. J. (2004). Promoting self-care and daily living skills among older widows and widowers: Evidence from the Pathfinders demonstration project. *OMEGA: The Journal of Death and Dying, 49,* 217–236.

Dratler, M. B., Burns, M. K., & Dratler, H. L. (2006). Conveying adverse news in end-of-life situations. *Gastroenterology Clinics of North America, 35,* 41–52.

Druzin, M. L., Smith, J. F., Gabbe, S. G., & Reed, K. L. (2007). Antepartum fetal evaluation. In S. G. Gabbe, J. R. Niebyl, & J. L. Simpson (Eds.), *Obstetrics: Normal and problem pregnancies* (5th ed.). Philadelphia: Churchill Livingstone.

Egan, K. A., & Arnold, R. L. (2003). Grief and bereavement care. *American Journal of Nursing, 103*(9), 42–53.

Engel, G. L. (1964). Grief and grieving. *American Journal of Nursing, 64,* 93–98.

Flannelly, K. J., Weaver, A. J., & Costa, K. G. (2004). A systematic review of religion and spirituality in three palliative care journals, 1990–1999. *Journal of Palliative Care, 20*(1), 50–56.

Gibbs, R. S., & Roberts, D. J. (2007). Case records of the Massachusetts General Hospital. Case 27-2007. A 30-year-old pregnant woman with intrauterine fetal death. *New England Journal of Medicine, 357*(9), 918–925.

Hartford Institute for Geriatric Nursing. (2008). *Best nursing practices in care for older adults.* Try this: The geriatric depression scale. Retrieved February 14, 2008, from http://www.hartfordign.org/trythis/issue04.pdf

Hinds, P. S., Schum, L., Baker, J. N., & Wolfe, J. (2005). Key factors affecting dying children and their families. *Journal of Palliative Medicine, 8*(Suppl. 1), S70–S78.

Kirwin, K., & Hamrin, V. (2005). Decreasing the risk of complicated bereavement and future psychiatric disorders in children. *Journal of Child and Adolescent Psychiatric Nursing, 18*(2), 62–78.

Kübler-Ross, E. (1969). *On death and dying.* New York: Macmillan.

Kübler-Ross, E. (1983). *On children and death.* New York: Macmillan.

Lindsey, J. L. (2006). Evaluation of fetal death. *E-medicine.* Retrieved November 27, 2007, from http://www.emedicine.com/med/topic3235.htm

Lobar, S. L., Youngblut, J. M., & Brooten, D. (2006). Cross-cultural beliefs, ceremonies, and rituals surrounding death of a loved one. *Pediatric Nursing, 32*(1), 44–50.

Macdonald, M. E., Liben, S., Carnevale, F. A., Rennick, J. E., Wolf, S. L., Meloche, D., et al. (2005). Parental perspectives on hospital staff members' acts of kindness and commemoration after a child's death. *Pediatrics, 116*(4), 884–890.

Martocchio, B. C. (1985). Grief and bereavement: Healing through hurt. *Nursing Clinics of North America, 20,* 327–341.

Meadors, P., & Lamson, A. (2008). Compassion fatigue and secondary traumatization: Provider self care on intensive care units for children. *Journal of Pediatric Health Care, 22*(1), 24–34.

Michels, T. C., & Tiu, A. Y. (2007). Second trimester pregnancy loss. *American Family Physician, 76*(9), 1341–1346.

NANDA International. (2007). *NANDA nursing diagnoses: Definitions and classification 2007–2008.* Philadelphia: Author.

National Center for Health Statistics. (2006). Chartbook on trends on the health of Americans. Retrieved November 14, 2007, from http://www.cdc.gov/nchs/hus.htm

National Consensus Project (NCP) for Quality Palliative Care. (2004). Clinical practice guidelines for quality palliative care. Retrieved July 7, 2007, from http://www.nationalconsensusproject.org

Prairie, B. A., Lauria, M. R., Kapp, N., Mackenzie, T., Baker, E. R., & George, K. E. (2007). Mifepristone versus laminaria: A randomized controlled trial of cervical ripening in midtrimester termination. *Contraception, 76*(5), 383–388.

Ramer-Chrastek, J., & Thygesen, N. V. (2005). A perinatal hospice for an unborn child with a life-limiting condition. *International Journal of Palliative Nursing, 11*(6), 274–276.

Rando, T. A. (1991). *How to go on living when someone you love dies.* New York: Bantam.

Rando, T. A. (1993). *Treatment of complicated mourning.* Champaign, IL: Research Press.

Rando, T. A. (2000). *Clinical dimensions of anticipatory mourning: Theory and practice in working with the dying, their loved ones, and their caregivers.* Champaign, IL: Research Press.

Ronda, E., Regidor, E., Garcla, A. M., & Domlnguez, V. (2005). Association between congenital anomalies and paternal exposure to agricultural pesticides depending on mother's employment status. *Journal of Occupational Environmental Medicine, 47*(8), 826–28.

Sanders, C. M. (1998). *Grief: The mourning after: Dealing with adult bereavement* (2nd ed.). New York: John Wiley & Sons.

Shevell, T., Malone, F. D., Vidaver, J., Porter, T. F., Luthy, D. A., Comstock, C. H., et al. (2005). Assisted reproductive technology and pregnancy outcome. *Obstetrics & Gynecology, 106*(5 Pt 1), 1039–1045.

Silver, R. M. (2007). Fetal death. *Obstetrics & Gynecology, 109*(1), 153–167.

Sperling, L., Kiil, C., Larsen, L. U., Ovist, Q., Schwartz, M., Jorgenson, C., et al. (2006). Naturally conceived twins with monochorionic placentation have the highest risk of fetal loss. *Ultrasound in Obstetrics & Gynecology, 5,* 644–652.

Tierney, L. M., McPhee, S. J., & Papadakis, M. A. (2004). *Current medical diagnosis & treatment* (43rd ed.). New York: McGraw Hill.

U.S. Surgeon General. (2003). *Executive summary. Mental health: Culture, race and ethnicity.* U.S. Department of Health and Human Services, U.S. Public Health Service. Retrieved September 27, 2003, from http://www.surgeongeneral.gov

Health, Wellness, and Illness

13

Concept at-a-Glance

Concept Learning Outcomes

After reading about this concept, you will be able to:

1. Define health, illness, wellness, and disease.
2. Explain the health-illness continuum and the concept of high-level wellness.
3. Define health promotion.
4. Describe the nurse's role in health promotion.
5. Identify characteristics of health, disease, and illness.
6. Differentiate illness from disease and acute illness from chronic illness.
7. Develop and evaluate plans for health promotion across the life span.

Concept Key Terms

Acute illness, *638*
Autonomy, *639*
Chronic illness, *638*
Disease, *638*
Exacerbation, *638*
Health, *636*
Health promotion, *639*
Illness, *638*
Illness behavior, *638*
Lifestyle, *645*
Modeling, *648*
Positive reinforcement, *648*
Remission, *638*
Risk factors, *645*
Well-being, *637*
Wellness, *637*
Wellness diagnoses, *647*

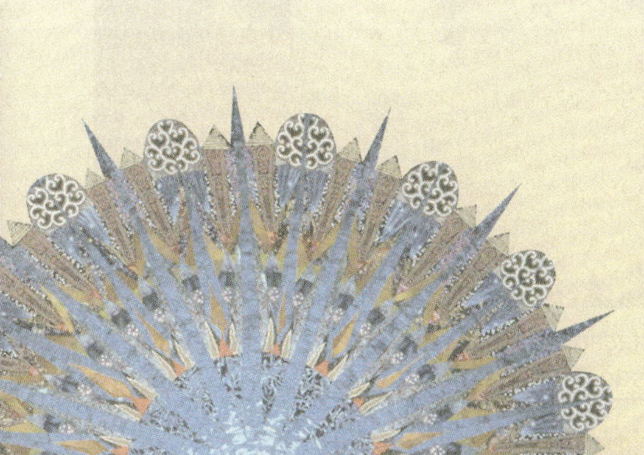

About Health, Wellness, and Illness

Nurses' understanding of health and wellness largely determines the scope and nature of nursing practice. Clients' health beliefs also influence health practices. Some people think of health and wellness (or well-being) as the same thing or, at the very least, as accompanying one another. However, health may not always accompany well-being: A person who has a terminal illness may have a sense of well-being; conversely, another person may lack a sense of well-being, yet be in a state of good health.

For many years the concept of disease was the yardstick by which health was measured. In the late 19th Century, the "how" of disease (pathogenesis) was the major concern of health professionals. The 20th Century focused on finding cures for diseases. Currently, health care providers are increasing their emphasis on promoting health and wellness in individuals, families, and communities. •

CONCEPTS OF HEALTH, WELLNESS, AND WELL-BEING

Health, wellness, and well-being have many definitions and interpretations. The nurse should be familiar with the most common aspects of these concepts and consider how they may be individualized with specific clients.

Health

Traditionally **health** has been defined in terms of the presence or absence of disease. Nightingale defined health as a state of being well and using every power the individual possesses to the fullest extent (Nightingale, 1860/1969). The World Health Organization (WHO) takes a more holistic view of health. Its constitution defines health as "a state of complete physical, mental, and social well-being, and not merely the absence of disease or infirmity" (WHO, 1948). This definition serves the following purposes:

- It reflects concern for the individual as a total person functioning physically, psychologically, and socially. Mental processes determine people's relationships with their physical and social surroundings, their attitudes about life, and their interaction with others.
- It places health in the context of environment. People's lives, and therefore their health, are affected by everything they interact with—not only environmental influences, such as climate and the availability of food, shelter, clean air, and water to drink, but also other people, including family, lovers, employers, coworkers, friends, and associates.

In 1980, the American Nurses Association (ANA) defined health in its social policy statement as "a dynamic state of being in which the developmental and behavioral potential of an individual is realized to the fullest extent possible" (ANA, 1980, p. 5). In this definition, health is more than a state or the absence of disease; it includes striving toward optimal functioning. In 2004, the ANA also stated that health was "An experience that is often expressed in terms of wellness and illness, and may occur in the presence or absence of disease or injury" (2004, p. 48).

PERSONAL DEFINITIONS OF HEALTH Health is a highly individual perception. Consider the following examples of individuals who would probably say they are healthy, even though they have physical impairments that some people would consider illnesses:

- A 15-year-old boy with diabetes takes injectable insulin each morning. He plays on the school soccer team and is editor of the high school newspaper.
- A 32-year-old man is paralyzed from the waist down and needs a wheelchair for mobility. He is taking accounting at a nearby college and uses a specially designed automobile for transportation.
- A 72-year-old woman takes antihypertensive medications to treat high blood pressure. She bowls once a week, is a member of the neighborhood golf club, makes handicrafts for a local charity, and travels 2 months each year.

Many people define and describe health as being free from symptoms of disease and pain as much as possible, being able to be active and to do what they want or must, and being in good spirits most of the time. These characteristics indicate that health is not something that a person achieves suddenly at a specific time. It is an ongoing process, a way of life through which a person develops and encourages every aspect of the body, mind, and feelings to interrelate harmoniously as much as possible (Figure 13–1 ■).

Many factors affect individual definitions of health—the individual's previous experiences, expectations of self, age, and sociocultural influences. Nurses should be aware of their own personal definitions of health and appreciate that other people have their individual definitions as well. How a person

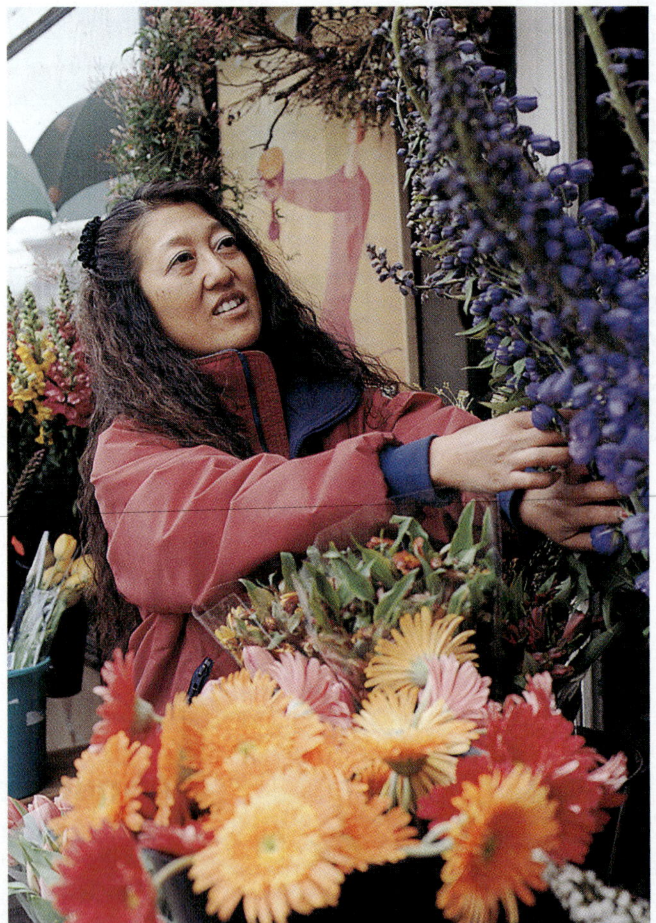

Figure 13–1 ■ Satisfaction with work enhances a sense of well-being and contributes to wellness.

defines health influences his or her behavior related to health and illness. By understanding clients' perceptions of health and illness, nurses can provide more meaningful assistance to help them regain or attain a state of health. For aid in developing a personal definition of health see Box 13–1.

Wellness and Well-Being

Wellness is a state of well-being. Basic aspects of wellness include self-responsibility; an ultimate goal; a dynamic, growing process; daily decision making in the areas of nutrition, stress management, physical fitness, preventive health care, and emotional health; and, most important, the whole being of the individual.

Anspaugh, Hamrick, and Rosato (2006) propose seven components of wellness (Figure 13–2 ■). To realize optimal health and wellness, people must deal with the factors within each component:

1. *Environmental:* The ability to promote health measures that improve the standard of living and quality of life in the community. This includes influences such as food, water, and air.
2. *Occupational:* The ability to achieve a balance between work and leisure time. A person's beliefs about education, employment, and home influence personal satisfaction and relationships with others.
3. *Intellectual:* The ability to learn and use information effectively for personal, family, and career development. Intellectual wellness involves striving for continued growth and learning to deal with new challenges effectively.
4. *Spiritual:* The belief in some force (nature, science, religion, or a higher power) that serves to unite human beings and provide meaning and purpose to life. It includes a person's own morals, values, and ethics.
5. *Physical:* The ability to carry out daily tasks, achieve fitness (e.g., pulmonary, cardiovascular, gastrointestinal), maintain adequate nutrition and proper body fat levels, avoid abusing drugs and alcohol or using tobacco products, and generally practice positive lifestyle habits.
6. *Emotional:* The ability to manage stress and to express emotions appropriately. Emotional wellness involves the ability to recognize, accept, and express feelings and to accept one's limitations.
7. *Social:* The ability to interact successfully with people and within the environment of which each person is a part, to develop and maintain intimacy with significant others, and to develop respect and tolerance for those with different opinions and beliefs.

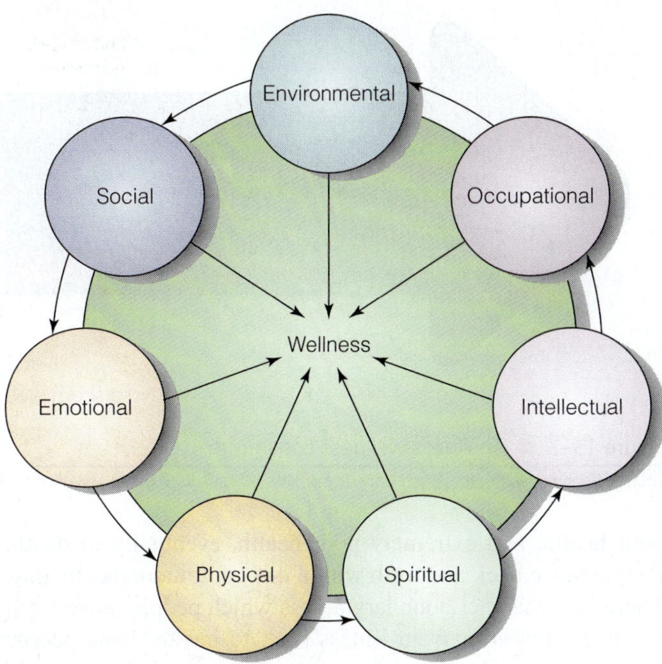

Figure 13–2 ■ The seven components of wellness.

Source: Reproduced with permission from Anspaugh, D. J., Hamrick, M. H., & Rosato, F. D. (2006). *Wellness: Concepts and applications* (6th ed., p. 4). New York: McGraw-Hill.

Box 13–1 **Developing a Personal Definition of Health**

Answering the following questions can help nurses develop a personal definition of health:

- Is a person more than a biophysiologic system?
- Is health more than the absence of disease symptoms?
- Is health the ability of an individual to perform work?
- Is health the ability of an individual to adapt to the environment?
- Is health a condition of a person's actualization?
- Is health a state or a process?
- Is health the effective functioning of self-care activities?
- Is health static or changing?
- Are health and wellness the same?
- Are disease and illness different?
- Are there levels of health?
- Are wellness, health, and illness separate entities or points along a continuum?
- Is health socially determined?
- How do you rate your health and why?

The seven components overlap to some extent, and factors in one component often directly affect factors in another. For example, a person who learns to control daily stress levels from a physiologic perspective is also helping to maintain the emotional stamina needed to cope with a crisis. Wellness involves working on all aspects of the model.

Well-being is a component of health. Hood and Leddy (2003) describe well-being as "a subjective perception of vitality and feeling well ...[that] can be described objectively, experienced, and measured ... and can be plotted on a continuum" (p. 264).

HEALTH-ILLNESS CONTINUA

Health-illness continua (grids or graduated scales) can be used to measure a person's perceived level of wellness. Health and illness or disease can be viewed as the opposite ends of a health continuum. Beginning at a high level of health, a person's condition can move through good health, normal health,

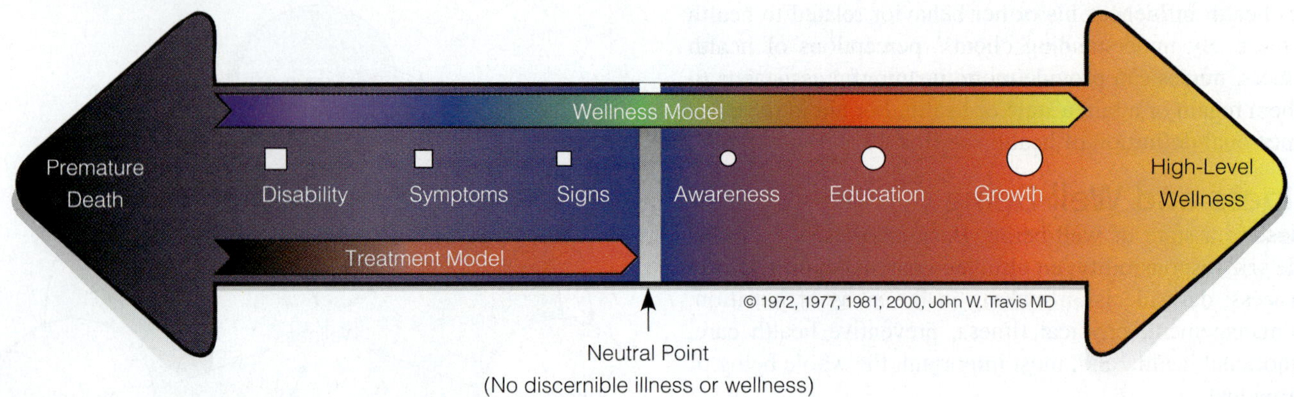

Figure 13–3 ■ An illness-wellness continuum.

Source: Reprinted with permission from Travis, J. W., & Ryan, R. S. (1988). *Wellness workbook.*, Berkeley, CA: Ten Speed Press.

poor health, and extremely poor health, eventually to death. People move back and forth within this continuum day by day. There is no distinct boundary across which people move from health to illness or from illness back to health. How people perceive themselves and how others see them in terms of health and illness will also affect their placement on the continuum. The ranges in which people can be thought of as healthy or ill are considerable (Figure 13–3 ■).

ILLNESS AND DISEASE

Illness is a highly personal state in which the person's physical, emotional, intellectual, social, developmental, or spiritual functioning is thought to be diminished. It is not synonymous with disease and may or may not be related to disease. An individual could have a disease, for example, a growth in the stomach, and not feel ill. Similarly a person can feel ill, that is, feel uncomfortable, and yet have no discernible disease.

Disease can be described as an alteration in body functions that results in a reduction of capacities or a shortening of the normal life span. Disease occurs when microorganisms produce a detectable alteration in normal tissue function that results in a reduction of capacities or a shortening of the normal life span. Primitive people thought "forces" or spirits caused disease. Later, this belief was replaced by the single-causation theory. Traditionally, the goal of intervention by primary care providers was to eliminate or ameliorate disease processes. Today, multiple factors are considered to interact in causing disease and determining an individual's response to treatment.

Illness and disease can be classified in many ways. The terms acute and chronic are commonly used. **Acute illness** is typically characterized by severe symptoms of relatively short duration. The symptoms often appear abruptly and subside quickly and, depending upon the cause, may or may not require intervention by health care professionals. Some acute illnesses are serious (for example, appendicitis may require surgical intervention), but many acute illnesses, such as colds, subside without medical intervention or with only the help of over-the-counter medications. Following an acute illness, most people return to their normal level of wellness.

A **chronic illness** is one that lasts for an extended period, usually 6 months or longer, and often for the duration of person's life. Chronic illnesses usually have a slow onset and often have periods of **remission**, when the symptoms disappear, and **exacerbation**, when the symptoms reappear. Some chronic diseases with intermittent or recurring symptoms may be termed persistent. For example, a client with severe asthma that is normally well-controlled may be diagnosed with severe persistent asthma.

Examples of chronic illnesses include arthritis, heart and lung diseases, and diabetes mellitus. Nurses are involved in caring for chronically ill individuals of all ages in all types of settings—homes, nursing homes, hospitals, clinics, and other institutions. Care needs to be focused on promoting the highest possible level of independence, sense of control, and wellness. Clients often need to modify their activities of daily living, social relationships, and perception of self and body image. In addition, many must learn how to live with increasing physical limitations and discomfort. Client teaching regarding compliance with medications and treatment plans, even when the client is feeling well, is an essential nursing intervention for individuals with chronic illnesses.

Illness Behaviors

When people become ill, they behave in certain ways that sociologists refer to as illness behavior. **Illness behavior**, a coping mechanism, involves ways that individuals describe, monitor, and interpret their symptoms, take remedial actions, and use the health care system. How people behave when they are ill is highly individualized and is affected by many variables such as age, sex, occupation, socioeconomic status, religion, ethnic origin, psychologic stability, personality, education, and modes of coping.

Effects of Illness on the Client and Family

Illness brings about changes in both the involved individual and the family. The changes vary depending upon the nature, severity, and duration of the illness; attitudes associated with the illness by the client and others; the financial costs associated with the illness; the lifestyle changes incurred; adjustments to usual roles; and so on.

Ill clients may experience behavioral and emotional changes, changes in self-concept and body image, and lifestyle changes. Behavioral and emotional changes associated with short-term illness are generally mild and short lived. The individual, for example, may become irritable and lack the energy or desire to interact with family members or friends in the usual fashion. More acute responses are likely with severe, life-threatening, chronic, or disabling illness. Anxiety, fear, anger, withdrawal, denial, a sense of hopelessness, and feelings of powerlessness are all common responses to severe or disabling illness. For example, a client experiencing a heart attack fears for his or her life and the financial burden it may place on the client's family. Another client informed about a diagnosis of cancer or AIDS or crippling neurologic disease may, over time, experience episodes of denial, anger, fear, and hopelessness. For a client with a lifelong chronic illness, these feelings can recur each time the client experiences an acute attack of the illness. Repeated acute attacks, the financial expense that they incur, and the emotional strain that they put on the client and family can cause both the client and family a great deal of stress.

Certain illnesses can also change the client's body image or physical appearance, especially if there is severe scarring or loss of a limb or special sense organ. The client's self-esteem and self-concept may also be affected. Many factors play a part in low self-esteem and a disturbance in self-concept and include: loss of body parts and function, pain, disfigurement, dependence on others, unemployment, financial problems, inability to participate in social functions, strained relationships with others, and spiritual distress. Nurses need to help clients express their thoughts and feelings, and to provide care that helps the client effectively cope with change.

Ill individuals are vulnerable to loss of **autonomy**—the state of being independent and self-directed without outside control. Family interactions may change so that clients are no longer involved in making family decisions or even in making decisions about their own health care. Nurses need to support clients' right to self-determination and autonomy as much as possible by providing them with sufficient information to participate in decision-making processes and to maintain a feeling of being in control.

Illness often necessitates a change in lifestyle. In addition to participating in treatments and taking medications, the ill person may need to change diet, activity and exercise, and rest and sleep patterns.

Nurses can help clients adjust their lifestyles in the following ways:

- Providing explanations about necessary adjustments
- Making arrangements wherever possible to accommodate the client's lifestyle
- Encouraging other health professionals to become aware of the person's lifestyle practices and to support healthy aspects of that lifestyle
- Reinforcing desirable changes in practices with a goal of making them a permanent part of the client's lifestyle.

HEALTH PROMOTION

The vision of **health promotion** was initially expressed in 1979 with the Surgeon General's report *Healthy People,* which emphasized health promotion and disease prevention. *Healthy People 2000* followed in 1990, providing a framework for national health promotion, health protection, and preventive service strategy. The current *Healthy People 2010: Understanding and Improving Health* (U.S. Department of Health and Human Services [USDHHS], 2000) presents a comprehensive 10-year strategy for promoting health and preventing illness, disability, and premature death. The two major goals of *Healthy People 2010* reflect the nation's changing demographics:

1. "Increase quality and years of healthy life" indicates the aging or "graying" of the population.
2. "Eliminate health disparities" reflects the diversity of the population.

To support these goals, *Healthy People 2010* is organized into 28 focus areas to improve health (Box 13–2). *Healthy People 2010* also establishes a set of leading health indicators that reflect the major public health concerns in the United States at the beginning of the 21st Century (Box 13–3). Each indicator relates to a number of the health objectives. It is

Box 13–2 The 28 Focus Areas in *Healthy People 2010*

1. Access to quality health services
2. Arthritis, osteoporosis, and chronic back conditions
3. Cancer
4. Chronic kidney disease
5. Diabetes
6. Disability and secondary conditions
7. Educational and community-based programs
8. Environmental health
9. Family planning
10. Food safety
11. Health communication
12. Heart disease and stroke
13. HIV
14. Immunization and infectious diseases
15. Injury and violence prevention
16. Maternal, infant, and child health
17. Medical product safety
18. Mental health and mental disorders
19. Nutrition and overweight
20. Occupational safety and health
21. Oral health
22. Physical activity and fitness
23. Public health infrastructure
24. Respiratory diseases
25. Sexually transmitted diseases
26. Substance abuse
27. Tobacco use
28. Vision and hearing

Source: U.S. Department of Health and Human Services. (2007). Retrieved July 6, 2009, from http://www.cdc.gov/nchs/about/otheract/hpdata2010/2010fa28.htm.

Box 13–3 The Leading Health Indicators in *Healthy People 2010*

- **Physical activity**
  Regular physical activity throughout life is important for maintaining a healthy body, enhancing psychological well-being, and preventing premature death (p. 26).
- **Overweight and obesity**
  Overweight and obesity are major contributors to many preventable causes of death. On average, higher body weights are associated with higher death rates. The number of overweight children, adolescents, and adults has risen over the past four decades (p. 28).
- **Tobacco use**
  Cigarette smoking is the single most preventable cause of disease and death in the United States (p. 30).
- **Substance abuse**
  Alcohol and illicit drug use are associated with many of this country's most serious problems, including violence, injury, and HIV infection (p. 32).
- **Responsible sexual behavior**
  Unintended pregnancies and sexually transmitted diseases (STDs), including infection with the human immunodeficiency virus that causes AIDS, can result from unprotected sexual behaviors (p. 34).
- **Mental health**
  Approximately 20% of the U.S. population is affected by mental illness during a given year; no one is immune. Of all mental illnesses, depression is the most common disorder. Major depression is the leading cause of disability and is the cause of more than two thirds of suicides each year (p. 36).
- **Injury and violence**
  More than 400 Americans die each day from injuries due primarily to motor vehicle crashes, firearms, poisonings, suffocation, falls, fires, and drowning (p. 38).
- **Environmental quality**
  An estimated 25% of preventable illnesses worldwide can be attributed to poor environmental quality. Two indicators of air quality are ozone (outdoor) and environmental tobacco smoke (indoor) (p. 40).
- **Immunization**
  Vaccines are among the greatest public health achievements of the 20th century. Immunizations can prevent disability and death from infectious diseases for individuals and can help control the spread of infections within communities (p. 42).
- **Access to health care**
  Strong predictors of access to quality health care include having health insurance, a higher income level, and a regular primary care provider or other source of ongoing health care. Use of clinical preventive services, such as early prenatal care, can serve as indicators of access to quality health care services (p. 44).

Source: U.S. Department of Health and Human Services. (2007). Retrieved July 6, 2009, from http://www.cdc.gov/nchs/about/otheract/hpdata2010/2010indicators.htm.

expected that these indicators will help develop action plans to improve the health of both individuals and communities.

The foundation for *Healthy People 2010* is the belief that individual health is closely linked to community health and the reverse. For example, community health is affected by the beliefs, attitudes, and behaviors of the individuals who live in the community. Thus, the vision for *Healthy People 2010* is "Healthy People in Healthy Communities" (USDHHS, 2000, p. 3). As a result, partnerships are important to improving individual and community health. Businesses, local government, and civic, professional, and religious organizations can all participate. Examples include sponsoring a health fair, establishing fitness programs, beginning community recycling, and printing immunization schedules.

Health Promotion, Health Protection, and Disease Prevention

Considerable differences appear in the literature regarding the use of the terms *health promotion, primary prevention, health protection,* and *illness/disease prevention.* Edelman and Mandle (2006) state that "prevention, in a narrow sense, means avoiding the development of disease in the future, and, in the broader sense, consists of all interventions to limit progression of a disease" (p. 13). Pender, Murdaugh, and Parsons (2006) consider health promotion to be different from disease prevention or health protection. They define *health promotion* as "behavior motivated by the desire to increase well-being and actualize human health potential," and *disease prevention* or *health protection* as "behavior motivated by a desire to actively avoid illness, detect it early, or maintain functioning within the constraints of illness" (p. 7). The individual's underlying motivation for the behavior is the major difference. Box 13–4 provides an overview of the differences between health promotion and health protection.

The difficulty in separating the terms *health promotion* and *disease prevention/health protection* lies in the fact that an activity may be carried out for numerous reasons. For example, a 40-year-old male may begin a program of walking 3 miles each day. If the goal of his program was to "decrease the risk of cardiovascular disease," then the activity would be considered disease prevention or health protection. By contrast, if the motivation for his walking regimen were to "increase his overall health and feeling of well-being," then

Box 13–4 Differences Between Health Promotion and Health Protection

HEALTH PROMOTION	HEALTH PROTECTION
■ Not disease oriented	■ Illness or injury specific
■ Motivated by personal, positive "approach" to wellness	■ Motivated by "avoidance" of illness
■ Seeks to expand positive potential for health	■ Seeks to thwart the occurrence of insults to health and well-being

Source: Pender, N. J., Murdaugh, C. L., & Parsons, M. A. (2006). *Health promotion in nursing practice* (5th ed., p. 8). Upper Saddle River, NJ: Prentice Hall. Reprinted with permission.

the activity would be considered a health promotion behavior. It is most helpful to think of health promotion and health protection as being complementary processes because both affect quality of health.

Health promotion can be offered to all clients regardless of their health and illness status or age. For example, weight-control measures can benefit both overweight clients without disease and clients with cardiac or joint disease. See Developmental Considerations feature for examples.

The Nurse's Role in Health Promotion

Health promotion is an important component of nursing practice. It is a way of thinking that revolves around a philosophy of wholeness, wellness, and well-being. In the past two decades, the public has become increasingly aware of and interested in health promotion. Many people are aware of the relationship between lifestyle and illness and have begun developing health-promoting habits, such as getting adequate exercise, rest, and relaxation; maintaining good nutrition; and controlling the use of tobacco, alcohol, and other drugs.

Individuals and communities that seek to increase their responsibility for personal health and self-care require health education. The trend toward health promotion has created new opportunities for nurses to strengthen the profession's influence on health promotion. Nurses also have more opportunity to disseminate information that promotes an educated public and to assist individuals and communities to change long-standing health behaviors. Today, nurses serve in a wide variety of organizations and committees.

A variety of programs can be used to promote health, including (a) information dissemination, (b) health risk appraisal and wellness assessment, (c) lifestyle and behavior change, and (d) environmental control programs.

Information dissemination is the most basic type of health promotion program. This method makes use of a variety of media to offer information to the public about the risk of particular lifestyle choices and personal behavior, as well as the benefits of changing that behavior and improving the quality of life. Billboards, posters, brochures, newspaper features, books, and health fairs all offer opportunities for disseminating health promotion information. Alcohol and drug abuse, driving under the influence of alcohol, hypertension, and the need for immunizations are some of the topics frequently discussed. Information dissemination is a useful strategy for raising the level of knowledge and awareness of individuals and groups about health habits.

When planning information dissemination, it is important to consider factors such as culture and age group. Knowing the best place and method for distributing information will increase the effectiveness. For example, churches often provide older Black individuals with social support while serving as a spiritual home. The church is often the appropriate place to hold health fairs or even small group discussions on various health topics. It offers a stepping-stone for providing information and suggesting resources for special needs—all done in a comfortable, nonthreatening environment.

It is just as critical to know where people get misinformation. Sending multiple mailings has become a marketing ploy for advertising "miracle" vitamins, herbs, and food supplements. These are heavily directed toward older adults, who may choose this route to purchase items if they have transportation problems.

DEVELOPMENTAL CONSIDERATIONS Health Promotion Topics Across the Life Span

INFANTS

- Infant-parent attachment/bonding
- Breast-feeding
- Sleep patterns
- Playful activity to stimulate development
- Immunizations
- Safety promotion and injury control

CHILDREN

- Nutrition
- Dental checkups
- Rest and exercise
- Immunizations
- Safety promotion and injury control

ADOLESCENTS

- Communicating with the teen
- Hormonal changes
- Nutrition
- Exercise and rest
- Peer group influences
- Self-concept and body image
- Sexuality
- Safety promotion and accident prevention

OLDER ADULTS

- Adequate sleep
- Appropriate use of alcohol
- Dental/oral health
- Drug management
- Exercise
- Foot health
- Health screening recommendations
- Hearing aid use
- Immunizations
- Medication instruction
- Mental health
- Nutrition
- Physical fitness
- Preventive health services
- Safety precautions
- Smoking cessation
- Weight control

Health risk appraisal and wellness assessment programs are used to teach individuals about the risk factors inherent in their lives and to motivate them to reduce specific risks and develop positive health habits. Wellness assessment programs are focused on more positive methods of enhancement, in contrast to the risk factor approach used in the health appraisal. A variety of tools are available to facilitate these assessments; some are computer based and can therefore be offered to educational institutions and industries at a reasonable cost.

Lifestyle and behavior change programs require the participation of the individual and are geared toward enhancing the quality of life and extending the life span. Individuals generally consider lifestyle changes after they have been informed of the need to change their health behavior and have become aware of the potential benefits of the process. Many programs are available to the public, on both a group and individual basis and may include topics such as stress management, nutrition awareness, weight control, smoking cessation, and exercise.

Environmental control programs have been developed in response to the continuing increase of contaminants of human origin being introduced into our environment. The amount of contaminants that are already present in the air, food, and water will affect the health of our descendants for several generations. The most common concerns of community groups are toxic and nuclear wastes, nuclear power plants, air and water pollution, and herbicide and pesticide use.

Health promotion activities, such as the variety of programs previously discussed, involve collaborative relationships with both clients and primary care providers. The role of the nurse is to work *with* people, not *for* them—that is, to act as a facilitator of the process of assessing, evaluating, and understanding health. The nurse may act as advocate, consultant, teacher, or coordinator of services. For examples of the nurse's role in health promotion, see Box 13–5.

In these roles, the nurse may work with individuals of all age groups and diverse family units or concentrate on a specific population, such as new parents, school-age children, or older adults. In any case, the nursing process is a basic tool for the nurse in a health promotion role. Although the process is the same, the nurse emphasizes teaching the client (either an individual or a family unit) self-care responsibility. Adult clients decide the goals, determine the health promotion plans, and take responsibility for the success of the plans.

As increasingly knowledgeable health care consumers, clients expect and deserve quality care. Whether assisting an individual, family, or an entire community, quality nursing care seeks to emphasize illness prevention and health promotion. Nurses recognize that a client's state of health and wellness encompasses many dimensions, including social, spiritual, cultural, sexual, environmental, physical, and psychological. Each client encounter affords the nurse an opportunity to influence and encourage both traditional and innovative health-seeking behaviors.

Assessing and planning health care of the individual client are enhanced when the nurse understands the concepts of individuality, holism, homeostasis, and human needs. The beliefs and values of each person and the support he or she receives come in large part from the family and are reinforced by the community. The reverse is also true—the health of a community is affected by the beliefs, attitudes, and behaviors of the individuals in the community.

Box 13–5 The Nurse's Role in Health Promotion

- Model healthy lifestyle behaviors and attitudes.
- Facilitate client involvement in the assessment, implementation, and evaluation of health goals.
- Teach clients self-care strategies to enhance fitness, improve nutrition, manage stress, and enhance relationships.
- Assist individuals, families, and communities to increase their levels of health.
- Educate clients to be effective health care consumers.
- Assist clients, families, and communities to develop and choose health-promoting options.
- Guide clients' development in effective problem solving and decision making.
- Reinforce clients' personal and family health-promoting behaviors.
- Advocate in the community for changes that promote a healthy environment.

VARIABLES INFLUENCING HEALTH

Many variables influence a person's health status, beliefs, and behaviors or practices. These factors may or may not be under conscious control. People can usually control their health behaviors and can choose healthy or unhealthy activities (external variables). In contrast, people have little or no choice over their genetic makeup, age, sex, culture, and sometimes their geographic environments (internal variables).

Internal variables include biologic, psychologic, and cognitive dimensions. They are often described as nonmodifiable variables because, for the most part, they cannot be changed. However, when internal variables are linked to health problems, the nurse must be even more diligent about working with the client to influence external variables (such as exercise and diet) that may assist in health promotion and illness prevention. Regular health exams and appropriate screening for early detection of health problems become even more important. See Table 13–1 for health screening guidelines across the life span.

Biologic Dimension

Genetic makeup, gender, age, and developmental level all significantly influence a person's health. Genetic makeup influences biologic characteristics, innate temperament, activity level, and intellectual potential. It can impact susceptibility to specific disease, such as diabetes and breast cancer. In some cases, genetic predisposition for health or illness is enhanced when parents are from the same ethnic genetic pool. For example, people of African heritage have a higher incidence of sickle-cell anemia and hypertension than the general population but may be less susceptible to malaria.

TABLE 13–1 Health Screenings and Immunization Guidelines Across the Life Span

AGE GROUP	RECOMMENDED SCREENINGS AND HEALTH PROMOTION
Newborn and infant	■ Screening of newborns for hearing loss; follow-up at 3 months and early intervention by 6 months if appropriate ■ Health examinations at 2 weeks and 2, 4, 6, and 12 months ■ Immunizations: diphtheria, tetanus, acellular pertussis (DTaP), inactivated poliovirus vaccine (IPV), pneumococcal, measles-mumps-rubella (MMR), *Haemophilus influenzae* type B (HIB), hepatitis B (HepB), varicella and influenza vaccines as recommended ■ Fluoride supplements if there is inadequate water fluoridation (less than 0.7 ppm) ■ Screening for tuberculosis ■ Screening for phenylketonuria (PKU) and other metabolic conditions ■ Denver II or other developmental screening
Toddler	■ Health examinations at 15 and 18 months and then as recommended by the primary care provider ■ Dental visit starting at age 3 or earlier ■ Immunizations: continuing DTaP, IPV series, pneumococcal, MMR, *Haemophilus influenzae* type B, hepatitis B, hepatitis A, and influenza vaccines as recommended ■ Screenings for tuberculosis and lead poisoning ■ Fluoride supplements if there is inadequate water fluoridation (less than 0.7 ppm)
Preschool	■ Health examinations every 1–2 years ■ Immunizations: continuing DTaP, IPV series, MMR, hepatitis, pneumococcal, influenza, and other immunizations as recommended ■ Screenings for tuberculosis ■ Vision and hearing screening ■ Regular dental screenings and fluoride treatment
School-age	■ Annual physical examination or as recommended ■ Immunizations as recommended (e.g., MMR, meningococcal, tetanus-diphtheria, adult preparation [Td]) ■ Screening for tuberculosis ■ Periodic vision, speech, and hearing screenings ■ Regular dental screenings and fluoride treatment
Adolescent	■ Health examination as recommended by the primary care provider ■ Immunizations as recommended, such as adult tetanus-diphtheria vaccine, MMR, pneumococcal, and hepatitis B vaccine ■ Screening for tuberculosis ■ Periodic vision and hearing screenings ■ Regular dental assessments
Young adults	■ Routine physical examination (every 1–3 years for females; every 5 years for males) ■ Immunizations as recommended, such as tetanus-diphtheria boosters every 10 years, meningococcal vaccine if not given in early adolescence (Bilukha & Rosenstein, 2005), and hepatitis B vaccine ■ Regular dental assessments (every 6 months) ■ Periodic vision and hearing screenings ■ Professional breast examination every 1–3 years ■ Papanicolaou smear annually within 3 years of onset of sexual activity ■ Testicular examination every year ■ Screening for cardiovascular disease (e.g., cholesterol test every 5 years if results are normal; blood pressure to detect hypertension; baseline electrocardiogram at age 35) ■ Tuberculosis skin test every 2 years ■ Smoking: history and counseling, if needed

(continued)

TABLE 13–1 Health Screenings and Immunization Guidelines Across the Life Span (continued)

AGE GROUP	RECOMMENDED SCREENINGS AND HEALTH PROMOTION
Middle-aged adults	■ Physical examination (every 3–5 years until age 40, then annually) ■ Immunizations as recommended, such as a tetanus booster every 10 years, and current recommendations for influenza vaccine ■ Regular dental assessments (e.g., every 6 months) ■ Tonometry for signs of glaucoma and other eye diseases every 2–3 years or annually if indicated ■ Breast examination annually by primary care provider ■ Testicular examination annually by primary care provider ■ Screenings for cardiovascular disease (e.g., blood pressure measurement; electrocardiogram and cholesterol test as directed by the primary care provider) ■ Screenings for colorectal, breast, cervical, uterine, and prostate cancer ■ Screening for tuberculosis every 2 years ■ Smoking: history and counseling, if needed
Older adults	■ Total cholesterol and high-density lipid protein measurement every 3–5 years until age 75 ■ Aspirin, 81 mg, daily, if in high-risk group ■ Diabetes mellitus screen every 3 years, if in high-risk group ■ Smoking cessation ■ Screening mammogram every 1–2 years (women) ■ Clinical breast exam annually (women) ■ Pap smear annually if there is a history of abnormal smears or previous hysterectomy for malignancy (U.S. Preventive Services Task Force, 2003) ■ Older women who have regular, normal Pap smears or hysterectomy for nonmalignant causes do NOT need Pap smears beyond the age of 65 (U.S. Preventive Services Task Force, 2003) ■ Annual digital rectal exam ■ Annual prostate-specific antigen (PSA) ■ Annual fecal occult blood test (FOBT) ■ Sigmoidoscopy every 5 years; colonoscopy every 10 years ■ Visual acuity screen annually ■ Hearing screen annually ■ Depression screen periodically ■ Family violence screen periodically ■ Height and weight measurements annually ■ Sexually transmitted disease testing, if in high-risk group ■ Annual flu vaccine if over 65 or in high-risk group ■ Pneumococcal vaccine at 65 and every 10 years thereafter ■ Td vaccine every 10 years

Gender influences the distribution of disease. Certain acquired and genetic diseases are more common in one sex than in the other. Disorders more common among women include osteoporosis and autoimmune diseases such as rheumatoid arthritis. Those more common among men are stomach ulcers, abdominal hernias, and respiratory diseases.

Age is also a significant factor in the distribution of disease. For example, arteriosclerotic heart disease is common in middle-aged men but occurs infrequently in younger people; communicable diseases such as whooping cough and measles are common in children but rare in older adults, who have acquired immunity to them.

Developmental level has a major impact on health status. Consider these examples:

- Because infants lack physiologic and psychologic maturity, their defenses against disease are lower during the first years of life.
- Toddlers who are learning to walk are more prone to falls and injury.
- Adolescents who need to conform to peers are more prone to risk-taking behavior and subsequent injury.
- Declining physical and sensory-perceptual abilities limit the ability of older adults to respond to environmental hazards and stressors.

Psychologic Dimension

Psychologic (emotional) factors influencing health include mind-body interactions and self-concept.

Mind-body interactions can affect health status positively or negatively. Emotional responses to stress affect body function. For example, a student who is extremely anxious before a test may experience urinary frequency or diarrhea. A person worried about the outcome of surgery or about the behavior of a teenager may chain smoke. Prolonged emotional distress may increase susceptibility to organic disease or precipitate it. Emotional distress may influence the immune system through central nervous system and endocrine alterations. Alterations in the immune system are related to the incidence of infections, cancer, and autoimmune diseases.

Increasing attention is being given to the mind's ability to direct the body's functioning. Relaxation, meditation, and biofeedback techniques are gaining wider recognition among individuals and health care professionals. For example, women often use relaxation techniques to decrease pain during childbirth. Other people may learn biofeedback skills to reduce hypertension.

Emotional reactions also occur in response to body conditions. For example, a person diagnosed with a terminal illness may experience fear and depression. *Self-concept* is how a person feels about self (self-esteem) and perceives the physical self (body image) and his or her needs, roles, and abilities. Self-concept affects how people view and handle situations. Such attitudes can affect health practices, responses to stress and illness, and when treatment is sought. An example is the anorexic woman who deprives herself of needed nutrients because she believes she is too fat even though she is well below an acceptable weight level. Self-perceptions are also associated with a person's definition of health. For example, a 75-year-old man who can no longer move large objects as he was accustomed to doing may need to examine and redefine his concept of health in view of his age and abilities.

Cognitive Dimension

Cognitive or intellectual factors influencing health include lifestyle choices and spiritual and religious beliefs. Some clients are better at problem solving and come equipped with better coping skills than others. Nurses must be aware of cognitive and intellectual factors that support or hinder a client's compliance with treatment.

Lifestyle refers to a person's general way of living, including living conditions and individual patterns of behavior that are influenced by sociocultural factors and personal characteristics. In brief, lifestyle is often considered as behavior and activities over which people have control. Lifestyle choices may have positive or negative effects on health. Practices that have potentially negative effects on health are often referred to as **risk factors**. For example, overeating, getting insufficient exercise, and being overweight are closely related to the incidence of heart disease, arteriosclerosis, diabetes, and hypertension. Excessive use of tobacco is clearly implicated in lung cancer, emphysema, and cardiovascular diseases. See Box 13–6 for examples of healthy lifestyle choices.

Box 13–6 Examples of Healthy Lifestyle Choices

- Regular exercise
- Weight control
- Avoidance of saturated fats
- Alcohol and tobacco avoidance
- Seat belt use
- Bike helmet use
- Immunization updates
- Regular dental checkups
- Regular health maintenance visits for screening examinations or tests

Spiritual and religious beliefs can significantly affect health behavior. For example, Jehovah's Witnesses oppose blood transfusions; some fundamentalists believe that a serious illness is a punishment from God; some religious groups are strict vegetarians; and religious Jews perform circumcision on the eighth day of a male baby's life. The influence of spirituality and religion is discussed further in the Spirituality concept.

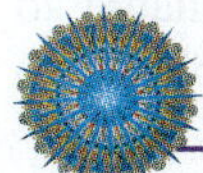

NURSING PROCESS

Health Promotion

A thorough assessment of the individual's health status is basic to health promotion. As nurses move toward greater autonomy in client care, expanded assessment skills are essential to providing the meaningful data needed for health planning.

Assessment

Components of this assessment are the health history and physical examination, physical fitness assessment, lifestyle assessment, spiritual assessment, social support systems review, health risk assessment, health beliefs review, and life-stress review.

HEALTH HISTORY AND PHYSICAL EXAMINATION The health history and physical examination provide a means for detecting any existing problems. The age of the individual must be considered when collecting data. For example, an environmental safety assessment and immunization history must be appropriate to the person's age. A nutritional assessment is another important part of the health history. The nurse must consider both age and body build of the client when gathering information on dietary patterns.

PHYSICAL FITNESS ASSESSMENT During an evaluation of physical fitness, the nurse assesses several components of the body's physical functioning: muscle endurance, flexibility, body composition, and cardiorespiratory endurance. See Exemplar 13.2, Physical Fitness and Exercise.

LIFESTYLE ASSESSMENT Lifestyle assessment focuses on the personal lifestyle and habits of the client as they affect health. Categories of lifestyle generally assessed include physical activity, nutritional practices, stress management, and such habits as smoking, alcohol consumption, and drug use. Other

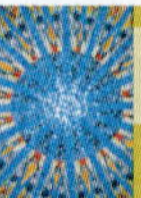

DEVELOPMENTAL CONSIDERATIONS Factors Affecting Health Promotion and Illness Prevention in Children and Older Adults

CHILDREN

Childhood obesity is becoming a serious health problem. Data collected by the Centers for Disease Control and Prevention (CDC) show that nearly 16% of American children are overweight, up from 6.5% in 1980 (National Center for Health Statistics, 2004). Obesity and overweight in children contribute to long-term health problems such as heart disease and diabetes mellitus.

Although specific causes of obesity and appropriate strategies to reduce weight will vary from child to child, healthy eating habits and adequate exercise patterns form the basis for healthy growth and prevention of obesity in children. It is the responsibility of parents and caregivers to provide children with healthy food choices and an environment that makes eating a pleasure. It is the responsibility of children to decide how much and what foods to eat. Adults must be role models for their children, eating well and exercising regularly themselves.

OLDER ADULTS

In older adults, health promotion and illness prevention are important, but often the focus is on learning to adapt to and live with increasing changes and limitations. Maximizing strengths continues to be of prime importance in maintaining optimal function and quality of life. Factors that may indicate a need for additional information or resources include the following:

- An increase in physical limitations
- Presence of one or more chronic illnesses
- Change in cognitive status
- Difficulty in accessing health care services due to transportation problems
- Poor support system
- Need for environmental modifications for safety and to maintain independence
- Attitude of hopelessness and depression, which decreases the motivation to use resources or learn new information

categories may be included. Several tools are available to assess lifestyle. The goals of lifestyle assessment tools are to provide the following:

- An opportunity for clients to assess the impact of their present lifestyle on their health
- A basis for decisions related to desired behavior and lifestyle change
- Special consideration may need to be given to the lifestyles of children and older adults (see the Developmental Considerations feature box).

SPIRITUAL HEALTH ASSESSMENT Spiritual health is the ability to develop one's inner nature to its fullest potential, including the ability to discover and articulate one's basic purpose in life; learn how to experience love, joy, peace, and fulfillment; and learn how to help ourselves and others achieve their fullest potential (Pender et al., 2006, p. 108). Spiritual beliefs can affect a person's interpretation of events in his or her life and, therefore, an assessment of spiritual well-being is a part of evaluating the person's overall health. (See the Spirituality concept for more information.)

SOCIAL SUPPORT SYSTEMS REVIEW Understanding the social context in which a person lives and works is important in health promotion. Individuals and groups, through interpersonal relationships, can provide comfort, assistance, encouragement, and information. Social support fosters successful coping and promotes satisfying and effective living.

Social support systems contribute to health by creating an environment that encourages healthy behaviors, promotes self-esteem and wellness, and provides feedback to ensure that the person's actions will lead to desirable outcomes. Examples of social support systems include family, peer support groups (including Internet-based support groups), community-organized religious support systems (e.g., churches), and self-help groups (e.g., Mended Hearts, Weight Watchers). The Focus on Diversity and Culture box addresses aspects of social support within the context of culture.

LIFE STRESS REVIEW There is abundant literature about the impact of stress on mental and physical well-being. A variety of stress-related instruments can be found in the literature.

Validating Assessment Data

Following the collection of assessment data, the nurse and client together need to review, validate, and summarize the information. During this process, the nurse verbally reviews the current practices and attitudes of the client. This allows

FOCUS ON DIVERSITY AND CULTURE Cultural Aspects of Social Support

It is important to understand how various subgroups of American society may define social support.

- In the Black community, the family and church traditionally are major providers of social support.
- Hispanic-Latin Americans and Asian Americans view the family as a major social support system.
- Asian Americans respect older adults and use shame and harmony in giving and receiving support.
- Native Americans live in social networks that foster mutual assistance and support.

Source: Pender, N. J., Murdaugh, C. L., & Parsons, M. A. (2006). *Health promotion in nursing practice* (5th ed., pp. 239–240). Upper Saddle River, NJ: Prentice Hall. Reprinted with permission.

validation of the information by the client and may increase awareness of the need to change behavior. The nurse and client need to consider the following:

- Any existing health problems
- The client's perceived degree of control over health status
- Key health beliefs
- Level of physical fitness and nutritional status
- Illnesses for which the client is at risk
- Current positive health practices
- Spirituality
- Sources of life stress and ability to handle stress
- Social support systems
- Information needed to enhance health care practices.

Diagnosis

Nursing diagnoses accepted by the North American Nursing Diagnosis Association (NANDA) have generally focused on impaired or imbalanced health patterns or problems. The NANDA **wellness diagnoses** definition, however, states "Describes human responses to levels of wellness in an individual, family, or community that have a readiness for enhancement" (2005, p. 277).

Wellness diagnoses can be applied at all levels of prevention but are particularly useful for healthy clients who require teaching for health promotion, disease prevention, and personal growth. When the nurse and client conclude that the client has positive function in a certain pattern area, such as adequate nutrition or effective coping, the nurse can use this information to help the client reach a higher level of functioning.

A wellness diagnosis is preceded by the modifier "readiness for enhanced." The following examples are included in the NANDA taxonomy:

- Readiness for Enhanced Spiritual Well-being
- Readiness for Enhanced Coping
- Readiness for Enhanced Nutrition
- Readiness for Enhanced Knowledge (Specify)
- Readiness for Enhanced Parenting
- Readiness for Enhanced Self-Concept
- Readiness for Enhanced Immunization Status
- Readiness for Enhanced Self-Care.

Wellness diagnoses provide a clear focus for planning interventions without indicating that a problem exists.

Plan

Health promotion plans need to be developed according to the needs, desires, and priorities of the client. The client decides on health promotion goals, the activities or interventions to achieve those goals, the frequency and duration of the activities, and the method of evaluation. During the planning process, the nurse acts as a resource person rather than as an advisor or counselor. The nurse provides information when asked, emphasizes the importance of small steps to behavioral change, and reviews the client's goals and plans to make sure they are realistic, measurable, and acceptable to the client.

STEPS IN PLANNING Pender et al. (2006, pp. 127–141) outline several steps in the process of developing a joint health promotion-prevention plan. These steps actively involve both the nurse and the client:

1. *Review and summarize data from assessment.* The nurse shares with the client a summary of the data collected from the various assessments (e.g., physical health and fitness, nutrition, sources of stress, spirituality, health practices).
2. *Reinforce strengths and competencies of the client.* The nurse and the client come to consensus about areas in which the client is doing well and areas that need further development.
3. *Identify health goals and related behavior-change options.* The client selects two or three top priority personal health goals, prioritizes them, and reviews behavior-change options.
4. *Identify behavioral or health outcomes.* For each of the selected goals or areas in step 1, the nurse and client determine what specific behavioral changes are needed to bring about the desired outcome. For example, to reduce the risk of cardiovascular disease, the client may need to stop smoking, lose weight, and increase activity level.
5. *Develop a behavior-change plan.* A constructive program of change is based on client "ownership" of those behavior changes selected for implementation within everyday life (Pender et al., 2006, p. 134). Nurses may need to assist clients in examining value-behavior inconsistencies and in selecting behavioral options that are most appealing and that clients are most willing to try. The client's priorities will reflect personal values, activity preferences, and expectations for success.
6. *Reiterate benefits of change.* The positive benefits will probably need to be reiterated by both the nurse and the client even though the client is committed to the change. The nurse should encourage the client to keep the health-related and non-health-related benefits before the client as central motivating factors.
7. *Address environmental and interpersonal facilitators and barriers to change.* Environmental and interpersonal factors that support positive change should be used to reinforce the client's efforts to change lifestyle. All people experience barriers, some of which can be anticipated and planned for, thereby making the change more likely to occur.
8. *Determine a time frame for implementation.* A time frame allows the client to develop the appropriate knowledge and skills before a new behavior is implemented. The time frame may be several weeks or months. Scheduling short-term goals and rewards can offer encouragement to achieve long-term objectives. Clients require help to be realistic and to deal with one behavior at a time.
9. *Formalize commitment to behavior-change plan.* Commitments to changing behaviors have usually been verbal. Increasingly, a formal, written behavioral contract is being used to motivate the client to follow

through with selected actions. Motivation to follow through is provided by a **positive reinforcement** or reward stated in the contract. Contracting is based on the belief that all people have the potential for growth and the right of self-determination, that is, to be able to make decisions independently without outside interference or compulsion, even though their choices may differ from the norm.

EXPLORING AVAILABLE RESOURCES Another essential aspect of planning is identifying support resources available to the client. These may be community resources such as a fitness program at a local gymnasium, or educational programs about important topics such as stress management, breast self-examination, nutrition, smoking cessation, and health lectures.

Implementation

Implementation is the "doing" part of behavior change. Self-responsibility is emphasized for implementing the plan. Depending on the client's needs, the nursing interventions may include supporting, counseling, facilitating, teaching, consulting, enhancing the behavior change, and modeling.

A major nursing role is to support the client. A vital component of lifestyle change is ongoing support that focuses on the desired behavior change and is provided in a nonjudgmental manner. Support can be offered by the nurse on an individual basis or in a group setting. The nurse can also facilitate the development of support networks for the client, including family members and friends.

INDIVIDUAL COUNSELING SESSIONS Counseling sessions may be routinely scheduled as part of the plan, or may be provided if the client encounters difficulty in carrying out interventions or meets insurmountable barriers to change. In a counseling relationship, the nurse and client share ideas. In this sharing relationship, the nurse acts as a facilitator, promoting the client's decision-making in regard to the health promotion plan.

TELEPHONE OR INTERNET COUNSELING Regular telephone sessions or Internet interaction may be provided to the client to help in answering questions, reviewing goals and strategies, and reinforcing progress. The client may find that scheduling a weekly interaction is helpful or may wish to initiate a call if a problem occurs. The nurse asks the client, "Is your plan working?" If the plan is not working, the nurse asks, "What would you like to do?" The client may wish to continue or may wish to change the plan to a more realistic one. Telephone or Internet support is efficient for the busy client who may not have the time for regular, in-person sessions.

GROUP SUPPORT Group sessions provide an opportunity for participants to learn from the experiences of others in changing behavior. Group contact gives individuals a renewed commitment to their goals. Groups can be scheduled at a variety of time intervals to best suit the group.

FACILITATING SOCIAL SUPPORT Social networks, such as family and friends, can facilitate or impede the efforts directed toward health promotion and prevention. The nurse's role is to assist the client to assess, modify, and develop the social support necessary to achieve the desired change. To provide the necessary support, families must communicate effectively, be aware of and support each other's needs and goals, and provide help and assistance to one another to achieve those goals. The client may wish the nurse to meet with the family or significant others to help enlist their understanding and support.

PROVIDING HEALTH EDUCATION Health education programs on a variety of topics discussed earlier can be provided to groups, individuals, or communities. Group programs need to be planned carefully before they are implemented. The decision to establish a health promotion program must be based upon the health needs of the people; also, specific health promotion goals must be set. After the program is implemented, outcomes must be evaluated.

ENHANCING BEHAVIOR CHANGE Whether people will make and maintain changes to improve health or prevent disease depends upon many interrelated factors. To help clients succeed in implementing behavior changes, the nurse needs to understand the stages of change and choose effective interventions that focus on helping the individual progress through the stages of change. Figure 13–4 ■ and the Client Teaching feature provide suggested strategies to assist clients depending upon their stage of change. As Saarmann, Daugherty, and Riegel (2000) point out, the nursing goal is not necessarily to change behavior but to advance the client to the next stage of change (p. 285).

MODELING In **modeling**, the client acquires ideas for behavior and coping strategies that can be used with specific problems by observing a model or role model. The client is not expected to mimic the sequence of actions or behavior patterns of the model, but can adapt them to fit with or modify the client's own behaviors. The nurse and client should mutually select models with whom the client can identify, since the cultural and ethnic backgrounds and age of the nurse and client often differ. Models should be people the client respects. Nurses should also serve as models of wellness. To model effectively, nurses need to adopt a personal philosophy and lifestyle that demonstrate good health habits.

Evaluation

Evaluation takes place on an ongoing basis as short-term goals are attained and after long-term goals have been completed. Goals are written during the planning phase, and a date is determined for attaining the specific results or behaviors that are desired to promote health or prevent illness. During evaluation, the client may decide to continue with the plan, reorder priorities, change strategies, or revise the health protection–promotion contract. Evaluation of the plan is a collaborative effort between the nurse and the client.

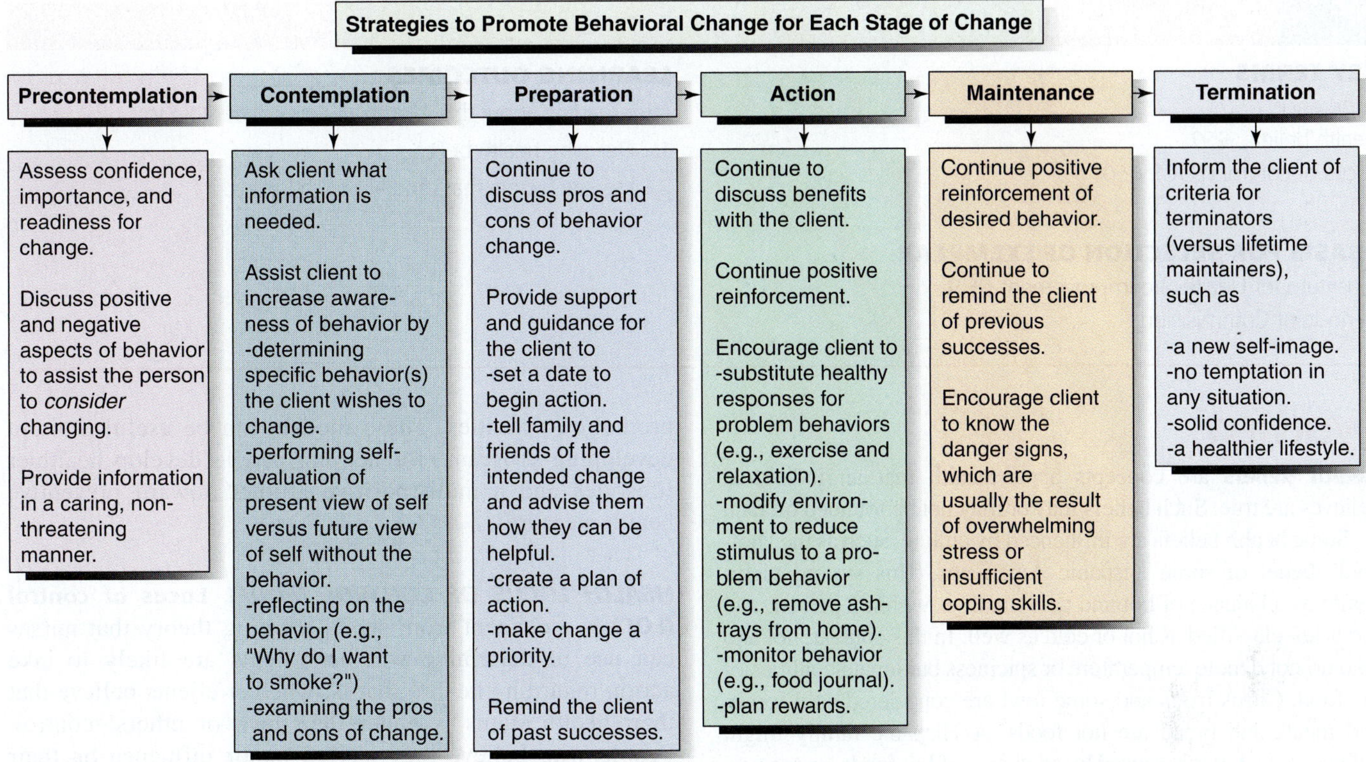

Strategies to Promote Behavioral Change for Each Stage of Change
Precontemplation
Contemplation
Preparation
Action
Maintenance
Termination
Assess confidence, importance, and readiness for change.
Discuss positive and negative aspects of behavior to assist the person to *consider* changing.
Provide information in a caring, non-threatening manner.
Ask client what information is needed.
Assist client to increase awareness of behavior by
-determining specific behavior(s) the client wishes to change.
-performing self-evaluation of present view of self versus future view of self without the behavior.
-reflecting on the behavior (e.g., "Why do I want to smoke?")
-examining the pros and cons of change.
Continue to discuss pros and cons of behavior change.
Provide support and guidance for the client to
-set a date to begin action.
-tell family and friends of the intended change and advise them how they can be helpful.
-create a plan of action.
-make change a priority.
Remind the client of past successes.
Continue to discuss benefits with the client.
Continue positive reinforcement.
Encourage client to
-substitute healthy responses for problem behaviors (e.g., exercise and relaxation).
-modify environment to reduce stimulus to a problem behavior (e.g., remove ashtrays from home).
-monitor behavior (e.g., food journal).
-plan rewards.
Continue positive reinforcement of desired behavior.
Continue to remind the client of previous successes.
Encourage client to know the danger signs, which are usually the result of overwhelming stress or insufficient coping skills.
Inform the client of criteria for terminators (versus lifetime maintainers), such as
-a new self-image.
-no temptation in any situation.
-solid confidence.
-a healthier lifestyle.

Figure 13–4 ■ Strategies to promote behavioral change for each stage of change.

CLIENT TEACHING Enhancing Behavior Change

ESTABLISH RAPPORT

- Provide privacy and a perception of a collaborative, equal-power relationship.
- If time allows, ask the client to describe a "typical" day. Usually the problematic behavior is described; however, even if it is not, the listening will strengthen rapport and the personal information may be helpful in understanding the client's current situation.

SET AGENDA

- Allow the client to identify concerns. If there are multiple concerns (e.g., smoking, exercise, diet, stress), it is best to focus on one specific behavior at a time. Ask the client which behavior he or she feels most ready to *think* about changing.

ASSESS IMPORTANCE, CONFIDENCE, AND READINESS

- A client's readiness to change is often influenced by his or her perception of importance and confidence.
- Importance refers to the personal value of change. Questions that elicit this information can include the following: "How do you feel at the moment about [state the change]?" "How important is it to you to [state the change]?" "On a scale of 1–10, with 1 being not important and 10 very important, what number would you give yourself?"
- Confidence relates to mastering the skills needed to achieve the behavior and the situations in which behavior change will be challenging to the client. A potential question to use to assess confidence is "If you decided right now to change, how confident would you feel about succeeding?"

EXCHANGE INFORMATION AND REDUCE RESISTANCE

- These two tasks are performed throughout the various stages of behavior change.
- Ask clients if they would like information; if so, ask what specific information they need.
- Present information in a neutral tone of voice, and avoid using the word "you" too much. Referring to other people (versus "you") and what happens to them makes the information less threatening to the client.
- After presenting the information, ask for the client's interpretation of the information.
- There are three *traps* that increase resistance. The traps and strategies to avoid them include the following:
  a. *Trap:* Taking control away. *Instead:* Emphasize personal choice and control.
  b. *Trap:* Misjudging importance, confidence, or readiness. Often this results in talking about action before the client is ready. *Instead:* It is important to reexamine the client's feelings about importance and confidence as they influence readiness to make a specific change.
  c. *Trap:* Meeting force with force (attacking or defending through argument). *Instead:* Sit back and use reflective listening. Try to understand how the client is feeling. The resistance usually subsides and the discussion can move in a different direction.

Source: Rollnick, S., Mason, P., & Butler, C. (1999). *Health behavior change: A guide for practitioners.* Philadelphia: Elsevier. Reprinted with permission.

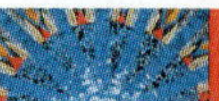

13.1 HEALTH BELIEFS

KEY TERMS
Adherence, *650*
Health beliefs, *650*
Locus of control (LOC), *650*

BASIS FOR SELECTION OF EXEMPLAR
Institute for Healthcare Improvement (IHI)
The Joint Commisision

LEARNING OUTCOMES
After reading about this exemplar, you will be able to:

1. Describe health belief.
2. Identify factors that modify health beliefs.

OVERVIEW

Health beliefs are concepts about health that an individual believes are true. Such beliefs may or may not be founded on fact.

Some health beliefs are influenced by culture, such as the "hot-cold" belief of some Hispanic Americans. This system views health as a balance of hot and cold qualities within a person, and foods are classified as hot or cold as well. In this context, hot and cold do not denote temperature or spiciness but innate qualities of the food. Citrus fruits and some fowl are considered cold foods, and meats and bread are hot foods. A Hispanic family might believe that a fever is caused by an excess of hot foods, so the person with a fever would be given cold foods as a remedy.

Another example of a culturally related health belief is the belief that health and illness are closely associated with the amount and quality of blood in the body. For example, some southerners say that "high blood," meaning too much blood in the body, causes headaches and dizziness. For additional information about cultural views of health and illness, see the Culture concept.

Health Beliefs Review

Clients' health beliefs must be clarified, particularly those that determine how clients perceive control of their own health status. Several instruments are available that assess a person's health-belief measures. Assessment of clients' health beliefs provides the nurse with an indication of how much the clients believe they can influence or control health through personal behaviors.

Several cultures have a strong belief in fate, that is, "Whatever will be, will be." When people hold this belief, they do not think they can do anything to change the course of their disease. An example is a client with diabetes who must make many lifestyle changes in diet and exercise and closely control glucose levels to prevent complications. If the diabetic client believes he or she has no control over the outcome, it is difficult to teach the client to make the necessary changes. These health beliefs can provide a better indication of the client's readiness and motivation to engage in healthy behaviors.

Health Belief Models

Several theories or models of health beliefs and behaviors have been developed to help determine whether an individual is likely to participate in disease prevention and health promotion activities. These models can be useful tools in developing programs for helping people develop healthier lifestyles and a more positive attitude toward preventive health measures.

HEALTH LOCUS OF CONTROL MODEL **Locus of control (LOC)** is a concept from social learning theory that nurses can use to determine whether clients are likely to take action regarding health, that is, whether clients believe that their health status is under their own or others' control. People who believe they have a major influence on their own health status—that health is largely self-determined—are called *internals.* People who exercise internal control are more likely than others to take the initiative in their own health care, be more knowledgeable about their health, and adhere to prescribed health care regimens such as taking medication, making and keeping appointments with primary care providers, maintaining diets, and giving up smoking. By contrast, people who believe their health is largely controlled by outside forces (e.g., chance or powerful others) are referred to as *externals.*

Research has shown that locus of control plays an important role in clients' choices about health behaviors. In some cases, externals demonstrate better **adherence** (compliance) to medical regimens, while in others, internals have increased adherence. For example, Leong, Molassiotis, and Marsh (2004) found externals adhered better to weight loss regimens whereas internals adhered better to exercise programs.

Locus of control is a measurable concept that can be used to predict which people are most likely to change their behavior. Many measurement instruments are available to assess LOC. One widely used example is the Multidimensional Health Locus of Control (MHLC) Scale (Wallston, Wallston, & DeVellis, 1978), most recently expanded to Form C (Wallston, Stein, & Smith, 1994). Nurses can use LOC results to plan internal reinforcement training if necessary to improve client efforts toward better health.

Nurses play a major role in helping clients implement healthy behaviors. They help clients monitor health, supply anticipatory guidance, and impart knowledge about health. Nurses can also reduce barriers to action (e.g., by minimizing inconvenience or discomfort) and support positive actions.

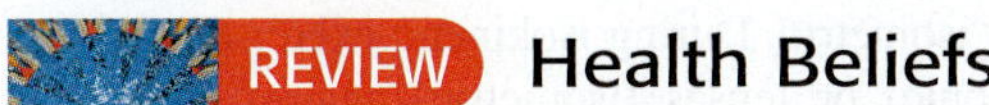

REVIEW Health Beliefs

RELATE: LINK THE CONCEPTS

Linking the exemplar of Health Beliefs with the concept of Development:

1. How would the client's locus of control vary at each stage of development?
2. How would you alter the way you assessed a client's health beliefs at each stage of development?

Linking the exemplar of Health Beliefs with the concept of Culture:

3. What role does culture play in forming a client's health beliefs?
4. You are caring for a client whose cultural beliefs negatively impact their health beliefs. How can you help this client to maintain their cultural beliefs while making healthier life choices?

REFER: GO TO MYNURSINGKIT

REFLECT: CASE STUDY

A home care nurse visits a 79-year-old woman client recently diagnosed with diabetes mellitus. The client takes her oral medication for diabetes only sporadically, and she is not following her new diet. The client says, "I don't really think I have diabetes. I feel fine, except that I'm always thirsty."

1. How is this client's health beliefs impacting her response to the diagnosis of diabetes mellitus?
2. How will you respond to the client's statement about not believing she has diabetes?
3. What is the nurse's role in advocating for this client's health needs?

13.2 PHYSICAL FITNESS AND EXERCISE

KEY TERMS

Activity-exercise pattern, *651*
Activity tolerance, *652*
Aerobic exercise, *652*
Anaerobic exercise, *652*
Exercise, *652*
Functional strength, *652*
Hypertrophy, *652*
Isokinetic exercise, *652*
Isometric exercise, *652*
Isotonic exercise, *652*
Physical activity, *652*

BASIS FOR SELECTION OF EXEMPLAR

Healthy People 2010

LEARNING OUTCOMES

After reading about this exemplar, you will be able to:

1. Differentiate isotonic, isometric, isokinetic, aerobic, and anaerobic exercise.
2. Describe the effects of exercise on body systems.
3. Assess activity-exercise pattern and activity tolerance.
4. Develop nursing diagnoses and outcomes related to activity and exercise.

OVERVIEW

Physical fitness is to the human body what fine-tuning is to an engine. It enables the body to perform to its potential. Fitness can be described as a condition that helps individuals look, feel, and do their best. More specifically, physical fitness is the ability to perform daily tasks vigorously and alertly, with energy left over for enjoying leisure-time activities and meeting emergency demands. It is the ability to endure, to bear up, to withstand stress, to carry on in circumstances where an unfit person could not continue, and it is a major basis for good health and well-being (President's Council on Physical Fitness and Sports, 2003).

Physical fitness involves the performance of the body's heart, lungs, and muscles. Fitness, to some degree, influences qualities such as mental alertness and emotional stability, because what humans do with their bodies also affects what they can do with their minds. To maintain fitness, one must meet the needs for exercise, nutrition, rest, and relaxation, and follow practices to promote and preserve health.

Many *Healthy People 2010* objectives pertain to exercise and activity. Following are some of these objectives:

- Increase the proportion of people who engage in moderate physical activity for at least 30 minutes a day
- Increase the proportion of adults and children who perform physical activities that enhance and maintain muscle strength, endurance, and flexibility
- Increase the proportion of work sites offering employer-sponsored physical activity and fitness programs
- Reduce activity limitation due to chronic back conditions
- Reduce the number of overweight people (Edelman & Mandle, 2006).

A strong, well-developed body of research evidence supports the role of exercise in improving the health status of individuals with cardiovascular disease, pulmonary dysfunction, disabilities of aging, and depression. Integrating well-researched exercise protocols with conventional nursing and medical approaches will result in optimal treatment of these common disorders. Evidence shows that exercise can prevent and even reverse many of the chronic diseases experienced by aging adults. A growing body of research supports the preventive and therapeutic effects of exercise for individuals with diabetes, cancer, arthritis, chronic fatigue syndrome, fibromyalgia, menopause, urinary incontinence, Parkinson's, Alzheimer's, and HIV/AIDS (Freeman, 2004; Micozzi, 2006).

An **activity-exercise pattern** refers to a person's routine of exercise, activity, leisure, and recreation. It includes (a) activities of daily living (ADLs) that require energy expenditure, such as hygiene, dressing, cooking, shopping, eating, working, and home maintenance; and (b) the type, quality, and quantity of exercise, including sports.

People often define their health and physical fitness by their activity because mental well-being and the effectiveness of body functioning depend largely on their mobility status. For example, when a person is upright, the lungs expand more easily, intestinal activity (peristalsis) is more effective, and the kidneys are able to empty completely. In addition, motion is essential for proper functioning of bones and muscles.

PHYSICAL ACTIVITY AND EXERCISE

The U.S. Department of Health and Human Services defines physical activity and exercise as follows (Edelman & Mandle, 2006):

- **Physical activity** is bodily movement produced by skeletal muscle contraction that increases energy expenditure.
- **Exercise** is a type of physical activity defined as a planned, structured, and repetitive bodily movement performed to improve or maintain one or more components of physical fitness.

People participate in exercise programs to decrease risk factors for cardiovascular disease and to increase their health and well-being. **Activity tolerance** is the type and amount of exercise or daily living activities an individual is able to perform without experiencing adverse effects. **Functional strength** is another goal of exercise, and it is defined as the body's ability to perform work.

Types of Exercise

Exercise involves the active contraction and relaxation of muscles. Exercises can be classified according to the type of muscle contraction (isotonic, isometric, or isokinetic) and the source of energy (aerobic or anaerobic).

Isotonic exercises, which are dynamic exercises, are those in which the muscle shortens to produce muscle contraction and active movement. Most physical conditioning exercises—running, walking, swimming, cycling, and other such activities—are isotonic, as are ADLs and active ROM (range of motion) exercises (those initiated by the client). Examples of isotonic bed exercises are pushing or pulling against a stationary object, using a trapeze to lift the body off the bed, lifting the buttocks off the bed by pushing with the hands against the mattress, and pushing the body to a sitting position.

Isotonic exercises increase muscle tone, mass, and strength and maintain joint flexibility and circulation. During isotonic exercise, both heart rate and cardiac output quicken to increase blood flow to all parts of the body.

Isometric exercises, which are static or setting exercises, are those in which muscles contract without moving the joint (muscle length does not change). These exercises involve exerting pressure against a solid object and are useful for strengthening abdominal, gluteal, and quadriceps muscles used in ambulation; for maintaining strength in immobilized muscles in casts or traction; and for endurance training. These are often called "quad sets." Isometric exercises produce a mild increase in heart rate and cardiac output, but no appreciable increase in blood flow to other parts of the body.

Isokinetic exercises, which are resistive exercises, involve muscle contraction or tension against resistance; thus, they can be either isotonic or isometric. During isokinetic exercises, the person moves (isotonic) or tenses (isometric) against resistance. Special machines or devices provide the resistance to the movement. These exercises are used in physical conditioning and are often done to build up certain muscle groups; for example, the pectorals (chest muscles) may be increased in size and strength by lifting weights. An increase in blood pressure and blood flow to muscles occurs with resistance training (Burke & Laramie, 2004).

Aerobic exercise is an activity during which the amount of oxygen taken into the body is greater than that used to perform the activity. Aerobic exercises use large muscle groups that move repetitively. Aerobic exercises improve cardiovascular conditioning and physical fitness. Aerobic exercise brings more oxygen into the body than is used to perform the activity.

1. *Target Heart Rate:* The goal is to work up to and sustain a target heart rate during exercise; the target rate is based on the person's age. To determine target heart rate, first calculate the person's maximum heart rate by subtracting his or her current age in years from 220. Then obtain the target heart rate by taking 60–85% of the maximum. Because heart rates vary among individuals, the Talk Test is one of several tests that is being used to replace this measure.
2. *Talk Test:* This test is easier to implement and keeps most people at 60% of maximum heart rate or higher. The test is simple: When exercising, the person should experience labored breathing, yet still be able to carry on a conversation.

Anaerobic exercise involves activity in which the muscles cannot draw out enough oxygen from the bloodstream, and anaerobic pathways are used to provide additional energy for a short time. This type of exercise, such as weight lifting and sprinting, is used in endurance training for athletes.

Benefits of Exercise

In general, regular exercise is essential for maintaining mental and physical health. Table 13–2 summarizes the benefits of exercise on body systems.

MUSCULOSKELETAL SYSTEM The size, shape, tone, and strength of muscles (including the heart muscle) are maintained with mild exercise and increased with strenuous exercise. With strenuous exercise, muscles **hypertrophy** (enlarge), and the efficiency of muscular contraction increases. Hypertrophy is commonly seen in the arm muscles of a tennis player, the leg muscles of a skater, and the arm and hand muscles of a carpenter.

Joints lack a discrete blood supply. It is through activity that joints receive nourishment. Exercise increases joint flexibility, stability, and range of motion. A growing number of randomized, controlled clinical trials have shown that exercise interventions significantly reduce weakness, frailty, depression, and the risk and incidence of falling in older adults (Burke & Laramie, 2004).

Bone density and strength is maintained through weight bearing. The stress of weight-bearing and high-impact movement maintains a balance between osteoblasts (bone-building cells) and osteoclasts (bone-resorption and breakdown cells). Weight-bearing activity is particularly important for individuals at risk for osteoporosis. Examples of weight-bearing activity

TABLE 13–2 **Benefits of Exercise by Body System**

BODY SYSTEM	BENEFITS
Musculoskeletal	■ Increases joint flexibility, stability, and range of motion ■ Maintains bone density and strength ■ Reduces weakness, frailty, and depression ■ Decreases risk and incidence of falling in older adults
Cardiovascular	■ Increases strength of heart muscle contraction and blood supply to heart and muscles ■ Mediates harmful effects of stress ■ Lowers resting heart rate ■ Raises HDL level ■ Lowers blood pressure ■ Improves circulation
Respiratory	■ Increases tidal volume ■ Increases vital capacity ■ Improves gas exchange ■ Increases oxygen to the brain ■ Improves stamina and immune function
Gastrointestinal	■ Facilitates peristalsis ■ Relieves constipation ■ May improve symptoms of conditions such as IBS
Metabolic/Endocrine	■ Elevates metabolic rate ■ Stabilizes blood sugar
Urinary	■ Promotes efficient blood flow and waste excretion
Psychoneurologic	■ Elevates mood ■ Relieves stress and anxiety ■ Relieves depressive symptoms

are walking, dancing, and weight lifting. Non-weight-bearing exercises offer great benefit for individuals with a variety of health considerations. Examples of non-weight-bearing exercise are swimming and bicycling.

CARDIOVASCULAR SYSTEM The American Heart Association's most recent guidelines for primary prevention of stroke and cardiovascular disease place great emphasis on physical activity (Freeman, 2004). Adequate moderate-intensity exercise (40–60% of maximum capacity such as walking a mile in 15–20 minutes) increases the heart rate, the strength of heart muscle contraction, and the blood supply to the heart and muscles through increased cardiac output. In two studies with male participants, levels of "good" (high-density lipoprotein [HDL]) cholesterol were increased through regular endurance (walking/jogging) exercise. Exercise also promotes heart health by mediating the harmful effects of stress. The types of exercise that provide cardiac benefit vary. They include aerobic exercise such as walking and cycling (Freeman, 2004). Recent research supports the benefits of yoga practice on cardiovascular health. Statistically significant effects include lowered systolic and diastolic blood pressure, improved oxygen uptake, improved heart rate variability, improved circulation, and self-reported stress reduction (Fontaine, 2005; Freeman, 2004; McCaffrey, Ruknui, Hatthakit, & Kasetsomboon, 2005).

RESPIRATORY SYSTEM Ventilation (air circulating into and out of the lungs) and oxygen intake increase during exercise, thereby improving gas exchange. More toxins are eliminated with deeper breathing, and problem solving and emotional stability are enhanced by increased oxygen to the brain. Adequate exercise also prevents pooling of secretions in the bronchi and bronchioles, decreasing breathing effort and risk of infection (Freeman, 2004). Attention to exercising muscles of respiration (by deep breathing) throughout activity as well as during rest enhances oxygenation (improving stamina) and circulation of lymph (improving immune function). A strong body of evidence supports the use of lower extremity exercise forms (e.g., walking, treadmill, stationary bike, stair climbing) for treating individuals with chronic obstructive pulmonary disease (COPD) (Freeman, 2004). Research reports citing the benefits of yogic breathing and postures for persons with asthma are increasing in the literature (Fontaine, 2005; Freeman, 2004; Micozzi, 2006).

GASTROINTESTINAL SYSTEM Exercise improves the appetite and increases gastrointestinal tract tone, facilitating peristalsis. Activities such as rowing, swimming, walking, and sit-ups work the abdominal muscles and can help relieve constipation (Fontaine, 2005). Abdominal compressive exercise, such as with twisting and forward bending yoga postures, has been shown to improve symptoms of irritable bowel syndrome (Fontaine, 2005; Micozzi, 2006).

METABOLIC/ENDOCRINE SYSTEM Exercise elevates the metabolic rate, thus increasing the production of body heat, waste products, and calorie use. During strenuous exercise, the metabolic rate can increase to as much as 20 times the normal rate. This elevation lasts after exercise is completed. Exercise increases the use of triglycerides and fatty acids, resulting in a reduced level of serum triglycerides and cholesterol. Weight loss and exercise stabilize blood sugar and make cells more responsive to insulin. The Diabetes Prevention Program a large 3-year study, showed that even a modest 5% decrease in body weight (about 10 pounds in most participants) achieved through exercise and dietary modification reduced the risk of diabetes by a striking 58%. In those over 60 years of age, the reduction was 71% (Freeman, 2004).

URINARY SYSTEM As adequate exercise promotes efficient blood flow, the body excretes wastes more effectively. In addition, adequate exercise usually prevents stasis (stagnation) of urine in the bladder.

IMMUNE SYSTEM As respiratory and musculoskeletal effort increase with exercise and as gravity is enlisted with postural changes, lymph fluid is more efficiently pumped from tissues into lymph capillaries and vessels throughout the body. Circulation through lymph nodes where destruction of pathogens and removal of foreign antigens can occur, is also improved. Research in older adults has shown benefits of moderate exercise on natural killer cell function, circulating T-cell function, and cytokine production, potentially increasing resistance to viral infections and preventing formation of malignant cells (Freeman, 2004).

While moderate exercise seems to enhance immunity, strenuous exercise may reduce immune function, leaving a window of opportunity for infection during the recovery phase. Adequate rest is important after vigorous training to allow the body to recover (Edelman & Mandle, 2006).

PSYCHONEUROLOGIC SYSTEM Mental or affective disorders such as depression or chronic stress may affect a person's desire to move. The depressed person may lack enthusiasm for taking part in any activity and may even lack energy for usual hygiene practices. Lack of visible energy is seen in a slumped posture with head bowed. Chronic stress can deplete the body's energy reserves to the point that the resulting fatigue discourages the desire to exercise, even though exercise can energize the person and facilitate coping. By contrast, individuals with eating disorders may exercise excessively in an effort to prevent weight gain.

A strong and growing body of evidence supports the role of exercise in elevating mood and relieving stress and anxiety across the life span. Solid data examining relationships between both aerobic and nonaerobic styles of exercise support the use of this modality to relieve symptoms of depression. The mechanism of action is thought to be a result of one or more of the following: Exercise increases levels of metabolites for neurotransmitters and serotonin exercise releases endogenous opioids, thus increasing levels of endorphins; exercise increases levels of oxygen to the brain and other body systems, inducing euphoria; and through muscular exertion (especially with movement modalities such as yoga and t'ai chi) the body releases stored stress associated with accumulated emotional demands. Regular exercise also improves quality of sleep for most individuals (Freeman, 2004).

COGNITIVE FUNCTION Current research supports the positive effects of exercise on cognitive functioning, in particular decision-making and problem-solving processes, planning, and paying attention. Physical exertion induces cells in the brain to strengthen and build neuronal connections. Research evidence demonstrates that athletic older adults have denser brains than their inactive counterparts (Freeman, 2004). Brain Gym (educational kinesiology) is a series of easy, mostly cross-lateral movements that enhance right- and left-brain integration, thus improving mood, learning, problem solving, and performance in persons of all ages. These contralateral movements have been shown to help individuals with attention deficit disorder (ADD), attention deficit/hyperactivity disorder (ADHD), learning disorders, and mood disorders. Recent research indicates that physical exercise also provides positive effects in individuals with Parkinson's and Alzheimer's diseases.

SPIRITUAL HEALTH Jackson (2003) found that a program of Pilates and yoga-style exercise significantly enhanced students' experiences of mind-body-spirit connection and relationship with God. The emphasis on breathing in both Pilates and yoga is thought to soothe the nervous and cardiorespiratory systems, promoting relaxation and preparedness for contemplative experience. Recitation of a word or phrase (mantra) and rosary prayer were both found to powerfully enhance and synchronize cardiovascular rhythms because of the resulting decrease in respiratory rate. Slow breathing enhances heart rate variability and baroreflex sensitivity, both beneficial for those with heart disease (Micozzi, 2006). (See the Spirituality concept.)

REVIEW Physical Fitness and Exercise

RELATE: LINK THE CONCEPTS

Linking the exemplar Physical Fitness and Exercise with the concept of Metabolism:

1. Identify the benefits of physical activity for a client with type 2 diabetes and osteoporosis.
2. What teaching plan will you implement for the obese client regarding exercise and nutrition?

Linking the exemplar Physical Fitness and Exercise with the concept Mobility:

3. A client with rheumatoid arthritis is interested in beginning a weight lifting program. What are your teaching priorities for this client?
4. You are caring for a client who normally exercises daily before fracturing his leg. How can you help to meet the client's exercise needs when he is placed in traction for six weeks?

REFER: GO TO MYNURSINGKIT

REFLECT: CASE STUDY

Mary Martin is a 75-year-old female who was recently widowed. She has limited income because her husband's pension terminated when he died, so she has moved in with her son, his wife, and their three teenage children. Mary has cataracts and glaucoma, for which she sees an ophthalmologist on a regular basis, but otherwise she is in good health. Mary recently learned she has low bone density.

1. What kind of physical activity and exercise is appropriate for Mary?
2. What are the benefits of these activities on body systems?
3. What are your expected outcomes for Mary?
4. What safety teaching will you provide Mary and her family?

13.3 ORAL HEALTH

KEY TERMS

Cheilosis, *658*
Dental caries, *656*
Gingiva, *656*
Gingivitis, *658*
Periodontal disease, *656*
Plaque, *656*
Pyorrhea, *658*
Tartar, *656*
Xerostomia, *660*

BASIS FOR SELECTION OF EXEMPLAR

Healthy People 2010

LEARNING OUTCOMES

After reading about this exemplar, you will be able to:

1. Identify factors influencing oral health.
2. Identify normal and abnormal assessment findings across the life span.
3. Describe the significance of oral hygiene across the life span.
4. Develop nursing diagnoses and outcomes related to oral health.

OVERVIEW

The mouth, also called the oral or buccal cavity, is lined with mucous membranes and is enclosed by the lips, cheeks, palate, and tongue (Figure 13–5 ■).

The lips and cheeks are skeletal muscle covered externally by skin. Their function is to keep food in the mouth during chewing. The palate consists of two regions: the hard palate and the soft palate. The hard palate covers bone in the roof of the mouth and provides a hard surface against which the tongue forces food. The soft palate, extending from the hard palate and ending at the back of the mouth as a fold called the uvula, is primarily muscle. When food is swallowed, the soft palate rises as a reflex to close off the oropharynx.

The tongue, composed of skeletal muscle and connective tissue, is located in the floor of the mouth. It contains mucous and serous glands, taste buds, and papillae. The tongue mixes food with saliva during chewing, forms the food into a mass (called a *bolus*), and initiates swallowing. Some papillae provide surface roughness to facilitate licking and moving food; other papillae house the taste buds.

Saliva moistens food so it can be made into a bolus, dissolves food chemicals so they can be tasted, and provides enzymes (such as amylase) that begin the chemical breakdown of starches. Saliva is produced by salivary glands, most of which lie superior or inferior to the mouth and drain into it. The salivary glands include the parotid, the submaxillary, and the sublingual glands.

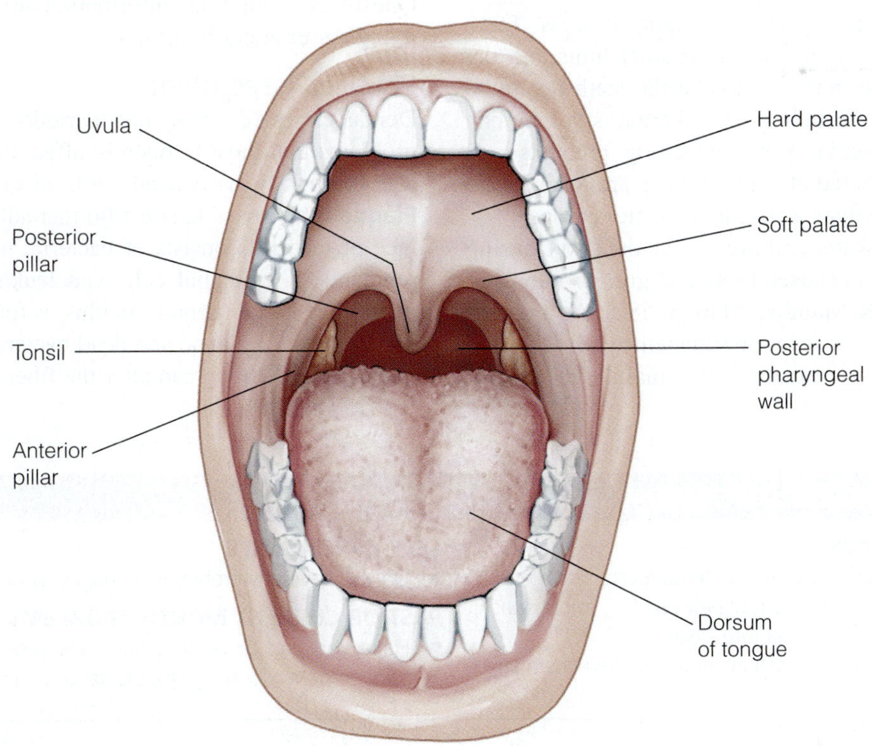

Figure 13–5 ■ Oral cavity.

The teeth chew (masticate) and grind food to break it down into smaller parts. As the food is masticated, it is mixed with saliva.

Each tooth has three parts: the crown, the root, and the pulp cavity. The crown is the exposed part of the tooth, which is outside the gum. It is covered with a hard substance called enamel. The ivory-colored internal part of the crown below the enamel is the dentin. The root of a tooth is embedded in the jaw and covered by a bony tissue called cementum. The pulp cavity in the center of the tooth contains the blood vessels and nerves.

DEVELOPMENTAL VARIATIONS

Teeth usually appear 5–8 months after birth. Baby-bottle syndrome may result in decay of all of the upper teeth and the lower posterior teeth (Pillitteri, 2003, p. 824). This syndrome occurs when an infant is put to bed with a bottle of sugar water, formula, milk, or fruit juice. The carbohydrates in the solutions cause demineralization of the tooth enamel, which leads to tooth decay.

By the time children are 2 years old, they usually have all 20 of their deciduous (temporary) teeth. At about age 6 or 7, children start losing their deciduous teeth, and these are gradually replaced by the 33 permanent teeth. By age 25, most people have all of their permanent teeth (Figure 13–6 ■).

The incidence of periodontal diseaseincreases during pregnancy because the rise in female hormones affects gingival tissue and increases its reaction to bacterial plaque. Many pregnant women experience more bleeding from the gingival sulcus during brushing and increased redness and swelling of the **gingiva** (the gum).

Teeth turn yellowish as a part of the aging process. Teeth are normally off-white. With age, the enamel thins and the yellow-gray color of the inner portion of the teeth begins to show. In addition, coffee drinking and cigarette smoking can stain the teeth. Commercial teeth whitening products and whitening treatments offered at dental offices are available to consumers who desire whiter teeth for cosmetic reasons.

Lack of fluoridated water and preventive dentistry during their developmental years caused tooth and gum problems in older adults (Edelman & Mandle, 2006, p. 582). As a result, some older adults may have few permanent teeth left, and some have dentures. Loss of teeth occurs mainly because of **periodontal disease** (gum disease) rather than **dental caries** (cavities); however, caries are also common in middle-aged adults.

Some receding of the gums and a brownish pigmentation of the gums occur with age. Because saliva production decreases with age, dryness of the oral mucosa is a common finding in older people.

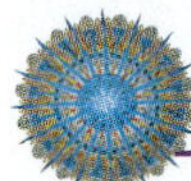

NURSING PROCESS

Assessment

Assessment of the client's mouth and hygiene practices includes (a) a nursing health history, (b) physical assessment of the mouth, and (c) identification of clients at risk for developing oral problems.

Health History

During the nursing health history, the nurse obtains data about the client's oral hygiene practices, including dental visits, self-care abilities, and past or current mouth problems. Data about the client's oral hygiene help the nurse determine learning needs and incorporate the client's needs and preferences in the plan of care. Assessment of the client's self-care abilities determines the amount and type of nursing assistance to provide. Clients whose hand coordination is impaired, whose cognitive function is impaired, whose illness alters energy levels and motivation, or whose therapy imposes restrictions on activities will need assistance from the nurse. Information about past or current problems alerts the nurse to specific interventions required or referrals that may be necessary. Questions to elicit this information are shown in the accompanying Assessment Interview.

Physical Assessment

Dental caries (cavities) and periodontal disease are the two problems that most frequently affect the teeth. Both problems are commonly associated with plaque and tartar deposits. **Plaque** is an invisible soft film that adheres to the enamel surface of teeth; it consists of bacteria, molecules of saliva, and remnants of epithelial cells and leukocytes. When plaque is unchecked, tartar (dental calculus) is formed. **Tartar** is a visible, hard deposit of plaque and dead bacteria that forms at the gum lines. Tartar buildup can alter the fibers that attach the teeth to

Assessment Interview Oral Hygiene

ORAL HYGIENE PRACTICES

- What are your usual mouth care and/or denture care practices?
- What oral hygiene products do you routinely use (e.g., mouthwash, type of toothpaste, dental floss, denture cleaner)?
- When was your last dental examination, and how often do you see your dentist?

SELF-CARE ABILITY

- Do you have any problems managing your mouth care?

PAST OR CURRENT MOUTH PROBLEMS

- Have you had or do you have any problems such as bleeding, swollen or reddened gums, ulcerations, lumps, or tooth pain?

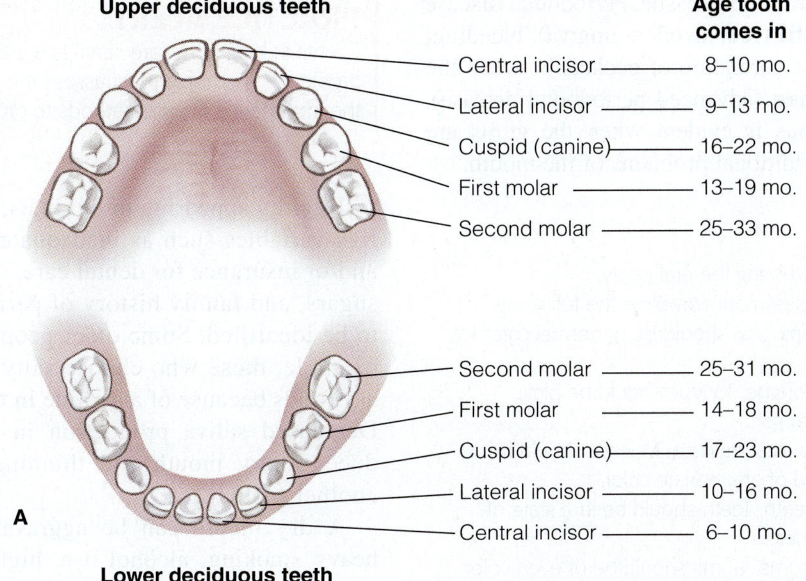
Upper deciduous teeth
Age tooth comes in
Central incisor 8–10 mo.
Lateral incisor 9–13 mo.
Cuspid (canine) 16–22 mo.
First molar 13–19 mo.
Second molar 25–33 mo.
Second molar 25–31 mo.
First molar 14–18 mo.
Cuspid (canine) 17–23 mo.
Lateral incisor 10–16 mo.
Central incisor 6–10 mo.
A
Lower deciduous teeth

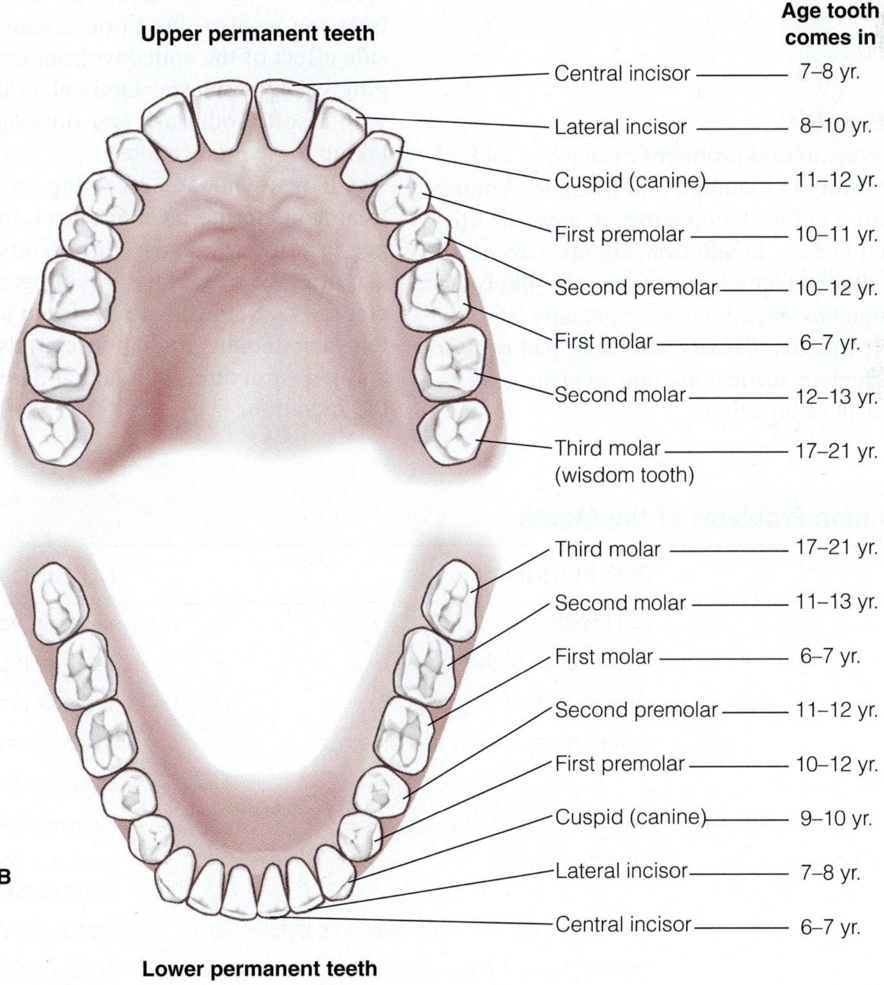
Upper permanent teeth
Age tooth comes in
Central incisor 7–8 yr.
Lateral incisor 8–10 yr.
Cuspid (canine) 11–12 yr.
First premolar 10–11 yr.
Second premolar 10–12 yr.
First molar 6–7 yr.
Second molar 12–13 yr.
Third molar (wisdom tooth) 17–21 yr.
Third molar 17–21 yr.
Second molar 11–13 yr.
First molar 6–7 yr.
Second premolar 11–12 yr.
First premolar 10–12 yr.
Cuspid (canine) 9–10 yr.
Lateral incisor 7–8 yr.
Central incisor 6–7 yr.
B
Lower permanent teeth

Figure 13–6 ■ Deciduous and permanent teeth.

the gum and eventually disrupt bone tissue. Periodontal disease is characterized by **gingivitis** (red, swollen gingiva), bleeding, receding gum lines, and the formation of pockets between the teeth and gums. In **pyorrhea** (advanced periodontal disease), the teeth are loose and pus is evident when the gums are pressed. Table 13–3 lists additional problems of the mouth.

PRACTICE ALERT

Always wear gloves when assessing the oral cavity.

To perform an oral health assessment complete the following:

- Inspect and palpate the lips. Lips should be of normal color for race without lesions.
- Inspect and palpate the tongue. Tongue should be pink, smooth, and have good turgor.
- Inspect and palpate the buccal mucosa. Mucosa should be moist, without lesions and of appropriate color.
- Inspect and palpate the teeth. Teeth should be in a state of good hygiene without caries.
- Inspect and palpate the gums. Gums should be of even color without swelling.
- Inspect the throat and tonsils. Tonsils (if present) should be of appropriate color and size.
- Note the client's breath. Breath should not have unusual or foul odors.

Identifying Clients at Risk

Certain clients are prone to oral problems because of lack of knowledge or the inability to maintain oral hygiene. Among these are seriously ill, confused, comatose, depressed, illiterate, and dehydrated clients. In addition, clients with nasogastric tubes and clients receiving oxygen are likely to develop dry oral mucous membranes, especially if they breathe through their mouths. Clients who have had oral or jaw surgery must maintain meticulous oral hygiene care to prevent the development of infections.

PRACTICE ALERT

Clients in long-term care settings are at high risk for oral health problems. The nurse must assess the client's oral health and teach the importance of and methods to promote oral hygiene.

Healthy appearing individuals, too, may be at risk. High-risk variables such as inadequate nutrition, lack of money and/or insurance for dental care, excessive intake of refined sugars, and family history of periodontal disease also need to be identified. Some older people may also be at risk, for example, those who choose salty and enamel-eroding sugary foods because of a decline in their number of taste buds. Decreased saliva production in older adults, which produces a dry mouth and thinning of the oral mucosa, is another factor.

A dry mouth can be aggravated by poor fluid intake, heavy smoking, alcohol use, high salt intake, anxiety, and many medications. Medications that can cause dryness of the mouth include diuretics; laxatives, if used excessively; and tranquilizers, such as chlorpromazine (Thorazine) and diazepam (Valium). Some chemotherapeutic agents used to treat cancer also cause oral dryness and lesions. A common side effect of the anticonvulsant drug phenytoin (Dilantin) is gingival hyperplasia. Optimal oral hygiene (e.g., brushing with a soft toothbrush and flossing) is necessary for clients taking these medications.

Clients who are receiving or have received radiation treatments to the head and neck may have permanent damage to salivary glands. This results in a very dry mouth and can often be treated by providing a thick liquid called artificial saliva. Some clients prefer to just sip on liquids to moisten their mouth. Radiation can also cause damage to teeth and jaw structure, with actual damage occurring years after the radiation.

TABLE 13–3 **Common Problems of the Mouth**

PROBLEM	DESCRIPTION	NURSING IMPLICATIONS
Halitosis	Bad breath	Teach or provide regular oral hygiene.
Glossitis	Inflammation of the tongue	Teach or provide regular oral hygiene.
Gingivitis	Inflammation of the gums	Teach or provide regular oral hygiene.
Periodontal disease	Gums appear spongy and bleeding	Teach or provide regular oral hygiene.
Reddened or excoriated mucosa		Check for ill-fitting dentures.
Excessive dryness of the buccal mucosa		Increase fluid intake as health permits.
Cheilosis	Cracking of lips	Lubricate lips, use antimicrobial ointment to prevent infection.
Dental caries	Darkened areas on teeth, may be painful	Advise client to see a dentist.
Sordes	Accumulation of foul matter (food, microorganisms, and epithelial elements) on the teeth and lips	Teach or provide regular cleaning.
Stomatitis	Inflammation of the oral mucosa	Teach or provide regular cleaning.
Parotitis	Inflammation of the parotid salivary glands	Teach or provide regular oral hygiene.

Diagnosis

Three nursing diagnoses are related to problems with oral hygiene and the oral cavity:

- Self-Care Deficit
- Impaired Oral Mucous Membrane
- Deficient Knowledge.

Note that the North American Nursing Diagnosis Association (NANDA, 2007) includes oral hygiene in the diagnostic label self-care deficit: bathing/hygiene. In this book, the diagnosis self-care deficit: oral hygiene will be used for clients unable to perform oral care independently. This includes the inability to brush or floss teeth or clean dentures.

The nursing diagnosis impaired oral mucous membrane refers to the state in which an individual experiences disruptions in the tissue layers of the oral cavity. Manifestations include a coated tongue, dry mouth, halitosis, gingivitis, oral pain, discomfort, erythema, oral lesions or ulcers, and dry mouth. These may be the result of ineffective oral hygiene, physical injury or drying effect (e.g., mouth breathing, oxygen therapy, dehydration), mechanical trauma (e.g., oral surgery, braces, or ill-fitting dentures), chemical trauma (e.g., side effects of medications), or radiation therapy.

Plan

In planning care, the nurse and, if appropriate, the client and/or family set outcomes for each nursing diagnosis. The nurse then performs nursing interventions and activities to achieve the client outcomes.

During the planning phase, the nurse also identifies interventions that will help the client achieve these goals. Specific, detailed nursing activities taken by the nurse may include the following:

- Monitor for dryness of the oral mucosa.
- Monitor for signs and symptoms of glossitis (inflammation of the tongue) and stomatitis (inflammation of the mouth).
- Assist dependent clients with oral care.
- Provide special oral hygiene for clients who are debilitated, are unconscious, or have lesions of the mucous membranes or other oral tissues.
- Teach clients about good oral hygiene practices and other measures to prevent tooth decay.
- Reinforce the oral hygiene regimen as part of health promotion and discharge teaching.

Implementation

Good oral hygiene includes daily stimulation of the gums, mechanical brushing and flossing of the teeth, and flushing of the mouth. The nurse is often in a position to help people maintain oral hygiene by helping or teaching them to clean the teeth and oral cavity, by inspecting whether clients (especially children) have done so, or by actually providing mouth care to clients who are ill or incapacitated. The nurse can also be instrumental in identifying problems that require the intervention of a dentist or oral surgeon and arranging a referral.

Promoting Oral Health Throughout the Life Span

A major role of the nurse in promoting oral health is teaching clients about specific oral hygienic measures.

INFANTS AND TODDLERS Most dentists recommend that dental hygiene begin when the first tooth erupts and be practiced after each feeding. Cleaning can be accomplished by using a wet washcloth or small gauze moistened with water.

Dental caries occur frequently during the toddler period, often as a result of the excessive intake of sweets or a prolonged use of the bottle during naps and at bedtime. The nurse should give parents the following instructions to promote and maintain dental health:

- Beginning at about 18 months of age, brush the child's teeth with a soft toothbrush. Use only a toothbrush moistened with water at first and introduce toothpaste later. Use a toothpaste that contains fluoride.
- Give a fluoride supplement daily or as recommended by the primary care provider or dentist, unless the drinking water is fluoridated.
- Schedule an initial dental visit for the child at about 2 or 3 years of age, as soon as all 20 primary teeth have erupted.
- Some dentists recommend an inspection type of visit when the child is about 18 months old to provide an early, pleasant introduction to the dental examination.
- Seek professional dental attention for any problems such as discoloring of the teeth, chipping, or signs of infection such as redness and swelling.

PRESCHOOLERS AND SCHOOL-AGE CHILDREN Because deciduous teeth guide the entrance of permanent teeth, dental care is essential to keep these teeth in good repair and to establish good dental habits early. Abnormally placed or lost deciduous teeth can cause misalignment of permanent teeth. Fluoride remains important at this stage to prevent dental caries. Preschoolers need to be taught to brush their teeth after eating and to limit their intake of refined sugars. Parental supervision may be needed to ensure the completion of these self-care activities. Regular dental checkups are required during these years when permanent teeth appear.

PRACTICE ALERT

Many parents are unaware of the importance of dental health in very young children. They may see their child's teeth as "baby teeth," and think they can put off dental visits until the child begins to lose his or her primary teeth. Nurses working with parents of very young children may need to provide teaching opportunities to help parents learn that care of primary teeth is essential to healthy permanent teeth.

ADOLESCENTS AND ADULTS Proper diet and tooth and mouth care should be evaluated and reinforced for adolescents and adults. Specific measures to prevent tooth decay and periodontal disease are listed in Client Teaching.

OLDER ADULTS Over 50% of older adults have their own teeth (Gooch, Eke, & Malvitz, 2004), and they are at risk for dental cavities and periodontal disease. Older adults who have

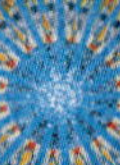

CLIENT TEACHING Measures to Prevent Tooth Decay

- Brush the teeth thoroughly after meals and at bedtime. Assist children or inspect their mouths to be sure the teeth are clean. If the teeth cannot be brushed after meals, vigorous rinsing of the mouth with water is recommended.
- Floss the teeth daily.
- Ensure an adequate intake of nutrients, particularly calcium, phosphorus, vitamins A, C, and D, and fluoride.
- Avoid sweet foods and drinks between meals. Take them in moderation at meals.
- Eat coarse, fibrous foods (cleansing foods), such as fresh fruits and raw vegetables.
- Have topical fluoride applications as prescribed by the dentist.
- Have a checkup by a dentist every 6 months.

self-care deficits are at an increased risk because they cannot maintain their oral hygiene practices and/or may not be able to visit the dentist on a routine basis. Furthermore, those who suffer the worst oral health and hygiene include older adults residing in nursing homes (Coleman, 2002, 2004). Coleman (2004) reported that poor oral hygiene among the frail and among dependent nursing home residents can place them at risk for serious illness such as pneumonia (p. 3). Nurses have an important role in promoting optimal geriatric oral health care.

Brushing and Flossing the Teeth Thorough brushing of the teeth is important in preventing tooth decay. The mechanical action of brushing removes food particles that can harbor and incubate bacteria. It also stimulates circulation in the gums, thus maintaining their healthy firmness. One of the techniques recommended for brushing teeth is called the sulcular technique, which removes plaque and cleans under the gingival margins. Fluoride toothpaste is often recommended because of its antibacterial protection.

Caring for Artificial Dentures Some people have artificial teeth in the form of a plate—a complete set of teeth for one jaw. A person may have a lower plate or an upper plate or both. When only a few artificial teeth are needed, the individual may have a bridge rather than a plate. A bridge may be fixed or removable. Artificial teeth are fitted to the individual and usually will not fit another person. People who wear dentures or other types of oral prostheses should be encouraged to use them. Ill-fitting dentures or other oral prostheses can cause discomfort and chewing difficulties. They may also contribute to oral problems as well as poor nutrition and enjoyment of food. Those who do not wear their prostheses are prone to shrinkage of the gums, which results in further tooth loss.

Like natural teeth, artificial dentures collect microorganisms and food. They need to be cleaned regularly, at least once a day. They can be removed from the mouth, scrubbed with a toothbrush, rinsed, and reinserted. Some people use a dentifrice for cleaning teeth, and others use commercial cleaning compounds for plates.

Assisting Clients With Oral Care When providing mouth care for partially or totally dependent clients, the nurse should wear gloves to guard against infections. Other required equipment includes a curved basin that fits snugly under the client's chin (e.g., a kidney basin) to receive the rinse water, and a towel to protect the client and the bedclothes.

Foam swabs are often used in health care agencies to clean the mouths of dependent clients. These swabs are convenient and effective in removing excess debris from the teeth and mouth but should be used infrequently and for short periods (i.e., less than 3 days) because they do not remove plaque that is at the base of the teeth.

Most people prefer privacy when they take their artificial teeth out to clean them. Many do not like to be seen without their teeth; one of the first requests of many postoperative clients is "May I have my teeth in, please?"

Clients With Special Oral Hygiene Needs For the client who is debilitated or unconscious or who has excessive dryness, sores, or irritations of the mouth, it may be necessary to clean the oral mucosa and tongue in addition to the teeth. Agency practices differ in regard to special mouth care and the frequency with which it is provided. Depending on the health of the client's mouth, special care may be needed every 2–8 hours; see Developmental Considerations for Oral Hygiene in Older Adults.

Mouth care for unconscious or debilitated people is important because their mouths tend to become dry, predisposing them to tooth decay and infections. Saliva has antiviral, antibacterial, and antifungal effects (Walton, Miller, & Tordecilla, 2001, p. 40). Dry mouth—also called **xerostomia**—occurs when the supply of saliva is reduced (American Dental Association, n.d.). This condition can be caused by certain medications (e.g., antihistamines, antidepressants, antihypertensives), oxygen therapy, tachypnea, and NPO status, where the client cannot take fluids by mouth (Anonymous, 2003).

DEVELOPMENTAL CONSIDERATIONS Oral Hygiene in Older Adults

- Oral care is often difficult for certain older adults to perform due to problems with dexterity or cognitive problems with dementia.
- Some long-term health care facilities have dentists who come on a regular basis to see clients with special needs.
- Dryness of the oral mucosa is a common finding in older adults. Because this can lead to tooth decay, advise clients to discuss it with their dentist or primary care provider.
- Decay of the tooth root is common among older adults. When the gums recede, the tooth root is more vulnerable to decay.
- Promoting good oral hygiene can have a positive effect on the older adults' ability to eat.

For clients with special oral hygiene needs, the nurse needs to focus on removing plaque and microorganisms as well as client comfort. If possible, a soft-bristled toothbrush should be used, as it provides the best means of removing plaque. A sodium bicarbonate toothpaste will help dissolve mucus and reduce the saliva's acidity, which helps decrease bacteria (Nainar & Mohummed, 2004). If the client cannot tolerate the use of a toothbrush, the nurse can use an oral swab or a gauze soaked with saline to swab the teeth and tongue. A foam swab can be used to provide oral hygiene for dependent clients. The swab, however, is not effective for plaque removal (Munro, Grap, & Kleinpell, 2004). Lemon-glycerin swabs are not recommended as they irritate and dry the oral mucosa and can decalcify teeth. Mouthwashes containing alcohol can irritate the oral mucosa as well as cause dryness. The Food and Drug Administration approves hydrogen peroxide as a mouth rinse (Anonymous, 2003, p. 12). It provides a cleaning action as well as an antimicrobial effect. Diluting the hydrogen peroxide with saline or a nonalcohol–based mouthwash will help decrease the potential for the client to experience a burning sensation. Mineral oil is contraindicated as a moisturizer for the lips or inside the mouth because aspiration of it can initiate an infection (lipid pneumonia). A water-soluble moisturizer, absorbed by the skin and tissue, provides important hydration. Saliva substitutes can also help moisturize the oral cavity.

Evaluation

Using data collected during care (e.g., status of oral mucosa, lips, tongue, and teeth), the nurse judges whether desired outcomes have been achieved.

If outcomes are not achieved, the nurse and client need to explore the reasons before modifying the care plan. Following are examples of questions to consider:

- Did the nurse overestimate the client's functional abilities?
- Is the client's hand coordination or cognitive function impaired?
- Did the client's condition change?
- Has there been a change in the client's energy level and/or motivation?

REVIEW Oral Health

RELATE: LINK THE CONCEPTS

Linking the exemplar of Oral Health with the concept of Development:

1. What are the different dental concerns of each developmental stage across the life span?
2. Design a teaching plan for a group of young mothers regarding oral health and nutrition for their toddlers?

Linking the exemplar of Oral Health with the concept of Comfort:

3. While working as a hospice nurse you are caring for a client requiring end-of-life care. What oral care will be of particular importance to provide this client?
4. What will you teach the client with chronic mouth pain about oral care?

READY: GO TO COMPANION SKILLS MANUAL

- Providing oral care
- Brushing and flossing the teeth
- Providing special oral care for the unconscious or debilitated client

REFER: GO TO MYNURSINGKIT

REFLECT: CASE STUDY

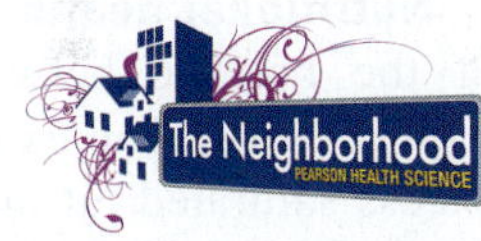

Tyler Martin is a 2-year-old boy. Since he was 4 weeks old, Tyler has been going to various babysitters while his parents worked. He and his father have recently moved in with Tyler's grandparents. Tyler loves living at his grandfather's home because of all the attention he gets. Tyler also no longer has to go to day care.

Tyler has generally been in good health; he is of normal weight and has a good appetite. Tyler still loves his bottle, and each night he is given a bottle of milk or juice to help him go to sleep. If he doesn't receive a bottle to sleep with, he screams until someone gives in and brings him one.

1. Are there any concerns that require intervention and teaching in this scenario?
2. What oral care needs does Tyler require in terms of dental visits and tooth care?
3. How would you teach Tyler to brush his teeth? Can he be taught how to floss at this stage? Explain your answer.

13.4 NUTRITION SCREENING

KEY TERMS

Diet recall, *663*
Malnutrition, *662*
Nutritional health, *662*
Overnutrition, *662*
Protein-calorie malnutrition, *662*
Undernutrition, *662*

BASIS FOR SELECTION OF EXEMPLAR

Healthy People 2010

LEARNING OUTCOMES

After reading about this exemplar, you will be able to:

1. Define nutritional health.
2. Outline risk factors that affect nutritional health status.
3. Identify physical and laboratory parameters utilized in a nutrition assessment.
4. Identify components of a diet history and techniques for gathering diet history data.
5. Describe existing validated nutritional assessment tools.
6. Identify specific nutritional assessment techniques and tools appropriate for unique stages in the life span.
7. Discuss strategies for integrating a complete nutritional assessment into the nursing care process.

OVERVIEW

Nutritional health is a crucial component of overall health across the life span. The nutritional health of a pregnant female will influence pregnancy outcome. Nutritional health in growing children plays a central role in growth and development. In adults and older adults, nutritional health can be associated with prevention or development of chronic disease in conditions involving both undernutrition and overnutrition. **Undernutrition**, also called **malnutrition**, is defined as health effects of insufficient nutrient intake or stores. **Overnutrition** results from excesses in nutrient intake or stores and can manifest itself in conditions such as obesity, hypertension, hypercholesterolemia, or toxic levels of stored vitamins or minerals.

The determination of an individual's nutritional status is based on a thorough nutritional assessment. The assessment portion of the nursing care process incorporates the gathering and interpretation of data often used as part of a nutritional assessment. These data then create the foundation for later development of appropriate nursing and nutritional interventions aimed at preserving or improving nutritional health.

Nutritional health can be defined as the physical result of the balance between nutrient intake and nutritional requirements. For example, an individual who consumes excess saturated fat may be at risk for elevated blood cholesterol and cardiovascular disease. This person may therefore be considered to have poor nutritional health due to overnutrition. A pregnant female who consumes less than the required amounts of folic acid may place her unborn child at risk for certain birth defects, such as neural tube defects, and could be considered in poor nutritional health due to undernutrition. A client who consumes adequate nutrition to meet individual needs and avoids habitual excesses and insufficiencies would be considered in good nutritional health.

Many factors can influence nutritional health. When gathering data for a nutritional assessment, it is important to know common risk factors for poor nutritional status. Overnutrition in the form of excess dietary intake of fat, especially saturated fat, has been associated with an increased risk of atherosclerosis. Overweight and obesity are linked to increased risk of hypertension, cardiovascular disease, type 2 diabetes, some cancers, degenerative joint disease, and other conditions. Additionally, excess body weight has been shown to increase the risk of all-cause mortality in adults 30–74 years of age. In the United States, 63% of males and 55% of females 20–74 years of age are considered overweight or obese, a statistic that has increased by 25% over the past 30 years. The prevalence of obesity and overweight has doubled in children and adolescents in the last 30 years to 13 and 14%, respectively. Excess alcohol intake is associated with chronic liver disease and cirrhosis, the 12th leading cause of death in the United States, according to the National Center for Health Statistics at the Centers for the CDC.

Undernutrition is less common than overnutrition in the United States, but it can have devastating physical health consequences when **protein-calorie malnutrition** or other nutrient deficiencies develop. Undernutrition can lead to growth faltering, compromised immune status, poor wound healing, muscle loss, physical and functional decline, and lack of proper development. Generally, individuals at risk for undernutrition include those who have a chronic illness or who are poor, elderly, hospitalized, restrictive eaters (from chronic dieting or disordered eating), or alcoholics. An individual can have both overnutrition and undernutrition, such as an overweight child who consumes no fruit or vegetables. Box 13–7 outlines additional risk factors for overnutrition and undernutrition to consider when conducting a nutrition assessment.

Healthy People 2010's objectives for targeting overweight, obesity, and issues of undernutrition are important reminders to the clinician of the central role nutrition plays in overall health across the life span. The increasing prevalence of overweight and obesity in the United States and the statistics on nutritional health disparities illustrate the importance of nutritional screening and assessment as the first step toward reaching these important goals. Box 13–8 outlines the cultural and socioeconomic influences that may affect nutritional health. And the Focus on Culture and Diversity lists cultural influences on diet.

Laboratory Data

Laboratory tests provide objective data for the nutritional assessment, but because many factors can influence these tests, no single test specifically predicts nutritional risk or

Box 13–7 **Risk Factors for Poor Nutritional Health**

UNDERNUTRITION

- Chronic disease, acute illness, or injury
- Multiple medications
- Food insecurity—lack of free access to adequate and safe food
- Restrictive eating due to chronic dieting, disordered eating, faddism, or food beliefs
- Alcohol abuse
- Depression, bereavement, loneliness, social isolation
- Poor dental health
- Decreased knowledge or skills about food preparation and recommendations
- Extreme age—premature infants or adults over 80 years of age

OVERNUTRITION

- Excess intake of fat, sugar, calories, or nutrients
- Alcohol abuse
- Sedentary lifestyle
- Decreased knowledge or skills about food preparation and recommendations

Box 13–8 Cultural and Socioeconomic Influences on Nutritional Health

OVERWEIGHT AND OBESITY

- More than than 60% of adults 20–74 years of age are overweight; 27% are classified as obese.
- Up to 15% of children 6–19 years of age are overweight.
- Prevalence of obesity has increased in the three major racial and ethnic groups.
- Prevalence of overweight is highest among Mexican American males.
- Prevalence of obesity is highest among Mexican American females.
- Hypertension, a comorbid condition of overweight and obesity, affects 23% of adults in the United States.
- Prevalence of hypertension is highest among Black persons.
- Adults of low socioeconomic status have twice the rate of overweight or obesity than those of medium and high socioeconomic status.

UNDERNUTRITION

- Undernutrition can contribute to growth retardation. By definition, 5% of children would be expected to be at the 5th percentile for height. However, up to 15% of Black children have growth retardation in the first year of life, and 11% of Asian and Pacific Islander children have growth retardation during the second year.
- Up to 60% of older adults in dependent care or hospitals are malnourished.
- Adequate folic acid and iron status are important for healthy outcomes during pregnancy. Pregnant Mexican American females are more likely than those of other ethnic groups to have iron deficiency and low folic acid levels. Females of lower economic status and those with less education are also more likely to have inadequate folic acid or iron status.
- Black women and adolescents under age 15 years are more likely to have insufficient gestational weight gain and deliver low-birth-weight babies than women of other populations.

POVERTY AND FOOD INSECURITY

- Poverty is a major risk factor for food insecurity and malnutrition. Public programs such as Women, Infants and Children (WIC) and the Supplemental Nutrition Assistance Program (formerly the Food Stamp program) assist families in poverty with accessing healthy food for their children.
- Among Americans, the prevalence of poverty was 12.5% in 2007.
- Children under age 18 experience a 17.6% poverty rate, although this rate is higher in some states.
- Prevalence of poverty is highest among Black (24.5%) and Hispanic populations (21.5%).

Sources: Healthy People 2010. 19. Nutrition and Overweight. Retrieved June 24, 2005, at www.healthypeople.gov/Document/HTML/VOLUME2/19Nutrition.htm; and *Income, Poverty, and Health Insurance Coverage in the United States: 2007.* Retrieved May 31, 2009 at www.census.gov/prod/2008pubs/p60-235.pdf.

measures the presence or degree of a nutritional problem. The tests most commonly used are serum proteins, urinary urea nitrogen and creatinine, and total lymphocyte count.

Food Guide Pyramid

Dietary Guidelines for Americans is published jointly every 5 years by the Department of Health and Human Services (HHS) and the Department of Agriculture (USDA). The most recent guidelines, released in January 2005, provide a new comprehensive Food Guide Pyramid and an interactive Web site that may be used for individual food guide planning and diet analysis. The nurse can compare the **diet recall** or nutrition history data to the distribution of food groups recommended and make a general assessment of diet adequacy. The benefit of the new pyramid is that it is flexible and molds to the individual. Instead of requiring special food pyramids

FOCUS ON DIVERSITY AND CULTURE Cultural Diet Influences

- Cultural and religious beliefs and traditions can affect food choices, beliefs, and practices in many ways from the number of meals eaten in a day to food choices, preparation methods, and overall food beliefs.
- Diversity exists within cultural and religious groups. It is important to avoid applying general knowledge about cultural and religious food practices to all people within a group; instead explore individual interpretation and influences.
- Assess common dietary staples as well as foods believed to be associated with health or symbolic benefits. Some food is thought to promote health or cure conditions, such as making a "hot" condition "colder." Other beliefs may be related to life span issues, such as the proper diet during pregnancy for easy delivery.
- Many religious groups have dietary laws that are observed differently by subgroups within the population. Consumption of kosher meats, fasting, and avoidance of certain foods such as pork, crustaceans, birds of prey, beef, or other animal products are examples.
- Ask about food practices and particular meals for special occasions and holidays. Some religious groups fast during parts of some holy days.
- Discuss food preparation methods. A variety of cultures make similar dishes but prepare them differently—for example, using different fats such as bacon drippings, lard, oils, or ghee clarified butter.
- Ask about medicinal herb use as this varies among cultures and is often an important aspect of health beliefs.
- Explore to what extent any acculturation has taken place and which traditional practices changed once the client was living in a new dominant culture. Ask whether new foods have been added to traditional foods, newer versions have been substituted for traditional foods, and any traditional foods have been omitted. In some cases, traditional diets are healthier than the diet in the new culture, and encouragement to maintain healthy traditions may be helpful.

for various age or culture groups, the new Web site (www.usda.gov) has the richness of choice to meet all needs.

The Minimum Data Set

The Minimum Data Set (MDS) is a component of the Residential Assessment Instrument mandated for all clients in Medicare-certified health care facilities. The MDS nutritional components are to be included in admission assessments for all residents as well as in quarterly and annual updates. Any changes in client status that involve a nutritional component of the MDS require a complete reassessment of nutritional status.

Mini Nutritional Assessment and Subjective Global Assessment

The Mini Nutritional Assessment (MNA) and Subjective Global Assessment (SGA) have both been validated for use in the nutritional assessment of older adults. The SGA has also been used in assessing other populations since its development over 20 years ago. The MNA is a newer tool with extensive data validating its use with older adults. The MNA can be included as a routine component of a physical examination or as a quick bedside tool.

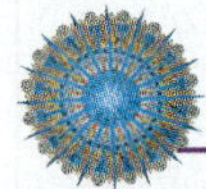

NURSING PROCESS

Assessment

Nurses assessing clients with suspected nutritional deficits should ask the following questions:

- Self-care abilities: Is the client able to feed self, purchase food, and prepare meals?
- Adaptive feeding aids: Does the client require special cups, plates, or feeding utensils?
- Instructional needs: What are the client's nutritional requirements, including special diet, availability of adaptive aids, cultural and religious preferences or considerations, and management of enteral/parenteral nutrition?
- Physical environment: Is there adequacy of water, electricity, refrigeration, and telephone facilities? If enteral/parenteral equipment is needed, is there a clean, secure area for storage and preparation?
- General eating patterns: How frequently does the client eat each day? What does a typical breakfast, lunch, and dinner consist of? When and what kind of snacks does the client eat?

Diagnosis

NANDA (2007) includes the following diagnostic labels for nutritional problems:

- Imbalanced Nutrition: More Than Body Requirements
- Imbalanced Nutrition: Less Than Body Requirements
- Readiness for Enhanced Nutrition
- Risk for Imbalanced Nutrition: More Than Body Requirements.

Many other NANDA nursing diagnoses may apply to certain individuals, because nutritional problems often affect other areas of human functioning. In this case, the nutritional diagnostic label may be used as the etiology of other diagnoses. Examples include the following:

- Activity Intolerance related to inadequate intake of iron-rich foods resulting in iron-deficiency anemia
- Constipation related to inadequate fluid intake and fiber intake
- Low Self-esteem related to obesity
- Risk for Infection related to immunosuppression secondary to insufficient protein intake.

Plan

Major goals for clients with or at risk for nutritional problems include the following:

- Maintain or restore optimal nutritional status.
- Promote healthy nutritional practices.
- Prevent complications associated with malnutrition.
- Decrease weight.
- Regain specified weight.

Specific nursing activities associated with each of these interventions can be selected to meet the individual needs of the client.

Implementation

Nursing interventions to promote optimal nutrition for hospitalized clients are often provided in collaboration with the primary care provider who writes the diet orders and the dietitian who informs clients about special diets. The nurse reinforces this instruction and, in addition, creates an atmosphere that encourages eating, provides assistance with eating, monitors the client's appetite and food intake, administers enteral and parenteral feedings, and consults with the primary care provider and dietitian about nutritional problems that arise.

In the community setting, the nurse's role is largely educational. For example, nurses promote optimal nutrition at health fairs, in schools, at prenatal classes, and with well or ill clients and support people in their homes. In the home setting, nurses also initiate nutritional screens, refer clients at risk to appropriate resources, instruct clients about enteral and parenteral feedings, and offer nutrition counseling as needed. Nutrition counseling involves more than simply providing information. The nurse must help clients integrate diet changes into their lifestyle and provide strategies to motivate them to change their eating habits.

Evaluation

The goals established in the planning phase are evaluated according to specific desired outcomes, also established in that phase. If the outcomes are not achieved, the nurse should explore the reasons. The nurse might consider the following questions:

- Were the outcomes unrealistic for this person?
- Were the client's food and religious preferences considered?
- Is anything interfering with digestion or absorption of nutrients (e.g., diarrhea)?
- Was the family included in the teaching plan? Are family members supportive?
- Is the client experiencing symptoms that cause loss of appetite (e.g., pain, nausea, fatigue)?

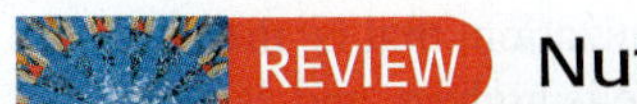

REVIEW Nutrition Screening

RELATE: LINK THE CONCEPTS

Linking the exemplar of Nutrition Screening with the concept of Culture:

1. You are caring for a client who has recently immigrated from another country. The client is unable to find foods from his homeland so he does not eat because he finds Western food distasteful. He is very malnourished. What client teaching and support can you provide to improve this client's nutritional status?
2. You are planning a seminar for African American clients living in the area about nutrition and risks associated with poor nutrition. What are your priority teaching points related to known risk factors faced by this racial group?

Linking the exemplar of Nutritional Screening with the concept of Cellular Regulation:

3. What are the important teaching points to provide a client in order to reduce the risk of colon cancer?
4. How would you assist the young mother with anemia to plan a healthy menu?

REFER: GO TO MYNURSINGKIT

READY: GO TO COMPANION SKILLS MANUAL

- Measuring body mass index
- Assessing height and weight

REFLECT: CASE STUDY

Madison, a 17-month-old, is brought to the Pediatric Clinic by her mother, who is worried because it seems Madison is eating less. Madison is always moving and doing something. The mother asks you what are some good snack foods to give Madison. Her mother says Madison wants milk and juice when she is "on the move."

1. Madison seems to eat less to her mother. What phenomenon is occuring?
2. What are the elements of a healthy diet for a toddler? What are examples of healthy snacks?
3. How much milk and juice should Madison be drinking?
4. Describe a typical daily dietary intake for Madison.

13.5 NORMAL SLEEP/REST PATTERNS

KEY TERMS

Biological rhythms, *666*
Nocturnal emissions, *668*
NREM (non-rapid-eye-movement) sleep, *666*
REM (rapid-eye-movement) sleep, *666*
Sleep, *666*
Sleep architecture, *666*
Somnology, *665*

LEARNING OUTCOMES

After reading about this exemplar, you will be able to:

1. Explain the functions and the physiology of sleep.
2. Identify the characteristics of the sleep states.
3. Describe variations in sleep patterns throughout the life span.
4. Describe interventions that promote normal sleep.

BASIS FOR SELECTION OF EXEMPLAR

Institute of Medicine (IOM)

OVERVIEW

Sleep is a basic human need; it is a universal biological process common to all people. Humans spend about one third of their lives asleep. We require sleep for many reasons: to cope with daily stresses, to prevent fatigue, to conserve energy, to restore the mind and body, and to enjoy life more fully. Sleep enhances daytime functioning. It is vital for not only optimal psychological functioning but also physiological functioning, as the rate of healing of damaged tissue is greatest during sleep (Robinson, Weitzel, & Henderson, 2005, p. 263).

Sleep is an important factor in a person's quality of life, yet a 2006 report from the Institute of Medicine (IOM) states that sleep disorders and sleep deprivation is an unmet public health problem. It is estimated that 50 million to 70 million Americans suffer from a chronic disorder of sleep and wakefulness that hinders daily functioning and adversely affects health (IOM, 2006, p. 24). Numerous *Sleep in America* polls by the National Sleep Foundation reflect that Americans, from infants to older adults, need more sleep. Furthermore, many members of the general public and health professionals are unaware of the consequences of chronic sleep loss (e.g., increased risk of hypertension, diabetes, obesity, depression, heart attack, and stroke). Almost 20% of all serious car crash injuries are associated with driver sleepiness (IOM, 2006, p. 25).

As a result of these studies, the IOM report made a number of recommendations, including to (a) increase financial investments in interdisciplinary **somnology** (the study of sleep) and sleep medicine research training; (b) increase public awareness by establishing a multimedia public education campaign; (c) increase education and training of health care professionals in somnology and sleep medicine; (d) develop new technologies for the diagnosis and treatment of sleep disorders; and (e) monitor the American population's sleep patterns and the prevalence and health outcomes associated with sleep disorders (IOM, 2006).

PHYSIOLOGY OF SLEEP

Historically, sleep was considered a state of unconsciousness. More recently, **sleep** has come to be considered an altered state of consciousness in which the individual's perception of and reaction to the environment are decreased. Sleep is characterized by minimal physical activity, variable levels of consciousness, changes in the body's physiologic processes, and decreased responsiveness to external stimuli. Some environmental stimuli, such as a smoke detector alarm, will usually awaken a sleeper, whereas many other noises will not. It appears that individuals respond to meaningful stimuli while sleeping and selectively disregard nonmeaningful stimuli. For example, a mother may respond to her baby's crying but not to the crying of another baby.

The cyclic nature of sleep is thought to be controlled by centers located in the lower part of the brain. Neurons within the reticular formation, located in the brainstem, integrate sensory information from the peripheral nervous system and relay the information to the cerebral cortex. The upper part of the reticular formation consists of a network of ascending nerve fibers called the reticular activating system (RAS) which is involved with the sleep-wake cycle. An intact cerebral cortex and reticular formation are necessary for the regulation of sleep and waking states.

Neurotransmitters, located within neurons in the brain, affect the sleep-wake cycles. For example, serotonin is thought to lessen the response to sensory stimulation and gamma-aminobutyric acid (GABA) to shut off the activity in the neurons of the RAS. Another key factor to sleep is exposure to darkness. Darkness and preparing for sleep cause a decrease in RAS stimulation. During this time, the pineal gland in the brain begins actively to secrete the natural hormone melatonin, and the person feels less alert. During sleep, the growth hormone is secreted and cortisol is inhibited.

With the beginning of daylight, melatonin is at its lowest level in the body and the stimulating hormone cortisol is at its highest. Wakefulness is also associated with high levels of acetylcholine, dopamine, and noradrenaline. Acetylcholine is released in the reticular formation, dopamine in the midbrain, and noradrenaline in the pons. These neurotransmitters are localized within the reticular formation and influence cerebral cortical arousal.

Circadian Rhythms

Biological rhythms exist in plants, animals, and humans. In humans, these are controlled from within the body and synchronized with environmental factors, such as light and darkness. The most familiar biological rhythm is the circadian rhythm. The term *circadian* is from the Latin *circa dies,* meaning "about a day." Although sleep and waking cycles are the best known of the circadian rhythms, body temperature, blood pressure, and many other physiologic functions also follow a circadian pattern.

Sleep is a complex biological rhythm. When a person's biological clock coincides with the sleep-wake cycles, the person is said to be in circadian synchronization; that is, the person is awake when the body temperature is highest, and asleep when the body temperature is lowest. Circadian regularity begins to develop by the sixth week of life, and by 3–6 months most infants have a regular sleep-wake cycle.

Types of Sleep

Sleep architecture refers to the basic organization of normal sleep. There are two types of sleep: **NREM (non-rapid-eye-movement) sleep** and **REM (rapid-eye-movement) sleep**. During sleep, NREM and REM sleep alternate in cycles. Irregular cycling and/or absent sleep stages are associated with sleep disorders (IOM, 2006, p. 42).

NREM SLEEP NREM sleep occurs when activity in the RAS is inhibited. About 75–80% of sleep during a night is NREM sleep. NREM sleep is divided into four stages, each associated with distinct brain activity and physiology. Stage I is the stage of very light sleep and lasts only a few minutes. During this stage, the person feels drowsy and relaxed, the eyes roll from side to side, and the heart and respiratory rates drop slightly. The sleeper can be readily awakened and may deny that he or she was sleeping.

Stage II is the stage of light sleep during which body processes continue to slow down. The eyes are generally still, the heart and respiratory rates decrease slightly, and body temperature falls. Stage II constitutes 44–55% of total sleep (IOM, 2006, p. 44). An individual requires more intense stimuli in stage II than in stage I to awaken.

Stages III and IV are the deepest stages of sleep, differing only in the percentage of delta waves recorded during a 30-second period. During *deep sleep* or *delta sleep,* the sleeper's heart and respiratory rates drop 20–30% below those exhibited during waking hours. The sleeper is difficult to arouse. The person is not disturbed by sensory stimuli, the skeletal muscles are very relaxed, reflexes are diminished, and snoring is most likely to occur. Even swallowing and saliva production are reduced during delta sleep (Orr, 2000). These stages are essential for restoring energy and releasing important growth hormones (Box 13–9).

PRACTICE ALERT

In a sleep-deprived client, the loss of NREM sleep causes immunosuppression, slows tissue repair, lowers pain tolerance, triggers profound fatigue, and increases susceptibility to infection (Lower, Bonsack, & Guion, 2003, p. 40D).

Box 13–9 Physiologic Changes During NREM Sleep

- Arterial blood pressure falls.
- Pulse rate decreases.
- Peripheral blood vessels dilate.
- Cardiac output decreases.
- Skeletal muscles relax.
- Basal metabolic rate decreases 10–30%.
- Growth hormone levels peak.
- Intracranial pressure decreases.

REM SLEEP REM sleep usually recurs about every 90 minutes and lasts 5–30 minutes. Most dreams take place during REM sleep but usually will not be remembered unless the person arouses briefly at the end of the REM period.

During REM sleep, the brain is highly active, and brain metabolism may increase as much as 20%. For example, during REM sleep, levels of acetylcholine and dopamine increase, with the highest levels of acetylcholine release occurring during REM sleep. Since both of these neurotransmitters are associated with cortical activation, it makes sense that their levels would be high during dreaming sleep. This type of sleep is also called paradoxical sleep because electroencephalogram (EEG) activity resembles that of wakefulness. Distinctive eye movements occur, voluntary muscle tone is dramatically decreased, and deep tendon reflexes are absent. In this phase, the sleeper may be difficult to arouse or may wake spontaneously, gastric secretions increase, and heart and respiratory rates often are irregular. It is thought that the regions of the brain used in learning, thinking, and organizing information are stimulated during REM sleep.

PRACTICE ALERT

In a sleep-deprived client, the loss of REM sleep causes psychologic disturbances such as apathy, depression, irritability, confusion, disorientation, hallucinations, impaired memory, and paranoia (Lower, Bonsack, & Guion, 2003, p. 40D).

Sleep Cycles

During a sleep cycle, people typically pass through NREM and REM sleep, with the complete cycle usually lasting about 90–110 minutes in adults. In the first sleep cycle, a sleeper usually passes through all of the first three NREM stages in a total of about 20–30 minutes. Then, stage IV may last about 30 minutes. After stage IV NREM, the sleeper passes back through stages III and II over about 20 minutes. Thereafter, the first REM stage occurs, lasting about 10 minutes, completing the first sleep cycle. It is not unusual for the first REM period to be very brief or even skipped entirely. The healthy adult sleeper usually experiences four to six cycles of sleep during 7–8 hours (Figure 13–7 ■). The sleeper who is awakened during any stage must begin anew at stage I NREM sleep and proceed through all the stages to REM sleep.

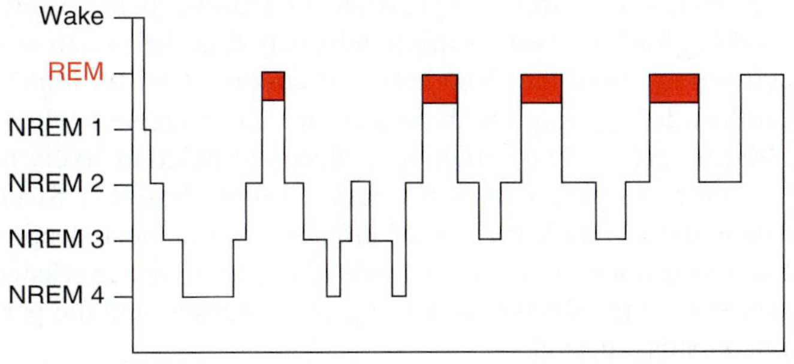

Figure 13–7 ■ Time spent in REM and non-REM stages of sleep in an adult.

The duration of NREM stages and REM sleep varies throughout the sleep period. During the early part of the night, the deep sleep periods are longer. As the night progresses, the sleeper spends less time in stages III and IV of NREM sleep. REM sleep increases and dreams tend to lengthen. Before sleep ends, periods of near wakefulness occur, and stages I and II NREM sleep and REM sleep predominate.

FUNCTIONS OF SLEEP

The effects of sleep on the body are not completely understood. Sleep exerts physiologic effects on both the nervous system and other body structures. Sleep in some way restores normal levels of activity and normal balance among parts of the nervous system. Sleep is also necessary for protein synthesis, which allows repair processes to occur.

The role of sleep in psychological well-being is best noticed by the deterioration in mental functioning related to sleep loss. Persons with inadequate amounts of sleep tend to become emotionally irritable, have poor concentration, and experience difficulty making decisions.

NORMAL SLEEP PATTERNS AND REQUIREMENTS

Although it used to be believed that maintaining a regular sleep-wake rhythm is more important than the number of hours actually slept, recent research has shown that sleep deprivation is associated with significant cognitive and health problems. Although reestablishing the sleep-wake rhythm (e.g., after the disruption of surgery) is an important aspect of nursing, it is not appropriate to curtail or decrease daytime napping in hospitalized clients.

Newborns

Newborns sleep 16–18 hours a day, on an irregular schedule with periods of 1–3 hours spent awake. Unlike older children and adults, newborns enter REM sleep (called active sleep during the newborn period) immediately. Rapid eye movements are observable through closed lids, and the body movements and irregular respirations may be observed. NREM sleep (also called quiet sleep during the newborn period) is characterized by regular respirations, closed eyes, and the absence of body and eye movements. Newborns spend nearly 50% of their time in each of these states, and the sleep cycle is about 50 minutes.

It is best to put newborns to bed when they are sleepy but not asleep. Newborns can be encouraged to sleep less during the day by exposing them to light and by playing more with them during the day hours. As evening approaches, the environment can be less bright and quieter, with less activity (National Sleep Foundation, n.d.d). It is important to teach new parents and caregivers of newborns to put the baby "back to sleep," to make sure the newborn who is lying down while sleeping is sleeping on the back, as babies who sleep on their stomachs are at greater risk for sudden infant death syndrome.

Infants

At first, infants awaken every 3 or 4 hours, eat, and then go back to sleep. Periods of wakefulness gradually increase during the first months. By 6 months, most infants sleep through the night (from midnight to 5 a.m.) and begin to establish a pattern of daytime naps. At the end of the first year, an infant usually takes two naps per day and should get about 14–15 hours of sleep in 24 hours.

About half of the infant's sleep time is spent in light sleep. During light sleep, the infant exhibits a great deal of activity, such as movement, gurgles, and coughing. Parents need to make sure that infants are truly awake before picking them up for feeding and changing. Putting infants to bed when they are drowsy but not asleep helps them to become "self-soothers." This means that they fall asleep independently, and if they do awake at night, they can put themselves back to sleep. Infants who become used to parental assistance at bedtime may become "signalers" and cry for their parents to help them return to sleep at night (National Sleep Foundation, n.d.a).

Toddlers

Between 12 and 14 hours of sleep are recommended for children 1–3 years of age. Most still need an afternoon nap, but the need for midmorning naps gradually decreases. The toddler may exhibit a great deal of resistance to going to bed and may awaken during the night. Nighttime fears and nightmares are also common. A security object such as a blanket or stuffed animal may help. Parents need assurance that if the child has had adequate attention from them during the day, maintaining a daily sleep schedule and consistent bedtime routine will promote good sleep habits for the entire family.

Preschoolers

The preschool child (3–5 years of age) requires 11–13 hours of sleep per night, particularly if the child is in preschool. Sleep needs fluctuate in relation to activity and growth spurts. Many children of this age dislike bedtime and resist by requesting another story, game, or television program. The 4–5-year-old may become restless and irritable if sleep requirements are not met.

Parents can help children who resist bedtime by maintaining a regular and consistent sleep schedule. It also helps to have a relaxing bedtime routine that ends in the child's room. Preschool children wake up frequently at night, and they may be afraid of the dark or experience night terrors or nightmares. Often limiting or eliminating TV will reduce the number of nightmares.

School-Age Children

The school-age child (5–12 years of age) needs 10–11 hours of sleep, but most receive less because of increasing demands (e.g., homework, sports, social activities). They may also be spending more time at the computer and watching TV. Some may be drinking caffeinated beverages. All of these activities can lead to difficulty falling asleep and fewer hours of sleep. Nurses can teach parents and school-age children about healthy sleep habits. A regular and consistent sleep schedule and bedtime routine need to be continued.

Adolescents

Adolescents (12–18 years of age) require 9–10 hours of sleep each night; however, few actually get that much sleep (IOM, 2006, p. 56). The National Sleep Foundation's 2006 *Sleep in America* poll found that teens are sleepy at times and places where they should be fully awake—at school, at home, and on the road. This can result in lower grades, negative moods (e.g., unhappy, sad, tense), and increased potential for car accidents. Interestingly, while more than half of the adolescents knew they were not getting enough sleep, 90% of the parents believed their adolescent was getting enough sleep. Nurses can teach parents to recognize signs and symptoms that indicate their teen is not getting enough sleep.

As children reach adolescence, their circadian rhythms tend to shift. Research in the 1990s found that later sleep and wake patterns among adolescents are biologically determined; the natural tendency for teenagers is to stay up late at night and wake up later in the morning (National Sleep Foundation, n.d.a). Many schools, however, start at 7 a.m., which is in conflict with adolescents' sleep patterns and needs and contribute to their sleep deprivation. As a result, some members of Congress have introduced resolutions to encourage schools and school districts to reconsider the early school start times.

During adolescence, boys begin to experience **nocturnal emissions** (orgasm and emission of semen during sleep), known as "wet dreams," several times each month. Boys need to be informed about this normal development to prevent embarrassment and fear.

Adults

Most healthy adults need 7–9 hours of sleep a night (National Sleep Foundation, n.d.b). However, there is individual variation as some adults may be able to function well (e.g., without sleepiness or drowsiness) with 6 hours of sleep and others may need 10 hours to function optimally. Signs that may indicate a person is not getting enough sleep include falling asleep or becoming drowsy during a task that is not fatiguing (e.g., listening to a boring or monotonous presentation), not being able to concentrate or remember information, and being unreasonably irritable with others.

The National Sleep Foundation (n.d.b) reports that certain adults are particularly vulnerable to getting insufficient sleep: students, shift workers, travelers, and persons suffering from acute stress, depression, or chronic pain. Adults working long hours or multiple jobs may find their sleep less refreshing. Also, the sleep habits of children have an impact on the adults caring for them. Parents and caregivers whose children get the least amount of sleep are twice as likely to say they sleep less than 6 hours a night (National Sleep Foundation, n.d.b). Parents of infants lose the most sleep—nearly an hour on a typical night. Women may experience more disrupted sleep during pregnancy, menses, and the perimenopausal period.

Nurses need to teach adults the importance of obtaining sufficient sleep and tips on how to promote sleep that result in the client waking up feeling restored or refreshed.

Older Adults

A hallmark change with age is a tendency toward earlier bedtime and wake times. Older adults (65–75 years) usually awaken 1.3 hours earlier and go to bed approximately 1 hour earlier than younger adults (ages 20–30). Older adults may show an increase in disturbed sleep that can create a negative impact on their quality of life, mood, and alertness. Although sleeping becomes more difficult, the need to sleep does not decrease with age (IOM, 2006, pp. 57–59).

The National Sleep Foundation's 2003 *Sleep in America* poll was the first poll to look at the sleep habits of Americans between the ages of 55 and 84. It found that older adults are sleeping 7–9 hours on both weeknights and weekends. Of interest, however, was the striking relationship between the older adult's health and quality of life and the person's sleep quantity and quality. The poll found that the better the health of older adults, the more likely they are to sleep well. And, conversely, the more diagnosed medical conditions, the more likely they were to report sleep problems (National Sleep Foundation, n.d.c). Older adults who have several medical conditions and complain of having sleeping problems should discuss this with their primary care provider: They may have a major sleep disorder that is complicating treatment of the other conditions. It is important for the nurse to teach about the connection between sleep, health, and aging.

Some older adult clients with dementia may experience *sundown syndrome*. Although not a sleep disorder directly, it refers to a pattern of symptoms (e.g., agitation, anxiety, aggression, and sometimes delusions) that occur in the late afternoon (thus the name). These symptoms can last throughout the night, further disrupting sleep (Arnold, 2004).

FACTORS AFFECTING SLEEP

Both the quality and the quantity of sleep are affected by a number of factors. *Sleep quality* is a subjective characteristic and is often determined by whether or not a person wakes up feeling energetic. *Quantity of sleep* is the total time the individual sleeps.

Following an irregular morning and nighttime schedule can affect sleep. Moderate exercise in the morning or early afternoon usually is conducive to sleep, but exercise late in the day can delay sleep. The person's ability to relax before retiring is an important factor affecting the ability to fall asleep. It is best, therefore, to avoid doing homework or office work before or after getting into bed.

Night shift workers frequently obtain less sleep than other workers and have difficulty falling asleep after getting off work. Wearing dark wraparound sunglasses during the drive home and light-blocking shades can minimize the alerting effects of exposure to daylight, thus making it easier to fall asleep when body temperature is rising.

Emotional Stress

Most sleep experts consider stress to be the number one cause of short-term sleeping difficulties (National Sleep Foundation, n.d.b). A person preoccupied with personal problems (e.g., school- or job-related pressures, financial difficulties, family or marriage problems) may be unable to relax sufficiently to get to sleep. Anxiety increases the norepinephrine blood levels through stimulation of the sympathetic nervous system. This chemical change results in less deep sleep and REM sleep and more stage changes and awakenings.

Stimulants and Alcohol

Caffeine-containing beverages act as stimulants of the central nervous system. Drinking beverages containing caffeine in the afternoon or evening may interfere with sleep. People who drink an excessive amount of alcohol often find their sleep disturbed. Although it may hasten the onset of sleep, alcohol disrupts REM sleep. While making up for lost REM sleep after some of the effects of the alcohol have worn off, people often experience nightmares. The alcohol-tolerant person may be unable to sleep well and become irritable as a result.

Diet

Weight gain has been associated with reduced total sleep time as well as broken sleep and earlier awakening. Weight loss, on the other hand, seems to be associated with an increase in total sleep time and less broken sleep. Dietary L-tryptophan—found, for example, in cheese and milk—may induce sleep, a fact that might explain why warm milk helps some people get to sleep.

Smoking

Nicotine has a stimulating effect on the body, and smokers often have more difficulty falling asleep than nonsmokers do. Smokers are usually easily aroused and often describe themselves as light sleepers. Refraining from smoking after the evening meal usually helps the person sleeps better; moreover, many former smokers report that their sleeping patterns improved once they stopped smoking.

Motivation

Motivation can increase alertness in some situations (e.g., a tired person can probably stay alert while attending an interesting concert or surfing the Web late at night). Motivation alone, however, is usually not sufficient to overcome the normal circadian drive to sleep during the night. Nor is motivation sufficient to overcome sleepiness due to insufficient sleep. Boredom alone is not sufficient to cause sleepiness, but when insufficient sleep combines with boredom, sleep is likely to occur.

Medications

Some medications affect the quality of sleep. Most hypnotics can interfere with deep sleep and suppress REM sleep. Beta-blockers have been known to cause insomnia and nightmares. Narcotics, such as meperidine hydrochloride (Demerol) and morphine, are known to suppress REM sleep and to cause frequent awakenings and drowsiness. Tranquilizers interfere with REM sleep. Although antidepressants suppress REM sleep, this effect is considered a therapeutic action. In fact, selectively depriving a depressed client of REM sleep will result in an immediate but transient improvement in mood. Clients accustomed to taking hypnotic medications and antidepressants may experience a REM rebound (increased REM sleep) when these medications are discontinued. Warning clients to expect a period of more intense dreams when these medications are discontinued may reduce their anxiety about this symptom.

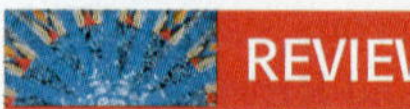

REVIEW Normal Sleep/Rest Patterns

RELATE: LINK THE CONCEPTS

Linking the exemplar of Normal Sleep/Rest Patterns with the concept of Cognition:

1. What expected outcome would you anticipate on the postpartum client's cognition when she is awakened every 2–4 hours by the newborn's cry and need to eat?
2. The daughter of an 80-year-old client who has early dementia complains to the nurse that the client is up and ready to go at 4:30 in the morning. She is concerned that lack of sleep will eventually impact her mother's dementia. What teaching would you provide this client's daughter?

Linking the exemplar of Normal Sleep/Rest Patterns with the concept of Infection:

3. What is your priority of care for the client with pneumonia who sleeps 4 hours a night?
4. What interventions will you initiate to promote normal sleep patterns for a client with septicemia who is in the ICU?

REFER: GO TO MYNURSINGKIT

REFLECT: CASE STUDY

Ms. Smith, a 70-year-old woman, reports that she is having difficulty falling asleep at night. This has been occurring more frequently over the past year. She says, "I am so tired in the mornings, I can hardly get out of bed."

1. Which assessment tools might be used to determine her problem?
2. Identify life span issues that might be influencing her condition.
3. What will Ms. Smith report if the interventions are successful?

13.6 CONSUMER EDUCATION

KEY TERMS

Health literacy, *671*
Teaching, *670*

BASIS FOR SELECTION OF EXEMPLAR

Healthy People 2010

LEARNING OUTCOMES

After reading about this exemplar, you will be able to:

1. Explain the importance of the teaching role of the nurse in consumer education.
2. Explain the implications of using the Internet as a source of health information.
3. Identify methods to evaluate learning.
4. Demonstrate effective documentation of teaching–learning activities.

OVERVIEW

Teaching client education is a major aspect of nursing practice and an important independent nursing function. In 1992, the American Hospital Association passed *A Patient's Bill of Rights*, mandating client education as a right of all clients. State nurse practice acts include client teaching as a function of nursing, thereby making teaching a legal and professional responsibility. In addition, the Joint Commission on Accreditation of Healthcare Organizations (JCAHO) recently expanded its standards of client education by nurses to include "evidence that patients and their significant others understand what they have been taught. This requirement means that providers must consider the literacy level, educational background, language skills, and culture of every client during the education process" (Bastable, 2003, p. 5).

Client education is multifaceted, involving promoting, protecting, and maintaining health. It involves teaching about reducing health risk factors, increasing a person's level of wellness, and taking specific protective health measures.

TEACHING

Teaching is a system of activities intended to produce learning. The teaching-learning process involves dynamic interaction between teacher and learner. Each participant in the process communicates information, emotions, perceptions, and attitudes to the other. The teaching process and the nursing process are much alike.

Nurses teach a variety of learners in various settings. They teach clients and their families or significant others in the hospital, primary care clinics, urgent care, managed care, the home, and assisted living and long-term care facilities. Nurses teach large and small groups of learners in community health education programs.

Nurses also teach professional colleagues and other health care personnel in academic institutions such as vocational schools, colleges, and universities, and in health care facilities such as hospitals or nursing homes.

Teaching Clients and Their Families

Nurses may teach individual clients in one-to-one teaching episodes. For example, the nurse may teach about wound care while changing a client's dressing or may teach about diet, exercise, and other lifestyle behaviors that minimize the risk of a heart attack for a client who has a cardiac problem. The nurse may also be involved in teaching family members or other support people who are caring for the client. Nurses working in obstetric and pediatric areas teach parents and sometimes grandparents how to care for children.

The Internet has become a source of information for many clients. See Box 13–10 for more information on how Americans are using the Internet for health care information.

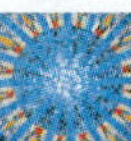

CLIENT TEACHING **Areas for Client Education**

PROMOTION OF HEALTH

- Increasing a person's level of wellness
- Growth and development topics
- Fertility control
- Hygiene
- Nutrition
- Exercise
- Stress management
- Lifestyle modification
- Resources within the community

PREVENTION OF ILLNESS/INJURY

- Health screening (e.g., blood glucose levels, blood pressure, blood cholesterol, Pap test, mammograms, vision, hearing, routine physical examinations)
- Reducing health risk factors (e.g., lowering cholesterol level)
- Specific protective health measures (e.g., immunizations, use of condoms, use of sunscreen, use of medication, umbilical cord care)
- First aid
- Safety (e.g., using seat belts, helmets, walkers)

RESTORATION OF HEALTH

- Information about tests, diagnosis, treatment, and medications
- Self-care skills or skills needed to care for family member
- Resources within health care setting and community

ADAPTING TO ALTERED HEALTH AND FUNCTION

- Adaptations in lifestyle
- Problem-solving skills
- Adaptation to changing health status
- Strategies to deal with current problems (e.g., home IV skills, medications, diet, activity limits, prostheses)
- Strategies to deal with future problems (e.g., fear of pain with terminal cancer, future surgeries, or treatments)
- Information about treatments and likely outcomes
- Referrals to other health care facilities or services
- Facilitation of strong self-image
- Grief and bereavement counseling

Teaching in the Community

Nurses are often involved in community health education programs. Such teaching activities may be voluntary, as part of the nurse's involvement in an organization such as the Red Cross or Planned Parenthood, or they may be compensated as part of the nurse's work role, such as school nurses. Community teaching activities may be aimed at large groups of people who have an interest in some aspect of health, such as nutrition classes, cardiopulmonary resuscitation (CPR) or cardiac risk factor reduction classes, and bicycle or swimming safety programs. Community education programs can also be designed for small groups or individual learners, such as childbirth or family planning classes.

Health Literacy

A 1993 National Adult Literacy Study reported that the average reading ability of many American adults is at the fifth-grade level (Edmunds, 2005). A report from the Institutes of Medicine (IOM, 2004) titled *Health Literacy: A Prescription to End Confusion* states that nearly half of all American adults—90 million people—have difficulty understanding and acting on health information (p. 1). Moreover, studies that assessed a variety of health-related materials found that the reading level exceeded the twelfth-grade level.

Health literacy is the ability to read, understand, and act on health information, and includes such tasks as comprehending prescription labels, interpreting appointment slips, completing health insurance forms, and following instructions for diagnostic tests (Redman, 2004, pp. 30–31). Limited health literacy skills are often greater among certain groups: older adults, people with limited education, poor people, minority populations, and people with limited English proficiency.

Low health literacy skills are associated with poor health outcomes and higher health care costs (IOM, 2004). For example, a client may not be able to read a prescription to know how many pills to take, and may take the wrong number of pills (e.g., "once" reads as "eleven" in Spanish). Clients with low literacy skills have less information about health promotion and/or management of a disease process for themselves and their families because they are unable to read the educational materials. As a result, they have higher rates of hospitalization than people with adequate health literacy.

It is a challenge for the nurse to teach clients with low or no reading and writing skills. However, such teaching is vital because clients with low literacy skills need learning opportunities to improve their health practices.

PRACTICE ALERT

The majority of people at the lowest reading levels will report that they "read well." Often clients will not admit to having difficulty reading because of the embarrassment it brings them. A nurse who suspects a client has difficulty reading may ask the client tactful questions, such as "Would you like me to go over it with you?"

It is difficult, however, to assess a client's literacy skills because the shame and stigma associated with limited health literacy skills are major barriers. Clients may be too embarrassed to admit they cannot read. The following client behaviors may cause a nurse to suspect a literacy problem:

- Pattern of noncompliance
- Insisting that they already know the information
- Having a friend or family member read the document for them
- Pattern of excuses for not reading the instructions (e.g., glasses broken, stating will read later or when they get home).

There are many formulas for assessing reading level of written material. Most word processing programs have a feature that will calculate the readability. Nurses involved in

Box 13–10 The Internet and Health Information

The Internet has become a part of the lives of many Americans, allowing them to communicate and obtain information quickly. Internet technology has dramatically changed the activities of business, including health care. The term *e-health* is defined as "the application of Internet and other related technologies in the healthcare industry to improve the access, efficiency, effectiveness, and quality of clinical and business processes utilized by healthcare organizations, practitioners, patients, and consumers in an effort to improve the health status of patients" (Healthcare Information and Management Systems Society E-Health Special Interest Group, 2003, p. 4). E-health includes many aspects such as online appointment access, billing review, e-mail access between the client and health care provider, online health information, and online support groups.

ONLINE HEALTH INFORMATION

The Pew Internet & American Life Project (2006) reports that 73% of American adults use the Internet. Using the Internet to locate health information is common. Health care online usage is growing twice as fast as any other online type of usage (Curran & Curran, 2005, p. 496). Eight out of 10 American Internet users have searched for information on at least one major health topic online. Certain groups of users are more likely to search the Internet for health information: women, adults younger than 65, college graduates, people with online experience, and those with broadband (high-speed) access (Pew Internet & American Life Project, 2005a, p. 1).

ACCESS

The Pew Internet & American Life Project (2005b, p. 7) reported on three groups of adults in the United States: those who do not use the Internet, those with a modest connection, and those highly engaged with the Internet. Each group has its distinct characteristics.

Twenty-two percent of American adults have never used the Internet. They tend to have a high school or less education or to be over the age of 65. Forty percent of adults have a loose connection to the Internet. That is, they have access (usually dial-up) but do not use the Internet regularly. They are younger and more educated than the previous group. Thirty-three percent of American adults are highly engaged by using the Internet daily. They tend to have college educations and are under age 50; however, there are "pockets" of older adults who are also highly engaged in Internet use.

OLDER ADULTS AND USE OF THE INTERNET

The Kaiser Family Foundation (2005, pp. 3–10) conducted a survey research study that provided the first close look at how older adults use the Internet for health information. Following are key findings of the report:

- Only 4 in 10 adults age 65 and over have used a computer.
- Seventy percent of "Baby Boomers" (age 50–64) use the Internet. Thus, the number of older adults using the Internet will increase over the next decade.
- There is a "digital divide" among older adults. Those whose annual income is under $20,000, those who have a high school degree or less, those who are older (e.g., 75 and above), and older women are less likely to use the Internet.
- One in five older adults (65 and over) use the Internet for health information. These elders are more likely to use TV and books for their health information.
- Many older adults do not trust the Internet as a source for health information except for the 50–64 age group, who trust the Internet "a lot."
- Seeking information on prescription drugs is the top reason for using the Internet for health information.
- Of those older adults who have used the Internet for health information, about half say it helped them and the other half say it wasn't helpful.
- Most older adults do not check the source of health information they find online.

IMPLICATIONS

The Internet is an important source of health information for many adult clients in the United States. Therefore, nurses need to know and be able to integrate this technology into the teaching plans for those clients who use the Internet. On the other hand, nurses also need to apply effective teaching strategies for those clients who do not use the Internet.

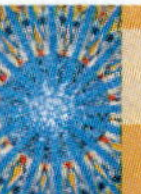

CLIENT TEACHING Developing Written Teaching Aids

- Keep language level at or below the fifth-grade level.
- Use active, not passive, voice.
- Use easy, common words of one or two syllables (e.g., *use* instead of *utilize*, or *give* instead of *administer*).
- Use the second person (*you*) rather than the third person (*the client*).
- Use a large type size (14–16 point).
- Write short sentences.
- Avoid using all capital letters.
- Place priority information first and repeat more than once.
- Use bold for emphasis.
- Use simple pictures, drawings, or cartoons, if appropriate.
- Leave plenty of white space.
- Obtain feedback from nurses and clients.

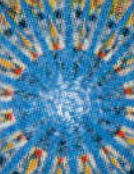

CLIENT TEACHING Teaching Clients With Low Literacy Levels

- Use multiple teaching methods: Show pictures. Read important information. Lead a small group discussion. Role play. Demonstrate a skill. Provide hands-on practice.
- Emphasize key points in simple terms and provide examples.
- Limit the amount of information in a single teaching session. Instead of one long session with a great deal of information, it is better to have more frequent sessions with a major point at each session.
- Associate new information with something the client already knows and/or associates with his or her job or lifestyle.
- Reinforce information through repetition.
- Involve the client in the teaching.
- Obtain feedback: Ask the client specific questions about the information presented or ask the client to repeat it in his or her own words.
- Avoid handouts with many pages and classroom lecture format with a large group.

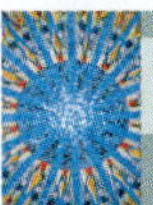

EVIDENCE-BASED PRACTICE Can Animated Cartoons Increase Knowledge of Educational Information?

Clinical Question

Printed client information may not be helpful to clients with low levels of English language literacy. The researchers in this study compared the gain of knowledge about polio vaccination from information presented in two formats: printed pamphlet and videotape of animated cartoons. Both formats contained the same information.

Evidence

The participants were parents/caretakers of pediatric clinic clients. Ninety-six participants were in the treatment group that watched the videotape in the clinic waiting room in the midst of intense client traffic. The comparison group consisted of 96 participants who were given a written pamphlet to read. Both groups completed a pretest that included demographics and five questions related to understanding polio vaccines. After the two groups finished reading the pamphlet or viewing the videotape, the participants completed a posttest that included the same five pretest questions and three additional questions.

There was no statistical difference between the two groups regarding demographic information or pretreatment knowledge. There was a significant statistical difference between the two groups in posttest knowledge. Both groups scored higher on the posttest in comparison to the pretest. However, 30% of the participants in the videotape group answered all of the posttest questions correctly, while none of the participants in the pamphlet group responded correctly to all of the questions.

Implications for Nursing II

Patient education about vaccinations is within the scope of nursing practice.

This study showed that animated cartoons can improve client knowledge independent of the level of literacy. It also showed that print material may not be sufficient to provide clients with complete information regarding vaccinations. Nurses should not rely only on pamphlets to provide patient education. Nurses should provide essential information at the level of understanding of the client in conjunction with pamphlets or other written materials.

Critical Thinking

1. What information regarding polio vaccines is most essential for parents to know?
2. Why might animated cartoons be a more effective way of sharing information with clients?
3. How can the nurse best present information about a vaccine to a client with a low level of English language literacy?
4. What side effects of polio vaccination should result in the parent calling the clinic office?

Note: Health Education Research by M. Leiner, G. Handal, and D. Williams. Copyright 2004 by Oxford University Press Journals. Reproduced with permission of Oxford University Press Journals in the format Textbook via Copyright Clearance Center.

developing written health teaching materials should write for lower reading levels (see Client Teaching). The goal is to have the education materials at a fifth- or sixth-grade level (Aldridge, 2004). People with good reading skills are not offended by simple reading material and prefer easy-to-read information. Even the simplest written directions, however, won't be helpful for the client with low or no reading skills. See the following Client Teaching box for suggestions on how to teach clients with low literacy levels; see also the following Evidence-Based Practice box.

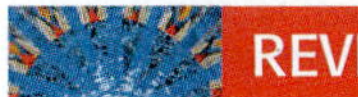

REVIEW Consumer Education

RELATE: LINK THE CONCEPTS

Linking the exemplar of Consumer Education with the concept of Development:

1. Select a developmental theorist, and identify the factors to consider when planning a literacy program for school-age children through older adulthood.
2. You admit an older adult who has begun to self-medicate with over-the-counter medications she saw advertised on TV. What interview questions will you ask this client and what risk factors will you address in her plan of care?

Linking the exemplar of Consumer Education with the concept of Metabolism:

3. You are caring for a client who has been diagnosed with type 2 diabetes mellitus who is refusing the prescription medication prescribed and is opting for herbals that have been advertised in magazines as blood sugar reducers. What will you plan to teach this client about using herbal supplements to treat this disease process?
4. You have been asked to present an educational program at a high school for obese students. Design a teaching plan for this program.

REFER: GO TO MYNURSINGKIT

REFLECT: CASE STUDY

Marge Loder is a 48-year-old client with diabetes. Her husband of 20 years recently died in a car crash; 2 days later, Marge was admitted with diabetic ketoacidosis. After she was stabilized, Marge told the nurse that she does not know how to read and her husband managed all of her care.

1. What are Marge's immediate needs?
2. How will you implement teaching?

PEARSON

EXPLORE mynursingkit™

MyNursingKit is your one stop for online chapter review materials and resources. Prepare for success with additional NCLEX®-style practice questions, interactive assignments and activities, web links, animations and videos, and more!

Register your access code from the front of your book at **www.mynursingkit.com**.

REFERENCES

Aldridge, M. D. (2004). Writing and designing readable patient education materials. *Nephrology Nursing Journal, 31*(4), 373–377.

American Dental Association. (n.d.). *Cleaning your teeth and gums (oral hygiene)*. Retrieved June 13, 2006, from http://www.ada.org/public/ topics/cleaning_faq.asp

American Dental Association. (n.d.). *Oral changes with age*. Retrieved June 13, 2006, from http://www.ada.org/public/ topics/oral_ changes_faq.asp

American Nurses Association. (1980). *Nursing: A social policy statement*. Kansas City, MO: Author.

American Nurses Association. (2004). *Nursing: Scope and standards of practice*. Washington, DC: Author.

Anonymous. (2003). Oral care update. *Nursing Management, 34*(5), S1–S16.

Anspaugh, D. J., Hamrick, M. H., & Rosato, F. D. (2006). *Wellness: Concepts and applications* (6th ed., p. 4). New York: McGraw-Hill.

Arnold, E. (2004). Sorting out the 3 D's: Delirium, dementia, and depression. *Nursing, 34*(6), 36–42.

Bastable, S. (2003). *Nurse as educator: Principles of teaching and learning for nursing practice* (2nd ed.). Boston: Jones & Bartlett.

Bilukha, O. O., & Rosenstein, N. (2005). Prevention and control of meningococcal disease. Recommendations of the Advisory Committee on Immunization Practices (ACIP). *Morbidity and Mortality Weekly Report, 54* (RR-7), 1–21.

Burke, M., & Laramie, J. (2004). *Primary care of the older adult: A multidisciplinary approach* (2nd ed.). Philadelphia: Mosby/Elsevier.

Coleman, P. R. (2002). Improving oral health care for the frail elderly: A review of widespread problems and best practices. *Geriatric Nursing, 23,* 189–199.

Coleman, P. R. (2004). Promoting oral health in elder care: Challenges and opportunities. *Journal of Gerontological Nursing, 30*(4), 3.

Curran, M. A., & Curran, K. E. (2005). The e-health revolution: Competitive options for nurse practitioners as local providers. *Journal of the American Academy of Nurse Practitioners, 17*(12), 495–498.

Edelman, C., & Mandle, C. (2006). *Health promotion throughout the life span* (6th ed.). St. Louis, MO: Mosby.

Edmunds, M. (2005). Health literacy a barrier to patient education. *Nurse Practitioner, 30*(3), 54.

Fontaine, K. L. (2005). *Complementary & alternative therapies for nursing practice* (2nd ed.). Upper Saddle River, NJ: Prentice Hall. *This practical guide covers the principles, techniques, research, and health promotion methods and healing practices of specific illnesses and symptoms. It discusses over 40 alternative therapies.*

Freeman, L. (2004). *Mosby's complementary & alternative medicine: A research-based approach* (2nd ed.). Philadelphia: Mosby/Elsevier.

Gooch, B. F., Eke, P. I., & Malvitz, D. M. (2004). Public health and aging: Retention of natural teeth among older adults–United States, 2002. *Journal of the American Medical Association, 291*(3), 292.

Healthcare Information and Management Systems Society E-Health Special Interest Group (SIG). (2003). *HIMSS e-health SIG white paper.* Retrieved June 9, 2006, from http://www. himss.org/content/files/ehealth_whitepaper.pdf

Hood, L., & Leddy, S. K. (2003). *Leddy & Pepper's conceptual bases of professional nursing* (5th ed.). Philadelphia: Lippincott Williams & Wilkins.

Institute of Medicine. (2004). *Health literacy: A prescription to end confusion*. Washington, DC: National Academies Press.

Institute of Medicine (IOM). (2006). *Sleep disorders and sleep deprivation: An unmet public health problem.* Washington, DC: Institute of Medicine.

Jackson, C. (2003). Movement, breathing and Christian meditation: Catalysts for spiritual growth. *International Journal of Healing and Caring On-Line, 3*(2), 1–24.

Kaiser Family Foundation. (2005). *E-health and the elderly: How seniors use the Internet for health information. Key findings from a national survey of older Americans.* Menlo Park, CA: Kaiser Family Foundation.

Leiner, M., Handal, G., & Williams, D. (2004). Patient communication: A multidisciplinary approach using animated cartoons. *Health Education Research, 19*(5), 591–595.

Leong, J., Molassiotis, A., & Marsh, H. (2004). Adherence to health recommendations after a cardiac rehabilitation programme in post-myocardial infarction patients: The role of health beliefs, locus of control and psychological status. *Clinical Effectiveness in Nursing, 8*(1), 26–38.

Lower, J., Bonsack, C., & Guion, J. (2003). Peace and quiet. *Nursing Management, 34*(4), 40A–40D. *The authors reviewed factors that make it difficult for clients to rest in hospitals and steps that are needed to help provide a healing environment (e.g., uninterrupted sleep, massage, music). They describe their vision, implementation, and outcomes of providing quiet time between 2 and 4 p.m. for clients in two ICUs.*

McCaffrey, R., Ruknui, P., Hatthakit, U., & Kasetsomboon, P. (2005). The effects of yoga on hypertensive persons in Thailand. *Holistic Nursing Practice, 19*(4), 173–180.

McCaffrey, Ruknui, Hatthakit, & Kasetsomboon (2005).

Micozzi, M. (2006). *Fundamentals of complementary and alternative medicine* (3rd ed.). Philadelphia: Mosby/Elsevier.

Munro, C. L., Grap, M. J., & Kleinpell, R. (2004). Oral health and care in the intensive care unit: State of the science. *American Journal of Critical Care, 13*(1), 25–34.

Nainar, S. M., & Mohummed, S. (2004). Role of infant feeding practices on the dental health of children. *Clinical Pediatrics, 43*(2), 129–133.

NANDA International. (2005). *NANDA nursing diagnoses: Definitions and classification 2005–2006.* Philadelphia: Author.

National Center for Health Statistics. (2004). *Health, United States, 2004. With chartbook on trends in the health of Americans.* Hyattsville, MD: National Center for Health Statistics.

National Sleep Foundation. (n.d.a). *A look at the school start times debate.* Retrieved June 29, 2006, from http://www .sleepfoundation.org/hottopics/index.php?secid=18&id=206

National Sleep Foundation. (n.d.b). *ABCs of ZZZZ–When you can't sleep.* Retrieved June 29, 2006, from http://www .sleepfoundation.org/sleeplibrary/index.php?secid=id=53

National Sleep Foundation. (n.d.c). *Aging gracefully and sleeping well.* Retrieved June 29, 2006, from http://www. sleepfoundation.org/hottopics/index.php?secid=12&id=225

National Sleep Foundation. (n.d.d). *Children's sleep habits.* Retrieved June 29, 2006, from http://www.sleepfoundation. org/hottopics/index.php?secid=11&id=39

National Sleep Foundation. (n.d.e). *Parents of teens: Recognize the signs and symptoms of sleep deprivation and sleep problems.* Retrieved July 2, 2006, from http://www .sleepfoundation.org/_content/hottopics/teensigns.pdf

National Sleep Foundation. (2006). National *Sleep Foundation 2006 Sleep in America poll highlights and key findings.* Retrieved July 4, 2006, from http://www.sleepfoundation .org/_content/hottopics/Highlights_facts_06.pdf

Nightingale, F. (1860; 1969). *Notes on nursing: What it is, and what it is not.* New York: Dover Books.

North American Nursing Diagnosis Association (NANDA). (2005). *Nursing diagnoses: Definitions & classification 2005–2006.* Philadelphia: NANDA.

North American Nursing Diagnosis Association (NANDA). (2007). *Nursing diagnoses: Definitions & classification 2007–2008.* Philadelphia: NANDA.

Orr, W. C. (2000). Editorial: Sleep and functional bowel disorders: Can bad bowels cause bad dreams? *American Journal of Gastroenterology, 95,* 1118–1121.

Pender, N. J., Murdaugh, C. L., & Parsons, M. J. (2006). *Health promotion in nursing practice* (5th ed.). Upper Saddle River, NJ: Prentice Hall.

Pew Internet & American Life Project. (2005a). *Health information online.* Retrieved June 9, 2006, from http://www.pewinternet.org/PPF/r/165/report_display.asp

Pew Internet & American Life Project. (2005b). *Digital sections.* Retrieved June 9, 2006, from http://www.pewinternet.org/ PPF/r/165/report_display.asp

Pew Internet & American Life Project. (2006). *Demographics of Internet users.* Retrieved June 9, 2006, from http://www .pewinternet. org/trends.asp

Pillitteri, A. (2003). *Maternal and child health nursing: Care of the childbearing and childrearing family* (2nd ed.). Philadelphia: Lippincott Williams & Wilkins.

President's Council on Physical Fitness and Sports. (2003). Washington, DC: U. S. Department of Health and Human Services.

President's Council on Physical Fitness and Sports. (2003). *Fitness Fundamentals: Guidelines for Personal Exercise Programs.* Washington DC.

Redman, B. K. (2004). *Advances in patient education.* New York: Springer.

Robinson, S. B., Weitzel, T., & Henderson, L. (2005). The sh-h-h-h project. Nonpharmacological interventions. *Holistic Nursing Practice, 19*(6), 263–266.

Rollnick, S., Mason, P., & Butler, C. (1999). *Health behavior change. A guide for practitioners.* Edinburgh: Churchill Livingstone.

Saarmann, L., Daugherty, J., & Riegel, B. (2000). Patient teaching to promote behavioral change. *Nursing Outlook, 48*(6), 281–287.

Travis, J. W., & Ryan, R. S. (1988). *Wellness workbook.* Berkeley, CA: Ten Speed Press.

U. S. Department of Health and Human Services. (2000). *Healthy people 2010: Understanding and improved health* (2nd ed.). Washington, DC: U. S. Government Printing Office.

U.S. Preventive Services Task Force. *Screening for Cervical Cancer. Recommendations and Rationale.* AHRQ Publication No. 03-515A. January 2003. Agency for Healthcare Research and Quality, Rockville, MD. Retrieved June 30, 2006, from, http://www.ahrq.gov/clinic/3rduspstf/cervcan/cervcanrr.htm

Wallston, K. A., Stein, M. J., & Smith, C. A. (1994). Form C of the MHLC scales: A condition-specific measure of locus of control. *Journal of Personality Assessment, 63,* 534–553.

Wallston, K. A., Wallston, B. S., & DeVellis, R. (1978, Spring). Development of the Multidimensional Locus of Control (MHLC) scales. *Health Education Monographs, 6,* 160–170.

Walton, J. C., Miller, J., & Tordecilla, L. (2001). Elder oral assessment and care. *Medsurg Nursing, 10*(1), 37–44.

World Health Organization. (1948). *Preamble to the constitution of the World Health Organization as adopted by the International Health Conference.* New York, June 19–22, 1946; signed on July 22, 1946, by the representatives of 61 states (Official Records of the World Health Organization, no. 2, p. 100) and entered into force on April 7, 1948.

Immunity 14

Concept at-a-Glance

Concept Learning Outcomes

After reading about this concept, you will be able to:

1. Summarize the structure and physiologic processes of the immune system.
2. List factors affecting immunity.
3. Identify commonly occurring alterations in immunity and their related treatments.
4. Explain common physical assessment procedures to examine the immune health of clients across the life span.
5. Outline diagnostic and laboratory tests used to determine an individual's immune status.
6. Explain management of immune health and prevention of illness.
7. Demonstrate the nursing process in providing culturally competent and caring interventions across the life span for individuals with common alterations in immunity.
8. Identify pharmacologic interventions in caring for an individual with alterations in immune function.

Concept Key Terms

Acquired immunity, *679*
Acquired immunodeficiency syndrome (AIDS), *676*
Active immunity, *682*
Antibodies, *680*
Antibody-mediated (humoral) immune response, *680*
Antigens, *676*
Autoimmune disorders, *676*
B lymphocytes (B cells), *679*
Cell-mediated (cellular) immune response, *681*
Cytokines, *681*
Eosinophils, *677*
Graft-versus-host disease, *692*
Hypersensitivity, *676*
Immunity, *676*
Immunization, *682*
Immunocompetent, *676*
Immunodeficiency, *676*
Immunoglobulins, *680*
Infection, *676*
Inflammation, *682*
Leukocytes, *676*
Leukocytosis, *676*
Leukopenia, *676*
Lymphocytes, *679*
Macrophages, *678*
Natural killer cells (NK cells, null cells), *679*
Opportunistic infections, *676*
Passive immunity, *682*
Phagocytosis, *681*
Primary immune response, *680*
Secondary immune response, *680*
T lymphocytes (T cells), *679*
Transplacental immunity, *683*
Vaccine, *682*

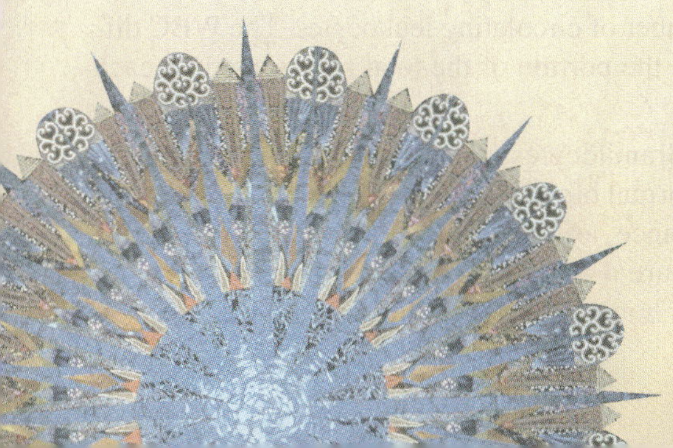

About Immunity

The human body is continually threatened by foreign substances, infectious agents, and abnormal cells. Recent years have seen the emergence of resistant microorganisms, such as methicillin-resistant *Staphylococcus aureus*, and altered strains of familiar diseases, such as multidrug-resistant tuberculosis. New diseases, such as Lyme disease, *Clostridium difficile,* and human immunodeficiency virus (HIV), also have emerged. The body's major weapon against these threats is the immune system.

The function of the immune system is to protect the body from invasion by foreign **antigens** (foreign substances that trigger the immune response), to identify and destroy potentially harmful cells, and to remove cellular debris. These actions are accomplished by the lymphoid organs and specifically designed lymphocytes through the processes of antibody-mediated immune response and cell-mediated immune response. The immune system recognizes any foreign substances within the body—in simple terms, it distinguishes "nonself" from "self"—and attempts to eliminate foreign substances as efficiently as possible.

Immunity, therefore, is the body's natural or induced response to infection and the conditions associated with its response. Clients who are **immunocompetent** have an immune system that identifies antigens and effectively destroys or removes them. When the immune system functions improperly, the result may be an overreaction or an immunodeficiency. Overreaction of the immune system to an antigen or antigens is termed **hypersensitivity**. In **autoimmune disorders**, for example, the immune system loses the ability to recognize and begins to attack its own tissues. An **immunodeficiency** can develop when the immune system is incompetent or unable to respond effectively, as is the case with **acquired immunodeficiency syndrome (AIDS)**, an immune system deficit that is induced by infection with HIV and is characterized by **opportunistic infections** (those that would normally not affect people with intact immune systems).

Our understanding of the components of the immune system and specific immune responses is growing, and having a thorough knowledge of the immune system increases understanding of the local and systemic inflammatory response, resistance to infectious disease, and the importance of immunization. This foundation can help the nurse teach clients and families to follow recommended treatment regimens, to promote and maintain health, and to prevent disease. In addition, the nurse can prescribe appropriate rehabilitative measures, such as increased rest and attention to optimal nutrition. It is vital that today's nurses understand the foundations of the immune system and the immune response. ●

NORMAL PRESENTATION

The immune system is a complex and intricate network of specialized cells, tissues, and organs. Cells of the immune system seek out and destroy damaged cells and foreign tissue yet recognize and preserve host cells (Porth, 2005). The immune system performs the following functions:

- Defends and protects the body from **infection** (an invasion of the body tissue by microorganisms).
- Removes and destroys damaged or dead cells.
- Identifies and destroys malignant cells, thereby preventing their further development into tumors.

The immune system is activated by external agents, such as microorganisms; minor injuries, such as small lacerations or bruises; or major injuries, such as burns, surgeries, and systemic diseases (e.g., pneumonia). The response of the immune system may be nonspecific or specific. Nonspecific responses prevent or limit the entry of invaders into the body, thereby limiting the extent of tissue damage and reducing the workload of the immune system. Inflammation is a nonspecific response. When the inflammatory process is unable to destroy invading organisms or toxins, a more specific response, called the immune response, is activated.

The effectiveness of the immune system depends on its ability to differentiate normal host tissue from abnormal or foreign tissue. Body cells, tissues, and fluids have unique antigenic properties that are recognized by the immune system as "self." External agents, such as microorganisms, cells and tissues from other humans or animals, and some inorganic substances, have antigenic properties that are recognized by the immune system as "nonself."

Components of the Immune System

The immune system consists of molecules, cells, and organs that produce the immune response (Table 14–1). These components may be involved in the nonspecific inflammatory response, the specific immunologic response, or both.

LEUKOCYTES **Leukocytes**, or white blood cells (WBCs), are the primary cells involved in both nonspecific and specific immune system responses. Like all blood cells, leukocytes derive from stem cells, the hemocytoblasts, in the bone marrow (Figure 14–1 ■). Unlike red blood cells (RBCs), which are confined to the circulation, leukocytes use the circulation to transport themselves to the site of an inflammatory or immune response. As the mobile units of the immune system, leukocytes detect, attack, and destroy anything that is recognized as "foreign." They are able to move through tissue spaces, where they locate damaged tissue and infection by responding to chemicals released by other leukocytes and damaged tissue.

The normal number of circulating leukocytes is 4,500 to 10,000 cells per cubic millimeter (mm^3) of blood. Many more leukocytes are marginated; that is, they adhere to vascular epithelial cells along the vessel walls, in other tissue spaces, or in the lymph system. In the presence of an attack such as an infection, additional WBCs are released from the bone marrow, and as WBCs move out of the bone marrow into the blood, the bone marrow increases its production of additional leukocytes. This leads to a WBC count of greater than $10{,}000/mm^3$, a condition known as **leukocytosis**. A decrease in the number of circulating leukocytes, known as **leukopenia**, occurs when bone marrow activity is suppressed or when leukocyte destruction increases.

Leukocytes are divided into three major groups: granulocytes, monocytes, and lymphocytes. The granulocytes and monocytes derive from the myeloid stem cells of the bone marrow and are instrumental in the inflammatory response. Lymphocytes derive from the lymphoid stem cells of the bone marrow and are the primary cells involved in the specific immune response. In laboratory tests, the WBC count indicates the total number of circulating leukocytes. The WBC differential identifies the portion of the total represented by each type of leukocyte.

Granulocytes Granulocytes constitute 60 to 80% of the total number of normal blood leukocytes. Their cytoplasm has a granular appearance, and their nuclei are distinctively multilobular (see Figure 14–1). Granulocytes have a short life span, measured in hours to days, compared with the life span

TABLE 14–1 **Cells and Tissues of the Immune System**

COMPONENT	LOCATION	FUNCTION
Leukocytes		
Granulocytes		
Neutrophils	Circulation	Phagocytosis and chemotaxis
Eosinophils	Circulation, respiratory tract, and gastrointestinal tract	Phagocytosis Protection against parasites Involved in allergic response
Basophils	Circulation	Release of chemotactic substances
Monocytes and macrophages	Circulation (monocytes) and body tissue, such as skin (histiocytes), liver (Kupffer cells), alveoli, spleen, tonsils, lymph nodes, bone marrow, and brain	Trapping and phagocytizing of foreign substances and cellular debris Secretion of interleukin-1 to stimulate lymphocyte growth
Lymphocytes	Circulation, lymph system, and tissues	Activation of T and B cells
T cells (mature in thymus gland)		Control of viral infections and destruction of cancer cells Involved in hypersensitivity reactions and graft tissue rejection
B cells (mature in bone marrow)	Circulation and spleen	Production of antibodies (immunoglobulins) to specific antigens
Natural killer (NK) cells	Circulation	Cytotoxic (killing of tumor cells, fungi, viral-infected cells, and foreign tissue)
Lymphoid Tissues		
Primary or central lymphoid structures	Bone marrow and thymus gland	Production of immune cells; sites for cell maturation
Secondary or peripheral lymphoid structures	Lymph nodes, spleen, tonsils, intestinal lymphoid tissue, and lymphoid tissue in other organs	Sites for activation of immune cells by antigens

of monocytes, which is measured in months to years. Granulocytes play a key role in protecting the body from harmful microorganisms during acute inflammation and infection. There are three types of granulocytes: neutrophils, eosinophils, and basophils.

- *Neutrophils,* also called polymorphonuclear leukocytes (or polys), are the most plentiful of the granulocytes, constituting 55 to 70% of the total number of circulating leukocytes. Neutrophils are phagocytic cells, responsible for engulfing and destroying foreign agents, particularly bacteria and small particles. Drawn by chemicals released by damaged tissue and invading organisms, neutrophils are the first phagocytic cells to arrive at the site of invasion. Neutrophils are produced in the bone marrow and released into the circulation when they mature. Segmented neutrophils (or segs) are mature forms and usually account for approximately 55% of total leukocytes. Bands are immature neutrophils and usually comprise 5% of leukocytes. As neutrophils mature, their nucleus changes from round to kidney-bean-shaped (banded), and then the nucleus separates into small, attached segments—thus the designations "banded" versus "segmented" neutrophils. It takes approximately 10 days for a neutrophil to mature and be released into the circulation. Once released, neutrophils have a circulating half-life of 6 to 10 hours. They cannot replicate and must be replaced constantly to maintain adequate numbers in the circulation. They do not return to the bone marrow.
- **Eosinophils** account for 1 to 4% of the total number of circulating leukocytes. They mature within the bone marrow in 3 to 6 days before being released into the circulation. Eosinophils have a circulating half-life of 30 minutes and a tissue half-life of 12 days. They too are phagocytic cells, but they are less efficient at this process than neutrophils. Eosinophils are found in large numbers in the respiratory and gastrointestinal tracts, where they are thought to be responsible for protecting the body from parasitic worms, including tapeworms, flukes, pinworms, and hookworms. Eosinophils surround the parasite and release toxic enzymes from their cytoplasmic granules. The parasite, although too large to be phagocytized, is destroyed. Eosinophils also are involved in a hypersensitivity response, inactivating some of the inflammatory chemicals released during the inflammatory response.
- *Basophils* constitute approximately 0.5 to 1% of the circulating leukocytes. These cells are not phagocytic. Granules within basophils contain proteins and chemicals, such as heparin, histamine, bradykinin, serotonin, and a slow-reacting substance of anaphylaxis (leukotrienes). These substances are released into the bloodstream during an acute hypersensitivity reaction or stress response.

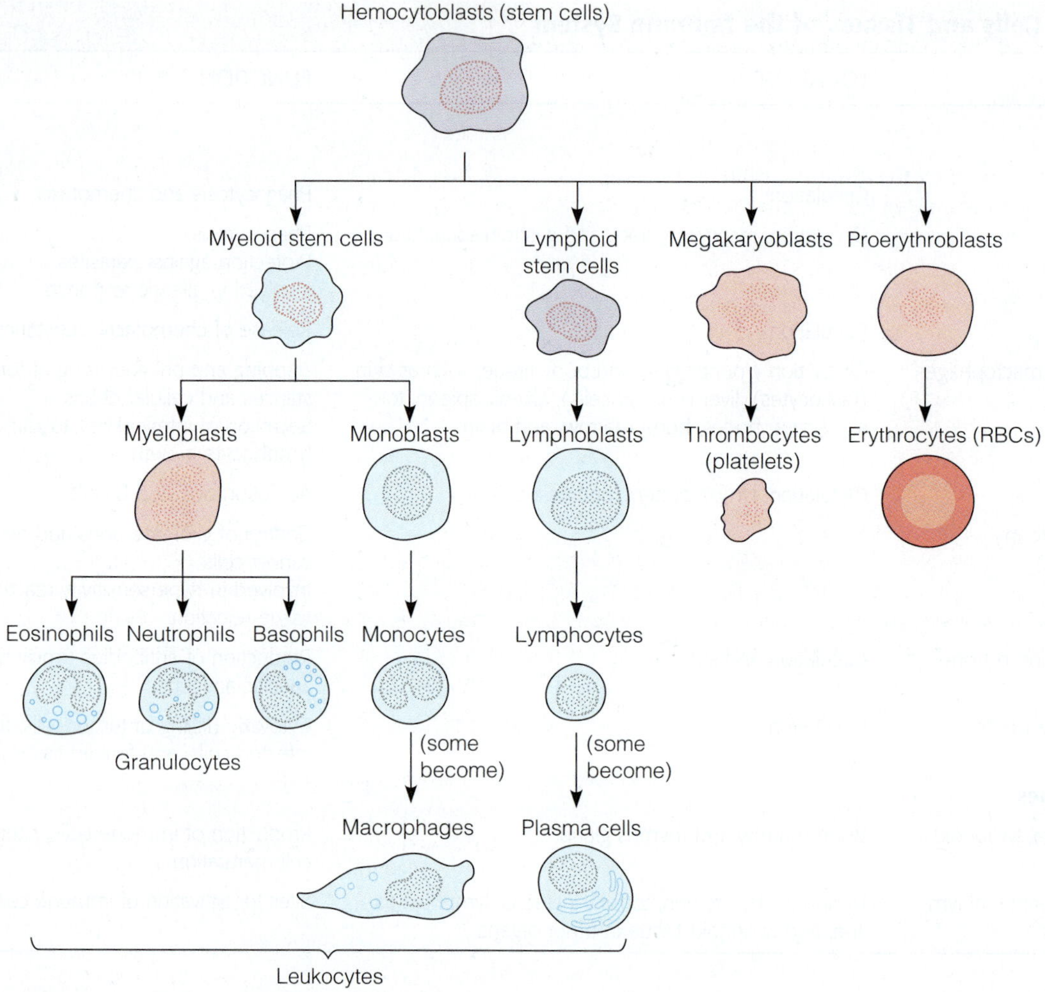

Figure 14–1 ■ The development and differentiation of leukocytes from hemocytoblasts.

Antigen-Presenting Cells Antigen-presenting cells (APCs), which activate immune responses in both B and T lymphocytes, are the mediators of immunity. They recognize foreign matter (from molecules to cells), initiate immune responses, and are actively phagocytic, with the capacity to phagocytize large foreign particles and cellular debris. There are three types of APCs: monocytes, macrophages, and dendritic cells.

- *Monocytes* are the largest of the leukocytes and constitute 2 to 3% of circulating leukocytes. After their release from the bone marrow, monocytes circulate in the serum for 1 to 2 days. They then migrate to various tissues throughout the body, attach themselves to the tissues, and remain for months or even years until they are activated. Monocytes activate the immune response against chronic infections such as tuberculosis, viral infections, and certain intracellular parasitic infections.
- After settling into the tissues, monocytes mature into **macrophages**, which are differentiated by the tissues in which they reside. Histiocytes are tissue macrophages in loose connective tissue, Kupffer cells are found in the liver, alveolar macrophages in the lungs, and microglia in the brain. Tissue macrophages also are found in the spleen, tonsils, lymph nodes, and bone marrow. Once they are in the tissue, macrophages can multiply to encapsulate and trap foreign matter that cannot be phagocytized. Like neutrophils, macrophages are drawn to an inflamed area by chemicals released from damaged tissue, a process known as chemotaxis. And like monocytes, macrophages activate the immune response against chronic infections such as tuberculosis, viral infections, and certain intracellular parasitic infections.
- *Dendritic cells* are star-shaped cells that originate in both the myeloid and the lymphoid cell lines. These APCs have long processes that can capture antigens and migrate to lymphoid tissue. They serve as sentinels for antigens in most organs, including the heart, lungs, liver, kidney, and gastrointestinal tract (Goldsby, Kindt, Osborne, & Kuby, 2003). Langerhans cells are specialized dendritic cells in the skin. Two specific types of dendritic cells develop from pluripotent stem cells in the bone marrow. DC1s arise from monocytes, myeloid-type immune cells; DC2s derive from lymphocyte precursors (DeMeyer & Buchsel, 2005). DC1s activate T cells against cancer cells. DC2s assist B lymphocytes to produce antibodies and to downregulate the immune system, which is very important to avoiding autoimmune disorders (Kimball, 2005).

Lymphocytes Like other leukocytes, **lymphocytes** derive from the stem cells in the bone marrow (Figure 14–2 ■). Small and nondescript, these cells account for 20 to 40% of circulating leukocytes and are the principal effector and regulator cells of specific immune responses to protect the body from microorganisms, foreign tissue, and cell mutations or alterations. Through a process known as immune surveillance, lymphocytes monitor the body for cancerous cells and attempt to destroy them.

Lymphocytes constantly circulate, then return in a "homing" pattern to concentrate in lymphoid tissues, where they often mature into memory cells. Memory cells stay inactive, sometimes for years, but activate immediately with subsequent exposure to the same antigen. They then proliferate rapidly, producing an intense immune response. Memory cells are responsible for providing **acquired immunity** (resistance to an antigen resulting from previous exposure to that antigen).

Although difficult to distinguish by appearance, lymphocyte types have distinct differences in how and where they mature as well as in life cycle, surface characteristics, and function. The three types of lymphocytes are **T lymphocytes (T cells)**, **B lymphocytes (B cells)**, and **natural killer cells (NK cells** or **null cells)**. None of these cells acts independently; their functions are closely interrelated.

- *T cells* mature in the thymus gland and are integral to the specific immune response. On contact with APCs, T lymphocytes mature into active helper T cells, cytotoxic T cells, or memory T cells.
- *B cells* complete their maturation in the bone marrow and, like T cells, are integral to the specific immune response. On contact with an antigen, B lymphocytes are activated and mature into either plasma cells, which secrete antibodies, or memory cells.
- *Natural killer cells* are large, granular cells found in the spleen, lymph nodes, bone marrow, and blood. They constitute 15% of circulating lymphocytes. NK cells provide immune surveillance and resistance to infection, and they play an important role in the destruction of early malignant cells. Like B cells and T cells, NK cells are cytotoxic, but unlike T cells, they do not require connection with an APC to become activated and kill cancer cells, virus-infected cells, and cells infected with microbes (Porth, 2005). Fortunately, NK cells are inhibited when contact is made with normal host cells.

ANTIGENS Antigens provoke a specific immune response when introduced into the body. Typically, antigens are large protein molecules, although polysaccharides, polypeptides, and nucleic acids also may be antigenic. Many antigens are proteins found on the cell membrane or cell wall of microorganisms or tissues (e.g., transplanted tissue or organs), incompatible blood cells, vaccines, pollen, egg white, animal dander, and insect or snake venom.

The portion of an antigen that incites a specific immune response is called its antigenic determinant site (or epitope). Complete antigens (also known as immunogens) typically are

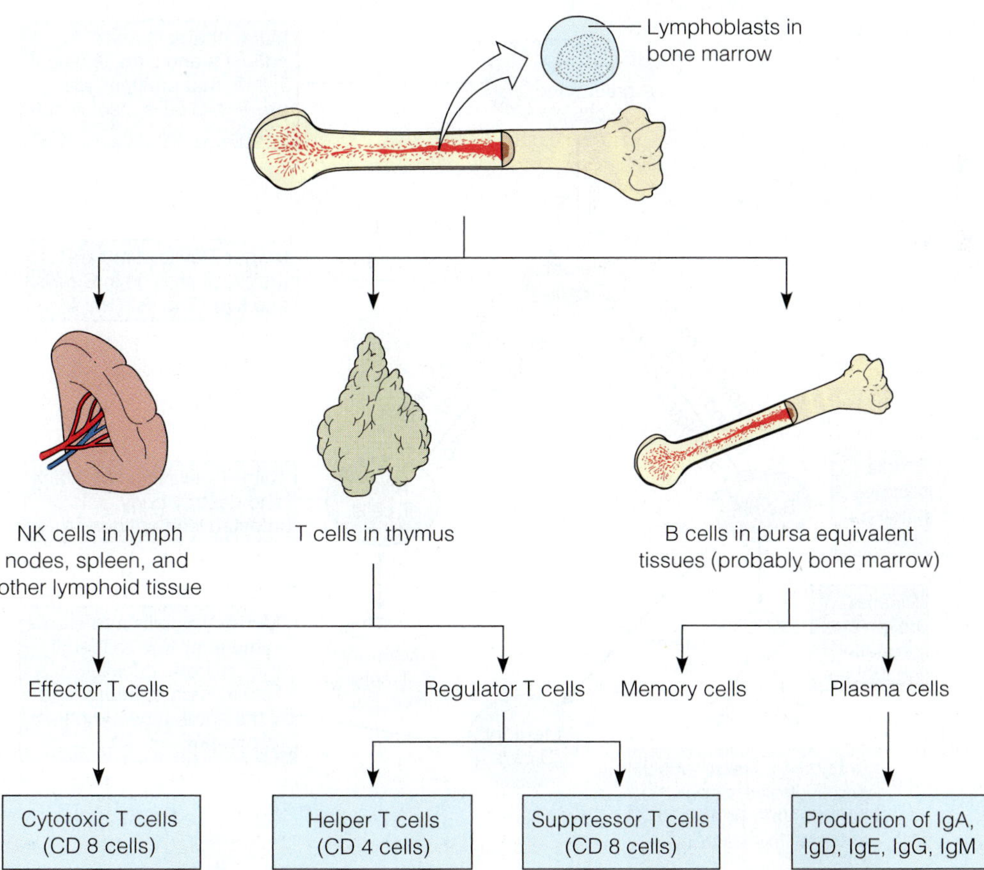

Figure 14–2 ■ The development and differentiation of lymphocytes from lymphoid stem cell (lymphoblasts).

large molecules with multiple antigenic determinant sites; examples include proteins and certain polysaccharides. Complete antigens have two characteristics:

1. *Immunogenicity*, or the ability to stimulate a specific immune response
2. *Specific reactivity*, or the ability to stimulate specific immune system components

Small molecules that cannot evoke an antigenic response alone (e.g., chemical toxins, drugs, and dust) may link to proteins to function as complete antigens. The proteins to which they link are known as haptens.

When an antigen is encountered in the body, two major groups of cells—lymphocytes and APCs—generate an effective immune response. APCs are recognized by a specific receptor on a lymphocyte, and an immune response is generated by those lymphocytes. Depending on the antigen itself and the type of immune cell activated by contact with the antigen, two separate but overlapping immune responses may occur. The B cell or humoral branch of the immune system mainly eliminates extracellular antigens, such as bacteria, bacterial toxins, and free viruses, through the production of **antibodies** (molecules that bind with the antigen and inactivate it). Antibodies are found in serum, body fluids, and certain tissues. When a person is first exposed to an antigen, the B lymphocyte system begins to produce antibodies that react specifically to that antigen (Figure 14–3 ■). It takes approximately 3 days for this process, known as the **primary immune response**, to occur. Subsequent encounters with the antigen trigger memory cells, resulting in a **secondary immune response** within 24 hours.

There are five classes of antibodies, called **immunoglobulins**: IgG, IgA, IgM, IgD, and IgE. One immunoglobulin in particular, IgM, forms natural antibodies, such as those for ABO blood group antigens. IgM is an important component of the immune system complexes seen in clients with autoimmune disorders. IgE is useful in combating parasitic infections and is part of the allergic response mechanism. The role of IgD is unknown. Together, these proteins make up the **antibody-mediated (humoral) immune response.**

The five major types of immunoglobulins and their functions are:

- IgG: IgG is the major immunoglobulin. IgG results from secondary exposure to the foreign antigen and is responsible for antiviral and antibacterial activity. This antibody passes through the placental barrier and provides early immunity for the newborn. The IgG response is longer and stronger than that of the other immunoglobulins.
- IgA: This immunoglobulin is found in the secretions of the respiratory, gastrointestinal, and genitourinary tracts; tears; and saliva. Its purpose is to protect mucous membranes from invading organisms (viruses, certain bacteria—*Escherichia coli* and *Clostridium tetani*). IgA does not pass the placental barrier. Those having congenital IgA deficiency are prone to autoimmune disease.

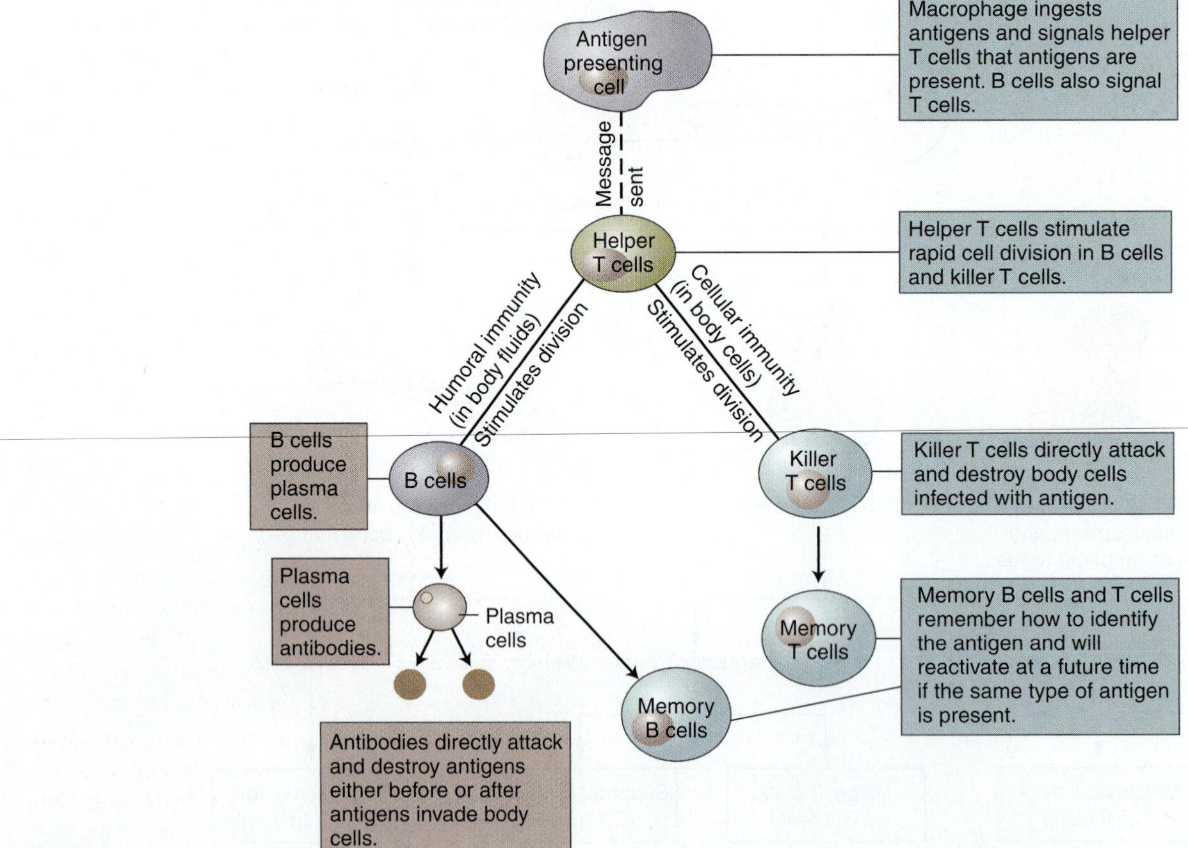

Figure 14–3 ■ The primary immune response encompasses a cascade of events that involve humoral immunity and cellular immunity.

- IgM: IgM antibodies are produced 48 to 72 hours after an antigen enters the body and are responsible for primary immunity. This immunoglobulin produces antibody activity against rheumatoid factors, gram-negative organisms, and the ABO blood group. IgM activates the complement system by destroying antigenic substances. Because it does not pass the placental barrier, the serum value is low in newborns; however, it is produced early in life and the level increases after 9 months of age.
- IgD: Unknown.
- IgE: This immunoglobulin increases during allergic reactions and anaphylaxis.

Intracellular pathogens, such as viral-infected cells, cancer cells, and foreign tissue, activate T lymphocytes, which are the primary agents of the **cell-mediated (cellular) immune response**. In this immune response, the lymphocytes themselves, in the form of helper T cells, cytotoxic T cells, and NK cells, inactivate the antigen, either directly or indirectly.

Cell-mediated immunity acts at the cellular level by attacking antigens directly and by activating B cells. T lymphocytes comprise the cell-mediated immune response and are subdivided into effector cells and regulator cells. The cytotoxic cell or killer T cell is the primary effector cell. Regulator T cells are divided into two subsets, known as helper T cells and suppressor T cells.

Helper T cells initiate the immune response, whereas suppressor T cells limit it. Helper T cells accomplish their role by promoting growth of additional T cells, by stimulating proliferation of B cells, and by activating killer T cells. Suppressor T cells are believed to be important in preventing autoimmune disorders. Proper immune system function depends on the correct balance between helper and suppressor T cells.

Complement is a component of blood serum consisting of 11 protein compounds. It is an inactive enzyme that activates in response to antigen-antibody functions, resulting in a generalized inflammatory reaction that kills foreign cells. It plays a role in causing some autoimmune disorders as well.

Immune cells also secrete proteins called **cytokines** that carry messages for immune system function. Lymphocytes, monocytes, and macrophages all secrete cytokines that have a variety of effects on the target cells. These effects may include stimulation of growth through cell proliferation, differentiation of cellular actions, production of inflammation, sensitization to pain, and other actions. Interleukins, a type of cytokine, were identified first in WBCs but are present in many cells. Many types of interleukins have been identified, and some are known to influence the function of the immune system.

In addition to destroying viruses and bacteria, cytotoxic T lymphocytes also attack malignant cells. They are responsible for the rejection of transplanted organs and grafted tissues as well.

LYMPHOID SYSTEM The lymphoid system consists of the lymph nodes, spleen, thymus, tonsils, lymphoid tissue scattered in connective tissues and mucosa, and bone marrow. The thymus and bone marrow, in which T cells and B cells mature, are considered to be central lymphoid organs. The spleen, lymph nodes, tonsils, and other peripheral lymphoid tissue are considered to be peripheral lymphoid organs (Figure 14–4 ■).

This system exists to recover proteins for the vascular system and to protect the bloodstream from invading organisms.

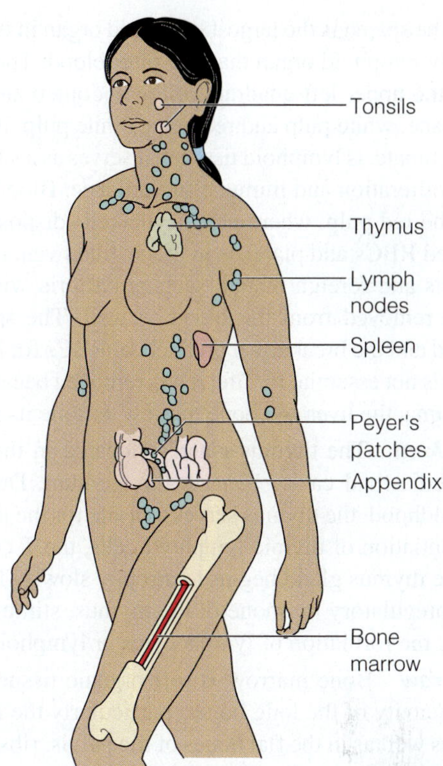

Figure 14–4 ■ The lymphoid system, showing the central organs of the thymus and bone marrow and the peripheral organs, including the spleen, tonsils, lymph nodes, and Peyer's patches.

Cells of the immune system, such as neutrophils, macrophages, and dendritic cells, carry antigens from the interstitial space to the lymph nodes for immune surveillance in the lymphatic circulation. Unlike the vascular tree, which has tight epithelial junctions, lymphatic epithelium is replete with open junctions that promote lymphocyte access and effectively protect the bloodstream from antigen entry.

Lymph Nodes Lymph nodes, the most numerous elements of the lymphoid system, are small, round, or bean-shaped, encapsulated bodies that vary in size from 1 mm to 2 cm. Distributed throughout the body, lymph nodes generally occur in groups at the junction of the lymphatic vessels. They can be found in the neck, axillae, abdomen, and groin and have two specific functions:

1. To filter foreign products or antigens from the lymph
2. To house and support proliferation of lymphocytes and macrophages.

Lymph, a clear, protein-containing fluid transported within lymph vessels, enters the node through afferent lymphatic vessels. Inside the node, the lymph flows through sinuses in the cortex of the lymph node, where T lymphocytes, B lymphocytes, and macrophages are abundant, and then through sinuses of the medulla of the lymph node, which contains macrophages and plasma cells. The presence of a foreign antigen stimulates lymphocytes and macrophages to proliferate in the lymph nodes. Macrophages destroy the antigen by **phagocytosis** (engulfing and then digesting the antigen). Immune cells and lymph then leave the lymph node through efferent vessels. An abundant blood supply to the node also facilitates lymphocyte movement.

Spleen The spleen is the largest lymphoid organ in the body—and the only lymphoid organ that can filter blood. The spleen is located in the upper left quadrant of the abdomen and has two kinds of tissue, white pulp and red pulp. White pulp, in which B cells predominate, is lymphoid tissue that serves as a site for lymphocyte proliferation and immune surveillance. Blood filtration occurs in the red pulp, where phagocytic cells dispose of damaged or aged RBCs and platelets in blood-filled venous sinuses. Other debris and foreign matter, such as bacteria, viruses, and toxins, are removed from the blood as well. The spleen also stores blood and the breakdown products of RBCs for future use. The spleen is not essential for life; if it is removed because of disease or trauma, the liver and bone marrow assume its functions.

Thymus Gland The thymus gland is located in the superior anterior mediastinal cavity beneath the sternum. During fetal life and childhood, the thymus serves as a site for the maturation and differentiation of thymic lymphoid cells, the T cells. After puberty, the thymus gland begins to atrophy slowly. Thymosin, an immunoregulatory hormone of the thymus, stimulates lymphopoiesis, the formation of lymphocytes or lymphoid tissue.

Bone Marrow Bone marrow is soft organic tissue found in the hollow cavity of the long bones, particularly the femur and humerus, as well as in the flat bones of the pelvis, ribs, and sternum. Bone marrow produces and stores hematopoietic stem cells, from which all cellular components of the blood are derived (see Figure 14–2).

Lymphoid Tissues Lymphoid tissues are located at key sites of potential invasion by microorganisms: the submucosa of the genitourinary, respiratory, and gastrointestinal tracts and the skin. Plasma cells in these lymphoid tissues defend the body against bacterial invasion at areas exposed to the external environment. In general, these tissues are known as mucosa-associated lymphoid tissue. Diffuse collections of lymphocytes, plasma cells, and phagocytes are scattered throughout the respiratory tract, concentrating at bifurcations of the bronchi and bronchioles. Peyer's patches, or gut-associated lymphoid tissue (GALT), comprise the largest collection of immune cells in the body (Bourlioux, Koletzko, Guarner, & Braesco, 2003). Ingestion and absorption of solid foodstuffs and liquids continually expose the lining of the gut to resident microflora and infectious pathogens. Unlike peripheral lymph nodes, which respond to pathogens with acute inflammatory responses, GALT processes common intestinal antigens without producing acute inflammation. Collections of immune cells make up GALT. Intraepithelial lymphocytes fill the spaces between mucosal epithelial cells. Beneath the basement membrane of gut epithelium lie abundant T cells and mature plasma cells, which are sources of IgA. Peyer's patches hold dense collections of lymphocytes in lymphoid nodules. As naïve B cells and T cells migrate through Peyer's patches, they are sensitized to specific antigens. In mesenteric lymph nodes, these sensitized cells proliferate and circulate throughout the vascular tree where they produce secretory IgA. Secretory IgA coats mucosal cells and prevents attachment of intraluminal bacteria in the intestine, upper respiratory tract, bronchi, mammary ducts, and salivary glands. Thus, the collection of immune cells in GALT effectively protects mucosa throughout the body that is exposed to resident and foreign pathogens.

Tonsils and Adenoids Tonsils and adenoids protect the body from inhaled or ingested foreign agents. These skin-associated lymphoid tissues contain lymphocytes and dendritic cells such as Langerhans cells in the epidermis, which transport antigens to regional lymph nodes for destruction and development of specific immunity to the antigen.

Nonspecific Inflammatory Response

Barrier protection is the body's first line of defense against infection. The skin is the primary barrier; when intact, it prevents invasion by external organisms. The membranes lining the inner surfaces of the body are protected by a barrier of mucus, which traps microorganisms and other foreign substances. These can then be removed by other protective mechanisms, such as ciliary movement or the washing action of tears or urine. In addition, many body fluids contain bactericidal substances that provide barrier protection. These include acid in gastric fluid, zinc in prostatic fluid, and lysozyme in tears, nasal secretions, saliva, and sweat (Porth, 2005; Rink & Gabriel, 2000).

When these first-line defenses are breached, the resulting tissue damage or foreign material entering the body induces a nonspecific immune response known as inflammation. **Inflammation** is an adaptive response to what the body sees as harmful. Inflammation brings fluid, dissolved substances, and blood cells into the interstitial tissues where the invasion or damage has occurred. (The inflammatory response is described in more detail in Concept 16, Inflammation.) The inflammatory response is called a nonspecific response because the same events occur regardless of what causes the inflammatory process. Through the inflammatory reaction, the invader is neutralized and eliminated, destroyed tissue removed, and the process of healing and repair initiated.

Immunizations

One of the great breakthroughs of modern medicine has been the development and widespread availability of vaccines. The average infant born today receives immunizations for 13 diseases by the age of 6 years. The diseases for which vaccines are routinely recommended include measles, mumps, rubella, polio, pertussis (whooping cough), diphtheria, tetanus, *Haemophilus influenzae* type b, hepatitis A and B, pneumococcus, varicella (chickenpox), and influenza. In 2006, the new rotavirus vaccine was approved for administration to infants. In addition, vaccines have been developed recently for older children, adolescents, and adults to protect against pertussis, meningococcus, and human papillomavirus. Administering these vaccines greatly improves health and reduces the parental burden of caring for ill children.

Immunization introduces an antigen into the body, allowing immunity against a disease to develop naturally. The immunized individual then produces antibodies in response to the antigens. In **active immunity** (immunity in which antibody production is stimulated without causing clinical disease), an antigen is given in the form of a **vaccine**. Information about each immunization commonly given to children and adults is listed in the Medications feature that follows.

When a child needs antibodies faster than the body can develop them, **passive immunity** may be induced. In this approach, antibodies are produced in another human or animal host and then given to the child. This approach also is used with at-risk children after a single exposure to a disease in an attempt to prevent the disease from occurring or to reduce its severity. For example, if a child who has never had a tetanus immunization steps on a rusty nail, the child needs immediate protection (passive immunity) from tetanus. Tetanus immunoglobulin is given by injection to combat the tetanus toxin produced when bacterial spores are introduced by the nail. Passive immunity does not confer lasting immunity, however, so the tetanus toxoid vaccine also is administered to start the process of antibody development (active immunity).

TYPES OF VACCINES Types of vaccines against childhood illnesses used in the United States include the following:

- *Killed virus vaccine:* A vaccine that contains a microorganism that has been killed but is still capable of inducing the human body to produce antibodies (e.g., inactivated poliovirus vaccine).
- *Toxoid:* A toxin that has been treated (by heat or chemical) to weaken its toxic effects but retain its antigenicity (e.g., tetanus toxoid).
- *Live virus vaccine:* A vaccine that contains a microorganism in live but attenuated (weakened) form (e.g., measles and varicella vaccines).
- *Recombinant forms:* An organism that has been genetically altered for use in vaccines (e.g., hepatitis B and acellular pertussis vaccine, which uses proteins from pertussis rather than the whole cell to stimulate the process of active immunity).
- *Conjugated forms:* An altered organism joined with another substance to increase the immune response (e.g., *Haemophilus influenzae* type b vaccine is conjugated with a protein-carrier like tetanus toxoid; however, this specific vaccine brand confers no immunity to tetanus).

Improvements in vaccine technology continue to increase the safety and efficacy of immunization against an increasing number of diseases. Today's vaccines often are produced synthetically by means of recombinant DNA technology or genetic engineering.

PRACTICE ALERT

Thimerosal, a bacteriostatic agent that contains ethyl mercury, was previously used to prevent contamination of vaccines in multidose vials. Because of the possible association between mercury poisoning and nerve and brain damage, vaccine manufacturers worked to remove thimerosal from vaccines. Many vaccines now have either no thimerosal or only trace amounts (American Academy of Pediatrics, 2006, p. 48).

RESPONSES TO VACCINES Children receiving vaccines can have a variety of responses as the body responds to the injected antigen stimulating the immune system. Depending on the specific immunization, up to 50% of vaccine recipients have a local reaction that includes erythema, swelling, pain, and induration at the site of the injection. Systemic reactions that often occur include fever, fussiness or irritability, malaise, and loss of appetite. With some vaccines, other systemic reactions include a rash or arthralgia. Provide guidelines for managing expected mild reactions at home, and make sure parents have the correct dosage information for the acetaminophen or ibuprofen formulation that is in the home.

Other serious reactions to vaccines occur in rare instances, for which the National Vaccine Injury Compensation Program was established. The range of illnesses and disabilities that may occur include anaphylaxis, encephalopathy, bacterial neuritis, chronic arthritis, thrombocytopenia purpura, and death. Each of these reactions is a reportable event.

Local allergic reactions, such as a wheal and urticaria, can occur in minutes to hours after the injection. A severe local allergic reaction is manifested by warmth, erythema, edema, petechiae, or ulceration occurring 2–8 hours after vaccination. A non-life-threatening systemic allergic reaction, such as generalized urticaria or transient petechiae, may occur within minutes. Anaphylaxis is a life-threatening allergic reaction that may result in shock and death. Its manifestations include hypotension, generalized urticaria, and angioedema. Laryngeal edema has occurred in rare cases with nearly every vaccine.

PRACTICE ALERT

Be prepared for potential vaccine anaphylaxis. Keep epinephrine (1:1,000) and resuscitation equipment immediately available. The dose for epinephrine (aqueous 1:1,000) is 0.01 mL/kg up to 0.5 mL intramuscularly. The dose can be repeated every 10–20 minutes, up to a total of three doses, until symptoms subside or other emergency care interventions are initiated (American Academy of Pediatrics, 2006, p. 65).

IMMUNIZATION SCHEDULE Vaccines should be administered at specific ages and intervals. The timing for first immunizations is determined by the age at which **transplacental immunity** (passive immunity transferred from mother to infant) decreases or disappears and when the infant or child develops the ability to make antibodies in response to the vaccine. Scientists also continue to study the duration of protection from vaccines. Some do not confer lifelong immunity. For example, it was determined recently that a second dose of varicella vaccine is necessary for immunity (Centers for Disease Control and Prevention [CDC], 2006a).

The recommended schedule for immunization is updated at least annually to reflect new vaccines and the need for repeat immunization. The Advisory Committee on Immunization Practices (ACIP) of the CDC, the American Academy of Pediatrics (AAP), and the American Academy of Family Practitioners (AAFP) collaborate to provide a uniform vaccination schedule. Figure 14–5 ■ gives the recommended schedule of immunizations in the United States for 2009. Because the vaccine schedule changes at least annually, visit the CDC website (www.cdc.gov/vaccines/recs/schedules/child-schedule.htm) for the most current recommendations.

Many missed opportunities to immunize children have been identified. Children (and any siblings present) should have their immunization status assessed during all health care visits, during hospitalizations, and in schools. Efforts to increase immunization levels among children also are supported by

Recommended Immunization Schedule for Persons Aged 0 Through 6 Years—United States • 2009

For those who fall behind or start late, see the catch-up schedule

Vaccine ▼ Age ▶	Birth	1 month	2 months	4 months	6 months	12 months	15 months	18 months	19–23 months	2–3 years	4–6 years
Hepatitis B[1]	HepB	HepB		*see footnote 1*		HepB					
Rotavirus[2]			RV	RV	*RV*[2]						
Diphtheria, Tetanus, Pertussis[3]			DTaP	DTaP	DTaP	*see footnote 3*	DTaP				DTaP
Haemophilus influenzae type b[4]			Hib	Hib	*Hib*[4]	Hib					
Pneumococcal[5]			PCV	PCV	PCV	PCV				PPSV	
Inactivated Poliovirus			IPV	IPV		IPV					IPV
Influenza[6]								Influenza (Yearly)			
Measles, Mumps, Rubella[7]						MMR			*see footnote 7*		MMR
Varicella[8]						Varicella			*see footnote 8*		Varicella
Hepatitis A[9]							HepA (2 doses)			HepA Series	
Meningococcal[10]										MCV	

Range of recommended ages

Certain high-risk groups

This schedule indicates the recommended ages for routine administration of currently licensed vaccines, as of December 1, 2008, for children aged 0 through 6 years. Any dose not administered at the recommended age should be administered at a subsequent visit, when indicated and feasible. Licensed combination vaccines may be used whenever any component of the combination is indicated and other components are not contraindicated and if approved by the Food and Drug Administration for that dose of the series. Providers should consult the relevant Advisory Committee on Immunization Practices statement for detailed recommendations, including high-risk conditions: http://www.cdc.gov/vaccines/pubs/acip-list.htm. Clinically significant adverse events that follow immunization should be reported to the Vaccine Adverse Event Reporting System (VAERS). Guidance about how to obtain and complete a VAERS form is available at http://www.vaers.hhs.gov or by telephone, 800-822-7967.

1. **Hepatitis B vaccine (HepB).** ***(Minimum age: birth)***
   At birth:
   - Administer monovalent HepB to all newborns before hospital discharge.
   - If mother is hepatitis B surface antigen (HBsAg)-positive, administer HepB and 0.5 mL of hepatitis B immune globulin (HBIG) within 12 hours of birth.
   - If mother's HBsAg status is unknown, administer HepB within 12 hours of birth. Determine mother's HBsAg status as soon as possible and, if HBsAg-positive, administer HBIG (no later than age 1 week).

   After the birth dose:
   - The HepB series should be completed with either monovalent HepB or a combination vaccine containing HepB. The second dose should be administered at age 1 or 2 months. The final dose should be administered no earlier than age 24 weeks.
   - Infants born to HBsAg-positive mothers should be tested for HBsAg and antibody to HBsAg (anti-HBs) after completion of at least 3 doses of the HepB series, at age 9 through 18 months (generally at the next well-child visit).

   4-month dose:
   - Administration of 4 doses of HepB to infants is permissible when combination vaccines containing HepB are administered after the birth dose.
2. **Rotavirus vaccine (RV).** ***(Minimum age: 6 weeks)***
   - Administer the first dose at age 6 through 14 weeks (maximum age: 14 weeks 6 days). Vaccination should not be initiated for infants aged 15 weeks or older (i.e., 15 weeks 0 days or older).
   - Administer the final dose in the series by age 8 months 0 days.
   - If Rotarix® is administered at ages 2 and 4 months, a dose at 6 months is not indicated.
3. **Diphtheria and tetanus toxoids and acellular pertussis vaccine (DTaP).** ***(Minimum age: 6 weeks)***
   - The fourth dose may be administered as early as age 12 months, provided at least 6 months have elapsed since the third dose.
   - Administer the final dose in the series at age 4 through 6 years.
4. ***Haemophilus influenzae* type b conjugate vaccine (Hib).** ***(Minimum age: 6 weeks)***
   - If PRP-OMP (PedvaxHIB® or Comvax® [HepB-Hib]) is administered at ages 2 and 4 months, a dose at age 6 months is not indicated.
   - TriHiBit® (DTaP/Hib) should not be used for doses at ages 2, 4, or 6 months but can be used as the final dose in children aged 12 months or older.
5. **Pneumococcal vaccine.** ***(Minimum age: 6 weeks for pneumococcal conjugate vaccine [PCV]; 2 years for pneumococcal polysaccharide vaccine [PPSV])***
   - PCV is recommended for all children aged younger than 5 years. Administer 1 dose of PCV to all healthy children aged 24 through 59 months who are not completely vaccinated for their age.
   - Administer PPSV to children aged 2 years or older with certain underlying medical conditions (see *MMWR* 2000;49[No. RR-9]), including a cochlear implant.
6. **Influenza vaccine.** ***(Minimum age: 6 months for trivalent inactivated influenza vaccine [TIV]; 2 years for live, attenuated influenza vaccine [LAIV])***
   - Administer annually to children aged 6 months through 18 years.
   - For healthy nonpregnant persons (i.e., those who do not have underlying medical conditions that predispose them to influenza complications) aged 2 through 49 years, either LAIV or TIV may be used.
   - Children receiving TIV should receive 0.25 mL if aged 6 through 35 months or 0.5 mL if aged 3 years or older.
   - Administer 2 doses (separated by at least 4 weeks) to children aged younger than 9 years who are receiving influenza vaccine for the first time or who were vaccinated for the first time during the previous influenza season but only received 1 dose.
7. **Measles, mumps, and rubella vaccine (MMR).** ***(Minimum age: 12 months)***
   - Administer the second dose at age 4 through 6 years. However, the second dose may be administered before age 4, provided at least 28 days have elapsed since the first dose.
8. **Varicella vaccine.** ***(Minimum age: 12 months)***
   - Administer the second dose at age 4 through 6 years. However, the second dose may be administered before age 4, provided at least 3 months have elapsed since the first dose.
   - For children aged 12 months through 12 years the minimum interval between doses is 3 months. However, if the second dose was administered at least 28 days after the first dose, it can be accepted as valid.
9. **Hepatitis A vaccine (HepA).** ***(Minimum age: 12 months)***
   - Administer to all children aged 1 year (i.e., aged 12 through 23 months). Administer 2 doses at least 6 months apart.
   - Children not fully vaccinated by age 2 years can be vaccinated at subsequent visits.
   - HepA also is recommended for children older than 1 year who live in areas where vaccination programs target older children or who are at increased risk of infection. See *MMWR* 2006;55(No. RR-7).
10. **Meningococcal vaccine.** ***(Minimum age: 2 years for meningococcal conjugate vaccine [MCV] and for meningococcal polysaccharide vaccine [MPSV])***
    - Administer MCV to children aged 2 through 10 years with terminal complement component deficiency, anatomic or functional asplenia, and certain other high-risk groups. See *MMWR* 2005;54(No. RR-7).
    - Persons who received MPSV 3 or more years previously and who remain at increased risk for meningococcal disease should be revaccinated with MCV.

The Recommended Immunization Schedules for Persons Aged 0 Through 18 Years are approved by the Advisory Committee on Immunization Practices (www.cdc.gov/vaccines/recs/acip), the American Academy of Pediatrics (http://www.aap.org), and the American Academy of Family Physicians (http://www.aafp.org).

DEPARTMENT OF HEALTH AND HUMAN SERVICES • CENTERS FOR DISEASE CONTROL AND PREVENTION

CS103164

Figure 14–5 ■ *A*, Recommended immunization schedule for children from birth to 6 years in the United States, 2009.

Source: CDC. (2008). *2009 Child and adolescent immunization schedules.* Retrieved July 14, 2009, from http://www.cdc.gov/vaccines/recs/schedules/child-schedule.htm#printable

Recommended Immunization Schedule for Persons Aged 7 Through 18 Years—United States • 2009

For those who fall behind or start late, see the schedule below and the catch-up schedule

Vaccine ▼ Age ▶	7–10 years	11–12 years	13–18 years
Tetanus, Diphtheria, Pertussis[1]	*see footnote 1*	Tdap	Tdap
Human Papillomavirus[2]	*see footnote 2*	HPV (3 doses)	HPV Series
Meningococcal[3]	MCV	MCV	MCV
Influenza[4]	Influenza (Yearly)		
Pneumococcal[5]	PPSV		
Hepatitis A[6]	HepA Series		
Hepatitis B[7]	HepB Series		
Inactivated Poliovirus[8]	IPV Series		
Measles, Mumps, Rubella[9]	MMR Series		
Varicella[10]	Varicella Series		

Range of recommended ages

Catch-up immunization

Certain high-risk groups

This schedule indicates the recommended ages for routine administration of currently licensed vaccines, as of December 1, 2008, for children aged 7 through 18 years. Any dose not administered at the recommended age should be administered at a subsequent visit, when indicated and feasible. Licensed combination vaccines may be used whenever any component of the combination is indicated and other components are not contraindicated and if approved by the Food and Drug Administration for that dose of the series. Providers should consult the relevant Advisory Committee on Immunization Practices statement for detailed recommendations, including high-risk conditions: http://www.cdc.gov/vaccines/pubs/acip-list.htm. Clinically significant adverse events that follow immunization should be reported to the Vaccine Adverse Event Reporting System (VAERS). Guidance about how to obtain and complete a VAERS form is available at http://www.vaers.hhs.gov or by telephone, 800-822-7967.

1. Tetanus and diphtheria toxoids and acellular pertussis vaccine (Tdap). ***(Minimum age: 10 years for BOOSTRIX® and 11 years for ADACEL®)***
- Administer at age 11 or 12 years for those who have completed the recommended childhood DTP/DTaP vaccination series and have not received a tetanus and diphtheria toxoid (Td) booster dose.
- Persons aged 13 through 18 years who have not received Tdap should receive a dose.
- A 5-year interval from the last Td dose is encouraged when Tdap is used as a booster dose; however, a shorter interval may be used if pertussis immunity is needed.

2. Human papillomavirus vaccine (HPV). ***(Minimum age: 9 years)***
- Administer the first dose to females at age 11 or 12 years.
- Administer the second dose 2 months after the first dose and the third dose 6 months after the first dose (at least 24 weeks after the first dose).
- Administer the series to females at age 13 through 18 years if not previously vaccinated.

3. Meningococcal conjugate vaccine (MCV).
- Administer at age 11 or 12 years, or at age 13 through 18 years if not previously vaccinated.
- Administer to previously unvaccinated college freshmen living in a dormitory.
- MCV is recommended for children aged 2 through 10 years with terminal complement component deficiency, anatomic or functional asplenia, and certain other groups at high risk. See *MMWR* 2005;54(No. RR-7).
- Persons who received MPSV 5 or more years previously and remain at increased risk for meningococcal disease should be revaccinated with MCV.

4. Influenza vaccine.
- Administer annually to children aged 6 months through 18 years.
- For healthy nonpregnant persons (i.e., those who do not have underlying medical conditions that predispose them to influenza complications) aged 2 through 49 years, either LAIV or TIV may be used.
- Administer 2 doses (separated by at least 4 weeks) to children aged younger than 9 years who are receiving influenza vaccine for the first time or who were vaccinated for the first time during the previous influenza season but only received 1 dose.

5. Pneumococcal polysaccharide vaccine (PPSV).
- Administer to children with certain underlying medical conditions (see *MMWR* 1997;46[No. RR-8]), including a cochlear implant. A single revaccination should be administered to children with functional or anatomic asplenia or other immunocompromising condition after 5 years.

6. Hepatitis A vaccine (HepA).
- Administer 2 doses at least 6 months apart.
- HepA is recommended for children older than 1 year who live in areas where vaccination programs target older children or who are at increased risk of infection. See *MMWR* 2006;55(No. RR-7).

7. Hepatitis B vaccine (HepB).
- Administer the 3-dose series to those not previously vaccinated.
- A 2-dose series (separated by at least 4 months) of adult formulation Recombivax HB® is licensed for children aged 11 through 15 years.

8. Inactivated poliovirus vaccine (IPV).
- For children who received an all-IPV or all-oral poliovirus (OPV) series, a fourth dose is not necessary if the third dose was administered at age 4 years or older.
- If both OPV and IPV were administered as part of a series, a total of 4 doses should be administered, regardless of the child's current age.

9. Measles, mumps, and rubella vaccine (MMR).
- If not previously vaccinated, administer 2 doses or the second dose for those who have received only 1 dose, with at least 28 days between doses.

10. Varicella vaccine.
- For persons aged 7 through 18 years without evidence of immunity (see *MMWR* 2007;56[No. RR-4]), administer 2 doses if not previously vaccinated or the second dose if they have received only 1 dose.
- For persons aged 7 through 12 years, the minimum interval between doses is 3 months. However, if the second dose was administered at least 28 days after the first dose, it can be accepted as valid.
- For persons aged 13 years and older, the minimum interval between doses is 28 days.

The Recommended Immunization Schedules for Persons Aged 0 Through 18 Years are approved by the Advisory Committee on Immunization Practices (www.cdc.gov/vaccines/recs/acip), the American Academy of Pediatrics (http://www.aap.org), and the American Academy of Family Physicians (http://www.aafp.org).

DEPARTMENT OF HEALTH AND HUMAN SERVICES • CENTERS FOR DISEASE CONTROL AND PREVENTION

CS103164

Figure 14–5 ■ *B*, Recommended immunization schedule for children and adolescents from 7–18 years in United States, 2009.

Source: CDC. (2008). *2009 Child and adolescent immunization schedules.* Retrieved July 14, 2009, from http://www.cdc.gov/vaccines/recs/schedules/child-schedule.htm#printable

managed care organizations that require contracted health care providers to comply with the pediatric immunization standards; client records are audited to ensure compliance. Lower immunization rates of children often are associated with economic factors, limited access to health care, lack of health care services at hours convenient for working parents, inadequate education regarding the importance of immunization, and religious prohibitions.

> **PRACTICE ALERT**
> Schedule the child's next appointment for a health supervision visit to complete needed immunizations for that child's age.

CONTRAINDICATIONS Contraindications for immunizations may include an acute illness with high fever, hypersensitivity reaction to specific vaccine components, immunoglobulin therapy in the last 3–6 months, cancer treatment, and pregnancy (AAP, 2006, pp. 45–50).

PARENTAL RIGHTS AND INFORMED CONSENT An increasing number of parents are choosing not to immunize their children for philosophical reasons. Some of these reasons include the following (Benin, Wisler-Scher, Colson, Shapiro, & Holmboe, 2006):

- Concerns that too many vaccines are dangerous and can be harmful to their child.
- Belief that vaccines do not work. (Even some vaccinated children get the infectious disease, so the vaccines are not completely protective.)
- Disagreement with government regulation and monitoring of immunizations.
- Belief that their child is not at risk, because the disease threat is low as a result of so many other children being immunized.
- Realization that the number of adverse events after vaccinations now exceeds the number of cases of vaccine-preventable diseases.
- Belief that they can control their child's susceptibility to disease and the outcome if their child becomes infected.
- Belief that it is better to get the disease to develop immunity.

All health care providers should be consistent in their message about the value of vaccines and should provide parents with an opportunity to have their questions answered before giving consent for immunization. It is important to understand that parents want to protect their child both from diseases and from any potential harm caused by vaccines. Federal legislation requires parental consent to be obtained before administering a vaccine, and a trusting relationship between the health care provider and the parents is an important factor in obtaining consent for immunizations (Benin et al., 2006).

In most health care settings, the nurse is responsible for informing the parents or the child's legal guardian, supplying literature, and obtaining written consent before the vaccine is administered. The nurse has a legal obligation to assure that consent is obtained from the proper person who has the legal authority to do so. The nurse also has the responsibility to make sure that the most current Vaccine Information Statement (VIS) is provided to the parents about the vaccines to be administered. When teaching about immunizations, make sure that the parents understand the information in the VIS, and answer any questions the parents might have. Identify the vaccines to be given at this visit and on the next visit so that the parents know their child's immunization status. It may save time to give parents the VIS about the next vaccines to take home and review before the next visit.

Discuss vaccine risks and benefits with parents. Parents often hear sensational stories about the consequences of vaccines, so correct information is needed to help them make informed decisions. For example, studies have repeatedly failed to find a relationship between the measles-mumps-rubella vaccine and the development of autism (DeStefano, Bhasin, Thompson, Yeargin-Allsopp, & Boyle, 2004; Smeeth, Cook, Fombonne et al., 2004). Other studies have not revealed a relationship between vaccines and disorders such as asthma (Destefano et al. 2002), inflammatory bowel disease (Taylor, Miller, Lingram et al., 2002), sudden infant death syndrome (Institute of Medicine Board of Health Promotion and Disease Prevention, 2003), and type 1 diabetes mellitus (Hviid, Stellfeld, Wohlfahrt, & Melbye, 2004). Despite the lack of evidence, much misinformation has been provided in the media, and parents sometimes come to conclusions about vaccines based on poor information.

Parents have the right to refuse immunizations, but if a disease outbreak occurs, the nonimmunized child must be kept out of child care or school. If the parent chooses not to have the child receive a particular vaccine, document an informed refusal. A form for documentation of informed refusal is available online at http://www.cispimmunize.org/pro/pdf/RefusaltoVaccinate.pdf.

HEALTHY PEOPLE 2010 *Healthy People 2010* is a nationwide effort to identify and eliminate the most serious preventable threats to health. Reducing the number of preventable childhood illnesses is one of the major goals, and nurses are important partners in this effort. The incidences of the following infectious diseases are targeted for reduction or elimination (U.S. Department of Health and Human Services, Office of Disease Prevention, 2000):

- *Elimination:* Rubella and congenital rubella syndrome, diphtheria, *Haemophilus influenza* type b, measles, mumps, polio, and tetanus.
- *Reduction:* Pertussis, hepatitis B, varicella, food-borne pathogens, and HIV infection.

To accomplish this, an effort to increase the numbers of children protected from vaccine-preventable diseases and to monitor immunization status is a national public health initiative. *Healthy People 2010* states important specific goals for the reduction of vaccine-preventable diseases:

- Adequately immunize 90% of U.S. children by their second birthday.
- Adequately immunize 95% of children in kindergarten and first grade.
- Have 95% of children younger than 6 years of age participating in a fully operational, population-based immunization registry. Once fully operational, the registries should meet 13 functional standards that will enable states or managed care organizations to monitor the immunization status of their population (CDC, 2002; U.S. Department of Health and Human Services, Office of Disease Prevention, 2000).

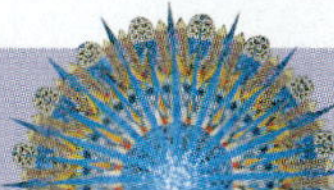

IMMUNIZATIONS Pediatric

Immunization Type	Side Effects	Contraindications	Nursing Considerations
Diphtheria and pertussis vaccines and tetanus toxoid (DTaP, Tdap)			
Type: Inactivated *Route:* Intramuscular *Dosage:* 0.5 mL *Age(s) given:* DTaP at 2, 4, 6, and 15–18 months, then again at 4–6 years (five doses total); Tdap at 11–12 years *Timing:* May give at same time as all other vaccines, but in a separate site. *Storage*: Store in body of refrigerator at 2–8°C (35–46°F). Do not freeze. *Product preparations:* Tripedia and Infanrix are licensed for all three doses. Daptacel is licensed for the first four doses. Pediarix is composed of DTaP, hepatitis B (HepB), and poliovirus vaccine (IPV) and can be given as the primary series. TriHiBit is composed of DTaP and *Haemophilus influenzae* type B (Hib). Pentacel is composed of Hib, DTaP, and IPV. BOOSTRIX and Adacel (Tdap vaccines) are approved for children over 10 years and adults.	*Common:* Redness, pain, swelling, and nodule at injection site; temperature up to 38.3°C (101°F); drowsiness, irritability, and fussiness; anorexia within 2 days of injection. Increase in frequency and magnitude of local reactions with fourth and fifth doses, (e.g., entire limb swelling). *Serious*: Allergic reaction or anaphylaxis; shock or collapse (hypotonic-hyperresponsive episode—sudden loss of muscle tone, pallor, fever, and unresponsiveness); fever > 38.8°C (>102°F); febrile seizure; persistent inconsolable crying; coma or permanent brain damage.	Hypersensitivity to vaccine component; for gelatin hypersensitivity, do not use Tripedia. Occurrence of a serious side effect after previous administration of DTaP, such as anaphylaxis or encephalopathy within 7 days after DTP or DTaP. Precautions with additional DTaP doses should be considered in children having the following reactions within 48 hours of the previous dose: ■ Fever ≥ 40.5°C (105°F) ■ Continuous inconsolable crying lasting ≥ 3 hours ■ Pale or limp episode or collapse ■ Convulsion within 3 days of dose Administration should be delayed for 1 month after immunosuppressive therapy and until moderate to severe febrile illnesses have resolved. Administration of immune serum globulin within last 90 days. Tdap is contraindicated in adolescents with a history of coma or prolonged seizures within 7 days of previous vaccination with pertussis.	■ Use same brand for all doses when feasible. Before vaccination, ask about previous reactions to immunization. ■ DTaP may coincide with or hasten the recognition of a seizure disorder. In children with a history of seizures with or without fever, give acetaminophen at the time of vaccine and then every 4 hours for 24 hours. ■ Shake vaccine before withdrawing. Solution will be cloudy. If it contains clumps that cannot be resuspended, do not use. ■ Daptacel stopper vial contains latex. Pediarix stopper vial is latex-free. When required, simultaneous administration of tetanus immune globulin or diphtheria antitoxin should be given in separate sites with a new needle and syringe. ■ Inform parents about the chance of increased reaction to the third and fourth doses. ■ When the child has a progressive neurologic problem, defer the vaccine until that child is stable. ■ DT is given to children older than 7 years who have had a serious reaction to the pertussis component of DTP or DTaP. ■ Td is given to children 7 years or older. ■ Adolescents (11–18 years) who received Td but not Tdap are encouraged to get a dose of Tdap to gain protection against pertussis (CDC, 2006c). ■ Carefully check vials of DTaP, DT, Td, and Tdap to ensure that the proper vaccine is administered for the child's age. ■ The series does not need to be restarted, no matter how long since the previous dose was given. ■ After the primary series of three is completed, a tetanus booster may be given in the case of a contaminated wound or burn if 5 or more years have passed since the last dose (American Academy of Pediatrics, 2006, p. 650).
Haemophilus influenzae type B (Hib)			
Type: Inactivated *Route*: Intramuscular *Dosage*: 0.5 mL *Age(s) given*: 2, 4, 6, and 12–15 months; (four doses for HbOC [HibTITER] and PRP-T [ActHIB] *or* 2, 4, and 12–15 months (three doses for PRP-OMP [PedvaxHIB]	*Common*: Pain, redness, or swelling at injection site *Serious*: Allergic reaction or anaphylaxis (extremely rare); fever	Previous anaphylactic reaction to this vaccine	■ Before immunizations, ask if child is immunosuppressed. ■ Solution is clear and colorless. ■ Refrigerate reconstituted PedvaxHIB, and discard within 24 hours. ■ Use or discard reconstituted ActHIB and OmniHIB within 30 minutes. ■ Because schedules for product preparations of different companies vary, it is important to read package inserts carefully.

(continued)

IMMUNIZATIONS Pediatric (continued)

Immunization Type	Side Effects	Contraindications	Nursing Considerations
Haemophilus influenzae type B (Hib) *(continued)*			
Timing: May give at same time as all other vaccines, but in a separate site. *Storage:* Store in body of refrigerator at 2–8°C (35–46°F). Do not freeze. *Product preparations:* HibTITER, ActHIB, and PedvaxHIB are single-vaccine preparations Comvax is a combination of PRP-OMP plus HepB. TriHIBit is composed of DTaP and Hib.			■ If the first dose is given at 7–11 months of age, three doses are needed. If the first dose was given at 12–14 months of age, give a booster dose in 8 weeks. If the first dose is given when the child is older than 15 months but younger than 5 years, only one dose is needed (American Academy of Pediatrics, 2006, p. 317). ■ Second and third doses can be given 4–8 weeks after the first dose. ■ Use the same vaccine preparation for all doses of the primary series, if possible. ■ The series does not need to be restarted, no matter how long since the previous dose was given.
Hepatitis A			
Type: Inactivated *Route*: Intramuscular *Dosage*: 0.5 mL (1.0 mL if client > 18 years) *Age(s) given*: 12–23 months; in areas with increased incidence, 2–18 years and then 6–12 months after the first dose (two doses total) *Timing:* May give at same time as all other vaccines, but in a separate site. *Storage*: Store in body of refrigerator at 2–8°C (35–46°F). Do not freeze; do not use if it has been frozen. *Product preparations:* Havrix and Vaqta are single-vaccine preparations.	*Common*: Pain, tenderness, soreness, redness, swelling, and warmth at injection site; rash; fever *Serious:* Rare reports of anaphylaxis/anaphylactoid reactions	Known hypersensitivity to any vaccine component Previous hypersensitivity reaction to the vaccine	■ Shake well; vaccine is a slightly opaque, white suspension. ■ No reconstitution is needed. ■ Can be given for postexposure prophylaxis against hepatitis A. ■ Immunoglobulin and vaccine can be given at the same time in different sites. ■ Do not restart the series, no matter how long since the previous dose. ■ Vaccine brands can be interchanged. ■ Vaqta vials have a latex stopper.
Hepatitis B (HepB)			
Type: Inactivated *Route*: Intramuscular *Dosage*: Engerix-B, 10 mcg, or Recombivax HB, 5 mcg *Age(s) given*: Birth–2 months, 1 month after first dose, and 6 months after first dose (three doses total) *or* Birth–2 months, 1–4 months, and 6–18 months(three doses total) *Timing:* May give at same time as all other vaccines, but in a separate site. *Storage*: Store in body of refrigerator at 2–8°C (35–46°F). Do not freeze. *Product preparations:* Engerix-B and Recombivax HB are single-vaccine preparations.	*Common*: Pain or redness at injection site *Serious*: Allergic reaction or anaphylaxis; fever	Previous anaphylaxis or liver abnormalities Serious hypersensitivity reaction to past dose Yeast hypersensitivity	■ Before immunization, check status of mother's HepB test and presence of other liver disease. If mother has positive or unknown hepatitis B surface antigen (HBsAg) status, give vaccine to infant within 12 hours of birth along with HepB immune globulin in another site. ■ Shake vaccine before withdrawing. Solution will appear cloudy. ■ Various formulations (pediatric, adult, and dialysis) are available in different strengths. Read package insert carefully to determine proper dosage for age for the formulation used. ■ A three-dose series can be started at any age. ■ Minimum spacing for children and teens is 4 weeks between first and second doses and 8 weeks between second and third doses. ■ The last dose in an infant series should not be given before 6 months of age.

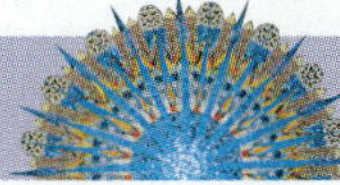

IMMUNIZATIONS Pediatric (continued)

Immunization Type	Side Effects	Contraindications	Nursing Considerations
Hepatitis B (HepB) *(continued)*			
Comvax is a combination of Hib and HepB. Newborn dose should be monovalent (single-vaccine) preparation.			■ Infants of mothers with positive HBsAg status should have anti-HBs levels checked after vaccine completion and be reimmunized if anti-HBs levels are less than 10 mU/mL (American Academy of Pediatrics, 2006, p. 347). ■ Vaccine brands can be interchanged for three-dose series. ■ The series does not need to be restarted, no matter how long since the previous dose was given.
Human papillomavirus vaccine (quadrivalent)			
Type: Recombinant *Route*: Intramuscular *Dosage*: 0.5 mL *Age(s) given*: Girls at 11–12 years, second dose 2 months later, and third dose 4 months later (three doses total over a 6-month period) *Timing:* May be administered with hepatitis B vaccine, but in a separate site. *Storage:* Store in body of refrigerator at 2–8°C (35–46°F). Do not freeze. *Product preparations:* Gardasil is a single-vaccine preparation.	*Common:* Pain, swelling, erythema at the injection site, pruritus, and fever *Serious:* Headache, gastroenteritis, bronchospasm, asthma, and arthritis	Hypersensitivity to any vaccine substances Not recommended for pregnant women Should not be given to individuals with a bleeding disorder. Use caution when administering to lactating women; it is not known if vaccine is excreted in human milk.	■ Shake well before use. ■ Solution is a white, cloudy liquid. ■ No dilution or reconstitution is needed. ■ Keep vaccine out of the light to protect its potency. ■ Vaccine is licensed for girls as young as 9 years old and for women up to 26 years old. Testing is ongoing for potential use in male clients. ■ Vaccine should be administered before sexual activity begins. ■ Discuss with parents the potential of this new vaccine to prevent cervical cancer as well as human papillomavirus infections. ■ The fact that human papillomavirus is transmitted by sexual activity may reduce acceptance of the vaccine by some parents during their child's preteen years.
Influenza			
Type: Trivalent inactivated vaccine (TIV), live attenuated vaccine for intranasal use (LAIV) *Route*: Intramuscular (all ages), intranasal (≥5 years) *Dosage*: 0.25 mL in infants (6–35 months), 0.5 mL beginning at 3 years *Age(s) given:* 6–59 months (all children) and again older, high-risk children *Timing:* May give at same time as all other vaccines, but in a separate site. *TIV storage*: Store in body of refrigerator at 2–8°C (35–46°F). Do not use if it has been frozen. *LAIV storage*: Keep frozen. May be thawed and kept in refrigerator at 2–8°C (35–46°F) for no more than 24 hours before use.	*Common after TIV*: May have soreness or swelling at injection site, fever, aches. Life-threatening allergic reactions are rare. *Common after LAIV*: Runny nose or nasal congestion, fever, headache or muscle aches, abdominal pain, and occasional vomiting. No life-threatening problems were detected during clinical trials.	Contraindicated in children with a history of anaphylactic reaction to egg or chicken protein, hypersensitivity to thimerosol, or known hypersensitivity to gentamicin or other aminoglycosides. LAIV is contraindicated in children who are on long-term aspirin therapy or who have reactive airway disease or other conditions considered to create a high risk for influenza, close contacts with severe immunosuppression, or known or suspected immune deficiency disorders. Should not be given within 3 days of pertussis vaccine (*Mosby's Drug Consult,* 2004).	■ Thawed LAIV is pale yellow and clear to slightly cloudy. ■ Administered annually in autumn at the time recommended by the CDC. ■ Intranasal dose is split (0.25 mL) with a dose-divider clip. Administer in each nostril while child is sitting in an upright position. Insert the tip of the sprayer inside the nose, and depress the plunger to spray. ■ Breast-feeding is not a contraindication for use of either vaccine in infants. ■ Children younger than 9 years who are receiving the influenza vaccine for the first time should get two doses separated by at least 4 weeks (injectable) or 6 weeks (intranasal). ■ Children at high risk are those who are on long-term aspirin therapy or who have chronic disorders of the cardiovascular or pulmonary system (including asthma), a condition that increases risk for aspiration, chronic metabolic disease, renal dysfunction, hemoglobinopathies, or immunodeficiency (CDC, 2006d, p. 2).

(continued)

IMMUNIZATIONS Pediatric (continued)

Immunization Type	Side Effects	Contraindications	Nursing Considerations
Influenza *(continued)*			
Product preparations: Flu Shield (TIV) and Flu Mist (LAIV)		Postpone vaccination in a child who has acute febrile illness until symptoms abate, but vaccine may be given to those with minor illness, with or without fever.	■ Must be reimmunized each year (one dose) as immunity wanes.
Measles, mumps, rubella vaccines (MMR)			
Type: Live attenuated *Route:* Subcutaneous *Dosage:* 0.5 mL *Age(s) given:* 12–15 months and 4–6 years (two doses total) *Timing:* May give at same time as all other vaccines, but in a separate site. *Storage:* Store in body of refrigerator at 2–8°C (35–46°F). When reconstituted, keep refrigerated and away from light; discard if unused within 8 hours. Diluent is stored at room temperature or in refrigerator. Do not freeze. *Product preparations:* ProQuad combines varicella vaccine with MMR	*Common:* Elevated temperature 1–2 weeks after immunization, redness or pain at injection site, noncontagious rash, and joint pain *Serious:* Allergic reaction or anaphylaxis, febrile seizure, meningitis (usually mild), encephalopathy, thrombocytopenia purpura, and rare cases of coma and permanent brain damage	Previous anaphylactic reaction to vaccine Hypersensitivity to neomycin or gelatin Severely impaired immune system caused by malignancy, immune deficiency disease, or immunosuppressive therapy Wait at least 3–11 months after administration of immune globulin or blood products (time determined by type) before giving vaccine. Pregnancy or possibility of pregnancy within 4 weeks Thrombocytopenia or history of thrombocytopenic purpura Tuberculosis or positive PPD	■ Reconstituted vaccine is a clear, yellow solution. ■ Give entire contents of reconstituted vial, even if more than 0.5 mL. ■ Before immunization, ask if child has allergy to neomycin or gelatin. ■ Observe the child with an egg allergy for 90 minutes after injection. Egg allergy is not a contraindication for the vaccine (Cox, 2006). ■ Inquire about immunosuppression. ■ MMR vaccine is recommended for those infected with human immunodeficiency virus. ■ Instruct adolescent girls of childbearing age to avoid pregnancy for 3 months after immunization. ■ Give tuberculosis test at same time as MMR vaccine or 4–6 weeks later. ■ If MMR and Varivax are not given on the same day, space them ≥28 days apart. ■ College students are at greater risk because of decreasing immunity, so make sure they have received a second MMR dose.
Meningococcal Tetravalent Conjugate Vaccine (MCV4)			
Type: Inactivated *Route*: Intramuscular *Dosage*: 0.5 mL in children 11 years and older *Timing:* May be given at same time as typhoid or Td vaccine. *Storage*: Store in body of refrigerator at 2–8°C (35–46°F) until use. Do not freeze. *Product preparations:* Menactra is a single-vaccine preparation.	*Common:* Pain at injection site, headache, and fatigue *Serious:* Less than 5% experienced a severe systemic reaction in vaccine trials (Bilukha & Rosenstein, 2005). A possible association between MCV4 (Menactra) and Guillain-Barré syndrome occurring 2–4 weeks after vaccination has been reported (U.S. Food and Drug Administration, 2005).	Hypersensitivity to any component of vaccine, including diphtheria toxoid. Clients at risk for hemorrhage should not receive vaccine. Pregnant women should receive vaccine only if clearly needed.	■ Protect vaccine from light. ■ May be given to children 11 years or older who are immunosuppressed by disease or medication. Use MPSV4 for younger children. ■ Recommended for control of meningococcal outbreaks caused by serogroups A, C, W-135, and Y. ■ Until an adequate supply exists, recommended for preadolescents and adolescents wishing to reduce health risks (e.g., those going to boarding school or college). ■ Vial stopper contains latex.
Pneumococcal Conjugate Vaccine (Heptavalent) (PCV7)			
Type: Inactivated *Route*: Intramuscular. *Dosage*: 0.5 mL *Age(s) given:* 2, 4, 6, and 12–15 months (four doses total) *Storage*: Store in body of refrigerator at 2–8°C (35–46°F). Do not freeze. *Product preparation:* Prevnar is a single vaccine preparation.	*Common*: Soreness, swelling, and redness at injection site; mild to moderate fever; irritability; drowsiness; restless sleep; decreased appetite; vomiting and diarrhea; and rash or hives *Severe*: Allergic reaction or anaphylaxis	Hypersensitivity to diphtheria toxoid	■ Clear, colorless, or slightly opalescent liquid. ■ May be given to children up to 9 years of age. ■ Use PPV23 for children 2 years and older who are at high risk for acquiring pneumococcal infection. ■ The series does not need to be restarted, no matter how long since the previous dose was given.

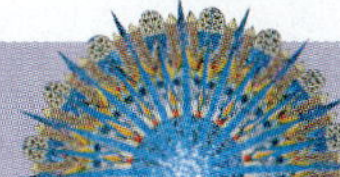

IMMUNIZATIONS **Pediatric (continued)**

Immunization Type	Side Effects	Contraindications	Nursing Considerations
Poliovirus Vaccine (IPV)			
Type: Inactivated *Route:* Subcutaneous or intramuscular, depending on vaccine used *Dosage:* 0.5 mL *Age(s) given:* 2, 4, and 12–18 months, then again at 4–6 years (four doses total) *Timing:* May give at same time as all other vaccines, but in a separate site. *Storage:* Store in body of refrigerator at 2–8°C (35–46°F). Do not freeze. *Product preparations:* Pediarix includes IPV, DTaP, and HepB Pentacel is composed of Hib, DTaP, and IPV. IPV may be given as single-vaccine preparation.	*Common:* Swelling and tenderness, irritability, and tiredness *Serious:* Allergic reaction or anaphylaxis	Hypersensitivity to vaccine components (neomycin, streptomycin, or polymyxin B) Anaphylactic response Pregnancy	■ Before immunization, ask if the child has an allergy to neomycin, streptomycin, or polymyxin B (whichever of these antibiotics the specific vaccine to be used contains). ■ Clear, colorless suspension. Do not use if it contains particulate matter, becomes cloudy, or changes color. ■ Recommended for use in all vaccine doses. ■ All doses must be separated by at least 4 weeks. ■ The series does not need to be restarted, no matter how long since the previous dose was given. ■ Giving IPV to an infant or child when a family member is immunocompromised is not contraindicated.
Rotavirus Vaccine (PRV)			
Type: Live *Route*: Oral *Dosage*: 2 mL *Age(s) given*: 2, 4, and 6 months (three doses total) *Timing:* May give at same time as all other vaccines. *Storage*: Store in body of refrigerator at 2–8°C (35–46°F). Do not freeze. *Product preparations:* RotaTeq is a single-vaccine preparation.	Data from vaccine trials *Common:* Vomiting, diarrhea, and irritability *Serious:* Seizures, bronchiolitis, gastroenteritis, pneumonia, fever, and urinary tract infection	Hypersensitivity to vaccine components Hypersensitivity after receiving a dose of vaccine Should not be given to infants with a known or suspected weakened immune system	■ Vaccine is pale yellow, clear liquid in single-dose tube for direct oral administration. ■ Protect vaccine from light. ■ Squeeze the liquid into the infant's mouth toward the inner cheek until the dosing tube is empty. ■ No restrictions on the infant's intake of formula, breast milk, or food before or after vaccination. ■ Discard the empty tube and cap into an approved biologic waste container. ■ All three doses should be completed by 32 months of age.
Varicella Virus Vaccine			
Type: Live attenuated *Route*: Subcutaneous *Dosage*: 0.5 mL *Age(s) given*: 12–15 months and 4–6 years (two doses total), and then two doses (4–8 weeks apart) at 13 years or older *Storage*: Frozen at −15°C (5°F) or colder. May be stored in refrigerator at 2–8°C (35–46°F) up to 72 hours before reconstitution. Do not refreeze. *Product preparations:* Varivax is a single-vaccine preparation. ProQuad combines varicella vaccine with MMR.	*Common*: Pain or redness at injection site; fever up to 38.8°C (102°F) in children or up to 37.7°C (100°F) in adults *Less common:* Vaccine-related rash (mild exanthem of 6–10 lesions that last 2–3 days) during first month after the injection *Severe*: Allergic reaction or anaphylaxis, thrombocytopenia, febrile seizure, and central nervous system manifestations	Previous anaphylactic reaction to vaccine Hypersensitivity to neomycin or gelatin Immunodeficiency or receiving immunosuppression therapy Administration of immune serum globulin or blood products in last 3–11 months Active, untreated tuberculosis Pregnancy Moderate or severe febrile illness	■ Before immunization, ask if child is immunodeficient, is on immunosuppression treatment, or has had an allergy to neomycin or gelatin. Determine if a family member is immunocompromised. ■ Clear, colorless to pale yellow liquid when reconstituted. ■ Once reconstituted, vaccine must be used within 30 minutes or discarded. ■ Give the entire contents of the vial, even if more than 0.5 mL. ■ Instruct adolescent girls of childbearing age to avoid pregnancy for 3 months after immunization. ■ The vaccine is effective. Only very mild cases of breakthrough varicella have occurred in immunized children, primarily caused by wild-type virus (American Academy of Pediatrics, 2006, p. 719).

Source: Data from American Academy of Pediatrics. (2006). *Red book: Report of the committee on infectious disease* (27th ed.). Elk Grove Village, IL; R. M. Bindler & L. B. Howry. (2005). *Pediatric drugs and nursing implications* (3rd ed.). Upper Saddle River, NJ: Prentice Hall Health; M. L. Buck. (2005). Meningococcal conjugate vaccine. *Pediatric pharmacology, 11*(5). Retrieved June 7, 2005, from http://www.medscape.com/viewarticle/505508_print; Immunization Action Coalition; Merck & Co. Inc. (2006). *Gardasil.* Retrieved June 13, 2006, from http://www.fda.gov/cber/label/hpvmer060806LB.pdf; Mosby. (2004). *Mosby's drug consult 2004.* St. Louis: Mosby.

Pediatric Differences

Immune system development is a complex and multifactorial process. Early in utero experiences, environmental exposures after birth, and other factors influence this important feedback system. While the immune system protects children from harmful diseases, it also can lead to conditions such as asthma, food allergies, or skin atopy.

Infants and children have differing amounts of some immunoglobulins. IgG is the only immunoglobulin that crosses the placenta; as a result, a newborn's levels are similar to those of the mother. This maternal IgG disappears by 6 to 8 months of age. The infant's IgG level then increases gradually, until mature levels are reached at 7 to 8 years. IgM levels are low at birth, rise markedly at 1 week of age, and then continue to increase until adult levels are reached at about 1 year. IgA and IgE are not present at birth. Manufacture of these immunoglobulins begins by 2 weeks of age; however, normal values are not achieved until 6 to 7 years. Considering this, it is easy to see why children under 6 years of age become ill so often—they do not have a full complement of immunoglobulins.

In contrast, cell-mediated immunity achieves full function early in life. Early in fetal life, the thymus begins producing T cells, and by birth, many of these cells are present. The thymus is large at birth, grows during childhood and adolescence, and decreases in size during adulthood (Chamley, Carson, Randall, & Sandwell, 2005). Other lymphoid tissues, such as the spleen and tonsils, also are comparatively large in young children. Because of the well-developed cellular immunity, any blood infused into newborns generally is irradiated to prevent **graft-versus-host disease** (a series of immunologic reactions in response to transplanted cells) as a result of transfused lymphocytes (Figure 14–6 ■).

Newborns are most prone to development of infection, particularly when born prematurely, because they have lower levels of their own immune protections as well as less IgG obtained from the mother. Specifically, newborns have somewhat lower numbers of NK cells than older children and adults, and this decreases their ability to respond to certain antigens. The levels of some complement proteins also are lower in newborns than in older children and adults, thus delaying and hampering response to certain infections. Levels of monocytes and macrophages are low as well (Marodi, 2006). Feeding newborns with human milk is protective against infections, however. Nurses also play an important role by following infection-control practices with newborns and promptly identifying infections in children of all ages.

Normal Changes of Aging

Immune function declines with aging, although many of the mechanisms leading to this decline are not clear. External factors, such as nutritional status and the effects of chemical exposure, ultraviolet radiation, and environmental pollution, affect the older adult's immune status. Internal factors, including genetics, the function of the neurologic and endocrine systems, chronic and prior illnesses, and individual anatomic and physiologic variations, affect it as well. These myriad influences make it difficult to determine the effect of aging on the immune system.

Although in some older individuals the immune system is as effective as that of younger persons, normal changes associated with aging demonstrate a decrease in immune response

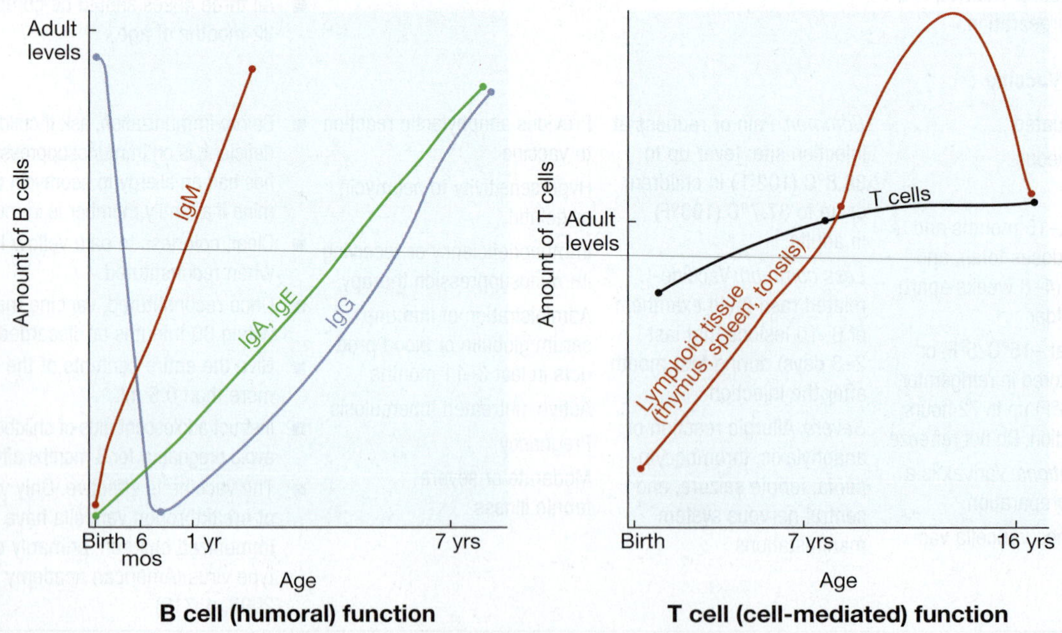

Figure 14–6 ■ Different types of immunoglobulins mature at variable times throughout childhood. Children have high levels of some types of immunoglobulins, whereas other types may be low at certain periods during development.

TABLE 14–2 **Selected Autoimmune Disorders**

ORGAN SPECIFICITY	DISORDER	DESCRIPTION
More organ specific	Hashimoto's thyroiditis	A chronic, progressive inflammatory disease of the thyroid, with lymphocyte infiltration and gradual destruction of the gland
	Addison's disease	Atrophy and hypofunction of the adrenal cortex, probably autoimmune in origin
	Goodpasture's syndrome	A type II hypersensitivity disorder, with pulmonary hemorrhage and progressive glomerulonephritis characterized by circulating antiglomerular basement membrane antibodies
	Active chronic hepatitis	A serious liver disease often resulting in hepatic failure and/or cirrhosis; may be autoimmune, with infiltration by T cells and plasma cells
Less organ specific	Ulcerative colitis	A chronic inflammatory disease of the colon mucosa, possibly of autoimmune origin
	Sjögren's syndrome	A systemic inflammatory disorder characterized by dryness of the mouth, eye, and other mucous membranes, with lymphocyte infiltration of affected tissues
	Scleroderma	Diffuse fibrosis, degenerative changes, and vascular abnormalities of the skin, joint structures, and internal organs; probably of autoimmune origin

and lowered resistance to infection, with poor response to immunizations. T cells are less responsive to antigens, while B cells produce fewer antibodies. Immune system changes may precipitate insulin resistance, and the hypersensitivity response is reduced or delayed.

Whereas the antibody response to foreign antigens is diminished in older persons, autoantibodies (antibodies that react to the client's own tissues) are more common. Immunologic theories of aging propose that a decrease in immune function may result in an increase in autoimmune responses, causing the body to produce antibodies that attack itself. The presence of autoantibodies in older adults does suggest impaired regulation of the immune system, but this change is not associated with an increased incidence of autoimmune disorders (Murasko & Gardner, 2003).

ALTERATIONS

Considering the complexity of the immune system, it is not surprising that abnormal or harmful responses occur. Altered immune system responses include those characterized by hyperresponsiveness of the immune system and those characterized by an impaired immune response.

ALTERATIONS AND TREATMENTS Immunity

Alteration	Description	Treatment
Hypersensitivity reaction	Hypersensitivity reaction is an altered immune response to an antigen, resulting in harm to the client ranging from an allergy to anaphylactic shock.	■ Antihistamines for mild reactions ■ Epinephrine and corticosteroids in life-threatening reactions ■ Assessment of airway with any hypersensitivity reaction
Rheumatoid arthritis	Rheumatoid arthritis is a chronic, systemic autoimmune disorder that causes inflammation of connective tissue.	■ Nonsteroidal anti-inflammatory drugs (NSAIDs) ■ Low-dose corticosteroids ■ Antirheumatic drugs, including immunosuppressive and cytotoxic drugs
Human immunodeficiency virus/acquired immunodeficiency syndrome (HIV/AIDS)	AIDS results from a retrovirus (HIV) that is transmitted by direct contact with infected blood and body fluids. AIDS weakens the immune system, leaving clients vulnerable to opportunistic infections.	■ Prevention of opportunistic infections ■ Ensuring adequate respiratory function and perfusion ■ Stimulating hematopoietic response ■ Antiviral treatment if CD4 count falls below 200/mm^3 or client exhibits severe disease symptoms
Systemic lupus erythematosus (SLE)	SLE is a chronic inflammatory disease that involves many organ systems.	■ Dependent on severity of the disease ■ Aspirin or NSAIDS for arthralgias, arthritis, fever, or fatigue ■ Antimalarial drugs ■ High-dose corticosteroids ■ Immunosuppressive agents

Box 14–1 Other Endocrine System Alterations

Other alterations related to the endocrine system that are not covered as a part of this concept include, but are not limited to, the following:

- Graves' disease
- Hashimoto's disease
- Myasthenia gravis
- Sjögren's syndrome
- Urticaria.

Allergies, autoimmune disorders, and reactions to organ or tissue transplants are all examples of hyperresponsive immune function. AIDS and other immunodeficiency disorders result from impairment of the immune system. Table 14–2 outlines selected autoimmune disorders; other endocrine system alterations are listed in Box 14–1.

PHYSICAL ASSESSMENT

Unlike body systems that are composed of a few closely related organs, the immune system is diverse and scattered. Optimal immune function depends on intact skin and mucous membrane barriers, adequate blood cell production and differentiation, a functional system of lymphatics and the spleen, and the ability to differentiate foreign tissue and pathogens from normal body tissue and flora. Because of this diversity of organs and function, assessment of the immune system often is integrated throughout the health history and physical examination.

Health History

Before conducting the interview, review the client's biographic data, including age, sex, race, and ethnic background. This information can provide valuable clues about possible immunologic disorders. For example, many autoimmune disorders are more prevalent in women than in men, and epidemiologic data show that certain social and racial groups have particular risks for HIV infection. Family history also is important, because the etiology of many disorders affecting the immune system includes a genetic component.

Many interview questions related to the immune system and the disorders that affect it are of a sensitive nature. Be sure to provide for privacy before the interview. If family members are present, request that they leave as well. Establish a trusting relationship with the client before asking the most sensitive questions (e.g., those related to the use of illicit drugs or sexual activity).

As with all history taking, the nurse must individualize the specific terms used, examples given to the client, and teaching techniques used to validate agreement on the meaning of words according to the client's culture, language spoken, and education or intellectual abilities. Cultural sensitivity is necessary for effective communication.

Physical Examination

The techniques of inspection and palpation are especially important in assessing a client's immune system:

- Assess the general appearance, and note whether the client's stated and apparent age coincide. Assess height, weight, and body type for apparent weight loss or wasting.
- Check vital signs. An elevated temperature may indicate an infection or inflammatory response.
- Inspect the mucous membranes of the nose and mouth for color and condition. Pale, boggy (edematous) nasal mucosa often is associated with chronic allergies. Petechiae, white patches, or lacy white plaques in the oral mucosa may indicate hemolysis or immunodeficiency.
- Assess skin color, temperature, and moisture. Pale or jaundiced skin may indicate a hemolytic reaction. Pallor also may indicate bone marrow suppression with accompanying immunodeficiency.
- Inspect the skin for evidence of rashes or lesions, such as petechiae, numerous bruises, purple or blue patches or lesions indicative of Kaposi's sarcoma, and wounds that are infected, inflamed, or unhealed. Note the location and distribution of any rashes or lesions.
- Inspect and palpate the cervical lymph nodes for evidence of lymphadenopathy (swelling) or tenderness. Palpate the nodes of the axillae and groin as well (Figure 14–7 ■).
- Assess the musculoskeletal system by inspecting and palpating the joints for redness, swelling, tenderness, or deformity. Such changes may indicate an autoimmune disorder, such as rheumatoid arthritis or systemic lupus erythematosus.
- Check joint range of motion (ROM), including that of the spine. Observe ease of movement, and note any evident stiffness or difficulty moving. Evident fatigue or weakness may indicate acute or chronic illness or immunodeficiency.

Assessment Interview Immunity

- When were you last immunized for diphtheria, tetanus, poliomyelitis, rubella, measles, influenza, hepatitis, and pneumococcal pneumonia? Do you have a record of your immunizations?
- When did you last have a tuberculin skin test?
- What infections have you had in the past, and how were these treated?
- Have any of these infections recurred?
- Are you taking any antibiotics; anti-inflammatory medications, such as aspirin or ibuprofen; or medications for cancer?
- Have you had any recent invasive procedures or radiologic examinations?
- Do you have any allergies to food, medications, or any other substance, such as latex, bees, pollen, and so on? If so, what happens when you come in contact with this substance?
- On a scale of 1 to 10, how would you rate the stress you have experienced during the last 6 months?
- Do you have any chronic conditions?

Immune System Assessments

Assessment Focus	Assessment Guidelines
Family history	■ Does a family member have a history of allergy? Does the mother or other family member have a history of HIV or other immune system disorder? ■ Has the child been treated prophylactically for HIV because of the mother's positive status?
Growth and development	■ Children's height and weight should be plotted on each visit to monitor steady and expected progress. The child should have a healthy appetite and consume normal amounts of food for age. Developmental milestones should emerge at expected times. Delayed growth and development, as well as lethargy and lack of energy, can indicate immune system malfunction.
Skin and mucous membranes	■ Is the skin intact? Are there lesions of the mucous membranes? ■ Are infections or allergic responses commonly occurring? ■ Do lesions heal quickly and without additional infection?
Evidence of disease	■ Frequently recurring infections and unusual infectious agents may signify immune system malfunction. Respiratory system infections, as well as frequent and untreatable ear infections, are common indicators of potential problems.

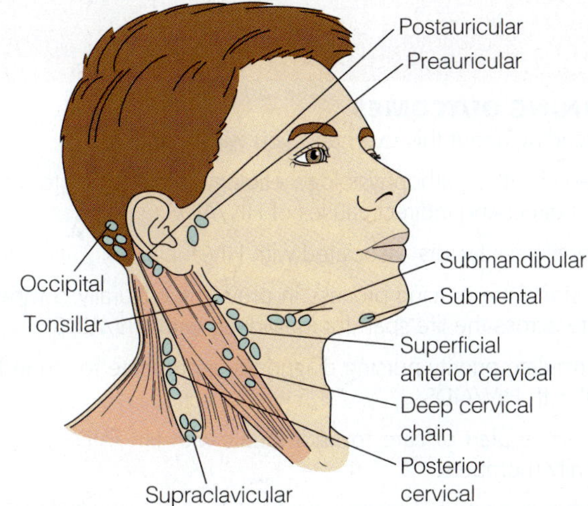

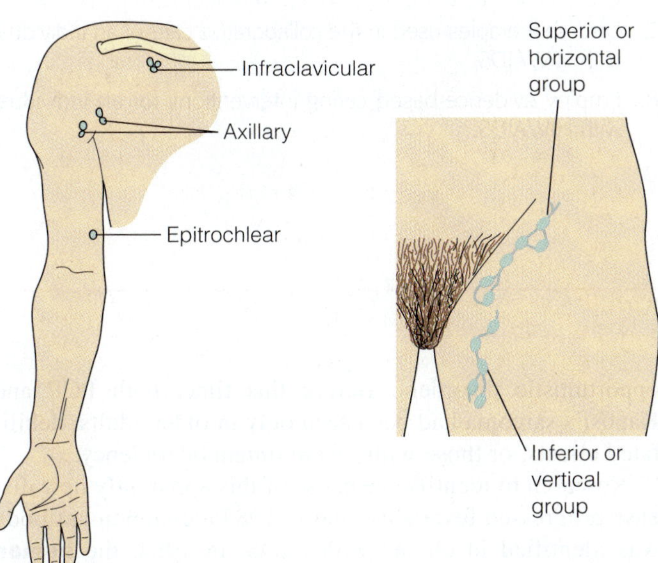

Figure 14–7 ■ Lymph nodes that can be assessed by palpation.

DIAGNOSTIC TESTS

Diagnostic and laboratory tests are ordered specific to the type of immune disorder that is suspected. Possible tests include:

- Enzyme immunoassay and enzyme-linked immunosorbent assay
- Immunoglobulins
- Polymerase chain reaction
- Rapid HIV tests
- Radioallergosorbent test
- Skin reactions
- Western blot test
- Complete blood count (CBC)
- Complement.

(See Diagnostic Tests appendix.)

CARING INTERVENTIONS

Simple as it may sound, proper nutrition, adequate exercise, and a good night's sleep are profoundly important in maintaining an effective immune system. Stress reduction and stress management also play a role. As respiratory and musculoskeletal effort increase with exercise, and as gravity is enlisted with postural changes, lymph fluid is more efficiently pumped from tissues into lymph capillaries and vessels throughout the body. Circulation through lymph nodes, where destruction of pathogens and removal of foreign antigens can occur, also improves with exercise. Research in older adults has shown benefits of moderate exercise on NK cell function, circulating T-cell function, and cytokine production, potentially increasing resistance to viral infections and preventing formation of malignant cells (Freeman, 2004). While moderate exercise seems to enhance immunity, strenuous exercise may reduce immune function, leaving a window of opportunity for infection during the recovery phase. Adequate rest is important after vigorous training to allow the body to recover (Edelman & Mandle, 2006).

PHARMACOLOGIC THERAPIES

The goals of medical management are to restore immune function and to prevent further stress on the immune system. Treatment may be supportive for those with only mild manifestations. Anti-inflammatories, such as nonsteroidal anti-inflammatory drugs (NSAIDs) and corticosteroids, are a staple in the management of alterations in immune function, because pain and swelling are frequent manifestations.

Prevention and prompt treatment of infection is essential. Antibiotic therapy is targeted at infectious agents. Antibiotic prophylaxis and specific immunization recommendations for immunodeficiency are needed. Children with T-cell deficiencies should receive cytomegalovirus-negative, irradiated blood products because of the risk of infection and graft-versus-host disease posed by lymphocytes in donor blood (Cooper, Pommering, & Koryani, 2003).

Intravenous immunoglobulin may be administered to provide protection until humoral immunity can be established. Hematopoietic stem cell transplantation may be considered if T-cell function cannot be restored by other methods. Gene transfer is showing optimistic results, and this experimental therapy is expected to be used more often in the future, particularly for certain defects (Bonilla & Geha, 2006; Champi, 2002).

COMPLEMENTARY THERAPIES

Many clients with immune disorders have begun trying complementary and alternative medicine to relieve symptoms. Johns Hopkins University reports that therapies such as dietary supplements, hydrotherapy, and acupuncture show promise for treating conditions like rheumatoid arthritis, but that relatively few studies have been done (Haaz, 2008). The use of acupuncture in alleviating side effects of antiretroviral medicines has become sufficiently popular that in Massachusetts, clients with AIDS can access acupuncture for free (Community Resources Information, Inc., 2009).

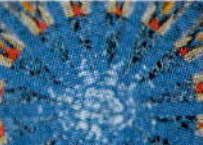

14.1 HUMAN IMMUNODEFICIENCY VIRUS AND ACQUIRED IMMUNODEFICIENCY SYNDROME

KEY TERMS

Acute retroviral syndrome, *702*
AIDS dementia complex, *704*
Antiretroviral therapy, *703*
Candidiasis, *704*
Epidemic, *697*
Helper T cells, *697*
Human immunodeficiency virus (HIV), *696*
Kaposi's sarcoma, *705*
Pneumocystis carinii pneumonia (PCP), *703*
Opportunistic infections, *704*
Seroconversion, *697*
Toxoplasmosis, *704*
Vertical transmission, *697*
Virions, *697*

BASIS FOR SELECTION OF EXEMPLAR

Centers for Disease Control
Healthy People 2010
Institute of Medicine

LEARNING OUTCOMES

After reading about this exemplar, you will be able to:

1. Describe the pathophysiology, etiology, clinical manifestations, and direct and indirect causes of HIV/AIDS.
2. Identify risk factors associated with HIV/AIDS.
3. Illustrate the nursing process in providing culturally competent care across the life span for individuals with HIV/AIDS.
4. Formulate priority nursing diagnoses appropriate for an individual with HIV/AIDS.
5. Create a plan of care for individuals with HIV/AIDS and their family members.
6. Assess expected outcomes for an individual with HIV/AIDS.
7. Discuss therapies used in the collaborative care of an individual with HIV/AIDS.
8. Employ evidence-based caring interventions for an individual with HIV/AIDS.

OVERVIEW

In 1981, 5 cases of *Pneumocystis carinii* pneumonia (PCP) and 26 cases of a rare cancer, Kaposi's sarcoma, were diagnosed in young, previously healthy gay men in Los Angeles and New York City. The term *acquired immunodeficiency syndrome (AIDS)* was given to this new phenomenon to describe the immune system deficits associated with these opportunistic disorders. Before this time, both PCP and Kaposi's sarcoma had been seen only in older adults, debilitated clients, or those with severe immunodeficiency.

Research to identify the cause of this apparently new disease progressed feverishly, and in 1983 a common antibody was identified in clients with AIDS. In 1984, the **human immunodeficiency virus (HIV)**, a retrovirus (meaning that it

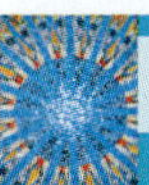

FOCUS ON DIVERSITY AND CULTURE
HIV/AIDS

An estimated 36.2 million people are infected with AIDS worldwide, with virtually every country in the world reporting cases of AIDS (Joint United Nations Programme on HIV/AIDS, 2000). The highest incidence is found in sub-Saharan Africa, South and Southeast Asia, the United States, Western Europe, South America, and Canada. Approximately 70% of all people infected with HIV or who have AIDS live in sub-Saharan Africa, and another 16% live in South and Southeast Asia, largely in Thailand and India. The most common mode of transmission is heterosexual intercourse. The cofactors of general health status, presence of genital ulcers, and number of sexual partners correlate with incidence (Tierney, McPhee, & Papadakis, 2005).

carries its genetic information in RNA) that is transmitted by direct contact with infected blood and body fluids, was isolated. It then became apparent that the chronic disease known as AIDS was the final, fatal stage of infection with HIV, which was being spread primarily through sexual contact with an infected person.

Human immunodeficiency virus is an example of an emerging infectious agent that jumped from animal to human, probably in the 1950s. Like so many previous **epidemics** (widespread outbreak of infectious disease with many infected people), HIV/AIDS began with a few isolated cases and has now become a worldwide concern. (See the accompanying Focus on Diversity and Culture feature.) The virus invades our lives in ways we never imagined—testing our scientific knowledge, probing our private values, and eluding a vaccine or a cure. The widespread organ involvement associated with the infection has caused much human suffering and death. Progression of HIV-positive status to AIDS has slowed, however, because of the effectiveness of highly active antiretroviral therapy (HAART) (CDC, 2006f). The change these medications cause in HIV's progression to AIDS makes monitoring of AIDS less useful as an indicator for infected cases. For this reason, the CDC has developed new surveillance methods based on infection rates in high-risk populations.

PATHOPHYSIOLOGY AND ETIOLOGY

Acquired immunodeficiency syndrome is caused by HIV (specifically, HIV-1). The best example of a primary immunodeficiency disorder, HIV destroys the body's ability to fight infection.

Significant concentrations of the virus are present in blood, semen, vaginal and cervical secretions, and cerebrospinal fluid of infected individuals. The virus also is found in breast milk and saliva. Sexual contact is the primary mode of transmission. However, HIV can be transmitted through contact with infected blood via needle sharing during injection drug use or by transfusion as well. Approximately 13 to 40% of infants born to HIV-positive mothers are infected perinatally. Breastfeeding also is a route of transmission postnatally and should be avoided by women infected with HIV (Tierney, McPhee, & Papadakis, 2005).

On entry into the body, the virus infects cells that have the CD4 antigen. Once inside the cell, the virus sheds its protein coat and uses an enzyme called reverse transcriptase to convert the viral RNA to DNA (Figure 14–8 ■). This viral DNA is then integrated into host cell DNA and duplicated during normal processes of cell division. Within the cell, the virus may remain latent or become activated to produce new RNA and to form **virions** (virus able to grow and reproduce outside a host). The virus then buds from the cell surface, disrupting its cell membrane and leading to destruction of the host cell.

Although the virus may remain inactive in infected cells for years, antibodies are produced to its proteins, a process known as **seroconversion**. These antibodies usually are detectable 6 weeks to 6 months after the initial infection. Although helper T or CD4 cells are the primary cells infected by HIV, the virus also infects macrophages and certain cells of the central nervous system (CNS). **Helper T cells** play a vital role in normal function of the immune system, recognizing foreign antigens and infected cells and activating antibody-producing B cells. They also direct cell-mediated immune activity and influence the phagocytic activity of monocytes and macrophages. The loss of these helper T cells leads to the immunodeficiencies seen with HIV infection (Porth, 2005). Figure 14–9 ■ illustrates the typical course of HIV infection.

Children can acquire HIV by a form of **vertical transmission** (perinatal transmission) from their mothers either transplacentally or during delivery. Transmission can occur during birth from blood, amniotic fluid, and exposure to genital tract secretions and after birth through breast milk from mothers who are HIV positive. However, risk for perinatal transmission is significantly reduced when mothers identified as infected receive zidovudine (Retrovir, AZT) during pregnancy, when deliveries are by cesarean section, and when their babies are given drug therapy after birth (Ramstead, 2003). Because of the high rate of transmission from mother to infant, HIV counseling and voluntary testing are encouraged for all pregnant women. (Box 14–2).

Before mandatory screening of blood and blood products was instituted in 1985, some children received HIV through transfusions of infected blood. Most of these children were

Box 14–2 HIV Screening in Prenatal Care

In 2001, the CDC recommended including HIV screening as a routine part of prenatal care. In 2006, the CDC recommended HIV screening for clients in all health care settings unless the client declines such testing. In areas with elevated HIV rates, pregnant women should be offered repeat HIV screening during the third trimester (CDC, 2006e).

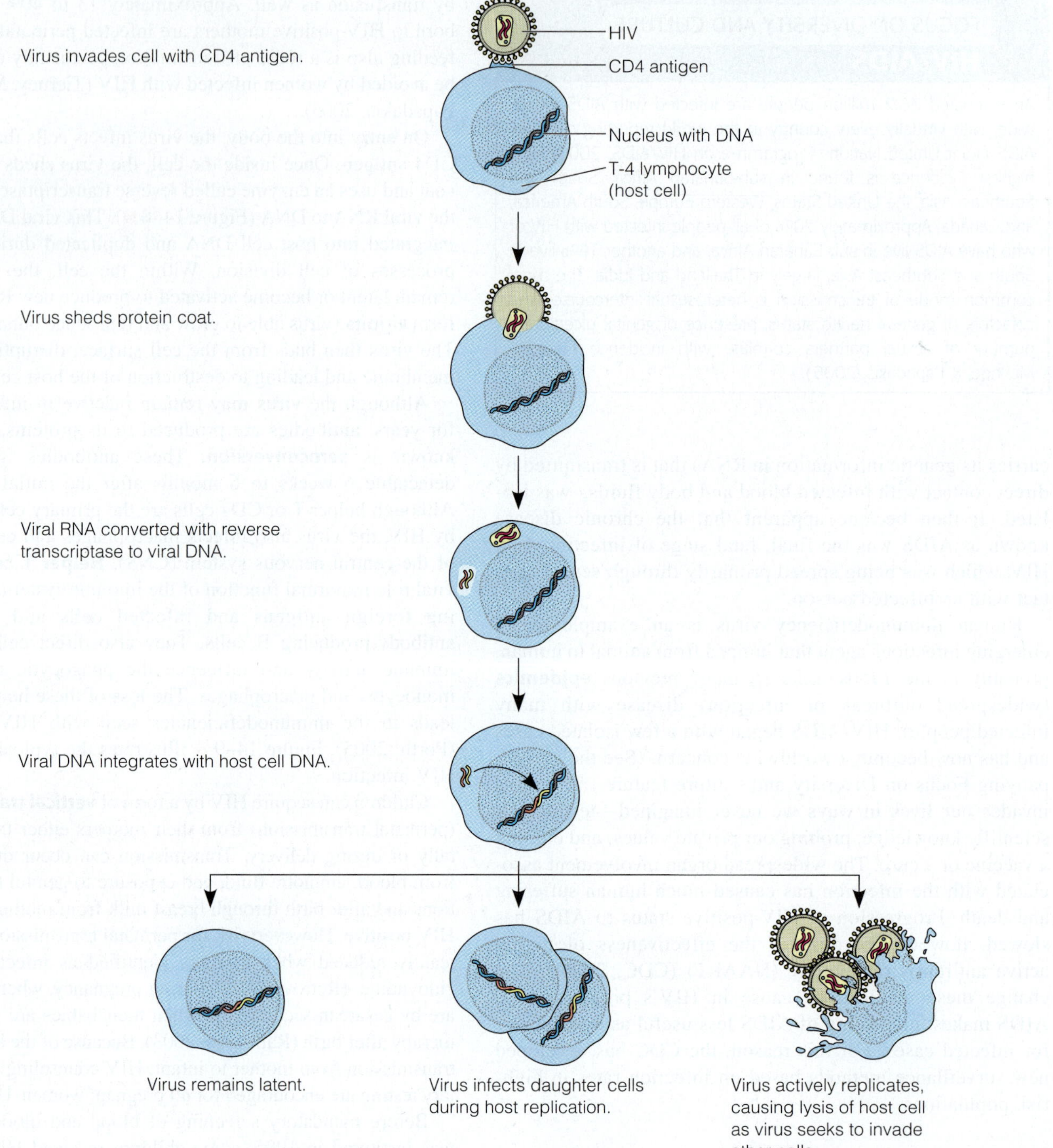
HIV
CD4 antigen
Virus invades cell with CD4 antigen.
Nucleus with DNA
T-4 lymphocyte
(host cell)
Virus sheds protein coat.
Viral RNA converted with reverse
transcriptase to viral DNA.
Viral DNA integrates with host cell DNA.
Virus remains latent.
Virus infects daughter cells
during host replication.
Virus actively replicates,
causing lysis of host cell
as virus seeks to invade
other cells.

Figure 14–8 ■ How HIV infects and destroys CD4 cells.

infected during treatment of hemophilia. Today, adolescents most commonly acquire HIV through unprotected sexual activities, less commonly through contact with blood from needle sharing, and very rarely, from blood transfusions (CDC, 2005).

Etiology

The estimated number of diagnosed AIDS cases in the United States from 1981 to 2006 was 982,498. In 2006, a total of 35,314 new cases of HIV/AIDS were diagnosed in the 33 states with long-term reporting data. Men still make up the majority of cases, whereas women account for approximately 26% (CDC, 2008d). The major transmission categories are identified in Figure 14–10 ■. Among females, 80% of the cases result from high-risk heterosexual contact, 19% from injection drug use, and 1% from other categories of transmission (CDC, 2008d). Although approximately 24% of U.S. women are African American or Latina, these groups accounted for 82% of all female AIDS

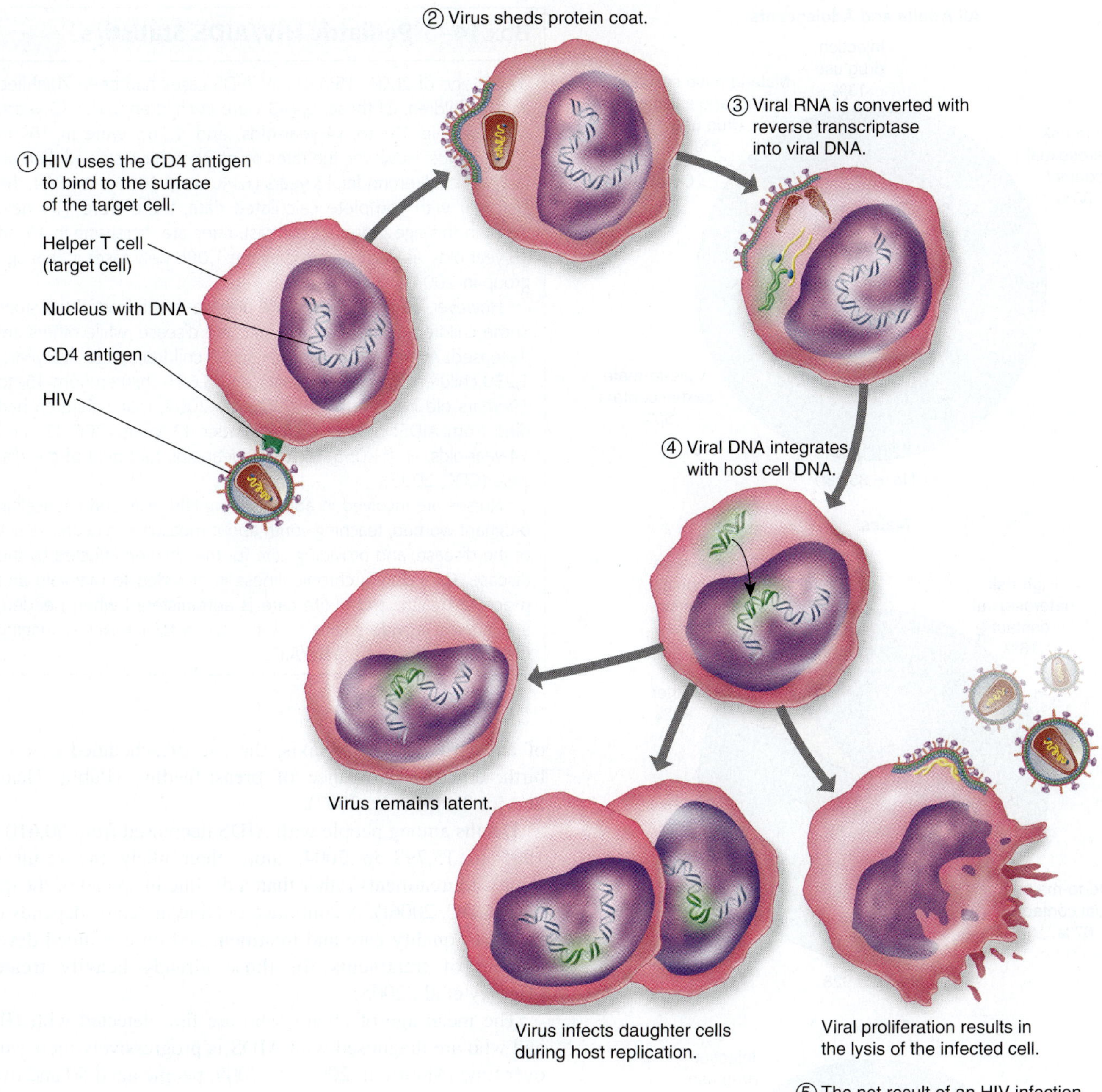

② Virus sheds protein coat.
③ Viral RNA is converted with reverse transcriptase into viral DNA.
① HIV uses the CD4 antigen to bind to the surface of the target cell.
Helper T cell (target cell)
Nucleus with DNA
CD4 antigen
HIV
④ Viral DNA integrates with host cell DNA.
Virus remains latent.
Virus infects daughter cells during host replication.
Viral proliferation results in the lysis of the infected cell.
⑤ The net result of an HIV infection is decreased cellular immunity.

Figure 14–9 ■ The HIV virus gains entry into helper T cells, uses the cell DNA to replicate, interferes with normal function of the T cells, and destroys the normal cells.

cases in 2005 (CDC, 2007). For the 4 years from 2001 to 2004, a total of 15,338 U.S. children and teens from birth to 19 years of age were diagnosed with HIV/AIDS (Box 14–3). Clients with hemophilia who require large amounts of intravenous clotting factors and people infected through blood transfusion account for a small number of cases, approximately 2% (CDC, 2004).

Among risk groups, the most rapid increases have been noted in young gay and bisexual men, women, and inner-city injection drug users, especially African Americans and Hispanics (CDC, 2004). In the United States, the rate of male adult/adolescent HIV/AIDS cases (per 100,000 population) reported was 131.6 among African Americans, 60.2 among Hispanics, 20.8 among American Indians/Alaska Natives, 18.7 among Whites, and 13.9 among Asians/Pacific Islanders (CDC, 2004). The rapid increase of AIDS cases among women is of special concern; those numbers increased from 7% of cases in 1985 to 27% of newly reported cases in 2003 (CDC, 2004). The rate of perinatal transmission in the United States has dropped dramatically, however, and is now less than 2% because of the implementation of recommendations for universal prenatal HIV counseling and testing, the availability

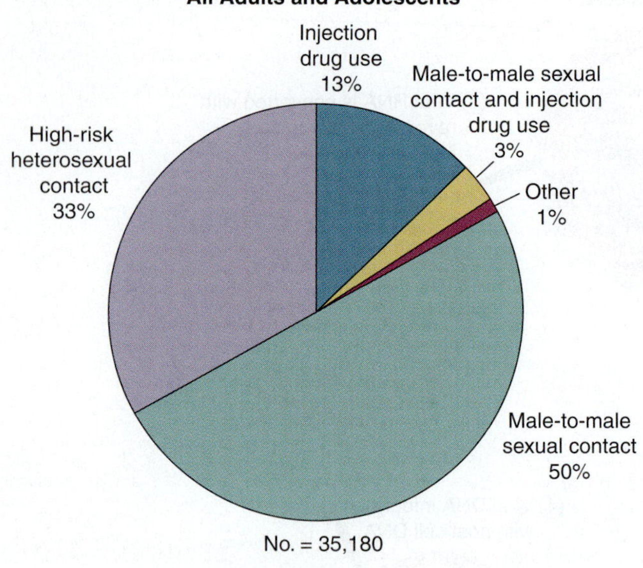

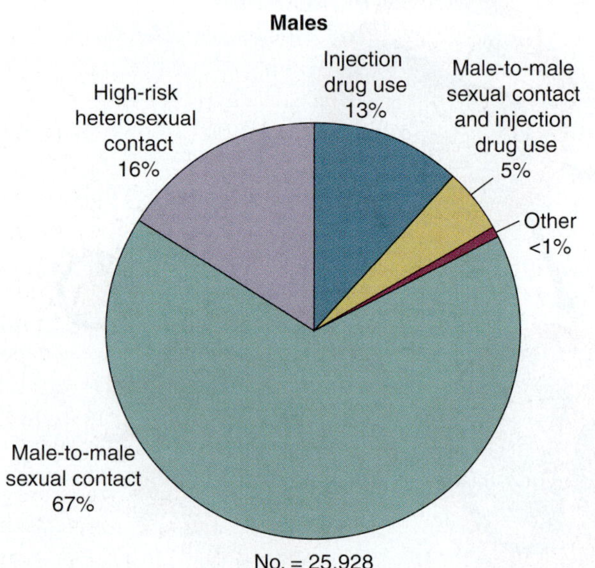

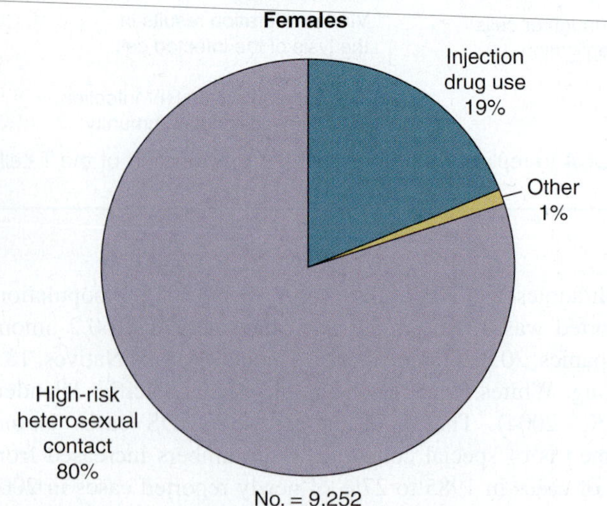

Figure 14–10 ■ Transmission categories of adults and adolescents diagnosed with HIV/AIDS during 2006.

Source: CDC. (2008). *HIV/AIDS in the United States.* CDC/HIV AIDS Facts. Retrieved April 29, 2008, from http://www.cdc.gov/hiv

Box 14–3 **Pediatric HIV/AIDS Statistics**

By the end of 2004, 15,338 HIV/AIDS cases had been identified in U.S. children. Of these, 9,443 were in children under 13 years, 959 were in 13- to 14-year-olds, and 4,963 were in 15- to 19-year-olds. However, the rates of infection have slowed dramatically for children under 13 years (61% since 2000). In 2004, the last year with complete calculated data, there were 174 new cases in this age group. In contrast, rates are increasing in 15- to 19 year olds, as demonstrated by the 1,080 new cases in that age group in 2004.

However, the incidence of the disease is only part of the story. Some children continue to live with the disease, while others are deceased. At present, there are 3,713 children under 13 years, 1,239 children from 13–14 years, and 3,683 children from 15- to 19 years old living with HIV/AIDS. By 2004, many children had died from AIDS: 5,094 children under 13 years, 266 13- and 14-year-olds, and 1,055 15- to 19-year-olds had died of the disease (CDC, 2005).

Nurses are involved in administering HIV tests and counseling pregnant women, teaching youth about measures to decrease risk of the disease, and providing care for the children affected by the disease. Care during chronic illness is provided to maintain and promote health, end-of-life care is administered when needed, and nurses provide solace and assistance for families managing the complex disease of HIV/AIDS.

of antiretroviral prophylaxis, the use of scheduled cesarean birth, and the avoidance of breast-feeding (Public Health Service Task Force, 2007).

Deaths among people with AIDS decreased from 50,610 in 1995 to 15,798 in 2004, more than likely the result of improved treatments rather than a decline in spread of the disease (CDC, 2006f). A continued decline in deaths depends on access to quality care and treatment and on continued development of treatments for those already heavily treated (Tierney et al., 2005).

The mean age of clients who are first detected with HIV and who are diagnosed with AIDS is progressively increasing over time (Manfredi, 2002). In 2005, people aged 50 and over accounted for 15% of new HIV/AIDS diagnoses (CDC, 2008c). This is the result of a number of factors. Survival rates for those infected with HIV have improved because of advances in diagnostic resources, antiviral treatment, and prophylaxis; those infected at a relatively young age are now becoming older. The entire senior population is increasing, and so are their expectations regarding their sex lives. Male sexual function has been enhanced by medications such as sildenafil citrate (Viagra), and medications to enhance female sexual drive and response are being developed. The sexually permissive baby boomers are entering the ranks of the older population. Some older persons continue their risky sexual behaviors and pay little attention to preventive measures, believing that HIV infection is not an issue for their age group. These factors have contributed not only to an increased incidence of HIV/AIDS in older adults but also to an increase in other sexually transmitted diseases, often among people who live in over-55 communities. Older people have been compared to teenagers in their knowledge of HIV. They have not known people who have been diagnosed with HIV/AIDS, so they have little knowledge, personal awareness, or interest in preventing the disease. However, many senior centers now have AIDS awareness programs that provide information about HIV prevention and safe sex. Clearly, a need exists for concisely presented, accurate, and culturally sensitive information that is appropriate for older people. The health section of newspapers and the Internet can be valuable resources.

Risk Factors

The risk factors for HIV infection primarily are behavioral. Other risk factors involve hemophilia and blood transfusions, health care as an occupation, poverty, pregnancy and breast-feeding, and older age.

BEHAVIOR Among adults in the United States, 60% of reported cases are in men who have sex with other men, including gays, bisexuals, and groups such as prison populations. Unprotected anal intercourse is the major route of transmission in these men. Injection drug use is the second leading risk factor, accounting for approximately 25% of cases. Among those cases, sharing of needles and other drug paraphernalia is the primary route of transmission. Heterosexual intercourse with an infected drug user and exchanging sex for drugs are major risk factors for women. In the United States, heterosexual contact accounts for 75% of these cases, with injection drug using accounting for the remaining 25% of cases.

HEMOPHILIA AND BLOOD TRANSFUSIONS Blood donation poses no risk for the donor of contracting HIV, because only new, sterile equipment is used. In addition, screening of voluntary blood donors (a process that generally excludes people with high-risk behavior) and of donated blood supplies has reduced the risk for transmission of HIV by transfusion to 1 in 100,000. Less than 0.04% of people voluntarily donating blood are found to be HIV positive.

Current blood-screening methods use antibody testing, and the small risk of HIV transmission through blood supplies arises from donors in the so-called *window period* between contracting the virus and development of detectable antibodies. This window period usually lasts from 6 weeks to 6 months; rarely, it may last up to 1 year. Those in the window period are able to transmit HIV to others even though they do not yet test positive for HIV.

HEALTH CARE AS AN OCCUPATION A small but real occupational risk exists for health care workers. Percutaneous exposure to infected blood or body fluids through a needle-stick injury or nonintact skin is the primary route of transmission. Documented evidence indicates that parenteral exposure poses a 0.3% risk of becoming HIV positive (Carrico, 2001; Tierney et al., 2005). Mucosal exposures, such as splashing in the eyes or mouth, pose a much smaller risk.

POVERTY Poverty increases an individual's risk for HIV/AIDS. Individuals living in poverty have less access to preventive health care and health care education. These individuals also are at risk for increased illiteracy, making print media less effective as a health promotion tool, and are less likely to have access to the Internet as a health promotion tool. Studies suggest that poverty among women, particularly African American women, increases their risk for sexually transmitted diseases overall, primarily because of the resulting power imbalance and related financial dependence on men (CDC, 2008d).

PREGNANCY AND BREAST-FEEDING Many women who are HIV positive choose to avoid pregnancy because of the risk of infecting the fetus and the increased risk of dying before the child is grown. Women who are asymptomatic and become pregnant should be advised that pregnancy is not believed to accelerate the progression of HIV/AIDS, that the use of antiretroviral therapy during pregnancy significantly reduces the risk of transmitting HIV-1 to the fetus, and that most medications used to treat HIV can be safely taken during the pregnancy. Pregnant women who are HIV positive should receive information about known risk factors for perinatal transmission and ways of reducing the risk. Risk factors for perinatal transmission include cigarette smoking, illicit drug use, genital tract infections, and unprotected sexual intercourse with multiple partners (Public Health Service Task Force, 2007).

Following birth, infants often have a positive antibody titer, which reflects the passive transfer of maternal antibodies and does not indicate HIV infection. However, HIV/AIDS may develop in infants whose mothers are seropositive, usually through perinatal transmission. Perinatal transmission can occur transplacentally, at birth (when the infant is exposed to maternal blood and vaginal secretions), and via breast milk. The CDC recommends that in developed countries, women infected with HIV not breast feed because of this risk for transmission. Therefore, if a viable alternative method of feeding is available, it should be used (Venkatesh et al., 2006).

Older Age Adults older than age 50 account for approximately 10% of all reported AIDS cases in the United States (CDC, 2004). Declining immune system function in older adults significantly increases their risk for contracting HIV/AIDS, along with the belief that they cannot be affected. Just as younger persons with HIV/AIDS contract the diseases primarily through sexual intercourse, so do older adults. Because older adults are beyond childbearing years, they often fail to use condoms when engaging in sexual activity. In addition, manifestations of HIV may be overlooked by health care professionals, leading to a delayed diagnosis and increased severity of the disease. As a result of these combined factors, HIV infection in the older adult is likely to be underdiagnosed and underreported. The CDC (2008c) recommends routine HIV screening for all people aged 13 to 64 who have risk factors for infection and counseling about HIV testing for adults aged 64 and older who are at risk. Clients who are uncertain of their risk potential should be counseled to obtain screening.

MYTHS AND MISCONCEPTIONS HIV is not transmitted by casual contact, nor is there any evidence of its transmission by vectors such as mosquitoes. HIV is only transmitted by contact with blood and body fluids. There have been no cases of mosquito- or vector-transmitted infections and the virus lives for a very short time in the body of an insect. Casual contact, in the form of touching, hugging, kissing or breathing the air of an HIV positive person cannot transmit the disease.

Some people believe they do not have to take personal responsibility for preventing the spread of HIV because they think newer antiretroviral medications can protect them. While newer drugs are improving the outcome for clients with HIV, they are not a vaccine to prevent the spread of the disease and the primary means of preventing the spread of infection is personal responsibility, including safer sex practices and avoiding exposure through shared needles or contact with blood and body fluids.

HIV is seen by many as a death sentence. However, newer medications are improving the longevity of people infected with the disease. Early detection of HIV-positive status is important because the antiretrovirals are most effective before the symptoms of AIDS begin. However, even after AIDS symptoms occur antiretrovirals are contributing to a longer and improved life span for infected individuals.

In some communities, a strongly held belief is that HIV is a government conspiracy aimed at eliminating minorities. As discussed in the exemplar on beliefs in the concept of culture, strongly held beliefs may be difficult, if not impossible, to dispel. However, it is believed that higher rates of HIV infection in specific communities may be due to the unavailability of health teaching, medical care, and reduced personal responsibility for behaviors that increase the risk of HIV infection such as unsafe sex practices or drug use with needle sharing.

Finally, many people think that if they don't use IV drugs and they are not homosexual they do not have to worry about HIV infection. However, HIV infection is significant in the heterosexual population, especially among women who are more likely to experience minor tissue tears in the vagina, which serve as portals of entrance for the HIV virus secreted in the semen.

CLINICAL MANIFESTATIONS

The clinical manifestations of HIV infection range from no symptoms at all to severe immunodeficiency with multiple opportunistic infections and cancers (Box 14–4). It appears that the majority of clients develop an acute, mononucleosis-type illness within days to weeks after contracting the virus. Typical manifestations include fever, sore throat, arthralgias and myalgias, headache, rash, and lymphadenopathy. The client also may experience nausea, vomiting, and abdominal cramping. Clients often attribute this initial manifestation of HIV infection to a common viral illness, such as influenza, upper respiratory infection, or stomach virus. Pathologic changes also are noted in the CNS of many infected individuals, although the mechanism of neurologic dysfunction is unclear.

Following this acute illness, clients enter a long-lasting, asymptomatic period. Although the virus is present and can be transmitted to others, the infected host has few or no symptoms. Clearly, the majority of HIV-infected persons are in this stage of the disease. The length of the asymptomatic period varies widely, but its mean duration is estimated to be 8–10 years.

Some clients with few other symptoms following HIV infection, develop persistent generalized lymphadenopathy. This is defined as enlargement of two or more lymph nodes outside the inguinal chain with no other illness or condition to account for the lymphadenopathy.

The move from asymptomatic disease or persistent lymphadenopathy to AIDS often is not clearly defined. The client may complain of general malaise, fever, fatigue, night sweats, and involuntary weight loss. Persistent skin dryness and rash may be a problem. Diarrhea is common, as are oral lesions, such as hairy leukoplakia, candidiasis, and gingival inflammation and ulceration. The development of advanced HIV typically occurs 10 to 11 years after initial infection; this

Box 14–4 **Manifestations of HIV/AIDS**

ACUTE RETROVIRAL SYNDROME OR PRIMARY HIV INFECTION
- Fever
- Sore throat
- Arthralgias and myalgias
- Headache
- Rash
- Nausea, vomiting, and abdominal cramping

ASYMPTOMATIC INFECTION
- None; converts to seropositive status

PERSISTENT GENERALIZED LYMPHADENOPATHY
- Enlargement of two or more extrainguinal sites for more than 3 months

OTHER ACUTE DISEASE SYMPTOMS
- General malaise, fatigue
- Low-grade fever
- Night sweats
- Involuntary weight loss
- Skin dryness or rashes

OTHER DISEASES AND AIDS
- AIDS dementia complex
- Secondary infectious diseases
  - *Pneumocystis carinii* pneumonia
  - *Mycobacterium tuberculosis*
  - *Mycobacterium avium* complex
  - Candidiasis
  - Cryptosporidiosis
  - Cryptococcosis
  - Toxoplasmosis
  - Herpes simplex or herpes zoster
  - Cytomegalovirus
- Secondary cancers
  - Kaposi's sarcoma
  - Non-Hodgkin's lymphoma
  - Cervical dysplasia and cervical cancer
- Other conditions
  - Pelvic inflammatory disease
  - Human papillomavirus

varies according to the viral load, rate of disease progression, and development of resistance to antiretroviral therapy (Kenny, 2004).

With the development of significant constitutional disease, neurologic manifestations, or opportunistic infections or cancers, the client has manifestations that are characteristic of AIDS and a very poor prognosis. HIV/AIDS may be classified by using the CDC's matrix classification system. Under this system, HIV disease is determined by the presence of clinical symptoms (clinical categories A, B, and C) and by T4 cell counts (categories 1, 2, and 3) (Box 14–5). When a client's T4 cell count falls to less than 200/mm³, he or she has late-stage AIDS; a T4 cell count of less than 50/mm³ is end-stage AIDS (Coyne, Lyne, & Watson, 2002).

When clinical manifestations develop, the outcome varies. With antiretroviral therapy, many clients are living longer after being diagnosed with AIDS. **Antiretroviral therapies** stop or suppress the activity of a retrovirus, preventing further weakening of the immune system and thereby minimizing opportunistic infections. Today ***Pneumocystis carinii*** **pneumonia (PCP)** (an opportunistic infection that is not pathogenic in those with intact immune systems) is most commonly diagnosed in those who are undiagnosed, have a late diagnosis of HIV infection, or fail to take prophylactic antibiotics when their CD4 count is less than 200/mm³. Antiretroviral therapy is credited with decreasing the incidence of opportunistic infections and with improving survival (CDC, 2004). The time of survival has increased from approximately 13 months at the start of the AIDS epidemic. Once AIDS is diagnosed in the HIV infected client, survival time is estimated to be 2–3 years; however, survival after diagnosis of HIV-related lymphomas still averages less than 8 months.

AIDS Dementia Complex and Neurologic Effects

Neurologic manifestations of HIV are common, affecting 40–60% of clients with AIDS and including dementia, delirium, and seizures. These manifestations result from both direct effects of the virus on the nervous system and opportunistic infections.

Box 14–5 Classification System for HIV Infection and Expanded AIDS Surveillance Case Definitions for Adolescents and Adults

DIAGNOSTIC CATEGORIES	CLINICAL CATEGORIES		
	A	B	C
CD4 + T-cell Conditions	Asymptomatic, Acute (Primary) HIV or Persistent Generalized Lymphadenopathy (PGL)	Symptomatic, Not (A) or (C) Conditions	AIDS-Indicator Categories
500/mm³	A1	B1	C1
200–499/mm³	A2	B2	C2
< 200/mm³	A3	B3	C3

As of January 1, 1993, people with AIDS-indicator conditions (clinical category C) and those in categories A3 or B3 were considered to have AIDS.

CLINICAL CATEGORY A

One or more of the following conditions in an adolescent or adult with documented HIV infection and without conditions in categories B and C:

- Asymptomatic HIV infection
- Persistent generalized lymphadenopathy
- Acute HIV infection with accompanying illness or history of acute HIV infection

CLINICAL CATEGORY B

Examples of conditions include but are not limited to the following:

- Candidiasis, oral (thrush) or vulvovaginal (persistent, frequent, or poorly responsive to therapy)
- Cervical dysplasia/cervical carcinoma in situ
- Constitutional symptoms, such as fever (38.5°C) or diarrhea exceeding 1 month in duration
- Hairy leukoplakia
- Herpes zoster involving at least two distinct episodes
- Pelvic inflammatory disease
- Peripheral neuropathy

CLINICAL CATEGORY C

- Candidiasis of bronchi, trachea, lungs or esophagus
- Coccidioidomycosis
- Cryptococcosis
- Cryptosporidiosis with persistent diarrhea
- Cytomegalovirus (CMV) infection (other than of liver, spleen, or lymph nodes)
- CMV retinitis
- HIV encephalopathy
- Herpes simplex: chronic ulcers or bronchitis, pneumonitis, or esophagitis
- *Mycobacterium avium* complex or disseminated
- *Mycobacterium tuberculosis*
- *Pneumocystis carinii* pneumonia
- Progressive multifocal leukoencephalopathy
- *Salmonella* septicemia
- Toxoplasmosis of the brain
- Kaposi's sarcoma
- Cervical cancer, invasive
- Lymphoma
- HIV wasting syndrome

Source: Adapted from "Revised Classification System for HIV Infection and Expanded Case Definition for AIDS Among Adolescents and Adults," 1993, *MMWR, CDC Recommendations and Reports, 41*(RR 17), pp. 1–19.

AIDS dementia complex is the most common cause of mental status changes for clients with HIV infection. This dementia results from a direct effect of the virus on the brain and impacts cognitive, motor, and behavioral functioning. Fluctuating memory loss, confusion, difficulty concentrating, lethargy, and diminished motor speed are typical manifestations of AIDS dementia complex. Clients become apathetic, losing interest in work as well as social and recreational activities. As the complex progresses, the client develops severe dementia with motor disturbances, such as ataxia, tremor, spasticity, incontinence, and paraplegia (Kasper et al., 2005; Porth, 2005).

Infections and lesions that are common in clients with AIDS also may affect the CNS. **Toxoplasmosis** and non-Hodgkin's lymphoma are space-occupying lesions that may cause headache, altered mental status, and neurologic deficits. Cryptococcal meningitis and cytomegalovirus infection also are common in people with AIDS. CNS complications have declined with the use of HAART therapy (Tierney et al., 2005).

Peripheral nervous system manifestations also are common in clients infected with HIV. Sensory neuropathies with manifestations of numbness, tingling, and pain in the lower extremities affect approximately 30% of clients with AIDS. A Guillain-Barré type of inflammatory demyelinating polyneuropathy can occur as well, resulting in progressive weakness and paralysis.

Opportunistic Infections

Opportunistic infections are the most common manifestations of AIDS and often occur simultaneously. The risk of opportunistic infections is predictable by the T4 or CD4 cell count. The normal CD4 cell count is greater than 1,000/mm^3. When the CD4 count falls below 500/mm^3, manifestations of immunodeficiency develop. With a CD4 count of less than 200/mm^3, opportunistic infections and cancers are likely.

PNEUMOCYSTIS CARINII PNEUMONIA *Pneumocystis carinii* pneumonia is the most common opportunistic infection affecting clients with AIDS. Approximately 75–80% of clients develop PCP at some point in their disease (Tierney et al., 2005). PCP tends to be recurrent and is the cause of death in approximately 20% of clients with AIDS. It is caused by a common environmental fungus that is not pathogenic in clients with intact immune systems.

Unlike those of many pneumonias, the manifestations of PCP are nonspecific and may progress insidiously. Clients often present with fever, cough, dyspnea, tachypnea, and tachycardia. Complaints of mild chest pain and sputum also may be present. Breath sounds initially may be normal. With severe disease, the client may present with cyanosis and significant respiratory distress.

TUBERCULOSIS An estimated 4% of clients with AIDS develop tuberculosis. In some clients, active tuberculosis results from reactivation of a previous infection; in others, it is a new, primary disease facilitated by impaired immune function. Rapid progression, diffuse pulmonary infiltrates, and disseminated disease occur more commonly in clients with AIDS. Multidrug-resistant strains of tuberculosis present a significant problem (Tierney et al., 2005).

Clients with pulmonary tuberculosis present with a cough productive of purulent sputum, fever, fatigue, weight loss, and lymphadenopathy. Disseminated disease affects the bone marrow, bone, joints, liver, spleen, cerebrospinal fluid, skin, kidneys, gastrointestinal tract, lymph nodes, brain, and other sites.

CANDIDIASIS *Candida albicans* infection, or **candidiasis**, is a common, opportunistic fungal infection in clients with AIDS. It usually manifests as oral thrush or esophagitis. Oral thrush presents as white, friable plaques on the buccal mucosa or tongue and, in the client with HIV infection, often is the first indication of progression to AIDS. Clients with esophagitis have difficulty swallowing as well as substernal pain or burning that increases with swallowing. In women with AIDS, vaginal candidiasis is frequent and often recurrent.

MYCOBACTERIUM AVIUM COMPLEX *Mycobacterium avium* complex (MAC) affects up to 25% of clients with AIDS and typically occurs late in the course of the disease, when CD4 cell counts are less than 50/mm^3. MAC is more common in women than in men. It is caused by organisms commonly found in food, water, and soil and is a major cause of "wasting syndrome" in persons with AIDS (Figure 14–11 ■).

Manifestations of MAC include chills and fever, weakness, night sweats, abdominal pain and diarrhea, and weight loss. Nearly every organ can be infected, and most people with MAC develop disseminated disease.

OTHER INFECTIONS Herpes virus infections are common in clients with AIDS and may be severe. Cytomegalovirus can affect the retina, gastrointestinal tract, or lungs. Disseminated herpes simplex or herpes zoster infection may occur, although severe mucocutaneous manifestations are more common.

Parasitic infections with *Toxoplasma gondii* and *Cryptococcus neoformans* commonly affect the CNS. Toxoplasmosis occurs as encephalitis or an intracerebral mass lesion. Changes in mental status, focal neurologic signs, and seizures may result. *Cryptococcus* infection may present as

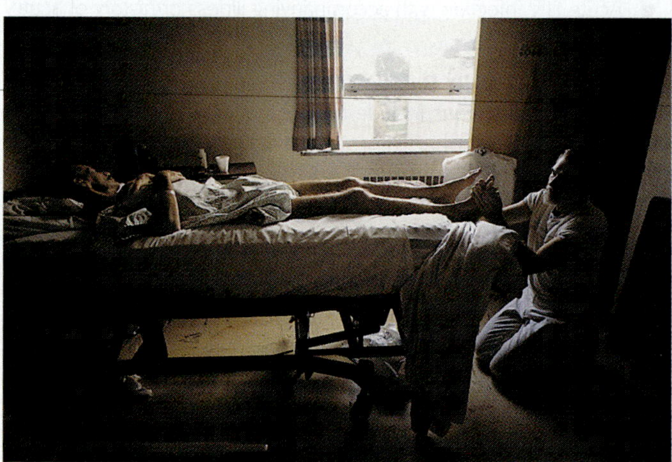

Figure 14–11 ■ Wasting syndrome in a client with AIDS.

either meningitis or disseminated disease, primarily affecting the lungs. *Cryptosporidium,* a protozoon affecting the gastrointestinal tract, is an important cause of prolonged diarrhea in clients with AIDS. Bacterial salmonella infections also are a relatively common cause of diarrhea.

Women with AIDS have a high incidence of pelvic inflammatory disease (PID). Although the pathogens appear to be the same as those in PID affecting women who are not infected with HIV, the disease is more severe. Inpatient treatment with intravenous antibiotics often is necessary.

Secondary Cancers

As cell-mediated immune function declines, the risk of malignancy increases. The CDC classification of AIDS currently includes four cancers: Kaposi's sarcoma, two lymphomas (non-Hodgkin's lymphoma and primary lymphoma of the brain), and invasive cervical carcinoma.

KAPOSI'S SARCOMA Often the presenting symptom of AIDS, **Kaposi's sarcoma (KS)** remains the most common cancer associated with the disease. KS may progress slowly or rapidly, and it is an indicator of late-stage HIV disease. The average survival time after diagnosis of KS is 18 months.

Kaposi's sarcoma is caused by a virus called the KS-associated herpesvirus, also known as human herpesvirus 8. This virus appears to be transmitted mainly through sexual contact, although cases have been reported in injection drug users. Men who have sex with men not only have a risk for HIV infection but also have a higher risk for infection with the virus responsible for KS. Women who have sex with these men have a risk for HIV infection and KS as well. People whose immune system is suppressed because they have received an organ transplant have a 1 in 200 risk of developing KS (American Cancer Society, 2008).

A tumor of the endothelial cells lining small blood vessels, KS presents as vascular macules, papules, or violet lesions affecting the skin and viscera (Figure 14–12 ■). A common site for skin lesions is the face, especially the tip of the nose and pinnae of the ears. Common sites for visceral disease include the gastrointestinal tract, lungs, and lymphatic system.

The lesions of KS usually are painless initially, but they may become painful as the disease progresses. Internally, the tumors may obstruct organ function or cause bleeding. When the lungs are involved, gas exchange may be severely impaired, resulting in pulmonary hemorrhage.

LYMPHOMAS Lymphomas are malignancies of the lymphoid tissue, including lymphocytes, lymph nodes, and the lymphoid organs, such as the spleen and bone marrow. In clients with AIDS, two lymphomas are common: non-Hodgkin's lymphoma (including Burkitt's lymphoma) and primary lymphoma of the brain. Hodgkin's disease also occurs five times more frequently in clients with HIV infection than in those without. The CNS is the usual site for these lymphomas, but they also may be found in the bone marrow, gastrointestinal tract, liver, skin, and mucous membranes. These malignancies are aggressive tumors that grow and spread rapidly. Headache and changes in mental status are common early symptoms of lymphomas affecting the CNS.

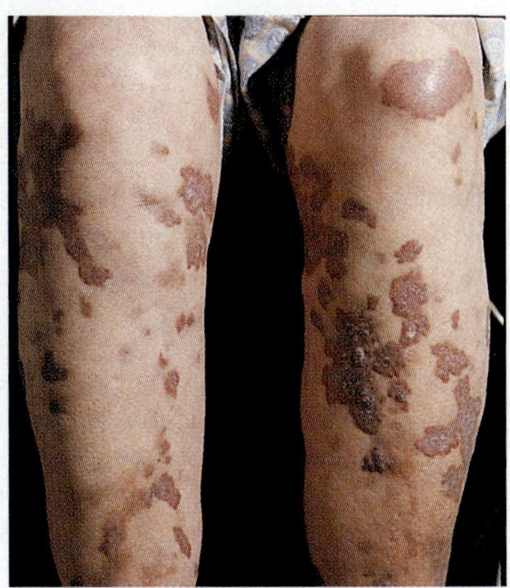

Figure 14–12 ■ Kaposi's sarcoma lesions.

Source: Zeva Oelbaum/Peter Arnold, Inc.

CERVICAL CANCER Of women infected with HIV, 40% have cervical dysplasia. Cervical cancer develops frequently and tends to be aggressive. Women with concurrent HIV infection and cervical cancer usually die of the cervical cancer, not AIDS. Therefore, it is recommended that women with HIV infection have Papanicolaou (Pap) smears every 6 months and aggressive treatment of cervical dysplasia with colposcopic examination and cone biopsy.

Pediatric Manifestations

The neonate with HIV infection is asymptomatic at birth. The time period for development of opportunistic infections varies; however, the interval from HIV infection to the onset of overt AIDS is shorter in children than in adults. This interval is even shorter in children infected perinatally than in those infected through transfusion.

Opportunistic diseases such as gram-negative sepsis and problems associated with prematurity are the primary causes of mortality in babies infected with HIV. Some infants infected by maternal-fetal transmission suffer from severe immunodeficiency, with HIV disease progressing more rapidly during the first year of life. Many newborns exposed to HIV/AIDS are premature, small for gestational age (SGA), or both and show evidence of failure to thrive during the neonatal and infant periods. They can show signs and symptoms of disease within days of birth. Signs that may be seen during early infancy include enlarged spleen and liver, swollen glands, recurrent respiratory infections, rhinorrhea, interstitial pneumonia (rarely seen in adults), recurrent gastrointestinal manifestations (diarrhea and weight loss) and urinary system infections, persistent or recurrent oral candidiasis infections, and loss of achieved developmental milestones (Venkatesh et al., 2006). A high risk of acquiring *Pneumocystis carnii* pneumonia also exists.

Most children with AIDS have nonspecific findings, including lymphadenopathy, hepatosplenomegaly, nephropathy, oral candidiasis, failure to thrive and weight loss, diarrhea, chronic eczema and dermatitis, and fever. Specific symptoms often appear within approximately 2 years of infection and include conjunctivitis, ear infections, and tonsillitis.

CLINICAL MANIFESTATIONS AND THERAPIES **HIV/AIDS**

ETIOLOGY	CLINICAL MANIFESTATION	CLINICAL THERAPIES
Opportunistic infections result from diminished immune response, including:	Manifestations are dependent on where the infection occurs and on the severity of infection, often related to effectiveness of immune response.	■ Therapy depends on the level of immune function and severity of disease as well as on consideration of comorbid conditions (e.g., liver or kidney disease).
Kaposi's sarcoma	Most common AIDS-related cancer, frequently seen in gay and bisexual men, usually manifests as red to purple lesions on the skin but also can be found on internal organs, including the lymph nodes, mouth, GI tract, and lungs. The CDC considers this an AIDS-defining condition.	■ Liposomal daunorubicin, liposomal doxorubicin ■ Recombinant human alpha interferon if CD4 $> 200/mm^3$ ■ Radiation therapy
Cytomegalovirus (CMV)	While 50% of adults are infected with CMV, the normal immune system usually can keep it under control. In clients with AIDS and with ineffective immune systems, CMV can infect the eyes, brain, throat, large intestines, stomach, or spinal cord.	■ Preventative therapy or treatment may include administration of cidofovir, ganciclovir, foscarnet, or fomivirsen. ■ Approximately 10% have a strain resistant to ganciclovir.
Candidiasis	Most common HIV-related fungal infection, involving the mucous membranes around the mouth, vagina, esophagus, and skin. Manifests as white bumps, dry mouth, difficulty swallowing, and altered sense of taste. The CDC considers this an AIDS-related complex (ARC) disease.	■ Oral thrush is treated with fluconazole, clotrimazole, ketoconazole, nystatin. ■ Esophageal candidiasis is treated with fluconazole, ketoconazole, itraconazole. ■ Vaginal candidiasis is treated with over-the-counter antifungal remedies, clotrimazole, miconazole.
Aspergillosis	A fungal pathogen found in soil and decaying plant life, more commonly seen in clients with cancer receiving chemotherapy and clients receiving a transplant but may be seen in clients with HIV infection. Manifests with cough, chest pain, shortness of breath, facial pain, fever, and night sweats.	■ Amphotericin B ■ Itraconazole
Histoplasmosis	Infection occurs by inhaling the fungus, infecting the lungs, but can also affect other internal organs. Symptoms include fever, skin lesions, breathing problems, weight loss, and liver enlargement. The CDC considers this an AIDS-defining condition.	■ Clinical trials are underway studying the effect of itraconazole as prophylaxis therapy. ■ Treatment may include amphotericin B or itraconazole and requires long-term maintenance therapy.
Mycobacterium avium complex	In clients who are not HIV positive, this infection normally involves only the lungs, but in clients with HIV infection, the disease usually disseminates and often is seen in those with late-stage AIDS involving the liver, spleen, and bone marrow. Resulting symptoms include night sweats, fevers, unintentional weight loss, diarrhea, low red and white blood cell counts, elevated alkaline phosphate, and painful intestines.	■ Clarithromycin ■ Azithromycin ■ Ethambutol ■ Rifampin ■ Rifabutin ■ Ciprofloxacin ■ Amikacin
Tuberculosis (TB)	Infection occurs from contact with clients who are TB positive and often occurs early in the course of HIV infection, often months or years before other opportunistic infections occur, and may be the first indication of HIV infection. In later stages of HIV infection, TB often infects other organs outside the lungs. Multidrug-resistant TB is of particular concern. Symptoms include cough, fever, night sweats, weight loss, and fatigue.	■ Prophylaxis usually is isoniazid. ■ Treatment may include multiple drug, including some combination of isoniazid, rifampin, pyrazinamide, and ethambutol.
Oral hairy leukoplakia	Often the first opportunistic infection to appear, symptoms include white lesions on the edges of the tongue caused by Epstein-Barr virus. Occurs almost exclusively in men and indicates serious damage to the immune system. The CDC considers this a category B-defining illness.	■ Acyclovir or topical podophyllin resin

CLINICAL MANIFESTATIONS AND THERAPIES **HIV/AIDS (continued)**

ETIOLOGY	CLINICAL MANIFESTATION	CLINICAL THERAPIES
NEUROLOGIC DISORDERS SEEN IN SOME CLIENTS DIAGNOSED WITH HIV/AIDS INCLUDE:		
AIDS dementia complex	Caused directly by the HIV infection, but the central nervous system also can be damaged by opportunistic infections or toxic effects of drug treatments. Early symptoms include dementia, apathy, and loss of interest in surroundings. Later symptoms involve cognitive and motor problems, resulting in memory loss and mobility issues. The CDC considerers HIV encephalopathy an AIDS-defining condition.	■ Zidovudine
Peripheral neuropathy	Severe burning, aching pain in the feet and legs that may prevent walking. Most commonly seen is sensory neuropathy (distal symmetric polyneuropathy). A less frequent but more severe type is acute or chronic inflammatory demyelinating polyneuropathy. Drug-induced or toxic neuropathies can be very painful. CMV-related neurologic syndromes include encephalitis, myelitis, and polyradiculopathy.	■ Acetyl-carnitine from vitamin stores may reduce symptoms.
GASTROESOPHAGEAL DISORDERS MAY INCLUDE:		
Diarrhea	May be caused by infection, lactose intolerance, pancreatic issues, medications, or emotional stress.	■ Avoid diarrhea-causing foods, such as dairy, fatty, or spicy foods and foods high in insoluble fiber. ■ Eat bananas, plain white rice, applesauce, cream of wheat, toasted white bread, crackers, plain pasta, boiled eggs, oatmeal, mashed potatoes, or yogurt. Soluble fiber has been proven to reduce therapy related diarrhea (Heiser, et. al. 2004), ■ Over-the-counter products such as l-glutamine, bismuth subsalicylate, attapulgite, or loperamide may help treat the symptoms. Acidophilus capsules, peppermint, ginger, and nutmeg are believed to help with digestive problems. Studies have shown calcium supplements also are helpful.
Malabsorption	Fairly common with advanced AIDS, reduces absorption of nutrients and medications taken orally. Results from gastrointestinal infections and other health problems, causing weight loss, fatigue, anemia, and malnutrition.	■ Careful monitoring of nutritional status, administration of vitamin supplements, increased intake of calories, and administration of IV total parenteral nutrition may help to improve nutritional status.

Source: AEGiS. (2006). *Opportunistic Infections*. Retrieved June 1, 2009, from http://www.aegis.com/topics/oi/

Bacterial and opportunistic infections, such as *Streptococcus*, *Haemophilus influenzae*, *Salmonella,* and PCP, as well as malignancies, such as lymphoma, frequently occur in children as the disease progresses. Lymphocytic interstitial pneumonitis is a common manifestation of pediatric AIDS, and children often develop encephalopathy, resulting in developmental delay or a deterioration of motor skills and intellectual functioning. Approximately 75% of new cases of HIV in adolescents occur in minority populations, such as Blacks and Hispanics, so teaching methods to avoid infection must be strongly emphasized in these groups (Rangel, Gavin, Reed, Fowler, & Lee, 2006).

CLINICAL MANIFESTATIONS AND THERAPIES **Pediatric HIV**

ETIOLOGY	CLINICAL MANIFESTATION	CLINICAL THERAPIES
Frequent, chronic, or unusual infections because of poor immune response	Chronic bilateral otitis media Oral candidiasis *Pneumocystis carinii* pneumonia (PCP) Skin disorders Fever	■ Vigorous antimicrobial therapy for treatment of infections ■ Limit exposure to groups of people ■ Obtain recommended immunizations
Poor nutritional intake because of lack of appetite resulting from disease and medications	Failure to thrive (eating disorder of childhood) Weight and body mass index below 10th percentile Chronic diarrhea Skin irritation	■ Monitor growth ■ Supplemental intake such as enteral feedings at night, and TPN if needed ■ Meticulous skin care to prevent breakdown
Immune system overgrowth to compensate for lack of proper immune response	Hepatosplenomegaly and lymphadenopathy	■ Assess abdomen frequently ■ Teach about safe transport to avoid injury to liver and spleen

COLLABORATION

Although multiple research studies to identify a cure for HIV/AIDS are underway, no cure is currently available. This fact, plus the apparent universally fatal nature of the disease, make prevention a vital strategy in HIV care. However, new treatments are under investigation (Box 14–6).

The goals of care for the client with HIV disease are as follows:

- Early identification of the infection
- Promoting health maintenance activities to prolong the asymptomatic period for as long as possible
- Prevention of opportunistic infections
- Treatment of disease complications, such as cancers
- Providing emotional and psychosocial support.

Collaboration among physicians and nurses treating clients with HIV/AIDS is essential. Because of the number of medications that some clients may need to take, regular consultation with a pharmacist will help to ensure a client is not taking any medications that are contraindicated. Nurses should encourage clients with HIV/AIDS to use a single pharmacy to fill prescriptions, which will decrease further the possibility of taking contraindicated medications.

Nurses may find themselves collaborating with homeless shelter directors and other nonprofits to provide preventive education to communities whose members have an unusually high risk for contracting HIV/AIDS. Counselors and religious leaders can provide support and leadership to clients with HIV infection and their families.

Box 14–6 **Investigational Immune-Based Treatment for HIV**

Infection with HIV progressively alters the function of and destroys CD4 lymphocytes. CD4+ cells are essential to proper functioning of the immune system, including the body's ability to respond to infections. These cells initiate, direct, and regulate immune responses and may directly attack infected cells as well. They also are a source of cytokines, the chemical messengers of the immune system.

Destruction of CD4+ cells by HIV devastates the immune system, facilitating the development of fatal infections and neoplasms in the infected person. Immune-based treatments indirectly affect HIV by improving the function of the immune system through actions that inhibit cytokines, replenish cytokines, or restore immune function. These treatments, used alone or in combination with antiretroviral drugs, are being investigated for use in the treatment of clients with HIV.

INHIBITING CYTOKINES

Tumor necrosis factor alpha (TNF-α) is a cytokine secreted by activated monocytes and macrophages in response to infection, infestation, or tumor growth. It causes a proliferation of B cells and T cells. However, high levels of this cytokine actually may facilitate the development of disease by blocking the normal inflammatory response. It is believed that blocking the effect of TNF-α can suppress HIV production, although caution must be used.

REPLENISHING CYTOKINES

Some cytokines (interleukin-2, interleukin-12, and interferon alpha) may be helpful in treating HIV infection by stimulating the production of killer cells as well as increasing the function of lymphocytes. The interferons are part of the body's first line of defense against viruses. All these agents have toxic side effects, however, and require careful nursing assessment and care.

RESTORING IMMUNE SYSTEM FUNCTION

Infection with HIV not only destroys CD4+ cells; it also eventually destroys the lymphoid organs, such as bone marrow and the thymus gland. Lymphocytes, including the CD4+ cells, are derived from stem cells in bone marrow and mature in the thymus. Two investigational treatments to restore the immune system are bone marrow transplant and thymus transplant. Bone marrow transplants have been used to correct other types of immune disorders (e.g., leukemia or lymphoma) but have yet to be effective in persons with HIV. A few thymus transplants have been done in persons infected with HIV but have provided only temporary benefits.

Nurses also may find themselves collaborating with day care directors and teachers, school staff, and even camp personnel to ensure the health and safety not only of a child with HIV/AIDS but also of center's personnel. Nurses should instruct staff in these centers about the use of standard precautions in handling blood and body fluids. Nurses also should assist child care centers in establishing procedures to notify all parents when a child with an infectious disease has been at the center. Parents of immunocompromised children can then take any necessary precautions to minimize the chances of their children becoming ill. Parents of children with HIV infection must be very cautious to limit the exposure of their children to infectious diseases.

Diagnostic Tests

Diagnostic testing is used to screen and identify HIV infection as well as to monitor the client's disease and immune status. The likelihood that a positive screening test truly indicates the presence of HIV infection decreases as HIV prevalence in the tested population becomes lower. Therefore, false-positive HIV test results are more likely in settings where the tested population prevalence is lower than in settings where the tested population prevalence is higher. When a preliminary, positive rapid test is explained to clients, phrases like "a good chance of being infected" or "very likely infected" can be used to indicate the likelihood of HIV infection and qualified based on the HIV prevalence in that particular setting and the client's individual risk.

RAPID DIAGNOSTIC TESTS The FDA has licensed more than one rapid test. These tests are widely used, because the results can be given immediately. Immediate notification of results is critical, because many clients who are tested for HIV do not return to learn the results. Also, many cannot be located to be given the test results and educated about safe behaviors whether they are positive or negative for HIV. Although confirmation of results is dependent on testing with a second source, such as an enzyme-linked immunosorbent assay or a Western blot test, learning the results immediately gives the client more information to make wise choices about his or her behaviors and self-care.

Further testing is always required to confirm a reactive or rapid screening test result. The following diagnostic tests may be ordered:

- *Enzyme-linked immunosorbent assay (ELISA):* This is the most widely used screening test for HIV infection. Developed in 1985 to screen blood donors, ELISA tests for HIV antibodies; it does not detect the virus itself. Therefore, a client may have a negative ELISA test early in the course of infection, before detectable antibodies have developed. The test has a sensitivity of 99.5% or higher when performed at least 13 weeks after infection. This means that more than 99.5% of tests performed on blood containing HIV antibodies will show a positive result. False-positives results can occur, however, so an initial positive result is always tested repeatedly and confirmed using a different method of antibody detection, usually the Western blot.
- *Western blot antibody testing:* This is more reliable than ELISA but is more time-consuming and more expensive. When combined with ELISA, however, a specificity of greater than 99.9% is achieved. Specificity is a measure of the probability that a negative test result indicates no antibodies are present. In this test, the client's serum is mixed with HIV proteins to detect a reaction. If antibodies to HIV are present, a detectable antigen–antibody response will occur.
- *HIV viral load tests:* These tests measure the amount of actively replicating HIV. Levels correlate with disease progression and with response to antiretroviral medications. Levels of greater than 5,000 to 10,000 copies/mL indicate the need for treatment.
- *CBC:* This test is performed to detect anemia, leukopenia, and thrombocytopenia, which often are present in clients with HIV infection. Lymphopenia (or low levels of lymphocytes) is especially common in those with this disease.
- *CD4 cell count:* This is the most widely used test to monitor progress of the disease and to guide therapy. The CD4 cell count correlates very closely with the immunodeficiency disorders seen in clients with AIDS. Today, AIDS is defined not only by the presence of opportunistic infections and other diseases indicative of immunodeficiency but also by HIV-seropositive status and a CD4 count of less than 200/mm^3 or a percentage of CD4 lymphocytes of less than 14%. CD4 counts are recommended every 3 to 6 months for all people with HIV disease.

Two screening tests also have been developed that are useful for assessing the HIV status of women who did not receive prenatal care before labor and for women in active labor who do not know their HIV status. These tests (OraQuick HIV-1 Antibody Test and the SUDS HIV-1 Test) require a small blood sample, can be read in 20 minutes, and are very sensitive and specific (Lachat, Scott, & Relf, 2006).

OTHER DIAGNOSTIC TESTS In addition to these widely used tests, several other diagnostic tests may be performed. These include the following:

- *Blood culture for HIV:* This provides the most specific diagnosis, but it is an expensive and cumbersome test and is not widely available in the United States.
- *Immune-complex-dissociated p24 assay:* This is a test for p24 (HIV) antigen in the blood. This antigen indicates active reproduction of HIV and tends to be positive before seroconversion and with advanced disease. It is most useful in monitoring disease progression and the antiviral activity of experimental medications (Pagana & Pagana, 2002; Tierney et al., 2005).

Still other diagnostic tests are used primarily to detect secondary cancers and opportunistic infections in the client with HIV. The tests ordered are both general and specific to the client's manifestations and may include the following:

- *Tuberculin skin testing* to detect possible tuberculosis infection
- *Magnetic resonance imaging* of the brain to identify lymphomas
- *Specific cultures and serologic examinations for opportunistic infections* such as PCP, toxoplasmosis, and others
- *Pap smears* every 6 months for early detection of cervical cancer in women with cervical dysplasia (Tierney et al., 2005).

PEDIATRIC TESTING Early identification of babies either with HIV infection or at risk for HIV/AIDS is essential during the newborn period. However, the currently available HIV serologic tests (ELISA and Western blot) cannot distinguish between maternal and infant antibodies. It may take up to 18 months for infected infants to form their own antibodies to HIV (Read & Committee on Pediatric AIDS, 2007); therefore, these tests are inappropriate for infants up to 18 months of age. Testing by HIV DNA polymerase chain reaction (PCR) is the preferred test. Results can be made available within 24 hours (Venkatesh et al., 2006). A viral culture also may be performed at birth, but this test is more expensive. The first DNA PCR test should be performed on the newborn of a mother with HIV infection during the first 48 hours after birth. Umbilical cord blood should not be used for HIV testing because of possible contamination with maternal blood (AAP Committee on Fetus and Newborn & ACOG, 2007). If PCR and viral culture are unavailable, the acid-dissociated p24 antigen may be used to assess HIV infection status in infants older than 1 month (Bernstein, 2007; Cloherty, Eichenwald, & Stark, 2008). A second test should be performed at 1–2 months of age, and a third test is recommended at 2–4 months of age. An infant is considered to be infected if two separate samples are positive (AAP Commitee on Fetus and Newborn & ACOG, 2007). Most clinicians confirm the absence of HIV infection with a negative HIV antibody assay result at 12–18 months of age (Read & Committee on Pediatric AIDS, 2007).

Most children with AIDS are diagnosed early in life. Serologic tests for detection of the virus, performed within 48 hours of birth, are monitored in infants born to mothers who are HIV positive. Infants with initially negative tests should be retested at 1–2 months. Tests are again repeated at 3 and 6 months, and then again at 15 and 18 months. The preferred test is the PCR; other tests include p24 antigen or HIV culture, which is not universally available. Any positive result is confirmed by retesting. When the infant has had two negative tests, testing with ELISA (for HIV antibody) should be done at 12, 15, and 18 months. After two consecutive negative ELISA results, the child is considered to be free of HIV. In addition, a CBC and CD4 T-cell subset is performed at 3 to 6 months of age. A quick-response HIV test using saliva is available for use in certain circumstances as well; positive results are checked with blood studies (Box 14–7). The CDC considers children under 13 years of age to be infected if their symptoms meet the CDC criteria for AIDS, if they have HIV in the blood or tissues, or if they have antibodies to HIV. The CDC criteria address two issues: the diagnosis of HIV and the clinical classification of children infected with HIV (Box 14–8).

Box 14–7 **HIV Testing**

Many people who are at risk of HIV infection may not have HIV testing readily available. To reduce barriers to early detection of the virus, rapid HIV tests have been developed. Specimens are obtained from saliva or fingerstick for a blood sample. Oral fluids are obtained by gently swabbing both the upper and lower outer gum of the mouth. Some options include OraQuick Rapid HIV-1/2 Antibody Test, Reveal Rapid HIV-1 Antibody Test, Uni-Gold Recombigen HIV Test, and Multispot HIV-1/HIV-2 Rapid Test. Because results are available in 1 hour or less, these tests require preparedness for counseling in the same session as the test is administered. Positive results are confirmed using traditional methods.

Source: CDC. (2006e); Greenwald, Burstein, Pincus, & Branson, 2006.

Box 14–8 **Clinical Staging of Pediatric HIV Infection**

DIAGNOSIS OF HIV INFECTION IN CHILDREN

- HIV infected (two or more positive tests for HIV or demonstrates AIDS)
- Perinatally exposed (born to a mother known to be infected with HIV)
- Seroconverter (born to a mother known to be infected with HIV but has had two negative HIV tests)

When Infected, the Child with HIV is Classified as

- Category N—not symptomatic
- Category A—mildly symptomatic with two or more of the following:
  - Lymphadenopathy
  - Hepatomegaly
  - Splenomegaly
  - Dermatitis
  - Parotitis
  - Recurrent or persistent upper respiratory infection, sinusitis, or otitis media
- Category B—moderately symptomatic with additional symptoms to those previously listed, such as:
  - Anemia
  - Bacterial meningitis, pneumonia, sepsis
  - Candidiasis
  - Cardiomyopathy
  - Cytomegalovirus
  - Diarrhea
  - Hepatitis
  - Herpes simplex virus, herpes zoster
  - Leiomyosarcoma
  - Nephropathy
  - Persistent fever
  - Toxoplasmosis
- Category C—severely symptomatic, manifested by
  - Multiple, recurrent infection
  - Encephalopathy
  - Kaposi's sarcoma
  - Lymphoma
  - Wasting syndrome

Note: From American Academy of Pediatrics, 2006.

Pharmacologic Therapies

As more antiretroviral medications have been developed, a wide array of options has emerged. Highly active antiretroviral therapy, or HAART, is a treatment approach that uses a minimum of three antiretroviral agents. It generally includes zidovudine (Retrovir, AZT), an NRTI, plus a second NRTI, such as didanosine or lamivudine, combined with a nonnucleoside reverse transcriptase inhibitor (NNRTI), such as nevirapine, or a protease inhibitor (PI), such as indinavir, ritonavir, or saquinavir.

Testing for HIV antiretroviral drug resistance is recommended before beginning treatment in pregnant women who are infected but who do not require treatment for their own health. When possible, treatment of these women is delayed until after the first trimester. Women who are infected with HIV and are already receiving HAART when they become pregnant are advised to continue their current regimen if it is effective, but they should not receive drugs such as efavirenz (EFV), which have known teratogenic effects (Public Health Service Task Force, 2007).

Treatment recommendations also have been developed for the mother and infant for the intrapartum and postpartum periods. The decision about which regimen is most appropriate should be determined following discussion with the woman about the risks and benefits based on her individual HIV status.

For term infants, AZT is started prophylactically 2 mg/kg po every 6 hours (Nash & Smith, 2008). If the infant is confirmed to be HIV positive, AZT is changed to a multidrug anti-retro-viral regimen.

Pharmacologic treatment of HIV disease has four primary foci:

1. To suppress the infection itself, decreasing symptoms and prolonging life
2. To provide prophylaxis of opportunistic infections
3. To stimulate hematopoietic response
4. To treat opportunistic infections and malignancies.

Effectiveness of treatment is monitored by viral load and CD4 cell counts; positive results are indicated by a reduction in viral load along with preserving the CD4 count above 350/mm^3. Treatment is recommended when the CD4 count falls below 200/mm^3. Clients with symptoms of severe disease are treated regardless of their CD4 level or viral load, so monitoring these individuals may reveal higher levels of CD4 or lower viral load. Initiating therapy in asymptomatic individuals with higher CD4 levels did not show a protective effect and was thought to perhaps increase viral resistance. Today, the drugs have been combined and the dosing schedules simplified, which helps clients to adhere to medication administration schedules. Currently, researchers are using clinical trials of asymptomatic clients receiving HAART to evaluate alternating-drug regimens to prevent drug resistance by the viral organisms (Martinez-Picado et al., 2003).

Four classes of drugs used in antiretroviral treatment include NRTIs, NNRTIs, PIs, and entry inhibitors. HAART combines three or four antiretroviral drugs to reduce the incidence of drug resistance. Combination therapies increase the likelihood of decreasing viral load and symptoms but also burden clients with complicated and expensive medication schedules. Clients beginning the HAART protocol must understand the benefits, risks, costs, and effects on daily life. HAART does not eradicate HIV infection, and the medications are expensive. The newer triple combinations, such as Trizivir, cost approximately $1,030 for a 30-day supply of 60 doses. This costs approximately $13,400 per year, and it does not include the costs of medications to prevent or treat opportunistic infections or cancer (Tierney et al., 2005). These medications also are scheduled for specific times throughout the day; therefore, leading a normal life becomes a challenge. In addition, all HAART medications cause major adverse reactions leading to less-than-perfect adherence, as with most chronic diseases. In this case, however, the outcome could be fatal.

Each client must be able to adhere to the treatment regimen. It may be preferable to delay initiating therapy until the client is able to agree to adhere so that irregular dosing does not lead to viral resistance. Some providers gauge client ability to follow the HAART regimen by the client's success with prophylaxis for an opportunistic infection.

Several methods to promote and ensure adherence are being used and studied. One such approach is the use of electronic monitoring devices (Bova et al., 2005). By placing a microprocessor in a medication cap, records are created of the time, date, and frequency of bottle opening. Although this method does not guarantee that the medication will be taken even if the cap is removed, the record created is a source for follow-up and discussion between the provider and the client. Whether the client is asked to keep a diary of taking the medication, using an electronic monitoring device, to keep a record or relying on pill count, adherence to the medication regimen is critically important.

Some clients undergoing HAART are developing body composition changes and metabolic abnormalities associated with the therapy, especially that involving the PIs. Increased fat deposition in the midsection, breasts, and neck with atrophy in the face, buttocks, and extremities describes the body composition changes; metabolic abnormalities include increased low-density lipoprotein cholesterol and triglycerides as well as insulin resistance. The combination of changes is consistent with metabolic syndrome, which increases the risk of cardiovascular disease and diabetes. These conditions commonly are treated with medications. Robinson (2005) has observed these serious changes in clients who are HIV positive and hopes to prevent and treat the changes with diet and exercise—that is, without adding to the polypharmacy already experienced by those undergoing HAART.

NUCLEOSIDE REVERSE TRANSCRIPTASE INHIBITORS The NRTIs (also called nucleoside analogues) inhibit the action of viral reverse transcriptase, a retroviral enzyme that catalyzes the substrates for conversion and copying of viral RNA to DNA sequences. This enzyme is necessary for viral integration into cellular DNA and replication. The nucleoside analogues act as a chemical decoy for building blocks in the formation of the DNA copy, preventing the RNA from being copied into DNA. Each drug substitutes for a particular nucleoside base at different points on the chain. See the guidelines in Box 14–9 for medication administration of this group of drugs.

Zidovudine was the first antiretroviral agent approved for use with HIV infection. It remains in widespread use and has been shown to decrease symptoms and prolong the lives of clients with AIDS. Zidovudine often is given to clients with a CD4 cell count of less than 500/mm^3 because of evidence that it slows the progression to severe disease (Tierney et al., 2005). Zidovudine also may be used prophylactically following a documented parenteral exposure to HIV. It is used in combination with didanosine, ddC, or 3TC.

- Didanosine (ddI, Videx) also inhibits reverse transcriptase and viral replication. It is used in combination therapy with AZT.

Box 14–9 Antiretroviral Nucleoside Analogues

ZIDOVUDINE (AZT, AZIDOTHYMIDINE)

Zidovudine was the first antiretroviral agent developed to treat HIV infection. It interferes with reverse transcriptase, thus inhibiting replication of the virus. The usual dose is 300 mg twice daily. It is administered orally. Dose-limiting side effects are anemia and neutropenia.

Nursing Responsibilities

- Assess for possible contraindications to therapy, including allergic response or a CD4 count of greater than 350/mm^3.
- Administer by mouth, instructing the client to swallow capsules whole.
- Assess for adverse effects. Nausea and headache are common. They may be self-limiting, decreasing with time, or significant and continuing, necessitating a change of therapy. Nausea and neutropenia are treated with erythropoietin (Epoetin Alfa) and granulocyte colony-stimulating factor (filgrastim).
- Assess CBC with differential and creatine phosphokinase. Notify the physician of significant changes.

Health Education for the Client and Family

- Zidovudine will not cure HIV infection, but it will slow its progress and reduce significant symptoms.
- Take the drug at least 0.5 hour before or 1 hour after meals if tolerated.
- As with all antiretroviral drugs, it is important to emphasize that the client is still infective and can pass the infection to others. Clients should use safer sex practices and other measures to prevent transmission to partners and should not donate blood or breast-feed.
- Notify the physician if signs of an infection or adverse response to zidovudine develop. These include sore throat, swollen lymph glands, and fever; unusual fatigue or weakness; easy bruising, bleeding gums, or an injury that will not heal; persistent or intractable nausea; and muscle pain or wasting.
- Continue all scheduled follow-up visits and laboratory studies to monitor for drug toxicity.
- Have the client check with the physician before taking any other prescription or over-the-counter drug.

DIDANOSINE (DDI, VIDEX)

As with zidovudine, didanosine does not kill HIV; rather, the drug inhibits its replication within the cells. Its activity is similar to that of zidovudine. Didanosine has been shown to increase CD4 cell counts and to lower p24 antigen levels (Tierney et al., 2005). Didanosine is used alone for clients who are intolerant or resistant to zidovudine. It also is used with zidovudine in combination therapy regimens. Didanosine does not cause the anemia associated with zidovudine, but it may cause neutropenia. Didanosine also is associated with an increased risk of pancreatitis, peripheral neuropathy, and dry mouth.

Nursing Responsibilities

- Assess for possible contraindications to didanosine therapy, including previous episodes of pancreatitis and impaired renal or liver function.
- Administer as directed. Tablets are to be chewed thoroughly or dissolved in 1 oz of water at room temperature. The powder form is dissolved in water before administration, and diarrhea is attributable to the buffering agent used in this formula.
- Administer with caution to clients taking vincristine, rifampin, pentamidine, ethambutol, or metronidazole; the action of both drugs may be affected by concurrent administration. Intravenous pentamidine and trimethoprim-sulfamethoxazole taken concurrently may increase the risk of acute and fatal pancreatitis.
- Didanosine interferes with the absorption of ketoconazole and dapsone. Doses of these drugs should be scheduled at least 2 hours apart from doses of didanosine.
- Evaluate for therapeutic response and possible adverse effects. Notify the physician if manifestations of peripheral neuropathy, diarrhea, depression, or other adverse effects develop.
- Stop the drug and notify the physician immediately if the client develops manifestations of pancreatitis or hepatic failure, including nausea and vomiting, severe abdominal pain, elevated bilirubin, or elevated serum enzymes (e.g., amylase, aspartate aminotransferase, and alanine aminotransferase).

Health Education for the Client and Family

- Take the drug as directed. The prescribed two-tablet dose always must be taken to get the required amount of antacid to prevent the drug from being destroyed by stomach acid.
- Take on an empty stomach, at least 1 hour before or 2 hours after meals.
- Do not use alcohol while taking didanosine; alcohol may increase the risk of pancreatitis.
- Stop the drug and call the doctor immediately if nausea, vomiting, abdominal pain, or diarrhea develops. These may indicate pancreatitis.
- Call the doctor if extremity pain, weakness, numbness, or tingling occurs. These side effects usually disappear when didanosine is discontinued.
- Other side effects to report to the physician include unusual bleeding or bruising, fatigue, weakness, fever, or persistent sore throat.

ABACAVIR

Abacavir is a nucleoside analogue with activity against some HIV strains that are resistant to other nucleoside drugs. It is prepared in combination with zidovudine and lamivudine (Trizivir), and one tablet is taken twice daily. This combination drug is composed exclusively of nucleoside analogues; it lacks NNRTIs or PIs. As such, it is less effective at decreasing viral load and allowing immune system enhancement, but the ease of administration makes it a useful drug for clients who cannot adhere to more complex regimens. The main toxicity is a hypersensitivity response in approximately 5% of clients, which manifests with flulike symptoms. Avoid repeated use in those individuals.

Nursing Responsibilities

- Assess for possible hypersensitivity reactions, anemia, and neutropenia.
- Evaluate for desired effect of increased CD4 counts and lower blood levels of p24 antigen.
- Notify the physician if the client develops evidence of pancreatitis, impaired hepatic function, or painful peripheral neuropathy.

Health Education for the Client and Family

- Take without regard to food or water.
- Have the client check with the physician before taking any other prescription or over-the-counter medication.
- Report all signs and symptoms of hypersensitivity to this drug.
- Report to the physician any signs of infection or changes in condition.

- Stavudine (d4T, Zerit) is a retroviral inhibitor that has been shown to increase CD4 cell counts and decrease serum p24 antigen levels. Current use is for clients who are intolerant of AZT.
- Lamivudine (3-TC, Epivir) is used for low CD4 cell counts or symptomatic disease as a first-line treatment in combination with AZT.
- Abacavir (Ziagen) is a potent inhibitor of reverse transcriptase; however, it may cause serious hypersensitivity reactions.
- Zidovudine plus lamivudine (Combivir) is a combination drug used to decrease zidovudine-resistant HIV strains.

PROTEASE INHIBITORS Protease is a viral enzyme necessary in the formation of specific viral protein needs for viral assembly and maturation. PIs bond chemically with protease to block the function of the enzyme and result in the production of immature, noninfectious viral particles. When combined with other antiviral drugs, these chemicals increase the chance of eliminating the virus by interfering with different stages of its life cycle. Viral resistance occurs rather quickly, however. PIs inhibit and induce metabolism of other drugs, so their use with other medications as well as the dose of those medications must be carefully planned. Some drugs will circulate longer because their metabolism is inhibited; others will be speedily metabolized and eliminated.

Protease inhibitors and nucleoside analogues are associated with serious metabolic derangements. These include elevated cholesterol and triglycerides, insulin resistance and diabetes mellitus, and changes in body fat composition, which are particularly distressing to clients. These body fat changes primarily are abdominal obesity and skeletal wasting, and this set of symptoms is referred to as lipodystrophy (Tierney et al., 2005). Elevated cholesterol should be treated with pravastatin or atorvastatin. Lovastatin and simvastatin react to PIs, so they need to be avoided. Reduction of dietary sources of cholesterol should be made.

- Saquinavir (Invirase) is used in combination with nucleoside analogues to treat progression of the disease.
- Ritonavir (Norvir) is used in combination with nucleoside analogues to treat progression of the disease.
- Indinavir (Crixivan) is used in combination with nucleoside analogues to treat progression of the disease.
- Nelfinavir (Viracept) is used in clients with failure of or intolerance to other PIs.
- Amprenavir (Agenerase) is the newest PI.
- Lopinavir/Ritonavir (Kaletra) is the first combination of PIs active against some HIV strains resistant to other PIs.

NONNUCLEOSIDE REVERSE TRANSCRIPTASE INHIBITORS Nevirapine (Viramune), delavirdine (Rescriptor), and efavirenz (Sustiva) are NNRTIs that may be used in combination with nucleoside analogues and PIs. However, one limitation to NNRTIs is the high incidence of cross-resistance to NRTIs. Some studies have shown that nevirapine and efavirenz may significantly reduce serum levels of the PIs. Only one NNRTI should be used at the same time. Nevirapine has a reported risk for liver toxicity and Stevens-Johnson syndrome (Bartlett & Weber, 2005).

ENTRY INHIBITORS Entry or fusion inhibitors, such as enfuvirtide (Fuzeon), prevent HIV from entering target cells by binding to the protein envelope that surrounds the virus. When bound to the drug, the virus cannot morph to fit and adhere to cell membranes (Covington, 2005). Adding this new class of drug, which became available in 2003, to the regimen of heavily pretreated individuals improves CD4 counts and lowers viral loads (Tierney et al., 2005).

AGENTS USED IN COMBINATION WITH ANTIRETROVIRAL THERAPY Other agents may be administered in combination with antiretroviral therapy. Interferons, which are naturally occurring lymphokines, have been used alone and in combination. Alpha-interferon may be used to treat KS and in combination with zidovudine to slow disease progression. Gamma-interferon also is used. As more drugs become available, the burden to choose the best regimen increases for the health care provider. As mentioned, the most important limiting factor when choosing a regimen is client adherence. Second to that is selecting an effective combination of drugs without overlapping toxicities or toxicities so debilitating that adherence will be further impaired.

A number of pharmacologic agents are used to prevent and treat opportunistic infections and malignancies in the client with HIV. These agents are outlined in Table 14–3.

It is recommended that all clients infected with HIV receive pneumococcal, influenza, hepatitis B, and *Haemophilus influenzae b* vaccines. Persons with a positive PPD and negative chest x-ray are given prophylactic isoniazid. When the client's CD4 cell count falls to less than 200/mm^3, prophylactic treatment for PCP is begun, usually with trimethoprim-sulfamethoxazole. Clients with a CD4 count of less than 100/mm^3 are started on prophylactic treatment for MAC.

Clinical Therapies

Clients may require an implanted venous access device, such as a Groshong catheter, to facilitate blood sampling, intravenous medication administration, transfusions, and parenteral nutrition when frequent intravenous access is needed. However, because of the client's altered immune response, it is of particular importance that strict infection control principles be followed to prevent the introduction of pathogens into the bloodstream.

The goal for antenatal care is identification of the pregnant woman at risk for HIV infection. Thus, the revised CDC HIV testing guidelines indicate that screening should be included in the routine panel of prenatal screening tests for all pregnant women, with the understanding that the woman is notified it is part of the testing and can "opt out" of the HIV screening if she chooses (Branson, Handsfield, Lampe, et al., 2006). Initial testing is done using ELISA. If the results are positive, the Western blot test is used to confirm the diagnosis. Women who test positive should be counseled about the implications of the diagnosis for themselves and their fetus to ensure an informed reproductive choice.

Women infected with HIV should be evaluated and treated for other sexually transmitted infections and for conditions

TABLE 14–3 Pharmacologic Treatment of Common Opportunistic Infections and Malignancies in HIV Disease

CONDITION	TREATMENT	POTENTIAL ADVERSE EFFECTS
Infections		
Pneumocystis carinii pneumonia	Trimethoprim/sulfamethoxazole	Rash, neutropenia, anemia, thrombocytopenia, and Stevens-Johnson syndrome
	Pentamidine	Hypotension, altered blood glucose levels, hypocalcemia, anemia and leukopenia, liver and renal toxicity, and pancreatitis
Tuberculosis	Combination drug therapy using isoniazid, rifampin, ethambutol, pyrazinamide, or streptomycin	Multiple (see Concept 15, Infection, for an exemplar on this diagnosis)
Candidiasis (oral thrush)	Clotrimazole troches	Few toxic responses noted
	Nystatin suspension	Few toxic responses noted
Esophagitis or recurrent vaginitis	Ketoconazole	Hepatitis and adrenal insufficiency
	Fluconazole	Hepatitis
	Amphotericin B	Bone marrow toxicity, acute renal or hepatic failure, nausea and vomiting, chills, fever, and headache
Mycobacterium avium complex	Combination therapy using:	
	Clarithromycin, plus	Hepatitis, nausea, diarrhea
	Clofazimine	Diarrhea, nausea and vomiting, skin discoloration, pruritus, and rash
	Ethambutol	Thrombocytopenia, hepatitis, and optic neuritis
	Rifampin	Bone marrow depression, renal failure, and hepatitis
	Ciprofloxacin	Nausea and rash
	Amikacin	Bone marrow depression, renal failure, ototoxicity, and hepatitis
Cytomegalovirus	Ganciclovir	Bone marrow depression and fever
	Foscarnet	Renal failure, electrolyte imbalances, and seizures
Herpes simplex or herpes zoster	Acyclovir	Nausea and vomiting, diarrhea, central nervous system effects, and renal failure
Toxoplasmosis	Pyrimethamine, plus sulfadiazine or clindamycin and folinic acid	Bone marrow depression, rash, respiratory failure, nausea and vomiting, abdominal pain, and hematuria
Malignancies		
Kaposi's sarcoma	Intralesional vinblastine	Inflammation and pain at injection site
Lymphoma	Combination chemotherapy	Nausea and vomiting, bone marrow toxicity, and alopecia

occurring more commonly in women with HIV, such as tuberculosis, cytomegalovirus, toxoplasmosis, and cervical dysplasia. Women infected with HIV and with no history of hepatitis B should receive the hepatitis vaccine, which is not contraindicated prenatally, as well as the pneumococcal vaccine and an annual flu shot. In addition to routine prenatal laboratory tests, a platelet count and a CBC with differential should be obtained at the first prenatal visit and repeated each trimester to identify anemia, thrombocytopenia, and leukopenia, which are associated both with HIV infection and with antiviral therapy.

The woman with HIV also should be assessed regularly for serologic changes that indicate the disease is progressing. This is determined by the absolute CD4 T-lymphocyte count, which provides the number of helper T4 cells. When CD4 counts fall to 200/mm³ or lower, opportunistic infections (e.g., PCP) are more likely to develop.

At each prenatal visit, women who are infected with HIV but are asymptomatic are monitored for early signs of complications, such as weight loss during the second or third trimester or fever. The woman is asked about signs of vaginal infection. Her mouth is inspected for signs of infections, such as thrush (candidiasis) or hairy leukoplakia; her lungs are auscultated for signs of pneumonia; and her lymph nodes, liver, and spleen are palpated for signs of enlargement. Each trimester, the woman should have a visual examination and a funduscopic examination to detect such complications as toxoplasmosis retinitis.

A pregnancy complicated by HIV infection, even if asymptomatic, is considered to be high risk, and the fetus is monitored closely. Weekly nonstress testing is begun at 32 weeks' gestation, and serial ultrasounds are done to detect intrauterine growth restriction. Biophysical profiles also are indicated. Invasive procedures such as amniocentesis are avoided when possible to prevent contamination of a noninfected infant. To reduce the risk of perinatal transmission, intrapartum intravenous zidovudine is indicated for all pregnant women regardless of their prenatal therapy regimen.

Scheduled cesarean birth at 38 weeks' gestation and before rupture of the membranes is recommended for women with elevated viral loads (Limpongsanurak, 2006). Women who are HIV positive have an increased risk for complications such as intrapartal or postpartal hemorrhage, postpartal infection, poor wound healing, and infections of the genitourinary tract. Thus, they need careful monitoring and appropriate therapy as indicated. Following childbirth, the women who is HIV positive should be referred to a physician knowledgeable about treating individuals with HIV infection. Because of the profound implications of HIV infection for the woman, her family, the fetus/newborn, and her health care providers, screening is recommended for all pregnant women but especially those at increased risk, including the following:

- Prostitutes
- Women with multiple sexual partners
- Women whose current or previous sexual partners have been bisexual, have abused injection drugs, had hemophilia, or tested positive for HIV
- Women who are or have been injection drug users
- Women from countries where heterosexual transmission is common.

In addition, clinics located in areas with a large HIV-positive population may require routine HIV screening of all prenatal clients.

Medical management begins with prevention of the spread of HIV from mother to newborn. Because of the rapidity of disease progression in perinatally transmitted HIV infection, early identification of infected infants is important to ensure the most effective treatment. Mothers infected with HIV should be identified during pregnancy, and their infants should undergo periodic laboratory testing as described previously. Pregnant women infected with HIV who are treated with zidovudine (AZT) and who deliver their babies by cesarean section reduce the chance of transmission to 1%. All infected mothers should receive oral zidovudine (AZT) after the first trimester of pregnancy and intravenous AZT during labor and delivery; in addition, the newborn of a mother with HIV infection should receive 6 weeks of oral AZT after birth.

All infants of infected mothers should start prophylaxis against PCP (a commonly serious or fatal outcome in infants) by 4 to 6 weeks of age. Prophylaxis should continue to 12 months or until two negative HIV tests have been documented (at 1 and 4 months of age).

The earlier the child develops AIDS, the poorer the prognosis. However, as treatment improves, more children are living longer with the disease. Younger children are more likely to die of pulmonary diseases or infection, while those who survive past 10 years of age are more likely to die of cardiac disease, wasting syndrome, encephalopathy, and infection with *Mycobacterium avium* complex. Many children who acquired HIV in perinatal transmission (before frequent testing during pregnancy and treatment during pregnancy and in neonates) are now entering the adolescent age group (Rangel et al., 2006).

Complementary Therapies

Complementary and alternative medicine has been shown to help decrease side effects of certain medical treatments and to increase client comfort related to acute exacerbations. However, the National Center for Complementary and Alternative Medicine (NCCAM) has issued warnings against the use of garlic supplements with HIV medications (NCCAM, 2000). The use of St. John's wort also is contraindicated for clients receiving antiretroviral therapy (NCCAM, 2000). Any client with HIV/AIDS should be encouraged to consult his or her treating physician before beginning any therapy involving complementary and alternative medicine.

NURSING PROCESS

The client with HIV/AIDS has many care needs, and requires both physical and psychosocial support (see the Evidence-Based Practice feature that follows). Because no cure or effective treatment currently exists for HIV disease, many of these needs fall within the realm of nursing to promote knowledge and understanding, self-care, comfort, and quality of life. As with many diseases with an ultimately fatal outcome, the course of HIV infection may well be affected by the client's social support systems, control, perceived self-efficacy in management, and coping mechanisms.

As the epidemic continues, nurses are providing care for increasing numbers of clients with HIV infection at various stages of disease. These clients are not only in special care settings but also in general units, maternal–child units, hospices, long-term care facilities, and home settings. As clients with HIV disease live longer, nurses will increasingly encounter those in whom HIV disease is a secondary diagnosis, with another primary diagnosis such as seizures, heart disease, diabetes mellitus, or an operative procedure.

Assessment

Assessment is the basis for differential diagnosis; fitting appropriate treatment to the correct etiology is critical. For example, delirium is an acute confusional state and, unlike dementia, is reversible. Effective nursing interventions are available for these conditions (Coyne et al., 2002).

Collect the following data through the health history and physical examination. Further focused assessments are described in the Implementation section that follows.

- *Health history.* Risk factors (transfusion, unprotected sex, and needle exposure), infections (sexually transmitted infections, hepatitis, and tuberculosis), medications, recreational drug use, foreign travel, and pets
- *Physical assessment.* Height, weight, nutrition, skin and mucous membranes, vision, lymph nodes, breath sounds, abdominal tenderness, motor strength, coordination, cranial nerves, gait, deep tendon reflexes, genitourinary examination, and mental status

Assessment centers on observation and evaluation of potential sites of infection. Assess breath sounds, respiratory status, arterial blood gases, level of consciousness, and mental status. Any evidence of lymphocytic interstitial pneumonitis or neurologic abnormalities should be reported. Assess the child's height and weight frequently. Observe for signs of failure to thrive and assess for anemia. Look for *Candida* infections in the mouth and the diaper area. Note any developmental delays in motor skills or intellectual functioning, which could result

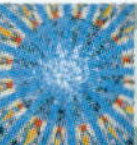

EVIDENCE-BASED PRACTICE Nurses' Willingness to Care for People With AIDS

Clinical Question

As reported by the Centers for Disease Control and Prevention, the number of deaths from AIDS has declined. This is believed to be the result of both slowing of the epidemic and improved treatment, which has lengthened the life span of people with AIDS. As treatment continues to improve survival, a key challenge will be the increasing number of people living with HIV/AIDS—and the additional resources needed for services, treatment, and care. Several studies have found that some professional nurses and students are resistant to caring for clients with AIDS.

Evidence

Sherman (1996) examined relationships among moral choices about one's own mortality (death anxiety), spirituality, and social support and nurses' willingness to care for these clients. In a survey of 220 registered nurses employed in eight hospitals in the New York Metropolitan area, Sherman found that willingness to care for clients with AIDS was positively correlated with spirituality and perceived social support and negatively correlated with death anxiety. It is suggested that nurses' willingness to care for people with AIDS may be related not only to nurses' personal values and beliefs (expressed in spirituality), but also to their professional identity and role expectations.

Addressing nursing reluctance to treat clients with HIV infection, nursing educators Valois, Turgeon, Godin, Blondeau, and Cote (2001) researched the impact of persuasive messages on nursing students' beliefs and attitudes about caring for these clients. Nursing education certainly increases knowledge about and awareness of the science of HIV infection, but it may not modify attitudes or behaviors. The underlying theory of this study was that individuals who receive evidence-based persuasive messages may develop favorable beliefs that will alter their willingness to perform a given behavior. Three main types of beliefs were considered in this study: behavioral belief (related to the expected consequences of adopting a behavior), normative belief (related to perceived social pressures by significant others resulting from adopting a behavior), and control belief (related to resources or barriers that seem to facilitate or hamper adoption of the behavior).

In three sessions, the student nurses in the experimental group were given positive persuasive messages about caring for clients with HIV infection. The persuasive messages were compelling and specific to caring for these clients, and case studies provided opportunities for the students to discuss the elements of the case within the framework of the persuasive messages. Students in the control group studied the science of caring for clients with HIV but did not receive the persuasive messages. When beliefs and attitudes about caring for these clients were compared, the researchers found significantly greater willingness to provide care in the experimental group. Nursing students proved to be well prepared and motivated to receive this information.

Best Practice

Standards of professional nursing clearly state that nurses will care for people with HIV/AIDS. To increase nurses' willingness to do so, students need to be better socialized into their roles and responsibilities. Providing information within an evidence-based framework, analyzing and defining effective nursing care in client cases, and using the standards of professional nursing help to promote the development of positive attitudes among nurses. Discussions within the classroom and clinical settings provide a safe means of bringing fears into the open and sharing experiences. Student groups can serve as support groups, improving communication, decreasing isolation and anxiety, and improving self-esteem and morale. Within the work setting, perceived support from colleagues and administrators as well as increased contact with people who have HIV/AIDS are important factors in making caring a rewarding and positive experience.

Critical Thinking

1. These studies were of student nurses and registered nurses and conducted a decade or more previously. What differences do you think might be found between the two groups today?
2. Carefully consider each of the following clients with AIDS, and write a brief paragraph about how you would feel if you were assigned to care for them:
   a. A heterosexual woman, age 25
   b. A gay man, age 35
   c. A newborn baby girl
   d. A 40-year-old single mother of three teenagers
   e. A 30-year-old homeless drug user
   f. A 17-year-old male client with hemophilia, infected by blood transfusions
   g. A heterosexual male, age 80

from encephalopathy and poor nutrition, and can signal an increasing severity in symptom level. These should be reported so that further medical evaluation can be carried out.

Assess family support systems and coping mechanisms. Support the family when they decide to inform a school-age child or adolescent of the diagnosis. When assessing an adolescent with AIDS, evaluate the teen's understanding of how AIDS is transmitted and the response to the diagnosis.

When conducting the physical assessment, remember that symptoms must be interpreted and reported by the client. Like pain, the presence and severity of dyspnea are determined and reported by the client. We must believe what the client tells us.

Diagnosis

Client needs change throughout the course of the disease, so the plan of care and nursing diagnoses are amended frequently, sometimes with every visit. Appropriate nursing diagnoses may include the following:

- Ineffective Coping
- Impaired Skin Integrity
- Imbalanced Nutrition: Less Than Body Requirements
- Risk for Deficient Fluid Volume
- Risk for Infection
- Anxiety
- Fear
- Deficient Knowledge.

Specific disease-related diagnoses may include the following:

- Diarrhea related to gastrointestinal infection, malignancy, or drug reactions
- Impaired Gas Exchange related to pulmonary disease
- Delayed Growth and Development related to chronic infection and poor nutrition
- Risk for Compromised Family Coping related to life-threatening illness.

Examples of nursing diagnoses that might apply to the pregnant woman who tests positive for HIV include the following:

- Risk for Ineffective Health Maintenance related to lack of information about HIV/AIDS and its long-term implications for the woman, her unborn child, and her family
- Risk for Infection related to altered immunity secondary to HIV infection
- Compromised Family Coping related to the implications of a positive HIV test in one of the family members.

Appropriate nursing diagnoses for the neonate exposed to HIV/AIDS include the following:

- Imblanced Nutrition: Less Than Body Requirements related to formula intolerance and inadequate intake
- Risk for Impaired Skin Integrity related to chronic diarrhea
- Risk for Infection related to perinatal exposure and immunoregulation suppression secondary to HIV/AIDS
- Impaired Physical Mobility related to decreased neuromuscular development
- Impaired Parenting related to diagnosis of HIV/AIDS and fear of future outcome.

Plan

The first step in dealing with HIV infection is prevention. Nurses must be active in evaluating test results and in teaching measures to prevent transmission of HIV to others. Adequate testing, prophylaxis for HIV and PCP, and follow-up visits to evaluate the general health of those at risk for the disease are advised. Guidelines from the AAP recommend that pediatricians offer HIV testing and counseling to adolescents who are sexually active or involved in substance abuse (AAP, Committee on Pediatric AIDS, 2001). Recommendations also have been made for inclusion of HIV/AIDS education in comprehensive health education for students from kindergarten through 12th grade (AAP, Committee on Pediatric AIDS, 1998) (Box 14–10). Nurses can implement these policies and counsel teens about the dangers of and prevention measures for HIV.

Nursing care needs for the client with HIV infection change over the course of the disease. Preventive health care measures, health maintenance activities, education, and support of coping mechanisms are important during the early stages of the disease. Counseling the client with a new diagnosis of HIV infection is vital. HIV/AIDS continues to carry a social stigma that may interfere with the client's usual support systems and coping mechanisms. As the disease progresses and the client experiences more physical symptoms, the need for psychosocial support continues, but direct care needs become more important. Acute exacerbation of opportunistic infections may necessitate hospitalization, but typically, the client is managed at home.

Box 14–10 **Teaching About AIDS**

The American Academy of Pediatrics recommends that HIV and AIDS education be part of health education in kindergarten through 12th grade. School nurses should be educated about HIV/AIDS, ethics, testing, and counseling. The particular roles defined for nurses in school settings include:

1. Participate in education programs for teachers.
2. Assist schools and other organizations to develop education programs.
3. Review, adapt, and develop educational materials.
4. Participate in public discussions about HIV/AIDS.
5. Take part in meetings with school administrators, staff, and parents.
6. Facilitate networking among parents and AIDS community groups.

Source: Adapted from American Academy of Pediatrics, Committee on Pediatric AIDS. (1998). Human immunodeficiency virus/acquired immunodeficiency syndrome education in schools. *Pediatrics, 101,* 933–935.

PRACTICE ALERT

Health care workers who come in contact with blood or other body fluids of clients infected with HIV are at risk for exposure to the virus. Standard precautions should be used in caring for all clients, because HIV status and presence of other infections may not be known.

Implementation

Implementations are directed toward specific nursing diagnoses selected on the basis of client needs. The following implementations are linked to nursing diagnoses.

Prevent Infection

Preventing infection involves preventing new cases of HIV infection as well as preventing and treating opportunistic infections in clients diagnosed with HIV to avoid conversion to AIDS. Client teaching is an important nursing intervention to meet this goal.

PREVENTING INFECTION WITH HIV To date, no safe immunization to protect against HIV infection has been developed. Education, counseling, and behavior modification are the primary tools for AIDS prevention. The benefit of education and behavior modification is evident in the gay male population. The incidence of new HIV infections within this population has declined dramatically in high-prevalence cities. Nurses play a vital role for individuals and communities in providing education about this epidemic and how to prevent infection.

Education Educate sexually active adolescents and adults about the importance of practicing safe sex and the ramifications of high-risk sexual behaviors and injection drug use. In fact, all sexually active individuals need to know how HIV is spread and how to practice safer sex (Box 14–11). Reducing the number of sexual partners—for example, by entering into and remaining in a long-term, mutually monogamous relationship with an uninfected partner—reduces the risk. Clients should not engage in unprotected sex, especially if the HIV status of the partner is unknown. Latex condoms have been

Box 14–11 Guidelines for Safer Sex

- Practice mutual monogamy; if you are not in a mutually monogamous relationship, limit the number of sexual partners.
- Do not engage in unprotected sex, especially if the HIV status of your partner is unknown. A person may be infected and infective for up to 6 months before converting to seropositive status.
- When entering into a new monogamous relationship, both partners should undergo HIV testing. If both are negative, practice abstinence or safer sex for 6 months, followed by retesting. If results still indicate that both partners are negative, sexual activity probably can be considered safe.
- Use latex condoms for oral, vaginal, or anal intercourse; avoid natural or animal skin condoms, which allow passage of HIV.
- For vaginal or anal sex, lubricate the condom with the spermicidal agent nonoxynol-9 for additional protection.
- Do not use an oil-based lubricant such as petroleum jelly, which can result in condom damage; water-based lubricants are acceptable.
- Women should carry and use a female condom.
- Remember that use of other means of birth control, such as oral contraceptives, provide no protection against HIV; barrier protection with a condom is necessary.
- Engage in safer sexual practices that are less damaging to sensitive tissues (e.g., mutual masturbation and avoiding anal or oral sex).
- Do not use drugs or alcohol.
- Do not share needles, razors, toothbrushes, sexual toys, or other items that may be contaminated with blood or body fluids.
- If HIV positive:
  a. Do not engage in unprotected sexual activity.
  b. Inform all current and former sexual partners of HIV status.
  c. Inform all health care personnel—primary care providers, physicians, and dentists in particular—of HIV status.
  d. Do not donate blood, plasma, blood products, sperm, organs, or tissue.
  e. If female, do not become pregnant.

shown to reduce the risk of transmitting HIV. Their effectiveness is improved when nonoxynol-9, a spermicide, is used for lubrication; however, nonoxynol-9 may cause genital ulcers, which can facilitate HIV transmission. To be effective, condoms must be used with every sexual encounter involving vaginal, oral, or anal intercourse. They also need to be applied and removed properly. A female condom also is available for use. However, the following are the only *totally* safe sex practices:

- No sex
- Long-term, mutually monogamous sexual relations between two uninfected people
- Mutual masturbation without direct contact.

The most difficult group of high-risk people to reach and educate is injection drug users. People in this group should never share needles, syringes, or other drug paraphernalia. Many cities have initiated needle-exchange programs, providing a sterile needle and syringe in return for a used one. A fresh solution of household bleach and water in a 1:10 ratio is effective to clean paraphernalia when sterile supplies are not available. It also is important to teach people in this population about safer sex practices, because most heterosexual HIV transmission occurs between injection drug users and their partners.

When possible, encourage clients to use autologous transfusion (donating their own blood before an anticipated surgery). Seeking donations from family members is not encouraged for several reasons. Family members may have engaged in high-risk behaviors but lie about their risk because of embarrassment or fear of discovery. Furthermore, the family member may have a different blood type or other contraindications to donating.

Encourage clients who are HIV positive to abstain from donating blood, organs, or sperm. They should understand tactics to avoid exchange of body fluids by not sharing needles or other drug paraphernalia, not sharing razors, and not getting a tattoo. Stress the importance of informing all medical personnel providing direct care (especially anyone performing a dental, surgical, or obstetric procedure) about the diagnosis.

Standard Precautions Health care workers can prevent most exposures to HIV by using standard precautions (Figure 14–13 ■). Testing to determine HIV status remains voluntary and relies on the use of antibody-screening methods; therefore, it remains

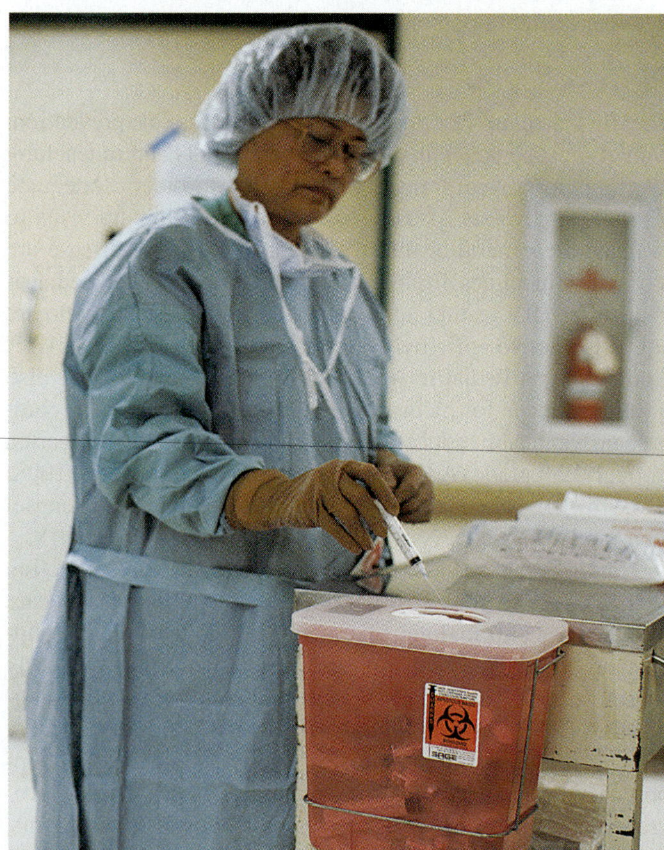

Figure 14–13 ■ This nurse is disposing of a needle and syringe in a special container, a necessary practice to avoid the transmission of HIV through needle sticks with contaminated needles.

impossible to identify every client who is HIV positive. With standard precautions, however, all clients are treated alike, eliminating the need to know the client's HIV status. All high-risk body fluids are treated as if they are infectious, and barrier precautions are used to prevent skin, mucous membrane, or percutaneous exposure to these fluids.

Nursing care of the newborn exposed to HIV/AIDS includes all the care normally given to any newborn in a nursery. In addition, the nurse must include care for a newborn suspected of having a bloodborne infection. Standard precautions should be used when caring for the newborn immediately after birth and when obtaining blood samples via vein puncture or heel stick. The blood of all newborns must be considered potentially infectious, because the status of the infant's blood often is not known until after the infant is discharged. As mentioned, a window of time exists before seroconversion occurs, and during this window, the baby is still considered infectious. Nursing care involves providing for comfort; keeping the newborn well nourished and protected from opportunistic infections; providing good skin care to prevent skin rashes; and facilitating growth, development, and attachment. Most institutions recommend that their caregivers wear gloves during all diaper changes and examination of babies. Disposable gloves are worn when changing diapers or cleaning the diaper area, especially in the presence of diarrhea, because blood may be in the stool; gloves should be considered part of standard precautions for hospital personnel (AAP Committee on Fetus and Newborn & American College of Obstetricians and Gynecologists [ACOG] Committee on Obstetrics, 2007). Table 14–4 outlines issues for caregivers of infants who are at risk for HIV/AIDS.

Postexposure Prophylaxis Health care workers exposed to HIV infection or adults who experience a high-risk exposure to HIV may choose postexposure prophylaxis. Risk of exposure for health care workers may be through needle sticks or cuts with a sharp object, contact with mucous membrane or nonintact skin, semen, vaginal secretions, and fluids contaminated with visible blood. Other possible risks include cerebrospinal fluid, synovial fluid, and pleural, peritoneal, pericardial, or amniotic fluids.

Some clinicians and facilities recommend prophylactic AZT therapy after needlestick or splash exposure. However, such therapy must be initiated immediately, and its effectiveness has yet to be established. CDC guidelines recommend treatment with HAART, which includes two nucleoside reverse transcriptase inhibitors (NRTIs) for lower-risk exposures and the addition of a third drug for higher-risk exposure. A 4-week course of treatment is recommended and should be

TABLE 14–4 **Issues for Caregivers of Infants at Risk for HIV/AIDS**

Resuscitation	For suctioning use a bulb syringe, mucus extractor, or meconium aspirator with wall suction on low setting. Use masks, goggles, and gloves.
Admission care	To remove blood from baby's skin, give warm water–mild soap bath using gloves as soon as possible after admission.
Handwashing	Thorough handwashing is indicated before and after caring for infant. Hands must be washed immediately if contaminated with blood or body fluids. Wash hands after removal of gloves.
Gloves	Gloves are indicated with touching blood or other high-risk fluids. Gloves should also be worn when handling newborns before and during their initial baths, cord care, eye prophylactics, and vitamin K administration.
Mask, goggle, and gown	Not routinely needed unless coming in contact with placenta or the blood and amniotic fluid on the skin of the newborn.
Needles and syringes	Used needles should not be recapped or bent; they should be disposed of in a puncture-resistant plastic container belonging specifically to that baby. After the newborn is discharged the container is discarded.
Specimens	Blood and other specimens should be double-bagged and/or sealed in an impervious container and labeled according to agency protocol.
Equipment and linen	Articles contaminated with blood or body fluids should be discarded or bagged according to isolation or institution protocol.
Body fluid spills	Blood and body fluids should be cleaned promptly with a solution of 5.25% sodium hypochlorite (household bleach) diluted 1:10 with water. Apply for at least 30 seconds then wipe after the minimum contact time.
Education and support	Provide education and psychologic support for family and staff. Caregivers who avoid contact with a baby at risk or who overdress in unnecessary isolation garb subtly exacerbate an already difficult family situation. Information resources include the National AIDS Hotline (1-800-342-2437) and HIV/AIDS Treatment Enforcement Service website http://www.hevatis.org
Exempted personnel	Immunologically compromised staff (pregnant women may be included in this group) and possibly infectious staff members should not care for these infants.

Source: Adapted from American Academy of Pediatrics, Committee on Pediatric AIDS and Committee on Infectious Diseases. (1999). Issues related to human immunodeficiency transmission in schools, child care, medical settings, the home, and community. *Pediatrics, 104*(2), 318–324; Mendez, H., & Jule, J. E. (1990). Care of the infant born exposed to AIDS. *Obstetric and Gynecologic Clinics of North America, 17*(3), 637; Krist, A. H., & Crawford-Faucher, A. (2002). Management of newborns exposed to maternal HIV infection. *American Family Physician*, *65*(10), 2049–2056.

started within 72 hours, but preferably within 2–3 hours of exposure (Bartlett & Weber, 2005).

Counseling and testing are provided to health care workers with a documented needlestick exposure.

PREVENTING INFECTIONS IN THOSE WITH HIV/AIDS Clients who are immunosuppressed become infected with bacteria as well as other organisms that are common in the environment. Frequent hand hygiene and limiting exposure of the client to individuals with upper respiratory or other infections are the best interventions to protect the client with HIV from acquiring other infections.

The child with HIV should be immunized as soon as he or she is at the recommended age for diphtheria, tetanus, and acellular pertussis; inactivated poliovirus; *Haemophilus influenzae* type b; hepatitis B; pneumococcal vaccine; and annual influenza vaccine. Live measles-mumps-rubella vaccine is administered at 12 months of age unless the child is severely immunocompromised, because the risk of serious outcomes for measles is great. Live varicella vaccine should be administered if the child has no or mild symptoms of HIV. If the infant is exposed to varicella, the parents should notify their health care professional, because the baby may need varicella zoster immunoglobulin (VZIG) within 96 hours of exposure or if exposed to measles (may need vaccination within 72 hours of exposure). Tuberculosis is more common in children with AIDS, so annual skin tests that are read by health professionals are recommended (AAP, 2006).

Protect the neonate from HIV-infected maternal secretions. Bathe the newborn as soon as possible after delivery, and wash the eyes and face before administration of prophylactic eyedrops or ointment. Avoid invasive procedures in the newborn, and encourage the mother to formula feed the baby rather than breast feed (Luxner, 2003).

Promote Adherence to Medication Regimen

The treatment regimen with the use of antiretroviral therapies for the client with HIV/AIDS may be complex and time-consuming, presenting an overwhelming challenge to the client and family. Nonadherence to the prescribed antiretroviral treatment regimen likely will result in increased morbidity and mortality. Some common reasons for nonadherence include frequent dosing, displeasure with medication (e.g., large pills, gritty powders, and bitter taste), and associated side effects including nausea and rashes (Brackis-Cott, Mellins, Abrams, Reval, & Dolezal, 2003).

Wroe and Thomas (2003) found it helpful to distinguish between intentional and unintentional nonadherence and to treat them as separate entities. Client beliefs and internal logic were found to impact intentional nonadherence; preparing the client for the effects of HAART therapy by focusing on lessening the client's reasons for not taking medication is believed to reduce intentional nonadherence. Enriquez and McKinsey (2004) emphasize the role of nursing in preventing drug resistance by assessing client readiness to adhere to the treatment regimen and by intervening to overcome identified barriers to adherence before initiating therapy.

Strategies for achieving optimal management of the treatment regimen include educating the client regarding the purpose of the medication, the benefits of adhering to the regimen, and the potential consequences of failing to adhere to the regimen. Behavior modification techniques, using positive reinforcement, can be very effective in promoting the child's adherence. Support should be provided to the client, and the medication regimen should be tailored to the client's routine. Praise should be offered for adhering to the regimen. Ingersoll and Heckman (2005), however, found the most effective provider–client relationship for fostering adherence is a balance of appropriate challenge and support. Providers who were never confrontational seem to be perceived by clients as giving permission to be less adherent. Although depression, substance use, and financial considerations undoubtedly influence a client's adherence to HAART therapy and need to be addressed, provider–client relationships seem to have the most influence on adherence behavior.

If problems exist in the management of the treatment regimen, carefully listen to the client to help determine the cause. Collaborate with the client in establishing goals to help meet the prescribed treatment regimen, and consider the effect of cultural beliefs on medication adherence. If further intervention is required, other options include direct observational therapy, home visits, or use of electronic monitoring devices, as described later in Pharmacologic Therapies.

CARE SETTINGS Home Care of the Newborn With HIV

- The baby should have his or her own skin care items, towels, and washcloths. Most clothing and linens can be washed with other household laundry. Linen that is visibly soiled with blood or body fluids should be kept and washed separately in hot, sudsy water with household bleach.
- Prompt diaper changing and perineal care can prevent or minimize diaper rash and promote comfort. Topical Mycostatin or Desitin ointment is used for diaper rashes. Soiled diapers should be placed in plastic bags, sealed, and disposed of daily. Diaper-changing areas should be cleaned with a 1:10 dilution of household bleach after each diaper change.
- If diarrhea occurs, the baby needs frequent perineal care as well as fluid replacement. Antidiarrheal medications often are ineffective.
- Toys should be kept as clean as possible, not shared with other children, and checked for sharp edges to prevent scratches.
- The nurse instructs the parents about signs of infection to be alert for and when to call their health care provider.
- The inability to feed without pain may indicate esophageal yeast infection and may require administration of nystatin (Mycostatin) for the oral thrush.

Address Ineffective Coping

On receiving the test results indicating seropositive status, the person with HIV infection is faced with multiple issues that only rarely affect other clients. First and foremost, HIV is a disease with no known cure, and one that is thought to be almost universally fatal. Social support systems, family relationships, and the ability to obtain and retain useful work and health insurance may be disrupted by the disease. In addition, the client may experience guilt about his or her lifestyle and how the disease was contracted. As the disease progresses, social isolation, fatigue, changes in body image, medication side effects, and multiple other issues also affect the client's abilities to cope.

- Assess social support network and usual methods of coping. This will help both the nurse and the client identify people and mechanisms that can help the client cope more effectively with the disease.
- If possible, assign a primary nurse, whether the setting is home health care, hospice, or acute care. This helps to promote the development of a therapeutic and trusting relationship, and it provides for continuity of care.
- Plan for consistent, uninterrupted time with the client. Time and a consistent presence encourage the client to express feelings and work through issues related to HIV infection.
- Interact at every opportunity outside of providing specific nursing care treatments. This purposeful interaction communicates caring and acceptance without fear of HIV disease.
- Support the client's social network. Nontraditional families may offer more support than the traditional family. This in turn may necessitate a liberal interpretation of the term *family* if unit policy is immediate family only.
- Promote interaction between the client, significant others, and family. Hospitalization and manifestations of HIV disease may bring about isolation from others and decrease the client's ability to cope.
- Encourage involvement in making care decisions. This gives clients a greater sense of self-worth and more control over the situation, increasing their coping abilities.
- Set and maintain limits on manipulative and other destructive behaviors. The client who is unable to limit inappropriate behaviors needs the external control established by the nurse setting limits.
- Assist the client to accept responsibility for actions without blaming others. Effective coping cannot occur without accepting responsibility for one's actions.
- Support positive coping behaviors, decisions, actions, and achievements. As self-esteem is enhanced, coping improves (Côté & Pepler, 2005).

Because of the stress and social isolation that a family caring for a baby or child with HIV/AIDS may face, emotional support for family members is essential. As a result of these stresses, parents may not bond with the baby or may fail to provide the baby with enough sensory and tactile stimulation. Parents and family members need to be reassured that there are no documented cases of people contracting HIV/AIDS from routine care of infected babies and encouraged to hold the baby during feedings, because the infant benefits from frequent, gentle touch. Auditory stimulation also may be provided by using music or tapes of parents' voices. The nurse offers families information about support groups, available counseling, and information resources. Current therapeutic information about HIV is available to both health care providers and families through the AIDS Clinical Trials Information Service (1-800-TRIALS-A).

Maintain Skin Integrity

Dryness, malnutrition, immobility from fatigue, and skin lesions on pressure sites contribute to impaired integrity of the skin for the client with HIV disease. Maintaining skin integrity is important because of the progressive and debilitating nature of the disease. It also is a consideration both as the first line of defense against infection in a client with immunosuppression and as a site for secondary manifestations (e.g., KS and herpes).

- Monitor the skin frequently for lesions and areas of breakdown. Early identification of impaired skin integrity allows prompt intervention.
- Monitor lesions for signs of infection or impaired healing. Infection or poor tissue perfusion not only impairs healing but also may lead to further skin breakdown.
- Turn the client at least every 2 hour, and more frequently if necessary. Turning decreases unrelieved pressure on bony prominences and improves circulation to the tissues.
- Use pressure-relieving devices, such as pressure and egg-crate mattresses, or sheepskin pads for elbows and heels. *These* devices provide prophylactic relief of pressure.
- Keep skin clean and dry using mild, nondrying soaps or oils for cleansing. Night sweats and diarrhea, if present, can cause breakdown and damage to the skin. Frequent cleansing with nondrying products discourages bacterial growth, reducing the risk of infection.
- Massage around, but not over, affected pressure sites to increase circulation to the surrounding tissue. Massaging over the affected area can cause skin breakdown.
- If blisters are noted, leave them intact, and dress with a hydrocolloid (DuoDERM) dressing. Blisters provide natural sterile coverings for damaged tissue, improving healing and preventing bacterial invasion.
- Caution against scratching. If the client is confused, trim his or her fingernails, and use mitts or soft restraints to prevent scratching. If mitts or restraints are used, check the circulation of hands and fingers frequently. Scratching and skin damage allow bacteria to be introduced into lesions, increasing the risk of infection. Tight or restrictive restraints or mitts may compromise circulation.
- Avoid the use of heat or occlusive dressings. Heat can further dry and damage the skin; occlusive dressings may impair circulation and lead to ulceration.
- Prevent skin shearing by using a turnsheet and adequate personnel when repositioning. Shearing causes tissue trauma that can lead to decubitus ulcers.
- Encourage ambulation if possible; if the client is confined to bed, encourage active or passive ROM exercises. Activity increases circulation, decreases pressure and skin breakdown, and helps to maintain muscle tone.

- Monitor nutritional intake and albumin levels. Maintenance of optimal nutrition decreases the risk of tissue breakdown and improves resistance to infection.

PRACTICE ALERT

Applying protective creams to reddened areas in the rectal area protects skin from the caustic effects of diarrhea.

Manage Imbalanced Nutrition: Less Than Body Requirements

Many factors associated with HIV disease, including manifestations of the disease itself, put the client at risk for altered nutrition and weight loss. Nausea and anorexia may be manifestations of the disease or the result of antiretroviral therapy. Chronic diarrhea is a common manifestation of constitutional HIV disease. Wasting syndrome also is common and is manifested by involuntary weight loss of greater than 10 to 15% of baseline weight, severe diarrhea, fever, and chronic fatigue and weakness. The exact cause of wasting syndrome is unclear, but the diarrhea and fatigue contribute, as does the increased metabolic rate associated with fever. Oral and esophageal candidiasis and KS of the gastrointestinal tract may cause painful swallowing, making eating difficult and thereby contributing to anorexia. Poor nutritional status in the client with HIV ultimately can result in altered comfort, change in body image, muscle wasting, increased risk for infection, and higher mortality and morbidity.

- Assess nutritional status, including weight, body mass, caloric intake, and laboratory studies, such as total protein and albumin levels, hemoglobin, and hematocrit. These factors provide a baseline to determine the effectiveness of interventions.
- Identify possible causes of altered nutrition. Identification of causes provides direction for planned interventions.
- Administer prescribed medications for candidiasis and other manifestations as ordered. Eliminating this opportunistic infection improves comfort and facilitates food intake. Topical viscous anesthetic can help to reduce pain and improve oral intake.
- Administer antidiarrheal medications after stools and antiemetics before meals. Provide antipyretics as needed to control fever. Reducing diarrhea will improve nutrient absorption; preprandial medication with an antiemetic reduces nausea and improves food intake. Reduction of fever lowers the body's metabolic demands.
- Provide a diet high in protein and kilocalories. A high-protein, high-kilocalorie diet provides the necessary nutrients to meet metabolic needs as well as requirements for tissue healing.
- Offer soft foods, and serve small portions. Soft foods are easily digested. Small portions are more appealing to the anorectic or nauseated client.
- Involve the client in meal planning, and encourage significant others to bring favorite foods from home. The client is more likely to consume adequate amounts of preferred foods. Allowing food choices enhances the client's sense of control.
- Assist with eating as needed. Fatigue and weakness can prevent the client from eating an adequate amount of food.
- Provide supplementary vitamins and enteral feedings, such as Ensure. This improves nutritional status and caloric intake.
- Provide or assist with frequent oral hygiene. Oral hygiene improves comfort and appetite and reduces the risk of mucosal lesions.
- Administer appetite stimulants, such as megestrol (Megace) and dronabinol (Marinol), as ordered. Both drugs may increase appetite and promote weight gain.

Address Ineffective Sexuality Patterns

The diagnosis of HIV infection can significantly alter the client's expressions of sexuality. Guilt over the diagnosis may interfere with libido, and the client may fear spreading the disease to others via sexual relations. The client also may be angry with a significant other or partner if that person was the probable source of infection.

As the disease progresses, its manifestations can affect body image and self-esteem, again impairing sexuality. Other symptoms, such as nausea, fatigue, and weakness, may interfere with libido and sexual satisfaction as well.

- Examine your own feelings about sexuality, your role in dealing with a client's sexuality, the client's lifestyle, and sexual preferences. To deal effectively with the client's concerns, it is vital that the nurse be comfortable with his or her own feelings of sexuality and be able to accept the client's lifestyle. Referring the client to another nurse or counselor may be necessary.
- Establish a trusting, therapeutic relationship through the use of time, active listening, caring, and self-disclosure. Maintain a nonthreatening, nonjudgmental attitude toward the client. Sexuality is a private issue that will be uncomfortable or impossible for the nurse and client to discuss without a mutually trusting relationship.
- Provide factual information about HIV infection and its effects. This helps the client to separate fears and myths from reality.
- Discuss safer sex practices, including hugging, cuddling, nonsexual contact, use of latex condoms and spermicidal lubricant, and mutual masturbation. Alternative forms of sexual activity and expressing affection can allow the client and significant other to remain close throughout the course of the disease.
- Encourage discussion of fears and concerns with the significant other, if any. Open communication helps a couple to deal with issues related to sexuality.
- For the client without a significant other, stress the need to continue meeting people and developing social relationships while practicing safer sex. The risk of isolation is high in the client with HIV infection, and relationships with others help the client to cope with the disease.
- Refer the client and significant other to local support groups for people and partners of people with HIV. Support groups provide a social and support network of people facing the same issues.

NURSING CARE PLAN **A Client With HIV Infection**

Sara Lu is a 26-year-old elementary school teacher who lives with her parents and two younger sisters. Ms. Lu is very close to her parents and sisters; they share everything with each other.

During the required physical for admission to graduate school, Ms. Lu tells her physician that lately she has felt fatigued. She also states that she has had a persistent sore throat, intermittent bouts of diarrhea, and mild shortness of breath for about a month. She takes no routine medications other than a daily multivitamin and an occasional acetaminophen tablet for a headache. She is active in a drama club in her community, and she jogs 3 miles three to four times a week. She is engaged to be married in 6 months, and her fiancé is the only person with whom she has had sexual relations. Her sexual activity has been unprotected. Ms. Lu also has a history of open heart surgery 7 years ago to correct a congenital valve defect. She has been physically healthy since that time until about a month or two ago.

The physician orders a mononucleosis test, enzyme-linked immunosorbent assay (ELISA), Western blot analysis, CD4 cell count, a p24 antigen test, and an erythrocyte sedimentation rate (ESR). She is asked to return in 1 week for follow-up.

ASSESSMENT

On Ms. Lu's follow-up visit, Carole Kee, RN, obtains her nursing history. Ms. Lu continues to have flulike symptoms but has improved somewhat. She states that she just has not been as active as usual and is worried about her health. Her appetite has decreased because of soreness in her mouth, and she has noted some whitish patches on her tongue and cheeks.

A chest film reveals no abnormality. The results of her laboratory tests are as follows:

- *ELISA:* positive for antibodies against HIV
- *Western blot analysis:* positive for antibodies against HIV
- *p24 antigen test:* positive for circulating HIV antigens
- *ESR:* increased to 25 mm/hr (normal range: women, 15–20 mm/hr; men, 10–15 mm/hr)
- *CD4 cell count:* 599/mm^3 (normal range, 600–1,200 mm^3)

Ms. Lu's physical examination reveals that she has enlarged lymph nodes in her neck and white patches on her oral mucosa. Her skin is warm to the touch. Her vital signs are as follows: T_O 99.9°F (37.7°C), P 84, R 20, and BP 120/78.

Ms. Lu is told of the results of her laboratory tests and the medical diagnosis of HIV infection. Ms. Lu is is obviously distressed and wants to know how this happened, its meaning, whether she has infected her loved ones, and whether she will get better.

DIAGNOSES

Nursing diagnoses that may be appropriate for Ms. Lu include the following:

- Imbalanced Nutrition: Less Than Body Requirements related to soreness in mouth
- Risk for Deficient Fluid Volume related to decreased fluid intake and diarrhea
- Risk for Infection related to altered immune protection
- Anxiety related to diagnosis and fear
- Deficient Knowledge about the HIV disease process

PLANNING

The goals for care specify that Ms. Lu will:

- Maintain adequate nutrition for optimal body and cellular function.
- Consume at least 2,500 mL of fluid per day.
- Remain free of infections and their complications.
- Verbalize anxiety and use appropriate coping mechanisms.
- Verbalize and demonstrate knowledge of HIV disease.
- Verbalize measures, including safer sex practices, to prevent transmission of HIV to others.

IMPLEMENTATION

The following nursing interventions may be appropriate for Ms. Lu:

- Monitor daily weight as well as intake and output.
- Monitor dietary habits and serum albumin levels.
- Teach Ms. Lu the importance of consuming a nutritionally balanced diet and of maintaining adequate fluid intake.
- Suggest strategies for coping with anorexia and nausea.
- Provide referral for dietary consultation.
- Encourage oral care before and after meals.
- Assess bowel sounds, and monitor elimination pattern.
- Administer antiemetic and antimotility medications as ordered.
- Monitor for signs of dehydration, such as poor skin turgor, oliguria, and orthostatic hypotension.
- Increase fluid intake to 2,500 mL daily.
- Use strict aseptic technique for all invasive procedures.
- Teach Ms. Lu to avoid exposure to infection and people with known illnesses.
- Administer antiretroviral medications and antibiotics as prescribed, and monitor response.
- Encourage maintenance of regular physical exercise.
- Provide opportunities for Ms. Lu to verbalize her feelings.
- Avoid false reassurances.
- Provide appropriate and adequate information about HIV/AIDS.
- Teach safer sex practices and other measures to prevent transmission of HIV.
- Teach anxiety-controlling techniques, such as deep breathing and meditation.

EVALUATION

Ms. Lu is eager to learn about her illness and wants her family to come with her for further explanation. She states that she is sure her fiancé will be available as well. Ms. Lu is taking home antifungal medication, diet plans, and a schedule for increased exercise. She will return in 1 week for counseling and in 1 month for a follow-up physical.

(continued)

NURSING CARE PLAN A Client With HIV Infection *continued*

CRITICAL THINKING

1. How does age affect the body's response to fighting HIV? What other factors affect the risk for HIV infection and its progression?
2. Are the laboratory results for Ms. Lu a true indication that she is HIV positive? What additional tests might be ordered?
3. What is the most likely source of Ms. Lu's infection? What measures could have been used to reduce this risk, and how did she contract HIV? What is another possible source of Ms. Lu's HIV infection?
4. Ms. Lu says that her fiancé would like to have a child. How will you counsel her regarding pregnancy and childbearing?

Address Knowledge Deficits

Teaching needs for both the client and significant other are extensive. The primary need is information about the disease, its spread, and its expected course. The client and family need current factual information to plan realistically and to combat myths, misperceptions, and prejudices. At the same time, it is important to include information about current research and progress in treating the disease to maintain a sense of hopefulness.

The following topics should be discussed with the client and family to prepare for home care:

- Guidelines for safer sex practices
- Nutrition, rest and exercise, stress reduction, lifestyle changes, and maintaining a positive outlook
- Infection prevention and transmission, including hand washing and wearing gloves when handling client's secretions or excretions
- Importance of regular medical follow-up and monitoring of immune status
- Signs and symptoms of opportunistic infections and malignancies, as well as other symptoms that should be reported
- Medications and adverse effects
- Use and care of implanted venous access devices, total parenteral nutrition, intravenous pumps and continuous medication delivery systems, and intravenous or aerosolized medications
- Cessation of smoking, alcohol, and recreational or illicit drug use
- Home health services
- Hospice and respite care services
- Community resources, such as support groups, social agencies, and counselors.

Evaluation

There are many desired outcomes of care for the client with HIV/AIDS. Expected outcomes of nursing care include the following:

- Number of cases of HIV infection will decrease.
- Interventions will be successful in preventing infectious diseases in clients with the virus.
- Client will have adequate respiratory function and perfusion.
- Nutritional intake of affected clients will support normal nutritional patterns and prevent malnutrition.
- Client will demonstrate adequate coping with the stress of chronic disease.
- The child with HIV will be able to attend school and receive other supports in the educational process.

Expected outcomes of nursing care for the childbearing woman include the following:

- The woman discusses the implications of her HIV infection (or diagnosis of AIDS), its implications for her unborn child and for herself, the method of transmission, and the treatment options.
- The woman uses information about social services (or other agency referral) for follow-up assistance and counseling.
- The woman begins to verbalize her feelings about her condition and its implications for her and her family.

Outcomes specific to care of the exposed newborn include the following:

- Parents are able to bond with their infant and have realistic expectations about the baby.
- Potential opportunistic infections are identified early and treated promptly.
- Parents verbalize their concerns about their baby's existing and potential health problems and long-term care needs, and they accept outside assistance as needed.

HEALTH CARE

Nurses need to understand a variety of concepts when providing care for the client with HIV/AIDS. Consider some of the following concepts and how they apply to nursing care.

Ethics

To keep medical information private, it is not unusual for facilities to code HIV status with terms that have nothing to do with the disease. Why do nurses carry an ethical obligation to the client to take special precautions to maintain the privacy of clients diagnosed as HIV positive?

Evidence-Based Practice

Why is maintaining an evidenced-based practice of particular significance when caring for clients with HIV/AIDS?

Health Policy

How has HIV/AIDS influenced health policy over the past few decades?

Legal Issues

What are the legal obligations of the nurse caring for a client with HIV/AIDS?

Safety

How can the nurse maintain safety to prevent self-infection when caring for a client whose HIV status is unknown?

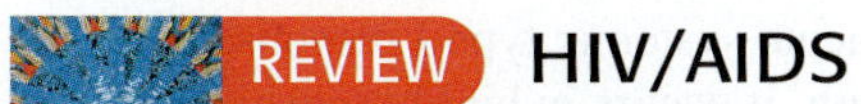

REVIEW HIV/AIDS

RELATE: LINK THE CONCEPTS

Linking the exemplar of HIV with the concept of Stress and Coping:

1. How might accessive stress impact the client with HIV and/or AIDS?
2. What nursing interventions could you implement to improve a client's coping methods in order to reduce complications related to HIV infection?

Linking the exemplar of HIV with the concept of Grief and Loss:

3. You are caring for a client who is newly diagnosed as being HIV positive with no symptoms of AIDS. Why might this client experience grief and loss?
4. What nursing interventions might you initiate to help the client through the grieving process?

READY: GO TO COMPANION SKILLS MANUAL

- Assessing the skin
- Latex precautions
- Donning and removing clean gloves
- Caring for the AIDS or HIV client in a home setting
- Teaching safer practices to HIV users

REFER: GO TO MYNURSINGKIT

REFLECT: CASE STUDY

Casey is a physically fit, 23-year-old man who had a troubled youth. His parents divorced when he was very young, and he bounced back and forth between them. Both parents remarried. Growing up, he often saw his father hit his stepmother when she made him angry. As an adolescent, Casey became involved with a gang and was arrested on a couple of occasions for petty crimes, such as shoplifting and vandalism. He never finished high school and moved out on his own at the age of 18. Since that time, he has held a number of odd jobs and has made an effort to stay out of trouble. He currently works for a landscape contractor. He hates his job because he has to work too hard and is underpaid, but he has not attempted to look for other jobs.

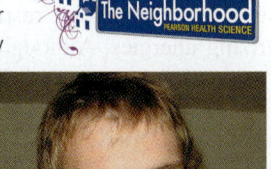

The Neighborhood
PEARSON HEALTH SCIENCE

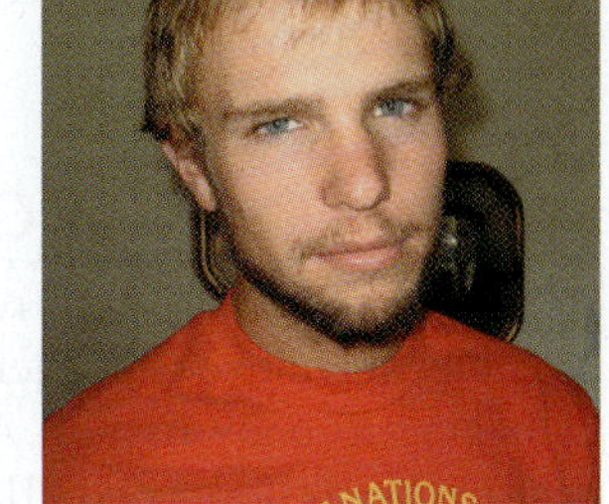

Casey lives with his pregnant girlfriend, Jessica Riley, and her 10-month-old son, Ryan. Casey does not particularly like Ryan and thinks that Jessica spoils him. However, he is very proud of the fact that Jessica is pregnant with his baby. He is controlling of Jessica and does not want anybody else looking at her.

On most days after work and into the evening, Casey drinks beer and smokes dope with his buddies. He is irritated that Jessica does not party with him as much as she did when they first met. Casey also uses other drugs when he can afford to buy them. He sometimes worries about the possibility of getting caught in a random drug screen but figures he can always get another job.

1. What factors in Casey's lifestyle place him at risk for HIV infection?
2. What teaching might you provide Casey to help him reduce his risk of HIV infection?
3. When caring for his pregnant girlfriend, what teaching might be indicated to reduce her risk of HIV infection related to her relationship with Casey?

14.2 HYPERSENSITIVITY

KEY TERMS

Allergen, *725*
Allergy, *725*
Anaphylaxis, *726*
Antigen, *725*
Cell-mediated immune responses, *730*
Hypersensitivity, *725*
Localized response, *726*
Serum sickness, *729*
Systemic response, *726*
Transfusion reaction, *727*

BASIS FOR SELECTION OF EXEMPLAR

Chronic Disease Management
Emergency room visits

LEARNING OUTCOMES

After reading about this exemplar, you will be able to:

1. Describe the pathophysiology, etiology, clinical manifestations, and direct and indirect causes of hypersensitivity.
2. Identify risk factors associated with hypersensitivity.
3. Illustrate the nursing process in providing culturally competent care across the life span for individuals with hypersensitivity.
4. Formulate priority nursing diagnoses appropriate for an individual with hypersensitivity.
5. Create a plan of care for individuals with hypersensitivity and their family members.
6. Assess expected outcomes for an individual with hypersensitivity.
7. Discuss therapies used in the collaborative care of an individual with hypersensitivity.
8. Employ evidence-based caring interventions for an individual with hypersensitivity.

OVERVIEW

Hypersensitivity is an altered immune response to an **antigen** (a foreign substance triggering the immune response) that results in harm to the client. When the antigen is environmental or exogenous, it is called an **allergy**, and the antigen is referred to as an **allergen**. The tissue response to a hypersensitivity reaction may be simply irritating or bothersome, causing a runny nose or itchy eyes, or it may be life-threatening, leading to blood cell hemolysis or laryngospasm.

Hypersensitivity reactions are classified primarily by the type of immune response that occurs on contact with the allergen. They also may be classified as immediate or delayed hypersensitivity responses. Anaphylaxis and transfusion reactions are examples of immediate hypersensitivity reactions; contact dermatitis is a typical delayed response. Allergies sometimes are referred to by the organ system affected (e.g., allergic rhinitis) or by the allergen involved (e.g., hay fever). However, classification by immunologic response is the preferred means of categorizing allergies. Although more than one type of reaction may occur simultaneously, it is practical and insightful to study and treat allergy by classified types (King, Mabry, Mabry, Godeon, & Marple, 2005).

PATHOPHYSIOLOGY AND ETIOLOGY

In a hypersensitivity reaction, an antigen–antibody or antigen–lymphocyte interaction causes a response that is damaging to body tissues. Antigen–antibody responses characterize types I, II, and III hypersensitivity, which are also known as immediate hypersensitivity responses (Table 14–5). Type IV hypersensitivity is an antigen–lymphocyte reaction, resulting in a delayed hypersensitivity response.

Type I (IgE-Mediated) Hypersensitivity

Common hypersensitivity reactions, such as allergic asthma, allergic rhinitis (hay fever), allergic conjunctivitis, hives, and anaphylactic shock, are typical of type I or IgE-mediated hypersensitivity. This type of hypersensitivity response is triggered when an allergen interacts with free IgE, causing IgE to bind to mast cells and basophils. This antigen–antibody complex prompts release of histamine and other chemical mediators, complement, acetylcholine, kinins, and chemotactic factors (Figure 14–14 ■).

Allergens can be ingested in food, injected as drugs, inhaled through the air, or absorbed through contact with unbroken skin. When a potent allergen enters the bloodstream and triggers a widespread antibody–antigen reaction and response to these chemical mediators, a **systemic response**, such as anaphylaxis, urticaria, or angioedema results. Common allergens in children include medications such as penicillin; animal dander; dust mites, mold, and plant pollens; and foods such as nuts, seafood, or egg white.

Anaphylaxis is an acute systemic type I response that may result in shock and death. It occurs in highly sensitive persons following exposure to a specific antigen, usually through injection or ingestion. The reaction begins within minutes of exposure to the allergen and may be almost instantaneous. The release of histamine and other mediators causes vasodilation and increased capillary permeability, smooth muscle contraction, and bronchial constriction. These chemical mediators cause the client to experience the typical manifestations of anaphylaxis. Initially, a sense of foreboding or uneasiness, light-headedness, and itching palms and scalp may be noted. Hives may develop, along with angioedema (localized tissue swelling) of the eyelids, lips, tongue, hands, feet, and genitals. Swelling also can affect the uvula and larynx, impairing breathing; this is further complicated by bronchial constriction. The client exhibits air hunger, stridor and wheezing, and a barking cough. These respiratory effects can be lethal if the reaction is severe and intervention is not immediately available. Vasodilation and fluid loss from the vascular system can lead to impaired tissue perfusion and hypotension, a condition known as *anaphylactic shock*. Substances known to trigger anaphylaxis are summarized in Box 14–12.

A **localized response** is a more common manifestation of type I hypersensitivity. Localized responses typically are atopic responses; that is, they have a strong genetic predisposition. Atopic reactions are the result of localized, rather than systemic, IgE-mediated responses to an allergen. They are prompted by contact of the allergen with IgE in the bronchial tree, nasal mucosa, and conjunctival tissues. Chemical mediators are released locally, producing symptoms such as asthma, allergic rhinitis (hay fever), conjunctivitis, or atopic dermatitis. Allergens commonly associated with atopic reactions of this type include pollens, fungal spores, house dust mites, animal dander, and feathers (Porth, 2005). Food allergens also may cause localized responses, such as diarrhea or vomiting. If the gastrointestinal mucosa is altered by a local allergic response, then the allergen may be absorbed, leading to a systemic reaction. Urticaria (hives) is the most common systemic response to food allergies.

TABLE 14–5 **Types of Hypersensitivity Reactions**

TYPE	ETIOLOGY	CLINICAL MANIFESTATIONS	EXAMPLES
Type I: Localized or systemic reactions	Antibodies bind to certain cells, causing release of chemical substances that produce an inflammatory reaction.	Hypotension, wheezing, gastrointestinal or uterine spasm, stridor, and urticaria	Extrinsic asthma, allergic rhinitis (hay fever), and food allergies
Type II: Tissue-specific reactions	Antibodies cause activation of a complement system, which leads to tissue damage.	Variable; may include dyspnea or fever	Transfusion reaction, ABO incompatibility, and hemolytic disease of the newborn
Type III: Immune complex–mediated reactions	Immune complexes are deposited in tissues, where they activate complement, which results in a generalized inflammatory reaction.	Urticaria, fever, and joint pain	Acute glomerulonephritis and serum sickness
Type IV: Delayed reactions	Antigens stimulate T cells, which release lymphokines that cause inflammation and tissue damage.	Variable; may include fever, erythema, and itching	Contact dermatitis, tuberculin skin test, and graft-versus-host disease

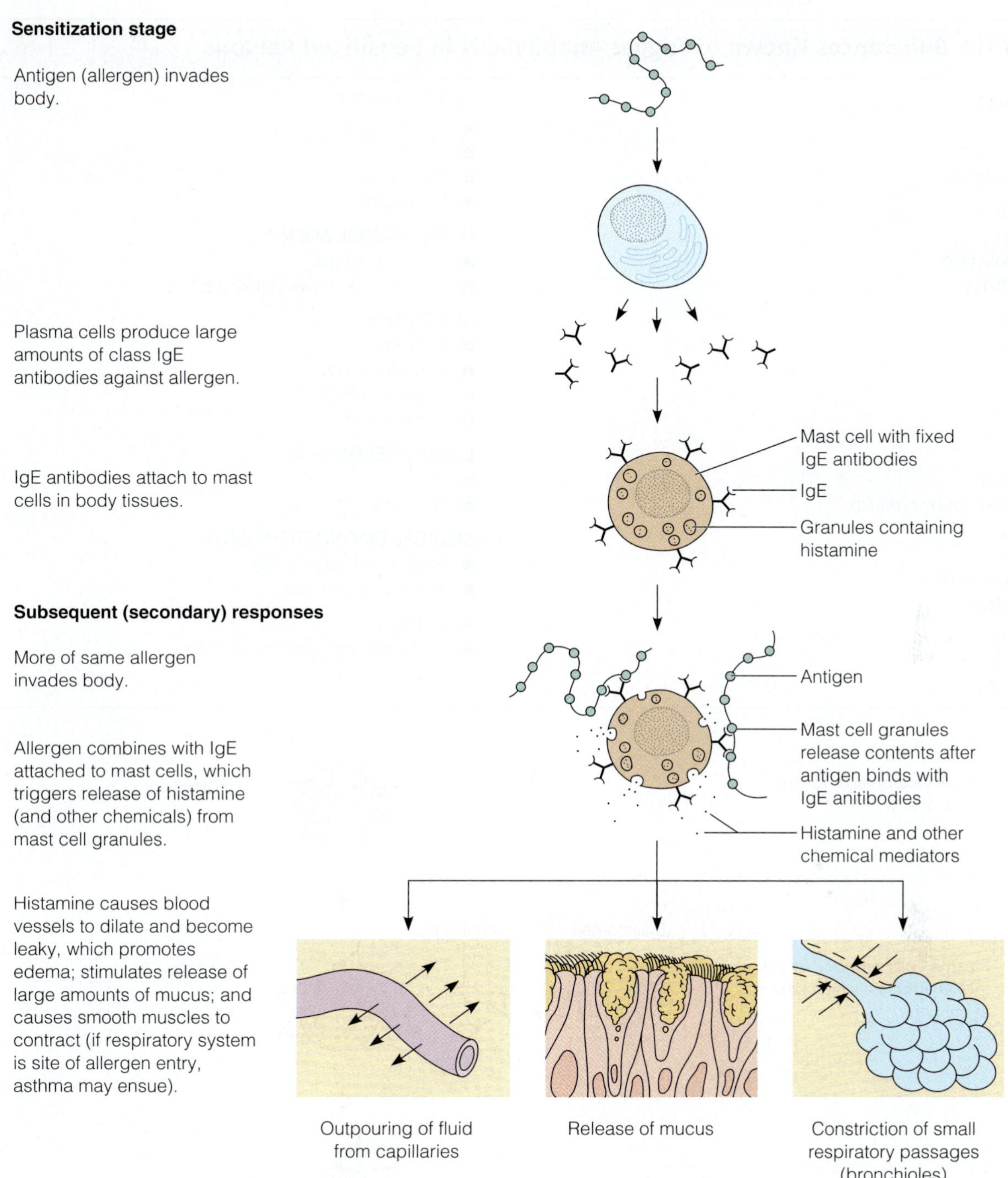
Sensitization stage
Antigen (allergen) invades body.
Plasma cells produce large amounts of class IgE antibodies against allergen.
IgE antibodies attach to mast cells in body tissues.
Mast cell with fixed IgE antibodies
IgE
Granules containing histamine
Subsequent (secondary) responses
More of same allergen invades body.
Allergen combines with IgE attached to mast cells, which triggers release of histamine (and other chemicals) from mast cell granules.
Antigen
Mast cell granules release contents after antigen binds with IgE anitibodies
Histamine and other chemical mediators
Histamine causes blood vessels to dilate and become leaky, which promotes edema; stimulates release of large amounts of mucus; and causes smooth muscles to contract (if respiratory system is site of allergen entry, asthma may ensue).
Outpouring of fluid from capillaries
Release of mucus
Constriction of small respiratory passages (bronchioles)

Figure 14–14 ■ Type I (IgE-mediated) hypersensitivity response.

Type II (Cytotoxic) Hypersensitivity

A hemolytic **transfusion reaction** to blood of an incompatible type is characteristic of a type II or cytotoxic hypersensitivity reaction. IgG- or IgM-type antibodies are formed to a cell-bound antigen, such as the ABO or Rh antigen. When these antibodies bind with the antigen, the complement cascade is activated, resulting in destruction of the target cell (Figure 14–15 ■). This type of reaction causes hemolytic disease of the newborn.

Type II reactions may be stimulated by an exogenous antigen, such as foreign tissue or cells, or by a drug reaction, in which the drug forms an antigenic complex on the surface of a blood cell, stimulating the production of antibodies. The resulting antigen–antibody reaction destroys the affected cell; for example, the administration of drugs such as penicillins, cephalosporins, and streptomycin may cause hemolytic anemia. Withdrawal of the drug stops the reaction and cell destruction (Goldsby et al., 2003).

Box 14–12 Substances Known to Trigger Anaphylaxis in Sensitized Persons

HORMONES
- Insulin
- Vasopressin
- Parathormone

ENZYMES
- Trypsin
- Chymotrypsin
- Penicillinase

POLLENS
- Ragweed
- Grass
- Trees

FOODS
- Eggs
- Seafoods
- Nuts and nut by-products
- Grains
- Beans
- Cottonseed oil
- Chocolate

VITAMINS
- Thiamine
- Folic acid

INSECT VENOM
- Yellow jacket
- Hornet
- Paper wasp
- Honey bee

OCCUPATIONAL AGENTS
- Rubber products
- Industrial chemicals (ethylenes)

ANTIBIOTICS
- Penicillins
- Cephalosporins
- Amphotericin B
- Nitrofurantoin

LOCAL ANESTHETICS
- Procaine
- Lidocaine

MEDICAL DIAGNOSTIC AGENTS
- Sodium dehydrocholate
- Sulfobromophthalein

ANTISERUM
- Antilymphocyte gamma globulin

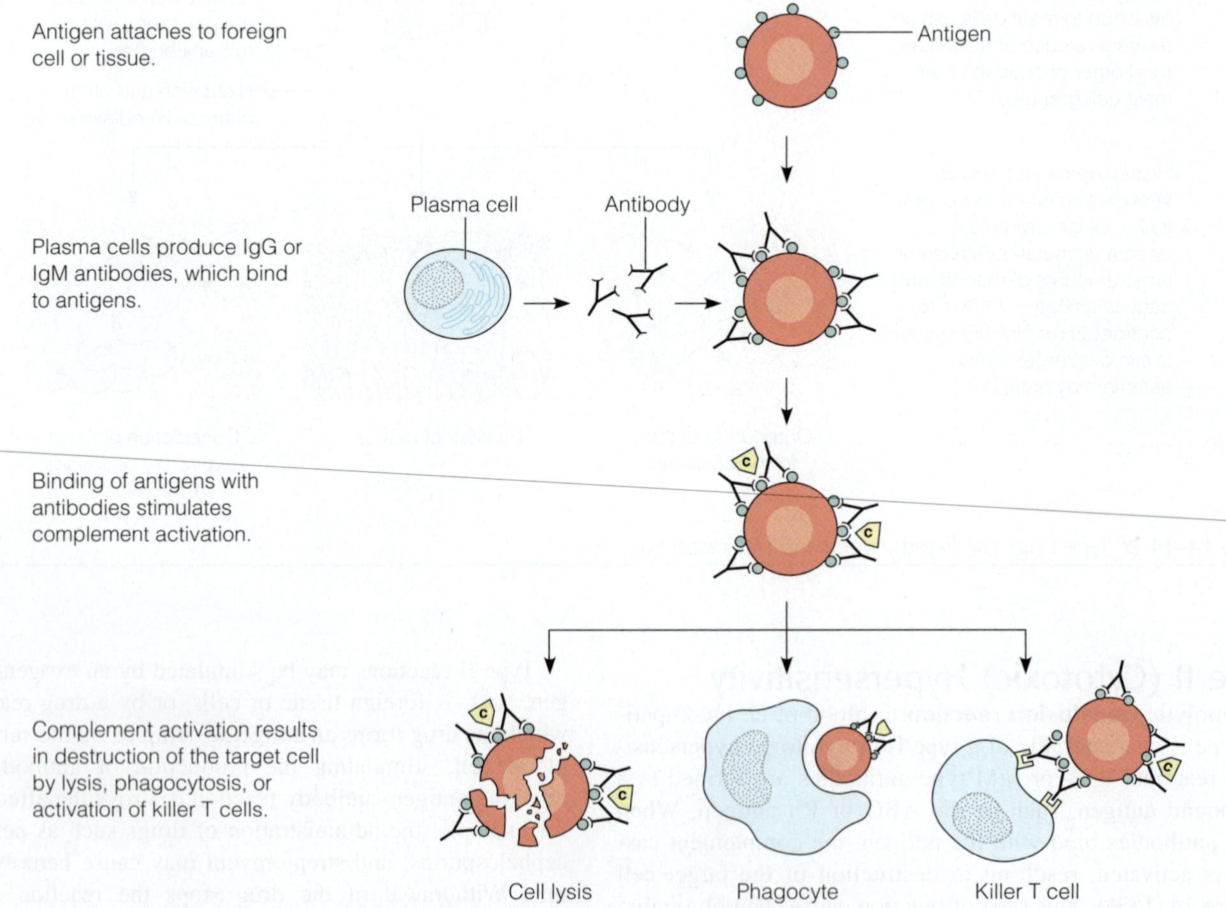

Antigen attaches to foreign cell or tissue.
Antigen
Plasma cell
Antibody
Plasma cells produce IgG or IgM antibodies, which bind to antigens.
Binding of antigens with antibodies stimulates complement activation.
C
Complement activation results in destruction of the target cell by lysis, phagocytosis, or activation of killer T cells.
Cell lysis
Phagocyte
Killer T cell

Figure 14–15 ■ Type II (cytotoxic) hypersensitivity response.

Endogenous antigens also can stimulate a type II reaction, resulting in an autoimmune disorder such as Goodpasture's syndrome, in which antigens are formed to specific tissues in the lungs and kidneys. Hashimoto's thyroiditis and autoimmune hemolytic anemia are additional examples of autoimmune type II reactions.

Type III (Immune Complex–Mediated) Hypersensitivity

Type III or immune complex–mediated hypersensitivity reactions result from the formation of IgG or IgM antibody–antigen immune complexes in the circulatory system. When these complexes are deposited in vessel walls and extravascular tissues, complement is activated, and chemical mediators of inflammation, such as histamine, are released. Chemotactic factors attract neutrophils to the site of inflammation. When neutrophils attempt to phagocytize the immune complexes, lysosomal enzymes are released, increasing tissue damage (Figure 14–16 ■).

Either systemic or local responses may be seen with type III reactions. For example, **serum sickness**, so named because it was first identified after administration of foreign serum (e.g., horse antitetanus toxin), is a systemic response. Immune complexes are deposited in walls of small blood vessels, the kidneys, and joints. Manifestations of serum sickness include fever, urticaria or rash, arthralgias, myalgias, and lymphadenopathy. Although foreign serums are no longer administered, serum sickness still occurs in response to some drugs, such as penicillin and sulfonamides.

Localized responses may occur at a number of different sites. As immune complexes accumulate in the glomerular basement membrane of the kidneys—for example, following a streptococcal infection or with systemic lupus erythematosus—glomerulonephritis develops. When an

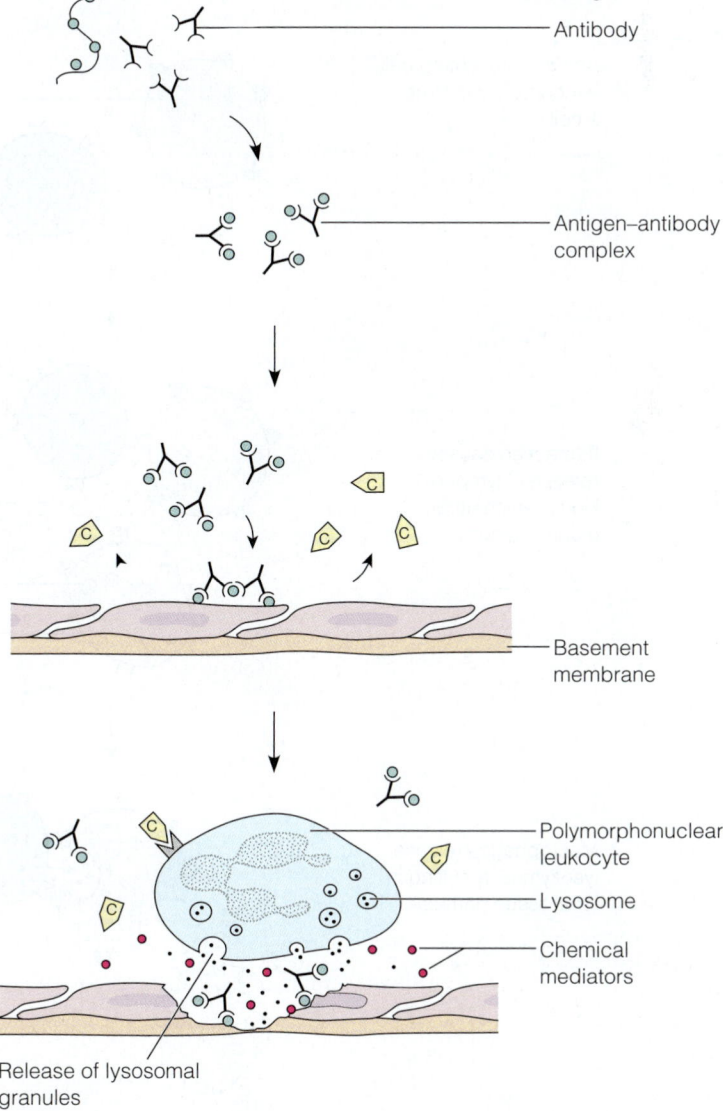

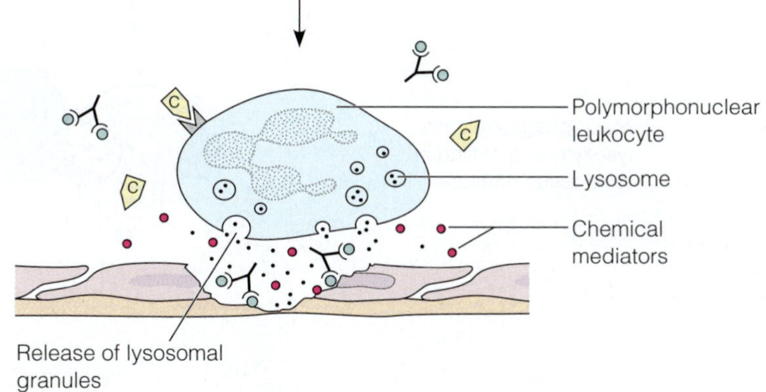

Figure 14–16 ■ Type III (immune complex–mediated) hypersensitivity response.

antigen such as dust from moldy hay is inhaled, an acute alveolar inflammatory response can occur. This condition can develop in agricultural workers.

Type IV (Delayed) Hypersensitivity

Type IV reactions differ from other hypersensitivity responses in two ways. First, these are **cell-mediated immune responses**, not antibody-mediated responses, and involve T cells of the immune system. Second, type IV reactions are delayed rather than immediate, developing 24–48 hours after exposure to the antigen.

Type IV hypersensitivity responses result from an exaggerated interaction between an antigen and normal cell-mediated mechanisms. This exaggerated interaction results in the release of soluble inflammatory and immune mediators (from the lysozymes within the macrophages) and recruitment of killer T cells, causing local tissue destruction (Figure 14–17 ■).

CONTACT DERMATITIS Contact dermatitis is a classic example of a type IV reaction. Intense redness, itching, edema, and thickening affect the skin in the area exposed to the antigen. Fragile vesicles often are present as well. Many antigens can provoke this response; poison ivy is a prime perpetrator. In the health care setting, an allergic response to latex also can produce contact dermatitis (see the section on latex allergy that follows). Other examples of cell-mediated responses include a positive tuberculin test and episodes of graft rejection.

LATEX ALLERGY Although the repetitive use of latex gloves is protective against infection, it also creates a persistent exposure to latex for health care workers. When gloves are powdered with cornstarch to facilitate donning and removing them, the cornstarch particles aerosolize when the gloves are removed. The arosolized cornstarch includes latex particles, and this creates a respiratory exposure as well as dermal exposure to latex. In addition, chemicals used in the manufacture of latex products may be irritating. Products such as balloons, condoms, and rubber bands commonly are made of latex.

Sensitivity to latex develops without the user being aware until a rash appears on the hands. Type IV hypersensitivity (contact dermatitis) can progress to type I systemic allergic

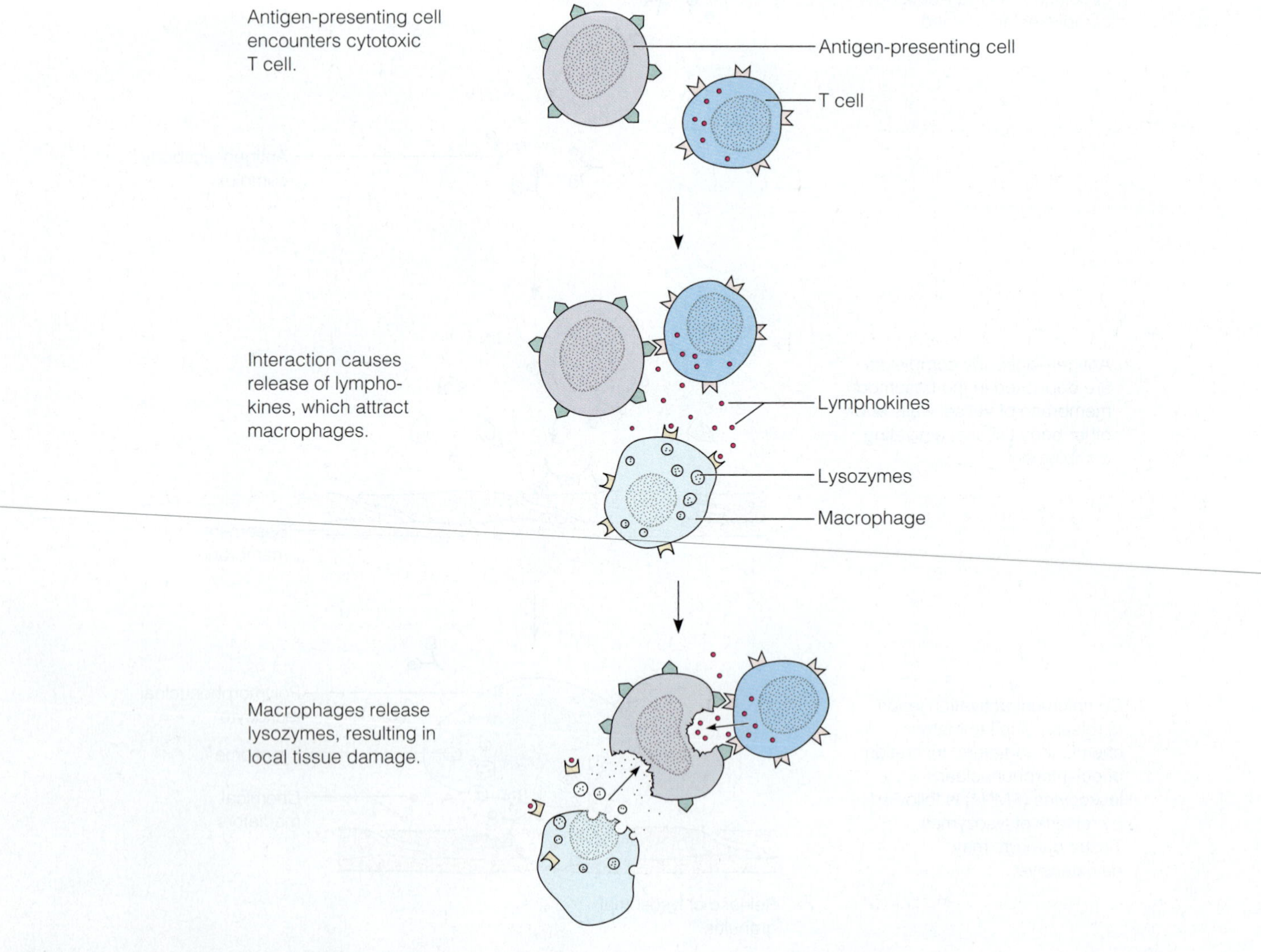
Antigen-presenting cell encounters cytotoxic T cell.
Antigen-presenting cell
T cell
Interaction causes release of lymphokines, which attract macrophages.
Lymphokines
Lysozymes
Macrophage
Macrophages release lysozymes, resulting in local tissue damage.

Figure 14–17 ■ Type IV (delayed) hypersensitivity response.

reactions without previous symptoms signaling an escalation. It is important to protect the client and the health care worker who is allergic to latex. Prevention is aided by employers who select products free of latex. Nonlatex gloves are recommended for use where there is no contact with infectious materials or blood. Workers should be screened periodically to detect symptoms of allergy and educated about latex sources. Hand washing after using latex products limits exposure (National Institute of Occupational Safety and Health [NIOSH], 2005).

An estimated 8–13% of health care workers are allergic to latex (NIOSH, 2005). Among health care workers with an allergic reaction to latex, sensitization to gloves is most prevalent (22%), 3.6% report contact urticaria, and 2.3% have asthma or rhinitis (Filon & Radman, 2006).

Latex allergy also is common among clients with certain health conditions. For example, approximately 50% of children with spina bifida and 34% of children with three or more surgeries are sensitive to latex (Bousquet et al., 2006; Reines & Seifert, 2005). Children most at risk for latex allergy include those with myelodysplasia and congenital urinary tract anomalies as well as those with bladder exstrophy (Hourihane, Allard, Wade, McEwan, & Strobel, 2002). Persons who have had repeated surgeries also are at higher risk because of high exposure to latex during surgery. Persons who are allergic to latex also have a high incidence of allergy to certain foods, most commonly kiwi fruit, bananas, and avocadoes (Taylor & Erkek, 2004).

Box 14–13 describes measures to protect against latex allergy. Table 14–6 addresses latex use in the hospital and home environments.

Box 14–13 **Measures to Protect Against Latex Allergy**

Health care personnel are at high risk of developing latex allergy because of intense exposure to products containing latex. An estimated 8–12% of health care workers are latex sensitive.

Nurses can protect themselves by using the following measures:

- Decrease exposure by using alternative products when available (use synthetic rubbers, polyethylene, nitrile, neoprene, and vinyl gloves).
- Use powder-free gloves if using latex gloves (the powder has high amounts of latex, which can be inhaled).
- Avoid use of oil-based hand creams and lotions before putting on latex gloves, because these preparations break down the latex.
- When symptoms of sensitivity to latex occur on exposure (e.g., rash, hives, nasal congestion, conjunctivitis, cough, or wheeze), contact the employee health department of your facility.
- If diagnosed as latex allergic, avoid all contact with latex, and wear a medical identification bracelet.

For more information, contact the National Institute for Occupational Safety and Health (NIOSH) at 1-800-346-4647 or the American Nurses Association at 1-800-637-0323 for more information.

PRACTICE ALERT

Starting in September 1998, the FDA ordered that medical products with latex carry a warning label that reads: "Caution: This product contains natural rubber latex, which may cause allergic reactions." Check the labels of products in your health care facility to find this label. What products do you expect to need the label? When children have latex allergy, have the family investigate all medical supplies for the warning label.

TABLE 14–6 **Latex in the Hospital and Home Environment**

FREQUENTLY CONTAIN LATEX	LATEX-SAFE ALTERNATIVES/BARRIERS
Latex in the Hospital	
Adhesives, skin (Smith+Nephew)	Mastisol (Ferndale)
Anesthesia circuits, bags, oxygen masks	Neoprene (Anesthesia Associates, Ohmeda adult), *some* Vital Signs
Band-Aids	Active Strip (3M), CURAD Neon, Readi-Bandages, NHP, *some* Airstrip
Blood pressure cuff, tubing (J&J)	Cleen Cuff (Vital Signs), nylon (*some* Trimline)
Bulb syringe	*Selected* Davol, Medline, Rusch, Premium, Baxter
Casts: Delta-Lite Podiatry, Orthoflex (J&J)	Scotchcast soft, Delta-Lites, *recent* Conformable (J&J), Caraglas Ultra, liners (Gore)
Catheters, condom	Clear Advantage, ProSys NL, *selected* Coloplast, Rochester, PolyTech (Hollister)
Catheters, indwelling & systems, urodynamic study (USD)	*Some* Am BioMed, Argyle, Bard, Cook, Dale, Kendall, Lifetech, Mentor, Rochester, Rusch, Vitaid, Adapters & plug (Addto)
Catheters, cardiac, vascular, pulmonary	*Some* World Medical, Am BioMed
Catheters, straight, coude	Mentor, RobNel (Sherwood), Coloplast, *selected* Bard, Rusch catheters
Catheters, feeding	Accumark feeding catheter (Sims Portex)
Cardiopulmonary resuscitation mannequins and medical training aids	*Most* Laerdal products

(continued)

TABLE 14–6 **Latex in the Hospital and Home Environment** **(continued)**

FREQUENTLY CONTAIN LATEX	LATEX-SAFE ALTERNATIVES/BARRIERS
Dressings: Dyna-flex, butterfly closures (J&J), BDF Elastoplast, Action Wrap, Coban (3M) Lyofoam (Acme), Spandage (Medi-tech), Telfa	Duoderm, Reston foam (3M), Opsite, Venigard, Comfeel, Sorbaview, Telfa (some) Xeroform, PinCare, Bioclusive, Montgomery strap (J&J), Webril, Metalline, Selopor, Opraflex, Centurion brief, *some* Airstrips, Rainbow Net (Surgilast), VAC
NOTE: latex in package only: Steri-strip wound closure system, Tegaderm, Tegasorb, Active Strips (3M), Nu-Derm (J&J), CURAD	
Ear plugs	Grainger (5F767)
Elastic wrap: ACE, Esmarch, Zimmer Dyna-flex, Elastikon (J&J)	E-Cotton, CEB elastic(coNco), Champ (Carolon), Adban Adhesive, X-Mark (Avcor) Co-Flex, PowerFlex (Andover), Comprilan (Jobst), Esmark (DeRoyal, NHP)
Electrode bulbs, pads, grounding	*Some* Baxter, Dantec EMG, Conmed, ValleyLab, Vermont Med, Staodyn, Neotrode
Endotracheal tubes, airways	*Selected* Berman, Mallinckrodt, Polamedco, Portex, Rusch, Sheridan, Shiley
Enemas	BabyLax, Theravac, Bowel Man't Tube (MIC), Pharmaseal set, all Fleet Ready-to-use, cone irrigation set (Convatec), silicone retention cuff tip (Lafayette)
G-tubes, buttons	Silicone (Bard, Flexiflo, MIC, Rusch, Stomate)
Gloves: sterile, clean, surgical, orthodontic	Allergard (J&J), dermaprene (Ansell), N-DEX (Best), Safeskin Nitrile, Neolon, SensiCare, Tru-touch (Maxxim), Nitrex, Tactyl 1,2 (SmartPractice), Duraprene (Allegiance Healthcare), Elastyren (Hermal, Center Labs), Boston Medical, Masel, Neotech
Incentive deep breathing exerciser	Voldyne 5000 (Sherwood David & Geck), Triflo II
IV access: injection ports, Y-sites, bags, pumps, buretrol ports, PRN adapters, needleless systems	*Cover Y-sites and bag ports—do not puncture. Use stopcocks for meds.* Polymer injection caps + burettes + Safsite (Braun), Abbot systems, Walrus, Gemini (IMED), *selected* Baxter (InterLink), Statlock, Ready Med, ConMed, Clave, Alaris, Hudson, *select sims,* IV boards (Avcor), Terumo Pumps: Mach II, ADS 100; Clic-Open (vial top remover [Sepha Pharm.])
Operating room/infection control masks, hats, shoe covers	*Some* by Kimberly Clark, TECNOL; OR and sterile packs (CML, DeRoyal) twill ties
Medication vial stoppers	*Some* AmRegent, Astra, Bedford Labs, Fujisawa, Gensia, Glaxo, Lilly, Roche
Miscellaneous items	Soft-Grip fabric clamp covers (Scanlan), Precision Dynamics I.D. bracelets
Penrose drains	Jackson-Pratt, Zimmer Hemovac
Pulse oximeters, thermometer probes	Nonin oximeters, *selected* Nellcor sensors, Diatec probe covers
Reflex hammers	Cover with plastic bag
Respirators	Advantage (MSA), HEPA-Tech (Uvex), PFR 95 (Tecnol), 3M 1860
Resuscitators, manual	*Certain* Ambu, Armstrong, Laerdal, Puriton Bennett, Vital Blue, Respironics, Rusch
Spacer (for metered dose inhalers)	ACE spacer (Center Labs), OptiHaler (HealthScan)
Stethescope tubing	PVC (*some* Littman) cover with ScopeCoat or latex-free stockinette (Albahealth)
Suction tubing	PVC (Davol, Laerdal, Mallinckrodt, Superior, Yankauer) Medline, Ballard
Syringes, disposable	Terumo Medical, Abbott PCA Abboject, Norm-Ject (Air-Tite), EpiPen, *selected* BD syringes, AdvantaJet (Activa)
Tapes: pink, Waterproof (3M), Zonas, Moleskin, cloth, Waterproof (J&J), adhesive felt (Acme)	Dermicel (J&J), Durapore, Microfoam, Micropore, Transpore (3M) Cath-Strip (Genetic Labs), Ice Tape (P.O.Pak), All-Felt (Universal Foot Care)
Tonopen disposable covers (glaucoma tester)	
Tourniquets	Children's Medical, Grafco, VelcroPedic, X-Tourn straps (Avcor), Free-Band (Kent)
Theraband (also strip, tube), other OT supplies	REP Bands & Cords (OPTP), Exercise putty (Rolyan), new Thera-Band Exercisers plastic tubing-Tygon LR-40 (Norton), elastic thread, sheets (JPS Elastomerics)
Tubing, sheeting	
Vascular stockings (Jobst)	Compriform Custom (Jobst)
Latex in the Home and Community	
Art supplies: paints, glue, erasers, fabric paints	Elmers (School Glue, Glue-All, GluColors, Carpenters Wood Glue, Sno-Drift paste) FaberCastel erasers, Crayola (*except* stamps, erasers), Liquitex paints, DickBlick Tempera & acrylic paints & soap erasers, Play-Doh

TABLE 14–6 **Latex in the Hospital and Home Environment** **(continued)**

FREQUENTLY CONTAIN LATEX	LATEX-SAFE ALTERNATIVES/BARRIERS
Balloons	Mylar balloons, self-sealing *Myloons*
Balls: Koosh balls, tennis balls, bowling balls	PVC (Headstrom Sports Ball), Nerf Foam Balls
Carpet backing, gym floor, basement sealant	Provide barrier—cloth or mat
Chewing gum	Bubblicious, Trident (Warner-Lambert), Wrigley gums (check new products)
Clothes: applique on Tees, elastic on socks, underwear, sneakers, sandals	Cloth-covered elastic, neoprene (Decent Exposures, NOLATEX Industries) Buster Brown elastic-free socks (Vermont Country Store)
Condoms, contraceptive sponges, diaphragm	Polyurethane (Avanti), female condom (Reality), Wideseal Silicone Diaphragms (Milex), Trojan Supra Condom
Crutches: tips, axillary pads, hand grips	Cover with cloth, tape
Dental dams, cups, bands, root canal material orthodontic rubber bands	PURO/M27 intraoral elastics (Midwest Orthodontic), wire springs, sealant (Delton) dams (Meer Dental, Hygenic Corp), John O Butler, Earloop masks (Richmond)
Diapers, incontinence pads, rubber pants	Huggies, First Quality, Gold Seal, Tranquility, Always, *some* Attends, Drypers Diapers (not training pants), Confidence (Paper-Pak), Pampers, Luvs
Feeding nipples	Silicone, vinyl (*selected* Gerber, Evenflo, MAM, Ross, Mead Johnson)
Food handled with latex gloves	Synthetic gloves for food handling
NOTE: Associated allergies are reported to banana, avocado, chestnut, kiwi, and other fruits.	
Handles on racquets, tools, bicycles	Vinyl, leather handles, or cover with cloth or tape
Infant toothbrush-massager	Soft bristle brush or cloth, Gerber/NUK
Kitchen cleaning gloves	PVC MYPLEX (Magla), cotton liners (Allerderm)
Miscellaneous items	*Some* medical stickers by MediBadge, UAL, Cushie Tushie Potty Seat
Newsprint, ads, coupons, lottery scratch tickets	
Pacifiers	Soothies (Children's Med Ventures), *selected* Binky, Gerber, Infa, Kip, MAM
Rubber bands, bungee cords	Plasti bands
Toys: Stretch Armstrong, old Barbies	Jurassic Park figures (Kenner), 1993 Barbie, Disney dolls (Mattel), many toys by Fisher Price, Little Tikes, Playschool, Discovery, Trolls (Norfin), Silly-putty
Water toys & equipment: beach thongs, masks, bathing suits, caps, scuba gear, goggles	PVC, plastic, nylon, Suits Me Swimwear
Wheelchair cushions, tires	Jay, ROHO cushions, use leather gloves, Sof Care bed/chair cushions (Gaymar)
Zippered plastic storage bags	Waxed paper, plain plastic bags, Ziploc bags

Source: From the Spina Bifida Association of America, www.sbaa.org, 4590 MacArthur Blvd NW, Suite 250, Washington, DC 20001–4226. Used with permission.

Etiology

An estimated 50 million people in the United States (or one in every five) are diagnosed with some form of hypersensitivity. The incidence of hypersensitivity has been noted to be on the increase since the early 1980s. Hypersensitivity is the fifth leading chronic disease in the United States among all age groups and the third most common in children under 18 years of age. More than 17 million outpatient office visits are scheduled as a result of hypersensitivity reactions. Each year, nearly 400 people die from penicillin reactions, 200 from food allergies, and 100 from allergies to insects. In 2008, 10 deaths were attributed to latex reactions (Asthma and Allergy Foundation of American, 2009).

As people age, the secondary immune response may show changes. In some individuals, the number of B cells in the circulation decreases. As a result, tissues are slower to repair and are more vulnerable to disease, especially infections. A decline in the production of IgE with aging leads to a decrease in allergic, or hypersensitivity, reactions.

Risk Factors

Anyone can have a hypersensitivity reaction. However, risk generally increases with previous exposure, because antigens must be formed with the first exposure before hypersensitivity is likely to occur. Hypersensitivity reactions are likely to increase in intensity with repeated exposure. Age, sex, concurrent illnesses, and previous reactions to related substances have been identified as having a role in risk for hypersensitivity (Gomes & Demoly, 2005). According to Viale (2009), factors that determine the development and severity of anaphylaxis include the antigen's route of entry, the amount of antigen introduced, the rate of absorption for the antigen, and the individual's degree of hypersensitivity.

Having a family member with an allergy increases the chance that a child will be affected, even to different allergens or by showing different bodily manifestations. If one parent has an allergy of any type, chances are one in three that each child will have an allergy (Asthma and Allergy Foundation of American, 2009).

CLINICAL MANIFESTATIONS

Hypersensitivity can manifest in a number of ways, including anaphylaxis, atopic disease, serum sickness, or contact dermatitis. Therefore, symptoms can range from mild to severe or life-threatening and be either localized or systemic. Characteristic findings in clients with hypersensitivity are summarized in Table 14–7.

Mild hypersensitivity responses can cause discomfort, fatigue, and even embarrassment to the client. These may last for a few hours to a day or two and normally resolve either by themselves or with over-the-counter treatments. Acute exacerbations of allergic rhinitis or asthma lasting beyond a day or two may result in a localized infection. Localized pain and inflammation, difficulty breathing, and loss of smell, taste, and appetite are associated with moderate to severe respiratory hypersensitivity responses. Moderate hypersensitive responses of the skin include urticaria and atopic and contact dermatitis. Moderate reactions from food allergies include urticaria and gastrointestinal symptoms. Severe reactions, regardless of the means of entry by the antigen or the location of the initial reaction, may lead to respiratory distress or death.

Care for clients with allergic responses focuses on minimizing exposure to the allergen, preventing a hypersensitivity response, and providing prompt, effective interventions for allergic responses when they occur. Identifying allergens for the individual to reduce the likelihood of exposure is a key aspect of management. A complete history of the client's allergies is obtained, including medications, foods, animals, plants, and other materials. The type of hypersensitivity

CLINICAL MANIFESTATIONS AND THERAPIES Hypersensitivity

ETIOLOGY	CLINICAL MANIFESTATION	CLINICAL THERAPIES
Serum sickness is a reaction to proteins in antiserum derived from animals.	Manifestations develop up to 2 weeks after exposure and include rash, pruritus, arthralgia, fever, lymphadenopathy, hypotension, splenomegaly, glomerulonephritis, or proteinuria.	■ Often does not require medical intervention. Severe reactions may be treated with corticosteroids, antihistamines, and/or plasmapheresis.
Allergic rhinitis is a seasonal response to pollens of specific plants but also may result from exposure to dust mites, danders, or molds at any time of year.	Rhinorrhea, watery eyes, itchy throat, hives, sore throat, nasal congestion, and headache are common manifestations. Facial edema; if the client does not respond to initial treatment, may result in a severe reaction.	■ Most effective treatment is reducing exposure to allergen by remaining indoors, showering on entering the house to remove pollen, keeping doors and windows closed, use of special filters on air conditioners, and maintaining a clean, dust-free environment. ■ Pharmacologic therapies include decongestants, antihistamines, antileukotrienes, and immunotherapy. A tapered dose of oral steroids may be necessary to resolve an acute exacerbation.
Graft-versus-host disease results as an immune response to organ, bone marrow, or stem cell transplants.	Acute in the first 100 days after transplant. Manifestations include a pruritic macular-papular rash beginning on extremities and progressing to the trunk, nausea, vomiting, anorexia, diarrhea, cramping, abdominal pain, and impaired liver function. Chronic after the first 100 days. Manifestations include recurrent infections, skin reactions, thrombocytopenia, mouth throat and esophageal ulcers, GI disorders, cholestasis, and eye irritation (Higman & Vogelsang, 2004).	■ Immunosuppressant drugs are the standard therapy. ■ Careful assessment of clients who have received a transplant. ■ Education of client regarding symptoms to report immediately.
Allergic asthma	Characterized by bronchoconstriction and airway inflammation. Clients may complain of having shortness of breath, chest pain, or a feeling like "an elephant is sitting on my chest."	■ Prevention and treatment are similar to that for allergic rhinitis, with inhaled medications such as albuterol and inhaled corticosteroids being among the most effective treatments. Clients with severe allergic asthma may require antibiotics and oral steroids if an exacerbation continues beyond 2–3 days, trapping mucus and resulting in an infection.

TABLE 14–7 **Characteristic Findings in Children with Allergies**

SYSTEM	CHARACTERISTIC FINDINGS
Respiratory	Asthma, rhinitis (seasonal and perennial), serous otitis media, cough, pneumonia, croup, and edema of glottis
Gastrointestinal	Abdominal pain and colic, stomatitis, constipation, diarrhea, bloody stools, geographic tongue, and vomiting
Skin	Angioedema, urticaria, eczema, atopic dermatitis, erythema multiforme, purpura, drug and food rashes, and contact dermatitis
Nervous	Headache, tension, fatigue, convulsions, Ménière's disease, and tremor
Eye	Conjunctivitis, cataract, ciliary spasm, and iritis
Blood	Thrombocytopenic purpura, hemolytic anemia, leukopenia, and agranulocytosis
Musculoskeletal	Arthralgia, myalgia, rheumatoid arthritis, and torticollis
Genitourinary	Dysuria, vulvovaginitis, and enuresis
Miscellaneous	Anaphylactic shock, serum sickness, and autoimmune disorders

response is documented, as is its onset, manifestations, and usual treatment.

When a documented or suspected hypersensitivity reaction occurs, the allergen (e.g., intravenous medication or transfusion) is withdrawn immediately. With a type I hypersensitivity response, managing the client's airway takes highest priority, followed by maintaining cardiac output. Type II hypersensitivity responses may necessitate aggressive management of bleeding or renal failure. A type III (immune complex–mediated) reaction is treated by removing the offending antigen and interrupting the inflammatory response.

With a hypersensitivity response, supportive care is important to relieve discomfort. This often involves the administration of selected antihistamine or anti-inflammatory medications. Other therapies, such as plasmapheresis, may be prescribed in selected instances.

COLLABORATION

Clients with recurrent moderate and severe hypersensitivity responses should be referred to a specialist. Clients with allergic rhinitis, asthma, and atopic dermatitis may be referred to an allergist for further evaluation and testing. Immunologists care for those with other, more complicated immune disorders. Clients with complicated respiratory issues may benefit from working with a respiratory therapist to learn appropriate posturing and breathing techniques. Physical therapists can help clients design an appropriate exercise regimen after surgery or transplantation. Dieticians can help clients with food allergies develop appropriately healthy, tasty recipes and menus.

For children with severe hypersensitivity reactions, nurses at the child's clinic or specialist's office should help the parents design and provide an action plan for the child's school. This ensures that teachers, nurses, and other school personnel know how to respond in the event the child has an exacerbation at school. Any medication being kept at school should also accompany the child on field trips. Day care centers and summer camps should receive copies of the child's action plan as well.

Severe allergies in children can be very frightening for the parents. Any parent who has witnessed a child experience a severe exacerbation or anaphylactic reaction lives in fear that it will happen again—and that the child's life will be at risk. These parents, as well as adult clients with severe hypersensitivity reactions, may benefit from support groups. Many hospitals and clinics offer such groups. The Food Allergy and Anaphylaxis Network (http://www.foodallergy.org) is a helpful resource for many, as are the websites of the American Academy of Allergy, Asthma, and Immunology (http://www.aaaai.org) and National Jewish Health (http://www.nationaljewish.org), one of the leading medical research centers in the United States. Many support groups also are available online through sites like *Web*MD (http://www.webmd.com) and Yahoo! (http://www.yahoo.com).

Diagnostic Tests

To identify possible allergens and hypersensitivity reactions, laboratory tests may be ordered. To determine causes of hypersensitivity reactions, skin tests may be ordered.

LABORATORY TESTING To identify possible allergens or hypersensitivity reactions, the following laboratory tests may be ordered:

- *White blood cell (WBC) count with differential:* This test can detect high levels of circulating eosinophils. Normally, eosinophils constitute a very small percentage (1–4%) of the total WBCs. Eosinophilia, however, often is present in clients with type I hypersensitivities.
- *Radioallergosorbent test (RAST):* This test measures the amount of IgE directed toward specific allergens. Test results are compared with control values and used to identify hypersensitivities. RAST poses no risk for an anaphylactic reaction. It is particularly useful in detecting allergies to some occupational chemicals and toxic allergens (Goldsby et al., 2003).
- *Blood type and crossmatch:* These tests are ordered before any anticipated transfusions. The client's ABO blood group and Rh status are determined. Two major antigens, designated A and B, may be present on RBCs. Clients with the A antigen are designated as blood type A; those with

the B antigen are designated as blood type B. When neither antigen is found on the RBCs, the person is identified as type O. A third major RBC antigen is the Rh antigen. Persons with this antigen are called Rh positive; those without are called Rh negative. Because a blood transfusion is actually a transplant of living tissue, antigen matching is vital to prevent significant hypersensitivity reactions. Once blood type is determined, a sample of the client's blood is mixed with a sample of matching donor blood and observed for antigen–antibody reactions in the crossmatch portion of this test. Although this procedure greatly reduces the risk of a hemolytic transfusion reaction (type II hypersensitivity), it does not totally eliminate it.

- *Indirect Coombs' test:* This test detects the presence of circulating antibodies (other than ABO antibodies) against RBCs. The client's serum is mixed with the donor's RBCs. If the client's serum contains antibodies to an RBC antigen, agglutination (clumping together) will occur. This is called a positive response. The normal value is negative (no agglutination). This test is also part of the crossmatch of a blood "type and crossmatch."
- *Direct Coombs' test:* This test detects antibodies on the client's RBCs that damage and destroy the cells. This test is used following a suspected transfusion reaction to detect antibodies coating the transfused RBCs. It also can identify hemolytic anemia when the cause is unknown. In the direct Coombs' test, the client's RBCs are mixed with Coombs' serum, which contains antibodies to IgG and several complement components. Agglutination will occur if the client's RBCs are coated with antibodies, resulting in a positive test. As with the indirect Coombs' test, the normal test result is negative (no agglutination).
- *Immune complex assays:* These tests may be performed to detect the presence of circulating immune complexes in suspected type III hypersensitivity responses. These assays are particularly useful in diagnosing suspected autoimmune disorders. Nonspecific assays of IgG-, IgM-, and IgA-containing immune complexes, which do not detect specific antibodies, as well as specific antibody assays may be done. The normal result is a test negative for circulating immune complexes. A negative test does not, however, rule out an immune complex hypersensitivity response. In some cases, a negative result may indicate that the disease process has reached a later stage, in which complexes are no longer circulating but have initiated extensive tissue damage, such as glomerulonephritis (Kasper et al., 2005).
- *Complement assay:* This test also is useful in detecting immune complex disorders. In these disorders, complement is, in effect, used up by the development of antigen–antibody complexes. Decreased levels are seen on examination. Both total complement level and amounts of individual components of the complement cascade can be determined.

SKIN TESTING Skin tests also are used to determine causes of hypersensitivity reactions. These tests can identify specific allergens to which a person may be sensitive. Allergens for testing are selected according to the client's history. Test solutions made from extracts of inhaled, ingested, or injected materials, such as pollens, mites, venoms, or some drugs, are used for the prick test and intradermal testing. Epicutaneous testing (prick testing) generally is done first to avoid a systemic reaction; it is followed by intradermal testing of allergens with a negative response to prick testing (Tierney et al., 2005). Performing the large-dose intradermal test first would place individuals who are highly allergic to a substance at increased risk for an anaphylactic reaction. Substances that cause a reaction to the prick test should not be tested intradermally.

Specific skin tests include the following:

- *Prick (epicutaneous or puncture) test:* A drop of diluted allergenic extract is placed on the skin, and the skin is then pricked or punctured through the drop. With a positive test, a localized pruritic wheal and erythema occur. The response is maximal at 15–20 minutes.
- *Intradermal test:* A small amount (just enough to create a wheal) of allergen extract at a 1:500 or 1:1,000 dilution is injected on the forearm or intrascapular area. If several allergens are being tested, injections are spaced 0.25–0.5 cm apart. As control measures, plain diluent (negative control) and histamine (positive control) also are injected. If no response to a particular allergen has occurred at 15–20 minutes, the test is negative. The appearance of a wheal and erythema, with a wheal diameter at least 5 mm greater than that produced by the control, indicates a positive response (Figure 14–18 ■).
- *Patch test:* A 1-inch patch impregnated with the allergen (e.g., perfume, cosmetics, detergents, or clothing fibers) is applied to the skin for 48 hours. Absence of a response indicates a negative test result. Positive responses are graded from mild (erythema in the exposed area) to severe (erythema, papules, vesicles, or ulceration).
- *Food allergy test:* This test is performed when a food allergy is suspected but the source or implicated food item has not been clearly identified. Symptoms of a food allergy typically are demonstrated within hours of eating. Initially, the client is asked to keep a diary of foods consumed and any allergic responses for a week. After this period, an elimination diet is prescribed. This diet excludes most common food allergens and all suspected foods for 1 week. Any

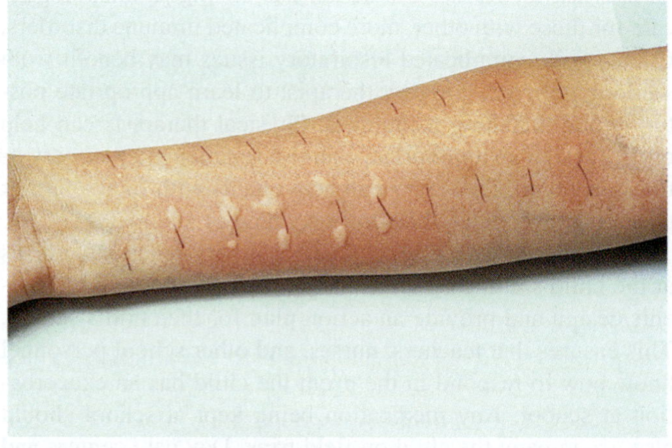

Figure 14–18 ■ Skin testing on the forearm, showing induration and erythema typical of a positive response to an antigen.

Source: Southern Illinois University/Photo Researchers, Inc.

foods that may contain allergens in combination, such as breads, also are eliminated. If symptoms do not improve, a different variation of the elimination diet is prescribed. If symptoms are relieved, foods are reintroduced to the diet one at a time until symptoms recur, indicating an allergy to that food.

Pharmacologic Therapies

Pharmacologic treatments are chosen based on the severity of the hypersensitivity reaction and the impact on the client's lifestyle. More severe reactions may require administration via the IV route in order to get the fastest possible action while mild reactions may be treated with oral medications. A thorough medication history should be collected before administering any medication, including medication allergies.

ANTIHISTAMINES Antihistamines are the major class of drugs used in treating the symptoms of hypersensitivity responses, particularly type I reactions. They also are useful to some extent in relieving manifestations (e.g., urticaria) of some type II and type III reactions.

Antihistamines block H_1-histamine receptors, acting as a competitive antagonist to histamine, but they do not affect the production or release of histamine. The prototype antihistamine is diphenhydramine (Benadryl). It and other antihistamines alleviate the systemic effects of histamine, such as urticaria and angioedema. They also are useful in relieving allergic rhinitis, but they are not effective in all clients. They also dry respiratory secretions through an anticholinergic effect.

Antihistamines are not effective in relieving asthmatic responses to allergens and may actually worsen symptoms by their drying effect on respiratory secretions. In addition, their use is limited by their side effects, especially drowsiness and dry mouth.

Antihistamines are available in both prescription and nonprescription preparations. The preferred route of administration is oral, although diphenhydramine and others can be given parenterally, particularly when immediate action is needed, as in anaphylaxis. Antihistamines often are combined with a sympathomimetic agent, such as pseudoephedrine, to improve their decongestant activity and counteract their sedative effect.

CROMOLYN SODIUM Cromolyn sodium (Intal, NasalCrom) is a drug used to treat allergic rhinitis and asthma. It acts by stabilizing the mast cell membrane, thus preventing chemical mediator release (Lehne, 2004), and it is most effective when applied directly to involved tissue by inhaler or nasal spray. Cromolyn sodium has few side effects and a wide margin of safety, making it a good choice for clients in whom it is effective (Tierney et al., 2005).

CORTICOSTEROIDS Corticosteroids (glucocorticoids) are used in both systemic and topical forms for many types of hypersensitivity responses. Their anti-inflammatory effects, rather than their immunosuppressive effects, are of most benefit. A short course of corticosteroid therapy often is used for severe asthma, allergic contact dermatitis, and some immune-complex disorders (Tierney et al., 2005). Corticosteroids in topical forms or delivered by inhaler may be used for longer periods of time with few side effects; however, systemic absorption can occur.

IMMUNOTHERAPY For clients who receive only minimal benefit from antihistamines and cromolyn sodium, or who require a course of oral steroids more than once a year, immunotherapy may be recommended. Also called hyposensitization, desensitization, or allergy shots, immunotherapy consists of injecting an extract of the allergen(s) in gradually increasing doses. Immunotherapy is used primarily for allergic rhinitis or asthma related to inhaled allergens. It also has been shown to be effective in preventing anaphylactic responses to insect venom. With weekly or biweekly subcutaneous injections of the allergen, the client develops IgG antibodies to the allergen that appear to effectively block the allergic IgE-mediated response. Once a therapy plateau is reached, injections are continued indefinitely, either monthly or bimonthly. Immunotherapy typically is provided by an allergist or immunologist.

EPINEPHRINE The immediate treatment for anaphylaxis is parenteral epinephrine, an adrenergic agonist (sympathomimetic) drug that has both vasoconstricting and bronchodilating effects. These qualities, combined with its rapid action, make epinephrine ideal for treating an anaphylactic reaction. For mild reactions with wheezing, pruritus, urticaria, and angioedema, a subcutaneous injection of 0.3–0.5 mL of 1:1,000 epinephrine generally is sufficient. For clients with an injected toxin such as a bee sting, an additional amount equivalent to half the above may be injected directly into the site of the sting and a tourniquet applied above it to prevent further systemic absorption. Intravenous epinephrine using a 1:100,000 concentration may be used in the client with a more severe anaphylactic reaction.

Clients who have experienced an anaphylactic reaction to insect venom or other potentially unavoidable allergens should carry a kit (commonly called a bee sting kit or EPI-Pen) for immediate treatment of future exposures. This kit typically includes a prefilled syringe of epinephrine and an epinephrine nebulizer, allowing prompt self-treatment.

OMALIZUMAB (XOLAIR) In 2003, the FDA approved omalizumab (Xolair), a new therapy that was originally tested and approved for use by clients with steroid-dependent asthma and high IgE values but who have been unresponsive to immunotherapy. Xolair inhibits type I hypersensitivity reactions by binding to free-floating IgE, thereby preventing IgE from binding to the mast cell. Since its introduction, Xolair has had wide success for its target client population—so much so that many physicians are trying it on clients with other type I hypersensitivities, including severe allergic dermatitis and severe allergic rhinitis.

Radioallergosorbent testing and approval from one's physician, insurance company, and the manufacturer are required before a client can receive Xolair. Administered by subcutaneous injection in a physician's office, clinic, or infusion center, Xolair is an incredibly expensive medication. It also is not an immediate solution: Some clients may not experience improvement in symptoms for several months to a year. The

FDA has issued a black box warning regarding the possibility of clients who take Xolair exhibiting anaphylactic reactions within 48 hours of receiving the medication, but these episodes are very rare.

Clinical Therapies

Other treatments used for hypersensitivity responses generally are dictated by the severity of the response and by the organ system affected. Airway management takes highest priority for the client with an acute anaphylactic reaction. Insertion of an endotracheal tube or emergency tracheostomy may be required to maintain airway patency with severe laryngospasm. Because anaphylaxis places the person at risk for vasomotor collapse and significant hypotension, it is necessary to insert an intravenous line and initiate fluid resuscitation with an isotonic solution, such as Ringer's lactate.

Plasmapheresis (removal of harmful components in the plasma) may be used to treat immune complex responses such as glomerulonephritis and Goodpasture's syndrome. Plasma and the glomerular-damaging antibody–antigen complexes are removed by passing the client's blood through a blood cell separator. The RBCs are then returned to the client along with an equal amount of albumin or human plasma. This procedure usually is done in a series rather than as a one-time treatment. It also is not without risk; informed consent is required. Potential complications of plasmapheresis include those associated with intravenous catheters, shifts in fluid balance, and alteration of blood clotting.

Complementary Therapies

Many people find a number of complementary and alternative medicine therapies soothing and comforting for a number of illnesses. However, clients with type I hypersensitivity should consult their physician before using herbal remedies, teas, and aromatherapy, because many of these may contain substances to which individuals can be allergic. Chamomile tea, widely used for its comforting properties, has not been studied thoroughly, but there have been sufficient reports of allergic reactions to chamomile to warrant concern. Like ragweed, it is a member of the daisy family, so individuals with ragweed allergies should avoid using chamomile products (NCCAM, 2008).

Many Asian Americans and Native Americans may rely on complementary and alternative medicine because such therapies are a part of their culture. Nurses working with clients from these cultures should ask appropriate questions to determine if the client practices any herbal medicine and should be sensitive to the importance that clients may place on traditional therapies from their cultures of origin.

NURSING PROCESS

Nursing care related to hypersensitivity reactions is directed primarily toward prevention, early identification, and the provision of prompt, effective treatment. Nurses are also responsible for teaching clients and families to alert school personnel, coworkers, and all health care personnel in hospitals and clinics to the client's allergy or condition.

Health promotion activities include helping clients to identify possible allergens that prompt a hypersensitivity response and discussing possible strategies to avoid these allergens. Anyone with severe food allergies may need assistance from a dietitian to discuss necessary dietary changes and ways to continue meeting nutrient needs. It is important that persons with hypersensitivities inform health care personnel of all allergens. People who experience or are at risk for anaphylactic reactions should wear a MedicAlert bracelet or tag at all times to identify the substance(s) that provokes this response.

Assessment

Collect the following data through the health history and physical examination:

- *Health history.* Risk factors, hypersensitivities (medications, household dust, bee stings, etc.), reaction (rash, hives, difficulty breathing), type of treatment for hypersensitivity reactions, allergy skin testing, and history of asthma, hay fever, or dermatitis
- *Physical assessment.* Mucous membranes of nose and mouth, skin for lesions or rashes, eyes (tearing and redness), respiratory rate, and adventitious breath sounds.

Further focused assessments are described in the Implementation section that follows.

Diagnosis

Priority nursing diagnoses will vary according to the type of hypersensitivity reaction experienced by the client. Because nurses are most likely to become involved with a client experiencing a type I or type II response, this section focuses on diagnoses for these clients.

Airway, breathing, and circulation (the ABCs) are of greatest importance for the client with an anaphylactic reaction. When a hemolytic reaction to an incompatible blood transfusion occurs, the client is at risk for injury. Priority nursing diagnoses include the following:

- Ineffective Airway Clearance
- Decreased Cardiac Output
- Risk for Injury
- Impaired Spontaneous Ventilation
- Risk for Shock.

Plan

Of key importance in planning nursing care is prevention of hypersensitivity reaction through thorough data collection to help the client avoid exposure to known allergens. Priority goals for the client with hypersensitivity may include the following:

- Client will avoid known substances that provoke hypersensitivity response.
- Client will describe self-care to reduce symptoms of seasonal allergies.
- Client will describe proper self-administration of medications prescribed by the physician.
- Client participates in determining substances that cause hypersensitivity by keeping an accurate food journal.

Implementation

Nursing implementations are dependent on the client's individualized needs and the nursing diagnoses selected. Actions in the following section are grouped by nursing diagnosis.

Ineffective Airway Clearance

Maintaining a patent airway (or establishing airway clearance in the event of anaphylactic shock) is the highest priority in caring for the client experiencing a hypersensitivity response. Placing the client in Fowler's to high-Fowler's position allows optimal lung expansion and ease of breathing (Figure 14–19 ■).

For mild to moderate reactions, the nurse will:

- Assess respiratory rate and pattern, level of consciousness and anxiety, nasal flaring, use of accessory muscles of respiration, chest wall movement, audible stridor; palpate for respiratory excursion; auscultate lung sounds and any adventitious sounds, such as wheezes. Extreme anxiety or agitation, nasal flaring, stridor, and diminished lung sounds indicate air hunger and possible airway obstruction, necessitating immediate intervention.

In anaphylactic reactions, the airway may be obstructed as a result of facial angioedema, bronchospasm, or laryngeal edema. In these cases, the nurse will:

- Administer oxygen per nasal cannula at a rate of 2–4 L/min. Apply oxygen emergently, and obtain a physician order for oxygen administration. This increases the alveolar oxygen and its availability to cells of the body.
- Insert a nasopharyngeal or oropharyngeal airway, and arrange for immediate intubation as indicated. Ensuring an adequate airway is vital to preserve life.
- Administer subcutaneous epinephrine 1:1,000, 0.3–0.5 mL, as prescribed. This may be repeated in 20–30 minutes if necessary. Also, administer parenteral diphenhydramine (deep intramuscular or intravenous) as prescribed. Epinephrine is a potent vasoconstrictor and bronchodilator, counteracting the effects of histamine. Diphenhydramine is an antihistamine that blocks histamine receptors and their effect. These medications can be effective in rapidly reversing manifestations of anaphylaxis (Box 14–14).
- Provide calm reassurance. Hypoxemia and air hunger are terrifying for the client. Anxiety can impair the client's ability to cooperate with treatment and increase the respiratory rate, making breathing less effective.

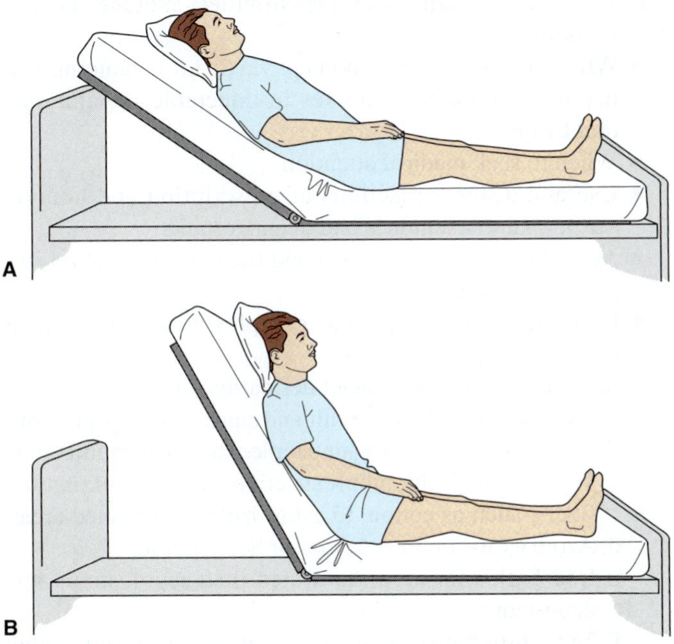

Figure 14–19 ■ *A*, Fowler's position and *B*, high-Fowler's position.

Decreased Cardiac Output

Peripheral vasodilation and increased capillary permeability resulting from the release of histamine can significantly impair cardiac output. In all cases in which a client is exhibiting a hypersensitive reaction, the nurse should:

- Monitor vital signs frequently, noting fall in blood pressure, decreasing pulse pressure, tachycardia, and tachypnea. These changes in vital signs may indicate shock.
- Assess skin color, temperature, capillary refill, edema, and other indicators of peripheral perfusion. As cardiac output falls, peripheral vessels constrict, and tissue perfusion is impaired.
- Monitor level of consciousness. A change in level of consciousness (lethargy, apprehension, or agitation) often is the first indicator of decreased cardiac output.

When cardiac output falls to the degree that tissue perfusion becomes impaired and hypoxia results, a state of anaphylactic shock exists. In this event, the nurse should:

- Insert one or more large-bore (≥18 gauge) intravenous catheters. It is important to insert intravenous catheters as soon as possible to provide sites for rapid fluid replacement.
- Administer warmed intravenous solutions of lactated Ringer's or normal saline as prescribed. These isotonic solutions help to maintain intravascular volume. Warmed solutions are used to prevent hypothermia from the rapid administration of large amounts of fluid at room temperature (~70°F [21.1°C]).

Box 14–14 **Using an EpiPen®**

If the client has had a severe or systemic reaction in the past, ensure that the client and family or caregivers know how to handle an anaphylactic reaction if another one occurs:

- Inform the client that kits with syringes of premeasured epinephrine are available by prescription.
- Ensure that client, family members, and caregivers understand how to use the kit.
- Encourage the client to wear a medical alert bracelet.
- Instruct the client and family on proper storage of the kit and to avoid exposing the kit to sun or high temperature.
- Instruct the client and family to frequently check the expiration date of the adrenaline.
- Emphasize to the client and family that a kit should be readily available in all settings where the client studies, works, or plays, including school, camp, work, and child care. In addition to the client, someone else should always be instructed in how to use the kit as well.

- Insert an indwelling catheter, and monitor urinary output frequently. As the cardiac output drops, the glomerular filtration rate falls. With an output of less than 30 mL/hr, the client is at risk for acute renal failure from ischemia.
- Place a tourniquet above the site of an injected venom (e.g., a bee sting), and infiltrate the site with epinephrine as prescribed. Use of a tourniquet and the vasoconstriction resulting from epinephrine infiltration reduce further absorption of the allergen.
- Once breathing is established, place the client flat with the legs elevated. This position enhances perfusion of the central organs, such as the brain, heart, and kidneys.

PRACTICE ALERT

Aggressive fluid therapy may lead to hypervolemia and pulmonary edema. Assess for shortness of breath and crackles in the lungs.

Risk for Injury

As noted, the potential for hypersensitivity responses is high in clients subjected to medical treatments. Because a blood transfusion is a transplant of living tissue, the risk for adverse immunologic response and injury is particularly significant.

- Obtain and record a thorough history of previous blood transfusions and any reactions experienced, *no matter how mild.* Alert the physician if previous transfusion reactions have occurred. The client who has received prior blood transfusions is at increased risk for a hypersensitivity reaction, because antibody production may have been stimulated by previous exposure to antigens.
- Check for a signed informed consent to administer blood or blood products. It is important to obtain informed consent for such invasive and risky procedures.
- Using two licensed health care professionals, double-check client identity, blood type, Rh factor, crossmatch, and expiration date for all blood and blood components received from the blood bank with the client's data. This is an important safety measure to reduce the risk of a hemolytic transfusion reaction as a result of incompatible blood types.
- Take and record vital signs within 15 minutes before initiating the blood infusion. This provides a baseline for evaluating any changes related to the blood transfusion.
- Acetaminophen and diphenhydramine are prescribed and administered prior to beginning a blood transfusion to decrease inflammation and increase client comfort. These medications will not mask serious reactions.
- Infuse blood into a site separate from that of any other intravenous infusion. Use a catheter of at least 20 gauge for the infusion to promote flow. This reduces the risk of damage to the blood cells because of incompatibility with other intravenous solutions or physical trauma.
- Administer with normal saline to prime intravenous tubing. When blood is administered with dextrose solutions (e.g., D_5W, D_5NS), blood cell hemolysis and aggregation occur; administration with lactated Ringer's can cause agglutination of cells.
- Administer 50 mL of blood during the first 15 minutes of the transfusion. Reactions generally occur within the first 15 minutes.
- During transfusion, monitor for complaints of back or chest pain, increase in the temperature of more than 1.8°F, chills, tachycardia, tachypnea, wheezing, hypotension, hives, rashes, or cyanosis. These signs may indicate an adverse reaction to the blood transfusion.
- Stop the blood transfusion immediately if a reaction occurs, no matter how mild. Remove the blood bag and the tubing with blood in it. Flush new intravenous tubing with normal saline, keeping the intravenous line open. Notify the physician and the blood bank.
- If a reaction is suspected, send the blood and administration set to the laboratory with a freshly drawn blood sample and urine specimen from the client. These will be used to identify the cause of the reaction as well as its effect on the client.
- If no adverse reaction occurs, administer the transfusion over 2–4 hours. This time frame is important to limit the risk of bacterial growth.

PRACTICE ALERT

To reduce bacterial contamination, begin a blood transfusion within 30 minutes of its delivery from the blood bank.

Community-Based Care

The vast majority of hypersensitivity responses are appropriately treated by the client or family members, with little or no medical intervention. Teaching therefore is a vital component of care. If the client is at risk for anaphylaxis, involving the family in teaching is essential because the response may occur with such rapidity that the client will be unable to provide self-care. When teaching the client and family about managing hypersensitivities, include the following points:

- When and how to use an anaphylaxis kit containing epinephrine and antihistamines in injectable, inhaler, and oral forms
- When to seek medical attention
- Use and adverse reactions of prescription and nonprescription antihistamines and decongestants
- Advantages of autologous blood transfusion if future surgery is scheduled
- Prevention of an immune complex reaction, such as glomerulonephritis
- Skin care to prevent contact dermatitis, including:
  a. Expose affected areas to air and sun as much as possible.
  b. Avoid direct contact with people who have an infection.
  c. Wear cool, light, nonrestrictive clothing of natural fibers, such as cotton, to avoid irritating affected areas.
  d. Avoid exposure to extremes of heat or cold.
  e. Use bath oils or plain water instead of soaps and detergents.
  f. Take tub baths in cool to lukewarm water rather than showers.

SPINE Spinal involvement usually is limited to the cervical vertebrae. Neck pain is common, and neurologic complications can occur.

Extra-Articular Manifestations

RA is a systemic disease with a variety of extra-articular manifestations. These are seen particularly in clients with high levels of circulating rheumatoid factor. As mentioned previously, fatigue, weakness, loss of appetite, weight loss, and low-grade fever are common when the disease is active. In addition, anemia resistant to iron therapy frequently affects clients with RA. Skeletal muscle atrophy also is common, usually being most apparent in the musculature around affected joints.

Rheumatoid nodules may develop, generally in the subcutaneous tissue of areas subject to pressure: on the forearm, olecranon bursa, over the MCP joints, and on the toes (Figure 14–22 ■). Rheumatoid nodules are granulomatous lesions that are firm and either movable or fixed. These nodules also may be found in viscera, including the heart, lungs, intestinal tract, and dura.

Other possible extra-articular manifestations of RA include subcutaneous nodules, pleural effusion, vasculitis, pericarditis, and splenomegaly (enlargement of the spleen). The effect of RA on the body can be seen in the following Multisystem Effects feature.

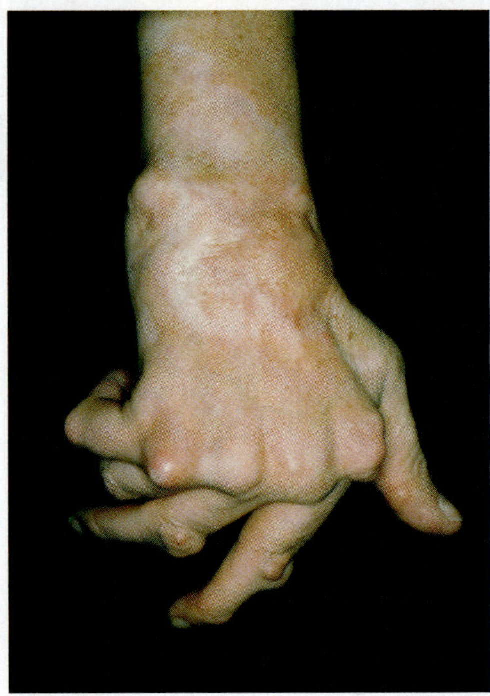

Figure 14–22 ■ Rheumatoid nodules.

Increased Risk of Coronary Heart Disease

People with RA have an increased risk of developing coronary heart disease. In turn, coronary heart disease increases the risk for myocardial infarction and death; in fact, RA is associated with a shortened life expectancy (Flynn & Johnson, 2005). RA affects the heart by:

- Direct effects on the blood vessels, with measures of C-reactive proteins (inflammatory markers) being more predictive of future cardiovascular disease than levels of low-density lipoprotein.
- Increased risk for having low high-density lipoprotein level, high cholesterol and triglyceride levels, high blood pressure, and high homocysteine levels—all of which increase the risk for coronary heart disease.
- The damaging side effects that many medications (e.g., methotrexate and steroids) often have on coronary vessels.

Juvenile Rheumatoid Arthritis

Similar to RA diagnosed in adults, **Juvenile rheumatoid arthritis (JRA)** is a chronic inflammatory autoimmune disorder diagnosed in children that is characterized by joint inflammation resulting in decreased mobility, swelling, and pain. JRA occurs slightly more often in girls than in boys. It may enter remission or occasionally continue as a chronic disease. Approximately 5–18 of every 100,000 children develop JRA each year (Ilowite, 2002). Treatment is similar to that provided for adults with RA.

Remission may last for months, years, or a lifetime. JRA affects joints and surrounding tissues in addition to possibly affecting other organs, such as the heart, lungs, liver, and eyes. During the course of this disease, the child may experience pain, impaired mobility, and interference with normal growth and development. However, 70% of children with JRA experience permanent remission by adulthood. In rare cases, the disease is unresponsive to treatment, or the child may suffer lasting impairment, such as bone and joint changes. Children with an early onset of JRA have a better prognosis for complete recovery.

There are three types of JRA: pauciarticular, systemic, and polyarticular. **Pauciarticular arthritis** primarily affects the knees, ankles, and elbows, and it occurs more frequently in female clients. **Systemic arthritis** affects male and female clients equally and characteristically manifests by high fever, polyarthritis, and rheumatoid rash. Systemic arthritis also affects internal organs and joints. **Polyarticular arthritis** involves many joints (five or more), particularly the small joints of the hands and fingers. It also may affect the hips, knees, feet, ankles, and neck.

As with RA, the cause of JRA is unknown, but it is thought to have an autoimmune basis. Inflammation begins in the joint and leads to pain and swelling. Scar tissue eventually develops, resulting in limited ROM. This may be restricted to a few joints or be systemic, with involvement of multiple joints. Symptoms can include fever, rash, lymphadenopathy, splenomegaly, and hepatomegaly. The child may develop a limp or obviously favor one extremity over the other. A slow rate of growth or uneven growth of extremities also may be noted. Pain, stiffness, loss of motion, and swelling occur in the large joints, such as the knees. Older children may develop symmetric involvement of the small joints of the hand. The disease frequently is chronic, extending over several years after an initial manifestation with pain and other symptoms. However, remissions and exacerbations are characteristic.

MULTISYSTEM EFFECTS OF **Rheumatoid Arthritis**

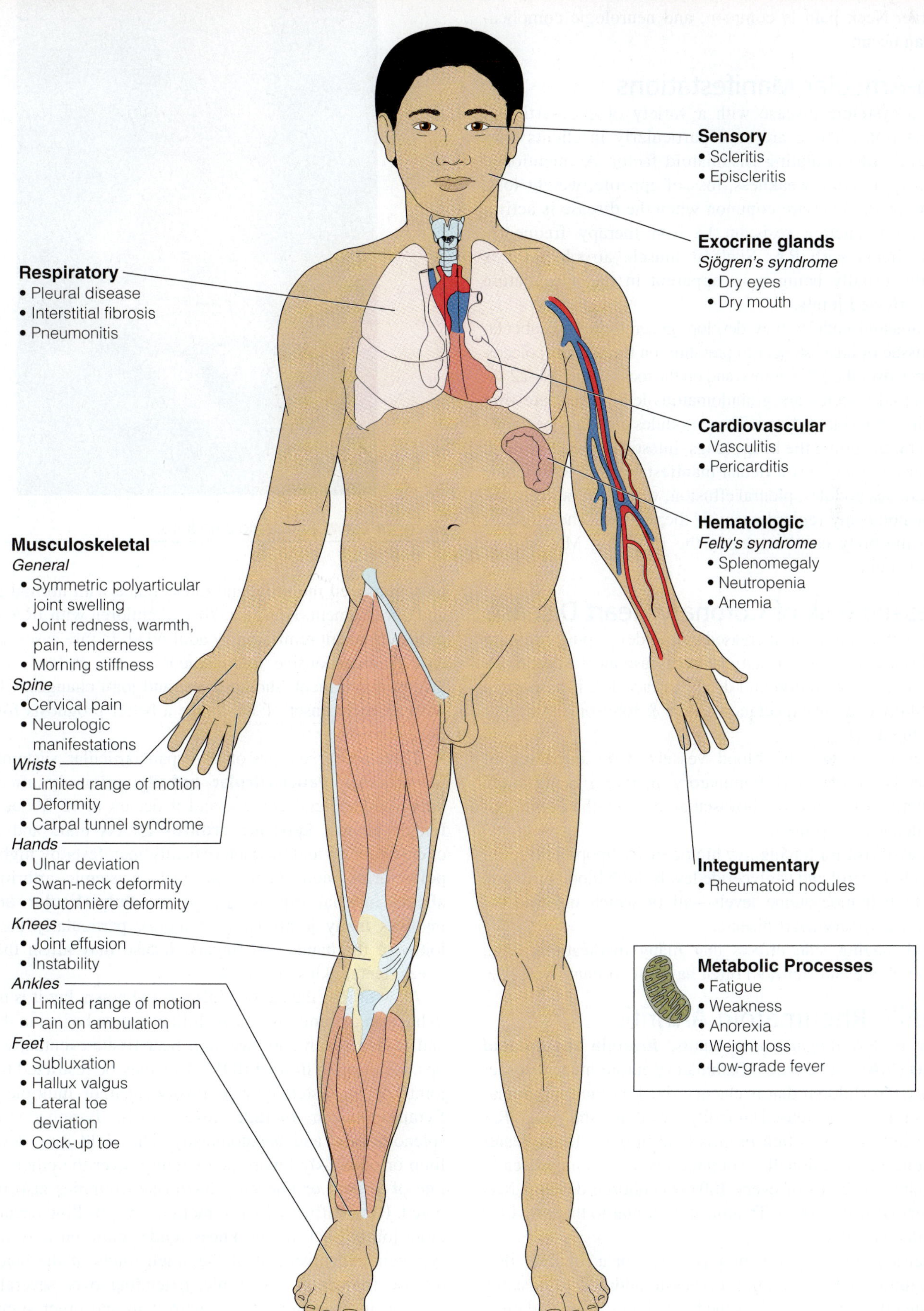

Sensory
• Scleritis
• Episcleritis
Exocrine glands
Sjögren's syndrome
• Dry eyes
• Dry mouth
Respiratory
• Pleural disease
• Interstitial fibrosis
• Pneumonitis
Cardiovascular
• Vasculitis
• Pericarditis
Hematologic
Felty's syndrome
• Splenomegaly
• Neutropenia
• Anemia
Musculoskeletal
General
• Symmetric polyarticular joint swelling
• Joint redness, warmth, pain, tenderness
• Morning stiffness
Spine
• Cervical pain
• Neurologic manifestations
Wrists
• Limited range of motion
• Deformity
• Carpal tunnel syndrome
Hands
• Ulnar deviation
• Swan-neck deformity
• Boutonnière deformity
Knees
• Joint effusion
• Instability
Ankles
• Limited range of motion
• Pain on ambulation
Feet
• Subluxation
• Hallux valgus
• Lateral toe deviation
• Cock-up toe
Integumentary
• Rheumatoid nodules
Metabolic Processes
• Fatigue
• Weakness
• Anorexia
• Weight loss
• Low-grade fever

CLINICAL MANIFESTATIONS AND THERAPIES Rheumatoid Arthritis

ETIOLOGY	CLINICAL MANIFESTATION	CLINICAL THERAPIES
Coronary heart disease (CHD)	Elevated C-reactive protein, low high-density lipoprotein, elevated cholesterol and triglycerides, and high homocysteine Hypertension	■ Treatment is similar to that of any client with CHD but must include management of rheumatoid arthritis (RA), with additional goal of reducing inflammation that exacerbates risk for worsening CHD
Pleural effusion (collection of fluid in the pleural space)	Shortness of breath and hypoxia Pain, fever, and heat at the site if fluid becomes infected	■ Therapeutic aspiration may be sufficient; may require chest tube insertion for continuous drainage ■ Chemical or surgical pleurodesis in which two pleural surfaces are scarred to each other, preventing recurrence of fluid accumulation ■ Placement of Pleurex catheter with one-way valve for daily drainage of fluid ■ Management of inflammatory process resulting from RA can reduce risk of development or reduce reaccumulation of fluid
Vasculitis (inflammation of veins and/or arteries)	Fever, weight loss, palpable purpura, livedo reticularis, myalgia or myositis, mononeuritis multiplex, stroke, myocardial infarction, hypertension, gangrene, nose bleeds, bloody cough, pulmonary infiltrates, abdominal pain, bloody stools, perforations, and glomerulonephritis	■ Reducing the inflammatory process ■ Immune suppression ■ Cortisone ■ Specific treatments aimed at the organ system involved
Pericarditis (inflammation of the pericardium)	Chest pain radiating to the back that is relieved by sitting up and leaning forward is worsened by lying down Dry cough, fever, and anxiety Auscultated friction rub, ST-segment elevation, PR-interval depression in all leads, cardiac tamponade, congestive heart failure, jugular vein distention, and peripheral edema	■ Pericardiocentesis ■ Antibiotics if cause is believed to be infectious (unlikely when associated with RA) ■ Steroids to reduce inflammation ■ Colchicine ■ Emergency surgery may be required to restore normal heart function if other treatments fail
Uveitis (inflammation of the middle layer of the eye; most commonly a complication of juvenile RA)	Redness of the eye, blurred vision, sensitivity to light, dark floating spots along the visual field, and eye pain	■ Good prognosis if treated promptly ■ Glucocorticoid steroids (oral or topical eye drops) after ruling out any corneal ulcers ■ Topical cycloplegics to reduce eye swelling ■ Antimetabolite medications are used for harder-to-treat or more aggressive cases

Diagnosis is made primarily on the basis of the history and assessment findings—in particular, arthritis having an onset before 17 years of age and persisting for at least 6 weeks, with no other identifiable cause. The disease may occur for a limited time and then improve (**monophasic**), may recur periodically (**polycyclic**), or may last for 3–6 months or longer (**persistent**) (Singh-Grewal, Schneider, Bayer, & Feldman, 2006). There are no specific laboratory tests for the disease. In some children, rheumatoid factor, human leukocyte antigen B27, and antinuclear antibody tests are positive, and the erythrocyte sedimentation rate may be elevated.

Complications such as eye chronic uveitis, which results from chronic inflammation, may occur in children with JRA, especially those with pauciarticular arthritis. Children with polyarticular and systemic JRA should be examined by an ophthalmologist for uveitis every 6 months, and children with pauciarticular arthritis should be examined every 3 months.

As mentioned, interference with normal growth is another potential complication. JRA may result in bone growth disturbance, such as contractures or effusions. The administration of corticosteroids as treatment can inhibit growth as well.

COLLABORATION

Once the diagnosis of RA has been established, the goals of therapy are to relieve pain, reduce inflammation, slow or stop joint damage, and improve well-being and ability to function. No cure currently exists for RA; the goal of treatment is to relieve its manifestations. An interdisciplinary approach is used, with a balance of rest, exercise, physical therapy, and suppression of the inflammatory processes.

Clients will benefit from collaboration among many health care providers, including physicians, nurses, physical and occupational therapists, and nutritionists or dieticians.

Working together, the health care team and client will be able to find a more effective combination of treatments that will result in minimum discomfort and maximum function for the client. Including the client's pharmacist as a member of the health care team can help to ensure that contraindicated medications are not being prescribed and minimize any potential side effects. Clients with RA should be encouraged to get all their prescriptions filled at a single pharmacy to reduce the chance of contraindicated medications being prescribed by multiple physicians.

Diagnostic Tests

Diagnostic tests are used to help establish the diagnosis of RA. Testing also is used to rule out other forms of arthritis and connective tissue disorders. Laboratory tests are used to measure rheumatoid factors and the erythrocyte sedimentation rate, which typically is elevated. CBC is done to identify anemia. Diagnosing RA in the early stages often is difficult, but a new blood test in which clients are tested for antibodies to cyclic citrullinated peptide is highly effective in accurately detecting early RA.

Examination of the synovial fluid will demonstrate changes associated with inflammation, including increased turbidity (cloudiness), decreased viscosity, and increased protein and WBC levels. X-rays of affected joints are the most specific test for diagnosis of RA. Early in the disease, few changes may be evident other than soft-tissue swelling and joint effusions. However, as the disease progresses, joint space narrowing and erosions are seen.

Pharmacologic Therapies

Four general approaches are used in the pharmacologic management of RA:

1. Aspirin and other NSAIDs and mild analgesics are used to reduce the inflammatory process and manage the manifestation of the disease. Although these drugs may relieve manifestations of RA, they appear to have little effect on disease progression.
2. Low-dose oral corticosteroids are used reduce pain and inflammation. Recent studies suggest that low-dose oral corticosteroids also may slow the development and progression of bone erosions associated with RA.
3. A diverse group of drugs classified as disease-modifying or slow-acting antirheumatic drugs may be employed to treat RA. These drugs, which include gold compounds, d-penicillamine, antimalarial agents, infliximab (Remicade), and sulfasalazine, appear to alter the course of the disease, reducing its destruction of joints. Immunosuppressive and cytotoxic drugs are included in this category as well.
4. Intra-articular corticosteroids may be used to provide temporary relief in clients for whom other therapies have failed to control inflammation.

ASPIRIN Unless its use is contraindicated for the client, aspirin often is the first drug prescribed in the treatment of RA. Aspirin, an NSAID, is an inexpensive and effective anti-inflammatory and analgesic agent. The dose of aspirin required to achieve a therapeutic blood level (15–30 mg/dL) and its full anti-inflammatory effect is approximately 4 g/day in divided doses (three or four 325-mg. tablets qid). This effective dose is just under the toxic dose, which produces tinnitus and hearing loss. The client may be instructed to increase the dose of aspirin gradually, until either maximal improvement or toxicity occurs. If tinnitus develops, the client should reduce the dose by two to three tablets per day until the tinnitus stops.

Gastrointestinal side effects and interference with platelet function are the greatest hazards of aspirin therapy. Clients are instructed to take aspirin with meals, milk, or antacids to minimize gastrointestinal distress and reduce the risk of gastrointestinal bleeding. Enteric-coated forms of aspirin and nonacetylated salicylate compounds produce less gastric distress than plain or buffered aspirin and reduce the risk of gastric ulceration, but they are more expensive. Salsalate (Disalcid, Mono-Gesic, Salflex) and choline magnesium trisalicylate (Trilisate, Tricosal) are examples of nonacetylated salicylate products. All salicylate products are contraindicated for clients with a history of aspirin allergy.

OTHER NONSTEROIDAL ANTI-INFLAMMATORY DRUGS A number of other NSAIDs are available for use in the management of RA if aspirin is not tolerated or effective. All NSAIDs act by inhibiting prostaglandin synthesis. Although the efficacy of all NSAIDs, including aspirin, is equivalent, client responses are individual. Several trials of different NSAIDs may be necessary to find the most effective drug.

Some NSAIDs are considerably more expensive than aspirin but may cause less gastrointestinal distress and require fewer doses per day. Gastric irritation, ulceration, and bleeding remain the most common toxic effects of NSAIDs. They also can affect the lower intestinal tract, leading to perforation or aggravation of inflammatory bowel disorders. All NSAIDs can be toxic to the kidneys.

Common NSAIDs prescribed for clients with RA are listed in Table 14–10. Nonprescription drugs also are available and include those containing ibuprofen, naproxen, and ketoprofen. The U.S. Food and Drug Administration (FDA) has initiated regulatory actions for both prescription and over-the-counter, nonselective NSAIDs. These actions include increased label warnings about the potential serious adverse cardiovascular and gastrointestinal effects of these drugs.

CORTICOSTEROIDS Systemic corticosteroids can dramatically relieve the symptoms of RA and appear to slow the progression of joint destruction. However, long-term use of corticosteroids is associated with multiple side effects, such as poor wound healing, increased risk of infection, osteoporosis, and gastrointestinal bleeding. In addition, severe rebound manifestations can occur when these medications are discontinued. For these reasons, the use of systemic corticosteroids is limited to low dosages daily. A client who discontinues use of systemic corticosteroids should wean off the medication over a period of several days or weeks.

DISEASE-MODIFYING DRUGS Disease-modifying drugs are a diverse group of medications including drugs that modify immune and inflammatory responses, gold salts, antimalarial agents, sulfasalazine, and d-penicillamine (Table 14–11). However, they share characteristics that make them useful in

g. To decrease pruritus, maintain a cool environment and avoid exercising.
h. Trim fingernails to reduce the risk of skin damage.

- Helpful resources:
  a. ALERT, Inc., Allergy to Latex Education and Resource Team
  b. Food Allergy Network.

Clients with type I hypersensitivities often are misunderstood and even mistreated by their families and community. "Are you really sick, or is it just your allergies?" is not an uncommon response to children returning to school or adults returning to work after being out sick because of an allergic reaction. Sometimes, even family members portray these negative attitudes. Nurses can help clients who are getting the "it's all in your head" treatment by giving them language, print media, and other resources to help clients teach family members, fellow students, and coworkers about this sometimes life-threatening condition.

Evaluation

Clients are evaluated based on their progress in meeting goals set during the planning stage. Potential outcomes may include the following:

- Client exhibits decreased symptoms and decreased frequency of hypersensitivity responses.
- Client demonstrates proper technique when administering medication using an EpiPen.
- Client provides accurate and thorough information in food or activity and symptom journal.

HEALTH CARE

If one in five Americans suffer from some form of hypersensitivity, the annual cost of treatment is $7 billion, and hypersensitivity is the fifth leading chronic disease and a major cause of absenteeism from work, what impact does hypersensitivity have on the health care system?

REVIEW Hypersensitivity

RELATE: LINK THE CONCEPTS

Linking the exemplar of Hypersentitivity with the concept of Oxygenation:

1. You are caring for a client who is having a severe hypersensitivity response. How will you assess the client's oxygenation statutes?
2. What nursing care can you provide to improve the client's oxygenation status?

Linking the exemplar of Hypersentitivity with the concept of Comfort:

3. You are caring for a client with seasonal hypersensitivity resulting in rhinorrhea, sore throat, and sinus congestion. What actions can you promote to improve comfort?
4. What client teaching would you provide in order to improve this client's comfort?

READY: GO TO COMPANION SKILLS MANUAL

- Administering an intradermal injection
- Administering a subcutaneous injection
- Mixing intradermal injections for skin tests
- Assessing the nose and sinuses
- Assessing the mouth and oropharynx
- Assessing the thorax and lungs

REFER: GO TO MYNURSINGKIT

REFLECT: CASE STUDY

Ron Jackson is a 12-month-old, African American child born to Martha Jackson. Martha has a history of multiple allergies, including drugs, food, pine pollen, and environmental hypersensitivities. Ron is brought to the clinic today for a well-baby checkup and to receive his 1-year immunizations. His vital signs are within normal limits, he is meeting developmental milestones, and his growth charts are within the 50th percentile. His mother reports that Ron has had several urinary tract infections this spring and that she has been treating them with over-the-counter medications, such as acetaminophen (Tylenol) for fever and discomfort and saline nasal spray to reduce nasal congestion. He is currently asymptomatic, bright and alert.

1. When administering immunizations, what special precautions would you initiate based on Ron's history?
2. What teaching would you provide to Ron's mother regarding his risk for hypersensitivity?
3. What symptoms related to potential hypersensitivity would you teach Ron's mother to report?

14.3 RHEUMATOID ARTHRITIS

KEY TERMS

Arthrodesis, *750*
Arthroplasty, *750*
Autoimmune disorder, *742*
Boutonnière deformities, *752*
Immunosuppression, *749*
Juvenile rheumatoid arthritis (JRA), *745*
Monophasic, *747*
Orthotic devices, *757*
Osteoarthritis, *742*
Pannus, *743*
Pauciarticular arthritis, *745*
Persistent, *747*
Plasmapheresis, *750*
Polyarticular arthritis, *745*
Polycyclic, *747*
Range of motion (ROM) exercises, *753*
Rheumatoid arthritis (RA), *742*
Swan-neck deformity, *744*
Synovectomy, *750*
Systemic arthritis, *745*
Total lymphoid irradiation, *751*

BASIS FOR SELECTION OF EXEMPLAR

Healthy People 2010

Institute of Medicine

LEARNING OUTCOMES

After reading about this exemplar, you will be able to:

1. Describe the pathophysiology, etiology, clinical manifestations, and direct and indirect causes of rheumatoid arthritis.
2. Identify risk factors associated with rheumatoid arthritis.
3. Illustrate the nursing process in providing culturally competent care across the life span for individuals with rheumatoid arthritis.
4. Formulate priority nursing diagnoses appropriate for an individual with rheumatoid arthritis.
5. Create a plan of care for individuals with rheumatoid arthritis and their family members.
6. Assess expected outcomes for an individual with rheumatoid arthritis.
7. Discuss therapies used in the collaborative care of an individual with rheumatoid arthritis.
8. Employ evidence-based caring interventions for an individual with rheumatoid arthritis.

OVERVIEW

Rheumatoid arthritis (RA) is a chronic systemic **autoimmune disorder** (a disease caused by abnormal, overactive functioning of the immune system that produces a response against the body's own cells and tissues, normally resulting in damage to the tissues). RA causes inflammation of connective tissue, primarily in the joints. The course and severity of the disease are variable. Manifestations of RA may be minimal, with mild inflammation of only a few joints and little structural damage, or relentlessly progressive, with multiple inflamed joints and marked deformity. RA contributes to disability and tends to shorten life expectancy. Most clients exhibit a pattern of symmetric involvement of multiple peripheral joints and periods of remission and exacerbation.

Rheumatoid arthritis is the most prevalent inflammatory arthritis of any age group, including children and adolescents; juvenile RA usually occurs between 2 and 5 or between 9 and 12 years of age. Clients diagnosed with RA must cope with chronic pain, experience alterations in body image, and often require specially modified tools to allow them to perform activities of daily living (ADLs). Holistic care is of particular importance in helping these clients meet physical, psychosocial, and safety needs.

PATHOPHYSIOLOGY AND ETIOLOGY

It is believed that long-term exposure to an unidentified antigen causes an aberrant immune response in a genetically susceptible host. As a result, normal antibodies (immunoglobulins) become autoantibodies and attack host tissues. These transformed antibodies, usually present in people with RA, are called rheumatoid factors. The self-produced antibodies bind with their target antigens in blood and synovial membranes, forming immune complexes.

Leukocytes are attracted to the synovial membrane from the circulation, where neutrophils and macrophages ingest the immune complexes and release enzymes that degrade synovial tissue and articular cartilage. Activation of B lymphocytes and T lymphocytes results in increased production of rheumatoid factors and enzymes that, in turn, increase and continue the inflammatory process.

The synovial membrane is damaged by the inflammatory and immune processes. It swells from infiltration of the leukocytes, and it thickens as cells proliferate and abnormally enlarge. The inflammation then spreads and involves synovial blood vessels. Small venules are occluded, and vascular flow to the synovial tissue decreases. As blood flow decreases and metabolic needs increase (from the increased number and size of cells), hypoxia and metabolic acidosis occur. Acidosis stimulates synovial cells to release hydrolytic enzymes into surrounding tissues, starting erosion of the articular cartilage and inflammation of the supporting ligaments and tendons. The damage to cartilage that occurs in RA is the result of at least three processes:

1. Neutrophils, T cells, and other synovial fluid cells are activated and degrade the surface layer of the articular cartilage.
2. Cytokines, especially interleukin-1 (IL-1) and tumor necrosis factor alpha (TNF-α), cause the chondrocytes to attack the cartilage.
3. The synovium digests nearby cartilage, releasing inflammatory molecules containing IL-1 and TNF-α.

The inflammation also causes hemorrhage, coagulation, and deposits of fibrin on the synovial membrane, in the intracellular matrix, and in the synovial fluid. Fibrin develops into granulation tissue (*pannus*) over denuded areas of the synovial membrane. The formation of pannus leads to scar tissue formation that immobilizes the joint (Figure 14–20 ■).

Etiology

RA is found worldwide, affecting from 1 to 2% of the total population and all races. RA affects three times as many women as men. However, men tend to have more severe articular disease symptoms. The onset of RA occurs most frequently between the ages of 40 and 60 years.

The cause of RA is unknown. A combination of genetic, environmental, hormonal, and reproductive factors is thought to play a role in its development. It is speculated that infectious agents, such as bacteria, mycoplasmas, and viruses (especially Epstein-Barr virus), may play a role in initiating the autoimmune processes in RA. The incidence of RA has decreased during the past 40 years, which supports the theory that environmental factors may change and either promote or protect against RA (Flynn & Johnson, 2005). Genetic predisposition is a major factor in both the susceptibility and the severity of RA.

RA is less common than osteoarthritis (Flynn & Johnson, 2005). **Osteoarthritis** is the most common form of arthritis in older adults. It is caused by chronic

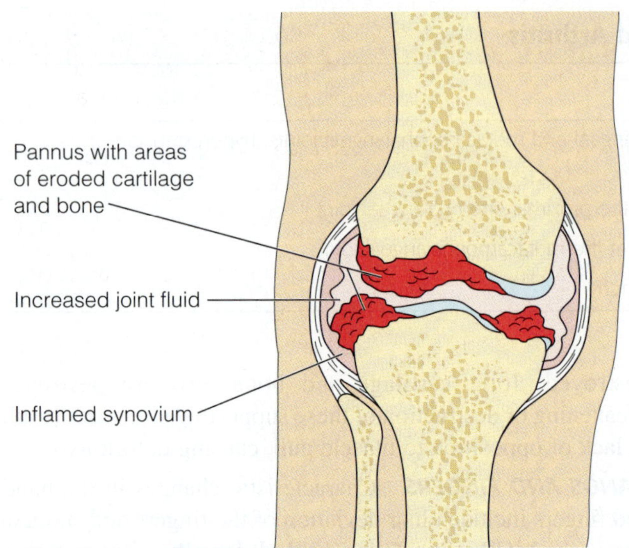

Figure 14–20 ■ Joint inflammation and destruction in rheumatoid arthritis. Note the synovial inflammation with pannus formation and the erosion of cartilage and underlying bone.

degenerative changes in the cartilage and synovial membranes of the joints. The incidence of RA increases with age up to approximately 70 years. Although the onset and manifestations of RA are much the same in older and younger clients, differentiating between RA and osteoarthritis in the older adult may be difficult at times. It is important to establish an accurate diagnosis, however, because the management of these disorders differs significantly. Clinical features distinguishing RA from osteoarthritis are listed in Table 14–8.

Risk Factors

While RA can be diagnosed in anyone, it is most commonly found in women between the ages of 40 and 60 years. People with a family history of RA may be at increased risk. Several studies have found that heavy smokers are at increased risk for developing RA, but that risk can be reduced if the client stops smoking. It is important to note that absence of risk factors does not preclude diagnosis of the disease.

CLINICAL MANIFESTATIONS

RA is a chronic condition that manifests clinically by symmetric inflammation of the peripheral joints, with marked pain (chiefly in the upper extremities), swelling, significant and often disabling morning stiffness, as well as general symptoms of fatigue and malaise. The course of RA may be slow and insidious, or it may present with an acute process affecting several joints (polyarticular). Disease progression is fastest during the first 6 years, slowing thereafter. The older person may experience the first symptoms of RA after the age of 65; this is known as de novo development of RA.

Rheumatoid arthritis causes tenderness and limitation of movement. The morning stiffness of RA lasts more than an hour and may occur after a period of rest as well. On assessment, the joints will have severe redness, swelling, and warmth of the soft tissue. These symptoms cause severe pain on movement, limitation of movement, and a disrupted sleep pattern (National Institute of Arthritis and Musculoskeletal and Skin Diseases, 2006). In the early stage of the disease, the older person may have symptoms that are severely disabling, but deformities are not present.

A second category of RA in older persons occurs in those who have been diagnosed with the disease before 65 years of age. Over time, RA becomes a symmetric, additive disease of the joints. The physical stresses and inflammatory changes of the disease result in the characteristic joint deformities (Table 14–9). Within 2 years of the establishment of the disease, more than 10% of clients with RA will develop deformities of the hands; after 10 years, most clients will experience these changes. As described previously, these deformities are caused by the development of a **pannus** (long-term, severe proliferation of the synovial intimal layer).

TABLE 14–8 Comparison of the Manifestations of Rheumatoid Arthritis and Osteoarthritis

FEATURE	RHEUMATOID ARTHRITIS	OSTEOARTHRITIS
Onset	Usually insidious, may be abrupt	Insidious
Course	Generally progressive, characterized by remissions and exacerbations	Slowly progressive
Pain and stiffness	Predominant on arising, lasting >1 hour; also occurs after prolonged inactivity	Pain with activity; stiffness following periods of immobility, generally relieved within minutes
Affected joints	Appear red, hot, and swollen; "boggy" and tender to palpation; decreased range of motion; weakness	Affected joints may appear swollen; cool and bony hard on palpation; decreased range of motion
	Multiple joints affected in symmetric pattern; proximal interphalangeal, metacarpophalangeal, wrists, knees, ankles, and toes often involved	One or several joints affected including hips, knees, lumbar and cervical spine, proximal interphalangeal and distal interphalangeal, wrist, and first metatarsophalangeal joint
Systemic manifestations	Fatigue, weakness, anorexia, weight loss, fever; rheumatoid nodules; anemia	Fatigue

TABLE 14–9 **Deformities of Chronic Advanced Rheumatoid Arthritis**

SITE	DEFORMITY	DESCRIPTION
Hands	Swan neck deformity	Flexion of the distal interphalangeal and metacarpophalangeal joints, hyperextension of the proximal interphalangeal joint
	Boutonnière deformity	Avulsion of extensor hood of the proximal interphalangeal joint
	Ulnar deformity	Ulnar deviation of the fingers at the metacarpophalangeal joint
Feet	Hallux valgus	Displaced toes, lateral angulation

Remissions are most likely to occur in the first year of the disease. Approximately 10% of people with RA go into long-term remission within 1 year, and another 50–60% go into remission within 2 years (Flynn & Johnson, 2005).

Many women diagnosed with RA will experience a remission during pregnancy, often followed by a relapse after delivery. Anemia may be present as a result of blood loss from salicylate therapy. The mother needs extra rest, particularly to relieve weight-bearing joints, but also needs to continue range-of motion exercises. During remission, she may stop medication usage, because salicylates may prolong labor and have the possibility of inducing teratogenic effects. It is not uncommon for women diagnosed with RA to have prolonged gestations.

For older clients, RA is managed much as it is for younger people. Prolonged bed rest or inactivity is not prescribed for acute episodes, however, because it may result in irreversible immobility in the older adult. Also, medications are used with greater caution in older adults because of the increased risk of toxicity. In many cases, less emphasis is placed on preventing joint deformity and more on maintaining functional status for the older client with RA.

Joint Manifestations

As mentioned, the onset of RA typically is insidious, although it may be acute (precipitated by a stressor, e.g., infection, surgery, or trauma). Joint manifestations often are preceded by systemic manifestations of inflammation, including fatigue, loss of appetite, weight loss, and nonspecific aching and stiffness. Clients report joint swelling with associated stiffness, warmth, tenderness, and pain.

The pattern of joint involvement typically is polyarticular (involving multiple joints) and symmetric, but the rate at which joint deformities develop can fluctuate. The proximal interphalangeal (PIP) and metacarpophalangeal (MCP) joints of the fingers, the wrists, the knees, the ankles, and the toes most frequently are involved, although RA can affect any joint. Stiffness is most pronounced in the morning, lasting more than 1 hour. It may also occur with prolonged rest during the day and may be more severe following strenuous activity. Swollen, inflamed joints feel "boggy" or spongelike on palpation because of synovial edema. ROM is limited in affected joints, and weakness may be evident.

The persistent inflammation of RA causes deformities of the joint itself and of the supporting structures, such as ligaments, tendons, and muscles. As the joint is destroyed, ligaments, tendons, and the joint capsule are weakened or destroyed. Joint cartilage and bone also are destroyed. Weakening or destruction of these supporting structures results in lack of opposition to muscle pull, causing deformity.

HANDS AND FINGERS Characteristic changes in the hands and fingers include ulnar deviation of the fingers and subluxation at the MCP joints. **Swan-neck deformity** is characterized by hyperextension of the PIP joints with compensatory flexion of the distal interphalangeal (DIP) joints. A flexion deformity of the PIP joints with extension of the DIP joints is called a boutonnière deformity (Figure 14–21 ■). The ability to affect a pinch is limited by hyperextension of the interphalangeal joint and flexion of the MCP joint of the thumb.

WRISTS AND ELBOWS Wrist involvement is nearly universal, leading to limited movement, deformity, and carpal tunnel syndrome. Inflammation of the elbows often causes flexion contracture.

KNEES The knees frequently are affected in RA, with visible swelling often obliterating normal contours. Instability of the knee joint along with quadriceps atrophy, contractures, and valgus (knock-knee) deformities can lead to significant disability.

ANKLES AND FEET Ambulation may be limited by pain and deformities when the ankles and feet are involved. Typical deformities of the feet and toes include subluxation, hallux valgus (deviation of the great toe toward the other digits of the foot), lateral deviation of the toes, and cock-up toes (turned-up toes).

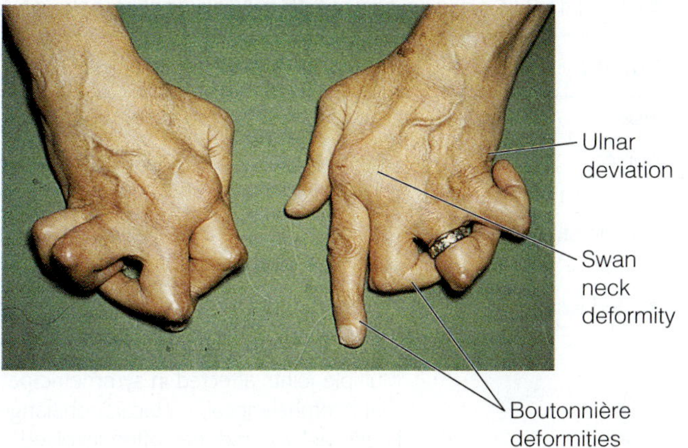

Figure 14–21 ■ Typical hand deformities associated with rheumatoid arthritis.

Source: Biophoto Associates/Photo Researchers, Inc.

TABLE 14–10 **Examples of Nonsteroidal Anti-Inflammatory Drugs (NSAIDs) Used to Treat Rheumatoid Arthritis**

DRUG	AVERAGE DOSE	COMMENTS AND PRECAUTIONS
Aspirin	600–900 mg given 4–6 times daily	Least expensive; associated with risk of gastrointestinal ulceration, bleeding, and possible hemorrhage; may cause hepatotoxicity
Diclofenac (Voltaren)	50 mg tid or qid, or 75 mg bid	Expensive; risk of hepatotoxicity
Etodolac (Lodine)	200–400 mg q6h	Expensive; may have less gastrointestinal toxicity
Fenoprofen (Nalfon)	300–600 mg tid or qid	Do not administer to clients with impaired renal function; risk of genitourinary effects (e.g., dysuria, cystitis, hematuria, acute interstitial nephritis, and nephrotic syndrome)
Flurbiprofen (Ansaid)	50–100 mg tid or qid, not to exceed 300 mg/day	Expensive
Ibuprofen (Motrin, Advil, others)	300 mg qid; 400–800 mg tid or qid	Available in prescription and over-the-counter forms; less gastric distress reported than with aspirin or indomethacin; discontinue if visual disturbances develop
Indomethacin (Indocin)	25–50 mg bid or tid	Potent NSAID used for moderate to severe RA and acute episodes of chronic disease; higher incidence of adverse gastrointestinal effects and central nervous system effects (e.g., headache, dizziness, and depression)
Ketoprofen (Orudis)	50–75 mg tid or qid	Expensive; older adults and clients with renal insufficiency require lower doses
Meclofenamate sodium (Meclomen)	100 mg bid to qid	Increased risk of adverse effects in older adults; gastrointestinal effects include diarrhea and abdominal pain; anemia may develop during therapy
Nabumetone (Relafen)	1,000–2,000 mg/day	Most common adverse effects include diarrhea, dyspepsia, and abdominal pain
Naproxen (Aleve, Anaprox, Naprosyn)	250–500 mg bid	Available in prescription and over-the-counter preparations
Oxaprozin (Daypro)	1,200 mg daily	Expensive; risk of severe hepatotoxicity; rash may occur
Piroxicam (Feldene)	20 mg daily in a single or divided dose	Expensive; gastrointestinal side effects, including stomatitis, loss of appetite, and gastric distress, may occur more frequently than with other NSAIDs
Sulindac (Clinoril)	150–200 mg bid	May be safer than other NSAIDs in clients with chronic renal disease; rare fatal hypersensitivity reaction with fever, liver function abnormalities, and severe skin reaction
Tolmetin (Tolectin)	200–600 mg tid	Expensive; may have higher rate of side effects, including gastrointestinal distress, headache, dizziness, elevated blood pressure, edema, and weight gain

the treatment of RA. Beneficial effects are not apparent for several weeks or months following the initiation of therapy, but these drugs can produce not only clinical improvement but also evidence of decreased disease activity. Because their anti-inflammatory effect is minimal, NSAIDs are continued during therapy with disease-modifying drugs. As many as two-thirds of clients taking these drugs show improvement, although such therapy has not been shown to slow bone erosion or facilitate healing. All of these drugs are fairly toxic, and close monitoring is necessary during the course of therapy.

Immune and Inflammatory Agents **Immunosuppression** helps to reduce the body's autoimmune response, thereby controlling the effects of the disease process, and immunosuppressive or cytotoxic drugs are increasingly employed in the management of RA. Indeed, many now consider methotrexate the treatment of choice for clients with aggressive RA. Methotrexate may be used along with NSAIDs in the initial treatment plan. A weekly dose can produce a beneficial effect in as few as 2 to 4 weeks. Gastric irritation and stomatitis are the most frequent side effects associated with methotrexate, but side effects may be better controlled if folic acid is taken at the same time. Alcoholism, diabetes, obesity, advanced age, and renal disease increase the risk of toxic effects (e.g., hepatotoxicity, bone marrow suppression, and interstitial pneumonitis). Other immunosuppressive agents, such as cyclosporine, azathioprine, and monoclonal antibodies, also have been employed in the treatment of clients with severe, progressive, and crippling disease who have failed to respond to other measures.

Drugs that modify the autoimmune and inflammatory responses in clients with RA include leflunomide (Arava) and etanercept (Enbrel). Leflunomide reversibly inhibits an enzyme involved in the autoimmune process, and etanercept inhibits the binding of tumor necrosis factor to receptor sites. Infliximab (Remicade) is a biologic response modifier and TNF-α receptor antagonist. Given by intravenous infusion, this drug is administered to reduce infiltration of inflammatory cells and production of TNF-α. Adalimumab (Humira) is a biologic response modifier that is given to people with RA to reduce the inflammatory events of polyarthritis and to slow the progression of joint damage. Given by subcutaneous injection, the drug cannot be administered if the person has an acute or chronic infection in any part of the body. Before initiating the drug, the client should be tested for tuberculosis.

TABLE 14–11 **Disease-Modifying Drugs Used to Treat Rheumatoid Arthritis**

CLASS/MEDICATIONS	USUAL DOSE	ADVERSE EFFECTS	COMMENTS/NURSING CONSIDERATIONS
Gold salts: Gold sodium thiomalate (Myochrysine) Aurothioglucose (Solganal) Auranofin (Ridaura Capsules)	Parenteral: 1st dose, 10 mg; 2nd dose, 25 mg; then 50 mg weekly im Oral: 6 mg daily	■ Pruritus, dermatitis ■ Stomatitis, metallic taste ■ Renal toxicity ■ Blood dyscrasias ■ Gastrointestinal distress	■ Frequent UA and CBC ■ Monitor client after injection for flushing, fainting, dizziness, sweating, and possible anaphylactic reaction
Antimalarial: Hydroxychloroquine (Plaquenil)	200–600 mg daily with meals	■ Central nervous system reactions, including irritability, nightmares, and psychoses ■ Retinopathy ■ Alopecia, pruritus ■ Blood dyscrasias ■ Gastrointestinal disturbances	■ Should not be used during pregnancy ■ Regular ophthalmologic examination required
Sulfasalazine (Azulfidine)	2 g/day in divided doses with meals	■ Anorexia, nausea, vomiting, gastric distress ■ Decreased sperm count ■ Headache ■ Rash ■ Blood dyscrasias ■ Hypersensitivity responses, including Stevens-Johnson syndrome ■ Central nervous system, liver, and renal toxicity	■ Administer in evenly divided doses ■ Maintain high fluid intake ■ May cause yellow-orange skin or urine discoloration ■ Regular CBCs necessary
D-Penicillamine (Cuprimine, Depen Titratable)	125–250 mg/day initially, then slowly increased to 1,000–1,500 mg/day	■ Skin rashes ■ Fever ■ Gastrointestinal distress ■ Oral ulcers, loss of taste ■ Fever ■ Bone marrow depression with thrombocytopenia, leukopenia, anemia ■ Renal toxicity ■ May induce immune complex disorders (e.g., Goodpasture's syndrome and myasthenia gravis)	■ Regular CBC and UA necessary ■ Administer on an empty stomach ■ Discontinue during pregnancy ■ May require 2–3 months of therapy before benefit is seen

Note. CBC = complete blood count; UA = urinalysis.

Gold Salts Gold salts may be administered by mouth, but the intramuscular route is more effective. The mode of action of gold is unknown, but it may produce clinical remission in some clients and decrease new bony erosions. Unless toxic reactions occur, weekly therapy is continued until significant improvement is noted. Clients experiencing benefit from gold therapy may be continued on monthly injections for several years. About one third of clients on gold therapy experience toxic reactions, including dermatitis, stomatitis, bone marrow depression, and proteinuria. Mild skin reactions do not always necessitate discontinuation of therapy. CBC and urinalysis are monitored throughout treatment with gold to assess for more severe toxic responses.

Antimalarial Agents Hydroxychloroquine (Plaquenil) is an antimalarial agent sometimes employed in the treatment of RA. Three to 6 months of therapy are required to achieve the desired response, and many clients do not experience significant benefit. Although hydroxychloroquine has a relatively low toxicity, it can cause pigmentary retinitis and vision loss. Clients receiving this drug require a thorough vision examination every 6 months.

Sulfasalazine Sulfasalazine, a drug regularly prescribed for chronic inflammatory bowel disease, also may be prescribed for RA. For clients not responding to the above preparations, penicillamine may be prescribed. Although this agent may be effective in the management of RA, toxic reactions, including bone marrow suppression, proteinuria, and nephrosis, are common and can be severe.

Surgery and Other Procedures

Surgical intervention may be employed for the client with RA at a variety of disease stages. Early in the course of the disease, **synovectomy** (excision of synovial membrane) can provide temporary relief of inflammation, relieve pain, and slow the destructive process, thus helping to preserve joint function. **Arthrodesis** (joint fusion) may be used to stabilize joints such as cervical vertebrae, wrists, and ankles. **Arthroplasty** (total joint replacement) may be necessary in cases of gross deformity and joint destruction.

Several newer treatments not yet in widespread use may be employed in clients with progressive RA. **Plasmapheresis** has been used to remove circulating antibodies, thereby moderating the autoimmune response. **Total lymphoid irradiation** decreases total lymphocyte levels, although serious adverse effects are associated with this treatment and its continued efficacy has not been established.

Other Therapies

The primary objectives in treating the client with RA are to reduce pain and inflammation, preserve function, and prevent deformity. Therapies in this area include rest and exercise, physical and occupational therapy, heat and cold, assistive devices and splints, and nutrition, as well as complementary and alternative medicines.

REST AND EXERCISE A balanced program of rest and exercise is an important component in the management of RA. During an acute exacerbation of the disease, the client may be hospitalized, or a short period of complete bed rest may be prescribed. For most clients, regular rest periods during the day are beneficial to reduce manifestations of the disease. In addition, splinting of inflamed joints reduces unwanted motion and provides local joint rest (see the following Orthotic and Assistive Devices section).

Rest must be balanced with a program of physical therapy and exercise to maintain muscle strength and joint mobility. ROM exercises are prescribed to maintain joint function and prevent contractures. Isometric exercises are used to improve muscle strength without increasing joint stress. Isotonic exercises also help to improve muscle strength and preserve function. Low-impact aerobic exercises, such as swimming and walking, have been shown to benefit clients with RA without adversely affecting joint inflammation or prompting acute episodes.

PHYSICAL AND OCCUPATIONAL THERAPY Physical and occupational therapists can design and monitor individualized programs of activity and rest. Physical therapy is aimed at improving mobility and preventing complications of inactivity. Occupational therapy works to create modifications to practices and tools needed to perform ADLs and promote as normal a lifestyle as possible.

HEAT AND COLD Heat and cold are used for their analgesic and muscle-relaxing effects. Moist heat generally is most effective and can be provided by a tub bath. Joint pain is relieved in some clients through the application of cold.

ORTHOTIC AND ASSISTIVE DEVICES A variety of **orthotic devices** (orthopedic devices that may include splints or braces applied to reduce strain on a joint) are available to help maintain function. Splints provide joint rest and prevent contractures. Night splints for the hands and/or wrists should maintain the extremity in a position of maximum function. The best "splint" for the hip is lying prone for several hours a day on a firm bed. In general, splints should be applied for the shortest period needed, be made of lightweight materials, and be easily removed to perform ROM exercises once or twice a day. Assistive devices, such as a cane, walker, or raised toilet seat, are most useful for clients with significant hip or knee arthritis.

NUTRITION For most clients with RA, an ordinary, well-balanced diet is recommended. Some clients may benefit from substitution of usual dietary fat with omega-3 fatty acids found in certain fish oils. Inactivity can lead to obesity, which places excess strain on the joints and can exacerbate pain. It is important the client receives adequate calories and nutrients for health while adapting calorie intake to meet activity levels.

COMPLEMENTARY AND ALTERNATIVE MEDICINE The client and health care team may consider complementary and alternative medicine if the client continues to experience discomfort from RA despite compliance with more traditional therapies. While many clients have reported improvement of pain and swelling with acupuncture or hydrotherapy, these have yet to be clinically proven as beneficial for clients. Nutritional supplements such as fish oils may be used if they are not contraindicated for the client. Nurses should ask the client at each health care interaction about any nontraditional therapies being used. Because a cure is not available and traditional therapies are not always fully effective, the client with RA is vulnerable to quackery. Many nontraditional treatments, including diets, topical preparations, vaccines, hormones, plant extracts, and copper bracelets, have been put forth. These treatments often are costly, and none has been shown to be effective.

FOCUS ON DIVERSITY AND CULTURE
Using Complementary and Alternative Medicine for RA

Clients of Asian origin may already be taking herbal remedies and using acupuncture to treat symptoms of rheumatoid arthritis by the time they seek assistance from a Western physician. It is important for the nurse to respect the client's desire to use Eastern medicine.

Nurses working with these clients may want to recommend that clients keep a medication and symptom journal that documents the times and dosages of any medications and remedies taken, including herbal teas, as well as the onset of both symptoms and side effects. This may assist the client and nurse with determining if a side effect or an improvement in the client's symptoms can be attributed to a specific treatment or a change in a specific treatment, regardless of the treatment's source.

NURSING PROCESS

Clients with chronic, progressive, systemic disorders such as RA have multiple nursing care needs involving many functional health patterns. Physical manifestations of the disease often result in acute and chronic pain, fatigue, impaired mobility, and difficulty performing routine tasks. The disease also has many psychosocial effects. The client has an incurable, chronic disease that may lead to severe crippling. Pain and fatigue can interfere with the client's ability to perform expected roles, such as home maintenance or job responsibilities. Even though the client's hands may appear swollen or deformed, other people may not understand the systemic nature of the disease or realize the difference between RA and osteoarthritis. Information about arthritis self-management is found in Box 14–15, and a Nursing Care Plan for a client with RA is found later in this section.

Box 14–15 Arthritis Self-Management

People with RA can take control of their lives by becoming arthritis self-managers. They can help to prevent deformities and the effects of arthritis by following prescriptions for exercise, rest, weight management, posture, and positioning. The following suggestions for clients with RA are outlined by the Moss Rehab Resource Net (2005):

- Never attempt an activity that cannot be stopped immediately if it proves beyond your power to complete it.
- Respect pain as a warning signal. When you experience pain, change your method of doing things, use equipment or tools if necessary, and take intermittent rest periods.
- Use the strongest joints available for an activity. For example, instead of your fingers, use the palm of your hand or the crook of your elbow for grasping while carrying.
- Avoid stress toward a position of deformity, such as when the fingers drift closer to the little finger. For example, open a jar with your right hand, and close a jar with your left hand.
- Avoid activities that need a tight grip, such as writing, wringing, and unscrewing.

Assessment

A careful history is important, because the history sometimes is the primary mode of diagnosis. Collect the following data through the health history and physical examination:

- *Health history.* Pain; stiffness; fatigue; joint problems, including location, duration, onset, and effect on function; fever; sleep patterns; past illnesses or surgery; and ability to carry out ADLs and self-care activities
- *Physical assessment.* Height/weight; gait; joints, including symmetry, size, shape, color, appearance, temperature, ROM, and pain; skin, including nodules and purpura; respiratory, including cough and crackles; and cardiovascular, including pericardial friction rub, apical bradycardia, and S_3 (third heart sound).

During the physical examination, look specifically for flexion contractures associated with RA, including swan-neck contractures, in which the PIP joints are hyperextended while the DIP joints are fixed in flexion, and **boutonnière deformities**, in which the PIP joint is flexed in conjunction with DIP joint hyperextension (see Figure 14–21). Also assess for joint swelling and deformities, fever, nodules under the skin, growth delays in children, and enlarged lymph nodes. Pain and tenderness along the calcaneal (Achilles) tendon may indicate tendinitis or bursitis. Small nodules sometimes occur in clients with RA. Palpate the metatarsophalangeal joints just below the ball of the foot. Pain and discomfort with this maneuver suggest early involvement of RA. Limited ROM and painful movement of the joint without signs of inflammation suggest degenerative joint disease.

Diagnosis

Many nursing diagnoses may be appropriate for the client with RA. Those focusing on predominant manifestations and their effect on the client's life include the following:

- Chronic Pain related to joint inflammation
- Fatigue related to chronic pain and complications of disease process
- Ineffective Role Performance related to pain and activity intolerance
- Disturbed Body Image related to joint deformities caused by disease process
- Impaired Physical Mobility related to joint stiffness
- Anxiety related to stress of chronic illness
- Activity Intolerance related to chronic pain.

The diagnosis of RA is based on the client's history, physical assessment, and diagnostic tests. Diagnostic criteria developed by the American Rheumatism Association are used as well. At least four of the following seven criteria must be present to establish the diagnosis:

1. Morning stiffness lasting for at least 1 hour and persisting for at least 6 weeks
2. Arthritis with swelling or effusion of three or more joints persisting for at least 6 weeks
3. Arthritis of wrist, MCP, or PIP joints persisting for at least 6 weeks
4. Symmetric arthritis with simultaneous involvement of corresponding joints on both sides of the body
5. Rheumatoid nodules
6. Positive serum rheumatoid factor
7. Characteristic radiologic changes of RA noted in hands and wrists.

Plan

Outcomes should be created for individualized client needs. These outcomes may include the following:

- Client reports effectiveness of pain management techniques, maintaining pain in tolerable levels by (*specific date*).
- Client performs ADLs independently (or with minimal assistance, depending on degree of impairment) using tools modified by occupational therapy.
- Client expresses feelings about diagnosis of chronic disease and displays progression through grieving process.

Implementation

Nursing care focuses on promoting mobility, encouraging adequate nutrition, and teaching the client and family about the disease and its management. Most care will occur in the community, including physical therapy, with only occasional hospitalizations at the time of an exacerbation of the disease.

Chronic Pain

Pain is a constant feature of RA when the disease is active. It accompanies both acute inflammation and lower levels of chronic inflammation. Some clients say the pain in joints and surrounding tissue is like a deep, constant toothache. Pain can significantly affect the client's ability to provide self-care and maintain daily activities. It also contributes to the client's fatigue.

- Monitor the level of pain and duration of morning stiffness. Pain and morning stiffness are indicators of disease activity. Increased pain may necessitate changes in the therapeutic treatment plan.
- Encourage the client to relate pain to activity level and adjust his or her activities accordingly. Teach the importance of joint and whole-body rest in relieving pain. Pain

is an indicator of excess stress on inflamed joints. Increasing pain indicates a need to decrease activity levels.

- Teach the use of heat and cold applications to provide pain relief. The client may apply heat by showering or taking tub baths, or by using warm compresses or other local applications, such as paraffin dips. For clients who find that heat increases pain and swelling during periods of acute inflammation, cold packs may be more effective. Both heat and cold have analgesic effects and can help to relieve associated muscle spasms.
- Teach about the use of prescribed anti-inflammatory medications and the relationship of pain and inflammation. Anti-inflammatory agents reduce chemical mediators of inflammation and swelling, relieving pain.
- Encourage the use of other, nonpharmacologic pain relief measures, such as visualization, distraction, meditation, and progressive relaxation techniques. These techniques can reduce muscle tension and help the client focus away from the pain, decreasing the intensity of the pain experience.

Fatigue

The pain and chronic inflammatory processes associated with RA lead to fatigue, but other factors contribute as well. Discomfort often disrupts the client's sleep patterns. Anemia, muscle atrophy, oxygenation, and poor nutrition play a role in the development of fatigue. The client with RA also may experience depression or hopelessness, with associated manifestations of fatigue.

- Encourage a balance of periods of activity with periods of rest. Both joint and whole-body rest are important to reducing the inflammatory response.
- Stress the importance of planned rest periods during the day. Rest is vital during acute exacerbations of the disease but also is important to maintain the client in remission.
- Help the client to prioritize activities, encouraging the client to perform the most important ones early in the day. Assigning priorities helps the client to avoid performing relatively unimportant activities at the expense of more meaningful and important ones.
- Encourage regular physical activity in addition to prescribed **range of motion (ROM) exercises** (exercises designed to take each joint through all possible movements to maintain flexibility and movement in the joint). Aerobic exercise promotes a sense of well-being and restful sleep patterns.
- Refer the client to counseling or support groups. Counseling and support groups can help the client to develop effective coping strategies and deal with depression and hopelessness.

Ineffective Role Performance

Fatigue, pain, and the crippling effects of RA can interfere with the client's ability to pursue an education or career and to fill other life roles, such as parent, spouse, or homemaker. As the client's role changes, so must the roles of other family members. This can contribute to changes in family processes, increased stress in the family, and further difficulty in coping with the effects of the disease.

- Discuss the effects of the disease on the client's career and other life roles. Encourage the client to identify changes brought on by the disease. Discussion helps the client to accept the changes and begin to identify strategies for coping with them.
- Encourage the client and family to discuss their feelings about role changes and to grieve over lost roles or abilities. Verbalization allows family members to validate and accept feelings about losses and changes, helping them to move into new roles.
- Listen actively to concerns expressed by the client and family members, and acknowledge the validity of concerns about the disease, prescribed treatment, and the prognosis. Demonstrating acceptance of these feelings and concerns promotes trust and validates their reality.
- Help the client and family to identify strengths they can use to cope with role changes. Identifying strengths helps the client and family to consider role changes that maintain self-esteem and dignity.
- Encourage the client to make decisions and assume personal responsibility for management of the disease. Clients who assume a personal and active role in managing their disease maintain a greater sense of self-control and self-esteem.

> **PRACTICE ALERT**
>
> Remember that grief resolution takes time and that clients may respond to loss with anger.

Disturbed Body Image

The acute and long-term effects of RA can affect the client's body image, leading to feelings of hopelessness and powerlessness, social withdrawal, and difficulty adapting to changes. When inflammation and joint deformity occur despite compliance, the client may have difficulty accepting the need to continue therapeutic measures, particularly those that have side effects or are costly or time-consuming. In addition, unproven alternative treatment strategies and quackery may become increasingly attractive to the client.

- Demonstrate a caring, accepting attitude toward the client. This attitude helps the client to accept the physical changes brought on by the disease.
- Encourage the client to talk about the effects of the disease, both the physical effects and the effects on life roles. Verbalization helps the client to identify feelings and gives the nurse an opportunity to validate these feelings.
- Encourage the client to maintain self-care and usual roles to the extent possible. Discuss the use of clothing and adaptive devices that promote independence. Independence enhances the client's self-esteem.
- Provide positive feedback for self-care activities and adaptive strategies. Positive reinforcement encourages the client to continue adaptive measures and maintain independence.
- Refer the client to self-help groups, support groups, and other agencies that provide assistive devices and literature. These groups and agencies can help the client develop adaptive strategies to cope with the effects of RA, enhancing the client's self-concept, body image, and independence.

- Encourage the child to maintain contact with peers and to attend school when possible. Children require social interaction and education in order to meet developmental milestones and changes in body image can make them feel self-conscious or awkward leading to isolation.

Impaired Mobility

Physical therapists play an essential role in the client's treatment. The goals of physical therapy are to maintain joint function, strengthen muscles, increase tone, maintain body alignment, and prevent permanent deformities, such as contractures. Range-of-motion exercises, stretching, hydrotherapy, and swimming all help to prevent deformities.

Nurses can help clients with impaired mobility by encouraging them to perform ADLs. Medications may be given to reduce joint swelling and inflammation. In addition, warm or cold compresses to involved joints may provide pain relief.

- Promote general health by encouraging a well-balanced diet. Periodically perform dietary and nutritional assessments. Reduced mobility may reduce metabolic needs, and excess weight causes additional muscle strain.
- For children with JRA, plot growth carefully and watch for changes in growth percentiles. Growth must be carefully monitored for early detection of problems and to prevent long-term complications.
- Teach the client and family about the condition, prognosis, and importance of optimizing activity levels. Typically, care is provided within the community; hospitalizations are rare. It is important the client understand that overexertion may lead to exacerbation of the disease and activities should be within tolerable limits.
- Refer to occupational therapy that can help the client to continue performing ADLs. Tools with larger handles can reduce the pain of gripping, and longer handles on implements reduce reaching, The goal is to maintain independence in performing daily activities.

Evaluation

RA typically is a chronic, progressive disease. As with most diseases of this nature, involvement of the client and family in its management is vital. Evaluation of nursing care is a continuous and ongoing part of meeting the client's needs to determine if the current plan of care is effective. Expected outcomes of nursing care for the client include the following:

- The client maintains joint mobility.
- The client expresses comfort and freedom from pain.
- The client develops or maintains a positive body image.
- The client is free from infection.
- Client and family display adequate understanding, support, and management of the therapeutic regimen.

HEALTH CARE

Weakened, painful joints can result in inactivity, which impacts strength, so clients with RA are at risk for injury secondary to falls. Home safety assessments may be indicated for these clients. A physical or occupational therapist working with the client will be able to suggest tools and assistive devices that can reduce the client's risk for injury.

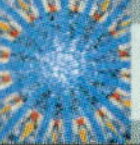

EVIDENCE-BASED PRACTICE Teaching the Client With Rheumatoid Arthritis

Clinical Question

Rheumatoid arthritis (RA) is a disease that can occur at any age, but it is seen most often in older adults. RA causes physical, emotional, and economic difficulties, but appropriate management can do much to reduce pain and disability, improve a sense of control, and improve quality of life. With recent advances in computer technology, the Internet has become a convenient means of providing information to people with RA. However, little is known about how many older adults use the computer to gain access to information.

Evidence

Tak and Hong (2005) examine the use of computers and the Internet by older adults with arthritis and described the characteristics of those who used the Internet to find health information. Although one of every four older adults who participated in the study owned a computer, only slightly more than half actually used the Internet. Lack of knowledge about using the computer or about accessing the Internet were given as possible reasons.

Best Practice

The Internet is a powerful method for providing health information to older adults. Although health history questions rarely contain questions about availability and use of the computer and the Internet, it may be equally important to ask about Internet use as to ask about other components of one's dwelling. If older adults have but do not use a computer, then referral to community resources that provide computer learning classes can facilitate their success in using the computer and doing online searches of the Internet for health information. In addition, before recommending an Internet-based health resource, nurses should review the site for content, readability, navigation features, credibility, organization, and graphic appearance.

Critical Thinking

1. You are designing an Internet site to teach older adults about RA. What topics would you include? How would your presentation be most effective for this age group?
2. You are conducting a computer-literacy course for older adults with RA at a local library. All of them have computers, but no one has used the Internet to find out about the disease. What sites would you recommend, and why?
3. Develop a plan to include assessment about computers on an agency's health history. What would you include to convince the agency personnel that this is important?

Source: Tak, S. H., & Hong, S. H. (2005). Use of the Internet for health information by older adults with arthritis. *Orthopaedic Nursing, 24*(2), 134–139.

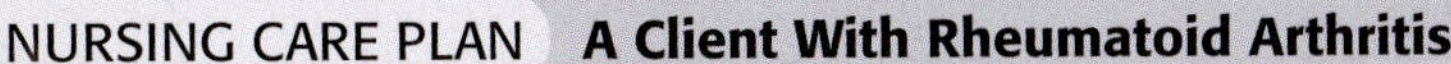

NURSING CARE PLAN A Client With Rheumatoid Arthritis

Janice James is a 42-year-old high school science teacher who began noticing vague joint pain, fatigue, poor appetite, and general malaise, which she initially attributed to a case of the flu. However, her symptoms continued, and she began to notice aching in her hands and wrists, which she attributed to the quilting she loves to do in the evenings. She made an appointment with her family physician when she noticed that her knuckles and finger joints were not just achy but also swollen and hot. She reports feeling very stiff in the mornings, often taking until 10:00 or 11:00 a.m. to begin to feel "normal."

Noting that Mrs. James has lost 10 lb since her last visit and has mild anemia and a significantly elevated erythrocyte sedimentation rate, the physician refers her to the rheumatology clinic for further evaluation. Following examination, laboratory, and radiologic testing, the rheumatologist establishes a diagnosis of rheumatoid arthritis and initiates a multidisciplinary team conference to plan the management of Mrs. James's condition.

ASSESSMENT

Cathy Greenstein, RN, completes an assessment of Mrs. James. She notes that Mrs. James is well groomed and answers questions readily. However, she appears fatigued and ill. Mrs. James relates that her job has been extremely stressful, because teacher layoffs have resulted in larger class sizes and fewer teaching assistants. Despite symptoms, she continues to teach full time but says she feels unable to keep up with all her responsibilities because of her fatigue.

Mrs. James states that she is allergic to penicillin. Her past medical history reveals only the usual childhood diseases and three uncomplicated pregnancies, resulting in the births of her children, ages 14, 11, and 9. Physical assessment findings include T_O 37.8°C (100.2°F), P 82 regular, R 18, BP 124/78. Hands: swelling of the proximal interphalangeal (PIP) and metacarpophalangeal (MCP) joints of both hands; second and third PIP and second MCP joints on right hand are red, shiny, hot, spongy, and tender to palpation; able to extend fingers to 180 degrees but cannot make a complete fist with either hand, with flexion limited to less than 90 degrees; grip strength is weak bilaterally; wrist ROM is limited in all directions. Knees are swollen, and flexion is slightly limited; positive bulge sign in the right knee. Diagnostic findings are an erythrocyte sedimentation rate of 52 mm/hr, a hematocrit of 30%, and positive for rheumatoid factor. Few changes other than soft-tissue swelling are evident on hand and wrist x-rays.

DIAGNOSES

Nursing diagnoses that may be appropriate for Mrs. James include the following:

- Chronic Pain related to joint inflammation
- Impaired Home Maintenance related to fatigue
- Activity Intolerance related to the effects of inflammation
- Deficient Knowledge regarding her therapeutic regimen.

PLANNING

The expected outcomes for the plan of care specify that Mrs. James will:

- Verbalize effective pain management strategies.
- Use assistive devices to minimize joint stress with ADLs.
- Verbalize a plan to reduce responsibilities for home maintenance.
- Express willingness to plan rest breaks during the day.
- Demonstrate understanding of the prescribed therapeutic regimen and its importance for both short- and long-term benefit.

IMPLEMENTATION

The following nursing interventions may be appropriate for Mrs. James:

- Teach techniques for relieving pain and morning stiffness, including:
  a. Schedule NSAIDs at equal intervals throughout the day.
  b. Take morning NSAID dose with milk and crackers approximately 30 minutes before rising.
  c. Perform ROM exercises in shower or bathtub.
  d. Apply local heat with paraffin dip or compress; use cold packs as needed.
  e. Teach techniques to minimize joint stress while performing ADLs.
- Provide Arthritis Foundation literature and information.
- Discuss ways to delegate household tasks to other family members.
- Explore ways to incorporate 30-minutes rest breaks into work schedule.
- Provide information about the disease process and its manifestations, prescribed medications and their desired and adverse effects, and the importance of balancing rest and activity.

EVALUATION

The initial treatment regimen of aspirin, rest, exercise, and physical therapy succeeded in partially relieving the acute manifestations of rheumatoid arthritis in Mrs. James. However, complete remission has not been achieved. She has had difficulty scheduling rest periods at work and has had to struggle to delegate household tasks. "I don't look sick to the kids, and they seem to think housecleaning is a terrible imposition on their time. It's often easier to just do it myself than to fight about it. Besides, that way it gets done right." Mrs. James has faithfully followed the prescribed medication regimen and exercise routines, and she has kept her scheduled appointments and maintained contact with the treatment team.

CRITICAL THINKING

1. Mrs. James is 42 years old. Would your nursing interventions differ if she were 72 years old? If so, how?
2. Rheumatoid arthritis is a chronic illness. What are the physical, emotional, and economic implications of an illness that results in chronic pain and deformity?
3. Develop a nursing care plan for Mrs. James using the nursing diagnosis Ineffective role performance.

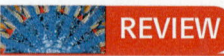

REVIEW Rheumatoid Arthritis

RELATE: LINK THE CONCEPTS

Linking the exemplar of Rheumatoid Arthritis with the concept of Inflammation:

1. What role does inflammation play in the disease process of RA?
2. What nursing care (independent or collaborative) can you provide that will slow the inflammatory process?
3. What signs and symptoms of RA indicate the inflammatory process?

Linking the exemplar of Rheumatoid Arthritis with the concept of Safety:

4. When caring for a client with RA impacting both knees, what nursing care can you provide to improve the client's safety?
5. What risks for injury would RA in both knees create?

READY: GO TO COMPANION SKILLS MANUAL

- Applying heat and cold
- Performing range of motion exercises
- Assessing home for safe environment

REFER: GO TO MYNURSINGKIT

REFLECT: CASE STUDY

Justine Belamo is a 48-year-old white female who has been married to Gil Belamo for 18 years. Justine has a daughter (Majel) from a previous marriage, and she has two teenage children (Mark and Maria) with Gil. Justine works as a grocery store clerk. Although she finds her job monotonous, she appreciates the steady income and family health insurance.

Justine is overweight and has tried to lose weight most of her adult life. She frequently diets and, in the past, has lost a great deal of weight, but she just can't seem to keep the weight off. She blames menopause for her most recent weight gain.

1. What factors place Justine at risk for development of RA?
2. When talking with Justine, what interview questions might you ask to determine if she has any early signs of RA?
3. If Justine were to be diagnosed with RA, what teaching might you provide to reduce joint damage?

14.4 SYSTEMIC LUPUS ERYTHEMATOSUS

KEY TERMS

Antigen–antibody complex, *760*
Autoantibodies, *756*
Cellular immune response, *756*
Connective tissue, *756*
Discoid lesions, *757*
Human leukocyte antigen (HLA), *757*
Humoral immune response, *756*
Inflammatory response, *757*
Systemic lupus erythematosus (SLE), *756*

BASIS FOR SELECTION OF EXEMPLAR

Chronic Disease Management

LEARNING OUTCOMES

After reading about this exemplar, you will be able to:

1. Describe the pathophysiology, etiology, clinical manifestations, and direct and indirect causes of systemic lupus erythematosus.
2. Identify risk factors associated with systemic lupus erythematosus.
3. Illustrate the nursing process in providing culturally competent care across the life span for individuals with systemic lupus erythematosus.
4. Formulate priority nursing diagnoses appropriate for an individual with systemic lupus erythematosus.
5. Create a plan of care for individuals with systemic lupus erythematosus and their family members.
6. Assess expected outcomes for an individual with systemic lupus erythematosus.
7. Discuss therapies used in the collaborative care of an individual with systemic lupus erythematosus.
8. Employ evidence-based caring interventions for an individual with systemic lupus erythematosus.

OVERVIEW

The generalized disorder known as **systemic lupus erythematosus (SLE)** is a chronic, inflammatory, **connective tissue** disease of unknown origin that affects almost all body systems, including the musculoskeletal system, and is characterized by remissions and exacerbations. It can range from a mild, episodic disorder to a rapidly fatal disease process. Manifestations are widely variable and are thought to result from cell and tissue damage caused by deposition of antigen–antibody complexes in connective tissues. The majority of cases are diagnosed during the teenage and early adult years.

PATHOPHYSIOLOGY AND ETIOLOGY

The pathophysiology of SLE involves production of a large variety of **autoantibodies** (antibodies that react to the client's own tissues) against normal body components, such as nucleic acids, erythrocytes, coagulation proteins, lymphocytes, and platelets. Autoantibody production results from hyperreactivity of B cells (**humoral immune response**) because of disordered T-cell function (**cellular immune response**). The most characteristic autoantibodies in SLE are produced in response to nucleic acids, including DNA, histones, ribonucleoproteins, and other components of the cell nucleus.

The SLE autoantibodies react with their corresponding antigen to form immune complexes, which are then deposited in the connective tissue of blood vessels, lymphatic vessels, and other tissues. These deposits trigger an **inflammatory response** (chain reaction leading to inflammatory described in detail in the concept of inflammation), which leads to local tissue damage. The kidneys are a frequent site of complex deposition and damage; other affected tissues include the musculoskeletal system, brain, heart, spleen, lung, gastrointestinal tract, skin, and peritoneum. The autoantibodies produced and their target tissues determine the manifestations of SLE.

Etiology

Although the exact etiology of SLE is unknown, genetic, environmental, and hormonal factors play a role in its development. Twin studies and a familial pattern of the disease point to a genetic component, as does an increased incidence of other connective tissue diseases in relatives of people with SLE. In addition, certain **human leukocyte antigen (HLA)** genes (a major histocompatabiltiy complex) are seen more frequently in people with SLE.

It is believed that an outside environmental agent causes the body to initiate an abnormal immune system response to its own tissues (Lupus Foundation of America, 2004; Pongmarutani, Alpert, & Miller, 2006). Environmental factors such as viruses, bacterial antigens, chemicals, drugs, or ultraviolet light may play a role in activating the pathologic mechanisms of the disease.

Sex hormones also are thought to influence the development of SLE. Women with SLE have reduced levels of several active androgens that are known to inhibit antibody responses. In addition, estrogens have been shown to enhance antibody responses and to have an adverse effect in clients with SLE.

Risk Factors

Approximately 1 person in 2,000 is affected by SLE (~500,000 people in the United States), with women predominating over men by a ratio of 9:1 (Pullen, Cannon, & Rushing, 2003; Stichweh, Arce, & Pascual, 2004). SLE usually affects women of childbearing age (when the incidence is 30 times greater than in men), but it can occur at any age. SLE is more common in African Americans, Hispanics, and Asians than it is in Caucasians (Porth, 2005).

In clients with no other risk factors for the disease, a number of drugs can cause a syndrome that mimics lupus (drug-induced lupus). Procainamide (Procan-SR, Pronestyl) and hydralazine (Apresoline, Hydralyn) are the most commonly implicated drugs, along with isoniazid (INH). Renal and CNS manifestations of SLE rarely occur with drug-induced lupus, but arthritic and other systemic symptoms are common. Manifestations of drug-induced lupus usually resolve when the medication is discontinued.

CLINICAL MANIFESTATIONS

There are three major classifications of SLE. The first, known as systemic lupus, involves one or more of the following systems: cardiovascular, central nervous, hematological, kidneys, lungs, and musculoskeletal. The second, known as drug-induced lupus, is associated with some antineoplastic drugs, isoniazid (INH), hydralazine (Apresoline), and others. Symptoms of drug-induced lupus generally subside after the drugs are discontinued. The third, known as discoid lupus, is limited to the skin.

The course of SLE is mild in most clients, with periods of remission and exacerbation. The number and severity of exacerbations tend to decrease with time. In some clients, however, SLE is a virulent disease, with significant organ system involvement.

Clients with active disease have an increased risk for infections, which often are opportunistic and severe. Infections such as pneumonia and septicemia are the leading cause of death in clients with SLE, followed by the effects of renal or CNS involvement (see the following Multisystem Effects feature).

Typical early manifestations of SLE mimic those of rheumatoid arthritis, including systemic manifestations of fever, loss of appetite, malaise, and weight loss, and musculoskeletal manifestations of multiple arthralgias and symmetric polyarthritis. Joint symptoms affect more than 90% of clients with SLE. Although synovitis may be present, the arthritis associated with SLE rarely is deforming.

Most people affected by SLE have skin manifestations at some point during their disease. In fact, SLE originally was described as a skin disorder and was named for the characteristic red butterfly rash across the cheeks and bridge of the nose (Figure 14–23 ■). Many clients with SLE are photosensitive; a diffuse, maculopapular rash on skin exposed to the sun is common. Other cutaneous manifestations include **discoid lesions**

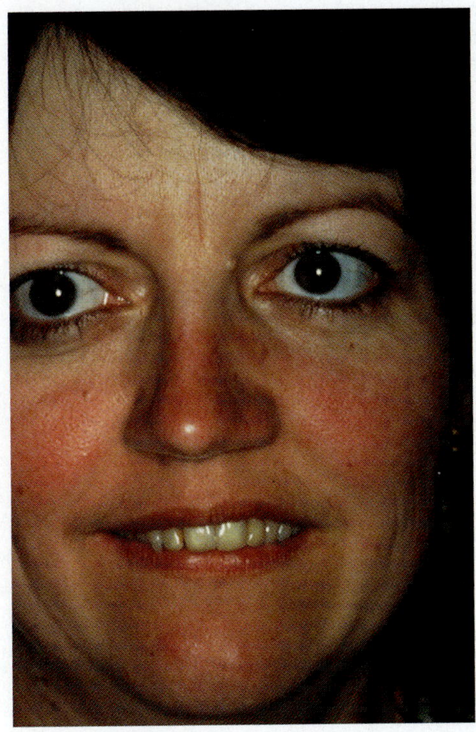

Figure 14–23 ■ The butterfly rash of systemic lupus erythematosus.

MULTISYSTEM EFFECTS OF **Lupus Erythematosus**

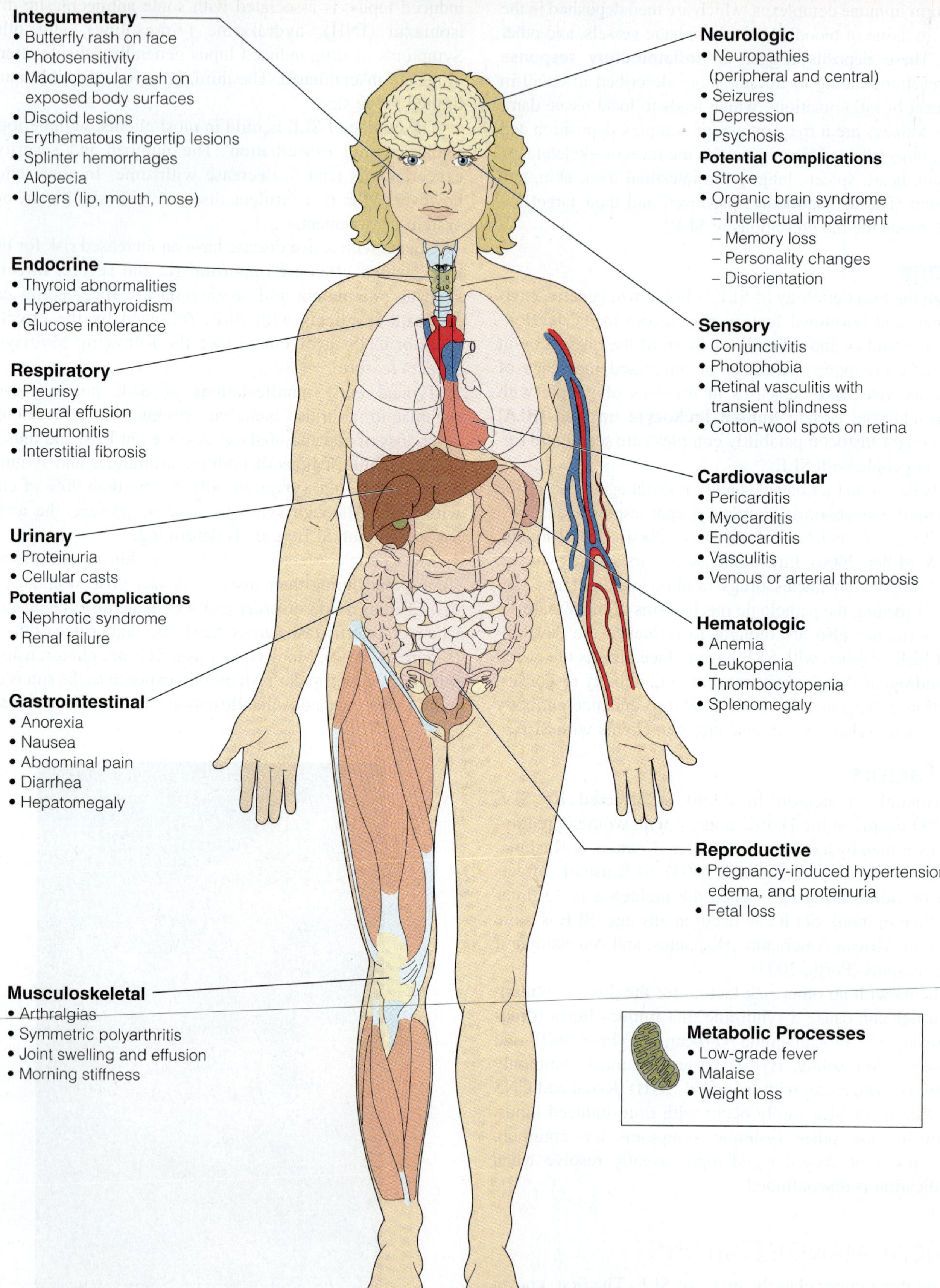

Integumentary
• Butterfly rash on face
• Photosensitivity
• Maculopapular rash on exposed body surfaces
• Discoid lesions
• Erythematous fingertip lesions
• Splinter hemorrhages
• Alopecia
• Ulcers (lip, mouth, nose)
Endocrine
• Thyroid abnormalities
• Hyperparathyroidism
• Glucose intolerance
Respiratory
• Pleurisy
• Pleural effusion
• Pneumonitis
• Interstitial fibrosis
Urinary
• Proteinuria
• Cellular casts
Potential Complications
• Nephrotic syndrome
• Renal failure
Gastrointestinal
• Anorexia
• Nausea
• Abdominal pain
• Diarrhea
• Hepatomegaly
Musculoskeletal
• Arthralgias
• Symmetric polyarthritis
• Joint swelling and effusion
• Morning stiffness
Neurologic
• Neuropathies (peripheral and central)
• Seizures
• Depression
• Psychosis
Potential Complications
• Stroke
• Organic brain syndrome
– Intellectual impairment
– Memory loss
– Personality changes
– Disorientation
Sensory
• Conjunctivitis
• Photophobia
• Retinal vasculitis with transient blindness
• Cotton-wool spots on retina
Cardiovascular
• Pericarditis
• Myocarditis
• Endocarditis
• Vasculitis
• Venous or arterial thrombosis
Hematologic
• Anemia
• Leukopenia
• Thrombocytopenia
• Splenomegaly
Reproductive
• Pregnancy-induced hypertension, edema, and proteinuria
• Fetal loss
Metabolic Processes
• Low-grade fever
• Malaise
• Weight loss

CLINICAL MANIFESTATIONS AND THERAPIES Systemic Lupus Erythematosus

ETIOLOGY	CLINICAL MANIFESTATIONS	CLINICAL THERAPIES
Organic brain syndrome may result from neurological involvement	General term referring to many disorders causing impaired mental function; manifestations include confusion with impaired memory, judgment, and cognition. Symptoms may include agitation, withdrawal, or depression.	Treatment varies and is aimed at treating the underlying cause of the condition, in this case SLE.
Anemia	Manifestations range from absence of clinical signs and symptoms to more life threatening, depending on the severity of the condition. Common manifestations include: ■ Weakness ■ Fatigue ■ Poor concentration ■ Shortness of breath ■ Dyspnea ■ Palpitations ■ Intermittent claudication ■ Symptoms of heart failure.	Initial treatment is aimed at restoring normal red blood cell counts as well as treating the underlying cause. Treatment to increase red blood cell count includes: ■ Increased iron intake in diet ■ Iron supplementation ■ Medications to stimulate red cell production such as erythropoietin. In severe cases blood transfusions may be administered.
Leukopenia	The most common manifestation is frequent infections resulting from inadequate immune response caused by low white blood cell counts.	Treatment to increase white blood cell count is predominantly aimed at treating the underlying cause of leukopenia. Supportive treatment to resolve infections and prevent further infection may include antibiotics, protective isolation, and strict aseptic technique.
Thrombocytopenia may occur spontaneously but it is more commonly associated with medications used to treat SLE.	Manifestations generally do not arise until platelet count falls to significant levels of less than 50,000. Common manifestations include: ■ Bruising ■ Petechia ■ Purpura ■ Nosebleeds ■ Bleeding gums.	Treatment is guided by etiology and severity and may include: ■ Corticosteroids ■ IV IgG ■ Splenectomy. Administration of IV platelet transfusion.
Pericarditis	■ Chest pain radiating to the back relieved by sitting forward and worsening when lying down ■ Dry cough ■ Fever ■ Fatigue ■ Anxiety ■ Friction rub ■ ST elevation and PR depression	■ Pericardiocentesis to remove fluid produced by inflammatory process, especially if it is restricting function ■ Antibiotics if infectious ■ Corticosteroids to reduce inflammation ■ Colchicine
Renal involvement	■ Proteinuria ■ Cellular casts ■ Nephrotic syndrome ■ Renal failure	Treatment is aimed at correcting the underlying cause and relieving stress on the kidney. Dialysis may be indicated if renal failure results.
Skin involvement is the most common result of SLE.	Photosensitivity with a diffuse maculopapular rash on skin exposed to the sun; discoid lesions, hives, erythematous fingertip lesions, alopecia, and splinter hemorrhages.	■ Avoid sunlight ■ Corticosteroids ■ Immunosuppressants ■ Disease modifying antirheumatic drugs Low fat, mostly vegetarian wholesome diet may lessen symptoms.

(raised, scaly, circular lesions with an erythematous rim), hives, erythematous fingertip lesions, and splinter hemorrhages. Alopecia is common in clients with SLE, although the hair usually grows back. Painless mucous membrane ulcerations may occur on the lips or in the mouth or nose. Common manifestations of SLE are listed in Box 14–16.

Approximately 50% of people with SLE experience renal manifestations of the disease, including proteinuria, cellular casts, and nephrotic syndrome. Up to 10% develop renal failure as a result of the disease.

Hematologic abnormalities, such as anemia, leukopenia, and thrombocytopenia, are common with SLE. Cardiovascular disorders, such as pericarditis, vasculitis, and Raynaud's phenomenon, often occur. Less frequently, myocarditis, endocarditis, and venous or arterial thrombosis may develop. Pleurisy, pleural effusions, and lupus pneumonitis are common pulmonary manifestations of SLE.

Many clients with SLE develop transient nervous system involvement, often within the first year of the disease. Manifestations of organic brain syndrome include decline in intellect, memory loss, and disorientation. Other possible neurologic manifestations include psychosis, seizures, depression, and stroke. Ocular manifestations of SLE include conjunctivitis, photophobia, and transient blindness due to retinal vasculitis.

Gastrointestinal manifestations of SLE, such as anorexia, nausea, abdominal pain, and diarrhea, may affect up to 45% of clients with the disease. The liver may be enlarged, and liver function tests may yield abnormal results.

Although SLE was once considered to be a fatal disease, the survival rate has been improved through earlier diagnosis and better treatment options. Prognosis depends on the severity of the internal organ involvement. Kidney failure is managed by hemodialysis or peritoneal dialysis. Renal transplantation has been very successful for treatment of renal failure secondary to lupus nephritis, a common complication of SLE.

Women who conceive when the disease is in remission appear to have little risk for adverse outcomes, whereas those who conceive when they have active disease experience less favorable outcomes. Pregnancy does not appear to alter the long-term prognosis of women with SLE (Molad et al., 2005).

Box 14–16 **Common Manifestations of Systemic Lupus Erythematosus**

- Painful or swollen joints and muscle pain
- Unexplained fever
- Red rash, especially on the face
- Unusual loss of hair
- Pale, cyanotic fingers or toes
- Sensitivity to the sun
- Edema in legs and around eyes
- Ulcers in the mouth
- Enlarged glands
- Extreme fatigue

There is an increased incidence of spontaneous abortion, stillbirth, prematurity, and intrauterine growth retardation. Infants born to women with SLE may have characteristic skin rash, which usually disappears by 12 months. However, these infants are at increased risk for complete congenital heart block, a condition that can be diagnosed prenatally. Fetal echocardiography is then performed to rule out other cardiac defects (Byron & Clancy, 2005). No known treatment exists for congenital heart block, although various therapies have been tried with varying degrees of success. The prognosis for the fetus varies, but because the heart damage is permanent, a pacemaker may be necessary if the newborn is to survive (Branch, Silver & Aagaard-Tillery, 2008).

COLLABORATION

As with rheumatoid arthritis, effective management of SLE requires teamwork, with active participation by both the client and members of the health care team. Although currently no cure exists for SLE, the 10-year survival rate is greater than 70% among clients with this disease, which was once considered fatal in most cases. Depending on the severity of a client's manifestations, nurses may want to collaborate with dieticians and physical therapists to help the client develop a nutrition and exercise plans. Referrals to counselors can help clients and caregivers learn to manage stress.

Diagnostic Tests

Because of the diversity of both organ system involvement and manifestations of SLE, diagnosis can be difficult. No one specific test is available to confirm the presence of this disease in all people suspected of having it. Instead, the diagnosis is based on the client's history and physical assessment, as well as laboratory studies.

The multiple autoantibodies produced in SLE cause a number of abnormalities in laboratory studies. The following tests may be helpful in confirming the presence of SLE:

- *Anti-DNA antibody testing:* This test is a more specific indicator of SLE, because these antibodies rarely are found in any other disorder.
- *Erythrocyte sedimentation rate:* This value typically is elevated, occasionally to 100 mm/hr or greater.
- *Serum complement levels:* These values usually are decreased as complement is consumed or "used up" by the development of **antigen–antibody complexes**.
- *Complete blood count (CBC):* Abnormalities in the CBC include moderate to severe anemia, leukopenia, lymphocytopenia, and possible thrombocytopenia.
- *Urinalysis:* This test shows mild proteinuria, hematuria, and blood cell casts during exacerbations of the disease when the kidneys are involved. Renal function tests including *serum creatinine* and *blood urea nitrogen (BUN)* may also be ordered to evaluate the extent of renal disease.
- *Kidney biopsy:* This test may be performed to assess the severity of renal lesions and guide therapy.

Pharmacologic Therapies

The client with mild or remittent SLE may need little or no therapy other than supportive care. Arthralgias, arthritis, fever, and fatigue often can be managed with aspirin or other NSAIDs. Aspirin is particularly beneficial for clients with SLE, because its antiplatelet effects help to prevent thrombosis. However, it may cause liver toxicity and hepatitis.

Skin and arthritic manifestations of SLE may be treated with antimalarial drugs, such as hydroxychloroquine (Plaquenil). Hydroxychloroquine also has been shown to be effective in reducing the frequency of acute episodes of SLE in people with mild or inactive disease. Retinal toxicity and possibly irreversible blindness are the primary concerns with this drug. For this reason, clients taking hydroxychloroquine should undergo an ophthalmologic examination every 6 months.

Clients with severe and life-threatening manifestations of SLE (e.g., nephritis, hemolytic anemia, myocarditis, pericarditis, or CNS manifestations) require corticosteroid therapy in high doses. Initially, such clients may need 40 to 60 mg of prednisone per day. The dosage is then tapered as rapidly as the client's disease allows, although lowering the dosage may precipitate an acute episode. Some clients with SLE require long-term corticosteroid therapy to manage symptoms and prevent major organ damage. These clients are at increased risk for corticosteroid side effects, such as cushingoid effects, weight gain, hypertension, infection, accelerated osteoporosis, and hypokalemia.

Immunosuppressive agents such as cyclophosphamide or azathioprine may be used, either alone or in combination with corticosteroids, to treat clients with active SLE or lupus nephritis (Box 14–17). When these agents are used in combination, lower, less toxic doses of each drug can be used. The client receiving immunosuppressive agents is at increased risk for infection, malignancy, bone marrow depression, and toxic effects specific to the drug prescribed.

Clinical Therapies

Because of the photosensitivity that is associated with SLE, the client should be cautioned to avoid sun exposure. Clients should use sunscreens with an SPF rating of 15 or higher when outdoors. Topical corticosteroids may be used to treat skin lesions. Some physicians recommend avoiding the use of oral contraceptives, because estrogen can trigger an acute episode. Clients with lupus nephritis who progress to develop end-stage renal disease are treated with dialysis (hemodialysis or peritoneal dialysis) and kidney transplantation.

Complementary Therapies

Exacerbations of SLE have been linked to stress. Stress-reducing techniques, such as guided imagery, yoga, massage, or aroma therapy, can reduce exacerbations. Because SLE is most common in adolescents, however, what stress reduction might be possible? Consider a busy teen who plays sports, has many social activities, and excels in school. How can you assist this teen to see the importance of identifying techniques for stress reduction, and then of using those techniques? How can stress reduction be integrated into the daily life of an active teen?

Box 14–17 **Immunosuppressive Agents for Systemic Lupus Erythematosus**

Certain cytotoxic or antineoplastic drugs are effective as immunosuppressive agents. They act by decreasing the proliferation of cells within the immune system and are widely used to prevent rejection following a tissue or organ transplant. Usually, they are administered concurrently with corticosteroid therapy, allowing lower doses of both preparations and resulting in fewer side effects. Such agents include:

- Azathioprine (Imuran)
- Cyclophosphamide (Cytoxan)
- Cyclosporine (Sandimmune)

NURSING RESPONSIBILITIES

- Monitor blood count, with particular attention to the WBC and platelet counts. Notify the physician if WBCs fall below 4,000 or platelets below 75,000.
- Monitor renal and liver function studies, including creatinine, blood urea nitrogen, creatinine clearance, and liver enzyme levels. Report any abnormal levels to the physician.
- Oral preparations should be administered with food to minimize gastrointestinal effects. Antacids may be ordered.
- Increase fluids to maintain good hydration and urinary output.
- Monitor intake and output.
- Monitor for signs of abnormal bleeding, such as bleeding gums, bruising, petechiae, joint pain, hematuria, and black or tarry stools.
- Use meticulous hand washing and other appropriate measures to protect the client from infection. Assess for signs of infection.
- Pulmonary fibrosis is a potential adverse effect of cyclophosphamide. Therefore, monitor the results of pulmonary function studies, and be alert to clinical signs of dyspnea or cough.

HEALTH EDUCATION FOR THE CLIENT AND FAMILY

- Avoid large crowds and situations where you might be exposed to infections.
- Report signs of infection, such as chills, fever, sore throat, fatigue, or malaise, to the physician.
- Use contraceptive measures to prevent pregnancy while you are taking these drugs, because they may increase the risk of birth defects.
- Avoid using aspirin or ibuprofen while taking these drugs. Report any signs of bleeding to the physician.
- Be aware that menstruation may stop while taking cyclophosphamide. The menses will resume after the drug is discontinued.
- Report difficulty breathing or cough to the physician if you are taking cyclophosphamide.

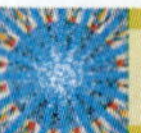

DEVELOPMENTAL CONSIDERATIONS Treatment of Systemic Lupus Erythematosus

CHILDREN

- The side effects of the corticosteroids, immunosuppressants, and antimalarial drugs used in the treatment of children with SLE are significant and include hair loss, susceptibility to infection, "moon face," retinal damage, and bone loss.
- These are significant side effects for adolescent clients, who commonly are concerned about appearance. Special teaching, guidance, and support may be needed for teens with SLE.
- Encourage the teen to find methods to explain the side effects and appearance. For example, a science or health teacher may allow the adolescent the opportunity to present information about the disease and treatment.
- The adolescent also may benefit from peer interaction with others who have similar experiences. Support groups or Internet chat rooms may be helpful.

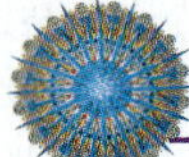

NURSING PROCESS

Nursing management focuses on thorough assessments (because of the multitude of systems that can be affected by SLE) and on teaching to enhance general health practices. The client with severe disease, however, has many diverse nursing needs, which vary according to the organ systems involved. Because of the close link between RA and SLE, many of the nursing diagnoses and interventions identified for the client with arthritis may be appropriate for the client with SLE. The client with lupus nephritis or end-stage renal disease has the nursing care needs outlined in the examplar on chronic renal failure in Concept 11, Fluid and Electrolytes, and in Exemplar 16.4, Nephritis, in Concept 16, Inflammation.

Assessment

Assess the client's nutritional status including baseline weight and history of recent weight loss or weight gain. The skin is assessed for rashes, ulcers, photosensitivity, ecchymosis, petechiae, cyanosis, and hair loss. Respiratory assessment includes breath sounds and respiratory rate as well as assessment for pleural effusion or pleuritis. Cardiovascular assessment includes vital signs, heart tones, and symptoms of pericarditis or friction rub. Musculoskeletal assessment includes joint pain, joint deformity, pain, weakness, and ability to perform ADLs. Neurologic assessment includes changes in affect or cognitive abilities and seizure activity. Gastrointestinal assessment includes splenomegaly.

Because SLE is a chronic disease that affects primarily adolescents, psychosocial assessment is indicated. Assess family interactions, and exploring stressful situations, such as divorce or trauma. Treatment-related restrictions and changes in appearance can lead to withdrawal, depression, and suicidal tendencies. Perform psychologic assessments periodically as the client grows and adapts to the disorder or faces new developmental challenges with a chronic disease.

Diagnosis

Nursing diagnoses will vary depending on severity of disease process and organ involvement but likely will include the following:

- Risk for Ineffective Management of Therapeutic Regimen (family) related to complexity of therapeutic regimen
- Risk for Ineffective Tissue Perfusion (renal) related to interrupted blood flow in kidneys
- Risk for Impaired Skin Integrity related to immunologic deficit
- Risk for Activity Intolerance related to chronic disease
- Risk for Disturbed Body Image related to side effects of medications and skin alterations
- Risk for Infection related to immunosuppressive medications
- Chronic Pain related to joint inflammation and injury
- Disturbed Body Image related to changes from the disease and medication treatment
- Compromised Family Coping related to demands of chronic illness with unknown outcome.

Plan

The goals of nursing care are to assist clients (especially children) to manage and cope with a chronic disease, prevent infection, promote nutrition, facilitate a remission, and recognize and avoid triggers for flares. Goals are created with input from the client based on needs, current status, and severity of disease, including organ involvement. Goals should be specific and contain a time frame for attainment. Goals may include the following:

- Client is able to verbalize skin care needs to reduce the risk of altered skin integrity at the end of the teaching session.
- Client demonstrates proper hand hygiene techniques before discharge.
- Client verbalizes the impact of the diagnosis when seen by the health care provider.
- Client verbalizes methods for preventing infection, including use of prophylactic antibiotics and home infection control measures.

Implementation

The priority nursing interventions for the client with SLE are focused on problems with impaired skin integrity, ineffective protection, and impaired health maintenance.

Promote Skin Integrity

Skin lesions are a common manifestation of SLE. A rash or discoid lesion interrupts the integrity of the skin and the first line of protection against infection, increasing the client's already high risk for infection. These lesions, which usually appear on exposed parts of the skin, also can be disfiguring and cause the client emotional distress.

- Assess the client's knowledge of SLE and its possible effects on the skin. Assessment allows the nurse to base teaching and information on the client's existing knowledge, thereby improving learning and retention.
- Discuss the relationship between sun exposure and disease activity, both dermatologic and systemic. It is important for the client to understand that sun exposure may not only cause dermatologic manifestations but also trigger an acute episode.
- Suggest the following strategies to limit sun exposure:
  a. Avoid being out of doors during hours of greatest sun intensity (10:00 a.m. to 3:00 p.m.).
  b. Use sunscreen with a sun protection factor (SPF) rating of 15 or higher when sun exposure cannot be avoided. Apply sunscreen 30 minutes before going out into the sun.
  c. Reapply sunscreen after swimming, exercising, or bathing.
  d. Wear loose clothing with long sleeves and wide-brimmed hats when outdoors.

These strategies can help the client to maintain a normal lifestyle while helping to prevent acute episodes.

- Keep skin clean and dry; apply therapeutic creams or ointments to lesions as prescribed. These measures promote healing and reduce the risk of infection.
- Encourage the use of good hygienic measures and a mild soap. This prevents infection resulting in stress that can lead to acute exacerbations.
- Recommend limited use of cosmetics. Cosmetics can irritate the skin and increase the risk of integumentary symptoms.
- Recommend the client avoid fluorescent lighting. Exacerbations of SLE have been reported following this exposure (Mulvihill, 2003).
- Provide instructions on oral care to maintain intact oral mucosa. Alterations in skin integrity, including those in the oral cavity, can increase the risk of acute exacerbations of SLE.
- Provide instructions on the care of the head if alopecia occurs. Alopecia, especially in women, can be very traumatic so care of the skin on the head is important because wigs cannot be worn when skin integrity is impacted.

Prevent Infection

Infections are a leading cause of death for clients with SLE. Prophylactic antibiotics may be required for dental work and surgical procedures. Instruct the client and family to inform all health care providers of the disease in order to plan for prophylactic measures. Educate the client and family on the importance of adhering to the immunization schedule and obtaining a yearly influenza vaccine to prevent infection. Instruct the client on hand hygiene and infection control measures in the home, and warn adolescents about the dangers of tattooing and body piercing because of the risk of infection.

Maintain Fluid Balance

Because many clients with SLE have renal involvement, it is important to monitor intake and output and frequently evaluate fluid and electrolyte status. Renal dysfunction can manifest itself by edema, muscle cramps, diarrhea, tetany, and convulsions.

Promote Adequate Nutrition

Currently, there are no specific dietary plans for the client with SLE; however, the diet may be restricted according to renal involvement, weight gain, weight loss, or other complications. The client is at risk for weight gain associated with treatment involving steroids and a decreased activity level during exacerbations of this disease. A well-balanced, nutritious diet as well as appropriate fluid intake should be encouraged.

Promote Rest and Comfort

Because of fatigue and joint pain, the client has little energy reserve during acute episodes of the disease. Encourage frequent rest periods and a nutritious diet to maximize energy stores. A physical therapist can plan a program to encourage mobility and increase muscle strength.

Manage Side Effects of Medications

Observe for any side effects of medications used for treatment, and teach the client and family about these effects. For example, immunosuppressant drugs can promote infection anywhere in the body, and NSAIDs commonly cause gastric distress and bleeding of the gastrointestinal tract. The antimalarial drug hydroxychloroquine can cause serious vision changes; thus, frequent eye examinations are needed.

Provide Emotional Support

Adolescents may have an altered body image as a result of rash, alopecia, arthritic changes in the joints, and chronic disease. Referral to a lupus support group, the local department of social services, or counseling may be helpful. The American Lupus Society and the Lupus Foundation of America (http://www.lupus.org) can provide information to help clients and family members adjust to the disease. The Arthritis Foundation (http://www.arthritis.org) also publishes a useful pamphlet: *Meeting the Challenge: A Young Person's Guide to Living with Lupus*. The client needs ongoing support and information to deal with the complexity of the disease.

Avoidance of Triggers for Disease Flares

Many clients can recognize the signs of an impending flare and the triggers that precede them. Partner with the client and family to implement measures to avoid these triggers. Discuss preventive behaviors, such as avoiding sun exposure and stressors. Clients should be warned that alcohol, smoking, and drugs also pose an increased risk because of the potential to stimulate flares. Female clients who are sexually active may be advised to avoid birth control pills that contain the hormone estrogen, because the extra estrogen may exacerbate symptoms. In addition, alternate birth control methods should be discussed.

Ineffective Protection

Ineffective protection can be a problem for the client with SLE, who is at increased risk for infection and multiple organ system problems because of the disease. In addition, treatment with corticosteroids or immunosuppressive agents further impairs immune responses and the ability to fight infection. The following interventions are for the client who is hospitalized.

- Wash hands before and after providing direct care. Hand washing removes transient organisms from the skin, reducing the risk of transmission to the client.

- Use strict aseptic technique in caring for intravenous lines and indwelling urinary catheters or performing any wound care. Aseptic technique offers protection against external and resident host microorganisms.
- Assess frequently for infection. Monitor temperature and vital signs every 4 hours. Assess for signs of cellulitis, including tenderness, redness, swelling, and warmth. Report signs of infection to the physician promptly. Therapy can suppress usual responses, such as elevated temperature and inflammation. The fever of infection may be mistaken for the fever commonly associated with SLE. The client receiving immunosuppressive therapy for the disease has an even higher risk for infection.
- Monitor laboratory values, including CBC and tests of organ function; report changes to the physician. An elevation in the WBC count with a shift to the left (increased numbers of immature leukocytes in the blood) may be an early indication of infection. Changes in liver function studies, renal function studies, myocardial enzymes, or other laboratory values may indicate organ system involvement.

Initiate reverse or protective isolation procedures as indicated by the client's immune status. These procedures provide further protection from infection for clients who are severely immunocompromised.

- Ensure an adequate nutrient intake, offering supplementary feedings as indicated or maintaining parenteral nutrition if necessary. Adequate nutrition is important for healing and immune system function.
- Teach the client the importance of good hand washing after using the bathroom and before eating. Hand washing reduces the risk of infection with endogenous organisms.
- Monitor for potential adverse effects of medications, including thrombocytopenia and possible bleeding, fluid retention with edema and possible hypertension, loss of bone density, osteoporosis, and possible pathologic fractures, renal or hepatic toxicity, and cardiac effects, particularly in the client with fluid retention and hypervolemia. Medications used to treat SLE have many potential adverse effects that can impair normal protective and homeostatic mechanisms.

PRACTICE ALERT

Hands must be washed before and after providing direct care, even if gloves are worn. A decrease in this type of medical asepsis is contributing to the increasing number of hospital-acquired infections that are resistant to antibiotics.

Impaired Health Maintenance

As with other chronic diseases, much of the responsibility for maintaining optimal health rests with the client. Disease manifestations such as fatigue, arthralgias, arthritis, and increased risk for infection can interfere with the client's ability to maintain health. Psychosocial issues also can be a significant factor in health maintenance for the client with SLE. These issues may include denial of the significance of the disease, poor coping, lack of financial and other resources, and an inadequate support system.

- Assess the client's ability to maintain optimal health, identifying physical and psychosocial factors that may affect health maintenance. Before intervening to improve the client's health maintenance, the nurse must identify and understand the factors affecting it.
- Provide care and teaching in a nonjudgmental manner. To intervene effectively, the nurse must accept the client and family as they are.
- Encourage the client and family members to discuss the effect of the disease on their lives. Open discussion helps the client and the nurse identify barriers to health maintenance and begin exploring alternative strategies.
- Initiate an interdisciplinary care conference with the client and family. In this care conference, a number of perspectives can be expressed, thus improving the planning of strategies for health maintenance activities.

CLIENT TEACHING **Self-Care of Systemic Lupus Erythematosus**

Teaching is a critical factor in preparing clients with SLE for self-care at home. Address the following topics:

- The disease and its potential effects. Promote an optimistic outlook, stressing that the majority of clients do not require long-term corticosteroid therapy and that the disease may improve over time.
- The importance of skin care.
- The importance of avoiding exposure to infection.
- The need to follow the prescribed treatment plan, including rest and exercise, medications, and follow-up appointments. Discuss manifestations of an acute episode (often called a flare), and stress the importance of contacting the physician promptly if any of these manifestations occur.
- The significance of wearing a MedicAlert tag that identifies their condition and therapy (e.g., corticosteroids or immunosuppressives).
- Family planning with the client and spouse. The use of oral contraceptives may be contraindicated for the client; if appropriate, provide information about alternative means of birth control. Pregnancy is not contraindicated for most women with SLE. However, the pregnant client requires close monitoring, because acute episodes sometimes accompany pregnancy.
- The need for preventive health care for both men and women with SLE. Women should have gynecologic and breast examinations and men should have prostate examinations each year. Both men and women should have regular screenings for cholesterol and blood pressure. Annual influenza vaccinations are important, as are pneumococcal vaccinations for older clients. If clients are taking corticosteroids or antimalarial medications, annual eye examinations should be conducted to screen for and treat any ocular problems.
- Helpful resources:
  a. National Institute of Arthritis and Musculoskeletal and Skin Diseases
  b. Lupus Foundation of America.

- Refer the client and family to counseling as needed. Counseling may help the client and family develop the coping skills necessary to accept and deal with the disease.
- Refer the client and family to community and social service agencies and to local support groups. These groups and agencies are valuable resources for the client and family.

PRACTICE ALERT

Warning signs of an acute episode (a flare) include increased fatigue, pain or abdominal discomfort, rash, headache, fever, and dizziness.

Evaluation

Successful outcomes of nursing care involve management of this chronic disease. Expected outcomes include the following:

- Client maintains normal intake and output levels, with demonstrated fluid and electrolyte balance.
- Client maintains healthy, intact skin.
- Client maintains a balance of rest and activity to promote health.
- Client maintains medication regimen to promote health and prevent side effects.
- Client develops or maintains a positive body image.

REVIEW Systemic Lupus Erythematosus

RELATE: LINK THE CONCEPTS

Link the exemplar of SLE with the concept of Inflammation:

1. Describe the inflammatory reaction and explain the role this process plays in SLE.
2. What types of treatment for inflammation would also be useful in treating SLE?

Link the exemplar of SLE with the concept of Health Behaviors:

3. Why would the client with SLE be less likely to have acute exacerbations if he or she made healthy lifestyle choices?
4. Create a teaching plan explaining health behaviors that can promote fewer acute exacerbations of SLE.

REFER: GO TO MYNURSINGKIT

REFLECT: CASE STUDY

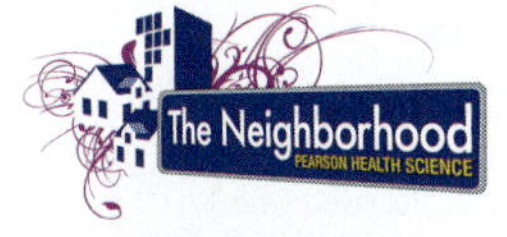

Yvonne Johnson is a 35-year-old African-American woman. She is a single parent to her 15-year-old son, Randall. Yvonne has had relationships with men off and on, but she is not currently involved with anybody. Yvonne completed a bachelor's degree in marketing 5 years ago but has been unable to break into the marketing field locally. Instead, she has been working full time as an administrative assistant for a large company. Her parents and siblings live nearby, and she maintains a close relationship with them.

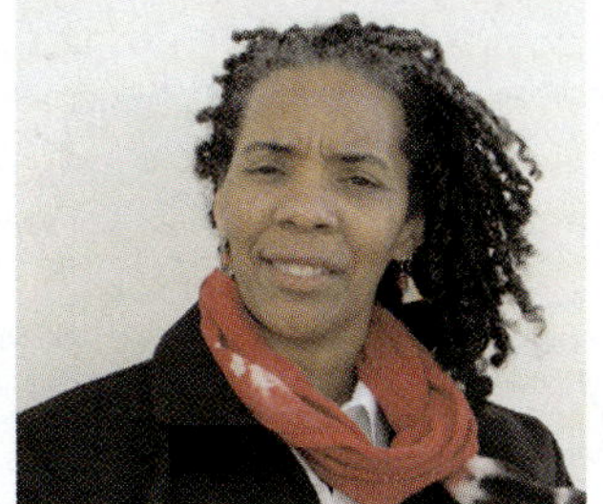

Over the past 4 years, Yvonne has noticed mild swelling in her hands and feet every morning. The symptoms began subtly not long after graduating from college and getting a job. She has always attributed the symptom to her sedentary lifestyle and being somewhat overweight. More recently, she has been experiencing pain along with the swelling in her hands and feet.

Yvonne sees her health care provider, Dr. Rowe, and tells her that she has had pain in her hands for the last several months. When asked about other symptoms, she mentions the swelling in her hands and feet for the past 4 years. Dr. Rowe believes the pain is occupational in nature (typing) and suggests that Yvonne take over-the-counter pain relievers, such as ibuprofen. Dr. Rowe notices that Yvonne's blood pressure is slightly elevated (134/92 mmHg) but attributes this to her race and diet. She suggests that Yvonne lose a little weight and reduce her salt intake.

Yvonne has been trying to follow the advice of Dr. Rowe for the past 3 months. Despite the fact that she has lost approximately 5 lbs, has avoided salty foods, and has been taking ibuprofen three times a day, she continues to have pain in her hands and swelling in her hands and feet. She also wonders if the symptoms are really associated with her work.

1. What diagnosis do you suspect for Yvonne? Explain the basis of your answer.
2. What diagnostic testing would you anticipate to confirm this diagnosis? Explain your answers.
3. If you are the nurse admitting Yvonne to her provider's office, what specific assessments would you perform to help you in confirming the suspected diagnosis?

EXPLORE PEARSON **mynursingkit**™

MyNursingKit is your one stop for online chapter review materials and resources. Prepare for success with additional NCLEX®-style practice questions, interactive assignments and activities, web links, animations and videos, and more!

Register your access code from the front of your book at **www.mynursingkit.com**.

REFERENCES

AegisAEGiS. (2006). *Opportunistic infections.* Retrieved June 1, 2009, from http://www.aegis.com/topics/oi/

American Academy of Pediatrics. (2006). *Red book: Report of the committee on infectious disease* (27th ed.). Elk Grove Village, IL: American Academy of Pediatrics.

American Academy of Pediatrics, Committee on Fetus and Newborn & American College of Obstetricians and Gynecologists Committee on Obstetrics. (2007). *Guidelines for perinatal care* (6th ed.). Elk Grove Village, IL: American Academy of Pediatrics Committee on Fetus and Newborn & American College of Obstetricians and Gynecologists Committee on Obstetrics.

American Academy of Pediatrics, Committee on Pediatric AIDS and Committee on Adolescence. (2001). Adolescents and human immunodeficiency virus infection: The role of the pediatrician in prevention and intervention (RE0031). *Pediatrics, 107*(1), 188–190

American Academy of Pediatrics, Committee on Pediatric AIDS. (1998). Human immunodeficiency virus/acquired immunodeficiency syndrome education in schools. *Pediatrics, 101*, 933–935.

American Cancer Society. (2008). *Infectious agents and cancer.* Retrieved October 25, 2009, from http://www.cancer.org/docroot/PED/content/PED_1_3X_Infectious_Agents_and_Cancer.asp?sitearea=PED

Asthma and Allergy Foundation of America (AAFA). (2009). *Allergy facts and figures.* Retrieved June 2, 2009, from http://www.aafa.org/display.cfm?id=9&sub=30

Bartlett, J. G., & Weber, D. J. (2005). *Management of adults exposed to HIV. Up to Date Online 13.2.* Retrieved October 14, 2005, from http://222.utdol.com

Benin, A. L., Wisler-Scher, D. J., Colson, E., Shapiro, E. D., & Holmboe, E.S. (2006). Qualitative analysis of mothers' decision-making about vaccines for infants: The importance of trust. *Pediatrics, 117* (5), 1532–1541.

Bernstein, H. (2007). Maternal and perinatal infection–viral. In S. G. Gabbe, J. R. Niebyl, & J. L. Simpson (Eds.), *Obstetrics: Normal and problem pregnancies* (5th ed., pp. 1203–1232). Philadelphia: Churchill Livingstone/Elsevier.

Bilukha, O. O. & Rosenstein, N. (2005). Prevention and control of meningococcal disease: Recommendations of the advisory committee on immunization practices. *Morbidity and Mortality Weekly Report 64*(7), 1–28.

Bindler, R. M., & Howry, L. B. (2005). *Pediatric drugs and nursing implications* (3rd ed.). Upper Saddle River, NJ: Prentice Hall Health.

Bonilla, F. A., & Geha, R. S. (2006). Update on primary immunodeficiency diseases. *Journal of Allergy and Clinical Immunology, 117*, S435–S441.

Bourlioux, P., Koletzko, B., Guarner, F., & Braesco, V. (2003). The intestine and its microflora are partners for the protection of the host: Report on the Danone Symposium "The Intelligent Intestine," held in Paris, June 14, 2002. *American Journal of Clinical Nutrition, 78*(4), 675–683.

Bousquet, J., Flahault, A., Vandenplas, O., Amielle, J., Duron, J. J., Pecquet, C., Chevrie, K., & Annesi-Maesano, I. (2006). Natural rubber latex allergy among health care workers: A systematic review of the evidence. *Journal of Allergy and Clinical Immunology, 118*, 447–454.

Bova, C. A., Fennie, K. P., Knafl, G. J., Dieckhaus, K. D., Wtrous, E., & Williams, A. B. (2005). Use of electronic monitoring devices to measure antiretroviral adherence: Practical considerations. *AIDS and Behavior, 9*(1), 103–110.

Brackis-Cott, E., Mellins, C. A., Abrams, E., Reval, T., & Dolezal, C. (2003). Pediatric HIV medication adherence: The views of medical providers from two primary care programs. *Journal of Pediatric Health Care, 17*, 252–260.

Branch, D. W., Silver, R. M., & Aagaard-Tillery, K. (2008). Immunologic disorders in pregnancy. In R. S. Gibbs, B. Y. Karlan, A. F. Haney, & I. E. Nygaard (Eds.), *Danforth's obstetrics and gynecology* (10th ed.). Philadelphia: Wolters Kluwer/Lippincott Williams & Wilkins.

Branson, B. M., Handsfield, H. H., Lampe, M. A., Janssen, R. S., Taylor, A. W., Lyss, S. B., et al. (2006). Revised recommendations for HIV testing of adults, adolescents, and pregnant women in health-care settings. *MMWR: Morbidity & Mortality Weekly Report, 55*(RR-14), 1–16.

Buck, M. L. (2005). Meningococcal conjugate vaccine. *Pediatric Pharmacology, 11*(5). Retrieved June 7, 2005, from http://www.medscape.com/viewarticle/505508_print

Byron, J. P., & Clancy, R. M. (2005). Neonatal lupus, basic research and clinical perspectives. *Rheumatic Diseases Clinics of North America, 31*(2), 299–313.

Carrico, R. M. (2001). What to do if you're exposed to a bloodborne pathogen. *Home Healthcare Nurse, 19*(6), 362–368.

Centers for Disease Control and Prevention (CDC). (2002). Immunization registry use and progress–United States, 2001. *Morbidity and Mortality Weekly Report, 51* (3), 53–56.

Centers for Disease Control and Prevention(CDC). (2004). Treating opportunistic infections among HIV-infected adults and adolescents. *MMWR Recommendations and Reports, 53*(RR-15), 1–113.

Centers for Disease Control and Prevention (CDC). (2005). *Cases of HIV infection and AIDS in the United States, 2004.* Retrieved April 22, 2006, from http://www.cdc.gov

Centers for Disease Control and Prevention (CDC). (2006a). *CDC's advisory committee recommends changes in varicella vaccinations.* Retrieved July 5, 2006, from Error! Hyperlink reference not valid.

Centers for Disease Control and Prevention (CDC). (2006b). *HIV and its transmission.* Retrieved October 25, 2009, from http://www.cdc.gov

Centers for Disease Control and Prevention (CDC). (2006c). Preventing tetanus, diphtheria, and pertussis among adolescents: Use of tetanus toxoid, reduced diphtheria toxoid, and acellular pertussis vaccines. *Morbidity and Mortality Weekly Report, 55*, 1–34.

Centers for Disease Control and Prevention (CDC). (2006d). Prevention and control of influenza: Recommendations of the Advisory Committee on Immunization Practices (ACIP). *Morbidity and Mortality Weekly Report, 55*, 1–44.

Centers for Disease Control and Prevention (CDC). (2006e). Revised recommendations for HIV testing of adults, adolescents and pregnant women in health-care settings. *Morbidity and Mortality Weekly Report, 55*(RR14), 1–17.

Centers for Disease Control and Prevention (CDC). (2006f). *Statistics and surveillance.* Retrieved March 14, 2006, from http://www.cdc.gov/hiv/topics/surveillance/index.htm

Centers for Disease Control and Prevention (CDC). (2007). HIV/AIDS Surveillance in Women. Retrieved July 31, 2009 from http://www.cdc.gov/hiv/topics/surveillance/resources/slides/women/

Centers for Disease Control and Prevention (CDC). (2008a). *HIV and AIDS in the United States: A Picture of Today's Epidemic.* CDC Surveillance Topics. Retrieved June 17, 2009, from http://www.cdc.gov/hiv/topics/surveillance/united_states.htm

Centers for Disease Control and Prevention (CDC). (2008b). *HIV prevalence estimate–United States, 2006.* Retrieved May 29, 2009, from http://www.cdc.gov/mmwr/preview/mmwrhtml/mm5739a2.htm

Centers for Disease Control and Prevention (CDC). (2008c). *HIV/AIDS among persons aged 50 and older.* Retrieved March 19, 2008, from http://www.cdc.gov/flu/professionals/vaccination/vax-summary.htm

Centers for Disease Control and Prevention (CDC). (2008d). HIV and AIDS in the United States: A picture of today's epidemic. Retrieved June 9, 2009, from http://www.cdc.gov

Chamley, C. A., Carson, P., Randall, D., & Sandwell, M. (2005). *Developmental anatomy and physiology of children.* St. Louis, MO: Elsevier.

Champi, C. (2002). Primary immunodeficiency disorders in children: Prompt diagnosis can lead to lifesaving treatment. *Journal of Pediatric Health, 17*, 17–21.

Cloherty, J. R., Eichenwald, E. C., & Stark, A. R. (2008). *Manual of neonatal care.* Philadelphia: Lippincott Williams & Wilkins.

Community Resources Information, Inc. (2009). *Acupuncture Treatment for HIV/AIDS.* Retrieved June 10, 2009, from http://www.massresources.org/pages.cfm?contentID=114&pageID=31&subpages=yes&dynamicID=902

Cooper, M. A., Pommering, T. L., & Koranyi, K. (2003). Primary immunodeficiencies. *American Family Physician, 68*, 2001.

Côté, J. K., & Pepler, C. (2005). Cognitive coping intervention for acutely ill HIV-positive men. *Journal of Clinical Nursing, 14*(3), 321–326.

Covington, L. W. (2005). Update on antiviral agents for HIV and AIDS. *Nursing Clinics of North America, 40*(1), 149–165.

Cox, J. E. (2006). Egg-based vaccines. *Pediatrics in Review, 27*(3), 118–119.

Coyne, P. J., Lyne, M. E., & Watson, A. C. (2002). Symptom management in people with AIDS. *American Journal of Nursing, 102*(9), 48–57.

DeMeyer, E. S., & Buchsel, P. C. (2005). A dendritic cell primer for oncology nurses. *Clinical Journal of Oncology Nursing, 9*(4), 460–464.

DeStefano, F., Bhasin, T. K., Thompson, W. W., Yeargin-Allsopp, M., & Boyle, C. (2004). Age at first measles-mumps-rubella vaccination in children with autism and school-matched control subjects: A population-based study in metropolitan Atlanta. *Pediatrics, 113*(2), 259–266.

DeStefano, F., Gu, D., Kramarz, P., Truman, B. I., Iademarco, M. F., Mullooly, J. P., et al. (2002). Childhood vaccinations and risk of asthma. *Pediatric Infectious Disease Journal, 21*(6), 498–504.

Edelman, C., & Mandle, C. (2006). *Health promotion throughout the lifespan* (6th ed.). Philadelphia: Mosby/Elsevier.

Enriquez, M., & McKinsey, D. (2004). Readiness for HIV treatment: Adherence is vital to managing disease and reducing resistance. *American Journal of Nursing, 104*(10), 81–84.

Filon, F. L., & Radman, G. (2006). Latex allergy: A follow up study of 1,040 healthcare workers. *Occupational and Environmental Medicine, 63*, 121–125.

Flynn, J., & Johnson, T. (2005). *The Johns Hopkins white papers: Arthritis.* Baltimore, MD: Johns Hopkins Medicine.

Freeman, L. (2004). *Mosby's complementary & alternative medicine: A research-based approach* (2nd ed.). Philadelphia: Mosby/Elsevier.

Goldsby, R. A., Kindt, T. J., Osborne, B. A., & Kuby, J. (2003). *Immunology* (5th ed.). New York: W. H. Freeman.

Gomes, E. R , & Demoly, P. (2005). Epdemiology of hypersensitivity drug reactions: Risk factors for hypersensitivity drug reactions)

Gomes, E. R., & Demoly, P. (2005). *Epidemiology of hypersensitivity drug reactions: Risk factors for hypersensitivity drug reactions.* Retrieved June 2, 2009, from http://www.medscape.com/viewarticle/508375_3

Haaz, S. (2008). *Complementary and alternative medicine for patients with rheumatoid arthritis.* Retrieved June 10, 2009, from http://www.hopkins-arthritis.org/patient-corner/disease-management/cam.htmlHah

Higman, M. A., & Vogelsang, G. B. (2004). Chronic graft-versus-host disease. *British Journal of Haematology, 125*, 435–454.

Heiser, C. R., Ernst, J. A., Barrett, J. T., French, N., Schultz, M., & Dube, M. P. (2004). Probiotics, soluble fiber, and L-glutamine (GLN) reduce nelfinavir (NFV) or lopinavir/ritonavir (LPV/r) related diarrhea. *Journal of International Associate Physicians AIDS Care (Chic, Ill), 3*, 121–129.

Hourihane, J. O., Allard, J. M., Wade, A. M., McEwan, A. I., & Strobel, S. (2002). Impact of repeated surgical procedures on the incidence and prevalence of latex allergy: A prospective study of 1263 children. *Journal of Pediatrics, 140*, 479–482.

Hviid, A., Stellfeld, M., Wohlfahrt, J., & Melbye, M. (2004). Childhood vaccination and type 1 diabetes. *New England Journal of Medicine, 350*(14), 1398–1404.

Ilowite, N. T. (2002). Current treatment of juvenile rheumatoid arthritis. *Pediatrics, 109*, 109–115.

Immunization Action Coalition. (2005). *Screening questionnaire for child and teen immunization.* Retrieved July 3, 2006, from http://www.immunize.org

Ingersoll, K. S., & Heckman, C. J. (2005). Patient-clinician relationships and treatment system effects on HIV medication adherence. *AIDS and Behavior, 9*(1), 89–101.

Institute of Medicine Board of Health Promotion and Disease Prevention. (2003). *Immunization safety review: Vaccinations and sudden unexpected death in infancy.* Retrieved September 25, 2003, from http://books.nap.edu/books/0309088860/html/1.html

Joint United Nations Programme on HIV/AIDS. (2000). *Men make a difference.* Press kit: World AIDS Day. HIV/AIDS in Africa. Retrieved from http://www.unaids.org/wac/2000/wad00/files/FS_Africa.htm

Kasper, D. L., Braunwald, E., Fauci, A., Hauser, S., Longo, D., & Jameson, J. L. (2005). *Harrison's principles of internal medicine* (16th ed.). New York: McGraw-Hill.

Kenny, P. E. (2004). The changing face of AIDs. *Nursing, 34*(8), 56–62.

Kimball, J. (2005). *Kimball's biology pages.* Retrieved October 25, 2009, from http://biology-pages.info

King, H. C., Mabry, R. L., Mabry, C. S., Gordon, B. R., & Marple, B. F. (2005). *Allergy in ENT practice: The basic guide* (2nd ed.). New York: Thieme Medical Publisher.

Lachat, S., & Relf. (2006). HIV and pregnancy: Considerations for nursing practice. *MCN: The American Journal of Maternal Child Nursing, 31*, 233–240.

Lehne, R. A. (2004). *Pharmacology for nursing care* (4th ed.). St. Louis, MO: Saunders/Elsevier.

Limpongsanurak S. (2006). Efficacy and safety of caesarean delivery for prevention of mother-to-child transmission of HIV-1: RHL commentary (last revised: 15 December 2006). *The WHO Reproductive Health Library*. Geneva: World Health Organization.

Lupus Foundation of America. (2004). Retrieved December 4, 2004, from http://www.lupus.org/education/types/html

Luxner, K. L. (2003). The complicated prenatal experience. In M. H. Hogan & R. S. Glazebrook, (Eds.), *Material newborn nursing.* Upper Saddle Creek, NJ: Prentice Hall.

Manfredi, R. (2002). HIV disease and advanced age: An increasing therapeutic challenge. *Drugs Aging, 19*(9), 647–669.

Marodi, L. (2006). Innate cellular immune response in newborns. *Clinical Immunology, 118*, 137–144.

Martinez-Picado, J., Negredo, E., Ruiz, L., Shintani, A., Fumaz, C. R., Zala, C., et al. (2003). Alternation of antiretroviral drug regimens for HIV infection: A randomized, controlled trial. *Annals of Internal Medicine, 139*(2), 81–89.

Merck & Co., Inc. (2006). *Gardasil.* Retrieved June 13, 2006, from http://www.fda.gov/cber/label/hpvmer060806LB.pdf

Molad, Y., Borkowski, T.,Monselise, A., Ben-Haroush, A., Sulkes, J., Hod, M., et al. (2005). Maternal and fetal outcome of lupus pregnancy: A prospective study of 29 pregnancies. *Lupus 14*(2), 145–151.

Mosby. (2004). *Mosby's drug consult 2004.* St. Louis, MO: Mosby.

Moss Rehab Resource Net. (2005). *Arthritis fact sheet.* Retrieved from http://www.mossresourcenet.org/arthritis/htm

Mulvihill, K. (2003). Systemic lupus erythematosus: Early identification, co-management are key KP contributions. *Advances for Nurse Practitioners, 11*, 32–36.

Murasko, D. M., & Gardner, E. M. (2003). Immunology of aging. In *Principles of geriatric medicine and gerontology* (5th ed.). New York: McGraw-Hill Professional.

Nash, P., & Smith, J. R. (2008). Common neonatal complications. In K. R. Simpson & P. A. Creehan (Eds.), *AWHONN perinatal nursing* (3rd ed., pp. 612–646). Philadelphia: Lippincott Williams & Wilkins.

National Center for Complementary and Alternative Medicine. (2000). *NIH Clinical Center Study Demonstrates Dangerous Interaction Between St. John's Wort and an HIV Protease Inhibitor.* Retrieved June 17, 2009, from http://nccam.nih.gov

National Center for Complementary and Alternative Medicine. (2008). *Herbs at a glance: Chamomile.* Retrieved June 17, 2009, from http://nccam.nih.gov/health/chamomile/

National Institute of Arthritis and Musculoskeletal and Skin Diseases, National Institutes of Health. (2006). *Health topics: Questions and answers about arthritis and rheumatic diseases.* Retrieved September 1, 2007, from http://www.niams.nih.gov/hi/topics/arthritis/artrheu.htm

National Institute of Occupational Safety and Health. (2005). *Occupational latex allergies.* Retrieved March 15, 2006, from http://www.cdc.gov/niosh/topics/latex

Pagana, K. D., & Pagana, T. J. (2002). *Mosby's manual of diagnostic and laboratory tests* (2nd ed.). St. Louis, MO: Mosby.

Pongmarutani, T., Alpert, P. T., & Miller, S.K. (2006). Pediatric systemic lupus erythematosus: Management issues in primary practice. *Journal of the American Academy of Nurse Practitioners, 18*, 258–267.

Porth, C. (2005). *Pathophysiology: Concepts of altered health states* (6th ed.). Philadelphia: Lippincott Williams & Wilkins.

Public Health Service Task Force. (2007, November 2). *Recommendations for use of antiretroviral drugs in pregnant HIV-infected women for maternal health and interventions to reduce perinatal HIV transmission in the United States.* Retrieved May 19, 2008, from http://aidsinfo.nih.gov/

Pullen, R. L., Cannon, J. D., & Rushing, J. D. (2003). Managing organ-threatening lupus erythematosus. *Medsurg Nursing, 12*, 368–379.

Ramstead, C. (2003). HIV counseling, testing, and referral: Putting revised guidelines to use. *Clinician Reviews, 13*, 58–64.

Rangel, M. C., Gavin, L., Reed, C., Fowler, M. G., & Lee, L. M. (2006). Epidemiology of HIV and AIDS among adolescents and young adults in the United States. *Journal of Adolescent Health, 39*, 156–163.

Read, J. S., & Committee on Pediatrics AIDS. (2007). Diagnosis of HIV-1 infection in children younger than 18 months in the United States. *Pediatrics, 120*(6), e1547–e1562.

Reines, H. D., & Seifert, P. C. (2005). Patient safety: Latex allergy. *Surgical Clinics of North America, 85*, 1329–1340.

Rink, L., & Gabriel, P. (2000). Zinc and the immune system. *Proceedings of the Nutrition Society, 59*(4), 541–552.

Robinson, F. P. (2005). Body composition changes in patients with HIV. *American Journal of Nursing, 105*(13), 69–72.

Sherman, D. (1996). Nurses' willingness to care for AIDS patients and spirituality, social support, and death anxiety. *Image: Journal of Nursing Scholarship, 28*(3), 205–213.

Singh-Grewal, D., Schneider, R., Bayer, N., & Feldman, B. M. (2006). Predictors of disease course and remission in systemic juvenile idiopathic arthritis. *Arthritis & Rheumatism, 54*, 1595–1601.

Smeeth, L., Cook, C., Fombonne, E., et al. (2004). MMR vaccination and pervasive developmental disorders: A case-control study. *Lancet, 364*(9438), 963–969.

Stichweh, D., Arce, E., & Pascual, V. (2004). Update on pediatric systemic lupus erythematosus. *Current Opinion in Rheumatology, 17*, 577–587.

Tak, S. H., & Hong, S. H. (2005). Use of the Internet for health information by older adults with arthritis. *Orthopaedic Nursing, 24*(2), 134–139.

Taylor, B., Miller, E., Lingram R., et al. (2002), Measles, mumps, and rubella vaccination and bowel problems or developmental regression in children with autism: Population study. *British Medical Journal, 324*, 393.

Taylor, S., & Erkek, E. (2004). Latex allergy: Diagnosis and management. *Dermatology Therapeutics, 17*, 289–301.

Tierney, L., McPhee, S., & Papadakis, M. (Eds). (2005). *Current medical diagnosis & treatment* (44th ed.). New York: Lange Medical Books/McGraw-Hill.

U.S. Department of Health and Human Services, Office of Disease Prevention and Promotion. (2000). *Healthy People 2010.* Retrieved July 14, 2009, from http://www.healthypeople.gov

U.S. Food and Drug Administration. (2005). *FDA and CDC issue alert on Menactra meningococcal vaccine and Guillain Barré Syndrome.* Retrieved January 6, 2006, from http://www.fda.gov/bbs/topics/NEWS/2005/NEW1238.htm

Valois, P., Turgeon, H., Godin, G., Blondeau, D., & Cote, F. (2001). Influence of a persuasive strategy on nursing students' beliefs and attitudes toward provisions of care to people living with HIV/AIDS. *Journal of Nursing Education, 40*(8), 354–358.

Venkatesh, M., Merenstein, G. B., Adams, K. M., & Weisman, L.E. (2006). Infection in the neonate. In G.B.Merenstein & S.L. Gardner (Eds.), *Handbook of neonatal intensive care* (6th ed., pp. 569–593). St. Louis, MO: Mosby.

Viale, P. H. (2009). Management of hypersensitivity reactions: A nursing perspective. *Oncology, 23*(21). Retrieved July 14, 2009, from http://www.cancernetwork.com/supplements/2009/infusion-reactions/display/article/10165/1382802

Wroe, A. L., & Thomas, M. G. (2003). Intentional and unintentional nonadherence in patients prescribed HAART treatment regimens. *Psychology Health & Medicine, 8*(4), 453–463.

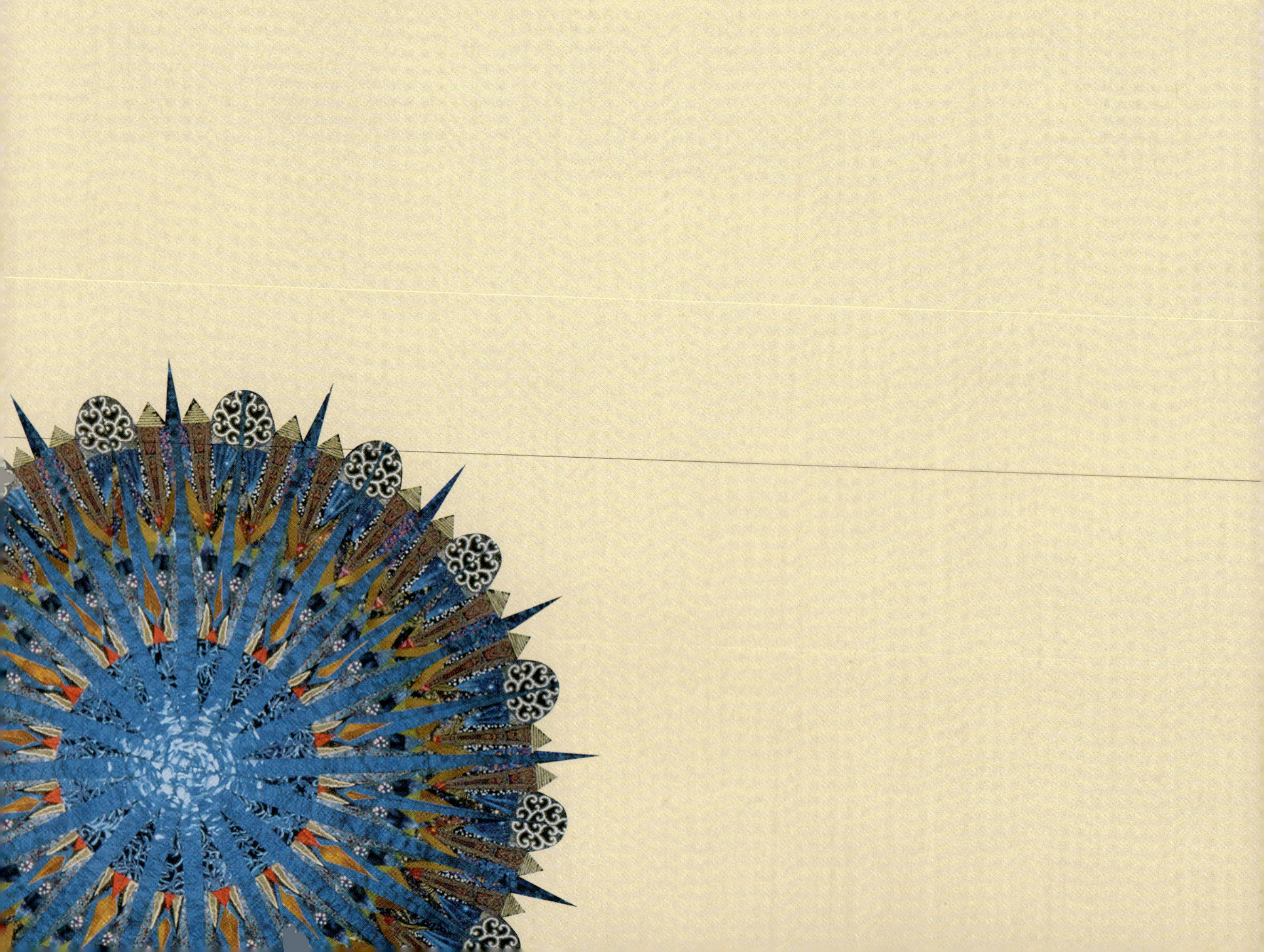

Infection 15

Concept at-a-Glance

Concept Learning Outcomes

After reading about this concept, you will be able to:

1. Summarize the structure and physiologic processes of the immune system related to infection prevention.
2. List factors that increase the risk for infection.
3. Identify commonly occurring alterations in the immune system that increase the risk for or occurrence of infection and their related treatments.
4. Explain common physical assessment procedures used to evaluate for the presence of infection in clients across the life span.
5. Outline diagnostic and laboratory tests and expected findings to determine whether an individual has an infection.
6. Explain the management of immune health and prevention of infection.
7. Demonstrate the nursing process in providing culturally competent care across the life span for individuals with infection.
8. Identify pharmacologic interventions used in caring for individuals with infection.

Concept Key Terms

Acute infections, *771*
Airborne precautions, *779*
Antibody, *777*
Antiseptics, *777*
Asepsis, *771*
Bacteremia, *771*
Bacteria, *771*
Bactericidal agent, *777*
Bacteriostatic agent, *777*
Bloodborne pathogens, *778*
Body substance isolation (BSI), *778*
Carrier, *772*
Chronic infections, *771*
Clean, *771*
Colonization, *771*
Communicable disease, *770*
Compromised host, *773*
Contact precautions, *779*
Cultures, *804*
Dirty, *771*
Disease, *770*
Disease surveillance, *791*
Disinfectants, *777*
Droplet nuclei, *773*
Droplet precautions, *779*
Endogenous, *787*
Endotoxins, *786*
Exogenous, *787*
Exotoxins, *786*
Fungi, *771*
Iatrogenic infections, *787*
Infection, *770*
Infectious disease, *770*
Isolation, *778*
Local infection, *771*
Medical asepsis, *771*
Nosocomial infections, *787*
Occupational exposure, *785*
Opportunistic pathogen, *771*
Parasites, *771*
Pathogenicity, *770*
Pathogens, *770*
Reservoirs, *772*
Sepsis, *771*
Septicemia, *771*
Specific defenses, *773*
Sterile field, *782*
Sterile technique, *771*
Sterilization, *778*
Surgical asepsis, *771*
Systemic infection, *771*
Universal precautions, *778*
Virulence, *770*
Viruses, *771*

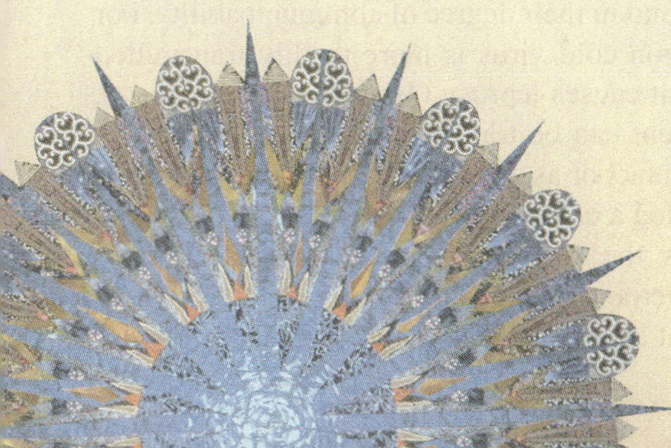

About Infection

Infection is the invasion of body tissue by microorganisms with the potential to cause illness or disease. The human body is continually threatened by foreign substances, infectious agents, and abnormal cells. Recent years have seen the emergence of resistant microorganisms, such as methicillin-resistant *Staphylococcus aureus,* and altered strains of familiar diseases, such as multiple-drug-resistant tuberculosis. New diseases have also emerged, including Lyme disease, *Clostridium difficile,* and HIV. •

The immune system is the body's major defense mechanism against infectious organisms and abnormal or damaged cells. Any illness or injury can result in an infection if it is left untreated or if the body's immune system is compromised in some way. More than any other group of health care providers, nurses think about infection prevention all the time: They know that if they move from client room to client room with contaminated hands or equipment, they risk infecting everyone they touch. It does not matter how effective the other care delivered might be if the nurse is not protecting the client against infection. As a result, nurses are directly involved in providing a biologically safe environment. Infection control is a central tenant to delivering quality nursing care. This concept explains the steps to take to prevent the spread of infection, how infection is shared, and the impact an infection can have on the human body.

Microorganisms exist everywhere: in water, in soil, and on body surfaces such as the skin, intestinal tract, and other areas open to the outside (e.g., mouth, upper respiratory tract, vagina, and lower urinary tract). Most microorganisms are harmless, and some are even beneficial because they perform essential functions in the body. Some microorganisms found in the intestines (e.g., enterobacteria) produce substances called bacteriocins, which are lethal to related strains of bacteria. Others produce substances that repress the growth of other microorganisms. Some microorganisms are normal resident flora (the collective vegetation in a given area) in one part of the body, yet produce infection in another. For example, *Escherichia coli* is a normal inhabitant of the large intestine, but a common cause of infection of the urinary tract. Table 15–1 provides a list of common resident microorganisms by body area.

Recall that an infection is an invasion of body tissue by microorganisms. If the microorganisms produce no clinical evidence of disease, the infection is *asymptomatic* or *subclinical*. **Disease** occurs when the microorganisms produce a detectable alteration in normal tissue function. A **communicable disease** is an illness that is directly transmitted from one person or animal to another by contact with body fluids, or indirectly transmitted by contact with contaminated objects or vectors (e.g., ticks, mosquitoes, other insects). An **infectious disease** is any communicable disease that is caused by microorganisms that are commonly transmitted from one person to another or from an animal to a person. Infectious and communicable diseases are a major cause of disease and death in infants and children in the United States. Some subclinical infections can cause considerable damage. For example, cytomegalovirus (CMV) infection in a pregnant woman can lead to significant disease in the unborn child.

TABLE 15–1 Examples of Common Resident Microorganisms

BODY AREA	RESIDENT MICROORGANISMS
Skin	*Staphylococcus epidermidis*
	Propionibacterium acnes
	Staphylococcus aureus
	Corynebacterium xerosis
	Pityrosporum oxale (yeast)
Nasal passages	*Staphylococcus aureus*
	Staphylococcus epidermidis
Oropharynx	*Streptococcus pneumoniae*
Mouth	*Streptococcus mutans*
	Lactobacillus
	Bacteroides
	Actinomyces
Intestine	*Bacteroides*
	Fusobacterium
	Eubacterium
	Lactobacillus
	Streptococcus
	Enterobacteriaceae
	Shigella
	Escherichia coli
Urethral orifice	*Staphylococcus epidermidis*
Urethra (lower)	*Proteus*
Vagina	*Lactobacillus*
	Bacteroides
	Clostridium
	Candida albicans

NORMAL PRESENTATION

Microorganisms vary in **virulence** (i.e., their ability to produce disease). Microorganisms also vary in the severity of the diseases they produce and in their degree of communicability. For example, the common cold virus is more readily transmitted than the bacillus that causes leprosy (*Mycobacterium leprae*). If the infectious agent can be transmitted to an individual by direct or indirect contact or as an airborne infection, the resulting condition is called a communicable disease.

Pathogenicity is the ability to produce disease; thus a **pathogen** is a microorganism that causes disease. Many microorganisms that are normally harmless can cause disease under certain circumstances. A "true" pathogen causes disease or infection in a healthy individual, whereas an **opportunistic pathogen** causes disease only in susceptible individuals.

Infectious diseases are a major cause of death worldwide. The spread of microorganisms is controlled and people are protected from communicable diseases and infections on the international, national, state, community, and individual levels. The World Health Organization (WHO) is the major regulatory agency at the international level. In the United States, the Centers for Disease Control and Prevention (CDC) is the principal public health agency concerned with disease prevention and control at the national level. State and county or city health departments track epidemics and illnesses as reports are made throughout those areas.

Asepsis is the absence of disease-causing microorganisms. Aseptic technique is used to decrease the possibility of transferring microorganisms from one place to another. There are two basic types of asepsis: medical and surgical. **Medical asepsis** includes all practices intended to confine a specific microorganism to a specific area, thus limiting the number, growth, and transmission of microorganisms. In medical asepsis, objects are referred to as **clean**, which means that almost all microorganisms are absent, or **dirty** (soiled, contaminated), which means that microorganisms are likely to be present, some of which may be capable of causing infection.

Surgical asepsis, or **sterile technique**, refers to those practices that keep an area or object free of all microorganisms; it includes practices that destroy all microorganisms and spores (microscopic dormant structures formed by some pathogens that are very hardy and often survive common cleaning techniques). Surgical asepsis is used for all procedures involving sterile areas of the body. **Sepsis** refers to the whole body inflammatory process, resulting in acute illness; however, the term is often used generally to refer to the state of infection.

Types of Microorganisms Causing Infections

Four major categories of microorganisms cause infection in humans: bacteria, viruses, fungi, and parasites. **Bacteria** are by far the most common infection-causing microorganisms. Several hundred species can cause disease in humans and can live and be transported through air, water, food, soil, body tissues and fluids, and inanimate objects. Most of the microorganisms listed in Table 15–1 are bacteria. **Viruses** consist primarily of nucleic acid and therefore must enter living cells in order to reproduce. Common virus families include the rhinovirus (causes the common cold), hepatitis, herpes, and HIV. **Fungi** include yeasts and molds. *Candida albicans* is a yeast considered to be normal flora in the human vagina. **Parasites** live on other organisms. They include protozoa, such as the one that causes malaria, helminths (worms), and arthropods (mites, fleas, ticks).

Types of Infections

Colonization is the process by which strains of microorganisms become resident flora. In this state, the microorganisms may grow and multiply, but they do not cause disease. Infection occurs when newly introduced or resident microorganisms succeed in invading a part of the body where the host's defense mechanisms are ineffective, and the pathogen causes tissue damage. The infection becomes a disease when the signs and symptoms of the infection are unique, can be differentiated from other conditions, and alter bodily function or processes.

Infections can be local or systemic. A **local infection** is limited to the specific part of the body where the microorganisms remain. If the microorganisms spread and damage different parts of the body, it is a **systemic infection**. When a culture of the person's blood reveals microorganisms, the condition is called **bacteremia**. When bacteremia results in systemic infection, it is referred to as **septicemia**. Unfortunately, these infections have become more common in recent times.

Infections are also classified as acute or chronic. **Acute infections** generally appear suddenly and last a short time. A **chronic infection** may develop slowly, over a very long period, and often persist for months and sometimes years.

It is important to note that a person does not need to have an identified infection in order to transmit potentially infective microorganisms to another person. Even microorganisms that are normal for one person can infect another person.

Chain of Infection

The chain of infection consists of six links (Figure 15–1 ■): the etiologic agent, or microorganism; the place where the organism naturally resides (reservoir); a portal of exit from the

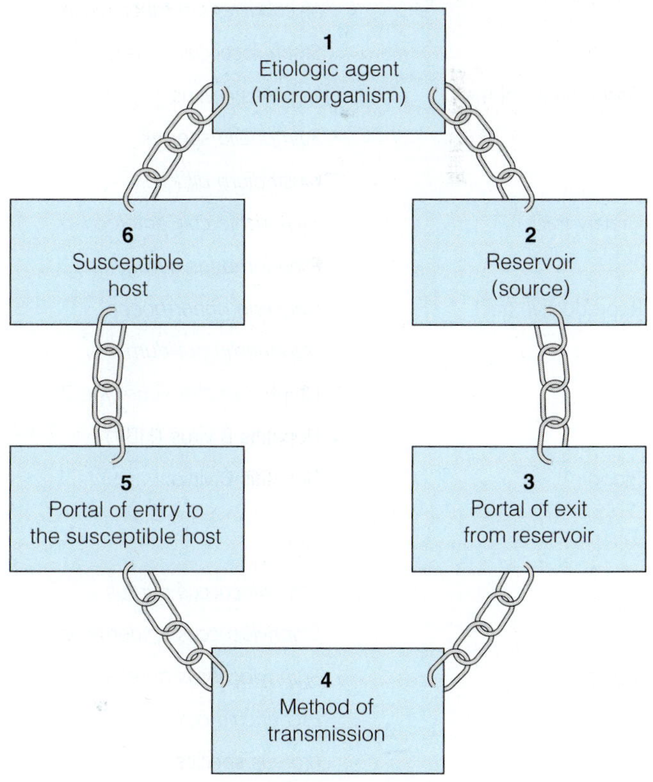

Figure 15–1 ■ The chain of infection.

reservoir; a method (mode) of transmission; a portal of entry into a susceptible host; and a susceptible host.

ETIOLOGIC AGENT The extent to which any microorganism is capable of producing an infectious process depends on the number of microorganisms present, the virulence and potency of the microorganisms (pathogenicity), the ability of the microorganisms to enter the body, the susceptibility of the host, and the ability of the microorganisms to live in the host's body.

Some microorganisms, such as the smallpox virus, have the ability to infect almost all susceptible people after exposure. By contrast, microorganisms such as the tuberculosis bacillus infect a relatively small number of the population who are susceptible and exposed. Those at risk are usually people who are poorly nourished or living in crowded conditions, or those whose immune systems are less competent (such as older adults and individuals with HIV or cancer).

RESERVOIR There are many **reservoirs**, or sources of microorganisms. Common sources are other humans, the client's own microorganisms, plants, animals, and the general environment. People are the most common source of infection for others and for themselves. For example, a person with an influenza virus frequently spreads it to others. A **carrier** is a human or animal reservoir of a specific infectious agent that usually does not manifest any clinical signs of disease. For example, the *Anopheles* mosquito reservoir carries the malaria parasite but is unaffected by it. The carrier state may also exist in individuals with a clinically recognizable disease, such as a dog with rabies. Under either circumstance, the carrier state may be of short duration (temporary or transient carrier) or long duration (chronic carrier). Food, water, and feces also can be reservoirs.

PORTAL OF EXIT FROM RESERVOIR Before an infection can establish itself in a host, the microorganisms must leave the reservoir. Common human reservoirs and their associated portals of exit are summarized in Table 15–2.

METHOD OF TRANSMISSION After a microorganism leaves its source or reservoir, it requires a means of transmission to reach another person or host through a receptive portal of entry. There are three modes of transmission:

1. *Direct transmission.* Direct transmission involves the immediate and direct transfer of microorganisms from person to person through touching, biting, kissing, or sexual intercourse. Droplet spread is also a form of direct

TABLE 15–2 **Human Body Area Reservoirs, Common Infectious Microorganisms, and Portals of Exit**

BODY AREA RESERVOIR	COMMON INFECTIOUS MICROORGANISMS	PORTALS OF EXIT
Respiratory tract	Parainfluenza virus	Nose or mouth through sneezing, coughing, breathing, or talking
	Mycobacterium tuberculosis	
	Staphylococcus aureus	
Gastrointestinal tract	Hepatitis A virus	Mouth: saliva, vomitus; anus: feces; ostomies
	Salmonella species	
	Clostridium difficile	Anus: feces, colostomies
Urinary tract	*Escherichia coli, enterococci*	Urethral meatus and urinary diversion
	Pseudomonas aeruginosa	
Reproductive tract	*Neisseria gonorrhoeae*	Vagina: vaginal discharge; urinary meatus: semen, urine
	Treponema pallidum	
	Herpes simplex virus type 2	
	Hepatitis B virus (HBV)	
Blood	Hepatitis B virus	Open wound, needle puncture site, any disruption of intact skin or mucous membrane surfaces
	HIV	
	Staphylococcus aureus	
	Staphylococcus epidermidis	
Tissue	*Staphylococcus aureus*	Drainage from cut or wound
	Escherichia coli	
	Proteus species	
	Streptococcus beta-hemolytic A or B	

transmission, but it can occur only if the source and the host are within 3 feet of each other. Sneezing, coughing, spitting, singing, or talking can project droplet spray into the conjunctiva or onto the mucous membranes of the eye, nose, or mouth of another person.

2. *Indirect transmission.* Indirect transmission can be either vehicle-borne or vector-borne.
   a. *Vehicle-borne transmission.* A *vehicle* is any substance that serves as an intermediate means to transport and introduce an infectious agent into a susceptible host through a suitable portal of entry. Fomites (inanimate materials or objects), such as handkerchiefs, toys, soiled clothes, cooking or eating utensils, and surgical instruments or dressings, can act as vehicles. Water, food, blood, serum, and plasma are also vehicles. For example, food can become contaminated by a food handler who carries the hepatitis A virus, and the food is then ingested by a susceptible host.
   b. *Vector-borne transmission.* A *vector* is an animal or flying or crawling insect that serves as an intermediate means of transporting the infectious agent. Transmission can occur by injecting salivary fluid during biting or by depositing feces or other materials on the skin through the bite wound or a traumatized skin area.
3. *Airborne transmission.* Airborne transmission can involve droplets or dust. **Droplet nuclei**, the residue of evaporated droplets emitted by an infected host, such as an individual with tuberculosis, can remain in the air for long periods of time. Dust particles containing the infectious agent (e.g., *Clostridium difficile,* commonly referred to as *C. difficile,* spores from the soil) can also become airborne. The material is transmitted by air currents to a suitable portal of entry on another person, usually the respiratory tract.

PORTAL OF ENTRY TO THE SUSCEPTIBLE HOST Before a person can become infected, microorganisms must enter the body. The skin is a barrier to infectious agents; however, any break in the skin can readily serve as a portal of entry. Often, microorganisms enter the body of a host by the same route they used to leave the source. For example, an airborne infection escapes its host or carrier via sneezing or coughing and is transmitted to a new host who inhales the microorganism through his or her nose or mouth. The mouth, throat, nose, ears, eyes, and genitalia are open to outside exposure, and thus are the most frequent portals of entry for microorganisms. Cuts and tears in the skin also provide portals through which microorganisms can enter and cause disease.

SUSCEPTIBLE HOST A susceptible host is any person who is at risk for infection. Infants and young children are often susceptible hosts. Their immune systems have not fully matured, and they have not yet developed antibodies to many agents. Therefore, they cannot defend themselves against infectious and communicable diseases as well as older children and adults. A **compromised host** is a person at increased risk, that is, an individual who for one or more reasons is more likely than others to acquire an infection. Impairment of the body's natural defenses and a number of other factors can also affect susceptibility to infection. Examples include age (the very young or the very old); individuals who receive immune suppression treatment for cancer or chronic illness, or following a successful organ transplant; and immune deficiency conditions.

Table 15–3 outlines nursing interventions that break the chain of infection, including their rationales.

Body Defenses Against Infection

Individuals normally have defenses that protect the body from infection. Nonspecific defenses include anatomic and physiological barriers and the inflammatory response. **Specific defenses** involve the immune system when an antigen induces a state of sensitivity and antibodies respond to contain or destroy the antigen.

Intact skin and mucous membranes are the body's first line of defense against microorganisms. Unless the skin and mucosa become cracked and broken, they act as an effective barrier against bacteria. Fungi can live on the skin, but they cannot penetrate it. The dryness of the skin also is a deterrent to bacteria. Bacteria are most plentiful in moist areas of the body, such as the perineum and axillae. Resident bacteria of the skin also prevent other bacteria from multiplying. They use up the available nourishment, and the end products of their metabolism inhibit other bacterial growth. Normal secretions make the skin slightly acidic, which also inhibits bacterial growth.

The nasal passages have a defensive function. As entering air follows the tortuous route of the passage, it comes in contact with moist mucous membranes and cilia. These structures trap microorganisms, dust, and foreign materials. The lungs have alveolar macrophages (large phagocytes). Phagocytes are cells that ingest microorganisms, other cells, and foreign particles.

Each body orifice also has protective mechanisms. The oral cavity regularly sheds mucosal epithelium to rid the mouth of colonizers. The flow of saliva and its partially buffering action help prevent infections. Saliva contains microbial inhibitors, such as lactoferrin, lysozyme, and secretory immunoglobulin A (IgA).

The eye is protected from infection by tears, which continually wash microorganisms away and contain inhibiting lysozyme. The gastrointestinal tract also has defenses against infection. The high acidity of the stomach normally prevents microbial growth. The resident flora of the large intestine help prevent the establishment of disease-producing microorganisms. Peristalsis also tends to move microbes out of the body.

The vagina also has natural defenses against infection. When a girl reaches puberty, lactobacilli ferment sugars in the vaginal secretions, creating a vaginal pH of 3.5–4.5. This low pH inhibits the growth of many disease-producing microorganisms. The entrance to the urethra normally harbors many microorganisms, including *Staphylococcus epidermidis coagulase* (from the skin) and *Escherichia coli* (from feces). It is believed that the urine flow has a flushing and bacteriostatic action that keeps the bacteria from ascending the urethra. An intact mucosal surface also acts as a barrier.

TABLE 15–3 **Nursing Interventions That Break the Chain of Infection**

LINK IN CHAIN OF INFECTION	INTERVENTIONS	RATIONALES
Etiologic agent (microorganism)	Ensure that articles are correctly cleaned and disinfected or sterilized before use.	Correct cleaning, disinfecting, and sterilizing reduce or eliminate microorganisms.
	Educate clients and support persons about appropriate methods to clean, disinfect, and sterilize articles.	Knowledge of ways to reduce or eliminate microorganisms reduces the numbers of microorganisms present and the likelihood of transmission.
Reservoir (source)	Change dressings and bandages when they are soiled or wet.	Moist dressings are ideal environments for microorganisms to grow and multiply.
	Assist clients to carry out appropriate skin and oral hygiene.	Hygienic measures reduce the numbers of resident and transient microorganisms and the likelihood of infection.
	Dispose of damp, soiled linens appropriately.	Damp, soiled linens harbor more microorganisms than dry linens.
	Dispose of feces and urine in appropriate receptacles.	Urine and feces in particular contain many microorganisms.
	Ensure that all fluid containers, such as bedside water jugs and suction and drainage bottles, are covered or capped.	Prolonged exposure increases the risk of contamination and promotes microbial growth.
	Empty suction and drainage bottles at the end of each shift, before they become full, or according to agency policy.	Drainage harbors microorganisms that, if left for long periods, proliferate and can be transmitted to others.
Portal of exit from the reservoir	Avoid talking, coughing, or sneezing over open wounds and sterile fields, and cover the mouth and nose when coughing and sneezing.	These measures limit the number of microorganisms that escape from the respiratory tract.
Method of transmission	Cleanse hands between client contacts, after touching body substances, and before performing invasive procedures or touching open wounds.	Hand cleansing is an important means of controlling and preventing the transmission of microorganisms.
	Instruct clients and support persons to cleanse hands before handling food or eating, after eliminating, and after touching infectious material.	Hand cleansing helps prevent the transfer of microorganisms from one person to another.
	Wear gloves when handling secretions and excretions.	Gloves and gowns prevent soiling of the hands and clothing.
	Wear gowns if there is danger of soiling clothing with body substances.	
	Place discarded soiled materials in moisture-proof refuse bags.	Moisture-proof bags prevent the spread of microorganisms to others.
	Hold used bedpans steadily to prevent spillage, and dispose of urine and feces in appropriate receptacles.	Feces in particular contain many microorganisms.
	Initiate and implement aseptic precautions for all clients.	All clients can harbor potentially infectious microorganisms that can be transmitted to others.
	Wear masks and eye protection when in close contact with clients who have infections transmitted by droplets from the respiratory tract.	Masks and eyewear reduce the spread of droplet-transmitted microorganisms.
	Wear masks and eye protection when sprays of body fluid are possible (e.g., during irrigation procedures).	Masks and eye protection provide protection from microorganisms in clients' body substances.
Portal of entry to the susceptible host	Use sterile technique for invasive procedures (e.g., injections, catheterizations).	Invasive procedures penetrate the body's natural protective barriers to microorganisms.

TABLE 15–3 **Nursing Interventions That Break the Chain of Infection (continued)**

LINK IN CHAIN OF INFECTION	INTERVENTIONS	RATIONALES
	Use sterile technique when exposing open wounds and handling dressings.	Open wounds are vulnerable to microbial infection.
	Place used disposable needles and syringes in puncture-resistant containers for disposal.	Injuries from needles contaminated by blood or body fluids from an infected client or carrier are a primary cause of HBV and HIV transmission to health care workers.
	Provide all clients with their own personal care items.	People have less resistance to another person's microorganisms than to their own.
Susceptible host	Maintain the integrity of the client's skin and mucous membranes.	Intact skin and mucous membranes protect against invasion by microorganisms.
	Ensure that the client receives a balanced diet.	A balanced diet supplies proteins and vitamins necessary to build and maintain body tissues.
	Educate the public about the importance of immunizations.	Immunizations protect people against virulent infectious diseases.

Factors Increasing Susceptibility to Infection

Whether or not a microorganism causes an infection depends on a number of factors that have been identified above. One of the most important factors is host susceptibility, which is affected by age, heredity, level of stress, nutritional status, current medical therapy, and preexisting disease processes.

Age influences the risk of infection. Newborns and older adults have reduced defenses against infection. Infections are a major cause of death in newborns, who have immature immune systems and are protected only for the first 2 or 3 months by immunoglobulins passively received from the mother. Between 1 and 3 months of age, infants begin to synthesize their own immunoglobulins. Immunizations against diphtheria, tetanus, and pertussis are usually started at 2 months, when the infant's immune system can respond (see Table 15–3).

With advancing age, the immune responses again become weak. Although there is still much to learn about aging, it is known that immunity to infection decreases with advancing age. Because of the prevalence of influenza and its potential for causing death, the CDC recommends annual immunization against influenza for older adults and persons with chronic cardiac, respiratory, metabolic, and renal disease. Pneumococcal vaccine is recommended for older adults who were last vaccinated more than 5 years previously.

Special considerations related to infection in children and older adults are further described in the following Developmental Considerations feature.

Heredity also influences the development of infection in that some people have a genetic susceptibility to certain infections. For example, some individuals are deficient in serum immunoglobulins, which play a significant role in the internal defense mechanism of the body.

The nature, number, and duration of physical and emotional stressors can influence susceptibility to infection. Stressors elevate blood cortisone, and the prolonged elevation of blood cortisone decreases anti-inflammatory responses, depletes energy stores, leads to a state of exhaustion, and decreases resistance to infection. For example, a person recovering from a major operation or injury is more likely to develop an infection than a healthy person.

Resistance to infection also depends on adequate nutritional status. Because antibodies are proteins, inadequate nutrition can impair the body's ability to synthesize them, especially when protein reserves are depleted (e.g., as a result of injury, surgery, or debilitating diseases such as cancer).

Some medical therapies may predispose a person to infection. For example, radiation treatments for cancer destroy not only cancerous cells but also some normal cells, thereby rendering the client more vulnerable to infection. Some diagnostic procedures may also predispose the client to infection, especially when the skin is broken or sterile body cavities are penetrated during the procedure.

Certain medications also increase susceptibility to infection. Antineoplastic (anticancer) medications can depress bone marrow function, resulting in the inadequate production of white blood cells necessary to combat infections. Anti-inflammatory medications such as adrenal corticosteroids inhibit the inflammatory response, which is an essential defense against infection. Even some antibiotics used to treat infections can have adverse effects. Antibiotics can kill resident flora, allowing for the proliferation of strains that would not grow and multiply in the body under normal conditions. An important example of this is *C. difficile*–associated disease, an infection of the colon that is almost always caused initially by treatment with an antibiotic for another infection (Sunenshine & McDonald, 2006).

Any disease that lowers the body's defenses against infection places the client at risk. Examples are chronic pulmonary disease, which impairs ciliary action and weakens the mucous barrier; peripheral vascular disease, which restricts blood flow; burns, which impair skin integrity; chronic or debilitating

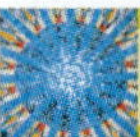

DEVELOPMENTAL CONSIDERATIONS **Infections**

CHILDREN

Infections are a normal part of childhood, with most children experiencing some kind of infection from time to time. The majority of these infections is caused by viruses, and for the most part they are transient, relatively benign, and can be overcome by the body's natural defenses and supportive care. Otitis media, or ear infection, is one of the most frequent reasons parents take children to the doctor. It is an excellent example of a typically transient infection that can be overcome by the body's defenses and supportive care. In some cases, however, severe and even life-threatening infections occur. Considerations related to children include the following:

- Newborns may not be able to respond to infections due to an underdeveloped immune system. As a result, in the first few months of life, infections may not be associated with typical signs and symptoms (e.g., an infant with an infection may not have a fever).
- Newborns have some naturally acquired immunity that is transferred from the mother across the placenta at birth.
- Breast-fed infants enjoy higher levels of immunity against infections than infants fed with formula.
- Fevers of less than 39°C (102.2°F) in children should not be treated, except for comfort of the child.
- Children between 6 months and 5 years of age are at higher risk for fever-induced (febrile) seizures. Febrile seizures are not associated with neurological seizure disorders (e.g., epilepsy).
- Children who are immune compromised (e.g., leukemia, HIV) or have a chronic health condition (e.g., cystic fibrosis, sickle cell disease, congenital heart disease) need additional precautions to prevent exposure to infectious agents.
- Hand hygiene, comprehensive immunizations, proper nutrition, adequate hydration, and appropriate rest are essential to preventing and/or treating infections in children.
- Handwashing and good hygiene in day care and schools are important to prevent the spread of infections.
- Adolescents are at high risk for sexually transmitted diseases and should be well educated about how to prevent infections.

OLDER ADULTS

Normal aging may predispose older adults to increased risk of infection and delayed healing. As the body ages, changes take place in the skin, respiratory tract, gastrointestinal system, kidneys, and immune system. If unchallenged, these systems work well to maintain homeostasis for the individual, but if compromised by stress, illness, infections, treatments, or surgeries, these defense systems cannot provide adequate protection. Special considerations for older adults include the following:

- Nutrition is often poor in older adults. Certain nutritional components, especially adequate protein, are necessary to build up and maintain the immune system.
- Diabetes mellitus, which occurs more frequently in older adults, increases the risk of infection and delayed healing by causing an alteration in nutrition and impaired peripheral circulation, which in turn decrease the oxygen transport to the tissues.
- The immune system reacts slowly to the introduction of an antigen, allowing the antigen to reproduce itself several times before the immune system recognizes it.
- The normal inflammatory response is delayed, which often causes atypical responses to infections with unusual presentations. Instead of exhibiting the redness, swelling, and fever that are usually associated with infections, atypical symptoms, such as confusion and disorientation, agitation, incontinence, falls, lethargy, and general fatigue, are often seen first in the older adult.

Recognizing these changes in older adults is important for the early detection and treatment of infections and delayed healing. Nursing interventions to promote prevention include the following:

- Provide and teach ways to improve nutritional status.
- Use strict aseptic technique to decrease the risk of infections (especially nosocomial infections in health care facilities).
- Encourage older adults to have regular immunizations for flu and pneumonia.
- Be alert to subtle, atypical signs of infection and act quickly to diagnose and treat them.

diseases, which deplete protein reserves; and immune system diseases such as leukemia and aplastic anemia, which alter the production of white blood cells. Diabetes mellitus is a major underlying disease that predisposes clients to infection because compromised peripheral vascular status and increased serum glucose levels increase susceptibility.

Infectious Process in Older Adults

Older adults, particularly individuals over the age of 75 years, are at greater risk of acquiring an infection than younger people. Although the incidence of septicemia in the United States is increasing in all age groups, the greatest increase is among people over the age of 65 years (Baine, Yu, & Summe, 2001). Physiologic changes of aging that put older adults at increased risk for infection include the following:

- Cardiovascular changes: Decreased cardiac output, loss of capillaries, and decreased tissue perfusion, delaying inflammatory response and healing
- Respiratory system changes: Decreased mucociliary escalator, decreased elastic recoil, and a diminished cough reflex, leading to decreased clearance of respiratory secretions
- Genitourinary changes: Loss of muscle tone, reduced bladder contractility, altered bladder reflexes, and prostatic hypertrophy in men, leading to reduced bladder capacity and incomplete emptying
- Gastrointestinal system changes: Impaired swallow reflex, decreased gastric acidity, and delayed gastric emptying, increasing the risk of aspiration
- Skin and subcutaneous tissue changes: Thinning of skin, decreased cushioning, and decreased sensation, leading to increased risk of injury and ulceration
- Immune changes: Decreased phagocytosis, reduced inflammatory response, slowed or impaired healing processes, leading to reduced immunity

In addition to these physiologic changes, the following are other factors that can contribute to an older adult's increased risk for infectious disease:

- Decreased activity level related to musculoskeletal, neurologic, or balance problems
- Poor nutrition and an increased risk of dehydration

- Chronic diseases, such as diabetes mellitus, cardiac disease, and renal disease
- Chronic medication use
- Lack of recent immunizations against preventable infectious diseases
- Altered mentation and dementias
- Hospitalization or residence in a long-term care facility
- Presence of invasive devices, such as indwelling urinary catheters and gastric tubes.

The thymus gland also atrophies, and by age 50–60 years, thymic hormone levels are undetectable. Although the exact relationship of these events to T-cell function is unclear, some T-cell populations decrease or decline in function as the person ages. The ability of T cells to proliferate following activation also declines with advancing age, and a portion of T cells cannot be activated in older adults (Porth, 2005). With these changes, cell-mediated immune function declines, and the client has reduced resistance to antigens, such as *M. tuberculosis,* influenza and varicella-zoster viruses, malignant cells, and tissue grafts.

Although immunoglobulin levels remain relatively stable, primary and secondary **antibody** responses decline with aging. This diminished antibody production has clinical implications in that immunizations (single-dose and booster) may not produce the expected protective immune response.

Older adults are not only at increased risk for infection, but also may not exhibit the classic manifestations of inflammation and infection. They are likely to take nonsteroidal anti-inflammatory drugs (NSAIDs) and corticosteroids, which interfere with inflammation and healing. The cardinal signs of inflammation—redness, heat, and swelling—tend to be diminished or absent in older adults. The classic signs of infection—fever and chills—may be absent altogether because of age-related changes in the immune system, loss of central temperature control mechanisms, decreased muscle mass, and loss of shivering ability. The older adult may have only subtle signs of sepsis, such as changes in mental status, disorientation, and tachypnea (Porth, 2005).

Supporting the Defenses of a Susceptible Host

People are constantly in contact with microorganisms in the environment. Normally a person's natural defenses ward off the development of an infection. Susceptibility is the degree to which an individual can be affected, that is, the likelihood of an organism causing an infection in that person. The following measures can reduce a person's susceptibility to infection:

- *Hygiene.* Intact skin and mucous membranes are one barrier against microorganisms entering the body. In addition, good oral care, including flossing the teeth, reduces the likelihood of an oral infection. Regular and thorough bathing and shampooing remove microorganisms and dirt that can result in an infection.
- *Nutrition.* A balanced diet enhances the health of all body tissues, helps keep the skin intact, and promotes the skin's ability to repel microorganisms. Adequate nutrition enables tissues to maintain and rebuild themselves and helps keep the immune system functioning well.
- *Fluid.* Fluid intake permits fluid output, which flushes out the bladder and urethra, removing microorganisms that could cause an infection.
- *Sleep.* Adequate sleep is essential to maintaining health and renewing energy.
- *Stress.* Excessive stress predisposes people to infections. Nurses can assist clients to learn stress-reducing techniques.
- *Immunizations.* The use of immunizations has dramatically decreased the incidence of infectious diseases. It is recommended that immunizations begin shortly after birth and be completed in early childhood (except for boosters). Immunizations may be given by injection, inhalation, oral solutions, or nasal sprays. They are frequently given in combination to minimize multiple injections. Because immunization schedules change frequently, it is advisable to update immunization schedules yearly.

PRECAUTIONS AND PRACTICES TO PREVENT AND MINIMIZE INFECTION

Disinfecting and Sterilizing

The first two links in the chain of infection, the etiologic agent and reservoir, are interrupted by the use of **antiseptics** (agents that inhibit the growth of some microorganisms) and **disinfectants** (agents that destroy pathogens other than spores), and by sterilization.

DISINFECTING A disinfectant is a chemical preparation, such as phenol or iodine compounds, used on inanimate objects. Disinfectants are frequently caustic and toxic to tissues. An antiseptic is a chemical preparation used on skin or tissue. Disinfectants and antiseptics often have similar chemical components, but disinfectants are more concentrated.

Both antiseptics and disinfectants have bactericidal or bacteriostatic properties. A **bactericidal agent** destroys bacteria, whereas a **bacteriostatic agent** prevents the growth and reproduction of some bacteria. An agent that is known to be effective against the specific bacteria should be selected. For example, spore-forming bacteria such as *C. difficile*, which is a frequent cause of nosocomial diarrhea, and *Bacillus anthracis* (anthrax) may be inhibited by only a few of the agents normally effective against other forms of bacteria. Table 15–4 lists commonly used antiseptics and disinfectants.

When disinfecting articles, nurses need to follow agency protocol and consider the following factors:

1. The type and number of infectious organisms. Some microorganisms are readily destroyed, whereas others require longer contact with the disinfectant.
2. The recommended concentration of the disinfectant and duration of contact.
3. The presence of soap. Some disinfectants are ineffective in the presence of soap or detergents.
4. The presence of organic materials. The presence of saliva, blood, pus, or excretions can readily inactivate many disinfectants.
5. The surface areas to be treated. The disinfecting agent must come into contact with all surfaces and areas.

TABLE 15–4 **Commonly Used Antiseptics and Disinfectants, Effectiveness, and Use**

	EFFECTIVE AGAINST					
AGENT	BACTERIA	TUBERCULOSIS	SPORES	FUNGI	VIRUSES	USE ON
Isopropyl and ethyl alcohol	X	X		X	X	Hands, vial stoppers
Chlorine (bleach)	X	X	X	X	X	Blood spills
Hydrogen peroxide	X	X	X	X	X	Surfaces
Iodophors	X	X	X	X	X	Equipment, intact skin and tissues if diluted
Phenol	X	X		X	X	Surfaces
Chlorhexidine gluconate (Hibiclens)	X				X	Hands
Triclosan (Bacti-Stat)	X					Hands, intact skin

STERILIZING **Sterilization** is a process that destroys all microorganisms, including spores and viruses. Four commonly used methods of sterilization are moist heat, gas, boiling water, and radiation.

- *Moist Heat.* To sterilize with moist heat (such as with an autoclave), steam under pressure is used to attain temperatures higher than the boiling point.
- *Gas.* Ethylene oxide gas destroys microorganisms by interfering with their metabolic processes. It is also effective against spores. Its advantages are good penetration and effectiveness for heat-sensitive items. Its major disadvantage is its toxicity to humans.
- *Boiling Water.* This is the most practical and inexpensive method for sterilizing in the home. The main disadvantage is that this method does not kill spores and some viruses. Boiling for a minimum of 15 minutes is advised to disinfect articles in the home.
- *Radiation.* Both ionizing (such as alpha, beta, and x-rays) and nonionizing (ultraviolet light) radiation are used for disinfection and sterilization. The main drawback to ultraviolet light is that the rays do not penetrate deeply. Ionizing radiation is used effectively in industry to sterilize foods, drugs, and other items that are sensitive to heat. Its main advantage is that it is effective for items difficult to sterilize, and its chief disadvantage is that the equipment is very expensive.

Isolation Precautions

Isolation refers to measures designed to prevent the spread of infection or potentially infectious microorganisms to health personnel, clients, and visitors. Several sets of guidelines have been used in hospitals and other health care settings.

Category-specific isolation precautions use seven categories: strict isolation, contact isolation, respiratory isolation, tuberculosis isolation, enteric precautions, drainage/secretions precautions, and blood/body fluid precautions.

Disease-specific isolation precautions do exactly that: provide precautions to protect against a specific disease. These precautions delineate use of private rooms with special ventilation, sharing of rooms only with other clients infected with the same organism, and gowning to prevent gross soilage of clothes for specific infectious diseases (Garner & Simmons, 1983).

Universal precautions (UP) are techniques to be used with all clients to decrease the risk of transmitting unidentified pathogens (CDC, 1987; U.S. Department of Health and Human Services [USDHHS], 1988). Universal precautions obstruct the spread of **bloodborne pathogens**, those microorganisms that are carried in blood and body fluids that are capable of infecting other persons with serious and difficult to treat viral infections, namely, hepatitis B virus, hepatitis C virus, and HIV. The CDC does not recommend that universal precautions replace disease-specific or category-specific precautions, but that they be used in conjunction with them.

The **body substance isolation (BSI)** system employs generic infection control precautions for all clients, except those with the few diseases transmitted through the air. The BSI system (Jackson, 1993) is based on three premises:

1. All people have an increased risk for infection from microorganisms entering through mucous membranes and nonintact skin.
2. All people are likely to have potentially infectious microorganisms in all of their moist body sites and substances.
3. An unknown portion of clients and health care workers will always be colonized or infected with potentially infectious microorganisms in their blood and other moist body sites and substances.

The term *body substance* refers to blood, some body fluids, urine, feces, wound drainage, oral secretions, and any other body product or tissue.

In addition to other actions and precautions discussed in this concept, significant emphasis is placed on avoiding injury from sharp instruments, taking measures in cases of exposure to bloodborne pathogens, and communicating information about biohazards to employees. In most cases, federal regulations require that warning labels be affixed to containers of regulated waste and to refrigerators and freezers containing blood or other potentially infectious materials. The labels required are fluorescent orange or orange-red and feature the biohazard legend shown in Figure 15–2 ■.

CDC (HICPAC) ISOLATION PRECAUTIONS (1996) The Hospital Infection Control Practices Advisory Committee (HICPAC) of the CDC presented new guidelines for isolation precautions in hospitals in 1996 (Garner & HICPAC, 1996). These guidelines designate two tiers of precautions:

1. Standard Precautions
2. Transmission-Based Precautions.

Standard Precautions are used in the care of all hospitalized persons regardless of their diagnosis or possible infection status. They apply to blood; all body fluids, secretions, and excretions except sweat (whether or not blood is present or visible); nonintact skin; and mucous membranes. Thus, they combine the major features of UP and BSI. Box 15–1 lists recommended isolation precautions for use in hospitals.

Transmission-Based Precautions are used in addition to standard precautions for clients with known or suspected infections that are spread by contact or by airborne or droplet transmission. The three types of transmission-based precautions may be used alone or in combination, but always *in addition to* standard precautions. They encompass all of the conditions or diseases previously listed in the category-specific or disease-specific classifications developed by the CDC in 1983.

Airborne precautions are used for clients who are known to have or suspected of having serious illnesses transmitted by airborne droplet nuclei smaller than 5 microns. Examples of such illnesses are measles (rubeola), varicella (including disseminated zoster), and tuberculosis. The CDC has prepared special guidelines for preventing the transmission of tuberculosis. The most current information can be found on the CDC Division of Tuberculosis Elimination website.

Droplet precautions are used for clients who are known or suspected to have serious illnesses transmitted by particle droplets larger than 5 microns. Examples of such illnesses are diphtheria (pharyngeal); *Mycoplasma* pneumonia; pertussis; mumps; rubella; streptococcal pharyngitis, pneumonia, and scarlet fever in infants and young children; and pneumonic plague.

Contact precautions are used for clients who are known or suspected to have serious illnesses that are easily transmitted by direct client contact or by contact with items in the client's environment. According to the CDC (Garner & HICPAC, 1996), such illnesses include gastrointestinal, respiratory, skin, or wound infections or colonization with multidrug-resistant bacteria; specific enteric infections, such as *C. difficile,* enterohemorrhagic *Escherichia coli 0157:H7, Shigella,* and hepatitis A, in diapered or incontinent clients; respiratory syncytial virus, parainfluenza virus, and enteroviral infections in infants and young children; and highly contagious skin infections, such as herpes simplex virus, impetigo, pediculosis, and scabies.

Figure 15–2 ■ Biohazard alert.

ISOLATION PRACTICES The initiation of practices to prevent the transmission of microorganisms is generally a nursing responsibility that is based on a comprehensive assessment of the client. This assessment takes into account the status of the client's normal defense mechanisms, the client's ability to implement necessary precautions, and the source and mode of transmission of the infectious agent. The nurse then decides whether to wear gloves, gown, mask, and protective eyewear. *In all client situations, nurses must cleanse their hands before and after providing care.*

In addition to the precautions cited within this concept, nurses implement aseptic precautions when performing many specific therapies that are described in this textbook. The following are examples of aseptic precautions:

- Use strict aseptic technique when performing any invasive procedure (e.g., inserting an intravenous needle or catheter) and when changing surgical dressings.
- Change intravenous tubing and solution containers according to hospital policy (e.g., every 48–72 hours).
- Check all sterile supplies for expiration date and intact packaging.
- Prevent urinary infections by maintaining a closed urinary drainage system with a downhill flow of urine. Keep the drainage bag and spout off the floor.
- Implement measures to prevent impaired skin integrity and accumulation of secretions in the lungs (e.g., encourage the client to move, cough, and breathe deeply at least every 2 hours).

PERSONAL PROTECTIVE EQUIPMENT All health care providers must apply clean or sterile gloves, gowns, masks, and protective eyewear according to the risk of exposure to potentially infective materials.

Gloves Gloves are worn for three reasons:

1. They protect the hands when the nurse is likely to handle any body substances.
2. Gloves reduce the likelihood of nurses transmitting their own endogenous microorganisms to individuals receiving care. Nurses who have open sores or cuts on the hands must wear gloves for protection.
3. Gloves reduce the chance that the nurse's hands will transmit microorganisms or a fomite from one client to another client.

In all situations, gloves are changed between client contacts. Nurses should clean their hands each time they remove gloves for two primary reasons: The gloves may have imperfections or be damaged during wearing, allowing microorganism entry, and the hands may become contaminated during glove removal.

Box 15–1 Recommended Isolation Precautions in Hospitals

STANDARD PRECAUTIONS

- Designed for all clients in hospital
- Apply to (a) blood; (b) all body fluids, excretions, and secretions except sweat; (c) nonintact (broken) skin; and (d) mucous membranes
- Designed to reduce the risk of transmission of microorganisms from recognized and unrecognized sources

1. Perform proper hand hygiene after contact with blood, body fluids, secretions, excretions, and contaminated objects, whether or not gloves are worn.
   a. Perform proper hand hygiene immediately after removing gloves.
   b. Use a nonantimicrobial product for routine hand cleansing.
   c. Use an antimicrobial agent or an antiseptic agent for the control of specific outbreaks of infection.
2. Wear clean gloves when touching blood, body fluids, secretions, excretions, and contaminated items (e.g., soiled gowns).
   a. Clean gloves can be unsterile unless their use is intended to prevent the entrance of microorganisms into the body. (See the following discussion of sterile gloves.)
   b. Remove gloves before touching noncontaminated items and surfaces.
   c. Perform proper hand hygiene immediately after removing gloves.
3. Wear a mask, eye protection, or a face shield if splashes or sprays of blood, body fluids, secretions, or excretions can be expected.
4. Wear a clean, nonsterile gown if client care is likely to result in splashes or sprays of blood, body fluids, secretions, or excretions. The gown is intended to protect clothing.
   a. Remove a soiled gown carefully to avoid the transfer of microorganisms to other individuals (e.g., clients or other health care workers).
   b. Cleanse hands after removing gown.
5. Carefully handle client care equipment that is soiled with blood, body fluids, secretions, or excretions to prevent the transfer of microorganisms to other individuals and the environment.
   a. Ensure reusable equipment is cleaned and reprocessed correctly.
   b. Dispose of single-use equipment correctly.
6. Handle, transport, and process linen that is soiled with blood, body fluids, secretions, or excretions in such a manner to prevent contamination of clothing and the transfer of microorganisms to other individuals and to the environment.
7. Prevent injuries from used scalpels, needles, and other equipment, and place in puncture-resistant containers.

TRANSMISSION-BASED PRECAUTIONS

AIRBORNE PRECAUTIONS

Use standard precautions, as well as the following:

1. Place client in a private room that has negative air pressure, 6–12 air changes per hour, and either discharge of air to the outside or a filtration system for the room air.
2. If a private room is not available, place client with another client who is infected with the same microorganism.
3. Wear a respiratory device (N95 respirator) when entering the room of a client who is known or suspected of having primary tuberculosis.
4. Susceptible people should not enter the room of a client who has rubeola (measles) or varicella (chickenpox). If they must enter, they should wear a respirator.
5. Limit movement of client outside the room to essential purposes. Place a surgical mask on the client during transport.

DROPLET PRECAUTIONS

Use standard precautions, as well as the following:

1. Place client in private room.
2. If a private room is not available, place client with another client who is infected with the same microorganism.
3. Wear a mask if working within 3 feet of the client.
4. Limit movement of client outside the room to essential purposes. Place a surgical mask on the client during transport.

CONTACT PRECAUTIONS

Use standard precautions, as well as the following:

1. Place client in private room.
2. If a private room is not available, place client with another client who is infected with the same microorganism.
3. Wear gloves as described in standard precautions.
   a. Change gloves after contact with infectious material.
   b. Remove gloves before leaving the client's room.
   c. Cleanse hands immediately after removing gloves, using an antimicrobial agent. Note: If the client is infected with *C. difficile*, do *not* use an alcohol-based hand rub, as it may not be effective on these spores. Use soap and water.
   d. After hand cleansing, do not touch possibly contaminated surfaces or items in the room.
4. Wear a gown (see standard precautions) when entering a room if there is a possibility of contact with infected surfaces or items, or if the client is incontinent, has diarrhea, a colostomy, or wound drainage that is not contained by a dressing.
   a. Remove gown in the client's room.
   b. Make sure uniform does not contact possible contaminated surfaces.
5. Limit movement of client outside the room.
6. Dedicate the use of noncritical client care equipment to a single client or to clients with the same infecting microorganisms.

Source: Adapted from Garner, J. S. and the Hospital Infection Control Practices Advisory Committee (HICPAC). (1996). Guidelines for isolation precautions in hospitals. *Infection Control Hospital Epidemiology, 17*, pp. 53–80, and 1996, *American Journal of Infection Control, 24*, pp. 24–52.

Some of the gloves used in infection control are made of latex rubber, as are various other items used in health care (e.g., catheters, blood pressure cuffs, rubber sheets, intravenous tubing, stockings and binders, adhesive bandages, and dental dams). Because of the frequent use of gloves, health care workers and some clients with chronic illnesses have increasingly reported allergic reactions to latex. Latex gloves that are lubricated by powder or cornstarch are particularly allergenic because the latex allergen adheres to the powder, which is aerosolized during glove use and inhaled by the user.

Latex gloves that are labeled "hypoallergenic" still contain measurable latex and should not be used by or on persons with known latex sensitivity. Recent studies show some level of latex allergy in 8–12% of health care personnel (Occupational Safety and Health Administration, 2005). The people at greatest risk for developing latex allergies are those with other allergic conditions and those who have had frequent or long-term exposure to latex. Even though most hospitals have eliminated latex products wherever possible and established a "latex-free environment" goal, clients and health care workers should be assessed for possible allergies to latex.

Gowns Clean or disposable impervious (water-resistant) gowns or plastic aprons are worn during procedures when the nurse's uniform is likely to become soiled. Sterile gowns may be indicated when the nurse changes the dressings of a client with extensive wounds (e.g., burns). *Single-use gown technique* (using a gown only once before it is discarded or laundered) is the usual practice in hospitals. After the gown is worn, the nurse discards it (if it is paper) or places it in a laundry hamper. Before leaving the client's room, the nurse cleanses his or her hands.

PRACTICE ALERT

Wearing a client hospital gown over your uniform does not serve any infection control purpose.

Face Masks Masks are worn to reduce the risk of transmitting organisms by the droplet contact and airborne routes, and by splatters of body substances. The CDC recommends that masks be worn by the following persons:

1. Individuals close to the client if the infection (e.g., measles, mumps, or acute respiratory diseases in children) is transmitted by large-particle aerosols (droplets). Large-particle aerosols are transmitted by close contact and generally travel short distances (about 1 m, or 3 feet).
2. All persons entering the room if the infection (e.g., pulmonary tuberculosis and SARS-CoV) is transmitted by small-particle aerosols (droplet nuclei). Small-particle aerosols remain suspended in the air and thus travel greater distances by air. Special masks that provide a tighter face seal and better filtration may be used for these infections.

Various types of masks differ in their filtration effectiveness and fit. Single-use disposable surgical masks are effective for use while the nurse provides care to most clients, but they should be changed if they become wet or soiled. These masks are discarded in the waste container after use. Disposable particulate respirators of different types may be effective for droplet transmission, splatters, and airborne microorganisms. Some respirators now available are effective in preventing inhalation of tuberculin organisms. The National Institute for Occupational Safety and Health (NIOSH) tests and certifies such respirators. Currently, the category "N" respirator at 95% efficiency (referred to as an N95 respirator) meets tuberculosis and SARS control criteria.

During performance of certain techniques requiring surgical asepsis (sterile technique), masks are worn (a) to prevent droplet contact transmission of exhaled microorganisms to the sterile field or to a client's open wound, and (b) to protect the nurse from splashes of body substances from the client.

Eyewear Protective eyewear (goggles, glasses, or face shields) and masks are indicated in situations in which body substances may splatter the face. If the nurse wears prescription eyeglasses, goggles must still be worn over the glasses to extend around the sides of the glasses.

DISPOSAL OF SOILED EQUIPMENT AND SUPPLIES Many pieces of equipment are supplied for single use only and disposed of afterward. Some items, however, are reusable. Agencies have specific policies and procedures for handling soiled equipment (e.g., disposal, cleaning, disinfecting, and sterilizing), and nurses need to become familiar with these practices in the employing agency. Appropriate handling of soiled equipment and supplies is essential to prevent inadvertent exposure of health care workers to articles contaminated with body substances and contamination of the environment.

Bagging Articles that are contaminated or likely to have been contaminated with infective material such as pus, blood, body fluids, feces, or respiratory secretions need to be enclosed in a sturdy bag impervious to microorganisms before they are removed from the room of any client. Some agencies use labels or bags of a particular color that designates them as infective wastes.

CDC guidelines recommend the following methods:

- A single bag, if it is sturdy and impervious to microorganisms, and if the contaminated articles can be placed in the bag without soiling or contaminating its outside
- Double-bagging if the above conditions are not met.

Follow agency protocol or use the following CDC guidelines to handle and bag soiled items:

- Place garbage and soiled *disposable* equipment, including dressings and tissues, in the plastic bag that lines the waste container. Some agencies separate dry and wet waste material and incinerate dry items, such as paper towels and disposable items. No special precautions are required for disposable equipment that is not contaminated.
- Place *nondisposable* or *reusable* equipment that is visibly soiled in a labeled bag before removing it from the client's room or cubicle, and then send it to a central processing area for decontamination. Some agencies may require that glass bottles or jars and metal items be placed in separate bags from rubber and plastic items. Glass and metal can be sterilized in an autoclave, but rubber and plastic are damaged by this process and must be cleaned by other methods, such as gas sterilization.
- Disassemble special procedure trays into component parts. Some components are disposable, whereas others need to be sent to the laundry or central services for cleaning and decontaminating.
- Bag soiled clothing before sending it home or to the agency laundry.

Linens Soiled linens should be handled as little as possible and with the least agitation possible before placing them in a laundry hamper. This prevents gross microbial contamination of the air and persons handling the linen. The bag is closed before sending it to the laundry in accordance with agency practice.

Laboratory Specimens Laboratory specimens, if placed in a leakproof container with a secure lid and labeled as a biohazard, need no special precautions. Care should be used when collecting specimens to avoid contaminating the outside of the container. Containers that are visibly contaminated on the outside should be placed inside a sealable plastic bag before they are sent to the laboratory to prevent personnel from having hand contact with potentially infective material.

Dishes Dishes require no special precautions. Soiling of dishes can largely be prevented by encouraging clients to cleanse their hands before eating. Some agencies use paper dishes for convenience, which are disposed of in the refuse container.

Blood Pressure Equipment Blood pressure equipment needs no special precautions unless it becomes contaminated with infective material. If it does become contaminated, the agency policy should be followed to decontaminate it. Cleaning procedures vary according to whether it is a wall or portable unit. In some agencies, a disposable cuff is used for clients placed on contact precautions.

Thermometers Nondisposable thermometers are generally disinfected after use. The nurse should check agency practice.

Disposable Needles, Syringes, and Sharps Place needles, syringes, and "sharps" (e.g., lancets, scalpels, and broken glass) into a puncture-resistant container. To avoid puncture wounds, use approved safety or needleless systems and do not detach needles from the syringe or recap before disposal.

PRACTICE ALERT

Federal rules protecting the privacy of personal health information may extend to the client labels placed on disposable supplies such as intravenous fluid containers. Agencies may require that these be returned to the pharmacy so that personal information can be removed before disposal. Check agency policy.

TRANSPORTING CLIENTS WITH INFECTION Avoid transporting clients with infections outside their own rooms unless it is absolutely necessary. If a client must be moved, the nurse follows agency protocol to implement appropriate precautions and measures to prevent soilage of the environment. For example, the nurse ensures that any draining wound is securely covered, or that the client who has an airborne infection wears a surgical mask during transport. In addition, the nurse notifies personnel at the receiving area of any infection risk so that they can maintain necessary precautions.

PSYCHOSOCIAL NEEDS OF ISOLATION CLIENTS Clients requiring isolation precautions can develop several problems as a result of the special precautions taken in their care and their separation from other people. Two of the most common are sensory deprivation and decreased self-esteem related to feelings of inferiority. Sensory deprivation occurs when the environment lacks normal stimuli for the client, such as communication with others. Nurses should therefore be alert to common clinical signs of sensory deprivation, such as boredom, inactivity, slowness of thought, daydreaming, increased sleeping, thought disorganization, anxiety, hallucinations, and panic.

A client's feeling of inferiority can stem from perception of the infection itself or from the required precautions and related isolation. In North America, many people place a high value on cleanliness, and the idea of being "soiled," "contaminated," or "dirty" can make clients feel as if they are at fault and substandard. Although this is obviously not true, infected individuals may feel "not as good" as others and blame themselves. An appropriate nursing diagnosis may be risk for situational low self-esteem.

Nurses need to provide care that prevents or addresses sensory deprivation and feelings of inferiority. Related nursing interventions include the following:

1. Assess the individual's need for stimulation.
2. Initiate measures to help meet the need for stimulation, including regular communication with the client and diversionary activities, such as toys for a child and books, television, or radio for an adult. Provide a variety of foods to stimulate the client's sense of taste, and stimulate the client's visual sense by providing a view or an activity to watch.
3. Explain the infection and the associated procedures to help clients, their families, and caregivers understand and accept the situation.
4. Demonstrate warm, accepting behavior. Avoid conveying to the client any sense of annoyance about the precautions or any feelings of revulsion about the infection.
5. Do not use stricter precautions than are indicated by the diagnosis or the client's condition.

Sterile Technique

An object is sterile only when it is free of all microorganisms. It is well known that sterile technique is practiced in operating rooms and special diagnostic areas. Less well known, perhaps, is that sterile technique is also employed for many procedures in general care areas, such as administering injections, changing wound dressings, performing urinary catheterizations, and administering intravenous therapy. In these situations, all of the principles of surgical asepsis are applied, as in the operating and delivery rooms; however, not all of the sterile techniques that follow are always required. For example, before an operating room procedure, the "scrub" nurse generally puts on a mask and cap, performs a surgical hand scrub, and then dons a sterile gown and gloves. In a general care area, the nurse may only perform hand cleansing and don sterile gloves. The basic principles of surgical asepsis and practices that relate to each principle are outlined in Table 15–5.

STERILE FIELD A **sterile field** is a microorganism-free area. Nurses often establish a sterile field by using the innermost side of a sterile wrapper or by using a sterile drape. When the field is established, sterile supplies and sterile solutions can be placed on it. Sterile forceps are often used to handle and transfer sterile supplies.

So that sterility can be maintained, supplies may be wrapped in a variety of materials. Commercially prepared items are frequently wrapped in plastic, paper, or glass. Liquids are preferably packaged in amounts adequate for one use only. Any leftover liquid is discarded.

TABLE 15–5 **Principles and Practices of Surgical Asepsis**

PRINCIPLES	PRACTICES
All objects used in a sterile field must be sterile.	All articles are sterilized appropriately before use by dry or moist heat, chemicals, or radiation. Always check a package containing a sterile object for intactness, dryness, and expiration date. Sterile articles can be stored only for a prescribed time; after that, they are considered unsterile. Any package that appears already open, torn, punctured, or wet is considered unsterile. Storage areas should be clean, dry, off the floor, and away from sinks. Always check chemical indicators of sterilization before using a package. The indicator is often a tape used to fasten the package or contained inside the package. The indicator changes color during sterilization, indicating that the contents have undergone a sterilization procedure. If the color change is not evident, the package is considered unsterile. Commercially prepared sterile packages may not have indicators but may be marked with the word *sterile*.
Sterile objects become unsterile when touched by unsterile objects.	Handle sterile objects that will touch open wounds or enter body cavities only with sterile forceps or sterile gloved hands. Discard or resterilize objects that come into contact with unsterile objects. Whenever the sterility of an object is questionable, assume the article is unsterile.
Sterile items that are out of vision or below the waist or table level are considered unsterile.	Once left unattended, a sterile field is considered unsterile. Sterile objects are always kept in view. Nurses do not turn their backs on a sterile field. Only the front part of a sterile gown, from shoulder to waist (or table height, whichever is higher), and the cuff of the sleeves to 2 inches above the elbows are considered sterile. Always keep sterile gloved hands in sight and above waist/table level; touch only objects that are sterile. Sterile draped tables in the operating room or elsewhere are considered sterile only at surface level.
Sterile objects can become unsterile by prolonged exposure to airborne microorganisms.	Keep doors closed and traffic to a minimum in areas where a sterile procedure is being performed, because moving air can carry dust and microorganisms. Keep areas in which sterile procedures are carried out as clean as possible by frequent damp cleaning with detergent germicides to minimize contaminants in the area. Keep hair clean and short or enclose it in a net to prevent hair from falling on sterile objects. Microorganisms on the hair can make a sterile field unsterile. Wear surgical caps in operating rooms, delivery rooms, and burn units. Refrain from sneezing or coughing over a sterile field. Droplets containing microorganisms from the respiratory tract can travel 1 m (3 feet), making a sterile field unsterile. Some agencies recommend that masks covering the mouth and the nose should be worn by anyone working over a sterile field or an open wound. Nurses with mild upper respiratory tract infections should refrain from carrying out sterile procedures or wear masks. When working over a sterile field, keep talking to a minimum. Avert the head from the field if talking is necessary. To prevent microorganisms from falling over a sterile field, refrain from reaching over a sterile field unless sterile gloves are worn. Refrain from moving unsterile objects over a sterile field.

(continued)

TABLE 15–5 Principles and Practices of Surgical Asepsis (continued)

PRINCIPLES	PRACTICES
Fluids flow in the direction of gravity.	Unless gloves are worn, always hold wet forceps with the tips below the handles. When the tips are held higher than the handles, fluid can flow onto the handle and become contaminated by the hands. When the forceps are again pointed downward, the contaminated fluid can flow back down and contaminate the tips.
	During a surgical hand wash, hold the hands higher than the elbows to prevent contaminants from the forearms from reaching the hands.
Moisture that passes through a sterile object draws microorganisms from unsterile surfaces above or below the sterile surface by capillary action.	Sterile, moisture-proof barriers are used beneath sterile objects. Liquids (sterile saline or antiseptics) are frequently poured into containers on a sterile field. If they are spilled onto the sterile field, the barrier keeps the liquid from seeping beneath it. Keep the sterile covers on sterile equipment dry. Damp surfaces can attract microorganisms in the air. Replace sterile drapes that do not have a sterile barrier underneath when they become moist.
The edges of a sterile field are considered unsterile.	A 2.5-cm (1-in.) margin at each edge of an opened drape is considered unsterile because the edges are in contact with unsterile surfaces.
	Place all sterile objects more than 2.5 cm (1 in.) inside the edges of a sterile field.
	Any article that falls outside the edges of a sterile field is considered unsterile.
The skin cannot be sterilized and is unsterile.	Use sterile gloves or sterile forceps to handle sterile items.
	Prior to a surgical aseptic procedure, cleanse the hands to reduce the number of microorganisms on them.
Conscientiousness, alertness, and honesty are essential qualities in maintaining surgical asepsis.	When a sterile object becomes unsterile, it does not necessarily change in appearance. The person who sees a sterile object become contaminated must correct or report the situation. Do not set up a sterile field ahead of time for future use.

STERILE GLOVES Sterile gloves may be donned by the open method or the closed method. The open method is most frequently used outside the operating room because the closed method requires that the nurse wear a sterile gown. Gloves are worn during many procedures to maintain the sterility of equipment and protect a client's wound.

Sterile gloves are packaged with a cuff of approximately 5 cm (2 in.) and with the palms facing upward when the package is opened. The package usually indicates the size of the glove (e.g., size 6 or 7½).

Latex and latex-free (e.g., nitrile and vinyl) sterile gloves are available to protect nurses from contact with blood and body fluids. Latex and nitrile are more flexible than vinyl, mold to the wearer's hands, allow freedom of movement, and have the added feature of resealing tiny punctures automatically. Therefore, wear latex or nitrile gloves when performing tasks that (a) demand flexibility, (b) place stress on the material (e.g., turning stopcocks, handling sharp instruments or tape), and (c) involve a high risk of exposure to pathogens. Choose vinyl gloves for tasks that are unlikely to stress the glove material, require minimal precision, and carry a minimal risk of exposure to pathogens.

STERILE GOWNS Sterile gowning and closed gloving are carried out chiefly in operating and delivery rooms, where surgical asepsis is necessary. The closed method of gloving can be used only when a sterile gown is worn because the gloves are handled through the sleeves of the gown. Before these procedures, the nurse dons a hair cover and a mask and performs a surgical hand wash.

Infection Control for Health Care Workers

NIOSH is part of the CDC and is a research agency of the U.S. Department of Health and Human Services. It investigates potentially hazardous working conditions and publishes recommendations for preventing workplace illnesses and injuries. For example, in 1999 NIOSH published a study on preventing needlestick injuries in health care settings that found that the majority of needlestick injuries were preventable. This, in part, led to the Needlestick Safety and Prevention Act, which went into effect in April 2001.

The Occupational Safety and Health Administration (OSHA), an agency of the U.S. Department of Labor, publishes and enforces regulations to protect health care workers from occupational injuries, including exposure to bloodborne pathogens in the workplace. **Occupational exposure** is defined as skin, eye, mucous membrane, or parenteral contact with blood or other potentially infectious materials that may result from the performance of an employee's duties.

There are three major modes of transmission of infectious materials in the clinical setting:

1. Puncture wounds from contaminated needles or other sharps
2. Skin contact, which allows infectious fluids to enter through wounds and broken or damaged skin
3. Mucous membrane contact, which allows infectious fluids to enter through mucous membranes of the eyes, mouth, or nose.

Using proper precautions with general medical asepsis, appropriately using personal protective equipment (PPE) (e.g., gloves, masks, gowns, goggles, special resuscitative equipment), and vigilance in the clinical area will place the caregiver at significantly less risk for injury. The chance of a health care worker becoming infected following exposure to pathogens varies widely—estimates range from 30% for hepatitis B (nonimmune workers), to 1.8% for hepatitis C, to 0.3% for HIV (CDC, 2003). Measures to be taken in cases of possible exposure to these viruses are delineated by the CDC. Hepatitis C, a worldwide epidemic greater than HIV, has become a significant concern to all health care workers, because there is currently no vaccine against the virus or postexposure prophylaxis. Prevention remains the primary goal.

OSHA requires that health care employers make the hepatitis B vaccine and vaccination series available to all employees. Other vaccinations may also be made available (e.g., nurses working in an obstetric area should be vaccinated against rubella to protect pregnant clients and their fetuses).

PRACTICE ALERT

Nurses should consider in advance whether they would want prophylaxis for HIV exposure, because it should optimally begin within 1 hour of exposure.

Role of the Infection Control Nurse

All health care organizations are required to have interdisciplinary infection control committees that may include representatives from the clinical laboratory, housekeeping, maintenance, dietary, and client care areas. One important member of this committee is the infection control nurse. This nurse is specially trained to be knowledgeable about the latest research and practices in preventing, detecting, and treating infections. All infections are reported to the infection control nurse in a manner that permits recording and analyzing statistics that can assist in improving infection control practices. In addition, the infection control nurse may be involved in employee education and implementation of the bloodborne pathogen exposure control plan mandated by OSHA.

ALTERATIONS

Microorganisms—including bacteria, viruses, fungi, and parasites—often invade the human body and proliferate when they are undetected, uncontrolled, or not eliminated by the inflammatory and immune responses. In most cases, contact between humans and microorganisms is incidental and may even be beneficial to both organisms. Resident bacteria of the skin, mucous membranes, and gastrointestinal tract are an important part of the body's defense system. However, many microorganisms are virulent; that is, they have the ability to cause disease. Pathogens are virulent organisms rarely found in the absence of disease. Some microorganisms, known as opportunistic pathogens, rarely, if ever, cause harm to people with intact immune systems, but are capable of producing infectious disease in immunocompromised hosts (Porth, 2005).

Modern medicine, antibiotic therapy, immunizations, and other public health measures to protect food and water supplies have significantly reduced the prevalence of infectious diseases in many parts of the world. In spite of these advances, many infections, including malaria, typhoid, and tuberculosis, remain prevalent in developing nations. Sexually transmitted infections rage through modern cities and industrialized populations. New varieties and strains of pathogens, such as HIV, evolve to cause disease.

To a certain extent, modern medicine has contributed to the development of infectious diseases caused by antibiotic-resistant strains of microorganisms. For example, tuberculosis is on the rise in the United States, partially because organisms have become resistant to standard therapies. Clients receive immunosuppressive therapy following organ or tissue transplant and in the treatment of neoplasms, making them more susceptible to infection. Metal and plastic prosthetic devices are implanted, providing potential sites for colonization of disease-producing organisms (Fauci et al., 1998). Many diseases that were long considered unrelated to microorganisms may also actually be infectious; for example, colonization of the gastric mucosa with *Helicobacter pylori* is the predominant cause of peptic ulcer disease and oncogenic viruses are able to transform normal cells into malignant cells.

Poor hygiene behaviors of young children and their caregivers facilitate transmission of infectious diseases in child care settings and other environments, including hospitals, clinics, and physician offices. The fecal-oral and respiratory routes are the most common modes of transmission in children. Children often do not wash their hands after toileting unless they are closely supervised. They put toys and their hands in their mouths, and then rub their nose and eyes. They often are unable to care for a runny nose without help. Diapers may leak stool and provide exposure to fecal organisms. In addition, caregivers in child care centers, other persons caring for children, and health care professionals may not use proper hand hygiene techniques. All of these behaviors promote the transmission of infection.

Pathogens

Pathogens capable of infecting and causing disease in susceptible hosts include bacteria, viruses, *Mycoplasma, Rickettsia, Chlamydia,* fungi, and parasites, such as protozoa, helminths (worms), and arthropods (Box 15–2). Each organism causes a different specific reaction in the host.

A number of mechanisms have evolved in pathogens to facilitate their transmission and increase their ability to invade the host and cause disease. Factors influencing the transmission of an organism include its resistance to drying and to variations in environmental temperature. For example, spore-forming organisms are extremely resistant to drying.

Many microorganisms are capable of producing toxins or enzymes to facilitate their invasion of the host, increase their resistance to host defenses, and increase their ability to cause disease. Adhesion factors produced by or incorporated into the cell wall or membrane of the pathogen improve its ability to attach and colonize the host. Pathogens may also produce enzymes to enhance their spread to local tissues, chemicals to block specific immune processes or deplete neutrophils and macrophages, or extracellular capsules to discourage phagocytosis.

Pathogens are often capable of producing toxins that alter or destroy the normal function of host cells and promote colonization, proliferation, and invasion by the pathogen. Toxins often increase the disease-producing capability of the pathogen and, in some cases, are totally responsible for it. For example, cholera, tetanus, and botulism result from bacterial toxins, not from the direct effects of the infection. **Exotoxins** are soluble proteins that the microorganisms secrete into surrounding tissue. Exotoxins are highly poisonous, causing cell death or dysfunction. **Endotoxins** are found in the cell wall of gram-negative bacteria and released only when the cell is disrupted. They have less specific effects than exotoxins, but can activate many human regulatory systems, producing fever, inflammation, and potentially clotting, bleeding, or hypotension when released in large quantities.

Stages of the Infectious Process

When infectious disease develops in a host, it typically follows a predictable course, with stages based on the progression and intensity of manifestations. Stages include

1. Incubation period
2. Prodromal stage
3. Acute stage
4. Convalescent stage

The initial stage is the *incubation period*, during which the pathogen begins active replication but does not yet cause symptoms. Depending on the organism and host factors, the incubation period may last from hours, as with *Salmonella*, to years, as with HIV infection.

In the *prodromal stage*, symptoms begin to appear. At this stage, symptoms are often nonspecific and include general malaise, fever, myalgias, headache, and fatigue.

Maximal impact of the infectious process occurs during the *acute stage* as the pathogen proliferates and disseminates rapidly. Toxic byproducts of microorganism metabolism and cell lysis, along with the immune response, produce tissue damage and

Box 15–2 Pathogenic Organisms

BACTERIA

Bacteria are single-celled organisms that are capable of autonomous reproduction. Bacteria have different characteristics and growth requirements: *Aerobes* require oxygen for survival, whereas *anaerobes* cannot survive in the presence of oxygen; *gram-positive* bacteria stain purple when subjected to crystal violet stain, whereas *gram-negative* bacteria do not stain with crystal violet stain, but turn red when subjected to safranin stain; and the colonies formed by replicating bacteria differ from one another.

VIRUSES

Viruses are obligate intracellular parasites that are incapable of reproducing outside of a living cell. Some viruses are shed continuously from infected cell surfaces; others, after inserting their genetic material into that of the infected cell, remain latent until they are stimulated to replicate. Viruses may or may not cause lysis and death of the host cell during replication. Oncogenic viruses are able to transform normal cells into malignant cells.

MYCOPLASMA

Although similar to bacteria, *Mycoplasma* are smaller and have no cell wall, making them resistant to antibiotics that inhibit cell wall synthesis, such as penicillins.

RICKETTSIA* AND *CHLAMYDIA

As obligate intracellular parasites with a rigid cell wall, *Rickettsia* and *Chlamydia* have some features of both bacteria and viruses. Rather than depending on the host cell for reproduction, they use vitamins, nutrients, and products of metabolism (e.g., ATP) from the host. *Chlamydia* are transmitted by direct contact, whereas many Rickettsiae infect the cells of arthropods (e.g., fleas, ticks, and lice) and are transmitted from these vectors to humans.

FUNGI

Fungi are prevalent throughout the world, but few are capable of causing disease in humans. Most fungal infections are self-limited, affecting the skin and subcutaneous tissue. Some fungi, such as *Pneumocystis carinii*, can cause life-threatening opportunistic infections in the immunocompromised host.

PARASITES

The term *parasite* is typically applied to members of the animal kingdom that infect and cause disease in other animals. Protozoa, helminths, and arthropods are considered parasites. Protozoa are single-celled organisms transmitted via direct or indirect contact or by an arthropod vector. Helminths are wormlike parasites: Roundworms, tapeworms, and flukes are examples. They gain entry into humans primarily through ingestion of fertilized eggs or penetration of larvae through the skin or mucous membranes. Arthropod parasites, such as scabies (mites), lice, and fleas, typically infest external body surfaces, causing localized tissue damage and inflammation. Transmission is by direct contact with the arthropod or its eggs.

Source: Data summarized from Porth, C. M. (2005). *Pathophysiology: Concepts of altered health states* (7th ed.). Philadelphia: Lippincott Williams & Wilkins.

inflammation during this stage (Porth, 2005). Manifestations are more pronounced and specific to the infecting organism and site. Fever and chills may be significant during this phase. However, alcoholic clients and the older adults may respond to severe infection by becoming hypothermic. A client in the acute stage of infection is often tachycardic and tachypneic because of increased metabolic demands. Localized manifestations include redness, heat, swelling, pain, and impaired function. When the infectious disease affects an internal organ, manifestations are related to inflammatory changes in that organ and surrounding tissue. The client may experience tenderness to palpation over the site or show signs of impaired function, such as the hematuria and proteinuria that are characteristic of renal infections.

If the infectious process is prolonged, manifestations of the continuing immune response may become apparent. Catabolic and anorexic effects of the infection can lead to loss of body fat and muscle wasting. Immune complexes may be deposited at sites other than the primary infection, resulting in an inflammatory process. Glomerulonephritis (e.g., following strep throat) and vasculitis are possible results. Another possible consequence of prolonged infection and immune response is the triggering of an autoimmune disease process, such as rheumatic cardiomyopathy or celiac disease. Type 1 diabetes mellitus is thought to be the result of such a response (Porth, 2005).

As the infection is contained and the pathogen eliminated, the *convalescent stage* of the disease occurs. During this stage, affected tissues are repaired and manifestations resolve. Resolution of the infection is total elimination of the pathogen from the body without residual manifestations.

If a balance between organism and host factors occurs, with neither predominating, chronic disease may develop, or the organism may be driven into a protected site, such as an abscess. A *carrier state* develops when host defenses eliminate the infectious disease, but the organism continues to multiply on mucosal sites (Fauci et al., 1998).

Complications of Infectious Diseases

Multiple and varied complications are associated with infectious diseases. They are typically specific to the infecting organism and the body system affected.

Acute invasion of the blood by certain microorganisms or their toxins can result in septicemia and septic shock. Although bacteremia, the presence of bacteria in the blood, may not have serious effects, in septicemia, systemic disease is associated with their presence or that of toxins. Septic shock indicates a state of hypotension and impaired organ perfusion resulting from sepsis. Unless treated aggressively, septic shock leads to diffuse cell and tissue injury, and potentially to organ failure.

Nosocomial Infections

Nosocomial infections, called health care–associated infections (HAIs), are classified as infections that are associated with the delivery of health care services in a facility such as a hospital or nursing home. HAIs add hospital days, reduce admissions by occupying available beds, and increase the cost of health care (Stone, Hedblom, Murphy, & Miller, 2005). Nosocomial infections can either develop during a client's stay in a facility or manifest after discharge. They typically manifest after 48 hours of hospitalization. Infections that manifest within 48 hours of hospitalization are attributed to community sources.

Urinary tract infection is the most common type of HAI and the most frequent cause of gram-negative septicemia in hospitalized clients. Pneumonia is the second most common hospital-acquired infection, with a mortality rate of 20–50%. It is associated with mechanical ventilators, tracheostomies, and endotracheal intubation (Porth, 2005). Bacteremia is associated with intravascular and urinary catheters. Because of the risk of infection, insertion of central lines and urinary catheters is conducted as a sterile procedure with careful attention to preventing contamination. *Clostridium difficile*-associated diarrhea is a frequently acquired nosocomial infection. Associated with antibiotic use, the risk of acquiring this infection increases with length of hospital stay, especially in an intensive care unit (ICU). Nosocomial microorganisms can also be acquired by health care personnel working in the facility, which can cause significant illness and time lost from work.

Nosocomial infections have received increasing attention in recent years. They are believed to involve approximately 2 million clients per year, cause 90,000 deaths, and add $4.5 billion in excess health care costs annually. The Joint Commission (formerly known as The Joint Commission on Accreditation of Healthcare Organizations), an independent, not-for-profit organization that accredits and certifies health care organizations and programs in the United States, included reducing the risk of health care–associated infections as one of the 2006 National Patient Safety Goals. The most common settings where nosocomial infections develop are hospital surgical and medical ICUs. The microorganisms that cause nosocomial infections can originate from the clients themselves (an **endogenous** source) or from the hospital environment and hospital personnel (**exogenous** sources). Most nosocomial infections appear to have endogenous sources. *Escherichia coli, Staphylococcus aureus,* and enterococci are the most common infecting microorganisms.

A number of factors contribute to nosocomial infections. **Iatrogenic infections** are the direct result of diagnostic or therapeutic procedures. One example of an iatrogenic infection is the bacteremia that results from insertion of an intravascular line. Not all nosocomial infections are iatrogenic, nor are all nosocomial infections preventable.

Another factor that contributes to the development of nosocomial infections is the compromised host, that is, a client whose normal defenses have been lowered by surgery or illness. Clients entering hospitals are often the least able to mount immune defenses to infection. Immunologic responses may be compromised and normal defenses impaired in clients with, for example, cancer or chronic diseases, pressure ulcers, or organ transplants (Tierney, McPhee, & Papadakis, 2006). Nosocomial infections also occur when antibiotic therapy has altered the body's natural defenses and impaired resistance to harmful microorganisms. Endogenous organisms outside their normal habitats (such as in *E. coli* in the urinary tract) become a threat to the client.

Other pharmacologic and therapeutic procedures, such as chemotherapy, the use of corticosteroids, and radiation therapy, also contribute to nosocomial infections. gram-negative enteric bacteria and gram-positive *S. aureus* are the most common bacteria responsible.

Invasive procedures and altered immune defenses are the main factors that contribute to infection. Urinary catheterization is the number one cause; cardiac catheterization, insertion of peripheral and central intravenous lines, respiratory care procedures, and surgical procedures are also closely linked to nosocomial infection. Consequently, the urinary tract, surgical wounds, the respiratory tract, and invasive catheter sites on the skin are most often affected by hospital-acquired infection. Hospital-acquired pneumonia is the second most common nosocomial infection, accounting for 15–20% of these serious infections. Sopena and Sabria (2005) found hospital-acquired pneumonia, usually associated with ICU residency and mechanical ventilation, in non-ICU clients with severe underlying disease and a hospital stay greater than 5 days. Organisms causing the infection are often resistant to many drugs and may not respond to antibiotics that are usually effective in treating infections acquired outside the hospital.

The hands of personnel are a common vehicle for the spread of microorganisms. Insufficient hand cleansing is an important factor contributing to the spread of nosocomial microorganisms.

PRACTICE ALERT

Since October 2002, alcohol-based hand rub has been recommended by the CDC as the preferred method for hand hygiene (CDC, 2002a). Antiseptic soaps and detergents are the next most effective agents, and nonantiseptic soaps are the least effective. A soap and water wash is recommended for visibly soiled hands. Wearing gloves does not eliminate the need for handwashing.

Table 15–6 outlines the most common microorganisms responsible for nosocomial infections and their causes.

PREVENTING NOSOCOMIAL INFECTIONS Prevention is the most important control measure for nosocomial infections. The pathogens causing these infections are transmitted primarily by contact with hospital personnel and contaminated inanimate objects (Posani, 2004). *Effective handwashing is the single most important measure in infection control.* Although infections can also be transmitted by the airborne route, via contaminated equipment, and from the environment, these are less significant routes. Invasive procedures and equipment should be used only when absolutely necessary; for example, it is not appropriate to insert an indwelling catheter when the only indication is incontinence. Peripheral intravenous equipment and sites must be kept clean and changed regularly: intravenous bags and bottles every 24 hours, tubing every 24–96 hours, and sites every 2–3 days according to agency policy (CDC, 2002b; Evans-Smith, 2005).

Meticulous use of medical and surgical asepsis is necessary to prevent transport of potentially infectious microorganisms. Many nosocomial infections can be prevented using proper hand hygiene techniques, environmental controls, sterile technique when warranted, and identification and management of clients at risk for infection. Many research studies have investigated the effectiveness of aseptic technique. Not all, however, show what might have been considered intuitive results. For example, no controlled studies have shown that removing nail polish or rings influences the rate of infection following surgical hand scrubbing and gloving (Arrowsmith, Maunder, Sargent, & Taylor, 2005). A number of studies have shown a link between artificial fingernails and infection transmission, especially fungal infections. In any case, nurses use critical thinking and agency policy in implementing infection control procedures.

Hand hygiene is important in every setting, including hospitals. It is considered one of the most effective infection control measures. Any client can harbor microorganisms that are currently harmless to the client yet potentially harmful to another person or to the same client if the microorganisms find a portal of entry. It is important that both the nurses' and clients' hands be cleansed at the following times to prevent the spread of microorganisms: before eating, after using the bedpan or toilet, and after the hands have come in contact with any

TABLE 15–6 Nosocomial Infections

MOST COMMON MICROORGANISMS	CAUSES
Urinary Tract	
Escherichia coli	Improper catheterization technique
Enterococcus species	Contamination of closed drainage system
Pseudomonas aeruginosa	Inadequate hand cleansing
Surgical Sites	
Staphylococcus aureus (including methicillin-resistant strains—MRSA)	Inadequate hand cleansing
Enterococcus species (including vancomycin-resistant strains—VRE)	Improper dressing change technique
Pseudomonas aeruginosa	
Bloodstream	
Coagulase-negative staphylococci	Inadequate hand cleansing
Staphylococcus aureus *Enterococcus* species	Improper intravenous fluid, tubing, and site care technique
Pneumonia	
Staphylococcus aureus	Inadequate hand cleansing
Pseudomonas aeruginosa	Improper suctioning technique
Enterobacter species	

body substances, such as sputum or drainage from a wound. In addition, health care workers should cleanse their hands before and after giving care of any kind.

For routine client care, the WHO (2005) recommends handwashing under a stream of water for at least 20 seconds using plain granule soap, soap-filled sheets, or liquid soap when hands are visibly soiled, after using the restroom, after removing gloves, before handling invasive devices (such as intravenous tubing), and after contact with medical equipment or furniture.

However, soap and water are inadequate to sufficiently remove pathogens. The CDC recommends use of alcohol-based antiseptic hand rubs (rinses, gels, or foams) before and after direct client contact. Recently, placement of alcohol-based antiseptic hand rub dispensers has been approved for agency corridors (Centers for Medicare and Medicaid Services, 2005). Previous concerns that this represented a fire hazard have been addressed in the regulations.

Antimicrobial soaps are usually provided in high-risk areas, such as the newborn nursery, and are frequently supplied in dispensers at the sink. Studies have shown that the convenience of antimicrobial foams and gels, which do not require soap and water, may increase health care workers' adherence to hand cleansing. The CDC recommends antimicrobial hand cleansing agents.

It is important to recognize that performing hand hygiene with either soap or alcohol-based cleansers can damage the skin through the drying effect of the detergents or chemicals. If the nurse develops dermatitis, the client may be at higher risk for infection, because handwashing does not decrease bacterial counts on skin with dermatitis. The nurse is also at higher risk because the normal skin barrier has been broken. Although lotions, moisturizers, and emollients have been tried, no research has yet confirmed their effectiveness in minimizing the problem.

Antibiotic-Resistant Bacteria

Antibiotic-resistant microorganisms are increasing at an alarming rate, primarily due to the prolonged and inappropriate use of antibiotic therapy. Although antibiotic therapy is expected to eradicate all targeted microorganisms, sometimes a few bacteria survive, leading to bacteria that reproduce with antibiotic resistance already encoded into their genetic makeup (Lehne, 2004). Other bacteria produce enzymes that inactivate drugs, change drug binding sites, or alter their cell membrane to prevent drug absorption.

Some of the current resistant strains include

- Methicillin-resistant *S. aureus* (MRSA)
- Multidrug-resistant tuberculosis (MDR-TB)
- Penicillin-resistant *Streptococcus pneumoniae* (PRSP)
- Vancomycin-resistant *Enterococcus* (VRE)
- Vancomycin-intermediate or -resistant *S. aureus* (VISA or VRSA)
- Extended-spectrum beta-lactamase (ESBL) (Kjonegaard & Myers, 2005)

MRSA is becoming more prevalent in community settings in which young people, such as children in day care and amateur and professional athletes, share equipment. MRSA colonizes in the nares and skin. Health care personnel often transmit *S. aureus* unknowingly on their hands, because it is transmitted primarily by direct physical contact, not through respiratory droplets (Kjonegaard & Myers, 2005). Most *S. aureus* strains resist treatment by methicillin and similar drugs, which are the treatment of choice for *S. aureus* infections. Vancomycin has been the only uniformly effective drug for hospital-acquired MRSA; however, community-acquired MRSA is sensitive to antibiotics such as tetracycline, doxycycline, clindamycin, sulfamethoxazole-trimethoprim, cephalexin, dicloxacillin, erythromycin, and quinolones. Soft-tissue infections with MRSA may manifest as abscesses, furuncles, or cellulites, and may be mistaken for spider bites.

In 1997, a new form of *S. aureus* emerged with resistance to vancomycin, known as vancomycin-intermediate or vancomycin-resistant *S. aureus.* (VISA or VRSA); both VISA and VRSA are resistant to methicillin. Clients with MRSA, VISA, or VRSA are isolated in a private room using contact precautions.

Enterococci are part of the normal flora of the gastrointestinal and female genital tracts. Frequent use of vancomycin caused *Enterococci* to develop resistance, leading to VRE.

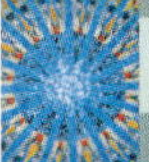

EVIDENCE-BASED PRACTICE **Does Frequency of Handwashing Vary According to Risk of Infection Transmission?**

In this Canadian study, all visits by nurses in an acute care hospital to selected client rooms were recorded for 3 days and 2 nights to assess compliance with handwashing. The highest level of infection transmission risk was contact with body fluids in 11% of visits and contact with skin in 40% of visits. The overall rate of handwashing was 46%; however, the rate for visits involving contact with body fluids was 81% and contact with skin was 61%. Nurses returned immediately to the same client 45% of the time. The rate of handwashing was higher for the last of a series of visits to a client's room. The researchers concluded that nurses adjusted their handwashing rates in accordance with the risk level of each visit.

Implications

Many studies have examined compliance with handwashing policies among health care workers. In almost every case, the compliance rates were far below what is recommended. This study suggests that raw data of compliance are less useful than examining the use and pattern of handwashing in those cases in which the care provider recognizes the highest risk of infection transmission. Education programs about hand hygiene may be more effective if patterns of care and levels of risk are incorporated into recommendations.

Source: Raboud J., Saskin, R., Wong, K., Moore, C., Parucha, G., Bennett, J., et al. (2004). Patterns of handwashing behavior and visits to patients on a general medical ward of healthcare workers. *Infection Control and Hospital Epidemiology, 25,* pp. 198–202.

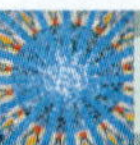

EVIDENCE-BASED PRACTICE Antibiotics and Infection

Nurses who discharge clients from outpatient and acute care settings frequently teach clients to take a complete prescribed dose of oral antibiotics to manage acute infectious illness. Ingesting less than complete doses exposes clients to the risk of resistant infections and can result in less than therapeutic outcomes. There are many potential barriers to the completion of antibiotic dosing: cost of purchase; difficulty swallowing the pills; multiple, frequent doses; and the potential for adverse, unpleasant side effects.

Aronson (2005) studied in depth the experience of 11 clients who had just completed a short-term antibiotic regimen to treat a variety of acute infectious illnesses with various antibiotic regimens. The 11 participants represented diverse gender and cultural backgrounds. They participated in 30-minute interviews within 2 weeks of completing their antibiotic regimen. The interviews were audiotaped and evaluated for themes. This qualitative study is the first part of a research program to evaluate an intervention that promotes adherence to taking antibiotics for a short-term period. The clients' descriptions, views, and experiences are the unique aspect of this research on adherence to antibiotic self-administration; most studies of adherence have been conducted from the prescribers' rather than the clients' perspective.

Aronson analyzed the client descriptions of their experiences taking their prescribed antibiotics by organizing the responses into categories of consistent themes. A second colleague experienced in qualitative research independently analyzed the data, and the results were compared until the categories were agreed upon. The central theme that emerged was successful antibiotic self-administration. The clients integrated the dosing into their daily schedules and adapted to any unplanned circumstances. The primary categories involved in self-administration were (1) medication-taking behaviors, (2) factors influencing adherence, and (3) attitudes and beliefs about the medication and the value of completing the prescribed dose. Subcategories were identified for each of these main categories.

Clients described methods for remembering to take the medication, methods of dealing with anticipated or experienced side effects, and factors that built trust in their relationship with the prescriber. Clients with a higher severity of symptoms leading to antibiotic prescription were more likely to report intention to adhere to the dosing regimen.

Implications for Nursing

Nurses teach clients about short-term antibiotic self-administration in outpatient and inpatient settings. The findings from this study can be used to guide educational interactions. Based on the findings in this study, nurses should encourage client involvement in the decision to take short-term antibiotic medications in order to strengthen the relationship with the prescriber. Nurses can ask clients to identify the method they will use to remind themselves to take each dose, and inquire about their knowledge of and plans to manage side effects from the medication.

Critical Thinking in Client Care

1. Identify methods that clients can use to remind themselves of dosing schedules.
2. An 86-year-old woman is being discharged to her home following a respiratory infection. Identify the information she will need to learn about short-term antibiotic medication when she is discharged.
3. Discuss potential side effects of short-term antibiotics on the gastrointestinal tract.
4. Discuss the interrelationship between malnutrition and immune system function.

Source: Data from Aronson, B. (2005). Medication management behaviors of adherent short-term antibiotic users. *Clinical Excellence for Nurse Practitioners, 9*(1), 23–30.

Direct transmission occurs on the hands of health care personnel and from contact with contaminated equipment. In cases of infection, stringent infection control measures are instituted, care is provided using contact precautions, and clients are placed either alone or with other VRE-infected clients.

Streptococcus pneumoniae, the most common cause of community-acquired pneumonia, has developed into its resistant form, penicillin-resistant *S. pneumoniae* (PRSP). Unlike MRSA and VRE, PRSP is transmitted by droplets from the respiratory tract and requires transmission-based droplet precautions.

C. difficile is an organism that has developed very resistant and highly morbid strains associated with frequent use of broad-spectrum antibiotics in hospitals. A common cause of nosocomial diarrhea, it is usually treated with metronidazole or vancomycin (Rao & Bradley, 2003). An even more virulent strain has been identified that is resistant to both metronidazole and vancomycin (Warny et al., 2005).

Extended-spectrum beta-lactamase–producing microorganisms are resistant to third-generation cephalosporins and include gram-negative *Klebsiella* and *E. coli*. These organisms colonize indwelling urinary catheters and gastrostomies, as well as mechanical ventilators. They spread by direct and indirect contact.

Universal precautions, most importantly handwashing, and modest use of antibiotics are critical actions for stopping the spread of antibiotic-resistant bacteria. Equipment such as stethoscopes, blood pressure cuffs, and thermometers should be restricted to use by each client identified with one of these diseases. Personal protective gear that is used and disposed of appropriately is another important safeguard.

Certain antibiotics can also induce resistance in some strains of organisms. This resistance has become so widespread that the CDC has created a 12-step Campaign to Prevent Antimicrobial Resistance in Healthcare Settings, which consists of four strategies: preventing infection, diagnosing and treating infection effectively, using antimicrobials wisely, and preventing transmission.

Biological Threat Infections

Since the terrorist attacks on September 11, 2001, and the development of anthrax cases in the United States, there is an increased level of concern about the possible use of biological

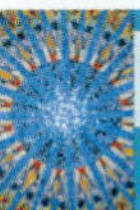

FOCUS ON DIVERSITY AND CULTURE
Beliefs About Disease Causation

In some cultures, infectious diseases are seen as punishment for sin or the result of curses or evil spirits. For example, Native Americans traditionally view illnesses as the result of disharmony or displeasing the spirits. They may not believe in the germ theory of disease causation.

weapons. The most likely pathogens to be used for this purpose include anthrax, smallpox, botulism, pneumonic plague, and viral hemorrhagic fevers.

As with any potential large-scale infectious disease, state public health systems are charged with the responsibility of identifing cases, controlling the spread of infection, and preparing the local and state responses for caring for the potential large numbers of ill adults and children. As a part of this responsibility, public health authorities conduct **disease surveillance**, monitoring patterns of disease occurrence from the cases of infectious and communicable diseases reported by health care workers to state health officials. Disease surveillance procedures may be followed for any type of communicable and infectious disease, from *shigella* to H1N1 influenza to a biological threat infection.

Pediatric Infectious and Communicable Diseases

Reducing the number of preventable childhood illnesses is a major national goal in *Healthy People 2010*, and nurses are important partners in this effort. Specific objectives targeted at reducing or eliminating specific infectious diseases (USDHHS, 2000) include

- *Elimination.* Rubella and congenital rubella syndrome, diphtheria, *Haemophilus influenza* type b, measles, mumps, polio, and tetanus.
- *Reduction.* Pertussis, hepatitis B, varicella, food-borne pathogens, and HIV infection. Common preventable infectious diseases are a significant public health problem. The national health objectives are a reflection of how significant these preventable diseases are as a public health problem. Table 15–7 lists selected infectious and communicable diseases in children.

TABLE 15–7 Selected Infectious and Communicable Diseases in Children

DISEASE	CLINICAL MANIFESTATIONS	CLINICAL THERAPY	NURSING MANAGEMENT
Diphtheria[*+] *Causal agent: Corynebacterium diphtheriae* *Epidemiology:* Occurs mostly in colder months in unimmunized or partially immunized children and immunized children with waning immunity. Cases of cutaneous and wound diphtheria occur sporadically in the tropics. Maternal immunity lasts up to 6 months after birth. The disease is endemic in areas where immunization is no longer routine, such as Russia. *Transmission:* Contact with nasal or eye discharge or skin lesion, or, less commonly, by indirect contact with contaminated items. Unpasteurized milk has served as a vehicle. *Incubation period:* 2–7 days or longer *Period of communicability:* Usually 2–4 weeks or until 4 days after antibiotics are started	Symptoms can be mild or severe with a gradual onset over 1–2 days. Low-grade fever, anorexia, malaise, rhinorrhea with a foul odor, cough, sore throat, hoarseness, stridor or noisy breathing, cervical lymphadenitis, and pharyngitis may be present. In more severe cases, the membranes of the tonsils, pharynx, and larynx are affected. The characteristic membranous lesion is a thick, bluish white to grayish black patch that covers the tonsils. It can spread to cover the soft and hard palates and the posterior portion of the pharynx. Attempts to remove the membrane result in bleeding. *Complications:* Produces an endotoxin that causes myocarditis and peripheral neuropathy (diplopia, slurred speech, difficulty swallowing, or paralysis of the palate) or ascending paralysis similar to Guillain-Barré syndrome.	Diagnostic tests include a culture from any mucosal or cutaneous lesion. Administer IV antitoxin and antibiotics within 3 days of onset of symptoms. The child must be tested for sensitivity to horse serum before giving the antitoxin. When diphtheria is suspected, antibiotic therapy (penicillin G or erythromycin) should be initiated without waiting for laboratory results. Removal of the membrane may be needed to treat airway obstruction. *Prognosis*: With treatment, prognosis is good. If untreated, death can occur due to airway obstruction. *Prevention*: Diphtheria is a vaccine-preventable disease. Booster doses are needed every 10 years after primary series. This is a reportable disease.	■ Use droplet precautions for pharyngeal disease and contact precautions for cutaneous disease. ■ Monitor closely for signs of increasing respiratory distress, as well as cardiac and neurologic complications. Provide humidified oxygen as necessary. ■ Have emergency airway equipment available. ■ Administer antibiotics. Give no medications containing caffeine or other stimulants. ■ Use oral suction gently as necessary. ■ Allow children to use mouthwash if desired. Gargling is not permitted because it can irritate the pharyngeal surfaces. ■ Encourage liquids as tolerated. Intravenous fluids may be necessary. ■ Provide emotional support to the family. ■ Initiate the search for client contacts to give antibiotics and immunization boosters.

(continued)

TABLE 15–7 **Selected Infectious and Communicable Diseases in Children** **(continued)**

DISEASE	CLINICAL MANIFESTATIONS	CLINICAL THERAPY	NURSING MANAGEMENT
Erythema Infectiosum (Fifth Disease) *Causal agent*: Human parvovirus B-19 *Epidemiology:* Occurs worldwide, most often in winter and spring. The disease also occurs in epidemics, with peak activity every 6 years. The incidence is highest in children between the ages of 5 and 14 years. *Transmission:* Respiratory secretions and blood *Incubation period:* 6–21 days *Period of communicability:* Believed to be highest the week before symptom onset 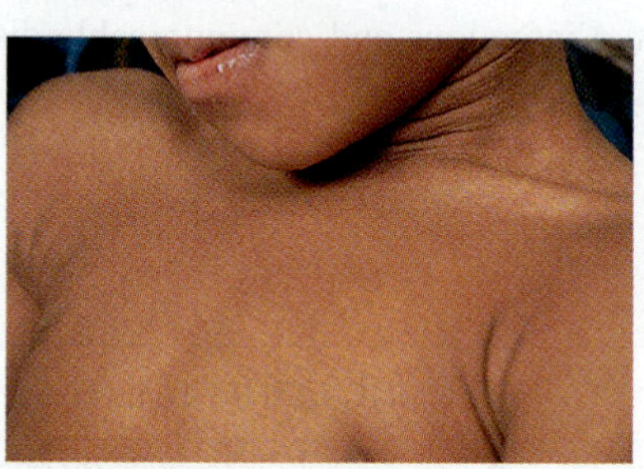 Figure 15–3 ■ Lace-like, erythematous, maculopapular rash with erythema infectiosum. *Source:* Courtesy of Maura Connor.	Stage 1 begins as a flu-like illness (headache, chills, malaise, nausea, body ache) lasting 2–3 days. A symptom-free period of 1–7 days follows. Stage 2 occurs 1 week later with a fiery-red rash on the cheeks, giving a "slapped face" appearance. Circumoral pallor is seen. In 1–4 days a lace-like, symmetric, erythematous, maculopapular rash appears on the trunk and limbs, spreading proximal to distal, but sparing the palms and soles (see Figure 15–3 ■). Stage 3 lasts 1–3 weeks as the rash fades, but can reappear if the skin is irritated or exposed to sunlight. The rash can be mildly pruritic. *Complications*: Children with hemolytic conditions can have transient aplastic crisis. Arthritis and arthralgia can occur.	Diagnosis is made by physical signs or a serologic test for immunoglobulin M (IgM) parvovirus B-19–specific antibody. Medical treatment is supportive, and recovery is usually spontaneous. Children with hemolytic conditions may need blood transfusions if an aplastic crisis occurs. Immunodeficient clients may develop a chronic infection for which IV immune globulin therapy is often effective (American Academy of Pediatrics, 2006). *Prognosis*: Fetal infection can occur, resulting in fetal hydrops or spontaneous abortion. *Prevention*: Avoid contact with infected persons.	■ Children with aplastic crisis are often hospitalized. ■ Use standard and droplet precautions. Isolation is needed only for children with aplastic crisis or who are immunosuppressed. ■ Nonaspirin antipyretics may be given to control fever. ■ Use soothing oatmeal or Aveeno baths if the rash is pruritic. Antipruritics may also help to relieve itching. ■ Encourage rest and offer frequent fluids. ■ Keep children out of direct sunlight if possible. Provide protective, light, loose clothing if exposure to sunlight cannot be avoided. ■ Provide quiet diversionary activity. There is no reason to keep the immune-competent child out of school or day care once he or she is no longer infectious. ■ Explain the three stages of rash development to parents.
Haemophilus Influenzae, *Type B*[+] *Causal agent:* Coccobacilli *H. influenzae* bacteria, which has several serotypes and can be encapsulated or nonencapsulated *Epidemiology:* Occurs most often in the spring and summer. Most commonly affected are infants and young children in child care centers. Low-birth-weight children and children with chronic illnesses have an increased susceptibility. *Transmission:* Direct contact or droplet inhalation. The organism is frequently asymptomatically colonized in the respiratory tract. *Incubation period*: Unknown *Period of communicability:* Three days from onset of symptoms	Begins with a viral upper respiratory infection. The organism passes through the mucosal barrier to directly invade the bloodstream. It can cause several severe invasive illnesses, including meningitis, epiglottitis, pneumonia, septic arthritis, and cellulitis. It is also a cause of sepsis in infants. Other illnesses include sinusitis, otitis media, bronchitis, and pericarditis. Each disease has very specific clinical manifestations. Invasive disease has decreased 99% since the introduction of the vaccine (American Academy of Pediatrics, 2006). *Complications*: Illness caused by *H. influenzae* type B responds to antibiotic therapy. Left untreated, severe sequelae and death, especially in young infants, can occur from conditions such as meningitis, epiglottitis, sinusitis, pneumonitis, and cellulitis.	Diagnosis is made by culture of blood, cerebrospinal fluid, or middle ear aspirate. Treatment consists of antibiotic therapy. Rifampin may be given to unprotected household contacts (not pregnant women), if another child has not completed immunizations, within 1 week after diagnosis. *Prognosis:* With rapid diagnosis and treatment, recovery is good, but highly dependent on the disease the organism has caused. When treatment is delayed, the prognosis for full recovery becomes much more guarded. *Prevention*: Immunization for *H. influenzae* type B	■ Use droplet precautions until 24 hours after the initiation of antibiotics. ■ Antibiotic therapy is administered intravenously for severe infections. Infections such as otitis media can be managed with oral antibiotics. ■ Unimmunized children under the age of 4 years are at increased risk for developing disease from *H. influenzae*. Specific prophylactic measures for susceptible children may be ordered by the physician. ■ Administer antipyretics to help the child feel more comfortable. ■ Closely monitor IV sites for patency and infiltration. ■ Perform nursing care measures specific to the illness. ■ Inform family members that rifampin turns urine and other body fluids orange, and it will cause stains.

TABLE 15–7 **Selected Infectious and Communicable Diseases in Children (continued)**

DISEASE	CLINICAL MANIFESTATIONS	CLINICAL THERAPY	NURSING MANAGEMENT
Influenza *Causal agent:* Orthomyxoviridae, types A and B *Epidemiology:* Prevalent in the United States from October to March, but the virus is active in other parts of the world year-round. During annual epidemics, 10–40% of healthy children are infected, and 1% are hospitalized (American Academy of Pediatrics, 2006). *Transmission:* Spreads by aerosolized particles and direct contact with respiratory secretions. *Incubation period:* 1–4 days *Period of communicability:* One day before symptoms until 5 days after onset of illness	Abrupt onset of fever (38–40°C), chills, cough, runny nose, sore throat, malaise, aches, headache, and anorexia. Children can have nausea and vomiting, diarrhea, and abdominal pain. Children may also present with croup, bronchiolitis, conjunctivitis, or other nonspecific febrile illness. *Complications:* Otitis media, exacerbations of chronic lung conditions such as asthma and cystic fibrosis. Pneumonia, croup, bronchiolitis, and wheezing can occur in up to 25% of children. Myositis, myocarditis, encephalitis, transverse myelitis, Reye's syndrome, and Guillain-Barré syndrome are all potential complications.	Diagnostic tests may include viral culture, rapid antigen testing from throat or nasopharynx, polymerase chain reaction, and immuno-fluorescence. Treatment is supportive. Antiviral therapy (oseltamivir, and zanamivir) may be given to children 1 year of age or older at high risk of complications. Relenza is approved for children 5 years and older (Food and Drug Administration, 2006). Amantadine and rimantadine should not be used due to viral resistance (Centers for Disease Control, 2006c, pp. 2–3). Follow updated antiviral therapy guidelines on http://www.cdc.gov/flu. When antiviral medication is initiated within 2 days of symptoms, the duration of symptoms may be reduced by 1–1 ½ days. *Prevention:* Influenza vaccine is now recommended for infants and children over 6 months of age.	■ Use droplet and contact precautions for hospitalized infants and children. ■ The child is usually cared for at home. Encourage parents to wash hands frequently and to reduce exposure of other family members to the infected child. ■ Provide fluids to keep nasal secretions moist and prevent dehydration. ■ Provide acetaminophen or ibuprofen for fever management and mild pain. ■ If antiviral medications are given, be alert for nausea and vomiting. Zanamivir can exacerbate asthma. ■ Provide rest and quiet diversional activities. ■ Teach parents to be alert to signs of complications from the viral infection. ■ Nurses should be familiar with pandemic influenza plans for the local area and state (http://www.pandemicflu.gov).
Measles (Rubeola)*+ *Causal agent:* Morbillivirus, a member of the paramyxovirus group *Epidemiology:* Occurrence peaks in the late winter and early spring. In developed countries, measles occurs mostly in outbreaks among unimmunized children, or possibly those with declining immunity. Spreads by direct contact with droplets or by airborne route. Passive maternal immunity lasts 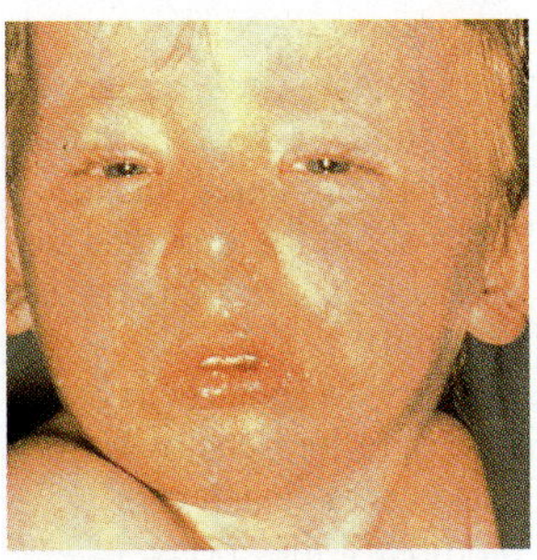 **Figure 15–4** ■ Confluent maculopapular rash with measles. *Source:* Courtesy of Centers for Disease Control and Prevention.	Children are quite ill in the 3–5 day prodromal phase, with symptoms including high fever, conjunctivitis, coryza, cough, anorexia, and malaise. Koplik's spots (small, irregular, bluish white spots on a red background) appear on the buccal mucosa about 2 days before and after the rash appears. The characteristic red, blotchy maculopapular rash that becomes confluent usually appears 2–4 days after onset of prodromal phase. The rash begins on the face and spreads to the trunk and extremities (Figure 15–4 ■). Symptoms gradually subside in 4–7 days. Other symptoms include anorexia, malaise, fatigue, and generalized lymphadenopathy.	Diagnosis can be made by a serologic test for IgM measles antibody. Treatment is supportive. No antiviral therapy is available. Antibiotics are used for secondary bacterial infections. *Prognosis*: Recovery is generally good with supportive care. *Prevention*: Measles is a vaccine-preventable disease. Immune globulin, administered up to 6 days after exposure, can be helpful in preventing the disease in susceptible persons (immunocompromised children, infants less than 1 year of age, pregnant women). All health care workers should have documented immunity.	■ If the child is hospitalized, maintain airborne precautions during the contagious period. ■ Use a cool-mist vaporizer to help clear respiratory passages. ■ Suction nose and oral cavity very gently as necessary. ■ Give nonaspirin antipyretics for fever and antipruritics for itching. ■ Assess lungs carefully, especially in young children in whom pneumonias are a common complication. ■ Antitussives may be ordered to control coughing. ■ Keep lights dim and cover windows if the child has photophobia. ■ Elevate the head of the bed. Keep the room cool with good air circulation. Provide light and nonirritating blankets.

(continued)

TABLE 15–7 **Selected Infectious and Communicable Diseases in Children** **(continued)**

DISEASE	CLINICAL MANIFESTATIONS	CLINICAL THERAPY	NURSING MANAGEMENT
Measles (Rubeola) **(continued)** until the infant is age 12–15 months. In developing countries, measles remains an endemic disease and is a significant cause of infant and child morbidity and mortality. *Transmission:* Airborne, respiratory droplets and contact with infected persons *Incubation period:* Aproximately 8–12 days *Period of communicability*: Begins 3–5 days before the rash until 4 days after the rash appears	*Complications*: Diarrhea, otitis media, pneumonia, bronchitis, laryngotracheo-bronchitis, encephalitis, and death. Complications and sequelae occur most often in children who are malnourished, medically fragile, and immunosuppressed. The younger the child, the greater the risk for complications.	This is a reportable disease. A total of 37 cases were reported in the United States in 2004, and many were imported from another country or secondary exposures to these infected children (Centers for Disease Control, 2005b).	■ Keep skin clean and dry. No soaps should be used. ■ Maintain fluid intake. Offer cool liquids frequently in small amounts. Blended, pureed, and mashed foods are most easily tolerated. ■ Maintain bedrest. Visitors should be immune to measles. ■ Provide diversions such as music, stories, and favorite toys.
Meningococcus *Causal agent:* *Neisseriameningitides,* a gram-negative diplococcus *Epidemiology:* Most often in winter or early spring. Spread by respiratory droplets from human carriers. Majority of infections in the United States are caused by serogroups B, C, and Y. Highest rates are in children under 2 years and 11 years and older (Bilukha & Rosenstein, 2005). African Americans and persons of low socioeconomic status are at higher risk. Outbreaks have occurred in child care centers, college dormitories, and military recruit camps. *Transmission:* Direct contact with droplet respiratory secretions *Incubation period:* 1–10 days *Period of communicability*: Until 24 hours after antibiotic started	Abrupt onset of flulike symptoms of fever, chills, malaise, muscle aches, vomiting, and prostration (extreme exhaustion). Meningitis neurologic signs include drowsiness, disorientation, hallucinations, and convulsions. Meningococcemia: An urticarial, maculopapular, or petechial rash also appears that may progress to purpura (Figure 15–5 ■). The condition may further deteriorate to shock, hypotension, disseminated intravascular coagulation, and coma. *Complications:* Loss of digits or limbs due to necrosis, hearing loss, arthritis, myocarditis, pericarditis, ataxia, seizures, hemiparesis, cranial nerve palsies, and obstructive hydrocephalus. Up to 10% of children and 25% of adolescents with invasive meningococcal disease die (American Academy of Pediatrics, 2006).	Diagnostic tests include cultures of the blood and cerebrospinal fluid. A Gram stain of petechial skin scrapings may also be done. *Treatment*: Penicillin G is given IV (cefotaxime, ceftriaxone, and ampicillin are alternate antibiotics). Chloramphenicol is used for children allergic to penicillin. The child is managed aggressively in the ICU to maintain the airway, assist ventilation, and manage shock with IV fluids and vasopressors. Plasma, blood, or platelets are used to treat the disseminated intravascular coagulation. *Prevention*: A vaccine has been approved for adolescents 11 years and older. A vaccine is available for children over 2 years old with asplenia and other high-risk conditions. Close contacts are given medication (rifampin, ceftriaxone, or ciprofloxacin) for prophylaxis. Health professionals exposed to oral secretions need prophylaxis (American Academy of Pediatrics, 2006). This is a reportable disease.	■ The child will be hospitalized. Use standard precautions and droplet precautions until the antibiotic has been administered for 24 hours. ■ Disease onset is abrupt and rapidly progresses to life threatening. Be alert for development of shock and respiratory compromise. Have emergency equipment available and be prepared to perform resuscitation. ■ When giving IV fluids and blood products, make sure the child does not get overloaded with fluids, and monitor for evidence of increased intracranial pressure. ■ Keep the family informed of the child's status and treatment as the disease progresses. Help the family to mobilize its support system. ■ The surviving child will likely need rehabilitation. Work with the social worker or case manager to transition the child to long-term care. ■ Help identify close contacts who should receive prophylactic antibiotics and educate them about the expected side effects (e.g., orange urine with rifampin). ■ Teach close contacts to be observant for signs of illness and to seek health care promptly if they occur.

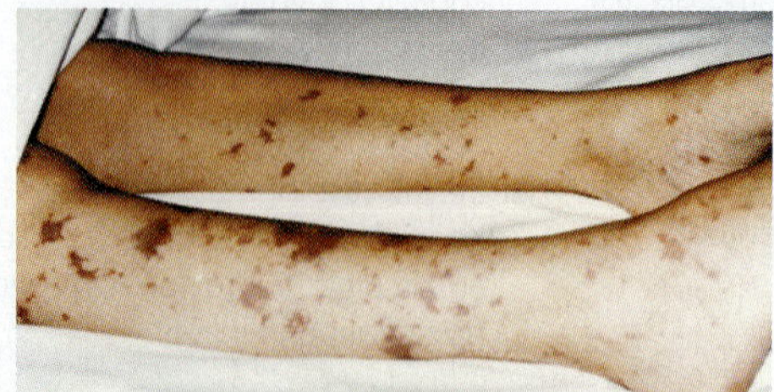

Figure 15–5 ■ Purpura with meningococcemia.

Source: Used with permission of the America Academy of Pediatrics. Retrieved June 20, 2004, from http://www.vaccineinformation.org/photos/variaapoo3.jpg.

TABLE 15–7 **Selected Infectious and Communicable Diseases in Children (continued)**

DISEASE	CLINICAL MANIFESTATIONS	CLINICAL THERAPY	NURSING MANAGEMENT
Mononucleosis *Causal agent*: Epstein-Barr virus (EBV), a member of the herpesvirus group *Epidemiology*: Occurs worldwide in no seasonal pattern. Infection commonly occurs early in life, and it often spreads among family members. *Transmission*: Direct contact with infected oropharyngeal and genital tract secretions. EBV can survive in saliva for several hours outside the body. EBV can also be transmitted by blood transfusion. *Incubation period*: Estimated to be 30–50 days *Period of communicability*: Indeterminate, asymptomatic carriage is common (American Academy of Pediatrics, 2006).	In very young children, mononucleosis can cause irritability, but be otherwise asymptomatic. A maculopapular rash may be seen in a few cases. In other children, the disease is characterized by malaise, headache, anorexia, abdominal pain, fatigue, and fever for 2–3 days, followed by lymphadenopathy and a sore throat. Hepatospleno-megaly can occur. Pain from swelling of the tonsils and lymph nodes may be significant. The syndrome typically lasts 2–3 weeks and is self-limited. Weakness and lethargy may continue for several months. *Complications*: Rare side effects include central nervous system symptoms, such as encephalitis, aseptic meningitis, and Guillain-Barré syndrome. Splenic rupture, respiratory failure, and hematologic complications such as thrombocytopenia can also occur. In immunodeficient children, fatal infections or lymphomas can develop.	Diagnostic tests include the serologic monospot test or a heterophil antibody response test. Greater than 10% atypical lymphocytes and a positive heterophil antibody response test are diagnostic (American Academy of Pediatrics, 2006). Treatment is supportive. Corticosteroids may be used to control tonsillar swelling and pain when there is impending airway obstruction, massive splenomegaly, myocarditis, or hemolytic anemia. Ampicillin and amoxicillin should be avoided, as a nonallergic rash often develops (American Academy of Pediatrics, 2006). *Prognosis*: After recovery, the virus remains latent in the lymphoid system. It can be reactivated during periods of immuno-suppression. *Prevention*: There is no known prevention.	■ Children are usually treated at home. Standard precautions should be used. ■ Give antipyretics and analgesics for fever and sore throat. Offer warm saltwater for gargling. Offer soft foods and encourage fluids. ■ Maintain bedrest during acute phase. ■ Give adolescents a sense of responsibility by involving them in decisions about care whenever possible. Be sure to include parents and adolescents in discussions. ■ Reassure adolescents who may be worried about keeping up with schoolwork that they can return to school when the fever is gone and swallowing is normal. ■ Teens should avoid kissing until the fever has been gone for several days. ■ Contact sports should be avoided until the liver and spleen are normal, usually in about 4 weeks. ■ If splenomegaly is present, alcohol should be avoided for 3 months after liver function test results return to normal.
Mumps (Parotitis)[+] *Causal agent:* Rubulavirus in the Paramyxoviridae family 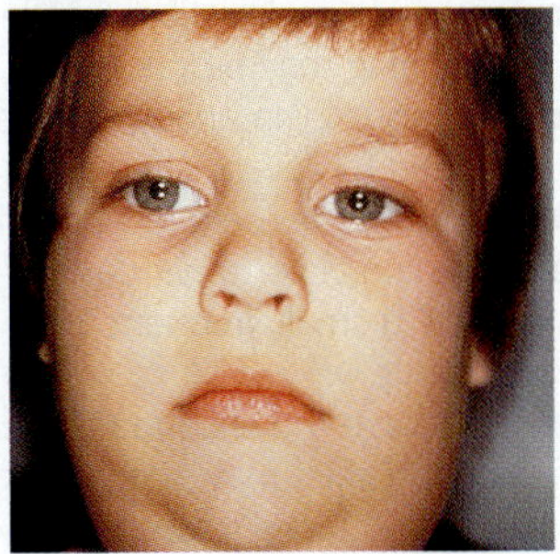 **Figure 15–6** ■ Parotid gland swelling with mumps. *Source:* Courtesy of Centers for Disease Control and Prevention.	Malaise, low-grade fever, earache, headache, pain with chewing, and decreased appetite and activity; followed by bilateral or unilateral parotid gland swelling (Figure 15–6 ■). Swelling peaks around the third day. Meningeal signs (stiff neck, headache, and photophobia) occur in about 15% of clients. *Complications*: Orchitis (inflammation of the epididymis, pain on testicular palpation, and scrotal swelling—most often unilateral) may occur in postpubertal males; sterility is relatively rare (American Academy of Pediatrics, 2006). Oophoritis, pancreatitis, glomerulonephritis, myocarditis, thrombocytopenia, cerebellar ataxia, and hearing impairment are sometimes seen.	Diagnostic tests include a viral culture from a throat washing, urine, or cerebrospinal fluid. Serum mumps IgM antibody titer may also be performed. Therapy is supportive, focused on symptom relief. *Prognosis*: Mumps is usually self-limiting. *Prevention*: Mumps is a vaccine-preventable disease. This is a reportable disease. In 2006 an outbreak of more than 2,500 cases of mumps in 11 states occurred in the United States. The infection was originally imported from Britain (Centers for Disease Control, 2006d).	■ Use standard and droplet precautions for hospitalized children while contagious. ■ Children are usually cared for at home. They are generally uncomfortable, but are rarely very ill. ■ Avoid exposure to immunocompromised or susceptible individuals. ■ Give nonaspirin analgesics and antipyretics to control fever and pain. ■ Encourage fluid intake. Swallowing and chewing may be painful. Offer soft and blended foods. Avoid foods and beverages that increase salivary flow (citrus, spices, and candies), because they cause pain.

(continued)

TABLE 15–7 Selected Infectious and Communicable Diseases in Children (continued)

DISEASE	CLINICAL MANIFESTATIONS	CLINICAL THERAPY	NURSING MANAGEMENT
Mumps (Parotitis) **(continued)** *Epidemiology:* Occurs worldwide in unvaccinated children, most often in winter and spring. Infection and vaccination induce lifelong immunity. Maternal antibodies begin to disappear in infants at the age of 12–15 months. *Transmission:* Contact with respiratory tract secretions *Incubation period:* 12–25 days *Period of communicability:* 1–2 days before parotid swelling until 9 days after swelling occurs			■ Talking may be painful. Provide a bell or other attention-getting device. ■ Apply warm or cool compresses, whichever is preferred, to the parotid area. ■ Be alert for signs of complications. Headache, stiff neck, vomiting, and photophobia may indicate meningeal irritation. ■ Provide scrotal supports if testicular swelling occurs. ■ Reassure children that the facial swelling will go away. ■ Keep children out of school or child care until 9 days after parotid swelling occurs. Encourage diversional activities.
Pertussis (Whooping Cough)[+] *Causal agent:* Bordetella pertussis *Epidemiology:* Occurs worldwide. Most common in children under 6 months of age. Epidemic cycles occur every 3–4 years. Pertussis can occur in health care workers, adolescents, and adults who have waning immunity, and these individuals can spread the disease to unimmunized children. Neither pertussis infection nor vaccine immunity is long lasting (Cherry, 2005). *Transmission:* Respiratory droplets and direct contact with discharge from the respiratory membranes *Incubation period*: 7–10 days *Period of communicability*: Begins about 1 week after exposure. Communicable for 5–7 days after antibiotic therapy is initiated. The disease is most contagious before the paroxysmal cough stage.	The onset is insidious. *Catarrhal stage:* The disease begins with nasal congestion, a runny nose, low-grade fever, and a mild nonproductive cough, lasting about 2 weeks. *Paroxysmal stage:* The cough is more severe at night, with coughing spasms when the child attempts to expel a thick mucoid plug. A forceful inspiration through a narrowed glottis and stridor, or "whooping," follows. Young infants may have apnea rather than the "whooping." Sucking on a bottle may trigger the coughing spell. Coughing may be accompanied by flushing; cyanosis; vomiting; and profuse drainage from the nose, eyes, and mouth. Paroxysmal coughing can last 1–6 weeks or more. Dehydration may result from decreased oral intake. *Convalescent stage:* Up to 6 weeks, when paroxysms gradually subside. Adolescents and adults often have symptoms of an upper respiratory infection with persistent coughing spasms lasting longer than 7 days. *Complications*: Pneumonia, atelectasis, otitis media, encephalopathy, seizures, and death. Highest mortality rate and complication rate is in infants under 1 year.	Diagnostic tests include culture and polymerase chain reaction (PCR) testing. Treatment with macrolide antibiotics (erythromycin, azithromycin, and clarithromycin); corticosteroids, if ordered; and supportive care. *Prognosis*: The disease is most severe in infants under 1 year of age, and most deaths occur in this age group. *Prevention*: Pertussis is a vaccine-preventable disease. Close contacts should be treated with macrolide antibiotics for prophylaxis (Tiwari, Murphy, & Moran, 2005). Vaccine protection wanes after 5–10 years. This is a reportable disease. An estimated 800,000–3.3 million cases occur in the United States per year in a cyclic pattern (Cherry, 2005).	■ Use droplet precautions until 5–7 days after antibiotics are initiated. Most hospitalized cases occur in children under the age of 5 years. ■ Use a cardiac monitor and pulse oximetry to continuously assess respirations and oxygen saturation. The smaller the child, the greater the risk for respiratory distress and apnea. ■ Remain with the child during coughing spells, when hypoxic and apneic episodes are most likely. Give oxygen if ordered. Have emergency equipment available. ■ Provide humidification. Gentle suctioning may be necessary. ■ Give nonaspirin antipyretics as needed for fever. ■ Encourage frequent rest periods. ■ Allow the child to eat desired foods in small, frequent feedings. ■ Encourage the child to take fluids. The child may need IV hydration if oral intake is not tolerated. ■ Provide emotional support to parents. ■ Teach parents to watch for signs of respiratory failure and dehydration if the child is managed at home.

TABLE 15–7 **Selected Infectious and Communicable Diseases in Children (continued)**

DISEASE	CLINICAL MANIFESTATIONS	CLINICAL THERAPY	NURSING MANAGEMENT
Pneumococcal infection[+] *Causative agent: Streptococcus pneumoniae,* a gram-positive diplococcus *Epidemiology*: The organism is found in the nasopharynx of healthy people. Outbreaks occur in the winter and spring among people in crowded settings. In temperate climates, 8 of 90 serotypes account for most of the invasive pediatric infections. The disease is more common in infants, young children, African Americans, Native Americans, and Alaskan Natives. Of particular concern is the development of penicillin- and multi-antibiotic-resistant strains. *Transmission*: Respiratory secretions and droplets *Period of communicability*: Unknown; probably less than 24 hours after beginning effective antibiotic therapy	The signs and symptoms are related to the focal area of infection. The organism causes otitis media, sinusitis, pharyngitis, laryngotracheo-bronchitis, pneumonia, meningitis, and bacteremia. In otitis media, upper respiratory infection, fever, ear pain, and decreased appetite are seen. In bacteremia, there is unexplained fever and no localized infection site. In pneumonia, fever, chills, chest pain, dyspnea, malaise, and a productive cough are seen. In meningitis, inconsolable crying, increased irritability, lethargy, refusal to eat, nausea, vomiting, diarrhea, myalgia, photophobia, and seizures are seen. *Complications*: Prior to the introduction of a vaccine, it caused 30–50% of acute otitis media, and was a major cause of sinusitis, meningitis, bacteremia, and pneumonia (Durbin, 2004). Other complications include septic arthritis, osteomyelitis, endocarditis, and brain abscess.	Diagnostic tests include bacterial culture from site of infection. Symptomatic care is provided. Antibiotic selection is based on susceptibility of organism to penicillin, macrolides, and other agents. Up to 50% of pneumococcal strains are penicillin resistant. Third-generation cephalosporins (cefotaxime or ceftriaxone) may be used. Vancomycin and rifampin are used in combination when strains are resistant to the antibiotics listed above (American Academy of Pediatrics, 2006). *Prevention*: Many serotypes are preventable with immunization. A significant reduction in invasive disease and antibiotic-resistant strains caused by serotypes in the vaccine has occurred since vaccination of infants was initiated (Durbin, 2004).	■ If the child is hospitalized, maintain standard precautions. ■ Provide nonaspirin antipyretics for control of fever and comfort. ■ Encourage fluids, and monitor intake and output. ■ Monitor vital signs and level of consciousness to identify signs of worsening condition. ■ Educate parents about the need for the vaccine, as the unimmunized child could become infected repeatedly with different serotypes. ■ Many children with mild disease are treated at home. Educate parents about signs indicating a need to seek additional medical care, the need for proper medication administration, and comfort measures for the child. ■ Individuals with congenital asplenia or traumatic splenectomy, malignancy, sickle cell disease, and nephrotic syndrome are at higher risk for invasive disease with this organism. ■ Additional factors that increase risk of pneumococcal disease include poverty, crowded housing, homelessness, and exposure to tobacco smoke.
Poliomyelitis[+] *Causal agent:* Poliovirus is an enterovirus with three serotypes. *Epidemiology*: Occurs worldwide. Polio primarily affects children and immuno-compromised or unimmunized adults caring for infants who received live poliovirus vaccine. The vaccine induces lifelong immunity. Since live poliovirus vaccine was discontinued in the United States, no vaccine-associated paralytic poliomyelitis has been reported since 2000 (American Academy of Pediatrics, 2006, p. 543). *Transmission*: Primarily by the fecal-oral route, but also the respiratory route *Incubation period*: Usually 7–10 days (range 3–21 days) *Period of communicability*: Greatest shortly before and right after clinical symptoms develop when the virus is in the throat; excreted in the feces for several weeks	Affects the central nervous system. Less severe infections may be limited to fever and stiffness in the neck and back, headache, vomiting, and sore throat. In other cases, fever, headache, stiff neck, Kernig or Brudzinski sign, decreased deep tendon reflexes, and progressive weakness occur. With cranial nerve involvement, there may be respiratory tract muscle paralysis. An increased respiratory rate may interfere with the ability to talk, because frequent pauses are needed. Onset of paralysis may be sudden, over hours, or gradual over 3–5 days. Paralysis results from damage to motor neurons. *Complications*: Permanent motor paralysis, respiratory arrest, myocardial failure, aseptic meningitis, and postpolio syndrome	Diagnosis is made by cell culture from stool or throat swabs. Treatment is supportive. No chemotherapeutic agents that directly kill the poliovirus are available. *Prognosis*: Respiratory complication is life threatening and involves 5–10% of all cases. Respiratory paralysis can lead to death, and motor paralysis can result in long-term disability. *Prevention*: Poliomyelitis is a vaccine-preventable disease. This is a reportable disease.	■ Use standard and contact precautions in the hospital and keep the child on strict bedrest. ■ Observe closely for respiratory paralysis (ineffective cough, talking with frequent pauses, shallow and rapid respiratory rate). Have emergency equipment at bedside. Assist ventilations as needed until mechanical ventilation is set up. ■ Administer sedatives and nonaspirin analgesics as ordered to allow for rest and comfort. Moist hot packs may relieve discomfort. ■ Encourage fluids. ■ Position the child to promote body alignment. ■ Perform range-of-motion exercises to prevent contractures after the acute phase. ■ Provide emotional support. ■ Clients are alert and aware. Tell them what is happening to them. ■ Long-term orthopedic (physical therapy) support may be needed by some children.

(continued)

TABLE 15–7 Selected Infectious and Communicable Diseases in Children (continued)

DISEASE	CLINICAL MANIFESTATIONS	CLINICAL THERAPY	NURSING MANAGEMENT
Roseola (Exanthem Subitum, Sixth Disease) *Causal agent:* Human herpesvirus type 6 (HHV-6) *Epidemiology:* Occurs worldwide, primarily in children 6–24 months of age (after maternal antibodies decline); no seasonal pattern *Transmission:* Likely to be from respiratory secretions of healthy individuals *Incubation period*: Appears to be 9–10 days *Period of communicability*: Lifelong persistent viral shedding in healthy individuals (American Academy of Pediatrics, 2006)	Sudden, high fever up to 40.5°C (105°F) for 3–8 days, during which the child does not appear toxic (normal appetite and behavior). The fever phase is followed by a characteristic pale pink, discrete, maculopapular rash that starts on the trunk and spreads to the face, neck, and extremities. The rash can last for 1–2 days. The child's appetite is normal. *Complications*: Children may have febrile seizures during high fever stage. Encephalopathy can develop in rare cases.	Roseola is self-limiting, and treatment is supportive. *Prognosis*: Roseola is benign in most cases. Nearly all children over 2 years of age have an antibody titer to HHV-6 (American Academy of Pediatrics, 2006).	■ Children are rarely hospitalized, but if they are, use standard precautions. ■ Give nonaspirin antipyretics to control fever. ■ Observe closely for any seizure activity, especially during the acute febrile periods. ■ Encourage fluids. ■ Reassure parents that the rash will disappear in a few days.
Rotavirus *Causal agent:* Group A, B, and C rotaviruses *Epidemiology:* Occurs during late fall to early spring in yearly diarrhea epidemics in the United States; it is the most common cause of severe diarrhea in children under 5 years. *Transmission:* Fecal-oral route *Incubation:* 2–4 days *Period of communicability:* Virus is present in stool before onset and may persist up to 21 days after onset of symptoms.	Acute onset of low-grade fever and vomiting followed by watery diarrhea 1–2 days later. Up to 10–20 diarrheal stools a day. Symptoms last 3–8 days. *Complications*: Dehydration and electrolyte disturbances. Death occurs in rare circumstances.	Diagnosis is by enzyme immunoassay or latex agglutination assay to detect group A rotavirus antigen. Treatment involves adequate fluid and electrolyte replacement with oral rehydration solution. Introducing a regular diet within a few hours of rehydration shortens the duration of the disease (Dennehy, 2005). In severe dehydration, IV fluid resuscitation is performed. No antiviral therapy is available. *Prevention*: Naturally acquired infection protects against reinfection that causes severe diseases. A new vaccine has been approved for infants.	■ Use standard and contact precautions. ■ Hand hygiene with soap and water removes 75% of virus from contaminated hands. Use of alcohol-based hand sanitizers after washing with soap and water increases effectiveness (Dennehy, 2005). ■ Clean contaminated surfaces followed by disinfection with an alcohol-containing disinfectant (Dennehy, 2005). ■ Assess hydration status frequently. ■ Breastfeeding is continued during oral rehydration therapy. Formula feeding can begin 12–24 hours after oral rehydration therapy is started. ■ Older children can be fed complex carbohydrates and lean meats, yogurt, fruits and vegetables 12–24 hours after oral rehydration therapy is started.
Rubella (German Measles)[+] *Causal agent:* An RNA virus, member of the family Togaviridae, genus *Rubivirus* *Epidemiology:* Occurs worldwide and is most prevalent in the winter and spring. Maternal antibodies disappear about 6–9 months after birth. Most U.S. cases occur among foreign-born children and adults from countries that do not have rubella vaccination programs. Congenital rubella syndrome is thought to occur due to lack of immunization. Four cases were reported from 2001–2004 in	Rubella is generally a mild disease with a characteristic pink, nonconfluent, maculopapular rash. The rash appears on the face; progresses to the neck, trunk, and legs; and disappears in the same order. Prodromal symptoms occur 1–5 days before the rash and include low-grade fever, headache, malaise, coryza, sore throat, and anorexia. Forchheimer spots (discrete, erythematous pinpoint or larger lesions on the soft palate) are seen during the prodromal phase. Generalized lymphadenopathy involving the	Diagnostic tests include cell culture from a nasal swab and detection of IgM or IgG antibodies. Treatment is supportive. Rubella is generally self-limiting in children. *Prognosis*: Disease is usually mild and benign. Major risk is for fetus if the mother is infected in the first trimester. Congenital rubella syndrome is associated with ophthalmologic, cardiac, auditory, and neurologic anomalies.	■ Maintain standard and droplet precautions for contagious children. ■ Maintain contact precautions for infants with congenital rubella syndrome until 1 year of age unless nasopharyngeal and urine cultures are repeatedly negative after 3 months of age (American Academy of Pediatrics, 2006). ■ Children are usually treated at home. They should be isolated from pregnant women.

(continued)

TABLE 15–7 **Selected Infectious and Communicable Diseases in Children (continued)**

DISEASE	CLINICAL MANIFESTATIONS	CLINICAL THERAPY	NURSING MANAGEMENT
Rubella (German Measles) **(continued)** the United States (Centers for Disease Control, 2005a). *Transmission:* Droplet spread, direct contact with infected persons, or contact with articles soiled by nasal secretions *Incubation period:* 14–21 days (most commonly 16–18 days) *Period of communicability:* Seven days before until 7 days after the onset of rash. Infants with congenital rubella may shed the virus for months after birth.	postauricular, suboccipital, and posterior cervical areas is common up to 7 days before the rash. Many cases are asymptomatic. Neonatal signs of congenital rubella syndrome include growth retardation, radiolucent bone disease, hepatosplenomegaly, thrombocytopenia, and purpuric skin lesions (giving a "blueberry muffin" appearance) (Figure 15–7 ■). *Complications*: Complications are rare, but include arthritis in adolescents, and encephalitis.	*Prevention*: Rubella is a vaccine-preventable disease. Females of childbearing age need to be immunized to reduce the risk for congenital rubella syndrome. All health care workers should have documented immunity. 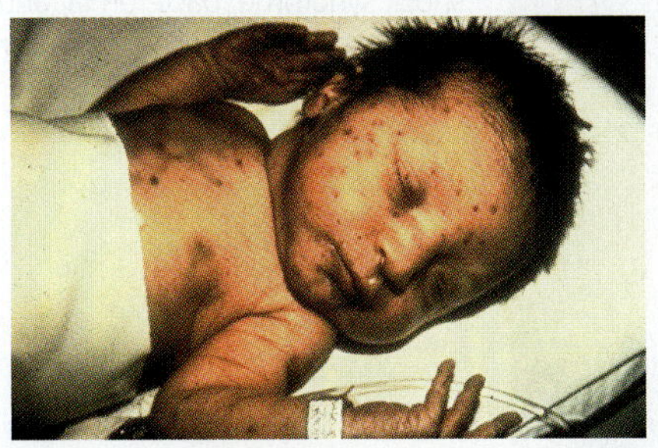 **Figure 15–7** ■ "Blueberry muffin" appearance in infant with congenital rubella syndrome. *Source:* Courtesy of Centers for Disease Control and Prevention.	■ Give nonaspirin analgesics and antipyretics for any pain and fever. ■ Allow children to choose what they would like to eat and drink. Encourage fluids. ■ Provide quiet activities. ■ Exclude children from child care or school for 7 days after onset of rash. School and child care facilities should be notified of the child's illness.
Streptococcus A *Causal agent*: Group A streptococci (GAS) *Epidemiology:* The illness is caused by various M-protein groups of group A beta-hemolytic streptococci. Different strains are associated with pharyngeal and pyodermal infections, and also rheumatic fever and acute glomerulonephritis (American Academy of Pediatrics, 2006). Pharyngeal infections tend to occur more in late fall, winter, and spring. Pyodermal infections tend to occur in warmer seasons because of the association with minor skin trauma and insect bites. *Transmission:* Contact with respiratory secretions for pharyngitis or skin lesions for pyoderma *Incubation period*: Pharyngeal: usually 2–5 days; Pyodermal: usually 7–10 days	*Pharyngeal:* Abrupt onset with a sore throat, dysphagia, malaise, high fever, chills, headache, abdominal pain, anorexia, and vomiting. A beefy red pharynx with exudate (strep throat) and tender cervical nodes are seen. Palatal petechiae may be seen. Cough and rhinitis are absent in most cases. *GAS respiratory tract infection:* Children under 3 years may develop serous rhinitis and a respiratory illness with moderate fever, irritability, and anorexia rather than pharyngitis. *Scarlet fever:* A characteristic erythematous, "sandpaper" rash that blanches with pressure appears in some cases 12–48 hours after onset of symptoms, concentrates in flexor skin creases, and spares the circumoral area. In 3–4 days, the rash begins to fade, and the tips of the toes and fingers begin to peel. The classic strawberry tongue is seen on days 4–5.	Diagnosis can be made by a rapid strep antigen test or culture of secretions from the pharynx and tonsils. Cultures of skin lesions are not indicated (American Academy of Pediatrics, 2006). Prompt antibiotic treatment is effective. Penicillin V is the drug of choice. Erythromycin is used if the child is allergic to penicillin. Uncomplicated impetigo is treated with mupirocin ointment. Invasive strains causing necrotizing fasciitis or myositis need IV antibiotics and surgical intervention (exploration and debridement of dead tissue). *Prognosis:* Recovery is usually good with antibiotic therapy. Up to 15% of healthy children become chronic carriers (American Academy of Pediatrics, 2006).	■ Children with uncomplicated infections are usually cared for at home. ■ Promote bedrest during the febrile stage. ■ Give nonaspirin antipyretics to control fever. Teach parents important signs of a worsening condition. ■ For pharyngeal infections, offer warm saltwater for gargling, a soft diet, and nonacidic beverages. Encourage fluids. Provide cool, clear liquids. Swallowing may be difficult. ■ Explain to parents the importance of giving the child the full course of antibiotics. ■ Encourage family members with sore throats to have throat cultures taken. ■ For impetigo, teach the parents to wash the skin, remove crusts, and apply antibiotic ointment. ■ If the child is hospitalized, maintain droplet precautions for pharyngeal infections and contact precautions for skin lesions for 24 hours after beginning antibiotics. Monitor vital signs, especially temperature. Administer antibiotics as ordered.

(continued)

TABLE 15–7 **Selected Infectious and Communicable Diseases in Children (continued)**

DISEASE	CLINICAL MANIFESTATIONS	CLINICAL THERAPY	NURSING MANAGEMENT
***Streptococcus A* (continued)** *Period of communicability:* Four weeks in untreated pharyngeal infections; noncontagious within 24 hours of starting antibiotics 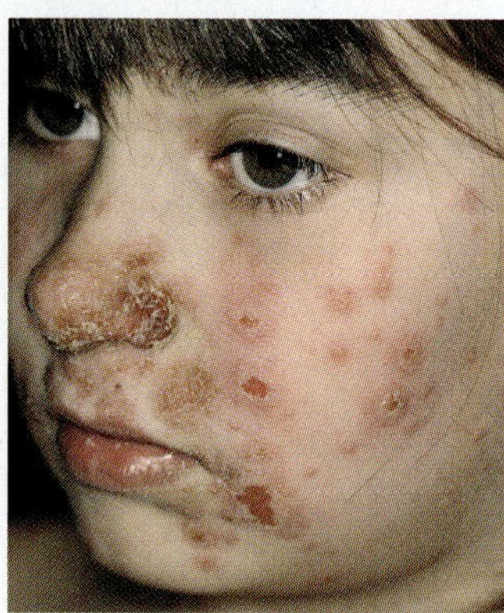 Figure 15–8 ■ Impetigo.	*Pyodermal:* Lesions (impetigo) are honey-colored crusts at the site of open lesions (Figure 15–8 ■). *Complications:* If untreated, acute otitis media, sinusitis, peritonsillar or retropharyngeal abscess, cervical lymphadenitis, acute rheumatic fever, acute glomerulonephritis occur. Invasive disease with toxic shock syndrome, bacteremia, and necrotizing fasciitis or myositis can be fatal.	*Prevention*: None	■ If the child develops invasive streptococcal infection, use standard precautions. The child with toxic shock syndrome will need intensive care to manage shock and fluid and electrolyte imbalances.
Tetanus *Causal agent: Clostridium tetani* or tetanus bacillus *Epidemiology:* The bacillus is common and exists as a spore in soil, dust, and animal excretions. The organism produces an endotoxin that affects the central nervous system. *Transmission:* The organism is transmitted to humans through puncture wounds or broken skin. Newborns can acquire tetanus via the umbilical cord if they are born in an unclean area, a contaminated implement is used to cut the cord, or clay is applied to the umbilical cord as a ritual in some Middle Eastern cultures. *Incubation period:* 3 days to 3 weeks (average 8 days) *Period of communicability:* Not communicable to other individuals except through skin wounds	Stiffness of the neck and jaw, with painful facial spasms and difficulty chewing and swallowing over a few days, and headache. Noise and sudden movements can stimulate spasms. Spasms of facial muscles may produce a grinning expression (risus sardonicus). Localized prolonged and painful muscle contraction may occur at the site of the wound. Eventually rigidity of the abdomen and trunk produce *opisthotonos* (rigid hyperextension of the entire body). Spasms and fever occur, along with difficulty swallowing the increased oral secretions. Respiratory muscles can be affected and cause airway obstruction and suffocation. Newborns have difficulty with sucking, progressing to an inability to suck, irritability, and nuchal rigidity. *Complications:* Laryngospasm, respiratory distress, or death	Tetanus immune globulin is given to unimmunized persons as soon as possible. Tetanus toxoid is given at the same time at a separate site. Medications are provided to treat muscle spasms. Intensive care is provided with cardiorespiratory monitoring, assisted ventilation, IV metronidazole or penicillin G, nutrition, and supportive care. Wound cleansing and debriding are performed. Survival beyond 4 days indicates an increased chance of recovery. Paroxysms become less frequent, and complete recovery may take weeks. *Prognosis:* 30% mortality; much higher in newborns. Intensive care has improved mortality. *Prevention:* Tetanus is a vaccine-preventable disease. Tetanus boosters are updated every 10 years, or, if a potentially contaminated wound occurs, in 5 years. Proper surgical debridement of wounds decreases the chance of infection.	■ Prevent disease by checking immunization records and administering immunizations as necessary. ■ Give immune globulin to unimmunized persons. ■ Assist with wound debridement. ■ Use standard precautions, as the child with tetanus is hospitalized. ■ Monitor the child's condition. Handle as little as possible. Reduce stimulation by placing the child in a quiet, darkened room. ■ Offer skin and respiratory care. The child may need an endotracheal tube, suctioning, and supplemental oxygen for airway support. ■ Provide feedings via total parenteral nutrition or feeding tube. ■ Maintain hydration with intravenous fluids and electrolytes. ■ Try to reduce the child's anxiety, as mental status may be unaffected. ■ Prepare the family for a possible poor prognosis.

Note: *Indicates that a vaccine or antitoxin is available for use in high-risk or as-needed situations. +Indicates that the disease has a safe and effective vaccine.

ALTERATIONS AND TREATMENTS **Infections**

The following summary table includes the most frequent infectious illnesses or diseases with which a nurse may come in contact. Others include, but are not limited to, bacterial meningitis, bacterial endocarditis, giardiasis, Chlamydia, tetanus, streptococcus A, shigella, hepatitis, and HIV.

Alteration	Description	Treatment
Cellulitis	Acute bacterial infection of the dermis and underlying connective tissue	■ Antibiotics ■ Antipyretics ■ Palliative care ■ Fluid administration
Urinary tract infection	Infection of any part of the urinary tract: kidneys, ureters, urinary bladder, or urethra	■ Antibiotics per culture results ■ Antipyretics ■ Fluid management
Viral pneumonia	Infection of the lung, often causing fluid accumulation in one or more lobe	■ Treatment based on symptoms ■ Cough suppressant, expectorant ■ Rest ■ Encouraging breathing ■ Support for respiratory effort may include oxygen, Fowler's position, respiratory toilet
Otitis Media	Inflammation of the middle ear	■ Palliative care ■ Antibiotics only if symptoms do not resolve after 48–72 hours
Influenza	Highly contagious viral respiratory disease	■ Antipyretics ■ Rest ■ Fluid management ■ Monitor for respiratory rate, pattern, and effective airway clearance ■ Antiviral medications can reduce duration and severity of symptoms ■ Prevention through vaccination of at-risk individuals
Conjunctivitis	Highly contagious inflammation of the conjunctiva	■ Antibiotics ■ Palliative care
Tuberculosis	Chronic, recurrent infectious disease caused by *Mycobacterium tuberculosis*	■ Fluid management ■ Monitoring vital signs, especially temperature, frequently ■ Administering antipyretics and analgesics ■ Antitubercular medications ■ Respiratory support as dictated by symptoms ■ Isolation
Sepsis	Whole body inflammatory process resulting in acute critical illness	■ Reverse underlying cause ■ Protect respiratory and cardiovascular systems ■ Fluid management ■ Monitor neurologic status, vital signs

ASSESSMENT

During the assessing phase of the nursing process, the nurse obtains the client's history, conducts the physical assessment, and gathers laboratory data.

Nursing History

During the nursing history, the nurse assesses the degree to which a client is at risk for developing an infection and any client complaints suggesting the presence of an infection. To identify clients at risk, the nurse reviews the client's chart and structures the nursing interview to collect data regarding the factors that influence the development of infection, especially existing disease process, history of recurrent infections, current medications and therapeutic measures, current emotional stressors, nutritional status, and history of immunizations (see the following Assessment Interview).

Physical Assessment

Signs and symptoms of an infection vary according to the body area involved. For example, sneezing, watery, or mucoid discharge from the nose and nasal stuffiness commonly occur with

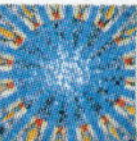

EVIDENCE-BASED PRACTICE **Medicating for Fever**

A recent study in Israel of 464 children ages 6–36 months compared the treatment of fever with acetaminophen (12.5 mg/kg) every 6 hours, ibuprofen (5 mg/kg) every 8 hours, and alternating doses of acetaminophen (12.5 mg/kg) and ibuprofen (5 mg/kg) every 4 hours. The group of children receiving the alternating therapy had a more rapid reduction of fever and a lower mean temperature than the two other groups (Sarrell, Wielunsky, & Cohen, 2006). This study did not effectively compare alternating doses of antipyretics with single antipyretics because the alternating medications were given more frequently than the single medication, and more antipyretic medication was in the bloodstream at one time. More study is needed before parents are routinely encouraged to alternate acetaminophen and ibuprofen for treating a fever.

an infection of the nose and sinuses, and urinary frequency and cloudy or discolored urine often occur with a urinary infection. Commonly, the skin and mucous membranes are involved in a local infectious process, resulting in the following:

- Localized swelling
- Localized redness
- Pain or tenderness with palpation or movement
- Palpable heat at the infected area
- Loss of function of the body part affected, depending on the site and extent of involvement.

In addition, open wounds may exude drainage of various colors. Signs of systemic infection include the following:

- Fever
- Increased pulse and respiratory rate if the fever is high
- Malaise and loss of energy
- Loss of appetite and, in some situations, nausea and vomiting
- Enlargement and tenderness of lymph nodes that drain the area of infection.

Table 15–8 lists the clinical manifestation of infection in infants and children by body system.

TABLE 15–8 Clinical Manifestation of Infection in Infants and Children

BODY SYSTEM	INFANTS	CHILDREN
Central nervous system	Irritable	Irritable or combative
	Decreased responsiveness	Stiff neck
	Lethargy	Back pain
	Bulging anterior fontanel	Decreased responsiveness
	High-pitched cry	Photophobia
	Muscle weakness	Brudzinski sign
	Additional Signs in Newborns:	Kernig sign
	Seizures	Malaise
	Subtle changes in muscle tone or hypotonia	
Cardiovascular system	Tachycardia	Tachycardia
	Decreased perfusion	Decreased perfusion
	Weak peripheral pulses	Weak peripheral pulses
	Pallor or mottled skin	Pallor or flushed, dry skin
	Flushed, dry skin	Delayed capillary refill time
	Delayed capillary refill time	
	Additional Signs in Newborns:	
	Cyanosis	
	Hypotension	
	Bradycardia	
Respiratory system	Tachypnea	Tachypnea
	Increased work of breathing with retractions, nasal flaring	Dyspnea

TABLE 15–8 Clinical Manifestation of Infection in Infants and Children (continued)

BODY SYSTEM	INFANTS	CHILDREN
	Crackles	Retractions
	Cough	Nasal flaring
	Stridor	Crackles
	Decreased oxygen saturation	Cough
	Irregular breathing	Stridor
	Additional Signs in Newborns:	Decreased oxygen saturation
	Apnea (new onset or increased episodes)	
	Increased or new-onset oxygen requirement	
	Grunting	
Gastrointestinal system	Vomiting	Nausea and vomiting
	Diarrhea	Diarrhea
	Abdominal distention	Abdominal discomfort
	Poor feeding	Abdominal distention
	Additional Signs in Newborns:	Poor appetite
	Abdominal wall discoloration	
	Paralytic ileus	
	Bloody stool	
	Jaundice or hepatosplenomegaly	
Renal system	WBCs and bacteria in urine	WBCs and bacteria in urine
	Additional Signs in Newborns:	
	Decreased urine output	
	Hematuria, proteinuria	
Hematopoietic system	Neutropenia	Leukocytosis
	Increased immature WBCs (bands) in bacterial infections	Increased immature WBCs (bands) in bacterial infections
	Lymphocytosis in viral infections	Lymphocytosis in viral infections
	Additional Signs in Newborns:	
	Fraction of band cells >0.2	
	Thrombocytopenia	
Metabolic system	Hyperthermia or hypothermia	Hyperthermia
	Hypoglycemia or hyperglycemia	Chills
		Hypothermic in septic shock
Other systems	Rash	Rash
	Dry mucous membranes	Petechiae and/or purpura
	Poor skin turgor	Dry mucous membranes
	Sunken anterior fontanel	Poor skin turgor
	Petechiae and/or purpura	

Assessment Interview Client at Risk for Infections

- When were you last immunized for diphtheria, tetanus, poliomyelitis, rubella, measles, influenza, hepatitis, and pneumococcal pneumonia?
- When did you last have a tuberculin skin test?
- What infections have you had in the past, and how were these treated?
- Have any of these infections recurred?
- Are you taking any antibiotics, anti-inflammatory medications such as aspirin or ibuprofen, or medications for cancer?
- Have you had any recent diagnostic procedure or therapy that penetrated your skin or a body cavity?
- What past surgeries have you had?
- How would you describe your eating habits? Do you eat a variety of types of foods?
- Do you take vitamins?
- On a scale of 1–10, how would you rate the stress you have experienced in the past 6 months?
- Have you experienced any loss of energy, loss of appetite, nausea, headache, or other signs associated with specific body systems (e.g., difficulty urinating, urinary frequency, or a sore throat)?

Note: As with all history taking, the nurse must individualize the specific terms used, examples given to the client, and teaching techniques used to validate agreement on the meaning of words according to the client's culture, language spoken, and education or intellectual abilities.

DIAGNOSTIC TESTS

To assess the client's response to infection, identify the infecting organism, and monitor the progress of therapy, the following diagnostic tests may be ordered:

- *WBC count* provides clues about the infecting organism and the body's immune response to it (Table 15–9).
- *WBC differential* is also ordered (see Table 15–9). Neutrophilia, or increased numbers of circulating neutrophils (or PMNs), is a common response to infection, as the bone marrow responds to an increased need for phagocytes. Along with neutrophilia, a shift to the left is common in acute infection. This means that there are more immature neutrophils in circulation than normal (Figure 15–9 ■), indicating an appropriate bone marrow response.
- *Procalcitonin (CTpr)* is a precursor of the hormone calcitonin. Procalcitonin increases dramatically during infection and sepsis, and is accepted as both a marker of sepsis and a harmful mediator in lower respiratory tract and systemic infections (Christ-Crain et al., 2004; Müller & Becker, 2001).
- ***Cultures*** *of the wound, blood, or other infected body fluids* are used to identify probable microorganisms by their characteristics, such as shape, growth patterns, and Gram-staining qualities. After the organism is cultured, it is subjected to various antibiotics known to be effective against its particular strain to determine which antibiotic is likely to be most effective. This is known as sensitivity testing. Generally, 24–48 hours are required to grow the organism, potentially delaying initiation of therapy. Because antibiotics (and possibly oxygen therapy) can alter the ability to culture an organism, specimens should be obtained before instituting therapy.

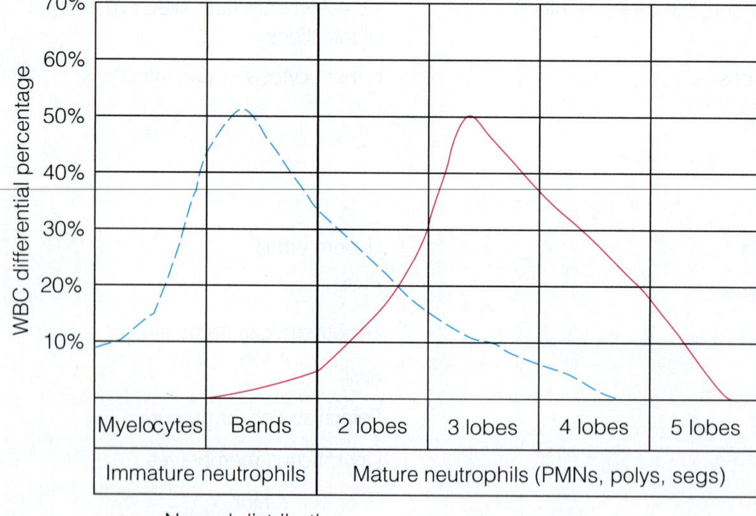

Type of WBC	Normal differential	Shift to left
Myelocytes	0%	Present
Band neutrophils (bands)	3–5%	Increased
Segmented neutrophils (segs, polys, PMNs)	50–65%	May be stable, increased, or decreased

Figure 15–9 ■ Neutrophils by stage of maturity and normal distribution in the blood.

TABLE 15–9 **White Blood Cell Count and Differential**

CELL TYPE AND NORMAL VALUE	INCREASED	DECREASED
Total WBCs: 4,000–10,000 per mm^3	*Leukocytosis:* Infection or inflammation, leukemia, trauma or stress, tissue necrosis	*Leukopenia:* Bone marrow depression, overwhelming infection, viral infections, immunosuppression, autoimmune disease, dietary deficiency
Neutrophils (segs, PMNs, or polys): 55–70%	*Neutrophilia:* Acute infection or stress response, myelocytic leukemia, inflammatory or metabolic disorders	*Neutropenia:* Bone marrow depression, overwhelming bacterial infection, viral infection, Addison's disease
Eosinophils (eos): 1–4%	*Eosinophilia:* Parasitic infections, hypersensitivity reactions, autoimmune disorders	*Eosinopenia:* Cushing's syndrome, autoimmune disorders, stress, certain drugs
Basophils (basos): 0.5–1%	*Basophilia:* Hypersensitivity responses, chronic myelogenous leukemia, chickenpox or smallpox, splenectomy, hypothyroidism	*Basopenia:* Acute stress or hypersensitivity reactions, hyperthyroidism
Monocytes (monos): 2–8%	*Monocytosis:* Chronic inflammatory disorders, tuberculosis, viral infections, leukemia, Hodgkin's disease, multiple myeloma	*Monocytopenia:* Bone marrow depression, corticosteroid therapy
Lymphocytes (lymphs): 20–40%	*Lymphocytosis:* Chronic bacterial infection, viral infections, lymphocytic leukemia	*Lymphocytopenia:* Bone marrow depression, immunodeficiency, leukemia, Cushing's syndrome, Hodgkin's disease, renal failure

Source: Data from Corbett, J. V. (2004). *Laboratory tests and diagnostic procedures with nursing diagnoses* (6th ed.). Upper Saddle River, NJ: Prentice Hall; and Pagana, K. D., & Pagana, T. J. (1997). *Diagnostic and laboratory test reference* (3rd ed.). St. Louis, MO: Mosby-Year Book.

- *Serologic testing* provides an indirect means of identifying infecting agents by detecting antibodies to the suspected organism. When the antibody titer against a specific organism rises during the acute phase of an infectious disease and begins to fall during convalescence, the diagnosis is supported. Although it is not as accurate as culture, serology is particularly useful for organisms that cannot easily be cultured, such as hepatitis B and HIV (Porth, 2005).
- *Direct antigen detection methods* are in the process of being developed. These tests use monoclonal antibodies, which are purified antibody forms, to detect antigens in specimens from a diseased host (Porth, 2005). See Box 15–3. These tests offer rapid and accurate identification of the offending microorganism.
- *Antibiotic peak and trough levels* monitor therapeutic blood levels of the prescribed medication(s). The therapeutic range, that is, the minimum and maximum blood levels at which the drug is effective, is known for a given drug. By measuring blood levels at the predicted peak (1–2 hours after oral administration, 1 hour after intramuscular administration, and 30 minutes after intravenous administration) and trough (lowest level, usually a few minutes before the next scheduled dose), health care personnel can determine that the client is maintaining a level within the therapeutic range at all times, ensuring maximal effect from the drug. Measuring blood levels of a prescribed medication also helps determine whether the drug is reaching a toxic or harmful level during therapy, an unintended result that can increase the likelihood of adverse effects.
- *Radiologic examination of the chest, abdomen, or urinary system* may be ordered to detect organ abnormalities that indicate an inflammatory response or tissue damage.
- *Lumbar puncture* is performed to obtain cerebrospinal fluid (CSF) for examination and culture if a central nervous system (CNS) infection, such as meningitis or encephalitis, is suspected.
- *Ultrasonic examination, such as an echocardiogram or renal ultrasonography,* is a noninvasive diagnostic test to evaluate organ function.
- *Urinalysis* is a noninvasive test to assess for the presence of bacteria or blood in the urine.

CARING INTERVENTIONS

The goals of care for the client with an infection are to identify the organ system affected by the infection, identify the causative agent, and achieve a cure by the least toxic, least expensive, and most effective means. Fortunately, most infectious diseases are self-limiting and will resolve with little or no medical care. However, medical treatment may be required for an overwhelming infection or immunocompromised host.

The body part or organ system affected by the infection is often obvious from the client's history and presenting signs and symptoms. Identifying the system allows the range of possible infecting organisms to be narrowed to those known to affect that system. The manner of presentation provides further clues as to the diagnosis. For example,

Box 15–3 Monoclonal Antibodies

Antigens typically have numerous antigenic determinant sites, each capable of stimulating a different subset of B cells. Each clone secretes a slightly different antibody from the others. The resulting immunoglobulin produced is therefore *polyclonal,* with multiple different antibodies. In 1975, researchers devised a technique for making a single clone of "immortal" B cells that could be maintained indefinitely in a laboratory and would produce a single antibody to a specific antigen (see Figure 15–10 ■). This pure antibody, known as a *monoclonal* antibody, offers the following advantages:

- It can target specific antigens.
- It has a single, constant binding affinity for the antigen.
- It can be diluted to a specific titer or concentration, because it is not mixed with other antibodies.
- It can be purified to avoid adverse responses (McCance & Huether, 2002).

In addition to providing passive protection from disease, monoclonal antibodies are being used in a variety of other ways, including the diagnosis and treatment of cancer, immunosuppression to prevent rejection of transplanted tissue or organs, immune response analysis, imaging techniques for diagnostic uses, and the early detection of viral infections (Lehne, 2004; McCance & Huether, 2002).

Source: Figure adapted from Becker, W., & Deane, D. (1986). *The world of the cell.* Redwood City, CA: Benjamin Cummings; Mahon, C. R., & Manuselis, G. Jr. (1995). *Textbook of diagnostic microbiology.* Philadelphia: W.B. Saunders. Reprinted with permission.

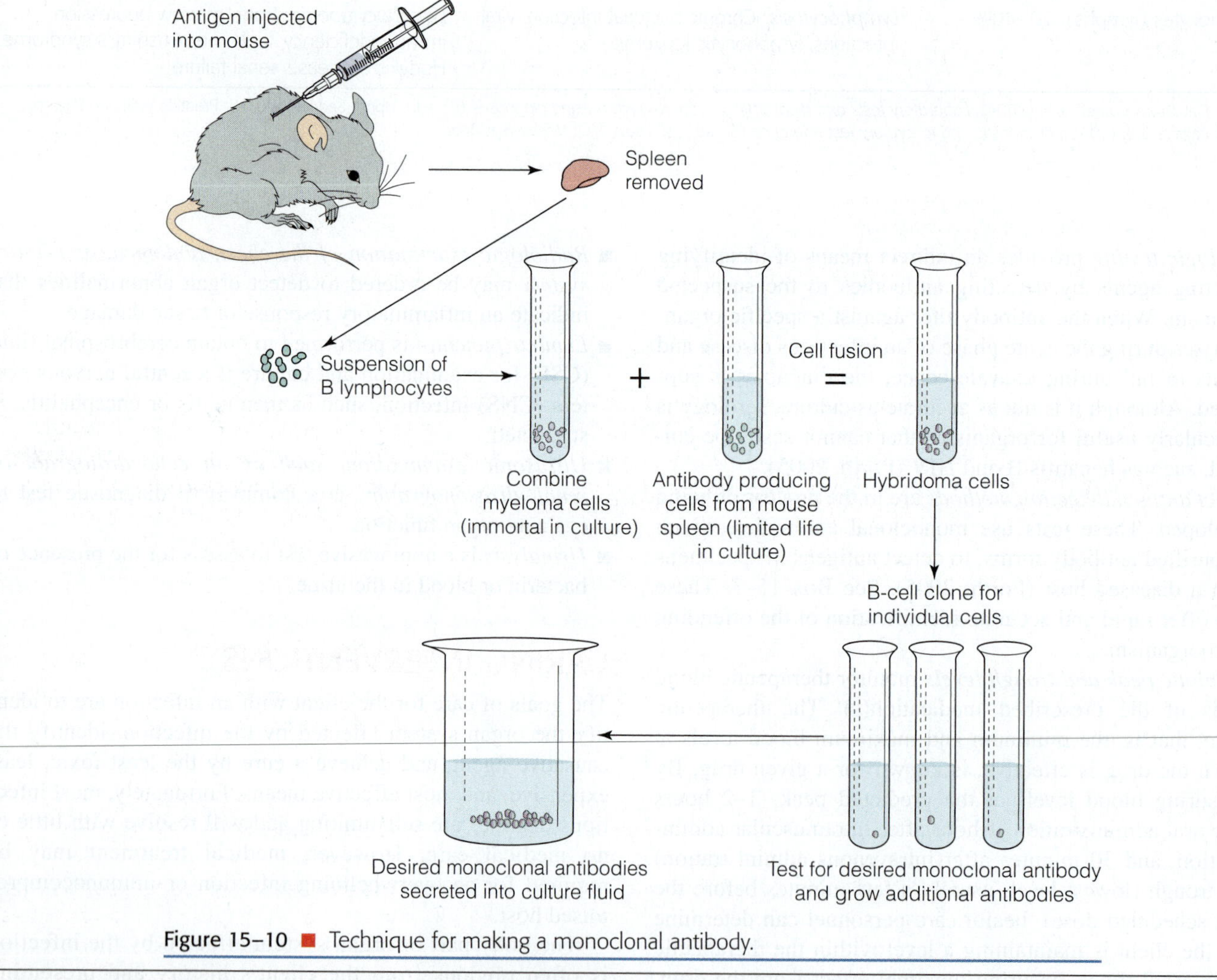

Figure 15–10 ■ Technique for making a monoclonal antibody.

pneumococcal pneumonia typically presents with the acute onset of chills, fever, and cough in a previously healthy adult, whereas a client with viral pneumonia relates a gradual onset of symptoms, with systemic manifestations such as muscle aches and headache often predominant. A history of recent activities also provides clues. Family members who all vomit and have diarrhea within 12 hours after a picnic probably do not have the flu.

Once the infecting agent has been identified, either positively or by probability, therapy can be specifically tailored to the client's needs. Viral infections often resolve without treatment other than supportive care, such as providing rest and fluids.

Skin infections may respond to a topical agent, avoiding the potential adverse effects of one administered systemically.

All skills and treatments, whether administering medications (see the following Medications feature) or preparing a client for discharge, are performed in a manner that prevents possible infection of clients. Some skills are specific to preventing infection, diagnosing infection, and treating the client with a diagnosed infection. Nursing skills used in preventing infection and caring for clients diagnosed with infection can be found in the skills manual and include the following:

- Hand hygiene
- Basic medical asepsis
- Use of standard precautions
- Isolation techniques
- Sterile field
- Culture specimen collection
- Use of personal protective equipment and decontamination.

MEDICATIONS Antimicrobial Agents

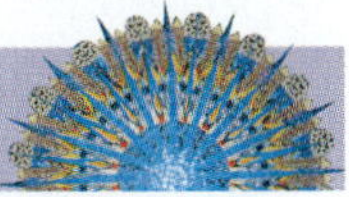

Once the infecting organism and affected body system have been identified, specific therapy to cure the infectious disease can begin. The number of antimicrobial agents available makes choosing the appropriate one seem overwhelming. The perfect anti-infective agent would destroy pathogens while preserving host cells, be effective against many organisms while not promoting the development of resistance, distribute to necessary tissues, and remain in the body for relatively long periods.

Because no available antimicrobial meets all these criteria, physicians look for an agent that will be effective, has little toxicity, can be administered with relative convenience, and is cost effective. Characteristics of both the host and the infecting organism are considered in making the selection.

Classification	Mechanism of Action	Generic Drug Examples	Nursing Considerations
Antibiotics ■ Amino-glycosides ■ Macrolides ■ Tetracyclines ■ Cephalosporins ■ Penicillins ■ Sulfonamides ■ Fluoro-quinolones	May be used prophylactically to prevent infection or treat existing bacterial infection. Specific antibiotic is chosen based on pathogen causing infection.	Cefaclor, erythromycin, penicillin, tobramycin, trimethoprim-sulfamethoxazole	■ Teach clients importance of taking the entire prescribed amount. ■ Encourage adequate fluid intake. ■ Monitor for signs of allergic reaction. ■ Assess renal and hepatic function and vital signs.
Antifungal	Selective for fungal plasma membranes, they inhibit ergosterol synthesis.	Amphotericin B, anidulafungin, caspofungin acetate, flucytosine, micafungin, fluconazole, nystatin	■ Carefully monitor client's condition. ■ Use cautiously in clients with renal impairment, severe bone marrow suppression, and pregnancy. ■ Closely monitor kidney function (intake and output, BUN, creatine, daily weights). ■ Monitor serum electrolytes.
Antipyretic/Analgesic	Relieves pain and reduces fever.	Acetaminophen	■ Monitor temperature. ■ Assess pain level. ■ Teach proper administration.
Antipyretic, Analgesic, Anti-inflammatory	Reduces fever and inflammation, in addition to relieving pain.	Aspirin, ibuprofen	■ Monitor temperature. ■ Assess pain level. ■ Teach proper administration.
Antimalaria	Interrupts the complex life-cycle of plasmodium, with greater success early in the course of the disease.	Atovaquone, proguanil, chloro-quine, hydroxychloro-quine sulfate, mefloquine, primaquine phosphate, pyrimethamine, quinine	■ Carefully monitor client's condition. ■ Provide education about prescribed drug treatment. ■ Contraindicated in clients with hematological disorders or severe skin disorders such as psoriasis, and during pregnancy. ■ Assess lab results (complete blood cell count [CBC], liver and renal function tests, G5PD deficiency). ■ Obtain a baseline electrocardiogram. ■ Monitor for gastrointestinal side effects and changes in cardiac rhythm.

(continued)

MEDICATIONS Antimicrobial Agents (continued)

Classification	Mechanism of Action	Generic Drug Examples	Nursing Considerations
Antihelminthic	Is targeted at killing the parasites locally in the intestine and systemically in the tissues and organs they have invaded.	Albendazole, diethyl-carbamazine, ivermectin, mebendazole, praziquantel, pyrantel	■ Monitor vital signs, CBC, and liver function studies after obtaining a baseline. ■ Specific worm or parasite must be identified before initiating therapy. ■ Educate on nature of parasite infestation to prevent future reinfestation. ■ Warn clients if bowel elimination of worm is anticipated. ■ Assess for GI symptoms. ■ Monitor for CNS side effects.
Antiretroviral ■ Nonnucleoside reverse transcriptase inhibitors ■ Nucleoside and nucleotide reverse transcriptase inhibitors ■ Protease inhibitors ■ Fusion and integrase inhibitors	Target specific phases of the HIV replication cycle, requiring multiple drugs taken concurrently.	Delavirdine, efavirenz, abacavir, didanosine, amprenavir, atazanavir, darunavir, enfuvirtide, raltegravir, acyclovir, cidofovir, docosanol, idoxuridine, penciclovir	■ Clients require extensive teaching regarding pharmacotherapy, disease process, and prevention of contaminating others. ■ Psychosocial issues must be addressed to improve compliance with treatment regimen. ■ Use nonjudgmental approach. ■ Assess for side effects that can dramatically affect the client's life. ■ Assess T-cell count and client response to pharmacotherapy.

15.1 CELLULITIS

KEY TERMS

Cellulitis, *808*
Erythema, *808*
Inflammation, *808*
Lymphadenopathy, *808*
Lymphangitis, *810*
Septicemia, *809*
Tinea pedis, *809*
White blood cell, *808*

BASIS FOR SELECTION OF EXEMPLAR

Centers for Disease Control and Prevention
Joint Commission
Institute for Healthcare Improvement

LEARNING OUTCOMES

After reading about this exemplar, you will be able to:

1. Describe the pathophysiology, etiology, and clinical manifestations of cellulitis.
2. Identify the risk factors associated with cellulitis.
3. Illustrate the nursing process in providing culturally competent care across the life span for individuals with cellulitis.
4. Formulate priority nursing diagnoses appropriate for an individual with cellulitis.
5. Create a plan of care for an individual with cellulitis.
6. Employ evidence-based caring interventions (or prevention) for an individual with cellulitis.
7. Assess expected outcomes for an individual with cellulitis.
8. Discuss therapies used in the collaborative care of an individual with cellulitis.

OVERVIEW

Infection can occur in a small localized area, affect an entire organ system, or attack the entire body, as in the case of septicemia. Cellulitis is an example of an infection that can be small and well contained, but, if not treated promptly, it can develop into a life-threatening septicemia.

Cellulitis is an acute bacterial infection of the dermis and underlying connective tissue. It is characterized by red or lilac, tender, warm, edematous skin that may have an ill-defined, nonelevated border. Cellulitis usually occurs on the face and lower extremities as a result of trauma or a compromised skin barrier. Its chief symptom is **inflammation**, which includes intense pain, heat, redness, and swelling. It may appear in a localized area as a complication of a wound infection, or it may involve an entire limb. In severe infections, fever may be present, as well as an increase in **white blood cells** (WBCs) and tender lymph nodes (**lymphadenopathy**). Elevated WBCs and fever, although common signs of infection, may not be present in frail, older clients.

PATHOPHYSIOLOGY AND ETIOLOGY

Normal flora gain entry into the dermis through a break in the skin. There, they multiply, causing an inflammatory response with classic signs of inflammation, including **erythema** (redness), pain, warmth at the site, and edema. The wound is generally irregular in shape with well-defined borders. As the organisms grow in number, they can overwhelm the immune response that normally contains and localizes inflammation. This allows cellular debris to accumulate, resulting in enlarged areas of involvement.

Erysipelas, a superficial cellulitis of the skin caused by group A *Streptococcus*, usually affects the lower extremities or the face (Figure 15–11 ■). The involved area is bright red and raised with well-defined borders. Skin infections such as this can predispose the individual to **septicemia** and septic shock. Although antibiotic therapy is effective, the most important method of therapy is prevention.

If treated promptly, the prognosis is generally very good. However, delays in treatment can result in septicemia as bacteria enter the circulating blood system.

Etiology

Common causative organisms are *Staphylococcus aureus, hemolytic Streptococci (group g Streptococci* and *Streptococcus pyogenes), Streptococcus pneumoniae, Haemophilus influenzae,* and beta-hemolytic and group A *Streptococcus* (Curtis, 2007). Cellulitis can also result from a nearby abscess or sinusitis. Onset is usually rapid.

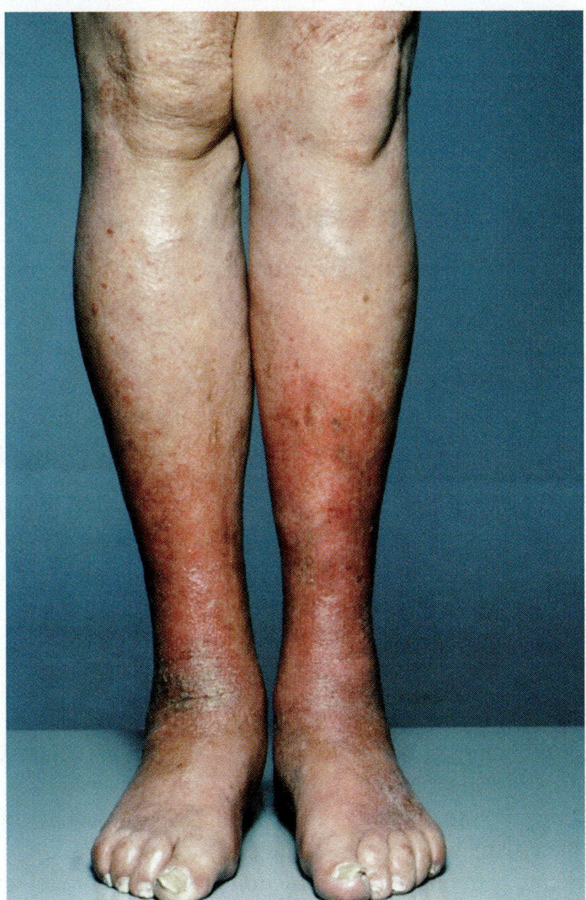

Figure 15–11 ■ Erysipelas, a superficial cellulitis of the skin caused by group A streptococcus.

Source: © Custom Medical Stock Photography.

Risk Factors

Children with cellulitis often have a history of trauma, impetigo, folliculitis, untreated tooth decay, or recent otitis media. As the skin becomes thinner and less elastic with age, older adults become more susceptible to injury and breakdown of tissue, which can result in cellulitis. Peripheral neuropathy with decreased sensation and circulation can lead to abrasions, burns, and stasis ulcers that can become infected. Reduced physical activity, malnutrition, dehydration, and other systemic illnesses are also predisposing factors. Any interruption of skin integrity can lead to infection, especially with organisms that are part of the normal skin flora.

Other factors that increase the risk of infection include any illness that compromises skin integrity such as diabetes mellitus, obesity, a previous history of cellulitis, peripheral vascular disease, tinea pedis, and alcohol abuse (Mayo Foundation for Medical Education and Research, 2006). Clients with **tinea pedis** (fungal infection of the feet) or lymphatic obstruction are most vulnerable to cellulitis and may experience recurrent infections over time.

CLINICAL MANIFESTATIONS

Clients with cellulitis experience a rapid onset and appear ill. Classic signs and symptoms include erythema, edema of the face or infected limb, warmth, and tenderness around the infected site (Figure 15–12 ■). Other symptoms include fever,

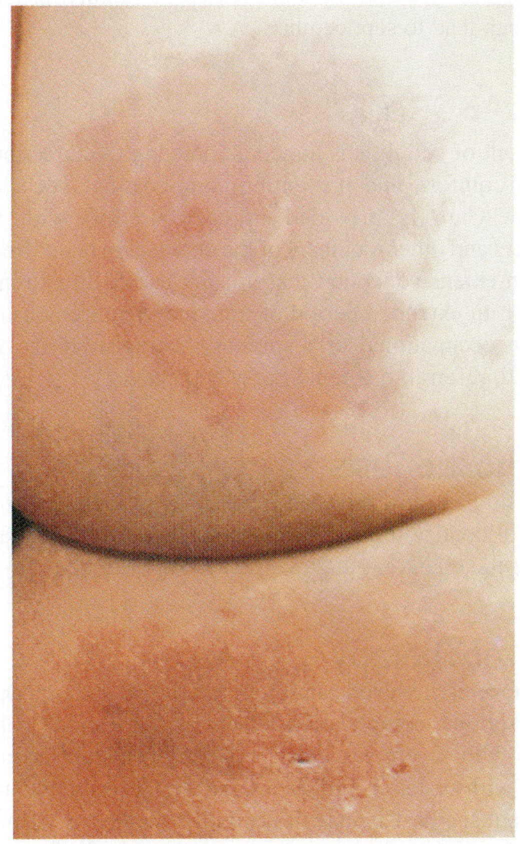

Figure 15–12 ■ Characteristic appearance of cellulitis.

CLINICAL MANIFESTATIONS AND THERAPIES Cellulitis

ETIOLOGY	CLINICAL MANIFESTATIONS	CLINICAL THERAPIES
Fever	Tachycardia, tachypnea, elevated temperature, lethargy	■ Maintain adequate hydration. ■ Administer antipyretics. ■ Treat underlying cause.
Skin inflammation	Redness, pain, warmth, edema	■ Administer antibiotics. ■ Maintain bedrest. ■ Provide adequate nutrition to promote healing. ■ Manage pain using both pharmacologic and nonpharmacologic therapies.
Septicemia	Whole-body inflammation manifested by fever, altered WBC count (may be high or low), and hemodynamic alterations (tachycardia, tachypnea, decreased cardiac output)	■ Monitor hemodynamic status. ■ Administer antibiotic therapy. ■ Provide fluid management. ■ Provide supportive care based on symptoms. ■ Measure vital signs frequently.

chills, malaise, and enlargement and tenderness of regional lymph nodes (also see the preceding Clinical Manifestations and Therapies). **Lymphangitis** (inflammation of a lymph vessel) may be present. In some cases, a rapidly progressive lesion can lead to septicemia.

COLLABORATION

Treatment of cellulitis is aimed at reducing the infection, promoting comfort, and preventing complications such as septicemia. Care is provided in collaboration with family members and other members of the health care team. Recovery from an extensive wound that impairs use of an extremity or limb for an extended period of time may require consultation with an occupational or respiratory therapist. If the face is involved, referral to a dentist may be necessary.

Diagnostic Tests

Blood studies may show an increase in WBCs. Cultures are taken to identify the causative organisms. Blood cultures are taken if the client has a toxic (very ill) appearance.

Clinical Therapy

If the face is involved, antibiotic therapy is administered to avoid serious complications such as periorbital cellulitis. Clients with severe cases or a large affected surface area are treated with systemic antibiotics and analgesics in the hospital to prevent sepsis. Clients with cellulitis on the trunk, limbs, or perianal area may be treated on an outpatient basis with oral antibiotics. Recovery begins within 48 hours, but therapy should continue for at least 10 days. Untreated cellulitis or cellulitis that does not respond to treatment can lead to osteomyelitis, arthritis, or serious systemic infection.

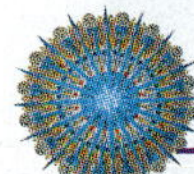

NURSING PROCESS

The nurse plays an important role in assessing the status of the client and teaching self-care to prevent complications.

Assessment

Assessment centers on recognition of infection, documentation of location and related symptoms, and monitoring of vital signs. The nurse assesses the wound frequently (at least every 2 hours), including tracing along the border with a marker to allow for any change in size to be clearly recognized. In the event of change, the nurse places a new mark so that future care providers can clearly see if the wound enlarges.

Diagnosis

Nursing diagnoses that may be appropriate for a client with cellulitis include the following:

- Impaired skin integrity related to mechanical factors (injury, the inflammatory process, and presence of infection)
- Acute pain related to destruction of tissue due to infection
- Interrupted family processes related to home care needs of the child with acute illness.

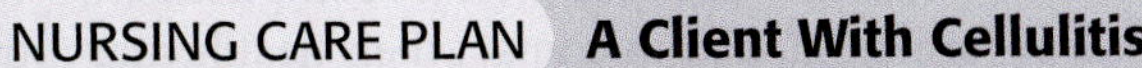

NURSING CARE PLAN A Client With Cellulitis

Maria Gonzalez is a 74-year-old widow who lives in an assisted living facility in a small town in central Pennsylvania. Her family includes three daughters and two sons who live out of state and a son who lives within 5 miles of Ms. Gonzalez's home. While visiting his mother, he notices a red area on her lower leg and asks her about it. She says it developed earlier today and is very painful. She's been treating it with wet compresses, but that does not seem to be helping much. Her son takes her to the local emergency department, where the nurse admits her to one of the examination rooms.

ASSESSMENT

Ms. Gonzalez speaks Spanish and is able to communicate only minimally in English. Her son acts as an interpreter when necessary. Ms. Gonzalez's history reveals diabetes mellitus with complications of peripheral vascular disease and neuropathy in the right leg, hypertension, coronary artery disease with angina, and cataracts in both eyes. She says she is allergic to penicillin and sulfa drugs. She denies ever having had a similar wound and describes the pain as a 7 on a 1–10 scale.

Physical examination of the painful right leg reveals an irregularly shaped, flat area that is red, warm, and painful, extending from just below the knee to mid-shin, and wrapping medially from midline to the back of the leg. The wound measures 6 in. by 5 in. at its widest point. Her vital signs are temperature 100.8°F oral, pulse 88 beats/min, respirations 16 breaths/min. and BP 122/74 mmHg.

The physician orders laboratory studies that reveal an elevated WBC count. Because of her age and medical history, the physician orders blood cultures and admits her to the facility for IV antibiotics and monitoring.

DIAGNOSES

- Altered Skin Integrity related to infectious process
- Acute Pain related to the inflammatory process secondary to cellulitis
- Deficient Knowledge of the cause of the skin disorder and recommended treatment
- Anxiety related to the need to be admitted to the hospital and inability to communicate with staff
- Impaired Verbal Communication related to the inability to speak English

PLAN

- Skin will heal without evidence of a secondary infection or complication of sepsis.
- Client will obtain relief of pain with the proper use of medications.
- Client will verbalize an understanding of the disease process and participate in the treatment plan.
- Client will describe proper home care, including self-administration of medication after discharge.
- Client anxiety will be reduced after orientation to the hospital environment and speaking with staff members who also speak Spanish.
- Communication will be improved after assigning a Spanish-speaking nurse and using translation services in the hospital.

IMPLEMENTATION

- Provide orientation to facility and treatment plan (IV therapy, warm soaks) in Spanish.
- Keep right leg elevated and explain the need to stay in bed.
- Trace outer border of wound with black marker and avoid washing off marks to allow for assessment every 2 hours. Report any increase in size to provider.
- Provide verbal and written instructions (in Spanish) for self-care after discharge, including the following:
  - a. Take all antibiotics prescribed until they are gone.
  - b. Take medications as prescribed for pain.
  - c. Take the antibiotic for your wound every 6 hours, even during nighttime hours, for 10 days.
  - d. Monitor the size of the wound and notify physician if there is any increase or if fever returns.
  - e. Apply warm, moist heat to wound four times a day.
  - f. Wash hands carefully before applying warm, moist compresses.
  - g. Reduce activity to bathroom privileges only and keep right leg elevated.
  - h. Monitor oral temperature and take two acetaminophen (Tylenol) for temperature higher than 100°F orally.

EVALUATION

Ms. Gonzalez's wound decreased in size over the next 48 hours. She was discharged with a prescription for antibiotics to be taken orally for 10 days and pain medication, although she reported that the pain was almost gone by the time she went home. Her fever subsided within 36 hours of beginning treatment. Ms. Gonzalez will see her physician at the completion of oral antibiotics and says she will call the office sooner if the wound increases in size or her fever returns.

CRITICAL THINKING

1. Identify barriers to care in this case. What nursing interventions can be initiated to overcome these barriers?
2. What further assessments and interventions might have been indicated had the wound shown little improvement or the pain remained severe?
3. If Ms. Gonzalez were unable to provide self-care after discharge, what options might the nurse have recommended for this client?

Plan

Planning care for the client with cellulitis is directed at pain management, client teaching related to self-care, and infection resolution without progression to systemic infection. Potential outcomes may include the following:

- Client will report pain of 3 or lower, on a scale of 1–10.
- Client will describe situations requiring contact with the provider.
- Client will explain how to take antibiotics and analgesics properly.

Implementation

Because of the risk of sepsis, cellulitis is managed carefully. Administer prescribed oral or intravenous antibiotics as scheduled. Supportive care includes warm compresses to the affected area four times daily, elevation of the affected limb, and bedrest. Outpatient follow-up is crucial to ensure positive response to therapy.

Advise clients about possible complications, such as abscess formation, and to contact their health care provider if any of the following signs develop:

- Spread of the infected area in the 24- to 48-hour period after the start of treatment
- Temperature over 38.3°C (101°F)
- Increased lethargy.

Reinforce to clients and caregivers the importance of compliance with the treatment regimen and the seriousness of the possible complications.

Evaluation

Outcomes developed in collaboration with the client will be evaluated to determine the client's progress. The nurse should trace the outer edges of the wound with a black marker to allow for better evaluation of changes in the size and area covered by the wound. The provider should be notified if the cellulitis enlarges or spreads.

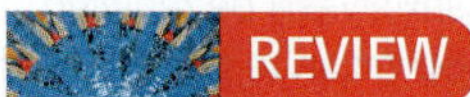

Cellulitis

RELATE: LINK THE CONCEPTS

Linking the exemplar of Cellulitis with the concept of Comfort:

1. What teaching interventions will you provide the client with cellulitis of the leg who is taking a narcotic for pain?
2. What nonpharmacological interventions will you implement for the client experiencing pain from cellulitis?

Linking the exemplar of Cellulitis with the concept of Perfusion:

3. How will you assess perfusion in the client with cellulitis of the thigh?
4. What symptoms will you teach the client with cellulitis to report to the provider immediately regarding perfusion?

READY: GO TO COMPANION SKILLS MANUAL

- Administering oral medications
- Preventing skin breakdown
- Assessing body temperature
- Assessing the client in pain
- Collecting a routine urine specimen
- Assessing vital signs
- Applying compresses and moist packs
- Performing surgical and antisepsis/scrubs
- Latex precautions

REFLECT: CASE STUDY

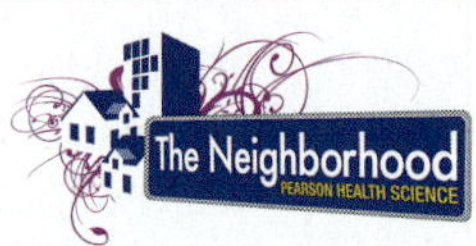

Norma James is a 65-year-old widow who lives alone. Although she has lived in the neighborhood for years, she is somewhat socially isolated. She has two adult sons with whom she has limited contact, because they live out of state and rarely call. She has only a few individuals she considers friends; she does not particularly like many people and prefers the company of her six cats.

Mrs. James has a long history of type 2 diabetes mellitus and hypertension. In more recent years, she has been diagnosed with atrial fibrillation. She has multiple physicians and takes multiple medications, including the following:

- Glucotrol: 10 mg, twice a day
- Captopril, 50 mg, twice a day
- Digoxin, 125 mcg, once a day
- Coumadin, 5 mg, once a day.

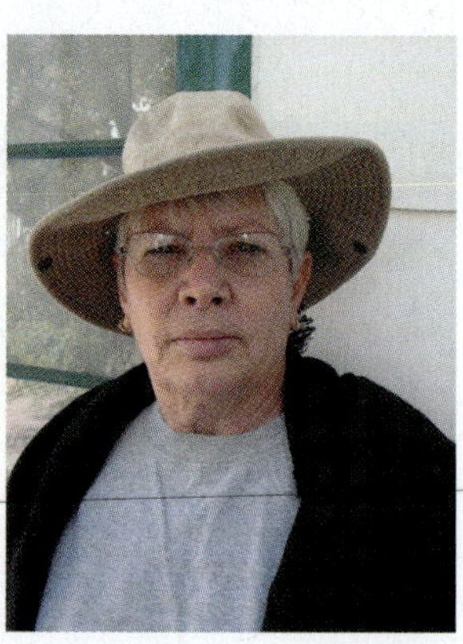

Mrs. James has a known drug allergy to penicillin.

Mrs. James does not work; she has very limited savings and relies on Social Security benefits for income. She smokes about half a pack of cigarettes a day and has been a smoker since she was in her 20s. She drinks alcohol "a couple times a year, usually a glass of wine at a special dinner."

She does not drive and relies on her friends, neighbors, or the city bus for transportation. She lives near a grocery store and prides herself in being able to get most things she needs without assistance. She spends most of her time alone at home and occupies herself by watching television, reading, and doing crossword and jigsaw puzzles.

Mrs. James noticed a small, tender area on her ankle yesterday and, remembering what the cashier at the convenience store told her, decided to apply butter to the wound.

1. What factors in Mrs. James history put her at risk for cellulitis?
2. What do you suspect the outcome of applying butter to this wound may be?
3. What client teaching would you provide Mrs. James?

15.2 CONJUNCTIVITIS

KEY TERMS

Conjunctivitis, *813*
Entropion, *814*
Photophobia, *814*
Trachoma, *814*
Uveitis, *815*

BASIS FOR SELECTION OF EXEMPLAR

Most common office-based visits

Most common eye disease

LEARNING OUTCOMES

After reading about this exemplar, you will be able to:

1. Describe the pathophysiology, etiology, clinical manifestations, and direct and indirect causes of conjunctivitis.
2. Identify risk factors associated with conjunctivitis.
3. Illustrate the nursing process in providing culturally competent care across the life span for individuals with conjunctivitis.
4. Formulate priority nursing diagnoses appropriate for an individual with conjunctivitis.
5. Create a plan of care for individuals with conjunctivitis and their family members.
6. Assess expected outcomes for an individual with conjunctivitis.
7. Discuss therapies used in the collaborative care of an individual with conjunctivitis.
8. Employ evidence-based caring interventions for an individual with conjunctivitis.

OVERVIEW

The conjunctiva—the thin, transparent membrane that covers the anterior surface of the eye and lines the inner surfaces of the eyelids—is vulnerable to inflammation and infection because of its constant exposure to the environment. **Conjunctivitis** (inflammation of the conjunctiva) is the most common eye disease. Its usual cause is a bacterial or viral infection. These infections can be transmitted to the eye by direct contact (e.g., hands, tissues, and towels). Allergens, chemical irritants, and exposure to radiant energy, such as ultraviolet light from the sun or tanning devices, can also lead to this common condition. Its severity can range from mild irritation with redness and tearing to conjunctival edema, hemorrhage, or a severe necrotizing process with tissue destruction.

All neonates born in the United States receive prophylactic treatment to prevent conjunctivitis. By federal law, all infants are given prophylactic eye treatment soon after delivery. The nurse is responsible for administering this eye ointment. Penicillin, tetracycline, erythromycin, or povidone-iodine ointments are most commonly used. Sometimes an infant can develop chemical conjunctivitis due to the prophylactic eye ointment. A chemical reaction should be considered as a possible cause when conjunctivitis develops within 24–48 hours after instillation of this medication.

PATHOPHYSIOLOGY AND ETIOLOGY

There are several types of conjunctivitis, depending on the cause of inflammation. Bacteria, viruses, allergies, trauma, or irritants cause the conjunctiva to become edematous, inflamed, and reddened with a yellow or white discharge (Figure 15–13 ■). Parents commonly refer to all conjunctivitis as "pink eye."

Conjunctivitis in an infant under 30 days of age is called *ophthalmia neonatorum*. These infections are usually acquired from the mother during vaginal delivery as a result of contact with infected vaginal discharge containing bacterial organisms such as *Chlamydia trachomatis* and *Neisseria gonorrhoeae*. Antibiotics usually are instilled into the eyes of newborns soon after birth as a prophylactic measure. In infants who have frequent tearing and mattering (eyelid discharge that has formed a crust) on awakening, a plugged lacrimal duct may mimic conjunctivitis.

Bacterial conjunctivitis is common in older children. It is characterized by edema of the eyelid, reddened conjunctiva, and enlarged preauricular lymph glands. Mucopurulent

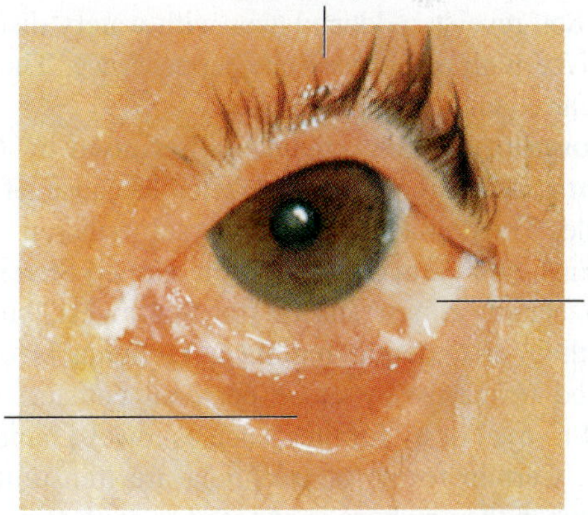

Figure 15–13 ■ Acute conjunctivitis. The major difference between bacterial and viral conjunctivitis is that bacterial conjunctivitis has a purulent discharge that may result in crusting whereas the discharge from viral conjunctivitis is serous (watery). Allergic conjunctivitis produces watery to thick drainage and is characterized by itching.

Source: Adapted from Newell, F.W. (1996). *Ophthalmology: Principles and concepts* (8th ed.). St. Louis, MO: Mosby Year-Book.

discharge causes matting and makes the eyes difficult to open upon awakening. Older children with conjunctivitis complain of itching or burning, mild photophobia, and a feeling of scratching under the lids.

Common infectious organisms include *Staphylococcus aureus, Haemophilus influenzae*, *Streptococcus pneumoniae*, *Moraxella catarrhalis,* and *Escherichia coli* (Mah, 2006; Stephenson, 2003). Most cases are caused by hand-to-eye contact. The disease can spread rapidly when groups of youth spend time together, such as young children and adolescents in schools and child care centers and college students in dormitories or on sports teams. The infection can be bilateral but is more commonly unilateral.

Other infections in newborns and children can be caused by viruses. Viral conjunctivitis is commonly bilateral. Adenovirus is a common cause and spreads from respiratory adenovirus infection in a hand-to-eye manner.

Herpes simplex virus (HSV) can also cause infections, either by transfer from a mother with herpes infection to a neonate during birth or by contact with an infected person in infants or children of any age. Ophthalmic herpes infection is often accompanied by characteristic vesicular lesions on the skin of the face. A culture of the lesion is performed for diagnosis, and any accompanying conjunctivitis is assumed to be caused by herpes virus. For the infection caused by HSV, prompt and vigorous treatment is needed to prevent eye injury or blindness, which can occur in children with recurrent herpes virus infections as a result of antibody reaction to the viral antigen. Herpes virus infections commonly recur, so periodic treatment and sometime prophylaxis may be needed.

Allergic conjunctivitis is a common cause of eye discomfort (Abelson & Granet, 2006). When conjunctivitis is caused by an allergy, the client complains of intense itching. Examination reveals reddened eyes with watery discharge and conjunctivae with a "cobblestone" appearance. The eyes may also appear edematous.

Trachoma (a chronic conjunctivitis caused by *Chlamydia trachomatis*) is a significant preventable cause of blindness worldwide. Trachoma is endemic in sub-Saharan Africa, the Middle East, and parts of Asia. In the United States, it can be found in Native Americans of the Southwest, but less frequently than in endemic regions. Trachoma is contagious, transmitted primarily by close personal contact (eye-to-eye and hand-to-eye) or by fomites, such as towels, handkerchiefs, and flies. Certain forms of trachoma are transmitted during delivery when the newborn is exposed to contaminated genital secretions of the mother (Kasper et al., 2005).

Etiology

Infectious conjunctivitis may be bacterial, viral, or fungal in origin. Bacterial conjunctivitis, also known as "pink eye," is highly contagious and often is caused by *Staphylococcus* and *Haemophilus* sp. Adenovirus infection is the leading cause of conjunctivitis in adults. Systemic infections that may affect the eyes include herpes simplex and other viral infections. Contact with genital secretions infected with *Gonococcus* sp. can cause gonococcal conjunctivitis, a medical emergency that can lead to corneal perforation.

Risk Factors

Clients who wear contact lenses, especially extended-wear lenses, are at higher risk for development of conjunctivitis. Others at risk include young children in school and day care settings and clients with compromised immune response. The most common occurrence of viral conjunctivitis is seen in children with viral upper respiratory infections.

CLINICAL MANIFESTATIONS

Redness and itching of the affected eye are common manifestations of acute conjunctivitis (Figure 15–14 ■). The client may also complain of a scratchy, burning, or gritty sensation. Pain is not common, and **photophobia** (sensitivity to light) may occur. Tearing and discharge accompany the inflammatory process. The discharge may be watery, purulent, or mucoid, depending on the cause of conjunctivitis. The client may have associated manifestations, such as pharyngitis, fever, malaise, and swollen preauricular lymph nodes.

Early manifestations of trachoma include redness, eyelid edema, tearing, and photophobia. Small conjunctival follicles develop on the upper lids. The inflammation also causes superficial corneal vascularization and infiltration with granulation tissue. Scarring of the conjunctival lining of the lid causes **entropion** (inversion of the eyelid) (Figure 15–15 ■). The lashes then abrade the cornea, eventually causing ulceration and scarring. The scarred cornea is opaque, resulting in loss of vision.

COLLABORATION

Collaboration with an ophthalmologist may be indicated if disruption to the cornea is suspected. If a nurse working in a pediatric practice observes a number of a children from a single school or day care setting presenting with conjunctivitis, the nurse may want to contact the school or day care nurse or health coordinator to discuss increased prevention and student education.

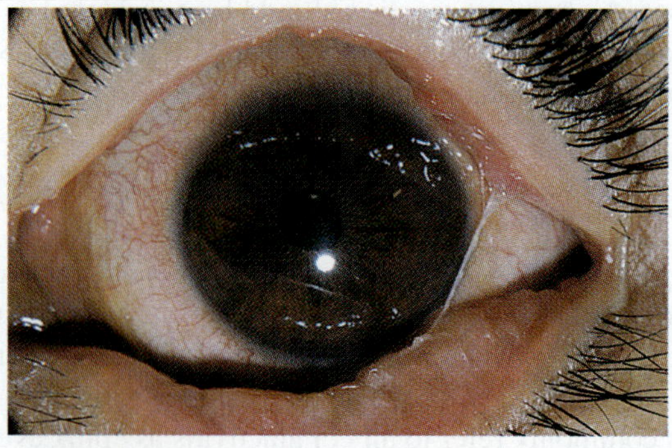

Figure 15–14 ■ The appearance of an eye with conjunctivitis.

Source: Buddy Crofton/Medical Images, Inc.

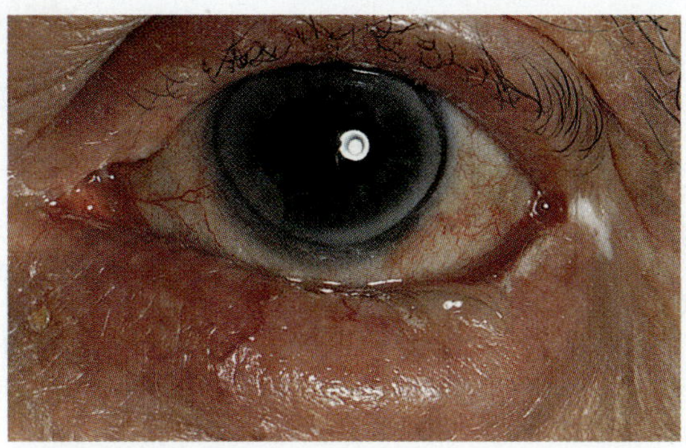

Figure 15–15 ■ Entropion.

Source: Science Photo Library/Photo Researchers, Inc.

Diagnostic Tests

Accurate diagnosis of conjunctivitis is especially important, because other potentially vision-threatening conditions, such as acute **uveitis** (inflammation of the middle layer of the eye, called the uvea) or acute angle-closure glaucoma, can also cause a red eye (Table 15–10). In most cases, a diagnosis of the cause of conjunctivitis is made based on the client's history and presenting symptoms.

Diagnostic procedures may include the following:

- *Culture and sensitivity* of exudates to determine presence of an infection and identify the infecting organism. Cultures can be taken, especially in infants or in cases suspected of being an unusual bacterial illness or involving herpes viruses. A Gram stain of discharge and conjunctival scraping for potential *Chlamydia* or herpes are performed. Cultures, if ordered, should be obtained before beginning treatment.
- *Fluorescein stain* with slit-lamp examination to identify possible corneal ulcerations or abrasions, which appear green with staining.
- *Conjunctival scrapings*, which are examined microscopically or cultured to identify the organisms.

Additional laboratory testing, such as blood counts or antibody titers, may be used to identify underlying infectious or autoimmune processes.

Pharmacologic Therapies

Conjunctivitis is treated with antibiotic, antiviral, or anti-inflammatory drugs as appropriate. Topical anti-infectives, applied as either eyedrops or ointment, may include erythromycin, gentamicin, penicillin, bacitracin, sulfacetamide sodium, amphotericin B, or idoxuridine. For severe infections or cellulitis, anti-infectives may be administered orally, by subconjunctival injection, or by systemic intravenous infusion.

When gonococcal conjunctivitis occurs in newborns, ceftriaxone is recommended, because that particular disease is resistant to penicillin. Chlamydial infections are treated with oral erythromycin or tetracycline. Careful total evaluation of the newborn with any conjunctivitis is also performed to watch for other signs of infection.

Herpes simplex virus infections of the eye are treated promptly by an ophthalmologist, neonatologist, or others who are trained in this serious disease. Topical drugs are used and often are combined with a systemic antiviral agent, such as acyclovir (Teoh & Reynolds, 2003). Neonatal HSV is treated vigorously with parenteral acyclovir for 14 days (or longer if central nervous system involvement is found upon lumbar puncture), and with topical ophthalmic medication (trifluridine, iododeoxyuridine, or vidarabine). Recurrent lesions may necessitate suppressive or prophylactic treatment with oral acyclovir (American Academy of Pediatrics, 2006).

Antihistamines are used to minimize symptoms of conjunctivitis when an allergic response underlies the inflammatory process. Topical steroids and vasoconstrictors may also be used (Abelson & Granet, 2006). Decongestants can be combined with systemic antihistamines for short-term therapy. More current treatment involves use of mast-cell stabilizers to decrease the activation of mast cells that accompanies allergic reactions. Most mast-cell stabilizers have been tested and found to be safe in children 3 years of age and older (Alexander, 2003).

Clinical Therapies

Adenoviral conjunctivitis may be treated with comfort measures, such as cleaning drainage away with a warm clean cloth, avoiding bright lights, and avoiding reading. Cool compresses applied to the eyes can help to relieve the feeling of eye irritation.

TABLE 15–10 **Possible Causes of Acute Red Eye**

	ACUTE CONJUNCTIVITIS	CORNEAL TRAUMA OR INFECTION	ACUTE UVEITIS	ACUTE ANGLE-CLOSURE GLAUCOMA
Incidence	Very common	Common	Common	Rare
Pain	Mild	Moderate to severe	Moderate	Severe
Vision	Normal	Blurred	Blurred	Markedly blurred
Discharge	May be copious	Watery, may be purulent	None	None
Conjunctival erythema	Diffuse	Primarily around cornea	Primarily around cornea	Primarily around cornea
Cornea	Clear	Depends on cause	Usually clear	Cloudy
Pupils	Normal size, response to light	Normal size, response to light	Small, minimal response to light	Moderately dilated, fixed

MEDICATIONS Conjunctivitis

Medication	Action/Indication	Nursing Implications
Fluoroquinolones (e.g., norfloxacin, ciprofloxacin, ofloxacin, levofloxacin, and sparfloxacin)	Antibiotics effective against a broad spectrum of gram-positive and gram-negative organisms; generally interfere with enzymes needed for DNA replication in bacteria causing eye infections.	■ If a culture and sensitivity test is ordered, perform the test before beginning the antibiotic. ■ Teach parents correct administration of drops or ointment. ■ Be alert for signs of reactivity to medication that might be manifested as local burning, crusting, itching, and edema.
Acyclovir	Antiviral drug effective against herpes simplex virus (HSV).	■ Most viral conjunctivitis infections are not treated; good hygiene practices are followed, and the infection clears without treatment by medication. However, HSV infections must be treated, because they can harm vision. Acyclovir is administered intravenously to neonates and some children with HSV; ongoing suppressive oral therapy is used for recurred infections. ■ Teach family to recognize characteristic herpes skin lesions and to report these and all eye redness immediately. Ensure that family and other care providers understand the possible chronic nature of HSV and engage in careful hygiene to prevent spread when infections are active. ■ Prepare and administer the intravenous form as ordered, over at least 1 hour. Shake oral suspension when that form is used for children.
Mast-cell stabilizers (e.g., cromolyn, nedocromil, and olopatadine)	Inhibit release of histamine from mast cells, thereby decreasing allergic response. Used to treat itching and other symptoms of allergic conjunctivitis.	■ Teach family the correct instillation of medication. Encourage other methods to decrease itching, such as cool compresses several times daily to the eyes. Avoid rubbing eyes, which can introduce bacteria or virus to the already inflamed eyes. If medication does not provide relief or additional eye symptoms appear, consult again with the health care provider.

Frequent eye irrigations may be ordered to remove the copious purulent discharge associated with conjunctivitis. Soaking the lids with warm saline compresses before cleansing promotes comfort and facilitates the removal of crusts and exudate in conjunctivitis.

NURSING PROCESS

The nursing role in treating conjunctivitis is primarily one of education to prevent both the disorder itself and its spread when it does occur. Education is a vital strategy for preventing conjunctivitis. Teach all clients about proper eye care, including the importance of not sharing towels, makeup, or contact lenses as well as avoiding rubbing or scratching the eyes. Instruct clients to avoid using old eye makeup, which can cause eye infections. Teach contact lens users appropriate care. Emphasize the need to follow cleaning instructions precisely to avoid bacterial contamination of lenses. If the eyes become red, irritated, or develop discharge, instruct the client to avoid wearing contact lenses until the inflammatory process has cleared.

Assessment

Collect the following data through the health history and physical examination:

- *Health history.* Presence of redness, discomfort, tearing, photophobia, and drainage; symptom onset; care measures; use of contact lenses; exposure to "pink eye" or recent travel; allergies; previous history of conjunctivitis; and presence of any chronic diseases
- *Physical assessment.* Visual acuity; inspect eyelids, conjunctiva, sclera, and cornea; vital signs, including temperature.

PRACTICE ALERT

During assessment, place a gloved index finger on the child's nose next to the inner corner of the eye, and apply gentle pressure for several seconds. If mucopurulent drainage is discharged from the eye, bacterial conjunctivitis may be present.

CLIENT TEACHING Contact Lens Care

- Wash hands thoroughly before handling contact lenses.
- Keep storage case clean.
- Remove lenses before sleep, and clean and store the lenses as recommended by the manufacturer.
- Use cleaning and wetting solutions recommended by an eye care professional or the lens manufacturer. Do not use water or home-made solutions for wetting or cleaning lenses.
- If eye redness, tearing, vision loss, or pain occurs, remove lenses and contact an eye care professional as soon as possible.
- Do not share contact lenses or allow another person to "try on" lenses.

Diagnosis

- Risk for Infection
- Risk for Disturbed Sensory Perception: Visual

Plan

Goals are created based on each individualized client's needs and may include:

- Client will demonstrate proper hand hygiene.
- Client will avoid contaminating unaffected eye or other family members.
- Client will experience no visual complications following recovery.

Implementation

Nursing care focuses primarily on preventing complications from the disorder and spread of infection to the other eye or to others in close contact with the client. Care should be individualized based on specific needs of the client.

Risk for Infection

Acute conjunctivitis is highly contagious. While most clients experience no more than discomfort from the disease, the infection carries a risk for scarring and damage to the delicate cornea of the eye. Preventing the spread of this infection is a vital nursing role.

When conjunctivitis is diagnosed in an infant in the neonatal intensive care unit, the infant is isolated to prevent the disease from spreading to other infants. Typically, however, clients with conjunctivitis are managed in the community, reinforcing the need for effective teaching for home care to prevent transmission of infection. Because bacterial infectious conjunctivitis is extremely contagious, tell parents that children should not return to child care or school until they have been taking an antibiotic for 24 hours. Infected clients should avoid sharing towels. Mittens may be applied to the young child to prevent rubbing the eye.

- Teach client to wash hands thoroughly before instilling eye medications. Instruct client to avoid touching or rubbing the eyes. Advise client to use a new, clean, cotton-tipped swab or cotton ball for cleaning each eye. Hand washing is the single most important measure to prevent transmission of infection to the eye. Touching or rubbing the eyes increases the risk of infection and corneal trauma. Using a new swab or cotton ball prevents cross-contamination between eyes.
- Teach client how to instill prescribed eyedrops as ordered. Prescribed medications reduce inflammation and eliminate infection.
- Discuss the importance of avoiding contact lens use until the infectious process has cleared; discuss the importance of completing the prescribed treatment. Use of contact lenses in the inflamed eyes can lead to further damage and impair healing.

Risk for Disturbed Sensory Perception: Visual

Conjunctivitis can potentially disrupt the integrity or clarity of the cornea. Because of its vital role in focusing light on the retina, corneal damage can impair visual acuity.

- Assess vision with and without corrective lenses. Assessment provides a baseline to evaluate possible changes in vision resulting from the infection.
- Instruct client to avoid activities requiring high visual acuity until the infection has cleared. The inflammatory process, edema of the conjunctiva, and local antibiotic applications can decrease visual acuity and cloud vision.
- Instruct client to use dark sunglasses with appropriate UV protection when out of doors, even on cloudy days. Photophobia, a common manifestation of conjunctivitis, causes eye pain with increased light intensity.

Home Care

As mentioned, clients with conjunctivitis typically are managed in the community, reinforcing the need for effective teaching for home care. Emphasize to the family ways to prevent transmission of infection. If the client is unable to administer eye medications, involve the family in teaching. Include the following topics:

- Safety and medical asepsis when cleansing the eye
- Instillation of prescribed eyedrops and ointments
- Comfort measures such as reducing lighting intensity and wearing sunglasses
- Avoidance of activities such as excessive reading while eye is inflamed.

Evaluation

Clients are evaluated based on the outcomes created during the planning process. Resolution of the infection is indicated by return of conjunctiva to a normal white color, absence of drainage, and elimination of symptoms.

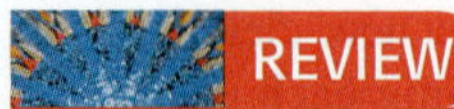

REVIEW Conjunctivitis

RELATE: LINK THE CONCEPTS

Linking the exemplar of Conjunctivitis with the concept of Development:

1. When caring for children with conjunctivitis, what prevention strategies can be used to keep children from different stages of development from rubbing their eyes?
2. What cognitive developmental issues will the nurse anticipate for a child with recurrent conjunctivitis?

Linking the exemplar of Conjunctivitis with the concept of Health, Wellness, and Illness:

3. What strategies could the school nurse teach students to prevent conjunctivitis?
4. When teaching infant care to a group of new parents, what important strategy will you demonstrate to reduce the risk of conjunctivitis?

READY: GO TO COMPANION SKILLS MANUAL

- Administration of ophthalmic medications

REFER: GO TO MYNURSINGKIT

REFLECT: CASE STUDY

Marcus is a 6-year-old boy who is the son of Angie and Steve Young. He is a pretty typical boy who is in enrolled in first grade at the elementary school. He likes his teacher at school and has many friends. He has a stable home life and is close to his parents and sister, Kelsey. He loves to read and to go to the park and play on the playground equipment. He is very interested in sports and wants to play football and baseball someday. He takes piano lessons but is not interested in this activity at all.

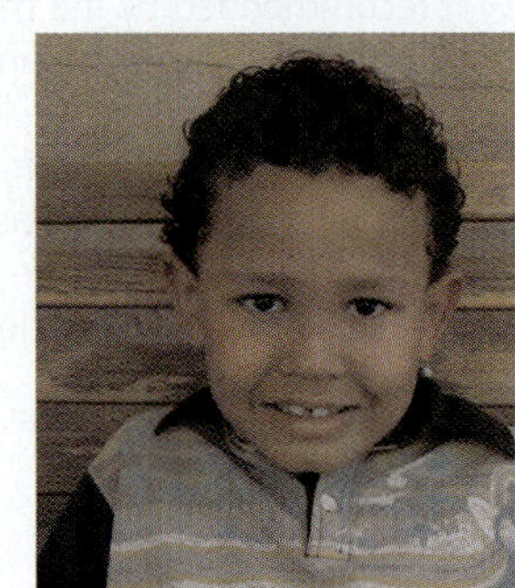

Marcus is normally healthy, is up to date on his immunizations, and sees a dentist every 6 months. His mother brings him to the clinic today because she noticed a white, milky discharge in both eyes this morning, and she says his eyes were crusted shut when he first woke up. He has had a cold for the past 3 days, with a low-grade fever, rhinorrhea, productive cough, and mild lethargy. The provider examines the boy's eyes and determines he has viral conjunctivitis.

1. What client teaching will you provide this family to prevent others from contracting this infection?
2. What teaching will you provide to Mrs. Young regarding how to care for Marcus's conjunctivitis?
3. Develop a nursing plan of care for Marcus.

15.3 INFLUENZA

KEY TERMS

Antigenic drift, *819*
Antigenic shift, *819*
Atelectasis, *822*
Avian influenza, *818*
Coryza, *818*
Epidemic, *818*
H1N1 influenza, *819*
Influenza, *818*
Malaise, *818*
Pandemic, *818*
Rhinorrhea, *819*

BASIS FOR SELECTION OF EXEMPLAR

Most common office-based visits
Number of annual U.S. hospitalizations
World Health Organization, Epidemic and Pandemic Alert & Response System

LEARNING OUTCOMES

After reading about this exemplar, you will be able to:

1. Describe the pathophysiology, etiology, clinical manifestations, and direct and indirect causes of influenza.
2. Identify risk factors associated with influenza.
3. Illustrate the nursing process in providing culturally competent care across the life span for individuals with influenza.
4. Formulate priority nursing diagnoses appropriate for an individual with influenza.
5. Create a plan of care for individuals with influenza and their family members.
6. Assess expected outcomes for an individual with influenza.
7. Discuss therapies used in the collaborative care of an individual with influenza.
8. Employ evidence-based caring interventions for an individual with influenza.

OVERVIEW

Influenza, or "the flu," is a highly contagious, viral respiratory disease characterized by **coryza** (inflammation of the mucous membranes lining the nose, usually associated with nasal discharge), fever, cough, and systemic symptoms, such as headache and **malaise** (a vague feeling of physical discomfort). Influenza usually occurs as an **epidemic** (widespread outbreak of an infectious disease) or a **pandemic** (global epidemic), although sporadic cases do occur. Localized outbreaks of influenza usually occur approximately every 1 to 3 years. Pandemics are less frequent, developing every 10 to 15 years until the past two decades.

Recently identified strains of **avian influenza** (bird influenza) and H1N1 influenza (popularly but incorrectly known as "swine flu") have raised concerns about a potential future pandemic. The avian flu virus has not yet demonstrated the ability to spread between humans; however, the possibility that it will mutate to allow person-to-person spread is a concern. This viral strain has a mortality rate of greater than 50% in people who have been infected as a result of close association with infected birds. (See Box 15–4 for more information about avian influenza.) **H1N1 influenza** is a form of the virus that consists of avian genes, human genes, and genes from flu viruses typically found in pigs from Asia and Europe. H1N1, like all flu viruses spreads from human to human via airborne droplets (Centers for Disease Control and Prevention [CDC], 2009).

Influenza tends to be mild and self-limited in healthy adults. Older adults, those with compromised immune systems, and people with chronic heart or pulmonary disease, however, have a high incidence of complications (e.g., pneumonia) and a higher risk for mortality related to the disease and its complications (Kasper et al., 2005).

PATHOPHYSIOLOGY AND ETIOLOGY

The incubation period for influenza is short, only 18–72 hours. The virus infects the respiratory epithelium. It rapidly replicates in infected cells and is released to infect neighboring cells. The resulting inflammation leads to necrosis and shedding of serous and ciliated cells of the respiratory tract. This allows extracellular fluid to escape, producing **rhinorrhea** (runny nose). With recovery, serous cells are replaced more rapidly than ciliated cells, leading to continued cough and coryza. Systemic symptoms of influenza are likely caused by release of inflammatory mediators (Kasper et al., 2005) as the influenza infection activates humoral and cell-mediated immune responses.

The respiratory epithelial necrosis caused by influenza increases the risk for secondary bacterial infections. Sinusitis and otitis media are frequent complications of influenza. Tracheobronchitis (inflammation of the trachea and bronchi) may develop. Although tracheobronchitis is not a serious health risk, its manifestations may persist for up to 3 weeks.

Influenza is clearly linked to an increased risk for pneumonia, particularly in young children and older adults. Narrower airways and underdeveloped alveoli increase the risk for pneumonia in young children. Changes in respiratory function associated with aging, including decreased effectiveness of cough and increased residual lung volume, pose little risk in the healthy older adult but greatly increase the risk for pneumonia when associated with influenza. Primary influenza viral pneumonia, while uncommon, is a serious complication that may be fatal. It typically develops within 48 hours of the onset of influenza, often in clients with preexisting heart valve or pulmonary disease. Influenza pneumonia progresses rapidly and can cause hypoxemia and death within a few days. Bacterial pneumonia is more likely to occur in older at-risk adults but also may affect otherwise healthy adults. It usually presents as a relapse of influenza, with a productive cough and evidence of pneumonia on the chest x-ray. (See the pneumonia exemplar for more information.) Other respiratory complications of influenza include exacerbation of chronic obstructive pulmonary disease (COPD), chronic bronchitis, or asthma.

Box 15–4 **Focus on Influenza and Its Potential for Pandemic**

Influenza viruses are common in nature, found in wild birds, such as ducks and shore birds, and in some animals, such as pigs. Although wild birds and animals carry the virus, they usually are not harmed by it. Movement of the virus into domesticated animals, however, can be devastating to that animal population.

Type A influenza viruses are subclassified by two proteins found on the surface of the virus: hemagglutinin (HA) and neuraminidase (NA). HA allows the virus to attach to a cell and initiate an infection, whereas NA allows the virus to exit the host cell after replicating. Currently, only three known subtypes of influenza A are circulating among humans (H1N1, H1N2, and H3N2). The H5N1 virus, commonly called avian influenza, is particularly virulent and is spread by migratory birds. Currently, it is not known to be spread from human to human. Both the H1N1 and H5N1 viruses raise fears of a potential human pandemic in the event of person-to-person transmission.

Influenza viruses are very changeable, undergoing small, continuous changes as well as occasional large and abrupt changes. **Antigenic drift** is the term for small changes that occur continuously as a virus makes copies of itself. These changes help a virus to elude the immune system, and necessitate the production of new vaccines every year. Sudden, dramatic changes occur when two different strains of influenza virus (e.g., avian influenza and human influenza) infect the same cell and exchange genetic material. These changes, called **antigenic shift**, create a new subtype of a virus to which people have little or no immunity.

On April 29, 2009, the World Health Organization raised its Influenza Pandemic Alert from Phase 4 to Phase 5 (indicating person-to-person contact of the virus in at least two countries of the same region) based on reported instances of H1N1 flu from around the world. By the next week, 23 countries had reported 1,490 cases of H1N1 flu. It is important to note that the cases being reported probably represent the most seriously ill people; milder infections may not be reflected in reported numbers. Early symptoms of H1N1 flu include runny nose, fever, cough, headache, muscle and joint pain, and in some cases, gastrointestinal symptoms, such as diarrhea (World Health Organization, 2009).

No vaccine to protect against either the H1N1 or the H5N1 virus has yet been developed for commercial use. Measures are being taken, however, to develop pre-pandemic vaccines based on current strains of both H1N1 and H5N1 influenza virus, to increase the capacity for vaccine production in the United States, and to research new types of vaccines. Some currently available antiviral medications may effectively treat the symptoms of H1N1 flu (CDC, 2009).

A severe pandemic of any type of influenza could disrupt all aspects of life, not only causing severe illness and death but also overwhelming the health care system, impacting social services, and causing significant economic loss. Advance preparations such as those currently being undertaken by the World Health Organization and the United States and other countries can reduce the impact of a pandemic.

Reye's syndrome is a rare but potentially fatal complication of influenza. A neurologic disease that typically occurs following a viral infection, it is more likely to affect children but also has been identified in older adults. It is associated with administration of aspirin products to children with any viral infection, including influenza. Most often associated with influenza B virus, Reye's syndrome develops within 2 to 3 weeks after the onset of influenza. It has a 30% mortality rate. Hepatic failure and encephalopathy develop rapidly in clients with Reye's syndrome.

Other potential complications of influenza, while uncommon, include myositis (inflammation of skeletal muscles), myocarditis (inflammation of the heart muscle), and central nervous system disorders, such as encephalitis and Guillain-Barré syndrome.

Etiology

Although vaccinations are offered either free or at very low cost at physicians' offices, pharmacies, community clinics, and local health departments, influenza remains one of the leading causes of morbidity and mortality in the United States. In the 2007–2008 flu season, approximately 200,000 hospitalizations and 36,000 deaths resulted from this preventable disease (Moyad & Robinson, 2008).

Influenza virus is transmitted by airborne droplet and direct contact. Three major strains of the virus have been identified as influenza A virus, influenza B virus, and influenza C virus. Influenza A is responsible for most infections and for the most severe outbreaks of influenza. This is primarily a result of its ability to alter its surface antigens, bypassing previously developed immune defenses to the virus. New strains of influenza virus are named according to the strain, geographic origin, and year the strain was identified (e.g., A/Taiwan/89). Surface antigens of the specific virus may be used to further differentiate influenza A viruses. Outbreaks of influenza B virus are generally less extensive and less severe than those caused by influenza A virus. Illness associated with influenza C virus is mild and often goes unrecognized.

Type A influenza viruses are found in birds, pigs, whales, and humans and are believed to have caused three pandemics (in 1918, 1957, and 1968). Type B influenza viruses are commonly found among humans and often are responsible for influenza outbreaks, but not pandemics. Type C influenza viruses, found in humans, pigs, and dogs, typically cause mild respiratory infections (National Institute of Allergy and Infectious Diseases, 2006).

Risk Factors

People at increased risk of influenza or its complications include infants, young children, and anyone age 50 or older. Residents of a nursing home or other long-term care facility are at increased risk because of their age as well as the increased risk of exposure from others (both residents and health care providers). Clients with chronic disorders, especially diabetes and cardiac, renal, or pulmonary diseases, are more susceptible as well. Pregnant women, particularly during the second and third trimesters, are also at increased risk of complications. As with any infection, clients with weakened or compromised immune systems, such as those diagnosed with AIDS, receiving treatment for cancer, or taking immunosuppressive medications, are at greatest risk. Health care providers who work in a facility where they are more likely to be exposed to the influenza virus and day care providers or others who have close contact with infants and young children also face greater risk.

CLINICAL MANIFESTATIONS

Infection with influenza virus produces one of three syndromes:

1. Uncomplicated nasopharyngeal inflammation
2. Viral upper respiratory infection followed by bacterial infection
3. Viral pneumonia.

The onset is rapid; profound malaise may develop in a matter of minutes.

Manifestations of influenza include abrupt onset of chills and fever, malaise, muscle aches, and headache. Respiratory manifestations include dry, nonproductive cough, sore throat, substernal burning, and coryza (see Box 15–5). Acute symptoms subside within 2 to 3 days, although fever may last as long as a week. The cough may be severe and productive. Along with fatigue and weakness, the cough can persist for days or several weeks.

COLLABORATION

Preventing community outbreaks and protecting vulnerable populations (e.g., older adults and people with chronic diseases) are the primary focus for interdisciplinary care related to influenza. Medical treatment of influenza focuses on establishing the diagnosis, providing symptomatic relief, and preventing complications. Collaborative partners include local health departments, hospitals and urgent care centers, primary care and infectious disease clinics, school nurses, and other medical providers.

Prevention

Influenza vaccine is recommended for high-risk populations. The predominant strain of influenza virus varies from year to year. Therefore, a new vaccine formulation is prepared yearly, which incorporates antigens of the influenza strains predicted

Box 15–5 Manifestations of Influenza

RESPIRATORY MANIFESTATIONS

- Coryza
- Cough, initially dry but becoming productive
- Substernal burning
- Sore throat

SYSTEMIC MANIFESTATIONS

- Fever and chills
- Muscle aches
- Malaise
- Fatigue

CLINICAL MANIFESTATIONS AND THERAPIES Influenza

ETIOLOGY	CLINICAL MANIFESTATION	CLINICAL THERAPIES
Reye's syndrome is linked to children with a virus who are receiving aspirin.	Acute noninflammatory encephalopathy with an altered level of consciousness, hepatic failure with liver biopsy showing fatty metamorphosis, increase in alanine aminotransferase and aspartate aminotransferase, cerebrospinal fluid with white blood cells, and cerebral edema with or without inflammation. Initial symptoms include the following: ■ Persistent or recurrent vomiting ■ Listlessness ■ Personality changes and alteration in level of consciousness ■ Seizures.	■ Initiate intravenous (IV) therapy with D10/NSS. ■ Maintain patent airway and brain oxygenation. ■ Monitor cardiorespiratory function; be prepared for potential cardiac arrest. ■ Assess for hyperventilation to reduce cerebral edema. ■ Administer osmotic diuretics to reduce intracranial pressure. ■ Consider possible liver transplantation if extensive liver damage results.
Guillain-Barré syndrome is a possible complication of influenza.	Progressive paralysis of the muscles that may include muscles of respiration.	■ Provide supportive care to prevent complications such as assistance with activities of daily living, frequent repositioning, and artificial airway with mechanical ventilation to support oxygenation. ■ Administer IV therapy as ordered. ■ Provide nasogastric tube to meet nutritional needs if swallowing is impaired. ■ Provide for rehabilitation after disease recovery to restore baseline functioning.

to be the most prevalent for the upcoming flu season (typically the winter months). The vaccine contains egg protein and is not recommended for people who have a severe allergy to eggs or have previously experienced a severe hypersensitivity response to the vaccine.

Immunization with polyvalent (containing antigens of several viral strains) influenza virus vaccine is approximately 85% effective in preventing influenza infection for several months to a year (Tierney et al., 2005). Annual immunization is recommended for at-risk clients, including people older than the age of 65, residents of nursing homes, adults and children with chronic cardiopulmonary disorders (e.g., asthma) or chronic metabolic diseases (e.g., diabetes), and health care workers who have frequent contact with high-risk clients. Additionally, family members of at-risk clients should be vaccinated to reduce the client's risk of exposure. The vaccine is given in the fall, before the annual winter outbreak. Live attenuated vaccine, administered by intranasal spray, is available for healthy people under age 50.

Although the vaccine is readily available and inexpensive, only about 30% of at-risk clients are vaccinated each year. Many may fear a reaction from the vaccine, even though these vaccines are highly purified and reactions are rare. Approximately 5% of people experience mild symptoms of low-grade fever, malaise, or myalgia for up to 24 hours after vaccination. Serious adverse reactions to influenza vaccine are rare. *Guillain-Barré syndrome*, an acute neurologic disorder characterized by muscle weakness and distal sensory loss, has been associated with certain batches of vaccine.

Diagnostic Tests

The diagnosis of influenza is based on history, clinical findings, and knowledge of an influenza outbreak in the community. A chest x-ray and white blood cell (WBC) count may be done to rule out complications, such as pneumonia. The WBC count is commonly decreased in clients with influenza; bacterial infections usually cause an increased WBC count.

Pharmacologic Therapies

The antiviral drugs amantadine (Symmetrel) or rimantadine (Flumadine) may be used for prophylaxis in people who have not been vaccinated but are exposed to the virus. If the drug is given before or within 48 hours of exposure, it inhibits viral shedding and prevents or decreases the symptoms of influenza. If possible, those who have not been vaccinated should receive the vaccine along with the antiviral drug. The drug is continued for several weeks or for the duration of the influenza outbreak. Some strains of type A influenza virus have been found to be resistant to amantadine and rimantadine, potentially limiting their effectiveness in preventing or treating an influenza outbreak.

Amantadine, rimantadine, and the antiviral drugs zanamivir (Relenza), oseltamivir (Tamiflu), and ribavirin (Virazole) also may be used to reduce the duration and severity of flu symptoms. Both zanamivir and ribavirin are administered by inhalation; the other drugs are given orally. Zanamivir can precipitate bronchospasm in clients with a history of asthma or COPD, so it is not recommended for use in these clients (U.S. Food and Drug Administration, 2000).

Over-the-counter analgesics, such as aspirin, acetaminophen, or nonsteroidal anti-inflammatory drugs, provide symptomatic relief of fever and muscle ache. However, aspirin should never be given to children because of the risk of Reye's syndrome. Antitussives may decrease cough, promoting rest. Antibiotics are not indicated unless secondary bacterial infection occurs.

NURSING PROCESS

Stress the importance of yearly influenza vaccination for clients in high-risk groups and their families. Teach about the spread of the disease, including measures to reduce the risk for contracting influenza, such as thorough and timely hand washing and avoiding crowds and people who are ill.

Assessment

Unless there is a known outbreak of influenza in the community, it can be difficult to differentiate the manifestations of influenza from those of other upper respiratory infections. A thorough nursing assessment should provide clues to help determine if a client's symptoms can be attributed to influenza. The assessment should include the following:

- *Health history.* Known exposure to virus; current symptoms, their onset, and their duration; presence of dyspnea, chest pain, productive cough, and facial pain or pressure in sinus areas; current medications; history of influenza vaccine; chronic diseases, such as heart disease, COPD, or diabetes; and known medication allergies
- *Physical examination.* General appearance; vital signs, including temperature; skin color; lung sounds; and abdominal exam.

Diagnosis

Nursing diagnoses may differ based on the client's comorbid conditions and any complications that may develop. Suggested nursing diagnoses for clients with influenza may include the following:

- Ineffective Breathing Pattern
- Ineffective Airway Clearance
- Disturbed Sleep Patterns
- Risk for Infection.

Plan

Outcomes are individualized based on each client's condition and baseline health patterns. Suggested outcomes may include the following:

- Temperature remains within normal limits.
- Client maintains normal fluid balance by increasing fluid intake.
- Oxygen saturation remains within acceptable limits.
- Client maintains patent airway.

Implementation

Although the symptoms of influenza are distressing, most people with the illness provide self-care and do not contact a health care provider. Encourage appropriate self-care for clients with influenza. Discuss the following topics related to home care:

- Increase rest during the acute, febrile phase of the illness.
- Maintain a liberal fluid intake, even if anorexic.
- Appropriately use over-the-counter medications for symptom relief.
- Employ hygiene measures, such as using disposable tissues and frequent hand washing, to reduce spread of the disease.
- Know the manifestations of potential complications of influenza to report to the primary care provider.

Severe disease or complications of influenza may necessitate hospitalization for respiratory support and management. For these clients, nursing care focuses on maintaining breathing patterns, airway clearance, adequate rest, and risk for infection.

Ineffective Breathing Pattern

Muscle aches, malaise, and elevated temperature may increase the respiratory rate and alter the depth of respirations, decreasing effective alveolar ventilation. Shallow respirations also increase the risk of **atelectasis** (the collapse of lung tissue affecting all or part of the lung, impacting the exchange of oxygen and carbon dioxide).

- Pace activities to provide for periods of rest. Tachypnea increases the work of breathing, causing fatigue; fatigue, in turn, can further impair ventilation and reduce the effectiveness of coughing.
- Elevate the head of the bed. The upright position improves lung excursion (movement from the resting position) and reduces the work of breathing by lowering the diaphragm, moving abdominal contents downward, creating less resistance to diaphragmatic excursion, and slightly decreasing venous return.

PRACTICE ALERT

Monitor respiratory rate and pattern. Tachypnea and/or rapid, shallow respirations may impair effective alveolar ventilation and gas exchange.

Ineffective Airway Clearance

Swelling and congestion of mucous membranes, extracellular fluid exudate, and impaired ciliary action as a result of cell damage increase the risk of impaired airway clearance during influenza. The older adult is at particular risk because of normally reduced ciliary activity and increased lung compliance.

- Maintain adequate hydration. Assess mucous membranes and skin turgor for evidence of dehydration. Fever and decreased oral fluid intake may lead to dehydration and increased viscosity of secretions. Thick, viscous secretions are more difficult to expectorate.

- Increase the humidity of inspired air with a bedside humidifier. Increasing the water content of inhaled air helps to loosen thick secretions and soothe mucous membranes.
- Teach effective cough techniques. Administer analgesics as ordered. The huff cough (a series of small, low-pressure coughs) is effective to maintain open airways, and it spares energy. Relieving muscle ache increases the ability to cough effectively.

PRACTICE ALERT

Monitor the effectiveness of cough and the ability to remove airway secretions. Fatigue and general malaise may impair the ability to cough effectively and mobilize secretions.

Disturbed Sleep Pattern

Airway congestion, malaise, muscle aches, and persistent cough may interfere with the ability to rest, increasing fatigue and prolonging recovery.

- Assess sleep patterns using subjective and objective information. The client may appear to be sleeping but not achieving normal sleep patterns because of influenza symptoms. Both subjective and objective data are important to accurately assess sleep.
- Provide antipyretic and analgesic medications at or shortly before bedtime. These drugs promote comfort by reducing fever and relieving muscle aches.

PRACTICE ALERT

If necessary, request a cough suppressant for nighttime use. Cough suppressants are not recommended during the day, because coughing promotes airway clearance. They may, however, be necessary at night to allow rest.

Risk for Infection

Infection control measures are recommended to prevent person-to-person transmission of influenza and to control influenza outbreaks in health care facilities.

- Use standard precautions, and encourage all staff and visitors to frequently wash their hands. Hand washing is a primary control measure for infections transmitted via respiratory secretions.
- Instruct clients and visitors to control respiratory secretions by using tissues and to maintain a distance of at least 3 feet from others when coughing or sneezing. Provide masks for clients and visitors who are unable to control secretions. Limiting the spread of aerosolized secretions by covering the nose and mouth and maintaining distance from other people can reduce the spread of the disease to vulnerable populations.
- Use droplet precautions for clients with suspected or confirmed influenza: private room, masks for caregivers and visitors, and a mask for the client when he or she is being transported within the facility. These measures limit the spread of respiratory secretions.

Evaluation

The client should be evaluated for airway patency, breathing pattern, oxygenation, and thermoregulation. Appropriate alterations to the plan of care should be considered if the client is not responding to therapy or develops complications.

CARE PLAN

Care of the client with influenza should follow the steps outlined in the Practice Alerts in this exemplar, with considerations given to chronic illnesses or diseases that may worsen symptoms.

REVIEW Influenza

RELATE: LINK THE CONCEPTS

Linking the exemplar of Influenza with the concept of Oxygenation:

1. Describe the pathophysiology that would cause influenza to potentially diminish the body's ability to meet oxygen demands?
2. Would an older adult with COPD be at any greater risk for complications from influenza? Why, or why not?

Linking the exemplar of Influenza with the concept of Cognition:

3. Why might the older adult client who develops influenza display alterations in cognition?
4. What caring interventions can the nurse implement to reduce this impact on cognition when working in a long-term care facility with older adults?

READY: GO TO COMPANION SKILLS MANUAL

- Sputum collection
- Measuring oxygen saturation using a pulse oximeter
- Oxygen administration
- Assessing body temperature
- Assessing vital signs
- Turning clients
- Assessment of the lungs
- Medication administration
- Performing chest physiotherapy
- Suctioning
- Intravenous therapy
- Monitoring intake and output
- Caring for the client on a mechanical ventilator

REFER: GO TO MYNURSINGKIT

REFLECT: CASE STUDY

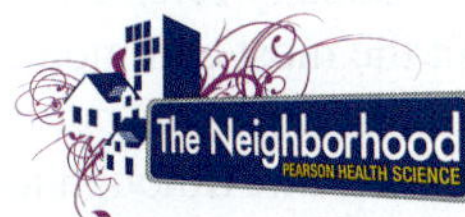

Norma James is a 65-year-old widow who lives alone. Although she has lived in the neighborhood for years, she is somewhat socially isolated. She has two adult sons with whom she has limited contact, because they live out of state and rarely call. She has only a few individuals she considers friends; she does not particularly like many people and prefers the company of her six cats.

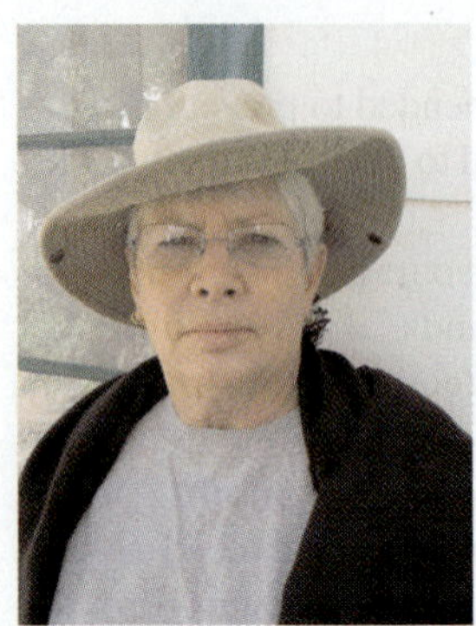

Mrs. James has a long history of type 2 diabetes mellitus and hypertension. In more recent years, she has been diagnosed with atrial fibrillation. She has multiple physicians and takes multiple medications. Mrs. James has a known drug allergy to penicillin.

Mrs. James does not work; she has very limited savings and relies on Social Security benefits for income. She smokes about half a pack of cigarettes a day and has been a smoker since she was in her 20s. She drinks alcohol "a couple times a year, usually a glass of wine at a special dinner."

Mrs. James does not drive and relies on her friends, neighbors, or the city bus for transportation. She lives near a grocery store and prides herself on being able to get most things she needs without any assistance. She spends most of her time alone at home and occupies herself by watching television, reading, and doing crossword and jigsaw puzzles.

1. Based on her biography, would you consider Mrs. James to be a candidate for influenza immunization? Explain your answer.
2. What information would you provide Mrs. James to assist her in making an informed decision about immunization?
3. If Mrs. James declines immunizations, what increased risks would you face if she contracted influenza based on her medical history?

15.4 OTITIS MEDIA

KEY TERMS

Audiologist, *828*
Eustachian tube, *824*
Hemotympanum, *826*
Labyrinthitis, *824*
Middle ear effusion, *825*
Myringotomy, *827*
Otitis externa, *824*
Otitis interna, *824*
Otitis media, *824*
Otoscope, *826*
Special gradient acoustic reflexometry, *828*
Tympanic membrane, *824*
Tympanocentesis, *829*
Tympanogram, *828*
Tympanostomy tubes, *829*
Vertigo, *826*

BASIS FOR SELECTION OF EXEMPLAR

Most common office-based visit

LEARNING OUTCOMES

After reading about this exemplar, you will be able to:

1. Describe the pathophysiology, etiology, and clinical manifestations of otitis media.
2. Identify risk factors associated with otitis media.
3. Illustrate the nursing process in providing culturally competent care across the life span for individuals with otitis media.
4. Formulate priority nursing diagnoses appropriate for an individual with otitis media.
5. Create a plan of care for an individual with otitis media.
6. Employ evidence-based caring interventions (or prevention) for an individual with otitis media.
7. Assess expected outcomes for an individual with otitis media.
8. Discuss therapies used in the collaborative care of an individual with otitis media.

OVERVIEW

The ear can become infected in any of the three chambers. **Otitis externa** is inflammation of the ear canal (often called swimmer's ear, because it is most frequently found in people who spend significant time in the water). **Otitis interna**, also called **labyrinthitis**, is inflammation of the inner ear. **Otitis media**, the topic of this exemplar, is inflammation of the middle ear.

Usually referred to as an ear "infection," otitis media is one of the most common childhood illnesses and a common reason for office visits, but it is not always accompanied by an actual infection. Although it is very common in young children under the age of 5 years, it can occur at any age. In the past decade, an increased number of cases have been observed, and recent changes have been made in recommendations for treatment (American Academy of Pediatrics, Subcommittee on Management of Acute Otitis Media, 2004; Pelton, 2005).

PATHOPHYSIOLOGY AND ETIOLOGY

The **tympanic membrane** (a thin, tense membrane that separates the middle ear from the external auditory canal) protects the middle ear from the external environment. However, the **eustachian tube** connects the middle ear with the nasopharynx to help equalize the pressure in the middle ear with the atmospheric pressure, and this connecting tube provides a route by which infectious organisms can enter the middle ear from the nose and throat, causing otitis media.

An upper respiratory infection often precedes the development of otitis media. This infection causes the mucous membranes of the eustachian tube to become edematous. As a result, air that normally flows to the middle ear is blocked, and the air in the middle ear is reabsorbed into the bloodstream. Fluid is pulled from the mucosal lining into the former air space, providing a medium for the rapid growth of pathogens. The tympanic membrane and the fluid behind it become infected.

The two primary forms of otitis media are serous and acute or suppurative; a chronic form can also develop. Both forms are associated with upper respiratory infection and eustachian tube dysfunction. The eustachian tube is narrow and flat, normally opening only during yawning and swallowing. Allergies or upper respiratory tract infections can cause edema of the tube lining, impairing its function.

Serous Otitis Media

Serous otitis media (also called *otitis media with effusion*) occurs when the eustachian tube is obstructed for a prolonged time, impairing equalization of air pressure in the middle ear. As the air within the middle ear space is gradually absorbed, the tube obstruction prevents more air from entering the middle ear. The resulting negative pressure in the middle ear causes sterile serous fluid to move from the capillaries into the space, which is known as **middle ear effusion**.

Acute Otitis Media

The eustachian tube also provides a route for the entry of pathogens into the normally sterile middle ear, resulting in acute, or suppurative, otitis media. Acute otitis media typically follows an upper respiratory infection. Edema of the eustachian tube impairs drainage of the middle ear, causing mucus and serous fluid to accumulate. This fluid is an excellent environment for the growth of bacteria, which may enter from the oronasopharynx via the eustachian tube.

Chronic Otitis Media

Chronic otitis media involves permanent perforation of the tympanic membrane, with or without recurrent pus formation. Changes in the mucosa and bony structures (ossicles) of the middle ear often accompany chronic otitis media. It usually is the result of recurrent acute otitis media and eustachian tube dysfunction, but it may also result from trauma or other diseases.

Marginal perforations, which usually occur in the posterosuperior portion of the tympanic membrane, are associated with more complications than central perforations. With marginal perforations, squamous epithelium may migrate from the ear canal into the middle ear, where it begins to desquamate and accumulate, forming a *cholesteatoma* (a cyst or mass filled with epithelial cell debris). Its incidence is highest in children and young adults. The desquamating epithelium continues to accumulate and remains infected, producing collagenases (enzymes) that destroy adjacent bone. The inflammatory process impairs the blood supply to the stapes, causing its destruction and conductive hearing loss. Cholesteatomas are benign and slow-growing tumors, which can enlarge to fill the entire middle ear. Untreated, the cholesteatoma can progressively destroy the ossicles and erode into the inner ear, causing profound hearing loss.

Tympanic membrane perforation can be repaired with a tympanoplasty to restore sound conduction and the integrity of the middle ear. A cholesteatoma may require delicate surgery to remove it. If at all possible, radical mastoidectomy with removal of the tympanic membrane, ossicles, and tumor should be avoided.

Etiology

Approximately 70% of infants have at least one case of acute otitis media during the first year of life, and 93% of children are diagnosed with the problem by 7 years of age. Peak incidence is during the first 2 years of life, particularly from 6 to 20 months of age (Bernius & Perlin, 2006).

The specific cause of otitis media is unknown, but it appears to be related to eustachian tube dysfunction. The most common causative organisms are *Streptococcus pneumoniae*, *Haemophilus influenzae*, and *Moraxella catarrhalis* (Pelton, 2005).

Upper respiratory infection or allergies (e.g., hay fever) predispose the client to serous otitis media. In addition, clients with narrowed or edematous eustachian tubes may also be subject to barotrauma or barotitis media. In these clients, the middle ear cannot adapt to rapid changes in barometric pressure, such as those that occur during air travel or underwater diving. Barotrauma tends to occur during descent in an airplane, because negative pressure within the middle ear causes the eustachian tube to collapse and lock. However, underwater diving places even greater stress on the eustachian tube and middle ear (Tierney et al., 2005).

Although a viral upper respiratory infection may predispose the client to acute otitis media, the bacteria *Streptococcus pneumoniae, Haemophilus influenzae,* and *Streptococcus pyogenes* account for most cases of otitis media in adults. Invasion and colonization of the middle ear by bacteria and the resultant migration of WBCs cause pus formation. Accumulated pus can increase middle ear pressure sufficient to rupture the tympanic membrane. The bacterial infection may also migrate internally, causing mastoiditis, brain abscess, or bacterial meningitis. A more common complication of otitis media is a persistent conductive hearing loss, which typically resolves when the middle ear effusion clears.

Risk Factors

Otitis media occurs more frequently among boys, children who attend child care centers, those with allergies, children exposed to tobacco smoke, and those who use pacifiers several hours daily. It is most common during the winter months. Children with conditions such as cleft lip and palate or Down syndrome more often experience otitis media. Breast-feeding appears to be protective against otitis media. Conditions such as enlarged adenoids or edema from allergic rhinitis can also obstruct the eustachian tube and lead to otitis media. Pacifier use raises the soft palate and thus alters dynamics in the eustacian tube, providing for entry of microorganisms from the nasopharynx (Neto, Hemb, & Silva, 2006). Recurrent otitis media has an increased frequency in children of parents who smoke (Brook & Gober, 2005). Children with multiple siblings and those who attend child care centers have increased rates of recurrent acute otitis media (Harrison, 2005). Parents should be taught not to put children to bed with a bottle and feed infants in an upright position to reduce the risk for otitis media.

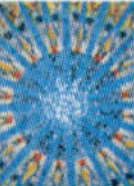

FOCUS ON DIVERSITY AND CULTURE
Otitis Media

Native American and Alaska Native children have a very high rate of otitis media, perhaps related to culture-specific bony structure of the ear, nose, and mouth. One study found that these children are seen about three times more frequently in outpatient clinics for otitis media than are other U.S. children (Curns et al., 2002). Nurses should be alert for the common incidence in these population groups, plan prevention programs, and ensure prompt care and teaching about treatments for families of children affected.

CLINICAL MANIFESTATIONS

Typical manifestations of serous otitis media in adults include decreased hearing in the affected ear and complaints of "snapping" or "popping" in the ear. On examination, the tympanic membrane demonstrates decreased mobility and may appear retracted or bulging. Fluid or air bubbles are often visible behind the drum. Severe pressure differences, such as those occurring with barotrauma, may cause acute pain, hemorrhage into the middle ear, rupture of the tympanic membrane, or even rupture of the round window, with sensory hearing loss and severe **vertigo** (a sensation of whirling or rotation). **Hemotympanum** (bleeding into or behind the tympanic membrane) may be observed when examining the ear with an **otoscope** (a hand-held instrument with a light and a cone-shaped attachment known as the "ear speculum"). Figure 15–16 ■ demonstrates the appearance of hemotympanum on otoscopic examination.

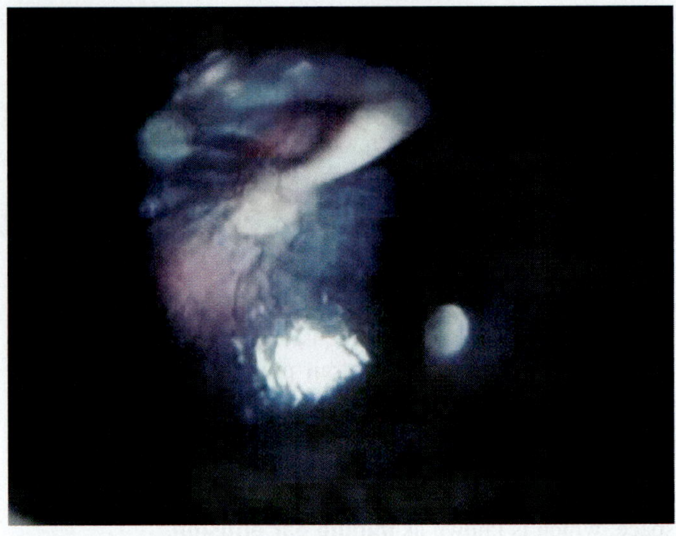

Figure 15–16 ■ Hemotympanum.

The client with acute otitis media typically experiences mild to severe pain in the affected ear. The client's temperature is

CLINICAL MANIFESTATIONS AND THERAPIES Otitis Media

ETIOLOGY	CLINICAL MANIFESTATION	CLINICAL THERAPY
Acute otitis media—bacterial infection in the middle ear from pathogens transferred from the nasopharynx; most common infectious agents are *Streptococcus. pneumoniae, Haemphilus influenzae, Moraxella catarrhalis*	*Behavioral*—ear pain, pulling at ear, rapid onset, irritability, malaise, and poor feeding	■ Treat ear pain with local anesthetic, local herbal pain products, or systemic acetaminophen or ibuprofen.
	Examination—bulging tympanic membrane; air or fluid bubbles present behind tympanic membrane; immobile or poorly mobile tympanic membrane; red tympanic membrane, or other color change (e.g., white, gray, or yellow) as long as bulging is present; and reduced visibility of tympanic membrane landmarks with displaced light reflex	■ Observe child's condition for 48–72 hours and, if not improved, treat with course of antibiotics.
Otitis media with effusion—collection of fluid in the middle ear behind the tympanic membrane, which is not infected with bacteria	*Behavioral*—difficulty hearing or responding as expected to sounds	■ Symptomatic treatment or pain
	Examination—signs of acute inflammation are NOT present; tympanic membrane is retracted or neutral; immobile or partly mobile tympanic membrane; yellow or gray tympanic membrane; opaque or thickened tympanic membrane with visibility of landmarks reduced	■ Careful observation of hearing acuity over several months ■ Speech assessment if loss of hearing acuity occurs ■ Developmental assessment

often elevated. Diminished hearing, dizziness, vertigo, and tinnitus are common associated complaints. Pus within the mastoid air cells often causes mastoid tenderness in acute otitis media. On otoscopic examination, the tympanic membrane appears red and inflamed or dull and bulging (Figure 15–17 ■). Decreased movement of the membrane is demonstrated by tympanometry or air insufflation. Spontaneous rupture of the tympanic membrane releases a purulent discharge, as seen in Figure 15–18 ■. A **myringotomy** (a surgical incision of the tympanic membrane) may be performed to relieve the pressure.

Acute otitis media is diagnosed in pediatric clients when the child has acute onset of ear pain, marked redness of the tympanic membrane on otoscopy, and middle ear effusion, as seen in Figure 15–19 ■. Recurrent acute otitis media refers to repeated bouts of acute otitis media, such as three in 6 months or four in 12 months. *Serous otitis media* is evidenced by fluid in the middle ear without inflammation, as demonstrated in Figure 15–20 ■. Serous otitis media sometimes becomes chronic (continuing for more than 3 months) and is more commonly associated with hearing loss.

Diarrhea, vomiting, and fever are typical of otitis media. Infants and young children also have characteristic behaviors that can indicate otitis media may be present. Pulling at the ear is a sign of ear pain (Figure 15–21 ■). Irritability and "acting out" may be signs of a related hearing impairment. The child with otitis media often awakens crying at night because of increased ear pressure when prone or supine. See the Clinical Manifestations of Therapies feature that follows for further details.

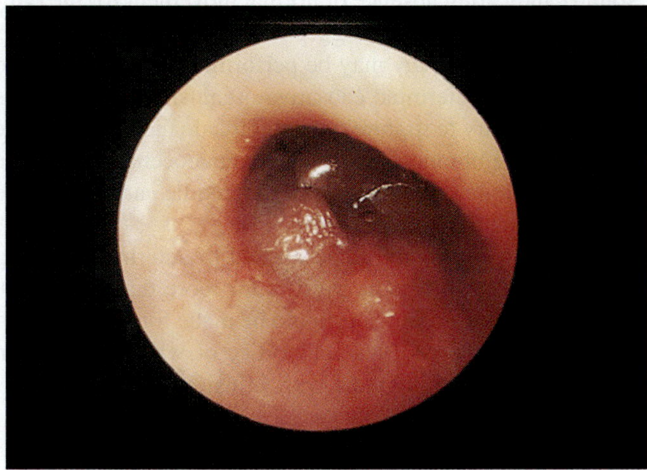

Figure 15–17 ■ A red, bulging tympanic membrane of otitis media.

Source: Janet Hayes/Medical Images, Inc.

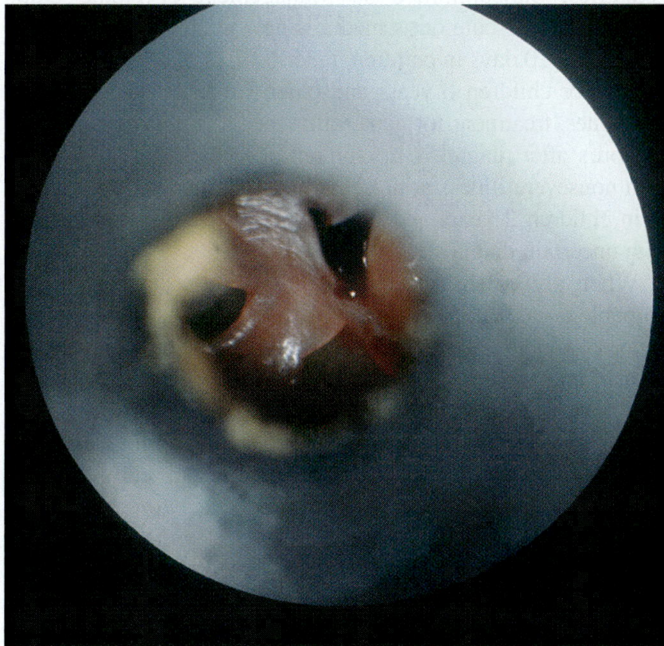

Figure 15–18 ■ Perforation of tympanic membrane.

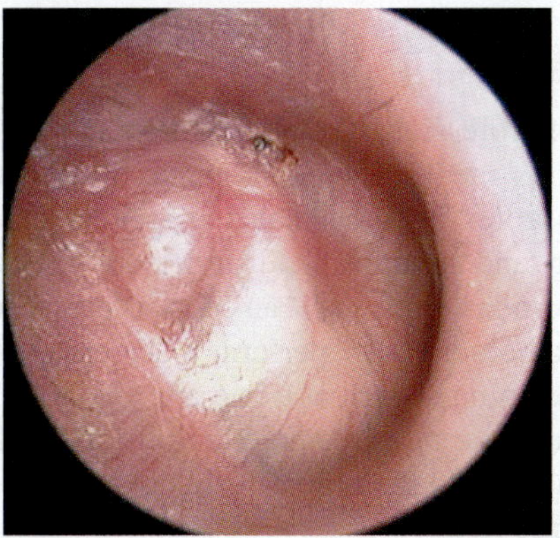

Figure 15–19 ■ Acute otitis media is characterized by abrupt onset, pain, middle ear effusion, and inflammation. Note the injected vessels and altered shape of the cone of light.

Courtesy of Kevin Kavanagh, MD, FACS.

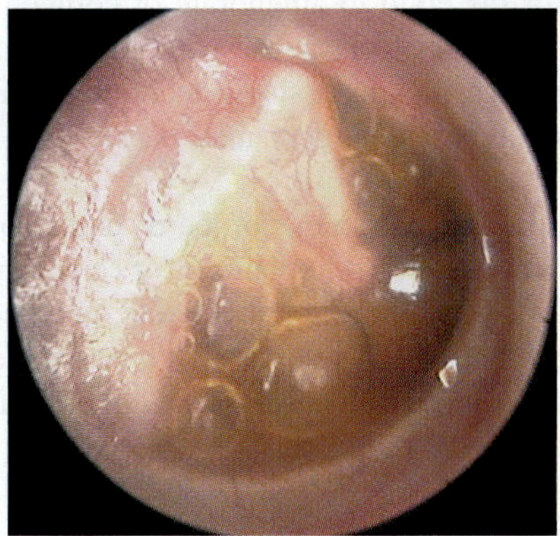

Figure 15–20 ■ Otitis media with effusion is noted on otoscopy by fluid line or air bubbles. Pneumatic otoscopy or tympanometry shows a nonmobile tympanic membrane. Note that the light reflex is not in the expected position due to a change in tympanic membrane shape from air bubbles. Where would you expect to see the cone of light?

Courtesy of Kevin Kavanagh, MD, FACS.

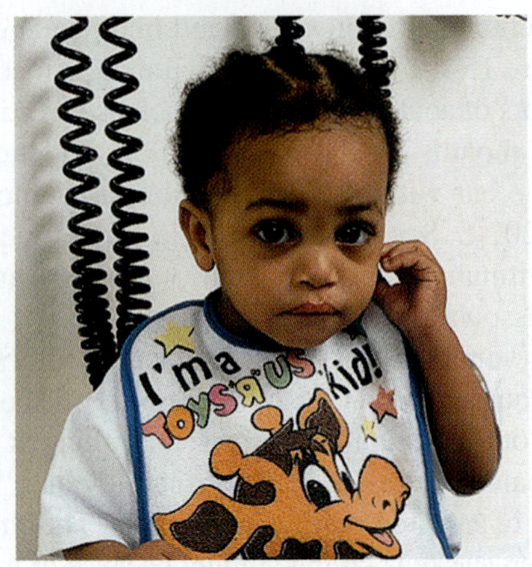

Figure 15–21 ■ This young child is pulling at the ear and acting fussy, two important signs of otitis media. Ask the parents about the presence of fever and night awakenings, additional signs that are often observed in children with this condition.

COLLABORATION

A number of professionals may provide support to a child with recurrent otitis media. Either the nurse or an **audiologist** (a health care professional specializing in identifying, diagnosing, treating and monitoring disorders of the auditory and vestibular portions of the ear) can conduct a hearing screening. A speech pathologist may perform a screening to ensure the child is developing speech at a rate appropriate for his age. If a child fails a hearing screening, the professional conducting the screening should then refer the client to an audiologist for further testing.

Either the nurse, the speech pathologist, or the child's classroom teacher can assist the parent with understanding the importance of maintaining verbal communication in the home and reading to the child on a regular basis. If a child does experience hearing or speech loss as a result of recurrent otitis media, the audiologist or speech pathologist can assist the parents and classroom teachers in developing an individual education plan for the child to ameliorate or compensate for any deficit. The audiologist or speech pathologist can also assist the parent in accessing any assistive technology the child may require. In some cases, surgery may be required to alleviate pressure in the ear.

The nurse in a pediatrician's office or family practice may collaborate with a child's school nurse (or center director if the child is in day care) about any preventive practices that may need to be emphasized in the child's classroom, such as frequent hand washing, or the need for the child to increase fluid intake or avoid water activities.

Diagnostic Tests

Diagnostic tests that may be conducted in addition to physical examination include the following:

- *Impedance audiometry,* also known as tympanometry, is an accurate diagnostic test for serous otitis media. An audiometer with a sealed probe tip delivers a continuous tone to the tympanic membrane. Compliance of the tympanic membrane and middle ear is measured by recording energy reflected from the membrane surface. With middle ear effusion, compliance is reduced.
- *Complete blood count (CBC)* may be done to assess for an elevated WBC count and increased numbers of immature cells indicative of acute bacterial infection.
- *Tympanocentesis or myringotomy* is performed if the tympanic membrane has ruptured. Drainage is cultured to determine the infecting organism.
- **Special gradient acoustic reflectometry** measures the condition of the middle ear by introducing a sound and then measuring the response of the tympanic membrane (Windmill & Windmill, 2006). A flat **tympanogram** (a test that provides a graph of the middle ear's ability to transmit sound), indicating absence of normal movement for the tympanic membrane, is also suggestive of otitis media.
- *Culture and sensitivity* may be performed on fluid from the middle ear to determine causative organisms if drainage is noted secondary to rupture of the tympanic membrane. If the tympanic membrane is intact, a tympanocentesis may be done to aspirate some fluid from the middle ear through the tympanic membrane.
- *Audiologic testing* may be performed to determine hearing loss if serous otitis media persists for more than 3 months. A referral to an audiologist should be made for children who fail testing in the pediatrician's office or who are less than 4 years of age (Otitis Media with Effusion, 2004).

Pharmacologic Therapies

Concern in the medical community has grown over the increasing appearance of drug-resistant microbials as causative agents in otitis media. The American Academy of Pediatrics and the American Academy of Family Physicians joined together to establish recommendations in 2004 (American Academy of Pediatrics, Subcommittee on Management of Acute Otitis Media, 2004). Acute otitis media is now treated with antibiotic therapy for 10 days in children under 6 years of age and for 5 to 7 days for children 6 years and older. Consistent with current guidelines, treatment for acute otitis media is delayed for 48 to 72 hours after diagnosis in children aged 6 months to 2 years with nonsevere illness at presentation AND uncertain diagnosis or in children 2 years and older without severe symptoms OR with uncertain diagnosis.

When prescribed, the choice of antibiotic depends on the probable organism, ease of administration, cost, previous effectiveness, and any history of allergies. First-line therapy for children is amoxicillin at a dose of 80 to 90 mg $\cdot$ kg^{-1} $\cdot$ day^{-1}. Amoxicillin with clavulanate or cefuroxime are second-line drugs. If an intramuscular drug is preferred, cefdinir at 14 mg $\cdot$ kg^{-1} $\cdot$ day^{-1}, cefpodoxime at mg $\cdot$ kg^{-1} $\cdot$ day^{-1}, or cefuroxime at 30 mg $\cdot$ kg^{-1} $\cdot$ day^{-1} can be prescribed (Zacharyczuk, 2004). When the tympanic membrane is intact, topical anesthetic eardrops are sometimes prescribed for several days to provide pain relief.

Acute otitis media in adults is usually treated with antibiotic therapy, especially amoxicillin, trimethoprim-sulfamethoxazole, cefaclor, or azithromycin, for 5 to 10 days. This course of treatment is long enough to ensure eradication of the infective organism yet short enough to reduce the incidence of bacterial resistance. Symptomatic relief may be provided by analgesics, antipyretics, antihistamines, and local application of heat. Referral to an audiologist may be necessary if the adult client reports loss of hearing following successful healing of infection.

Serous otitis media is not treated with antibiotics but is evaluated periodically to be sure there is not an additional acute otitis media that needs treatment. Children with serous otitis media generally improve within 3 months. Since this type of otitis is more commonly associated with hearing loss and cochlear damage, follow-up with audiology is essential. If hearing is abnormal, speech testing should also be performed (Otitis Media with Effusion, 2004). When eustachian tube dysfunction and serous otitis media do not spontaneously resolve or when they lead to hearing loss, a short course of an anti-inflammatory drug (e.g., oral prednisone for 7 days) is prescribed to reduce mucosal edema of the tube and improve its patency.

Neither decongestants nor antihistamines have been shown to be effective in the treatment of otitis media with or without effusion. Steroids also do not appear to have any long-term beneficial effect. If infection recurs despite antibiotic treatment for acute otitis media or if serous otitis media continues 4 months or more with persistent hearing loss present, myringotomy may be performed, and **tympanostomy tubes** (pressure-equalizing tubes) may be inserted to drain fluid from the middle ear.

The *Haemophilus influenzae* type B (Hib) vaccine, which is routinely given to children beginning at 2 months of age, has been influential in reducing the incidence of diseases, such as otitis media, that are caused by *H. influenzae* type B. Another, more recently recommended immunization for pneumococcal disease has also decreased cases of otitis media from that pathogen.

Surgery

A myringotomy or tympanocentesis may be performed to relieve excess pressure in the middle ear and prevent spontaneous rupture of the eardrum. To perform a **tympanocentesis**, the physician inserts a 20-gauge spinal needle through the inferior portion of the tympanic membrane, allowing aspiration of fluid and pus from the middle ear to relieve pressure and, if necessary, obtain a specimen for culture. Myringotomy may be performed to relieve severe pain or when complications of acute otitis media, such as mastoiditis, are present. As soon as the pressure is released, pain subsides and hearing improves.

Clients who do not respond to antibiotic therapy may require myringotomy with insertion of tympanostomy tubes. Small tubes are inserted into the inferior portion of the tympanic membrane, providing for ventilation and drainage of the middle ear during healing. The tube is eventually extruded from the ear, and the tympanic membrane heals. While the tube is in place, it is important to avoid getting any water in the ear canal, because the water may then enter the middle ear space.

Alternative Therapies

Because many children with otitis media experience ear pain that can disrupt their sleep, as well as that of family members, anesthetic eardrops have been used for their analgesic effect on the tympanic membrane. Because some families might prefer to use natural remedies for ear pain, a study comparing Naturopathic Herbal Extract Ear Drops (a naturopathic herbal extract of *Allium sativum*, *Verbascum thapsus*, *Calendula flores*, and *Hypericum perforatum,* lavender, and vitamin E) with a local anesthetic of amethocaine and phenazone was conducted. About half of the total of 171 children were given the naturopathic pain treatment, with the remaining children receiving the anesthetic. Parents rated the children after training with a pain tool. Both treatments were effective in decreasing ear pain over the 3 days of the study. No significant difference in success rates of local anesthetic and naturopathic agent was found; in fact, the naturopathic agent was as effective as, or even more effective than, the anesthetic at each measurement period. It was concluded that herbal pain control may be very beneficial for treatment of ear pain and can help to decrease the need for antibiotic treatment of otitis media (Sarrell, Cohen, & Kahan, 2003). However, in a collective analysis of several studies, it was concluded that insufficient evidence currently exists to describe whether naturopathic treatment is effective for treatment of ear pain in children (Foxlee et al., 2006).

NURSING PROCESS

Clients with otitis media are commonly treated in outpatient and community settings. The nursing role is primarily one of support and education. Health promotion for otitis media focuses on educating clients about the importance of seeking medical care for prolonged, severe ear pain, with or without drainage, combined with an upper respiratory tract infection. Untreated or repeated attacks of otitis media can progress to a chronic form of otitis media, acute mastoiditis, or eardrum perforation.

Assessment

Collect assessment data through a health history and physical examination. The data collected should include the following:

- *Health history.* Recent upper respiratory infection; presence, intensity, and nature of pain in affected ear; sense of fullness or pressure in the ear; change in hearing; snapping or popping sensation in the affected ear; and presence of vertigo
- *Physical examination.* Temperature; hearing test; inspect tympanic membrane at each health promotion visit and during examinations for illness; examine the color, transparency, mobility, presence of landmarks, and light reflex; with pediatric clients, ask parents if the child has had a fever, been fussy, or been pulling at the ears; observe for signs of impaired hearing, such as difficulty hearing a whisper or soft sounds.

During the physical examination, have parents assist with holding the head steady of young or uncooperative children (Figure 15–22 ■) Young children have more narrow auditory canals that angle downward. To assess the tympanic membrane of children under the age of 4 years, pull the tragus of the external ear down and back. Carefully insert the speculum of the otoscope into the ear following the curve of the auditory canal. Assess the tympanic membrane for the following: color, opacity, mobility, position, and the presence of fluid or other abnormal findings. Use a speculum that fits tightly into the ear canal, and gently press the bulb insufflator to assess tympanic membrane mobility. Look for dimpling, or inward movement, of the tympanic membrane lateral to the umbo. Normal tympanic membranes are pearly-gray, transparent, mobile, and neutrally positioned. The tympanic membrane is a vascular organ; it will redden with conditions that cause flushing (e.g., fever and crying). Reddening of the tympanic membrane in the absence of purulent discharge does not indicate the presence of middle ear infection. Otitis media causes full, orange-yellow tympanic membranes with decreased motility. Serous otitis media results in tympanic membranes that are amber-colored, immobile, and in neutral to full positions.

Diagnosis

Nursing diagnoses that may apply to the client with otitis media include the following:

- Acute Pain related to inflammation and pressure on tympanic membrane
- Infection related to presence of pathogens
- Risk for Caregiver Role Strain related to sleep deprivation and/or chronic condition
- Knowledge Deficit related to preventative strategies
- Risk for Delayed Growth and Development related to hearing loss
- Risk for Imbalanced Body Temperature: Hyperthermia related to infectious process
- Fatigue (child and parent) related to sleep deprivation
- Disturbed Sensory Perception: Auditory related to chronic ear infections and altered hearing reception.

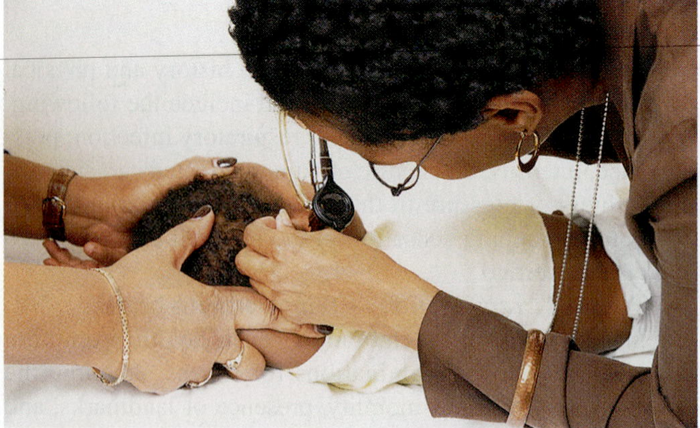

Figure 15–22 ■ Parent restraint of a young child during examination of the ear.

Plan

Most clients with otitis media do not require hospitalization; therefore, nursing management centers on planning care in the home. Potential outcomes may include the following:

- The client or parent will indicate absence of pain.
- The client will be infection free following the course of treatment.
- Caregivers will manage the child's condition with minimal stress.
- The client or parents will state their understanding of preventive measures.
- The child will have normal hearing.
- The child will have normal motor and language development.

Implementation

Nursing care is individualized based on the diverse needs presented by clients. Care is focused on pain management, client and family teaching, and preventing recurrence of infection. Screening for potential hearing loss is of particular importance in clients who contract repeated otitis media.

Acute Pain

Tissue edema, effusion of the middle ear, and the resulting inflammatory response can affect the pain-sensitive tissues of the middle ear in otitis media, causing acute discomfort. This discomfort is increased by pressure changes, such as those that occur during air travel or underwater diving. A nurse working with a client who reports pain associated with otitis media should:

- Assess client's pain for severity, quality, and location. A thorough assessment is important to determine the source of the pain. The pain of otitis media, unlike that of external otitis, is not aggravated by movement of the external ear.
- Encourage client to use mild analgesics, such as ibuprofen or acetaminophen every 4 hours, as needed to relieve pain and fever. These nonprescription medications are effective in reducing the perception of pain. Ibuprofen also has anti-inflammatory properties that may help to relieve inflammation of the ear.
- Advise client to apply heat to the affected side unless contraindicated. Heat dilates blood vessels, promoting the reabsorption of fluid and reducing swelling.
- Instruct client to avoid air travel, rapid changes in elevation, or diving. A rapid change in barometric pressure can increase the client's pain significantly.
- Instruct client to report promptly an abrupt relief of pain to the primary care provider. Pain that subsides abruptly may indicate spontaneous perforation of the tympanic membrane with relief of pressure within the middle ear.

Risk for Caregiver Role Strain

The chronic nature of otitis media in some children can create many problems for the family. Parents often become frustrated and disillusioned because of the inability of the health care system to cure the child, and they may fear a permanent hearing impairment.

NURSING CARE PLAN A Client With Otitis Media

Melinda Jeffries is a 2-year-old, African American toddler who lives with her mother, father, and 6-year-old sister. She attends child care every day, because both parents work outside the home. The child care center is a large building with multiple classrooms for different age groups and approximately 15 to 20 students in her class on a given day. Melinda has had recurrent diagnoses of otitis media, with four infections diagnosed over the course of the winter thus far.

Her mother has brought her to the pediatric nurse practitioner's office today because Melinda has a temperature of 102.6°F axillary, has been pulling at her ear, and was awake most of last night crying in pain. The nurse practitioner diagnoses a left otitis media with effusion and prescribes amoxicillin and corticosteroid eardrops and informs the mother to administer ibuprofen every 6 hours for pain and fever control. Melinda's mother is concerned that these recurrent ear infections will result in hearing loss and asks about insertion of tubes to prevent further infections. The nurse practitioner explains that the occurrence of ear infections tends to be highest during winter months; she recommends waiting to see if Melinda improves when the weather gets warmer. Ms. Jeffries agrees, saying she noticed that with her older child when she was this age.

ASSESSMENT

Melinda is admitted to the provider's office by Sarah McKinney, RN. In her assessment, she finds Melinda irritable and less tolerant of separation from her mother than usual. Examination finds an orange-yellow tympanic membrane with decreased motility, warm dry skin, and vital signs 99.8_{AX}°F– 108 -20; blood pressure is deferred at this time secondary to age and general good health. Neurologic, respiratory, cardiovascular, and abdominal assessments are essentially normal. Auditory examination reveals a slight decrease in hearing, most likely caused by the collection of fluid in the middle ear. Further testing will need to be done when Melinda is asymptomatic.

DIAGNOSES

- Disturbed Sensory Perception: Auditory related to otitis media
- Pain related to tympanic pressure secondary to fluid accumulation in the middle ear
- Deficient Knowledge related to lack of information regarding indications for myringotomy and administration of eardrops
- Risk for Fluid Volume Deficit related to hyperthermia

PLANNING

Goals for Melinda's care include:

- Melinda will demonstrate improved hearing with resolution of otitis media.
- Melinda will demonstrate reduced level of pain and increased ability to sleep at night.
- Melinda's mother can describe indications for performing myringotomy and demonstrate administration of eardrops.
- Melinda will take in fluid adequate to maintain hydration.

IMPLEMENTATION

- Schedule a return visit to retest hearing in 2 to 3 weeks.
- Encourage the mother to call the office if Melinda shows signs of discomfort uncontrolled by ibuprofen.
- Teach the mother nonpharmacologic pain relief measures, such as application of heat and elevation of the head of the bed at night to promote drainage from the middle ear via the eustachian tube.
- Instruct the mother on the importance of administering the entire dispensed quantity of antibiotics, calling the office if a rash or other sign of allergic reaction occurs, and encouraging fluid intake.
- Demonstrate the technique for administering eardrops, and then have the mother provide a return demonstration.
- Provide verbal and written instructions about ear care, including scheduled follow-up examinations.
- Teach parents about potential complications, actions to take in response and when to call the provider.

EVALUATION

Melinda returns in 2 weeks and is found to be infection free. Her tympanic membrane is normal in appearance, and she is her usual happy self. Hearing tests reveal that her hearing is within the normal range and consultation with an audiologist is not indicated.

CRITICAL THINKING

1. What are the indications for performance of a myringotomy? Why was this client not a candidate?
2. What other medications might have been prescribed to treat Melinda's ear infection?
3. Had Melinda's hearing not improved after resolution of the infection, what actions could the audiologist have recommended to improve hearing?
4. Develop a plan of care related to caregiver role strain secondary to Melinda's inability to sleep because of pain.

- Reassure parents that as the child grows older, the recurrent infections eventually will cease.
- Provide pain relief techniques, such as teaching correct administration of eardrops, oral administration of acetaminophen, and positioning the baby or child with the head slightly elevated, which often decreases pressure and pain.

Knowledge Deficit

Both the client who has otitis media and the family need teaching about the disorder, its causes and prevention, and any specific treatment that is recommended or prescribed.

- Discuss with the client and family the antibiotic therapy and potential side effects (if prescribed), the importance of completing all ordered doses (if prescribed), the follow-up examinations in 2 to 4 weeks, the importance of avoiding swimming, diving, or submerging the head while bathing (if ventilation tubes are in place).
- Emphasize preventive measures. Exposure to secondhand smoke in the home increases the incidence of otitis media in children; therefore, parents who smoke should be encouraged to avoid smoking near the child or in the home. Wood burning stoves should also be avoided when possible. Breast-feeding provides some protection from the disease. Placing babies to sleep with a pacifier may increase the incidence of otitis media and should be avoided in the infant with prior infections (Pelton, 2005).
- Teach the client and family members about the surgery and postoperative care (if surgical intervention is necessary). Provide instruction about any special postoperative precautions, such as avoiding water in the ear canals and sudden changes in air pressure.
- Inform parents that the child who is having tympanostomy tubes inserted is generally treated in a day surgery setting. Teach the child and parents about what to expect, and provide instructions for safe care upon discharge.
- Explain to them the problem of developing resistant strains of bacteria. Parents may not understand why the child with a possible infection is not given antibiotics. New research indicates that most children improve after 48–72 hours even without antibiotics, and that overuse of antibiotics contributes to drug resistance.
- Explain to parents of children with serous otitis media that antibiotics, steroids, and antihistamines/decongestants have not been effective and that most children improve in 3 months without medication. Assure parents that if the effusion continues beyond that time, the child will be tested for hearing acuity and, if indicated, for speech development.
- Encourage parents to bring the child back for care if the condition worsens or has not improved in the recommended time.

Risk for Delayed Growth and Development

For the child with some hearing loss as a result of serous otitis media, a home environment that fosters math, reading, and verbal skills can overcome the effects of lowered hearing during the time of infection. Nurses should focus interventions on helping parents to read and talk frequently with children who have serous otitis media.

Fatigue

Both child and parents experience fatigue when a child awakens in the night with ear pain.

Disturbed Sensory Perception: Auditory

Provide hearing and language examinations at regular intervals, inform parents of results, and refer to an audiology specialist if hearing problems are identified.

Evaluation

Expected outcomes of nursing care for the child with otitis media include the following:

- The child will return to normal sleep and feeding patterns.
- The child will maintain normal hearing and speech development.
- The child will free of pain and fever.
- The parents will indicate adequate understanding of treatment regimen.

REVIEW Otitis Media

RELATE: LINK THE CONCEPTS

Linking the exemplar of Otitis Media with the concept of Evidence-Based Practice:

1. What peer-reviewed research can you find supporting the evidence-based practice of not prescribing antibiotics routinely for all diagnosed otitis media?
2. Based on your findings, how would this impact your practice when caring for clients with otitis media?

Linking the exemplar of Otitis Media with the concept of Health Policy:

3. How has health policy changed in the treatment of otitis media?
4. Does this change in policy seem reasonable? Why, or why not?

READY: GO TO COMPANION SKILLS MANUAL

- Administration of eardrops
- Restraint of infants and toddlers
- Assessing the ears and hearing

REFER: GO TO MYNURSINGKIT

REFLECT: CASE STUDY

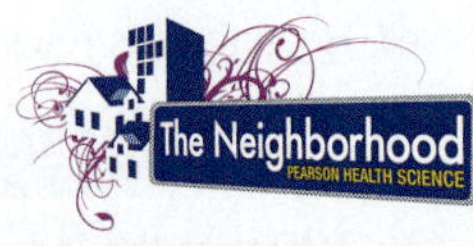

Ryan Riley is the 1-year-old son of Jessica Riley. They live in a one-bedroom apartment with Jessica's boyfriend, Casey. Ryan has a history of hospital admission for dehydration, respiratory syncytial virus, and failure to thrive. Because he was found to be underweight and undernourished, Social Services made arrangements for him to attend Peanut Butter and Jelly day care during the day and to stay with his grandmother, Evelyn, in the evenings when his mother is working. He is seen for

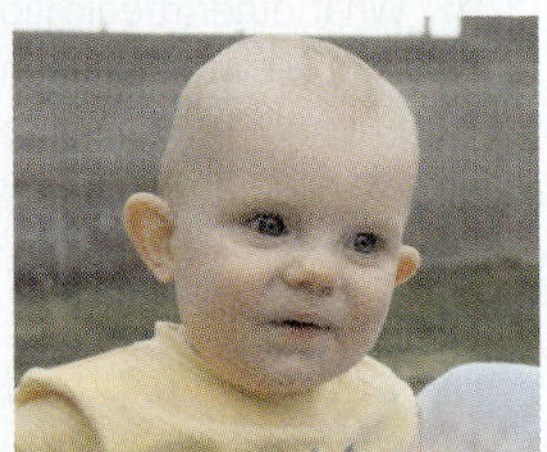

his 12-month immunizations and well-child exam, and his weight is 20 pounds, demonstrating good progress.

Fifteen-month-old Ryan has been running a fever and has a great deal of nasal drainage and congestion. He does not feel well at all. Worried about how ill he was last time he was sick, Evelyn takes him to Neighborhood Pediatrics to be examined. Ryan is diagnosed with an upper respiratory infection. Evelyn is instructed to give him plenty of fluids and to give him children's Tylenol for the fever.

1. What factors place Ryan at risk for developing otitis media?
2. What teaching would you provide Ryan's grandmother to reduce the risk of otitis media?
3. While teaching Ryan's grandmother about his care, what symptoms would you tell her need to be reported to the provider should they occur?

15.5 PNEUMONIA

KEY TERMS

Apnea, *840*
Atelectasis, *841*
Bronchiectasis, *837*
Consolidation, *835*
Cyanosis, *839*
Dyspnea, *839*
Empyema, *835*
Hemoptysis, *839*
Hypoxemia, *846*
Lung abscess, *835*
Pleural effusion, *835*
Pleuritic pain, *836*
Pleuritis, *835*
Pneumonia, *833*
Retractions, *839*
Tachypnea, *840*
Thoracentesis, *835*
Unilateral lobar pneumonia, *834*
Ventilation, *833*
Virulence, *834*

BASIS FOR SELECTION OF EXEMPLAR

Centers for Disease Control and Prevention
Top 20 reasons to be admitted through the emergency department
Agency for Health Care Research and Quality
National Center for Health Statistics

LEARNING OUTCOMES

After reading about this exemplar, you will be able to:

1. Describe the pathophysiology, etiology, and clinical manifestations of pneumonia.
2. Identify risk factors associated with pneumonia.
3. Illustrate the nursing process in providing culturally competent care across the life span for individuals with pneumonia.
4. Formulate priority nursing diagnoses appropriate for an individual with pneumonia.
5. Create a plan of care for an individual with pneumonia.
6. Employ evidence-based caring interventions (or prevention) for an individual with pneumonia.
7. Assess expected outcomes for an individual with pneumonia.
8. Discuss therapies used in the collaborative care of an individual with pneumonia.

OVERVIEW

Inflammation of the lung parenchyma (the respiratory bronchioles and alveoli) is known as **pneumonia**. Despite significant advances in antibiotic therapy, pneumonia remains the seventh-leading cause of death in the United States overall—and the leading cause of death from infectious disease (Porth, 2005). In 2003, more than 65,000 deaths in the United States were attributed to pneumonia and influenza (Hoyert, Heron, Murphy, & Kung, 2006). Its incidence and mortality are highest in older adults and people with debilitating diseases. Pneumonia currently accounts for approximately 10% of adult hospital admissions in the United States.

The respiratory system is constantly open to the possibility of infection. The respiratory tree is exposed to the environment as air moves into and out of the lower respiratory tract. In addition, huge numbers of microorganisms in the oropharynx may be aspirated into the bronchial tree. Both anatomic and physiologic defenses help to maintain the sterility of the lower respiratory tract. When these defenses are impaired, the risk for infection increases. For example, drugs, alcohol, or neuromuscular disease may suppress the cough reflex; asthma can both narrow and inflame airways, trapping mucus and impairing oxygenation; and the influenza virus can leave the respiratory epithelium vulnerable to bacterial infection. Even in healthy people, microorganisms and other foreign material occasionally enter the bronchial tree and lung parenchyma.

PATHOPHYSIOLOGY AND ETIOLOGY

Disorders affecting the lower respiratory system (below the larynx) can affect the ability to effectively move air into and out of the lungs (**ventilation**), the exchange of oxygen and carbon dioxide across the alveolar-capillary membrane (respiration), as well as the ability to maintain clear and patent airways and to ventilate the lungs. Organisms causing such

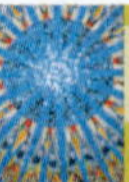

DEVELOPMENTAL CONSIDERATIONS

Pneumonia in the Older Adult

Several changes associated with aging and disease affect respiratory function and airway clearance. As a person ages, the number of cilia decreases, and the gag and cough reflexes diminish. The older adult is at greater risk for dehydration, leading to thick, viscous mucus that is difficult to expectorate. Immune function declines with aging as well. These factors increase the risk of pulmonary infection and reduce the older adult's ability to respond effectively to infectious processes.

Other factors also may increase the risk for and severity of lower respiratory infections in the older adult. These factors include immobility, smoking history, surgical procedures, use of multiple medications, malnutrition, and diseases such as chronic obstructive pulmonary disease and heart disease.

disorders can enter the lung in several ways. The most common means of entry is aspiration of microbe-containing secretions from the oropharynx. Microorganisms may be inhaled following release when an infected person coughs, sneezes, or talks. Inhalation of contaminated aerosolized water can result in viral and some other types of pneumonia. Bacteria also may spread to the lungs through the bloodstream from infection elsewhere in the body. Regardless of the means of entry, host defenses must be overwhelmed either by the number of organisms or by their **virulence** (disease-causing ability) for an infection to develop.

When invading microorganisms colonize the alveoli, they initiate an inflammatory and immune response. The antigen–antibody response and endotoxins released by some organisms damage bronchial and alveolar mucous membranes, causing inflammation with vascular congestion and edema. Infectious debris and exudate can fill alveoli, interfering with ventilation and gas exchange (Figure 15–23 ■). Pneumonia may develop in any one of four distinct patterns (Table 15–11):

1. Lobar pneumonia
2. Bronchopneumonia
3. Interstitial pneumonia
4. Miliary pneumonia.

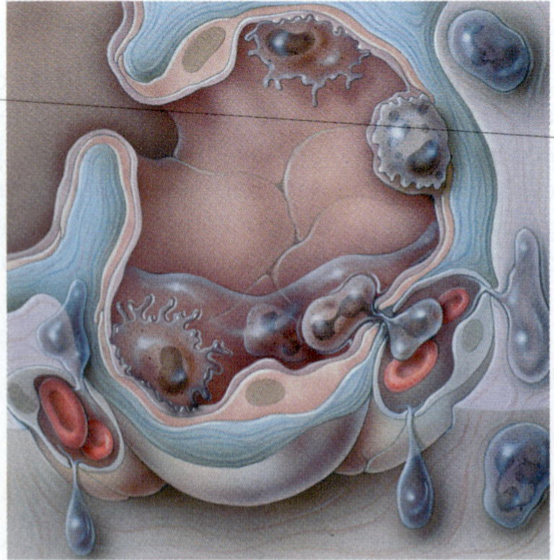

Figure 15–23 ■ In pneumonia, the inflammatory response causes fluid to accumulate in the alveoli and edema to form as alveolar capillaries dilate and allow fluid to leak into interstitial tissues.

Source: Kevin A. Somerville, Phototake NYC.

The pathologic process, anatomic location, and manifestations of pneumonia vary according to the infective organism. Bacterial and viral pathogens act differently within the lungs:

- Bacterial pathogens circulate through the bloodstream to the lungs, where they damage cells. Cellular debris and mucus cause airway obstruction. Bacteria tend to be distributed evenly throughout one or more lobes of a single lung, a pattern termed **unilateral lobar pneumonia**.
- Viruses frequently enter from the upper respiratory tract, infiltrating the alveoli nearest the bronchi of one or both lungs. There, they invade the cells, replicate, and burst out forcefully, killing the cells and sending out cell debris. They rapidly invade adjacent areas, distributing themselves in the scattered, patchy pattern referred to as bronchopneumonia.
- Aspiration of food, emesis, gastric reflux, or hydrocarbons causes a chemical injury and an inflammatory response. Materials with a lower pH cause more inflammation, which sets the stage for bacterial invasion.

Pneumonia may be either infectious or noninfectious. Bacteria, viruses, fungi, protozoa, and other microbes can lead to infectious pneumonia. Noninfectious causes include aspiration of gastric contents and inhalation of toxic or irritating gases. Pneumonias often are classified as community acquired, nosocomial (hospital acquired), or opportunistic. Different organisms are implicated in each of these classifications (Table 15–12). The most common causative organism for community-acquired pneumonia is *Streptococcus pneumoniae* (also called pneumococcus), a gram-positive bacterium. This organism causes approximately 50% of the cases of community-acquired pneumonia leading to hospital admission. *Mycoplasma pneumoniae, Chlamydia pneumoniae, Haemophilus influenzae*, and the influenza virus are also leading causes of community-acquired pneumonia (Kasper et al., 2005). *Staphylococcus aureus* and gram-negative bacteria such as *Klebsiella pneumoniae, Pseudomonas aeruginosa*, and enteric bacilli, including *Escherichia coli*, are often implicated as nosocomial causes of pneumonia. Organisms such as *Pneumocystis carinii* generally cause infections only in those who are immunocompromised (opportunistic infections).

In children older than 5 years, pneumonia is caused by bacteria, such as *Streptococcus pneumoniae*. Children with a condition such as cystic fibrosis or immunosuppression are susceptible to many other bacterial, parasitic, or fungal infections.

Acute Bacterial Pneumonia

Of the bacterial pneumonias, the pathogenesis of pneumococcal (*Streptococcus pneumoniae*) pneumonia is best understood (Figure 15–24 ■). These bacteria reside in the

TABLE 15–11 Patterns of Lung Involvement in Pneumonia

PATTERN OF INVOLVEMENT	DESCRIPTION
Lobar pneumonia	Typically involves an entire lobe of a lung. Early in the process, when the immune response is minimal, bacteria spread throughout the affected lobe by rapid accumulation of fluid exudate. As the immune and inflammatory responses develop, red blood cells and neutrophils, damaged epithelial cells, and fibrin accumulate in the alveoli. Purulent exudate containing neutrophils and macrophages forms. As alveoli and respiratory bronchioles fill with exudate, blood cells, fibrin, and bacteria, **consolidation** (solidification) of lung tissue occurs. The process finally resolves as enzymes destroy the exudate and residual debris is reabsorbed, phagocytized, or coughed out.
Bronchopneumonia	Usually involves dependent portions of lung tissue; characterized by patchy consolidation. Exudate tends to remain primarily in the bronchi and bronchioles, with less edema and congestion of the alveoli than with lobar pneumonia.
Interstitial pneumonia	The inflammatory process primarily involves the interstitium (the alveolar walls and connective tissue supporting the bronchial tree). Involvement may be patchy or diffuse as lymphocytes, macrophages, and plasma cells infiltrate the alveolar septa. While alveoli typically do not contain significant exudates, protein-rich hyaline membranes may line the alveoli, interfering with gas exchange.
Miliary pneumonia	In miliary pneumonia, the spread of the pathogen to the lungs via the bloodstream causes the development of numerous discrete inflammatory lesions. Miliary pneumonia is primarily seen in people who are severely immunocompromised. Because the immune response is poor, damage to pleural tissue may be significant.

upper respiratory tract of up to 70% of adults. They may be spread by direct person-to-person contact via droplets. In many cases, infection results from aspiration of resident bacteria. The inflammatory response initiated by these organisms in the lower respiratory tract causes alveolar edema and the formation of exudate. As alveoli and respiratory bronchioles fill with serous exudate, blood cells, fibrin, and bacteria, *consolidation* of lung tissue occurs. The lower lobes of the lungs are usually affected because of gravity. The typical pattern for pneumococcal pneumonia is lobar pneumonia, although it may present in a pattern more typical of bronchopneumonia. The process resolves when macrophages predominate, digesting and removing inflammatory exudate from the infected lung.

Pneumococcal pneumonia typically resolves uneventfully; normal lung structure is restored on completion of the process. Local extension of the infection to involve the pleura (**pleuritis**) is the most common complication. Pneumonias caused by *Staphylococcus aureus* and gram-negative bacteria often cause extensive parenchymal damage, with necrosis, lung abscess, and empyema or **pleural effusion** (accumulation of excess fluid in the pleural cavity). Progressive destruction of lung tissue and functional impairment is a possible consequence of *Klebsiella* pneumonia.

A **lung abscess** is a local area of necrosis and pus formation within the lung itself and is relatively uncommon. The manifestations of lung abscess develop slowly and include weight loss, malaise, night sweats, fever, and a productive cough. Sputum is foul smelling and tasting. Rupture of the abscess into a larger airway is heralded by production of copious amounts of purulent sputum.

Empyema is accumulation of purulent exudate in the pleural cavity. It is identified by chest x-ray or computed tomography. **Thoracentesis** (insertion of a needle into the pleural space to remove fluid accumulation) may be done, or a chest tube can be inserted to allow continuous drainage of purulent exudates.

TABLE 15–12 Common Organisms Causing Pneumonia in Adults

COMMUNITY ACQUIRED	HOSPITAL ACQUIRED	OPPORTUNISTIC
Streptococcus pneumoniae	*Staphylococcus aureus*	*Pneumocystis carinii*
Mycoplasma pneumoniae	*Pseudomonas aeruginosa*	*Mycobacterium tuberculosis*
Haemophilus influenzae	*Klebsiella pneumoniae*	Cytomegalovirus
Influenza virus	*Escherichia coli*	Atypical mycobacteria
Chlamydia pneumoniae		Fungi
Legionella pneumophila		

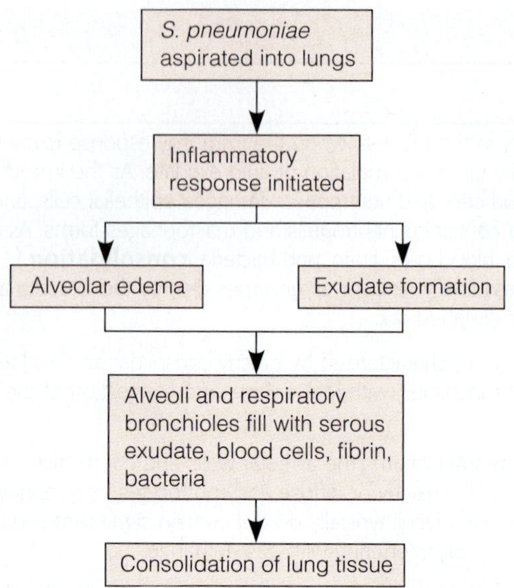

Figure 15–24 ■ The pathogenesis of pneumococcal pneumonia.

The presentation of bacterial pneumonia is usually acute, with rapid onset of shaking chills, fever, and cough that produces rust-colored or purulent sputum. Chest aching or **pleuritic pain** (sharp, localized chest pain that increases with breathing and coughing) is common. Limited breath sounds and fine crackles or rales are heard over the affected area of lung. A pleural friction rub may be audible. If the involved area is large and gas exchange is impaired, dyspnea and cyanosis may be noted.

A more insidious onset with low-grade fever, cough, and scattered crackles is more typical of bronchopneumonia. However, dyspnea is less common with bronchopneumonia. The older adult or debilitated client may have atypical manifestations of pneumonia, with little cough, scant sputum, and minimal evidence of respiratory distress. Fever, tachypnea, and altered mentation or agitation may be the primary presenting symptoms.

Legionnaires' Disease

Legionnaires' disease is a form of bronchopneumonia caused by *Legionella pneumophila*, a gram-negative bacterium widely found in water, particularly warm, standing water. Legionnaires' disease occurs sporadically and in outbreaks, such as that which occurred at an American Legion convention in 1976, when the disease was first recognized. Contaminated water-cooled air conditioning systems and other water sources have been implicated in its spread. Smokers, older adults, and people with chronic diseases or impaired immune defenses are most susceptible to Legionnaires' disease.

Symptoms of Legionnaires' disease develop gradually, beginning 2 to 10 days after exposure. Dry cough, dyspnea, general malaise, chills and fever, headache, confusion, diminished appetite and diarrhea, myalgias, and arthralgias are common manifestations. Consolidation of lung tissue is patchy or lobar. The mortality rate in Legionnaires' disease is up to 31% without treatment in otherwise healthy people and up to 80% in people who are immunocompromised (Kasper et al., 2005).

Primary Atypical Pneumonia

Pneumonia caused by *Mycoplasma pneumoniae* is generally classified as *primary atypical pneumonia*, because its presentation and course significantly differ from those of other bacterial pneumonias. Mycoplasma infection often causes pharyngitis or bronchitis. When this type of pneumonia develops, patchy inflammatory changes in the alveolar septum and interstitial tissue of the lung occur. Alveolar exudate and consolidation of lung tissue are not features of atypical pneumonia. Young adults—college students and military recruits in particular—are the primary affected populations.

Primary atypical pneumonia is highly contagious. Its manifestations resemble those of viral pneumonia; systemic manifestations of fever, headache, myalgias, and arthralgias often predominate. The cough associated with atypical pneumonia is dry, hacking, and nonproductive. Because of the typically mild nature and predominant systemic manifestations, mycoplasmal and viral pneumonia are often referred to as walking pneumonias.

Viral Pneumonia

Approximately 10% of pneumonias in adults are viral. Influenza and adenovirus are the most common organisms; however, the incidence of cytomegalovirus pneumonia in those who are immunocompromised is on the rise. Other viruses, such as herpes viruses and measles virus, also may cause viral pneumonia. As in primary atypical pneumonia, lung involvement in viral pneumonia is limited to the alveolar septum and interstitial spaces.

Viral pneumonia is typically a mild disease that often affects older adults and people with chronic conditions. It usually occurs in community epidemics. Flulike symptoms of headache, fever, fatigue, malaise, and muscle aching are common, along with a dry cough.

Pneumocystis carinii Pneumonia

People with AIDS and others with significant immunocompromise are at risk for developing an opportunistic pneumonia caused by *Pneumocystis carinii*, a common parasite found worldwide. Immunity to *P. carinii* is nearly universal, except in those who are immunocompromised. Opportunistic infection may develop in people treated with immunosuppressive or cytotoxic drugs for cancer or organ transplant and in people with genetic or acquired immunodeficiency. People with AIDS account for most cases (60%) of *P carinii* pneumonia (PCP) (Copstead & Banasik, 2005).

Infection with *P. carinii* produces patchy involvement throughout the lungs, causing affected alveoli to thicken, become edematous, and fill with foamy, protein-rich fluid. Gas exchange is severely impaired as the disease progresses. PCP has an abrupt onset, with fever, tachypnea, shortness of breath, and a dry, nonproductive cough. Respiratory distress can be significant, with intercostal retractions and cyanosis.

Table 15–13 compares the manifestations of infectious pneumonias.

TABLE 15–13 **Manifestations of Infectious Pneumonias**

TYPE	ONSET	RESPIRATORY MANIFESTATIONS	SYSTEMIC MANIFESTATIONS
Pneumococcal or lobar pneumonia	Abrupt	Cough productive of purulent or rust-colored sputum; pleuritic or aching chest pain; decreased breath sounds and crackles over affected area; possible dyspnea and cyanosis	Chills and fever
Bronchopneumonia	Gradual	Cough, scattered crackles; minimal dyspnea and respiratory distress; low-grade fever	
Legionnaires' disease	Gradual	Dry cough; dyspnea	Chills and fever; general malaise; headache; confusion; diminished appetite and diarrhea; myalgias and arthralgias
Primary atypical pneumonia	Gradual	Dry, hacking, nonproductive cough	Fever, headache, myalgias, and arthralgias predominate
Viral pneumonia	Sudden or gradual	Dry cough	Flulike symptoms
Pneumocystis carinii pneumonia	Abrupt	Dry cough; tachypnea and shortness of breath; significant respiratory distress	Fever

Aspiration Pneumonia

Aspiration of gastric contents into the lungs results in a chemical and bacterial pneumonia known as *aspiration pneumonia*. Major risk factors for aspiration pneumonia include emergency surgery or obstetric procedures, depressed cough and gag reflexes, and impaired swallowing. Older surgical clients and those with advanced dementia are at significant risk. Enteral nutrition by either nasogastric or gastric tube also increases the risk for aspiration pneumonia. Vomiting is not always apparent; silent regurgitation of gastric contents may occur when the level of consciousness is decreased. Measures to reduce the risk for aspiration pneumonia include minimizing the use of preoperative medications, promoting anesthetic elimination from the body, and preventing nausea and gastric distention.

The low pH of gastric contents causes a severe inflammatory response when aspirated into the respiratory tract. Pulmonary edema and respiratory failure may result. Common complications of aspiration pneumonia include abscesses, **bronchiectasis** (chronic dilation of the bronchi and bronchioles), and gangrene of pulmonary tissue.

Pediatric Differences

A child's airway is shorter and narrower than an adult's. These differences create a greater potential for obstruction (Figure 15–25 ■). The infant's airway is approximately 4 mm in diameter, about the width of a drinking straw, in contrast to the adult's airway diameter of 20 mm. The child's little finger is a good estimate for the child's tracheal diameter and can be used for a quick assessment of airway size.

The trachea primarily increases in length rather than diameter during the first 5 years of life. Also, the tracheal division of the right and left bronchi is higher in a child's airway and at a different angle than in an adult's (Figure 15–26 ■). The cartilage that supports the trachea is more flexible and has the potential to compress the airway if the head and neck are not appropriately positioned. The child's narrower airway causes a greater increase in airway resistance (the effort or force needed to move oxygen through the trachea to the lungs) in any condition causing edema of the airway or accumulation of secretions (Figure 15–27 ■).

At birth, the lung tissue contains only 25 million alveoli, which are not fully developed, and the distal bronchioles that extend to the alveoli are narrow and fewer in number than in an adult. After 8 years of age, the alveoli begin increasing in size and complexity. The number of alveoli increases to 300 million by adulthood (Brashers, 2006). As a result, disease of a small number of alveoli can have a much larger impact on a child's clinical condition because of the increased proportion of lung involvement. For example, involvement of 1 million alveoli secondary to pneumonia would be 4% of the lung in a pediatric client but only 0.33% of an adult's lung.

Pneumonia in children often resolves much sooner than in adults. The key is early recognition, enabling the child to be managed at home rather than in the hospital.

Risk Factors

The immature immune systems of infants and young children increase their risk for pneumonia. Older adults are at greater risk because of diminished cough and gag reflexes as well as diminishing immune response. Anyone with a compromised immune system, such as those diagnosed with HIV/AIDS, individuals on medication to prevent rejection of a transplanted organ, or those receiving treatment for cancer such as chemotherapy or radiation therapy, is at increased risk for infection—and for pneumonia in particular. Clients in a debilitated or weakened condition from any cause also face increased risk.

Research indicates a high rate of pneumonia in clients with frequent exposure to cigarette smoke and alcohol or drug abuse. Smoking injures tissues in the airways and decreases the action of cilia. Chemicals in cigarettes have a numbing effect on the cough reflex. All of these actions diminish the

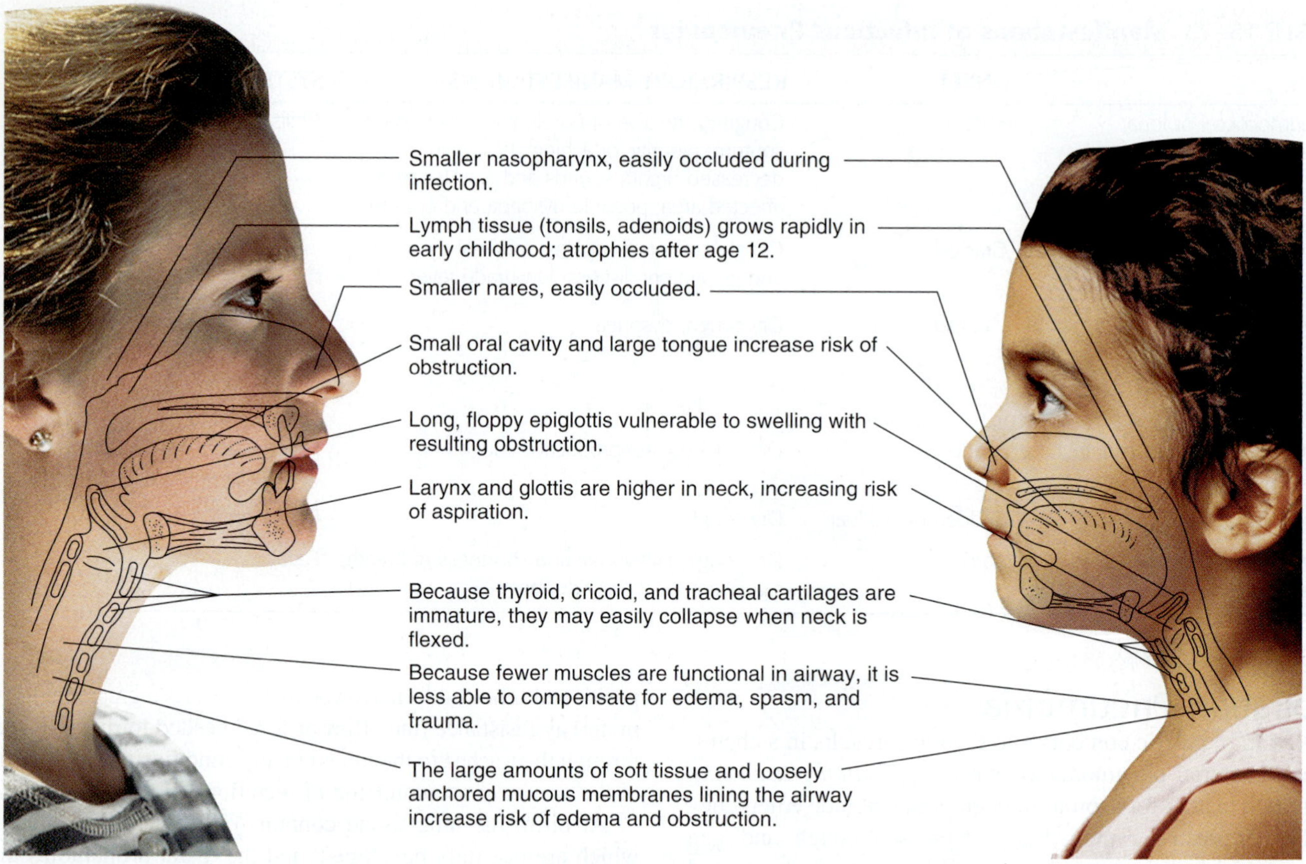

Smaller nasopharynx, easily occluded during infection.
Lymph tissue (tonsils, adenoids) grows rapidly in early childhood; atrophies after age 12.
Smaller nares, easily occluded.
Small oral cavity and large tongue increase risk of obstruction.
Long, floppy epiglottis vulnerable to swelling with resulting obstruction.
Larynx and glottis are higher in neck, increasing risk of aspiration.
Because thyroid, cricoid, and tracheal cartilages are immature, they may easily collapse when neck is flexed.
Because fewer muscles are functional in airway, it is less able to compensate for edema, spasm, and trauma.
The large amounts of soft tissue and loosely anchored mucous membranes lining the airway increase risk of edema and obstruction.

Figure 15–25 ■ It is easy to see that a child's airway is smaller and less developed than an adult's airway, but why is this important? An upper respiratory tract infection, allergic reaction, positioning of the head and neck during sleep, and the small objects children play with can have serious consequences in the child.

Bifurcation of trachea in children is at T3 level.
Right mainstem bronchus in children has a steeper slope than in adults.
Bifurcation in adults is at T6 level.

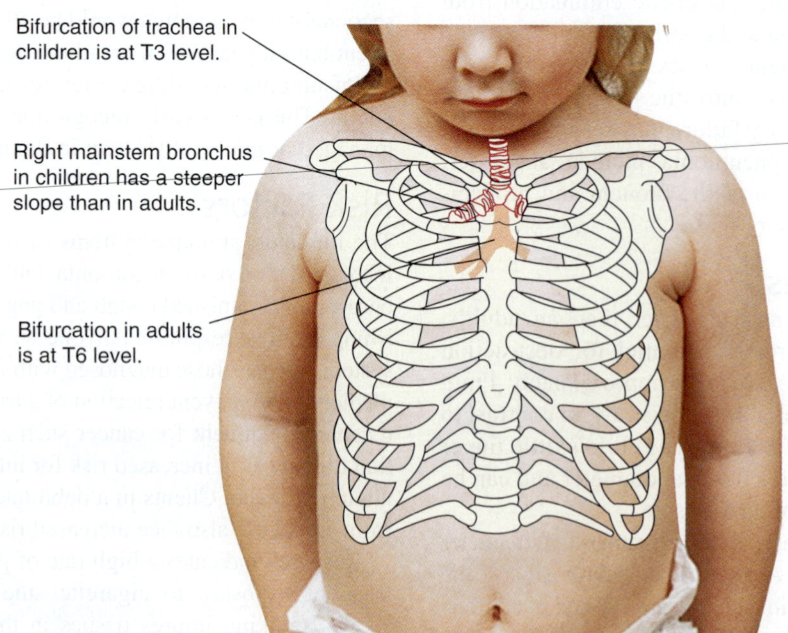

Figure 15–26 ■ In children, the trachea is shorter and the angle of the right bronchus at bifurcation is more acute than in the adult. When you are resuscitating or suctioning, you must allow for the differences. Do you think that this difference is significant in respiratory infection? Why?

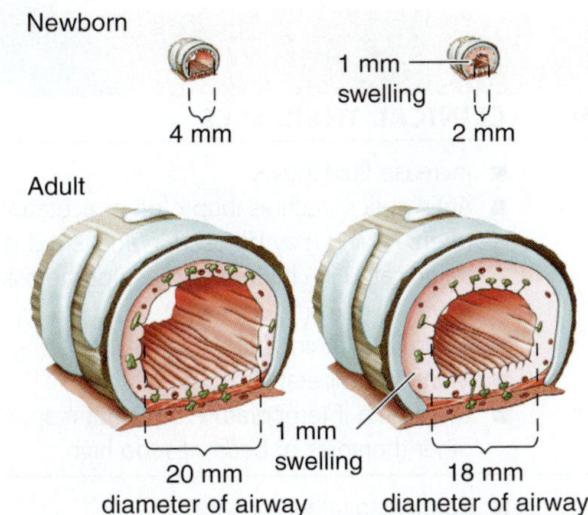

Figure 15–27 ■ The diameter of an infant's airway is approximately 4 mm, in contrast to an adult's airway diameter of 20 mm. An inflammatory process in the airway causes swelling that narrows the airway, and airway resistance increases. Note that swelling of 1 mm reduces the infant's airway diameter to 2 mm, but the adult's airway diameter is only narrowed to 18 mm. Air must move more quickly in the infant's narrowed airway to get the same amount of air to the lungs. The friction of the quickly moving air against the side of the airway increases airway resistance. The infant must use more effort to breathe and breathe faster to get adequate oxygen.

lung's natural protective mechanisms. Alcohol interferes with the actions of macrophages, while injection drug users are at risk from infections that originate at the injection site and then spread through the bloodstream to the lungs.

People who have a high risk of adverse outcome from bacterial pneumonias include those older than 65 years; those with chronic cardiac or respiratory conditions, diabetes mellitus, alcoholism, or other chronic diseases; and those who are immunocompromised.

CLINICAL MANIFESTATIONS

Infection of the lower respiratory tract has both local and systemic effects. Local effects include cough, excess mucous production, shortness of breath or **dyspnea** (difficult or labored breathing), **hemoptysis** (bloody sputum), and chest pain. Systemic effects may include fever, diminished appetite and malaise, **cyanosis** (gray to blue or purple skin color caused by deoxygenated hemoglobin), and other manifestations of impaired gas exchange.

Pediatric Differences

Children under 6 years of age use the diaphragm to breathe, because the intercostal muscles are immature. By 6 years of age, the child uses the intercostal muscles more effectively. The ribs are primarily cartilage and very flexible, and in cases of respiratory distress, the negative pressure that results from the diaphragm movement causes the chest wall to be drawn inward, producing **retractions** (visible sinking of the chest wall). While often a late sign of respiratory distress in adults and older children, retractions in infants and young children can often be a much earlier manifestation of alteration in breathing patterns and gas exchange (Figure 15–28 ■).

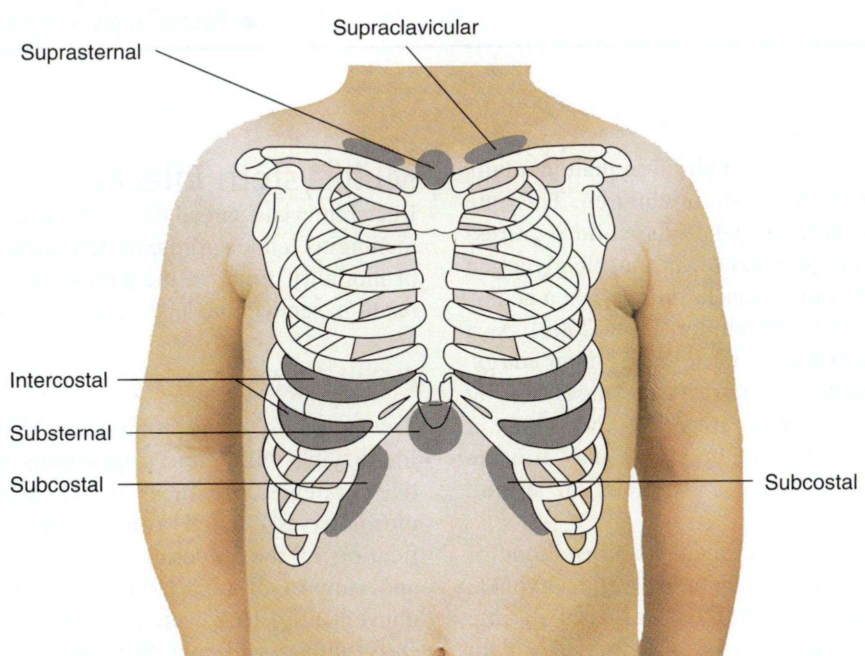

Figure 15–28 ■ Retractions may occur in the very young infant in the suprasternal area. In the older infant and child, retractions occur when the airway is severely obstructed, as in croup. The depth and location of retractions is associated with the severity of respiratory distress. Isolated intercostal retractions indicate mild distress. Subcostal, suprasternal, and supraclavicular retractions indicate moderate distress. These retractions accompanied by use of accessory muscles indicate severe distress.

CLINICAL MANIFESTATIONS AND THERAPIES Pneumonia

ETIOLOGY	CLINICAL MANIFESTATIONS	CLINICAL THERAPIES
Presence of pathogens causes the hypothalamus to increase the set point of body temperature in an attempt to kill the invader.	Fever	■ Increase fluid intake. ■ Antipyretics, such as ibuprofen or acetaminophen. Aspirin may be used in adults but is contraindicated in children because of the risk for Reye's syndrome. ■ Minimize clothing and coverings. ■ Monitor temperature frequently. ■ Tepid bath if temperature does not respond to other therapies or becomes too high.
The child has fewer muscle glycogen reserves, leading to more rapid muscle fatigue when accessory muscles must be used for breathing (Froh, 2006).	Apnea	■ Cardiorespiratory monitor. ■ Measures to reduce the work of breathing may include assistance with airway clearance, positioning, and oxygen administration. ■ Recurrent or severe episodes of apnea indicate the need for intubation and mechanical ventilation.
Accumulation of fluid and debris in the airways	Cough	■ Increase fluid intake to liquefy secretions. ■ Frequently change position to prevent atelectasis and help drain different airways. ■ Chest physiotherapy to promote airway clearance. ■ Airway suctioning to promote airway clearance if the cough is weak or ineffective. ■ Mucolytics to promote sputum expectoration and bronchodilators to open airways, allowing movement of sputum may be administered.
Fluid accumulation in the airways impairing gas exchange	Hypoxia	■ Administer oxygen. ■ Encourage coughing and deep breathing to clear airways and promote gas exchange. ■ Monitor vital signs and oxygen saturation. ■ Position to promote airway clearance.

Oxygen consumption is higher in children than in adults because of the greater metabolic rate in children. This rate of oxygen consumption increases when the child is in respiratory distress. The child also has fewer muscle glycogen reserves, leading to more rapid muscle fatigue when accessory muscles must be used for breathing (Froh, 2006). As a result, children become hypoxic more quickly than adults. **Tachypnea** (rapid respirations), retractions, nasal flaring (opening of the nares on inspiration in an attempt to draw in more air), and increased effort of breathing may tire the infant or young child, resulting in periods of **apnea** (absence of breathing).

These differences impact the clinical manifestations of pneumonia in children. Symptoms include fever, tachypnea, rhonchi, crackles, wheezes, cough, dyspnea, nasal flaring, restlessness, chest pain, and malaise. Decreased breath sounds may be present if consolidation exists. The child also may have poor oral intake, nausea, vomiting, and abdominal pain.

Multisystem Effects

Bacteremia can spread the infection to other tissues, leading to meningitis, endocarditis, or peritonitis and increasing the risk of mortality. Entry of the pathogens into the bloodstream can result in septicemia, leading to septic shock.

COLLABORATION

Prevention is a key component in managing pneumonia. Identifying vulnerable populations and instituting preventive strategies are measures to reduce the mortality and morbidity associated with the condition. With early identification of the infecting organism, appropriate treatment, and support of respiratory function, most clients recover uneventfully. However, pneumonia remains a serious disease with significant mortality, especially in aged and debilitated populations.

Collaboration in caring for an individual with pneumonia may include nurses, doctors, phlebotomists, respiratory therapists, and radiologists. In some cases, consultation with an infectious disease specialist or a pulmonologist may be necessary. Clients who are gravely ill and their families may want the opportunity to talk with the hospital chaplain or their own minister, rabbi, or other religious leader.

Diagnostic Tests

The history and physical examination, along with diagnostic testing, are used to establish the diagnosis, determine the extent of lung involvement, and identify the causative organism.

COMMON DIAGNOSTIC TESTS Diagnostic tests include the following:

- *Chest x-ray* is obtained to determine the extent and pattern of lung involvement. Fluid, infiltrates, consolidated lung tissue, and **atelectasis** (areas of alveolar collapse) appear as densities on the film.
- *Computed tomography* provides a more detailed image of pulmonary tissue and may be used when the chest x-ray is not diagnostic.
- *Sputum Gram stain* rapidly identifies the infecting organisms as gram-positive or gram-negative bacteria. Antibiotic therapy can then be directed at the predominant type of organism until culture and sensitivity results are obtained.
- *Sputum culture and sensitivity* is ordered to identify the infecting organism and determine the most effective antibiotic therapy. When obtaining sputum for culture, it is important to obtain secretions from the lower respiratory tract, not from the mouth and nasal passages.
- *Complete blood count (CBC) with WBC differential* shows an elevated WBC ($\geq$11,000/mm^3) with increased circulating immature leukocytes (a left shift) in response to the infectious process. WBC changes are minimal in viral and other pneumonias.
- *Serology testing* (blood tests to detect antibodies to respiratory pathogens) may be used to identify the infecting organism when blood and sputum cultures are negative.
- *Pulse oximetry,* a noninvasive method of measuring arterial oxygen saturation (SaO_2), is ordered to continuously monitor gas exchange. The SaO_2 normally is 95% or higher. An SaO_2 of less than 95% may indicate impaired alveolar gas exchange.
- *Arterial blood gas* may be ordered to evaluate gas exchange. Respiratory secretions or pleuritic pain can interfere with alveolar ventilation. Alveolar inflammation can interfere with gas exchange across the alveolar-capillary membrane, especially if exudate or consolidation is present. An arterial partial pressure of oxygen (PaO_2) of less than 75 to 80 mmHg indicates impaired gas exchange or alveolar ventilation.
- *Fiberoptic bronchoscopy* may be done to obtain a sputum specimen or remove secretions from the bronchial tree.

PEDIATRIC DIFFERENCES In children over 12 months of age who have clinical manifestations associated with pneumonia, a respiratory rate greater than 50/minute and an oxygen saturation of 96% or less are more likely to be associated with a positive chest x-ray. In children under 12 months of age, nasal flaring is an important finding that is more likely to be associated with a positive chest x-ray (Mahabee-Gittens, et al., 2005). The older child may have dullness to chest percussion, increased fremitus, and egophony. There is no clinical way to differentiate bacterial and viral cause, because it is difficult to get a sputum culture from a child. Blood cultures may be taken instead. The child's age, severity of symptoms, and presence of an underlying lung, cardiac, or immunodeficiency disease can create varying responses.

Immunizations

Vaccines offer some degree of protection against the most common bacterial and viral pneumonias. Pneumococcal vaccine, made of antigens from 23 types of pneumococcus, usually imparts lifetime immunity with a single dose. The vaccine is recommended for people who have a high risk of adverse outcome from bacterial pneumonias. A one-time revaccination is recommended for selected populations, including people over age 65 who were immunized more than 5 years previously and before age 65, people with chronic renal failure or immunosuppressive conditions (e.g., malignancy), and people receiving chemotherapy with selected agents (CDC, 2005d).

PRACTICE ALERT

Annual influenza vaccination helps prevent pneumonia. Inquire about allergic responses to eggs or previous influenza vaccinations before administering influenza vaccine. A significant hypersensitivity response may occur in clients who are allergic to egg protein.

Pharmacologic Therapies

Medications used to treat pneumonia may include antibiotics to eradicate the infection and bronchodilators to reduce bronchospasm and improve ventilation. Initial antibiotic therapy is based on the results of sputum Gram stain and the pattern of lung involvement shown on a chest x-ray. Considerations such as the presence of cardiovascular disease or residence in a long-term care facility are also considered in the initial antibiotic choice. Typically, a broad-spectrum antibiotic, such as a macrolide (e.g., clarithromycin, azithromycin, or erythromycin), a penicillin or a second- or third-generation cephalosporin, or a fluoroquinolone (e.g., ciprofloxacin), is ordered until the results of sputum culture and sensitivity tests are available. Table 15–14 lists commonly prescribed antibiotics for selected pneumonias.

When an inflammatory response to the infection causes bronchospasm and constriction, bronchodilators may be ordered to improve ventilation and reduce hypoxia. Bronchodilators generally belong to one of two major groups: the sympathomimetic drugs, such as albuterol sulfate (Proventil) and metaproterenol (Alupent), or the methylxanthines, such as theophylline and aminophylline.

TABLE 15–14 Antibiotic Therapy for Selected Pneumonias

CAUSATIVE ORGANISM	ANTIBIOTIC OF CHOICE	ALTERNATIVE ANTIBIOTICS
Streptococcus pneumoniae	Penicillin G; amoxicillin	Erythromycin, cephalosporins, doxycycline, fluoroquinolone, clindamycin, vancomycin, trimethoprim-sulfamethoxazole (TMP-SMZ), linezolid
Haemophilus influenzae	Second- or third-generation cephalosporins, doxycycline, azithromycin, TMP-SMZ	Fluoroquinolones, clarithromycin
Staphylococcus aureus	Penicillinase-resistant penicillin (e.g., nafcillin); vancomycin for methicillin-resistant organisms	Cephalosporins, vancomycin, clindamycin; ciprofloxacin, fluoroquinolones, TMP-SMZ
Mycoplasma pneumoniae	Erythromycin, doxycycline	Clarithromycin, azithromycin, fluoroquinolone
Klebsiella pneumoniae	Third-generation cephalosporin (with aminoglycoside if severe); metronidazole	Aztreonam, imipenem-cilastatin, fluoroquinolone
Legionella pneumophila	Macrolide + rifampin; fluoroquinolone	TMP-SMZ, doxycycline + rifampin
Pneumocystis carinii	TMP-SMZ, pentamidine + prednisone	Dapsone + trimethoprim, clindamycin + primaquine, trimetrexate + folinic acid
Chlamydia pneumoniae	Doxycycline	Macrolide, fluoroquinolone

An agent to "break up" mucus or reduce its viscosity may be prescribed. Acetylcysteine (Mucomyst), potassium iodide, and guaifenesin (a common ingredient in expectorant cough syrups) help to liquefy mucus, making it easier to expectorate. For many clients, however, increasing fluid intake is an effective means of liquefying mucus.

Clinical Therapies

Clinical management for all types of pneumonia includes symptomatic therapy (pain and fever control) and supportive care through airway management, fluids, and rest. When mucous secretions are thick and viscous, increasing fluid intake to between 2,500 and 3,000 mL/day helps to liquefy secretions, making them easier to cough up and expectorate. If the client is unable to maintain an adequate oral intake, intravenous fluids and nutrition may be required.

Incentive spirometry may be used to promote deep breathing, coughing, and clearance of respiratory secretions. Endotracheal suctioning may be required if the cough is ineffective. On occasion, bronchoscopy is used to perform pulmonary toilet and remove secretions.

OXYGEN THERAPY Oxygen therapy may be indicated for the client who is tachypneic or hypoxemic. Inflammation of the alveolar-capillary membrane interferes with diffusion of gases across the membrane. Diffusion is affected by several other factors, including the partial pressure of gases on each side of the membrane. Increasing the percentage of inspired oxygen above that of room air (21%) increases the partial pressure of oxygen in the alveoli and enhances its diffusion into the capillaries. Supplemental oxygen therefore improves oxygenation of the blood and tissues in clients with pneumonia.

Depending on the degree of hypoxia, oxygen may be administered by either a low-flow or a high-flow system. Low-flow systems include the nasal cannula, simple face mask, partial rebreathing mask, and nonrebreathing mask (Figure 15–29 ■). A nasal cannula can deliver 24–45% oxygen concentrations with flow rates of 2–6 L/minute. The nasal cannula is comfortable and does not interfere with eating or talking. A simple face mask delivers 40–60% oxygen concentrations with flow rates of 5–8 L/minute. Up to 100% oxygen can be delivered by the

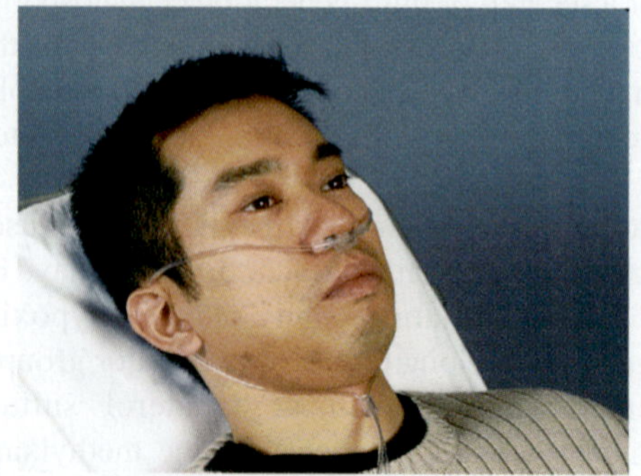
A

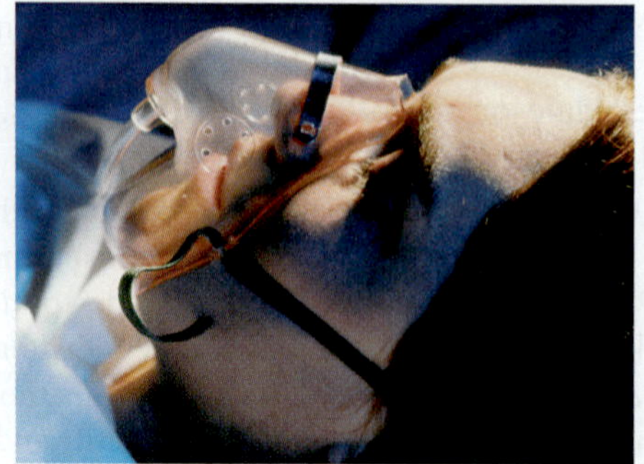
B

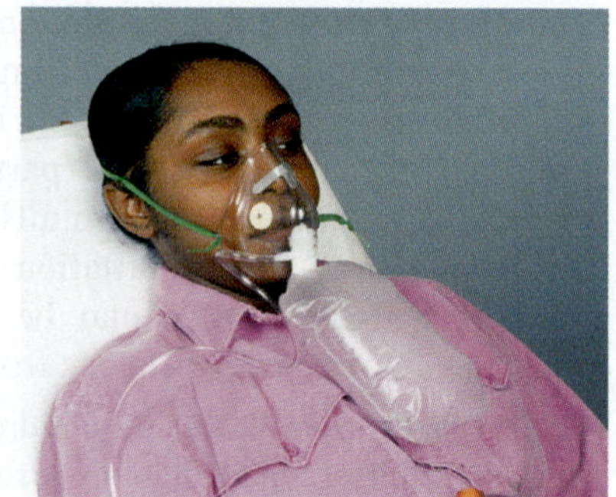
C

Figure 15–29 ■ Low-flow oxygen delivery devices: *A,* nasal cannula; *B,* simple face mask; *C,* nonrebreather mask.

Source: A, C, Michal Heron, Person Education/PH College; B, Tony McConnell, Photo Researchers, Inc.

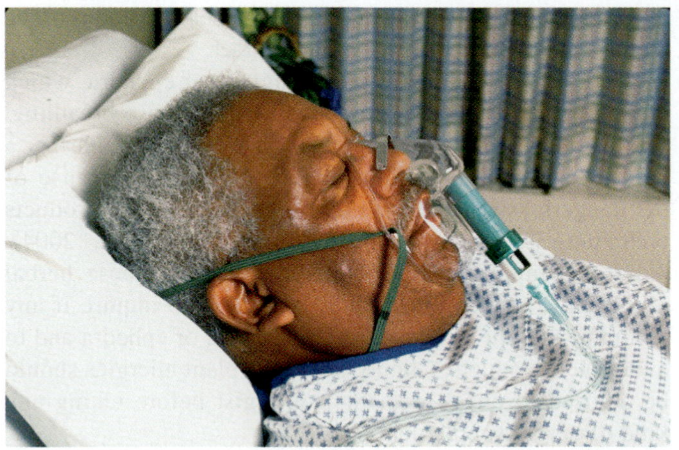

Figure 15–30 ■ Venturi mask, a high-flow oxygen delivery system.
Source: Michal Heron, Pearson Education/PH College.

nonrebreather mask, the highest concentration possible without mechanical ventilation. When the amount of oxygen delivered must be precisely regulated, a high-flow system, such as a Venturi mask, is used (Figure 15–30 ■). The Venturi mask regulates the ratio of oxygen to room air, allowing precise regulation of the oxygen percentage delivered, from 24–50%. Severe hypoxia may necessitate intubation and mechanical ventilation.

CHEST PHYSIOTHERAPY Chest physiotherapy, including percussion, vibration, and postural drainage, may be prescribed to reduce lung consolidation and prevent atelectasis. *Percussion* is performed by rhythmically striking or clapping the chest wall with cupped hands (Figure 15–31A ■), using rapid wrist flexion and extension. Cupping traps air between the palm and the client's skin, setting up vibrations through the chest wall that loosen respiratory secretions. The trapped air also provides a cushion, preventing injury. When performed correctly, percussion produces a hollow, popping sound. Percussion may also be done using a mechanical percussion cup. The breasts, sternum, spinal column, and kidney regions are avoided during percussion.

Vibration facilitates the movement of secretions into larger airways. It usually is combined with percussion, although it may be used when percussion is contraindicated or poorly tolerated. Vibration is performed by repeatedly tensing the arm and hand muscles while maintaining firm but gentle pressure over the affected area with the flat of the hand (Figure 15–31B).

Percussion and vibration are done in conjunction with *postural drainage*, which uses gravity to facilitate removal of secretions from a particular lung segment. The client is positioned with the segment to be drained superior to or above the trachea or mainstem

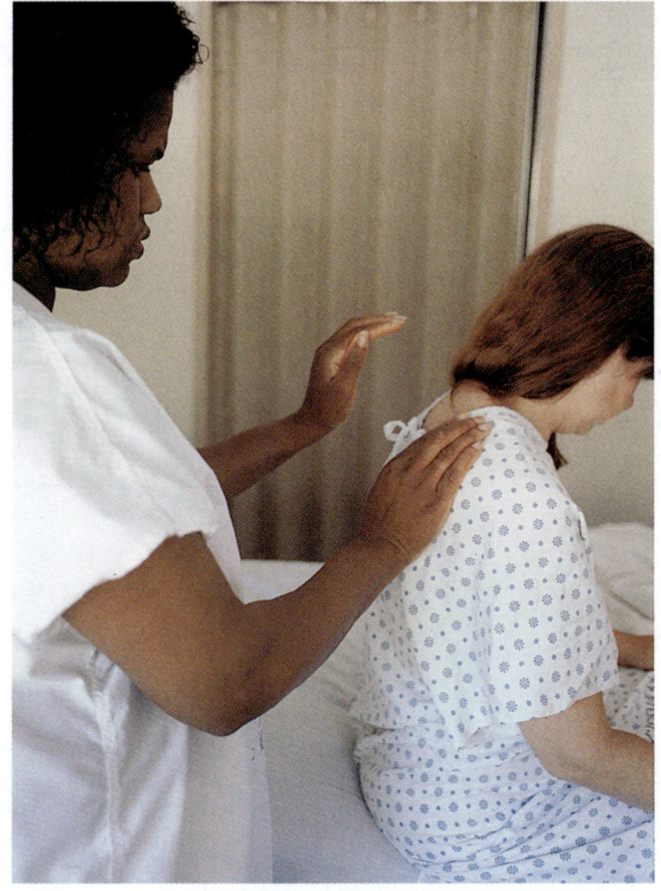

A

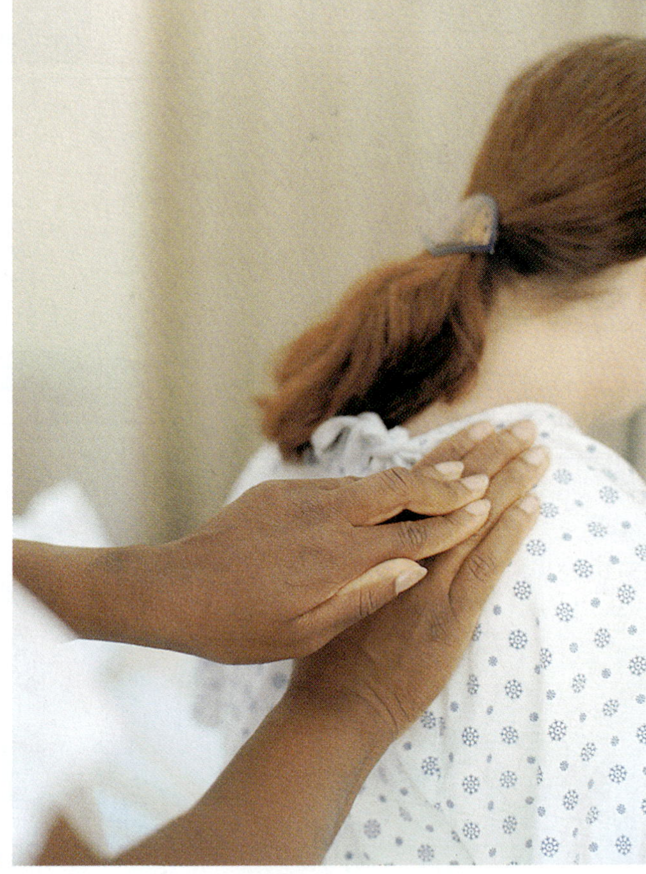

B

Figure 15–31 ■ *A,* Percussing (clapping) the upper posterior chest. Notice the cupped position of the nurse's hands. *B,* Vibrating the upper posterior chest.

bronchus. Drainage of all lung segments requires a variety of positions (Figure 15–32 ■); rarely do all segments require drainage. Bronchodilators or nebulizer treatments are administered as ordered before postural drainage. It is best to perform postural drainage before meals to avoid nausea and vomiting.

Complementary Therapies

Although complementary therapies do not replace conventional treatment for pneumonia, they often promote comfort and speed recovery. The herb echinacea is widely used to stimulate immune function and treat upper respiratory infections. Because viral upper respiratory infections often precede pneumonia, echinacea may be helpful in preventing pneumonia. Recent research, however, shows mixed results for the effectiveness of echinacea in reducing the duration and severity of an upper respiratory infection (National Center for Complementary and Alternative Medicine [NCCAM], 2005). Goldenseal, which often is sold in combination with echinacea, is used to treat bacterial, fungal, and protozoal infections of the mucous membranes of the respiratory tract.

Ma huang contains the active ingredient ephedra, which has been used to relieve bronchospasm and ease breathing. The primary active ingredient in ephedra is epinephrine, a cardiac and central nervous system stimulant. Because of the dangers associated with its use, sale of herbal products containing ephedra has been banned (NCCAM, 2004). Advise clients inquiring about the use of Chinese herbal remedies to reduce pneumonia symptoms to inquire if any recommended product contains ma huang or ephedra and to avoid such products. Clients who have plant allergies should be advised to check with their allergist before taking any kind of herbal supplement.

Some clients with respiratory disease find that symptoms can be alleviated with the help of acupuncture. Clients seeking symptom relief through acupuncture should be advised to get approval from their treating physician first.

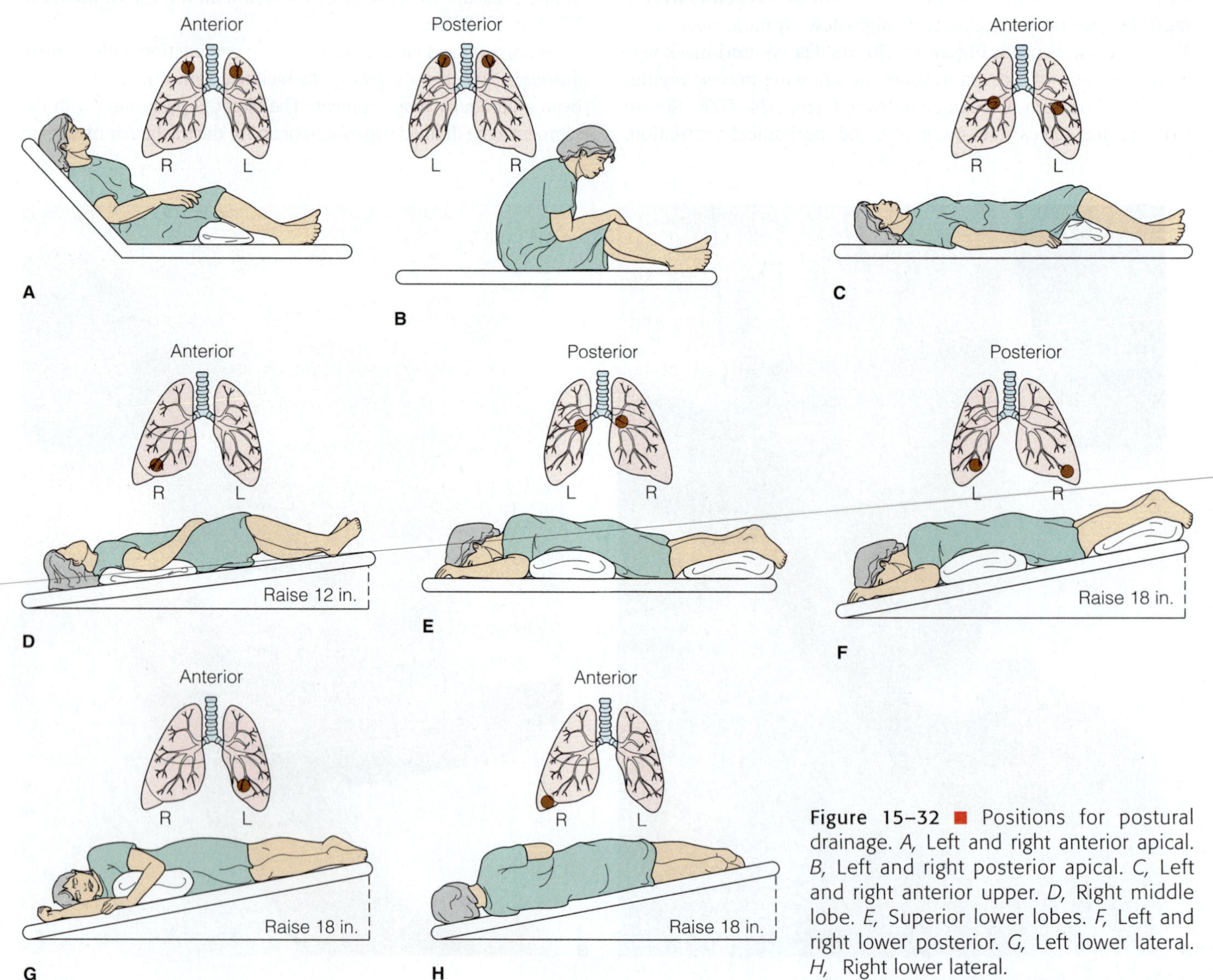

Figure 15–32 ■ Positions for postural drainage. *A,* Left and right anterior apical. *B,* Left and right posterior apical. *C,* Left and right anterior upper. *D,* Right middle lobe. *E,* Superior lower lobes. *F,* Left and right lower posterior. *G,* Left lower lateral. *H,* Right lower lateral.

NURSING PROCESS

Health promotion activities focus on pneumonia prevention. Make clients in high-risk groups aware of the benefits of immunizations against influenza and pneumococcal pneumonia. A single dose of pneumococcal vaccine usually produces immunity to most strains of pneumococcal pneumonia, although repeat doses may be needed for older adults and people who are immunosuppressed. (Pneumococcal vaccine is contraindicated for people receiving immunosuppressive therapy.) Annual influenza vaccine helps to prevent pneumonia, because pneumonia often occurs as a sequela to influenza.

Additional measures to screen for and detect pneumonia in older adults are appropriate. Frequent pulmonary assessment and aggressive interventions help to prevent problems. Restoring and maintaining mobility improves ventilation and helps to mobilize secretions. Promoting adequate fluid intake is necessary, because fluid helps to liquefy secretions, making them easier to expectorate.

Assessment

Focused assessment of the client with pneumonia includes the following:

- *Health history.* Current symptoms and their duration; presence of shortness of breath or difficulty breathing, chest pain and its relationship to breathing; cough, productive or nonproductive, color and consistency of sputum; other symptoms; recent upper respiratory or other acute illness; chronic diseases, such as diabetes, chronic lung disease, or heart disease; current medications; and medication allergies
- *Physical examination.* Presentation, apparent distress; level of consciousness; vital signs, including temperature; skin color and temperature; respiratory excursion, use of accessory muscles of respiration; and lung sounds.

Assessment of the pediatric client is different secondary to their anatomic and physiologic differences, resulting in presentation of a different clinical picture. Assessment guidelines for pediatric clients are given in Table 15–15).

TABLE 15–15 Assessment Guidelines for the Child with a Respiratory Condition

ASSESSMENT FOCUS	ASSESSMENT GUIDELINES
Position of comfort	■ Is the child comfortable lying down? ■ Does the child prefer to sit up or be in the tripod position (sitting forward with arms on knees for support and extending the neck)?
Vital signs	■ Assess the rate, depth, and ease of respirations. See Table 22–5 in Concept 22, Perfusion, for expected respiratory rate ranges by age. ■ Assess the pulse for rate and strength. See Table 22–5 in Concept 22, Perfusion, for expected heart rate ranges by age.
Lung auscultation	■ Are breath sounds bilateral, diminished, or absent? ■ Are adventitious sounds (wheezes, crackles, or rhonchi) present?
Respiratory effort (work of breathing)	■ Are there audible inspiratory and expiratory breath sounds or stridor? Is there grunting with expiration? ■ Is breathing labored? ■ Are retractions (visible appearance of the chest being drawn on inspiration) present or are accessory muscles used to breathe? ■ Is nasal flaring present? ■ Is tachypnea (abnormally rapid rate of respirations) present? ■ Can the child say a full sentence or is a breath needed every few words? Is the cry strong or weak? ■ Do the chest and abdomen rise simultaneously with inspiration or is paradoxical breathing present in which the chest and abdomen do not simultaneously rise?
Color	■ What is the color of the mucous membranes (pink, pale, mottled, cyanotic)? ■ Does crying improve or worsen the color?
Cough	■ Is the cough dry (nonproductive), wet (productive, mucousy), brassy (noisy, musical), or croupy (barking, seal-like)? ■ Is the coughing effort forceful or weak?
Behavior change	■ Note any sudden behavior changes such as irritability, restlessness, or change in level of responsiveness.
Family history	■ Is there a family history of asthma or cystic fibrosis?

Ongoing respiratory assessments are important to the care of all clients with pneumonia. Frequency of assessment is determined by the clinical acuity of the client and severity of the symptoms displayed. Auscultation of breath sounds, measurement of vital signs and oxygen saturation, and general assessment should be performed at a minimum of every 4 hours for the clinically stable client.

Diagnosis

Clients with lower respiratory disorders such as pneumonia may have multiple nursing care needs, depending on the severity of the illness. Possible nursing diagnoses related to pneumonia include the following:

- Ineffective Airway Clearance
- Ineffective Breathing Pattern
- Hyperthermia related to fever
- Activity Intolerance
- Anxiety related to hypoxia
- Imbalanced Nutrition: Less Than Body Requirements related to altered breathing pattern
- Disturbed Sleep Pattern related to orthopnea.

Plan

The goal of nursing care is to restore optimal respiratory function. Outcomes are determined in conjunction with client and family and may include the following:

- The client maintains normal temperature for 24 hours.
- The client obtains adequate sleep and rest without interruption from coughing or orthopnea.
- The client maintains adequate fluid and caloric intake.
- The client demonstrates strong cough sufficient to clear airway.
- The client maintains oxygen saturation greater than 90%.
- The client does not require supplemental oxygen to maintain oxygen saturations of greater than 90%.

Implementation

Nursing care focuses on supporting optimal respiratory function, such as maintaining airway patency and an effective breathing pattern, and promoting rest to reduce metabolic and oxygen needs. Nursing interventions are prioritized based on the most important nursing diagnoses of *ineffective airway clearance, ineffective breathing pattern,* and *activity intolerance.*

Ineffective Airway Clearance

- Assess respiratory status, including vital signs, breath sounds, SaO_2, and skin color at least every 4 hours. Early identification of respiratory compromise allows intervention before tissue hypoxia is significant.
- Assess cough and sputum (amount, color, consistency, and possible odor). Assessment of the cough and nature of sputum produced allows evaluation of the effectiveness of respiratory clearance and the response to therapy.
- Monitor arterial blood gas results; report increasing **hypoxemia** (deficient blood oxygenation) and other abnormal results to the physician. Blood gas changes may be an early indicator of impaired gas exchange caused by airway narrowing or obstruction.
- Place in Fowler's or high-Fowler's position. Encourage frequent position changes and ambulation as allowed. The upright position promotes lung expansion; position changes and ambulation facilitate the movement of secretions.
- Assist to cough, deep breathe, and use assistive devices. Provide endotracheal suctioning using aseptic technique as ordered. Coughing, deep breathing, and suctioning help to clear airways.
- Provide a fluid intake of at least 2,500–3,000 mL/day for the adult client. See Table 15–16 for fluid requirements of the pediatric client. A liberal fluid intake helps to liquefy secretions, facilitating their clearance.
- Work with the physician and respiratory therapist to provide pulmonary hygiene measures, such as postural drainage, percussion, and vibration. These techniques help to mobilize and clear secretions.
- Administer prescribed medications as ordered, and monitor their effects. If the infecting organism is resistant to the prescribed antibiotic, little improvement may be seen with treatment. Bronchodilators help to maintain open airways but may have adverse effects such as anxiety and restlessness.

TABLE 15–16 Daily Maintenance Fluid Requirements for the Pediatric Client

For the first 0–10 kg of body weight	100 mL · kg^{-1} · day^{-1}
For the next 11–20 kg of body weight	50 mL · kg^{-1} · day^{-1}
For all additional body weight over 20 kg	20 mL · kg^{-1} · day^{-1}
Example: A child weighs 66 lbs, which is equal to 30 kg	
For the first 0–10 kg of body weight	100 mL · kg^{-1} · day^{-1} 3 10 kg = 1,000 mL/day
For the next 11–20 kg of body weight	50 mL · kg^{-1} · day^{-1} × 10 kg = 500 mL/day
For all additional body weight over 20 kg	30 kg – 20 kg = 10 kg over 20 kg 10 kg × 20 mL · kg^{-1} · day^{-1} = 200 mL/day
Total daily requirement of fluid	1,000 + 500 + 200 = 1,700 mL/day

This 66-lb child requires 1,700 mL of fluid to be administered throughout the day.

NURSING CARE PLAN **A Client With Pneumonia**

Mary O'Neal is a 35-year-old executive assistant and part-time college student. On returning home from class one evening, she begins to chill. She alternates between chills and sweats all night. Staying home from work, she remains in bed most of the next day. Her fever continues, and she develops a cough and dull, aching chest pain. When the cough becomes productive of rust-colored sputum the following day, she seeks medical treatment from her family doctor.

ASSESSMENT

Debby Kowalski, RN, the family practice clinic nurse, admits Mrs. O'Neal to the clinic and obtains the nursing assessment. Mrs. O'Neal denies any previous history of respiratory diseases "other than the usual colds, flu, and such." She also denies any history of smoking or medication allergies. She says her symptoms began abruptly, with the onset of the chills. She describes her chest pain as a dull ache that was initially substernal but now is localized in her lower lateral right chest. The pain increases with deep breathing, coughing, and moving. Her cough is increasing in frequency and severity, and her sputum appears rusty brown. Her vital signs are BP 116/74 mmHg, pulse 104 bpm and regular, respirations 26/minute, and temperature 101.8°F (38.7°C). Her skin is warm and flushed, with no evidence of cyanosis. Her respirations shallow and unlabored; respiratory excursion is equal. Diminished breath sounds are noted in bases bilaterally, with crackles noted in the right posterior and lateral base. A faint pleural rub heard at right midaxillary line.

A STAT CBC shows a WBC of 18,900/mm^3; differential shows increased numbers of neutrophils and immature WBCs (bands). Ms. Kowalski has Mrs. O'Neal rinse with an antiseptic mouthwash and then collects a sputum specimen for culture and Gram stain before seeing the physician.

The physician orders a chest x-ray after examining Mrs. O'Neal. Based on her history, examination, and the chest x-ray, he makes the diagnosis of acute bacterial pneumonia, probably pneumococcal. He prescribes oral penicillin V, 500 mg every 6 hours for 10 days. He asks Mrs. O'Neal to return for a follow-up appointment in 10 days and refers her back to Ms. Kowalski for appropriate teaching.

DIAGNOSES

- Ineffective Breathing Pattern related to pleuritic chest pain
- Hyperthermia related to inflammatory process
- Deficient Knowledge about pneumonia and its treatment

PLANNING

Goals for Mrs. O'Neal's care include:

- The client will maintain normal pulmonary function.
- The client will describe measures to minimize elevations in body temperature.
- The client will identify a schedule for taking her medication that will facilitate compliance with the regimen.
- The client will describe manifestations that should be reported to the physician.

INTERVENTIONS

- Assess knowledge and understanding of pneumonia and its effects.
- Assist to develop a medication schedule that coordinates with normal daily routine.
- Teach client and family about the following:
  a. Importance of avoiding use of a cough suppressant except at night to facilitate rest
  b. Ways to increase fluid intake to reduce fever and maintain thin mucus for easy expectoration
  c. Beneficial effects of rest, especially during the acute phase of her illness
  d. Safe use of aspirin and acetaminophen to reduce fever
  e. Importance of taking all prescribed medication doses as scheduled
  f. Common side effects of penicillin V and their management
  g. Early manifestations of penicillin allergy that necessitate stopping the medication and notifying the physician
  h. Signs of complications or worsening pneumonia to report.

EVALUATION

The sputum culture confirms *Streptococcus pneumoniae* as the cause of Mrs. O'Neal's pneumonia. When she returns for her follow-up appointment, she reports that she began to feel better after 2 days on the penicillin and returned to work the following Monday. Her examination reveals good breath sounds throughout, with no adventitious sounds. The follow-up sputum culture is free of pathogens.

CRITICAL THINKING

1. Do any of the factors identified in the case study increase Mrs. O'Neal's risk for acute bacterial pneumonia?
2. Mrs. O'Neal's WBC differential showed increased neutrophil and band counts. Describe the reason for and effect of this change.
3. Even though Mrs. O'Neal has no history of medication allergies, anaphylactic shock remains a potential risk. Describe the sequence of events leading to anaphylactic shock, its initial symptoms, and immediate nursing interventions.
4. Had Mrs. O'Neal required hospitalization to treat her acute pneumonia, interruption of her usual activities and responsibilities could lead to anxiety. Develop a care plan for this situation, using the nursing diagnosis ineffective role performance related to hospitalization.

PRACTICE ALERT

Assess respiratory rate, depth, and lung sounds at least every 4 hours. Tachypnea and diminished or adventitious breath sounds may be early indicators of respiratory compromise.

Ineffective Breathing Pattern

- Provide for rest periods. Rest reduces metabolic demands, fatigue, and the work of breathing, promoting a more effective breathing pattern.
- Assess for pleuritic discomfort. Provide analgesics as ordered. Adequate pain relief minimizes splinting and promotes adequate ventilation. Analgesics, such as ibuprofen or acetaminophen, can have the added benefit of fever control and may aid in sleep.
- Teach the client how to splint the chest by hugging a small pillow, or a teddy bear for the pediatric client, to make coughing less painful. Pain may result from coughing and deep breathing as well as from accessory muscle fatigue.
- Provide reassurance during periods of respiratory distress. Hypoxia and respiratory distress produce high levels of anxiety, which tend to further increase tachypnea and fatigue and decrease ventilation.
- Administer oxygen as ordered. Oxygen therapy increases the alveolar oxygen concentration and facilitates its diffusion across the alveolar–capillary membrane, reducing hypoxia and anxiety.
- Teach slow abdominal breathing. This breathing pattern promotes lung expansion.
- Teach use of relaxation techniques, such as visualization and meditation. These techniques help to reduce anxiety and slow the breathing pattern.

Activity Intolerance

- Assess activity tolerance, noting any increase in pulse, respirations, dyspnea, diaphoresis, or cyanosis. These assessment findings may indicate limited or impaired activity tolerance.
- Assist with self-care activities, such as bathing. Assistance with activities of daily living reduces energy demands.
- Schedule activities, planning for rest periods. Rest periods minimize fatigue and improve activity tolerance.
- Provide assistive devices, such as an overhead trapeze. These assistive devices facilitate movement and reduce energy demands.
- Enlist the family's help to minimize stress and anxiety levels. Stress and anxiety increase metabolic demands and can decrease activity tolerance.
- Perform active or passive range-of-motion exercises. Exercises help to maintain muscle tone and joint mobility and to prevent contractures if bedrest is prolonged.
- Provide emotional support and reassurance that strength and energy will return to normal when the infectious process has resolved and the balance of oxygen supply and demand is restored. The client may be concerned that activity intolerance will continue to be a problem after the acute infection is resolved.

PRACTICE ALERT

Activity intolerance may be an early sign of cardiorespiratory compromise, particularly in the older adult or client with preexisting heart disease. New or worsening manifestations of activity intolerance should be reported to the physician.

Home Care

Discuss the following topics when preparing the client and family for home care:

- The importance of completing the prescribed medication regimen as ordered; potential drug side effects and their management, including manifestations that necessitate stopping the drug and notifying the physician
- Recommendations for limiting activities and increasing rest
- The importance of maintaining adequate fluid intake to keep mucus thin for easier expectoration
- Ways to maintain adequate nutritional intake, such as small, frequent, well-balanced meals
- The importance of avoiding smoking or exposure to secondhand smoke to prevent further irritation of the lungs
- Manifestations to report to the physician, such as increasing shortness of breath, difficulty breathing, increased fever, fatigue, headache, sleepiness, or confusion
- The importance of keeping all follow-up appointments to ensure disease cure.

Evaluation

Clients with pneumonia are usually treated in the community unless their respiratory status is significantly compromised (e.g., altered mental status, tachypnea, tachycardia, hypotension, hypo- or hyperthermia, and altered blood gases) or if risk factors (e.g., advanced age and/or coexisting heart, kidney, or liver disease) are present. As a result, caregivers must be taught to evaluate the outcome of care and the signs and symptoms requiring immediate consultation with the primary care provider.

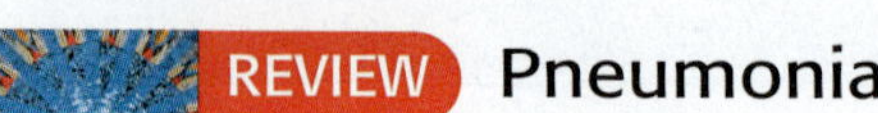

REVIEW Pneumonia

RELATE: LINK THE CONCEPTS

Linking the exemplar of Pneumonia with the concept of Oxygenation:

1. Describe the pathophysiology of pneumonia related to how it impacts oxygenation.
2. What measures could you implement when caring for a client with pneumonia to improve oxygenation?

Linking the exemplar of Pneumonia with the concept of Development:

3. When caring for a 2-year-old diagnosed with pneumonia requiring use of an oxygen tent, what developmentally appropriate activities might you provide to occupy him and keep the child in the tent as much as possible?

4. You are caring for a 6-year-old child diagnosed with cystic fibrosis who is hospitalized for recurrent pneumonia diagnoses. How can you promote this child's normal development during hospitalization?

READY: GO TO COMPANION SKILLS MANUAL

- Sputum collection
- Measuring oxygen saturation using a pulse oximeter
- Oxygen administration
- Assessing body temperature
- Oral hygiene
- Turning clients
- Assessing the lungs and thorax
- Medication administration
- Performing chest physiotherapy
- Suctioning
- Intravenous therapy
- Monitoring intake and output
- Caring for the client on a mechanical ventilator

REFER: GO TO MYNURSINGKIT

REFLECT: CASE STUDY

Jimmy Bley is a 78-year-old, Native American man with moderate emphysema and hearing loss. He is a retired veteran who served as an electronics technician in the army for his entire career. In his retirement, Jimmy has taken an interest in computers. He spends most of his time surfing the Internet or playing games on the computer; he also likes to build computers. Jimmy has been married for 56 years to his wife, Cecelia. They argue a lot, but they would not know what to do without one another just the same. They have several grown children, grandchildren, and great-grandchildren who live within the community. Jimmy often goes with his wife to the Neighborhood Senior center for bingo night.

Jimmy considers himself to be healthy. He describes his hearing loss as mild. He has a hearing aid, but he does not like to wear it and thus does not make changing the batteries a priority. He does not perceive his hearing loss to be much of a problem. Likewise, Jimmy describes his emphysema as "not that bad." However, he becomes short of breath with most activities; thus, it takes time for him to complete tasks. He compensates by taking his time to do most things. He has learned that he must pace himself; if he does not, he becomes exhausted and needs several days to recover. He continues to smoke and knows he should quit, but he just can't seem to get interested in quitting because he enjoys it.

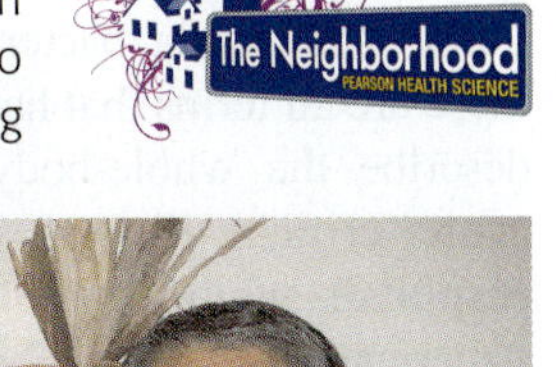

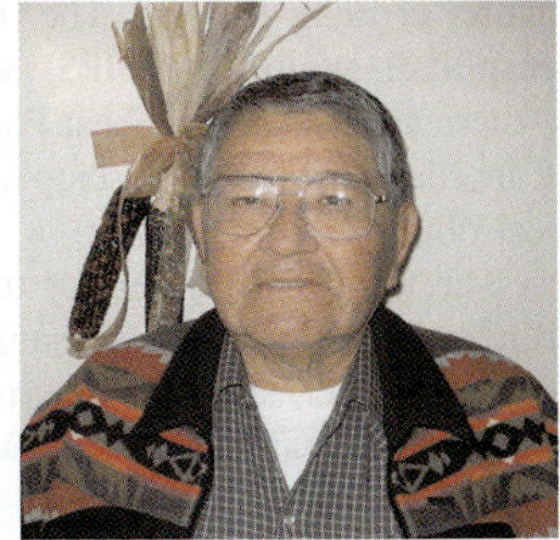

Today, Jimmy is awakened from sleep feeling like he can't catch his breath. He sits up, and his breathing becomes a little easier and he feels slightly less anxious. However, he also notices he is hot. When he takes his temperature, he gets a reading of 101.2°F orally. He still feels a little bit short of breath and decides he will call the clinic in the morning. In the meantime, he goes downstairs, sits in the recliner, and naps fitfully. When he gets to the clinic the doctor performs a chest x-ray (patchy infiltrates in left lower lobe), CBC with differential (elevated WBC count, with differential showing a shift to the left, indicating a bacterial infection), and arterial blood gas (pH 7.32, PaO_2 52, $PaCO_2$ 48, HCO_3 30) and diagnoses Jimmy with pneumonia. Jimmy is taken to the local hospital and admitted with orders for intravenous (IV) fluids; a high-calorie, low-salt, low-fat diet; oxygen via nasal cannula at 2 L/minute; cefaclor (Keflex, Ceclor), 500 mg IV q8h; aminophylline, 100 mg po q8h; and Atrovent HFA 2 puffs qid.

1. What factors contributed to the decision to hospitalize Jimmy instead of treating him at home?
2. Why would the physician order oxygen at only 2 L/minute instead of a 100% mask at 6 L/minute? Provide a physiological explanation for this order.
3. Develop a nursing plan of care for this client.

15.6 SEPSIS

KEY TERMS

Bacteremia, *850*
Ischemia, *854*
Refractory septic shock, *850*
Sepsis, *850*
Septicemia, *850*
Septic shock, *850*
Severe sepsis, *850*
Systemic inflammatory response syndrome (SIRS), *850*

BASIS FOR SELECTION OF EXEMPLAR

Top 20 reasons to be admitted through the emergency department
Agency for Health Care Research and Quality

LEARNING OUTCOMES

After reading about this exemplar, you will be able to:

1. Describe the pathophysiology, etiology, clinical manifestations, and direct and indirect causes of sepsis.
2. Identify risk factors associated with sepsis.
3. Illustrate the nursing process in providing culturally competent care across the life span for individuals with sepsis.
4. Formulate priority nursing diagnoses appropriate for an individual with sepsis.
5. Create a plan of care for individuals with septicemia and their family members.
6. Assess expected outcomes for an individual with sepsis.
7. Discuss therapies used in the collaborative care of an individual with sepsis.
8. Employ evidence-based caring interventions for an individual with sepsis.

OVERVIEW

Sepsis, septicemia, bacteremia, septic shock, blood poisoning—these are all terms that have been used at one time or another to describe the whole-body inflammatory process resulting in acute critical illness. The term **systemic inflammatory response syndrome (SIRS)** was coined in 1992 when the American College of Chest Physicians and Society of Critical Care Medicine met to develop a consensus definition of this critical illness.

The term SIRS describes the body's response to a critical illness that can result from an infectious or noninfectious (e.g., burns, trauma, and pancreatitis) cause precipitating a whole-body inflammatory process. Other common terms can be differentiated as follows:

- **Sepsis** is defined as SIRS resulting from an infection.
- **Severe sepsis** is defined as sepsis with acute associated organ failure.
- **Septic shock** is defined as a persistently low mean arterial blood pressure despite adequate fluid resuscitation.
- **Refractory septic shock** is a persistently low mean arterial blood pressure despite vasopressor therapy and adequate fluid resuscitation (LaRosa, 2008).

For the purpose of this exemplar, we will use the term sepsis, because this exemplar address SIRS resulting from infection.

Sepsis can occur as a complication of virtually any infection of any body tissue if the pathogen causing the infection enters the bloodstream and travels to other tissues. When pathogens enter the bloodstream, they can travel throughout the body, spreading the infection from organ to organ and creating a multisystem response. The whole-body inflammatory response results in symptoms of shock, reduced organ perfusion, multiple-organ dysfunction syndrome, and ultimately, death. Clients with sepsis are very ill and require attentive monitoring and rapid intervention in response to sometimes subtle changes in condition. Nurses play a pivotal role in caring for these clients, because they are with the clients constantly and are most competent to monitor their condition.

PATHOPHYSIOLOGY AND ETIOLOGY

Septic shock begins with **septicemia** (the presence of pathogens and their toxins in the blood). More specifically, septic shock generally begins with **bacteremia** (the presence of bacteria and their toxins in the blood). As pathogens are destroyed, their ruptured cell membranes allow endotoxins to leak into the plasma. The endotoxins disrupt the vascular system, coagulation mechanism, and immune system and trigger an immune and inflammatory response (see the concept on Inflammation, for more information). For this reason, the initial effects of septic shock differ from those of hypovolemic and cardiogenic shock, because cardiac output is high and systemic vascular resistance is low.

Endotoxins directly damage the endothelial lining of small blood vessels first; the small blood vessels of the kidneys and lungs are most susceptible. Cellular damage stimulates the release of vasoactive proteins and activates coagulation factor XII. The vasoactive proteins stimulate peripheral vasodilatation and increase capillary permeability; the activation of coagulation factors results in the production of multiple intravascular blood clots.

As a result of the increased capillary permeability and vasodilatation, fluid shifts from the intravascular space to the interstitial space. Hypovolemia results as fluid volume is lost from the circulating blood. Hypovolemia and intravascular coagulation alter oxygenation and cellular metabolism, leading to anaerobic metabolism, lactic acidosis, and cellular death.

Toxic shock syndrome is an especially virulent form of septic shock and occurs most frequently in menstruating women who use tampons improperly. It is thought that bacterial toxins diffuse from the site of infection in the vagina into the circulation. The toxins then trigger a widespread inflammatory response and septic shock. The manifestations of toxic shock syndrome include extreme hypotension, hyperpyrexia, headache, myalgia, confusion, skin rash, vomiting, and diarrhea (Porth, 2005).

Disseminated intravascular coagulation, a generalized response to injury, is a potential risk in septic shock. This condition is characterized by simultaneous bleeding and clotting throughout the vasculature. Sepsis injures blood cells, causing platelet aggregation and decreased blood flow. As a result, blood clots form throughout the microcirculation. The clotting slows circulation further while stimulating excess fibrinolysis. As the body's stores of clotting factors are depleted, generalized bleeding begins. See Figure 15–33 ■ for an illustration of the pathophysiology of sepsis that develops into septic shock.

Etiology

Sepsis is the leading cause of death in noncoronary intensive care units and the tenth leading cause of death in the United States overall. More than 70% of clients with sepsis have comorbidities, and more than 60% of cases occur in people over the age of 65. Sepsis is most often the result of gram-negative bacterial infections (i.e., *Pseudomonas* sp. *Escherichia coli,* and *Klebsiella* sp.) but may also follow gram-positive infections from *Staphylococcus* and *Streptococcus* bacteria. Six percent of cases are related to fungal infections.

The incidence of gram-negative sepsis has greatly increased over the past 10 years, with a 60% mortality rate despite treatment. The incidence of sepsis is increasing the most in older adults and nonwhite populations. This is believed to be the result of an increase in invasive procedures, immunosuppressive therapy, and antimicrobial resistance (LaRosa, 2008).

Portals of entry for infection that may lead to septic shock are as follows:

- *Urinary system:* catheterizations, suprapubic tubes, and cystoscopy.
- *Respiratory system:* suctioning, aspiration, tracheostomy, endotracheal tubes, respiratory therapy, and mechanical ventilators.
- *Gastrointestinal system:* peptic ulcers, ruptured appendix, peritonitis.
- *Integumentary system:* surgical wounds, intravenous catheters, intra-arterial catheters, invasive monitoring, decubitus ulcers, burns, and trauma.

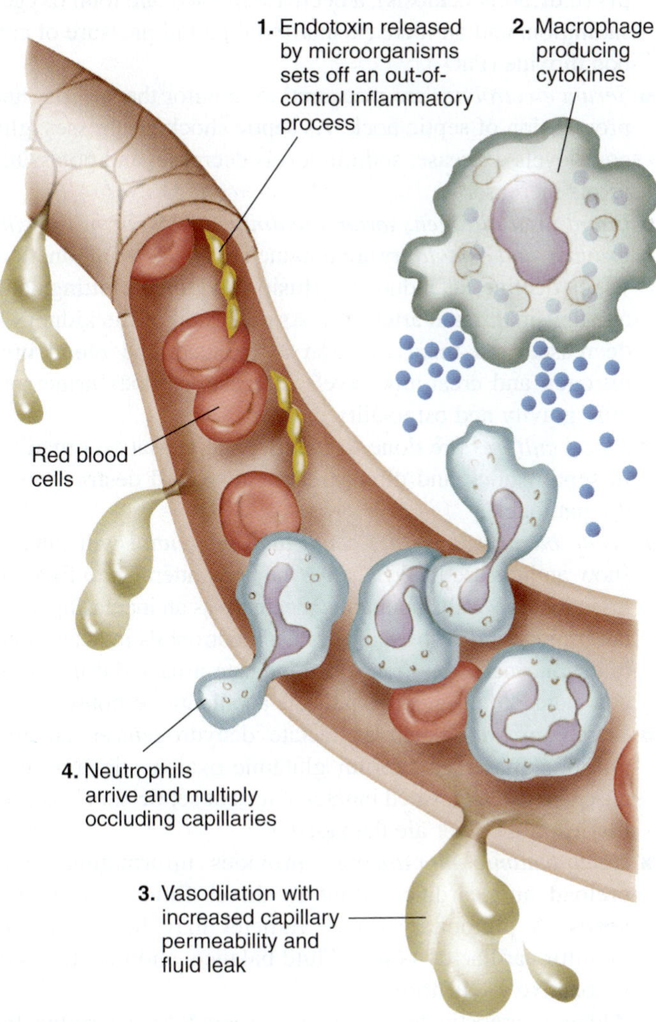
1. Endotoxin released by microorganisms sets off an out-of-control inflammatory process
2. Macrophage producing cytokines
Red blood cells
4. Neutrophils arrive and multiply occluding capillaries
3. Vasodilation with increased capillary permeability and fluid leak

Figure 15–33 ■ In septic shock, blood pools in the extremities. Blood flow is sluggish and amounts of oxygen inadequate for cell metabolism are received by the tissues.

- *Female reproductive system:* elective surgical abortion, ascending infections from transmission of bacteria during the intrapartal and postpartal periods, tampon use, and sexually transmitted infections.

Risk Factors

Clients at risk for developing infections leading to septic shock include those who are hospitalized, have debilitating chronic illnesses, or have poor nutritional status. The risk is heightened after invasive procedures or surgery. Other clients at risk of septic shock include older adults and those who are immunocompromised.

Any infant with an infectious process must be watched carefully for early signs of sepsis; thorough teaching of parents and regular caregivers is indicated. Children with cancer, especially those undergoing treatment with chemotherapy or radiation therapy, must be carefully monitored for symptoms of sepsis and may be placed on prophylactic antibiotics because their risk is so great. During periods of immune suppression, the child is vulnerable to overwhelming infection, resulting in circulatory failure, hypothermia or hyperthermia, tachypnea, mental changes, inadequate tissue perfusion, and hypotension. Factors contributing to massive infection include inadequate neutrophil production, abnormal granulocytes (not able to be actively phagocytic), erosions through normal barriers (e.g., blood vessels and mucous membranes), and altered bone marrow production caused by chemotherapy and some forms of radiation. Such infections must be vigorously treated with antimicrobial therapy and hydration management.

CLINICAL MANIFESTATIONS

Manifestations of sepsis include fever or hypothermia, tachycardia, tachypnea, peripheral vasodilation, septic shock, and mental status changes. Hemodynamic monitoring shows an increase in cardiac output. Lab results show an abnormal CBC (leukocytosis or leukopenia), alteration in clotting factors (thrombocytosis or thrombopenia), and elevated liver enzyme, C-reactive protein, and creatinine levels are likely. Hypophosphatemia and positive blood culture are anticipated.

Septic shock has an early phase and a late phase. In early septic shock (sometimes called the *warm phase*), vasodilation results in weakness and warm, flushed skin, and septicemia often causes high fever and chills. In late septic shock (sometimes called the *cold phase*), hypovolemia and activity of the compensatory mechanisms result in typical shock manifestations, including cold, moist skin; oliguria; and changes in

CLINICAL MANIFESTATIONS AND THERAPIES **Sepsis**

ETIOLOGY	CLINICAL MANIFESTATION	CLINICAL THERAPIES
Disseminated intravascular coagulation may develop as a result of altered coagulation.	Varies from increased tendency to bleed to hemorrhage. Small clots may reduce blood flow to major organs; manifestations will be determined by organs affected. Prolonged clotting times, reduced fibrinogen and platelet levels. Often see spider angiomas or purpura on the client's skin and the affected person is acutely ill.	■ Only effective treatment is to reverse the underlying cause (i.e., sepsis). ■ Platelet transfusions ■ Fresh-frozen plasma administration ■ Antithrombin administration may be considered. ■ Activated protein C is given only in the intensive care unit to clients with severe sepsis.

mental status. Death may result from respiratory failure, cardiac failure, and/or renal failure. Manifestations of septic shock are listed in Box 15–6.

Manifestations of sepsis in infants include temperature instability, abdominal distention, poor feeding, lethargy, respiratory distress, hepatomegaly, vomiting, and/or jaundice. Children under 3 months of age with a temperature of greater than 100.4°F (38°C) rectally will require diagnostic testing to rule out sepsis, because they are at increased risk secondary to immature immune systems and inadequate immune response to infection.

COLLABORATION

Septic shock can be fatal, but early and aggressive therapy improves outcomes (Haut, 2005). Collaborative care of the client with sepsis includes active participation by a number of specialists, such as infectious disease specialists, phlebotomists, and when clients experience impaired oxygenation, respiratory therapists. Gerontologists and pediatricians may be required for clients in those respective age groups, especially in determining safety and side effects when multiple medications are recommended.

Diagnostic Tests

The following diagnostic tests can help to identify the cause of sepsis and assess the client's physical status:

- *Hemoglobin and hematocrit* are performed, because changes in hematocrit concentrations usually occur in clients with septic shock as fluid leaks from the intravascular to the extravascular spaces. These changes reflect the body's response to endotoxins. In septic shock resulting from intravascular fluid loss, the hemoglobin and hematocrit concentrations are higher than normal.
- *Arterial blood gas* is performed to determine oxygen and carbon dioxide levels and pH. The effects of septic shock and of the body's compensatory mechanisms cause a decrease in pH (indicating acidosis), a decrease in PaO_2 and total oxygen saturation, and an increase in arterial partial pressure of carbon dioxide (PaO_2).
- *Serum electrolytes* are measured to monitor the severity and progression of septic hock. As septic shock progresses, glucose levels decrease, sodium levels decrease, and potassium levels increase.
- *Blood urea nitrogen, serum creatinine levels, urine specific gravity, and osmolality* are obtained to check renal function, which declines as reduced perfusion and microclotting damage the small renal arterioles. As perfusion of the kidneys is decreased and renal function is reduced, the blood urea nitrogen and creatinine levels increase, as does urine specific gravity and osmolality.
- *Blood cultures* are done to identify the causative organism in septic shock and direct treatment toward destruction of the pathogen.
- *White blood cell (WBC) count and differential* will initially show an increase in WBCs. As the body attempts to fight the infection, the WBC count may decrease as an increasing number of them are destroyed. Elevated neutrophils indicate acute infection, increased monocytes indicate a bacterial infection, and increased eosinophils indicate an allergic response.
- *Serum enzymes,* such as lactate dehydrogenase, creatine phosphokinase, and serum glutamic-oxaloacetic transaminase, are often elevated in later stages of septic shock as capillaries in the liver are damaged.
- *Hemodynamic monitoring* provides information about preload and cardiac output to direct fluid resuscitation needs. A pulmonary artery catheter may be inserted to monitor cardiac dynamics, fluid balance, and the effects of vasoactive medications.

Other diagnostic tests may be ordered to determine the extent of injury or damage. These tests might include x-ray studies, computed tomography, magnetic resonance imaging, endoscopic examinations, and echocardiograms. Newer diagnostic methods for hypoperfusion include gastric tonometry and sublingual $Paco_2$. Gastric tonometry measures the partial pressure of carbon dioxide in the gastric lumen. The measurement of sublingual carbon dioxide correlates well with decreased mean arterial pressure (MAP) (Sole, Lamborn, & Hartshorn, 2001).

Box 15–6 Manifestations of Septic Shock

EARLY (WARM) SEPTIC SHOCK

- *Blood pressure:* normal to hypotension
- *Pulse:* increased, thready
- *Respirations:* rapid and deep
- *Skin:* warm, flushed
- *Mental status:* alert, oriented, anxious
- *Urine output:* normal
- *Other:* increased body temperature; chills; weakness; nausea, vomiting, diarrhea; decreased CVP

LATE (COLD) SEPTIC SHOCK

- *Blood pressure:* hypotension
- *Pulse:* tachycardia, arrhythmias
- *Respirations:* rapid, shallow, dyspneic
- *Skin:* cool, pale, edematous
- *Mental status:* lethargic to comatose
- *Urine output:* oliguria to anuria
- *Other:* normal to decreased body temperature; decreased CVP

Pharmacologic Therapies

Antimicrobials are a primary pharmacologic treatment if the infection is caused by bacteria or fungi. Generally, broad-spectrum antibiotics are used. The client may be placed on several antibiotics to ensure adequate coverage of the pathogen until culture and sensitivity results return in 72 hours to indicate the best antibiotic of choice. As antibiotics begin to take effect, the client's condition may actually worsen initially as increasing numbers of toxins are released into the circulating bloodstream because of pathogen destruction, further activating the immune response.

When fluid replacement alone is not sufficient to reverse shock, vasoactive drugs (drugs causing vasoconstriction or vasodilatation) and inotropic drugs (drugs improving cardiac contractility) may be administered. When used to treat shock, these drugs increase venous return through vasoconstriction of peripheral vessels; they also improve the pumping ability of the heart by facilitating myocardial contractility and dilating coronary arteries to increase perfusion of the myocardium. More information on pharmacologic treatment for shock can be found in the concept on Perfusion.

Oxygen Therapy

Establishing and maintaining a patent airway and ensuring adequate oxygenation are critical interventions in reversing septic shock. All clients in septic shock (even those with adequate respirations) should receive oxygen therapy (usually by mask or nasal cannula) to maintain the PaO_2 at greater than 80 mmHg during the first 4–6 hours of care. If the client's unassisted respiration cannot maintain PaO_2 at this level, ventilatory assistance may be necessary. Care of the client requiring ventilatory assistance is discussed in the concept on Oxygenation.

Fluid Replacement

The most effective treatment for the client in septic shock is the administration of intravenous fluids or blood. Various fluids may be administered alone or in combination as part of fluid replacement therapy. Whole blood or blood products increase the oxygen-carrying capacity of the blood and thus increase the oxygenation of cells. Fluid replacements, such as crystalloid and colloid solutions, increase circulating blood volume and tissue perfusion. Fluid replacements are administered in massive amounts through two large-bore peripheral lines or, most often, through a central line. More information about types of fluids can be found in the concept on Fluid and Electrolytes.

NURSING PROCESS

Nursing assessments are critical in reducing the complications associated with sepsis. Identifying clients at risk and performing focused assessments are essential. Although septic shock may occur at any age, the physiologic changes of the aging process place the older adult at higher risk. Clients who are hospitalized, are debilitated, are chronically ill, or have undergone invasive procedures or tube insertions are at high risk for septic shock. Nursing care to prevent septic shock includes careful and consistent hand washing, use of aseptic techniques for procedures (e.g., catheterizations, suctioning, changing dressings, and starting and maintaining intravenous fluids or medications), and monitoring for early local and systemic manifestations of infection.

Assessment

Sepsis involves the entire body. Therefore, assessment of the client most importantly includes frequent vital signs, hemodynamic assessment if a central line is in place, and focused assessments evaluating perfusion, renal function, and pulmonary competence.

Baseline vital signs are necessary to determine trends in subsequent findings. As septic shock progresses, blood pressure decreases, and pulse becomes rapid, weak, and thready. As perfusion of the lungs decreases, crackles, wheezes, and dyspnea are commonly assessed. Capillary refill is prolonged, and peripheral pulses are weak or nonpalpable. Neck veins that cannot be seen when the client is in the supine position indicate decreased intravascular volume. CVP is an accurate means of determining fluid status in the client in shock; the findings will be low (5–15 cm of water is normal) in hypovolemic shock because of the decreased blood volume.

Diagnosis

Nursing diagnoses for the client with sepsis may include the following:

- Ineffective Tissue Perfusion
- Altered Gas Exchange
- Deficient Fluid Volume
- Interrupted Family Processes
- Death Anxiety
- Risk for Electrolyte Imbalance
- Risk for Ineffective Renal Perfusion
- Hyperthermia
- Impaired Mobility
- Imbalanced Nutrition: Less Than Body Requirements.

Plan

Planning care for the client with sepsis is very fluid, because the client's condition and needs can change very quickly. Because the client is critically ill, reassessment findings will often redirect the plan of care. Potential outcomes that may be appropriate for the client with sepsis include the following:

- Client maintains adequate renal perfusion to produce a minimum of 30 mL of urine per hour.
- Client maintains oxygen saturation greater than 90% and PaO_2 within normal limits.
- Client responds to fluid resuscitation with mean arterial blood pressure that returns to normal range.

DEVELOPMENTAL CONSIDERATIONS Variations in Assessment Findings in Older Adults

- Cardiac changes may include a thickened left ventricular wall, decreased elasticity of the myocardium, and more rigid valves. These changes result in a decreased stroke volume and cardiac output, thus decreasing responses to septic shock.
- Decreased arterial wall elasticity and vasomotor tone reduce the older adult's ability to respond to a decrease in oxygenation.
- Decreased elasticity and turgor of the skin make assessments of skin turgor more difficult.
- Decreased immune system response increases the risk of septic shock.

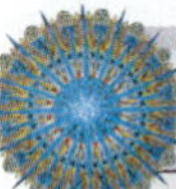

NURSING CARE PLAN A Client With Septic Shock

Huang Mei Lan is a 43-year-old, unmarried woman who lives alone in a major West Coast city. Ms. Huang came to America 15 years ago from China and now speaks English well. Her family still lives in China. She worked in a neighborhood sewing shop until 3 years ago, when she was diagnosed with breast cancer. Her treatment included mastectomy of the affected breast and follow-up chemotherapy.

Last month, Ms. Huang experienced a recurrence of cancer in the lymph glands of the affected side. Surgery to remove the glands was performed and chemotherapy started. Ms. Huang has a central line, a urinary catheter, and a surgical incision. She is underweight, weak, and depressed. Although she has multiple physical problems, she never complains or asks for any kind of medication.

ASSESSMENT

Ms. Huang's primary nurse, Robert O'Brien, enters her room early in the morning to make an initial assessment. He finds Ms. Huang huddled in the middle of the bed, shivering violently. Her vital signs are temperature 104°F, pulse 110 bpm, respirations 30/minute, and BP 106/66 mmHg. Her skin is hot, dry, and flushed with poor turgor. She is alert and oriented but is restless and appears anxious. Ms. Huang states she is nauseated and suddenly begins vomiting and is incontinent of liquid stool. Laboratory data indicate leukocytosis, respiratory alkalosis, and reduced platelet count. Blood cultures, as well as cultures of Ms. Huang's sputum, urine, and wound drainage, are conducted. She is diagnosed as having septic shock.

Hetastarch is ordered per intravenous line, and intravenous broad-spectrum antibiotics are begun until the organism and its portal of entry can be determined. Despite treatment, Ms. Huang's condition worsens. Her blood pressure continues to drop, her skin becomes cool and cyanotic, and she begins to have periods of disorientation. She is transferred to the critical care unit. As she is being prepared for the transfer, she begins to cry and asks, "Am I going to die?"

DIAGNOSES

- Deficient Fluid Volume related to vomiting, diarrhea, high fever, and shift of intravascular volume to interstitial spaces
- Ineffective Breathing Pattern related to rapid respirations and progression of septic shock
- Ineffective Tissue Perfusion related to progression of septic shock with decreased cardiac output, hypotension, and massive vasodilatation
- Anxiety related to feelings that illness is worsening and is potentially life-threatening and the transfer to the critical care unit

PLANNING

Goals for Mrs. Huang's care include:

- The client will maintain adequate circulating blood volume.
- The client will regain and maintain blood gas parameters within normal limits.
- The client will regain and maintain stable hemodynamic levels.
- The client will verbalize increased ability to cope with stressors.

INTERVENTIONS

- Monitor neurologic status, including mental status and level of consciousness.
- Monitor cardiovascular status, including arterial blood pressure; rate, rhythm, and quality of pulses; central venous pressure; pulmonary artery pressure; and cardiac output.
- Monitor color and character of skin.
- Monitor results of arterial blood gas, blood counts, clotting times, and platelet counts.
- Monitor respiratory status, including respiratory rate, rhythm, and breath sounds.
- Monitor body temperature every 2 hours.
- Monitor urinary output hourly, reporting any output of less than 30 mL/hours.
- Explain procedures, and provide comfort measures (e.g., oral care, skin care, turning, and positioning).

EVALUATION

Despite intensive nursing and medical care, Ms. Huang's condition remains critical. The interventions are continued.

CRITICAL THINKING

1. Vasopressors may be used in the treatment of septic shock. Explain the rationale for their use.
2. While monitoring Ms. Huang's arterial blood gas, the nurse notes that her PaO_2 is less than 60 mmHg and her $PaCO_2$ is greater than 50 mmHg. What do these findings indicate, and why have they occurred?
3. Ms. Huang has been given large amounts of colloids intravenously. Hemodynamic monitoring indicates a higher-than-normal CVP and pulmonary artery pressure. What do these findings indicate? What physical assessments would you make to confirm the changes?

Implementation

Diminished tissue perfusion causes **ischemia** (inadequate blood supply) and hypoxia (insufficient oxygen) of major organ systems, with the potential for significant impact on the kidneys, brain, heart, lungs, and gastrointestinal tract. Nurses working with clients who have sepsis should:

- Monitor skin color, temperature, turgor, and moisture. Decreased tissue perfusion is evidenced by the skin becoming pale, cool, and moist; as hemoglobin concentrations decrease, cyanosis occurs.

- Monitor cardiopulmonary function by assessing/monitoring the following:
  a. Blood pressure (by auscultation or hemodynamic monitoring)
  b. Rate and depth of respirations
  c. Lung sounds
  d. Pulse oximetry
  e. Peripheral pulses (brachial, radial, dorsalis pedis, and posterior tibial); include presence, equality, rate, rhythm, and quality (if unable to palpate pulses, use a device such as a Doppler ultrasound flowmeter to assess peripheral arterial blood flow).
- Monitor jugular vein distention.
- Take CVP measurements.
- Monitor body temperature. An elevated body temperature increases metabolic demands, depleting reserves of bodily energy. It also increases myocardial oxygen demand and may place the client with previous cardiac problems at even greater risk for hypoperfusion.
- Monitor urinary output per Foley catheter hourly, using a urometer. Urine output is a reliable indicator of renal perfusion.
- Assess mental status and level of consciousness. The appropriateness of the client's behavior and responses reflects the adequacy of cerebral circulation. Restlessness and anxiety are common early in septic shock; in later stages, the client may become lethargic and progress to a comatose state. Altered levels of consciousness are the result of both cerebral hypoxia and the effects of acidosis on brain cells.

Other nursing interventions appropriate for the client with sepsis can be found in the concept on Perfusion, Exemplar 22.9, Shock.

Evaluation

Clients with sepsis must be continuously and frequently reevaluated, sometimes as often as every few minutes, because their condition changes quickly. Following fluid administration, the client's blood pressure and perfusion may improve. As fluid leaves the intravascular space, however, the client's condition may decline again. As perfusion declines, renal, cardiac, pulmonary, and neurovascular status may change quickly.

REVIEW Sepsis

RELATE: LINK THE CONCEPTS

Linking the exemplar of Sepsis with the concept of Perfusion:

1. How is perfusion impacted by sepsis?
2. What nursing implementations could you initiate to promote perfusion in the client diagnosed with sepsis?

Linking the exemplar of Sepsis with the concept of Acid–Base Balance:

3. When analyzing the arterial blood gas of a client in septic shock, what changes would you anticipate?
4. What interventions (both nursing and collaborative) could you implement to promote acid–base balance in the client diagnosed with sepsis?

READY: GO TO COMPANION SKILLS MANUAL

- Pulmonary artery pressure monitoring
- Arterial blood pressure monitoring
- Caring for the client on a mechanical ventilator
- Assessing appearance and mental status
- Total parenteral nutrition
- Blood transfusions
- Assisting with insertion of a central line
- Intravenous therapy

REFER: GO TO MYNURSINGKIT

REFLECT: CASE STUDY

Frank Lauer is a 72-year-old man with moderate emphysema and hearing loss. He is a retired veteran who served as a medic in the army for his entire career. In his retirement, Frank has taken an interest in electronics. Mr. Lauer has been married for 49 years to his wife Marie. They have several grown children, grandchildren, and great-grandchildren who live within a few miles. Mr. Lauer occasionally goes with his wife to the Senior Center for bingo night or to the local movies.

Mr. Lauer's daughter tells him about free flu shots being provided at the local clinic, but he is afraid it will make him sick so he declines. A few weeks later, he feels tired and develops a nagging cough. He gets short of breath very easily. His children want him to see the physician immediately but Mr. Lauer says it's just a cold and he'll feel better in a few days without seeing the doctor. His cough becomes more severe at night and he begins having trouble breathing but finds that sleeping in the recliner makes him feel better.

A few nights later Mr. Lauer's cough is so severe he feels like he can't catch his breath between coughing episodes. Marie sets up a humidifier next to his chair and encourages him to drink more fluids and see the doctor in the morning. He just laughs and tells her she's a worrier. His breathing improves and he falls asleep in the chair. In the morning he feels so weak he has trouble walking to the bathroom. His temperature is elevated again and his breathing is rapid and he feels awful. He consents to visiting the doctor where he is diagnosed with bacterial pneumonia. Blood cultures are drawn and the results indicate septicemia.

1. What factors increased Mr Lauer's likelihood of being diagnosed with sepsis?
2. How would you explain his condition to both Mr. and Mrs. Lauer?
3. Develop a nursing plan of care listing all potential nursing diagnoses and developing two of them to include goals, interventions, and expected outcomes.

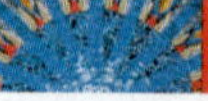

15.7 TUBERCULOSIS

KEY TERMS

Anergic, *862*
Bacilli, *856*
Caseation necrosis, *856*
Cavitation, *857*
Dormant, *857*
Droplet nuclei, *857*
Encapsulated, *856*
Extrapulmonary tuberculosis, *857*
Hematogenous spread, *857*
Hemoptysis, *860*
Miliary tuberculosis, *857*
Mycobacterium tuberculosis, *856*
Negative airflow room, *868*
Pneumothorax, *861*
Purified protein derivative (PPD), *861*
Tine test, *861*
Tubercle, *856*
Tuberculosis, *856*

BASIS FOR SELECTION OF EXEMPLAR

Centers for Disease Control and Prevention
World Health Organization

LEARNING OUTCOMES

After reading about this exemplar, you will be able to:

1. Describe the pathophysiology, etiology, clinical manifestations, and direct and indirect causes of tuberculosis.
2. Identify risk factors associated with tuberculosis.
3. Illustrate the nursing process in providing culturally competent care across the life span for individuals with tuberculosis.
4. Formulate priority nursing diagnoses appropriate for an individual with tuberculosis.
5. Create a plan of care for individuals with tuberculosis and their family members.
6. Assess expected outcomes for an individual with tuberculosis.
7. Discuss therapies used in the collaborative care of an individual with tuberculosis.
8. Employ evidence-based caring interventions for an individual with tuberculosis.

OVERVIEW

Tuberculosis is a chronic, recurrent, infectious disease caused by **Mycobacterium tuberculosis**, a relatively slow-growing, slender, rod-shaped, acid-fast organism with a waxy outer capsule that increases its resistance to destruction. Because tuberculosis most often affects the lungs, many people think of it as a pulmonary disease, but primary or secondary tuberculosis lesions may affect other body systems, such as the kidneys, genitalia, bone, and brain.

Tuberculosis was a major public health concern earlier in this century, before the development of effective sanitation measures and drug treatment. Currently, it is uncommon in the United States, especially among young adults of European descent. However, the development of drug-resistant strains, susceptibility of people with HIV/AIDS, and inadequate access to health care for high-risk populations contribute to the continuing significance of tuberculosis as a public health threat.

PATHOPHYSIOLOGY AND ETIOLOGY

Pulmonary Tuberculosis

Minute droplet nuclei containing one to three **bacilli** (rod-shaped bacteria) may elude upper airway defense systems, enter the lungs, and implant in an alveolus or respiratory bronchiole, usually in an upper lobe. As these bacteria multiply, they cause a local inflammatory response. The inflammatory response brings neutrophils and macrophages to the site. These phagocytic cells then surround and engulf the bacilli, isolating them and preventing their spread. The *M. tuberculosis* organisms continue to slowly multiply, however, and some of these bacilli enter the lymphatic system to stimulate a cellular-mediated immune response. Neutrophils and macrophages isolate the bacteria but, again, cannot destroy them. A granulomatous lesion called a **tubercle** (a sealed-off colony of bacilli) is formed. Within the tubercle, infected tissue dies, forming a cheeselike center, a process called **caseation necrosis**. These tubercle bacilli grow slowly, dividing within the macrophage, and after 2–12 weeks, once the organisms number from 1,000 to 10,000, cellular immune response can be elicited with the tuberculosis skin test.

In infants and children, infection may progress to active tuberculosis even before the skin test becomes reactive in infants and children because of their immature immune system (Reznik & Ozuah, 2005). If the immune response is adequate, however, scar tissue develops around the tubercle, and the bacilli remain **encapsulated** (enclosed). These lesions eventually calcify and become visible on x-ray, but the client with an adequate immune response, while still infected by *M. tuberculosis*, does not develop tuberculosis disease. If the immune response is inadequate to contain the bacilli, the disease of tuberculosis can develop. If a tubercle ruptures, the bacilli spread, leading to tuberculosis pneumonia. Occasionally, the infection can progress, leading to extensive destruction of lung tissue. In *primary tuberculosis*, granulomatous tissue may erode into a bronchus or a blood vessel, allowing the disease to spread throughout the lung or other organs. This severe form of tuberculosis is uncommon in healthy adults (Kasper et al., 2005).

A previously healed tuberculosis lesion may be reactivated. *Reactivation tuberculosis* occurs when the immune system is suppressed because of age, disease, or use of immunosuppressive drugs. The extent of lung disease can vary from small lesions to extensive cavitation of lung tissue. Tubercles rupture, spreading bacilli into the airways to form satellite lesions and produce tuberculosis pneumonia. Without treatment, massive lung involvement can lead to death, or a more chronic process of tubercle formation and **cavitation** (formation of a cavity or bubble) may result. People with chronic disease continue to spread *M. tuberculosis* into the environment, potentially infecting others. Figure 15–34 ■ illustrates the pathogenesis of tuberculosis.

Extrapulmonary Tuberculosis

When primary disease or reactivation allows live bacilli to enter the bronchi, the disease may spread through the blood and lymph system to other organs and become **extrapulmonary tuberculosis**. These distant disease metastases may produce an active lesion, or they may become **dormant** (temporarily inactive but not dead) and reactivate at a later time. Extrapulmonary tuberculosis is especially prevalent in people with HIV/AIDS.

Miliary tuberculosis results from **hematogenous spread** (through the blood) of the bacilli throughout the body. Miliary tuberculosis causes chills and fever, weakness, malaise, and progressive dyspnea. Multiple lesions evenly distributed throughout the lungs are noted on x-ray, but the sputum rarely contains organisms. The bone marrow is usually involved, causing anemia, thrombocytopenia, and leukocytosis. Without appropriate treatment, the prognosis is poor.

The kidney and genitourinary tract are common extrapulmonary sites for tuberculosis. The organism spreads to the kidney through the blood, initiating an inflammatory process similar to that which occurs in the lungs. Reactivation can occur years after the original infection. As the lesion then enlarges and caseates, a large portion of the renal parenchyma is destroyed. The infection then can spread to the rest of the urinary tract, including the ureters and bladder. Scarring and strictures commonly result. In men, the prostate, seminal vesicles, and epididymis may be involved. In women, tuberculosis may affect the fallopian tubes and ovaries. Manifestations of genitourinary tuberculosis develop insidiously. Symptoms of a urinary tract infection, including malaise, dysuria, hematuria, and pyuria, develop. Flank pain may be present. Men may develop manifestations of epididymitis or prostatitis: perineal, sacral, or scrotal pain and tenderness; difficulty voiding; and fever. Women may have manifestations of pelvic inflammatory disease, impaired fertility, or ectopic pregnancy.

Tuberculosis meningitis results when tuberculosis spreads to the subarachnoid space. In the United States, this complication most often affects older adults, usually from reactivation of latent disease. Manifestations develop gradually, including listlessness, irritability, diminished appetite, and fever. Headache and behavioral changes are common early symptoms in the older adult. As the disease progresses, the headaches increase in intensity, vomiting develops, and the level of consciousness decreases. Convulsions and coma may follow. Without appropriate treatment, neurologic effects may become permanent.

Tuberculosis of the bones and joints is most likely to occur during childhood, when bone epiphyses are open and their blood supply is rich. The organisms spread via the blood to vertebrae, the ends of long bones, and joints. Immune and inflammatory processes isolate the bacilli, and the disease often becomes evident years or even decades later. Tuberculous spondylitis usually involves the thoracic vertebrae, eroding vertebral bodies and causing them to collapse. Significant kyphosis (concave curvature of the spinal column) develops, and the spinal cord may be compressed. The large, weight-bearing joints (hips and knees) are most often affected by tuberculous arthritis, although other joints can also be affected, particularly if they have been previously damaged. The involved joint is painful, warm, and tender.

Etiology

As mentioned, tuberculosis is caused by the organism *M. tuberculosis*. It is transmitted by **droplet nuclei** (airborne droplets produced when an infected person coughs, sneezes, speaks, or sings). The tiny droplets can remain suspended in air for several hours. Infection may develop when a susceptible host breathes in air containing droplet nuclei and the contaminated particle eludes the normal defenses of the upper respiratory tract to reach the alveoli.

Thanks to improved sanitation, surveillance, and treatment of people with active disease, the incidence of tuberculosis fell steadily until the mid-1980s. The late 1980s and early 1990s, however, saw a resurgence of the disease, attributed primarily to the HIV/AIDS epidemic, the emergence of multidrug-resistant (MDR) strains of tuberculosis, and social factors, such as immigration, poverty, homelessness, and drug abuse. Today, the number of people affected in the United States continues to decline, with a total of 14,093 cases reported in 2005, the lowest number recorded since national reporting began in 1953 (CDC, 2006g). This decline can be attributed to tuberculosis-control programs that emphasize promptly identifying new cases and initiating and completing appropriate therapy.

Worldwide, tuberculosis continues to be a significant health problem, with an estimated 2 billion people (one third of the world's population) infected by *M. tuberculosis*. An estimated 9 million cases of tuberculosis develop annually, with the vast majority (95%) occurring in the developing countries of Asia, Africa, the Middle East, and Latin America. The disease accounts for an estimated 2 million deaths each year (CDC, 2006i).

In the United States, more than 50% of new cases occur in individuals who are foreign born (CDC, 2004d). The number of tuberculosis cases in children was 1.5 cases per 100,000 in 2001, compared to 2.9 cases per 100,000 in 1993. More children have latent infection (the organism has replicated in the lungs, but no signs of disease are present) than have active disease. In young children, the disease develops as an immediate complication of the primary infection.

Risk Factors

Today, tuberculosis in the United States is a disease primarily affecting immigrants, those with HIV/AIDS, and disadvantaged populations. Children under 5 years of age, racial and ethnic

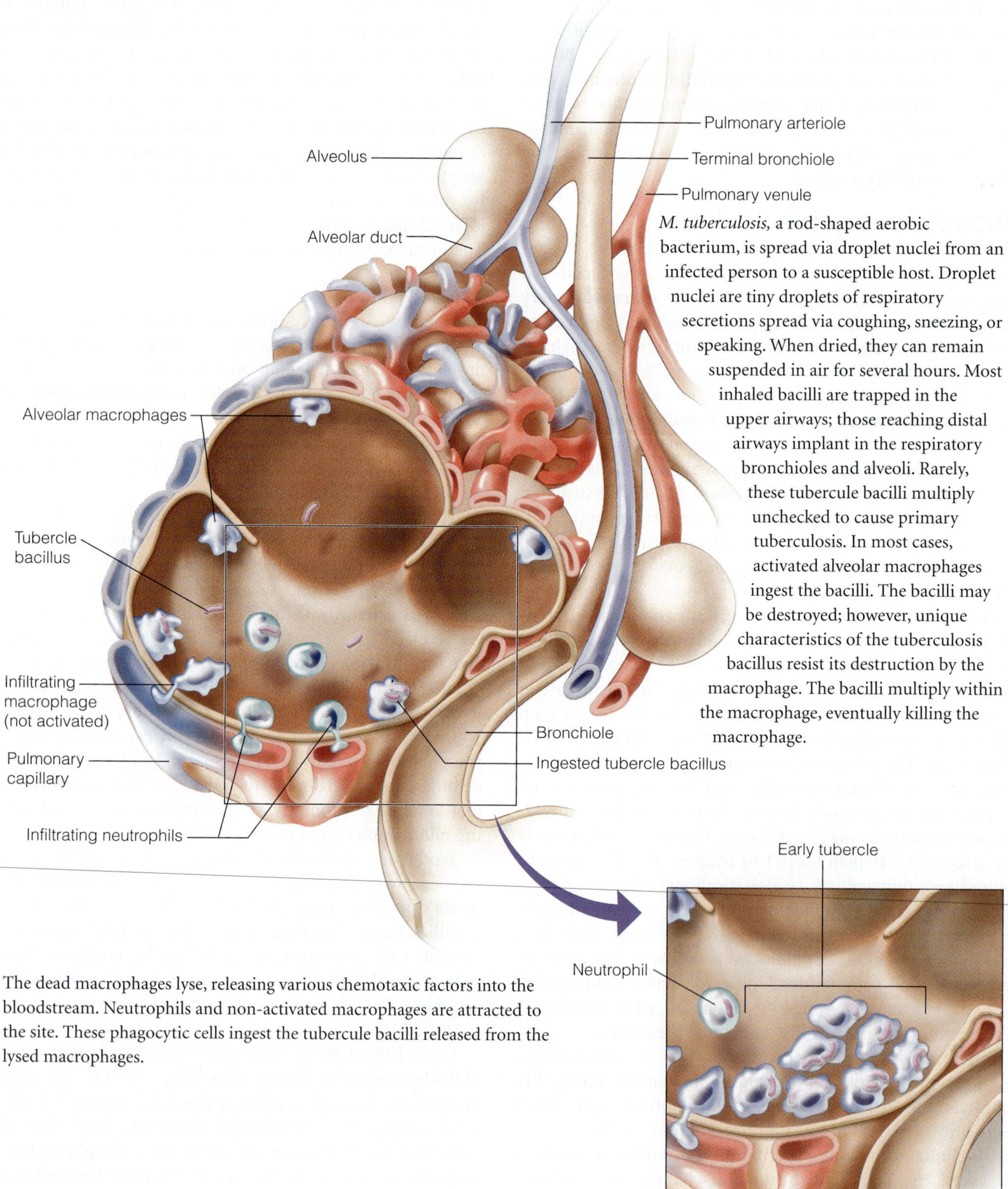

M. tuberculosis, a rod-shaped aerobic bacterium, is spread via droplet nuclei from an infected person to a susceptible host. Droplet nuclei are tiny droplets of respiratory secretions spread via coughing, sneezing, or speaking. When dried, they can remain suspended in air for several hours. Most inhaled bacilli are trapped in the upper airways; those reaching distal airways implant in the respiratory bronchioles and alveoli. Rarely, these tubercule bacilli multiply unchecked to cause primary tuberculosis. In most cases, activated alveolar macrophages ingest the bacilli. The bacilli may be destroyed; however, unique characteristics of the tuberculosis bacillus resist its destruction by the macrophage. The bacilli multiply within the macrophage, eventually killing the macrophage.

The dead macrophages lyse, releasing various chemotaxic factors into the bloodstream. Neutrophils and non-activated macrophages are attracted to the site. These phagocytic cells ingest the tubercule bacilli released from the lysed macrophages.

Figure 15–34

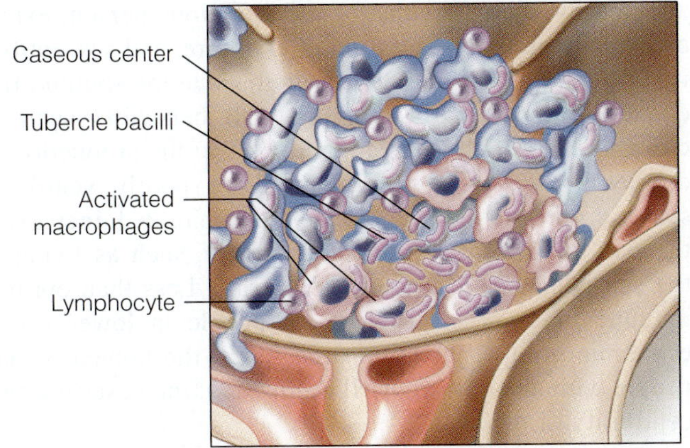

After several weeks, a delayed hypersensitivity response to bacterial antigens destroys many of the macrophages. Concurrently, a cell-mediated immune response activates additional macrophages, which ingest and destroy the bacilli. The lysed macrophages and bacilli are surrounded by a mass of live, activated macrophages and lymphocytes. Scar (granulomatous) tissue forms, encapsulating the primary lesion. Most lesions calcify and are visible on x-ray. These lesions may remain dormant for a year or more (in some cases, many years) before being reactivated to produce secondary or reactivation tuberculosis.

When the immune and macrophage-activating responses are weakened by age or disease (e.g., HIV disease), the tuberculosis bacilli continue to multiply within the lesion. The caseous material at the center of the lesion liquefies, and the lesion grows.

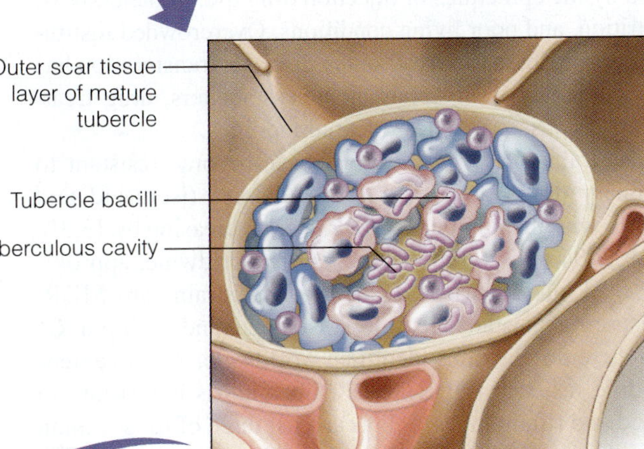

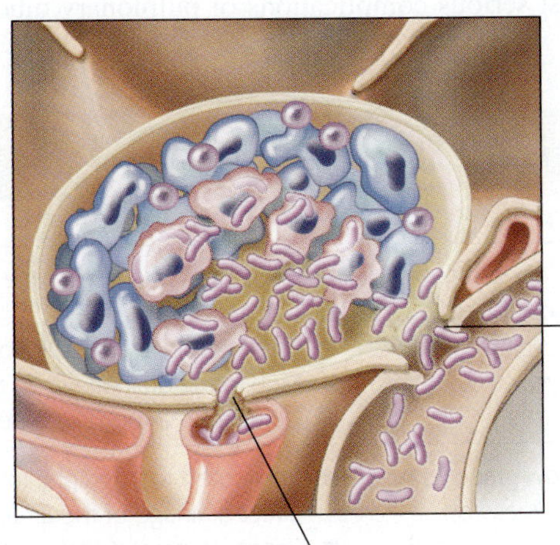

The enlarging lesion damages surrounding bronchial walls and blood vessels. Granulomatous tissue surrounding the lesion can erode into a bronchus, forming an air-filling cavity. Within this cavity, the bacilli multiply, spreading into the airways and the environment via infected sputum. Bacilli multiply, spreading into the airways and the environment via infected sputum. Bacilli also spread via the blood and within macrophages to regional lymph nodes, and from there to many organs and tissues. Resulting extrapulmonary lesions evolve in the same sequence as pulmonary lesions.

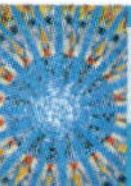

FOCUS ON DIVERSITY AND CULTURE

Tuberculosis

- The case rate for foreign-born U.S. residents is 8.7 times higher than that for people born in the United States (CDC, 2006g).
- Asians and Pacific Islanders living in the United States have the highest case rates, nearly 20 times higher than that for whites.
- Case rates for blacks and Hispanics in the United States are 7 to 8 times that for whites.

minorities, and foreign-born children are more likely to develop tuberculosis than older children (Nelson, Schneider, Wells, & Moore, 2004). People with altered immune function, including older adults and people with HIV/AIDS, are at particular risk.

Poor urban areas are hit the hardest—areas that are also affected by the epidemics of injection drug use, homelessness, malnutrition, and poor living conditions. Overcrowded institutions also contribute to spread of the disease. Transmission has been documented in hospitals, homeless shelters, drug treatment centers, prisons, and residential facilities.

Some strains of *M. tuberculosis* have become resistant to the primary drugs used to treat the disease (isoniazid and rifampin), with the number of MDR cases increasing by 13.3% between 2004 and 2005 (CDC, 2006b). Worldwide, approximately 39% of identified *M. tuberculosis* strains are MDR, demonstrating resistance to at least isoniazid and rifampin. Of MDR tuberculosis strains identified worldwide, 7% are extensively drug resistant (XDR). XDR tuberculosis is resistant to isoniazid and rifampin, as well as at least three of the six main classes of second-line antituberculosis drugs (CDC, 2006b). The prevalence of MDR and XDR tuberculosis in the United States is lower, with 1.6% of cases reported from 1993 through 2004 identified as MDR. Of these, 4.1% were resistant to three or more classes of antituberculosis drugs, qualifying as XDR tuberculosis (CDC, 2006b).

The risk for a new infection by *M. tuberculosis* is affected by characteristics of the infectious person, extent of air contamination, duration of exposure, and susceptibility of the host. The number of microbes in the sputum, frequency and force of coughing, and behaviors such as covering the mouth when coughing affect the production of droplet nuclei. In a small, closed, or poorly ventilated space, droplet nuclei become more concentrated, increasing the risk of exposure. Prolonged contact, such as living in the same household, increases the risk. Less-than-optimal immune function, a problem for people in lower socioeconomic groups, injection drug users, the homeless, and people with alcoholism or HIV infection, increases the susceptibility of the host.

Once infection with *M. tuberculosis* has occurred, clients with HIV/AIDS are at high risk for developing active tuberculosis. HIV infection suppresses cellular immunity, which is vital to limiting the replication and spread of the bacilli.

CLINICAL MANIFESTATIONS

Initial infection causes few symptoms and typically goes unnoticed until the tuberculin test becomes positive or calcified lesions are seen on a chest x-ray. Manifestations of primary progressive or reactivation tuberculosis often develop insidiously and are initially nonspecific. Fatigue, weight loss, diminished appetite, low-grade afternoon fever, and night sweats are common. A dry cough develops, which later becomes productive of purulent and/or blood-tinged sputum (**hemoptysis**). It is often at this stage that the client first seeks medical attention.

Tuberculosis empyema and bronchopleural fistula are the most serious complications of pulmonary tuberculosis. When

CLINICAL MANIFESTATIONS AND THERAPIES Tuberculosis

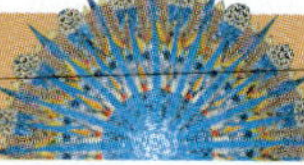

ETIOLOGY	CLINICAL MANIFESTATION	CLINICAL THERAPIES
Rupture of tuberculosis lesion with contamination of the pleural space resulting in pneumothorax	Shortness of breath, hypoxia, dry cough, cyanosis, chest pain, and subcutaneous emphysema	■ Placement of a chest tube to water seal ■ Analgesics ■ Continuous cardiorespiratory monitoring ■ Monitoring drainage from chest tube ■ Isolation in a room with negative airflow
Empyema and bronchopleural fistula are the most serious complications of tuberculosis. Empyema is a collection of pus within the pleural space that initiates an inflammatory response, leading to fibrous peel and trapped lung parenchyma. After resection of lung tissue, bronchopleural fistulas may develop because of inadequate healing of the stump, allowing bacteria to move into the pleural space and risking infection of the other lung.	Dyspnea with little exertion, low-grade fever, pleuritic chest pain, chest heaviness on affected side, purulent sputum, decreased breath sounds on involved side of chest, hemithorax, and opacification of the affected side on chest x-ray	■ Computed tomography to locate and direct drainage of the area ■ Priority to protect the healthy lung ■ May require intubation ■ Antibiotics may be given both intravenously and directly into the infected cavity ■ Analgesics for pain related to condition and treatment may be required

a tuberculosis lesion ruptures, bacilli may contaminate the pleural space. Rupture also may allow air to enter the pleural space from the lung, causing **pneumothorax** (a partial lung collapse caused by air or gas collecting in the lung or pleural space that surrounds the lungs).

Infants, children, and adolescents with latent infection will have no symptoms. Clinical manifestations of active tuberculosis in infants include a persistent cough, weight loss or failure to gain weight, and low-grade fever. Wheezing and decreased breath sounds may be present. Children with active disease may have fatigue, cough, diminished appetite, weight loss or growth delay, night sweats, chills, a low-grade fever, and enlarged lymph nodes.

COLLABORATION

Interdisciplinary care focuses on the following:

- Early detection
- Accurate diagnosis
- Effective disease treatment
- Preventing the spread of tuberculosis to others.

To support the client with active infection, collaboration with an infectious disease specialist may be necessary. A client whose tuberculosis negatively impacts oxygenation may need to see a respiratory therapist, who can serve the client either at home or in an institutional setting. Clients who are homeless may need additional medical care, because the diagnosis and treatment of tuberculosis may lead to the diagnoses of other illnesses that have not been previously identified or for which the client has not been receiving treatment.

Screening

The tuberculin test is used to screen for tuberculosis infection. A cellular, or delayed hypersensitivity, response to *M. tuberculosis* develops within 3 to 10 weeks after the infection. Injecting a small amount of **purified protein derivative (PPD)** of tuberculin any time thereafter activates this response, attracting macrophages to the area and causing a pronounced local inflammatory response. The amount of induration surrounding the injection site is used to determine infection (see Table 15–17 and Figure 15–35 ■). It is important to remember that a positive response indicates that infection and a cellular (T-cell) response have developed; however, it does not mean that active disease is present or that the client is infectious to others.

Several methods are currently available for tuberculin testing:

- *Intradermal PPD test (Mantoux test):* 0.1 mL of PPD (5 tuberculin units) is injected intradermally into the dorsal aspect of the forearm. This test is read within 48–72 hours (the peak reaction period) and recorded as the diameter of induration (raised area, not erythema) in millimeters.
- *Multiple-puncture test (**tine test**):* A multiple-puncture device is used to introduce tuberculin into the skin. This test is less accurate than other testing methods. A vesicular reaction is considered to be positive; any other reaction must be confirmed using a Mantoux test.

TABLE 15–17 **Interpreting Tuberculin Test Results**

AREA OF INDURATION	SIGNIFICANCE
<5 mm	Negative response; does not rule out infection.
5–9 mm	Positive for people who: ■ Are in close contact with a client who has infectious tuberculosis ■ Have an abnormal chest x-ray ■ Have HIV infection or are immunocompromised ■ Have an organ transplant. Negative for all others.
10–15 mm	Positive for people who have other risk factors: ■ Birth in a high-incidence country ■ African American, Hispanic, or Asian American in poverty areas ■ Injection drug use ■ Residence in a long-term care facility, correctional institution, residential care setting, homeless shelter ■ Medical risk factors (e.g., malnutrition, diabetes, others).
>15 mm	Positive for all people.

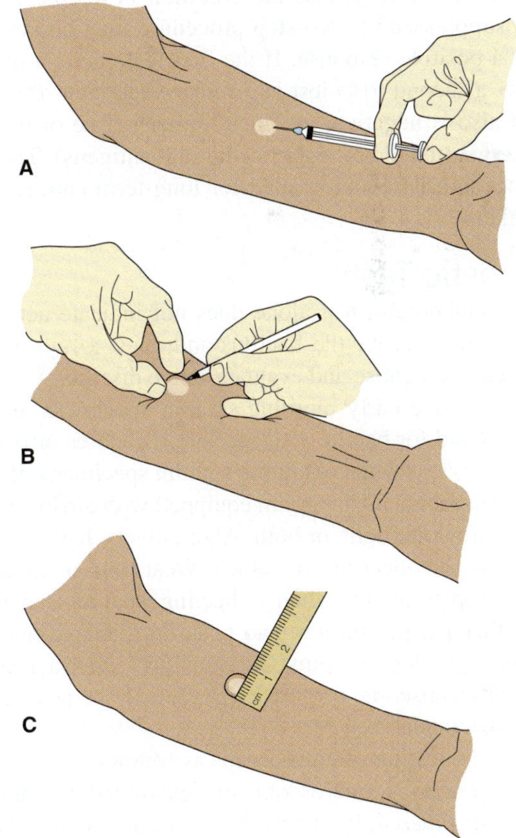

Figure 15–35 ■ *A,* Intradermal injection for tuberculin testing. *B,* The injection causes a local inflammatory response (wheal). *C,* Measurement of induration following tuberculin testing.

Although it is impractical and unnecessary to screen the entire population, the CDC recommends screening people in the following risk groups:

- People with or at high risk for HIV infection
- Close contacts of people who have or are suspected of having infectious tuberculosis
- People with medical risk factors, such as silicosis, chronic malabsorption, end-stage renal failure, diabetes mellitus, immunosuppression, and hematologic and other malignancies
- People born in countries with a high prevalence of tuberculosis
- Medically underserved, low-income populations, including racial and ethnic minorities
- People with alcoholism and injection drug users
- Residents and staff of long-term residential facilities, such as long-term care facilities, correctional institutions, and mental health facilities.

Only children who have one or more risk factors should have an intradermal tuberculin skin test with PPD (the Mantoux test) applied. Children should not be routinely tested for tuberculosis for entry to child care, camp, or school (Taylor, Nolan, & Blumberg, 2005). Children with a positive PPD then have further diagnostic testing to determine if active disease is present. Children who are immunocompromised (e.g., HIV infection, organ transplantation, and malignancies) are at greater risk for rapid progression from latent infection to active tuberculosis (Taylor, 2005).

False-negative responses are common in people who are immunosuppressed. A two-step procedure may be necessary to elicit a positive response. If the first test elicits a negative response, a second PPD test is given 1 week later. If the second test also is negative, the client either is free of infection or is **anergic** (unable to react to common antigens). This two-step procedure is recommended for long-term care residents and workers.

Diagnostic Tests

A positive tuberculin test alone does not indicate active disease. Sputum tests for the bacillus and chest x-rays are routinely used to diagnose and evaluate active disease. A series of three consecutive early morning sputum specimens are typically examined for bacilli. Use special procedures or personal protective devices when obtaining sputum specimens. If possible, collect specimens in a room equipped with airflow control devices, ultraviolet light, or both. Alternatively, have the client step outside to collect the specimen. Wear a mask capable of filtering droplet nuclei when collecting sputum specimens. Aerosol therapy, percussion, and postural drainage may help the client to produce sputum. Occasionally, endotracheal suctioning, bronchoscopy, or gastric lavage may be necessary to obtain a specimen.

Diagnostic testing often proceeds as follows:

- *Sputum smear* is microscopically examined for acid-fast bacilli. *M. tuberculosis* resists decolorizing chemicals after staining. This property is called *acid fast*. The acid-fast smear provides a rapid indicator of the tubercle bacillus.
- *Sputum culture* positive for *M. tuberculosis* provides the definitive diagnosis. However, *M. tuberculosis* is slow growing, requiring 4–8 weeks before it can be detected using traditional culture techniques. Automated radiometric culture systems (e.g., Bactec) allow detection of *M. tuberculosis* in several days.
- Once the organism is detected, *sensitivity testing* is performed to identify appropriate drug therapy.
- *Polymerase chain reaction* permits rapid detection of DNA from *M. tuberculosis*.
- *Chest x-ray* is ordered to diagnose and evaluate tuberculosis. Typical findings in pulmonary tuberculosis include dense lesions in the apical and posterior segments of the upper lobe and possible cavity formation.

Before initiating antituberculosis drug therapy, several additional diagnostic tests may be done to establish baseline data for monitoring potential adverse effects of the drugs:

- *Liver function tests* are obtained before treatment with isoniazid, because this drug is hepatotoxic.
- A thorough *vision examination* is done before treatment with ethambutol, a commonly used antituberculosis medication. Optic neuritis is a potential adverse effect of this drug. Periodic eye examinations are scheduled during the course of therapy.
- *Audiometric testing* is performed before streptomycin therapy is initiated. Ototoxicity is a significant adverse effect of streptomycin and other aminoglycoside antibiotics. Hearing also is evaluated periodically during the course of therapy to detect any hearing loss.

Pharmacologic Therapies

Chemotherapeutic medications are used both to prevent and to treat tuberculosis infection. Goals of the pharmacologic treatment of tuberculosis are as follows:

- To make the disease noncommunicable to others
- To reduce symptoms of the disease
- To effect a cure in the shortest possible time.

PROPHYLAXIS Prophylactic treatment is used to prevent active tuberculosis. Clients with a recent skin test conversion from negative to positive are often started on prophylactic therapy, especially when other risk factors are present. Prophylactic therapy also is used for people in close household contact with a person whose sputum is positive for bacilli. Single-drug therapy is effective for prophylactic treatment, whereas treatment of active disease always involves two or more chemotherapeutic medications. For adults, isoniazid, 300 mg per day for a period of 6–12 months, is commonly used to prevent active tuberculosis.

When isoniazid prophylaxis is contraindicated, Bacille Calmette-Guérin (BCG) vaccine may be prescribed. This vaccine is widely used in developing countries. BCG is made from an attenuated strain of *Mycobacterium bovis*, a closely related bacillus that causes tuberculosis in cattle. In the United States, BCG vaccine is recommended only for infants, children, and health care workers with a negative tuberculin test who are repeatedly exposed to untreated or ineffectively treated people who have active disease. After vaccination with BCG, a positive reaction to tuberculin testing is common. Periodic chest x-rays may be required for screening purposes.

TREATMENT OF ACTIVE DISEASE The tuberculosis bacillus mutates readily to drug-resistant forms when only one anti-infective agent is used. Active disease is always treated with concurrent use of at least two antibacterial medications to which the organism is sensitive. The primary antituberculosis drugs can prevent development of resistance, because all act by different mechanisms. However, the organism is protected within the tubercle, and 6 or more months of treatment are necessary to eradicate it.

Newly diagnosed tuberculosis is typically treated with an initial regimen of four oral antituberculosis drugs—isoniazid, rifampin, pyrazinamide, and ethambutol daily (or several times per week on a decreasing schedule of frequency)—for the first 2 months of treatment. This initial regimen is followed by at least 4 additional months of therapy with isoniazid and rifampin, given daily, twice per week, or weekly. In the presence of HIV infection, treatment is continued for at least 9 months. The most common antituberculosis drugs are outlined in Table 15–18. Nursing implications are outlined in Box 15–7. If a drug-resistant strain is suspected, therapy is tailored to the resistance. In some cases, four or more anti-infective drugs may be used.

ADVERSE EFFECTS Antituberculosis medications have many adverse and toxic effects. While isoniazid crosses the placenta, most studies show no teratogenic effects. Rifampin crosses the placenta, and the possibility of teratogenic effects is still being studied. Close monitoring during therapy is necessary. Most antituberculosis medications have some degree of, or risk for, hepatotoxicity. For this reason, clients should avoid using alcohol and other drugs (e.g., acetaminophen) or chemicals that can damage the liver. Baseline liver and renal function studies are done before initiating therapy. Audiometric testing also may be done before treatment is started, because several commonly used medications can affect hearing. Regular visits to a health care provider are necessary to evaluate regularly for adverse effects. Although none of these drugs has been proved to be teratogenic, potential adverse effects on the fetus are weighed against the benefit to the mother before they are prescribed during pregnancy.

COMPLIANCE Compliance with the prescribed regimen is evaluated during follow-up visits. The urine can be examined for color changes characteristic of rifampin and tested for metabolites of isoniazid. When compliance is a problem, medications are administered under direct supervision. Twice-weekly therapy is more cost effective in this instance, with a public health nurse watching the client take and swallow the prescribed medication.

FOLLOW-UP Repeat sputum specimens and chest x-rays are used to evaluate the effectiveness of therapy. In most cases, sputum cultures for *M. tuberculosis* are negative within 2 months of therapy; virtually all clients have negative sputum cultures within 3 months. If cultures remain positive at 3 months and beyond, treatment failure and drug resistance are suspected. In this case, cultures of the organism are tested for susceptibility to antituberculosis agents, and two or three previously unused drugs are added to the treatment regimen (Kasper et al., 2005).

With adherence to prescribed treatment, virtually all clients should have negative sputum cultures for *M. tuberculosis* within 3 months. The relapse rate for current treatment regimens is less than 5%. The principal cause of treatment failure is noncompliance (Tierney et al., 2005).

TABLE 15–18 **Antituberculosis Medications**

DRUG AND DOSAGE	ADVERSE EFFECTS	NURSING IMPLICATIONS
Isoniazid (INH), oral: 300 mg daily or 900 mg one, two, or three times weekly	Peripheral neuropathy Hepatitis	Administer pyridoxine (vitamin B_6) concurrently. Monitor liver function studies (aspartate aminotransferase [AST] and alanine aminotransferase [ALT]); avoid other hepatotoxins.
Rifampin, oral: 600 mg daily or two or three times weekly	Hepatitis Flulike syndrome Fever	As for INH. Do not miss or skip doses; flulike syndrome and fever occur when drug is resumed.
	Colors body fluids—including sweat, urine, saliva, tears, and cerebrospinal fluid—orange-red	Contact lenses may become discolored and should not be worn.
Pyrazinamide, oral: 1–2 g daily or 2–4 g twice weekly	Hyperuricemia Hepatotoxicity	Monitor uric acid levels. Monitor AST and ALT; avoid other hepatotoxins.
Ethambutol, oral: 800–1,600 mg daily or 2–4 g twice weekly	Optic neuritis	Monitor red-green color discrimination and visual acuity.
Streptomycin, intramuscular: 15 mg/kg, up to 1 g daily; or 25–30 mg/kg twice weekly	Ototoxicity, vertigo Nephrotoxicity Have periodic audiometric examinations conducted.	Monitor renal function studies, including blood urea nitrogen and serum creatinine.

Box 15–7 Nursing Considerations for Antituberculosis Drugs

ISONIAZID (INH, LANIAZID, NYDRAZID)

Isoniazid is the drug of choice for tuberculosis prophylaxis and a first-line drug for treating active disease. It is effective against both intracellular and extracellular organisms. Isoniazid is used alone as a prophylactic medication and in combination with rifampin, ethambutol, or both. A fixed-dose combination form with 150 mg of INH and 300 mg of rifampin (Rifamate) is available as well.

Nursing Responsibilities

- Administer on an empty stomach 1 hour before or 2 hours after meals for maximal effect if tolerated; may be given with meals to reduce gastrointestinal effects.
- Monitor for adverse effects:
  a. Numbness and tingling of the extremities (most likely to occur in clients who are malnourished, alcoholic, or diabetic)
  b. Hepatotoxicity, as evidenced by abnormal liver function studies and scleral jaundice
  c. Hypersensitivity reactions, such as rash, drug fever, or evidence of anemia, bruising, bleeding, or infection related to agranulocytosis.
- Isoniazid interferes with the metabolism of diazepam (Valium), phenytoin (Dilantin), and carbamazepine. Doses of these drugs may need to be reduced to prevent toxicity.

Health Education for the Client and Family

- Take the medication as prescribed for the entire treatment period to prevent incomplete eradication of the bacteria and development of resistant strains.
- Take the medication on an empty stomach. If nausea and vomiting occur, take with meals.
- If diminished appetite, nausea, vomiting, and jaundice (yellowing of the skin and the whites of the eyes) develop, notify your doctor immediately.
- Take pyridoxine as prescribed to prevent peripheral neuropathy.
- Avoid alcohol and other agents that may be harmful to the liver.
- Notify your doctor if you develop signs of an allergic reaction, such as rash, fever, easy bruising, bleeding gums, or fatigue.
- Use measures to prevent pregnancy while taking INH; this drug may be harmful to the developing fetus.

RIFAMPIN (RIFADIN, RIMACTANE)

Rifampin is commonly used in combination with INH and other antituberculosis drugs. It is relatively low in toxicity, although it can cause hepatitis, a flulike immune response, and rarely, renal failure. Rifampin stimulates the microsomal enzymes of the liver, increasing the rate of metabolism of many drugs and decreasing their effectiveness.

Nursing Responsibilities

- Administer on an empty stomach.
- Monitor CBC, liver function studies, and renal function studies for evidence of toxicity.
- Rifampin reduces the effect of oral contraceptives, quinidine, corticosteroids, warfarin, methadone, digoxin, and hypoglycemics. Monitor for the effectiveness of these drugs.

Health Education for the Client and Family

- Rifampin causes body fluids, including sweat, urine, saliva, and tears, to turn red-orange. This is not harmful. Avoid wearing soft contact lenses, because they may be permanently stained.
- Aspirin may interfere with rifampin absorption and should not be taken concurrently.
- Fever, flulike symptoms, excessive fatigue, sore throat, or unusual bleeding may indicate an adverse reaction to the drug and should be reported to your doctor.

PYRAZINAMIDE (TEBRAZID)

Pyrazinamide typically is given with INH and rifampin for the first 2 months of tuberculosis treatment. Concurrent use of pyrazinamide allows a shorter course of therapy. As with many of the antituberculosis agents, pyrazinamide is toxic to the liver. Its other principal adverse effect is hyperuricemia. Gout, however, rarely develops.

Nursing Responsibilities

- Administer with meals to reduce gastrointestinal side effects.
- Monitor liver function studies and serum uric acid levels. Notify the physician if changes are noted.

Health Education for the Client and Family

- Notify your doctor if you develop loss of appetite, nausea, vomiting, jaundice, or symptoms of gout (a painful, red, hot, swollen joint, often the great toe or elbow).
- While taking this drug, avoid using alcohol or other substances that may be harmful to the liver.

ETHAMBUTOL (MYAMBUTOL)

Ethambutol is added to the initial treatment regimen or substituted for INH when an INH-resistant strain of tuberculosis is suspected. Ethambutol is a bacteriostatic drug that reduces the development of resistance to the bactericidal first-line agents. Its principal toxic effect is optic neuritis; fortunately, this is reversible. Early signs of optic neuritis include decreased visual acuity and loss of red-green discrimination. This drug may be safe for use in pregnancy.

Nursing Responsibilities

- Record a baseline visual examination before therapy. Schedule periodic eye exams during the course of treatment.
- Administer with meals to reduce gastrointestinal side effects.
- Monitor liver and renal function studies and neurologic status while taking this drug. Notify the physician of abnormal findings or significant changes.

Health Education for the Client and Family

- Monitor vision daily by reading newspapers and looking at the same blue object (using usual corrective lenses, if appropriate). Notify your doctor if changes in vision or color perception occur.

STREPTOMYCIN

An aminoglycoside antibiotic, streptomycin is highly effective in treating most mycobacterial infection. Resistance may develop if it is used alone. There are two primary drawbacks to streptomycin: First, it must be administered parenterally, because it is not absorbed in the gastrointestinal tract. Second, it has toxic effects on the kidneys and ears.

Nursing Responsibilities

- Administer by deep intramuscular injection into a large muscle mass, rotating sites to minimize tissue trauma.
- Monitor urine output, weight, and renal function studies (including blood urea nitrogen and serum creatinine) to detect early signs of nephrotoxicity. Report significant changes to the physician.
- Maintain fluid intake at 2,000 to 3,000 mL per day to minimize the concentration of drug in the kidney tubules.
- Assess hearing and balance frequently. Have audiometric testing performed as indicated.

Box 15–7 Nursing Considerations for Antituberculosis Drugs (continued)

Health Education for the Client and Family

- Maintain a daily fluid intake of at least 2.5–3 quarts.
- Weigh yourself on the same scale at least twice a week. Report any significant weight gain to your doctor.
- Notify your doctor if hearing acuity decreases, ringing or buzzing sensations in the ear develop, or dizziness occurs.

NURSING PROCESS

Today, tuberculosis presents a greater threat to public health than it does to individuals. Nurses play a key role in maintaining public health. Education and tuberculosis screening are major nursing strategies to prevent tuberculosis. Nurses have an important role in identifying children with one or more risk factors for infection, such as foreign-born children and children residing in states with a higher incidence of tuberculosis (California, Texas, New York, Illinois, Georgia, and Florida) (Reznik & Ozuah, 2005).

Public health teaching includes increasing awareness of tuberculosis as a reemerging threat. Teach clients in all settings how to reduce the spread of tuberculosis by covering their mouths when coughing or sneezing and disposing of sputum appropriately. The benefit of screening programs to identify infected (though not necessarily infective) people also needs to be included in public health education.

The best tuberculosis prevention is early diagnosis of infection and appropriate treatment to achieve cure. BCG vaccine is recommended for infants born in countries where tuberculosis is prevalent, but the vaccine is not widely used in the United States. It may be administered to health care workers in settings where the risk of infection with MDR strains of *M. tuberculosis* is high despite rigorous infection control measures (Kasper et al., 2005).

The primary preventive strategy used in the United States is treating people with latent tuberculosis infection demonstrated by a positive tuberculin test. A 9- to 10-month course of treatment with isoniazid reduces the risk of active disease by 90% or more (Kasper et al., 2005). Isoniazid is also prescribed prophylactically for people with HIV infection who have been exposed to tuberculosis.

Assessment

Focused assessment for the client with suspected tuberculosis includes the following:

- *Health history.* Complaints of fatigue, weight loss, night sweats, difficulty breathing, cough (productive or nonproductive), hemoptysis, or chest pain; known exposure to tuberculosis; most recent tuberculin test and results; living circumstances; and alcohol and other recreational drug use
- *Physical examination.* Vital signs, including temperature; general appearance; respiratory rate and lung sounds; and weight and appearance of malnutrition.

Screening questions (Box 15–8) should be used to identify infants and children at risk for latent infection during health visits every 6 months until 2 years of age and then annually (American Academy of Pediatrics, 2006, p. 682).

Diagnosis

Nursing diagnoses for the client with the medical diagnosis of tuberculosis may include the following:

- Deficient Knowledge
- Ineffective Therapeutic Regimen Management
- Risk for Infection.

Plan

Care planning is based on the needs of the client, the resources and support available, the client's general health status, and the client's environment. Suggested outcomes may include the following:

- The client demonstrates behaviors that reduce the risk of contamination of others.
- The client describes required treatment and follow-up care required.
- The client has adequate resources available to obtain necessary medications and supplies.

Implementation

Nursing care related to tuberculosis focuses primarily on infection control and compliance with prescribed treatment. See the Nursing Care Plan feature that follows.

Deficient Knowledge

Adequate knowledge and information are necessary to manage the disease and prevent its transmission to others. The client needs to understand reasons for prolonged drug therapy and the importance of complying with treatment and follow-up.

Box 15–8 Screening Questions to Identify Risk for Latent Tuberculosis Infection

- Determine client's understanding of tuberculosis
- Collect demographic information so follow up can be provided if needed
- Review the client's medical record including laboratory and radiology findings
- Question the client's past tuberculosis history and exposure to others diagnosed with tuberculosis
- Does the client have any symptoms of tuberculosis
- Determine history of present illness and social history
- If the client was previously treated for tuberculosis were they compliant with the treatment regimen
- Was the client born outside the country or traveled outside the country? Have immediate family members recently traveled outside the country?

Source: http://www.cdc.gov/tb/education/ssmodules/module8/ss8reading4.htmhttp://www.cdc.gov/tb/education/ssmodules/module8/ss8reading4.htm.

Antituberculosis drugs are relatively toxic. The client needs to know how to minimize toxicity.

- Assess the client's knowledge about the disease process, and identify misperceptions and emotional reactions. Teaching based on previous learning enhances understanding and retention of information.
- Assess the client's ability and interest in learning, developmental level, and obstacles to learning. Assessment allows presentation of information in a manner tailored to the learning needs and style of the client, promoting learning.
- Identify the client's support systems, and include significant others in teaching. A knowledgeable significant other provides reinforcement of learning, confirmation of understanding, and encouragement for the client. Including significant others also reduces the risk of inadvertent sabotage of the treatment plan.

DEVELOPMENTAL CONSIDERATIONS Nursing Care of the Older Adult With Tuberculosis

The prevalence of active tuberculosis is significantly higher among older white adults in the United States than it is among young adults (Kasper et al., 2005). Of cases among older adults, approximately 90% occur because of reactivation of a dormant bacterium. Older adults are at increased risk for reactivation tuberculosis as a result of age-related decreases in cell-mediated immunity. Chronic illnesses, poor nutrition, gastrectomy, alcoholism, or the long-term use of steroids and immunosuppressive agents may also reactivate dormant tuberculosis lesions.

Presenting symptoms of tuberculosis in the older adult are often vague, including coughing, weight loss, diminished appetite, or periodic fevers. These signs and symptoms should not be dismissed as a normal part of aging.

Residents of nursing homes are at increased risk for acquiring tuberculosis because of their close proximity to each other. Yearly tuberculin skin testing with purified protein derivative (PPD) is often required by state health departments for nursing home residents. If the initial test is negative, a repeat PPD in 1–2 weeks is recommended. This improves sensitivity to the test so that silent cases of tuberculosis are not missed. A chest x-ray and sputum culture for acid-fast bacilli are obtained if the PPD is positive.

Successful treatment for tuberculosis includes taking at least two drugs for at least 6–9 months to totally eradicate the organism. Older adults usually do not develop drug-resistant forms of tuberculosis, because they often acquired the disease before emergence of drug-resistant strains.

ASSESSING FOR HOME CARE

Community-dwelling older adults as well as those in care facilities are susceptible to tuberculosis. The older adult with respiratory symptoms often is treated presumptively for pneumonia, without a sputum smear and Gram stain. Older adults living in the community may not have had a tuberculin test or chest x-ray for many years.

Nurses working with these clients will typically assess risk factors for tuberculosis, such as the following:

- General health and nutritional status, including intake of specific nutrients, such as vitamin D (lack of vitamin D is associated with a higher risk of developing active tuberculosis)
- Presence of a chronic disease (e.g., silicosis, diabetes, alcoholism, or HIV infection) or past history of a gastrectomy
- Past history of a positive tuberculin test that now has converted to negative
- Medications, such as corticosteroids or other immunosuppressive drugs.

Nurses may also assess living and social situations, such as the following:

- Natural light and ventilation in the home
- Access to clean water, cooking facilities, grocery stores, and other services
- Possible exposure to infected people, such as sharing a household with someone who has active tuberculosis, crowded living facilities, homelessness, frequent participation in senior activities, and volunteer work in residential care facilities or other institutional settings
- Access to health care.

Tuberculosis is typically treated in the community; hospitalization or institutionalization is rarely necessary or desirable. For the older adult being treated for active tuberculosis in the community, the nurse should assess the following:

- Knowledge and understanding of the disease and the prescribed treatment regimen
- Mental status and ability to follow both the prescribed regimen and precautions to avoid exposing others to the disease
- Transportation and ability to access health care services on a regular basis
- Financial resources to complete treatment and follow-up care
- Need for home health or social services to ensure adequate treatment.

HEALTH EDUCATION FOR THE CLIENT AND FAMILY

Teaching focuses on improving the older adult's ability to self-manage the disease and on treatment. Teach about tuberculosis and how it is spread. Emphasize the importance of taking all medications as prescribed and complying with follow-up appointments and testing. Discuss the importance of:

- Using disposable tissues to contain respiratory secretions, especially during the first 2 weeks of treatment, when the disease may be transmitted to others
- Avoiding exposure to crowds or people with infectious diseases
- Eating a well-balanced diet with adequate nutrients
- Getting adequate rest, sleep, and exercise to maintain good general health
- Ensuring that housemates or others having frequent contact with the client are tested and receive prophylactic treatment if indicated.

Teach about possible side effects of the prescribed medications and the importance of reporting these to health care providers. Possible side effects include the following:

- Peripheral neuropathy (numbness, tingling, or a burning sensation of the extremities) may occur with isoniazid (INH). Pyridoxine (vitamin B_6) often is prescribed to prevent this adverse effect.
- Both INH and rifampin may cause hepatitis. Avoid alcohol while taking these drugs, and report any manifestations, such as nausea and diminished appetite, jaundice, a change in urine or stool color, or pain in the upper right quadrant.
- Rifampin may cause an orange-red coloration of saliva and urine.
- Streptomycin can affect hearing and balance. Promptly report any changes, because they may be irreversible.
- Ethambutol may affect red-green color discrimination and visual acuity. Use caution when driving or walking in unfamiliar areas and promptly report any vision changes.

- Establish a relationship of mutual trust with the client and significant others. An atmosphere of trust increases receptiveness to teaching and learning.
- Develop mutually acceptable learning goals with the client and significant other. Working together to identify learning needs and establish goals increases the client's "ownership" and interest in the process.
- Select appropriate teaching strategies, using learning aids such as literature and visual materials that are appropriate for age, level of education, and intellect. Teaching tailored to the client is more effective and results in better learning.
- Teach about tuberculosis and the prescribed treatment, including:
  a. Nature of the disease and its spread
  b. Purpose of treatment and follow-up procedures
  c. Measures to prevent spreading the disease to others
  d. Importance of maintaining good general health by eating a well-balanced, high-protein, high-carbohydrate diet; balancing exercise with rest; and avoiding crowds and people with upper respiratory infections
  e. Names, doses, purposes, and adverse effects of prescribed medications
  f. Importance of avoiding alcohol and other substances that may damage the liver while taking chemotherapeutic drugs
  g. Fluid intake needs of 2.5–3.0 quarts of fluid per day
  h. Manifestations to report to the physician: chest pain, hemoptysis, or difficulty breathing; diminished appetite, nausea, or vomiting; yellow tint to skin or sclera; sudden weight gain, swollen feet, ankles, legs, or hands; hearing loss, tinnitus, or vertigo; and change in vision or difficulty discriminating colors.

Tuberculosis is a chronic disease requiring lengthy treatment with antitubercuosis medications. A good understanding of the disease, its treatment, and potential adverse effects of therapy prepares the client to manage care.

- Document teaching and level of understanding. Reinforce teaching and learning as needed. Teaching is not complete until the client can demonstrate learning of the information.

Ineffective Therapeutic Regimen Management

The populations at highest risk for developing active tuberculosis—the homeless and members of lower socioeconomic groups—are also at high risk for being unable to manage its complex treatment regimen. Three or more costly medications that may have unpleasant or even dangerous side effects are prescribed. Frequent medical follow-up is required. Infectious diseases such as tuberculosis also carry a stigma that may lead to denial of the disease or its seriousness. Those with alcoholism and who use injection drugs need to withdraw from their addiction to be successful in treating the disease, and the client with HIV infection faces a potentially fatal disease and costly treatment that may well override concerns about tuberculosis management.

- Assess self-care abilities and support systems. Assessment is used to help determine the client's ability to follow the prescribed regimen.
- Assess knowledge and understanding of the disease, its complications, treatment, and risks to others. Provide additional teaching and reinforcement as indicated. Lack of understanding is a barrier to compliance with and management of the treatment regimen.
- Work collaboratively to identify barriers or obstacles to managing the prescribed treatment. Working collaboratively with the client and other members of the health care team provides insight for overcoming identified barriers to effective treatment.
- Assist the client, significant others (if available), and health care team members to develop a plan for managing the prescribed regimen. Including the client in developing a plan to manage care increases the sense of control and ownership and helps to ensure that personal, cultural, and lifestyle factors are considered. This increases the likelihood of compliance.
- Provide verbal and written instructions that are clear and appropriate for the client's level of literacy, knowledge, and understanding. Clearly written directions provide support and reinforcement for the client.
- Provide active intervention for homeless people, including shelter placement or other housing and ongoing follow-up by easily accessed health care providers (clinics and public health workers in the neighborhood that do not present transportation or access problems, either real or perceived). Simple referral will not ensure compliance, especially among disenfranchised populations. Active intervention is needed to help ensure treatment compliance.
- Refer clients who are unlikely to comply with the treatment regimen to the public health department for management and follow-up. *B*ecause tuberculosis presents a significant public health risk, public health follow-up is essential. In some cases, it is necessary for nurses to administer medications, observing the client swallow all pills.

PRACTICE ALERT

Children with active tuberculosis should receive "directly observed drug therapy" administered by a nurse or other health care provider to ensure the drug is being taken. Direct observation should occur at least twice a week for the duration of treatment (Reznik & Ozuah, 2005). Children with latent tuberculosis should also receive "directly observed drug therapy" twice a week (American Academy of Pediatrics, 2006, p. 686).

Risk for Infection

The spread of tuberculosis is a risk in any facility housing many people. The risk is especially high in residential care facilities for older clients and for people with AIDS. The increasing incidence of tuberculosis among homeless people and members of lower socioeconomic groups increases the risk in hospitals, emergency departments, and public and urgent care clinics. Respiratory precautions are necessary to prevent the spread of the disease via microscopic airborne droplets to other clients and to health care workers.

- Place the client in a private room with airflow control that prevents air within the room from circulating into the hallway or other rooms. A **negative airflow room** (a room where air flows out of the room) in which air is diluted by at least six fresh-air exchanges per hour is recommended. A negative flow room and multiple fresh-air exchanges dilute the concentration of droplet nuclei within the room and prevent their spread to adjacent areas.

- Use standard precautions and tuberculosis isolation techniques as recommended by the CDC, including wearing masks and gowns when caring for clients who do not reliably cover the mouth when coughing. These measures are important to prevent the spread of tuberculosis to others.
- Discuss the reasons for and importance of respiratory isolation procedures during initial hospitalization. When treatment is provided as an outpatient, instruct the client to avoid crowds and close physical contact and to maintain ventilation in living facilities, particularly during the first 3 weeks of treatment. These measures help to protect others during initial treatment, when sputum is still likely to contain significant numbers of bacilli.
- Place a mask on the client when transporting to other parts of the facility for diagnostic or treatment procedures. Covering the client's nose and mouth during transport minimizes air contamination and the risk to visitors and personnel.
- Inform all personnel having contact with the client of the diagnosis. This allows personnel to take appropriate precautions.
- Assist visitors to mask before entering the room. Providing visitors with appropriate masks or respirators reduces their risk of infection.
- Teach the client how to limit transmitting the disease to others:
  a. Always cough and expectorate into tissues.
  b. Dispose of tissues properly, placing them in a closed bag.
  c. Wear a mask if you are sneezing or unable to control respiratory secretions.
  d. The disease is not spread by touching inanimate objects, so no special precautions are required for eating utensils, clothing, books, or other objects used.
  Teaching appropriate precautions helps to prevent the spread of tuberculosis to others while allowing as much freedom from restraints as possible.
- Teach the client how to collect sputum specimens. If necessary, have the client step outside to collect a sputum specimen. This minimizes the risk of exposure to health care personnel and provides for rapid dilution of any droplet nuclei produced and their exposure to ultraviolet light, which kills the bacteria.
- Teach the client the importance of complying with the prescribed treatment for the entire course of therapy. Completion of the entire treatment regimen is important to reduce the risk of relapse and creation of drug-resistant organisms.

PRACTICE ALERT

Use personal protective devices to reduce the risk of transmission during client care. The U.S. Occupational Safety and Health Administration (OSHA) requires use of a HEPA-filtered respirator for protection against occupational exposure to tuberculosis. Surgical masks are ineffective to filter droplet nuclei, necessitating the use of protective devices capable of filtering bacteria and particles smaller than 1 micron.

EVIDENCE-BASED PRACTICE Clients With Risk for Tuberculosis

Homeless people and those living in homeless shelters have several identified risk factors for tuberculosis: high incidence of drug and alcohol abuse, lowered immune status, and crowded living conditions. Access to and participation in tuberculosis screening, however, often is problematic. Swigart and Kolb (2004) identified factors contributing to homeless persons' decisions to participate in free screening. Contrary to the beliefs of many health care providers, many homeless people chose to participate in the screening out of a desire to maintain good health and a recognition that homelessness and shelter life increased their risk of developing tuberculosis. The desire to maintain good health was particularly noted as a reason among those participants in early recovery from drug or alcohol addiction. Other major factors cited for participating included a history of lung problems, a desire to identify possible problems related to smoking, and encouragement by shelter personnel. Fear of the results and a desire "not to be bothered" had negative effects on participation. Women with children were least likely to participate in screening in this study, citing fear of a diagnosis resulting in a loss of child custody.

Implications for Nursing

Outreach to homeless populations for health services, while difficult, has personal and public health benefits. The homeless often lack access to preventive and health promotion services, instead interacting with health care providers only when urgent care is needed. This study suggests, however, that a portion of this population desires to maintain good health and is receptive when screening and health promotion services are accessible. Shelter personnel were instrumental in getting many of the study participants to the screening. Recruiting the support of these workers can improve resident participation. Regularly scheduling a nurse in a shelter can allow trust to develop and can also improve participation in health promotion activities. This may be a particularly important strategy in shelters for women with children—bringing services to the residents to reduce the fear of being perceived as unable to care for dependent children.

Critical Thinking in Client Care

1. What factors contribute to the perception of many health care providers that homeless people and shelter residents do not care about maintaining good health?
2. The participants in this study were screened for their ability to understand English and to read or hear and comprehend the interview and process. How might the health care team need to alter its approach to reach homeless people who have mental illnesses that affect thinking and cognition?
3. Design a tuberculosis screening program using a multidisciplinary team to reach a specific population. Identify members of the team and discuss your rationale for their inclusion on the team.

NURSING CARE PLAN A Client With Tuberculosis

Harry Facée, age 53, arrives at a metropolitan public health clinic complaining of aching chest pain that has lasted for the past few days. He says that his sputum also is bloody. He is afraid he might have lung cancer, so he came in to see a doctor.

ASSESSMENT

Raj Kamil, RN, the public health nurse at the clinic, obtains an admission history and physical examination of Mr. Facée. Mr. Kamil notes that Mr. Facée is a homeless person who has lived on the streets and in various shelters for the past "10 years or so." He usually prefers to sleep outdoors, taking refuge in shelters only during very cold or very wet weather. He has a small disability income, but usually scrounges for food or eats with other homeless people at soup kitchens. Mr. Facée states that he has had a cough for a long time, which has become worse recently. It is now productive, especially in the mornings. He also admits that he has recently been waking up drenched with sweat in the middle of the night and is more tired than usual.

Although Mr. Facée's clothes are tattered, he is fairly clean. He answers questions appropriately and intelligently. Mr. Kamil does not detect any odor of alcohol on his breath. He is very thin, almost emaciated. Mr. Facée's vital signs are BP 152/86 mmHg, pulse 92 bpm, respirations 20/minute, and temperature 100.2°F (37.8°C).

Suspecting tuberculosis, Mr. Kamil obtains a sputum specimen for Gram stain and culture, administers a tuberculin test, and sends Mr. Facée for a chest x-ray before he sees the clinic physician. Although the chest x-ray is inconclusive, the Gram stain is positive for acid-fast bacilli. The diagnosis of probable active pulmonary tuberculosis is made. The physician prescribes isoniazid, 300 mg orally; rifampin, 600 mg orally; and pyrazinamide, 1,500 mg orally daily for 2 months, to be followed by twice-weekly isoniazid, 900 mg orally, and rifampin, 600 mg orally. The physician also orders weekly sputum cultures for the first month.

DIAGNOSES

- Ineffective Health Maintenance related to homelessness
- Risk for Noncompliance With Prescribed Treatment related to lack of understanding and resources
- Imbalanced Nutrition: Less Than Body Requirements related to increased metabolic needs associated with infection
- Risk for Disturbed Sensory Perception: Kinesthetic, related to effects of isoniazid therapy

PLANNING

Goals for Mr. Facée's care include:

- The client will keep all follow-up appointments as scheduled.
- The client will verbalize an understanding of his disease and its treatment.
- The client will follow the prescribed plan of care.
- The client will demonstrate measures to prevent spread of the organism to others.
- The client will gain 1–2 lb of weight per week.
- The client will promptly report symptoms of peripheral neuropathy, including numbness, tingling, or burning sensations.

IMPLEMENTATION

- Teach about tuberculosis, and provide a client education pamphlet about the disease.
- Instruct about the prescribed medications, potential adverse effects, and importance of completing the entire prescribed regimen.
- Emphasize the importance of continued follow-up.
- Teach and demonstrate sputum and droplet control measures.
- Escort to the local incentive shelter program for directly observed medical therapy and meals.
- Identify verbally and in writing manifestations to report to the physician.

EVALUATION

Mr. Kamil successfully enrolls Mr. Facée in the local incentive shelter program. In this program, a health care worker administers Mr. Facée's medications daily, watching him swallow them. He is assigned a small individual room and can eat three daily meals at the shelter. He still prefers to sleep outside when the weather permits, but he complies with the requirement for supervised medication administration because he "likes the food there." Always a clean person, Mr. Facée is able to demonstrate appropriate sputum control measures and practices them faithfully. The sputum culture done after 2 months of treatment is negative for tubercle bacilli, and his chest x-ray indicates no disease progression.

CRITICAL THINKING

1. Many homeless people have schizophrenia or other mental diseases. How would you adapt the care plan for a homeless client with schizophrenia and active tuberculosis?
2. Mr. Kamil was fortunate in having access to an incentive shelter with health care workers to supervise medication compliance. Identify available resources in your area for homeless clients infected with tuberculosis.
3. Develop a care plan for the nursing diagnosis ineffective airway clearance related to mucopurulent sputum and weak cough.

Most clients with tuberculosis are managed in community settings; few require institutionalization. In addition to the teaching topics and strategies identified above, discuss the following topics when preparing the client and significant others for home care:

- Importance of screening close contacts for infection and, possibly, prophylactic treatment
- Effect, dose, and timing for all medications as well as potential side effects and their management
- Importance of long-term therapy in eradicating the disease
- Principles of good nutrition, dietary guidelines for a client with tuberculosis, and other measures to help maintain good health, such as balancing rest with exercise
- Signs and symptoms of complications to report to the physician or healthcare provider.

Provide referrals as appropriate:

- Smoking cessation clinics or support groups
- Alcohol treatment facilities, Alcoholics Anonymous, and other treatment programs or support groups
- Drug treatment facilities, Narcotics Anonymous, and other outpatient or inpatient treatment programs or support groups
- Low-cost community clinics and incentive programs for people with tuberculosis
- Counseling, support groups, and other community resources that provide additional assistance and support.

When caring for the pregnant or recently delivered woman, the nurse must consider both the woman and the baby. If a newly delivered woman is found to have tuberculosis, it is important to prevent direct contact with the newborn until the woman is noninfectious. If maternal tuberculosis is inactive or the mother has been on therapy long enough to prevent infection of the newborn, the mother may breast-feed and care for her baby. Because the newborn has an immature immune response, it is the nurse's responsibility to teach the mother how to reduce the infant's risk of infection.

Evaluation

Compliance with prescribed therapies, resolution of symptoms, and improvement on chest x-ray are all positive evaluation findings. Clients are evaluated on progress toward outcomes, and the plan of care is amended as indicated. Expected outcomes of nursing care include the following:

- The client with latent infection completes therapy and does not develop active tuberculosis.
- The client's contacts are evaluated for tuberculosis and those infected are treated.

HEALTH CARE

Advocacy

Because clients diagnosed with tuberculosis are frequently from medically underserved populations, what role does the nurse play in advocating for their needs?

Health Policy

What role does the government play in determining policies to mandate tuberculosis testing of those traveling to the United States from other countries, especially those countries with the highest number of cases?

Legal Issues

You are working in a clinic and read a PPD skin test done 2 days ago as positive. While providing routine teaching, you inform the client of the need to test those who have been in contact with the client, and the client says, "No, I will not tell you who I've been in contact with, and you have no right to share my personal medical information with others, especially the government." What legal rights does this client have regarding privacy of information, and how would you handle this situation?

REVIEW Tuberculosis

RELATE: LINK THE CONCEPTS

Linking the exemplar of Tuberculosis with the concept of Oxygenation:

1. How would the diagnosis of active tuberculosis impact oxygenation?
2. What factors could increase or decrease the severity of the impact on oxygenation?

Linking the exemplar of Tuberculosis with the concept of Immunity:

3. What natural protections does the body have to reduce the risk of tuberculosis?
4. Describe factors that could limit immune response and increase the risk of contracting tuberculosis?

READY: GO TO COMPANION SKILLS MANUAL

- Administration of intradermal injections
- Care of the client with a chest tube
- Isolation precautions
- Use of personal protective equipment
- Oxygen administration

REFER: GO TO MYNURSINGKIT

REFLECT: CASE STUDY

Ngong Lee is a 62-year-old female who has been married to Daniel for 50 years. Born and raised in Vietnam, Ngong came to the United States after marrying Daniel when she was 20. Their only child, John, was killed at age 22 in an automobile accident. His death devastated Ngong, but over time, she adequately adjusted and coped with the loss. All of Ngong's brothers and sisters have passed away, but she has a few nieces and nephews who still live in Vietnam. She and Daniel have no relatives nearby.

Ngong has noticed a steady weight loss and lack of appetite over the past few weeks, ever since they returned from visiting relatives in Vietnam. At first, she was delighted with her new, slender figure, but as she continued to lose weight, she started to wonder if she had cancer. This week, she has been waking at night wet with perspiration, and this afternoon, she took her temperature and realized she has a slight fever. As she thinks about it, she realizes she's been tired lately and decides it's time to see her doctor. She makes an appointment at the local clinic and tells the nurse she has lost 12 pounds in the past 3 weeks and describes her other symptoms. The nurse notices Ngong coughing and asks when the cough started. Ngong looks surprised and said she hadn't noticed she'd been coughing. The physician orders a chest x-ray, CBC with differential, PPD, and sputum specimen for culture. The physician advises the nurse to take appropriate precautions, because tuberculosis is the suspected diagnosis.

1. How will the nurse collect the sputum specimen to reduce the spread of infection?
2. When Ngong comes back in 48 hours, her PPD is negative. The chest x-ray ordered by the physician shows dense lesions in the apical and posterior segments consistent with a diagnosis of tuberculosis. Sputum culture results have not returned yet. What does the nurse anticipate will be ordered for this client?
3. If Ngong is confirmed to have tuberculosis, what teaching will the nurse provide?
4. The sputum culture returns positive for the presence of bacilli. Why did her PPD come back negative? Will her family in Vietnam need to be tested? How will that be arranged? Who else will need to be tested secondary to exposure to Ngong?

15.8 URINARY TRACT INFECTION

KEY TERMS

Cystitis, *872*
Cystoscopy, *876*
Dysuria, *874*
Enuresis, *880*
Gram stain, *875*
Hematuria, *874*
Hydronephrosis, *873*
Intravenous pyelography (IVP), *876*
Neurogenic bladder, *873*
Nocturia, *874*
Nosocomial, *872*
Persistent bacteriuria, *882*
Pyelonephritis, *872*
Pyuria, *874*
Reflux, *872*
Reinfection, *882*
Unresolved bacteriuria, *882*
Ureteral stent, *876*
Ureteroplasty, *876*
Urgency, *874*
Urinary drainage system, *871*
Vesicoureteral reflux, *872*
Voiding cystourethrography, *876*

BASIS FOR SELECTION OF EXEMPLAR

Centers for Disease Control and Prevention
Joint Commission
Institute for Healthcare Improvement

LEARNING OUTCOMES

After reading about this exemplar, you will be able to:

1. Describe the pathophysiology, etiology, and clinical manifestations of urinary tract infection.
2. Identify the risk factors associated with urinary tract infection.
3. Illustrate the nursing process in providing culturally competent care across the life span for individuals with urinary tract infection.
4. Formulate priority nursing diagnoses appropriate for an individual with urinary tract infection.
5. Create a plan of care for an individual with urinary tract infection.
6. Employ evidence-based caring interventions (or prevention) for an individual with urinary tract infection.
7. Assess expected outcomes for an individual with urinary tract infection.
8. Discuss therapies used in the collaborative care of an individual with urinary tract infection.

OVERVIEW

The urinary tract includes the kidneys, ureters, urinary bladder, and urethra. Any part of this system can be affected by pathogens. A severe infection may involve multiple components of the urinary tract. Kidney infections can affect urine production and waste elimination, resulting in renal failure (explained in the Fluids and Electrolytes concept). Infection can interrupt the **urinary drainage system** (those organs required to drain urine from the kidneys, including the ureters, urinary bladder, and urethra), obstructing urine flow and affecting elimination.

- When caring for clients with urinary tract infections, it is important to consider the client's modesty in voiding, possible difficulty in discussing the genitals, potential embarrassment about being exposed for examination and testing, and fear of changes in body function. These psychosocial issues can interfere with the client's willingness to seek help, discuss treatment, and learn about preventive measures.
- Nursing interventions for clients with urinary tract infections are directed toward primary prevention, early detection, and management of the disorder through health teaching and nursing care.
- Bacterial infections of the urinary tract are a common reason for seeking health services, second only to upper respiratory infections. More than 8 million people are treated annually for urinary tract infection (UTI) (Porth, 2005). Community acquired UTIs are common in young women, but unusual in men under the age of 50.
- Most community-acquired UTIs are caused by *Escherichia coli*, common gram-negative enteral bacteria. Approximately 10–15% of symptomatic UTIs are caused by *Staphylococcus saprophyticus*, a gram-positive organism. Catheter-associated UTIs often involve other gram-negative bacteria, such as *Proteus*, *Klebsiella*, *Serratia*, and *Pseudomonas*.

PATHOPHYSIOLOGY AND ETIOLOGY

The urinary tract is normally sterile above the urethra. Adequate urine volume, a free flow from the kidneys through the urinary meatus, and complete bladder emptying are the most important mechanisms of maintaining sterility. Pathogens that enter and contaminate the distal urethra are washed out during voiding. Other defenses for maintaining sterile urine include the normal acidity of urine itself and the bacteriostatic properties of the bladder and urethral cells.

The peristaltic activity of the ureters and a competent vesicoureteral junction help to maintain sterility of the upper urinary tract. As the ureter enters the bladder, the distal portion tunnels between the mucosa and muscle layers of the bladder wall (Figure 15–36 ■). During voiding, increased intravesicular (within the bladder) pressure compresses the ureter, preventing **reflux**, or the backflow of urine toward the kidneys. In males, a long urethra and the antibacterial effect of zinc in prostatic fluid also help prevent contamination of this normally sterile environment.

UTIs can be bacterial, viral, or fungal, and may be categorized in several ways. Anatomically, UTIs may affect the lower or the upper urinary tract. Lower urinary tract infections include *urethritis*, inflammation of the urethra; *prostatitis*, inflammation of the prostate gland; and **cystitis**, inflammation of the urinary bladder. The most common upper urinary tract infection is pyelonephritis, inflammation of the kidney and renal pelvis. The infection can involve superficial tissues, such as the bladder mucosa, or invade other tissues, such as prostate or renal tissues.

Epidemiologically, UTIs are identified as community acquired or **nosocomial** (often associated with catheterization). UTIs can be further categorized as acute or chronic, with the latter being either recurrent or persistent.

Cystitis is the most common UTI. This infection tends to remain superficial, involving the bladder mucosa. The mucosa becomes hyperemic (red) and may hemorrhage. The inflammatory response causes pus to form, a process that causes the classic manifestations associated with cystitis.

Pyelonephritis is inflammation of the renal pelvis and parenchyma, the functional kidney tissue. *Acute pyelonephritis* is a bacterial infection of the kidney, and *chronic pyelonephritis* is associated with nonbacterial infections and inflammatory processes that can be metabolic, chemical, or immunologic in origin (see the Inflammation concept).

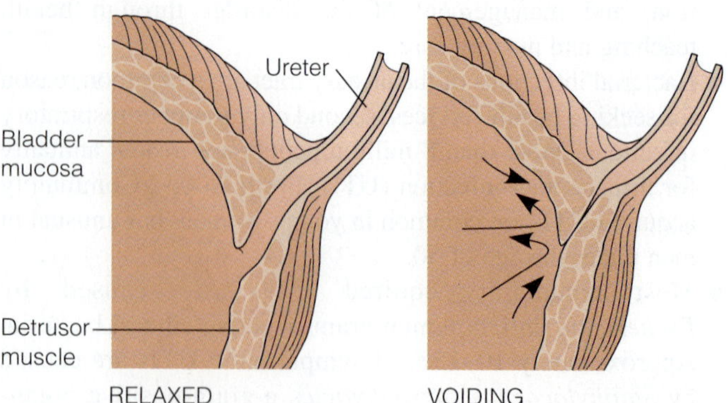

Figure 15–36 ■ A competent vesicoureteral junction. Note how increased intravesicular pressure during voiding occludes the distal portion of the ureter, preventing reflux.

Acute pyelonephritis usually results from an infection that ascends to the kidney from the lower urinary tract. Asymptomatic bacteriuria or cystitis can lead to acute pyelonephritis. Risk factors include pregnancy (due to slowed ureteral peristalsis), urinary tract obstruction, and congenital malformation. Urinary tract trauma, scarring, calculi (stones), kidney disorders such as polycystic or hypertensive kidney disease, and chronic diseases such as diabetes can also contribute to pyelonephritis. **Vesicoureteral reflux**, a condition in which urine moves from the bladder back toward the kidney, is a common risk factor in children who develop pyelonephritis that is also seen in adults when bladder outflow is obstructed.

The infection spreads from the renal pelvis to the renal cortex. The pelvis, calyces, and medulla of the kidney are primarily affected, with WBC infiltration and inflammation. The kidney becomes grossly edematous. Localized abscesses may develop on the cortical surface of the kidney. As with cystitis, *E. coli* is the organism responsible for 85% of the cases of acute pyelonephritis. Other organisms commonly found include *Proteus* and *Klebsiella*, bacteria that normally inhabit the intestinal tract.

The onset of acute pyelonephritis is typically rapid, with chills and fever, malaise, vomiting, flank pain, costovertebral tenderness, and urinary frequency. Symptoms of cystitis also may be present. The older adult may present with a change in behavior, acute confusion, incontinence, or a general deterioration in condition.

Etiology

UTIs are the second most common infections in children, after otitis media. An estimated 3% of girls and 1% of boys will have a UTI by age 11 years (National Kidney and Urological Diseases Information Clearinghouse, 2003). Most UTIs among newborns and young infants occur in boys, as obstructive structural defects that predispose infants to infection have a higher incidence in males. The incidence of UTIs in older infants and children is higher in girls because the shorter female urethra (2 cm [1 in.] in young girls) has closer proximity to the anus and vagina, increasing the risk of contamination by fecal bacteria.

Pathogens usually enter the urinary tract by ascending from the mucous membranes of the perineal area into the lower urinary tract. Bacteria that have colonized the urethra, vagina, or perineal tissues are the usual source of infection (Porth, 2005). From the bladder, bacteria can continue to ascend the urinary tract, eventually infecting the *parenchyma* (functional tissue) of the kidneys (Kasper et al., 2005). Hematogenous spread of infection to the urinary tract is rare; infections introduced in this manner are usually associated with previous damage or scarring of the urinary tract. Bacteria introduced into the urinary tract can cause asymptomatic bacteriuria or an inflammatory response with manifestations of UTI.

At least 10–15% of hospitalized clients with indwelling urinary catheters develop bacteriuria. The longer the catheter remains in place, the greater the risk for infection. Bacteria, including *E. coli*, *Proteus*, *Pseudomonas*, and *Klebsiella*, reach the bladder either by migrating through the column of urine within the catheter or moving up the mucous sheath of the urethra outside the catheter (Kasper et al., 2005). Bacteria enter the catheter system at the connection between the catheter and drainage system or through the emptying tube of the drainage bag. Colonization of perineal skin by bowel flora is a common source of infection in catheterized women.

Another cause of UTI is vesicoureteral reflux, the backflow of urine from the bladder into the ureters during voiding. Bacteria in the urine can be swept up to the kidneys, leading to pyelonephritis. Vesicoureteral reflex also prevents complete emptying of the bladder and, because urine returns to the bladder, it creates a reservoir for bacterial growth (Huether, 2006). Vesicoureteral reflux can also result from a structural anomaly in which the ureters insert into the bladder in an abnormal position.

Renal scarring can result from **hydronephrosis** (accumulation of urine in the renal pelvis as a result of obstructed outflow) or pyelonephritis, due to the inflammatory and ischemic effects of the infection. Scars have been associated with hypertension, proteinuria, and kidney failure. The risk of kidney damage increases in the following cases:

- UTI in an infant less than 1 year of age
- Delay in diagnosis and effective antibacterial treatment for an upper UTI
- Anatomic obstruction or nerve supply interruption
- Recurrent episodes of upper UTIs.

Risk Factors

Clients can be predisposed to UTI by a variety of factors (Box 15–9). Some risk factors cannot be changed (e.g., aging and a female's short urethra). Cystitis occurs most frequently in adult females, usually because of colonization of the bladder by bacteria that are normally found in the lower gastrointestinal tract. These bacteria gain entry by ascending the short, straight female urethra. Wiping from back to front after urination can transfer bacteria from the anorectal area to the urethra.

In women, sexual activity increases the risk for UTI, because bacteria can be introduced into the bladder via the urethra during sexual intercourse. Use of spermicidal compounds with a diaphragm, cervical cap, or condom alters the normal bacterial flora of the vagina and perineal tissues and further increases the risk for UTI. Diaphragms are not recommended for women with a history of UTIs because pressure from the diaphragm on the urethra can interfere with complete bladder emptying and lead to recurrent UTIs.

Some females lack a normally protective mucosal enzyme and have decreased levels of cervicovaginal antibodies to enterobacteria, further increasing their risk. Personal hygiene practices and voluntary urinary retention can contribute to the risk for UTI in women. Up to three UTIs annually is considered to be within normal limits for sexually active women and does not usually warrant additional diagnostic tests beyond urine culture.

Prostatic hypertrophy and bacterial prostatitis are risk factors among males. Circumcision appears to have a protective effect. Anal intercourse also is a risk factor for men. In healthy adult men, UTIs are unusual and may prompt additional diagnostic testing.

Urinary stasis increases the risk of UTI. Stasis may be caused by abnormal anatomic structures or abnormal function (e.g., a **neurogenic bladder** in which an interrupted nerve supply from meningomyelocele or spinal cord trauma impairs bladder voiding function and leads to incomplete bladder emptying). Children typically void five to six times a day. Infrequent voiding, which is common in school-age children, results in incomplete emptying of the bladder and urinary stasis. Voluntarily suppressing the desire to urinate is a predisposing factor, as retention overdistends the bladder and can lead to an infection. Other factors associated with increased risk of UTI include an irritated perineum, uncircumcised male in the first 6 months of life, constipation, masturbation, sexual abuse, and sexual activity in adolescent females (Dulczak & Kirk, 2005).

Asymptomatic bacteriuria (ASB) (bacteria in the urine that actively multiply without accompanying clinical symptoms) is a condition that becomes significant if a woman is pregnant, because about 30% of pregnant women with untreated ASB will develop symptomatic UTIs (Smail, 2007). ASB is almost always caused by a single organism, typically *E. coli*. If more than one type of bacteria is cultured, the possibility of urine-culture contamination must be considered.

Box 15–9 **Risk Factors for UTI**

FEMALE

- Short, straight urethra
- Proximity of urinary meatus to vagina and anus
- Sexual intercourse
- Use of diaphragm and spermicidal compounds for birth control
- Pregnancy

MALE

- Uncircumcised
- Prostatic hypertrophy
- Anal intercourse

BOTH MALES AND FEMALES

- Aging
- Urinary tract obstruction
- Neurogenic bladder dysfunction
- Vesicoureteral reflux
- Genetic factors
- Catheterization

A woman who has had a UTI is susceptible to recurrent infection. If a pregnant woman develops an acute UTI, especially with a high temperature, amniotic fluid infection can develop and retard the growth of the placenta.

Congenital and acquired factors that contribute to the risk of infection include urinary tract obstruction by tumors or calculi, structural abnormalities such as strictures, impaired bladder innervation, bowel incontinence, and chronic diseases such as diabetes mellitus. Instrumentation of the urinary tract (e.g., catheterization or cystoscopy) is a major risk factor for UTI. Even when performed under strict aseptic conditions, catheterization can result in bladder infection. Research indicates that the risk for catheter-associated UTI is reduced when anesthetic lubricating gels are inserted into the urethra prior to catheter insertion (Bardsley, 2005). The placement of the catheter prevents the flushing action of voiding, and bacteria can ascend to the bladder through the catheter lumen or via exudate between the urethral mucosa and the catheter.

Older clients have an increased incidence of UTI. The greatest increase is seen in men, as the ratio of female-to-male UTI in older adults changes from 50:1 to less than 5:1. Although the bacteriostatic effect of prostatic fluid and a longer urethra provide an effective barrier to bladder infection for adult males, the hypertrophy of the prostate that is commonly associated with aging increases the risk of cystitis in older males. An enlarged prostate can impede urine flow, leading to incomplete bladder emptying and urinary stasis. Bacteria are not completely flushed with voiding, allowing colonization of the bladder. An increased risk of urinary stasis, chronic disease states (such as diabetes mellitus), and an impaired immune response also contribute to the higher incidence of UTI in older adults. In older women, loss of tissue elasticity and weakening of perineal muscles often contribute to the development of a cystocele or rectocele. Resulting changes in bladder and urethral position increase the risk of incomplete bladder emptying.

The risk for UTI increases during pregnancy, particularly during the second trimester, secondary to the pressure of the fetus, which causes urinary stasis and incomplete bladder emptying. The diagnosis of UTI in the pregnant client carries significant risks for the mother and fetus. UTIs are associated with an increased risk of preeclampsia (Conde-Agudelo, Villar, & Lindheimer, 2008). An increased risk of premature birth and intrauterine growth restriction is associated with acute pyelonephritis, which is often caused by asymptomatic bacteriuria (ASB). Although the exact cause is unknown, there is an increased risk of premature rupture of membranes associated with UTI. If urine stasis exists, the risk of UTI increases, because of bacteriuria and the presence of dilated ureters and renal pelves, which persist for about 6 weeks after delivery.

The postpartal woman is at increased risk of developing urinary tract problems caused by the normal postpartal diuresis, increased bladder capacity, and decreased bladder sensitivity from stretching or trauma. Possible inhibited neural control of the bladder following the use of general or regional anesthesia and contamination from catheterization also put the postpartal woman at risk for UTIs. These factors make it essential that the mother empty her bladder completely with each voiding. UTI in the newborn predisposes the neonate to hyperbilirubinemia (elevated serum bilirubin).

CLINICAL MANIFESTATIONS

The symptoms of UTI depend on the infection's location as well as the client's age. Symptoms in a newborn tend to be nonspecific—unexplained fever, failure to thrive, poor feeding, vomiting and diarrhea, strong-smelling urine, and irritability. Any child younger than 2 years of age with a fever of unknown origin should be tested for a UTI. The more "classic" symptoms of lower UTI are not seen until the toddler years, as shown in the following Clinical Manifestations and Therapies. Approximately 40% of UTIs are asymptomatic.

Typical presenting symptoms of cystitis include **dysuria** (painful or difficult urination), urinary frequency and **urgency** (a sudden, compelling need to urinate), and **nocturia** (voiding two or more times at night). In addition, the urine may have a foul odor and appear cloudy (**pyuria**) or bloody (**hematuria**) because of mucus, excess white cells in the urine, and bleeding of the inflamed bladder wall. Suprapubic pain and tenderness also may be present. See Box 15–10 for manifestations of cystitis.

Older clients may not experience the classic symptoms of cystitis. Instead, they often present with nonspecific manifestations, such as nocturia, incontinence, confusion, behavior change, lethargy, loss of appetite, or "just not feeling right." Fever may be present; however, hypothermia also may develop in an older adult. Particularly in a long-term care setting, a change in behavior may be the only indicator of a UTI (Bentley et al., 2001). This can be frustrating for the family members and health care team, who may easily suspect any number of other possible causes when an older adult presents with these symptoms.

The symptoms usually seen in younger adults with UTIs—urgency and frequency—are common age-related changes in the older adult and therefore lack diagnostic usefulness. If, however, an older adult has not previously experienced urinary urgency, and presents with a shortened period of time between the urge to void and actual urination, or urinary frequency of more than seven voids per 24-hour period, his or her symptoms should be thoroughly investigated.

The majority of UTIs in older adults are asymptomatic (Nicolle, 2003). Some authors term this condition *asymptomatic UTI*, whereas others apply the term *UTI* only to those older adults with symptoms, and use *bacteriuria* to define the presence of bacteria in the urine with no concomitant symptoms (Nicolle, 2003). Asymptomatic UTI does not require

Box 15–10 **Manifestations of Cystitis**

- Dysuria
- Pyuria
- Frequency
- Hematuria
- Urgency
- Suprapubic discomfort
- Nocturia

CLINICAL MANIFESTATIONS AND THERAPIES Urinary Tract Infection

ETIOLOGY	CLINICAL MANIFESTATION	CLINICAL THERAPIES
Lower UTI—cystitis	Frequency, dysuria, urgency, enuresis, strong-smelling urine, cloudy urine, hematuria, abdominal or suprapubic pain	Administer 5- to 7-day course of trimethoprim or sulfamethoxazole or antibiotic matching organism sensitivity, encourage oral fluids, administer analgesic such as acetaminophen or Pyridium.
Upper UTI—pyelonephritis	High fever, chills, abdominal pain, flank pain, costovertebral angle tenderness, persistent vomiting, moderate to severe dehydration Infants may have nonspecific signs such as poor appetite, failure to thrive, lethargy, irritability. Older children may have signs of cystitis.	Administer antipyretics and intravenous antibiotics initially, and then transition to oral antibiotics matching organism sensitivity for a total of 7–10 days. Rehydration is essential.

treatment. In fact, treatment does not improve the morbidity or mortality in affected older persons (Gandhi, 2006; Krogh & Bruskewitz, 1998; McCue, 1999; Nicolle, 2003; Steers, 1999). Routine urinalysis for older adults without symptoms is neither appropriate nor cost effective.

Cystitis is usually uncomplicated and readily responds to treatment. When left untreated, the infection can ascend to involve the kidneys. Severe or prolonged infection can lead to sloughing of bladder mucosa and ulcer formation. Chronic cystitis can lead to bladder stones.

Catheter-associated UTIs often are asymptomatic. Gram-negative bacteremia is the most significant complication associated with these UTIs. Most catheter-associated UTIs resolve quickly when the catheter is removed and a short course of antibiotic is administered. Intermittent catheterization carries a lower risk of infection than does an indwelling catheter, and is preferred for clients who are unable to empty their bladder by voiding. UTIs in catheterized older adults tend to be polymicrobial and difficult to eradicate. Before an indwelling catheter is used, the potential benefits to the older adult must be carefully weighed against the serious risks posed.

Instillation of anesthetic lubricating gel into the urethra prior to catheter insertion further reduces the risk by dilating the urethra and reducing trauma to fragile urethral tissues (Bardsley, 2005).

COLLABORATION

Collaborative treatment of UTI focuses on eliminating the causative organism, preventing relapse or reinfection, and identifying and correcting any contributing factors. Drug treatment with antibiotics and urinary anti-infectives is commonly used. In some cases, surgery may be indicated to correct contributing factors.

Diagnostic Tests

- Urinalysis to assess for pyuria, bacteria, and blood cells in the urine. A bacteria count greater than 100,000 (10^5) per milliliter is indicative of infection. Rapid tests for bacteria in the urine include using a *nitrite dipstick* (which turns pink in the presence of bacteria) and the *leukocyte esterase test*, an indirect method of detecting bacteria by identifying lysed or intact WBCs in the urine.
- Urine should be a midstream clean-catch specimen; if necessary, straight catheterization or "mini-cath," with strict aseptic technique, may be used. Catheterization is avoided if possible to reduce the risk of further infection. Routine urinalysis for older adults without symptoms is neither appropriate nor cost effective.

PRACTICE ALERT

Urine obtained from infants using urine collection bags may be used for urinalysis and to screen for UTI, but the specimen collection procedure is not sterile. Confirmation of a UTI must be made with urine collected by a clean-catch or catheterization procedure (Raszka & Khan, 2005).

- **Gram stain** of the urine may be done to identify the infecting organism by shape and characteristic (gram-positive or gram-negative).
- Urine culture and sensitivity tests may be ordered to identify the infecting organism and the most effective antibiotic. Culture requires 24–72 hours, so treatment to eliminate the most common organisms often is initiated without culture. Urine cultures do not distinguish between upper and lower UTIs (Raszka & Khan, 2005). UTI in an older person with an indwelling catheter is considered to be complicated and may include a variety of microorganisms.

PRACTICE ALERT

Urine specimens collected for culture must be delivered to the laboratory within 1 hour or the specimen must be refrigerated to prevent the growth of organisms that occur with prolonged room temperature exposure.

- WBC with differential may be done to detect the typical changes associated with infection, such as leukocytosis (elevated WBC) and increased numbers of neutrophils.

In clients with recurrent infections or persistent bacteriuria, additional diagnostic testing may be ordered to evaluate for structural abnormalities, renal scarring, and other contributing factors. These tests include the following:

- ***Intravenous pyelography (IVP)***, also known as *excretory urography,* is used to evaluate the structure and excretory function of the kidneys, ureters, and bladder. As the kidneys clear an intravenously injected contrast medium from the blood, the size and shape of the kidneys, their calyces and pelvises, the ureters, and the bladder can be evaluated, and structural or functional abnormalities, such as vesicoureteral reflux, can be detected.
- ***Voiding cystourethrography*** involves instilling contrast medium into the bladder, and then using x-rays to assess the bladder and urethra when filled and during voiding. This study can detect structural and functional abnormalities of the bladder and urethral strictures. This test has a lower risk of allergic response to the contrast dye than IVP.
- ***Cystoscopy***, direct visualization of the urethra and a bladder through a cystoscope, can be used to diagnose conditions such as prostatic hypertrophy, urethral strictures, bladder calculi, tumors, polyps, diverticula, and congenital abnormalities. A tissue biopsy may be obtained during the procedure, and other interventions may be performed (e.g., stone removal or stricture dilation).
- *Manual pelvic* or *prostate examinations* are done to assess for structural changes of the genitourinary tract, such as prostatic enlargement, cystocele, or rectocele.
- *Renal and bladder ultrasound and DMSA scanning* are used to detect pyelonephritis and renal scarring (Dulczak & Kirk, 2005).

Pharmacologic Therapy

Most uncomplicated infections of the lower urinary tract can be treated with a short course of antibiotic therapy. Upper urinary tract infections, in contrast, usually require longer treatment (2 or more weeks) to eradicate the infecting organism. Treatment should be initiated as soon as the diagnosis of UTI is made.

Antibiotics are selected based on the age of the client, sensitivity of the cultured organism, renal function, and the client's signs and symptoms. Gender is a consideration in treatment choices, because men require longer periods of treatment than women. The longer urethra in men makes it less likely that bacteria can ascend into the bladder. When bacteria do reach the older man's bladder, the infection is considered to be complicated and requires a longer course of treatment. The antibiotic is changed if necessary after culture sensitivity is determined.

Follow-up cultures may be obtained 48–72 hours after drug therapy is started in the pediatric client who is still febrile (Raszka & Khan, 2005). Children with pyelonephritis should be maintained on antibiotic prophylaxis until radiologic tests are performed to detect any structural defects.

Short-course therapy (either a single antibiotic dose or a 3-day course of treatment) reduces treatment cost, increases compliance, and has a lower rate of side effects. Single-dose therapy is associated with a higher rate of recurrent infection and continued vaginal colonization with *E. coli*, making a 3-day course of treatment the preferred option for uncomplicated cystitis. Oral TMP-SMZ, TMP, or a quinolone antibiotic such as ciprofloxacin (Cipro) or enoxacin (Penetrex) may be ordered.

Men and women with pyelonephritis, urinary tract abnormalities or stones, or a history of previous infections with antibiotic-resistant infections require a 7- to 10-day course of TMP-SMZ, ciprofloxacin, ofloxacin (Floxin), or an alternative antibiotic. The client with severe illness may need hospitalization. Intravenous ciprofloxacin, gentamicin, ceftriaxone (Rocephin), or ampicillin may be prescribed for severe illness or sepsis associated with UTI.

Children who appear ill and cannot tolerate oral antibiotics are often hospitalized because they need rehydration and parenteral antibiotic treatment until they have been afebrile for 24 hours. Infants can develop permanent kidney damage or generalized sepsis if the UTI is not treated aggressively. If a structural defect is identified, surgical correction may be necessary to prevent recurrent infections that could lead to renal damage.

Clients who experience frequent symptomatic UTIs may be treated with prophylactic antibiotic therapy. Drugs such as TMP-SMZ, TMP, and nitrofurantoin (Furadantin, Macrodantin, Macrobid) do not achieve effective plasma concentrations at recommended doses, but do reach effective concentrations in the urine. Nitrofurantoin also may be used to treat UTI in pregnant women.

Antibiotics and urinary anti-infectives generally are not recommended to treat asymptomatic bacteriuria in catheterized clients. The preferred treatment for catheter-associated UTI is removal of the indwelling catheter, followed by a 10- to 14-day course of antibiotic therapy to eliminate the infection.

Surgery

Surgery may be indicated for recurrent UTI if diagnostic testing indicates calculi, structural anomalies, or strictures that contribute to the risk of infection. Stones, or *calculi,* in the renal pelvis or bladder are an irritant and provide a matrix for bacterial colonization. Treatment may include surgical removal of a large calculus from the renal pelvis or cystoscopic removal of bladder calculi. *Percutaneous ultrasonic pyelolithotomy* or *extracorporeal shock wave lithotripsy* (see the Elimination concept) may be used instead of surgery to crush and remove stones.

Ureteroplasty, the surgical repair of a ureter, may be indicated for structural abnormality or stricture of a ureter. This may be combined with a ureteral reimplantation if vesicoureteral reflux is present. The client returns from these surgeries with an indwelling urinary catheter (Foley or suprapubic) and a **ureteral stent** (a thin catheter inserted into the ureter to provide for urine flow and ureteral support), which remains in place for 3–5 days. Box 15–11 describes nursing care of the client with a ureteral stent in place.

Box 15–11 Ureteral Stent

Ureteral stents are used to maintain patency and promote healing of the ureters (see Figure 15–37 ■). A stent may be temporary, used during and after a surgical procedure, or it may be used for longer periods in clients with ureteral obstruction due to tumors, strictures, or other causes.

Stents may be positioned during surgery or cystoscopy. They are made of a nontoxic material such as silicone or polyurethane, with side drainage holes placed along the length of the stent. Stents are radiopaque for easy radiographic identification. One or both ends of the stent may be pigtail or J shaped to prevent migration.

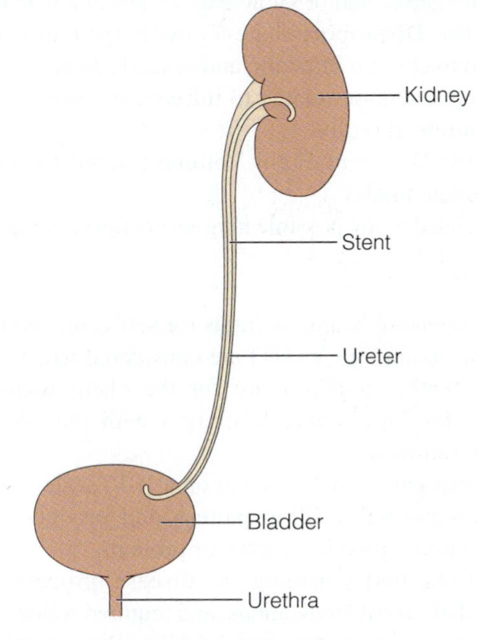

Figure 15–37 ■ A ureteral stent.

In caring for a client with a ureteral stint, the nurse should do the following:

- Label all drainage tubes, including stents, for easy identification. Attach each catheter and stent to a separate closed drainage system. Careful labeling allows close monitoring of output from all sources and reservoirs. Separate drainage systems minimize the risk of infection.
- If the stent has been brought to the surface, secure it and maintain its position. The stent is usually placed in the renal pelvis. It is important to secure it well to prevent trauma to the kidney, inadvertent removal of the stent, and ureter obstruction.
- Monitor urine output, including color, consistency, and odor. Monitor for signs of infection or bleeding, including fever, tachycardia, pain, hematuria, and cloudy or malodorous urine. The stent facilitates urine flow, but can become obstructed due to bleeding, calculi, or sediment. Obstruction can result in hydronephrosis and kidney damage. The stent itself is a foreign body in the urinary tract and can increase the risk of UTI.
- Maintain fluid intake, encouraging fluids that acidify urine, such as low-sugar apple, cranberry, and blueberry juice. The stent can precipitate calculus formation as well as UTI. Increasing fluid intake and acidifying the urine help prevent these complications.
- For an indwelling stent, stress the need for regular follow-up to monitor for and prevent complications such as UTI and calculi. The client with an indwelling stent may tend to forget that the stent is in place and become noncompliant with follow-up and preventive measures.

Follow-up urine cultures should be obtained according to the frequency specified by agency guidelines. Clients with pyelonephritis may have repeat urine cultures monthly for 3 months, every 3 months for 6 months, and then annually. Most reinfections occur within 1 year, and subsequent infections may be asymptomatic. For children with VUR or recurrent infections, a long-term, suppressive dose of an antibiotic may be ordered in an attempt to keep the urine sterile and prevent subsequent pyelonephritis and renal scarring, but there is limited evidence that this is effective (Raszka & Khan, 2005). Children with renal scarring should have their blood pressure monitored.

Complementary Therapies

Complementary therapies, such as aromatherapy or herbal preparations, may be used in conjunction with antibiotics to treat UTI. Low-sugar cranberry juice or extract and blueberry juice also are commonly used to prevent and treat UTI. Adding bergamot, sandalwood, lavender, or juniper oil to bath water may help relieve the discomfort of UTI. Herbal supplements such as saw palmetto have a urinary antiseptic effect, and may be beneficial in treating or preventing UTI. Consult a qualified herbologist for recommended doses and appropriate use. Some

EVIDENCE-BASED PRACTICE VUR and Prophylactic Antibiotics

A randomized control trial of 218 children, ages 3 months to 18 years, who were diagnosed with pyelonephritis and mild or moderate vesicoureteral reflux (VUR), evaluated the effect of prophylactic antibiotics on outcomes. One-half of the children received antibiotics, and the remainder did not. Children were seen every 3 months for the year of the study, and each had a urine culture at each visit. Results indicated that the presence of mild or moderate VUR did not increase the incidence of UTI, pyelonephritis, or renal scarring following an acute episode of pyelonephritis. The children who did not receive prophylactic antibiotics had no more infections or renal scarring than the children who did receive antibiotics (Garin, Olavarria, Nieto et al., 2006).

aromatherapy and herbal preparations are contraindicated in clients with allergies; those clients should check with their allergist before participating in these types of therapies.

NURSING PROCESS

The nursing process for UTI generally focuses on returning the client to maximum health. In order to maintain optimum urinary health, nurses should be alert for opportunities to provide health promotion. Teach measures to prevent UTI to all clients, particularly to young, sexually active women. Encourage clients to maintain a generous fluid intake of 2.0–2.5 quarts per day, increasing intake during hot weather and strenuous activity. Discuss the need to avoid voluntary urinary retention, emptying the bladder every 3–4 hours. Instruct women to cleanse the perineal area from front to back after voiding and defecating. Teach to void before and after sexual intercourse to flush out bacteria introduced into the urethra and bladder. Teach measures to maintain the integrity of perineal tissues, such as avoiding bubble baths, feminine hygiene sprays, and vaginal douches; wearing cotton briefs; and avoiding synthetic materials. Unless contraindicated, suggest the following measures to maintain acid urine: Drink two glasses of low-sugar cranberry juice daily, take ascorbic acid (vitamin C), and avoid excess intake of milk and milk products, other fruit juices, and sodium bicarbonate (baking soda).

Assessment

Focused assessment data for the client with a suspected UTI includes the following:

- *Health history.* Current symptoms, including frequency, urgency, burning on urination, and number of voidings per night; color, clarity, and odor of urine; other manifestations, such as lower abdominal, back, or flank pain, nausea or vomiting, or fever; duration of symptoms and any treatment attempted; history of previous UTIs and their frequency; possibility of pregnancy and type of birth control used; chronic diseases such as diabetes; current medications; and any known allergies
- *Physical examination.* General health; vital signs including temperature; abdominal shape, contour, and tenderness to palpation (especially suprapubic); and percuss for costovertebral tenderness.

Nursing assessment for a child with a suspected UTI involves assessing the infant or child for signs of acute or chronic illness, examining the genitourinary system, and collecting a urine specimen for culture. Assess the infant for toxic (very ill) appearance, fever, and oral fluid intake. Evaluate the child's oral fluid intake. Assess for quality, quantity, and frequency of voiding. Measure the child's height and weight, and plot the data on a growth curve to identify any change in growth pattern associated with a chronic illness. Take the infant's or child's blood pressure. Palpate the abdomen and suprapubic and costovertebral areas for masses, tenderness, and distention.

Sexually active adolescents may deny having symptoms for fear of disclosing their sexual activity to their parents. Careful questioning may be necessary to elicit a response despite these concerns. The nurse should be open and approachable, and give the client and family the chance to address their concerns.

Diagnosis

Priority nursing diagnoses focus on comfort, urinary elimination, and teaching/learning needs and may include the following:

- Acute Pain related to dysuria, systemic discomforts, or renal pain secondary to upper UTI
- Impaired Urinary Elimination related to UTI
- Deficient Knowledge related to self-care, medication administration, and/or knowledge of preventative measures
- Risk for Disproportionate Growth (pediatric clients) related to chronic infection and renal damage
- Urinary Retention related to infrequent voiding habits or vesicoureteral reflux
- Risk for Deficient Fluid Volume related to fever and inadequate intake
- Fear related to the possible long-term effects of the disease.

Plan

The client's general health, abilities for self-care, and risk factors that may contribute to UTI are considered when planning and implementing nursing care for the client with a UTI. Outcomes, developed in collaboration with the client, may include the following:

- Describes pain as a 3 or lower on a 1–10 scale.
- Regains normal voiding pattern and produces normal urine without blood, bacteria, or protein.
- Verbalizes understanding of disease process, proper method of taking medications, and required follow-up care.
- Provides strategies for reducing the risk of another UTI.

Implementation

Nursing care for the hospitalized client with a complicated UTI focuses on administering prescribed medications, promoting rehydration, assessing renal function, and teaching the client and family how to minimize the risk of future infection.

Pain

Pain is a common manifestation of both lower and upper UTIs. Urinary tract pain is caused primarily by distention and increased pressure within the urinary tract. The severity of the pain is related to the rate at which inflammation and distention develop, not their degree.

PRACTICE ALERT

The older adult with a UTI may not complain of dysuria. Be alert for other manifestations of UTI, such as incontinence or cloudy or malodorous urine. Inflammatory and immune responses tend to diminish with aging, reducing the irritative symptoms of UTI.

In cystitis, inflammation causes a sensation of fullness; dull, constant suprapubic pain; and possibly low back pain. The inflamed bladder wall and urethra cause dysuria, pain, and

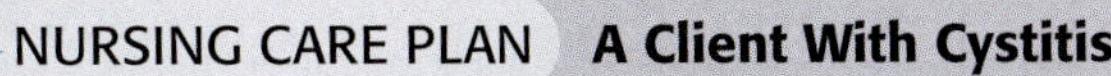

NURSING CARE PLAN A Client With Cystitis

Miija Waisanen is a 25-year-old second-year nursing student. She was recently married, and she and her husband live in an apartment near the college she attends. Mrs. Waisanen has never been pregnant, and she is using a diaphragm for birth control. She presents at the local urgent care clinic complaining of low back pain, frequency, urgency, and burning on urination, which began the day before.

ASSESSMENT

Patrice Ramiros, RN, admits Mrs. Waisanen to the clinic. Mrs. Waisanen denies having had similar symptoms in the past or ever having been diagnosed with a urinary tract infection. She describes her pain as a constant, dull ache that does not change with movement. She feels the need to urinate almost constantly, but experiences difficulty in starting her stream, and burning pain, and cramping when voiding. She reports getting up four times the night before to urinate. She denies painful intercourse and states that her last menstrual period began only 2 weeks ago. Physical examination reveals: BP 112/68 mmHg; pulse 90 beats/minute and regular, and afebrile. Suprapubic tenderness is noted, but there is no flank or costovertebral angle tenderness. Clean-catch urine specimen shows hematuria, multiple WBCs, and a bacteria count greater than 10^5 /mL.

The nurse practitioner prescribes trimethoprim-sulfamethoxazole (TMP-SMZ) 160 mg/800 mg po two times a day for 3 days, and aspirin or acetaminophen gr × po every 4 hours as needed for pain. Mrs. Waisanen is instructed to return to the clinic in 7 days for a follow-up urine culture, or sooner if her symptoms do not improve.

DIAGNOSES

- Pain related to infection and inflammatory process in tthe urinary tract
- Impaired Urinary Elimination related to inflammation, as evidenced by frequency, urgency, nocturia, and dysuria
- Deficient Knowledge related to lack of information about risk factors for UTI

PLANNING

- Client reports relief of low back pain and burning on urination.
- Client reports a normal voiding pattern without frequency, urgency, nocturia, and abnormal urine characteristics.
- Client verbalizes understanding of the disease process, related risk factors, follow-up instructions, and symptoms of recurrence that indicate the need for medical attention.

IMPLEMENTATION

- Teach comfort measures: warm sitz baths, a heating pad on low heat applied to the lower back or abdomen, rest, increased fluid intake, avoiding caffeinated beverages, and aspirin or acetaminophen as ordered.
- Advise client to refrain from sexual intercourse until infection and inflammation have cleared to avoid further irritation of inflamed tissues.
- Discuss the possible relationship between using a diaphragm for birth control and UTIs in women.
- Discuss dietary and hygiene practices to prevent UTI symptoms.
- Discuss symptoms indicating the need for further intervention and the risks of undertreatment.

EVALUATION

Six months later, Mrs. Waisanen rotates through the urgent care clinic for her community-based nursing experience. When Ms. Ramiros asks how she is doing, Mrs. Waisanen reports that her symptoms and urine cleared within about a day after starting the antibiotic, and she has had no further problems. She has seen her women's health care nurse practitioner to change her birth control to oral contraceptives, increased her intake of fluid and vitamin C, and no longer puts off urinating until she "has time to go!"

CRITICAL THINKING

1. What physiologic and psychosocial factors put Mrs. Waisanen at risk for UTI?
2. Compare the benefits and drawbacks to short-course therapy versus conventional therapy for UTI.
3. Why was it appropriate for the nurse practitioner to use short-course therapy with the advice to return if symptoms did not clear?
4. Develop a care plan for Mrs. Waisanen for the nursing diagnosis Ineffective Health Maintenance.

burning on urination. Bladder spasms may develop, causing periodic severe, stabbing discomfort. Pain associated with pyelonephritis is often steady and dull, localized to the outer abdomen or flank region. Urologic disorders rarely cause central abdominal pain.

Nursing interventions for the client experiencing pain include the following:

- Assess pain: timing, quality, intensity, location, duration, and aggravating and alleviating factors. A change in the nature, location, or intensity of the pain could indicate an extension of the infection or a related but separate problem.
- Teach or provide comfort measures, such as warm sitz baths, warm packs or heating pads, and balanced rest and activity. Systemic analgesics, urinary analgesics, or antispasmodic medication should be used as ordered. Warmth relaxes muscles, relieves spasms, and increases local blood supply. Because pain can stimulate a stress response and delay healing, it should be relieved when possible.
- Increase fluid intake unless contraindicated. Increased fluid dilutes urine, reducing irritation of the inflamed bladder and urethral mucosa.

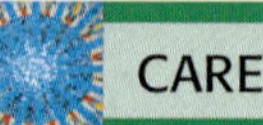

CARE SETTINGS Community-Based Care for Prevention of UTIs

Because both upper and lower urinary tract infections are usually managed in the community, teaching is the most important nursing intervention. Provide instruction on the following topics:

- Risk factors for UTI and how to minimize or eliminate these factors through increased fluid intake, regular elimination, and personal hygiene measures
- Early manifestations of UTI and the importance of seeking medical intervention promptly
- Maintaining optimal immune system function by attending to physical and psychosocial stressors, such as lack of adequate rest, poor nutrition, and high levels of emotional stress
- The importance of completing the prescribed treatment and keeping follow-up appointments
- Minimizing the risk of UTI when an indwelling urinary catheter is necessary:
  a. Use alternatives to an indwelling catheter when possible. For urinary incontinence, try scheduled toileting, incontinence pads or diapers, and external catheters if possible. For urinary retention, teach the client or a family member to perform straight catheterization every 3–4 hours using clean technique.
  b. When an indwelling catheter is necessary, teach care measures such as perineal care, managing and emptying the collection chamber, maintaining a closed system, and bladder irrigation or flushing if ordered.

- Instruct the client to notify the primary care provider if pain and discomfort continue or intensify after therapy is initiated. Pain and discomfort in voiding typically are relieved within 24 hours of initiating antibiotic therapy. Continued discomfort may indicate a complicated UTI or other urinary tract disorder.

Impaired Urinary Elimination

Inflammation of the bladder and urethral mucosa affects the normal process and patterns of voiding, causing frequency, urgency, and burning on urination, as well as nocturia. Urine may be blood tinged, cloudy, and malodorous. The client with short- or long-term urinary retention requires additional measures to assess for and prevent UTI.

Because bladder training is such an important milestone for young children, any disorder that affects voiding can have developmental implications. A toddler who has been toilet trained may regress and require diapers temporarily due to incontinence related to the UTI. An older child may develop **enuresis** (the involuntary passage of urine after control has been established) after a prolonged period of being dry at night. A preschooler may perceive the infection as punishment for an imagined wrong, such as masturbation. Reassure parents that this temporary period of urinary incontinence is normal when associated with UTI and emphasize that they should offer the child support rather than disapproval.

PRACTICE ALERT

Nurses who work with clients in hospitals and other institutional settings should provide easy access to a bedpan, urinal, commode, or bathroom. Make sure that lighting is adequate and that pathways are free from obstacles for clients getting up to use the bathroom. Frequency, urgency, and nocturia increase the risk of urinary incontinence and injury due to falls, particularly in older or debilitated clients.

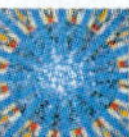

EVIDENCE-BASED PRACTICE Male Catheterization

Insertion of an indwelling (retention) catheter is a commonly performed procedure in hospitals and long-term care facilities. Although the location of the female urethral meatus presents a challenge to maintaining catheter sterility during insertion, the anatomy of the male urethra presents a different set of challenges. Little research is available to support evidence-based practice for male urethral catheterization. In addition, reports of urethral injury in men related to catheter insertion and balloon inflation are not uncommon.

A multidisciplinary team of researchers at the University of Colorado Hospital conducted a study to determine the correct urethral catheter placement in male adults (Daneshgari, Krugman, Bahn, & Lee, 2002). Their research showed that inserting the catheter to the bifurcation (attachment of the arm for balloon inflation) always placed the retention balloon well within the urinary bladder prior to its inflation. Insertion to any lesser distance was inadequate to ensure safe balloon inflation without potential damage to the urethra.

Implications for Nursing

Nursing fundamentals and skills texts recommend inserting the retention catheter from 6–10 inches into the male urethra before inflating the balloon. Some texts recommend inserting the catheter 1–2 inches beyond the point at which urine is obtained before inflating the balloon. This study (Daneshgari et al., 2002) showed that these recommendations could result in an attempt to inflate the balloon while that portion of the catheter is still in the urethra, not fully into the bladder. To ensure safe practice and reduce the risk for injury and discomfort, insert a retention catheter to the bifurcation before inflating the balloon.

Critical Thinking in Client Care

1. Why is insertion of a urinary catheter frequently a more uncomfortable and difficult procedure for a male client than a female client? What nursing measures or techniques can be used to reduce this discomfort?
2. Sterile technique generally is used when catheterizing clients in acute care settings. However, clients who require intermittent catheterization to empty their bladder typically use clean technique. Would clean technique be appropriate in an acute or long-term care setting? Why or why not?

Source: Daneshgari, F., Krugman, A., Bahn, A., & Lee, R. S. (2002). Evidence-based multidisciplinary practice: Improving the safety and standards of male bladder catheterization. *Medsurg Nursing, 11*(5), 236–241, 246.

PRACTICE ALERT

Unless contraindicated, instillation of an anesthetic lubricating gel into the urethra (10 mL for a male and 6 mL for a female) promotes comfort during the procedure, protects fragile urethral tissues from trauma, and reduces the risk for catheter-associated UTI (Bardsley, 2005).

Nursing interventions for clients with impaired urinary elimination include the following:

- Monitor (or instruct the client to monitor) color, clarity, and odor of urine. Urine should return to clear yellow within 48 hours, unless drug therapy causes a change in the color of urine. If clarity does not return, further investigation may be necessary.
- Instruct clients with impaired urinary elimination to avoid caffeinated drinks, including coffee, tea, and cola; citrus juices; drinks containing artificial sweeteners; and alcoholic beverages. Caffeine, citrus juices, and artificial sweeteners irritate bladder mucosa and the detrusor muscle, and can increase urgency and bladder spasms.
- Use strict aseptic technique and a closed urinary drainage system when inserting a straight or indwelling urinary catheter. Insert indwelling catheters to the full recommended length (4 inches or more in women and to the bifurcation in men) before inflating the balloon. Bacteria colonizing the perineal tissues or on the nurse's hands can be introduced into the bladder during catheterization. Aseptic technique reduces this risk. Inflating the balloon while it is in the urethra damages urethral tissues and can cause significant discomfort for the client.
- When possible, use intermittent straight catheterization to relieve urinary retention. Remove indwelling urinary catheters as soon as possible. Using intermittent straight catheterization allows the bladder to fill and completely empty in a more normal manner, maintaining physiologic function. The risk of infection associated with an indwelling catheter is about 3–5% per day of catheterization (Kasper et al., 2005).
- Maintain the closed urinary drainage system, and use aseptic technique when emptying the catheter drainage bag. Maintain gravity flow to prevent reflux of urine into the bladder from the drainage system. Bacteria can enter the drainage system when its integrity is interrupted (e.g., disconnecting the catheter from the drainage system) or during emptying of the drainage bag. These bacteria can ascend the column of urine to the bladder, causing UTI.

EVIDENCE-BASED PRACTICE Clean Catch

Cleansing with nonsterile gauze, moistened with tap water and soap, is as effective for clean-catch specimen collection as prepackaged sterile towelettes, and is gentler to the mucous membranes (Ünlü, Sardan, & Ülker, 2007).

- Provide perineal care on a regular basis and following defecation. Use antiseptic preparations only as ordered. Regular cleansing of perineal tissues reduces the risk of colonization by bowel or other bacteria. Although antiseptic solutions may be ordered for catheter care, they can dry perineal tissues and reduce normal flora, increasing the risk of colonization by pathogens, and should not be used routinely.

Ineffective Health Maintenance

Because clients with UTIs are at increased risk for future UTIs, they need to understand the disease process, risk factors, measures to prevent recurrent infection, diagnostic procedures, and best practices for home care. In addition, clients need to understand that, even when the manifestations of UTI are relieved, the treatment plan needs to continue. Failure to complete the full course of therapy and recommended follow-up can lead to continued bacteriuria and recurrent infections.

Nurses who work with clients with ineffective health maintenance should do the following:

- Teach clients how to obtain a midstream clean-catch urine specimen. Cleansing of the urinary meatus and perineal area reduces contamination of the specimen by external cells and bacteria. Ninety percent of urethral bacteria are cleared in the first 10 mL of voided urine, so a midstream specimen is representative of urine in the bladder.
- Assess knowledge about the disease process, risk factors, and preventive measures. The client may have little understanding of UTI, its causes, and contributing factors.
- Discuss the prescribed treatment plan and the importance of taking all prescribed antibiotics.
- Help the client develop a plan for taking medications, such as taking them with meals (unless contraindicated) or setting out all doses for the day in the morning. Missed doses of antibiotic can result in subtherapeutic blood levels and reduced effectiveness. Taking medication in association with a regular daily activity such as meals helps clients remember doses.
- Instruct clients to keep appointments for follow-up and urine culture. Follow-up urine culture, often scheduled 7–14 days after completion of antibiotic therapy, is vital to ensure complete eradication of bacteria and prevent relapse or recurrence.
- Teach measures to prevent future UTI, as discussed at the beginning of this exemplar. Keeping urine dilute and acidic and voiding regularly help to flush bacteria out of the bladder and urethra. The proximity of the female urethral meatus to the vagina and anus increases the risk of bacterial contamination, especially during intercourse. Bubble baths, feminine hygiene sprays, synthetic fibers, and douches can dry and irritate perineal tissues, promoting bacterial growth.

See Box 15–12 for information about avoiding cystitis for women.

Evaluation

The outcome of treatment for UTI may be determined by follow-up urinalysis and culture. Cure, as evidenced by the absence of pathogens in the urine, is the desired outcome.

Box 15–12 Key Facts to Remember

INFORMATION FOR WOMEN ABOUT WAYS TO AVOID CYSTITIS

- If you use a diaphragm for contraception, try changing methods or using another size of diaphragm.
- Avoid bladder irritants such as alcohol, caffeine products, and carbonated beverages.
- Increase fluid intake, especially water, to a minimum of six to eight glasses per day.
- Make regular urination a habit; avoid long waits.
- Practice good genital hygiene, including wiping from front to back after urination and bowel movements.
- Be aware that vigorous or frequent sexual activity may contribute to UTI.
- Urinate before and after intercourse to empty the bladder and cleanse the urethra.
- Complete medication regimens even if symptoms decrease.
- Do not use medication left over from previous infections.
- Drink cranberry juice to acidify the urine. This has been found to relieve symptoms in some cases.

When therapy fails to eradicate bacteria in the urine, it is known as **unresolved bacteriuria**. **Persistent bacteriuria**, or *relapse*, occurs when a persistent source of infection causes repeated infection after the initial cure. **Reinfection** is the development of a new infection with a different pathogen following successful UTI treatment (Tierney, McPhee, & Papadakis, 2005). Clients are generally required to submit a urinalysis for culture 7–10 days after completing a course of antibiotics to ensure that bacteria have been eliminated.

Expected outcomes of nursing care include the following:

- The client increases fluid intake and number of voidings each day.
- Client completes prescribed course of antibiotic therapy.
- Urine is free from bacteria following treatment.
- Client experiences no recurrent UTIs for 1 year.
- Client incorporates preventative self-care measures into daily regimen.

HEALTH CARE

Research indicates the best practice is not to treat asymptomatic bacteruria. If you were caring for a client with bacteria in the urine who denied any symptoms or problems, how would you explain the decision not to treat this? Would best practice change if the client wanted a prescription for an antibiotic? What would you tell the client who adamantly demands a prescription for an antibiotic after being informed that it is not in his or her best interest?

REVIEW Urinary Tract Infection

RELATE: LINK THE CONCEPTS

Linking the exemplar of Urinary Tract Infection with the concept of Elimination:

1. What are your teaching priorities for the client who has a urinary tract infection accompanied by urinary retention?
2. What teaching would you provide related to urinary elimination for the young adult woman who has experienced recurrent urinary tract infections over the past year?

Linking the exemplar of Urinary Tract Infection with the concept of Mobility:

3. What factors put the 90-year-old client who is wheelchair bound at risk for a urinary tract infection?
4. What preventive measures will you implement for the elderly client who is confined to bed to reduce the risk of urinary tract infections?

READY: GO TO COMPANION SKILLS MANUAL

- Providing perineal-genital care
- Assessing the client in pain
- Administering medication
- Collecting a midstream urine specimen
- Collecting urine externally
- Performing urinary catheterization

REFER: GO TO MYNURSING KIT

REFLECT: CASE STUDY

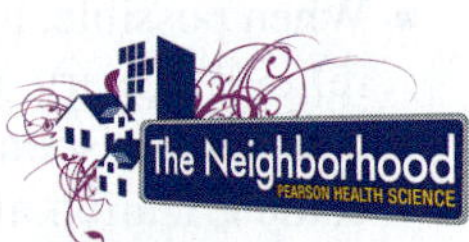

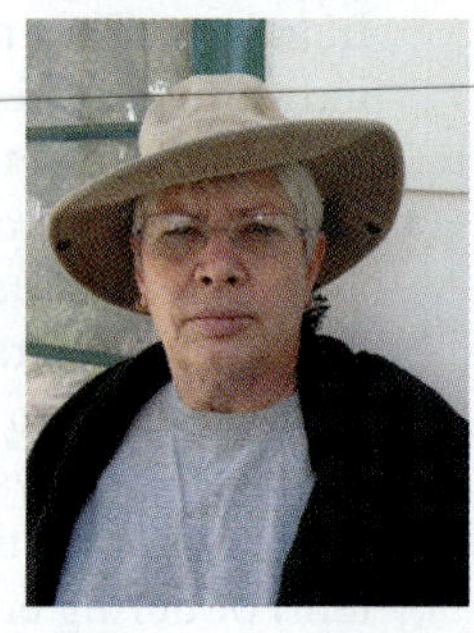

Mrs. James, who was introduced under the exemplar of Cellulitis within this concept, wakes up one day and does not feel well. She is taken by ambulance to the Neighborhood Hospital, where a diagnosis of stroke is made. She has a feeding tube and indwelling catheter placed, and later develops a fever and confusion. Urine in the drainage bag is cloudy. A urine specimen is collected and sent to the laboratory for urinalysis and culture and sensitivity. Results confirm the diagnosis of UTI.

1. How will Mrs. James' history of diabetes mellitus affect her risk for UTI and response to treatment?
2. What risk factors does Mrs. James have that place her at increased risk for UTI?
3. After removing the indwelling catheter and treating the UTI with antibiotics for 7 days, urine culture reveals the bacteria remain in the urine. What does the nurse anticipate will be done next if the client still experiences symptoms? How would the treatment differ if the client did not have symptoms?

PEARSON
EXPLORE mynursingkit™

MyNursingKit is your one stop for online chapter review materials and resources. Prepare for success with additional NCLEX®-style practice questions, interactive assignments and activities, web links, animations and videos, and more!

Register your access code from the front of your book at **www.mynursingkit.com**.

REFERENCES

Abelson, M.B., & Granet, D. (2006). Ocular allergy in pediatric practice. *Current Allergy and Asthma Reports, 6,* 306–311.

Alexander, M. (2003). Ocular allergy: Treatment options for children. *Contemporary Pediatrics* (Suppl.), 3–6.

American Academy of Pediatrics. (2006). *Red book: 2006 Report of the Committee on Infectious Diseases* (27th ed.). Elk Grove Village, IL: American Academy of Pediatrics.

American Academy of Pediatrics, Subcommittee on Management of Acute Otitis Media. (2004). Diagnosis and management of acute otitis media. *Pediatrics 113,* 1451–1465.

Aronson, B. (2005). Medication management behaviors of adherent short-term antibiotic users. *Clinical Excellence for Nurse Practitioners, 9*(1), 23–30.

Arrowsmith, V.A., Maunder, J.A., Sargent, R.J., & Taylor, R. (2005). Removal of nail polish and finger rings to prevent surgical infection. *The Cochrane Library* (Oxford) (ID #CD003325).

Baine, W.B., Yu, W., & Summe, J.P. (2001). The epidemiology of hospitalization of elderly Americans for septicemia or bacteremia in 1991–1998. Application of Medicare claims data. *Annals of Epidemiology, 11*(2), 118–126.

Barbacane, J.L. (2004). Back to the basics: Hand washing. *Geriatric Nursing, 25*(2), 90–92.

Bardsley, A. (2005). Use of lubricant gels in urinary catheterization. *Nursing Standard, 20*(8), 41–46.

Becker, W., & Deeane, D. (1986) *The World of the Cell,* Redwood City, CA: Benjamin Cummings.

Bentley, D.W., Bradley, S., High, K., Schoenbaum, S., Taler, G., & Yoshikawa, T. (2001). Practice guidelines for evaluation of fever and infection in long-term care facilities. *Journal of the American Geriatrics Society, 49,* 210–222.

Bernius, M., & Perlin, D. (2006). Pediatric ear, nose, and throat emergencies. *Pediatric Clinics of North America, 53,* 195–214.

Bilukha, O.O., & Rosenstein, N. (2005). Prevention and control of meningococcal disease. *Morbidity and Mortality Weekly Report, 54*(RR-7), 1–21.

Boyce, J.M., & Pittet, D. (2002). Guideline for hand hygiene in health-care settings: Recommendations of the Healthcare Infection Control Practices Advisory Committee and the HICPAC/SHEA/APIC/IDSA Hand Hygiene Task Force. *Morbidity and Mortality Weekly Report, 51*(RR-16), 1–44.

Brashers, V.L. (2006). Structure and function of the pulmonary system. In K.L. McCance & S.E. Huether, *Pathophysiology: The biologic basis for disease in adults and children* (5th ed., pp. 1181–1204). St. Louis, MO: Elsevier Mosby.

Brook, I., & Gober, A. (2005). Recovery of potential pathogens and interfering bacteria in the nasopharynx of otitis media-prone children and their smoking and non-smoking patients. *Archives of Otolaryngology and Head & Neck Surgery, 131,* 509–512.

Carr, M.P. (2004). Waterless hand washing: A new era in hand hygiene. *Journal of Practical Hygiene, 13*(2), 33–36.

Centers for Disease Control and Prevention. (1987). Recommendations for prevention of HIV transmission in health-care settings. *Morbidity and Mortality Weekly Report, 36*(2s), 1S–18S.

Centers for Disease Control and Prevention. (1997). 1997 USPHS/IDSA guidelines for the prevention of opportunistic infections in persons infected with human immunodeficiency virus. *Morbidity and Mortality Weekly Report, 46*(RR-12), 1–46.

Centers for Disease Control and Prevention. (2001). Updated U.S. Public Health Service guidelines for the management of occupational exposures to HBV, HCV, and HIV and recommendations for postexposure prophylaxis. *Morbidity and Mortality Weekly Report, 50*(RR-11), 1–67.

Centers for Disease Control and Prevention. (2002a). Guidelines for hand hygiene in health-care settings. *Morbidity and Mortality Weekly Report, 51*(RR-16), 1–56.

Centers for Disease Control and Prevention. (2002b). Immunization registry use and progress—United States, 2001. *Morbidity and Mortality Weekly Report, 51*(3), 53–56.

Centers for Disease Control and Prevention. (2003). *Exposure to blood: What health care personnel need to know.* Atlanta, GA: Centers for Disease Control and Prevention.

Centers for Disease Control and Prevention. (2004a). Fact sheet. Basic information about SARS. Retrieved from http://www.cdc.gov/ncidod/sars/pdf/factsheet.pdf

Centers for Disease Control and Prevention. (2004b). *Sequence for donning and removing personal protective equipment.* Retrieved July 16, 2006, from http://www.cdc.gov/ncidod/dhqp/ppe.html

Centers for Disease Control and Prevention. (2004c). Vaccines for Children program. Retrieved May 12, 2006, from http://www.cdc.gov/PROGRAMS/IMMUN10.HTM

Centers for Disease Control and Prevention (2004d). Trends in Tuberculosis—United States, 1998–2003. *Morbidity and Mortality Weekly Report,* 53(10), 209–214.

Centers for Disease Control and Prevention. (2005a). Achievements in public health: Elimination of rubella and congenital rubella syndrome—United States, 1969–2004. *Morbidity and Mortality Weekly Report, 54*(11), 279–282.

Centers for Disease Control and Prevention. (2005b). Measles—United States, 2004. *Morbidity and Mortality Weekly Report, 54*(48), 1229–1231.

Centers for Disease Control and Prevention. (2005c). National, state, and urban area vaccination coverage among children aged 19–35 months—United States, 2004. *Morbidity and Mortality Weekly Report, 54*(29), 717–721.

Centers for Disease Control and Prevention. (2005d). *Public health guidance for community-level preparedness and response to severe acute respiratory syndrome (SARS) version 2: Supplement I: Infection control in healthcare, home, and community settings.* Retrieved June 3, 2006, from http://www.cdc.gov/ncidod/sars/guidance/I/healthcare.htm

Centers for Disease Control and Prevention. (2006a). CDC's advisory committee recommends changes in varicella vaccinations. Retrieved July 5, 2006, from http://cdc.gov/od/media/pressrel/r060629-b.htm

Centers for Disease Control and Prevention. (2006b). Emergence of *Mycobacterium tuberculosis* with extensive resistance to second-line drugs—Worldwide, 2000–2004. *Morbidity and Mortality Weekly Report, 55*(11), 301–305.

Centers for Disease Control and Prevention. (2006c). Preventing tetanus, diphtheria, and pertussis among adolescents: Use of tetanus toxoid, reduced diphtheria toxoid, and acellular pertussis vaccines. *Morbidity and Mortality Weekly Report, 55,* 1–34.

Centers for Disease Control and Prevention. (2006d). Prevention and control of influenza: Recommendations of the Advisory Committee on Immunization Practices (ACIP). *Morbidity and Mortality Weekly Report, 55,* 1–44.

Centers for Disease Control and Prevention. (2006e). *Recommended adult immunization schedule, United States, 2006.* Retrieved June 1, 2006, from http://www.cdc.gov/nip/recs/adult-schedule.htm#print

Centers for Disease Control and Prevention. (2006f). *Recommended childhood and adolescent immunization schedule, United States, 2005.* Retrieved June 1, 2006, from http://www.cdc.gov/nip/recs/child-schedule.htm#printable

Centers for Disease Control and Prevention. (2006g). Trends in tuberculosis—United States, 2005. *Morbidity and Mortality Weekly Report, 55*(11), 305–308.

Centers for Disease Control and Prevention. (2006h). Update: Multistate outbreak of mumps—United States, January 1–May 2, 2006. *Morbidity and Mortality Weekly Dispatch, 55,* 1–5.

Centers for Disease Control and Prevention (2006i). World TB day—March 24, 2006. *Morbidity and Mortality Weekly Report, 55*(11), 301.

Centers for Disease Control and Prevention. (2009). Fact Sheet. H_1N_1 Flu. Retrieved from http://www.cdc.gov/h1n1flu/

Centers for Medicare and Medicaid Services. (2005). Alcohol based hand rub solutions TIA 00-1 (101). *Federal Register, 70*(57), 15229–15239.

Centers for Disease Control And Prevention. (2009). *2009 H1N1 flu (Swine flu).* Retrieved from http://www.cdc.gov/H1N1FLU/

Cherry, J.D. (2005). The epidemiology of pertussis: A comparison of the epidemiology of the disease pertussis with the epidemiology of *Bordatella pertussis* infection. *Pediatrics, 115*(5), 1422–1427.

Christ-Crain, M., Jaccard-Stolz, D., Bingisser, R., Gencay, M.M., Huber, P.R., Tamm, M., et al. (2004). Effect of procalcitonin-guided treatment on antibiotic use and outcome in lower respiratory tract infections: Cluster-randomized, single-blinded intervention trial. *Lancet, 363*(9409), 600–607.

Conde-Agudelo, A.,Villar, J., & Lindheimer, M. (2008). Maternal infection and risk of preeclampsia: Systematic review and meta-analysis. *American Journal of Obstetrics & Gynecology, January,* 7–22.

Copstead, L.C., & Banasik, J.L. (2005). *Pathophysiology* (3rd ed.). St. Louis, MO: Elsevier/Saunders.

Curns, A.T., Holman, R.C., Shay, D.K., Cheek, J.E., Kaufman, S.F., Singleton, R.J., & Anderson, L.J. (2002). Outpatient and hospital visits associated with otitis media among American Indian and Alaska Native children younger than 5 years. *Pediatrics, 109*(3). Retrieved October 2, 2006, from http://www.pediatrics.org/cgi/content/full/109/3/e41

Curtis, D. (2007). *Cellulitis.* Retrieved October 2007 from http://www.emedicine.com/EMERG/topic88.htm

Daneshgari, F., Krugman, M., Bahn, A., & Lee, R.S. (2002). Evidence-based multidisciplinary practice: Improving the safety and standards of male bladder catheterization. *Medsurg Nursing, 11*(5), 236–241, 246.

Dennehy, P.H. (2005). Update on a high-morbidity infection: Rotavirus. *Contemporary Pediatrics, 22*(12), 34–40.

Dulczak, S., & Kirk, J. (2005). Overview of the evaluation, diagnosis, and management of urinary tract infections in infants and children. *Urologic Nursing, 25*(3), 185–191.

Durbin, W.J. (2004). Pneumococcal infections. *Pediatrics in Review, 25*(12), 418–423.

Evans-Smith, P. (Ed.). (2005). *Taylor's clinical nursing skills: A nursing process approach.* Philadelphia: Lippincott Williams & Wilkins.

Fauci, A., et al. (1998). *Harrison's principles of internal medicine* (14th ed.). New York: McGraw-Hill.

Foxlee, R., Johansson, A., Wejfalk, J., Dawkins, J., Dooley, L., & Del Mar, C. (2006). Topical anesthesia for acute otitis media. *Cochrane Database of Systematic Reviews* Issue 3. Art. No.: CD005657.DOI:10.1002/14651858.CD005657.pub2.

Froh, D.L. (2006). Alterations in pulmonary function in children. In K.L. McCance & S.E. Huether (Eds.), *Pathophysiology: The biologic basis for disease in adults and children* (5th ed., pp. 1249–1278). St. Louis, MO: Elsevier Mosby.

Gandhi, M. (2006). *Asymptomatic bacteruria*. Retrieved July 1, 2008, from http://www.nlm.nih.gov/medlineplus/ency/article/000520.htm

Garcia-Martin, M., Lardelli-Claret, P., Jimenez-Moleon, J.J., Bueno-Cavanillas, A., de Dios Luna del Castillo, J., & Galvez-Vargas, R. (2001). Proportion of hospital deaths potentially attributable to nosocomial infection. *Infection Control and Hospital Epidemiology, 22,* 708–714.

Garin, E.H., Olavarria, F., Nieto, V.G., Valenciano, B., Campos, A., & Young, L. (2006). Clinical significance of primary vesicoureteral reflux and urinary antibiotic prophylaxis after acute pyelonephritis: A multicenter, randomized controlled study. *Pediatrics, 117* (3), 626–632.

Garner, J.S., & Hospital Infection Control Practices Advisory Committee. (1996). Guidelines for isolation precautions in hospitals. *Infection Control Hospital Epidemiology, 17,* 53–80, and *American Journal of Infection Control, 24,* 24–52.

Garner, J.S., & Simmons, B.P. (1983). *CDC guideline for isolation precautions in hospitals* (HHS Publication No. CDC 83-8314). Atlanta, GA: U.S. Department of Health and Human Services, Public Health Service, Centers for Disease Control.

Goldrick, B.A. (2003). Adult respiratory infections. *American Journal of Nursing, 103* (10), 65–66.

Goldrick, B.A. (2004a). 21st century emerging and reemerging infections. *American Journal of Nursing, 104* (1), 67–70.

Goldrick, B.A. (2004b). MRSA, VRE, and VRSA: How do we control them in nursing homes? *American Journal of Nursing, 104* (8), 50–51.

Harrison, C.J. (2005). The microbiology of acute otitis media: Past, present, and future. *Contemporary Pediatrics, 22* (12), 8–16.

Haut, C. (2005). Oncological emergencies in the pediatric intensive care unit. *AACN Clinical Issues, 16,* 232–245.

Hospital Infection Control Practices Advisory Committee. (1995). Recommendations for preventing the spread of vancomycin resistance. *American Journal of Infection Control, 23,* 87–94; *Infection Control and Hospital Epidemiology, 16,* 105–113; and *Morbidity and Mortality Weekly Report, 44* (RR-12), 1–13.

Houghton, D. (2006). HAI prevention: The power is in your hands. *Nursing Management, 37* (Suppl.), 1–7.

Hoyert, D.L., Heron, M., Murphy, S.L., & Kung, H.C. (2006). Deaths: Final data for 2003. Health & Stats. Retrieved from http://www.cdc.gov/nchs/products/pubs/pubd/hestats/finaldeaths03

Huether, S.E. (2006). Alterations of renal and urinary tract function in children. In K.L. McCance & S.E. Huether, *Pathophysiology: The biologic basis for disease in adults and children* (5th ed., pp. 1337–1352). St. Louis, MO: Elsevier Mosby.

Jackson, M.M. (1993). Infection precautions: What works and what does not. *CRNA: The Clinical Forum for Nurse Anesthetists, 4* (2), 77–82.

Jarvis, J.R. (2001). Infection control and changing health-care delivery systems. *Emerging Infectious Diseases, 7,* 170–173.

Joint Commission on Accreditation of Healthcare Organizations. (2006). *National patient safety goals.* Retrieved June 3, 2006, from http://www.jointcommission.org/Standards/NationalPatientSafetyGoals/

Kasper, D.L., Braunwald, E., Fauci, A.S., Hauser, S.L., Longo, D.L., & Jameson, J.L. (Eds.). (2005). *Harrison's principles of internal medicine* (16th ed.). New York: McGraw-Hill.

Kjonegaard, R., & Myers, F.E., III. (2005). Arresting drug-resistant organisms. *Nursing 2005, 35* (6), 48–50.

Krogh, R.H., & Bruskewitz, R.C. (1998). Disorders of the lower genitourinary tract. *Clinical Geriatrics, 6* (13), 19–25.

LaRosa, S.P. (2008). *Sepsis*. Retrieved April 20, 2009, from http://www.clevelandclinicmeded.com/medicalpubs/diseasemanagement/infectious-disease/sepsis/

Lehne, R.A. (2004). *Pharmacology for nursing care* (4th ed.). St. Louis, MO: Saunders/Elsevier.

Mah, F. (2006). Bacterial conjunctivitis. *Pediatric Clinics of North America, 53* (Suppl. 1), 7–10.

Mahabee-Gittens, E.M., Grupp-Phelan, J., Brody, A.S., Donnelly, L.F., Bracey, S.E.A., Duma, E.M., et al. (2005). Identifying children with pneumonia in the emergency department. *Clinical Pediatrics, 44,* 427–435.

Mahon, C.R., & Manuselis, G., Jr. (1995). *Textbook of diagnostic microbiology.* Philadelphia: W.B. Saunders.

Markenson, D. (2005). The treatment of children exposed to pathogens linked to bioterrorism. *Infectious Diseases of North America, 19,* 731–745.

Mayo Foundation for Medical Education and Research, (2006). *Recurrent ceullulitis: What causes it?* Retrieved October 15, 2007, from http://ww.nlm.nih.gov/medlineplus/cellulitis.html

McCance, K., & Huether, S. (2002). *Pathophysiology: The biologic basis for disease in adults and children* (4th ed.). St. Louis, MO: Mosby.

McCue, J.D. (1999). Treatment of urinary tract infections in long-term care facilities: Advice, guidelines, and algorithms. *Clinical Geriatrics, 7* (8), 11–17.

Moyad, M.A., & Robinson, L.E. (2008). Lessons learned from the 2007–2008 cold and flu season: What worked and what was worthless. *Urological Nursing, 28* (2), 146-150.

Müller, B., & Becker, K.L. (2001). Procalcitonin: How a hormone became a marker and mediator of sepsis. *Swiss Medical Weekly, 131,* 595–602.

National Center for Complementary and Alternative Medicine. (2004). Consumer advisory. Ephedra. Retrieved from http://www.nccam.nih.gov/health/alerts/ephedra/consumeradvisory

National Center for Complementary and Alternative Medicine (2005). Herbs at a glance. Echinacea. Retrieved from http://www.nccam.nih.gov/health/echinacea/

National Center for HIV, STD, and TB Prevention, Division of Tuberculosis Elimination. (2004). *Self-study modules on tuberculosis*. Retrieved July 16, 2006, from http://www.phppo.cdc.gov/phtn/tbmodules/Default.htm

National Institute of Allergy and Infectious Diseases, National Institutes of Health. (2006). Focus on the flu. Retrieved from http://www3.niaid.nih.gov/news/focuson/flu/research/primer/default.htm

National Institute for Occupational Safety and Health. (1999). *Preventing needlestick injuries in health care settings.* (DHHS Publication No. 2000-108) Cincinnati, OH: U.S. Department of Health and Human Services, Public Health Service, Centers for Disease Control and Prevention, National Institute for Occupational Safety and Health.

National Kidney and Urological Diseases Information Clearinghouse, (2003). Urinary tract infections in children. NIH Publication No. 04-4246. Retrieved December 13, 2004, from http://www.kidney.niddk.nih.gov/kudiseases/pubs/uitchildren/index.htm

Nelson, L.J., Schneider, E., Wells, C.D., & Moore, M. (2004). Epidemiology of childhood tuberculosis in the United States, 1993–2001: The need for continued vigilance. *Pediatrics, 114* (2), 333–341,

Neto, J.F., Hemb, L., & Silva, D.B. (2006). Systematic literature review of modifiable risk factors for recurrent acute otitis media in childhood. *Journal of Pediatrics (Rio J), 82,* 87–96.

Nicolle, L.E. (2003). Urinary tract infections in the elderly. In W.R. Hazzard, J.P. Blass, J.B. Halter, J.G. Ouslander, & M.E. Tinetti (Eds.), *Principles of geriatric medicine and gerontology* (5th ed., pp. 1107–1116). New York: McGraw-Hill.

Otitis Media with Effusion. (2004). Clinical practice guideline. *Pediatrics, 113,* 1412–1429.

Pagana, K.D., & Pagana, T.J. (2002). *Mosby's manual of diagnostic and laboratory tests* (2nd ed.). St. Louis, MO: Mosby.

Peate, I. (2004). Infection control. Occupational exposure of staff to HIV and prophylaxis therapy. *British Journal of Nursing, 13,* 1146–1150.

Pelton, S.I. (2005). Otitis media: Re-evaluation of diagnosis and treatment in the era of antimicrobial resistance, pneumococcal conjugate vaccine, and evolving morbidity. *Pediatric Clinics of North America, 52,* 711–728.

Porth, C. (2005). *Pathophysiology: Concepts of altered health states* (6th ed.). Philadelphia: Lippincott Williams & Wilkins.

Posani, T. (2004). *Clostridium difficile:* Causes and interventions. *Critical Care Nursing Clinics of North America, 16* (4), 547–551.

Raboud, J., Saskin, R., Wong, K., Moore, C., Parucha, G., Bennett, J., et al. (2004). Patterns of handwashing behavior and visits to patients on a general medical ward of health care workers. *Infection Control and Hospital Epidemiology, 25,* 198–202.

Rao, A.S., & Bradley, S.F. (2003). *Clostridium difficile* in older adults and residents of long-term care facilities. *Annals of Long-Term Care, 11* (5), 42–47.

Raszka, W.V., & Khan, O. (2005). Pyelonephritis. *Pediatrics in Review, 26* (10), 364–369.

Reznik, M., & Ozuah, P.O. (2005). A prudent approach to screening for and treating tuberculosis. *Contemporary Pediatrics, 22* (11), 73–88.

Sarrell, E.M., Cohen, H.A., & Kahan, E. (2003). Naturopathic treatment for ear pain in children. *Pediatrics, 111,* e574–e579.

Sarrell, E.M., Wielunsky, E., & Cohen, H.A. (2006). Antipyretic treatment in young children with fever. *Archives of Pediatric and Adolescent Medicine, 160* (2), 197–202.

Sehulster, L.M., Chinn, R.Y.W., Arduino, M.J., Carpenter, J., Donlan, R., Ashford, D., et al. (2004). *Guidelines for environmental infection control in health-care facilities. Recommendations from CDC and the Healthcare Infection Control Practices Advisory Committee (HICPAC).* Chicago: American Society for Healthcare Engineering/American Hospital Association.

Smail, F. (2007). Asymptomatic bacteriuria in pregnancy. *Best Practice & Research Clinical Obstetrics and Gynaecology, 21* (3), 439–450.

Sole, M.L., Lamborn, M.L., & Hartshorn, J.C. (Eds.). (2001). *Introduction to critical care nursing* (3rd ed.). Philadelphia: Saunders.

Sopena, N., & Sabria, M. (2005). Multicenter study of hospital-acquired pneumonia in non-ICU patients. *Chest, 127* (1), 213–219.

Srinivasan, A., McDonald, L.C., Jernigan, D., Helfand, R., Ginsheimer, K., Jernigan, J., et al. (2004). Foundations of the severe acute respiratory syndrome preparedness and response plan for healthcare facilities. *Infection Control and Hospital Epidemiology, 25,* 1020–1025.

Steers, W.D. (1999). Meeting the urologic needs of the aging population. *Clinical Geriatrics, 7* (5), 62–64, 73.

Stephenson, M. (2003). Mucopurulent discharge is good sign conjunctivitis is bacterial. *Infectious Diseases in Children, 3,* 32–33.

Stirling, B., Littlejohn, P., & Willbond, M.L. (2004). Nurses and the control of infectious disease: Understanding epidemiology and disease transmission is vital to nursing care. *The Canadian Nurse, 100*(9): 16-20.

Stone, P.W., Hedblom, E.C., Murphy, D.M., & Miller, S.B. (2005). The economic impact of infection control: Making the business case for increased infection control resources. *American Journal of Infection Control, 33* (9), 542–547.

Sunenshine, R.H., & McDonald, L.C. (2006). *Clostridium difficile*-associated disease: New challenges from an established pathogen. *Cleveland Clinical Journal of Medicine, 73,* 187–197.

Swigart, V., & Kolb, R. (2004). Homeless persons' decisions to accept or reject public health disease-detection services. *Public Health Nursing, 21* (2), 162–170.

Taylor, Z. (2005). Guidelines for the investigation of contacts of persons with infectious tuberculosis. *Morbidity and Mortality Weekly Report, 54* (RR15), 1–37.

Taylor, Z., Nolan, C.M., & Blumberg, H.M. (2005). Controlling tuberculosis in the United States: Recommendations from the American Thoracic Society, CDC, and Infectious Diseases Society of America. *Morbidity and Mortality Weekly Report, 54* (RR12), 1–81.

Teoh, D.L., & Reynolds, S. (2003). Diagnosis and management of pediatric conjunctivitis. *Pediatric Emergency Care, 19,* 48–55.

Tierney, L.M., Jr., McPhee, S.J., & Papadakis, M.A. (Eds.). (2005). *Current medical diagnosis & treatment* (44th ed.). New York: McGraw-Hill.

Tierney, L., McPhee, S., & Papadakis, M. (Eds). (2007). *Current medical diagnosis & treatment 2007* (46th ed). Stamford, CT: Appleton & Lange.

Tiwari, T., Murphy, T.V., & Moran, J. (2005). Recommended antimicrobial agents for the treatment and postexposure prophylaxis of pertussis: 2005 CDC guidelines. *Morbidity and Mortality Weekly Report, 54* (RR-14), 1–16.

Ünlü, H., Sardan, Y.C., & Ülker, S. (2007). Comparison of sampling methods for urine cultures. *Journal of Nursing Scholarship, 39* (4), 325–329.

U.S. Department of Health and Human Services, Office of Disease Prevention and Promotion. (2000). *Healthy People 2010.* Washington, D.C. Retrieved from http://www.healthypeople.gov

U.S. Department of Health and Human Services, Public Health Service. (1988). Update: Universal precautions for prevention of transmission of human immunodeficiency virus, hepatitis B virus, and other bloodborne pathogens in health care settings. *Morbidity and Mortality Weekly Report, 37* (24), 377–388.

U.S. Food and Drug Administration. (2000). *Relenza consumer information.* Retrieved from http://www.fda.gov/cder/consumerinfo/druginfo/relenza.HTM

U.S. Food and Drug Administration. (2006). FDA approves a second drug for prevention of influenza A and B in adults and children. Retrieved April 3, 2006, from http://www.fda.gov/bbs/topics/news/2006/new01231.html

U.S. Occupational Safety & Health Administration. (2005). *Latex allergy.* Retrieved June 3, 2006, from http://www.osha.gov/SLTC/latexallergy/

Warny, M., Pepin, J., Fang, A., Killgore, G., Thompson, A., Brazier, J., et al. (2005). Toxic production by an emerging strain of *Clostridium difficile* associated with outbreaks of severe disease in North America and Europe. *Lancet, 366,* 1079–1083.

Windmill, S., & Windmill, I.M. (2006). The status of diagnostic testing following referral from universal newborn hearing screening. *Journal of the American Academy of Audiology, 17,* 367–378.

World Health Organization. (2005). *WHO guidelines on hand hygiene in health care*. Geneva, Switzerland: World Health Organization.

World Health Organization. (2009). *Influenza A(H1N1) – update 5.* Retrieved August 7, 2009, from http://www.who.int/csr/don/2009_04_29/en/index.html

Yetman, R.J., Parks, D., & Taft, E. (2002). Management of patients exposed to biologic weapons. *Journal of Pediatric Health Care, 16* (5), 256–261.

Zacharyczuk, C. (2004). New guidelines outline AOM management options. *Infectious Diseases in Children,* (April), 24.

Inflammation 16

Concept at-a-Glance

Concept Learning Outcomes

After reading about this concept you will be able to:

1. Summarize the physiologic process required to mount an inflammatory response and describe the response's contribution to homeostasis.
2. List factors affecting inflammation.
3. Identify commonly occurring alterations in inflammatory response and related treatments.
4. Explain common physical assessment procedures used to examine inflammation in clients across the life span.
5. Outline diagnostic and laboratory tests and expected findings to determine the individual's inflammatory response.
6. Explain management of inflammatory disorders aimed at limiting the response and supporting the helpful effects.
7. Demonstrate nursing process in providing culturally competent and caring interventions across the life span for individuals with inflammatory disorders.
8. Identify pharmacologic interventions in caring for the individual with inflammatory disorders.

Concept Key Terms

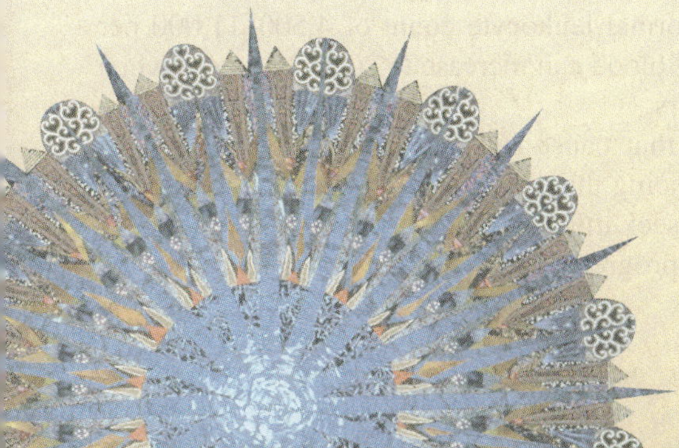

About Inflammation

Inflammation is a nonspecific but complex response to reduce the effects of what the body sees as harmful. Inflammation may result from an injury such as an ankle sprain. It may also result from an underlying infection. Autoimmune diseases frequently cause inflammation sufficient to result in tissue damage. Other harmful agents include pathogens, damaged cells, and irritants.

Under normal circumstances, inflammation acts as a protective process that stimulates healing and prevents further damage or progressive deterioration. The occasional uncomfortable symptoms of normal inflammation are usually successfully treated with palliative care. However, the inflammatory process can get carried away, leading to problems such as autoimmune disorders (e.g., rheumatoid arthritis, psoriasis, asthma, and allergies). These conditions may require more aggressive care, including pharmacotherapy. •

NORMAL PRESENTATION

Inflammation is an adaptive response to injury or illness that brings fluid, dissolved substances, and blood cells into the interstitial tissues where the invasion or damage has occurred. The response is called *nonspecific* because the same events occur regardless of the cause of the inflammatory process. Through the inflammatory reaction, the invader is neutralized and eliminated, destroyed tissue is removed, and the process of healing and repair is initiated. Inflammation is the first phase of the healing process. During the inflammatory process, particulate matter, bacteria, damaged cells, and inflammatory exudate are removed through phagocytosis. This process, called **debridement**, prepares the wound for healing. Adequate nutrition is essential for inflammation and healing to proceed. Through the process of inflammation, a large number of potentially damaging chemicals and microorganisms may be neutralized.

Inflammation is an adaptive mechanism that destroys or dilutes the injurious agent, prevents further spread of the injury, and promotes the repair of damaged tissue. It is characterized by five signs: (a) pain, (b) swelling, (c) redness, (d) heat, and (e) impaired function of the part, if the injury is severe. Commonly, words with the suffix *-itis* describe an inflammatory process. For example, *appendicitis* means inflammation of the appendix; *gastritis* means inflammation of the stomach.

Injurious agents can be categorized as physical agents, chemical agents, and microorganisms. *Physical agents* include mechanical objects causing trauma to tissues, excessive heat or cold, and radiation. *Chemical agents* include external irritants (e.g., strong acids, alkalis, poisons, and irritating gases) and internal irritants (substances manufactured within the body, such as excessive hydrochloric acid in the stomach). Microorganisms that can cause inflammation include bacteria and viruses.

The Function of Inflammation

The human body has developed many complex ways to defend itself against injury and invasion by microorganisms. Inflammation is one of these defense mechanisms. The central purpose of inflammation is to contain the injury or destroy the microorganism. By neutralizing the foreign agent and removing cellular debris and dead cells, inflammation allows repair of the injured area to proceed at a faster pace. Signs of inflammation include swelling, pain, warmth, and redness of the affected area.

Inflammation may be classified as *acute* or *chronic*. During acute inflammation, such as that caused by minor physical injury, 8–10 days are normally needed for the symptoms to resolve and repair to begin. If the body cannot contain or neutralize the damaging agent, inflammation may continue for long periods and become chronic. In chronic autoimmune disorders, such as lupus and rheumatoid arthritis, inflammation may persist for years with symptoms becoming progressively worse. Other disorders such as seasonal allergies occur at predictable times during each year, and the resulting inflammation may produce only minor, annoying symptoms.

Stages of Inflammation

A series of dynamic events is commonly referred to as the three stages of the inflammatory response:

First stage: Vascular and cellular responses
Second stage: Exudate production
Third stage: Reparative phase.

VASCULAR AND CELLULAR RESPONSES At the start of the first stage of inflammation, blood vessels at the site of injury or infection constrict. The injured tissues release histamines, kinins, and prostaglandins in response to the injury or infection. These substances serve as chemical mediators to dilate blood vessels and contract smooth muscle, causing more blood to flow to the injured area. This marked increase in blood supply is referred to as **hyperemia** and is responsible for the characteristic sign of redness and the heat that accompanies inflammation.

Vascular permeability increases at the site with dilation of the vessels. Fluid, proteins, and **leukocytes** (white blood cells) leak into the interstitial spaces, causing the signs of inflammatory swelling (edema) and pain to appear. Pain is caused by the pressure of accumulating fluid on nerve endings and the irritating chemical mediators. Fluid pouring into areas such as the pleural or pericardial cavity can seriously affect organ function. In other areas, such as joints, mobility is impaired by accumulating fluid.

Blood flow slows in the dilated vessels, allowing more leukocytes to arrive at the injured tissues. The leukocytes aggregate or line up along the inner surface of the blood vessels. This process is known as **margination**. Leukocytes then move through the blood vessel wall into the affected tissue spaces, a process called **emigration**.

In response to the exit of leukocytes from the blood, the bone marrow produces more leukocytes in even larger numbers and releases them into the bloodstream. This process is called **leukocytosis**. A normal leukocyte count of 4,500–11,000 per cubic millimeter of blood can increase to 20,000 or more when inflammation occurs.

All conditions that cause inflammation will result in an individual experiencing this first stage of inflammation. Often individuals do not seek medical treatment for an inflammatory response unless it progresses to the second stage and exudate results. Typical injuries for which an individual will seek treatment for stage 1 inflammation include sprained ankles and wrists, broken bones, and minor blunt force injuries (e.g., two children running into each other on a playground).

EXUDATE PRODUCTION In the second stage of inflammation, inflammatory **exudate** is produced. The term *exudate* comes from the Latin word meaning "exude" or "to ooze." Exudate consists of fluid that escaped from the blood vessels, dead phagocytic cells, and dead tissue cells and the products they release.

The nature and amount of exudate vary according to the tissue involved and the intensity and duration of the inflammation. The major types of exudate are serous, purulent, and hemorrhagic (sanguineous). Serous exudate typically accompanies mild inflammation and presents as clear or straw colored with a thin, watery consistency. Purulent exudate is usually opaque, or milky. Commonly referred to as "pus," purulent exudate normally indicates the presence of infection and contains a large quantity of cells and necrotic debris. Because hemorrhagic exudate contains blood from ruptured blood vessels, it is red and thick. This type of exudate exudes from tissue or its capillaries as a result of infection or injury.

Whether the presence of exudate should be reported depends primarily on the underlying cause and the amount and degree of the exudate. A minor cut that exhibits either serous or hemorrhagic exudate may resolve with simple first aid. Exudate over a larger surface or that appears in conjunction with other symptoms, such as fever, will warrant a greater degree of medical care.

REPARATIVE PHASE The third stage of the inflammatory response involves the repair of injured tissues by regeneration or replacement with fibrous tissue (scar) formation. **Regeneration** is the replacement of destroyed tissue cells by cells that are identical or similar in structure and function. Damaged cells are replaced one by one, and new cells are organized so that the architectural pattern and function of the tissue are restored. The ability to regenerate cells varies considerably from one type of tissue to another. For example, epithelial tissues of the skin and the digestive and respiratory tracts have a good regenerative capacity, as long as their underlying support structures are intact. The same holds true for osseous, lymphoid, and bone marrow tissues. Tissues that have little regenerative capacity include nervous, muscular, and elastic tissues.

When regeneration is not possible, repair occurs by fibrous (scar) tissue formation. The inflammatory exudate with its interlacing network of fibrin provides the framework for this tissue to develop. Damaged tissues are replaced with the connective tissue elements of collagen, blood capillaries, lymphatics, and other tissue-bound substances. In the early stages of this process, the tissue is called **granulation tissue**. It is a fragile, gelatinous tissue that appears pink or red because of the many newly formed capillaries. Later in the process, the tissue shrinks (the capillaries are constricted, even obliterated) and the collagen fibers contract, leaving a firmer fibrous tissue. This is called cicatrix, or scar tissue.

Histamine is a key chemical mediator of inflammation (Table 16–1). It is stored primarily within mast cells located in tissue spaces under epithelial membranes such as the skin, bronchial tree, and digestive tract and along blood vessels. **Mast cells** detect foreign agents or injury and respond by releasing histamine, which initiates the inflammatory response within seconds. In addition to its role in inflammation, histamine also directly stimulates pain receptors. Both mast cells and histamine are important components of theallergic process.

When released at an injury site, histamine dilates nearby blood vessels, causing capillaries to become more permeable. Plasma, complement proteins, and phagocytes can then enter the area to neutralize foreign agents. The affected area may become congested with blood, which can lead to significant swelling and pain. Figure 16–1 ■ illustrates the fundamental steps in acute inflammation.

Rapid release of the chemical mediators of inflammation on a large scale throughout the body is responsible for **anaphylaxis**, a life-threatening allergic response that may result in shock and death (Box 16–1). A number of chemicals, insect stings, foods, and some therapeutic drugs can cause this widespread release of histamine from mast cells if the person has an allergy to any of these substances.

TABLE 16–1 **Chemical Mediators of Inflammation**

MEDIATOR	DESCRIPTION
Bradykinin	Present in an inactive form in plasma and mast cells; vasodilator that causes pain; effects are similar to those of histamine
Complement	Series of at least 20 proteins that combine in a cascade fashion to neutralize or destroy an antigen
Histamine	Stored and released by mast cells; causes dilation of blood vessels, smooth-muscle constriction, tissue swelling, and itching
Leukotrienes	Stored and released by mast cells; effects are similar to those of histamine
Prostaglandins	Present in most tissues and stored and released by mast cells; increase capillary permeability, attract white blood cells to site of inflammation, and cause pain

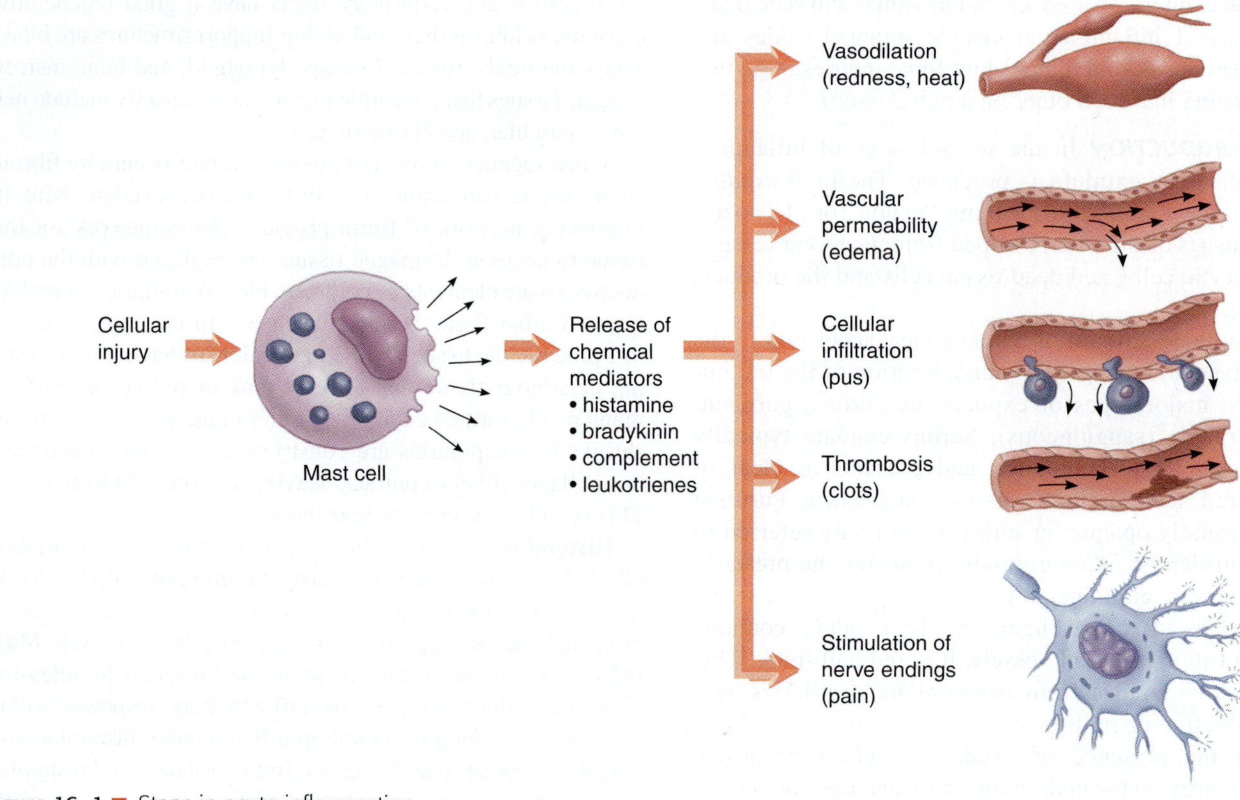

Figure 16–1 ■ Steps in acute inflammation.

Histamine Receptors

Histamine works by combining with specific cellular histamine receptors. There are four classified receptors, with the H_1 receptors and H_2 receptors participating in the inflammatory process. **H_1 receptors** are present in the smooth muscle of the vascular system, the bronchial tree, and the digestive tract. Stimulation of these receptors results in itching, pain, edema, vasodilation, bronchoconstriction, and the characteristic symptoms of inflammation and allergy. In contrast, **H_2 receptors** are present primarily in the stomach, and their stimulation results in the secretion of large amounts of hydrochloric acid.

Box 16–1 **Symptoms and Treatment of Anaphylaxis**

Anaphylaxis is a life-threatening allergic reaction that necessitates immediate emergency medical treatment. Anaphylaxis develops extremely rapidly—in seconds to minutes—and requires immediate initiation of the Emergency Medical System (EMS). Signs and symptoms of anaphylaxis include the following:

- Wheezing sounds, labored breathing
- Nausea, vomiting, or diarrhea
- Weakness, light-headedness, dizziness
- Blue skin as a result of oxygenation impairment or pale skin resulting from shock (advanced signs)
- Inflammation of the airways, swelling of the throat (this can become severe enough to block the airway)
- Hives, itching
- Low blood pressure
- Abnormal heart rhythm.

Epinephrine is the first line of treatment for an individual experiencing an anaphylactic reaction. Given by subcutaneous or intramuscular injection, epinephrine dilates the airways and narrows the blood vessels, essentially counteracting the allergic response. Some allergic individuals carry EpiPens™, self-injectors with epinephrine, to use in the case of an anaphylactic response. EMS should be called for an individual having an anaphylactic reaction even if he or she is carrying and uses an EpiPen™. During and immediately following an anaphylactic response, airway protection is critical, so adjunctive medications may include beta-agonists, antihistamines, and corticosteroids. A severe reaction resulting in laryngeal swelling sufficient to close the airway may require a tracheotomy.

ALTERATIONS

Inflammation can occur in virtually any tissue, organ, or system. The suffix *-itis* indicates inflammation such as in appendic*itis*, arthr*itis* or pancreat*itis*. Many autoimmune disorders involve the inflammatory response and result from the body misinterpreting its own tissues as harmful and needing to be destroyed or limited. Rheumatoid arthritis, systemic lupus erythematosus, and Guillain Barré syndrome are a few examples of autoimmune responses involving inflammation. The following are some common diseases that have an inflammatory component:

- Allergic rhinitis
- Anaphylaxis
- Ankylosing spondylitis
- Appendicitis
- Arthritis (the most common inflammatory disorder, and the leading cause of disability in the United States)
- Contact dermatitis
- Crohn's disease
- Gallbladder disease
- Hashimoto's thyroiditis
- Inflammatory bowel disease (affecting 300,000–500,000 Americans each year)
- Nephritis
- Peptic ulcers
- Rheumatoid arthritis
- Systemic lupus erythematosus
- Ulcerative colitis.

ALTERATIONS AND TREATMENTS Inflammation

Alteration	Description	Treatment
Anaphylaxis	A severe and acute systemic allergic reaction proceeds to anaphylactic shock after large quantities of immunological mediators are released. Acute inflammation can result in edema of the airways and anoxia.	Epinephrine, dexamethasone, and diphenhydramine are usually the medications of choice. Nursing care includes maintaining a patent airway, removing allergens causing reaction if possible, and reducing client anxiety. If treatment is not initiated quickly enough, a tracheostomy may be performed to open the airway and prevent or treat respiratory arrest.
Ankylosing spondylitis	Chronic painful inflammatory arthritis primarily affects the spine and sacroiliac joints, causing fusion of the spine.	No cure is available but treatments include physical therapy, exercise, and medications including NSAIDs, immunosuppressants, and biologicals that are tumor necrosis factor (TNF) blockers.
Appendicitis	The appendix is inflamed.	The inflamed appendix is surgically removed.
Crohn's disease	Inflammatory disease of the anus.	No cure is known. Exacerbations can be treated and prevented with changes to lifestyle (changes in diet, smoking cessation, and proper hydration), antibiotics for infections, aminosalicylate, and anti-inflammatory drugs. If exacerbations do not respond to medical treatment, surgical removal of the inflamed area may be required.
Glomerulonephritis	The glomeruli in the kidneys are inflamed.	Acute form may improve spontaneously with treatment of cause, often antibiotics for strep infection. Other treatments for acute and chronic form may include diuretics, ACE inhibitors, calcium channel blockers, and beta blockers. Temporary dialysis may be needed to support kidney function if kidney failure occurs.
Ulcerative colitis	Inflammatory bowel disease usually affects the large bowel and is characterized by ulcerated areas causing bloody diarrhea.	Treatment depends on extent of bowel involvement and disease severity. Aminosalicylates, corticosteroids, immunosuppressive drugs, and surgery are the most common treatments. Oatmeal and fiber from Brassica may be recommended because they seem to reverse ulceration.

Inflammation Assessment

Local Manifestations	Systemic Manifestations
■ Erythema ■ Warmth ■ Pain ■ Edema ■ Functional impairment	■ T > 100.4°F (38°C) or < 96.8°F (36°C) ■ P > 90 beats/min ■ R > 20 breaths/min (tachypnea) ■ WBC > 12,000/mm³ or >10% bands

ASSESSMENT

During the assessment phase of the nursing process, the nurse obtains the client's history, conducts the physical assessment, and gathers laboratory data. Assessment for inflammation, which can impact any of the body's tissues, will be guided by the area of the body involved. Classic signs to assess for are indicated in the Inflammation Assessment feature.

When taking the patient's medical history, the nurse assesses (a) the degree to which a client is at risk of developing inflammation and (b) any client self-reports that suggest the presence of inflammation. To identify clients at risk, the nurse reviews the client's chart and structures the nursing interview to collect data regarding the factors influencing the development of inflammation, especially existing conditions. Because inflammation can involve any organ or organ system, a thorough history of the patient's systems is required.

Signs and symptoms of inflammation vary according to the body area involved. Appendicitis may involve abdominal pain, rigid abdomen, and elevated white blood cell (WBC) count. Arthritis may involve joints that are warm, red, edematous, and painful. As a result, physical assessment may be focused on any area of the body, depending on where the inflammation is suspected or noted. Localized inflammation requires assessment for localized edema, pain or tenderness with palpation or movement, redness or palpable heat at the inflamed area, and reduced or absent function in the body part involved. Conditions causing more widespread inflammation, such as nephritis or allergies, may cause more diverse symptoms.

DIAGNOSTIC TESTS

A primary laboratory test ordered to detect the presence of inflammation is the erythrocyte sedimentation rate (ESR). ESR measures how far the erythrocyte settles in a tube over a given period of time, usually 1 hour. Normal sedimentation rate for males is 0–15 mm/h, 0–20 mm/h for women. It is not unusual to see the sedimentation rate slightly elevated in older adults. When an inflammatory process is active, the increased proportion of fibrinogen causes red blood cells to stick to one another and settle faster, resulting in a higher reading.

Another important diagnostic laboratory test is the C-reactive protein (CRP). CRP is a protein found in the blood that is produced by the liver and fat cells in response to the inflammatory process. In the absence of liver failure, a rise in CRP levels indicates an inflammatory process is occurring somewhere in the body. CRP can also be used to evaluate the effectiveness of treatment for inflammation. Research also indicates the CRP can be used to assess risk for cardiac disease, as it elevates in response to arterial damage.

Other laboratory tests for inflammation are ordered based on the cause, location, and type of inflammation suspected. A WBC with differential may be ordered to determine the presence of an infection (Table 16–2); serum protein electrophoresis may reveal increased gamma globulin and decreased albumin, indicating systemic lupus erythematosus; and routine chemistry panels may reveal kidney involvement, abnormal liver function, or increased muscle enzymes if the muscle is involved.

Assessment Interview Inflammation

- Do you have any pain? If the client reports pain, the nurse should assess the pain for location, intensity, type, severity, current treatments, and effectiveness of treatment.
- Are you taking any anti-inflammatory medications such as aspirin or ibuprofen, or medications for chronic conditions?
- Have you had any recent diagnostic procedure or therapy that penetrated your skin or a body cavity?
- What past surgeries have you had?
- How would you describe your eating habits? Do you eat a variety of types of foods?
- Do you take vitamins or dietary supplements?
- On a scale of 1–10, how would you rate the stress you have experienced in the last 6 months?
- Have you experienced any loss of energy, loss of appetite, nausea, headache, or other signs associated with specific body systems (e.g., difficulty urinating, urinary frequency, or a sore throat)?

Note: As with all history taking, the nurse must individualize the specific terms used; give examples to the client; and use teaching techniques to validate agreement on the meaning of words according to the client's culture, language spoken, and education or intellectual abilities.

TABLE 16–2 **The White Blood Cell Count and Differential**

CELL TYPE AND NORMAL VALUE	INCREASED	DECREASED
Total white blood cells (WBCs): 4,000–10,000 per mm^3	*Leukocytosis:* Infection or inflammation, leukemia, trauma or stress, tissue necrosis	*Leukopenia:* Bone marrow depression, overwhelming infection, viral infections, immunosuppression, autoimmune disease, dietary deficiency
Neutrophils (segs, PMNs, or polys): 55–70%	*Neutrophilia:* Acute infection or stress response, myelocytic leukemia, inflammatory or metabolic disorders	*Neutropenia:* Bone marrow depression, overwhelming bacterial infection, viral infection, Addison's disease
Eosinophils (eos): 1–4%	*Eosinophilia:* Parasitic infections, hyper-sensitivity reactions, autoimmune disorders	*Eosinopenia:* Cushing's syndrome, autoimmune disorders, stress, certain drugs
Basophils (basos): 0.5–1%	*Basophilia:* Hypersensitivity responses, chronic myelogenous leukemia, chickenpox or smallpox, splenectomy, hypothyroidism	*Basopenia:* Acute stress or hypersensitivity reactions, hyperthyroidism
Monocytes (monos): 2–8%	*Monocytosis:* Chronic inflammatory disorders, tuberculosis, viral infections, leukemia, Hodgkin's disease, multiple myeloma	*Monocytopenia:* Bone marrow depression, corticosteroid therapy
Lymphocytes (lymphs): 20–40%	*Lymphocytosis:* Chronic bacterial infection, viral infections, lymphocytic leukemia	*Lymphocytopenia:* Bone marrow depression, immunodeficiency, leukemia, Cushing's syndrome, Hodgkin's disease, renal failure

Source: Data from Corbett, J. V. (2004). *Laboratory tests and diagnostic procedures with nursing diagnoses* (6th ed.). Upper Saddle River, NJ: Prentice Hall; Pagana, K. D. and Pagana, T. J. (1997). *Diagnostic and laboratory test reference* (3rd ed.). St. Louis, MO: Mosby-Year Book.

CARING INTERVENTIONS

Management of inflammation due to injury is generally aimed at reducing mobility of the involved area, elevation to reduce edema, antipyretics if fever is involved, and anti-inflammatory medications. Other causes of inflammation will necessitate other, more specific treatments. For example, surgery will be indicated in most cases for appendicitis and gallbladder disease, antibiotics may be required to treat inflammation caused by infection, and steroids may be indicated for severe systemic inflammation. A client's diet should be evaluated to ensure that he or she is receiving adequate nutrients to support healing, including adequate protein, carbohydrates, and vitamins. Vitamins important in cellular repair include vitamin C.

Nurses working with clients experiencing inflammation should be sure to emphasize the importance of preventing further injury, taking medications as prescribed to treat or prevent illness, and maintaining adequate intake of liquids and nutrients. Family teaching may be necessary if the client needs assistance with changing dressings, preventing the inflamed area from exposure to water while bathing, or any other aspects of daily living until healing occurs. Additional client teaching during the reparative phase may be necessary to ensure that the client does not resume activity too quickly and that the client continues treatment until healing is complete and the client is released by the physician.

PHARMACOLOGIC THERAPIES

Pharmacological therapies are aimed at reducing the inflammatory response and reducing pain associated with the symptoms of inflammation. Common medications include nonsteroidal anti-inflammatory drugs (NSAIDs), which have fewer adverse effects than the more powerful anti-inflammatory corticosteroids. Corticosteroids are normally administered when inflammation is more severe or is life threatening. NSAIDs, in addition to their anti-inflammatory actions, are also analgesics and antipyretics that help not only to reduce inflammation but also to minimize its effects.

MEDICATIONS Inflammation

Classification	Actions	Common drugs	Nursing considerations
NSAIDs	Analgesic, antipyretic, and anti-inflammatory properties act by inhibiting the synthesis of prostaglandins (lipids found in all tissues with potent physiological effects in addition to promoting inflammation depending on the tissue where they are found). NSAIDs block inflammation by inhibiting cyclooxygenase (COX), the key enzyme in the biosynthesis of prostaglandins.	Ibuprofen, naproxen sodium, aspirin, indomethacin, celecoxib	■ Give on an empty stomach if tolerated or with food if nausea, vomiting, or abdominal pain occurs. ■ Give for pregnancy category B. ■ Do not administer to clients with peptic ulcer disease. ■ Avoid NSAIDs with anticoagulants. ■ Actions of some diuretics can be reduced with NSAIDs. ■ May increase bleeding time. ■ Monitor client response to treatment. ■ Use with caution in the elderly because of potential reduction in kidney and liver function.
Glucocorticoids	Natural hormones are released by the adrenal cortex with potent anti-inflammatory actions on nearly every cell in the body that can suppress severe cases of inflammation. Generally reserved for short-term treatment due to serious potential side effects.	Betamethasone, cortisone, dexamethasone, hydrocortisone	■ If administered im, administer deep im to avoid atrophy or abscesses. ■ Do not use in presence of systemic infection due to reduced immune response. ■ Do not discontinue abruptly. ■ Use in pregnancy category C. ■ Carefully monitor condition, blood glucose levels, WBC count, changes in mood, or signs of Cushing's syndrome if used long term. ■ Use cautiously in clients with gastrointestinal ulcers, renal disease, hypertension, osteoporosis, varicella, diabetes mellitus, heart failure, mental instability, or any disease that reduces immune response (HIV, cancer, etc.).
Analgesics	Give to treat the pain associated with inflammation if NSAID analgesic effect is not sufficient alone.	Morphine, oxycodone	■ Monitor pain status for adequate relief of pain. ■ If administering a narcotic, monitor respiratory rate. ■ See concept of pain for further information about analgesics.
Natural therapies	Eicosapentaenoic acid (EPA) and docosahexaenoic acid (DHA) have anti-inflammatory actions in addition to their triglyceride-lowering activity.	Fish oils	■ Interactions may occur between fish oil supplements and aspirin and other NSAIDs. While rare, interactions may be manifested by increased susceptibility to bruising, nosebleeds, hemoptysis, hematuria, and blood in the stool.

16.1 APPENDICITIS

KEY TERMS

Appendectomy, *894*
Appendicitis, *893*
Dehiscence, *898*
Elective surgery, *895*
Emergency surgery, *895*
Evisceration, *898*
Fecalith, *893*
Perforation, *893*
Perioperative nursing care, *894*
Peritonitis, *893*

BASIS FOR SELECTION OF EXEMPLAR

Top 20 reasons to be admitted through the emergency department

Agency for Health Care Research and Quality

LEARNING OUTCOMES

After reading about this exemplar, you will be able to:

1. Describe the pathophysiology, etiology, clinical manifestations, and direct and indirect causes of appendicitis.
2. Identify risk factors associated with appendicitis.
3. Illustrate the nursing process in providing culturally competent care across the life span for individuals with appendicitis.
4. Formulate priority nursing diagnoses appropriate for an individual with appendicitis.
5. Create a plan of care for individuals with appendicitis and their family members.
6. Assess expected outcomes for an individual with appendicitis.
7. Discuss therapies used in the collaborative care of an individual with appendicitis.
8. Employ evidence-based caring interventions for an individual with appendicitis.

OVERVIEW

Appendicitis, inflammation of the vermiform appendix, is a common cause of acute abdominal pain. It is the most common reason for emergency abdominal surgery, affecting 10% of the population (Tierney, McPhee, & Papadakis, 2005). Appendicitis can occur at any age, but it is more common in adolescents and young adults and slightly more common in adolescent boys (10–19 years of age) than girls.

Children account for one fourth to one third of the appendectomies performed every year in more than 250,000 Americans (Ziegler, 2004). The incidence of a ruptured appendix is much higher in children less than 4 years of age as compared to older children and adolescents. Infants and young children are unable to verbalize the presence of symptoms such as pain and nausea. They also may have symptoms that are not specific to appendicitis (Kwok, Kim, & Gorelick, 2004). These factors may lead to a delayed diagnosis of appendicitis, increasing the risk of perforation.

PATHOPHYSIOLOGY AND ETIOLOGY

The appendix is a tubelike pouch attached to the cecum just below the ileocecal valve. It is usually located in the right iliac region, at an area designated as McBurney's point (Figure 16–2A ■). The function of the appendix is not fully understood, although it regularly fills with and empties digested food.

Obstruction of the proximal lumen of the appendix is apparent in most acutely inflamed appendices. Following obstruction, the appendix becomes distended with fluid secreted by its mucosa. Pressure within the lumen of the appendix increases, impairing its blood supply and leading to inflammation, edema, ulceration, and infection. Purulent exudate forms, further distending the appendix. Within 24–36 hours, tissue necrosis and gangrene result, leading to **perforation** (rupture) if treatment is not initiated. Perforation allows the contents of the gastrointestinal (GI) tract to flow into the peritoneal space of the abdomen, resulting in inflammation and bacterial infection of the entire abdominal area known as **peritonitis**. Appendicitis can be classified as simple, gangrenous, or perforated depending on the stage of the process. In simple appendicitis, the appendix is inflamed but intact. When areas of tissue necrosis and microscopic perforations are present in the appendix, the disorder is called gangrenous appendicitis. A perforated appendix shows evidence of gross perforation and contamination of the peritoneal cavity.

Etiology

Appendicitis almost always results from an obstruction in the appendiceal lumen. The obstruction is often caused by a **fecalith**, or hard mass of feces. Other obstructive causes include a calculus or stone, a foreign body, inflammation, a tumor, parasites (e.g., pinworms), edema of lymphoid tissue, or a tumor. Continued secretion of mucus following acute obstruction of the lumen increases pressure, causing ischemia, cellular death, and ulceration.

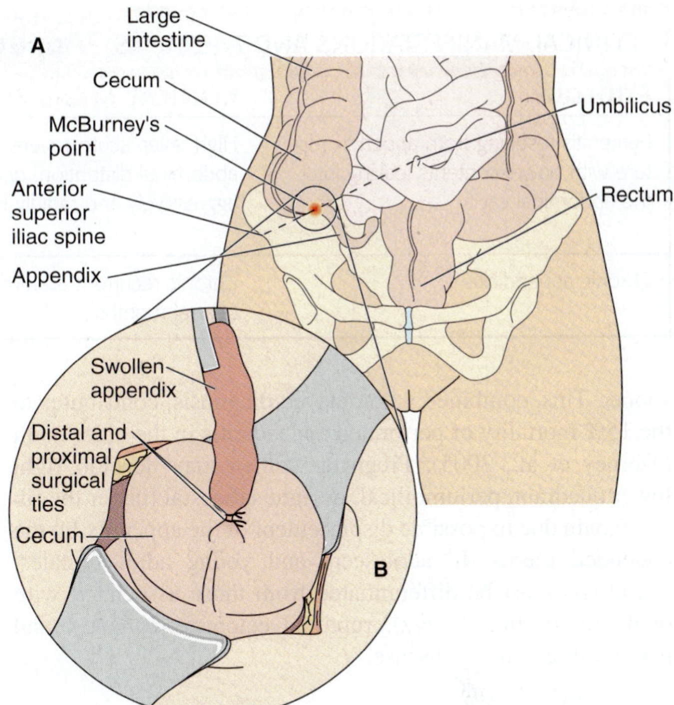

Figure 16–2 ■ *A* McBurney's point, located midway between the umbilicus and the anterior iliac crest in the right lower quadrant. It is the usual side for localized pain and rebound tenderness due to appendicitis. *B* In an appendectomy, the appendix and cecum are brought through the incision to the surface of the abdomen. The base of the appendix is clamped and ligated; the appendix is then removed.

Risk Factors

Adolescent males are at greatest risk, although fecaliths can occur in both genders at any age. Individuals whose diet is low in fiber or high in carbohydrates are at greater risk for developing fecaliths. Most cases of appendicitis seem to occur in the winter months between October and May, perhaps related to reduced activity levels that result in slowed peristalsis. GI infections also can promote appendicitis.

CLINICAL MANIFESTATIONS

The initial characteristic manifestation of acute appendicitis is continuous, mild generalized or upper abdominal pain. Over the next 4 hours, the pain intensifies and localizes in the right lower quadrant of the abdomen. Pain associated with appendicitis is aggravated by moving, walking, or coughing. On palpation, localized and rebound tenderness are noted at McBurney's point. Rebound tenderness is demonstrated by relief of pain with direct palpation of McBurney's point followed by pain on release of pressure. Extension or internal rotation of the right hip increases the pain. In addition to pain, a low-grade temperature, anorexia, nausea, and vomiting are often present.

Pain and local tenderness may be less acute in older adults, delaying the diagnosis. Because the course of acute appendicitis is more virulent in older adults, complications can develop

CLINICAL MANIFESTATIONS AND THERAPIES **Appendicitis**

ETIOLOGY	CLINICAL MANIFESTATIONS	CLINICAL THERAPIES
Peritonitis resulting from appendix rupture with bowel contents leaking into the abdominal cavity	High fever, acute severe abdominal pain, abdominal distention; death may result if not aggressively and rapidly treated	■ Removal of the ruptured appendix ■ Antibiotics ■ Fluid resuscitation ■ Supportive treatment to maintain vital signs
Chronic appendicitis	Chronic recurrent abdominal pain over several months	■ Appendectomy ■ Pain management

sooner. This, combined with delayed diagnosis, contributes to the 15% mortality of perforated appendicitis in the older adult (Tierney et al., 2005). Pregnant women may develop right lower quadrant, periumbilical, or right subcostal (under the rib cage) pain due to possible displacement of the appendix by the distended uterus. In adolescent and young adult females, symptoms must be differentiated from those associated with ovulation (mittelschmerz), ruptured ectopic pregnancy, and pelvic inflammatory disease.

Complications

Perforation, peritonitis, and abscess (accumulation of pus) are possible complications of acute appendicitis. Perforation is manifested by increased pain and a high fever. It can lead to a small, localized abscess; local peritonitis; or significant generalized peritonitis.

A less common disorder is chronic appendicitis, characterized by chronic abdominal pain and recurrent acute attacks at intervals of several months or more. Other conditions, such as inflammatory bowel disease (IBD) and renal disorders, often cause manifestations attributed to chronic appendicitis.

COLLABORATION

The acutely inflamed appendix can perforate within 24 hours, so rapid diagnosis and treatment is important. Because of this urgency and the low incidence of surgical complications, diagnostic testing and preoperative treatment are limited. The client is admitted to the hospital, and intravenous fluids are initiated. Oral food and fluids are withheld until a diagnosis is confirmed.

Diagnostic Tests

Diagnostic and laboratory tests help confirm the diagnosis and rule out other possible causes for the manifestations. Abdominal ultrasound is the most effective test for diagnosing acute appendicitis. Ultrasound examination has reduced the incidence of exploratory surgery. It is particularly useful with clients who have atypical symptoms (e.g., older adults). Other diagnostic tests used to diagnose appendicitis and rule out other possible conditions include abdominal x-rays, intravenous pyelogram, urinalysis, and pelvic examination. In addition, a white blood cell (WBC) count with differential is obtained. With appendicitis, the total white count is elevated, with an increased number of immature WBC (bands).

Pharmacologic Therapies

Prior to surgery, intravenous fluids are given to restore or maintain vascular volume and prevent electrolyte imbalance. Antibiotic therapy with a third-generation cephalosporin effective against many gram-negative bacteria, such as cefoperazone (Cefobid), cefotaxime (Claforan), ceftazidime (Fortaz), and ceftriaxone (Rocephin), is initiated prior to surgery. Antibiotic administration is repeated during surgery and continued for at least 48 hours postoperatively. The sudden disappearance of pain is an indication that the appendix has ruptured, so administration of strong analgesics is withheld preoperatively in order to assess for this indicator. Once the diagnosis is established, an appendectomy is performed and analgesics are administered to maintain comfort as ordered.

Surgery

The treatment of choice for acute appendicitis is an **appendectomy**, surgical removal of the appendix. Either a laparoscopic approach (insertion of an endoscope to view abdominal contents) or laparotomy (surgical opening of the abdomen) may be used for appendectomy. Laparoscopic appendectomy requires a very small incision through which the laparoscope is inserted. This procedure has several advantages: (1) Direct visualization of the appendix allows definitive diagnosis without laparotomy, (2) postoperative hospitalization is short, (3) postoperative complications are infrequent, and (4) recovery and resumption of normal activities is rapid.

An open appendectomy is performed by laparotomy. A small transverse incision is made at McBurney's point (Figure 16–2A); the appendix is isolated and ligated (tied off) to prevent contamination of the site with bowel contents and then removed (Figure 16–2B). Laparotomy generally is used when the appendix has ruptured. It allows removal of contaminants from the peritoneal cavity by irrigation with sterile normal saline. Occasionally, the wound may be left unsutured for periodic irrigation. Recovery is generally uneventful.

PERIOPERATIVE NURSING CARE

Perioperative nursing care refers to nursing care provided during any or all of the three phases of surgery: the preoperative period, the intraoperative period, and the postoperative period. Perioperative nursing diagnoses are provided in Table 16–3 to

TABLE 16–3 **Examples of Perioperative Nursing Diagnoses**

PREOPERATIVE	INTRAOPERATIVE	POSTOPERATIVE
■ Knowledge, Deficient	■ Knowledge, Deficient	■ Knowledge, Deficient
■ Anxiety	■ Anxiety	■ Pain
■ Fear	■ Fear	■ Breathing Pattern, Ineffective
■ Decisional Conflict	■ Airway Clearance, Ineffective	■ Airway Clearance, Ineffective
■ Coping, Ineffective	■ Aspiration, Risk for	■ Skin Integrity, Impaired
■ Sexuality Patterns, Ineffective	■ Cardiac Output, Decreased	■ Nutrition Imbalanced: Less than Body Requirements
■ Sleep Pattern, Disturbed	■ Hypothermia	■ Sexuality Patterns, Ineffective
■ Thought Processes, Disturbed	■ Infection, Risk for	■ Sleep Pattern, Disturbed
■ Family Processes, Interrupted	■ Thought Processes, Disturbed	■ Fatigue
■ Spiritual Distress	■ Gas Exchange, Impaired	■ Urinary Retention
	■ Urinary Elimination, Impaired	■ Urinary Elimination, Impaired
	■ Fluid Volume, Deficient	■ Adjustment, Impaired
	■ Fluid Volume, Excess	■ Body Image, Disturbed
	■ Communication: Verbal, Impaired	■ Mobility: Physical, Impaired
		■ Activity Intolerance, Risk for
		■ Injury, Risk for
		■ Health Maintenance, Ineffective
		■ Diversional Activity, Deficient
		■ Social Isolation
		■ Spiritual Distress

assist in identifying the needs of the surgical client. This is not an exhaustive list, but it can serve as a guide in identifying possible nursing diagnoses.

Surgery is classified by its urgency and necessity to preserve the client's life, body part, or body function. **Emergency surgery** is performed immediately to preserve function or the life of the client. Surgeries to control internal hemorrhage or repair a fracture are examples of emergency surgeries. Because of the dangers associated with peritonitis, an appendectomy is considered emergency surgery. **Elective surgery** is performed when surgical intervention is the preferred treatment for a condition that is not imminently life threatening (but may ultimately threaten life or well-being) or to improve the client's life. Examples of elective surgeries include cholecystectomy for chronic gallbladder disease, hip replacement surgery, and plastic surgery procedures such as breast reduction surgery.

Preoperative Nursing Care

The client's response to planned surgery varies greatly. When planning and implementing nursing care, consider individual psychologic and physical differences, the type of surgery, and the circumstances surrounding the need for surgery. A thorough nursing assessment is needed to determine the most appropriate care for each client undergoing surgery.

Before planning and implementing care for the surgical client, gather assessment information by taking a nursing history and performing a physical examination. Use this information to establish baseline data, identify physical needs, determine teaching needs and emotional and spiritual support for the client and family, and prioritize nursing care. The type of surgical procedure directs the assessment and intervention planned by the nurse.

PRACTICE ALERT

Be sure to assess information about use of over-the-counter medications including herbal supplements. These drugs can interact with medications administered in the perioperative period.

Surgery is a significant and stressful event. Regardless of the nature of the surgery, the client and family will be anxious. Some clients and their families seek care from a spiritual provider during this time. The degree of anxiety they will feel is not necessarily proportional to the magnitude of the surgical procedure.

The nurse's ability to listen actively to both verbal and nonverbal messages is imperative to establishing a trusting relationship with the client and family. Therapeutic communication can help the client and family identify fears and concerns. The nurse can then plan nursing interventions and supportive care to reduce the client's anxiety level and assist the client to cope successfully with the stressors encountered during the perioperative period.

PREOPERATIVE CLIENT AND FAMILY TEACHING Client teaching is an essential nursing responsibility in the preoperative period. Client education and emotional support have a positive effect on the client's physical and psychologic well-being, both before and after surgery. In an analysis of 102 studies, surgical clients receiving client education and/or supportive interventions had less pain and anxiety, experienced fewer complications, were discharged sooner, were more satisfied with their care, and returned to normal activities sooner than clients who did not receive this type of care (Yount, Edgell & Jakovec, 1990). These positive outcomes may be attributed in part to the sense of control the client gains through the nurse's teaching.

Client teaching should begin as soon as the client learns of the upcoming surgery. Teaching may begin as early as in the physician's office or at the time of preadmission testing. Although education continues during postoperative care, most teaching is done before surgery, because pain and the effects of anesthesia can greatly diminish the client's ability to learn.

The amount of information desired varies from client to client. Therefore, assess the client's need for and readiness to accept information. The teaching will be directed in part by the particular surgical procedure that is being performed and by the type of anesthesia being provided.

In addition to teaching the client and family about measures that will decrease the risk of complications, provide other preoperative information to prepare the client and family for surgery. This information should include the following:

- Diagnostic tests—reasons, preparations (e.g., fasting), and what to expect (i.e., dark room, confined space, blood draw, etc.)
- Arrival time if surgery is scheduled in early morning
- Preparations for surgery after midnight prior to a morning surgery, skin preparation, indwelling catheter or bladder elimination, start of intravenous infusion, preoperative medication, handling of valuables (rings, watch, money)
- Sedative/hypnotic medication to be taken the night before surgery to promote rest and sleep
- Counseling on whether to take significant medications the morning of surgery
- Informed consent
- Expected timetable for surgery and the recovery room
- Method to inform family of progress throughout surgery
- Transfer to the surgery department
- Location of the surgical waiting room
- Transfer to recovery room
- Anticipated postoperative routine and devices or equipment (drains, tubes, equipment for IV infusions, oxygen or humidifying mask, dressings, splints, casts)
- Plans for postoperative pain control.

Preoperative Fasting Researchers report that many clients experience unnecessarily long preoperative fasts. The American Society of Anesthesiologists provides guidelines for preoperative fasting in healthy clients undergoing elective procedures; they are available online. Withdrawal from caffeine in beverages such as coffee or colas may cause headaches and irritability. Dehydration, hypovolemia, and hypoglycemia are other recognized side effects. Thirst, worry, and hunger are reported by clients to be related to fasting. Fasting does not ensure that the stomach will be empty or that the gastric contents will be less acidic.

PREOPERATIVE CLIENT PREPARATION A preoperative surgical checklist serves as an outline for finalizing preparation of the client for surgery in most institutions. Complete the checklist before the client is transported to surgery. Nursing responsibilities the day of surgery are as follows:

- Assist with bathing, grooming, and changing into operating room gown.
- Ensure that the client takes nothing by mouth (NPO). Provide additional teaching, and reinforce prior teaching.
- Remove nail polish, lipstick, and makeup to facilitate circulatory assessment during and after surgery.
- Ensure that identification, blood, and allergy bands are correct, legible, and secure.
- Remove hair pins and jewelry; a wedding ring may be worn if it is removed from the finger, covered with gauze, replaced, and then taped to the finger.
- Complete skin or bowel preparation as ordered.
- Insert an indwelling catheter, intravenous line, or nasogastric tube as ordered.
- Remove dentures, artificial eye, and contact lenses, and store them in a safe place.
- Leave a hearing aid in place if the client cannot hear without it, and notify the operating room nurse.
- Verify that the informed consent has been signed prior to administering preoperative medications.
- Weigh the client and record height and weight in the chart (for dosage of anesthesia).
- Administer preoperative medication as ordered.
- Ensure the safety of the client once the medication has been given by placing the client on bed rest with raised side rails and by placing the call light within reach.
- Verify that all ordered diagnostic test reports are in the chart.
- Have the client empty the bladder immediately before the preoperative medication is administered (unless an indwelling catheter is in place).
- Obtain and record vital signs.
- Provide ongoing supportive care to the client and the client's family.
- Document all preoperative care in the appropriate location, such as the preoperative surgical checklist, the medication record, and the narrative preoperative nursing notes.
- Verify with the surgical personnel the client's identity, and verify that all client information is documented appropriately.
- Help the surgical personnel transfer the client from the bed to the stretcher.
- Prepare the client's room for postoperative care, including making the surgical bed and ensuring that the anticipated supplies and equipment are in the room.

Intraoperative Nursing Care

The intraoperative phase of surgery begins when the client enters the operating room and ends when the client is transferred to the postanesthesia care unit (PACU). Nursing care in this phase focuses on keeping the client and the environment safe and providing physiologic monitoring and psychologic support. Circulating nurses and scrub nurses, according to specific role definitions, support and care for the client and assist the surgeons. Nurses working in the operating room need specialized training after licensure. Maintaining a sterile field, sterile gowning and gloving, and surgical asepsis are discussed in Concept 15.

PRACTICE ALERT

Objects on the sterile drape are considered sterile. Remain a minimum of 12 inches away from draped tables and sterile fields to avoid contamination if you are not attired in sterile gown and gloves.

Postoperative Nursing Care

Immediate postoperative care begins when the client has been transferred from the operating room to the PACU. The PACU nurse is part of the surgical team and monitors the client's vital signs and surgical site to determine the response to the surgical procedure and to detect significant changes. Assessing mental status and level of consciousness is another ongoing nursing responsibility, and the client may require repeated orientation to time, place, and person. Emotional support also is essential because the client is in a vulnerable and dependent position. Assessing and evaluating hydration status by monitoring intake and output is crucial to detecting cardiovascular or renal complications. In addition, the PACU nurse assesses the client's pain level. Careful administration of analgesics provides comfort without compounding the potential side effects from the anesthesia.

CARE WHEN THE CLIENT IS STABLE When awake and after being stabilized, the client is transferred to his or her room. The PACU nurse communicates information about the client's condition and postoperative orders to the floor nurse prior to the client's arrival. This prepares the floor nurse for additional problems or needed equipment.

Immediate and continuing assessment is essential to detect and/or prevent complications. In documenting assessment findings, the nurse completes a flow record of the individual client's situation. Baseline data are obtained and compared with preoperative data. A postoperative head-to-toe assessment includes, but may not be limited to, the following:

- General appearance
- Vital signs
- Level of consciousness
- Emotional status
- Quantity of respirations
- Skin color and temperature
- Discomfort/pain
- Nausea/vomiting
- Type of intravenous fluids and flow rate
- Dressing site
- Drainage on the dressing and/or bed linen
- Urinary output (catheter or ability to urinate)
- Ability to move all extremities.

The hospital policy or physician's orders dictate the frequency of follow-up assessments. After major surgery, the nurse generally assesses the client every 15 minutes during the first hour and, if the client is stable, every 30 minutes for the next 2 hours, and then every hour during the subsequent 4 hours. Assessments are then carried out every 4 hours, subject to change according to the client's condition and protocol for the particular surgical procedure. It is critically important to inform the surgeon immediately if the assessment reveals any signs of impending shock or other life-threatening changes.

After carrying out the initial assessment and ensuring the client's safety by lowering the bed, raising the side rails, and placing the call light within reach, the nurse notes the physician's postoperative orders. These orders guide the nurse in the care of the postoperative client. For example, the orders specify activity level, diet, medications for pain and nausea, antibiotics, continuation of preoperative medications, frequency of vital sign assessments, administration of intravenous fluids, and laboratory tests such as hemoglobin and potassium level. In most institutions, orders written prior to surgery must be reordered following surgery because the client's condition is presumed to have changed.

NURSING CARE OF COMMON POSTOPERATIVE COMPLICATIONS Several factors place the client at risk for postoperative complications. Nursing care before, during, and after surgery is aimed at preventing and/or minimizing the effects of these complications.

Common postoperative cardiovascular complications include shock, hemorrhage, deep venous thrombosis, and pulmonary embolism. Nursing considerations for these complications can be found in Concept 22, Perfusion.

Common postoperative respiratory complications include pneumonia and atelectasis. Nursing considerations for pneumonia can be found in Concept 15, Infection. More information regarding prevention and treatment of atelectasis can be found in Concept 21, Oxygenation.

Common postoperative complications associated with elimination include urinary retention, altered bowel elimination, and the absence of peristalsis. Nursing considerations for these conditions are discussed in Concept 9, Elimination.

Effective pain management is essential in caring for the postoperative client. The Nursing Process in the next section and Concept 5, Comfort, provide detailed information regarding pain management.

Care of the Client With a Surgical Wound Nursing care of the postoperative client with a surgical wound focuses on preventing and monitoring for wound complications. The nurse assumes a leading role in supporting the wound healing process, providing emotional support to the client and teaching wound care to the client. Wound care is discussed in more detail in Concept 30.

Dehiscence is a separation in the layers of the incisional wound (Figure 16–3A ■). Treatment depends on the extent of wound disruption. If the dehiscence is extensive, the incision must be resutured in surgery. **Evisceration** is the protrusion of body organs from a wound dehiscence (Figure 16–3B). These serious complications may result from delayed wound healing or may occur immediately following surgery. They also may occur after forceful straining (coughing, sneezing, or vomiting). When dehiscence occurs, immediately cover the wound with a sterile dressing moistened with normal saline. Emergency surgery is performed to repair these conditions.

Either the nurse, physician, physician assistant (PA), or nurse practitioner (NP) removes sutures or staples after the wound has healed sufficiently (usually 5 to 10 days after surgery). Removal is performed using medical aseptic technique. Additional support may be provided to the incision by applying strips of tape (or Steri-Strips) as directed by institutional policy or by the physician. More information about wound care and wound healing can be found in Exemplar 30.4, Wound Healing.

SPECIAL CONSIDERATIONS FOR OLDER ADULTS Physiologic, cognitive, and psychosocial changes associated with the aging process place the older adult at increased risk for postoperative complications. These age-related changes and selected nursing interventions are summarized in Table 16–4. With an ever-increasing population of older adults, particularly the very old, the nurse must be aware of these normal changes and modify nursing care accordingly in an effort to provide safe, supportive care.

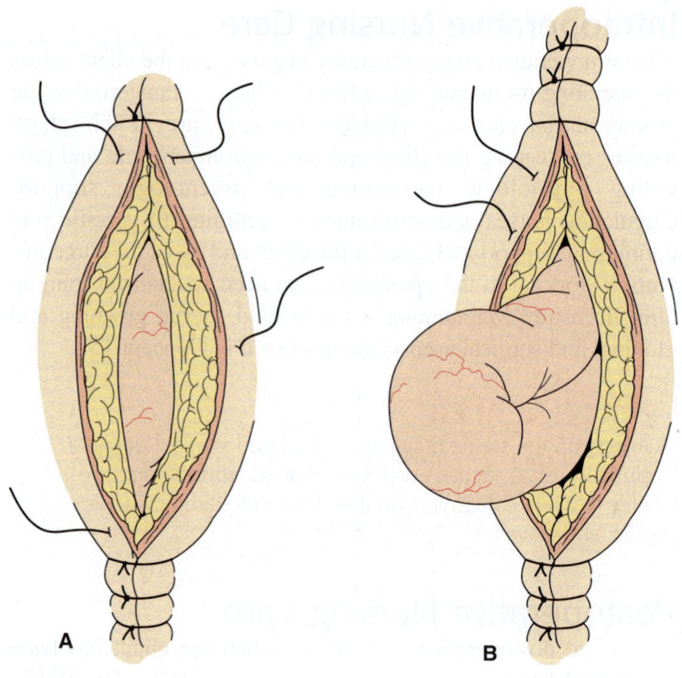

Figure 16–3 ■ Wound complications. *A* Dehiscence is a disruption in the incision resulting in a separation of the layers of the wound. *B* Evisceration is a protrusion of a body organ through a surgical incision.

TABLE 16–4 **Nursing Interventions for Older Surgical Clients**

SYSTEM	AGE-RELATED CHANGES	NURSING INTERVENTIONS
General appearance	Change in height, weight, and fat distribution	Assess physical parameters. Provide for warmth. Turn frequently.
Integument	Diminished integrity secondary to loss of subcutaneous fat and decreased oil production, elasticity, and hydration	Provide careful preoperative preparation to avoid trauma. Use other means to assess oxygenation and hydration, such as evaluation of mucous membranes, laboratory studies, and urine output.
Sensory-perceptual	Decline in vision and hearing ability; dryness of mouth	Compensate for sensory deficits: speak low, not loud; minimize noise in environment; provide adequate room light; stay within client's field of vision when speaking; encourage client to wear hearing aid to the operating room. Provide comfort measures when NPO.
Respiratory	Decreased efficiency of cough reflex and decreased aeration of lung fields	Teach and encourage coughing and diaphragmatic breathing exercises. Assess baseline parameters. Constantly monitor lung sounds and respiratory status.
Cardiovascular	Less efficient, decreased adaptation to stress	Monitor for hypotension and shock. Assess for thrombus formation, cardiac dysrhythmias, peripheral pulses, and edema.
Gastrointestinal	Decline in gastric motility	Encourage intake of adequate fluids, nutritious meals, soft diet. Assist with feeding; monitor bowel function.
Genitourinary	Decreased efficiency of kidney; loss of bladder control	Monitor I&O and electrolyte levels. Assess for drug side effects. Assist with voiding as needed.
Musculoskeletal	Stiffness of joints; decrease in strength; brittleness of bones	Carefully position on OR table. Move carefully and gently. Prevent pressure sores.
Cognitive-psychosocial	Decreased reaction time; stable intellectual ability; proneness to delirium and altered mental status while in hospital	Provide ample time for making decisions. Implement safety measures. Talk to client as adult, not as child. Orient frequently.

Source: Adapted from Burgunder, C. and Dellasea, C. (1991). Perioperative nursing care for the elderly surgical patient. *Today's O.R. Nurse, 13*(6), 12–17.

NURSING PROCESS

Nursing management of the client with appendicitis includes collaborative assessment, preoperative and postoperative care, and prevention of complications. As previously discussed, preoperative teaching is an important nursing responsibility.

Assessment

Because appendicitis can rapidly progress from inflammation to perforation, prompt assessment is vital. Obtain the following assessment data:

- *Health history.* Current manifestations, including onset, duration, progression, and aggravating or relieving factors; most recent food or fluid intake; known medication or other allergies; current medications; and history of chronic diseases
- *Physical examination.* Vital signs, including temperature; apparent general health; abdominal shape and contour, bowel sounds, tenderness to light palpation.

PRACTICE ALERT

Keep the client with suspected appendicitis NPO. Do not administer laxatives or enemas, which may cause perforation of the appendix. Do not apply heat to the abdomen, as this may increase circulation to the appendix and also cause perforation.

Diagnosis

Among the nursing diagnoses that may apply to the client with appendicitis are as follows:

- Acute Pain
- Risk for Deficient Fluid Volume
- Anxiety
- Fear
- Risk for Infection
- Risk for Ineffective Airway Clearance.

Plan

The plan of care developed in collaboration with the client and family may include the following:

- The client will articulate any concerns about surgery prior to the event.
- The client will articulate an understanding of the procedure, the reasons for it, and any preoperative instructions prior to arrival for surgery.
- The client will verbalize relief from pain following administration of pain management.
- The client will receive appropriate postoperative wound care.
- The client will verbalize instructions for self-care prior to being discharged.

Implementation

Nursing management focuses on promoting comfort, maintaining hydration, providing emotional support, supporting respiratory function, providing care of the surgical site, and monitoring for symptoms of infection.

Acute Pain

The client with appendicitis experiences pain before and after surgery. Analgesia is limited until the diagnosis is established. Postoperative pain is controlled by narcotic or nonnarcotic analgesics.

- Assess pain, including its character, location, severity, and duration. Report any unexpected changes in the nature of pain. Both preoperatively and postoperatively, the client's pain provides important clues about the diagnosis and possible complications, such as rupture of the appendix or peritonitis.
- Administer analgesics as ordered. Preoperatively, pain medication can be given after a diagnosis is established. Postoperatively, provide analgesics to maintain comfort and enhance mobility.
- Assess effectiveness of medication 30 minutes after administration. Report unrelieved pain. Pain unrelieved by prescribed analgesic may indicate a complication or the need for further assessment. For example, continued abdominal discomfort and distention may indicate excess intestinal gas that may be better relieved by ambulation.

PRACTICE ALERT

Be alert to the child who does not complain of postoperative pain following surgery for a ruptured appendix. This child will need pain medication. While the child may not verbally complain of pain, he or she will cry when approached and will resist or refuse to move in the bed. Proper pain management will facilitate the child's recovery and will help prevent respiratory complications related to immobilization.

Risk for Deficient Fluid Volume

- Monitor and continue the intravenous infusion that was initiated preoperatively until bowel function returns after surgery.

CARE SETTINGS Home Care for the Client With Appendicitis

Preoperative teaching may be limited by pain and the emergent nature of surgery. Explain why food and fluids are not permitted during this time. If time allows, teach postoperative turning, coughing, deep breathing, and pain management.

With uncomplicated appendectomy, the client often is discharged the day of surgery or the day following surgery. Postoperative teaching includes the following:

- Wound or incision care, including hand washing and dressing change procedures as indicated
- Instructions to report to the physician fever, increased abdominal pain, swelling, redness, drainage, bleeding, or warmth of the operative site
- Activity limitations (e.g., lifting, driving), if any
- Return to work if appropriate.

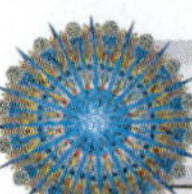

NURSING CARE PLAN **A Client With Acute Appendicitis**

Jamie Lynn is a 19-year-old college student majoring in physical therapy. Ms. Lynn arrives at the emergency department at 1 a.m. complaining of general lower abdominal pain that started the previous evening. By midnight, the pain was more localized over the right lower quadrant. She also reports nausea and vomiting.

ASSESSMENT	DIAGNOSES	PLANNING
Sue Grady, RN, completes the admission assessment in the emergency department. Ms. Lynn is complaining of nausea and severe abdominal pain, stating, "Walking makes my stomach hurt worse." Physical assessment findings include T_O 37.8°C (100.2°F), P 84, R 16, BP 110/70; skin warm to touch; abdomen flat and guarded, with marked tenderness in right lower quadrant. Ms. Lynn's complete blood count (CBC) shows WBC 14,000/mm³; neutrophils 81.1%; lymphocytes 12.5%. The diagnosis of acute appendicitis is made, and Ms. Lynn is transferred to surgery for a laparoscopic appendectomy.	■ Impaired Skin Integrity related to surgical incision ■ Acute Pain related to surgical intervention ■ Anxiety related to situational crisis	■ Incision will heal without infection or complications. ■ Client will verbalize adequate pain relief. ■ Client will verbalize decreased anxiety. ■ Client will return to preoperative activities.

IMPLEMENTATION

- Provide analgesics as needed.
- Teach pain management.
- Teach abdominal splinting during coughing, turning, or ambulating as needed.
- Teach home care of incision.
- Discuss activity limitations as ordered.
- Instruct to report fever or warmth, redness, or drainage from the incision.

EVALUATION

On discharge the following evening, Ms. Lynn is fully ambulatory. Her appetite has returned, and she is tolerating food and fluids well. Her temperature is normal. The nurse provides Ms. Lynn with written and verbal information on postoperative care following an appendectomy.

CRITICAL THINKING

1. What is the pathophysiologic basis for Ms. Lynn's elevated WBC?
2. How would Ms. Lynn's postoperative care and teaching differ if she had undergone a laparotomy instead of a laparoscopic appendectomy?
3. Outline a teaching plan to give to clients for home care following an appendectomy.
4. Develop a care plan for Ms. Lynn for the nursing diagnosis Anxiety related to a situational crisis.

- Once bowel sounds return and after the nasogastric tube has been removed (if needed), offer water in small amounts, then other clear fluids.
- Closely monitor the client after giving oral fluids to ensure he or she does not become nauseated.
- Monitor intake and output. If the client had a ruptured appendix and has a nasogastric tube after surgery, accurate assessment of the amount of output from the nasogastric tube is essential. The client may have orders for the amount of fluid lost from the nasogastric tube to be replaced with additional intravenous fluids. The nurse should be alert to an increase in nasogastric drainage postoperatively, as this drainage should decrease over time. Promptly report any concerns to the physician.

Anxiety

For many clients, this may be their first hospitalization and their first experience with health care personnel beyond their usual provider. The nurse must do the following:

- Elicit a history, perform a physical examination, coordinate diagnostic tests, and prepare the client for surgery in a short period of time.
- Provide emotional support for both client and family.
- Provide good preoperative education to reduce anxiety.
- Encourage and answer any questions the client or family may have.

Risk for Ineffective Airway Clearance

General anesthesia during surgery compromises respiratory function.

- It is important for the client to turn, cough, and breathe deeply to prevent atelectasis.
- While the client with uncomplicated appendicitis is usually willing to get out of bed and walk soon after surgery, the client with a ruptured appendix is generally hesitant to move and may need to be repositioned by family or staff. The client must get out of bed as soon as his or her condition allows and walk 2 or 3 times a day to decrease the risk of pulmonary complications and decrease recovery time.
- The nurse should encourage the client to splint the incision area with a pillow during coughing to decrease pain.
- Incentive spirometry is frequently ordered for the client. Young children may be resistant to (or too young to understand) this procedure. An effective alternative approach is to give the child bubbles to blow. Giving praise and rewards such as stickers each time the child completes the task will likely increase compliance with the procedure and decrease the likelihood of complications.

Risk for Infection

Preventing complications during the preoperative and postoperative periods is a primary nursing care goal. Perforation and peritonitis are the most likely preoperative complications;

postoperative complications include wound infection, abscess, and possible peritonitis.

- Monitor vital signs, including temperature. Tachycardia and rapid, shallow respirations may indicate perforation of the appendix with resulting peritonitis. Fever may develop as well; a decrease in blood pressure may indicate the presence of sepsis.
- Maintain intravenous infusion until oral intake is adequate. Intravenous fluids are given to maintain vascular volume and to provide a route for antibiotic administration.
- Assess wound, abdominal girth, and postoperative pain. Swelling of the wound, increased abdominal girth, or an increase in pain may indicate infection or peritonitis.

Discharge Planning and Home Care Teaching

For a client with an appendix that did not rupture, the client is discharged once bowel function returns and he or she has a bowel movement.

- Give instructions on slowly reestablishing a nutritious diet as tolerated.
- Teach client or parents to recognize the signs and symptoms of infection and to seek early treatment.

If the appendix was ruptured, the client will be hospitalized for several days for intravenous antibiotics. If the wound was left open, it is generally closed after a few days and prior to discharge. Prepare the client and family for this procedure. Sedation or anesthesia is used to decrease the client's anxiety and discomfort. Prior to discharge, the nurse should provide client teaching and ensure that the client (or parents, if the client is a child) can verbalize the following:

- How to care for the wound
- The signs and symptoms of wound infection and when to call the physician
- Method and frequency of taking temperature
- Activity limitations and restrictions, including when to return to work or school
- Pain management, including medication instructions and possible side effects.

Evaluation

Expected outcomes of nursing care include the following:

- The client's pain is managed effectively.
- The client will not develop a secondary infection.
- The client and family verbalize understanding of the condition and treatment.
- Effective airway clearance is maintained.
- Adequate hydration is achieved and maintained.
- Restoration of normal nutritional intake will occur.
- The client experiences decreased fear and anxiety associated with the hospitalization and procedures.

REVIEW Appendicitis

RELATE: LINK THE CONCEPT

Linking the exemplar of Appendicitis with the concept of Infection:

1. How would you change or anticipate changing your nursing care for a client whose appendix is believed to have ruptured preoperatively?
2. How would the pathophysiology of a client with a ruptured appendix differ from a client whose appendix is removed without rupturing?

Linking the exemplar of Appendicitis with the concept of Mobility:

3. When caring for a client who required a laparoscopic appendectomy yesterday, what teaching would you provide to stress the importance of mobility?
4. The 14-year-old client who is 1 day postoperative following an appendectomy is reluctant to ambulate for fear of pain. What strategies would you use to encourage ambulation?

READY: GO TO COMPANION SKILLS MANUAL

- Applying bandages and binders
- Cleaning a sutured wound and changing a dressing on a wound with a drain
- Monitoring intake and output
- Establishing intravenous infusions
- Maintaining infusions
- Performing surgical and antisepsis/scrubs
- Deep breathing and coughing
- Assessing the abdomen
- Assessing blood pressure
- Assessing body temperature
- Assessing the client in pain
- Administering oral medications
- Removing sutures

REFER: GO TO MYNURSINGKIT

REFLECT: CASE STUDY

Mike Mortimer is a healthy, active 9-year-old boy who lives with his father. His mother died six months ago from metastatic breast cancer. At first, everyone at school was really nice to him, but lately they've been teasing him about being a motherless orphan. He's come to wishing he didn't have to go to school. This morning he told his dad that he had a stomachache and asked to stay home, but his dad said he didn't have a fever so he needed to get dressed and get going. The school nurse called his father at 11:30 to report that Mike had a fever and was feeling sick to his stomach. The nurse encouraged his dad to take him to the doctor.

When Mike arrives at the doctor's office, he reports severe pain in his lower left quadrant, nausea, and one emesis at school. The nurse measures his vital signs and obtains the following reading: T_O 100.2°F, P 96, R 12, BP 110/74. Rebound tenderness is noted in McBurney's point. CBC reveals a WBC count of 11,000 mm^3, and an ultrasound reveals an inflamed appendix. He is scheduled for surgery and admitted to the local acute care facility.

1. As you admit Mike to the pediatric unit, his father asks you to please give him something for pain. How do you respond?
2. Mike is scheduled to leave the unit for the operating room in 1 hour. What information will you gather to prepare him for surgery?
3. When Mike returns from the operating room, what priority assessments will you perform?
4. What teaching will you provide Mike and his dad prior to discharge?

16.2 GALLBLADDER DISEASE

KEY TERMS

Biliary colic, *902*
Cholangitis, *902*
Cholecystitis, *902*
Cholelithiasis, *902*
Empyema, *902*
Gallstone ileus, *902*
Laparoscopic cholecystectomy, *905*

BASIS FOR SELECTION OF EXEMPLAR

Healthy People 2010
Institute of Medicine
Top 20 reasons to be admitted through the emergency department
Agency for Health Care Research and Quality

LEARNING OUTCOMES

After reading about this exemplar, you will be able to:

1. Describe the pathophysiology, etiology, clinical manifestations, and direct and indirect causes of gallbladder disease.
2. Identify risk factors associated with gallbladder disease.
3. Illustrate the nursing process in providing culturally competent care across the life span for individuals with gallbladder disease.
4. Formulate priority nursing diagnoses appropriate for an individual with gallbladder disease.
5. Create a plan of care for individuals with gallbladder disease and their family members.
6. Assess expected outcomes for an individual with gallbladder disease.
7. Discuss therapies used in the collaborative care of an individual with gallbladder disease.
8. Employ evidence-based caring interventions for an individual with gallbladder disease.

OVERVIEW

Altered bile flow through the hepatic, cystic, or common bile duct is a common problem. It often leads to inflammation and other complications. Gallstones are the most common cause of obstructed flow. Tumors and abscesses also may obstruct bile flow.

Cholelithiasis is the formation of stones (*calculi* or *gallstones*) in the gallbladder or biliary duct system. Cholelithiasis is a common problem in the United States, affecting more than 10% of men and 20% of women by age 65 (Tierney et al., 2005).

PATHOPHYSIOLOGY AND ETIOLOGY

Most gallstones are formed in the gallbladder. They may migrate into the ducts (Figure 16–4 ■), leading to **cholangitis** (duct inflammation). Although some people with cholelithiasis are asymptomatic, many develop manifestations. Early manifestations of gallstones may be vague: epigastric fullness or mild gastric distress after eating a large or fatty meal. Stones that obstruct the cystic duct or common bile duct lead to distention and increased pressure behind the stone. This causes **biliary colic**, a severe, steady pain in the epigastric region or right upper quadrant (RUQ) of the abdomen. The pain may radiate to the back, right scapula, or shoulder. The pain often begins suddenly following a meal and may last as long as 5 hours. It often is accompanied by nausea and vomiting.

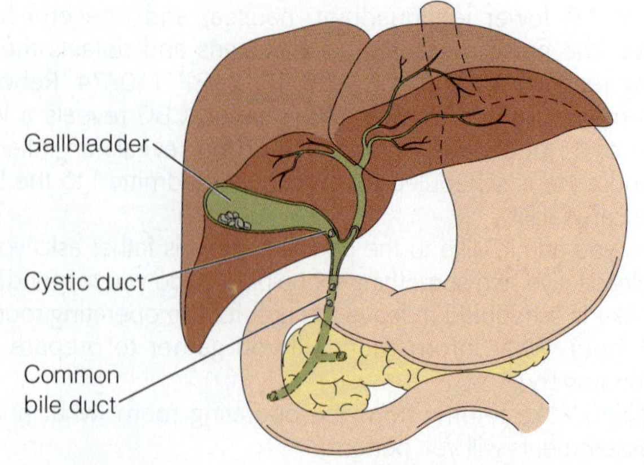

Figure 16–4 ■ Common locations of gallstones.

Obstruction of the common bile duct may cause bile reflux into the liver, leading to jaundice, pain, and possible liver damage. If the common duct is obstructed, pancreatic enzymes are unable to enter the small intestine, and pancreatitis becomes a potential complication.

Cholecystitis

Cholecystitis is inflammation of the gallbladder. *Acute cholecystitis* usually follows obstruction of the cystic duct by a stone. The obstruction increases pressure in the gallbladder, leading to ischemia of the gallbladder wall and mucosa. Chemical and bacterial inflammation often follows. The ischemia can lead to necrosis and perforation of the gallbladder wall.

Acute cholecystitis usually begins with an attack of biliary colic. The pain involves the entire RUQ and may radiate to the back, right scapula, or shoulder. Movement or deep breathing may aggravate the pain. The pain usually lasts longer than biliary colic, continuing for 12–18 hours. Anorexia, nausea, and vomiting are common. Fever often is present and may be accompanied by chills. The RUQ is tender to palpation.

Chronic cholecystitis may result from repeated bouts of acute cholecystitis or from persistent irritation of the gallbladder wall by stones. Bacteria may be present in the bile as well. Chronic cholecystitis often is asymptomatic.

Complications of cholecystitis include **empyema**, a collection of infected fluid in the gallbladder; gangrene and perforation with resulting peritonitis or abscess formation; formation of a fistula into an adjacent organ (such as the duodenum, colon, or stomach); or obstruction of the small intestine by a large gallstone (**gallstone ileus**).

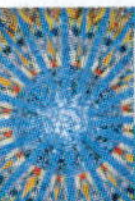

FOCUS ON DIVERSITY AND CULTURE

Gallstones

Native Americans in both the Northern and Southern Hemisphere—and those of the Pima tribe in particular—have a higher incidence of gallstones than do Caucasians of American or European heritage. This is thought to result from genes that promote efficient calorie use and fat storage—a beneficial trait when the availability of adequate food varies over time. Gallstones composed of cholesterol are less common in African Americans; Asians have a low incidence of the disease (Tierney et al., 2005).

Box 16–2 Risk Factors for Gallstones

- Age
- Family history of gallstones
- Race or ethnicity: Native American (either Northern or Southern Hemisphere); Northern European heritage
- Obesity, hyperlipidemia
- Rapid weight loss
- Female gender; use of oral contraceptives
- Biliary stasis: pregnancy, fasting, prolonged parenteral nutrition
- Diseases or conditions: cirrhosis; ileal disease or resection; sickle cell anemia; glucose intolerance

Etiology

Gallstones form when several factors interact: abnormal bile composition, biliary stasis, and inflammation of the gallbladder. Most gallstones (80%) consist primarily of cholesterol; the rest contain a mixture of bile components. Excess cholesterol in bile is associated with obesity, a high-calorie and high-cholesterol diet, and drugs that lower serum cholesterol levels. When bile is supersaturated with cholesterol, it can precipitate out to form stones. Biliary stasis, or slowed emptying of the gallbladder, contributes to cholelithiasis. Stones do not form when the gallbladder empties completely in response to hormonal stimulation. Slowed or incomplete emptying allows cholesterol to concentrate and increases the risk of stone formation. Finally, inflammation of the gallbladder allows excess water and bile salt reabsorption, increasing the risk for lithiasis.

Risk Factors

The incidence of gallstones varies among people of different ethnic backgrounds and other characteristics. Risk factors are listed in Box 16–2.

CLINICAL MANIFESTATIONS

Table 16–5 compares the manifestations and complications of acute cholelithiasis with those of cholecystitis.

COLLABORATION

Treatment of the client with cholelithiasis or cholecystitis depends on the acuity of the condition and the client's overall health status. When gallstones are present but asymptomatic and the client has a low risk for complications, conservative treatment is indicated. However, when the client experiences frequent symptoms, has acute cholecystitis, or has very large stones, the gallbladder and stones are usually surgically removed.

Diagnostic Tests

Diagnostic tests are ordered to identify the presence and location of stones, identify possible complications, and help differentiate gallbladder disease from other disorders.

- *Serum bilirubin* is measured. Elevated direct (conjugated) bilirubin may indicate obstructed bile flow in the biliary duct system (Box 16–3).
- *CBC* may indicate infection and inflammation if the WBC count is elevated.
- *Serum amylase* and *lipase* are measured to identify possible pancreatitis related to common duct obstruction.
- *Abdominal x-ray* (flat plate of the abdomen) may show gallstones that have a high calcium content.

TABLE 16–5 Manifestations and Complications of Cholelithiasis and Cholecystitis

MANIFESTATIONS	CHOLELITHIASIS	CHOLECYSTITIS
Pain	■ Abrupt onset ■ Severe, steady ■ Localized to epigastrium and RUQ of abdomen ■ May radiate to back, right scapula, and shoulder ■ Lasts 30 minutes to 5 hours	■ Abrupt onset ■ Severe, steady ■ Generalized in RUQ of abdomen ■ May radiate to back, right scapula, and shoulder ■ Lasts 12–18 hours ■ Aggravated by movement, breathing
Associated symptoms	■ Nausea, vomiting	■ Anorexia, nausea, vomiting ■ RUQ tenderness and guarding ■ Chills and fever
Complications	■ Cholecystitis ■ Common bile duct obstruction with possible jaundice and liver damage ■ Common duct obstruction with pancreatitis	■ Gangrene and perforation with peritonitis ■ Chronic cholecystitis ■ Empyema ■ Fistula formation ■ Gallstone ileus

Box 16–3 Sorting Out Total, Direct, and Indirect Bilirubin Levels

When serum bilirubin levels are drawn, the results usually are reported as the total bilirubin, direct bilirubin, and indirect bilirubin levels. Most bilirubin is formed from hemoglobin as aging or abnormal red blood cells (RBCs) are removed from circulation and destroyed. It is then bound to protein and transported to the liver. This protein-bound bilirubin is called *indirect* or *unconjugated* bilirubin. Once in the liver, bilirubin is separated from the protein and converted to a soluble form, *direct* or *conjugated* bilirubin. Conjugated bilirubin is then excreted in the bile.

- Total (serum) bilirubin, the total bilirubin in the blood, includes both indirect and direct forms. In adults, the normal total bilirubin is 0.3–1.2 mg/dL. Total bilirubin levels increase when more is being produced (e.g., RBC hemolysis) or when its metabolism or excretion are impaired (e.g., liver disease or biliary obstruction).
- Direct (conjugated) bilirubin levels, normally 0–0.2 mg/dL in adults, rise when its excretion is impaired by obstruction in the liver (e.g., in cirrhosis, hepatitis, exposure to hepatotoxins) or in the biliary system.
- Indirect (unconjugated) bilirubin levels, normally <1.1 mg/dL in adults, rise in RBC hemolysis (e.g., sickle cell disease or transfusion reaction).

- *Ultrasonography of the gallbladder* is a noninvasive exam that can accurately diagnose cholelithiasis. It also can be used to assess emptying of the gallbladder.
- *Oral cholecystogram* is performed using a dye administered orally to assess the gallbladder's ability to concentrate and excrete bile.
- *Gallbladder scans* use an intravenous radioactive solution that is rapidly extracted from the blood and excreted into the biliary tree to diagnose cystic duct obstruction and acute or chronic cholecystitis.

Pharmacologic Therapies

Clients who refuse surgery or for whom surgery is inappropriate may be treated with a drug to dissolve the gallstones. Ursodiol (Actigall) and chenodiol (Chenix) reduce the cholesterol content of gallstones, leading to their gradual dissolution. These drugs act by reducing cholesterol production in the liver, thus reducing the cholesterol content of bile. Consequently, these drugs are most effective in treating stones with high cholesterol content. They are less effective in treating radiopaque stones with high calcium salt content. Ursodiol is generally well tolerated with few side effects, whereas chenodiol has a high incidence of diarrhea at therapeutic doses. Chenodiol also is hepatotoxic, so periodic liver function studies are required during therapy. The primary disadvantages of pharmacologic treatment for gallstones include its cost, its long duration (2 years or more), and the high incidence of recurrent stone formation when treatment is discontinued.

If infection is suspected, antibiotics may be ordered to cure the infection and reduce associated inflammation and edema.

EVIDENCE-BASED PRACTICE Client Undergoing Laparoscopic Cholecystectomy

Following ambulatory surgery procedures such as laparoscopic cholecystectomy, clients must self-manage their pain after discharge. In a study of pain severity and management among ambulatory surgery clients, Watt-Watson, Chung, Chan, and McGillion (2004) found that while the most severe pain was experienced within the first 72 hours, some clients reported severe pain episodes up to a week after surgery. For most clients undergoing laparoscopic cholecystectomy, however, by 72 hours postoperatively the worst pain reported was moderate and the interference with usual activities was minimal. Clients tended to reduce their use of analgesics significantly by 72 hours after surgery, perhaps because many experienced adverse effects such as constipation, nausea, and/or drowsiness. Overall, analgesic use was found to be inadequate and inappropriate among study participants (Watt-Watson et al., 2004). Most clients used acetaminophen with codeine, an analgesic with known dose-related adverse effects. Some clients did not fill their prescription for the analgesic or stopped taking it early in the postoperative course because of nausea or constipation. Preoperative teaching about pain management was inadequate for a number of participants in this study.

Implications for Nursing

Effective pain relief is known to promote healing and immune function following surgery. This study indicates a crucial need to carefully prepare clients undergoing ambulatory surgery, including laparoscopic cholecystectomy, for pain management strategies. Effective postoperative pain management requires a combination of good preoperative education, discharge planning related to the client's expectations of pain, and postoperative pain management.

Critical Thinking in Client Care

1. Some clients in this study reported purposely not filling their analgesic prescription due to anticipated adverse effects of the drug. How can the nurse intervene to prevent this and to promote effective postoperative pain management? What teaching can the nurse provide to help clients manage adverse effects of the prescribed drug?
2. Few clients in this study reported use of adjunctive pain relief measures (nonsteroidal anti-inflammatory drugs (NSAIDs), application of heat or cold, etc.). What adjunctive pain relief measures would be appropriate for the nurse to teach clients undergoing laparoscopic cholecystectomy?
3. Some clients in this study expressed concern about becoming addicted to opioid analgesics, citing this as a reason to discontinue their use within 48–72 hours after surgery. How should the nurse respond to a client who expresses this as a concern?

Source: Data from Watt-Watson, J., Chung, F., Chan, V. W. S., and McGillion, M. (2004). Pain management following discharge after ambulatory same-day surgery. *Journal of Pain Management, 12*(3), 153–161.

Clients with pruritus (itching) due to severe obstructive jaundice and an accumulation of bile salts on the skin may be given cholestyramine (Questran). This drug binds with bile salts to promote their excretion in the feces. A narcotic analgesic such as morphine may be required for pain relief during an acute attack of cholecystitis.

Surgery

Laparoscopic cholecystectomy (removal of the gallbladder) is the treatment of choice for symptomatic cholelithiasis or cholecystitis. This minimally invasive procedure has a low risk of complications and generally requires a hospital stay of less than 24 hours. Not all clients are candidates for laparoscopic cholecystectomy, however, and there is a risk that a laparoscopic cholecystectomy may be converted to a *laparotomy* (surgical opening into the abdomen) during the procedure.

When stones are lodged in the ducts, a cholecystectomy with common bile duct exploration may be done. A T-tube (Figure 16–5 ■) is inserted to maintain patency of the duct and to promote bile passage while the edema decreases. Excess bile is collected in a drainage bag secured below the surgical site. If it is suspected that a stone has been retained following surgery, a postoperative cholangiogram via the T-tube or direct visualization of the duct with an endoscope may be performed. See Box 16–4 for nursing care for a client with a T-tube.

Some clients who are poor surgical risks and for whom laparoscopic cholecystectomy is inappropriate may have a *cholecystostomy* to drain the gallbladder or a *choledochostomy* to remove stones and position a T-tube in the common bile duct.

Nutrition

Food intake may be eliminated during an acute attack of cholecystitis and a nasogastric tube inserted to relieve nausea and vomiting. Dietary fat intake may be limited, especially if the client is obese. If bile flow is obstructed, fat-soluble vitamins (A, D, E, and K) and bile salts may need to be administered.

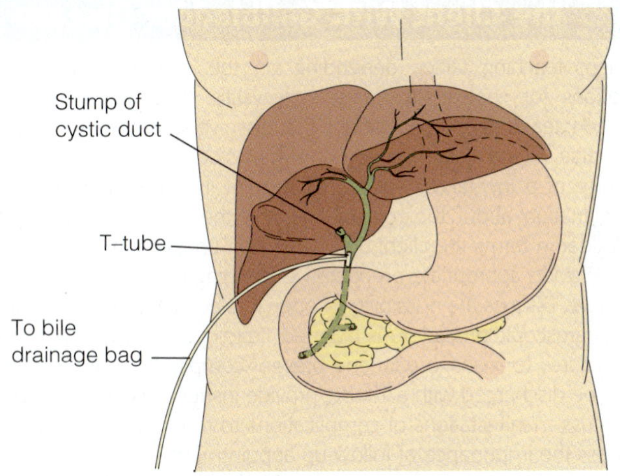

Figure 16–5 ■ T-tube placement in the common bile duct. Bile fluid flows with gravity into a drainage collection device below the level of the common bile duct.

Box 16–4 Nursing Care of the Client With a T-Tube

- Ensure that the T-tube is properly connected to a sterile container; keep the tube below the level of the surgical wound. This position promotes the flow of bile and prevents backflow or seepage of caustic bile onto the skin. The tube itself decreases biliary tree pressure.
- Monitor drainage from the T-tube for color and consistency; record as output. Normally, the tube may drain up to 500 mL in the first 24 hours after surgery; drainage decreases to less than 200 mL in 2–3 days and is minimal thereafter. Drainage may be blood-tinged initially, changing to green-brown. Report excessive drainage immediately. (After 48 hours, drainage greater than 500 mL is considered excessive.) Stones or edema and inflammation can obstruct ducts below the tube, requiring treatment.
- Place in Fowler's position. This promotes gravity drainage of bile.
- Assess skin for bile leakage during dressing changes. Bile irritates the skin; it may be necessary to apply skin protection with karaya or another barrier product.
- Teach client how to manage the tube when turning, ambulating, and performing activities of daily living. Direct pulling or traction on the tube must be avoided.
- If indicated, teach client how to take care of the T-tube, how to clamp it, and to recognize the signs of infection. Clients may be discharged home with the tube in place. Reporting early signs of infection facilitates prompt treatment.

Clinical Therapies

In some cases, shock wave lithotripsy may be used with drug therapy to dissolve large gallstones. In *extracorporeal shock wave lithotripsy,* ultrasound is used to align the stones with the source of shock waves and the computerized lithotripter. Positioning is of prime importance throughout the procedure, which usually takes an hour. Mild sedation may be given during the procedure. Nursing care after the procedure includes monitoring for biliary colic, which can result from the gallbladder contracting to remove stone fragments; nausea; and transient hematuria. *Percutaneous cholecystostomy,* ultrasound-guided drainage of the gallbladder, may be done in high-risk clients to postpone or even eliminate the need for surgery.

Complementary Therapies

The herb goldenseal has been used in treating cholecystitis. Berberine, one of the active ingredients in goldenseal, stimulates secretion of bile and bilirubin. It also inhibits the growth of many common pathogens, including those known to infect the gallbladder. A study of the effectiveness of berberine in clients with cholecystitis demonstrated relief of all symptoms. Goldenseal can stimulate the uterus, so it is contraindicated for use during pregnancy. It also should not be used by nursing mothers.

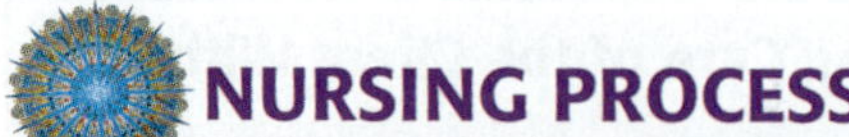

NURSING PROCESS

Although most risk factors for cholelithiasis cannot be controlled or modified, several can. Modifiable risk factors include obesity, hyperlipidemia, extremely low-calorie diets, and diets high in cholesterol. Encourage clients who are obese to increase their activity level and follow a low-carbohydrate, low-fat, low-cholesterol diet to promote weight loss and reduce their risk for developing gallstones. Discuss the dangers of yo-yo dieting, with cycles of weight loss followed by weight gain, and of extremely low-calorie diets. Encourage clients with high serum cholesterol levels to discuss using cholesterol-lowering drugs with their primary care provider.

Nursing care of the client with gallbladder disease is focused on client teaching, pain management, and instruction on healthy nutrition.

Assessment

Assessment data related to cholelithiasis and cholecystitis include the following:

- *Health history.* Current manifestations, including right upper quadrant pain, its character and relationship to meals, duration, and radiation; nausea and vomiting; other symptoms; duration of symptoms; risk factors or previous history of symptoms; chronic diseases such as diabetes, cirrhosis, or inflammatory bowel disease; current diet; use of oral contraceptives or possibility of pregnancy
- *Physical assessment.* Current weight; color of skin and sclera; abdominal assessment including light palpation for tenderness; color of urine and stool.

Diagnosis

Priority nursing diagnoses for the client with cholelithiasis or cholecystitis often include the following:

- Pain
- Imbalanced Nutrition
- Risk for Infection.

Plan

Goals of nursing care, developed in collaboration with the client, may include the following:

- Client will obtain adequate pain relief to allow for comfort.
- Client will demonstrate understanding of low-fat diet with adequate intake of fat-soluble vitamins.
- Client will verbalize symptoms to report immediately.
- Client will not contract an infection.

Implementation

Nursing interventions for the client who has undergone a laparoscopic or open cholecystectomy are similar to those for other clients who have had abdominal surgery.

Pain

The pain associated with cholelithiasis can be severe. Sometimes a combination of interventions is indicated.

- Discuss the relationship between fat intake and the pain. Teach ways to reduce fat intake (Box 16–5). Fat entering the duodenum initiates gallbladder contractions, causing pain when gallstones are present in the ducts.
- Withhold oral food and fluids during episodes of acute pain. Insert nasogastric tube and connect to low suction if ordered. Emptying the stomach reduces the amount of chyme entering the duodenum and the stimulus for gallbladder contractions, thus reducing pain.
- For severe pain, administer morphine, meperidine, or another narcotic analgesia as ordered. Recent research indicates that morphine is no more likely to cause spasms of the sphincter of Oddi than meperidine.
- Place in Fowler's position. Fowler's position decreases pressure on the inflamed gallbladder.
- Monitor vital signs, including temperature, at least every 4 hours. Bacterial infection often is present in acute cholecystitis and may cause an elevated temperature.

Imbalanced Nutrition: Less Than Body Requirements

The client with severe gallbladder disease may develop nutritional imbalances related to anorexia, pain, nausea following meals, and impaired bile flow that alters absorption

Box 16–5 Examples of High-Fat Foods

- Whole-milk products (e.g., cream, ice cream, cheese)
- Doughnuts, deep-fried
- Avocados
- Sausage, bacon, hot dogs
- Gravies with fat, cream
- Most nuts (e.g., pecans, cashews)
- Corn chips and potato chips
- Butter and cooking oils
- Fried foods (e.g., cheeseburgers, hamburgers, French fries)
- Peanut butter
- Chocolate candy

CARE SETTINGS Community Care for the Client With Gallbladder Disease

Client teaching varies depending on the choice of treatment options for cholelithiasis and cholecystitis. If surgery is not an option, teach about medications that dissolve stones; their use and adverse effects (diarrhea is a common side effect); and maintenance of a low-fat, low-carbohydrate diet if indicated. Include an explanation about the role of bile and the function of the gallbladder in terms the client and family can understand.

Provide appropriate preoperative teaching for the planned procedure. Discuss the possibility of open cholecystectomy even when a laparoscopic procedure is planned. Teach postoperative self-care measures to manage pain and prevent complications. If the client will be discharged with a T-tube, provide instructions about its care. Discuss manifestations of complications to report to the physician. Stress the importance of follow-up appointments.

Following cholecystectomy, a low-fat diet may be recommended initially. Refer the client and food preparer to a dietitian to review low-fat foods. (See Box 16–5 for examples of high-fat foods to avoid.) Higher-fat foods may be added to the diet gradually as tolerated.

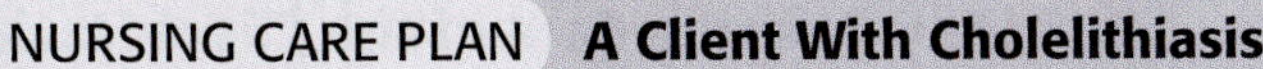

NURSING CARE PLAN A Client With Cholelithiasis

Joyce Red Wing is a 44-year-old married mother of three children. A member of the Chickasaw tribe, she is active in tribal activities and works part-time as a cook at a community kitchen. Recently, Mrs. Red Wing has noticed a dull pain in her upper abdomen that gets worse after eating fatty foods; nausea and sometimes vomiting accompany the pain. She had a similar pain after the birth of her last child. She is diagnosed with cholelithiasis and is admitted for a laparoscopic cholecystectomy.

ASSESSMENT

David Corbin, RN, takes Mrs. Red Wing's admission history. It includes intolerance to fatty foods and intermittent "stabbing" abdominal pain that radiates to her back. Her usual diet includes tacos or fried bread and biscuits with gravy for breakfast. She reports "not wanting to eat much of anything lately." She states that she has never had surgery before and hopes "everything goes well." Physical assessment includes T_O 37.7°C (100°F), P 88, R 20, and BP 130/84. She has had a recent 5 lb weight loss, currently weighing 130 lb (59 kg). She is 63 inches (160 cm) tall. Abdominal examination elicits tenderness in the right upper abdominal quadrant. She has no jaundice, chills, or evidence of complications.

DIAGNOSES

- Imbalanced Nutrition: Less Than Body Requirements related to anorexia and recent weight loss
- Pain related to inflamed gallbladder and surgical incisions
- Risk for Infection related to potential bacterial contamination of abdominal cavity
- Anxiety related to lack of information about perioperative experience

PLANNING

- Maintain present weight within 5 lb (2.3 kg) over the next 3 weeks.
- Resume regular diet, decreasing intake of foods high in fat.
- Verbalize adequate pain control after surgery and with activity resumption.
- Remain free of infection.
- Verbalize a decrease in anxiety before surgery.

IMPLEMENTATION

- Teach about the gallbladder and the function of bile.
- Discuss pre- and postoperative care, including self-care following discharge.
- Promote mobility as soon as allowed after surgery.
- Teach home care of incisions and recognition of signs of infection.
- Review specific high-fat foods to avoid and ways to maintain her weight.
- Provide analgesia as needed postoperatively. Teach appropriate analgesic use after discharge.

EVALUATION

Mrs. Red Wing is discharged the morning after her surgery. She is afebrile, has no signs of infection, and is able to appropriately care for her incisions. She identifies signs of infection and talks about ways to reduce her fat intake while keeping her weight stable. She verbalizes understanding of initial activity restrictions and resumption of normal activities. Mrs. Red Wing states, "It wasn't as bad as I thought it would be at first." She has an appointment to see her surgeon in 1 week.

CRITICAL THINKING

1. What is the rationale for a low-fat diet with cholelithiasis? Discuss nutritional practices as they relate to the medical problem and Mrs. Red Wing's culture.
2. How would your discharge teaching for Mrs. Red Wing differ if she had had an open cholecystectomy instead of a laparoscopic cholecystectomy?
3. Design a nursing care plan for Mrs. Red Wing for the nursing diagnosis fatigue.

of fat and fat-soluble vitamins (A, D, E, and K) from the gut.

- Assess nutritional status, including diet history, height and weight, and skinfold measurements. Clients with gallbladder disease may have an imbalanced diet or may have specific vitamin deficiencies, particularly the fat-soluble vitamins.
- Evaluate laboratory results, including serum bilirubin, albumin, glucose, and cholesterol levels. Report abnormal results to the primary care provider. Elevated serum bilirubin may indicate impaired bilirubin excretion due to obstructed bile flow. A low serum albumin may indicate poor nutritional status. Glucose intolerance and hypercholesterolemia are risk factors for cholelithiasis.
- Refer to a dietitian or nutritionist for diet counseling to promote healthy weight loss and to reduce pain episodes. A low-carbohydrate, low-fat, higher-protein diet reduces symptoms of cholecystitis. While fasting and very low-calorie diets are contraindicated, a moderate reduction in calorie intake and increased activity levels promote weight loss.
- Administer vitamin supplements as ordered. Clients who do not absorb fat well due to obstructed bile flow may require supplements of the fat-soluble vitamins.

Risk for Infection

An acutely inflamed gallbladder may become necrotic and rupture, releasing its contents into the abdominal cavity. While the resulting infection often remains localized, peritonitis can result from chemical irritation and bacterial contamination of the peritoneal cavity.

Following open cholecystectomy (*laparotomy*), the risk for pulmonary infection is significant due to the high abdominal incision.

- Monitor vital signs, including temperature, every 4 hours. Promptly report vital sign changes or temperature elevation.

Tachycardia, increased respiratory rate, or an elevated temperature may indicate an infectious process.

- Assess abdomen every 4 hours and as indicated (e.g., when pain level changes abruptly). Increasing abdominal tenderness or a rigid, boardlike abdomen may indicate rupture of the gallbladder with peritonitis.
- Assist with coughing and deep breathing or use incentive spirometer every 1–2 hours while awake. Splint abdominal incision with a blanket or pillow during coughing. The high abdominal incision of an open cholecystectomy interferes with effective coughing and deep breathing, increasing the risk of atelectasis and respiratory infections such as pneumonia.
- Place in Fowler's position and encourage ambulation as allowed. Fowler's position and ambulation promote lung expansion and airway clearance, reducing the risk of respiratory infections.
- Administer antibiotics as ordered. Antibiotics may be given preoperatively to reduce the risk of infection from infected gallbladder contents; they may be continued postoperatively to prevent infection.

Evaluation

Client progress toward goals may be evaluated based on the following expected outcomes:

- Client reports adequate pain control to maintain comfort.
- Client demonstrates food choices reflecting diet low in fat and high in fat-soluble vitamins.
- Client's temperature remains within normal limits, and client displays no symptoms of infection.

Box 16–6 Nursing Care of the Client Having Laparoscopic Cholecystectomy

PREOPERATIVE CARE

- Provide routine preoperative care as ordered.
- Reinforce teaching about the procedure and postoperative expectations, including pain management, deep breathing, and mobilization. Preoperative teaching reduces anxiety and promotes rapid postoperative recovery.

POSTOPERATIVE CARE

- Provide routine postoperative recovery care.
- Assist to chair at bedside as allowed. Early mobilization promotes lung ventilation and circulation, reducing the potential for postoperative complications.
- Advance oral intake from ice chips to regular diet as tolerated. Oral intake can be rapidly resumed due to minimal disruption of the gastrointestinal (GI) tract during surgery.
- Provide and reinforce teaching regarding pain management, incision care, activity level, and postoperative follow-up appointments. With early discharge, the client and family assume responsibility for the majority of postoperative care. A clear understanding of this care and expected needs reduces anxiety and the risk of postoperative complications.
- Initiate follow-up contact 24–48 hours after discharge to evaluate adequacy of pain control, incision management, and discharge understanding. Contact following discharge provides an opportunity to evaluate care and reinforce teaching.

REVIEW Gallbladder Disease

RELATE: LINK THE CONCEPTS

Linking the exemplar of Gallbladder Disease with the concept of Fluids and Electrolytes:

1. How might gallbladder disease affect fluid homeostasis?
2. What nursing care might you initiate with the client who reports severe, acute abdominal pain secondary to cholelithiasis to avoid fluid and electrolyte imbalance?

Linking the exemplar of Gallbladder Disease with the concept of Health, Wellness, and Illness:

3. What health promotion topics might you teach adults to prevent the development of cholelithiasis?
4. What group would you consider most at risk for development of gallbladder disease?

READY: GO TO COMPANION SKILLS MANUAL

- Assessing the abdomen
- Assessing the client in pain
- Inserting a nasogastric (NG) tube
- Removing a nasogastric tube
- Using an incentive spirometer
- Deep breathing and coughing
- Using the narcotic control system
- Administering oral medications

REFER: GO TO MYNURSINGKIT

REFLECT: CASE STUDY

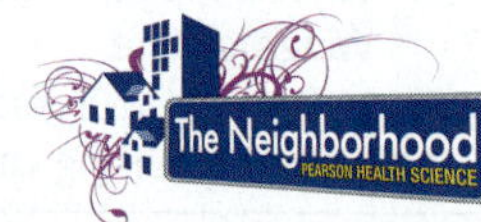

Helen Martin is a 48-year-old Caucasian female who is married to Gil Martin. They have been married for 18 years. Helen has a daughter (Tracie) from a previous marriage, and she has two teenage children with Gil (Anthony and Kristina). Helen works as a teller at a bank. Although she finds her job monotonous, she appreciates the steady income and family health insurance.

Helen is overweight and has tried to lose weight most of her adult life. She frequently diets and, in fact, has lost a great deal of weight in the past but has been unable to keep the weight off. She blames menopause for her most recent weight gain.

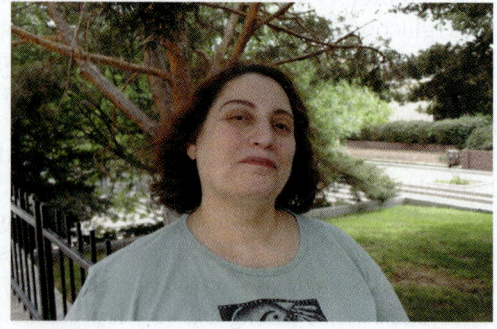

Helen experiences indigestion following a few meals. Over several weeks, the severity and frequency increases. She takes an antacid, believing the problem is just heartburn. The discomfort is usually located in the upper right side of her abdomen, and sometimes it is quite painful. The pain may last up to a couple of hours and then subsides. Occasionally, she feels nauseous as well. After putting up with this for several weeks, she makes an appointment with her physician.

Based on Helen's symptoms, her physician suspects that Helen has cholelithiasis and orders an ultrasound scan of her abdomen. The ultrasound confirms the presence of gallstones. The physician tells Helen that she has two options: (1) conservative therapy that would involve dietary modification involving a low-fat, reduced-calorie diet or (2) surgery to remove her gallbladder. Helen decides to try dietary modification.

1. What information would you include in your teaching plan for Helen about low-fat, low-calorie diets?
2. Based on your own likes and dislikes, design a 1-week diet plan, including all meals and snacks, that would meet the low-fat low calorie requirements for Helen.
3. What rationale exists for beginning with conservative treatment as opposed to immediately initiating surgical intervention?
4. How will you evaluate the effectiveness of conservative treatment for Helen?

16.3 INFLAMMATORY BOWEL DISEASE

KEY TERMS

Chronic intermittent colitis, *909*
Colectomy, *916*
Crohn's disease, *909*
Fulminant colitis, *909*
Ileostomy, *917*
Inflammatory bowel disease (IBD), *909*
Stoma, *916*
Ulcerative colitis, *909*

BASIS FOR SELECTION OF EXEMPLAR

Centers for Disease Control and Prevention
Chronic Disease Management
Health People 2010
Institute of Medicine

LEARNING OUTCOMES

After reading about this exemplar, you will be able to:

1. Describe the pathophysiology, etiology, clinical manifestations, and direct and indirect causes of inflammatory bowel disease.
2. Identify risk factors associated with inflammatory bowel disease.
3. Illustrate the nursing process in providing culturally competent care across the life span for individuals with inflammatory bowel disease.
4. Formulate priority nursing diagnoses appropriate for an individual with inflammatory bowel disease.
5. Create a plan of care for individuals with inflammatory bowel disease and their family members.
6. Assess expected outcomes for an individual with inflammatory bowel disease.
7. Discuss therapies used in the collaborative care of an individual with inflammatory bowel disease.
8. Employ evidence-based caring interventions for an individual with inflammatory bowel disease.

OVERVIEW

As many as 1 million Americans have **inflammatory bowel disease (IBD)**, chronic inflammation of the bowel, with that number divided about equally between ulcerative colitis and Crohn's disease (Crohn's & Colitis Foundation of America, 2005). **Ulcerative colitis** is a chronic inflammatory bowel disorder that affects the mucosa and submucosa of the colon and rectum.

Chronic intermittent colitis (recurrent ulcerative colitis) is the most common form of the disease and affects 250,000–500,000 people in the United States each year, resulting in steep hospital and drug costs as well as lost work (Hellekson, 2005). Its onset is insidious, with attacks lasting 1–3 months and occurring at intervals of months to years. Typically, only the distal colon is affected, with few systemic manifestations of the disease.

Approximately 15% of people with ulcerative colitis develop **fulminant colitis**, an acute form of the disease that involves the entire colon. Manifestations include severe bloody diarrhea, acute abdominal pain, and fever. Clients with fulminant disease are at high risk for complications.

Like ulcerative colitis, **Crohn's disease** is a chronic, relapsing inflammatory disorder affecting the gastrointestinal (GI) tract. Crohn's disease, also known as regional enteritis, can affect any portion of the GI tract from the mouth to the anus, but it usually affects the terminal ileum and ascending colon. About 30–40% of clients with Crohn's disease experience only small bowel involvement. The disease is limited to the colon only in 15–20% of those affected. Both the small and large intestine are involved in the majority of clients (Porth, 2005). A comparison of ulcerative colitis and Crohn's disease is found in Table 16–6.

PATHOPHYSIOLOGY AND ETIOLOGY

The inflammatory process of ulcerative colitis begins at the rectosigmoid area of the anal canal and progresses proximally. In most clients, the disease is confined to the rectum and sigmoid colon. It may progress to involve the entire colon, stopping at the ileocecal junction.

Ulcerative colitis begins with inflammation at the base of the crypts of Lieberkühn in the distal large intestine and rectum.

TABLE 16–6 **Characteristics of Ulcerative Colitis and Crohn's Disease**

	CHARACTERISTIC	ULCERATIVE COLITIS	CROHN'S DISEASE
Clinical	Gender	Equal	Equal
	Age at onset	15–35 years; secondary peak between 50 and 70 years	10–30 years
	Course of disease	Typically chronic and intermittent	Slowly progressive, relapsing
	Diarrhea	5–30 stools per day with blood and mucus	Common, usually less severe than colitis, with no obvious blood or mucus in stool
	Abdominal pain	Cramping in left lower quadrant; relieved by defecation	Cramping or steady right lower quadrant or periumbilical pain; tenderness and mass noted in right lower quadrant
	Nutritional deficit	Common; involves anemia, hypoalbuminemia, and weight loss	Common and significant; involves anemia, weight loss, and multiple vitamin and mineral deficits
	Constitutional manifestations	Fever rare; may have associated arthritic, skin, or other organ involvement such as erythema nodosum or uveitis	Fever, malaise, fatigue; may have some associated conditions and urinary complications
Pathologic	Depth of involvement	Mucosa and submucosa	Transmural (entire bowel wall)
	Portion of bowel involved	Typically rectum and sigmoid colon; may extend to involve entire large bowel	Any portion of GI tract; terminal ileum and ascending colon involvement predominates
	Distribution	Continuous from rectum	Patchy; skip lesions
	Appearance of mucosa	Granular, dull, hyperemic, friable; disease uniform in affected bowel; pseudopolyps may be seen	Cobblestone appearance, with areas of normal tissue surrounded by ulceration and fissures
Complications	Acute	Toxic megacolon, perforation, massive hemorrhage	Obstruction, fistulization, abscess formation, malabsorption
	Long-term	Colorectal cancer	Colon cancer

Microscopic, pinpoint mucosal hemorrhages occur, and crypt abscesses develop (Figure 16–6 ■). These abscesses penetrate the superficial submucosa and spread laterally, leading to necrosis and sloughing of bowel mucosa. Further tissue damage is caused by inflammatory exudates and the release of inflammatory mediators such as prostaglandins and other cytokines. The mucosa becomes red and edematous due to vascular congestion, friable (easily broken), and ulcerated. It bleeds easily, and hemorrhage is common. Edema creates a granular appearance. Pseudopolyps, tonguelike projections of bowel mucosa into the lumen, may develop as the epithelial lining of the bowel regenerates. Chronic inflammation leads to atrophy, narrowing, and shortening of the colon, with loss of its normal haustra (small pouches or recesses into which the large intestine is divided).

Crohn's disease typically begins as a small inflammatory *aphthoid lesion* (a shallow ulcer with a white base and elevated margin, similar to a canker sore) of the mucosa and submucosa of the bowel. These initial lesions may regress, or the inflammatory process can progress to involve all layers of the intestinal wall. Deeper ulcerations, granulomatous lesions, and fissures (knifelike clefts that extend deeply into the bowel wall) develop. The inflammatory process involves the entire bowel wall (transmural).

The lumen of the affected bowel assumes a cobblestone appearance as fissures and ulcers surround islands of intact mucosa over edematous submucosa. The inflammatory lesions of Crohn's disease are not continuous; rather, they often occur as "skip" lesions with intervening areas of normal-appearing bowel. Some evidence suggests that despite its normal appearance, the entire bowel is affected by this disorder.

As the disease progresses, fibrotic changes in the bowel wall cause it to thicken and lose flexibility, taking on a rubber hoselike appearance. The inflammation, edema, and fibrosis can lead to local obstruction, the development of abscesses, and the formation of fistulas between loops of bowel or between bowel and other organs (Figure 16–7 ■). Fistulas between loops of bowel are known as enteroenteric fistulas; fistulas that occur between bowel and bladder are known as enterovesical fistulas; and fistulas that occur between bowel and skin are known as enterocutaneous fistulas. Perineal fistulas are relatively common, originating in the ileum.

Depending on the severity and extent of the disease, malabsorption and malnutrition may develop as the ulcers prevent absorption of nutrients. When the jejunum and ileum are affected, the absorption of multiple nutrients (including carbohydrates, proteins, fats, vitamins, and folate) may be impaired. Disease in the terminal ileum can lead to vitamin B_{12} malabsorption and bile salt reabsorption. The ulcerations also can lead to protein loss and chronic, slow blood loss with consequent anemia.

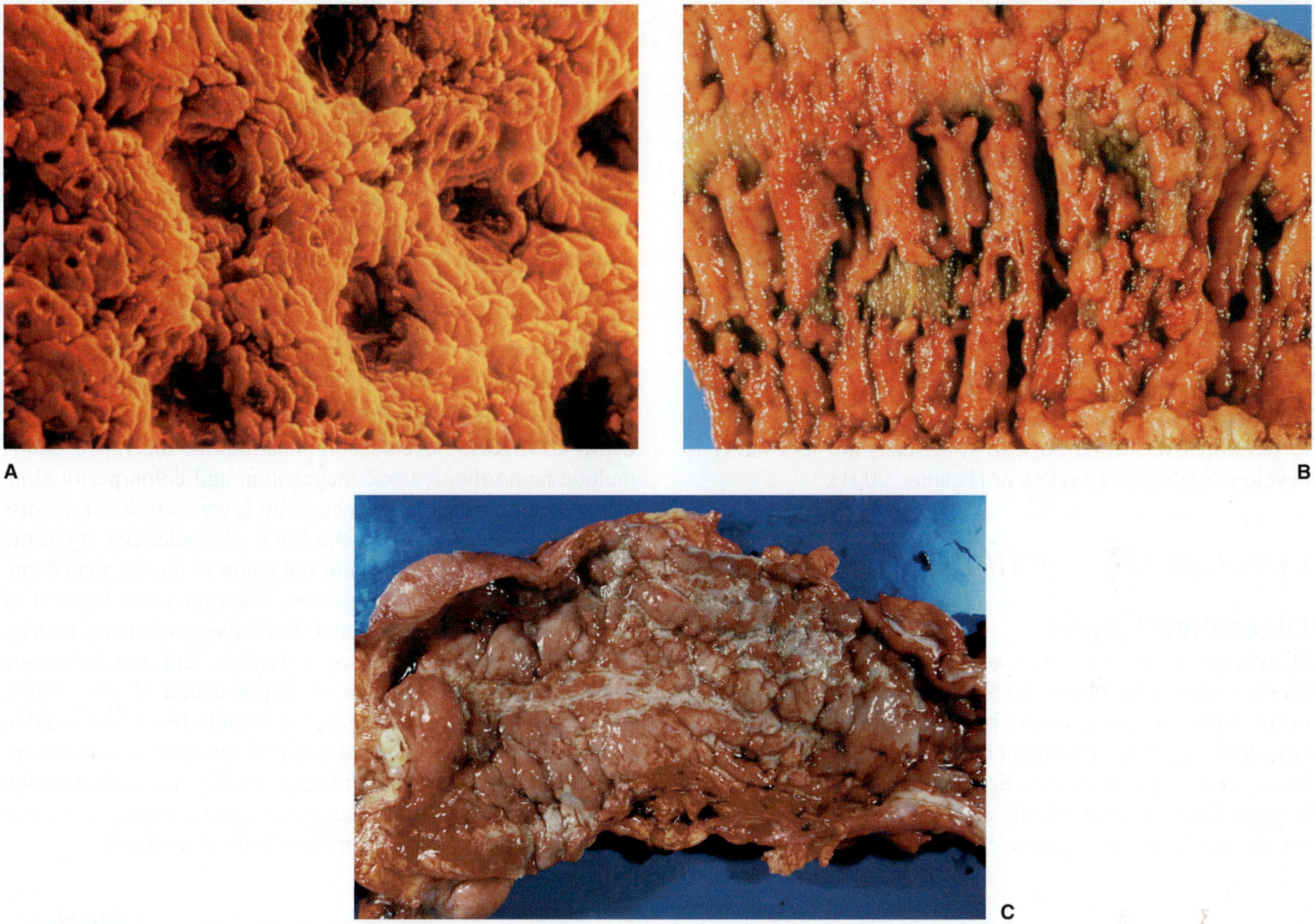

A

B

C

Figure 16–6 ■ *A* Photomicrograph of the mucosa of the large intestine showing the entrances to the crypts of Lieberkühn. The crypts are the focal points for *B* ulcerative colitis and *C* Crohn's disease.

Source: B, Dr. E. Walker/Photo Researchers, Inc., C, Javier Domingo/Photo Researchers, Inc.

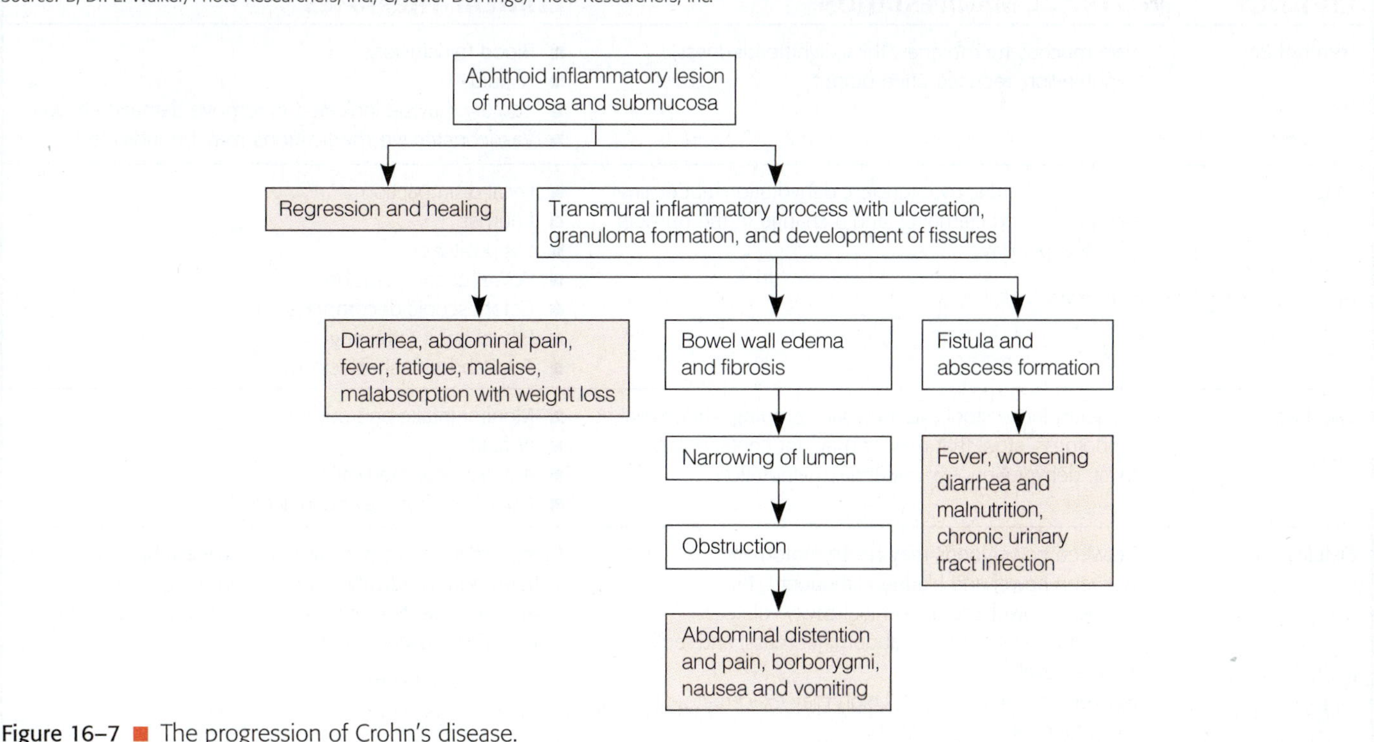

Figure 16–7 ■ The progression of Crohn's disease.

Etiology

The etiology of both ulcerative colitis and Crohn's disease is unknown. Genetic and environmental factors have been implicated in the development of IBD. Factors such as an infectious agent and altered immune responses are thought to play a role in the development of IBD. Autoimmunity is thought to play a role, and lifestyle factors (such as smoking) also may affect its development.

Risk Factors

Inflammatory bowel disease occurs more frequently in the United States and in northern European nations than it does in southern Europe and countries in the Southern Hemisphere. American Jews of European descent are 4–5 times more likely to develop IBD, while African Americans are less likely to develop the disease (Bayless & Hanauer, 2001).

CLINICAL MANIFESTATIONS

Ulcerative Colitis

Diarrhea is the predominant manifestation of ulcerative colitis. Stools contain both blood and mucus. Nocturnal diarrhea may occur. Mild ulcerative colitis is characterized by fewer than five stools per day, intermittent rectal bleeding and mucus, and few systemic manifestations. Severe ulcerative colitis can lead to more than six to ten bloody stools per day, extensive colon involvement, anemia, hypovolemia, and malnutrition. Rectal inflammation causes fecal urgency and tenesmus (a painful but ineffective urge to defecate). Left lower quadrant cramping relieved by defecation is common. Other manifestations include fatigue, anorexia, and weakness.

Clients with severe disease may have systemic manifestations such as arthritis involving one or several joints, skin and mucous membrane lesions, or *uveitis* (inflammation of the uvea, the vascular layer of the eye, which may involve the sclera and cornea as well). Some clients develop thromboemboli, with blood vessel obstruction due to clots carried from the site of their formation. Sclerosing cholangitis (inflammation and scarring of the bile ducts) may occur; it is more common in men than women, occurring most frequently in the third to fifth decade of life (Porth, 2005).

COMPLICATIONS Acute complications of ulcerative colitis include hemorrhage, toxic megacolon, and colon perforation. Massive hemorrhage may occur with severe attacks of the disease. *Toxic megacolon,* a condition characterized by acute motor paralysis and dilation of the colon to greater than 6 cm, may affect part or all of the colon. The transverse segment of the bowel is most often affected. Toxic megacolon may be triggered by the use of laxatives, narcotics, and anticholinergic drugs and by the presence of hypokalemia (Porth, 2005). Manifestations of toxic megacolon include fever, tachycardia, hypotension, dehydration, abdominal tenderness and cramping, and a change in the number of stools per day. Perforation is rare, but the risk of this dangerous complication is increased with toxic megacolon. Perforation leads to peritonitis.

CLINICAL MANIFESTATIONS AND THERAPIES Inflammatory Bowel Disease

ETIOLOGY	CLINICAL MANIFESTATION	CLINICAL THERAPIES
Hemorrhage	Pale mucous membranes, thirst, lightheadedness, hypotension, reduced urine output	■ Blood transfusions ■ IV fluid ■ Surgery may be indicated to remove damaged bowel ■ Vasoconstrictive medications may be indicated
Megacolon	Fever, tachycardia, hypotension, dehydration, abdominal tenderness and cramping, and a change in the number of stools per day	■ Fecal disimpaction ■ Enemas ■ Suppositories ■ Bowel decompression ■ Colonoscopic decompression ■ Bowel habit retraining ■ Total abdominal colectomy
Diarrhea	Frequent loose stools, abdominal cramping, abdominal tenderness, stool that may or may not contain blood, thirst, dehydration, hypovolemia, malnutrition	■ Monitor intake and output ■ IV fluid ■ Antidiarrheal medications ■ Guaiac testing may be indicated
Fistulas	Between bowel loops may be asymptomatic. Between bowel and bladder–Frequent UTIs. Between bowel and abdominal cavity–abscess, chills and fever, a tender abdominal mass, and leukocytosis develop. Between small bowel and colon may exacerbate diarrhea, weight loss, and malnutrition.	Symptomatic treatment may include antibiotics, antidiarrheal medication, and IV fluid support. Dissection of section of bowel with fistula may be indicated if tissue cannot be repaired.

MULTISYSTEM EFFECTS OF **Inflammatory Bowel Disease**

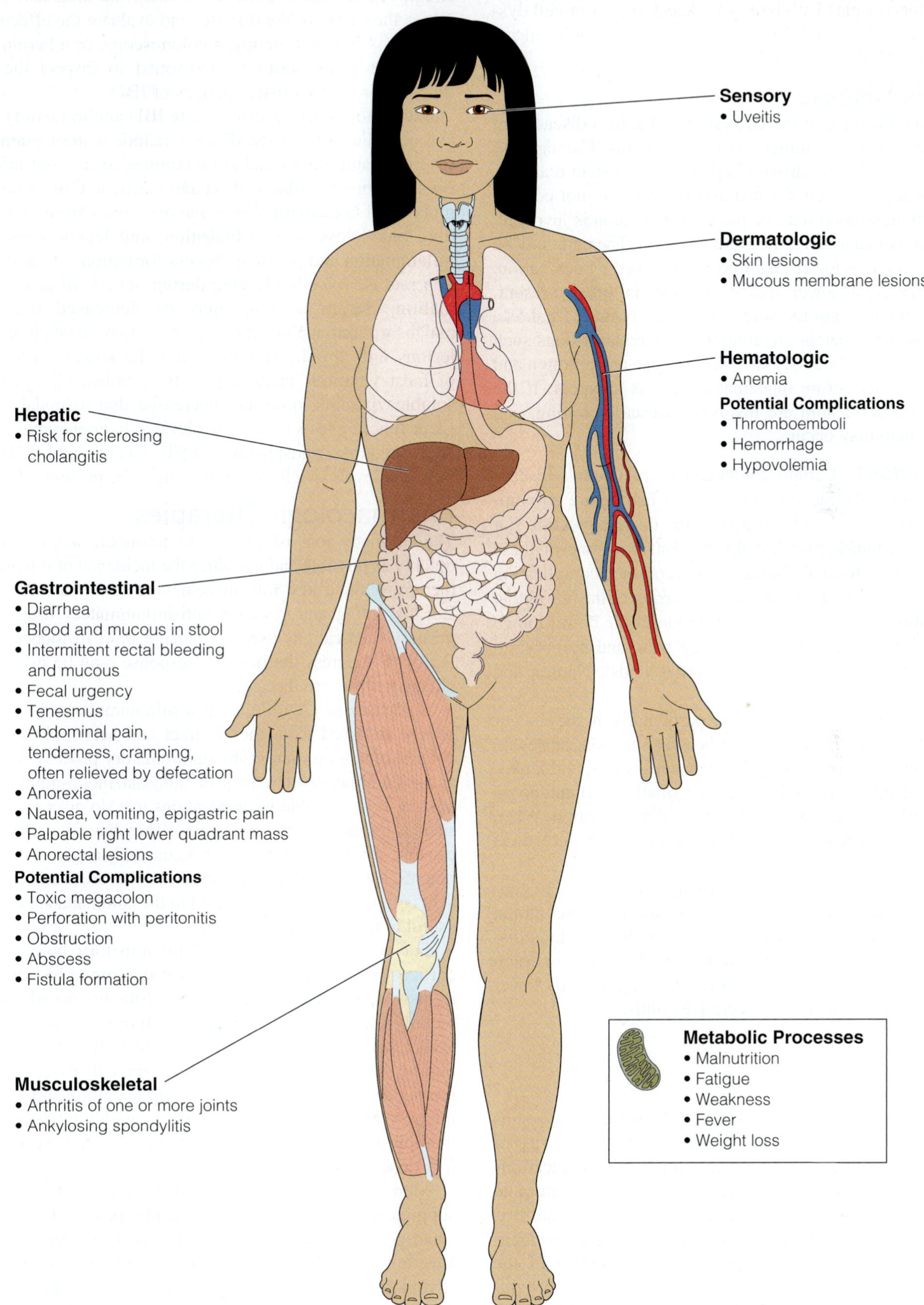

Sensory
• Uveitis
Dermatologic
• Skin lesions
• Mucous membrane lesions
Hematologic
• Anemia
Potential Complications
• Thromboemboli
• Hemorrhage
• Hypovolemia
Hepatic
• Risk for sclerosing cholangitis
Gastrointestinal
• Diarrhea
• Blood and mucous in stool
• Intermittent rectal bleeding and mucous
• Fecal urgency
• Tenesmus
• Abdominal pain, tenderness, cramping, often relieved by defecation
• Anorexia
• Nausea, vomiting, epigastric pain
• Palpable right lower quadrant mass
• Anorectal lesions
Potential Complications
• Toxic megacolon
• Perforation with peritonitis
• Obstruction
• Abscess
• Fistula formation
Musculoskeletal
• Arthritis of one or more joints
• Ankylosing spondylitis
Metabolic Processes
• Malnutrition
• Fatigue
• Weakness
• Fever
• Weight loss

Clients with ulcerative colitis are at increased risk for colorectal cancer. Beginning 8–10 years after the diagnosis, yearly colonoscopies with biopsy to detect masses or cell dysplasia are recommended for clients who have extensive ulcerative colitis (Hellekson, 2005).

Crohn's Disease

Because involvement of the GI system in Crohn's disease can be so diverse, manifestations vary among clients. The majority of people with Crohn's disease experience persistent diarrhea. Stools are liquid or semiformed and typically do not contain blood, although blood may be passed if the colon is involved. Abdominal pain and tenderness are common. The pain may be located in the right lower quadrant and relieved by defecation. A palpable right lower quadrant mass is often present. Systemic manifestations such as fever, fatigue, malaise, weight loss, and anemia are common. Anorectal lesions such as fissures, ulcers, fistulas, and abscesses also are common and may occur years before intestinal disease is apparent. If the stomach and duodenum are involved, nausea, vomiting, and epigastric pain may occur.

COMPLICATIONS Certain complications of Crohn's disease (e.g., intestinal obstruction, abscess, and fistula) are so common that they are considered part of the disease process. For many clients, the disease initially presents with one of these complications. Intestinal obstruction is a common complication caused by repeated inflammation and scarring of the bowel that leads to fibrosis and stricture. Obstruction of the bowel lumen causes abdominal distention, cramping pain, and borborygmi (excessive loud and hyperactive bowel sounds). Nausea and vomiting may occur.

Fistulas may be asymptomatic, particularly if they occur between loops of small bowel. When fistulization causes an abscess, chills and fever, a tender abdominal mass, and leukocytosis develop. A fistula between the small bowel and colon may exacerbate diarrhea, weight loss, and malnutrition. When the bladder is involved, recurrent urinary tract infections (UTIs) occur.

Perforation of the bowel is uncommon, but can lead to generalized peritonitis. Massive hemorrhage also is an uncommon complication of Crohn's disease. Long-standing Crohn's disease increases the risk of cancer of the small intestine or colon by 5–6 times. This cancer risk, however, is significantly lower than the risk associated with ulcerative colitis.

COLLABORATION

Interdisciplinary care for inflammatory bowel disease begins by establishing the diagnosis and the extent and severity of the disease. Treatment is supportive, including medications and dietary measures to decrease inflammation, promote intestinal rest and healing, and reduce intestinal motility. Many clients with IBD require surgery at some point to manage the disease or its complications. As a member of the health care team, the nurse plays an essential role by providing client teaching about disease management, diagnostic tests, and surgical or other treatments.

Diagnostic Tests

Diagnostic testing is used to establish the diagnosis of IBD, assess the extent of the disease, and evaluate the effects of the disorder. A sigmoidoscopy, a colonoscopy, or a barium upper and lower x-ray series is performed to inspect the bowel mucosa for characteristic changes of IBD.

Laboratory tests to differentiate IBD and to identify effects and complications of the disease include a stool examination for blood and mucus and stool cultures to rule out infectious causes of bowel inflammation and diarrhea. CBC with hemoglobin and hematocrit shows anemia from chronic inflammation, blood loss, and malnutrition, and leukocytosis due to inflammation and possible abscess formation. The sedimentation rate is typically elevated during periods of acute inflammation. Serum albumin may be decreased because of malabsorption, malnutrition, protein loss through intestinal lesions, and chronic inflammation. Folic acid and serum levels of most vitamins, including A, B complex, C, and the fat-soluble vitamins, often are decreased due to malabsorption. Liver function tests may show elevated liver enzymes (such as ALT, alkaline phosphatase, AST, GGTP, and LDH) and bilirubin levels if sclerosing cholangitis is present.

Pharmacologic Therapies

The ultimate goal of care is to terminate acute attacks as quickly as possible and to reduce the incidence of relapse. Drug therapy plays a key role in achieving this goal (Box 16–7). Locally acting and systemic anti-inflammatory drugs are the primary medications used to manage mild to moderate IBD. Drugs to suppress the immune response may be used to treat clients with severe disease.

Sulfasalazine (Azulfidine) is a sulfonamide antibiotic that is poorly absorbed from the GI tract and acts topically on the colonic mucosa to inhibit the inflammatory process. The active anti-inflammatory ingredient in sulfasalazine, 5-aminosalicylic acid, also is available in preparations that do not contain sulfa, such as olsalazine and mesalamine. They have the advantage of causing fewer adverse effects than sulfasalazine. Azo compounds, such as balsalazide and olsalazine, are 5-aminosalicylic acid compounds that are released in the colon and are especially useful to treat ulcerative colitis.

For acute exacerbations of inflammatory bowel disease, corticosteroids are given to reduce inflammation and induce remission. For ulcerative colitis, the drug may be administered rectally for its local effect and to minimize systemic effects. Hydrocortisone can be administered rectally. Intravenous corticosteroids may be required to treat severe disease; oral preparations are used for less severe manifestations and long-term therapy. Many clients are unable to withdraw from steroid therapy without experiencing relapse and may need chronic low-dose therapy.

Mercaptopurine (6-MP, Purinethol) and other immunosuppressive agents such as azathioprine (Imuran) and cyclosporine (Sandimmune) can be used to treat clients who have not responded to other treatments or who require chronic steroid therapy. These drugs may allow withdrawal from corticosteroids, maintain remission, and facilitate healing. Long-term therapy may be required to produce a beneficial effect.

Box 16–7 Medication Administration: Inflammatory Bowel Disease

SULFASALAZINE (AZULFIDINE)

Sulfasalazine is an anti-inflammatory drug used for its local effect on the intestinal mucosa in IBD. The active part of the drug is 5-aminosalicylic acid, which inhibits prostaglandin production in the bowel. Prostaglandin is an important mediator of the inflammatory process; blocking its production reduces inflammation.

Nursing Responsibilities

- Assess for contraindications, including pregnancy or a history of hypersensitivity to sulfonamides or salicylates.
- Assess baseline values for renal function tests (serum creatinine, blood urea nitrogen (BUN), urinalysis), liver function tests, and CBC.
- Administer as ordered. Suppositories or retention enemas may be administered at bedtime. Administer oral forms with a full glass of water.
- Have resuscitation equipment available; anaphylactic responses may occur.
- Evaluate for therapeutic response, including reduced number of stools, reduced mucus and blood, and improved stool consistency.
- Monitor for the following possible adverse responses:
  a. Skin rash, dermatitis, urticaria, or pruritus
  b. Evidence of blood dyscrasias such as bleeding, easy bruising, or fever
  c. Leukopenia, thrombocytopenia, hemolytic anemia, or angranulocytosis
  d. Changes in urinary output or renal function studies
  e. Evidence of hepatitis or myocarditis.

Health Education for the Client and Family

- Take oral preparations after meals to decrease gastric distress.
- Drink at least 2 quarts of fluid per day to reduce the risk of kidney damage.
- Use sunscreen to prevent burns; this drug increases sensitivity to sun.
- Do not take aspirin, vitamin C, or any other over-the-counter medications containing aspirin or vitamin C without consulting your doctor.
- Use alternative methods of contraception; this medication may interfere with the effectiveness of oral contraceptives.
- Notify your doctor if you develop skin rash or hives, sore throat or mouth, bleeding gums, joint pain, easy bruising, or fever.

MESALAMINE (ASACOL, ROWASA) AND OLSALAZINE (DIPENTUM)

Mesalamine and olsalazine also contain 5-aminosalicylic acid, but they cause fewer adverse effects than sulfasalazine. Their mechanism of action is the same as that of sulfasalazine. These drugs are available as suppositories, suspension for enema, or oral tablets.

Nursing Responsibilities

- Assess for possible contraindications such as pregnancy, lactation, or hypersensitivity to these drugs or to aspirin.
- Administer as ordered. If more than one dose per day is ordered, space doses evenly over the 24-hour period.
- Evaluate for desired effects (as for sulfasalazine) and potential adverse effects, including the following:
  a. Nausea, diarrhea, abdominal cramps, or flatulence
  b. Central nervous system (CNS) effects including headache, dizziness, insomnia, weakness, or fatigue
  c. Rash or itching
  d. Flulike symptoms, general malaise.

Health Education for the Client and Family

- Teach the recommended method of administration, including how to insert rectal suppositories or administer a retention enema.
- Shake suspension forms well before using.
- Notify your doctor if adverse effects occur. Diarrhea is the most common side effect of these drugs.

CORTICOSTEROIDS

Methylprednisolone (Medrol, Solu-Medrol)
Prednisolone (Delta-Cortef), Prednisone

Glucocorticoids are hormones produced by the adrenal cortex. These hormones are necessary for the stress response. Cortisol, the main glucocorticoid, has potent anti-inflammatory effects. Corticosteroids are used to treat acute episodes of IBD. Because of their multiple and significant side effects, they are not used to maintain remission.

Nursing Responsibilities

- Assess for conditions that may be adversely affected by corticosteroid drugs: peptic ulcer disease, glaucoma or cataracts, diabetes, or psychiatric disorders.
- Obtain baseline vital signs and weight; monitor both routinely during therapy. Hypertension and weight gain may result from salt and water retention.
- Monitor for edema.
- Administer as ordered. For daily or alternate-day dosing, administer in the morning, when physiologic glucocorticoid levels are highest, to reduce adrenal cortisone suppression.
- Administer oral preparations with food to decrease GI side effects. Antacids or histamine H_2-receptor blocking agents such as cimetidine (Tagamet) may be prescribed during corticosteroid therapy.
- Monitor for desired effects: reduced diarrhea, less blood and mucus in the stool, and less abdominal cramping.
- Monitor for adverse effects:
  a. Increased susceptibility to infection and masking of early signs of infection
  b. Hyperglycemia
  c. Hypokalemia, as manifested by muscle weakness, nausea, vomiting, and cardiac rhythm disturbances
  d. Edema, hypertension, and signs of heart failure
  e. Peptic ulcer formation and possible GI hemorrhage (abdominal pain, black or tarry stools, and signs of bleeding)
  f. Changes in mental status, including depression, euphoria, aggression, and behavioral changes
  g. With long-term use: Cushingoid effects such as abnormal fat deposits in the face (moon faces) and trunk (buffalo hump), muscle wasting and thin extremities, thinning of the skin, and osteoporosis.

Health Education for the Client and Family

- Take as prescribed; do not change the dose or time of day. Do not stop the medication abruptly. The dose will be tapered gradually when the drug is discontinued.
- Notify the physician if adverse or Cushingoid effects occur.
- Take with food or at mealtimes to decrease the GI effects.
- Monitor weight. If a gain of more than 5 pounds is noted, notify the physician.
- Moderate salt intake and avoid foods and snacks high in sodium, such as processed meats and potato chips. Increase intake of foods high in potassium, such as fruits, vegetables, and lean meats.
- Carry a card or wear a bracelet or tag at all times identifying corticosteroid use.

Newer treatments for IBD employ other immune response modifiers, such as the monoclonal antibody infliximab (Remicade), to suppress tumor necrosis factor (TNF, an inflammatory mediator substance) in clients who have not responded to standard therapies. Mesalamine (Canasa, Rowasa) is an orally or rectally administered anti-inflammatory medication that provides topical anti-inflammatory action in the colon of clients with ulcerative colitis.

Although antibiotic therapy generally is not indicated in IBD, metronidazole (Flagyl) has active anti-inflammatory effects. It may be prescribed to help prevent remission after ileal resection in Crohn's disease. Ciprofloxacin (Cipro) is an alternative to metronidazole.

Antidiarrheal agents, such as loperamide and diphenoxylate, may be given to slow gastrointestinal motility and reduce diarrhea. These drugs are safe for clients with mild, chronic manifestations, but they are not given during acute attacks because they may precipitate toxic dilation of the colon.

When working with clients who are prescribed pharmacologic therapy for IBD, reinforce the importance of adhering to a strict medication regimen. Emphasize that medications should be continued even when the client is asymptomatic. Discuss the side effects of the drugs and what to do if any of the symptoms occur. Teach the client and family members how to recognize and respond to side effects of medications. Because immune status may be altered by steroid use, have families should avoid situations that pose a risk for contact with infectious diseases when the client is taking steroids. Instruct them to report any diseases and fevers the client experiences, as well as, and to report the use of steroids to all health care providers. Immunization schedules for pediatric clients may need to be altered.

Nutrition

Antigens in the diet may stimulate the immune response in the bowel, exacerbating inflammatory bowel disease. As a result, dietary management for IBD should be individualized. Some clients benefit from eliminating all milk and milk products from the diet. Increased dietary fiber may help reduce diarrhea and relieve rectal manifestations, but it is contraindicated for clients with intestinal strictures caused by repeated inflammation and scarring.

All food may be withheld to promote bowel rest during an acute exacerbation of Crohn's disease. Nutritional status during this time is maintained using enteral or total parenteral nutrition (TPN). TPN carries a higher risk of complications than does enteral nutrition. An elemental diet such as Ensure, which contains all essential nutrients in a residue-free formula, may be prescribed. Enteral diets provide essential nutrients to the small intestine to support cell growth, but they are not always palatable.

Surgery

Surgical interventions for inflammatory bowel disease differ depending on the primary disease process and the portion of the bowel affected. Generally, surgery is performed only when necessitated by complications of the disease or failure of conservative treatment measures.

Bowel obstruction is the leading indication for surgery in Crohn's disease. Other complications that may require surgical intervention include perforation, internal or external fistula, abscess, and perianal complications. Resection of the affected portion of bowel with an end-to-end anastomosis to preserve as much bowel as possible is the usual treatment. The disease process tends to recur in other areas following removal of affected bowel segments. There is an increased risk of fistula formation following surgery. Bowel strictures may be treated with a *strictureplasty*. In this procedure, longitudinal incisions are made in the narrowed segment to relieve the stricture while preserving bowel.

COLECTOMY Clients with extensive chronic ulcerative colitis may require a total **colectomy** (surgical resection and removal of the colon) to treat the disease itself; to eliminate complications such as toxic megacolon, perforation, or hemorrhage; or to serve as a prophylactic measure due to the high colon cancer risk associated with extensive ulcerative colitis.

The surgical procedure of choice for extensive ulcerative colitis is a *total colectomy with an ileal pouch-anal anastomosis (IPAA)*. In this procedure, the entire colon and rectum are removed; a pouch is formed from the terminal ileum; and the pouch is brought into the pelvis and anastomosed (connected) to the anal canal (Figure 16–8 ■). A temporary or loop ileostomy (described in the next section) is generally performed at the same time and is maintained for 2–3 months to allow the anal anastomosis to heal. When the healing is complete, the ileostomy is closed, and the client has six to eight daily bowel movements through the anus. Advanced age, obesity, or other factors may preclude an IPAA. For these clients, a permanent ileostomy or continent ileostomy may be created.

OSTOMY An intestinal ostomy is a surgically created opening between the intestine and the abdominal wall that allows the passage of fecal material. The surface opening is called a **stoma** (Figure 16–9 ■). The precise name of the ostomy

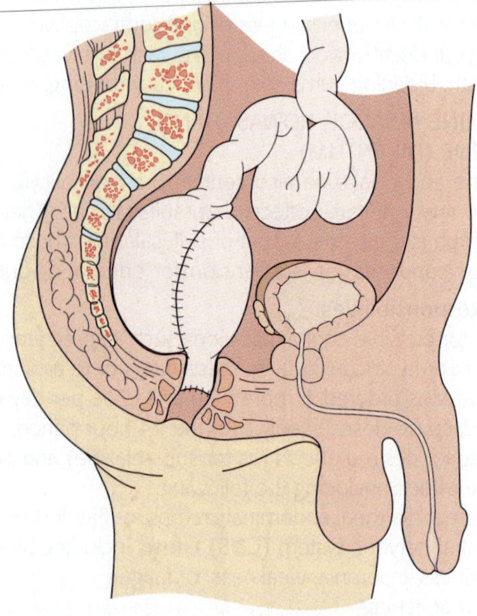

Figure 16–8 ■ Ileal pouch-anal anastomosis (IPAA).

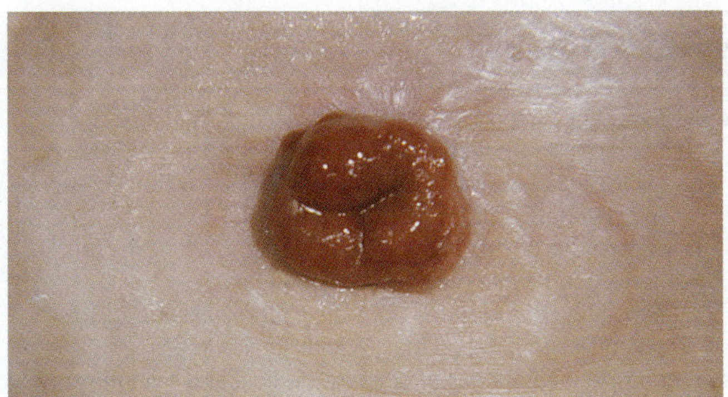

Figure 16–9 ■ A healthy-appearing stoma.

Courtesy of Carol Williams, RN, BS, UC Davis Medical Center.

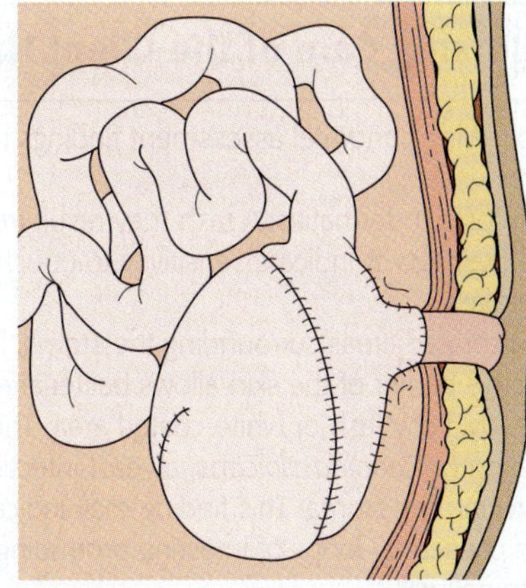

Figure 16–10 ■ Continent (Kock's) ileostomy.

depends on the location of the stoma. An **ileostomy** is an ostomy made in the ileum of the small intestine. In an ileostomy, the colon, rectum, and anus are usually completely removed (*total proctocolectomy with permanent ileostomy*). The anal canal is closed, and the end of the terminal ileum is brought to the body surface through the right abdominal wall to form the stoma. A temporary or *loop ileostomy* may be formed to eliminate feces and allow tissue healing for 2–3 months following an IPAA. A loop of ileum is brought to the body surface to form a stoma and allow stool drainage into an external pouch. When the ileostomy is no longer necessary, a second surgery is performed to close the stoma and repair the bowel, restoring fecal elimination through the anus.

In a *continent ileostomy* (Figure 16–10 ■), an intra-abdominal reservoir is constructed and a nipple valve formed (the ileum folded back on itself) from the terminal ileum before it is brought to the surface of the abdominal wall. Stool collects in the internal pouch; the nipple valve prevents it from leaking through the stoma. A catheter is inserted into the pouch to drain the stool.

Nursing care of the client with an ileostomy is outlined in Box 16–8.

Box 16–8 Nursing Care of the Client Having an Ileostomy

PREOPERATIVE CARE

- Provide routine preoperative care and teaching as outlined in the Appendicitis exemplar.
- Refer client to an enterostomal therapist for marking and teaching about the stoma location, ostomy care, and options for ostomy appliances. It is important to begin teaching prior to surgery to facilitate learning and postoperative acceptance of the ostomy.
- Discuss the availability of a local chapter of the United Ostomy Association and provide a referral as necessary or desired. Local chapters often have members with ostomies who are willing to provide both preoperative and postoperative teaching, listening, and support.
- Provide preoperative bowel preparation as ordered. Cathartics, enemas, and preoperative antibiotics are often ordered to reduce the risk of abdominal contamination and infection after surgery.

POSTOPERATIVE CARE

- Provide routine postoperative care and teaching as outlined in the Appendicitis exemplar.
- Apply an ostomy pouch over the stoma. Stool from an ileostomy is expressed continuously or irregularly and is liquid in nature; continuous use of a pouch to collect the drainage is necessary.
- Assess frequently for bleeding, stoma viability, and function. In the early postoperative period, small amounts of blood in the pouch are expected. A healthy stoma appears pink or red and moist as a result of mucous production (see Figure 16–9 ■). It should protrude approximately 2 cm from the abdominal wall. Frequent assessment in the initial postoperative period is particularly important to ensure stoma health and to monitor for possible complications. A dusky, brown, black, or white stoma indicates circulatory compromise. Other possible stoma complications include retraction (indentation or loss of the external portion of the stoma) or prolapse (outward telescoping of the stoma, that is, an abnormally long stoma).
- As the stoma starts to function, empty the pouch, explaining the procedure to the client. Initial drainage is dark green, viscid, and usually odorless. Drainage gradually thickens and becomes yellow-brown. Empty the pouch when it is one-third full. Measure drainage and include it as output on intake and output records. Rinse the pouch and reapply the clamp. Emptying the pouch when it is no more than one-third full helps prevent the skin seal from breaking as a result of the weight of the pouch. Because of the potential for excess fluid loss through ileostomy drainage, it is important to include it as fluid output.
- Assess the peristomal skin. Skin around the stoma should remain clean and pink and free of irritation, rashes, inflammation, or excoriation. Skin complications may arise from appliance irritation or hypersensitivity; excoriation from a leaking appliance; or *Candida albicans*, a yeast infection.
- Protect peristomal skin from enzymes and bile salts in the ileostomy effluent. Using a skin barrier on the pouch is essential. Change the pouch if leakage occurs or if the client complains of burning or itching skin. Enzymes and bile salts normally reabsorbed in the large intestine are irritating to the skin. Excoriation of skin surrounding the stoma impairs the first line of defense against microorganisms and can interfere with the ability to achieve a tight skin seal and prevent pouch leakage.

(continued)

Box 16–8 Nursing Care of the Client Having an Ileostomy (continued)

- Report the following abnormal assessment findings to the physician:
  a. Allergic or contact dermatitis. A rash may result from contact with fecal drainage or indicate sensitivity to pouch, paste, tape, or sealant.
  b. Purulent ulcerated areas surrounding the stoma. Disruption of the protective barrier of the skin allows bacterial entry.
  c. A red, bumpy, itchy rash or white-coated area. This is a manifestation of *Candida albicans*, a yeast infection.
  d. Bulging around the stoma. This finding may indicate herniation caused by loops of intestine protruding through the abdominal wall.
- Apply protective ointments to the perirectal area of clients with newly functioning ileoanal reservoirs and anastomoses. This helps protect the skin from the initial stools. As stools thicken and become fewer per day, the client experiences less perirectal irritation.

HEALTH EDUCATION FOR THE CLIENT AND FAMILY

- While caring for the ostomy, explain procedures to the client. Teaching is immediate and ongoing to facilitate acceptance of the ostomy and self-care.
- Teach client to manage the pouch clamp and to empty, rinse, and perform pouch changes. Self-care is vital to independence and self-esteem.
- Instruct client how to use an electric razor to shave the peristomal hair if necessary. An electric razor prevents accidental cutting of the stoma with a razor blade.
- Teach client to check the stoma and peristomal skin with each pouch change. Ongoing assessment is important for optimal health and function of the stoma and surrounding skin. Stripping of tape or excessively frequent pouch removal may cause mechanical trauma to peristomal skin. Chronic skin irritation by ileostomy effluent may lead to pseudoverrucous lesions, or wartlike nodules.
- Instruct client to report abnormal appearance of the stoma or surrounding skin (as noted previously and below) to the physician.
  a. Narrowing of the stoma lumen. This indicates stenosis and may interfere with fecal elimination.
  b. Lacerations or cuts in the stoma. The stoma contains no nerves, so trauma may occur without pain.
  c. Separation of the stoma from the abdominal surface. This potential complication may require surgical repair.
- Emphasize the importance of adequate fluid and salt intake. Discuss that the risk for dehydration and hyponatremia is increased particularly during hot weather, when fluid is lost through perspiration as well as ileostomy drainage. Water intake should be sufficient to maintain pale urine and an output of at least 1 quart per day. When exercising in hot weather, the client should consume extra water and salt. High-potassium foods such as bananas and oranges may be recommended. Loss of the reabsorptive surface of the large bowel increases the amount of water and sodium loss in the stool. If the ileostomy is high (more proximal in the ileum), additional potassium losses also may occur.
- Discuss the following manifestations of fluid and electrolyte imbalances:
  a. Extreme thirst
  b. Dry skin and oral mucous membrane
  c. Decreased urine output
  d. Weakness, fatigue
  e. Muscle cramps
  f. Abdominal cramps, nausea, vomiting
  g. Shortness of breath
  h. Orthostatic hypotension (feeling faint when suddenly changing positions).
- Discuss dietary concerns. A low-residue diet is recommended initially (Table 16–7). Foods that may cause excessive odor or

TABLE 16–7 Low-Residue Diet

FOOD GROUP	ALLOWED	AVOID
Beverages	Coffee, teas, juices, carbonated beverages; milk limited to 2 cups per day	Alcohol, prune juice
Breads and cereals	Products made from refined flours (white bread, crackers) or finely milled grains (e.g., corn flakes, crisp rice cereal, puffed wheat)	Whole-grain breads, rolls, or cereal; breads or rolls with seeds, nuts, or bran
Desserts	Gelatins, tapioca, plain custards, or puddings; angel-food or sponge cake; ice cream or frozen desserts without fruit or nuts	Any desserts containing dried fruits, nuts, seeds, or coconut; rich pastries, pies
Fruits	Fruit juices and strained fruits; cooked or canned apples, apricots, cherries, peaches, pears; bananas	All other raw or cooked fruits
Meats and other protein sources	Roasted, baked, or broiled tender or ground beef, veal, pork, lamb, poultry, or fish; smooth peanut butter; cottage, cream, American, or mild cheddar cheeses in small amounts	Tough or spiced meats and those prepared by frying; highly flavored cheeses; nuts
Potatoes, rice, and pasta	Peeled potatoes; white rice; most pasta products	Potato skins, potato chips, or fried potatoes; brown rice; whole-grain pasta products
Sweets	Sugar, honey, jelly, hard candy and gumdrops, plain chocolates	Jam, marmalade; candy made with seeds, nuts, coconut
Vegetables	Vegetable juices and strained vegetables; cooked or canned vegetables	Raw or whole cooked vegetables
Other	Salt, ground seasonings; cream sauce and plain gravy	Chili sauce, horseradish; popcorn, seeds of any kind; whole spices, olives, vinegar

Box 16–8 Nursing Care of the Client Having an Ileostomy (continued)

gas are typically avoided as well. Because food blockage is a potential problem, high-fiber foods are limited. Foods that may cause blockage, such as popcorn, corn, nuts, cucumbers, celery, fresh tomatoes, figs, strawberries, blackberries, and caraway seeds, are avoided. Symptoms of food blockage include abdominal cramping, swelling of the stoma, and absence of ileostomy output for more than 4–6 hours.

- Teach the following self-care measures to relieve food blockage:
  a. Take a warm shower or tub bath. This can help relax the abdominal muscles.
  b. Assume a knee–chest position. The knee–chest position reduces intra-abdominal pressure.
  c. Drink warm fluids or grape juice if not vomiting. This provides a mild cathartic effect.
  d. Massage peristomal area. Massage may stimulate peristalsis and fecal elimination.
  e. Remove pouch if the stoma is swollen and apply a pouch with a larger opening. If the stoma swells, the pouch may create a mechanical obstruction to output.
- Notify the physician or enterostomal therapy nurse if the following is observed:
  a. The above measures fail to relieve the obstruction.
  b. Signs of a partial obstruction persist, including output of high-volume odorous fluid, abdominal cramps, nausea, and vomiting.
  c. There is no ileostomy output for 4–6 hours.
  d. Signs of fluid and electrolyte imbalance occur, such as weakness, dizziness, lightheadedness, or headache.

Complementary and Alternative Therapies

The chronic nature of inflammatory bowel disease and the adverse effects of many prescribed treatments lead many clients with IBD to seek or use complementary and alternative therapies. Chiropractic care, megavitamin therapy, dietary supplements, and herbal medicine have been reported as common complementary and alternative therapies for IBD (Heuschkel et al., 2002; Verhoef, Rapchuk, Liew, Weir, & Hilsden, 2002). A study by Langmead et al. (2002) concluded that herbal remedies such as slippery elm, fenugreek, devil's claw, Mexican yam, termentil, and wei tong ning have antioxidant effects and may provide an effect similar to that of 5-aminosalicylic acid preparations. Peppermint tea is an excellent tonic for reducing nausea, relieving abdominal pain, and providing a calming effect. Chamomile tea helps to reduce intestinal inflammation (Balch & Stengler, 2004). Many complementary and alternative therapies for IBD may interact with prescribed medications. Nurses should instruct the client to discuss all potential therapies with the primary care provider. Accupressure, body massage, reflexology, aromatherapy, and stress reduction therapies also may help reduce manifestations of IBD.

NURSING PROCESS

Although at this time inflammatory bowel disease cannot be predicted or prevented, effective management may help the client avoid complications of the disease. Stress the importance of complying with the prescribed treatment regimen and promptly reporting manifestations of exacerbations to the physician.

Assessment

A thorough assessment of the client with inflammatory bowel disease should include the following:

- *Health history.* Current manifestations, including onset, duration, severity (number of stools per day, presence of blood or mucus in stool, abdominal pain or cramping, tenesmus); usual diet, ability to maintain weight and nutrition, food intolerances; associated manifestations such as arthralgias, fatigue, malaise; current medications; previous treatment and diagnostic tests
- *Physical examination.* General appearance; weight; vital signs, including orthostatic vitals and temperature; abdominal assessment, including shape, contour, bowel sounds, palpation for tenderness and masses, presence of stoma or scars.

Diagnosis

When planning nursing care for the client with IBD, it is vital to consider the chronic, recurrent nature of the disorder. Potential nursing diagnoses include the following:

- Diarrhea
- Disturbed Body Image
- Imbalanced Nutrition: Less Than Body Requirements.

Plan

In planning care for the client with IBD, many considerations must be reviewed concerning client needs, including severity of disease process, age, frequency of exacerbations, and physical condition. Potential goals of care include the following:

- Client will achieve resolution of discomfort from symptoms such as diarrhea.
- Client will maintain adequate hydration.
- Client will maintain optimal nutritional status.
- Client will demonstrate positive, healthy coping skills.
- Client will describe appropriate home self-care, including administering medication, making dietary choices, and preventing exacerbations.

Implementation

Teaching is a major aspect of care. Diarrhea and disturbed body image are significant problems for the client with IBD. Children and adolescents often have specific needs, especially related to body image and the desire to fit in with peers. With severe disease, impaired nutrition must be considered a priority problem as well.

Diarrhea

During an acute exacerbation of IBD, diarrhea can be frequent and painful. The frequency of defecation and associated abdominal pain and cramping may interfere with activities of daily living (ADLs) and increase the risk for fluid volume deficit and impaired skin integrity.

- Use a stool chart to record the frequency, amount, and color of stools. Measure and record liquid stool as output. The severity of diarrhea is an indicator of the severity of the disease and helps determine the need for fluid replacement.
- Monitor vital signs every 4 hours. Tachycardia, tachypnea, and fever may be indicators of fluid volume deficit.
- Weigh daily and record. Rapid weight loss (over days to a week) usually indicates fluid loss, whereas weight loss over weeks to months may indicate malnutrition.
- Assess for other indications of fluid deficit: warm, dry skin; poor skin turgor; dry, shiny mucous membranes; weakness; lethargy; complaints of thirst. The extent of fluid loss may not be readily evident with diarrhea, particularly if the client uses the bathroom without assistance. Systemic manifestations of fluid volume deficit may be the first indicators of the problem.
- Maintain bowel rest by keeping NPO or limiting oral intake to elemental feedings as indicated. Bowel rest during an acute exacerbation of IBD promotes healing and reduces diarrhea and other manifestations.
- Administer prescribed anti-inflammatory and antidiarrheal medications as indicated. Anti-inflammatory medications reduce the extent of bowel inflammation and diarrhea. Unless contraindicated, antidiarrheal medications help reduce fluid loss and increase comfort.
- Maintain fluid intake by mouth or intravenously as indicated. The client with IBD requires fluid to replace ongoing losses, as well as fluid to meet the usual daily needs of the body. If an elemental diet or total parenteral nutrition (TPN) is prescribed, additional fluids may be required to meet fluid intake needs.
- Provide good skin care. Fluid deficit and tissue dehydration increase the risk for skin excoriations or breakdown.
- Assess perianal area for irritation or denuded skin from the diarrhea. Use gentle cleansing agents such as Peri-Wash or Tucks, diaper wipes, or cotton balls saturated with witch hazel. Apply a protective cream, such as a zinc oxide–based preparation, to protect skin from the irritating effects of diarrheal stool. Digestive enzymes in the stool are very corrosive, increasing the risk of skin breakdown when exposed to diarrheal stool.

PRACTICE ALERT

Observe stools for obvious blood and test for occult blood as indicated. Report grossly bloody stools, which may indicate hemorrhage and necessitate emergency surgery.

Disturbed Body Image

The client with inflammatory bowel disease may experience frustration at not being able to control, or even predict, fecal elimination, particularly when the disease is severe. Diarrhea can interfere with the ability to complete tasks; maintain employment or engage in social activities; and even meet basic needs such as eating, sleeping, and having sex. Body image can suffer as a result. Treatment of IBD, be it total colectomy with IPAA, ileostomy or chronic corticosteroid therapy, also can affect the client's self image.

Body image is a major concern for children and adolescents with IBD. Corticosteroid therapy causes growth retardation and delayed sexual maturation. Encourage the client to discuss feelings about these side effects. If a permanent colostomy or ileostomy is required, the nurse can assist the client and family in understanding the need for surgical treatment.

- Accept the client's feelings and perception of self. Negating or denying the reality of the client's perception impairs trust.
- Encourage discussion of physical changes and their consequences as they relate to self-concept. This demonstrates acceptance and provides an opportunity for the client to express the personal impact of the disease and its treatment.
- Encourage discussion about concerns regarding the effect of the disease or treatment on close personal relationships. This demonstrates understanding and provides an opportunity for the client to express feelings about the impact of the disease on relationships and significant others.
- Encourage the client to make choices and decisions regarding care. This increases the client's sense of control over the disease and his or her future.
- Discuss possible treatment options and their effects openly and honestly. Open discussion allows for more informed decisions.
- Involve the client in care, teaching and demonstrating as needed. This encourages and facilitates independence and decision making.
- Provide care in an accepting, nonjudgmental manner. Acceptance of the client despite potential embarrassment about odors or diarrhea enhances self-esteem.
- Arrange for interaction with other clients or groups of people with IBD or ostomies. The client may think that unless someone has experienced a similar problem, that person cannot understand the client's feelings.
- Teach coping strategies (e.g., odor control and dietary modifications) and support their use. This facilitates healthy adaptation to the disease.

PRACTICE ALERT

Provide emotional support and counseling to help the pediatric client adjust to feeling "different" from peers. Inability to compete with peers and frequent absences from school can affect the client's self-esteem. Collaborate care with parents and assist them in contacting their child's school to arrange for tutoring or home schooling in case extended absences from school become necessary.

CLIENT TEACHING Dietary Instructions for Children with Inflammatory Bowel Disease

- Provide several small feedings each day, which may be better tolerated than three meals.
- Limit fiber intake to decrease intestine motility and inflammation. Peel fruits and avoid large quantities of whole grains and nuts.
- Offer high-calorie meals if the child is not eating well. If lactose intolerance is not a problem for the child, offer cream soups, milkshakes, puddings, and custards.
- Provide liquid dietary supplements to ensure that protein and caloric requirements are met.
- Watch for foods that cause intestinal problems for the individual child and avoid them in the future.
- Prevent mealtimes from becoming a reason for family strife. Seek help of nurses and dietitians if needed.

Imbalanced Nutrition: Less Than Body Requirements

Crohn's disease can significantly alter the bowel's ability to absorb nutrients. In both forms of IBD, blood and protein-rich fluid may be lost in diarrheal stools. With malabsorption and continuing nutrient losses, multiple nutrient deficits can develop, affecting growth and development, healing, muscle mass, bone density, and electrolyte balances.

- Monitor laboratory results, including hemoglobin and hematocrit, serum electrolytes, and total serum protein and albumin levels. These studies provide an indicator of nutritional status.
- Provide the prescribed diet: high-kilocalorie, high-protein, low-fat diet with restricted milk and milk products if lactose intolerance is present. Calories and protein are important to replace lost nutrients. Fat restriction helps reduce diarrhea and nutrient loss, particularly when significant portions of the terminal ileum have been resected.
- Provide parenteral nutrition as necessary if the client is unable to absorb enteral nutrients. Parenteral nutrition can help reverse nutritional deficits and promote weight gain and healing in the client with acute manifestations.
- Arrange for dietary consultation. Consider food preferences as allowed. Providing preferred foods in the prescribed diet increases intake and supports nutritional status.
- Provide or administer elemental enteral nutrition and supplements as ordered. Elemental enteral nutritional supplements support healing while providing for bowel rest. They can replace losses and improve nutritional status more rapidly than diet alone.
- Include family members, the primary food preparer in particular, in teaching and dietary discussions. Families can reinforce teaching and help the client maintain required restrictions or kilocalorie intake.

PRACTICE ALERT

Clients and family members will require instructions for total parenteral nutrition if it is used, as well as information about care of a central venous catheter, including dressing changes, sterile and nonsterile techniques. Instructions should also include how to recognizes signs of infection, how to handle infusion pumps and tubing, and how to measure the client's intake and output. Assist clients in obtaining equipment and supplies necessary for care. During home visits and appointments for health care, have clients or parents demonstrate their mastery of care for the central venous catheter and their understanding of TPN techniques.

CARE SETTINGS Home Care for the Client With IBD

Inflammatory bowel disease is a chronic condition for which the client provides daily self-management. For this reason, teaching is a vital component of care. Teach the client and family about the following topics:

- The type of IBD affecting the client, including the disease process, short- and long-term effects, relationship of stress to disease exacerbations, and manifestations of complications
- Prescribed medications, including drug names, desired effects, schedules for tapering the doses if ordered (as with corticosteroids), and possible side effects or adverse reactions and their management
- Recommended diet and the rationale for any specific restrictions
- Use of nutritional supplements such as Ensure to maintain weight and nutritional status
- Indicators of malabsorption and impaired nutrition; recommendations for self-care and the need to seek medical intervention
- If discharged with a central catheter and home parenteral nutrition, written and verbal instructions on catheter care, troubleshooting, and TPN administration (Have the client and a family member demonstrate catheter care and TPN maintenance.)
- Importance of maintaining a fluid intake of at least 2–3 quarts per day, increasing fluid intake during warm weather, exercise, or strenuous work, and when fever is present
- Increased risk for colorectal cancer and importance of regular bowel exams
- Risks and benefits of various treatment options.

If surgery is planned or has been done, include the following topics in home care instructions:

- IPAA or ileostomy care as indicated
- Suppliers from which to obtain ostomy supplies
- Use of nonprescription drugs (e.g., enteric-coated and timed-release capsules) that may not be adequately absorbed before being eliminated through the ileostomy
- Community and national ostomy support groups.

Provide referrals to a dietary consultant or nutritionist, a community health care agency, home care services, and home intravenous care services as indicated. In addition, suggest the following resources:

- Crohn's and Colitis Foundation of America
- The Israel Foundation for Crohn's Disease and Ulcerative Colitis
- United Ostomy Associations of America, Inc.

Providing adequate stress reduction may be helpful in the control of IBD. Teach relaxation techniques such as deep breathing, progressive tensing and relaxing of muscles, and visualization of favorite places. Encourage busy school-age children and teens to have quiet and restful times each day, in addition to periods of physical activity.

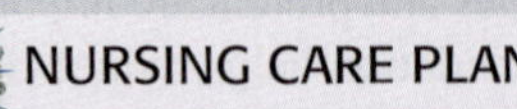

NURSING CARE PLAN A Client With Ulcerative Colitis

Cortez Lewis is a 42-year-old real estate agent and mother of three school-age children. She has had ulcerative colitis for 18 years and has been treated with prednisone and sulfasalazine. Over the past 4 months, she has been having abdominal pain and cramping and frequent bloody diarrhea stools. During the same period, she lost 20 lb (9 kg), and she has had difficulty maintaining her career. She recently developed several lesions of the lower leg, identified as erythema nodosum. A recent colonoscopy revealed extensive involvement of the entire colon. On admission, Mrs. Lewis states, "I'm tired of fighting this disease. I'm a prisoner in my home because of the diarrhea." She is admitted for a total proctocolectomy and IPAA.

ASSESSMENT

Janet Wheeler, RN, completes the admission assessment. Mrs. Lewis now weighs 115 lb (52.2 kg). She complains of abdominal cramping, pain, and frequent bloody diarrhea stools. Several reddened lesions are noted on her lower legs. Physical assessment findings include T_O 36.6°C (98°F), P 72, R 20, and BP 104/72. Skin is cool and pale. Abnormal laboratory findings include hemoglobin 7.3 g/dL (normal 11.7–15.7 g/dL), hematocrit 23.3% (normal 35–47%), WBC 15,580/mm^3 (normal 3500–11,000/mm^3), platelet count 995,000/mm^3 (normal 150,000–450,000/mm^3), serum protein 4.6 g/dL (normal 6–8 g/dL), and serum albumin 2.4 g/dL (normal 3.5–5.0 g/dL). Preparation for surgery is begun.

DIAGNOSES

- Imbalanced Nutrition: Less Than Body Requirements related to impaired absorption
- Diarrhea related to inflammation of bowel
- Risk for Deficient Fluid Volume related to abnormal fluid loss
- Risk for Impaired Tissue Integrity related to drainage from temporary ileostomy
- Acute Pain related to surgical intervention
- Risk for Sexual Dysfunction related to temporary ileostomy.

PLANNING

- Resume prescribed diet within 5 days after surgery.
- Demonstrate normal fecal elimination through the temporary ileostomy.
- Maintain adequate fluid balance.
- Demonstrate appropriate ostomy care prior to discharge.
- Report a tolerable level of discomfort.
- Verbalize feelings about sexuality and acknowledge importance of discussing sexual issues with husband.

IMPLEMENTATION

- Discuss dietary modifications related to nutritional status and presence of ileostomy. Provide referral to dietitian for diet planning and teaching.
- Teach importance of maintaining a high fluid intake and manifestations of dehydration.
- Teach how to empty and change ostomy, pouch of choice.
- Teach stoma and peristomal skin assessment with each pouch change.
- Teach food blockage management.
- Refer to local chapter of the United Ostomy Association.
- Provide list of local medical suppliers for ostomy appliances.

EVALUATION

On discharge, Mrs. Lewis is caring for her ileostomy by demonstrating her ability to empty, rinse, and change the pouch. The enterostomal therapy (ET) nurse has provided written and verbal instructions on ileostomy care. Mrs. Lewis verbalizes her understanding of the recommended diet and the need to limit high-fiber food intake and avoid enteric-coated and timed-release medications. The ET nurse has discussed sexual aspects of having an ileostomy and has given Mrs. Lewis a booklet, "Sex and the Female Ostomate," available through the United Ostomy Association. Mrs. Lewis is looking forward to the planned surgery to close the temporary ileostomy.

CRITICAL THINKING

1. Why is the client with an ileostomy at risk for dehydration? How can Mrs. Lewis monitor her fluid status at home?
2. Why were Mrs. Lewis's hemoglobin and hematocrit low on admission? If her hemoglobin had been low but her hematocrit normal on admission, what might be the explanation?
3. Outline a teaching plan that could be given to clients for home care of an ileostomy.
4. Develop a care plan for Mrs. Lewis for the nursing diagnosis risk for impaired skin integrity.

Evaluation

Expected outcomes of nursing care for the client with IBD include the following:

- The client demonstrates absence of GI distress.
- The client and family demonstrate successful management of medications without side effects.
- The client remains free from infection due to central line.
- A positive body image is achieved.
- The client demonstrates integration of relaxation techniques into daily life.

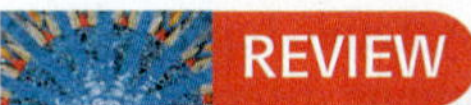

REVIEW Inflammatory Bowel Disease

RELATE: LINK THE CONCEPTS

Linking the exemplar of Irritable Bowel Disease with the concept of Stress and Coping:

1. What stress management techniques might you teach to an adolescent diagnosed with IBD?
2. You are caring for a client diagnosed with IBS who was just informed of the need for a colectomy with creation of an ileostomy. The client is very upset and tells the doctor that death is preferable to walking around with "poop coming out of my stomach." What can you do to help this client cope with the idea of an ileostomy?

Linking the exemplar of Irritable Bowel Disease with the concept of Elimination:

3. The client with IBD is about to have surgery to create an ileostomy. The client asks, "Will I need to wear a bag all of the time?" How do you respond? Explain your answer.
4. If the client with IBD is to have a colostomy instead of an ileostomy, how do you respond to the same question "Will I need to wear a bag all of the time?" Explain your answer

READY: GO TO COMPANION SKILLS MANUAL

- Applying a fecal ostomy pouch
- Measuring weights
- Assessing the skin
- Monitoring intake and output
- Providing total parenteral nutrition

REFER: GO TO MYNURSINGKIT

REFLECT: CASE STUDY

Jodi Thompson is a 17-year-old who is a junior in high school. She is a cheerleader for the school, is on the debate team, and an honor student. Jodi lives with her mother, Marie, and her two brothers, George aged 10 and Joe aged 8. Jodi's mom works full time, so Jodi is responsible for their care after school or for arranging care. Jodi's dad died of cirrhosis of the liver when Jodi was 10. Jodi is also responsible for caring for her brothers when her mom works weekends and she is responsible for getting them off to school in the morning. Jodi is planning to take the SAT exam in a few weeks because she is interested in becoming a dentist. Jodi has come to the clinic today because she has been having abdominal pain and frequent loose stools.

1. What risk factors for inflammatory bowel disease are apparent in Jodi's history?
2. What nutritional teaching will you plan for Jodi?
3. Create a plan of care for Jodi.

16.4 NEPHRITIS

KEY TERMS

Acute postinfectious glomerulonephritis, *923*
Glomerulonephritis, *923*
Goodpasture's syndrome, *924*
Lupus nephritis, *924*
Nephritis, *923*
Plasmapheresis, *927*

BASIS FOR SELECTION OF EXEMPLAR

Burden of Chronic Diseases
Centers for Disease Control and Prevention
Healthy People 2010
Institute of Medicine

LEARNING OUTCOMES

After reading about this exemplar, you will be able to:

1. Describe the pathophysiology, etiology, clinical manifestations, and direct and indirect causes of nephritis.
2. Identify risk factors associated with nephritis.
3. Illustrate the nursing process in providing culturally competent care across the life span for individuals with nephritis.
4. Formulate priority nursing diagnoses appropriate for an individual with nephritis I.
5. Create a plan of care for individuals with nephritis and their family members.
6. Assess expected outcomes for an individual with nephritis.
7. Discuss therapies used in the collaborative care of an individual with nephritis.
8. Employ evidence-based caring interventions for an individual with nephritis.

OVERVIEW

Nephritis is an inflammation of the kidneys. There are different classifications of nephritis based on area of involvement or etiology. One example is **glomerulonephritis**, which is an inflammation of the glomerular capillary membrane. Another is **acute postinfectious glomerulonephritis (APIGN)**, which may develop as a response to a group A beta-hemolytic streptococcal infection of the skin or pharynx or as a result of infection by the *Staphylococcus, Pneumococcus,* or *Coxsackie* virus.

PATHOPHYSIOLOGY AND ETIOLOGY

In *acute proliferative glomerulonephritis*, glomerular damage occurs as a result of an immune complex reaction that localizes on the glomerular capillary wall. Antibody–antigen complexes become lodged in the glomeruli, leading to inflammation and obstruction. The glomerular membranes are thickened and capillaries in the glomeruli are obstructed by damaged tissue cells, leading to a decreased glomerular filtration rate (GFR). Vascular permeability increases, allowing protein, red blood cells, and red cell casts to be excreted.

Sodium and water are retained, expanding the intravascular and interstitial compartments and resulting in the characteristic finding of edema (Figure 16–11 ■).

Chronic glomerulonephritis is typically the end stage of other glomerular disorders such as rapidly progressive glomerulonephritis (RPGN), lupus nephritis, and diabetic nephropathy. In many cases, however, no previous glomerular disease has been identified. Slow, progressive destruction of the glomeruli and a gradual decline in renal function are characteristic of chronic glomerulonephritis. The kidneys decrease in size symmetrically, and their surfaces become granular or roughened. Eventually, entire nephrons are lost. Symptoms develop insidiously, and the disease often is not recognized until signs of renal failure develop.

Lupus nephritis is a consequence of systemic lupus erythematosus (SLE), an inflammatory autoimmune disorder affecting the connective tissue of the body. Between 40% and 85% of clients with SLE develop manifestations of nephritis (Kasper et al., 2005). Immune complexes that form in the glomerular capillary wall are the usual trigger for glomerular injury in SLE. Manifestations of lupus nephritis range from microscopic hematuria to massive proteinuria. Its progression may be slow and chronic or fulminant, with a sudden onset and the rapid development of renal failure.

Goodpasture's syndrome is a rare autoimmune disorder of unknown etiology. It is characterized by formation of antibodies to the glomerular basement membrane. These antibodies also may bind to alveolar basement membranes,

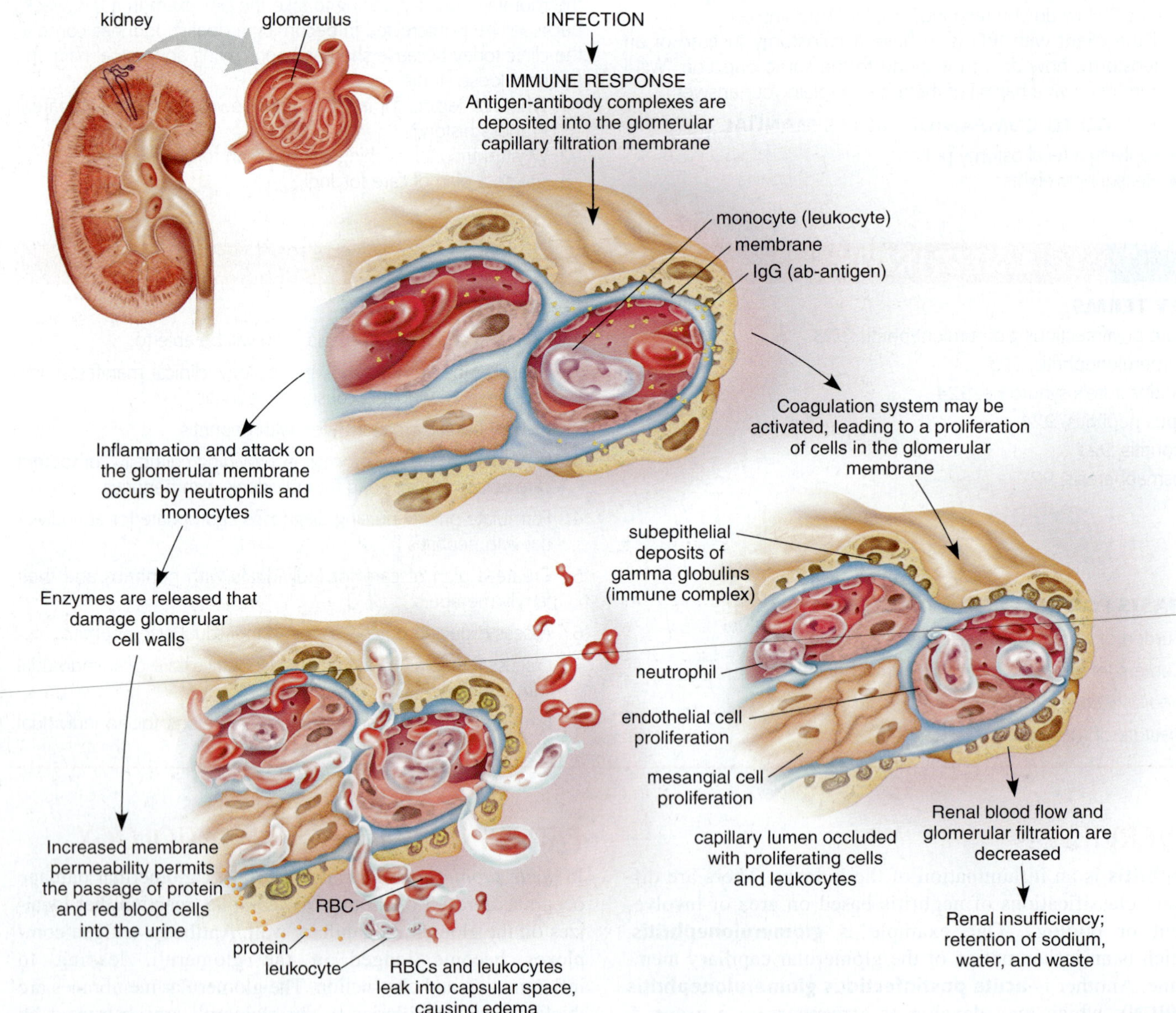
kidney
glomerulus
INFECTION
IMMUNE RESPONSE
Antigen-antibody complexes are deposited into the glomerular capillary filtration membrane
monocyte (leukocyte)
membrane
IgG (ab-antigen)
Inflammation and attack on the glomerular membrane occurs by neutrophils and monocytes
Coagulation system may be activated, leading to a proliferation of cells in the glomerular membrane
subepithelial deposits of gamma globulins (immune complex)
Enzymes are released that damage glomerular cell walls
neutrophil
endothelial cell proliferation
mesangial cell proliferation
capillary lumen occluded with proliferating cells and leukocytes
Renal blood flow and glomerular filtration are decreased
Renal insufficiency; retention of sodium, water, and waste
Increased membrane permeability permits the passage of protein and red blood cells into the urine
RBC
protein
leukocyte
RBCs and leukocytes leak into capsular space, causing edema

Figure 16–11 ■ Infection from group A beta-hemolytic *Streptococcus* leads to an immune response that causes inflammation and damage to glomeruli. Protein and red blood cells are allowed to pass through the glomeruli. Blood flow to the glomeruli is reduced due to obstruction, with damaged cells and renal insufficiency leading to retention of sodium, water, and waste.

damaging alveoli and causing pulmonary hemorrhage. Goodpasture's syndrome usually affects young men between the ages of 18 and 35, although it can occur at any age and affect women as well.

Although the glomeruli may be nearly normal in appearance and function in Goodpasture's syndrome, extensive cell proliferation and crescent formation characteristic of RPGN are common. Renal manifestations include hematuria, proteinuria, and edema. Rapid progression to renal failure may occur. Alveolar membrane damage can lead to mild or life-threatening pulmonary hemorrhage. Cough, shortness of breath, and hemoptysis (bloody sputum) are early respiratory manifestations.

Etiology

Each form of nephritis often has a distinct etiology. Lupus nephritis is the result of the inflammatory process caused by SLE and is an autoimmune disorder. Glomerulonephritis can result from infection, diabetes mellitus, or SLE. Tubulointerstitial nephritis results from injury to the renal tubules and interstitium often secondary to glomerular damage and renovascular disease.

Risk Factors

Clients with diabetes mellitus and/or hypertension are at much higher risk for nephritis secondary to vascular damage to the fragile vessels in the nephron. Infections can travel from the bladder to the kidney or cause scarring that results in urine retention that can damage the nephron. Overuse of over-the-counter painkillers and drug abuse increases risk of nephritis as well.

Nephritis also can result from prematurity, trauma, or family history of kidney disease. Diseases such as sickle cell anemia, AIDS, and congestive heart failure can damage the kidney, resulting in nephritis.

CLINICAL MANIFESTATIONS

Many clients are asymptomatic. In other clients, the onset is abrupt, with flank or midabdominal pain, irritability, malaise, and fever. Microscopic hematuria is present in nearly all cases, and gross hematuria, resulting in tea-colored urine, is found in up to 50% of cases and may last for 1–2 weeks. Mild periorbital edema occurs early, along with dependent edema of the feet and ankles. Edema may progress in severity to cause ascites (excessive fluid in the peritoneal cavity) or a pulmonary effusion manifested as dyspnea, cough, and crackles (Gray, Huether, & Forshee, 2006). Acute hypertension may cause an encephalopathy that includes headache, nausea, vomiting, irritability, lethargy, and seizures. Oliguria may or may not be present.

Acute postinfection glomerulonephritis is characterized by an abrupt onset of hematuria, proteinuria, salt and water retention, and evidence of azotemia occurring 10–14 days after the initial infection. The urine often appears brown or cola-colored. Salt and water retention increases extracellular fluid volume, leading to hypertension and edema. The edema is noted primarily in the face, particularly around the eyes. Dependent edema, affecting the hands and upper extremities in particular, also may be noted. Other manifestations may include fatigue, anorexia, nausea and vomiting, and headache.

The older adult may have fewer apparent symptoms. Nausea, malaise, arthralgias, and proteinuria are common manifestations; hypertension and edema are seen less often. Pulmonary infiltrates may occur early in the disorder, often due to worsening of a preexisting condition such as heart failure.

COLLABORATION

Collaborative care of the client with nephritis may include a nephrologists, primary care provider, nurses, pharmacists, dieticians or nutritionists, and (in the case of school-age children)

CLINICAL MANIFESTATIONS AND THERAPIES Nephritis

ETIOLOGY	CLINICAL MANIFESTATIONS	CLINICAL THERAPIES
Salt and water retention	■ Hypertension ■ Mild to moderate edema ■ Hematuria	■ Antihypertensives ■ Diuretics ■ Sodium restriction
Severe hypertension	■ Extremely high blood pressure with cerebral dysfunction	■ Emergency care to include IV diazoxide or hydralazine
Progressive edema, acute inflammatory processes	■ Ascites ■ Pulmonary effusion	■ Immunosuppressive therapy (prednisone, cyclophosphamide, azathroprine) ■ Sodium restriction
Encephalopathy resulting from acute hypertension	■ Headache ■ Nausea and vomiting ■ Irritability	■ Antihypertensives ■ Additional therapies as warranted
Presence of infection	■ Salt and water retention ■ Fever ■ Malaise ■ Edema	■ Antibiotics ■ Bed rest ■ Sodium restriction

parents, teachers, and the school nurse. The nurse's role includes providing client teaching, providing follow up, and coordinating referral services and communication between members of the health care team. Treatment focuses on relief of symptoms and supportive therapy. Bed rest is a key component of the treatment plan during the acute phase. Edema and mild to moderate hypertension should be treated with sodium restriction and a diuretic such as furosemide (Lau & Wyatt, 2005). Immediate emergency care is needed for severe hypertension with cerebral dysfunction; medication such as diazoxide or hydralazine is administered intravenously. For APIGN, a course of antibiotics may be given to ensure eradication of the original infectious agent.

Fluid requirements are determined by careful monitoring of urinary output, weight, blood pressure, and serum electrolytes. Initially, only insensible fluid losses are replaced until the status of renal function is known. Dietary restriction of sodium and potassium intake may be necessary; with severe azotemia, protein intake may have to be limited.

Diagnostic Tests

Laboratory and diagnostic testing is valuable for identifying the cause of nephritis and to evaluate kidney function.

The following studies may be ordered to help identify the underlying cause or etiology:

- *Throat or skin cultures* detect infection by group A beta hemolytic streptococci. Although poststreptococcal glomerulonephritis typically follows the acute infection by 1–2 weeks, treatment to eradicate any remaining organisms is initiated to minimize antibody production.
- *Antistreptolysin O (ASO) titer* and other tests detect streptococcal *exoenzymes* (bacterial enzymes that stimulate the immune response in acute postinfection glomerulonephritis). Other titers such as antistreptokinase (ASK) and antideoxyribonuclease B (ADNAase B) may be obtained as well.
- *Erythrocyte sedimentation rate (ESR)* is a general indicator of inflammatory response. It may be elevated in acute postinfection glomerulonephritis and in lupus nephritis.
- *KUB* (kidney, ureter, bladder) *abdominal x-ray* may be done to evaluate kidney size and to rule out other causes of the client's manifestations. The kidneys may be enlarged in acute nephritis, whereas bilateral small kidneys are typical of late chronic glomerulonephritis.
- *Kidney scan,* a nuclear medicine procedure, allows visualization of the kidney after intravenous administration of a radioisotope. In glomerular diseases, the uptake and excretion of the radioactive material are delayed.
- *Biopsy,* microscopic examination of kidney tissue, is the most reliable diagnostic procedure for glomerular disorders. Biopsy helps determine the type of nephritis, the prognosis, and appropriate treatment. Renal biopsy is usually done percutaneously, by inserting a biopsy needle through the skin into the kidney to obtain a tissue sample. Open biopsy, which requires surgery, may also be done.

The following studies are used to evaluate kidney function:

- *BUN* measures urea nitrogen, the end product of protein metabolism. It is created by the breakdown and metabolism of both dietary and body proteins. Urea is eliminated from the body by filtration in the glomerulus; minimal amounts are reabsorbed in the renal tubules. Glomerular diseases interfere with filtration and elimination of urea nitrogen, causing blood levels to rise. Increased protein catabolism (destruction), which may occur with GI bleeding or tissue breakdown, also can raise the BUN. Normal BUN values are listed in Appendix B. Levels up to 50 mg/dL or 17.7 mmol/L indicate mild azotemia, and levels higher than 100 mg/dL or 35.7 mmol/L indicate severe renal impairment.
- *Serum creatinine* measures the amount of creatinine in the blood. Creatinine also is a metabolic by-product, produced in relatively constant amounts by skeletal muscles. It is excreted entirely by the kidneys, making the serum creatinine a good indicator of kidney function. Normal values are lower in the older adult because of decreased muscle mass. Levels greater than 4 mg/dL indicate serious impairment of renal function.
- *Urine creatinine* also is an indicator of renal function and the glomerular filtration rate (GFR). Urine creatinine levels decrease when renal function is impaired because it is not effectively eliminated from the body.
- *Creatinine clearance* is a specific indicator of renal function used to evaluate the GFR. The *clearance,* or amount of blood cleared of creatinine in 1 minute, depends on the amount and pressure of blood being filtered and the filtering ability of the glomeruli. Levels normally decline with age as the GFR decreases in the older adult. Disorders such as nephritis affect glomerular filtration, decreasing the creatinine clearance.
- *Serum electrolytes* are evaluated because impaired kidney function alters their excretion. Monitoring serum electrolytes is particularly important to prevent complications associated with imbalances.
- *Urinalysis* often shows RBCs and proteins in the urine of clients with a glomerular disorder. These substances, normally too large to enter glomerular filtrate, escape due to increased porosity of glomerular capillaries in glomerular disorders. A 24-hour urine specimen is used to determine the amount of protein in the urine.

Pharmacologic Therapies

Although no drugs are available to cure glomerular disorders, medications are used to treat underlying disorders, reduce inflammation, and manage the symptoms.

Antibiotics are prescribed for the client with acute postinfection glomerulonephritis to eradicate any remaining bacteria, removing the stimulus for antibody production. Nephrotoxic antibiotics, such as the aminoglycoside antibiotics, streptomycin, and some cephalosporins, are avoided.

Aggressive immunosuppressive therapy is used to treat acute inflammatory processes such as RPGN, Goodpasture's syndrome, and exacerbations of SLE. When begun early, immunosuppressive therapy significantly reduces the risk of end-stage renal disease and renal failure. Prednisone, a glucocorticoid, is prescribed in relatively large doses of 1 mg per kilogram of body weight per day (e.g., a 160-pound man would receive 70–75 mg per day). Other immunosuppressive agents such as cyclophosphamide (Cytoxan) and azathioprine (Imuran) are prescribed in conjunction with corticosteroids. Corticosteroid use in acute postinfection glomerulonephritis may actually worsen the condition, so it is avoided.

Oral glucocorticoids such as prednisone also are used in high doses to induce remission of nephrotic syndrome. When glucocorticoids alone are ineffective, other immunosuppressive agents such as cyclophosphamide or chlorambucil (Leukeran) may be used to induce or maintain remission.

ACE inhibitors may be ordered to reduce protein loss associated with nephrotic syndrome. These drugs reduce proteinuria and slow the progression of renal failure. They have a protective effect on the kidney in clients with diabetic nephropathy. NSAIDs also reduce proteinuria in some clients, but can increase salt and water retention (Kasper et al., 2005).

Antihypertensives may be prescribed to maintain the blood pressure within normal levels. Blood pressure management is important because systemic and renal hypertension is associated with a poorer prognosis in clients with glomerular disorders.

Clinical Therapies

Bed rest may be ordered during the acute phase of acute postinfection glomerulonephritis. When the edema of nephrotic syndrome is significant or the client is hypertensive, sodium intake may be restricted to 1–2 g per day. Dietary protein may be restricted if azotemia is present. When proteins are restricted, those included in the diet should be complete or high-value proteins. Complete proteins supply the essential amino acids required for growth and tissue maintenance. Complete and incomplete proteins are compared in Table 16–8.

Plasma exchange therapy (**plasmapheresis**), a procedure to remove damaging antibodies from the plasma, is used in conjunction with immunosuppressive therapy to treat RPGN and Goodpasture's syndrome. Plasma and glomerular-damaging antibodies are removed using a blood cell separator. The RBCs are then returned to the client along with albumin or human plasma to replace the plasma removed. This procedure is usually done in a series of treatments. It is not without risk, and informed consent is required. Potential complications of plasma exchange therapy include those associated with intravenous catheters, fluid volume shifts, and altered coagulation.

TABLE 16–8 **Complete and Incomplete Protein Sources**

	COMPLETE PROTEINS	INCOMPLETE PROTEINS
Definition	Provide all essential amino acids needed for growth and tissue maintenance	Lack one or more essential amino acids or contain inadequate proportions
Examples	Milk, eggs, cheese, meats, poultry, fish, and soy	Vegetables, breads, cereals and grains; legumes, seeds, and nuts

NURSING PROCESS

Nursing care is supportive and educational. Monitoring renal function and fluid volume status are key components of care, as is protecting the client from infection. Both manifestations of glomerular disorders and their treatment can interfere with a client's ability to maintain usual roles and responsibilities.

Assessment

Focused assessment data related to glomerular disorders include the following:

- *Health history.* Complaints of facial or peripheral edema or weight gain, fatigue, nausea and vomiting, headache, general malaise, abdominal or flank pain; cough or shortness of breath; changes in amount, color, or character of urine (e.g., frothy urine); history of skin or pharyngeal streptococcal infection, diabetes, SLE, or kidney disease; current medications
- *Physical examination.* General appearance; vital signs; weight; presence of periorbital, facial, or peripheral edema; skin for lesions, infection; throat to obtain culture as indicated; urine specimen for color, character, and odor.

Diagnosis

Nursing diagnoses that may apply to the client with nephritis include the following:

- Excess Fluid Volume
- Risk for Infection
- Risk for Impaired Skin Integrity
- Risk for Imbalanced Nutrition: Less Than Body Requirements
- Fatigue
- Ineffective Role Performance.

Plan

Goals of nursing care are designed to be developmentally appropriate and may include the following:

- Client maintains or regains normal urine output.
- Client is able to meet nutritional needs.
- Client avoids infection.
- Client maintains skin integrity.

For pediatric clients, additional goals that may be appropriate include the following:

- Client maintains education to remain current with classmates.
- Client participates in diversional activities during period of bed rest.

Implementation

Bed rest is required during the acute phase. Nursing care focuses on monitoring fluid status, preventing infection, preventing skin breakdown, meeting nutritional needs, and providing emotional support to the client and family.

Excess Fluid Volume

Monitor vital signs, fluid and electrolyte status, and intake and output. Hypovolemia can occur as a result of fluid shifting from vascular to interstitial spaces despite the outward clinical signs of excess fluid retention. Monitor the degree of ascites by measuring abdominal girth. Document urine specific gravity.

Maintain fluid restriction as ordered. Offer ice chips (in limited and measured amounts) and frequent mouth care to relieve thirst. Make sure family members and visitors understand the need to limit fluids to prevent excessive intake. Arrange dietary consultation regarding sodium- or protein-restricted diets.

> **PRACTICE ALERT**
> Carefully monitor and regulate intravenous infusions; include fluid used to dilute IV medications as intake. Significant "hidden" fluid intake can occur with intravenous medication administration.

Risk for Infection

Impaired renal function puts the client at risk for infection. Immunosuppressive drugs may mask the presence of infection. Monitor for signs of infection, including fever, increased malaise, and an elevated WBC count, which may be an early indicator of infection.

Avoid or minimize invasive procedures. If catheterization is required, use sterile intermittent straight catheterization or maintain a closed drainage system for an indwelling catheter. Prevent urine reflux from the drainage system to the bladder or the bladder to the kidneys by ensuring a patent gravity flow system.

Instruct the family in good hand hygiene. Limit visitors and screen for upper respiratory infections. Screen family members for the presence of streptococcal infection and, if necessary, refer for treatment.

> **PRACTICE ALERT**
> Monitor vital signs, temperature, and mental status every 4 hours. An elevated temperature may indicate infection; anti-inflammatory drugs, however, may moderate this response. Tachycardia, increasing lethargy, or confusion may be the initial signs of infection.

Risk for Impaired Skin Integrity

Dependent areas or areas prone to pressure are vulnerable to skin breakdown. Turn the hospitalized client frequently. Pad bony prominences or susceptible areas with sheepskin or protect skin with a transparent dressing. Make sure the client's bed is free of crumbs. Keep sheets tight and free of wrinkles.

Risk for Imbalanced Nutrition: Less Than Body Requirements

A team approach is often needed to meet the client's nutritional needs. In most cases, the client follows a "no added salt" and low-protein diet. Anorexia presents the greatest challenge to meeting daily nutritional requirements during the acute phase of the disease. To increase the client's appetite, encourage family members to bring the client's favorite foods from home, serve age-appropriate quantities to children, and allow the client to eat with other clients or with family members.

Fatigue

Fatigue is a common manifestation. Anemia, loss of plasma proteins, headache, anorexia, and nausea compound this fatigue. The ability to maintain usual physical and mental activities may be impaired.

Schedule activities and procedures to provide adequate rest and energy conservation. Prevent unnecessary fatigue. Assist with ADLs as needed. Reduce energy demands with frequent small meals and short periods of activity. Limit the number of visitors and visit length. Discuss with the client and family the relationship between fatigue and the disease process.

Ineffective Role Performance

The manifestations and treatment of nephritis can affect the ability to maintain usual roles and activities. Fatigue and muscle weakness may limit physical and social activities. Bed rest or activity limitations may be ordered to minimize the degree of proteinuria. If azotemia is present, malaise, nausea, and mental status changes can interfere with role function. Facial and periorbital edema affects the client's self-esteem and may lead to isolation.

Encourage client self-care and participation in decision making. Support coping skills, helping the client identify personal strengths. Discuss the effect of the disease and treatments on roles and relationships, helping the client identify potential changes in roles, relationships, and lifestyle. Help the client and family develop a plan for alternative behaviors and relationships, encouraging the client to maintain usual roles to the extent possible.

Provide accurate and optimistic information about the disorder and its short- and long-term effects. Evaluate the need for additional support and social services for the client and family. Provide referrals as indicated.

> **CARE SETTINGS Home Care for Clients With Acute Nephritis**
>
> Acute postinfectious glomerularnephritis typically resolves following appropriate treatment. Other types of nephritis, however, may be progressive. Regardless, the course of the disorder is difficult and may be lengthy, sometimes ranging from months to years. Self-management is essential. Provide instructions for the client and family, including the following topics:
>
> - Information about the disease and the prognosis
> - Prescribed treatment, including activity and diet restrictions; the use and potential effects, both beneficial and adverse, of all medications
> - Risks, manifestations, prevention, and management of complications such as edema and infection
> - Signs, symptoms, and implications of improving or declining renal function
> - Measures to prevent further kidney damage, such as avoiding nephrotoxic drugs
> - Community resources such as home care providers, support groups, and (for children) home school teachers or tutoring programs.

NURSING CARE PLAN **A Client With Acute Nephritis**

Jung-Lin Chang is a 23-year-old graduate student in biology. He presents at the university health center with brown and foamy urine. The physician admits him to the infirmary and orders a throat culture, ASO titer, CBC, BUN, serum creatinine, and urinalysis.

ASSESSMENT

Connie King, the nurse admitting Mr. Chang, notes that his history is essentially negative for past kidney or urinary problems. He relates having had a "pretty bad" sore throat a couple of weeks before admission. However, it was during midterms, so he took a few antibiotics he had from a previous bout of strep throat, increased his fluids, and did not see a doctor. The sore throat resolved and he felt well until noticing the change in his urine. He admits that his eyes seemed a little puffy, but he thought this was due to lack of sleep and fatigue. He has eaten little the past 2 days, but was not alarmed because his food intake is irregular most of the time.

Physical assessment findings include T_O 37.1°C (98.8°F) PO, P 98, R 18, and BP 136/90. Weight 165 pounds (75 kg), up from his normal of 160 (72.5 kg). Mod N 42 mg/dL, serum creatinine 2.1 mg/dL. Urinalysis reveals the presence of protein, RBCs, and RBC casts. A subsequent 24-hour urine protein analysis shows 1025 mg of protein (normal 30–150 mg/24 hours).

The physician diagnoses acute postinfection glomerulonephritis and places Mr. Chang on bed rest with bathroom privileges. The physician orders fluid restriction (1200 mL/day) and a restricted sodium and protein diet.

DIAGNOSES

- Excess Fluid Volume related to plasma protein deficit and sodium and water retention
- Risk for Imbalanced Nutrition: Less Than Body Requirements related to anorexia
- Anxiety related to prescribed activity restriction
- Risk for Ineffective Therapeutic Regimen Management related to lack of information about nephritis and treatment

PLANNING

- Maintain blood pressure within normal limits.
- Return to usual weight with no evidence of edema.
- Consume adequate calories following prescribed dietary limitations.
- Verbalize reduced anxiety regarding ability to continue studies.
- Demonstrate an understanding of acute nephritis and prescribed treatment regimen.

IMPLEMENTATION

- Take vital signs every 4 hours; notify physician of significant changes.
- Weigh daily; monitor and record intake and output.
- Schedule fluids, allowing 650 mL on day shift, 450 mL on evening shift, and 100 mL on night shift.
- Arrange dietary consultation to plan a diet that includes preferred foods as allowed.
- Provide small meals with high-carbohydrate between-meal snacks.
- Encourage Mr. Chang to talk about his condition and its potential effects.
- Assist with problem solving and exploring options for maintaining studies.
- Enlist friends and family to listen and provide support.
- Teach Mr. Chang and his family about acute nephritis and prescribed treatment.
- Instruct in appropriate antibiotic use.

EVALUATION

Mr. Chang is released from the infirmary after 4 days. He decides to return to his parents' home for the 6–12 weeks of convalescence prescribed by his doctor. Mr. Chang's renal function gradually returns to normal with no further azotemia and minimal proteinuria after 4 months. He verbalizes understanding of the relationship between the strep throat, his inappropriate use of antibiotics, and the nephritis. He says, "I may not always remember to take every pill on time in the future, but I sure won't save them for the next time again!"

CRITICAL THINKING

1. How did Mr. Chang's use of "a few" previously prescribed antibiotics to treat his sore throat affect his risk for developing acute postinfection glomerulonephritis?
2. What additional risk factors did Mr. Chang have for developing nephritis?
3. The initial manifestations of acute postinfection glomerulonephritis and RPGN are very similar. What diagnostic test would the physician use to make the differential diagnosis? Develop a plan of care for a client undergoing this examination.

Evaluation

Expected outcomes of nursing care include the following:

- The client receives appropriate fluid volume each day and maintains or regains normal urine output.
- The client develops no areas of redness, abrasions, or skin breakdown over pressure points.
- The client's temperature remains within normal limits, and client is free of secondary infection.
- The client maintains pre-illness weight and tolerates daily intake that meets nutritional requirements.
- The client administers medications as prescribed.
- The client's sodium and potassium levels reflect adherence to dietary restrictions.

REVIEW Nephritis

RELATE: LINK THE CONCEPTS

Linking the exemplar of Nephritis with the concept of Fluids and Electrolytes:

1. If you are caring for a client with nephritis whose kidney function is insufficient to eliminate adequate fluid and waste products from the body, what nursing care might you provide to maintain fluid and electrolyte homeostasis?
2. While caring for a client with acute nephritis and reduced urine output, you review laboratory studies and find that the client's serum potassium is elevated greater than 6 mg/dL. What are your priorities of care? What orders would you anticipate receiving when you notify the primary provider?

Linking the exemplar of Nephritis with the concept of Mobility:

3. If the client with nephritis is required to maintain bed rest, how will you promote a return to ambulation when the time comes?
4. To promote future mobility, what nursing care can you provide the client who requires bed rest?

READY: GO TO COMPANION SKILLS MANUAL

- Monitoring intake and output
- Establishing intravenous infusions
- Maintaining infusions
- Hand hygiene (medical asepsis)
- Turning a client to the lateral or prone position in bed
- Measuring weights
- Measuring abdominal girth

REFER: GO TO MYNURSINGKIT

REFLECT: CASE STUDY

Marina McCullough, 13 years old, comes home from school and tells her mother she that doesn't feel well. She complains of feeling tired, having pain in her left flank, and feeling warm. Her mother goes into the bathroom to get the electronic thermometer to check Marina's temperature and notices that Marina forgot to flush the toilet. When she reaches over to flush the toilet, she notices that the water looks like iced tea. She checks Marina's oral temperature and gets a reading of 100.8°F. She suspects a possible UTI and wonders if Marina is sexually active, but she decides not to approach the subject when Marina isn't feeling well.

Mrs. McCullough makes an appointment with Marina's pediatrician and takes her in later that afternoon. The nurse admits her, notes mild periorbital edema and +2 pitting edema in both feet, and collects a urine specimen that tests positive for blood and protein. Mrs. McCullough administered acetaminophen earlier in the afternoon to treat both the fever and pain. Marina's vital signs upon arrival to the pediatrician's office are 99.4°F taken tympanically, P 92, R 18, and BP 138/86. Her weight is 132 lbs, which Marina reports is an 8 pound weight gain since she last checked it 3 days ago. Breath sounds reveal mild crackles in bases bilaterally, and the nurse notes a rattling productive cough. Marina reports pain rated 7 in the right flank area, a persistent headache, and nausea and feeling tired.

Marina is diagnosed with nephritis and is admitted to the acute care facility on the adolescent unit. The doctor orders serum electrolytes, CBC with differential, BUN, serum creatinine, creatinine clearance, KUB, urine culture, and kidney scan. Also ordered is fluid restriction to 750 mL per day.

1. How will you ration Marina's fluids throughout a 24-hour day?
2. You are starting a 24-hour urine collection for creatine. How will you instruct the client to begin? What actions will you take to improve accuracy of 24-hour collection?
3. What priority assessments will you perform when admitting Marina?

16.5 PEPTIC ULCER DISEASE

KEY TERMS

Duodenal ulcers, *931*
Gastric outlet obstruction, *932*
Gastric ulcers, *931*
Hemorrhage, *932*
Peptic ulcer disease (PUD), *930*
Peptic ulcers, *930*
Perforation, *932*
Steatorrhea, *933*
Ulcer, *930*
Zollinger-Ellison syndrome, *932*

LEARNING OUTCOMES

After reading about this exemplar, you will be able to:

1. Describe the pathophysiology, etiology, clinical manifestations, and direct and indirect causes of peptic ulcer.
2. Identify risk factors associated with peptic ulcer.
3. Illustrate the nursing process in providing culturally competent care across the life span for individuals with peptic ulcer.
4. Formulate priority nursing diagnoses appropriate for an individual with peptic ulcer.
5. Create a plan of care for individuals with peptic ulcer and their family members.
6. Assess expected outcomes for an individual with peptic ulcer.
7. Discuss therapies used in the collaborative care of an individual with peptic ulcer.
8. Employ evidence-based caring interventions for an individual with peptic ulcer.

BASIS FOR SELECTION OF EXEMPLAR

Centers for Disease Control and Prevention
Healthy People 2010
Institute of Medicine

OVERVIEW

Peptic ulcer disease (PUD), a break in the mucous lining of the GI tract where it comes in contact with gastric juice, is a chronic health problem. PUD affects approximately 10% of the population, or 4 million people in the United States every year (Kasper et al., 2005; Tierney et al., 2005).

An **ulcer** is a break in the GI mucosa. **Peptic ulcers** may occur in any area of the GI tract exposed to acid-pepsin secretions, including the esophagus, stomach, and duodenum.

Duodenal ulcers are those that occur in the duodenum and are the most common. They usually develop between the ages of 30 and 55 and are more common in men than in women. **Gastric ulcers**, which occur in the stomach, more often affect older clients between the ages of 55 and 70. Ulcers are more common in people who smoke and who are chronic users of NSAIDs. Alcohol and dietary intake do not seem to cause PUD, and the role of stress is uncertain. Although the incidence of PUD has decreased dramatically, the incidence of gastric ulcers is increasing, believed due to the widespread use of NSAIDs (Tierney et al., 2005).

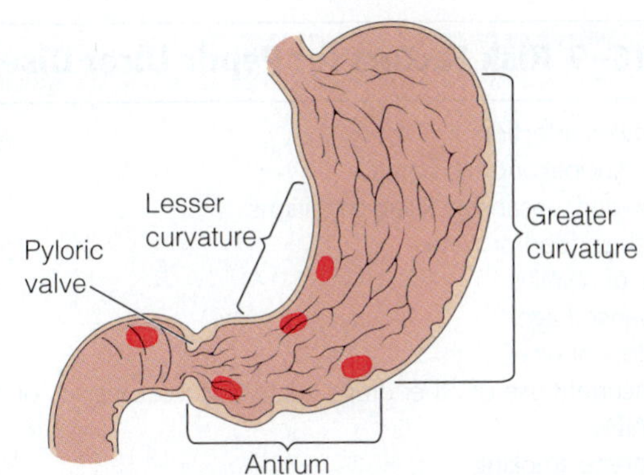

Figure 16–12 ■ Common sites affected by peptic ulcer disease.

PATHOPHYSIOLOGY AND ETIOLOGY

The innermost layer of the stomach wall, the gastric mucosa, consists of columnar epithelial cells supported by a middle layer of blood vessels and glands and a thin outer layer of smooth muscle. The mucosal barrier of the stomach, a thin coating of mucous gel and bicarbonate, protects the gastric mucosa. The mucosal barrier is maintained by bicarbonate secreted by the epithelial cells, by mucous gel production stimulated by prostaglandins, and by an adequate blood supply to the mucosa. An ulcer develops when the mucosal barrier is unable to protect the mucosa from damage by hydrochloric acid and pepsin, the gastric digestive juices.

Helicobacter pylori infection, found in about 70% of people who have PUD, is unique in colonizing the stomach. It is spread person to person (oral–oral or fecal–oral) and contributes to ulcer formation in several ways. The bacteria produce enzymes that reduce the efficacy of mucous gel in protecting the gastric mucosa. In addition, the host's inflammatory response to *H. pylori* contributes to gastric epithelial cell damage without producing immunity to the infection. Although the gastric mucosa is the usual site for *H. pylori* infection, this infection also contributes to duodenal ulcers. This may be related to increased production of gastric acid associated with *H. pylori* infection.

NSAIDs contribute to PUD through both systemic and topical mechanisms. Prostaglandins are necessary for maintaining the gastric mucosal barrier. NSAIDs interrupt prostaglandin synthesis by disrupting the action of the enzyme cyclooxygenase (COX). The two forms of this enzyme are COX-1 and COX-2. The COX-1 enzyme is necessary to maintain the integrity of the gastric mucosa, but the anti-inflammatory effects of NSAIDs are due to their ability to inhibit the COX-2 enzyme. The COX-2–selective NSAIDs may be less damaging to the gastric mucosa because they have less effect on the COX-1 enzyme. In addition to their systemic effect, aspirin and many NSAIDs cross the lipid membranes of gastric epithelial cells, damaging the cells themselves.

The ulcers of PUD may affect the esophagus, stomach, or duodenum. They may be superficial or deep, affecting all layers of the mucosa. Duodenal ulcers, the most common, usually develop in the proximal portion of the duodenum, close to the pylorus (Figure 16–12 ■). They are sharply demarcated and usually less than 1 cm in diameter (Figure 16–13 ■). Gastric ulcers often are found on the lesser curvature and the area immediately proximal to the pylorus. Gastric ulcers are associated with an increased incidence of gastric cancer.

PUD may be chronic, with spontaneous remissions and exacerbations. Exacerbations of the disease may be associated with trauma, infection, or other physical or psychologic stressors.

Etiology

It is now known that ulcers in both adults and children are often caused by *H. pylori,* a gram-negative rod (Vaira et al., 2005). Infections often occur in several members of a family, especially when the family's water supply is contaminated. Diet is usually not a major factor in the development of peptic ulcers, although caffeine and alcohol consumption may exacerbate the disease.

Risk Factors

Chronic *H. pylori* infection and use of aspirin and NSAIDs are the major risk factors for PUD. Contributing risk factors are listed in Box 16–9. Overall, an estimated one in six clients infected with *H. pylori* develops PUD. Of the NSAIDs, aspirin is the most ulcerogenic. A strong familial pattern suggests a genetic factor in the development of PUD. Cigarette smoking is a significant risk factor, doubling the risk of PUD. Cigarette smoking inhibits the secretion of bicarbonate by the pancreas and may cause more rapid transit of gastric acid into the duodenum.

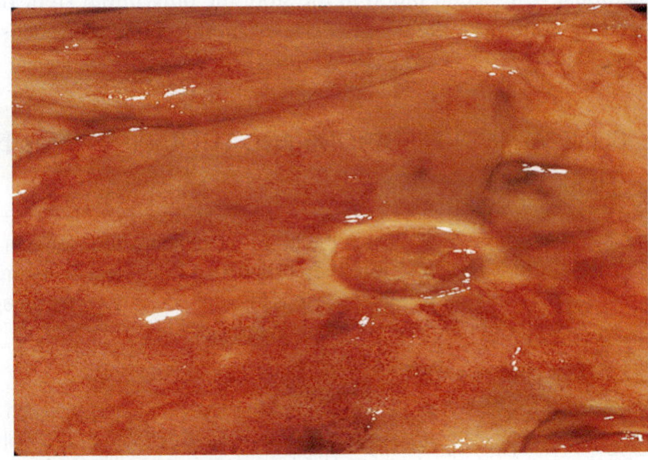

Figure 16–13 ■ A superficial peptic ulcer.

Source: SPL/Photo Researchers, Inc.

Box 16–9 Risk Factors for Peptic Ulcer Disease

- *H. pylori* infection
- Low socioeconomic status
- Crowded, unsanitary living conditions
- Unclean food or water
- Use of NSAIDs
- Advanced age
- History of ulcer
- Concurrent use of other drugs, such as glucocorticoids or other NSAIDs
- Cigarette smoking
- Family history of PUD

CLINICAL MANIFESTATIONS

Pain is the classic symptom of peptic ulcer disease. The pain is typically described as gnawing, burning, aching, or hunger-like, and is experienced in the epigastric region, sometimes radiating to the back. The pain occurs when the stomach is empty (2–3 hours after meals and in the middle of the night) and is relieved by eating, with a classic "pain–food–relief" pattern. The client may complain of heartburn or regurgitation and may vomit.

The presentation of PUD in the older adult is often less clear, with vague and poorly localized discomfort, perhaps chest pain or dysphagia, weight loss, or anemia. In the older adult, a complication of PUD, such as upper GI hemorrhage or perforation of the stomach or duodenum, may be the presenting symptom.

Complications

The complications associated with peptic ulcers include hemorrhage, obstruction, and perforation. See Box 16–10 for the manifestations of these complications.

Among people with PUD, 10% to 20% experience **hemorrhage** (rapid or excessive bleeding) as a result of ulceration and erosion into the blood vessels of the gastric mucosa. In the older adult, bleeding is the most frequent complication. When small blood vessels erode, blood loss may be slow and insidious, with occult blood in the stool the only initial sign. If bleeding continues, the client becomes anemic and experiences symptoms of weakness, fatigue, dizziness, and orthostatic hypotension. Erosion into a larger vessel can lead to sudden and severe bleeding with hematemesis, melena, or hematochezia (blood in the stool), and signs of hypovolemic shock.

Gastric outlet obstruction (obstruction of the pyloric region of the stomach and duodenum that impairs gastric outflow) may result from edema surrounding the ulcer, smooth muscle spasm, or scar tissue. Generally, obstruction is a gradual rather than acute process. Symptoms include a feeling of epigastric fullness, accentuated ulcer symptoms, and nausea. If the obstruction becomes complete, vomiting occurs. Hydrochloric acid, sodium, and potassium are lost in vomitus, potentially leading to fluid and electrolyte imbalance and metabolic alkalosis.

The most lethal complication of PUD is **perforation**, penetration of the ulcer through the mucosal wall. When perforation occurs, gastric or duodenal contents enter the peritoneum, causing an inflammatory process and peritonitis. Chemical peritonitis from the hydrochloric acid, pepsin, bile, and pancreatic fluid is immediate; bacterial peritonitis follows within 6–12 hours from gastric contaminants entering the normally sterile peritoneal cavity. When an ulcer perforates, the client has immediate, severe upper abdominal pain radiating throughout the abdomen and possibly to the shoulder. The abdomen becomes rigid and boardlike, with absent bowel sounds. Signs of shock may be present and include diaphoresis; tachycardia; and rapid, shallow respirations. Classic symptoms of perforation may not be present in an older adult. Instead, the older adult may present with mental confusion and other nonspecific symptoms. This atypical presentation can lead to delays in diagnosis and treatment, increasing the associated mortality rate.

Zollinger-Ellison syndrome

Zollinger-Ellison syndrome is a form of peptic ulcer disease caused by a gastrinoma, or gastrin-secreting tumor of the pancreas, stomach, or intestines. Gastrinomas may be benign, although 50–70% are malignant. Gastrin is a hormone that stimulates the secretion of pepsin and hydrochloric acid. The increased gastrin levels associated with these tumors result in hypersecretion of gastric acid, which in turn causes mucosal ulceration.

CLINICAL MANIFESTATIONS AND THERAPIES Peptic Ulcer Disease

ETIOLOGY	CLINICAL MANIFESTATIONS	CLINICAL THERAPIES
H. pylori infection	■ Pain in the epigastric region when stomach is empty. ■ Client may experience heartburn or regurgitation. ■ Manifestations in older adults may not be apparent until complications arise.	■ Protein-pump inhibitor (PPI) in combination with antibiotics to eliminate infection ■ H_2 Receptor agonists to decrease gastric acid contents ■ Mucosa-protecting agents such as sucralfate, bismuth, antacids, and prostaglandin analogs
NSAIDs	■ Pain in the epigastric region when stomach is empty. ■ Client may experience heartburn or regurgitation. ■ Manifestations in older adults may not be apparent until complications arise.	■ Discontinue NSAID use if possible ■ Twice-daily PPIs ■ H_2-receptor agonists ■ Mucosa-protecting agents

Box 16–10 Manifestations of PUD Complications

HEMORRHAGE
- Occult or obvious blood in the stool
- Hematemesis
- Fatigue
- Weakness, dizziness
- Orthostatic hypotension
- Hypovolemic shock

OBSTRUCTION
- Sensations of epigastric fullness
- Nausea and vomiting
- Electrolyte imbalances
- Metabolic alkalosis

PERFORATION
- Severe upper abdominal pain radiating to the shoulder
- Rigid, boardlike abdomen
- Absence of bowel sounds
- Diaphoresis
- Tachycardia
- Rapid, shallow respirations
- Fever

The peptic ulcers of Zollinger-Ellison syndrome may affect any portion of the stomach or duodenum, as well as the esophagus or jejunum. Characteristic ulcerlike pain is common. The high levels of hydrochloric acid entering the duodenum also may cause diarrhea and **steatorrhea** (excess fat in the feces) from impaired fat digestion and absorption. Complications of bleeding and perforation are often seen with Zollinger-Ellison syndrome. Fluid and electrolyte imbalances also may result from persistent diarrhea, with resultant losses of potassium and sodium in particular.

COLLABORATION

Treatment for PUD focuses on treating its cause. Primary treatments include eradicating *H. pylori* infection and treating or preventing ulcers related to use of NSAIDs. The nurse plays an essential role in the health care team by providing ongoing assessment and client teaching.

Diagnostic Tests

- *Upper GI series* using barium as a contrast medium can detect 80–90% of peptic ulcers. It commonly is the diagnostic procedure that is chosen first because it is less costly and less invasive than gastroscopy. Small or very superficial ulcers may be missed, however.
- *Gastroscopy* allows visualization of the esophageal, gastric, and duodenal mucosa and direct inspection of ulcers. Tissue also can be obtained for biopsy.
- Biopsy specimens obtained during a gastroscopy can be tested for the presence of *H. pylori* using several different methods. In the *biopsy urease test,* the specimen is put to a gel containing urea. If *H. pylori* is present, the urease that it produces changes the color of the gel, often within minutes. Biopsy specimen cells also can be microscopically examined or cultured for evidence of *H. pylori.* Although these tests are highly specific for *H. pylori* infection, their invasiveness, cost, and lack of availability in some areas limits their usefulness.
- Noninvasive methods of detecting *H. pylori* infection include *serologic testing* (to detect IgG antibodies through ELISA), fecal antigen immunoassays (to detect antigens to *H. pylori* in the feces), and the *urea breath test.* In this test, radiolabeled urea is given orally. The urease produced by *H. pylori* bacteria converts the urea to ammonia and radiolabeled carbon dioxide, which can then be measured as the client exhales. This test, as well as fecal antigen testing, also can be used to evaluate the effectiveness of treatment to eradicate *H. pylori.* Treatment with proton pump inhibitors (PPIs) interferes with urea breath test and fecal antigen test results, so these drugs should be discontinued for 1–2 weeks prior to testing (Tierney et al., 2005).
- If Zollinger-Ellison syndrome is suspected, *gastric analysis* may be performed to evaluate gastric acid secretion. Stomach contents are aspirated through a nasogastric tube and analyzed. In Zollinger-Ellison syndrome, gastric acid levels are very high.

Pharmacologic Therapies

The medications used to treat PUD include agents to eradicate *H. pylori,* drugs to decrease gastric acid content, and agents that protect the mucosa.

Eradication of *H. pylori* is often difficult. Combination therapies that use two antibiotics with a proton-pump inhibitor (PPI), are necessary. Possibilities include the combination of a PPI with clarithromycin and amoxicillin, or a PPI combined with bismuth subsalicylate, tetracycline, and metronidazole. With complete eradication of *H. pylori,* reinfection rates are less than 0.5% per year.

In clients who have NSAID-induced ulcers, the NSAID in use should be discontinued if at all possible. If that is not possible, twice-daily PPIs enable ulcer healing.

Medications that decrease gastric acid content include PPIs and the H_2-receptor antagonists.

- PPIs bind the acid-secreting enzyme (H^+, K^+ ATPase) that functions as the proton pump, disabling it for up to 24 hours. These drugs are very effective, resulting in more than 90% ulcer healing after 4 weeks. Compared to the H_2-receptor blockers, the PPIs provide faster pain relief and more rapid ulcer healing.
- Histamine$_2$-receptor blockers inhibit histamine binding to the receptors on the gastric parietal cells to reduce acid secretion. These drugs are well tolerated and have few serious side effects; however, drug interactions can occur. These drugs must be continued for 8 weeks or longer for ulcer healing.

Agents that protect the mucosa include sucralfate, bismuth, antacids, and prostaglandin analogs.

- Sucralfate binds to proteins in the ulcer base, forming a protective barrier against acid, bile, and pepsin. Sucralfate also stimulates the secretion of mucus, bicarbonate, and prostaglandin.
- Bismuth compounds (Pepto-Bismol) stimulate mucosal bicarbonate and prostaglandin production to promote ulcer healing. In addition, bismuth has an antibacterial action against *H. pylori.* There are very few side effects, other than a harmless darkening of stools.
- Antacids stimulate gastric mucosal defenses, thereby aiding in ulcer healing. They provide rapid relief of ulcer symptoms and are often used as needed to supplement other antiulcer medications. Antacids are inexpensive, but clients often have difficulty with a regular regimen because the drugs must be taken frequently and may cause constipation (from the aluminum-type antacids) or diarrhea (from the magnesium-based antacids). Antacids also interfere with the absorption of iron, digoxin, some antibiotics, and other drugs.
- Prostaglandin analogs (misoprostol) promote ulcer healing by stimulating mucus and bicarbonate secretions and by inhibiting acid secretion. Although not as effective as the other drugs discussed, misoprostol is used to prevent NSAID-induced ulcers.

Nutrition

In addition to pharmacologic treatment, clients are encouraged to maintain good nutrition, consuming balanced meals at regular intervals. It is important to teach clients that bland or restrictive diets are no longer necessary. Mild alcohol intake is not harmful. Smoking should be discouraged because it slows the rate of healing and increases the frequency of relapses.

Surgery

The identification of *H. pylori* as a cause of PUD and the availability of drugs to treat the infection and heal peptic ulcers has all but eliminated surgery as a treatment option for PUD. Older clients, however, may have undergone gastric resection surgery for PUD and may have long-term complications related to the surgery.

Treatment for Complications

The client hospitalized with a complication of PUD (e.g., bleeding, GI obstruction, or perforation and peritonitis) requires additional interventions to restore homeostasis.

In hemorrhage associated with PUD, initial interventions focus on restoring and maintaining circulation. Normal saline, lactated Ringer's, or other balanced electrolyte solutions are administered intravenously to restore intravascular volume if signs of shock (tachycardia, hypotension, pallor, low urine output, and anxiety) are present. Whole blood or packed RBCs may be administered to restore hemoglobin and hematocrit levels. A nasogastric tube is inserted to prevent aspiration of vomited gastric contents.

Gastroscopy with direct injection of a clotting or sclerosing agent into the bleeding vessel may be performed. Laser photocoagulation, which uses light energy, or electrocoagulation, which uses electric current to generate heat, also can be performed via gastroscopy to seal bleeding vessels.

The client is kept NPO until bleeding is controlled. PPIs are administered intravenously (e.g., 40 mg of pantoprazole (Protonix) per intravenous push or admixture daily) to reduce the risk of rebleeding. Surgery may be necessary if medical measures are ineffective in controlling bleeding. Older adults who experience bleeding as a complication of PUD are more likely to rebleed or require surgery to control the hemorrhage.

Repeated inflammation, healing, scarring, edema, and muscle spasm can lead to gastric outlet (pyloric) obstruction. Initial treatment includes gastric decompression with nasogastric suction and administration of intravenous normal saline and potassium chloride to correct fluid and electrolyte imbalance. H_2-receptor blockers are given intravenously as well. Balloon dilation of the gastric outlet may be done via upper endoscopy. If these measures are unsuccessful in relieving obstruction, surgery may be required.

Gastric or duodenal perforation resulting in contamination of the peritoneum with GI contents often requires immediate intervention to restore homeostasis and minimize peritonitis. Intravenous fluids maintain fluid and electrolyte balance. Nasogastric suction removes gastric contents and minimizes peritoneal contamination. Placing the client in Fowler's or semi-Fowler's position allows peritoneal contaminants to pool in the pelvis. Intravenous antibiotics aggressively treat bacterial infection from intestinal flora. Laparoscopic surgery or an open laparotomy may close the perforation.

NURSING PROCESS

Nurses may identify clients with peptic ulcer disease by looking for the symptoms and noting family history of *H. pylori* infection. Nursing care centers on interventions to promote adequate nutritional intake, promote healing, and prevent recurrences.

Although it is difficult to predict which clients will develop PUD, nurses can promote health by advising clients to avoid risk factors such as excessive aspirin or NSAID use and cigarette smoking. In addition, nurses should encourage clients to seek treatment for manifestations of gastroesophageal reflux disease (GERD) or chronic gastritis, both of which also are associated with *H. pylori* infection.

Assessment

Collect the following subjective and objective data when assessing the client with PUD:

- *Health history.* Complaints of epigastric or left upper quadrant pain, heartburn, or discomfort; its character, severity, timing, and relationship to eating; measures used for relief; nausea or vomiting, presence of bright blood or "coffee-grounds" appearing in vomitus; current medications, including use of aspirin or other NSAIDs; cigarette smoking and use of alcohol or other drugs
- *Physical examination.* General appearance, including height and weight relationship; vital signs, including

orthostatic measurements; abdominal examination, including shape and contour, bowel sounds, and tenderness to palpation; presence of obvious or occult blood in vomitus and stool.

Diagnosis

Nursing diagnoses that are frequently appropriate for clients with PUD include the following:

- Pain
- Disturbed Sleep Pattern
- Imbalanced Nutrition: Less Than Body Requirements
- Deficient Fluid Volume.

Plan

Goals of treatment are developed in collaboration with the client and may include the following:

- The client will reduce risk factors to prevent recurrence.
- The client will experience a reduction in discomfort related to PUD.
- The client will maintain adequate nutritional intake.
- The client will maintain hydration.

Implementation

The priorities of nursing care for the client with PUD are reducing discomfort, maintaining nutritional status, and preventing or rapidly identifying and intervening for potential complications.

Pain

The pain of PUD is often predictable and preventable. Pain is typically experienced 2–4 hours after eating, as high levels of gastric acid and pepsin irritate the exposed mucosa. Measures to neutralize the acid, minimize its production, or protect the mucosa often relieve this pain, minimizing the need for analgesics.

- Assess pain, including location, type, severity, frequency, and duration. Assess the relationship of pain to food intake or other contributing factors.
- Administer PPIs, H_2-receptor antagonists, antacids, or mucosal protective agents as ordered. Monitor for effectiveness and side effects or adverse reactions. The pain associated with PUD is generally caused by the effect of gastric juices on exposed mucosal tissue. These medications reduce pain and promote healing by reducing acid production, neutralizing acid, or providing a barrier for the damaged mucosa.
- Teach relaxation, stress reduction, and lifestyle management techniques. Refer for stress management counseling or classes as indicated. Although there is no clear relationship between stress and PUD, measures to relieve stress and promote physical and emotional rest help reduce the perception of pain and may reduce ulcer genesis.

PRACTICE ALERT

Avoid making assumptions about pain. Acute pain may indicate a complication, such as perforation (often manifesting as sudden, severe epigastric pain and a rigid, boardlike abdomen) or it may be totally unrelated to PUD (e.g., angina, gallbladder disease, or pancreatitis).

Disturbed Sleep Pattern

Nighttime ulcer pain, which typically occurs between 1 and 3 a.m., may disrupt the sleep cycle and result in inadequate rest. Anticipation of pain may lead to insomnia or other sleep disruptions.

- Emphasize the importance of taking medications as prescribed. The bedtime dose of PPI or H_2-receptor blocker minimizes hydrochloric acid production during the night, reducing nighttime pain.
- Instruct the client to limit food intake after the evening meal, eliminating any bedtime snack. Eating before bedtime can stimulate the production of gastric acid and pepsin, increasing the likelihood of nighttime pain.
- Encourage the use of relaxation techniques and comfort measures such as soft music as needed to promote sleep. Once the pain associated with PUD has been controlled, these measures help reduce anxiety and reestablish a normal sleep pattern.

Imbalanced Nutrition: Less Than Body Requirements

In an attempt to avoid discomfort, the client with PUD may gradually reduce food intake, sometimes jeopardizing nutritional status. Anorexia and early satiety are additional problems associated with PUD.

- Assess current diet, including pattern of food intake, eating schedule, and foods that precipitate pain or are being avoided in anticipation of pain. The client may not realize the extent of self-imposed dietary limitations, especially if symptoms have persisted for an extended time. Assessment increases awareness and helps identify the adequacy of nutrient intake.
- Refer to a dietitian for meal planning to minimize PUD symptoms and meet nutritional needs. Consider normal eating patterns and preferences in meal planning. Although no specific diet is recommended for PUD, clients should avoid foods that increase pain. Six small meals per day often helps increase food tolerance and decrease postprandial discomfort.
- Monitor for complaints of anorexia, fullness, nausea, and vomiting. Adjust dietary intake or medication schedule as indicated. PUD and resultant scarring can lead to impaired gastric emptying, necessitating a treatment change.
- Monitor laboratory values for indications of anemia or other nutritional deficits. Monitor for therapeutic effects and side effects of treatment measures such as oral iron replacement. Instruct the client taking oral iron replacement to avoid using an antacid within 1–2 hours of taking the iron preparation. Anemia can result from poor nutrient absorption or chronic blood loss in clients with PUD. Oral iron supplements may cause GI distress, nausea, and vomiting. If these side effects are intolerable, notify the physician for a possible change of therapy. Antacids bind with oral iron preparations, blocking absorption.

PRACTICE ALERT

Advise the client to report increasing or persistent symptoms of anorexia, nausea and vomiting, or fullness to the health care provider.

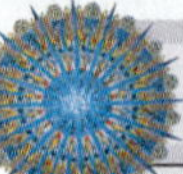

NURSING CARE PLAN **A Client With Peptic Ulcer Disease**

Sean O'Donnell is a 47-year-old police officer who lives and works in a metropolitan area. Mr. O'Donnell has had "heartburn" and abdominal discomfort for years, but thought it went along with his job. Last year, after becoming weak, light-headed, and short of breath, he was found to be anemic and was diagnosed as having a duodenal ulcer. He took omeprazole (Prilosec) and ferrous sulfate for 3 months before stopping both, saying he had "never felt better in his life." Mr. O'Donnell has now been admitted to the hospital with active upper GI bleeding.

ASSESSMENT	DIAGNOSES	PLANNING
Rachel Clark is Mr. O'Donnell's admitting nurse and case manager. On initial assessment, Mr. O'Donnell is alert and oriented, although very apprehensive about his condition. Skin pale and cool; BP 136/78, P 98; abdomen distended and tender with hyperactive bowel sounds; 200 mL bright red blood obtained on nasogastric tube insertion. Hemoglobin 8.2 g/dL and hematocrit 23% on admission. Mr. O'Donnell is taken to the endoscopy lab, where his bleeding is controlled using laser photocoagulation. On his return to the nursing unit, he receives 2 units of packed RBCs and intravenous fluids to restore blood volume. A 5-day course of high-dose oral omeprazole (40 mg bid) is ordered to prevent rebleeding, and Mr. O'Donnell is allowed to begin a clear liquid diet 24 hours after his endoscopy. Tissue biopsy obtained during endoscopy confirms the presence of *H. pylori* infection.	■ Deficient Fluid Volume related to acutely bleeding duodenal ulcer ■ Risk for Injury related to acute blood loss ■ Fear related to threat to well-being ■ Ineffective Therapeutic Regimen Management related to lack of knowledge regarding PUD and its treatment	■ Maintains normal blood pressure, pulse, and urine output (>30 mL/h) ■ Remains free of injury ■ Seeks information to reduce fear ■ Identifies and uses coping strategies to manage fear ■ Describes prescribed therapeutic regimen ■ Verbalizes ability to manage prescribed regimen

IMPLEMENTATION

- Place call light within reach and encourage client to ask for help when getting up or ambulating. Remind client to rise slowly from lying to sitting and from sitting to standing.
- Discuss situation and provide information about all procedures and treatments.
- Reassure about the effectiveness of treatment in reducing the risk for further bleeding.
- Discuss current and planned treatment measures; stress the importance of completing the prescribed treatment to reduce the risk of further ulcer development.
- Encourage client to avoid using aspirin or NSAIDs in the future; suggest alternative medications such as acetaminophen.
- Discuss stress reduction techniques and refer for stress reduction counseling or workshops as indicated.

EVALUATION

Mr. O'Donnell is discharged 48 hours after admission. He has had no further evidence of bleeding and has resumed a regular diet. His hemoglobin and hematocrit remain low, and he has a prescription for ferrous sulfate. He will complete the prescribed high-dose omeprazole regimen at home, then begin treatment with omeprazole, amoxicillin, and clarithromycin (Biaxin) to eradicate the *H. pylori* infection detected during endoscopy. After 2 weeks of this regimen, he will continue taking omeprazole at bedtime for 4–8 weeks. He verbalizes a good understanding of his treatment and the importance of completing the entire regimen. Mr. O'Donnell expresses concern about his ability to "keep his cool on the inside" when under stress. Ms. Clark, his case manager, gives him the names of several resources to help with stress management in case he wants help.

CRITICAL THINKING

1. How does *H. pylori* infection contribute to the development of peptic ulcers?
2. Describe the physiologic responses to fear and anxiety. Why is it important to alleviate fear and its physical consequences in clients with PUD?
3. What suggestions can you make to help Mr. O'Donnell manage his complex treatment regimen during the next 3 months?
4. Develop a teaching plan that includes stress reduction techniques that Mr. O'Donnell can use while performing his duties as a police officer.

Deficient Fluid Volume

Erosion of a blood vessel with resultant hemorrhage is a significant risk for the client with PUD. Acute bleeding can lead to hypovolemia and fluid volume deficit, which can lead to a decrease in cardiac output and impaired tissue perfusion.

- Monitor stools and gastric drainage for overt and occult blood. Assess gastric drainage (vomitus or drainage from a nasogastric tube) to estimate the amount and rapidity of hemorrhage. Drainage is bright red with possible clots in acute hemorrhage and is dark red or the color of coffee grounds when blood has been in the stomach for a period of time. Hematochezia (stool containing red blood and clots) is present in acute hemorrhage; melena (black, tarry stool) is an indicator of less acute bleeding. When small vessels are disrupted, bleeding may be slow and not overtly evident. With chronic or slow GI bleeding, the risk of a fluid volume deficit is minimal; anemia and activity intolerance are more likely.
- Maintain intravenous therapy with fluid volume and electrolyte replacement solutions; administer whole blood or packed cells as ordered. Both fluids and electrolytes are lost through vomiting, nasogastric drainage, and diarrhea in an episode of acute bleeding. To prevent shock, it is essential to maintain a blood volume and cardiac output sufficient to perfuse body tissues. Whole blood and packed cells replace both blood volume and RBCs, providing additional oxygen-carrying capacity to meet cell needs.

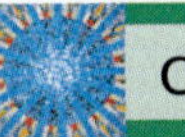

CARE SETTINGS Community and Home Care for Clients With PUD

Peptic ulcer disease is managed in home and community-based settings; only its complications typically require treatment in an acute care setting. Provide the following information when preparing the client for home care:

- Prescribed medication regimen, including desired and potential adverse effects
- Importance of continuing therapy even when symptoms are relieved
- Relationship between peptic ulcers and factors such as NSAID use and smoking; if indicated, refer to a smoking cessation clinic or program.
- Importance of avoiding aspirin and other NSAIDs; stress the necessity of reading the labels of over-the-counter medications for possible aspirin content
- Manifestations of complications that should be reported to the care provider, including increased abdominal pain or distention, vomiting, black or tarry stools, light-headedness, or fainting
- Stress and lifestyle management techniques that may help prevent exacerbation; refer to resources for stress management, such as classes, counseling, and formal or informal groups

- Insert a nasogastric tube and maintain its position and patency. Initially, measure and record gastric output every hour, then every 4–8 hours. Nasogastric suction removes blood from the GI tract, preventing vomiting and possible aspiration. Gastric output is replaced milliliter for milliliter with a balanced electrolyte solution to maintain homeostasis.
- Monitor hemoglobin and hematocrit, serum electrolytes, BUN, and creatinine values. Report abnormal findings. Hemoglobin and hematocrit are lower than normal with acute or chronic GI bleeding. In acute hemorrhage, initial results may be within normal range because both cells and plasma are lost. Loss of fluids and electrolytes with gastric drainage and diarrhea will alter normal levels. Digestion and absorption of blood in the GI tract may result in elevated BUN and creatinine levels.
- Assess abdomen, including bowel sounds, distention, girth, and tenderness, every 4 hours and record findings. Borborygmi or hyperactive bowel sounds with abdominal tenderness are common with acute GI bleeding. Increased distention; increasing abdominal girth; absent bowel sounds; or extreme tenderness with a rigid, boardlike abdomen may indicate perforation.
- Maintain bed rest with the head of the bed elevated. Ensure safety. Loss of blood volume may cause orthostatic hypotension with resultant syncope or dizziness upon standing.

Evaluation

Client care may be evaluated using the following expected outcomes:

- Client obtains pain control adequate to promote rest and sleep.
- Client describes actions that will reduce the risk of recurrence of PUD.
- Client maintains fluid volume homeostasis.
- Client obtains adequate rest and sleep to promote health.

REVIEW Peptic Ulcer Disease

RELATE: LINK THE CONCEPTS

Linking the exemplar of Peptic Ulcer Disease with the concept of Addiction Behavior:

1. When admitting a client with acute PUD, you learn that the client has a 20+ year history of smoking. How might this behavior contribute to PUD?
2. What teaching would you provide to motivate and support the client to quit smoking?

You are caring for a client with acute PUD who has had profuse hemoptysis secondary to ulceration of the stomach lining. The client has had significant blood loss, with approximately 3 liters of bloody emesis measured over the past 24 hours. The provider orders iced lavages, which seem to have stopped the bleeding for now.

Linking the exemplar of Peptic Ulcer Disease with the concept of Perfusion:

3. How will you assess this client related to shock?
4. What actions, independent or collaborative, can you take to promote the client's hemovascular stability?

READY: GO TO COMPANION SKILLS MANUAL

- Inserting a nasogastric tube
- Flushing/maintaining a nasogastric tube
- Removing a nasogastric tube
- Measuring abdominal girth
- Measuring weights
- Initiating intravenous infusion
- Administering blood components

REFER: GO TO MYNURSINGKIT

REFLECT: CASE STUDY

Raymond Combs, 38 years old, owns a chain of neighborhood convenience stores. He is married to his third wife, and they have two children by this marriage and are raising three children from former relationships. Raymond often jokes that he prefers to stay at work because it is less stressful than being at home with the children and his wife.

For the past month, Raymond has been noticing pain in his left upper abdomen approximately 2–3 hours after meals. He describes the pain as a burning, gnawing pain that goes away when he eats. He and his wife make plans to go out for dinner with their next door neighbors. Raymond's wife suggests that he talk to the neighbor, who is a nurse, about the discomfort he's been feeling.

1. You are Raymond's neighbor. When you go out for dinner with Raymond and his wife, he describes the pain and asks what you think is happening. How do you respond?
2. Raymond asks you what he can do to make his problem go away if it is, in fact, an ulcer. How do you respond?
3. Raymond's wife says that she heard that a milk and dairy diet is good for ulcers. How do you respond?

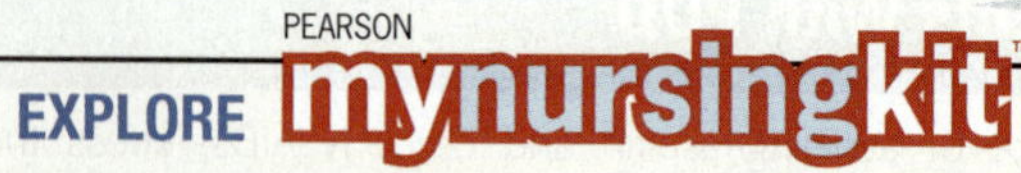

MyNursingKit is your one stop for online chapter review materials and resources. Prepare for success with additional NCLEX®-style practice questions, interactive assignments and activities, web links, animations and videos, and more!

Register your access code from the front of your book at **www.mynursingkit.com**.

REFERENCES

Adams, M.P., Holland, Jr., L.N., & Bostwick, P.M. (2008). *Pharmacology for nurses: A pathophysiologic approach* (2nd ed.). Upper Saddle River, NJ: Pearson Education.

Balch, J. F., & Stengler, M. (2004). *Prescription for natural cures: A self-care guide for treating health problems with natural remedies including diet and nutrition, nutritional supplements, bodywork, and more.* Hoboken, NJ: Wiley & Sons.

Bayless, T. M. and Hanauer, S. B. (2001). *Advanced therapy of inflammatory bowel disease.* Hamilton, Ontario: BC Decker Inc.

Berman, A., Snyder, S.J., Kozier, B., & Erb, G. (2008). *Kozier & Erb's fundamentals of nursing: Concepts, process, and practice* (8th ed.). Upper Saddle River, NJ: Pearson Education.

Crohn's & Colitis Foundation of America. (2005). *About Crohn's disease.* Retrieved from http://www.ccfa.org/info/about/crohns

Gray, M., Huether, S. E., & Forshee, B. A. (2006). Alterations of renal and urinary tract function. In K. L. McCance & S. E. Huether, *Pathophysiology: The biologic basis for disease in adults and children* (5th ed., pp. 1301–1335). St. Louis: Elsevier Mosby.

Hellekson, K. (2005). ACG releases updated practice guidelines for ulcerative colitis in adults. *American Family Physician, 71*(3), 604–606.

Heuschkel, R., Afzal, N., Wuerth, A., Zurakowski, D., Leichtner, A., Kemper, K., et al. (2002). Complementary medicine use in children and young adults with inflammatory bowel disease. *American Journal of Gastroenterology, 97*(2), 382–388.

Kasper, D. L., Braunwald, E., Fauci, A. S., Hauser, S. L., Longo, D. L., & Jameson, J. L. (2005). *Harrison's principles of internal medicine* (16th ed.). New York: McGraw-Hill.

Kwok, M. Y., Kim, M. K., & Gorelick, M. H. (2004). Evidence-based approach to the diagnosis of appendicitis in children. *Pediatric Emergency Care, 20,* 690–698.

Langmead, L., Dawson, C., Hawkins, C., Banna, N., Loo, S., & Rampton, D. S. (2002). Antioxidant effects of herbal therapies used by clients with inflammatory bowel disease: An *in vitro* study. *Alimentary Pharmacologic Therapy, 16*(2), 197–205.

Lau, K. K., & Wyatt, R. J. (2005). Glomerulonephritis. *Adolescent Medicine Clinics, 16*(1), 67–85.

LeMone, P., & Burke, K. (2008). *Medical-surgical nursing: Critical thinking in client care* (4th ed.). Upper Saddle River, NJ: Pearson Education.

Porth, C. M. (2005). *Pathophysiology: Concepts of altered health states* (7th ed.). Philadelphia: Lippincott.

Tierney, L. M., McPhee, S. J., & Papadakis, M. A. (2005). *Current medical diagnosis & treatment* (44th ed.). New York: Lange Medical Books/McGraw-Hill.

Vaira, D., Gatta, L., Ricci, C., Tampieri, A., Cavina, M., & Bernabucci V. (2005). Symposium on peptic acid disease. Peptic ulcer and *Helicobacter pylori*: Update on testing and treatment. *Postgraduate Medicine, 117*(6), 17–22, 46.

Verhoef, M. J., Rapchuk, I., Liew, T., Weir, V., & Hilsden, R. J. (2002). Complementary practitioners' views of treatment for inflammatory bowel disease. *Canadian Journal of Gastroenterology, 16*(2), 95–100.

Yount, S.T., Edgell, J., & Jakovec, V. (1990). Preoperative teaching: A study of nurses' perceptions. *AORN J, 51*(2), 574–575, 577–579.

Ziegler, M. M. (2004). The diagnosis of appendicitis: An evolving paradigm. *Pediatrics, 113,* 130–132.

Intracranial Regulation 17

Concept at-a-Glance

Concept Learning Outcomes

After reading about this concept, you will be able to:

1. Summarize the structure and physiologic processes of the neurologic system related to intracranial regulation.
2. List factors affecting intracranial regulation.
3. Identify commonly occurring alterations in intracranial regulation and their related treatments.
4. Explain common physical assessment procedures used to examine intracranial regulation in clients across the life span.
5. Outline diagnostic and laboratory tests to determine the individual's intracranial regulation.
6. Explain the management of intracranial regulation and prevention of intracranial disease.
7. Demonstrate the nursing process in providing culturally competent care across the life span for individuals with common alterations in intracranial regulation.
8. Identify pharmacologic interventions in caring for the individual with alterations in intracranial regulation.

Concept Key Terms

Aphasia, *951*
Brain death, *948*
Brainstem, *941*
Central nervous system, *940*
Cerebellum, *941*
Cerebrum, *940*
Consciousness, *946*
Decerebrate posturing, *945*
Decorticate posturing, *945*
Dermatome, *943*
Fasciculations, *954*
Increased intracranial pressure (IICP), *948*
Intracranial regulation, *939*
Kinesthesia, *954*
Locked-in syndrome, *948*
Meninges, *940*
Neuron, *940*
Peripheral nervous system, *940*
Persistent vegetative state, *948*
Reflexes, *941*
Seizures, *948*
Spinal cord, *941*
Tremors, *955*

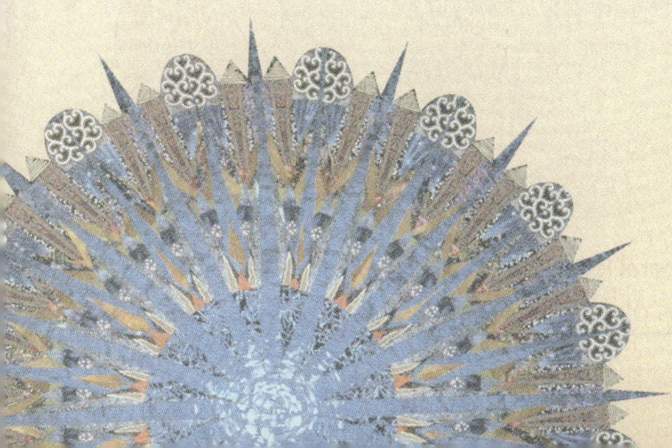

About Intracranial Regulation

Intracranial regulation refers to the processes that affect intracranial compensation and adaptive neurologic function. The neurologic system regulates and integrates all body functions, muscle movements, senses, mental abilities, and emotions. It collects, as sensory input, information from the internal and external environments, processes and interprets the input, and causes responses that are manifested as motor or sensory output. A threat to any aspect of neurologic function is a threat to the whole person. •

NORMAL PRESENTATION

The neurologic system is divided into two principal parts: the central nervous system (CNS) and the peripheral nervous system (PNS). The **central nervous system** consists of the brain and the spinal cord; the **peripheral nervous system** consists of the cranial nerves and the spinal nerves. The two systems work together to receive an impulse, interpret it, and initiate a response, enabling the individual to maintain a high level of adaptation and homeostasis. The nervous system is responsible for control of cognitive function and both voluntary and involuntary activities.

The basic cell of the nervous system is the **neuron**. This highly specialized cell sends impulses throughout the body. Myelin sheaths cover many of the larger diameter and longer nerves in order to help speed the rate of conduction of the nerve impulse. Without this covering nerve impulses would take a much longer time to travel. For example, if you place your hand on a hot surface, a sensory impulse travels to your brain, reporting that the surface is hot, and then a motor impulse travels back to your fingers so you'll pull them away. Myelin allows the impulse to travel quickly so the fingers are removed before serious damage is done. Myelin is white in color, hence the term *white matter of the nervous system.*

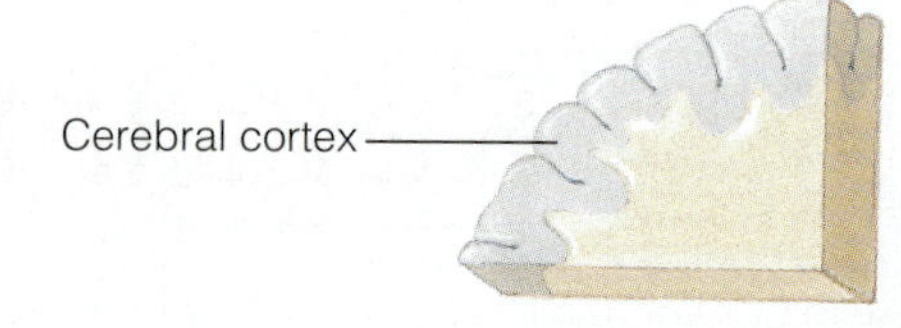

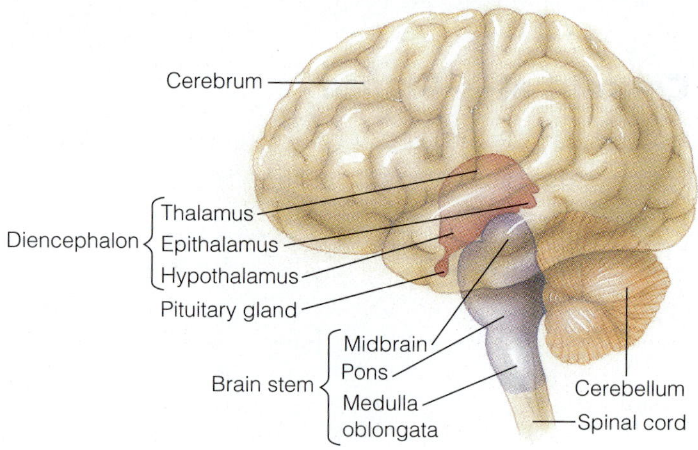

Figure 17–1 ■ Regions of the brain.

Central Nervous System (CNS)

The central nervous system includes the brain and spinal cord. These structures will be described in the following sections.

BRAIN The brain is the largest portion of the central nervous system. It is covered and protected by the meninges, the cerebrospinal fluid (CSF), and the bony structure of the skull. The **meninges** are three connective tissue membranes that cover, protect, and nourish the CNS. Cerebrosinal fluid also helps to nourish the central nervous system; however, the primary function of CSF is to cushion the brain and prevent injury to the brain tissue. The brain is made up of the cerebrum, diencephalon, cerebellum, and brainstem (Figure 17–1 ■).

Cerebrum The **cerebrum** is the largest portion of the brain. The outermost layer of the cerebrum, the *cerebral cortex,* is composed of gray matter. Responsible for all conscious behavior, the cerebral cortex enables the individual to perceive, remember, communicate, and initiate voluntary movements. The cerebrum consists of the frontal, parietal, occipital, and temporal lobes. The lobes of the cerebrum are illustrated in Figure 17–2 ■.

The frontal lobe of the cerebrum helps to control voluntary skeletal movement, speech, emotions, and intellectual activities. The prefrontal cortex of the frontal lobe controls intellect, complex learning abilities, judgment, reasoning, concern for others, and creation of abstract ideas.

The parietal lobe of the cerebrum is responsible for conscious awareness of sensation and somatosensory stimuli, including temperature, pain, shapes, and two-point discrimination (e.g., the ability to sense a round versus a square object placed in the hand or hot versus cold materials against the skin. The visual cortex, located in the occipital lobe, receives stimuli from the retina and interprets the visual stimuli in relation to past experiences.

The temporal lobe of the cerebrum is responsible for interpreting auditory stimuli. Impulses from the cochlea are transmitted to the temporal lobe and are interpreted regarding pitch, rhythm, loudness, and perception of what the individual hears. The olfactory cortex is also in the temporal lobe and transmits impulses related to smell.

Diencephalon The diencephalon is composed of the thalamus, hypothalamus, and epithalamus. The thalamus is the gateway to the cerebral cortex. All input channeled to the cerebral cortex is processed by the thalamus.

The hypothalamus, an autonomic control center, influences activities such as blood pressure; heart rate; force of heart contraction; digestive motility; respiratory rate and

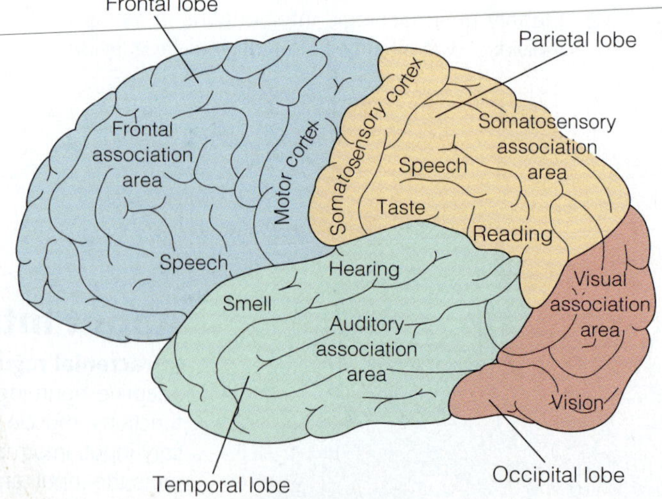

Figure 17–2 ■ Lobes of the cerebrum.

depth; and perception of pain, pleasure, and fear. Body temperature, food intake, water balance, and sleep cycles also are regulated by the hypothalamus.

The epithalamus helps control moods and sleep cycles. It contains the choroid plexus, where the CSF is formed.

Cerebellum The **cerebellum** is located below the cerebrum and behind the brainstem. It coordinates stimuli from the cerebral cortex to provide precise timing for skeletal muscle coordination and smooth movements. The cerebellum also assists with maintaining equilibrium and muscle tone.

Brainstem The **brainstem** contains the midbrain, pons, and medulla oblongata. Located between the cerebrum and spinal cord, the brainstem connects pathways between the higher and lower structures. Ten of the 12 pairs of cranial nerves originate in the brainstem. As an autonomic control center, the brainstem influences blood pressure by controlling vasoconstriction. It also regulates respiratory rate, depth, and rhythm as well as vomiting, hiccupping, swallowing, coughing, and sneezing.

SPINAL CORD The **spinal cord** is a continuation of the medulla oblongata. About 42 cm (17 in.) in length, it passes through the skull at the foramen magnum and continues through the vertebral column to the first lumbar vertebra. The meninges, CSF, and bony vertebrae protect the spinal cord. The spinal cord has the ability to transmit impulses to and from the brain via the ascending and descending pathways. Some reflex activity takes place within the spinal cord; however, for this activity to be useful, the brain must interpret it.

REFLEXES **Reflexes** are stimulus–response activities of the body. They are fast, predictable, unlearned, innate, and involuntary reactions to stimuli. The individual is aware of the results of the reflex activity but not the activity itself. The reflex activity may be simple and take place at the level of the spinal cord, with interpretation at the cerebral level. For example, if the tendon of the knee is sharply stimulated with a reflex hammer, the impulse follows the afferent (sensory) nerve fibers. A synapse occurs in the spinal cord, and the impulse is transmitted to the efferent nerve fibers (motor nerve), leading to an additional synapse and stimulation of muscle fibers. As the muscle fibers contract, the lower leg moves, causing the knee-jerk reaction. The individual is aware of the reflex after the lower leg moves and the brain has interpreted the activity. Figure 17–3 ■ illustrates two simple reflex arcs, the two-neuron reflex arc and the three-neuron reflex arc. In part A, the stimulus is transferred from the sensory neuron directly to the motor neuron at the point of synapse in the spinal cord. In part B, the stimulus travels from the sensory neuron to an interneuron in the spinal cord and then to the motor neuron.

Peripheral Nervous System (PNS)

The peripheral nervous system includes the 12 pairs of cranial nerves and the paired spinal nerves. They will be described in the following paragraphs.

CRANIAL NERVES The 12 pairs of cranial nerves originate in the brain and serve various parts of the head and neck (Figure 17–4 ■). The first 2 pairs originate in the anterior brain, and the remaining 10 pairs originate in the brainstem. The vagus nerve (cranial nerve X) is the only cranial nerve to serve a muscle and body region below the neck. The cranial nerves are numbered using Roman numerals and many times are discussed by number rather than name. Composition of the cranial nerve fibers varies, producing sensory nerves, motor nerves, and mixed nerves. A summary of the name, number, function, and activity of the cranial nerves is presented in Table 17–1.

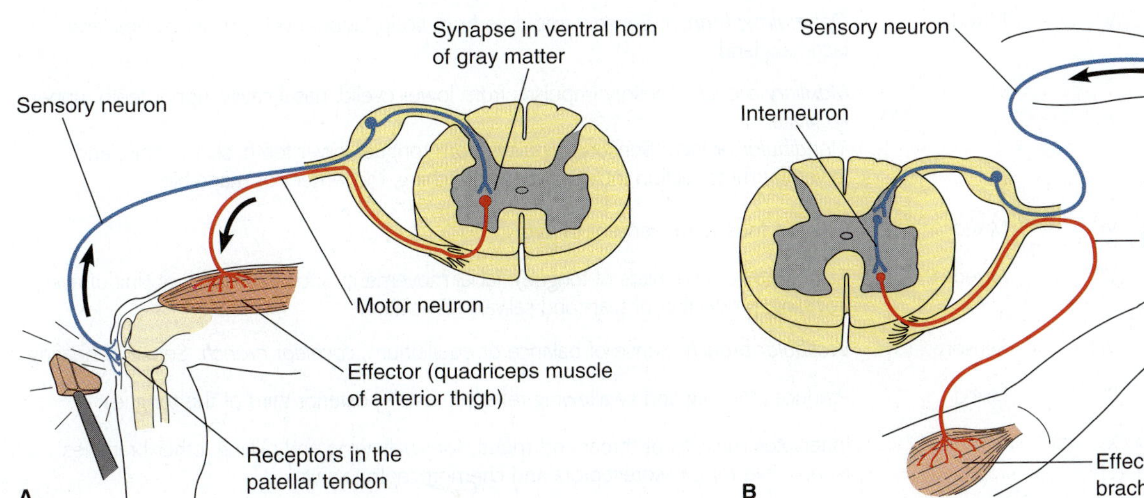

Figure 17–3 ■ Two simple reflex arcs. *A*, In the two-neuron reflex arc, the stimulus is transferred from the sensory neuron directly to the motor neuron at the point of synapse in the spinal cord. *B*, In the three-neuron reflex arc, the stimulus travels from the sensory neuron to an interneuron in the spinal cord and then to the motor neuron. (Sensory nerves are shown in blue; motor nerves are shown in red.)

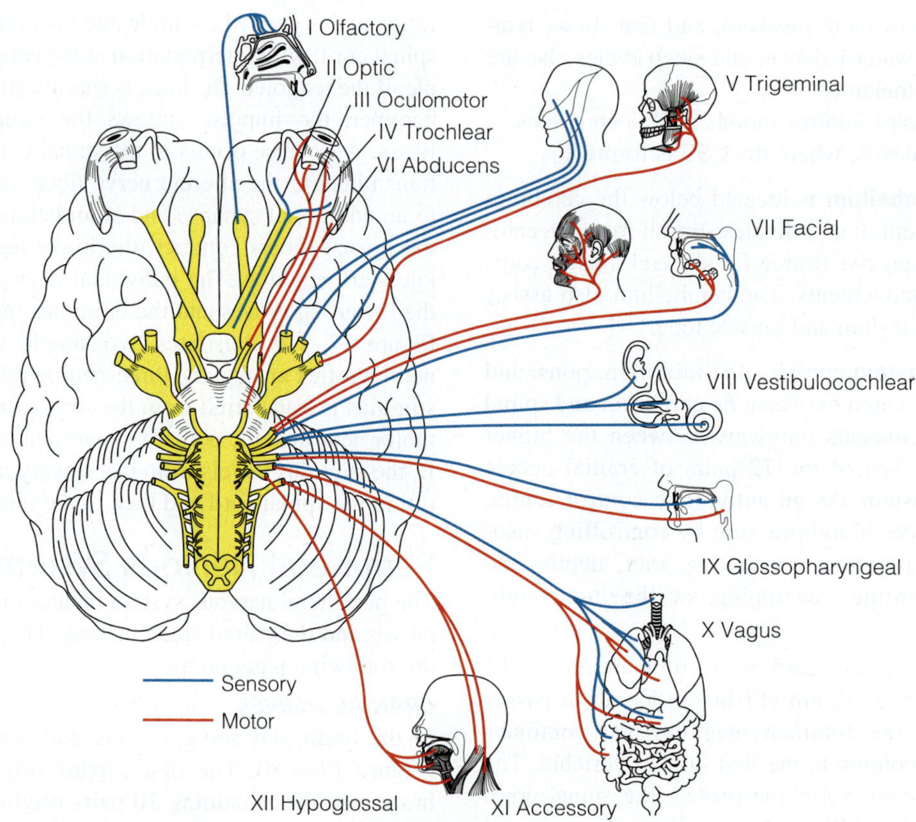

Figure 17–4 ■ Cranial nerves and their target regions. (Sensory nerves are shown in blue; motor nerves are shown in red.)

TABLE 17–1 Cranial Nerves

NAME	NUMBER	FUNCTION	ACTIVITY
Olfactory	I	Sensory	Sense of smell
Optic	II	Sensory	Vision
Oculomotor	III	Motor	Pupillary reflex, extrinsic muscle movement of eye
Trochlear	IV	Motor	Eye-muscle movement
Trigeminal	V	Mixed	*Ophthalmic branch:* Sensory impulses from scalp, upper eyelid, nose, cornea, and lacrimal gland
			Maxillary branch: Sensory impulses from lower eyelid, nasal cavity, upper teeth, upper lip, alate *Mandibular branch:* Sensory impulses from tongue, lower teeth, skin of chin, and lower lip; motor action includes teeth clenching, movement of mandible.
Abducens	VI	Mixed	Extrinsic muscle movement of eye
Facial	VII	Mixed	Taste (anterior two thirds of tongue); facial movements such as smiling, closing of eyes, frowning; production of tears and salivary stimulation
Vestibulocochlear	VIII	Sensory	*Vestibular branch:* Sense of balance or equilibrium; *cochlear branch:* Sense of hearing
Glossopharyngeal	IX	Mixed	Produces the gag and swallowing reflexes; taste (posterior third of the tongue)
Vagus	X	Mixed	Innervates muscles of throat and mouth for swallowing and talking; other branches responsible for pressoreceptors and chemoreceptor activity
Accessory	XI	Motor	Movement of the trapezius and sternocleidomastoid muscles; some movement of larynx, pharynx, and soft palate
Hypoglossal	XII	Motor	Movement of tongue for swallowing, movement of food during chewing, and speech

SPINAL NERVES The spinal cord supplies the body with 31 pairs of spinal nerves that are named according to the vertebral level of origin as shown in Figure 17–5 ■.

There are 8 pairs of cervical nerves, 12 pairs of thoracic nerves, 5 pairs of lumbar nerves, 5 pairs of sacral nerves, and 1 pair of coccygeal nerves. At the cervical level, the nerves exit superior to the vertebra except for the eighth cervical nerve. This nerve exits inferior to the seventh cervical vertebra. All remaining descending nerves exit the spinal cord and vertebral column inferior to the same-numbered vertebrae. All spinal nerves are classified as mixed nerves because they contain motor and sensory pathways that produce motor and sensory activities. Each pair of nerves is responsible for a particular area of the body. The nerves provide some overlap in terms of the body segments they serve. This overlap is more complete on the trunk than on the extremities.

A **dermatome** is an area of skin innervated by the cutaneous branch of one spinal nerve. All spinal nerves except the first cervical (C_1) serve a cutaneous region. The anterior and posterior views of the dermatomes of the body are shown in Figure 17–6 ■.

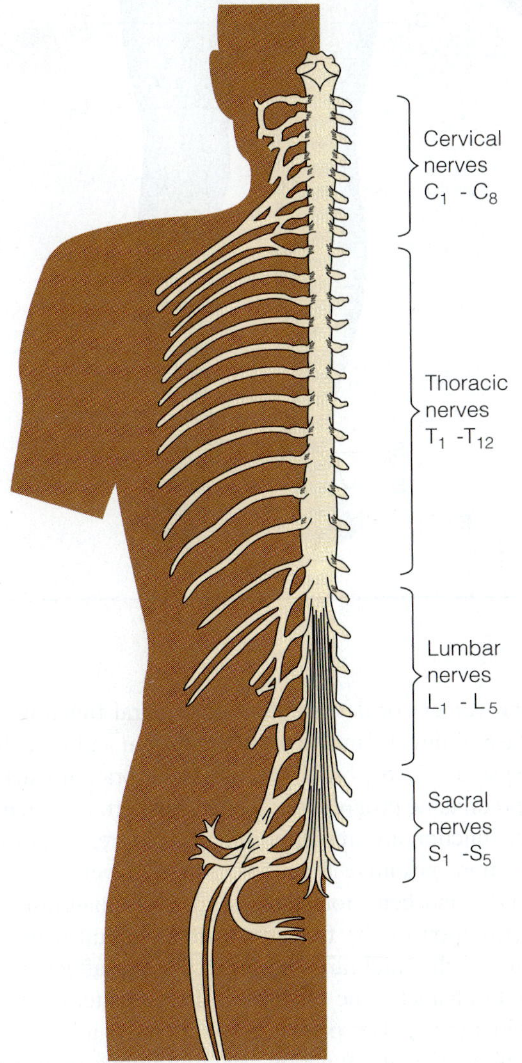

Figure 17–5 ■ Spinal nerves.

Age-Related Changes

INFANTS AND CHILDREN The growth of the nervous system is very rapid during the fetal period. This rate of growth does not continue during infancy. Some research indicates that no neurons are formed after the third trimester of fetal life. It is believed that the neurons mature during infancy, allowing for more complete actions to take place. The cerebral cortex thickens, brain size increases, and myelinization occurs. The maturational advances in the nervous system are responsible for the cephalocaudal and proximal-to-distal refinement of development, control, and movement.

The neonate has several primitive reflexes at birth. These include, but are not limited to, sucking, stepping, rooting, startle (Moro), and Babinski's reflex, in which stimulation of the sole of the foot from the heel toward the toes results in dorsiflexion of the great toe and fanning of other toes. Babinski's reflex is normal until around 2 years of age. By about 1 month of age, the various reflexes begin to disappear and the child takes on more controlled and complex activity.

The cry of the newborn helps place the infant on the health–illness continuum. *Strong* and *lusty* are terms used to describe the cry of a healthy newborn. An absent, weak, "catlike," or shrill cry usually indicates cerebral disease.

Head circumference is a measurement of the head above the level of the ears and across the forehead. Because the cranial sutures are not sealed in infancy, the head may increase in size to accommodate intracranial edema or bleeding. By measuring circumference of the head in the same spot every time, the nurse will obtain data early in the process that will allow for intervention before damage to neurons becomes acute.

Throughout infancy and the early childhood years, it is important to assess the child's fine and gross motor skills, language, and personal/social skills. The nurse identifies benchmarks or milestones related to age and level of functioning of the child, comparing the child's actual functioning to an anticipated level of functioning. Developmental delays or learning disabilities may or may not be related to neurologic conditions such as fetal alcohol syndrome, autism, and attention deficit disorder. (See Concept 2, Addiction Behavior, and Concept 7, Development.)

THE OLDER ADULT As the individual ages, many neurologic changes occur. Some of these changes are readily visible, whereas others are internal and are not easily detected. In general, the aging process causes a subtle, slow, but steady decrease in neurologic function. These changes can be more pronounced and more troublesome for the individual when they are accompanied by a chronic illness such as heart disease, diabetes, or arthritis. As individuals age, impulse transmission decreases, as does reaction to stimuli. Reflexes are diminished or disappear, and coordination is not as strong as it once was. Deep tendon reflexes are not as brisk. Coordination and movement may be slower and not as smooth as they were at an earlier age.

The senses—hearing, vision, smell, taste, and touch—are not as acute as they once were. Because the sense of taste is not as sensitive, older adults tend to use more seasonings on

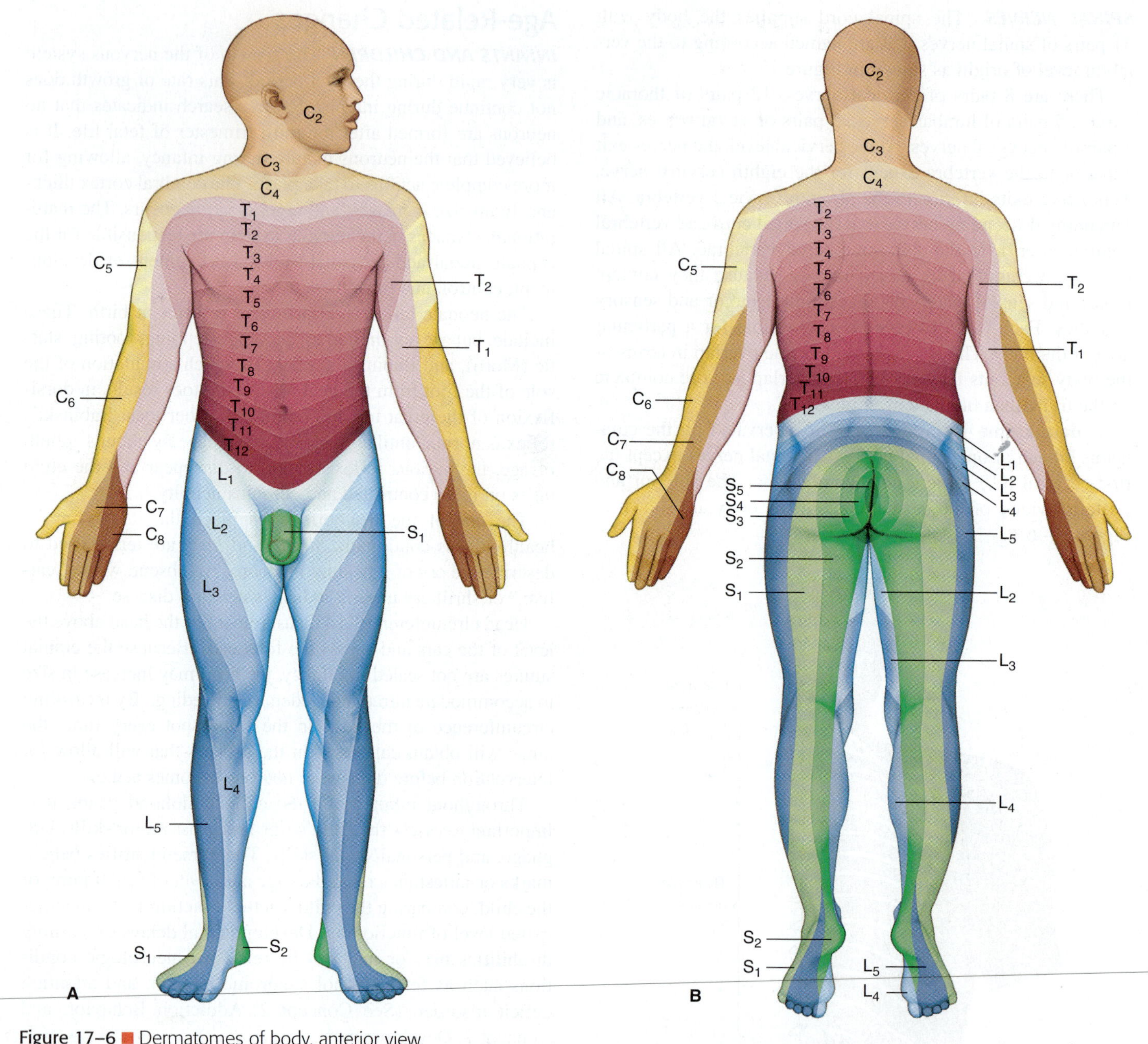

Figure 17–6 ■ Dermatomes of body, anterior view.

food. Visual acuity and hearing also begin to diminish as the individual ages. (See Concept 25, Sensory Perception.)

As muscle mass decreases, the older individual moves and reacts more slowly than during youth. The client's gait may now include short, shuffling, uncertain, and perhaps unsteady steps. The posture of the older adult demonstrates more flexion than in earlier years.

ALTERATIONS

The manifestations of altered cerebral function occur as a result of illness or injury. Assessment of the patterns of those manifestations helps determine the extent of the cerebral dysfunction and improvement or deterioration of cerebral function. Except in the case of direct damage to the brainstem and reticular activating system (RAS), brain function deterioration usually follows a predictable progression, that is, a pattern in which higher levels of function are impaired initially, progressing to impairment of more primitive functions. Altered level of consciousness (LOC) and behavior changes are early manifestations of the deterioration of the function of the cerebral hemispheres. Structures in the midbrain and brainstem are affected sequentially, with characteristic changes in LOC; patterns of respiration, widening pulse pressure, pupillary, and oculomotor responses; and motor function. Manifestations of progressive deterioration of cerebral function are outlined in Table 17–2.

TABLE 17–2 Progression of Deteriorating Brain Function

LEVEL OF CONSCIOUSNESS	PUPILLARY RESPONSE	OCULOMOTOR RESPONSES	MOTOR RESPONSES	BREATHING
Is alert; oriented to time, place, and person	Brisk and equal; pupils regular	Eyes move as head turns. Caloric testing (ear irrigation) produces nystagmus.	Purposeful movement; responds to commands	Regular pattern with normal rate and depth
Responds to verbal stimuli; shows decreased concentration; agitation, confusion, lethargy; is disoriented	Small and reactive	Roving eye movements; doll's eyes positive (Figure 17–7 ■), with gaze fixed straight ahead; eye deviation away from cold caloric stimulus and toward warm stimulus	Purposeful movement in response to pain stimulus	Yawning, sighing respirations

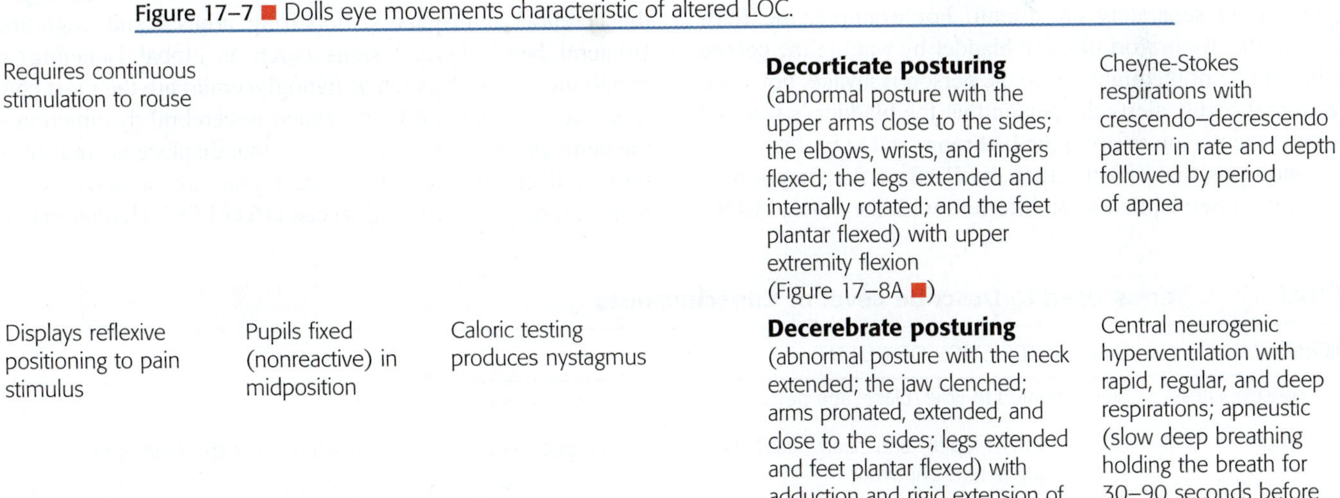
Head in neutral position
Head rotated to client's left
Eyes midline
Doll's eyes present:
Eyes move right in relation to head.
Doll's eyes absent:
Eyes do not move in relation to head.
Direction of vision follows head to left.

Figure 17–7 ■ Dolls eye movements characteristic of altered LOC.

LEVEL OF CONSCIOUSNESS	PUPILLARY RESPONSE	OCULOMOTOR RESPONSES	MOTOR RESPONSES	BREATHING
Requires continuous stimulation to rouse			**Decorticate posturing** (abnormal posture with the upper arms close to the sides; the elbows, wrists, and fingers flexed; the legs extended and internally rotated; and the feet plantar flexed) with upper extremity flexion (Figure 17–8A ■)	Cheyne-Stokes respirations with crescendo–decrescendo pattern in rate and depth followed by period of apnea
Displays reflexive positioning to pain stimulus	Pupils fixed (nonreactive) in midposition	Caloric testing produces nystagmus	**Decerebrate posturing** (abnormal posture with the neck extended; the jaw clenched; arms pronated, extended, and close to the sides; legs extended and feet plantar flexed) with adduction and rigid extension of upper and lower extremities (see Figure 17–8B)	Central neurogenic hyperventilation with rapid, regular, and deep respirations; apneustic (slow deep breathing holding the breath for 30–90 seconds before rapid exhalation) breathing with prolonged inspiration and pauses at full inspiration and following expiration

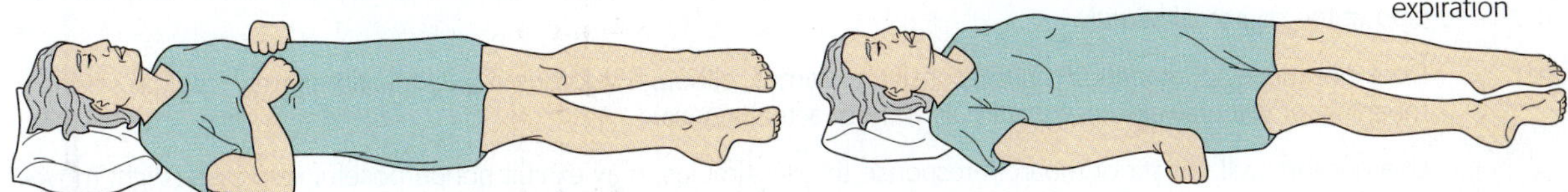

Figure 17–8 ■ *A*, Decorticate posturing, characterized by rigid flexion, is associated with lesions above the brainstem in the corticospinal tracts. *B*, Decerebrate posturing, distinguished by rigid extension, is associated with lesions of the brainstem.

(continued)

TABLE 17–2 Progression of Deteriorating Brain Function (continued)

LEVEL OF CONSCIOUSNESS	PUPILLARY RESPONSE	OCULOMOTOR RESPONSES	MOTOR RESPONSES	BREATHING
Shows no response to stimuli	Fixed pupils in midposition	No spontaneous eye movement or nystagmus	Extension of upper extremities with flexion of lower extremities; flaccidity	Cluster or ataxic breathing with irregular pattern and depth of respirations; gasping respirations or apnea

Alterations in Level of Consciousness

Consciousness is a condition in which the person is aware of self and environment and is able to respond appropriately to stimuli. Full consciousness requires both normal arousal and full cognition.

- *Arousal*, or alertness, depends on the reticular activating system (RAS), a diffuse system of neurons in the thalamus and upper brainstem.
- *Cognition* is a complex process by which an individual learns, stores, retrieves, and uses information. Cognitive processing involves all mental activities controlled by the cerebral hemispheres, including thought processes, memory, perception, communication, problem solving, and emotion.

These two components of consciousness depend on the normal physiologic functions of and connections between the arousal mechanisms of the reticular formation and the cognitive functions of the cerebral hemispheres. Because arousal and cognition are independent components of consciousness, each can act separately on stimuli. For example, the RAS reacts to the discomfort of a full bladder by waking the person in the middle of the night. Once the person is awake, however, the frontal cortex alerts the person that the bladder is full and prompts the person to go to the bathroom and empty it.

Conditions that affect either the RAS or the function of the cerebral hemispheres can interfere with the normal LOC. Terms describing altered LOC are listed and defined in Table 17–3. Nurses should remember that consciousness is a dynamic state: A client may pass from full consciousness to coma within hours or experience a slow diminishment of consciousness that does not become evident for weeks or months. The nurse can help provide effective care for a client with an altered LOC by looking beyond the diagnostic labels of consciousness and accurately assessing the client's behavior and response to stimuli.

An individual's LOC may be altered by processes that affect the arousal functions of the brainstem, the cognitive functions of the cerebral hemispheres, or both. The major causes of altered LOC are (1) lesions or injuries that affect the cerebral hemispheres directly and widely or that compress or destroy the neurons of the RAS, (2) metabolic disorders, and (3) medications.

The function of the brain, especially the cerebral hemispheres, depends on continuous blood flow with unimpeded supplies of oxygen and glucose. Processes that disrupt this flow of blood and nutrients may cause widespread damage to the cerebral hemispheres, impairing arousal and cognition. Bilateral hemispheric lesions (such as global ischemia) or metabolic disorders (such as hypoglycemia) are the most common causes of altered LOC related to cerebral dysfunction of the hemispheres. Localized masses that displace normal structures and cause direct or indirect pressure on the opposite hemisphere or brainstem also can affect LOC. Hematoma and

TABLE 17–3 Terms Used to Describe Level of Consciousness

TERM	CHARACTERISTICS OF CLIENT
Full consciousness	Alert; oriented to time, place, and person; comprehends spoken and written words
Confusion	Unable to think rapidly and clearly; easily bewildered, with poor memory and short attention span; misinterprets stimuli; judgment is impaired
Disorientation	Not aware of or not oriented to time, place, or person
Obtundation	Lethargic, somnolent; responsive to verbal or tactile stimuli but quickly drifts back to sleep
Stupor	Generally unresponsive; may be briefly aroused by vigorous, repeated, or painful stimuli; may shrink away from or grab at the source of stimuli
Semicomatose	Does not move spontaneously; unresponsive to stimuli, although vigorous or painful stimuli may result in stirring, moaning, or withdrawal from the stimuli, without actual arousal
Coma	Unarousable; will not stir or moan in response to any stimulus; may exhibit nonpurposeful response (slight movement) of area stimulated but makes no attempt to withdraw
Deep coma	Completely unarousable and unresponsive to any kind of stimulus, including pain; absence of brainstem reflexes, corneal, papillary, and pharyngeal reflexes and tendon and plantar reflexes

ALTERATIONS AND TREATMENTS Intracranial Regulation

Alteration	Description	Treatments
Seizure disorder	Periods of abnormal electrical discharges in the brain that cause involuntary movement as well as behavior and sensory alterations; can be partial (focal) or generalized	■ Maintain airway patency. ■ Ensure safety. ■ Administer medications as ordered. ■ Provide emotional support. ■ Identify and treat the underlying cause of the disorder.
Status epilepticus	A continuous seizure that lasts for more than 30 minutes or a series of seizures during which time consciousness is not regained	■ Maintain airway patency. ■ Keep suction equipment at the bedside for excessive secretions. ■ Give oxygen by mask. ■ Monitor vital signs and circulation. ■ Perform neurologic assessment. ■ Establish an intravenous line. ■ Insert a nasogastric tube. ■ Ensure safety. ■ Manage thermoregulation. ■ Administer medications as ordered; cumulative doses of drugs may produce apnea, so be prepared to assist ventilations.
Increased intracranial pressure (IICP) (also labeled *intracranial hypertension*)	Sustained elevated pressure (10 mmHg or higher) in the cranial cavity; a medical emergency	■ Maintain airway patency. ■ Monitor neurologic status; assessment areas include LOC, behavior, motor/sensory functions, pupillary size and reaction to light, and vital signs. ■ Monitor IICP monitor or ventilator. ■ Raise pads and bed rails; seizures may occur. ■ Monitor arterial blood gases. ■ Elevate HOB 30 degrees unless otherwise indicated. ■ Prevent complications associated with immobility. ■ Monitor fluid and electrolytes. ■ Monitor bladder distention and bowel constipation. ■ Provide emotional support as needed. ■ Reduce stimuli, coughing, sneezing, and vagal maneuvers that increase ICP. ■ Identify and treat the underlying cause of the disorder. ■ Realize that surgery may be performed to remove a tumor, lesion, or portion of the brain that has been identified as causing the seizures, particularly when seizures are not responsive to medication.

cerebral edema are just two examples of such masses. The client who has widespread damage to the cerebral hemispheres but an intact RAS has sleep–wake cycles and may rouse in response to stimuli; the client cannot be said to be alert, however, because cognition is impaired.

DISORDERS AFFECTING LEVEL OF CONSCIOUSNESS Both localized neurologic processes and systemic disorders can alter LOC. Processes occurring in the brain that may directly destroy or compress neurologic structures include the following:

- Increased intracranial pressure (IICP)
- Cerebral infarction
- Hematoma
- Intracranial hemorrhage
- Tumors
- Infections
- Injury from excitatory amino acids
- Demyelinating disorders.

Any systemic condition that affects the delivery of blood, oxygen, and glucose to the brain or that alters cell membranes also may alter LOC. If cerebral blood flow is impaired or the client becomes hypoxic or hypoglycemic, cerebral metabolism is impaired and LOC often declines rapidly. Severe hypoxia quickly leads to ischemia. Ischemia may be focal (for example, following a stroke) or global (as from cardiac arrest or hypovolemic shock). Widespread global ischemia causes almost immediate unconsciousness (Porth, 2005). Clients at particular risk include those with poorly controlled diabetes and those with cardiac or respiratory failure.

Other metabolic alterations that can affect LOC include fluid and electrolyte imbalances such as hyponatremia (an abnormally low level of sodium in the blood) or hyperosmolality (increased osmotic concentration of a solution expressed as osmoles of solute per kilogram of serum water) and acid–base alterations such as hypercapnia (an elevated arterial carbon dioxide level). Accumulated waste products and toxins from liver or renal failure can affect neuronal and neurotransmitter function, altering LOC. Drugs that depress the central nervous system (e.g., alcohol, analgesics, and anesthetics) suppress metabolic and membrane activities in the RAS and cerebral hemispheres, thereby affecting LOC. Glutamate, the main excitatory neurotransmitter in the brain, may accumulate during prolonged ischemia, resulting in acute glutamate toxicity and cell death.

Increased Intracranial Pressure **Increased intracranial pressure (IICP)** is sustained elevated pressure (10 mmHg or higher) in the cranial cavity (Wilensky & Bloom, 2005). Like blood pressure, ICP can be affected by routine activities such as sneezing, coughing, or even something as simple as sitting up. The body's compensatory mechanisms control for these minor alterations. However, when ICP raises dramatically or for sustained periods of time significant tissue ischemia and damage to delicate neural tissue may result. The cranial vault is of a fixed size (except in infants whose suture lines remain open allowing for expansion) and only have room for a prescribed amount of blood, cerebrospinal fluid (CSF), and brain matter. As pressure increases, room is made by reducing CSF first, then blood perfusion begins to decrease and this results in diminished oxygenation of neurons Because the neurons in the cerebral cortex are the most sensitive to oxygen deficit, changes in cortical function are the earliest manifestations of ICP, demonstrated by personality changes as well as impaired memory and judgement.

Seizures Seizure activity commonly affects level of consciousness. **Seizures** are periods of abnormal electrical discharges in the brain that may cause involuntary movement and/or behavior and sensory alterations. It appears that the spontaneous, disordered discharge of activity that occurs during a seizure exhausts energy metabolites or produces locally toxic molecules, altering LOC for a time after the seizure. Consciousness returns when the metabolic balance of the neurons is restored.

As the impairment of brain function progresses, more stimuli are required to elicit a response from the client. Initially, the client may rouse to verbal stimuli and respond appropriately to questions, remaining oriented to time, place, and person. With deterioration of neurologic function, the client becomes more difficult to rouse and may become agitated and confused when awakened. Orientation to time is lost initially, followed by orientation to place and then to person. Continuous stimulation or vigorous shaking is required to maintain wakefulness as LOC decreases. Eventually, the client does not respond even to deep, painful stimuli.

OUTCOMES OF ALTERED LEVEL OF CONSCIOUSNESS

Possible outcomes of altered LOC and coma include full recovery with no long-term residual effects, recovery with residual damage (e.g., learning deficits, emotional difficulties, or impaired judgment), and more severe consequences such as persistent vegetative state (cerebral death) or brain death.

Persistent Vegetative State **Persistent vegetative state** (also called *irreversible coma*) is a permanent condition of complete unawareness of self and the environment and loss of all cognitive functions. Usually the result of severe brain trauma or global ischemia, this condition results from death of the cerebral hemispheres with continued function of the brainstem and cerebellum. While the homeostatic regulatory functions of the brain continue, the ability to respond meaningfully to the environment is lost. The diagnosis of persistent vegetative state requires that the condition has continued for at least 1 month (Porth, 2005).

The client in a persistent vegetative state has sleep–wake cycles and retains the ability to chew, swallow, and cough but cannot interact with the environment. When the person is awake, the eyes may wander back and forth across the room, but they cannot track an object or a person. In a minimally conscious state, the client is aware of the environment and can follow simple commands, manipulate objects, gesture or verbalize to indicate yes/no responses, and make meaningful movements (such as blinking or smiling) in response to a stimulus. With appropriate supportive care, the client may remain in this state for years.

Locked-in Syndrome **Locked-in syndrome** is distinctly different from persistent vegetative state in that the client is alert and fully aware of the environment and has intact cognitive abilities but is unable to communicate through speech or movement because of blocked efferent pathways from the brain. Motor paralysis affects all voluntary muscles, although the upper cranial nerves (I through IV) may remain intact, allowing the client to communicate through eye movements and blinking. In essence, the client is "locked" inside a paralyzed body while remaining fully conscious of self and environment.

Infarction or hemorrhage of the pons that disrupts outgoing nerve tracts but spares the RAS is the usual cause of locked-in syndrome. This condition also may result when the corticospinal tracts between the midbrain and pons are interrupted. Disorders of the lower motor neurons or muscles (e.g., acute polyneuritis, myasthenia gravis, and amyotrophic lateral sclerosis [ALS]), also may paralyze motor responses, leading to locked-in syndrome.

Brain Death **Brain death** is the cessation and irreversibility of all brain functions, including the brainstem. Although the exact legal criteria for establishing brain death may vary somewhat from state to state, it is generally agreed that brain death has occurred when there is no evidence of cerebral or brainstem function for an extended period (usually 6–24 hours) in a client who has a normal body temperature and is not affected by a depressant drug or alcohol poisoning. Generally recognized criteria are as follows:

- Unresponsive coma with absent motor and reflex movements
- No spontaneous respiration (apnea)
- Pupils fixed (unresponsive to light) and dilated
- Absent ocular responses to head turning and caloric stimulation. (Caloric stimulation is performed by irrigating the ear with ice cold water to test the oculovestibular reflex, a reflex controlled by the brainstem. Normally, the cold causes the eyes to move first toward the irrigated side, followed by a return to midline.)

- Flat electroencephalogram (EEG) and no cerebral blood circulation present on angiography (if performed)
- Persistence of these manifestations for 30 minutes to 1 hour and for 6 hours after onset of coma and apnea.

Apnea in the comatose client is determined by the apnea test. The ventilator is removed while oxygenation is maintained by tracheal cannula and allowing the PCO_2 to increase to 60 mmHg or higher. This level of carbon dioxide is high enough to stimulate respiration if the brainstem is functional. The EEG may be used to establish the absence of brain activity when brain death is suspected. A flat (isoelectric) EEG over a period of 6–12 hours in a client who is not hypothermic or under the influence of drugs that depress the CNS is generally accepted as an indicator of brain death.

Prognosis

The prognosis for clients with altered LOCs and coma varies according to the underlying cause and pathologic process. Age and general medical condition also play a role in determining outcome. Young adults may fully recover following deep coma from head injury, drug overdose, or other causes. Recovery of consciousness within 2 weeks is associated with a favorable outcome. In general, the prognosis is poor for clients who lack pupillary reaction or reflex eye movements 6 hours after the onset of coma.

ASSESSMENT

A health assessment to determine problems with neurologic structure and/or function may be conducted during a health screening, may focus on a chief complaint (such as headaches), or may be part of a total health assessment. If the client's LOC is altered, the nurse may need to rely on family members for information. The client's LOC can be assessed by using the Glasgow Coma Scale (Table 17–4).

If the client has problems with neurologic structure or function, analyze its onset, characteristics, course, severity, precipitating and relieving factors, and any associated symptoms, noting the time and circumstances.

Assessment techniques for children require developmental considerations. Assessment techniques used with the older adult are the same as those used with the younger or middle-aged adult. However, because the older adult tires more easily, the nurse may need to do the total assessment in more than one visit, and the nurse should allow more time than usual. It is also imperative to obtain a detailed health history of the client because chronic health problems can influence the findings.

TABLE 17–4 **Glasgow Coma Scale for Assessment of Coma in Infants, Children, and Adults**

CATEGORY	SCORE	INFANT AND YOUNG CHILD CRITERIA	OLDER CHILD AND ADULT CRITERIA
Eye opening	4	Spontaneous opening	Spontaneous
	3	To loud noise	To verbal stimuli
	2	To pain	To pain
	1	No response	No response
Verbal response	5	Smiles, coos, cries to appropriate stimuli	Oriented to time, place, and person; uses appropriate words and phrases
	4	Irritable; cries	Confused
	3	Inappropriate crying	Inappropriate words or verbal response
	2	Grunts, moans	Incomprehensible words
	1	No response	No response
Motor response	6	Spontaneous movement	Obeys commands
	5	Withdraws to touch	Localizes pain
	4	Withdraws to pain	Withdraws to pain
	3	Abnormal flexion (decorticate)	Flexion to pain (decorticate)
	2	Abnormal extension (decerebrate)	Extension to pain (decerebrate)
	1	No response	No response

Add the score from each category to get the total. The maximum score is 15, indicating the best level of neurologic functioning. The minimum is 3, indicating total neurologic unresponsiveness.

Source: From Teasdale, G., & Jennett, B. (1974). Assessment of coma and impaired consciousness. *Lancet*, 2, 81–84; and James, H. E. (1986). Neurologic evaluation and support in the child with acute brain insult. *Pediatric Annals*, *15*(1), 16–22.

Assessment Interview Neurologic Assessment

GENERAL QUESTIONS

1. Have you had a change in your ability to carry out your daily activities?
   - If so, describe the change.
   - Do you know what is causing the change? What do you do about the problem?
   - How long has this been happening?
2. Do you have any chronic diseases such as diabetes or hypertension?
   - If so, is the condition well controlled?
   - What, if any, medications do you take?
3. Do any members of your family now have or have they ever had a neurologic problem or disease?
   - If so, what is the disease or problem?
   - Who in the family has the problem? When was it diagnosed?
   - How has it been treated? How effective has the treatment been?

ILLNESS, INFECTION, OR INJURY

1. Have you ever been diagnosed with a neurologic illness?
   - If so, when were you diagnosed with the problem?
   - What treatment was prescribed for the problem?
   - What kinds of things do you do to help with the problem?
   - Has the problem ever recurred (acute)?
   - How are you managing the disease now (chronic)?
2. Have you ever had an infection of the neurologic system such as meningitis?
3. Have you ever had an injury to your head or back?
   - If so, explain what happened and when.
   - What treatments did you receive?
   - As a result of this injury, what problems do you have today?

SYMPTOMS OR BEHAVIORS

1. Do you have fainting spells? Do you have a history of seizures or convulsions?
   - If so, when did you have your first episode?
   - What happens to you immediately before the seizure?
   - What have you been told about what your body does during the seizure?
   - How do you feel after the seizure?
   - What medications do you take? Do you take your medications regularly?
   - When was the last time you had a seizure?
2. Has your vision changed in any way?
   - If so, do you ever see two objects when you know there is just one?
   - Are you able to see off to the sides without turning your head?
   - When you go from a bright room to a darker room, do your eyes adjust to the change rapidly?
3. What changes, if any, have you noticed in your hearing?
   - Have you noticed any ringing in the ears?
4. Have you noticed any change with your ability to smell or taste?
5. Describe your balance.
   - Are you steady on your feet?
   - Are you able to function without difficulty?
   - Is one leg stronger than the other?
   - Do you notice any tremors?
   - Could you bend down to pick up a straight pin and stand up again?
   - Do you drop things easily? Do you find yourself being clumsy—tripping, spilling things, and knocking things over?
   - If so, how long have the symptoms been present? Are they continuous?
   - Are they getting worse? What do you do to control or limit the symptoms?
6. Do you have numbness or tingling in any part of your body?
   - If so, how long have you had this?
   - Do you know what causes it?
   - Have you sought treatment? What do you do to relieve the problem?

PAIN

1. Are you having any pain?
   - If so, where?
   - When did the pain begin?
   - Is the pain constant or intermittent?
   - What relieves or decreases the pain? What increases the pain?
   - Does the pain interfere with your daily activities?
   - How would you describe the pain–sharp, dull, acute, burning, stabbing, or stinging?
   - On a scale of 1 to 10, with 10 being the worst pain, how would you rate the pain?
2. Do you get headaches?
   - If so, describe them.
   - Where are they located? Are they always in the same area?
   - How often do they occur?
   - Are you able to function with these headaches?
   - What do you think causes your headaches?
   - What do you do to help relieve the pain? Does this remedy work?
   - On a scale of 1 to 10, rate the severity of your headaches.
   - Are your headaches accompanied by nausea or vomiting?

BEHAVIORS

1. Do you now use or have you ever used recreational drugs or alcohol?
   - If so, what was the drug or substance?
   - When and how long did you use it?
   - Have you experienced problems as a result of this drug?
   - How much alcohol do you consume? How long have you consumed that much alcohol?
2. Describe your memory.
   - Do you need to make a list or write things down so you won't forget?
   - Do you lose things easily?
   - What did you do today before you came here?

INFANTS AND CHILDREN

1. Describe, if you can, the pregnancy with this child, including any health problems, medications taken, or alcohol or drugs used.
   - Was the child premature, at term, or late?
   - Describe the birth of the child, including any complications during or shortly after the birth.
2. Has the child ever had a seizure?
   - If so, how often has this happened?
   - Describe what happens when the child has a seizure.
   - Has the child had a high fever when the seizures occurred?
3. Have you noticed any clumsiness in the child's activities? For example, does the child frequently drop things, have difficulty

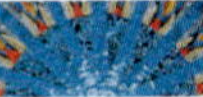

Assessment Interview Neurologic Assessment

manipulating toys, bump into things, have problems walking or climbing stairs, or fall frequently?

4. Are you aware of any surfaces in the home that are painted with lead-based paint?
   - Have you ever seen the child eating paint chips?
   - Have you observed the child eating anything that is not food?
5. How is the child doing in school?
   - Does the child seem to be able to concentrate on homework assignments and complete them on time?
   - Have you ever been told that the child has a learning disability or is hyperactive?
   - Do you agree with this assessment? Why or why not?
   - Have any medications or therapies been prescribed for the hyperactivity?

PREGNANT FEMALE

1. Do you have a history of seizures?
   - Have you had any seizures during this pregnancy or previous pregnancies?
   - If so, how often?
   - Describe the seizures.
2. Are you taking any vitamins or other nutritional supplements?

OLDER ADULT

1. Do you require more time to perform tasks today than perhaps 2 years ago? Explain.
2. When you stand up, do you have trouble starting to walk?
3. Do you notice any tremors?
4. What safety features have you added to your home?

ENVIRONMENT

1. Describe your daily diet.
   - Do you have problems eating or drinking certain products?
2. Are you currently taking any medications?
   - What are the medications? Do you use prescribed, over-the-counter, herbal, or culturally derived medications? Do you use home remedies?
3. Are you now or have you ever been exposed to environmental hazards such as insecticides, organic solvents, lead, toxic wastes, or other pollutants?
   - If so, which one, when, and for what period of time were you exposed?
   - What treatment did you seek?
   - Are you left with any problems because of the exposure?

Neurologic Assessment

Assessment Focus	Technique	Normal Findings	Abnormal Findings
Mental status	Assess appearance, including dress, hygiene, grooming, gait, and posture.	The client should be appropriately dressed and clean, with normal gait and posture.	Unilateral neglect (inattention to one side of body) may occur in some clients who have had a stroke. Poor hygiene and grooming may be seen in clients with dementia. Abnormal gait and posture may be seen in transient ischemic attacks (TIAs), strokes, and Parkinson's disease.
	Assess behavior, including actions and affect, content and quality of speech, and LOC. Use the Glasgow Coma Scale (Table 17–4) to document findings.	A score of 15 on the Glasgow Coma Scale indicates that the client is alert and oriented.	Emotional swings or changes in personality may be observed in clients who have had a stroke. The face appears masklike (very little expressive movement of facial muscles) in clients experiencing the later stages of Parkinson's disease. Apathy is seen in clients with dementing disorders. **Aphasia** (defective or absent language function) may occur in clients who experience TIAs and strokes. Aphasias are seen in cliens with damage to the left cerebral cortex. Aphasias are more often seen in clients with strokes of the left hemisphere rather than the right hemisphere. *Dysphonia* (change in the tone of the voice) is common in clients who have had strokes. Dysphonia is seen in clients with paralysis of the vocal cords (cranial nerve X). *Dysarthria* (difficulty speaking) is seen in clients with lesions of upper and lower motor neurons, the cerebellum, and the extrapyramidal tract. Damage to the brainstem and/or cerebral cortex may alter the client's LOC. Drowsiness and decreased LOC may be associated with brain trauma, infections, TIAs, stroke, and brain tumors. LOC ranging from confusion to coma is usually altered in a client who with a stroke.

(continued)

Neurologic Assessment (continued)

Assessment Focus	Technique	Normal Findings	Abnormal Findings
	Assess cognitive function. Note orientation to time, place, and person. Note attention span and recent and remote memory. Ask the client to: 1. Repeat five to seven numbers 2. Recall three items after 5 minutes 3. Recall his or her address, breakfast, or birthday. Assess thought processes (both content and perceptions) by noting responses to questions. Note ability to understand what is said and to express thoughts. Note ability to make logical and safe judgments.	The client should be oriented to time, place, and person; demonstrate attention and ability to remember recent and past events; respond appropriately to questions; and be able to make judgments.	Disorientation to time and place may occur in clients with stroke of the right cerebral hemisphere and in clients with dementing disorders. Memory deficits are often seen in clients who have had a stroke. Perceptual deficits may be seen in clients who have had strokes. These same deficits may occur after brain trauma and in dementing disorders. Impaired cognition is often noted in clients with strokes, cerebral trauma, brain tumors, and dementing disorders.
Cranial nerves	Test CN I (olfactory). Note client's ability to smell scents (e.g., soap, coffee) with each nostril. This test is usually done only if a problem with the ability to smell is reported.	Sense of smell should be equal in both nostrils.	*Anosmia* (inability to smell) may be seen in clients with lesions of the frontal lobe and may occur in clients with impaired blood flow to the middle cerebral artery.
	Test CN II (optic). Assess vision in each eye with Snellen chart.	Based on previous ability to see and use of visual aids, client should be able to see with both eyes.	Blindness in one eye may be seen in clients with strokes or TIAs. Impaired vision or blindness in one side of both eyes (homonymous hemianopia) is associated with stroke. Impaired vision may be seen in clients with strokes and brain tumors. Blindness or double vision may be noted in clients with strokes and TIAs.
	Test CN III, IV, and VI (oculomotor, trochlear, and abducens, respectively). Assess extraocular movements by asking the client to follow your finger as you write an *H* in the air. Assess PERRL (pupils equal, round, and reactive to light) by covering one eye at a time and shining a bright light directly into the uncovered eye using a penlight or the ophthalmoscope.	Extraocular movements should be present bilaterally, and pupils should be equal, round, and reactive to light.	*Nystagmus* (involuntary eye movement) may be seen in clients with strokes. Constricted pupils are associated with impaired blood flow from a stroke.
	Assess for *ptosis* (drooping eyelids).	Eyelids should not droop.	Ptosis occurs in clients with strokes, myasthenia gravis, and palsy of CN III.

Neurologic Assessment (continued)

Assessment Focus	Technique	Normal Findings	Abnormal Findings
	Test CN V (trigeminal). Assess ability to feel light, dull, and sharp sensations on the face. With the client's eyes closed, check whether sensation is the same on both sides of the face. Stroke the cheek with a wisp of cotton for light touch, with a closed safety pin for dull touch, and with a tongue depressor for sharp touch. If the sharp point of a safety pin is used to assess sharp touch, avoid scratching the surface of the skin and discard the pin after it is used. Assess the corneal reflex by touching the corneal surface with a wisp of sterile cotton. The reflex may be absent or decreased in clients who wear contact lenses.	Ability to feel light, dull, and sharp sensations should be intact. Normally the client blinks.	Changes in facial sensations are noted with impaired blood flow to the carotid artery. Decreased sensations to the face and cornea on the same side of the body, as well as numbness of the lip and mouth, occur in clients with strokes. Loss of facial sensation or contraction of the masseter and temporal muscles is seen in clients with lesions of CN V. Severe facial pain is seen in clients with trigeminal neuralgia (tic douloureux). The corneal reflex may be impaired in clients with lesions of CN V or VII.
	Test CN VII (facial). Assess ability to taste sweet, sour, and salt on the anterior two thirds of the tongue by asking the client to stick out the tongue and applying a salty, sweet, or sour substance. Assess ability to frown, show teeth, blow out cheeks, raise eyebrows, smile, and close eyes tightly.	Ability to taste sweet, sour, and salt should be intact. Client should be able to frown, show teeth, blow out cheeks, raise eyebrows, smile, and close eyes tightly. Muscle movement should be equal bilaterally.	Loss of ability to taste may occur in clients with brain tumors or nerve impairment. Asymmetry or decreased movement of facial muscles is noted in clients with lesions of the upper and lower motor neurons. Paralysis of the lower motor neurons from injury to CN VII results in inability to close eyes, a flat nasolabial fold, paralysis of lower face, and inability to wrinkle forehead. Paralysis of the upper motor neurons from a stroke results in weakness of eyelids and paralysis of lower face. Pain, paralysis, and sagging of facial muscles is seen on the affected side in Bell's palsy.
	Test CN VIII (acoustic). Assess ability to hear the ticking of a watch and whispered and spoken words.	Client should be able to hear with both ears.	Decreased hearing or deafness may occur in clients with strokes and/or tumors of CN VIII.
	Test CN IX and X (glossopharyngeal and vagus, respectively). If gag reflex is intact, observe client swallowing a small drink of water. Observe for a symmetric rise of soft palate and uvula as the client says "ah." Assess gag reflex by touching back of client's throat with tongue depressor. Assess ability to taste salty, sweet, and sour substances on the posterior third of the tongue. (See previous description.)	Client should be able to swallow without difficulty, have symmetrical rise of the soft palate, have intact gag reflex, and taste appropriately.	*Dysphagia* (difficulty swallowing) is common in clients with impaired blood flow to the brain. Unilateral loss of the gag reflex occurs in clients with lesions of CN IX and X.

(continued)

Neurologic Assessment (continued)

Assessment Focus	Technique	Normal Findings	Abnormal Findings
	Test CN XI (spinal accessory). Assess the client's ability to shrug the shoulders and turn the head against resistance: Ask the client to turn the head to one side against the resistance of your hand; ask the client to shrug the shoulders while you exert downward pressure. Observe symmetry, strength, and size of muscles.	Client should be able to shrug shoulders and turn head against resistance.	Muscle weakness is noted in clients with lower motor neuron disease. *Contralateral hemiparesis* (muscle weakness on the side opposite the lesion or trauma) is seen with strokes.
	Test CN XII (hypoglossal). Assess the client's ability to stick out the tongue and move the tongue from side to side against resistance of a tongue depressor. See Table 17–5 for assessment of cranial nerves in the unconscious client.	Client should be able to stick out the tongue and move it from side to side against resistance.	Atrophy and **fasciculations** (twitches) of the tongue are seen in clients with lower motor neuron disease. The tongue may deviate toward the involved side of the body.
	Assess ability to perceive various sensations. Touch both sides of various parts of the body (chest, abdomen, arms, and legs) with one or more of the following: ■ Cotton wisp ■ Sharp object ■ Dull object. Place vibrating tuning fork on bony prominences.	Client can differentiate between soft and sharp and can feel vibrations appropriately.	Decreased sensation of pain occurs in clients with injury to the spinothalamic tract. Decreased vibratory sensations are seen in clients with injuries to the posterior column tract. Transient numbness of face, arm, or hand is seen in clients with TIAs. Sensory loss on one side of the body is seen in clients with lesions of higher pathways to the spinal cord. Bilateral sensory loss is seen in polyneuropathy (a disease in which multiple peripheral nerves are affected, such as Guillain-Barré syndrome and diabetes mellitus). Sensations are impaired in clients with strokes, brain tumors, and spinal cord trauma or compression.
	Assess sense of position (**kinesthesia**). Move the client's finger or big toe up or down. Ask the client to describe the movement.	Client can accurately describe position of finger or toe when moved up or down.	Lesions of the posterior column of the spinal cord may affect sense of position.
	Assess ability to discriminate fine touch. Ask the client to identify: 1. Object in hand, such as a coin or key (tests stereognosis) 2. Number written on hand (tests graphesthesia) (Figure 17–9 ■)		

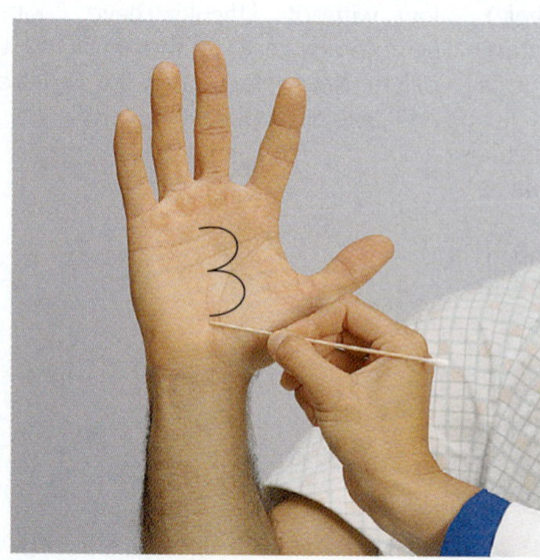

Figure 17–9 ■ Testing graphesthesia.

Neurologic Assessment (continued)

Assessment Focus	Technique	Normal Findings	Abnormal Findings
	3. Two points of simultaneous pinpricks on the hand (tests two-point discrimination) (Figure 17–10 ■) 4. Where he or she is being touched (tests localization) 5. How many sensations are felt when the client is touched simultaneously on both sides of the body (tests extinction).	Client can identify and discriminate fine touch.	Inability to discriminate fine touch (stereognosis, graphesthesia, two points, point localization, and extinction) may occur in clients with injury to the posterior columns or sensory cortex.
	Assess bilateral symmetry and size of muscles. Assess for **tremors** (rhythmic movements) and fasciculations (irregular movements). Observe movements as client is at rest (not making a purposeful movement) and with activity (making a purposeful movement such as reaching for a glass of water).	Muscles are bilaterally symmetrical and of equal size. Tremors or fasciculations are not present.	Atrophy of muscles is seen in clients with disease of the lower motor neurons. Tremors that occur with activity are seen in clients with multiple sclerosis and diseases of the cerebellar system. Tremors that occur at rest and disappear with movement are common in clients with Parkinson's disease. Fasciculations occur in clients with disease or trauma to the lower motor neurons, as a side effect of medications, in fever, in sodium deficiency, and in uremia.
	Assess muscle tone.	Muscle tone is appropriate.	Muscle tone is decreased (*flaccidity*) in clients with disease or trauma of the lower motor neurons and early stroke. Muscle tone is increased (*spasticity*) in clients with disease of the corticospinal motor tract. Muscles are rigid in clients with disease of the extrapyramidal motor tract. Muscles move in small, regular, jerky movements (known as *cogwheel rigidity*) in clients with Parkinson's disease.
	Assess bilateral muscle strength and movement. Ask the client to: 1. Squeeze your hands. 2 Push feet against the resistance of your hands. 3. Raise both legs off the bed.	Muscle strength and movement are bilaterally equal and strong.	Weakness of the arms, legs, or hands is often seen in clients with TIAs. Hemiplegia (paralysis of one half of the body vertically) is noted in clients with strokes. Flaccid paralysis is noted in clients with strokes. Paralysis or decreased movement is seen in clients with multiple sclerosis and myasthenia gravis. There is total loss of motor function below the level of injury in complete spinal cord transection and in injuries to the anterior portion of the spinal cord. Spasticity of muscles may occur as a result of incomplete spinal cord injuries.

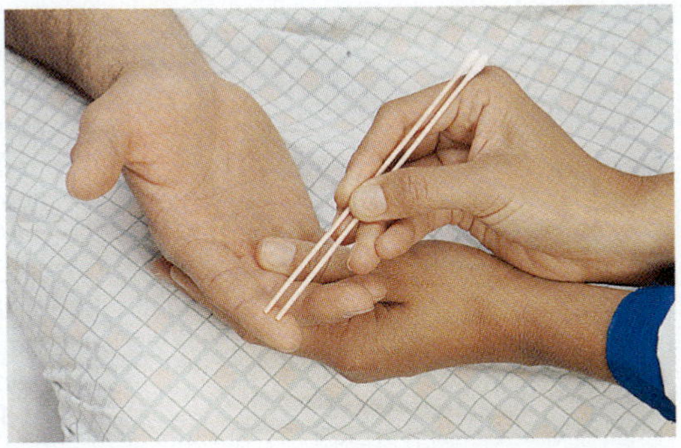

Figure 17–10 ■ Testing two-point discrimination.

(continued)

Neurologic Assessment (continued)

Assessment Focus	Technique	Normal Findings	Abnormal Findings
Cerebellar function	Assess the gait. Ask the client to walk normally, then in a heel-to-toe fashion, then on toes, and finally on heels. Perform Romberg's test: Ask the client to stand with feet together and eyes closed. (Stand close to the client to prevent falling.)	Client has appropriate gait and can walk heel to toe, on toes, and on heels. There should be minimal swaying for up to 20 seconds.	*Ataxia* is a lack of coordination and a clumsiness of movements, with staggering, wide-based, and unbalanced gait. Ataxia is often seen in clients with strokes and cerebellar tumors. Swaying and falling are seen in clients with cerebellar ataxia. Inability to walk on toes, then heels, may indicate disease of the upper motor neurons. Spastic hemiparesis is often associated with strokes or upper motor neuron disease. The client walks with one leg stiffly dragging while the other leg circles out and forward. One arm is held flexed and close to the side. Steppage gait is noted with disease of the lower motor neurons. The client drags or lifts the foot high, then slaps the foot onto the floor. The client cannot walk on the heels. Sensory ataxia may be associated with polyneuropathy or damage to the posterior columns. The client walks on the heels before bringing down the toes, and the feet are held wide apart. Gait worsens with the eyes closed. Parkinsonian gait is often seen in clients with Parkinson's disease. In Parkinsonian gait, the client stoops over while walking and shuffles the feet. The arms are held close to the side. A positive Romberg's test may be seen in clients with cerebellar ataxia.
	Assess coordination. Observe ability to pat knees, alternating front and back of hands and increasing speed. Observe ability to touch each finger of one hand to the thumb. Observe ability to touch the nose, then one of your fingers, then the nose again. Observe ability to run each heel down each shin while in a supine position (Figure 17–11 ■).	Client demonstrates coordinated movements.	Ataxic movements are apparent in clients with cerebellar disease.

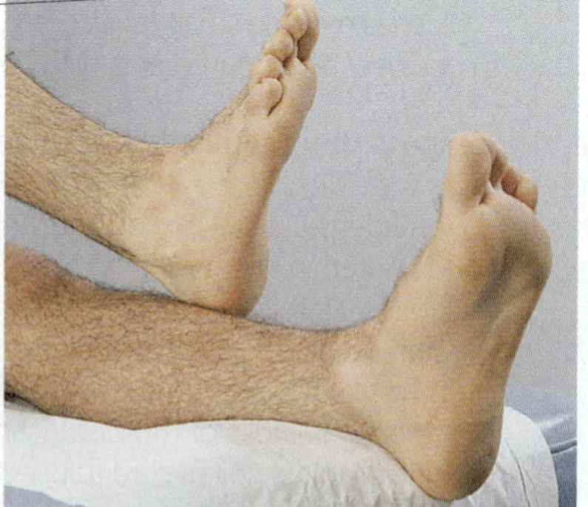

Figure 17–11 ■ Heel-to-shin test.

Neurologic Assessment (continued)

Assessment Focus	Technique	Normal Findings	Abnormal Findings
	Assess for Brudzinski's sign: With the client supine, flex the client's head to the chest (Figure 17–12 ■). Assess for Kernig's sign: With the client supine, flex the knees and hips, then straighten the knee (Figure 17–13 ■).	There should be no pain, resistance, or flexion of the hips or knees.	Pain, resistance, and flexion of hips and knees occur in clients with meningeal irritation. Excessive pain and/or resistance occurs in clients with meningeal irritation.

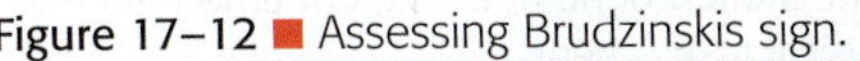

Figure 17–12 ■ Assessing Brudzinskis sign.

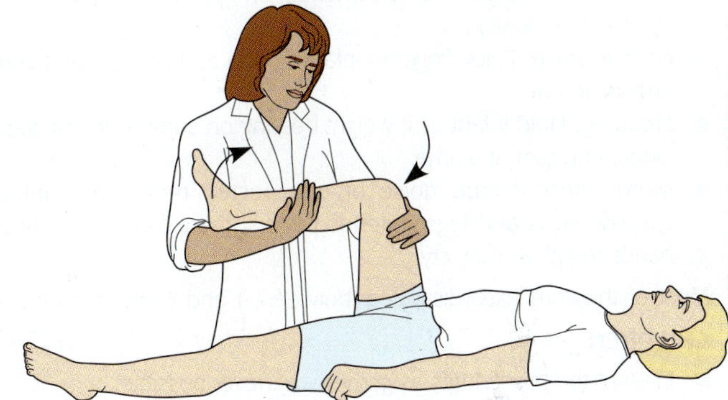

Figure 17–13 ■ Assessing Kernigs sign.

Assessment Focus	Technique	Normal Findings	Abnormal Findings
	Assess for abnormal postures in clients who are unconscious.	There should be no abnormal posturing.	Observe for decorticate posturing, in which the upper arms are close to the sides; the elbows, wrists, and fingers are flexed; the legs are extended with internal rotation; and the feet are plantar. (see Figure 17–8A). Observe for decerebrate posturing, in which the neck is extended, with the jaw clenched; the arms are pronated, extended, and close to the sides; the legs are extended straight out; and the feet are plantar (see Figure 17–8B). Decorticate posturing occurs with lesions of the corticospinal tracts. Decerebrate posturing occurs with lesions of the midbrain, pons, or diencephalons.

TABLE 17–5 Assessment of Cranial Nerves in the Unconscious Client

CRANIAL NERVES	REFLEX	ASSESSMENT PROCEDURE	NORMAL FINDINGS
II, III	Pupillary	Shine a light source in the eye.	Rapid, concentrically constricting pupils indicates intact cranial nerves II, III.
II, IV, VI	Oculocephalic	Should be performed with eyes held open (doll's eyes) and head turned from side to side. *Precaution:* Cervical spine injury must be ruled out before this assessment is performed.	Eyes gazing straight up or logging slightly behind head motion indicate intact cranial nerves.
III, VIII	Oculovestibular	Place the head in a midline and slightly elevated position. Inject ice water into the ear canal. *Precautions:* Cervical spine injury must be ruled out before this assessment is performed. Tympanic membrane must be intact; otherwise, brain may be filled with bacteria-laden fluid. *Note:* This assessment is usually performed by a physician.	Eyes deviating toward the irrigated ear indicate intact cranial nerves III, VIII.
V, VII	Corneal	Cornea is gently swabbed with sterile cotton swab.	A blink indicates intact cranial nerves V, VII.
IX, X	Gag	Pharynx is irritated with tongue depressor or cotton swab.	Gagging response indicates intact cranial nerves IX, X.

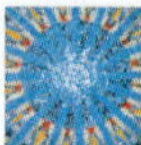

DEVELOPMENTAL CONSIDERATIONS Assessing the Neurologic System

INFANTS

Reflexes commonly tested in newborns include the following:

- *Rooting:* Stroke the side of the face near mouth; infant opens mouth and turns to the side that is stroked.
- *Sucking:* Place nipple or finger 3–4 cm into mouth; infant sucks vigorously.
- *Tonic neck:* Place infant supine, turn head to one side; arm on side to which head is turned extends; on opposite side, arm curls up (fencer's pose).
- *Palmar grasp:* Place finger in infant's palm and press; infant curls fingers around.
- *Stepping:* Hold infant as if weight bearing on surface; infant steps along, one foot at a time.
- *Moro:* Present loud noise or unexpected movement; infant spreads arms and legs, extends fingers, then flexes and brings hands together; may cry.

Most of these reflexes disappear between 4 and 6 months of age.

CHILDREN

- Present the procedures as games whenever possible.
- Positive Babinski's reflex is abnormal after the child ambulates or at 2 years of age.
- For children under 5 years of age, the Denver Developmental Screening Test II (DDSTII) provides a comprehensive neurologic evaluation, particularly for motor function. (Concept 7 describes the DDSTII in more detail)
- Note the child's ability to understand and follow directions.
- Assess immediate recall or recent memory by using names of cartoon characters. Normal recall in children is one less than age in years.
- Assess for signs of hyperactivity or abnormally short attention span.
- Children should be able to walk backward by 2 years of age, balance on one foot for 5 seconds by 4 years of age, heel-toe walk by 5 years of age, and heel-toe walk backward by 6 years of age.
- The Romberg test is appropriate over 3 years of age.

OLDER ADULTS

- A full neurologic assessment can be lengthy. Conduct the assessment in several sessions if indicated and cease the tests if the client is noticeably fatigued.
- A decline in mental status is not a normal result of aging. Changes are more the result of physical or psychologic disorders (e.g., fever, fluid and electrolyte imbalances, medications). Acute, abrupt-onset mental status changes are usually caused by delirium. These changes are often reversible with treatment. Chronic subtle insidious mental health changes are often caused by dementia and are usually irreversible.
- Intelligence and learning ability are unaltered with age. Many factors, however, inhibit learning (e.g., anxiety, illness, pain, cultural barrier).
- Short-term memory is often less efficient. Long-term memory is usually unaltered.
- Because old age is often associated with loss of support people, depression is a common disorder. Mood changes, weight loss, anorexia, constipation, and early morning awakening may manifest it.
- The stress of being in unfamiliar situations can cause confusion in older adults.
- As a person ages, reflex responses may become less intense.
- Because older adults tire more easily than younger clients, a total neurologic assessment is often done at a different time than the other parts of the physical assessment.
- Although there is a progressive decrease in the number of functioning neurons in the CNS and in the sense organs, older adults usually function well because of abundant reserves in the number of brain cells.
- Impulse transmission and reaction to stimuli are slower.
- Many older adults have some impairment of hearing, vision, smell, temperature and pain sensation, memory, and mental endurance.
- Coordination changes, including a reduced speed of fine finger movements. Standing balance remains intact, and Romberg's test remains negative.
- Reflex responses may slightly increase or decrease. Many show loss of Achilles reflex, and the plantar reflex may be difficult to elicit.
- When testing sensory function, the nurse needs to give older adults time to respond. Normally, older adults have unaltered perception of light touch and superficial pain, decreased perception of deep pain, and decreased perception of temperature stimuli. Many also reveal a decrease or absence of position sense in the large toes.

DIAGNOSTIC TESTS

Although the client's history and physical examination often indicate the cause of alterations in LOC, several diagnostic tests may be useful in establishing the diagnosis. The results of diagnostic tests of neurologic structure and function are used to support the diagnosis of a specific injury or disease, to provide information to identify or modify the appropriate medications or therapy used to treat the disease, and to help nurses monitor the client's responses to treatment and nursing care interventions.

Prior to the day of any test, the nurse should make sure the client understands the purpose of the test and explain to the client what will take place during testing. The nurse should provide the client with specific instructions, such as fasting and wearing appropriate clothes. Diagnostic tests to assess the structures and functions of the neurologic system are described in Appendix B and may include the following:

- Cat scan of the head with or without contrast
- Magnetic resonance imaging (MRI)
- X-rays
- Echoencephelogram
- EEG
- Ultrasonography of the brain
- Brain echogram
- Cerebral angiography
- Positron emission tomography
- Nerve conduction studies

- Myelogram
- Thermography
- Oculoplethysmography
- Serum electrolytes
- Intracranial pressure (ICP) monitoring
- Therapeutic drug levels
- Antidiuretic hormone levels
- Serum electrolytes
- CSF assessment
- Serum glucose
- Serum protein.

CARING INTERVENTIONS

Management of the client with an altered LOC must begin immediately. The focus of management is to identify the underlying cause, preserve function, and prevent deterioration if possible. Airway and breathing must be maintained during the initial acute stage until the diagnosis and prognosis can be established. Intravenous fluids are used to support circulation and to correct fluid, electrolyte, and acid–base imbalances. Treatment protocols to reduce IICP or to control seizure activity may be initiated. Changes in LOC associated with craniocerebral trauma, such as hematomas, often require immediate surgical intervention.

Specific interventions initiated and performed by the nurse may include the following:

- Assessing LOC
- Monitoring fluid intake and output
- Reducing environmental stimuli
- Positioning client
- Taking precautions for seizures, including padding side rails
- Monitoring ICP
- Assessing pupils for response to light
- Using hyperventilation to reduce ICP
- Measuring vital signs
- Administering IV fluids.

Fluid Management

An intravenous catheter is inserted, and fluid balance is maintained using isotonic or slightly hypertonic solutions such as normal saline and lactated Ringer's solution. The nurse should closely monitor the client's response to fluid administration for evidence of increased cerebral edema.

Any underlying fluid and electrolyte imbalance is corrected by administering IV fluid containing appropriate electrolytes. For the client who is hyponatremic and has a low serum osmolality, furosemide (Lasix) or an osmotic diuretic such as mannitol may be administered to promote water excretion, and fluid infusion may be minimized.

Surgery

Although surgery is not indicated for most clients with altered LOC, it may be used in the event of coma caused by intracerebral tumor, hemorrhage, or hematoma. When there is a risk of IICP, the client is monitored continuously. (See Exemplar 17.1.)

Other Treatments

Support of the airway and respirations is vital in the client with altered LOC. The client who is drowsy but arousable may need little more than an oral pharyngeal airway. With more severe alterations in consciousness, the client may need endotracheal intubation to maintain airway patency, particularly if the cough and gag reflexes are absent. Mechanical ventilation is indicated when hypoventilation or apnea is present. Unless a do-not-resuscitate (DNR) order is in effect, mechanical ventilation should be initiated even if it has not been established that the disorder is reversible. Without ventilatory support, cerebral anoxia develops rapidly, and brain death may ensue. Arterial blood gases are monitored frequently to determine the adequacy of ventilation. Cautious hyperventilation may be used to reduce $PaCO_2$ and promote cerebral vasoconstriction to reduce cerebral edema.

Nutrition

In clients with long-term alterations in consciousness (e.g., persistent vegetative state or locked-in syndrome), measures to maintain nutritional status are initiated. Enteral feedings with a gastrostomy tube are preferred if the client is unable to take enough food by mouth without aspirating. In some cases, total parenteral nutrition may be used.

PHARMACOLOGIC THERAPIES

Antiepileptic drugs (AEDs) (also called anticonvulsant drugs) can reduce or control most seizure activity. More than 20 drugs are available for use in the treatment of epilepsy. These medications do not cure the disorder; they only manage its manifestations. AEDs generally act in one of two ways: by raising the seizure threshold or by limiting the spread of abnormal activity in the brain.

The goals of medications for epilepsy are to protect the client from harm and to reduce or prevent seizure activity without impairing cognitive function or producing undesirable side effects. Ideally, the lowest possible dose of a single medication that will control the client's seizures is prescribed. Often, however, several medications must be tried before the most effective one is identified, and a combination of drugs may be needed to manage the client's seizures.

Status epilepticus requires immediate intervention to preserve life. Establishing and maintaining the airway is a priority. A solution of 50% dextrose is administered intravenously to prevent hypoglycemia. Diazepam or lorazepam is given intravenously, and the dose is repeated in 10 minutes, if necessary, to stop seizure activity. Phenytoin (Dilantin) is administered intravenously for longer-term control of seizures. Phenobarbital also may be administered to clients in status epilepticus.

Medications play an important role in the management of IICP. Diuretics, particularly osmotic diuretics, are commonly used to reduce ICP and are the mainstays of pharmacologic treatment. Loop diuretics such as furosemide (Lasix, typically the drug of choice) and ethacrynic acid (Edecrin) may be prescribed for some clients with IICP. Sedation and paralysis are used as chemical restraints to control restlessness and agitation

MEDICATIONS Seizure Disorders

Drug Classifications	Mechanism of Action	Commonly Prescribed Drugs	Nursing Considerations
AEDs	These drugs act in the motor cortex of the brain to reduce the spread of electrical discharges from the rapidly firing epileptic foci in this area. These agents control seizures without impairing the normal functions of the CNS.	Phenytoin (Dilantin) Phenobarbital Primidone (Mysoline) Carbamazepine (Tegretol) Valproic acid (Depakene) Ethosuximide (Zarontin) Clonazepam (Klonopin) Gabapentin (Neurontin) Lamotrigine (Lamictal) Tiagabine HCL (Gabitril)	■ Monitor blood pressure, pulse, and respirations. ■ Note evidence of CNS side effects such as blurred vision, dimmed vision, slurred speech, nystagmus, or confusion. Gingival hyperplasia may be noted in clients taking phenytoin. ■ Recognize that if clients are to be on prolonged therapy, they may need a diet rich in vitamin D. ■ Monitor the serum calcium level as ordered; phenytoin can contribute to demineralization of bone. ■ When administering anticonvulsants intravenously, monitor closely for respiratory depression and cardiovascular collapse. ■ Administer gabapentin 2 hours after antacids. ■ Administer tiagabine HCL with food.

because these movements increase blood pressure, ICP, and cerebral metabolism. Antipyretics such as acetaminophen are used alone or in combination with a hypothermia blanket to treat hyperthermia. (Hyperthermia increases the cerebral metabolic rate and exacerbates an existing increase in ICP.) Anticonvulsants are often required to manage seizure activity associated with brain injury and IICP. Gastrointestinal prophylaxis with intravenous histamine H_2 antagonists or proton pump inhibitors are often used because clients with IICP are at increased risk for developing stress gastritis and ulcers (Tierney, McPhee, & Papadakis, 2005). Corticosteroids may be administered to reduce inflammation.

Intravenous fluids are usually necessary to maintain the client's fluid and electrolyte balance as well as vascular volume. If the client's blood pressure is unstable, vasoactive medications may be administered to maintain the mean arterial pressure (MAP) in a range that supports cerebral perfusion while minimizing increases in ICP. When enteral feeding is not possible, total parenteral nutrition may be administered.

MEDICATIONS Increased Intracranial Pressure

Drug Classifications	Mechanism of Action	Commonly Prescribed Drugs	Nursing Considerations
Osmotic diuretics	Osmotic diuretics work by increasing the osmolarity of the blood, thereby drawing water out of edematous brain tissue and into the vascular system for elimination via the kidneys. The effects of these drugs vary with the type of injury.	Mannitol, glucose, urea, or glycerol	■ Monitor vital signs, urinary output, central venous pressure (CVP), and pulmonary artery pressure (PAP) before and every hour throughout administration. ■ Assess client for manifestations of dehydration. ■ Assess client for muscle weakness, numbness, tingling, paresthesia, confusion, and excessive thirst. ■ Monitor neurologic status and ICP readings. ■ Monitor renal function and serum electrolytes throughout therapy. ■ Do not discontinue medication abruptly. Rebound migraine headaches may occur.
Loop diuretics	Loop diuretics inhibit sodium and chloride reabsorption at the ascending loop of Henle. They cause a reduction in the rate of CSF production, thus reducing the ICP.	Furosemide or ethacrynic acid	■ Monitor vital signs and electrolyte values. ■ Assess fluid status throughout therapy. ■ Use infusion pump to ensure accurate fluid administration.

17.1 INCREASED INTRACRANIAL PRESSURE

KEY TERMS

Cerebral perfusion pressure (CPP), *964*
Compliance, *961*
Increased intracranial pressure, *961*
Intracranial hypertension, *961*
Monro-Kelli hypothesis, *961*

BASIS FOR SELECTION OF EXEMPLAR

Centers for Disease Control and Prevention
Standards of Nursing Practice

LEARNING OUTCOMES

After reading about this exemplar, you will be able to:

1. Describe the pathophysiology, etiology, clinical manifestations, and direct and indirect causes of increased intracranial pressure.
2. Identify risk factors associated with increased intracranial pressure.
3. Illustrate the nursing process in providing culturally competent care across life span for individuals with increased intracranial pressure.
4. Formulate priority nursing diagnoses appropriate for an individual with increased intracranial pressure.
5. Create a plan of care for individuals with increased intracranial pressure and their family members.
6. Assess expected outcomes for an individual with increased intracranial pressure.
7. Describe therapies used in the collaborative care of an individual with increased intracranial pressure.
8. Employ evidence-based caring interventions for an individual with increased intracranial pressure.

OVERVIEW

Increased intracranial pressure (IICP) (also labeled *intracranial hypertension*) is sustained elevated pressure (10 mmHg or higher) in the cranial cavity (Wilensky & Bloom, 2005). Transient increases in ICP occur with normal activities such as coughing, sneezing, straining, and bending forward. These transient increases are not harmful; however, sustained IICP can result in significant tissue ischemia and damage to delicate neural tissue. Cerebral edema is the most frequent cause of sustained increases in ICP. Other causes include head trauma, tumors, abscesses, stroke, inflammation, and hemorrhage.

PATHOPHYSIOLOGY AND ETIOLOGY

In the adult, the rigid cranial cavity created by the skull is normally filled to capacity with three essentially noncompressible elements: the brain (80%), cerebral spinal fluid (8%), and blood (12%). A state of dynamic equilibrium exists; if the volume of any of the three components increases, the volume of the others must decrease to maintain normal pressures in the cranial cavity. This is known as the **Monro-Kellie hypothesis**. The normal ICP is 5–10 mmHg (measured intracranially with a pressure transducer while the client is lying with the head elevated 30 degrees) or 60–180 cm H_2O (measured with a water manometer while the client is lying in a lateral recumbent position).

Cerebral blood flow and perfusion are important concepts for understanding the development and effects of IICP. Whereas blood and CSF contribute nearly equal percentages to normal intracranial volume, vascular factors account for twice the amount of increase in ICP that CSF does. The brain requires a constant supply of oxygen and glucose to meet its metabolic demands; 15–20% of the resting cardiac output goes to the brain to meet its metabolic needs. Interruption of the cerebral blood flow leads to ischemia and disruption of the cerebral metabolism.

Pressure and chemical autoregulation are compensatory mechanisms in which cerebral arterioles change diameter to maintain cerebral blood flow when ICP increases. In pressure autoregulation, stretch receptors in small blood vessels of the brain cause smooth muscle of the arterioles to contract. Increased arterial pressure stimulates these receptors, leading to vasoconstriction; when arterial pressure is low, stimulation of these receptors decreases, causing relaxation and vasodilation. Chemical, or metabolic, autoregulation works in much the same way as pressure autoregulation. In this case, the stimulus is a buildup of metabolic by-products of cell metabolism, including lactic acid, pyruvic acid, carbonic acid, and carbon dioxide. Carbon dioxide and increased hydrogen ion concentration are potent cerebral vasodilators that may act locally or systemically to increase cerebral blood flow. Conversely, a fall in $PaCO_2$ causes cerebral vasoconstriction. Arterial oxygen tension (PaO_2) also affects cerebral blood flow, although it is a less powerful mechanism than that exerted by carbon dioxide and hydrogen ions.

IICP may result from an increase in intracranial contents from a space-occupying lesion, hydrocephalus, cerebral edema (swelling), excess cerebrospinal fluid, or intracranial hemorrhage. Displacement of some CSF to the spinal subarachnoid space and increased CSF absorption are early compensatory mechanisms. The low-pressure venous system is also compressed, and cerebral arteries constrict to reduce blood flow. Brain tissue's ability to accommodate change is relatively restricted. The relationship between the volume of the intracranial components and intracranial pressure is known as **compliance**. When the capacity to compensate for IICP is exceeded, intracranial hypertension develops. **Intracranial hypertension** is a sustained state of IICP and is potentially life threatening.

Autoregulatory mechanisms have a limited ability to maintain cerebral blood flow. When autoregulation fails, cerebrovascular tone is reduced and cerebral blood flow becomes dependent on changes in blood pressure. Autoregulation may be lost either locally or globally because of several factors, including increasing ICP, local or diffuse cerebral tissue ischemia or inflammation, prolonged hypotension, and hypercapnia or hypoxia.

Etiology

Increased intracranial pressure most commonly results from head trauma, but other disease processes also may be implicated. Head trauma results from different causes throughout the life span. Infants and young children may experience IICP as the result of falling, being abused, or bumping their heads as a result of poor head control or depth perception. Preschool and school-aged children are at risk for bicycle, swimming, or activity-related accidents that cause head trauma. Adolescents and young adults are at risk for motor vehicle-related accidents, addiction behavior, and trauma resulting from violence. Older adults are prone to falls that may result in IICP.

Abnormal cellular growth such as intracranial tumors, either benign or malignant, may compete for space in the cranial vault, resulting in IICP. Increases in CSF production as seen in hydrocephalus or tissue necrosis as the result of cerebrovascular accidents or aneurysms also may lead to IICP.

Risk Factors

Any factor that increases the client's risk of trauma increases the risk of cerebral trauma resulting in IICP. These factors include use of medications that alter balance, perception, or reflex response; weakness resulting from lack of muscle strength, poor nutrition, or illness; and unhealthy lifestyle choices such as use of drugs or alcohol, violent behavior, or participation in contact sports without use of proper protective equipment.

The premature infant is at increased risk for IICP as a result of intracranial hemorrhage secondary to fragile cranial blood vessels. Caution should be taken when caring for the preemie to avoid rough handling, to provide adequate support of the head, and to avoid hypoxia.

CLINICAL MANIFESTATIONS

With loss of autoregulation, ICP continues to rise and cerebral perfusion falls. Cerebral tissue becomes ischemic, and manifestations of cellular hypoxia appear. Because the neurons of the cerebral cortex are most sensitive to oxygen deficit, changes in cortical function are the earliest manifestations of increasing

CLINICAL MANIFESTATIONS AND THERAPIES Increased Intracranial Pressure

ETIOLOGY	CLINICAL MANIFESTATIONS	CLINICAL THERAPIES
Cerebral edema, head trauma, tumors, abscesses, stroke, inflammation, and hemorrhage	■ Decreased LOC: *Early:* Confusion; restlessness, lethargy; disorientation, first to time, then to place and person: *Late:* Comatose with no response to painful stimuli ■ Pupillary dysfunction: Sluggish response to light, progressing to fixed pupils; with a localized process, pupillary dysfunction is first noted on the ipsilateral side. ■ Oculomotor dysfunction: Inability to move eye(s) upward; ptosis (drooping) of the eyelid. ■ Visual abnormalities: Decreased visual acuity, blurred vision, diplopia. ■ Papilledema (may be late sign). ■ Motor impairment: *Early:* Hemiparesis or hemiplegia of the contralateral side. *Late:* Abnormal responses such as decorticate or decerebrate positioning; flaccidity. ■ Headache: Uncommon but may occur with processes that slowly increase ICP; worse upon rising in the morning and with position changes. ■ Projectile vomiting without nausea. ■ Cushing's triad/response: Increased systolic blood pressure, widening pulse pressure, bradycardia. ■ Respirations: Altered respiratory pattern related to level of brain dysfunction. ■ Temperature (may be significantly elevated as compensatory mechanisms fail).	■ Maintain airway patency. ■ Monitor neurologic status; assessment areas include LOC, behavior, motor/sensory functions, pupillary size and reaction to light, and vital signs. ■ Monitor IICP monitor or ventilator. ■ Decrease stimuli. ■ Raise pads and bed rails; seizures may occur. ■ Elevate head of bed 30 degrees unless otherwise indicated. ■ Monitor arterial blood gases. ■ Position client as prescribed. ■ Prevent complications associated with immobility. ■ Monitor fluid and electrolytes. ■ Monitor bladder distention and bowel constipation. ■ Provide emotional support as needed. ■ Administer medications as ordered such as diuretics and steroids.

ICP (Porth, 2005). Behavior and personality changes occur; the client may become irritable and agitated. Memory and judgment are impaired, and changes in speech pattern may be noted. Additionally, the client's LOC decreases. As cerebral hypertension and hypoxia progress, LOC continues to decrease in a predictable pattern to coma and unresponsiveness.

COLLABORATION

Management of the client with IICP is directed toward identifying and treating the underlying cause of the disorder and controlling ICP to prevent herniation syndrome. IICP is a medical emergency, and there is little time to complete lengthy diagnostic tests. The diagnosis must be made on the basis of observation and neurologic assessment; even subtle changes may be clinically significant. The nurse, who often spends the most time caring for the client, is most likely to assess any subtle change in condition and must advocate for the client's needs.

Diagnostic Tests

A computed tomography (CT) scan or MRI is generally the initial test used to identify the possible causes of IICP (such as space-occupying lesions or hydrocephalus) and to evaluate therapeutic options. In general, a lumbar puncture is not performed when IICP is suspected because the sudden release of the pressure in the skull may cause cerebral herniation. Serum osmolality and arterial blood gases also are ordered and monitored.

Pharmacologic Therapy

Medications play an important role in the management of IICP. Diuretics, particularly osmotic diuretics, are commonly used to reduce ICP and are the mainstays of pharmacologic treatment. Loop diuretics such as furosemide (Lasix) (the drug of choice) and ethacrynic acid (Edecrin) may be prescribed for some clients with IICP. Sedation and paralysis are used as chemical restraints to control restlessness and agitation because these movements increase blood pressure, ICP, and

MEDICATIONS Increased Intracranial Pressure

Drug Classifications	Mechanism of Action	Commonly Prescribed Drugs	Nursing Considerations
Osmotic diuretics	Osmotic diuretics work by increasing the osmolarity of the blood, thereby drawing water out of edematous brain tissue and into the vascular system for elimination via the kidneys. The effects of these drugs vary with the type of injury. Regardless of the agent used, the optimal dose is the lowest that reduces ICP.	Mannitol is the most commonly employed osmotic diuretic. Glucose, urea, and glycerol are other osmotic diuretics that may be used. Mannitol therapy is often initiated if the client's ICP has exceeded 15–20 mmHg for at least 10 minutes. Both intravenous bolus and continuous infusion techniques are used. Repeated use of mannitol can lead to continual elevations in serum osmolality, with attendant risk of seizures and serious fluid and electrolyte imbalance. Urea is seldom administered intravenously because a severe local reaction may result if leakage occurs at the injection site. Mannitol and urea are used cautiously if renal disease is present.	■ Monitor vital signs, urinary output, CVP, and PAP before and every hour throughout administration. ■ Assess client for manifestations of dehydration. ■ Assess client for muscle weakness, numbness, tingling, paresthesia, confusion, and excessive thirst. ■ Assess client for pulmonary edema while administering the medication. ■ Monitor neurologic status and intracranial pressure readings. ■ Monitor renal function and serum electrolytes throughout therapy. ■ Do not administer the medication if crystals are present in solution. Administer with an in-line filter. Observe infusion site frequently for infiltration. ■ Do not administer mannitol solution with blood products. ■ Do not discontinue medication abruptly. Rebound migraine headaches may occur.
Loop diuretics	Loop diuretics such as furosemide and ethacrynic acid inhibit sodium and chloride reabsorption at the ascending loop of Henle. They cause a reduction in the rate of CSF production, thus reducing the ICP.	Furosemide (Lasix) Ethacrynic acid (Edecrin)	■ Monitor vital signs and electrolyte values closely. ■ Assess fluid status throughout therapy. ■ Monitor blood pressure and pulse before and during administration. ■ Monitor renal laboratory studies closely. ■ Use infusion pump to ensure accurate dosage.

cerebral metabolism. Antipyretics, such as acetaminophen, are used alone or in combination with a hypothermia blanket to treat hyperthermia. (Hyperthermia increases the cerebral metabolic rate and exacerbates an existing increase in ICP.) Anticonvulsants are often required to manage seizure activity associated with brain injury and IICP. Gastrointestinal prophylaxis with intravenous histamine H_2 antagonists or proton pump inhibitors are often used because clients with IICP are at increased risk for developing stress gastritis and ulcers (Tierney et al., 2005).

Intravenous fluids are usually necessary to maintain the client's fluid and electrolyte balance and vascular volume. If the client's blood pressure is unstable, vasoactive medications may be administered to maintain the mean arterial pressure in a range that supports cerebral perfusion while minimizing increases in ICP. When enteral feeding is not possible, total parenteral nutrition may be administered.

Surgery

Clients with IICP may undergo various intracranial surgical techniques to treat the underlying cause. In addition, infarcted or necrotic tissue may be resected to reduce brain mass. A drainage catheter or shunt may be inserted laterally via a burr hole into a ventricle to drain excess CSF and reduce hydrocephalus. The removal of even a small amount of CSF may dramatically reduce IICP and restore cerebral perfusion pressure.

ICP Monitoring

Critical to preserving brain function and preventing secondary brain damage from IICP are careful assessments and monitoring with ICP monitors, measuring cerebral blood flow and cerebral perfusion pressure, and measuring oxygen levels of brain tissue. ICP monitors facilitate continual assessment of ICP and the effects of medical therapy and nursing interventions on ICP. In addition, cerebral perfusion pressure (the difference between mean arterial pressure [MAP] and ICP) can be readily calculated, allowing more precise manipulation of therapeutic measures to maintain cerebral perfusion and thereby prevent ischemia. The criteria for ICP monitoring depends on the client's condition, but in general, clients who are comatose and have a Glasgow Coma Score of 8 or lower should be monitored.

Basic monitoring systems include an intraventricular catheter, a subarachnoid bolt or screw, and an epidural probe (Figure 17–14 ■). Intraventricular fluid-filled catheters are placed in the anterior horn of the lateral ventricle (most often in the right side). Ventricular catheters can drain CSF and measure ICP. The ICP value is measured deep in the brain and is considered most reflective of the whole brain pressure. Subarachnoid devices are placed in the subarachnoid space. A fiber-optic transducer-tipped catheter can be placed in the epidural, subdural, or parenchymal space, with ICP values considered very accurate. Once the intracranial sensor is implanted, it is connected to a transducer that converts the impulses to a signal that the recording device can translate into an oscilloscope tracing, digital value, or graphic recording. Factors that increase the risk for infection during ICP monitoring are listed in Table 17–6.

Transcranial blood flow is monitored with transcranial Doppler studies to measure the velocity of blood flow in the cerebral vessels. **Cerebral perfusion pressure (CPP)** is the pressure it takes for the heart to provide the brain with blood and is calculated by subtracting the ICP from MAP (normal CPP is 70–95 mmHg). Monitoring of brain oxygenation may be conducted using a jugular bulb oxygen saturation (Sjo_2) monitor connected to a small fiber-optic catheter inserted into the jugular vein. (Normal Sjo_2 is 50–75%.) Another device used to monitor brain tissue oxygenation is the LICOX system, which includes information about oxygen status and temperature status in the brain tissue itself (Brettler, 2004). In addition, cerebral microdialysis catheters can provide information about the nature of the cerebral interstitial fluid.

Mechanical Ventilation

Clients with IICP often require intubation and are placed on a ventilator for respiratory management. Mechanical ventilation may be used to maintain partial pressure of oxygen and carbon dioxide, thus preventing hypoxemia and hypercapnia, both of which can increase ICP. It is important to maintain adequate oxygenation with a partial pressure of arterial oxygen at about 100 mmHg and a partial pressure of arterial carbon dioxide of about 35 mmHg. The client with IICP and signs of impending herniation may be judiciously hyperventilated to cause cerebral vasoconstriction; however, this also increases cerebral ischemia. Mechanical ventilation is discussed in greater detail in Exemplar 21.1, Acute Respiratory Distress Syndrome.

TABLE 17–6 **Risk Factors for Infection With Intracranial Pressure Monitoring**

FACTOR	RATIONALE
Intraventricular catheter	Is more invasive than other monitoring devices
Open head trauma or neurosurgery	Disrupts protective skin and skeletal barriers
Intracranial hemorrhage	Necessitates frequent flushing of catheter to maintain patency
Older adult	Tends to have impaired immune defenses
Monitoring for more than 3–5 days or using open system or frequent irrigation	Offers increased opportunity for pathogens to enter and grow

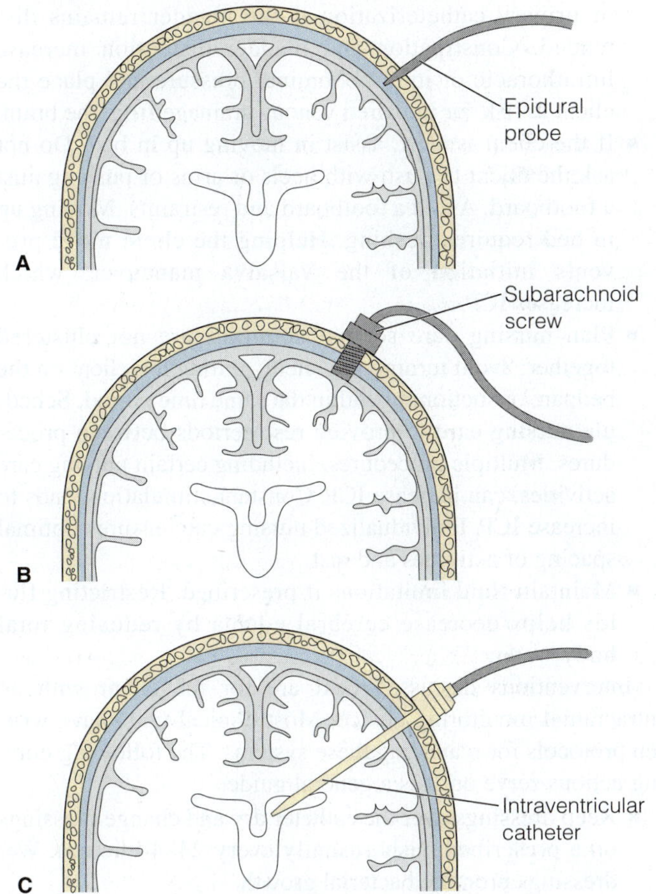

Figure 17–14 ■ Types of ICP monitoring. *A*, Epidural probe. *B*, Subarachnoid screw. *C*, Intraventricular catheter.

Other Therapies

Physical therapy to prevent muscle atrophy may be necessary for a client who is unconscious or bedridden for more than a few days. Respiratory therapy is usually necessary after a client is weaned from a mechanical ventilator. Families of clients who have ICP may benefit from spiritual or psychologic counseling. Nurses can provide much-needed support by contacting a hospital chaplain or making a referral to an experienced counseling professional.

NURSING PROCESS

The nursing care of clients with IICP involves identifying those at risk and managing factors known to increase intracranial pressure. A major focus is protecting the client from sudden increases in ICP or a decrease in cerebral blood flow.

Assessment

Assess for and report manifestations of IICP every 15 minutes to 1 hour and as necessary. Clients with unstable ICP may require continuous or more frequent monitoring. Assessment areas include LOC; behavior; motor/sensory functions; pupillary size and reaction to light; and vital signs, including temperature. Look for trends because vital signs alone do not correlate well with early deterioration. Assessment of neurologic status establishes the client's clinical condition and provides a baseline for measuring changes. Sudden changes in neurologic signs often indicate deterioration. An elevated temperature with increased oxygen consumption further increases ICP. Pupillary responses mirror the status of the midbrain and pons. Pressure on the brainstem may compromise the function of cranial nerves IX and X and protective mechanisms such as the gag and cough reflexes. The nurse needs to be alert to even the most subtle change as it may indicate early signs of a declining neurological condition.

Monitor pulse oximetry and arterial blood gas measurements. Adequate air exchange to keep oxygen and carbon dioxide levels within normal ranges and maintenance of acid–base balance are critical to reduce the risk of hypoxemia and IICP. If adequate respiratory effort cannot be maintained, mechanical ventilation will be necessary.

PRACTICE ALERT

Often the earliest manifestations of a change in ICP are alterations in LOC and respirations.

Diagnosis

Nursing diagnoses for the client with IICP may include the following:

- Ineffective Tissue Perfusion: Cerebral
- Ineffective Breathing Pattern
- Risk for Aspiration
- Risk for Infection.

Plan

Planning nursing care for the client with IICP is highly individualized and depends on the cause, treatment, and prognosis. Common goals include the following:

- Client will maintain ICP less than 20 mmHg.
- Client will experience no further complications as the result of IICP.
- Family members will demonstrate ability to maintain a low-stimuli environment.

CARE SETTINGS Increased Intracranial Pressure

- Provide a quiet environment, limiting noxious stimuli.
- Avoid jarring the bed.
- Try to limit situations that cause emotional upset; maintain a calm, reassuring manner; caution family members to refrain from unpleasant conversations or conversations that may be emotionally stimulating to the client.
- Remember that noxious stimuli and emotional upsets cause an elevation in ICP.

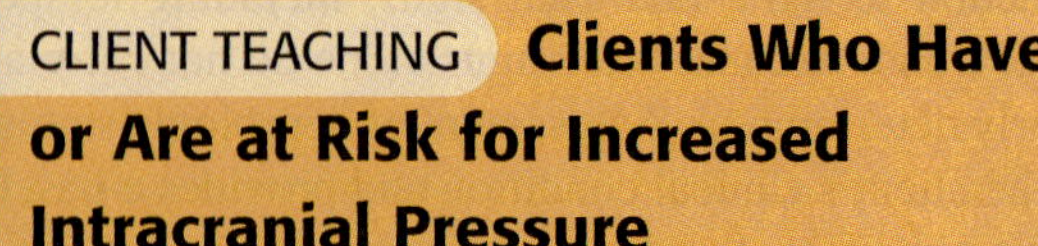

CLIENT TEACHING Clients Who Have or Are at Risk for Increased Intracranial Pressure

- Teach the client who is able to follow instructions to avoid coughing, blowing the nose, straining to have a bowel movement, pushing against the bed rails, or performing isometric (muscle contracting) exercises.
- Advise the client to maintain head and neck alignment when turning in bed and to take rest periods.
- Encourage the family to talk to the client but to maintain a quiet environment with a minimum of stimuli.
- Inform family members that upsetting the client may increase ICP and that they should avoid discussions that may distress the client.
- For clients unable to make decisions about treatment and to sign informed consent, contact the family, who must carry out these functions.

- Client will not experience infection as the result of ICP monitoring.
- Client will maintain adequate cerebral perfusion to prevent further cellular damage.

Implementation

Nursing interventions include performing neurologic assessments, maintaining airway patency, ensuring adequate ventilation, positioning and moving, instituting seizure precautions, and monitoring fluids and electrolytes. Additionally, both client and family need emotional support during this period.

- For the client on a ventilator: Maintain airway patency; preoxygenate with 100% oxygen before suctioning; limit suctioning to 10 seconds as suctioning increases ICP; suction gently. Preoxygenation helps maintain oxygen levels during suctioning. Suctioning stimulates the cough reflex and Valsalva maneuver. Correct suctioning minimizes the risk of hypoxemia.
- Monitor arterial blood gases. They provide a reliable indicator of oxygen and carbon dioxide levels. If oxygen concentration is low, oxygen may be given or increased.
- Elevate the head of the bed to 30 degrees in most cases, as prescribed (if neck trauma is involved the bed may need to be kept flat until x-rays of the cervical spine show no fractures); maintain alignment of the head and neck to avoid hyperextension or exaggerated neck flexion; avoid prone position. Keeping the head of the bed elevated facilitates venous drainage from the cerebrum. Obstruction of jugular veins can impede venous drainage from the brain.
- Monitor bladder distention and bowel constipation. Administer stool softeners and use Credé's method (the method of applying pressure to the suprapubic region with the fingers of one or both hands) to empty the bladder. If Credé's method is not effective, evaluate the pros and cons of urinary catheterization if the bladder remains distended. Constipation and bladder distention increase intrathoracic or intra-abdominal pressure and place the client at risk for impaired venous drainage from the brain.
- If the client is alert, assist in moving up in bed. Do not ask the client to push with heels or arms or push against a footboard. Avoid a footboard and restraints. Moving up in bed requires pushing. Helping the client move prevents initiation of the Valsalva maneuver, which increases ICP.
- Plan nursing care so that activities are not clustered together; avoid turning the client, getting the client on the bedpan, or suctioning within the same time period. Schedule nursing care to provide rest periods between procedures. Multiple procedures, including certain nursing care activities, can increase ICP. Constant stimulation tends to increase ICP. Individualized nursing care ensures optimal spacing of activities and rest.
- Maintain fluid limitations if prescribed. Restricting fluids helps decrease cerebral edema by reducing total body water.

Interventions discussed next are for the client with an intracranial monitoring device. Most clinical units have written protocols for managing these systems. The following nursing actions serve only as a general guide.

- Keep dressings over the catheter dry and change dressings on a prescribed basis (usually every 24–48 hours). Wet dressings promote bacterial growth.
- Monitor the insertion site for leaking CSF, drainage, or infection. Monitor for manifestations of infection, including changes in vital signs, chills, increased white blood counts (WBCs), lack of clarity in CSF, or positive cultures of drainage. Close monitoring helps detect the earliest signs of infection and helps prevent major complications. Fever is usually considered the key assessment. However, fever in a client with a neurologic disorder may be due to damage to the hypothalamus. Headache, generalized muscle aches, shivering, and chills also may be seen in the client with infection.
- Use strict aseptic technique when in contact with the device. Check drainage system for loose connections. Using aseptic technique and monitoring drainage systems for loose connections help prevent nosocomial infections.

Evaluation

The client is evaluated based on the plan of care developed. Potential expected outcomes may include the following:

- ICP returns to acceptable limits following treatment.
- Client's LOC improves with reduction of ICP.
- Client experiences no infection as the result of ICP monitoring.
- Family describes appropriate outcome expectations related to amount of cellular damage resulting from IICP.

REVIEW Increased Intracranial Pressure

RELATE: LINK THE CONCEPTS

The nurse is caring for a client who experienced severe head trauma in a motor vehicle accident. The client is placed on a mechanical ventilator set to 28 breaths per minute and is completely nonresponsive to deep, painful stimuli. The client's vital signs are T_O 101.2°F, P 112, R 28, BP 100/88. ICP readings are currently 16 but increase to 34–38 mm Hg when touched and 52 mm Hg when the endotracheal tube is suctioned.

Linking the exemplar of Increased Intracranial Pressure with the concept of Perfusion:

1. What nursing interventions can the nurse perform to optimize brain perfusion?
2. How would you interpret the client's blood pressure and ICP readings to determine brain perfusion?

The family of the client in the preceding scenario are told that if the client survives, he is likely to experience significant neurologic losses and may remain in a chronic vegetative state. The client's wife says, "I know him. He's a fighter, and he won't settle for anything less than full recovery." She then relates the story of a television show she saw the other day. The character on the show received this same prognosis and was back to normal within a few weeks.

Linking the exemplar of Increased Intracranial Pressure with the concept of Grief and Loss:

3. In what stage of the grieving process is this family member?
4. What nursing care can you provide to support this woman's grieving process and to help her accept the likelihood of a less than complete recovery?

READY: GO TO COMPANION SKILLS MANUAL

When caring for clients with IICP, the following nursing skills may be useful and can be found in your skills manual:

- Assessing appearance and mental status
- Assessing the neurologic system
- Assisting with chest tube insertion
- Maintaining chest tube drainage
- Assisting with chest tube removal
- Caring for a client on a mechanical ventilator
- Weaning a client from a mechanical ventilator
- Glasgow Coma Scale

REFER: GO TO MYNURSINGKIT

REFLECT: CASE STUDY

Antwan, 7 years old, was injured when he was struck by a car and thrown several feet into the air. He was unconscious upon admission to the emergency department and showed some signs of IICP (dilated and fixed pupils, lack of response to painful stimuli, irregular breathing pattern). Antwan was treated for shock, and his neurologic status and vital signs were assessed frequently. The initial evaluation revealed that Antwan had sustained several contusions of the brain but no skull fracture. He was intubated and medicated to manage the airway and IICP. After 7 days in the intensive care unit, he was moved to a general care floor. He is still not fully conscious but quiets when his parents speak to him. He is moving all extremities, but he does not yet follow commands.

1. Describe the neurologic nursing assessment that should be performed on Antwan at regular intervals in the general care unit.
2. Identify age-appropriate sensory stimulation strategies that may help promote Antwan's awareness and improvement in LOC.
3. What would you teach Antwan's family to help promote neurologic improvement?
4. What changes in Antwan's condition would require immediate notification of the primary provider?

17.2 SEIZURE DISORDERS

KEY TERMS

Aura, *970*
Automatisms, *969*
Clonic phase, *970*
Epilepsy, *968*
Febrile seizures, *968*
Focal seizures, *968*
Generalized seizures, *968*
Intractable seizures, *971*
Postictal period, *970*
Status epilepticus, *971*
Tonic phase, *968*

BASIS FOR SELECTION OF EXEMPLAR

Centers for Disease Control and Prevention
Chronic Disease Management
Standards of Nursing Practice

LEARNING OUTCOMES

After reading about this exemplar, you will be able to:

1. Describe the pathophysiology, etiology, clinical manifestations, and direct and indirect causes of seizures.
2. Identify risk factors associated with seizures.
3. Illustrate the nursing process in providing culturally competent care across life span for individuals with seizures.
4. Formulate priority nursing diagnoses appropriate for an individual with seizures.
5. Create a plan of care for individuals with seizures and their family members.
6. Assess expected outcomes for an individual with seizures.
7. Discuss therapies used in the collaborative care of an individual with seizures.
8. Employ evidence-based caring interventions for an individual with seizures.

OVERVIEW

Seizures are defined as periods of abnormal electrical discharges in the brain that may cause involuntary movement or behavior or sensory alterations. Seizure disorders affect over 3 million Americans of all ages in the United States. Approximately 2–4% of children have one or more seizures during childhood from a variety of causes, most often during infancy. **Epilepsy** is a chronic disorder characterized by recurrent, unprovoked seizures secondary to a central nervous system (CNS) disorder.

PATHOPHYSIOLOGY AND ETIOLOGY

Seizures are believed to be the result of abnormal excessive concurrent electrical discharges from the cortical neuronal network of cells on the surface of the brain. Chemical changes in the neurons create an electrical negativity that enables the transfer of information between neurons. When an excessive number of these cells become excited, they discharge abnormally. These cells can be triggered by environmental or physiologic stimuli (e.g., emotional stress, anxiety, fatigue, infection, or metabolic disturbances). Acute insults such as a CNS infection, hypoxia, and brain trauma are the most common causes of seizures in children.

Focal seizures (also known as *partial seizures)* are caused by abnormal electrical activity in one hemisphere or in a specific area of the cerebral cortex, most often the temporal, frontal, or parietal lobes. The seizure may spread regionally, and the symptoms are related to the region of the cortex that is affected.

In contrast, **generalized seizures** are the result of diffuse electrical activity that often begins in both hemispheres of the brain simultaneously, then spreads throughout the cortex into the brainstem. As a result, movements and spasms displayed by the client are bilateral and symmetric.

Etiology

Some seizures are idiopathic, that is, not provoked by known stimuli. Genetic factors may lower the seizure threshold by making brain cells more vulnerable to abnormal electrical discharges. Acquired seizures may be caused by underlying pathologic conditions such as trauma, infection, hypoglycemia, hypotonic dehydration, electrolyte imbalance, endocrine dysfunction, toxins, tumors, or lesions that may be manifested at any time.

Febrile seizures are generalized seizures that usually occur in children as the result of rapid temperature rise above 39°C (102°F), usually in association with an acute illness. No evidence of intracranial infection or other defined cause is found. Febrile seizures are usually seen between 3 months and 5 years of age, with a peak incidence between 17 and 24 months of age. There is often a family history of febrile seizures. In addition, children who have one febrile seizure have a 30–50% greater chance of having future seizures (Gill & Gieron-Korthals, 2002). The lower convulsive threshold of infants may explain this type of seizure.

Risk Factors

Infants are susceptible to developing epilepsy in the first year of life, with an incidence of 1 per 1,000. The incidence decreases with age. The median age for the development of epilepsy is 5–6 years of age. In the United States, approximately 150,000 to 325,000 children between 5 and 14 years of age have epilepsy (Blair & Selekman, 2004).

Other risk factors include an infant who is small for gestational age, presence of underlying neurologic conditions, brain tumors or infections of the brain, stroke, cerebral palsy, autistic disorder, family history, or abuse of drugs. Risk factors and other considerations for older adults are described in the Developmental Considerations feature.

CLINICAL MANIFESTATIONS

The length of a seizure, especially of a generalized seizure, is important because the airway may be compromised during the tonic phase. The initial manifestations of the **tonic phase** of a generalized seizure are unconsciousness and continuous muscular contraction. The basal metabolic rate rises during the peak of seizure activity, increasing the body's demand for oxygen and glucose. The client may become pale or cyanotic as a result of hypoxia. The client also may become hypoglycemic if glucose demand is excessive.

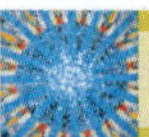

DEVELOPMENTAL CONSIDERATIONS **Epilepsy in Older Adults**

For years, epilepsy was believed to be a disease that principally affected children. Research has now found that the incidence of epilepsy in adults age 75 and over is higher than that in the first 10 years of life, with 7% of all older adults having epilepsy (Spitz, 2005). These data have important implications for nursing assessments and care.

- The most common cause of epilepsy in older adults is arteriosclerosis of the cerebrovascular system (with up to 80% of the older population having arteriosclerosis).
- The manifestations of epilepsy in older adults are different than those in younger adults and children. Although 60% of younger people have generalized tonic–clonic seizures, only 30% of older adults have generalized tonic–clonic seizures. The most common type of seizure in older adults is a complex partial seizure.
- Older adults tend to have longer post-seizure manifestations than do younger adults.
- Epilepsy that begins in older adults is often easier to control with antiepileptic drugs (AEDs) than that in younger people. However, some AEDs decrease the effect of statins used to treat arteriosclerosis (the most common cause of epilepsy in older adults).

CLINICAL MANIFESTATIONS AND THERAPIES **Seizure Disorders**

ETIOLOGY	CLINICAL MANIFESTATIONS	CLINICAL THERAPIES
Simple partial seizures involve activation of only a restricted part of one cerebral hemisphere	No alteration in consciousness. Typically only motor portion of cortex is affected causing recurrent muscle contractions of face or contralateral part of body. Motor movement may be confined to one area. If it spreads sequentially to adjacent parts it is called a Jacksonian march of Jacksonian seizure. If sensory portion is involved manifestations may include abnormal sensations or hallucinations. Disruption in autonomic nervous system may result in tachycardia, flushing, hypotension, or hypertension. Psychic symptoms such as a sense of déjà vu or inappropriate fear or anger may be experienced.	■ Antiepileptic medications ■ Maintain client safety during seizure ■ Assess exact manifestations experienced by client and document fully ■ Vagal nerve stimulation therapy
Complex partial seizures involve activation of only a restricted part of one cerebral hemisphere, usually originating in the temporal lobe	Often proceeded by an aura which may be visual, auditory, odd smell, or psychic in nature. Impaired consciousness lasting for several hours before full consciousness regained. Repetitive nonpurposeful activity such as lip smacking, aimless walking, or picking at clothing called **automatisms**. Amnesia is common after seizure.	■ Antiepileptics ■ Maintain client safety ■ Vagal nerve stimulation ■ Resection of epileptogenic focus, such as the temporal lobe, may be considered
Absence seizures (petit mal) involve both hemispheres of the brain as well as deeper structures such as thalamus, basal ganglia, and upper brainstem.	Impaired level of consciousness. Sudden brief cessation of all motor activity accompanied by blank stare and unresponsiveness. More common in children. Usually lasts 5–10 seconds, sometimes as long as 30 seconds. Vary from occasional to several hundred per day. Seizures are best described by others who witnessed the event because the client is.	■ Antiepileptic medications ■ Maintain client safety
Tonic-clonic seizures are the most common type seen in adults	Warning aura may proceed seizure activity (visual, gustatory, auditory, visceral, or sense of uneasiness). Sudden loss of consciousness. Tonic Phase: ■ Sharp tonic muscle contraction forcing air out of the lungs which may cause client to cry out.	■ Antiepileptic medications ■ Maintain client safety ■ Suspension of driving privileges until seizure activity is controlled and client is seizure free for a period of time determined by state statutes ■ Helmets may be recommended to prevent head injury until seizure activity is controlled

(continued)

CLINICAL MANIFESTATIONS AND THERAPIES Seizure Disorders (continued)

ETIOLOGY	CLINICAL MANIFESTATIONS	CLINICAL THERAPIES
	■ Loss of postural control causing client to fall in opisthotonic posture. ■ Muscles are rigid with arms and legs extended and jaw clenched. ■ Urinary incontinence is common and may be accompanied by bowel incontinence. ■ Breathing ceases and cyanosis develops. ■ Pupils fixed and dilated. ■ Lasts 15–60 seconds. The clonic phase follows characterized by: ■ Alternating contraction and relaxation of muscles in all extremities ■ Hyperventilation ■ Eyes roll back ■ Client froths at the mouth ■ Varies in duration and subsides gradually generally 60–90 seconds. Postictal phase: ■ Client remains unconscious and unresponsive to stimuli ■ Relaxed and breathes quietly ■ Regains consciousness gradually and may be confused and disoriented on waking ■ Headache, muscle ache, fatigue often reported ■ May sleep for several hours ■ Amnesia is usual both for the seizure and several minutes before seizure activity	■ Do not restrain client ■ Pad bedrails ■ Diazepam, lorazepam, or phenobarbital may be administered during seizure to limit time
Status epilepticus	Continuous seizure activity with only very short periods of calm between intense and persistent seizures. Seizures may be any type but most often are generalized tonic–clonic. Client in great danger of hypoxia, acidosis, hypoglycemia, hyperthermia, and exhaustion if seizure activity is not halted.	■ Immediate interventions to preserve life ■ Establish and maintain an airway ■ Administer 50% glucose to prevent hypoglycemia ■ Diazepam or lorazepam administered IV and repeated every 10 minutes until seizure activity stops ■ Antiepileptics such as phenytoin ■ Phenobarbital may also be administered

The symptoms of a seizure depend on its type and duration. Seizures are classified into two types: *partial (focal) seizures* and *generalized seizures*. Tonic–clonic seizures are the most common seizure type in children, characterized by alternating repetitive tonic–clonic activity (Weinstein, 2002). The tonic phase is followed by the **clonic phase**, characterized by alternating muscular contraction and relaxation. During the **postictal period** following seizure activity, LOC is decreased and the client is often sleepy but arousable. The length of the postictal period varies. An **aura** may provide an early warning sign of a seizure and may be manifest as any type of seonsory alteration ranging from odor, taste, or vision. When the client recognizes the pattern of an aura, he or she may have time to avoid injury by getting to the floor.

Febrile seizures involve generalized tonic–clonic movements that last less than 15 minutes.

COLLABORATION

The health care team, composed of the nurse, physician, and (in the case of children) the parents, teacher, and school nurse, work together to ensure that parents and adults working with the child understand care and prevention requirements. Many seizures are self-limiting and require no emergency intervention.

Diagnostic Tests

Laboratory tests that may be ordered include a complete blood cell count, blood chemistry, urine culture, and lumbar puncture. If the child is taking any anticonvulsants, the serum drug level is monitored regularly. An EEG is often performed at a follow-up visit between seizures. A lead level, toxicology screening, and radiologic tests such as a CT scan or MRI and angiography may be performed to identify a cerebral lesion or metabolic disorder in the brain.

Pharmacologic Therapy

AEDs (also called *anticonvulsant drugs*) can reduce or control most seizure activity (see Medications: Seizure Disorders on page 960 in the About section). More than 20 drugs are available for use in the treatment of epilepsy. These medications do not cure the disorder; they only manage its manifestations. AEDs generally act in one of two ways: by raising the seizure threshold or by limiting the spread of abnormal activity in the brain.

The goals of medications for epilepsy are to protect the client from harm and to reduce or prevent seizure activity without impairing cognitive function or producing undesirable side effects. Ideally, the lowest possible dose of a single medication that will control the client's seizures is prescribed; often, however, several medications must be tried before the most effective one is identified, and a combination of drugs may be needed to manage the client's seizures.

Status epilepticus is a continuous seizure that lasts for more than 30 minutes or a series of seizures during which time consciousness is not regained. It requires immediate intervention to preserve life. Establishing and maintaining the airway is a priority. A solution of 50% dextrose is administered intravenously to prevent hypoglycemia. Diazepam (Valium) or lorazepam (Ativan) is given intravenously, and if necessary, the dose is repeated in 10 minutes to stop seizure activity. Phenytoin (Dilantin) is administered intravenously for longer-term control of seizures. Phenobarbital also may be administered to clients in status epilepticus.

Clinical Therapies for Children

Children with febrile seizures are usually not treated with an anticonvulsant at the time of the seizure because of the side effects. Long-term anticonvulsants are not recommended for simple febrile seizures (Shinnar & O'Dell, 2004). Instead, parents should be taught to lower fevers by using antipyretics and keeping the child cool with light clothing. They also must protect the child from injury if there is another seizure. As 30–40% of children experience a second febrile seizure, rectal diazepam or diazepam gel may be prescribed for the parents to have at home for treatment of a future febrile seizure, especially when the family lives a long distance from medical care (Shinnar & O'Dell, 2004).

Any child with a generalized seizure lasting longer than 10 minutes needs to be monitored for electrolytes, glucose, blood gases, increasing fever, and abnormal blood pressure. Anticonvulsants may be given intravenously or rectally to control the seizure: The longer the seizure lasts, the harder it is to stop (Wheless, 2004). The child should be monitored for continued motor activity and the potential for status epilepticus (a continuous seizure that lasts for more than 30 minutes or a series of seizures during which consciousness is not regained). The postictal period ranges from 30 minutes to 2 hours. Management of status epilepticus is described in Table 17–7.

The physician should provide a seizure action plan for any child with a history of seizure activity who attends school or day care or who is cared for outside the home while the parents work. Nurses can assist parents in making sure that teachers and caregivers understand the action plan and know when and how to use it.

Most seizure disorders are treated with anticonvulsants. A single medication (monotherapy) is preferred for seizure control to minimize side effects such as sleepiness, decreased attention and memory, difficulty with speech, ataxia, and diplopia (double vision). When necessary, other medications may be added to control seizures. Serum drug levels are monitored to achieve therapeutic levels or to identify whether toxicity is possible. When tolerated, therapeutic ranges of medications may be exceeded to control seizures. Medication dosage adjustments are often needed in pediatric clients as the child grows.

Approximately 25–30% of children have refractory or **intractable seizures**, seizures that continue to occur even with optimal medical management (Danielpour & Peacock, 2000).

TABLE 17–7 Management of Status Epilepticus

TYPE OF CARE	CLINICAL THERAPY
Emergency assessment and management	■ Maintain a patent airway. Muscle rigidity may compromise the airway. ■ Perform a jaw thrust maneuver if the airway is obstructed. ■ Keep suction equipment at the bedside in case secretions are excessive. ■ Give oxygen by mask, as increased metabolic demands deplete oxygen stores. ■ Monitor vital signs and circulation with pulse oximeter and cardiorespiratory monitor. ■ Perform neurologic assessment.
Ongoing urgent medications	■ Establish an intravenous line to administer any necessary fluids or management. ■ Administer glucose if the child is hypoglycemic; the physical stress of the seizure may result in declining glucose levels. ■ Insert a nasogastric tube. ■ Protect the child from injury. ■ Manage thermoregulation.
Medications	■ Administer benzodiazepines such as diazepam, lorazepam, or midazolam. If there is no response, the dose may be repeated. Phenytoin or phenobarbital may be necessary if seizure activity continues. Cumulative doses of drugs may produce apnea, so be prepared to assist ventilations.

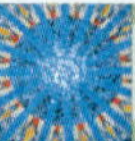

ALTERNATIVE THERAPIES Gingko

Families should be cautioned that herbal preparations with ginkgo may increase the risk of seizures in individuals with a history of seizures. In animal studies, ginkgo has been found to decrease the effectiveness of anticonvulsants such as valproic acid and carbamazepine (National Standard Research Collaboration, 2006).

These children are often treated with multiple anticonvulsants. Regular blood testing is performed to identify any developing hematologic or liver problems, as well as to determine if therapeutic ranges of medications are maintained.

A ketogenic diet is occasionally used for children under the age of 8 years with myoclonic and absence seizures. This diet involves a high intake of fat (90%), an adequate intake of protein (1 g/kg), and a very low intake of carbohydrates. Caloric intake is calculated at 75%, and fluids are restricted to 80% of usual (Freeman, 2003). The ketosis caused by the diet is believed to produce anticonvulsant effects. The diet is customized to the child to maintain the ideal body weight, maximize ketosis, and achieve optimal seizure control. Motivation must be high for the family to prepare the food and maintain the child on the diet for several years. The child's urine ketone values are monitored weekly or more frequently. The most common complications are constipation, hyperlipidemia, and kidney stones. Constipation is treated with medium chain triglycerides (MCT oil) and increased fluids. Kidney stones are treated by increasing fluid intake and alkalinizing the urine. Some children discontinue the diet after becoming seizure-free and require no antiepileptic medications. Other children have a dramatically reduced incidence of seizures (Rubenstein et al. 2005).

PRACTICE ALERT

Infants who are started on the ketogenic diet for infantile spasms may use a formula that is a mixture of Ross Carbohydrate Free formula with Ross Polycose and Novartis Microlipid (Rubenstein et al., 2005).

A trial of antiepileptic medication withdrawal is often attempted for children who have been seizure-free for 2 years (Goldstein, 2004). Approximately 60–70% of children are successfully weaned from antiepileptic medications and have no seizures (Blair & Selekman, 2004).

Surgery

Surgery may be performed occasionally to remove a tumor, lesion, or portion of the brain that has been identified as causing the seizures, particularly when seizures are not responsive to medication. Cerebral hemispherectomy is sometimes performed for a child with intractable epilepsy (Jonas et al., 2004). A vagal nerve stimulator is another option for children who are unable to tolerate multiple medications and are not candidates for surgery (Blair & Selekman, 2004).

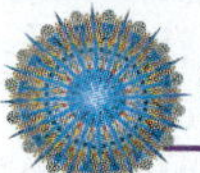

NURSING PROCESS

Assessment

After the client's first seizure, a thorough history must be taken from the parent, primary caretaker, or witnesses to the event. A description of the seizure and its length should be noted, in addition to whether an aura was present and whether the client lost consciousness. This information helps to identify the type of seizure according to the International Classification of Epileptic Seizures (Table 17–8).

TABLE 17–8 **Nursing Assessments Before, During, and After a Seizure**

ASSESSMENT	RATIONALE
What was the client's LOC? If consciousness was lost, at what point?	Indicates area of brain involved and type of seizure.
What was the client doing just before the attack?	May suggest precipitating factors.
In what part of the body did the seizure start?	May indicate the site of seizure activity in the brain tissue; for example, if jerking movements were first observed in the right hand, the seizure focus may be in the left motor cortex.
Was there an epileptic cry?	Usually indicates the tonic stage of a generalized tonic–clonic seizure.
Were any automatisms observed, such as eyelid fluttering, chewing, lip smacking, or swallowing?	Often seen in complex, partial, and absence seizures.
How long did movements last? Did the location or character change (tonic to clonic)? Did movements involve both sides of the body or just one side?	Indicates areas in which focal activity originated.
Did the head and/or eyes turn to one side? If so, which side?	Helps localize the focus of the seizure; during the seizure, the head and eyes typically turn away from the side of the epileptogenic focus.
Were there changes in pupillary reactions?	Indicates involvement of the autonomic nervous system.
If the client fell, was the head hit?	Skull x-ray studies may be needed to rule out subdural hematoma or fracture.
Was there foaming or frothing from the mouth?	Usually indicates a tonic–clonic seizure.

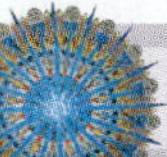

NURSING CARE PLAN A Client With Seizure Disorder

ASSESSMENT

Janet Carlson is a 19-year-old college student who lives with her parents and one younger sister. Although Janet had seizures while she was in grade school, they have been controlled with medication. However, she had a tonic–clonic seizure yesterday and immediately made an appointment with her family physician. She is currently taking phenytoin (Dilantin) 300 mg/day as a maintenance medication to prevent seizures.

Evita Farias, RN, completes a health history for Ms. Carlson. During the history, Ms. Carlson says that she has been under stress because of difficulties in completing her course requirements this semester. She has not been sleeping as many hours at night, and sometimes she forgets to take her medication. Her serum phenytoin level is 8 mg/mL. Her therapeutic level is 10–20 mg/mL.

DIAGNOSES

- Risk for Injury related to recurrence of generalized tonic–clonic seizure activity and low serum phenytoin levels
- Deficient Knowledge of activities that may trigger seizure occurrence, the effect of stress on seizures, and medication information

PLANNING

- Verbalize precipitating and triggering factors related to the onset of seizures.
- Verbalize the relationship between emotional and physical stress and seizures.
- Verbalize the importance of taking AEDs.

IMPLEMENTATION

Teach the client and her family the following:

- Current information about seizures
- Care during and after a seizure
- Medication protocols
- Factors and activities that can trigger seizures
- The importance of follow-up care.

Refer the client and her family to a local epilepsy support group.

Recommend that the client purchase and wear a medical ID bracelet.

EVALUATION

Ms. Carlson is instructed to continue taking Dilantin 300 mg/day. Ms. Farias states the importance of nutrition, rest, and measures to reduce stress. She also discusses with Ms. Carlson the importance of maintaining the proper blood levels of her medication, stating that too little or too much of the medication could cause problems. Ms. Carlson understands that the seizures had recurred during a busy time in school when she had forgotten to take her medication. She is now wearing a medical ID bracelet. Ms. Farias provides the Carlsons with the telephone number of the Epilepsy Foundation of America.

CRITICAL THINKING

1. If you were Ms. Carlson's nurse, would your teaching differ if Ms. Carlson were living alone? If so, how? If not, why not?
2. Ms. Carlson tells you that although she knows she should not drive a car, she often drives her friend to work. How would you approach this problem?
3. Ms. Carlson states, "It's embarrassing to wear a medical ID bracelet." How would you respond? What recommendation(s) would you make?

Perform a complete physical and neurologic examination. Assess and monitor the client's physiologic status. Observe the specific seizure activity, LOC, vital signs, and signs of hypoxia. During the postictal period, monitor vital signs, perform neurologic checks, and ensure safety. Once the client is stable, a more definitive assessment can be made. LOC is one of the most important indicators of neurologic function. Remember that a lack of response may be the result of the postictal state.

To help determine the type of seizure, collect and analyze historical information about the seizure activity, clustering, the aura, the motor activity or changes in muscle tone, automatisms, and any changes in developmental performance.

Assess the family's adaptation to the seizure disorder, including how well the family is coping with the uncertainty of when the next seizure will occur.

FOCUS ON DIVERSITY AND CULTURE Seizures

Seizures may have a special meaning for some cultural groups. For example, the Hmong believe that the child is experiencing *quag dab peg,* which means the "spirit catches you and you fall down." Hmong view the condition as serious, but there is a sense of pride that the child has the condition. In 1997, Anne Fadiman wrote *The Spirit Catches You and You Fall Down,* a compelling story about the cultural conflict between a Hmong family and health care providers over treatment of its daughter's seizures (Fadiman, 1997).

Diagnosis

Common nursing diagnoses for an individual with a seizure disorder include the following:

- Ineffective Breathing Pattern related to neuromuscular dysfunction during the tonic phase of a seizure
- Ineffective Airway Clearance related to inability to control or manage secretions during the seizure

- Risk for Trauma related to fall with onset of seizure activity
- Chronic Low Self-Esteem related to seizures and loss of bowel and bladder control during seizure activity
- Anxiety related to unpredictable nature of seizure disorder
- Ineffective Therapeutic Regimen Management related to poor adherence with medications
- Readiness for Enhanced Family Processes related to care of a child with a chronic disorder.

Plan

Nursing care focuses on maintaining airway patency, ensuring safety, administering medications, and providing emotional support. Both acute care and long-term management are involved. Planning also may include developing a seizure action plan for the client, particularly for children, so that family, close friends, teachers, and other caregivers or even professional colleagues know how to respond appropriately in the event the client has a seizure. Sample seizure action plans and other resources can be found at the Epilepsy Foundation's website: www.epilepsyfoundation.org.

Implementation

Nursing interventions during seizures include the following:

- Place nothing in the client's mouth during a seizure; loose teeth may be knocked out and aspirated. Position the client on his or her side so secretions can drain. Monitor to ensure adequate oxygenation: Mucus membranes should be pink, the heart rate should be at a normal or slightly elevated rate for age, and the pulse oximetry reading should be greater than 95%. Oxygen is usually administered when the pulse oximetry reading (SpO_2) falls below 95%.
- Protect the client from self-harm during violent seizures (Figure 17–15 ■). If the client is in bed, the side rails should be padded to prevent injury. Children who have frequent, recurrent seizures should wear helmets to protect their heads during falls. All clients with seizure disorders should wear some form of medical alert identification. Maintain functioning suction at the bedside to clear the airway as necessary.
- Take special precautions when administering intravenous medications (diazepam, lorazepam, or phenytoin) for the emergency management of status epilepticus. Give these

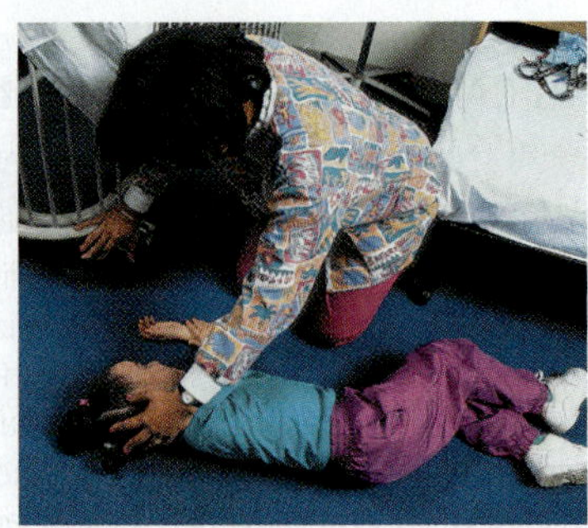

Figure 17–15 ■ A client who has a seizure when standing should be gently assisted to the floor and placed in a side-lying position. Clear the area of any objects that might cause harm.

DEVELOPMENTAL CONSIDERATIONS Seizures

CHILDREN

- Children and adolescents need to have medications adjusted as they grow and medication plasma levels monitored carefully in order to maintain the level within therapeutic range to obtain obtimal effects.
- The child and parents need to be educated about medication regimens. Explain the purpose of each drug, schedule for administration, side effects, and importance of giving all doses. Teaching the older child to take medications without parental intervention gives the child a feeling of control.
- Regular dental care is important because of the effect of phenytoin on the gingiva.
- The parents of children with recurrent febrile seizures should be taught how to administer antipyretics properly. Parents need to know, however, that antipyretics may not prevent a febrile seizure associated with an acute illness. The potential toxicity of an anticonvulsant in a child with febrile seizures is often considered greater than the risk of the seizures, and parents can be reassured that complications from febrile seizures are rare.
- The family should receive help in working with school administrators to develop an Individual Health Plan so the child can receive needed medications and care during school hours.
- Physical activity and exercise are important for all children. Encourage the child's participation in sports when adequate supervision is provided. Children who are prone to seizures require one-to-one supervision during swimming and water activities.
- The child may be afraid of having a seizure in front of friends. Reassure the child and family that taking medications regularly should control seizures.
- Summer camps for children with seizures can be a safe and comfortable place for the child to enjoy outdoor activities. Talk with parents about communicating with camp administrators and sharing health and action plans as they do with school administers.

ADOLESCENTS AND ADULTS

- Depending on state laws, most clients with seizure disorders can drive after they have been seizure-free for at least 2 years.
- Adolescent females need to be educated about the potential teratogenicity of some anticonvulsants, such as valproic acid and carbamazepine that are associated with neural tube defects and heart defects. Until pregnancy is desired, contraception should be used when the adolescent is sexually active.
- Some antiepileptic medications cause a drug interaction with oral contraceptive pills that can lead to contraceptive failure. Effective contraception may require increasing the amount of estrogen in the contraceptive hormones or using medroxyprogesterone injections (Marin, 2005).
- Families should be taught about safety guidelines. Families of clients with severe seizure disorders need to develop an emergency care plan so that emergency personnel know about the need for care in advance.

medications very slowly over several minutes to minimize the risk of respiratory or circulatory collapse.

- Give medications for the ongoing management of seizures orally. Crushing pills and mixing them in a teaspoonful of applesauce, pudding, or other soft food make them more palatable and easier for a child or older adult to swallow if the pill is one that may be crushed.
- Understand that the loss of control of body movements and possible loss of consciousness make seizures frightening and difficult to accept. Parents often feel guilty about a child's seizure disorder and compensate by not disciplining or restricting the child appropriately. Stress the need to treat the child as normally as possible. Refer the child and family to support groups and counseling services if indicated.
- Encourage clients and their families to express their fears and anxieties. Answer questions honestly and refer to organizations such as the Epilepsy Foundation of America, where clients and family can get more information about the disorder. Make sure parents know how to administer medications and keep their child safe.

PRACTICE ALERT

When the child on a ketogenic diet is hospitalized, it is important to limit glucose and dextrose from all sources. Normal saline intravenous fluid should be used. Medications in elixirs or syrups cannot be used because of the sugar content. Alternatively, medications can be obtained in pill form, crushed, and mixed with an allowable food that has been approved by the pharmacy.

Evaluation

Expected outcomes of nursing management include the following:

- The client achieves good seizure control with medication, ketogenic diet, or surgical intervention.
- The client's self-esteem is enhanced through participation in well-supervised sports and activities.
- Client maintains patent airway during seizure activity.
- Client's safety is maintained during seizure activity.
- Medication administration reduces frequency of seizure recurrence.
- Appropriate seizure management plan is created by client and family in conjunction with healthcare team.

REVIEW Seizure Disorders

RELATE: LINK THE CONCEPTS

Linking the exemplar of Seizures with the concept of Legal Issues:

1. When caring for an adult client newly diagnosed with recurrent seizures, what legal obligation does the nurse have regarding the client's driving privileges versus the obligation to client privacy?
2. If the client says, "You don't have to report this to the DMV—I promise not to drive until I get medical clearance," is it permissible for the nurse to take the client's word for it?

Linking the exemplar of Seizures with the concept of Thermoregulation:

3. The nurse is caring for a 14-month-old infant with a fever whose mother reports the two older siblings both experienced febrile seizures. What nursing interventions would you initiate with this child?
4. What would differ in your plan of care for a child with a fever if the child had a history of febrile seizures?

READY: GO TO THE COMPANION SKILLS MANUAL

Skills required for the care of clients diagnosed with seizures can be found in your skills manual and include the following:

- Implementing seizure precautions

REFER: GO TO MYNURSINGKIT

REFLECT: CASE STUDY

Joe Hill is a 77-year-old white male admitted with a diagnosis of new onset seizure. His heart rate is 78, his blood pressure is 154/90, his temperature is 97°F, and his O2 sat is 99%. He appears confused and is unable to respond to questions. Mr. Hill's wife reports that he has a history of hypertension, but he is otherwise healthy. He is placed on seizure precautions, and his vital signs are monitored.

1. On the basis of this description, what kind of seizure might Mr. Hill have experienced?
2. What factors may have contributed to Mr. Hill's seizure?
3. When examining the client what will the nurse assess for?
4. What are the priority nursing interventions?

PEARSON

EXPLORE mynursingkit™

MyNursingKit is your one stop for online chapter review materials and resources. Prepare for success with additional NCLEX®-style practice questions, interactive assignments and activities, web links, animations and videos, and more!

Register your access code from the front of your book at **www.mynursingkit.com**.

REFERENCES

Blair, J., & Selekman, J. (2004). Epilepsy. In P. J. Allen & J. A. Vessey (Eds.), *Primary care of the child with a chronic condition* (4th ed., pp. 469–497). St. Louis: Mosby.

Brettler, S. (2004). Trauma nursing: Traumatic head injury. *RN, 67*(4), 32–38.

Danielpour, M., & Peacock, W. J. (2000). Epilepsy surgery in children. *Clinical Neurosurgery, 47,* 400–421.

Fadiman, A. (1997). *The spirit catches you and you fall down.* New York: Farrar, Strauss, Giroux.

Freeman, J. M. (2003). What every pediatrician should know about the ketogenic diet. *Contemporary Pediatrics, 20*(5), 113–127.

Gill, J. K., & Gieron-Korthals, M. (2002). What pediatricians—and parents—need to know about febrile convulsions. *Contemporary Pediatrics, 19*(5), 139–144.

James, H. E. (1986). Neurologic evaluation and support in the child with acute brain insult. *Pediatric Annals, 15*(1), 16–22.

Jonas, R., Nguyen, S., Hu, B., Asarnow, R. F., LoPresti, C., Curtiss, S., et al. (2004). Cerebral hemispherectomy: Hospital course, seizure, developmental, language, and motor outcomes. *Neurology, 62*(10), 1712–1721.

Kossoff, E. H., & Mankad, D. N. (2006). Medication-overuse headache in children: Is initial preventive therapy necessary? *Journal of Child Neurology, 21*(1), 45–48.

Marin, S. (2005). The impact of epilepsy on the adolescent. *Maternal Child Nursing, 30*(5), 321–326.

National Standadrd Research Collaboration. (2006). *Ginkgo (Ginkgo biloba L.).* Retrieved May 2, 2008, from http://www.nlm.nih.gov/medlineplus/druginfo/natural/patient-ginkgo.html

Porth, C. M. (2005). *Pathophysiology: Concepts of altered health states* (7th ed.). Philadelphia: Lippincott.

Rubenstein, J. E., Kossoff, E. H., Pyzik, P. L., Vining, E. P. G., McGrogan, J. R., & Freeman, J. M. (2005). Experience in the use of the ketogenic diet as early therapy. *Journal of Child Neurology, 20*(1), 31–34.

Shinnar, S., & O'Dell, C. (2004). Febrile seizures. *Pediatric Annals, 33*(6), 394–401.

Spitz. M. (2005). *Review and commentary on epilepsy and the elderly.* Retrieved from http://professionals.epilepsy.com/page/ar_1110476473.html

Teasdale, G., & Jennett, B. (1974). Assessment of coma and impaired consciousness. *Lancet, 2,* 81–84.

Tierney, L., McPhee, S., & Papadakis, M. (Eds.). (2005). *Current medical diagnosis & treatment* (44th ed.). New York: McGraw-Hill.

Weinstein, S. (2007). Epilepsy. In M. L. Batshaw (Ed.), *Children with disabilities* (6th ed., pp. 439–460). Baltimore: Paul H. Brookes Publishing Co.

Wheless, J. W. (2004). Treatment of status epilepticus in children. *Pediatric Annals, 33*(6), 376–383.

Wilensky, E., & Bloom, S. (2005). Monitoring brain tissue oxygenation after severe brain injury. *Nursing, 35*(2), 32cc1–32cc4.

Metabolism 18

Concept-at-a-Glance

Concept Learning Outcomes

After reading about this concept, you will be able to:

1. Summarize the structure and physiological process of the body related to metabolism.
2. List factors affecting metabolism.
3. Identify commonly occurring alterations in metabolism and their related treatments.
4. Explain common physical assessment procedures used to examine metabolism in clients across the life span.
5. Outline diagnostic and laboratory tests to determine an individual's metabolic status.
6. Explain management of metabolic health and prevention of metabolic disorders.
7. Demonstrate the nursing process in providing culturally competent and caring interventions across the life span for individuals with common alterations in metabolism.
8. Identify pharmacologic interventions in caring for the individual with alterations in metabolisim.

Concept Key Terms

Acromegaly, *985*
Carpal spasm, *986*
Chvostek's sign, *986*
Dwarfism, *986*
Exophthalmos, *985*
Goiter, *985*
Hormones, *977*
Insulin, *980*
Metabolism, *977*
Tetany, *986*
Trousseau's sign, *986*

About Metabolism

After nutrients (carbohydrates, fats, and proteins) are ingested, digested, absorbed, and transported across cell membranes, they must be metabolized into individual chemicals that can be utilized by the cells to maintain life. **Metabolism** describes the processes of biochemical reactions occurring in the body's cells that are necessary to produce energy, repair cells, and maintain life. Through the release of hormones, the endocrine system controls the cellular activity that regulates growth and body metabolism. **Hormones** are chemical messengers secreted by various glands that exert controlling effects on the cells of the body. Hormones regulate such varied functions as growth, reproduction, fluid and electrolyte balance, and gender differentiation. •

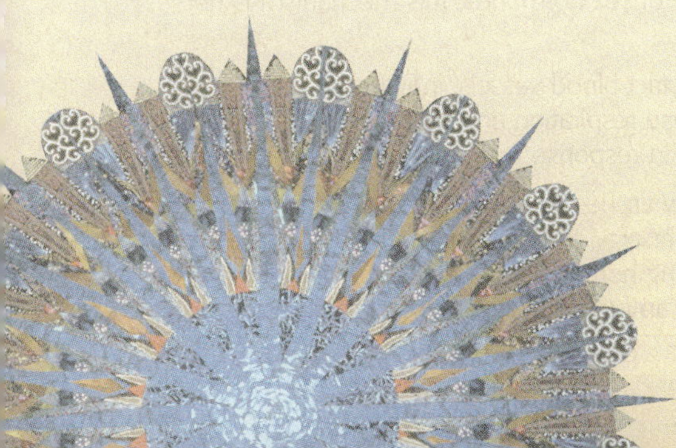

NORMAL PRESENTATION

The major endocrine organs are the pituitary gland, thyroid gland, parathyroid glands, adrenal glands, pancreas, and gonads (reproductive glands). The locations of these glands are illustrated in Figure 18–1 ■. Table 18–1 summarizes the functions of the endocrine organs and their hormones.

Pituitary Gland

The pituitary gland (hypophysis) is located in the skull beneath the hypothalamus of the brain. It often is called the "master gland," because its hormones regulate many body functions. The pituitary gland has two parts: the anterior pituitary (or adenohypophysis) and the posterior pituitary (or neuro hypophysis). The anterior pituitary is composed of glandular tissue, whereas the posterior pituitary is actually an extension of the hypothalamus.

Anterior Pituitary

The anterior pituitary has several types of endocrine cells and secretes at least six major hormones (Figure 18–2 ■):

1. Somatotropic cells secrete growth hormone (also called somatotropin), which stimulates growth of the body by signaling cells to increase protein production and by stimulating the epiphyseal plates of the long bones.
2. Lactotropic cells secrete prolactin, which stimulates the production of breast milk.
3. Thyrotropic cells secrete thyroid-stimulating hormone (TSH), which stimulates the synthesis and release of thyroid hormones from the thyroid gland.
4. Corticotropic cells secrete adrenocorticotropic hormone (ACTH), which stimulates release of hormones, especially glucocorticoids, from the adrenal cortex.
5. Gonadotropic cells secrete the gonadotropin hormones, follicle-stimulating hormone and luteinizing hormone (LH). These hormones stimulate the ovaries and testes (the gonads). (See Concept 23, Reproduction, for more information on the reproductive system.)

Posterior Pituitary

The posterior pituitary is made of nervous tissue. Its primary function is to store and release antidiuretic hormone and oxytocin, which are produced in the hypothalamus:

- Antidiuretic hormone (also called vasopressin) decreases urine production by causing the renal tubules to reabsorb water from the urine and return it to the circulating blood.
- Oxytocin induces contraction of the smooth muscles in the reproductive organs. In women, oxytocin stimulates the myometrium of the uterus to contract during labor. It also induces milk ejection from the breasts.

TABLE 18–1 **Organs, Hormones, Functions, and Feedback Mechanisms of the Endocrine System**

ENDOCRINE ORGAN	HORMONES SECRETED	TARGET ORGANS, FUNCTIONS, AND FEEDBACK MECHANISMS
Thyroid gland	Thyroid hormone: Thyroxine (T_4) is the major hormone secreted by the thyroid gland. It is converted to triiodothyronine (T_3) at the target tissues.	Maintains metabolic rate and growth and development of all tissues. Both T_3 and T_4 are secreted in response to thyroid-stimulating hormone.
	Calcitonin	Maintains serum calcium levels by decreasing bone resorption and decreasing resorption of calcium in the kidneys whenever levels of plasma calcium are elevated.
Parathyroid gland	Parathyroid hormone	Maintains serum calcium levels by stimulating bone resorption and formation and by stimulating kidney resorption of calcium in response to falling levels of plasma calcium.
Adrenal cortex	Mineralocorticoids (e.g., aldosterone)	Promote kidney tubule reabsorption of sodium and water and excretion of potassium in response to elevated levels of potassium and low levels of sodium, thereby increasing blood pressure and blood volume.
	Glucocorticoids (e.g., cortisol)	Help regulate metabolism of carbohydrates, fats, and proteins. Activate anti-inflammatory responses to stressors. Low cortisol levels stimulate hypothalamic secretion of corticotropin-releasing hormone, which stimulates the anterior pituitary gland to release adrenocorticotropic hormone, which in turn stimulates the adrenal cortex to secrete cortisol.
	Gonadocorticoids (androgens and small amounts of estrogen and progesterone)	Produce a small quantity of sex hormones; this mechanism is not well understood.
Adrenal medulla	Catecholamines (epinephrine and norepinephrine)	Stimulate the heart, constrict blood vessels, inhibit visceral muscles, dilate bronchioles, increase respiration and metabolism, and promote hyperglycemia. Secreted in response to physical or psychologic stress.
Anterior pituitary (adenohypophysis)	Growth hormone (GH)	Promotes growth of body tissues by enhancing protein synthesis and promoting use of fat for energy, thus conserving glucose. Release is stimulated by GH-releasing hormone in response to low GH levels, hypoglycemia, increased amino acids, low fatty acids, and stress.

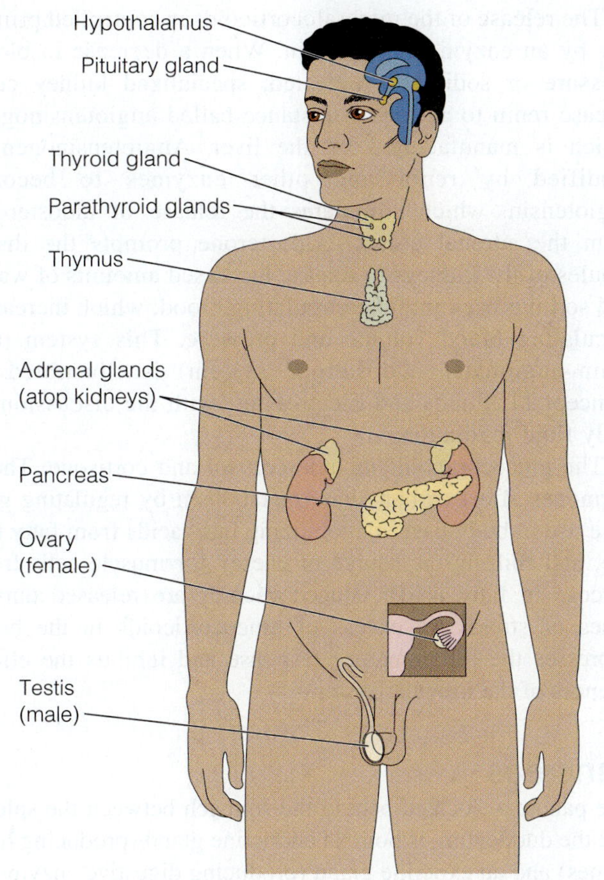

Figure 18–1 ■ Location of the major endocrine glands.

Thyroid Gland

The thyroid gland (Figure 18–3 ■) is anterior to the upper part of the trachea and just inferior to the larynx. This butterfly-shaped gland has two lobes connected by a structure called the isthmus.

The glandular tissue of the thyroid consists of follicles filled with a jellylike, colloid substance called thyroglobin, a glycoprotein–iodine complex. Cells within the follicles secrete thyroid hormone, a general name for two similar hormones: thyroxine (T_4) and triiodothyronine (T_3). The primary role of thyroid hormones in adults is to increase metabolism. Secretion of thyroid hormone is initiated by the release of TSH from the pituitary gland and is dependent on an adequate supply of iodine.

The thyroid gland also secretes calcitonin, a hormone that decreases excessive levels of calcium in the blood by slowing the calcium-releasing activity of bone cells. Although calcitonin also serves as a marker for sepsis and is believed to be a mediator of inflammatory responses, its functions are not fully understood. When the thyroid gland is totally removed and thyroid hormone replaced, calcium homeostasis and bone density remain relatively unchanged without replacing calcitonin.

Parathyroid Glands

The parathyroid glands (usually four to six in number) are embedded on the posterior surface of the lobes of the thyroid gland. They secrete parathyroid hormone (PTH), or parathormone. When calcium levels in the plasma fall, secretion of PTH increases in response. This increased secretion acts to maintain calcium levels by stimulating bone resorption and formation and by stimulating kidney resorption of calcium.

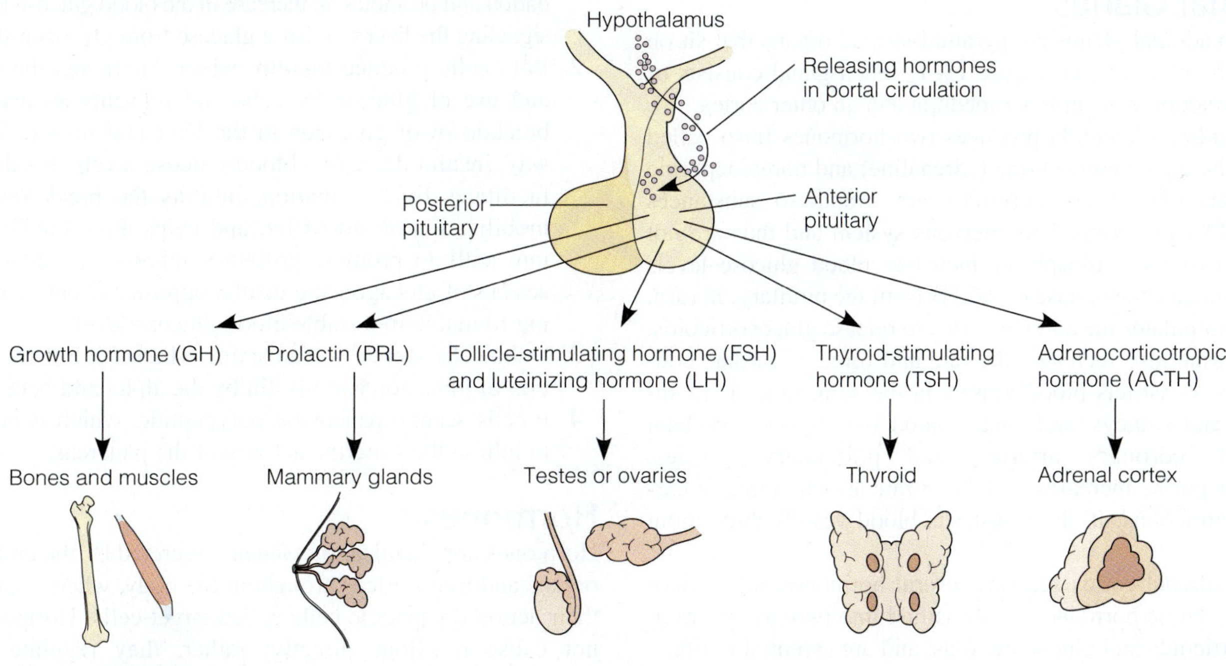

Figure 18–2 ■ Actions of the major hormones of the anterior pituitary gland.

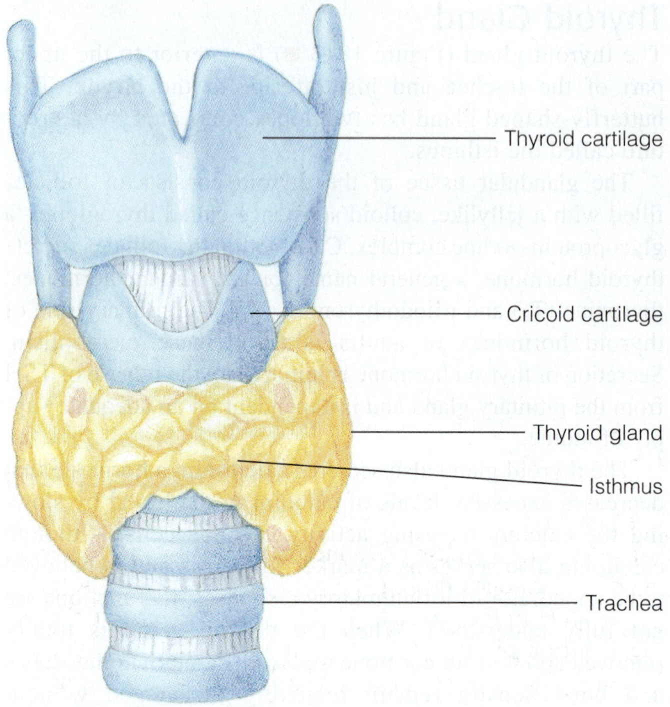

Figure 18–3 ■ The thyroid gland.

Source: Dorling Kindersley Media Library.

PTH also controls phosphate metabolism. It acts primarily by increasing renal excretion of phosphate in the urine, by decreasing the excretion of calcium, and by increasing bone reabsorption to cause the release of calcium from bones. Normal levels of vitamin D are necessary for PTH to exert these effects on bone and kidneys.

Adrenal Glands

The two adrenal glands are pyramid-shaped organs that sit on top of the kidneys (see Figure 18–1). Each gland consists of two distinct organs: an inner medulla and an outer cortex.

The adrenal medulla produces two hormones (also called catecholamines): epinephrine (adrenaline) and norepinephrine (noradrenaline). These hormones are similar to substances released by the sympathetic nervous system and thus are not essential to life. Epinephrine increases blood glucose levels and stimulates the release of ACTH from the pituitary; in turn, ACTH stimulates the adrenal cortex to release glucocorticoids. Epinephrine also increases the rate and force of cardiac contractions; constricts blood vessels in the skin, mucous membranes, and kidneys; and dilates blood vessels in the skeletal muscles, coronary arteries, and pulmonary arteries. Norepinephrine increases both heart rate and the force of cardiac contractions. It also constricts blood vessels throughout the body.

The adrenal cortex secretes several hormones, all corticosteroids. These hormones are classified into two groups, mineralocorticoids and glucocorticoids, and are essential to life.

The release of the mineralocorticoids is controlled primarily by an enzyme called renin. When a decrease in blood pressure or sodium is detected, specialized kidney cells release renin to act on a substance called angiotensinogen, which is manufactured by the liver. Angiotensinogen is modified by renin and other enzymes to become angiotensin, which stimulates the release of aldosterone from the adrenal cortex. Aldosterone prompts the distal tubules of the kidneys to release increased amounts of water and sodium back into the circulating blood, which increases circulating blood volume and pressure. This system (the renin–angiotensin–aldosterone system) is illustrated in Concept 11, Fluids and Electrolytes, with the discussion of body fluid regulation.

The glucocorticoids include cortisol and cortisone. These hormones affect carbohydrate metabolism by regulating glucose use in body tissues, mobilizing fatty acids from fatty tissue, and shifting the source of energy for muscle cells from glucose to fatty acids. Glucocorticoids are released during times of stress. An excess of glucocorticoids in the body depresses the inflammatory response and inhibits the effectiveness of the immune system.

Pancreas

The pancreas, located behind the stomach between the spleen and the duodenum, is both an endocrine gland (producing hormones) and an exocrine gland (producing digestive enzymes).

The endocrine cells of the pancreas produce hormones that regulate carbohydrate metabolism. They are clustered in bodies called pancreatic islets (or islets of Langerhans) scattered throughout the gland. Pancreatic islets have at least four different cell types:

1. Alpha cells produce glucagon, which decreases glucose oxidation and promotes an increase in the blood glucose level by signaling the liver to release glucose from glycogen stores.
2. Beta cells produce **insulin**, which facilitates the uptake and use of glucose by cells and prevents an excessive breakdown of glycogen in the liver and muscle. In this way, insulin decreases blood glucose levels. Insulin also facilitates lipid formation, inhibits the breakdown and mobilization of stored fat, and helps amino acids move into cells to promote protein synthesis. In general, the actions of glucagon and insulin oppose one another, helping to maintain a stable blood glucose level.
3. Delta cells secrete somatostatin, which inhibits the secretion of glucagon and insulin by the alpha and beta cells.
4. F cells secrete pancreatic polypeptide, which is believed to inhibit the exocrine activity of the pancreas.

Hormones

Hormones are chemical messengers secreted by the endocrine organs and transported throughout the body, where they exert their action on specific cells called target cells. Hormones do not cause reactions directly; rather, they regulate tissue responses. They may produce either generalized effects or local effects.

Hormones are transported from endocrine gland cells to target cells in the body in one of four ways:

1. Endocrine glands release most hormones, including thyroid hormone and insulin, into the bloodstream. Some hormones require a protein carrier.
2. Neurons release some hormones, such as epinephrine, into the bloodstream. This is called the neuroendocrine route.
3. The hypothalamus releases its hormones directly to target cells in the posterior pituitary by nerve cell extension.
4. With the paracrine method, released messengers diffuse through the interstitial fluid. This method of transport involves a number of hormonal peptides that are released throughout various organs and cells and act locally. An example is endorphins, which act to relieve pain.

Hormones that are released into the bloodstream circulate as either free, unbound molecules or as hormones attached to transport carriers. Peptide and protein hormones (e.g., insulin) circulate unbound, whereas steroid and thyroid hormones are carried by specific transport carriers synthesized by the liver. Hormone receptors are complex molecular structures located on or inside target cells. They act by binding to specific receptor sites located on the surfaces of the target cells. These receptors recognize a specific hormone and translate the message into a cellular response. The receptor sites are structured so that they respond only to a specific hormone; for example, receptors in the thyroid gland are responsive to TSH but not to LH. Drugs that compete with a hormone for binding to transport carrier molecules increase hormone action by increasing the availability of the free, unbound hormone.

Hormone levels are controlled by the pituitary gland and by feedback mechanisms. Although most feedback mechanisms are negative, a few are positive. Negative feedback is controlled much as the thermostat in a house regulates temperature. Sensors in the endocrine system detect changes in hormone levels and adjust hormone secretion to maintain normal body levels. When the sensors detect a decrease in hormone levels, they begin actions to cause an increase in hormone levels; when hormone levels rise above normal, the sensors cause a decrease in hormone production and release. For example, when the hypothalamus or anterior pituitary gland senses increased blood levels of thyroid hormone, it releases hormones, causing a reduction in the secretion of TSH, which in turn prompts a decrease in the output of thyroid hormone by the thyroid gland. For an illustration of negative feedback, see Figure 18–4 ■.

In positive-feedback mechanisms, increasing levels of one hormone cause another gland to release a hormone. For example, the increased production of estradiol (a female ovarian hormone) during the follicular stage of the menstrual cycle in turn stimulates increased FSH production by the anterior pituitary gland. Estradiol levels continue to increase until the ovarian follicle disappears, eliminating the source of the stimulation for FSH production, which then decreases.

Stimuli for hormone release may also be classified as hormonal, humoral, or neural (Figure 18–5 ■). In hormonal release, hypothalamic hormones stimulate the anterior pituitary to release hormones. Fluctuations in the serum level of these hormones in turn prompt other endocrine glands to release hormones. In humoral release, fluctuations in the serum levels of certain ions and nutrients stimulate specific endocrine glands to release hormones to bring these levels back to normal. In neural release, nerve fibers stimulate the release of hormones.

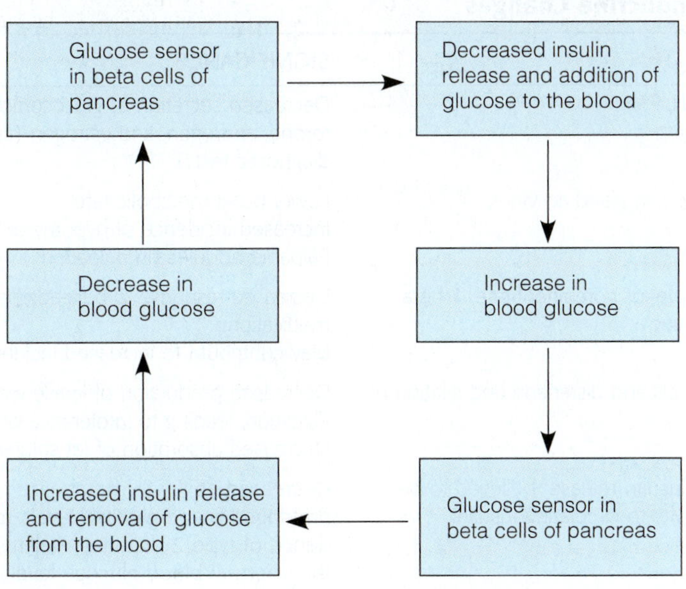

Figure 18–4 ■ Negative feedback.

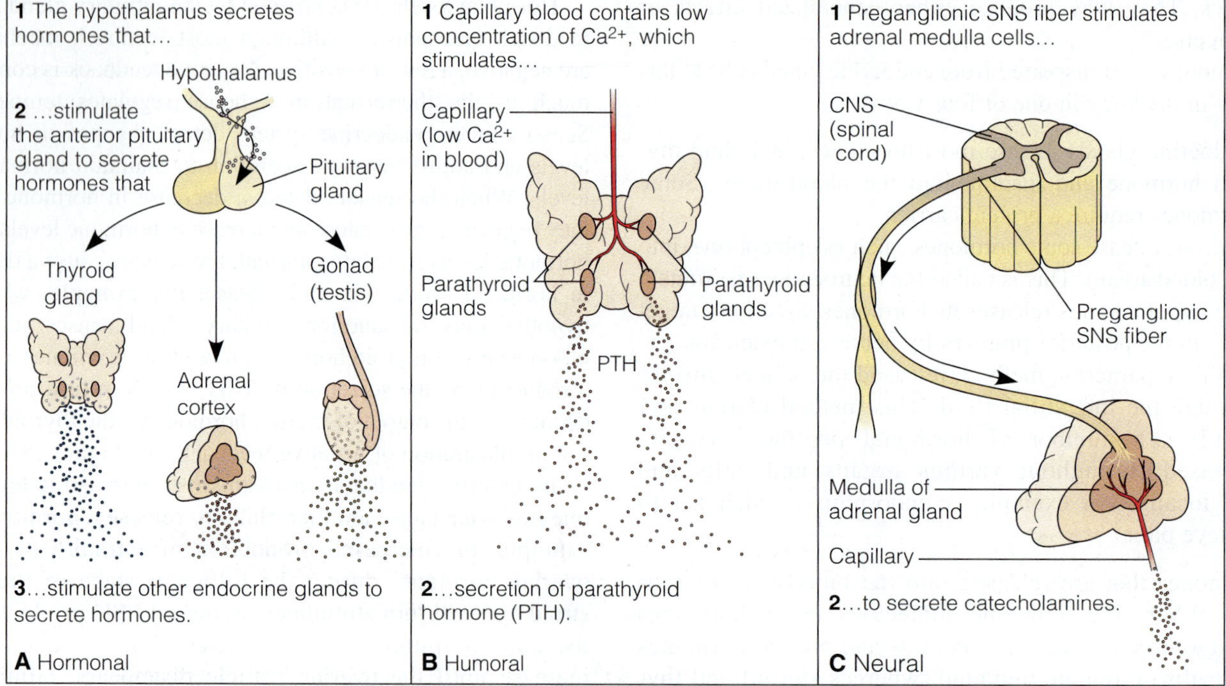

Figure 18–5 ■ Examples of three mechanisms of hormone release: *A*, hormonal; *B*, humoral; or *C*, neural. CNS = central nervous system; SNS = sympathetic nervous system.

AGE-RELATED CHANGES

The endocrine system is responsible for sexual differentiation during fetal development and for stimulating growth and development during childhood and adolescence. Growth hormone, produced by the anterior pituitary gland, is secreted in pulses when the child is in Stage 4 sleep. Growth hormone stimulates the growth of muscles and improves bone mineralization (Grimberg & De León, 2005). Multiple hormones in the endocrine system, including growth hormone, thyroid hormone, adrenal and gonadal androgens, and estrogen, are responsible for skeletal growth and maturation, including the appearance of secondary ossification centers in the bones

TABLE 18–2 **Age-Related Endocrine Changes**

AGE-RELATED CHANGE	SIGNIFICANCE
Pituitary: ↓ production of ACTH, TSH, FSH	Decreased secretion of glucocorticoids, 17-ketosteroids, progesterone, androgen, and estrogen (and thus lower levels on diagnostic tests)
Thyroid: ↑ in fibrosis and nodularity, ↓ in gland activity	Lower basal metabolic rate Increased incidence of hypothyroidism Palpable nodules on palpation
Adrenal medulla: ↑ secretion and level of norepinephrine, ↓ beta-adrenergic response to norepinephrine	Decreased response to beta-adrenergic and receptor-blocking medications May contribute to increased incidence of hypertension
Pancreas: calcification of blood vessels and distention and dilation of pancreatic ducts	Decreased production of lipase with reduced fat absorption and digestion, leading to intolerance of fatty foods and indigestion Decreased absorption of fat-soluble vitamins
Pancreas: delayed and decreased insulin release; believed to be accompanied by decreased sensitivity to circulating insulin	Decreased ability to metabolize glucose with higher and more prolonged blood glucose levels may contribute to increased incidence of type 2 diabetes mellitus with aging (however, higher-than-normal blood glucose levels are not unusual in older adults without diabetes)

(Carroll, 2006). Estrogen secretion associated with puberty is a dominant stimulator of increased skeletal maturity that can be detected by examining the child's bone age (Lee & Kulin, 2005). See Table 18–2 for normal age-related changes to the endocrine system in adults.

ALTERATIONS

Disorders of the structure and function of the endocrine glands alter normal hormone levels and the way that body tissues use those hormones. When hormone production increases or decreases, people experience alterations in health such as diabetes, obesity, osteoporosis, and glandular disorders.

Other alterations related to the endocrine system that are not covered as a part of this concept include, but are not limited to, the following:

- Leukodistrophies
- Menkes' disease
- Niemann-Pick disease
- Phenylketonuria
- Porphyria
- Tay-Sachs disease
- Zellweger's syndrome
- Maple syrup urine disease.

ALTERATIONS AND TREATMENTS Endocrine and Metabolic Disorders

Alteration	Description	Treatment
Diabetes mellitus	A disorder of hyperglycemia resulting from defects in insulin secretion, insulin action, or both, leading to abnormalities in carbohydrate, protein, and fat metabolism (American Diabetes Association, 2006).	■ Blood glucose monitoring ■ Maintain stable serum glucose levels
Type 1	Beta cells are destroyed, usually leading to absolute insulin deficiency.	■ Insulin ■ Dietary management ■ Exercise
Type 2	May range from predominantly insulin resistance with relative insulin deficiency to a predominantly secretory defect with insulin resistance.	■ Dietary management ■ Exercise ■ Weight management ■ Oral medication to improve insulin sensitivity
Obesity	Occurs when excess calories are stored as fat. It can result from excess energy intake, decreased energy expenditure, or a combination of both. Several hormones are involved in regulating obesity, including thyroid hormone, insulin, and leptin. Genetics also may have a role.	■ Individualized program of exercise, diet, and behavior modification ■ Pharmacotherapy ■ Bariatric surgery (usually limited to clients with morbid obesity: BMI > 40 kg/m^2, or $>200\%$ of ideal body weight)
Graves' disease	An autoimmune disorder, the most common cause of hyperthyroidism; occurs when immunoglobulins produced by B lymphocytes stimulate oversecretion of thyroid hormones.	■ Pharmacotherapy ■ Radioactive iodine therapy ■ Surgery (subtotal or total thyroidectomy)
Hypothyroidism	Results when the thyroid gland produces an insufficient amount of thyroid hormone; may be congenital or acquired.	■ Pharmacotherapy ■ Subtotal thyroidectomy (if goiter is large enough to cause respiratory difficulties or dysphagia)
Osteoporosis	Characterized by loss of bone mass, increased bone fragility, and increased risk of fractures.	■ Pharmacotherapy, including hormonal agents, biophosphonates, and selective estrogen receptor modulators (SERMs) ■ Weight-bearing exercises
Cirrhosis	In this end-stage liver disease, functional liver tissue is gradually destroyed and replaced by fibrous scar tissue, which forms constrictive bands that disrupt blood flow to liver lobules.	■ Pharmacotherapy to address manifestations ■ Procedures such as paracentesis, central line insertion, or balloon tamponade as necessary to treat manifestations and complications

PHYSICAL ASSESSMENT

Endocrine gland functions are assessed using findings from diagnostic tests, a health assessment interview to collect subjective data, and a physical assessment to collect objective data. Because hormones affect all body tissues and organs, manifestations of dysfunction often are nonspecific, sometimes making assessment of endocrine function more difficult than assessment of other body systems.

When conducting a health assessment interview and a physical assessment, it is important for the nurse to consider genetic influences on the health of the adult. During the health assessment interview, ask if any immediate family members have or have had endocrine disorders and, if so, the family member's age of onset and gender. Also ask the client about a family history of such diseases as diabetes mellitus, diabetes insipidus, thyroid disease, growth problems, hypertension, and obesity.

During the physical assessment, assess for any manifestations that might indicate a genetic disorder. If data are found to indicate genetic risk factors or alterations, ask if the client is willing to undergo genetic testing and, if so, refer for appropriate genetic counseling and evaluation.

A health assessment interview to determine problems with the endocrine system may be part of a health screening or a total health assessment, or it may focus on a chief complaint (e.g., increased urination or changes in energy levels). If the client has a problem with endocrine function, the nurse analyzes its onset, characteristics and course, severity, precipitating and relieving factors, and any associated symptoms, noting the timing and circumstances.

The health history includes information about the client's medical history, family history, and social and personal history. Ask the client about any changes in normal growth and development and in height and weight. Changes in the size of extremities often can be detected by asking whether the client has had to have rings enlarged or to buy increasingly larger gloves and shoes. Enlargement of the neck may be identified by asking whether the client has difficulty finding shirts or blouses with a collar that fits. Nurses also should explore such changes as difficulty swallowing; increased or decreased thirst, appetite, and/or urination; visual changes; sleep disturbances; altered patterns of hair distribution (e.g., increased facial hair in women); changes in menstruation; changes in memory or ability to concentrate; and changes in hair and skin texture. Ask the client about any blow to the head or previous hospitalizations, chemotherapy, radiation (especially to the neck), and use of medications (especially hormones or steroids).

Ask about the client's occupational and social history as well. Include questions about the client's satisfaction with his or her occupation, personal relationships, and lifestyle. Other areas of assessment include the client's usual means of coping; use of alcohol, smoking, or drugs; diet (including weight gain

Assessment Interview Endocrine System

GENERAL

- Have you had any problems with an endocrine gland (pituitary, thyroid, parathyroid, adrenal, pancreas, ovaries, testes)?
- If you had a problem with any of these glands, how was it treated (medications, surgery, diet, hormone replacement)?
- Does anyone in your family have an endocrine disorder? If so, when did it begin, and how does it affect them? What family member is affected, and at what age did it begin?
- Do you smoke, drink alcohol, or use recreational drugs? If so, how much and what kind?
- Have you ever been tested for high or low blood sugar?

NUTRITION AND METABOLISM

- Describe what you eat as well as how much (and what type of) fluid you drink in a 24-hour period.
- Do you take any nutritional supplements, herbs, or vitamins?
- Have you noticed any change in your hunger or thirst?
- Has your weight changed? If so, by how many pounds and over what time period?
- Have you noticed any change in your energy level? If so, explain.
- Have you noticed any change in your ability to tolerate heat or cold?
- Have you noticed any difficulty swallowing? If so, explain.
- Have you noticed any change in the texture of your skin? If so, what were they?
- Have you noticed any change in the color, odor, amount, or frequency of urination? If so, describe it.
- Describe your physical activities in a usual day.
- Has your energy level increased or decreased? If so, explain.
- Do some activities make you very tired? Explain how you feel.
- How many hours of sleep do you get each night?
- Do you feel nervous and unable to rest?
- Do you sweat at night?
- Have you noticed any change in the color or condition of your skin and hair (color, dryness, oiliness, bruises)?

COGNITION AND SENSORY PERCEPTION

- Have you noticed any problem with your memory?
- Do you feel restless, anxious, or confused?
- Have you noticed any change in your voice?
- Have you had any headaches, memory loss, changes in sensation, or depression? If so, describe them.
- Have you noticed any change in your vision? If so, describe it.
- Have you had any heart palpitations?
- Have you had any abdominal pain? If so, what is it like, and where is it located?
- Have you had any pain or stiffness in your muscles and joints?

STRESS AND COPING

- How does this condition make you feel about yourself?
- How do you feel about taking medications?
- How does this condition affect your relationships with others? with your work?
- Does stress seem to make your condition worse? Explain.
- Describe what you do when you feel stressed.
- Describe any social or community pressures or activities that affect how you care for and feel about this condition.
- Are there any specific treatments that you would not use to treat this condition?

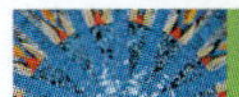

Endocrine Assessments

Techniques and Normal Findings	Abnormal Findings
Skin Assessments with Abnormal Findings	
Inspect skin color. *Skin color should be even and appropriate to the age and race of the client.*	■ Hyperpigmentation may be seen in clients with Addison's disease or Cushing's syndrome. ■ Hypopigmentation may be seen in clients with diabetes mellitus, hyperthyroidism, or hypothyroidism. ■ A yellowish cast to the skin might indicate hypothyroidism. ■ Purple striae over the abdomen and bruising may be present in clients with Cushing's syndrome.
Palpate the skin, assessing texture, moisture, and the presence of lesions. *Skin should be appropriate to the client's race, smooth, warm, dry, and intact, without abnormal lesions.*	■ Rough, dry skin often is seen in clients with hypothyroidism, whereas smooth and flushed skin can be a sign of hyperthyroidism. ■ Lesions (e.g., ulcerations) on the lower extremities might indicate diabetes mellitus.
Nails and Hair Assessment With Abnormal Findings	
Assess texture, distribution, and condition of the nails and hair. *Hair should be of normal texture and appropriately distributed for gender; nails surfaces should have even color with smooth surfaces.*	■ Increased pigmentation of the nails often is seen in clients with Addison's disease. ■ Dry, thick, brittle nails and hair may be apparent in clients with hypothyroidism; thin, brittle nails and thin, soft hair may be apparent in clients with hyperthyroidism. ■ Hirsutism (excessive facial, chest, or abdominal hair) may be seen in clients with Cushing's syndrome.
Facial Assessments With Abnormal Findings	
Inspect the symmetry and form of the face. *Face should be bilaterally symmetric.*	■ Variations of form and structure may indicate growth abnormalities, such as **acromegaly** (continued growth of bone from growth hormone hypersecretion).
Inspect position of eyes. *Eyes should be equal in position on both sides of the face. Eyelids should close over the eyes.*	■ **Exophthalmos** (protruding eyes) may be seen in clients with hyperthyroidism.
Thyroid Gland Assessment with Abnormal Findings	
Palpate the thyroid gland for size and consistency. Stand behind the client, and place your fingers on either side of the trachea below the thyroid cartilage (Figure 18–6 ■). Ask the client to tilt the head to the right. Now ask the client to swallow. As the client swallows, displace the left lobe while palpating the right lobe. Repeat to palpate the left lobe. *The thyroid gland is not usually palpable. If it is, the lobes should feel smooth, rubbery, and free of nodules.*	■ The thyroid may be enlarged in clients with Graves' disease or a **goiter** (enlarged thyroid gland). ■ Multiple nodules may be seen in clients with metabolic disorders, whereas the presence of only one nodule may indicate a cyst or a benign or malignant tumor. ■ One enlarged nodule suggests malignancy.
Motor Function Assessment With Abnormal Findings	
Assess the deep tendon reflexes. Deep tendon reflexes are assessed with the reflex hammer and include the biceps reflex, brachioradialis reflex, triceps reflex, patellar reflex, and Achilles reflex. *Normal values range from 1+ (present but decreased) to 2+ (normal) to 3+ (increased).*	■ Increased reflexes may be seen in clients hyperthyroidism; decreased reflexes may be seen in those with hypothyroidism.

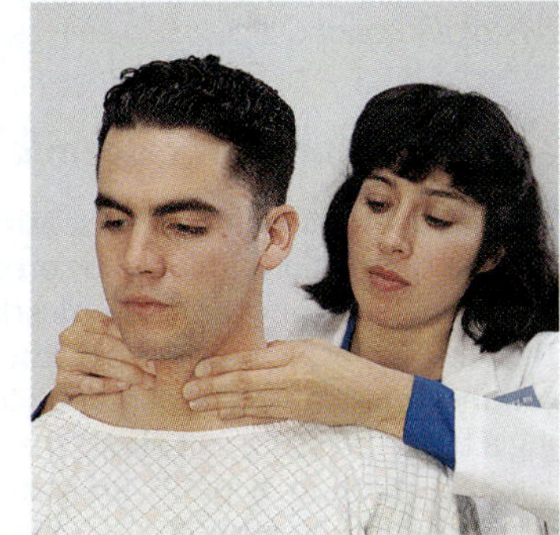

Figure 18–6 ■ Palpating the thyroid gland from behind the client.

(continued)

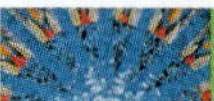

Endocrine Assessments (continued)

Techniques and Normal Findings | **Abnormal Findings**

Sensory Function Assessment With Abnormal Findings

Test the client's sensitivity to pain, temperature, vibration, light touch, and stereognosis (the ability to identify an object merely by touch). Ask the client to close his or her eyes. Then, compare symmetric areas on both sides of the body, and compare the distal to the proximal regions of the extremities:

- To test pain, use the blunt and sharp ends of a new safety pin. Discard the pin after use.
- To test temperature, use cups or other containers of cold and hot water.
- To test vibration, use a tuning fork over one of the client's finger or toe joints.
- To test light touch, use a cotton wisp.
- To test stereognosis, place in the client's hand a simple, familiar object, such as a rubber band, cotton ball, or button. Ask the client to identify the object.

Sensory function should be bilaterally intact.

- Peripheral neuropathy and paresthesias (altered sensations) may occur in clients with diabetes, hypothyroidism, or acromegaly.

Musculoskeletal Assessment With Abnormal Findings

Inspect the size and proportions of the client's body structure. *Size and proportion of body structures should be bilaterally equal.*

- Extremely short stature may indicate **dwarfism**, which is caused by insufficient growth hormone.
- Extremely large bones may indicate acromegaly, which is caused by excessive growth hormone.

Assessing for Hypocalcemic Tetany

Assess for **Trousseau's sign** (spasmodic muscle contractions induced by pressure on the nerves going to those muscles; a test for hypocalcemia) with resulting **tetany** (tonic muscle spasms) by inflating a blood pressure cuff above the antecubital space to a point greater than systolic blood pressure for 2–5 minutes. *A normal finding is no carpal spasm in response to compression of the arm by the blood pressure cuff.*

- Decreased calcium levels cause the client's hand and fingers to contract (**carpal spasm**).

Assess for **Chvostek's sign** (facial grimacing caused by repeated contractions of the facial muscle; a test for hypocalcemia) by tapping your finger in front of the client's ear at the angle of the jaw. *A normal finding is no facial grimacing in response to tapping the client's face in front of the ear.*

- Decreased calcium levels cause the client's lateral facial muscles to contract.

or loss); exercise patterns; and sleep patterns. Although the client may not recognize changes in behavior, family members may be able to provide important information.

Physical assessment of the endocrine system may be performed as part of a total health assessment, or it may be a focused assessment of clients who have known or suspected problems with endocrine function. The only endocrine organ that can be palpated is the thyroid gland; however, other assessments that provide information about endocrine problems include inspection of the skin, hair, nails, facial appearance, reflexes, and musculoskeletal system. Measuring and monitoring trends in height and weight and in vital signs also provide clues to altered function of the endocrine system.

DIAGNOSTIC TESTS

The results of diagnostic tests are used to support the diagnosis of a specific disease, to provide information to identify or modify the appropriate medication or therapy used to treat the disease, and to help nurses monitor the client's responses to treatment and nursing care interventions. Specific diagnostic tests to assess the structure and function of the glands of the endocrine system are described in the Diagnostic Tests feature regarding the endocrine system in the Appendix and may include, but are not limited to:

- Serum blood sugarA1c
- T3, T4, TSH
- Individual hormone levels—parathyroid, catecholamines, estrogen, progesterone, growth hormone, etc
- Serum electrolytes
- Liver enzymes (AST, ALT, SGOT, LDH)
- Bilirubin
- Serum albumin
- Serum calcium.

CARING INTERVENTIONS

Clients with the disorders discussed in this concept—diabetes, obesity, thyroid disease, osteoporosis, and liver disease—require multidisciplinary care for multiple problems. They often face exhausting diagnostic tests, changes in physical appearance and emotional responses, and permanent alterations in lifestyle. Nursing care is directed toward meeting physiologic needs of the client, providing education, and ensuring psychologic support for the client and family. A holistic approach to the complex needs of clients with metabolic disorders is an essential component of nursing care.

PHARMACOLOGIC THERAPIES

The goals of hormone pharmacotherapy vary widely. In many cases, a hormone is administered as replacement therapy for clients who are unable to secrete sufficient quantities of their own endogenous hormones. Examples of replacement therapy include administering thyroid hormone after the thyroid gland has been surgically removed or supplying insulin to clients whose pancreas is not functioning. Replacement therapy supplies the same physiologic, low-level amounts of the hormone that would normally be present in the body.

MEDICATIONS Metabolic and Endocrine Disorders

Classification	Mechanism of Action	Common Drugs	Nursing Considerations
Insulin	Replacement therapy; insulin is an endogenous hormone secreted by the beta cells of the pancreas. It lowers the blood glucose level by stimulating passage of glucose across cell membranes and uptake into the cells. It also promotes the conversion of glucose to glycogen and inhibits the production of hepatic glucose from glycogen.	Insulin available in short-acting (Humalog R), intermidiate-acting (NPH), and long-acting(insulin detemir) forms	■ Monitor for and discard vials past the expiration date. ■ Refrigerate, but do not freeze, extra insulin vials not currently in use. ■ Store insulin in a cool place, and avoid exposure to temperature extremes or sunlight. ■ Store compatible mixtures of insulin for no longer than 1 month at room temperature or 3 months at 36–46°F (2–8°C). ■ Discard any vials with discoloration, clumping, granules, or solid deposits on the sides.
Antithyroid agents	Inhibit thyroid hormone (TH) synthesis and release	■ Potassium iodide (Thyro-Block) ■ Methimazole (Tapazole) ■ Propylthiouracil ■ Radioactive iodide (I-131, Iodotope)	■ Assess for hypersensitivity to iodine before giving medication (e.g., ask client about allergies to shellfish). ■ Dilute liquid iodine sources in water or orange juice to disguise bitter taste. ■ Monitor for increased bleeding tendencies if the client is also taking anticoagulants (iodine increases their effect). ■ Administer drugs at the same time each day with meals to maintain stable blood levels.

(continued)

MEDICATIONS Metabolic and Endocrine Disorders (continued)

Classification	Mechanism of Action	Common Drugs	Nursing Considerations
Thyroid agents	Increase blood levels of TH, raising the metabolic rate	■ Levothyroxine sodium (T_4; Levoxyl, Levothroid, Synthroid) ■ Liothyronine sodium (T_3; Cytomel) ■ Liotrix (T_3–T_4; Euthyroid, Thyrolar)	■ For best absorption give 1 hour before meals or 2 hours after meals. ■ Thyroid preparations potentiate the effect of anticoagulant drugs. ■ Thyroid medications potentiate the effect of digitalis. ■ The effect of insulin may change as thyroid function increases. ■ During dose adjustment, take the client's pulse before administering the drug. Report a pulse > 100 bpm.
Hormonal agents	Selective estrogen-receptor modulators (SERMs) appear to prevent bone loss by mimicking estrogen's beneficial effects on bone density in postmenopausal women. Synthetic parathyroid hormone, administered subcutaneously stimulates new bone formation and mass.	Calcitonin: ■ Calcitonin—human (Cibacalcin) ■ Calcitonin—salmon (Calciman, Miacalcin) SERMs: ■ Raloxifene hydrochloride (Evista) Synthetic parathyroid hormones: ■ Teriparatide (Forteo)	■ Parenteral and nasal spray forms may cause an anaphylactic-type allergic response. ■ Alternate nostrils daily when administering calcitonin nasal spray. ■ Observe for side effects. ■ Teach the client the proper technique for handling and injecting the drug at home. ■ Hot flashes are a common side effect.
Bisphosphonates	Bisphosphonates are potent inhibitors of bone resorption that may be used to prevent and treat osteoporosis. They inhibit bone breakdown, preserve bone mass, and increase bone density in the hip and vertebrae.	■ Alendronate sodium (Fosamax) ■ Etidronate disodium (Didronel) ■ Ibandronate (Boniva) ■ Pamidronate disodium (Aredia) ■ Risedronate sodium (Actonel) ■ Tiludronate disodium (Skelid).	■ Should not be taken by a woman with a history of blood clots. ■ Take on an empty stomach, first thing in the morning, with water. ■ Remain upright for 30 minutes, and do not eat or drink anything else for 30 minutes to avoid esophagitis ■ Monitor for pathological fractures and bone pain. ■ Monitor for GI side effects. ■ Monitor calcium lab values. ■ Monitor kidney function, especially creatinine level. ■ Monitor BUN, vitamin D, urinalysis, and serum phosphate and magnesium levels. ■ Monitor dietary habits for adequate intake of vitamin D, calcium, and phosphate.)

18.1 DIABETES

KEY TERMS

BASIS FOR SELECTION OF EXEMPLAR

Institute of Medicine

Healthy People 2010

LEARNING OUTCOMES

After reading about this exemplar, you will be able to:

1. Describe the pathophysiology, etiology, clinical manifestations, and direct and indirect causes of diabetes mellitus.
2. Identify risk factors associated with diabetes mellitus.
3. Illustrate the nursing process in providing culturally competent care across the life span for individuals with diabetes mellitus.
4. Formulate priority nursing diagnoses appropriate for an individual with diabetes mellitus.
5. Create plan of care for individuals with diabetes mellitus and their family members.
6. Assess expected outcomes for an individual with diabetes mellitus.
7. Discuss therapies used in the collaborative care of an individual with diabetes mellitus.
8. Employ evidence-based caring interventions for an individual with diabetes mellitus.

OVERVIEW

Diabetes mellitus (also referred to more simply as diabetes) is a disorder of hyperglycemia resulting from defects in insulin secretion, insulin action, or both, leading to abnormalities in carbohydrate, protein, and fat metabolism (American Diabetes Association, 2006). There are four major types of diabetes: type 1 diabetes mellitus (type 1 DM; 5–10% of diagnosed cases), type 2 diabetes mellitus (type 2 DM; 90–95% of diagnosed cases), gestational diabetes (2–5% of all pregnancies), and other specific types of diabetes (1–2% of diagnosed cases).

Role of Hormones

The endocrine pancreas produces hormones necessary for the metabolism and cellular utilization of carbohydrates, proteins, and fats. The cells that produce these hormones are clustered in groups of cells called the islets of Langerhans. These islets have three different types of cells:

1. Alpha cells produce the hormone **glucagon**, which stimulates the breakdown of glycogen in the liver, the formation of carbohydrates in the liver, and the breakdown of lipids in both the liver and adipose tissue. The primary function of glucagon is to decrease glucose oxidation and to increase blood glucose levels. Through **glycogenolysis** (the breakdown of liver glycogen) and **gluconeogenesis** (the formation of glucose from fats and proteins), glucagon prevents blood glucose from decreasing below a certain level when the body is fasting or between meals. The action of glucagon is initiated in most people when blood glucose falls below approximately 70 mg/dL.
2. Beta cells secrete the hormone **insulin**, which facilitates the movement of glucose across cell membranes into cells, thus decreasing blood glucose levels. Insulin prevents the excessive breakdown of glycogen in the liver and in muscle, facilitates the formation of lipid while inhibiting the breakdown of stored fats, and helps to move amino acids into cells for protein synthesis. After secretion by the beta cells, insulin enters the portal circulation, travels directly to the liver, and is then released into the general circulation. Circulating insulin is rapidly bound to receptor sites on peripheral tissues (especially muscle and fat cells) or is destroyed by the liver or kidneys. Insulin release is regulated by blood glucose: It increases when blood glucose levels increase, and it decreases when blood glucose levels decrease. When a person eats food, insulin levels begin to rise in minutes, peak in 30 to 60 minutes, and return to baseline in 2–3 hours.
3. Delta cells produce **somatostatin**, which is believed to be a neurotransmitter that inhibits the production of both glucagon and insulin.

Blood Glucose Homeostasis

All body tissues and organs require a constant supply of glucose; however, not all tissues require insulin for glucose uptake. The brain, liver, intestines, and renal tubules do not require insulin to transfer glucose into their cells. Skeletal muscle, cardiac muscle, and adipose tissue require insulin for glucose movement into the cells.

Normal blood glucose is maintained in healthy people primarily through the actions of insulin and glucagon. Increased blood glucose levels, amino acids, and fatty acids stimulate pancreatic

FOCUS ON DIVERSITY AND CULTURE **Risk and Incidence of Diabetes**

- *Non-Hispanic whites:* 13.1 million (8.7%) of those aged 20 years or older have diabetes.
- *Non-Hispanic African Americans:* 3.2 million (13.3%) have diabetes. This group is 1.8 times as likely to have diabetes as non-Hispanic whites of similar age. In addition, African Americans with type 2 diabetes mellitus have higher rates of coronary heart disease, cerebrovascular accident, and end-stage renal disease than do whites with the disease.
- *Hispanic/Latino Americans:* 2.5 million (9.5%) have diabetes. This group is 1.7 times as likely to have diabetes as non-Hispanic whites of similar age, and Mexican Americans are twice as likely to have diabetes as non-Hispanic whites of similar age.
- *American Indians and Alaska Natives:* This group is 2.2 times as likely to have diabetes as non-Hispanic whites, and diabetes is especially prevalent in American Indians who are middle-age or older. Diabetes is most common among Native Americans of the southern United States (27.8%) and is least common among Alaska natives (8.1%) (Centers for Disease Control and Prevention, 2005).

beta cells to produce insulin. As the cells of cardiac muscle, skeletal muscle, and adipose tissue take up glucose, plasma levels of nutrients decrease, which suppresses the stimulus to produce insulin. If blood glucose falls, glucagon is released to raise hepatic glucose output, which raises glucose levels. Epinephrine, growth hormone, T_4, and glucocorticoids (often referred to as glucose counterregulatory hormones) also stimulate an increase in glucose in times of hypoglycemia, stress, growth, or increased metabolic demand. The regulation of blood glucose levels by insulin and glucagon is illustrated in Figure 18–7 ■.

TYPE 1 DIABETES MELLITUS

Type 1 DM, formerly called juvenile-onset diabetes or insulin-dependent diabetes mellitus, is the result of pancreatic islet cell destruction and a total deficit of circulating insulin.

Pathophysiology and Etiology

Type 1 DM results from destruction of the beta cells of the islets of Langerhans in the pancreas—the only cells in the body that make insulin. When beta cells are destroyed, insulin is no longer produced. Although type 1 DM may be classified as either an autoimmune or an idiopathic disorder, 90% of the cases are immune mediated. The disorder begins with insulinitis, a chronic inflammatory process that occurs in response to the autoimmune destruction of islet cells. This process, which slowly destroys beta cell production of insulin, usually occurs over a long preclinical period, with the onset of hyperglycemia occurring when 80–90% of beta cell function is lost. It is believed that both alpha-cell and beta-cell functions are abnormal, with a lack of insulin and a relative excess of glucagon resulting in hyperglycemia.

ETIOLOGY Type 1 DM most often occurs in childhood and adolescence, but it may occur at any age, even in the 80s and 90s. The actual cause and exact sequence are not completely understood.

Genetic predisposition plays a role in the development of type 1 DM (see the Focus on Diversity and Culture feature earlier in this exemplar), and environmental factors are believed to trigger development of the disorder. The trigger can be a viral infection (e.g., mumps, rubella, or coxsackievirus B4) or a chemical toxin (e.g., those found in smoked and cured meats). As a result of exposure to the virus or chemical, an abnormal autoimmune response occurs in which antibodies respond to normal islet beta cells as though they were foreign substances—in other words, by destroying them.

RISK FACTORS Although the risk in the general population ranges from 1 in 400 to 1 in 1,000, the child of a person with diabetes has a risk of 1 in 20 to 1 in 50. Genetic markers that determine immune responses have been found in 95% of people diagnosed with type 1 DM. The presence of these markers does not guarantee that the person will develop type 1 DM, but it does indicate increased susceptibility (Porth, 2005).

Clinical Manifestations

Type 1 DM is characterized by **hyperglycemia** (elevated blood glucose levels), a breakdown of body fats and proteins, and development of **ketosis** (an accumulation of ketone bodies produced

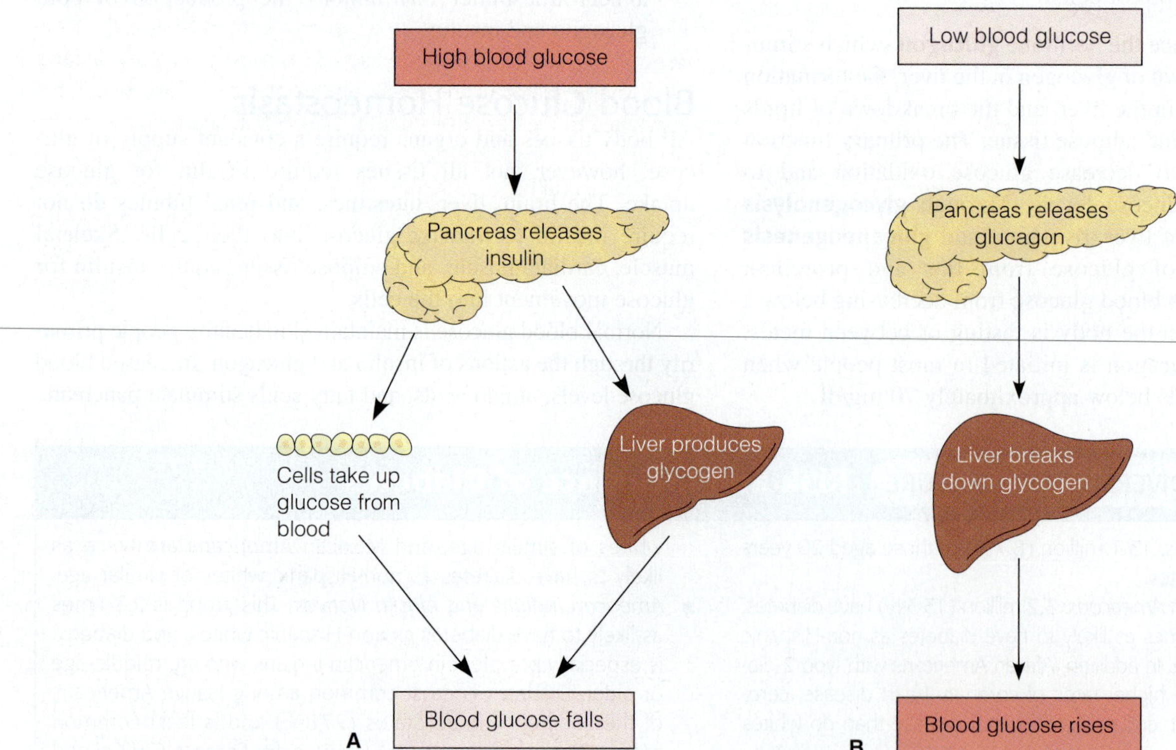

Figure 18–7 ■ Regulation (homeostasis) of blood glucose levels by insulin and glucagon. *A,* High blood glucose is lowered by insulin release. *B,* Low blood glucose is raised by glucagon release.

CLINICAL MANIFESTATIONS AND THERAPIES Type 1 Diabetes Mellitus

ETIOLOGY	CLINICAL MANIFESTATION	CLINICAL THERAPIES
Immune-mediated insulin deficiency caused by pancreatic beta-cell destruction	Polyuria, polydipsia Recent weight loss, but client may be overweight Ketoacidosis on initial presentation in 30–40% of cases, at continued risk for ketoacidosis Short duration of symptoms Ketosis Initial period of decreased insulin requirement, then need of insulin for survival	■ Blood glucose monitoring ■ Insulin ■ Dietary management, balancing carbohydrate intake to insulin ■ Exercise

during oxidation of fatty acids). As mentioned, the manifestations of type 1 DM appear when approximately 90% of the beta cells are destroyed. However, manifestations may appear at any time during the loss of beta cells if an acute illness or stress increases the demand for insulin beyond the reserves of the damaged cells.

The clinical manifestations of type 1 DM result from a lack of insulin to transport glucose across the cell membrane into the cells. Glucose molecules accumulate in the circulating blood, resulting in hyperglycemia. Hyperglycemia causes serum hyperosmolality, drawing water from the intracellular spaces into the general circulation. The increased blood volume increases renal blood flow, and the hyperglycemia acts as an osmotic diuretic. The resulting osmotic diuresis increases urine output (**polyuria**). When the blood glucose level exceeds the renal threshold for glucose—usually approximately 180 mg/dL—glucose is excreted in the urine (**glucosuria**). The decrease in intracellular volume and the increased urinary output cause dehydration. The mouth becomes dry, and thirst sensors are activated, causing the person to drink increased amounts of fluid (**polydipsia**).

Because glucose cannot enter the cell without insulin, energy production decreases. This decrease in energy stimulates hunger, causing the individual to eat more food (**polyphagia**). Despite increased food intake, the person loses weight as the body loses water and breaks down proteins and fats in an attempt to restore energy sources. Malaise and fatigue accompany the decrease in energy. Blurred vision also is common, resulting from osmotic effects that cause the lenses of the eyes to swell.

Thus, the classic manifestations of type 1 DM are polyuria, polydipsia, and polyphagia, accompanied by weight loss, malaise, and fatigue. Depending on the degree of insulin lack, the manifestations vary from slight to severe. People with type 1 DM require **exogenous insulin** (insulin from a source outside the body) to maintain life.

TYPE 2 DIABETES MELLITUS

Type 2 DM was formerly labeled non-insulin-dependent diabetes mellitus or adult-onset diabetes; however, a disturbingly large number of children are being diagnosed with type 2 diabetes believed to be related to the increase in childhood obesity. Type 2 DM results from insulin resistance with a defect in compensatory insulin secretion.

Pathophysiology and Etiology

Type 2 DM is a condition of fasting hyperglycemia that occurs despite the availability of **endogenous insulin** (insulin that is produced by one's own body). The level of insulin produced varies in type 2 DM, and despite the availability of insulin, its function is impaired by insulin resistance. Insulin resistance forces the pancreas to work harder and produce more insulin, but when demand exceeds supply, type 2 DM results (Saudek & Margolis, 2005). Whatever the cause, there is sufficient production of insulin to prevent the breakdown of fats with resultant ketosis; thus, type 2 DM is characterized as a nonketotic form of diabetes. However, the amount of insulin available is not sufficient to lower blood glucose levels through the uptake of glucose by muscle and fat cells.

ETIOLOGY Type 2 DM can occur at any age, but it usually is seen in those who are middle-age and older. Heredity plays a role in its transmission (see the Focus on Diversity and Culture feature earlier in this exemplar). In the United States, the incidence of type 2 DM has increased 33% during the past decade.

A major factor in the development of type 2 DM is cellular resistance to the effect of insulin. This resistance is increased by obesity, inactivity, illnesses, medications, and increasing age. In obesity, insulin has a decreased ability to influence glucose metabolism and uptake by the liver, skeletal muscles, and adipose tissue. The exact reason for this is not clear, but weight loss and exercise may improve the mechanism responsible for insulin receptor binding or postreceptor activity (McCance & Huether, 2002).

Risk Factors

The major risk factors for type 2 DM are as follows:

- History of diabetes in parents or siblings. Although no HLA linkage has been identified, the children of a person with type 2 DM have a 15% chance of developing type 2 DM and a 30% risk of developing a glucose intolerance (the inability to metabolize carbohydrate normally).
- Obesity, defined as being at least 20% over the desired body weight or having a body mass index of at least 27 kg/m^2. Obesity, especially of the upper body, decreases the number of available insulin receptor sites in cells of skeletal muscles and adipose tissues, a process called peripheral insulin resistance. In addition, obesity impairs the ability of the beta cells to release insulin in response to increasing glucose levels.

- Physical inactivity.
- Race/ethnicity.
- In women, a history of gestational diabetes, polycystic ovary syndrome, or delivering a baby weighing more than 9 lb.
- Hypertension (≥130/85 mmHg in adults), high-density lipoprotein (HDL) cholesterol of ≥35 mg/dL, and/or a triglyceride level of ≥250 mg/dL.
- Metabolic syndrome, which is a cluster of manifestations associated with type 2 DM and thought to link cardiovascular disease with insulin resistance (Larsen, Kronenberg, Melmed, & Polonsky, 2003). Hypertension, abdominal obesity, dyslipidemia, elevated C-reactive protein, and a fasting blood glucose greater than 110 mg/dL increase the risk of type 2 DM, coronary heart disease, and stroke (Porth, 2005; Saudek & Margolis, 2005). This syndrome is thought to exist in more than half of all Americans who are older than 50 years. Although there is widespread acknowledgment that these manifestations are associated with type 2 DM, clinicians differ about the appropriate treatment (Larsen et al., 2003; Tierney, McPhee, & Papadakis, 2005).

Clinical Manifestations

The client with type 2 DM experiences a slow onset of manifestations and often is unaware of the disease until he or she seeks health care for some other problem. Hyperglycemia increases gradually and may exist for a long time before diabetes is diagnosed; thus, approximately half of those with newly diagnosed type 2 DM already have complications (Capriotti, 2005).

The hyperglycemia in type 2 DM usually is not as severe as that in type 1, but similar symptoms occur, especially polyuria and polydipsia. Polyphagia is not often seen, and weight loss is uncommon. Other manifestations that result from hyperglycemia include blurred vision, fatigue, paresthesias, and skin infections. If available insulin decreases, especially during times of physical or emotional stress, the person with type 2 DM may develop diabetic ketoacidosis, but this is uncommon.

Treatment usually begins with prescriptions for weight loss and increased activity. If these changes can be sustained, no further treatment will be necessary for many individuals. Hypoglycemic medications are begun when lifestyle changes are insufficient. Often, a combination of insulin and hypoglycemic medication is used to achieve the best glycemic control in the client with type 2 DM.

COMPLICATIONS OF DIABETES

The person with diabetes, regardless of type, is at increased risk for complications involving many body systems. Alterations in blood glucose levels, alterations in the cardiovascular system, neuropathies, increased susceptibility to infection, and periodontal disease are common. In addition, the interaction of several complications can cause problems of the feet. The Multisystem Effects feature that follows shows the progression from cardinal signs to acute and late complications for the client with diabetes. A discussion of each of these complications follows; nursing care and related collaborative care are discussed later.

Acute Complications

The following discussion provides additional information about hyperglycemia and hypoglycemia. Table 18–3 compares diabetic ketoacidosis, hyperosmolar hyperglycemic state, and hypoglycemia.

HYPERGLYCEMIA The major problems resulting from hyperglycemia in the person with diabetes are diabetic ketoacidosis and hyperosmolar hyperglycemic state. Two other problems are the dawn phenomenon and the Somogyi phenomenon.

Dawn Phenomenon The **dawn phenomenon** is a rise in blood glucose between 4 a.m. and 8 a.m. that is not a response to hypoglycemia. This condition occurs in people with both type 1 and type 2 DM. The exact cause is unknown, but it is believed to relate to nocturnal increases in growth hormone, which decrease peripheral uptake of glucose.

CLINICAL MANIFESTATIONS AND THERAPIES Type 2 Diabetes Mellitus

ETIOLOGY	CLINICAL MANIFESTATION	CLINICAL THERAPIES
Insulin resistance with relative insulin secretory defect	Obese, little or no weight loss, or may have significant recent weight loss Acanthosis nigricans Long duration of symptoms Polyuria, polydipsia; may be mild or absent Glycosuria without ketonuria on initial presentation in 33% of cases Ketoacidosis on initial presentation in 5–25% of cases Lipid disorders Hypertension Androgen-mediated problems (e.g., acne, hirsutism, menstrual disturbances, polycystic ovary disease) Excessive weight gain and fatigue caused by insulin resistance	■ Diet with decreased calories and low-fat foods ■ Decrease sedentary activity time, or increase routine physical activity ■ Blood glucose monitoring ■ Oral medication (metformin) to improve insulin sensitivity

TABLE 18–3 Comparison of Diabetic Ketoacidosis (DKA), Hyperosmolar Hyperglycemic State (HHS), and Hypoglycemia

		DKA	HHS	HYPOGLYCEMIA
Diabetes type		Primary type 1	Type 2	Both
Onset		Slow	Slow	Rapid
Cause		↓ Insulin	↓ Insulin	↑ Insulin
		Infection	Older age	Omitted meal/snack
				Error in insulin dose
Risk factors		Surgery	Surgery	Surgery
		Trauma	Trauma	Trauma
		Illness	Illness	Illness
		Omitted insulin	Dehydration	Exercise
		Stress	Medications	Medications
			Dialysis	Lipodystrophy
			Hyperalimentation	Renal failure
				Alcohol intake
Assessments	Skin	Flushed, dry, warm	Flushed, dry, warm	Pallor, moist, cool
	Perspiration	None	None	Profuse
	Thirst	Increased	Increased	Normal
	Breath	Fruity	Normal	Normal
	Vital signs	↓ BP	↓ BP	↓ BP
		↑ P	↑ P	↑ P
		R Kussmaul's	R normal	R normal
	Mental status	Confused	Lethargic	Anxious; restless
	Thirst	Increased	Increased	Normal
	Fluid intake	Increased	Increased	Normal
	Gastrointestinal effects	Nausea/vomiting	Nausea/vomiting	Hunger
		Abdominal pain	Abdominal pain	
	Fluid loss	Moderate	Profound	Normal
	Level of consciousness	Decreasing	Decreasing	Decreasing
	Energy level	Weak	Weak	Fatigue
	Other	Weight loss	Weight loss	Headache
		Blurred vision	Malaise	Altered vision
			Extreme thirst	Mood changes
			Seizures	Seizures
Laboratory findings	Blood glucose	>300 mg/dL	>600 mg/dL	<50 mg/dL
	Plasma ketones	Increased	Normal	Normal
	Urine glucose	Increased	Increased	Normal
	Urine ketones	Increased	Normal	Normal
	Serum potassium	Abnormal	Abnormal	Normal
	Serum sodium	Abnormal	Abnormal	Normal
	Serum chloride	Abnormal	Abnormal	Normal
	Plasma pH	<7.3	Normal	Normal
	Osmolality	>340 mOsm/L	>340 mOsm/L	Normal
Treatment		Insulin	Insulin	Glucagon
		Treatment	Intravenous fluids	Rapid-acting carbohydrate
		Intravenous fluids	Electrolytes	Intravenous solution of 50% glucose
		Electrolytes		

Note: BP = blood pressure; P = pulse; R = respiration.

MULTISYSTEM EFFECTS OF **Diabetes**

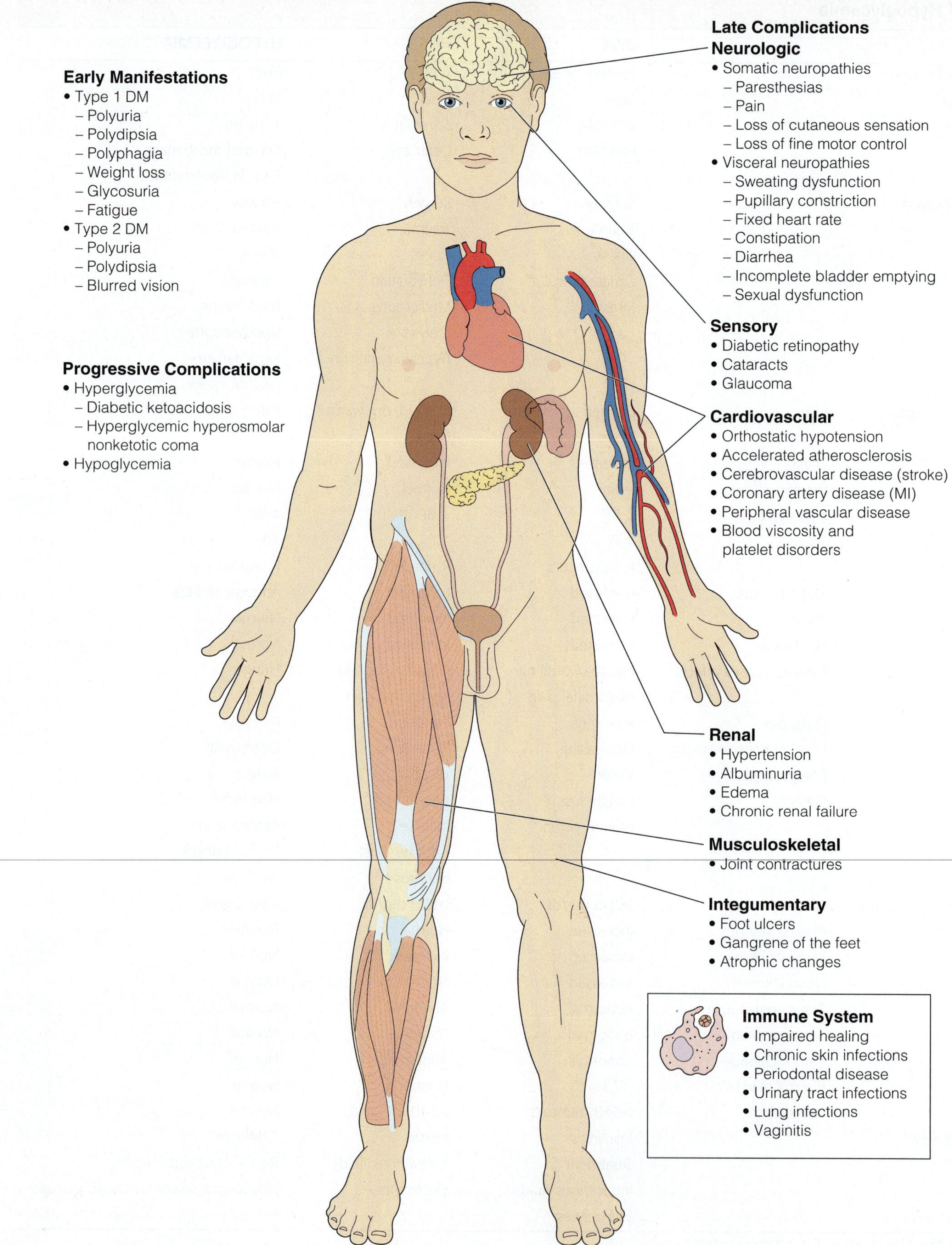

Early Manifestations
• Type 1 DM
– Polyuria
– Polydipsia
– Polyphagia
– Weight loss
– Glycosuria
– Fatigue
• Type 2 DM
– Polyuria
– Polydipsia
– Blurred vision
Progressive Complications
• Hyperglycemia
– Diabetic ketoacidosis
– Hyperglycemic hyperosmolar nonketotic coma
• Hypoglycemia
Late Complications
Neurologic
• Somatic neuropathies
– Paresthesias
– Pain
– Loss of cutaneous sensation
– Loss of fine motor control
• Visceral neuropathies
– Sweating dysfunction
– Pupillary constriction
– Fixed heart rate
– Constipation
– Diarrhea
– Incomplete bladder emptying
– Sexual dysfunction
Sensory
• Diabetic retinopathy
• Cataracts
• Glaucoma
Cardiovascular
• Orthostatic hypotension
• Accelerated atherosclerosis
• Cerebrovascular disease (stroke)
• Coronary artery disease (MI)
• Peripheral vascular disease
• Blood viscosity and platelet disorders
Renal
• Hypertension
• Albuminuria
• Edema
• Chronic renal failure
Musculoskeletal
• Joint contractures
Integumentary
• Foot ulcers
• Gangrene of the feet
• Atrophic changes
Immune System
• Impaired healing
• Chronic skin infections
• Periodontal disease
• Urinary tract infections
• Lung infections
• Vaginitis

Somogyi Phenomenon The **Somogyi phenomenon** is a combination of hypoglycemia during the night with a rebound morning rise in blood glucose to hyperglycemic levels. The hyperglycemia stimulates the counterregulatory hormones, which in turn stimulate gluconeogenesis and glycogenolysis and inhibit peripheral glucose use. This may cause insulin resistance for 12–48 hours (McCance & Huether, 2002).

Diabetic Ketoacidosis As the pathophysiology of untreated type 1 DM continues, the insulin deficit causes fat stores to break down, resulting in continued hyperglycemia and mobilization of fatty acids with a subsequent ketosis. **Diabetic ketoacidosis (DKA)** develops when there is an absolute deficiency of insulin and an increase in the insulin counterregulatory hormones. Glucose production by the liver increases, peripheral glucose use decreases, fat mobilization increases, and ketogenesis (ketone formation) is stimulated. Increased glucagon levels activate the gluconeogenic and ketogenic pathways in the liver. In the presence of insulin deficiency, hepatic overproduction of beta-hydroxybutyrate and acetoacetic acids (ketone bodies) causes increased ketone concentrations and increased release of free fatty acids. Because of a loss of bicarbonate, which occurs when the ketone is formed, bicarbonate buffering does not occur, and a metabolic acidosis—namely, DKA—occurs. Depression of the central nervous system from the accumulation of ketones and the resulting acidosis may cause coma and death if left untreated (Porth, 2005). For additional details, see Figure 18–8 ■.

Diabetic ketoacidosis also may occur in a person with diagnosed diabetes when energy requirements increase during physical or emotional stress. Stress states initiate the release of gluconeogenic hormones, resulting in the formation of carbohydrates from protein or fat. The person who is sick, who has an infection, or who decreases or omits insulin doses is at a greatly increased risk for developing DKA.

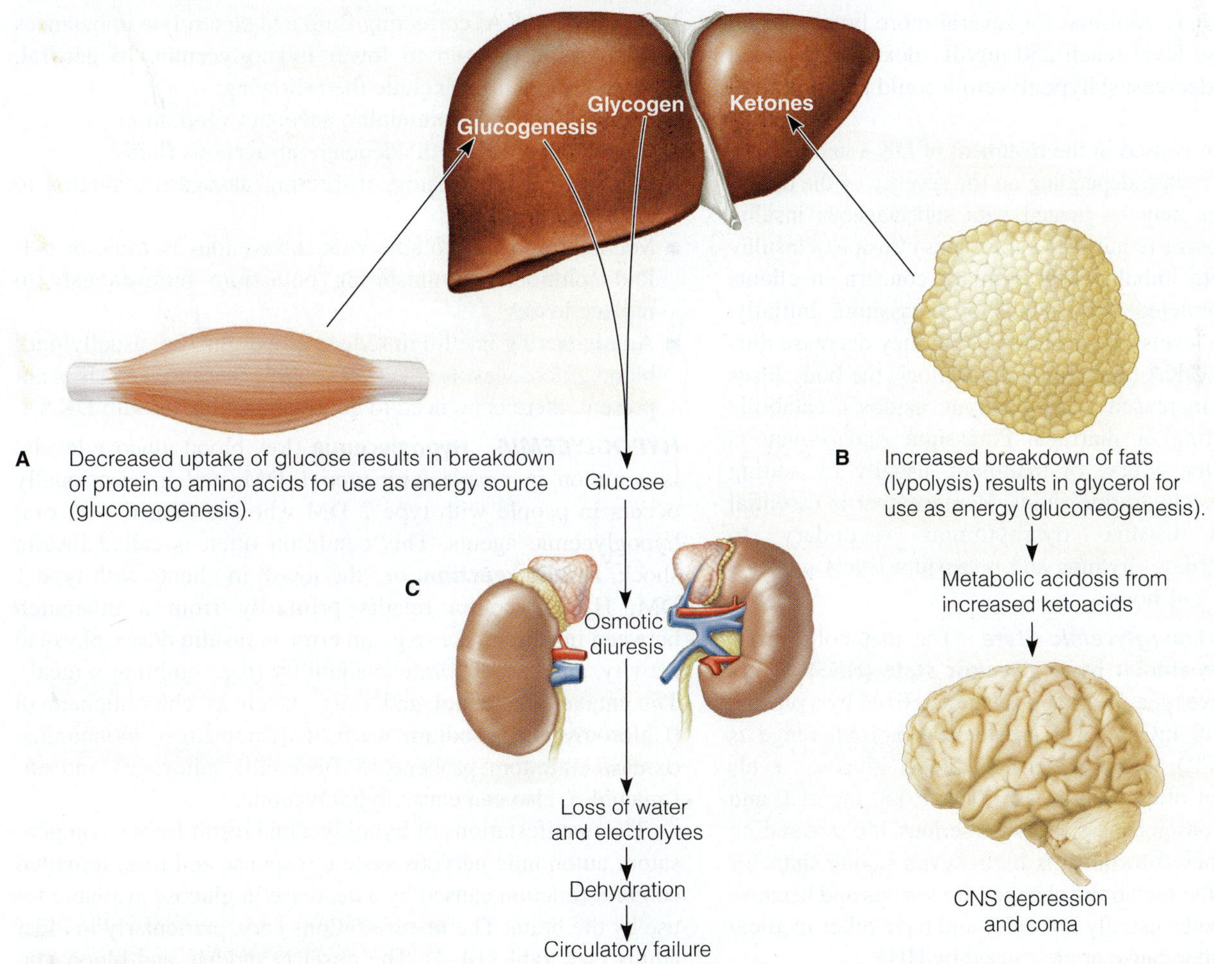
Glycogen
Glucogenesis
Ketones
A
Decreased uptake of glucose results in breakdown of protein to amino acids for use as energy source (gluconeogenesis).
Glucose
B
Increased breakdown of fats (lypolysis) results in glycerol for use as energy (gluconeogenesis).
C
Osmotic diuresis
Metabolic acidosis from increased ketoacids
Loss of water and electrolytes
Dehydration
Circulatory failure
CNS depression and coma

Figure 18–8 ■ In type 1 diabetes mellitus, without adequate insulin, muscle *A*, and fat *B*, cells are metabolized to provide sources of energy. Amino acids from skeletal muscle are converted to glucose in the liver; glycerol from fat cells is converted to glucose and fatty acids (ketoacids), which cause central nervous system (CNS) depression and coma. Increased glucose *C*, causes osmotic diuresis, leading to dehydration and decreased circulatory volume. These processes create the symptoms of diabetic ketoacidosis. The symptoms can be reversed with intravenous insulin to lower blood glucose. Blood pressure is raised to prevent circulatory failure by administering intravenous fluids; electrolytes are monitored and corrected.

Diabetic ketoacidosis involves four metabolic problems:

1. Hyperosmolarity from hyperglycemia and dehydration
2. Metabolic acidosis from an accumulation of ketoacids
3. Extracellular volume depletion from osmotic diuresis
4. Electrolyte imbalances (e.g., loss of potassium and sodium) from osmotic diuresis.

Manifestations of DKA result from severe dehydration and acidosis, and DKA requires immediate medical attention. Admission to the hospital is appropriate when the person has a blood glucose level of greater than 250 mg/dL, a decreasing pH, and ketones in the urine. If the client is alert and conscious, fluids may be replaced orally. In the first 12 hours of treatment, adults usually require 8–10 L of fluid to replace losses from polyuria and vomiting (Lehne, 2004). However, alterations in level of consciousness, vomiting, and acidosis are common, necessitating intravenous fluid replacement. The initial fluid replacement may be accomplished by administering 0.9% saline solution at a rate of 500–1,000 mL/hr. After 2–3 hours (or when blood pressure is returning to normal), administration of 0.45% saline at 200–500 mL/hr may continue for several more hours. When the blood glucose level reach 250 mg/dL, dextrose is added to prevent rapid decreases; hypoglycemia could result in fatal cerebral edema.

Regular insulin is used in the treatment of DKA and may be given by various routes, depending on the severity of the condition. Mild ketosis may be treated with subcutaneous insulin, whereas severe ketosis requires an intravenous infusion of insulin.

The electrolyte imbalance of primary concern in clients with DKA is depleted body stores of potassium. Initially, serum potassium levels may be normal, but they decrease during treatment. In DKA (and from rehydration), the body loses potassium from increased urinary output, acidosis, catabolic state, and vomiting or diarrhea. Potassium replacement is begun early in the course of treatment, usually by adding potassium to the rehydration fluids. Replacement is essential for preventing cardiac dysrhythmias secondary to hypokalemia. Cardiac rhythms and potassium levels must be monitored every 2–4 hours.

Hyperosmolar Hyperglycemic State The metabolic problem called **hyperosmolar hyperglycemic state (HHS)** occurs in people who have type 2 DM and is characterized by a plasma osmolarity of 340 mOsm/L or greater (the normal range is 280–300 mOsm/L), greatly elevated blood glucose levels (>600 mg/dL and often as high as 1,000–2,000 mg/dL), and altered levels of consciousness. HHS is a serious, life-threatening medical emergency. Mortality is high—even higher than for DKA—because the metabolic changes are serious and because people with diabetes usually are older and have other medical problems that either cause or are caused by HHS.

The precipitating factors associated with HHS include infection, therapeutic agents, therapeutic procedures, acute illness, and chronic illness. The most common precipitating factor is infection. The manifestations of this disorder may be slow to appear, with onset ranging from 24 hours to 2 weeks. The manifestations are initiated by hyperglycemia, which causes increased urine output, and with increased output, plasma volume decreases and glomerular filtration rate drops. As a result, glucose is retained, and water is lost. Glucose and sodium accumulate in the blood and increase serum osmolarity.

Serum hyperosmolarity results in severe dehydration, which reduces intracellular water in all tissues, including the brain. The person has dry skin and mucous membranes, extreme thirst, and altered levels of consciousness (progressing from lethargy to coma). Neurologic deficits may include hyperthermia, motor and sensory impairment, positive Babinski's sign, and seizures. Metabolic acidosis is not part of the pathology; despite elevated blood glucose, sufficient insulin is present to prevent metabolism of fats with the resulting fatty acids and ketones of DKA. Treatment is directed toward correcting fluid and electrolyte imbalances, lowering blood glucose levels with insulin, and treating underlying conditions.

The client admitted to the intensive care unit (ICU) for treatment of HHS typically manifests blood glucose levels greater than 700 mg/dL, increased serum osmolarity, and altered levels of consciousness or seizures. Treatment is similar to that of DKA: correcting fluid and electrolyte imbalances and providing insulin to lower hyperglycemia. In general, treatment modalities include the following:

- Establishing and maintaining adequate ventilation
- Correcting shock with adequate intravenous fluids
- If the client is comatose instituting nasogastric suction to prevent aspiration
- Maintaining fluid volume with intravenous isotonic or colloid solutions, administering potassium intravenously to replace losses
- Administering insulin to reduce blood glucose, usually until blood glucose levels reach 250 mg/dL (because ketosis is not present, there is no need to continue insulin, as with DKA).

HYPOGLYCEMIA **Hypoglycemia** (low blood glucose levels) is common in people with type 1 DM, and it occasionally occurs in people with type 2 DM who are treated with oral hypoglycemic agents. This condition often is called insulin shock, **insulin reaction**, or "the lows" in clients with type 1 DM. Hypoglycemia results primarily from a mismatch between insulin intake (e.g., an error in insulin dose), physical activity, and carbohydrate availability (e.g., omitting a meal). The intake of alcohol and drugs, such as chloramphenicol (Chloromycetin), sodium warfarin (Coumadin), monoamine oxidase inhibitors, probenecid (Benemid), salicylates, and sulfonamides, also can cause hypoglycemia.

The manifestations of hypoglycemia result from a compensatory autonomic nervous system response and from impaired cerebral function caused by a decrease in glucose available for use by the brain. The manifestations vary, particularly in older adults (see Table 18–3). The onset is sudden, and blood glucose usually is less than 45–60 mg/dL. Severe hypoglycemia may cause death.

People who have type 1 DM for 4 or 5 years fail to secrete glucagon in response to a decrease in blood glucose. These clients then depend on epinephrine to serve as a counterregulatory response to hypoglycemia. However, this compensatory response can become absent or blunted, and the person then develops a syndrome called *hypoglycemia unawareness.* In this syndrome, the person does not experience symptoms of hypoglycemia, even though it is present. Because treatment is not initiated in the absence of symptoms, the person is likely to have episodes of severe hypoglycemia.

When mild hypoglycemia occurs, immediate treatment is necessary. People experiencing hypoglycemia should take approximately 15 g of a rapid-acting sugar. This amount of sugar is found, for example, in three glucose tablets, half a cup of fruit juice or regular soda, 8 oz of skim milk, five Life Savers candies, three large marshmallows, or 3 tsp of sugar or honey. Sugar should not be added to fruit juice. Adding sugar to the fruit sugar already in the juice could cause a rapid rise in blood glucose, with persistent hyperglycemia.

If the manifestations continue, the 15/15 rule should be followed: Wait 15 minutes, monitor blood glucose, and if the blood glucose is low, eat another 15 g of carbohydrate. This procedure can be repeated until blood glucose levels return to normal (Haire-Joshu, 1996). People with diabetes should have some source of carbohydrate readily available at all times so that hypoglycemic symptoms can be quickly reversed. If hypoglycemia occurs more than two or three times a week, the individual's diabetes management plan should be adjusted.

Clients with diabetes who have severe hypoglycemia often are hospitalized. The criteria for hospitalization are one or more of the following:

- Blood glucose is less than 50 mg/dL, and the prompt treatment of hypoglycemia has not resulted in recovery of sensorium.
- The client has coma, seizures, or altered behavior.
- The hypoglycemia has been treated, but a responsible adult cannot be with the client for the following 12 hours.
- The hypoglycemia was caused by a sulfonylurea drug.

If the client is conscious and alert, 10–15 g of an oral carbohydrate may be given. If the client has altered levels of consciousness, administer parenteral glucose or glucagon.

Glucose is administered intravenously as a 25–50% solution, usually at a rate of 10 mL over 1 minute by intravenous push, followed by an intravenous infusion of 5% dextrose in water (D_5W) at 5–10 g/hr (Haire-Joshu, 1996). This is the most rapid method of increasing blood glucose levels.

Glucagon is an antihypoglycemic agent that raises blood glucose by promoting the conversion of hepatic glycogen to glucose. It is used in severe insulin-induced hypoglycemia and may be given in the recommended dose of 1 mg by the subcutaneous, intramuscular, or intravenous route. Glucagon has a short period of action; an oral (if the client is conscious) or intravenous carbohydrate should be administered following the glucagon to prevent a recurrence of hypoglycemia. If the client has been unconscious, glucagon may cause vomiting when consciousness returns.

Chronic Complications

Chronic complications of diabetes include alterations in the cardiovascular system, the peripheral and autonomic nervous systems, and mood as well as increased susceptibility to infection, periodontal disease, and complications involving the feet.

ALTERATIONS IN THE CARDIOVASCULAR SYSTEM The macrocirculation (large blood vessels) in people with diabetes undergoes changes as a result of atherosclerosis; abnormalities in platelets, red blood cells, and clotting factors; and changes in arterial walls. Atherosclerosis has an increased incidence and earlier age of onset in people with diabetes (although the reason is unknown). Other risk factors that contribute to the development of macrovascular disease of diabetes are hypertension, hyperlipidemia, cigarette smoking, and obesity. Alterations in the vascular system increase the risk of the long-term complications of coronary artery disease, cerebral vascular disease, and peripheral vascular disease.

Alterations in the microcirculation in the person with diabetes involve structural defects in the basement membrane of smaller blood vessels and capillaries. (The basement membrane is the structure that supports and serves as the boundary around the space occupied by epithelial cells.) These defects cause the capillary basement membrane to thicken, eventually resulting in decreased tissue perfusion. Changes in basement membranes are believed to be caused by one or more of the following: presence of increased amounts of sorbitol (a substance formed as an intermediate step in the conversion of glucose to fructose), formation of abnormal glycoproteins, or problems in the release of oxygen from hemoglobin (Porth, 2005). The effects of alterations in the microcirculation impact all body tissues but are seen primarily in the eyes and the kidneys.

Coronary Artery Disease Coronary artery disease is a major risk factor for the development of myocardial infarction in people with diabetes, especially the middle-age to older adult with type 2 DM. Coronary artery disease is the most common cause of death in people with diabetes (National Institutes of Health, 2004). People with diabetes who have myocardial infarction are more prone to develop congestive heart failure as a complication of the infarction and also are less likely to survive in the period immediately following the infarction.

Hypertension Hypertension (blood pressure $\geq$ 140/90 mmHg) is a common complication of diabetes. It affects 20–60% of all people with diabetes and is a major risk factor for cardiovascular disease and microvascular complications such as retinopathy and nephropathy. Hypertension may be reduced by weight loss, exercise, and decreased sodium intake and alcohol consumption. If these methods are not effective, treatment with antihypertensive medications is necessary.

Stroke (Cerebrovascular Accident) People with diabetes, especially older adults with type 2 DM, are two to six times more likely to have a stroke. Although the exact relationship between diabetes and cerebral vascular disease is unknown, hypertension (a risk factor for stroke) is a common health problem in those who have diabetes. In addition, atherosclerosis of the cerebral vessels develops at an earlier age and is more extensive in people with diabetes (Porth, 2005).

The manifestations of impaired cerebral circulation are similar to those of hypoglycemia or HHS—namely, blurred vision, slurred speech, weakness, and dizziness. People with these manifestations have potentially life-threatening health problems and require constant medical attention.

Peripheral Vascular Disease Peripheral vascular disease of the lower extremities accompanies both types of diabetes, but the incidence is greater in people with type 2 DM. Atherosclerosis of vessels in the legs of people with diabetes begins at an earlier age, advances more rapidly, and is equally common in both men and women. Impaired peripheral vascular circulation leads to peripheral vascular insufficiency with intermittent claudication (pain) in the lower legs and ulcerations of the feet. Occlusion and thrombosis of large vessels and small arteries and arterioles, as well as alterations in neurologic function and infection, result in gangrene (necrosis, or the death of tissue). Gangrene from diabetes is the most common cause of nontraumatic amputations of the lower leg. In people with diabetes, dry gangrene is most common, which is manifested by cold, dry, shriveled, and black tissues of the toes and feet. The gangrene usually begins in the toes and moves proximally into the foot.

DIABETIC RETINOPATHY **Diabetic retinopathy** refers to the changes in the retina that occur in the person with diabetes. The retinal capillary structure undergoes alterations in blood flow, leading to retinal ischemia and breakdown in the blood–retinal barrier. Diabetic retinopathy is the leading cause of blindness in people between 20 and 74 years of age (National Institutes of Health, 2004). Retinopathy has three stages:

1. *Stage I: nonproliferative retinopathy.* Dilated veins, microaneurysms, edema of the macula, and presence of exudates characterize this stage.
2. *Stage II: preproliferative retinopathy.* Retinal ischemia causes infarcts of the nerve fiber layer, with characteristic "cotton wool" patches on the retina. Shunts form between occluded and patent vessels.
3. *Stage III: proliferative retinopathy.* As fibrous tissue and new vessels form in the retina or optic disc, traction on the vitreous humor may cause hemorrhage or retinal detachment.

After 20 years of diabetes, almost all clients with type 1 DM and more than 70% of clients with type 2 DM will have some degree of retinopathy, in most cases without vision loss (Saudek & Margolis, 2005). If exudate, edema, hemorrhage, or ischemia occurs near the fovea, the person experiences visual impairment at any stage. In addition, the person with diabetes is at increased risk for developing cataracts (opacity of the lens) as a result of increased glucose levels within the lens itself. Screening for retinopathy is important, because laser photocoagulation surgery has proven to be beneficial in preventing loss of vision.

DIABETIC NEPHROPATHY **Diabetic nephropathy** is a disease of the kidneys characterized by the presence of albumin in the urine, hypertension, edema, and progressive renal insufficiency. In the United States, this disorder accounts for 44% of new cases of end-stage renal disease requiring dialysis or transplantation. Nephropathy occurs in 30–40% of people with type 1 DM and in 20% of those with type 2 DM (Saudek & Margolis, 2005).

The exact pathologic origin of diabetic nephropathy is unknown. It has been established, however, that thickening of the basement membrane of the glomeruli eventually impairs renal function, and it has been suggested that an increased intracellular concentration of glucose supports the formation of abnormal glycoproteins in the basement membrane and mesangium. The accumulation of these large proteins stimulates glomerulosclerosis (fibrosis of the glomerular tissue). Glomerulosclerosis thickens the basement membrane and simultaneously makes it functionally leaky, allowing large molecules (e.g., proteins) to be lost in the urine. Kimmelstiel-Wilson syndrome is a type of glomerulosclerosis found only in people with diabetes. In advanced nephropathy, tubular atrophy occurs, and end-stage renal disease results. (See Concept 11, Fluids and Electrolytes, for a discussion of renal failure.)

The first indication of nephropathy is **microalbuminuria** (a low but abnormal level of albumin in the urine). Without specific interventions, people with type 1 DM and sustained microalbuminuria will develop overt nephropathy, accompanied by hypertension, over a period of 10–15 years. Because type 2 DM may go undetected for years, people with this type often have microalbuminuria and overt nephropathy shortly after diagnosis.

Because hypertension accelerates the progress of diabetic nephropathy, aggressive antihypertensive management should be instituted. Management includes control of hypertension with angiotensin-converting enzyme inhibitors (e.g., captopril [Capoten]), weight loss, reduced salt intake, and exercise.

ALTERATIONS IN THE PERIPHERAL AND AUTONOMIC NERVOUS SYSTEMS Peripheral and visceral neuropathies are disorders of the peripheral nerves and the autonomic nervous system. In people with diabetes, these disorders often are called **diabetic neuropathies** The manifestations depend on the locations of the lesions.

The etiology of diabetic neuropathies involves the following:

- A thickening of the walls of the blood vessels that supply nerves, causing a decrease in nutrients
- Demyelinization of the Schwann cells that surround and insulate nerves, slowing nerve conduction
- Formation and accumulation of sorbitol within the Schwann cells, impairing nerve conduction.

Peripheral Neuropathies The peripheral neuropathies (also called somatic neuropathies) include polyneuropathies and mononeuropathies. Polyneuropathies, the most common type of neuropathy associated with diabetes, are bilateral sensory disorders. The manifestations appear first in the toes and feet and then progress upward. The fingers and hands also may be involved, but usually only in later stages of diabetes. The manifestations of polyneuropathy depend on which nerve fibers are involved.

The person with polyneuropathy commonly has distal paresthesias (a subjective feeling of a change in sensation; e.g., numbness or tingling); pain described as aching, burning, or shooting; and feelings of cold feet. Other manifestations may include impaired sensations of pain, temperature, light touch, two-point discrimination, and vibration. There is no specific treatment for polyneuropathies.

Mononeuropathies are isolated peripheral neuropathies that affect a single nerve. Depending on the nerve involved, manifestations may include the following:

- Palsy of the third cranial (oculomotor) nerve, with headache, eye pain, and inability to move the eye up, down, or medially
- Radiculopathy, with pain over a dermatome and loss of cutaneous sensation, most often located in the chest
- Diabetic femoral neuropathy, with motor and sensory deficits (e.g., pain, weakness, and areflexia) in the anterior thigh and medial calf
- Entrapment or compression of the medial nerve at the wrist, resulting in carpal tunnel syndrome with pain and weakness of the hand; of the ulnar nerve at the elbow, resulting in weakness and loss of sensation over the palmar surface of the fourth and fifth fingers; and of the peroneal nerve at the head of the fibula, resulting in foot drop.

Visceral Neuropathies The visceral neuropathies (also called *autonomic neuropathies*) cause various manifestations, depending on which area of the autonomic nervous system is involved. These neuropathies may include the following:

- Sweating dysfunction, with an absence of sweating (anhydrosis) on the hands and feet and increased sweating on the face or trunk.
- Abnormal pupillary function, most commonly seen as constricted pupils that dilate slowly in the dark.
- Cardiovascular dysfunction, resulting in such abnormalities as a fixed cardiac rate that does not change with exercise, postural hypotension, and a failure to increase cardiac output or vascular tone with exercise.
- Gastrointestinal dysfunction, with changes in upper gastrointestinal motility (gastroparesis) resulting in dysphagia, loss of appetite, heartburn, nausea and vomiting, and altered blood glucose control. Constipation is one of the most common gastrointestinal symptoms associated with diabetes, possibly as a result of hypomotility of the bowel. Diabetic diarrhea is not as common, but it does occur and often is associated with fecal incontinence during sleep because of a defect in internal sphincter function.
- Genitourinary dysfunction, producing changes in bladder function and sexual function. Changes in bladder function include inability to empty the bladder completely, loss of sensation of bladder fullness, and increased risk of urinary tract infections. Sexual dysfunctions in men include ejaculatory changes and impotence. Sexual dysfunctions in women include changes in arousal patterns, vaginal lubrication, and orgasm. Alterations of sexual function in people with diabetes are the result of both neurologic and vascular changes.

ALTERATIONS IN MOOD Persons with type 1 or type 2 DM endure the chronic strains of living with complex self-care and have an increased risk for depression, which can negatively affect management of diabetes. Treatment of depression in these clients has been associated with better control of serum glucose, so screening for depression is an important part of assessing the individual's ability to manage the disease. Tests to identify the scope of depression are available (Harper-Jacques, 2004).

Interventions for helping clients with depression include a combination of antidepressant medications and psychotherapy focused on restoring logical thinking and problem-solving skills (Williams et al., 2004). Nurses can assist these clients by correcting misconceptions about depression, identifying individual strengths in managing diabetes, acknowledging negative feelings that may be expressed, and suggesting problem-solving behaviors to better manage the disease.

INCREASED SUSCEPTIBILITY TO INFECTION The person with diabetes has an increased risk of developing infections. The exact relationship between infection and diabetes is not clear, but many dysfunctions that result from diabetic complications predispose the person to develop an infection (Aragon, Ring, & Covelli, 2003). Vascular and neurologic impairments, hyperglycemia, and altered neutrophil function are believed to be responsible (Porth, 2005).

The person with diabetes may have sensory deficits that result in inattention to trauma and vascular deficits that decrease circulation to the injured area. In this situation, the normal inflammatory response is diminished, and healing is slowed.

Nephrosclerosis and inadequate bladder emptying with retention of urine predispose the person with diabetes to pyelonephritis (inflammation of the kidney and its pelvis) and urinary tract infections. Bacterial and fungal infections of the skin, nails, and mucous membranes are common, and tuberculosis is more prevalent in people with diabetes than in the general population. Hospitalized clients with a blood glucose greater than 220 mg/dL have higher infection rates (American Diabetes Association, 2005).

PERIODONTAL DISEASE Although periodontal disease does not occur more often in people with diabetes, it does progress more rapidly, especially if the diabetes is poorly controlled. This more rapid progression is believed to be caused by microangiopathy, with changes in vascularization of the gums. As a result, gingivitis (inflammation of the gums) and periodontitis (inflammation of the bone underlying the gums) occur.

COMPLICATIONS INVOLVING THE FEET The high incidence in people with diabetes of problems with and amputations of the feet is the result of angiopathy, neuropathy, and infection. People with diabetes are at high risk for amputation of a lower extremity, with an even greater risk in those who have had diabetes for more than 10 years, are male, have poor glucose control, or have cardiovascular, retinal, or renal complications.

Vascular changes in the lower extremities of the person with diabetes result in arteriosclerosis. Diabetes-induced arteriosclerosis tends to occur at an earlier age, has an equal incidence in men and women, is usually bilateral, and progresses more rapidly. The blood vessels most often affected are located below the knee. Blockages form in the large, medium, and small arteries of the lower legs and feet. Multiple occlusions with decreased blood flow result in the manifestations of peripheral vascular disease (see Concept 22, Perfusion, for more details).

Diabetic neuropathy of the foot produces multiple problems. Because the sense of touch and perception of pain are absent, the person with diabetes may have some type of foot trauma without being aware of it. This increases the risk for trauma to the tissues of the feet, leading to ulcer development. Infections commonly occur in traumatized or ulcerated tissue.

Despite the many potential sources of foot trauma in the person with diabetes, the most common are cracks and fissures caused by dry skin or infections (e.g., athlete's foot), blisters caused by improperly fitting shoes, pressure from stockings or shoes, ingrown toenails, and direct trauma (e.g., cuts, bruises, or burns). It is important to remember that the person with diabetic neuropathy who has lost the perception of pain may not be aware these injuries have occurred. In addition, when a part of the body loses sensation, the person tends to dissociate from or ignore that part, so an injury may go unattended for days or weeks—or even be forgotten entirely.

Foot lesions usually begin as a superficial skin ulcer. In time, the ulcer extends deeper, into muscles and bone, leading to an abscess or osteomyelitis. Gangrene can develop on one or more toes; if untreated, the whole foot eventually becomes gangrenous. (Care of the feet, an essential part of client and family education, is discussed in the Client Teaching feature later in the chapter.)

COLLABORATION

The results of a 10-year Diabetes Control and Complications Trial, sponsored by the NIH, have significant implications for the management of type 1 DM. People in the study who kept their blood glucose levels close to normal by frequent monitoring, several daily insulin injections, and lifestyle changes that included exercise and a healthier diet reduced by 60% their risk for the development and progression of complications involving the eyes, the kidneys, and the nervous system. The DIGAMI study of 1995 stimulated interest in greater glycemic control in clients with type 2 DM (Cummings et al., 1999; Malmberg et al., 1995). Treatment of the client with diabetes focuses on maintaining blood glucose at levels as nearly normal as possible through medications, dietary management, and exercise. Type 2 DM benefits from similar levels of control.

Diagnostic Tests

Diagnostic tests are conducted for screening purposes to diagnose diabetes, and ongoing laboratory tests are conducted to evaluate the effectiveness of diabetic management. Definitions of normal blood glucose levels vary in clinical practice, depending on the laboratory that performs the assay.

DIAGNOSTIC SCREENING Three diagnostic tests may be used to diagnose DM, and each must be confirmed, on a subsequent day, with one of the three tests. The following diagnostic criteria are recommended by the ADA (2005):

1. Symptoms of diabetes plus casual plasma glucose (PG) concentration > 200 mg/dL (11.1 mmol/L). Causal is defined as any time of day without regard to time since last meal.
2. Fasting plasma glucose (FPG) > 126 mg/dL (7.0 mmol/L). Fasting is defined as no caloric intake for 8 hours.
3. Two-hour PG > 200 mg/dL (11.1 mmol/L) during an oral glucose tolerance test (OGTT). The test should be performed with a glucose load containing the equivalent of 75 anhydrous glucose dissolved in water.

When using these criteria, the following levels are used for the FPG:

- Normal fasting glucose = 100 mg/dL (6.1 mmol/L)
- Impaired fasting glucose (IFG) > 100 (6.1 mmol/L) and <126 mg/dL (7.0 mmol/L)
- Diagnosis of diabetes > 126 mg/dL (7.0 mmol/L).

When using these criteria, the following levels are used for the OGTT:

- Normal glucose tolerance = 2-h PG < 140 mg/dL (7.8 mmol/L)
- Impaired glucose tolerance (IGT) = 2-h PG ≥ 140 (7.8 mmol/L) and < 200 mg/dL (11.1 mmol/L)
- Diagnosis of diabetes = 2-h PG ≥ 200 mg/dL (11.1 mmol/L).

Note that although either method may be used to diagnose diabetes, in a clinical setting the FPG is the recommended screening test for nonpregnant adults (ADA, 2002).

PREDIABETES *Prediabetes* is a term used to describe people who are at increased risk of developing diabetes. Prediabetes is characterized by blood sugar between 100 and 126 mg/dL after fasting overnight, which is high but not high enough to be classified as diabetes. In 2000, an estimated 41 million adults ages 40–74 had prediabetes. These test results indicate there is a risk for progression to diabetes, but it is not inevitable. Studies suggest that weight loss and increased physical activity among people with prediabetes prevent or delay diabetes and may return blood glucose levels to normal. People with prediabetes are already at increased risk for other adverse health outcomes such as heart disease and stroke (CDC, 2005).

DIABETES MANAGEMENT MONITORING The following diagnostic tests may be used to monitor diabetes management:

- *Fasting blood glucose (FBG).* This test is often ordered, especially if the client is experiencing symptoms of hypoglycemia or hyperglycemia. In most people, the normal range is 70–110 mg/dL.
- *Glycosylated hemoglobin (c) (A1c).* This test determines the average blood glucose level over approximately the previous 2–3 months. When glucose is elevated or control of glucose is erratic, glucose attaches to the hemoglobin molecule and remains attached for the life of the hemoglobin, which is about 120 days. The normal level depends on the type of assay done, but values above 7–9% are considered elevated. The ADA recommends that A1c be performed at the initial

assessment, and then at regular intervals, individualized to the medical regimen used.

- *Urine glucose and ketone levels.* These are not as accurate in monitoring changes in blood glucose as blood levels. The presence of glucose in the urine indicates hyperglycemia. Most people have a renal threshold for glucose of 180 mg/dL; that is, when the blood glucose exceeds 180 mg/dL, glucose is not reabsorbed by the kidney and spills over into the urine. This number varies highly, however. Ketonuria (the presence of ketones in the urine) occurs with the breakdown of fats and is an indicator of DKA; however, fat breakdown and ketonuria also occur in states of less than normal nutrition.
- *Urine test* for the presence of protein as albumin (*albuminuria*). If albuminuria is present, a 24-hour urine test for creatinine clearance is used to detect the early onset of nephropathy.
- *Serum cholesterol and triglyceride levels.* These are indicators of atherosclerosis and an increased risk of cardiovascular impairments. The ADA (2005) recommends treatment goals to lower LDL cholesterol to <100 mg/dL, raise HDL cholesterol to >45 mg/dL, and lower triglycerides to <150 mg/dL.
- *Serum electrolytes.* Levels are measured in clients who have DKA or hyperosmolar hyperglycemic state (HHS) to determine imbalances.

Monitoring Blood Glucose

People with diabetes must monitor their condition daily by testing glucose levels. Two types of tests are available. The first type, long used prior to the development of devices to directly measure blood glucose, is urine testing for glucose and ketones. Urine testing is less commonly used today. The second type, direct measurement of blood glucose, is widely used in all types of health care settings and in the home.

Urine testing for glucose and ketones was at one time the only available method for evaluating the management of diabetes. An inexpensive, noninvasive, and painless test, it has unpredictable results and cannot be used to detect or measure hypoglycemia. In the healthy state, glucose is not present in the urine because insulin maintains serum glucose below the renal threshold of 180 mg/dL. The accuracy of this measurement is not reliable in diabetes because the renal threshold may rise with aging or secondary to diabetes. Urine testing is recommended to monitor hyperglycemia and ketoacidosis in people with type 1 DM who have unexplained hyperglycemia during illness or pregnancy. Ketones may be detected through urine testing and reflect the presence of DKA. Urine testing may also be used by people who choose not to self-monitor blood glucose by other methods.

Self-monitoring of blood glucose (SMBG) allows the person with diabetes to monitor and achieve metabolic control and decrease the danger of hypoglycemia. The ADA recommends that all clients with diabetes must be taught some method of monitoring glycemic control (Figure 18–10). The timing of SMBG is highly individualized, depending on the person's diagnosis, general disease control, and physical state. SMBG is recommended three or more times a day for clients with type 1 DM; for clients with type 2 DM, testing should be sufficient to help them reach glucose goals. When adding or modifying therapy, clients with both types of DM should test more often than usual. SMBG is also useful when the person is ill or pregnant, or has symptoms of hypoglycemia or hyperglycemia (ADA, 2006).

The ADA annually publishes a comprehensive list of currently available blood glucose monitoring machines and strips with approximate prices in *Diabetes Forecast.* Most medical insurance policies cover the cost of these machines. A new technology for continuous blood glucose monitoring is now available and clients are learning to use these monitors, especially if they use insulin pumps. A new insulin pump receives transmitted data from a continuous glucose monitor (CGM) worn on the skin. Like the insulin pump, the CGM has a sensor that is inserted under the skin. This sensor continuously sends data to the transmitter, which sends the information to the pump by radiofrequency wireless technology. This data can warn of high or low glucose levels. Fingerstick measurements are required before making therapy adjustments (Medtronic MiniMed, 2006). The CGM is also used for diagnostic evaluation; clients wear the pump for 3 days under the supervision of physicians and nurses. The data reveal patterns of glycemic control useful for clinical recommendations.

Following is the equipment needed for SMBG:

- Some type of lancet device to perform a fingerstick for obtaining a drop of blood (such as an Autolet, Penlet, or Soft Touch).
- Chemically impregnated test strips that change color when they come into contact with glucose or that can be read by machine (e.g., Glucostix and Chemstrip bG). The strip may also be read by comparing its color with a color chart on the side of the container or on an insert.
- A blood glucose monitor (e.g., the Glucometer, the Accu-Chek, or the One Touch) if the most accurate measurement is desired or recommended. The manufacturer's instructions must be followed carefully. If the timing of the blood on the strip is not exact, the test will not be accurate. In addition, the machine must be cleaned according to the manufacturer's directions to ensure accuracy. Monitors that use no-wipe technology improve the accuracy of glucose measurement. Other monitors are computerized and/or include a memory of previous glucose readings to show a pattern of control. The stored information is useful for clinicians to review and determine therapeutic needs.

According to the U.S. Food and Drug Administration (FDA), several factors affect the accuracy of blood glucose test results. The quality of the meter and test strips, and training to use the meter contribute to the degree of accuracy. Other factors can create false positive or negative readings.

Clients with higher hematocrit values will usually test falsely low in blood glucose and clients with lower hematocrit will test falsely higher. Anemia and sickle cell anemia are two conditions that can affect hematocrit values.

Overdoses of many medications will cause inaccurate results. Meters and supplies vary in sensitivity to medications. Uric acid (a natural substance in the body that can be more concentrated in some people with diabetes), glutathione (an antioxidant also called *GSH*), and ascorbic acid (vitamin C) are known to interfere. Check the package insert for each meter to find what substances might affect its testing accuracy (U.S. FDA, 2005).

Be sure the test strips are compatible with the glucose meter and that they are not outdated or exposed to air and humidity, which can alter strip sensitivity. Insufficient amounts of blood on the testing strip cause inaccurate results. Although a meter may indicate a sufficient amount of blood on the test strip, it is best to observe that the receptacle is full of capillary blood. Yared et al. (2005) found that meters read significantly smaller than reference volumes and gave results varying 40–68% from the reference volume results. The erroneous results underestimated the true glucose value.

Pharmacologic Therapies

The pharmacologic treatment for diabetes mellitus depends on the type of diabetes. People with type 1 DM must have insulin; those with type 2 DM are usually able to control glucose levels with an oral hypoglycemic medication, but they may require insulin if control is inadequate.

INSULIN The person with type 1 DM requires a lifelong exogenous source of the insulin hormone to maintain life. Insulin is not a cure for diabetes; rather, it is a means of controlling hyperglycemia. Insulin is also necessary in other situations, such as these:

- People with diabetes who are unable to control glucose levels with oral antidiabetic drugs and/or diet. Introduced when beta cell function declines, insulin maintains glycemic control and prevents complications (Funnell, Kruger, & Spencer, 2004).
- People with diabetes who are experiencing physical stress (such as an infection or surgery) or who are taking corticosteroids.
- Women with gestational diabetes who are unable to control glucose with diet.
- People with DKA or HHS.
- People who are receiving high-calorie tube feedings or parenteral nutrition.

Preparations of insulin are derived from animal (pork pancreas) or synthesized in the laboratory from either an alteration of pork insulin or recombinant DNA technology, using strains of *Escherichia coli* to form a biosynthetic human insulin. Insulin analogs have been developed by modifying the amino acid sequence of the insulin molecule. Although different types are prescribed on an individualized basis, it is standard practice to prescribe human insulin.

Insulins are available in rapid-acting, short-acting, intermediate-acting, and long-acting preparations. The trade names and times of onset, peak, and duration of action are listed in Table 18–4.

Insulin lispro (Humalog) is a human insulin analog that is derived from genetically altered *E. coli* that includes the gene for insulin lispro. It is classified as a rapid-acting or ultra-short-acting insulin. Compared to regular insulin, insulin lispro has a more rapid onset (<15 minutes), an earlier peak of glucose lowering (30–60 minutes), and a shorter duration of activity (3–4 hours). This means that lispro should be administered 15 minutes before a meal, rather than 30–60 minutes before as recommended for regular insulin. Clients with type 1 DM usually also require concurrent use of a longer acting insulin product. Lispro is much less likely than regular insulin to cause tissue changes and may lower the risk of nocturnal hypoglycemia in clients with type 1 DM.

Regular insulin is unmodified crystalline insulin, classified as a short-acting insulin. Regular insulin is clear in appearance and is the only insulin preparation that can be given by the intravenous route; the other types are suspensions and could be harmful if given by this route. Regular insulin is also used to treat DKA, to initiate treatment for newly diagnosed type 1 DM, and in combination with intermediate-acting insulins to provide better glucose control.

The onset and peak and duration of action of insulin can be changed by adding acetate buffers and protamine. Zinc and protamine are added to NPH insulin to prolong their action, and they are classified as intermediate- or long-acting insulins. These preparations appear cloudy when properly mixed prior

TABLE 18–4 **Insulin Preparations**

PREPARATION	NAME	ONSET (H)	PEAK (H)	DURATION (H)
Rapid acting	Lispro	0.25	1–1.5	3–4
	Aspart (NovoLog)	0.25	40–50 minutes	3–5
	Glulisine (Apidra)	0.25	1–1.5	3–5
Short acting	Regular (Novolin-R, Humulin-R)	0.5–1.0	2–3	4–6
Intermediate acting	NPH Humulin (N)	2	6–8	12–16
	NPH			
Long acting	Lantus	2	16–20	24+
		(Onset and peak not defined)		24
Combinations	Humulin 50/50	0.5	3	22–24
	Humulin 70/30	0.5	4–8	24
	Novolin 70/30	0.5	4–8	24

to injection. Protamine and zinc are foreign substances and may cause hypersensitivity reactions. As of July 6, 2005, Lilly discontinued manufacture of pork insulins and Humulin U and Humulin Lente insulin.

Insulin glargine (Lantus) is a 24-hour, long-acting rDNA human insulin analog that is given subcutaneously once a day, usually at bedtime, to treat clients with both type 1 and type 2 diabetes. It has a relatively constant effect (meaning it does not have a peak time of effect). It is not recommended for use in pregnancy. Do not mix this with other insulins; the pH is incompatible (Lehne, 2004; Tierney et al., 2005).

PRACTICE ALERT

Insulin glargine is clear unlike other intermediate or long-acting insulins. Do not mistake this for regular insulin. Do not mix with **any** other insulins. Do not inject intravenously, only subcutaneously.

Insulin is dispensed as 100 unit/mL (U-100) and 500 unit/mL (U-500) in the United States. U-100 is the standard insulin concentration used. U-500 insulin is only used in rare cases of insulin resistance when clients require very large doses. U-500 and the insulin analog lispro are the only insulins that require a prescription.

Nursing implications for administering insulin are outlined in Box 18–1 and further discussion follows in the chapter. The considerations for administering insulin include routes of administration, syringe and needle selection, preparing the injection, sites of injection, mixing insulins, and insulin regimens (see Box 18–1).

Box 18–1 Medication Administration: Insulin

- Discard vials of insulin that have been open for several weeks or whose expiration date has passed.
- Refrigerate extra insulin vials not currently in use, but do not freeze them.
- Store insulin in a cool place, and avoid exposure to temperature extremes or sunlight.
- Store compatible mixtures of insulin for no longer than 1 month at room temperature or 3 months at 36°–46°F (2°–8°C).
- Discard any vials with discoloration, clumping, granules, or solid deposits on the sides.
- If breakfast is delayed, also delay the administration of rapid-acting insulin.
- Monitor and maintain a record of blood glucose readings 30 minutes before each meal and bedtime (or as prescribed).
- Monitor food intake, and notify the physician if food is not being consumed.
- Monitor electrolytes (especially potassium), blood urea nitrogen (BUN) levels, and creatinine.
- Observe injection sites for manifestations of hypersensitivity, lipodystrophy, and lipoatrophy.
- If symptoms of hypoglycemia occur, confirm by testing blood glucose level, and administer an oral source of a fast-acting carbohydrate, such as juice, milk, or crackers. Hypoglycemic symptoms may vary but commonly include feelings of shakiness, hunger, and/or nervousness accompanied by sweating, tachycardia, or palpitations.
- If symptoms of hyperglycemia occur, confirm by testing blood glucose level, and notify the physician.

CLIENT TEACHING Diabetes Mellitus

- The manifestations of diabetes mellitus.
- Self-administration of insulin, with a return demonstration.
  a. Wash hands carefully.
  b. Have a vial of insulin, the insulin syringe with needle, and alcohol pads ready to use.
  c. Remove the cover from the needle.
  d. Fill the syringe with an amount of air equal to the number of units of insulin, and insert the needle into the vial.
  e. Push air into the vial, invert the vial, and withdraw the prescribed units of insulin.
  f. Replace the cover over the needle.
  g. Wipe the selected site with alcohol. The injection is less likely to be painful if the alcohol is allowed to dry.
  h. Pinch up a fold of skin, and insert the needle into the tissue at the recommended angle.
  i. Insert the insulin.
  j. Withdraw the needle; if desired, apply firm pressure to the site for a few seconds.
  k. Recap the needle. Many people with diabetes reuse disposable syringes with attached needles without adverse effects. The primary reason for discarding after several uses is that the needle becomes dull and makes the injection painful.
- Follow instructions for mixing insulins.
- Always keep an extra vial of insulin available.
- Always have a vial of regular insulin available for emergencies.
- Be aware of the signs of hypersensitivity responses, hypoglycemia, and hyperglycemia.
- Keep candy or a sugar source available at all times to treat hypoglycemia, if it occurs. Eat within 15 minutes of injecting rapid-acting insulins.
- Vision may be blurred during the first 6–8 weeks of insulin therapy; this is the result of fluid changes in the eye and should clear up in 8 weeks.
- Avoid alcoholic beverages, which may cause hypoglycemia.
- Follow these guidelines for sick days:
  a. Never omit insulin.
  b. Always monitor blood glucose and/or urine ketones at least every 2–4 hours.
  c. Always drink plenty of fluids, try to drink at least one glass of water or other calorie-free, caffeine-free liquid each hour.
  d. Get as much rest as possible.
  e. Contact the physician if there is persistent fever, vomiting, shortness of breath, severe pain in the abdomen, dehydration, loss of vision, chest pain, persistent diarrhea, blood glucose levels above 250, or ketones in the urine.
- Establish a plan for rotating injection sites, and observe closely for changes in tissues such as hardness, dimpling, or sunken areas.

All insulins are given parenterally, although current research is investigating the development of a nasal spray and an oral preparation of insulin. Only regular insulin is given by both subcutaneous and intravenous routes; all others are given only subcutaneously. If the intravenous route is not available, regular insulin may also be administered intramuscularly in an emergency situation.

Regular or rapid-acting insulins are used in continuous subcutaneous insulin infusion (CSII) devices, often called *insulin pumps* (e.g., MiniMed and Disetronic pumps). CSII devices have a small pump that holds a syringe of insulin, connected to a subcutaneous needle by tubing. The pump is about the size of a pager and can be worn on a belt or tucked into a pocket. The needle is placed in the skin, usually in the abdomen, and is changed every 3 days. This device delivers a constant amount of programmed insulin throughout each 24-hour period. It also can be used to deliver a bolus of insulin manually (e.g., before meals).

Type 2 diabetics cannot be managed with oral medications during hospitalization because of the risk of hypoglycemia from not eating and the slow response of these medications to correct hyperglycemia. There is growing acceptance of the need to achieve tighter control of blood sugar in individuals who are hospitalized with hyperglycemia, whether they are diagnosed with diabetes, have unrecognized diabetes, or have hospital-related diabetes (Clement et al., 2004; Magee, 2006).

In a study of 1,200 medical ICU patients, Van den Berghe et al. (2006) compared those receiving intensive insulin therapy with patients receiving conventional therapy (insulin administered when the blood glucose reached 215 mg/dL). Those in the intensively treated group who were in the ICU for 3 days or more had significantly reduced morbidity, slightly more incidents of hypoglycemia (although significantly less mortality related to hypoglycemia than those treated conventionally), and significantly reduced acquired kidney injury (defined as a serum creatinine level at least twice the admission level).

Maintaining normal blood glucose during hospitalization decreases the risk of postoperative infections and shortens hospital stays. Healing is impaired when hemoglobin is glycosylated (hemoglobin A_{1c}); glycosylated Hgb has increased affinity for oxygen, putting tissues at risk for ischemia (McCance & Huether, 2002). Further, diabetes leads to small-vessel disease, which impairs circulation and oxygenation of tissue for healing.

Intravenous insulin infusions are preferable for maintaining normal blood glucose during hospitalization, although their use depends on frequent blood glucose monitoring and intensive nursing care. Supplements of regular insulin following sliding scale prescriptions (relative to monitored blood glucose levels) are ineffective management protocols, risking both hyperglycemia and hypoglycemia. These supplements treat hyperglycemia after it has occurred rather than preventing it.

Many people with diabetes believe the pump allows more normal regulation of blood glucose and provides greater lifestyle flexibility. Pumps are as safe as multiple-injection therapy when recommended procedures are followed. A potential complication is an undetected interruption in insulin delivery, which may result in a rapid onset of DKA. The needle site must be kept clean and changed on a regular basis (usually every 2–3 days) to prevent inflammation and infection.

Other special injection products are available for people with physical handicaps. These products include automatic injectors and jet spray injectors. Prefilled syringes are useful for people who are visually impaired or traveling. Prefilled syringes are stable for up to 30 days if stored in the refrigerator.

The vial of insulin in use may be kept at room temperature for up to 4 weeks. Stored vials should be kept in the refrigerator and brought to room temperature prior to administration.

Regular insulin does not require mixing. If the solution is cloudy or discolored, the vial should be discarded. The other types of insulin must be mixed to disperse the particles evenly throughout the solution. Mix the vial by gently rolling it between the hands; vigorous shaking causes bubble formation and frothing, which makes the dose inaccurate. It is critical that no air bubbles remain in the prepared dose, because even a small bubble can displace several units of insulin.

Although in theory any area of the body with subcutaneous tissue can be used for injections of insulin, certain sites are recommended (Figure 18–9 ■). The rate of absorption and peak of action of insulin differ according to the site. The site that allows the most rapid absorption is the abdomen, followed by the deltoid muscle, then the thigh, and then the hip. Because of the rapid absorption, the abdomen is the recommended site. See Box 18–2 for techniques to minimize painful injections.

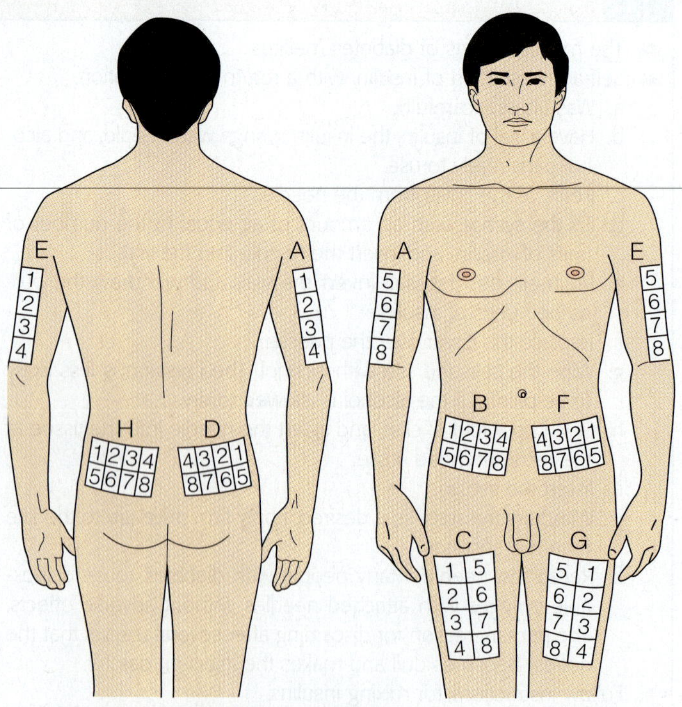

Figure 18–9 ■ Sites of insulin injection.

Box 18–2 Techniques to Minimize Painful Injections

- Inject insulin that is at room temperature.
- Make sure no air bubbles remain in the syringe before the injection.
- Wait until alcohol on the skin completely dries before the injection.
- Relax muscles in the injection area.
- Penetrate the skin with the needle quickly.
- Don't change the direction of the needle during insertion or withdrawal.
- Don't reuse dull needles.

Source: Adapted from "Insulin Administration" by the American Diabetes Association, 1998, *Diabetes Care, 21* (Supplement 1), 572–575.

Do not massage the site after administering the injection, because this may interfere with absorption; pressure, however, may be applied for about 1 minute. Insulin should not be injected into an area to be exercised (such as the thigh before a vigorous walk) or to which heat will be applied; exercise or heat may increase the rate of absorption and cause a more rapid onset and peak of action.

Lipodystrophy (hypertrophy of subcutaneous tissue) or lipoatrophy (atrophy of subcutaneous tissue) may result if the same injection sites are used repeatedly, especially with pork and beef insulins. The tissues become hardened and have an orange-peel appearance. The use of refrigerated insulin may trigger the development of tissue atrophy or hypertrophy. These problems rarely occur with the use of human insulins. Lipodystrophy and lipoatrophy alter insulin absorption, delaying its onset or retaining the insulin in the tissue for a period of time instead of allowing it to be absorbed into the body. Lipodystrophy usually resolves if the area is unused for a minimum of 6 months.

HYPOGLYCEMIC AGENTS Hypoglycemic agents are used to treat people with type 2 DM. These medications lower blood sugar by stimulating or increasing insulin secretion, preventing breakdown of glycogen to glucose by the liver, and increasing peripheral uptake of glucose by making cells less resistant to insulin. Peripheral uptake refers to uptake by muscles and fat in the arms and legs rather than in the trunk. Some hypoglycemics keep blood sugar low by blocking absorption of carbohydrates in the intestines. A new hypoglycemic that is not insulin but is available only as an injectable is exenatide (Byetta). It has several modes of action: (1) signals the pancreas to make insulin when nutrients are ingested and stop insulin release as blood sugar normalizes, (2) stops liver conversion of glycogen to glucose, and (3) decreases absorption of sugar from the intestines. The goal of therapy with these agents is to reduce glycosylated hemoglobin and lower fasting and postprandial glucose (Capriotti, 2005).

ASPIRIN THERAPY People with diabetes are up to four times more likely to die from cardiovascular disease. It is recommended that a once-daily dose of 81–325 mg of enteric-coated aspirin be given to reduce atherosclerosis in clients with vascular disease or increased cardiovascular risk factors. Aspirin therapy is contraindicated for clients with aspirin allergy, bleeding tendency, anticoagulant therapy, recent gastrointestinal bleeding, or active liver disease (ADA, 2003).

Nutrition

The management of diabetes requires a careful balance between the intake of nutrients, the expenditure of energy, and the dose and timing of insulin or oral antidiabetic agents. Although everyone has the same need for basic nutrition, the person with diabetes must eat a more structured diet to prevent hyperglycemia. The goals for dietary management for adults with diabetes, based on guidelines established by the ADA (2002), are as follows:

- Maintain as near normal blood glucose levels as possible by balancing food intake with insulin or oral glucose.
- Achieve optimal serum lipid levels.
- Provide adequate calories to maintain or attain reasonable weights, and to recover from catabolic illness.
- Prevent and treat the acute complications of insulin-treated DM, short-term illnesses, and exercise-related problems; or the long-term complications of diabetes.
- Improve overall health through optimal nutrition, using Dietary Guidelines for Americans and the Food Guide Pyramid.

The ADA recommends that carbohydrates should be individualized to the client's needs, with recommended allowances of 45–65% of the daily diet. Carbohydrates contain 4 kcal/g and intake should not be restricted to less than 130 g/day (Sheard et al., 2004). This group of nutrients consists of plant foods (grains, fruits, vegetables), milk, and some dairy products. Carbohydrates can be divided into simple sugars and complex carbohydrates. Glycemic index is the rate a food raises blood glucose and, thus, insulin. Proponents of low-carbohydrate diets use glycemic index as the scientific foundation for decreasing intake of foods with a high glycemic index. However, many factors affect the digestion of carbohydrates; to date research does not support using glycemic index as a basis for therapy. The ADA does not recommend reliance on glycemic index as a method to treat or prevent diabetes (ADA, 2006).

The use of sucrose as part of the total carbohydrate content in the diet does not impair blood glucose control in people with diabetes. Sucrose and sucrose-containing foods must be substituted for other carbohydrates gram for gram. Dietary fructose (from fruits and vegetables or from fructose-sweetened foods) produces a smaller rise in plasma glucose than sucrose and most starches, so it may offer an advantage as a sweetening agent. However, large amounts of fructose have potentially adverse effects on serum cholesterol and LDL cholesterol, so amounts used should be controlled.

The recommended daily protein intake is 15–20% of total daily kilocalorie intake. Protein has 4 kcal/g. Sources of protein should be low in fat, low in saturated fat, and low in cholesterol. Although this amount of protein is much less than most people normally consume, it is recommended to help prevent or delay renal complications. To help the client accept the decrease in the amount of protein, the nurse may suggest a less severe restriction at diagnosis with a gradual decrease to take place over a period of years.

Dietary fats should be low in saturated fat and cholesterol. Saturated fats should be no higher than 10% of the total kilocalories allowed per day, with dietary cholesterol less than 300 mg/day. Fat has 9 kcal/g. Sources of the different types of fat include:

- *Saturated fat.* Sources are animal meats (meat and butter fats, lard, bacon), cocoa butter, coconut oil, palm oil, and hydrogenated oils.
- *Polyunsaturated fat.* Sources are oils of corn, safflower, sunflower, soybean, sesame seed, and cottonseed.
- *Monosaturated fat.* Sources are peanut oil, olive oil, and canola oil.

Limiting fat and cholesterol intake may help prevent or delay the onset of atherosclerosis, a common complication of diabetes.

Dietary fiber may be helpful in treating or preventing constipation and other gastrointestinal disorders, including colon cancer. It also helps provide a feeling of fullness, and large amounts of soluble fiber may be beneficial to serum lipids. Soluble fiber is found in dried beans, oats, barley, and in some vegetables and fruits (e.g., peas, corn, zucchini, cauliflower, broccoli, prunes, pears, apples, bananas, oranges). Insoluble fiber, which is found in wheat, corn, and in some vegetables and fruits (e.g., carrots, brussels sprouts, eggplant, green beans, pears, apples, strawberries), does facilitate intestinal motility and give a feeling of fullness.

The ideal level of fiber has not been determined, but an intake of 20–35 g/day is recommended. An increase in fiber may cause nausea, diarrhea, or constipation, and increased flatulence, especially if the person does not also increase fluid intake. Fiber in the diet should therefore be increased gradually.

Although the body requires sodium, most people consume much more than is needed each day, especially in processed foods. The recommended daily intake is 1,000 mg of sodium per 1,000 kcal, not to exceed 3,000 mg. The primary concern with sodium is its association with hypertension, a common health problem in people with diabetes. It is suggested that table salt (which is 40% sodium) and processed foods high in sodium be avoided in the diabetes meal plan.

The diet plan for people with diabetes restricts the amount of refined sugars. As a result, many people use noncaloric sweeteners and foods or drinks made with noncaloric sweeteners. Commercially produced nonnutritive sweeteners are approved for use by the FDA. Although questions have been raised about the safety of these substances in laboratory animal studies, they are considered safe for use by humans. Included in this category of sweeteners are saccharin (Sweet & Low), aspartame or neotame (Nutrasweet, Equal), sucralose (Splenda), and acesulfame potassium (Sunnette). The nonnutritive sweeteners have negligent amounts of or no kilocalories, do not produce dental caries, and produce very little or no changes in blood glucose levels.

People with diabetes also use nutritive sweeteners, including fructose, sorbitol, and xylitol. The kilocalorie content of these substances is similar to that of table sugar (sucrose), but they cause less elevation in blood glucose. They are often included in foods labeled as "sugar free." Sorbitol may cause flatulence and diarrhea.

Researchers are continuing to study the safety and effectiveness of the sweeteners. In addition, the FDA recommends that the food industry label products with the amount of each ingredient in milligrams per serving and the number of servings per container. When teaching clients about diet, the nurse should include information about the kilocalorie content of sweeteners and the meaning of such phrases as *sugar free* and *dietetic* on labels.

Although drinking alcoholic beverages is not encouraged, neither is it totally prohibited for the client with diabetes. Alcohol consumption may potentiate the hypoglycemic effects of insulin and oral agents. The ADA recommends that men with diabetes consume no more than two drinks and women with diabetes no more than one drink per day. In the following list are guidelines for people who include alcohol in their diet plan:

- The signs of intoxication and hypoglycemia are similar; thus, the person with type 1 DM is at increased risk for an insulin reaction.
- Two oral hypoglycemic agents (chlorpropamide and tolbutamide) may interact with the alcohol, causing headache, flushing, and nausea.
- Liqueurs, sweet wines, wine coolers, and sweet mixes contain large amounts of carbohydrate.
- Light beer is the recommended alcoholic drink.
- Alcohol should be consumed with meals and added to the daily food intake. In most instances, the alcohol is substituted for fat in calculating the diet; a drink with 1.5 oz of alcohol is the equivalent of two fat exchanges (90 kcal).

Several systems for meal planning are available to the person with diabetes. These systems include a consistent-carbohydrate diabetes meal plan, exchange lists, point systems, food groups, carbohydrate counting, and calorie counting. No matter what system is used, however, it must take into account the person's individualized eating habits, diet history, food values, and special needs. Altering foods and meal patterns is often one of the most difficult parts of diabetes management; careful consideration of individualized preferences enhances compliance with the diet. Although the ADA recommends that a registered dietitian provide the nutrition prescription, nurses must know what is prescribed and be able to reinforce teaching and answer questions.

Sick-Day Management

When the person with diabetes is sick or has surgery, blood glucose levels increase, even though food intake decreases. The person often mistakenly alters or omits the insulin dose, causing further problems. The guidelines for dietary management during illness focus on preventing dehydration and providing nutrition for promoting recovery. In general, sick-day management includes the following:

- Monitoring blood glucose at least four times a day throughout an illness
- Testing urine for ketones if blood glucose is greater than 240 mg/dL
- Continuing to take the usual insulin dose or oral hypoglycemic agent
- Sipping 8–12 oz of fluid each hour
- Substituting easily digested liquids or soft foods if solid foods are not tolerated. (The substituted liquids and foods should be carbohydrate equivalents, for example, 1/2 cup sweetened gelatin, 1/2 cup fruit juice, one Popsicle, 1/4 cup sherbet, and 1/2 cup regular soft drink.)

- Calling the health care provider if the client is unable to eat for more than 24 hours or if vomiting and diarrhea last for more than 6 hours.

Exercise

The third component of diabetes management is a regular exercise program. The benefits of exercise are the same for everyone, with or without diabetes: improved physical fitness, improved emotional state, weight control, and improved work capacity. In people with diabetes, exercise increases the uptake of glucose by muscle cells, potentially reducing the need for insulin. Exercise also decreases cholesterol and triglycerides, reducing the risk of cardiovascular disorders. People with diabetes should consult their primary health care provider before beginning or changing an exercise program. The ability to maintain an exercise program is affected by many factors, including fatigue and glucose levels. It is as important to assess the person's usual lifestyle before establishing an exercise program as it is before planning a diet. Factors to consider include the client's usual exercise habits, living environment, and community programs. The exercise that the person enjoys most is probably the one that he or she will continue throughout life.

Use proper footwear, inspect the feet daily and after exercise, avoid exercise in extreme heat or cold, and avoid exercise during periods of poor glucose control. Stress electrocardiogram (EKG) tests to detect ischemia are no longer recommended in asymptomatic individuals at low CAD risk (<10% risk of a cardiac event over 10 years) (Sigal, Kenny, Wasserman, & Castaneda-Sceppa, 2004).

In the person with type 1 DM, glycemic responses to exercise vary according to the type, intensity, and duration of the exercise. Other factors that influence responses include the timing of exercise in relation to meals and insulin injections, and the time of day of the activity. Unless these factors are integrated into the exercise program, the person with type 1 DM has an increased risk of hypoglycemia and hyperglycemia. Following are general guidelines for an exercise program:

- People who have frequent hyperglycemia or hypoglycemia should avoid prolonged exercise until glucose control improves.
- The risk of exercise-induced hypoglycemia is lowest before breakfast, when free-insulin levels tend to be lower than they are before meals later in the day or at bedtime.
- Low-impact aerobic exercises are encouraged.
- Exercise should be moderate and regular; brief, intense exercise tends to cause mild hyperglycemia, and prolonged exercise can lead to hypoglycemia.
- Exercising at a peak insulin action time may lead to hypoglycemia.
- Self-monitoring of blood glucose levels is essential both before and after exercise.
- Food intake may need to be increased to compensate for the activity.
- Fluid intake, especially water, is essential.

Young adults may continue participating in sports with some modifications in diet and insulin dosage. Athletes should begin training slowly, extend activity over a prolonged period, take a carbohydrate source (such as a drink consisting of 5–10% carbohydrate) after about 1 hour of exercise, and monitor blood glucose levels for possible adjustments. In addition, a snack should be available after the activity is completed. It may be necessary to omit the usual regular insulin dose prior to an athletic event; even if the athlete is hyperglycemic at the beginning of the event, blood glucose levels will fall to normal after the first 60–90 minutes of exercise.

An exercise program for the person with type 2 DM is especially important. The benefits of regular exercise include weight loss in those who are overweight, improved glycemic control, increased well-being, socialization with others, and a reduction of cardiovascular risk factors. A combination of diet, exercise, and weight loss often decreases the need for oral hypoglycemic agents. This decrease is due to an increased sensitivity to insulin, increased kilocalorie expenditure, and increased self-esteem. Regular exercise may prevent type 2 DM in high-risk individuals (Roberts & Barnard, 2005).

Following are general guidelines for an exercise program:

- Before beginning the program, have a medical screening for previously undiagnosed hypertension, neuropathy, retinopathy, and nephropathy.
- Begin the program with mild exercises, and gradually increase intensity and duration.
- Self-monitor blood glucose before and after exercise.
- Exercise at least three times a week or every other day, for at least 20–30 minutes.
- Include muscle-strengthening and low-impact aerobic exercises in the program.

Surgery

Surgical management of diabetes involves replacing or transplanting the pancreas, pancreatic cells, or beta cells. Although it is still in the investigative stage, many researchers believe that transplantation of the tail of the pancreas is the most promising technique for achieving long-term disease control. Islet cell transplantation has had moderate success, and research is continuing. Other research is being conducted in the use of an internally implanted artificial pancreas, or closed-loop artificial beta cell.

Surgery is a stressor that often alters self-management and glycemic control in people with diabetes. In response to stress, levels of catecholamines, cortisol, glucagon, and growth hormones increase, as does insulin resistance. Hyperglycemia occurs, and protein stores are decreased. In addition, diet and activity patterns change, and medication types and dosages vary. As a result, surgical clients who have diabetes are at increased risk for postoperative infection, delayed wound healing, fluid and electrolyte imbalances, hypoglycemia, and DKA (Aragon et al., 2003).

Preoperatively, all clients should be in the best possible metabolic state. Screening for complications and regular blood glucose monitoring are part of preoperative preparation. Oral hypoglycemic agents may be withheld for 1 or 2 days before surgery, and regular insulin is often administered to the client with type 2 DM during the perioperative period. The client with type 1 DM follows a carefully prescribed insulin regimen individualized to specific needs.

The insulin regimen in the preoperative, intraoperative, and immediate postoperative periods is individualized and may involve any of the following:

- No intermediate- or long-acting insulin is given the day of surgery; regular insulin is given with intravenous glucose. When the client is npo, short-acting insulin should not be given without intravenous glucose.
- Half of the usual intermediate- or long-acting insulin is given before surgery and the remaining half is given in the recovery room.
- The total daily dose of insulin is divided into four equal doses of regular insulin, and one dose is administered subcutaneously every 6 hours. An intravenous solution of 5% dextrose in 0.45% normal saline is administered for fluid replacement, and blood glucose monitoring precedes each insulin dose (Guthrie & Guthrie, 1997).
- Clients with type 1 DM or type 2 DM with preoperative blood glucose greater than 200 receive IV glucose and insulin infusion. The target blood glucose level during surgery is between 125 and 200 mg/dL. This avoids hypoglycemia, which is difficult to detect under anesthesia, and prevents glycosuria, dehydration, and impaired wound healing. IV infusion of glucose, insulin, and added potassium is appropriate for all hyperglycemic patients undergoing surgery (Amiel & Alberti, 2005; Mabrey, 2004).

The surgical procedure should be scheduled for as early as possible in the morning to minimize the length of fasting. If there is no food intake after surgery, intravenous dextrose should be administered, accompanied by subcutaneous regular insulin every 6 hours. The dose can be adjusted to blood glucose levels. Although kilocalorie intake is decreased postoperatively, stress can increase insulin requirements. Glucose control is also affected postoperatively by nausea and vomiting, anorexia, and gastrointestinal suction.

During the postoperative period, the client with type 2 DM may continue to require insulin or may resume oral medications, depending on glucose control. The client with type 1 DM may require reduced insulin as healing progresses and stress diminishes. Regular blood glucose monitoring is essential, as are assessments for hypoglycemia.

NURSING PROCESS

The responses of clients with diabetes to their illness often are complex and individual, involving multiple body systems. Assessments, planning, and implementation differ for the client with newly diagnosed diabetes, the client with long-term diabetes, and the client with acute complications of diabetes. The plan of care and the content of teaching also differ according to the type of diabetes and the client's age, culture, and intellectual, psychologic, and social resources.

Teaching the client (and family) to self-manage diabetes is a nursing responsibility. Even if a formal teaching plan is developed and implemented by advanced practice nurses, all nurses must be able to reinforce this knowledge and answer questions. Teaching is necessary for both the person who is newly diagnosed and for the person who has had diabetes for years. In fact, the latter may need almost as much teaching as the newly diagnosed client. Products for diabetes care, especially insulins, have changed dramatically, and knowledge about risk reduction to prevent complications has increased.

The American Diabetes Association recommends that teaching be carried out on three levels. The first level focuses on survival skills, with the person learning basic knowledge and skills to provide diabetes management for the first week or two, while he or she adjusts to the idea of having the disease. The second level deals with home management, emphasizing self-reliance and independence in the daily management of diabetes. The third level aims at improving lifestyle and educating clients to individualize self-management of the illness.

Health promotion activities primarily focus on preventing the complications of diabetes. Clients should prevent or decrease excess weight, follow a sensible and well-balanced diet, and maintain a regular physical exercise program. Blood glucose screening at 3-year intervals beginning at age 45 is recommended for those in high-risk groups. These same activities, when combined with medications and self-monitoring, also are beneficial in reducing the onset of complications.

Assessment

The following data are collected through the health history and physical examination:

- *Health history.* Family history of diabetes; history of hypertension or other cardiovascular problems; history of any change in vision (e.g., blurring) or speech, dizziness, and numbness or tingling in hands or feet; pain when walking; frequent voiding; change in weight, appetite, infections, and healing; problems with gastrointestinal function or urination; or altered sexual function
- *Physical assessment.* Height/weight ratio, vital signs, visual acuity, cranial nerves, sensory ability of extremities (e.g., touch, hot/cold, and vibration), peripheral pulses, and skin and mucous membranes (e.g., hair loss, appearance, lesions, rash, itching, and vaginal discharge).

Further focused assessments are described later in the Caring Interventions section.

Older Adults

When assessing older clients, be aware of normal aging changes in all body systems that may alter interpretation of findings.

Children

Children generally are admitted to the hospital at the time of diagnosis. Assess the child's physiologic status; focus on vital signs and level of consciousness. Also, assess hydration by checking mucous membranes, skin turgor, and urine output. Blood initially is collected hourly to monitor blood gases, glucose, and electrolytes. Once the child is stable, assess dietary and caloric intake and the ability of the child or family to manage care.

If parents waited to seek care until the child began to experience symptoms of DKA, they may feel guilty at the time of diagnosis. Assess coping mechanisms, family strengths and resources, ability to manage the disease, and the educational needs of both the child and parents. Identify family stressors that will cause challenges in the long-term management of diabetes, including access to health insurance and other financial considerations.

Diagnosis

The goals of care are to maintain function, prevent complications, and teach self-management. Although many NANDA nursing diagnoses are appropriate for the person with diabetes, the following address some of the more common problems:

- Knowledge Deficit
- Risk for Impaired Skin Integrity
- Risk for Infection
- Risk for Injury
- Risk for Deficient Fluid Volume
- Sexual Dysfunction
- Ineffective Coping.

Plan

The nursing plan of care is focused on helping the client learn to provide self-care and reduce the risk of complications. Goals of care include, but are not limited to the following:

- Client describes how to administer medications and respond to side effects appropriately.
- Client demonstrates meal planning compliant with the American Diabetic Association diet.
- Client demonstrates proper foot care and inspection.
- Client demonstrates proper procedure for monitoring blood sugar levels.
- Client describes strategies for reducing risk of infection.

Implementation

Nursing care is individualized and focuses on teaching the client and family about the disease and its management, planning dietary intake, providing emotional support, and creating strategies for daily management in the community. Some hospitals have developed clinical pathways to streamline and standardize diabetes care. Include the following when teaching the client and family about care at home:

- Information about normal metabolism, diabetes, and how diabetes changes metabolism
- How diet helps keep blood glucose in the normal range; the number of kilocalories required and why; the amount of carbohydrates, meats, and fats allowed and why; and how to calculate the diet while integrating personal food preferences
- Exercise helps lower blood glucose, the importance of a regular exercise program, types of exercise, integrating personal exercise preferences, and how to handle increased activity

DEVELOPMENTAL CONSIDERATIONS **Diabetes**

CHILDREN

- The child's developmental stage and cognitive level influence his or her readiness to take on responsibility for self-care—for example, to obtain and read a blood glucose sample or inject insulin. Children usually can perform some tasks with supervision by 6–8 years of age.
- Caution parents to check the blood glucose level of a toddler who is extremely sleepy or irritable, because these can be signs of hypoglycemia or hyperglycemia.
- The preschool child's need for autonomy and control can be met by allowing the child to choose snacks or pick which finger to stick for glucose testing and by helping parents to gather necessary supplies.
- School-age children need to learn how to recognize the signs of hypoglycemia and hyperglycemia and to understand the importance of carrying a rapidly absorbed sugar product.
- Adolescents in particular are present-time oriented and may rebel against the daily regimen of insulin injections, the food plan, and the exercise plan. The desire to be like peers may interfere with their adherence to treatment.
- When the child with diabetes is sick, parents need to be extra attentive to the child's glycemic control.
- Record growth measurements and vital signs in the child's chart. Puberty may be delayed if diabetic control is inadequate.
- The child with type 1 DM may develop circulatory and neurologic changes over time. Emphasize the importance of good foot care from an early age.
- The child with diabetes needs an Individual Health Plan (IHP) for management of diabetes while in school or child care. The IHP should include when blood glucose testing needs to be performed, insulin administration and storage, meals and snacks needed, and symptoms and management of hypoglycemia and hyperglycemia.

OLDER ADULTS

- The prevalence of diabetes becomes greater with age, increasing from 8.2% with diagnosed diabetes in those age 20 years or older to 18.4% for those equal to or older than age 65 (ADA, 2005).
- Although most older adults with diabetes have type 2 DM, the improved survival rates for people with diabetes have resulted in an increased number of older adults with type 1 DM. The picture is further complicated by the fact that blood glucose levels increase with age, beginning in the 50s. For this reason, it is more difficult to diagnose diabetes in older adults, because these clients may be mistakenly diagnosed with the disease simply for exhibiting essentially normal age-related changes in glucose. The relationship between normal increases in glucose levels and the presence of diabetes is not yet understood.
- The normal physiologic changes of aging may mask manifestations of the onset of diabetes. Signs and symptoms of diabetes in older adults may not include the classic symptoms of polyuria and thirst. Conditions such as orthostatic hypotension, periodontal disease, infections, stroke, gastric hypotony, impotence, neuropathy, confusion, and glaucoma should be considered as potential indicators of diabetes (Eliopoulos, 2005), and these condition also may increase the potential for complications from the disease or its treatment.
- The older adult with diabetes has multiple, complex health care problems and needs, including risks for polypharmacy, depression, cognitive impairment, urinary incontinence, injurious falls, and persistent pain (ADA, 2005).
- The older adult with diabetes also has a longer recovery period after surgery or serious illness, often requiring insulin to maintain blood glucose levels. The benefits and risks of treatment to maintain glycemic control as well as blood pressure and lipid management must be carefully balanced.

- Self-monitoring of blood glucose, how to care for equipment, and what to do about a high or low blood glucose level
- Medications:
  a. *Insulin: intravenous agents.* Type, dosage, mixing instructions (if necessary), times of onset and peak actions, how to get and care for equipment, how to give injections, and where to give injections
  b. *Insulin: oral agents.* Type, dosage, side effects, and interaction with other drugs.
- Manifestations of acute complications of hypoglycemia and hyperglycemia, and what to do when they occur
- Hygiene, including skin care, dental care, and foot care
- What to do about food, fluids, and medications when the client is sick
- Helpful resources.

Teaching may have to be adapted to the special needs and developmental level of a child or older adult. However, because 40% of all people with diabetes are over the age of 65, considering the special needs of the older population is particularly essential. Uncontrolled diabetes in the older adult increases the potential for functional loss, social disengagement, and increased morbidity and mortality. Education for self-care allows the older adult to be more actively involved in diabetes management and decreases the potential for acute and chronic complications from the disease. Considerations for teaching the older adult with diabetes include the following:

- Changes in diet may be difficult to implement for many reasons. Favorite foods are difficult to give up. Balanced meals at regular intervals may not have been part of the client's lifestyle. Purchasing, storing, and preparing foods may be a problem. Dentures may not fit well. Changes in taste sensation often cause the client to increase the use of salt and sugar. (For more information on nutrition and the older adult, see the nutrition exemplar in Concept 13, Health, Illness and Wellness.)
- Exercise of any type may not have been part of the activities of daily living. An exercise plan must be individualized for any physical limitations imposed by other chronic illnesses, such as arthritis, Parkinson's disease, chronic respiratory diseases, and/or cardiovascular diseases.
- Diagnosis of a chronic illness threatens a client's independence and self-worth. After years of taking care of self, the older adult with diabetes may now have to depend on others for help in meeting self-care needs. This change of circumstance often leads to withdrawal from social interactions with others.
- Money to purchase medications and supplies often must be taken out of a fixed income.
- Visual deficits may make insulin administration difficult or impossible. Visual deficits also can interfere with blood glucose monitoring, food preparation, exercises, and foot care.

Caring interventions may also focus on the risks for impaired skin integrity, infection, and injury as well as on sexual dysfunction and ineffective coping. Interventions for each diagnosis is discussed in the following section.

Risk for Impaired Skin Integrity

The client with diabetes is at increased risk for altered skin integrity as a result of decreased or absent sensation from neuropathies, decreased tissue perfusion from cardiovascular complications, and infection. In addition, poor vision increases the risk of trauma, and an open lesion is more prone to infection and delayed healing.

Impaired skin and tissue integrity, with resultant gangrene, is especially common in the feet and lower extremities. In fact, people with diabetes are at significant risk for lower-extremity gangrene. Conduct baseline and ongoing assessments of the feet, including the following:

- Musculoskeletal assessment that includes foot and ankle joint range of motion, bone abnormalities (e.g., bunions, hammertoes, and overlapping digits), gait patterns, use of assistive devices for walking, and abnormal wear patterns on shoes
- Neurologic assessment that includes sensations of touch and position, pain, and temperature
- Vascular examination that includes assessment of lower extremity pulses, capillary refill, color and temperature of skin, and edema
- Assessment of hydration status, including dryness or excessive perspiration
- Assessment for lesions, fissures between toes, corns, calluses, plantar warts, ingrown or overgrown toenails, redness over pressure points, blisters, cellulitis, or gangrene.

Peripheral neuropathies may result in altered perception of pain, loss of deep tendon reflexes, loss of cutaneous pressure and position sensation, foot drop, changes in the shape of the foot, and changes in bones and joints. Peripheral vascular disease may cause intermittent claudication, absent pulses, delayed venous filling on elevation, dependent rubor, and gangrene. Injuries, lesions, and changes in skin hydration potentiate infections, delayed healing, and tissue loss in the person with diabetes.

- Teach foot hygiene. Wash the feet daily with lukewarm water and mild hand soap. Pat dry, and dry well between the toes. Apply a very thin coat of lubricating cream if dryness is present (but not between the toes). Proper hygiene decreases the chance of infection. Temperature receptors may be impaired, so the water should always be tested before use.
- Discuss the importance of not smoking if client smokes. Nicotine in tobacco causes vasoconstriction, further decreasing the blood supply to the feet.
- Discuss the importance of maintaining blood glucose levels through prescribed diet, medication, and exercise. Hyperglycemia promotes the growth of microorganisms.
- Conduct foot care teaching sessions (see the Client Teaching feature that follows) as often as necessary. Foot care is a priority in diabetes management to prevent serious problems. Many people with diabetes are unaware of lesions or injury until infection and compromised circulation are

far advanced. The hows and whys of each component must be included in teaching. A variety of methods may be used, including demonstration, return demonstration, audiovisual aids, and written lists. If the person is wearing shoes and socks, ask him or her to remove them to practice foot care effectively.

Risk for Infection

The person with diabetes is at increased risk for infection. The risk of infection is believed to result from vascular insufficiency that limits the inflammatory response, neurologic abnormalities that limit the awareness of trauma, and a predisposition to bacterial and fungal infections.

- Use and teach meticulous hand washing. Hand washing is the single most effective method for preventing the spread of infection.
- Monitor for manifestations of infection: increased temperature, pain, malaise, swelling, redness, discharge, and cough. Early diagnosis and treatment of infections can control their severity and decrease complications.
- Discuss the importance of skin care. Using lukewarm water and mild soap, keep the skin clean and dry. People with diabetes are more prone to develop furuncles and carbuncles; the infection often increases the need for insulin. Clean, intact skin and mucous membranes are the first line of defense against infection.
- Teach dental health measures:
  a. Obtain a dental examination every 4–6 months.
  b. Maintain careful oral hygiene, which includes brushing the teeth with a soft toothbrush and fluoridated toothpaste at least twice a day and flossing as recommended.
  c. Be aware of symptoms requiring dental care: bad breath; unpleasant taste in the mouth; bleeding, red, or sore gums; and tooth pain.
  d. Monitor for the need to make adjustments in insulin if dental surgery is necessary.

  All people with diabetes need to be taught proper oral hygiene, the risk of periodontal disease, and the importance of obtaining dental care for symptoms of oral or dental problems.
- Teach women with diabetes the symptoms and preventive measures for vaginitis caused by Candida albicans. The symptoms are an odorless, white or yellow cheese-like discharge and itching. Sexual transmission is unlikely, but discomfort may cause the client to avoid sexual activity. Diabetes is a predisposing factor for C. albicans vaginitis, the most common form of vaginitis. Poor personal hygiene and clothing that keeps the vaginal area warm and moist increase the risk of vaginitis. The infection may spread to the urinary tract, resulting in urinary tract infections; preventing and treating vaginitis decrease this risk.

CLIENT TEACHING **Foot Care**

GENERAL INFORMATION

- Never go barefoot. Wear slippers when leaving the bed during the night.
- Do not use commercial corn medicines or pads, chemicals (e.g., boric acid, iodine, or hydrogen peroxide), or over-the-counter cortisone medications on the feet.
- Do not put heating pads, hot-water bottles, or ice packs on the feet. If the feet become cold at night, wear socks, or use extra blankets.
- Do not allow the feet to become sunburned.
- Do not put tape on the feet.
- Do not sit with the legs crossed at the knees or ankles.

BUYING AND WEARING SHOES AND STOCKINGS

- Shoes that allow 1/2–3/4 in. of toe room are best; there should be room for toes to spread out and wiggle. The lining and inside stitching should be smooth and the insole soft. The sole should be flexible and cushion the foot. The heel should fit snugly, and good arch support should be present.
- Do not wear open-toed shoes, sandals, high heels, or thongs; these increase the risk of trauma.
- Buy shoes late in the afternoon, when feet are at their largest; always buy shoes that feel comfortable and do not need to be "broken in."
- Shoes made of natural fibers (e.g., leather and canvas) allow perspiration to escape.
- Check the shoes before each wearing for foreign objects, wrinkled insoles, and cracks that might cause lesions.
- Stockings made of wool or cotton allow perspiration to dry.
- Do not wear garters, knee stockings, or pantyhose; these may interfere with circulation.
- Wear insulated boots in the winter.

INSPECTING THE FEET

- Check the feet daily for red areas, cuts, blisters, corns, calluses, or cracks in the skin. Check between the toes for cracks or reddened areas.
- Check the skin of the feet for dry or damp areas.
- Use a mirror to check each sole and the back of each heel.
- If you are unable to inspect the feet daily, be sure that someone else does.

CARE OF TOENAILS

- Cut the toenails after washing, when they are softer and easier to trim.
- Cut the nails straight across with a clipper, and smooth edges and corners with an emery board.
- Do not use razor blades to trim the toenails.
- If you are unable to see well or to reach the feet easily, have someone else trim the nails. If the nails are very thick or ingrown, if the toes overlap, or if circulation is poor, get professional care from a podiatrist.

Risk for Injury

The client with diabetes is at risk for injury from multiple factors. Neuropathies may alter sensation, gait, and muscle control. Cataracts or retinopathy may cause visual deficits. Hyperglycemia often causes osmotic changes in the lenses of the eye, resulting in blurred vision. In addition, changes in blood glucose alter levels of consciousness and may cause seizures. The impaired mobility, sensory deficits, and neurologic effects of complications of diabetes increase the risk of accidents, burns, falls, and trauma.

- Assess for the presence of contributing or causative factors that increase the risk of injury: blurred vision, cataracts, decreased adaptation to dark, decreased tactile sensitivity, hypoglycemia, hyperglycemia, hypovolemia, joint immobility, and unstable gait. A knowledge base is necessary to develop an individualized plan of care. The risk of injury increases with the number of factors identified.
- Reduce environmental hazards in the health care facility, and teach the client about safety in the home and in the community.
- Monitor for and teach the client and family to recognize and seek care for the manifestations of DKA in the client with type 1 DM: hyperglycemia, thirst, headaches, nausea and vomiting, increased urine output, ketonuria, dehydration, and decreasing level of consciousness. Blood glucose levels increase if the need for insulin is unmet or insufficiently met, because the cellular use of fats for fuel results in ketosis. Osmotic diuresis increases urinary output, resulting in thirst and dehydration.
- Monitor for and teach the client and family to recognize and seek care for the manifestations of HHS in the client with type 2 DM: extreme hyperglycemia, increased urinary output, thirst, dehydration, hypotension, seizures, and decreasing level of consciousness. HHS is a life-threatening condition requiring recognition and treatment.
- Monitor for and teach the client and family to recognize and treat the manifestations of hypoglycemia: low blood glucose, anxiety, headache, uncoordinated movements, sweating, rapid pulse, drowsiness, and visual changes. Teach client and family to carry some form of rapid-acting sugar source at all times. Severe hypoglycemia causes a decrease in the level of consciousness. The decrease in blood glucose most often results from too much insulin, too little food, or too much exercise.
- Recommend wearing a MedicAlert bracelet or necklace that identifies the client as a person with diabetes. In case of sudden, severe illness or accident, a MedicAlert bracelet can allow immediate medical attention for diabetes.

PRACTICE ALERT

Make frequent assessments to monitor for symptoms of HHS in the older adult who has had major surgery.

Sexual Dysfunction

Sexuality is a complex and inseparable part of every person. It involves not only physical sexual activities but also a person's self-perception as male or female, roles and relationships, and attractiveness and desirability. Changes in sexual function and sexuality have been identified in both men and women with diabetes.

Alterations in erectile ability occur in approximately 50% of all men with diabetes. The incidence of impotence increases with the duration of the diabetes and often is associated with peripheral neuropathy. Libido usually is unaffected, even when impotence is present.

PRACTICE ALERT

Sexual function is a private matter, and clients rarely share concerns unless the nurse initiates the discussion.

Women with diabetes may have alterations in sexual function, although the reason is less clear. The problems reported by women involve decreased desire and decreased vaginal lubrication. Women with diabetes are at increased risk for vaginitis as well. These symptoms often make sexual intercourse painful, which may be the source of alterations in libido.

- Include a sexual history as a part of the initial and ongoing assessment of the client with diabetes. A specific history form may be used that addresses sexual development, personal and family values, current sexual practices and concerns, and the changes desired. To elicit information, ask a nonthreatening, open-ended question, such as "Tell me about your experience with sexual function since you have been diagnosed with diabetes." Obtaining accurate information to assess the sexual health of a client is necessary before counseling can begin or referrals can be made.
- Provide information about the actual and potential physical effects of diabetes on sexual function. Include the effect of poor control of blood glucose on sexual function as part of any teaching plan. Clients benefit from basic information about male and female anatomy, the sexual response cycle, and how diabetes can affect this part of the body. Changes in blood glucose levels not only may cause changes in desire and physical response but also may alter sexual responses as a result of depression, anxiety, and fatigue.
- Provide counseling, or make referrals as appropriate. The nurse is responsible for knowing about sexuality and sexual health throughout the life span and provides information based on knowledge about the effects of illness and treatment on sexual function. The nurse may make specific suggestions to facilitate positive sexual functioning and, as necessary, refer the client to the appropriate health care provider for intensive therapy.

Ineffective Coping

Coping is the process of responding to internal or environmental stressors or potential stressors. When coping responses are ineffective, the stressors exceed the individual's available

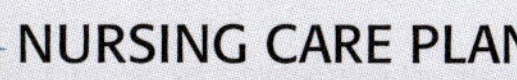

NURSING CARE PLAN A Client With Type 1 Diabetes Mellitus

Jim Meligrito, age 24, is a third-year nursing student at a large midwestern university. Mr. Meligrito also works 20 hours a week as a campus student security guard. His working hours are 8 p.m. to midnight, five nights a week. He lives with his father, who also is a student. Neither of the two men likes to cook, and they usually eat "whatever is handy." Mr. Meligrito has smoked 8–10 cigarettes a day for 5 years.

Mr. Meligrito was diagnosed with type 1 DM at age 12. Although his insulin dosage has varied, he currently takes a total of 32 U of insulin each day, 10 U of NPH, and 6 U of regular insulin each morning and evening. He monitors his blood glucose about three times a week. He feels that he is too busy for a regular exercise program and that he gets enough exercise in clinicals and in weekend sports activities. He has not seen a health care provider for over a year.

One day during a 6-hour clinical laboratory in pediatrics, Mr. Meligrito notices that he is urinating frequently, is thirsty, and has blurred vision. He also is very tired, but he blames all his symptoms on drinking a couple of beers and having had only 4 hours of sleep the night before while studying for an examination and on the stress he has been under lately from school and work. When he remembers that he had forgotten to take his insulin that morning, he realizes he must have hyperglycemia but decides that he will be all right until he gets home in the afternoon. Around noon, he begins having abdominal pain, feels weak, has a rapid pulse, and vomits. When he reports his physical symptoms to his clinical instructor, she immediately sends him, accompanied by another student, to the hospital emergency department.

ASSESSMENT

As soon as Mr. Meligrito arrives at the emergency room, his blood glucose level is measured at 300 mg/dL. Urine samples and additional blood samples are sent to the laboratory for analysis. Blood glucose is 330 mg/dL, hemoglobin A1c (HgbA1c) is 9.5%, urine shows the presence of ketones, electrolytes are normal, and pH is 7.1. His vital signs are as follows: T 99°F (37.2°C), P 140, R 28, and BP 102/52. An intravenous infusion of 1,000 mL of normal (0.9%) saline with 40 mEq of KCl is started at a rate of 400 mL/hr. Intravenous regular insulin at 5 U/hr (diluted in 0.9% saline) is begun. Hourly blood glucose monitoring also is initiated. Mr. Meligrito is nauseated and lethargic but remains oriented. Three hours later, he has a blood glucose level of 160 mg/dL, and his pulse and blood pressure are normal. He is dismissed from the emergency department after making an appointment for the next morning with the hospital's diabetes nurse educator. When he meets with the diabetes educator, he says that he no longer feels in control of the diabetes or his future goal of becoming a nurse anesthetist.

DIAGNOSES

Nursing diagnoses that may be appropriate for Mr. Meligrito include the following:

- Powerlessness related to a perceived lack of control of diabetes because of present demands on time
- Deficient Knowledge of self-management of diabetes
- Risk for Ineffective Role Performance related to uncertainty about capacity to achieve desired role as registered nurse.

PLANNING

The expected outcomes for the plan of care specify that Mr. Meligrito will:

- Identify those aspects of diabetes that can be controlled, and participate in making decisions about self-managing care.
- Demonstrate an understanding of diabetes self-management through planned medication, diet, exercise, and blood glucose self-monitoring activities.
- Explore and clarify his perceptions of his role as a student nurse, and verbalize his ability to meet his expectations.

IMPLEMENTATION

The following interventions may be appropriate for Mr. Meligrito:

- Mutually establish specific and individualized short-term and long-term goals for self-management to control blood glucose.
- Provide opportunities to express his feelings about himself and his illness.
- Explore perceptions of his own ability to control his illness and his future, and clarify these perceptions by providing information about resources and support groups.
- Facilitate decision-making abilities in self-managing his prescribed treatment regimen.
- Provide positive reinforcement for increasing involvement in self-care activities.
- Provide relevant learning activities about insulin administration, dietary management, exercise, self-monitoring of blood glucose, and healthy lifestyle.

EVALUATION

After taking an active part in the weekly educational meetings for 2 months, Mr. Meligrito has greatly enhanced his understanding of and compliance with self-management of his diabetes. He states that he finally understands how insulin, food, and exercise affect his body, having previously thought they were "just things I should do when I wanted to." He decides to perform self-management activities 1 week at a time rather than think too far into (and thereby feel overwhelmed by) the future. Both son and father have developed a workable meal schedule and weekly grocery list, and they have begun eating breakfast and dinner together. Jim and a friend have arranged to walk 2–3 miles three times a week on a community hiking trail. To gain a sense of control over his illness, he has also worked out a schedule that allows time for school, health care, and himself.

(continued)

NURSING CARE PLAN **A Client With Type 1 Diabetes Mellitus** *continued*

CRITICAL THINKING

1. What is the pathophysiologic basis for the changes in temperature, pulse, respiration, and blood pressure that were recorded on Mr. Meligrito's admission to the hospital emergency department?
2. How can smoking and poor self-management of diabetes increase the risk of long-term complications?
3. Is powerlessness a common response to a chronic illness? Why, or why not?
4. Consider that you are teaching Mr. Meligrito and another client, Mr. McDaniel (age 75, newly diagnosed with type 2 DM). What components of your teaching plan would be the same, and what components would be different?
5. What does the HgbA1c of 9.5% suggest about Mr. Meligrito's control of his diabetes?

resources for responding. The client diagnosed with diabetes is faced with lifelong changes. Diet, exercise habits, and medications must be integrated into his or her lifestyle and carefully controlled. Daily injections may be a reality. Fear of potential complications and of negative effects on the future is common.

If the client is unable to cope successfully with these changes or lacks a strong support system, emotional stress can interfere with glycemic control. In addition, unsuccessful coping often results in noncompliance with prescribed treatments, further impairing glycemic control and increasing the potential for acute and chronic complications.

- Assess the client's psychosocial resources, including emotional resources, support resources, financial resources, lifestyle, and communication skills. Chronic illness affects all dimensions of a person's life, as well as the lives of family members and significant others. A comprehensive assessment of strengths and weaknesses is the first step in developing an individualized plan of care to facilitate coping.
- Explore with the client and family the effects (actual and perceived) of the diagnosis and treatment of diabetes on finances, occupation, energy levels, and relationships. Common frustrations associated with diabetes are the disease itself, the treatment modalities, and the health care system. Effective coping involves maintaining a healthy self-concept and satisfying relationships, emotional balance, and handling emotional stress.
- Teach constructive problem-solving techniques. Problem-focused behaviors include setting attainable and realistic goals, learning about all aspects of the problem, learning new procedures or skills that increase self-esteem, and reaching out to others for support.
- Provide information about support groups and resources, such as suppliers of products, journals, books, and cookbooks for people with diabetes. Clients living on limited incomes or without health insurance may need assistance in accessing special programs offered by pharmaceutical companies or local clinics to help them pay for their prescriptions. Sharing with others who have similar problems provides opportunities for mutual support and problem solving. Using available resources improves the ability to cope.

Evaluation

Expected outcomes of nursing care are individualized based on the nursing care plan and the goals established during the planning phase. These outcomes may include the following:

- Client will demonstrate an age-appropriate understanding of diabetes self-management through medication, diet, exercise, and blood glucose self-monitoring activities.
- Skin integrity will remain intact.
- Client will remain free of infection.
- Client will remain free of injury.

REVIEW Diabetes

RELATE: LINK THE CONCEPTS

Linking the exemplar of Diabetes with the concept of Development:

1. In consideration of development, how would you approach diabetes teaching for an 8-year-old?
2. When teaching a 15-year-old about diabetes, how would teaching differ from an adult based on developmental level?

Linking the exemplar of Diabetes with the concept of Sensory Perception:

3. When caring for a client with diabetic neuropathy, what teaching would you provide to reduce the risk of injury?
4. When caring for a client with diabetic retinopathy, what strategies would you teach in order to facilitate a normal standard of living for the client?

READY: GO TO COMPANION SKILLS MANUAL

- Preparing for medication administration
- Preparing medications from vials
- Mixing insulins
- Administering a subcutaneous injection
- Assisting a client with eating
- Assisting a visually impaired client to eat
- Providing foot care
- Collecting a routine urine specimen
- Performing urine testing

REFER: GO TO MYNURSINGKIT

REFLECT: CASE STUDY

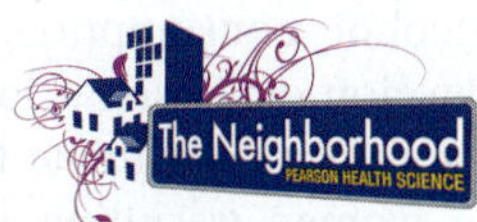

Norma James is a 65-year-old widow who lives alone. She has a long history of type 2 DM and hypertension. Mrs. James does not work; she has very limited savings and relies on Social Security benefits for income. She smokes about half a pack of cigarettes a day and has been a smoker since she was in her 20s. She drinks alcohol "a couple times a year, usually a glass of wine at a special dinner."

Mrs. James has a sore on her ankle that she has noticed for the last several months. The sore does not really hurt all that much, but she has been unable to get it to heal. The cashier at the convenience store tells her that she should use butter to help heal wounds, because the butter keeps the wound moist and helps to enhance healing.

Mrs. James decides to follow the cashier's advice and applies butter to her wound for about a week. The wound does not seem to be getting any better; in fact, it looks worse. It now has a yellowish drainage, and the skin around the wound has become red. Her foot also hurts when she walks on it. Mrs. James stops the butter treatment and goes to the emergency department.

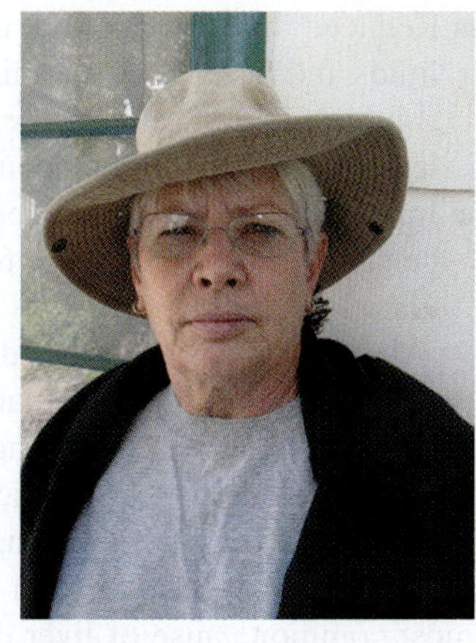

1. What are the priority nursing diagnoses for Mrs. James?
2. What discharge teaching will you provide to the client?
3. How can you advocate for Mrs. James regarding required medical equipment, supplies, and medications and their cost on a limited budget?
4. What expectation would you anticipate for Mrs. James regarding follow-up care?

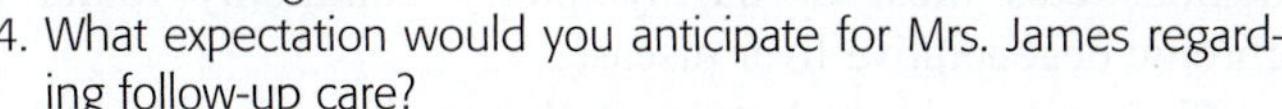

18.2 LIVER DISEASE

KEY TERMS

Alcoholic cirrhosis, *1016*
Balloon tamponade, *1024*
Cirrhosis, *1016*
Gastric lavage, *1024*
Hematochezia, *1021*
Laënnec's cirrhosis, *1016*
Paracentesis, *1022*
Transjugular intrahepatic portosystemic shunt, *1024*

BASIS FOR SELECTION OF EXEMPLAR

Centers for Disease Control and Prevention

LEARNING OUTCOMES

After reading about this exemplar, you will be able to:

1. Describe the pathophysiology, etiology, clinical manifestations, and direct and indirect causes of liver disease.
2. Identify risk factors associated with liver disease.
3. Illustrate the nursing process in providing culturally competent care across the life span for individuals with liver disease.
4. Formulate priority nursing diagnoses appropriate for an individual with liver disease.
5. Create a plan of care for individuals with liver disease and their family members.
6. Assess expected outcomes for an individual with liver disease.
7. Discuss therapies used in the collaborative care of an individual with liver disease.
8. Employ evidence-based caring interventions for an individual with liver disease.

OVERVIEW

The liver is a complex organ with multiple metabolic and regulatory functions. Optimal liver function is essential to health. Because of the significant amount of blood in the liver at all times, it is exposed to the effects of pathogens, drugs, toxins, and possibly malignant cells. As a result, liver cells may become inflamed or damaged, or cancerous tumors may develop.

The essential functions of the liver include the metabolism of proteins, carbohydrates, and fats. It also is responsible for the metabolism of steroid hormones and most drugs. It synthesizes essential blood proteins, including albumin and clotting factors in particular. The liver detoxifies alcohol and other toxic substances. Ammonia, a toxic by-product of protein metabolism, is converted to urea in the liver for elimination by the kidneys. The liver produces bile, an essential substance for absorbing fats and eliminating bilirubin from the body. Minerals and fat-soluble vitamins are stored in the liver, as is glycogen (stored carbohydrate for energy reserves). The Kupffer cells that line the sinusoids phagocytize foreign cells and damaged blood cells.

The liver is vital to digestion and metabolism of nutrients; the production of plasma proteins, including those involved in clotting; and the metabolism and excretion of compounds such as bilirubin, steroid hormones, and ammonia, as well as toxins (such as alcohol) and drugs. Impaired function of liver cells has multiple effects, including:

- Impaired protein metabolism with decreased production of albumin and clotting factors. Low albumin levels contribute to edema in peripheral tissues and *ascites*, accumulation of fluid in the abdomen, as plasma oncotic pressure is reduced. Impaired clotting factor production increases the risk for bleeding.
- Disrupted glucose metabolism and storage with resulting alterations in blood glucose levels (either hyperglycemia or hypoglycemia).

- Reduced bile production that impairs the absorption of lipids and fat-soluble vitamins. Inadequate vitamin K, a fat-soluble vitamin, affects the production of clotting factors, leading to a bleeding tendency.
- Impaired metabolism of steroid hormones (including estrogen and testosterone) leads to feminization in men and irregular menses in women.

Although many different disorders can disrupt liver function, their manifestations relate to three primary effects: disrupted liver cell function, impaired bilirubin conversion and excretion leading to jaundice, and disrupted blood flow through the liver, with resulting portal hypertension. Cirrhosis of the liver will be examined in more detail because it is the most common cause of liver disease in the United States and demonstrates most of the symptoms commonly found in chronic degenerative liver disease.

Cirrhosis is the end stage of chronic liver disease. It is a progressive, irreversible disorder, eventually leading to liver failure. **Alcoholic cirrhosis** (or **Laënnec's cirrhosis**) is the most common type of cirrhosis in North America and many parts of Europe and South America (Kasper et al., 2005). Cirrhosis also may result from chronic hepatitis B or C; prolonged obstruction of the biliary (bile drainage) system; long-term, severe right heart failure; and other uncommon liver diseases.

PATHOPHYSIOLOGY AND ETIOLOGY

In cirrhosis, functional liver tissue is gradually destroyed and replaced by fibrous scar tissue. As hepatocytes and liver lobules are destroyed, the metabolic functions of the liver are lost. Structurally abnormal nodules encircled by connective tissue form. This fibrous connective tissue forms constrictive bands that disrupt blood and bile flow within liver lobules. Blood no longer flows freely through the liver to the inferior vena cava. This restricted blood flow leads to portal hypertension (increased pressure in the portal venous system).

Etiology

The incidence and mortality attributable to cirrhosis and chronic liver disease vary significantly among populations.

ALCOHOLIC CIRRHOSIS Alcoholic (or Laënnec's) cirrhosis is the end result of alcoholic liver disease. Its development is directly related to alcohol consumption—specifically, total amount of alcohol consumed, number of years of excessive alcohol consumption, and blood alcohol levels. Women develop cirrhosis at lower overall levels of alcohol use than men. This may relate to less effective metabolism of alcohol in women, resulting in higher blood alcohol levels (Mann et al., 2003).

Alcohol causes metabolic changes in the liver: Triglyceride and fatty acid synthesis increases, and formation and release of lipoproteins decrease, leading to fatty infiltration of hepatocytes (fatty liver). At this stage, abstinence from alcohol can allow the liver to heal. However, with continued alcohol abuse, the disease continues to progress. Inflammatory cells infiltrate the liver (alcoholic hepatitis), causing necrosis, fibrosis, and destruction of functional liver tissue. In the final stage of alcoholic cirrhosis, regenerative nodules form, and the liver shrinks and develops a nodular appearance. Malnutrition commonly accompanies alcoholic cirrhosis.

BILIARY CIRRHOSIS When bile flow is obstructed within the liver or in the biliary system, the retained bile damages and destroys liver cells close to the interlobular bile ducts. This leads to inflammation, fibrosis, and formation of regenerative nodules.

POSTHEPATIC CIRRHOSIS Advanced progressive liver disease resulting from chronic hepatitis B or C or from an unknown cause is known as posthepatic or postnecrotic cirrhosis. Chronic viral hepatitis appears to be the leading cause of posthepatic cirrhosis in the United States (Kasper et al., 2005). In clients with this type of cirrhosis, the liver is shrunken and nodular, with extensive loss of liver cells and fibrosis.

Risk Factors

For most clients, high-risk behaviors are the risk factors for cirrhosis. While many clients tolerate alcohol use in moderation with no adverse effects on the liver, excess alcohol use is the leading cause of cirrhosis. Injection drug use also is a significant risk factor, increasing the risk for contracting bloodborne hepatitis (B, C, or D). These types of viral hepatitis can lead to chronic hepatitis and, ultimately, to cirrhosis.

CLINICAL MANIFESTATIONS

Early in the course of cirrhosis, few manifestations may be present. The liver usually is enlarged and may be tender. A dull, aching pain in the right upper quadrant may be present.

FOCUS ON DIVERSITY AND CULTURE Cirrhosis

- Although cirrhosis/chronic liver disease is the 12th leading cause of death overall in the United States, it is the sixth leading cause of death for people of Native American (including Alaska Natives) and Hispanic (or Latino) origin.
- Native American men have the highest incidence and mortality rate from cirrhosis and chronic liver disease, followed by Native American women, Hispanic men, and women of Hispanic or Latino origin (National Center for Health Statistics, 2005).
- At this time, there is no clear explanation for these differences. Contributory factors may include:
  a. Socioeconomic factors that lead to greater stress and alcohol consumption among certain populations
  b. Patterns of alcohol consumption (e.g., consuming alcohol without food calories)
  c. Variations in alcohol metabolism among populations (Mann, Smart, & Govoni, 2003).

Other early signs include weight loss, weakness, and anorexia. Bowel function is disrupted with diarrhea or constipation (Porth, 2005).

As the disease progresses, manifestations related to liver cell failure and portal hypertension develop. Impaired metabolism causes such manifestations as bleeding, ascites, gynecomastia (breast enlargement) in men and infertility in women, jaundice, and neurologic changes. Portal hypertension accounts from such manifestations as ascites, peripheral edema, anemia, and low white blood cell (WBC) and platelet counts.

Treatment of cirrhosis is supportive and directed at slowing the progression to liver failure and reducing complications. It can include medications to help regulate protein metabolism, maintenance of fluid and electrolyte balance, and supportive therapies, including treatment of underlying problems (e.g., malnutrition, anemia, bleeding, encephalopathy, renal failure, and infections).

PORTAL HYPERTENSION Portal hypertension causes blood to be rerouted to adjoining, lower-pressure vessels. This *shunting* of blood involves collateral vessels. Affected veins, which become engorged and congested, are located in the esophagus, rectum, and abdomen. Portal hypertension increases the hydrostatic pressure in vessels of the portal system. Increased hydrostatic pressure in the capillaries pushes fluid out, contributing to ascites formation.

SPLENOMEGALY Because portal hypertension causes blood to be shunted into the splenic vein, the spleen enlarges (splenomegaly). Splenomegaly increases the rate at which red blood cells (RBCs), WBCs, and platelets are removed from circulation and destroyed. This increased destruction of blood cells leads to anemia (low RBC count), leukopenia (low WBC count), and thrombocytopenia (low platelet count) (Porth, 2005).

ASCITES Ascites is the accumulation of plasma-rich fluid in the abdominal cavity. Although portal hypertension is the primary cause of ascites, decreased serum proteins and increased aldosterone also contribute to the fluid accumulation. *Hypoalbuminemia* low serum albumin) decreases the colloidal osmotic pressure of plasma. This pressure normally holds fluid in the intravascular compartment, but when the plasma colloidal osmotic pressure decreases, fluid escapes into extravascular compartments. *Hyperaldosteronism* an increase in aldosterone) causes sodium and water retention, contributing to ascites and generalized edema.

CLINICAL MANIFESTATIONS AND THERAPIES **Liver Disease**

ETIOLOGY	CLINICAL MANIFESTATION	CLINICAL THERAPIES
Impaired plasma protein synthesis (hypoalbuminemia) Disrupted hormone balance and fluid retention Increased pressure in portal venous system	Edema, ascites	■ Diuretics ■ Sodium and fluid restrictions ■ Paracentesis ■ Transjugular intrahepatice portosystemic shunt (TIPS)
Decreased clotting factor synthesis Increased platelet destruction by enlarged spleen Impaired vitamin K absorption and storage	Bleeding, bruising	■ Ferrous sulfate, folic acid to treat anemia ■ Vitamin K to reduce risk of bleeding ■ For acute bleeding, packed RBCs, fresh frozen plasma, or platelets may be administered to promote hemostasis ■ Institute bleeding precautions
Increased pressure in portal venous system with collateral vessel development	Esophageal varices	■ Beta-blocker nadolol with isosorbide mononitrate ■ For bleeding esophageal varices, central line insertion; monitor central venous and pulmonary artery pressures ■ Upper endoscopy with gastric lavage ■ Balloon tamponade ■ Transjugular intrahepatic portosystemic shunt (TIPS)
Engorged veins in gastrointestinal system Alcohol ingestion Impaired bile synthesis and fat absorption	Gastritis, anorexia, diarrhea	
Impaired bilirubin metabolism and excretion	Jaundice	
Impaired nutrient metabolism Impaired fat absorption Impaired hormone metabolism	Malnutrition, muscle wasting	■ Arranging for consultation with a dietician for meal planning
Accumulated metabolic toxins Impaired ammonia metabolism and excretion	Asterixis, encephalopathy	■ Medications to reduce nitrogenous load and lower serum ammonia levels ■ Protein restrictions in acute encephalopathy ■ Parenteral nutrition as needed

MULTISYSTEM EFFECTS OF **Cirrhosis**

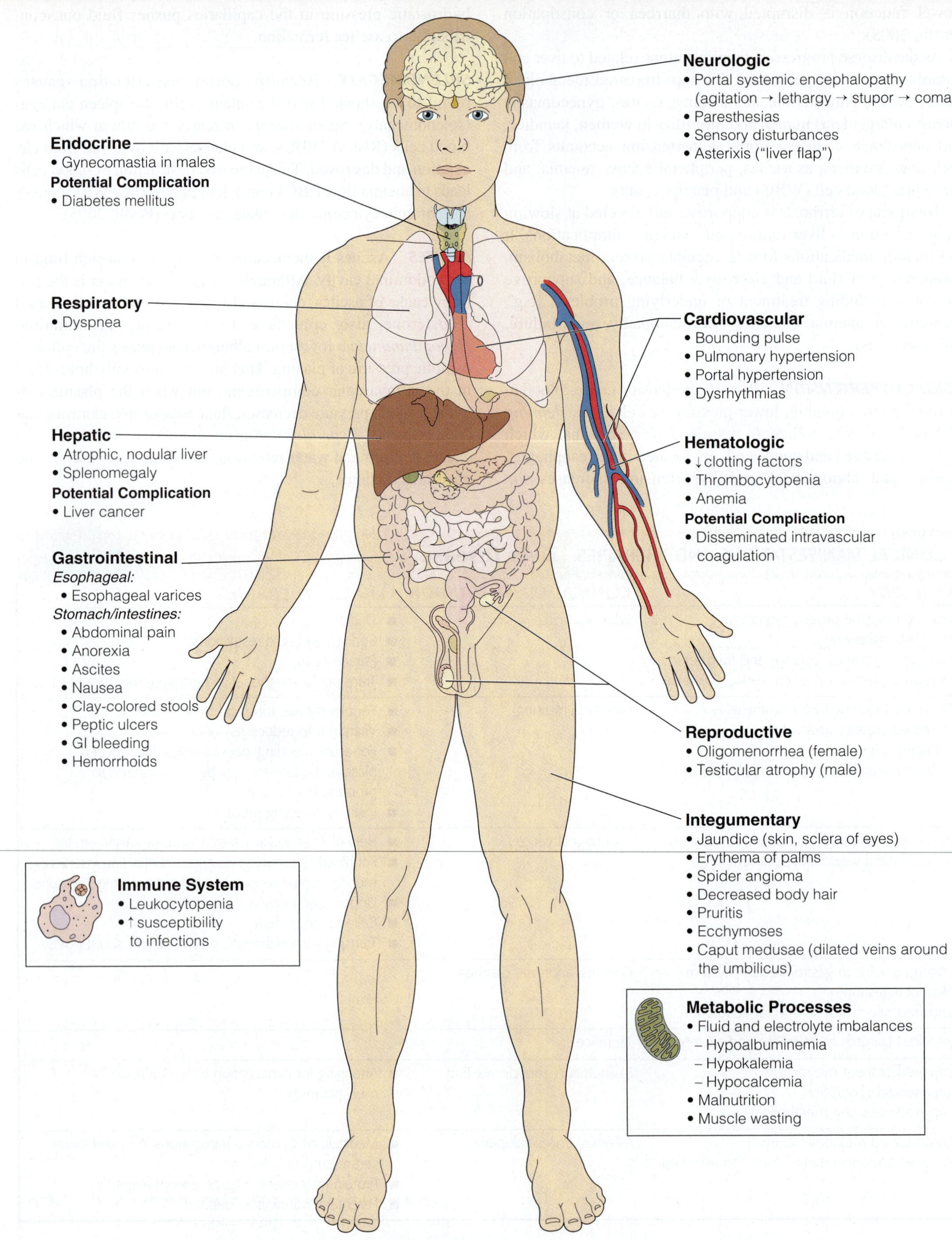
Neurologic
• Portal systemic encephalopathy (agitation → lethargy → stupor → coma)
• Paresthesias
• Sensory disturbances
• Asterixis ("liver flap")
Endocrine
• Gynecomastia in males
Potential Complication
• Diabetes mellitus
Respiratory
• Dyspnea
Cardiovascular
• Bounding pulse
• Pulmonary hypertension
• Portal hypertension
• Dysrhythmias
Hepatic
• Atrophic, nodular liver
• Splenomegaly
Potential Complication
• Liver cancer
Hematologic
• ↓ clotting factors
• Thrombocytopenia
• Anemia
Potential Complication
• Disseminated intravascular coagulation
Gastrointestinal
Esophageal:
• Esophageal varices
Stomach/intestines:
• Abdominal pain
• Anorexia
• Ascites
• Nausea
• Clay-colored stools
• Peptic ulcers
• GI bleeding
• Hemorrhoids
Reproductive
• Oligomenorrhea (female)
• Testicular atrophy (male)
Integumentary
• Jaundice (skin, sclera of eyes)
• Erythema of palms
• Spider angioma
• Decreased body hair
• Pruritis
• Ecchymoses
• Caput medusae (dilated veins around the umbilicus)
Immune System
• Leukocytopenia
• ↑ susceptibility to infections
Metabolic Processes
• Fluid and electrolyte imbalances
– Hypoalbuminemia
– Hypokalemia
– Hypocalcemia
• Malnutrition
• Muscle wasting

ESOPHAGEAL VARICES Esophageal varices are enlarged, thin-walled veins that form in the submucosa of the esophagus. These collateral vessels form when blood is shunted from the portal system because of portal hypertension. The thin-walled varices may rupture, causing massive hemorrhage, and even eating high-roughage foods can precipitate bleeding in these clients. Thrombocytopenia, platelet deficiency, and impaired production of clotting factors by the liver contribute to the risk for hemorrhage.

PORTAL SYSTEMIC ENCEPHALOPATHY Portal systemic encephalopathy (also known as *hepatic encephalopathy*) results from accumulation of neurotoxins in the blood and cerebral edema. Ammonia, a by-product of protein metabolism, contributes to hepatic encephalopathy. Ammonium ion is produced as proteins and amino acids are broken down by bacteria in the intestinal tract. Normally, the ammonia produced is then converted by the liver to urea before entering the general circulation. However, as functional liver tissue is destroyed, ammonia can no longer be converted to urea, and it accumulates in the blood. Other nervous system depressants, such as narcotics and tranquilizers, also may contribute to hepatic encephalopathy. Accumulation of other metabolic toxins is thought to contribute as well. Additional factors are constipation, blood transfusions, gastrointestinal bleeding, hypoxia, high-protein diet, severe infection, and surgery.

Asterixis (also known as liver flap) is a muscle tremor that interferes with the ability to maintain a fixed position of the extremities and causes involuntary jerking movements. It also is an early sign of portal systemic encephalopathy. Asterixis primarily affects the upper extremities, but it may affect the tongue and feet. Asterixis is elicited by instructing the client to extend the arms and dorsiflex the wrists; if present, asterixis causes a downward flapping of the hands.

People with portal systemic encephalopathy also develop changes in personality and mentation. Agitation, restlessness, impaired judgment, and slurred speech are early manifestations; as the condition progresses, confusion, disorientation, and incoherence develop. Cerebral edema that leads to increased intracranial pressure and cerebral hypoxia is the leading cause of death in people with portal systemic encephalopathy and liver failure.

HEPATORENAL SYNDROME Although the cause is unclear, renal failure with azotemia (excess nitrogenous waste products in the blood), sodium retention, oliguria, and hypotension may develop in clients with advanced cirrhosis and ascites. Hepatorenal syndrome appears to be the result of imbalanced blood flow, leading to constriction of vessels leading to and within the kidneys. The syndrome may be precipitated by gastrointestinal bleeding, aggressive diuretic therapy, or by an unknown cause.

SPONTANEOUS BACTERIAL PERITONITIS Clients with cirrhosis and ascites may develop bacterial peritonitis even in the absence of known contamination of the peritoneal cavity or other specific risk factors (e.g., paracentesis). The inflammatory response to peritonitis worsens ascites by increasing the permeability of capillaries in the mesentery. The manifestations of spontaneous bacterial peritonitis may be subtle, with increased abdominal discomfort or pain, fever, increasing ascites, worsening encephalopathy, and an overall decline in condition.

COLLABORATION

Care for the client with cirrhosis is holistic, addressing physiologic, psychosocial, and spiritual needs, and the nurse is responsible for coordinating care among providers. The importance of including the family in the plan of care cannot be overemphasized, particularly if alcohol abuse is identified as the cause. Counseling, job coaching, and behavioral therapy may be helpful. Consultation with a nutritionist can help to reinforce any client teaching the nurse has provided as well as give the client an additional resource in this area.

Diagnostic Tests

Studies to confirm the diagnosis of cirrhosis and identify its cause and effects are performed. Diagnostic tests may include the following:

- *Liver function studies:* These include *alanine aminotransferase, aspartate aminotransferase, alkaline phosphatase,* and *gamma-glutamyltransferase.* All four may be elevated in clients with cirrhosis, but usually not as severely as in clients with acute hepatitis. Elevations in these enzymes may not correlate well with the extent of liver damage in cirrhosis.
- *Complete blood count (CBC) with platelets:* A low RBC count, hemoglobin, and hematocrit demonstrate anemia related to bone marrow suppression, increased RBC destruction, bleeding, and deficiencies of folic acid and vitamin B_{12}. Platelets are low, related to increased destruction by the spleen. Leukopenia (low WBC count) also relates to splenomegaly.
- *Coagulation studies:* A prolonged prothrombin time results from impaired production of coagulation proteins and lack of vitamin K.
- *Serum electrolytes:* Hyponatremia is common, resulting from hemodilution. Hypokalemia, hypophosphatemia, and hypomagnesemia also frequently are seen, related to malnutrition and altered renal excretion of these electrolytes.
- *Bilirubin:* Both direct (conjugated) and indirect (unconjugated) bilirubin usually are elevated in clients with severe cirrhosis.
- *Serum albumin:* Hypoalbuminemia results from impaired liver production.
- *Serum ammonia:* Levels are elevated, because the liver fails to effectively convert ammonia to urea for renal excretion.
- *Serum glucose* and *cholesterol:* These levels frequently are abnormal in clients with cirrhosis.
- *Abdominal ultrasound:* This test is performed to evaluate liver size, detect ascites, and identify liver nodules. Ultrasound may be used in conjunction with *Doppler studies* to evaluate blood flow through the liver and spleen (Tierney et al., 2005).
- *Esophagoscopy:* Upper endoscopy may be done to determine the presence of esophageal varices.

- *Liver biopsy:* This test is not always necessary to diagnose cirrhosis, but it may be done to distinguish cirrhosis from other forms of liver disease. Biopsy may be deferred if the bleeding time is prolonged (e.g., prothrombin time >3 sec over the control).

Pharmacologic Therapies

Medications are used to treat the complications and effects of cirrhosis; they do not reverse or slow the process of cirrhosis itself. Known hepatotoxic drugs and alcohol are avoided, as are drugs metabolized by the liver (e.g., barbiturates, sedatives, hypnotics, and acetaminophen). Several groups of drugs are commonly prescribed:

- Diuretics reduce fluid retention and ascites. Spironolactone (Aldactone) is frequently the drug of first choice, because it addresses increased aldosterone levels, one of the causes of ascites. If additional diuresis is necessary, a loop diuretic, such as furosemide (Lasix), may be added to the regimen.
- Medications to reduce the nitrogenous load and lower serum ammonia levels are added when manifestations of hepatic encephalopathy develop. Two commonly administered medications are lactulose and neomycin. Both exert their effects locally, in the bowel. Lactulose reduces the number of ammonia-forming organisms in the bowel and increases the acidity of colon contents, converting ammonia into ammonium ion. Ammonium ion is not absorbable and is excreted in the feces. Neomycin sulfate is a locally acting antibiotic that also reduces the number of ammonia-forming bacteria in the bowel.
- The beta-blocker nadolol (Corgard) may be given together with isosorbide mononitrate (Ismo, Imdur, Monoket) to prevent rebleeding of esophageal varices. This drug combination also lowers hepatic venous pressure.
- Ferrous sulfate and folic acid are given as indicated to treat anemia. Vitamin K may be ordered to reduce the risk of bleeding. When bleeding is acute, packed RBCs, fresh frozen plasma, or platelets may be administered to restore blood components and promote hemostasis.
- Antacids are prescribed as indicated. A drug regimen to treat *Helicobacter pylori* infection also may be effective.
- Oxazepam (Serax), a benzodiazepine antianxiety/sedative drug, is not metabolized by the liver and may be used to treat acute agitation.

Nutritional Therapies

Dietary support is an essential part of care for the client with cirrhosis. Dietary needs change as hepatic function fluctuates. Nutritional therapy often involves the following:

- Sodium intake is restricted to less than 2 g/day, and fluids are restricted as necessary to reduce ascites and generalized edema. Fluids often are limited to 1,500 mL/day. Fluid needs are calculated based on response to diuretic therapy, urine output, and serum electrolyte values.
- Unless serum ammonia levels are high, a palatable diet with adequate calories and protein is recommended. If hepatic encephalopathy is acute, protein may initially be eliminated from the diet; for chronic hepatic encephalopathy, protein generally is restricted to 60 g/day (Kasper et al., 2005). When encephalopathy resolves and serum ammonia levels stabilize, protein intake is allowed as tolerated. The diet is high in calories and includes moderate fat intake to promote healing. Parenteral nutrition is used as needed to maintain nutritional status when food intake is limited.
- Vitamin and mineral supplements are ordered based on laboratory values. Deficiencies in the B-complex vitamins, particularly thiamin, folate, and B_{12}, and in the fat-soluble vitamins A, D, and E are common. These vitamins may need to be administered in a water-soluble form. Clients with alcohol-induced cirrhosis are at high risk for magnesium deficiency, which requires replacement therapy.

Surgery

Liver transplantation is indicated for some clients with irreversible, progressive cirrhosis. A decline in functional status, increasing bilirubin levels, falling albumin levels, and increasing problems with complications that respond poorly to treatment are indications for liver transplantation. Malignancy, active alcohol or drug abuse, and poor surgical risk are contraindications for the surgery.

NURSING PROCESS

Nursing care of clients with cirrhosis is aimed at reducing further liver damage, teaching the client to make healthier lifestyle choices, and minimizing the symptoms of the disease. In addition to the nursing care discussed in this section, see the Nursing Care Plan for a client with alcoholic cirrhosis.

Assessment

Assessment data related to cirrhosis include the following:

- *Health history.* Current manifestations, including abdominal pain or discomfort, recent weight loss, weakness, and anorexia; altered bowel elimination; excess bleeding or bruising; abdominal distention; jaundice; pruritus (itching); altered libido or impotence; duration of symptoms; history of liver or gallbladder disease; pattern and extent of alcohol or injection drug use; and use of other prescription and nonprescription drugs
- *Physical assessment.* Vital signs; mental status; color and condition of skin and mucous membranes; peripheral pulses and presence of peripheral edema; and abdominal assessment, including appearance, shape and contour, bowel sounds, abdominal girth, percussion for liver borders, and palpation for tenderness and liver size.

Diagnosis

Nursing care of the client with cirrhosis presents many challenges, because liver function affects all body systems. Many NANDA nursing diagnoses may apply. Those diagnoses discussed in this section focus on problems with fluid and electrolyte balance, disturbed thought processes, risk for bleeding, skin integrity, and nutrition and include the following:

- Excess Fluid Volume
- Disturbed Thought Processes
- Ineffective Protection
- Impaired Skin Integrity
- Imbalanced Nutrition: Less Than Body Requirements.

Plan

Expected outcomes for a client with cirrhosis may include any of the following:

- Client will maintain proper hydration levels as indicated by urine specific gravity tests.
- Client will maintain appropriate diet.
- Client will report regular bowel elimination pattern.
- Client will be oriented to surroundings, person, and place.
- Client will maintain vital signs within normal limits.
- Client will avoid alcohol.

Implementation

With all clients (including children and young adults), stress the relationship between alcohol and drug abuse and liver diseases. Specific interventions include those dealing with excess fluid volume, disturbed thought processes, ineffective protection, impaired skin integrity, and imbalanced nutrition.

Excess Fluid Volume

Cirrhosis affects water and salt regulation because of portal hypertension, hypoalbuminemia, and hyperaldosteronism. Signs of fluid volume overload and portal hypertension may develop, such as ascites, peripheral edema, internal hemorrhoids and varices, and prominent abdominal wall veins. Careful monitoring is necessary, because treatment measures can lead to further fluid and electrolyte imbalances.

- Weigh daily. Assess for jugular vein distention, measure abdominal girth daily, check for peripheral edema, and monitor intake and output. Careful assessment is important to detect fluid shifts.
- Assess urine specific gravity. Specific gravity measures the concentration of urine, an indicator of hydration.
- Provide a low-sodium diet (500–2,000 mg/day), and restrict fluids as ordered. Excess sodium leads to water retention and can increase fluid volume, ascites, and portal hypertension.

PRACTICE ALERT

Monitor the client with cirrhosis for signs of impaired renal function, such as oliguria, a fixed specific gravity of approximately 1.012, central edema (around the eyes and of the face), and increasing serum creatinine and blood urea nitrogen levels. Such signs may indicate hepatorenal syndrome or acute renal failure from another cause.

Disturbed Thought Processes

Accumulated nitrogenous waste products and other metabolites affect mental status and thought processes. Effects of hepatic encephalopathy can range from mild confusion to agitation to coma.

- Assess neurologic status, including level of consciousness and mental status. Observe for signs of early encephalopathy, such as changes in handwriting, speech, and asterixis. Early identification of evidence of encephalopathy allows prompt intervention. Subtle changes in neurologic functioning are important.
- Avoid factors that may precipitate hepatic encephalopathy. Avoid hepatotoxic medications and drugs that depress the central nervous system. Cautious use of medications and close monitoring can eliminate iatrogenic causes of encephalopathy.
- Plan for consistent nursing care assignments if possible. Consistent care providers facilitate early identification of subtle neurologic changes that indicate hepatic encephalopathy.
- Provide low-protein diet as prescribed; teach the family the importance of maintaining diet restrictions. Nitrogenous by-products from dietary protein increase serum ammonia levels.
- Administer medications or enemas as ordered to reduce nitrogenous products. Monitor bowel function, and provide measures to promote regular elimination and prevent constipation. Oral or rectally administered (per enema) medications are ordered to reduce intestinal bacteria and the ammonia they produce. Regular bowel elimination promotes protein and ammonia elimination in the feces.
- Orient the client to surroundings, person, and place; provide simple explanations and reassurance. Modification of verbal interactions to the level of understanding and mental status of the client may reduce anxiety and agitation.

PRACTICE ALERT

Closely monitor clients who have experienced gastrointestinal bleeding for signs of hepatic encephalopathy. Blood in the intestinal tract is digested as a protein, which increases serum ammonia levels and the risk for hepatic encephalopathy.

Ineffective Protection

Impaired coagulation, esophageal varices, and possible acute gastritis place the client with cirrhosis at significant risk for hemorrhage. Clotting is altered by vitamin K deficiency; impaired manufacture of coagulation factors II, VII, IX, and X; and increased platelet destruction because of splenomegaly.

- Monitor vital signs, and report tachycardia or hypotension. Increased pulse and decreasing blood pressure may indicate hypovolemia caused by hemorrhage.
- Institute bleeding precautions. Preventive measures can decrease the risk for active bleeding.
- Monitor coagulation studies and platelet count, and report abnormal results. Coagulation studies help to determine the risk for bleeding and the need for treatment.
- Carefully monitor the client who has had bleeding esophageal varices for evidence of rebleeding, such as hematemesis (blood in the vomit), **hematochezia** (bright blood in the stool) or tarry stools, and signs of hypovolemia or shock. Rebleeding is common following variceal hemorrhage, especially within the first week.

PRACTICE ALERT

Carefully monitor the respiratory status of the client with a Sengstaken-Blakemore or Minnesota tube, which sometimes are used in the treatment of esophageal varices. Displacement of the tube can obstruct the airway unless an endotracheal tube is in place. The esophageal balloon prevents the client from swallowing oral secretions, increasing the risk for aspiration. Keep the head of the bed elevated to 45° to reduce the risk of aspiration and promote gas exchange.

Impaired Skin Integrity

Severe jaundice with bile salt deposits on the skin may cause pruritus. Scratching related to the pruritus damages the skin and impairs its integrity. Malnutrition, particularly protein deficiency, and edema also increase the risk for tissue breakdown and impaired skin integrity.

- Use warm water rather than hot water when bathing. Hot water increases pruritus.
- Use measures to prevent dry skin: Apply an emollient or lubricant as needed to keep skin moist, avoid soap or preparations with alcohol, and do not rub the skin. Dry skin contributes to pruritus.
- If indicated, apply mittens to the hands to prevent scratching. Clients with encephalopathy may not understand the need to refrain from scratching.
- Institute measures to prevent skin and tissue breakdown: Turn the client at least every 2 hours, use an alternating pressure mattress, and frequently assess skin condition. Frequent position changes relieve pressure and promote circulation and tissue oxygenation.
- Administer a prescribed antihistamine (to relieve pruritus) cautiously. Decreased liver function increases the risk for altered drug responses.

Imbalanced Nutrition: Less Than Body Requirements

The client with cirrhosis is at risk for malnutrition for a number of reasons. These reasons include possible chronic alcohol use, anorexia, impaired vitamin and mineral absorption, and impaired protein metabolism. In addition, salt and protein restrictions may make the diet less palatable and appealing to the client.

- Weigh daily. Instruct the client to weigh self at least weekly at home. Weight is a good indicator of both nutritional status and fluid balance. Short-term weight fluctuations tend to reflect fluid balance, while longer-term changes in weight are more reflective of nutritional status.
- Provide small meals with between-meal snacks. A small meal is more appealing for a client with anorexia. Between-meal snacks help to maintain adequate calorie and nutrient intake.
- Unless protein is restricted because of impending hepatic encephalopathy, promote protein and nutrient intake by providing nutritional supplements, such as Ensure or instant breakfasts. The sodium and protein content of all meals and snacks must be calculated when maintaining restrictions of these nutrients.
- Arrange consultation with a dietitian for diet planning while hospitalized and at home. The dietitian can provide detailed instructions, sample menus, and suggestions for improving the palatability of the diet and promoting intake.

Management of Complications

Paracentesis (aspiration of fluid from the peritoneal cavity) may be a diagnostic or a therapeutic procedure (to relieve severe ascites that does not respond to diuretic therapy). The goal of paracentesis is to relieve respiratory distress caused by excess fluid in the abdomen. Ascites fluid may be withdrawn in moderate amounts of 500 mL to 1 L daily to reduce the risk of fluid and electrolyte imbalances. Large-volume paracentesis (withdrawal of 4–6 L of fluid at one time) may be used. Albumin often is administered intravenously during large-volume paracentesis to maintain intravascular volume as the pressure of the ascites fluid in the abdomen is relieved.

Bleeding esophageal varices are life-threatening and require intensive care management. Restoration of hemodynamic stability is the first priority. A central line is inserted, and central venous and pulmonary artery pressures are monitored. Blood is given to restore blood volume, and fresh frozen plasma may be administered to restore clotting factors. Somatostatin or octreotide, which constrict blood vessels in the gut, are given intravenously to reduce blood flow in the portal venous system. Vasopressin, which produces generalized vasoconstriction, also may be used.

When the blood pressure and cardiac output have stabilized, upper endoscopy is performed to evaluate and treat the

CLIENT TEACHING The Client With Cirrhosis of the Liver

Cirrhosis is a chronic, progressive disease. As such, the client and family assume major roles in managing the disease and its manifestations and in preventing complications. Teaching topics for home care include the following:

- The absolute necessity of avoiding alcohol and other hepatotoxic drugs. Suggest inpatient or community-based alcohol treatment programs and Alcoholics Anonymous as indicated.
- Diet and fluid intake restrictions and recommendations. Include suggestions to promote nutritional intake and increase the flavor of food when sodium is restricted.
- Prescribed medications. Include their timing, intended and adverse effects, and manifestations to report to the primary care provider.
- Bleeding precautions.
- Manifestations of potential complications to be reported to the primary care provider. Stress the importance of promptly reporting evidence of gastrointestinal bleeding for prompt intervention for potential hemorrhage.
- Skin care techniques to reduce pruritus and the risk of damage.
- Ways to manage fatigue and conserve energy.

Provide referrals for home health services, dietary consultation, social services, and counseling as needed by the client and family. Suggest local support groups where available. If appropriate, suggest hospice services for the client with end-stage liver disease.

NURSING CARE PLAN **A Client With Alcoholic Cirrhosis**

Richard Wright is a 48-year-old, divorced father of two teenagers. Mr. Wright has been admitted to the community hospital with ascites and malnutrition. He has had three previous hospital stays for cirrhosis, with the most recent 6 months ago.

ASSESSMENT

Mr. Wright is lethargic but responds appropriately to verbal stimuli. He complains of "spitting up blood the past week or so," and he says, "I'm just not hungry." He has lost 20 lb (9 kg) since his previous admission. He is jaundiced and has petechiae and ecchymoses on his arms and legs. Liz Mowdi, Mr. Wright's nurse, notes pitting pretibial edema. Abdominal assessment reveals a tight, protuberant abdomen with caput medusae. The liver margin is not palpable, and the spleen is enlarged. Vital signs are T 100°F (37.7°C), P 110, R 24, and BP 110/70.

Abnormal laboratory results include the following: WBC, 3,700/mm^3 (normal range, 4,300–10,800/mm^3); RBC, 4.0 million/mm^3 (normal range, 4.6–5.9 million/mm^3); platelets, 75,000/mm^3 (normal range, 150,000–350,000/mm^3); serum ammonia, 105 μm/dL (normal range, 35–65 μm/dL); total bilirubin, 4.9 mcg/dL (normal range, 0.1–1.0 mcg/dL); and serum sodium, 150 mEq/L (normal range, 135–145 mEq/L). Potassium, hemoglobin, hematocrit, total protein, and albumin levels are markedly decreased. Hepatic enzymes are elevated. Blood urea nitrogen and creatinine levels are marginally elevated. Oxygen saturation is 88% (normal range, 96–100%) per pulse oximetry.

Endoscopy shows bleeding from a gastric ulcer, and the diagnosis of alcoholic cirrhosis with gastritis is made. Mr. Wright is started on Aldactone, 25 mg po q8h; Riopan, 30 mL 2 h pc and hs; lactulose, 30 mL qh until onset of diarrhea, then 15 mL tid; a low-protein, 800-mg sodium diet; and fluid restriction of 1,500 mL/day.

DIAGNOSES

Nursing diagnoses that may be appropriate for Mr. Wright include the following:

- Impaired Gas Exchange related to pressure of ascites fluid on the diaphragm as manifested by tachypnea and decreased oxygen saturation
- Excess Fluid Volume related to electrolyte imbalance and hypoalbuminemia as manifested by ascites and peripheral edema
- Imbalanced Nutrition: Less Than Body Requirements related to anorexia and possible alcohol abuse as manifested by weight loss and low serum protein levels
- Disturbed Thought Processes related to effects of high ammonia levels as manifested by lethargy
- Ineffective Protection related to impaired platelet formation and malnutrition.

PLANNING

The goals for the plan of care for Mr. Wright include the following:

- Have respiratory rate and oxygen saturation within normal limits.
- Have a decrease in abdominal girth of 1–2 cm/day and a decrease in peripheral edema decrease.
- Gain 1 lb (0.45 kg) per week without evidence of increased fluid retention.
- Have serum albumin levels return to normal range.
- Be alert and oriented.
- Have serum ammonia levels within the normal range.
- Demonstrate no further evidence of active bleeding.
- Verbalize willingness to join a community support group.

IMPLEMENTATION

The following nursing interventions may be appropriate for Mr. Wright:

- Weigh daily.
- Provide high-calorie, low-salt, low-protein diet with between-meal snacks.
- Maintain stool chart.
- Assign the same nurses as much as possible to facilitate evaluation of mental status, and promptly report changes in status or laboratory values.
- Measure abdominal girth every 8 hours, marking level of measurement.
- Institute bleeding precautions.
- Elevate head of bed; assist client to chair with legs elevated three times a day as tolerated.
- Include significant others in care and teaching, and refer to community agencies for discharge follow-up.

EVALUATION

A week after admission, Mr. Wright's ascites has decreased, and no further active bleeding is noted. His serum protein levels have increased, and his laboratory values are improving. No further bruising is noted during hospitalization. Although he shows a 5-lb weight loss as excess water is eliminated, he is consuming 100% of his diet. His serum ammonia levels have returned to normal. On discharge, oxygen saturation is 96%; respirations are 18. Lactulose will be continued on discharge.

Ms. Mowdi provides both written and verbal information about the medication and cirrhosis, including measures to prevent complications. Mr. Wright and his children express interest in Alcoholics Anonymous and Al-Anon and are referred to those agencies. Before discharge, follow-up appointments are made with a psychiatric social worker and a primary caregiver.

CRITICAL THINKING

1. Describe the relationship between portal hypertension, liver dysfunction, and ascites.
2. Outline a 1-day menu for a low-protein, low-sodium, high-calorie diet.
3. What is the pathophysiologic basis for hepatic encephalopathy?
4. What are the nursing responsibilities related to lactulose and neomycin?
5. Design a nursing care plan for Mr. Wright for the diagnosis *ineffective coping*.

varices. A large nasogastric tube is inserted before endoscopy, and **gastric lavage** (irrigation of the stomach with large quantities of normal saline) is performed to improve visualization. During endoscopy, the varices may be banded or sclerosed to reduce the risk of recurrent bleeding. In *banding* (*variceal ligation*) small rubber bands are placed on varices to occlude blood flow. *Endoscopic sclerosis* involves injecting a sclerosing agent directly into the varices to induce inflammation and clotting.

Balloon tamponade of bleeding varices may be used if bleeding cannot be controlled through vasoconstriction or if endoscopy is unavailable. A multiple-lumen nasogastric tube (e.g., a Sengstaken-Blakemore or a Minnesota tube) is inserted, and the gastric and esophageal balloons are inflated to apply direct pressure on the bleeding varices. Tension is applied to the tube to further compress the varices. Balloon tamponade carries a number of risks, including aspiration, airway obstruction, and tissue ischemia and necrosis. An endotracheal tube is inserted before nasogastric intubation to support the airway and reduce the risk of aspiration. This short-term measure is used only until more definitive treatment can be performed.

PRACTICE ALERT

When caring for a client with a multiple-lumen nasogastric tube, always deflate the esophageal balloon before the gastric balloon. This practice prevents the balloon from becoming misplaced and occluding the airway. Always keep an appropriate syringe at the bedside to deflate the esophageal balloon should the client develop respiratory distress.

Transjugular intrahepatic portosystemic shunt (TIPS) is used to relieve portal hypertension and its complications of esophageal varices and ascites. A channel is created through the liver tissue using a needle inserted transcutaneously. An expandable metal stent is inserted into this channel to allow blood to flow directly from the portal vein into the hepatic vein, bypassing the cirrhotic liver. The shunt relieves pressure in esophageal varices and allows better control of fluid retention with diuretic therapy. Stenosis and occlusion of the shunt are frequent complications. TIPS also increases the risk of developing hepatic encephalopathy (because of decreased perfusion of the liver and impaired ammonia metabolism), and it may reduce long-term survival. It generally is used as a short-term measure until a liver transplant can be performed.

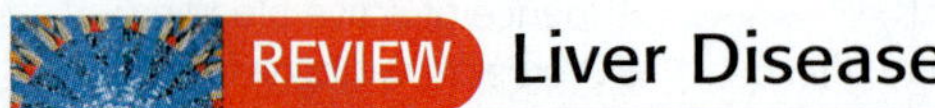

REVIEW Liver Disease

RELATE: LINK THE CONCEPTS

Linking the exemplar of Liver Disease with the concept of Addiction Behaviors:

1. What strategies might the nurse employ to help the client with alcohol addiction experiencing symptoms of liver disease find the motivation to abstain from alcohol?
2. The family of a client who is addicted to alcohol and has liver disease informs the nurse that the client has relapsed and returned to regular alcohol use after discharge from an alcohol treatment center. What assessment data would the nurse collect from the client?

Linking the exemplar of Liver Disease with the concept of Tissue Integrity:

3. When caring for a client with jaundice resulting from liver disease, what specific skin care measures might the nurse initiate to reduce the risk of altered skin integrity?
4. What factors increase the risk of altered skin integrity in the client with chronic or acute liver disease?

READY: GO TO COMPANION SKILLS MANUAL

- Assessing height and weight
- Collecting a urine specimen
- Performing a urine test
- Assessing appearance and mental status
- Assessing the neurologic system
- Obtaining a capillary blood specimen and measuring blood glucose

REFER: GO TO MYNURSINGKIT

REFLECT: CASE STUDY

Saul Mendato is a 60-year-old male who was found unconscious by his wife and brought to the emergency department; he has a history of alcohol-induced cirrhosis. The nurse evaluating his laboratory values notes the following: total bilirubin, 4.6 mg/dL; serum ammonia, 95 mm/dL; platelets, 68,000/mm^3; and RBC, 4.2 million/mm^3.

1. Based on the laboratory reports, Mr. Mendato is at most risk for which complication of cirrhosis?
2. What are the priorities of nursing care?
3. What outcomes would be appropriate for this client?

18.3 OBESITY

KEY TERMS

Basal metabolic rate (BMR), *1025*
Body mass index (BMI), *1026*
Lower body obesity, *1026*
Metabolic syndrome, *1027*
Morbid obesity, *1027*
Nutrients, *1025*
Obesity, *1025*
Satiety, *1025*
Triglycerides, *1025*
Upper body obesity, *1026*
Very-low-calorie diets, *1029*

BASIS FOR SELECTION OF EXEMPLAR

Healthy People 2010

LEARNING OUTCOMES

After reading about this exemplar, you will be able to:

1. Describe the pathophysiology, etiology, clinical manifestations, and direct and indirect causes of obesity.
2. Identify risk factors associated with obesity.
3. Illustrate the nursing process in providing culturally competent care across the life span for individuals with obesity.
4. Formulate priority nursing diagnoses appropriate for an individual with obesity.
5. Create a plan of care for individuals with obesity and their family members.
6. Assess expected outcomes for an individual with obesity.
7. Discuss therapies used in the collaborative care of an individual with obesity.
8. Employ evidence-based caring interventions for an individual with obesity.

OVERVIEW

Obesity (an excess of adipose tissue) is one of the most prevalent, preventable health problems in the United States. Obesity has serious physiologic and psychologic consequences and is associated with increased morbidity and mortality. It contributes to poor health-related quality of life to a greater extent than smoking, excess alcohol use, or poverty. If current trends continue, obesity will soon replace tobacco use as the leading preventable cause of death in the United States (Uphold & Graham, 2003).

Obesity is a major public health issue. More than 30% of the adult population in the United States is obese, and nearly two thirds of all adults in the United States are overweight. The incidence of obesity is higher in women, in African Americans, and in economically disadvantaged people of all races (Kasper et al., 2005; Tierney et al., 2005). While the prevalence of overweight has been increasing since 1960, the prevalence of obesity is increasing to an even greater extent, especially during the past 10–15 years (National Heart, Lung, and Blood Institute [NHLBI], 2000). Of particular concern is the increasing incidence of obesity in children and young adults. The incidence of overweight and obesity varies among ethnic and cultural groups.

PATHOPHYSIOLOGY AND ETIOLOGY

All body activities, including activities of daily living as well as those necessary to maintain cell and tissue function, require energy. **Nutrients** in food (or enteral or parenteral feedings) provide energy and are the building blocks for growth and tissue repair. The body stores excess nutrients and energy (measured as kilocalories) to meet the body's needs when required nutrients are unavailable. This ability to store and release energy is important to maintaining body function. More than 70% of the energy expended each day goes to maintaining the **basal metabolic rate (BMR)**—essentially, the "cost" (in kilocalories) of being alive. Physical activity accounts for only 5–10% of the energy spent daily.

Energy is stored primarily as fat in adipose tissue. Although mature fat cells (adipocytes) do not multiply, the immature cells in adipose tissue can multiply, particularly when exposed to estrogen during puberty, in late adolescence, during breastfeeding, and in middle-age adults who are overweight. Fat cells store excess energy as **triglycerides**, which are formed from dietary fats and carbohydrates. The body breaks down the triglycerides in fat cells when needed to provide energy (Porth, 2005).

Etiology

Obesity occurs when excess calories are stored as fat. It can result from excess energy intake, decreased energy expenditure, or a combination of both. The etiology of obesity is not, however, as simple as excess kilocalorie intake in relation to energy expenditure. The systems that regulate food intake, energy storage, and energy expenditure are complex and not fully understood.

Appetite, which affects food intake, is regulated by the central nervous system and by emotional factors. The hunger center in the hypothalamus stimulates appetite in response to stimuli such as hypoglycemia. As nutrient levels rise, the satiety center (also in the hypothalamus) sends the message to stop eating. Gastrointestinal filling and hormonal factors also signal **satiety** (a sensation of fullness). Appetite may have little relationship to hunger: People may eat to relieve depression or anxiety.

Several hormones are involved in regulating obesity; these include thyroid hormone, insulin, and leptin (a peptide produced by fatty tissue that suppresses appetite and increases energy expenditure). Some studies suggest that leptin resistance is a cause of obesity. Insulin is associated with body fat distribution.

Risk Factors

Many factors, including genetic, physiologic, psychologic, environmental, and sociocultural factors, contribute to obesity. Heredity may contribute as much as 25–40% of the risk for obesity (NHLBI, 1998). The inheritance of obesity does not usually follow a clear mendelian pattern, and it is difficult to separate the role of environment from genetic factors. However, a strong correlation exists between the weight of adopted children and their biologic parents. In addition, identical twins tend to have similar body mass indexes, whether raised together or apart, providing further evidence of a genetic link to obesity. While several genes that contribute to appetite and fat deposition have been identified, obesity as a purely genetic condition is rare (Kasper et al., 2005).

Physical inactivity is probably the most important factor contributing to obesity. Inactive people may consume fewer calories than active people do but continue to gain weight because of a lack of energy expenditure. Cultural and environmental factors, such as labor-saving devices, reliance on the automobile for transportation, and increased time spent using the computer, contribute to decreased energy expenditure among adults in the United States. Increased time spent watching television is seen as a major contributing factor to the increased incidence of obesity among children and adolescents (Kasper et al., 2005).

Environmental influences, such as an abundant and readily accessible food supply, fast-food restaurants, advertising, and vending machines, contribute to increased food intake. Sociocultural influences that contribute to obesity include overeating at family meals, rewarding behavior with food, religious and family gatherings that promote food intake, and sedentary lifestyles. Socioeconomic status also tends to correlate with the risk for overweight and obesity: In the United States, women with low incomes or low educational levels are more likely to be obese than are those with higher socioeconomic status (NHLBI, 1998). However, the association between socioeconomic status and obesity is less clear in men.

Psychologic factors, such as low self-esteem, also play a role in obesity. Low self-esteem may precipitate unhealthy eating behaviors, and the resulting weight gain may diminish self-image even further. A person may overeat as a result of anxiety, depression, guilt, or boredom; overeating also may be a means of getting attention. Some experts characterize overeating as a food addiction and as a mechanism for coping with stressful life events.

CLINICAL MANIFESTATIONS

While obesity often is defined by weight, it is more accurately defined by the **body mass index (BMI)**, which is an indirect measure of the amount of body fat, or adipose tissue. Adipose tissue is created when energy consumption exceeds energy expenditure. A BMI of 25–29.9 kg/m² is classified as *overweight*; a BMI of 30 kg/m² or greater is classified as obesity (National Institutes of Health, 2004). The terms *overweight* and *obese* are not mutually exclusive; a client who is obese also is overweight (Table 18–5).

The two major types of body fat distribution are upper body and lower body obesity. **Upper body obesity** (also called *central obesity*) is identified by a waist-to-hip ratio of greater than 1 in men or 0.8 in women. People with upper body obesity tend to have more intra-abdominal fat and higher levels of circulating free fatty acids (Porth, 2005). As a result, upper body obesity is associated with a greater risk of complications such as hypertension, abnormal blood lipid levels, heart disease, stroke, and elevated insulin levels. Men tend to have more intra-abdominal fat than women, although women develop a central fat distribution pattern after menopause.

Lower body obesity (also known as *peripheral obesity*) is identified by a waist-to-hip ratio of less than 0.8 and is more commonly seen in women. The risk for hyperinsulinemia, abnormal lipids, and heart disease is lower in people with lower body obesity than in those with upper body obesity. Lower body obesity may be more difficult to treat, however.

Because obesity has many contributing factors, its treatment is far more complex than just reducing the amount of food consumed. Treatment is an ongoing process requiring a number of strategies. Most experts recommend an individualized program of exercise, diet, and behavior modification designed to meet the client's specific needs. Pharmacotherapy usually is recommended only as an adjunct when traditional therapies have been unsuccessful. Surgical treatment (bariatric surgery) generally is limited to clients with morbid obesity (BMI ≥ 40 kg/m², or >200% of ideal body weight) who are unable to lose weight through diet and exercise or have serious obesity-related problems, such as metabolic syndrome, hypertension, or heart disease (Weight-Control Information Network [WIN], 2004).

TABLE 18–5 **Classification of Overweight and Obesity by BMI, Waist Circumference, and Associated Disease Risks**

			DISEASE RISK RELATIVE TO NORMAL WEIGHT AND WAIST CIRCUMFERENCE[a]	
	BMI (KG/M²)	OBESITY CLASS	MEN 102 CM (40 IN.) OR LESS, WOMEN 88 CM (35 IN.) OR LESS	MEN > 102 CM (40 IN.). WOMEN > 88 CM (35 IN.)
Underweight	<18.5		–	–
Normal	18.5–24.9		–	–
Overweight	25.0–29.9		Increased	High
Obesity	30.0–34.9	I	High	Very high
	35.0–39.9	II	Very high	Very high
Extreme obesity	≥40.0	III	Extremely high	Extremely high

Source: National Heart, Lung, and Blood Institute. Retrieved May 6, 2009, from http://www.nhlbi.nih.gov/health/public/heart/obesity/lose_wt/bmi_dis.htm

[a] Disease risk for type 2 DM, hypertension, and cardiovascular disease. Increased waist circumference also can be a marker for increased risk even in persons of normal weight.

CLINICAL MANIFESTATIONS AND THERAPIES Obesity

CLINICAL MANIFESTATION	THERAPIES
BMI of 25–26.9 with two or more comorbidities	■ Diet, exercise, and behavior modification
BMI of 27–29.9 with two or more comorbidities	■ Diet, exercise, and behavior modification ■ Pharmacotherapy
BMI of 30–34.9 with two or more comorbidities (obesity class 1)	■ Diet, exercise, and behavior modification ■ Pharmacotherapy ■ Surgery
BMI of 35–39.9 with two or more comorbidities (obesity class 2)	■ Diet, exercise, and behavior modification ■ Pharmacotherapy ■ Surgery
BMI of ≥40 (obesity class 3)	■ Diet, exercise, and behavior modification ■ Pharmacotherapy ■ Surgery

Source: Adapted from National Institutes of Health, National Heart, Lung, and Blood Institute, North American Association for the Study of Obesity. (2000). *The Practical guide: Identification, evaluation, and treatment of overweight and obesity in adults.* Bethesda, MD: National Institutes of Health; Department of Health and Human Services, National Heart, Lung, and Blood Institute. Retrieved June 24, 2005, from http://www.nhLbi.nih.gov/health/public/heart/obesity

Note: Diet, exercise, and behavior modification can be appropriate for clients with hypertension, hyperlipidemia, diabetes, and other obesity-related complications. Consider surgery when 6 months of combined therapy has not produced a loss of 1 lb/week. BMI = body mass index.

COMPLICATIONS OF OBESITY

As obesity increases, adverse consequences of obesity increase. Individuals with **morbid obesity** (>200% of ideal body weight) have a risk of dying 12 times greater than that of people who are not obese (Kasper et al., 2005).

Obesity is a significant risk factor for cardiovascular disease, including hypertension, coronary heart disease (CHD), and heart failure. The prevalence of hypertension in obese men and women is approximately twice that in people with a BMI of less than 25 (NHLBI, 1998). The increases in blood pressure seen with obesity increase the risk for CHD and stroke. Approximately 60% of obese individuals have **metabolic syndrome**, including three or more of the following: increased waist circumference, hypertension, elevated blood triglycerides and fasting blood glucose, and low HDL cholesterol (Tierney et al., 2005). Metabolic syndrome is an identified risk factor for atherosclerosis and CHD. The Nurses' Health Study showed that the relative risk for CHD in women increases with a BMI of 25 or higher (NHLBI, 1998). Obesity also increases the risk for developing heart failure: Left ventricular muscle mass increases, and the ventricle dilates in obese individuals, possibly related to increased blood volume and cardiac output. Obesity-associated obstructive sleep apnea also contributes to the risk for heart failure.

Obesity increases the risk of insulin resistance and type 2 DM. Both weight gain in adulthood and abdominal (central) obesity are positively correlated with the risk for developing type 2 DM (NHLBI, 1998).

Obesity affects reproductive function in both men and women. Androgen (male sex hormone) levels are reduced in obese men; menstrual irregularities and polycystic ovarian syndrome are more common in obese women. (Polycystic ovarian syndrome is an additional risk factor for hyperinsulinemia and insulin resistance as well.)

Increased weight also increases the risk for developing gallstones in both men and women. The risk for developing several types of cancer, including colon, breast, and endometrial, increases in obesity as well. Increased weight places abnormal stress on joints, increasing the prevalence of joint pain and osteoarthritis, particularly in weight-bearing joints (especially the knee joints). Other health-related problems associated with obesity are listed in Table 18–6.

COLLABORATION

Successful treatment of obesity—that is, sustained achievement of normal body weight without adverse consequences—rarely is achieved. Treatment often is interdisciplinary and focuses on reducing the health risks associated with obesity by changing both eating and exercise habits.

Diagnostic Tests

Diagnostic tests that may be part of the physical assessment include the following:

- *Body mass index:* Used to identify excess adipose tissue. The BMI is calculated by dividing the weight (in kg) by the height (in m^2). Calculations may not reflect as accurately the extent of adipose tissue in people who are highly muscular (e.g., body builders) or in those who have lost muscle mass (e.g., older adults).

TABLE 18–6 Health-Related Problems Associated With Obesity

BODY SYSTEM	OBESITY-RELATED PROBLEMS
Cardiovascular	Atherosclerosis, hypercholesterolemia Coronary heart disease Heart failure Hypertension Stroke Varicosities Venous thrombosis
Respiratory	Sleep disorders Sleep apnea
Gastrointestinal	Gallbladder disease Hiatal hernia Colon cancer
Genitourinary	Cancers of the breast, uterus, prostate, and colon Complications of pregnancy Stress incontinence
Musculoskeletal	Low back pain Muscle strains and sprains Osteoarthritis
Endocrine and reproductive	Type 2 diabetes mellitus Endometrial cancer Polycystic ovarian syndrome
Other	Depression Binge-eating disorder Postoperative complications

- *Anthropometry:* Includes measurements of height, weight, bone size, and skinfold measurements to estimate subcutaneous fat.
- *Underwater weighing (hydrodensitometry):* Considered to be the most accurate way to determine body fat. This technique involves submerging the whole body and then measuring the amount of displaced water.
- *Bioelectrical impedance:* Uses a low-energy electrical impulse to determine the percentage of body fat by measuring the electrical resistance of the body.
- *Waist circumference:* Measured to determine body fat distribution. Men with a waist measurement of 40 in. (102 cm) or greater and women with a waist measurement of 35 in. (88 cm) or greater have a higher risk for complications of obesity.

Other diagnostic tests may be done to help identify a physiologic cause or complications related to obesity. These tests include:

- *Thyroid profile:* Includes a total T_3 and T_3 uptake, free T_4 and total T_4, free T_4 index, and TSH and is done to rule out thyroid disease.
- *Serum glucose:* Measured to identify coexisting diabetes.
- *Serum cholesterol:* Measured to assess for elevated levels.
- *Lipid profile:* HDL levels may be reduced in clients with obesity, whereas low-density lipoprotein (LDL) levels are elevated.
- *Electrocardiography:* Performed to detect effects of obesity on the heart (e.g., rate or rhythm disruptions, myocardial infarction, or heart enlargement).

Pharmacologic Therapies

Many prescription and over-the-counter drugs have been used to help people lose weight. When used in combination with diet and exercise, drugs can help to promote weight loss. Their long-term efficacy, however, is questionable; rebound weight gain following the cessation of drug use is common. In addition, tolerance, addiction, and side effects may occur. These products usually are recommended only as an adjunct to therapy and only when traditional therapies have been unsuccessful.

Amphetamines, which have a high potential for abuse, and nonamphetamine appetite suppressants (e.g., phentermine) may be used for a short time to promote weight loss. Phentermine is believed to act directly on the appetite control center in the central nervous system. As with amphetamines, nonamphetamine appetite suppressants stimulate the central nervous system, with resulting increased alertness, nervousness, and insomnia. They reduce fatigue and can interfere with sleep. They are used with caution in clients who have pre-existing heart disease, because they can increase blood pressure and heart rate and cause anginal pain.

Sibutramine (Meridia) is an appetite suppressant that acts on the central nervous system. Sibutramine also may increase the metabolic rate, promoting weight loss. It has the additional benefit of lowering cholesterol and triglyceride levels. However, sibutramine increases both pulse rate and blood pressure, potentially limiting its appropriateness for use in clients with hypertension, CHD, or heart failure.

Orlistat (Xenical) has a different mechanism of action: It inhibits fat absorption from the gastrointestinal tract, leading to weight loss. It has the added benefit of lowering blood glucose and cholesterol. The adverse effects of orlistat relate to its inhibition of fat absorption: oily stools, flatulence, and fecal urgency. These effects tend to diminish, however, when dietary fat intake is limited.

Over-the-counter products such as benzocaine and bulk-forming agents also commonly are used in weight management efforts. Methylcellulose and other bulk-forming products may decrease appetite by producing a sensation of fullness. Clients taking these products may experience flatulence or diarrhea and may need to increase fluid intake.

Exercise

Exercise is a critical element in weight loss and maintenance. Physical activity increases energy consumption and promotes weight loss while preserving lean body mass. Such activity improves physical fitness, decreases appetite, promotes self-esteem, and increases the BMR. Clients may benefit from consulting with a physical therapist or personal trainer to help them develop an exercise plan that reflects the client's physical condition, interests, lifestyle, and abilities.

If a client is under the care of a physician for another condition, such as asthma or diabetes, the client should consult with the treating physician, but evaluation by a health care practitioner is important for any client before beginning an exercise program. The practitioner instructs the client to increase the duration and intensity of activity and to stop exercising and report symptoms if chest pain or shortness of breath occurs. An aerobic exercise program of 30–40 minutes of exercise five or more days a week promotes weight loss while reducing adipose tissue, increasing lean body mass, and promoting long-term weight control. (See Concept 13, Health, Wellness, and Illness, for more details.)

Nutrition

Collaboration with a nutritionist will help clients to identify healthy foods that appeal to them and that can make up a diet plan to create a daily 500- to 1,000-kcal deficit. Ideally, the recommended diet should be low in kilocalories and fat, contain adequate nutrients and minerals, and be high in dietary fiber. The client should eat regular meals with small servings. A gradual, slow weight loss of no more than 1–2 lb/week is recommended. For most people, this means a diet of 1,000–1,200 kcal/day for most women and 1,200–1,600 kcal/day for men. Fewer than 1,200 kcal each day may lead to loss of lean tissue and nutritional deficiencies. Excessive calorie restrictions also can lead to failure to follow the prescribed diet, feelings of guilt, and overeating.

"Yo-yo" dieting (repeated cycles of weight loss and gain) may lead to a metabolic deficiency that makes subsequent weight loss efforts increasingly difficult. Therefore, it is critical that dieters take any weight loss effort seriously and include plans for long-term maintenance. The best approach is to modify dietary intake without severe restrictions, eating a well-balanced, low-fat diet and developing improved eating habits.

Very-low-calorie diets generally are reserved for clients who have a BMI of greater than 30 (WIN, 2003b). This type of program offers a protein-sparing modified fast (400–800 kcal/day or less) under close medical supervision. In a typical program, the client consumes 45–70 g of high-quality protein, 30–50 g of carbohydrate, and approximately 2 g of fat per day for a 1- to 2-month period. Exercise, nutrition, and behavior modification counseling should accompany the diet. The client generally experiences a dramatic and rapid weight loss while maintaining lean body mass. Suppression of hunger brought on by ketone production associated with fat metabolism is an added benefit of the diet. Complications generally are minor, and benefits include decreased blood pressure, blood glucose, and cholesterol and triglyceride levels along with improved exercise tolerance (Kasper et al., 2005). Very-low-calorie diets may not be appropriate for use in people over age 50 because of normal loss of lean body mass and adverse effects of the diet. Adverse effects generally are minor but can include fatigue, constipation, nausea, diarrhea, and gallstone formation (WIN, 2003b).

Behavior Modification

Behavior modification is a critical component of successful weight management. Strategies such as keeping food records, eliminating cues that precipitate eating, and changing the act of eating often are helpful.

Recording food intake, amount, location of eating, and situations that induce eating often help the dieter to gain self-control. These strategies generally are most effective when used in combination with other behavior modification approaches.

Researchers have found that for most overweight people, eating is regulated by external cues, such as the proximity to food and the time of day. In contrast, hunger and satiety are the cues that regulate eating in adults of normal weight. Strategies to control food cues include keeping food out of view, eliminating snack foods, and eating only in designated areas.

Other behavior modification approaches focus on helping clients to examine factors that affect eating behaviors. Examining lifestyle, personality, and environment helps the client to understand eating behaviors and their consequences. The goal is to empower the person who is stimulated to eat to choose activities that are not related to food.

Social support and group programs such as Weight Watchers, Overeaters Anonymous, and Take Off Pounds Sensibly promote weight loss success through peer support. Most organized programs require participants to pay a fee, which may improve compliance.

Surgery

Surgical treatment of obesity (bariatric surgery) generally is limited to clients who are morbidly obese (BMI > 40 kg/m^2, or >200% of ideal body weight) and unable to lose weight through diet and exercise or have serious obesity-related problems, such as metabolic syndrome, hypertension, or heart disease (WIN, 2004). In addition, clients must be able to tolerate surgery and be free of addiction to alcohol or other drugs. A thorough psychologic evaluation is done before surgery. The benefits of surgery include major weight loss and improved blood pressure, plus a reduced risk of diabetes, sleep apnea, angina, heart failure, blood lipid levels, and venous disease (Kasper et al., 2005). Bariatric surgery, is not without risk, however, and the decision to undergo surgery is a significant one.

RESTRICTIVE/MALABSORPTIVE PROCEDURES The most commonly used bariatric surgical procedures in the United States are combined restrictive/malabsorptive surgeries. These surgeries restrict stomach capacity, thus limiting food intake, and bypass a portion of the small intestine to restrict the absorption of calories and nutrients. In the Roux-en-Y gastric bypass (Figure 18–10A ■), a small stomach pouch is created to restrict food intake. A Y-shaped section of the jejunum is then attached to the pouch to allow food to bypass the lower stomach and duodenum. As a result, calorie and nutrient absorption is limited. A more complex procedure, the biliopancreatic diversion, carries a higher risk of nutritional deficiencies and is used less frequently. In biliopancreatic diversion, a portion of the stomach is removed to reduce its capacity. The duodenum and jejunum are bypassed by connecting the ileum either directly to the stomach pouch or just distal to the pyloric valve.

These combined restrictive/malabsorptive surgeries have the advantage of resulting in rapid weight loss that is maintained over time. Many clients maintain a 60–70% weight loss for 10 years or more following Roux-en-Y gastric bypass surgery (WIN, 2004). These surgeries also help to improve obesity-associated health problems, such as type 2 DM, hypertension, and sleep apnea. Because these procedures allow food to bypass the duodenum and jejunum, nutrient deficiencies, particularly of iron, calcium, vitamin B_{12}, and possibly, the fat-soluble vitamins, are common.

RESTRICTIVE PROCEDURES Restrictive procedures, which are safer but generally less effective in the long term, include adjustable gastric banding and the vertical banded gastroplasty. In adjustable gastric banding (Figure 18–10B), a hollow band of silicone rubber is placed around the upper (proximal) portion of the stomach. The band is inflated with saline solution to create a small stomach pouch with a narrow passage through to the rest of the stomach. The amount of band inflation can be adjusted using a port implanted under the skin. The vertical banded gastroplasty (Figure 18–10C) uses both a band and staples to create a small stomach pouch. Both procedures may be performed laparoscopically and can be reversed if necessary. Few nutritional deficiencies are associated with restrictive bariatric procedures. Vomiting is a common postoperative risk with restrictive procedures. The band may slip or break, necessitating a return to surgery. Approximately 15–20% of clients undergoing vertical banded gastroplasty procedures may require a second procedure. Because of this and the increased complexity of the vertical banded procedure, it is performed less commonly than adjustable gastric banding (WIN, 2004). While clients typically lose approximately 50% of their excess body weight within the first year after these procedures, less than one quarter maintain that weight loss over a 10-year period (WIN, 2004).

COMPLICATIONS OF SURGERY Although the risk for postoperative complications is high, the mortality rate for bariatric procedures is low (<1% for restrictive surgeries and up to 5% for combination procedures). Possible postoperative complications include anastomosis leak with peritonitis, abdominal wall hernia, gallstones, wound infections, deep venous thrombosis, nutritional deficiencies, and gastrointestinal symptoms (Tierney et al., 2005). Dumping syndrome, which can be precipitated by a meal that is high in simple carbohydrates, may develop following combined bariatric surgeries such as Roux-en-Y gastric bypass and biliopancreatic diversion. In dumping syndrome, stomach contents move rapidly through the small intestine, drawing fluid into the intestine by osmosis. The client experiences nausea, bloating, abdominal pain, weakness, sweating, and possibly syncope.

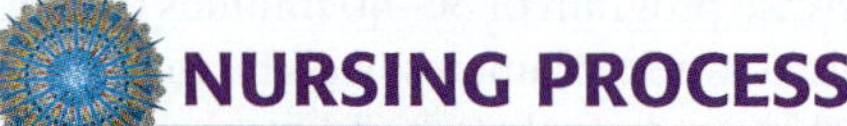

NURSING PROCESS

Maintaining a healthy weight throughout the life span begins in childhood. Obese children and teenagers become obese adults. Promote healthy eating, including a diet rich in whole grains, fruits, and vegetables and low in fat. The U.S. Department of Agriculture Food Guide Pyramid and the Healthy Eating Pyramid provide visual guidance for appropriate food choices to maintain a healthy, well-balanced diet. Encourage all children and adults to maintain an active lifestyle, engaging in at least 30 min of aerobic activity daily. Encourage parents to limit the time that children spend watching television, using the computer, and playing video games. Discuss the effects of smoking and excess alcohol use on nutrition and activity.

Adults commonly gain approximately 20 pounds between early and middle adulthood. Encourage clients to reduce the amount of calories consumed as their energy needs change.

Assessment

Collect the following data through the health history and physical examination:

- *Health history.* Risk factors; current and usual weight; recent weight gains or losses; perception of weight and effect on health; usual diet and food intake; exercise/activity patterns; previous weight loss efforts and results; current medications; coexisting disorders, such as cardiovascular disease and diabetes; tobacco use; and family history of overweight, diabetes, and weight-related morbidity
- *Physical examination.* Vital signs, weight and height, skinfold measurements, waist-to-hip ratio, and inspection of skin under the breasts and abdominal folds.

PRACTICE ALERT

Use of an inappropriate-size sphygmomanometer is a common source of error in measuring blood pressure in clients with obesity. Choose a cuff on which the width of the bladder is 40% of the circumference of the arm and the length of the bladder is sufficient to cover at least 65% of the arm circumference.

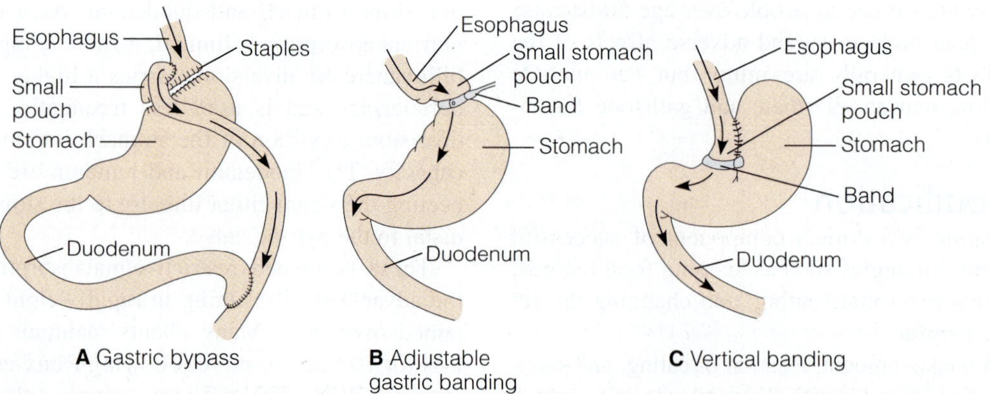

Figure 18–10 ■ Types of surgical procedures to treat obesity: *A*, Roux-en-Y gastric bypass surgery; *B*, adjustable gastric banding; and *C*, Vertical banded gastroplasty.

Although body weight may be used to identify obesity, measures of body fat are more accurate. Male clients at ideal body weight have 10–20% body fat, whereas female clients at ideal body weight have 20–30% body fat.

Diagnosis

Nursing care for clients who are overweight or obese is community based and holistic, focusing on both physiologic and psychologic responses to weight and appearance. Appropriate NANDA nursing diagnoses may include the following:

- Imbalanced Nutrition: More Than Body Requirements
- Chronic Low Self-Esteem
- Ineffective Therapeutic Regimen Management
- Activity Intolerance.

Plan

Although many factors contribute to obesity, this condition always involves an imbalance of kilocalorie consumption to energy expenditure. Client education will include exercise, diet, and behavior modification. Goals will be individualized based on classification of obesity, risk factors, and treatments and may include:

- Client will make sensible dietary choices in order to plan meals within the caloric limitations chosen by the collaborative team.
- Client will follow an exercise routine planned in collaboration with health care team.
- Client will relate strategies to deal with hunger and making unhealthy food choices.
- Client will attend support group meetings to help him or her meet weight loss goals.
- Client will demonstrate appropriate weight loss, attending regular weigh-in appointments.

Implementation

Caring interventions focus on diet, exercise, and behavior modification.

- Encourage the client to identify the factors that contribute to excess food intake. Identification of cues for eating helps the client to eliminate or reduce these cues.
- Establish realistic weight loss goals and exercise/activity objectives. Small, reasonable goals, such as loss of 1–2 lb/week, increase the likelihood of success.
- Assess the client's knowledge, and discuss well-balanced diet plans. Provide necessary teaching about diet. Knowledge empowers the client to participate and make appropriate diet choices.
- Discuss behavior modification strategies, such as self-monitoring and environmental management. Behavior modification, diet, and exercise are critical to promoting successful, long-term weight loss.
- Monitor weight loss, blood pressure, and laboratory data, including blood glucose and lipid levels. Continuing assessment not only is important to evaluate the safety of weight loss strategies but also to reinforce positive benefits of weight loss.

Exercise Program

Clients with obesity may experience excess fatigue, tachycardia, and shortness of breath with activity. These symptoms result from the physiologic effects of excess weight as well as a sedentary lifestyle. A medical evaluation may be needed before beginning an exercise program.

- Assess the client's current activity level and tolerance of that activity. Assess vital signs. *This provides baseline information to plan an activity program and assess the client's response to that activity.*
- After medical clearance, plan with the client a program of regular, gradually increasing exercise. Consider a consultation with an exercise physiologist. *An individualized exercise program promotes activities within the client's physical capabilities.*

Weight-Loss Program

Most clients who are overweight or obese experience some difficulty integrating all the components of a weight loss program into a daily routine. For a weight loss and maintenance program to be successful, the overweight client must modify dietary intake in a world of daily temptations. There may be many obstacles to exercise, including a busy schedule, activity intolerance, impaired physical mobility, lack of equipment, and the embarrassment of being fat.

- Discuss the client's ability and willingness to incorporate changes into daily patterns of diet, exercise, and lifestyle. This provides data from which to set realistic goals with the client.
- Help the client to identify behavior modification strategies and support systems for weight loss and maintenance. Weight loss and maintenance are most successful if the client establishes lifestyle patterns that promote interest and motivation and, thus, exercise and diet management. Family and social support is critical for successful adherence to the therapeutic regime.
- Have the client establish strategies for dealing with "stress" eating or interruptions in the therapeutic regime. A sense of failure associated with overeating or lack of exercise can lead to further overeating. Identifying positive strategies to deal with these situations promotes self-acceptance and limits self-punishment through overeating.

Self-Esteem

Although many clients with obesity may have accepted their weight and body appearance on some level, most overweight and obese individuals verbalize the experience of "fat prejudice" in their family, workplace, or community. These clients may experience ridicule, prejudice, and health problems attributed to being "fat." These experiences, coupled with day-to-day problems such as finding attractive clothing or a chair large enough to sit on, can affect self-esteem. Many clients report that "fat" jokes or comments contribute to a sense of negative self-worth.

- Encourage the client to verbalize the experience of being overweight, and validate the client's experience. This

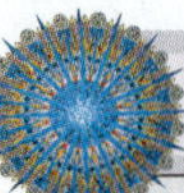

NURSING CARE PLAN **A Client With Obesity**

Sam Elliott, age 57, has gained 30 lb since his retirement 2 years ago. The most active things he does each day are "puttering around" and "walking to the end of the driveway to get the mail." His diet includes juice, oatmeal, a muffin, and coffee with cream for breakfast; donuts and coffee with friends midmorning; a bologna-and-cheese sandwich with chips and a root beer for lunch; and cheese, crackers, and wine before a dinner of meat, potatoes, vegetables, and dessert. He tells the nurse, "I have never had to diet. I just don't know how to get this weight off."

ASSESSMENT

Mr. Elliott is 5′8″ (173 cm) tall and weighs 201 lb (91.2 kg). His BMI is 30.1 kg/m^2. His cholesterol is 240 mg/dL (normal, 150–200 mg/dL), with an HDL of 37 mg/dL (normal male value, >45 mg/dL) and an LDL of 180 mg/dL (normal, v130 mg/dL). His BP is 138/90 mmHg. His fasting blood glucose is normal at 103 mg/dL. His electrocardiogram shows normal sinus rhythm. He reports fatigue and shortness of breath with activity. His health care provider has advised a weight loss of 30 lb and a regular exercise program.

DIAGNOSES

Nursing diagnoses that may be appropriate to Mr. Elliot include the following:

- Imbalanced Nutrition: More Than Body Requirements related to food intake in excess of energy expenditure
- Risk for Ineffective Therapeutic Regimen Management related to knowledge deficit
- Activity Intolerance related to sedentary lifestyle.

PLANNING

The goals for the plan of care specify that Mr. Elliot will:

- Lose 1 lb each week.
- Walk 30 minutes 5 days each week.
- Verbalize an understanding of the relationship between weight loss, weight control, and exercise.
- Identify behavior modification strategies to avoid overeating.
- Identify support systems for behavior modification.

IMPLEMENTATION

The following nursing interventions may be appropriate for Mr. Elliot:

- Assess weight and blood pressure once or twice each week.
- Discuss current eating habits and strategies to reduce fat and calorie intake.
- Discuss cues that promote eating, and identify strategies to eliminate or reduce these cues.
- Teach how to keep a food diary to examine and change eating habits.
- Discuss the role of regular exercise in weight loss and weight control. Instruct to maintain an exercise record to track the intensity and duration of activity.
- Discuss lifestyle and behavior modification strategies to promote successful weight loss and control.

EVALUATION

Two weeks after changing his diet and beginning to exercise, Mr. Elliott has lost 2 lb. He has maintained a food diary. He has identified boredom as a cue to eating. In light of this, he has started volunteering at the local hospital, where he is working with children. He is walking for 30 minutes 5 days a week. He plans to increase his activity periods to 45 minutes. He verbalizes commitment to a lifelong plan of exercising and eating a low-fat diet. His BP has ranged from 132/76 to 136/84 mmHg. He plans to have the employee health nurse at the hospital check his weight and BP each week and to join Weight Watchers for ongoing support.

CRITICAL THINKING

1. What are some possible pathophysiologic bases for Mr. Elliott's abnormal cholesterol, HDL, and LDL levels?
2. Develop a teaching plan for a group of overweight men and women.
3. Identify potential barriers to losing weight and strategies to reduce or eliminate these barriers.

provides baseline data to use in developing individualized interventions to address self-esteem issues.

- Set small goals with the client, and offer positive feedback and encouragement. Small goals provide more opportunities for success. Positive feedback and encouragement provide a comfortable environment in which to develop self-esteem.
- Refer the client for counseling as appropriate. Many clients benefit from counseling for issues related to self-esteem.

Evaluation

Expected outcomes of nursing care are individualized based on the nursing care plan. These outcomes may include the following:

- Identification and understanding of factors contributing to weight gain
- Understanding and application of behavioral modification techniques to reduce weight
- Accomplishment of desired weight loss at a rate of 1–2 lb/week
- Incorporation of physical activity into routines.

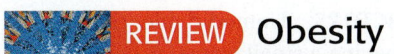

REVIEW Obesity

RELATE: LINK THE CONCEPTS

Linking the exemplar of Obesity with the concept of Culture:

1. Research perceptions about obesity and overweight in several cultures, and identify cultural differences.
2. How would you teach a client from a culture that values obesity as a sign of status to make healthier food choices?

Linking the exemplar of Obesity with the concept of Health, Wellness, and Illness:

3. What teaching would you provide an adolescent client who is obese to promote health and reduce the risk of complications in later life?
4. Is it possible to be obese and still maintain optimal health? Explain your answer.

READY: GO TO COMPANION SKILLS MANUAL

- Assessing height and weight
- Measuring waist circumference
- Assessing blood pressure
- Measuring body mass index

REFER: GO TO MYNURSINGKIT

REFLECT: CASE STUDY

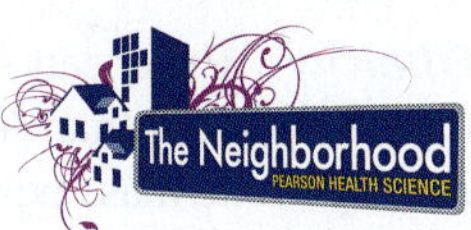

Jenna Riley is a healthy but overweight 14-year-old girl who lives with her mother Evelyn and her brother Jason. Her older sister Jessica lives a short distance away in her own apartment with her new infant son Ryan. Jenna misses having her older sister around, and she looks up to Jessica. Jenna has had minimal contact with her father during the last 10 years and does not really even know him. Because her mother works a few evenings a week, Jenna is responsible for her younger brother. She gets along okay with Jason, but she thinks he is such a weirdo.

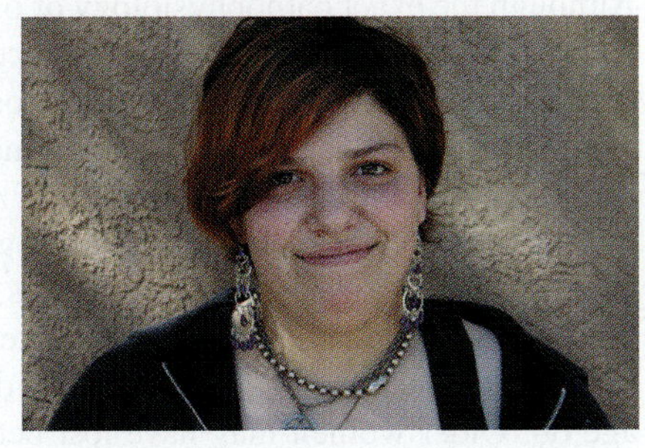

Jenna is a good student in the eighth grade at the local middle school. She has many friends and spends a great deal of time on the phone or in computer chat rooms talking with them each evening. Jenna is self-conscious about her weight, however. She knows she should try to lose weight, but she doesn't really know how and does not have much discipline when it comes to resisting snacks. She finds it very hard to not join in with her friends when they eat.

1. What risk factors does Jenna face as a result of obesity?
2. What client teaching will you provide Jenna?
3. What support groups might you recommend for Jenna?
4. Plan a one week meal plan reflecting healthy eating for Jenna that would promote sensible weight loss.

18.4 OSTEOPOROSIS

KEY TERMS

Cancellous bone, *1034*
Diaphysis, *1034*
Metaphysis, *1034*
Osteoporosis, *1033*

BASIS FOR SELECTION OF EXEMPLAR

Centers for Disease Control and Prevention
Healthy People 2010
Most common condition

LEARNING OUTCOMES

After reading about this exemplar, you will be able to:

1. Describe the pathophysiology, etiology, clinical manifestations, and direct and indirect causes of osteoporosis.
2. Identify risk factors associated with osteoporosis.
3. Illustrate the nursing process in providing culturally competent care across the life span for individuals with osteoporosis.
4. Formulate priority nursing diagnoses appropriate for an individual with osteoporosis.
5. Create a plan of care for individuals with osteoporosis and their family members.
6. Assess expected outcomes for an individual with osteoporosis.
7. Discuss therapies used in the collaborative care of an individual with osteoporosis.
8. Employ evidence-based caring interventions for an individual with osteoporosis.

OVERVIEW

Osteoporosis (literally defined as "porous bones") is a metabolic bone disorder characterized by loss of bone mass, increased bone fragility, and increased risk of fractures. The reduced bone mass is caused by an imbalance of the processes that influence bone growth and maintenance. Although osteoporosis may result from an endocrine disorder or malignancy, it most often is associated with aging as a result of inadequate calcium intake. Children, however, can have osteoporosis related to imbalanced nutrition or other pathological conditions.

PATHOPHYSIOLOGY AND ETIOLOGY

Although the exact pathophysiology of osteoporosis is unclear, it is known to involve an imbalance in the activity of osteoblasts that form new bone and osteoclasts that resorb bone. Until age 35, when peak bone mass occurs, formation occurs more rapidly than reabsorption. After peak bone mass is achieved, slightly more is lost than is gained (~0.3–0.5% per year); this loss is accelerated if the diet is deficient in vitamin D and calcium. In women, bone loss increases after menopause (with loss of estrogen), then slows but does not stop at about age 60. Older women may have lost between 35 and 50% of their bone mass; older men may have lost between 20 and 35% (Mayo Clinic, 2002).

Osteoporosis affects the **diaphysis** (shaft of the bone) and the **metaphysis** (portion of the bone between the diaphysis and the epiphysis). The diameter of the bone increases, thinning the outer supporting cortex. As osteoporosis progresses, trabeculae are lost from **cancellous bone** (the spongy tissue of bone), and the outer cortex thins to the point that even minimal stress will fracture the bone (Porth, 2005).

Etiology

The National Osteoporosis Foundation (2006) has found that osteoporosis is a health threat for an estimated 44 million Americans: 10 million people have osteoporosis, and 34 million have low bone mass, increasing their risk for the disease. Although osteoporosis can occur at any age and in both men and women, 80% of those with osteoporosis are women. One in two women and one in four men over age 50 will have an osteoporosis-related fracture in his or her remaining lifetime.

Risk Factors

The risk for developing osteoporosis depends on how much bone mass is achieved between ages 25 and 35 and, afterward, on how much bone mass is lost. Certain diseases, lifestyle habits, and ethnic backgrounds increase the risk of developing osteoporosis. Different variables affect one's risk of osteoporosis. Some of these variables can be modified, but others cannot.

FOCUS ON DIVERSITY AND CULTURE The Client with Osteoporosis

- Significant risk is reported for people of all ethnic backgrounds, but the highest percentage of cases involve non-Hispanic and Asian women age 50 or older, with 20% estimated to have osteoporosis and 52% estimated to have low bone mass. Ten percent of Hispanic women age 50 or older are affected, with 49% estimated to have low bone mass.
- The lowest incidence is in non-Hispanic black women over the age of 50, with an estimated 5% having osteoporosis and 35% having low bone mass.
- In men, 7% of those affected are non-Hispanic white and Asian, 4% are non-Hispanic black, and 3% are Hispanic (all age 50 or older).

Source: National Osteoporosis Foundation. (2008). *Fast facts on osteoporosis.* Retrieved July 13, 2009, from http://www.nof.org/osteoporosis/diseasefacts.htm

UNMODIFIABLE RISK FACTORS Unmodifiable risk factors include being thin and/or having a small frame. A personal history of fracture after age 50 also is a risk factor. Other unmodifiable risk factors include family history, age, ethnicity, female athletes, other chronic diseases, and current low bone mass.

Family History Those with a family history of osteoporosis are at increased risk for developing osteoporosis themselves. Those with a history of fracture in a first-degree relative also are at higher risk.

Age Both men and women are susceptible to osteoporosis as they age, because the osteoblasts and osteoclasts undergo alterations that diminish their activity. Women (especially white and Asian women), however, have a significantly higher risk for the manifestations and complications of osteoporosis, because their peak bone mass is 10–15% less than that of men. In addition, age-related bone loss begins earlier and proceeds more rapidly in women, beginning in their 30s and accelerating before menopause. Age-related bone loss in men occurs 15–20 years later than in women and at a slower rate. Estrogen in women and testosterone in men appear to help prevent osteoporosis; the decreasing levels of these hormones associated with aging contribute to bone loss.

Ethnicity European Americans and Asians are at a higher risk for osteoporosis than African Americans, who have greater bone density (bone mass positively correlates with the amount of skin pigmentation). As mentioned, this is especially true for women.

Female Athletes Premature osteoporosis is increasing in female athletes, who have a greater incidence of eating disorders and amenorrhea. Poor nutrition combined with intense physical training can result in a deficient production of estrogen. In turn, decreased estrogen, combined with a lack of calcium and vitamin D, results in a loss of bone density (Porth, 2005).

PRACTICE ALERT

The combination of eating disorders, amenorrhea, and osteoporosis in female athletes has come to be known as the Female Athlete Triad. More information on this disorder can be found at http://www.femaleathletetriad.org.

Other Chronic Diseases Clients who have an endocrine disorder, such as hyperthyroidism, hyperparathyroidism, Cushing's syndrome, or diabetes, are at high risk for osteoporosis. These disorders affect the metabolism, which in turn affects nutritional status and bone mineralization. Clients with moderate to severe persistent asthma or severe allergies who take steroids frequently also are at greater risk for osteoporosis.

Current Low Bone Mass Children who may show signs of osteoporosis include those with decreased mechanical loading. Children with spina bifida or cerebral palsy that interferes with ambulation have limited pressure on their bones; therefore, bones in the affected extremities and the spine have lower mass. Some other conditions associated with lower bone mass include Turner's syndrome, growth hormone deficiency, osteogenesis imperfecta, juvenile rheumatoid arthritis, and diabetes. Children who are treated for disorders or injuries with casting and bracing also are at high risk of osteoporosis because of immobilization. Children who are treated for some types of cancer have increased rates of osteoporosis.

MODIFIABLE RISK FACTORS Modifiable risk factors include behaviors that place a person at risk for developing osteoporosis. These factors also include physical changes for which the contribution to osteoporosis can be modified by preventive strategies (e.g., menopause).

Menopause With menopause and decreasing estrogen levels, bone loss accelerates in women. Estrogen promotes the activity of osteoblasts, increasing new bone formation. In addition, estrogen enhances calcium absorption and stimulates the thyroid gland to secrete calcitonin, a hormone that suppresses osteoclast activity and increases osteoblast activity.

Calcium Deficiency Calcium is an essential mineral in the process of bone formation and other significant body functions. When the intake of calcium through the diet is insufficient, the body compensates by removing calcium from the skeleton, weakening the bone tissue. A high intake of diet soda with a high phosphate content also can deplete calcium stores.

Acidosis Acidosis, which may result from a high-protein diet, contributes to osteoporosis in two ways. First, acidosis may result in calcium being withdrawn from the bone as the kidneys attempt to buffer the excess acid. Second, acidosis may directly stimulate osteoclast function.

Substance Abuse Both cigarette smoking and excess alcohol intake are risk factors for osteoporosis. Smoking decreases the blood supply to bones, and nicotine slows the production of osteoblasts and impairs the absorption of calcium, contributing to decreased bone density. Alcohol has a direct toxic effect on osteoblast activity, suppressing bone formation during periods of alcohol intoxication. In addition, heavy alcohol use may be associated with nutritional deficiencies that contribute to osteoporosis. Interestingly, moderate alcohol consumption in postmenopausal women actually may increase bone mineral content, possibly by increasing levels of estrogen and calcitonin.

Sedentary Lifestyle Weight-bearing exercises, such as walking, influence bone metabolism in several ways. The stress of this type of exercise causes an increase in blood flow to bones, which brings growth-producing nutrients to the cells. Walking causes an increase in osteoblast growth and activity.

Medications Prolonged use of medications that increase calcium excretion, such as aluminum-containing antacids and anticonvulsants, increase the risk of developing osteoporosis. Heparin therapy increases bone resorption, and prolonged use of heparin is associated with osteoporosis. Antiretroviral therapy for people with AIDS or HIV infection may cause decreased bone density and osteoporosis (Porth, 2005).

Anyone who takes a glucocorticoid medication for more than 3 months is at risk for glucocorticoid-induced osteoporosis. These medications, often prescribed to control many rheumatic diseases, include prednisone (Deltasone, Orasone), prednisolone (Prelone), dexamethasone (Decadron, Hexadrol), and cortisone (Cortisone Acetate). These medications can directly affect bone cells, slowing the rate of bone formation. They also interfere with how the body uses calcium and affect levels of sex hormones, leading to bone loss. The problems that result, such as increased possibility of fractures, can be prevented by a daily regimen of calcium supplements with added vitamin D and one multivitamin (American College of Rheumatology, 2004).

CLINICAL MANIFESTATIONS

The most common manifestations of osteoporosis are loss of height, progressive curvature of the spine, low back pain, and fractures of the forearm, spine, or hip. Osteoporosis often is called the "silent disease," because bone loss occurs without symptoms; the problem may not become apparent until the client has a fracture or radiologic studies reveal the condition.

The loss of height occurs as vertebral bodies collapse. Acute episodes generally are painful, with radiation of the pain around the flank into the abdomen. Vertebral collapse can occur with little or no stress; minimal movements, such as bending, lifting, or jumping, may precipitate the pain. In some clients, vertebral collapse may occur slowly, accompanied by little discomfort.

Along with loss of height, characteristic dorsal kyphosis and cervical lordosis develop, accounting for the "dowager's hump" often associated with aging. The abdomen tends to protrude and the knees and hips flex as the body attempts to maintain its center of gravity (Figure 18–11 ■).

Fractures are the most common complication of osteoporosis, with the disease being responsible for more than 1.5 million fractures each year. These include 700,000 vertebral compression fractures, 300,000 hip fractures, 250,000 wrist fractures, and 300,000 fractures at other sites (National Osteoporosis Foundation, 2006). There may be no obvious manifestations of osteoporosis until fractures occur. Some fractures are spontaneous; others may result from everyday activities. Wrist and vertebral fractures have not been shown to increase client disability or mortality, but the persistent pain and associated changes in posture may restrict the client's activities or interfere with activities of daily living.

Pharmacotherapy is used for prevention and treatment of osteoporosis. Medications used include hormonal agents, biophosphonates, and selective estrogen receptor modulators. Estrogen replacement therapy reduces bone loss, increases bone density in the spine and hip, and reduces the risk of fractures in postmenopausal women. It is particularly recommended for women who have undergone surgical menopause before age 50, and it often is prescribed for women with other risk factors. Estrogen therapy alone is associated with an increased risk of endometrial cancer, so it usually is prescribed in combination with progestin (hormone replacement therapy).

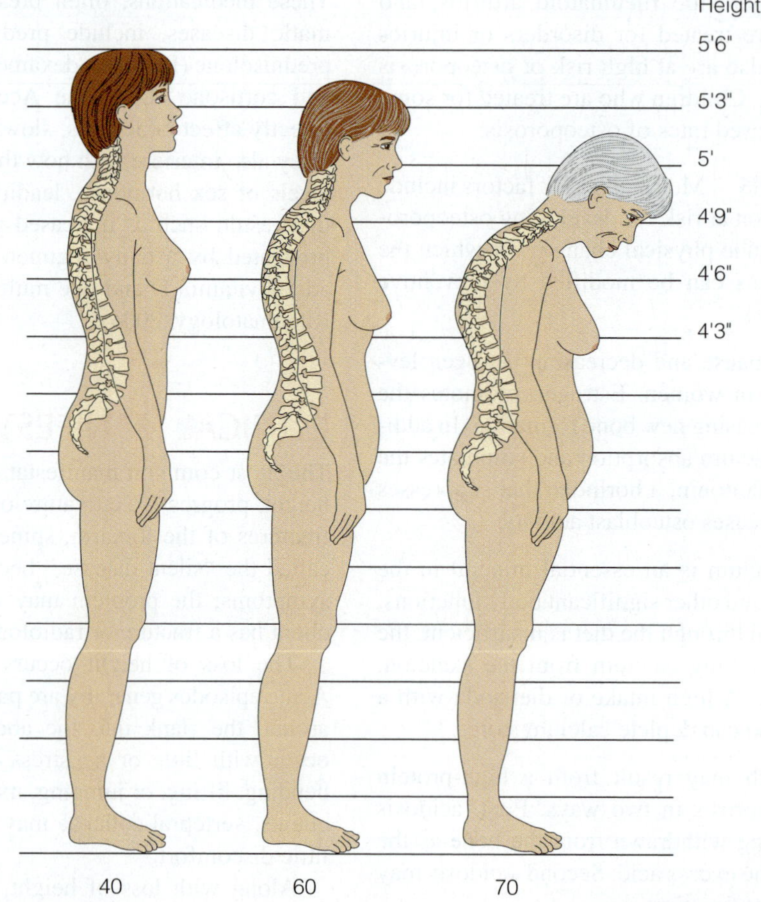

Figure 18–11 ■ Spinal changes caused by osteoporosis. As the condition progresses, height can be reduced by as much as 7 in.

COLLABORATION

Care of the client with osteoporosis focuses on stopping or slowing the process, alleviating the symptoms, and preventing complications. Proper nutrition and exercise are important components of the treatment program.

Diagnostic Tests

The manifestations of osteoporosis can mimic those of other bone disorders. Therefore, diagnostic tests are needed to differentiate osteoporosis from other problems.

Dual-energy x-ray absorptiometry (DEXA) measures bone density in the lumbar spine or hip and is considered to be highly accurate. Ultrasound transmits painless sound waves through the heel of the foot to measure bone density. This 1-minute test is not as sensitive as DEXA, but it is accurate enough for screening purposes.

Laboratory tests include alkaline phosphatase, which may be elevated following a fracture, and serum bone Glaprotein (osteocalcin), which can be used as a marker of osteoclastic activity and, therefore, is an indicator of the rate of bone turnover. This test is most useful to evaluate the effects of treatment rather than as an indicator for the severity of the disease.

Physical Therapy

Nurses may collaborate with physical therapists to design appropriate exercises for clients with osteoporosis. This may be particularly helpful for clients who have a comorbid condition that limits exercise, such as chronic obstructive pulmonary disease or asthma. Clients who have problems with balance may benefit from tai chi or yoga, both of which can be of benefit to individuals with osteoporosis. If a nurse working with a female athlete suspects an eating disorder or amenorrhea, the nurse should discuss counseling and nutrition referrals with the client.

Dietary Management

Clients with osteoporosis or at risk for later development of the disease will benefit from choosing healthier menu items, particularly those high in calcium and vitamin D. Calcium rich foods include dairy, vegetables, and beans. Food supplemented with extra calcium includes orange juice, breakfast cereals, and breads. Foods rich in vitamin D include fish and those with vitamin D added include milk, cereal and breads. If inadequate calcium and vitamin D are found in the diet, supplements may be taken to assure the body has an adequate supply of these nutrients.

Pharmacologic Therapies

Selected drugs for osteoporosis are listed in Table 18–7. Calcium gluconate and other calcium compounds are used to treat and prevent osteoporosis. Oral calcium supplements are best taken with meals or within 1 hour following meals. The most common adverse effects is hypercalcemia caused by taking too much of the supplement. Symptoms include lethargy, drowsiness, weakness, headache, anorexia, nausea and vomiting, increased urination, and thirst. Calcium supplementation is contraindicated in clients with ventricular fibrillation, metastatic bone cancer, renal calculi, or hypercalcemia. Caution should be taken in administering calcium supplements with digoxin, tetracyclines, and calcium channel blockers.

The most common drug class for treating osteoporosis is the bisphosphonates. These drugs are structural analogs of pyrophosphate, a natural substance that inhibits bone resorption. Bisphosphonates inhibit bone resorption by suppressing osteoclast activity, thus increasing bone density and reducing the incidence of fractures by about 50%. Examples include etidronate (Didronel), alendronate (Fosamax), tiludronate (Skelid), and pamidronate (Aredia), which is available as an injectable drug. Adverse effects include GI problems such as nausea, vomiting, abdominal pain, and esophageal irritation. Because these drugs are poorly absorbed, they should be taken on an empty stomach, as tolerated by the client. Recent studies suggest that once-weekly dosing with bisphosphonates may give the same bone density benefits as daily dosing because of the extended duration of drug action.

NURSING PROCESS

Osteoporosis is both preventable and treatable; therefore, nursing care focuses primarily on planning and implementing interventions to prevent the disease, its manifestations, and the resulting injuries. An important aspect of preventing osteoporosis is educating clients under age 35. Health promotion activities to prevent or slow osteoporosis focus on calcium intake, exercise, and health-related behaviors.

TABLE 18–7 Selected Drugs for Osteoporosis

DRUG	ROUTE AND ADULT DOSE (MAX DOSE WHERE INDICATED)	ADVERSE EFFECTS
Hormonal Agents		
Calcitonin—human (Cibacalcin)	Paget's disease: subcutaneous; human, 0.5 mg/day; subcutaneous/IM; salmon, 100 international units/day	*Nausea, inflammation at infection site, and flushing of face*
Calcitonin—salmon	Hypercalcemia: subcutaneous/IM; salmon, 4 international units/kg bid	
(Calciman, Miacalcin)	Osteoporosis: intranasal; 1 spray/day (200 international units)	Anaphylaxis
Raloxifene hydrochloride (Evista)	po; 60 mg/day	*Hot flashes, sinusitis, flulike symptoms, nausea* Breast pain, vaginal bleeding, pneumonia, and chest pain
Teriparatide (Forteo)	Subcutaneous; 20 mcg/day	*Dizziness, depression, insomnia, vertigo, rhinitis, increased cough, leg cramps, nausea, and arthralgia* Syncope, angina
BISPHOSPHONATES		
Alendronate sodium (Fosamax)	Osteoporosis treatment: po; 10 mg/day Osteoporosis prevention: po; 5 mg/day Paget's disease: po; 40 mg/day for 6 months	*Nausea, dyspepsia, diarrhea, bone pain, back pain*
Etidronate disodium (Didronel)	po; 5–10 mg/kg/day for 6 months or 11–20 mg/kg/day for 3 months	Bone fractures, nephrotoxicity, hypocalcemia, hypophosphatemia, gastric ulcer, esophagitis, dysrhythmias (pamidronate)
Ibandronate (Boniva)	po; 2.5 mg/day or one 150-mg tablet per month, taken on the same date each month	
Pamidronate disodium (Aredia)	IV; 15–90 mg in 1,000 ml normal saline or D5W over 4–24 hours	
Risedronate sodium (Actonel)	po; 30 mg/day at least 30 minutes before the first drink or meal of the day for 2 months	
Tiludronate disodium (Skelid)	po; 400 mg/day taken with 6–8 oz of water 2 hours before or after food for 3 months	

Note: Italics indicate common adverse effects; underlining indicates serious adverse effects.

Assessment

Collect the following data through the health history and physical examination:

- *Health history.* Age; risk factors; history of fractures; smoking history; alcohol intake; medications; usual diet; menstrual history, including menopause; usual exercise/activity level; and low back pain
- *Physical examination.* Height and spinal curves.

Diagnosis

While there may be some variance among clients who are at risk for or have osteoporosis regarding appropriate NANDA nursing diagnoses, the following should be considered:

- Risk for Injury
- Imbalanced Nutrition: Less Than Body Requirements
- Acute Pain.

Plan

Planning should be structured around self-care strategies that clients can use to reduce their risk for developing osteoporosis and/or minimize its symptoms and effects. Appropriate goals for clients may include:

- Client participates in weight-bearing exercises for approximately 30 minutes a day at least 4 days per week.
- Client's bone density is evaluated at least every other year.
- Client gets sufficient nutrition, particularly calcium and vitamin D, through diet or diet in combination with dietary supplements.
- Client is able to discuss risk factors for osteoporosis and how to prevent or minimize them.
- Clients with a high risk for injury modify their home and work environments to minimize such risk.

Implementation

Nursing care of clients who have osteoporosis focuses on teaching about the disease process, helping to maintan physical mobility and nutrition, and solving problems associated with pain and injury.

Risk for Injury

Falls that would result in little or no injury in the healthy adult may cause fractures in the client with osteoporosis. Even normal movements, such as twisting, bending, lifting, or rising from bed, can precipitate a vertebral fracture.

- Implement safety precautions as necessary for the client who is hospitalized or in a long-term care facility. Maintain the bed in low position; use side rails if indicated to prevent the client from getting up alone. Provide nighttime lighting to toilet facilities. Most falls are preventable, particularly in hospitals and long-term care facilities.
- Avoid using restraints on the client who is hospitalized or a resident in a long-term care facility if at all possible. Restraints may actually increase the client's risk of falling and the risk of injury associated with a fall.
- Encourage older adults to use assistive devices to maintain independence in activities of daily living. Walking sticks, canes, and other assistive devices encourage client independence and support activities that promote bone growth.
- Teach older clients about safety and fall precautions. An assessment of the client's home for safety and fall risks may reduce the risk of fractures and, in turn, the cost of hospitalization and potential disability and/or death.

Imbalanced Nutrition: Less Than Body Requirements

Most Americans do not maintain their recommended daily intake of calcium. Clients therefore must be made aware of the relationship between an adequate calcium intake and maintaining strong bones.

- Teach adolescents, pregnant or lactating women, and adults through age 35 to eat foods that are high in calcium and to maintain a daily calcium intake of 1,200–1,500 mg. The National Institutes of Health recommend a daily calcium intake of 1,200–1,500 mg/ day for adolescents and young adults as well as for pregnant and lactating women.
- Encourage postmenopausal women to maintain a calcium intake of 1,000–1,500 mg daily, either through diet or a calcium supplement. Calcium needs for postmenopausal women vary depending on age.
- Teach clients taking calcium supplements the importance of taking the medication at the proper time and about the side effects that may occur. Free hydrochloric acid is needed for calcium absorption. Calcium carbonate supplement (e.g., Tums) should be taken 30–60 minutes before meals to allow adequate absorption. Calcium citrate supplements should be taken with meals to prevent gastrointestinal distress.
- Inform clients that calcium absorption requires sufficient levels of vitamin D. Clients who are at risk for insufficient levels of vitamin D may need to take a vitamin D supplement in combination with their calcium supplement. The National Institutes of Health recommend 400–800 IU of vitamin D daily for those under 50 years of age and 800–1,000 IU for those 50 years and older.

PRACTICE ALERT

Calcium supplements should be taken in divided doses (two to three times daily) for improved distribution, because the body requires calcium 24 hours per day.

Acute Pain

Advanced stages of osteoporosis can result in pain and immobilization. Acute pain usually results from a complicating fracture, especially a compression fracture of the vertebrae.

- Suggest the application of heat to relieve pain. A heating pad may offer temporary pain relief. To avoid the "rebound effect," the heat should be removed every 20–30 minutes.
- Suggest the client take over-the-counter anti-inflammatory pain medications for treatment of both acute and chronic pain. Clients should be instructed in the amount and frequency as noted on the manufacturer's labels. Continuous administration of ibuprofen or other nonsteroidal anti-inflammatory drugs (NSAIDs) can be useful to provide relief from pain, but clients must be cautioned not to exceed dosage recommendations.

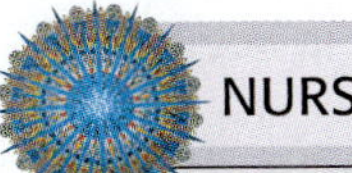

NURSING CARE PLAN A Client With Osteoporosis

Nancy Bauer is a 53-year-old schoolteacher. She has been married for 36 years and has two children. Mrs. Bauer is 65 in. tall. She has smoked one pack of cigarettes a day for 30 years and drinks one to two glasses of wine with dinner each evening. She does not exercise routinely. Mrs. Bauer has had symptoms of menopause for 8 years, including hot flashes in the early years and mood swings more recently. She has never been on hormone replacement therapy.

Mrs. Bauer is currently seeking medical advice for continuous low back pain. The pain is not relieved with an over-the-counter analgesic, and she frequently wakes up during the night because of the pain. She is diagnosed with osteoporosis.

ASSESSMENT

The nurse practitioner notes that Mrs. Bauer's vital signs are within normal limits. She has full range of motion of all extremities and is able to stand and bend over, but she reports discomfort when returning to the upright position. Mrs. Bauer has a slightly pronounced "hump" on her upper back and is 1 in. shorter than her stated height on admission. Her muscle strength is symmetric and strong.

DIAGNOSES

Nursing diagnoses that may be appropriate for Mrs. Bauer include the following:

- Acute Pain of the Lower Spine related to vertebral compression
- Deficient Knowledge related to osteoporosis and treatment to prevent further damage
- Imbalanced Nutrition: Less Than Body Requirements related to inadequate intake of calcium
- Risk for Injury related to effects of change in bone structure secondary to osteoporosis.

PLAN

The goals for the plan of care specify that Mrs. Bauer will:

- Verbalize a decrease in back pain.
- Be able to describe ways to treat her osteoporosis and prevent further complications.
- Verbalize an understanding of the current research and treatment regarding osteoporosis.
- Verbalize how stopping smoking can help to prevent further progression of osteoporosis.
- Seek consultation for supplements and medications to prevent further bone loss.
- Design a program of physical activity to prevent complications of osteoporosis.
- Verbalize safety precautions to prevent fractures resulting from falls.

IMPLEMENTATION

The following nursing interventions may be appropriate for Mrs. Bauer:

- Teach back-strengthening exercises.
- Refer to an osteoporosis support group if available.
- Provide realistic, yet optimistic, feedback about loss of height and bone integrity and the potential outcomes of treatment.
- Assess the client's current knowledge base, and correct any misconceptions regarding treatment of osteoporosis.
- Provide current educational literature regarding treatment of osteoporosis.
- Instruct in dietary and calcium supplements that help to prevent the effects of osteoporosis.
- Discuss physical exercises that help to prevent complications resulting from osteoporosis.
- Review safety and fall precautions, and provide literature regarding how to create a safe home environment.

EVALUATION

On her return visit 6 months later, Mrs. Bauer reports that she feels much better. She is no longer irritable and does not experience mood swings, because she has been taking her prescribed hormone replacements for 6 months: She is eating products rich in calcium and is taking a twice-daily supplement of calcium with vitamin D. Mrs. Bauer has reduced her wine intake to one glass in the evening and now drinks decaffeinated coffee and tea. She also states that since she stopped smoking, she has been walking 30 to 45 min every day.

CRITICAL THINKING

1. What is the rationale for stopping smoking and limiting caffeine and alcohol intake in the treatment of osteoporosis?
2. What foods would you encourage for clients at high risk for osteoporosis and whose serum cholesterol and LDL/HDL ratios indicate a high risk for cardiovascular disease?
3. What physical activities would you consider to be beneficial in helping to prevent the effects of osteoporosis in the female client who is wheelchair bound or has limited mobility?
4. Develop a care plan for Mrs. Bauer for the nursing diagnosis risk for trauma.

PRACTICE ALERT

Teach clients on long-term anti-inflammatory medications to watch for bright red bleeding from the stomach (in vomitus) or dark black bowel movements.

Exercise

Teach clients the importance of physical activity and weight-bearing exercises in preventing and slowing bone loss. Inform clients that swimming and pool aerobic exercises are not as beneficial for maintaining bone density because of the lack of weight-bearing activity.

- Teach clients who are able to participate in weight-bearing exercises to perform such exercises for a sustained period of 30–40 minutes at least three times a week. The mechanical force of weight-bearing exercises promotes bone growth. Bones weaken and demineralize without exercise. Walking is an easy, low-impact form of exercise. Swimming (including walking on the bottom of the pool) does not provide the needed weight-bearing activity.
- Prior to beginning teaching related to exercise, determine client's preexisting health problems and consult with primary provider to determine safety in beginning an exercise regime.
- Determine client's interests and plan an exercise regimen in keeping with the client's preferences.

Healthy Behaviors

Behaviors that help to prevent osteoporosis include not smoking, avoiding excessive alcohol intake, and limiting caffeine intake to two or three cups of coffee each day.

Evaluation

Nurses should evaluate outcomes when planning with the client at the client's annual check up. Nurses should ask clients about any pharmacologic therapies at each health care visit to ensure clients are taking their medications and provide the opportunity to discuss any possible side effects.

Expected outcomes for the client with osteoporosis include the following:

- Client will identify and implement strategies to change or modify lifestyle factors such as smoking cessation, weight-bearing exercise, and alcohol use.
- Client will achieve adequate calcium intake.
- Client will identify and eliminate safety hazards.
- Client will experience relief from acute pain.

REVIEW Osteoporosis

RELATE: LINK THE CONCEPTS

Linking the exemplar of Osteoporosis with the concept of Fluid and Electrolytes:

1. Create a flow chart diagramming the relationship between calcium and osteoporosis.
2. In addition to calcium, explain what other electrolytes are required in order for calcium to be properly metabolized and absorbed into the bone, explaining the physiology involved.

Linking the exemplar of Osteoporosis with the concept of Safety:

3. What safety issues will the nurse address in caring for a client with osteoporosis?
4. What strategies will the nurse recommend to reduce the risk of fractures for a client with osteoporosis?

READY: GO TO COMPANION SKILLS MANUAL

- Assessing height and weight
- Assessing home for safe environment
- Assessing the musculoskeletal system

REFER: GO TO MYNURSINGKIT

REFLECT: CASE STUDY

Mary Martin is a 75-year-old female who was recently widowed. She has a limited income because her husband's pension terminated when he died, and has moved in with her son, his wife, and their three teenage children. Mary has cataracts and glaucoma, for which she sees an ophthalmologist on a regular basis; otherwise, she is in good health.

Mary goes to the community health fair with her friend. While at the fair, she has a bone density screening performed and is told that she needs further evaluation for low bone density, a finding commonly associated with osteoporosis. In a follow-up visit with her primary care provider, Mary is told her bone scan shows evidence of decreased bone mineral density consistent with osteoporosis. She is told to increase her activity for weight-bearing exercise, to increase her calcium intake to 1,500 mg/day, and to take vitamin D supplements. She also is given a prescription for alendronate (Fosamax).

1. What teaching will the nurse provide Mary?
2. What outcomes are appropriate for Mary?
3. What recommendations will the nurse make to reduce the risk of injury when assessing Mary's home?

18.5 THYROID DISEASE

KEY TERMS

Euthyroid, *1041*
Exophthalmos, *1043*
Goiter, *1041*
Graves' disease, *1041*
Hashimoto's thyroiditis, *1048*
Hyperthyroidism, *1041*
Hypothyroidism, *1047*
Myxedema, *1047*
Myxedema coma, *1048*
Pretibial myxedema, *1043*
Proptosis, *1043*
Thyroid crisis, *1043*
Thyroidectomy, *1045*
Thyroiditis, *1043*
Thyroid storm, *1043*
Thyrotoxicosis, *1041*
Toxic multinodular goiter, *1043*

BASIS FOR SELECTION OF EXEMPLAR

Centers for Disease Control and Prevention

Most common condition

LEARNING OUTCOMES

After reading about this exemplar, you will be able to:

1. Describe the pathophysiology, etiology, clinical manifestations, and direct and indirect causes of thyroid disease.
2. Identify risk factors associated with thyroid disease.
3. Illustrate the nursing process in providing culturally competent care across the life span for individuals with thyroid disease.
4. Formulate priority nursing diagnoses appropriate for an individual with thyroid disease.
5. Create a plan of care for individuals with thyroid disease and their family members.
6. Assess expected outcomes for an individual with thyroid disease.
7. Discuss therapies used in the collaborative care of an individual with thyroid disease.
8. Employ evidence-based caring interventions for an individual with thyroid disease.

OVERVIEW

The thyroid gland is a small saddle-shaped gland that wraps around the anterior portion of the trachea. Altered production or use of thyroid hormone (TH) affects all major organ systems. In the adult, TH changes primarily affect metabolism, cardiovascular function, gastrointestinal function, and neuromuscular function. Thyroid disorders are among the most common endocrine disorders and if left untreated can result in cardiac disease and ultimately death.

Hyperthyroidism

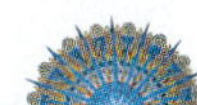

Hyperthyroidism (also called **thyrotoxicosis**) is a disorder caused by excessive delivery of TH to the peripheral tissues. Because the primary effect of TH is to increase metabolism and protein synthesis, hyperthyroidism affects all major organ systems of the body.

PATHOPHYSIOLOGY AND ETIOLOGY

The effects of hyperthyroidism are the result of increased circulating levels of TH. This hormonal excess increases the metabolic rate and heightens the sympathetic nervous system's physiologic response to stimulation. The sensitizing effect of abnormally elevated TH levels increases the cardiac rate and stroke volume. As a result, cardiac output and peripheral blood flow increase. Elevated TH levels also increase carbohydrate, protein, and lipid metabolism. Lipids are depleted, glucose tolerance decreases, and protein degradation increases, resulting in a negative nitrogen balance. Over time, the hypermetabolic effects of excess TH result in caloric and nutritional deficiencies.

Etiology

Hyperthyroidism results from many different factors, including autoimmune stimulation (as in Graves' disease), excess secretion of TSH by the pituitary gland, thyroiditis, neoplasms (e.g., toxic multinodular goiter), and an excessive intake of thyroid medications. The most common etiologies of hyperthyroidism are Graves' disease and toxic multinodular goiter.

Risk Factors

Women are at increased risk for hyperthyroidism, being five times more likely to develop the condition. Genetic factors, such as a family history of Graves' disease also contributes to increased risk. Other risk factors include increased iodine intake and age between 20 and 40 years.

CLINICAL MANIFESTATIONS

The client with hyperthyroidism typically has an increased appetite yet loses weight and may have hypermotile bowels (characterized by increased peristalsis, bloating, and pain) and diarrhea. Additional manifestations related to hypermetabolism include heat intolerance, insomnia, palpitations, and increased sweating. The skin is smooth and warm, hair may become fine, and hair loss in the scalp, eyebrow, axillary, or pubic areas of the body are common. Emotional lability also is common.

Treatment of hyperthyroidism focuses on reducing the production of TH by the thyroid gland, thus establishing a **euthyroid** (normal thyroid) state, and preventing or treating complications. Depending on the client's age and physical status, either medications, radioactive iodine (RAI) therapy, or surgery may be used.

Graves' Disease

Graves' disease, the most common cause of hyperthyroidism, is an autoimmune disorder sometimes associated with the presence of other autoimmune disorders, such as myasthenia gravis and pernicious anemia (Porth, 2005). More than 80% of clients with Graves' disease have an antibody in their serum that binds to TSH receptors in the thyroid follicles and causes the thyroid cells to hyperfunction (Tierney et al., 2005). When this antibody binds to the TSH receptors on the thyroid gland, it stimulates hormone synthesis and secretion, enlarging the gland. The cause is unknown, but there is a hereditary link. The incidence of Grave's disease is similar to that of hyperthyroidism.

Clients with Graves' disease have an enlarged thyroid gland (**goiter**) and manifestations of hyperthyroidism. The goiter can result from excess TSH stimulation (when the amount of circulating TH is deficient), abnormal growth-stimulating immunoglobulins, or substances that inhibit TH synthesis. A goiter may be present in clients with hyperthyroidism or hypothyroidism.

MULTISYSTEM EFFECTS OF **Hyperthyroidism**

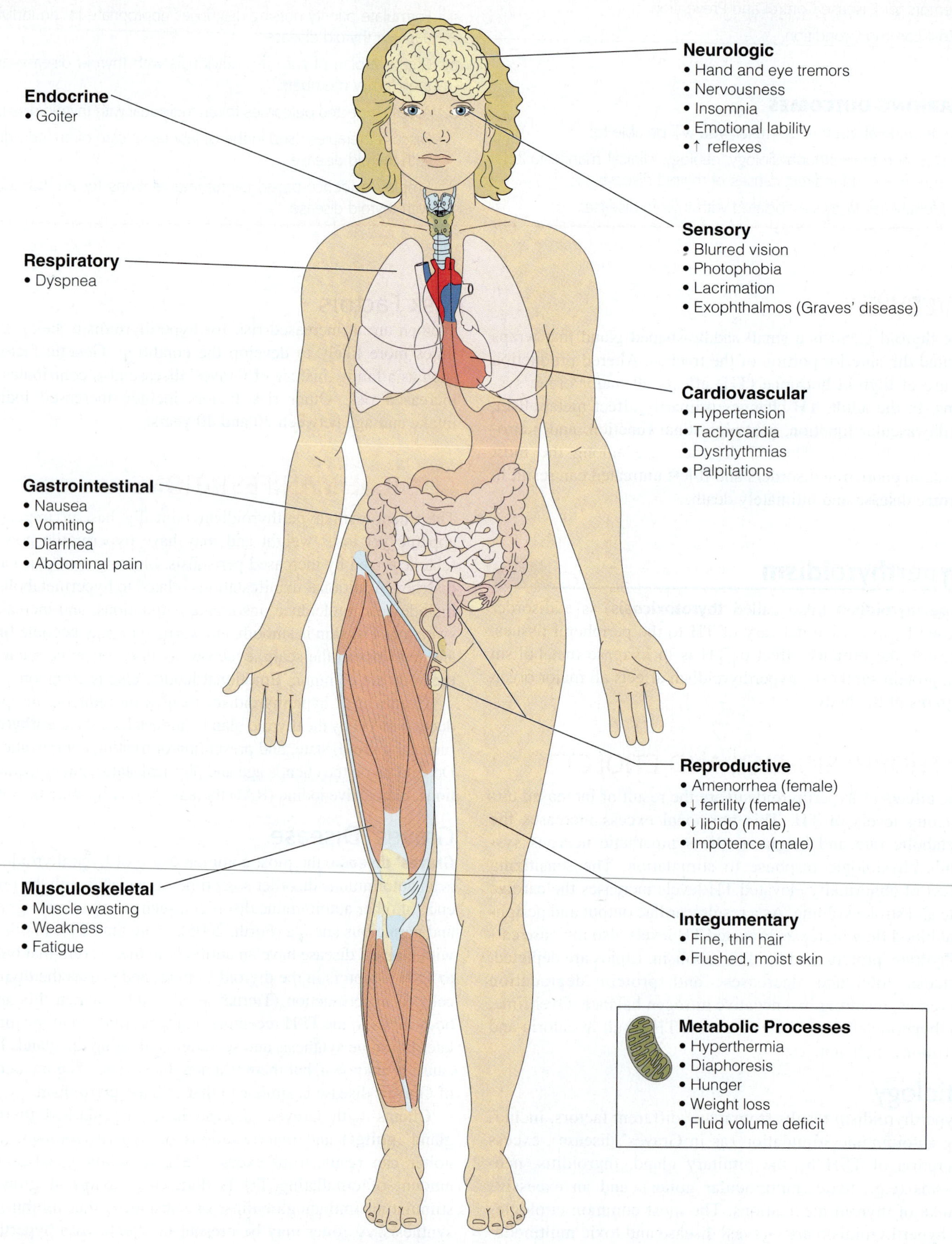

Neurologic
• Hand and eye tremors
• Nervousness
• Insomnia
• Emotional lability
• ↑ reflexes
Endocrine
• Goiter
Sensory
• Blurred vision
• Photophobia
• Lacrimation
• Exophthalmos (Graves' disease)
Respiratory
• Dyspnea
Cardiovascular
• Hypertension
• Tachycardia
• Dysrhythmias
• Palpitations
Gastrointestinal
• Nausea
• Vomiting
• Diarrhea
• Abdominal pain
Reproductive
• Amenorrhea (female)
• ↓ fertility (female)
• ↓ libido (male)
• Impotence (male)
Musculoskeletal
• Muscle wasting
• Weakness
• Fatigue
Integumentary
• Fine, thin hair
• Flushed, moist skin
Metabolic Processes
• Hyperthermia
• Diaphoresis
• Hunger
• Weight loss
• Fluid volume deficit

The ophthalmopathy (disease of the eye) of Graves' disease is manifested as proptosis and visual dysfunction. **Proptosis** (forward displacement of the eye) occurs in about one third of cases (Porth, 2005). This forward protrusion of the eyeballs (also known as **exophthalmos**) results from an accumulation of inflammation by-products in the retro-orbital tissues. Many times, the sclera is visible above the iris. The upper lids often are retracted, and the person has a characteristic unblinking stare (Figure 18–12 ■). Proptosis usually is bilateral, but it may involve only one eye. The client may experience blurred vision, diplopia, eye pain, lacrimation, and photophobia. The inability to close the eyelids completely over the protruding eyeballs increases the risk of corneal dryness, irritation, infection, and ulceration. Infiltration of the muscles that move the eye and of the optic nerve leads to paralysis and vision loss. The treatment of Graves' disease may stabilize these symptoms but generally does not reverse the changes in the eyes.

A rare, characteristic dermopathy (disease of the skin) of Graves' disease is **pretibial myxedema**, in which plaques and nodules develop bilaterally over the shins and dorsal surface of the feet. These plaques are edematous, erythematous, and sometimes, hyperpigmented. Like the ophthalmopathy, the skin changes often persist despite successful treatment of Graves' disease (Levin & Greer, 2001).

Other manifestations of Graves' disease include fatigue, difficulty sleeping, hand tremors, and changes in menstruation ranging from decreased flow to amenorrhea. Older clients may present with atrial fibrillation, angina, or congestive heart failure.

Toxic Multinodular Goiter

Toxic multinodular goiter (Figure 18–13 ■) is a tumor characterized by small, discrete, independently functioning nodules in the thyroid gland tissue that secrete excessive amounts of TH. How these nodules grow or become independent is not known, but a genetic mutation of follicle cells is suspected. Despite elevated TH levels, the resulting manifestations of hyperthyroidism develop slowly; neither ophthalmopathy nor

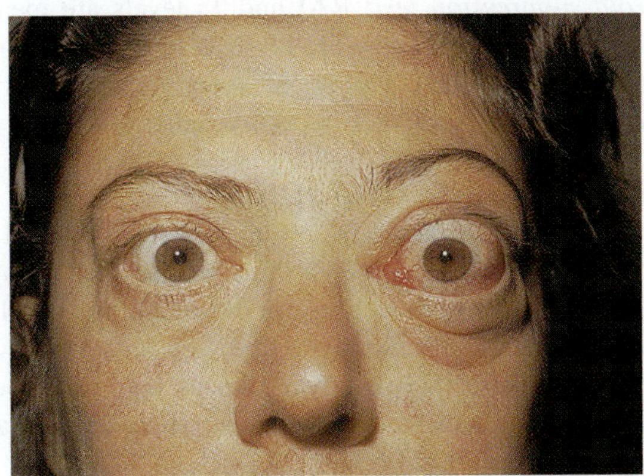

Figure 18–12 ■ Exophthalmos in a client with Graves' disease. The disease causes edema of fat deposits behind the eyes and inflammation of the extraocular muscles. The accumulating pressure forces the eyes outward from their orbits.

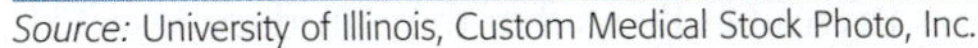

Source: University of Illinois, Custom Medical Stock Photo, Inc.

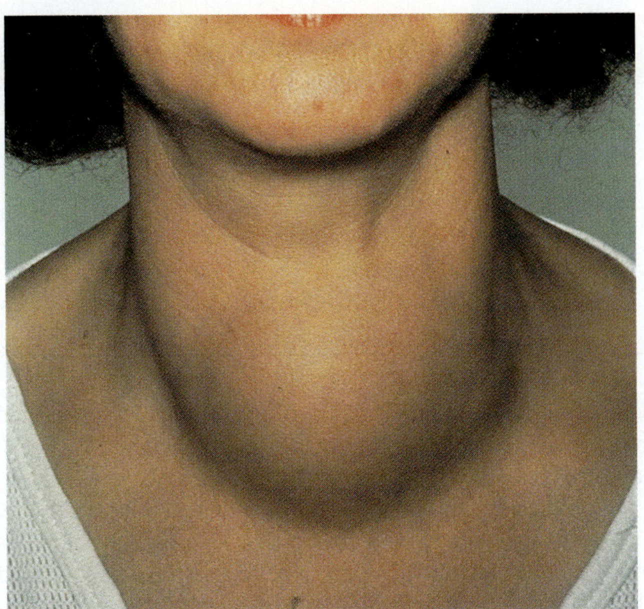

Figure 18–13 ■ Toxic multinodular goiter. The formation and growth of numerous nodules in the thyroid gland cause the characteristic massive enlargement of the neck.

Source: Custom Medical Stock Photo, Inc.

dermopathy develop (McCance & Huether, 2002). The client with this type of hyperthyroidism usually is a woman in her 60s or 70s who has had a goiter for a number of years.

Excess TSH Stimulation

Overproduction of TSH by the pituitary usually stimulates the thyroid gland to produce excess TH. The elevation in TSH secretion often results from a pituitary adenoma. This secondary form of hyperthyroidism is rare.

Thyroiditis

Thyroiditis (inflammation of the thyroid gland) most often is the result of a viral infection of the thyroid gland. The symptoms of thyroiditis are those of acute inflammation and the effects of increased TH. Thyroiditis is an acute disorder that may become chronic, resulting in a hypothyroid state as repeated infections destroy gland tissue. (See the discussion of Hashimoto's thyroiditis later in this exemplar.)

Thyroid Storm

Thyroid storm (also called **thyroid crisis**) is an extreme state of hyperthyroidism that is rare today because of improved diagnosis and treatment methods (Porth, 2005). When it does occur, those affected usually are people with untreated hyperthyroidism (most often Graves' disease) and people with hyperthyroidism who have experienced a stressor, such as an infection, trauma, untreated DKA, or manipulation of the thyroid gland during surgery. Thyroid storm is a life-threatening condition.

The rapid increase in metabolic rate that results from the excessive TH causes the manifestations of thyroid storm. These manifestations include hyperthermia, with body temperatures ranging from 102–106°F (39–41°C); tachycardia; systolic hypertension; and gastrointestinal symptoms (e.g., abdominal

CLINICAL MANIFESTATIONS AND THERAPIES **Hyperthyroidism**

ETIOLOGY	CLINICAL MANIFESTATION	CLINICAL THERAPIES
Autoimmune stimulation (as in Graves' disease) Excess secretion of thyroid-stimulating hormone by the pituitary gland Thyroiditis Neoplasms (e.g., toxic multinodular goiter) Excessive intake of thyroid medications.	■ Increased appetite accompanied by weight loss ■ Hypermotile bowels and diarrhea ■ Heat intolerance ■ Insomnia ■ Palpitations ■ Increased sweating ■ Emotional lability	■ Pharmacotherapy ■ Radioactive iodine therapy ■ Surgery (subtotal or total thyroidectomy)

pain, vomiting, and diarrhea). Agitation, restlessness, and tremors are common, progressing to confusion, psychosis, delirium, and seizures. The mortality rate is high.

Rapid treatment of thyroid storm is essential to preserve life. Treatment includes cooling without aspirin (which increases free TH) or inducing shivering; replacing fluids, glucose, and electrolytes; relieving respiratory distress; stabilizing cardiovascular function; and reducing TH synthesis and secretion.

COLLABORATION

The focus of care is aimed at preventing complications until the thyroid hormone levels can be brought into normal range. Because hyperthyroidism is generally treated by destroying all or part of the thyroid gland, thereby reducing or eliminating the production of thyroid hormone, it is important for clients to recognize the need for lifelong thyroid supplementation to replace the hormone that will no longer be produced by the thyroid gland following treatment. Clients should understand symptoms to report immediately to their provider and signs and symptoms of both hyperthyroidism and hypothyroidism.

Diagnostic Tests

Hyperthyroidism is diagnosed according to the manifestations of the specific disorders causing excessive TH and by diagnostic test results (Table 18–8). Elevated levels of TH (both T_3 and T_4) and increased RAI uptake are diagnostic criteria of hyperthyroidism.

TABLE 18–8 **Laboratory Findings in Hyperthyroidism**

TEST	NORMAL VALUES	FINDINGS
Serum TA	Negative to 1:20	Increased
Serum TSH (sensitive assay)	2–10 mU/mL (mU = microunits)	Decreased in primary hyperthyroidism
Serum T_4	512 mcg/dL (mcg = microgram)	Increased
Serum T_3	80–200 ng/dL	Increased
T_3 uptake	25–35 relative percentage	Increased
Thyroid suppression		Increased RAI uptake and T_4 levels

The following diagnostic tests may be ordered:

- *Thyroid antibodies (TA) test:* Serum TA is measured to determine whether a thyroid autoimmune disease is causing the client's symptoms. TA is elevated in Graves' disease.
- *TSH test (sensitive assay):* Serum TSH levels are measured and compared with T_4 levels to differentiate pituitary from thyroid dysfunction. The best indicator of primary hyperthyroidism (e.g., in Graves' disease) is suppression of TSH below 0.1 mcg/mL. When the sensitive TSH is not suppressed, the hyperthyroidism is caused by a TSH-secreting pituitary tumor.
- *T_4 test:* Serum T_4 levels are measured to determine TH concentration and to test thyroid gland function. T_4 levels are elevated in hyperthyroidism and in acute thyroiditis.
- *T_3 test:* Serum T_3 is measured by radioimmunoassay, which measures bound and free forms of this hormone. This test is effective for the diagnosis of hyperthyroidism. T_3 levels also may be elevated in thyroiditis.
- *T_3 uptake test:* T_3 uptake is measured by an in vitro test in which the client's blood is mixed with radioactive T_3; the results are elevated in hyperthyroidism.
- *RAI uptake test:* An RAI uptake test (thyroid scan) measures the absorption of ^{131}I or ^{123}I by the thyroid gland. A calculated dose of RAI is given orally or intravenously, and the thyroid is then scanned (often after 24 hours). The distribution of radioactivity in the gland is recorded (increased uptake of RAI is seen in Graves' disease). In addition, the scan reveals the size and shape of the gland.
- *Thyroid suppression test:* RAI and T_4 levels are measured first. The client then takes TH for 7 to 10 days, after which the tests are repeated. Failure of hormone therapy to suppress RAI and T_4 indicates hyperthyroidism.

Pharmacologic Therapies

Hyperthyroidism is treated by administering antithyroid medications that reduce TH production. Because these drugs do not affect the release or activity of hormone that is already formed, therapeutic effects may not be seen for several weeks. To rapidly decrease the cardiovascular symptoms associated with hyperthyroidism, a beta-blocker, such as propanolol (Inderal), is part of initial treatment.

Radioactive Iodine Therapy

Because the thyroid gland takes up iodine in any form, radioactive iodine (RAI or ^{131}I) concentrates in the thyroid gland and damages or destroys thyroid cells so that they produce less TH.

The RAI is given orally. Results typically occur in 6–8 weeks. In most instances, the client is not hospitalized during treatment and does not require radiation precautions. This type of therapy is contraindicated in pregnant women, because RAI crosses the placenta and can have negative effects on the developing fetal thyroid gland. Because the amount of gland destroyed by this therapy is not readily controllable, the client may become hypothyroid and require lifelong TH replacement. Adverse reactions include thyroiditis and cardiac instability caused by liberation of stored TH in the gland (Holcomb, 2006). Clients should be taught to measure their pulse rate and notify the provider if the rate exceeds 100 following therapy until released stores of TH diminish.

Surgery

Some clients with hyperthyroidism have such enlarged thyroid glands that pressure on the esophagus or trachea causes problems with breathing or swallowing. In these clients, a **thyroidectomy** (removal of all or part of the gland) is indicated. A subtotal thyroidectomy usually is performed; this procedure leaves enough of the gland in place to produce an adequate amount of TH. A total thyroidectomy is performed to treat cancer of the thyroid; the client then requires lifelong hormone replacement (Kumrow & Dahlen, 2002).

Before surgery, the client should be in as nearly a euthyroid state as possible. The client may be given antithyroid drugs to reduce hormone levels and iodine preparations to decrease the vascularity and size of the gland (which also reduces the risk of hemorrhage during and after surgery).

NURSING PROCESS

Nursing care of the client is focused on providing client education regarding disease process, treatment options, and posttreatment self care. When caring for the client with hyperthyroidism it is important to recognize the impact increased metabolism rates will have on the client's ability to concentrate on information presented by the nurse.

Assessment

The following data are collected through the health history and physical examination:

- *Health history.* Other diseases, family history of thyroid disease, when symptoms began, severity of symptoms, intake of thyroid medications, menstrual history, changes in weight, bowel elimination
- *Physical assessment.* Muscle strength, tremors, vital signs, cardiovascular and peripheral vascular systems, integument, size of thyroid, presence of bruit over thyroid, eyes and vision.

Diagnosis

For the client with hyperthyroidism, the nurse must consider the client's responses to the systemic effects of the disorder. Although each client may have different needs, the NANDA diagnoses discussed in this exemplar focus on the most common problems:

- Risk for Decreased Cardiac Output
- Disturbed Sensory Perception: Visual
- Imbalanced Nutrition: Less Than Body Requirements
- Disturbed Body Image.

Plan

Care is directed at symptom resolution, client teaching related to self-care, and appropriate treatment modalities. Potential goals may include the following:

- Client will report improvement related to manifestations.
- Client will describe situations requiring contact with the provider.
- Client will explain how to take prescribed medications.

Implementation

Hyperthyroidism is often treated on an outpatient basis so it is important that the client understand how to provide self care, symptoms to monitor for, and when to call the provider. Emphasis should be placed on teaching clients about the importance of taking medications daily and not skipping a dose due to absence of symptoms.

Risk for Decreased Cardiac Output

The client with hyperthyroidism is at risk for alterations in cardiac output. Excess TH directly affects the heart, resulting in increased heart rate and stroke volume. Increases in the metabolic demands and oxygen requirements of peripheral tissues increase the demands on the heart, and systolic hypertension, angina, arrhythmias, or cardiac failure may occur. The client often has palpitations and shortness of breath and is easily fatigued. The risk of complications is greater in clients with preexisting cardiovascular disorders.

- Monitor blood pressure, pulse rate and rhythm, respiratory rate, and breath sounds. Assess for peripheral edema, jugular vein distention, and increased activity intolerance. Higher TH level increases cardiac rate, stroke volume, and tissue demand for oxygen, causing stress on the heart. This may result in hypertension, arrhythmias, tachycardia, and congestive heart failure.
- Suggest keeping the environment as cool and free of distractions as possible. Decrease stress by explaining interventions and by teaching relaxation procedures. A physically comfortable and psychologically calm environment can reduce stimuli and stressors. Stress increases circulating catecholamines, which further increase cardiac workload.
- Encourage the client to balance periods of activity with periods of rest. Rest periods decrease energy expenditure and tissue requirements for oxygen, which decrease demands on the heart by lowering the cardiac workload.

Disturbed Sensory Perception: Visual

Visual changes that occur in clients with hyperthyroidism include difficulty in focusing, diplopia (double vision), or visual loss. If the client is unable to close the eyelids because of exophthalmos, the risk of corneal dryness with resultant infection or

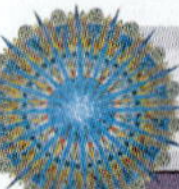

NURSING CARE PLAN **A Client With Graves' Disease**

ASSESSMENT

Mrs. Juanita Manuel is a 33-year-old mother of four small children. She is a second-year student at the local community college and is within one semester of completing the requirements for an associate degree in child care. For the past 3 months, Juanita has been constantly hungry and has eaten more than usual, but she has still lost 15 lb (6.8 kg). She has repeated bouts of diarrhea and often feels nauseated. Her hands shake, she can feel her heart beating rapidly, and she finds herself laughing or crying for no apparent reason.

Mrs. Manuel makes an appointment with her family physician. The nurse at the office completes a health history and physical assessment. When asked how she has been feeling, Mrs. Manuel replies, "Well, I don't know what's wrong with me—but I keep losing weight and I cry at the drop of a hat. I am also just so hot all the time, and I've never had that problem before. I hope I find out what's wrong and it's nothing serious."

The health history indicates that although her appetite has increased, Mrs. Manuel has lost 15 lb (6.8 kg). Mrs. Manuel states that she has had diarrhea, nausea, palpitations, heat intolerance, and mood changes. Physical assessment findings include the following: T 101°F (38.3°C), P 110, R 24, and BP 162/86. Her skin is moist and warm, and her hair is thin and fine. She has visible tremors in her hands. Her eyeballs protrude, and she is unable to close her eyelids completely. Her thyroid is enlarged and palpable. Diagnostic tests reveal the following abnormal results: T_3, 350 g/dL (normal range: 80–200 ng/dL); T_4, 15.1 mg/dL (normal range: 5–12 mg/dL). A thyroid scan demonstrates an enlarged thyroid with increased iodine uptake. After the medical diagnosis of Graves' disease is made, Mrs. Manuel is started on the antithyroid medication propylthiouracil at 150 mg orally every 8 hours.

DIAGNOSES

Nursing diagnoses that may be appropriate for Mrs. Manuel include the following:

- Risk for Imbalanced Nutrition: Less Than Body Requirements related to weight loss of 15 lb (6.8 kg), with present weight 10% less than normal for height
- Diarrhea related to increased peristalsis, as evidenced by 8–10 liquid stools per day
- Risk for Disturbed Sensory Perception: Visual related to an inability to close the eyelids completely
- Anxiety related to a lack of knowledge about disease process.

PLAN

The goals for the plan of care specify that Mrs. Manuel will:

- Gain at least 1 lb (0.45 kg) every 2 weeks
- Regain normal bowel elimination patterns
- Maintain normal vision (with no evidence of corneal damage), and verbalize measures to protect her eyes
- Verbalize medical treatment and self-care needs
- Verbalize a decrease in anxiety.

IMPLEMENTATION

The following nursing interventions may be appropriate for Mrs. Manuel:

- Request that she keep a record of daily weight.
- Discuss adopting a high-kilocalorie diet. Identify food likes and dislikes, as well as foods that increase diarrhea, before instituting a plan to increase food intake.
- Request that she keep a stool chart, noting the time, type, and precipitating factors for diarrhea stools.
- Teach comfort measures for irritated anal area (clean washcloth and soap, nonirritating ointment).
- Teach how to apply eyedrops (artificial tears).
- Explain the need to elevate the head of the bed to 45° at night and to tape eye shields over the eyes before sleep.
- Teach about Graves' disease, the medication's effects and side effects, and the need for continued medical care.

EVALUATION

By her next office visit, Mrs. Manuel has gained 1 lb (0.45 kg) and has discussed her dietary needs with the nurse and her husband. She is having diarrhea less often. She has safely applied the eyedrops and states that she uses the eye shields and elevates the head of her bed at night. The office nurse reviewed the written and verbal information about Graves' disease and the medication prescribed. Mrs. Manuel verbalizes her understanding, stating, "I'll always take my medicine—I never want to feel like that again!" She also says that she feels much less anxious now that she understands what has happened.

CRITICAL THINKING

1. What is the pathophysiologic basis for Mrs. Manuel's abnormal vital signs?
2. What is the rationale for having the client with exophthalmos elevate the head of the bed at night?
3. Outline a teaching plan that could be given to clients for home care following a subtotal thyroidectomy.

injury increases. Visual deficits also may result from pressure on the optic nerve from retro-orbital edema and shortening of the eye muscles. Although treatment of hyperthyroidism may stop the progression of eye changes, not all symptoms are reversible.

- Monitor visual acuity, photophobia, integrity of the cornea, and lid closure. The cornea is at risk for dryness, injury, conjunctivitis, and corneal infections. Injury and infection of the cornea can result in further loss of visual acuity.
- Teach measures for protecting the eye from injury and maintaining visual acuity:
  a. Use tinted glasses or shields as protection.
  b. Use artificial tears to moisten the eyes.
  c. Use cool, moist compresses to relieve irritation.
  d. Cover or tape the eyelids shut at night if they do not close.
  e. Elevate the head of the bed to 45° to promote periorbital fluid decrease.
  f. Have the client promptly report any pain or changes in vision.

These measures decrease the risk of injury, provide comfort, decrease periorbital edema that can compromise vision further, and ensure immediate care for problems, thereby minimizing the risk of further visual loss.

Imbalanced Nutrition: Less Than Body Requirements

The hypermetabolic state that occurs in hyperthyroidism causes gastrointestinal hypermotility, with nausea, vomiting, diarrhea, and abdominal pain. Although the client may have an increased appetite and eat more than usual, weight loss continues.

- Monitor nutritional status through results of laboratory tests. Serum albumin, transferrin, and total lymphocyte counts commonly are lower than normal in clients with nutritional deficits. A negative nitrogen balance signifies a catabolic state in which protein is lost and metabolic demands are not being met.
- Ask the client to check his or her weight daily (at the same time each day) and to keep a record of results. Regular monitoring detects continued weight loss, which can result from not meeting the body's metabolic demands.
- In collaboration with a dietitian, teach the client about the need for a diet high in carbohydrates and protein that includes between-meal snacks. Six small meals a day may be more desirable than three large meals. Caloric intake may need to be increased to 4,000 kcal/day if weight loss exceeds 10–17% for height and frame. Increased nutrients as part of a well-balanced diet are necessary to meet metabolic demands. Clients often are better able to increase food intake by eating frequent, small meals. A 1-lb weight gain requires approximately 3,500 extra kilocalories.

Disturbed Body Image

Physical changes that are common in hyperthyroidism include exophthalmos, goiter, tremors, hair loss, increased perspiration, loss of strength, fatigue, weight loss, and changes in reproductive and sexual function (amenorrhea in women, impotence in men, and increased libido in both men and women). In addition, the client often has mood changes and insomnia and is constantly nervous and anxious. There may even be periods of psychosis. These changes are frightening not only for the client but also for family members.

- Establish a trusting relationship, and encourage the client to verbalize feelings about self and to ask questions about the illness and treatment. Provide reliable information, and clarify misconceptions. *Establishing trust facilitates open sharing of feelings and perceptions.*

Evaluation

Expected outcomes for the client with hyperthyroidism include the following:

- Client's cardiac status will stabilize.
- Client will regain or maintain visual acuity.
- Client will take in an appropriate amount of calories per day and will exhibit no further weight loss.
- Client will communicate feelings about changes in body image and will verbalize coping mechanisms.
- Client will explain importance of daily medications and proper self-administration.

Hypothyroidism

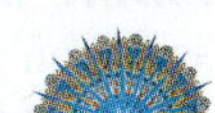

Hypothyroidism is a disorder that results when the thyroid gland produces an insufficient amount of TH.

PATHOPHYSIOLOGY AND ETIOLOGY

When TH production decreases, the thyroid gland enlarges in a compensatory attempt to produce more hormone. The goiter that results is usually a simple or nontoxic form. Older clients have a decrease in T_4 production of approximately 30%, but serum levels usually are maintained because of the age-related decrease in T_4 degradation (Weissel, 2006).

The hypothyroid state in adults is sometimes called **myxedema**. The term reflects the characteristic accumulation of nonpitting edema in the connective tissues throughout the body. The edema is the result of water retention in mucoprotein (hydrophilic proteoglycans) deposits in the interstitial spaces. The face of a client with myxedema appears puffy, the tongue is enlarged, and the voice is hoarse and husky (Porth, 2005).

Etiology

Hypothyroidism may be either primary or secondary. Primary hypothyroidism, which is more common, may be caused by congenital defects in the gland, loss of thyroid tissue following treatment of hyperthyroidism with surgery or radiation, antithyroid medications, thyroiditis, or endemic iodine deficiency. Secondary hypothyroidism may result from pituitary TSH deficiency or peripheral resistance to TH.

The cardiac drug amiodarone (Cordarone), which contains 75 mg of iodine per 200-mg tablet, is increasingly being implicated in causing thyroid problems (Porth, 2005). Clofibrate, estrogens, methadone, amiodarone, and birth control pills increase T_4 measurement; anabolic steroids, androgens, lithium, phenytoin, propanolol, interferon alpha, and interleukin-2 decrease T_4 measurement in thyroid tests. Of course, the drugs propylthiouracil and methimazole, which are used to treat hyperthyroidism, decrease T_4 measurement as well (Medline Plus, 2006).

The disorder can occur at any stage of life, but it is common in women between the ages of 30 and 60. The incidence rises after age 50. Therefore, careful evaluation of symptoms is important in the older adult, because manifestations of hypothyroidism often are thought to be the result of aging instead of a pathologic process.

Risk Factors

Anyone can develop hypothyroidism; however, it is more common among women older than 50 years, among those who have a close relative with an autoimmune condition, and among those who have had thyroid surgery, received radiation to the neck, or been treated with RAI or antithyroid medication. Other factors that result in decreased TH include iodine deficiency and Hashimoto's thyroiditis.

IODINE DEFICIENCY Iodine is necessary for synthesis and secretion of TH. Iodine deficiency may result from certain goitrogenic drugs, which block TH synthesis; lithium carbonate, which is used to treat bipolar mental disorders; and antithyroid drugs. Goitrogenic compounds in foods such as turnips, rutabagas, and soybeans also may block TH synthesis if consumed in sufficient quantities.

In areas of the world where the soil is deficient in iodine, dietary intake of iodine may be inadequate. People living in these areas are more prone to become hypothyroid and to develop simple goiter. In the United States, the use of iodized salt has reduced this risk.

HASHIMOTO'S THYROIDITIS **Hashimoto's thyroiditis** is the most common cause of goiter and primary hypothyroidism in adults and children. In this autoimmune disorder, antibodies develop that destroy thyroid tissue. Functional thyroid tissue is replaced with fibrous tissue, and TH levels decrease. In addition, decreasing levels of TH during the early stages of the disease prompt the gland to enlarge in an attempt to compensate, causing a goiter. However, as the disease progresses, the thyroid gland becomes smaller. This disorder is more common in women and has a familial link.

CLINICAL MANIFESTATIONS

Hypothyroidism has a slow onset, with manifestations occurring over months or even years. Clients with hypothyroidism characteristically have goiter, fluid retention and edema, decreased appetite, weight gain, constipation, dry skin, dyspnea, pallor, hoarseness, and muscle stiffness. Many clients have a decreased sense of taste and smell, menstrual disorders, anemias, and cardiac enlargement. The pulse typically is slow in clients with hypothyroidism, and sleep apnea is more common.

Deficient amounts of TH cause abnormalities in lipid metabolism, with elevated serum cholesterol and triglyceride levels. As a result, the client is at increased risk for atherosclerosis and cardiac disorders. Decreased renal blood flow and glomerular filtration rate reduce the kidney's ability to excrete water, which may cause hyponatremia.

Because a decrease in TH levels will lower metabolic rate and heat production, hypothyroidism affects all body systems. Treatment of the client with hypothyroidism focuses on diagnosis, prevention or treatment of complications, and replacement of the deficient TH. With early and continued treatment, the mental and physical symptoms rapidly reverse in clients of all ages, and both appearance and mental function return to normal.

MYXEDEMA COMA **Myxedema coma** is a life-threatening complication of long-standing, untreated hypothyroidism usually triggered by an acute illness or trauma (Tierney et al., 2005). It is characterized by severe metabolic disorders (e.g., hyponatremia, hypoglycemia, and lactic acidosis); hypothermia; a shallow edema, especially around the eyes, hands, and feet; cardiovascular collapse; impaired mentation; and coma. Although rare, myxedema coma most commonly occurs during the winter months in older women with chronic hypothyroidism (Porth, 2005).

Myxedema coma may be precipitated by trauma, infection, failure to take thyroid replacement medications, use of central nervous system depressants, and exposure to cold temperatures (Porth, 2005). The treatment of myxedema coma addresses the precipitating factors and manifestations and involves maintaining a patent airway; maintaining fluid, electrolyte, and acid–base balance; maintaining cardiovascular status; increasing body temperature; and increasing TH levels. If untreated, the mortality rate is high (Tierney et al., 2005).

COLLABORATION

Collaboration with the client's pharmacist will help minimize any side effects and ensure the client is not taking any medications prescribed by different doctors that are contraindicated. If the client has an existing comorbid condition, collaboration with the client's other physicians' offices may be necessary to ensure optimal care.

CLINICAL MANIFESTATIONS AND THERAPIES **Hypothyroidism**

ETIOLOGY	CLINICAL MANIFESTATION	CLINICAL THERAPIES
Decrease in TH production May be primary or secondary	Hypothermia Decreased appetite accompanied by weight gain Systemic edema	■ Pharmacotherapy ■ Subtotal throidectomy if goiter is large enough to cause respiratory difficulties or dysphagia

MULTISYSTEM EFFECTS OF **Hypothyroidism**

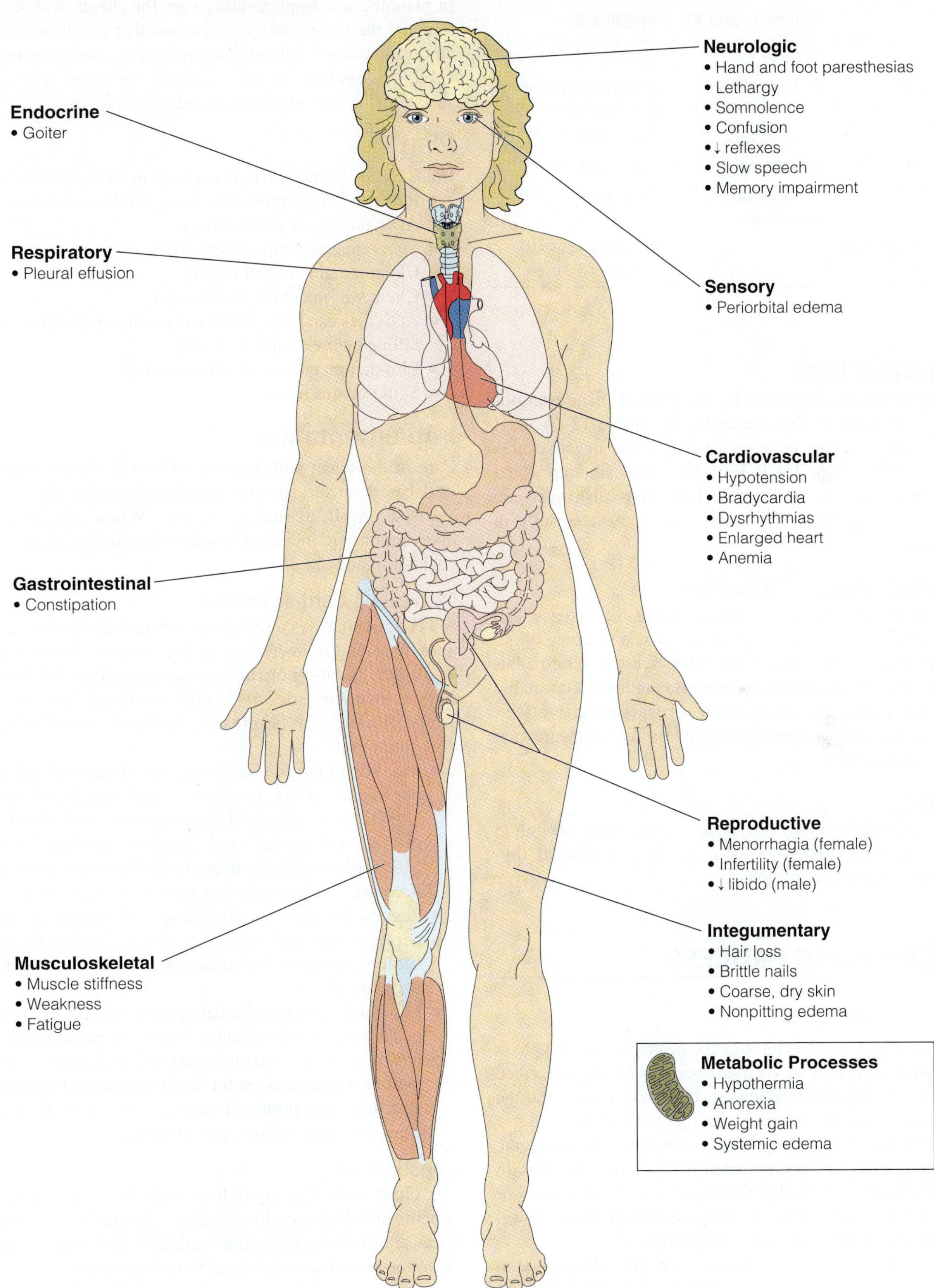
Neurologic
• Hand and foot paresthesias
• Lethargy
• Somnolence
• Confusion
• ↓ reflexes
• Slow speech
• Memory impairment
Endocrine
• Goiter
Respiratory
• Pleural effusion
Sensory
• Periorbital edema
Cardiovascular
• Hypotension
• Bradycardia
• Dysrhythmias
• Enlarged heart
• Anemia
Gastrointestinal
• Constipation
Reproductive
• Menorrhagia (female)
• Infertility (female)
• ↓ libido (male)
Integumentary
• Hair loss
• Brittle nails
• Coarse, dry skin
• Nonpitting edema
Musculoskeletal
• Muscle stiffness
• Weakness
• Fatigue
Metabolic Processes
• Hypothermia
• Anorexia
• Weight gain
• Systemic edema

TABLE 18–9 **Laboratory Findings in Hypothyroidism**

TEST	NORMAL VALUES	FINDINGS
Serum TA	None to 1:20	Normal
Serum TSH	2–10 mU/mL (mU = microunit)	Increased in primary hypothyroidism
Serum T_4	5–12 mcg/dL	Decreased
Serum T_3	80–200 ng/dL	Decreased
T_3 uptake	25–35 relative percentage	Decreased
Thyroid suppression		No change in RAI uptake or T_4 levels

Diagnostic Tests

Hypothyroidism is diagnosed by the clinical manifestations and by a decrease in TH, especially T_4 (Table 18–9). TSH concentration often is increased, because the negative hormonal feedback from TH is lost. The same laboratory and diagnostic tests used to diagnose hyperthyroidism also are used to diagnose hypothyroidism, with opposite results in most cases.

Pharmacologic Therapies

Hypothyroidism is treated with medications that replace TH. Levothyroxine (T_4) is the treatment of choice (Tierney et al., 2005). In older clients, an age-related decrease in serum albumin and renal excretion can increase the amount of available drug and cause an exaggerated pharmacologic effect. Therefore, the older client may require less thyroid medication than a younger client.

Surgery

If the client with hypothyroidism has a goiter large enough to cause respiratory difficulties or dysphagia, a subtotal thyroidectomy may be performed.

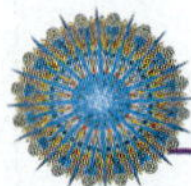

NURSING PROCESS

Assessment

Collect the following data through the health history and physical examination. Further focused assessments are described later in the Caring Interventions section. When assessing the older client, be aware of normal changes with aging.

- *Health history.* Pituitary diseases, when symptoms began, severity of symptoms, treatment of hyperthyroidism with medications or RAI, thyroid surgery, treatment of head or neck cancer with radiation, diet, use of iodized salt, bowel elimination, and respiratory difficulties
- *Physical assessment.* Muscle strength, deep tendon reflexes, vital signs, cardiovascular and peripheral vascular systems, integument, thyroid gland, and weight

Diagnosis

In planning and implementing care for clients with hypothyroidism, the nurse takes into account that the disorder affects all organ systems. Although many nursing diagnoses might be valid, this section focuses on client problems with cardiovascular function, elimination, and skin integrity.

Plan

Goals for the client with hypothyroidism include the following:

- Pulse and blood pressure remain within established limits.
- Arrhythmias are not exhibited.
- Skin remains warm and dry to touch.
- Client remains free of edema.
- Client will maintain visual acuity.
- Activities can be resumed without heart rate exceeding or falling below established limits.
- Elimination pattern returns to normal.
- Skin remains intact.

Implementation

Care of the client with hypothyroidism is always individualized based on the specific manifestations the client experiences as well as unique needs. When planning care, interventions are indicated based on the nursing diagnosis and goals of treatment.

Decreased Cardiac Output

A TH deficit causes a reduction in heart rate and stroke volume, resulting in decreased cardiac output. There also may be an accumulation of fluid in the pericardial sac (from the edema characteristic of hypothyroidism), and coronary artery disease may be present, further compromising cardiac function.

- Monitor blood pressure, rate and rhythm of apical and peripheral pulses, respiratory rate, and breath sounds. Hypotension indicatesdecreasing peripheral blood. Fluid in the pericardial sac restricts cardiac function. Monopolysaccharide deposits in the respiratory system decrease vital capacity and cause hypoventilation.
- Suggest the client avoid chilling (e.g., increase room temperature, use additional bed covers, and avoid drafts). Chilling increases metabolic rate and puts increased stress on the heart.
- Explain the need to alternate periods of activity with periods of rest. Ask the client to report any breathing difficulties, chest pain, heart palpitations, or dizziness. Activity increases demands on the heart and should be balanced with rest. Symptoms of cardiac stress include dyspnea, chest pain, palpitations, and dizziness.

Constipation

The client with hypothyroidism is likely to have a reduced appetite and decreased food intake, a diminished activity level because of muscle aches and weakness, and reduced peristalsis to the point that fecal impactions may occur.

- Encourage a fluid intake of up to 2,000 mL/day. Discuss preferred liquids and the best times of day to drink fluids.

NURSING CARE PLAN **A Client With Hypothyroidism**

ASSESSMENT

Jane Lee is a 60-year-old, retired nurse living with her husband and daughter on a farm that has been in the family for four generations. Mrs. Lee has gained 10 lb (4.5 kg) in the past few months, even though she is rarely hungry and eats much less than normal. She is always tired and weak—so tired that she has not even been able to help with the chores on the farm or do housework. She is concerned about her appearance and the way she sounds when she talks. Her face is puffy, and her tongue always feels thick. Mr. Lee convinces his wife to make an appointment at a health center in a nearby town.

Brian Henning, RN, completes the health assessment for Mrs. Lee at the health center. He finds that she now weighs 150 lb (68 kg), an increase of 10 lb (4.5 kg) over her weight at her last visit 6 months earlier. Mrs. Lee states that she always feels cold, tired, and weak. She also states that she is constipated, has difficulty remembering things, and looks different. Physical assessment findings include a palpable and bilaterally enlarged thyroid; dry, yellowish skin; nonpitting edema of the face and lower legs; and slow, slurred speech. Diagnostic tests reveal the following abnormal findings: T_3, 56 ng/dL (normal range, 80–200 ng/dL); T_4, 3.1 (normal range, 5–12 mg/dL); TSH increased. The medical diagnosis of hypothyroidism is made, and Mrs. Lee is started on levothyroxine at 0.05 mg daily.

DIAGNOSES

Nursing diagnoses that may be appropriate for Mrs. Lee include the following:

- Constipation related to decreased peristalsis, as evidenced by hard, formed stools every 4 days
- Impaired Verbal Communication related to changes in speech patterns and enlarged tongue
- Low Self-Esteem related to changes in physical appearance and activity intolerance.

PLAN

The client goals based on the plan of care for Mrs. Lee include:

- Regain normal bowel elimination patterns, having a soft, formed stool at least every other day
- Experience improvement in verbal communication
- Regain positive self-esteem as medication reduces physical changes and fatigue.

IMPLEMENTATION

The following nursing interventions may be appropriate for Mrs. Lee:

- Teach to increase fluids, bulk, and fiber in the diet to help regain a normal bowel elimination pattern of a soft, formed stool every other day.
- Take medication as prescribed and do not expect immediate reversal of symptoms affecting speech.
- Plan activities around rest periods. Encourage husband and daughter to help with housecleaning and cooking.

EVALUATION

On return to the health center 2 months later, Mrs. Lee reports that she is no longer constipated but is continuing to drink six glasses of water and eating oatmeal every day. She no longer feels cold, is regaining her normal energy, and even feels well enough to plant her garden. Her speech is clear and easy to understand. As she leaves the examining room, Mrs. Lee says, "It's hard to believe that I have changed so much—now I look and feel like the 'old' me!"

CRITICAL THINKING

1. What physical changes that normally occur with aging are similar to the manifestations of hypothyroidism?
2. Describe the factors that put Mrs. Lee's safety at risk. What alterations in her home environment would you suggest to promote safety until the prescribed medication takes effect?
3. The client taking oral thyroid medications may become hyperthyroid. List the manifestations you would include in a teaching plan to signal this condition.

If kilocalorie intake is restricted, ensure that liquids have no kilocalories or are low in kilocalories. *Sufficient fluid intake is necessary to promote proper stool consistency.*

- Discuss ways to maintain a high-fiber diet. *Diets high in fiber and fluid produce soft stools. Fiber that is not digested absorbs water, which adds bulk to the stool and assists in the movement of fecal material through the intestines.*
- Encourage activity as tolerated. *Activity influences bowel elimination by improving muscle tone and stimulating peristalsis.*

PRACTICE ALERT

High-fiber foods include beans, potatoes, fruits, breads, cereal, crackers, popcorn, and rice.

Risk for Impaired Skin Integrity

The client with hypothyroidism is at risk for impaired skin integrity related to the accumulation of fluid in the interstitial spaces and to dry, rough skin. Decreased peripheral circulation, decreased activity levels, and slow wound healing further

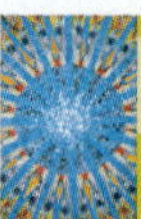

DEVELOPMENTAL CONSIDERATIONS
Hypothyroidism

NORMAL CHANGES WITH AGING

- The thyroid gland undergoes some degree of atrophy, fibrosis, and nodularity.
- Hair growth decreases.
- Nails are often thick, brittle, and yellow.
- Facial skin sags, and bones become more prominent.
- Deep tendon reflexes decrease.
- Response to questions may be slower.

increase the risk. The following interventions are for the older client who is hospitalized for surgery or severe hypothyroidism.

- Monitor skin surfaces for redness or lesions, especially if the client's activity is greatly reduced. Use a pressure ulcer risk assessment scale to identify clients at risk. Hypothyroidism causes dry, rough, edematous skin conditions that increase the risk of skin breakdown.
- Provide or teach the immobile client measures to promote optimal circulation:
  a. Use a turning schedule if the client is on bedrest, or teach the client to change position every 2 hours.
  b. Limit the time for sitting in one position; shift weight or lift the body using arm rests every 20–30 minutes.
  c. Use pillows, pads, or sheepskin or foam cushions for bed and/or chair.

  Prolonged pressure, especially in clients with edema and circulatory impairment, can occlude capillaries and cause hypoxic tissue damage.
- Teach and implement a schedule of range-of-motion exercises.
- Provide or teach the client measures to maintain skin integrity:
  a. Take baths only as necessary; use warm (not hot) water.
  b. Use gentle motions when washing and drying skin.
  c. Use alcohol-free skin oils and lotions.

  Dry skin and edema increase the risk of skin breakdown. Hot water, rough massage, and alcohol-based preparations may increase skin dryness, further impairing the body's ability to maintain skin integrity.

PRACTICE ALERT

Lift the client up in bed to prevent tissue damage from shearing forces.

Evaluation

Evaluation involves determining if the client has met expected outcomes and, in the event that outcomes have not been met, modifying outcomes or making changes to the nursing care plan. Any diagnostic tests should be repeated to ensure that medications are at appropriate levels.

REVIEW Thyroid Disease

RELATE: LINK THE CONCEPTS

Linking the exemplar of Thyroid Disease with the concept of Mood and Affect:

1. What strategies might you employ when teaching a client diagnosed with hypothyroidism and disturbed body image?
2. What impact might hypothyroidism have on the client's mood and affect and how would this alter the nursing plan of care?

Linking the exemplar of Thyroid Disease with the concept of Stress and Coping:

3. What stressors would you assess the client diagnosed with hypothyroidism for?
4. The time between initial diagnosis of hyperthyroidism and symptom relief may be several weeks to months as additional diagnostic testing is performed and treatments are decided upon. What might you teach the client to help him or her cope with the symptoms of hyperthyroidism?

READY: GO TO COMPANION SKILLS MANUAL

- Assessing body temperature
- Assessing the skin
- Assessing blood pressure
- Assessing the heart rate
- Moving a client up in bed
- Performing range-of-motion exercises

REFER: GO TO MYNURSINGKIT

REFLECT: CASE STUDY

Judy Smith is a 55-year-old female who has recently returned to the United States after a lengthy missionary assignment in South Africa. Judy arrives at the provider's office today requesting a "head to toe" physical examination, including a Pap smear and mammogram. Judy has been reassigned to serve in the Fiji Islands, where health care is scarce, so she would like a full workup. Vital signs: BP 134/92, P 112, R 22, T 99; weight: 101 lb; height: 5 ft 2 in.; overall physical appearance: thin, older woman who looks older than stated age, with wispy gray hair in matted bun. You note that Judy has a visible goiter, and as you question her about it, she says, "Oh, I've had that for a long time; my mother had one too." She states that she has been going through "the change of life" (for the past 5 years) and is having frequent hot flashes. She has lost 10 lb over the past few years from what she describes as "self-imposed caution" when eating in Third World countries.

As she is talking, you note she has slight tremors as she pushes her hair from her eyes. Her face is flushed, and she is fanning herself throughout the interview. She is anxious and fidgits a lot. Her hair is thin and shiny, and her goiter is palpable, which has caused an enlargement of her neck. She denies sleep apnea but states she snores.

1. What focused health history would be appropriate to elicit from Judy?
2. What physical assessment will you perform to obtain a complete picture of Judy's status?
3. Based on physical assessment, what nursing diagnosis best describes Judy's health?

PEARSON

EXPLORE mynursingkit™

MyNursingKit is your one stop for online chapter review materials and resources. Prepare for success with additional NCLEX®-style practice questions, interactive assignments and activities, web links, animations and videos, and more!

Register your access code from the front of your book at **www.mynursingkit.com**.

REFERENCES

American College of Rheumatology. (2004). *Glucocorticoid-induced osteoporosis.* Retrieved from http://www.rheumatology.org/public/factsheets/gi_osteopor_new.asp?aud=mem

American Diabetes Association. (2002). Evidence-based nutrition principles and recommendations for the treatment and prevention of diabetes and related complications. *Diabetes Care, 25,* 202–212.

American Diabetes Association. (2005). Standards of medical care in diabetes. *Diabetes Care, 28* (S1), S4–S36.

American Diabetes Association. (2006). Diagnosis and classification of diabetes mellitus. *Diabetes Care, 29* (S1), S43–S48.

Amiel, S. A., & Alberti, K. G. (2005). Diabetes and surgery. In S. Inzucchi, D. Porte, R. S. Sherwin, & A. Baron (Eds.), *The diabetes mellitus manual: A primary care companion to Ellenberg & Rifkin's* (6th ed., pp. 231–242). New York: McGraw-Hill.

Aragon, D., Ring, C.A., & Covelli, M. (2003). The influence of diabetes mellitus on postoperative infections. *Critical Care Nursing Clinics of North America, 15,* 125–135.

Capriotti, T. (2005). Type 2 diabetes epidemic increases use of oral antidiabetic agents. *MEDSURG Nursing, 14* (5), 341–347.

Carroll, K. L. (2006). Alterations of musculoskeletal function in children. In K.L. McCance & S. E. Huether (Eds.), *Pathophysiology: The biologic basis for disease in adults and children* (5th ed., pp. 1547–1571). St. Louis, MO: Elsevier Mosby.

Centers for Disease Control and Prevention. (2005). National Diabetes Fact Sheet. Retrieved from http://www.cdc.gov/diabetes/pubs/factsheet05.htm

Clement, S., Braithwaite, S. S., Magee, M. F., Ahmann, A., Smith, E. P., Schafer, R. G., & Hirsch, I. R., on behalf of the diabetes in hospitals writing committee. (2004). Management of diabetes and hyperglycemia in hospitals. *Diabetes Care, 27,* 553–591.

Cummings, J., Mineo, K., Levy, R., & Josephson, R. (1999). A review of the DIGAMI Study: Intensive insulin therapy during and after myocardial infarctions in diabetic patients. *Diabetes Spectrum, 12*(2), 84–88.

Eliopoulos, C. (2005). *Gerontological nursing* (6th ed.). Philadelphia: Lippincott Williams & Wilkins.

Funnell, M. M., Kruger, D. F., & Spencer, M. (2004). Self-management support for insulin therapy in type 2 diabetes. *The Diabetes Educator, 30*(2), 274–280.

Grimberg, A., & De León, D. D. (2005). Disorders of growth. In T.M. Moshange (Ed.), *Pediatric endocrinology: The requisites for pediatrics* (pp. 127–167). St. Louis, MO: Elsevier Mosby.

Guthrie, D., & Guthrie, R. (1997). *Nursing management of diabetes mellitus* (4th ed.). New York: Springer.

Haire-Joshu, D. (Ed.). (1996). *Management of diabetes mellitus: Perspectives of care across the life span* (2nd ed.). St. Louis, MO: Mosby.

Harper-Jacques, S. (2004). Diabetes and depression: Addressing the depression can improve glycemic control. *American Journal of Nursing, 104* (9), 56–59.

Holcomb, S .S. (2006). Do the clues add up to Addison's disease? *Nursing, 36*(3), 64hn1-64hn4.

Kasper, D. L., Braunwald, E., Fauci, A. S., Hauser, S. L., Longo, D. L., & Jameson, J. L. (Eds.). (2005). *Harrison's principles of internal medicine* (16th ed.). New York: McGraw-Hill.

Kumrow, D., & Dahlen, R. (2002). Thyroidectomy: Understanding the potential for complications. *MEDSURG Nursing, 11*(5), 228-235.

Larsen, P. R., Kronenberg, H. M., Melmed, S., & Polonsky, K. S. (2003). *Williams textbook of endocrinology* (10th ed.). Philadelphia: Saunders.

Lee, P. A., & Kulin, H. E. (2005). Normal pubertal development. In T. M. Moshange (Ed.), *Pediatric endocrinology: The requisites for pediatrics* (pp. 63–71). St. Louis, MO: Elsevier Mosby.

Lehne, R. A. (2004). *Pharmacology for nursing care* (4th ed.). St. Louis, MO: Saunders/Elsevier.

Levin, N. A., & Greer, K. E. (2001). Cutaneous manifestations of endocrine disorders. *Dermatology Nursing, 13* (3), 185–196.

Mabrey, M. E. (2004). Using insulin to prevent hyperglycemia in surgical patients. *Nursing, 34*(10), 22.

Malmberg, K., Ryden, L., Hamsten, A., Herlitz, J., Waldenstrom, A., Wedel, H., et al. (1995). Randomized trial of insulin-glucose infusion followed by subcutaneous insulin treatment in diabetic patients with acute myocardial infarction (DIGAMI study): Effects on mortality at 1 year. *Journal of the American College of Cardiology, 26,* 56–65.

Magee, M. (2006). Insulin therapy for intensive glycemic control in hospital patients. *Hospital Physician, 42*(4), 17–27, 38.

Mann, R. E., Smart, R. G., & Govoni, R. (2003). The epidemiology of alcoholic liver disease. *Alcohol Research & Health, 27* (3), 209–219.

Mayo Clinic. (2002). *Osteoporosis.* Retrieved from http://www.mayoclinic.com/invoke.cfm?id=DS00128

McCance, K., & Huether, S. (2002). *Pathophysiology: The biologic basis for disease in adults and children* (4th ed.). St. Louis, MO: Mosby.

Medline Plus. (2006). T_4 tests. U.S. National Library of Medicine and the National Institutes of Health. Retrieved March 22, 2006, from http://www.nlm.nih.gov/medlineplus/ency/article/003517.htm

Medtronic MiniMed, Inc. (2006). MiniMed Paradigm® REAL-Time Insulin Pump and Continuous Glucose Monitoring System. Retrieved April 24, 2006, from http://www. minimed.com/products/insulinpumps/realtime/index.html

National Center for Health Statistics. (2005). *Health, United States, 2005, with chartbook on trends in the health of Americans.* Hyattsville, MD: Author.

National Heart, Lung, and Blood Institute. (1998). *Clinical guidelines on the identification, evaluation, and treatment of overweight and obesity in adults: The evidence report.* National Institutes of Health: Publication No. 98-4083. Retrieved from http://www.nhlbi.nih.gov

National Heart, Lung, and Blood Institute. (2000). *The practical guide. Identification, evaluation, and treatment of overweight and obesity in adults.* National Institutes of Health Publication No. 00-4084. Retrieved from http://www.nhlbi.nih.gov

National Institutes of Health. (2004). *Diabetes statistics in the United States.* Retrieved from http://diabetes.niddk.nih.gov/dm/pubs/statistics/

National Osteoporosis Foundation. (2006). *Fast facts on osteoporosis.* Retrieved from http://www.nof.org/osteoporosis/diseasefacts.htm

Porth, C. (2005). *Pathophysiology: Concepts of altered health states* (7th ed.). Philadelphia: Lippincott.

Roberts, C. K., & Barnard, R. J. (2005). Effects of exercise and diet on chronic disease. *Journal of Applied Physiology, 98,* 3–30.

Saudek, C. D., & Margolis, S. (2005). *Diabetes. The Johns Hopkins White Papers.* Baltimore, MD: Johns Hopkins Medicine.

Sheard, N. F., Clark, N. G., Brand-Miller, J. C., Franz, M. J., Pi-Sunyer, F. X., Mayer-Davis, E., et al. (2004). Dietary carbohydrate (amount and type) in the prevention and management of diabetes: ADA statement. *Diabetes Care, 27,* 2266–2271.

Sigal, R. J., Kenny, G. P., Wasserman, D. H., & Castaneda-Sceppa, C. (2004). Physical activity/exercise and type 2 diabetes. *Diabetes Care, 27,* 2518–2539.

Tierney, L. M., McPhee, S. J., & Papadakis, M. A. (Eds.). (2005). *Current medical diagnosis & treatment* (44th ed.). New York: Lange Medical Books/McGraw-Hill.

U.S. Food and Drug Administration. (2005). *Diabetes information: Glucose meters and diabetes management.* Retrieved April 24, 2006, from http://www.fda.gov/diabetes/glucose.html#8

Uphold, C. R., & Graham, M. V. (2003). *Clinical guidelines in adult health* (3rd ed.). Gainesville, FL: Barmarrae Books.

Van den Berghe, G., Wilmer, A., Hermans, G., Meersseman, W., Wouters, P. J., Milants, I., Van Wijngaerden, E., Bobbaers, H., & Bouillon, R. (2006). Intensive insulin therapy in the medical ICU. *The New England Journal of Medicine, 354*(5), 449–461.

Weight-Control Information Network. (2003b). *Very-low-calorie diets.* National Institutes of Health Publication No. 03-3894. Bethesda, MD: National Institutes of Health.

Weight-Control Information Network. (2004). *Gastrointestinal surgery for severe obesity.* National Institutes of Health Publication No. 04-4006. Bethesda, MD: National Institutes of Health.

Weissel, M. (2006). Disturbances of thyroid function in the elderly. *The Middle European Journal of Medicine, 118* (1–2), 16–20.

Williams, J. W., Katon, W., Lin, E., Nöel, P., Worchel, J., Cornell, J., et al. (2004). The effectiveness of depression care management on diabetes-related outcomes in older patients. *Annals of Internal Medicine, 140* (12), 1015–1024.

Yared, Z., Aljaberi, K., Renouf, N., & Yale, J. (2005). The effect of blood sample volume on 11 glucose monitoring systems. *Diabetes Care, 28,* 1836–1837.

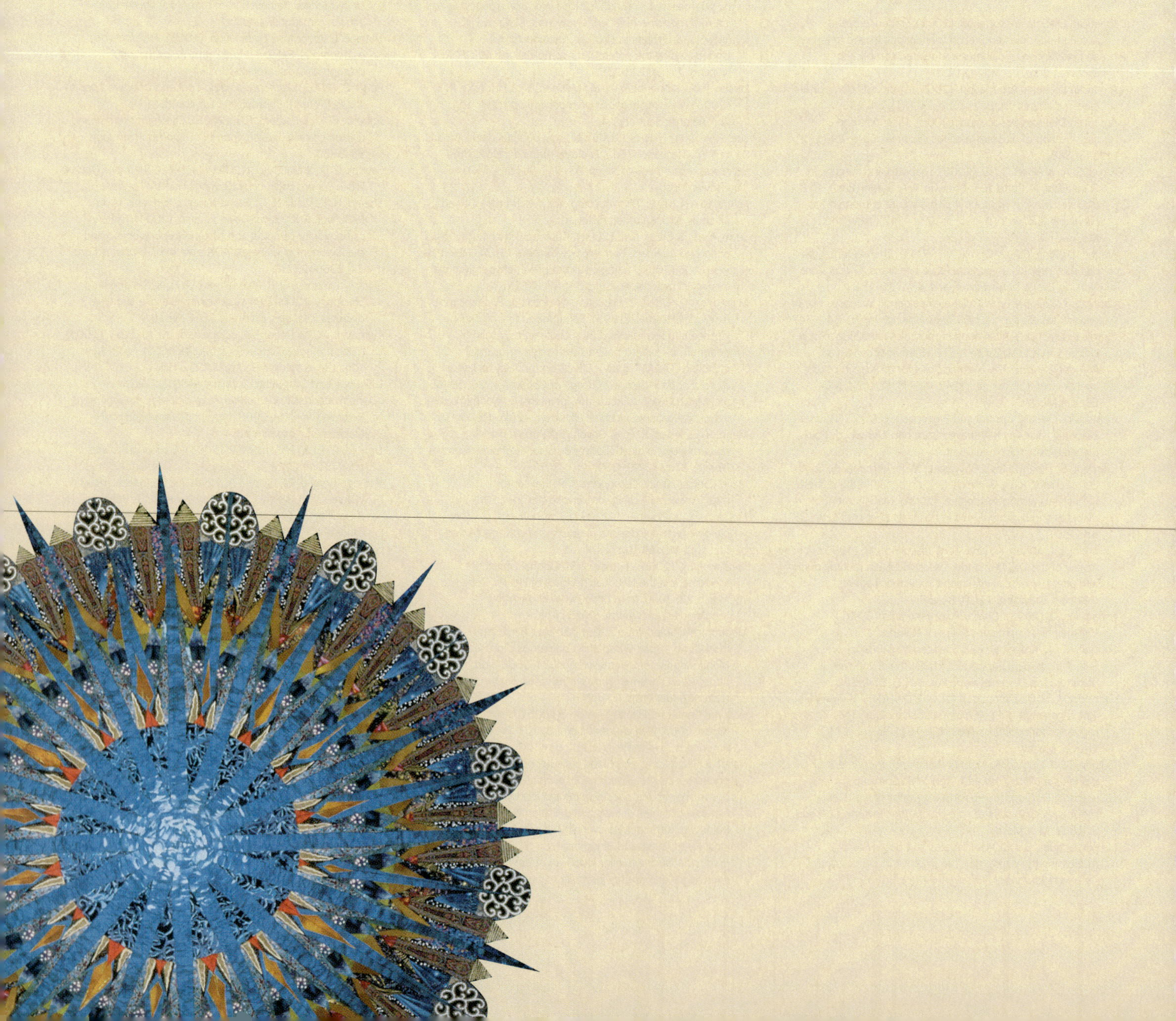

Mobility 19

Concept at-a-Glance

Concept Learning Outcomes

After reading about this concept, you will be able to:

1. Summarize the structure and physiologic processes of the musculoskeletal system related to mobility.
2. List factors affecting mobility.
3. Identify commonly occurring alterations in mobility and their related treatments.
4. Explain common physical assessment procedures used to examine musculoskeletal health of clients across the life span.
5. Outline diagnostic and laboratory tests to determine the individual's mobility status.
6. Explain management of musculoskeletal health and prevention of mobility-related illness.
7. Demonstrate the nursing process in providing culturally competent and caring interventions across the life span for individuals with common alterations in mobility.
8. Identify pharmacologic interventions in caring for the individual with alterations in mobility.

Concept Key Terms

Activities of daily living (ADLs), *1067*
Atrophy, *1061*
Bradykinesia, *1066*
Crepitation, *1071*
Fracture, *1066*
Gout, *1067*
Hematopoiesis, *1056*
Hip fracture, *1066*
Multiple sclerosis, *1066*
Ossification, *1058*
Osteoarthritis, *1066*
Osteoblasts, *1056*
Osteoclasts, *1056*
Osteocytes, *1056*
Parkinson's disease, *1066*
Parkinsonism, *1066*
Range of motion (ROM), *1065*
Sarcopenia, *1063*
Scoliosis, *1065*
Sprain, *1063*
Synovitis, *1073*
Temporomandibular joint (TMJ) syndrome, *1066*
Tendonitis, *1073*

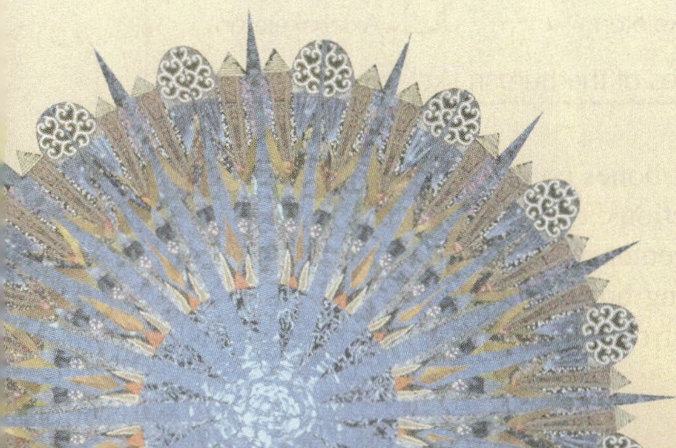

About Mobility

The tissues and structures of the musculoskeletal system perform many functions, including support, protection, and movement. The musculoskeletal system has two subsystems: the bones and joints of the skeleton and the skeletal muscles. These subsystems work together to allow the body to perform both gross simple movements such as closing a door, and fine complex movements such as repairing a watch.

While the musculoskeletal system is primarily responsible for movement, the importance of the other body systems should also be considered. The neurologic system controls the movements of these subsystems. At a cellular level, movement of electrolytes in and out of cells creates the electrical activity required to make muscles contract. Perfusion of oxygen-rich blood to the muscles and bones is required to maintain tissue integrity.

An alteration of mobility can have severe consequences for the client experiencing impairment. Regardless of the etiology—injury, infection, neurologic or cellular dysfunction—an impairment in mobility can affect the client's activities of daily living, ability to communicate with others, and ability to participate in a range of recreational and occupational activities. Impairments in mobility can also cause embarrassment, frustration, and pain. •

NORMAL PRESENTATION

The musculoskeletal system is composed of the bones of the skeletal system; the ligaments, tendons, and muscles of the muscular system; and the joints. The bones serve as the framework for the body and for the attachment of muscles, tendons, and ligaments. Innervated by the nervous system, contraction and relaxation of muscles permit movement at joints.

The Skeleton

Bones form the body's structure and provide support for soft tissues. They also protect vital organs from injury and serve to move body parts by providing points of attachment for muscles. Bones also store minerals and serve as a site for **hematopoiesis** (blood cell formation).

The human skeleton is made up of 206 bones (Figure 19–1 ■). Bones of the skeletal system are divided into the axial skeleton and the appendicular skeleton. The axial skeleton includes the bones of the skull, the ribs and sternum, and the vertebral column. The appendicular skeleton consists of all bones of the limbs, the shoulder girdles, and the pelvic girdle.

BONE STRUCTURE Bone cells include **osteoblasts** (cells that form bone), **osteocytes** (cells that maintain bone matrix), and **osteoclasts** (cells that resorb bone). Bone matrix is the extracellular element of bone tissue; it consists of collagen fibers, minerals (primarily calcium and phosphate), proteins, carbohydrates, and ground substance. Ground substance is a gelatinous material that facilitates diffusion of nutrients, wastes, and gases between the blood vessels and bone tissue. Bones are covered with periosteum, a double-layered connective tissue. The outer layer of the periosteum contains blood vessels and nerves; the inner layer is anchored to the bone.

Bones consist of a rigid connective tissue called osseous tissue, of which there are two types: Compact bone, which is smooth and dense; spongy bone, which contains spaces between meshworks of bone. Both types contain the same elements and are found in almost all bones of the body.

The basic structural unit of compact bone is the Haversian system (also called an osteon). The Haversian system consists of a central canal, called the Haversian canal; concentric layers of bone matrix, called lamellae; spaces between the lamellae, called lacunae; osteocytes within the lacunae; and small channels called canaliculi (Figure 19–2 ■).

Spongy bone has no Haversian systems. Instead, the lamellae are arranged in concentric layers called trabeculae that branch and join to form meshworks. The spongy sections of long bones and flat bones contain tissue for hematopoiesis. In the adult, these sections, called red marrow cavities, are present in the spongy center of flat bones (especially the sternum) and in only two long bones: the humerus and the head of the femur. This red marrow is active in hematopoiesis in adults.

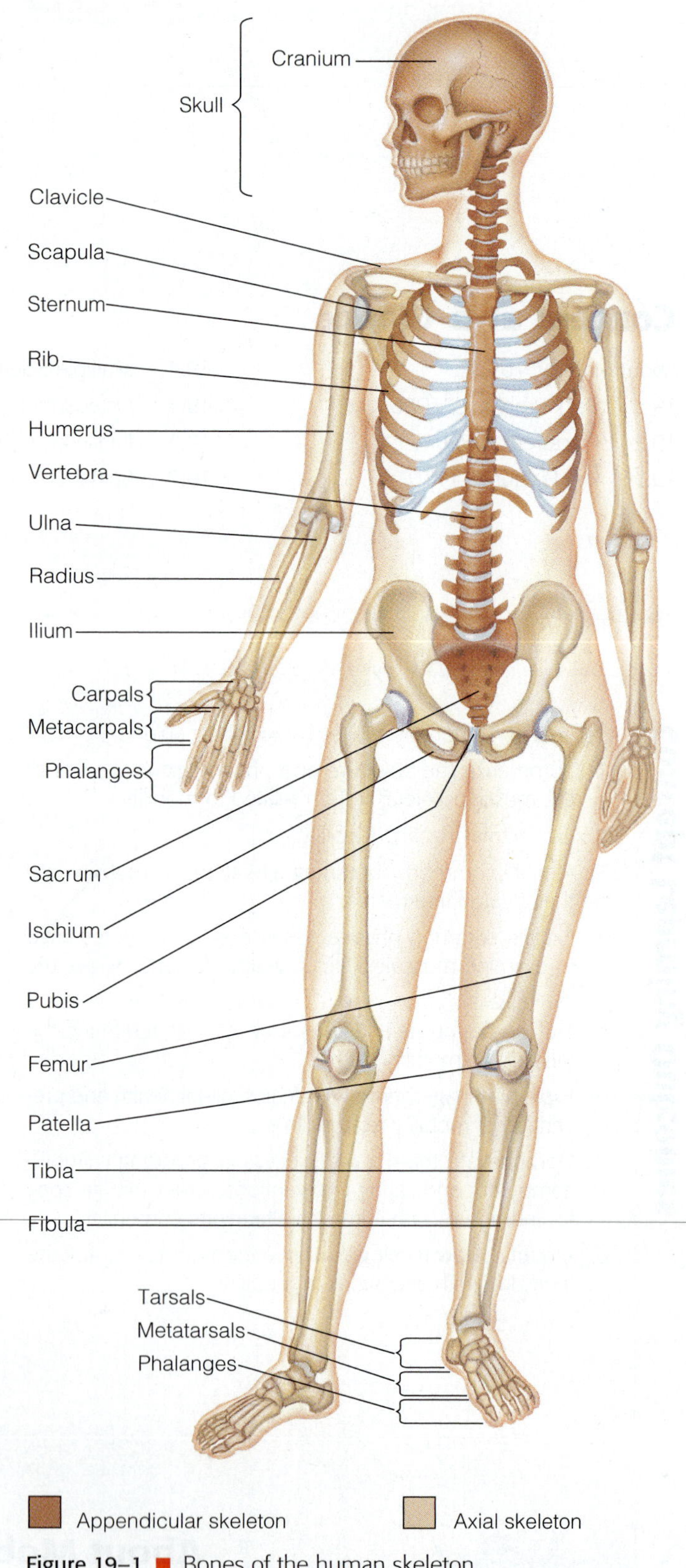

Figure 19–1 ■ Bones of the human skeleton.

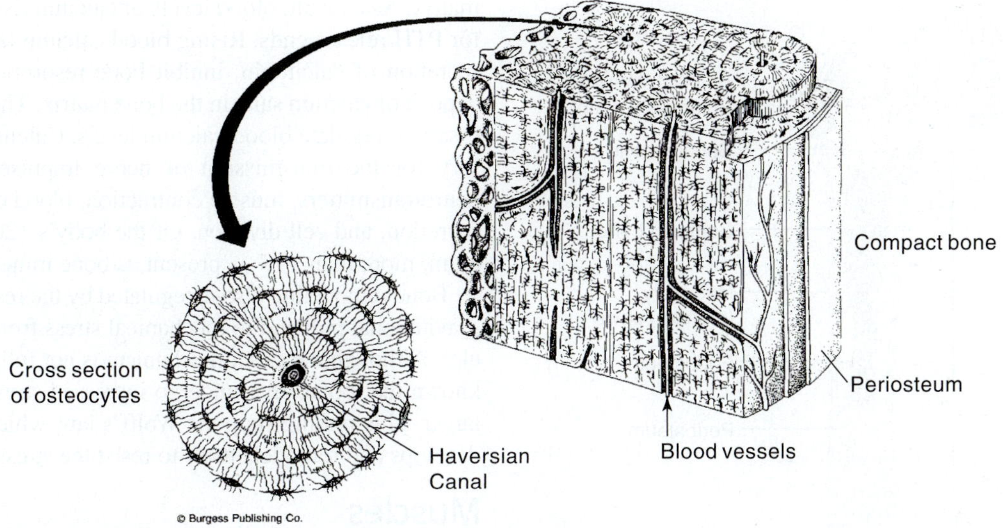

Figure 19–2 ■ The microscopic structure (Haversian system) of compact bone.

BONE SHAPES Bones are classified by shape (Figure 19–3 ■), as follows:

- *Long bones* are longer than they are wide. They have a midportion, or shaft, called a diaphysis and two broad ends, called epiphyses (Figure 19–4 ■). The diaphysis is compact bone that contains the marrow cavity, which is lined with endosteum. Each epiphysis is spongy bone covered by a thin layer of compact bone. Long bones include the bones of the arms, legs, fingers, and toes.

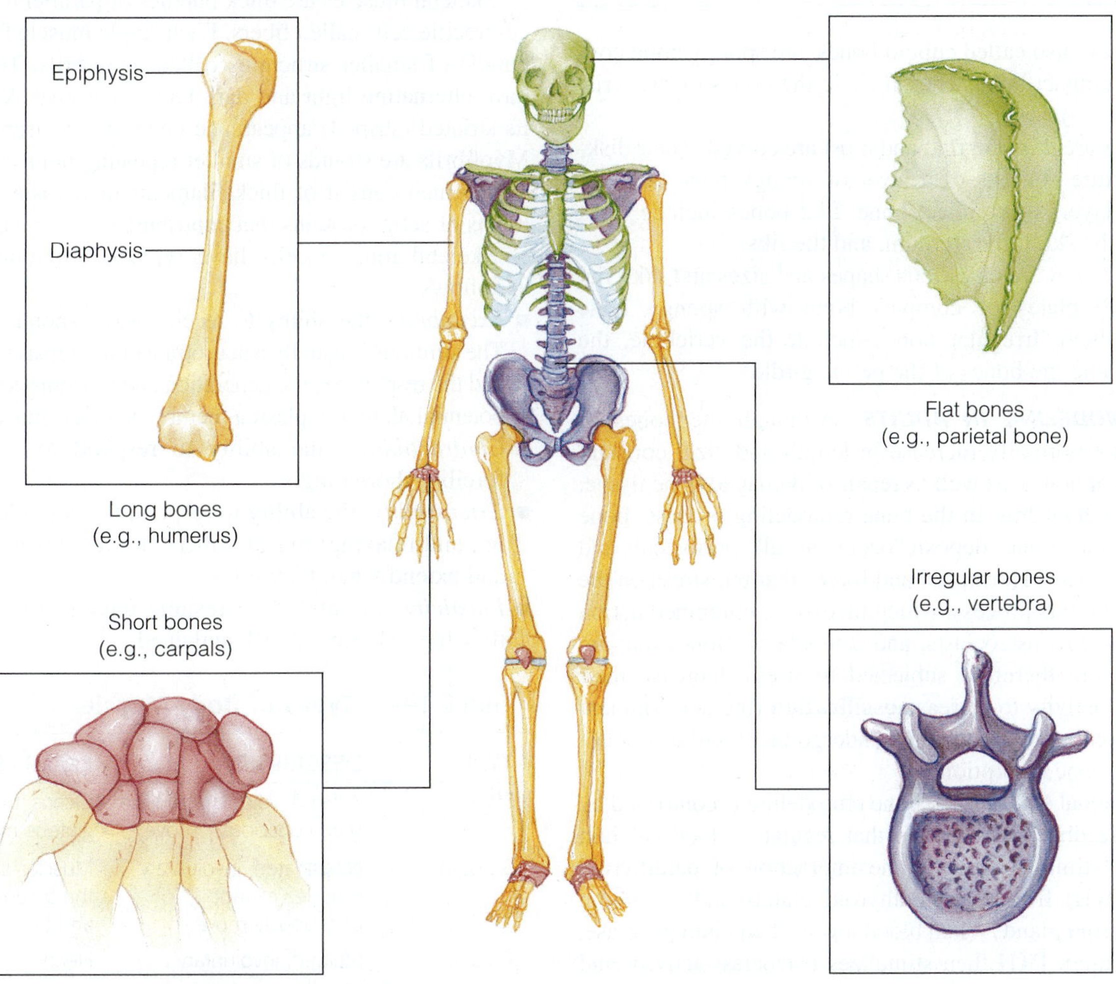

Figure 19–3 ■ Classification of bones according to shape.

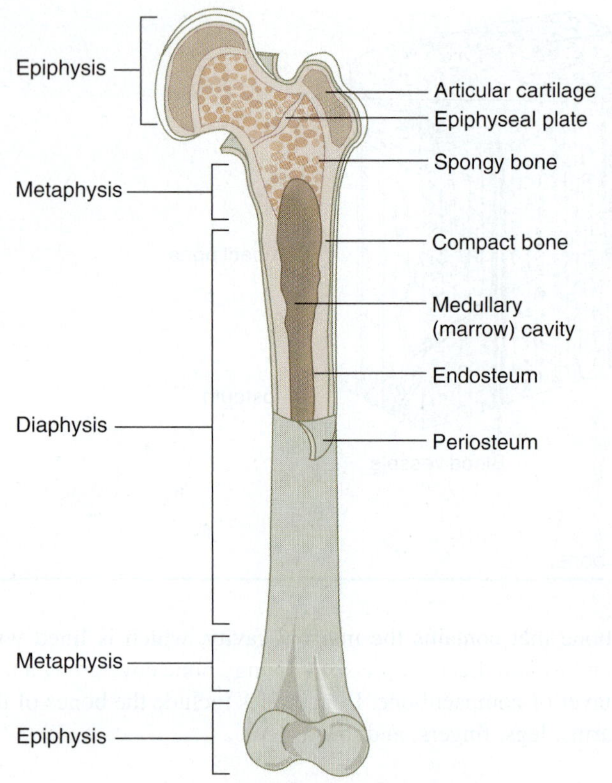

Figure 19–4 ■ Parts of a long bone.

- *Short bones,* also called cuboid bones, are spongy bone covered by compact bone. They include the bones of the wrist and ankle.
- *Flat bones* are thin and flat, and most are curved. Their disk-like structure consists of a layer of spongy bone between two thin layers of compact bone. Flat bones include most bones of the skull, the sternum, and the ribs.
- *Irregular bones* are of various shapes and sizes and, like flat bones, are plates of compact bone with spongy bone between them. Irregular bones include the vertebrae, the scapulae, and the bones of the pelvic girdle.

BONE REMODELING IN ADULTS Although the bones of adults do not normally increase in length and size, constant remodeling of bones, as well as repair of damaged bone tissue, occurs throughout life. In the bone remodeling process, bone resorption and bone deposit occur at all periosteal and endosteal surfaces. Hormones and forces that put stress on the bones regulate this process, which involves a combined action of the osteocytes, osteoclasts, and osteoblasts. Bones that are in use, and are therefore subjected to stress, increase their osteoblastic activity to increase **ossification** (the development of bone). Bones that are inactive undergo increased osteoclast activity and bone resorption.

The hormonal stimulus for bone remodeling is controlled by a negative feedback mechanism that regulates blood calcium levels. This stimulus involves the interaction of parathyroid hormone (PTH) from the parathyroid glands and calcitonin from the thyroid gland. When blood levels of calcium decrease, PTH is released; PTH then stimulates osteoclast activity and bone resorption so that calcium is released from the bone matrix. As a result, blood levels of calcium rise and the stimulus for PTH release ends. Rising blood calcium levels stimulate the secretion of calcitonin, inhibit bone resorption, and cause the deposit of calcium salts in the bone matrix. Thus, bones are necessary to regulate blood calcium levels. Calcium ions are necessary for the transmission of nerve impulses, the release of neurotransmitters, muscle contraction, blood clotting, glandular secretion, and cell division. Of the body's 1200–1400 g of calcium, more than 99% is present as bone minerals.

Bone remodeling also is regulated by the response of bones to gravitational pull and to mechanical stress from the pull of muscles. Although the exact mechanism is not fully understood, it is known that bones that undergo increased stress are heavier and larger. This finding supports Wolff's law, which states that bone develops and remodels itself to resist the stresses placed on it.

Muscles

The three types of muscle tissue in the body are skeletal muscle, smooth muscle, and cardiac muscle (Table 19–1). This discussion focuses on skeletal muscle, the only muscle that allows musculoskeletal function. Skeletal muscles attach to and cover the bones of the skeleton. Skeletal muscles promote body movement, help maintain posture, and produce body heat. They may be moved by conscious, voluntary control or by reflex activity. The body has approximately 600 skeletal muscles (Figure 19–5 ■).

Skeletal muscles are thick bundles of parallel multinucleated contractile cells called fibers. Each single muscle fiber is itself a bundle of smaller structures called myofibrils. The myofibrils have alternating light and dark bands that give skeletal muscle its striated (striped) appearance under an electron microscope. Myofibrils are strands of smaller repeating units called sarcomeres, which consist of thick filaments of myosin and thin filaments of actin, proteins that contribute to muscle contraction.

Skeletal muscle cells have typical functional properties, as follows:

- *Excitability:* the ability to receive and respond to a stimulus. The stimulus is usually a neurotransmitter released by a neuron, and the response is the generation and transmission of an action potential along the plasma membrane of the muscle cell.
- *Contractibility:* the ability to respond to a stimulus by forcibly shortening.
- *Extensibility:* the ability to respond to a stimulus by extending and relaxing; muscle fibers shorten when they contract and extend when they relax.
- *Elasticity:* the ability to resume their resting length after they have shortened or lengthened.

TABLE 19–1 **Types of Body Muscle**

TYPE	DESCRIPTION	EXAMPLES
Skeletal	Striated, voluntary muscle (can consciously move)	Biceps, triceps, deltoid, gluteus maximus
Smooth	Nonstriated, involuntary muscle (cannot consciously move)	Muscles in the walls of the bladder, stomach, and bronchi
Cardiac	Striated, involuntary muscle	Heart muscle

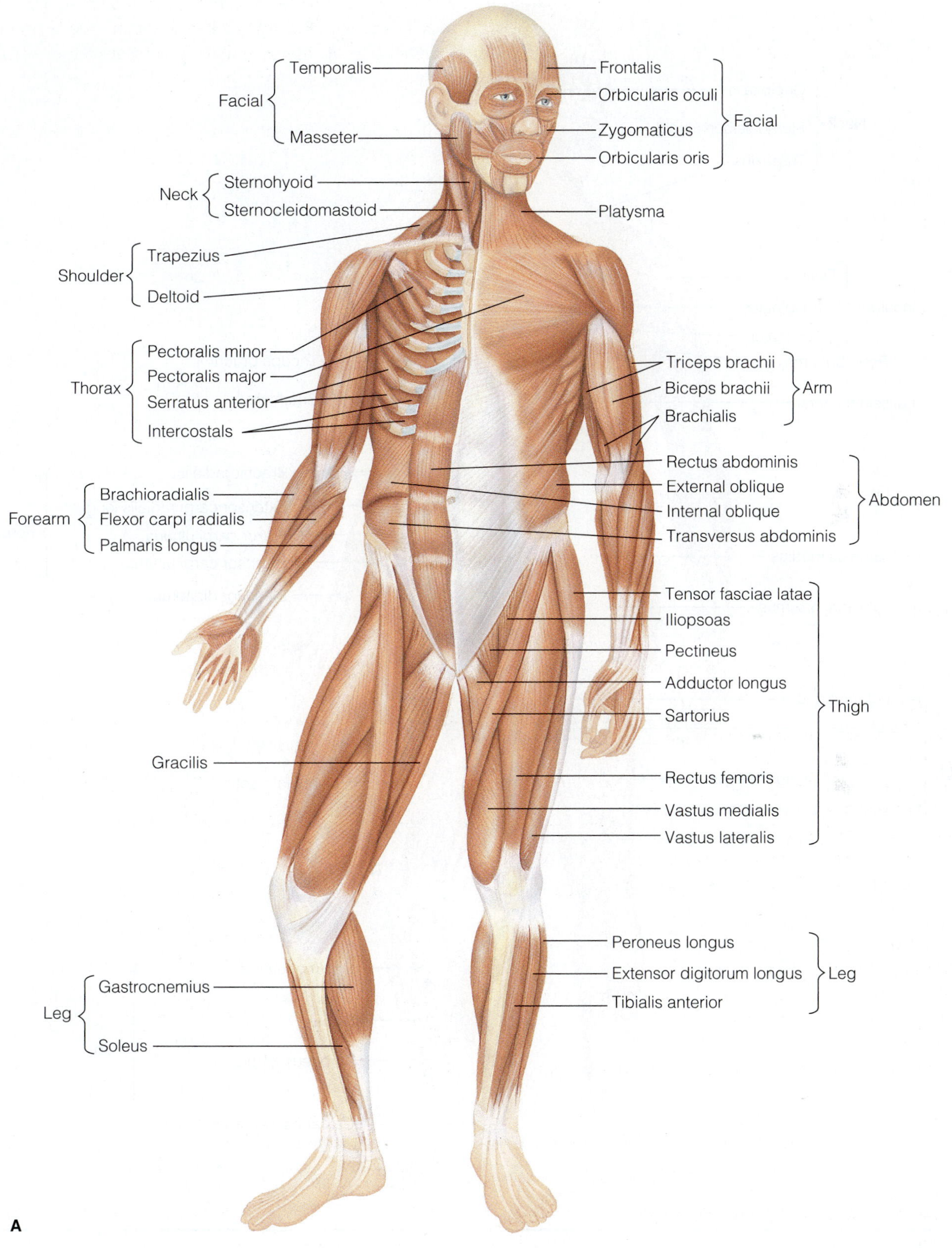

Figure 19–5 ■ *A*, Muscles of the anterior body.

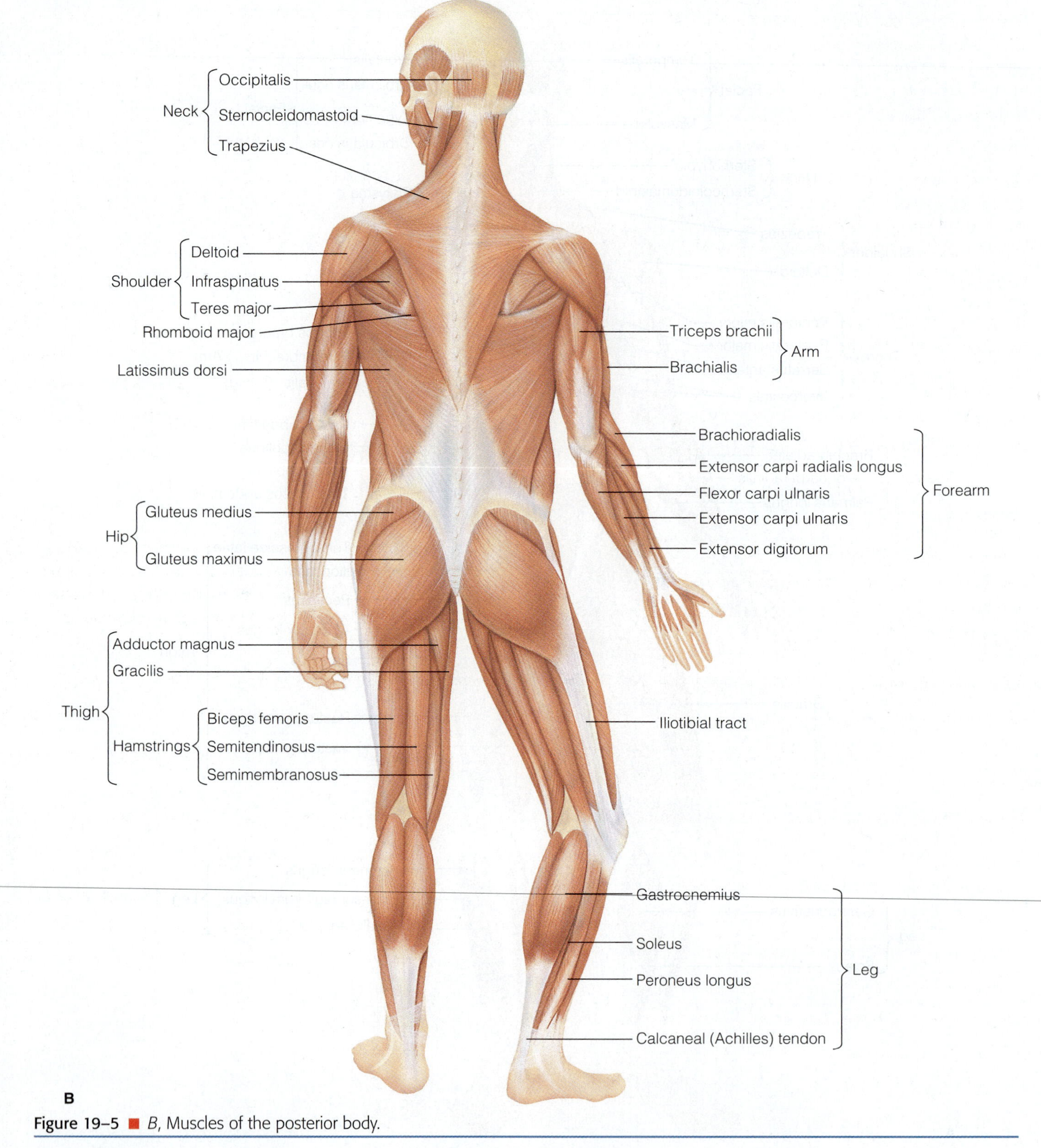

Figure 19–5 ■ *B*, Muscles of the posterior body.

Skeletal muscle movement is triggered when motor neurons release acetylcholine, a neurotransmitter that crosses the neuromuscular junction and alters the permeability of the muscle fiber. Sodium ions enter the fiber, producing an action potential that causes muscle contraction. The more fibers contract, the stronger the contraction of the entire muscle.

Prolonged strenuous activity causes continuous nerve impulses and eventually results in a buildup of lactic acid and reduced energy in the muscle, or muscle fatigue. However, continuous nerve impulses also are responsible for maintaining muscle tone. Lack of use results in muscle **atrophy**, the wasting away or decrease in size of an organ, muscle, or tissue; regular exercise increases the size and strength of muscles.

Joints, Ligaments, and Tendons

Joints, or articulations, are regions where two or more bones meet. Joints hold the bones of the skeleton together while allowing the body to move. Joints may be classified by function as synarthroses, amphiarthroses, or diarthroses. Table 19–2 describes each of these types. Joints also are classified by structure as fibrous, cartilaginous, or synovial.

FIBROUS JOINTS Fibrous joints permit little or no movement because the articulating bones are joined either (1) by short connective tissue fibers that bind the bones together, as with the sutures of the skull; or (2) by short cords of fibrous tissue called ligaments, which permit slight give but no true movement.

CARTILAGINOUS JOINTS Some cartilaginous joints, such as the sternocostal joints of the rib cage, are composed of hyaline cartilage growths that fuse together the articulating bone ends. These joints are immobile. In other cartilaginous joints, such as the intervertebral disks, the hyaline cartilage fuses to an intervening plate of flexible fibrocartilage. This structural feature accounts for the flexibility of the vertebral column.

SYNOVIAL JOINTS Bones in synovial joints are enclosed by a cavity that is filled with synovial fluid, a filtrate of blood plasma (Figure 19–6 ■). Synovial joints are freely movable, allowing many kinds of movements, as listed and described in Table 19–3 Synovial joints are found at all articulations of the limbs. They have several characteristics:

- The articular surfaces are covered with articular cartilage.
- The joint cavity is enclosed by a tough, fibrous, double-layered articular capsule; internally, the cavity is lined with a synovial membrane that covers all surfaces not covered by the articular cartilage.
- Synovial fluid fills the free spaces of the joint capsule, enhancing the smooth movement of the articulating bones.

TABLE 19–2 Functional Classification of Joints

TYPE	DESCRIPTION	EXAMPLES
Synarthrosis	Immovable joint	Skull sutures Epiphyseal plates Joint between first rib and manubrium of sternum
Amphiarthrosis	Slightly movable joint	Vertebral joints Joint of the pubic symphysis
Diarthrosis	Freely movable joint	Joints of the limbs Shoulder joints Hip joints

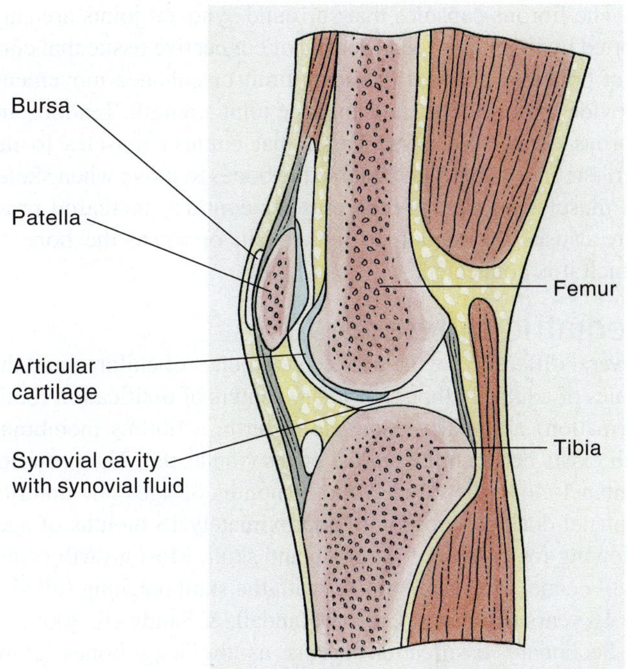

Figure 19–6 ■ Structure of a synovial joint (knee).

Bursae are small sacs of synovial fluid that cushion and protect bony areas that are at high risk for friction, such as the knee and the shoulder. Tendon sheaths are a form of bursae, but they are wrapped around tendons in high-friction areas.

TABLE 19–3 Movements Allowed by Synovial Joints

MOVEMENT	DESCRIPTION
Abduction	Move limb away from body midline
Adduction	Move limb toward body midline
Extension	Straighten limbs at joint
Flexion	Bend limbs at joint
Dorsiflexion	Bend ankle to bring top of foot toward shin
Plantar flexion	Straighten ankle to point toes down
Pronation	Turn forearm to place palm down
Supination	Turn forearm to place palm up
Eversion	Turn out
Inversion	Turn in
Circumduction	Move in circle
Internal rotation	Move inward on a central axis
External rotation	Move outward on a central axis
Protraction	Move forward and parallel to ground
Retraction	Move backward and parallel to ground

The fibrous capsules that surround synovial joints are supported by ligaments, dense bands of connective tissue that connect bones to bones. Ligaments limit or enhance movement, provide joint stability, and enhance joint strength. Tendons are fibrous connective tissue bands that connect muscles to the periosteum of bones and enable the bones to move when skeletal muscles contract. When muscles contract, increased pressure causes the tendon to pull, push, or rotate the bone to which it is connected.

Pediatric Differences

Several differences exist between the bones of children and the bones of adults. Although primary centers of ossification (bone formation) are nearly complete at birth, a fibrous membrane still exists between the cranial bones (fontanels). The posterior fontanel closes between 2 and 3 months of age. The anterior fontanel does not close until approximately 18 months of age, allowing for growth of the brain and skull. Most growth of the skull occurs by 2 years of age, with the skull reaching full size by 16 years (Chamley, Carson, Randall, & Sandwell, 2005).

Secondary ossification occurs as the long bones grow. Cartilage cells at the epiphyses (an area enriched with blood cells) are replaced by osteoblasts (immature bone cells), which push the end of the bone away from the shaft and engineer the deposition of calcium in the newly formed bone. Calcium intake during childhood and adolescence is essential to provide adequate bone density that will prevent osteoporosis and fractures in adulthood. Because growth takes place at the epiphyseal plates, injuries to this portion of a long bone are of particular concern in young children. The rapid bone growth of childhood facilitates healing after fractures, but also may lead to "growing pains," as muscles are pulled when bones grow quickly. The ends of the long bones (epiphyses) remain cartilaginous, allowing growth, until approximately age 20, when skeletal maturation is complete. At this time, the epiphyseal plate closes, cartilage at the site is replaced by bone, and only an epiphyseal line remains (Figure 19–7 ■).

The long bones of children are porous and less dense than those of adults. For this reason, children's bones can bend, buckle, or break as a result of a simple fall. In addition to the structural differences between the bones of children and adults, there are functional differences in the skeletal system of children. Before birth, the thoracic and sacral regions of the spine are convex curves. As the infant learns to hold up the head, the cervical region becomes concave. When the child learns to stand, the lumbar region also becomes concave. Failure of the spine to assume these final curves results in an abnormal curvature of the spine (kyphosis or lordosis).

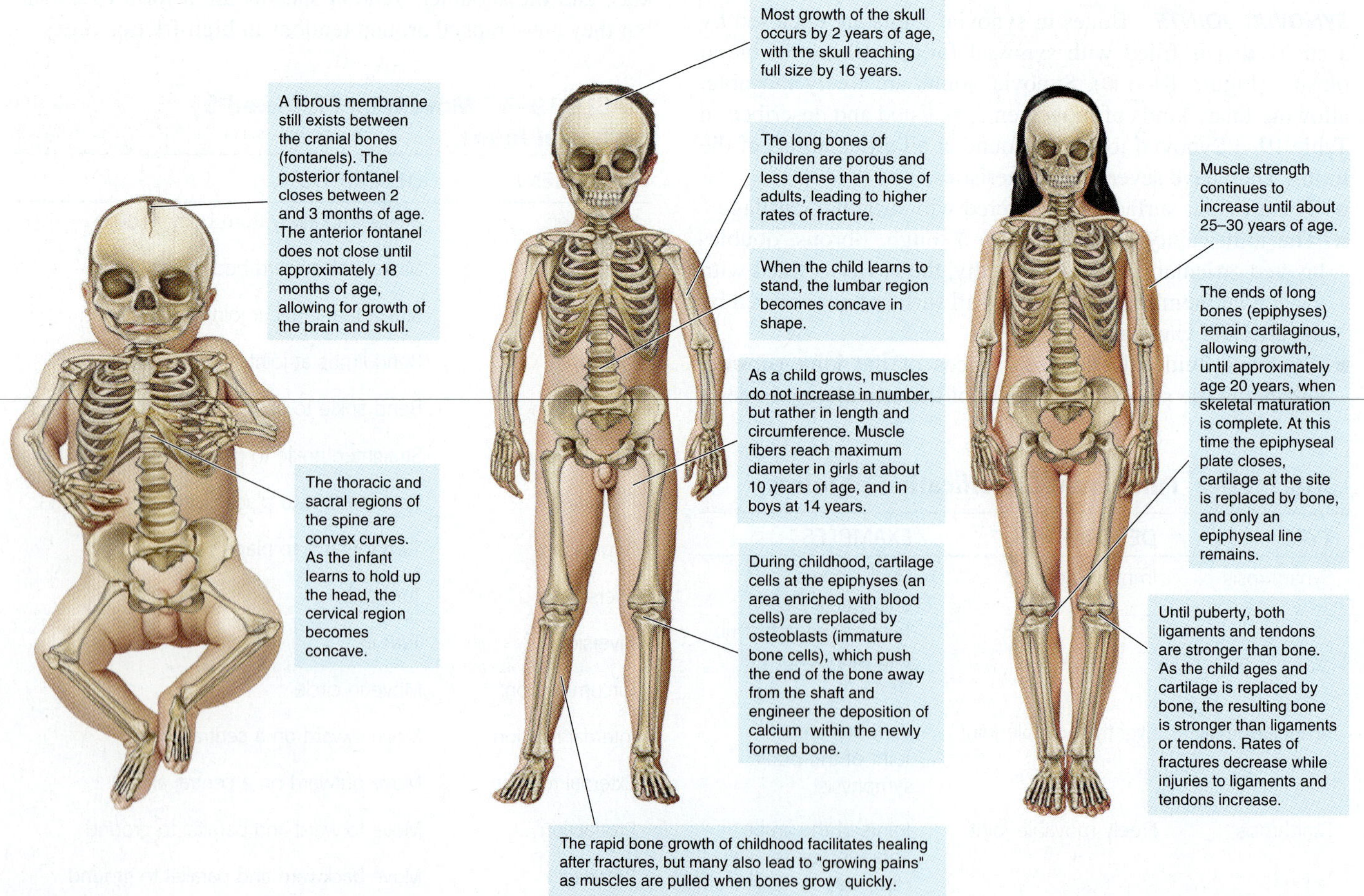
A fibrous membranne still exists between the cranial bones (fontanels). The posterior fontanel closes between 2 and 3 months of age. The anterior fontanel does not close until approximately 18 months of age, allowing for growth of the brain and skull.
The thoracic and sacral regions of the spine are convex curves. As the infant learns to hold up the head, the cervical region becomes concave.
Most growth of the skull occurs by 2 years of age, with the skull reaching full size by 16 years.
The long bones of children are porous and less dense than those of adults, leading to higher rates of fracture.
When the child learns to stand, the lumbar region becomes concave in shape.
As a child grows, muscles do not increase in number, but rather in length and circumference. Muscle fibers reach maximum diameter in girls at about 10 years of age, and in boys at 14 years.
During childhood, cartilage cells at the epiphyses (an area enriched with blood cells) are replaced by osteoblasts (immature bone cells), which push the end of the bone away from the shaft and engineer the deposition of calcium within the newly formed bone.
The rapid bone growth of childhood facilitates healing after fractures, but many also lead to "growing pains" as muscles are pulled when bones grow quickly.
Muscle strength continues to increase until about 25–30 years of age.
The ends of long bones (epiphyses) remain cartilaginous, allowing growth, until approximately age 20 years, when skeletal maturation is complete. At this time the epiphyseal plate closes, cartilage at the site is replaced by bone, and only an epiphyseal line remains.
Until puberty, both ligaments and tendons are stronger than bone. As the child ages and cartilage is replaced by bone, the resulting bone is stronger than ligaments or tendons. Rates of fractures decrease while injuries to ligaments and tendons increase.

Figure 19–7 ■ Skeletal and muscle development throughout childhood.

MUSCLES, TENDONS, AND LIGAMENTS The muscular system, unlike the skeletal system, is almost completely formed at birth, with any remaining increase achieved in the first year of life. As a child grows, muscles do not increase in number, but rather in length and circumference. Muscle fibers reach maximum diameter in girls at about 10 years of age and in boys at 14 years. Muscle strength continues to increase until about 25–30 years of age (Chamley et al., 2005).

Until puberty, both ligaments and tendons are stronger than bone. When these structural differences are not recognized, a childhood fracture is sometimes mistaken for a sprain. A **sprain** is a tearing of ligaments, the structural support connecting bones, usually caused when a joint is twisted or otherwise traumatized. Tendons, which connect bones to muscles, grow in length, and fibrous tissue as mechanical pressure is placed on them.

Changes of Aging

Significant alterations in human structure, function, biochemistry, and genetic patterns are responsible for changes in the muscles, tendons, bones, and joints of the older person. These changes contribute to the appearance of aging in many older people (e.g., decreased height, stooped shoulders, and rigid movements). Figure 19–8 ■ and Table 19–4 illustrate the normal changes of aging and the musculoskeletal system.

BONE: NORMAL CHANGES OF AGING The bone loss of normal aging has been described in two distinct phases (Manolagas, 2006). Type I, or menopausal bone loss, and type II, senescent bone loss. Menopausal bone loss is a rapid phase of bone loss that affects women in the first 5–10 years after menopause. Senescent bone loss is a slower phase that affects both sexes after midlife. These two phases are distinct in their clinical features, but in women, there is eventual overlap, which leads to increased difficulty in differentiating the two phases. Other conditions also may contribute to skeletal deterioration in the older adult and may alter the clinical symptoms.

In the older adult, bones become stiff, weaker, and more brittle. Changes in appearance are evident after the fifth decade, and changes in height are most obvious. At about 50 years of age, the long bones of the arms and legs appear disproportionate in size due to the adult's shrinking stature. An average loss of height is 1–2 cm every two decades, from about 20–70 years of age. This change in height is due to various processes that result in shortening of the vertebral column. Thinning of the vertebral disks occurs more commonly in midlife; in later years, there is a decrease in the height of individual vertebrae. As the older person enters the eighth and ninth decades, there is a more rapid decrease in vertebral height due to osteoporotic collapse of the vertebrae. The result is a shortening of the trunk and the appearance of long extremities. Additional postural changes are kyphosis and a backward tilt of the head to make eye contact. The result is a forward bent, or "jutting out" posture, with the hips and knees assuming a flex position.

MUSCLES: NORMAL CHANGES OF AGING There is a great deal of variation in muscle function in the older person. Muscle function remains trainable well into advanced age, and the regenerative function of muscle tissue remains normal in the older person.

By age 75, most people lose one half of the skeletal muscle mass they had at the age of 30 (Metter, Lynch, Conwit et al., 1999). This process is known as **sarcopenia**. Muscle tone and tension decreases steadily after the third decade. Some muscles

TABLE 19–4 **Age-Related Changes in the Musculoskeletal System**

AGE-RELATED CHANGE	SIGNIFICANCE
Bones and Joints	
■ ↓bone mass and minerals ■ ↓calcium reabsorption, a slow resorption of the interior of long bones, and slower production of new bone on the outside surface of bones ■ ↓Shortening of vertebrae and thinning of intervertebral disks; kyphosis often occurs. ■ ↓Deterioration of cartilage on bone surfaces in joints; bone spurs may occur.	Decreased bone mass as well as decreased calcium absorption contributes to bones that are often thinner and weaker, with an increased risk of fractures with trauma. As the spinal column shortens, height decreases. Loss of joint cartilage and formation of bone spurs makes movement more painful and may even limit mobility.
Muscles	
■ Muscle fibers atrophy, and fibrous tissue slowly replaces muscle tissue. ■ ↓muscle mass and strength ■ ↓muscle movements, especially in the arms and legs ■ Decreased range of motion (ROM) ■ Shrinking and hardening of tendons ■ Muscle cramping is common.	Regular exercise is important in decreasing the loss associated with aging in terms of maintaining muscle mass, strength, and agility.

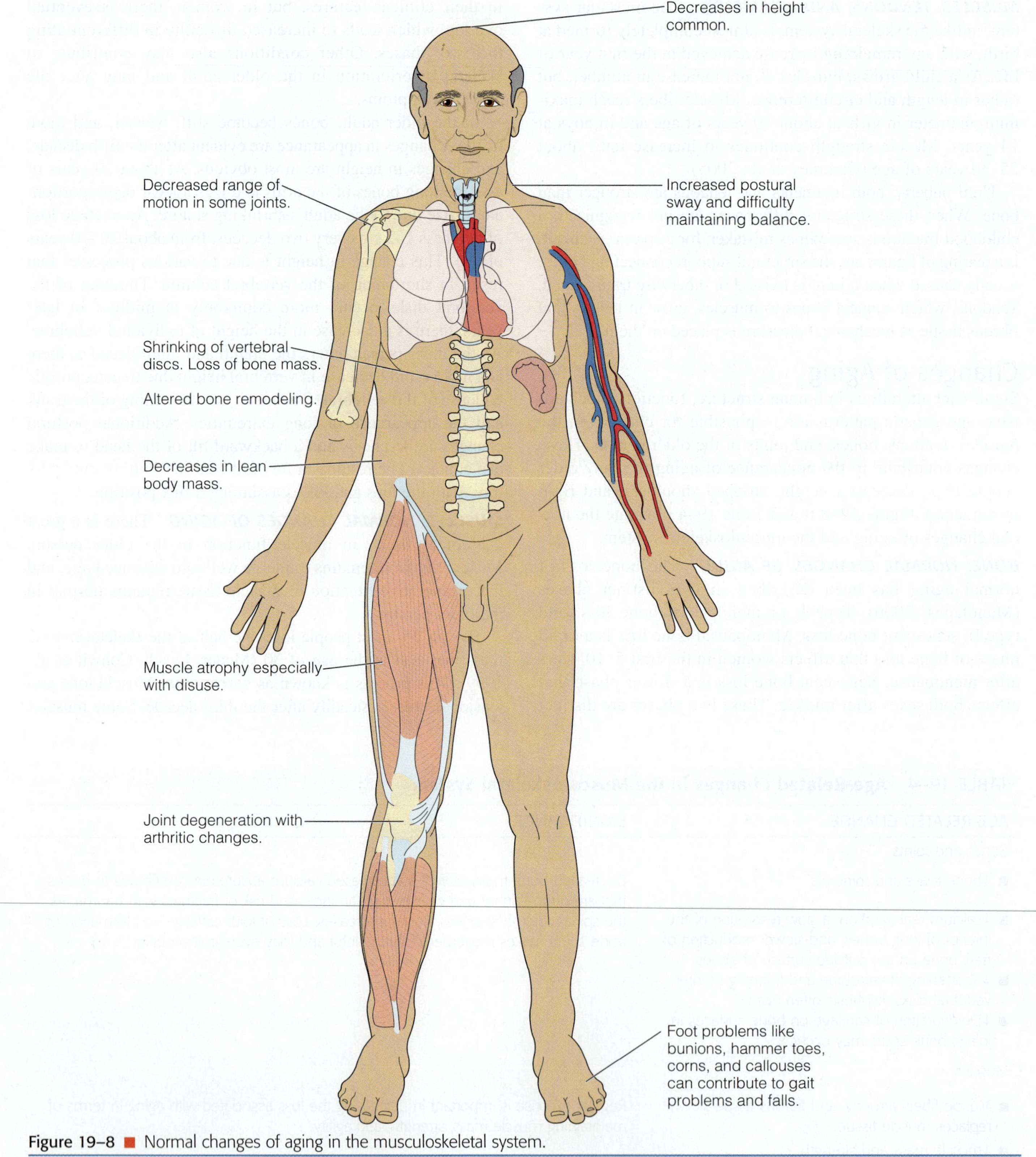
Decreases in height common.
Decreased range of motion in some joints.
Increased postural sway and difficulty maintaining balance.
Shrinking of vertebral discs. Loss of bone mass.
Altered bone remodeling.
Decreases in lean body mass.
Muscle atrophy especially with disuse.
Joint degeneration with arthritic changes.
Foot problems like bunions, hammer toes, corns, and callouses can contribute to gait problems and falls.

Figure 19–8 ■ Normal changes of aging in the musculoskeletal system.

decrease in size, resulting in weakness. The shape of muscles becomes more prominent and feels more distinct. Maximum muscle strength is achieved between 20 and 35 years of age. Muscle strength declines slowly, but by 50 years of age, a decline in stamina is often noticed. By 80 years of age, the maximum muscle strength that the individual had in the mid-20s has decreased 65–85% (Metter, Lynch, Conwit, et al., 1999).

The lower extremity muscles tend to atrophy earlier than those of the upper extremity. Routine daily activities most likely keep the upper extremities functioning on a regular basis. By comparison, walking may be limited to a small living area and for short periods of time. Despite age-related change in muscle strength, the older adult can usually perform functional activities of daily living (ADLs) and demonstrate adequate muscle function when climbing stairs, walking a straight line, and rising from a sitting or squatting position.

JOINTS, LIGAMENTS, TENDONS, AND CARTILAGE: NORMAL CHANGES OF AGING Hyaline cartilage, which lines the joints, erodes and tears with advancing age, allowing bones to be in direct contact with one another. Knee cartilage is subjected to a great deal of wear and tear, and the result is a thinning of about 0.25 mm per year. Thinning, damaged cartilage and diminished lubricating fluid result in discomfort and slowness of joint movement.

Ligaments, tendons, and joint capsules lose elasticity and become less flexible. There is a decrease in the **range of motion (ROM)** of the joints due to changes in ligaments and muscles. Nonarticular cartilage, such as the ears and nose, grows throughout life, which may cause the nose to look large in relation to the face.

ALTERATIONS

Alterations in the musculoskeletal system may result in rheumatic disease, abnormalities of the spine, joint disorders, or trauma-induced disorders. This section introduces the alterations in mobility that are discussed in the exemplars that follow and offers a brief overview of other disorders that can affect mobility.

Back Problems

Back problems can arise from a variety of causes, including trauma or sudden injury, degenerative disorders, gastrointestinal causes, and pregnancy. Upper back pain can result from muscular irritation or joint dysfunction. Strain over time and

ALTERATIONS AND TREATMENTS Mobility

ALTERATION	DESCRIPTION	TREATMENT
Back problems Herniated intervertebral disk	A rupture of the cartilage surrounding the intervertebral disk with protrusion of the nucleus pulposus. Herniated disks cause excrutiating pain and limited mobility, which in turn cause alterations in role function, coping, and the ability to perform ADLs.	■ Pharmacologic therapy to relieve pain and reduce swelling and muscle spasms. ■ Surgery for clients who do not respond to conservative management or who have neurologic deficits. The type of surgery depends on the location of the disk and the stability of the spinal column.
Scoliosis	A lateral S- or C-shaped curvature of the spine that is often associated with a rotational deformity of the spine and ribs.	■ *(Mild)* Exercises to improve posture, muscle tone, and flexibility of the spine. Reevaluation by the treating physician necessary every 3 months. ■ *(Moderate)* Bracing to prevent further increase of curvature; electrical stimulation. ■ *(Severe)* Spinal fusion.
Fracture	Trauma causes a partial or complete break in the continuity of the bone.	■ Emergency care includes immediate immobilization, maintaining tissue perfusion, and preventing infection; splinting to relieve pain and prevent further damage. ■ Pharmacologic therapies focus on relieving pain. ■ Closed reduction or open reduction depending on the type of fracture, followed by casting, pinning, and/or traction.
Hip Fractures	Fracture of the femur at the femoral head, neck, or trochanteric regions.	■ Immediate immobilization to prevent further damage. ■ Traction to decrease muscle spasm. ■ Surgery (within 24 hours) to reduce and stabilize the fracture.
Multiple Sclerosis	A chronic demyelinating neurologic disease of the CNS associated with an abnormal immune response to an environmental factor.	■ Pharmacologic therapies to slow the progression of MS and decrease the number of attacks. ■ Antinflammatories during an exacerbation to reduce inflammation, inhibit manifestations, and induce remission.
Osteoarthritis	In osteoarthritis, the joint cartilage erodes, resulting in pain and stiffness. Disability is associated with osteoarthritic changes in the spine, knees, and hips.	■ Nonsteroidal anti-inflammatory drugs (NSAIDs) ■ Application of warm moist heat ■ Gentle exercise and ROM
Parkinson's disease	A progressive, degenerative neurologic disease characterized by tremors, muscle rigidity, and bradykinesia.	■ Pharmacologic therapies to control manifestations ■ Deep brain stimulation ■ Surgery ■ Physical, occupational, and speech therapy

poor posture also can cause upper back pain, a growing problem for those who sit at computers for long hours (Sellers, 2002). Two common causes of back pain, herniated disks and scoliosis, are discussed in the exemplar that follows.

Fractures

A **fracture** is any break in the continuity of a bone. Fractures can greatly impair mobility and cause a great deal of pain for the client. Two factors that affect the severity of the fracture are the nature of the event (e.g., a fall) and the strength of the bone. Falls, blunt trauma, motor vehicle accidents, child abuse, and repetitive forces are all common causes of fractures.

Hip Fractures

A **hip fracture** refers to a fracture of the femur at the head, neck, or trochanteric regions. Hip fractures are most common in adults over the age of 65, although they can occur at any age. Women are at greater risk of hip fracture than men because women lose bone density at a younger age and greater rate than do men. In an older adult, hip fracture is more likely to result from a traumatic event such as a fall. In younger individuals, hip fractures more commonly result from sports injuries and motor vehicle accidents. Chronic medical conditions such as osteoporosis and lack of physical activity are two of the risk factors for hip fractures (Mayo Clinic, 2008).

Multiple Sclerosis

Multiple sclerosis (MS) is a chronic demyelinating neurologic disease of the CNS (brain, optic nerves, and spinal cord) associated with an abnormal immune response to an environmental factor. More simply, the disease causes the immune system to attack the myelin sheath covering the nerves, impairing the brain's ability to communicate with the rest of the body. Symptoms vary widely and can include numbness or weakness of a limb, visual impairments, tremors, fatigue, and dizziness. In severe cases the client can lose the ability to speak or walk. In the early stages, symptoms can disappear for months at a time, making multiple sclerosis difficult to diagnose (Mayo Clinic, 2009).

Osteoarthritis

Osteoarthritis (OA), the most common type of arthritis, is due to excessive wear and tear of articular cartilage of the weight-bearing joints; the knee, spine, and hip are particularly affected. Symptoms include localized pain and stiffness, joint and bone enlargement, and limitations in movement. OA is not accompanied by the degree of inflammation associated with other forms of arthritis.

Parkinson's Disease

Parkinson's disease is a degenerative disorder of the CNS caused by death of neurons that produce the brain neurotransmitter dopamine. It is the second most common degenerative disease of the nervous system, affecting more than 1.5 million Americans. Pharmacotherapy is the first line of treatment, often reducing some of the distressing symptoms of this disease.

Parkinson's disease affects primarily clients older than 50 years of age; however, even teenagers and younger adults can develop the disorder. Men are affected slightly more than women. The disease is progressive, with the expression of full symptoms often taking many years. The symptoms of Parkinson's disease, or **parkinsonism**, include tremors, muscle rigidity, postural instability, and **bradykinesia** (slowed movements due to muscle rigidity). Early symptoms may go unnoticed for months at a time and may include lack of facial expressions or slow and mumbling speech, sometimes accompanied by drooling.

Spinal Cord Injuries

Spinal cord injuries typically result in permanent disability or paralysis. Risk factors include age, gender, and alcohol or drug abuse. While motor vehicle accidents account for approximately 55% of spinal cord injuries, a number of other events and activities can result in this type of injury. Christopher Reeve, an actor and perhaps the most famous American affected by spinal cord injury, fell off his horse in 1995. He sustained severe damaged to his spinal cord and was paralyzed from the waste down. Detailed information on spinal cord injuries is provided in the exemplars that follow. Additional information regarding research and quality of life issues for clients with spinal cord injuries can be found at the website of the Christopher and Dana Reeve Foundation, www.christopherreeve.org.

Other Alterations That Affect Mobility

A number of other disorders can greatly impair mobility (see Figures 19–9 through 19–26 on pages 1068–1070). Rheumatoid arthritis, for example, is discussed in detail in Exemplar 14.3. A number of abnormalities of the spine and various joint disorders also cause a great deal of discomfort and frustration by reducing mobility and causing pain for the client.

ABNORMALITIES OF THE SPINE Abnormalities of the fine that impair mobility include the following:

- *Kyphosis*, an exaggeration of the normal convex curve of the thoracic spine
- *Scoliosis*, a lateral curvature of the spine
- *Lordosis*, an exaggeration of the normal lumbar curve.

JOINT DISORDERS One of the more common joint disorders of the head and neck is **temporomandibular joint (TMJ) syndrome**, which is characteristically manifested by pain on the opening and closing of the mouth. In the shoulder, *rotator cuff tears* arise from repeated impingement, injury, or falls. Rotator cuff tears are more common after the age of 40 and among athletes, such as pitchers, whose positions require frequent throwing.

A number of joint disorders cause impairment of mobility in the wrist and hand. These include the following:

- Joint effusion
- Rheumatoid nodules

- Carpal tunnel syndrome
- Dupuytren's contracture.

A number of disorders of the foot can also impair mobility. These include:

- **Gout**
- Bunion
- Hallux valgus, a condition in which the great toe is abnormally adducted at the metatarsophalangeal joint
- Hammertoe.

ASSESSMENT

Structures and functions of the musculoskeletal system are assessed using findings from diagnostic tests, a health assessment interview to collect subjective data, and a physical assessment to collect objective data.

The primary manifestations of altered function of the musculoskeletal system are pain and limited mobility. Specific descriptors of the pain, its location, and its nature are important. Acute and chronic pain are discussed in detail in Exemplar 5.1. Significant information also includes related manifestations such as fever, fatigue, changes in weight, rash, and/or swelling. Other important information includes details about the client's lifestyle—type of employment, ability to carry out **activities of daily living (ADLs)** and to provide self-care, exercise or participation in sports, use of alcohol or drugs, and nutrition. The nurse should explore past injuries and measures to self-treat pain (such as OTC medications, prescribed medications, application of heat or cold, splinting, wrapping, or rest).

Physical Assessment

Physical assessment of the musculoskeletal system may be performed as part of a total assessment or as a single examination of a client with known or suspected problems. The techniques used to assess the musculoskeletal system are inspection, palpation, and measurement of muscle mass and ROM. The client should be comfortably dressed in clothing that lets the examiner clearly see the movement of all joints. The client may be standing, sitting, or lying down; the sequence of the examination should be such that the client does not to change positions frequently. An assessment of the older adult, the client in pain, or the client who is weak may take extra time. Normal age-related findings for the older adult are summarized in Table 19–4.

Prior to the examination, collect all equipment and explain the techniques to decrease the client's anxiety. The sequence for a musculoskeletal examination follows:

1. Begin the examination with an assessment of gait and posture. Observe how the client walks, sits, and/or moves about in bed.
2. Inspect and palpate the bones for any obvious deformity, changes in size or shape, tenderness, or pain upon palpation.

TABLE 19–5 Muscle Grading Scale

GRADING SCALE	ASSESSMENT DESCRIPTION
0	No visible contraction; paralysis
1	Can feel contraction of muscle, but there is no movement of limb
2	Passive ROM
3	Full ROM against gravity
4	Full ROM against some resistance
5	Full ROM against full resistance

3. Measure the extremities for length and circumference. Before taking measurements, make sure the client is lying in a comfortable position. Remember to compare limbs bilaterally.
4. Assess muscle mass by inspecting for obvious increase or decrease in size. Assess and document muscle strength on a scale of 0–5 (Table 19–5). Box 19–1 provides instructions for testing the strength of various muscles.

Box 19–1 Guidelines for Assessing Muscle Strength

In adults, muscles are usually strong and equally strong bilaterally. However, neuromuscular diseases, disuse, metabolic disorders, or infections can cause muscle weakness. Muscle strength is expected to be greater in the dominant arm and leg. In most instances (and especially when moving digits and extremities), the nurse provides resistance by pushing in the opposite direction.

The muscles listed below are routinely tested. Instructions for clients also are provided.

MUSCLE	CLIENT INSTRUCTIONS
Ocular muscles and lids	Close eyes tightly.
Finger muscles	Shake hands. Make a fist. Spread fingers.
Facial muscles	Blow out cheeks. Stick out tongue.
Hip muscles	Raise straight leg while supine.
Neck muscles	Bend head forward and backward.
Gluteal and leg muscles	Alternately cross legs while sitting.
Deltoid muscles	Hold arms up.
Biceps muscle	Bend the arm.
Quadriceps muscle	Straighten leg.
Triceps muscle	Straighten the arm.
Wrist muscles	Bend hand forward and backward.
Ankle and foot muscles	Bend foot up and down.

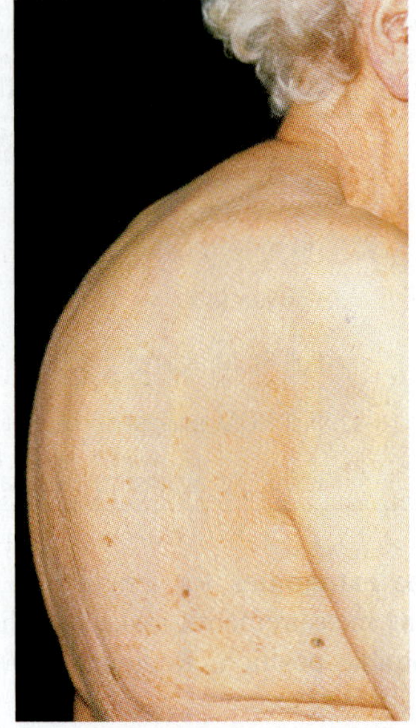

Figure 19–9 ■ Kyphosis (hunchback).

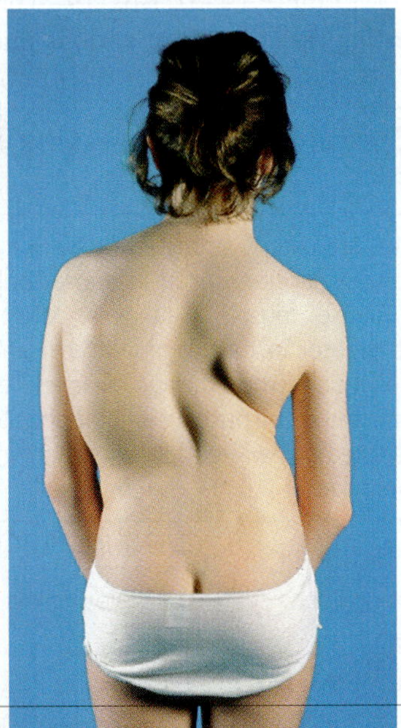

Figure 19–10 ■ Scoliosis.

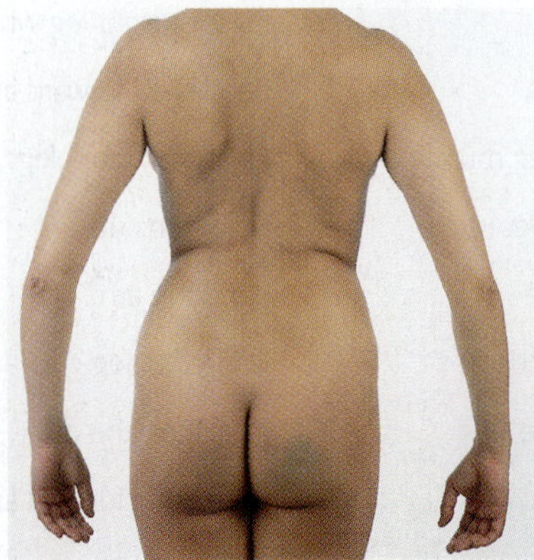

Figure 19–11 ■ Lumbar lordosis.

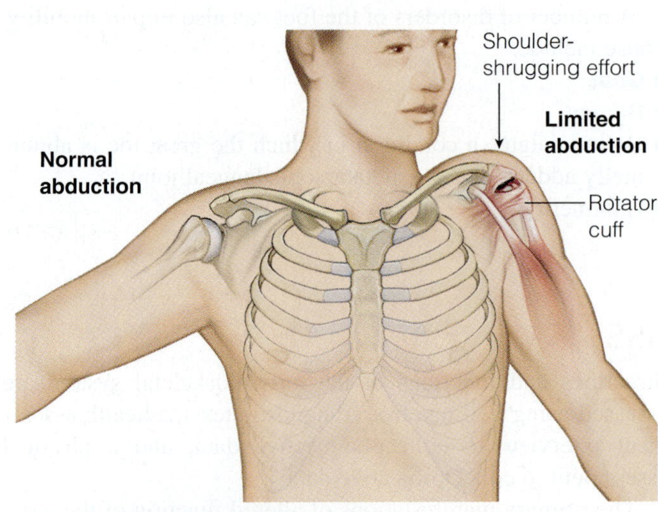

Figure 19–12 ■ Rotator cuff tear.

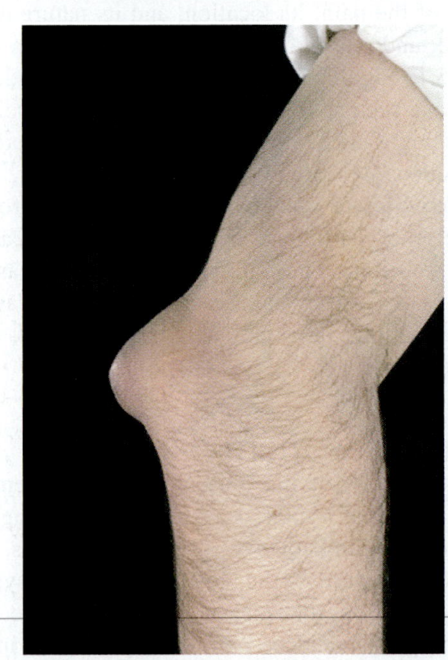

Figure 19–13 ■ Olecranon bursitis.

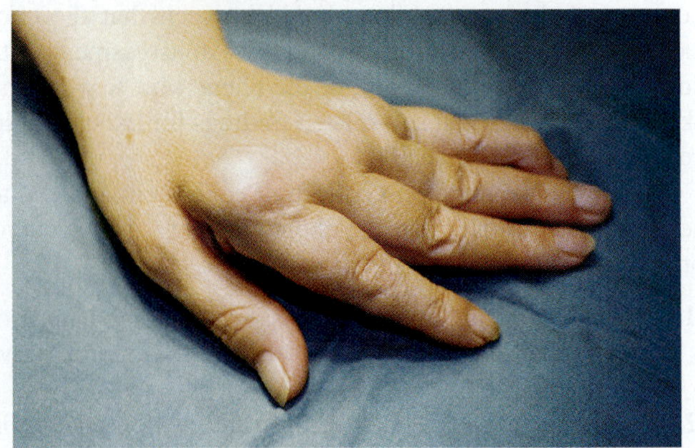

Figure 19–14 ■ Joint effusion of the hand.

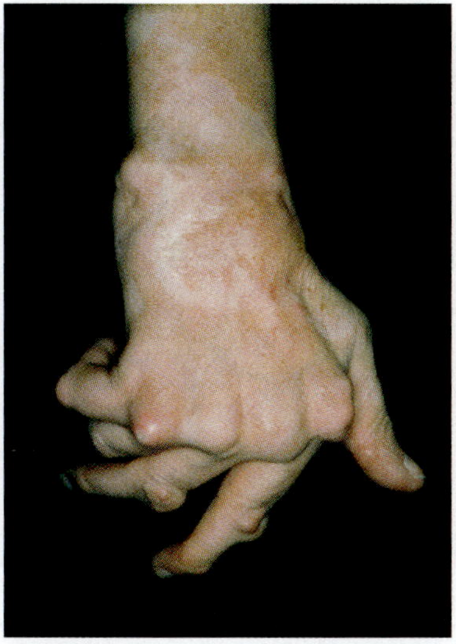

Figure 19–15 ■ Rheumatoid nodules.

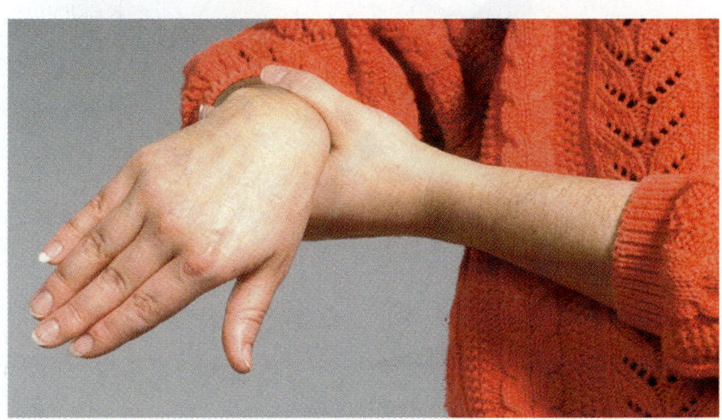

Figure 19–18 ■ Ulnar deviation.

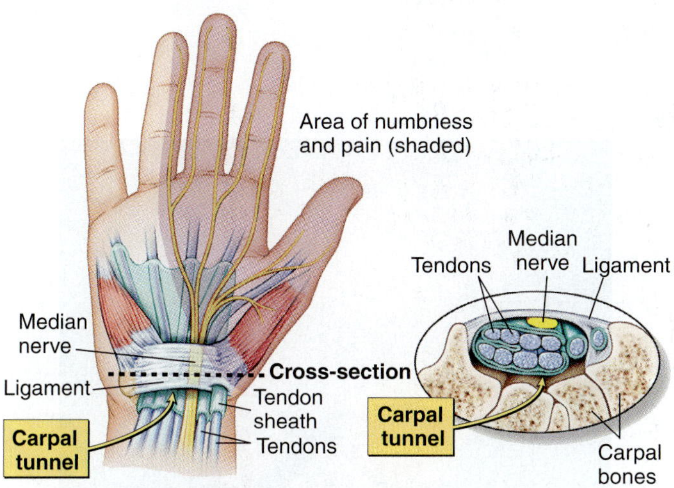

Figure 19–16 ■ Carpal tunnel syndrome.

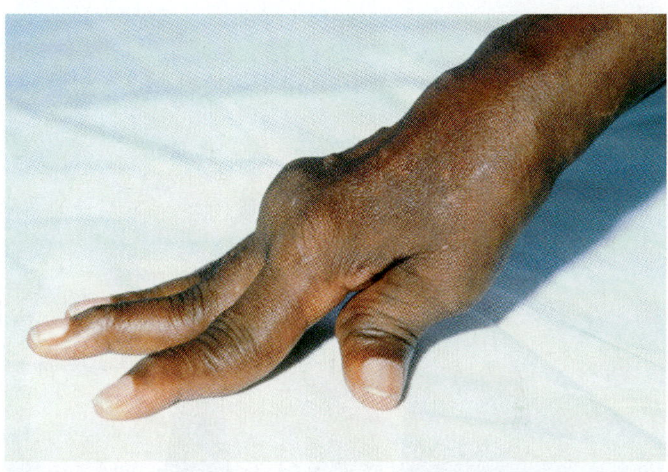

Figure 19–19 ■ Swan-neck and boutonnière deformities.

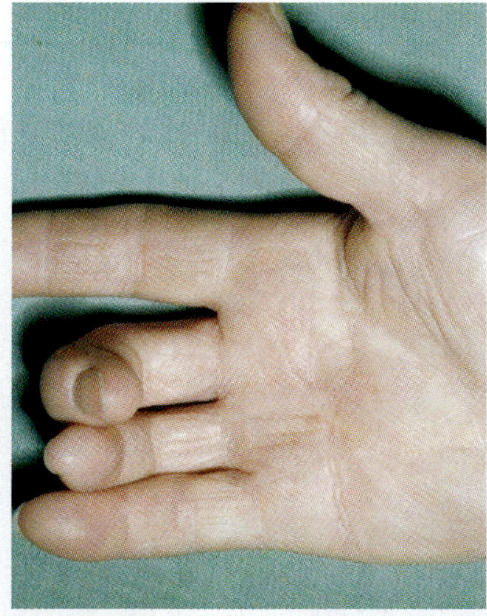

Figure 19–17 ■ Dupuytren's contracture.

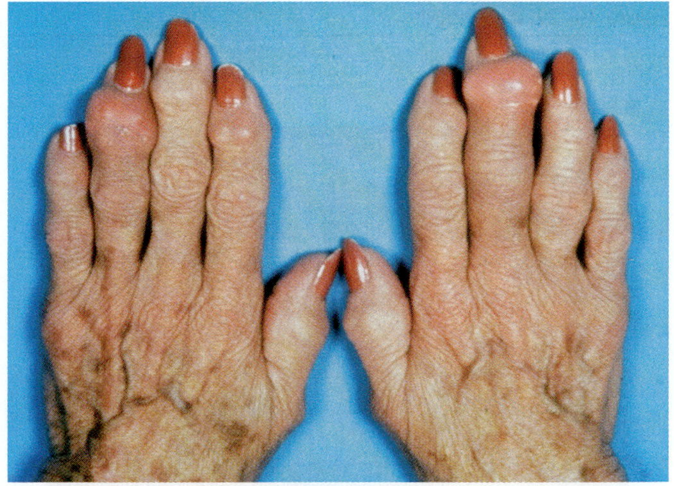

Figure 19–20 ■ Osteoarthritis.

Source: © 1972–2004 American College of Rheumatology Clinical Slide Collection. Used with permission.

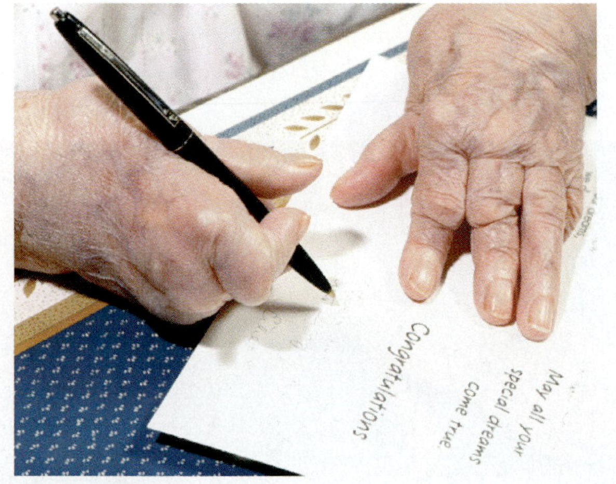

Figure 19–21 ■ Rheumatoid arthritis.

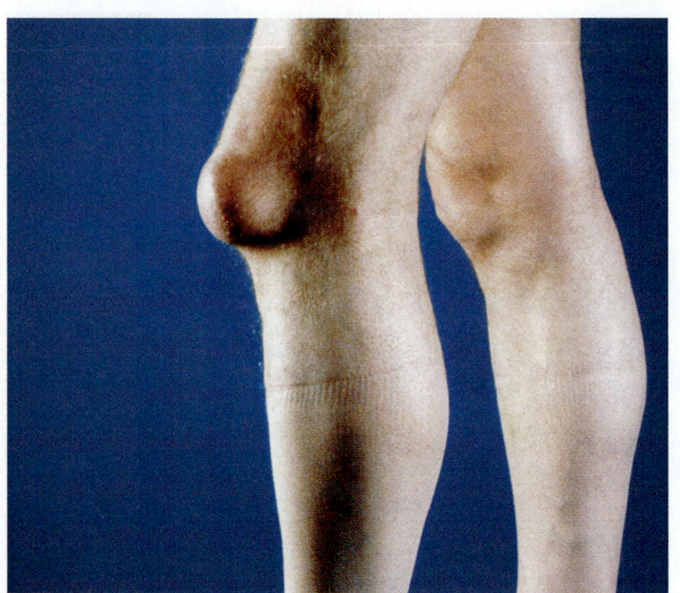

Figure 19–22 ■ Synovitis.

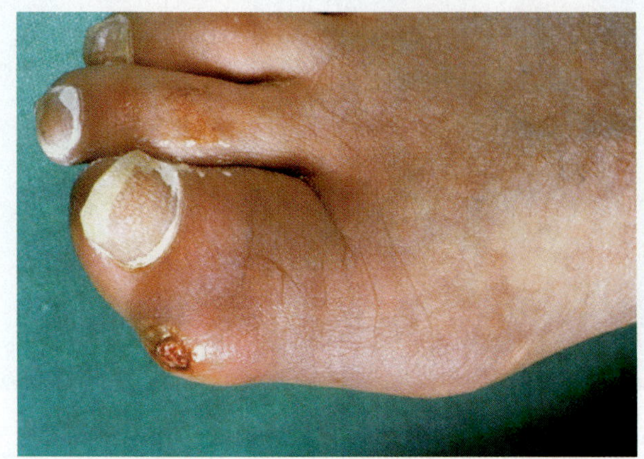

Figure 19–23 ■ Gout.

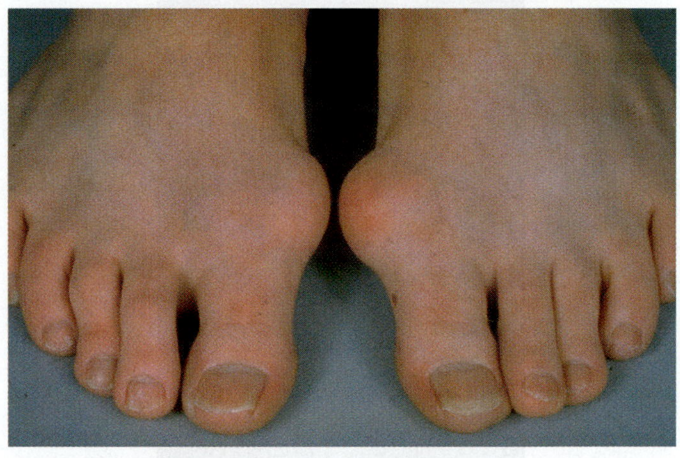

Figure 19–24 ■ Bunion.

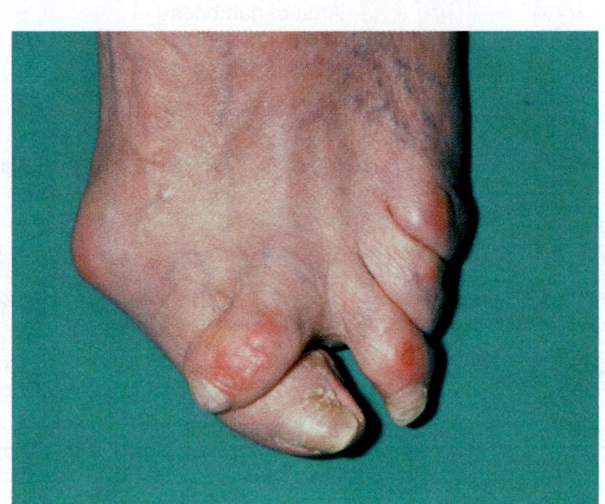

Figure 19–25 ■ Hallux valgus.

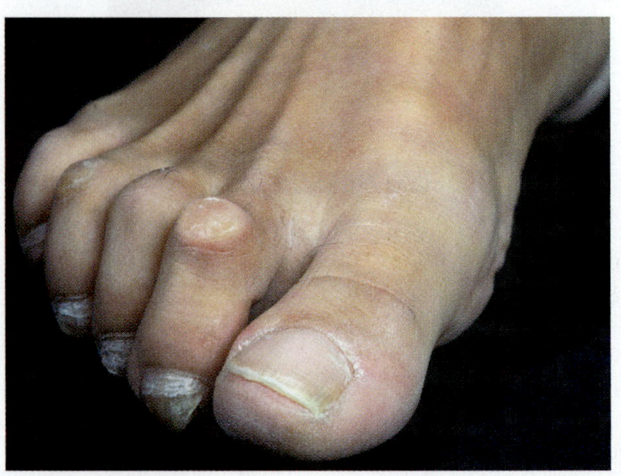

Figure 19–26 ■ Hammertoe.

5. Assess joints for swelling, pain, redness, warmth, crepitus, and ROM. Assessing the ROM of one or more joints is a common part of nursing care; every joint should be assessed if the client has or is suspected of having a specific musculoskeletal problem. Use a goniometer for precise measurements of joint ROM (Figure 19–27 ■). This device has a pointer joined to a protractor at 0 degrees. These two arms are placed along articulating bones, and the angle of joint movement is recorded in degrees.

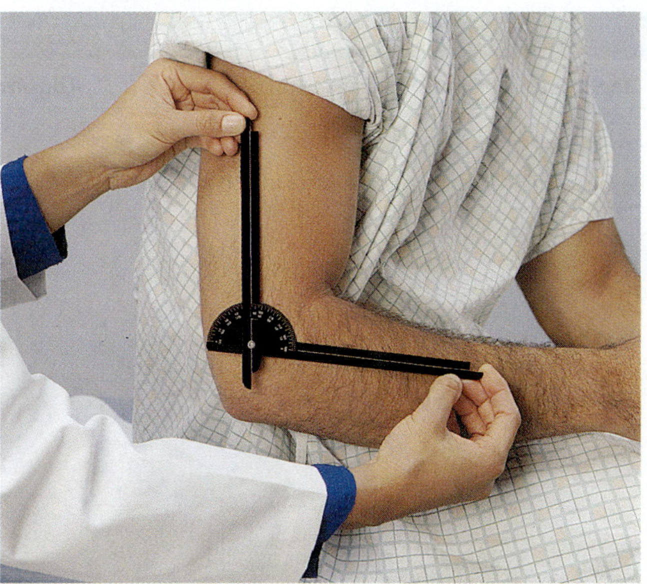

Figure 19–27 ■ Using a goniometer to measure joint ROM.

Health Assessment Interview

A health assessment interview to determine problems with musculoskeletal structure and/or function may be conducted during a health screening, may focus on a chief complaint (such as joint pain), or may be part of a total health assessment. Health problems affecting the neurologic system may manifest as problems with musculoskeletal function, and an assessment of both systems may be necessary. (See Concept 17, Intracranial Regulation, for assessment of the neurologic system.) If the client has a problem with musculoskeletal structure or function, analyze its onset, characteristics, course, severity, precipitating and relieving factors, and any associated symptoms, noting the timing and circumstances. For example, ask the client the following questions:

- Describe the pain you have had in your elbow. Does the pain increase with movement? Have you noticed any redness or swelling?
- Did you injure your ankle before you began to experience difficulty walking?
- Is your pain worse in the morning, or does it get worse throughout the day?

Musculoskeletal Assessments

Technique/Normal Findings	Abnormal Findings
Gait and Body Posture Assessment	
Inspect body posture and gait. *Body posture should be upright; gait should be smooth and steady.*	■ Joint stiffness, pain, deformities, and muscle weakness can cause changes in gait and posture.
Inspect the spine for curvature. Ask the client to stand and bend back slowly as far as possible, bend slowly to the right and then to the left as far as possible, turn slowly to the right and left in a circular motion, and bend forward slowly and try to touch fingers to toes. *When viewed from the back, the cervical and lumbar spine are concave, the thoracic spine is convex, and the spine is straight.*	■ With herniated lumbar disks, the lumbar curve flattens and spinal mobility is decreased. ■ An increased lumbar curve, called lordosis, may be seen in obesity or pregnancy. ■ A lateral S-shaped curvature of the spine is called scoliosis. Functional scoliosis usually is a compensatory response to painful paravertebral muscles, herniated disks, or discrepancy in leg length. It disappears with forward flexion. Structural scoliosis is often congenital and tends to appear during adolescence. It is accentuated with forward bending. ■ Kyphosis is an exaggerated thoracic curvature of the spine common in older adults.
Joint Assessment	
Inspect the joints for deformity, swelling, and redness. *There should be no visible deformity, swelling, or redness of joints.* Palpate the joints for tenderness, warmth, crepitation, consistency, and muscle mass. *Joints should be nontender and consistent bilaterally without visible or palpable excess warmth, crepitation, or masses.*	■ Diseases of the joints may be manifested by deformities such as tissue loss, tissue overgrowth, contractures, or irreversible shortenings of muscles and tendons. ■ Edema in a joint may cause obvious bulging. ■ Redness, swelling, and pain are evidence of an inflammation or infection in the joint. ■ Inflammation and injury cause joint pain. ■ Arthritis, bursitis, tendonitis, and osteomyelitis (infection of a bone) result in painful, hot joints. ■ **Crepitation** (a grating sound) is present in a joint when the articulating surfaces have lost their cartilage, such as in arthritis.

(continued)

Musculoskeletal Assessments (continued)

Technique/Normal Findings	Abnormal Findings
Range-of-Motion Assessment	
Assess joint ROM by asking the client to perform activities specific to each joint, as follows: *All bilateral joints should move through full ROM.*	
Temporomandibular joint: "Open your mouth wide and then close your mouth." (As the client opens and closes the mouth, palpate the temporomandibular joints with your index and middle fingers, as shown in Figure 19–28 ■).	■ Clicking or popping noises, decreased ROM, pain, and swelling may indicate TMJ syndrome or, in rare cases, osteoarthritis.

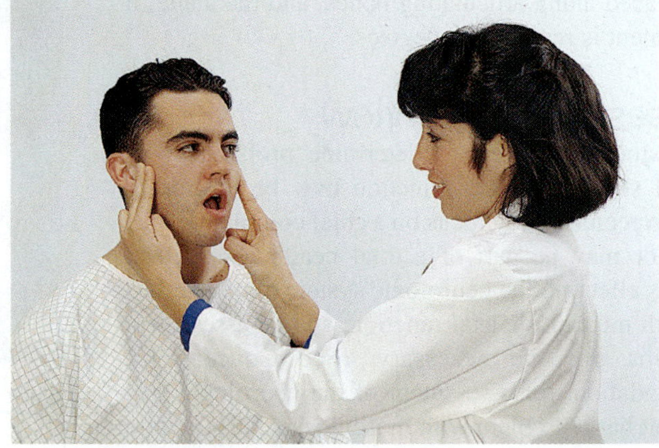

Figure 19–28 ■ Palpating the temporomandibular joints.

Technique/Normal Findings	Abnormal Findings
Cervical spine: 45-degree flexion: "Touch your chin to your chest." 55-degree extension: "Look at the ceiling." 40-degree lateral bending: "Try to touch your right ear to your right shoulder." Repeat with the left side. 70-degree rotation: "Try to touch your chin to each shoulder."	■ Neck pain and limited extension with lateral bending are seen with herniated cervical disks and in cervical spondylosis. ■ An immobile neck with head and neck thrust forward is seen with ankylosing spondylitis.
Lumbar spine: 75- to 90-degree flexion: "Touch your toes with your fingers" (Figure 19–29A ■). 30-degree extension: "Bend backward slowly." 35-degree lateral bending: "Bend right and left" (Figure 19–29B). 30-degree rotation: "Twist your shoulders right and left" (Figure 19–29C).	■ Decreased movement or pain with movement may indicate an abnormal spinal curvature, arthritis, herniated disk, or spasm of paravertebral muscles.

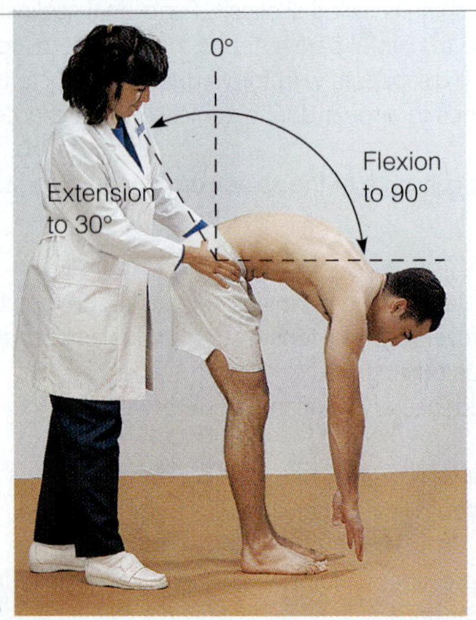

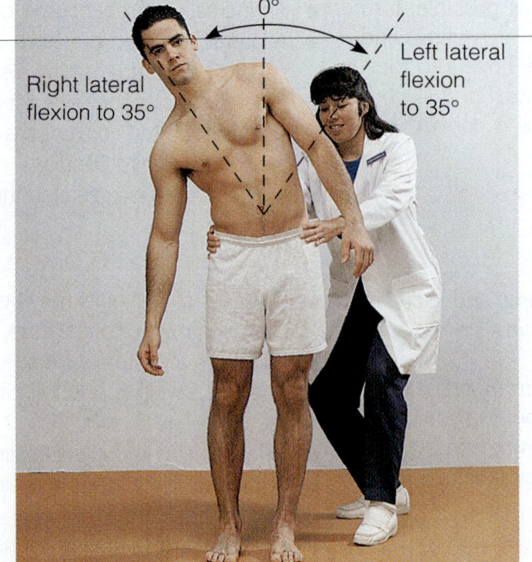

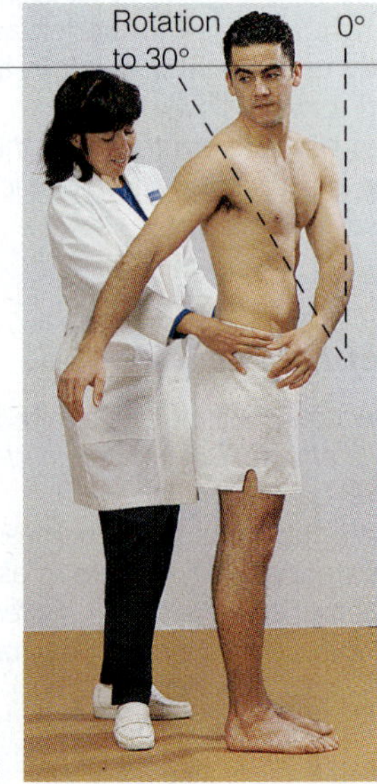

Figure 19–29 ■ *A*, Forward flexion of spine. *B*, Lateral flexion of spine. *C*, Rotation of spine.

Musculoskeletal Assessments (continued)

Technique/Normal Findings	Abnormal Findings
Fingers: Flexion: "Make a fist." Extension: "Open your hand." Abduction: "Spread your fingers." Adduction: "Close your fingers."	■ Flexion and extension of fingers are decreased in arthritis. ■ Heberden's nodes and Bouchard's nodes are hard, nontender nodules on the dorsolateral parts of the distal and proximal interphalangeal joints, respectively. They are common in osteoarthritis. ■ Stiff, painful, swollen finger joints are seen in acute RA. ■ Boutonnière and swan-neck deformities are seen in chronic RA. ■ Swollen finger joints with a white chalky discharge may be seen in chronic gout.
Wrists: 90-degree flexion: "Bend wrist down." 70-degree extension: "Bend wrist up." 55-degree ulnar deviation: "Bend wrist toward little finger." 20-degree radial deviation: "Bend wrist toward thumb."	■ Bilateral chronic swelling in the wrist is seen in arthritis.
Elbows: 160-degree flexion: "Touch your hands to your shoulders." 180-degree extension: "Straighten your elbows." 90-degree supination: "Bend your elbows 90 degrees and turn hands palm up." 90-degree pronation: "Bend your elbows 90 degrees and turn fists down."	■ Swollen, tender, inflamed elbows are apparent in gouty arthritis and RA. ■ Pain and tenderness at the lateral epicondyle occur in tennis elbow.
Shoulders: 180-degree flexion: "Hold your arms straight up and out." 50-degree hyperextension: "Put your straight arm behind your back." 90-degree internal rotation: "Put your forearm behind your lower back." 180-degree abduction: "Raise your straight arm up and out to your side." 50-degree adduction: "Put your straight arm across your chest."	■ Pain and tenderness over the biceps tendon occurs with **tendonitis** (inflammation of a tendon). ■ The arm cannot be abducted fully when the supraspinatus tendon of the shoulder is ruptured. ■ Pain and limited abduction also is seen with bursitis (inflammation of a bursa) and calcium deposits in this area.
Toes: 90-degree flexion: "Walk on your toes."	■ The great toe is excessively abducted in hallux valgus. ■ The joint above the great toe is swollen, inflamed, and painful in gouty arthritis. ■ There is hyperextension of the metatarsophalangeal joint and flexion of the proximal interphalangeal joint with hammer toes.
Ankles: 20-degree dorsiflexion: "Point your foot to the ceiling." 45-degree plantar flexion: "Point your foot to the floor." 30-degree inversion: "Walk on the outside of your feet." 20-degree eversion: "Walk on the inside of your feet."	■ Contractures of the Achilles tendon may occur in clients with RA or after prolonged bed rest.
Knees: 130-degree flexion: "Do a deep knee bend." 180-degree extension: "Sit down and hold your legs straight out in front of you."	■ Swelling over the suprapatellar pouch is seen with inflammation and fluid in the articular capsule of the knee. **Synovitis** is inflammation of the synovial membrane lining the articular capsule of a joint. It is common with knee trauma. ■ Swelling over the patella is seen in bursitis.
Hips: (The client is lying down.) 120-degree flexion: "Bring bent knee up to your chest." 30-degree hyperextension: "Lie on the abdomen and lift one leg at a time." 45-degree abduction: "Hold your leg straight and move it out to the side." 40-degree internal rotation: "Bend your knee and swing it toward your other leg." 45-degree external rotation: "Bend your knee and swing it out to the side."	■ Movement of the hip is limited and/or painful in arthritis.

(continued)

Musculoskeletal Assessments (continued)

Technique/Normal Findings	Abnormal Findings

Special Assessments

Perform Phalen's test. Ask the client to hold the wrist in acute flexion for 60 seconds (Figure 19–30 ■). *There should be no tingling, numbness, or pain.*

- Numbness and burning in the fingers during Phalen's test may indicate carpal tunnel syndrome.

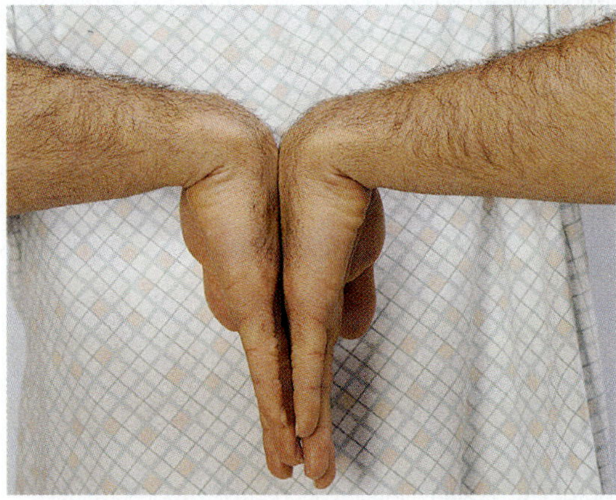

Figure 19–30 ■ Phalen's test.

Check for small amounts of fluid on the knee by conducting the bulge test. Milk upward on the medial side of the knee and then tap the lateral side of the patella (Figure 19–31 ■). *No bulge of fluid should appear on the medial side of the knee.*

- A fluid bulge indicates increased fluid in the knee joint rather than soft tissue swelling.

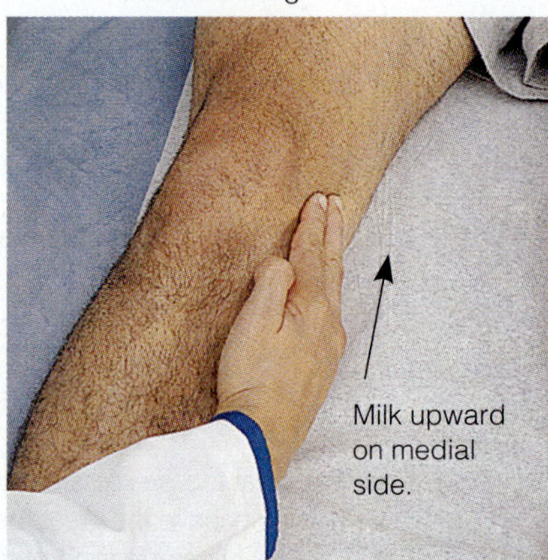
Milk upward on medial side.

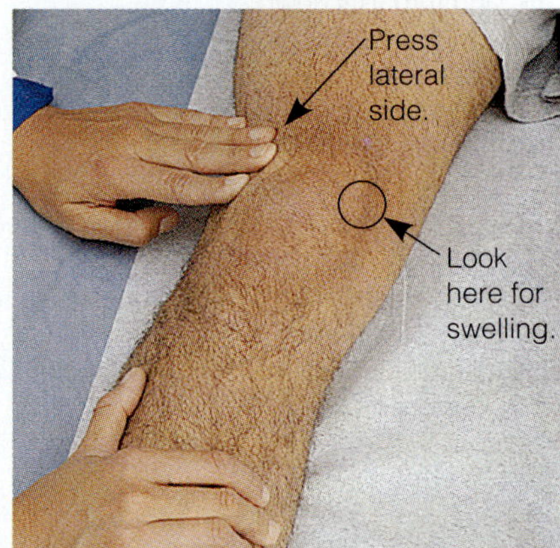
Press lateral side.
Look here for swelling.

Figure 19–31 ■ Checking for the bulge sign.

Check for large amounts of fluid in the knee by conducting the ballottement test. Apply downward pressure on the knee with one hand while pushing the patella backward against the femur with the other hand (Figure 19–32 ■). *There should be no movement of the patella. The patella should rest firmly over the femur.*

- Increased fluid will cause a tapping sound as the patella displaces the fluid and hits the femur.

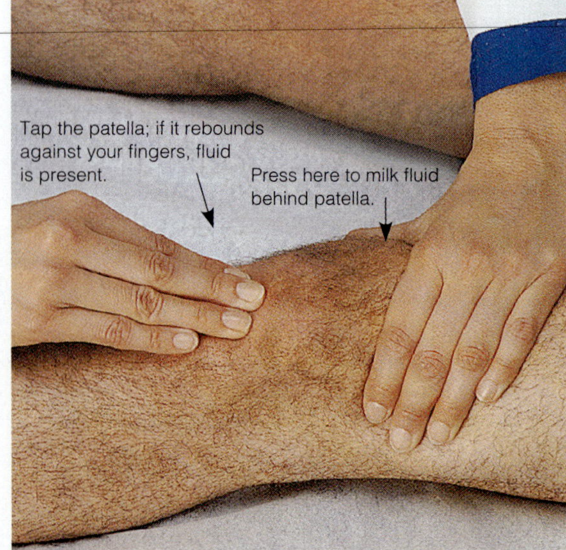
Tap the patella; if it rebounds against your fingers, fluid is present.
Press here to milk fluid behind patella.

Figure 19–32 ■ Checking for ballottement.

Musculoskeletal Assessments (continued)

Technique/Normal Findings	Abnormal Findings
Perform McMurray's test. While the client is reclining, ask the client to turn the flexed knee toward the center of the body. Stabilize the knee with one hand and apply pressure on the lower leg with the other hand (Figure 19–33 ■). *There should be no pain or clicking.*	■ Pain, locking (inability to fully extend the knee), or a popping sound may indicate an injury to a meniscus, a disk of cartilaginous tissue in the knee. 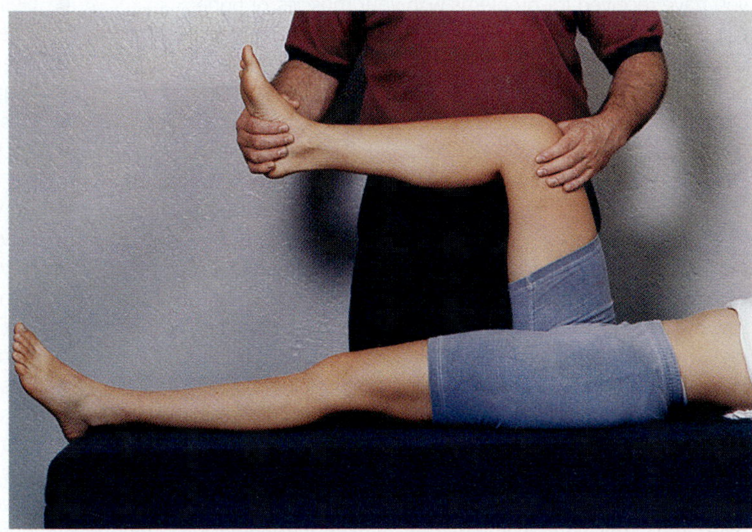 **Figure 19–33** ■ McMurray's test.
Perform the Thomas test. Ask the client to lie down and extend one leg while bringing the knee of the opposite leg to the chest (Figure 19–34 ■). *The extended leg should not rise off the table.*	■ A hip flexion contracture will cause the extended leg to rise off the table. 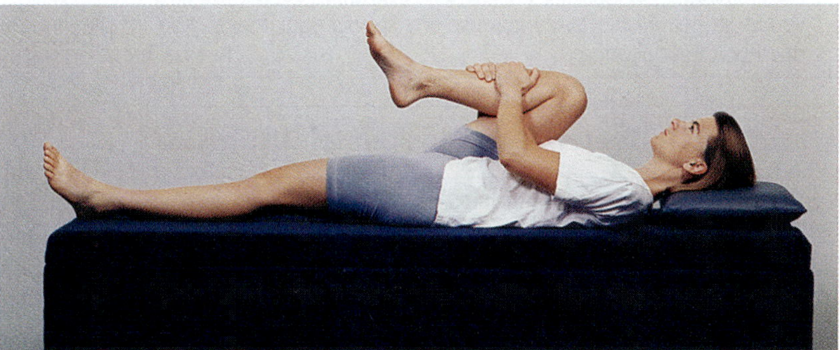 **Figure 19–34** ■ Thomas test for hip contracture.

Genetic Considerations

When conducting a health assessment interview and a physical assessment, it is important for the nurse to consider genetic influences on health of the adult. During the health assessment interview, ask about family members with health problems affecting musculoskeletal structure or function. In addition, ask about a family history of arthritis, abnormally long bones, children with muscular dystrophy, and amyotrophic lateral sclerosis (ALS) (Box 19–2). During the physical assessment, assess for any manifestations that might indicate a genetic disorder. If data are found to indicate genetic risk factors or alterations, ask about genetic testing and refer for appropriate genetic counseling and evaluation.

Assessment Interview Musculoskeletal System

INTERVIEW QUESTIONS AND LEADING STATEMENTS

- Have you ever had any muscle or bone diseases or injuries? If so, describe them.
- Describe any surgery, physical therapy, heat, or other treatments you have received for problems with your muscles or bones.
- List any medications such as muscle relaxants or prescribed or OTC medications and ointments that you use for musculoskeletal problems.
- Do you take any herbal or nutritional supplements for musculoskeletal problems? If so, what and how often?
- Describe your dietary intake in a typical 24-hour period. Does your diet include milk, cheese, cottage cheese, and vegetables? If so, how often?
- Do you take vitamins and/or additional calcium supplements? If so, what type and how often?
- Have you had a recent weight gain or loss? What do you see as your ideal weight?
- Have you had any redness or swelling in your joints?
- Does your musculoskeletal problem make it difficult for you to get to the bathroom?
- Describe your usual activities for a 24-hour period.
- Describe any musculoskeletal problems (e.g., weakness, stiffness, pain) that limit your ADL, such as driving, gardening, dressing, bathing, walking, climbing stairs, cooking, or cleaning.
- Has there been a change in your usual ability to move around? If so, describe the change.
- Do you regularly exercise or take part in strenuous activities such as heavy lifting? If so, describe the exercise/activity. If your job requires you to lift heavy objects, do you use any special equipment? If so, describe the equipment.
- Do you use any assistive devices (such as a cane or walker) to help you move around?
- Does having this problem with your musculoskeletal system interfere with your ability to rest and sleep? If so, how and what do you do?
- Describe any muscle, bone, or joint pain that you have. What relieves it or makes it worse?
- Describe any changes in the color, temperature, or sensations in your extremities.
- Describe any muscle weakness you are experiencing.
- Do you have stiffness in your joints when you wake up? Does it get better with movement?
- Do you ever have muscle cramps?
- How does having this condition make you feel about yourself?
- How has having this condition affected your relationships with others?
- Has having this condition interfered with your ability to work? If so, how?
- Has anyone in your family had problems with bone, joint, or muscle disease? If so, explain.
- Has this condition interfered with your usual sexual activity?
- Has having this condition created stress for you?
- Have you experienced any kind of stress that makes the condition worse? If so, explain.
- Describe what you do when you feel stressed.
- Describe how specific relationships or activities help you cope with this problem.
- Describe specific cultural beliefs or practices that affect how you care for and feel about this problem.
- Are there any specific treatments that you would not use to treat this problem?

Box 19–2 Inherited Musculoskeletal Disorders

- Myotonic dystrophy is an inherited disorder in which the muscles become weak, have a decreased ability to relax, and eventually waste away. Other parts of the body affected are mental deficiency, hair loss, and cataracts. Although rare, the disease does increase in severity with each successive generation.
- Marfan's syndrome, an autosomal dominant disorder of connective tissue, affects the bones, lungs, eyes, heart, and blood vessels. It is characterized by abnormally long extremities and is believed to have affected Abraham Lincoln. The aspect of the disease that is most life-threatening is the effect on the cardiovascular system. The average life span of a person with Marfan's syndrome is 30–40 years (Porth, 2005).
- Ellis-van Creveld syndrome is a rare genetic disorder characterized by a variety of physical alterations, including short-limb dwarfism, additional fingers or toes, malformed wrists, cardiac abnormalities, and partial tooth eruption.
- Duchenne muscular dystrophy, an X-linked disorder, affects primarily males. It is one of the most common muscular dystrophies and is characterized by rapid muscle degeneration early in life.
- Amyotropic lateral sclerosis (ALS) is a neurologic disease that affects the motor neurons in the spinal cord and brain, eventually resulting in paralysis and death.
- Other musculoskeletal diseases believed to have a genetic component include RA, osteoarthritis, gout, muscular dystrophy, ankylosing spondylitis, lupus erythematosus, and scleroderma.

DIAGNOSTIC TESTS

The results of diagnostic tests of musculoskeletal structure and function are used to support the diagnosis of a specific injury or disease, to provide information to identify or modify the appropriate medications or therapy used to treat the disease, and to help nurses monitor the client's responses to treatment and nursing care interventions. Diagnostic tests to assess the structures and functions of the musculoskeletal system are described in Appendix B and summarized in the bulleted list that follows.

- Blood tests are used to monitor levels of alkaline phosphatase, calcium, uric acid, and creatine kinase, which commonly are increased in bone and joint diseases and with muscle trauma (Table 19–6).
- Radiologic examinations, including x-rays, computed tomography (CT) scans, magnetic resonance imaging (MRI), and bone scans, identify and evaluate bone density and structure in conditions such as arthritis, intervertebral disk disease, musculoskeletal trauma, muscle tears, osteomyelitis, and bone tumors.
- Bone density examinations (dual energy x-ray absorptiometry [DEXA], quantitative ultrasound [QUS], and bone mineral density [BMD]) evaluate bone mineral density and evaluate the degree of osteoporosis.
- An arthroscopy uses a fiber-optic endoscope to examine the joint interior, to diagnose diseases, and to perform surgery.

TABLE 19–6 **Blood Tests With Purposes Specific to the Musculoskeletal System**

NAME OF TEST	PURPOSE
Alkaline phosphatase (ALP)	To identify bone diseases; increased in bone cancer, Paget's disease, healing fractures, RA, and osteoporosis
Calcium (Ca)	To monitor calcium levels and detect calcium imbalances; decreased with lack of calcium and vitamin D intake and with malabsorption from the gastrointestinal (GI) tract; increased in bone cancer and multiple fractures
Phosphorus (P)	To assess phosphorus levels; increased with bone tumors and phosphate (PO_4) healing fractures
Rheumatoid factor (RF)	To diagnose RA (positive for RA at >1:80); also increased in lupus erythematosus and scleroderma
Uric acid	To diagnose and monitor the treatment of gout; panic level considered >12 mg/dL
Human leukocyte antigen	To diagnose diseases such as juvenile RA and ankylosing spondylitis
Creatine kinase (CK)	To diagnose muscle trauma or disease; increased in muscular dystrophy and traumatic injuries (specifically, CPK-MM isoenzyme)

An arthrocentesis withdraws fluid from a joint by needle aspiration.

- Both electromyogram (EMG) and somatosensory evoked potential (SSEP) are tests of the electrical activity of skeletal muscle.

Regardless of the type of diagnostic test, the nurse is responsible for explaining the procedure and any special preparation needed, for assessing for medication use that may affect the outcome of the tests, for supporting the client during the examination as necessary, for documenting the procedures as appropriate, and for monitoring the results of the tests.

CARING INTERVENTIONS

Rehabilitative nursing is the process of restoring a person's ability to live and work in as normal a manner as possible. Rehabilitative nursing involves the prevention and correction of alterations in the musculoskeletal system. To assist clients to achieve and maintain optimal mobility, both preservative and restorative methods are used.

Preservative methods, such as exercises and assisted ambulation, include those interventions that are needed to help clients maintain their normal mobility. Hospitalization adds another level of care to rehabilitative nursing. Because the changes that occur in the human body when a person is hospitalized are varied and subtle, preservative methods are used with every client. Restorative methods, such as crutch walking and splinting, are used with clients who have decreased mobility caused by factors such as debilitating illness or major surgery. Restorative methods are applied to assist the client in achieving the level of mobility enjoyed before becoming ill.

The general goals for using these methods are to assist the client to strive for optimal function, to prevent further injury, and to restore normal function. To achieve these goals of care, it is important for the nurse to embrace the philosophy underlying rehabilitative nursing: that every illness is accompanied by the intrinsic threat of disability and that this part of total client care must begin with the initial client contact. Finally, it is important for the nurse to accept that the principles of rehabilitation are basic to the care of all clients and that rehabilitation must begin early in the client's hospitalization.

Being hospitalized and immobile seriously affects a person's body image, behavior, and overall adaptation and adjustment. The greater the disability, the more these aspects of a person's life are affected. The nurse's responsibility in providing total client care is to be aware of these responses and to take them into account when developing a client care plan.

Exercise

Muscles that are not used become weak and shortened. During prolonged bed rest, strength and endurance decrease rapidly. Clients can regain muscle strength and mobility by practicing specific groups of exercises daily. Promoting exercise, both passive and active, is one of the most important nursing functions. The purpose of exercises is to promote proper alignment, prevent contractures, stimulate circulation, and prevent thrombophlebitis and pressure ulcers. Exercise reduces joint pain and stiffness and increases flexibility and endurance. Exercise also prevents edema of the extremities and promotes lung expansion.

The nurse both performs and teaches several types of exercises as a component of providing total client care. Passive exercises are carried out by the therapist or nurse without assistance from the client. These exercises enable the client to retain as much joint ROM as possible, as well as stimulating circulation. Active exercises, although supervised by the nurse, are performed by the client. These exercises increase muscle strength when the client is partially immobile.

Resistive exercises, another rehabilitative measure, provide resistance in order to increase muscle power. These active exercises are performed by the individual working against resistance. Isometric or muscle-setting activities are similar to resistive exercises. These exercises maintain strength in a muscle when the joint is immobilized. They are performed by the individual without assistance.

Range-of-motion exercises are the most common form of exercises for maintaining joint mobility and increasing maximal motion of a joint when the client is totally or partially immobilized. These exercises are completed by the nurse or physical therapist (PT). The therapist puts an extremity through its full range so that the joint is moved through all of the appropriate planes. Before beginning these exercises, it is important that the therapist and/or nurse assess the client's condition and the baseline ROM capabilities, establish the extent of ROM to be carried out, and ensure that the client is comfortable. Because clients may be fearful of this type of exercise, a full explanation of what is going to be done is helpful for allaying clients' fears. Enlist the cooperation of the client for maximum benefit. Discontinue all ROM exercises if the client complains of pain because at this point the exercises become counterproductive.

Ambulation

Ambulation, or walking, is an important function that most people accomplish automatically, that is, without thinking or conscious effort. When a person has been immobilized, confined to bed following surgery or an injury, or unable to ambulate, this seemingly simple activity can become a major hurdle to overcome. The longer a person is immobilized, the more difficult it is to regain ambulatory ability; likewise, the sooner a person begins to ambulate after being bedridden, the more easily the person will regain preimmobilization status. Early ambulation decreases hospitalization time and prevents complications such as paralytic ileus and thrombophlebitis.

The human body functions best when it is frequently placed in a vertical position. Ambulation improves physical and mental well-being. Ambulation increases muscle strength and joint mobility. It also increases respiratory exchange, GI muscle tone, and circulation. Without stress on bones, calcium deposits occur and renal problems increase from calcium-based calculi.

Balance, coordination, and good body alignment are important aspects for walking. One must be able to move forward and maintain an upright balance; use muscles, bones, and joints correctly for coordination; and keep the head erect and vertebral column fairly straight with feet and knee caps pointed forward in order to maintain good body alignment.

The major muscle groups used for walking are the thigh and leg muscles. If these muscles have not been used or exercised because the client has been in bed for a long time, ambulation must be accomplished step-by-step. Weak muscles cannot support a human frame for the mechanics of walking. It is important, then, to begin the process of ambulation by administering muscle-strengthening exercises. Several different types of exercises were described previously; however, the most important preambulatory preparation is quadriceps-setting and gluteal-setting exercises. Carried out several times a day, these exercises restore muscle strength and prepare the legs for weight bearing.

Before assisting the client with walking, explain precisely what you are going to do and prepare the client by completing the ambulatory procedure in stages. For example, begin with the muscle-strengthening exercises. Then assist the client with sitting up in bed to determine whether vertigo ensues. Have the client move to the side of the bed with legs down, and only when the client is ready and feels comfortable doing so, assist the client to stand beside the bed. You may decide to take the client's vital signs after dangling to determine if they are stable. Allow the client to remain standing with the bed as support until he or she feels secure. Finally, and with the assistance of one or two nurses (depending on the assessment of the client's ability and readiness to ambulate), have the client walk by taking short steps and walking only as long as tolerated. By doing this several times a day, it will not be long before the client's legs are strengthened and the client can graduate to one assistant, a walker, or a cane. Throughout this procedure, do not allow the client to lose confidence in the ability to walk or your ability to support and assist while regaining the client's independence of action.

Assistive Devices

A variety of assistive devices are available to give the client support when ambulating. Assistive devices are used to relieve the client's body weight to enable the client to ambulate. Canes relieve about 40% of the weight mainly attributable to the lower limb. Walkers and crutches allow for complete non-weight-bearing ambulation. Such devices may give the client confidence (especially important with the elderly), stability, or support for a weak limb or may reduce the pressure on a limb. These devices may include canes (standard cane, T-handled cane, tripod cane, and quad cane) and walkers (standard, with wheels, or a hemi-walker). Crutches are another type of assistive device used to lessen or remove weight from one or both legs.

CRUTCHES Crutches aid walking by providing support during ambulation when the lower extremities are unable to support the body weight. It is hoped that this situation is temporary, but even if it is permanent, crutches allow independence of movement that otherwise could not occur.

There are three main types of crutches: the axillary (most common for short-term use); the Lofstrand, or Canadian (a forearm crutch with a metal band and handle); and the platform, for clients who are unable to use their wrists to bear weight.

Several safety factors should be taken into account before assisting the client in using crutches. The measurement should be 5 cm (2 inches) from the axillary fold to the crutch bar. The handpiece should be adjusted to allow 20–30° elbow flexion, and rubber suction tips should be placed on the bottom of the crutches. Finally, the client should be informed that while using crutches, well-fitting shoes with nonslip soles should be worn.

The type of crutch the client will use depends on the ability to ambulate, the muscle strength needed for support, and the individual needs of the client.

WALKERS Walkers assist the client with balance and with walking. The client's arms are used to support all or part of the client's body and take weight off the lower limbs while ambulating.

Walkers are a necessary assistive device for postoperative clients requiring help with ambulation. These clients include those with major spinal cord surgery or hip replacement surgery or those who were/are debilitated from major surgery and are unsteady with ambulation.

Walkers are constructed with or without wheels, or platforms. Wheels are on only the front legs of the walker to prevent falls and possible injury. All walkers have rubber tips that must be observed frequently to ensure that they are in good repair.

The height of the walker is adjusted by lowering or raising the legs of the extension piece to properly fit the client's height.

CANES Canes are used to protect clients from falls. Clients who are unsteady, lose their balance, are weak, or have a leg(s) that cannot hold them in an upright position are candidates for canes.

Using a cane affords the client the confidence to ambulate and maintain independence. Canes, like crutches, are measured for a proper fit. The cane is turned upside down with the handle on the floor, and the rubber tip is removed. Instruct the client to stand with arms at the sides of the body. The correct measurement is marked with the tip of the cane facing upward at the level of the wrist. The cane is cut (if a wooden cane) 1/2 inch shorter than the mark. Aluminum canes can be adjusted within 1 inch of the desired height.

PHARMACOLOGIC THERAPIES

Medications used to treat musculoskeletal disorders are often focused on palliative rather than curative care. Pain relief, reduction of inflammation, and relieving muscle spasm are the primary goals of pharmacological therapy.

MEDICATIONS Musculoskeletal Disorders

Classification	Mechanism of Action	Generic Names	Nursing Considerations
Centrally acting skeletal muscle relaxants	Act at various levels of the central nervous system (CNS) by inhibiting upper motor neuron activity, causing CNS depressant effects or altering simple spinal reflexes	cyclobenzaprine hydrochloride, diazepam, lorazepam, metaxalone, methocarbamol	Provide education regarding medication usage and monitor compliance. Avoid in clients with liver disease. Monitor for sedation effects and caution clients to avoid driving or using heavy equipment while taking. Because of CNS depressant activity, monitor respirations when client is first beginning therapy.
Direct acting antispasmodic drugs	May interfere with release of calcium ions in skeletal muscles (dantrolene) or block the release of acetylcholine from cholinergic nerve terminals	dantrolene sodium, botulinum toxin type A	Remember that these may be contraindicated in clients with liver disease, compromised pulmonary functions, or cardiac dysfunction. Assess for jaundice and monitor liver enzymes. Understand that caregiver assistance may be needed if client is unable to self-medicate.
Analgesics—both narcotic and nonnarcotic	Narcotic analgesics are CNS depressants, and both types act by the "gate control" mechanism described in the concept that discusses comfort.	Nonnarcotic: acetaminophen, NSAIDs such as ibuprofen or naproxen Narcotic: morphine sulfate, oxycodone, meperidine	Monitor pain levels, vital signs, and response to analgesic. Monitor respiratory status when administering narcotic analgesics. Teach proper self-administration. Monitor for GI side effects.
NSAIDs	Inhibit pain mediators at the nociceptor level, inhibiting prostaglandins	ibuprofen, indomethacin, aspirin, tramadol	Administer oral versions with food to reduce potential GI side effects. Avoid use in clients with liver, kidney, or peptic ulcer disease. Teach proper self-administration.

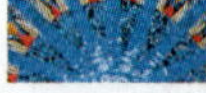

19.1 BACK PROBLEMS

KEY TERMS

BASIS FOR SELECTION OF EXEMPLAR

Healthy People 2010
Institute of Medicine

LEARNING OUTCOMES

After reading about this exemplar, you will be able to:

1. Describe the pathophysiology, etiology, clinical manifestations, and direct and indirect causes of back problems.
2. Identify risk factors associated with back problems.
3. Illustrate the nursing process in providing culturally competent care across the life span for individuals with back problems.
4. Formulate priority nursing diagnoses appropriate for an individual with back problems.
5. Create a plan of care for individuals with back problems and their family members.
6. Assess expected outcomes for an individual with back problems.
7. Discuss therapies used in the collaborative care of an individual with back problems.
8. Employ evidence-based caring interventions for an individual with back problems.

OVERVIEW

Back problems are one of the most common alterations in mobility. They are a source of great pain and frustration. Individuals with chronic back problems often find themselves losing some degree of quality of life, including lost work hours.

When back problems arise, people typically try to attribute the cause to activity or movement at the time of injury or appearance of pain. However, back problems often result from years of improper bending, lifting, and standing over time, culminating in acute exacerbation or injury when one event acts as "the straw that broke the camel's back." Due to the variety of causes of back problems, it is difficult to estimate accurately the number of people who experience back problems or injury each year. For the same reason, it is important not to underestimate the prevalence of back problems and their affect on individuals.

A number of physical conditions can result in back problems. More than 50% of women experience backache during pregnancy due primarily to exaggeration of the lumbosacral curve that occurs as the uterus enlarges and becomes heavier (Johnson, Gregory, & Niebyl, 2007). Common occurrences such as bad posture and sleeping habits, poor physical conditioning, and bad workplace ergonomic conditions often lead to aching backs. Scoliosis, or curvature of the spine, is most often diagnosed in school-age and adolescent children. Herniated disk can occur at any age but is most commonly diagnosed in adulthood. Low back pain can be the result of mechanical injury or trauma that causes strains in the muscles and tendons of the back, with the potential to cause muscle spasms that can be extremely painful. Low back pain also can result from degenerative disorders (spondylosis, spinal stenosis, or osteoarthritis), systemic disorders (osteomyelitis, osteoporosis, or neoplasms), referred pain (GI, genitourinary [GU], or gynecologic disorders; abdominal aortic aneurysm; or hip pathology), and other disorders such as fibromyalgia. This exemplar will deal with two common causes of back problems—herniated disk and scoliosis.

Herniated Disk

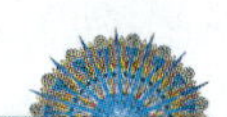

A **herniated intervertebral disk** (also called a ruptured disk, a herniated nucleus pulposus, or a slipped disk) is a rupture of the cartilage surrounding the intervertebral disk with protrusion of the nucleus pulposus (Figure 19–35 ■). Perhaps few neuro-orthopedic disorders are as challenging as those involving the intervertebral disks. Clients with herniation (rupture) of a disk experience excruciating pain and limited mobility. These problems may in turn cause alterations in role function, coping, and the ability to perform ADL.

PATHOPHYSIOLOGY AND ETIOLOGY

The intervertebral disks, located between the vertebral bodies, are made of an inner nucleus pulposus and an outer collar (the annulus fibrosus). The disks allow the spine to absorb compression by acting as shock absorbers. A herniated intervertebral disk occurs when the nucleus pulposus protrudes through

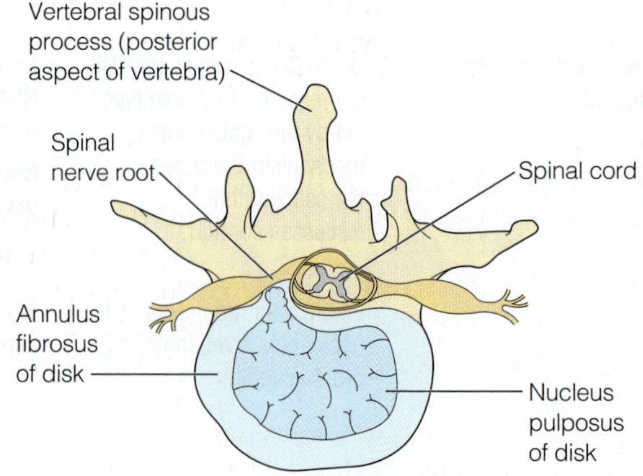

Figure 19–35 ■ A herniated intervertebral disk. The herniated nucleus pulposus is applying pressure against the nerve root.

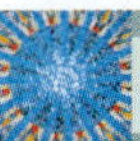

EVIDENCE-BASED PRACTICE Backpack Use and Pain

Problem

Many children wear backpacks that are heavy and that they carry for large parts of the day. Lower back, neck, and shoulder pain seem to be increasing in children, and a possible connection with backpacks has been suggested. About half of youth report back and shoulder pain, most of which is associated with carrying heavy items (Rateau, 2004).

Evidence

Several studies have investigated the relationship between backpack use and complaints of pain. In one study, 1,126 youth from 12–18 years completed a questionnaire about backpack use and their health. They also had physical measurements completed. Almost 75% of the youth had back pain, and the pain was associated with being in poor general health, being overweight, being female, and carrying heavier backpacks (Sheir-Neiss, Kruse, Rahman, Jacobsen, & Pelli, 2003). In another study of 745 adolescents, 45% had back pain and 6% suffered severe neck and shoulder pain. The weight of backpacks was not associated with incidence of pain reports in this study (van Gent, Dols, de Rover, Hira Sing, & de Vet, 2003).

Implications

A clear association between complaints of pain and backpack use and weight is not evident. Therefore, nurses should ask about backpack use at health promotion visits and advise youth how to wear their backpacks. The American Academy of Pediatrics lists the following recommendations for backpack use:

- Have wide, padded shoulder straps and wear the pack on both shoulders, close to the body.
- Use a padded back and waist strap.
- Wear the backpack over both shoulders and evenly distribute its weight.
- Make sure the backpack is lightweight (no more than 10–20% of the youth's weight) or consider a rolling pack.
- Practice back strengthening exercises and learn to bend at the knees.

Critical Thinking

How will you partner with youth who participate in after-school sports to plan how to carry school items and sports gear safely? What exercises can you recommend to help strengthen the back and thighs for carrying a pack?

a weakened or torn annulus fibrosus of an intervertebral disk (Figure 19–35 ■). This protrusion may occur anywhere along the vertebral column, but herniation of thoracic disks is uncommon. The protrusion may occur spontaneously or as a result of trauma, with trauma (e.g., lifting heavy objects or falling) causing about half of all cases. Rupture of the disk allows herniation of the nucleus pulposus in a posterolateral direction, with compression of the associated nerve root. The resulting pressure on adjacent spinal nerves causes characteristic manifestations, which vary with the location and the amount of protruding disk material. Occasionally, the herniation is central rather than posterolateral, with pressure on the spinal cord.

The herniation may be abrupt or gradual. Lifting incorrectly or suddenly twisting the spine can cause rupture with immediate intense pain and muscle spasms. Gradual herniation is the result of degenerative changes, osteoarthritis, or ankylosis spondylitis. Clients with a gradual herniation have a slow onset of pain and neurologic deficits.

Etiology

As the body ages, the nucleus pulposus of the intervertebral disk loses fluid content and the disks are less able to absorb shocks. The disks become smaller and slip out of place more easily. Aging causes degeneration in the annulus fibrosus and the posterior longitudinal ligaments, and the vertebrae and disks are less able to respond to movement and are more easily injured. The majority of herniated disks occur in the lumbar region (L4 or L5 to S1); when disks herniate in the cervical region, they most commonly do so at C6 to C7. Multiple herniations are not common, occurring in only about 10% of all clients (Hickey, 2003).

Risk Factors

A herniated intervertebral disk may occur at any adult age. However, it is more common as people enter middle age and age-related changes occur. Herniated intervertebral disks are more common in men than women. Most clients are between the ages of 30 and 50.

CLINICAL MANIFESTATIONS

Lumbar Disks

The classic manifestation of a ruptured lumbar disk is recurrent episodes of pain in the lower back. The pain typically radiates across the buttock and down the posterior leg, although it may be experienced only in the leg. **Sciatica** is a term used to describe lumbar back pain that radiates down the posterior leg to the ankle and is increased by sneezing or coughing (the result of pressure on nerve roots L4, L5, S1, S2, or S3, which give rise to the sciatic nerve). Sciatica may be elicited by straight-leg raising: The client feels pain when lifting one leg while dorsiflexing the foot of that leg. Sciatica pain varies in intensity, ranging from mildly uncomfortable to excruciating. It is aggravated by a variety of positions and activities, including sitting, straining, coughing, sneezing, climbing stairs, walking, and riding in a car.

Other manifestations include postural deformity, motor deficits, sensory deficits, and changes in reflexes. In about 60% of clients with ruptured lumbar disks, the normal lumbar lordosis is absent. When standing, the client typically has a slight forward tilt to the trunk, scoliosis of the lumbar spine, slight flexion of the hip and knee on the affected side, and paravertebral muscle spasms (Hickey, 2003). Motor deficits include weakness and in some clients problems with sexual function and urinary elimination. Sensory deficits include paresthesia and numbness. Knee and ankle reflexes are decreased or absent.

Cervical Disk Manifestations

Cervical disks that herniate laterally cause pain in the shoulder, neck, and arm. Other manifestations of lateral cervical herniation include paresthesia, muscle spasms and stiff neck, and decreased or absent arm reflexes (Box 19–3). Central cervical herniations result in mild, intermittent pain; however, the client also may experience lower extremity weakness, unsteady gait, muscle spasms, urinary elimination problems, altered sexual function, and hyperactive lower extremity reflexes.

PRACTICE ALERT

Maintaining good posture and using proper body mechanics throughout pregnancy can help prevent backache. The pregnant woman is advised to avoid bending over at the waist to pick up objects and should bend from the knees instead (Figure 19–36 ■). She should place her feet 12–18 inches apart to maintain body balance. If the woman uses work surfaces that require her to bend, the nurse can advise the woman to adjust the height of the surfaces.

COLLABORATION

Considerations for the client with a ruptured intervertebral disk include identifying the location of herniation and determining whether conservative treatment or surgery is indicated. Nursing care is directed toward preparing clients for diagnostic tests and providing teaching and care for the client who has either medical or surgical intervention. Collaborative care for the client with a ruptured intervertebral disk may include any of the following: nurses, physicians, chiropractors, pharmacists, physical therapists, massage therapists, and acupuncturists.

Diagnostic Tests

Diagnostic tests differentiate the cause of back pain; for example, back and leg pain also may be caused by spinal tumors, degenerative processes, and abdominal diseases. The tests include x-rays and CT scans of the lumbosacral or cervical area to identify skeletal deformities and narrowing of the disk spaces. Electromyography (EMG), which measures electrical activity of skeletal muscles at rest and during voluntary contraction, may be conducted to identify specific muscles affected by the pressure of the herniation on the nerve roots.

A myelogram with contrast medium is done to illustrate areas of herniation, although it does not provide the detail found with CT or MRI. However, myelography is diagnostic in 80–90% of all cases and is used to rule out tumors and locate the herniation.

Pharmacologic Therapies

The client with a ruptured intervertebral disk is treated with medications to relieve pain and reduce swelling and muscle spasms. Pain is usually managed with NSAIDs. Muscle spasms are treated with muscle relaxants. Nurses working with the clients should teach them about side effects, contraindications, and avoiding over the counter medications that include similar medications that can result in toxicity.

Treatment

A ruptured intervertebral disk may be treated through conservative means or with surgery.

CONSERVATIVE TREATMENT A ruptured intervertebral disk is usually managed conservatively unless the client is experiencing severe neurologic deficits. The goals of treatment are relieving pain and healing the involved disk by fibrosis. Conservative treatment is usually prescribed for 2–6 weeks. If the client continues to have pain after that time, surgery may

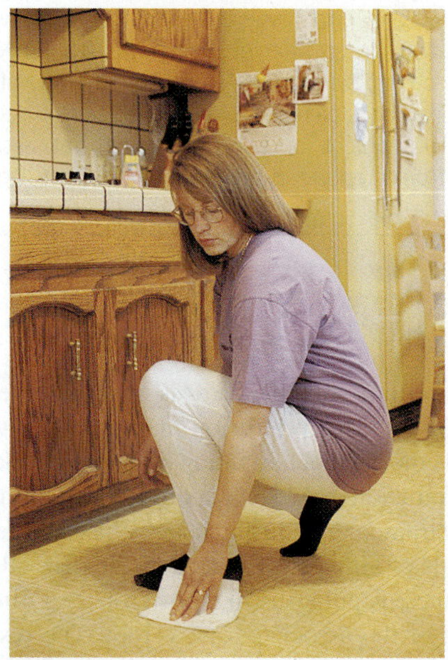

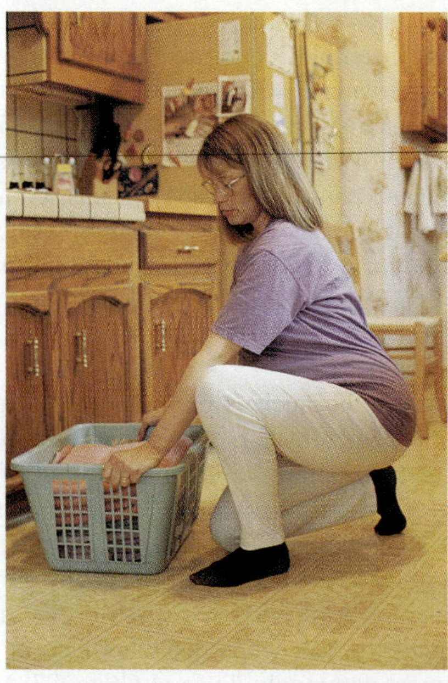

Figure 19–36 ■ When picking up objects from floor level or lifting objects, the pregnant woman needs to use proper body mechanics.

Box 19–3 Manifestations of a Ruptured Intervertebral Disk

L4 TO L5 LEVEL (AFFECTS FIFTH LUMBAR NERVE ROOT)

- Pain in hip, lower back, posterolateral thigh, anterior leg, dorsal surface of foot, great toe
- Muscle spasms in affected areas
- Paresthesia over lateral leg and web of great toe
- Foot drop (rare)
- Decreased or absent ankle reflex
- Cauda equina syndrome (with complete nerve root compression): bowel and bladder incontinence, paralysis of lower extremities

L5 TO S1 LEVEL (AFFECTS FIRST SACRAL NERVE ROOT)

- Pain in midgluteal region, posterior thigh, calf to heel, plantar surface of the foot to the fourth and fifth toes
- Paresthesia in posterior calf and lateral heel, foot, and toes
- Difficulty walking on toes

C5 TO C6 LEVEL (AFFECTS SIXTH CERVICAL NERVE ROOT)

- Pain in neck, shoulder, anterior upper arm, radial area of forearm, thumb
- Paresthesia of forearm, thumb, forefinger, and lateral arm
- Decreased biceps and supinator reflex
- Triceps reflex normal to hyperactive

be considered. The treatment regimen depends on the severity of the manifestations. Decreasing activity level with bed rest is no longer recommended. In many cases, the client is advised to continue with normal activities while taking prescribed medications for pain, inflammation, and muscle spasms.

Medications used to treat back pain include nonnarcotic analgesics, anti-inflammatory drugs such as the NSAIDs, muscle relaxants, and sedatives/tranquilizers.

SURGERY Surgery is indicated for clients who do not respond to conservative management or who have serious neurologic deficits. Several surgical interventions are used to treat a ruptured intervertebral disk. The type of surgery chosen depends on the location of the disk and the stability of the spinal column.

- A **laminectomy**, the type of surgery most often performed, is the removal of a part of the vertebral lamina. The surgery is done to relieve pressure on the nerves. It is often combined with removal of the protruding nucleus pulposus (**nuclectomy**). A **diskectomy** is the removal of the nucleus pulposus of an intervertebral disk. A diskectomy may be performed alone or along with a laminectomy.
- **Spinal fusion** is the insertion of a wedge-shaped piece of bone or bone chips between the vertebrae to stabilize them. The bone is usually taken from a client donor site such as the iliac crest. A spinal fusion also may be performed through a spinal implant with a device called a BAK (a hollow titanium cylinder with holes), which is packed with grafted bone from a donor site and placed in the space where a disk is removed. Although not appropriate for all clients requiring a spinal fusion, this does facilitate a short hospital stay and convalescence.
- **Foraminotomy** is an enlargement of the opening between the disk and the facet joint to remove bony overgrowth compressing the nerve. The location and size of the incision vary according to the surgeon's preference and the location and size of the ruptured disk. The posterior approach is taken for lumbar surgery. Either the posterior or anterior approach may be taken for cervical disks.

CLINICAL MANIFESTATIONS AND THERAPIES Back Problems

ETIOLOGY	CLINICAL MANIFESTATION	CLINICAL THERAPIES
Pregnancy changes the center of gravity as the fetus grows in the uterus, exaggerating the lumbar curvature and resulting in low back pain.	Waddling gait, difficulty standing or walking for extended periods of time without pain	Pregnant women should be encouraged to use good posture when sitting and standing.
Low back pain often results from herniation of the disk due to pressure placed on nerves exiting the spinal column or to postural abnormalities	Pain in the area of herniation may radiate to other areas depending on location. Most commonly, sciatica is experienced when herniation occurs in a lumbar disk, causing pain that radiates across the buttocks and down the leg.	Medical management may include: ■ Application of heat or cold ■ Analgesics ■ Proper positioning and posture ■ Use of firm, supportive mattress. If medical management is insufficient, surgery may be performed to correct or remove the herniated disk or to stabilize the vertebrae and remove pressure from surrounding nerves.
Scoliosis	Curvature of the spine is visible upon assessment	■ Braces to maintain straight posture ■ Surgical repair

- **Intradiscal electrothermal therapy (IDET)** uses thermal energy to treat pain from a bulging spinal disk. A special needle is inserted into the disk and heated to a high temperature. The heat thickens and seals the disk wall and decreases bulging of the disk.
- A microdiskectomy, in which microsurgical techniques are used, is performed through a very small incision. This type of surgery decreases the possibility of trauma to surrounding structures during surgery and allows early postoperative mobility and a short hospital stay.

Complementary and Alternative Therapies

Many clients with back problems will seek complimentary and alternative therapies in an attempt to alleviate pain and prevent surgery. Chiropractice, massage therapy and acupuncture are forms of complimentary alternative medicine frequently used by clients with back problems.

CHIROPRACTIC THERAPY Back pain is a leading cause of disability and the second most common reason (after the common cold) people visit a doctor. Chiropractors have two times the number of visits for back pain as conventional physicians. Most chiropractors also treat peripheral joints—elbows, knees, and shoulders. In 1994, a panel for the Agency for Health Care Policy and Research of the U.S. Department of Health and Human Services concluded that spinal manual therapy speeds recovery from acute low back pain and recommended it either in combination with or as a replacement for nonsteroidal anti-inflammatory drugs.

MASSAGE THERAPY **Massage therapy**, the scientific manipulation of the soft tissues of the body, is a healing art, an act of physical caring, and a way of communicating without words. Massage, a hands-on touch therapy, has reached out to an ever-widening U.S. audience. Massage is now the third most common form of alternative treatment in the United States, after chiropractic and relaxation techniques. The goal of massage therapy is to achieve or increase health and well-being and to help the body heal itself. Although massage therapists may hold general views of health and well-being, massage therapy has no specific theoretical framework or diagnostic system of disease. The physical benefits that massage therapy may provide to clients with ruptured disks include the following:

- Relief of muscle tension and stiffness
- Reduction in muscle spasms and tension
- More efficient recovery from exertion
- Improvement in joint flexibility and range of motion
- Improvement in posture
- Stimulation of lymphatic circulation, which decreases edema.

ACUPUNCTURE Acupuncture is effective in the treatment of acute and chronic pain and motion disabilities. Acupuncture involves stimulating specific anatomic points called *hsueh* where each meridian passes close to the skin surface. Puncturing the skin with very fine needles is the usual method but practitioners may also use pressure (shiatsu), friction, suction, heat, or electromagnetic energy to stimulate points. The primary goal of acupuncture is the manipulation of energy flow throughout the body following a thorough assessment by a practioner of Traditional Chinese Medicine.

CLIENT TEACHING Proper Body Mechanics

Proper body mechanics may help prevent the occurrence of a ruptured intervertebral disk. Teaching the proper method of lifting and moving heavy objects should begin when children enter school. This information also should be given to workers (including nurses) who have lifting as part of their responsibilities. The guidelines for proper body mechanics are as follows:

- Begin activities by spreading the feet apart to broaden the base of support.
- Use the large muscles of the arms to lift and the legs to push when lifting.
- Work as closely as possible to the object that is to be lifted or moved.
- Slide, roll, push, or pull an object rather than lift it.
- When lifting, bend the knees and lift up over your center of gravity.
- When lifting, use a back support belt.

NURSING PROCESS

Nursing care for the client with a ruptured intervertebral disk may be provided through information in community and work settings, during conservative treatment, and during pre- and postoperative treatment. The pain of the ruptured disk is often discouraging and debilitating and is likely to affect the client's ability to work.

Assessment

The following data are collected through the health history and physical examination.

- *Health history.* Type of employment, risk factors, characteristics of pain (location, duration, intensity), history of previous injury, types of sports and recreational activities
- *Physical assessment.* Muscle strength and coordination, sensation, reflexes

Diagnosis

Nursing diagnoses for the client with a herniated disk include the following:

- Acute pain
- Chronic pain
- Constipation.

Plan

Goals of nursing care include the following:

- Client will report diminished pain to a tolerable level that allows for performance of ADLs.

- Client explains proper use of medications prescribed for pain control.
- Client maintains quality of life and is able to maintain normal activities.

Implementation

Nursing care for clients with a herniated intervertebral disk focuses largely on pain management, both during conservative management and after surgery (Box 19–4).

Acute Pain

Clients with a ruptured intervertebral disk experience acute back and leg pain. Acute pain may be related to preoperative muscle spasms or nerve root compression. After surgery, the client may have pain at the site of the incision and in the surgical area.

- Assess the degree of pain on a scale of 0–10 (10 being the greatest pain) and identify contributing and relieving factors. *Pain is a subjective experience. The nurse needs to assess it thoroughly before initiating interventions.*
- Use a firm mattress or place a board under the mattress. *A firm bed supports the spinal column and muscles.*
- Teach the client to avoid turning or twisting the spinal column and to assume positions that decrease stress on the vertebral column (e.g., when in the supine position, flex the hips slightly). A small pillow may be placed under the knees (for clients with a herniated lumbar disk) or under the neck (for clients with a herniated cervical disk). *Correct body positions can decrease intradisk pressure.*
- Provide analgesic medications around the clock. *Intense pain can increase muscle spasms; maintaining serum levels of analgesics often prevents severe pain.*

Chronic Pain

The client with a ruptured intervertebral disk often has pain for an extended period of time. Despite conservative treatment or previous surgery, pain may be ongoing or intermittent. If previous surgery has not relieved the pain, the client may be depressed or angry. Caring for a client with chronic pain is frustrating, and the client is often regarded as difficult.

- Treat the client's reports of pain with respect. *The client is the person experiencing the pain and thus is the expert about it.*
- Do not refer to the client as being addicted to pain medication. *All types of pain medications may be used legitimately to manage pain.*
- Monitor the client carefully for any changes in condition. *Significant changes in the client's condition may go unrecognized when pain is present for a prolonged period of time.*
- Maintain individualized written plans of care for pain management and ensure continuity of care. *When the client makes several visits (for instance, to an emergency department [ED] or a pain clinic), written records help caregivers determine what is and is not effective in managing pain.*
- Teach the client alternative methods of pain management. Consider the client's coping style when recommending methods. *Clients who have a passive coping style are often better able to manage pain by depending on others, taking medications, and resting. Clients with an active coping style are probably better able to manage pain by learning self-management methods, taking part in activities, and staying busy.*
- Develop effective methods of improving rest and sleep. *Problems with rest and sleep make pain management more difficult. Sleeping poorly at night contributes to decreased motivation, confused thinking, depression, and muscle aches.*
- If appropriate, refer the client to a physical therapist for an exercise program. *The client needs to know what exercises to do, how many repetitions are recommended, and how long and how often to do them. The client should not exercise to the point that increased pain results.*
- Assess the need for referrals (and make them if necessary) for the client who is depressed or anxious. *Anxiety and depression often are a part of long-term chronic pain, making pain management more difficult. Suggest that referrals for help with the frustration (rather than the depression) may make a significant difference in the client's ability to manage pain.*

Constipation

The client with a ruptured intervertebral disk often has problems with constipation because of reduced mobility. Nursing interventions to alleviate and prevent constipation are important because straining to have a bowel movement can increase intradisk pressure, thus increasing pain.

- Assess the client's usual bowel routine, including diet, fluid intake, and the use of laxatives or enemas. *Effective interventions are based on the client's individual needs.*
- Encourage a fluid intake of 2500–3000 mL per day unless contraindicated by the presence of renal or cardiac disease. *Adequate fluid intake facilitates the passage of feces.*
- Increase fiber and bulk in the diet. If the client is unable to tolerate increased fiber, consult with the physician about the use of stool softeners or bulk-forming agents. *Bulk and fiber promote regularity by retaining water in the large intestine.*

Evaluation

Client outcomes are evaluated based on the goals established for care as well as the client's satisfaction with recovery. Potential expected outcomes may include the following:

- Client reports pain as a 3 or less with adequate relief from pain management strategies.
- Client is able to maintain an acceptable quality of life, including participation in daily activities.
- Client maintains normal bowel elimination patterns.

Box 19–4 Perioperative Care for the Client Having a Posterior Laminectomy

PREOPERATIVE TEACHING

- Demonstrate and ask the client to practice logrolling. Explain that it will be done by the nurses for the first day or two; then the client can do it alone. To ensure healing, the spinal column must remain in alignment when the client is turning and moving.
- Explain the importance of taking pain medications regularly and of asking for them before the pain becomes severe. Include information about the possibility of the pain being much the same after surgery. Pain is easier to control if medications are taken before the pain becomes severe. Pain may be the same following surgery for a herniated intervertebral disk because edema due to surgery irritates and compresses the nerve roots.
- Demonstrate the use of a fracture bedpan and ask the client to practice using it. The client usually must remain flat in bed for a period of time following surgery. A fracture bedpan is more comfortable for clients who must lie flat.
- Explain that the client may need to eat while lying flat. This position prevents flexion of the spine.
- Demonstrate and ask the client to demonstrate deep breathing, the use of the incentive spirometer, and leg exercises. These measures prevent respiratory and circulatory complications.

POSTOPERATIVE CARE

- Maintain the client in a position that minimizes stress on the surgical wound. For clients with cervical laminectomy:
  a. Elevate the head of the bed slightly.
  b. Position a small pillow under the neck.
  c. Maintain the position of the cervical collar.

  For clients with lumbar laminectomy:
  a. Keep the bed flat or elevate the head of the bed slightly.
  b. Place a small pillow under the head.
  c. Place a small pillow under the knees or use a pillow to support the upper leg when the client lies on one side.

These positions minimize stress on the surgical wound and suture line. A cervical collar provides stability and prevents flexing or twisting the neck.

- Turn the client every 2 hours using the logrolling technique. Teach the client not to use the side rails to change position. Maintain proper body alignment in all positions. The client's body is turned as a single unit (usually with a turning sheet) to avoid movement of the operative area. Pulling on the side rails puts stress on the operative area and may cause misalignment of the vertebral column.
- Monitor the client for signs of nerve root compression:
  a. Cervical laminectomy: Assess hand grips and arm strength, ability to move the fingers, and ability to detect touch.
  b. Lumbar laminectomy: Assess leg strength, ability to wiggle the toes, and ability to detect touch.

Compare bilateral findings. Report muscle weakness or sensory impairment to the physician immediately. Loss of motor and sensory function may indicate nerve root compression.

- Assess for hematoma formation as manifested by severe incisional pain that is not relieved by analgesics and by decreased motor function. Report these findings immediately. A hematoma may form at the surgical site. If untreated, it may cause irreversible neurologic deficits including paraplegia and bowel/bladder dysfunctions (Hickey, 2003).
- Assess for leakage of cerebrospinal fluid. Assess the dressing for increased moisture. Check the sheets for wetness when the client is lying supine; check for clear liquid running down the back when the client is sitting or standing. Gently palpate the sides of the wound to detect a bulge. Use a Dextrostrix strip to assess any leakage for the presence of glucose, a positive indicator of cerebrospinal fluid. Although uncommon, leakage of cerebrospinal fluid greatly increases the risk for infection of the wound and the meninges.
- Assess for nerve root injury. Assess the client's ability to dorsiflex the foot (lumbar laminectomy) and the client's grip strength (cervical laminectomy). Assess the client who has had a cervical laminectomy for hoarseness. Report hoarseness and further assess the client's ability to swallow. Nerve root compression may cause permanent damage, resulting in footdrop (in lumbar laminectomy clients) and hand weakness (in cervical laminectomy clients). Damage to the laryngeal nerve may cause permanent hoarseness. Impaired ability to swallow puts the client at risk for aspiration.
- Assess for urinary retention. The client should void within 8 hours after surgery. If the physician allows, let males stand to void. Compare intake and output for each 8-hour period. All clients who have received a general anesthetic are at risk for urinary retention. The client who has had a lumbar laminectomy may have even more difficulty voiding as a result of stimulation of sympathetic nerves during surgery.
- Assess for pain using a scale from 0 (no pain) to 10 (severe pain). Administer prescribed analgesics on a regular basis or teach the client to use **patient-controlled analgesia (PCA)** if prescribed. Discuss client concerns about pain that is unrelieved by surgery. Compression of the nerve root over time results in edema and inflammation. Because of surgery-induced edema, the client is likely to experience the same pain or perhaps more severe pain in the period immediately after surgery. This pain usually persists for several weeks after surgery. In addition, many clients who have had a lumbar laminectomy experience muscle spasms in the lower back, abdomen, and thighs for the first few days after surgery.
- Assess for infection by taking and recording vital signs at least every 4 hours; report increased body temperature. Assess the wound and dressing for signs of infection—increased redness, drainage, pain, and pus. Use sterile technique to change dressings. The surgical client is at risk for infection; the client with a laminectomy also is at risk for arachnoiditis. This inflammation of the arachnoid layer of the spinal meninges results from wound infection or contamination during surgery and may cause the formation of painful adhesions.
- Encourage deep breathing and the use of the incentive spirometer every 2 hours; discourage coughing. Anesthesia and immobility depress respiratory function. Coughing is discouraged because it can disrupt healing tissues, especially in clients who had a cervical laminectomy.
- Increase mobility as prescribed. (The time frame for ambulation is prescribed by the physician; the routine here is representative.) Clients often sit on the side of the bed and dangle their legs the evening after surgery or the first day thereafter. Many clients ambulate the first or second postoperative day. To help the client out of bed, elevate the head of the bed. Then bring the client's legs over the side of the bed at the same time the upper body moves to an upright position. Clients should ambulate without assistance only when they are no longer dizzy or weak. Early ambulation increases respiratory and circulatory function and decreases the risk of thrombophlebitis of the lower extremities. The vertebral column should remain in alignment while the client sits and stands. Client safety must be considered throughout care.

Scoliosis

Scoliosis is a lateral S- or C-shaped curvature of the spine that is often associated with a rotational deformity of the spine and ribs.

PATHOPHYSIOLOGY AND ETIOLOGY

Many individuals exhibit some degree of spinal curvature, but curvatures of more than 10 degrees are considered abnormal. Curves are either structural or compensatory, as the spine curves to compensate for a structural deformity along its length.

Etiology

The cause of scoliosis is complex. Structural scoliosis may be congenital, idiopathic, or acquired (associated with neuromuscular disorders such as muscular dystrophy and myelodysplasia or secondary to spinal cord injuries).

In idiopathic structural scoliosis (the most common type), the spine for unknown reasons begins to curve laterally, with vertebral rotation. The most common curve is a right thoracic and left lumbar deformity. As the curve progresses, structural changes occur. The ribs on the concave side (inside of the curve) are forced closer together, while the ribs on the convex side separate widely, causing narrowing of the thoracic cage and formation of the rib hump. The lateral curvature affects the vertebral structure. Disk spaces are narrowed on the concave side and spread wider on the convex side, resulting in an asymmetric vertebral canal (Figure 19–37 ■).

Scoliosis also can occur in congenital diseases involving the spinal structure and in the musculoskeletal changes seen in conditions such as myelomeningocele, cerebral palsy, and muscular dystrophy. It also can be acquired after injury to the spinal cord. The child in Figure 19–38 ■ acquired scoliosis after chemotherapy and radiation to the chest during treatment for cancer.

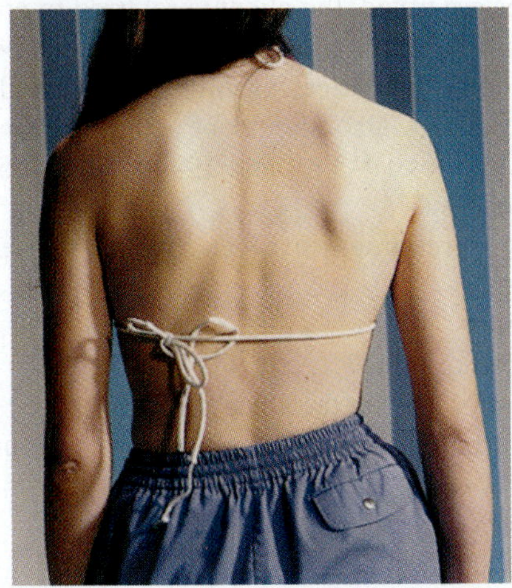

Figure 19–37 ■ A child may have varying degrees of scoliosis. For mild forms, treatment focuses on strengthening and stretching. Moderate forms require bracing. Severe forms may necessitate surgery and fusion. Clothes that fit at an angle, such as this teenage girl's shorts, and anatomic asymmetry of the back provide clues for early detection.

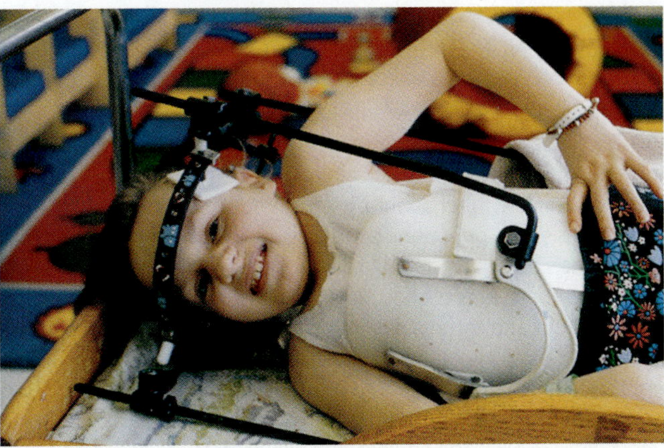

Figure 19–38 ■ In severe scoliosis, the child may wear a halo brace, shown here, to hold the body in position after surgery.

Risk Factors

Idiopathic scoliosis occurs most often in girls, especially during the growth spurt between the ages of 10 and 13 years. Early onset of idiopathic scoliosis occurs before 10 years of age and comprises 15% of cases (Thompson, 2004a).

CLINICAL MANIFESTATIONS

The classic signs of scoliosis include truncal asymmetry, uneven shoulders and hips, a one-sided rib hump, and a prominent scapula. Typically the client does not complain of pain or discomfort. If diagnosis does not occur before the curvature reaches about 40 degrees, some compensatory problems may develop. Hip and back pain can result, and lung compromise can lead to fatigue or dyspnea with exertion.

COLLABORATION

The goal of medical management is to limit or stop progression of the curvature. School and office nurses often screen children for scoliosis and refer abnormalities for further evaluation. Many professionals such as physical therapists, physicians, and nurses partner with families to treat the adolescent with scoliosis.

Diagnostic Tests

Generally, observation and radiographic examination are used to diagnose scoliosis. An inclinometer (scoliometer) can be placed on the spine with the client bent forward; a variation from one side to the other of greater than 5–7 degrees warrants referral for further evaluation (Hart & Grottkau, 2006). Additional diagnostic studies include MRI, CT scan, and bone scan, which are used occasionally to assess the degree of curvature.

Clinical Therapy

Early detection is essential to successful treatment. Adequate treatment and follow-up maximize the client's chances for proper spinal alignment. The treatment regimen depends on

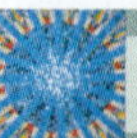

EVIDENCE-BASED PRACTICE Adolescent Self-Image and Braces

A comparison of 150 adolescents who wore a brace for scoliosis with 150 adolescents without scoliosis revealed that those wearing the brace had poorer perception of self-image when completing the Piers-Harris scale "How I feel about myself." In addition, only 5% of youth with scoliosis had opportunities to discuss their feelings with health professionals and 90% stated that they wanted more opportunities to do so (Sapountzi-Krepia et al., 2001). Another study using interviews to learn about adolescents' feelings related to brace wear had similar findings. The youth expressed feelings of stress, anger, denial, and shame. They received support from family and friends but did not receive adequate support from health care professionals (Sapountzi-Krepia et al., 2006). The findings that adolescents are concerned with body image is not surprising, considering it is a developmental stage that focuses on appearance and fitting in with others. It is surprising that this is not acknowledged and discussed sufficiently during health care. Health care professionals should realize that wearing a brace can be difficult for adolescents and should provide a chance for youth to discuss how they feel about the diagnosis and treatment. Interventions that aid in improving body image should be considered. For example, some department stores sponsor fashion shows for adolescents with scoliosis who wear braces. Children with braces model and demonstrate how popular clothing can be worn to disguise the brace. These events can have a positive impact on the self-esteem of adolescents who participate in and view the fashion shows.

the degree and progression of the curvature and the response of the client and family to medical management.

MILD SCOLIOSIS Treatment of children with mild scoliosis (curvatures of 10–20 degrees upon radiographic study) consists of exercises to improve posture and muscle tone and to maintain, or possibly increase, flexibility of the spine. Emphasis is placed on building strength toward the outside of the curve while stretching the inside of the curve. These exercises are not a cure, however, and the client should be evaluated by a physician at 3-month intervals, with radiographic evaluation every 6 months.

MODERATE SCOLIOSIS Medical management of moderate scoliosis (curvatures of 20–40 degrees) includes bracing, most commonly with a Boston brace. The goal of wearing a brace is to maintain the existing spinal curvature with no increase. Brace wear begins immediately after diagnosis. To achieve maximum effectiveness, the brace should be worn 23 hours per day. Brace treatment is lengthy and requires a high degree of compliance, which can be difficult for adolescents who view body image and/or sports involvement as important. (See Evidenced-Based Practice: Adolescent Self-Image and Braces.)

Electrical stimulation is used occasionally as an alternative treatment. An electric current stimulates the back muscles to contract, thus helping to correct the spinal curvature. This treatment, which is performed at night, eliminates the need for bracing.

SEVERE SCOLIOSIS Children with severe scoliosis (curvatures of 40–50 degrees or more) require surgery, which involves spinal fusion. The majority of spinal fusions are performed using segmental instrumentation of the spinal cord. Examples of surgical approaches include Luque wires, Cotrel-Dubosset (CD) instrumentation, the Texas Scottish Rite Hospital system, and the Moss-Miami system (Lonstein, 2006). These treatments stabilize the spine during surgery, may be accompanied by bone grafting to the spine, and require no long-term therapy or postoperative casting. Following surgery with wires or instrumentation, the child is on bed rest during a recovery period and may be fitted with anteroposterior plastic shells (also called thoracolumbar sacral orthotics) that are worn for several months to provide stability for the spine. The wires remain in the back forever. Occasionally, in severe cases, halo traction is used postoperatively to provide support for the unstable spine (Figure 19–38 ■).

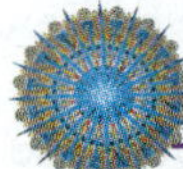

NURSING PROCESS

The nurse—whether the school nurse or the nurse working with pediatric clients—is often the first person to notice scoliosis. Care is aimed at teaching client and family and providing postoperative care if surgery is indicated.

Assessment

School nurses often screen children for scoliosis, generally in the fifth and seventh grades. Although screeing for scoliosis is mandated by law in several states, it is not universally recommended (U.S. Preventive Services Task Force, 2006). When abnormalities are noted, the client is referred to an orthopedic center for further evaluation. Children should be examined every 6–9 months thereafter. If scoliosis is detected, the child's brothers and sisters also should be examined and observed closely. See Figures 19–39 ■ and 19–40 ■ for photographs of scoliosis screening.

Scoliosis screening involves visual observation of the following:

From the Front

- Is the head midline?
- Are the shoulders at the same height?
- Do the arms and body have the same amount of space between them on each side?

From the Back

- Is the head midline?
- Are the shoulders at the same height?
- Are the scapulae equally prominent and at the same height?
- Is the spine straight?
- Do the arms and body have the same amount of space between them on each side?
- Are the hips at the same height?

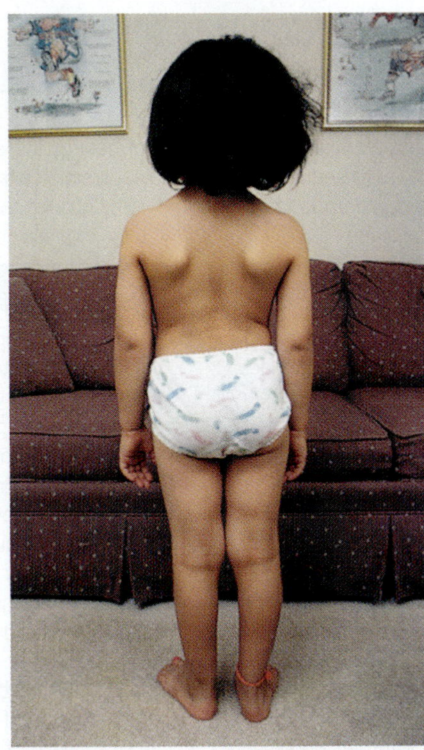

Figure 19–39 ■ Does this child have legs of different lengths or scoliosis? Look at the level of the iliac crests and shoulders to see if they are level. See the more prominent crease at the waist on the right side? This child could have scoliosis.

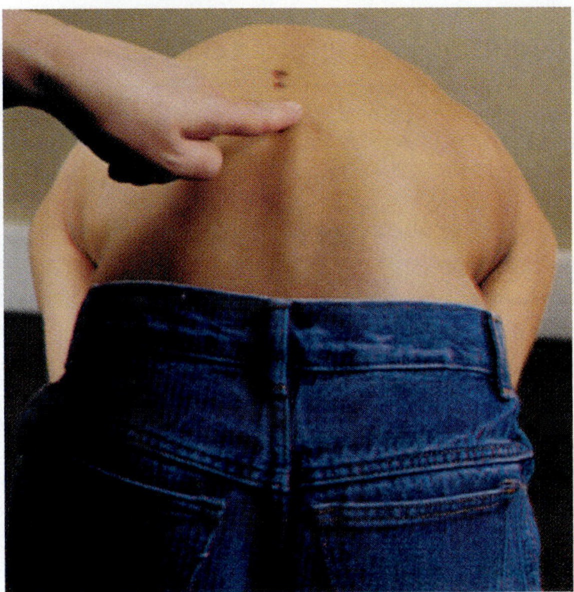

Figure 19–40 ■ Inspection of the spine for scoliosis. Ask the child to slowly bend forward at the waist, with arms extended toward the floor. Run your forefinger down the spinal processes, palpating each vertebra for a change in alignment. A lateral curve to the spine or a one-sided rib hump is an indication of scoliosis.

With the Adolescent Holding Hands Together and Bent Over Slightly

- Are the scapular humps even?

With the Adolescent Holding Hands Together and Bent Over Toward Floor

- Are the flank humps even?
- Is the spine straight?
- Is there a marked roundness when viewing the client from the side (evidence of kyphosis)?

Diagnosis

The following nursing diagnoses may apply to the client with scoliosis who is *not* undergoing surgery:

- Risk for Impaired Adjustment to the exercise program related to duration and intensity of exercise
- Impaired Physical Mobility related to brace
- Risk for Impaired Skin Integrity related to brace
- Ineffective Breathing Pattern related to rib cage deformity
- Health-Seeking Behaviors (child and parent) related to unfamiliarity with disease process
- Disturbed Body Image related to deformity and brace wear.

Common nursing diagnoses for the client who is having surgery can be found in the accompanying Nursing Care Plan.

Plan

Goals of nursing care often include the following:

- Client and family describe the selected treatment regimen and their role in maintaining compliance.
- Client and family accurately describe the condition and the stages of treatment.
- Client requiring surgery can describe the procedure to be performed.
- Client demonstrates proper use of a PCA pump and describes the importance of reporting any pain to the nurse.

Other considerations for the child requiring surgery also may be addressed by the nurse. Often the child donates blood prior to surgery. The family also may donate so the child's or a family member's blood is transfused in surgery. The adolescent will benefit from learning about deep breathing, positioning, surgical incision, and all other aspects of postoperative care. The accompanying Nursing Care Plan summarizes nursing care for the client who is undergoing surgery for scoliosis.

Implementation

Promote Understanding and Acceptance of the Treatment Plan

Provide instructions about exercises that will help decrease the severity of the spinal curvature. Demonstrate the exercises and explain their purpose (e.g., to strengthen back muscles). Help the client adjust to wearing a brace. Adolescents, in particular, may be reluctant to wear an external device such as a brace. To

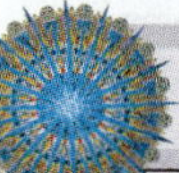

NURSING CARE PLAN A Child Undergoing Surgery for Scoliosis

Frances Bomgardner is an 11-year-old girl who was discovered to have scoliosis during a routine screening at her middle school. Conservative treatment was attempted, although her pediatrician warned that it might not work due to the severity of her curvature. As anticipated, adequate results were not obtained, so Frances is admitted to the local hospital where she is to undergo spinal fusion. Both Frances and her family are anxious for the procedure to be over, and Frances' mother pulls the nurse aside to ask if there is any chance that Frances could end up paralyzed as a result of the surgery.

ASSESSMENT

Frances displays a 35% lateral curvature with vertebral rotation. She is currently wearing a brace, and skin around and under the brace is intact with no indication of interruption of integrity. She and her parents express anxiety related to the upcoming procedure. Frances' oxygen saturation is 93%, and breath sounds are reduced in the bases bilaterally. Respiratory rate is 18 and shallow.

DIAGNOSES

- Deficient Knowledge (child and parents) related to lack of information about surgery
- Ineffective Breathing Pattern related to hypoventilation syndrome
- Risk for Injury related to neurovascular deficit secondary to instrumentation
- Pain related to spinal fusion with instrumentation
- Impaired Physical Mobility related to movement restrictions and pain
- Risk for Disturbed Body Image related to treatment
- Risk for Deficient Knowledge (child and parent) related to lack of information about home care

PLANNING

- The child and parents will verbalize understanding of the disease, its treatment, and the surgical procedure.
- The child will show no signs of respiratory compromise.
- The child's neurovascular system will remain intact as evidenced by circulation, sensation, and motor checks. The child will feel no numbness or tingling.
- The child will verbalize an adequate level of comfort or show absence of pain behavior within 1 hour of a specific nursing intervention.
- The child will maintain proper body alignment and progress with activity as ordered by the physician. If no anteroposterior shell bracing is required, the child will have active mobility by the third to fifth postoperative day.
- The child will verbalize feelings about body image and self-esteem in relation to the disease and its treatment. The child will be informed about available support services and use them as needed.
- The child and family will verbalize reduced anxiety about home care. The child will demonstrate knowledge of self-care and permitted activities.

IMPLEMENTATION

- Teach the child and family about the course of the disease, its signs and symptoms, and treatment. Provide appropriate handouts. Encourage the child and parents to ask questions.
- Begin preoperative teaching at the time of admission. Orient the child to the hospital and postoperative procedures. Before surgery, have the child demonstrate logrolling, ROM exercises, and the use of an incentive spirometer. Discuss pain management.
- Monitor respiratory status, especially after the administration of analgesics. Apply pulse oximeter.
- Administer oxygen if ordered.
- Have the child use an incentive spirometer.
- Monitor intake and output.
- Reposition the child at least every 2 hours.
- Monitor the child's color, circulation, capillary refill, warmth, sensation, and motion in all extremities. Perform neurovascular checks every 2 hours for the first 24 hours and then every 4 hours for the next 48 hours. Record presence of pedal and distal tibial pulses every hour for 48 hours. Report changes and abnormal findings immediately.

NURSING CARE PLAN A Child Undergoing Surgery for Scoliosis *continued*

- Have the child wear antiembolism stockings until ambulatory. The stockings may be removed for 1 hour 2 or 3 times daily.
- Check for pain, swelling, or a positive Homans' sign in the legs. Record any evidence of edema.
- Encourage and assist the child with ROM exercises, both passive and active.
- Assess the level of pain and initiate pain management strategies as soon as possible. Use patient-controlled analgesics if ordered.
- Administer pain medication around the clock to help ensure pain relief, especially during the first 48 hours. Monitor epidural blocks and PCA or other methods used for pain control.
- Use nonpharmacologic pain management techniques such as imagery, relaxation, touch, music, application of heat and cold, and reduced environmental stimulation to supplement medications.
- Document pain assessment, interventions, and the child's reactions.
- Reassure the child that some discomfort is expected and that a variety of measures can be tried to reduce discomfort.
- Reposition the child every 2 hours using the logrolling technique. Support the back, feet, and knees with pillows.
- Have the child perform passive and active ROM exercises every 2 hours for 48 hours and then every 4 hours while awake. Have the child dangle the legs at bedside by the second to fourth postoperative day or as ordered by surgeon. Begin ambulation generally by the third to fifth postoperative day. Note pallor and any complaints of dizziness. Proceed slowly.
- Encourage independence in daily activities within allowable limits. Use positive reinforcements. Encourage the child to participate in community activities if possible. Involve the child in scoliosis support groups.
- Provide contact with a peer resource person who has undergone treatment for scoliosis.
- Teach cast or brace care as appropriate. Provide oral and written instructions and a list of activity limitations. Have the child and family demonstrate adequate knowledge.
- Arrange for follow-up appointments as ordered by the physician. Encourage the child and family to notify the nurse or physician if they have any questions or concerns.

EVALUATION

Care is evaluated based on the following expected outcomes:

- The child and family accurately verbalize knowledge about the disease and its treatment.
- The child and family ask appropriate questions about postoperative care.
- The child has no respiratory complications.
- The child exhibits only temporary alteration. (Pale skin, faint pulse, and edema occur, but then resolve within the initial postoperative phase.)
- The child returns to the preoperative baseline state by discharge.
- The child experiences pain relief early in the postoperative period.
- The child is mobile as appropriate for condition within 3–5 days after surgery.
- The child has a positive self-image and is involved in community activities or support groups.
- The child and family demonstrate home care and implementation of discharge teaching.

CRITICAL THINKING

1. How would you respond to the mother's question related to potential paralysis after surgery?
2. What nursing care can you provide to reduce the client's preoperative anxiety?
3. What specific client and family teaching would you provide to prepare Frances for discharge and for meeting home care needs?

CLIENT TEACHING Home Care for Clients Who Had Spinal Surgery

Home care needs should be identified and addressed well in advance of client's discharge after spinal surgery. The client must learn to adapt to a new set of body mechanics. Show the client how to do simple tasks without bending or twisting the torso. Before discharge from the hospital, have the client demonstrate the ability to perform ADLs. Collaborate with physical therapy/rehabilitation to plan for the youth's needs related to safe and effective movement with the brace.

Activities for the client who has had spinal surgery are commonly limited for a period of time. Depending on the type of surgery and the surgeon, activities are usually restricted for 6–8 months. Emphasize to both the client and family the importance of compliance; give them written discharge instructions. Follow-up visits are important. The client should be examined 4–6 weeks after discharge, then every 3–4 months for 1 year and every 1–2 years thereafter.

promote a sense of control, allow the adolescent to choose when to exercise and when to be out of the brace, within the treatment guidelines. Provide reassurance and encouragement and promote interaction with peers. Suggesting that the adolescent work with a peer support person who is being treated for scoliosis or who had the condition in the past may be beneficial. Provide information about fashionable clothing that can be worn with the brace.

Several organizations provide information and assistance to families of children with scoliosis. Appropriate referrals can be made.

Evaluation

Expected outcomes of nursing care for the client with scoliosis treated by brace often include the following:

- Client maintains intact skin under brace.
- Client wears brace as directed.

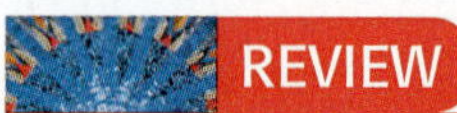

REVIEW Back Problems

RELATE: LINK THE CONCEPTS

Linking the exemplar of Back Problems with the concept of Addiction Behaviors:

1. What focused assessment will you plan for the client with chronic back problems who has been taking Percocet for pain?
2. Your assigned client diagnosed with back problems was admitted last evening with an alcohol overdose. What is your priority of care for this client?

Linking the exemplar of Back Problems with the concept of Elimination:

3. Describe the risk factors for altered urinary elimination in a client with back problems who leads a sedentary lifestyle.
4. The client with back problems is experiencing chronic constipation. What are your teaching priorities for the client to reduce this issue?

READY: GO TO COMPANION SKILLS MANUAL

- Assessing the musculoskeletal system
- Assessing the client in pain
- Applying body mechanics
- Supporting the client's position in bed
- Supporting a client in Fowler's position
- Turning the client to the lateral or prone position in bed
- Logrolling a client
- Using a turn or lift sheet

REFER: GO TO MYNURSINGKIT

REFLECT: CASE STUDY

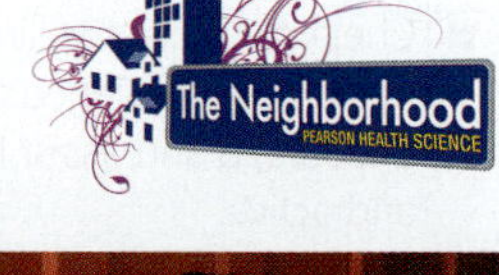

Gilbert Martin is a 53-year-old Hispanic male who is married to Helen Martin. Gil has a son from a previous marriage and a step-daughter whom he has raised since she was three. Gil's father has recently passed away, so he has been helping his mother manage her affairs.

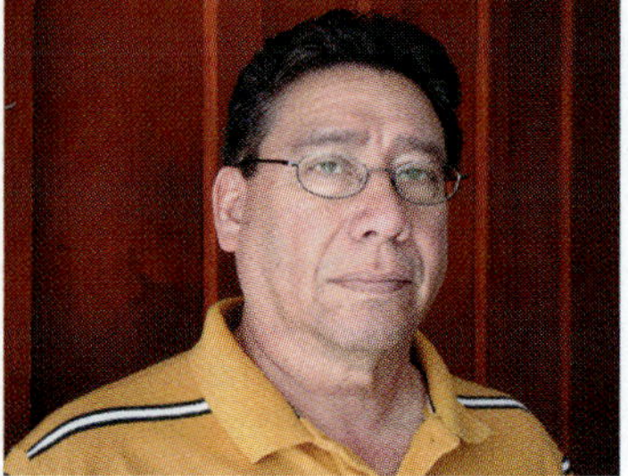

Gil works as a local delivery truck driver for a construction company. His job includes assisting with the loading and unloading of construction materials. Gil considers himself to be in good health with the exception of chronic back pain. Gil also has hyperlipidemia for which he takes atorvastatin (Lipitor) 20 mg/day. Gil sees his primary care provider once a year for triglyceride and liver function tests and has also been encouraged to follow a low-fat diet.

1. What non-pharmacological interventions will you initiate for Gil to reduce his chronic back pain?
2. What factors place Gil at risk for exacerbation of his back problems?
3. Describe how the stress in Gil's life may be affecting his chronic low back pain.

19.2 FRACTURES

KEY TERMS

Cast, *1100*
Closed (simple) fracture, *1093*
Compartment syndrome, *1094*
Deep venous thrombosis (DVT), *1096*
Delayed union, *1097*
5 P's of neurovascular assessment, *1104*
Fracture, *1093*
Nonunion, *1097*
Open (compound) fracture, *1093*
Open reduction and internal fixation (ORIF), *1101*
Paresis, *1096*
Paresthesia, *1096*
Pathologic fracture, *1093*
Stress fracture, *1093*
Traction, *1099*

BASIS FOR SELECTION OF EXEMPLAR

Most common ER visit

LEARNING OUTCOMES

After reading about this exemplar, you will be able to:

1. Describe the pathophysiology, etiology, clinical manifestations, and direct and indirect causes of fractures.
2. Identify risk factors associated with fractures.
3. Illustrate the nursing process in providing culturally competent care across the life span for individuals with a fracture.
4. Formulate priority nursing diagnoses appropriate for an individual with a fracture.
5. Create a plan of care for individuals with fractures and their family members.
6. Assess expected outcomes for an individual with a fracture.
7. Discuss therapies used in the collaborative care of an individual with a fracture.
8. Employ evidence-based caring interventions for an individual with a fracture.

OVERVIEW

A **fracture** is any break in the continuity of a bone. Fractures vary in severity according to the location and type. Although fractures occur in all age groups, they are more common in people who have sustained trauma and in older clients.

PATHOPHYSIOLOGY AND ETIOLOGY

Any of the 206 bones in the body can be fractured. A fracture occurs when the bone is subjected to more kinetic energy than it can absorb. Fractures may result from a direct blow, a crushing force (compression), a sudden twisting motion (torsion), a severe muscle contraction, or disease that has weakened the bone (called a **stress** or **pathologic fracture**). Two basic mechanisms produce fractures: direct force and indirect force. With direct force, the kinetic energy is applied at or near the site of the fracture. The bone cannot withstand the force. With indirect force, the kinetic energy is transmitted from the point of impact to a site where the bone is weak. The fracture occurs at the weak point.

Fractures in adults are classified in the following ways:

- If the skin is intact, the fracture is considered a **closed (simple) fracture**. If the skin integrity is interrupted, the fracture is considered an **open (compound) fracture** (Figure 19–41 ■). An open fracture allows bacteria to enter the injured area and increases the risk of complications.
- The fracture line may be *oblique* (at an angle to the bone) or *spiral* (curves around the bone). An *avulsed* fracture occurs when the fracture pulls bone and other tissues away from the point of attachment. It also may be described as *comminuted* (the bone breaks in many pieces), *compressed* (the bone is crushed), *impacted* (the broken bone ends are forced into each other), or *depressed* (the broken bone is forced inward) (Figure 19–42 ■).
- *Complete* fractures involve the entire width of the bone, whereas *incomplete* fractures involve only a part of the width of the bone.
- In a *stable* (nondisplaced) fracture, the bones maintain their anatomic alignment. An *unstable* (displaced) fracture occurs when the bones move out of correct anatomic alignment. If a fracture is displaced, immediate interventions are required to prevent further damage to soft tissue, muscle, and bone.

Fractures also may be classified by point of reference on the bone, such as midshaft, middle third, and distal third. The point of reference also may be specific, such as intra-articular and diaphyseal.

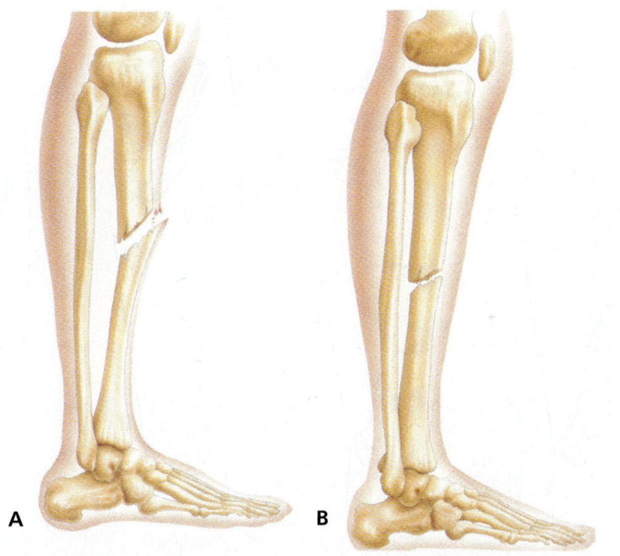

Figure 19–41 ■ *A*, An open fracture. *B*, A closed fracture.

Etiology

Fractures in children may result from direct trauma to a bone (falls, sports injuries, abuse, motor vehicle crashes) or bone diseases (osteogenesis imperfecta) that result in weakening of the bone. Clients with osteoporosis or osteopenia are more prone to fractures. Trauma may be caused by an acute injury, a direct and forceful impact, or overuse such as in chronic and repetitive activities. Due to their porous nature, the bones of children may bow, leading to more common greenstick or spiral fractures (Table 19–7). Abuse is a cause of fracture and should be suspected when the type of fracture is uncommon for a given age.

Risk Factors

Osteoporosis, osteogenesis imperfecta, and bone cancer increase risk of fracture because the bone becomes more porous and brittle. Inadequate intake of vitamin D, calcium, and phosphorous also contribute to risk of bone fractures. Other risk factors include aging, Caucasian race, low bone mass, and history of previous fracture. Any factor that increases risk of trauma, such as driving while taking substances that impact reaction time, unsteady gait, or weakness, can increase the likelihood of a fracture.

Fracture Healing

Regardless of classification or type, fracture healing progresses over three phases: the inflammatory phase, the reparative phase, and the remodeling phase. The bleeding and inflammation that

DEVELOPMENTAL CONSIDERATIONS Stress Fractures

Stress fractures are becoming more common in adolescents who limit their intake of calories and calcium in an attempt to remain lean for sports such as distance running and gymnastics. These fractures may present with chronic pain that changes in intensity. Be alert to this possibility when teenagers' diets and athletic activities place them at risk.

The risk of bone fractures is significantly increased with higher cola consumption and more television viewing time and with lower levels of physical activity and lower milk intake (Ma & Jones 2004; Manias, McCabe, & Bishop, 2006).

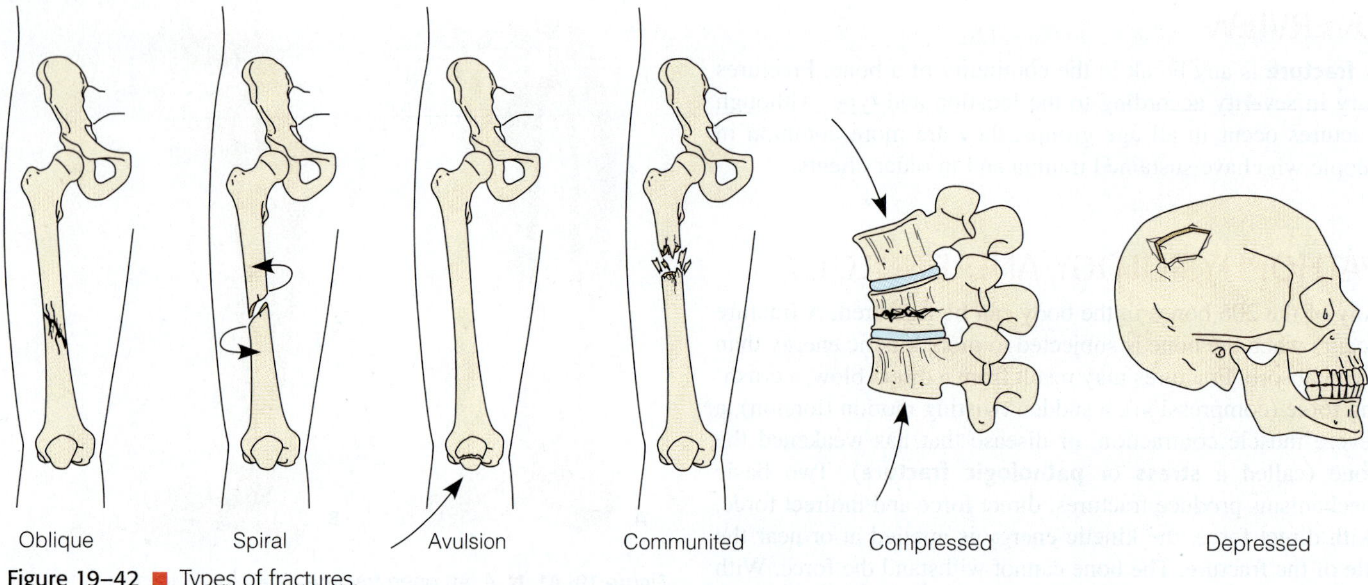

Figure 19–42 ■ Types of fractures.

develop at the site of the fracture initiate the inflammatory phase. A hematoma forms between the fractured bone ends and around the bone surfaces. The osteocytes at the bone ends die as the hematoma clots, obstructing blood flow and depriving the osteocytes of oxygen and nutrients. Necrosis of the cells heightens the inflammatory response, which in turn leads to vasodilation and edema. In addition, fibroblasts, lymphocytes, macrophages, and even osteoblasts from the bone migrate to the fracture site. Fibroblasts form a fibrin meshwork and promote the growth of granulation tissue and capillary buds. The lymphocytes and macrophages wall off the area, localizing and containing the inflammation. The capillary buds invade the fracture site and supply a source of nutrients to promote the formation of collagen. The collagen allows calcium to be deposited.

Once calcium is deposited, a callus begins to form. In this reparative phase, osteoblasts promote the formation of new bone and osteoclasts destroy dead bone and assist in the synthesis of new bone. Collagen formation and calcium deposition continue. During the remodeling phase, excess callus is removed and new bone is laid down along the fracture line. Eventually, the fracture site is calcified and the bone is reunited.

The age, physical condition of the client, and type of fracture sustained influence the healing of fractures. Other factors influence bone healing positively or negatively and may be grouped according to their local or systemic influence (Box 19–5). Healing time varies with the individual. An uncomplicated fracture of the arm or foot can heal in 6–8 weeks. A fractured vertebra will take at least 12 weeks to heal. Healing of a fractured hip may take from 12–16 weeks.

CLINICAL MANIFESTATIONS

Fractures are often accompanied by soft tissue injuries that involve muscles, arteries, veins, nerves, or skin (Table 19–8). The degree of soft tissue involvement depends on the amount of energy or force transmitted to the area.

Complications

Complications of musculoskeletal trauma are associated with pressure from edema and hemorrhage, development of fat emboli, deep venous thrombosis (DVT), infection, loss of skeletal integrity, or involvement of nerve fibers. Bone fragments also may result in further injury or complications.

COMPARTMENT SYNDROME A compartment is a space enclosed by a fibrous membrane or fascia. The fascia lines the compartment in the limbs and is nonexpandable. Compartments in the limbs may enclose and support bones, nerves, and blood vessels. **Compartment syndrome** occurs when excess pressure in a limited space constricts the structures in a compartment, reducing circulation to muscles and nerves. *Acute compartment syndrome* may result from hemorrhage and edema in the compartment following a fracture or from a crush injury or from external compression of the limb by a cast that is too tight. Increased pressure in the confined space of the compartment results in entrapment of nerves, blood vessels, and muscles.

Entrapment of the blood vessels limits tissue perfusion, beginning a cycle of events that may result in the loss of the limb. Inadequate oxygen supply causes cellular acidosis, which intensifies as cellular energy requirements are met through anaerobic metabolism. The capillaries inside the compartment dilate in an attempt to increase the supply of blood and oxygen. Additional blood and oxygen are not available, and plasma proteins leak into the interstitial tissues. The interstitial tissue then pulls fluid in to balance the protein load. As a result, edema in the compartment increases. The edema causes further compression of the vascular network, and the cycle continues. Uninterrupted, this cycle threatens the client's limb and increases the risk of sepsis. Compartment syndrome usually develops within the first 48 hours of injury, when edema is at its peak. Manifestations of compartment syndrome are listed in Box 19–6. It is important to note that arterial pulses may remain normal, even when pressure within the compartment is high enough to significantly impair tissue perfusion.

TABLE 19–7 Common Fractures

FRACTURE TYPE	DESCRIPTION	COMMENTS
Closed	Bone breaks cleanly but does not penetrate the skin.	Also called a simple fracture.
Open	Broken ends of bone protrude through soft tissues and skin.	Serious; may result in osteomyelitis. Also called a compound fracture.
Comminuted	Bone fragments into many pieces.	Common in those with conditions causing brittle bones, such as osteogenesis imperfecta.
Compression	Bone is crushed.	Common in clients with osteoporosis.
Impacted	Broken ends of bone are forced into each other.	Commonly results from falls; also common in hip fracture.
Depressed	Broken bone is pressed inward.	Common in skull fractures.
Spiral	Jagged break due to twisting force applied to bone.	Common fracture due to sports injuries.
Greenstick	Bone breaks incompletely, in much the way a green twig breaks.	Common in children whose bones have proportionally more organic matrix and are more flexible than those of adults.

Source: Drawings adapted from Marieb, E. N. (1998). *Human anatomy and physiology* (4th ed., p. 180). Menlo Park, CA: Benjamin Cummings.

If compartment syndrome develops, interventions to alleviate pressure will be implemented, one of which may include removal of a tightly fitting cast. If the pressure is internal, a *fasciotomy*, a surgical intervention in which muscle fascia is cut to relieve pressure in the compartment, may be necessary. After a fasciotomy, the incision is left open and passive ROM exercises are performed on the extremity.

VOLKMANN'S CONTRACTURE Volkmann's contracture, a common complication of elbow fractures, can result from unresolved compartment syndrome. Arterial blood flow decreases, leading to ischemia, degeneration, and contracture of the muscle. Arm mobility is impaired, and the client is unable to extend the arm completely.

Box 19–5 Factors Influencing Bone Healing

POSITIVE FACTORS

Local

- Immobilization
- Timely correction of displacement
- Application of ice
- Electrical stimulation

Systemic

- Adequate amounts of growth hormone, vitamin D, and calcium
- Adequate blood supply
- Absence of infection or diseases
- Younger age
- Moderate activity level prior to injury

NEGATIVE FACTORS

Local

- Delay in correction of displacement
- Open fracture (increases risk of infection)
- Presence of foreign body at fracture site

Systemic

- Immunocompromised status
- Decreased circulation (as in diabetes and peripheral vascular disease)
- Malnutrition
- Osteoporosis
- Advanced age

TABLE 19–8 Manifestations of Fracture

MANIFESTATION	CAUSE
Deformity	Abnormal position of bones secondary to fracture and muscles pulling on fractured bone
Swelling	Edema from localization of serous fluid and bleeding
Pain/tenderness	Muscle spasm, direct tissue trauma, nerve pressure, movement of fractured bone
Numbness	Nerve damage or nerve entrapment
Guarding	Pain
Crepitus	Grating of bones or entrance of air into an open fracture. *Note:* Do not manipulate the extremity to elicit crepitus; doing so may cause additional damage.
Hypovolemic shock	Blood loss or associated injuries
Muscle spasms	Muscle contraction near the fracture
Ecchymosis	Extravasation of blood into the subcutaneous tissue

FAT EMBOLISM SYNDROME (FES) Fat emboli occur when fat globules lodge in the pulmonary vascular bed or peripheral circulation. Fat embolism syndrome (FES) is characterized by neurologic dysfunction; pulmonary insufficiency; and a petechial rash on the chest, axilla, and upper arms. Long bone fractures and other major trauma are the principal risk factors for fat emboli; hip replacement surgery also poses a risk for FES.

When a bone is fractured, pressure in the bone marrow rises and exceeds capillary pressure; as a result, fat globules leave the bone marrow and enter the bloodstream. Another contributing factor may be the stress-induced release of catecholamine, which causes the rapid mobilization of fatty acids. Once the fat globules are released, they combine with platelets and travel to the brain, lungs, kidneys, and other organs, occluding small blood vessels and causing tissue ischemia.

Manifestations usually develop within a few hours to a week after injury. The manifestations result from the occlusion of the blood supply and the presence of fatty acids. Altered cerebral blood flow causes confusion and changes in level of consciousness. Pulmonary circulation may be disrupted, and free fatty acids damage the alveolar-capillary membrane. Pulmonary edema, impaired surfactant production, and atelectasis can result in significant respiratory insufficiency and manifestations of acute respiratory distress syndrome. (See Concept 21, Exemplar 21.1, Acute Respiratory Distress Syndrome.) Fat droplets activate the clotting cascade, causing thrombocytopenia. Petechiae (pin-sized purplish areas from bleeding under the skin) appearing on the skin, buccal membranes, and conjunctival sacs are thought to result from either microvascular clotting or the accompanying thrombocytopenia.

Early stabilization of long bone fractures is preventive for FES. Prompt identification and treatment of the syndrome are necessary to maintain adequate pulmonary function. In severe cases, the client may require intubation and mechanical ventilation to prevent hypoxemia. Fluid balance is closely monitored. Corticosteroids may be administered to decrease the inflammatory response of lung tissues, stabilize lipid membranes, and reduce bronchospasm (Porth, 2005).

DEEP VENOUS THROMBOSIS (DVT) A **deep venous thrombosis (DVT)** is a blood clot that forms along the intimal lining of a large vein. Three precursors linked to DVT formation are (1) venous stasis, or decreased blood flow; (2) injury to blood vessel walls; and (3) altered blood coagulation

Box 19–6 Manifestations of Compartment Syndrome

EARLY MANIFESTATIONS

- Pain
- Normal or decreased peripheral pulse

LATER MANIFESTATIONS

- Cyanosis
- Tingling, loss of sensation (**paresthesia**)
- Weakness (**paresis**)
- Severe pain, especially when the extremity is passively flexed
- Eventual renal failure (due to release of myoglobin into the bloodstream; myoglobin molecule is too large for effective filtration and excretion by kidney, and renal failure results)

(Table 19–9). Any or all of these precursors can cause a DVT to form. Damage to the lining of the vein causes the platelets to aggregate, or clump together, forming the thrombus. Fibrin, white blood cells (WBCs), and red blood cells (RBCs) begin to cling to the thrombus, and a tail forms. This tail or the entire thrombus may dislodge and move to the brain, lungs, or heart. Five percent of DVTs dislodge and enter the pulmonary circulation to form a pulmonary embolus. If the thrombus remains in the vein, venous insufficiency may result from scarring and valve damage.

If a DVT is present, there may be swelling, leg pain, tenderness, or cramping. Not all clients experience manifestations, however. For this reason, diagnostic tests such as a venogram or Doppler ultrasound of lower extremities may be required. A venogram, performed in the radiology department, requires intravenous administration of dye, whereas a Doppler ultrasound study is noninvasive and can be performed at the client's bedside. Doppler ultrasonography uses sound waves to form an image on a computer screen.

The best treatment for DVT is prevention. Early immobilization of the fracture and early ambulation of the client are imperative. The extremity should be elevated above the level of the heart. Frequent assessments of the injured extremity may lead to early recognition of DVT and prevent the formation of pulmonary embolus. Prophylactic anticoagulant administration is beneficial. Antiembolism stockings and compression boots increase venous return and prevent stasis of blood. Constrictive clothing should be avoided.

The diagnosis of DVT requires rapid intervention. The client is placed on bed rest for 5–7 days to prevent dislodgment of the clot. Fibrinolytic agents, which dissolve the clot, may be administered. Heparin may be administered intravenously to prevent more clots from forming. Placement of a vena cava filter may prevent the existing clot from entering the pulmonary circulation and forming a pulmonary embolus. In extreme cases in which anticoagulation therapy is contraindicated, a thrombectomy (surgical removal of the clot) may be necessary.

INFECTION Infection is more likely to occur in an open fracture than a closed fracture, but any complication that decreases blood supply increases the risk of infection. Infection may result from contamination at the time of injury or during surgery. *Pseudomonas, Staphylococcus,* or *Clostridium* organisms may invade the wound or bone. *Clostridium* infection is particularly serious because it may lead to severe gas gangrene and cellulitis, but any infection can delay healing and result in osteomyelitis, infection in the bone that can lead to tissue death and necrosis.

DELAYED UNION AND NONUNION **Delayed Union** is the prolonged healing of bones beyond the usual time period. Many factors inhibit bone healing, including poor nutrition, inadequate immobilization, prolonged reduction time, infection, necrosis, age, immunosuppression, and severe bone trauma resulting in multiple fragments. Delayed union is diagnosed by means of serial x-ray studies. It is important to note that x-ray findings may lag 1–2 weeks behind the healing process; for example, a client may be completely healed by week 13, but this fact may not be apparent on the x-ray until week 14.

Delayed union may lead to **nonunion**, or failure of the ends of the fracture to heal together, which can cause persistent pain and movement at the fracture site. Nonunion may require surgical interventions such as internal fixation and bone grafting. If infection is present, the bones are surgically debrided. Electrical stimulation of the fracture site may be as effective as bone grafting.

REFLEX SYMPATHETIC DYSTROPHY *Reflex sympathetic dystrophy* may occur after musculoskeletal or nerve trauma. This term refers to a group of poorly understood posttraumatic conditions involving persistent pain, hyperesthesia, swelling, changes in skin color and texture, changes in temperature, and decreased motion. Diagnosis is made by the client's history and physical examination. X-rays may demonstrate spotty osteoporosis, and bone scans may reveal increased uptake of radionuclide. Treatment with a sympathetic nervous system blocking agent often alleviates the manifestations.

COLLABORATION

A fracture requires treatment to stabilize the fractured bone(s), maintain bone immobilization, prevent complications, and restore function. The diagnosis of a fracture is based primarily on physical assessments and x-rays. Collaborative care of the client begins with emergency care, sometimes initiated by Emergency Medical System professionals, and continues through the healing process which may or may not require the assistance of a physical or occupation therapist. The nurse's role is to assist with procedures, maintain client's comfort, provide client education, ongoing assessments for potential complications, and facilitation of referrals as necessary.

TABLE 19–9 **Precursors of Deep Venous Thrombosis**

PRECURSOR	IMPLICATIONS FOR FRACTURES
Decreased blood flow	Common in fracture clients who are immobilized and less active. Bed rest alone can decrease venous flow by 50%.
Injury to blood vessel wall	May occur as a direct result of the force that caused the fracture or from surgical manipulation.
Altered blood coagulation	May result from active blood loss. The body's attempt to maintain homeostasis leads to increased production of platelets and clotting factor.

CLINICAL MANIFESTATIONS AND THERAPIES Fractures

ETIOLOGY	CLINICAL MANIFESTATIONS	CLINICAL THERAPIES
Infection		■ Debridement, drainage, culture, treatment with antibiotics
Acute (may occur with open fractures)	Fever, pain at the site, purulent drainage, redness, edema, heat	
Chronic (osteomyelitis)		
Neurovascular injury resulting from physical nerve damage	Loss of sensation, numbness or tingling, electric acute pain, loss of motor function	■ Nerve repair
Vascular injury	Pale, cool skin; acute severe pain; loss of pulses distal to injury; necrosis of tissue if severe	■ Vascular repair, amputation, tendon lengthening
Malunion (undesired healed alignment of bone) or delayed union	Abnormal appearance of extremity, x-ray demonstrates poor approximation of bone ends, loss of function, pain with movement of distal joint	■ Corrective osteotomy, prolonged immobilization
Nonunion	Abnormal appearance of extremity, x-ray demonstrates poor approximation of bone ends, loss of function, pain with movement of distal joint	■ Surgical intervention, internal fixation
Leg length discrepancy	Client walks with a noticeable limp and may complain of back pain or pain in the hip of involved leg	■ Shoe lift

Emergency Care

Emergency care of the client with a fracture includes immobilizing the fracture, maintaining tissue perfusion, and preventing infection. In the case of serious trauma, normal body alignment must be maintained and may involve cervical immobilization. Once the client is in a secure location, instability or deformity of the bone is assessed. If any deformity or instability is detected, the extremity is rapidly immobilized. Open wounds are covered with sterile dressings, and bleeding may be controlled with a pressure dressing. The extremities are assessed for the presence of pulses, movement, and sensation. The joint above and below the deformity is immobilized. Pulses, movement, and sensation are reevaluated after splinting.

The fracture is splinted to maintain normal anatomic alignment and to prevent it from dislocating. Splinting relieves pain and prevents further damage to the arteries, nerves, and bones. Splinting can be accomplished with air splints. If equipment is not available, the limb may be secured to the body. For example, the client's arm may be secured to the torso with a sling or one leg may be strapped to the other leg.

Diagnostic Tests

Diagnosis of a fracture begins with the history and initial assessment and usually is confirmed by radiographic tests. x-rays and bone scans are used to identify fractures (Figure 19–43 ■). Blood chemistry studies, complete blood count (CBC), and coagulation studies may be used to assess blood loss, renal function, muscle breakdown, and the risk of excessive bleeding or clotting. Diagnostic tests are described in Appendix B.

Pharmacologic Therapies

Most clients with a fracture require pharmacologic interventions. The priority intervention focuses on relieving pain. In the case of multiple fractures or fractures of large bones, narcotics are administered initially and then may be controlled later by nonnarcotic analgesics. Pain management for the client with a fracture is described in Box 19–7.

Stool softeners may be administered to decrease the risk of constipation secondary to narcotics and immobility. Clients who have sustained trauma are often placed on antiulcer medications or antacids. NSAIDs may be prescribed to decrease inflammation. Antibiotics may be

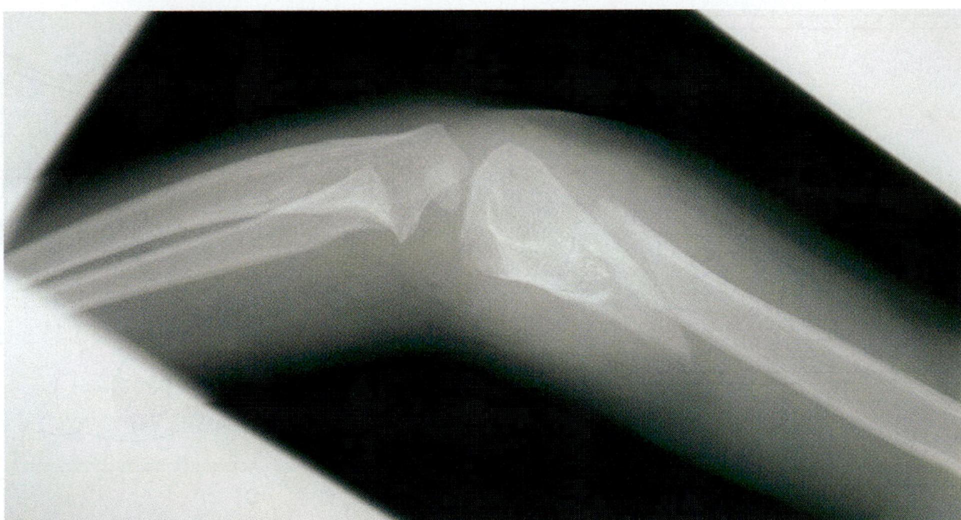

Figure 19–43 ■ X-ray of an oblique fracture of the femur.

Source: Charles Stewart and Associates.

administered prophylactically, particularly to clients with open or complex fractures. Anticoagulants may be prescribed to prevent DVT.

Treatment

Fracture treatment may involve a closed reduction and the application of a cast, or it may include one or more of the following: traction, casts, surgery, and electrical bone stimulation.

TRACTION Muscle spasms usually accompany fractures and may pull bones out of alignment. **Traction** is the application of a straightening or pulling force to return or maintain the fractured bones in normal anatomic position. Weights are applied to maintain the necessary force (Figure 19–44 ■). Types of traction are as follows:

- In *manual traction,* the hand applies the pulling force directly.
- *Skin traction* (also called straight traction) is used to control muscle spasms and to immobilize a part of the body before surgery, with traction exerting its grabbing and pulling force through the client's skin. The most common type of skin traction is Buck's traction, in which traction tape or a foam boot is applied to the lower portion of a client's leg and a free-hanging weight is attached to the taped or booted area

Box 19–7 **Pain Management in the Client With a Fracture**

The client who has had musculoskeletal trauma experiences pain from many different causes:

- The interruption in the continuity of the bone itself
- Damage to ligaments and tendons
- Swelling of tissues around the trauma site
- Muscle spasms
- Tissue anoxia from swelling inside a cast, a splint, or the muscle fascia sheath
- Hematoma formation
- Pressure over bony prominences from casts or splints

The pain is often severe and may be described as sharp, aching, or burning. Carefully assess any complaint of pain; pain may be an indication of a serious complication such as compartment syndrome, decreased tissue perfusion and neurovascular impairment, or pressure ulcers. Do not administer analgesics until the location, character, and duration of pain have been assessed carefully and thoroughly. After the cause of the pain has been identified, the following nursing interventions may be implemented:

1. Administer prescribed analgesics, which may include NSAIDs and narcotic analgesics. For serious fractures or following orthopedic surgery, patient-controlled analgesia (PCA) or epidural methods of providing pain relief may be used. If medications are used on an as-needed basis, tell the client to request the medication before the pain is severe; alternatively, offer the medications at regular intervals for the first 24–48 hours. Reassure the client that addiction does not result from taking medications to relieve fracture or surgical pain. Most clients require only oral analgesics by the third or fourth day after orthopedic surgery.
2. Elevate the involved extremity and apply cold (if prescribed) to help decrease swelling.
3. Monitor and drain the accumulated fluids in any drainage devices to ensure patency and to decrease the possibility of hematoma formation.
4. Encourage the client to wiggle fingers or toes of an extremity in a cast or in traction to improve venous return and decrease edema.
5. Assist the client to change positions to relieve pressure and use pillows to provide support.
6. Teach the client alternative methods of pain management, such as relaxation and guided imagery.
7. Notify the physician of unrelieved pain, which may indicate a serious complication such as compartment syndrome or neurovascular impairment.

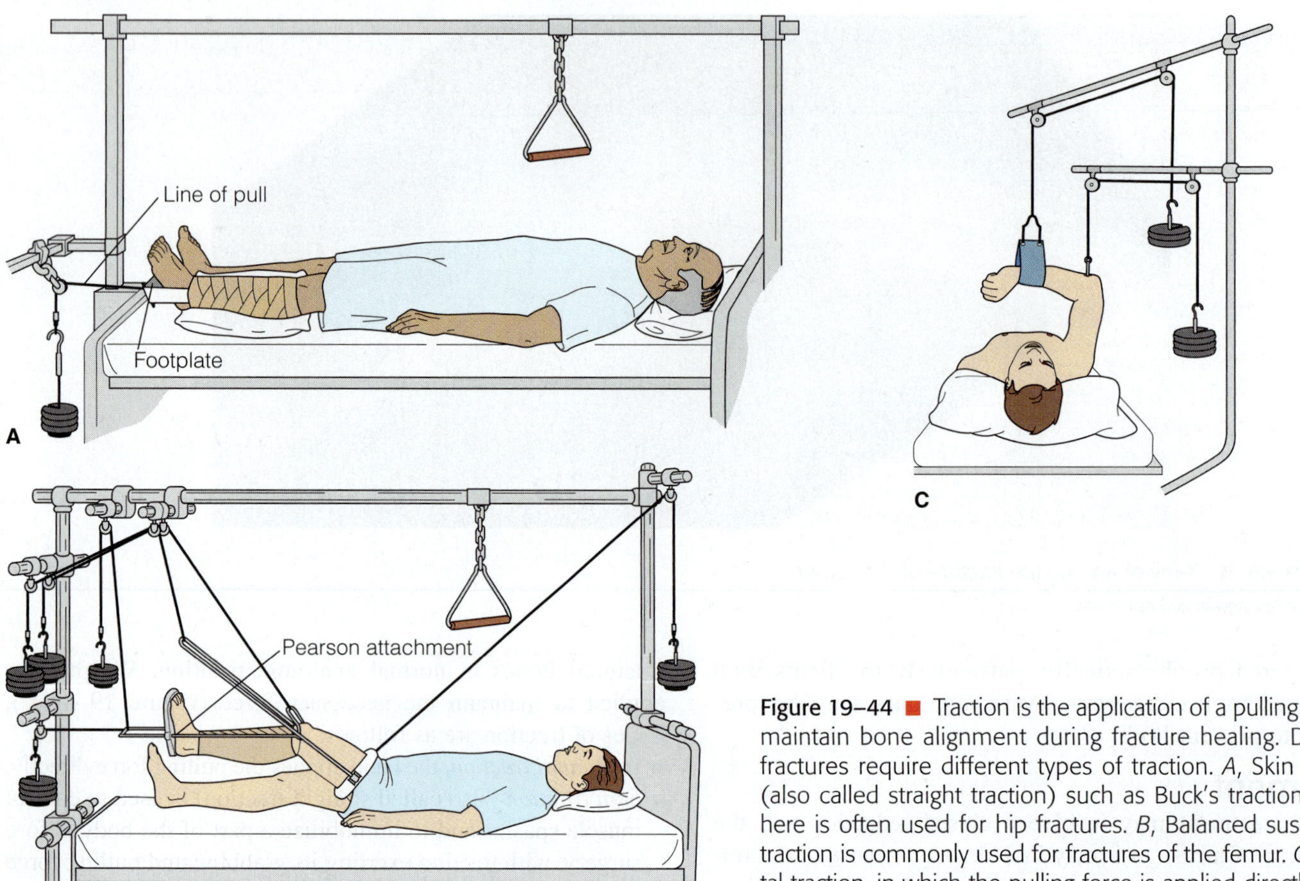

Figure 19–44 ■ Traction is the application of a pulling force to maintain bone alignment during fracture healing. Different fractures require different types of traction. *A*, Skin traction (also called straight traction) such as Buck's traction shown here is often used for hip fractures. *B*, Balanced suspension traction is commonly used for fractures of the femur. *C*, Skeletal traction, in which the pulling force is applied directly to the bone, may be used to treat fractures of the humerus.

(Figure 19–44A). Buck's traction is used to immobilize the leg before surgery to repair a fracture of the proximal femur. The advantage of skin traction is the relative ease of use and ability to maintain comfort. The disadvantage is that the weight required to maintain normal body alignment or fracture alignment cannot exceed the tolerance of the skin (about 6 lb per extremity). It is important to ensure that the weights hang freely; they should never rest on the bed or the floor. The nurse may have to reposition the client or the weights if this occurs.

- *Balanced suspension traction* involves more than one force of pull. Several forces work in unison to raise and support the client's injured extremity off the bed and pull it in a straight line away from the body (Figure 19–44B). The advantage of this type of traction is that it increases mobility without threatening joint continuity. The disadvantage is that the increased use of multiple weights makes the client more likely to slide down in the bed.
- *Skeletal traction* is the application of a pulling force through placement of pins into the bone (Figure 19–44C). The client may receive a local, spinal, or general anesthetic, and the pins are inserted into the bone. This type of traction must be applied under sterile conditions because of the increased risk of infection. One or more pulling forces may be applied with skeletal traction. The advantage of this type of traction is that more weight can be used to maintain the proper anatomic alignment if necessary. The disadvantages include increased anxiety, increased risk of infection, and increased discomfort. The weights used for skeletal traction are not removed by the nurse. Nursing interventions for clients receiving traction are described in Box 19–8.

CASTS A **cast** is a rigid device applied to immobilize the injured bones and promote healing. The cast immobilizes the joint above and the joint below the fractured bone so that the bone will not move during healing. A fracture is first reduced manually (by hand), and then a cast is applied. Casts are applied on those clients who have relatively stable fractures.

The cast, which may be composed of plaster or fiberglass, is applied over a thin cushion of padding and is molded to the normal contour of the body. The cast must be allowed to dry before any pressure is applied to it; simply palpating a wet cast with the fingertips will leave dents that can cause pressure ulcers. A plaster cast may require up to 48 hours to dry, whereas a fiberglass cast dries in less than 1 hour. The type of

Box 19–8 Nursing Interventions for Clients in Traction

- In skeletal traction, never remove the weights.
- In skin traction, remove weights only when intermittent skin traction has been ordered to alleviate muscle spasm.
- For traction to be successful, a countertraction is necessary. In most instances, the countertraction is the client's weight. Therefore, do not wedge the client's foot or place it flush with the footboard of the bed.
- Maintain the line of pull as follows:
  a. Center the client on the bed.
  b. Ensure that weights hang freely and do not touch the floor.
- Ensure that nothing is lying on or obstructing the ropes. Do not allow the knots at the end of the rope to come in contact with the pulley.
- If a problem is detected, assist in repositioning. The area of the fracture must be stabilized when the client is repositioned.
- In skin traction:
  a. Frequently assess skin for evidence of pressure, shearing, or pending breakdown.
  b. Protect pressure sites with padding and protective dressings as indicated.
- In skeletal traction:
  a. Include pin care per policy in frequent skin assessments.
  b. Report signs of infection at the pin sites, such as redness, drainage, and increased tenderness.
  c. Administer more frequent analgesic if needed.
- Perform neurovascular assessments frequently.
- Assess for common complications of immobility, including formation of pressure ulcers, formation of renal calculi, DVT, pneumonia, paralytic ileus, and loss of appetite.
- Teach the client and family about the type and purpose of the traction.

cast applied is determined by the location of the fracture (Figure 19–45 ■). Nursing care of the client with a cast is discussed in Box 19–9. During follow-up appointments, the physician may x-ray the bone to assess alignment and healing and may remove the cast for skin assessment.

SURGERY Surgery is indicated for a fracture that requires direct visualization and repair, a fracture with common long-term complications, or a fracture that is severely comminuted and threatens vascular supply.

The simplest form of surgery is done by external fixation with an external fixator device. An external fixator consists of a frame connected to pins that are inserted perpendicular to the long axis of the bone (Figure 19–46 ■). The number of pins inserted varies with the type and site of the fracture, but in all cases, the same number of pins is inserted above and below the fracture line. The pins require care similar to that of skeletal traction pins. The client is monitored for infection, and frequent neurovascular assessment is performed. The fixator increases independence while maintaining immobilization.

Box 19–9 Nursing Care of the Client With a Cast

NURSING INTERVENTIONS

- Perform frequent neurovascular assessments.
- Palpate the cast for "hot spots" that may indicate the presence of underlying infection.
- Report any drainage promptly.

HEALTH EDUCATION FOR THE CLIENT AND FAMILY

- Do not place any objects in the cast.
- If the cast is made of plaster, keep it dry.
- If the cast is made of fiberglass and it becomes wet, dry it with a blow dryer on the cool setting.
- Assess the injured extremity for coolness, changes in color, increased pain, increased swelling, and/or loss of sensation.
- Use a blow dryer on the cool setting to relieve itching by blowing cool air into the cast.
- If a sling is used, check that it distributes the weight of the cast evenly around the neck. Do not roll the sling; this can impair circulation to the neck.
- If crutches are used, arrange for a physical therapist to teach correct crutch walking.
- When the cast is removed, an oscillating cast remover will be used. A guard prevents the cast remover from penetrating past the depth of the cast so it will not cut the client. The machine is noisy, and the client will feel vibration.

Internal fixation can be accomplished through a surgical procedure called an **open reduction and internal fixation (ORIF)**. In this procedure, the fracture is reduced (placed in correct anatomic alignment) and nails, screws, plates, or pins are inserted to hold the bones in place (Figure 19–47 ■). Open fractures of the arms and legs are most commonly repaired this way. Hip fractures in older clients are usually repaired with ORIF to prevent complications and to allow early rehabilitation. Interventions for postoperative nursing care are presented in Box 19–10.

Box 19–10 Nursing Interventions for Clients With Internal Fixation

- Expect the client to have sutures and at least one Hemovac drain.
- Perform neurovascular assessments frequently.
- Assess the following:
  a. Wounds for drainage
  b. Hemovac for drainage of serosanguineous fluid
  c. Bowel sounds
  d. Lung sounds
- Administer medications such as analgesics and antibiotics per physician's orders.
- In hip fractures, place an abductor pillow between client's legs to prevent dislocation of the hip joint.
- Arrange for physical and occupational therapy as ordered.
- Assist with weight-bearing program, if ordered.
- Encourage early mobilization, coughing, and deep breathing as appropriate to help prevent complications.

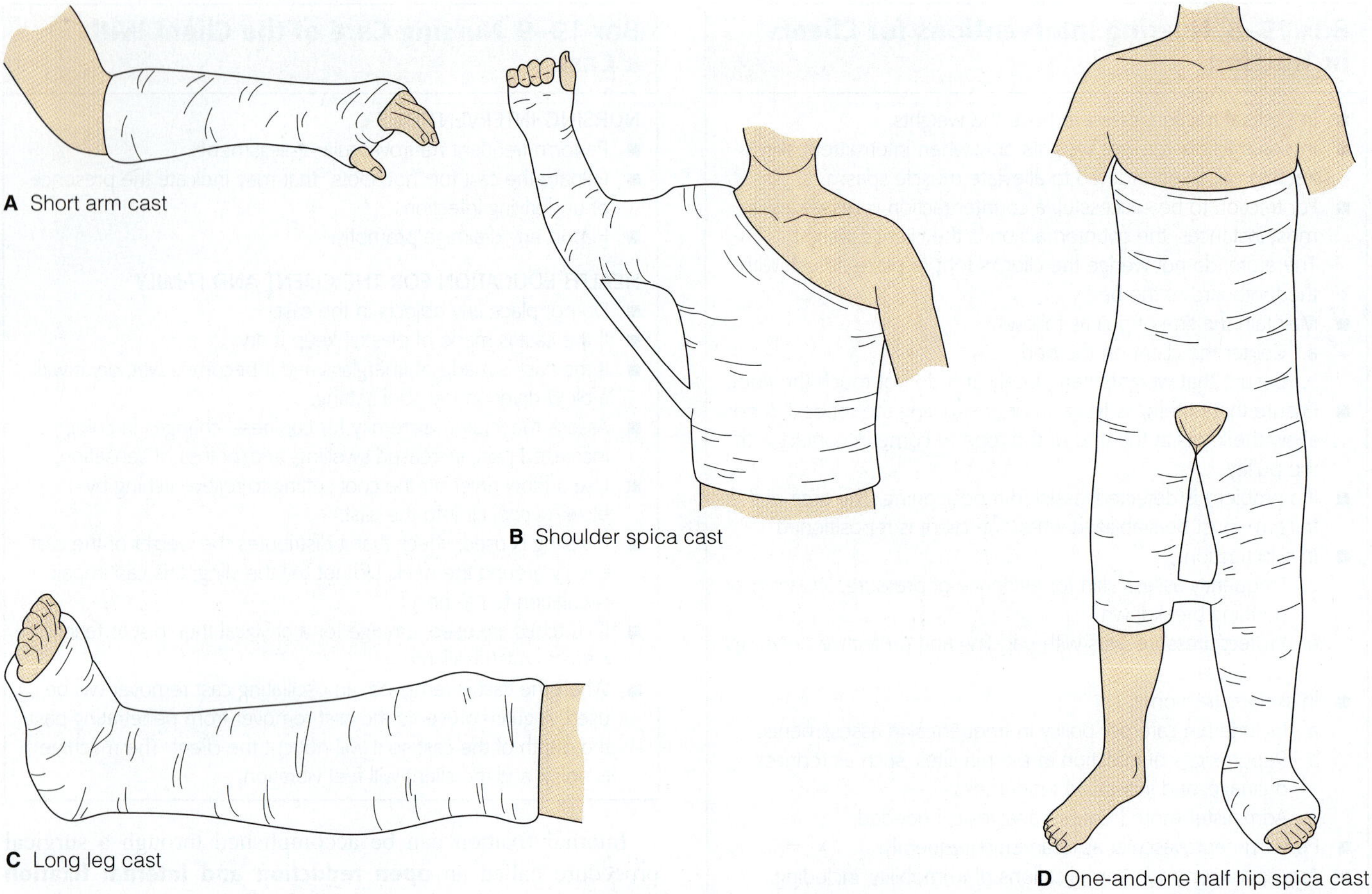

A Short arm cast

B Shoulder spica cast

C Long leg cast

D One-and-one half hip spica cast

Figure 19–45 ■ Examples of types of casts used to immobilize fractures.

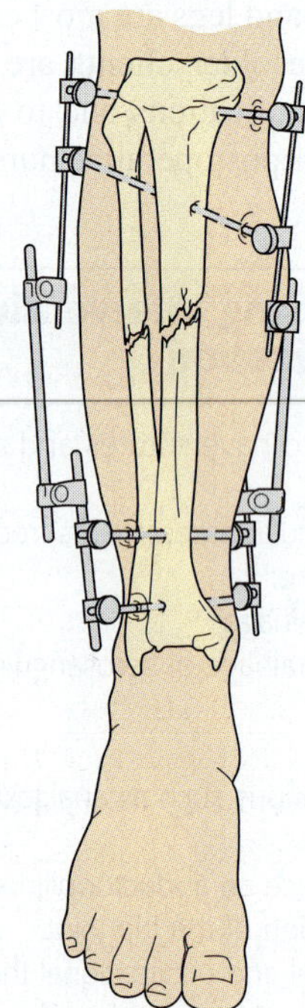

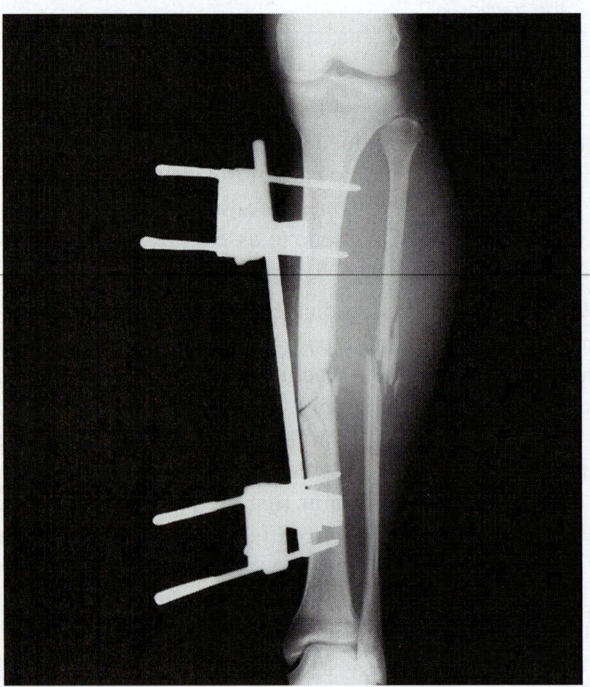

Figure 19–46 ■ In external fixation, pins are placed through the bone above and below the fracture site to immobilize the bone. External fixation rods hold the pins in place.

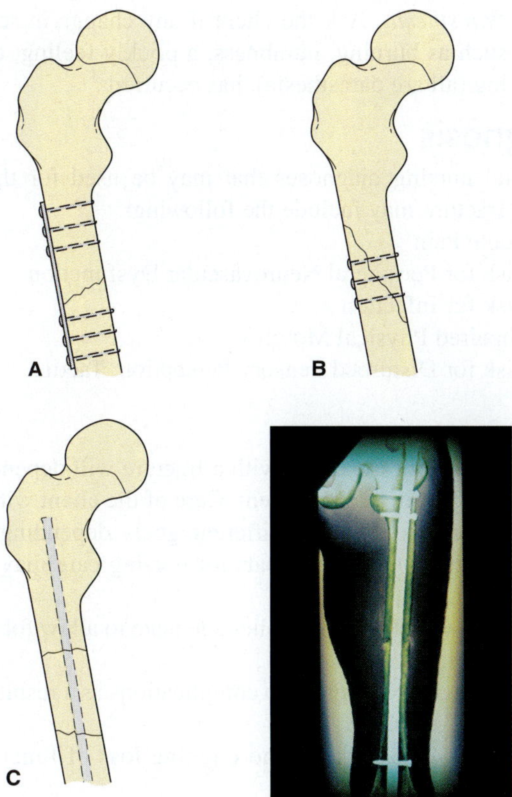

Figure 19–47 ■ Internal fixation hardware is entirely within the body. *A*, Fixation of a short oblique fracture using a plate and screws above and below the fracture. *B*, Fixation of a long oblique fracture using screws through the fracture site. *C*, Fixation of a segmental fracture using a medullary nail.

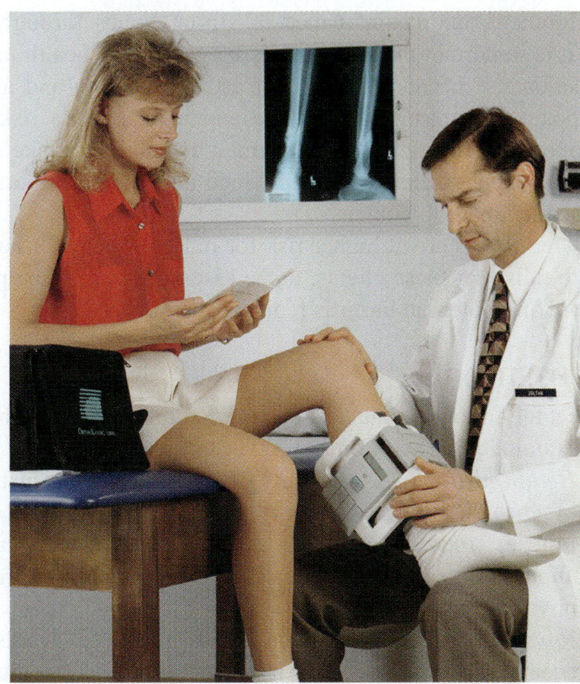

Figure 19–48 ■ External electrical bone growth stimulator.
Courtesy of Orthologic, Inc.

ELECTRICAL BONE STIMULATION Electrical bone stimulation is the application of an electric current at the fracture site. It is a painless method of treating fractures that are not healing appropriately. The electrical stress increases the migration of osteoblasts and osteoclasts to the fracture site. Mineral deposition increases, promoting bone healing. Electrical bone stimulation can be accomplished invasively or noninvasively (Figure 19–48 ■). In invasive stimulation, the surgeon inserts a cathode and a lead wire at the fracture site. The lead wire is attached to an internal or external generator, which delivers electricity through the lead wire to the cathode 24 hours a day. In noninvasive inductive stimulation, a treatment coil encircles the cast or skin directly over the fracture site. The coil is attached to an external generator that runs on batteries. The electricity goes through the skin to the fracture site. The time period for external stimulation can vary from 3–10 hours per day. The client may be taught to self-administer the noninvasive electrical stimulation. Electrical bone stimulation is contraindicated in the presence of infection and for upper extremities if the client has a pacemaker.

NURSING PROCESS

In planning and implementing nursing care for the client with fractures, the nurse should consider the client's response to the traumatic experience. Although each client has individual needs, nursing care commonly focuses on client problems with pain, impaired physical mobility, impaired tissue perfusion, and neurovascular compromise.

Trauma prevention can save lives. Many communities are educating people of all ages—from grade-schoolers to older adults—in trauma prevention. Young adults face a high risk of sustaining trauma. They need to be taught the importance of safety equipment—automobile seat belts, bicycle and motorized vehicle helmets, football pads, proper footwear, protective eyewear, and hard hats—in preventing or decreasing the severity of injury from trauma. Older adults should have regular screenings for osteoporosis (with a bone density test), activity level, cognitive and affective disorders, vision impairments, and risk for falls. Older adults can reduce their risk of falling by increasing lower body strength and balance through regular physical activity and by asking their health care provider or pharmacist to review their medications. Educational programs about workplace and farm safety, including information about ergonomic principles, also can help prevent musculoskeletal injuries.

Exercising regularly and avoiding obesity are important factors in maintaining good bone health in all adults. An adequate intake of calcium is essential to ensure proper growth, development, and maintenance of strong bones throughout life. It is important that women ensure good bone health prior to menopause because the loss of estrogen during and after menopause decreases calcium use and increases the risk of osteoporosis. Strong bones are formed by calcium intake and weight-bearing exercise, both of which are equally important in postmenopausal women.

Older clients are at higher risk for musculoskeletal trauma due to falls. For these clients, home assessments must be performed and potential hazards removed.

Assessment

Collect the following data through the health history and physical examination. (See Concept 32.)

- *Health history*. Age, history of traumatic event, history of chronic illnesses, history of prior musculoskeletal injuries, medications (ask the older adult specifically about anticoagulants and calcium supplements), normal physical activity level
- *Physical assessment*. Pain with movement, pulses, edema, skin color and temperature, deformity, ROM, touch. These assessments include the **5 P's of neurovascular assessment**, as follows, which are included in both the initial assessment and ongoing focused assessments:
  a. *Pain:* Assess pain in the injured extremity by asking the client to grade it on a scale of 0–10, with 10 being the most severe pain.
  b. *Pulses:* Assess distal pulses beginning with the unaffected extremity. Compare the quality of pulses in the affected extremity to those of the unaffected extremity.
  c. *Pallor:* Observe for pallor and skin color in the injured extremity. Paleness and coolness may indicate arterial compromise, whereas warmth and a bluish tinge may indicate venous blood pooling.
  d. *Paralysis/Paresis:* Assess ability to move body parts distal to the fracture site. Inability to move indicates paralysis. Loss of muscle strength (weakness) when moving is paresis. A finding of limited range of motion may lead to early recognition of problems such as nerve damage and paralysis.
  e. *Paresthesia:* Ask the client if any change in sensation, such as burning, numbness, a prickly feeling, or stinging (all are paresthesia), has occurred.

Diagnosis

Potential nursing diagnoses that may be used for the client with a fracture may include the following:

- Acute Pain
- Risk for Peripheral Neurovascular Dysfunction
- Risk for Infection
- Impaired Physical Mobility
- Risk for Disturbed Sensory Perception: Tactile.

Plan

Planning care for the client with a fracture will depend on the severity, location, and treatment. Care of the client with multiple fractures will require different goals depending on the bones involved. Common goals for nursing care may include the following:

- Client will obtain pain relief adequate to allow for rest and comfort.
- Client will experience no complications as a result of fracture or treatment.
- Client will experience no ongoing loss of function as a result of fracture.

Implementation

Nursing care for clients with fractures ranges from teaching to home care treatments provided in the emergency or urgent care department (such as manual reduction and cast application) to providing interventions to maintain health and decrease the risk of complications in clients with complex or multiple fractures.

Nurses who work in community settings may need to provide emergency care and arrange for transport for a client who experiences a fracture. Emergency personnel are informed of the assessment data to provide for safe care. In addition, nurses are aware that repeated fractures in the same person can be a sign of other health care conditions, such as child or elder abuse.

CLIENT TEACHING Teaching Older Adults to Prevent Falls

- Begin a regular exercise program; lack of exercise leads to weakness and an increased chance of falling. Exercises that improve balance and coordination (such as tai chi) are most beneficial.
- Make your home safer to reduce the risk of injury, by implementing the following:
  - Remove any items in your pathway, including from stairs, to avoid tripping.
  - Remove small throw rugs or use double-sided tape to keep rugs from slipping.
  - Place frequently used items within easy reach to avoid use of a step stool.
  - Install grab bars next to the toilet and in the tub or shower.
  - Use nonslip mats in the bathtub and on shower floors.
  - Improve lighting, using lamp shades or frosted bulbs to reduce glare.
  - Install handrails and lights in all staircases.
- Wear shoes that provide good support and that have thin, nonslip soles. Avoid wearing slippers and athletic shoes with deep treads.
- Ask your health care provider to review your medications, including prescriptions and OTC medications. Some medications or a combination of medications may cause dizziness or drowsiness, leading to falls.
- Have your vision checked by an eye doctor. Your glasses may no longer have the correct prescription, or you may have developed an eye condition such as cataracts or glaucoma that limits your vision.

Nursing care focuses on care of the client before and after fracture reduction, encouraging mobility as ordered, maintaining skin integrity, preventing infection, and teaching the client and family how to care for the fracture. When caring for a client who has undergone fracture reduction, it is important to watch for signs of complications (Table 19–10). Notify the physician immediately if these signs occur. The most serious complication is compartment syndrome, which compromises circulation and nervous innervation (Altizer, 2004). Compartment syndrome is a medical emergency and needs to be reported immediately to the primary health care provider or medical personnel on hand. A cast cutter should be available so the cast can be removed if needed.

Maintain Proper Alignment

Immobilization maintains proper alignment of the fracture. Casts and traction are used to immobilize both the joint above and the joint below the fracture because muscles attach to bones above and below the joint and any motion can impact the integrity of the bone as it heals.

Different types of traction are used depending on the location and type of fracture (Box 19–11).

Monitor Neurovascular Status

Neurovascular assessment is used for early detection of compartment syndrome, which may occur with a crush injury or when a fracture is reduced. Swelling associated with inflammation reduces blood flow to the affected area, and casting causes further constriction of blood flow. Monitor the client's sensation to touch, temperature, movement, pulse strength, and capillary refill time in the extremity distal to the injury. Monitor every 15 minutes after the cast is applied for at least 2 hours and then every 1–2 hours depending on the care facility's policy and the client's condition. Keep the cast elevated above heart level to minimize edema.

Promote Mobility

The physician orders the amount of mobility the client is allowed. Restrictions depend on the extent and site of the fracture. Fractures of the hip or pelvis may involve body casts, and providing wheeled carts makes mobility possible. Clients with leg fractures can sometimes bear weight on the cast. If they cannot bear weight, they move around with crutches, walkers, or wheelchairs. See the Skills Manual for information on crutch walking.

Discharge Planning and Home Care Teaching

Most fractures can be easily managed at home. Activities are generally limited for approximately 8 weeks. Teach the client and family cast care, activity restrictions, and identification of problems that should be reported. Help parents to identify any modifications that may be needed at home and school. The client who must manage steps at home or school may need special training with crutches or a temporary ramp. For pediatric clients, refer parents to home health nurses or home teaching services if indicated. Provide pertinent teaching to prevent future injuries.

Acute Pain

Pain is caused by soft tissue damage and is compounded by muscle spasms and swelling.

- Monitor vital signs. Some analgesics decrease respiratory effort and blood pressure.
- Ask the client to rate the pain on a scale of 0–10 (with 10 being the most severe pain) before and after any intervention. This facilitates objective assessment of the effectiveness of the chosen pain relief strategy. Pain that increases in intensity or remains unrelieved with analgesics can indicate compartment syndrome.
- For the client with a hip fracture, apply Buck's traction per physician's orders. Keep the traction weights hanging freely. Buck's traction immobilizes the fracture and decreases pain and additional trauma.
- Move the client gently and slowly. Gentle movement helps prevent the development of severe muscle spasms.
- Elevate the injured extremity above the level of the heart. Elevating the extremity promotes venous return and decreases edema, which decreases pain.
- Encourage distraction or other noninvasive methods of pain relief, such as deep breathing and relaxation. Distraction, deep breathing, and relaxation help decrease the focus on the pain and may lessen the intensity of pain.
- Administer pain medications as prescribed. For home care, explain the importance of taking pain medications before the pain becomes severe. Analgesics alleviate pain by stimulating opiate receptor sites.

TABLE 19–10 **Complications of Fracture Reduction**

COMPLICATION	CLINICAL THERAPY
Infection Acute (may occur with open fractures) Chronic (osteomyelitis)	Debridement, drainage, culture, treatment with antibiotics
Neurovascular injury resulting from physical nerve damage	Nerve repair
Vascular injury	Vascular repair, amputation, tendon lengthening
Malunion (undesired healed alignment of bone) or delayed union	Corrective osteotomy, prolonged immobilization
Nonunion	Surgical intervention, internal fixation
Leg length discrepancy	Shoe lift

Box 19–11 Types of Traction

SKIN TRACTION
Pull is applied to the skin surface, which puts traction directly on the bones and muscles. Traction is attached to the skin with adhesive materials or straps or with foam boots, belts, or halters.

DUNLOP TRACTION (EITHER SKELETAL OR SKIN)
Used for fracture of the humerus. The arm, which is flexed, is suspended horizontally with straps placed on both the upper and lower portion for pull from both sides.

BRYANT TRACTION (Figure 19–49 ■)
Used specifically for the child under 3 years of age and weighing less than 17.5 kg (35 lb) who has developmental dysplasia of the hip or a fractured femur. This bilateral traction is applied to the child's legs and kept in place by wrapping the legs from foot to thigh with elastic bandages. The hips are flexed at a 90-degree angle, with knees extended. This position is maintained by attaching the traction appliance to weights and pulleys, which are suspended above the crib. The buttocks do not rest on the mattress, but are slightly elevated off the bed.

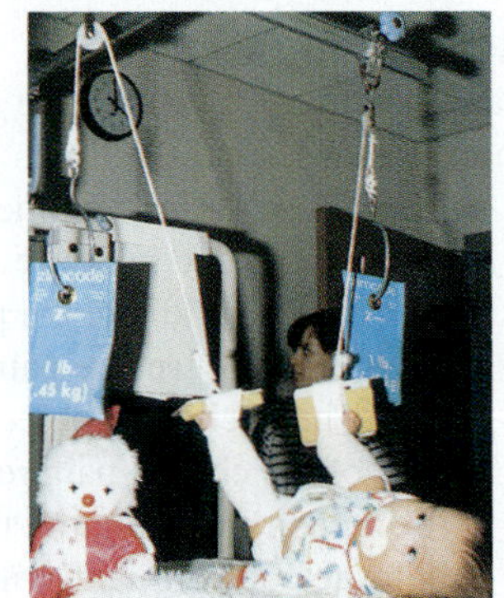

Figure 19–49 ■ Bryant traction.

BUCK TRACTION (Figure 19–50 ■)
Used for knee immobilization, for correcting contractures or deformities, and for short-term immobilization of a fracture. It keeps the leg in an extended position without hip flexion. Traction is applied to the extremity in one direction (straight line) with a single pulley system.

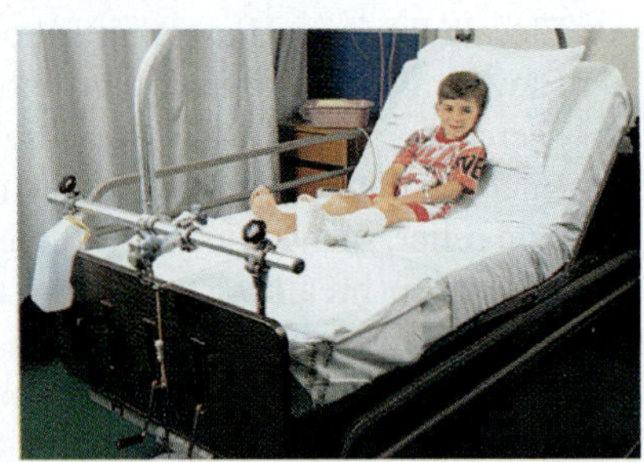

Figure 19–50 ■ Buck traction.

RUSSELL TRACTION (Figure 19–51 ■)
Used for fractures of the femur and lower leg. Traction is placed on the lower leg while the knee is suspended in a padded sling. The hips and knees, which are slightly flexed, are immobilized. One force is applied by a double pulley to the foot, and another force is applied upward using a sling under the knee and an overhead pulley.

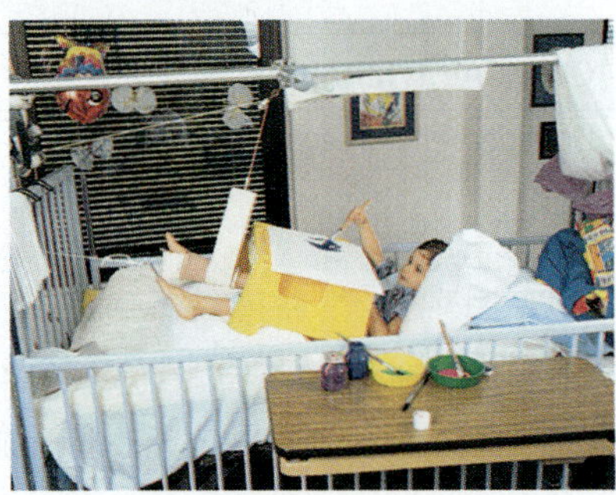

Figure 19–51 ■ Russell traction.

SKELETAL TRACTION
Pull is directly applied to the bone by pins, wires, tongs, or other apparatus that have been surgically placed through the distal end of the bone.

SKELETAL CERVICAL TRACTION
Used for cervical spine injuries to reduce fractures and dislocations. Crutchfield, Gardner-Wells, or Vinke tongs are placed in the skull with burr holes. Weights are attached to the apparatus with a rope-and-pulley system to the hyperextended head.

HALO TRACTION
Used to immobilize the head and neck after cervical injury or dislocation. Also used for positioning and immobilization after cervical injury.

90-90 TRACTION (Figure 19–52 ■)
Used for fractures of the femur or tibia. A skeletal pin or wire is surgically placed through the distal part of the femur, while the lower part of the extremity is in a boot cast. Traction ropes and pulleys are applied at the pin site and on the boot cast to maintain the flexion of the hip and knee at 90 degrees. This traction also can be used for treatment of an upper extremity fracture.

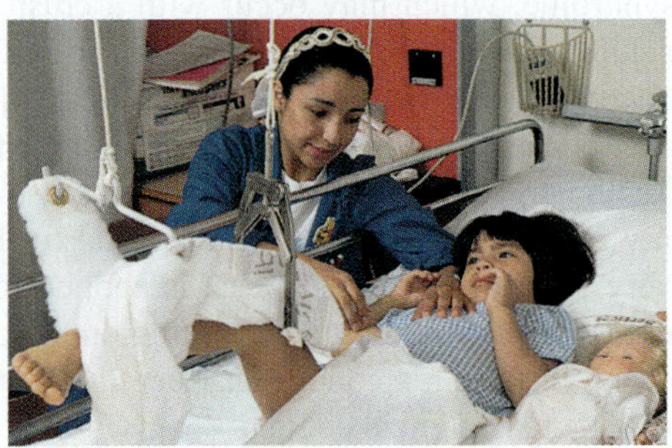

Figure 19–52 ■ 90-90 traction.

EXTERNAL FIXATORS (Figure 19–53 ■)
These devices can be used in the treatment of simple fractures, both open and closed; complex fractures with extensive soft tissue involvement; correction of bony or soft tissue deformities; pseudoarthroses; and limb length discrepancy. They are attached to the extremity by percutaneous transfixing of pins or wires to the bone.

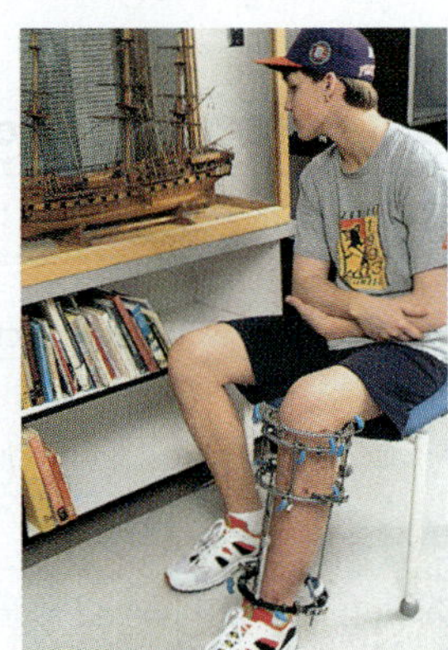

Figure 19–53 ■ External fixators.

Risk for Peripheral Neurovascular Dysfunction

In the client with a fracture, compartment syndrome or DVT can impair circulation and, in turn, tissue perfusion.

- Assess the 5 P's every 1–2 hours. Report abnormal findings immediately. Unrelenting pain, pallor, diminished distal pulses, paresthesia, and paresis are strong indicators of compartment syndrome.
- Assess nail beds for capillary refill. If nails are too thick or discolored, assess the skin around the nail. Delayed capillary refill may indicate decreased tissue perfusion.
- Monitor the extremity for edema and swelling. Excessive swelling and hematoma formation can compromise circulation.
- Assess for deep, throbbing, unrelenting pain. Pain that is not relieved by analgesics may indicate neurovascular compromise.
- Monitor the tightness of the cast. Edema can cause the cast to become tight; a tight-fitting cast may lead to compartment syndrome or paralysis.
- If the cast is tight, be prepared to assist the physician with bivalving (Figure 19–54 ■). Bivalving, the process of splitting the cast down both sides, alleviates pressure on the injured extremity.
- If compartment syndrome is suspected, assist the physician in measuring compartment pressure. Normal compartment pressure is 10–20 mmHg. Compartment pressure greater than 30 mmHg indicates compartment syndrome.
- Elevate the injured extremity above the level of the heart. Elevating the extremity increases venous return and decreases edema.
- Administer anticoagulant per physician's order. Prophylactic anticoagulation decreases the risk of clot formation.

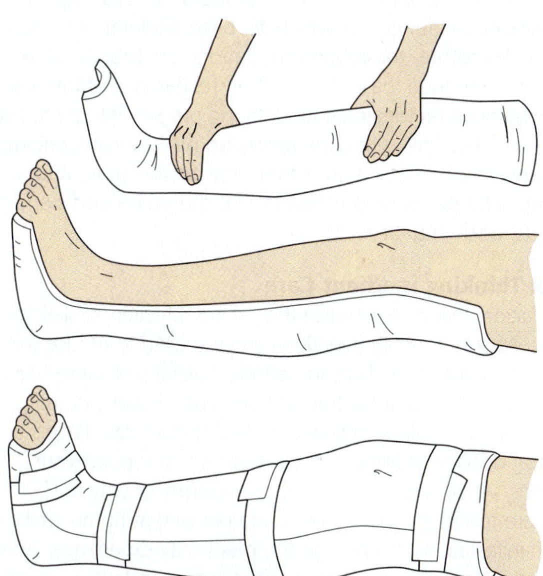

Figure 19–54 ■ Bivalving is the process of splitting the cast down both sides to alleviate pressure on or allow visualization of the extremity.

Risk for Infection

The client who undergoes surgical repair will have a postoperative wound. Any break in skin integrity must be monitored for infection. Wound healing in orthopedic clients is affected by the cause of the wound as well as the therapies used to repair musculoskeletal structures. It is important for nurses to understand processes of normal wound healing; characteristics of musculoskeletal wounds, contamination, and drainage; and potential complications for which to plan and implement appropriate interventions (Harvey, 2005). Exemplar 30.4, Wound Healing provides a detailed discussion of the processes of and alterations in wound healing.

- For clients with skeletal pins, follow established guidelines for skeletal pin site care, as outlined in the Evidenced-Based Practice box. Pins or wires attached to traction, casts, or external fixators stabilize a segment of bone so optimal healing can occur. However, pin infections of varying severity do occur (Holmes & Brown, 2005).
- Monitor vital signs and lab reports of WBCs. Increases in pulse rate, respiratory rate, temperature, and WBCs may indicate infection.
- Use sterile technique for dressing changes. The surgeon will change the initial postoperative dressing. The nurse must change all subsequent dressings without introducing organisms to the operative site.
- Assess the wound for size and color and the presence of any drainage. Redness, swelling, and purulent drainage indicate infection.
- Administer antibiotics per physician's orders. Prophylactic antibiotic administration inhibits bacterial reproduction, thereby helping to prevent skin flora from entering the wound. In the case of "dirty wounds," such as those occurring from vehicular crashes, antibiotics are routinely administered.

Impaired Physical Mobility

The client who has experienced a fracture requires immobilization of the fractured bone(s). Immobilization alters normal gait and mobility. The client will need to use assistive devices such as crutches, canes, slings, or walkers.

- Teach or assist client with ROM exercises of the unaffected limbs. ROM exercises help prevent muscle atrophy and maintain strength and joint function. Flexion and extension exercises prevent the development of foot drop, wrist drop, and frozen joints.
- Teach isometric exercises and encourage the client to perform them every 4 hours. Isometric exercises help prevent muscle atrophy and force synovial fluid and nutrients into the cartilage.
- Encourage ambulation when client is able; provide assistance as necessary. Ambulation maintains and improves circulation, helps prevent muscle atrophy, and helps maintain bowel function.
- Teach and observe the client's use of assistive devices (such as canes, crutches, walkers, and slings) in conjunction with the physical therapist. Proper use of devices is necessary for safe ambulation and helps prevent the loss of joint function secondary to complications and falls.

- Turn the client on bed rest every 2 hours. If the client is in traction, teach the client to shift his or her weight every hour. Turning and shifting weight increases circulation and helps prevent skin breakdown.

Risk for Disturbed Sensory Perception: Tactile

The client who has sustained a fracture is at risk for nerve injury from the initial trauma, as well as from complications such as compartment syndrome.

- Assess the ability to differentiate between sharp and dull touch and the presence of paresthesia and paralysis every 1–2 hours. Paresthesia develops as a result of pressure on nerves and may indicate compartment syndrome.
- Elevate the injured extremity above the level of the heart. Elevating the extremity decreases swelling and the risk of compartment syndrome and nerve entrapment. Check the cast for fit. A tightly fitting cast can decrease blood flow to distal tissues, compress nerves, and cause compartment syndrome.
- Support the injured extremity above and below the fracture site when moving the client. Supporting the injured extremity above and below the fracture site helps prevent displacement of bony fragments and decreases the risk of further nerve damage.

Clients who have experienced a fracture or who have had orthopedic surgery often wear a cast and require an extended period of immobilization or limited activities. Address the following topics for home care:

- Do not use a sharp object to try to scratch under a cast.
- Do not get a plaster cast wet.
- Follow the physician's order for weight bearing.
- Physical therapists often can evaluate the home environment for safety and suggest modifications as needed. Physical therapists also teach crutch walking, limited weight bearing, transferring, and other activities.
- Home care agencies also can teach wound care and provide ongoing monitoring of wound healing.
- Local medical equipment and supply sources rent or sell durable equipment such as crutches, walkers, wheelchairs, overhead trapeze units, shower chairs, elevated toilet seats, grab bars, and bedside commodes. Slings and braces may be purchased through medical equipment dealers.
- Local pharmacies are good sources for dressing supplies such as antiseptic solutions and ointments, dressings, and tape.
- Fitness equipment suppliers may be able to provide rehabilitation equipment such as hand and ankle weights to use for strengthening exercises.

PRACTICE ALERT

When in doubt about the nature of an injury, apply a splint. Splinting immobilizes the site, prevents further damage, and decreases pain. Be sure to immobilize the joint directly above and directly below the injury.

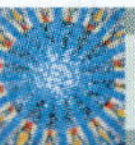

EVIDENCE-BASED PRACTICE The Client With Skeletal Pins

Clinical guidelines for specific client care interventions, such as skeletal pin care, should be based on research in order to provide the most appropriate evidence-based practice. The recommendations contained in this report from the National Association of Orthopaedic Nurses were based on published research and are for skin care of areas surrounding the pin insertion sites. Data from the studies provided beginning guidelines, but were not conclusively useful as there were few experimental studies, and the studies were diverse in definitions and variables. However, the following recommendations were made:

- Pins located in areas with considerable soft tissue should be considered at greater risk for infection.
- For the first 48–72 hours (when drainage may be heavy), pin site care should be done daily. Once drainage declines and the site is mechanically stable (bone-pin interface) weekly pin site care may be adequate.
- Chlorhexidine (2 mg/mL) solution may be the most effective cleansing solution for pin site care.
- Clients and their families should be taught pin site care before discharge from the hospital. They should be required to demonstrate whatever care needs to be done and should be provided with written instructions that include signs and symptoms of infection.

Implications for Nursing

Evaluation of the literature by members of this expert panel found scanty evidence on which to base skeletal pin site interventions. Therefore, the recommendations are broadly stated, but they do serve as a base for further research. Future research should examine factors such as defining pin site infection, risk for pin site infection, pin site care versus no pin site care, showering, management of crusts, skin adherence to the pins, and use of dressings. The panel recommends that the guidelines be individualized to each situation.

Critical Thinking in Client Care

1. List factors that may increase the risk for infection of skeletal pin sites. What nursing interventions may be used to reduce this risk?
2. You are caring for a client for whom skeletal pins were used for external fixation of a fracture of bones of a lower extremity. There is dried yellow drainage around the pin site. Based on clinical decision making without research to support your actions, would you remove the crusts? Why or why not?
3. You are teaching a client how to do pin care at home. Make a list of manifestations of infection the client may experience. What would you recommend if any of these manifestations occur?

Data from Holmes, S. B., & Brown, S. J. (2005). Skeletal pin site care. National Association of Orthopaedic Nurses guidelines for orthopaedic nursing. *Orthopaedic Nursing, 24*(2), 99–108.

NURSING CARE PLAN **A Client With an Arm Fracture**

Frank Dexter, 14 years old, is an active, healthy adolescent who lives part-time with his mother and the rest of the time with his father. His parents divorced 2 years ago, and he still secretly hopes they'll work things out. Frank enjoys skateboarding with his friends at the local park and was attempting to do some tricks he saw on television when he fell and fractured his left radius. His friends helped him home, and his mother washed the laceration on his arm and took him to the emergency department, where he was diagnosed with a compound fracture. After analgesics and anesthesia were administered, a closed reduction was performed and the laceration on his arm was sutured. A cast was applied with a window cut to allow observation of the laceration. The orthopedist wrote a prescription for oxycodone for pain relief prior to Frank's being discharged from the ED.

ASSESSMENT

During the initial assessment at the ED, abnormal findings are that Frank's left arm has a 2-inch laceration on the dorsal aspect of the arm with visible bone. Frank is pale and moaning in pain and fear. Distal pulses are present and strong. His fingers are warm and pink with brisk capillary refill. Frank complains of severe pain but states that no numbness or burning is present. He is unable to wiggle his fingers. Initial vital signs are as follows: T_O 98.0°F (36.6°C), P 100, R 18, BP 120/58. An x-ray of the left arm is performed. He denies hitting his head or pain in any other area other than his left arm. The x-ray reveals a fracture of the left radius.

Frank is taken to the orthopedic room where he is given analgesics and adequate sedation to perform a closed reduction, and the laceration is sutured. A cast is applied with a window cut to allow observation of the laceration. He is now alert but drowsy and denies pain. He tells his mother that he is going to have all of his friends sign his cast and that they need to save it when it's removed.

DIAGNOSES

- Acute Pain related to fractured left radius
- Risk for Ineffective Tissue Perfusion related to unstable bones and swelling
- Risk for Disturbed Sensory Perception: Tactile related to the risk of nerve impairment
- Risk for Infection related to contaminated laceration and exposure of bone to pathogens

PLAN

Goals include the following:

- Verbalize a decrease in pain.
- Verbalize the essential cast assessments and signs and symptoms to report immediately.
- Maintain normal neurovascular status.
- Demonstrate appropriate cast and laceration care.

IMPLEMENTATION

- Assess pain on a scale of 0–10 before and after measures are implemented to reduce pain.
- Administer narcotics per the physician's order.
- Teach mother to perform neurovascular assessment every 2–4 hours.
- Teach mother to elevate arm higher than level of heart and to apply ice for 48 hours.
- Teach mother and client how to handle cast to prevent denting or malformation.

EVALUATION

Seven days after being casted, Frank is seen at his pediatrician's office. His fingers are warm and pink, and he is able to move his fingers appropriately. The laceration is healing well, and sutures are removed. Frank has not needed narcotics for pain relief and has been taking ibuprofen, obtaining adequate comfort. His cast is removed 4 weeks later, and he is taught exercises to perform for regaining full mobility in his left arm.

CRITICAL THINKING

1. Why was it necessary to cut a window in the cast? What might have happened if the window had not been cut?
2. What specific client teaching would you have given regarding cast care?
3. When teaching Frank and his mother how to assess the left arm, what would you have told them to look for and what symptoms would you have taught them to report immediately?

Evaluation

Evaluation of client care is determined based on the goals of care, the client's specific needs, the location of the fracture, and the treatment received. Potential client outcomes may include the following:

- Client regains prior level of function when fracture resolves.
- Client experiences no complications as a result of treatment.
- Client explains home cast care.
- Client lists symptoms to report to provider immediately.

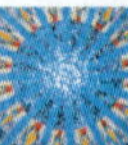

CLIENT TEACHING Home Care for the Client With a Fracture

Client and family teaching focuses on the client's needs. The type of fracture and its location determine how much teaching the client and family will require. For example, the client who has a simple nondisplaced tibial fracture may need to be taught only cast care and crutch walking. By contrast, the older client who sustained a hip fracture and requires surgical intervention has a wider array of teaching needs, including the use of an abduction pillow, proper bending, and proper sitting. Address the following topics for home care of the client who has fractured a hip:

Encourage independence in ADLs as follows:

- Explain that the client should sit only on high chairs to prevent excess flexion of the hip; a high toilet seat can be added to a regular toilet seat.
- Encourage the client and family to install a rail in the shower to aid in stability and to prevent falls.
- If a walker is needed, teach the client its proper use: Do not carry the walker, but lift it, advance it, and then take two steps, or use a rolling walker.
- If a cane is needed, instruct the client to use it on the affected side.
- Stress the importance of well-balanced meals and explain all prescribed medications.

REVIEW Fractures

RELATE: LINK THE CONCEPTS

Linking the exemplar of Fractures with the concept of Safety:

1. In the preceding Care Plan, what safety risks does Frank have as a result of his fracture?
2. What teaching would you provide to reduce Frank's risk of further injury or complications?

Linking the exemplar of Fractures with the concept of Perfusion:

3. List the precursors to deep vein thrombosis (DVT) formation for a client with a compound fracture of the left femur.
4. What are the nursing priorities to initiate in order to reduce the risk of DVT in the client in traction with a broken femur?

READY: GO TO COMPANION SKILLS MANUAL

- Assessing the musculoskeletal system
- Assessing the client in pain
- Transferring a client with an injured lower extremity
- Assisting the client to use crutches
- Assisting the client to use a walker
- Applying a splint
- Performing initial (wet) cast care
- Performing ongoing cast care
- Performing care for a child with a cast

REFER: GO TO MYNURSINGKIT

REFLECT: CASE STUDY

Saul Genmar is a 21-year-old man who has graduated from Harvard and is working as a car salesman. He is engaged to Joanne who is 19 and a sophomore at Smith College. Joanne lives at home when she is not in school and Saul has an apartment with three friends. Saul and his buddies were out drinking and were involved in an auto accident at 0300 last night. Saul has a compound fracture of his right tibia and has returned from surgery with an external fixation device and is in traction. Joanne came to visit and is lying on the bed next to Saul.

1. What is your priority of care for Saul as you begin your shift?
2. How will you address Saul and Joanne when you enter the room to deliver care?
3. What teaching interventions will you initiate for both Saul and Joanne?

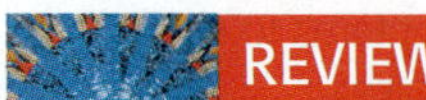

19.3 HIP FRACTURES

KEY TERMS

Arthroplasty, *1112*
Extracapsular fractures, *1111*
Hemiarthroscopy, *1112*
Intracapsular fractures, *1111*

BASIS FOR SELECTION OF EXEMPLAR

Most common ER visit

LEARNING OUTCOMES

After reading about this exemplar, you will be able to:

1. Describe the pathophysiology, etiology, clinical manifestations, and direct and indirect causes of hip fractures.
2. Identify risk factors associated with hip fractures.
3. Illustrate the nursing process in providing culturally competent care across the life span for individuals with a hip fracture.
4. Formulate priority nursing diagnoses appropriate for an individual with a hip fracture.
5. Create a plan of care for individuals with a hip fracture and their family members.
6. Assess expected outcomes for an individual with a hip fracture.
7. Discuss therapies used in the collaborative care of an individual with a hip fracture.
8. Employ evidence-based caring interventions for an individual with a hip fracture.

OVERVIEW

A hip fracture refers to a fracture of the femur at the head, neck, or trochanteric regions (Figure 19–55 ■). While a hip fracture is most often associated with older adults, it can occur at any age. Hip fractures often are seen in younger adults involved in high-speed automobile accidents when seat belts were improperly placed or shoulder restraints were not worn with lap belts.

PATHOPHYSIOLOGY AND ETIOLOGY

Hip fractures are classified as intracapsular or extracapsular. **Intracapsular fractures** involve the head or neck of the femur; **extracapsular fractures** involve the trochanteric region. The majority of hip fractures involve the neck or trochanteric regions. The femoral head and neck lie within the joint capsule and are not covered in periosteum; thus, they do not have a large blood supply. Fractures at this location usually fragment, further decreasing blood supply and increasing the risk of nonunion and avascular necrosis. The trochanteric region is covered in periosteum and therefore has more of a blood supply than the head or neck.

Intracapsular fractures frequently impair the flow of blood to the femoral head. A displaced femoral neck fracture can completely disrupt the blood supply to the femoral head, which may result in avascular necrosis and nonunion of the fracture. Extracapsular fractures cause acute blood loss from the vascular cancellous bone surfaces, but rarely cause avascular necrosis (Gerhart, 2003).

Etiology

Hip fractures are typically caused by trauma, such as a fall or motor vehicle collision. Some conditions, such as osteoporosis, contribute to the tendency of bone to fracture. More than one third of all adults over the age of 65 fall each year. Of those, white men have the highest fall-related death rates, followed by white women, black men, and black women. Older adults most often fracture the hip from falls; in contrast, motor vehicle crashes are the most common cause in young and middle adults.

Risk Factors

Hip fractures are common in older adults as a result of decreases in bone mass and the increased tendency to fall. Hip fractures are the most common injury in the older population, requiring hospitalization of more than 300,000 older adults each year in the United States. Hip fractures result in the greatest number of deaths and are the most serious health problem of all fractures for people 65 years and older (Centers for Disease Control and Prevention, 2005). By the year 2040, the number of hip fractures is expected to exceed 500,000, which reflects society's increasing older population. Factors contributing to falls include problems with gait and balance, neurologic and musculoskeletal impairments, dementia, psychoactive medications, and visual impairments. Modifiable risk factors, identified through research, include experiencing lower body weakness, having problems with walking and balance, and taking four or more medications or any psychoactive medications. The risk for a fractured hip increases with each decade of life, especially in white postmenopausal women, who have the highest incidence

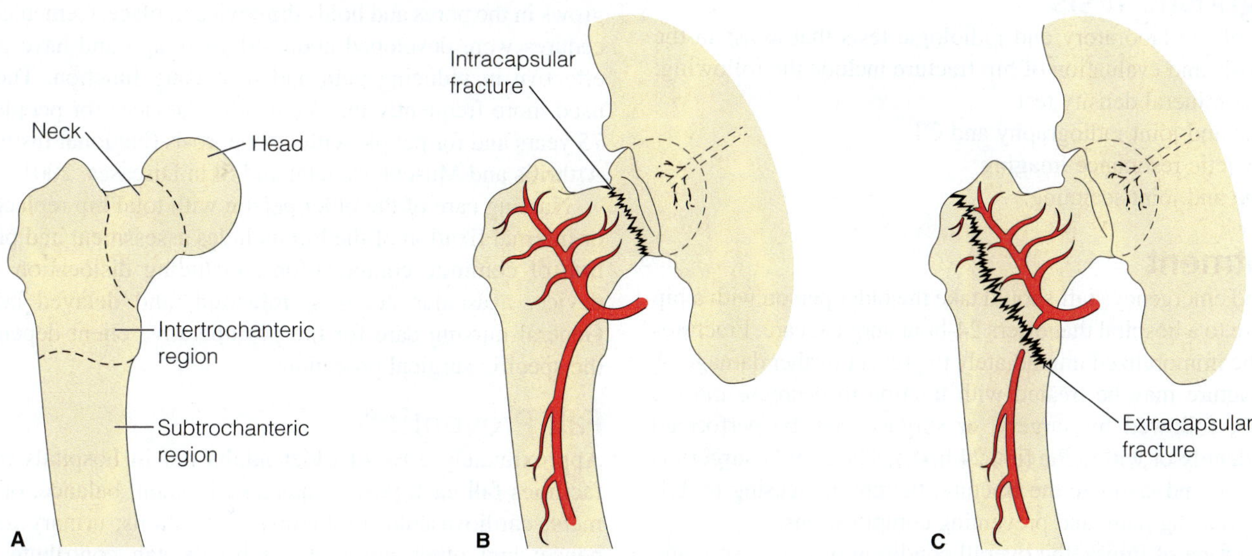

Figure 19–55 ■ Regions where hip fractures may occur: *A*, The head of the femur, the neck of the femur, and the trochanteric regions of the femur. *B*, Intracapsular fractures occur across the head or neck of the femur. *C*, Extracapsular fractures occur across the trochanteric regions. Note how both intracapsular and extracapsular fractures disrupt the blood supply to the bone.

of osteoporosis. Women have about 80% of all hip fractures (Centers for Disease Control and Prevention, 2005). Women who smoke are at greater risk because smoking reduces bone density among menopausal women (CDC, 2005).

CLINICAL MANIFESTATIONS

Clients with a hip fracture may be unable to walk, stand, or bear weight on the affected side. Clients often experience acute pain. The extreme pain of the fracture prevents any movement; and the older client often cannot even crawl to reach a phone. The force of gravity and the pull of muscles cause the affected leg to appear shortened and externally rotated.

Complications are related to both the fracture and the resulting treatment. Only a small number of clients retain their previous mobility, while about 20% require nursing home care. Half of all older adults hospitalized for a hip fracture cannot return home or live independently after the fracture (Centers for Disease Control and Prevention, 2005).

COLLABORATION

Collaborative care is essential to optimizing client outcomes. The health care team may include nurses, treating physicians (e.g., orthopedic surgeon and the client's general practioner), pharmacists, and physical and occupational therapists. For the older client who has an existing respiratory or cardiac condition, consultation with the treating specialist is recommend. Social service referrals may be indicated to help the client receive the rehabilitative care required after being discharged from the acute care facility.

Diagnostic Tests

Some of the laboratory and radiologic tests that assist in the diagnosis and evaluation of hip fracture include the following:

- Bone mineral density test
- Bone and joint radiography and CT
- Magnetic resonance imaging
- Bone and joint scanning.

Treatment

Trained emergency staff should take the older person with a hip fracture to a hospital that offers 24-hour surgical care. Fractures must be immobilized immediately to prevent further damage. A hip fracture may be treated with traction to decrease muscle spasms, followed by surgery, or surgery may be performed immediately or within the first 24 hours. The goal of surgery is to reduce and stabilize the fracture, thereby increasing mobility, decreasing pain, and preventing complications.

The type of injury, the overall condition of the person, and any preexisting orthopedic conditions will determine the type of surgical procedure. In general, the more invasive the surgical procedure, the more risk involved for the older person. For some older people with acute or chronic disease, the risk of surgery may be too great, in which case medical management may be the preferred course. For example, a person with severe osteoporosis who has been bedridden may not benefit from surgical interventions. Examples of fracture type and common surgical procedures include the following:

- *Nondisplaced subcapital and femoral neck fractures*: Surgical procedure is internal fixation with multiple pins.
- *Displaced fractures of subcapital and femoral neck*: Surgical procedure includes ORIF, with any of the following: intramedullary rod, pins, prosthesis, or a fixed sliding plate such as a compression screw.
- *Open reduction and internal fixation* is the surgical preference for active elderly adults who are able to use crutches with partial weight bearing.
- *Moore's prosthesis* (**hemiarthroscopy**, replacement of the femoral head with a smooth metal sphere) is preferred for the less active older person. It allows full weight bearing and return to active function. Figure 19–56 ■ illustrates the repair of a hip fracture using Moore's prosthesis
- *Total hip replacement* is done only when severe arthritis is present.

Total joint replacement, or **arthroplasty**, involves removing the damaged part of the joint and replacing it with a prosthetic device made of metal or polyethylene. Joint replacements are indicated when pain, decreased ROM, and increased disability interfere with daily function. The most common reason for a joint replacement is osteoarthritis, but other conditions such as rheumatoid arthritis, avascular necrosis, injury, and bone tumors also may require joint replacement.

The goals of joint replacement surgery are to decrease pain and increase joint function. In a total hip replacement, surgeons replace the head of the femur (the ball) and the acetabulum (the socket) with new parts that allow a natural gliding motion of the joint. The surgeon may use a cemented or uncemented prosthetic device. In the uncemented device, the person's bone grows in the pores and holds the device in place. Cemented procedures were developed about 40 years ago and have proven effective in reducing pain and increasing function. They are used more frequently than cementless devices for people over 75 years and for people with osteoporosis (National Institute of Arthritis and Musculoskeletal and Skin Diseases, 2001).

Nursing care of the older person with total hip replacement or internal fixation of the hip includes assessment and prevention of common complications, including dislocation of the device, avascular necrosis, infection, and delayed healing. General nursing care for the postoperative client depends on the specific surgical procedure.

Fall Prevention

Approximately 30% of older adults not in hospitals or care facilities fall each year. Changes in vision, balance, or judgment; cardiovascular problems; medications; urinary incontinence; and other physical conditions can contribute to an increased risk of falling (Brown et al., 2000). Vigorous prevention measures are needed to limit the numbers of injuries to the aging population (Box 19–12). Many of the so-called safety measures used in the past, such as restraints and side rails, have not been found to be effective and may even cause injury (Capezuti, 2002). Assessment of functional mobility,

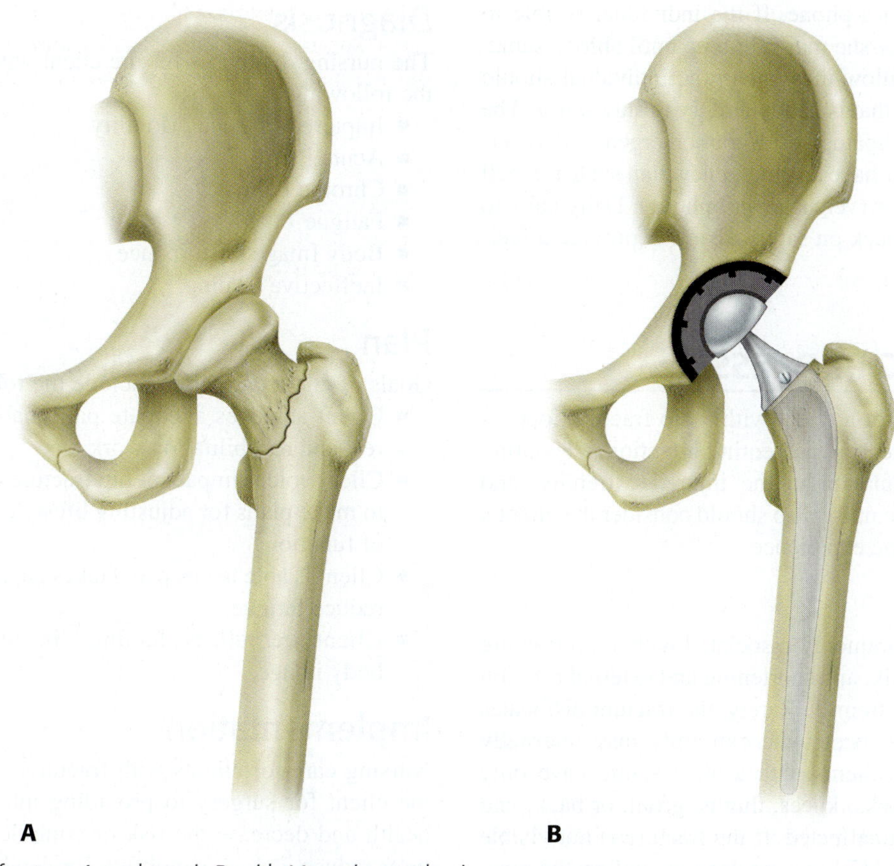

Figure 19–56 ■ A hip fracture *A*, and repair *B*, with Moore's prosthesis.

such as gait, balance, and position changes, provides valuable clues regarding a person's risk for future falls.

> **PRACTICE ALERT**
>
> A simple assessment of routine mobility tasks can provide clinical information to determine fall risk. Observe the older client while he or she is doing the following activities: (1) getting up from a chair, (2) turning while walking, (3) raising the foot completely off the floor, and (4) sitting down. Difficulty with any of these activities often points to an increased risk for falls. The nurse should develop an individualized plan to increase muscle strength and prevent falls.

Difficulty with any routine mobility task, such as walking or sitting down, points to an increased risk for falls. The more difficulties the older adult has, the greater the risk for falls. Many functional and performance assessment tools provide quantitative data (a score) on an older adult's limitation in mobility and risk for falls (Alexander, 2003; Patrick, Leber, Scrim, Gendron, & Eisener-Parche, 1999; Tinetti, 2003). Many exercise options are available to help the older adult regain and maintain muscle strength and improve general fitness (Bernick & Bretholz, 1999).

The older adult should be taught how to get up from a fall and how to get help. One method is to turn over on the stomach and crawl to a phone. Another option is to scoot on the

Box 19–12 **Fall Prevention Advice for Older Persons**

GENERAL ADVICE

- Have your vision and hearing checked regularly.
- Talk to your doctor or nurse about side effects of medications.
- Keep your intake of alcoholic beverages to a minimum.
- Wear rubber-soled shoes that fit well and support your feet.
- Avoid walking on icy sidewalks.
- Avoid slippery floor surfaces.
- Wear nonslip shoes at all times.
- Wear hip protectors.
- Keep temperature at a comfortable level.

HOME SAFETY ADVICE

- Clean the house and remove clutter.
- Clean spills immediately.
- Keep lighting adequate and make sure switches are easy to reach.
- Have handrails installed where needed.
- Remove scatter rugs and mats.
- Ensure that bathtub and bathroom areas have nonskid mats.
- Secure all electrical cords.

Source: Adapted from National Osteoporosis Foundation, 2007b; National Center for Injury Prevention and Control, 2006; Minnesota Safety Council , 2008.

bottom or side to reach a phone. If the individual is able to crawl to a stairway, he or she may climb up until able to stand. If the injury does not allow movement, the individual should cover up with anything that is handy and try to stay warm. The older adult should participate in a 24-hour emergency alert service, such as Lifeline, or have an emergency plan such as a bell or a phone near the floor (versus a wall phone). Daily calls to the elderly person to check on safety also will provide a feeling of reassurance.

NURSING PROCESS

Nursing care for a client with a hip fracture focuses on maintaining skin integrity, preventing infection, alleviating pain, maintaining circulation to the injured extremity, and increasing mobility. The nurse also should consider the client's response to the traumatic experience.

Assessment

Assessment findings commonly associated with a hip fracture are pain, inability to walk, and shortening and external rotation of the affected lower extremity. Rarely, the fracture dislocates posteriorly; if that does occur, the extremity may internally rotate. However, some clients with a hip fracture have only vague pain in the buttocks, knees, thighs, groin, or back, and their ability to walk is unaffected. If the fracture is not visible on x-ray, a bone scan or MRI may be done to confirm the presence of the fracture.

- *Health history.* Age, history of traumatic event, history of chronic illnesses, history of prior musculoskeletal injuries, medications (ask the older adult specifically about anticoagulants and calcium supplements)
- *Physical assessment.* Pain with movement, pulses, edema, skin color and temperature, deformity, ROM, touch. These assessments include the 5 P's of neurovascular assessment, as follows, which are included in both the initial assessment and ongoing focused assessments:
  a. *Pain:* Assess pain in the injured hip by asking the client to grade it on a scale of 0–10, with 10 being the most severe pain.
  b. *Pulses:* Assess distal pulses beginning with the unaffected hip. Compare the quality of pulses in the affected extremity to those of the unaffected extremity.
  c. *Pallor:* Observe for pallor and skin color in the injured extremity. Paleness and coolness may indicate arterial compromise, whereas warmth and a bluish tinge may indicate venous blood pooling.
  d. *Paralysis/Paresis:* Assess ability to move body parts distal to the fracture site. Inability to move indicates paralysis. Loss of muscle strength (weakness) when moving is paresis. A finding of limited ROM may lead to early recognition of problems such as nerve damage and paralysis.
  e. *Paresthesia:* Ask the client if any change in sensation, such as burning, numbness, prickly feeling, or stinging (all are paresthesia), has occurred.

Diagnosis

The nursing diagnoses for the client with hip fracture include the following:

- Impaired Physical Mobility
- Acute Pain
- Chronic Pain
- Fatigue
- Body Image Disturbance
- Ineffective Coping.

Plan

Goals of client care often include the following:

- Client achieves adequate pain management to allow for rest and rehabilitation work.
- Client voices impact of hip fracture on lifestyle and begins to make plans for adjusting lifestyle based on residual loss of function.
- Client is able to sleep and takes naps throughout the day to reduce fatigue.
- Client verbalizes feelings in regard to changes in body image.

Implementation

Nursing care for clients with fractures ranges from preparing the client for surgery to providing interventions to maintain health and decrease the risk of complications when hip fractures reduce a client's mobility for significant periods of time. Teaching also is necessary for caregivers of the older adult who is discharged home or to a long-term care or rehabilitation facility following a fractured hip.

Acute Pain

Pain is caused by soft tissue damage and is compounded by muscle spasms and swelling.

- Monitor vital signs. *Some analgesics decrease respiratory effort and blood pressure.*
- Ask the client to rate the pain on a scale of 0–10 (with 10 being the most severe pain) before and after any intervention. This facilitates objective assessment of the effectiveness of the chosen pain relief strategy. Pain that increases in intensity or remains unrelieved with analgesics can indicate compartment syndrome.
- For the client with a hip fracture, apply Buck's traction per physician's orders. Keep the traction weights hanging freely. Buck's traction immobilizes the fracture and decreases pain and additional trauma.
- Administer pain medications as prescribed. For home care, explain the importance of taking pain medications before the pain becomes severe. Analgesics alleviate pain by stimulating opiate receptor sites.

PRACTICE ALERT

Do not let weights lie on the bed or floor. The weights can be removed long enough to move the client up or down in bed to ensure that weights are hanging freely.

- Move the client gently and slowly. Gentle movement helps prevent the development of severe muscle spasms.

Risk for Peripheral Neurovascular Dysfunction

In the client with a fracture, DVT can impair circulation and, in turn, tissue perfusion.

- Assess the 5 P's every 1–2 hours. Report abnormal findings immediately. Unrelenting pain, pallor, diminished distal pulses, paresthesia, and paresis indicate reduced perfusion.
- Monitor the extremity for edema and swelling. Excessive swelling and hematoma formation can compromise circulation.
- Assess for deep, throbbing, unrelenting pain. Pain that is not relieved by analgesics may indicate neurovascular compromise.
- Administer anticoagulant per physician's order. Prophylactic anticoagulation decreases the risk of clot formation.

Risk for Infection

The client who undergoes surgical repair will have a postoperative wound. Any break in skin integrity must be monitored for infection. Wound healing in orthopedic clients is affected by the cause of the wound as well as the therapies used to repair musculoskeletal structures. It is important for nurses to understand processes of normal wound healing; characteristics of musculoskeletal wounds, contamination, and drainage; and potential complications for which to plan and implement appropriate interventions (Harvey, 2005).

- Monitor vital signs and lab reports of WBCs. *Increases in pulse rate, respiratory rate, temperature, and WBCs may indicate infection.*
- Use sterile technique for dressing changes. *The surgeon will change the initial postoperative dressing. The nurse must change all subsequent dressings without introducing organisms to the operative site.*
- Assess the wound for size and color and the presence of any drainage. *Redness, swelling, and purulent drainage indicate infection.*
- Administer antibiotics per physician's orders. *Prophylactic antibiotic administration inhibits bacterial reproduction, thereby helping to prevent skin flora from entering the wound. In the case of "dirty wounds," such as those occurring from vehicular crashes, antibiotics are routinely administered.*

Impaired Physical Mobility

The client who has experienced a fracture requires immobilization of the fractured bone(s). Immobilization alters normal gait and mobility. The client will need to use assistive devices such as crutches, canes, or walkers.

- Teach or assist client with ROM exercises of the unaffected limbs. *ROM exercises help prevent muscle atrophy and maintain strength and joint function. Flexion and extension exercises prevent the development of foot drop and frozen joints.*
- Teach isometric exercises and encourage the client to perform them every 4 hours. *Isometric exercises help prevent muscle atrophy and force synovial fluid and nutrients into the cartilage.*
- Encourage ambulation when the client is able; provide assistance as necessary. *Ambulation maintains and improves circulation, helps prevent muscle atrophy, and helps maintain bowel function.*
- Teach and observe the client's use of assistive devices (such as canes, crutches, and walkers) in conjunction with the PT. *Proper use of devices is necessary for safe ambulation and helps prevent the loss of joint function secondary to complications and falls.*
- Turn the client on bed rest every 2 hours. If the client is in traction, teach the client to shift his or her weight every hour. *Turning and shifting weight increases circulation and helps prevent skin breakdown.*

Risk for Disturbed Sensory Perception: Tactile

The client who has sustained a fracture is at risk for nerve injury.

- Assess every 1–2 hours the ability to differentiate between sharp and dull touch and the presence of paresthesia and paralysis. *Paresthesia develops as a result of pressure on nerves and may indicate compartment syndrome.*

PRACTICE ALERT

Paralysis is a late sign of nerve entrapment and requires that the physician be notified immediately.

- Support the injured extremity above and below the fracture site when moving the client. *Supporting the injured extremity above and below the fracture site helps prevent displacement of bony fragments and decreases the risk of further nerve damage.*

Client and family teaching focuses on the client's needs. The type of fracture and its location determine how much teaching the client and family will require. For example, an older client who has sustained a hip fracture and requires surgical intervention has a wider array of teaching needs, including the use of an abduction pillow, proper bending, and proper sitting. Address the following topics for home care of the client who has fractured a hip.

Encourage independence in ADL as follows:

- Explain that the client should sit only on high chairs to prevent excess flexion of the hip; a high toilet seat can be added to a regular toilet seat.
- Encourage the client and family to install a rail in the shower to aid in stability and to prevent falls.
- If a walker is needed, teach the client its proper use: Do not carry the walker, but lift it, advance it, and then take two steps, or use a rolling walker.
- If a cane is needed, instruct the client to use it on the affected side.
- Stress the importance of well-balanced meals and explain all prescribed medications.

Address the following topics for home care:

- Follow the physician's order for weight bearing.

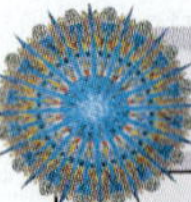

NURSING CARE PLAN A Client With a Hip Fracture

Stella Carbolito is a 74-year-old Italian American with a history of osteoporosis. She is a widow who lives alone in a two-story row home. Mrs. Carbolito is retired and depends on a pension check and Social Security for her income. She takes pride in making her own food from scratch. While walking to the market one day, Mrs. Carbolito falls and fractures her left hip. She is transported by ambulance to the nearest hospital ED.

ASSESSMENT	DIAGNOSES	PLANNING
During the initial assessment at the ED, abnormal findings are that Mrs. Carbolito's left leg is shorter than her right leg and is externally rotated. Distal pulses are present and bilaterally strong; both legs are warm. Mrs. Carbolito complains of severe pain but states that no numbness or burning is present. She is able to wiggle the toes on her left leg and has full movement of her right leg. Initial vital signs are as follows: T_O 98.0°F (36.6°C), P 100, R 18, BP 120/58. Diagnostic tests include CBC, blood chemistry, and x-ray studies of the left hip and pelvis. The CBC reveals a hemoglobin of 11.0 g/dL and a normal WBC count. Blood chemistry findings are within normal limits. The x-ray reveals a fracture of the left femoral neck. Mrs. Carbolito is admitted to the hospital with an order for 10 lb of straight leg traction. An ORIF is planned for the following day.	■ Acute Pain related to fractured left femoral neck and muscle spasms ■ Impaired Physical Mobility related to bed rest and fractured left femoral neck ■ Risk for Ineffective Tissue Perfusion related to unstable bones and swelling ■ Risk for Disturbed Sensory Perception: Tactile related to the risk of nerve impairment	■ Verbalize a decrease in pain. ■ Verbalize the purpose of traction and surgery. ■ Maintain normal neurovascular status. ■ Demonstrate postoperative exercises.

IMPLEMENTATION

- Assess pain on a scale of 0–10 before and after measures are implemented to reduce pain.
- Administer narcotics per the physician's order.
- Perform neurovascular assessment every 2–4 hours and document findings.
- Apply straight leg traction per physician's order.
- Encourage deep breathing and relaxation techniques.
- Teach the purpose of traction and surgery.
- Teach the purpose of and the procedure for performing isometric and flexion/extension exercises.

EVALUATION

Three days after surgery, Mrs. Carbolito is out of bed and in a chair. She verbalizes a decrease in pain. There have been no abnormal neurovascular assessments. She is able to independently perform isometric and flexion/extension exercises in both lower extremities. Discharge planning includes referrals for home care. A home health nurse will visit, and the social worker at the hospital has ordered a trapeze for her bed, an elevated toilet seat, an elevated cushion for her chair, and a walker.

CRITICAL THINKING

1. What factors placed Mrs. Carbolito at risk for a hip fracture?
2. Mrs. Carbolito says, "I don't understand why they had to put that heavy thing on my leg before I went to surgery to get my hip fixed." What would you tell her? What preoperative factors might have decreased teaching effectiveness?
3. Describe how each of the following, if manifested by Mrs. Carbolito, would increase her risk for postoperative complications: urinary incontinence, weight more than 20% under normal for her height, and chronic constipation. What nursing diagnoses and interventions would you include in her plan of care to decrease the risk?

- Physical therapy departments and offices often can evaluate the home environment for safety and suggest modifications as needed. Physical therapists also teach crutch walking, limited weight bearing, transferring, and other activities.
- Home care agencies can teach wound care and provide ongoing monitoring of wound healing.
- Local medical equipment and supply sources rent or sell durable equipment such as crutches, walkers, wheelchairs, overhead trapeze units, shower chairs, elevated toilet seats, grab bars, and bedside commodes. Braces may be purchased through medical equipment dealers.
- Local pharmacies are good sources for dressing supplies such as antiseptic solutions and ointments, dressings, and tape.
- Fitness equipment suppliers may be able to provide rehabilitation equipment such as ankle weights to use for strengthening exercises.

Evaluation

Client outcomes are evaluated for the following:

- Attains greatest possible return of mobility
- Reports that pain is controlled, allowing the client to rest and attend to rehabilitation needs
- Copes with loss in mobility by altering lifestyle/living arrangements to accommodate needs.

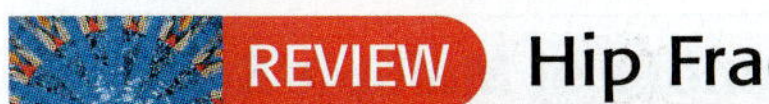

REVIEW Hip Fractures

RELATE: LINK THE CONCEPTS

Linking the exemplar of Hip Fractures with the concept of Health, Wellness, and Illness:

1. Describe the modifiable risk factors and teaching interventions for those clients at risk for hip factors.
2. What nutritional screening findings assessed from an elderly female client would indicate an increased risk for hip fractures? What teaching would you provide to lower this risk?

Linking the exemplar of Hip Fractures with the concept of Safety:

3. What priority safety interventions will you initiate for the client with osteoporosis that will help reduce the risk of hip fracture?
4. What client teaching will you provide an aging adult with declining muscle strength to reduce the risk of hip fracture?

READY: GO TO COMPANION SKILLS MANUAL

- Assessing the musculoskeletal system
- Assessing the client in pain
- Moving a client up in bed
- Turning a client to the lateral or prone position in bed
- Using a sliding board
- Transferring between bed and stretcher
- Caring for a client with posteriolateral approach hip arthroplasty

REFER: GO TO MYNURSINGKIT

REFLECT: CASE STUDY

Maria Haley is 65 years old and lives alone in her two-story house. Maria's husband Del passed away two years ago but left her financially comfortable if she is careful. Maria has two grown children who are both married, but no grandchildren as yet. Her children both live in another state. Maria is active at the senior center in town, is an avid bridge player, and enjoys relatively good health. She is taking simvastatin 20 mg/day for a slightly elevated cholesterol level. Maria also takes 10 mg of lisinopril once a day for borderline hypertension with good control. Since Maria is alone, she doesn't bother to cook much and fixes frozen dinners or soup for her meals at night. As active as Maria is, she does not do much exercising and weighs 140 pounds, which is a 10 pound increase over last year's weight. Maria drives but admits to the nurse that things seem blurry at night.

1. What factors put Marie at risk for hip fracture?
2. During her annual check-up, what safety teaching regarding risks for hip fracture will you address with Maria?
3. What nutritional suggestions might you implement to help with the prevention of hip fractures?
4. What recommendations regarding exercise will you make to Maria?

19.4 MULTIPLE SCLEROSIS

KEY TERMS

Multiple sclerosis (MS), *1117*
Myelin sheaths, *1118*

BASIS FOR SELECTION OF EXEMPLAR

Chronic Disease Management

LEARNING OUTCOMES

After reading about this exemplar, you will be able to:

1. Describe the pathophysiology, etiology, clinical manifestations, and direct and indirect causes of multiple sclerosis.
2. Identify risk factors associated with multiple sclerosis.
3. Illustrate the nursing process in providing culturally competent care across the life span for individuals with multiple sclerosis.
4. Formulate priority nursing diagnoses appropriate for an individual with multiple sclerosis.
5. Create a plan of care for individuals with multiple sclerosis and their family members.
6. Assess expected outcomes for an individual with multiple sclerosis.
7. Discuss therapies used in the collaborative care of an individual multiple sclerosis.
8. Employ evidence-based caring interventions for an individual with multiple sclerosis.

OVERVIEW

Multiple sclerosis (MS) is a chronic demyelinating neurologic disease of the CNS (brain, optic nerves, and spinal cord) associated with an abnormal immune response to an environmental factor. The manifestations of MS vary according to the area of the nervous system affected. The initial onset may be followed by a total remission, making diagnosis difficult. In about 60% of clients, MS is characterized by periods of exacerbation, when manifestations are highly pronounced, followed by periods of remission, when manifestations are not obvious. The end result, however, is progression of the disease with increasing loss of function.

Diagnosis of MS is challenging because the disease does not present uniformly. A diagnosis requires that the client have one of the following: (1) two or more exacerbations separated by 1 month or more and lasting more than 24 hours, followed by recovery; (2) a history of repeated exacerbations and remissions with or without complete recovery, followed by progressively more severe manifestations lasting for 6 months or more; or (3) slowly increasing manifestations for at least 6 months.

PATHOPHYSIOLOGY AND ETIOLOGY

Myelin sheaths are fatty, segmented wrappings that normally protect and insulate nerve fibers and increase the speed of transmission of nerve impulses. In MS, these myelin sheaths of the white matter of the spinal cord, brain, and optic nerve are destroyed in patches, called *plaques,* along the axon. The demyelination of nerve fibers slows and distorts the conduction of nerve impulses and sometimes results in the total absence of impulse transmission. The neurons usually affected by MS are located in the spinal cord, brainstem, cerebral and cerebellar areas, and optic nerve.

Both plaques and diffuse lesions form as demyelinating lesions. Plaques typically are scattered through the white matter of the CNS, although they may extend into adjacent gray matter. Early manifestations are the result of inflammatory edema in and around the plaque and partial demyelination. These manifestations typically disappear within weeks after the initial episode. With progression of the disease, the demyelination and plaque formation result in scarring of glia (*gliosis*) and degeneration of axons. Continued loss of function leads to permanent disability, usually over about 20 years.

Etiology

MS is believed to occur as a result of an autoimmune response to a prior viral infection in a genetically susceptible person. The infection, which is thought to occur early in life, activates T cells. T cells usually move in and out of the CNS across the blood–brain barrier, but for an unknown reason, they remain in the CNS in people with MS. The T cells facilitate infiltration by other leukocytes, and an inflammatory process follows. Inflammation destroys myelin and oligodendrocytes (myelin-producing cells), leading to axon dysfunction.

Risk Factors

The onset of MS is usually between 20 and 50 years of age, with a peak at age 30. MS is the most prevalent CNS demyelinating disorder and is a leading cause of neurologic disability in young adults. Although all races are affected, MS is primarily a disease of people of northern European ancestry; however, MS does occur in people of African, Asian, and Hispanic descent. A definite genetic factor has not been established, but studies suggest that genetic factors may make some individuals more susceptible than others (National MS Society, 2005).

CLINICAL MANIFESTATIONS

There are four classifications of MS: relapsing-remitting, primary progressive, secondary progressive, and progressive-relapsing (Box 19–13). Most individuals with MS present with the relapsing-remitting type.

Various stressors have been suggested as triggers for MS. These stressors include febrile states, pregnancy, extreme physical exertion, and fatigue. These precipitating factors also can cause a relapse of the manifestations during the course of the disease.

Box 19–13 Classifications of Multiple Sclerosis

- **Relapsing-remitting:** The most common clinical course of MS, it is characterized by exacerbations (acute attacks) with full recovery or with partial recovery with disability.
- **Primary progressive:** Steady worsening of disease from the onset with occasional minor recovery.
- **Secondary progressive:** Begins as with relapsing-remitting, but the disease steadily becomes worse between exacerbations.
- **Progressive-relapsing:** This rare form continues to progress from the onset but also has exacerbations.

The manifestations of MS vary according to the areas destroyed by demyelination and the affected body system. (See Multisystemic Effects of MS on page 1119.) Fatigue, one of the most disabling manifestations, affects almost all clients with MS. The manifestations, which are categorized by the established syndromes of MS, are listed in Box 19–14.

Brief attacks of manifestations are described as short-lived or paroxysmal. Short-lived attacks of neurologic deficits indicate the appearance or worsening of manifestations. Conditions that cause short-lived attacks include (1) minor increases in body temperature or serum calcium concentrations (both increase the leakage of current through demyelinated neurons) and (2) functional demands that exceed conduction capacity. Paroxysmal attacks are sensory or motor

Box 19–14 Manifestations of Multiple Sclerosis

MIXED OR GENERALIZED TYPE (50% OF CASES)

- Visual deficits with visual blurring, fogginess, or haziness; impaired color perception, decreased central visual acuity, area of diminished vision in the visual fields, acquired color vision deficit (especially to red and green), and an altered pupillary reaction to light
- Brainstem lesions (cranial nerves III–XII) with nystagmus, dysarthria, deafness, vertigo, vomiting, tinnitus, facial weakness, decreased sensation, diplopia, and eye pain and cognitive dysfunctions involving concentration, short-term memory, word finding, and planning
- Mood alterations manifested as depression more often than euphoria

SPINAL TYPE (25% OF CASES)

- Weakness and/or numbness in one or both extremities (most often the legs)
- Upper motor neuron involvement manifested by stiffness, slowness, weakness (spastic paresis)
- Bladder dysfunctions: urgency, hesitancy, and incontinence
- Bowel dysfunction most often seen as constipation
- Neurogenic impotence noted

CEREBELLAR TYPE (5% OF CASES)

- Manifestations of nystagmus, ataxia, and hypotonia

AMAUROTIC FORM (5% OF CASES)

- Blindness

MULTISYSTEM EFFECTS OF **Multiple Sclerosis**

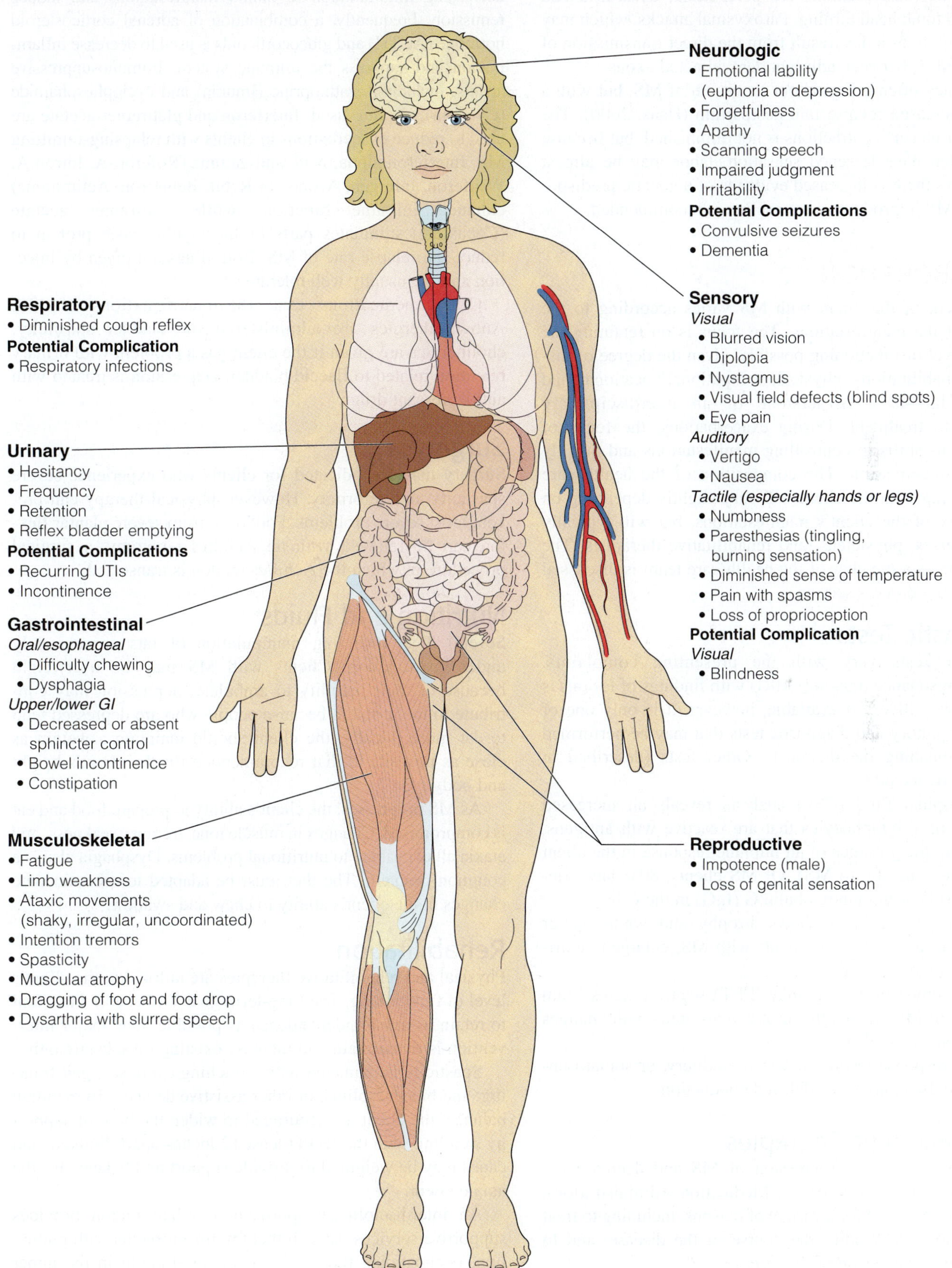

Neurologic
• Emotional lability (euphoria or depression)
• Forgetfulness
• Apathy
• Scanning speech
• Impaired judgment
• Irritability
Potential Complications
• Convulsive seizures
• Dementia
Sensory
Visual
• Blurred vision
• Diplopia
• Nystagmus
• Visual field defects (blind spots)
• Eye pain
Auditory
• Vertigo
• Nausea
Tactile (especially hands or legs)
• Numbness
• Paresthesias (tingling, burning sensation)
• Diminished sense of temperature
• Pain with spasms
• Loss of proprioception
Potential Complication
Visual
• Blindness
Respiratory
• Diminished cough reflex
Potential Complication
• Respiratory infections
Urinary
• Hesitancy
• Frequency
• Retention
• Reflex bladder emptying
Potential Complications
• Recurring UTIs
• Incontinence
Gastrointestinal
Oral/esophageal
• Difficulty chewing
• Dysphagia
Upper/lower GI
• Decreased or absent sphincter control
• Bowel incontinence
• Constipation
Musculoskeletal
• Fatigue
• Limb weakness
• Ataxic movements (shaky, irregular, uncoordinated)
• Intention tremors
• Spasticity
• Muscular atrophy
• Dragging of foot and foot drop
• Dysarthria with slurred speech
Reproductive
• Impotence (male)
• Loss of genital sensation

manifestations that occur abruptly and last for only seconds or minutes; the manifestations are paresthesia, dysarthria and ataxia, and tonic head turning. Paroxysmal attacks, which may occur many times a day, result from the direct transmission of nerve impulses between adjacent demyelinated axons.

Pregnancy often brings about remission of MS, but with a slightly increased relapse rate postpartum (Haas, 2000). The strength of uterine contractions is not diminished, but because clients often have lessened sensation, labor may be almost painless. As there is increased evidence of a genetic predisposition for MS, reproductive counseling is recommended.

COLLABORATION

Management of the client with MS varies according to the severity of the manifestations. The focus is on retaining the optimal level of functioning possible, given the degree of disability. Rehabilitation—physical, occupational/vocational, and psychosocial—is a cornerstone of an interdisciplinary approach to treatment. During exacerbations, the focus of interventions shifts to controlling manifestations and quickly returning to remission. The composition of the health care team working with the client will vary slightly depending on the severity of the client's manifestations, but will typically include nurses, physicians, and rehabilitative therapists. The nurse's role as a member of the health care team is discussed in the nursing process section.

Diagnostic Tests

Diagnostic tests vary with the presenting complaints. Magnetic resonance imaging (MRI) with findings of lesions is the most definitive test available; however, it is only one of several laboratory and diagnostic tests that may be performed when establishing the diagnosis. Other tests (described in Appendix B) include:

- Cerebrospinal fluid (CSF) analysis reveals an increased number of T lymphocytes that are reactive with antigens, indicating the presence of an immune response in the client (but is not specific to MS). Of MS clients, 80% have elevated levels of immunoglobulin G (IgG) in the CSF.
- CT scan of the brain shows atrophy and white matter lesions. In about 25% of clients with MS, enlarged ventricles are visible on CT.
- Positron emission tomography (PET) scan measures brain activity. In MS clients, the scan reveals areas with changes in glucose metabolism.
- Evoked response testing of visual, auditory, or somatosensory impulses may show delayed conduction.

Pharmacologic Therapies

Medications slow the progression of MS and decrease the number of attacks (Box 19–15, Medication Administration). Medications are used for a variety of reasons, including to treat manifestations, to modify the course of the disease, and to interrupt the progression of the disease.

The medications used during an exacerbation are aimed at decreasing inflammation to inhibit manifestations and induce remission. Frequently, a combination of adrenal corticosteroid hormone (ACTH) and glucocorticoids is used to decrease inflammation and suppress the immune system. Immunosuppressive agents, including azathioprine (Imuran) and cyclophosphamide (Cytoxan), also are used. Interferon and glatiramer acetate are used to reduce exacerbations in clients with relapsing-remitting MS. Interferon alpha, beta, and gamma (Roferon-A, Intron A, Wellferon, Infergen, Avonex or Rebif, Betaseron, Actimmune) enhance immune function, while glatiramer acetate (Copaxone) stimulates parts of the myelin basic protein to reduce the relapse rate of MS. Both drugs are given by injection and are usually well tolerated.

Other medications treat the manifestations of MS. Anticholinergics are administered for bladder spasticity; cholinergics are given if the client has a problem with urinary retention related to flaccid bladder. Depression is treated with antidepressant drugs.

Surgery

Surgery may be indicated for clients who experience severe spasticity and deformity. However, physical therapy can prevent most severe problems. Foot drop from severe plantar flexion can be relieved with an Achilles tenotomy, a surgical procedure in which the Achilles tendon is transected.

Nutrition and Fluids

Several diets involving manipulation of fats are currently under investigation. Clients with MS may be overweight because of their inability to ambulate; depression may contribute to the problem because people who are depressed tend to eat more. Ideally, the client should maintain a weight as close as possible to that recommended for the client's height and body type.

As MS progresses, the client's ability to prepare food and eat is compromised. Changes in muscle tone, tremor, weakness, and ataxia all contribute to nutritional problems. Dysphagia also is a common problem. The diet must be adapted to accommodate changes in the client's ability to chew and swallow.

Rehabilitation

Physical and rehabilitative therapies are tailored to the client's level of functioning. The long-term goal is to enable the client to retain as much independence as possible. One major intervention is to maintain and increase existing muscle strength.

Spasticity is managed with stretching exercises; gait training; and braces, splints, or other assistive devices. To maintain balance, the client is encouraged to widen the base of support by standing with the feet at least 12 inches apart. Walkers and canes may be weighted to provide support and balance for the ataxic client.

An interdisciplinary approach to rehabilitation provides supportive services: speech therapy for problems with phonation, occupational therapy to maintain strength in the upper

Box 19–15 **Medication Administration for the Client With Multiple Sclerosis**

IMMUNOMODULATORS

- **Interferon beta-1a (Avonex)**
- **Interferon beta-1b (Betaseron)**
- **Glatiramer acetate (Copaxone, Copolymer-1)**

Interferon beta-la, interferon beta-1b, and glatiramer acetate are administered to clients with relapsing-remitting MS to prolong the time of onset to disability. Their use is based on the assumption that MS is an immunologically mediated disease. Interferon beta-1b produces a decrease in the MS lesions in some clients. Some clients, however, develop a decrease in the absolute neutrophil count and increases in the levels of liver enzymes. Anxiety, confusion, and depression with suicidal tendencies also have been reported. Other adverse reactions include pain, inflammation, hypersensitivity at the injection site, and generalized flulike manifestations. Some women experience menstrual disorders. Pregnant women should not take these medications.

Nursing Responsibilities

- Assess baseline parameters to evaluate drug side effects: psychologic profile, liver function tests, and CBC with differential.
- Monitor CBC and liver function tests every 3 months or as prescribed.
- Assess injection site and report ulceration promptly. (Pain and redness are common reactions.)
- Evaluate client's baseline neurologic, sensory, and motor function. Monitor changes in condition and function.
- Report if client is pregnant or breastfeeding.

Health Education for the Client and Family

- These drugs may cause depression and thoughts of suicide; report these feelings to the physician immediately.
- Administer medication within 3 hours of reconstitution. Rotate injection sites and avoid any areas that are red or show other skin reactions.
- Seek follow-up care to monitor neurologic changes, CBC, and liver function.
- Avoid prolonged exposure to sunlight.

ADRENALCORTICOSTEROID THERAPY

- **Adrenocorticotropic hormone (ACTH) (Acthar)**
- **Prednisone (Deltasone, Meticorten, Orasone)**
- **Methylprednisolone (Medrol, Solu-Medrol)**

Adrenalcorticosteroids are used to sustain a remission and to treat exacerbations of MS. ACTH is usually given to induce a remission. It is administered intravenously for 1 week and may be followed by oral prednisone therapy. Another protocol involves administering ACTH intravenously for 3 days followed by intramuscular injections every 12 hours for 1 week (Hickey, 2003). The drugs are given to suppress the immune system, which is implicated in the etiology of MS. If the drug is used long-term, the usual steroid precautions are indicated, such as monitoring for glucose intolerance, osteoporosis, and cataract formation. The drugs are used with caution in pregnant and lactating women.

MUSCLE RELAXANTS

- **Baclofen (Lioresal)**
- **Dantrolene (Dantrium)**
- **Diazepam (Valium)**

Muscle relaxants are given to clients with MS to relieve muscle spasms. Baclofen and diazepam act by suppressing CNS reflexes that regulate muscle activity; neither drug affects muscle strength. Baclofen therapy should be discontinued over 1–2 weeks; sudden withdrawal may cause seizures and paranoid ideation. In contrast to diazepam and baclofen, dantrolene acts directly on skeletal muscles, and it may affect muscle strength. Dantrolene may cause hepatotoxicity and should not be administered when hepatitis or cirrhosis is present.

Nursing Responsibilities

- Evaluate baseline muscle strength and spasticity, ROM, and dexterity.
- Maintain safety or fall precautions; dizziness and drowsiness are common side effects.
- For the client taking dantrolene, monitor liver function tests (enzymes and bilirubin) for signs of hepatotoxicity.

Health Education for the Client and Family

- These drugs may cause sedative effects. Take appropriate safety measures (e.g., avoid driving).
- Avoid CNS depressants (antihistamines, alcohol); they can increase the sedative effects of the medication.
- Continue follow-up care; if you are taking dantrolene, for example, monitoring of liver function will be necessary.
- If you are taking baclofen, do not suddenly stop the medication.
- Increase fiber and fluids in the diet to prevent constipation.
- Change positions slowly to minimize dizziness and other effects of orthostatic hypotension.

IMMUNOSUPPRESSANTS

- **Azathioprine (Imuran)**
- **Cyclophosphamide (Cytoxan)**

Immunosuppressants are given to clients with MS because of the autoimmune component of the disease. Both medications can cause bone marrow suppression and increase the risk of cancer. Azathioprine may produce hepatitis. Toxic effects of cyclophosphamide include hemorrhagic cystitis, sterility, and stomatitis.

Nursing Responsibilities

- Monitor baseline parameters: CBC with platelet count and differential, urinalysis, liver function tests, hepatitis profile.
- Assess for anemia: fatigue, lethargy, pallor.
- Watch for bleeding.
- Protect against and observe for subtle signs of infection.

Health Education for the Client and Family

- Report infection, bleeding, and anemia immediately.
- Drink at least 2 L (2 quarts) of fluid a day and observe urine for blood.
- Report jaundice immediately.
- Check oral cavity daily for changes or ulcers.
- Avoid becoming pregnant while taking these drugs.
- Obtain follow-up care, including frequent blood tests.

extremities and to carry out ADL, and occupational counseling. Referrals to a urologist are indicated for problems with urinary incontinence, urinary tract infections, retention, and impotence. Consultation with a respiratory therapist may be needed if the client develops chronic respiratory infections from inability to cough, move secretions, or breathe deeply, especially with increased debilitation.

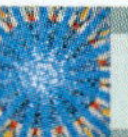

NURSING PROCESS

Because the disease most often affects young adults in the prime of life, the psychosocial and economic effects can be devastating. People with MS have to make adjustments to body image changes while simultaneously adapting to the altered relationships and decreased earnings usually encountered with the disease. A once-healthy spouse becomes wheelchair-bound; a person once independent may eventually become dependent for even the most basic ADL. The unpredictable course of MS is a challenge for long-term planning.

Following an overview of the disorder, the client needs to understand how to prevent fatigue and exacerbations. Teach the client to avoid stress, extremes of cold and heat, high humidity, physical overexertion, and infections. Because pregnancy can exacerbate manifestations, counseling about this risk is indicated. Also address preventive measures to avoid risk of respiratory and urinary tract infections.

Assessment

The assessment of the client involves taking a thorough nursing history and conducting a physical assessment. These findings will indicate what additional information may need to be gained from diagnostic testing and will inform the client's plan of care.

- *Health history.* History of childhood viral illnesses, children's geographic residence, exposure to physical or emotional stressors (pregnancy/delivery, extremes of heat), medications, symptom onset, severity of manifestations.
- *Physical assessment.* Affect, mood, speech, eye movements, gait, tremors, vision and hearing, reflexes, muscle strength and movement, sensation.

Diagnosis

Many nursing diagnoses relate to the inability to perform ADLs. Others reflect problems with musculoskeletal changes or altered nerve conduction. The following nursing diagnoses are discussed in this section:

- Fatigue
- Self-Care Deficit.

Plan

Goals of nursing care include the following:

- Client takes rest breaks several times a day to reduce fatigue.
- Client maintains maximum level of autonomy possible.

Implementation

Interventions for the client with MS vary with the acuity of exacerbations and the presenting problems.

Fatigue

Fatigue is defined by NANDA as an overwhelming sustained sense of exhaustion and decreased capacity for physical and mental work at the usual level. Fatigue affects every aspect of the MS client's life: the ability to remain independent and perform self-care, sexual function, mobility, airway clearance, and ultimately self-concept and coping. The client and family need a great deal of teaching to understand fatigue and how to

---

EVIDENCE-BASED PRACTICE Aging Clients With MS

MS is a chronic, debilitating disease, but it does not reduce life expectancy. Most clients are diagnosed with the disease as young or middle-age adults; they must learn how to live with the disease for the rest of their lives. However, little research has been published regarding the experiences and health-related concerns of people who are aging with MS. Finlayson and colleagues (2004) conducted a study to initiate dialogue about the role of nurses in addressing those concerns. The study's subjects perceived two major differences between their experience of aging with MS and the experiences of people aging without MS: less freedom (restrictions on travel and social activities, limitations of physical accessibility of buildings, and financial limitations) and needing more assistance (with housework, shopping, hygiene, cooking, and transportation).

Implications for Nursing

The findings of this study support the need for nurses to consider issues of daily living for clients with chronic disabilities, including MS. Nurses have the knowledge and ability to include information in client teaching that facilitates quality of life, ways to cope with a disability, and symptom management. By working closely with members of the interdisciplinary health team, nurses select and implement appropriate interventions to enable clients with MS to age in place and to continue to be active and involved members of the family and community as they age.

Critical Thinking in Client Care

1. How would your teaching differ for the following clients with MS?
   a. A 45-year-old woman who is married and has family nearby
   b. A 70-year-old woman who is widowed and has no family
   c. A man who has been a farmer all his life and lives in an isolated rural area
   d. A man who has always lived in an urban area with access to public transportation
2. You are making a home visit to an older woman who has had MS for 30 years. She tells you, "I never leave my condo anymore because I can't control my urine, and I'm so afraid I will have an accident." What can you do to help her resolve this problem?
3. Design a plan of care focused on the nursing diagnosis of fatigue for a 73-year-old man who is living independently but says, "Some days I am just too tired to cook anything to eat."

NURSING CARE PLAN **A Client With MS**

George McMurphy, a 45-year-old from northern Minnesota, was diagnosed with MS approximately 5 years ago. He states that he probably had mild symptoms as long ago as 10 years. He works as a manager for a large grocery store chain near his home. He lives at home with his wife and two children, ages 12 and 15. Recently, Mr. McMurphy has had increasing problems with urinary incontinence, lack of energy, weakness, extreme fatigue, and altered mobility from spasticity in his leg muscles. He also has a fever, chest congestion, and a cough productive of green sputum. He is admitted to the hospital for evaluation and treatment of pneumonia and exacerbation of his MS.

ASSESSMENT	DIAGNOSES	PLANNING
Denise Miller, RN, primary care nurse, is assigned to care for Mr. McMurphy. His major complaint is the inability to "... bring up all this sputum; I feel rotten from being so congested. I hate not being able to get to work and for my wife having to tend to my personal needs." Vital signs are as follows: T_O 102°F (38.8°C), P 94, R 30, BP 134/84. Mr. McMurphy is admitted for an acute exacerbation of the disorder, probably triggered by pneumonia. He will be treated with ACTH and intravenous antibiotics during this admission.	■ Ineffective Airway Clearance related to lung infection and thick mucus ■ Activity Intolerance related to fatigue and spasticity ■ Self-Care Deficit: Toileting, Feeding, and Grooming related to muscle weakness	■ Be able to clear airway ■ Have breath sounds clear to auscultation and pulse oximetry readings above 95% ■ Be able to ambulate using assistive devices if needed ■ Perform self-care activities without becoming overly fatigued and tired ■ Verbalize methods to adapt daily routine to level of tolerance

IMPLEMENTATION

- Initiate pulmonary hygiene measures (e.g., incentive spirometry, turning, deep breathing and coughing, breathing exercises, and postural drainage) at least every 2 hours. Assess lung sounds, oxygen saturation, and ability to clear airway.
- Teach the importance of maintaining an oral fluid intake of at least 2000 mL per day to prevent tenacious sputum and urinary tract infections. Teach signs and symptoms of urinary and respiratory infections.
- Encourage participation in decision making about care.
- Assist with ADLs only as needed and based on level of fatigue and muscle weakness.
- Plan self-care activities to be performed during periods of peak level of energy; intersperse rest periods throughout the day.
- Refer to an MS support group.
- Refer to physical and occupational therapists for counseling regarding control of spasticity and possible splinting of spastic muscles.
- Consult a urologist for assessment of bladder incontinence; teach intermittent catheterization. Alternatively, the use of an external condom catheter may be indicated.
- Suggest performing tasks in the morning hours. *Biorhythm studies indicate that people usually have greater energy reserves in the morning hours and diminished reserves in the afternoon.*
- Advise to avoid temperature extremes such as hot showers and exposure to cold. *Maintaining a relatively constant body temperature may avoid exacerbation of the disorder. Heat can delay impulse transmission across demyelinated nerves, which contributes to fatigue.*
- Refer to the appropriate professionals to manage fatigue: stress management groups, support groups, and occupational or PT as indicated. *Support groups and therapy can facilitate self-management and improve coping.*

adapt. Clients and families also need assistance managing fatigue in a society in which energy level is highly valued.

- Assess degree of fatigue and identify contributing factors. Fatigue is a subjective experience that must be evaluated thoroughly before planning can begin.
- Arrange daily activities to include rest periods. Rest is essential to manage feelings of fatigue; periods of relaxation may help replenish energy reserves.
- Ask the client to consider which activities are necessary and to set priorities. Prioritizing activities promotes independence and self-control.

Self-Care Deficit

Clients with MS may need assistance with bathing, toileting, dressing, grooming, and feeding. The client may need just minimal guidance or may be totally dependent. The client's ability to perform self-care activities is the gauge by which family members and caregivers need to adjust assistance. Self-care encompasses the decisions about the extent and provision of care; most clients are capable of making decisions even after physical limitations prevent physical self-care. The need to maintain self-determination cannot be overemphasized and must be incorporated into each intervention. As the client with MS ages, there may be even more need for teaching to provide self-care, as described in the Evidenced-Based Practice box.

- Assess the extent of the client's self-care deficit; refer to other health team members for assessment as appropriate. For example, if indicated, refer to a speech pathologist to assess swallowing and gag reflex. An accurate assessment is crucial to individualizing interventions.
- Suggest adaptive devices such as arm and wrist braces as needed. Meeting hygiene needs and feeding self are essential for positive self-concept, self-esteem, and socialization.

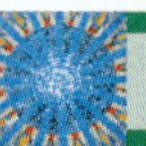

CARE SETTINGS Community Care for Clients With MS

The inconsistent and erratic nature of MS can make teaching for self-care difficult. Initial teaching focuses on a realistic explanation of MS. Referral to a support group early in the course of the disease is indicated. Social support can make a positive difference in a client's ability to cope with MS. Address the following topics in preparing the client for home care:

- Various treatment options and their side effects
- Information about medications, particularly steroid use, and about possible interactions with prescription and OTC medications
- Ongoing care from nurses; counselors; physical, occupational, and speech therapists; and the physician and community health nurse
- Helpful resources:
  a. National Multiple Sclerosis Society
  b. National Institute of Neurological Disorders and Stroke.

- Teach to use assistive devices such as plate guards, to modify consistency of foods, and to eat when energy level is higher. If unable to buy and prepare meals, provide referral to Meals on Wheels. Proper nutrition is basic to health; adapting utensils and foods can facilitate meeting nutritional needs.
- Teach interventions related to altered bowel and bladder function: fluid intake of at least 2000 mL daily, bowel routine as indicated to prevent constipation, and self-catheterization skills as necessary. Maintaining optimal bowel and bladder function decreases the risk of urinary tract infection and bowel impaction.

PRACTICE ALERT

It is important to remember that fatigue from chronic illnesses such as MS is very different from being "tired," and that rest and sleep may not result in improvement.

Evaluation

Expected outcomes used to evaluate nursing care include the following:

- Client adapts lifestyle to reduce fatigue.
- Client uses assistive devices to optimize autonomy.

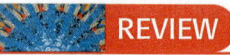

REVIEW Multiple Sclerosis

RELATE: LINK THE CONCEPTS

Linking the exemplar of Multiple Sclerosis with the concept of Sensory Perception:

1. What assessment findings would you anticipate for the client with multiple sclerosis regarding alterations in visual acuity?
2. If the demyelination from multiple sclerosis is affecting the brainstem, what physical assessment data is a priority for the nurse to gather related to sensory perception?

Linking the exemplar of Multiple Sclerosis with the concept of Mood and Affect:

3. How will the administration of interferonbeta-1a (Avonex) put the client with MS at risk for alterations in mood and affect?
4. What mental health data is a priority for the nurse to assess before planning care for the client with MS?

READY: GO TO COMPANION SKILLS MANUAL

- Assessing the neurologic system
- Assessing the musculoskeletal system
- Providing morning care
- Providing evening care
- Assisting an adult to eat
- Assessing home for safe environment
- Bathing an adult client
- Providing special oral care to a debilitated client

REFER: GO TO MYNURSINGKIT

REFLECT: CASE STUDY

Elena Jones is a 48-year-old nurse who works in a busy pediatric ICU as a charge nurse. She works three days a week doing 12-hour shifts and attends management and committee meetings on her days off. Elena lives with her husband Brett and their three children, Debbie 16, Jason 11, and Ryan 8. Debbie is busy visiting colleges who are interested in recruiting her as she is a star soccer player. She has been sneaking out of the house at night to visit her boyfriend. Jason has been in trouble in school for sassing teachers and has mild ADHD. Ryan has just discovered an interest in playing football after school. Brett is a remodeler whose runs his business out of the home.

Elena began having symptoms of neck pain and blurred vision. She has consulted a number of doctors but did not receive a satisfactory diagnosis until she saw a neurologist who ordered an MRI and diagnosed her with multiple sclerosis. She quickly enters a period of remission following treatment that lasted for a few weeks. From that time on she has experienced 3–4 exacerbations per year. She has had to quit her job because she is unable to walk and has blurred vision that precludes driving. Her doctor begins prednisone infusions five times a week for one week during flare-ups of MS.

1. What role might stress be playing in exacerbating her MS? What strategies can you promote to reduce stress?
2. How might you guide Elena's family to contribute to improving her condition?
3. What are your expected outcomes for Elena's care?

19.5 OSTEOARTHRITIS

KEY TERMS

BASIS FOR SELECTION OF EXEMPLAR

Healthy People 2010
Institute of Medicine

LEARNING OUTCOMES

After reading about this exemplar, you will be able to:

1. Describe the pathophysiology, etiology, clinical manifestations, and direct and indirect causes of osteoarthritis.
2. Identify risk factors associated with osteoarthritis.
3. Illustrate the nursing process in providing culturally competent care across the life span for individuals with osteoarthritis.
4. Formulate priority nursing diagnoses appropriate for an individual with osteoarthritis.
5. Create a plan of care for individuals with osteoarthritis and their family members.
6. Assess expected outcomes for an individual with osteoarthritis.
7. Discuss therapies used in the collaborative care of an individual with osteoarthritis.
8. Employ evidence-based caring interventions for an individual with osteoarthritis.

OVERVIEW

Osteoarthritis (OA) (also labeled *degenerative joint disease*) is the most commonly occurring form of arthritis and is a leading cause of pain and disability in older adults (Porth, 2005). This disease is characterized by loss of articular cartilage in articulating joints and hypertrophy of the bones at the articular margins. Osteoarthritis may be idiopathic (without known cause) or secondary (associated with known risk factors). It affects more than 12% of Americans between the ages of 25 and 74, with about 90% of people having x-ray evidence of OA in the weight-bearing joints by age 40 (American College of Rheumatology, 2005; Flynn & Johnson, 2005). The joints most affected are in the hands, wrists, neck, lower back, hip, knees, anklse, and feet. Racial and ethnic effects on the development of OA are outlined in the following Focus on Diversity and Culture.

Localized OA affects only one or two joints. Generalized OA affects three or more joints. Generalized OA also may be classified as nodal (involving the hand) or nonnodal (not involving the hand). Nodal OA also may affect the knees, hips, cervical spine, and lumbar spine. Idiopathic OA most commonly affects the terminal interphalangeal joints (*Heberden's nodes*) and less often affects the proximal interphalangeal joints (*Bouchard's nodes*) (Figure 19–57 ■); the joints of the thumb, hip, and knee; the metatarsophalangeal joint of the big toe; and the cervical and lumbar spine. Secondary OA may occur in any joint from an articular injury.

FOCUS ON DIVERSITY AND CULTURE
The Client With Osteoarthritis

- White women are more likely to have hand OA.
- Black women are more likely to have knee OA.
- Hip OA incidence is less in Chinese people.

PATHOPHYSIOLOGY AND ETIOLOGY

Osteoarthritis is characterized by progressive erosion of the joint articular cartilage with formation of new bone in the joint space (Figure 19–57 ■). The joints most commonly involved in OA are joints of the hands, the weight-bearing joints of the knee and hip, and the central joints of the cervical and lumbar spine.

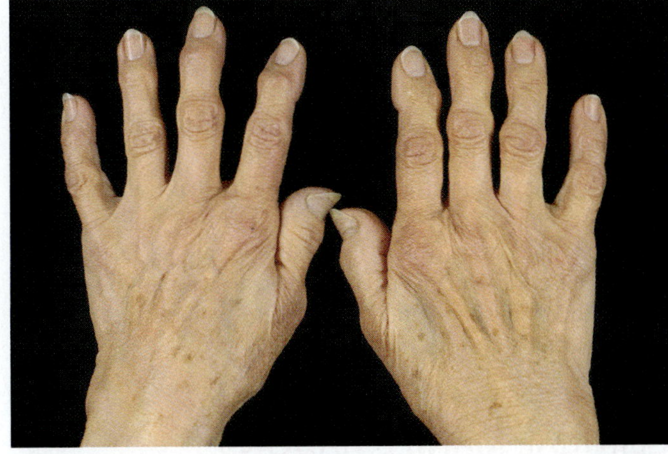

Figure 19–57 ■ Typical interphalangeal joint changes associated with osteoarthritis.

Source: L. Samsuri/Custom Medical Stock Photo.

The normal joint cartilage covers the joint and bone ends and provides a cushioning structure to reduce the mechanical force of the joint. In OA, the cartilage thins and erodes. The underlying bone (subchondral bone) is no longer protected, particularly in areas of increased stress. Without the cartilage performing as a buffer, the subchondral bone becomes irritated, which leads to degeneration of the joint. As cartilage deteriorates, subchondral bone cells hypertrophy and eventually cause bony spurs (**osteophytes**). These bony spurs grow and enlarge and often change the contour of the joint. Small pieces may break off (joint mice) and irritate the synovial membrane, causing a joint effusion and further limitation of movement.

Etiology

Primary or idiopathic OA has no single clear cause. The disease is likely a group of similar disorders that involve various complex biomedical, biochemical, and cellular processes. The typical changes can occur in several joints but have various causes. Secondary arthritis has an underlying condition, such as trauma, bone disease, or inflammatory joint disease.

Risk Factors

Idiopathic OA is associated with increasing age. OA affects more than 50% of people over the age of 65 and is the leading cause of disability for this age group (Agency for Healthcare Research and Quality, 2002). Findings suggest that OA may be inherited as an autosomal recessive trait, with genetic defects causing premature destruction of the joint cartilage. The causes of secondary OA include trauma; mechanical stress; and inflammation of joint structures, joint instability, neurologic disorders, endocrine disorders, and selected medications.

Excessive weight contributes to the development of OA, especially in the hip and knee. Excess fat may have a direct metabolic effect on the development of the disease. Primary OA of the knee is almost 4 times more common in obese women and 5 times more common in obese men (Flynn & Johnson, 2005). Inactivity is another risk factor. Moderate recreational exercise has been shown to decrease both the chance of developing OA and the progression of manifestations when OA is present. People involved in strenuous repetitive exercise (e.g., participating in sports) have an increased risk of developing secondary OA.

Other risk factors linked to OA are hormonal factors such as decreased estrogen in menopausal women, excessive growth hormone, and increased PTH. Women are affected more than men.

CLINICAL MANIFESTATIONS

The onset of OA is usually gradual and insidious and the course slowly progressive. Pain and stiffness in one or more joints (usually weight-bearing) are the first manifestations of OA. The pain is localized to the affected joints and may be described as a deep ache. Typically, the pain is aggravated by use or motion of the joint and relieved by rest, although it may become persistent as the disease progresses. Pain at night may be accompanied by paresthesia (numbness, tingling). Pain also may be referred to other parts of the body; for example, OA of the lumbosacral spine may cause severe pain along the path of the sciatic nerve. Following periods of immobility, such as after sleeping all night or after a taking long automobile ride, involved joints may stiffen. Usually, only a few minutes of activity are necessary to relieve the stiffness. Range of motion of the joint decreases as the disease progresses, and grating or crepitus may be noted during movement. Bony overgrowth may cause joint enlargement, and flexion contractures may occur because of joint instability. In OA, enlarged joints are characteristically bony-hard and cool on palpation. Manifestations specific to affected joints are outlined in Table 19–11.

TABLE 19–11 Manifestations of Osteoarthritis

AFFECTED SITE	MANIFESTATIONS
Interphalangeal joints	■ *Heberden's nodes*—bony enlargements of distal joints; may cause pain, redness, and swelling
	■ *Bouchard's nodes*—bony enlargement of proximal joints
First carpometacarpal	■ Swelling, tenderness at base of thumb
	■ Crepitus with movement
	■ "Squared" appearance of joint
Spine	■ Localized pain and stiffness
	■ Muscle spasm
	■ Limited ROM
	■ Nerve root compression with radicular pain and motor weakness
Hips	■ Pain referred to inguinal area, buttock, thigh, or knee
	■ Loss of internal rotation
	■ Limited extension, adduction, and flexion
Knees	■ Pain and bony enlargement
	■ Effusions
	■ Crepitus
	■ Instability and deformity with advanced disease

Complications

Osteoarthritis of the spine may involve the vertebral bodies and intervertebral disks, the diarthrodial joints, or both. *Spondylosis* is degenerative disk disease. As the intervertebral disks degenerate, disk space between the vertebrae is lost. Degenerative disk disease may be complicated by herniated disk, the protrusion of the nucleus pulposus of the disk. Herniation usually occurs in a lateral direction, potentially compressing nerve roots and causing radicular (pertaining to distribution along the nerve) pain and muscle weakness.

Disk degeneration and joint space narrowing alter the mechanics of the spinal column, promoting osteoarthritic changes in the articular processes (facet joints) of the vertebrae. The cartilage covering the inferior and superior articular processes degenerates, causing localized pain, stiffness, muscle spasm, and limited ROM. Osteophytes may form on articular processes, further contributing to pain and muscle spasm.

The presentation of OA in older clients is similar to that in younger adults. However, in the older population, the risk of debilitation due to OA is greater and the disease may progress faster. In addition, pain, stiffness, and limited ROM increase the risk of falls and fractures.

COLLABORATION

At this time, no treatment is available to stop the process of joint degeneration. Appropriate collaborative management is important to relieve pain and maintain the client's function and mobility. Ongoing research is occurring on a new class of medications called disease-modifying osteoarthritis drugs (DMOADs) and gene therapy.

An important part of treatment of the older person with a chronic disease such as arthritis is learning how to live with the disease and attain the best quality of life. The *Healthy People 2010* website provides the nation's goals and objectives for improved health for 2000–2010. One objective for arthritis clients is stated as follows: "Increase the proportion of persons with arthritis who have had effective, evidence based arthritis education as an integral part of the management of their condition" (Centers for Disease Control and Prevention, 2009). Many arthritis self-help programs have been offered in the United States in the past decade. Strategies such as self-help groups, online courses, telephone support, and one-to-one instruction have been found to be effective. Client benefits include decreased pain, increased knowledge about arthritis, and an increase in the frequency of exercise. An additional benefit is fewer physician visits, which results in costs savings for both RA and OA clients (Boutaugh & Brady, 2001). Technology-supported arthritis programs also show promise for the future.

For the older person with OA, early treatment can significantly affect outcomes and improve overall quality of life. Older clients should be offered a variety of cognitive-behavioral modalities (relaxation, imagery) to help them cope with adjusting to a chronic illness. The nonpharmacologic strategies are applicable to most types of arthritis. Each strategy must be individualized to the older person's needs. Nonpharmacologic treatment of OA includes:

- Education about the disease
- Weight reduction to decrease stress on joints
- Exercise to relieve pain and stiffness (along with many other benefits)
- General and specific rest as needed to control symptoms
- The use of canes, crutches, and walkers to protect joints
- The use of assistive technology to help with functional ability
- Surgical intervention for joint replacement (hips and knees).

Diagnostic Tests

The diagnosis of OA is generally based on the client's history, physical examination, and x-rays of affected joints. Diagnostic tests are described in Appendix B.

Characteristic changes of OA are visible in x-ray studies of affected joints. Initially, narrowing of irregular joint space is seen. Progressive changes include increased density of subchondral (under cartilage) bone, osteophyte formation at the joint periphery, and formation of cysts in the bone. Examination of synovial fluid from involved joints can identify the type of arthritis. In addition, research of the blood level of **hyaluronic acid (HA)** (a lubricating substance in cartilage and joint synovial fluid) suggests that HA may be a useful biochemical marker indicating the presence and severity of OA (National Institute of Arthritis and Musculoskeletal and Skin Diseases, 2005).

Pharmacologic Therapies

The pain of OA often can be managed through the use of analgesics such as aspirin and acetaminophen. Acetaminophen (Tylenol) is generally preferred for use in older clients because it has fewer toxic side effects. NSAIDs such as ibuprofen (Motrin), naproxen (Aleve), and ketoprofen (Orudis KT) also may be prescribed.

Topical medications include counterirritants, salicylates, and capsaicin, sold without prescription as creams, gels, sprays, patches, and ointments to relieve pain. Counterirritants include Flexall 454 Maximum Strength Gel, ArthriCare, Bengay, and Icy Hot; salicylates include Aspercreme and Sportscreme, and capsaicin is included in Capzasin and Zostrix. The client should be taught to keep the medications away from their eyes, nose, mouth, and any open skin and not to bandage or apply heat to the treated area. The products should be used no more than three or four times a day and discontinued immediately if severe irritation occurs.

Medications that are effective in decreasing the pain and stiffness of OA are the NSAID COX-2 inhibitors. However, because of the increased risk of adverse cardiovascular effects (heart attack and strokes) and GI effects (bleeding) of most drugs in this category, several have been recalled by the FDA. The only COX-2 inhibitor being prescribed as of 2006 is celecoxib (Celebrex).

Potent anti-inflammatory medications such as systemic corticosteroids are seldom prescribed for clients with OA, although intra-articular corticosteroid injections may be used. With intra-articular injections, a long-acting corticosteroid medication, often mixed with a local anesthetic such as lidocaine, is injected directly into the joint space of the affected joints. Although this procedure may provide marked pain relief, it can hasten the rate of cartilage breakdown if performed more frequently than every 4–6 months.

Weight Loss

The most important risk factor for OA that can be modified is obesity. Reducing weight can improve quality of life and reduce health care costs associated with OA. Karlson et al. (2003) studied 568 participants from the ongoing Nurses Health Study who received a hip replacement to treat OA. The researchers examined the following risk factors for hip replacement: body mass index (estimates body fat), use of hormone replacement therapy after menopause, age, alcohol consumption, physical inactivity, and cigarette smoking. Of all of the risk factors, body mass index and age were associated with the need for hip replacement. Participants with a high body mass index had double the risk for hip replacement compared to participants with a low body mass index. The risk from obesity seems to begin early in life and established by age 18. This is one of the first long-term prospective studies to show an association between a modifiable risk factor and OA.

PRACTICE ALERT

To prevent OA, the obese elderly person should lose weight. An obese person is 5 times more likely to have OA of the knees and twice as likely to have OA of the hips.

Exercise to Relieve Pain and Stiffness

Many older people with OA (and other joint diseases) believe that exercise will cause a flare-up of their arthritis and lead to more pain. As a result, many are afraid to partake in activities that they previously enjoyed. Contrary to that misconception, exercise is an important part of treatment for the older person with arthritis. In fact, joints are dependent upon the surrounding muscles for strength, joint protection, and weight bearing. If the muscles are not used, atrophy may result and lead to weakness, falls, and mobility limitations. (See the exercise guidelines in Client Teaching: Exercise Guidelines for Older People With Arthritis.) Physical therapy referrals are often indicated to help clients learn the best approach to exercise.

Rest to Control Symptoms

Rest also is an important part of an overall plan for the older person with arthritis. Teaching the older person about rest must include both general rest and rest for the specific joints involved. General rest includes adequate sleep at night and rest periods to ensure overall health and to prevent the excessive fatigue that often occurs with inflammatory conditions. Rest should be done at specific times with proper positioning and should be limited to prevent disuse that occurs with prolonged immobility. Frequent short rest periods are better than long ones to prevent stiffness.

Specific rest relates to rest of joints that are painful or inflamed. This includes inflammatory arthritis (RA and gout) and OA. While maintaining overall physical activity and preserving function, this type of rest gives affected joints time to recover and prevents additional pain and injury.

The older person should rest an acutely painful or inflamed joint by limiting particular activities and using assistive devices. It is important not to overstretch damaged tissues. During inflammation, tensile strength of the tissue is reduced by up to 50%; thus, overstretching and tearing can more easily occur (Minor & Westby, 2001). However, daily ROM exercises of the remaining joints should continue because strong muscles support the damaged joint. It is important to rest painful joints to prevent overuse, provide support, and maintain function. (See the preceding Client Teaching feature.) Resting the joint should result in decreased pain, swelling, and fatigue.

CLIENT TEACHING Exercise Guidelines for Older People With Arthritis

- Stretching of all muscle groups (prevent overstretching) 10 minutes daily.
- Active ROM daily for all joints.
- Isometric exercises. Keep intensity low. Extremely forceful muscle contractions may cause intra-articular pressure and promote damage.
- Isotonic exercises. Move the joint in an arc. Start gently and progress to weights. Attempts should be made to do full ROM.
- Resistive exercises twice a week. Increase weights gradually.
- Aerobic exercises (aquatic, walking) are usually well tolerated by older adults with mild to moderate lower extremity OA. For some older people with moderate to severe OA, walking as aerobic exercise may not be well tolerated. Alternative exercises such as swimming, biking, and water walking can be offered. Aerobics and strength training improve strength, exercise capacity, gait, functional performance, and balance (Resnick, 2001).

Conservative Treatment

Osteoarthritis is initially treated conservatively, but as pain increases and joint function decreases, surgery often becomes necessary. The goals of OA treatment are to relieve pain and maintain as much normal joint function as possible. Conservative treatment may include any or all of the following:

- *Apply heat to painful joints.* Applying heat to a painful joint decreases pain and improves flexibility. Hot packs can be applied for about 20 minutes to elevate skin temperature; then they should be removed. Clients sometimes find hot showers and tub baths to be soothing. Moist heat is more effective than dry heat because it penetrates deeper (Robbins, Burckhardt, Hannan, & Dehoratius, 2001).
- *Use cold applications to reduce pain and swelling.* Cold is applied to the skin with ice packs or cold packs, usually for 10–30 minutes depending on the intensity of the cold source and depth of the tissue (Hayes, 2001). Mild cold is used for swelling; deeper cold, for pain. Care should be taken not to frost the skin.
- *Use canes, crutches, and walkers to protect joints.* These devices are important for joint rest and safety, especially during times of acute joint pain and inflammation. The nurse should teach the client the correct use of the device or consult with a PT or an occupational therapist (OT) for client follow-up.

- *Use assistive technology.* Assistive devices are used to maintain, increase, or improve function. They may be bought commercially or be custom-made for the client. The device may be as simple as a kitchen grip, an enlarged pen, a specialized motor scooter, or a dressing aid such as a sock holder. Assistive devices are available for general daily living, home management, school, and work activities. Compliance with their use increases when the client has been adequately taught. Specific guidelines are available for environmental accessibility. The Job Accommodation Network (a service of the U.S. Department of Labor Office of Disability Employment Policy) is a helpful resource for working with a client in need of modification of environment.

Viscosupplementation

Viscosupplementation is a new treatment for OA of the knee. Hyaluronan, a natural component of synovial fluid, is injected directly into the knee joint. Four hyaluronan derivatives have been approved for use: Hyalgan, Supartz, Orthovisc, and Synvisc. The injection may provide pain relief and improvement in knee function for up to 1 year, but its long-term effects are unknown (Flynn & Johnson, 2005).

Surgery

Surgical procedures can provide dramatic results for clients with significant chronic pain and loss of joint function. Although elective surgical procedures are frequently avoided in the older adult, even older clients will see significant benefits as long as they do not have a chronic medical condition that contraindicates surgery.

ARTHROSCOPY An **arthroscopy** is a surgical procedure in which an arthroscope (a thin tube that is lighted and has a camera in one end) is inserted into a joint. It may be done to diagnose the type of arthritis or to perform debridement by smoothing rough cartilage and flushing out the joint to remove debris. Although arthroscopic debridement and lavage of involved joints have been used, arthroscopy has not proven effective in the treatment of knee OA. It may be useful to remove large pieces of debris or to repair a torn cartilage (Flynn & Johnson, 2005).

OSTEOTOMY An **osteotomy**, an incision into or transection of the bone, may be performed to realign an affected joint, particularly when significant bony overgrowth or osteophyte formation has occurred. This procedure also may be used to shift the joint load toward areas of less severely damaged cartilage. Although osteotomy does not halt the process of OA, it may have a beneficial effect on joint function and pain, delaying the need for a joint replacement by several years.

JOINT ARTHROPLASTY A **joint arthroplasty** is the reconstruction or replacement of a joint. Arthroplasty is usually indicated when the client has severely restricted joint mobility and pain at rest. Pain is virtually eliminated, and the function of the joint is generally improved. Arthroplasty may involve partial joint replacement or reshaping of the bones of a joint. For most clients with OA, both surfaces of the affected joint are replaced with prosthetic parts in a procedure known as a *total joint replacement.* Joints that may be replaced include the hip, knee, shoulder, elbow, ankle, and wrist and joints of the fingers and toes.

In a total joint replacement, some or all of the synovium, cartilage, and bone on both sides of the joint are removed. A metallic prosthesis is inserted to replace one joint surface (generally the load-end or distal portion of a weight-bearing joint). The other joint surface is replaced by a silicone-lined ceramic or plastic prosthesis.

Most prosthetic joints are uncemented, that is, made of porous ceramic and metal components inserted so that they fit tightly into existing bone. The implant is secured by new bone growth into the prosthesis, a process that requires approximately 6 weeks. Although a longer non–weight-bearing period is necessary initially until the prosthesis is fixed in place by the bony growth, the implant appears to have a longer useful life span than cemented prostheses. In a cemented joint replacement, methyl methacrylate (a pliable polymer that hardens to hold the prosthesis in place) is used to secure the prosthesis to existing bone. Although the client can resume normal activities more rapidly following a cemented joint replacement, methyl methacrylate initiates an inflammatory response, and the joint eventually loosens.

In a *total hip replacement,* the articular surfaces of the acetabulum and femoral head are replaced. The entire head of the femur and part of the femoral neck are removed and replaced with a prosthesis (Figure 19–58 ■). The acetabulum is remodeled, and a prosthesis of high molecular-weight polyethylene is inserted. The success rate for total hip replacement is reported to be greater than 90%. Approximately 150,000 total hip replacements are done each year in the United States; most are for treatment of OA (Boston Total Joint Association, 2004). Most hip replacements last 10–15 years, after which a second joint replacement, called a revision, can be performed. Potential problems

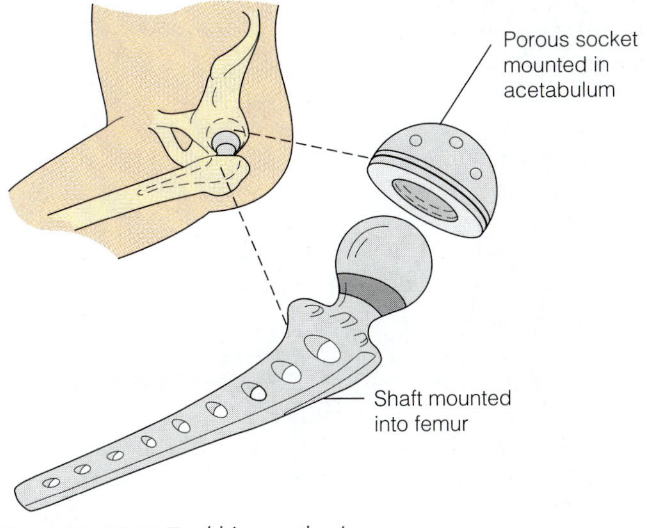

Figure 19–58 ■ Total hip prosthesis.

associated with a total hip replacement include blood clots in leg veins, dislocation within the prosthesis, loosening of joint components from surrounding bone, and infection. If recurrent or ineffectively treated, these complications may necessitate removal of the prosthesis, resulting in severe shortening of the extremity and an unstable hip joint.

Total knee replacement is performed if the client has intractable pain and x-ray films show evidence of arthritis of the knee. More than 350,000 knee replacements are performed in the United States each year (Flynn & Johnson, 2005). Several prosthetic devices involving removal of varying amounts of bone are available for knee joint replacement (Figure 19–59 ■). The femoral side of the joint is replaced with a metallic surface; the tibial side, with polyethylene. More than 80% of clients obtain significant or total relief of pain after having a total knee replacement. However, they must engage in a vigorous program of rehabilitation to achieve the best results. Joint failure is more common with knee replacement than with a total hip replacement. Loosened joint components, often on the tibial side, are the most common cause of failure. The possible complications following a total knee replacement are the same as for a total hip replacement.

Total shoulder replacement is indicated for unremitting pain and marked limitation of ROM because of arthritic involvement of the humeral and glenoid joint surfaces of the shoulder. The joint is immobilized in a sling or an abduction splint for 2–3 weeks following arthroplasty. Dislocation, loosening of the prosthesis, and infection are potential problems associated with total shoulder replacement.

Total elbow replacement involves replacement of the humeral and ulnar surfaces of the elbow joint with a metal and polyethylene prosthesis. Pain and disabling stiffness of the joint are indications for an elbow arthroplasty. Complications, including dislocation, fracture, triceps weakness, loosening, and infection, occur frequently.

Infection is the major complication associated with total joint replacement. Infection not only interferes with healing and prolong recovery, but also may necessitate removal of the prosthesis and may lead to loss of joint function. Other potential complications include circulatory impairment to the affected limb, thromboembolism, nerve damage, and dislocation of the joint.

Physical Therapy and Rehabilitation

Recovery from all types of joint replacement requires postoperative physical therapy, focusing on building strength and regaining joint flexibility. Rehabilitation begins in the hospital, most often the day following surgery, and may be continued during home care. Recovery from a hip replacement is 80% complete in 4 weeks and 100% complete in 6 months. Recovery from a knee replacement is 80% complete in 4 weeks and 100% complete after 1 year. During rehabilitation, the client must follow a regimen of exercise, rest, and medication (Flynn & Johnson, 2005).

Complementary and Alternative Therapies

The following complementary therapies are examples of therapies that people with OA may use to relieve pain and stiffness. These therapies also are used by people with RA.

- Biomagnetic therapy
- Acupuncture
- Elimination of nightshade foods such as potatoes, tomatoes, peppers, eggplant, and tobacco
- Nutritional supplements such as glucosamine, chondroitin, boron, zinc, copper, selenium, manganese, flavonoids, and SAM-e
- Herbal therapy
- Massage therapy
- Osteopathic manipulation
- Vitamin therapy
- Yoga.

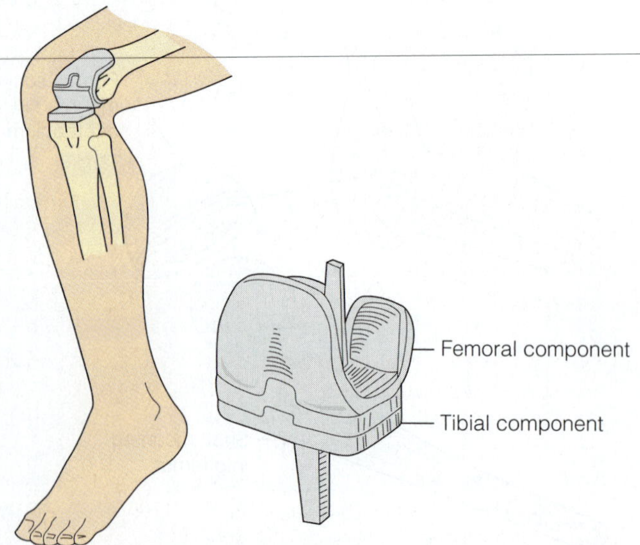

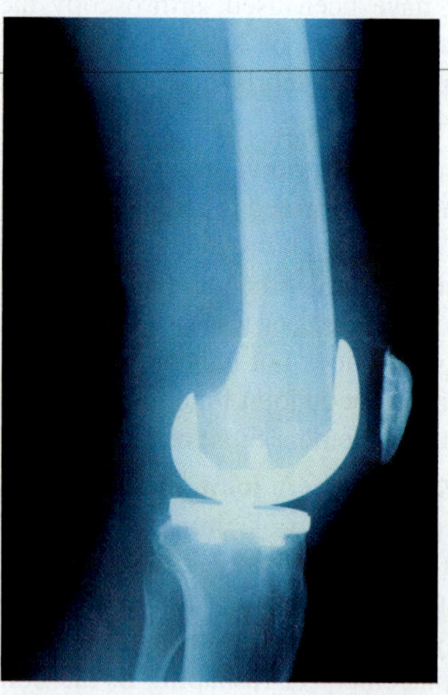

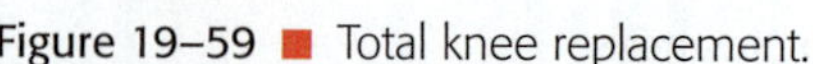
Figure 19–59 ■ Total knee replacement.

NURSING PROCESS

Osteoarthritis is a chronic process for which there is no cure. The focus of nursing care for the client with OA is providing comfort, helping to maintain mobility and ADL, and assisting with adaptations to maintain life roles.

Although OA cannot be prevented, maintaining a normal weight and having a program of regular moderate exercise reduces risk factors. Glucosamine and chondroitin are nutritional supplements for OA that are increasingly popular and have been found to be of benefit in reducing manifestations. Clients should discuss these supplements with their health care provider before using them.

Assessment

The nursing assessment includes a thorough health history and physical examination.

- *Health history.* Family history of OA, occupation, recreational activities, joint pain and stiffness, ability to carry out ADL and self-care activities
- *Physical assessment.* Height/weight; gait; joints: symmetry, size, shape, color, appearance, temperature, pain, crepitus, ROM, Heberden's nodes, Bouchard's nodes

Diagnosis

The nursing diagnoses addressed in this section include the following:

- Chronic Pain
- Impaired Physical Mobility
- Self-Care Deficit.

Plan

The plan of care will be designed in collaboration with the client. Some goals that may be appropriate include the following:

- Client will articulate strategies for reducing pain.
- Client will maintain maximum ROM of involved joints.
- Client will minimize the impact of osteoarthritis on his or her lifestyle.
- Client will use assistive devices to maintain autonomy in performing ADL.

Implementation

The priority nursing interventions for clients with OA are directed toward managing chronic pain, facilitating physical mobility, and improving ability to provide self-care.

Chronic Pain

Pain is a primary manifestation of OA. As joint tissues degenerate and changes in joint structure occur, the amount of discomfort generally increases. The pain associated with OA increases with activity and tends to be relieved with rest. Nonpharmacologic comfort measures are appropriate, with mild analgesics used to supplement these as needed.

- Monitor the level of pain, including intensity, location, quality, and aggravating and relieving factors. Accurate assessment of pain provides a basis for evaluation of the effect of interventions.
- Teach clients to take prescribed analgesic or anti-inflammatory medication as needed. Analgesics reduce the perception of pain and may decrease muscle spasm as well. Anti-inflammatory medication may be ordered to decrease local inflammatory response in affected joints.
- Encourage rest of painful joints. The pain of OA is often relieved by joint rest.
- Suggest applying heat to painful joints using the shower; a tub or sitz bath; warm packs; hot wax baths; heated gloves; or **diathermy**, which uses high-frequency electrical currents to generate heat. The application of heat reduces accompanying muscle spasm, relieving pain. Moist heat penetrates deeper than dry heat; diathermy delivers heat directly to lesions in deeper body tissues.
- Emphasize the importance of proper posture and good body mechanics for walking, sitting, lifting, and moving. Good body mechanics and posture reduce stress on affected joints.
- Encourage the overweight client to lose weight. Excess weight places abnormal stress on joints, particularly the knees.
- Encourage the use of nonpharmacologic pain relief measures such as progressive relaxation, meditation, visualization, and distraction. These adjunctive pain relief measures can reduce the client's reliance on analgesics and increase comfort.

CARE SETTINGS Community Care for the Client With Osteoarthritis

Because of the chronicity of OA, clients and their families need appropriate teaching to manage the disease and its consequences effectively. Much of the teaching focus is on preservation of joint function and mobility. Discuss the following topics:

- Safeguard against hazards of safe mobility, such as scatter rugs. Encourage installation of safety devices such as handrails and grab bars.
- Understand the disease process and its chronic degenerative nature.
- Learn exercise techniques, including ROM, isometric, postural, stretching, and strengthening to maintain healthy cartilage, preserve ROM, and develop supportive muscles and tendons. A walking program is beneficial for clients with OA of the knee.
- Do not overuse or stress affected joints with heavy lifting, excessive stair climbing or bending, or other repetitive actions.
- Sit in a straight chair without slumping; avoid soft chairs or recliners and sleep on a firm mattress or use a bed board.
- Use pain relief measures including prescribed or OTC analgesic medications and nonpharmacologic pain relief measures such as heat, rest, massage, relaxation, and meditation.

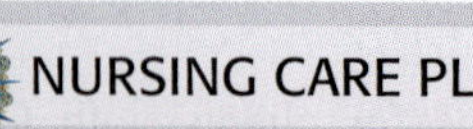

NURSING CARE PLAN A Client With Osteoarthritis

Robert Cerulli is a 72-year-old retired commercial fisherman who has experienced arthritic pain in his hips for the past 10–15 years. During the past year, the pain in his right hip has become severe, prompting him to seek medical attention. Significant degenerative changes in both hip joints are noted on x-ray films. The physician recommends a total replacement of the right hip, with total replacement of the left hip to follow in 6–12 months. Mr. Cerulli has preoperative teaching and tests the afternoon prior to his surgery, scheduled for 0800 the following morning.

ASSESSMENT

Christie Phlaugh, RN, completes a health history and examination of Mr. Cerulli on admission. Reviewing his medical record, she notes that Mr. Cerulli has mild Parkinson's disease (PD) and is taking carbidopa-levodopa (Sinemet 25-100) four times a day to control his symptoms. No other chronic medical conditions have been reported. Mr. Cerulli says that essentially he has been healthy his entire life. He has no known allergies to medications, has never smoked, and consumes only small amounts of alcohol.

On examination of Mr. Cerulli, Ms. Phlaugh notes that he is alert and oriented. His vital signs are T_O 97.4°F (36.3°C), P 68 regular, R 18, BP 116/64. Peripheral pulses are strong and equal in the upper extremities and slightly weaker but equal in the lower extremities. His feet are cool to touch but have immediate capillary refill. He has full ROM of his shoulders, elbows, and wrists. The ROM of both hips is significantly restricted. Hip flexion beyond 90 degrees prompts pain on both sides. Both flexion and extension of the knees are limited slightly. Mr. Cerulli walks with a limp, favoring his right hip, and has a shuffling gait.

Preoperative laboratory studies including CBC, coagulation studies, chemistry panel, and urinalysis show a serum creatinine of 1.7 mg/dL and blood urea nitrogen (BUN) of 30 mg/dL, with no other abnormal values noted. His electrocardiogram (ECG) and chest x-ray show no apparent pathologies. Cefazolin (Ancef) 500 mg is to be administered intravenously at 0600 prior to surgery, and Mr. Cerulli is to shower and shampoo with antibacterial soap at bedtime. The PT meets with Mr. Cerulli to evaluate his mobility and to begin teaching him about postoperative weight-bearing restrictions.

DIAGNOSES (POSTOPERATIVE)

- Acute Pain related to surgical incision
- Impaired Physical Mobility related to activity and weight-bearing restrictions
- Risk for Infection related to disruption in skin integrity
- Risk for Ineffective Tissue Perfusion, Right Leg related to vascular disruption and edema

PLANNING

Goals of client care include the following:

- Maintain an adequate level of comfort postoperatively as demonstrated by:
- The ability to move easily within restrictions
- Compliance with instructions to cough and breathe deeply
- Verbal expressions of comfort
- No adverse consequences of immobility such as pneumonia, pressure areas, thromboembolism, or contracture.
- Remain free of infection.
- Maintain adequate perfusion of affected leg.
- Remain free of injury postoperatively.

IMPLEMENTATION

- Assess pain at least hourly during first 24–48 hours postoperatively and as needed thereafter.
- Instruct in the use of PCA and monitor its effectiveness.
- Help change position at least every 2 hours; encourage the use of the overhead trapeze to shift positions frequently.
- Maintain sequential compression device and antiembolic stocking as ordered; remove for 1 hour daily.
- Encourage the use of the incentive spirometer hourly for first 24 hours, then at least every 2 hours while awake.
- Assist out of bed three times a day after the first 24 hours.
- Maintain abduction of the right hip with pillows.
- Perform passive ROM exercises of unaffected extremities every shift.
- Encourage frequent quadriceps-setting exercises and plantar and dorsiflexion of feet.
- Assess the surgical site frequently; report signs of excess bleeding or inflammation.
- Monitor temperature every 4 hours.
- Assess pulses, color, movement, and sensation of right foot hourly for the first 24 hours, then every 2 hours for 24 hours, then every 4 hours.

EVALUATION

Mr. Cerulli returns to the orthopedic unit from the postanesthesia care unit. He becomes confused and disoriented during the first 36 hours after surgery, but his orientation and thought processes gradually clear. His family has stayed with him, and he has not experienced injury or other adverse consequences from his confusion. Otherwise, Mr. Cerulli has had an uneventful postoperative recovery. Six days after surgery he is transferred to an extended care rehabilitation facility for further therapy until he can ambulate with partial weight bearing on his affected leg. He returns home 5 weeks after surgery, able to use a walker for ambulation. Arrangements are made for an overbed trapeze, elevated toilet seat, and shower chair in his home. A home health nurse and PT visit Mr. and Mrs. Cerulli weekly for a month following his discharge. During that time, he gradually resumes full weight bearing. Mr. Cerulli expresses pleasure with the relief of his hip pain and says that he has no fear of having his left hip replaced in the future.

NURSING CARE PLAN **A Client With Osteoarthritis** *continued*

CRITICAL THINKING

1. Mr. Cerulli's preoperative laboratory work showed a modest elevation in his serum creatinine and BUN. What do those studies indicate? How might those changes have affected nursing responsibilities related to medication administration for Mr. Cerulli?
2. Mr. Cerulli became confused postoperatively. What factors in his history might have alerted the nurses to this possibility? How might anesthesia and postoperative analgesics have contributed to his confusion?
3. Develop a care plan for Mr. Cerulli using the nursing diagnosis acute confusion.

Impaired Physical Mobility

As intra-articular cartilage degenerates and joint structures are altered, the client with OA experiences pain, stiffness, and decreased ROM in affected joints. When the spine, large weight-bearing joints of the hips and knees, or the ankles and feet are affected, physical mobility can be reduced significantly.

- Assess the ROM of affected joints. Assessing joint mobility is important as a basis for planning appropriate interventions.
- Perform a functional mobility assessment, evaluating gait, ability to sit and rise from a sitting position, ability to step in and out of the tub or shower, and negotiation of stairs. The functional assessment provides vital data about the client's ability to maintain ADL.
- Teach active and passive ROM exercises as well as isometric, progressive resistance, and low-impact aerobic exercises. Active ROM exercises help maintain muscle tone and mobility of affected joints and prevent contractures. Isometric and progressive resistance exercises improve muscle tone and strength; aerobic exercise improves endurance and cardiovascular fitness.

Self-Care Deficit

Just as OA of the lower extremities can reduce the client's mobility, OA of the upper extremities (the wrist, hand, and finger joints in particular) can significantly interfere with performance of ADL such as cooking and brushing one's hair. When the lower extremities are affected, bathing and toileting can be difficult.

- Perform a functional assessment of the upper and lower extremities. For upper extremities, assess the ability to touch the back of the head and to hold and use small items such as eating utensils. The functional assessment provides important data about the client's ability to provide self-care.
- Assess the home setting to determine the need for assistive devices such as handrails, grab bars, a walk-in shower stall, or a shower chair and handheld showerhead. Many assistive devices are relatively easy and inexpensive to obtain and can significantly improve the client's independence in performing ADLs.
- Assist in obtaining other assistive devices such as long-handled shoehorns, zipper grabbers, long-handled tongs or grippers for retrieving items from the floor, jar openers, and special eating utensils. These devices can prolong independence in performing ADLs.

Evaluation

The client's progress in meeting goals is often based on the following expected outcomes:

- Client maintains autonomy in performing ADL.
- Client's lifestyle is not significantly impacted by OA.
- Client reports pain control adequate to allow for rest and sleep.

REVIEW Osteoarthritis

RELATE: LINK THE CONCEPTS

Linking the exemplar of Osteoarthritis with the concept of Comfort:

1. What assessment data will you gather to help you plan for chronic pain relief in the client with osteoarthritis?
2. Compare and contrast the various complementary and alternative therapies for pain relief for the client with osteoarthritis.

Linking the exemplar of Osteoarthritis with the concept of Safety:

3. Create a safety plan for the client with severe osteoarthritis in both hands who lives alone.
4. What teaching interventions will you initiate for the client with osteoarthritis of the knees who is learning to use a walker?

READY: GO TO COMPANION SKILLS MANUAL

- Assessing the musculoskeletal system
- Assessing the client in pain
- Applying body mechanics
- Transferring from bed to wheel chair
- Performing passive range-of-motion exercises
- Assisting the client to use a walker

REFER: GO TO MYNURSINGKIT

REFLECT: CASE STUDY

Maureen Murphy is a 68-year-old woman who has recently been diagnosed with osteoarthritis in her right hip. Maureen lives with her husband Marty who is 75 and has been diagnosed with early dementia. Marty has a descending aortic aneurysm that required surgery 5 months ago. He has not recovered as well as expected and is frequently confused and forgetful as well as weak. Maureen is retired and carries good health insurance for she and Marty. Each have an IRA as well as social security benefits.

Maureen is extremely organized, pays attention to detail, and gets very agitated when her routine is interrupted. Maureen and Marty belong to a small community church and have many caring friends and neighbors.

Maureen's provider recommends hip replacement which she has readily agreed to. She has been limping and in pain which is causing problems as she attempts to care for Marty. The doctor has told Maureen that she will be in the hospital for one week after surgery and then two weeks at a rehabilitation hospital. Before surgery, Maureen is trying to arrange for Marty's care as well as her own.

1. What priorities of care do you see for Maureen prior to surgery?
2. What safety concerns do you anticipate for Maureen and Marty when Maureen is discharged from rehabilitation?
3. What resources will you recommend for Maureen's home care after discharge from rehabilitation?

19.6 PARKINSON'S DISEASE

KEY TERMS

Bradykinesia, *1134*
Bradyphrenia, *1136*
Pallidotomy, *1137*
Parkinson's disease (PD), *1134*
Stereotaxic thalamotomy, *1137*

BASIS FOR SELECTION OF EXEMPLAR

Centers for Disease Control and Prevention

LEARNING OUTCOMES

After reading about this exemplar, you will be able to:

1. Describe the pathophysiology, etiology, clinical manifestations, and direct and indirect causes of Parkinson's disease.
2. Identify risk factors associated with Parkinson's disease.
3. Illustrate the nursing process in providing culturally competent care across the life span for individuals with Parkinson's disease.
4. Formulate priority nursing diagnoses appropriate for an individual with Parkinson's disease.
5. Create a plan of care for individuals with Parkinson's disease and their family members.
6. Assess expected outcomes for an individual with Parkinson's disease.
7. Discuss therapies used in the collaborative care of an individual with Parkinson's disease.
8. Employ evidence-based caring interventions for an individual with Parkinson's disease.

OVERVIEW

Parkinson's disease (PD) is a progressive, degenerative neurologic disease characterized by tremors (shaking), muscle rigidity, and **bradykinesia** (slowness of movement) (Porth, 2005). People with PD are faced with multiple problems involving independence in ADL, emotional well-being, financial security, and relationships with caregivers.

PATHOPHYSIOLOGY AND ETIOLOGY

Coordinated, voluntary body movement is achieved through the actions of neurotransmitters in the basal ganglia of the brain. Some neurotransmitters facilitate the transmission of excitatory nerve impulses, while other neurotransmitters inhibit their transmission. Together, this system allows control of movement. A disturbed balance between excitatory and inhibitory neurotransmitters causes disorders of voluntary motor function, such as PD.

In PD, neurons in the cerebral cortex atrophy and are lost, the dopaminergic nigrostriatal (pigmented) pathway degenerates, and the number of specific dopamine receptors in the basal ganglia decreases. These pathologic processes cause a decrease in the production of dopamine (a neurotransmitter that helps regulate nerve impulses involved in motor function) from the substantia nigra. The usual balance of dopamine (an inhibitory neurotransmitter) and acetylcholine (an excitatory neurotransmitter) in the brain is disrupted, and dopamine no longer inhibits acetylcholine. The failure to inhibit acetylcholine is the underlying basis for the manifestations of the disorder.

Parkinson's disease has five stages, outlined in Box 19–16.

Etiology

The exact cause of PD is unknown, but it is hypothesized that exposure to environmental toxins or a genetic predisposition lead to PD.

Risk Factors

Parkinson's disease is a disorder for which the risk increases dramatically with age. It occurs at similar rates in all ethnic groups, is equally distributed in males and females, and has a prevalence of 1 or 2 per 1,000 people in the general population, which increases to 2% of adults over age 65. Inheritable

Box 19–16 Stages of Parkinson's Disease

1. Unilateral involvement only, usually with minimal or no functional impairment.
2. Bilateral or midline involvement, without impairment of balance.
3. First sign of impaired righting reflexes, evidenced as unsteadiness as the client turns or demonstrated when the client is pushed from standing equilibrium with the feet together and eyes closed. Functionally, the client is somewhat restricted in activities but may have some employment potential depending on the type of employment. Clients are physically capable of leading independent lives, and their disability is mild to moderate.
4. Fully developed, severely disabling disease; the client is still able to walk and stand unassisted but is markedly incapacitated.
5. Client is confined to bed or wheelchair unless aided.

factors may influence the risk of PD. First-degree relatives of clients are twice as likely to develop PD as are controls.

CLINICAL MANIFESTATIONS

Parkinson's disease begins with subtle manifestations. Clients complain of feeling tired and seem to move more slowly; a slight tremor may accompany the fatigue. Over time, the manifestations progressively increase in severity. The manifestations and complications of PD are presented in Box 19–17.

Tremor

Tremor at rest is usually the first manifestation experienced, with one of the upper extremities affected more often. Resting tremors of the hand show a "pill-rolling" motion of the thumb and fingers. (This name reflects the way in which medicinal pills were formed in the early days of medicine.) The tremor may be controlled with purposeful voluntary movement and is worsened by stress and anxiety. Clients have progressive impairment in performing skills that require dexterity and fine muscle control, such as writing and eating.

Box 19–17 Manifestations and Complications of Parkinson's Disease

RELATED TO MOTOR DYSFUNCTION

- Nonintentional tremor
- Bradykinesia or akinesia
  a. Slowed movements; inability to initiate voluntary movements
  b. Slowed speech, low amplitude
  c. Poor articulation
  d. Decreased eye movements (i.e., blinking)
  e. Masklike, expressionless face
- Rigidity
- Posture and gait disturbances
  a. Forward tilt of trunk
  b. Shuffling gait, propulsive at times
  c. Retropulsion
- Complications: falls, fractures, impaired communication, social isolation

RELATED TO AUTONOMIC SYSTEM DYSFUNCTION

- Skin problems
  a. Seborrhea
  b. Excess sweating on face and neck, absence of sweating of trunk and extremities
  c. Mottled skin
- Heat intolerance
- Postural hypotension
- Constipation
- Complications: skin breakdown, dizziness, falls, constipation

RELATED TO COGNITIVE AND PSYCHOLOGIC DYSFUNCTION

- Dementia
  a. Memory loss
  b. Lack of insight and problem-solving ability
  c. Declining intellectual abilities
- Anxiety
- Depression
- Complications: loss of ability to function, social isolation

Rigidity and Bradykinesia

Manifestations related to motor and postural effects include rigidity, bradykinesia, and uncoordinated movements. Rigidity (resulting from involuntary contraction of all skeletal muscles) makes both active and passive movement difficult. It is manifested as increased resistance to passive ROM. Although the extremity moves, it does so in a jerky motion, called *cogwheel rigidity*. The first manifestation of rigidity may be muscle cramps in the toes or hands, but most often the client describes stiffness, heaviness, or aching in muscles.

Bradykinesia, experienced as difficulty in starting, continuing, or coordinating movements, is the most common and crippling manifestation. All striated muscles are affected, including those that involve chewing, swallowing, and speaking. Slowed or delayed movements affect the eyes, mouth, and voice, causing a masklike face and a softened or muffled voice. Disorders of swallowing result in problems with eating and with drooling. Clients have a staring gaze with minimal change in expression (Figure 19–60 ■). Clients describe being "frozen" in place as voluntary movement is lost, and they sit or lie in one position without movement for long periods of time. Movement is interspersed with freezing, brought about by turning, which increases the effort to move or to make visual or touch contact.

Abnormal Posture

The loss of normal postural reflexes results in postural abnormalities, including disorders of postural fixation, equilibrium, and righting. Involuntary flexion of the head and shoulders means that the person with PD cannot maintain an upright

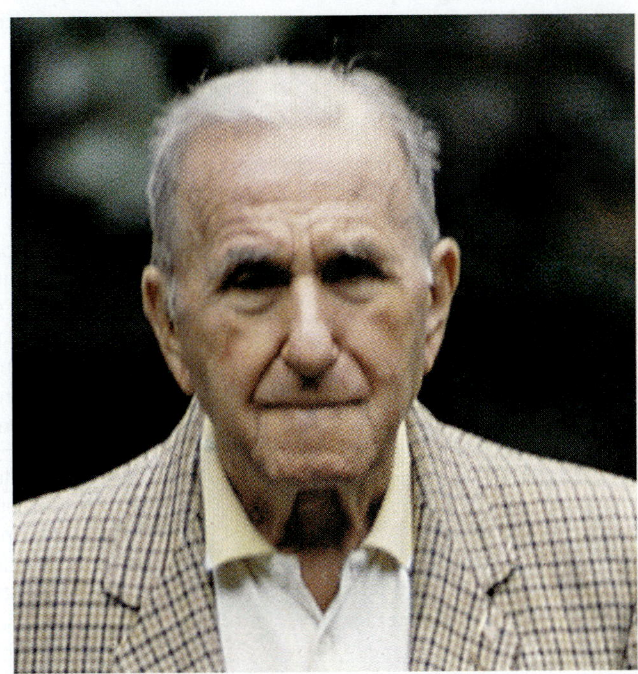

Figure 19–60 ■ In Parkinson's disease, the client's face lacks expression or animation.

Source: Yoav Levy/Phototake NYC.

position of the trunk when sitting or standing. This problem of postural fixation results in the characteristic stooped, leaning-forward position. Disorders of equilibrium follow loss of postural fixation with an inability to make adjustments when leaning or falling, increasing the risk of injury from falls. (The person usually falls backward.) The client takes short, accelerated steps to try to maintain an upright position when walking.

Autonomic and Neuroendocrine Effects

Many manifestations result from the loss of functions controlled by the autonomic nervous system. Elimination problems include constipation and urinary hesitation or frequency. Clients may experience problems related to orthostatic hypotension, including dizziness with position change. Eczematous skin changes and seborrhea are related to the increase in sweat gland activity secondary to increased sebotrophic hormone production.

Mood and Cognition

Both depression and dementia are pathologies associated with PD. Depression occurs in half of all clients, and a third have dementia. Dementia, resulting from loss of cholinergic cells, loss of neurons, senile plaques, neurofibrillary tangles, and amyloid changes in small blood vessels, occurs in 20% of clients with PD and develops later in the disease (Porth, 2005). The client has manifestations similar to the person with Alzheimer's disease, including confusion, disorientation, memory loss, distractibility, and changes in abstraction and judgment. **Bradyphrenia** also may occur, resulting in slow thinking and a decreased ability to form thoughts, to plan, or to make decisions.

CLINICAL MANIFESTATIONS AND THERAPIES **Parkinson's Disease**

ETIOLOGY	CLINICAL MANIFESTATIONS	CLINICAL THERAPIES
Constipation may result from immobility, tremors, dietary changes, lack of fluid intake, and lack of peristalsis	■ Infrequent, hard stool ■ Abdominal pain, distention ■ Flatus ■ Hemorrhoids	■ Increase fluid and fiber intake. ■ Give occasional laxatives, stool softeners, and fiber supplements. ■ Administer enemas and/or disimpact impacted stool.
Dementia resulting from loss of cholinergic cells, loss of neurons, senile plaques, neurofibrillary tangles, and amyloid changes in small blood vessels	■ Confusion, disorientation, memory loss, distractibility, bradyphrenia and changes in abstraction and judgment	■ Surround with familiar items. ■ Promote reorientation through use of calendars, clocks, and photographs. ■ Provide support to caregivers to avoid caregiver stress.
Loss of functions controlled by the autonomic nervous system	■ Constipation and urinary hesitation or frequency Orthostatic hypotension Eczematous skin changes and seborrhea	■ Teach client to change positions slowly to prevent injury. ■ Assess for urinary retention, hesitancy, or frequency and suggest strategies for management. ■ Promote use of lotions to avoid alteration in skin integrity.
Loss of normal postural reflexes	■ Postural abnormalities including disorders of postural fixation, equilibrium, and righting; involuntary flexion of the head and shoulders ■ Inability to maintain an upright position of the trunk when sitting or standing; stooped, leaning-forward position ■ Disorders of equilibrium with an inability to make adjustments when leaning or falling ■ Short, accelerated steps	■ Reduce risk of falls by removing barriers such as throw rugs and electrical cords on the floor. ■ Provide client with mobility-assistive devices as needed. ■ Provide physical therapy to help clients compensate for postural changes.
Bradykinesia	■ Difficulty in starting, continuing, or coordinating movements ■ Difficulty chewing, swallowing, and speaking; slowed or delayed movements affecting the eyes, mouth, and voice ■ Masklike face and softened or muffled voice ■ Staring gaze with minimal change in expression ■ Loss of voluntary movement ■ Movement interspersed with freezing	■ Assist with frequent repositioning. ■ Assess for ability to swallow prior to feeding. ■ Provide adequate time for client to verbalize thoughts. ■ Assess for and prevent drying of the eye. ■ Listen carefully when the client is speaking.

Sleep Disturbances

Clients with PD commonly have sleep disturbances, although they may experience decreased manifestations during sleep in the early stages. The ability to fall and stay asleep is affected by acetylcholine. Muscle rigidity may compromise sleep because of the inability to change position. This lack of muscle movement causes the client to awaken and consciously shift position.

Interrelated Effects

Some of the manifestations that clients with PD experience have multiple contributing factors. For example, constipation is common because of decreased peristalsis. However, decreased peristalsis is not the only cause: Immobility, tremors (resulting in being unable to drink easily from a glass), and dietary changes from dysphagia all contribute to the problem of constipation.

Complications

The following complications are associated with PD:

- Oculogyric crisis, in which the eyes become fixed with a lateral and upward gaze
- Paranoia and hallucinations, which may accompany dementia
- Impaired communication due to changes in speech, handwriting, and expressiveness
- Falls from balance, posture, and motor changes
- Infections such as pneumonia related to immobility
- Malnutrition related to dysphagia and inability to prepare meals
- Altered sleep patterns due to loss of dopamine and L-dopa side effects (nightmares, dreams) or side effects of anticholinergics (hyperreflexia, muscle twitching) and depression
- Skin breakdown and pressure ulcers associated with urinary incontinence, malnutrition, and sweat reflex changes
- Depression and social isolation.

COLLABORATION

Prognosis is poor, owing to the progressive degeneration that ultimately affects multiple physiologic systems and their function. Psychosocial effects are equally devastating, and the family needs more support as the client's debilitation increases. Total disability usually results 10–20 years after diagnosis. The leading cause of death is pneumonia.

Diagnostic Tests

Diagnostic studies may support a potential diagnosis of PD; no test clearly differentiates Parkinson's disease from other neurologic disorders (Hickey, 2003). However, a PET scan will show decreased uptake of 6-[18F]-fluorodopa.

Pharmacologic Therapies

The goal of drug therapy is to control manifestations as much as possible. Generally, medications vary with the stage of the disease; however, response is individualized and guides the selection of medications. The types of drugs used include monoamine oxidase (MAO) inhibitors, dopaminergics, dopamine agonists, and anticholinergics. Information about these drugs is presented in Box 19–18.

Initially, clients are treated with selegiline (Carbex, Eldepryl), amantadine (Symmetrel), or anticholinergics. As the disease progresses, levodopa (Dopar, Larodopa) in combination with carbidopa (Lodosyn) is used in the medication carbidopa-levodopa (Sinemet). Because levodopa eventually loses its effectiveness, dopamine agonists are added to increase the effectiveness of levodopa. Eventually, pharmacotherapeutic agents lose their efficacy, and the disease continues to progress despite treatment. Response to the drugs fluctuates, a phenomenon called the "on–off" response.

Bromocriptine (Parlodel) and pergolide (Permax), agents that inhibit the breakdown of dopamine, are used to delay progression of the disease. Catechol-*O*-methyltransferase (COMT) inhibitors (tolcapone [Tasmar] and entacapone [Comtan]) are used in conjunction with carbidopa-levodopa therapy to reduce the metabolism of levodopa, leading to more sustained dopaminergic stimulation of the brain. Selegiline (Deprenyl) increases dopaminergic activity and is used as an adjunctive therapy for clients who have fluctuations in response or become unresponsive to levodopa.

Other medications may be used to treat problems related to PD. Antidepressants may be prescribed. Propranolol (Inderal), which may be administered to treat tremors, should be used cautiously when clients have orthostatic hypotension. Botulism toxin injections may be given to treat eyelid spasms and abnormal posturing (dystonia) involving the extremities.

Deep Brain Stimulation

Activa TM tremor control therapy uses an implanted pacemaker-like device to deliver mild electrical stimulation to block the brain impulses that cause tremor, rigidity, stiffness, slowed movement, and problems with walking. In this procedure, an insulated wire is surgically placed in the thalamus and is connected to an implanted pulse generator (similar to an advanced cardiac pacemaker) near the clavicle. It is used only for clients who cannot adequately control manifestations with medications (National Institute of Neurological Disorders and Stroke, 2005c).

Surgery

Pallidotomy is a surgical technique for PD, and its results have been helpful for many clients. In this procedure, the neurosurgeon locates the affected areas of the globus pallidus and destroys the involved tissue. As a result, clients who could not previously ambulate are able to walk and tremors cease. The long-term effects are still being evaluated.

Stereotaxic thalamotomy (an x-ray taken during neurosurgery to guide the insertion of a needle into a specific area of the brain) has been used only for clients who do not respond to medications—generally, younger people with extreme unilateral tremor. The surgeon destroys a small amount of tissue by creating a lesion in the ventrolateral nucleus of the thalamus. This surgery decreases tremors and rigidity in the contralateral extremity.

Fetal tissue transplantation is a controversial surgical procedure limited to a few medical centers. In this procedure,

Box 19–18 Medication Administration: The Client With Parkinson's Disease

DOPAMINERGICS

- **Levodopa (Larodopa, Dopar)**
- **Carbidopa-levodopa (Sinemet)**
- **Amantadine (Symmetrel)**

These drugs have a major effect on the akinesia of PD, improving mobility while decreasing muscle rigidity and tremor. Levodopa is a metabolic precursor of dopamine, but unlike dopamine, it can cross the blood–brain barrier. Levodopa is converted to dopamine in the brain by decarboxylase, a catalytic enzyme, and stimulates dopamine receptors to balance the dopamine/acetylcholine concentrations. Carbidopa prevents decarboxylase from converting levodopa to dopamine in the peripheral tissues; therefore, carbidopa is frequently given in combination with levodopa. Amantadine, used to treat dyskinesia, also elevates mood.

Levodopa is avoided in clients with narrow-angle glaucoma, severe angina pectoris, transient ischemic attacks, or melanoma. The "on–off" phenomenon occurs after the client takes levodopa for several years; this phenomenon is characterized by unexpected dyskinesias and lack of symptom control.

Common side effects are nausea and vomiting; darkening of urine and sweat; dyskinesias, especially in the first few months of therapy; dysrhythmias; orthostatic hypotension; and psychologic reactions such as hallucinations and vivid dreams. Older adults are particularly susceptible to psychologic disturbances.

Nursing Responsibilities

- Establish the client's baseline functional abilities in performing ADL and administering medication; assess motor control and coordination.
- To avoid adverse reactions, assess the client's overall health status before initiating therapy.
- Monitor medications known to cause adverse drug interactions: Anticholinergics, pyridoxine, and antipsychotic agents alter the effectiveness of levodopa; MAO-B inhibitors can cause severe hypertension because of their vasoconstrictive effects.
- Withhold levodopa for 8 hours prior to administering Sinemet to avoid potentiating the effects of the circulating levodopa.

Health Education for the Client and Family

- Levodopa may not take effect for several weeks to months.
- Clients should not alter dosages of medications; taking more of a medication may not result in better symptom control and can cause severe side effects.
- Protein intake should be divided into equal amounts for the day's meals. Clients should avoid foods high in pyridoxine, such as pork, beef, ham, avocados, beans, and oatmeal.
- Levodopa may cause a darker color of urine; this is harmless, however.
- To prevent side effects:
  - Prevent nausea by taking medication with food.
  - Change position slowly to avoid a drop in blood pressure and risk of falling.
- Prevent constipation by increasing fluid intake and exercising regularly.
- Notify practitioner if you begin to have difficulty making voluntary movements or cardiac or psychologic symptoms develop.
- Watch for the "on–off" phenomenon in which periods of symptom control alternate with periods when the drug fails to control symptoms.

MONOAMINE OXIDASE INHIBITORS

- **Selegiline (Eldepryl, Carbex)**

Selegiline works by selectively inhibiting the enzyme that inactivates dopamine in the brain. It may be administered alone or used as an adjunct therapy with levodopa. Selegiline inhibits the enzyme system that would otherwise break down and destroy dopamine. This synergistic effect lasts approximately 1–2 years. Because the combination of selegiline and levodopa increases the adverse reactions of dopamine, nurses must be alert for orthostatic hypotension, changes in movement, hallucinations, and confusion. These responses can be modified by lowering the dose of levodopa. Because it is highly selective for the MAO-A enzyme, selegiline does not have antidepressant effects like the MAO-B inhibitors. The risk of severe hypertension is low.

Nursing Responsibilities

- Establish baseline functional abilities: motor control and movements, position changes, mental status.
- Monitor problems with insomnia.
- Assess for orthostatic hypotension; look for unsteadiness with position change and complaints of dizziness.
- Assess for hypertension, which can occur with higher-than-usual doses.

Health Education for the Client and Family

- Take the medication only as directed, especially dose and time of administration.
- Notify the practitioner if insomnia occurs.
- Report signs of dizziness when changing positions or standing, changes in ability to move, or psychologic changes.
- Change positions slowly, especially when moving from a sitting to standing position.
- Keep follow-up appointments for evaluation of the medication's effectiveness.

DOPAMINE AGONISTS

- **Bromocriptine (Parlodel)**
- **Pergolide (Permax)**
- **Pramipexole (Mirapex)**
- **Ropinirole (Requip)**

Dopamine agonists act by directly activating dopamine receptors in the brain. They are frequently used in combination with levodopa therapy. When dopamine agonists are given with levodopa, they increase the therapeutic effects of levodopa and reduce fluctuations in motor symptoms. Adverse reactions are similar to those of levodopa: nausea, orthostatic hypotension, and psychologic disturbances. Nursing responsibilities and client and family teaching information are similar to those for the dopaminergics.

COMT INHIBITORS

- **Tolcapone (Tasmar)**
- **Entacapone (Comtan)**

COMT inhibitors inhibit catechol-*O*-methyltransferase (COMT), which is responsible for metabolizing dopamine. The concurrent administration of a COMT inhibitor with levodopa increases the amount of levodopa available to the brain to control PD.

Box 19–18 Medication Administration: The Client With Parkinson's Disease (continued)

Nursing Responsibilities

- Monitor liver function test results and manifestations of liver impairment (dark urine, jaundice).
- Administer with food.
- If given concurrently with warfarin, monitor prothrombin time (PT) and international normalized ratio (INR).

Health Education for the Client and Family

- Avoid using alcohol and sedatives.
- Rise slowly from a sitting or lying position to avoid falling.
- Know that nausea is common at the beginning of therapy.
- Do not abruptly stop taking the medication.
- Report increased loss of muscle control, yellow skin or eyes, dark urine, hallucinations, and severe diarrhea.

ANTICHOLINERGICS

- **Trihexyphenidyl (Artane)**
- **Benztropine (Cogentin)**
- **Biperiden (Akineton)**
- **Cycrimine (Pagitane)**
- **Procyclidine (Kemadrin)**
- **Chlorphenoxamine (Phenoxine)**

Anticholinergics are effective in PD because they block the excitatory action of the neurotransmitter acetylcholine. They are frequently used during the early stages of the disease or when the client can no longer take levodopa. They may be given in combination with carbidopa-levodopa therapy. These medications ease drooling, tremors, and rigidity. However, side effects are common and may include blurred vision, dry mouth, constipation, delayed gastric emptying, urinary retention, photophobia, and tachycardia. Older adults are especially susceptible to heat stroke and psychologic side effects including confusion, depression, delusions, and hallucinations. Anticholinergics should be tapered slowly when discontinued to avoid enhancing parkinsonian symptoms.

Nursing Responsibilities

- Perform baseline assessment for presence of glaucoma, cardiac dysfunction, and prostatic hypertrophy.
- Note other medications, including OTC medications that have anticholinergic effects (e.g., antihistamines and tricyclic antidepressants).
- Monitor for side effects, especially changes in vision, elimination, gastric emptying, and mentation.

brain cells from aborted fetuses are implanted into the client's brain in the hopes that the new cells will grow and produce enough dopamine to restore some lost mobility.

Rehabilitation

Depending on individual needs, clients frequently benefit from rehabilitation therapy with a PT, social worker, psychologist, and/or speech therapist.

Physical therapists (PTs) can implement an individual exercise program to improve coordination, balance, gait, and transfers. Preventing contractures is an important goal of exercise therapy. It is crucial that family and health care personnel permit the client adequate time to perform exercise regimens as well as ADL. Activities should not be rushed.

An OT helps the client adapt to changing abilities pertinent to work, self-care, and recreational activities. Some rehabilitation centers assign OT personnel the responsibility of addressing the client's upper extremity functions while assigning PT personnel to manage lower extremity problems. For example, skills related to cooking and grooming would be supervised by the OT, whereas mobility and posture skills would be supervised by the PT.

Speech therapists frequently address not only the client's speech, but also chewing and swallowing. These therapists evaluate clients and plan treatment regimens. The challenge with clients who have PD is that in addition to vocalization problems, they also have dexterity deficits; Therefore, speech therapists must evaluate the potential benefits of assistive devices such as a magic slate, voice synthesizer, or computer for each client.

NURSING PROCESS

The chronic and eventually debilitating nature of PD poses many challenges to clients, families, and health care professionals. Dependence due to declining physical and mental abilities is of major concern. In the early stages, most clients are able to remain at home, with the family assisting with or providing many of the client's ADL needs. As the disease progresses and the burden of care increases, the client and family may prefer placing the client in a long-term care facility.

Teaching preventive measures is extremely important when caring for clients who have PD. Preventing malnutrition, falls and other environmental accidents, constipation, skin breakdown from incontinence or immobility, and joint contracture requires teaching and reinforcement.

In addition to incorporating information about safety needs, teach ways to prevent orthostatic hypotension when the client changes positions; some clients also may benefit from wearing individually fitted compression hose. In addition, address safety considerations about proper administration of medications.

Assessment

When assessing the older client, be aware of normal changes with aging. Collect the following data through the health history and physical examination:

- *Health history.* Brain trauma, stroke, infection, exposure to heavy metals or carbon monoxide, medication and drug use, incontinence, constipation, weight loss, sweating, sleep problems, muscle pain, mood

- *Physical assessment.* Affect; appearance; speech, scalp, eyelashes, and skin; drooling; tremors; coordination; posture; gait; muscle rigidity; mental status.

Diagnosis

Clients with PD have complex and, ultimately, multisystem needs. Deficits in mobility and self-care are common, and the clients' psychosocial needs are considerable. Potential nursing diagnoses include the following:

- Impaired Physical Mobility
- Impaired Verbal Communication
- Imbalanced Nutrition: Less Than Body Requirements
- Disturbed Sleep Pattern.

Plan

Goals of nursing care may include the following:

- The client will maintain autonomy as long as possible.
- The client will employ strategies to prevent injury from falls or loss of mobility.
- The client will implement strategies to promote communication.
- The client will maintain adequate nutrition and fluid intake.
- The client will get adequate sleep and rest.
- The client will use positive coping skills to reduce anxiety.

Implementation

Nursing interventions require holistic considerations of client's needs. The degenerative process (with gradual loss of function), as well as the disease process itself, increases the likelihood of depression, anxiety, and fear. Nursing care must include meeting the psychosocial as well as the physical needs of the client.

Impaired Physical Mobility

Clients with PD have impaired mobility for several reasons. Mobility impairments include tremors, gait pattern disturbances, and alterations in body positioning (e.g., forward bending of the trunk). Poor self-esteem may contribute to the client's lack of motivation and willingness to be mobile.

- Suggest referral to a PT to develop an individualized exercise program. A program specific to the client provides motivation and helps the client maintain muscle tone, flexibility, and mobility.
- Request that the PT teach caregivers how to do ROM exercises at least twice a day, emphasizing the trunk, neck, arms, hips, and legs. Maintaining joint mobility promotes better function and strength, improving gait pattern. Consistent ROM exercises can prevent contractures.
- Ask caregivers to ambulate the client at least four times a day if possible. Exercise fosters independence and self-esteem.
- Recommend assistive devices such as lift chairs, canes, splints, and braces as indicated. Adaptive equipment improves balance, protects joints, and promotes proper anatomic positioning.
- To promote mobility and safety:
  - Slightly elevate the back legs of chairs and raise the toilet seat to help in rising from a sitting to a standing position.
  - Wear shoes with Velcro closures.
  - Remove potential hazards such as unanchored throw rugs.
  - Install handrails and nonskid surfaces in bath tubs and showers.
  - Ensure adequate lighting throughout the home and in outside areas, especially in areas where transfers are common.

Safety measures prevent potential complications that may result from falls or other accidents and promote self-esteem through self-care.

Impaired Verbal Communication

Diminished vocal amplitude and loss of muscle control can impair the client's ability to speak. Both caregivers and family members must give clients enough time for self-expression; an unhurried approach is recommended. Seek input from family members when determining alternative methods of communicating with the client.

- Assess current communication abilities in speech, hearing, and writing. Communication involves both sending and receiving messages.
- Develop methods of communication appropriate to coordination abilities, such as using a magic slate; using flash cards with common phrases; and pointing to objects. Individualizing a method of communication decreases anxiety and isolation.
- Suggest referral to a speech pathologist to develop oral exercises and interventions that will facilitate speaking. The muscles of speech and swallowing are affected by the PD process.
- Remind client to speak louder if possible. A low, monotonous voice is characteristic of the client with PD.

Imbalanced Nutrition: Less Than Body Requirements

Tremors, altered gait, and impaired chewing and swallowing can cause nutritional problems in the client with PD. As the disorder progresses, interventions for ensuring optimal nutrition need to be adapted to the client's functional abilities. Assess the

CLIENT TEACHING Strategies to Minimize the Effects of Parkinson's Disease

- Inform your practitioner if you begin taking any new medications or notice any new symptoms.
- Avoid overexposure to heat and take precautions to avoid heat stroke: Drink fluids, stay cool, and avoid strenuous activity on hot days.
- Drink adequate amounts of fluid to minimize constipation.
- Practice home safety to prevent falls associated with blurred vision.
- Avoid taking OTC antihistamines or sleeping aids, which have anticholinergic activity.
- Have the eyes examined annually to check for glaucoma; wear dark glasses if photophobia develops.
- Do not suddenly stop taking anticholinergics.

NURSING CARE PLAN A Client With PD

Walter Avneil, aged 78, was diagnosed with PD at age 64. His wife died 5 years ago, and he has no other family living. Mr. Avneil worked for more than 40 years as a mechanic in a large factory. He is a resident of a long-term care facility. During his last clinic visit for a review of his medications, the following assessment was made.

ASSESSMENT	DIAGNOSES	PLAN
White male with history of PD for the past 14 years. Skin oily and damp. Tremors in both hands and the lips. Gait is slow and shuffling, with a forward leaning posture. Speech slow and slurred. Face expressionless. Has lost 10 lb since last visit 3 months ago. Has been on levodopa with carbidopa since diagnosis. States major problems are "eating problems, bowel problems, walking problems."	■ Constipation related to lack of exercise, decreased food intake, and effects of medications ■ Impaired Verbal Communication related to lip tremors, slow/slurred speech, and facial muscle involvement of PD ■ Imbalanced Nutrition: Less Than Body Requirements related to difficulty swallowing and chewing ■ Impaired Physical Mobility related to rigidity and bradykinesia	Goals for client care include the following: ■ Have a soft stool at least every other day. ■ Practice exercises provided by speech therapist twice a day. ■ Increase number of calories, fluids, and fiber in diet provided at long-term facility. ■ Improve joint mobility and ability to ambulate.

IMPLEMENTATION

- Discuss with staff at long-term facility his problems with bowel elimination; suggest increasing fluids to 3000 mL per day and increasing fiber in the diet with oatmeal for breakfast and more fruits and vegetables at meals.
- Encourage exercises provided by speech therapist to improve speech and swallowing. If these are not effective, make a referral for another evaluation.
- Discuss diet plan with dietitian at the long-term care facility, including consistency of foods and number of calories. Suggest that dietitian be a part of swallowing evaluation by the speech therapist.
- Refer for physical therapy and occupational therapy for a program to improve gait and joint mobility and to decrease risk of falling.

EVALUATION

In a return visit 3 months later, Mr. Avneil reports that "my bowels are working better." He has gained 7 lb, and the staff report that this is related to multiple factors, including practicing his swallowing exercises, getting more exercise that stimulated his appetite, and changing his diet to six small meals a day of soft or pureed foods. The staff is offering him liquids at meals and snack times, and he usually drinks all that they give him. His speech is not much improved. His posture and gait are somewhat better, and he is doing the exercises provided by the PT and OT. Mr. Avneil's functional abilities have improved so much that the staff is considering training sessions specific to care of residents with PD.

CRITICAL THINKING

1. Although Mr. Avneil did not mention it, the staff reports that he is frustrated by not being able to dress himself. What suggestions could you make to facilitate his independence?
2. Mr. Avneil spends most of his time alone, although he enjoys the company of the other residents. List assessments and interventions you might provide to increase his diversionary activity.
3. The loss of his wife and the debilitating effects of his disease increase Mr. Avneil's risk for the nursing diagnosis of chronic sorrow. What might you suggest that the long-term staff do to reduce this risk?

client's swallow reflex before starting any feeding program. During the initial stages of the disorder, some clients may have the nursing diagnosis imbalanced nutrition: more than body requirements if kilocalorie intake exceeds energy expenditure.

- Assess nutritional status and self-feeding abilities; suggest referral to an occupational or speech therapist if needed. An initial assessment of abilities ensures that interventions are personalized to the client's current functional abilities.
- Teach caregivers how to prepare foods of proper consistency as determined by swallowing function. The client may aspirate food that is too liquid.
- Weigh weekly. Early recognition of weight loss allows for intervention.

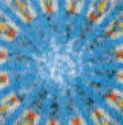

CARE SETTINGS Community Care for the Client With Parkinson's Disease

It is important for both the client and family to maintain independence and self-care as long as possible. To maintain function and quality of life, the following topics should be addressed:

- Realistic expectations
- Equipment suppliers
- Home environment that is conducive to using equipment
- Referrals to speech therapist, OT, PT, and dietitian
- Gait training and exercises for improving ambulation, speech, swallowing, and self-care
- Increased fluid intake of 3000 mL/day and increased fiber in every meal
- Stool softeners or laxatives as needed for bowel elimination
- Ability to swallow during eating and practice of taking prescribed medications (Have suction equipment available and know the Heimlich maneuver in case choking occurs.)
- Foods that can be easily swallowed (pureed or soft) and six small meals a day if possible.

- Teach eating methods to decrease tremors, such as holding a piece of bread in the hand that is not holding an eating utensil. Nonintentional tremor may be reduced through purposeful activity.
- Encourage diet that is high in bulk and fluids. Several anti-Parkinson's medications and inactivity can cause constipation.

Disturbed Sleep Pattern

Rigidity and weakness can cause clients with PD to lose the ability to move and change positions during sleep. The resulting discomfort causes periods of wakefulness. Medications to treat PD contribute to sleep pattern disturbance; for example, levodopa can cause vivid dreams. Nurses can help assess the sleep pattern disturbance and plan interventions to improve or increase sleep time.

- Assess sleep pattern and existing conditions that may affect sleep, such as depression or pain. Clients experiencing anxiety, depression, and dementia have a difficult time falling asleep and may wake up more often during the night.
- Explain the disease process and the effects of decreased dopamine on the sleep–wake cycle. Depending on the dosage, levodopa causes less REM sleep and deep sleep.
- Review the client's medication. Bromocriptine and levodopa, especially when used with an anticholinergic, can cause vivid dreams. Other medications (diuretics, theophylline, and hypnotics) also may interfere with sleep.
- Teach how to modify lifestyle activities that affect sleep, as follows:
  - Institute a routine of activities with limited rest periods during the day; avoid napping close to bedtime. Avoid strenuous exercise in the evening. Daytime sleeping may contribute to decreased nighttime sleeping. Vigorous exercise just before bedtime may act as a stimulant.
  - Incorporate diet modifications such as limiting caffeine and alcohol intake. Caffeine is a stimulant, and alcohol may cause early morning awakenings, increased daytime sleepiness, and nightmares.
  - Drink a glass of milk before bedtime. Milk contains L-tryptophan, which produces sedative effects by shortening the time it takes to fall asleep (sleep latency).
  - Adapt the environment to aid in sleep (e.g., darken the room and decrease noise). Reducing environmental stimuli decreases external sleep disturbances.

Evaluation

Evaluation of client response to nursing care is dependent upon the specific needs and goals of the client. Expected outcomes used to evaluate care may include the following:

- Client is able to communicate effectively.
- Client maintains optimal and realistic levels of autonomy in performing ADL.
- Client avoids injury.
- Client maintains adequate nutritional status.

REVIEW Parkinson's Disease

RELATE: LINK THE CONCEPTS

Linking the exemplar of Parkinson's disease with the concept of Cognition:

1. Relate the impact of Parkinson's disease on cognition.
2. What safety measures will you initiate for the client with Parkinson's disease who has alterations in cognition?

Linking the exemplar of Parkinson's disease with the concept of Elimination:

3. What factors associated with Parkinson's disease put the client at risk for constipation?
4. What nursing interventions might you implement for the client with Parkinson's disease to reduce the risk of urinary retention?

READY: GO TO COMPANION SKILLS MANUAL

- Assessing the musculoskeletal system
- Assessing the neurologic system
- Assessing the home for safe environment
- Assisting client to use a walker
- Performing passive range-of-motion exercises
- Monitoring intake and output

REFER: GO TO MYNURSINGKIT

REFLECT: CASE STUDY

Kody Manuel is a 65-year-old male who was diagnosed with Parkinson's disease 1 year ago. Kody is retired from the railroad where he worked in management. He lives with his daughter

Susan and her husband Val. Susan and Val both work and have one infant daughter. Kody has been able to care for himself at home while Susan and Val work. The baby is taken to a daycare center in the morning by Susan and Val picks her up in the evening. Kody was started on Levadopa one month ago.

Kody has been reading about Parkinson's disease online and is very disturbed by what he learned. He tells Susan and Val that he needs to move out in order to prevent disruption of their home as the disease progresses. While visiting the doctor today he tells the nurse about his plans to move.

1. What data will you need to get from Kody before continuing the discussion about his decision to move out of his daughter's home?
2. What are your concerns for Kody's mental health status today?
3. How do you respond to Kody's report that the Levadopa is not working for him?

19.7 SPINAL CORD INJURY

KEY TERMS

Areflexia, *1146*
Autonomic dysreflexia, *1147*
Autonomic hyperreflexia, *1147*
Axial loading, *1144*
Deformation, *1144*
Hyperextension, *1144*
Hyperflexion, *1144*
Neuron deficits, *1147*
Paraplegia, *1147*
Quadriplegia, *1147*
Spinal cord injury (SCI), *1143*
Spinal shock, *1146*
Tetraplegia, *1147*

BASIS FOR SELECTION OF EXEMPLAR
Most common ER visits

LEARNING OUTCOMES

After reading about this exemplar, you will be able to:

1. Describe the pathophysiology, etiology, clinical manifestations, and direct and indirect causes of spinal cord injury.
2. Identify risk factors associated with spinal cord injury.
3. Illustrate the nursing process in providing culturally competent care across the life span for individuals with spinal cord injury.
4. Formulate priority nursing diagnoses appropriate for an individual with spinal cord injury.
5. Create a plan of care for individuals with spinal cord injury and their family members.
6. Assess expected outcomes for an individual with spinal cord injury.
7. Discuss therapies used in the collaborative care of an individual with spinal cord injury.
8. Employ evidence-based caring interventions for an individual with spinal cord injury.

OVERVIEW

A **spinal cord injury (SCI)** usually results from trauma. Motor vehicle crashes account for 55% of cases, either pedestrian-vehicular, bicycle-vehicular, passenger, or driver-related (Vitale et al., 2006). Other causes of spinal cord injuries, especially in toddlers and young children, include falls, pedestrian injury, and child abuse. Recreation or sports-related trauma accounts for more injuries as children grow older. Penetrating injuries such as stabbing and gunshot wounds are becoming more prevalent.

PATHOPHYSIOLOGY AND ETIOLOGY

The spinal cord provides a two-way pathway for the conduction of impulses and information to and from the brain and the body, serves as a major reflex center, and (through its attached spinal nerves) is involved in the sensory and motor innervation of the entire body below the head. It consists of an outer region of white matter and an inner region of gray matter. The gray matter comprises the central canal of the cord, the posterior horns, the anterior horns, and the lateral horns. It is divided into a sensory half (dorsally) and a motor half (ventrally) and innervates somatic and visceral regions of the body. The white matter consists of tracts, or pathways, that convey information. The ascending (sensory) pathways carry information about proprioception, fine touch, discrimination, pain, temperature, deep pressure, and touch. The descending (motor) pathways carry information about movement. The pyramidal tracts control skilled voluntary movements such as writing. The extrapyramidal tracts (all tracts other than the pyramidal tracts) bring about all other body movements.

When the spinal cord is injured, the primary injury causes microscopic hemorrhages in the gray matter of the cord and edema of the white matter of the cord. These initial pathologic changes are followed by the secondary injury, with mechanisms that increase the area of injury. The hemorrhages extend, eventually involving the entire gray matter. Microcirculation to the cord is impaired by edema and hemorrhage. The injured tissue releases norepinephrine, serotonin, dopamine, and histamine; these vasoactive substances cause vasospasm and further decrease microcirculation. As a result, vascular perfusion and oxygen tension of the affected area are decreased, which leads to ischemia.

When ischemia is prolonged, necrosis of both gray and white matter begins within a few hours, and within 24 hours, the function of nerves passing through the injured area is lost. Although circulation returns to the white matter of the cord in about 24 hours, decreased circulation in the gray matter continues. Because edema extends the level of injury for two cord segments above and below the affected level, the extent of injury cannot be determined for up to 1 week.

Tissue repair occurs over a period of 3–4 weeks. Phagocytes enter the area in 36–48 hours after the initial injury. Neurons degenerate and are removed by microphages in the first 10 days after the injury. RBCs disintegrate, and the hemorrhages are reabsorbed. Eventually, the area of injury is replaced by acellular collagenous tissue, and the meninges thicken.

Forces Resulting in Spinal Cord Injury

Spinal cord injuries result from the application of excessive force to the spinal column. The most common cause of abnormal spinal column movements are acceleration and deceleration (forces that are applied to the body, for example, in automobile crashes and falls). *Acceleration* occurs when external force is applied in a rear-end collision; the upper torso and head are forced backward and then forward. *Deceleration* occurs in a head-on collision; the external force is applied from the front. The head and body move forward until they meet a stationary object and then are forced backward. The following forces and movements (Figure 19–61 ■) may cause a variety of spinal cord injuries, with the extent of injury depending on the amount and direction of motion and the rate of application of force.

- **Hyperflexion**, or forcible forward bending, may compress vertebral bodies and disrupt ligaments and intervertebral disks.
- **Hyperextension**, or forcible backward bending, often disrupts ligaments and causes vertebral fractures. A whiplash injury is a less severe form of hyperextension, with injury to soft tissues but no vertebral or spinal cord damage.
- **Axial loading**, a form of compression, is the application of vertical force to the spinal column (for instance, by falling and landing on the feet or buttocks or by diving into shallow water).
- *Excessive rotation,* in which the head is excessively turned, may tear ligaments, fracture articular surfaces, and cause compression fractures.

The alteration of the spinal cord and soft tissues caused by these abnormal movements is called **deformation**. Bullets and other foreign objects (e.g., sharp objects used as weapons and shrapnel from explosions) may penetrate the spinal cord. Penetrating injuries may cause vertebral fractures, tear ligaments and muscles, or cut through a part or all of the spinal cord. Complete severing of the cord is rare.

SITES OF PATHOLOGY Injuries occur most often in the lumbar and cervical regions. The most frequent sites of injury of the cord are at the first, second, and fourth to sixth cervical vertebrae (C1, C2, and C4 to C6, respectively) and at the eleventh thoracic to second lumbar vertebrae (T11 to L2). Because the cervical spine has a wider range of movement than the rest of the spine, the cervical portion is more likely to be affected by externally applied forces. In addition, the cord fills most of the vertebral canal in the cervical and lumbar regions and thus is more easily injured. Damage to the vertebrae and ligaments causes the spinal column to become unstable, increasing the possibility of compression or stretching of the spinal cord with any further movement.

CLASSIFICATION OF SPINAL CORD INJURY Spinal cord injuries may be classified as complete or incomplete, by cause of injury, and by level of injury. In clinical practice, these classifications often overlap. In a *complete SCI* (about 45% of all

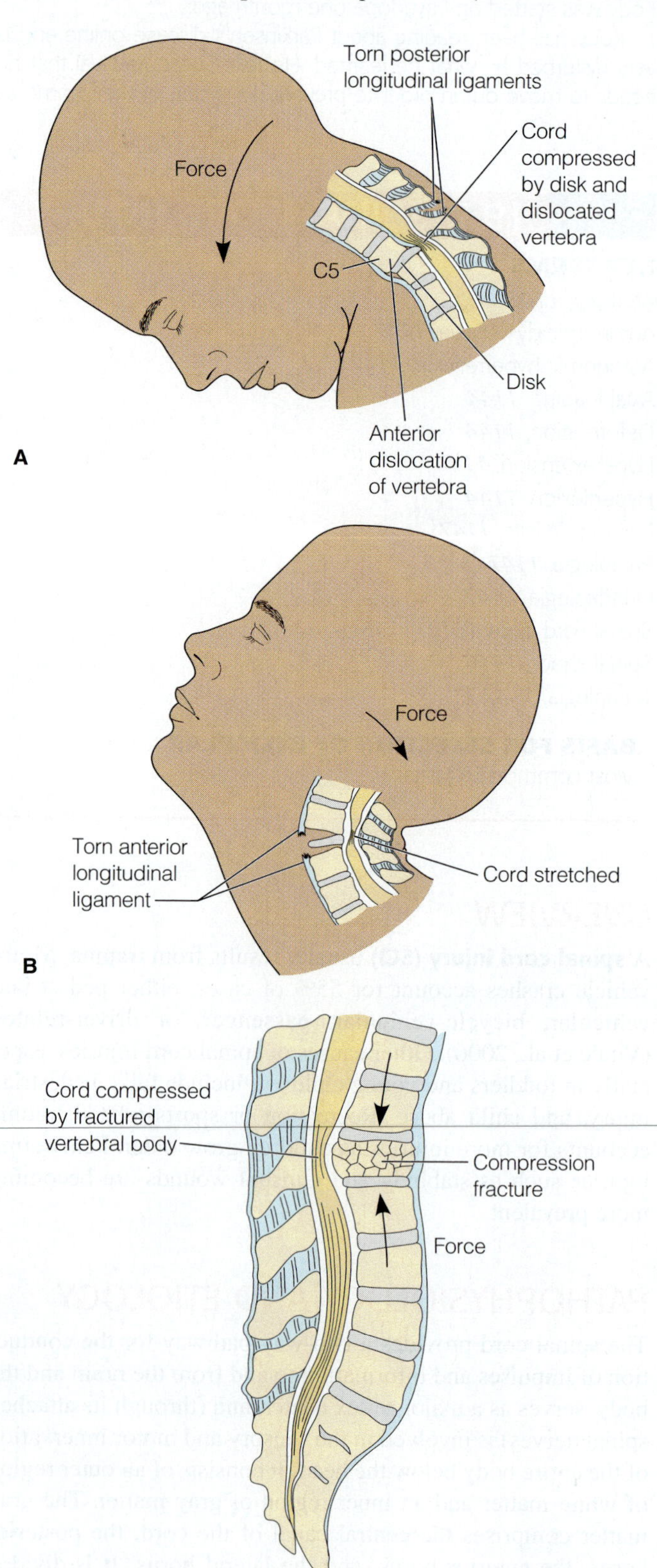

Figure 19–61 ■ Spinal cord injury mechanism. *A*, Hyperflexion. *B*, Hyperextension. *C*, Axial loading, a form of compression.

injuries), the motor and sensory neural pathways are completely interrupted (transected), resulting in total loss of motor and sensory function below the level of the injury. However, "complete" does not necessarily mean that the spinal cord has been severed. In an *incomplete SCI* (about 55% of all injuries), the motor and sensory pathways are only partially interrupted, with variable loss of function below the level of injury. Incomplete spinal cord injuries are further classified into syndromes, as outlined in Table 19–12. Both complete and incomplete injuries can occur in paraplegia and quadriplegia (The National Spinal Cord Injury Association, 2006). The alterations in function that occur as the result of an SCI injury vary greatly depending on the amount of tissue damage and the level of injury.

Etiology

The major causes of SCI are contusion, laceration, transection, hemorrhage, and damage to blood vessels that supply the spinal cord. If vertebrae are fractured and ligaments torn, bony fragments can damage the cord and make the spinal column unstable. Injury to blood vessels supplying the cord can cause permanent damage. The injury is identified by vertebral level. For example, a C6 SCI is at the sixth cervical vertebra.

The mechanism of injury and the direction of forces determine the type of lesion that occurs (Figure 19–62 ■). Hyperflexion injuries (e.g., extreme bending that occurs with whiplash or around a safety belt) produce tears or avulsions and fractures of vertebral bodies as well as subluxation and dislocation. Rotation may cause joint dislocations or unstable spinal fractures. Hyperextension may result in a hangman's fracture, ligament tears, avulsion fractures of vertebral bodies, and central or posterior spinal cord syndrome (damage to the center of the cord only). Compression fractures may result from falling from a height.

Risk Factors

The three major risk factors for SCIs are age, gender, and alcohol or drug abuse. Young men are more prone to risk-taking behaviors than are women. Older adults are more likely to have a cord injury from even minor trauma as a result of age-related vertebral degeneration. Motor vehicle crashes that occur while the driver is under the influence of alcohol or drugs are a major source of trauma to people of all ages.

TABLE 19–12 **Incomplete Spinal Cord Injury Syndromes**

TYPE	CAUSE	LOCATION	DEFICITS
Central syndrome	Cord transection	Cervical	Spastic paralysis of the upper extremities
	Hyperextension		Variable paralysis of the lower extremities
			Variable effects on the bowel, the bladder, and sexual function
Anterior syndrome	Damage to the anterior spinal artery	Anterior two thirds of the cord	Paralysis below the level of injury
	Infarction of the anterior spinal artery		Loss of temperature and pain sensation below the level of injury
	Hyperflexion		
Posterior syndrome	Vertebral dislocation	Nerve roots	Weakness in isolated muscle groups
	Herniated disk		Tingling, pain
	Compression		Decreased or absent reflexes in the involved area
			Bowel or bladder dysfunction
Brown-Séquard's syndrome	Penetrating trauma	Hemisection of the anterior and posterior cord	Paralysis below the level of injury on the ipsilateral (same) side of the body
			Contralateral loss of temperature and pain sensation below the level of injury
			Ipsilateral loss of proprioception below the level of injury
Homer's syndrome	Incomplete cord transection	Cervical sympathetic nerves	Ipsilateral ptosis of the eyelid, constricted pupil, and facial anhidrosis (inability to perspire)

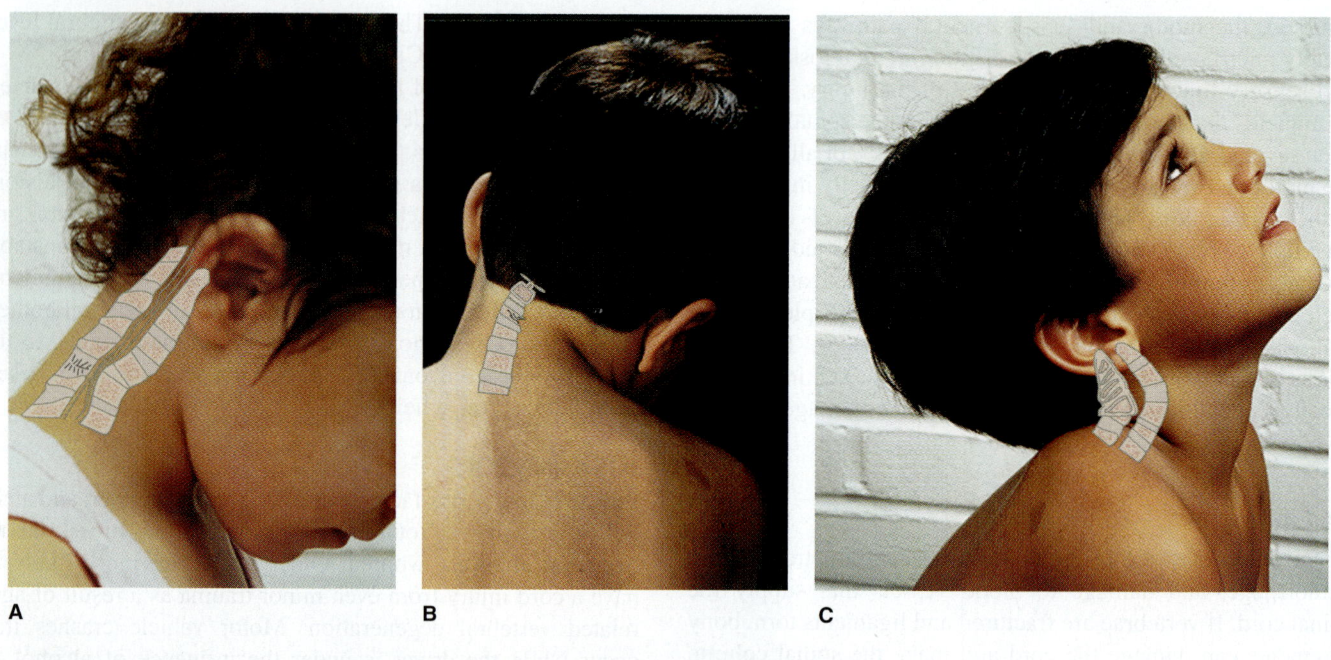

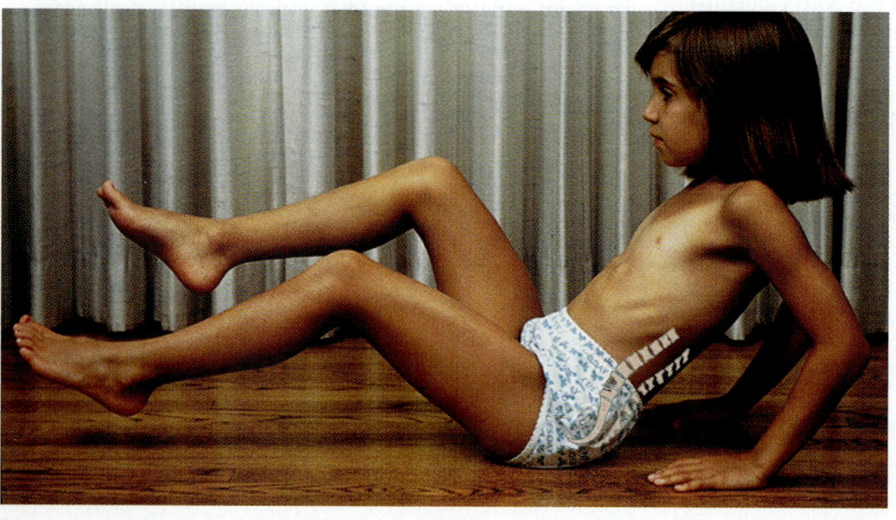

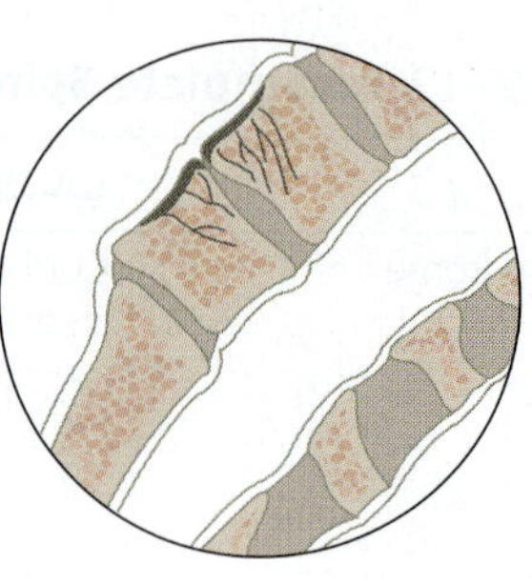

Figure 19–62 ■ Mechanics of injury to the spinal cord: *A*, Hyperflexion often due to diving and frontal motor vehicle crashes. *B*, Rotation in which the head and neck are twisted. *C*, Hyperextension often due to rear-end motor vehicle crashes and falls. *D*, Compression due to falls that put vertical pressure on the spinal column. Infants and young children are at higher risk for injury to the brain and spinal cord because of developing bones and muscles.

CLINICAL MANIFESTATIONS

Spinal cord injuries are classified as complete or incomplete. Complete lesions are irreversible and involve a loss of sensory, motor, and autonomic function below the level of the injury. Incomplete lesions involve varying degrees of sensory, motor, and autonomic function below the level of injury. Hypotension, loss of bladder and bowel control, and loss of environmental thermoregulatory function are associated with autonomic dysfunction. The higher the level of SCI, the more severe the neurologic damage.

Injuries of the spinal cord have the potential to affect movement, perception, sensation, sexual function, and elimination.

Spinal shock is the temporary loss of reflex function (called **areflexia**) below the level of injury. This response begins immediately after complete transection of the spinal cord, when connections between the brain and the spinal cord are interrupted and the cord does not function at all. The response also occurs (although in varying degrees) after partial transection as well as after spinal cord contusions, compression, and ischemia.

Normal activity of the spinal cord is dependent on constant impulses from the higher centers of the brain. When damage from an injury stops these impulses, spinal shock follows. There is loss of motor function, tendon reflexes, and autonomic function. Spinal shock may begin within 1 hour of the injury. The condition may last from a few minutes to several months (although it usually lasts from 1–6 weeks); then reflex activity returns. Spinal shock ends slowly, with the gradual reappearance of reflexes, hyperreflexia (increased reflex responses), muscle spasticity, and reflex bladder emptying.

The manifestations of acute spinal shock (which vary in degree) include the following:

- Flaccid paralysis of skeletal muscles below the level of injury
- Loss of all spinal reflexes below the level of injury
- Loss of sensations of pain, touch, temperature, and pressure below the level of injury
- Absence of visceral and somatic sensations below the level of injury
- Bowel and bladder dysfunction
- Loss of the ability to perspire below the level of injury.

A person with a cervical or upper thoracic SCI also may have neurogenic shock, which results in cardiovascular changes. These changes are due to the inability of higher centers in the brainstem to modulate reflexes. As a result, vascular beds below the level of injury dilate and the cardiac accelerator reflex is suppressed. The client experiences hypotension and bradycardia. Other manifestations may include respiratory insufficiency due to loss of innervation of the diaphragm in C1 to C4 injuries, hypothermia, paralytic ileus, urinary retention, and oliguria.

Both bradycardia and hypotension may persist even after the spinal shock resolves. In addition to losing sympathetic control of the heart rate, the client with a high-level SCI experiences decreased peripheral resistance and loss of muscle activity. These changes result in sluggish blood flow and decreased venous return, increasing the risk for thrombophlebitis.

Complications

The complications of an SCI involve many different body systems and often result in permanent disability and loss of functional health status. The complications include but are not limited to upper and lower motor neuron deficits, paraplegia and quadriplegia, and autonomic dysreflexia. Depending on the level and severity of the injury, other complications may include ineffective respirations; altered skin integrity; increased risk of thrombosis; and alterations in bowel elimination, urinary elimination, and sexual pattern.

***UPPER AND LOWER MOTOR* Neuron Deficits** Injuries to the spinal cord are often classified as *upper motor neuron lesions or lower motor neuron lesions*. Motor neurons are functional units that carry motor impulses. The upper motor neurons (located in the cerebral cortex, thalamus, brainstem, and corticospinal and corticobulbar tracts) are responsible for voluntary movement. When these motor pathways are interrupted, the client experiences spastic paralysis and hyperreflexia and may be unable to carry out skilled movement.

Lower motor neurons (located in the anterior horn of the spinal cord, the motor nuclei of the brainstem, and the axons that reach the motor end plate of skeletal muscles) are responsible for innervation and contraction of skeletal muscles. Interruption of lower motor neurons results in muscle flaccidity and extensive muscle atrophy, with loss of both voluntary and involuntary movement. If only some of the motor neurons supplying a muscle are affected, the client experiences partial paralysis (paresis); if all motor neurons to a muscle are affected, the client experiences complete paralysis. Hyporeflexia is also present.

PARAPLEGIA AND QUADRIPLEGIA Two common neurologic deficits resulting from an SCI are paraplegia and quadriplegia (Figure 19–63 ■). **Paraplegia** is paralysis of the lower portion of the body, sometimes involving the lower trunk. Paraplegia occurs when the thoracic, lumbar, and sacral portions of the spinal cord are injured, causing loss or impairment of sensory and/or motor function. **Quadriplegia**, also called **tetraplegia**, occurs when cervical segments of the cord are injured, impairing function of the arms, trunk, legs, and pelvic organs.

AUTONOMIC DYSREFLEXIA **Autonomic dysreflexia** (also called **autonomic hyperreflexia**) is an exaggerated sympathetic response that occurs in clients with SCIs at or above the T6 level. This response, which is seen only after recovery from spinal shock, occurs as a result of lack of control of the autonomic nervous system by higher centers. When stimuli are unable to ascend the cord, mass reflex stimulation of the sympathetic nerves below the level of the injured cord area occurs, triggering massive vasoconstriction. In response, the vagus nerve causes bradycardia and vasodilation above the level of injury. If untreated, autonomic dysreflexia can cause seizures, a stroke, or a myocardial infarction and is potentially fatal (Hickey, 2003).

Autonomic dysreflexia is triggered by stimuli that would normally cause abdominal discomfort (a full bladder is the most common cause), by stimulation of pain receptors, and by visceral contractions (Porth, 2005). Causes include fecal impaction, bladder infections or stones, intrauterine contractions, ejaculation, peritonitis, and stimulation from pressure ulcers or ingrown toenails. The most common precipitating event is a blocked urinary catheter.

The manifestations of this condition include pounding headache; bradycardia; hypertension (with readings as high as

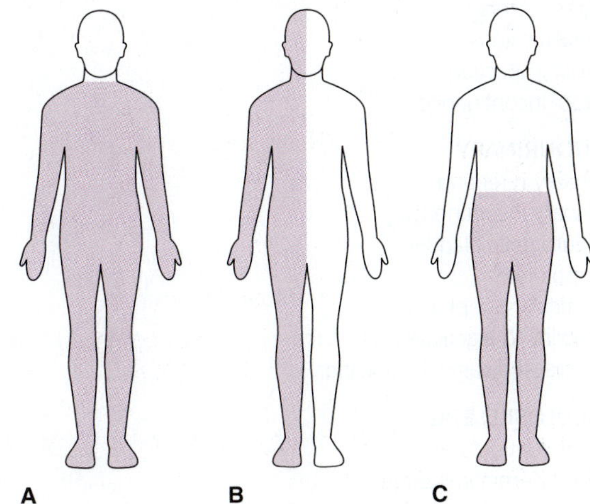

Figure 19–63 ■ Types of paralysis. *A*, Complete quadriplegia or partial paralysis of the upper extremities and complete paralysis of the lower part of the body. *B*, Hemiplegia is paralysis of one half of the body when it is divided along the median sagittal plane. *C*, Paraplegia is paralysis of the lower part of the body.

300/160); flushed, warm skin with profuse sweating above the lesion and pale, cold, and dry skin below it; and anxiety (Porth, 2005). Dysreflexia is a neurologic emergency and requires immediate treatment.

The manifestations and complications of SCI are summarized by body system in Box 19–19.

COLLABORATION

The client with an acute SCI requires emergency assessment and care along with prompt administration of medications; sometimes the client also requires immobilization and surgery. The client is assessed and stabilized at the scene of the accident, initially treated in the ER, and then admitted to the hospital intensive care unit. The nurse's role as a member of the collaborative healthcare team is discussed in the nursing process section.

Box 19–19 Manifestations and Complications of Spinal Cord Injury by Body System

INTEGUMENT
- Decubitus (pressure) ulcers

NEUROLOGIC
- Pain
- Areflexia
- Hypotonia
- Autonomic dysreflexia

CARDIOVASCULAR
- Spinal shock
- Paroxysmal hypertension
- Orthostatic hypotension
- Cardiac dysrhythmias
- Decreased venous return
- Hypercalcemia

RESPIRATORY
- Limited chest expansion
- Decreased cough reflex
- Decreased vital capacity

GASTROINTESTINAL
- Stress ulcers
- Paralytic ileus
- Stool impaction
- Stool incontinence

GENITOURINARY
- Urinary retention
- Urinary incontinence
- Neurogenic bladder
- Impotence
- Testicular atrophy
- Inability to ejaculate
- Decreased vaginal lubrication

MUSCULOSKELETAL
- Joint contractures
- Bone demineralization
- Osteoporosis
- Muscle spasms
- Muscle atrophy
- Pathologic fractures
- Paraplegia
- Quadriplegia

Emergency Care

The danger of death from SCI is greatest when there is damage to or transection of the upper cervical region. When the injury is at the C1 to C4 level, respiratory paralysis is common and the client who survives requires ventilator assistance to breathe. Injuries below C4 may increase the risk of respiratory failure if edema ascends the cord. It is of critical importance not to complicate the initial injury by allowing the fractured vertebrae to damage the cord further during transport to the hospital. Although at one time injuries to the high cervical cord were almost always fatal, advances in trauma care have greatly improved the survival rate.

All people who have sustained trauma to the head or spine or who are unconscious should be treated as though they have an SCI. Prehospital management includes rapidly assessing the ABCs (airway, breathing, circulation), immobilizing and stabilizing the head and neck, removing the person from the site of injury, stabilizing other life-threatening injuries, and rapidly transporting the person to the appropriate facility. Guidelines for emergency care are as follows:

- Avoid flexing, extending, or rotating the neck.
- Immobilize the neck using rolled towels or blankets or apply a cervical collar before moving the client onto a backboard.
- Secure the head by placing a belt or tape across the forehead and securing it to the stretcher.
- Maintain the client in the supine position.
- Transfer directly from the stretcher with backboard still in place to the type of bed that will be used in the hospital.

Assessment findings at the scene of the accident or in the ER vary according to the level of injury. The assessment findings common to the level of injury and spinal shock are outlined in Box 19–20. The client in the ED with a suspected or identified SCI also is treated for respiratory problems, paralytic ileus, atonic bladder, and cardiovascular alterations. Respiratory distress in the client with a cervical-level injury is treated by placing the client on a ventilator. Oxygen is administered to the client with a thoracic-level injury. Paralytic ileus (obstruction of the intestines due to lack of peristalsis) is common in clients with an SCI and is treated by the insertion of a nasogastric tube with connection to suction. To prevent overdistention of an atonic bladder, an indwelling catheter is inserted and connected to dependent drainage. Cardiovascular status is assessed on a continuous basis by inserting an invasive monitoring device such as a Swan-Ganz catheter and attaching the client to a cardiac monitor; or it is assessed by arterial monitoring to identify hypotension and to draw ABGs.

Diagnostic Tests

Diagnosis is made by observation, neurologic examination, and radiographic studies. Tests are ordered to identify the level and extent of injury and to detect any complications. Radiographic studies include lateral cervical spine and anteroposterior and

Box 19–20 Assessment Findings in Acute Spinal Cord Injury

CERVICAL INJURY
- Paralysis or weakness of extremities
- Respiratory distress manifested by changes in ABG studies, cyanosis, flaring of the nostrils, use of accessory muscles of respiration, and restlessness
- Pulse rate below 60 and systolic BP below 80
- Decreased peristalsis

THORACIC AND LUMBAR INJURY
- Paralysis or weakness of extremities

SPINAL SHOCK
- Loss of skin sensation
- Flaccid paralysis, areflexia
- Absent bowel sounds
- Bladder distention
- Decreasing blood pressure
- Absence of the cremasteric reflex in males (retraction of the left or right testicle in response to stimulation of the skin of the inner left or right thigh, respectively)

lateral views of the thoracic and lumbosacral spine to determine if a vertebral fracture or compression on the spinal cord is present. The client's immobilized position is unchanged until radiographs are read by a radiologist and the spine is declared uninjured. In addition, CT scanning, MRI, fluoroscopy, or myelography may be performed. Somatosensory evoked potential studies (SSEP) locate the level of SCI by stimulating peripheral nerves and measuring response times. Arterial blood gases are measured to establish a baseline or to identify problems due to respiratory insufficiency.

Pharmacologic Therapies

The pharmacologic treatment of the client with SCI is symptomatic. It is directed primarily toward decreasing edema from the injury, treating hypotension and bradycardia, and treating spasticity. High-dose steroid protocol using methylprednisolone (Medrol) must be implemented within 8 hours of the injury to improve neurologic recovery. Clinical research indicates that the use of this adrenocorticosteroid is effective in preventing secondary spinal cord damage from edema and ischemia. Treatment with G_{M1} ganglioside for 3–4 weeks is an experimental approach that has been effective for some clients (Tierney, McPhee, & Papadakis, 2005).

- Vasopressors are used in the immediate acute care phase to treat bradycardia or hypotension due to spinal and neurogenic shock. Examples of drugs are dopamine (Intropin) to treat hypotension in neurogenic shock and dobutamine (Dobutrex) to support cardiac function. Atropine should be available at the bedside to treat bradycardia.
- Antispasmodics are used to treat spasticity in clients with SCI. Both baclofen (Lioresal) and diazepam (Valium) may be used. A discussion of nursing implications of treatment with antispasmodics is found in Medication Administration (Box 19–21).
- Analgesics such as NSAIDs and narcotics are administered to reduce pain.
- Proton pump inhibitors such as omeprazole (Prilosec), rabeprazole (Aciphex), and pantoprazole (Protonix) are often administered to prevent stress-related gastric ulcers, a common complication in SCI.
- Unless contraindicated, anticoagulants (heparin or warfarin) may be given to prevent thrombophlebitis.
- Stool softeners may be administered as part of a bowel training program.

Treatment

Spinal injuries are managed aggressively as the spinal injury extends upward 1–2 levels during the immediate hours and days after the injury (Hayes & Arriola, 2005). The treatments used in the management of an SCI include surgery, stabilization, and immobilization.

Box 19–21 Medication Administration: Antispasmodics in Spinal Cord Injury

- **Baclofen (Lioresal)**
- **Chlorzoxazone (Paraflex)**
- **Cyclobenzaprine hydrochloride (Flexeril)**
- **Diazepam (Valium)**
- **Orphenadrine citrate (Norflex)**

These drugs depress the CNS and inhibit the transmission of impulses from the spinal cord to skeletal muscle. They are used to control muscle spasm and pain associated with acute or chronic musculoskeletal conditions. They are not always effective in controlling spasticity resulting from cerebral or spinal cord conditions.

NURSING RESPONSIBILITIES
- Assess the client's spasticity and involuntary movements to obtain baseline data for comparison of results of therapy.
- Do not expect therapy to have effects for 1 week.
- Administer oral medications with food to decrease GI symptoms.

HEALTH EDUCATION FOR THE CLIENT AND FAMILY
- Know that these drugs may cause drowsiness, diplopia, and impotence.
- Take your medications with meals to decrease gastric irritation.
- Understand that physical improvement may take several weeks.
- Report slurred speech, drooling, or inability to carry out usual functions to the physician.
- Do not stop taking the medication without consulting your health care provider.

SURGERY Early surgical treatment may be necessary if there is evidence of compression of the spinal cord by bone fragments or a hematoma. Surgery also may be done to stabilize and support the spine. However, many clients are treated with stabilization devices and do not require surgery. Possible surgeries include a decompression laminectomy, a spinal fusion, and insertion of metal rods.

STABILIZATION AND IMMOBILIZATION As a result of one or more dislocations or fractures of the cervical vertebrae, the client with an SCI may be immobilized in some type of traction or external fixation device to stabilize the vertebral column and prevent any further damage (Figure 19–64 ■). For clients who are not yet in a condition to have surgery or who have severe bleeding and edema of the injured cord, traction may be used to stabilize the spinal column. The physician applies the traction or fixation device; the nurse is responsible for assessments and interventions following the application.

Although used less frequently today, various devices provide cervical traction. For example, Gardner-Wells tongs may be used (Figure 19–65 ■). In this type of traction, the physician applies pins to the skull approximately 1 cm above each ear and weights are attached to the device.

The halo external fixation device is often used to provide stabilization when there is no significant involvement of the ligaments (Figure 19–66 ■). It is used most often to provide stability for fractures of the cervical and high thoracic vertebrae without cord damage. This device allows greater mobility, self-care, and participation in rehabilitation programs. The device is secured with four pins inserted into the skull, two in the frontal bone and two in the occipital bone. The halo ring is then attached to a rigid plastic vest lined with sheepskin.

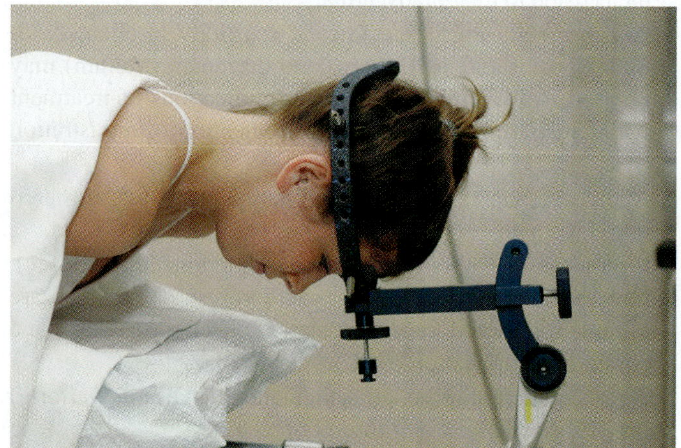

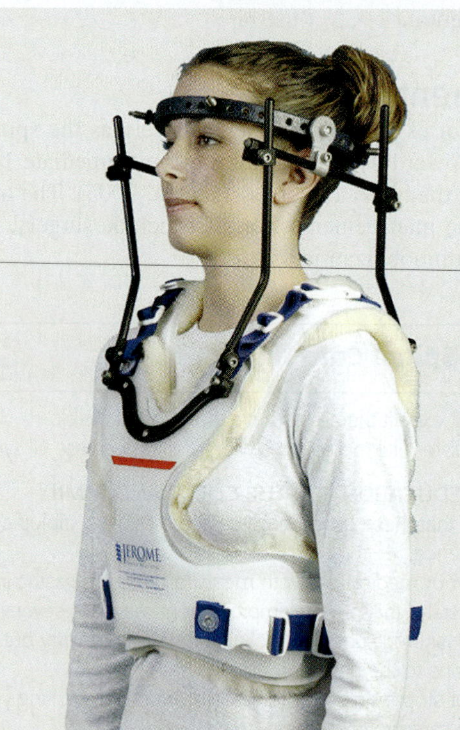

Figure 19–64 ■ Examples of traction or external fixation devices.

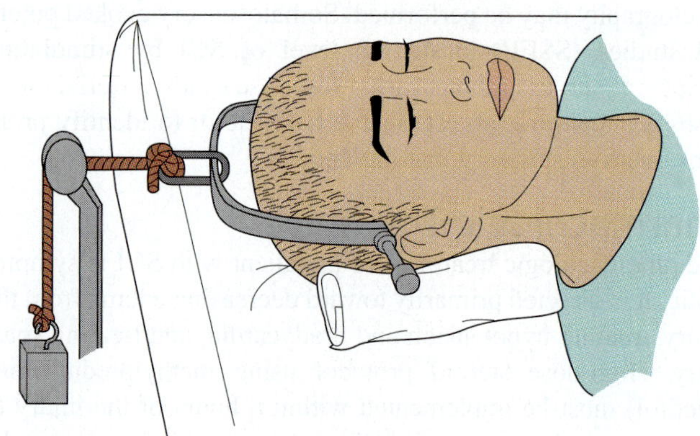

Figure 19–65 ■ Cervical traction may be applied by several methods, including Gardner-Wells tongs.

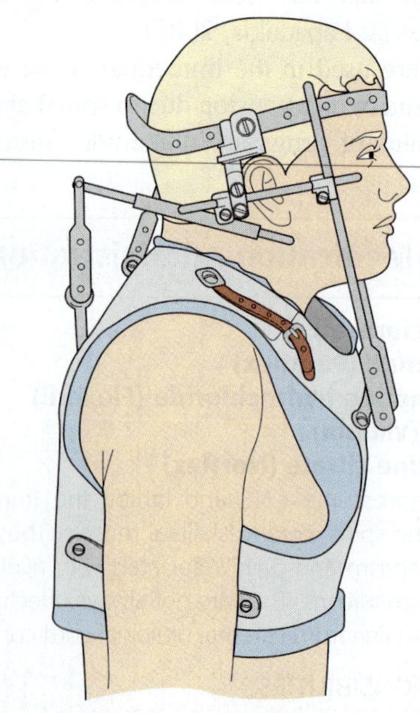

Figure 19–66 ■ The halo external fixation device.

NURSING PROCESS

During both the acute and rehabilitative phase, the client with a spinal cord injury has complex needs that involve all members of the health care team. Because these injuries are more common in younger clients, the impact of lifelong effects on both the client and the family must be considered. The nurse coordinates client care and develops and implements a care plan that is individualized to each client and family. The focus of the plan is to prevent the secondary complications of immobility and altered body functions, to promote self-care, and to educate the client and family.

Health promotion for SCI primarily involves preventing injuries. Nurses can provide valuable information in the community and the workplace to prevent SCI. Programs that focus on wearing seat belts and using approved infant seats and child booster seats in automobiles can do a great deal to help decrease the number of SCIs each year. Educational programs that promote workplace and farm safety should include information on preventing falls and using heavy equipment safely.

Assessment

The following data are collected through the health history and physical examination:

- *Health history*. Time, location, and type of event-causing injury; location, duration, quality, and intensity of pain; dyspnea; sensation; paresthesia
- *Physical examination*. Vital signs, motor strength, movement, spinal reflexes, bowel sounds, bladder distention.

Diagnosis

Because the possible effects of an SCI are varied, many nursing diagnoses are appropriate. Common nursing diagnoses often include the following:

- Impaired Physical Mobility
- Impaired Gas Exchange
- Ineffective Breathing Patterns
- Altered Perfusion: Tissue
- Impaired Urinary Elimination and Constipation
- Sexual Dysfunction
- Low Self-Esteem
- Fear
- Anxiety
- Caregiver Role Strain.

Plan

Goals of nursing care include the following:

- The client will remain free of complications such as pressure ulcers and contractions.
- The client will maintain adequate nutrition.
- The client will regain bowel and bladder control.
- The client will achieve maximum self-care.
- The client and family will adapt to the disability.

Implementation

Nursing care is determined based on specific needs of the client, level of injury, and sensory or motor loss. Each client will have unique requirements. It is essential that the nurse care for the client's psychosocial, spiritual, and emotional needs as well as physical needs.

Impaired Physical Mobility

After the initial period of spinal shock and areflexia, the client regains spinal reflex activity and muscle tone that is not under the control of higher centers. Clients with injuries above the level of T12 experience involuntary spastic movements of skeletal muscles. These movements reach a peak about 2 years after the injury and then gradually subside (Porth, 2005). Spasms impair the ability to carry out the activities of daily life and work. In addition, the paraplegia or quadriplegia increases the potential for impaired skin integrity, thrombophlebitis, and contractures.

The goals of care for clients with impaired mobility related to an SCI are to reduce the effects of spasticity and to prevent complications involving the skin, the cardiovascular system, and joint function.

- Perform passive range of motion (ROM) exercises for all extremities at least twice a day. Identify stimuli that cause spastic movements and avoid the stimuli (e.g., certain exercises) or teach the client to expect the movements. ROM exercises help prevent contractures and stretch spastic muscles, promoting rehabilitation.
- Maintain skin integrity by turning every 2 hours, assessing pressure points at least once each shift, and using a special bed if necessary. The client may be placed on a regular or special bed (e.g., a kinetic bed). Immobility compresses soft tissues and promotes the development of decubitus ulcers. The lack of sensory warning mechanisms and of voluntary motor control of skin dermatomes further increases the risk for altered skin integrity. Special beds allow movement or turning while keeping the spinal column aligned.
- Assess the lower extremities each shift for manifestations of thrombophlebitis. Observe for redness and for increased heat every shift; measure thigh and calf circumference daily. If antiembolic stockings (TEDs) are ordered, remove for 30–60 minutes each shift. Assess for skin impairment and provide skin care while TEDs are removed. Clients with neurologic deficits are at high risk for deep venous thrombosis (DVT) as a result of immobility, vasomotor dysfunction, and decreased venous return with venous stasis. Antiembolic stockings help to prevent the pooling of blood in the lower extremities and increase venous return, lessening the risk for venous stasis and thrombus formation.

Impaired Gas Exchange

Injuries at the level of T1 to T7 leave the phrenic nerve intact, but the innervation of intercostal muscles is affected, compromising respiratory function. In addition, because the abdominal muscles are paralyzed, the client cannot expel secretions by coughing. Clients with cord injuries at C3 or above have paralysis of the respiratory muscles and cannot breathe without a ventilator.

- Monitor vital capacity and respiratory effectiveness, assessing for tachycardia, restlessness, PaO_2 less than 60 mmHg, $PaCO_2$ greater than 50 mmHg, and vital capacity less than 1 L. Clients with cervical cord injuries frequently require ventilatory support because of reduced vital capacity and inability to expel secretions by coughing.
- Monitor for signs of ascending edema of the spinal cord, including difficulty swallowing or coughing, respiratory stridor, use of accessory muscles of respiration, bradycardia, and increased motor and sensory loss. Hemorrhage and edema can further impair respiratory function.
- Help the client cough as follows: Place the hand between the umbilicus and xiphoid process and push in and up as the client exhales and coughs. The client who is unable to cough effectively and has decreased ventilatory capacity may develop atelectasis, pneumonia, and respiratory failure.

Ineffective Breathing Patterns

Respiratory function is impaired in the client with SCI in the cervical and thoracic levels if the diaphragm (innervated at C3 to C5), the intercostal muscles (innervated at T1 to T7), and the abdominal muscles are affected. In clients with injury at higher levels, assisted ventilation and a tracheostomy are necessary; when the injury is at lower levels, the client's ability to take a deep breath and cough is diminished. The goal of nursing interventions is to maintain normal respiratory rate (12–20 breaths per minute) and to prevent pulmonary complications such as atelectasis and pneumonia.

- Assess respiratory rate, rhythm, and depth every 4 hours (or more frequently if needed). Auscultate breath sounds as a part of respiratory assessment. Injury to the cord in the cervical or thoracic regions can decrease respiratory function and increase the risk for respiratory problems.
- Monitor results of oxygen saturation with pulse oximetry and ABG studies. ABG studies provide information about gas exchange; decreasing pH, oxygen, and oxygen saturation levels, and increasing carbon dioxide levels signal respiratory acidosis.
- Administer supplemental oxygen as prescribed. Oxygen saturation must be maintained at 100% with supplemental oxygen to prevent hypoxemia and secondary SCI in all acute SCI clients.
- Help the client turn, cough, and deep breathe at least every 2 hours. Use assisted coughing as necessary. Paralysis of intercostal or abdominal muscles decreases the ability to expel secretions by coughing; retained secretions increase the risk for pneumonia. The inability to breathe deeply may result in atelectasis.
- Increase fluids given by mouth to 3000 mL per day (if oral intake is approved) according to client preference for type of liquids and predicated on the client's ability to swallow. Increased fluid intake thins secretions, which can more easily be expelled and expectorated.

Alteration in Perfusion

Autonomic dysreflexia is an emergency that requires immediate assessment and intervention to prevent complications of extremely high blood pressure with reduced perfusion of the tissues including the brain causing symptoms of loss of consciousness, seizure, and even death.

- Elevate the head of the client's bed and remove TEDs or sequential compression boots. These measures increase pooling of blood in the lower extremities and decrease venous return, thus decreasing blood pressure.
- Assess blood pressure every 2–3 minutes while at the same time assessing for stimuli that initiated the response (such as a full bladder, impacted stool, or skin pressure). The most serious danger in dysreflexia is elevated blood pressure, which could precipitate a stroke, myocardial infarction, dysrhythmias, or seizures. If the client has a Foley catheter, ensure that there are no kinks in the tubing. If the client does not have a Foley catheter, drain the bladder with a straight catheter. If manifestations persist, assess for a fecal impaction. If an impaction is present, insert Nupercaine cream into the anus, wait 10 minutes, and manually remove the impaction.
- If blood pressure remains dangerously elevated, the physician may prescribe intravenous administration of diazoxide (Hyperstat). Other medications that may be used include nifedipine (Procardia) and hydralazine (Apresoline). Diazoxide is an antihypertensive drug used in emergency situations to lower blood pressure in adults with dangerously high readings. Nifedipine and hydralazine are peripheral vasodilators that are administered to decrease elevated blood pressure.

Impaired Urinary Elimination and Constipation

Depending on the level of the injury, the client with an SCI may have alterations in bowel and bladder function. Clients with injuries to the cord at or above the S2 to S4 levels will have a neurogenic bladder, with deficits in control of micturition. Voluntary and involuntary bowel control is affected in the client with a lower motor neuron injury. Both bowel and bladder retraining are possible; if not, some form of assisted elimination is necessary. Although an indwelling catheter may be used in the acute phase of care, the goal is to reestablish a catheter-free state.

- Monitor for manifestations of a full bladder. Overdistention stretches the bladder and can lead to backflow of urine into the ureters and kidney; stasis of urine in an incompletely emptied bladder increases the risk for infection.
- Teach client to use trigger voiding techniques prior to straight catheterization. These techniques include stroking the inner thigh, pulling the pubic hair, tapping on the abdomen over the bladder, and (in females) pouring warm water over the vulva. These trigger voiding techniques stimulate parasympathetic nerve fibers to cause reflex activity and may facilitate voiding.
- Teach self-catheterization to clients who will be able to carry out the procedure alone or with minimal assistance. Straight catheterization at regular intervals is part of bladder training because periodic distention and relaxation of

the muscles of the bladder promote reflex bladder activity. In addition, self-care fosters independence.

- Monitor residual urine throughout the bladder retraining program. A residual urine amount of less than 80 mL after a triggered voiding is considered satisfactory.
- Institute a bowel retraining program as follows:
  - Assess usual patterns of bowel elimination to establish best times for an individualized program.
  - Maintain a high-fluid, high-fiber diet.
  - Use stool softeners as prescribed; rectal suppositories and enemas may be used 30 minutes after meals to stimulate stronger peristalsis and facilitate evacuation.
  - Maintain upright position if at all possible and ensure privacy.
  - If client is unable to evacuate, digital stimulation or manual removal on a regular basis may be the most effective long-term management.

A bowel retraining program to regulate the bowel through reflex activity may be instituted in clients with upper motor neuron injuries. The client with a lower motor neuron injury loses the defecation reflex, and bowel retraining is more difficult (if not impossible).

Sexual Dysfunction

Sexual intercourse is often possible for the client with an SCI. In men, the general rule is that the higher the level of injury the greater the potential to have reflexogenic erections, although ejaculation or orgasm may not occur. Fertility is usually lower as a result of a lack of temperature control of the testes. However, ejaculation may be stimulated and the sperm used to inseminate the client's partner so that fatherhood is a possibility. Men who have sacral-level injuries do not have reflexogenic erections but may have psychogenic erections. They also are more likely to remain fertile.

Women with an SCI generally do not have sensation during sexual intercourse, but pregnancy is possible. However, pregnant women with an SCI are at increased risk for autonomic dysreflexia during labor and delivery. Birth control options should be discussed prior to discharge from the acute care setting.

A client with an SCI may be deeply concerned about alterations in sexual function. These concerns may lead to lowered self-esteem, altered self-image, or changes in feelings about being an attractive and desirable person. Assess concerns and provide a climate that is receptive to discussion about sexuality. Examples of objectives for sexual counseling for the client with an SCI are that the client will understand how the injury has altered sexual functioning, be aware of alternative ways of achieving sexual pleasure, and have a positive self-concept and body image.

- Include data about sexuality when obtaining the nursing history and database. Sexuality is a private matter for most people, and the client may not discuss it unless the nurse introduces the topic.
- Provide accurate information about the effect of the SCI on sexual function. Accurate information gives the client a realistic picture of how the injury will affect sexuality.
- Initiate a discussion with the client and partner of alternative means of gaining sexual satisfaction; these include the use of vibrators and oral–genital and manual stimulation. Alternatives to intercourse can meet sexual needs and help maintain the relationship with a significant other.
- Refer for sexual counseling if appropriate or to local support groups where others with similar experiences can answer questions. Knowing that others have had similar experiences can decrease social isolation and provide a means of learning alternative methods of sexual functioning.

Low Self-Esteem

An SCI is often the result of sudden trauma. Within moments, a formerly independent, fully functioning individual is suddenly unable to move and faces enormous adjustments in social, economic, and personal roles and relationships. Body image, self-esteem, and role performance are all affected by the damage. As a result, the client often demonstrates behaviors that may be difficult for the nurse to handle—depression,

CARE SETTINGS Community Care for the Client With a Spinal Cord Injury

Rehabilitation of the client with an SCI is an ongoing process that moves from intensive care through intermediate care to rehabilitation and then community-based and home care. Nursing interventions are necessary at all points in the process to prevent the complications of altered physical mobility and body functions and to teach the client and family measures that promote independence in self-care.

Discharge planning should be addressed in the initial plan of care while the client is in the critical care setting. Advance planning ensures continuity of care when the client leaves the hospital setting.

The following topics should be included in teaching the client and family about care at home:

- Self-care activities (ADL, exercises, bowel and bladder programs, skin care)
- Mobility (use of assistive devices: wheelchair, crutches, special automobiles)
- Preparation of the home environment
- If the client is in a wheelchair, will steps, stairs, doors, or carpeted floors present physical barriers?
- If a special bed is necessary, have arrangements been made and is it in the home?
- Psychologic support
- Independent activities
- Community resources such as Lifeline (emergency alerting systems through a local hospital or agency), support groups, career centers for job retraining, counseling
- Coping skills for client and caregiver
- Referral to a home health agency and PT for the client who is returning home
- Helpful resources:
  a. The National Spinal Cord Injury Association
  b. American Paralysis Association
  c. Christopher & Dana Reeve Foundation
  d. Paralyzed Veterans of America.

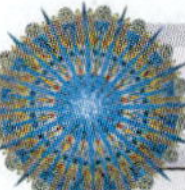

NURSING CARE PLAN **A Client With a Spinal Cord Injury**

Jim Valdez, a 19-year-old college sophomore, is admitted to the hospital by ambulance following an automobile crash. His family (father, mother, and sister) live 100 miles away and cannot visit often, although they are very concerned. On admission to the hospital, a CT scan of the spine shows a fracture and partial laceration of the cord at the C7 level. Mr. Valdez is in halo traction. One night he tells the nurse, "I wish I had just died when I got hurt. I don't think I can live like this."

ASSESSMENT

When Mr. Valdez is admitted to the intensive care unit, he has flaccid paralysis involving all extremities. He has no sensation below the clavicle or in portions of his arms and legs. His bladder is distended, and bowel sounds are absent. Other assessment findings include T_O 97°F (36.1°C), P 50, BP 90/56, ABGs pH 7.4, PaO_2 96, $PaCO_2$ 37, SaO_2 96%. Oxygen per nasal cannula is given at 2 L/min, and halo traction is applied. A Foley catheter is inserted into his bladder, and a nasogastric tube is inserted and attached to low-pressure continuous suction.

After 7 days, Mr. Valdez is moved from the intensive care unit to the neurosurgical unit for continuing care and planning for transfer to a rehabilitation hospital in his home town. His vital signs have stabilized and are normal for his age; respirations and oxygenation are normal. Other neurologic assessments remain the same.

DIAGNOSES

- Impaired Physical Mobility related to paralysis of lower and upper extremities
- Bowel Incontinence related to lack of voluntary sphincter control
- Dysfunctional Grieving related to denial of loss

PLANNING

- Be actively involved in exercise programs.
- Have a soft, formed stool every second or third day.
- Verbally express his grief to parents and staff.

IMPLEMENTATION

- Conduct passive exercises on all extremities four times a day.
- Provide progressive mobilization by initially raising the head of the bed 90 degrees (repeat two or three times during the first day of movement); if blood pressure remains normal, dangle for 5 minutes before transferring him to a chair.
- His usual time for a bowel movement is after breakfast; schedule retraining program for that time.
- Encourage a diet high in fiber and fluids. He likes whole wheat bread, orange juice, and cola; does not like water.
- Promote grief work by providing time to express feelings. Explain to the family that his denial and anger are part of the grieving process.
- Determine food likes and dislikes and order preferred foods from the menu. Encourage his friends to bring in his favorite foods periodically.
- Take and record weight every third day using the bed scales.

EVALUATION

By the time Mr. Valdez is transferred to the rehabilitation hospital, he is looking forward to learning how to use special equipment and getting his own motorized wheelchair. He is able to sit up in a chair without dizziness or hypotension. The use of ordered stool softeners combined with a high-fiber diet and fluid intake of 2000–3000 mL per day has maintained bowel elimination. Mr. Valdez and his parents have spent 3 hours talking about their feelings related to the accident and the future. Although the discussion is emotionally difficult, all three say that they now feel much better. Mr. Valdez still has episodes of angry outbursts and tears, but he is more optimistic about what can be done and believes he can finish college. He selects foods from the menu each day and eats most of his meals, but he especially enjoys the times his friends bring in pizza or hamburgers.

CRITICAL THINKING

1. Considering Mr. Valdez's age and developmental level, do you think his emotional responses to his injury were appropriate? Explain.
2. Issues of sexuality are obviously important for the client with an SCI. How would you approach Mr. Valdez about this topic?
3. What would be your response as a male or female nurse if Mr. Valdez would allow only male nurses to provide care?
4. Outline a teaching program to help Mr. Valdez meet long-term urinary elimination needs.

denial, and anger are seen in the period immediately after the injury. In addition to these responses, the young adult client may act out by making sexually overt statements.

- Encourage discussion about all aspects of physical function and care. Talking provides a safe outlet for fears and frustrations and increases self-awareness. Acceptance of self facilitates rehabilitation.
- Encourage self-care and independent decision making. Participating in self-care can promote positive coping; making decisions decreases feelings of powerlessness.
- Help identify strategies to increase independence in desired roles; include both short- and long-term goals. Discuss assistive devices (such as hand-operated automobiles). Identifying strategies to increase independence in the future fosters a positive self-concept and motivates the client to achieve rehabilitation goals.
- Include family members and important others in discussions. The realization that others do care and will continue to provide support is important in fostering positive self-regard.

- Refer the client and family to support groups or for psychologic counseling. Adjustment to change is more likely when the client and family seek peer and professional assistance.

Evaluation

Client response to nursing care is evaluated based on the goals established during the planning phase. Expected outcomes may include the following:

- Client attains appropriate bowel and bladder elimination habits.
- Client maintains healthy nutritional status.
- Client optimizes remaining motor and sensory function.
- Client and family accept limitations of disability.
- Caregiver finds adequate support to reduce role strain.

REVIEW Spinal Cord Injury

RELATE: LINK THE CONCEPTS

You are caring for an adult client with a C-2 fracture of the vertebrae that left him ventilator-dependent. He is 4 days post trauma and will require a tracheostomy for long-term ventilator support. The surgeon describes the procedure to be performed and requests the client's consent for the procedure. The client writes a one-word answer: "NO!!!" While exploring the client's reasoning, it becomes clear that the client is alert and oriented and does not want the procedure performed, saying he wants to be removed from the ventilator and allowed to die. The client's wife tries to persuade him to change his mind, but he is adamant about not consenting to the tracheotomy.

Linking the exemplar of Spinal Cord Injury with the concept of Ethics:

1. What is the health care team's ethical responsibility to this client?
2. Is it ethical to remove the client's endotracheal tube knowing that he will die within a few minutes due to complete lack of respiratory effort? The other option is to allow the endotracheal tube to remain in place knowing it will damage his trachea to the point of causing blockage of the airway if left in place too long? What would you recommend?

Linking the exemplar of Spinal Cord Injury with the concept of Legal Issues:

3. Can the wife legally give permission for the procedure?
4. Can a court order be obtained forcing the client to undergo the procedure?

READY: GO TO COMPANION SKILLS MANUAL

- Assessing the musculoskeletal system
- Assessing the neurologic system
- Assessing the client in pain
- Assessing respirations
- Oxygen saturation using a pulse oximeter
- Administering oxygen by cannula
- Using an oxygen analyzer
- Using an oxygen cylinder
- Caring for the client on a mechanical ventilator
- Turning a client to the lateral or prone position in bed
- Using a lift or turn sheet
- Performing passive range-of-motion exercises

REFER: GO TO MYNURSINGKIT

REFLECT: CASE STUDY

Robert Morris is a 25-year-old male who is in rehabilitation following a spinal cord injury that resulted from falling from his parents' roof while cleaning gutters. He lost his balance and fell two stories to the ground fracturing his L1 vertebrae. Robert had a job in the marketing department of a large department store in a town 15 miles away but he doesn't think he'll be able to remain in the job following his injury. He is currently on medical leave of absence.

Robert is engaged to Laura, 25 years old, and a newly graduated occupational therapist employed by a local hospital. They have dated since high school and always planned to marry. Laura has been very supportive of Robert during his convalescence but Robert has been noticeably cool and withdrawn toward her. Robert plans to live with his parents, Marcia and John, when he is discharged. They are concerned about Robert's treatment of Laura, whom they love very much. Robert's 18-year-old sister has been giving him a hard time about how he is treating his fiance.

Robert is paralyzed from the waist down and the doctor's don't seem to be sure if the paralysis is permanent or not. Robert spent four weeks in the rehabilitation hospital and is planning for discharge where he will receive physical therapy in the home. You are the home health nurse visiting Robert in the rehabilitation center to obtain a current assessment and begin developing his plan of care.

1. How will you respond to Robert if he confides his concerns that he will never be able to hold a decent job or have a family?
2. What assumptions do you have about why Robert is pushing Laura away? How can you help him deal with this?
3. Design Robert's initial plan of care for his first week at home.

PEARSON

EXPLORE mynursingkit™

MyNursingKit is your one stop for online chapter review materials and resources. Prepare for success with additional NCLEX®-style practice questions, interactive assignments and activities, web links, animations and videos, and more!

Register your access code from the front of your book at **www.mynursingkit.com**.

REFERENCES

Agency for Healthcare Research and Quality. (2002). Managing osteoarthritis: Helping the elderly maintain function and mobility. *Research in Action,* Issue 3. Retrieved July 19, 2002, from http://www.ahrq.gov

Alexander, N. (2003). Falls. In M. Beers & R. Berkow (Eds.), *The Merck manual of geriatrics* (Chap. 20). Whitehouse Station, NJ: Merck Research Laboratories.

Altizer, L. (2004). Compartment syndrome. *Orthopedic Nursing, 23,* 391–396.

American College of Rheumatology. (2005). *Background information on arthritis and rheumatology: Prevalence statistics.* Retrieved from http://www.rheumatology.org/press/index.asp?uad=mem

Bernick, L., & Bretholz, I. (1999). Safe mobility program: A comprehensive falls prevention program for a multilevel geriatric setting. *Journal of the Gerontological Nursing Association, 23*(3), 4–11.

Boston Total Joint Association. (2004). *Total hip replacement surgery.* Retrieved from http://www.bostontotaljoint.com/thr.html

Boutaugh, M.L., & Brady, T.J. (2001). Patient education for self-management. In: *Clinical Care in the Rheumatic Diseases,* (2nd ed.),. L. Robbins, C.S Burckhardt, M.T. Hannan, & R.J. DeHoratius (Eds.). Atlanta: American College of Rheumatology, pp.155–161.

Brown, J., Vittinghoff, E., Wyman, J., Stone, K., Nevitt, M., Ensrud, K., et al. (2000). Urinary incontinence: Does it increase risk for falls and fractures. *Journal of the American Geriatrics Society, 48*(7), 721–725.

Capezuti, E. (2002). Side rail use and bed-related fall outcomes among nursing home residents. *Journal of the American Geriatrics Society, 50*(1), 90–96.

Centers for Disease Control and Prevention. (2005). Bone health. Retrieved from http://www.cdc.gov/nccdphp/dnpa/bonehealth

Centers for Disease Control and Prevention, National Institutes of Health (2009). Arthritis, osteoporosis, and chronic back conditions. Retrieved October 9, 2009, from http://www.healthypeople.gov/Document/HTML/Volume1/02Arthritis.htm#_Toc490538008

Chamley, C. A., Carson, P., Randall, D., & Sandwell, M. (2005). *Developmental anatomy and physiology of children.* St. Louis, MO: Elsevier.

Finlayson, M., Van Denend, T., & Hudson, E. (2004). Aging with multiple sclerosis. *Journal of Neuroscience Nursing, 36*(5), 245–251, 259.

Flynn, J., & Johnson, T. (2005). *The Johns Hopkins white papers: Arthritis.* Baltimore: Johns Hopkins Medicine.

Gerhart, T. (2003). Fractures. In M. Beers & R. Berkow (Eds.), *The Merck manual of geriatrics* (Chap. 22). Whitehouse Station, NJ: Merck Research Laboratories.

Haas, J. (2000). High dose IVIG in the postpartum period for prevention of exacerbations in MS. *Multiple Sclerosis, 6*(Suppl. 2), 518–520.

Hart, E. S., & Grottkau, B. E. (2006). *Clinical Advisor,* February, 43–47.

Harvey, C. (2005). Wound healing. *Orthopaedic Nursing, 24*(2), 143–160.

Hayes, J. S., & Arriola, T. (2005). Pediatric spinal injuries. *Pediatric Nursing, 31*(6), 464–467.

Hayes, K. (2001). Physical modalities. In L. Robbins, C. Burckhardt, & R. Dehoratius (Eds.), *Clinical care in the rheumatic diseases* (pp. 185–189). Atlanta, GA: Association of Rheumatology Health Professionals.

Hickey, J. (2003). *The clinical practice of neurological and neurosurgical nursing* (4th ed.). Philadelphia: Lippincott.

Holmes, S., & Brown, S. (2005). Skeletal pin site care. National Association of Orthopaedic Nurses guidelines for orthopaedic nursing. *Orthopaedic Nursing, 24*(2), 99–108.

Hwang, M. Y., Glass, R., & Moher, J. (1999a). Falling and the elderly. *Journal of the American Medical Association, 281*(20), 1962.

Hwang, M. Y., Glass, R., & Moher, J. (1999b). Living with arthritis. *Journal of the American Medical Association, 282*(20), 1982.

Johnson, T. R. B., Gregory, K. D., & Niebyl, J. R. (2007). Preconception and prenatal care: Part of the continuum. In S. G. Gabbe, J. R. Niebyl, & J. L. Simpson (Eds.), *Obstetrics: Normal and problem pregnancies* (5th ed.). New York: Churchill-Livingstone.

Karlson, E., Mandl, L., Aweh, G., Sangha, O., Liang, M., & Grodstein, F. (2003). Total hip replacement due to osteoarthritis: The importance of age, obesity, and other modifiable risk factors. *American Journal of Medicine, 114*(2), 93–98.

Lonstein, J. E. (2006). Scoliosis: Surgical versus nonsurgical treatment. *Clinical Orthopaedics and Related Research, 443,* 248–259.

Ma, D., & Jones, G. (2004). Soft drink and milk consumption, physical activity, bone loss, and upper limb fractures in children: A population-based case-control study. *Calcified Tissue International, 75,* 286–291.

Manias, K., McCabe, D., & Bishop, N. (2006). Fractures and recurrent fractures in children: Varying effects of environment factors as well as bone size and mass. *Bone, 39,* 652–657.

Manolagas, S. (2006). Aging and the musculoskeletal system. In M. Beers (Ed.), The Merck manual of geriatrics. Retrieved September 14, 2007, from http://www.merck.com/mkgr/mmg/tables/48t1.jsp

Mayo Clinic. (2008). *Hip fracture.* Retrieved October 14, 2009 from http://www.mayoclinic.com/health/hip-fracture/DS00185/DSECTION=risk-factors

Mayo Clinic. (2009). *Multiple sclerosis.* Retrieved October 14, 2009 from http://www.mayoclinic.com/health/multiple-sclerosis/DS00188

Metter, E.J., Lynch, N., Conwit, R., Lindle, R., Tobin, J., & Hurley, B. (1999). Muscle quality and age: cross-sectional and longitudinal comparisons. *Journals of Gerontology Series A: Biological Sciences and Medical Sciences, 54*(5), B207-B218.

Minnesota Safety Council. (2008). *Fall prevention checklist.* Retrieved October 14, 2008, from http://www.minnesotasafetycouncil .org/seniorsafe/falls

Minor, M., & Westby, M. (2001). Rest and exercise. In L. Robbins, C. Burckhardt, M. Hannan, & R. Dehoratius (Eds.), *Clinical care in rheumatic disease* (2nd ed., pp. 179–184). Atlanta, GA: Association of Rheumatology Health Professionals.

National Center for Injury Prevention and Control (NCIPC), Centers for Disease Control and Prevention. (2006). *Falls and hip fractures among older adults.* Retrieved September 15, 2007, from http://www.cdc.gov/ncipc/factsheets/adulthipfx.htm

National Institute of Arthritis and Musculoskeletal and Skin Diseases. (2001). *National Institutes of Health, health topics: Questions and answers about hip replacement.* Retrieved November, 2002, from http://www.niams.nih.gov/hi/topics/hip/hiprepqa.htm

National Institute of Arthritis and Musculoskeletal and Skin Diseases. (2005). *Hyaluronic acid shows potential as biomarker for osteoarthritis.* Retrieved from http://www.niams.nih.gov/ne/highlights/spotlight/2005/hyaluronic_acid.htm

National Institute of Neurological Disorders and Stroke. (2005c). *Deep brain stimulation for Parkinson's disease information page.* Retrieved from http://www.ninds.nih.gov/disorders/deep_brain_stimulation/deep_brain_stimulation_pr.htm

National MS Society. (2005). *Just the facts: 2005–2006.* Retrieved from http://www.nationalmssociety.org/Brochures-Just%20the.asp

National Osteoporosis Foundation (NOF). (2007b). *Beat the break: Home safety checklist.* Retrieved September 19, 2007, from http://www.nof.org

The National Spinal Cord Injury Association. (2006). *More about spinal cord injury.* Retrieved from http://www.spinalcord.org/html/factsheets/spinstat.php

Patrick, L., Leber, M., Scrim, C., Gendron, I., & Eisener-Parche, P. (1999). A standardized assessment and intervention protocol for managing risk for falls on a geriatric rehabilitation unit. *Journal of Gerontological Nursing, 25*(4), 40–46.

Porth, C. (2005). *Pathophysiology: Concepts of altered health states* (7th ed.). Philadelphia: Lippincott.

Rateau, M. R. (2004). Use of backpacks in children and adolescents. *Orthopaedic Nursing, 23,* 101–105.

Resnick, B. (2001). Promoting health in older adults: A four-year analysis. *Journal of the American Academy of Nurse Practitioners, 13*(1), 23–33.

Robbins, L., Burckhardt, C., Hannan, M., & Dehoratius, R. (Eds.), (2001). *Clinical care in the rheumatic diseases.* Atlanta, GA: Association of Rheumatology Health Professionals.

Sapountzi-Krepia, D., Psychogiou, M., Peterson, D., Zafari, B., Iordanopoulou, E., Michailidou, F., et al. (2006). The experience of brace treatment in children/adolescents with scoliosis. *Scoliosis, 22,* 8.

Sapountzi-Krepia, D. S., Valavanis, J., Panteleakis, G. P., Zangana, D. T., Vlachojiannis, P. C., & Sapkas, G. S. (2001). Perceptions of body image, happiness and satisfaction in adolescents wearing a Boston brace for scoliosis treatment. *Issues and Innovations in Nursing Practice, 35,* 683–690.

Sellers, J. T. (2002) Causes of upper back pain. Retrieved October 14, 2009 from http://www.spine-health.com/conditions/upper-back-pain/causes-upper-back-pain

Sheir-Neiss, G. I., Kruse, R. W., Rahman, T., Jacobsen, L. P., & Pelli, J. A. (2003). Association of backpack use and back pain in adolescents. *Spine, 28,* 922–930.

Thompson, G. H. (2004a). The spine. In R. E. Behrman, R. M. Kliegman, & H. B. Jenson, *Nelson textbook of pediatrics* (17th ed.). Philadelphia: Saunders.

Tierney, L., McPhee, S., & Papadakis, M. (Eds.), (2005). *Current medical diagnosis & treatment* (43rd ed.). Stamford, CT: Appleton & Lange.

Tinetti, M. (2003). Chronic dizziness and postural instability. In M. Beers & R. Berkow (Eds.), *The Merck manual of geriatrics* (Chap. 19). Whitehouse Station, NJ: Merck Research Laboratories.

U.S. Preventive Services Task Force. (2006b). *The guide to clinical preventive services.* Agency for Healthcare Research and Quality. Retrieved August 10, 2008, from http://www.preventiveservices.ahrq.gov

Van Gent, C., Dols, J. J., de Rover, C. J., Hira Sing, R. A, & de Vet, H. C. (2003). The weight of schoolbags and the occurrence of neck, shoulder, and back pain in young adolescents. *Spine, 28,* 916–921.

Vitale, M. G., Goss, J. M., Matsumoto, H., & Roye, D. P. (2006). Epidemiology of pediatric spinal cord injury in the United States, years 1997 and 2000. *Journal of Pediatric Orthopedics, 26*(6), 745–749.

Mood and Affect 20

Concept at-a-Glance

Concept Learning Outcomes

After reading about this concept, you will be able to:

1. Summarize the structure and physiological processes of the neurological system related to mood and affect.
2. List factors affecting mood and affect.
3. Identify commonly occurring alterations in mood and affect and their related treatments.
4. Explain common assessment procedures used to examine the mood and affect of clients across the life span.
5. Outline diagnostic and laboratory tests used to determine causes of alterations in an individual's mood and affect.
6. Explain prevention and management strategies for alterations in mood and affect.
7. Demonstrate the nursing process in providing culturally competent and caring interventions across the life span for individuals with alterations of mood and affect.
8. Identify pharmacologic interventions used in caring for the individual with alterations of mood and affect.

Concept Key Terms

Adjustment disorder, *1159*
Affect, *1157*
Aggressive behavior, *1169*
Assertive behavior, *1169*
Biological rhythms, *1162*
Bipolar disorders, *1160*
Double depression, *1159*
Dysthymic disorder, *1159*
Electroconvulsive therapy (ECT), *1175*
Emotions, *1157*
Major depressive disorder, *1159*
Mania, *1160*
Monoamine oxidase inhibitors (MAOIs), *1172*
Mood, *1157*
Mood stabilizers, *1173*
Passive behavior, *1169*
Postpartum blues, *1159*
Postpartum depression, *1159*
Postpartum psychosis, *1159*
Recovery, *1158*
Recurrence, *1158*
Relapse, *1158*
Remission, *1158*
Seasonal affective disorder (SAD), *1162*
Selective serotonin reuptake inhibitors (SSRIs), *1171*
Situational depression, *1159*
Somatization, *1167*
Switching, *1158*
Tricyclic antidepressants (TCAs), *1170*
Unipolar disorder, *1159*

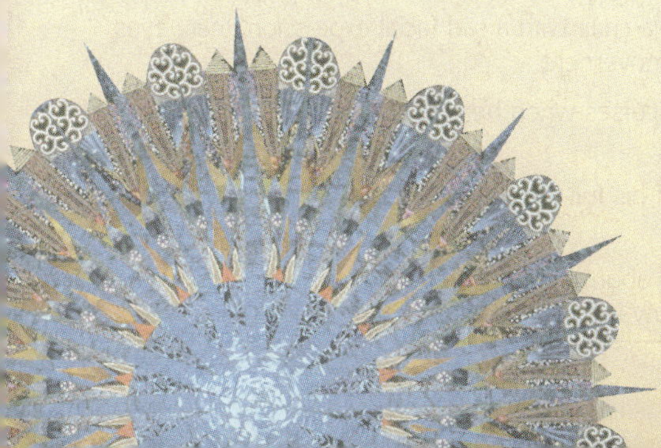

About Mood and Affect

Emotions are feeling responses to a wide variety of stimuli. Positive emotions such as joy stimulate the individual to remain in the situation, while negative emotions such as fear stimulate the individual to avoid or withdraw from the situation. **Mood** is defined as "a sustained emotional state and how one feels subjectively." The way in which people communicate mood to others is called affect. **Affect** is the immediate and observable emotional expression of mood that people communicate verbally and nonverbally. People may use *verbal cues* to describe an emotional state with words such as *elation, happiness, pleasure,* *frustration, anger,* and *hostility. Nonverbal cues* to emotions include facial expressions such as smiling, frowning, and looking blank; motor activities such as clenching hands into fists and pacing; and physiologic responses such as sweating profusely and experiencing increased respirations. Although an individual may choose not to communicate verbally to another person, it is almost impossible to prevent nonverbal expression of feelings. •

A variety of descriptors of affect are used to facilitate communication among health care professionals. Table 20–1 gives definitions of affect descriptors and behavioral examples. Emotions, mood, and affect can be pictured along a continuum ranging from depression through normal to mania. The normal range of mood is stable and appropriate to the situation. Emotions, mood, and affect become dysfunctional when they occur in inappropriate situations or when the response is out of proportion to the stimulus. People diagnosed with mood disorders experience disrupting disturbances at varying points along the continuum.

Mood disorders tend to be chronic in nature. As many as 85% of people who have one major depressive episode will experience another episode, and 35% experience residual symptoms between acute episodes. Relapse rates for bipolar disorders range from 44% in 1 year to 73–89% over 4–5 years. Between 30% and 60% of individuals with bipolar disorders do not fully recover between episodes. In addition, bipolar disorder has the highest suicide risk of all psychiatric disorders (Steinhauer, 2003; Tohen et al., 2005; Valdivia & Rossy, 2004). Descriptions of the course of these disorders include the following (Tohen et al., 2003):

- **Recovery**: Return to or exceed pre-illness levels of functioning
- **Remission**: Sustained recovery of at least 8 weeks
- **Switching**: A new illness phase (manic or depressed) without recovery
- **Relapse**: Return of disorder soon after recovery
- **Recurrence**: A later recurrence after recovery.

The high rate of mood disorders makes these disorders a major concern for nurses. Clients with mood disorders are found in the community and in all types of clinical settings and are not restricted to psychiatric settings. It is vital that the nurse be alert to cues because one of the tragic results in untreated depression is suicide.

COMORBID DISORDERS

Severe depression and *anxiety disorders* frequently occur at the same time. Studies indicate that as many as 40% of those suffering from agoraphobia, 50% of those experiencing panic attacks, 44% of those with obsessive-compulsive disorder, and 17% of those with generalized anxiety disorder are also clinically depressed. An estimated 85% of adults with depression experience significant symptoms of anxiety. Compared to the general population, individuals with bipolar disorders are more likely to have concomitant panic disorder and generalized anxiety disorder. Major depression increases the risk of developing post-traumatic stress disorder. People with both mood and anxiety disorders have fewer personal and social resources and demonstrate poorer overall functioning (Ghaemi, 2004; Oquendo et al., 2005; Steinhauer, 2003).

The rate of comorbidity between mood disorders and *substance-related disorders* is high. In some cases, the primary diagnosis is a mood disorder, with substance abuse being an attempt to self-medicate. In other situations, the substance-related disorder is the primary diagnosis. An example is the person who becomes depressed during withdrawal from amphetamines or cocaine. A third possibility is that the person has both disorders as primary diagnoses.

TABLE 20–1 **Descriptors of Affect**

AFFECT	DEFINITION	BEHAVIORAL EXAMPLE
Appropriate	Mood is congruent with the immediate situation.	Juan cries when learning of the death of his father.
Inappropriate	Mood is not related to the immediate situation.	When Sue's husband tells her about his terrible pain, Sue begins to laugh out loud.
Stable	Mood is resistant to sudden changes when there is no provocation in the environment.	During a party, Dan smiles and laughs at the appropriate social interchanges.
Labile	Mood shifts suddenly in a way that cannot be understood in the context of the situation.	During a friendly game of checkers, Dorothy, who has been laughing, suddenly knocks the board off the table in anger. She then begins to laugh and wants to continue the game.
Elevated	Mood is one of euphoria not necessarily related to the immediate situation.	Sean bounces around the dayroom, laughing, singing, and telling other clients how wonderful everything is.
Depressed	Mood is one of despondency not necessarily related to the immediate situation.	Leo sits slumped in a chair with a sad facial expression, teary eyes, and minimal body movement.
Overreactive	Mood is appropriate to the situation but out of proportion to the immediate situation.	Karen screams and curses when her child spills a glass of milk on the kitchen floor.
Blunted	Mood is a dulled response to the immediate situation.	When Tom learns of his full-tuition scholarship, he responds with only a small smile.
Flat	There are no visible cues to the person's mood.	When Juanita is told about her best friend's death, she says "Oh" and does not give any indication of an emotional response.

Research reports that major depression tends to come before alcohol problems in women, while the opposite is true for men. Unfortunately, the use of alcohol to relieve depression can aggravate the depression by causing other problems for the drinker and by intensifying the level of the depression. Thirty-two percent of all depressed adolescents have a comorbid substance abuse disorder. As stated earlier, people with bipolar disorders have the highest rate of comorbid substance abuse disorder of all major psychiatric illnesses. Treatment for both mood and substance abuse disorders should be concurrent (Baethge et al., 2005; Davis et al., 2005; Wilens et al., 2004).

ALTERATIONS

The mood spectrum disorders are characterized by changes in feelings ranging from severe depression to inordinate elation. They are best understood as syndromes with a core cluster of symptoms. We are beginning to understand that there are many different subtypes of mood disorders, each with different patterns and probably a different prognosis. These subtypes of depressive and bipolar disorders are just now becoming clear.

Depression

What most Americans think of as depression is **major depressive disorder** (MDD, also called **unipolar disorder**). MDD is diagnosed when, along with a loss of interest in life, a person experiences a depressed mood that moves from mild to severe, with the severe phase lasting at least 2 weeks. MDD often has a chronic course with lengthy episodes or incomplete remission between episodes. Another depressive disorder, dysthymic disorder, is also commonly referred to as "depression" but is different from MDD. **Dysthymic disorder** is a chronic disorder in which periods of depressed mood are interspersed with normal mood. With this disorder, people experience a depressed mood for most of the day more days than not for at least 2 years. Symptoms in dysthymic disorder tend to be less severe than those in MDD, and there are fewer physiologic symptoms (disturbed sleep, altered appetite, and weight loss or gain). Most people with dysthymic disorder also experience one or more episodes of MDD. When this occurs, it is referred to as **double depression**. Individuals with double depression have more severe symptoms and higher rates of suicide than clients with MDD (Klein, Shankman, Lewinsohn, Rohde, & Seeley, 2004).

POSTPARTUM DEPRESSION Although 10–15% of pregnant women meet criteria for depression, they often remain undiagnosed because the symptoms of depression are similar to the somatic changes of pregnancy. The prevalence of depression among pregnant adolescents is almost twice as high as among adult pregnant women and is more severe between the second and third trimester. Untreated maternal mood disorders are associated with poor prenatal care, preterm delivery, small infant size, postpartum depression or mania, and maternal suicide (Suppaseemanont, 2006; Yonkers et al., 2004).

Mood disorders in women after delivering a child are fairly common. During pregnancy, levels of estrogens, glucocorticoids, and amino acids increase by as much as 200 times, only to drop sharply within 24 hours after delivery. This results in a hypoactive hypothalamic–pituitary axis that may last for months. Symptoms can be described along a continuum from postpartum blues to postpartum depression to the rare form, postpartum psychosis. These disorders may be complicated by postpartum panic disorder and postpartum obsessive–compulsive disorder (Bailara et al., 2005).

Postpartum blues begin within the first 10 days postpartum and last a few days to 2 weeks with symptoms disappearing spontaneously. The mood may be unstable, accompanied by sadness, weepiness, irritability, anxiety, and fatigue. As many as 70% of new mothers may experience these symptoms, which are thought to be caused by hormonal fluctuations. Most of these women have not had previous emotional problems (Ugarriza, 2004; Varney, Kriebs, & Gegor, 2004).

Postpartum depression is a severe form of depression that is estimated to occur in 13% of new mothers. It often begins within 3 months of delivery but may strike at any time during the first year after having had a child. Women who give birth to multiple children and/or to preterm children are at higher risk for postpartum depression. Symptoms include insomnia, loss of energy, inability to concentrate, anxiety, mood swings, periods of crying, and feelings of despair as the person ruminates over perceived inadequacies as a mother. If depression is untreated, it will affect the ability to parent and to cope with stressful situations. These symptoms are more intense and last longer than those of postpartum blues. Any symptoms lasting longer than 2 weeks qualify as postpartum depression. Contributing factors are hormonal changes, family history of depression, feelings of being overwhelmed by parenting tasks, changes in family dynamics, and inadequate support. Those who develop postpartum depression are at an increased risk for depression after subsequent pregnancies (Beck, 2003; Ugarriza, 2004; Wisner et al., 2004).

One to 2 women in 1,000 with no history of a mood disorder experiences a **postpartum psychosis**—a medical emergency. The incidence of relapse for women who have a diagnosed bipolar disorder is 25–40% during postpartum, or 260 women per 1,000 deliveries. The symptoms usually occur between the first 2–6 weeks after delivery but may occur as early as 48 hours postpartum. Symptoms develop rapidly and include insomnia, mood lability, delusions, hallucinations, agitation, and bizarre feelings or behavior. An inordinate concern with the baby's health, guilt about lack of love, and delusions about the infant's being dead or defective also may be present. The mother may deny having given birth or hear voices that command her to hurt the baby. In extreme cases, the mother may even kill the child and/or herself. Unlike other types of psychoses, the woman with postpartum psychosis may alternate between lucid states and a "zombie-like" psychotic state (Spinelli, 2004; Ugarriza, 2004).

SITUATIONAL DEPRESSION People often experience dramatic life changes because of losses due to death, relocation, loss of autonomy, illness, and financial stress. One or a combination of life changes and losses may contribute to the development of **situational depression**, also known as **adjustment disorder**. The essential feature of situational depression is a maladaptive reaction to an identifiable psychosocial stressor or stressors that occurs within 3 months after the onset of the stressor and has persisted for no longer than 6 months (APA, 2000). Symptoms of situational depression are similar to the other depressive disorders, although a higher level of anxiety may be present.

Bipolar Disorders

The medical diagnosis of **bipolar disorders** is given when a person's mood alternates between the extremes of depression and elation (**mania**), with interspersing periods of normal mood. *Bipolar I disorder* is characterized by the occurrence of one or more manic episodes and one or more depressive episodes. *Bipolar II disorder* is characterized by one or more hypomanic episodes (less severe) and one or more depressive episodes. There is evidence that some individuals experience a unipolar mania with no depressive episodes. Data suggest that unipolar disorder and bipolar disorders are not two separate disorders but rather the same disorder with fluctuations in mood (Cassano et al., 2004; Schneck et al., 2004; Solomon et al., 2003).

Bipolar disorders are further classified as follows:

- *Mixed:* The person has rapidly alternating moods.
- *Manic:* The person is presently in the manic phase.
- *Depressed:* The person is in the depressed phase but has a history of manic episodes.

Rapid cycling describes the course for some people with a bipolar disorder. It is defined as four or more episodes of illness within a 12-month period. A person with rapid cycling could be diagnosed as bipolar I; bipolar II; or mixed, manic, or depressed. Rapid cycling occurs in 10–20% of people with bipolar disorder, with 70–90% of rapid cyclers being women. This form of the disorder tends to be more resistant to treatment than the nonrapid-cycling course (Schneck et al., 2004)

THEORIES OF DEPRESSION

Multiple theories have been developed to explain the cause of mood disorders. Depression, like schizophrenia, is considered a spectrum disorder. At one end of the spectrum is an incapacitating illness such as a double depression or bipolar disorder with psychosis. At the other end is a depressive personality characterized only by a pessimistic outlook on life or mood swings that are mild in nature. Most cases fall somewhere between these two extremes.

In understanding people with mood disorders, the nurse must look at how factors interacted in the person's past and how they interact in present circumstances. A person may have a genetic predisposition to abnormalities in neurotransmission. The abnormalities may occur only when certain psychological mechanisms are present, and these mechanisms may operate only when particular social interactions occur. Many factors in the individual and the environment increase or decrease the risk of mood disorders. Different forms of the illness may have different risk factors. In some forms, predisposition may have a stronger role, and in other forms, stressors may play more of a role. Mood disorders likely represent a common final pathway of multiple underlying factors. By applying genetic, neurobiologic, intrapersonal, learning, cognitive, social, and gender bias theories, the nurse can approach the client from a holistic perspective.

Genetics

Some evidence suggests that people who experience mood disorders have a genetic predisposition to them. It is not yet clear what is inherited, neurobiologic vulnerability, cognitive vulnerability, or social vulnerability. The inheritability of major depression is

ALTERATIONS AND TREATMENTS Mood and Affect

Alteration	Description	Treatment
Depression (including major depressive disorder and dysthymic disorder)	Depressed mood that varies from mild to severe with severe phases lasting longer than six weeks. Symptoms include: ▪ Feelings of sadness, hopelessness, powerlessness ▪ Sleep disturbances ▪ Deterioration of functioning ▪ Inability to concentrate.	▪ Antidepressants ▪ Electroconvulsive therapy ▪ Cognitive-behavioral therapy (CBT)
Bipolar disorders	Extreme alterations in mood with intermittent periods of normal mood	Mood stabilizers may be prescribed concurrently with an antidepressant to prevent onset of manic phase.
Postpartum depression	Severe depression appearing within the first year following birth of a child. Symptoms include: ▪ Insomnia ▪ Fatigue ▪ Crying ▪ Feelings of despair ▪ Anxiety ▪ Mood swings.	Combination of antidepressants and psychosocial interventions are most effective. Sertraline (Zoloft) and paroxetine (Paxil) are first-line pharmacologic treatments for breastfeeding mothers.
Situational depression	Hyperreaction to an identifiable, life-altering (but not life-threatening) stressor that occurs within 3 months after the onset of the stressor and has persisted for no more than 6 months; symptoms similar to those of depression	Psychosocial interventions (e.g., CBT) alone may be sufficient to relieve symptoms and return client to normal.

40–50%. The more severe the depression, the stronger the genetic link. The rate of recurrent unipolar depression in the general population is 8%. Children of depressed parents (top-down sampling as shown in Figure 20–1 ■) have twice the risk, or about 16% over a lifetime. If both parents have depression, the risk rises to 75%. First-degree relatives of depressed children (bottom-up sampling as depicted in Figure 20–2 ■) also have twice the risk of depression. Studies of the incidence in twins show that in 60% of monozygotic twins, both twins developed a unipolar depression, compared with only 12% of dizygotic twins (Faraone, Glatt, Su, & Tsuang, 2004).

Bipolar disorders have the greatest inheritability; about 85% of the risk appears to be inherited. Early onset of the disorder may be the result of a particularly strong genetic effect. Studies of the incidence in twins demonstrate that in 50–80% of monozygotic twins, both twins developed bipolar disorders, compared with only 17–24% of dizygotic twins (Badner, 2003; Fisfalen et al., 2005).

Studies suggest that rather than a single dominant gene, a complex mode of inheritance exists. The individual mix of these multiple genes likely determines differences such as age of onset, symptoms, severity, and course of the mood disorders.

Neurobiology

The *prefrontal cortex* has been the subject of increasing research on mood disorders. Studies of depressed people have shown lower-than-normal activity, low glucose metabolism, and decreased blood flow in the anterior cingulate cortex. These abnormalities may be associated with abnormal processing of emotion. Neuroimaging findings in bipolar disorders include ventricular enlargement and smaller volumes in the posterior hippocampus, left amygdala, and temporal lobe. The amygdala plays a role in keeping social and emotional behavior within bounds, both of which are impaired in manic episodes (Caetano et al., 2006; Frazier et al., 2005; Neumeister, Charney, & Drevets, 2005).

The *neurotransmission hypothesis* is specifically concerned with the levels of serotonin (5-HT), dopamine (DA), norepinephrine (NE), and acetylcholine (ACh) in the central nervous system (CNS). It is believed that there is a functional deficiency of these neurotransmitters during a depressive episode and a functional excess during a manic episode (Meyer et al., 2003).

Most likely there are different combinations of problems with the neurotransmitter systems. Both DA and the balance between DA and ACh are responsible for difficulties with motivation. ACh is implicated in the sleep disturbances of both bipolar and unipolar disorders. NE is important in motor arousal, movement, energy, concentration, and motivation. The principal neurotransmitter for mood states is 5-HT, which is associated with anxiety and aggression, especially self-destructive behavior. A newly found protein named p11 appears to regulate how brain cells respond to 5-HT by increasing the number of receptors. Compared to people who are not depressed, people who are depressed have lower levels of p11. In addition, endogenous opioids are necessary to moderate sad moods. The interactions between these different neurotransmitters explain how clinical features tend to vary from client to client (Svenningsson et al., 2006).

One way this imbalance may occur is through the action of the enzyme *monoamine oxidase (MAO)*, which is responsible for deactivating neurotransmitters after they have been released from the receptor sites. If there is an excess of MAO, neurotransmitter levels will be low, resulting in decreased impulse transmission. If there is insufficient MAO to deactivate the neurotransmitters, they will accumulate at the synapse and increase the transmission of impulses.

This hypothesis may be one explanation for the higher incidence of depression in women and older people. Throughout life, women and older adults have consistently higher levels of MAO than do men and younger people. The result may be a functional decrease in the necessary neurotransmitters.

Another part of the hypothesis concerns the *sensitivity of the receptors* to the neurotransmitters. During depression, the receptors may be subsensitive, so fewer impulses are transmitted. During the manic state, receptors may be supersensitive, resulting in an increase in the transmission of impulses.

Although peripheral *thyroid hormone levels* may be normal, 35% of people with depression experience CNS thyroid dysfunction, which has a major effect on 5-HT, DA, and gamma-aminobutyric acid (GABA). It is believed that people who are depressed have a lower level of transthyretin, a protein important for transporting thyroid hormones in the brain. Current or past hypothyroidism may be associated with rapid-cycling bipolar disorder (Mayberg, Keightley, Mahurin, & Brannan, 2004).

Continuing research into the relationship between stress and mood disorders indicates that the limbic system of the brain is the major site of stress adaptation. With stress, neurotransmitter production in the limbic system increases. When the stress becomes chronic or recurrent, the body can no longer adapt as efficiently, and a shortage of neurotransmitters results. During

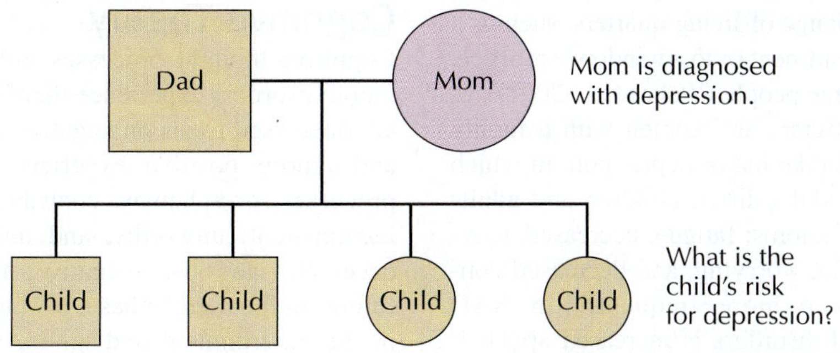

Figure 20–1 ■ Top-down sampling.

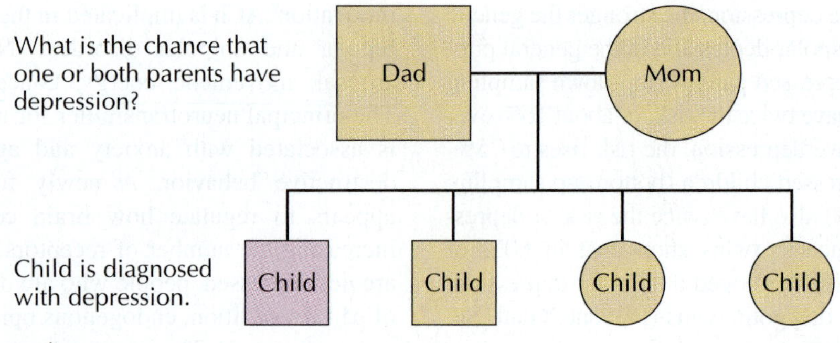
What is the chance that one or both parents have depression?
Dad
Mom
Child is diagnosed with depression.
Child
Child
Child
Child

Figure 20–2 ■ Bottom-up sampling.

manic episodes, there appears to be a defective feedback mechanism in the limbic system. Even after the stressful event has been resolved, the limbic system continues to produce excessive neurotransmitters; the increased transmission of impulses continues. Different areas of the limbic system play a major role in the regulation of emotions such as fear, rage, excitement, and euphoria. The signs and symptoms of limbic dysfunction correlate to the characteristics seen in the mood disorders.

Another hypothesis involves biological rhythms. **Biological rhythms** are regular fluctuations of a variety of physiologic factors over a period of time. In some individuals, internal desynchronization may result in depression. The tendency toward internal desynchronization is probably inherited, but stresses, lifestyle, and normal aging also influence it. It is unclear, however, whether changes in circadian rhythms cause mood disturbances or whether changes in mood alter circadian rhythms. (See Concept 13, Health, Wellness, and Illness, for a more detailed discussion of circadian rhythms.)

The *sleep–wake cycle* has an important role in mood disorders. In 50–75% of adults and 90% of older adults with depression, there is an earlier onset of REM sleep and alternations in brain activity during REM sleep. For those with bipolar disorders, lack of sleep can trigger a manic episode (Rao, 2003).

Some forms of mood disorders are related to the time of year and the amount of available sunlight. In **seasonal affective disorder (SAD)**, the individual typically experiences depression during fall and winter, returning to normal mood in spring and summer. The depressive state appears to be directly related to the amount of light because symptoms disappear when the person is exposed to more sunlight. Light has an inhibiting effect on the production of melatonin, a hormone that affects mood, sensations of fatigue, and sleepiness. Seasonal light changes are not the only trigger. A change of living quarters, such as a move to a darker basement apartment or to a windowless office, can trigger the disorder in some people (Wehr et al., 2001).

The majority of SAD sufferers are women with a family history of mood disorders. Unlike major depression, in which symptoms for children and adults differ, children and adults with SAD exhibit similar symptoms: fatigue, decreased activity, irritability, sadness, crying, worrying, and decreased concentration. A symptom seen more frequently in SAD compared to the other mood disorders is increased appetite, carbohydrate craving, and weight gain.

Intrapersonal Factors

Intrapersonal theory focuses on the theme of loss, either real or symbolic. The loss may be of another person, a relationship, an object, self-esteem, or security. When grief concerning the loss is unrecognized or unresolved, depression may result. A normal feeling accompanying all loss is anger, a compensatory response to feelings of powerlessness. People who have been taught that it is inappropriate to experience and express anger learn to repress it. The result is that anger is turned inward and against the self. Some theorists believe that the repressed anger and aggression against the self are the cause of depressive episodes. Other theorists believe that the cause of depression is an inability to achieve desired goals, the loss of those goals, and a feeling of lack of control in life.

People who are unusually sensitive to loss or abandonment issues are said to have dependent traits. People who are unusually sensitive to failure to achieve their goals are said to have self-critical traits. Both of these cognitive-personality features increase the likelihood that environmental stressors will lead to depression.

Learning Theory

Learning theory states that people learn to be depressed in response to an external locus of control, as they perceive themselves lacking control over their life experiences. Throughout life, depressed people experience little success in achieving gratification and little positive reinforcement for their attempts to cope with negative incidents. These repeated failures teach them that what they do has no effect on the final outcome. The more stressful life events that occur, the more their sense of helplessness is reinforced. When people reach the point of believing they have no control, they no longer have the will or energy to cope with life, and a depressive state results.

Cognitive Theory

Cognitive thought processes influence the way people with mood disorders experience themselves and others. Those who are depressed focus on negative messages in the environment and ignore positive experiences. These negative thought processes, or schemas, contribute to a view of the self as incompetent, unworthy, and unlikable. All present experiences are viewed as negative, and there is no hope for the future. In the manic phase, people focus on positive messages in the environment and ignore negative experiences. These positive schemas contribute to manic clients' grandiose view of themselves. Everything that occurs is seen as positive, and the future holds no limits. When people get caught up in this process, a number of cognitive distortions may occur.

Sociocultural Factors

A variety of sociocultural conditions may contribute to a person's depressive feelings of powerlessness, hopelessness, and low self-esteem. Racism, classism, sexism, ageism, and homophobia are predominant sociocultural characteristics in the United States. Whatever way *minorities* are defined, they experience discrimination psychologically, educationally, vocationally, and economically. When someone is the subject of cultural stereotypes in comments or jokes, it is difficult not to feel inadequate and shameful. When education has been substandard, a person cannot expect to be successful without remedial work. When promotions are based on race, gender, age, or sexual orientation, it is difficult to feel hopeful about advancing in one's career. It also is difficult to combat the feeling of helplessness when one's financial compensation is clearly inadequate for the job being done.

There is a much higher rate of depression among women than men. One of the contributing factors in Western society may be the stress of being a single parent. Approximately 85% of single parents are women. These women must deal with financial hardships, parenting problems, loneliness, and lack of a supportive adult relationship. A major predisposing factor for depression in women is having three or more children under the age of 14 living at home. When the children grow up and leave, the rate of depression decreases. This is contrary to the theory that depression results from the empty-nest syndrome. It appears that being responsible for children is a source of stress that contributes to depression (Peden, Rayens, Hall, & Grant, 2005; Peden, Rayens, Hall, & Grant, 2004).

Another sociocultural factor that may contribute to depression is the occurrence of stressful life events. Some events cause expansion of the family system: marriage, births, adoptions, and other people moving into the home. Other events cause a reduction of the family system: children leaving, marital separations, divorce, and death. Some life events involve a threat, as in job problems, difficulties with the police, and illness. Others can be emotionally exhausting, such as celebrating holidays, changing residences, and arguing with family and friends. Many people who experience stressful events do not become depressed. However, for people who are vulnerable to depression, stressors may play a significant role in the exacerbation and course of the disorder.

A number of factors influence the degree of stress that accompanies significant life events. Figure 20–3 ■ illustrates the relationship between life events and depression. The presence of a social support network can decrease the impact that an event may have on a person. People who have developed adaptive coping patterns such as problem solving, direct communication, and use of resources are more likely to maintain their normal mood. Those who feel out of control, are unable to problem-solve, and ignore available resources are more apt to feel depressed. Thus, an individual's perception and interpretation of significant events may contribute to depression.

Childhood sexual abuse is a significant risk factor for depression during both childhood and adulthood. Although the depressive episodes do not seem to be more severe, the onset is often earlier and the survivors are more likely to self-mutilate and attempt suicide (Weili, Mueser, Rosenberg & Jankowski, 2008).

FOCUS ON DIVERSITY AND CULTURE Native Americans and Mental Illness

Native Americans living in rural areas or tribal territories who suffer from mental illness face a number of barriers to treatment and recovery. These include lack of culturally competent, trained mental health professionals; a higher than average rate of uninsured individuals; discrimination and social stigmas; transportation issues; and lack of preventive health programs. In addition, Native Americans suffer from high rates of substance abuse, suicide, homelessness, and unemployment (Mental Health America, n.d.).

Gender Bias Theory

In the definition of mental health, there has, in the past, been a double standard for women and men. A healthy woman has been described as acquiescent, subdued, dependent, and emotionally expressive. A healthy man, on the other hand, has been described as logical, rational, independent, aggressive, and unemotional. These stereotypes have had unfortunate consequences for both women and men. There is, however, movement toward an androgynous definition of mental health. This perspective stresses positive human qualities such as assertiveness, self-reliance, sensitivity to others, intimacy, and open communication—qualities that legitimately belong in the repertoire of both women and men.

Throughout the world, women experience more depression than do men. Certainly, there are cross-cultural similarities in the way women are socialized and in the inferior status they experience in many societies. Psychosocial stressors, including multiple work and family responsibilities, poverty, sexual and

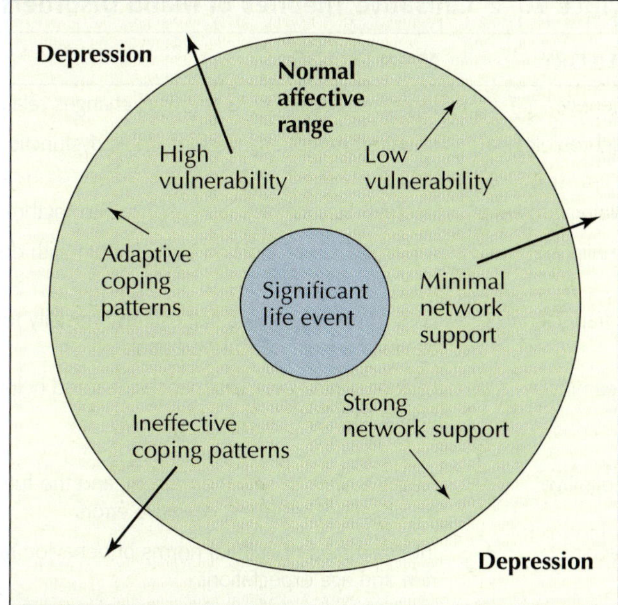

Figure 20–3 ■ The relationship between life events and depression.

physical abuse, gender discrimination, lack of social supports, and traumatic life experiences, may contribute to women's increased vulnerability to depression. In the United States and Canada, African American women are at higher risk for depression than Euro-American women are. Research suggests that additional risk factors include minority status, socioeconomic stress, and multiple roles (Schreiber, Stern, & Wilson, 2000).

Gender socialization differences may be a factor in the higher rate of depression in women. It starts early, when many girls are encouraged to play with dolls and help take care of other children in the family. Girls are taught to be "nice," nonargumentative, and docile. They become more concerned than boys about fitting in and backing down in the face of conflict. Gradually, they begin to question the worth of their abilities and opinions, which decreases self-esteem. Boys are socialized to be individualistic, to speak up, to raise their hand in class. Gradually, they begin to see themselves as autonomous individuals with good self-esteem (Brommelhoff, Conway, Merikangas, & Levy, 2004).

Rigid expectations about gender roles continue to linger and contribute to higher rates of depression among women. Women who are full-time homemakers may develop no identity other than that of wife and mother. The tremendous duties of managing a household are often invisible to others and lack prestige. Positive feedback or positive reinforcement such as compliments, a paycheck, and retirement benefits are uncommon. And the position is continuous, 24 hours a day. Because the homemaker lives in the workplace, there is no stimulation from a change in environment. Indeed, being a full-time homemaker is one of the most isolating professions in society today.

Women who are employed outside the home, in both professional and blue-collar positions, are less depressed than women who remain at home. This is true even for women who must assume the responsibility of two full-time jobs with minimal or no support from other family members. Employed women often must accept lower pay, inferior jobs, and fewer opportunities for career advancement. The legal system has been slow to redress employment discrimination, which increases women's frustration, anger, and distress. Thoughts of the future focus on the helplessness of their situations and contribute to depression.

Gender bias theory can also be applied to the situation in which some older adults find themselves. In a society that places a premium on youth, older people feel useless, unimportant, incapable, and at times even repulsive. Role changes and losses may threaten their self-esteem. With aging, physiologic changes may lead to a self-perception of being unfit, which then extends to further thoughts of being ineffectual and inferior. All of these changes may contribute to despair about one's life and a sense of hopelessness about the limited future. Considering these effects, it is not surprising to find a higher rate of depression among older people. See Table 20–2 for an overview of the etiologies of mood disorders, with specific relevance to women and older adults.

ASSESSMENT

Assessing clients with mood disorders is often done in segments of 15–20 minutes each. Individuals who are depressed do not have the energy to talk for longer periods, and those who are in a manic phase are unable to concentrate and sit still for longer periods. The nurse must exercise a great deal of patience when assessing these clients. Clients who are depressed may take a long time to answer questions; the nurse may need to repeat questions. If family members are present, the nurse should discourage them from answering questions for the client who is responding slowly. Clients in a manic phase with flight of ideas must be refocused frequently on the topic at hand. Their elevated mood may interfere with their ability to give accurate information. The nurse may want to use the Beck Depression Inventory (Table 20–3). This is a self-rating scale that measures levels of depression.

TABLE 20–2 **Causative Theories of Mood Disorders**

THEORY	MAIN POINTS	RELEVANCE TO WOMEN AND OLDER ADULTS
Genetic	Increased sensitivity to chemical changes related to stress	
Neurobiologic	Impaired neurotransmission; limbic dysfunction	There are higher levels of MAO in the central nervous system of women and older people.
Biologic rhythms	Internal desynchronization of circadian rhythms	
Sunlight	A decrease in production of melatonin with decreased exposure to sunlight	Older people do not go outside as much during the winter months.
Intrapersonal	Loss of person, object, self-esteem; hostility turned against the self; unachieved goals	Women are more dependent on others for self-esteem; older people suffer multiple losses.
Learning	Lack of control over experiences; learned helplessness; failure to adapt	Expectation of women's dependency reinforces helplessness; older people have increased stress with decreased resources, which contributes to loss of control.
Cognitive	Negative view of self, the present, and the future; focus on negative messages; cognitive errors	
Feminist	Internalization of cultural norms of behavior; rigid gender role and age expectations	Women's identity may be limited to the role of homemaker; employment positions are less prestigious; women may hold two full-time jobs. Older people suffer from the cultural value on youth and endure many role changes and losses.

TABLE 20–3 **Beck Depression Inventory**

The Beck Depression Inventory is a self-rating scale that measures depression. The client can complete the questionnaire in about 10 minutes. The total score provides an estimate of the degree of severity of the depressed mood. Add the raw scores. The mean scores can be interpreted as follows.

TOTAL SCORE	LEVELS OF DEPRESSION
1–10	Normal ups and downs
11–16	Mild mood disturbance
17–20	Borderline clinical depression
21–30	Moderate depression
31–40	Severe depression
Over 40	Extreme depression

(A persistent score of 17 or above indicates that professional treatment might be necessary.)

1. 0 I do not feel sad.
   1 I feel sad.
   2 I am sad all the time and I can't snap out of it.
   3 I am so sad or unhappy that I can't stand it.

2. 0 I am not particularly discouraged about the future.
   1 I feel discouraged about the future.
   2 I feel I have nothing to look forward to.
   3 I feel that the future is hopeless and that things cannot improve.

3. 0 I do not feel like a failure.
   1 I feel I have failed more than the average person.
   2 As I look back on my life, all I can see is a lot of failures.
   3 I feel I am a complete failure as a person.

4. 0 I get as much satisfaction out of things as I used to.
   1 I don't enjoy things the way I used to.
   2 I don't get real satisfaction out of anything anymore.
   3 I am dissatisfied or bored with everything.

5. 0 I don't feel particularly guilty.
   1 I feel guilty a good part of the time.
   2 I feel quite guilty most of the time.
   3 I feel guilty all of the time.

6. 0 I don't feel I am being punished.
   1 I feel I may be punished.
   2 I expect to be punished.
   3 I feel I am being punished.

7. 0 I don't feel disappointed in myself.
   1 I am disappointed in myself.
   2 I am disgusted with myself.
   3 I hate myself.

8. 0 I don't feel I am worse than anybody else.
   1 I am critical of myself for any weaknesses or mistakes.
   2 I blame myself all the time for my faults.
   3 I blame myself for everything bad that happens.

9. 0 I don't have any thoughts of killing myself.
   1 I have thoughts of killing myself, but I would not carry them out.
   2 I would like to kill myself.
   3 I would kill myself if I had the chance.

(continued)

TABLE 20–3 Beck Depression Inventory (continued)

10. 0 I don't cry any more than usual.
    1 I cry more now than usual.
    2 I cry all the time now.
    3 I used to be able to cry, but now I can't even though I want to.

11. 0 I am no more irritated by things than I ever am.
    1 I am slightly more irritated now than usual.
    2 I am quite annoyed or irritated a good deal of the time.
    3 I feel irritated all the time now.

12. 0 I have not lost interest in other people.
    1 I am less interested in other people than I used to be.
    2 I have lost most of any interest in other people.
    3 I have lost all of my interest in other people.

13. 0 I make decisions about as well as I ever could.
    1 I put off making decisions more than I used to.
    2 I have greater difficulty in making decisions than before.
    3 I can't make decisions at all anymore.

14. 0 I don't feel that I look any worse than I used to.
    1 I am worried that I am looking old or unattractive.
    2 I feel that there are permanent changes in my appearance that make me look unattractive.
    3 I believe that I look ugly.

15. 0 I can work about as well as before.
    1 I take an extra effort to get started doing something.
    2 I have to push myself very hard to do anything.
    3 I can't do any work at all.

16. 0 I can sleep as well as usual.
    1 I don't sleep as well as I used to.
    2 I wake up 1–2 hours earlier than I used to and cannot get back to sleep.
    3 I wake up several hours earlier than I used to and cannot get back to sleep.

17. 0 I don't get more tired than usual.
    1 I get tired more easily than I used to.
    2 I get tired from doing almost anything.
    3 I am too tired to do anything.

18. 0 My appetite is no worse than usual.
    1 My appetite is not as good as it used to be.
    2 My appetite is much worse now.
    3 I have no appetite at all anymore.

19. 0 I haven't lost much weight, if any, lately.
    1 I have lost more than 5 pounds.
    2 I have lost more than 10 pounds.
    3 I have lost more than 15 pounds.

20. 0 I am no more worried about my health than usual.
    1 I am worried about physical problems such as aches and pains, or upset stomach, or constipation.
    2 I am very worried about physical problems and it's hard to think of much else.
    3 I am so worried about my physical problems that I cannot think about anything else.

21. 0 I have not noticed any recent change in my interest in sex.
    1 I am less interested in sex than I used to be.
    2 I am much less interested in sex now.
    3 I have lost interest in sex completely.

Source: Reprinted with permission from Beck, A. T., Ward, C. H., Mendelson, M., Mock, J., & Erbaugh, J. (1961). Inventory for measuring depression. *Archives of General Psychiatry, 4,* 561–571.

People with mood disorders display a variety of characteristics involving changes in behavior, affect, cognition, and physiology. Somewhat similar changes occur for people experiencing grief. Table 20–4 differentiates between depression and grief during the assessment process.

The nurse conducting an assessment of the client who is suspected of having a mood disorder must remember that these disorders affect individuals in a variety of ways. The nurse should be aware that individuals with mood disorders may display changes in a number of characteristics, including behavioral, cognitive, and physiologic. Table 20–5 lists some of the most common characteristics of mood disorders.

Cultural Considerations

Appropriate expressions of mood are largely culturally determined. For example, situations in which people are expected to experience sadness, anger, loneliness, frustration, joy, or happiness are defined by the culture. Culture also determines how people are to behave when experiencing a variety of feelings. For example, cultural expectations of grieving individuals may be self-control and a "stiff upper lip" or may be loud mourning and ripping of clothing. Extreme pleasure may be expressed with a nod and a smile or may be expressed with loud laughter and exuberant behavior.

The Western interpretation of feelings is that emotions are intrapersonal. In contrast, in Micronesia, emotions are considered to be not within a person, but rather between people. In some Middle Eastern, African, Hispanic, and Chinese cultures, emotions are viewed and expressed in somatic (bodily) terms. The process by which psychological distress is experienced and communicated in the form of somatic symptoms is called **somatization**. Because these cultures are not subject to the mind–body dualism of Western thinking, psychological distress is viewed as arising from bodily imbalances (Chou, 2005).

Emotions of suffering and depression have dramatically different meaning and forms of expression in different cultures. Many Americans view suffering as unexpected or unacceptable and perceive depression as something to overcome through personal striving. Latin American cultures associate suffering with a deep sense of tragedy. Shi'ite Muslims view suffering within a religious context of martyrdom, while Buddhist cultures view suffering as a positive feature of life. Throughout the entire world, most cases of depression are experienced and expressed in bodily terms such as fatigue, headaches, heart distress, and dizziness. Only in Western cultures is that depression considered to be a mental disorder (Sethabouppha & Kane, 2005).

When nurses assess clients from cultures different from their own, they must understand that the expression of depression is culturally determined. Immigrants are at higher risk for depression as they cope with multiple stressors such as long-distance family relationships, unemployment or underemployment, discrimination, language problems, and a new environment. Immigrant children are at risk for depression as they are often expected to interpret the concerns of adult family members to outside authority figures such as doctors, nurses, teachers, and government officials (Aroian & Norris, 2002; Heilemann, Coffey-Love, & Frutos, 2004).

Rather than seeking professional help, African Americans and Latinos often look to their family and faith communities for help. There is a strong fear of hospitalization and involuntary commitment, both of which are more likely for African Americans and Latinos than for Euro-Americans. Children are less likely to receive outpatient treatment when compared to their Euro-American peers. Among older adults, African Americans are less likely to receive treatment for depression (37%) compared to 24% of Hispanics, 22% of Euro-Americans, and 14% of Asians. African Americans and Latinos who experience mood disorders are often misdiagnosed as having schizophrenia. As a result of this misdiagnosis, they may receive antipsychotic medication and no antidepressants. Thus, appropriate treatment is delayed, resulting in poorer therapeutic response (Draucker, 2005; Strothers et al., 2005).

TABLE 20–4 **Differences Between Depression and Grief**

TRAIT	DEPRESSION	GRIEF
Trigger	Specific trigger not necessary	Trigger usually loss or multiple losses
Active/passive	Passive behavior tends to keep them "stuck" in sadness	Actively feel their emotional pain and emptiness
Emotions	Generalized feeling of helplessness, hopelessness	Experience a range of emotions that are usually intense
Ability to laugh	Likely to be humorless and incapable of being happy or even temporarily cheered up; likely to resist support	Sometimes will be able to laugh and enjoy humor; more likely to accept support
Activities	Lack of interest in previously enjoyed activities	Can be persuaded to participate in activities, especially as they begin to heal
Self-esteem	Low self-esteem, low self-confidence; feels like a failure	Self-esteem usually remains intact; does not feel like a failure unless it relates directly to the loss
Feeling of failure	May dwell on past failures; catastrophize	Any self-blame or guilt relates directly to the loss; feelings resolve as they progress toward healing.

TABLE 20–5 **Characteristics of Mood Disorders**

CHARACTERISTIC	DEPRESSED STATE	MANIC STATE
Behavioral		
Desire to participate in activities	Decreased to absent	Interested in all activities; increase in high-risk behaviors
Interaction with others	Limited; client withdraws	Talkative, gregarious
Affiliation needs	Increased dependency	Independent, self-sufficient
Affective		
Mood	Despair, desolation	Unstable: euphoric and irritable
Guilt	High level	Unable to experience guilt
Crying spells	Frequent crying to inability to cry	May have brief episodes
Gratification	Loss of interest in pleasurable activities	Constantly seeking fun and excitement
Emotional attachments	Indifference to others	Forms intense attachments rapidly
Cognitive		
Self-evaluation	Focuses on failures; sees self as incompetent; catastrophizes and personalizes	Grandiose beliefs about self
Expectations	Believes present and future are hopeless; over generalizes one experience or fact	Inordinate positive expectations; unable to see potential negative outcomes
Self-criticism	Harshly critical of self; is a perfectionist; anticipates disapproval from others	Approves of own behavior; irate if criticized by others
Concentration	Decreased	Decreased
Decision-making ability	Decreased ability or inability to make decisions	Difficulty due to distractibility and impulsiveness
Flow of thought	Decreased rate and number of thoughts	Flight of ideas; can't be interrupted
Body image	Believes self unattractive or ugly	Believes self unusually beautiful
Delusions	Somatic delusions	Delusions of grandeur
Hallucinations	Occur in 15–25% of cases	Occur in 15–25% of cases
Sociocultural		
Sexual desire	Loss of desire	Increase in activity and partners
Physiologic		
Appetite	Increased or decreased in mild and moderate depression; decreased in severe depression	Difficulty eating due to inability to sit still
Amount of sleep	Increased or decreased in mild and moderate depression; decreased in severe depression	Sleeps only 1 or 2 hours a night
Activity level	Impaired motor activity; loss of energy	Hyperactivity; high energy
Bowel activity	Constipation	Constipation
Physical appearance	Unkempt; poor hygiene	Bright clothing; frequently changes clothing

CARING INTERVENTIONS

Nurses are in the singular position to provide a number of caring interventions for depressed clients and their families. The most important of these are preventing client suicide and promoting client and family safety.

Preventing Suicide and Promoting Safety

There are few times when *always* and *never* are applicable. Client safety, however, *always* takes priority over other nursing care concerns. Clients experiencing severe depression are at a high risk for suicide and violent behaviors. When the risk for self-directed violence is high, immediate intervention is necessary. The risk of suicide increases as the severest stage of depression is alleviated because clients then have sufficient energy and cognitive ability to plan and successfully implement a suicide plan. See Box 20–1 for guidelines to help prevent inpatient suicide and promote safety.

Encourage clients to discuss all of their feelings. Clients need to know that all feelings are valid and that it benefits them to express their emotions—particularly anger and hopelessness—rather than act them out through maladaptive behaviors. Having the feeling is always acceptable. Acting on the feeling,

Box 20–1 Preventing Inpatient Suicide and Promoting Safety

Check the policy and procedures of the individual inpatient treatment facility and implement those guidelines as well.

- Evaluate the level of suicide intent regularly and institute the appropriate level of staff supervision following unit protocol.
- Let suicidal clients know that the environment is safe for them. Remove sharp objects, razors, breakable glass items, mirrors, matches, and straps or belts and explain why these objects are being removed. Monitor the use of scissors, razors, and other potential weapons.
- Place suicidal clients in a centrally located room near the nurses' station to facilitate ease of observation.
- Avoid establishing a predictable pattern of observation during the day and especially at night.
- Be particularly alert during change of shifts and on holidays or other times when staffing is limited and during times of distraction, such as mealtimes and visiting hours.
- Examine items brought by visitors and monitor for safety.
- Encourage clients to seek you or another staff member when bothered by suicidal thoughts or impulses. Discussing these thoughts and impulses may be sufficient to diminish them and prevent a suicidal crisis from occurring. Avoid discussing suicidal ruminations in repetitious detail, as this may reinforce maladaptive behavior.

however, may be problematic. What counts in the long run is what a person decides to do about the feeling. Nurses should assist in the transition from hospital to home by helping clients identify people in their usual environments to whom they can express feelings candidly without being judged.

Use a calm, reassuring approach and teach calming measures such as time-outs and controlled breathing. Provide safe physical outlets for expression of anger or increasing tension.

Collaborate with clients to identify community resources to which they can turn if suicidal thoughts recur outside the treatment setting. Most communities provide hotlines that are staffed around the clock with trained volunteers or professionals who are available to discuss feelings before they reach crisis proportions. Collaborate with families to determine the risks for injury in the home (e.g., the presence of firearms) and to understand how the family plays a role in the client's illness.

Assertive Behavior

Assertiveness is a learned behavior. Everyone has assertiveness potential, but not everyone is born knowing how to be assertive. Children learn patterns of communicating from the adults around them. People can unlearn poor communication patterns that don't work and learn new ones, which is the idea behind assertiveness training. The goal is to help people express themselves without fear of disapproval from others. Being assertive does not guarantee that others will agree, but it does provide an individual the satisfaction of offering a personal opinion without ignoring the opinions of others.

Aggressive behavior is directed toward getting what one wants without considering the feelings of others. Aggressive communicators want to get their own way at any cost. They want others to "back off," and they use intimidation to convey this message. An example of aggressive behavior is insisting on going to a certain movie even though you know your companion does not enjoy that type of movie. The outcome of aggressive behavior is that although you may get what you want in the short run, others feel discredited and tend to avoid you.

Passive behavior consists of avoiding conflict at any cost, even at the expense of one's own happiness. An example of passive behavior is agreeing to go to a movie you don't want to see because your friend pressures you to go. Passive communicators hold their feelings in and allow anger to build up. Anger can explode suddenly or can be expressed in passive–aggressive behavior. An example of passive–aggressive behavior is taking a long time to get ready to go out while your friend is waiting because you are angry at him for insisting on seeing a movie you don't want to see. The outcome is that the passive person gives up control and is left with resentment, which usually emerges in other ways that damage relationships.

Assertive behavior consists of expressing one's wishes and opinions, or taking care of oneself, but not at the expense of others. An example of assertive communication is saying, "I really don't care for violent movies. Let's look at the movie listings and see if there is something playing that we can both enjoy." The outcome of assertive behavior is self-confidence and self-esteem. Helpful references include these books that can be obtained through a local library or bookseller: *The Assertiveness Handbook (Overcoming Common Problems),* by Mary Hartley, 2007; *Peace at Any Price: How to Overcome the Please Disease,* by Deborah Day Poor, 2005; and *Civilized Assertiveness for Women: Communication with Backbone . . . Not Bite,* by Judith Selee McClure, 2007.

Minimizing Maladaptive Dependence

Hopeless clients have a tendency to form dependent relationships. Nurses must work from the first contact with these clients to minimize the likelihood that maladaptive dependence occurs in the nurse–client relationship. Strategies to minimize maladaptive dependence include the following:

- Emphasize the short-term nature of the relationship.
- Recognize that a client who singles out one staff member exclusively and refuses to relate to others is developing dependence.
- Avoid giving dependent clients the hope that the nurse–client relationship can continue after therapy has ended.
- Refuse (kindly but firmly) requests for your address or telephone number.
- Remind clients that social contact will not be allowed.

If you find yourself wanting to continue relationships with certain clients, discuss these feelings with your instructor (if you are a student), your supervisor, or a respected professional peer (if you are a practicing nurse). It is essential that you separate your professional life from your social life.

DIAGNOSTIC TESTS

While no laboratory studies definitively diagnose mood disorders, some abnormal findings are noted more often in individuals with mood disorders than in control subjects. These findings are as follows:

- Sleep abnormalities in 40–60% of outpatients and up to 90% of inpatients with major depressive episode and in 25–50% of adults with dysthymic disorder; decreased need for sleep and abnormal polysomnographic (sleep study) findings in people with manic episode (sleep abnormalities may precede the onset of a mood disorder and may persist in the absence of other symptoms)
- Neurotransmitter and neuropeptide dysregulation in major depressive episode and manic episode
- Hormonal disturbances (blunted growth hormone and thyroid-stimulating hormone); elevated urinary free cortisol; dexamethasone nonsuppression of prolactin; elevated plasma cortisol
- Brain imaging studies that show increased blood flow in limbic and paralimbic regions and decreased blood flow in the lateral prefrontal cortex in depression; increased rates of right hemispheric lesions or bilateral subcortical or preventricular lesions in people with bipolar I disorder
- Preventricular vascular changes when depression begins late in life
- Urine and blood drug screens that may indicate a substance-induced mood disorder.

PHARMACOLOGIC THERAPIES

A number of medications are available for the treatment of mood disorders. Often they achieve greatest effect when used in combination with psychotherapy.

Antidepressants

Drugs used to treat depression are categorized as antidepressants. Antidepressants treat major depression by enhancing mood. Antidepressants are also sometimes prescribed to treat anxiety disorders. Recent studies link depression and anxiety to similar neurotransmitter dysfunction, and both seem to respond to treatment with antidepressant medications. Antidepressants are also beneficial in treating psychological and physical signs of pain, especially in clients without MDD (e.g., when mood problems are associated with debilitating conditions such as fibromyalgia or muscle spasticity).

There is one important warning about antidepressants: In 2004, the U.S. Food and Drug Administration (FDA) issued an advisory "black box warning" to be included at the beginning of drug package inserts and drug information sheets. The advisory was issued to clients, families, and health professionals to closely monitor adults and children taking antidepressants for warning signs of suicide, especially when treatment begins and when doses are changed. The FDA further advised that some signs might be expected in certain clients, including anxiety, panic attacks, agitation, irritability, insomnia, impulsivity, hostility, and mania. The warning applies especially to children, who are at a greater risk for suicidal ideation.

Depression is associated with dysfunction of neurotransmitters in certain regions of the brain. Although medication does not completely restore normal chemical balance, it may help reduce depressive symptoms while the client develops effective means of coping.

It is thought that antidepressants exert their effect through their action on certain neurotransmitters in the brain, including norepinephrine, DA, and 5-HT. The two basic mechanisms of action are blocking the enzymatic breakdown of norepinephrine and slowing the reuptake of serotonin. The four primary classes of antidepressant drugs are as follows:

- Tricyclic antidepressants (TCAs)
- Selective serotonin reuptake inhibitors (SSRIs)
- Monoamine oxidase inhibitors (MAOIs)
- Atypical antidepressants including the serotonin–norepinephrine reuptake inhibitors (SNRIs) and other atypical antidepressants.

TRICYCLIC ANTIDEPRESSANTS Named for their three-ring chemical structure, **tricyclic antidepressants (TCAs)** were the mainstay of depression pharmacotherapy from the early 1960s until the 1980s. They are still used today, although less frequently.

TCAs act by inhibiting the reuptake of both norepinephrine and serotonin into presynaptic nerve terminals. TCAs are used mainly for major depression and occasionally for milder situational depression.

Shortly after their approval as antidepressants in the 1950s, it was found that the TCAs produced fewer side effects and were less dangerous than MAOIs. However, TCAs have some unpleasant and serious side effects. The most common side effect is orthostatic hypotension, which is due to $alpha_1$ blockade on blood vessels. The most serious adverse effect occurs when TCAs accumulate in cardiac tissue. Although rare, cardiac dysrhythmias can occur.

Sedation is a frequently reported complaint at the initiation of therapy, though clients may become tolerant to this effect after several weeks of treatment. Most TCAs have a long half-life, which increases the risk of side effects for clients with delayed excretion. Anticholinergic effects such as dry mouth, constipation, urinary retention, excessive perspiration, blurred vision, and tachycardia are common. These effects are less severe if the drug is gradually increased to the therapeutic dose over 2–3 weeks. Significant drug interactions can occur with CNS depressants, sympathomimetics, anticholinergics, and MAOIs. Since the advent of newer antidepressants that have fewer side effects, TCAs are less frequently used as first-line drugs in the treatment of depression and/or anxiety.

Nursing Considerations The role of the nurse in TCA therapy involves careful monitoring of a client's condition and providing education as it relates to the prescribed drug treatment. The therapeutic effects of TCAs may take 2–6 weeks to occur. Suicide potential increases as blood levels of a TCA increase but have not yet reached their peak therapeutic levels. Monitor the client closely for symptoms of suicidal ideation throughout treatment. As clients begin to recover from both psychological and physical depression (psychological depression slows all body processes), their energy level rises.

Assessing previous health history is essential. Tricyclic antidepressants are contraindicated in clients in the acute recovery phase of an MI, with heart block, or with a history of dysrhythmias because of the effects of TCAs on cardiac tissue. Because TCAs lower the seizure threshold, carefully monitor clients with epilepsy. Clients with urinary retention, narrow-angle glaucoma, or prostatic hypertrophy may not be good candidates for TCAs because of anticholinergic side effects. Annoying anticholinergic effects, coupled with the weight gain effect of TCAs, may lead to noncompliance. Tricyclics must be given with extreme caution to clients with asthma, cardiovascular disorders, gastrointestinal disorders, alcoholism, and other psychiatric disorders including schizophrenia and bipolar disorders. Most TCAs are pregnancy category C or D, so they are used during pregnancy or lactation only when medically necessary.

Significant drug interactions may occur with TCAs. Oral contraceptives may decrease the efficacy of tricyclics. Cimetidine (Tagamet) interferes with their metabolism and excretion. Tricyclics affect the efficacy of clonidine (Catapres) and guanethidine (Ismelin). The nurse should observe clients for the effects of drugs that enhance the effects of TCAs, such as antidysrhythmics, antihistamines, antihypertensives, and CNS depressants. Clients who take cimetidine and atropine also should be monitored. Some drugs increase the rate of TCA metabolism and excretion from the body. These include carbamazepine (Tegretol), phenytoin (Dilantin), and rifampin (Rifadin). Cigarette smoking also diminishes the effect of TCAs.

Client Teaching Client education as it relates to TCAs should include the goals of therapy, the reasons for obtaining baseline data such as vital signs and the existence of underlying cardiac and renal disorders, and possible drug side effects. Include the following points when teaching clients about TCAs:

- Be aware that it may take several weeks or more to achieve the full therapeutic effect of the drug.
- Keep all scheduled follow-up appointments with your health care provider.
- Understand that sweating, along with anticholinergic side effects, may occur.
- Take the medication exactly as prescribed and report side effects if they occur.
- Do not take other prescription drugs, over-the-counter (OTC) medications, or herbal remedies without notifying your health care provider.
- Avoid using alcohol and other CNS depressants.
- Change positions slowly to avoid dizziness.
- Do not drive or engage in hazardous activities until the drug's sedative effect is known.
- Take the drug at bedtime if sedation occurs.
- Immediately discuss with your health care provider an intention or desire to become pregnant because these drugs must be withdrawn over several weeks and not discontinued abruptly.

SELECTIVE SEROTONIN REUPTAKE INHIBITORS Drugs that slow the reuptake of serotonin into presynaptic nerve terminals are called **selective serotonin reuptake inhibitors (SSRIs)**. They have become drugs of choice in the treatment of depression because of their favorable side-effect profile.

Serotonin is a natural neurotransmitter in the CNS, found in high concentrations in certain neurons in the hypothalamus, limbic system, medulla, and spinal cord. Serotonin is important to several body activities, including the cycling between NREM and REM sleep, pain perception, and emotional states. Lack of adequate serotonin in the CNS can lead to depression. Serotonin is metabolized to a less active substance by the enzyme monoamine oxidase (MAO). Serotonin is also known by its chemical name, 5-hydroxytryptamine (5-HT).

In the 1970s, it became increasingly clear that serotonin had a more substantial role in depression than was once thought. Clinicians knew that the TCAs altered the sensitivity of serotonin to certain receptors in the brain, but they did not know how this change was connected with depression. Ongoing efforts to find antidepressants with fewer side effects led to the development of a third category of medications, the selective serotonin reuptake inhibitors (SSRIs).

Whereas the tricyclic class inhibits the reuptake of both norepinephrine and serotonin into presynaptic nerve terminals, the SSRIs selectively target serotonin. Increased levels of serotonin in the synaptic gap induce complex neurotransmitter changes in presynaptic and postsynaptic neurons in the brain. Presynaptic receptors become less sensitive, and postsynaptic receptors become more sensitive.

Nursing Considerations The role of the nurse in SSRI therapy involves careful monitoring of a client's condition and providing education as it relates to the prescribed drug treatment. Assess the client's needs for antidepressant therapy by noting the intensity and duration of symptoms and identifying factors that led to depression, such as life events and health changes. Obtain a careful drug history, including the use of CNS depressants, alcohol, and other antidepressants, especially MAOI therapy, because these may interact with SSRIs. Assess for hypersensitivity to SSRIs. Also ask the client about suicidal ideation because the drugs may take several weeks before full therapeutic benefit is obtained. Because these drugs have a high incidence of sexual side effects, obtain a history of any disorders of sexual function. Note any history of eating disorders; SSRIs commonly cause weight gain, which may contribute to noncompliance in clients with distortions and concerns about body image.

Although the SSRIs are safer than other antidepressants, serious adverse effects can still occur. Obtain baseline liver function tests because SSRIs are metabolized in the liver and hepatic disease can result in higher serum levels. Obtain a baseline body weight to monitor weight gain.

Client Teaching Client education as it relates to SSRIs should include the goals of therapy, the reasons for obtaining baseline data such as vital signs and the existence of underlying disorders or concurrent medication use, and possible drug side effects. Include the following points when teaching clients about SSRIs:

- Know that SSRIs may take up to 5 weeks to reach their maximum therapeutic effectiveness.
- Do not take any prescription drugs, OTC drugs, or herbal products without notifying your health care provider.
- Keep all follow-up appointments with your health care provider.
- Report side effects, including nausea, vomiting, diarrhea, sexual dysfunction, and fatigue.
- Do not drive or engage in hazardous activities until the drug's sedative effect is known.
- Do not stop taking the drug suddenly after long-term use because withdrawal symptoms can occur. Although these symptoms are not life-threatening, they are uncomfortable.
- Take most SSRIs in the morning with food to avoid gastrointestinal upset and insomnia. Lexapro and Zoloft may be taken in the morning or evening. Take Remerron at bedtime because it usually causes excessive drowsiness, especially at lower doses.
- Exercise and restrict caloric intake to avoid weight gain.

MONOAMINE OXIDASE INHIBITORS The group of drugs called **monoamine oxidase inhibitors (MAOIs)** inhibit monoamine oxidase, the enzyme that terminates the actions of neurotransmitters such as DA, norepinephrine, epinephrine, and serotonin. Because of their low safety margin, these drugs are reserved for clients who have not responded to TCAs or SSRIs.

The MAOIs were the first drugs approved to treat depression, introduced in the 1950s. They are as effective as TCAs and SSRIs in treating depression. However, because of drug–drug and food–drug interactions, hepatotoxicity, and the development of safer antidepressants, MAOIs are now reserved for clients who are not responsive to other antidepressant classes.

Common side effects of the MAOIs include orthostatic hypotension, headache, insomnia, and diarrhea. A primary concern is that these agents interact with a large number of foods and other medications—sometimes with serious effects. A hypertensive crisis can occur when an MAOI is used concurrently with other antidepressants or sympathomimetic drugs. Combining an MAOI with an SSRI can produce serotonin syndrome. If MAOIs are given with antihypertensives, the client can experience excessive hypotension. MAOIs also potentiate the hypoglycemic effects of insulin and oral antidiabetic drugs. Hyperpyrexia is known to occur in clients taking MAOIs with meperidine (Demerol), dextromethorphan (Pediacare and others), and TCAs.

A hypertensive crisis also can result from an interaction between MAOIs and foods containing tyramine, a form of the amino acid tyrosine. Tyramine is usually degraded by MAO in the intestines. If a client is taking MAOIs, however, tyramine enters the bloodstream in high amounts and displaces norepinephrine in presynaptic nerve terminals. The result is a sudden release of norepinephrine, causing acute hypertension. Symptoms usually occur within minutes of ingesting the food and include occipital headache, stiff neck, flushing, palpitations, diaphoresis, and nausea. Myocardial infarctions (MIs) and cerebral vascular accidents, although rare, are possible consequences as well. Calcium channel blockers may be given as an antidote. Because of their serious side effects when taken with food and drugs, MAOIs are rarely used and are limited to clients with symptoms that are resistant to the more typical antidepressants and who are likely to comply with the restrictions regarding foods and drugs. Examples of foods containing tyramine are listed in Table 20–6.

Nursing Considerations The role of the nurse in MAOI therapy involves careful monitoring of a client's condition and providing education as it relates to the prescribed drug treatment. A client taking an MAOI must refrain from foods that contain tyramine, which is found in many common foods. Assess cardiovascular status because these agents may affect blood pressure. Phenelzine (Nardil) is contraindicated in cardiovascular disease, heart failure, CVA, hepatic or renal dysfunction, and

TABLE 20–6 **Foods Containing Tyramine**

FRUITS	DAIRY PRODUCTS	ALCOHOL	MEATS
avocados	cheese (cottage cheese is okay)	beer	beef or chicken liver
bananas	sour cream	wines (especially red wines)	paté
raisins	yogurt		meat extracts
papaya products, including meat tenderizers			pickled or kippered herring or pepperoni
canned figs			salami
			sausage
			bologna/hot dogs
VEGETABLES	**SAUCES**	**YEAST**	**OTHER FOODS TO AVOID**
pods of broad beans (fava beans)	soy sauce	all yeast or yeast extracts	chocolate

paranoid schizophrenia. Obtain a CBC because MAOIs can inhibit platelet function. Assess for the possibility of pregnancy because these agents are pregnancy category C and enter breast milk. Use MAOIs with caution in epilepsy because they may lower the seizure threshold.

Take a careful drug history; common drugs that may interact with an MAOI include other MAOIs, insulin, caffeine-containing products, other antidepressants, meperidine (Demerol), and possibly opioids and methyldopa (Aldomet). There must be at least a 14-day interval between the use of MAOIs and these other drugs.

Some clients may not achieve the full therapeutic benefits of an MAOI for 4–8 weeks. Because depression continues during this time, clients may discontinue the drug if they believe it is not helping them. Symptoms of sleep disorder or anxiety are treated with short-term antianxiety agents and sleep aids until the therapeutic effects of the medication are achieved.

Because of the serious side effects that are possible with MAOIs, client education is vital. The client's ability to comprehend restrictions and be compliant with them may be impaired when the client is in a severely depressed state.

Client Teaching Client education as it relates to MAOIs should include the goals of therapy, the reasons for obtaining baseline data such as vital signs and the existence of underlying disorders, and possible drug side effects. Include the following points when teaching clients and their caregivers about MAOIs:

- Strictly observe dietary restrictions for foods containing tyramine.
- Do not take any prescription, OTC drugs, or herbal products without notifying your health care provider.
- Avoid caffeine.
- Wear a medic alert bracelet identifying the MAOI medication.
- Be aware that it may take several weeks or more to obtain the full therapeutic effect of the drug.
- Keep all follow-up appointments with your health care provider.
- Do not drive or engage in hazardous activities until the drug's sedative effect is known; it may be taken at bedtime if sedation occurs.
- Observe for and report signs of impending stroke or MI.

ATYPICAL ANTIDEPRESSANTS The atypical antidepressants do not fit into the three major drug classes. Duloxetine (Cymbalta) and venlafaxine (Effexor), examples of atypical antidepressants, are SNRIs. They inhibit the reabsorption of serotonin and norepinephrine and elevate mood by increasing the levels of serotonin, norepinephrine, and DA in the CNS. Venlafaxine (Effexor), more recently used to relieve the symptoms of depression, is available in an intermediate-release form that requires two or three doses a day and an extended-release form that allows the client to take the medication just once a day.

Bupropion (Wellbutrin) not only inhibits the reuptake of serotonin, but may also affect the activity of norepinephrine and DA. It should be used with caution in clients with seizure disorders because it lowers the seizure threshold. Mirtazapine (Remeron), used for depression, blocks presynaptic serotonin and norepinephrine receptors, thereby enhancing release of neurotransmitters from nerve terminals. Nefazodone (Serzone) is similar to Remeron. It was originally designed to treat depression while causing minimal cardiovascular effects, fewer anticholinergic effects, less sedation, and less sexual dysfunction than the other antidepressants.

Drugs for Bipolar Disorders

Drugs for bipolar disorders are called **mood stabilizers** because they have the ability to moderate extreme shifts in emotions between mania and depression. Some antiseizure drugs also are used for mood stabilization in bipolar clients. Table 20–7 lists medications more commonly prescribed for the treatment of bipolar disorders. Further information about pharmacologic therapies for bipolar disorders is provided in Exemplar 20.1.

PRACTICE ALERT

People with bipolar disorders who are in the depressive phase and prescribed *only* an antidepressant are at high risk for switching to a manic episode. For that reason, mood stabilizers are always prescribed at the same time (Brown, 2004).

NURSING CONSIDERATIONS The role of the nurse in lithium therapy involves carefully monitoring a client's condition and providing education as it relates to prescribed drug treatment. Because lithium is a salt, clients with a history of cardiovascular and kidney disease should not take it. Clients frequently experience dehydration and sodium depletion; therefore, clients on a low-salt diet should not be prescribed lithium. Assess for and identify signs and symptoms of lithium toxicity, which includes diarrhea, lethargy, slurred speech, muscle weakness, ataxia, seizures, edema, hypotension, and circulatory collapse.

CLIENT TEACHING Client education as it relates to lithium therapy should include the goals of therapy, the reasons for obtaining baseline data such as vital signs and the existence of cardiac and renal disorders, and possible drug side effects. Include the following points when teaching clients about lithium:

- Take medication as ordered because compliance is the key to successful treatment.
- Keep all scheduled laboratory visits to monitor lithium levels.
- Do not change diet or decrease fluid intake because any changes in diet and fluid status can affect therapeutic drug levels.
- Avoid alcohol use.
- Do not take other prescription medications, OTC drugs, or herbal products without notifying your health care provider.

PRACTICE ALERT

Aripiprazole (Abilify) is an antipsychotic that may be prescribed for clients with manic or mixed episodes of schizophrenia. It is sometimes prescribed for depressed clients along with an antidepressant when the client's depression is not controlled by an antidepressant alone. Aripiprazole carries a black box warning because older adults with dementia who take antipsychotics are at a greater risk for stroke or death while being treated with aripiprazole. As with other antidepressants, aripiprazole carries an increased risk for suicidal behaviors (Medline Plus, 2008).

TABLE 20–7 **Drugs for Bipolar Disorders**

DRUG	ROUTE AND ADULT DOSE (MAXIMUM DOSE WHERE INDICATED)	ADVERSE EFFECTS
lithium (Eskalith)	po; initial: 600 mg tid; maintenance: 300 mg tid (max: 2.4 g/day)	*Headache, lethargy, fatigue, recent memory loss, nausea, vomiting, anorexia, abdominal pain, diarrhea, dry mouth, muscle weakness* Peripheral circulatory collapse
aripiprazole	Poor injection; dosages vary.	*Akathisia, headache, nausea, vomiting, constipation, dizziness, anxiety, restlessness* Increased risk of stroke and mortality in older adults; as with other antidepressants, increased risk of suicidal behavior
ANTISEIZURE DRUGS		
carbamazepine (Tegretol)	po; 200 mg bid, gradually increased to 800–1200 mg/day in 3 to 4 divided doses	*Dizziness, ataxia, somnolence, headache, nausea, diplopia, blurred vision, sedation, drowsiness, nausea, vomiting, prolonged bleeding time*
lamotrigine (Lamictal)	po; 50 mg/day for 2 weeks, then 50 mg bid for 2 weeks; may increase gradually up to 300–500 mg/day in 2 divided doses (max: 700 mg/day)	Heart block, aplastic anemia, respiratory depression, exfoliative dermatitis, Stevens-Johnson syndrome, toxic epidermal necrolysis, deep coma, death (with overdose), liver failure, pancreatitis
valproic acid (Depakene)	po; 250 mg tid (max: 60 mg/kg/day)	

Italics indicate common adverse effects; underlining indicates serious adverse effects.

Developmental Considerations

To date, no psychotropic medication has been approved by the FDA for use during pregnancy. On the other hand, abrupt discontinuation of maintenance medications including antipsychotics, antidepressants, and mood stabilizers has been associated with a high, early relapse risk. The practice of abrupt discontinuation of these medications to minimize potential birth defects can place a woman and her fetus at risk due to impulsive or self-injurious behavior, substance abuse, or inattention to prenatal care. Untreated mood disorders during pregnancy have been associated with premature delivery, low birth weight, and infant's lower Apgar score.

Tricyclic antidepressants (TCAs) and SSRIs have not generally been associated with a high risk of major birth defects. Lamotrigine (Lamictal) appears to be safer than the other anticonvulsants. Lithium doses should be decreased at the onset of labor to avoid maternal toxicity at delivery. Divalproex (Depakote) should be switched to another mood stabilizer before conception because of the higher-than-average risk for neural tube defects. Carbamazepine (Tegretol) should be used during pregnancy only when there are no other options, as this medication is associated with craniofacial defects and developmental delay (Yonkers et al., 2004).

Women who are breastfeeding and need antidepressant medication can usually take the SSRIs and anticonvulsants safely, although the infant should be monitored periodically. Taking medication immediately after breastfeeding minimizes the amount present in milk and maximizes clearance before the next feeding. Dosage should be as low as possible while still being clinically effective (Gjerdingen, 2003; Yonkers et al., 2004).

Women with postpartum depression have a 25% risk of recurrence with future pregnancies. It is suggested that at-risk women be treated with antidepressants after birth for as long as 26 weeks.

Medication is considered for children and adolescents in the following situations:

- Severe symptoms that prevent effective psychotherapy
- Psychosis
- Chronic or recurrent episodes.

The mood stabilizers lamotrigine (Lamictal) and gabapentin (Neurontin) should never be used in clients younger than 16 due to the risk of developing Stevens-Johnson syndrome.

The clinical response to antidepressant medications in older depressed clients is often delayed. The average time for easing of symptoms is 12–13 weeks. Studies show that while only 30% of older adults responded by week 6 of treatment, the number jumped to 55% at week 12. This suggests that longer treatment periods may be important in evaluating the effectiveness in older adults (Bondareff et al., 2000).

NONPHARMACOLOGIC THERAPIES

A number of nonpharmacologic therapies are available to those clients experiencing depression. Psychotherapy is used most frequently, often in combination with pharmacologic therapy. Electroconvulsive therapy is typically reserved for clients who are difficult to treat, while alternative therapies are often tried by clients in addition to more traditional therapies.

Psychotherapy

While medication alone may be adequate to treat situational or acute onset depression, chronic depression often requires both medication and psychotherapy. One of the most successful forms of psychotherapy is CBT. However, there are a number of different forms of psychotherapy that may be considered. The best approach to psychotherapy is chosen based on the cause and symptoms of the depressive condition as well as the client's needs and personality.

COGNITIVE-BEHAVIORAL THERAPY Cognitive-behavioral therapy (CBT) is a combination therapy. The behavioral aspect helps people identify habitual reactions to troublesome situations. It also teaches them how to relax and calm their bodies. The *cognitive* aspect focuses on distorted thinking patterns that cause unpleasant feelings or symptoms of mental disorders. The role of the therapist is that of a coach or tutor, and there is shared responsibility to work as a team to explore problems. The goal of CBT is accurate and rational thinking based on logic and available facts.

When participating in CBT, clients initially identify the most troubling problems in their lives. The therapist then helps them problem-solve by asking the following questions:

- What happens? What do you *think* when this happens? What do you *feel?* What do you *do?*
- When does this happen? Where? With whom? What are the consequences?
- Why do you think this happens to you?
- How does this relate to your ideas about how things are or ought to be in your world?
- How often do you expect similar problems to happen to you in the future?
- How can you change this situation or learn to accept it?

Cognitive-behavioral therapists utilize various techniques. One is *cognitive modification* of negative automatic thoughts or maladaptive schemas. Every person has automatic thoughts, some of which are helpful and some of which are negative. An example is that a person's teenage daughter is 1 hour late for her curfew and has not called. The person's automatic thought might be one of the following: "She must have been in an accident and can't call." "She cares so little for me that she can't call even though she knows how much I worry." "She is just trying to 'push my buttons' and rebel against the rules." "She is usually very responsible, so I am sure she will be home soon and will be able to tell me what happened."

Automatic thoughts that have a theme are called *schemas.* They are basic assumptions or beliefs about oneself and the world. Examples of maladaptive schemas are "Nobody in my life has ever respected me," "I am not lovable," or "My mother was right—I really am stupid." Cognitive-behavioral therapists help clients identify these patterns of irrational thinking and find ways to replace them with more logical and fact-based patterns of thinking.

Relaxation training is one of the behavioral techniques used in this type of therapy. It is difficult to think clearly when one is anxious, angry, or resentful. *Behavioral activation* involves strategies that get clients actively involved in their treatment. For example, a person with depression may develop lists of pleasurable activities, schedule some of these, actually participate in the activity, and then evaluate the impact of the activity on thoughts and feelings.

Most often people go through daily routines with little awareness or attention. People read while they eat, exercise while watching television, or cook while talking to their children, and the nuances of these experiences are lost. This situation might be called living mindlessly by ignoring present moments. *Mindfulness,* another technique, is the opposite of living on "automatic pilot." It is the art of conscious living by focusing one's full attention on the activity at hand. While it may be simple to practice mindfulness, it is not necessarily easy. Habitual unawareness is persistent, and mindfulness requires effort and discipline. Cognitive-behavioral therapists believe that the way for people to start changing their minds is not to force the change, but to watch it. Through the process of mindfulness, people can learn to identify destructive thought patterns, simply label them, and watch them pass by whenever they come to mind. As people learn how their brains "tell stories," they can begin to change their negative automatic thoughts and schemas.

Cognitive-behavioral group therapy is often the treatment of choice for clients experiencing depression. The group setting allows people the opportunity to practice new ways of interacting with others while receiving immediate feedback (Chen, Lu, Chang, Chu, & Chou, 2006).

Electroconvulsive Therapy

Electroconvulsive therapy (ECT), a treatment procedure during which an electric current is passed through the brain, is useful to clients with severe depression, acute mania, some psychotic conditions, and those who are acutely suicidal. It is usually given several times a week until a course of 12 treatments is completed. Caution is advised when ECT is administered to clients with increased intracranial pressure and those who have had recent MIs.

Electroconvulsive therapy may be useful for a variety of clients. It is a safer alternative for highly suicidal clients, those who suffer from psychotic depression, and those who are medically deteriorated. In addition, it is a safe alternative for children and adolescents. Electroconvulsive therapy is safe in all trimesters of pregnancy and may be less harmful to the fetus than psychotropic medications. Clients who do not respond to medications or cannot tolerate the side effects often respond positively to ECT. Because of concurrent medications, poor tolerance of the side effects of psychotropic medications, and marked disability with depression, ECT is often the treatment of choice in older clients (Valdivia & Rossy, 2004).

During a course of ECT, a transient short-term memory loss is expected. This is distressing to some clients, and they need to be reassured that memory is usually completely restored. Because ECT is not curative, ongoing psychotherapy and pharmacotherapy are often continued to prevent relapse.

Alternative Therapies

In community surveys, depression, fatigue, insomnia, and anxiety are among the most commonly reported reasons for the use of alternative therapies. The following are some alternative therapies used for mood disorders.

TRANSCRANIAL MAGNETIC STIMULATION Repetitive transcranial magnetic stimulation (rTMS) is the use of a magnetic field that passes through the skull, causing cells in the cerebral cortex to fire. Repetitive transcranial magnetic stimulation in depression is the most-studied clinical application in psychiatry. The target area is the left prefrontal cortex, which is the brain area thought to be disrupted in depression. Targeting the opposite lobe, the right prefrontal cortex, has therapeutic effects in manic episodes. This therapy has a rapid onset of action of 1–2 weeks, which is faster than most psychotropic medications. Electroconvulsive therapy and rTMS have the same effectiveness in depression without psychosis, while depression with psychosis is best treated with ECT. There are several ongoing studies using oscillating magnetic fields similar to those used in functional magnetic resonance imaging (fMRI), especially with people having bipolar disorders (Brown, 2004; Rohan et al., 2004).

VAGUS NERVE STIMULATION Vagus nerve stimulation (VNS) has been used successfully with hard-to-treat seizure disorders and has FDA approval for this use. Noticing an improvement in subjects' moods, researchers are now studying VNS for people suffering from treatment-resistant depression. A cookie-size generator that is surgically implanted under the skin in the chest conveys electrical impulses via a connecting wire to the vagus nerve. The nerve is a leading provider of information from the heart and other organs to the brain; it also affects areas of the brain involved with mood. It provides continuous therapy for 8–12 years, which is the life of the implant's battery. Vagus nerve stimulation is most effective in people who have low to moderate, but not severe, resistance to antidepressants (Brown, 2004).

EXERCISE There have been numerous studies on the effect of exercise on depression. Short periods of vigorous aerobic exercise or longer periods of nonaerobic exercise for at least several weeks is most helpful in mild to moderate depression. Exercise raises levels of endorphins, which enhance one's feelings of well-being. Exercise also increases levels of DA, 5-HT, and NE, which are related to feelings of reward, motivation, and attention.

Yoga has been found to improve wellness and prevent disorders such as depression. The gentle nature of the exercises allows its use in almost any condition. People who practice yoga on a regular basis report improved life satisfaction, alertness, enthusiasm, and mental and physical energy, all of which are the opposite of the symptoms of depression (Kabat-Zinn, 2003).

ST. JOHN'S WORT St. John's wort (*Hypericum perforatum*) has been the most widely publicized alternative treatment for mild to moderate depression. The side effects of St. John's wort in higher doses are similar to that of SSRIs. The dosage is 300–600 mg/day of 0.3% hypericin, the active component in St. John's wort. It should *not* be combined with prescription antidepressants. It also may interfere with the action of anticonvulsants. There are insufficient data to recommend this herb for children. St. John's wort has been found to reduce the effectiveness of birth control pills, HIV treatment medications, and the asthma medication theophylline (Basch & Ulbricht, 2005).

SAME A nutritional supplement called SAMe (pronounced "sammy") has been used by more than 1 million people in Europe, primarily for depression and arthritis. SAMe (S-adenosylmethionine), a compound made by every cell in the body, helps produce DA, 5-HT, and NE. Numerous trials have found SAMe to be effective in treating depression, postpartum depression, and postmenopausal depression. It may, however, worsen bipolar depression. Its rapid onset (10–12 days), low side effects (no weight gain or sexual dysfunction), and ability to boost antioxidants give it many advantages in the treatment of depression. The dose is 800–1,600 mg/day and is best taken 30 minutes before meals. It has been successfully used as augmentation of all categories of antidepressants without adverse effects, and there is no evidence that it interacts with other medications. Side effects are generally mild and temporary (headaches, loose bowels, anxiety, and insomnia). Like TCAs, SAMe should be used with caution in people who have a history of cardiac arrhythmia. Infants normally have a three to four times naturally higher level of SAMe than do adults. Given this knowledge, the amount of SAMe passing to infants through breast milk may be inconsequential (Goren, Stoll, Damico, Sarmiento, & Cohen, 2004).

VITAMIN B Vitamin B is necessary for the production of DA, 5-HT, and NE, as well as for the natural synthesis of SAMe. One study found that individuals with a significant vitamin B deficiency were at twice the risk of depression than those who had normal levels. Depression itself could cause low levels through decreased appetite and resulting decreased food intake. In addition, many of the TCAs deplete the body of vitamin B (Hvas, Juul, Bech, & Nexo, 2004).

TYROSINE Tyrosine, an amino acid, is the precursor for DA and NE and, as such, acts as a mood elevator. Supplemental tyrosine has been used in depression, stress reduction, anxiety, and chronic fatigue. People taking MAOIs should not take any supplements containing tyrosine, as it may lead to a hypertensive crisis. Tyrosine combined with vitamin B_6 and vitamin C will provide better absorption.

MELATONIN Insomnia is a frequent complaint among people suffering from depression. Melatonin, a hormone secreted by the pineal gland, plays a critical role in the regulation of the day–night cycle. Studies have shown that melatonin is effective in inducing sleep and has no notable side effects. Slow-release melatonin combined with standard antidepressant treatment often improves the sleep pattern in depressed individuals.

OMEGA-3 FATTY ACIDS A number of studies have been done on the effects of omega-3 fatty acids from concentrated fish oils on mood disorders. Omega-3 fatty acids are thought to act on cells similar to lithium, to block calcium channels as do the other mood stabilizers, and to help regulate 5-HT. It appears to be an antidepressant, an antimanic, and a mood stabilizer. Research shows significantly low levels of omega-3 fatty acids in depression, and the lower the levels, the more severe the depression. The recommended dose is 5 grams per day, which is usually seven or eight capsules. The maximum dose is 15 grams daily. Taking the capsules at night with orange juice cuts down on the fishy aftertaste (Basch & Ulbricht, 2005).

ACUPUNCTURE Acupuncture is helpful in relieving feelings of depression and anxiety, most likely related to the rise in endorphin levels as a result of the treatment. Adding electrostimulation to acupuncture needles usually increases the effectiveness of the treatment. After only a single session, many people report a sense of well-being. Two rigorous studies found acupuncture to be as effective as TCAs. It is unclear how helpful acupuncture is for bipolar disorders. Client response appears to be quite variable at the present time (Larzelere & Wiseman, 2002).

ANIMAL-ASSISTED THERAPY Companionship with animals is associated with people experiencing less depression and loneliness. Animals provide meaningful and substantial comfort for many individuals. Studies show that older women (who are at higher risk for depression) who live alone tend to be in better emotional health when they live with an animal. They were less lonely, more optimistic, and more interested in the future than women who lived alone without a pet (Hart, 2000).

MUSIC THERAPY Music has often been used in healing—from the ancient sounds of the drum, rattle, bone flute, and other primitive instruments to the current use of music as a prescription for good health. In a study of 54 people who were clinically depressed and on medication, there was meaningful clinical improvement following 2 weeks of music therapy (Hsu & Lai, 2004).

Care of the client experiencing depression requires an individualized plan of care that is revised based on the client's response. Different treatment options may need to be tried before the one that works best for the client is found. Careful assessment of the client's mental status, screening for suicidal ideation, and ongoing evaluation to determine client response to treatment is a primary focus of nursing care. It is also important to reassure the client that depression is often successfully treated because hope can help the client focus on the future.

20.1 BIPOLAR DISORDERS

KEY TERMS

Bipolar disorders, *1177*
Cyclothymic disorder, *1180*
Flight of ideas, *1179*
Hypomania, *1179*
Mania, *1179*

BASIS FOR SELECTION OF EXEMPLAR

Healthy People 2010
National Institute of Mental Health

LEARNING OUTCOMES

After reading about this exemplar, you will be able to:

1. Describe the pathophysiology, psychopathology, and clinical manifestations of bipolar disorder.
2. Identify risk factors associated with bipolar disorders.
3. Illustrate the nursing process in providing culturally competent care across the life span for individuals with bipolar disorder.
4. Formulate priority nursing diagnoses appropriate for an individual with bipolar disorder.
5. Create a plan of care for individuals with bipolar disorder and their family members.
6. Assess expected outcomes for an individual with bipolar disorder.
7. Discuss therapies used in the collaborative care of an individual with bipolar disorder.
8. Employ evidence-based caring interventions for an individual with bipolar disorder.

OVERVIEW

The **bipolar disorders** are a group of mood disorders that include manic episodes, hypomanic episodes, mixed episodes, depressed episodes, and cyclothymic disorder. The *DSM-IV TR* diagnostic criteria for these disorders are listed in Box 20–2. Although only 1% of the population is diagnosed with bipolar disorders, the disorders can have a tremendous impact on those closest to the person with the disorder.

Bipolar I disorder consists of one or more manic or mixed episodes, and the course of illness can be accompanied by major depressive episodes. *Bipolar II disorder* consists of one or more major depressive episodes accompanied by at least one hypomanic episode.

Bipolar disorders tend to be recurrent and have the unusual tendency to increase in frequency as the individual ages. The majority of bipolar I disorder clients do not have the chance to experience a baseline mood—called *euthymic*—because a major depressive episode quickly follows. Many clients return to normal functioning during remissions, but approximately 20–30% have residual mood symptoms, and as many as 60% have continuing interpersonal and occupational difficulties. Of clients with bipolar II disorder, 5–10% have four or more mood episodes in a given year and approximately 15% experience continuing mood lability and interpersonal and occupational difficulties (APA, 2000).

Bipolar disorders typically appear between the ages of 15 and 30. Risk factors include a family history of bipolar disorders, drug abuse, periods of very high stress, and a major life-altering event. Women and men are at equal risk of having bipolar disorders.

Box 20–2 *DSM-IV TR* Diagnostic Criteria for Bipolar Disorders

MANIC EPISODE

A. A distinct period of abnormally and persistently elevated, expansive, or irritable mood, lasting at least 1 week (or any duration if hospitalization is necessary).

B. During the period of mood disturbance, three (or more) of the following symptoms have persisted (four if the mood is only irritable) and have been present to a significant degree:

1. inflated self-esteem or grandiosity
2. decreased need for sleep (e.g., feels rested after only 3 hours of sleep)
3. more talkative than usual or pressure to keep talking
4. flight of ideas or subjective experience that thoughts are racing
5. distractibility (i.e., attention too easily drawn to unimportant or irrelevant external stimuli)
6. increase in goal-directed activity (either socially, at work or school, or sexually) or psychomotor agitation
7. excessive involvement in pleasurable activities that have a high potential for painful consequences (e.g., engaging in unrestrained buying sprees, sexual indiscretions, or foolish business investments)

C. The symptoms do not meet criteria for a Mixed Episode.

D. The mood disturbance is sufficiently severe to cause marked impairment in occupational functioning or in usual social activities or relationships with others, or to necessitate hospitalization to prevent harm to self or others, or there are psychotic features.

E. The symptoms are not due to the direct physiological effects of a substance (e.g., a drug of abuse, a medication, or other treatment) or a general medical condition (e.g., hyperthyroidism).

Note: Manic-like episodes that are clearly caused by somatic antidepressant treatment (e.g., medication, electroconvulsive therapy, light therapy) should not count toward a diagnosis of Bipolar I Disorder.

HYPOMANIC EPISODE

A. A distinct period of persistently elevated, expansive, or irritable mood, lasting throughout at least 4 days, that is clearly different from the usual nondepressed mood.

B. During the period of mood disturbance, three (or more) of the following symptoms have persisted (four if the mood is only irritable) and have been present to a significant degree:

1. inflated self-esteem or grandiosity
2. decreased need for sleep (e.g., feels rested after only 3 hours of sleep)
3. more talkative than usual or pressure to keep talking
4. flight of ideas or subjective experience that thoughts are racing
5. distractibility (i.e., attention too easily drawn to unimportant or irrelevant external stimuli)
6. increase in goal-directed activity (either socially, at work or school, or sexually) or psychomotor agitation
7. excessive involvement in pleasurable activities that have a high potential for painful consequences (e.g., the person engages in unrestrained buying sprees, sexual indiscretions, or foolish business investments)

C. The episode is associated with an unequivocal change in functioning that is uncharacteristic of the person when not symptomatic.

D. The disturbance in mood and the change in functioning are observable by others.

E. The episode is not severe enough to cause marked impairment in social or occupational functioning, or to necessitate hospitalization, and there are no psychotic features.

F. The symptoms are not due to the direct physiological effects of a substance (e.g., a drug of abuse, a medication, or other treatment) or a general medical condition (e.g., hyperthyroidism).

Note: Hypomanic-like episodes that are clearly caused by somatic antidepressant treatment (e.g., medication, electroconvulsive therapy, light therapy) should not count toward a diagnosis of Bipolar II Disorder.

MIXED EPISODE

A. The criteria are met both for a Manic Episode and for a Major Depressive Episode (except for duration) nearly every day during at least a 1-week period.

B. The mood disturbance is sufficiently severe to cause marked impairment in occupational functioning or in usual social activities or relationships with others, or to necessitate hospitalization to prevent harm to self or others, or there are psychotic features.

C. The symptoms are not due to the direct physiological effects of a substance (e.g., a drug of abuse, a medication, or other treatment) or a general medical condition (e.g., hyperthyroidism).

Note: Mixed-like episodes that are clearly caused by somatic antidepressant treatment (e.g., medication, electroconvulsive therapy, light therapy) should not count toward a diagnosis of Bipolar I Disorder.

CYCLOTHYMIC DISORDER

A. For at least 2 years, the presence of numerous periods with hypomanic symptoms and numerous periods with depressive symptoms that do not meet criteria for a Major Depressive Episode.

Note: In children and adolescents, the duration must be at least 1 year.

B. During the above 2-year period (1 year in children and adolescents), the person has not been without the symptoms in Criterion A for more than 2 months at a time.

C. No Major Depressive Episode, Manic Episode, or Mixed Episode has been present during the first 2 years of the disturbance.

Note: After the initial 2 years (1 year in children and adolescents) of Cyclothymic Disorder, there may be superimposed Manic or Mixed Episodes (in which case both Bipolar I Disorder and Cyclothymic Disorder may be diagnosed) or Major Depressive Episodes (in which case both Bipolar II Disorder and Cyclothymic Disorder may be diagnosed).

D. The symptoms in Criterion A are not better accounted for by Schizoaffective Disorder and are not superimposed on Schizophrenia, Schizophreniform Disorder, Delusional Disorder, or Psychotic Disorder Not Otherwise Specified.

E. The symptoms are not due to the direct physiological effects of a substance (e.g., a drug of abuse, a medication) or a general medical condition (e.g., hyperthyroidism).

F. The symptoms cause clinically significant distress or impairment in social, occupational, or other important areas of functioning.

Source: Reprinted with permission from American Psychiatric Association. (2000). *Diagnostic and statistical manual of mental disorders* (4th ed., Text Revision).

CLINICAL MANIFESTATIONS

The manifestations experienced by the individual define the type of bipolar disorder. Nurses must recognize these manifestations, understand how clients respond during various stages, and provide client and family teaching regarding symptoms and treatments.

Mania and Hypomania

Mania is characterized by an abnormal and persistently elevated, expansive, or irritable mood lasting at least one week, significantly impairing social or occupational functioning, and generally requiring hospitalization. This disturbance in mood must be accompanied by at least three additional symptoms, such as "inflated self-esteem or grandiosity, decreased need for sleep, pressure of speech, **flight of ideas** (rapidly changing, fragmentary thoughts), distractibility, increased involvement in goal-directed activities or psychomotor agitation, and excessive involvement in pleasurable activities with a high potential for painful consequences" (APA, 2000). Psychotic symptoms such as delusions or hallucinations may be a feature of severe mania. The *DSM-IV-TR* diagnostic criteria for a manic episode are listed in Box 20–2.

> **PRACTICE ALERT**
>
> Health care providers often use language that is unfamiliar to clients and their families. To help clients and family members understand manic episodes, explain "flight of ideas," one possible symptom.

Hypomania is a less extreme form of mania that is not severe enough to markedly impair functioning or require hospitalization. Individuals experiencing hypomania feel wonderful, "on top of the world," and do not recognize changes in themselves. Those who know them well, however, are aware of the changes in mood and behavior. There are no psychotic features in hypomania.

The onset of manic episodes usually occurs in the person's early twenties but may begin at any time. It often follows a severe disappointment, embarrassment, or other psychic stressor. The mood of clients experiencing a manic episode is euphoric, or "high." Their behavior is excessive and out of bounds. It is characterized by overly enthusiastic involvement in projects of an interpersonal, political, religious, or occupational nature. When someone or something gets in the way or appears to put a snag in their way, they become irritable. Moods alternate between euphoria and irritability. Increased sexual behaviors are often seen, including flirting, making sexual overtures, having inappropriate sexual relationships, and feeling compelled to seduce and be seduced. Women may dress in an uncharacteristically flashy or seductive manner and wear garish makeup. Speech is pressured, and racing thoughts or flight of ideas are often present. Grandiosity can reach delusional proportions. Clients with mania rarely believe they are sick, even when they are in financial or legal trouble, and may vehemently protest the need for treatment. The characteristics of a manic episode are illustrated in Figure 20–4 ■.

Depressed Episodes

A diagnosis of bipolar disorder does not always mean that manic or hypomanic behaviors will be manifested in the current illness. There are several types of bipolar disorders in which manic or hypomanic episodes have occurred in the past but the features of the client's current episode are purely depressive. This stage in the course of the disorder is termed a *depressed episode.* Treatment of the client experiencing a depressed episode is similar to treatment of depression, with the exception that pharmacologic treatment adds a mood stabilizer to antidepressant treatment in order to prevent recurrence of mania.

Recent studies explain why many clinicians struggle when treating people who are not responsive to antidepressant pharmacotherapy. People who have already been diagnosed with major depression and have these five features—anxiety, tendency to experience people as unfriendly, a family history of bipolar

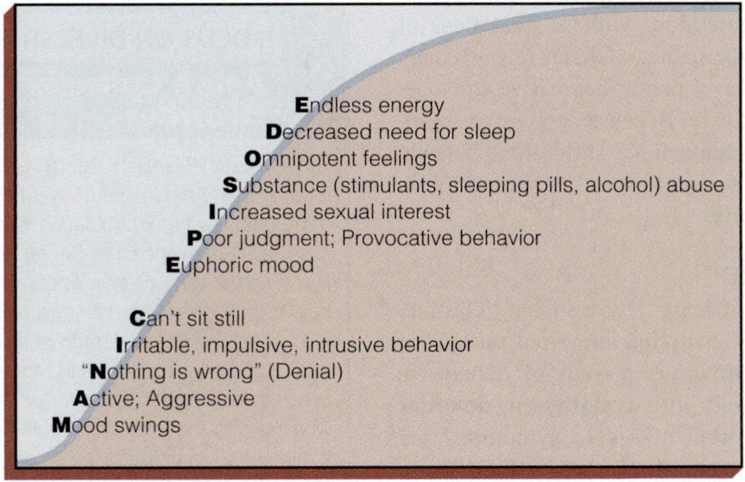

Figure 20–4 ■ Characteristics of a manic episode.

CLINICAL MANIFESTATIONS AND THERAPIES **Bipolar Disorders**

ETIOLOGY	CLINICAL MANIFESTATIONS	CLINICAL THERAPIES
Mania/manic episode	Characterized by elevated, expansive, or irritable mood that significantly impairs social or occupational functioning and is accompanied by at least three of the following: ■ Increased self-esteem ■ Decreased need for sleep ■ Pressure of speech ■ Flight of ideas ■ Distractibility ■ Increased involvement in goal-directed activities ■ Psychomotor agitation ■ Excessive involvement in pleasurable activities that carry a high risk of painful consequences	■ Mood stabilizers such as lithium ■ Remove or limit environmental stimuli ■ Set limits; teach limit setting ■ Orient to self, place, and time
Hypomania	Less extreme than mania; individuals describe themselves as feeling "wonderful" and do not recognize changes in their behavior, although friends and family will observe changes.	■ Mood stabilizers such as lithium ■ Remove or limit environmental stimuli ■ Set limits or teach limit setting
Depressed episode	Symptoms of depression	Antidepressant with mood stabilizer

disorder, a recent diagnosis of depression, and legal problems—may very well have bipolar disorder rather than depression. The probability that these features predict bipolar disorder risk in those unsuccessfully treated with antidepressants is high (Perlis, Brown, Baker, & Nierenberg, 2006). Previous research has shown that nearly half of all people who have bipolar disorders are first diagnosed with major depression.

Many clients with bipolar disorders are not correctly diagnosed in a timely manner. This can mean that an individual loses years to an illness that could have been successfully managed if it had been correctly diagnosed and treated.

Mixed Episodes

In a *mixed episode,* symptoms of both mania and depression are present nearly every day in rapidly alternating succession over a period of at least a week. These clients are often agitated, are suffering from insomnia and appetite disturbances, and may exhibit suicidal and psychotic thinking. The presentation also can resemble depression, with a great deal of energy and animation behind the sadness. Clients recently may have had a manic episode or a major depressive episode, although this is not always the case. Because depressive symptoms are part of the clinical picture, clients suffer more psychic pain than do individuals who are in a state of mania and therefore may seek help more readily.

Cyclothymic Disorder

When clients have suffered at least 2 years from "chronic, fluctuating mood disturbances involving numerous periods of hypomanic symptoms and numerous periods of depressive symptoms," they are diagnosed with **cyclothymic disorder** (APA, 2000). They must be free of severe symptoms that qualify for the diagnosis of manic disorder or MDD. These individuals are often considered to be moody, unpredictable, or temperamental, and they may go on to develop an overlay of symptoms that are of major depressive or manic intensity. Figure 20–5 ■ compares mood in MDD, bipolar disorders, dysthymia, and cyclothymia.

Cyclothymic disorder begins early, usually in adolescence or early adulthood. Although not common, with a lifetime risk of only 0.4–1.0% of the general population, cyclothymic disorder is thought to predispose the person to other mood disorders. The incidence is approximately equal between males and females.

Bipolar Disorders in Children and Adolescents

Children with bipolar disorders often present with irritability or hyperactivity. About 1% of children and adults suffer from bipolar disorders, with a high rate of onset from 15–19 years (Lansford, 2005). The disorder has been diagnosed in children

FOCUS ON DIVERSITY AND CULTURE

Asian Cultures and Mood Disorders

The National Research Center on Asian American Mental Health reports that Asian Americans underutilize mental health services more than any other population. Some Asian cultures view mental illness as an imbalance that can be restored through diet and exercise. Many Asians view mental illness as a stigma and frown on seeking help from Western practitioners, although this may vary according to level of education and length of time in the United States. It is common among Asian peoples to report physical symptoms when experiencing depression, mania, or another mental illness. Nurses working with these clients should be especially alert to conduct culturally sensitive, holistic assessments and not simply assume that the physical symptom is related exclusively to a biophysical alteration (HealthyPlace.com, 2008).

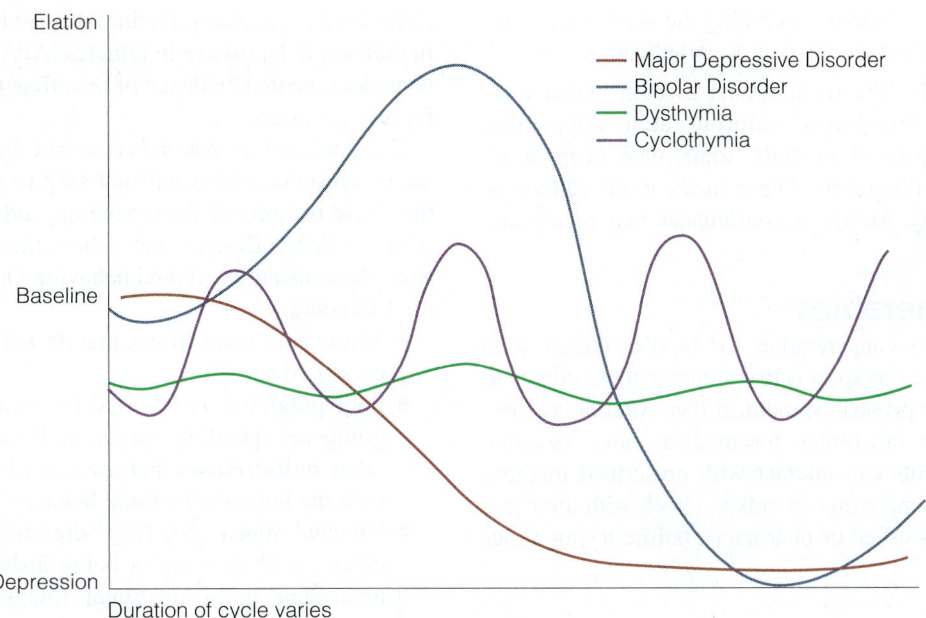

Figure 20–5 ■ Comparison of affect (mood) in major depressive disorder, bipolar disorder, dysthymia, and cyclothymia.

as young as preschool age (Apps, Winkler, & Jandrisevits, 2008). There is a high rate of attempted suicide in those with bipolar disorders, as well as co-occurrence with other disorders such as ADHD, anxiety, and substance abuse, all of which complicates diagnosis (Kowatch, et al., 2005).

When parents or close relatives are affected, the child is more likely to have the disorder. The manic phase of childhood bipolar disorder is characterized by hyperactivity and high energy, irritability, aggression, and sometimes hallucinations. In the depressive phase, the child is sad, has alterations in sleep and eating patterns, feels worthless, lacks energy, and is socially withdrawn, similar to any depressive illness. Mania may be the persistent symptom in children, or rapid cycles of mania and depression can occur throughout the day (Lansford, 2005). The individual prefers the manic phase, but it is followed by depression; the cycling and instability of moods is distressing.

COLLABORATION

Care of the client with a bipolar disorder requires a multidisciplinary effort that includes the nurse, the client, the primary care provider, a mental health specialist, and possibly a pharmacist as the team works to find a successful therapeutic regimen. The nurse should take special care to encourage the client to track feelings, behaviors, and side effects, especially during the first few weeks of trying a new medication.

Pharmacologic Therapies

Hyperactive and agitated behavior usually responds fairly rapidly to antipsychotic mood stabilizers such as risperidone (Risperdal) and olanzapine (Zyprexa). The atypical antipsychotics, effective as mood-stabilizing medications, are often given in conjunction with anticonvulsive mood stabilizers. Because lithium takes 1–3 weeks before it is effective, typical antipsychotics are used to help manage the symptoms of mania when individuals have begun lithium carbonate therapy.

Nursing interventions include monitoring clients for adverse side effects of antipsychotic medications. Side effects include sedation, agitation, postural hypotension, dizziness, dry mouth, and blurry vision. Several psychopharmacologic agents have proven effective in the long-term treatment of mania. One effective and widely used agent is lithium carbonate.

LITHIUM CARBONATE Lithium carbonate is a potentially dangerous alkali metal that has been used in the treatment and prevention of acute manic episodes since the 1960s. It is now used in preventing the recurrence of bipolar disorders as well.

Lithium alters neurotransmission in the CNS. It is thought to interfere with the ionic pump mechanism in brain cells, but its exact mode of action is unknown. Its use is not recommended during pregnancy and breastfeeding or in clients with impaired renal function, congestive heart failure, sodium-restricted diets, organic brain disease, and impaired CNS functioning.

Administered orally, the onset of action ranges from 1–3 weeks. The dosage is gradually increased until the recommended therapeutic blood level of 1.0–1.5 mEq/L is achieved. Once the desired effect is achieved, the dosage is adjusted downward to the maintenance blood level of 0.6–1.2 mEq/L. There are cultural considerations to the therapeutic blood level: People of Asian descent may have toxic reactions at dosages as low as 0.6 mEq/L. Monitor therapeutic effect as well as side effects.

Toxic symptoms begin appearing at blood levels above 1.5 mEq/L. Because there is such a narrow margin of safety, serum concentrations must be closely monitored until stabilized. The need for close monitoring means that clients are often hospitalized when lithium therapy is initiated. Before discharge, both clients and families must learn how to continue lithium therapy safely at home, including the need to maintain hydration in order to reduce the risk of complications.

ANTICONVULSANTS The main agents used in mania therapy are the anticonvulsants valproic acid (Depakote, Depakene), lamotrigine (Lamictal), topiramate (Topamax), and carbamazepine (Tegretol). These medications cannot be discontinued abruptly. Abrupt discontinuance may precipitate a seizure.

Alternative Therapies

The primary nursing consideration for bipolar clients who want to try alternative therapies is to encourage these clients to continue taking their prescribed medications. Alternative therapies should not be substituted for medical care. As some herbs and supplements can interact with prescribed medications, nurses should encourage clients to check with their primary care provider's office or pharmacist before trying either of these therapies.

NURSING PROCESS

Because the nursing care of clients experiencing depressive symptoms is the same whether the diagnosis is MDD, dysthymic disorder, or depressed episode bipolar disorder, this section will focus on hypomania and mania, which constitute the other half of the bipolar continuum of behaviors.

Assessment

The onset of a hypomanic or manic episode may be gradual or dramatic. Affect is euphoric or elated but can change quickly to irritability or hostility if the person is confronted with limits or is otherwise frustrated. The signs and symptoms range in severity from mild (in hypomania) to extreme (in a frank manic episode).

Subjective Data

Nurses should be alert for clients exhibiting the following manic behaviors:

- Changes in the client's thought processes, evidenced by statements such as "I feel like my thoughts are racing."
- Inflated self-esteem, sometimes to the extent of having delusions of grandeur. Delusions of persecution also may be a feature.
- Clients ignoring fatigue, hunger, and even hygiene, being too involved in activity to focus on physiologic sensations.
- Distractibility. The client experiencing a manic episode often suffers from an inability to concentrate and is easily distracted by the slightest stimulus in the environment.
- Hallucinations.
- A surprising sense of well-being. Hypomanic individuals and those early in manic episodes feel wonderful and do not understand why people are upset with their behavior.

Objective Data

Clients who are experiencing their first mania are most likely to be young people in their twenties, although adolescents are sometimes affected. Although bipolar disorders appear to have little gender specificity, the initial episode is likely to be manic in males and depressive in females (APA, 2000). To date, there is no documented evidence of the effect of race or ethnicity on bipolar disorders.

The hallmark of mania is constant motor activity. During a manic episode, clients will not stop to eat. They do not rest, they have disordered sleep patterns, and they may go for days without sleep. Bruises and other injuries sometimes result from the constantly agitated behavior. Other indicators include the following:

- Manic communications, manifested in a flight of ideas or pressured speech
- Poor judgment as reported by family members, such as going on spending sprees and committing sexual and other indiscretions that are completely out of character with the individual's usual behavior
- Unusual appearance (e.g., dressing inappropriately and using garish makeup or being disheveled and unkempt).

Impairment in occupational functioning may result in being laid off from work, being placed on a leave of absence, or being fired because the behavior is disruptive in the workplace. People who have mania cause interpersonal chaos by behaving manipulatively, testing limits, and playing one person against another. If their attempts at manipulation fail, they become irritable or hostile, and such behavior further alienates others.

Clients who have mania are not usually able to cooperate fully in the assessment process. In many cases, nurses find it necessary to rely on their own assessment skills and secondary sources such as family members to obtain essential assessment data. Family members often can provide detailed information about the onset and progression of symptoms, as well as information about any previous episodes.

Diagnosis

Several nursing diagnoses are common in the care of clients who have mania. These include the following:

- Risk for Injury related to impairment of adaptive and defensive abilities. Because of their hyperactivity and agitation, manic clients often lose control of their movements and bump into objects, fall, and otherwise injure themselves. Their impulsivity, poor judgment, and propensity toward hostile outburst also places them at risk for injury.
- Disturbed Thought Processes related to biochemical alteration, genetic predisposition, sleep deprivation, a severe blow to self-esteem, or denial of depression.
- Impaired Social Interaction resulting from efforts to manipulate others to meet their own wishes and needs (egocentrism), impulsiveness, poor personal hygiene, and unwillingness to accept responsibility for the effect of their own behaviors.
- Self-Care Deficit related to impaired ability to perform self-care activities such as feeding and bathing.
- Sleep Deprivation related to hyperactivity, agitation, and possibly biochemical alterations.

Plan

Outcomes for mood disorders include the expectation of a return to premorbid functioning. While these will vary by client, appropriate outcomes for a client with bipolar disorder include the following:

- The client will remain free of injury.
- The client will remain oriented.
- The client will be able to focus on a specific stimulus for more than 10 minutes at a time.
- The client will be able to choose between two or more alternatives.
- The client will use appropriate behaviors in a variety of social settings.
- The client will maintain self-care.
- The client will no longer experience sleep disturbances.

Implementation

With clients who are manic, maintain a calm, relaxed, but firm and matter-of-fact demeanor, particularly when communicating limits. The nurse's behavior serves as a model and can be reassuring to out-of-control clients. As with all clients, building a trusting relationship is important (Box 20–3).

Promoting Client Safety

Taking steps to ensure the safety of clients and others in the environment is a priority.

- Provide a safe environment by reducing environmental stimuli. For inpatient clients, this means providing a simply furnished private room that has had all unnecessary items removed. It should be in a quiet location to reduce noise stimulation. Low lighting also can be calming to the hyperactive client. Some hospitals have "quiet units." From there, clients can be transferred to milieu units when they are better able to deal with the distractions of community living.
- Remove or prohibit smoking materials. These are particularly hazardous in the hands of agitated clients. They may burn themselves or leave burning cigarettes lying around when they become distracted by other stimuli. While not an issue in most institutions, allow the client who is experiencing mania to smoke only under supervision.
- Monitor activities. Scheduling a program of appropriate activity interspersed with rest periods helps provide an outlet for tension while protecting clients from exhaustion. Appropriate activities include walking, exercising, or dancing with the supervision of an activity therapist and supervised vacuuming or sweeping chores. Avoid highly competitive activities that bring out hostility and overtly aggressive behaviors.
- Set and enforce limits on unsafe or socially inappropriate behavior when clients are unable to control their impulses. Matter-of-fact intervention rather than angry scolding is the most effective approach. Clients may respond to verbal reminders, or you can use their distractibility to redirect them into safer and more appropriate activities. Remember to reward appropriate behavior with positive reinforcement such as "I enjoyed our walk today because you were able to walk with me rather than running ahead."

Promoting Reality-Based Thinking

Present reality by spending time with clients. Identify yourself, the time and day, the location, and other orienting information as needed. Engage clients in reality-based, somewhat concrete activities (e.g., discussing a current event).

Consistency is reassuring to clients with altered thought processes. Establish consistency by following a schedule to help clients understand what is expected of them. Consistency also is enhanced by assigning the same caregivers to work with the same clients whenever possible.

When dealing with delusional or hallucinating clients, the nurse should communicate acceptance of their need for false beliefs while clearly stating that he or she does not share their perceptions. A statement such as "I understand that you believe you are the owner of this facility, but I see it differently" conveys acceptance without supporting delusional thinking.

It is not therapeutic to argue or try to reason with delusional clients. Arguing with a client often serves to harden the belief system and can impair the development of trust. Instead, use statements such as "I find that hard to believe" or "That is extremely unusual" to instill reasonable doubt as a therapeutic intervention.

Box 20–3 Potential Reactions of Nurses Working With Clients Who Have Mania

Working with clients who have mania will challenge your maturity, self-control, and professionalism. When you work with clients who have mania, you may experience some of the following feelings. Think about and discuss with your classmates and instructor how you might handle each of these reactions in order to maintain a positive nurse–client relationship.

- I feel annoyed by the client's demanding behavior.
- I feel outsmarted and outmaneuvered. I question whether my judgments and actions are appropriate.
- I develop rescue fantasies in response to a client's flattery and think I am the only one who understands this client.
- I become defensive and angry when colleagues point out a client's manipulative behavior.
- I feel anxious and insecure when a client turns on me, saying, "I'm not progressing because you're cold and mean."
- I have difficulty being objective about clients who have manic symptoms.
- I disagree emphatically with colleagues about how to handle a client's manipulative behavior. The client sits back and watches nurses fight with each other.
- I become angry and unsure of my judgment when a client consistently exceeds established limits.
- I withdraw and avoid clients who have mania so I do not feel embarrassed or experience self-doubt.

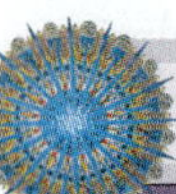

NURSING CARE PLAN A Client With Bipolar Disorder

ASSESSMENT

Mr. Grey, a 52-year-old engineer, is brought to the emergency psychiatric clinic by two adult sons at 2 a.m. Their mother called them to come help with their father, who has not slept in 3 days. When they arrived at their parents' home, they found their father working on a large landscaping project in the backyard that involved stonework, a waterfall, a fish pond, and extensive plantings of trees, shrubs, and flowers.

According to the sons, Mr. Grey has had three prior episodes of manic behavior, beginning when he was in the army many years ago. He was stabilized on lithium carbonate for years but stopped taking it about a year ago because he felt so good. The current episode began about 1 week ago, after he was passed over for a promotion at work. He then took a leave of absence from his job to create what he called "the world's first home-based theme park." Any attempt by his wife to talk him out of the project has been met with anger and renewed resolve. Mr. Grey angrily tells the admitting nurse, "I don't know why these boys brought me here. I need to get back to work! I'm going to get millions for this franchise."

DIAGNOSES

- Disturbed Thought Processes
- Sleep Deprivation
- Caregiver Role Strain
- Interrupted Family Processes
- Ineffective Therapeutic Regimen Management

PLANNING

Goals for care include:

- The client will comply with instructions for taking medications as ordered.
- The client will sleep through the night.
- The client will be oriented to time and place.
- Family members will return to normal activities.
- Family members will support medication administration.

IMPLEMENTATION

- With Mr. Grey and family members, develop a plan of activity that will help Mr. Grey disperse energy at appropriate times.
- Help family members set and enforce limits. For example, "From 8 p.m. until 6 a.m., Mr. Grey will remain indoors, engaged in sleep-promoting activities or sleeping."
- Refer Mr. Grey and his family to a therapist who can help them learn how to orient Mr. Grey to reality when his mind begins to stray.
- Help Mr. Grey and his wife learn how to promote sleep by decreasing environmental stimuli in the bedroom and engaging in good sleep hygiene.

EVALUATION

Expected outcomes to evaluate the client's care include:

- Client maintains therapeutic drug levels indicating compliance with medication regimen.
- Client and family report Mr. Grey obtains 6–8 hours of sleep per night.
- Client demonstrates orientation to time and place.
- Family reports a return to normal daily routine.
- Client regularly attends counseling sessions.

CRITICAL THINKING

1. What client teaching can the nurse provide to reduce the risk of medication noncompliance once Mr. Grey feels well and is no longer symptomatic?
2. What teaching will the nurse provide the family to help them cope with the client's diagnosis?
3. How can the nurse assist the client to meet his nutritional needs during manic phases of the illness?

When clients communicate perceptions of altered reality, reflect their statements back to them for validation. For example, asking "Are you saying that your husband is trying to poison you with monosodium glutamate?" can help a client understand how her perceptions sound to others. You will recognize that clients are becoming less delusional when they make statements such as "I know this sounds bizarre, but. . . ." Remember to give positive reinforcement when clients begin to focus on reality.

Enhancing Socialization

Nursing activities are designed to facilitate the client's ability to interact with others by identifying needed behavior changes and assigning tasks that will improve the client's interactions with others. This may require mediating between the client and others when the client exhibits negative behavior. Nursing actions should encourage and demonstrate honesty and respect for others' rights.

Manipulation, a maladaptive behavior of clients who are manic, significantly impairs social interactions. This may take a simple form, such as borrowing money from other clients rather than using their own, or it may be highly complex, such as pitting staff members against one another by giving them false information about each other.

Manipulation meets a need for the client. It serves the purpose of increasing the client's sense of control and interpersonal power. (The mania can be frightening as it spins out of control.) Nursing interventions such as setting limits promote client security and often enable clients to curb their manipulative behavior or give it up entirely. Nurses should be aware of their own need for control and provide opportunities for clients to be in control when appropriate. Forming a therapeutic alliance with the client, discovering his or her expectations, and providing opportunities for interpersonal interactions have been linked with positive long-term outcomes for people with bipolar disorders (Gaudiano & Miller, 2006).

Setting Limits

Out-of-control manipulative behavior requires setting limits. All staff members must agree on the established limits and enforce them consistently. Violations of limits must have established consequences, also agreed upon by all staff members. Clients must know what behaviors are expected and what consequences will result if they exceed the limits. Inconsistent application of consequences will cause failure in efforts to decrease manipulative behavior.

Nurses should expect clients to give charming explanations of why they exceeded this or that limit, but should not be disarmed by these explanations. They are another form of manipulative behavior. Matter-of-fact limit enforcement and the consistent application of consequences are essential in promoting adaptive behaviors.

Promoting Improved Self-Care

Well-being is compromised when clients do not receive sufficient nourishment and fluids for extended periods of time, particularly during periods of hyperactivity. Monitoring intake and output is an important nursing activity. The hyperactive client who is unable to sit down and eat is most likely to consume frequent small snacks that can be eaten on the go. For the inpatient client, work with a dietitian to ensure that high-calorie finger foods and nutritious liquids are available on the nursing unit until the client is able to attend regular meals. For outpatient clients or those preparing for discharge, collaborate with the client and dietician to determine client preferences and create a list of easily prepared foods that the client finds palatable and can make or eat on the go.

A minimal level of personal hygiene is needed to ensure health, self-esteem, and healthy social interactions. Assist hyperactive clients who are unwilling or unable to bathe, brush their teeth, shave, wash their hair, change clothes, or use the toilet. Autonomy is desirable, so allow clients to do as much for themselves as possible with verbal encouragement. Reinforce any attempts at self-care with recognition; for example, "I see you shaved today, Mr. Adams."

Incontinence of urine or feces is occasionally seen in severely regressed clients during mania. This can be very disturbing to other clients and staff and insults the dignity of the client who is experiencing incontinence. Nursing activities include establishing a schedule of frequent, regular toileting. Accompany the client to the bathroom every hour or half hour until "accidents" no longer occur.

A more common elimination problem is constipation. Hyperactive clients suppress the urge to defecate and may become severely constipated. The anticholinergic effect of some medications also may exacerbate constipation. Frequent fluid intake and a a high-fiber diet can reduce constipation.

Enhancing Rest and Sleep

Clients in the manic phase of bipolar disorder appear deceptively energetic when they may actually be nearing the point of exhaustion. Design nursing activities to facilitate regular sleep–wake cycles. Monitor clients closely for signs of fatigue and make provisions for rest periods. Promote nighttime sleeping by limiting extended daytime naps.

Sleep may promote the rapid resolution of first episodes of mania. Prior to bedtime, decrease light and noise and encourage quiet activities and presleep routines such as listening to soothing music. A warm bath and snack may aid relaxation, as may a backrub. Administer medications that do not suppress REM sleep, such as zolpidem tartrate (Ambien), as prescribed.

If clients experience extended nighttime wakefulness, avoid engaging them in long conversations or otherwise stimulating them or giving extra attention at night. Firmly encourage clients to stay in their darkened room with the expectation that they will fall asleep. If they will not stay in their room, assign a monotonous, repetitive task such as folding towels or sorting papers to encourage drowsiness.

When clients are able to sleep, avoid waking them for nonessential care or activities. Allow for sleep cycles of at least 90 minutes.

Evaluation

Specific client behaviors indicate that nursing interventions have been successful. Evaluation and outcome criteria answer the question "How do we know that the client's condition has improved?"

REVIEW Bipolar Disorders

RELATE: LINK TO CONCEPTS

Linking the exemplar of Bipolar Disorders with the concept of Family:

1. How might bipolar disorder affect parenting styles?
2. How might different family processes affect a child's treatment for bipolar disorder?

Linking the exemplar of Bipolar Disorders with the concept of Health, Wellness, and Illness:

3. How might bipolar disorder affect a client's nutritional status?
4. What consumer education resources are available to clients with bipolar disorders and their families to help them maintain their health during periods of relapse?

READY: GO TO COMPANION SKILLS MANUAL

- Assessing appearance and mental status
- Evaluating client's safety
- Assessing caregiver's safety

REFER: GO TO MYNURSINGKIT

REFLECT: CASE STUDY

Pam Mathews, 21 years old and attending college, has been diagnosed with bipolar disorder and is in the manic phase. Since admission 2 days ago, she has been averaging 2 hours of sleep a night. The rest of the night she spends pacing the hallways and talking to staff. She is in constant motion and brags about how much energy she has. Her clothing consists of startling bright miniskirts, low-cut sweaters, and high heels. Every few hours she changes clothes and reapplies her makeup to match.

1. What strategies might the nurse implement to maintain Pam's safety at this time?
2. How might the diagnosis of bipolar disorder impact Pam's ability to meet her developmental milestones and what actions can the nurse implement to reduce developmental delays?
3. What risks to health does Pam face during the manic phase of her illness and how can the nurse reduce these risks?

20.2 DEPRESSION

KEY TERMS

Anergy, *1188*
Anhedonia, *1188*
Hypersomnia, *1188*
Insomnia, *1188*
Major depressive disorder (MDD), *1188*
Major depressive episode, *1186*
Psychomotor retardation, *1188*

BASIS FOR SELECTION OF EXEMPLAR

Emergency room admissions
Healthy People 2010
Institute of Medicine
National Institute of Mental Health
Office-based physician visits

LEARNING OUTCOMES

After reading about this concept, you will be able to:

1. Describe the pathophysiology, psychopathology, and clinical manifestations of depressive disorders.
2. Identify risk factors associated with depression.
3. Illustrate the nursing process in providing culturally competent care across the life span for individuals with depression.
4. Formulate priority nursing diagnoses appropriate for an individual with depression.
5. Create a plan of care for individuals with depression and their family members.
6. Assess expected outcomes for an individual with depression.
7. Discuss therapies used in the collaborative care of an individual with depression.
8. Employ evidence-based caring interventions for an individual with depression.

OVERVIEW

Depression is a disorder characterized by a sad or despondent mood. Many symptoms are associated with depression, including lack of energy; sleep disturbances; abnormal eating patterns; and feelings of despair, guilt, and hopelessness. Depression is the most common mental health disorder of older adults, encompassing a variety of physical, emotional, cognitive, and social considerations.

The majority of depressed clients are not found in psychiatric hospitals, but in mainstream everyday settings. For proper diagnosis and treatment to occur, recognition of depression is a collaborative effort among health care providers. Because depressed clients are present in multiple settings and in all areas of practice, every nurse should be proficient in the assessment and nursing care of clients afflicted with this disorder.

Risk factors for depression include the following:

- History of child abuse or neglect, spousal abuse, loss of a close family member or intimate friend, other significant loss
- Dysfunctional family relationships, with or without the presence of substance abuse
- Family history of mental illness or substance abuse.

CLINICAL MANIFESTATIONS

Some of the clinical manifestations of depression seem fairly obvious: feelings of sadness and despair and sleep disturbances, for example. Others may not be as obvious, such as anger and physical complaints. Manifestations of depression also can differ according to culture. It is important for nurses involved with all levels of depression to know and recognize the symptoms.

Major Depressive Disorder

A **major depressive episode** is characterized by a change in several aspects of a person's life and emotional state consistently over a period of 14 days or longer. The most important factor is the client's mood, which the client may not describe in terms of "depression." Instead, the client may describe feelings of sadness, discouragement, or hopelessness. Or the client may complain of having no feelings at all or of feeling blah. Some clients may report vague somatic (physical) complaints such as aches and pains; other clients may report increased anger, frustration, and irritability, with uncharacteristic outbursts over minor matters. It is not difficult to imagine that someone who looks and feels sad or empty is depressed. A diagnosis of depression is more likely to be missed when a person simply seems anxious or irritable.

Box 20–4 *DSM-IV TR* Diagnostic Criteria for Depressive Disorders

MAJOR DEPRESSIVE EPISODE

A. Five (or more) of the following symptoms have been present during the same 2-week period and represent a change from previous functioning; at least one of the symptoms is either (1) depressed mood or (2) loss of interest or pleasure.

Note: Do not include symptoms that are clearly due to a general medical condition, or mood-incongruent delusions or hallucinations.

1. Depressed mood most of the day, nearly every day, as indicated by either subjective report (e.g., feels sad or empty) or observation made by others (e.g., appears tearful). Note: In children and adolescents, can be irritable mood.
2. Markedly diminished interest or pleasure in all, or almost all, activities most of the day, nearly every day (as indicated by either subjective account or observation made by others)
3. Significant weight loss when not dieting or weight gain (e.g., a change of more than 5% of body weight in a month), or decrease or increase in appetite nearly every day. Note: In children, consider failure to make expected weight gains.
4. Insomnia or hypersomnia nearly every day
5. Psychomotor agitation or retardation nearly every day (observable by others, not merely subjective feelings of restlessness or being slowed down)
6. Fatigue or loss of energy nearly every day
7. Feelings of worthlessness or excessive or inappropriate guilt (which may be delusional) nearly every day (not merely self-reproach or guilt about being sick)
8. Diminished ability to think or concentrate, or indecisiveness, nearly every day (either by subjective account or as observed by others)
9. Recurrent thoughts of death (not just fear of dying), recurrent suicidal ideation without a specific plan, or a suicide attempt or a specific plan for committing suicide

B. The symptoms do not meet criteria for a Mixed Episode.

C. The symptoms cause clinically significant distress or impairment in social, occupational, or other important areas of functioning.

D. The symptoms are not due to the direct physiological effects of a substance (e.g., a drug of abuse, a medication) or a general medical condition (e.g., hypothyroidism).

E. The symptoms are not better accounted for by bereavement (i.e., after the loss of a loved one), the symptoms persist for longer than 2 months or are characterized by marked functional impairment, morbid preoccupation with worthlessness, suicidal ideation, psychotic symptoms, or psychomotor retardation.

MAJOR DEPRESSIVE DISORDER, SINGLE EPISODE

A. Presence of a single Major Depressive Episode.

B. The Major Depressive Episode is not better accounted for by Schizoaffective Disorder and is not superimposed on Schizophrenia, Schizophreniform Disorder, Delusional Disorder, or Psychotic Disorder Not Otherwise Specified.

C. There has never been a Manic Episode, a Mixed Episode, or a Hypomanic Episode.

Note: This exclusion does not apply if all of the manic-like, mixed-like, or hypomanic-like episodes are substance or treatment induced or are due to the direct physiological effects of a general medical condition.

MAJOR DEPRESSIVE DISORDER, RECURRENT

A. Presence of two or more Major Depressive Episodes.

Note: To be considered separate episodes, there must be an interval of at least 2 consecutive months in which criteria are not met for a Major Depressive Episode.

B. The Major Depressive Episodes are not better accounted for by Schizoaffective Disorder and are not superimposed on Schizophrenia, Schizophreniform Disorder, Delusional Disorder, or Psychotic Disorder Not Otherwise Specified.

C. There has never been a Manic Episode, a Mixed Episode, or a Hypomanic Episode.

Note: This exclusion does not apply if all of the manic-like, mixed-like, or hypomanic-like episodes are substance or treatment induced or are due to the direct physiological effects of a general medical condition.

DYSTHYMIC DISORDER

A. Depressed mood for most of the day, for more days than not, as indicated either by subjective account or observation by others, for at least 2 years.

Note: In children and adolescents, mood can be irritable and duration must be at least 1 year.

B. Presence, while depressed, of two (or more) of the following:

1. Poor appetite or overeating
2. Insomnia or hypersomnia
3. Low energy or fatigue
4. Low self-esteem
5. Poor concentration or difficulty making decisions
6. Feelings of hopelessness.

C. During the 2-year period (1 year for children or adolescents) of the disturbance, the person has never been without the symptoms in Criteria A and B for more than 2 months at a time.

D. No Major Depressive Episode has been present during the first 2 years of the disturbance (1 year for children and adolescents) (i.e., the disturbance is not better accounted for by chronic Major Depressive Disorder, or Major Depressive Disorder, in Partial Remission).

Note: There may have been a previous Major Depressive Episode provided there was a full remission (no significant signs or symptoms for 2 months) before development of the Dysthymic Disorder. In addition, after the initial 2 years (1 year in children or adolescents) of Dysthymic Disorder, there may be superimposed episodes of Major Depressive Disorder, in which case both diagnoses may be given when the criteria are met for a Major Depressive Episode.

E. There has never been a Manic Episode, a Mixed Episode, or a Hypomanic Episode, and criteria have never been met for Cyclothymic Disorder.

F. The disturbance does not occur exclusively during the course of a chronic Psychotic Disorder, such as Schizophrenia or Delusional Disorder.

G. The symptoms are not due to the direct physiological effects of a substance (e.g., a drug of abuse, a medication) or a general medical condition (e.g., hypothyroidism).

H. The symptoms cause clinically significant distress or impairment in social, occupational, or other important areas of functioning.

(continued)

Box 20–4 *DSM-IV TR* Diagnostic Criteria for Depressive Disorders (continued)

SEASONAL PATTERN SPECIFIER

Specify if:

With Seasonal Pattern (can be applied to the pattern of Major Depressive Episodes in Bipolar I Disorder, Bipolar II Disorder, or Major Depressive Disorder, Recurrent)

A. There has been a regular temporal relationship between the onset of Major Depressive Episodes in Bipolar I or Bipolar II Disorder or Major Depressive Disorder, Recurrent, and a particular time of the year (e.g., regular appearance of the Major Depressive Episode in the fall or winter).

Note: Do not include cases in which there is an obvious effect of seasonal-related psychosocial stressors (e.g., regularly being unemployed every winter).

B. Full remissions (or a change from depression to mania or hypomania) also occur at a characteristic time of the year (e.g., depression disappears in the spring).

C. In the last 2 years, two Major Depressive Episodes have occurred that demonstrate the temporal seasonal relationships defined in Criteria A and B, and no nonseasonal Major Depressive Episodes have occurred during that same period.

D. Seasonal Major Depressive Episodes (as described previously) substantially outnumber the nonseasonal Major Depressive Episodes that may have occurred over the individual's lifetime.

Source: Reprinted with permission from American Psychiatric Association. (2000). *Diagnostic and statistical manual of mental disorders*(4th ed.,Text Revision). (Copyright 2000). American Psychiatric Association.

Major depressive disorder (MDD) may consist of a single episode or may exhibit as recurrent major depression at various points in life. The description of the diagnostic criteria for single-episode and recurrent major depression is found in Box 20–4. Key facts about MDD are listed in Box 20–5.

PRACTICE ALERT

Health care providers often use language that is unfamiliar to clients and their families. To help clients and families understand the symptoms of a major depressive episode, reword the DSM statement that symptoms may be characterized by "psychomotor retardation."

Individuals with a history of a manic or hypomanic episode are considered to have a bipolar disorder and are not classified under the categories of depressive disorders.

When a person experiences an MDD, activities that previously gave pleasure, such as socializing, hobbies, sports, and sex, often are no longer enjoyed. This is a condition known as **anhedonia**. Changes in appetite, usually experienced as a reduction or loss of interest in food, are often seen, although increased appetite and cravings are also reported.

Sleep disturbances, particularly **insomnia** (not being able to fall asleep or stay asleep or awakening early in the morning), are common in depressed individuals. Two types of insomnia are most often experienced by people having a major depressive episode. *Middle insomnia* refers to waking up during the night and having difficulty falling asleep again. *Terminal insomnia* refers to waking at the end of the night and being unable to return to sleep. Depressed clients also may report **hypersomnia**, in which the individual sleeps for prolonged periods at night as well as during the day but still wakes up tired or fatigued. These sleep disturbances are discussed at length in Concept 5, Comfort.

Fatigue and decreased energy, which are characteristic symptoms of depression, may be referred to as **anergy** or *anergia.* Anergic individuals report being tired upon awakening regardless of how long they have slept. Even the smallest task seems insurmountable, and routine activities require substantial effort and take longer to accomplish. Decreased energy may be manifested in **psychomotor retardation**, in which thinking and body movements are noticeably slowed and speech is slowed or absent. Psychomotor agitation also may occur, in which the person cannot sit still; paces; wrings the hands; and picks at the fingernails, skin, clothing, bedclothes, or other objects.

Other common symptoms in significantly depressed individuals include guilt or a sense of worthlessness, self-blame, impaired concentration and decision-making ability (even about trivial things), and suicidal ideation. The characteristics of a major depressive episode are illustrated in Figure 20–6 ■.

Dysthymic Disorder

The term *dysthymic disorder* describes chronic depression for the majority of most days for at least 2 years (1 year for children and adolescents). Throughout those 2 years, no more than 2 months can be described as symptom-free. The symptoms of

Box 20–5 Key Facts About Major Depressive Disorder

- The average age of onset of MDD is the mid-twenties, although the disorder can begin at any age and seems to be occurring in younger people.
- The risk of developing MDD during one's lifetime ranges from 15–25% for females and from 8–15% for males, making depression twice as likely for women as for men.
- First-degree biologic relatives (parents or siblings) of people with MDD are up to three times as likely to develop depression as are members of the general population (APA, 2000).
- Symptoms of MDD usually develop over a period of time. The person may experience anxiety and mild depression for several days, weeks, or months before the onset of a full major depressive episode.
- If untreated, major depression lasts 6 or more months. In about 20–30% of cases, some depressive symptoms persist for longer periods ranging from months to years. This is considered a partial remission and thought to be predictive of later depressive episodes and the development of chronic depression.

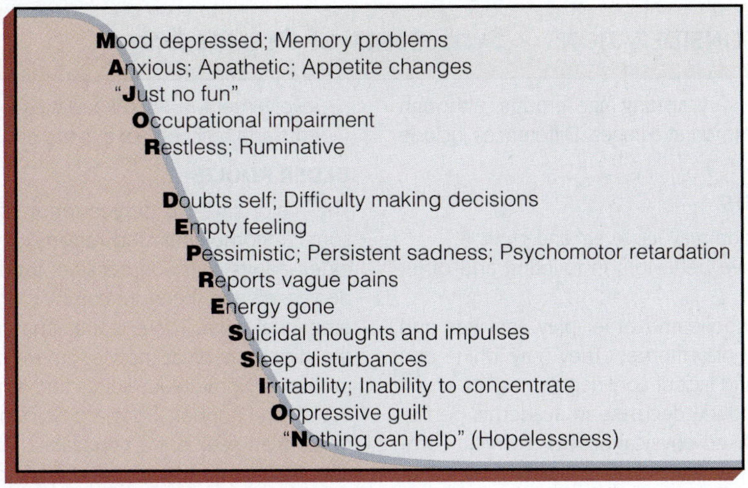

Mood depressed; Memory problems
Anxious; Apathetic; Appetite changes
"Just no fun"
Occupational impairment
Restless; Ruminative

Doubts self; Difficulty making decisions
Empty feeling
Pessimistic; Persistent sadness; Psychomotor retardation
Reports vague pains
Energy gone
Suicidal thoughts and impulses
Sleep disturbances
Irritability; Inability to concentrate
Oppressive guilt
"Nothing can help" (Hopelessness)

Figure 20–6 ■ Characteristics of major depression.

dysthymic disorder, while distressing, tend to be less severe than those in MDD, with fewer physiologic symptoms. Dysthymic disorder tends to predispose people to the development of MDD. According to the *DSM-IV TR*, 10–25% of individuals diagnosed with dysthymic disorder will develop MDD within the next year (APA, 2000).

Dysthymic disorder often occurs in childhood, adolescence, or early adulthood and tends to be chronic. While both females and males are equally affected as children, there are 2–3 times as many adult females as males with dysthymic disorder. The lifetime risk of developing dysthymic disorder is approximately 6% in the general population.

The symptoms of dysthymic disorder are similar to those of chronic major depressive disorder. This similarity makes it difficult, even for experienced clinicians, to make an accurate differential diagnosis. In clinical practice, nursing care of the dysthymic client is similar to that of depressed clients.

Seasonal Affective Disorder

Natural light is frequently taken for granted, and most people may be unaware of how it influences the human experience. As early as the days of Hippocrates, observers of human behavior noticed that some people suffer mood changes as the seasons change.

The relationships between light, biological rhythms, and mood have been the subject of robust and thorough scientific study. This research focuses on the use of light in the treatment of seasonal affective disorder (SAD), a depressive disorder

CLINICAL MANIFESTATIONS AND THERAPIES **Depressive Disorders**

ETIOLOGY	CLINICAL MANIFESTATIONS	CLINICAL THERAPIES
Major depressive disorder	Symptoms must last 14 days or longer and may include: ■ Feelings of sadness and hopelessness ■ Somatic complaints such as pain, stomachaches ■ Anxiety, anger, irritability ■ Loss of interest in pleasurable activities ■ Sleep disturbances	Pharmacologic therapies include: ■ Selective serotonin reuptake inhibitors (SSRIs) ■ Tricyclic antidepressants (TCAs) ■ Other antidepressants ■ Electroconvulsive therapy (most often used for those who are treatment-resistant to medications) ■ Cognitive-behavioral therapy ■ Suicide precautions
Dysthymic disorder	Symptoms are not as severe as those of major depressive disorder but last beyond 2 years with period of relief lasting less than 2 months.	Pharmacologic therapies include: ■ Selective serotonin reuptake inhibitors (SSRIs) ■ Tricyclic antidepressants (TCAs) ■ Other antidepressants ■ Electroconvulsive therapy (most often used for those who are treatment-resistant to medications) ■ Cognitive-behavioral therapy ■ Suicide precautions
Seasonal affective disorder	Depressive symptoms occur in relation to the seasons; usually during the winter months, when days are shorter.	■ Bupropion extended-release ■ Light therapy ■ Cognitive-behavioral therapy

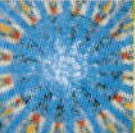

DEVELOPMENTAL CONSIDERATIONS Symptoms of Depression

Symptoms of depression can vary among age groups, although sadness and anhedonia are common at all ages. Differences include the following:

CHILDREN AND ADOLESCENTS

- Infants experiencing depression may fail to eat and grow.
- Toddlers can show regressive behaviors in toileting and other activities.
- Preschoolers have less symbolic and other play activities and demonstrate self-destructive play themes. They may whine and show irritability, disinterest, and lack of confidence.
- School-age children may show a decrease in academic performance, increased or decreased physical activity, somatic complaints, and loss of friends. The older school-age child may talk of running away or show signs of boredom and low self-esteem.
- The adolescent can have a wide array of symptoms (e.g., decreased social contact, poor school performance, lack of involvement in typical activities, poor self-care, difficulty with parents and teachers, or a focus on violence).

OLDER ADULTS

The major clues to depression in the older adult include multiple somatic complaints and reports of persistent chronic pain. Many older adults with depression tend not to consider themselves depressed and therefore complain more of physical symptoms than emotional ones. There is a stigma among many older adults about the diagnosis or acknowledgment of mental illness or psychiatric problems. Some older adults find it more socially acceptable to seek advice and support from a physician or nurse for a physical reason rather than seek out a psychiatrist for mental health problems. Only about 20% of older depressed clients seek advice and counseling from a mental health professional.

Source: Dopheide, 2006; Luby, Heffelfinger, Koenig-McNaught, Brown, & Spitznagel, 2004; Pruett & Luby, 2004.

that occurs in relation to the seasons, usually during winter months. Natural light may help modulate daily rhythms that influence sleep and activity patterns, neuroendocrine functions, and brain chemical systems.

Many antidepressants are typically used to treat the depressive features of SAD, but only one is currently indicated for this diagnosis by the FDA. Bupropion extended-release (Wellbutrin ER) may prevent major depressive episodes in people with SAD. Treatment for SAD has entered areas well beyond therapy and medication. Researchers are exploring the application of different forms of light to the skin and eyes at different times of the day, and the results indicate a reduction of fatigue and depression as well as improved alertness (Joseph, 2006). The exact relationship between SAD and light, biologic rhythms, and events at the cellular level has not yet been determined. Information on SAD and the clinical application of light therapy is available through the Society for Light Treatment and Biological Rhythms (www.sltbr.org) and the Seasonal Affective Disorder Association (www.sada.org.uk).

COLLABORATION

The health care team for a client with a depressive disorder will normally include nurses, the client's treating physician, a psychiatrist or psychologist (or a psychiatrist working with a licensed mental health therapist), and family members. The nurse's role as a member of the health care team is detailed in the Nursing Process section.

Pharmacologic Therapies

Antidepressant medications are often prescribed for clients with depression. Because individuals experience depletion of different neurotransmitters, different individuals respond differently to various antidepressants. A period of trial and error may be necessary to determine which medication is most effective for the client. Approximately 30% of clients do not respond to their antidepressant after a trial of 4–6 weeks. At that point, the primary care provider may try a different antidepressant or augment with other medications such as antipsychotics or mood stabilizers. Maintenance continues until clients are free of symptoms for 4 months to 1 year; then the drugs are slowly discontinued. See the About section of this concept for a more detailed discussion of these medications (Quitkin et al., 2005; Trivedi et al., 2006).

Antidepressants now come with FDA warning labels that describe a link between the drugs and increased suicidal thoughts and behavior in children and youth, especially during the first several months of administration. In contrast, many mental health professionals are worried that not medicating seriously ill children also can lead to an increase in suicidal behavior. In addition, the consequences of not treating with medications may in itself be detrimental to neurodevelopment in children with mood disorders (Pruett & Luby, 2004).

Psychotherapy

Psychotherapy is usually used in addition to medication therapy for major depression. Some of the psychosocial problems associated with depression (ability to relate to others, motivation, problem-solving ability) can be resolved with medications. Psychotherapy may be used in addition to medications to help the client learn to live with a chronic depressive disorder, to manage the specific symptoms that plague the specific client, to promote effective coping skills, and to change habitual negative thinking patterns or behaviors or for psychosocial rehabilitation. Some clients experiencing a mild to moderate depressive episode without psychotic symptoms may benefit from psychotherapy alone.

COGNITIVE-BEHAVIORAL THERAPY Cognitive-behavioral therapy (CBT) is the most effective psychotherapeutic approach for depression. The objective of CBT is twofold: (1) to reduce symptoms by identifying and correcting the client's distorted, negative thinking (Quilty, McBride, & Bagby, 2008) and (2) to determine which behaviors the client needs to change. By identifying the client's erroneous negative thinking and developing new thinking patterns and by helping the client learn to act in a positive, self-confident way, CBT enables the client to feel positive and self-confident. Reinforcement of the client's successes will promote the persistence of effective positive thinking and behavior for coping.

INTERPERSONAL PSYCHOTHERAPY The interpersonal psychotherapy approach involves identifying and resolving the client's interpersonal difficulties. Interpersonal problems are viewed as causal or aggravating factors of depression. According to the interpersonal theorists, the difficulties that lead to depression may be social isolation, prolonged grief, or early development of dysfunctional social behavior. The treatment focus is on interpersonal relationships and social functioning.

Electroconvulsive Therapy

Electroconvulsive therapy is the application of electric current to the brain, which induces a generalized seizure. The procedure is conducted while the client is under general anesthesia with muscle relaxation. The exact mechanism of action is not known, but ECT does increase circulating levels of brain neurotransmitters, which may explain how it relieves depression. Figure 20–7 ■ shows a client prepared for ECT.

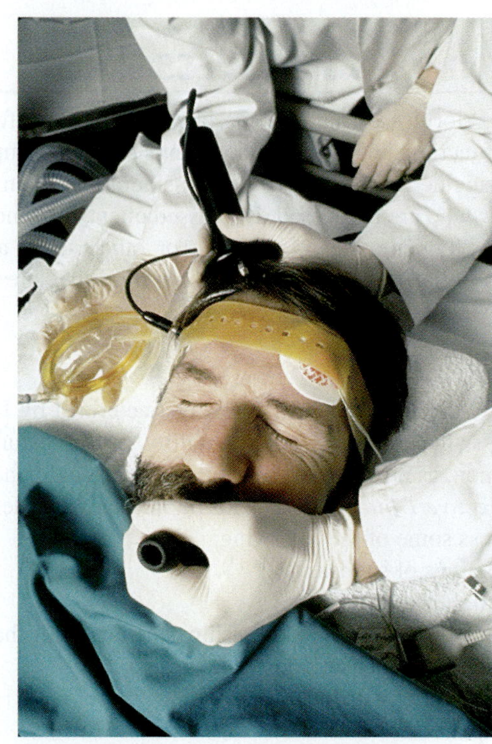

Figure 20–7 ■ A client prepared for electroconvulsive therapy (ECT).

Electroconvulsive therapy is not recommended as a first treatment for uncomplicated nonpsychotic major depression because less invasive treatments are available. It is used for clients who have intense, prolonged symptoms with marked disability, especially when the client has not responded to adequate trials with medications or when psychotic features are present. Electroconvulsive therapy has been successful in inducing remission in people with severe psychomotor retardation. It also may be used for clients who cannot take medications, who are at imminent risk of suicide, or who have dangerous delusions. Clients tend to respond more quickly to ECT than they do to medication therapy. Because of the history of misuse of ECT, a negative stigma is associated with its use (Mendelowitz, Dawkins, & Lieberman, 2000). Nursing considerations for clients receiving ECT are found in Box 20–6.

Box 20–6 **Nursing Considerations for Clients Receiving Electroconvulsive Therapy**

- Prepare the client by explaining the procedure and answering all questions as completely as possible.
- If part of responsibility, have client sign a separate consent for treatment because ECT requires the administration of anesthesia. While informing clients and obtaining consent forms is legally a medical responsibility, in practice, it is often shared by nurses.
- Keep clients npo for at least 4 hours before treatment.
- Just prior to treatment, request that the client void the ladder and remove contact lenses, jewelry, hairpins, and dentures.
- Assess vital signs.
- The anesthetic preparation usually consists of the following:
  a. Generally, an atropine-like medication such as glycopyrrolate (Robinul) is given to decrease secretions and block cardiac vagal reflexes during the seizure.
  b. A short-acting anesthetic such as methohexital sodium (Brevital) is administered intravenously.
  c. Following induction, a skeletal muscle relaxant such as succinylcholine chloride (Anectine) is administered to prevent injuries during the seizure.
  d. The client must be artificially ventilated until the muscle relaxant is fully metabolized, usually in 2–3 minutes. Oxygen is administered with a rubber bite block in place. If necessary, oxygen may be administered by positive pressure.
- An electric current is passed through the brain by means of unilateral or bilateral electrodes placed on the temples. This causes a generalized (or tonic–clonic) seizure, the effects of which are masked by the muscle relaxant. Often the only observable signs of seizure are a fluttering of the eyelids and carpopedal spasms.
- Clients are recovered in the lateral recumbent position to facilitate drainage and to prevent aspiration. Upon awakening, they will be confused and somewhat disoriented. After they are fully recovered and have been reoriented by the nurse, they may eat breakfast. Memory loss may be short term or permanent.

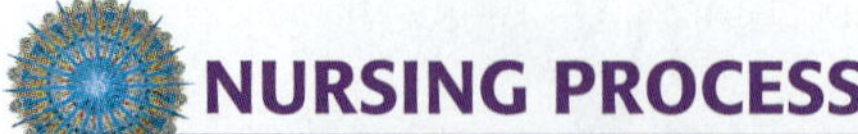

NURSING PROCESS

Priorities of nursing care are focused on safety and meeting functional needs until the client's condition improves. Risk of suicide must always be a consideration when caring for clients who are depressed. Depressed clients may not meet their daily hygiene, sleep, nutrition, or other needs and the nurse can initiate strategies to help them until they are able to function autonomously.

Assessment

As already discussed, depression is characterized by feelings of sadness, hopelessness, and irritability. Sleep disturbances are common, as are changes in eating patterns and behaviors.

- *Subjective Data:* Clients with depressive disorders may express some of the following:
  a. Feelings of sadness
  b. Fatigue
  c. Lack of interest in relationships and activities that were previously pleasurable
  d. Feelings of worthlessness
  e. Impaired concentration
  f. Impaired decision-making ability
  g. Sleep disturbances
  h. Appetite changes; weight loss or weight gain
  i. Excessive sleep.

Clients will often describe how long it takes them to complete activities that they formerly accomplished easily, such as preparing a simple meal. Tearfulness and emotional outbursts also may be a part of their description of the problem. Clients may or may not mention a loss or disappointment that they relate to the feelings.

- *Somatic Concerns:* Somatic concerns are often the presenting complaint. Depressed clients may complain of abdominal pains, headaches, and vague bodily aches. A problem with sexual functioning or lack of desire also may be a presenting complaint. Constipation is a common result of the general slowing of metabolism due to inactivity. Clients from some cultures are more likely to express symptoms of depression through complaints about body function and discomfort. See Box 20–7 for information on how depression evidenced by somatic concerns can be detected in other settings.
- *Suicide Assessment:* Assess all clients who describe depressive symptoms for suicide risk by using direct questioning. Ask about suicidal thinking and history of suicide attempts and whether the client has a specific suicide plan. This aspect of assessment is reassuring, not alarming, to clients. Ask these questions in a direct fashion; for example, "Tell me how you plan to kill yourself. Do you have or can you get the gun/pills/poison?" It is important to know whether the client has actually planned the suicide or it is a vaguely formed thought. The more organized the plan, the more concern it generates, particularly when the client has access to a lethal weapon or chemical or another means of self-injury.

Box 20–7 Physical Complaints and Depression

Frequently, individuals will feel aches and pains more acutely when they are depressed. The natural reaction to pain is to seek help from a primary medical health care provider. One out of every six clients going to a medical office is depressed. Out of *those* clients, only one in six is actually diagnosed and treated for depression. It is important for individuals who are suffering from depression to talk to their health care providers about other experiences and symptoms during their lifetime.

People seldom self-diagnose depression. They are more likely to assume that not enjoying their usual activities, experiencing changes in eating or sleeping habits, and feeling bad in one way or another are caused by a medical problem. Determining the real cause of distress will help to ensure effective responses to treatment.

- *Objective Data:* Depressed clients are most likely to be females under the age of 40. They often have had prior episodes of depression and may have a family history of depression or bipolar disorders. A history of a recent stressful event and the lack of social support are also common features.
- *Objective Signs:* Objective signs and symptoms of depression are few. Psychomotor agitation or retardation may be observable if it is profound or if the nurse is familiar with the client's usual level of functioning. Family members may report observations of the client's agitation or apathy and lack of pleasure in usual activities. They may describe a pattern of social withdrawal and lack of social participation, combined with an intense preoccupation with the client's own feelings. Be alert to a change in behavior.
- *Depression Inventory Checklists:* During assessment, many clinicians find it useful to provide a list of symptoms and ask clients to check the ones they are experiencing. A widely used and highly regarded self-reporting instrument designed to assess mood state is the Beck Depression Inventory (Table 20–3 in the About section of this concept). In use for over 35 years, the Beck Depression Inventory has been revised several times on the basis of clinical research. It is useful for detecting depression, anxiety, apathy, and irritability. Several different types of Beck inventories are now available; see Table 20–3 for one example (Beck, Steer, & Brown, 1996).
- *Medical Illnesses:* Other objective information to obtain during the nursing assessment includes concurrent general medical illnesses. Autoimmune, neurologic, metabolic, oncologic, and endocrine disorders often trigger depression. For example, hypothyroidism may be accompanied by depressive symptoms due to the underlying medical disease, while a client with AIDS or cancer may become depressed as a result of the diagnosis, prognosis, or disability connected with the disease.
- *Substance Use and Abuse:* Alcohol, which is a CNS depressant, and certain legal and illegal drugs can cause or complicate depression. Through matter-of-fact questioning, obtain a complete list of all substances and medications the

client uses. A few prescription medications have depression as a side effect, and they should not be overlooked in the complete assessment. Birth control pills, sedatives, reserpine, glucocorticoids, and anabolic steroids have all been associated with the development of depression.

Assessment of the Older Adult

The Geriatric Depression Scale (GDS) is a screening instrument used in many clinical settings to assess depression in older adults (Box 20–8). The GDS is a 30-item (long version) or 15-item (short version) instrument with questions that can be answered "yes" or "no." An older adult can complete the GDS by circling the correct answer, or a health care professional can read it to an older adult. In tests of various groups of older adults, the GDS was found to distinguish successfully between depressed and nondepressed older adults (Yesavage et al., 1983). The GDS can be used to screen older adults regardless of physical health status and may be used to screen those with cognitive impairment (Mini-Mental State Examination (MMSE) score above 15) (Hartford Institute for Geriatric Nursing, 2008). Older adults scoring above 10 on the GDS should be referred for further assessment. The Cornell Depression Scale (CDS) can be used to screen for depression in older adults with severe cognitive impairments (MMSE below 15). The CDS does not rely on client responses; rather, it is based on observations of behaviors and functional measures. People who score 12 or above on the CDS should be referred for further assessment. Because the CDS requires client observations, it takes slightly longer to administer than the GDS.

Assessment of Children

Careful and thorough assessment of a child suspected of having depression is necessary to rule out physical illness that can be linked to depressive symptoms. These may include diabetes, cancer, and some other conditions (Sheikh, Weller, & Weller, 2006). Initial psychiatric assessment is performed by a child psychologist or child psychiatrist. A variety of scales and techniques are used; however, very little guidance is available relating to evaluation of children under 6 years of age. Following are examples of useful tools:

- Children's Depression Inventory (CDI)
- Revised Children's Manifest Anxiety Scale
- Beck Depressive Inventory
- Preschool Feelings Checklist
- Reynolds Child Depression Scale
- Reynolds Adolescent Depression Scale
- Center of Epidemiological Studies Depression Scale of Children (CES-DC).

The child is tested for various mental health problems because comorbidities (appearance with other disorders) are common. Examples of these include a history of bullying or substance abuse.

Diagnosis

A number of nursing diagnoses may be appropriate for the depressed client, including the following:

- Risk for Self-Directed Violence related to negative thought processes and feelings of hopelessness
- Situational Low Self-Esteem or Chronic Low Self-Esteem related to feelings of abandonment, repeated failures or losses, lack of positive feedback from others, or negative thought processes
- Hopelessness related to believing his or her own actions cannot influence an outcome or that there is no solution to his or her problems
- Social Isolation due to inadequate social skills, self-absorption, and fear
- Ineffective Health Maintenance related to not complying with medication administration or therapy.

Plan

Together with the client, the nurse will design a plan of care that may include any of the following objectives:

- The client will remain free of injury.
- The client will refrain from attempts to injure self or others.
- The client will participate in recreational activities.

Box 20–8 **Geriatric Depression Scale, Short Form**

Choose the best answer for how you have felt over the past week:

1. Are you basically satisfied with your life? YES / **NO**
2. Have you dropped many of your activities and interests? **YES** / NO
3. Do you feel that your life is empty? **YES** / NO
4. Do you often get bored? **YES** / NO
5. Are you in good spirits most of the time? YES / **NO**
6. Are you afraid that something bad is going to happen to you? **YES** / NO
7. Do you feel happy most of the time? YES / **NO**
8. Do you often feel helpless? **YES** / NO
9. Do you prefer to stay at home, rather than going out and doing new things? **YES** / NO
10. Do you feel you have more problems with memory than most? **YES** / NO
11. Do you think it is wonderful to be alive now? YES / **NO**
12. Do you feel pretty worthless the way you are now? **YES** / NO
13. Do you feel full of energy? YES / **NO**
14. Do you feel that your situation is hopeless? **YES** / NO
15. Do you think that most people are better off than you are? **YES** / NO

Answers in **bold** indicate depression. Score 1 point for each bolded answer.

A score > 5 points is suggestive of depression.

A score ≥ 10 points is almost always indicative of depression.

A score > 5 points should warrant a follow-up comprehensive assessment.

Source: Sheikh, J. I., Yesavage, J. A., Brooks, J. O., III, Friedman, L. F., Gratzinger, P., Hill, R. D., et al. (1991). Proposed factor structure of the Geriatric Depression Scale. *International Psychogeriatrics 3,* 23–28.

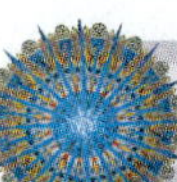

NURSING CARE PLAN A Client With Depression

ASSESSMENT	DIAGNOSES	PLANNING
You are the hospice nurse assigned to Pam Allen, who is dying of cancer. During your assessment of her husband, Cliff, he discloses the following: ■ He was diagnosed with depression years ago but is not currently receiving treatment. ■ Years ago his brother committed suicide. ■ He feels helpless about Pam's situation. He says that he has been a terrible husband and father. ■ He is not currently receiving any treatment for depression. ■ He has 2 or 3 alcoholic drinks every night after Pam goes to bed. ■ He is not sure how he is going to cope with caring for their disabled son, Gary, after Pam is gone.	■ Powerlessness ■ Anticipatory Grieving ■ Situational Low Self-Esteem ■ Risk for Caregiver Role Strain ■ Ineffective Health Maintenance ■ Anxiety	The next day the hospice nurse talks further with Cliff. Together they create a plan of care that will help Cliff: ■ Investigate resources for helping him care for Gary ■ Develop a plan of exercise and recreation ■ Stop drinking ■ Begin treatment for depression as recommended by a mental health professional.

IMPLEMENTATION

- Provide teaching Cliff about the need to begin treatment for depression again in order to prevent deterioration in mood and affect.
- Refer Cliff to a mental health professional for diagnosis and treatment.
- Encourage Cliff to explore his feelings regarding Pam's terminal condition and what his life will be like after her death.
- Encourage Cliff to talk with Pam about her wishes regarding her death and funeral care in order to take a more active role in meeting her needs.
- Support Cliff's need to grieve for his wife and help him to recognize that sadness is a normal part of the process.
- Encourage Cliff to see that maintaining his own health is an important contribution to both Pam and Gary's care.
- Refer Cliff to agencies serving the disabled to determine what assistance may be available to help him care for Gary.
- Help Cliff develop a plan of exercise and recreation.
- Support Cliff's need to obtain assistance in caring for Pam and Gary to reduce caregiver role strain.

EVALUATION

Cliff demonstrates improvement by meeting the following expected outcomes:

- Cliff begins seeing a mental health professional to treat depression.
- Cliff is taking medications as prescribed.
- Cliff finds a day care program that specializes in treating adults with Down's Syndrome.
- Pam and Cliff discuss her terminal condition, her desires for end of life care, and her post mortem wishes.
- Cliff learns that his medical insurance will pay for someone to come to the home to provide for Pam's care 4 hours a day and initiates these visits immediately.

CRITICAL THINKING

1. What expected outcome would you anticipate for Cliff if he fails to obtain treatment for depression?
2. What community programs might you suggest to Cliff to help him care for Gary and Pam?
3. What follow up care can the hospice nurse provide Cliff when making daily visits to Pam?

- The client will articulate steps to feeling better, such as engaging in recreational activities or exercise *before* beginning to feel better.
- The client will protect personal rights while respecting those of others.
- The client will comply with medication regimens.

Implementation

When implementing interventions designed to help depressed clients, keep two general principles in mind:

1. It is impossible to make depressed clients feel better by being cheerful. In fact, an overly cheerful attitude tends to make them feel even worse because it trivializes or minimizes the impact of their feelings. Try to adopt a more emotionally neutral attitude while maintaining confidence that they will feel better.
2. Recognize that working with depressed clients may eventually lower your own mood and make you feel "down" yourself. This is called *emotional contagion.* The nurse should be aware of personal feelings and, if necessary, ask to be assigned to a different type of client for a time.

Self-Esteem

While low self-esteem is a chronic problem, the nurse can take a number of actions to reduce negative thinking, thereby promoting improved self-esteem.

- Provide distraction from self-absorption by involving the client in recreational activities and pleasant pastimes. Simple conversation with a staff member or another client helps interrupt the pattern of negative thoughts. Use care to select activities that are not too complex for the client's current level of functioning. Experiences of success, not more failures, are needed. Increase the complexity of activities as the client progresses.

- Dispel the notion that clients often have that *when* they feel better, they will want to engage in activities. Explain that they must begin doing things *in order* to feel better. Being active promotes a more balanced feeling state. Acknowledge that it takes self-discipline and energy to do something when one doesn't really feel like it.
- Recognize accomplishment, but do not use flattery or excessive praise. Give positive, matter-of-fact reinforcement such as "I notice that you combed your hair," rather than overly enthusiastic compliments such as "What a great hairstyle!" Appropriate recognition increases the likelihood that the client will continue the positive behavior, while insincerity can be perceived as ridicule or infantilizing.
- Be accepting of clients' negative feelings, but set limits on the amount of time spent discussing accounts of past failures. Be alert for opportunities to interrupt negative conversational patterns with more neutral ones.
- Teach assertiveness techniques such as the ability to say no to protect one's rights while respecting the rights of others. Clients with low self-esteem often allow others to take advantage of them. Defining passive, aggressive, and assertive behavior and giving examples of each also are helpful when teaching assertiveness. (See the discussion in the About section of this concept for more information.) Practice these new techniques with the client, providing feedback on how it feels to the recipient of assertive communication or an assertive action.

Hopelessness

It is equally important to help clients identify the aspects of their lives that are not within their control. Being able to accept what *cannot* be changed is just as essential as developing the ability to bring about positive change. This skill is particularly helpful in reorienting clients from feelings of hopelessness to a more hopeful aspect. Other interventions to help clients combat hopelessness include the following:

- Help clients identify their personal strengths. It may be useful to write these down. Recognize that it often takes time for clients to realize that they have any strengths. Recognizing strengths helps a client design an activity or engagement plan that the client is more likely to enjoy and find successful.
- Engage clients in setting goals for themselves. Try to direct clients to focus on small goals at first. For example, instead of the goal of "going to yoga twice a week," the initial goal might be to go to the yoga center and get a list of class times and teachers or sit in on a class.
- Help clients weigh and choose alternatives. Taking responsibility even for small choices such as when or where to eat a meal helps the client begin to regain self esteem.
- Explore problem-solving models with the client, including practicing problem solving. "When you found out the toaster was broken, you threw it against the wall. You said all that did was put a dent in the wall and make a mess for you to clean up. What might you do differently next time that might be more helpful?"
- Help clients to identify resources such as family, community, or friends who can provide support and encouragement in overcoming problems they identify.

Planning for discharge should begin with the first client contact and is particularly important with hopeless, dependent clients. Help them and their families and significant others to identify resources in the community they can use to build support systems. Support groups, therapy groups, and social groups can help clients separate from caregivers more readily when the time comes to end therapy.

Evaluation

Client progress is evaluated based on the ability to meet the following suggested expected outcomes, although these should be modified based on each client's unique situation.

- Client meets daily functional needs appropriately such as eating three meals a day, bathing regularly, or sleeping 8 hours per night.
- Client does not demonstrate or express suicidal ideation.
- Client describes hopefulness for the future.
- Client is able to resume normal activity patterns such as returning to work or school.

REVIEW Depression

RELATE: LINK THE CONCEPTS

Linking the exemplar of Depression with the concept of Substance Abuse:

1. Why might dependence on alcohol promote depression?
2. What impact might dependence on nicotine have on mood and affect?

Linking the exemplar of Depression with the concept of Elimination:

3. What aspects of depression increase the risk for constipation?
4. How might alterations in elimination put an older client at risk for depression?

READY: LINK TO COMPANION SKILLS MANUAL

- Assessing appearance and mental status
- Evaluating client safety
- Assessing home for safe environment

REFER: GO TO MYNURSINGKIT

REFLECT: CASE STUDY

Melvin Thomas is a 14-year-old African American male whose mother brings him to their family doctor's office because this is the third day in a row that Melvin "hasn't felt well." Melvin has been getting in trouble at school for arguing with teachers, and he has missed a lot of school, complaining of stomachaches. Melvin's mother says that he rarely sees his dad but that her second husband tries to spend time with Melvin when he can. When they do spend time together, they go shooting at the gun range or play video games. Melvin's expression at the doctor's office is sullen, and he keeps his arms crossed in front of him. He answers the nurse by giving one-syllable responses or by nodding or shaking his head.

1. What assessment findings would make you suspect Melvin is depressed?
2. What priority assessment and teaching would you want to provide Melvin's mother if the diagnosis of depression is confirmed?
3. What impact is depression having on Melvin's ability to meet developmental milestones?

20.3 POSTPARTUM DEPRESSION

KEY TERMS

Acquaintance phase, *1198*
Adjustment reaction to depressed mood, *1200*
Engrossment, *1198*
Maternal role attainment (MRA), *1196*
Phase of mutual regulation, *1198*
Postpartum major mood disorder, *1201*
Puerperium, *1196*

BASIS FOR SELECTION OF EXEMPLAR

Emergency room admissions
Healthy People 2010
Institute of Medicine
National Institute of Mental Health
Office-based physician visits

LEARNING OUTCOMES

After reading about this exemplar, you will be able to:

1. Describe the pathophysiology, etiology, clinical manifestations, and direct and indirect causes of postpartum depression.
2. Identify risk factors associated with postpartum depression.
3. Illustrate the nursing process in providing culturally competent care across the life span for women with postpartum depression.
4. Formulate priority nursing diagnoses appropriate for a woman with postpartum depression.
5. Create a plan of care for women with postpartum depression and their family members.
6. Assess expected outcomes for a woman with postpartum depression.
7. Discuss therapies used in the collaborative care of a woman with postpartum depression.
8. Employ evidence-based caring interventions for a woman with postpartum depression

OVERVIEW

The postpartal period is a time of readjustment and adaptation for the entire family, but especially for the mother. The woman experiences a variety of responses as she adjusts to a new family member, postpartal discomforts, changes in her body image, and the reality that she is no longer pregnant. Postpartum blues is a transient period of depression that occurs during the first few days of the puerperium in 70% of all postpartal women (Varney et al., 2004). The **puerperium** is that time immediately following childbirth when physiologic changes that occurred in the mother during pregnancy begin to return to normal. Postpartum blues are a common occurrence that usually resolves within 10–14 days. Some women, however, are unable to resolve these feelings and are at risk for postpartum psychiatric disorders. This exemplar discusses the psychologic struggles that women face after giving birth and how nurses can support them during this critical time.

NORMAL PRESENTATION

During the first day or two after birth, the woman tends to be passive and somewhat dependent. She follows suggestions, hesitates to make decisions, and is still rather preoccupied with her needs. She may have a great need to talk about her perceptions of the labor and birth. This helps her work through the process, sort out the reality from her fantasized experience, and clarify anything that she does not understand. Food and sleep are major needs. In her early work, Rubin (1961) labeled this the *taking-in* period.

By the second or third day after birth, the new mother is observed to be ready to resume control of her body, her mothering, and her life in general. Rubin (1961) labeled this the *taking-hold* period. This period can be a time of great anxiety for the new mother. If she is breastfeeding, she may worry about her technique or the quality of her milk. If her baby spits up after a feeding, she may view it as a personal failure. She also may feel demoralized by the fact that the nurse or an older family member handles her baby proficiently while she feels unsure and tentative. She requires assurance that she is doing well as a mother. Today's mothers seem to be more independent and adjust more rapidly, exhibiting behaviors of "taking-in" and "taking-hold" in shorter time periods than those previously identified.

Maternal Role Attainment

Maternal role attainment (MRA) is the process by which a woman learns mothering behaviors and becomes comfortable with her identity as a mother. Formation of a maternal identity occurs with each child a woman bears. As the mother grows to know this child and forms a relationship, the mother's maternal identity gradually and systematically evolves and she "binds in" to the infant (Rubin, 1984).

Maternal role attainment often occurs in four stages (Mercer, 1995):

1. The *anticipatory stage* occurs during pregnancy. The woman looks to role models, especially her own mother, for examples of how to mother.
2. The *formal stage* begins when the child is born. The woman is still influenced by the guidance of others and tries to act as she believes others expect her to act.

3. The *informal stage* begins when the mother starts making her own choices about mothering. The woman begins to develop her own style of mothering and finds ways of functioning that work well for her.
4. The *personal stage* is the final stage of maternal role attainment. When the woman reaches this stage, she is comfortable with the notion of herself as "mother."

In most cases, MRA occurs within 3–10 months after birth. Social support, the woman's age and personality traits, the marital relationship, the presence of underlying anxiety or depression, the woman's previous child care experiences, the temperament of her infant, and the family's socioeconomic status all influence the woman's success in attaining the maternal role.

The postpartum woman faces a number of challenges as she adjusts to her new role (Mercer, 1995):

- For many women, finding time for themselves is one of the greatest challenges of motherhood. It is often difficult for the new mother to find time to read a book, talk to her partner, or even eat a meal without interruption.
- Women also report feelings of incompetence because they have not mastered all aspects of the mothering role. Many times mothers find themselves unsure of what to do in a given situation.
- The next greatest challenge involves fatigue resulting from sleep deprivation. The demands of nighttime care are tremendously draining, especially when the woman has other children.
- Another challenge for the new mother involves the feeling of responsibility that having a child brings. Women experience a sense of lost freedom, an awareness that they will never again be quite as carefree as they were before becoming a mother.
- Finding time for older children following the birth of a new baby also presents challenges. Many women feel guilty because the new baby takes up so much of their time. Sibling rivalry or ill feelings about the baby from other children can put additional stress on the mother.
- Mothers sometimes cite the infant's behavior as a challenge, especially when the child is about 8 months old. The baby develops stranger anxiety, begins crawling and getting into things, and may be fussy from teething. In addition, the baby's tendency to put things in his or her mouth requires constant vigilance by the parent.

In 2004, Mercer proposed replacing the term *maternal role attainment* (MRA) with the term *becoming a mother* (BAM). She stated that BAM "more accurately encompasses the dynamic transformation and evolution of a woman's persona than does MRA, and the term MRA should be discontinued" (Mercer, 2004). BAM more accurately reflects the transition process of becoming a mother that changes throughout the maternal–child relationship.

Postpartal nurses need to be aware of the long-term adjustments and stresses that the family faces as its members adjust to new and different roles. Nurses can help by providing anticipatory guidance about the realities of being a parent and by giving the postpartal family parenting literature for reference at home. Ongoing parenting groups give parents an opportunity to discuss problems and become comfortable in new roles.

FOCUS ON DIVERSITY AND CULTURE

Middle Eastern Initial Postpartum Experience

In many countries in the Middle East that follow a patriarchal system, the new mother and her infant stay with the husband's family following the birth of the infant. Frequent visits from the woman's family are discouraged and may even be viewed as burdensome by the husband's family. Typically, only women visit the new mother during the postpartum period. For the birth of the first baby, the wife's parents are expected to purchase all of the baby's supplies and clothing.

Development of Family Attachment

A mother's first interaction with her infant is influenced by many factors, including her involvement with her family of origin, her relationships, the stability of her home environment, the communication patterns she has developed, and the degree of nurturing she received as a child. These factors shaped the person she has become. The following personal characteristics are also important:

- *Level of trust.* What level of trust has this mother developed in response to her life experiences? What is her philosophy of childrearing? Will she be able to treat her infant as a unique individual with changing needs that should be met as much as possible?
- *Level of self-esteem.* How much does she value herself as a woman and a mother? Is she generally able to cope with the adjustments of life?
- *Capacity for enjoying herself.* Is the mother able to find pleasure in everyday activities and human relationships?
- *Adequacy of knowledge about childbearing and childrearing.* What beliefs about the course of pregnancy, the capabilities of newborns, previous experiences with infants or children, and the nature of her emotions may influence her behavior at first contact with her infant and later?
- *Prevailing mood or usual feeling tone.* Is the woman predominantly content, angry, depressed, or anxious? Is she sensitive to her own feelings and those of others? Will she be able to accept her own needs and to obtain support in meeting them?
- *Reactions to the present pregnancy.* Was the pregnancy planned? Did it go smoothly? Were there ongoing life events that enhanced her pregnancy or depleted her reserves of energy? How have other life roles changed because of her pregnancy and motherhood?

By the time of birth, each mother has developed some kind of emotional orientation to the baby based on these factors.

Initial Maternal Attachment Behavior

After labor and birth, a new mother demonstrates a fairly regular pattern of maternal behaviors as she continues to familiarize herself with her newborn. In a progression of touching activities, the mother proceeds from fingertip exploration of the newborn's extremities toward palmar contact with larger body areas and finally to enfolding the infant with the whole hand and arm. The time she takes to accomplish these steps varies from minutes to days. The mother increases the proportion of time spent in the *en face* position (Figure 20–8 ■). She arranges herself or the newborn so that she has direct face-to-face and eye-to-eye contact. There is an intense interest in having the infant's eyes open. When the infant's eyes are open, the mother characteristically greets the newborn and talks to the baby in high-pitched tones.

In most instances, the mother relies heavily on her senses of sight, touch, and hearing in getting to know what her baby is really like. She also tends to respond verbally to any sounds emitted by the newborn, such as cries, coughs, sneezes, and grunts. The sense of smell may be involved as well.

PRACTICE ALERT

Newborns are sometimes taken from their parents immediately after birth and placed in a special care or intensive care nursery. This separation can interfere with the normal attachment process. If this occurs, take the parents to the nursery as soon as possible to interact with their infant and allow them to hold and care for their infant as much as possible. If the infant is in an incubator and cannot be held, encourage the parents to stroke the infant's hand, foot, or cheek. Provide reassurance that this will not hurt the infant and is actually beneficial.

While interacting with her newborn, the mother may be experiencing shock, disbelief, or denial. She may state, "I can't believe she's finally here" or "I feel like he is a stranger." On the other hand, feelings of connectedness between the newborn and the rest of the family can be expressed in positive or negative terms: "She's got your cute nose, Daddy" or "Oh, no! He looks just like Matthew, and he was an impossible baby." A mother's facial expressions or the frequency and content of her questions may demonstrate concerns about the infant's general condition or normality, especially if her pregnancy was complicated or if a previous baby was not healthy.

During the first few days after her child's birth, the new mother applies herself to the task of getting to know her baby.

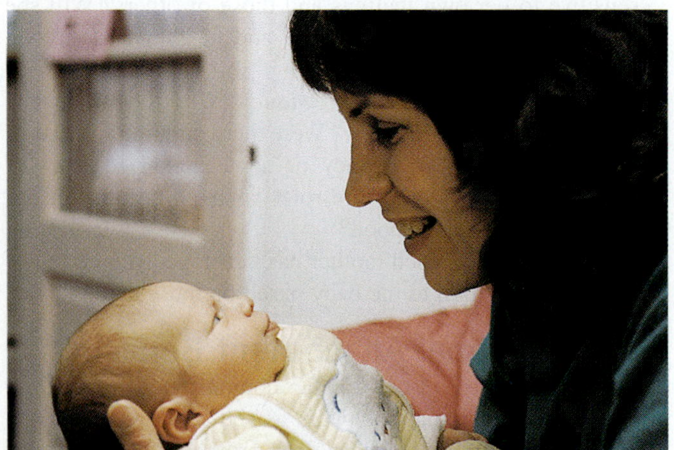

Figure 20–8 ■ The mother has direct face-to-face and eye-to-eye contact in the en face position.

Source: Stella Johnson (www.stellajohnson.com).

This is termed the **acquaintance phase**. If the infant gives clear behavioral cues about needs, the infant's responses to mothering will be predictable, which will make the mother feel effective and competent. Other behaviors that make an infant more attractive to caretakers are smiling, grasping a finger, nursing eagerly, and being easy to console.

During this time, the newborn also is becoming acquainted. Within a few days after birth, infants show signs of recognizing recurrent situations and responding to changes in routine. To the extent that their mother is their world, it can be said that they are actively acquainting themselves with her.

During the **phase of mutual regulation**, mother and infant seek to determine the degree of control each will exert in their relationship. In this phase of adjustment, a balance is sought between the needs of the mother and the needs of the infant. The most important consideration is that each should obtain a good measure of enjoyment from the interaction. During this phase, negative maternal feelings are likely to surface or intensify. Because "everyone knows that mothers love their babies," these negative feelings often go unexpressed and are allowed to build up. If they are expressed, the response of friends, relatives, or health care personnel is often to deny the feelings to the mother: "You don't mean that." Some negative feelings are normal in the first few days after birth, and the nurse should be supportive when the mother vocalizes these feelings.

When mutual regulation arrives at the point where both mother and infant primarily enjoy each other's company, reciprocity has been achieved. Reciprocity is an interactional cycle that occurs simultaneously between mother and infant. It involves mutual cuing behaviors, expectancy, rhythmicity, and synchrony. The mother develops a new relationship with an individual who has a unique character and evokes a response entirely different from the fantasy response of pregnancy. When reciprocity is synchronous, the interaction between mother and infant is mutually gratifying and is sought and initiated by both partners.

FATHER–INFANT INTERACTIONS In Western cultures, commitment to family-centered maternity care has fostered interest in understanding the feelings and experiences of the new father. Evidence suggests that the father has a strong attraction to his newborn and that the feelings he experiences are similar to the mother's feelings of attachment (Figure 20–9 ■). The father's characteristic sense of absorption, preoccupation, and interest in the infant demonstrated during early contact is termed **engrossment**. Differences in involvement still exist among fathers in Western culture and may be influenced by factors other than culture (e.g., previous experience with paternal role or exposure to male/father role models).

SIBLINGS AND OTHERS Infants are capable of maintaining a number of strong attachments without loss of quality. These attachments may include siblings, grandparents, aunts, and uncles. The social setting and personality of the individual seem to be significant factors in the development of multiple attachments. Birth centers are especially geared toward the family's inclusion in the birth process. In the hospital setting, the advent of open visiting hours and rooming-in permits siblings and others to participate in the attachment process.

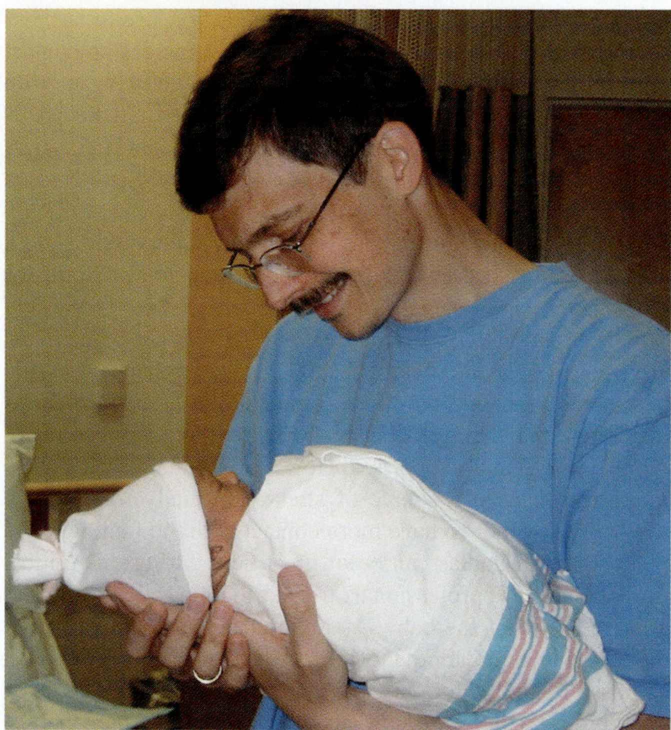

Figure 20–9 ■ The father experiences strong feelings of attraction.

Cultural Influences in the Postpartal Period

Whereas Western culture places primary emphasis on the events of birth, many other cultures place greater emphasis on the postpartum period. For women who are not from the dominant American culture, the new mother's culture and personal values influence her beliefs about her postpartal care. Her expectations about food, fluids, rest, hygiene, medications and relief measures, support, and counsel—as well as other aspects of her life—are influenced by the beliefs and values of her family and cultural group. Sometimes a new mother's preferences differ from the expectations of the certified nurse-midwife (CNM), physician, or nurse.

Nurses belong to a particular ethnoculture and share in the culture of health care. Thus, their nursing care may include practices that support the general beliefs of these groups, such as offering food and fluids in the recovery period after birth, expecting the woman to ambulate as soon as possible, and assuming the woman will want to shower and wash her hair soon after giving birth. Nurses must recognize that they are approaching their client's care from their own perspective and that to individualize care for each mother, they need to assess the woman's preferences, her level of acculturation and assimilation to Western culture, her linguistic abilities, and her educational level (Kim-Goodwin, 2005). In addition, with the help of cultural awareness and a sound knowledge base, the nurse should let the mother exercise her choices whenever possible and should support those choices.

> **FOCUS ON DIVERSITY AND CULTURE**
> **Muslim Paternal Attachment**
>
> In some cultures, the father may have little involvement in newborn care. In the Muslim culture, for example, emphasis on childrearing and infant care is on the mother and extended female family members. Nurses need to be aware of cultural differences when evaluating a father's interaction with his newborn.

Although describing particular practices of different cultural groups involves some generalization, it is helpful for nurses to understand some of the possible differences in beliefs and practices. Women of European heritage may expect to eat a full meal and have large amounts of iced fluids after the birth, in the belief that the food restores energy and the fluids help replace fluid lost during labor. They may want to ambulate shortly after the birth, shower, wash their hair, and put on a fresh gown. They may expect a short stay in the hospital and may or may not be interested in educational classes. Women of the Islamic faith may have specific modesty requirements: The woman must be completely covered, with only her feet and hands exposed, and no man, other than the husband or a family member, may be alone with her (Al-Oballi Kridli, 2002; Lauderdale, 2008).

Some cultures emphasize certain postpartal routines or rituals for mother and baby that are designed to restore the hot–cold balance of the body. Some women of Hispanic, African, and Asian cultures may avoid cold after birth. This prohibition includes cold air, wind, and all water (even if heated). On the other hand, some women of traditional Mexican descent may avoid eating "hot" foods such as pork just after the birth of a baby (considered a "hot" experience). It is important to note that individual or cultural groups may define hot and cold conditions and foods differently. The nurse should ask each woman what she can eat and what foods she thinks would be helpful for healing. The nurse may encourage family members to bring preferred foods and drinks for the mother.

In many cultures, the extended family plays an essential role during the puerperium. The grandmother is often the primary helper to the mother and newborn. She brings wisdom and experience, allowing the new mother time to rest and giving her ready access to someone who can help with problems and concerns as they arise. It is important to ensure that all family members have access to the mother and newborn. Visiting hours may be waived to allow family members or authority figures access to the mother and newborn. These practices show respect and foster a blending of old and new behaviors to meet the goals of all concerned (Purnell & Paulanka, 2008). African American mothers model their mothering skills after their older female relatives. In addition, these same older female relatives usually provide needed child care (Purnell & Paulanka, 2008). People of Jewish faith observe a Sabbath from sundown Friday to sundown Saturday. During this time, Orthodox Jews do not perform any manual labor; for the postpartal woman, this includes turning the lights on and off, pressing the call bell, or raising/lowering the head of the bed (De Sovo, 1997). Jewish clients also may request a kosher diet. Some traditional Jewish couples avoid physical contact while the woman is experiencing vaginal discharge; unfortunately, the staff may view the man following this custom as being unsupportive (D'Avanzo & Geissler, 2008).

Postpartum Blues

As stated previously, postpartum blues is a state of a transient period of depression that occurs in many women during the first few days following labor. Also referred to as **adjustment reaction to depressed mood**, it is sometimes classified as a postpartum psychiatric disorder despite the fact that it is such a common occurrence. Postpartum blues may be manifested by mood swings, anger, weepiness, anorexia, difficulty sleeping, and a feeling of letdown. This mood change frequently occurs while the woman is still hospitalized, but it may occur at home as well. Changing hormone levels are a factor; psychological adjustments, an unsupportive environment, and insecurity also have been identified as potential causes. In addition, fatigue, discomfort, and overstimulation may play a role. The postpartum blues usually resolve naturally within 10–14 days, but if symptoms persist or worsen, the woman may need evaluation for postpartum depression. Ideally, a depression assessment should be completed each trimester to update a pregnant woman's risk status (Beck, 2002). If one was not done previously, the nurse assesses the woman for predisposing factors during labor and the postpartum stay. Several depression scales are available for assessing postpartum depression. The routine use of a screening tool such as the Edinburgh Postnatal Depression Scale or Postpartum Depression Predictors Inventory-Revised significantly increases the diagnosis (Beck, 2008).

A key feature of postpartum blues is episodic tearfulness, often without an identifiable cause. Often when the woman is asked why she is crying, she responds that she does not know. Cunningham et al. (2005) speculate that several factors contribute to the blues:

- Emotional letdown that follows labor and childbirth
- Physical discomfort typical in the early postpartum period
- Fatigue
- Anxiety about caring for the newborn after discharge
- Fears about her physical attractiveness.

Validating the existence of this phenomenon, labeling it as a real but normal adjustment reaction, and providing reassurance can offer a measure of relief. Assistance with self- and infant care, rest, good nutrition, information, and family support aids recovery. The partner should be encouraged to watch for and report signs that the new mother is not returning to a normal mood, but is slipping into a deeper depression. Most affected women reported that they did not seek help because they believed that their depression was caused by the stress of becoming a mother, thought it was a normal reaction, and/or feared that they would be labeled mentally ill and considered unfit mothers (Driscoll, 2008).

IMPORTANCE OF SOCIAL SUPPORT The psychological outcomes of the postpartal period are far more positive when the parents have access to a support network. Women and their partners may find that family relationships become increasingly important, but the increased family interaction itself can be a source of stress. New parents also may have increasing contact with other parents of small children but find that contact with coworkers declines. Of great concern are women and their partners who have no family or friends with whom to form a social network. Isolation at a time when the woman feels an increased need for support can result in tremendous stress and is often a contributing factor in situations of postpartum depression, child neglect, or abuse. New mother support groups are helpful for women who lack a social support system.

The attention that their infant receives from family members is a source of satisfaction to the new parents. In many cases, the ties to the woman's family become especially good. Fathers may report that their relationships with their in-laws become far more positive and supportive. However, the increased family interaction can be a source of stress, especially for the new mother, who tends to have more contact with the families.

Postpartum doulas can be of great help during this critical time. Doulas are professionals trained to help the new mother after the birth of the baby. As a "mother helper," postpartum doula services are tailored to help the new mother feel as rested as possible and well-nourished and to place her household in good order so that she can focus her energy on her new baby.

POSTPARTUM PSYCHIATRIC DISORDERS

The relationship of affective disorders to childbirth is reflected in the fact that the rate of admission to a psychiatric hospital is greater during the year after childbirth than at any other time in a woman's life.

The classification of postpartum psychiatric disorders is a subject of some controversy. The *Diagnostic and Statistical Manual of Mental Disorders* (APA, 2000) has added a postpartum onset specifier to the mood disorder diagnostic category of psychiatric disorders. An alternative method of classification that has been proposed is for the postpartum psychiatric disorders to be considered as one diagnosable syndrome with three subclasses: (1) adjustment reaction with depressed mood, (2) postpartum psychosis, and (3) postpartum major mood disorder. The incidence, etiology, symptoms, treatment, and prognosis vary with each subclass.

Postpartum Psychosis

Postpartum psychosis, which has an incidence of 1–2 per 1,000, usually becomes evident within the first 1–3 months following birth (Beck, 2006). Although relatively rare, new onset postpartum psychosis gains considerable national attention in the media when an incident of infanticide is associated with it. Symptoms include agitation, hyperactivity, insomnia, mood lability, confusion, irrationality, difficulty remembering or concentrating, poor judgment, delusions, and hallucinations that tend to be related to the infant. With appropriate treatment, 95% of women experience improvement of symptoms within 2–3 months. Surprisingly, postpartum psychosis is not associated with depression during the antepartal period (Haessler & Rosenthal, 2007). Recurrence in subsequent pregnancies may be as high as 20–30%.

CLINICAL MANIFESTATIONS AND THERAPIES Postpartum Depression

ETIOLOGY	CLINICAL MANIFESTATIONS	CLINICAL THERAPIES
Postpartum depression	Severe depression that occurs within the first year of giving birth, with increased incidence at about the fourth week postpartum, just before menses resumes, and upon weaning.	■ Sertraline (Zoloft) or paroxetine (Paxil) ■ Support groups ■ Assistance with care of the newborn taking care to promote self-confidence in mothering ■ Mental health counseling ■ Assist to build self-esteem and self-confidence in mothering skills
Postpartum psychosis	■ Agitation ■ Hyperactivity ■ Insomnia ■ Mood lability ■ Confusion ■ Irrationality ■ Difficulty remembering or concentrating ■ Delusions and hallucinations that tend to be related to the infant	■ Lithium or antipsychotics ■ Should be supervised at all times when caring for infant or other children ■ Support groups ■ Short term institutionalization may be required

Postpartum psychosis is considered an emergency because of the risk of suicide and/or infanticide (Beck, 2006). The psychotic woman may experience delusions or hallucinations that support her perceptions that the infant should not be allowed to live. Illogical thinking or evidence of bonding difficulties may serve as cues to infanticide and suicide risk; however, this assessment is often challenging because of the lucidity seen in some psychotic clients.

Postpartum Major Mood Disorder

Postpartum major mood disorder, also known as postpartum depression, refers to severe depression that occurs within the first year of giving birth, with increased incidence at about the fourth week postpartum, just before menses resume, and upon weaning although it may occur at any time during the first year. Postpartum depression develops in about 3–30% of all postpartum women in North America (Beck & Driscoll, 2006).

RISK FACTORS Risk factors for postpartum depression include the following:

- Primiparity (first pregnancy)
- Ambivalence about maintaining the pregnancy
- History of postpartum depression or bipolar illness
- Lack of social support
- Lack of a stable and supportive relationship with parents or partner
- The woman's lack of a supportive relationship with her parents, especially her father, as a child
- The woman's dissatisfaction with herself, including body image problems and eating disorders.

Women with postpartum depression are at risk for suicide, most prominently as they enter or exit the deeply depressed state. In a deep depression, the woman is unlikely to be able to plan and carry out suicide. For that reason, signs of improvement in depression should be celebrated with some caution. Whereas the woman with postpartal psychosis may attempt suicide because of illogical thought processes, the woman with major depression attempts suicide because her suffering is so great that dying seems a more favorable option than continuing to live in such pain. She also may attempt suicide to save her newborn from some perceived or real threat—including the possibility that she herself might harm the baby. The risk of suicide is greater in women who have attempted suicide previously, have a specific plan, and can access the means or weapon identified in the plan. The more specific the plan, the greater the probability of an attempt.

COLLABORATION

Women with a history of postpartum psychosis or depression or other risk factors should be referred to a mental health professional for counseling and biweekly visits between the second and sixth week postpartum for evaluation. Medication, individual or group psychotherapy, and practical assistance with child care and other demands of daily life are common treatment measures for both disorders; however, specific therapies may vary. Treatment of postpartum depression is not unlike treatment of any other significant depression: psychotherapy and antidepression medications, usually the selective serotonin reuptake inhibitors. The nurse's responsibilities as part of the health care team are discussed in detail in the Nursing Process section.

Pharmacologic Therapies

Based on an expert consensus guideline for breastfeeding mothers, it is recommended that sertraline (e.g., Zoloft and Lustral) be the first-line treatment for PPD, with paroxetine (e.g., Paxil, Seroxat, and Deroxat) as an alternative first-line treatment (Beck, 2008). Recommendations are that a combination of antidepressants and psychosocial interventions be used regardless of whether the woman is breastfeeding. Many of the drugs used in treating postpartum psychiatric conditions may be contraindicated in breastfeeding women. Fluoxetine (e.g., Prozac and Sarafem) is not recommended for lactating women because of its long half-life (Beck, 2008). Some of the antidepressive drugs have been linked to an increase in congenital defects, so birth control also should be emphasized. The woman and her partner should be reminded that antidepressants may take several weeks to have an effect. Providers may prefer to start antidepressants before the birth of the baby (usually at 36 weeks gestation) so that a therapeutic blood level is achieved before the birth of the baby.

Support Groups

Support groups have proved to be successful adjuncts to such treatment. In a support group of postpartal women and their partners, a couple may feel consolation that they are not alone in their experience. Moreover, the group provides a forum for exchanging information about postpartum depression, learning stress reduction measures, and experiencing renewed self-esteem and support. The most effective support groups provide for safe child care to facilitate attendance. If a support group is not available locally, the woman and her family may be encouraged to contact Depression After Delivery (DAD), now a national Web-based support network that provides education and volunteers, or Postpartum Support International. The Mills Depression and Anxiety Symptom-Feeling Checklist also is available online.

Other Therapies

Treatment of postpartum psychosis is directed at the specific type of psychotic symptoms displayed and may include lithium, antipsychotics, or electroconvulsive therapy in combination with psychotherapy, removal of the infant, and social support. It is important that the nurse realize that many of the drugs used in treating postpartum psychiatric conditions are contraindicated in breastfeeding women.

NURSING PROCESS

The priority of nursing care for the client with postpartum depression is to maintain safety of both the client and her family. Nurses may hesitate to assess clients for risk of harm to themselves or others for fear of introducing an idea that hadn't occurred to the client. Not only is this not true, but questioning the client's thoughts of harming herself or others can actually contribute to saving lives and should be a component of care for any client experiencing depression.

Assessment

Assessment for factors predisposing a client to postpartal depression or psychosis should begin prenatally (Beck, 2002). Questions designed to detect problems can be included as part of the routine prenatal history interview or questionnaire. Women with a personal or family history of psychiatric disease, particularly postpartum depression or psychosis, need prenatal instructions on the signs and symptoms of depression and may need additional emotional support. Ideally, a depression assessment should be completed each trimester to update a pregnant woman's risk status (Beck, 2002). If one was not done previously, the nurse assesses the woman for predisposing factors during labor and the postpartum stay.

Several depression scales are available for assessing postpartum depression. The routine use of a screening tool in a matter-of-fact approach significantly improves the diagnosis. The Edinburgh Postnatal Depression Scale (Box 20–9) is the most widely used screening tool for postpartum depression in large populations of women. The tool has been validated, computerized, and used in telephone screening. Mothers who score above 12 are likely to be suffering from postpartum depression. Another tool is Beck's (2002) Postpartum Depression Predictors Inventory Revised (PDPI-R). This tool also is a practical and simple screening checklist for use during routine care with all postpartum women to identify those who might be experiencing postpartum depression, ensuring that early management can be initiated (Box 20–10).

No matter what approach the nurse uses to assess for postpartum depression, enabling the woman to voice her feelings of maternal role transition and how she is adjusting in this vulnerable time is of inestimable value (Beck, 2008). Listening to her story provides a critical emic (insider's) view of her circumstances as opposed to an etic (outsider's) view.

In providing daily care, the nurse observes the woman for objective signs of depression—anxiety, irritability, poor concentration, forgetfulness, sleep difficulties, appetite change, fatigue, and tearfulness—and listens for statements indicating feelings of failure and self-accusation. Severity and duration of symptoms should be noted. Behavior and verbalizations that are bizarre or seem to indicate a potential for violence against herself or others, including the infant, are reported as soon as possible for further evaluation.

The nurse needs to be aware that many normal physiologic changes of the puerperium are similar to symptoms of depression (lack of sexual interest, appetite change, fatigue). It is essential that observations be as specific and as objective as possible and that they are carefully documented. Beck and Indman (2005) found that anxiety was a prominent feature of illness for some women and suggested that women be assessed for their level of anxiety, particularly regarding infant care. Because of the strong association of interrupted sleep and postpartum depression and the finding that severe fatigue was an excellent predictor of postpartum depression (Corwin, Brownstead, Barton, Heckard, & Morin, 2005), assessing fatigue level at 2 weeks postpartum by telephone may be helpful in predicting depression risk early. Restorative sleep improves a woman's ability to cope and make decisions, thereby producing a sense of better self-control. A central challenge for nursing is identifying women at risk of suicide. Family members of the depressed woman also should be alert to signals that she may be intent on self-harm; they must be advised that threats be taken seriously. Family members should be told to be especially vigilant for suicide when the woman seems to be feeling better.

Box 20–9 **Edinburgh Postnatal Depression Scale**

In the past 7 days:

1. I have been able to laugh and see the funny side of things.
   As much as I always could
   Not quite so much now
   Definitely not so much now
   Not at all
2. I have looked forward with enjoyment of things.
   As much as I ever did
   Rather less than I used to
   Definitely less than I used to
   Hardly at all

*3. I have blamed myself unnecessarily when things went wrong.
   Yes, most of the time
   Yes, some of the time
   Not very often
   No, never

4. I have been anxious or worried for no good reason.
   No, not at all
   Hardly ever
   Yes, sometimes
   Yes, very often

*5. I have felt scared or panicky for no very good reason.
   Yes, quite a lot
   Yes, sometimes
   No, not much
   No, not at all

*6. Things have been getting on top of me.
   Yes, most of the time I haven't been able to cope at all
   Yes, sometimes I haven't been coping as well as usual
   No, I have been coping quite well
   No, I have been coping as well as ever

*7. I have been so unhappy that I have had difficulty sleeping.
   Yes, most of the time
   Yes, sometimes
   Not very often
   No, not at all

*8. I have felt sad or miserable.
   Yes, most of the time
   Yes, quite often
   Not very often
   No, not at all

*9. I have been so unhappy that I have been crying.
   Yes, most of the time
   Yes, quite often
   Only occasionally
   No, never

*10. The thought of harming myself has occurred to me.
   Yes, quite often
   Sometimes
   Hardly ever
   Never

Note: Response categories are scored 0, 1, 2, and 3 according to increased severity of the symptoms. Items marked with an asterisk are reverse-scored (3, 2, 1, 0). The total score is calculated by adding together the scores for each of the 10 items. A score above the threshold of 12 to 13 out of 30 indicates with 86% sensitivity that the woman is suffering from postpartum depression.

Source: Cox, J. L., Holden, J. M., & Sagovsky, R. (1987). Detection of postnatal depression: Development of the 10-item Edinburgh Postnatal Depression Scale. *British Journal of Psychiatry, 150,* 782–786. Users may reproduce the scale without further permission provided they respect copyright by quoting the names of the authors, the title, and the source of the paper in all reproduced copies.

Box 20–10 **Postpartum Depression Predictors Inventory (PDPI)—Revised and Guide Questions for Its Use**

DURING PREGNANCY

Marital status	**Check One**	
1. Single	❍	
2. Married/cohabitating	❍	
3. Separated	❍	
4. Divorced	❍	
5. Widowed	❍	
6. Partnered	❍	
Socioeconomic status		
Low	❍	
Middle	❍	
High	❍	
Self-esteem	**Yes**	**No**
Do you feel good about yourself as a person?	❍	❍
Do you feel worthwhile?	❍	❍
Do you feel you have a number of good qualities as a person?	❍	❍

(continued)

Box 20–10 Postpartum Depression Predictors Inventory (PDPI)—Revised and Guide Questions for Its Use (continued)

	Yes	No
Prenatal depression		
1. Have you felt depressed during your pregnancy?	❍	❍
If yes, when and how long have you been feeling this way?		
If yes, how mild or severe would you consider your depression?		
Prenatal anxiety		
Have you been feeling anxious during your pregnancy?	❍	❍
If yes, how long have you been feeling this way?		
Unplanned/unwanted pregnancy		
Was the pregnancy planned?	❍	❍
Is the pregnancy unwanted?	❍	❍
History of previous depression		
1. Before this pregnancy, have you ever been depressed?	❍	❍
If yes, when did you experience this depression?		
If yes, have you been under a physician's care for this past depression?	❍	❍
If yes, did the physician prescribe any medication for your depression?	❍	❍
Social support		
1. Do you feel you receive adequate emotional support from your partner?	❍	❍
2. Do you feel you receive adequate instrumental support from your partner (e.g., help with household chores or baby-sitting)?	❍	❍
3. Do you feel you can rely on your partner when you need help?	❍	❍
4. Do you feel you can confide in your partner? (repeat same questions for family and again for friends)	❍	❍
Marital satisfaction		
1. Are you satisfied with your marriage (or living arrangement)?	❍	❍
2. Are you currently experiencing any marital problems?	❍	❍
3. Are things going well between you and your partner?	❍	❍

Life stress	Yes	No
1. Are you currently experiencing any stressful events in your life such as:		
Financial problems	❍	❍
Marital problems	❍	❍
Death in the family	❍	❍
Serious illness in the family	❍	❍
Moving	❍	❍
Unemployment	❍	❍
Job change	❍	❍

AFTER DELIVERY, ADD THE FOLLOWING ITEMS

Childcare stress	Yes	No
1. Is your infant experiencing any health problems?	❍	❍
2. Are you having problems with your baby feeding?	❍	❍
3. Are you having problems with your baby sleeping?	❍	❍
Infant temperament		
1. Would you consider your baby irritable or fussy?	❍	❍
2. Does your baby cry a lot?	❍	❍
3. Is your baby difficult to console or soothe?	❍	❍
Maternity blues		
1. Did you experience a brief period of tearfulness and mood swings during the 1st week after delivery?	❍	❍

Comments:

Source: AWHONN. (2002). Beck, C. T. Revision of the Postpartum Predictors Inventory. *Journal of Obstetric, Gynecologic, and Neonatal Nursing, 31*(4), 394–402 (Table 2 on PDPI, pp. 399–400). Washington, DC: Author. © 2002 by the Association of Women's Health, Obstetric and Neonatal Nurses. All rights reserved.

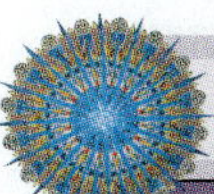

NURSING CARE PLAN **A Client With Postpartum Depression**

ASSESSMENT	DIAGNOSES	PLANNING
Salma al-Hussein, a 30-year-old woman who was born in Jordan but has lived in the United States for nearly 20 years, is brought to her primary care provider's office by her mother. Salma gave birth to her third child nearly 6 weeks ago. Her mother is worried because Salma is showing almost no interest in the baby and very little interest in her older children. Salma's mother and sister have been providing most of the care for the children. At first, Salma is slow to answer the nurse's questions and keeps her eyes on the floor during the assessment. Salma's mother says that Salma is not normally like this, that she is usually full of life and outgoing and polite with others, even those she does not know well. With the encouragement of her mother, Salma becomes more cooperative. The nurse uses the Edinburgh Postnatal Depression Scale; Salma scores 14 out of 30.	■ Impaired Parenting ■ Risk for Powerlessness ■ Impaired Social Interaction ■ Ineffective Coping	■ Salma will commit to safety. ■ Salma will express her feelings. ■ Salma will agree to participate in mental health counseling. ■ Family will continue to provide care for the children and support Salma as she begins the treatment process.

IMPLEMENTATION

- Refer to mental health professional.
- Attempt to persuade Selma to commit to safety for both herself and the children.
- Teach family to supervise mother's interaction with the infant and other children at all times to promote safety.
- Explain impact of postpartum depression to the family and help them cope with the impact on the family.
- Identify community resources for assisting with treatment.
- Encourage family to continue providing care for the infant and other children.
- Help Selma to recognize the signs of depression and accept the diagnosis of postpartum depression.
- Explain to both Selma and the family that postpartum depression is not uncommon and can be successfully treated but risk for reoccurrence is high if she has other children.

EVALUATION

Selma's care is evaluated based on the following expected outcomes:

- Selma begins treatment with a mental health counselor and is taking her prescribed medications regularly.
- Family members continue to provide supervision and care of the children until Selma's condition improves.
- Selma commits to safety for herself and her children.

CRITICAL THINKING

1. How would you persuade Selma to commit to safety for herself and her children?
2. What specific questions would you ask to determine if Selma is thinking about harming herself or her children?
3. If Selma admitted having fantasies of harming her children how could you advocate for the family?

Diagnosis

Possible nursing diagnoses that may apply to a woman with a postpartum psychiatric disorder include the following:

- Ineffective Individual Coping related to postpartum depression
- Risk for Altered Parenting related to postpartal mental illness
- Risk for Violence against self (suicide), newborn, and other children related to depression.

Plan

Appropriate goals for the woman experiencing postpartum depression may include the following:

- Maintain safety for the mother and family.
- Appropriate care for the newborn is provided by the family or support persons.
- Encourage the client to express feelings and concerns.
- Promote compliance with the agreed upon plan of care.
- Assist the client to integrate the newborn into the family.

Implementation

Nurses working in antepartal settings or teaching childbirth classes play indispensable roles in helping prospective parents appreciate the lifestyle changes and role demands associated with parenthood. Offering realistic information and anticipatory guidance and debunking myths about the perfect mother or perfect newborn may help prevent postpartum depression. Social support teaching guides are available for nurses to use in helping postpartum women explore their needs for postpartum support.

- Alert the mother, spouse, and other family members to the possibility of postpartum blues in the early days after birth and reassure them of the short-term nature of the condition.
- Describe symptoms of postpartum depression and encourage the mother to call her health care provider if symptoms become severe, if they fail to subside quickly, or if at any time she feels she is unable to function.

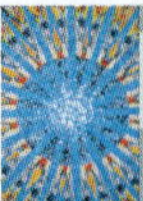

EVIDENCE-BASED PRACTICE Prevention of, Identification of, and Intervention for Postpartum Depression

Clinical Questions

How can the risk of postpartum depression be identified early in a pregnancy? What is the most effective way to prevent postpartum depression? When it occurs, how can it be treated?

The Evidence

Postpartum depression is a serious condition that occurs in the first 12 weeks after birth; approximately 13% of new mothers will experience it. Untreated, the condition may have consequences for mothers, infants, and their families. It often goes undetected, as symptoms may be hidden or misinterpreted. A team of advanced practice nurses developed recommendations for AWHONN, the professional association for nurses practicing in women's and neonatal health. Their recommendations focused on identification and prevention of depression and were based on a systematic review of research and expert opinion. Other evidence included a meta-analysis of studies focused on effective treatment of postnatal depression. This type of integrative review provides the strongest evidence for practice.

What Is Effective?

The strongest evidence supported individualized, flexible postpartum care that focused on the identification of risk for depression and/or signs of depression early in the pregnancy. Routine screening for depression should be part of the prenatal and postnatal assessment. The best outcomes are achieved when early preventive strategies accompany depression screening. When depression symptoms appear, supportive weekly interactions and ongoing assessment focused on mental health needs should be part of the routine postnatal treatment plan. Peer support (via technology or group) can help mediate depressive symptoms and encourage problem solving. Standard instruments should be used to identify mothers who are at risk for depression so that they can be referred to their primary care physician or a specialist in mental health for treatment.

What Is Inconclusive?

No best screening tool for depression during the perinatal period was definitively recommended. Several tools were used in these studies to determine risk of depression. Although various methods were shown to be effective in treating postnatal depression, no one therapy emerged as a definitive treatment.

Best Practice

Nurses are in a particularly good position to screen mothers for depression during the prenatal period and for at least 12 weeks after birth. You should use a standard instrument for screening at each encounter, and increased risk of depression should be cause for referral to a medical provider. Early detection and prevention will produce better outcomes for the mother, baby, and family. Diverse treatments—both pharmaceutical and counseling-based—have been shown to be effective in mediating the symptoms of depression. The treatment program should be matched to the specific client characteristics and needs.

References

Bledsoe, S., & Grote, N. (2006). Treating depression during pregnancy and the postpartum: A preliminary meta-analysis. *Research on Social Work Practice, 16,* 109–120.

McQueen, K., Montgomery, P., Lappan-Gracon, S., Evans, M., & Hunter, J. (2008). Evidence-based recommendations for depressive symptoms in postpartum women. *JOGNN: Journal of Obstetric, Gynecologic, and Neonatal Nursing, 37,* 127–136.

- Encourage the mother to plan how she will manage at home and provide concrete suggestions on how to cope in her adjustment to motherhood.

Community-Based Nursing Care

Home visits, especially for early-discharge families, are essential for fostering positive adjustments for the new family constellation (Box 20–11). Telephone follow-up at 2–3 weeks postpartum to ask whether the mother is experiencing difficulties is also helpful. If a mother calls with a seemingly innocuous question, she should be asked two or three open-ended questions about her general status (Katz, 2007). These questions allow the woman to open up if there is an underlying depression that she is too guilty/afraid to express initially; for example:

1. How do you feel things are going?
2. How are things going?
3. Are you feeling like you expected?

Monitoring for signs of depression or performing brief screening at well-child follow-ups also can be valuable for early identification and timely intervention (Katz, 2007).

In all postpartum women, the presence of three symptoms of depression on 1 day or one symptom for 3 days may signal serious depression and requires immediate referral to a mental health professional. Make an immediate referral if rejection of the infant or threatened or actual aggression against the infant has occurred. In such cases, the newborn is never left unattended with the mother. Depression does appear to interfere with optimal mothering; there is less interaction between mother and child, an increased incidence of mood and cognitive development problems, and more visits to the doctor in these children (Beck, 2002).

A diagnosis of postpartum depression or other psychiatric disorder poses major problems for the family, especially the father. The symptoms of these disorders are difficult to witness and may be harder to understand than physical problems such as hemorrhage and infection. The father may feel hurt by his partner's hostility; worry that she is becoming insane; or be baffled by her mood swings and lack of concern about herself, the newborn, or household responsibilities. He may be troubled by their lack of intimacy or deteriorating communication. Certainly, he has cause for concern about how the newborn and any other children are being affected. Very real practical matters—running the household; managing the children, including the totally dependent newborn; and caring for the mother—may be added to his usual routines and work responsibilities. It is not surprising that even in the most supportive families, relationships may suffer in response to these circumstances. It is often the father or another close family member who, in desperation, makes contact with

Box 20–11 Primary Prevention Strategies for Postpartum Depression

- Celebrate childbirth but appreciate that it is a life-changing transition that can be stressful—at times it can seem overwhelming. Share your feelings with each other and/or others.
- Consider keeping a journal in which you write down feelings. It not only is emotionally cathartic, but also provides a great memory book.
- Appreciate that you do not have to know everything to be a good parent—it is okay to seek advice during this transition.
- Connect to others who are parents—use them as a support and information network.
- Set a daily schedule and follow it even if you do not feel like it. Structuring activity helps counteract inertia that comes with feeling sad or unsettled.
- Prioritize daily tasks. Decide what must be done and what can wait. Try to get one major thing done every day. Remember, you do not always have to look like a magazine fashion model.
- Remember that you do not have to entertain or care for everyone who drops by. Doing something for someone else, however, often tends to make you feel better.
- If someone volunteers to lend a hand with tasks or baby care, accept the person's help. While your volunteer is in action, do something pleasurable or get some rest.
- Maintain outside interests. Plan some time every day—even if it's just 15 minutes—to do something exclusively for you that is pleasurable.
- Eat a healthful diet. Limit alcohol. Quit smoking. Get some exercise. (All of these can positively affect the immune system.)
- Get as much sleep as possible. Rest whenever you can, such as when the baby is napping. If you have other young children, bring them onto your bed to read or play quietly while you lie down.
- If possible, limit major changes (moves, job changes, etc.) the first year.
- Spend time with others.
- If things get overwhelming and you feel yourself slipping into depression, reach out to someone for help.
- Attend a postpartum support group if one is available. Also consider an international program such as Postpartum Support International which provides an emergency contact phone number at 1-800-944-4PPD as well as a website at http://postpartum.net).

the health care agency. This is especially difficult when the mother is reluctant to admit she is suffering emotional difficulty or is too ill to recognize her own needs.

The integration of the newborn into the family and care of the newborn and other children can be further compromised by concurrent postpartum depression in fathers. An examination of research studies that cite incidences of paternal postpartum depression indicate 24–50% incidence of depression among men whose partners were experiencing postpartum depression (Goodman, 2004).

Information, emotional support, and assistance in providing or obtaining care for the infant may be needed. The nurse can assist family members by identifying community resources, making referrals to public health nursing services and social services, and providing a list of telephone numbers as well as emergency services that the mother may need. Postpartum follow-up is especially important, as are visits from a psychiatric home health nurse.

Evaluation

Expected outcomes of nursing care include the following:

- The client's signs of depression are identified and she receives prompt intervention.
- The newborn is effectively cared for by the father or other support persons until the mother is able to provide care.
- The mother and newborn remain safe.
- The newborn is successfully integrated into the family unit.

REVIEW Postpartum Depression

RELATE: LINK TO CONCEPTS

Linking the exemplar of Postpartum Depression with the concept of Development:

1. How might a mother's postpartum depression impact the development of her 3-year-old daughter?
2. What is your priority developmental concern for the newborn when the mother has severe postpartum depression?

Linking the exemplar of Postpartum Depression with the concept of Comfort:

3. What are your concerns for the mother who has postpartum depression regarding sleep and rest?
4. How will fatigue impact postpartum depression and the care of the newborn?

REFER: GO TO MYNURSINGKIT

REFLECT: CASE STUDY

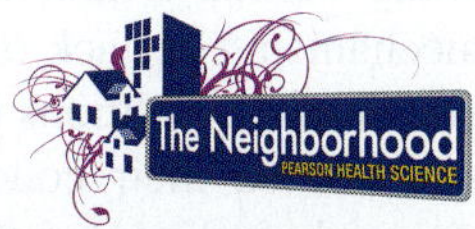

Jessica Riley is a single 17-year-old new mother of a 1-month-old infant son named Ryan whose father ended his relationship with Jessica when she was 4 months pregnant. Jessica's relationship with her mother has been strained for the last few years and worsened when she became pregnant. Because she was constantly fighting with her mother, Jessica moved to a small apartment when she was 6 months pregnant. Jessica's father left the family when Jessica was 7 years old. She recently completed her GED and is now trying to go to

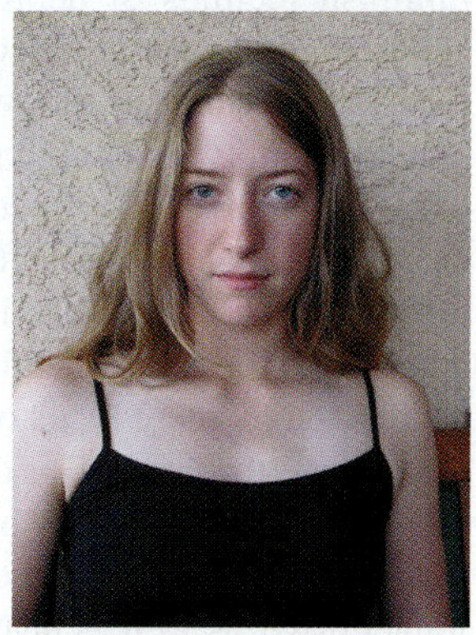

school part time for an associate's degree in cosmetology. She also works nearly full time as a waitress, but because she is supporting herself and her baby, she struggles financially.

1. What information in Jessica's history puts her at risk for postpartum depression?
2. How would you assess Jessica for potential postpartum depression?
3. What interventions can you implement to reduce Jessica's risk of postpartum depression?

20.4 SITUATIONAL DEPRESSION

KEY TERMS

Relaxation response, *1209*
Resilience, *1208*

BASIS FOR SELECTION OF EXEMPLAR

Emergency room admissions
Healthy People 2010
Institute of Medicine
Most common conditions
National Institute of Mental Health
Office-based physician visits

LEARNING OUTCOMES

After reading about this concept, you will be able to:

1. Describe the features, clinical manifestations, and direct and indirect causes of situational depression.
2. Identify risk factors associated with situational depression.
3. Illustrate the nursing process in providing culturally competent care across the life span for individuals with situational depression.
4. Formulate priority nursing diagnoses appropriate for an individual with situational depression.
5. Create a plan of care for individuals with situational depression and their family members.
6. Assess expected outcomes for an individual with situational depression.
7. Discuss therapies used in the collaborative care of an individual with situational depression.
8. Employ evidence-based caring interventions for an individual with situational depression.

OVERVIEW

As stated in the About section of this concept, an individual may develop situational depression after a developing a serious illness, being a victim of a crime, losing or changing jobs, or experiencing some other life-altering event. Symptoms generally begin 3 months after the event and typically last no more than 6 months. In contrast to post-traumatic stress disorder, which is a reaction to a life-threatening event and has a longer duration, situational depression is response to a situation or stressor that is greater than what is usually expected for such an event.

Risk Factors

Any life-altering event can create risk for the occurrence of situational depression. This risk is further increased by a preexisting mental health issue, ineffective or unhealthy coping mechanisms, or lack of a support network. Clients with these preexisting conditions may find that situational depression has exacerbated their condition. For example, in an attempt to diminish feelings of depression, a client who has remained sober after a history of alcohol abuse may resume drinking as a coping mechanism following a life-altering event.

Older adults are at high risk for situational depression, especially when they experience two or more life-altering events in close proximity. Loss of independence, be it cognitive, physical, or otherwise, often results in situational depression in the older adult. Even those older adults who "see the glass as half full" are challenged by these types of stressors. The loss of driving privileges (due to physical or cognitive changes) is a huge loss to older adults, often putting a great deal of strain on family members who must accommodate the older person who can no longer drive, as well as hear the individual complain about it.

Resilience Factors

The capacity to respond to stressors successfully is called **resilience**. Resilience is the ability not only to survive and bounce back from difficult and traumatic experiences, but also to continue to grow and develop emotionally and psychologically. The notion of resilience encompasses the biologic and psychologic characteristics intrinsic to an individual, such as personality style and quality of interpersonal relationships, that confer protection against the development of psychopathology (Hoge, Austin, & Pollack, 2007). Resilience probably explains why not all maltreated children experience mental health problems as adults (Collishaw et al., 2007). Researchers and clinicians alike have been surprised by the prevalence of the capacity for resilience (Mancini & Bonanno, 2006), and clinicians are beginning to focus on uncovering and energizing pathways to resilience in their clients.

Individuals who do not have a history of mental illness can succumb to situational depression following a major event. Resilience factors can make a great deal of difference in preventing the situational depression from becoming a depressive disorder. Nurses working with clients experiencing situational depression should help them determine their resilience factors and to use those factors as supportive mechanisms during this critical time. Resilience factors may include a close-knit family, close friends, a good job with benefits, membership in a volunteer organization, or any other number of factors.

CLINICAL MANIFESTATIONS

The symptoms of situational depression are similar to those of the other depressive disorders and include sleep disturbances, feelings of hopelessness and sadness, loss of self-esteem, irritability,

CLINICAL MANIFESTATIONS AND THERAPIES **Situational Depression**

ETIOLOGY	CLINICAL MANIFESTATIONS	CLINICAL THERAPIES
Sleep disturbances	Insomnia, hypersomnia	■ Improved sleep hygiene ■ Short-term sedative
Feelings of sadness, despair Loss of self-esteem Irritability	■ Crying ■ Avoiding pleasurable activities ■ Avoiding family and friends	■ Cognitive-behavioral therapy alone may be sufficient to help the individual return to normal. ■ Alternative therapies such as massage therapy or acupuncture may provide relief. ■ Antidepressant therapy
Behavioral changes	■ Ignoring financial responsibilities ■ Performing poorly at work and school ■ Fighting, behaving recklessly	■ Cognitive behavior therapy ■ Family therapy ■ Antidepressant therapy

difficulty concentrating, and anhedonia. Behaviors that may occur include ignoring financial responsibilities; arguing and fighting; performing poorly at work or school; and behaving recklessly, such as driving while intoxicated or vandalizing others' property.

COLLABORATION

As was previously stated, cognitive-behavioral therapy is often sufficient to help the client put things in perspective and return to a normal state. If the client exhibits behavioral changes that are affecting the family, such as ignoring financial responsibilities, direct intervention by a key family member may be helpful. Family therapy also may be helpful depending on how close or involved the family is as a whole.

The nurse's responsibilities as part of a collaborative team is discussed in detail in the Nursing Process section.

Pharmacologic Therapy

An antidepressant or antianxiety medication may be prescribed for the client with situational depression. Some of these medications require several weeks to take full effect, and clients suffering from situational depression are at a high risk for self-medicating with alcohol or other drugs. Client teaching regarding prescribed medications as well as the need to refrain from self-medicating is critical. Similarly, nurses also should provide client teaching regarding good sleep hygiene to any client who is prescribed a sedative or is self-medicating to treat a sleep disturbance.

Exercise

Mental or affective disorders such as depression or chronic stress may affect a person's desire to move. The depressed person may lack enthusiasm for taking part in any activity and may even lack energy for usual hygiene practices. Lack of visible energy is seen in a slumped posture with head bowed. Chronic stress can deplete the body's energy reserves to the point at which fatigue diminishes the desire to exercise, even though exercise can energize the person and facilitate coping. By contrast, individuals with eating disorders may exercise excessively in an effort to prevent weight gain.

A strong and growing body of evidence supports the role of exercise in elevating mood and relieving stress and anxiety across the life span. Solid data examining relationships between both aerobic and nonaerobic styles of exercise support the use of this modality to relieve symptoms of depression. The mechanism of action is thought to be a result of one or more of the following: Exercise increases levels of metabolites for neurotransmitters such as NE and 5-HT; exercise releases endogenous opioids, thus increasing levels of endorphins; exercise increases levels of oxygen to the brain and other body systems, inducing euphoria; and through muscular exertion (especially with movement modalities such as yoga and tai chi), the body releases stored stress associated with accumulated emotional demands. Regular exercise also improves the quality of sleep for most individuals (Freeman, 2004).

By eliciting the relaxation response, exercise is beneficial for counteracting some of the harmful effects of stress on the body and mind. First described by Dr. Herbert Benson, the **relaxation response** is a healthful physiologic state that can be elicited through deep relaxation breathing with emphasis on a prolonged exhalation phase (Edelman & Mandle, 2006). Emphasis on the exhalation recruits parasympathetic nervous system response, the "rest and digest" reflex. Progressive muscle relaxation techniques involve contracting and then releasing groups of muscles throughout the body until all parts of the body feel relaxed. These movements are subtle and, along with relaxation breathing, can be done by almost anyone at any time, regardless of mobility or fitness status, providing potent stress relief and neurocardiovascular health benefits.

Current research also supports the positive effects of exercise on cognitive functioning, in particular decision-making and problem-solving processes, planning, and paying attention. Physical exertion induces cells in the brain to strengthen and build neuronal connections. Research evidence demonstrates that athletic older adults have denser brains than their inactive counterparts (Freeman, 2004). Brain Gym (educational kinesiology) is a series of easy, mostly cross-lateral movements that enhance right- and left-brain integration, thus improving mood, learning, problem solving, and performance in people of all ages. These contralateral movements have been shown to help individuals with mood disorders, attention deficit disorder (ADD), attention deficit/hyperactivity disorder (ADHD), and learning disorders.

Exercise and muscle relaxation can be particularly helpful to clients with situational depression. Nurses should encourage these clients to maintain their regular exercise regimens, despite lack of enthusiasm, to ward off depressed feelings and maintain physical health. Maintaining exercise schedules during situational depression also helps clients maintain focus and orientation to time, increasing the likelihood that they will meet other schedule requirements, such as paying bills on time.

NURSING PROCESS

The client who is experiencing a life crisis with resulting situational depression often needs support and help to understand that his or her feelings are a normal result of the problems faced and assistance with effective problem solving strategies. Priorities of care are focused on maintaining the clients' safety, encouraging them to work through the grieving process or feelings of loss related to the problem, and encouragement to identify their strengths to help them overcome their feelings of hopelessness and fear.

Assessment

Assessment of the client with situational depression includes a nursing history to determine the precipitating stressor and symptoms the client is experiencing. The nurse also should assess the client's risk factors for depression, as well as the presence of resilience factors. If the precipitating stressor was a physical assault or accident, such as a motor vehicle accident, a physical examination may be necessary to confirm healing of any injuries. Depression scales or inventories may be used, such as those described in the About section and in Exemplar 20.2.

Diagnosis

The following nursing diagnoses may be appropriate for the client with situational depression:

- Helplessness
- Disturbed Sleep Pattern
- Disrupted Family Processes
- Situational Low Self-Esteem
- Ineffective Coping.

NURSING CARE PLAN A Client With Situational Depression

ASSESSMENT

Pearl G. is a 70-year-old African American widowed woman who is a resident in a long-term care facility. She had a stroke a year ago and has hemiplegia on her right side. She is right-handed. She does not feed herself and has little appetite. Ms. G. is alert and oriented to person and place. She cooperates with having her activities of daily living (ADL) done for her, but she does not try to help. When she talks, it is only one or two words at a time. Her face always seems to look sad. The nurse has worked with Ms. G. for the 11 months she has been in this facility. The nurse thinks Ms. G. is depressed. The nurse assessed her with the GDS. Ms. G. scored 12. In the conversation they had about the depression scale, Ms. G. said that she missed her family.

DIAGNOSES

Three priority nursing diagnoses were identified for this client:

- Powerlessness
- Self-Care Deficit in bathing/hygiene, dressing/grooming, feeding, and toileting
- Impaired Social Interaction

PLANNING

The goals for her plan of care are as follows:

- Client will identify two areas in which she feels some control.
- Client will assist with all her ADLs, feeding herself independently within 2 weeks.
- Client will interact with the staff, her peers, and her family.

IMPLEMENTATION

- Gradually relinquish control of ADLs by offering Ms. G simple choices regarding dressing, bathing, prioritizing care needs, and activities.
- Provide positive reinforcement for Ms. G as she takes a more active part in her self care and socializing.
- Encourage self care. Help Ms. G use her left hand to feed and bathe herself.
- Encourage social contact by promoting involvement in facility social gatherings. and introducing her to other residents with similar interests.
- Discuss Ms. G's care with her primary provider to determine her ability to participate in rehabilitation activities to regain function in her right side.

EVALUATION

Within two weeks Ms. G has begun to assist in bathing herself and has learned to eat with her left hand when the foods are easy to stab and bring to her mouth. Her primary provider has discussed rehabilitation with her and she has readily agreed to participate in the hopes of becoming more independent. She has developed a few friendships with other residents and seems more happy.

CRITICAL THINKING

1. Why might Ms. G's nurses have provide for her care without requiring her participation for an entire year?
2. What factors promoted Ms. G's depression?
3. When a client like Ms. G experiences situational depression can the depression only be resolved by removing the situation that caused it? Explain your answer.

Plan

Appropriate goals for the client with situational depression may include the following:

- Assist the client to obtain adequate sleep and rest.
- Promote avoidance of reckless or irresponsible behaviors.
- Encourage the client to return to normal daily routines.
- Maintain the client's safety as the priority goal of care.

Implementation

When initiating interventions it is important to prioritize care to meet the client's most immediate needs first. Involving the client, when possible, in planning priorities can promote independence and a feeling of control.

Helplessness

Nursing interventions to counteract helplessness and hopelessness include exploring clients' previous achievements of success, encouraging them to identify their strengths and abilities, and facilitating the evaluation of their behavior. Help clients to identify ways in which they have control of their lives. The nurse can help clients problem-solve situations in which they can become more autonomous, especially through vocational, social, and community activities.

Many people with mood disorders believe they have lost control over their lives, rights, and responsibilities and have lost the ability and right to effectively advocate for themselves. Nursing activities designed to help clients advocate for themselves provide them with hope and self-esteem. The nurse may assist clients in the following ways:

- Encourage them to believe in themselves.
- Inform them of their rights.
- Help them clarify what they need and want by setting clear goals.
- Provide them with accurate information, preferably in writing.
- Help them strategize by using the problem-solving process.
- Facilitate their identification of resources such as friends, family, self-help groups, and advocacy organizations.
- Encourage them to identify the best person(s) to assist them with this problem.
- Foster effective communication so they can get their message across; use suggestions such as these: Be brief, stick to the point, don't get diverted, and state the concern and how things should be changed.
- Promote firmness and persistence so clients can get what they need for themselves.

Disrupted Family Processes

Mood disorders affect not only the client, but also family and friends. Nurses must provide care to the family as well as to the depressed client. During acute episodes, clients may be dependent and needy or may need firm direction and limit setting. Help caregivers acknowledge clients' dependency and assume appropriate responsibility. Provide information about clients' condition in accordance with client preferences, remembering the importance of confidentiality. Provide the family with a list of community resources and encourage them to participate in support groups.

In some cases, the stressor that causes the client's situational depression also directly disrupts family processes. For example, a mother who is injured in a motor vehicle accident and confined to bed rest for more than a few days requires someone to step in and assume her normal roles until she is able to perform them again. In cases like this in which family processes and patterns are disrupted, the nurse can support the family by providing referrals to outside resources and by helping the father or another adult family member come up with a plan to "cover the bases" until the mother returns to health.

Families who have experienced a loss or stressor that disrupts family processes are at increased risk for family conflict. Nurses working with these families should encourage them to resolve disagreements in a healthy manner and not allow the situation to overrun their family strengths. Box 2–3 in Concept 2, Addiction Behaviors outlines eight steps to resolving family disagreements.

REVIEW Situational Depression

RELATE: LINK TO CONCEPTS

Linking the exemplar of Situational Depression with the concept of Family:

1. How might the client with situational depression be at risk for impaired parenting?
2. Other than a motor vehicle accident, what events in a family's life might increase the risk of a family member developing situational depression?

Linking the exemplar of Situational Depression with the concept of Health, Wellness, and Illness:

3. How might situational depression impact a client's nutritional status?
4. What client teaching should the nurse provide to the client with situational depression regarding nutrition?

REFER: GO TO MYNURSINGKIT

REFLECT: CASE STUDY

Jill Adkins is an 18-year-old African American woman in her second semester at the University of North Carolina at Chapel Hill, where she is a Morehouse scholar. Just before midterms, she gets a call from her aunt, who informs Jill that her mother, who has diabetes, has taken a turn for the worse and requires a kidney transplant. Jill phones her mother, who tells her to study hard and take her midterms. Jill tries to study, but she keeps thinking about her mother. She has trouble sleeping, and her roommate has to encourage her to eat. The weekend after midterms, Jill's uncle comes to take her home to see her mother, who looks very ill and is very weak but is in good spirits. Jill's mother convinces her to return to school, where Jill learns that she did poorly on her midterms. Jill feels poorly over the next couple of days. She decides to go to the student health center at the urging of her roommate.

1. What are the priority nursing considerations for Jill? What nursing diagnoses are appropriate?
2. What risk factors does Jill have for situational depression? What resilience factors does she have?
3. If you were the nurse at the student health center, what would your plan of care for Jill include?

PEARSON
EXPLORE mynursingkit™

MyNursingKit is your one stop for online chapter review materials and resources. Prepare for success with additional NCLEX®-style practice questions, interactive assignments and activities, web links, animations and videos, and more!

Register your access code from the front of your book at **www.mynursingkit.com**.

REFERENCES

Al-Oballi Kridli, S. (2002). Health beliefs and practices among Arab women. *American Journal of Maternal Child Nursing, 27*(3), 178–182.

American Psychiatric Association (APA). (2000). *Diagnostic and statistical manual of mental disorders: DSM-IV-TR* (4th ed., text rev.). Washington, DC: Author.

Apps, J., Winkler, J., & Jandrisevits, M. D. (2008). Bipolar disorders: Symptoms and treatment in children and adolescents. *Pediatric Nursing, 34*, 84–88.

Aroian, K. J., & Norris, A. (2002). Assessing risk for depression among immigrants at two-year follow-up. *Archives of Psychiatric Nursing, 16*(6), 245–253.

Badner, J. A. (2003). The genetics of bipolar disorder. In B. Geller & M. P. Delbello (Eds.), *Bipolar disorder in childhood and early adolescence* (pp. 247–254). New York: Guilford Press.

Baethge, C., Baldessarini, R. J., Khalsa, H. K., Hennen, J., Salvatore, P., & Tohen, M. (2005). Substance abuse in first-episode bipolar I disorder. *American Journal of Psychiatry, 162*(5), 1008–1010.

Bailara, K. M., Henry, C., Lestage, J., Launay, J. M., Parrot, F., Swendsen, J., et al. (2005). Decreased brain tryptophan availability as a partial determinant of post-partum blues. *Psychoneuroendocrinology, 31*(3), 407–413.

Basch, E. M., & Ulbricht, C. E. (2005). *Natural standard: Herb & supplement handbook.* St. Louis, MO: Elsevier Mosby.

Beck, A. T., Ward, C. H., Mendelson, M., Mock, J., & Erbaugh, J. (1961). Inventory for measuring depression. *Archives of General Psychiatry, 4*, 561–571.

Beck, A. T., Steer, R. A., & Brown, G. K. (1996). *Manual for the Beck depression inventory-II.* San Antonio, Texas: Psychological Corporation.

Beck, C. T. (2002). Revision of the postpartum depression predictors inventory. *Journal of Obstetric, Gynecologic, and Neonatal Nursing, 31*(4), 394–402.

Beck, C. T. (2003). Recognizing and screening for postpartum depression in mothers of NICU infants. *Advances in Neonatal Care, 3*(1), 37–46.

Beck, C. T. (2006). Postpartum depression: It isn't just the blues. *American Journal of Nursing, 106*(5), 40–51.

Beck, C. T. (2008). *Postpartum mood and anxiety disorders: Case studies, research, and nursing care* (2nd ed.). Washington, DC: Association of Women's Health, Obstetric and Neonatal Nurses.

Beck, C. T., & Driscoll, J. W. (2006). *Postpartum mood and anxiety disorders: A clinician's guide.* Sudbury, MA: Jones and Bartlett Publishers.

Beck, C. T., & Indman, P. (2005). The many faces of depression. *Journal of Obstetric, Gynecologic, and Neonatal Nursing, 34* (5), 569–576.

Bledsoe, S., & Grote, N. (2006). Treating depression during pregnancy and the postpartum: A preliminary meta-analysis. *Research on Social Work Practice, 16*, 109–120.

Bondareff, W., Alpert, M., Friedhoff, A. J., Richter, E. M., Clary, C., & Batzar, E. (2000). Comparison of sertraline and nortriptyline in the treatment of major depressive disorder in late life. *American Journal of Psychiatry, 157*(5), 729–736.

Brommelhoff, J. A., Conway, K., Merikangas, K., & Levy, B. R. (2004). Higher rates of depression in women: Role of gender bias within the family. *Journal of Women' Health, 13*(1), 69–76.

Brown, A. B. (2004). New strategies for treatment-resistant depression. *National Alliance for Research on Schizophrenia and Depression Research Newsletter, 15*(4), 37–40.

Caetano, S. C., Kaur, S., Brambilla, P., Nicoletti, M., Hatch, J. P., Sassi, R. B., et al. (2006). Smaller cingulated volumes in unipolar depressed patients. *Biological Psychiatry, 59*(8), 702–706.

Cassano, G. B., Rucci, P., Frank, E., Fagiolini, A., Dell'Osso, L., Shear, M. K., et al. (2004). The mood spectrum in unipolar and bipolar disorder: Arguments for a unitary approach. *American Journal of Psychiatry, 161*(7), 1264–1269.

Chen, T. H., Lu, R. B., Chang, A. J., Chu, D. M., & Chou, K. R. (2006). The evaluation of cognitive-behavioral group therapy on patient depression and self-esteem. *Archives of Psychiatric Nursing, 20*(1), 3–11.

Chou, J. C. Y. (2005). Eastern vs Western perspectives on depression. *Medscape Psychiatry & Mental Health, 10*(1), 1–4. Retrieved April 6, 2005, from http://www.medscape.com/viewarticle/501758

Collishaw, S., Pickles, A., Messer, J., Rutter, M., Shearer, C., & Maugham, B. (2007). Resilience to adult psychopathology following childhood maltreatment: Evidence from a community sample. *Child Abuse and Neglect, 31*(3), 211–229.

Corwin, E. J., Brownstead, J., Barton, N., Heckard, S., & Merin, K. (2005). The impact of fatigue on the development of postpartum depression. *Journal of Obstetric, Gynecologic, and Neonatal Nursing, 34* (5), 577–586.

Cunningham, F. G., Leveno, K. J., Bloom, S. L., Hauth, J. C., Gilstrap, L. C., & Wenstrom, K. D. (2005). *Williams obstetrics* (22nd ed.). New York: McGraw-Hill.

D'Avanzo, C. E., & Geissler, E. M. (2008). *Cultural health assessment* (4th ed.). St. Louis, MO: Mosby.

Davis, L. L., Rush, J. A., Wisniewski, S. R., Rice, L., Cassano, P., Jewell, M. E., et al. (2005). Substance use disorder comorbidity in major depressive disorder. *Comprehensive Psychiatry, 46*(2), 81–90.

De Sovo, M. R. (1997, August). Keeping the faith: Jewish traditions in pregnancy and childbirth. *Lifelines, 1*(4), 46–49.

Dopheide, J. A. (2006). Recognizing and treating depression in children and adolescents. *American Journal of Health-Systems Pharmacy, 63*, 233–243.

Draucker, C. B. (2005). Processes of mental health service use by adolescents with depression. *Journal of Nursing Scholarship, 37*(2), 155–162.

Driscoll, J. W. (2008). Psychosocial adaptation to pregnancy and postpartum. In K. R. Simpson & P. A. Creehan, *AWHONN perinatal nursing* (3rd ed., pp. 78–87). Philadelphia: Lippincott Williams & Wilkins.

Edelman, C., & Mandle, C. (2006). *Health promotion throughout the lifespan* (6th ed.). Philadelphia: Mosby/Elsevier.

Faraone, S. V., Glatt, S. J., Su, J., & Tsuang, M. T. (2004). Three potential susceptibility loci shown by a genome-wide scan for regions influencing the age at onset of mania. *American Journal of Psychiatry, 161*(4), 625–630.

Fisfalen, M. E., Schulze, T. G., DePaulo, J. R., DeGroot, L. J., Badner, J. A., & McMahon, F. J. (2005). Familial variation in episode frequency in bipolar affective disorder. *American Journal of Psychiatry, 162*(7), 1266–1272.

Frazier, J. A., Chiu, S., Breeze, J. L., Makris, N., Lange, N., Kennedy, D. N., et al. (2005). Structural brain magnetic resonance imaging of limbic and thalamic volumes in pediatric bipolar disorder. *American Journal of Psychiatry, 162*(7), 1256–1265.

Freeman, L. (2004). *Mosby's complementary & alternative medicine: A research-based approach* (2nd ed.). Philadelphia: Mosby/Elsevier.

Gaudiano, B. A., & Miller, I. W. (2006). Patients' expectancies, the alliance in pharmacotherapy, and treatment outcomes in bipolar disorder. *Journal of Consulting and Clinical Psychology, 74*(4), 671–676.

Ghaemi, S. N. (2004). Anxiety and bipolar disorder. *Medscape Primary Care, 6*(2), 1–4. Retrieved November 18, 2004, from http://www.medscape.com/viewarticle/492123

Gjerdingen, D. (2003). The effectiveness of various postpartum depression treatments and the impact of antidepressant drugs on nursing infants. *Journal of the American Board of Family Practice, 16*(5), 372–382.

Goodman, J. H. (2004). Paternal postpartum depression, its relationship to maternal postpartum depression, and implications for family health. *Journal of Advanced Nursing, 45*(1), 26–35.

Goren, J. L., Stoll, A. L., Damico, K. E., Sarmiento, I. A., & Cohen, B. M. (2004). Bioavailability and lack of toxicity of s-adenosyl-l-methionine (SAMe) in humans. *Pharmacotherapy, 24*(11), 1501–1507.

Haessler, A., & Rosenthal, M. B. (2007). Psychological aspects of obstetrics & gynecology. In A. H. DeCherney, L. Nathan, T. M. Goodwin, & N. Laufer (Eds.), *Current obstetric & gynecologic: Diagnosis & treatment* (10th ed., pp. 1003–1024). New York: Lange Medical Books/McGraw-Hill.

Hart, L. A. (2000). Psychosocial benefits of animal companionship. In A. H. Fine (Ed.), *Handbook on animal-assisted therapy* (pp. 59–78). San Diego, CA: Academic Press.

Hartford Institute for Geriatric Nursing. (2008). *Best nursing practices in care for older adults.* Try this: The geriatric depression scale. Retrieved February 14, 2008, from http://www.hartfordign.org/trythis/issue04.pdf

HealthyPlace.com. (2008). Cultural considerations in treating Asians with depression. Retrieved September 4, 2009, from http://www.healthyplace.com/depression/minorities/cultural-considerations-in-treating-asians-with-depression/menu-id-68

Heilemann, M. V., Coffey-Love, M., & Frutos, L. (2004). Perceived reasons for depression among low income women of Mexican descent. *Archives of Psychiatric Nursing, 18*(5), 185–192.

Hoge, E. A., Austin, E. D., & Pollack, M. H. (2007). Resilience: Research evidence and conceptual considerations for posttraumatic stress disorder. *Depression and Anxiety, 24*(2), 139–152.

Hsu, W. C., & Lai, H. L. (2004). Effects of music on major depression in psychiatric inpatients. *Archives of Psychiatric Nursing, 18*(5), 193–199.

Hvas, A. M., Juul, S., Bech, P., & Nexo, E. (2004). Vitamin B6 level is associated with symptoms of depression. *Psychotherapy and Psychosomatics, 73*(6), 340–343.

Joseph, A. (2006). *The impact of light on outcomes in healthcare settings.* Concord California Center for Health Design, Issue Paper #2.

Kabat-Zinn, J. (2003). Mindful yoga movement & meditation. *Yoga International, 70*, 86–93.

Katz, V. L. (2007). Postpartum care. In S. G. Gabbe, J. R. Niebyl, & J. L. Simpson (Eds.), *Obstetrics: Normal and problem pregnancies* (5th ed., pp. 566–585). Philadelphia: Churchill Livingstone/Elsevier.

Kim-Goodwin, Y. S. (2005). Postpartum beliefs & practices among non-Western cultures. *American Journal of Maternal-Child Nursing, 28*(2), 75–80.

Klein, D. N., Shankman, S. A., Lewinsohn, P. M., Rohde, P., & Seeley, J. R. (2004). Family study of chronic depression in a community sample of young adults. *American Journal of Psychiatry, 161*(4), 646–653.

Kowatch, R., Fristad, M., Birmaher, B., Wagner, K. D., Findling, R. L., Hellander, M., et al. (2005). Treatment guidelines for children and adolescents with bipolar disorder. *Journal of the American Academy of Child and Adolescent Psychiatry, 44*, 236–239.

Lansford, A. H. (2005). The importance of recognizing a child with bipolar disorder. *Contemporary Pediatrics, 22*(2), 69–78.

Larzelere, M. M., & Wiseman, P. (2002). Anxiety, depression, and insomnia. *Primary Care, 29*(2), 339–360.

Lauderdale, J. (2008). Transcultural perspectives in childbearing. In M. M. Andrews & J. S. Boyle, *Transcultural concepts in nursing care* (5th ed.). Philadelphia: Lippincott Williams & Wilkins.

Luby, J. L., Heffelfinger, A., Koenig-McNaught, A. L., Brown, K., & Spitznagel, E. (2004). The Preschool Feelings Checklist: A brief and sensitive screening measure for depression in young children. *Journal of the American Academy of Child and Adolescent Psychiatry, 43*, 708–717.

Mancini, A. D., & Bonanno, G. A. (2006). Resilience in the face of potential trauma: Clinical practices and illustrations. *Journal of Clinical Psychology, 62*(8), 971–985.

Mayberg, H. S., Keightley, M., Mahurin, R. K., & Brannan, S. K. (2004). Neuropsychiatric aspects of mood and affective disorders. In S. C. Yudofsky & R. E. Hales (Eds.), *Essentials of neuropsychiatry and clinical neurosciences* (pp. 489–517). Washington, DC: American Psychiatric Publishing.

McQueen, K., Montgomery, P., Lappan-Gracon, S., Evans, M., & Hunter, J. (2008). Evidence-based recommendations for depressive symptoms in postpartum women. *JOGNN: Journal of Obstetric, Gynecologic, and Neonatal Nursing, 37*, 127–136.

Medline Plus, a service of the National Library of Medicine. (2008). Aripiprazole. Retrieved September 4, 2009, from http://www.nlm.nih.gov/medlineplus/druginfo/meds/a603012.html

Mendelowitz, A. J., Dawkins, K., & Lieberman, J. A. (2000). Antidepressants. In J. A. Lieberman & A. Tasman (Eds.), *Psychiatric drugs*. Philadelphia: W. B. Saunders.

Mental Health America. (n.d.) Mental Health America Awarded Grant To Deliver Culturally Appropriate Support For Native Americans With Serious Mental Illness. Retrieved September 4, 2009, from http://www.nmha.org/index.cfm?objectid=5DBFF7A5-1372-4D20-C89022A71B5E615E

Mercer, R. T. (1995). *Becoming a mother*. New York: Springer.

Mercer, R. T. (2004). Becoming a mother versus maternal role attainment. *Journal of Nursing Scholarship, 36*(3), 226–232.

Meyer, J. H., McMain, S., Kennedy, S. H., Brown, G. M., DaSilva, J. N., Wilson, A. A., et al. (2003). Dysfunctional attitudes and 5-HT2 receptors during depression and self-harm. *American Journal of Psychiatry, 160*(1), 90–99.

Neumeister, A., Charney, D. S., & Drevets, W. C. (2005). Depression and the hippocampus. *American Journal of Psychiatry, 162*(6), 1057.

Oquendo, M., Brent, D. A., Birmaher, B., Greenhill, L., Kolko, D., Stanley, B., et al. (2005). Posttraumatic stress disorder comorbid with major depression. *American Journal of Psychiatry, 162*(3), 560–566.

Peden, A. R., Rayens, M. K., Hall, L. A., & Grant, E. (2004). Negative thinking and the mental health of low-income single mothers. *Journal of Nursing Scholarship, 36*(4), 337–344.

Peden, A. R., Rayens, M. K., Hall, L. A., & Grant, E. (2005). Testing an intervention to reduce negative thinking, depressive symptoms, and chronic stressors in low-income single mothers. *Journal of Nursing Scholarship, 37*(3), 268–274.

Perlis, R. H., Brown, E., Baker, R. W., & Nierenberg, A. A. (2006). Clinical features of bipolar depression versus major depressive disorder in large multicenter trials. *American Journal of Psychiatry, 163*(2), 225–231.

Pruett, J. R., & Luby, J. L. (2004). Recent advances in prepubertal mood disorders. *Current Opinions in Psychiatry, 17*(1), 31–36.

Purnell, L. D., & Paulanka, B. J. (2008). *Transcultural health care: A culturally competent approach* (3rd ed.). Philadelphia: F. A. Davis.

Quilty, L. C., McBride, C., & Bagby, R. M. (2008). Evidence for the cognitive mediational model of cognitive behavioural therapy for depression. *Psychological Medicine, 38*, 1531–1541. doi:10.1017/S0033291708003772

Quitkin, F. M., McGrath, P. J., Stewart, J. W., Deliyannides, D., Taylor, B. P., Davies, C. A., et al., (2005). *Journal of Clinical Psychiatry, 66*(6), 670–676.

Rao, U. (2003). Sleep and other biological rhythms. In B. Geller & M. P. Delbello (Eds.), *Bipolar disorder in childhood and early adolescence* (pp. 215–246). New York: Guilford Press.

Rohan, M., Parow, A., Stoll, A. L., Demopulos, C., Friedman, S., Dager, S., et al. (2004). Low-field magnetic stimulation in bipolar depression using an MRZ-based stimulator. *American Journal of Psychiatry, 161*(1), 93–98.

Rubin, R. (1961). Puerperal change. *Nursing Outlook, 9*, 753.

Rubin, R. (1984). *Maternal identity and the maternal experience*. New York: Springer.

Schneck, C. D., Miklowitz, D. J., Calabrese, J. R., Allen, M. H., Thomas, M. R., Wisniewski, S. R., et al. (2004). Pheomenology of rapid-cycling bipolar disorder. *American Journal of Psychiatry, 161*(10), 1902–1908.

Schreiber, R., Stern, P. N., & Wilson, C. (2000). Being strong: How Black West-Indian Canadian women manage depression and its stigma. *Journal of Nursing Scholarship, 32*(1), 39–45.

Sethabouppha, H., & Kane, C. (2005). Caring for the seriously mentally ill in Thailand: Buddist family caregiving. *Archives of Psychiatric Nursing, 19*(2), 44–57.

Sheikh, J. I., Yesavage, J. A., Brooks, J. O., III, Friedman, L. F., Gratzinger, P., Hill, R. D., et al. Proposed factor structure of the Geriatric Depression Scale. *International Psychogeriatrics 3*, 23–28, 1991.

Sheikh, R. M., Weller, E. B., & Weller, R. A. (2006). Prepubertal depression: Diagnostic and therapeutic dilemmas. *Current Psychiatry Reports, 8*, 121–126.

Solomon, D. A., Leon, A. C., Endicott, J., Coryell, W. H., Mueller, T. I., Posternak, M. A., et al. (2003). Unipolar mania over the course of a 20-year follow-up study. *American Journal of Psychiatry, 160*(11), 2049–2051.

Spinelli, M. G. (2004). Maternal infanticide associated with mental illness. *American Journal of Psychiatry, 161*(9), 1548–1557.

Steinhauer, E. (2003). Current topic review: Psychosocial treatment of bipolar disorder. *Medscape Psychiatry & Mental Health, 8*(1), 1–3. Retrieved June 30, 2003, from http://www.medscape.com/viewarticle/457054

Strothers, H. S. 3rd, Rust, G., Minor, P., Fresh, E., Druss, B., Satcher, D., et al. (2005). Racial disparities in depression care seen in elderly Medicare patients. *Journal of the American Geriatric Society, 53*(3), 456–461.

Suppaseemanont, W. (2006). Depression in pregnancy. *The American Journal of Maternal Child Nursing, 31*(1), 10–15.

Svenningsson, P., Chergui, K., Rachleff, I., Flajolet, M., Zhang, X., Yacoubi, M. E., et al. (2006). Alterations in 5-HT1B receptor function by p11 in depression-like states. *Science, 6*(5757), 77–80.

Tohen, M., Greil, W., Calabrese, J. R., Sachs, G. S., Yatham, L. N., Oerlinghausen, B. M., et al. (2005). Olanzapine versus lithium in the maintenance treatment of bipolar disorder. *American Journal of Psychiatry, 162*(7), 1281–1290.

Tohen, M., Zarate C. A., Hennen, J., Khalsa, H. K., Strakowski, S. M., Gebre-Medhin, P., et al. (2003). The McLean-Harvard first-episode mania study. *American Journal of Psychiatry, 160*(12), 2099–2107.

Trivedi, M. H., Fava, M., Wisniewski, S. R., Thase, M. E., Quitkin, F., Warden, D., et al. (2006). Medication augmentation after the failure of SSRIs for depression. *New England Journal of Medicine, 354*(12), 1243–1252.

Ugarriza, D. N. (2004). Group therapy and its barriers for women suffering from postpartum depression. *Archives of Psychiatric Nursing, 18*(2), 39–48.

Valdivia, I., & Rossy, N. (2004). Brief treatment strategies for major depressive disorder. *Topics in Advanced Practice Nursing eJournal, 4*(1), 1–12.

Varney, H., Kriebs, J. M., & Gegor, C. L. (2004). *Varney's midwifery* (4th ed.). Sudbury, MA: Jones & Bartlett.

Wehr, T. A., Duncan, W. C., Sher, L., Aeschback, D., Schwartz, P. J., Turner, E. H., et al. (2001). A circadian signal of change of season in patients with seasonal affective disorder. *Archives of General Psychiatry, 58*(12), 1108–1114.

Weili, L., Mueser, K. T., Rosenberg, S., & Jankowsi, M. K. (2008). Correlates of adverse childhood experiences among adults with severe mood disorders. *Psychiatric Services, 59*(9), 1018–1026.

Wilens, T. E., Biederman, J., Kwon, A., Ditterline, J., Forkner, P., Moore, H., et al. (2004). Risk of substance use disorders in adolescents with bipolar disorder. *Journal of the American Academy of Child & Adolescent Psychiatry, 43*(11), 1380–1386.

Wisner, K. L., Perel, J. M., Peindl, K. S., Hanusa, B. H., Piontek, C. M., Findling, R. L., et al. (2004). Prevention of postpartum depression. *American Journal of Psychiatry, 161*(7), 1290–1292.

Yesavage, J., Brink, T., Rose, T., Lum, O., Huang, V., Adey, M., et al. (1983). Development and validation of a geriatric depression screening scale: A preliminary report. *Journal of Psychiatric Research, 17*, 37–49.

Yonkers, K. A., Wisner, K. L., Stowe, Z., Leibenluft, E., Cohen, L., Miller, L., et al. (2004). Management of bipolar disorder during pregnancy and the postpartum period. *American Journal of Psychiatry, 161*(4), 608–620.

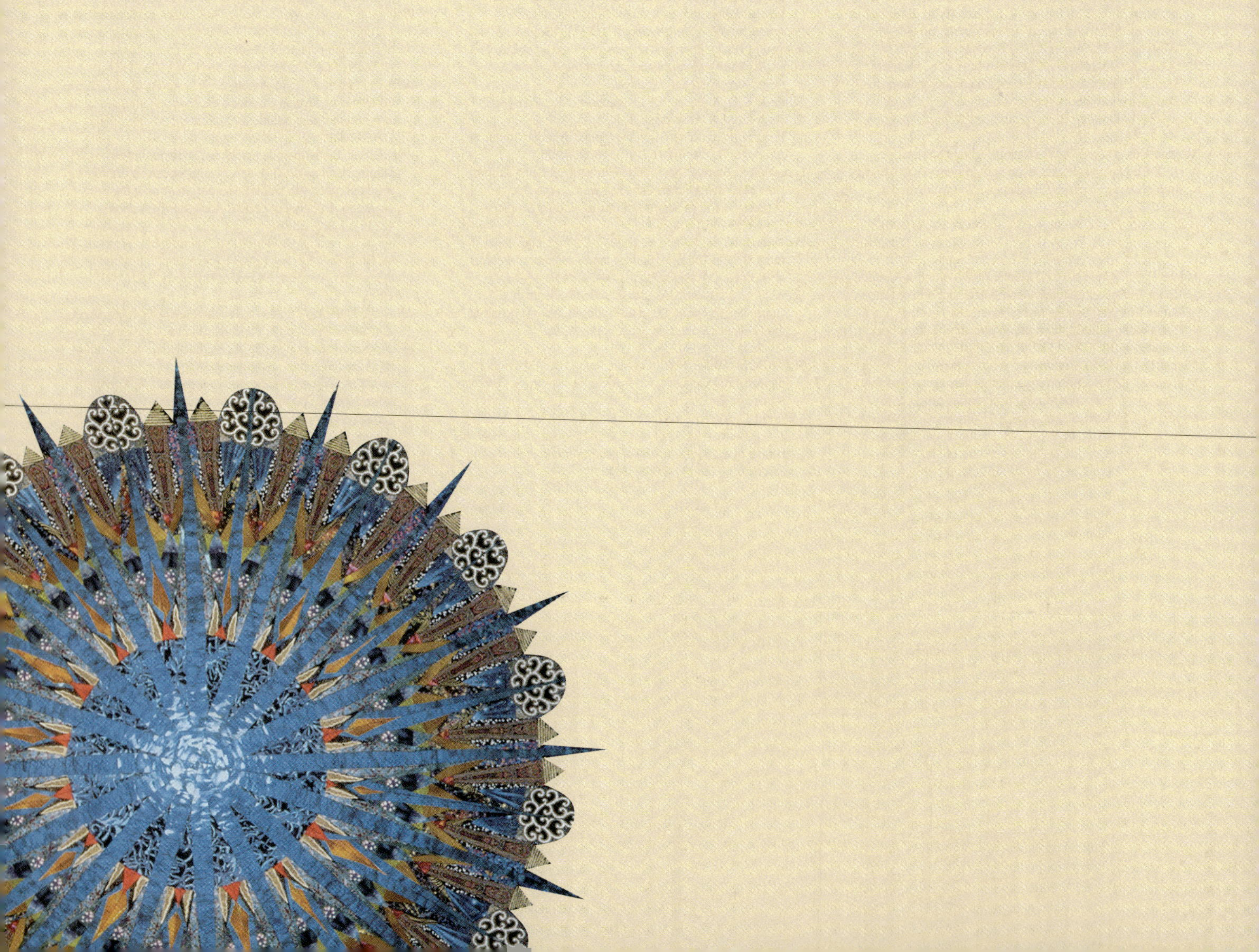

Oxygenation 21

Concept at-a-Glance

Concept Learning Outcomes

After reading about this concept, you will be able to:

1. Summarize the structure and physiologic processes of the respiratory system related to oxygenation.
2. List factors affecting oxygenation.
3. Identify commonly occurring alterations in oxygenation and their related treatments.
4. Explain common physical assessment procedures used to evaluate respiratory health of clients across the life span.
5. Outline diagnostic and laboratory tests to determine the individual's oxygenation status.
6. Explain management of respiratory health and prevention of alterations in oxygenation.
7. Demonstrate the nursing process in providing culturally competent and caring interventions across the life span for individuals with common alterations in oxygenation.
8. Identify pharmacologic interventions in caring for the individual with alterations in oxygenation.

Concept Key Terms

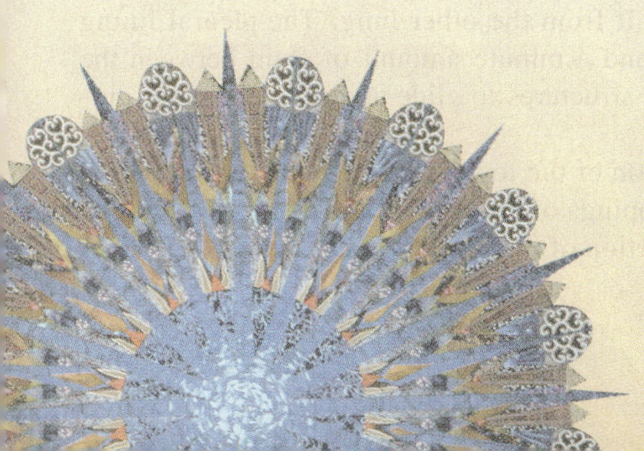

About Oxygenation

Oxygenation can be defined as the mechanisms that facilitate or impair the body's ability to supply oxygen to all cells of the body. The function of the respiratory system is to obtain oxygen from atmospheric air, to transport this air through the respiratory tract into the alveoli, and ultimately to diffuse oxygen into the blood that carries oxygen to all the cells of the body. **Ventilation** is the process of moving air into and out of the lungs, while **respiration** is the actual exchange of gases between the alveoli and pulmonary capillaries. Ventilation involves the process of inhaling (**inspiration**) air into the alveoli and exhaling (**expiration**) air from the lungs out into the environment.

The respiratory system is divided into two parts: the upper respiratory tract and the lower respiratory tract. The upper respiratory tract begins with the nose and ends in the pharynx. The lower respiratory tract begins at the epiglottis and ends in the alveoli. The alveoli are the functional portion of the respiratory system where the exchange of oxygen and carbon dioxide occurs by diffusion at the alveoli-pulmonary capillary bed interface. Adequate oxygenation within the body depends on a healthy, intact respiratory system. ●

Breathing is often an unnoticed activity that contributes to vital oxygenation of the cells and tissues. When oxygen status changes, breathing usually compensates to bring more air into the lungs. Changes in breathing patterns should be taken seriously and acted upon promptly because alterations in oxygen delivery can cause serious consequences.

Mrs. Lee presents at the emergency room where she reports that she has been breathing rapidly and deeply for the past 2 hours. She reports, "I cannot breathe. Get some fresh air in here." While still being interviewed by the triage nurse, her respiratory rate goes from 40 breaths per minute to 30 breaths per minute. Her respiratory quality changes from deep to shallow. The triage nurse follows protocol, summoning additional registered nurses, a respiratory therapist, a physician, a radiology technologist, and a phlebotomist to the room.

Although other indicators of hemodynamic instability also existed for Mrs. Lee, the sudden change in breathing was most important in determining whether a more aggressive approach to her care was necessary.

NORMAL PRESENTATION

Adequate oxygenation of the body depends on a healthy, intact respiratory system. The respiratory system obtains oxygen from atmospheric air and transports it into the alveoli, where oxygen diffuses into a capillary and is carried by the blood to all the cells of the body. The respiratory system also passes carbon dioxide from the body.

The upper respiratory system is the inlet for air into the body. The nose is the typical inlet. The nose is midline on the face, with the same color as facial skin. The nose is divided into two nares that are moist, pink, mucosa-lined passageways. The purpose of the nares is to warm, humidify, and filter air as it is breathed into the nose. The upper respiratory tract has two protective mechanisms to prevent foreign matter from entering the lower respiratory tract: sneezing and cilia. Foreign matter that enters the nose irritates the nasal passages and induces sneezing. Sneezing is a reflexive action that clears the upper airway. This reflexive action is active even in the neonatal period. Cilia are microscopic fine hairs within the posterior portion of the nares that trap small particles of foreign matter to prevent their entry into the lower respiratory tract. The cilia propel foreign matter into the pharynx to be coughed out or swallowed.

Breathing also happens through the mouth, which allows air to enter the respiratory system through the pharyngeal cavity. The respiratory system shares this cavity with the gastrointestinal system, providing passage for air during breathing and for food or drink during swallowing.

A protective mechanism within the pharyngeal cavity prevents food or drink from entering the lower respiratory tract. The glottis is the opening into the lower respiratory tract. The epiglottis is pendulous tissue that covers the tracheal opening during swallowing or any time foreign matter contacts the glottis. The closure of the epiglottis is a reflexive response.

The lower respiratory tract is enclosed in the musculoskeletal structures of the neck and thoracic cavity. The trachea, which sits midline in the neck, is the entrance way for air into the lungs. During normal breathing, the muscular structures of the neck are relaxed and the larynx easily rises and falls with a swallow. The chest wall effortlessly and symmetrically rises and falls with each equally spaced breath. Inspiration is half the rate of expiration. **Eupnea** describes breathing within the expected respiratory rates. **Auscultation**, listening to the body's sounds with a stethoscope, is an important diagnostic tool. Auscultation of the trachea will reveal a **tubular** sound of air movement, as if produced through a tube, when airways are clear and functioning.

The trachea bifurcates (divides in two) into two bronchi to access the right and left lungs (Figures 21–1 ■ and 21–2 ■). The right bronchus is shorter and wider than the left. Each bronchus further divides into bronchioles that terminate in the alveoli sacs. These passageways for air dilate and contract. The trachea and larger bronchi are supported by C-shaped cartilage rings, as well as by smooth muscle. The smaller bronchioles are supported by smooth muscles only. Bronchioles deliver air to the alveoli. These air passageways dilate and contract as the autonomic nervous system regulates the smooth muscles supporting them. The movement of air within the bronchial tree creates a mixture of sounds of air flowing through a tube and the breeziness of the open alveolar lung fields. This is termed **bronchovesicular** sound.

The lungs are also described in terms of their lobes. The lobes lie obliquely in the thoracic cavity. The right lung has three lobes; the left lung has two lobes. The inferior lobes are the largest. Most of the inferior lobes lie in the posterior thoracic cavity. Each lung has a pleural lining to aid respiration and separate it from the other lung. The pleural lining has two layers, and a minute amount of fluid between the layers allows the structures to glide across one another during respiration.

The final portion of the lower respiratory system is the air sacs. The outcroppings of the air sacs are called alveoli. The alveoli are the portion of the lungs that fulfill the function of

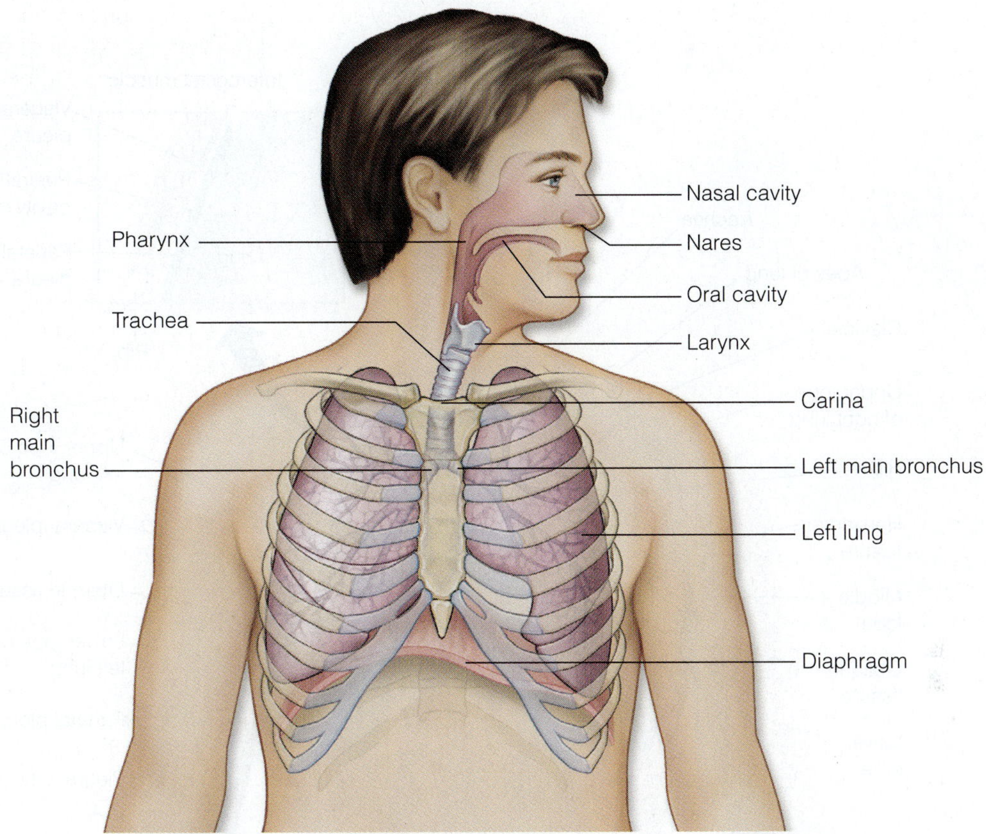

Figure 21–1 ■ Anatomy of the respiratory system.

the respiratory system. Alveoli are not directly connected to a specific bronchiole, but are interconnected to the terminal airways and to each other. This facilitates the filling of each alveoli with air. The sounds of air moving into and out of the lobes at the alveolar level are soft and breezy, defined as **vesicular**.

The alveoli have specialized cells that produce surfactant. **Surfactant** controls surface tension and keeps the alveoli from collapsing and sticking to itself. Surfactant is produced only with adequate oxygenation. Alveolar macrophages keep the alveoli region free of microbes and are swept upward from the alveolar region by cilia in the airway passages. Macrophages are large cells of the immune system that remove waste and harmful microorganisms from the alveoli and from other areas of the body. Mast cells in the alveoli mediate the immune response within the airways.

Alveoli have a simple squamous epithelial lining and basement that interface with the basement and epithelial lining of pulmonary capillaries. This interface is where oxygen and carbon dioxide diffusion occurs. The concentration of oxygen is greater in the alveoli than in the blood in the capillaries, so oxygen diffuses across the membranes into the blood. The concentration of carbon dioxide is greater in the blood, so it diffuses into the alveoli. Figure 21–3 ■ shows the alveolar-capillary membrane interface.

The typical drive to breathe occurs due to **hypercarbia**. Hypercarbia is an increased level of carbon dioxide in the blood. Receptor sites within the medulla and pons are sensitive to carbon dioxide levels in the blood. Elevated levels of carbon dioxide induce inhalation of air into the lungs. Yawns and sighs are induced after periods of shallow breathing or breath holding. Exhalation is a passive response to relaxation of the muscles of respiration. The typical breathing rate is regularly spaced, with inspiration half as long as expiration (I:E = 1:2).

TABLE 21–1 **Respirations Throughout the Life Span**

VALUE RANGES BY AGE GROUP	RATE (BREATHS/MIN)
Newborns	30–60
Infants	20–40
Toddlers	20–30
Preschooler	20–26
School aged	12–24
Adolescence	14–20
Adults	10–20
Older adults	12–24

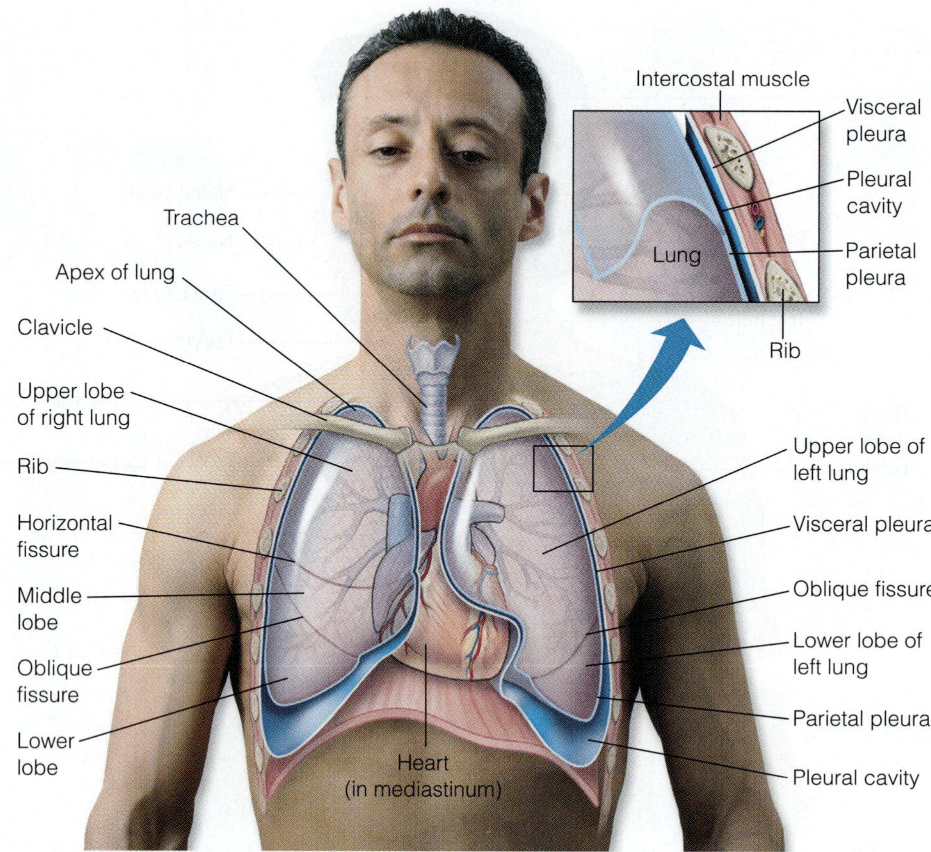

Figure 21–2 ■ Anterior view of thorax and lungs.

The normal respiratory rate in an adult ranges from 10 to 20 breaths per minute. Table 21–1 shows normal ranges for various age groups. Depth of normal inspiration is about 500 mL of air with each breath. The expansion of the chest wall is observable, but is neither shallow nor great. Quality of breathing refers to the effort involved in taking a breath and the sounds that may occur with inspiration or expiration. Quality of breathing requires a **patent airway**, one that is open and free of obstruction.

Receptor sites in the aortic arch and carotid arteries monitor oxygen. These receptors will induce inspiration with low enough levels of oxygen. Stretch receptors with the lungs control the volume of air inhaled with each breath. During relaxed states, the lungs will fill to approximately one half a liter. Strenuous activities of exercise result in deeper breaths of increasing volume to meet the oxygen demands of skeletal muscles.

The ability of the respiratory system to deliver oxygen to the blood depends on an inflated and well-oxygenated alveolus and an associated capillary with freely flowing blood at an adequate blood pressure. The movement of oxygen across the alveolar-capillary membrane into a well-perfusing capillary is defined as the **ventilation-perfusion (V-Q)** ratio. The concentration levels of oxygen and carbon dioxide dictate the movement of each gas across the alveolar-capillary membrane.

ALTERATIONS

The typical drive to breathe occurs due to hypercarbia. Hypercarbia interferes with the body's ability to respond appropriately to increased levels of carbon dioxide. When this happens, instead of hypercarbia initiating the breathing response, decreased levels of oxygen initiate the drive to breathe. This is commonly seen in individuals with **chronic obstructive pulmonary disease (COPD)**, resulting from prolonged cigarette smoking, as smoking is the primary cause of prolonged elevated levels of carbon dioxide.

Hypoxemia is defined as a decreased level of oxygen. Chest wall in-drawing is an early indicator of hypoxemia. **Cyanosis** is a late sign of hypoxemia and is seen as a blue tinge to the skin in fair individuals. In individuals with darker pigmentation, cyanosis may present as gray coloration of the skin. An indicator of chronic hypoxemia is clubbed nail beds. Clubbed nail beds have an angle of 180°

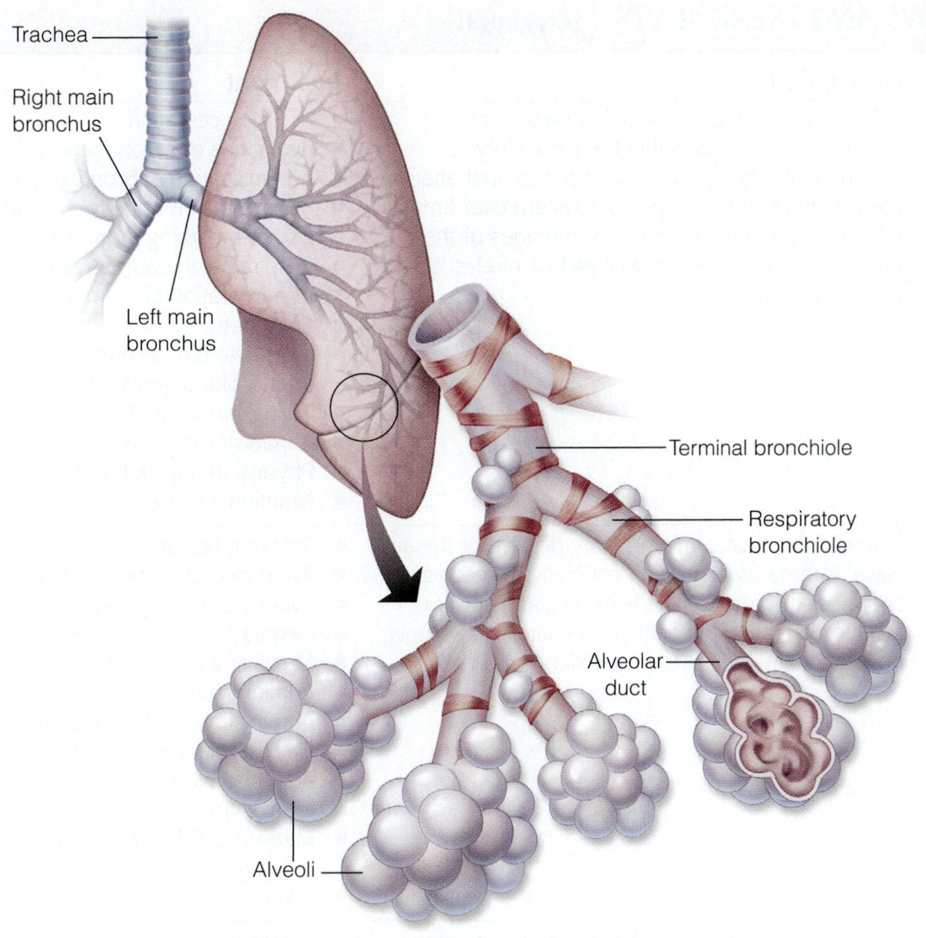

Figure 21–3 ■ Respiratory bronchioles, alveolar ducts, and alveoli.

or greater, depending on the duration of time an individual has had hypoxemia.

A number of factors affect a healthy respiratory system. The air an individual breathes, either indoors or outdoors, may be polluted. Exposure to airborne irritants may produce an inflammatory response within the airways. Infectious illnesses of the respiratory tract and hemoglobin disorders such as sickle cell anemia interfere with effective respiratory function. Lifestyle behaviors may affect respiratory health. Some medications affect respiratory rate and depth. Generally, inflammation, infection, sputum production, and compromised airflow contribute to alterations in respiratory health. *Healthy People 2010* has several directives related to maintaining or attaining respiratory health. These include the following:

- Management of environmental air quality is necessary to decrease the concentration of respiratory irritations affecting asthma and COPD in the United States. Environmental air quality includes interior and external air sources. A decrease in the use of tobacco products is necessary to stop the unnecessary damage to the health of tobacco users and those exposed secondhand to tobacco smoke. Tobacco smoking is the primary cause of COPD in Western countries such as the United States. Exposure to polluted air in homes and workplaces and to tobacco smoke exacerbates COPD, asthma, and respiratory synctial virus and is associated with sudden infant death syndrome.
- Vaccination is encouraged to decrease transmission of preventable diseases, many of which are transmitted by respiratory secretions. Many illnesses historically seen in children now are prevented by immunization. Immunization for influenza and pneumonia protects adults from serious respiratory illness. Respiratory syncytial virus (RSV) is a highly contagious respiratory infection that affects all age groups, but that is most serious for children younger than 2 years of age. Sudden infant death syndrome (SIDS) is the major cause of death with unknown cause for infants older than 1 month of age.

ALTERATIONS AND TREATMENTS Oxygenation

Alteration	Description	Treatment
Chronic obstructive pulmonary disease (COPD)	COPD is a preventable, treatable disease of compromised airflow within the respiratory system. COPD is a progressive disorder that alters the structures of the respiratory system over time. Inflammation of the mucous membranes of the bronchial tubes occurs as well as loss of elasticity in lung parenchyma.	■ Smoking cessation ■ Avoidance of secondhand smoke ■ Administration of bronchodilators ■ Administration of corticosteroids ■ Use of breathing exercises ■ Respiratory therapy consult ■ Administration of pulmonary function tests ■ Spirometry ■ Complete blood count (CBC), chemistries, and arterial blood gases ■ Taking sputum specimen ■ Administration of oxygen ■ Physical therapy consult ■ Nutritional consult
Asthma	Asthma is a chronic inflammatory disease of the airways. Asthma presents with coughing, wheezing, shortness of breath, chest tightness, and sputum production. Asthma is defined in relation to severity and control as well as to impairments and risk.	■ Smoking cessation ■ Avoidance of secondhand smoke ■ Avoidance of aggravating factors ■ Respiratory therapy consult ■ Measuring daily peak expiratory flow rate ■ Administration of maintenance bronchodilators ■ Administration of maintenance corticosteroids ■ Exercise planning by physical therapy ■ Administration of short-acting bronchodilators for exercise ■ Measuring CBC, chemistry panels, and arterial blood gases ■ Taking a sputum specimen
Respiratory syncytial virus (RSV)	RSV is a highly contagious lower respiratory infection that affects nearly 100% of children younger than 2 years of age. Repeated infections of RSV occur throughout the life span, though subsequent infections tend to be milder.	■ Avoidance of secondhand smoke ■ Separating sick individuals from well individuals ■ Observation of breathing pattern including, rate, rhythm, and quality ■ Teaching the parents or caregiver how to observe breathing patterns ■ Maintaining adequate fluid volume and calories ■ Oral and nasal suctioning ■ Possible use of bronchodilators and corticosteroids
Sudden infant death syndrome (SIDS)	SIDS is the leading cause of death of infants beyond the neonatal period. SIDS occurs most often between the first and the fourth months of life, but may occur up to 1 year of age. The cause of SIDS is not known. Infants who appear healthy are found dead by parents or caregivers. Preventive measures have reduced the incidence of SIDS in developed countries, including the United States.	■ Placing infant on his or her back to sleep ■ Smoking cessation by caregivers ■ Avoidance of secondhand smoke ■ Ensuring a totally smoke-free environment ■ Co-sleeper or same-room sleeping of infant and parents ■ Avoiding bed sharing ■ Maintaining adult-comfort room temperature ■ Breastfeeding ■ Using a pacifier
Acute respiratory distress syndrome (ARDS)	ARDS is a disorder with rapid onset of progressive malfunction of the lungs' ability to take in oxygen. Extensive lung tissue inflammation and small blood vessel injury occurs, followed by malfunction of other organs.	■ Measuring CBC, chemistry panels, and arterial blood gases ■ Testing sputum specimen ■ Administration of oxygen ■ Providing ventilator support ■ Administration of intravenous fluid to maintain hemodynamic status

Alterations in oxygenation can be described in relation to changes in breathing patterns, patency of airway, or interference with gas exchange. Damage to the supporting thoracic structure, either by injury or disease, can contribute to interference in effective respiration. Irritation or inflammation of the respiratory mucosa also affects the ability of the respiratory system to obtain adequate oxygenation for the cells within the body.

The airway of an infant is very small in diameter. It can be occluded with minimal amounts of sputum or swelling from inflammation. Infants are obligatory nose breathers; therefore, even stuffy noses can interfere with the infant's breathing process. Children, especially infants and toddlers, learn about their world by placing things into their mouths and noses. Small objects may become caught in their airways, interfering with breathing.

Adults also may be at risk of catching a foreign object in their airways. Large bites of food that are improperly chewed and swallowed can become lodged in the throat, interfering with the passage of air into the lungs. Older adults are at even greater risk of choking on food because their cough reflex response is decreased. The incidence of gastroesophageal reflux disease increases with age, increasing the risk of aspiration of food into the lower respiratory tract.

Loss of airway patency can result from increased sputum production from upper and lower respiratory infection or irritation. Thick sputum secretions are of special concern in relation to blocking large and small airways. Inflammation of airways due to infections or irritants narrows airways, decreasing the movement of air through the respiratory system.

Respiratory rate, rhythm, depth, and quality determine adequate oxygenation to the cells. A respiratory rate greater than 20 breaths per minute in adults is called **tachypnea**. Anxiety or stress may cause an individual to breathe very rapidly, inhaling and exhaling deeply. Hyperventilation is rapid and deep inhalation and exhalation of air from the lungs. In hypoventilation, a reduced amount of air enters the alveoli, resulting in a decrease of oxygen and an increase of carbon dioxide. A respiratory rate of less than 10 breaths per minute in adults is called **bradypnea**. **Apnea** is the absence of breathing. Continuous apnea is termed *respiratory arrest* and is life-threatening.

Dyspnea, labored breathing or shortness of breath that is uncomfortable or painful, also occurs when breathing is insufficient to meet oxygen demand. Exertional dyspnea occurs with activity. **Orthopnea** is difficulty breathing when a person is supine. The nurse's ability to differentiate changes in respiratory rate is critical when working with any individual, but particularly critical when working with elder patients because pulmonary function declines with age. Chest walls and airways become more rigid, losing their elasticity, and musculoskeletal strength decreases and the effort to breathe increases.

Several breathing patterns with irregular rates, rhythms, depth, and quality indicate abnormalities within other body systems. Kussmaul's breathing occurs in the presence of metabolic acidosis and results in very deep and rapid breaths. These deep, rapid exhalations rid the body of large amounts of carbon dioxide, which affects the acid–base balance. Cheyne-Stokes respirations exhibit as deep, rapid breathing and slow, shallow breathing with periods of apnea. Cheyne-Stokes is seen in individuals with congestive heart failure, increased intracranial pressure, and drug overdoses. Biot's respirations are seen in individuals with central nervous system disorders. Biot's presents as shallow breathing with periods of apnea. Benzodiazepines, barbiturates, and opioids may cause decreased depth and rate of breathing due to their oxygenation-compromising central nervous system effects.

Abnormalities within the alveolar-capillary bed system alter V-Q ratios. Airflow in an alveolus blocked by sputum, inflammation with its complementary swelling, atelectasis, or fluid volume excesses can cause decreased ventilation. Blood clots, plaque buildup, and emphysemic adjacent alveolus interfere with capillary blood flow. Each of these V-Q mismatches results in inadequate oxygenation of body cells. Any and all of these types of V-Q mismatch may occur simultaneously (Figure 21–4 ■).

Any alteration that impairs the oxygenation process can be life-threatening. In addition to determining and then treating the presenting alteration, it is critical to determine its cause. A mild case of exercise-induced asthma may only require administration of an albuterol inhaler prior to the individual participating in exercise or sports activities. By contrast, COPD is much more difficult to treat.

In addition to the exemplars detailed in this concept, other diseases and some injuries, such as a fractured pleural rib, can cause impairment in oxygenation. One disease that presents multiple problems for clients and their physicians is sickle cell anemia. An inherited blood disorder, sickle cell anemia impairs the transport of oxygen through the blood. Sickle cell can cause a variety of complications, including organ failure.

Pneumothorax, or a partial lung collapse resulting from air or gas collecting in the lung or in the pleural space that surrounds the lungs, is a respiratory emergency. A pneumothorax that appears without any known cause is termed a *spontaneous pneumothorax*. Risk factors for this type of pneumothorax include emphysema, cystic fibrosis, and tuberculosis. A tension pneumothorax results from injury (e.g., a fractured rib) or as a result of a progressive lung disease, such as asthma or emphysema. Tension pneumothorax is more difficult to treat than pneumothorax and can result in heart failure. Signs and symptoms of a pneumothorax include sudden sharp pleuritic pain, worsened by movement such as breathing and coughing; asymmetrical chest wall movement; shortness of breath; and cyanosis.

Impaired oxygenation can be frightening and frustrating. It is frightening in that it may be life-threatening. It is frustrating in that shortness of breath and other symptoms common to impairment of oxygenation cause fatigue and can affect so many other bodily processes, which in turn affect quality of life.

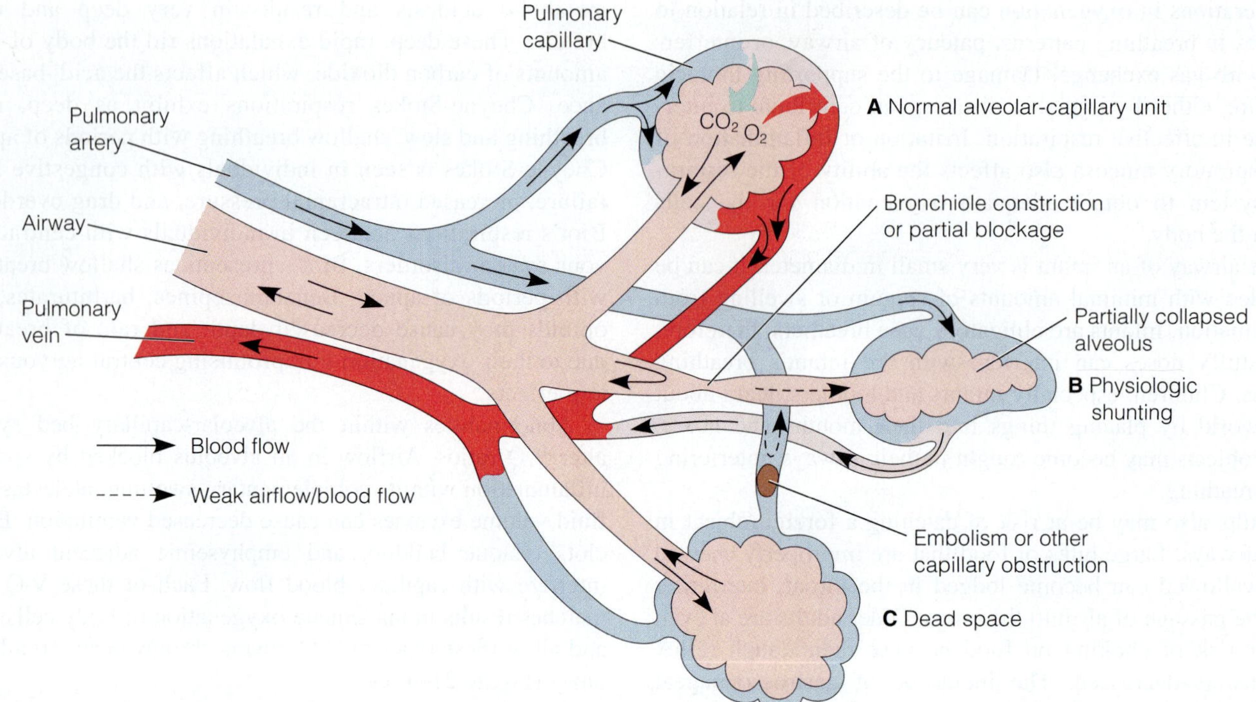

Figure 21–4 ■ Ventilation-perfusion relationships. *A*, Normal alveolar-capillary unit with an ideal match of ventilation and blood flow. Maximum gas exchange occurs between alveolus and blood. *B*, Physiologic shunting: A unit with adequate perfusion but inadequate ventilation. *C*, Dead space: A unit with adequate ventilation but inadequate perfusion. In the latter two cases, gas exchange is impaired.

PHYSICAL ASSESSMENT

The respiratory system health history and physical assessment include subjective and objective data. Lifestyle behaviors and current problems with breathing, including the presence of a cough and sputum, are determined. Any risk factors associated with compromised respiratory health are noted.

The assessment of any body system requires a systematic approach to ensure that no area or aspect of the body system is missed. The nurse uses all five senses to assess an individual. With inspection the nurse uses his or her eyes to observe expected and unexpected findings. Then with **palpation**, the nurse uses the hands to feel the areas related to the body system for **symmetry**, equality of the size, shape, or condition of opposite sides of the body. Next, the nurse uses **percussion**, a method of tapping the chest or back to assess underlying structures; tones heard during percussion determine solid-filled or air-filled spaces at the area percussed. Finally, the nurse uses auscultation to hear the sounds within the respiratory system (Box 21–1). Use of a stethoscope facilitates the hearing of sounds within the body. Any assessment is best supported by obtaining a full set of vital sign measurements with pulse oximetry.

The client presenting with breathing problems may provide a number of objective and subjective indicators that confirm the report. Self-posturing (leaning forward or against a

Box 21–1 Adventitious Breathing Sounds

A number of adventitious sounds can be heard while auscultating the lower respiratory tract.

- **Stridor** is a high-pitched sound within the trachea and larynx that suggests narrowing of the tracheal passage.
- **Crackles** are high-pitched popping sounds, much like when one pours milk over crisped rice cereal. Crackles are heard on inspiration, due to fluid associated with or resulting from inflammation, or exudates, within the lung fields or localized atelectasis. **Atelectasis** is the collapse of lung tissue affecting all or part a lung, impacting the exchange of oxygen and carbon dioxide. The primary cuase of atelectasis is the obstruction of the bronchus serving the affected area.
- **Rhonchi** is a long, low-pitched sound that continues throughout inspiration. Rhonchi suggests blockage of large airway passages, which can sometimes be cleared with coughing.
- **Wheezing** is a high-pitched whistling sound most often heard on expiration and caused by the narrowing of bronchi, but wheezes can also be heard on inspiration.
- When inflamed pleural surfaces rub together, they can make a low-pitched, grating sound. This occurs more during inspiration, but can also occur during expiration.

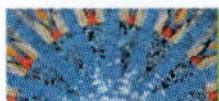

Oxygenation Assessment

Technique/Normal Findings	Abnormal Findings
Nasal assessment	
Inspect the nose symmetry. Inspect the nasal cavity using a flashlight. The septum should fall midline and intact. The mucosa of the nares is pink and moist without drainage. Both nares should be patent. (See Figure 21–5 ■)	■ Asymmetry indicates trauma or surgery. ■ Redness and/or swelling is observed. ■ Deviated septum narrows or occludes one naris. ■ Foreign bodies may be found in the nares, especially of infants, toddlers, and preschoolers. ■ Purulent drainage occurs. ■ Watery nasal drainage occurs. ■ Pale turbinates are seen.
Respiratory rate assessment	
Count respiratory rate for one full minute counting one inspiration and one expiration as one breath. Normal respiratory rate is eupnea (see Table 21–1 for development impact on rate)	■ Bradypnea ■ Tachypnea ■ Apnea ■ Cheyne-Stokes respirations
Assess quality of breathing: Determine regularity in timing I:E ratio is 1:2. Assess depth of inspiration. Observe effort to breathe.	■ Shortness of breath ■ Dyspnea ■ Orthopnea
Inspection of thoracic cavity	
Anteroposterior diameter is half the transverse diameter. *Normal ratio is 1:2*. (See Figures 21–6 ■ and 21–7 ■)	■ Anteroposterior equals transverse thoracic diameter measurements, called a barrel chest.
Inspection of the muscles of breathing	
The chest walls gently rise and fall with each breath. The muscles in the neck are relaxed. The trachea is midline. The intercostal muscles raise the chest upward and outward with inhalation, then calmly relax with exhalation.	■ Retraction of the intercostals occurs. ■ Sternocleidomastoid muscles of the neck contract. ■ Posturing occurs.
Inspection and palpation of the thoracic wall for symmetry	
Symmetrical movement of the hands is observed with symmetrical hand placement on the chest wall. The trachea is midline.	■ Asymmetry of movement occurs. ■ Decreased expansion occurs. ■ The trachea shifts from midline.
Skin assessment in relation to the respiratory system	
Pink skin indicates adequate oxygenation of the cell throughout the body. Nail beds are an extension of the finger and are normally curved with a 160° angle of the nail bed to the finger.	Cyanosis is a blue tinge to the skin in fair individuals and gray coloration of the skin in darker pigmented individuals. Clubbed nail beds have an angle of 180° or greater, depending on the duration of time an individual has had hypoxemia.

table or wall to breathe) may be evident. A client may have difficulty speaking, taking breaths in the middle of sentences. The individual's voice may be raspy. In the absence of a productive cough, repeated throat clearing may indicate the presence of phlegm. Individuals who cannot breathe well often become frustrated when answering questions because the effort to answer further impairs breathing, and the effort to breathe quickly brings on fatigue. When working with any individual, as well as with someone with impaired breathing, the nurse should be patient and sympathetic. A pulse oximetry reading above 90% may not be a true indicator of the level of respiratory distress if the client has used an albuterol inhaler within 30–60 minutes of presenting at the clinic or emergency room. Increased frequency of use of albuterol inhalers or nebulizer treatments indicates a severe respiratory episode.

Clients who present with impairment at or near respiratory failure will not be able to respond to questions. Assessment questions should be tailored and asked of any

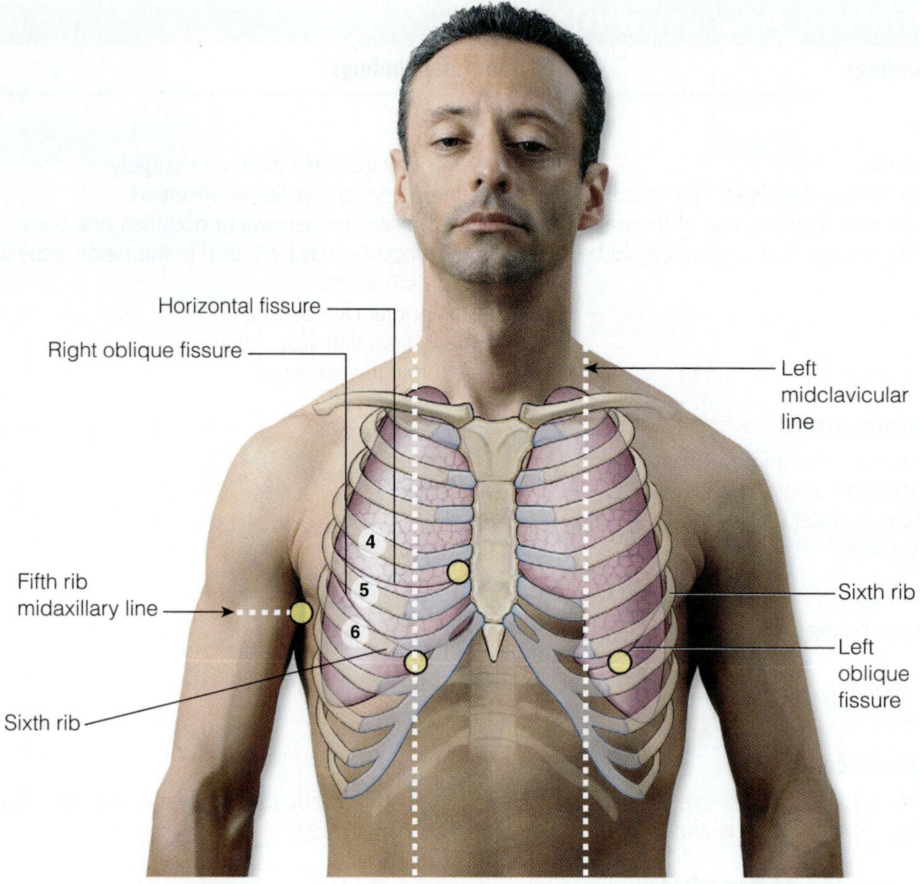

Figure 21–5 ■ Lobes of the lungs: anterior view.

Assessment Interview Oxygenation

CURRENT RESPIRATORY PROBLEMS

- Have you noticed any changes in your breathing pattern (e.g., shortness of breath, difficulty in breathing, need to be in upright position to breathe, or rapid and shallow breathing)?
- If so, which of your activities might cause these symptoms to occur?
- How many pillows do you use to sleep at night?

HISTORY OF RESPIRATORY DISEASE

- Have you had colds, allergies, asthma, tuberculosis, bronchitis, pneumonia, or emphysema?
- How frequently have these occurred? How long did they last? And how were they treated?
- Have you been exposed to any pollutants?

LIFESTYLE

- Do you smoke? If so, how much? If not, did you smoke previously, and when did you stop?
- Does any member of your family smoke?
- Is there cigarette smoke or other pollutants (e.g., fumes, dust, coal, asbestos) in your workplace?
- Do you drink alcohol? If so, how many drinks (mixed drinks, glasses of wine, or beers) do you usually have per day or per week?
- Describe your exercise patterns. How often do you exercise and for how long?

PRESENCE OF COUGH

- How often and how much do you cough?
- Is it productive, that is, accompanied by sputum, or nonproductive, that is, dry?
- Does the cough occur during certain activity or at certain times of the day?

DESCRIPTION OF SPUTUM

- When is the sputum produced?
- What is the amount, color, thickness, and odor of the sputum?
- Is it ever tinged with blood?

PRESENCE OF CHEST PAIN

- How does going outside in the heat or the cold affect you?
- Do you experience any pain with breathing or activity?
- Where is the pain located?
- Describe the pain. How does it feel?
- Does it occur when you breathe in or out?
- How long does it last, and how does it affect your breathing?
- Do you experience any other symptoms when the pain occurs (e.g., nausea, shortness of breath or difficulty breathing, lightheadedness, palpitations)?
- What activities precede your pain?
- What do you do to relieve the pain?

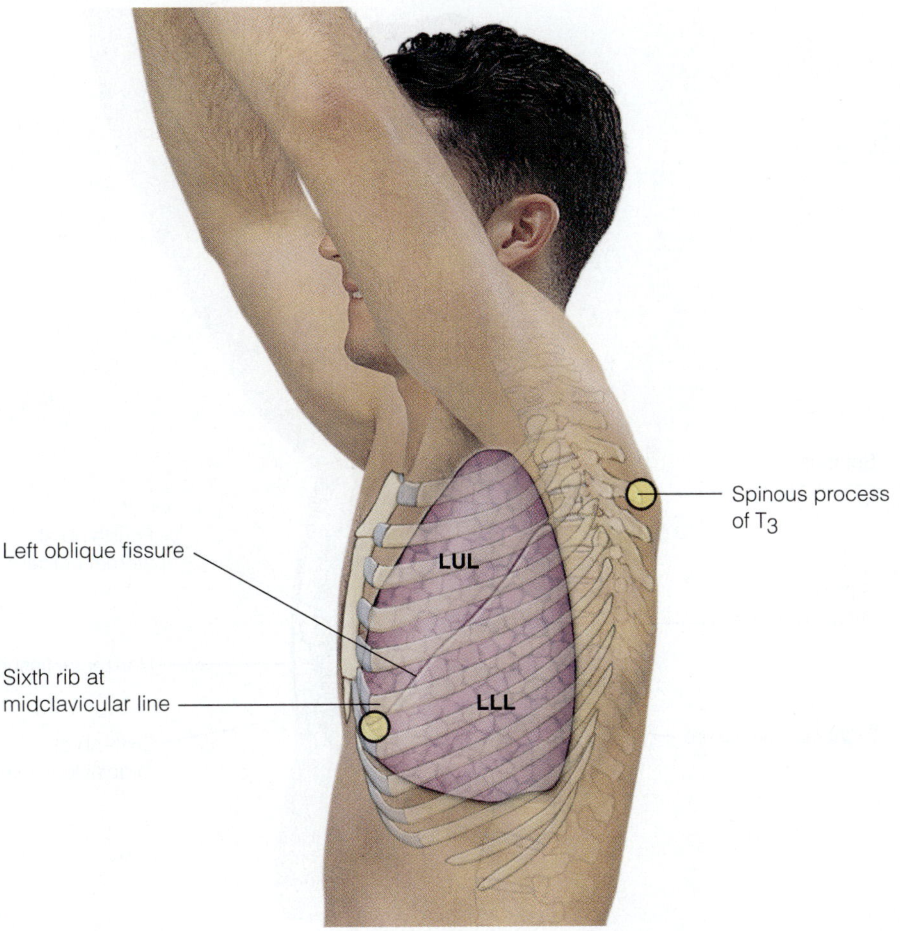

Figure 21–6 ■ Lateral view of lobes of the left lung.

Assessment Interview Oxygenation (continued)

PRESENCE OF RISK FACTORS

- Do you have a family history of lung cancer, cardiovascular disease (including strokes), or tuberculosis?
- The nurse should also note the client's weight, activity pattern, and dietary assessment. Risk factors include obesity, sedentary lifestyle, and diet high in saturated fats.

MEDICATION HISTORY

- Have you taken or do you take any over-the-counter or prescription medications for breathing (e.g., bronchodilator, inhalant, narcotic)?
- If so, which ones? And what are the dosages, times taken, and results, including side effects? Are you taking them exactly as directed?

family member or friend accompanying the client to the emergency room. The client's physician should be notified immediately on the client's arrival at the hospital. The immediate concern is to return respiratory status as near to normal as possible. Adrenaline may be given in the case of respiratory failure related to anaphylaxis or allergic reaction. Chest tubes and ventilators may be necessary. Support for family is also important at this time, as is an understanding of the client's religious and cultural preferences. The Roman Catholic Church, as well as other denominations, have prayers that are said over those who are very sick, which may bring comfort to the family when the client is diagnosed with a critical respiratory illness.

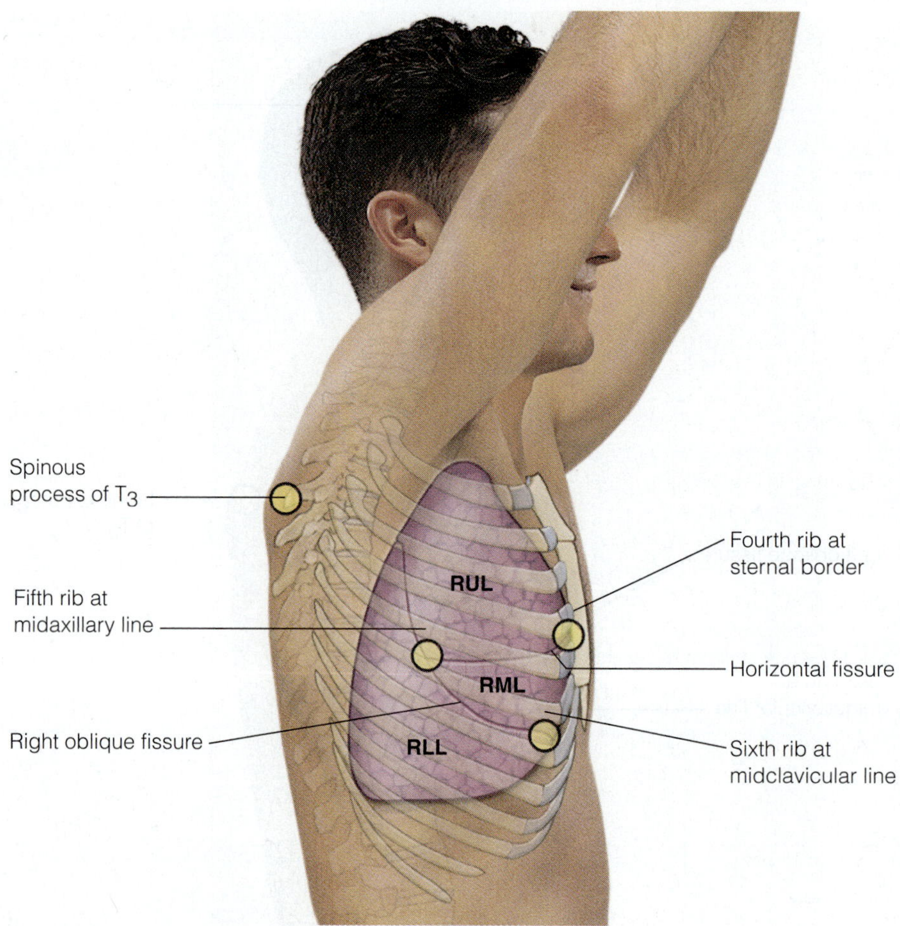

Figure 21–7 ■ Lateral view of lobes of the right lung.

DIAGNOSTIC TESTS

Specific diagnostic tests are used to assess for abnormalities of the respiratory system and to monitor for changes in individuals with chronic oxygenation impairment. Tests include those that determine the presence of inflammation or infection and changes in acid–base balance, and tests for viewing thoracic structures.

A sputum specimen may be used to identify the presence of microbes, metabolites of inflammation, and immunoglobulins. A sputum culture is used to identify specific microbes within the lower respiratory tract. Sputum is expectorant matter that may contain all or some mucus, cellular debris, blood, microorganisms, and purulent matter from the respiratory tract. It is important to ensure that the liquid obtained from an individual is from the lung fields and not from spit from his or her mouth. The proper identification of the microbe facilitates the selection of the appropriate antibiotic, antiviral, or antifungal agents to treat the inflammation. Excessive use of antibiotics for inflammatory processes that do not respond to the prescribed antibiotic has contributed to the emergence of drug-resistant microbes.

Arterial blood gas (ABG) provides a direct indication of oxygen and carbon dioxide exchange and the acid–base balance within the blood. The major chemical components monitored by ABG are hydrogen ions (pH), carbon dioxide (CO_2), oxygen (O_2), and bicarbonate (HCO_3). See Table 21–2 for normal ABG laboratory values. Each ABG component is reviewed in turn.

Initial assessment focuses on the oxygen values of the ABG. The oxygen value is defined by the amount of oxygen bound to hemoglobin (SaO_2) and the amount of oxygen dissolved in blood serum (PaO_2). An oxygen saturation value (SaO_2) in a healthy individual without any respiratory abnormalities is greater than 95%. The values of oxygen dissolved in blood serum (PaO_2) ranges from 80 to 100 mmHg. Oxygen levels that indicate hypoxemia should be treated by administering oxygen. Mild hypoxemia ranges from 60 to 79 mmHg, moderate hypoxemia ranges from 40 to 59 mmHg, and severe hypoxemia is less than 40 mmHg (Pruitt & Jacobs, 2004).

TABLE 21–2 **Arterial Blood Gas Values**

pH	7.35–7.45
CO_2	35–45
O_2	80–100
HCO_3	22–26

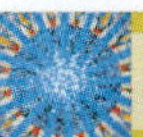

DEVELOPMENTAL CONSIDERATIONS Respiratory Development

INFANTS

- Respiratory rates are highest and most variable in newborns. The respiratory rate of a neonate is 40–80 breaths per minute.
- Infant respiratory rates average about 30 breaths per minute.
- Because of the structure of the ribcage infants rely almost exclusively on diaphragmatic movement for breathing. This is seen as abdominal breathing, as the abdomen rises and falls with each breath.

CHILDREN

- The respiratory rate gradually decreases, averaging around 25 breaths per minute in the preschooler and reaching the adult rate of 12–18 breaths per minute by late adolescence.
- During infancy and childhood, upper respiratory infections are common but usually not serious. Infants and preschoolers also are at risk for airway obstruction by foreign objects, such as coins and small toys. Cystic fibrosis, a chronic disease usually identified in early childhood, is a congenital disorder that affects the lungs, causing them to become congested with thick, tenacious (sticky) mucus. Asthma is another chronic disease often identified in childhood. The airways of the asthmatic child react to stimuli such as allergens, exercise, or cold air by constricting, becoming edematous, and producing excessive mucus. Airflow is impaired, and the child may wheeze as air moves through narrowed air passages.

OLDER ADULTS

- Older adults are at increased risk for acute respiratory diseases such as pneumonia and chronic diseases such as emphysema and chronic bronchitis. COPD may affect older adults, particularly after years of exposure to cigarette smoke or industrial pollutants.
- Pneumonia may not present with the usual symptom of a fever, but may present with atypical symptoms, such as confusion, weakness, loss of appetite, and increased heart rate and respiration.

Nursing interventions should be directed toward achieving optimal respiratory effort and gas exchange:

- Always encourage wellness and prevention of disease by reinforcing the need for good nutrition, exercise, and immunizations, such as for influenza and pneumonia.
- Increase fluid intake, if not contraindicated by other problems such as cardiac or renal impairment.
- Encourage proper positioning and frequent changing of position to allow for better lung expansion and air and fluid movement.
- Teach the client to use breathing techniques for better air exchange.
- Pace activities to conserve energy.
- Encourage the client to eat more frequent, smaller meals to decrease gastric distention, which can cause pressure on the diaphragm.
- Teach the client to avoid extreme hot or cold temperatures that will further tax the respiratory system.
- Teach actions and side effects of drugs, inhalers, and treatments.

The pH level is then assessed. The normal pH range is narrow, from 7.35 to 7.45; pH values less than 7.35 indicate acidosis and values greater than 7.45 indicate alkalosis.

Carbon dioxide values are assessed. Carbon dioxide is an acid expired from the lungs; changes in carbon dioxide are regulated by respiratory patterns. Carbon dioxide values range from 35 to 45 mmHg; values less than 35 mmHg indicate alkalosis and values greater than 45 mmHg indicate acidosis (Pruitt & Jacobs, 2004).

Bicarbonate is a base excreted via the kidneys; changes in bicarbonate are metabolic responses of the kidneys. Bicarbonate values range from 22 to 26 mEq/L. Values less than 22 mEq/L indicate acidosis and values greater than 26 mEq/L indicate alkalosis (Pruitt & Jacobs, 2004).

The body's natural inclination is to maintain a homeostatic balance. In relation to ABGs or acid–base, this means that the body will alter the carbon dioxide and bicarbonate levels to return the pH level to within normal range. Altering the individual components within acid–base balance is called *compensation*. A blood gas that has a pH greater than 7.45 indicates acidosis. If the same blood gas has a carbon dioxide greater than 45 mmHg, it indicates respiratory acidosis. The next value to be assessed is the bicarbonate level. If the value is in the normal range, the blood gas has not compensated. If the bicarbonate level is elevated, and the pH remains elevated the blood gas is partially compensated. A compensated blood gas will have carbon dioxide levels and bicarbonate levels that cause the pH to be in its normal range (Pruitt & Jacobs, 2004). A pH within normal range allows the body to achieve homeostasis.

Pulse oximetry is a noninvasive method of assessing arterial blood oxygenation. A clip or adhesive device with an infrared probe analyzes blood as it perfuses past the view of the two opposing sensors of the probe. Expected SaO_2 values in a healthy individual (one who has no alterations in pulmonary function) are greater than 95%.

Diagnosis of and differentiation of reactive airway diseases necessitates the use of **pulmonary function tests (PFTs)**. PFTs provide information about ventilation airflow, lung volume, and capacity and the diffusion of gas, and PFTs incorporate spirometry, peak flow meters, and the body plethysmograph. PFTs include measurement of inspired and expired air, as well as the diffusion ability of the alveolar-capillary membrane. A spirometer is used to measure airflow and lung volumes. **Incentive spirometry** measures the forced emptying of alveolar gas. Simply put, spirometry measures air exhaled from the lungs. Spirometry tests may be carried out in a primary care provider office or clinic. Levels for forced expiratory volume over 1 second (FEV1) and the ratio of forced vital volume over 1 second compared to forced expiratory volume (FEV1/FCV) are used to screen for pulmonary function deficits. Box 21–2 diagrams all the pulmonary function tests.

Peak expiratory flow rate (PEFR) is used to monitor the ability of an individual to exhale a specific volume of air related to the individual's age, gender, height, and weight.

Box 21–2 **Pulmonary Function Tests**

Pulmonary function tests (PFTs) are performed in a pulmonary function laboratory. After preparing the client, a nose clip is applied and the unsedated client breathes into a spirometer or body plethysmograph, a device for measuring and recording lung volume in liters versus time in seconds. The client is instructed how to breathe for specific tests: for example, to inhale as deeply as possible and then exhale to the maximal extent possible. Using measured lung volumes, respiratory capacities are calculated to assess pulmonary status. The specific values determined by PFT and illustrated in Figure 21–8 ■ include the following:

- *Total lung capacity (TLC)* is the total volume of the lungs at their maximum inflation. Four values are used to calculate TLC.
  a. *Total volume (TV)*, the volume inhaled and exhaled with normal quiet breathing (also called tidal volume)
  b. *Inspiratory reserve volume (IRV)*, the maximum amount that can be inhaled over and above a normal inspiration
  c. *Expiratory reserve volume (ERV)*, the maximum amount that can be exhaled following a normal exhalation
  d. *Residual volume (RV)*, the amount of air remaining in the lungs after maximal exhalation
- *Vital capacity (VC)* is the total amount of air that can be exhaled after a maximal inspiration. It is calculated by adding together the IRV, TV, and ERV.
- *Inspiratory capacity* is the total amount of air that can be inhaled following a normal quiet exhalation. It is calculated by adding the TV and IRV.
- *Functional residual capacity (FRC)* is the volume of air left in the lungs after a normal exhalation. The ERV and RV are added to determine the FRC.
- *Forced expiratory volume (FEV1)* is the amount of air that can be exhaled in 1 second.
- *Forced vital capacity (FVC)* is the amount of air that can be exhaled forcefully and rapidly after maximum air intake.
- *Minute volume (MV)* is the total amount or volume of air breathed in 1 minute.

In older clients, residual capacity is increased, and vital capacity is decreased. These age-related changes result from the following:

- Calcification of the costal cartilage and weakening of the intercostal muscles, which reduce movement of the chest wall
- Vertebral osteoporosis, which decreases spinal flexibility and increases the degree of kyphosis, further increasing the anterior-posterior diameter of the chest
- Diaphragmatic flattening and loss of elasticity.

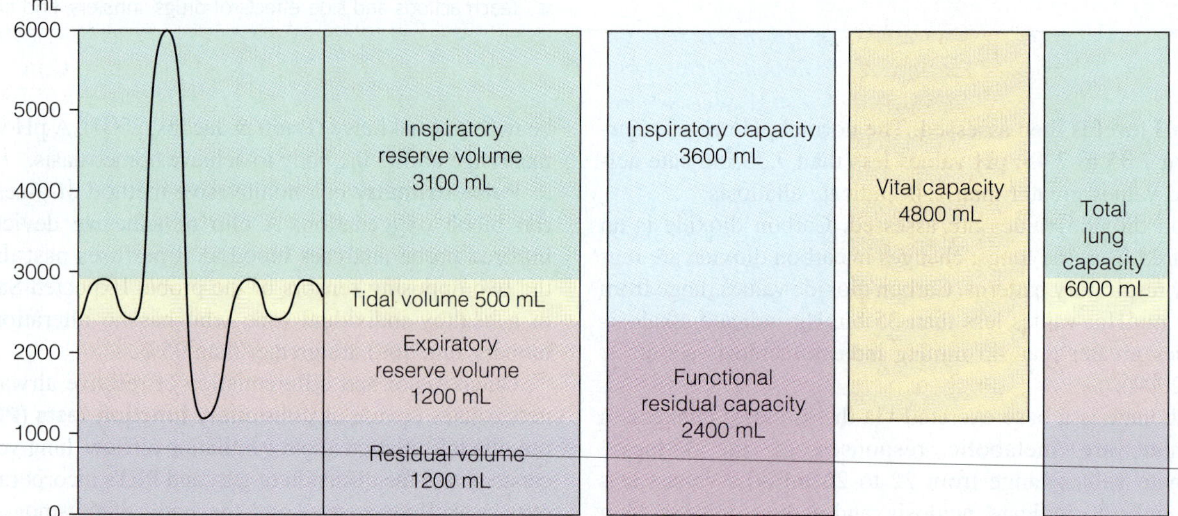

Figure 21–8 ■ The relationship of lung volumes and capacities. Volumes (mL) shown are for an average adult male.

PEFR allows individuals with asthma to monitor the reactivity of their lungs and adjust asthma treatments by the plan developed by the primary care provider and the individual. PEFR is not diagnostic for reactive airway diseases such as asthma and COPD.

Anterior-posterior **chest x-ray (CXR)** allows for two-dimensional visualization of the contents of the thoracic cavity. Thoracic computed tomography (CT) produces cross-sectional images of the contents of the chest. Thoracic CT may be used with dye to determine the presence of pulmonary embolism. Magnetic resonance imaging (MRI) allows for assessment of pulmonary embolism without the use of dye and is best for visualizing soft tissue and vascular structures. MRI is contraindicated in the individual who has implanted metal devices.

A pulmonary angiogram is used to identify structural changes in the pulmonary vasculature. Structural changes that cause occlusions may include blood clots, tumors, aneurysms, and overinflated alveoli. A pulmonary ventilation-perfusion scan (V-Q scan) uses radioactive isotopes to identify defects of ventilation and perfusion. Injected radioactive albumin helps identify defects of perfusion, whereas inhaled radioactive gas identifies defects of ventilation.

Bronchoscopy, a procedure that allows direct visualization of the lungs, is usually performed by a pulmonologist but may be performed by a primary care or emergency care physician. A bronchoscope is inserted orally into the trachea and advanced to the bronchi bifurcation. Biopsies, clearing of mucus plugs, and photographic identification of internal lung structures can be carried out. Sedation is necessary for client comfort.

Thoracentesis is both an intervention and a test. Thoracentesis is performed to drain excessive pleural fluid from between the pleural linings. The fluid drained is often analyzed for blood, fiber, and microbe content.

Chest x-rays reveal the presence of fluids, exudates, or masses within the thoracic cavity. CT and MRIs provide more information about the structures within the thoracic cavity. Pulmonary angiography and pulmonary V-Q scans demonstrate the ventilation and perfusion activities of the respiratory system. Individuals who respond poorly to bronchodilators may benefit from assessment of their pulmonary function. PFTs demonstrate changes in pulmonary health. Results outside the anticipated range for the individual's age, gender, height, and weight may indicate the need to alter care interventions. The respiratory therapist carries out PFTs. Bronchoscopy may be used for direct visualization of pulmonary structures, suctioning of mucus plugs from larger bronchials, and collection of lung tissue biopsy specimens.

PHARMACOLOGIC THERAPIES

Therapeutic management related to maintaining or attaining the health of the respiratory system focuses on the individual's ability to maintain a patent airway through the automatic protective mechanisms in the upper and lower respiratory tracts. The ability of the individual to maintain breathing patterns within the acceptable rates and quality for his or her particular age group is also assessed. Inspiration and expiration must provide adequate ventilation of the lung fields (Figure 21–9 ■). Individuals also must demonstrate an ease of breathing without the use of positioning or accessory muscles. Individuals demonstrate their respiratory patterns to define adequate gas exchange. A collaborative assessment with the health care team helps support the indication of excessive increases or decreases in oxygen or carbon dioxide levels.

An individual whose lung sounds indicate narrowing of the airways will benefit from a bronchodilator and possibly an anti-inflammatory agent to improve airway patency. The administration of bronchodilators, as ordered by the primary care provider relaxes the muscles around the airway, improving airflow. Common bronchodilators of short duration (short-acting beta-agonists, or SABAs) are levalbuterol (Xenopenex). Inflammation of the airways also contributes to impairment of oxygenation. The administration of corticosteroids (various adrenal cortex steroids, such as prednisone) in the presence of inflammation, as ordered by the primary care provider, aids in opening the air passageways by reducing the inflammation. Because oral steroids have a number of side effects, they are usually administered for a short period of time. Dosages are tapered, with the individual slowly decreasing the amount taken over the course of the prescription.

Individuals with chronic respiratory problems such as COPD and asthma usually benefit from use of a long-acting beta agonist (LABA) in combination with an inhaled corticosteroid (ICS). Commonly prescribed preparations include Symbicort and Advair. Because LABAs may be contraindicated in some individuals, inhaled corticosteroids are available without the addition of the LABA; common examples are Pulmocort and Asmanex.

Short-acting beta agonists and corticosteroids can be administered through a nebulizer. Nebulizers are machines that aerosolize a solution of medication so that it can be directly inhaled by the client by a mouthpiece or mask.

Anticholinergic medications relax the smooth muscles of the airways and decrease mucous secretions by blocking parasympathetic effect. The most commonly prescribed anticholinergic for impaired respiratory function is an ipatromium bromide inhaler (e.g., Atrovent). Inhaled anticholinergics are a good alternative for patients who cannot tolerate beta-agonists, and can be effective in relieving bronchospasm resulting from use of beta-blocker medications. Xanthines are another type of drug sometimes used to treat asthma, chronic bronchitis, and emphysema. Xanthines cause small airway dilation and increase heart rate and renal blood flow. Theophylline (Slo-Bid) is one of the more generic names used for this type of medication. Because of the narrow therapeutic range of this type of medication and the potential for serious side effects, patients taking xanthines should have periodic blood tests to ensure they are maintaining optimal therapeutic levels and to guard against risk of toxicity.

Additional medications may be prescribed. These can vary depending on the nature of the respiratory impairment. Allergic asthmatic individuals, for example, may take immunotherapy (allergy shots) or other medications for allergies to prevent attacks.

Medication compliance in individuals with chronic or recurrent respiratory impairment is critical. Some medications used for treating respiratory diseases are fairly expensive. Although albuterol and corticosteroids are reasonably inexpensive, LABAs usually are more expensive and are associated with higher insurance copayments. For individuals who require multiple prescription medications to maintain respiratory health, the combined costs of these medications may be overwhelming. Most pharmaceutical companies have programs to assist clients who lack health insurance or whose standard of living is at or close to the poverty level. Most free clinics are able to provide free medication to qualifying individuals. Usually, individuals are not required to see the doctor at the free clinic to receive free medication; a prescription from the treating physician is sufficient.

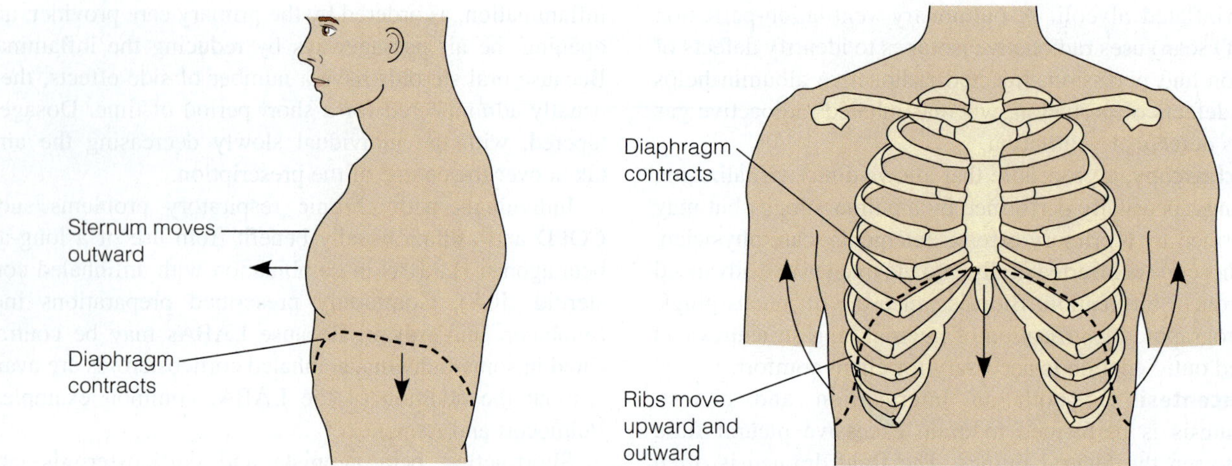

Figure 21–9 ■ Respiratory inspiration: Lateral and anterior views. Note the volume expansion of the thorax as the diaphragm flattens.

Teenagers often do not take medications as prescribed, either because they are embarrassed to be seen taking medication or because their hectic schedules do not make it possible for them to be home at certain times to take medication. Additional client teaching may be necessary when working with teenagers.

Older adults may be at risk for accidental noncompliance with medication administration schedules. A nurse working with an older adult exhibiting signs of confusion or early dementia should consult with the client or family members to determine whether additional support is available regarding medication administration.

CLINICAL THERAPIES

Encouraging Smoking Cessation

Individuals are assessed for tobacco use. Tobacco smoke exposure causes increased mucus production and reduced cilia action within the airway passages. Individuals who smoke present with a chronic cough and sputum production in the early years of tobacco use. Prolonged exposure to tobacco smoke yields a decline in pulmonary function. Because the capacity of the respiratory system to compensate is great, the sense of pulmonary decline occurs well after irreversible damage has occurred. All health care providers should encourage smoking cessation and advise nonsmoking individuals to avoid secondary smoke.

Cessation of smoking and use of spit tobacco contributes to an individual's overall health. Individuals who would like to quit should be offered nicotine replacement therapies, as ordered by the primary care provider. Table 21–3 lists strategies to decrease tobacco use. Reducing secondhand exposure of children to tobacco smoke within their homes and decreasing the exposure to secondhand smoke in public buildings will diminish the detrimental effects of tobacco for nonsmoking individuals.

Secretion Clearance

Lung sounds that indicate the presence of fluids or exudates necessitate encouragement of deep breaths and coughing to clear pulmonary secretions. Suction is needed to clear secretions in individuals unable to clear their own secretions. Individuals who are producing sputum with a cough may require the collection of a sputum specimen. They may benefit from postural drainage to clear secretions from various lung fields. (See Companion Skills Manual text for these skills.)

Oxygen Administration

Decreases in oxygen saturation in arterial blood indicate a need for supplemental oxygen. A variety of devices can be used to administer oxygen to an individual. The selection of a device depends on the amount of oxygen needed to relieve hypoxemia. Noninvasive devices require patent airways to be effective.

The most common and comfortable device is the nasal cannula (Figure 21–10 ■). The nasal cannula delivers flow rates from 2 to 6 L/min that administers 24–44% fraction of inspired oxygen (FiO_2). An Oxymizer also entrails air through the nasal passage, but it has an added reservoir for oxygen (Figure 21–11 ■). This additional reservoir increases the amount of oxygen inhaled with each breath. A Vapotherm delivers oxygen via a nasal cannula, but it warms and filters oxygen and increases the positive end expiratory pressure of oxygen delivery via the cannula (Figure 21–12 ■). A simple mask covers the mouth and nose. It is fitted to the individual's face size. The mask itself provides an additional gas reservoir to that provided by the nasopharynx alone (Figure 21–13 ■). Flow rates may be set from 5 to 10 L/min. The FiO_2 delivered is from 30 to 50%. To attain FiO_2 levels of 60% or more, masks that have an attached reservoir are necessary

TABLE 21–3 **Interventions for Tobacco Cessation**

ASK	ADVISE	ASSESS	ASSIST	ARRANGE
Identify and document tobacco use status for every individual at every health care interaction.	Urge every tobacco user to quit in a clear, strong, and personalized manner.	Determine if the tobacco user is willing to attempt to quit tobacco use at this time.	Request tobacco cessation medication order from primary care provider. Provide resources for counseling and support groups for the individual willing to attempt to quit tobacco use.	Establish a plan for follow-up contact for the individual willing to attempt to quit tobacco use within one week of quit date. Continue to ask tobacco users about quitting tobacco use at each visit.
Nurses document tobacco use with admission history and physical assessment.	Nurses provide tobacco cessation publications and teach about physiologic consequences of tobacco use with daily care interactions such as taking vital signs.	Nurses ask if individuals have attempted quitting tobacco before, what was effective, what did not work, and encourage trying with present visit.	Nurses seek nicotine replacement during hospitalizations and encourage individuals who have had nicotine replacement during hospitalization that they are on their way to quitting.	Nurses collaborate with individuals who desire to quit to arrange tobacco cessation support group contacts and request in-hospital tobacco cessation teaching.

Source: Adapted from the Tobacco Cessation Clinical Practice Guidelines as established by the U.S. Department of Health and Human Services. Used with permission.

to provide adequate oxygen. The nonrebreather mask has a one-way valve between the attached reservoir and the face mask (Figure 21–14 ■). This ensures that appropriate levels of oxygen are inhaled, with no carbon dioxide from exhaled gases. Oxygen delivery at a specified flow rate requires the use of a venturi mask (Figure 21–15 ■). Venturi masks are set with a specific oxygen flow rate and specific jet adaptor device. Flow rates of 24–40% may be set with the venturi mask. Table 21–4 summarizes the types of oxygen devices, along with flow rates and oxygen delivery amounts.

Nursing care for the client receiving supplemental oxygen includes ensuring that flow is sufficient as required, that the client is reasonably comfortable with the manner of oxygen administration, and that indwelling catheters (lines) remain clear. For the client being discharged to home with supplemental oxygen, both the nurse and the respiratory therapist delivering the oxygen to the home must teach the client how to use the devices properly, the importance of checking oxygen levels in tanks, the need for a portable device for trips outside of the house, and the need to maintain the lines and keep them clear of obstruction.

Clients prescribed supplemental oxygen for the first time may feel as though they have lost their quality of life. The nurse can assist the client in understanding that supplemental oxygen will help him or her maintain quality of life, and that the client can still participate in any number of activities. The nurse should be alert to any possible signs of depression in a client whose oxygen impairment is sufficient to warrant supplemental oxygen. Frustration, rising medical costs, and other issues can contribute to depression in a client with respiratory impairment.

Thoracic Catheter

A chest tube, or thoracic catheter, is used to treat conditions in which fluid enters the pleural cavity, causing lung collapse. Inserted under emergency conditions, and treated as a surgical procedure, a chest tube will typically remain in place for 2–5 days, until the client's x-rays indicate that all fluid from the pleural cavity has been removed.

There are many nursing considerations in working with a client who has a thoracic catheter, some of which will be specific to the underlying cause of the lung collapse. Typically, however, the nurse will need to do the following:

- Ensure oxygen therapy is immediately available at all times, if not already ordered and in place.
- Monitor dressings for drainage and air leakage; follow agency protocol for replacing or securing dressings.
- Monitor tubing to make sure it is free of kinks or other impediments.
- Monitor and record client vital signs as ordered.
- Monitor for and report any decrease in oxygen saturation, any changes in breath sounds, or any tympany or hollow sound with chest percussion.
- Assess for pain; administer pain medications as needed (PRN), notifying physician of any increase in client restlessness or anxiety.
- Monitor and report any changes in respiration or any excessive bleeding.

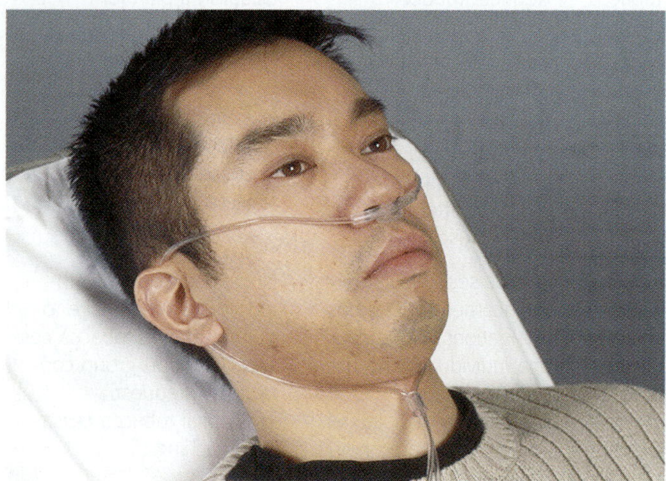

Figure 21–10 ■ A nasal cannula.

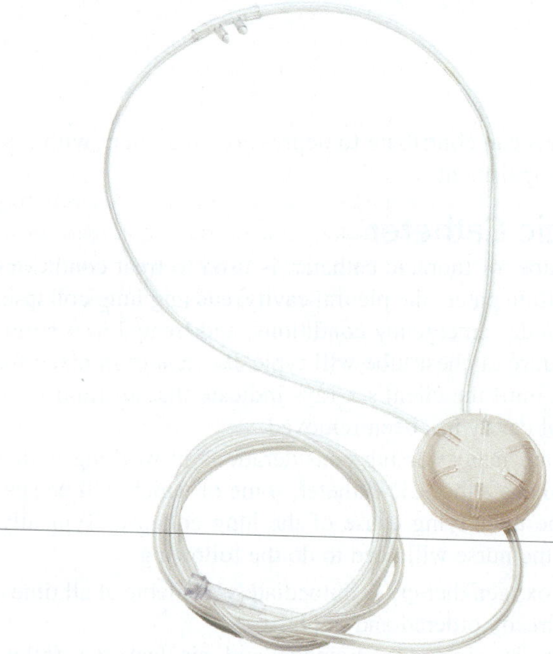

Figure 21–11 ■ Oxymizer.

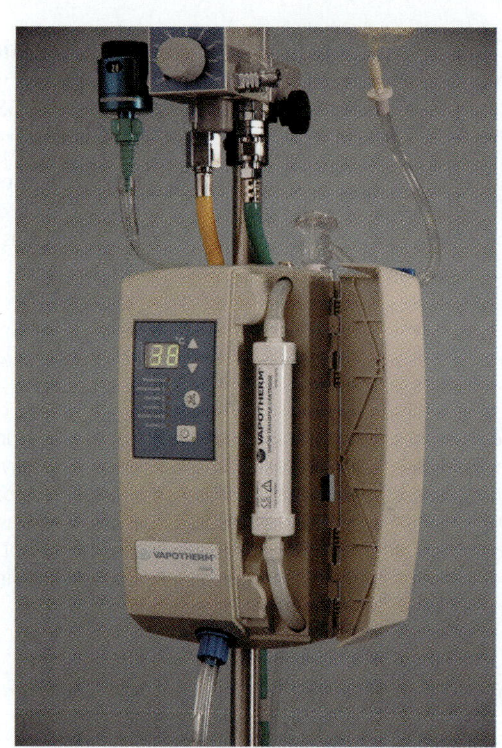

Figure 21–12 ■ Vapotherm.

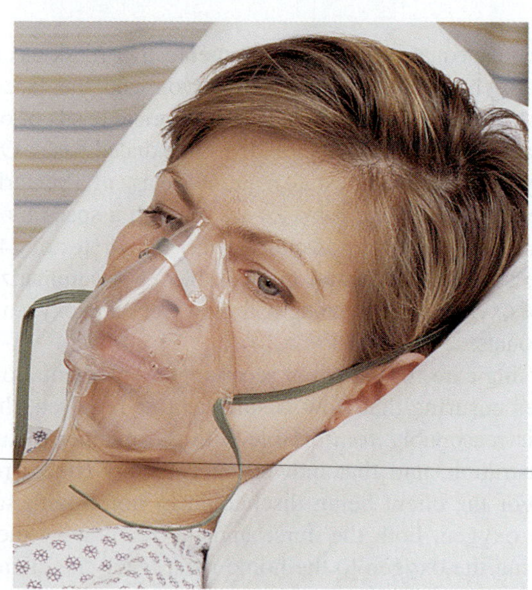

Figure 21–13 ■ A simple face mask.

Photographer: Jenny Thomas

Monitoring Activity Tolerance

Alterations in the respiratory system can affect an individual's activity levels. An individual may have insufficient physiologic or psychologic energy to endure or complete required or desired daily activities. For the individual with poor oxygenation, fatigue or weakness can occur from scheduling too many activities too close together. Dyspnea or shortness of breath occurs at varying points in the exercise program, depending on the individual's endurance level. Periods of activity should be spaced with periods of rest if the individual is unable to carry out many consecutive activities. A physical therapist will develop an exercise program to improve musculoskeletal function and endurance.

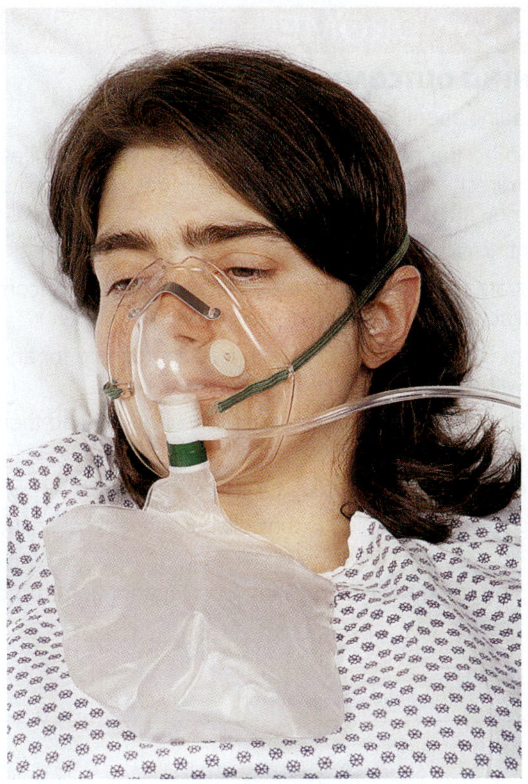

Figure 21–14 ■ A nonrebreather mask.
Photographer: Elena Dorfman

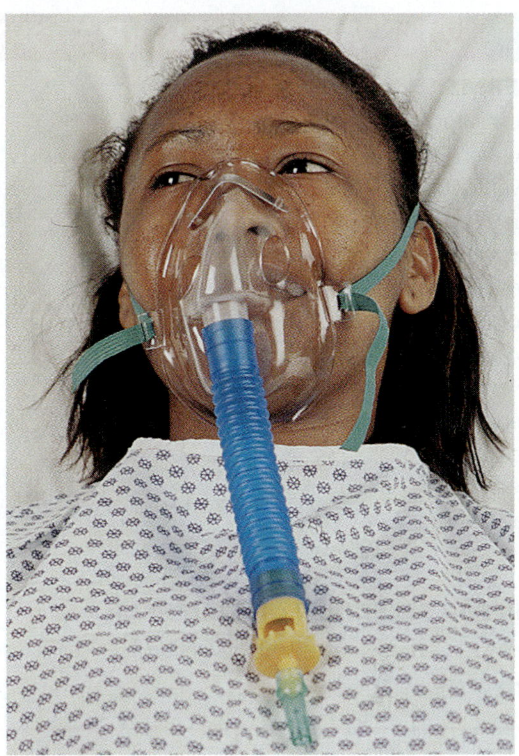

Figure 21–15 ■ A Venturi mask.
Photographer: Jenny Thomas

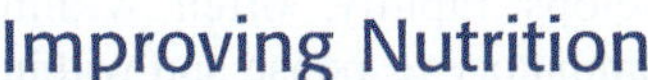

Improving Nutrition

Individuals with respiratory alterations often need an increased calorie intake but lack the endurance to consume adequate nutrition. A nutritionist is able to aid the individual in choosing foods and supplements to meet daily caloric and nutritional needs. A nutritionist can guide the individual in developing menus of frequent, small, nutritious meals.

Assisting With Activities of Daily Living

Individuals who are too weak to provide their own care may need assistance in activities of daily living (ADLs). An individual with compromised oxygenation may have very poor endurance for activities. Personal care must be provided for individuals too weak or too fatigued to carry out their own ADLs. The family and the health care team must collaborate to provide sufficient support to the individual with compromised oxygenation, while encouraging the individual to do as much as possible to maintain appropriate physical strength and prevent deteriorating mental condition.

TABLE 21–4 **Oxygen Delivery Systems**

DEVICE	FLOW RATE SETTING	OXYGEN CONCENTRATION (FIO_2)
Nasal cannula	1–6 L/min	24–44%
Oxymizer	1–6 L/min	24–88%
Vapotherm	1–40 L/min	24–100%
Face mask	5–10 L/min	30–50%
Nonrebreather	10–15 L/min	Greater than 60%
Venturi mask	Set with jet adaptor for flow rate and FiO_2	

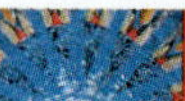

21.1 ACUTE RESPIRATORY DISTRESS SYNDROME

KEY TERMS

Acute respiratory distress syndrome (ARDS), *1234*
Barotrauma, *1241*
Bilevel ventilator (BiPAP), *1241*
Continuous positive airway pressure (CPAP), *1239*
Negative pressure ventilator, *1238*
Noninvasive ventilation (NIV), *1239*
Pneumomediastinum, *1242*
Pneumopericardium, *1242*
Positive end-expiratory pressure (PEEP), *1241*
Positive-pressure ventilators, *1238*
Refractory hypoxemia, *1234*
Suctioning, *1245*
Terminal weaning, *1242*
Weaning, *1242*

BASIS FOR SELECTION OF EXEMPLAR

Centers for Disease Control and Prevention
Institute of Medicine

LEARNING OUTCOMES

After reading about this exemplar, you will be able to:

1. Describe the pathophysiology, etiology, clinical manifestations, and direct and indirect causes of acute respiratory distress syndrome (ARDS).
2. Identify risk factors associated with ARDS.
3. Illustrate the nursing process in providing culturally competent care across the life span for individuals with ARDS.
4. Formulate priority nursing diagnoses appropriate for an individual with ARDS.
5. Create a plan of care for individuals with ARDS and their family members.
6. Assess expected outcomes for an individual with ARDS.
7. Discuss therapies used in the collaborative care of an individual with ARDS.
8. Employ evidence-based caring interventions for an individual with ARDS.

OVERVIEW

Acute respiratory distress syndrome (ARDS) is a disorder with rapid onset characterized by noncardiac pulmonary edema and progressive **refractory hypoxemia** (the decrease of particle arterial oxygen despite administration of oxygen at high flow rates). First identified in 1967, ARDS has been known by various names, including shock lung and adult hyaline membrane disease. It is widely recognized as a severe form of acute respiratory failure. The mortality rate associated with acute respiratory distress syndrome, while declining, remains around 30–40% (American Lung Association, 2006).

Extensive lung tissue inflammation and small blood vessel injury occur, with malfunction of other organs following. The onset of ARDS is rapid, with an arterial blood gas (ABG) showing respiratory failure. The initial admitting diagnoses of individuals who develop ARDS are varied, with most individuals presenting to the hospital with another critical event and being admitted to intensive care. Both direct and indirect injuries to the body can result in ARDS. Table 21–5 features some of the conditions commonly associated with the development of ARDS.

PATHOPHYSIOLOGY AND ETIOLOGY

The underlying pathology in ARDS is acute lung injury resulting from an unregulated systemic inflammatory response to acute injury or inflammation. Inflammatory cellular responses and biochemical mediators damage the alveolar-capillary membrane. This damage develops rapidly, often within 90 minutes of the systemic inflammatory response and within 24 hours of the initial insult.

Damaged capillary membranes allow plasma and blood cells to escape into the interstitial space. Increased interstitial pressure and damage to the alveolar membrane allow fluid to enter the alveoli. Within the alveolus, the fluid dilutes and inactivates surfactant. The inflammatory process damages surfactant-producing cells, leading to a deficit of surfactant, increased alveolar surface tension, and alveolar collapse with atelectasis. The lungs become less compliant, and gas exchange is impaired. As the syndrome progresses, hyaline membranes form, further reducing gas exchange and compliance. Finally, fibrotic changes occur in the lungs. Intra-alveolar septa thicken, and alveolar surface area for gas exchange is reduced. Hypoxemia becomes refractory or resistant to improvement with supplemental oxygen, and the $PaCO_2$ rises as diffusion is further impaired.

Figures 21–16 ■ and 21–17 ■ illustrate the pathogenesis and pathophysiology of ARDS. As ARDS progresses, tissue hypoxia becomes significant, and metabolic acidosis develops. Carbon dioxide exchange is impaired, as is oxygen exchange, leading to combined respiratory and metabolic acidosis. Sepsis and multiple organ system dysfunction of the kidneys, liver, gastrointestinal tract, central nervous system, and cardiovascular system are the leading causes of death in ARDS. If the process is halted before sepsis or organ system dysfunction occurs, the long-term prognosis for recovery is good.

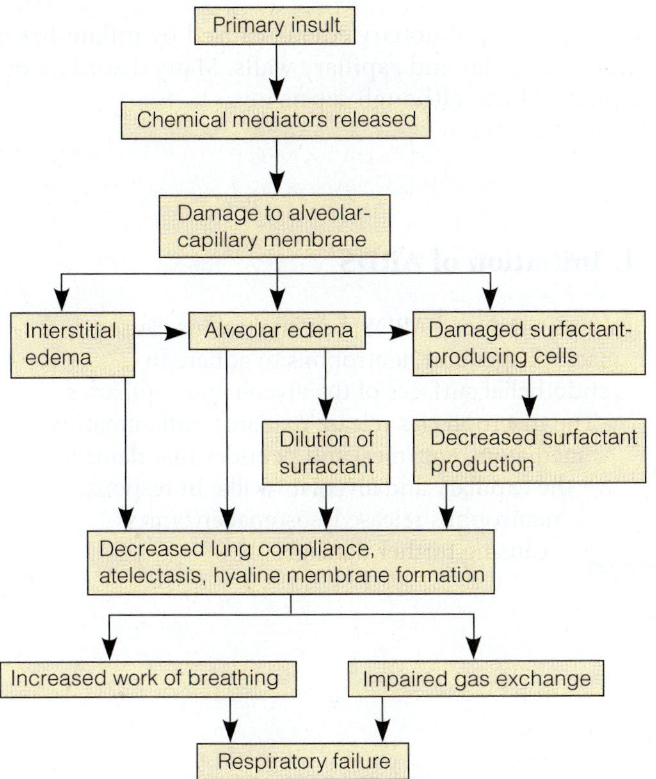

Figure 21–16 ■ Pathogenesis of acute respiratory distress syndrome.

Etiology

Approximately 190,000 Americans are affected by ARDS each year. ARDS affects all ages (American Lung Association, 2008; National Heart, Lung, and Blood Institute [NHLBI], 2007). The mortality rate ranges from 25 to 45%. Men and African Americans have a greater risk of dying of ARDS compared to women and people from other races. Clients who develop ARDS from sepsis have poorer outcomes than those who develop ARDS from pulmonary infections or trauma. Clients who develop ARDS as a complication of an acute lung injury or condition are more likely to recover fully compared to clients with chronic conditions (NHLBI, 2006).

Risk Factors

Direct and indirect insults to the lungs may result in ARDS. Pulmonary infections are a direct insult to lung tissue. Aspiration of gastric contents and inhalation injuries, such as smoke inhalation and saltwater inhalation from near-drowning in saltwater, can result in ARDS. Pulmonary contusions, fat embolism, and reperfusion pulmonary edema can cause ARDS. Indirect insults, including overall body sepsis, trauma, and gastrointestinal infections such as pancreatitis, also may result in ARDS. Drug overdoses, especially with tricyclic antidepressants, are associated with ARDS. Multiple blood transfusions have caused the development of ARDS, as has cardiopulmonary bypass. Sepsis is the most common cause of ARDS. Mortality is highest in those individuals who are older than 70 years, who are immunocompromised, and who have chronic liver failure. Increased incidence is seen in people who smoke.

CLINICAL MANIFESTATIONS

Initial manifestations of ARDS typically develop 24–48 hours after the initial insult. Dyspnea and tachypnea are early manifestations. Laboratory findings are consistent with the presenting illness. ABG values may be within the normal range. Chest x-ray (CXR) will often be clear of infiltrates, with the exception of direct pulmonary illness. Baseline laboratory data as well as diagnostic tests aid in identifying the change in pulmonary status.

Progressive respiratory distress develops, with increasing respiratory rate, intercostal retractions, and use of accessory muscles of respiration. Tachycardia occurs as the demands for oxygen to the cells of the body decrease. CXR will show interstitial changes with patchy infiltrates. Pulse oximetry and ABG levels may demonstrate hypoxemia refractory to oxygen administration. Cyanosis develops that may not improve with oxygen administration. Breath sounds are initially clear, but crackles (rales) and rhonchi develop later. As respiratory failure progresses, mental status changes, such as agitation, confusion, and lethargy, occur.

TABLE 21–5 Conditions Associated With Development of Acute Respiratory Distress Syndrome

CONDITIONS	EXAMPLES
Shock	Hemorrhagic shock, septic shock
Inhalation injuries	Aspiration of gastric contents, smoke and toxic gases, near-drowning, oxygen toxicity
Infections	Gram-negative sepsis, viral pneumonias, *Pneumocystis carinii* pneumonia, miliary tuberculosis
Drug overdose	Heroin, methadone, propoxyphene, aspirin
Trauma	Burns, head injury, lung contusion, fat emboli
Other	Disseminated intravascular coagulation, pancreatitis, uremia, amniotic fluid and air emboli, multiple transfusions, open heart surgery with cardiopulmonary bypass

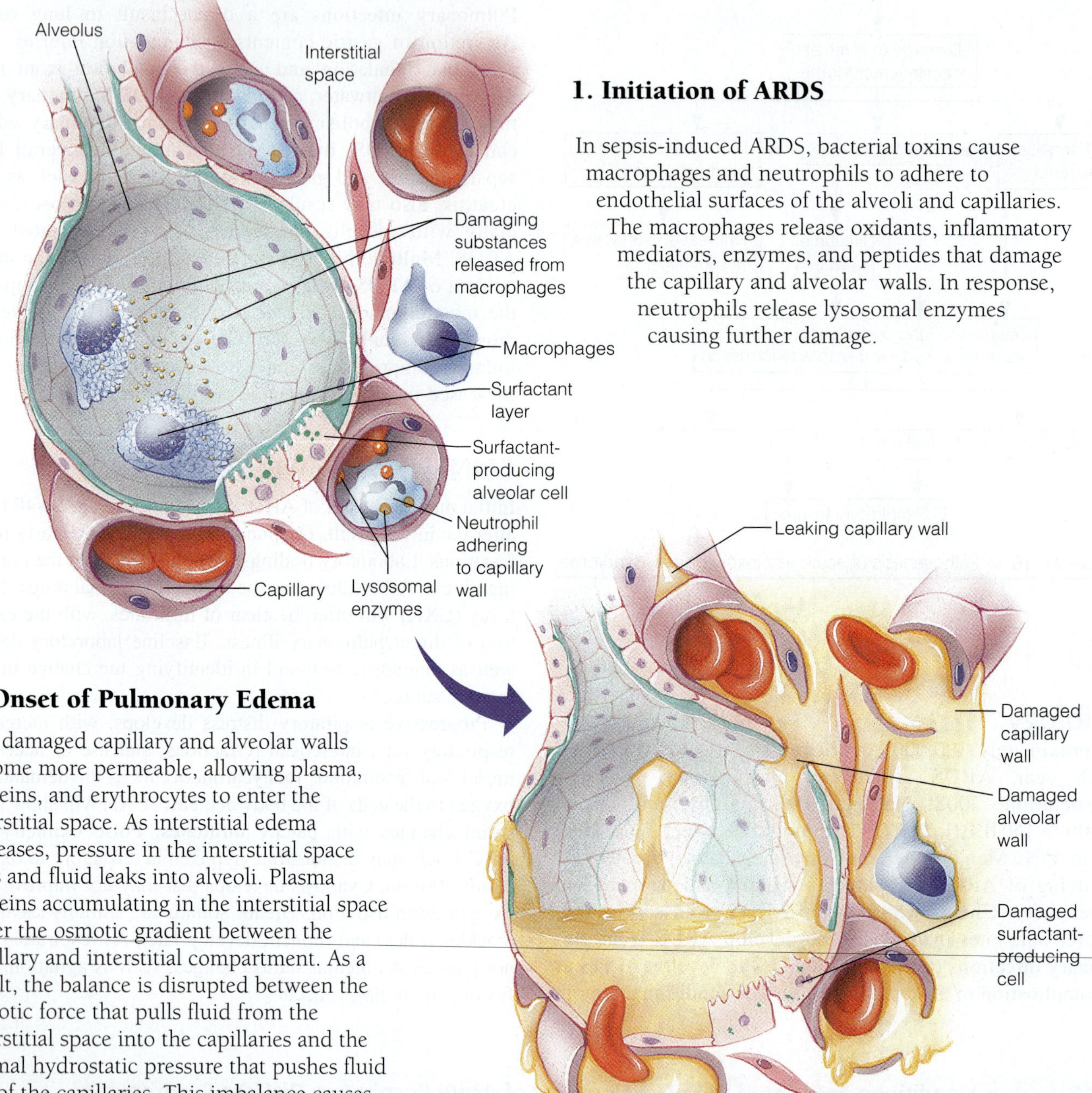

Acute respiratory distress syndrome (ARDS) is a severe form of acute respiratory failure that occurs in response to pulmonary or systemic insults. ARDS is characterized by noncardiogenic pulmonary edema caused by inflammatory damage to alveolar and capillary walls. Many disorders may precipitate ARDS, although sepsis is the most common.
Alveolus
Interstitial space
Damaging substances released from macrophages
Macrophages
Surfactant layer
Surfactant-producing alveolar cell
Neutrophil adhering to capillary wall
Lysosomal enzymes
Capillary
1. Initiation of ARDS
In sepsis-induced ARDS, bacterial toxins cause macrophages and neutrophils to adhere to endothelial surfaces of the alveoli and capillaries. The macrophages release oxidants, inflammatory mediators, enzymes, and peptides that damage the capillary and alveolar walls. In response, neutrophils release lysosomal enzymes causing further damage.
Leaking capillary wall
2. Onset of Pulmonary Edema
The damaged capillary and alveolar walls become more permeable, allowing plasma, proteins, and erythrocytes to enter the interstitial space. As interstitial edema increases, pressure in the interstitial space rises and fluid leaks into alveoli. Plasma proteins accumulating in the interstitial space lower the osmotic gradient between the capillary and interstitial compartment. As a result, the balance is disrupted between the osmotic force that pulls fluid from the interstitial space into the capillaries and the normal hydrostatic pressure that pushes fluid out of the capillaries. This imbalance causes even more fluid to enter alveoli.
Damaged capillary wall
Damaged alveolar wall
Damaged surfactant-producing cell

Figure 21–17 ■ Pathophysiology of acute respiratory distress syndrome.

4. End-Stage ARDS

Fibrin and cell debris from necrotic cells combine to form hyaline membranes, which line the interior of the alveoli and further reduce alveolar compliance and gas exchange. Because CO_2 cannot diffuse across hyaline membranes, $PaCO_2$ levels now begin to rise while PaO_2 levels continue to fall. Rising $PaCO_2$ levels can lead to respiratory acidosis. Without respiratory support, respiratory failure will develop. Even with aggressive treatment, almost 50% of clients with ARDS die.

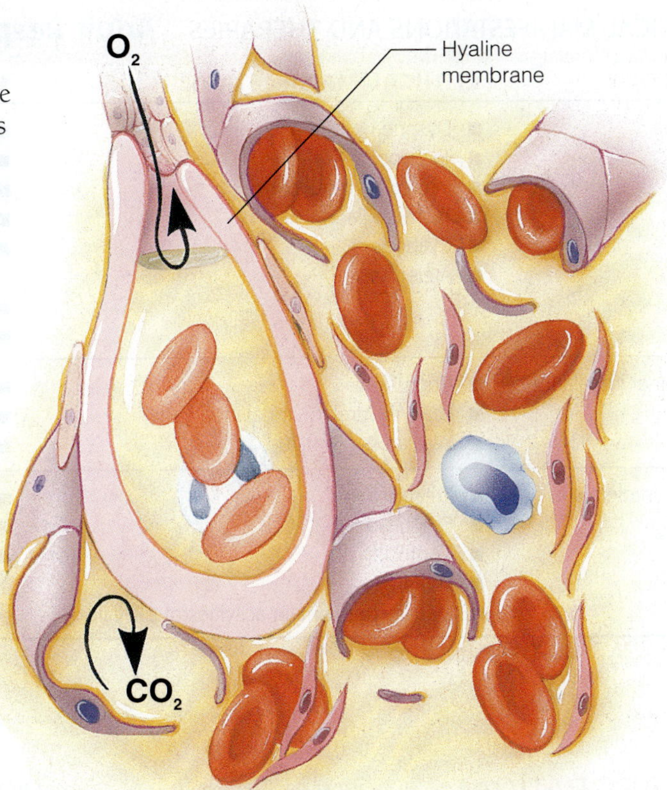

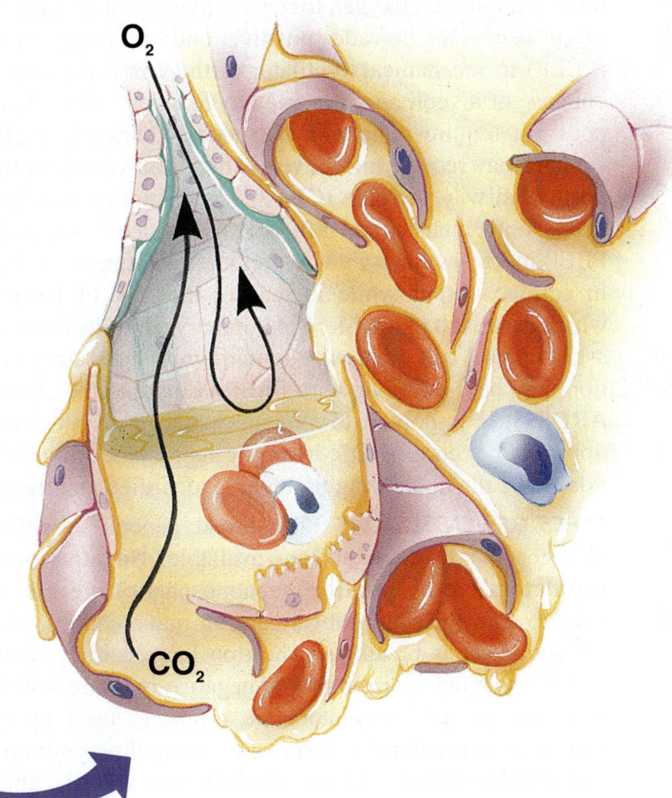

3. Alveolar Collapse

Protein-rich fluid accumulates in the alveoli, inactivating surfactant and damaging type II alveolar cells that produce surfactant. (Surfactant is important in maintaining alveolar compliance—the ability of tissue to stretch or distend.) As active surfactant is lost, the alveoli stiffen and collapse, leading to atelectasis, which increases breathing effort.

Decreased alveolar compliance, atelectasis, and fluid-filled alveoli interfere with gas exchange across the alveolar-capillary membrane. Blood oxygen (PaO_2) levels fall. Because carbon dioxide diffuses more readily than oxygen, however, blood carbon dioxide ($PaCO_2$) levels also fall initially as tachypnea causes more CO_2 to be expired.

CLINICAL MANIFESTATIONS AND THERAPIES Adult Respiratory Distress Syndrome

ETIOLOGY	CLINICAL MANIFESTATION	CLINICAL THERAPIES
Hypoxia	■ Dyspnea ■ Tachypnea ■ Intercostal retractions ■ Tachycardia ■ Cyanosis ■ Atelectasis	■ Bronchodilators, beta-agonists, corticosteroids ■ Oxygen administration ■ Monitor pulmonary artery pressures and cardiac output ■ Mechanical ventilation ■ Continuous positive airway pressure (CPAP), bilevel ventilator (BiPAP), or positive end-expiratory pressure (PEEP) as necessary ■ Prone positioning ■ Surfactant therapy
Nutritional imbalance	■ Confusion ■ Fluid/electrolyte imbalance ■ Weakness or fatigue	■ Fluid replacement ■ Total parenteral/enteral nutrition or enteral feedings ■ Nutritional analysis
Activity intolerance	■ Irritability ■ Fatigue ■ Confusion ■ Lethargy ■ Inability to maintain activities of daily living	■ Care may need to be split to prevent overtaxing the client ■ Assess level of consciousness as indicated ■ Severe activity intolerance resulting in significant hypoxia may require administration of paralytics and sedation to reduce oxygen demands

COLLABORATION

Clients with ARDS are seriously ill and require contributions from many members of the health care team. In addition to nurses, respiratory therapists, dieticians, physical therapists, and physicians may all play a significant role in the provision of health care services to the client. The role of the nurse is to constantly monitor the client's condition, respond to subtle cues indicating a change, and react appropriately. Focus of nursing care is discussed in more detail in the nursing process.

Pharmacologic Therapy

Although no definitive drug therapy currently exists for ARDS, a number of medications may be used. Inhaled nitric oxide reduces intrapulmonary shunting and improves oxygenation by dilating blood vessels in better-ventilated areas of the lungs. Surfactant therapy may be prescribed.

Interventions to block the inflammatory response, such as using nonsteroidal anti-inflammatory agents and corticosteroids, are under investigation. Corticosteroids may be used late in the course of ARDS to improve oxygenation and lung mechanics when fibrotic changes occur.

Mechanical Ventilation

The mainstay of ARDS management is endotracheal intubation and mechanical ventilation. With ARDS, it is rarely possible to maintain adequate tissue oxygenation with oxygen therapy alone.

With mechanical ventilation, the FIO_2 (fraction of inspired oxygen—the percentage of oxygen administered) is set at the lowest possible level to maintain a PaO_2 higher than 60 mmHg and oxygen saturation of approximately 90%. When the PaO_2 cannot be maintained with less than 50% inspired oxygen, there is a risk that oxygen toxicity will accentuate ARDS. It is often necessary to add positive end-expiratory pressure (PEEP) to mechanical ventilator settings in order to prevent collapse of alveoli and promote oxygenation. The client who does not require intubation but needs additional respiratory support may receive bilevel ventilation (BiPAP) or continuous positive airway pressure (CPAP). Maintaining open airways and alveoli enhances gas diffusion and reduces V-Q mismatch. PEEP increases intrathoracic pressure resulting in a decrease in cardiac output while increasing the risk of barotrauma which can result in long-term pulmonary complications. Either assist-control or synchronized intermittent mandatory ventilation may be used along with PEEP in treating the client with ARDS. It is important to remember that mechanical ventilation does not cure ARDS; it simply supports respiratory function while the underlying problem is identified and treated.

TYPES OF VENTILATORS Two broad, general classifications of mechanical ventilators are available. **Negative-pressure ventilators** create negative (subatmospheric) pressure externally to draw the chest outward and air into the lungs, mimicking spontaneous breathing. The iron lung, cuirass ventilator, and PulmoWrap are examples of negative-pressure ventilators. Negative-pressure ventilators are primarily used by clients with neuromuscular disorders (e.g., postpolio syndrome and amyotrophic lateral sclerosis) that interfere with the ability to maintain adequate ventilation. They also may be used by clients who primarily require ventilator support during sleep.

Positive-pressure ventilators are used more often than negative-pressure ones, especially in treating clients with acute respiratory failure (Figure 21–18 ■). These ventilators push air into the lungs rather than drawing it in like negative-pressure

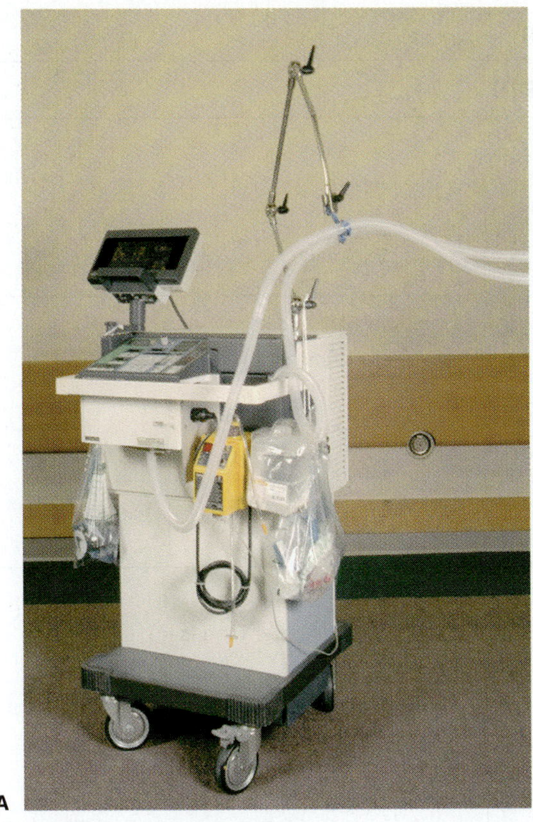

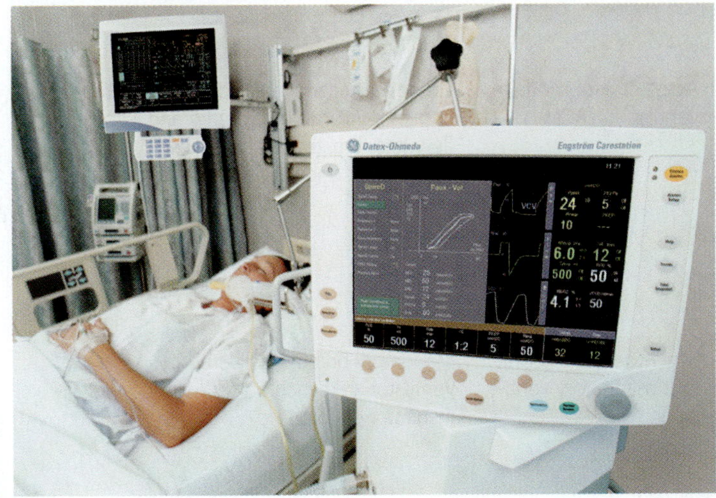

Figure 21–18 ■ Positive-pressure ventilators. *A*, Positive pressure ventilator. *B*, The control panel used to set the mode, rate, limits, and percentage of oxygen delivered.

ventilators. The amount of air delivered with each breath can be delivered in mL (volume ventilator) or until a specific pressure is reached (pressure ventilators). Either invasive ventilation using an endotracheal tube or tracheostomy or noninvasive positive-pressure ventilation may be used. Increasingly, noninvasive techniques, which use a nasal or face mask, nasal plugs, or an oral mouthpiece, are being used (Fenstermacher & Hong, 2004).

Noninvasive ventilation (NIV) provides ventilator support using a tight-fitting face mask, thus avoiding intubation. Its primary use is to support clients with obstructive sleep apnea, neuromuscular disease, or impending respiratory failure (e.g., advanced COPD). NIV also may be used for clients in respiratory failure who refuse intubation. The degree of success varies, primarily limited by client intolerance as a result of the physical and psychologic discomfort of wearing a mask when dyspneic (Kasper et al., 2005). NIV tends to be more successful in clients without significant underlying lung disease (e.g., respiratory failure related to neuromuscular disease).

Several variables are used to trigger, cycle, and limit airflow with positive-pressure ventilators. The trigger prompts the ventilator to deliver a breath. The client's inspiratory effort triggers ventilator-assisted breaths. Ventilator-controlled breaths usually are triggered by a preset time interval (e.g., a breath is delivered every 5 sec for a rate of 12 breaths/minute). The ventilator cycle, or duration of inspiration, can be limited by volume, pressure, flow, or time. Volume-cycled ventilators deliver air until a preset volume is delivered. Pressure-cycled ventilators cycle off when a preset pressure is achieved within the airways. Flow-cycled ventilators are cycled by a preset inspiratory flow rate, and time-cycled ventilatorsdeliver air for a set time interval. Airflow delivered by the ventilator also can be limited by factors such as airway pressure (e.g., a volume-cycled ventilator can be set to immediately stop inspiratory flow if airway pressure exceeds a preset value).

MODES OF VENTILATION A number of different modes or patterns of ventilation may be used with positive-pressure ventilators. The mode determines whether a breath is initiated by the client or the ventilator and the pattern of airway support provided by the ventilator. CPAP, bilevel airway pressure support, assist-control mode ventilation, synchronized intermittent mandatory ventilation, PEEP, pressure-support ventilation, and pressure-control ventilation are common modes of ventilation in use today (Table 21–6).

Continuous Positive Airway Pressure **Continuous positive airway pressure (CPAP)** applies positive pressure to the airways of a client who is breathing spontaneously. CPAP may be used with either endotracheal intubation or a tight-fitting face mask. All breathing is spontaneous (client triggered) and pressure controlled. CPAP is used to help maintain open airways and alveoli, decreasing the work of breathing.

TABLE 21–6 Modes of Positive-Pressure Ventilator Operation

MODE	DESCRIPTION	PATTERN
Spontaneous breathing	Client has full control of rate, tidal volume, pressures.	
Assist-control mode ventilation (ACMV)	Client can trigger ventilator to deliver breaths at preset volume or pressure and inspiratory flow rate; breaths will be delivered at preset rate if client does not initiate.	
Synchronized intermittent mandatory ventilation (SIMV)	Mandatory breaths delivered by ventilator are synchronized with client's inspiratory effort.	
Continuous positive airway pressure (CPAP)	Positive pressure is maintained in airways; all breaths are spontaneous.	
Positive end-expiratory pressure (PEEP)	Used in conjunction with other ventilator modes; positive airway pressure is maintained throughout respiratory cycle.	
Pressure support ventilation (PSV)	Pressurized inspiratory flow supports the client's inspiratory effort, decreasing the work of breathing.	

Bilevel Ventilators A **bilevel ventilator (BiPAP)** provides inspiratory positive airway pressure as well as airway support during expiration. Bilevel ventilation is primarily used at night with a tight-fitting mask (nasal, facial, or oral). Three modes of ventilation can be used with BiPAP: (1) spontaneous breathing (S); (2) timed mode (T), in which pressure-supported breaths are delivered at a predetermined rate; and (3) spontaneous/timed (S/T), in which the ventilator switches to timed mode if spontaneous breathing falls below a preset rate (International Ventilator Users Network, 2009).

Assist-Control Mode Ventilation Assist-control mode ventilation (ACMV) is frequently used to initiate mechanical ventilation and when the client is at risk for respiratory arrest (e.g., overdose or head injury). Assisted breaths are triggered by inspiratory effort; however, if the respiratory rate falls below a preset number (e.g., 14 breaths/minute), ventilator-controlled breaths are delivered. All breaths, assisted and controlled, are delivered at a specific tidal volume or pressure and inspiratory flow rate.

Synchronized Intermittent Mandatory Ventilation Synchronized intermittent mandatory ventilation (SIMV) allows the client to breathe spontaneously, without ventilator assistance, between delivered ventilator breaths. Mandatory or ventilator-controlled breaths are delivered at a preset rate, volume, and/or pressure, coordinated with the client's inspiratory efforts. This mode of ventilation is used to support ventilation, to exercise respiratory muscles between ventilator-assisted breaths, and during the weaning process (Kasper et al., 2005).

Positive End-Expiratory Pressure **Positive end-expiratory pressure (PEEP)** requires intubation and can be applied to any of the previously described ventilator modes. With PEEP, a positive pressure is maintained in the airways during exhalation and between breaths. Keeping alveoli open between breaths improves V-Q relationships and diffusion across the alveolar-capillary membrane. This reduces hypoxemia and allows use of lower percentages of inspired oxygen. PEEP is particularly useful for treating the client with ARDS.

Pressure-Support Ventilation Pressure-support ventilation (PSV) delivers ventilator-assisted breaths when the client initiates an inspiratory effort. The cycle is flow limited; inspiration is terminated when inspiratory airflow falls below a preset rate. This mode decreases the work of breathing. It can be used in combination with SIMV when the respiratory drive is depressed. Ventilator support can be gradually withdrawn during weaning.

Pressure-Control Ventilation Pressure-control ventilation controls pressure within the airways to reduce the risk of airway trauma (e.g., following thoracic surgery). Ventilation is time triggered and time cycled, but pressure is limited. The ventilator maintains a preset airway pressure throughout inspiration. Because all breaths are controlled by the ventilator, heavy sedation may be required to prevent competition between inspiratory effort and ventilator control.

VENTILATOR SETTINGS In addition to choosing the mode of ventilation, other parameters are set to meet individual client needs when positive-pressure ventilation is used (Table 21–7). The most important of these parameters are rate, tidal volume, and oxygen concentration.

For most adult clients, the rate is initially set between 12 and 15 ventilator breaths per minute. With ACMV or SIMV, the client's respiratory rate often is higher than the ventilator setting because of spontaneous breathing. Exhaled carbon dioxide ($ETCO_2$) or the $PaCO_2$ may be used to determine the rate. A $PaCO_2$ of less than 38 mmHg indicates hyperventilation and respiratory alkalosis; the set rate is reduced. A $PaCO_2$ above 42 mmHg or an $ETCO_2$ greater than 45 mmHg indicates hypoventilation and a need to increase the rate.

The tidal volume setting controls the amount of gas delivered with each ventilator breath. The normal adult tidal volume at rest is approximately 7 mL/kg body weight, or 400–550 mL. The tidal volume delivered by mechanical ventilation is slightly higher (500–750 mL) to compensate for tubing dead space. Higher tidal volumes can cause lung tissue trauma.

The percentage of oxygen delivered with ventilator breaths is adjusted to maintain the oxygen saturation and PaO_2 within acceptable ranges. Because prolonged delivery of high oxygen concentrations increases the risk of oxygen toxicity and pulmonary fibrosis, the FIO_2 is set at the lowest possible level for adequate tissue oxygenation. For most clients, the goal is to maintain an oxygen saturation of greater than 90%. Lower oxygen saturation levels may be appropriate for clients with long-standing COPD.

COMPLICATIONS Although endotracheal intubation and mechanical ventilation can be life-saving in respiratory failure, they are not without risk. Improper endotracheal tube placement or advancement of the tube into a mainstem bronchus can result in ventilation of one lung only. The inflated lung becomes overdistended and traumatized, and the uninflated lung develops atelectasis. In NIV, associated complications include gastric dilation, aspiration, facial skin necrosis, drying of the eyes and mucous membranes, stress, and claustrophobia (Fenstermacher & Hong, 2004).

Nosocomial Pneumonia Infection is a significant risk associated with intubation and mechanical ventilation. Normal upper respiratory tract defense mechanisms are bypassed, with loss of air humidification and trapping of pathogens. Oral secretions and gastric contents can enter the respiratory tree through the open epiglottis. Frequent, meticulous oral hygiene is vital in preventing ventilator-associated pneumonia. Often, the cough reflex is inhibited or impaired by the underlying disease process and the continued presence of the endotracheal tube. Even when strict asepsis is used for suctioning and other respiratory procedures, the lower airways are contaminated within 24 hours of intubation (Urden, Stacy, & Sough, 2006). Secretions often become thick and tenacious, increasing the risk of atelectasis.

Barotrauma **Barotrauma** (also called volutrauma) is lung injury caused by alveolar overdistention. Both the volume of delivered gas and the pressures under which it is delivered can contribute to barotraumas. As a result, overdistended alveoli rupture, allowing air to escape into the pulmonary interstitial

TABLE 21–7 Ventilator Settings

PARAMETER	DESCRIPTION
Rate (*f*)	Number of ventilator breaths per minute: usually 12–15 in adults using assist-control mode ventilation; may be lower in synchronized intermittent mandatory ventilation
Tidal volume (V_t)	Amount of gas delivered with each ventilator breath; usually 8–10 mL/kg body weight
Oxygen concentration (FIO_2)	Percentage of oxygen delivered with ventilator breaths; can be set between 21% (room air) and 100%
I:E ratio	Duration of inspiration to expiration: usually 1:2–1:1.5
Flow rate	Speed at which air is delivered
Sensitivity	Effort required by client to initiate ventilator-assisted breath
Pressure limit	Maximal pressure within airways that will terminate a ventilator breath

spaces and the mediastinum, pleural space, and other tissues. Subcutaneous emphysema, pneumothorax, and pneumomediastinum are possible results of barotrauma. Subcutaneous emphysema, or air in the subcutaneous tissue, causes tissue swelling of the chest, neck, and face. A "crackling" or air bubble-popping sensation is felt on palpation of subcutaneous emphysema. Swelling may be massive. Once the cause is corrected, the air is gradually reabsorbed.

Pneumothoraxis identified by signs of unequal chest expansion, a sudden loss or significant decrease in breath sounds on the affected side, and a hyperresonant percussion tone. Rapid chest tube insertion is necessary to prevent tension pneumothorax and cardiovascular compromise. **Pneumomediastinum** is the presence of air in the mediastinum (the space between the lungs that contains the heart, great vessels, trachea, and esophagus). Air in the mediastinal space can interfere with the function of all of these organs and lead to such complications as **pneumopericardium** (air in the pericardial sac). Pneumomediastinum may have few manifestations, but the CXR shows widening of the mediastinal space.

Cardiovascular Effects Positive-pressure ventilation increases intrathoracic pressure, which can interfere with venous return to the heart and ventricular filling. As a result, cardiac output falls. Use of PEEP increases the effects of mechanical ventilation on cardiac output. The decreased cardiac output can affect liver and kidney function secondarily.

Gastrointestinal Effects Gastrointestinal complications are commonly associated with prolonged mechanical ventilation. Stress ulcers (erosive gastritis) may develop, leading to painless gastrointestinal hemorrhage. Histamine H_2-receptor blockers or sucralfate are often used to prevent stress ulcers. Air leaks around the endotracheal tube can cause gastric distention; a nasogastric tube often is inserted to prevent vomiting. Sedation and other medications used during mechanical ventilation can slow intestinal motility, leading to constipation.

WEANING FROM VENTILATOR SUPPORT The process of removing ventilator support and reestablishing spontaneous, independent respirations is called **weaning**. Weaning begins only after the underlying process causing respiratory failure has been corrected or stabilized. The process and time required for weaning depend on factors such as preexisting lung condition, duration of mechanical ventilation, and the client's general condition, both physical and psychological. In all cases, the vital signs, respiratory rate, extent of dyspnea, blood gases, and clinical status are used to evaluate weaning and its progress.

Following a brief period of mechanical ventilation, a T-piece unit or CPAP may be used for weaning. In T-piece weaning, the ventilator is removed for brief periods during which oxygen is delivered using a T-piece (Figure 21–19 ■). The duration of periods off the ventilator is gradually increased until the client can maintain adequate independent respirations for several hours. Vital signs, oxygen saturation, $ETCO_2$, and PaO_2 are carefully monitored during the process. If signs of respiratory distress develop, the client is placed back on the ventilator at previous settings. When mechanical ventilation is no longer needed, the endotracheal tube is removed. CPAP weaning follows a similar process, with trials of spontaneous breathing supported by the ventilator in CPAP mode.

Both SIMV and PSV are used for weaning when the duration of mechanical ventilation has been longer and reconditioning of respiratory muscles is needed. When SIMV is used, the number of mandatory ventilator-assisted breaths is gradually decreased as ABG, $ETCO_2$, and the respiratory rate are monitored. When the client is able to tolerate SIMV at 4 breaths per minute without rest periods of greater ventilatory support, CPAP or T-piece weaning is attempted before extubation (Kasper et al., 2005).

Weaning is the primary use for PCV. Initially, PSV is set slightly below the peak inspiratory pressures required during volume-cycled ventilation. Pressure support levels are gradually decreased, often in a cyclic pattern of periods of minimal support alternating with period of higher support to recondition respiratory muscles. When the PSV level is just enough to overcome endotracheal tube resistance, support is discontinued and the client is extubated (Kasper et al., 2005).

When an illness is terminal or irreversible with a poor prognosis, terminal weaning may be requested by the client or family. **Terminal weaning** is the gradual withdrawal of mechanical ventilation when survival without assisted ventilation is not expected. Unlike weaning when recovery is

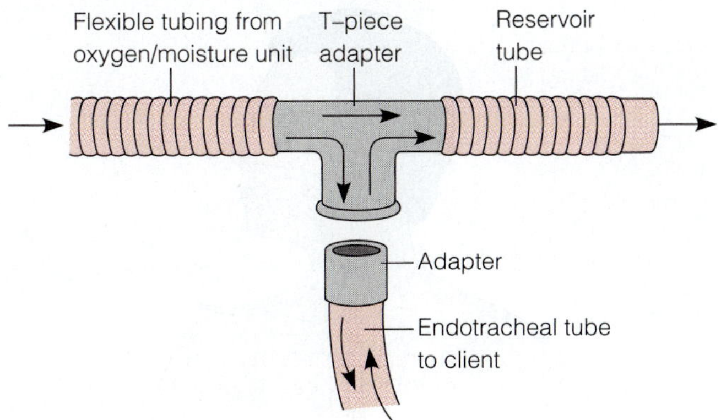

Figure 21–19 ■ A T-piece, or "blow-by," unit for weaning from mechanical ventilation.

expected, which usually occurs in an intensive care unit, the client is moved to a quiet medical-surgical room, a hospice room, or even the client's home before terminal weaning is initiated. Family members are encouraged to remain with the client throughout the process. If possible, decisions about sedation and analgesia before and during weaning are made with the client, as are decisions about hydration and nutritional support following weaning. Ventilator support is gradually withdrawn using the same modes described earlier (SIMV or PSV). Analgesia and sedation are given to promote comfort during weaning.

NUTRITION AND FLUIDS Monitoring fluid and electrolyte status and providing adequate nutrition during mechanical ventilation are vital to client health and outcomes. Mechanical ventilation promotes sodium and water retention as a result of its effects on cardiac output. Renal perfusion is decreased, stimulating the renin–angiotensin–aldosterone system to retain sodium and water. A Swan-Ganz catheter is often inserted to monitor pulmonary artery pressures and cardiac output. An arterial line allows repeated blood gas analysis and continuous arterial pressure monitoring. Serum electrolytes are drawn frequently, and intake, output, and daily weight are carefully monitored. Enteral or parenteral nutrition are provided during mechanical ventilation because the endotracheal tube prohibits eating. A nasogastric, gastrostomy, or jejunostomy feeding tube is placed for enteral nutrition. A jejunostomy tube may be used to reduce the risk of regurgitation and aspiration.

Artificial Airways

Artificial airways are inserted to maintain a patent air passage for a client whose airway has become or may become obstructed. A patent airway is necessary so that air can flow to and from the lungs. Four of the more common types of airways are oropharyngeal, nasopharyngeal, endotracheal, and tracheostomies.

OROPHARYNGEAL AND NASOPHARYNGEAL AIRWAYS Oropharyngeal and nasopharyngeal airways are used to keep the upper air passages open when they may become obstructed by secretions or by the tongue. These airways are easy to insert and have a low risk of complications. Sizes vary and should be appropriate to the size and age of the client. The airway should be well lubricated with water-soluble gel before insertion of the airway.

Oropharyngeal airways (Figure 21–20 ■) stimulate the gag reflex and are used only for clients with altered levels of consciousness (e.g., because of general anesthesia, overdose, or head injury). Nasopharyngeal airways are tolerated better by alert clients and are inserted through the nares, terminating in the oropharynx (Figure 21–21 ■). When caring for a client with a nasopharyngeal airway, provide frequent oral and nares care, repositioning the airway in the other naris every 8 hours or as ordered to prevent necrosis of the mucosa.

ENDOTRACHEAL TUBES Endotracheal tubes are most commonly inserted in clients who have had general anesthetics or who are in emergency situations where mechanical ventilation is required. An endotracheal tube is inserted by the primary care provider, nurse, or respiratory therapist with specialized education. It is inserted through the mouth or the nose and into the trachea with the guide of a laryngoscope (Figure 21–22 ■). The tube terminates just superior to the bifurcation of the trachea into the bronchi. The tube may have an air-filled cuff to prevent air leakage around it. Because an endotracheal tube passes through the epiglottis and glottis, the client is unable to speak while the tube is in place.

TRACHEOSTOMIES Clients who need long-term airway support may have a tracheostomy. A tracheostomy is an opening into the trachea through the neck. A tube is usually inserted through this opening, and an artificial airway is created. Tracheostomy is done using one of two techniques: the traditional open surgical method or a percutaneous insertion. The percutaneous method can be done at the bedside in a critical care unit. The open technique is done in the operating room: A surgical incision is made in the trachea just below the larynx, and a curved tracheostomy tube is inserted to extend through the

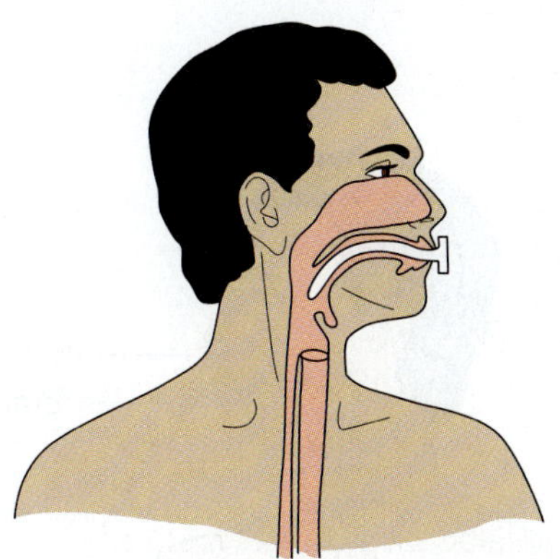

Figure 21–20 ■ An oropharyngeal airway in place.

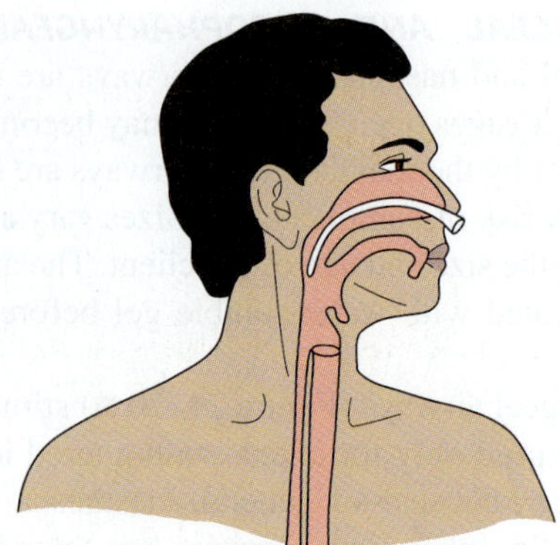
Figure 21–21 ■ A nasopharyngeal airway in place.

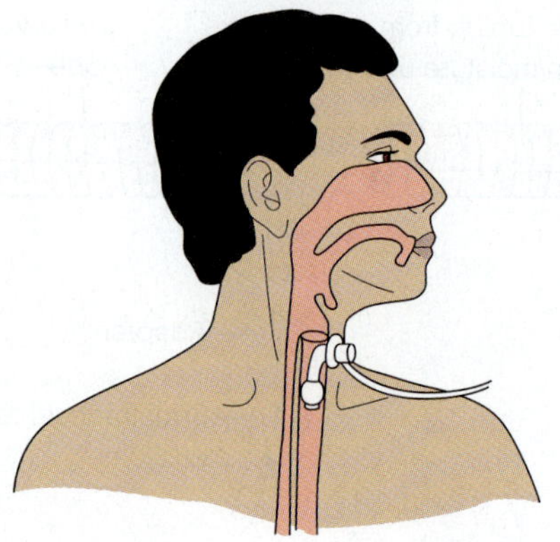
Figure 21–23 ■ A tracheostomy tube in place.

stoma into the trachea (Figure 21–23 ■). Tracheostomy tubes can be either plastic or metal and are available in different sizes with and without cuffs. Fenestrated tracheostomy tubes are available to allow the client to speak with the tube in place.

Tracheostomy tubes have an outer cannula that is inserted into the trachea and a flange that rests against the neck and allows the tube to be secured in place with tape or ties. All tubes also have an obturator, which is used to insert the outer cannula and is then removed. The obturator is kept at the client's bedside in case the tube becomes dislodged and needs to be reinserted. Some tracheostomy tubes have an inner cannula that may be removed for periodic cleaning.

Cuffed tracheostomy tubes are surrounded by an inflatable cuff that produces an airtight seal between the tube and the trachea. This seal prevents aspiration of oropharyngeal secretions and air leakage between the tube and the trachea. Cuffed tubes are often used immediately after a tracheostomy and are essential when ventilating a client with a tracheostomy using a mechanical ventilator. Children do not require cuffed tubes, because their tracheas are resilient enough to seal the air space around the tube.

Low-pressure cuffs (Figure 21–24 ■) are commonly used to distribute a low, even pressure against the trachea, thus decreasing the risk of tracheal tissue necrosis. They do not need to be deflated periodically to reduce pressure on the tracheal wall. Foam-cuffed tracheostomy tubes (Figure 21–25 ■) do not require injected air; instead, when the port is opened, ambient air enters the balloon, which then conforms to the client's trachea. Air is removed from the cuff before insertion or removal of the tube.

The nurse provides tracheostomy care for the client with a new or recent tracheostomy to maintain patency of the tube and reduce the risk of infection. Initially a tracheostomy may need to be suctioned (see the section on suctioning that follows) and cleaned as often as every 1–2 hours. After the initial inflammatory response subsides, tracheostomy care may only need to be done once or twice a day, depending on the client.

When the client breathes through a tracheostomy, air is no longer filtered and humidified as it is when passing through the upper airways; therefore, special precautions are necessary. Humidity may be provided with a mist collar. Clients with long-term tracheostomies may wear a light scarf or a 4-in. × 4-in. gauze held in place with a cotton tie over the stoma to filter air as it enters the tracheostomy.

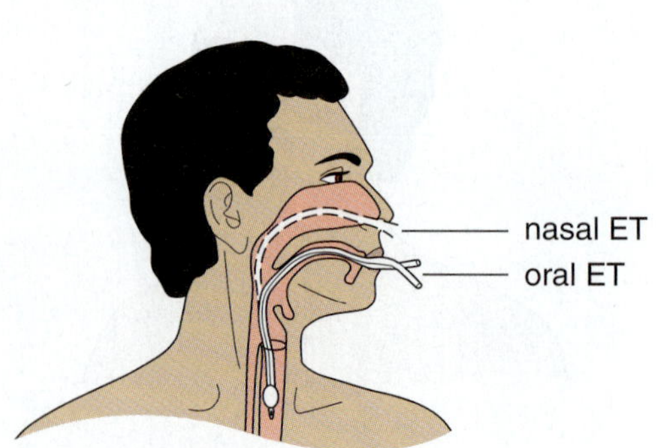

Figure 21–22 ■ An endotracheal tube.

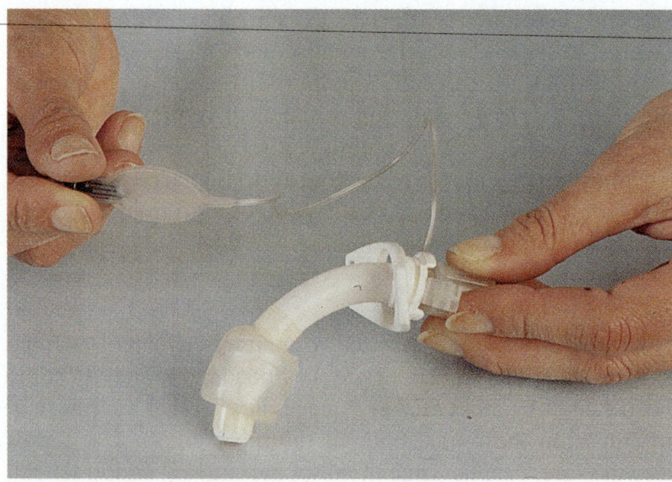
Figure 21–24 ■ A tracheostomy tube with a low-pressure cuff.

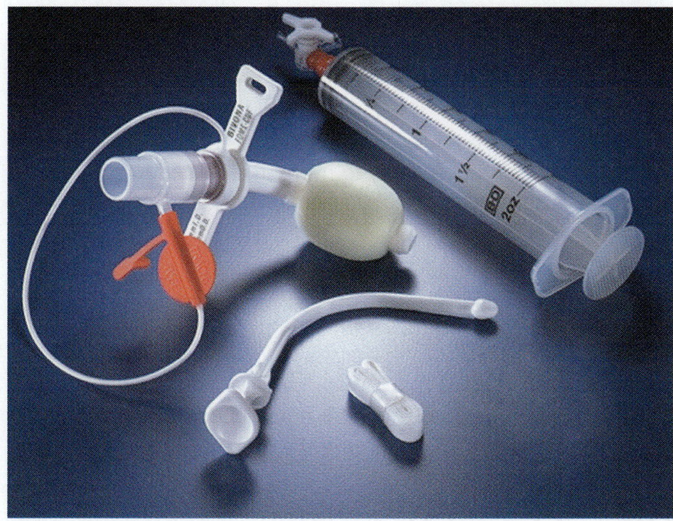

Figure 21–25 ■ A tracheostomy tube with a foam cuff.

Courtesy of Portex Inc., Keene, NH.

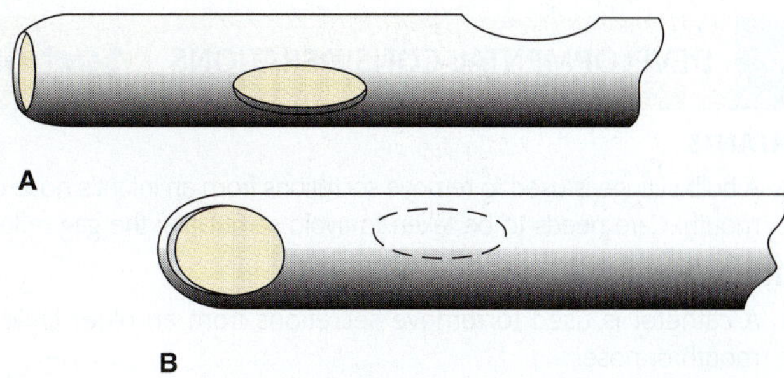

Figure 21–26 ■ Types of suction catheters. *A*, Open tipped. *B*, Whistle tipped.

Suctioning

When clients have difficulty handling their secretions or an airway is in place, suctioning may be necessary to clear air passages. **Suctioning** is aspirating secretions through a catheter connected to a suction machine or wall suction outlet. Even though the upper airways (the oropharynx and nasopharynx) are not sterile, sterile technique is recommended for all suctioning to avoid introducing pathogens into the airways.

Suction catheters may be either open tipped or whistle tipped (Figure 21–26 ■). The whistle-tipped catheter is less irritating to respiratory tissues, although the open-tipped catheter may be more effective for removing thick mucous plugs. An oral suction tube, or Yankauer device, is used to suction the oral cavity (Figure 21–27 ■). Most suction catheters have a thumb port on the side to control the suction. The catheter is connected to suction tubing, which in turn is connected to a collection chamber and suction control gauge.

The nurse decides when suctioning is needed by assessing the client for signs of respiratory distress or evidence that the client is unable to cough up and expectorate secretions. Dyspnea, bubbling or rattling breath sounds, poor skin color (cyanosis), or decreased oxygen saturation (also called O_2 sat) levels may indicate the need for suctioning. Good nursing judgment is necessary, because suctioning irritates mucous membranes and can increase secretions if performed too frequently. In other words, suctioning is based on clinical need, not a fixed schedule.

Oral and oropharyngeal suctioning removes secretions from the upper respiratory tract. Nasopharyngeal and nasotracheal suctioning provides closer access to the trachea and requires sterile technique.

Following endotracheal intubation or a tracheostomy, the trachea and surrounding respiratory tissues are irritated and react by producing excessive secretions. Sterile suctioning is necessary to remove these secretions from the trachea and bronchi to maintain a patent airway. The frequency of suctioning depends on the client's health and how recently the intubation was done. Additionally, suctioning may be necessary in clients who have increased secretions because of pneumonia or inability to clear secretions because of altered level of consciousness (LOC).

Suctioning is associated with several complications: hypoxemia, trauma to the airway, nosocomial infection, and cardiac dysrhythmia, which is related to the hypoxemia. The following techniques are used to minimize or decrease these complications:

- *Hyperinflation.* This involves giving the client breaths that are 1–1.5 times the tidal volume set on the ventilator through the ventilator circuit or via a manual resuscitation bag. Three to five breaths are delivered before and after each pass of the suction catheter.
- *Hyperoxygenation.* This can be done with a manual resuscitation bag or through the ventilator and is performed by increasing the oxygen flow (usually to 100%) before suctioning and between suction attempts.

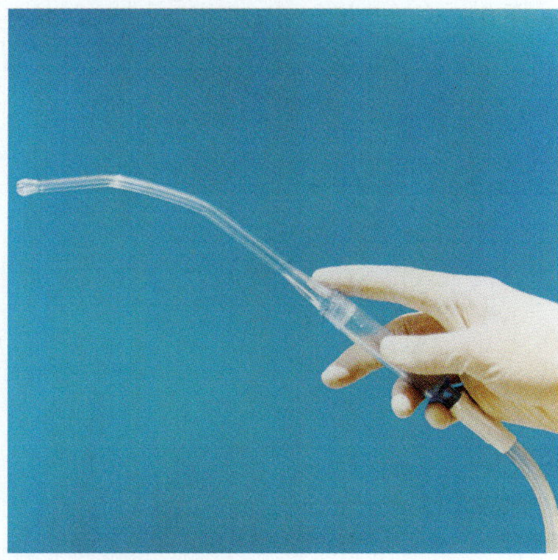

Figure 21–27 ■ Oral (Yankauer) suction tube.

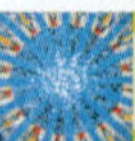

DEVELOPMENTAL CONSIDERATIONS Suctioning

INFANTS

- A bulb syringe is used to remove secretions from an infant's nose or mouth. Care needs to be taken to avoid stimulating the gag reflex.

CHILDREN

- A catheter is used to remove secretions from an older child's mouth or nose.

OLDER ADULTS

- Older clients may have cardiac and/or pulmonary disease, increasing their susceptibility to hypoxemia related to suctioning. Watch closely for signs of hypoxemia. If noted, stop suctioning and hyperoxygenate.

For tracheostomy and endotracheal suctioning, the outer diameter of the suction catheter should not exceed one half the internal diameter of the tracheostomy or endotracheal tube so that hypoxia can be prevented (St. John & Malen, 2004). The nurse uses sterile techniques to prevent infection of the respiratory tract. The traditional method of suctioning an endotracheal tube or tracheostomy is sometimes referred to as the *open method.* If a client is connected to a ventilator, the nurse disconnects the client from the ventilator, suctions the airway, reconnects the client to the ventilator, and discards the suction catheter. Drawbacks to the open airway suction system include the nurse needing to wear personal protective equipment (e.g., goggles or face shield and a gown) to avoid exposure to the client's sputum and the potential cost of one-time catheter use, especially if the client requires frequent suctioning.

With the *closed airway/tracheal suction system* (in-line suctioning) (Figure 21–28 ■), the suction catheter attaches to the ventilator tubing and the client does not need to be disconnected from the ventilator. The nurse is not exposed to any secretions, because the suction catheter is enclosed in a plastic sheath. The catheter can be reused as many times as necessary until the system is changed. The nurse needs to inquire about the agency's policy for changing the closed suction system.

Other Clinical Therapies

Atelectasis frequently occurs in dependent lung regions in clients with ARDS. Prone positioning in conjunction with mechanical ventilation reduces the pressure of surrounding tissue on dependent regions and improves oxygenation.

Other management strategies include careful fluid replacement, attention to nutrition, treatment of any infection, and correction of the underlying condition. A Swan-Ganz line is used to monitor pulmonary artery pressures and cardiac output. Fluid replacement is carefully tailored to avoid fluid imbalances, which may worsen hypoxia and ARDS. Enteral or parenteral feeding is necessary to maintain nutritional status and prevent tissue catabolism.

Infections are treated with intravenous antibiotic therapy tailored to the causative organism. Low-molecular-weight heparin may be ordered to prevent thrombophlebitis and possible pulmonary embolus or disseminated intravascular coagulation, a possible complication of ARDS.

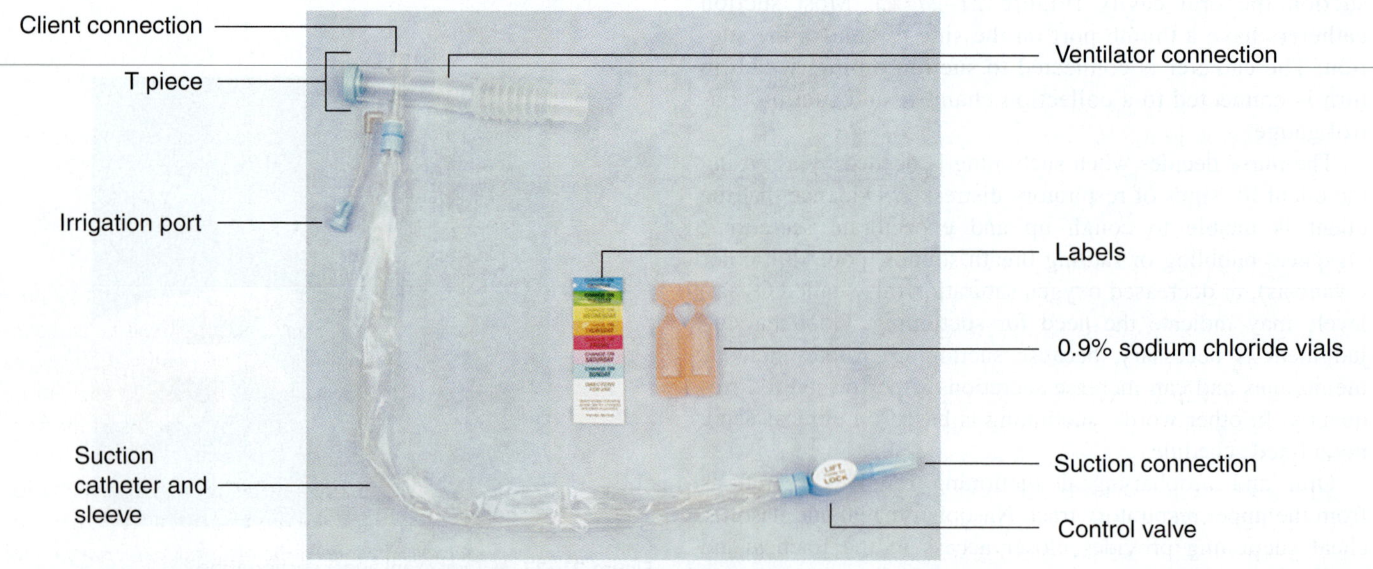

Figure 21–28 ■ A closed airway suction (in-line) system.

NURSING PROCESS

Caring for the client with ARDS requires careful and continuous monitoring of airway, breathing, and circulation. Changes in level of consciousness, oxygenation, or perfusion require rapid nursing interventions to maintain life. The focus of nursing care is on meeting these essential client needs.

Assessment

Collect assessment data through the health history and physical assessment:

- *Health history.* Previous respiratory alterations, previous illnesses and surgeries, and any direct or indirect injury in the previous 3–4 days
- *Physical assessment.* Respiratory rate and rhythm; auscultation of the lungs; level of consciousness, including orientation; baseline vital signs, peripheral perfusion.

Confusion, agitation, or anxiety are early signs of hypoxemia, especially in older clients. Changes from baseline vital signs alert the nurse to subtle changes in cardiac or respiratory status. Individuals developing ARDS may express desperate anxiety because of the inability of get enough air to relieve their shortness of breath.

Diagnosis

Any combination of the following NANDA diagnoses may be appropriate for the individual with ARDS:

- Risk for Acute Confusion
- Ineffective Airway Clearance
- Ineffective Breathing Pattern
- Impaired Spontaneous Ventilation
- Impaired Gas Exchange
- Decreased Cardiac Output
- Dysfunctional Ventilatory Weaning Response
- Risk for Imbalanced Fluid Volume
- Imbalanced Nutrition: Less Than Body Requirements
- Risk for Infection
- Acute Pain
- Anxiety.

Additional NANDA diagnoses may be appropriate depending on the underlying condition causing the acute respiratory distress.

Plan

The goal of care for individuals with ARDS is to protect the lungs from fibrotic damage while providing adequate oxygenation to the body systems. Expected outcomes may include the following:

- The client will be oriented to name, place, and time with each health care personnel individual interaction.
- The client will receive adequate ventilatory support to maintain oxygenation of body cells.
- The client will be free of pulmonary tissue damage.
- The client will maintain patent airways.
- The client will maintain cardiac output adequate to perfuse all body systems.
- The client will receive adequate nutrition to maintain body process.
- The client will be free of any sign or symptom of infection.
- The client will have no development of thrombosis.
- The client will manage pain successfully.
- The client will cope with or be free from anxiety.

Implementation

All body systems are at risk of failure caused by poor oxygenation and alterations in perfusion. The health care team will identify and treat the causative agent, as this is critical to returning the client to normal. Common interventions for the client with ARDS include the following:

- CBC, chemistry panel, ABG, blood cultures, sputum cultures, and gastric and stool cultures as indicated by symptoms.
- Monitor vital signs at least hourly. Continual monitoring may be required.
- Monitor oxygenation status with ABG and pulse oximetry.
- Monitor neurologic status, including orientation and LOC.
- Auscultate lung and heart sounds.
- Provide analgesia, anxiolytics, and sedation medications as ordered.
- Provide beta-agonist to maintain patent airways as ordered.
- Maintain head of bed at 30° or higher.
- Position the individual prone for 30 minutes to an hour as tolerated three or four times a day. This will recruit posterior alveoli and facilitate posterior drainage.
- Suction airways as needed.
- Monitor hemodynamic status with central venous catheters or pulmonary artery catheter as ordered.
- Monitor renal function by intake and output as well as blood urea nitrogen and creatinine levels.
- Place Foley catheter.
- Administer intravenous fluids as needed, but avoid fluid overload.
- Monitor glucose levels, and maintain levels within normal limits.
- Assess peripheral pulses.

PRACTICE ALERT

Provide sedation and antianxiety medications as needed, especially when neuromuscular blockade is used. Although neuromuscular blockade paralyzes voluntary muscles, the LOC is unimpaired.

Ineffective Airway Clearance

Ineffective airway clearance may either cause respiratory failure or occur as a result of interventions. Impaired ventilation frequently leads to acute respiratory failure. Although intubation and mechanical ventilation can be life-saving measures, they also increase the risk of respiratory infection and ineffective secretion management.

- Suction as needed to maintain a patent airway. Indicators for suctioning include crackles and rhonchi on auscultation, frequent coughing or setting off of the high-pressure alarm, and increasing restlessness or anxiety. Although clients with a tracheostomy can usually cough up secretions, the length and diameter of endotracheal tubes makes this extremely difficult. Even with humidification, secretions often become thick and tenacious, further inhibiting their removal.

- Obtain sputum for culture if it appears purulent or is odorous. Culture is necessary to identify pathogens and guide antibiotic therapy.
- Perform percussion, vibration, and postural drainage as ordered. These techniques help loosen secretions and move them into larger airways for removal by coughing or suctioning.
- Firmly secure the endotracheal or tracheostomy tube. Provide adequate slack on ventilator tubing to prevent tension on the tube when turning, positioning, or transferring the client to a chair or stretcher. If necessary, loosely restrain hands. These measures are important to ensure proper airway placement and prevent its inadvertent removal.
- Assess fluid balance, and maintain adequate hydration. Adequate hydration helps liquefy secretions.

PRACTICE ALERT

Frequently assess respiratory rate, chest movement, lung sounds, oxygen saturation, $ETCO_2$, and ABG. Intubation and mechanical ventilation do not ensure adequate oxygenation and ventilation. Displacement of the endotracheal tube or obstruction by respiratory secretions impairs ventilation.

Impaired Spontaneous Ventilation

In ARDS, the client's ability to maintain adequate ventilation is impaired. This is a concern both before initiation of mechanical ventilation and during the weaning process.

- Assess and document respiratory rate, vital signs, and oxygen saturation every 15–30 minutes. Close monitoring is vital to detect early signs of increasing respiratory distress and inability to sustain adequate breathing.
- Promptly report worsening ABG and oxygen saturation levels. Close assessment of these values allows timely intervention as needed.
- Administer oxygen as ordered, monitoring response. Observe closely for respiratory depression, especially in the client with COPD. Oxygen administration reduces the hypoxemic respiratory drive. Chronically high $PaCO_2$ levels depress the respiratory center; hypoxemia may provide the only respiratory drive.
- Place in Fowler's or high-Fowler's position. Sitting positions decrease pressure on the diaphragm and chest, improving lung ventilation and decreasing the work of breathing.
- Minimize activities and energy expenditures by assisting with ADLs, spacing procedures and activities, and by allowing uninterrupted periods of rest. Rest is vital to reduce oxygen and energy demands.

PRACTICE ALERT

Promptly report signs of respiratory distress, including tachypnea, tachycardia, nasal flaring, use of accessory muscles, intercostal retractions, cyanosis, increasing restlessness, anxiety, or decreased LOC. These may be early manifestations of respiratory failure and inability to maintain ventilatory effort.

Decreased Cardiac Output

With positive-pressure ventilation, increased intrathoracic pressure decreases cardiac output. When PEEP is applied, intrathoracic pressure increases further; this can significantly decrease venous return, ventricular filling, stroke volume, and cardiac output. Manifestations of decreased cardiac output include hypotension and compensatory tachycardia as the heart attempts to maintain cardiac output despite decreased stroke volume. In the client who is already hypoxic because of ARDS, this drop in cardiac output can increase tissue damage. Urine output falls, and dysrhythmias may develop.

- Monitor and record vital signs, including apical pulse, at least every 2 hours (more frequently immediately following initiation of mechanical ventilation or addition of PEEP). Frequent assessment is vital to detect early signs of decreased cardiac output.
- Assess LOC at least every 4 hours. Altered LOC, confusion, and restlessness are early signs of cerebral hypoxia resulting from decreased cardiac output.
- Monitor pulmonary artery pressures, central venous pressure, and cardiac output readings every 1–4 hours. Changes in these measurements may indicate worsening cardiac status.
- Assess heart and lung sounds frequently. Increasing crackles or abnormal heart sounds may indicate heart failure.
- Weigh daily at the same time. Accurate daily weights are the best indicator of fluid volume status.
- Frequently provide good skin care, keeping skin clean and dry and protecting pressure points. Tissue hypoxia increases the risk of skin breakdown, which in turn increases the risk of infection and sepsis.
- Maintain intravenous fluids as ordered. Intravenous fluids are given to maintain vascular volume and prevent dehydration.
- Administer analgesics, sedatives, and neuromuscular blockers as needed. These medications may be prescribed to decrease cardiac workload.

PRACTICE ALERT

Record urine output hourly. Because a significant portion of the cardiac output goes directly to the kidneys, a fall in urine output to less than 30 mL/hour is often the first sign of decreased cardiac output.

Dysfunctional Ventilatory Weaning Response

Assessment findings indicative of dysfunctional weaning include the following:

- Dyspnea, apprehension, or agitation
- Decreasing oxygen saturation level
- Cyanosis or pallor, diaphoresis
- Increased blood pressure, pulse, and respiratory rate
- Diminished or adventitious breath sounds, use of accessory muscles
- Decreased LOC
- Deteriorating ABG values
- Shallow, gasping breaths or paradoxic abdominal breathing.

PRACTICE ALERT

Frequently monitor oxygen saturation, $ETCO_2$, and ABG following changes in ventilator settings. These values are used to assess the adequacy of ventilation and gas exchange during the weaning process.

The client with dysfunctional ventilatory weaning response has difficulty adjusting to reduced mechanical ventilator support, prolonging the weaning process. Airway congestion, inadequate rest or nutrition, pain, anxiety, and a nonsupportive environment are factors that can contribute to difficulty weaning. With ARDS, the pathologic processes of the disease and its effects on gas exchange may be responsible for a prolonged or ineffective weaning process.

- Assess vital signs every 15–30 minutes following changes in ventilator settings and during T-piece trials. Vital signs (heart and respiratory rates in particular) can provide early signs of hypoxemia and poor tolerance of the weaning process.
- Place in Fowler's or high-Fowler's position. Fowler's position facilitates lung expansion and reduces the work of breathing.
- Fully explain all weaning procedures, along with expected changes in breathing. Adequate explanations help reduce anxiety and improve the ability to cooperate.
- Remain with the client during initial periods following changes of ventilator settings or T-piece trials. This provides reassurance and allows close monitoring of the response.
- Limit procedures and activities during weaning periods. Reducing energy expenditures and cardiac work facilitates the weaning process.
- Provide diversion, such as television or radio. Diversion helps distract the focus from breathing.
- Begin weaning procedures in the morning, when the client is well rested and alert; weaning may be discontinued overnight to provide rest. The work of breathing increases during the weaning process; adequate rest is important.
- When SIMV is used for weaning, decrease the SIMV rate by increments of two breaths per minute. Slow reduction of ventilator support allows respiratory muscle reconditioning and gradual resumption of the work of breathing.
- Avoid administering drugs that may depress respirations during the weaning process (except as ordered at night to facilitate rest when ventilator support is provided). Sedatives or analgesics that depress respirations can impair the weaning process.
- Keep oxygen at the bedside following weaning and extubation. Supplemental oxygen may be necessary to maintain adequate blood and tissue oxygenation.
- Provide pulmonary hygiene with percussion and postural drainage. Maintaining patent airways and adequate alveolar ventilation is vital during the weaning process.

PRACTICE ALERT

Frequently assess respiratory status following weaning and extubation. Keep an intubation kit readily available following extubation; be prepared for emergency reintubation. Laryngeal spasm or laryngeal edema may develop following extubation, necessitating reintubation to maintain respirations.

EVIDENCE-BASED PRACTICE The Client Who Is Intubated

Clinical Question

Clients who are intubated cannot communicate verbally. Subjective experiences such as pain may not be recognized and effectively treated in these clients.

Evidence

This retrospective study by Gélinas, Fortier, Viens, Fillion, & Puntillo (2004) used a standardized instrument to look at the assessment and management of pain as documented in the records of 52 clients undergoing mechanical ventilation. A total of 183 pain episodes were analyzed. In the majority of episodes, observable indicators of pain (e.g., restlessness, changes in vital signs, muscle tension) were recorded. Subjective reports were recorded only 29% of the time. Following intervention, pain was reassessed only approximately 60% of the time, usually using objective data and rarely (8%) using subjective information. The study concluded that documentation of pain and its management was incomplete or inadequate for clients who are intubated.

Best Practice

Pain is now considered to be the fifth vital sign, necessitating frequent assessment and monitoring. Unrelieved pain is known to reduce healing and prolong recovery. Observable indicators of pain are not always present; some clients deal with pain by attempting to relax muscles and doze. When neuromuscular blockers or other anesthetic agents are administered to clients who are intubated and mechanically ventilated, objective pain indicators are lost, as is the ability to subjectively report pain. However, it is important to remember that nursing practice standards dictate that pain level be assessed regularly and both before and following interventions to reduce or relieve pain.

Critical Thinking

1. What tools are available to assist the nurse in evaluating the client's subjective perception of pain?
2. How can the nurse adapt these tools for use with a client under neuromuscular blockade (consciousness intact but unable to move voluntary muscles)?
3. What factors might contribute to pain in the client who is intubated and mechanically ventilated?
4. Identify five nonpharmacologic measures the nurse could implement to reduce or relieve pain in clients who are intubated and ventilated.

NURSING CARE PLAN A Client With Acute Respiratory Distress Syndrome

Peggy Adamson is a 36-year-old, single woman admitted to the hospital following a near-drowning in a local lake. On admission to the emergency department, Ms. Adamson is alert and oriented, having been rescued and resuscitated within 2 minutes of submersion. Rescuers report that she seemed to have aspirated "a lot" of water. She was water-skiing when the accident occurred. She is admitted to the intensive care unit for observation. Oxygen is started per nasal cannula at 6 L/minute, intravenous fluids are administered to correct electrolyte imbalances, and 40 mg of furosemide (Lasix) are given intravenously for hypervolemia.

ASSESSMENT

Throughout her admission, Ms. Adamson has remained alert and oriented, with stable vital signs. Her respiratory rate has been 20–24 breaths/minute with scattered crackles, oxygen saturations of around 94%, and a PaO_2 of 75–80 mmHg on 6 L/minute of oxygen. Her pulse has been 96–100 bpm and regular. Tonight, Ms. Adamson seems apprehensive and anxious. Although her blood pressure is 116/74 mmHg, unchanged from previous levels, her heart rate is up to 106 bpm, and her respiratory rate is 28/minute. Her lungs have scattered crackles but good breath sounds throughout, unchanged from previous assessments. Ms. Adamson's oxygen saturation has dropped to 84%. The provider orders an ABG and increases the oxygen to 8 L/minute. ABG results show the following: pH 7.48 - PaO_2, 65 mmHg - $PaCO_2$, 32 mmHg. Portable chest x-ray reveals scattered infiltrates and a normal heart size. The physician orders a nonrebreather mask at 8 L/minute and repeat ABGs in 1 hour. Ms. Adamson's oxygen saturation continues to fall, and subsequent blood gases show a PaO_2 of 55 mmHg. The attending physician diagnoses probable ARDS and orders nasotracheal intubation and mechanical ventilation.

DIAGNOSES

- Ineffective Breathing Pattern related to hyoxia
- Impaired Gas Exchange related to effects of near-drowning
- Anxiety related to hypoxemia
- Risk for Decreased Cardiac output related to mechanical ventilation
- Risk for Infection related to endotracheal intubation

PLANNING

- Client will breathe effectively with the mechanical ventilator.
- Client will demonstrate improved oxygen saturation, $ETCO_2$, and ABG values.
- Client will express fears related to intubation and mechanical ventilation.
- Client will demonstrate reduced anxiety levels.
- Client will maintain adequate cardiac output and tissue perfusion.
- Client will tolerate endotracheal intubation and mechanical ventilation without evidence of infection or barotrauma.

IMPLEMENTATION

- Obtain all necessary supplies and notify respiratory therapy and radiology in preparation for intubation and mechanical ventilation.
- Explain the purpose and procedure of intubation.
- Provide an opportunity to express fears related to intubation and mechanical ventilation. Answer questions, and provide reassurance.
- Discuss communication strategies while intubated; obtain a magic slate.
- Administer analgesics and/or sedatives as ordered.
- Monitor oxygen saturation and $ETCO_2$ levels continuously initially after instituting mechanical ventilation; report changes to the physician.
- Obtain ABG as ordered or indicated; monitor and report results.
- Perform suction via endotracheal tube as needed to maintain clear airway.
- Allow periods of uninterrupted rest.
- Monitor vital signs at a minimum of every 1–2 hours.
- Assess skin color, capillary refill, and extremity pulses every 4 hours.
- Monitor urine output hourly; report output of less than 30 mL/hour.
- Assess for the presence of edema every 4 hours.
- Promote client communication through use of signals or magic slate
- Assess lung sounds and chest excursion at a minimum of every 1–2 hours.
- Continuous cardiorespiratory monitoring while requiring mechanical ventilation and until condition stabilizes after extubation.

EVALUATION

Ms. Adamson is intubated and placed on a volume-cycled ventilator at 50% FIO_2 and a tidal volume of 700 mL in the assist-control mode at 16 breaths per minute. She has difficulty working with the ventilator initially, so a fentanyl drip is ordered to reduce her anxiety.

Ms. Adamson's oxygen saturation, $ETCO_2$, and ABG results do not begin to improve until 5 mm Hg of PEEP is added to ventilator settings. After 3 days of mechanical ventilation with PEEP and aggressive fluid and diuretic therapy, Ms. Adamson begins to improve. She is placed on SIMV, and over the course of another 3 days, she is gradually weaned off the ventilator to a face mask with CPAP. She eventually recovers fully, with minimal apparent long-term effects.

CRITICAL THINKING

1. Endotracheal intubation and mechanical ventilation were effective in supporting Ms. Adamson's respiratory status as she recovered from ARDS. Discuss a possible sequence of events had it not been possible to wean her from the ventilator.
2. How might the presentation and management of an acute episode of respiratory failure caused by ARDS differ from respiratory failure related to COPD?
3. What measures can nurses take to prevent the development of ARDS?
4. Develop a nursing care plan for Ms. Adamson for the nursing diagnosis Powerlessness related to endotracheal intubation and mechanical ventilation.

Anxiety

Critical illness creates anxiety for any client. In ARDS, this anxiety is compounded by the presence of an endotracheal tube or tracheostomy, mechanical ventilator, numerous monitors and equipment, and potentially, neuromuscular blockade and paralysis of voluntary muscles. Fear of continued dependence on the mechanical ventilator and inability to return to a normal life may compound this anxiety.

- Remain with the client as much as possible. The frequent and continuing presence of a caregiver provides reassurance that help is readily available.
- Explain all monitors, procedures, unusual sounds, and machinery. Understanding the environment and the various sounds and alarms reduces anxiety. Have patience with multiple requests for explanation from clients or family members; they are under extreme stress during this time and may not initially remember explanations.
- Provide a simple means of communication, such as a slate, picture board, or alphabet board. If neuromuscular blockade is used, use methods such as looking to the right for "yes" and to the left for "no." Reassure that endotracheal tube removal restores the ability to speak. The inability to speak and call out for help is frightening for the client. Providing an alternate means of communication helps reduce anxiety.
- Encourage frequent family visits, especially if the time of visitations is being limited. Encourage family participation in care. Family visits help reduce anxiety and feelings of abandonment. Allowing family members to participate in care helps reduce their anxiety as well.
- Explain to the family that the client can hear and understand. Emphasize the importance of talking to the client, not over or about the client. The family may not understand that the client may be mentally alert although unable to respond. Talking to the client about everyday things reduces the client's sense of isolation and fear.
- Provide distraction with radio or television if allowed. Distraction helps reduce the focus on machines and unusual sounds of monitors and alarms.
- Attend to physical needs promptly and completely. This provides reassurance that needs will be met even though the client is unable to ask for assistance.
- Reassure that intubation and mechanical ventilation is a temporary measure to allow the lungs to rest and heal. Reinforce that the client will be able to breathe independently again. The client may fear continued dependence on mechanical ventilation.

PRACTICE ALERT

Frequently monitor anxiety level. High levels of anxiety increase oxygen use and often interfere with the ability to work with the respirator. This can increase hypoxemia and further increase anxiety; intervention is necessary to break this cycle. See the accompanying Evidence-Based Practice feature for information about assessing and managing pain in clients who are intubated.

Community-Based Care

Provide referrals to home health and respiratory care services as indicated, as well as for occupational therapy and counseling as needed. When preparing the client who has recovered from ARDS and the family for home care, discuss the following topics:

- ARDS developed as a consequence of serious illness, not as a consequence of client or family action or inaction. Provide factual information about ARDS.
- Maximal respiratory function following ARDS is usually achieved within 6 months, although respiratory function may remain significantly impaired. This may necessitate changes in occupation, lifestyle, and family roles.
- Avoid smoking and exposure to secondhand smoke and environmental pollutants in order to prevent further lung damage.
- Obtain immunization for pneumococcal pneumonia and annual influenza immunizations to prevent further episodes of serious respiratory disease.

Evaluation

The client's response to nursing care is evaluated often and nursing care is adjusted accordingly. Expected outcomes for the client with ARDS often include:

- Client maintains oxygen saturation greater than 90%.
- Vital signs remain within acceptable limits.
- Client's airway remains clear.
- Client experiences no complications secondary to hypoxia.
- Arterial blood gas results indicate acid–base balance is maintained.

REVIEW Acute Respiratory Distress Syndrome

RELATE: LINK THE CONCEPTS

Linking the exemplar of Acute Respiratory Distress Syndrome with the concept of Acid–Base Balance:

1. What impact will ARDS likely have on acid–base balance and how can the nurse intervene to promote normal balance?
2. Are the symptoms of ARDS entirely the result of acid–base imbalance, or are other factors involved? Explain your answer.

Linking the exemplar of Acute Respiratory Distress Sydnrome with the concept of Grief and Loss:

3. When caring for a client with acute respiratory distress syndrome who is not responding to treatments as anticipated, what nursing care might the family require as it deals with the possibility of the client's death?
4. How might you, as the nurse, help to support the family in this process?

READY: GO TO COMPANION SKILLS MANUAL

- Inserting an oropharyngeal airway
- Inserting a nasopharyngeal airway
- Assisting with endotracheal intubation
- Inflating a tracheal tube cuff
- Providing care for the client with an endotracheal tube
- Extubating an endotracheal tube
- Oropharyngeal, nasopharyngeal, and nasotracheal suctioning
- Suctioning a tracheostomy or endotracheal tube
- Providing tracheostomy care
- Capping a tracheostomy tube with speaking valve
- Caring for the client on a mechanical ventilator
- Weaning the client from a ventilator
- Assisting with chest tube insertion
- Maintaining chest tube drainage
- Chest tube removal
- Clearing an obstructed airway
- Performing rescue breathing
- Administering external cardiac compressions
- Administering automated external defibrillation
- Administering a nasogastric feeding
- Monitoring administration of total parenteral nutrition

REFER: GO TO MYNURSINGKIT

REFLECT: CASE STUDY

Mr. Michaels is a 75-year-old man with emphysema, asthma, high blood pressure, and almost complete hearing loss. A lifelong smoker, he quit smoking a few years ago when he was diagnosed with emphysema. For some time, he has been on oxygen therapy at night. He takes several medications daily, including 10 mg of prednisone, a corticosteroid inhaler, albuterol by nebulizer, and high-blood-pressure medication with a diuretic.

Two days ago, Mr. Michaels felt sick and was running a temperature. Mrs. Michaels, his wife, took him to his primary care provider's office where he was diagnosed with an upper respiratory infection and sent home with an oral antibiotic. Mr. Michaels woke up in the middle of the night in respiratory distress. Mrs. Michaels called 911, and Bobby was transported by ambulance to the emergency department, where he is diagnosed with pneumonia and acute respiratory distress syndrome. Bobby is placed on mechanical ventilation and admitted to the critical care unit.

1. What are the nursing priorities for Bobby?
2. What considerations need to be given to Bobby related to his hearing loss?
3. What factors are likely to exacerbate his respiratory function?
4. How can you promote oxygenation for this client?

21.2 ASTHMA

KEY TERMS

Airway remodeling, *1252*
Airway resistance, *1253*
Asthma, *1252*
Edema, *1253*
Hyperresponsiveness, *1253*
Hyperventilation, *1253*
Orthopneic position, *1264*
Retractions, *1254*
Status asthmaticus, *1253*

BASIS FOR SELECTION OF EXEMPLAR

Centers for Disease Control and Prevention
Healthy People 2010
Institute of Medicine

LEARNING OUTCOMES

After reading about this exemplar, you will be able to:

1. Describe the pathophysiology, etiology, clinical manifestations, and direct and indirect causes of asthma.
2. Identify risk factors associated with asthma.
3. Illustrate the nursing process in providing culturally competent care across the life span for individuals with asthma.
4. Formulate priority nursing diagnoses appropriate for an individual with asthma.
5. Create a plan of care for individuals with asthma and their family members.
6. Assess expected outcomes for an individual with asthma.
7. Discuss therapies used in the collaborative care of an individual with asthma.
8. Employ evidence-based caring interventions for an individual with asthma.

OVERVIEW

Asthma is a chronic inflammatory disease of the lungs characterized by recurrent episodes of wheezing, breathlessness, chest tightness, and coughing. While most episodes or asthma "attacks" are relatively brief, some clients with asthma may experience longer episodes with some degree of airway impairment daily. Mild, brief episodes may resolve spontaneously, but most asthma attacks require treatment. Asthma in early life may lead to an irreversible decline of pulmonary function in adulthood, as it can cause permanent, structural changes called **airway remodeling**. These changes can result in progressive or permanent loss of lung function.

PATHOPHYSIOLOGY AND ETIOLOGY

In asthma, the airways are in a persistent state of inflammation. During symptom-free periods, airway inflammation in asthma is subacute or quiet. Even during these periods, however, inflammatory cells, such as eosinophils, neutrophils, and lymphocytes, may be found in airway tissues, and

edema (swelling caused by excess fluid in bodily tissue) may be present.

An acute inflammatory response, during which resident inflammatory cells interact with inflammatory mediators, cytokines, and additional infiltrating inflammatory cells, may be triggered by a variety of factors. Common triggers for an acute asthma attack include exposure to allergens, respiratory tract infection, exercise, inhaled irritants, and emotional upsets. The inflammatory response resulting from exposure to one of these triggers leads to bronchoconstriction, airway edema, and impaired clearance of secretions. Airway narrowing limits airflow and increases the work of breathing; trapped air mixes with inhaled air, impairing gas exchange.

When a trigger such as inhalation of an allergen or irritant occurs, an acute or early response develops in the airways. The airways of clients with asthma are hyperreactive and predisposed to bronchospasm. Sensitized mast cells in the bronchial mucosa release inflammatory mediators, such as histamine, prostaglandins, and leukotrienes. Resident and infiltrating inflammatory cells also produce inflammatory mediators, such as cytokines, bradykinin, and growth factors. These mediators stimulate parasympathetic receptors and bronchial smooth muscle to produce bronchoconstriction. They also increase capillary permeability, which allows plasma to escape and leads to mucosal edema. Production of mucus is stimulated; excess mucus collects in the narrowed airways.

The asthma attack is prolonged by the late-phase response, which develops 4–12 hours after exposure to the trigger. Inflammatory cells, such as basophils and eosinophils, are activated, and they damage airway epithelium, produce mucosal edema, impair mucociliary clearance, and produce or prolong bronchoconstriction. The degree of hyperreactivity depends on the extent of inflammation. Together, bronchoconstriction, edema, and mucous secretion narrow the airway. Airway resistance increases, limiting airflow and increasing the work of breathing (Figure 21–29 ■).

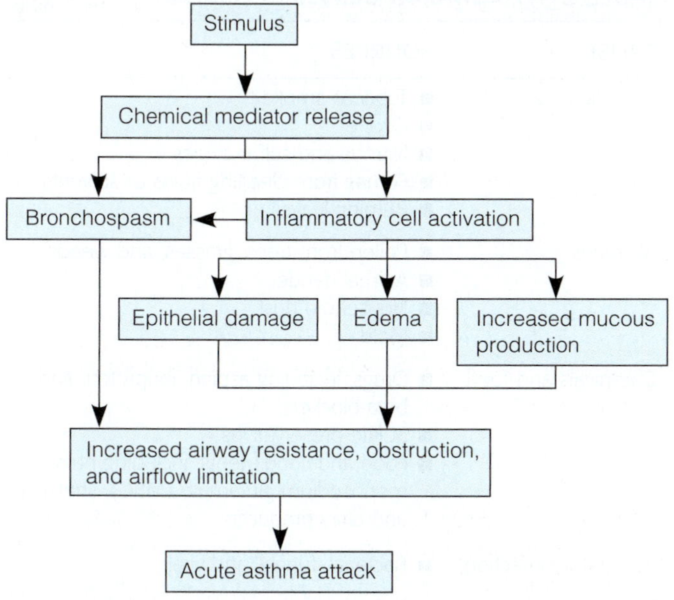

Figure 21–29 ■ Pathogenesis of an acute episode of asthma.

If an asthma attack goes untreated, limited expiratory airflow traps air distal to the spastic, narrowed airways. Trapped air mixes with inspired air in the alveoli, reducing oxygen tension and gas exchange across the alveolar-capillary membrane. Blood flow is reduced, further affecting gas exchange. As a result, hypoxemia develops. Hypoxemia and increased lung volume caused by trapping stimulate the respiratory rate. **Hyperventilation** (unusually fast respiration, or overbreathing) causes the $PaCO_2$ (the amount of pressure exerted by dissolved carbon dioxide) to fall, leading to respiratory alkalosis. (See Concept 1 for more information about acid–base imbalances.)

To summarize, in an acute asthma attack, inflammatory mediators are released from sensitized airways, causing activation of inflammatory cells. This progression leads to bronchoconstriction, airway edema, and impaired mucociliary clearance. Airway narrowing limits airflow and increases the work of breathing; trapped air mixes with inhaled air, impairing gas exchange.

Etiology

Asthma triggered by allergies accounts for as much as 50% of asthma attacks in the United States. Common allergens that can cause airway inflammation include pollens, weeds, molds, dust mites, and animal dander. Allergic asthma is an alteration of type I hypersensitivity, which is explained in more detail in Concept 14, Immunity.

Asthma may occur from exposure to aspirin and other nonsteroidal drugs. It may result from exercise, cold or hot air, viral infections, and even stress. Genetic involvement seems to be a component, but the role played by genetics in asthma is not clear. Occupational asthma arises from exposure to respiratory irritants in the workplace.

In an individual with asthma, any combination of these stimuli may result in airway **hyperresponsiveness** (an exaggerated bronchoconstrictor response) and airway obstruction from overproduction of mucus and edema of the airway mucosa (Figure 21–30 ■). **Status asthmaticus** is a severe, prolonged form of asthma that is difficult to treat. Untreated asthma or asthma that is unresponsive to treatment is a medical emergency that can result in respiratory failure.

According to the American Academy of Allergy, Asthma, and Immunology (2007), asthma affects some 5 million children in the United States, making it the most common serious chronic childhood illness. Overall, asthma affects some 20 million Americans, resulting in millions of lost work days each year, either for adult clients with asthma or for parents staying home with asthmatic children (American Academy of Allergy, Asthma, and Immunology, 2009).

PEDIATRIC DIFFERENCES The child's narrower airway causes a greater increase in **airway resistance** (the effort or force needed to move oxygen through the trachea to the

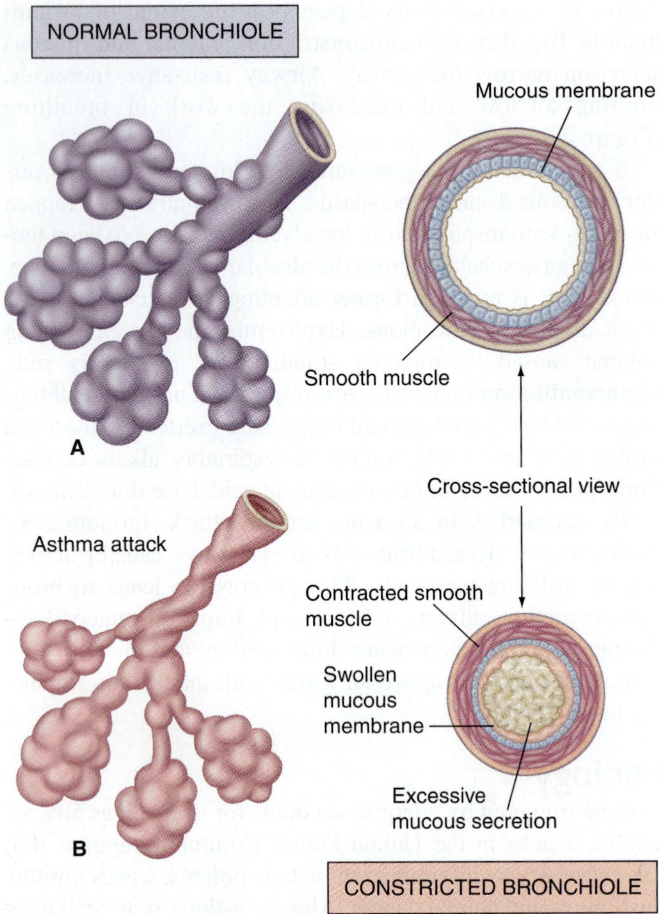

Figure 21–30 ■ Changes in bronchioles during an asthma attack. *A*, Normal bronchiole. *B*, In asthma attack.

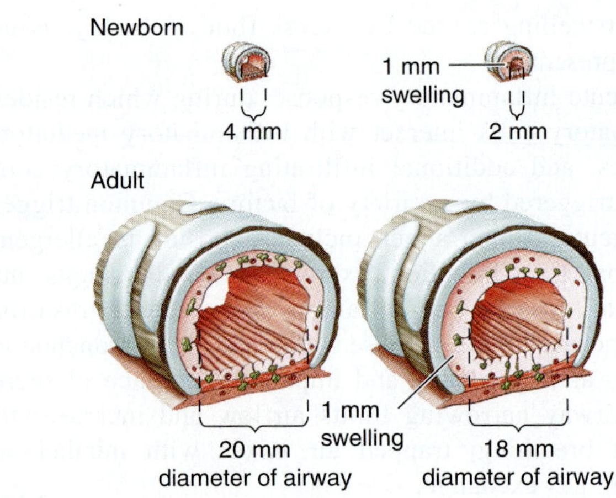

Figure 21–31 ■ Differences in airway diameter.

lungs). As air moves from the child's nares down the trachea to the distal airways (alveoli), it must flow through a relatively small area. Friction and increasing resistance are generated as air passes through the airway. When edema and swelling of the trachea occur in response to a virus, bacterium, or other irritant, the airway is further narrowed, and air is inspired more quickly to maintain oxygenation status (Figure 21–31 ■). The resulting negative pressure in the airway draws tissues closer together, further narrowing the airway and increasing airway resistance.

Children under 6 years of age use the diaphragm to breathe, because the intercostal muscles are immature. By 6 years of age, the child uses the intercostal muscles more effectively. The ribs are primarily cartilage and very flexible. In cases of respiratory distress, the negative pressure caused by movement of the diaphragm draws the chest wall inward, causing **retractions** (sunken areas seen between the ribs during inspiration). See Figure 21–32 ■ for sites of retractions associated with respiratory distress.

Oxygen consumption is higher in children than in adults because of their greater metabolic rate. This rate of oxygen consumption increases when the child is in respiratory distress. The child also has fewer muscle glycogen reserves, leading to more rapid muscle fatigue when accessory muscles must be used for breathing (Froh, 2006).

RISK FACTORS

Risk factors include genetic factors, exposure to certain infections early in life, air pollution, and allergies (Table 21–8). Early childhood exposure to respiratory syncytial virus (RSV), parainfluenza virus, adenovirus, mycoplasma, and chlamydia has been associated with the development of asthma. Atmospheric air can be polluted by ozone, industrial gaseous wastes, and particulate matter, such as pollens or tobacco smoke. Obesity, maternal smoking, and premature birth also increase the risk for asthma.

TABLE 21–8 **Common Causes of Asthma**

CAUSE	SOURCES
Air pollutants	■ Tobacco smoke ■ Ozone ■ Nitrous and sulfur oxides ■ Fumes from cleaning fluids or solvents ■ Burning leaves
Allergens	■ Pollen from trees, grasses, and weeds ■ Animal dander ■ Household dust ■ Mold
Chemicals and food	■ Drugs, including aspirin, ibuprofen, and beta-blockers ■ Sulfite preservatives ■ Food and condiments, including nuts, monosodium glutamate (MSG), shellfish, and dairy products
Respiratory infections	■ Bacterial, fungal, and viral
Stress	■ Emotional stress/anxiety ■ Exercise in dry, cold climates

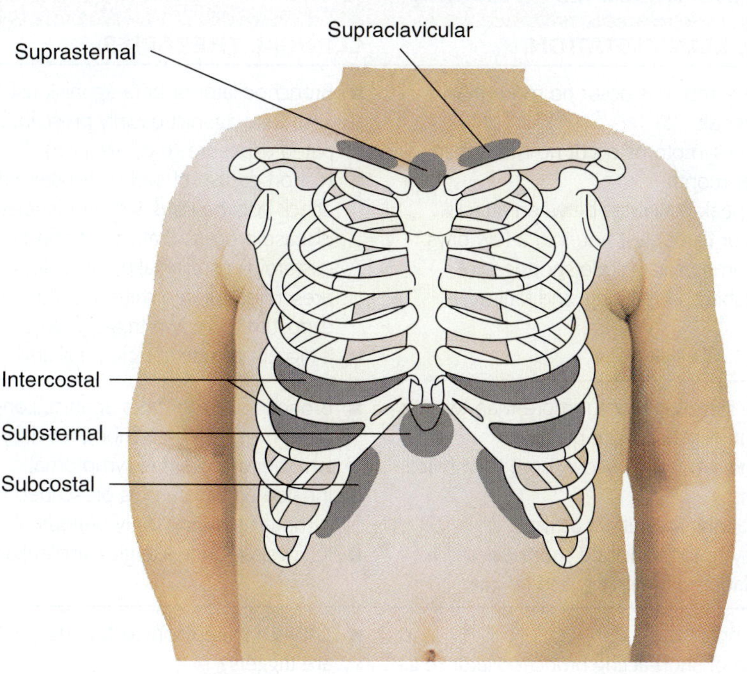

Figure 21–32 ■ Retraction sites.

CLINICAL MANIFESTATIONS

Clinical manifestations of asthma include coughing, wheezing, shortness of breath, chest tightness, tachypnea and tachycardia, and anxiety and apprehension. Asthma is defined by severity and control as well as by the frequency of exacerbations. Asthma that is not well controlled is evident by daytime symptoms, nocturnal awakenings because of symptoms, frequent use of a short acting beta agonist (SABA), and inability or difficulty performing normal activities, including exercise.

The onset of symptoms may be either abrupt or insidious, and an attack may subside rapidly or persist for hours or days. During an attack, tachycardia, tachypnea, and prolonged expiration are common. Diffuse wheezing may be heard on auscultation. With more severe attacks, use of accessory muscles for respirations, retractions, loud wheezing, and distant breaths sounds may be noted. Fatigue, anxiety, apprehension, and severe dyspnea that allows speaking only one or two words between breaths may occur with persistent severe episodes. The onset of respiratory failure is marked by inaudible breath sounds with reduced wheezing and an ineffective cough. Without careful assessment, this apparent relief of symptoms can be misinterpreted as improvement.

The frequency of attacks and the severity of symptoms vary greatly from person to person. Although some people have infrequent, mild episodes, or flares, others have nearly continuous manifestations.

Certain audible manifestations may offer a clue as to the location of airway obstruction. Table 21–9 lists the signs associated with obstructions in various locations of the airway.

TABLE 21–9 **Clinical Manifestations of Airway Obstructions in Different Locations**

LOCATION OF AIRWAY OBSTRUCTION	CLINICAL MANIFESTATION
Nasopharyngeal obstruction, enlarged tonsils or adenoids	Sonorous snoring
Partially obstructed upper airway (in or above the larynx, and upper trachea)	Inspiratory stridor
Obstruction of the mid to lower trachea and central bronchus	Expiratory stridor or wheeze, croupy or low-pitched cough
Fixed obstruction at site of larynx or subglottic space	Inspiratory and expiratory stridor
Obstructed vocal cords	Hoarseness, weak cry

Source: Data from Froh, D. K. (2006). Alterations in pulmonary function in children. In K. L. McCance & S. E. Huether (Eds.), *Pathophysiology: The biologic basis for disease in adults and children* (5th ed., p. 1252). St. Louis, MO: Mosby.

CLINICAL MANIFESTATIONS AND THERAPIES Asthma

SEVERITY	CLINICAL MANIFESTATION	CLINICAL THERAPIES
Mild intermittent	■ Daytime symptoms occur no more than twice a week. ■ Nighttime symptoms occur no more than twice per month. ■ Normal peak flow rates between attacks. ■ Attacks (or flares) last hours to a few days. ■ Typical symptoms include shortness of breath, labored breathing, and fatigue.	■ Bronchodilator or beta-agonist, usually via inhaler or nebulizer. Beta-agonist usually prescribed for use before anticipated exposure (e.g., exercise). ■ A short course of oral corticosteroids may be prescribed if attack lasts beyond 1 day or is related to infection or other disease process that may extend recovery time. Inhaled corticosteroids usually take a few days to work and may not be prescribed for intermittent asthma except during periods of exposure to known triggers (e.g., ragweed). ■ If triggers include allergies, oral antihistamine may be prescribed.
Mild persistent	■ Daytime symptoms occur more than twice a week but less than once per day. ■ Nighttime symptoms occur more than twice a month. ■ Exacerbations may affect activity. ■ Typical symptoms include shortness of breath, labored breathing, and fatigue.	■ Bronchodilator or beta-agonist. Long-acting beta-agonist (LABA) may be prescribed for daily use regardless of whether the client is symptomatic. ■ Inhaled corticosteroids prescribed for daily use to prevent symptoms during likely periods of exacerbation. ■ If triggers include allergies, antileukotrienes may be prescribed.
Moderate persistent	■ Daily symptoms. ■ Daily use of short-acting bronchodilator (e.g., albuterol inhaler). ■ Nighttime symptoms occur more than once a week. ■ Exacerbations may last for days. ■ Exacerbations affect activity. ■ Symptoms of exacerbations include shortness of breath, labored and painful breathing, and chest tightness; may include coughing, wheezing, tachypnea, tachycardia, and fatigue.	■ LABAs, inhaled corticosteroids, antileukotrienes (if allergies are triggers). ■ Immunotherapy may be tried if triggers include allergies. ■ Cromolyn sodium or theophylline (long-acting bronchodilators) may be prescribed. ■ A nebulizer may be prescribed for use during exacerbations. ■ Oral corticosteroids may be prescribed for use during exacerbations lasting more than 1–2 days.
Severe persistent	■ Continuous symptoms occur with frequent exacerbations. ■ Limited physical activity. ■ Symptoms include shortness of breath, labored and painful breathing, chest tightness, coughing, wheezing, tachypnea, tachycardia, difficulty speaking without pausing for breathing, and extreme fatigue.	■ LABA inhalers, inhaled corticosteroids, antileukotriene (if allergies are triggers). ■ Immunotherapy may be tried if triggers include allergies. ■ Cromolyn sodium or theophylline (long-acting bronchodilators) may be prescribed. ■ Oral corticosteroids may be prescribed for use during exacerbations lasting more than 1–2 days. ■ Steroids and beta-agonists delivered via nebulizer may be prescribed and used daily. ■ Steroid-dependent asthmatics with high IgE scores who do not receive relief from immunotherapy may be prescribed omalizulab (Xolair).

Disease Monitoring

Severity of asthma symptoms can be difficult for the client to describe and for the nurse to assess. A method of monitoring the disease using the peak expiratory flow reading (PEFR) provides an objective measure of lung function that allows clients to monitor symptoms and communicate their severity to others. Using small, inexpensive PEFR meters, clients take readings at varying times of day over several weeks to establish their personal best or normal PEFR. This value is then used to evaluate the severity of the airway obstruction. Traffic colors are used for simplicity: Green (80–100% of personal best) indicates asthma that is under control; yellow (50–80%) is caution, indicating a need for medication or treatment; and red (≤50%) signals an immediate need for a bronchodilator and further medical treatment if the level does not return to the yellow range immediately following administration of the bronchodilator.

Preventive Measures

Asthma attacks often can be prevented by avoiding allergies and environmental triggers. Modifying the home environment by controlling dust, removing carpets, covering mattresses and pillows to reduce dust mite populations, and installing air-filtering

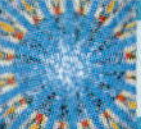

FOCUS ON DIVERSITY AND CULTURE Asthma Management

Asthma occurs in all racial and ethnic groups, but these groups differ in the use of preventive medications for asthma. A recent study investigated these disparities and found a difference in preventive medications used for asthma. Findings also revealed that differences in health beliefs, fear of steroids, or communication issues rather than financial barriers may play a role in the use of preventive asthma medications (Lieu et al., 2002). Learn about the family's cultural beliefs and practices. Parents of children from different cultures may have concerns about daily medication regimens. Individualize care through education based on "an assessment of the child's and family's resources, health care beliefs, access to health care services, and management styles" (Swartz, Cantey-Banasiak, & Meadows-Oliver, 2005).

systems may be useful. Pets may need to be removed from the household. Stuffed animals provide wonderful living spaces for dust mites and should be removed from bedrooms. Eliminating all tobacco smoke in the house is vital. Wearing a mask that retains humidity and warm air while exercising in cold weather may help prevent attacks of exercise-induced or cold-triggered asthma. Early treatment of respiratory infections is vital to prevent exacerbations.

The client with moderate or severe asthma who is prescribed controller medications to prevent asthma attacks must take these daily in order for the medicine to be effect. Compliance with medication regimens varies greatly among those with asthma, as some will stop taking the medication once they've started feeling better, increasing the likelihood of another asthma attack. Client teaching about prevention must include the issue of compliance with medication regimens.

Asthma in Children

An asthma attack can be frightening for both the child and the parent. Asthma interferes with a child's ability to sleep, concentrate in school, and play, causing multiple frustrations for both the child and the family. An understanding by parents of how, when, and why to give children their medications is crucial to the child's asthma management. The nurse plays an essential role by taking time to understand the parents' understanding of their child's asthma management and by providing important client teaching regarding use of asthma medications and avoidance of triggers.

Children with asthma should have written asthma action plans that both parents and caregivers (including classroom teachers) can follow. Action plans ensure that medications are given in a timely manner without risk of overdose, and they ensure successful outcomes for the child and family.

If a child with asthma has a parent or caregiver who smokes, that person should be made aware of the danger secondhand smoke poses to those with asthma. Nurses should provide parents and caregivers with information about smoking cessation programs and therapies available in their area. Additional resources for parents can be found at the following websites:

- American Academy of Allergy, Asthma, and Immunology: http://www.aaaai.org
- Allergy and Asthma Network: Mothers of Asthmatics: http://www.aanma.org

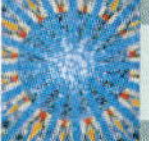

EVIDENCE-BASED PRACTICE Improving Asthma Management

Clinical Question

Many children with asthma have less-than-optimal medication management to control their symptoms and have increased asthma episodes. What information regarding the family's knowledge and perceptions about managing the child with asthma could help nurses collaborate more effectively with families to improve asthma management?

Evidence

Recent research on parental beliefs, knowledge, experience of living with a child who has asthma, and attitudes about controller medication was conducted through interviews with 18 mothers of children and adolescents with asthma. Parents indicated that they learned to manage the child's asthma through "trial and error." Even though they learned about medications one at a time, they still had gaps in knowledge about medication actions. Parents also wished to have health professionals listen to them regarding their child's health care needs. The parents reported that daily medication management was the most difficult aspect of asthma care, but they saw a good response in the child when it was used (Peterson-Sweeney, McMullen, Yoos, & Kitzman, 2003).

Another study involving the parents of 109 children with asthma explored their attitudes and understanding of asthma. Only 27 of the 78 children with persistent asthma had an appropriate medication regimen, and 17 parents reported using no anti-inflammatory medication even when the child had moderate to severe asthma. Some parents believed inhaled steroids should be a last-resort therapy or that if steroids were used for a while, they would not work when needed. These parents also anticipated that their children would have activity limitations and episodic emergency department visits (Yoos, Kitzman, & McMullen, 2003).

Best Practice

Demonstrating respect for the parent's knowledge of the child's health status and response to asthma management is an essential step in developing an effective partnership with the parent. It is also important to talk with parents regarding their beliefs about daily medications for asthma management, use of inhaled steroids, and their expectations of how asthma will affect their child. Gaining an understanding of the family's beliefs can help guide nursing education and collaborative development of a plan to manage the child's asthma.

Critical Thinking

Consider the possible perceptions and beliefs of parents and children with asthma in your practice setting. Develop an education program that integrates these beliefs and perceptions to help improve families' understanding of medication actions, the differences between inhaled and oral corticosteroids, and collaboration with health professionals to improve the control of their child's asthma.

Asthma and Pregnancy

Asthma is the most common respiratory disease found in pregnancy; it complicates 1–4% of all pregnancies (Davidson, Doyle, & Ramin, 2005). During pregnancy, in approximately one third of clients with asthma, their asthma improves; in one third, it remains unchanged; and in the remaining one third, the conditions worsens. The highest incidence of exacerbation occurs between 24 and 36 weeks of gestation. Asthma is often dormant during labor and birth, but PEFR should be monitored to detect changes in maternal respiratory status (Davidson et al., 2005).

Prematurity and low birth weight are more common among infants of women who have asthma (Dombrowski, 2006). Asthma has also been linked with higher rates of hyperemesis gravidarum, preeclampsia, uterine hemorrhage, and perinatal mortality. The goal of therapy is to prevent maternal exacerbations, because even a mild exacerbation can cause severe hypoxia-related complications in the fetus. If an exacerbation occurs, it should be managed in the same way as for a nonpregnant woman, because the asthma drugs used are less of a threat to the fetus than a serious asthma attack (Davidson et al., 2005).

Caring for a woman who is pregnant and has asthma calls for a multidisciplinary effort. If the client is not already in the care of a pulmonologist, the nurse should make a referral. The nurse should encourage the client to talk with the pulmonologist about a stepwise action plan so that the client knows what to do in the event of an exacerbation. The nurse should encourage the client to use her peak flow meter daily as a method of monitoring her condition.

COLLABORATION

Respiratory therapists are often essential members of the health care team caring for the client with asthma. The role of the nurse is discussed in more detail in the nursing process section.

Diagnostic Tests

An important diagnostic tool for a client with persistent asthma is the peak expiratory flow reading (PEFR). Nurses should encourage all clients to use their peak flow meters daily and to keep a log recording their readings, even on days when they are in the green zone (80–100% of personal best). Nurses should remind clients with persistent asthma of this at each health care interaction.

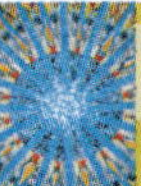

DEVELOPMENTAL CONSIDERATIONS

Children With Asthma

Growing children will have gradually increasing peak flow readings as their lungs grow and they exhale larger volumes of air with each breath. Daily use of peak flow monitors is particularly important in pediatric clients in order to track baseline or "normal" expiratory flow. Baseline should be reestablished as recommended by the physician.

For clients who are suspected of having allergic asthma, scratch or patch testing and IgE testing allow the physician to determine the severity of the client's allergies as well as specific triggers to which the client reacts. Allergy testing normally is available only through an allergist or immunologist and is described in more detail in Concept 14, Immunity.

Other diagnostic tests that may be useful for the client with asthma are described in more detail in Appendix B and may include the following:

- CBC with differential if infection is suspected
- ABG to monitor acid–base balance
- Pulmonary function studies
- CXR
- Oxygen saturation monitoring
- Transcutaneous oxygen and carbon dioxide monitoring.

Pharmacologic Therapy

Medications are used to prevent and control asthma symptoms, reduce the frequency and severity of exacerbations, and reverse airway obstruction. Drugs used for long-term control of asthma are taken daily to maintain control of the disease. The primary drugs in this group are anti-inflammatory agents, short-acting and long-acting bronchodilators, and leukotriene modifiers. Quick-relief medications provide prompt relief of bronchoconstriction and airflow obstruction with associated wheezing, cough, and chest tightness. Short-acting adrenergic stimulants (rapid-acting bronchodilators), anticholinergic drugs, and methylxanthines fall into this category.

A stepwise approach for managing asthma is recommended. This approach is based on the severity of disease (Table 21–10). For all clients, an inhaled SABA is recommended for quick relief of acute symptoms. Up to three treatments at 20-minute

TABLE 21–10 Stepwise Approach to Asthma Management for Adults

STEP/DISEASE SEVERITY	PREFERRED TREATMENT	ALTERNATE OR AS NEEDED TREATMENT
Step 1: mild intermittent	No daily medication needed	Systemic corticosteroids for severe exacerbations
Step 2: mild persistent	Low-dose inhaled corticosteroids	Cromolyn, leukotriene modifier, nedocromil, or sustained-release theophylline
Step 3: moderate persistent	Low-to-moderate dose inhaled corticosteroids *and* long-acting inhaled β_2 – agonist	Increase inhaled corticosteroid dose *or* combine inhaled corticosteroid with leukotriene modifier or theophylline
Step 4: severe persistent	High-dose inhaled corticosteroid *and* long-acting inhaled β_2 – agonist	Add systemic corticosteroid

Source: Adapted from *Expert Panel Report 2: Guidelines for the Diagnosis and Management of Asthma, Update on Selected Topics 2002,* Publication No. 02-5074 by National Education and Prevention Program, 2003, Bethesda, MD: National Institutes of Health.

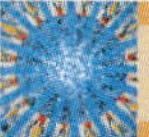

CLIENT TEACHING Using a Metered-Dose or Dry Powder Inhaler

- Firmly insert a charged metered-dose inhaler canister into the mouthpiece unit or spacer (if used).
- Remove mouthpiece cap. Shake canister vigorously for 3–5 seconds.
- Exhale slowly and completely.
- Holding the canister upside down, place the mouthpiece in the mouth, closing lips around it if a spacer is being used. When no spacer is used, hold the mouthpiece directly in front of the mouth.
- Press and hold the canister down while inhaling deeply and slowly for 3–5 seconds (see Figure 21–33 ■).
- Hold breath for 10 seconds, release pressure on the container, remove from mouth, and exhale. Wait 20–30 seconds before repeating the procedure for a second puff.
- Rinse the mouth after using the inhaler to minimize systemic absorption and drying of the mucous membranes.
- Rinse the inhaler mouthpiece and spacer after use; store in a clean location.

DRY POWDER INHALER

- Keep the inhaler and medication in a clean, dry location. Do not refrigerate or store in a humid place (for example, the bathroom).
- Remove the cap and hold the inhaler upright. Inspect to be sure that the mechanism is clean and the mouthpiece is clear.
- If necessary, load the dose into the inhaler, following manufacturer's directions.
- Hold the inhaler level with the mouthpiece end facing down.
- Breathe slowly and completely. Tilt your head back slightly.
- Place the mouthpiece in your mouth with your teeth over the mouthpiece. Seal your lips around the mouthpiece. Do not block the inhaler with your tongue.
- Breathe in rapidly and deeply through your mouth over 2–3 seconds to activate the flow of medication.
- Remove the inhaler from your mouth and hold your breath for 10 seconds.
- Exhale slowly through pursed lips to allow the medication to enter distal airways. Never exhale into the inhaler mouthpiece to prevent clogging.
- Rinse your mouth or brush your teeth after using the inhaler to avoid a bad taste from the medication and to prevent a yeast infection (if a corticosteroid medication is being used).
- Store the inhaler in a clean, sealed plastic bag; do not wash the inhaler unless so directed by the manufacturer. The mouthpiece should be cleaned weekly using a dry cloth.

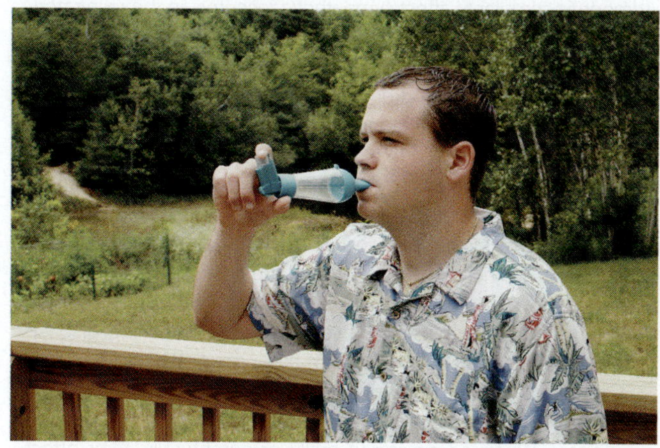

Figure 21–33 ■ Proper use of a metered-dose inhaler.

Source: Michal Heron, Pearson Education/PH College.

intervals or a single nebulizer treatment may be used as needed. Strategies for long-term control may need to be modified if a short-acting bronchodilator is needed more than twice a week (NHLBI, 2003).

Many of the drugs used for continued asthma management and relief of an acute attack can be administered by a metered-dose inhaler (MDI), dry powder inhaler (DPI), or nebulizer. The advantages of administering medications locally by inhalation include rapid onset and reduced systemic effects. In an MDI, a chemical propellant is used to deliver the medication when the canister is depressed. In contrast, a DPI contains no propellant. Instead, the medication is released by inhaling rapidly through the mouthpiece.

BRONCHODILATORS Most clients with asthma need bronchodilator therapy to relieve bronchoconstriction by relaxing the smooth muscles of the airway. Inhalation of nebulized medication is the preferred means of administration.

The primary bronchodilators used include adrenergic stimulants, methylxanthines, and anticholinergic agents. These drugs often are administered in combination with an anti-inflammatory agent. Adrenergic stimulants (beta$_2$-agonists) affect receptors on smooth muscle cells of the respiratory tract, causing smooth muscle relaxation and bronchodilation. Long-acting adrenergic stimulants, such as inhaled salmeterol and oral sustained-release albuterol, are used in conjunction with anti-inflammatory drugs to control symptoms but are not appropriate to treat an acute episode of asthma. Inhaled SABAs, such as albuterol, bitolterol, pirbuterol, and terbutaline, administered by MDI or DPI, are the treatment of choice for quick relief. They act within minutes, but their duration generally is short, lasting only 4–6 hours. Tachycardia and muscle tremors (common side effects of adrenergic agonists) are minimal with inhalation therapy.

Anticholinergic medications prevent bronchoconstriction by blocking parasympathetic input to bronchial smooth muscle. Ipratropium bromide, an anticholinergic drug administered by MDI, is useful when asthma symptoms are poorly controlled by adrenergic stimulants alone. Anticholinergic drugs act more slowly than adrenergic stimulants, requiring as much as 60–90 minutes to achieve maximal effect.

Theophylline is a methylxanthine used as adjunctive treatment for asthma. It relaxes bronchial smooth muscle and may also inhibit the release of chemical mediators of the inflammatory response. Regular monitoring of serum theophylline levels is necessary because of wide individual variations in metabolism and elimination of the drug and its toxic effects. Serum levels of 10–20 mcg/mL or lower are recommended. Theophylline may

Box 21–3 Medication Administration: Asthma

ADRENERGIC STIMULANTS

Epinephrine
Isoproterenol (Isuprel)
Metaproterenol (Alupent, Metaprel)
Terbutaline (Brethaire, Brethine)
Isoetharine (Bronkosol, Bronkometer)
Albuterol (Proventil, Ventolin)
Bitolterol (Tornalate)
Pirbuterol (Maxair)
Salmeterol (Serevent)
Formoterol (Foradil)
Combination products: albuterol/ipratropium (Combivent); salmeterol/fluticasone (Advair)

Adrenergic stimulants affect sympathetic receptors in the respiratory tract. Administered by metered-dose inhalers or dry powder inhalers, these drugs are the treatment of choice for acute bronchial asthma. Nearly all of the drugs in this class (epinephrine and isoproterenol being the exceptions) selectively activate β_2 – receptors at the doses typically used to treat asthma. β_2 – receptors activation results in smooth muscle relaxation and bronchodilation. Formoterol and salmeterol are highly selective to β_2 – receptors, resulting in fewer adverse effects. Formoterol and salmeterol have been shown to increase the risk of serious asthma exacerbations and death, however. The U.S. Food and Drug Administration (FDA, 2005b) recommends using these drugs only when the disease cannot be adequately controlled with other medications.

Oral forms of adrenergic agonists may be used for prophylaxis but are not effective in treating an acute attack because of their slow onset. When administered orally or parenterally, their effect on sympathetic nervous system receptors can produce undesirable side effects such as nervousness, irritability, tachycardia, and cardiac dysrhythmias.

Nursing Responsibilities

- Use with caution in clients with hypertension, cardiovascular disease or dysrhythmias, hyperthyroidism, or diabetes.
- When given to a client who is hypoxemic and acidotic, these drugs may cause potentially dangerous cardiac stimulation.
- When given by MDI, wait 1–2 minutes between puffs to allow airways to dilate, permitting the second dose to reach distal airways.
- Observe for desired effect of reduced dyspnea and wheezing. Central nervous system stimulation (anxiety, irritability, and insomnia) and tremor are common side effects.

Health Education for the Client and Family

- Use the prescribed inhaler or nebulizer as directed.
- If you are taking a bronchodilator along with another medication by inhalation, use the bronchodilator first to open airways and enhance the effectiveness of the second medication.
- Rinse the mouth after using inhalers to reduce systemic absorption of the medication.
- Keep a log to track your bronchodilator use. If the drug becomes less effective, or if you need a higher dosage or more frequent doses than prescribed, contact your physician.
- Report palpitations, irregular pulse, and other side effects to the physician.

METHYLXANTHINES

Theophylline (Bronkotabs, Quibron, Slo-Phyllin Theolair, Theo-Dur, others)
Aminophylline (Somophyllin)

The methylxanthines are central nervous system (CNS) stimulants chemically related to caffeine. These drugs produce bronchodilation through relaxation of bronchial smooth muscle. As CNS stimulants, they produce adverse effects such as nervousness, insomnia, and tremors. When administered in large doses, convulsions may result. Once the drugs of choice for preventing and treating asthma attacks, they are now used primarily to prevent nocturnal asthma in affected adult clients. Theophylline has a narrow margin of safety and high potential for toxicity. Because the metabolism and excretion of theophylline vary significantly from person to person—affected by such factors as age, smoking, genetic factors, alcoholism, and other chronic diseases—monitoring of serum levels is vital.

Nursing Responsibilities

- The therapeutic blood level for theophylline is 10–20 mcg/mL.
- Monitor for manifestations of toxicity. Anorexia, nausea, vomiting, restlessness, insomnia, cardiac dysrhythmias, and seizures are early manifestations. Other manifestations include epigastric pain, hematemesis, diarrhea, headache, irritability, muscle twitching, palpitations, tachycardia, flushing, and circulatory failure.
- Administer with meals or a full glass of water or milk to minimize gastric irritation.
- Monitor effect closely when administering concurrently with other medications such as barbiturates, anticonvulsants, thyroid hormone, beta blockers, bronchodilators, and others.
- Aminophylline is incompatible with many other intravenous drugs. Use a separate line or flush the line with normal saline before and after administering any other preparation.

Health Education for the Client and Family

- Oral methylxanthines are ineffective to treat an acute asthma attack; do not delay other treatment by using these drugs.
- Check with the physician before taking any over-the-counter medications or other prescription drugs while on theophylline.
- Do not smoke while using this drug.
- Report adverse effects to the physician.

ANTICHOLINERGICS

Atropine
Ipratropium bromide (Atrovent)
Tiotropium bromide (Spiriva)
Combination products: albuterol/ipratropium (Combivent)

Anticholinergics are potent bronchodilators, blocking muscarinic receptors of the parasympathetic nervous system. Activation of muscarinic receptors produces smooth muscle contraction and bronchoconstriction; blockade of these receptors facilitates smooth muscle relaxation and bronchodilation. Atropine is used infrequently because of its tendency to dry secretions of the mucous membranes and other side effects. Ipratropium and tiotropium bromide are available as inhalers and have fewer side effects than atropine.

Box 21–3 Medication Administration: Asthma (continued)

Nursing Responsibilities

- Assess for possible contraindications to the drug, including hypersensitivity, glaucoma, prostatic hypertrophy, or bladder-neck obstruction.
- Assess for desired and/or adverse effects: improving or worsening symptoms; nausea, vomiting, abdominal cramping, anxiety, dizziness; headache.
- Provide ice chips, fluids, or hard candy to relieve dry mouth.

Health Education for the Client and Family

- To prevent overdose, take no more than the prescribed number of doses per day.
- If the drug becomes less effective over time, notify the physician; an adjustment in dosage may be needed.

CORTICOSTEROIDS

Beclomethasone dipropionate (Vanceril, Beclovent)
Triamcinolone acetonide (Azmacort)
Flunisolide (AeroBid)
Fluticasone propionate (Flovent)
Dexamethasone sodium phosphate (Decadron Phosphate Respihaler)
Combination products: salmeterol/fluticasone (Advair)

The anti-inflammatory effect of corticosteroids helps both prevent and treat acute episodes. Corticosteroids are used to reduce the frequency and severity of asthma attacks and allow reduced dosages of other drugs. The beneficial effects of corticosteroids for asthma result from their ability to decrease the synthesis and release of inflammatory mediators (such as histamine and leukotrienes), reduce inflammatory cell activation and infiltration, and decrease airway edema. Corticosteroids also decrease mucous production in the airways and increase the number and receptivity of β_2 – receptors (Lehne, 2004). The cushingoid side effects of corticosteroids, always a major concern with their use, are minimized when they are inhaled. Note that the combination product salmeterol/fluticasone is associated with an increased risk of serious asthma exacerbations and death. It is a second-line drug, recommended for use only when asthma is inadequately controlled using other preparations (FDA, 2005a).

Nursing Responsibilities

- Administer inhaler doses after bronchodilators to facilitate transit of the medication to distal airways.
- Assess for common side effects: sore throat; hoarseness; and oropharyngeal or laryngeal *Candida albicans* infection.
- Administer antifungal medications or gargles as ordered.

Health Education for the Client and Family

- Rinse the mouth after using the inhaler and maintain good oral hygiene to reduce the risk of fungal infections.
- These medications should not be used to alleviate the symptoms of an acute attack.
- Several weeks of continued therapy may be required before a beneficial effect is noticed.
- Notify the physician if you develop weight gain, fluid retention, muscle weakness, redistribution of fat, or mood changes.

MAST CELL STABILIZERS

Cromolyn sodium (Intal, NasalCrom)
Nedocromil (Tilade)

Cromolyn sodium and nedocromil inhibit inflammatory cells in the airway, blocking early and late responses to inhaled antigens. Both drugs also prevent bronchoconstriction in response to inhaling cold air. These drugs act primarily by stabilizing the cytoplasmic membrane of mast cells, preventing the cells from releasing inflammatory mediators such as histamine (Lehne, 2004). These drugs are used only for preventing asthma attacks, not to treat an acute attack. They are administered by metered-dose inhaler, and have a wide margin of safety. Clients using nedocromil may complain of an unpleasant taste.

Nursing Responsibilities

- Evaluate for potential adverse effects of wheezing and bronchoconstriction.

Health Education for the Client and Family

- Gargling or sipping water can decrease the throat irritation associated with nebulizer treatment.
- Use appropriate technique. Inhale deeply with head tipped back to open airways, hold breath, and then exhale. Repeat until all of the drug has been inhaled.
- These drugs are used only to prevent asthma attacks; they are not effective in treating an acute attack.
- Several weeks may be required before a beneficial effect is noted.

LEUKOTRIENE MODIFIERS

Montelukast (Singulair)
Zafirlukast (Accolate)
Zileuton (Zyflo)

Leukotriene modifiers interfere with the inflammatory process in the airways by suppressing the effects of leukotrienes, a group of inflammatory mediators. Leukotrienes are powerful bronchoconstrictors and vasodilators; blocking their synthesis or their receptors improves airflow, decreases symptoms, and reduces the need for short-acting bronchodilators. They are used for maintenance therapy in adults and children over the age of 12 as an alternative to inhaled corticosteroid therapy. They are not used to treat an acute attack.

Nursing Responsibilities

- Administer at least 1 hour before or 2 hours after meals.
- These drugs inhibit some liver enzymes, affecting the metabolism of warfarin and possibly terfenadine and theophylline. Monitor prothrombin times and theophylline blood levels.
- Monitor liver enzymes, because these drugs may be toxic to the liver.

Health Education for the Client and Family

- Take the drugs as prescribed on an empty stomach.
- Notify the physician if a change in color of stools or urine is noted or if jaundice.

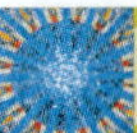

DEVELOPMENTAL CONSIDERATIONS Medication Administration in Children With Asthma

Inhalation is the preferred method of administration for asthma medication, because it rapidly delivers the medication to the lungs for prompt onset of action. Other benefits are reduced risk of adverse effects and lower dosing compared to the oral route. However, inhalers are relatively inefficient and have special challenges for infants and young children. Effective medication delivery to the lung is affected by respiratory rate, degree of airflow obstruction, the medication being administered, and the device being used. Many devices require cooperation, coordination, and appropriate technique (Pongracic, 2003).

- Children older than 5 years usually have the ability to use a metered-dose inhaler (MDI), coordinating medication release and inspiration; however, they may prefer to use a holding chamber or spacer with a valve. Spacers help increase the proportion of particles in the range that can reach the lungs. They also trap larger particles, preventing them from reaching the mouth and being swallowed, which can cause local and systemic side effects. Valves prevent the escape of medication during use. With proper technique, 12–15% of the dose may reach the lower airways. The plastic spacer should be washed with a household detergent and permitted to air dry. This action reduces the electrostatic charge and frees more of the drug for delivery (Meadows-Oliver & Banasiak, 2005). When teaching the child to use an MDI without a spacer, let the child learn to breathe in slowly with straws.
- Spacers have a mouthpiece or mask attachment. When selecting a spacer for infants and children up to 4 years of age, choose one with a mask, because children in this age range tend to be nasal breathers. Choose a mask size that fits the child's face and that has a flexible seal to prevent air from leaking around the facial features. When the young child is uncooperative, it may still be difficult to maintain a seal. Work with young children to improve cooperation for medication delivery using play and distraction. Crying leads to prolonged exhalation and short inspiratory efforts, which reduce lung deposition.
- Some inhaler and spacer brands have a whistle on inhalation that indicates a breath is too fast or too shallow; in others, the whistle signifies an adequate breath has been taken. When teaching the child and family about inhaler use, make sure you know what the whistle means.
- With nebulizers, no coordination of breathing is required, making them easier for young children to use. An added benefit is the humidification provided during treatment. A mask or mouthpiece is used. While nebulizers are not more effective than MDIs with a spacer, they may lead to better outcomes, because the child only needs to breathe in and out normally. Nebulizers should not be used with the mouthpiece held away from the mouth, because lung deposition of the medication is significantly reduced and because this increases the risk of depositing some medication in the eyes (Meadows-Oliver & Banasiak, 2005). Nebulizers are expensive, need a power source, and take 8–10 minutes to complete the treatment. Infants and young children may have difficulty cooperating for the duration of the nebulizer treatment. Crying and a face mask that is too large for the child's face can further decrease delivery of the medication to the lower airways.
- Dry powder inhalers (DPIs) are activated when the client takes a breath, so puffs do not need to be coordinated with inhalation. No spacer is required, and no propellant is used. DPIs can be used by children 5 years and older. Delivery to the lower airway varies between 15 and 30%, depending upon the type of inhaler. Children with severe asthma may not be able to produce enough airflow to get an adequate dose of medication.

Source: Data from Dolovich, M.B., Ahrens, T.C., Hess, D.R., et al. (2005). Device selection and outcomes of aerosol therapy: Evidence-based guidelines. *Chest, 127*, 335–371; Marshik, P.L. (2004). Pharmacologic treatment of pediatric asthma. *Advance for Nurse Practitioners, 12*(3), 35–36, 41–46; Meadows-Oliver, M., & Banasiak, N.C. (2005). Asthma medication delivery devices. *Journal of Pediatric Health Care, 19*(2), 121–123; and Pongracic, J.A. (2003). Asthma delivery devices: Age-appropriate use. *Pediatric Annals, 32*(1), 50–54.

be used as a long-term bronchodilator, given once or twice daily. A related drug, aminophylline, may be administered intravenously to treat an acute, severe exacerbation of the disease.

ANTI-INFLAMMATORY AGENTS Corticosteroids and two nonsteroidal anti-inflammatory agents, cromolyn sodium and nedocromil, are used to suppress airway inflammation and reduce asthma symptoms. Corticosteroids block the late response to inhaled allergens and reduce edema and bronchial hyperresponsiveness. The preferred route of administration is by MDI or DPI to minimize systemic absorption and reduce the many adverse effects of prolonged steroid use (cushingoid effects). For a severe acute attack, corticosteroids may be given systemically to alleviate symptoms and induce remission. Cromolyn sodium and nedocromil are used to prevent acute episodes of asthma. They reduce airway hyperreactivity and inhibit the release of mediator substances. These drugs are used for long-term control of asthma, not quick relief. They have a wide margin of safety and few side effects.

LEUKOTRIENE MODIFIERS The leukotriene modifiers montelukast (Singulair), zafirlukast (Accolate), and zileuton (Zyflo Filmtab) are oral medications that reduce the inflammatory response in clients with asthma. They appear to improve lung function, diminish symptoms, and reduce the need for short-acting bronchodilators. These drugs affect the metabolism and excretion of other medications, such as warfarin and theophylline, and they may cause liver toxicity. Nursing implications for medications used to treat asthma are outlined in the Medication feature.

Complementary Therapy

A number of herbal preparations and other complementary therapies have been shown to be helpful in treating asthma. Dietary therapies, environmental medicine, and nutritional supplements are the complementary therapies most widely recommended by health care professionals (Spencer & Jacobs, 2003).

Nutritional and dietary therapies may include elimination of certain foods or food additives (e.g., sulfite) from the diet, often in the absence of a documented food allergy or relationship between consumption and the onset of asthma symptoms. Although the evidence is inconsistent, some studies suggest that increasing intake of ascorbic acid (an antioxidant), zinc, and magnesium may help alleviate manifestations of asthma.

People with mild asthma may benefit from addition of omega-3 polyunsaturated fatty acids to the diet, experiencing less severe and fewer acute attacks (Spencer & Jacobs, 2003).

Herbal preparations that include *Atropa belladonna* (the natural form of atropine) or ephedra (also called ma huang), an herb that contains ephedrine, should not be used, as they can interact with prescribed medications. Because of the dangers associated with its use, sale of herbal products containing ephedra has been banned (National Center for Complementary and Alternative Medicine, 2004). Advise clients asking about the use of Chinese herbal remedies to treat asthma to inquire if any recommended product contains ma huang or ephedra—and to avoid such products. Capsaicin also may relieve acute asthma symptoms. Other herbal preparations include quercetin and grape seed extract. Refer clients interested in using natural preparations to a qualified herbalist, and emphasize the importance of talking to the physician before using these preparations along with conventional treatment.

In addition to herbals, other complementary therapies, such as biofeedback, yoga, breathing techniques, acupuncture, homeopathy, and massage have been found to alleviate or help control asthma symptoms.

NURSING PROCESS

The immediate priority for nursing care is to help the client maintain oxygenation and a patent airway. The long-term goal of care is to improve an individual's ability to function, ability to participate in ADLs and exercise, and ultimately, quality of life.

Assessment

Assessment of the client experiencing an acute asthma attack must be very focused and timely. Collect assessment data through the health history and physical assessment:

- *Health history.* Current symptoms, including chest tightness, shortness of breath, dyspnea; duration of current attack; measures used to relieve symptoms and their effect; identified precipitating factors for the attack; frequency of attacks; current medications; and known allergies
- *Physical examination.* Apparent level of distress; color; vital signs; respiratory rate and excursion; breath sounds throughout lung fields; apical pulse.

During the physical examination, the nurse also auscultates lung sounds, inspects and palpates the chest for symmetry, and assesses for use of accessory muscles, which indicates an increased need for oxygen at the alveolar level. In addition, the nurse assesses for thickness of pulmonary secretions (thinned secretions are easier to expectorate than thick mucus) and for tobacco use. The nurse also observes the position or posturing of the individual. Self-posturing (e.g., a child may take a tripod stance) may indicate respiratory distress.

During the health history, the nurse also assesses how effectively asthma is being controlled through how often exacerbation of symptoms requires use of SABA and how often the client requires emergency care from the primary care provider or emergency department. In addition, the nurse may ask about symptoms and control issues over the past 2–4 weeks to understand the affect of asthma on the client. The client also may be asked to monitor PEFR and keep a daily log. This may help the client recognize airflow obstruction earlier and use pharmacologic interventions and may also reveal which factors trigger or aggravate asthma symptoms.

Diagnosis

Appropriate diagnoses will vary depending on the severity of the asthma, its etiology, and the age and developmental level of the client. In many cases, the following diagnoses will be appropriate:

- Ineffective Breathing Pattern
- Ineffective Airway Clearance
- Impaired Gas Exchange
- Activity Intolerance
- Anxiety
- Ineffective Therapeutic Regimen Management.

Plan

Information obtained during the assessment process and the client's current condition will guide the planning process. Together, the nurse and client will develop a plan of care that may include the following goals:

- The client will experience decreased number and frequency of exacerbations.
- The client will require fewer unscheduled visits to the primary care provider or emergency department.
- The client will reduce his or her exposure to irritants that aggravate asthma symptoms.
- The client will have a reduced the need for SABA.
- The client will show improved asthma control.
- The client will experience improved quality of life.

Implementation

Asthmatic clients require careful monitoring and rapid intervention during exacerbations in order to prevent hypoxia and promote oxygenation. Because of the chronic nature of the disorder, clients are often the best source of information regarding the implementations that work best for them, and they should be consulted when planning and implementing care.

PRACTICE ALERT

The following signs and symptoms signal hypoxia:

- Increasing restlessness, irritability, or unexplained sudden confusion
- Rapid heart rate accompanied by a rapid respiratory rate.

Ineffective Airway Clearance

Bronchospasm and bronchoconstriction, increased mucous secretion, and airway edema narrow the airways and impair airflow during an acute attack of asthma. Both inspiratory and expiratory volume are affected, decreasing the oxygen available at the alveolus for the process of respiration. Narrowed air passages increase the work of breathing, increasing the metabolic rate and tissue demand for oxygen.

- Monitor skin color and temperature and LOC. Cyanosis, cool clammy skin, and changes in LOC (e.g., agitation, lethargy, and confusion) indicate worsening hypoxia.
- Assess ABG results and pulse oximetry readings; notify the physician of abnormal values or changes in status. These values provide information about gas exchange and the adequacy of alveolar ventilation. A fall in oxygen saturation levels is an early indicator of impaired gas exchange.
- Place in Fowler's, high-Fowler's, or **orthopneic position** (with head and arms supported on the overbed table) to facilitate breathing and lung expansion. These positions reduce the work of breathing and increase lung expansion, especially of basilar areas.
- Administer oxygen as ordered. If a mask is used, monitor closely for feelings of claustrophobia or suffocation. Supplemental oxygen reduces hypoxemia. Small children may require use of a pediatric tent. Oxygen therapy via mask or tent can be frightening; monitor client for anxiety during administration.
- Administer nebulizer treatments and provide humidification as ordered. Nebulizer treatments are used to administer bronchodilators and other medications; humidity helps loosen secretions.
- Increase fluid intake. Increasing fluids helps keep secretions thin.

PRACTICE ALERT

Frequently assess respiratory status (at least every 1–2 hours): respiratory rate and depth, chest movement or excursion, breath sounds, and PEFR. Respiratory status can change rapidly during an acute asthma attack and its treatment. Decreasing PEFRs indicate worsening airflow restriction. Slowed, shallow respirations with significantly diminished breath sounds and decreased wheezing may indicate exhaustion and impending respiratory failure. Immediate intervention is necessary.

Ineffective Breathing Pattern

The physiologic changes in lung ventilation that occur during an acute asthma attack impair both lung expansion and emptying. Hypoxia and dyspnea can also cause anxiety, compounding the problem by increasing the respiratory rate. Collaborative and nursing interventions can help restore a more normal breathing pattern and adequate lung ventilation.

- Monitor vital signs and laboratory results. Tachypnea, tachycardia, elevated blood pressure, and increasing hypoxemia and hypercapnia are signs of compromised respiratory status.
- Assist with ADLs as needed. This conserves client energy and reduces fatigue.
- Provide rest periods between scheduled activities and treatments. Scheduled rest is important to prevent fatigue and reduce oxygen demands.
- Administer medications, including bronchodilators and anti-inflammatory drugs, as ordered. Monitor for desired and possible adverse effects. Medications are used to improve airway status and facilitate breathing.

PRACTICE ALERT

Frequently assess respiratory rate, pattern, and breath sounds. Note manifestations of ineffective breathing, including rapid rate, shallow respirations, nasal flaring, use of accessory muscles, intercostal retractions, and diminished or absent breath sounds. Early identification of ineffective respirations allows timely initiation of interventions to prevent a decline in condition resulting in more severe complications.

Anxiety

Acute exacerbations of asthma can produce significant anxiety. Fear of being unable to breathe and feelings of suffocation associated with acute asthma are significant. Financial or other concerns may cause the client to want to avoid hospitalization. Increasingly frequent and severe episodes may cause fear for the future. Hypoxia contributes to anxiety as well, stimulating the sympathetic nervous system and the fight-or-flight response.

- Assess level of anxiety. Interventions for severe anxiety or panic differ from those for mild or moderate anxiety.
- Assist the client to identify coping skills that have been successful in the past. Successful coping helps the client regain control of the situation, reducing anxiety.
- Listen actively to concerns; do not deny or negate the fear of dying or of being unable to breathe. Active listening promotes trust and helps the client express concerns.
- Include the client in care planning and decisions as appropriate, without making excessive demands. Participating in decision making increases the client's sense of control. Because high levels of anxiety interfere with the ability to make decisions, it is important to avoid placing

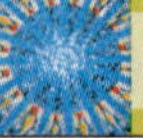

DEVELOPMENTAL CONSIDERATIONS Life-Threatening Total Airway Obstruction in Children

When a life-threatening total airway obstruction occurs, efforts to clear the obstruction include back blows and chest thrusts in an infant or abdominal thrusts in older children. In the emergency department, oxygen is administered. Efforts are made to visualize the foreign body with a laryngoscope and remove it with Magill forceps. Whenever possible, the child is taken to the operating room so that optimal conditions exist to protect and maintain the child's airway during removal of the foreign body. When a partial airway obstruction exists, fluoroscopy and fiber-optic bronchoscopy may be used to identify, locate, and extract the foreign body.

Following removal of the foreign body, the child is stabilized and observed for a few hours in a short-stay unit. Depending on the type of object, location of the object, and degree of obstruction, surgical removal and hospitalization may be required.

In some cases, children are initially treated for the complication or for asthma without recognizing that a foreign body was the cause of the respiratory distress. This occurs more often when the AFB is not visualized on an x-ray. When the child is nonresponsive to medications, further diagnostic testing may reveal the foreign body (Seth, Kamat, & Pansare, 2007).

NURSING CARE PLAN **A Client With Asthma**

Sarah Mitchell is a 35-year-old working mother with moderate persistent asthma. Her known triggers are allergies to dust mites, cockroach feces, grass and tree pollens, and some molds. She takes immunotherapy once a week and takes maintenance medications daily. She works as a full-time preschool teacher.

Mrs. Mitchell calls her allergist's office asking to be seen because she is having a bad asthma flare. She reports having to use her rescue inhaler every 3–4 hours , that her chest is very tight, and that she is having trouble breathing. She has used her home peak flow meter three times since late yesterday and has been in the yellow zone each time. She did not sleep last night because of her asthma symptoms.

ASSESSMENT

The nurse, Clancy O'Hara, admits Mrs. Mitchell when she arrives at the allergist's office. During the health history Mrs. Mitchell confirms she is compliant with her medication regimen. She takes a LABA in combination with a low-dose corticosteroid, a daily antihistamine, and montelukast. In checking Mrs. Mitchell's medical record, Clancy notes that the client is maintaining her scheduled immunotherapy appointments. Mrs. Mitchell reports that she is not aware of any unusual allergy exposure but says that several of her students have a cold this week.

On physical examination, Clancy notes that Mrs. Mitchell's vital signs are as follows: T_O 98.6°F (37°C), P 96, R 36, BP 128/86. Other assessment data include needing to pause frequently while speaking, use of accessory muscles for respirations, and scattered wheezes audible over both lung fields with stethoscope. ABG results are pH 7.32, PaO_2 of 88, $PaCO_2$ of 47, and HCO_3 of 38. Pulses are strong and equal bilaterally, and the client expectorates small amount of white mucus into a tissue.

DIAGNOSES

- Ineffective Breathing Pattern
- Impaired Gas Exchange
- Fatigue
- Activity Intolerance

PLANNING

Together Clancy and Mrs. Mitchell agree on the following outcomes:

- Mrs. Mitchell's breathing will return to the green zone within 24 hours.
- Mrs. Mitchell's need for rescue inhaler will decline within 3 days and return to baseline within 1 week.
- Mrs. Mitchell will maintain baseline respiratory rate and pattern sufficient to meet her ADLs within 72 hours.

IMPLEMENTATION

Mrs. Mitchell's provider prescribes a higher-dose inhaled steroid to use 10–15 minutes after she uses her LABA. The provider also gives Mrs. Mitchell a short, tapered course of prednisone. Clancy initiates the following implementations:

- Teaches Mrs. Mitchell how to properly self-administer medications and about possible side effects associated with steroid use, including those that should be reported immediately.
- Explains the importance of taking the steroid as ordered and not stopping the medication suddenly.
- Provides strategies for managing fatigue, including a handout with written instructions.
- Teaches Mrs. Mitchell the importance of proper nutrition and hydration in asthma management.
- Observes Mrs. Mitchell's technique when measuring peak flow.
- Reviews signs and symptoms indicating worsening condition, and instructs Mrs. Mitchell to call the provider if these occur.
- Schedules Mrs. Mitchell to return in 6 weeks for a further evaluation, but tells her to call the office if her symptoms worsen or if she sees no meaningful improvement in 3–4 days.

EVALUATION

Mrs. Mitchell returns in 6 weeks for her follow-up appointment and reports improvement of symptoms and no further recurrence. She expresses a desire to continue on the higher-dose steroid until school is out. Clancy assesses that Mrs. Mitchell's breathing rate and pattern have returned to baseline. Peak flow measurements indicate Mrs. Mitchell's breathing is within her green zone, and breath sounds are clear and equal bilaterally.

CRITICAL THINKING

1. Why is the prescription of the short, tapered course of oral prednisone appropriate for Mrs. Mitchell? Why is the continued use of the higher-dose inhaled corticosteroid appropriate? What special teaching will the client taking steroids require?
2. What role does nutrition and hydration have related to asthma management that required client teaching on this subject?
3. What signs and symptoms would you want Mrs. Mitchell to report to the provider immediately?

demands on the client that may further increase the level of anxiety.

- Reduce excessive environmental stimuli, and maintain a calm demeanor. This promotes rest.
- Allow supportive family members to remain with the client. Significant others provide additional support and can help reduce anxiety.
- Assist to use relaxation techniques, such as guided imagery, muscle relaxation, and meditation. These techniques help restore psychologic balance and reduce sympathetic stimulation and responses.

Ineffective Therapeutic Regimen Management

Once acute asthma is under control and effective respirations have been reestablished, it is important to help the client identify factors contributing to the attack. This helps the client prevent future episodes.

- Assess the client's level of understanding about asthma and the prescribed treatment regimen. Provide additional information and teaching as indicated. Assessment helps identify and clarify misperceptions and difficulties with disease management.
- Discuss the client's perception of the illness and its effect on his or her lifestyle. Open discussion can help identify conflicts between lifestyle and the treatment regimen.
- Assist the client and significant others to identify problems or difficulties integrating the treatment regimen into their lifestyle. Asthma and its management may necessitate lifestyle modifications to prevent acute exacerbations, which can significantly impact family members. Examples include eliminating cigarette smoking or pets from the household, removing carpets, or daily damp-dusting to remove dust mites.
- Assess knowledge and understanding of prescribed medications and use of over-the-counter preparations. This is important to determine misperceptions or possible misuse of medications.
- Provide verbal and written instructions at the client's level of understanding. Written instructions reinforce teaching and allow future reference.
- Refer to counseling, support groups, or self-help organizations. Counseling, support groups, and self-help organizations can help the client and family adapt to living with asthma and the treatment regimen.

Activity Intolerance

Clients with mild asthma may not experience any activity intolerance except during and immediately following a flare. For the client with moderate to severe asthma, however, activity intolerance can greatly limit quality of life.

- Teach the client how to monitor cardiopulmonary response to activity by taking his or her own pulse and blood pressure.
- Teach the client how to monitor and record peak flow rates before and after activities.
- Help the client assess his or her capacity to sustain activities and determine activities in which the client can participate and exercise.
- Assess the need for short-acting bronchodilators before activity or exercise.
- Teach the client to space periods of activity with periods of rest.
- Assist the client with ADLs as needed.

Evaluation

The nurse evaluates the client's response to treatment, which may be compared to the following common expected outcomes:

- Client maintains oxygen saturation greater than 90%.
- Client demonstrates proper use of inhalant medications.
- Client lists common triggers for asthmatic exacerbation and strategies to avoid triggers.
- Client and family member list symptoms requiring immediate notification of primary provider.
- Client responds appropriately to asthma flare-up.
- Client maintains optimal nutrition to promote health.
- Client describes appropriate follow up care to control condition.

REVIEW Asthma

RELATE: LINK THE CONCEPTS

The client has a history of severe persistent asthma, taking a daily LABA in combination with an inhaled corticosteroid, montelukast, and albuterol in both oral, inhaler, and nebulizer form for emergencies. Oral prednisone is prescribed approximately twice a year for severe flare-ups.

Linking the exemplar of Asthma with the concept of Metabolism:

1. What risk factors does this client have for osteoporosis? Explain the rationale for your answer
2. What risk factors does this client have for diabetes and obesity? Explain the rationale for your answer.

Linking the exemplar of Asthma with the concept of Acid–Base Balance:

3. When caring for a client in status asthmaticus, what would you anticipate finding when analyzing ABG? Explain the pathophysiology resulting in these findings.
4. What nursing interventions could be initiated to promote acid–base balance?

READY: GO TO COMPANION SKILLS MANUAL

- Using a pulse oximeter
- Using an incentive spirometer
- Measuring peak expiratory flow
- Performing chest percussion

- Assessing the thorax and lungs
- Assessing respiratory rate and pattern
- Administering MDI medications (with or without spacers)
- Administering DPI medications
- Administering medications by nonpressurized (nebulized) aerosol
- Applying and monitoring transcutaneous oxygen and carbon dioxide monitors
- Care of the client requiring an artificial airway and/or mechanical ventilation

REFER: GO TO MYNURSINGKIT

REFLECT: CASE STUDY

Hannah McGregor, a 9-year-old with asthma, lives at home with her parents and two brothers, who are 6 and 4 years old. Hannah developed asthma at approximately 5 years of age and has had wheezing episodes that were generally controlled by rescue medications. Two weeks ago, Hannah had a severe asthma episode that started at school and was possibly associated with the paint or glue used on a project. She did not have any quick-relief medications at school, and she delayed going to the school nurse so that she could finish her project. By the time her mother arrived to pick her up, Hannah was in respiratory distress. After receiving treatment in the emergency department, Hannah was admitted to the pediatric intensive care unit.

Hannah and her mother are in the health center to meet with the provider to learn more about asthma management. At today's visit, Hannah's lungs are clear to auscultation, and her peak expiratory flow reading is in the green zone. Mrs. McGregor reports that she has given all prescribed medications since the hospitalization. Both Hannah and her mother are motivated to prevent a future hospital admission if possible. The nurse uses a model to show Hannah how asthma narrows her airway and makes it difficult to breathe. The nurse then works with Mrs. McGregor and Hannah to develop a plan for asthma control with daily medications.

1. What are the current recommendations for managing Hannah's asthma and to help prevent asthma episodes?
2. How should Hannah handle future episodes that start at school?
3. What arrangements are needed for Hannah to have access to her medications at school?

21.3 CHRONIC OBSTRUCTIVE PULMONARY DISEASE

KEY TERMS

Air trapping, *1268*
Barrel chest, *1270*
Bronchitis, *1268*
Chronic obstructive pulmonary disease (COPD), *1267*
Chronic bronchitis, *1268*
Emphysema, *1268*
Expectorate, *1276*
Forced expiratory volume in 1 second (FEV_1), *1269*
Percussion, *1273*
Postural drainage, *1273*
Pursed-lipped breathing, *1270*
Sputum, *1267*
Tripod position, *1270*
Vibration, *1273*

BASIS FOR SELECTION OF EXEMPLAR

Centers for Disease Control and Prevention
Evidence-Based Criteria for Oxygenation
Healthy People 2010
Institute of Medicine

LEARNING OUTCOMES

After reading about this exemplar, you will be able to:

1. Describe the pathophysiology, etiology, clinical manifestations, and direct and indirect causes of chronic obstructive pulmonary disease (COPD).
2. Identify risk factors associated with COPD.
3. Illustrate nursing process in providing culturally competent care across the life span for individuals with COPD.
4. Formulate priority nursing diagnoses appropriate for an individual with COPD.
5. Create a plan of caring interventions for individuals with COPD and their family members.
6. Assess expected outcomes for an individual with COPD.
7. Discuss therapies used in the collaborative care of an individual with COPD.
8. Employ evidence-based caring interventions for an individual with COPD.

OVERVIEW

Obstructive pulmonary diseases are those that cause obstruction of the airways, usually through a combination of bronchoconstriction and inflammation. These include asthma, bronchitis (chronic or acute), and emphysema.

The term **chronic obstructive pulmonary disease (COPD)** is used to describe a specific progressive disorder that slowly alters the structures of the respiratory system over time, irreversibly affecting lung function. The disease is one of periodic exacerbations, often related to respiratory infection, with increased symptoms of dyspnea and **sputum** (mucus or mucopurulent matter expectorated from the lungs) production. Unlike acute processes in which lung tissues recover, airways and lung parenchyma do not return to normal following an exacerbation; instead, they demonstrate progressive destructive changes. COPD is not curable, but it can be managed (and sometimes prevented) with appropriate medical interventions and lifestyle choices.

Although one or the other may predominate, COPD typically includes components of both chronic bronchitis and emphysema, two distinctly different processes. Small airways disease, narrowing of small bronchioles, is also part of the COPD complex. Through different mechanisms, these processes cause airways to narrow, resistance to airflow to increase, and expiration to become slow or difficult (Figure 21–34 ■). The result is a mismatch between alveolar ventilation and blood flow or perfusion, leading to impaired gas exchange.

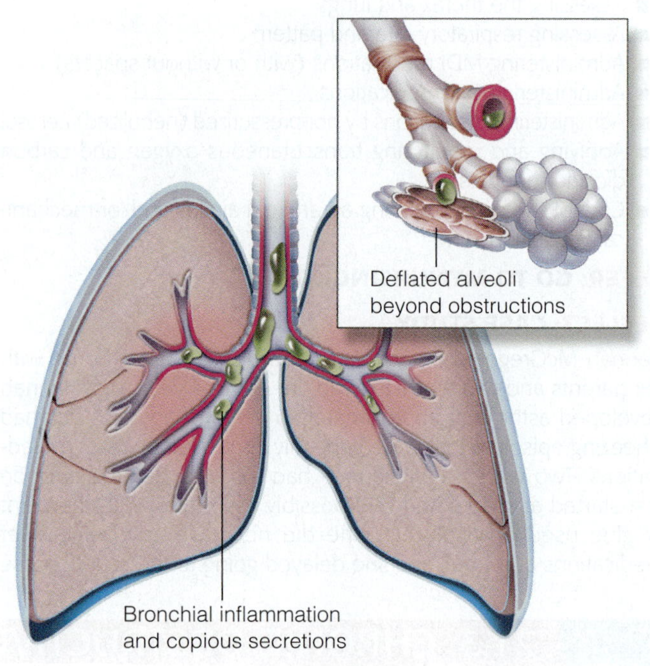

Figure 21–35 ■ Chronic bronchitis.

PATHOPHYSIOLOGY AND ETIOLOGY

Chronic obstructive pulmonary disease results from repeated exposure to respiratory irritants that begin to damage the structures within the lungs. Damage to the large and small airway passages causes increased mucus production, causing arrest in cilia action. Excessive amounts of fluid accumulate with the lung mucosal cells, causing edema. In turn, edema causes narrowing of airway passages, resulting in airflow limitation, **air trapping** (decreased airflow with exhalation), and ultimately, hyperinflation of the lungs. This process leads to **bronchitis** (best defined as inflammation of the mucous membranes of the bronchial tubes).

Chronic bronchitis is a disorder of excessive bronchial mucus secretion (Figure 21–35 ■). It is characterized by a productive cough lasting 3 or more months in two consecutive years (Porth, 2005). Cigarette smoke is the major factor implicated in the development of chronic bronchitis. Inhaled irritants lead to a chronic inflammatory process with vasodilation, congestion, and edema of the bronchial mucosa. Goblet cells increase in size and number, and mucous glands enlarge. Thick, tenacious mucus is produced in increased amounts. Changes in bronchial squamous cells impair the ability to clear mucus (Kasper et al., 2005). Narrowed airways and excess secretions obstruct airflow; expiration is affected first, then inspiration. Because ciliary function is impaired, normal defense mechanisms are unable to clear the mucus and any inhaled pathogens. Recurrent infection is common in chronic bronchitis.

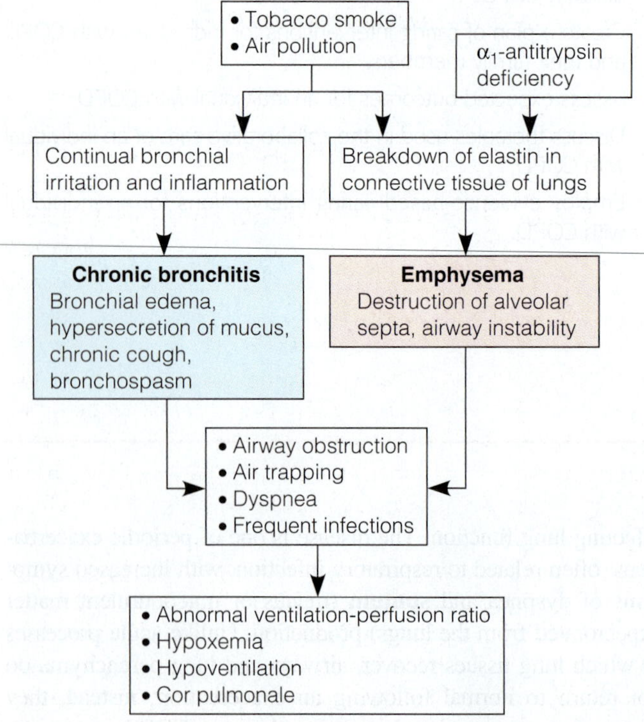

Figure 21–34 ■ Pathogenesis of chronic obstructive pulmonary disease.

Emphysema is characterized by destruction of the walls of the alveoli, with resulting enlargement of abnormal air spaces (Figure 21–36 ■). Deficiency of α_1-antitrypsin, an enzyme that normally inhibits the activity of proteolytic enzymes and tissue destruction in the lungs, contributes to the development of emphysema in some individuals, especially when combined with exposure to cigarette smoke. Inflammatory cells that collect in distal airway tissues appear to lead to destruction of elastic fibers in the respiratory bronchioles and alveolar ducts. Alveolar wall destruction causes alveoli and air spaces to enlarge, with loss of corresponding portions of the pulmonary capillary bed. As a result, the surface area for alveolar–capillary diffusion is reduced, affecting gas exchange. Elastic recoil is lost, reducing the volume of air that is passively expired. The loss of support tissue also affects airways, increasing the risk of expiratory collapse and further air trapping. Anatomically, either respiratory bronchioles or alveoli may be the primary tissue involved. As in chronic bronchitis, cigarette smoking is strongly implicated as a causative factor in most cases of emphysema.

Asthma often exists as a comorbid disease in the client with COPD. Clients who have lived with moderate to severe persistent asthma for most of their lives may develop COPD as a result of airway remodeling and damage to alveoli over time. Asthma is discussed in detail in Exemplar 21.2.

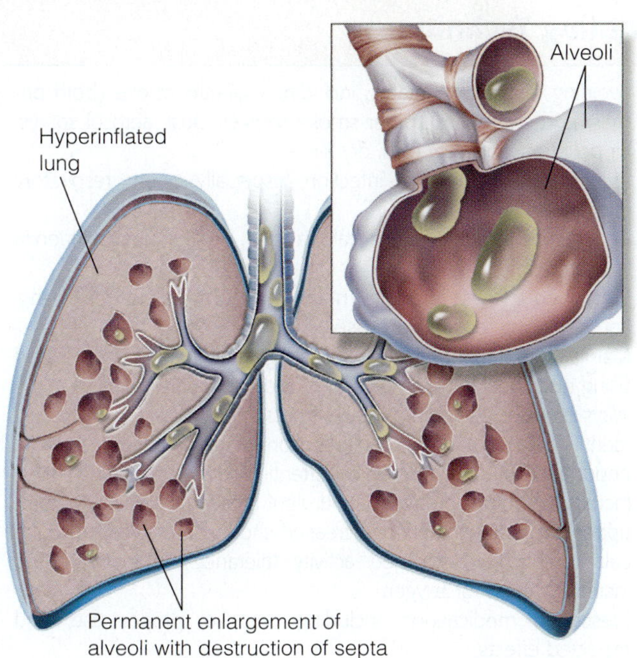

Figure 21–36 ■ Emphysema.

To summarize, COPD is a progressive, nonreversible process of airway narrowing and loss of supporting tissue. Three separate processes typically are involved:

1. Chronic bronchitis with persistent airway edema, excessive mucus production, and impaired airway clearance
2. Emphysema with loss of interstitial membranes and airway support tissue, resulting in airway collapse and loss of alveolar surface area for gas exchange
3. Small airways disease with bronchoconstriction.

The result of these processes and their combined effects is increased work of breathing, impaired expiration with air trapping, and impaired gas exchange.

Etiology

Chronic obstructive pulmonary disease is a leading cause of death, illness, and disability in the United States. COPD is often thought to be a disease that affects older adults, but 70% of individuals with COPD are under 65 years of age. Mortality rates are nearly equal for women and men, though rates for women have significantly increased since 1970. The direct costs of care in the United States are $18 billion annually, and indirect costs related to disability and loss of productive work is estimated at $14.4 billion annually. Although COPD is not curable, the symptoms of the disease can be managed. (Boyle & Locke, 2004; Centers for Disease Control and Prevention (CDC), 2009; Corbridge & Berry, 2007; Global Initiative for COPD, 2007).

Cigarette smoking is the greatest risk factor for COPD in the United States and other developed nations, accounting for approximately 80% of cases. Other causes that have contributory effects of COPD on the lungs include exposures to occupational respiratory irritants and air pollution (both indoors and outdoors) in industrialized nations. The use of wood, coal, or animal dung for cooking fires in close quarters in underdeveloped nations increases the risk of COPD in women from those countries. Accounting for less than 1% of the population with COPD are those with α-antitrypsin deficiency (a lack of a protein produced by the liver that protects the integrity of lung tissue). This lack of protein synthesis is genetic and most commonly seen in individuals of northern European origin. α-Antitrypsin deficiency causes individuals to develop COPD at earlier ages than those who develop the disease from chronic airway irritations (Boyle & Locke, 2004; CDC, 2007; Corbridge & Berry, 2007; Global Initiative for COPD, 2007).

Risk Factors

Smoking is the greatest risk factor for COPD: The more a person smokes, the greater the risk of acquiring the disease. Frequent exposure to smoke also increases an individual's risk for COPD. Long-term exposure to chemical irritants in the workplace or through a hobby also increases risk for COPD. Some evidence indicates that clients with asthma are more likely to develop COPD compared with the general population.

While short-term exposure to respiratory irritants normally does not pose a risk for COPD, there are indications that short-term exposure to high levels of highly irritating substances can result in impairment of lung function, leading to COPD and other respiratory disorders. A longitudinal study of first responders and workers at the World Trade Center following the terrorist attacks of September 11, 2001, found that these individuals experienced significantly decreased lung function within the first year following the attacks. The exposure-related decrease in lung function within that year of the study participants was equivalent to 12 years of aging-related decline in lung function (Banauch et al., 2006).

CLINICAL MANIFESTATIONS

The clinical presentation of COPD varies from simple chronic bronchitis without disability to chronic respiratory failure and severe disability. **Forced expiratory volume in 1 second (FEV_1)** is the amount of air that can be exhaled in 1 second as measured by a spirometer. A client's FEV_1 reading combined with symptom manifestations determines the client's level of COPD severity. Box 21–4 outlines the classifications of COPD severity.

Manifestations are typically absent or minor early in the disease. Initial symptoms are a chronic cough and sputum production, which tend to begin long before changes in pulmonary function. No incidence of shortness of breath occurs in the early stages of pulmonary decline as a result of COPD. When the client finally seeks care, chronic productive cough, dyspnea, and exercise intolerance often have been present for as long as 10 years. The cough typically occurs in the mornings and often is attributed to "smoker's cough." Initially, dyspnea occurs only on extreme exertion; as the disease progresses, dyspnea becomes more severe and accompanies mild activity. Manifestations characteristic of chronic bronchitis and emphysema develop. Manifestations of chronic bronchitis include a cough that produces copious amounts of thick,

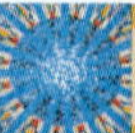

CLIENT TEACHING Effective Coughing and Breathing Techniques

Pursed-lipped and diaphragmatic breathing techniques help minimize air trapping and fatigue. Have the client repeat these exercises as often as necessary until the techniques become incorporated into normal breathing.

Pursed-lipped breathing helps maintain open airways by maintaining positive pressures longer during exhalation. Teach the client to:

1. Inhale through the nose with the mouth closed.
2. Exhale slowly through pursed lips, as though whistling or blowing out a candle, making exhalation twice as long as inhalation.

Diaphragmatic or abdominal breathing helps conserve energy by using the larger and more efficient muscles of respiration. Teach the client to:

1. Place one hand on the abdomen and the other on the chest.
2. Inhale, concentrating on pushing the abdominal hand outward while the chest hand remains still.
3. Exhale slowly, while the abdominal hand moves inward and the chest hand remains still.

Several coughing techniques may be useful. For controlled cough technique, teach the client to:

1. Following prescribed bronchodilator treatment, inhale deeply, and hold breath briefly.
2. Cough twice, the first time to loosen mucus and the second to expel secretions.
3. Inhale by sniffing to prevent mucus from moving back into deep airways.
4. Rest. Avoid prolonged coughing to prevent fatigue and hypoxemia.

For huff coughing, teach the client to:

1. Inhale deeply while leaning forward.
2. Exhale sharply with a "huff" sound to help keep airways open while mobilizing secretions.

In addition, include the following topics when teaching for home care:

- Maintaining adequate fluid intake (at least 2.0–2.5 quarts of fluid daily)
- Avoiding respiratory irritants, including cigarette smoke (both primary and secondary), other smoke sources, dust, aerosol sprays, air pollution, and very cold, dry air
- Preventing exposure to infection, especially upper respiratory infections
- Importance of pneumococcal vaccine and annual influenza immunization
- Prescribed exercise program, maintaining activities of daily living, and balancing rest and exercise
- Maintaining nutrient intake (e.g., eating small, frequent meals and using nutritional supplements to provide adequate calories)
- Ways of reducing sodium intake if prescribed
- Identifying early signs of an infection or exacerbation, and the importance of seeking medical attention for the following: fever, increased sputum production, purulent (green or yellow) sputum, upper respiratory infection, increased shortness of breath or difficulty breathing, decreased activity tolerance or appetite, and increased need for oxygen
- Prescribed medications, including purpose, proper use, and expected effects
- Avoiding use of over-the-counter medications unless approved by the physician
- Other prescribed therapies, such as use of home oxygen, percussion, postural drainage, and nebulizer treatments
- Use, cleaning, and maintenance of any required special equipment
- Importance of wearing an identification band and carrying a list of medications at all times in case of an emergency.

Provide referrals to home care services, such as home health, assistance with activities of daily living as needed, home maintenance services, respiratory therapy and home oxygen services, and other agencies such as Meals-on-Wheels and senior services as indicated.

tenacious sputum; cyanosis; and evidence of right-sided heart failure, including distended neck veins, edema, liver engorgement, and an enlarged heart. Adventitious lung sounds, including loud rhonchi, and possible wheezes are prominent on auscultation.

Box 21–4 Classification of Chronic Obstructive Pulmonary Disease by Severity

Stage I: Mild: usually, but not always, chronic cough and sputum production. Mild airflow limitation; FEV_1/forced vital capacity (FVC) < 70%; FEV_1 of >80% predicted.

Stage II: Moderate: usually worse symptoms, with shortness of breath typically developing on exertion; FEV_1/FVC < 70%; FEV1 of between 80 and 50% predicted.

Stage III: Severe: worse symptoms, with noticeable shortness of breath; FEV_1/FVC < 70%; FEV1 of between 50 and 30% predicted.

Stage IV: Very severe: severe symptoms; FEV_1/FVC < 70%; FEV_1 of <30% predicted or FEV1 of <50% predicted plus respiratory failure or clinical signs of right heart failure.

Source: Global Initiative for COPD (2009).

Emphysema is insidious in onset. Dyspnea is the first symptom. Initially occurring only with exertion, dyspnea may progress to become severe even at rest. Cough is minimal or absent. Air trapping and hyperinflation increase the anteroposterior chest diameter, a condition called **barrel chest**. The client often is thin, is tachypneic, uses accessory muscles of respiration, and often assumes a **tripod position** (a position of sitting and leaning forward) (Figure 21–37 ■). On auscultation, breath sounds are diminished, and the percussion tone is hyperresonant. The client may utilize **pursed-lipped breathing** to prolong the expiratory phase in an effort to promote more alveolar emptying while maintaining open alveoli. Purse-lipped breathing is exhaling through a narrow opening between the lips to prolong the expiratory phase in an effort to promote more alveolar emptying while maintaining open alveoli. See the Client Teaching feature for more information.

Prolonged impairment of gas exchange as a result of COPD eventually results in cardiac dysfunction. Chest pain and hypertension may be the earliest manifestations, indicating that the heart is having to work harder to provide oxygen through the bloodstream. Eventually, congestive heart failure

CLINICAL MANIFESTATIONS AND THERAPIES Chronic Obstructive Pulmonary Disease

ETIOLOGY	CLINICAL MANIFESTATION	CLINICAL THERAPIES
Bronchitis	■ Chronic cough with mucous production ■ Dyspnea ■ Tachycardia ■ Narrowed airway passages ■ Wheezing ■ Air trapping	■ Smoking cessation ■ Bronchodilators ■ Corticosteroids ■ Fluids to thin secretions ■ Elevate the head of the bed ■ Low-flow oxygen ■ Monitoring arterial blood gases and oxygen ■ Mechanical ventilation may be necessary if client cannot meet oxygen demands.
Emphysema	■ Air trapping ■ Possible wheezing ■ Dyspnea ■ Barrel chest ■ Pursed-lipped breathing ■ Posturing	■ Oxygen administration as needed ■ Pursed-lipped breathing technique ■ Teach posture changes to improve ventilation. ■ Low-flow oxygen ■ Monitoring arterial blood gases and oxygen ■ Mechanical ventilation may be necessary if client cannot meet oxygen demands. ■ Nutritional assessment and increased calorie intake
Cardiac dysfunction	■ Chest pain ■ Poor perfusion ■ Arrhythmias, particularly premature ventricular contractions ■ Hypertension ■ Cardiac hypertrophy ■ Congestive heart failure	■ Medications: a. Positive inotropics b. Calcium blockers c. Antiarrhythmic medications d. Diuretics e. Nitrites f. Antihypertensives ■ Monitor exercise tolerance ■ Holter monitoring ■ Antiembolism stockings to improve venous return ■ Fluid restrictions may be necessary if not medically managed.

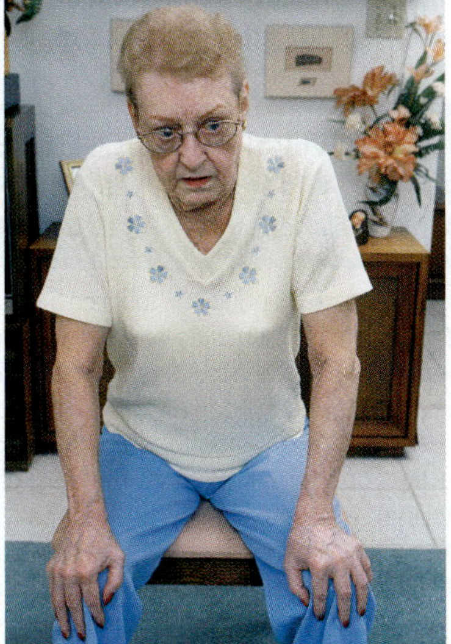

Figure 21–37 ■ Typical appearance of a client with emphysema. Note the client's anxious expression and assumption of the tripod position, leaning forward with the hands on the knees.

Source: Michal Heron, Pearson Education/PH College.

may result. Clients with COPD should be seen by their specialist or primary care provider at least every 6 months in order for their disease progression to be evaluated and therapies to be modified or added.

PRACTICE ALERT

Chronic cough and sputum is not a normal occurrence. An individual experiencing chronic cough and sputum beyond 3–4 days should consult with a health care professional. Individuals with a smoking history as well as chronic cough and sputum production should have PFTs to determine lung function.

The work of breathing requires calories. Caloric demand increases as the effort to breathe increases. Tachypnea makes eating more difficult. Increased caloric demand with decreased caloric intake often occurs in the latter stages of COPD, often resulting in weight loss and possibly anemia.

Anxiety related to increasing periods of dyspnea occurs with exacerbations in moderate and severe COPD. Severe COPD can result in impairment of other bodily systems because of insufficient airflow, further restricting quality of life.

COLLABORATION

Nurses will find it helpful to collaborate with physical therapists, nutritionists, pharmacists, family members, and sometimes, counselors to help clients achieve outcomes and improve their quality of life. In particular, nurses should be aware of who is caring for the client with COPD who continues to live at home and should discuss with the client and family the need for those persons to have sufficient information and training so they can provide care that meets best-practice guidelines.

Diagnostic Tests

Diagnostic tests are used to help establish the diagnosis of COPD and identify the predominant component, emphysema or chronic bronchitis. These procedures also are used to assess respiratory status and monitor treatment effectiveness. (See Appendix B for more detailed information about related diagnostic tests.)

PULMONARY FUNCTION TESTING Pulmonary function testing is performed to establish the diagnosis and evaluate the extent and progression of COPD. Results are based on calculated norms for each person by age, height, sex, and weight; note these as well as all current medications on the requisition. In clients with COPD, the total lung capacity and residual volume typically are increased. The FEV_1 and FVC are decreased as a result of narrowed airways and resistance to airflow.

VENTILATION-PERFUSION SCANNING Ventilation-perfusion scanningmay be performed to determine the extent of V-Q mismatch—that is, the extent to which lung tissue is ventilated but not perfused (dead space), or perfused but inadequately ventilated (physiologic shunting). A radioisotope is injected or inhaled to illustrate areas of shunting and absent capillaries.

SERUM α_1-ANTITRYPSIN LEVELS Serum α_1-antitrypsin levels may be drawn to screen for deficiency, particularly in clients with a family history of obstructive airway disease, those with an early onset, women, and those who do not smoke. Normal adult serum α_1-antitrypsin levels range from 80 to 260 mg/dL. Fasting is not required before this test.

ARTERIAL BLOOD GAS Arterial blood gas values are used to evaluate gas exchange, particularly during acute exacerbations of COPD. Clients with emphysema as the predominant component often have mild hypoxemia and normal or low carbon dioxide tension. Respiratory alkalosis may be present as a result of an increased respiratory rate. Clients with chronic bronchitis and airway obstruction as the predominant component may have marked hypoxemia and hypercapnia with respiratory acidosis. Oxygen saturation levels are low because of marked hypoxemia.

PRACTICE ALERT

Hypercapnia (elevated $PaCO_2$ levels) often is chronic in clients with COPD (CO_2 retainers). In these clients, administering oxygen can actually increase the $PaCO_2$, leading to somnolence and acute respiratory failure. While oxygen is the drug of choice for treating clients with COPD, close monitoring is necessary during oxygen therapy.

PULSE OXIMETRY Pulse oximetry is used to monitor oxygen saturation of the blood. Marked airway obstruction and hypoxemia often cause oxygen saturation levels of less than 95%. Pulse oximetry may be continuously monitored to assess the need for supplemental oxygen.

EXHALED CARBON DIOXIDE Exhaled carbon dioxide (capnogram or $ETCO_2$) may be measured to evaluate alveolar ventilation. The normal $ETCO_2$ reading is 35–45 mmHg; it is elevated when ventilation is inadequate and decreased when pulmonary perfusion is impaired. $ETCO_2$ monitoring can reduce the frequency of ABG determinations.

COMPLETE BLOOD COUNT WITH WHITE BLOOD CELL DIFFERENTIAL Complete blood count with white blood cell (WBC) differential often shows increased red blood cells and hematocrit (erythrocytosis) as chronic hypoxia stimulates increased erythropoiesis to improve the oxygen-carrying capacity of the blood. Polycythemia (increased numbers of all blood cells) may be evident. Increased WBC count and a higher percentage of immature WBCs (bands) are often indicative of bacterial infection.

CHEST X-RAY Chest x-rays of a client with COPD will show small white patches indicative of the hyperinflated alveolar sacs filled with secretions that are common in emphysema. Clients with more advanced chronic bronchitis will have long fields with larger areas of white, indicating the secretions. A CXR also may show flattening of the diaphragm because of hyperinflation and evidence of pulmonary infection if present.

Pharmacologic Therapy

Immunization against pneumococcal pneumonia and a yearly influenza vaccine are recommended to reduce the risk of respiratory infections. A broad-spectrum antibiotic may be prescribed if infection is suspected. Recent studies indicate that clients with purulent sputum and increased dyspnea will likely benefit from antibiotic therapy, even if no other signs of infection are present. Prophylactic antibiotics may be ordered for

FOCUS ON DIVERSITY AND CULTURE

Smoking and the U.S. Hispanic Population

Among the U.S. Hispanic population, tobacco use is the leading preventable cause of death. Issues associated with this high rate of tobacco use appear to include acculturation, education levels, and alcohol and substance abuse (Rodríguez-Esquivel, Cooper, Blow, & Resor, 2009). A 2007 study found that Hispanic clients with chronic obstructive pulmonary disease (COPD) do not receive referral to smoking cessation classes as frequently as clients of other ethnicities (Adams et al., 2008). Nurses working with Hispanic clients who exhibit chronic cough and sputum or who are diagnosed with COPD should inquire about nicotine and alcohol use and provide client teaching and appropriate referrals in these areas. Nurses should also be able to provide referrals to mental health resources that serve Spanish-speaking clients. Materials about COPD and that encourage smoking cessation should also be provided in Spanish wherever Hispanic clients are being served.

clients who experience four or more disease exacerbations per year (Kasper et al., 2005).

Bronchodilators improve airflow and reduce air trapping in clients with COPD, resulting in improved dyspnea and exercise tolerance. These agents accomplish this by relaxing bronchial smooth muscle, thus widening the airway and making breathing easier for the client; they have no anti-inflammatory properties. Bronchodilators may be given by MDI, DPI, nebulizer, or orally. Oral administration may promote adherence but is associated with much higher rates of adverse effects. A spacer or holding chamber may facilitate effective use of an MDI. Ipratropium bromide, an anticholinergic agent administered by MDI, is frequently prescribed. It has a longer duration of action than the short-acting $beta_2$-adrenergic stimulant bronchodilators and few side effects. Salmeterol, a LABA, may be used in combination therapy. Oral theophylline, a methylxanthine, is a weak bronchodilator and has a narrow therapeutic range, but it often is prescribed for its other effects. Theophylline stimulates the respiratory drive, strengthens diaphragmatic contractions, and improves cardiac output. As a result, dyspnea, exercise tolerance, and quality of life improve for the client with COPD. Bronchodilators are discussed in further detail, including their nursing implications, in Exemplar 21.2.

Corticosteroid therapy may be used when asthma is a major component of COPD. It also improves symptoms and exercise tolerance and may reduce the severity of exacerbations and the need for hospitalization. Oral corticosteroids, such as prednisone, are used initially. If a beneficial response occurs, the amount is reduced to the lowest effective dose. Every-other-day dosing or administration by inhaler is preferred to minimize steroid side effects, such as cushingoid effects, mood swings, and increased risk for osteoporosis and vertebral fractures.

New research indicates that the use of statins may result in significant improvement for the client with COPD. Data indicate that statins are associated with a decrease in all-cause mortality as well as a reduction in the rate of respiratory-related emergency care. Furthermore, it appears in addition to targeting systemic inflammation, statins may also target airway inflammation (Reuters Health Information, 2009).

Surgery

When medical therapy is no longer effective, lung transplantation may be an option. Both single and bilateral transplants have been performed successfully, with a 2-year survival rate of 75%. Lung reduction surgery is an experimental surgical intervention for advanced diffuse emphysema and lung hyperinflation. The procedure reduces the overall volume of the lung, reshapes it, and improves elastic recoil. As a result, pulmonary function and exercise tolerance improve, and dyspnea is reduced.

Oxygen Therapy

Long-term oxygen therapy is used for severe and progressive hypoxemia. Oxygen therapy improves exercise tolerance, mental functioning, and quality of life in clients with advanced COPD. It also reduces the rate of hospitalization and increases the length of survival. Oxygen may be used intermittently, at night, or continuously. Clients with severe hypoxemia see the greatest benefit with continuous oxygen. Home oxygen may be supplied as liquid oxygen, compressed gas cylinders, or oxygen concentrators. An acute exacerbation of COPD may necessitate oxygenation and inspiratory positive-pressure assistance with a face mask or intubation and mechanical ventilation. Oxygen administered without intubation and mechanical ventilation requires caution: Administering oxygen to clients with chronic elevated carbon dioxide levels in the blood can actually increase the $PaCO_2$, leading to increased somnolence and even respiratory failure. Close monitoring of LOC and ABG values during oxygen therapy is vital (Simmons & Simmons, 2004).

Percussion, Vibration, and Postural Drainage

Percussion, vibration, and postural drainage (PVD) are dependent nursing functions performed according to a primary care provider's order. **Percussion**, sometimes called *clapping,* is forceful striking of the skin with cupped hands. Mechanical percussion cups and vibrators are also available. When the hands are used, the fingers and thumb are held together and flexed slightly to form a cup, as one would to scoop up water. Percussion over congested lung areas can mechanically dislodge tenacious secretions from the bronchial walls. Cupped hands trap the air against the chest, and the trapped air sets up vibrations through the chest wall to the secretions. When done correctly, the percussion action should produce a hollow, popping sound. Percussion is avoided over the breasts, sternum, spinal column, and kidneys.

Vibration is a series of vigorous quiverings produced by hands that are placed flat against the client's chest wall. Vibration is used after percussion to increase the turbulence of the exhaled air and thus loosen thick secretions. It is often done alternately with percussion.

Postural drainage is the drainage by gravity of secretions from various lung segments. Secretions that remain in the lungs or respiratory airways promote bacterial growth and subsequent infection. They also can obstruct the smaller airways and cause atelectasis. Secretions in the major airways, such as the trachea and the right and left main bronchi, are usually coughed into the pharynx, where they can be expectorated, swallowed, or effectively removed by suctioning.

A wide variety of positions is necessary to drain all segments of the lungs, but not all positions are required for every client. Only those positions that drain specific affected areas are used. The lower lobes require drainage most frequently, because the upper lobes drain by gravity. Before postural drainage, the client may be given a bronchodilator medication or nebulization therapy to loosen secretions. Postural drainage treatments are scheduled two or three times daily, depending on the degree of lung congestion. The best times include before breakfast, before lunch, in the late afternoon, and before bedtime. It is best to avoid hours shortly after meals, because postural drainage at these times can be tiring and may induce vomiting.

The nurse needs to evaluate the client's tolerance of postural drainage by assessing the stability of the client's vital signs, particularly the pulse and respiratory rates, and by noting signs of intolerance, such as pallor, diaphoresis, dyspnea, nausea, and fatigue. Some clients do not react well to certain drainage positions, and the nurse must make appropriate adjustments. For example, some become dyspneic in Trendelenburg's position and require only a moderate tilt or a shorter time in that position.

The sequence for PVD is usually as follows: positioning, percussion, vibration, and removal of secretions by coughing or suction. Each position is usually assumed for 10–15 minutes, although beginning treatments may start with shorter times and gradually increase.

Following PVD, the nurse should auscultate the client's lungs, compare the findings to the baseline data, and document the amount, color, and character of expectorated secretions.

Other Interventions

Smoking cessation not only can prevent COPD from developing but also can improve lung function once the disease has been diagnosed. With smoking cessation, FEV_1 improves, and survival is prolonged, largely because of lower rates of lung cancer and heart disease. Sustained quitting is difficult; only 6% of smokers succeed in long-term abstinence from smoking (Kasper et al., 2005). Use of nicotine patches or gum and an antidepressant, such as bupropion (Wellbutrin, Zyban), improves the chances of success. More information about nicotine abuse can be found in the Behavior and Addiction concept in Exemplar 2.2, Nicotine Abuse.

In addition to refraining from smoking, exposure to other airway irritants and allergens should be avoided. The client should remain indoors during periods of significant air pollution to prevent exacerbations of the disease. Air-filtering systems or air conditioning may be useful.

Pulmonary hygiene measures, including hydration, effective coughing, percussion, and postural drainage, are used to improve clearance of airway secretions. Cough suppressants are usually ineffective, and sedatives are generally avoided because they may cause retention of secretions.

EXERCISE Unless disabling cardiac disease is present, a regular exercise program is beneficial for the following:

- Improving exercise tolerance
- Enhancing ability to perform ADLs
- Preventing deterioration of physical condition.

A program of regular aerobic exercise (e.g., walking for 20 minutes at least three times weekly) designed to gradually increase exercise tolerance is recommended. Activities that strengthen the muscles used for breathing and ADLs, such as swimming and golf, are also beneficial. Breathing exercises are used to slow the respiratory rate and relieve accessory muscle fatigue. Pursed-lipped breathing slows the respiratory rate and helps maintain open airways during exhalation by keeping positive pressure in the airways. Abdominal breathing relieves the work of accessory muscles of respiration.

HYDRATION Adequate hydration maintains the moisture of the respiratory mucous membranes. Normally, respiratory tract secretions are thin and therefore are moved readily by ciliary action. However, when the client is dehydrated or the environment has a low humidity, the respiratory secretions can become thick and tenacious. Fluid intake should be as great as the client can tolerate.

Humidifiers are devices that add water vapor to inspired air. Room humidifiers provide cool mist to room air. Nebulizers are used to deliver humidity and medications. They may be used with oxygen delivery systems to provide moistened air directly to the client. Humidifiers prevent mucous membranes from drying and becoming irritated and loosen secretions for easier expectoration.

Complementary Therapy

Complementary therapies may be useful to help manage symptoms of COPD. Dietary measures, such as minimizing intake of dairy products and salt, may help reduce mucus production and keep mucus more liquefied. Be sure to recommend measures to replace the protein and calcium in dairy products to help maintain nutritional balance. Herbal teas made with peppermint and yarrow, coltsfoot, or comfrey may act as expectorants to help relieve chest congestion. Licorice root, which may be taken in several forms, also has expectorant and anti-inflammatory effects that may be beneficial. Licorice root can, however, cause toxicity when used for extended periods of time (Spencer & Jacobs, 2003). Refer clients to a qualified herbalist for treatment.

Acupuncture may help the client with smoking cessation; it has also has been used to treat asthma and other respiratory conditions. Hypnotherapy and guided imagery may be used to assist with smoking cessation. These techniques also can help the client control anxiety and breathing patterns. Refer clients to a trained professional. Nurses, physicians, psychologists, counselors, social workers, and others can take professional training in hypnotherapy and guided imagery (Fontaine, 2005).

NURSING PROCESS

The priority of nursing care is focused on promoting oxygenation. Health promotion activities include smoking cessation, reducing the risk of infection, and maintaining client safety. Because of the chronic nature of this disease process, teaching the client how to maximize self-care while knowing when to notify the healthcare team is another important role of the nurse.

Assessment

Focused assessment for the client with COPD includes collecting the following data:

- *Health history.* Current symptoms, including cough, sputum production, shortness of breath or dyspnea, activity tolerance; frequency of respiratory infections, and most recent episode; previous diagnosis of emphysema, chronic bronchitis, or asthma; current medications; smoking history in pack-years (packs per day times number of years smoked); and history of exposure to secondhand smoke and to occupational or other pollutants

- *Physical examination.* General appearance, weight for height, mental status; vital signs, including temperature; skin color and temperature; anteroposterior:lateral chest diameter; use of accessory muscles, nasal flaring, or pursed-lip breathing; respiratory excursion and diaphragmatic excursion; percussion tone; breath sounds throughout; neck veins, apical pulse and heart sounds, peripheral pulses, and edema.

Auscultation of the chest may yield very little information to aid in establishing the diagnosis of COPD. Often, lung sounds are distant or reduced, although occasionally, wheezes or inspiratory crackles may be heard. However, these sounds are also associated with other diagnoses. Heart sounds may be difficult to hear if the client has a barrel chest. Auscultation over the xiphoid process (the lowest portion of the sternum) makes it easier to hear heart tones.

The nurse inspects and palpates the chest for symmetry. Increased anteroposterior diameter indicates chronic respiratory effort. The use of accessory muscles during breathing is also assessed. The position of the individual is observed. Upright posturing is an effective aid for ease of breathing. Self-posturing may indicate respiratory distress. An individual with COPD may sit upright with support of an overbed table.

Because COPD is a progressive and deteriorating illness, many clients with COPD reach the point at which they can no longer continue to live successfully at home. The nurse working with the client with COPD at home may want to use a Home Care Assessment for Oxygenation for COPD (Box 21–5).

Diagnosis

Clients with COPD, whether hospitalized or in the community, have multiple nursing care needs. Because of the obstructive nature of the disease, airway clearance is a high priority. Nutritional deficit is common, particularly when emphysema is predominant. Because this chronic disease affects all functional health patterns, psychosocial issues are also of concern in planning nursing care. NANDA diagnoses appropriate for the client with COPD include the following:

- Ineffective Breathing Pattern
- Ineffective Airway Clearance
- Activity Intolerance
- Imbalanced Nutrition: Less Than Body Requirements
- Compromised Family Coping
- Decisional Conflict: Smoking.

Plan

Nursing care of the client with COPD, especially in later stages, requires careful planning in order to meet the client's oxygenation demands. Possible outcomes for this client may include the following:

- The client will adapt breathing patterns to meet oxygenation demands adequately.
- The client will experience ease of respirations with the use of positioning and pursed-lipped breathing.
- The client will maintain a patent airway, allowing adequate oxygenation.
- The client will maintain oxygen saturation levels above 90%.
- The client will tolerate activity levels, allowing completion of ADLs.

Implementation

The highest priorities of nursing implementation are aimed at promoting oxygenation, which includes monitoring and promoting airway clearance and effective breathing patterns. Ongoing reassessment to determine effectiveness of interventions will help to guide the nursing plan of care.

Box 21–5 **Home Care Assessment: Oxygenation**

CLIENT

- *Self-care abilities:* ability to ambulate and perform activities of daily living (ADLs) independently
- *Exercise and activity pattern:* type and regularity of usual exercise, perceived and actual energy for desired and required leisure activities
- *Assistive devices required:* supplemental oxygen, humidifier, nebulizer treatments, or inhalers; walker, cane, or wheelchair; grab bars, shower chair, and other devices to promote safety and minimize energy expenditure; scale to monitor weight on a regular basis
- *Home environment:* factors that impair airway clearance, gas exchange, or activity tolerance; indoor pollutants, such as cigarette smoke, dust, and allergens (e.g., pets); lack of humidity in the air; barriers, such as stairs
- *Current level of knowledge:* importance of avoiding smoking and other pollutants; dietary salt and other restrictions if appropriate; recommended activities; medications; need to limit exposure to respiratory infections; use of prescribed nebulizer, multidose inhaler, powdered dose inhaler, or home oxygen; activity level

FAMILY

- *Caregiver availability, skills, and responses:* ability and willingness to provide care as needed (help with ADLs, providing meals, assisting with transportation and shopping, caring for dependents, and performing treatments, such as percussion and postural drainage)
- *Family role changes and coping:* effect on financial status, parenting and spousal roles, sexuality, social roles
- *Alternate potential primary or respite caregivers:* other family members, volunteers, church members, paid caregivers or housekeeping services, and available community respite care (e.g., adult day care or senior centers)

COMMUNITY

- *Environment:* usual temperature and humidity; presence of air pollutants, such as automobile exhaust, industrial smoke and pollutants, and smoke from field burning
- *Current knowledge of and experience with community resources:* medical and assistive equipment and supply companies, respiratory and physical therapy services, home health agencies, local pharmacies, available financial assistance, and support and educational organizations, such as the local lung association and chronic obstructive pulmonary disease support groups

Ineffective Airway Clearance

Both chronic bronchitis and emphysema affect the ability to maintain open airways. In chronic bronchitis, copious amounts of thick, tenacious mucus impair ciliary action, making it difficult to clear mucus from the airways. The loss of supporting tissue caused by emphysema increases the risk for airway collapse. In both cases, air is trapped distally, and less oxygen is available to the alveoli for diffusion. Normal respiratory defense mechanisms are impaired, and mucus-plugged airways provide an ideal environment for bacterial growth. Respiratory infection further impairs airway clearance and is often the cause of an acute exacerbation.

- Assess respiratory status every 1–2 hours or as indicated. Assess rate and pattern; cough and secretions (color, amount, consistency, and odor); and breath sounds, both normal and adventitious. Frequent assessment is vital to monitor current status and response to treatment. Adventitious sounds should decrease with effective intervention. Diminished or absent breath sounds may indicate increasing airway obstruction and possible atelectasis.
- Monitor ABG results. Increasing hypoxemia, hypercapnia, and respiratory acidosis may indicate increasing airway obstruction.
- Weigh daily, monitor intake and output, and assess mucous membranes and skin turgor. Dehydration causes respiratory secretions to become thicker, more tenacious, and difficult to **expectorate** (expel or spit out); fluid overload can further compromise respiratory status.
- Encourage a fluid intake of at least 2,000–2,500 mL/day unless contraindicated. Adequate fluid intake helps keep mucous secretions thin.
- Place in Fowler's, high-Fowler's, or orthopneic position (with head and arms supported on the overbed table); encourage movement and activity to tolerance. Upright positions improve ventilation and reduce the work of breathing. Activity helps mobilize secretions and prevent them from pooling.
- Assist with coughing and deep breathing at least every 2 hours while awake. Position the client seated upright and leaning forward during coughing. The upright position promotes chest expansion, increasing the effectiveness of coughing and reducing the work involved.
- Provide tissues and a paper bag to dispose of expectorated sputum. This important infection-control measure reduces the spread of respiratory organisms to other people.
- Refer to a respiratory therapist, and assist with or perform percussion and postural drainage as needed. Percussion helps loosen secretions in airways; postural drainage facilitates movement of these secretions out of the respiratory tract.
- Administer expectorant and bronchodilator medications as ordered. Correlate timing with respiratory treatments. Using expectorants and bronchodilators before coughing, percussion, and postural drainage increases their effectiveness in clearing airways.
- Provide supplemental oxygen as ordered. Supplemental oxygen helps maintain adequate blood and tissue oxygenation.

PRACTICE ALERT

Promptly report changes in oxygen saturation, skin color, or mental status. A drop in oxygen saturation levels, increasing cyanosis, or altered LOC indicates hypoxemia, possibly related to airway obstruction. Provide endotracheal, oral, or nasopharyngeal suctioning as necessary to stimulate cough and help clear secretions.

Ineffective Breathing Pattern

- Monitor vital signs and laboratory results. Tachypnea, tachycardia, an elevated blood pressure, and increasing hypoxemia and hypercapnia are signs of compromised respiratory status.
- Assist with ADLs as needed. This conserves client energy and reduces fatigue.
- Provide rest periods between scheduled activities and treatments. Scheduled rest is important to prevent fatigue and reduce oxygen demands.
- Teach and assist to use techniques to control breathing pattern:
  a. Pursed-lipped breathing
  b. Abdominal breathing
  c. Relaxation techniques including visualization and meditation.

  Breathing exercises are frequently indicated for clients with restricted chest expansion, such as people with COPD or clients recovering from thoracic surgery. Pursed-lipped breathing helps keep airways open by maintaining positive pressure, and abdominal breathing improves lung expansion. Relaxation techniques reduce anxiety and its effect on the respiratory rate.
- Administer medications, including bronchodilators and anti-inflammatory drugs, as ordered. Monitor for desired and possible adverse effects. Medications are used to improve airway status and facilitate breathing.

PRACTICE ALERT

Prepare for intubation and mechanical ventilation if respiratory status deteriorates (increasing hypoxemia and hypercapnia, decreased LOC, cyanosis, or worsening airway obstruction). Respiratory failure is a possible complication of an acute exacerbation of COPD and requires immediate intervention to preserve life.

Activity Intolerance

Clients with COPD, especially the more advanced stages, are at high risk for activity intolerance, especially if they do not intake sufficient fluids and nutrition.

- Assess at each health care interaction how the client is meeting ADLs.
- Discuss the importance of spacing periods of activity with periods of rest as well as other strategies, including trying to accomplish more important tasks early in the day.
- Design, together with the physician, physical therapist, and client, an exercise plan that meets the client's current level of performance but also helps build the client's stamina and strength. Regular exercise is critical to maintain lung function and quality of life.

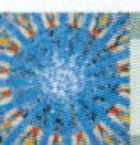

EVIDENCE-BASED PRACTICE Chronic Obstructive Pulmonary Disease

Clinical Question

The correlation between physical activity and performance of essential activities of daily living, quality of life, and higher-level functioning is well established. This is particularly true for older adults and for people with disease-related impairment in physical abilities. Physical inactivity is both a cause and an effect of declining physical function in older adults as well as in clients with chronic obstructive pulmonary disease (COPD).

Evidence

A study by Yang and Chen (2005) looked at change processes involved in moving from inactivity to activity in clients with COPD. This study found that those who adopted more behavioral change processes (counterconditioning, helping relationships, reinforcement management, and self-liberation) were more likely to engage in and maintain regular exercise (defined as at least 20 minutes of exercise of any intensity performed more than three times a week, usually walking). Most of these clients were aware of the benefits of exercise and the link between exercise and illness. Even so, 15% of study participants who achieved exercise maintenance returned to a more sedentary, inactive lifestyle.

Best Practice

This study and others support a program of regular physical activity to maintain functional status and reduce symptom progression. Additionally, this study suggests the importance of providing support and tools to help the client incorporate exercise into daily routines rather than simply recommending an exercise program and discussing the benefits of exercise. Strategies such as regular telephone follow-ups and creation of support groups help promote self-care responsibility. Encourage clients with COPD to enroll in a pulmonary rehabilitation program if one is available. If there is no organized program in the area, work with the client, family, and social support network to develop an exercise routine that can and will be maintained.

Critical Thinking

1. Consider other populations for whom regular exercise is recommended (e.g., clients who are overweight and clients with heart failure). What strategies have been shown to improve compliance with recommendations for regular exercise in these groups? How could these strategies be adapted for clients with COPD?
2. Use the physiologic and psychologic effects of regular exercise to explain its correlation with improved symptoms in the client with COPD.
3. Consider the age of most clients with COPD. What other physical or psychosocial factors commonly limit physical activity in this population? How can you use this information in designing an appropriate exercise program?

Imbalanced Nutrition: Less Than Body Requirements

With advanced COPD, minimal activity, including eating, can cause fatigue and dyspnea. The client may be unable to consume a full meal without resting. At the same time, the increased work of breathing increases metabolic demands, and more calories are required. The client may appear cachectic (thin and wasted). Poor nutritional status further impairs immune function and increases the risk of a complicating infection.

- Assess nutritional status, including diet history, appropriate weight for height (use reference tables of desired weights), and anthropometric (skinfold) measurements. It is important to differentiate nutritional status from body type rather than assume a nutritional impairment.
- Observe and document food intake, including types, amounts, and caloric intake. This information can provide direction for supplementation if needed.
- Monitor laboratory values, including serum albumin and electrolyte levels. These values provide information about the adequacy of nutritional intake, including protein.
- Consult with a dietitian to plan meals and nutritional supplements that meet caloric needs. More concentrated sources of high-energy foods may be required to maintain caloric intake without excess fatigue. A diet high in proteins and fats without excess carbohydrates is recommended to minimize carbon dioxide production during metabolism (carbohydrates are metabolized to form CO_2 and water).
- Provide frequent, small feedings with between-meal supplements. Frequent, small meals help maintain intake and reduce fatigue associated with eating.
- Place the client in a seated or high-Fowler's position for meals. An upright position promotes lung expansion and reduces dyspnea.
- Assist to choose preferred foods from the menu; encourage family members to bring food from home if allowed. Providing preferred foods encourages eating.
- Keep snacks at the bedside. Snacks provide additional caloric intake.
- Provide mouth care before meals. This helps enhance the appetite.
- If unable to maintain oral intake, consult with the physician about enteral or parenteral feedings. Maintenance of caloric and nutrient intake is vital to prevent catabolism.

Compromised Family Coping

Chronic illness affects the entire family structure. Roles and relationships change; additional demands are placed on the family. Family members may blame the client for causing the illness or have distorted perceptions about it, even denying its existence. They may refuse to assist or participate in care. The client may develop an attitude of helplessness or dependence or may demonstrate anger, hostility, or aggression.

- Assess interactions between client and family. Assessment helps identify desired and potential destructive behaviors.

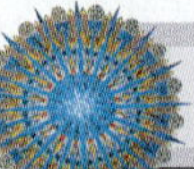

NURSING CARE PLAN A Client With Chronic Obstructive Pulmonary Disease

Anna Mercurio, known as "Happy" to all her friends, is an 83-year-old widow who lives with her two adult sons. During the past 15 years, Mrs. Mercurio has become increasingly short of breath while gardening and walking, two of her favorite activities. She also has developed a chronic cough that is particularly bad in the mornings. Ten years ago, her family physician told her that she had emphysema. She is admitted to the hospital with possible pneumonia and acute exacerbation of COPD.

ASSESSMENT

Jeff Harris, RN, admits Mrs. Mercurio to the medical unit. In the nursing history, Mr. Harris notes that she denies ever smoking but says that her husband and two sons have been smokers "for practically their whole lives." She says she lived an active life before developing lung disease, but her breathing and cough have progressed so that she now must rest after just a few minutes of housework or other activity. Her cough is productive of moderate to large amounts of sputum, particularly in the mornings. She developed increasing shortness of breath and sputum 2 days ago. This morning, she could not complete her morning activities without resting, so she contacted her doctor.

On physical examination, Mr. Harris notes the following: skin very warm and dry, color dusky. Pauses frequently while speaking to breathe. Respirations 36/minute, fairly shallow; coughs frequently, producing large amounts of thick, tenacious green sputum. Other vital signs: pulse 115 bpm and irregular, BP 186/60 mmHg, temperature 102.4°F (39°C). Appears very thin; weight 96 lb (43.6 kg), height 63 inches (160 cm). Anteroposterior:lateral chest diameter approximately 1:1; moderate kyphosis noted. Chest hyperresonant to percussion. Auscultation reveals distant breath sounds with scattered wheezes and rhonchi throughout lung fields. Chest x-ray shows flattening of diaphragm, slight cardiac enlargement, prominent vascular and bronchial markings, and patchy infiltrates. Initial laboratory work reveals moderate erythrocytosis, leukocytosis, and low serum albumin. ABG results: pH 7.19; PaO_2, 54 mmHg; $PaCO_2$, 59 mmHg; HCO_3, 30 mg/dL; and oxygen saturation, 88%. Admitting orders include sputum specimen for culture; intravenous penicillin G, 2 million units every 4 hours; albuterol/ipratropium (Combivent) inhaler, two puffs every 6 hours; salmeterol/fluticasone (Advair) dry powder inhaler, twice a day; bedrest with bathroom privileges; oxygen per nasal cannula at 2 L/minute continuously; and regular diet.

DIAGNOSES

- Ineffective Airway Clearance related to pneumonia and COPD
- Impaired Gas Exchange related to acute and chronic lung disease
- Risk for Impaired Spontaneous Ventilation related to loss of hypoxemic respiratory drive and respiratory muscle fatigue
- Impaired Home Maintenance related to activity intolerance

PLANNING

- The client expectorates secretions effectively.
- The client returns to a level of pulmonary function prior to acute exacerbation.
- The client demonstrates improved ABG and oxygen saturation values.
- The client maintains spontaneous respirations without excess fatigue.
- The client verbalizes willingness to allow sons or a housekeeper to assist with daily household tasks.

IMPLEMENTATION

- Assess respiratory status and LOC every 1–2 hours until stable, then at least every 4 hours.
- Closely monitor response to oxygen therapy, including skin color, oxygen saturation, sputum consistency, and respiratory drive.
- Increase fluid intake to at least 2,500 mL/day, and provide a bedside humidifier.
- Elevate head of bed to at least 30° at all times.
- Teach "huff" coughing technique.
- Administer medications as ordered, providing ipratropium inhaler before beclomethasone inhaler. Provide mouth care after inhalers.
- Contact respiratory therapy for percussion and postural drainage following inhaler treatments.
- Provide for uninterrupted rest periods following treatments and procedures.
- Meet with Mrs. Mercurio and her sons to develop a postdischarge care plan.
- Refer to home health department for nursing follow-up.
- Refer to social services for possible assistance with home maintenance.

EVALUATION

After the first day in the hospital, Mrs. Mercurio's condition begins to improve slowly. On discharge 6 days later, she is able to provide self-care with less fatigue and dyspnea. She is using oxygen at night only, admitting that it is just for security. Although a few scattered wheezes and rhonchi are still present in her lungs, Mrs. Mercurio's sputum is thinner, white, and easily expectorated. She will continue taking oral penicillin V for an additional 10 days at home. She will also continue using the Advair and Combivent inhalers as prescribed at home. Although Mrs. Mercurio's sons admit they will probably never be able to quit smoking, they have agreed to smoke only in the garage or outside. A home health nurse will initially evaluate Mrs. Mercurio's progress three times weekly. Arrangements have been made for a housekeeper to come twice a week for cleaning and laundry. Mrs. Mercurio is glad to be returning home and grateful for the arrangements that have been made.

NURSING CARE PLAN A Client With Chronic Obstructive Pulmonary Disease *continued*

CRITICAL THINKING

1. Mrs. Mercurio has never been a smoker but has had long-term exposure to secondhand smoke. How does secondhand smoke contribute to lung diseases in adults and children?
2. Mr. Harris's nursing care plan included the nursing diagnosis risk for impaired spontaneous ventilation related to loss of hypoxemic respiratory drive and respiratory muscle fatigue. Identify the normal physiologic events that stimulate breathing, and describe how these differ for the client with chronic hypoxemia and hypercapnia.
3. The client with an acute exacerbation of COPD is at risk for respiratory failure. What changes in Mrs. Mercurio's assessment findings could indicate this complication?
4. Develop a nursing care plan for Mrs. Mercurio for the nursing diagnosis deficient diversional activities related to inability to continue preferred activities.

- Assess the effect of the illness on the family. Assessment of family interactions, roles, and relationships assists in planning appropriate interventions.
- Help the client and family identify strengths for coping with the situation. Identifying personal and family strengths helps the family regain a sense of control.
- Provide information and teaching about COPD. Education helps the family gain an understanding of the client's condition and needs.
- Encourage expression of feelings. Avoid judging feelings that the client or family expresses, and avoid judging family members as "good" or "bad," "right" or "wrong." It is important that the nurse remain objective to maintain the therapeutic relationship.
- Help family members recognize behaviors and attitudes that may hinder effective treatment, such as continuing to smoke in the house. Family members may be unaware of the effect of their behavior on the client's ability to change habits and cope with a disabling disease.
- Encourage family members to participate in care. This helps develop skills for use at home.
- Initiate a care conference involving the client, family, and health care team members from a variety of disciplines. A wide range of perspectives and areas of expertise aids in problem solving and facilitates communication.
- If dysfunctional family relationships interfere with measures to enhance coping, advocate for the client, reaffirming his or her right to make decisions. Dysfunctional family relationships are not likely to change simply because of illness. The nurse can better meet the client's needs by accepting his or her limitations in dealing with family members.
- Refer the client and family to support groups and pulmonary rehabilitation programs as available. Support groups and structured rehabilitation programs enhance coping abilities.
- Arrange a social services consultation. This can help the client and family identify care and support service needs.
- Refer to community agencies or services such as home health, homemaker services, or Meals-on-Wheels as appropriate. Agencies or community services can provide additional support beyond the family's means or capability.

Decisional Conflict: Smoking

Smoking is more than a habit; it is an addiction. The client who must quit is facing a significant loss, not only of nicotine but also of a lifestyle. Although the client may fully comprehend the consequences of continuing to smoke, the decision to give up a part of his or her life is not easy. This fear may be expressed in such concerns as "I'll gain weight" or "What will I do with my hands?" In addition to providing practical information, a plan, and assistance with nicotine withdrawal, the nurse must support the client's decision-making process to comply with an order to stop smoking.

- Assess the client's knowledge and understanding of the choices involved and the possible consequences of each. The decision to quit smoking ultimately belongs to the client. He or she needs a full understanding of the consequences of quitting or continuing to smoke.
- Acknowledge concerns, values, and beliefs; listen without making judgments. The nurse needs to avoid imposing his or her values and beliefs about smoking on the client.
- Spend time with the client, encouraging expression of feelings. This demonstrates acceptance of the client and his or her right to make the decision.
- Help plan a course of action for quitting smoking, and adapt it as necessary. When the client develops the plan, he or she has more ownership in it and interest in making it work.
- Demonstrate respect for decisions and the right to choose. Respect supports self-esteem and the ability to cope.
- Provide referral to a counselor or other professional as needed. Counselors or other people trained to assist with smoking cessation can help with decision making.

Evaluation

Observe and record the rate, rhythm, and quality of breathing patterns, focusing on the trends of the client's vital signs and breathing patterns. Compare the actual respiratory parameters of the individual to the outcome goal established. Document and record the outcome of each intervention, its effectiveness, and plan. Some interventions may need to be carried out over a longer period of time before progress toward the goal is seen. For example, improving the ease of coughing may occur readily with increased fluid intake, while exercise programs established by the physical therapist may take several days to weeks to achieve effect.

Potential outcomes used to evaluate the effectiveness of nursing care may include the following:

- The client consistently maintains oxygen saturation greater than 90%.
- The client demonstrates appropriate modifications to ADLs as required based on activity tolerance.
- The client is able to maintain a patent airway adequate to allow for sufficient oxygenation.
- The family is able to describe resources available to reduce caregiver role strain and improve family coping.

REVIEW Chronic Obstructive Pulmonary Disease

RELATE: LINK THE CONCEPTS

Linking the exemplar of Chronic Obstructive Pulmonary Disease with the concept of Fluids and Electrolytes:

1. Why is it important for the client with COPD to drink sufficient fluids?
2. Why might a bedridden client with COPD choose to drink less and how can the nurse promote hydration in this client?

Linking the exemplar of Chronic Obstructive Pulmonary Disease with the concept of Safety:

3. Why is it important for the nurse to assess the client with COPD for risk for injury related to the use of oxygen?
4. What teaching would you provide a client who is to be discharged with home oxygen therapy for the first time?

READY: GO TO COMPANION SKILLS MANUAL

- Deep breathing and coughing
- Collecting a sputum specimen
- Using a pulse oximeter
- Administering oxygen by cannula, face mask, or face tent
- Using an oxygen cylinder
- Preparing client for chest physiotherapy
- Performing chest percussion
- Performing chest vibration
- Assisting with chest tube insertion
- Maintaining chest tube drainage
- Chest tube removal
- Clearing an obstructed airway
- Measuring respiratory rate
- Care of the ventilator-dependent client
- Care of a tracheostomy
- Care of an endotracheal tube

REFER: GO TO MYNURSINGKIT

REFLECT: CASE STUDY

James Winston is a 58-year-old white man living in North Carolina. Before retiring this past fall, he worked on a heavy-machinery production line most of his adult life. He served in the Marines during the Vietnam War. Throughout his work years, he was a weekend gardener. He has smoked a pack of cigarettes a day since high school, and he has increased to two packs a day since retirement. "I have been lying around the house waiting for spring so I can garden," he says.

Now that spring has arrived, trees are blooming, grass is again in need of mowing, and Mr. Winston is admitted to the medical unit with shortness of breath. The initial assessment demonstrates an afebrile man with vital signs as follows: temperature 98.9°F, pulse 88 bpm, respirations 32/minute, BP 164/96 mmHg, and pulse oximetry reading of 89%. Mr. Winston is tachypneic, sitting upright and forward with his hands on his knees. He has removed his oxygen face mask because "it smothers me," he says.

1. What other assessment data are needed before providing care for this individual?
2. What interventions are needed immediately for Mr. Winston?
3. What diagnostic examination would confirm this is COPD?
4. What interventions may be necessary for Mr. Winston to resume the healthy behaviors in his life?

21.4 RESPIRATORY SYNCYTIAL VIRUS/BRONCHIOLITIS

KEY TERMS

Apnea, *1281*
Atelectasis, *1281*
Bronchiolitis, *1281*
Comorbidity, *1282*
Play therapist, *1282*
Respiratory syncytial virus (RSV), *1281*
Rhinorrhea, *1282*

BASIS FOR SELECTION OF EXEMPLAR

American Academy of Pediatrics
Centers for Disease Control and Prevention
Most common condition

LEARNING OUTCOMES

After reading about this exemplar, you will be able to:

1. Describe the pathophysiology, etiology, clinical manifestations, and direct and indirect causes of respiratory syncytial virus (RSV)/bronchiolitis.
2. Identify risk factors associated with RSV/bronchiolitis.
3. Illustrate the nursing process in providing culturally competent care across the life span for individuals with RSV/bronchiolitis.
4. Formulate priority nursing diagnoses appropriate for an individual with RSV/bronchiolitis.
5. Create a plan of care for individuals with RSV/bronchiolitis and their family members.
6. Assess expected outcomes for an individual with RSV/bronchiolitis.
7. Discuss therapies used in the collaborative care of an individual with RSV/bronchiolitis.
8. Employ evidence-based caring interventions for an individual with RSV/bronchiolitis.

OVERVIEW

Respiratory syncytial virus (RSV) is a highly contagious respiratory infection that affects almost all children before 2 years of age. While persons of any age can contract the disease, in those older than 2 years it is likely to present as a simple cold or be asymptomatic. Only those 2 years old and younger will normally experience the more severe form of the disease. Older adults who are already at risk for impaired oxygenation may also be at risk for acquiring the more severe form of RSV, although they are at lower risk than young children. Because acquired immunity to the virus is weak, individuals may have repeated infections of RSV throughout their life span, although the symptoms tend to be less severe with repeated exposure.

Bronchiolitis is a lower respiratory tract illness that occurs when an infecting agent (virus or bacterium) causes inflammation and obstruction of the small airways (the bronchioles). Bronchiolitis is associated with a hospital admission rate of 30 per 1,000 infants under 1 year of age and with a mortality rate of 2 per 100,000 live births (Smyth & Openshaw, 2006). Children with bronchiolitis have an increased incidence of reactive airway disease and asthma later in childhood (Willis, 2007).

The most common cause of bronchiolitis is infection with RSV. Adenovirus, parainfluenza virus, influenza virus, and human meta pneumovirus are other potential causes. RSV occurs in annual epidemics from October to March. It is transmitted through direct contact with respiratory secretions or indirectly through contaminated surfaces. The virus is shed by the infected child for 3–8 days, and the incubation period is 2–8 days (American Academy of Pediatrics [AAP], 2006, p. 561). Nearly all children have been infected with RSV by 2 years of age, and reinfection (via siblings or close family contacts) throughout life is common (AAP Subcommittee on Diagnosis and Management of Bronchiolitis, 2006). RSV is a common cause of lower respiratory tract infections in infants and children. Infants at risk for severe infection with RSV include those under 24 months of age with chronic lung disease who have required medical therapy within 6 months of RSV season onset, those with significant congenital heart disease, and preterm infants under 35 weeks of gestation (Fowlkes & Fry, 2006).

PATHOPHYSIOLOGY AND ETIOLOGY

Respiratory syncytial virus infects the squamous epithelial cells of the bronchioles and alveoli. Infected cells merge with adjacent cells, creating large masses of cells, or "syncytia," that subsequently burst and die. The resulting debris clogs the minute airways of the lower respiratory tract, irritating the airway and resulting in edema and mucosal secretions. Partial airway obstruction and bronchospasms follow.

The cycle is repeated throughout both lungs as the airway cells are invaded by the virus. The partially obstructed airways allow air in, but the mucus and airway swelling block expulsion of the air. This creates the wheezing and crackles in the airways. Acute rhinorrhea also appears. **Atelectasis** (collapse of alveoli or section of alveoli) occurs in some areas, and air trapping and hyperinflation in others. Hypoxemia results because of the V-Q mismatch. The client with RSV is therefore at risk for respiratory failure as the oxygen level decreases and the carbon dioxide level increases. **Apnea** (absence of respirations) and pulmonary edema may occur.

This highly contagious viral infection is spread by direct physical contact with respiratory secretions or an infected individual. Virus droplets have also been detected in air as many as 22 feet from the infected individual.

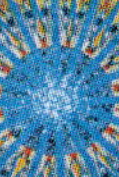

FOCUS ON DIVERSITY AND CULTURE

Alaskan Native Infants

RSV is a major cause of hospitalization among Alaskan Native infants and is responsible for one third of hospitalizations of children younger than 3 years in Alaska. Alaskan children hospitalized with RSV at any age are at a high risk for rehospitalization as a result of respiratory infection. Alaskan Native children living in rural areas have a higher rate of chronic lung disease; however, the relationship between RSV and chronic lung disease remains unclear (NCPDCID, 2009).

Etiology

Respiratory syncytial virus is a primary cause of respiratory infections among both children younger than 2 years and older adults. Between 75,000 and 125,000 children are hospitalized each year because of RSV. Worldwide, RSV affects some 64 million people and causes more than 150,000 deaths each year (NIAID, 2008). Approximately 14,000 high-risk adults and older adults die from RSV infections annually, with more than 170,000 adults being infected by the virus each year, at a cost of over $1 billion dollars (*Medical News Today*, 2005). Bronchiolitis results approximately 149,000 hospitalizations per year, with the frequency much higher for children younger than 1 year, males, and nonwhites.

Risk Factors

The risk of infection with RSV is higher for infants and toddlers who are not breastfed or who live in homes with secondary cigarette exposure, attend daycare, live in crowded conditions, or are socioeconomically disadvantaged. (APA, 2006: CDC, 2003; Cooper, Banasiak, & Allen, 2003; Goldmann, 2001).

Risk of infection is higher when the parent or caregiver smokes. Tobacco smoke increases mucus production and reduces the action of cilia within the airway passages. Exposure to secondhand smoke is thought to alter maturation of the respiratory epithelium.

Infants and toddlers who have a history of prematurity, chronic lung disease, acyanotic congenital heart disease, or reduced immunity are at greater risk for complications from RSV and may require hospitalized care. As mentioned, all children under the age of 2 have smaller airways, so they are risk for serious complications from RSV/bronchiolitis compared with older children and adults. In adults, high-risk populations include the older adults, those with chronic pulmonary disease, and those with congestive heart failure.

CLINICAL MANIFESTATIONS

The typical clinical presentation in otherwise healthy children begins 3–5 days after exposure to the virus. The early signs of a mild infection include **rhinorrhea** (drainable of mucus from the nose), cough, irritability, and a low-grade fever for 1–3 days. Copious mucous secretions occur in the lung fields and nasal passages and are usually green in color. The fever can lead to dehydration.

Signs and symptoms of a more serious infection may occur even in infants and toddlers with no history of **comorbidity** (the presence of one or more additional disease processes). These signs and symptoms, which call for medical care, include increased irritability, excessive coughing, wheezing, and observable retractions of the ribcage. Of even more concern are marked retractions of the ribcage, nasal flaring, rapid respiratory rate, blue skin, listlessness, and most important, periods without breathing. The emergency medical system should be called to provide transport to the hospital when a child presents with these symptoms.

COLLABORATION

Infants who demonstrate signs of respiratory distress while infected with RSV will require hospitalization. The plan of care includes monitoring breathing patterns, maintaining patent airways, maintaining adequate fluid and caloric intake, as well as supporting appropriate developmental behaviors. The respiratory therapist and nurse collaborate to monitor breathing patterns and keep airways clear of secretions. Infants who need endotracheal intubation will be closely cared for by the respiratory therapist.

Rapid breathing rates may require delivery of fluids and nutrition via an intravenous line. A nutritionist collaborates with the health care team to assure caloric intake meets the needs of the infant with RSV. A **play therapist** (a therapist educated in recreational activities related to the multiple age groups of people) is available in larger health care facilities to induce age-appropriate activities for children's play needs.

Diagnostic Tests

Laboratory tests that are used to identify the virus causing bronchiolitis include immunofluorescent or enzyme immunoassay techniques from a posterior nasopharyngeal specimen (CDC 2008). Viral cell culture and/or antigen detection testsmay also be performed. CXRs show hyperinflation, patchy atelectasis, and other signs of inflammation. Arterial blood gases indicate effectiveness of gas exchange.

CLINICAL MANIFESTATIONS AND THERAPIES RSV/Bronchiolitis

ETIOLOGY	CLINICAL MANIFESTATION	CLINICAL THERAPIES
Increased airway secretions	■ Rhinorrhea ■ Cough ■ Shortness of breath	Treatment at home may include: ■ Fluids ■ Rest ■ Antipyretics ■ Nasal suctioning using bulb syringe in children too young to clear their own airway.
Partial airway obstruction caused by increased secretions and resulting edema	■ Wheezing and crackles ■ Fever ■ Irritability ■ Anorexia ■ Poor fluid intake ■ Tachypnea ■ Grunting ■ Retractions	Evaluation by primary provider; treatment may include: ■ Increase fluid intake ■ Antipyretics ■ Suctioning the airway to relieve obstructions ■ Positioning to optimize oxygenation ■ Administration of oxygen via oxygen tent or oxyhood.
Hypoxia	■ Apnea ■ Tachypnea ■ Marked retractions of the ribcage ■ Use of accessory muscles ■ Listlessness ■ Cyanosis ■ Respiratory acidosis	Treatment at the emergency department may include: ■ Hydration with intravenous or oral fluids to prevent insensible fluid loss ■ Humidified oxygen therapy ■ Bronchodilators, steroids, beta-agonists ■ Suctioning to remove excess secretions if child cannot cough or swallow ■ Cardiopulmonary monitoring and pulse oximetry ■ Intubation and mechanical ventilation.

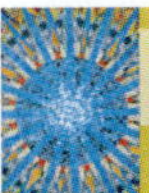

DEVELOPMENTAL CONSIDERATIONS

Diagnostic Tests for RSV Infection

Antigen detection tests and cultures are generally reliable in young children. They are less reliable in older children and adults, however, because of the lower viral loads in their respiratory specimens. Real-time polymerase chain reaction assays are more useful in these populations, because these tests are able to multiply the existing DNA/RNA so that it can be detected more easily (CDC, 2009).

Pharmacologic Therapy

Few medications are prescribed for RSV infection and bronchiolitis. The use of inhaled bronchodilators remains controversial, because most studies have not demonstrated improvement in symptoms over time (AAP Subcommittee on Diagnosis and Management of Bronchiolitis, 2006). A recent randomized, controlled trial investigating the use of dexamethasone for bronchiolitis in 600 infants revealed that there was no benefit to the medication in terms of hospital admission rate, respiratory status after 4 hours of observation, hospital length of stay, or subsequent emergency department visits (Corneli et al., 2007). Antipyretics may be used. Antibiotics, however, are not used routinely unless the child also has a bacterial infection.

Ribavirin is an antiviral drug specifically available for treatment of RSV infection. Its use remains controversial, however, because it has only marginal benefit. It is expensive, requires a cumbersome delivery, and has potential health risks for caregivers. Its use is reserved for cases of severe disease, such as infants with complicated congenital heart disease or who are immunocompromised (AAP Subcommittee on Diagnosis and Management of Bronchiolitis, 2006).

Clinical Therapy

No effective therapy for RSV infection and bronchiolitis exists. Hospitalized children are isolated, roomed together, or placed on the same unit to minimize the spread of the virus to other hospitalized children. Humidified oxygen using a hood, face tent, mask, or nasal cannula is provided to maintain pulse oximetry oxygen saturation readings at greater than 90% (Willis, 2007). The delivery method chosen is based upon the desired concentration of oxygen, degree of humidity, and the child's response. Other supportive care includes hydration with oral or intravenous fluids and nasal suctioning to facilitate breathing. Benefits of chest physiotherapy have not been documented by research (AAP Subcommittee on Diagnosis and Management of Bronchiolitis, 2006). CPAP may be used in the child with moderate to severe bronchiolitis. The child with apnea or respiratory failure will be cared for in the critical care unit, usually intubated and ventilated when too fatigued to breathe effectively.

NURSING PROCESS

Nursing management focuses on maintaining respiratory function, supporting overall physiologic function and hydration, reducing the child's and the family's anxiety, and preparing the family for home care. Prevent the transmission of RSV and other organisms by using airborne and standard precautions.

Assessment

Assessment allows the nurse to determine the severity of symptoms. Collect assessment data through the health history and physical assessment:

- *Health history.* Symptoms and behaviors for the previous 2 weeks, eating habits, fluid intake, any previous breathing problems or illnesses, birth history, and a list of those who provide care for the child other than the parents (e.g., grandparents, day care providers, and baby sitters)
- *Physical examination.* Breathing pattern, including rate, rhythm, and quality; inspection and palpation of the chest; use of accessory muscles when breathing, which indicates an increased need for oxygen; self-posturing.

Most children continue to play despite illness. Increased fatigue levels will interfere with play. Lack of play is an indication of severe illness in children.

Infants who are premature, have cardiac or respiratory disorders, or are immunocompromised have the greatest risk of severe RSV requiring hospital care. Assess for a more pronounced cough, wheezing, fevers to 102°F, and poor feeding. Also assess for signs of increased respiratory effort: marked retractions with nasal flaring, rapid respiratory rate, cyanosis, listlessness, and most important, periods without breathing.

Teach the parents or caregiver how to assess breathing patterns at home. Use of accessory muscles when breathing indicates an increased need for oxygen. A tripod stance, in which the client leans forward, resting arms on a table or the client's knees, indicates respiratory distress.

PRACTICE ALERT

Signs of life-threatening illness in the infant with bronchiolitis include central cyanosis, respiratory rate greater than 70 breaths per minute, listlessness, and apneic episodes. The chest is hyperinflated, and air exchange is so poor that breath sounds are very diminished on auscultation.

Diagnosis

Likely NANDA diagnoses for the infant or child with RSV infection include the following:

- Ineffective Breathing Pattern
- Ineffective Airway Clearance
- Impaired Gas Exchange
- Fluid and Electrolyte Imbalance: Less Than Body Requirements
- Impaired Nutrition: Less Than Body Requirements
- Activity Intolerance.

Plan

Care of the infant with RSV infection requires collaboration between the parents and the health care team. Goals often include the following:

- The client's breathing patterns will remain or return to regular rate, rhythm, and quality for the individual's age group.

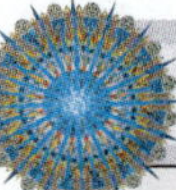

NURSING CARE PLAN A Client With Respiratory Syncytial Virus

Deborah Coley brings her 14-month-old son, Tyshawn, to the emergency department. Ms. Coley reports that Tyshawn has had a runny nose and a slight fever for 3 or 4 days and that he woke up coughing and crying during the night with a fever of 102°F. She says that she gave him some more children's Motrin and some juice and that she was able to stop him crying, but also that he is "not breathing right." She says that he had a slightly wet diaper this morning, but not as bad as it usually is.

ASSESSMENT	DIAGNOSES	PLANNING
Nurse Williams notices that Tyshawn has marked retractions of his ribcage. He is secreting green mucus from his nose, and he coughs frequently. His respiratory rate is 42/minute, and his oxygen saturation is 78%. Tyshawn is irritable, not wanting to comply with the initial physical examination. The attending physician suspects infection with RSV and prescribes a bronchodilator via nebulizer and oxygen therapy using a pediatric tent, after which Tyshawn's symptoms will be reassessed. His nasal secretions are sent to the lab to confirm the presence of RSV.	■ Ineffective Breathing Pattern ■ Impaired Gas Exchange ■ Ineffective Airway Clearance ■ Anxiety	■ The client will return to normal breathing rate and pattern. ■ The client will maintain adequate oxygenation. ■ The client will experience no further complications from the disease process. ■ The client will meet his nutritional needs.

IMPLEMENTATION

- The nurse administers a bronchodilator via nebulizer as ordered by the attending physician, then sets up the pediatric tent to provide oxygen therapy.
- The nurse reevaluates Tyshawn's oxygenation saturation levels and respiratory rate following the nebulizer treatment and again following the oxygen therapy.
- The nurse provides client teaching to Mrs. Coley related to RSV and the possibilities of recurrence.

EVALUATION

During administration of the oxygen therapy, Tyshawn falls asleep. After the oxygen therapy, his respiratory rate is 32/minute, and his oxygen saturation is at 92%. He is breathing through his mouth, indicating his nose is still stuffy.

CRITICAL THINKING

1. Why was the administration of the bronchodilator and oxygen therapy effective?
2. If Tyshawn's oxygen saturation did not improve following therapy, what would be the next step?
3. Develop a home care plan for Mrs. Coley to follow until Tyshawn's symptoms disappear and he returns to wellness.

- The client's airways will remain clear of secretions; swelling of mucosal linings will decrease to normal for the individual's age group.
- The client's fluid intake will meet daily requirements for the individual's age group.
- The client's daily nutritional needs will be meet as required for the individual's age group.
- If a child, the client will return to play activities as expected for the individual's age group.

Implementation

The priority of nursing care is maintaining a clear airway and promoting oxygenation. Parents of children requiring hospitalization are normally very anxious and protective. Including them in providing care and teaching the importance of interventions may help reduce that anxiety and allow them a measure of control in their child's life.

Ineffective Airway Clearance

The nurse working with a client who cannot clear the airway effectively should:

- Monitor temperature, pulse, respiration, blood pressure and pulse oximetry.
- Auscultate lung sounds.
- Encourage oral fluids to maintain thinned pulmonary secretions. Thinned secretions are easier to expectorate than thick, tenacious mucous. Intravenous fluids may be needed for the child with respiratory rates too great to safely feed orally or for the child who is too weak to consume adequate fluid volumes.
- Suction the mouth and nose. This maintains a patent airway.
- Teach parents the procedure to clear oral and nasal passages with a bulb syringe. Neonates are obligatory nose breathers, so their nasal passages do need to be kept clear of secretions.

- Teach parents and caregivers the signs and symptoms that indicate the need to return the child to the primary care provider or hospital. These signs and symptoms include increased irritability, cough, wheeze, and observable retractions of the ribcage.
- Teach parents and caregivers the sighs and symptoms that indicate the need to call emergency medical system to transport the child to the hospital. These signs and symptoms include marked retractions with nasal flaring, rapid respiratory rate, blue coloring of the skin, listlessness, and most importantly, periods without breathing.
- Teach parents not to smoke around infants and children. Encourage smoking cessation by parents and caregivers of children.
- Administer medications as ordered.

Ineffective Breathing Pattern

The nurse working with a client with an ineffective breathing pattern should:

- Continue to monitor breathing pattern, including rate, rhythm, and quality.
- Teach the parents or caregiver how to observe breathing patterns. Observable retractions of the ribcage indicate respiratory distress. If these are observed, the child should be brought to the hospital.
- Inspect and palpate chest for use of accessory muscles. Use of accessory muscles may indicate an increased need for oxygen.
- Assess for self-posturing. A tripod stance indicates respiratory distress.
- Administer bronchodilators and oxygen therapy as ordered.

Impaired Gas Exchange

The nurse working with a client at risk for impaired gas exchange should:

- Monitor temperature, pulse, respirations, blood pressure, and pulse oximetry.
- Monitor breathing patterns closely.
- Assess for bluish skin color.
- Collect a sputum specimen to identify causative agent.
- Collect ABG, CBC, and chemistry levels.
- Administer oxygen as ordered.

Impaired Nutrition: Less Than Body Requirements

The nurse working with a client at risk for impaired nutrition should:

- Monitor dietary intake. Adequate calories support healing.
- Take daily weight measurements, if in hospital setting.
- Offer foods that the client prefers.
- Offer small, frequent feedings.
- Encourage parents to continue to feed the child and provide liquids as normal. The child should not be forced to eat. If not eating or drinking as much as normal, the child may need more frequent feedings.

Fluid Volume Deficit

Nursing interventions for fluid volume deficit related to fever and poor oral intake include the following:

- Assess for poor skin elasticity, dry mucous membranes, and decreased urinary output.
- Record intake and output.
- Weigh each diaper for accurate output.
- Teach parents to count diapers per day.
- Encourage oral intake.
- Monitoring intravenous fluid rate if such fluids are ordered.

Activity Intolerance

Nursing interventions for activity intolerance include the following:

- Assess capacity to play. Even children who are ill play. Children who do not exert themselves to play may be experiencing increased fatigue levels. Increased levels of fatigue may indicate the disease is more severe. A follow-up by the primary care provider may be indicated.
- Organize care to allow for rest periods.

Evaluation

The rate, rhythm, and quality of breathing patterns are observed and recorded, focusing on the changes in vital signs and breathing patterns. Airway patency remains clear either through suctioning or by the individual's ability to cough and clear airways. Fluid and caloric intake are monitored to meet the needs of the age of the individual. Play fits the appropriate developmental stage of the child.

REVIEW Respiratory Syncytial Virus/Bronchiolitis

RELATE: LINK THE CONCEPTS

Linking the exemplar of Respiratory Synctial Virus/Bronchiolitis with the concept of Comfort:

1. What can you do to help a 3-month-old baby with RSV infection feel more comfortable?
2. What would you do differently to provide comfort to a 2-year-old with RSV infection?

Linking the exemplar of Respiratory Synctial Virus/Bronchiolitis with the concept of Stress and Coping:

3. How can you help parents to cope with the fear and anxiety related to hospitalization of their child?
4. When assessing the parents of a hospitalized child, how can you determine if they are coping in a healthy manner?

READY: GO TO COMPANION SKILLS MANUAL

- Collecting a sputum specimen
- Obtaining a nasal culture
- Providing oxygen via a pediatric tent
- Administering oxygen by cannula, face mask, or face tent
- Using an oxygen cylinder
- Assessing the thorax and lungs
- Assessing respiratory rate

REFER: GO TO MYNURSINGKIT

REFLECT: CASE STUDY

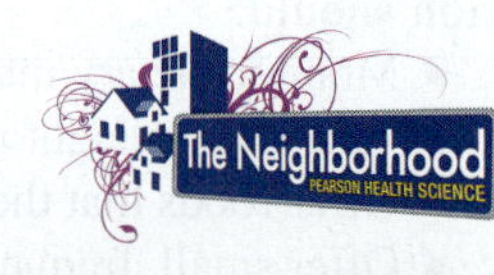

Ryan Riley is 9 months old. He has been sick off and on for the past week with a cold. He is not interested in eating or playing and has no energy. Ryan's mother, Jessica, leaves him in the care of her boyfriend, Casey, while she goes to work. Casey puts Ryan in his crib and leaves him alone all evening. During the course of the evening, Ryan gets worse and has nothing to drink. When Jessica comes home later that evening, Ryan feels very sick and is having problems breathing. Jessica immediately takes him to the hospital.

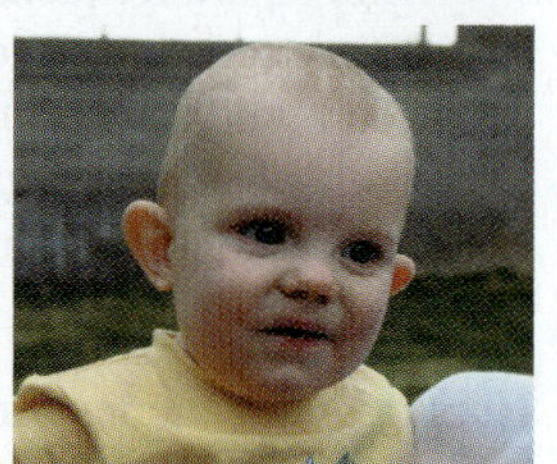

At the emergency department, Dr. Gordon asks Jessica how long Ryan has been sick, how many wet diapers he had in the past day, and when he last ate. Jessica tells Dr. Gordon that Ryan has had a cold for a week or so, but got sick just today. She admits that she doesn't know when he last ate or the number of wet diapers he has had. She tells Dr. Gordon that she has been working a lot of hours during the past several days. Dr. Gordon diagnoses Ryan with RSV infection and dehydration.

1. What signs and symptoms are priorities for the nursing assessment?
2. What are the priority nursing interventions for Ryan?
3. What are likely NANDA diagnoses for Ryan?
4. What tests or therapies is Dr. Gordon likely to order for Ryan?

21.5 SUDDEN INFANT DEATH SYNDROME

KEY TERMS

Prone, *1287*
Sudden infant death syndrome (SIDS), *1286*
Supine, *1287*

BASIS FOR SELECTION OF EXEMPLAR

Centers for Disease Control and Prevention
Evidence-Based Criteria for Oxygenation

LEARNING OUTCOMES

After reading about this exemplar, you will be able to:

1. Describe the pathophysiology, etiology, and direct and indirect contributing factors related to sudden infant death syndrome.
2. Identify risk factors associated with sudden infant death syndrome.
3. Illustrate the nursing process in providing culturally competent care for infants, parents, and caregivers to reduce the risk of sudden infant death syndrome.
4. Formulate priority nursing diagnoses appropriate for an infant at risk for sudden infant death syndrome.
5. Create a plan of care for infants at risk for sudden infant death syndrome and their family members.
6. Assess expected outcomes for the family who loses a child to sudden infant death syndrome.
7. Discuss therapies used in the collaborative care of an infant at risk for sudden infant death syndrome.
8. Employ evidence-based caring interventions to prevent the occurrence of, or reduce the risk for, sudden infant death syndrome (SIDS).

OVERVIEW

Sudden infant death syndrome (SIDS) is the sudden death of an apparently healthy infant that remains unexplained after other possible causes have been ruled out through autopsy, death scene investigation, and review of the medical history. SIDS is the third leading cause of infant mortality in the United States, accounting for 7.7% of all infant deaths; most SIDS deaths occur in infants between 2 and 4 months of age (CDC, 2006). It is currently unpredictable and, in some cases, unpreventable.

PATHOPHYSIOLOGY AND ETIOLOGY

There is no confirmed causative factor or pathophysiology for SIDS; it can be diagnosed only after a review of the child's clinical history, examination of the scene of death, and an autopsy that fails to find a cause of death. Sudden and unexplained infant deaths are investigated for cause. The CDC tabulates data to determine trends and similarities in relation to infant deaths. Nurses must be aware that data related to infant deaths are gathered and reported for research purposes and must know the procedures for gathering and reporting such data in the clinic or hospital where they work.

Etiology

Sudden infant death syndrome is referred to as a syndrome because of the many and varied autopsy and clinical findings that characterize most children who die of the disorder. The autopsy does not identify a disease process that caused the death.

A recent theory is that three factors occur simultaneously and lead to the sudden unexpected death of the infant. First, the infant has a vulnerability, a brainstem abnormality that controls respiratory and autonomic responses to stressors during sleep. Second, significant stressors contributing to SIDS are prone or side sleeping, face-down sleeping, and bed sharing. Infants in the prone or side-lying positions are vulnerable because the brainstem abnormality compromises their protective reflexes, such as arousal and head turning, when experiencing asphyxia. Third, infants are in a critical developmental period within the first 6 months of life (Paterson, Trachtenberg, Thompson, et al., 2006).

Covert homicide may be associated with 1–5% of cases designated as SIDS (Hymel & Committee on Child Abuse and Neglect, 2006). Other proposed causes include respiratory illness (potentially as a stress factor on a vulnerable infant) and long QT syndrome, a cardiac dysrhythmia (Daley, 2004). It is also possible that gene mutations or polymorphisms could make an infant more vulnerable to SIDS (Opdal & Rognum, 2004). SIDS has not been found to be associated with newborn apnea or immunizations (AAP Task Force on Sudden Infant Death Syndrome, 2005).

Risk Factors

Some infant and maternal risk factors have been associated with an increased incidence of SIDS. These are summarized in Box 21–6.

Infants placed **prone** (face-down) to sleep are at greatest risk. Infants should always be placed **supine** (on the back). The side-lying position also increases risk. Risk increases if a baby who has consistently been placed prone is placed supine for a nap or nighttime sleep. This often occurs when a caregiver other than a parent cares for the child. Grandparents, child care workers, and health care workers should be told to consistently place infants supine.

Premature and low-birth-weight babies have an increased risk of SIDS. Supine positioning for sleeping has been found to be an even greater protection against SIDS for the premature infant.

Maternal smoking during pregnancy and exposure to secondhand smoke during infancy have been correlated with an increased incidence of SIDS. The death rate from SIDS is nearly twice that for babies who are exposed to smoke compared to those who are not (Anderson, Johnson, & Batal, 2005). Smoking outside, away from babies, does not decrease the risk, because smoky hair and clothes also affect babies' respiratory status.

A previous case of SIDS in the family increases the risk for SIDS recurrence. Other risk factors associated with SIDS involve infant sleeping environments. Babies placed on soft sleeping surfaces with loose bedding are at increased risk, as are babies who are overheated or who share a bed with adults or other children. Sleeping with a baby on the couch, a recliner chair, or soft bedding places the baby at risk. Although bed sharing appears to be harmful, babies who sleep in the same room or in a separate co-sleeper that facilitates breast-feeding have a lower incidence of SIDS. Infants who are dressed in sleeper pajamas instead of being covered with blankets have less risk. Babies who sleep in bedrooms that are heated to the comfort level of typical adults also have less incidence of SIDS.

> **FOCUS ON DIVERSITY AND CULTURE**
> **Sudden Infant Death Syndrome**
>
> Rates of SIDS are highest for African Americans and American Indians and lowest for Asians and Hispanics. In 2001, the rate of SIDS among African Americans was more than twice that of whites, and the rate among American Indians was more than three times greater than that among whites (Health Resources Services Administration, 2004).
>
> To promote the use of supine sleeping position for African American babies, the Back to Sleep campaign joined with the National Black Child Development Institute and other historically black organizations to develop materials for a new initiative to reduce SIDS in African American communities. Another culturally competent effort to reduce SIDS deaths among American Indians and Alaskan Natives is a tool titled "Face Up to Wake Up,"™ which is used by health and medical service providers to expand SIDS risk reduction activities in Native American communities.

Breast-feeding appears to be protective, perhaps because breastfed babies are more easily aroused from sleep than formula-fed babies. Offering a pacifier at sleep times appears to support ease of arousal from sleeping and is considered to be protective.

CLINICAL MANIFESTATIONS

There are no warning signs or early clinical manifestations to indicate that a baby will die of SIDS. The first symptom is cardiopulmonary arrest. Clinical findings after the death include evidence of a struggle or change in position and the presence of frothy, blood-tinged secretions from the mouth and nares. Most deaths are unobserved. Typically, parents find the infant dead in the crib in the morning or after a nap, and they report having heard no cries or disturbances during the sleep interval.

COLLABORATION

All members of the health care team must work together to promote safety for the infant in order to reduce the occurrence of SIDS. All new parents should be taught the importance of "back to sleep" for their infants. Clients who purchase used older cribs and linens need to be taught how to assess them for safety because guidelines at the time of manufacture were different than those for bedding designed today. Infants at increased risk should be identified as early as possible to initiate precautions.

Box 21–6 Risk Factors for Sudden Infant Death Syndrome

- Preterm and low birth weight
- Race (in decreasing order of frequency): most common in American Indians and Alaska Natives, followed by non-Hispanic Blacks, non-Hispanic whites, Asian or Pacific Islanders, and Hispanics
- Gender: more common in males than in females
- Age: most common in infants between 2 and 4 months of age
- Sleeping in a prone or side-lying position
- Exposure to environmental tobacco smoke or mother who smoked during pregnancy
- Overheating (e.g., overdressing or too many bed covers)
- Bed sharing, especially with people who smoke or are under the influence of alcohol or drugs
- Loose bedding: use of pillows, comforters, quilts, and blankets
- Sleeping on soft surfaces: waterbed, sofa, pillows, with stuffed toys

Source: Adapted from Centers for Disease Control and Prevention. (2006). *October 2006 is SIDS (sudden infant death syndrome) awareness month.* Retrieved July 27, 2007, from http://www.cdc.gov/omh/Highlights/2006/HOct06SIDS.htm

Modeling Protective Behaviors

Members of the health care team are in a perfect position to teach new families to care for their baby. Protective behaviors should be modeled as well as taught. All members of the health care team need to place the newborn on its back for sleep. Because many nurses and physicians were educated that the appropriate sleep position for babies was prone, some health care providers may find it difficult to alter behaviors from what they learned to the positioning that is now supported by research. Supine positioning for sleeping has been found to be even more protective of SIDS for the premature infant. Neonatal health care workers, nursery, and pediatric health care personnel need to be conscious of their positioning behaviors, particularly since parents observe positioning behaviors of health care workers and then copy those behaviors.

Psychosocial Needs of the Family

Sudden infant death may occur despite following all the precautions. The sudden, unexpected nature of the infant's death is confirmed in the emergency department. Nurses are part of an interdisciplinary team that supports the family through their grief.

The nurse's role is to be empathetic and provide support during one of the greatest crises a family must face. The focus is on supporting the family during the acute grieving period. Guidelines for the support of families experiencing SIDS should include baptism services, religious support, grief counseling, assistance with funeral arrangements, and counseling on cessation of breastfeeding when appropriate. A spiritual leader of the family's particular belief system is asked to come to the family's aid in coping with grief. Other health care providers involved with the infant's care may also provide emotional support during the family's time of grief; some health care providers attend the funeral services to emotionally support to the grieving family.

Reassure the parents that they are not responsible for the infant's death, and assist them in contacting other family members and mobilizing support. Giving parents information about the potential reactions of siblings can help them respond to their needs. Older children may need reassurance that SIDS will not happen to them. They may also believe that bad thoughts or wishes about their baby brother or sister caused the death.

Nurses in perinatal or pediatric care as well as social workers may direct the family to a support group for those who have suffered the death of a child. Support groups can help parents, siblings, and other family members express these fears and work through their feelings about the infant's death. The First Candle organization can help families locate a support group in their geographic area (http://www.firstcandle.org). Local hospice organizations also provide supportive services to families grieving the loss of a child. Parents may need extra support at a later time with the birth of a subsequent newborn.

NURSING PROCESS

Nursing care is focused on prevention. When caring for the family who lost an infant to SIDS, the priority of care is to support the parents in the grieving process, reduce feelings of guilt, provide referrals to support groups, and help them cope with their loss.

Assessment

Nurses that provide care during pregnancy and early infancy should assess for risk for SIDS and not hesitate to ask appropriate questions. Collect assessment data through the health history and physical assessment:

- *Health history.* Does the mother or any other member of the household smoke? How and where does the mother put the child to sleep? What other caregivers put the child to sleep? What are the child's breathing patterns? Will the mother breastfeed or use formula? Has there been a previous death of an infant within the family?
- *Physical examination.* Respiratory rate and patterns.

Diagnosis

The following NANDA diagnoses are appropriate for the infant at risk for SIDS and immediate family members:

- Risk for SIDS
- Knowledge Deficit related to risk factors associated with SIDS
- Enhanced Parenting related to preventative measures associated with SIDS.

The following NANDA diagnoses may be appropriate for those families who have just lost a baby to SIDS:

- Grieving
- Compromised Family Coping
- Risk for Spiritual Distress.

Plan

Nurses collaborate with families and prospective family to design appropriate outcomes with the goal of decreasing the infant's risk for SIDS. These outcomes may include the following:

- Parents and other adults living in the household will describe appropriate habits to lower the risk for SIDS, including putting the infant back to sleep.
- Any adult in the household who smokes will participate in a smoking cessation program.
- Parents who lose a baby to SIDS will participate in grief counseling or a support group.

Parents who lose a baby may not feel ready to participate in counseling or support groups. The nurse should encourage, not push, parents to seek help, offering referral sources and calling to check on the parents at appropriate intervals following the death. The nurse on duty when the baby is brought to the emergency department should determine if the family has spiritual support and notify the hospital chaplain or offer to call the family's spiritual leader.

Implementation

Client teaching is an important nursing intervention. By educating parents of newborns on preventive strategies, it is possible to continue to reduce the number of SIDS deaths occurring annually.

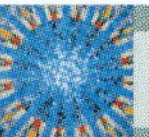

EVIDENCE-BASED PRACTICE Infant Sleep Positioning

Clinical Question

In spite of evidence that the supine position for newborns and infants reduces the risk for SIDS, this position is not consistently used by nurses in hospitals.

Evidence

A survey of 58 Missouri hospitals was conducted to examine nurses' knowledge, attitude, and practice in positioning healthy newborns for sleep in the hospital. While nurses no longer used prone positioning for newborns, 75% of 528 responding nurses used side-lying or a mixture of side-lying and supine positioning. Almost all nurses (96%) reported awareness of guidelines for newborns to sleep on their backs. Reasons given by nurses for the sleep position used included fear of aspiration, increasing the infant's comfort, and improving the infant's sleep. The majority of nurses reported having encountered an infant in supine position that was in distress at some time (Bullock, Mickey, Green, et al., 2004)

Another survey was conducted in eight California hospitals, with respondents including 96 newborn nursery staff (predominantly nurses) and 579 mothers. The majority of nurses (68.4%) reported placing infants on their side, and 65.3% of nurses advised mothers to use either the side or back positioning for sleep. Aspiration was the primary reason given for the side-lying position. Most nursery staff (72%) reported awareness of guidelines for infant positioning for sleep. The majority of mothers (72%) reported seeing their newborn placed in a nonsupine position by nursery staff, and 44% of mothers were not given recommendations for a sleep position for their newborn. Mothers receiving a recommendation for newborn sleep position were told to use the side or back (Stastny, Ichinose, Thayer, et al., 2004).

Best Practice

The Back to Sleep campaign has been very successful in increasing awareness regarding the importance of placing infants to sleep in a supine position. Nurses may feel that a side-lying position is safer and prevents aspiration but not be aware that this position increases the infant's risk for SIDS, especially if the infant rolls to a prone position. Up to 80% of mothers were more likely to use supine positioning for their infant when nurses gave that advice and modeled the position at the hospital (Stastny et al., 2004). Nurses have an important opportunity to model appropriate sleep positioning for newborns and to educate parents about reducing the risk for SIDS.

Critical Thinking

1. Identify methods to increase the use of supine positioning for newborns and infants who are hospitalized and to promote safe sleep for newborns and infants in the home.

Knowledge Deficit Related to Risk Factors Associated With SIDS

Caring interventions focus on teaching parents how to reduce risks. For caring interventions related to loss, see the Concept 12, Grief and Loss.

The most important teaching can be summed up by the phrase, "Back to sleep, tummy to play." "Back to sleep" should be applied to all sleeping sessions, whether a nap or at night. Protective behaviors should be modeled as well as taught.

Specifically, nurses will model and teach:

- "Back to sleep"
- Tummy for play time while awake
- Cuddle time for loving, upright position on lap or chest
- Cease smoking during pregnancy and around infants
- Use bedding that is firm
- Crib or co-sleeper in parents' room
- Sleeper or warm pajamas
- Blankets secured lower than infant's chest
- Avoid overheating sleeping room
- Parents need to tell caregivers "Back to sleep only."

CLIENT TEACHING The Back to Sleep Campaign

The single most important method of preventing SIDS is putting the infant to sleep on the back. The Back to Sleep campaign was launched in June 1994 to increase parents' and caregivers' understanding of this crucial issue. The campaign is a collaboration by the National Institutes of Health, the American Academy of Pediatrics, First Candle/SIDS Alliance, and Association of SIDS and Infant Mortality Programs. The campaign is credited with widespread success: As of 2002, the National Center for Health Statistics reported a more than 50% drop in SIDS death rates (National Institute for Child Health and Human Development, 2009). This campaign saturates hospitals, pediatricians' offices, clinics, child care programs, local health departments and other agencies serving mothers with young children with resources that demonstrate the importance of putting babies to sleep on their backs.

Evaluation

Nurses evaluate understanding of infant care to protect against risk for SIDS by discussion during follow-up visits and during perinatal care. Nurses determine if families understand the importance of supine sleeping and nonsmoking behaviors. Nurses ask if the sleeping arrangements for an infant include a separate, firm surface and whether dressing and heating arrangements provide for adequate warmth without overheating. A final evaluation may be related to SIDS occurring despite families following all the precautions. Nurses are part of an interdisciplinary team that supports the family through their grief.

HEALTH CARE

The assessment carried out after the death of an infant in the home is completed by a medical examiner and law enforcement agents. Other potential causes have to be ruled out. Sudden, unexplained infant deaths may be the result of homicide, undiagnosed genetic disorders, accidents, or other cardiopulmonary pathologies. Investigative questions are utilized to establish the cause and manner of the death or to support investigator's findings in court.

Families who have suddenly lost a baby are interviewed. The purpose of the interview is to determine any cause, clinical or accidental, and to rule out homicide. The CDC stresses balancing investigation with supporting a grieving family. Often, the investigation has the positive effect of demonstrating the family's innocence to friends and neighbors.

The physical address of the location where the death occurred is recorded. An assessment of the scene, including orientation of fixtures and body placement as well as body appearance, is completed. A health history of the infant, including diet, metabolic disorders, birth defects, and maternal pregnancy history, is recorded. A pathologist will summarize the findings from the autopsy and investigations reports to determine the cause of death.

REVIEW Sudden Infant Death Syndrome

RELATE: LINK THE CONCEPTS

The parents of an infant who has died of SIDS ask the emergency department nurse for ideas on how they can tell the 2-year-old sibling that the baby has died.

Linking the exemplar of Sudden Infant Death Syndrome with the concept of Development:

1. Based on the typical developmental stages of a 2-year-old's language, what suggestions might the nurse make?
2. How would the nurse's suggestions differ if the family asks for ideas for how to tell a 10-year-old sibling what has happened?

Linking the exemplar of Sudden Infant Death Syndrome with the concept of Family:

3. What resources could you recommend to the family of an infant who died of SIDS in your community?
4. What strategies might you suggest to help the family of an infant who died from SIDS who are displaying unhealthy coping strategies?

REFER: GO TO MYNURSINGKIT

REFLECT: CASE STUDY

Susan Miller is a 24-year-old, gravida 2 para 2 woman in the postpartum unit. Her son died at the age of 4 months because of SIDS. Mrs. Miller expresses fear that her newborn daughter, Grace, could also die from SIDS. She has heard that if SIDS occurs in a family, the likelihood of recurrence is greater.

1. What are possible nursing diagnoses for Mrs. Miller? for Grace?
2. Create a teaching plan that includes typical infant care, stressing behaviors that can reduce the risk of SIDS for this mother and child.
3. What coping strategies might you suggest to Ms. Miller to help her reduce her anxiety related to a reoccurance of SIDS with her new daughter?

EXPLORE PEARSON **mynursingkit**™

MyNursingKit is your one stop for online chapter review materials and resources. Prepare for success with additional NCLEX®-style practice questions, interactive assignments and activities, web links, animations and videos, and more!

Register your access code from the front of your book at **www.mynursingkit.com**.

REFERENCES

Adams, S. G., Hospenthal, A. C., Baillargeon, G. M., Kazis, L. E., Pugh, J. A., & Anzueto, A. (2008). Hispanic patients with chronic obstructive pulmonary disease did not receive referral to smoking cessation courses as commonly as patients of other ethnicities. *American Journal of Respiratory and Critical Care Medicine*, *177*(5) 473–478.

American Academy of Allergy, Asthma, and Immunology. (2007). *Tips to remember: Childhood asthma.* Retrieved July 8, 2009, from http://www.aaaai.org/patients/publicedmat/tips/childhoodasthma.stm

American Academy of Allergy, Asthma, and Immunology. (2009). *Diseases 101: Adult asthma.* Retrieved July 8, 2009, from http://www.aaaai.org/patients/gallery/adultasthma.asp

American Academy of Pediatrics. (2006). *Diagnosis and management of bronchiolitis*. Retrieved from http://www.pediatrics.org/cgi/doi/10.1542/peds.2006-2223

American Academy of Pediatrics Subcommittee on Diagnosis and Management of Bronchiolitis. (2006). Diagnosis and management of bronchiolitis. *Pediatrics, 118*(4), 1774–1793.

American Academy of Pediatrics Task Force on Sudden Infant Death Syndrome. (2005). The changing concept of sudden infant death syndrome: Diagnostic coding shifts, controversies regarding the sleeping environment, and new variables to consider in reducing risk. *Pediatrics, 116*(5), 1245–1255.

American Lung Association. (2006). *Lung disease data: 2006.* Retrieved from http://www.lungusa.org

American Lung Association. (2008). Acute respiratory distress syndrome (ARDS) in *Lung Disease Data: 2008*. Retrieved December 25, 2008, from http://www.lungusa.org

Anderson, M. E., Johnson, D. C., & Batal H. A. (2005). Sudden infant death syndrome and prenatal maternal smoking: Rising attributed risk in the Back to Sleep Era. *BMC Med, 3*(1), 4. Retrieved August 7, 2009 from http://www.firstcandle.org/FC-PDF4/Research_Recent%20Studies/Prenatal%20Maternal%20Smoking.pdf

American Academy of Pediatrics (AAP) Subcommittee on Diagnosis and Management of Bronchiolitis. (2006). Diagnosis and management of bronchiolitis. *Pediatrics, 118*(4), 1774–1793.

Banauch, G. I., Hall, C., Weiden, M., Cohen, H. W., Aldrich, T. K., Christodoulou, V., et al. (2006). Pulmonary function after exposure to the World Trade Center collapse in the New York City Fire Department. *American Journal of Respiratory Care and Critical Care Medicine, 174*, 312–319.

Boyle, A. H., & Locke, D. L. (2004). Update on chronic obstructive pulmonary disease. *Medical-Surgical Nursing, 13*(1).

Bullock, L. F. C., Mickey, K., Green, J., & Heine, A. (2004). Are nurses acting as role models for the prevention of SIDS? *Maternal Child Nursing, 29*(3), 172–177.

Centers for Disease Control and Prevention. (2003a). Respiratory diseases. *Healthy People 2010*. Retrieved from http://www.healthypeople.gov/Document/HTML/Volume2/24Respiratory.htm#_Toc489704826

Centers for Disease Control and Prevention. (2003b). Respiratory diseases: Chronic obstructive pulmonary disease. *Healthy People 2010*. Retrieved from http://http://www.healthypeople.gov/Document/HTML/Volume2/24Respiratory.htm#_Toc489704826

Centers for Disease Control and Prevention. (2006). *October 2006 is SIDS (sudden infant death syndrome) awareness month*. Retrieved July 27, 2007, from http://www.cdc.gov/omh/Highlights/2006/HOct06SIDS.htm

Centers for Disease Control and Prevention. (2008). *Respiratory syncytial virus: Laboratory testing*. Retrieved June 30, 2009, from http://www.cdc.gov/rsv/clinical/labtesting.html

Centers for Disease Control and Prevention. (2009). *Facts about chronic obstructive pulmonary disease*. Retrieved October 29, 2009, from http://www.cdc.gov/copd/copdfaq.htm

Cooper, A. C., Banasiak, N. C., & Allen, P. J. (2003). Management and prevention strategies for respiratory syncytial virus (RSV) bronchiolitis in infants and young children: A review of evidenced-based practice interventions. *Pediatric Nursing*, 29(6), 452–456.

Corbridge, S. J., & Berry, J. K. (2007). Chronic obstructive pulmonary disease. *AAOHN Journal, 55*(5). Retrieved August 7, 2009, from http://www.aaohnjournal.com/showAbst.asp?thing=34104

Corneli, H. M., Zorc, J. J., Mahajan, P., Shaw, K., Holubkov, R., et al. (2007). A multicenter, randomized controlled trial of dexamethasone for bronchiolitis. *New England Journal of Medicine, 357*(4), 331–339.

Daley, K. C. (2004). Update on sudden infant death syndrome. *Current Opinion in Pediatrics, 16*, 227–232.

Davidson, C. M., Doyle, N. M., & Ramin, S. M. (2005). Don't undertreat asthma in pregnancy. *Contemporary OB/GYN, 50*(8), 34–41.

Dolovich, M. B., Ahrens, T. C., Hess, D. R., et al. (2005). Device selection and outcomes of aerosol therapy: Evidence-based guidelines. *Chest, 127*, 335–371.

Dombrowski, M. P. (2006). Asthma and pregnancy. *Obstetrics and Gynecology, 108*, 667–681.

Fenstermacher, D., & Hong, D. (2004). Mechanical ventilation: What have we learned? *Critical Care Nursing Quarterly, 27*(3), 256–294.

Fontaine, K. L. (2005). *Healing practices: Alternative therapies for nursing* (2nd ed.). Upper Saddle River, NJ: Prentice Hall Health.

Fowlkes, A. L., & Fry, A. M. (2006). Respiratory syncytial virus activity–United States, 2005–2006. *Morbidity and Mortality Weekly Report, 55*(47), 1277–1279.

Froh, D. K. (2006). Alterations in pulmonary function in children. In K. L. McNance & S. E. Heuther (Eds.), *Pathophysiology: The biologic basis for disease in adults and children* (5th ed., pp. 1249–1278). St. Louis, MO: Elsevier Mosby.

Gélinas, C., Fortier, M., Viens, C., Fillion, L., & Puntillo, K. (2004). Pain assessment and management in critically ill intubated patients: A retrospective study. *American Journal of Critical Care, 13*(2), 126–135.

Global Initiative for COPD. (2009). *Global Initiative for Chronic Obstructive Lung Disease*. Retrieved August 7, 2009, from http://www.goldcopd.com/Guidelineitem.asp?l1=2&l2=1&intId=2002

Goldmann, D. A. (2001). Epidemiology and prevention of pediatric viral respiratory infections in health-care institutions. Retrieved August 4, 2008, from http://www.cdc.gov/ncidod/eid/vol7no2/goldmann.htm

Health Resources Services Administration, U. S. Department of Health and Human Services. (2004). *SIDS deaths by race and ethnicity 1995–2001*. Vienna, VA: National Sudden Infant Death Resource Center.

Hymel, K. P., & Committee on Child Abuse and Neglect. (2006). Distinguishing sudden infant death syndrome from child abuse fatalities. *Pediatrics, 118*(1), 421–427.

International Ventilator Users Network. (2009). *Home ventilator guide*. Post-Polio Health International (PHI). Retrieved October 29, 2009, from http://www.ventusers.org/edu/HomeVentGuide.pdf

Kasper, D. L., Braunwald, E., Fauci, A. S., Hauser, S. L., Longo, D. L., & Jameson, J. L. (Eds.). (2005). *Harrison's principles of internal medicine* (16th ed.). New York: McGraw-Hill.

Lieu, T. A., Lozano, P., Finkelstein, J. A., Chi, F. W., Jensvold, N. G., et al. (2002). Racial/ethnic variations in asthma status and management practices among children in managed Medicaid. *Pediatrics, 109*(5), 857–865.

Marshik, P. L. (2004). Pharmacologic treatment of pediatric asthma. *Advance for Nurse Practitioners, 12*(3), 35–36, 41–46.

Meadows-Oliver, M., & Banasiak, N. C. (2005). Asthma medication delivery devices. *Journal of Pediatric Health Care, 19*(2), 121–123.

Medical News Today. (2005). *Respiratory synctial virus poses a significant threat in the elderly*. Retrieved August 7, 2009, from http://www.medicalnewstoday.com/articles/23514.php

National Center for Complementary and Alternative Medicine. (2004). *Consumer advisory. Ephedra*. Retrieved from http://www.nccam.nih.gov/health/alerts/ephedra/consumeradvisory

National Center for Preparedness, Detection, and Control of Infectious Diseases. (2009). *RSV in Alaskan Children*. Retrieved June 30, 2009, from http://www.cdc.gov/ncidod/aip/research/rsv.html#rsv_ak

National Heart, Lung, and Blood Institute. (2003). *Expert panel report: Guidelines for the diagnosis and management of asthma. Update on selected topics 2002*. (NIH Publication No. 02-5074). Bethesda, MD: Author.

National Heart, Lung, and Blood Institute. (2006). *ARDS*. Retrieved August 7, 2009, from http://www.nhlbi.nih.gov/health/dci/Diseases/Ards

National Heart, Lung and Blood Institute. (2007). *Expert Panel Report 3: Guidelines for the diagnosis and management of asthma. National Asthma Education and Prevention Program*. Retrieved July 7, 2009, from http://www.nhlbi.nih.gov/guidelines/asthma/asthgdln.pdf

National Institute for Allergies and Infectious Diseases. (2008). *Respiratory Synctial Virus: NIAID's role in addressing RSV*. Retrieved August 7, 2009, from http://www3.niaid.nih.gov/topics/rsv/

National Institute of Child Health and Human Development. (2009). *SIDS: Back to Sleep Campaign*. Retrieved July 6, 2009, from http://www.nichd.nih.gov/sids/

Opdal, S. H., & Rognum, T. O. (2004). A sudden infant death syndrome gene: Does it exist? *Pediatrics, 114*(4), e506–512.

Paterson, D. S., Trachtenberg, F. L., Thompson, E. G., Belliveau, R. A., Beggs, A. H., et al. (2006). Multiple serotonergic brainstem abnormalities in sudden infant death syndrome. *Journal of the American Medical Association, 296*(17), 2124–2132.

Peterson-Sweeney, K., McMullen, A., Yoos, H. L., & Kitzman, H. (2003). Parental perceptions of their child's asthma: Management and medication use. *Journal of Pediatric Nursing, 17*(3), 118–125.

Pongracic, J. A. (2003). Asthma delivery devices: Age-appropriate use. *Pediatric Annals, 32*(1), 50–54

Porth, C. M. (2005). *Pathophysiology: Concepts of altered health states* (7th ed.). Philadelphia: Lippincott Williams & Wilkins.

Pruitt, W. C., & Jacobs, M. (2004). Interpreting arterial blood gases: Easy as A B C. *Nursing, 34*(8), 50–53.

Reuters Health Information. (2009). COPD patients may derive significant benefit from statin therapy. Retrieved August 6, 2009, from http://cme.medscape.com/viewarticle/706421?src=cmenews

Rodríguez-Esquivel, D., Cooper, T. V., Blow, J., & Resor, M. (2009). Characteristics associated with smoking in a Hispanic sample. *Addictive Behaviors 34*, 593–598.

Seth, D., Kamat, D., & Pansare, M. (2007). Foreign-body aspiration: A guide to early detection, optimal therapy. *Consultant for Pediatricians, 6*(1), 13–18.

Simmons, P., & Simmons, M. (2004). Informed nursing practice: The administration of oxygen to patients with COPD. *Medsurg Nursing, 13*(2), 82–85.

Smyth, R. L., & Openshaw, P. J. M. (2006). Bronchiolitis. *Lancet, 368*, 312–322.

Spencer, J. W., & Jacobs, J. J. (2003). *Complementary and alternative medicine: An evidence-based approach* (2nd ed.). St. Louis, MO: Mosby.

St. John, R. E., & Malen, J. F. (2004). Contemporary issues in adult tracheostomy management. *Critical Care Nursing Clinics of North America, 16*(3), 413–430.

Stastny, P. F., Ichinose, T. Y., Thayer, S. D., Olson, R. J., & Keens, T. G. (2004). Infant sleep positioning by nursery staff and mothers in newborn hospital nurseries. *Nursing Research, 53*(2), 122–129.

Swartz, M., Cantey-Banasiak, N., & Meadows-Oliver, N. (2005). Barriers to effective pediatric asthma care. *Journal of Pediatric Health Care, 19*(2), 71–79.

Urden, L. D., Stacy, K. M., & Sough, M. E. (2006). *Thelan's critical care nursing* (5th ed.). St. Louis, MO: Mosby.

Willis, K. C. (2007). Bronchiolitis: Advanced practice focus in the emergency department. *Journal of Emergency Nursing, 33*(4), 346–351.

Yang, P. S., & Chen, C. H. (2005). Exercise stage and processes of change in patients with chronic obstructive pulmonary disease. *Journal of Nursing Research, 13*(2), 97–104.

Yoos, H. L., Kitzman, H., & McMullen, A. (2003). Barriers to anti-inflammatory medication use in childhood asthma. *Ambulatory Pediatrics*, *3*(July), 181–190.

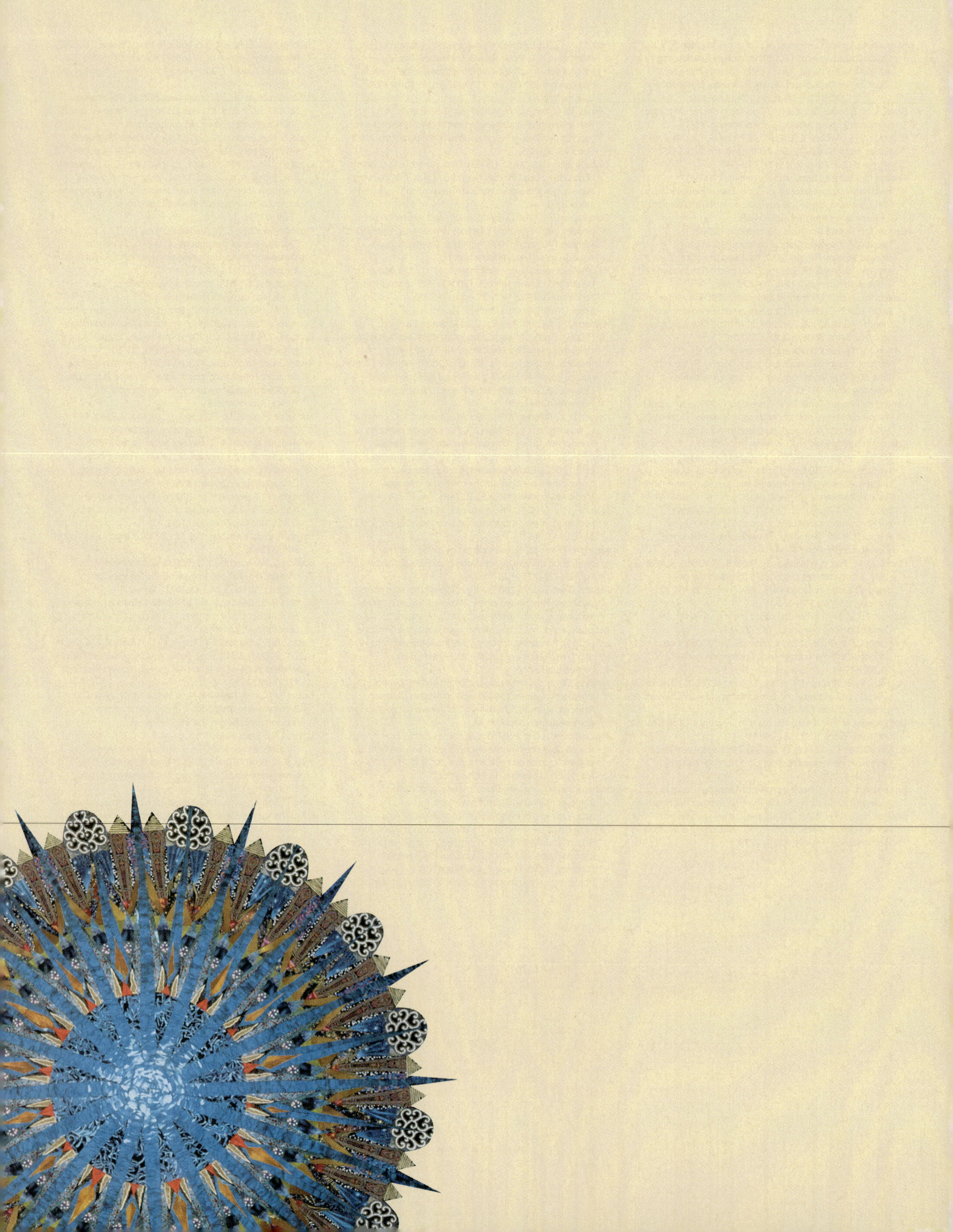

Perfusion 22

Concept at-a-Glance

Concept Learning Outcomes

After reading about this concept, you will be able to:

1. Summarize the structure and physiology of the cardiovascular system related to perfusion.
2. List factors affecting perfusion.
3. Identify commonly occurring alterations in perfusion and their related treatments.
4. Explain common physical assessment procedures used to examine cardiovascular health across the life span.
5. Outline diagnostic and laboratory tests to determine the individual's perfusion status.
6. Explain management of cardiovascular health and prevention of cardiovascular illness.
7. Demonstrate the nursing process in providing culturally competent and caring interventions across the life span for individuals with common alterations in perfusion.
8. Identify pharmacologic interventions in caring for the individual with alterations in perfusion.

Concept Key Terms

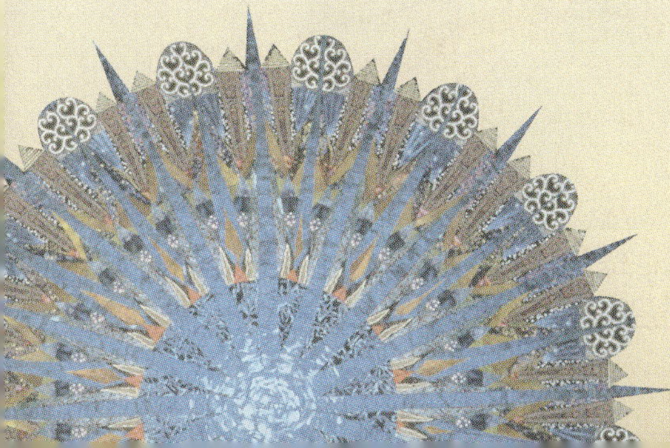

About Perfusion

The essential function of the cardiovascular and pulmonary systems is to provide a continuous supply of oxygenated blood to every cell in the body. Changes in perfusion affect all human functions, including self-care, mobility, fluid volume status, respiration, tissue integrity, and comfort. Impaired perfusion may also affect self-concept, sexuality, and role performance. •

NORMAL PRESENTATION

The heart is a hollow, cone-shaped organ, approximately the size of an adult's fist and weighing less than 1 lb. It is located in the mediastinum of the thoracic cavity, between the vertebral column and the sternum, and is flanked laterally by the lungs. Two-thirds of the heart mass lies to the left of the sternum; the upper base lies beneath the second rib, and the pointed apex is approximate with the fifth intercostal space (ICS), midpoint to the clavicle (Figure 22–1 ■).

The Pericardium

The heart is covered by the pericardium, a double layer of fibroserous membrane (Figure 22–2 ■). The pericardium encases the heart and anchors it to surrounding structures, forming the pericardial sac. The snug fit of the pericardium prevents the heart from overfilling with blood. The outermost layer is the parietal pericardium, and the visceral pericardium (or epicardium) adheres to the heart surface. The small space between the visceral and parietal layers of the pericardium is called the pericardial cavity. A serous lubricating fluid produced in this space cushions the heart as it contracts.

Layers of the Heart Wall

The heart wall consists of three layers of tissue: the epicardium, the myocardium, and the endocardium (see Figure 22–2). The epicardium covers the entire heart and great vessels, and then folds over to form the parietal layer that lines the pericardium and adheres to the heart surface. The myocardium, which is the middle layer of the heart wall, consists of specialized cardiac muscle cells (myofibrils) that provide the bulk of the contractile heart muscle. The endocardium, which is the innermost layer, is a thin membrane composed of three layers; the innermost layer is made up of smooth endothelial cells that line the inside of the heart's chambers and great vessels. The myocardium is the muscular layer of the heart that contracts during each heart beat. The epicardium is the outermost layer of the heart.

Chambers and Valves of the Heart

The heart has four hollow chambers, two atria (a left and a right) and two ventricles (also a left and a right). They are separated longitudinally by the interventricular septum (Figure 22–3 ■).

The right atrium receives deoxygenated blood from the veins of the body: The superior vena cava returns blood from the body area above the diaphragm, the inferior vena cava returns blood from the body below the diaphragm, and the coronary sinus drains blood from the heart. The left atrium receives freshly oxygenated blood from the lungs through the pulmonary veins.

The right ventricle receives deoxygenated blood from the right atrium and pumps it through the pulmonary artery to the pulmonary capillary bed for oxygenation. The newly oxygenated

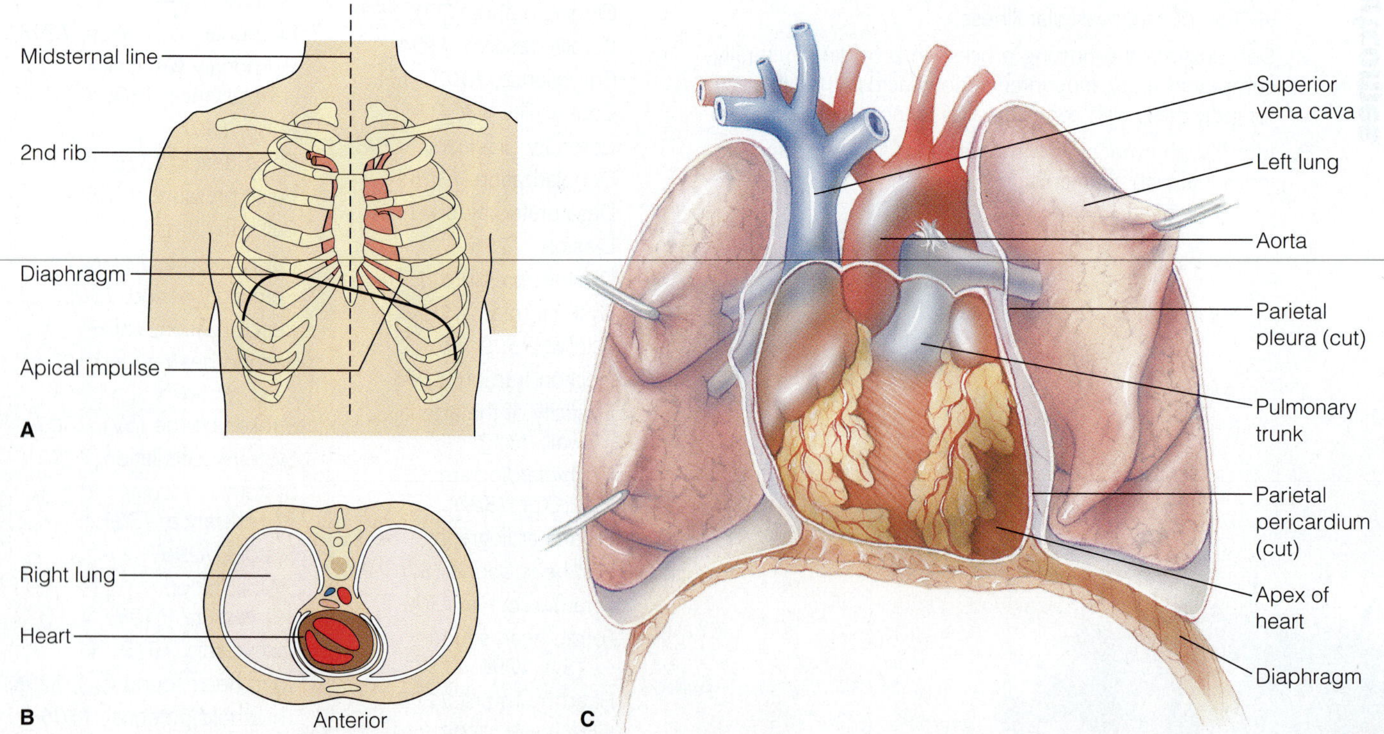

Figure 22–1 ■ Location of the heart in the mediastinum of the thorax. *A*, Relationship of the heart to the sternum, ribs, and diaphragm. *B*, Cross-sectional view showing relative position of the heart in the thorax. *C*, Relationship of the heart and great vessels to the lungs.

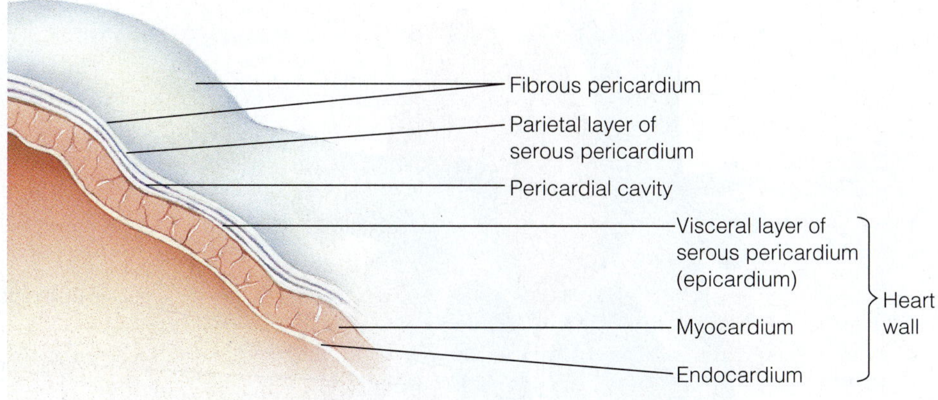

Figure 22–2 ■ Coverings and layers of the heart.

blood then travels through the pulmonary veins to the left atrium. Blood enters the left atrium and crosses the mitral (bicuspid) valve into the left ventricle. Blood is then pumped out of the aorta to the arterial circulation.

Each chamber of the heart is separated by a valve that allows unidirectional blood flow to the next chamber or great vessel (see Figure 22–3). The atria are separated from the ventricles by the two atrioventricular (AV) valves: the tricuspid valve is on the right side, and the bicuspid (or mitral) valve is on the left. The flaps of each of these valves are anchored to the papillary muscles of the ventricles by the chordae tendineae. These structures control the movement of the AV valves to prevent backflow of blood. The ventricles are connected to their great vessels by the semilunar valves. On the right, the pulmonary (pulmonic) valve joins the right ventricle with the pulmonary artery. On the left, the aortic valve joins the left ventricle to the aorta.

NORMAL HEART SOUNDS Closure of the valves of the heart gives rise to heart sounds (Figure 22–4 ■). These are heard as the "lub-dub" of the heart when auscultated over the precordium (the area of the chest that lies over the heart). Closure of the AV

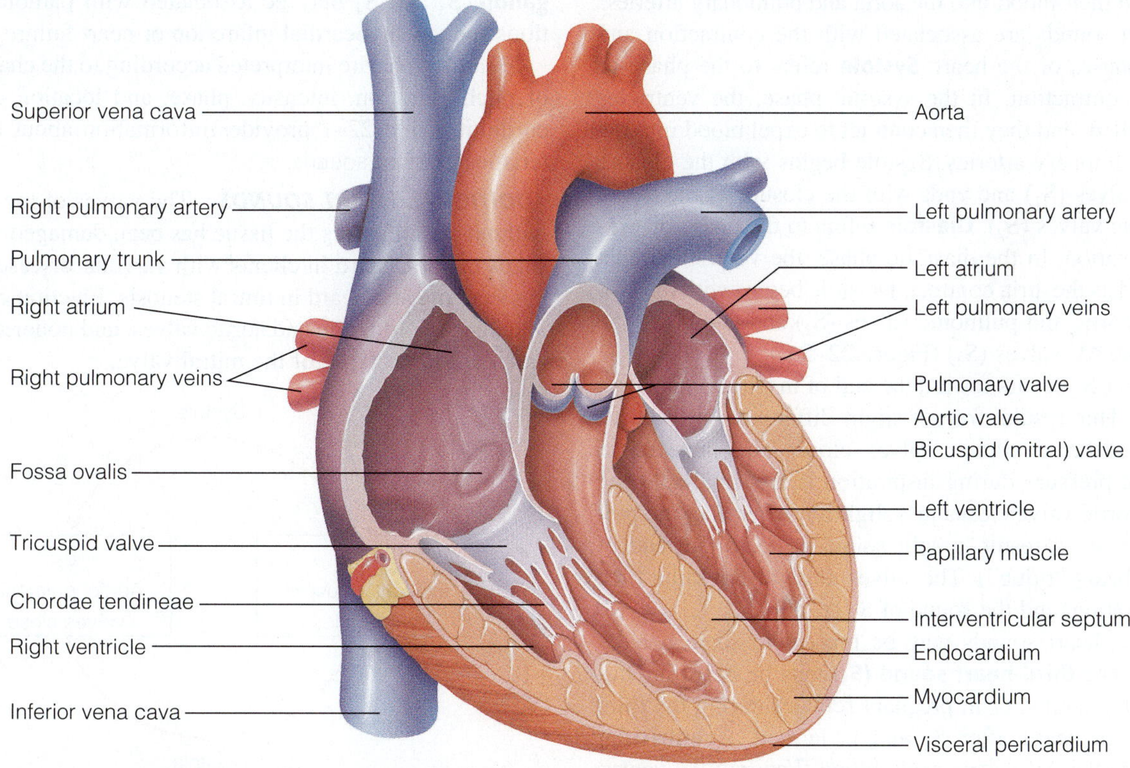

Figure 22–3 ■ The internal anatomy of the heart, frontal section.

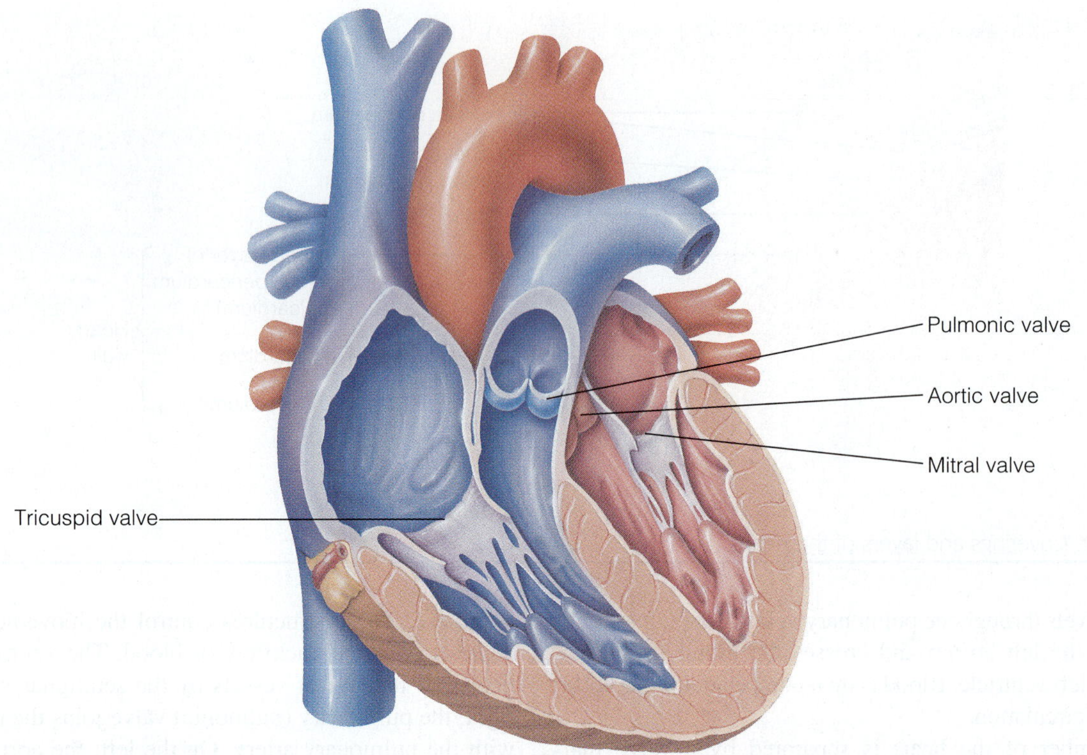

Figure 22–4 ■ Valves of the heart.

valves produces the **first heart sound (S_1)**, which is characterized by the syllable "lub." The AV valves close when the ventricles have been filled. Closure of the semilunar valves produces the **second heart sound (S_2)**, which is characterized by the syllable "dub." The semilunar valves close when the ventricles have emptied their blood into the aorta and pulmonary arteries.

The heart sounds are associated with the contraction and relaxation phases of the heart. **Systole** refers to the phase of ventricular contraction. In the systolic phase, the ventricles have been filled, and they then contract to expel blood into the aorta and pulmonary arteries. Systole begins with the closure of the AV valves (S_1) and ends with the closure of the aortic and pulmonic valves (S_2). **Diastole** refers to the phase of ventricular relaxation. In the diastolic phase, the ventricles relax and are filled as the atria contract. Diastole begins with the closure of the aortic and pulmonic valves (S_2) and ends with the closure of the AV valves (S_1) (Figure 22–5 ■).

Splitting of S_2 occurs toward the end of inspiration in some individuals. This results from a slight difference in the time that it takes the semilunar valves close. The increase in intrathoracic pressure during inspiration is a normal splitting of S_2. The aortic valve closes just slightly earlier than the pulmonic valve. As a result, a split sound is heard (instead of "dub," one hears "t-dub"). The valves close at the same time during expiration, and the sound of S_2 is "dub."

Two other heart sounds may be present in some healthy individuals. The **third heart sound (S_3)** may be heard in children, in young adults, or in pregnant females during the third trimester. It is heard after S_2 and is termed a **ventricular gallop**. When the AV valves open, blood flow into the ventricles may cause vibrations. These vibrations create the S_3 sound during diastole. The **fourth heart sound (S_4)** may also be heard in children, well-conditioned athletes, and even healthy older adults without cardiac disease. S_4 is caused by atrial contraction and ejection of blood into the ventricles in late diastole. S_4 is heard before S_1 and is termed an **atrial gallop**. S_3 and S_4 may be associated with pathologic conditions such as myocardial infarction or heart failure.

Heart sounds are interpreted according to the characteristics of pitch, duration, intensity, phase, and location on the precordium. Table 22–1 provides information about the characteristics of heart sounds.

ADDITIONAL HEART SOUNDS The valves of the heart open without sound unless the tissue has been damaged. Clicks and snaps may be heard in clients with valvular disease. An opening snap may be heard in mitral stenosis. Ejection clicks occur in damaged pulmonic and aortic valves, and nonejection clicks are heard in prolapse of the mitral valve.

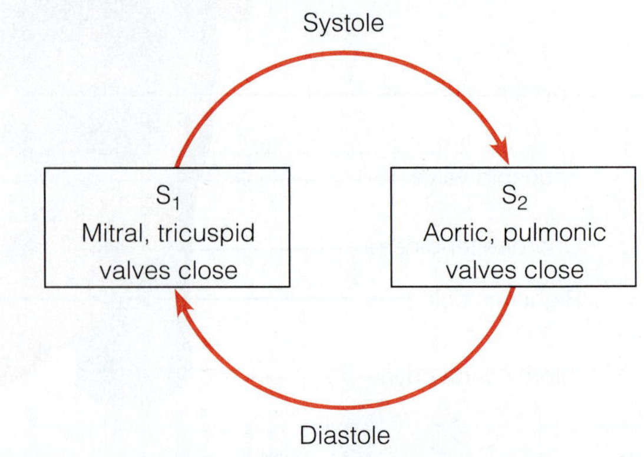

Figure 22–5 ■ Heart sounds in systole and diastole.

TABLE 22–1 Characteristics of Heart Sounds

HEART SOUNDS	CARDIAC CYCLE TIMING	AUSCULTATION SITE	POSITION	PITCH
S_1 (S_1 S_2; LUB — dub)	Start of systole	Apex with diaphragm	Position does not affect the sound	High
S_2 (S_1 S_2; lub — DUB)	End of systole	Both at 2nd intercostal space (ICS); pulmonary component best at left sternal border (LSB); aortic component best at right sternal border (RSB) with diaphragm	Sitting or supine	High
Split S_1 (S_1 S_2; T)	Beginning of systole	If normal, at 2nd ICS, LSB; abnormal if heard at apex	Best heard in the supine position	High
Fixed split S_2 (S_1 S_2)	End of systole	Both at 2nd ICS; pulmonary component best at LSB; aortic component best at RSB with diaphragm	Best heard in the supine position	High
Paradoxic split S_2 (S_1 S_2; P_2 A_2)	End of systole	Both at 2nd ICS; pulmonary component best at LSB; aortic component best at RSB with diaphragm	Best heard in the supine position	High
Wide split S_2 (S_1 S_2)	End of systole	Both at 2nd ICS; pulmonary component best at LSB; aortic component best at RSB with diaphragm	Best heard in the supine position	High
S_3 (S_1 S_2 S_3)	Early diastole right after S_2	Apex with the bell	Auscultated best in left lateral position or supine	Low
S_4 (S_4 S_1 S_2)	Late diastole right before S_1	Apex with the bell	Auscultated best in left lateral position or supine	Low

Friction rubs result from inflammation of the pericardial sac. The surfaces of the parietal and visceral layers of the pericardium cannot slide smoothly and produce the rubbing or grating sound. Table 22–2 includes information regarding interpretation of additional heart sounds.

Heart murmurs are harsh, blowing sounds caused by disruption of blood flow into the heart, between the chambers of the heart, or from the heart into the pulmonary or aortic systems. Methods to distinguish murmurs and the classification of heart murmurs are provided in Tables 22–3 and 22–4, respectively.

Systemic, Pulmonary, and Coronary Circulation

Because each side of the heart both receives and ejects blood, the heart is often described as a double pump. Blood enters the right atrium and moves to the pulmonary bed at almost the exact same time that blood is entering the left atrium. The circulatory system has two parts: the pulmonary circulation, which moves blood through the capillary bed surrounding the lungs to link with the gas exchange system of the lungs, and the systemic circulation, which supplies blood to all other body tissues. In addition, the heart muscle itself is supplied with blood via the coronary circulation.

PULMONARY CIRCULATION The **pulmonary circulation** consists of the right side of the heart, the pulmonary artery, the pulmonary capillaries, and the pulmonary vein. Because it is located in the thorax near the heart, the pulmonary circulation is a low-pressure system. Pulmonary circulation begins with the right side of the heart. Deoxygenated blood from the venous system enters the right atrium through two large veins (the superior vena cava and the inferior vena cava) and is transported to the lungs via the pulmonary artery and its branches (Figure 22–6 ■). After oxygen and carbon dioxide are exchanged in the pulmonary capillaries, oxygen-rich blood returns to the left atrium through several pulmonary veins. Blood is then pumped out of the left ventricle through the aorta and its major branches to supply all body tissues. This second circuit of blood flow is called the systemic circulation.

SYSTEMIC CIRCULATION The **systemic circulation** consists of the left side of the heart, the aorta and its branches, the capillaries that supply the brain and peripheral tissues, the systemic venous system, and the vena cava. The systemic system, which must move blood to peripheral areas of the body, is a high-pressure system.

CORONARY CIRCULATION The **coronary circulation** is a network of vessels that supply the heart muscle itself. The left and right coronary arteries originate at the base of the aorta and branch out to encircle the myocardium (Figure 22–7A ■), supplying blood, oxygen, and nutrients to the myocardium. The left main coronary artery divides to form the anterior descending and circumflex arteries. The anterior descending artery supplies the anterior interventricular septum and the left ventricle. The

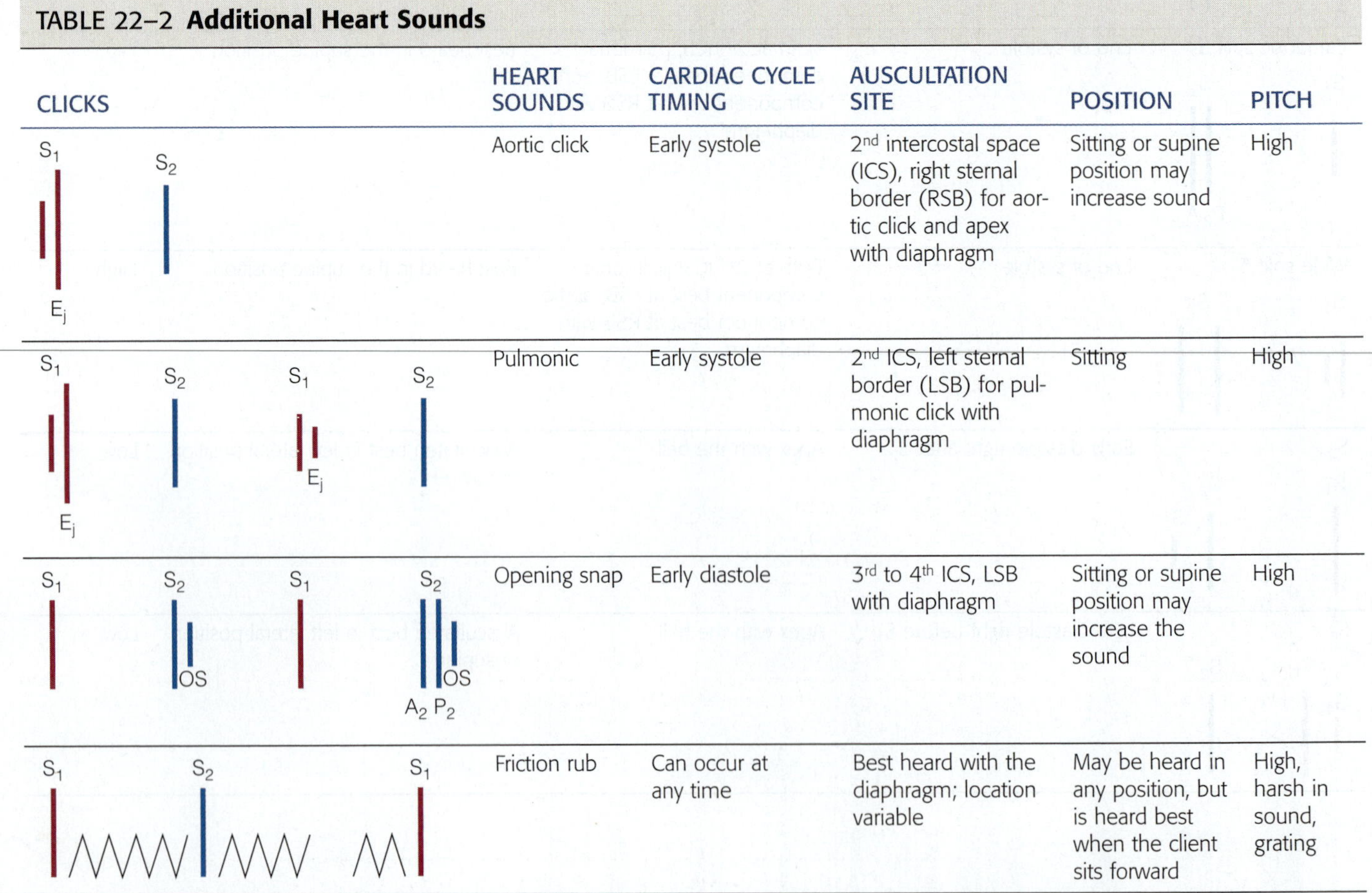

TABLE 22–2 **Additional Heart Sounds**

CLICKS	HEART SOUNDS	CARDIAC CYCLE TIMING	AUSCULTATION SITE	POSITION	PITCH
S_1 S_2 E_j	Aortic click	Early systole	2nd intercostal space (ICS), right sternal border (RSB) for aortic click and apex with diaphragm	Sitting or supine position may increase sound	High
S_1 S_2 S_1 S_2 E_j E_j	Pulmonic	Early systole	2nd ICS, left sternal border (LSB) for pulmonic click with diaphragm	Sitting	High
S_1 S_2 S_1 S_2 OS OS A_2 P_2	Opening snap	Early diastole	3rd to 4th ICS, LSB with diaphragm	Sitting or supine position may increase the sound	High
S_1 S_2 S_1	Friction rub	Can occur at any time	Best heard with the diaphragm; location variable	May be heard in any position, but is heard best when the client sits forward	High, harsh in sound, grating

TABLE 22–3 **Distinguishing Heart Murmurs**

ASK YOURSELF	INFORMATION
1. How loud is the murmur?	Murmurs are graded on a scale of 1–6: ■ Grade 1: Barely audible with stethoscope; often considered physiologic, not pathologic. Requires concentration and a quiet environment. ■ Grade 2: Very soft but distinctly audible. ■ Grade 3: Moderately loud; no thrill or thrusting motion is associated with the murmur. ■ Grade 4: Distinctly loud, in addition to a palpable thrill. ■ Grade 5: Very loud, can actually hear with part of the diaphragm of the stethoscope off the chest; palpable thrust and thrill are present. ■ Grade 6: Loudest, can hear with the diaphragm off the chest; visible thrill and thrust.
2. Where does it occur in the cardiac cycle: systole, diastole, or both?	Location in cardiac cycle: ■ Systole: early systole, midsystole, late systole ■ Diastole: early diastole, mid-diastole, late diastole ■ Both
3a. Is the sound continuous throughout systole, diastole, or only heard for part of the cycle?	Duration of murmur: ■ Continuous through systole only ■ Continuous through diastole only ■ Continuous through systole and diastole Systolic murmurs may be of two types: ■ Midsystolic: Murmur is heard after S_1 and stops before S_2. ■ Pansystolic/holosystolic: Murmur begins with S_1 and stops at S_2. Diastolic murmurs may be one of three types: ■ Early diastolic: Murmur auscultated immediately after S_2 and then stops. There is a gap between when this murmur stops and S_1 is heard. ■ Mid-diastolic: Murmur begins a short time after S_2 and stops well before S_1 is auscultated. ■ Late diastolic: This murmur starts well after S_2 and stops immediately before S_1 is heard.
3b. What does the configuration of the sound look like? *Potential configurations:* Pansystolic/holosystolic S_1 S_2 Continuous S_1 S_2 S_1 Crescendo (systolic represented) S_1 S_2	 Decrescendo (diastolic represented) S_2 S_1 Crescendo–decrescendo (systole represented) S_1 S_2 Rumble S_2 S_1
4. What is the quality of the sound of the murmur?	■ Blowing ■ Harsh ■ Musical ■ Raspy ■ Rumbling
5. What is the pitch or frequency of the sound?	■ Low ■ Medium ■ High
6. In which landmarks do you best hear the murmur?	Use the five landmarks for auscultation: ■ Pulmonic areas 1 and 2 ■ Aortic area ■ Tricuspid area ■ Mitral area ■ Apex

(continued)

TABLE 22–3 Distinguishing Heart Murmurs (continued)

ASK YOURSELF	INFORMATION
7. Does it radiate?	■ To the throat, neck, or back? ■ To the axilla or arm?
8. Is there any change in pattern with respirations?	■ Increases/decreases with inspiration ■ Increases/decreases with expiration
9. Is it associated with variations in heart sounds?	■ Associated with split S_1? ■ Associated with split S_2? ■ Associated with S_3? ■ Associated with S_4? ■ Associated with a click or ejection sound?
10. Does the intensity of the murmur change with position?	■ Increases/decreases with squatting? ■ Increases/decreases with client in the left lateral position?

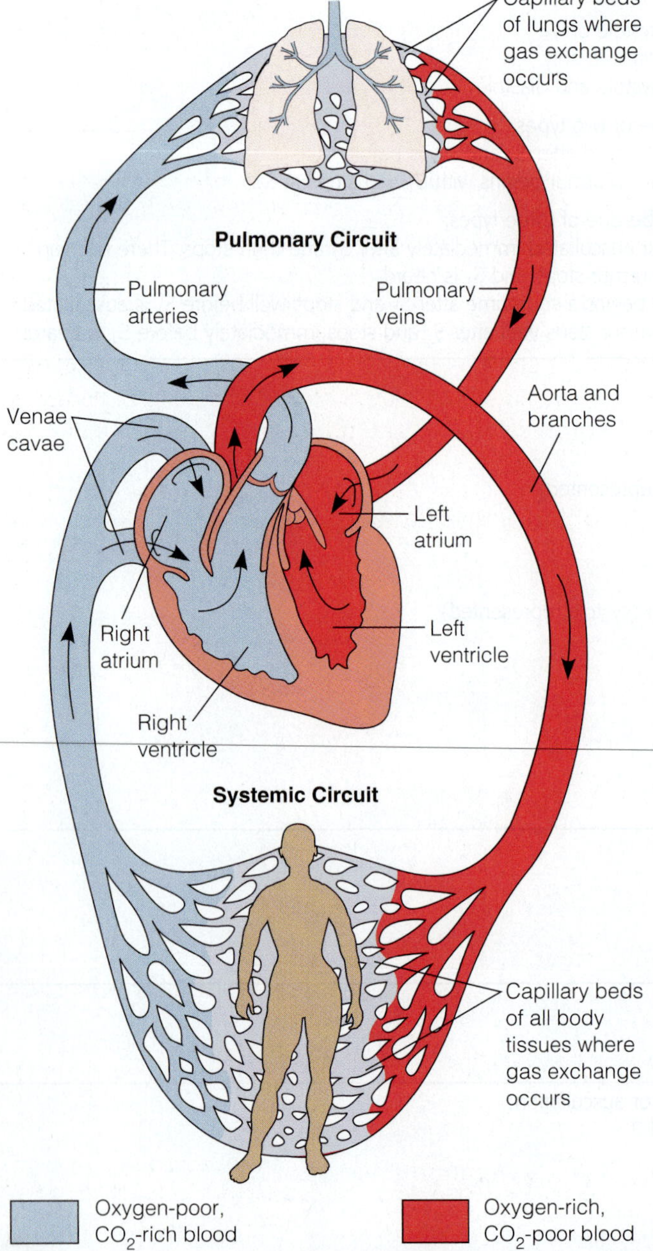

Figure 22–6 ■ Pulmonary and systemic circulations.

circumflex branch supplies the left lateral wall of the left ventricle. The right coronary artery supplies the right ventricle and forms the posterior descending artery. The posterior descending artery supplies the posterior portion of the heart. While ventricular contraction delivers blood through the pulmonary circulation and the systemic circulation, it is during ventricular relaxation that the coronary arteries fill with oxygen-rich blood. After the blood perfuses the heart muscle, the cardiac veins drain the blood into the coronary sinus, which empties into the right atrium of the heart (Figure 22–7B).

Blood flow through the coronary arteries is regulated by several factors. Aortic pressure is the primary factor. Other factors include the heart rate (most flow occurs during diastole, when the muscle is relaxed), metabolic activity of the heart, and blood vessel tone (constriction).

Transition From Fetal to Pulmonary Circulation

Blood flows from the placenta to the fetus through the umbilical vein to the ductus venosus (the fetal vascular channel between the umbilical vein and the inferior vena cava) and into the right atrium of the heart. The **foramen ovale** (an opening between the atria of the fetal heart) allows blood to flow from the right atrium to the left atrium and then into the left ventricle. Blood is then pumped into the aorta and systemic circulation. Some blood returns from the head and upper extremities to the superior vena cava and right atrium, and some blood travels to the right ventricle, where it is pumped into the pulmonary artery. The majority of the blood from the pulmonary artery passes through the ductus arteriosus, the vascular channel between the pulmonary artery and the aorta, and into the systemic circulation. A small amount of the blood from the pulmonary artery goes to the lungs. Blood eventually returns to the placenta by way of the umbilical arteries.

After the umbilical cord has been cut, the newborn must quickly adapt to receiving oxygen from the lungs. The transition from fetal to pulmonary circulation occurs in just a few hours. The first breath expands the lungs, and blood that previously flowed through the ductus arteriosus to the aorta begins flowing to the lungs. Increased pulmonary blood flow and decreased **pulmonary vascular resistance** (pressure

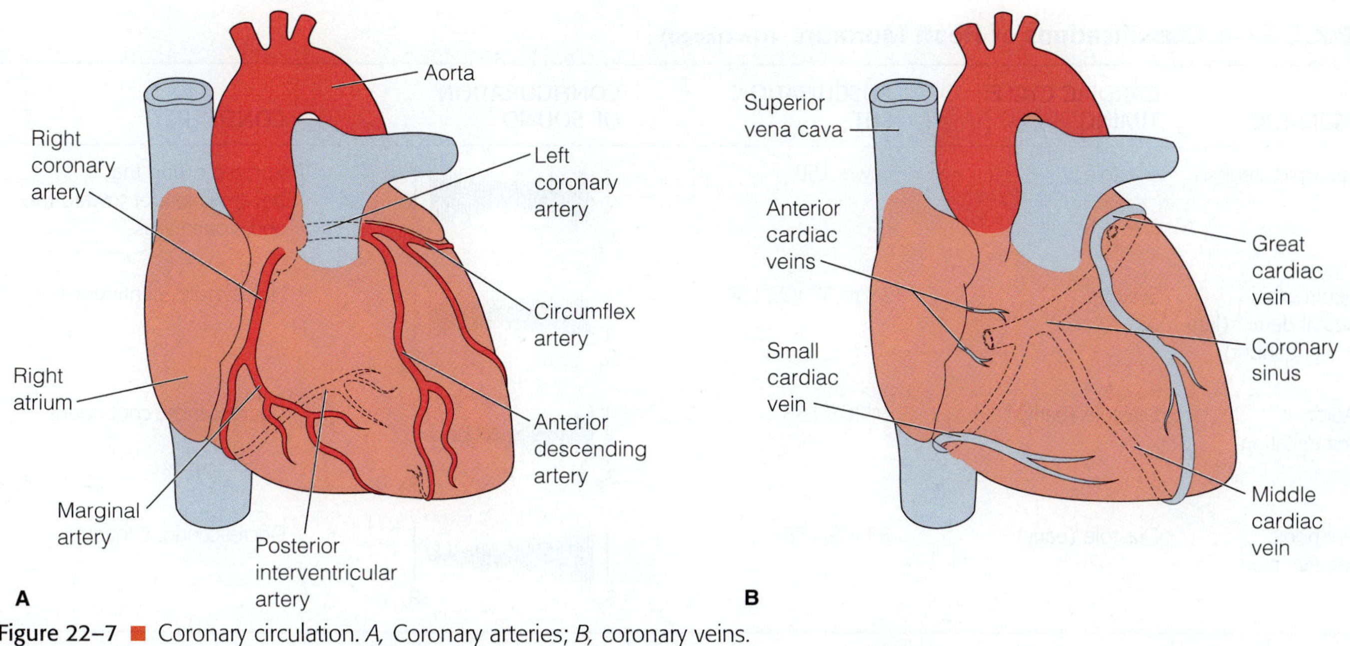

Figure 22–7 ■ Coronary circulation. *A,* Coronary arteries; *B,* coronary veins.

within the pulmonary blood vessels that must be overcome in order for blood to flow through the vessel) result. Pressure in the left atrium increases as increased blood flow is returned from the lungs through the pulmonary veins.

Systemic vascular resistance (the force or resistance of the blood in the body's blood vessels that helps return blood to the heart) increases and right atrial pressure falls after the umbilical cord is cut. Increased pressure in the left atrium stimulates closure of the foramen ovale. The flaps of the foramen ovale close, and fibrin deposits permanently seal the opening unless there is excess pressure on the right side of the heart. The ductus arteriosus, responding to higher oxygen saturation, normally constricts and closes within 10–15 hours after birth. Permanent closure occurs 10–21 days after birth, unless oxygen saturation remains low. Fetal tissues are accustomed to low oxygen saturation. This may explain why newborns with

TABLE 22–4 **Classifications of Heart Murmurs**

MURMUR	CARDIAC CYCLE TIMING	AUSCULTATION SITE	CONFIGURATION OF SOUND	CONTINUITY
Aortic stenosis	Midsystolic	Right sternal border (RSB), 2nd intercostal space (ICS)	S_1 S_2	Crescendo–decrescendo, continuous
Pulmonary stenosis	Midsystolic	Left sternal border (LSB), 2nd to 3rd ICS	S_1 S_2	Crescendo–decrescendo, continuous
Mitral regurgitation	Systole	Apex	S_1 S_2	Holosystolic, continuous
Tricuspid regurgitation	Systole	4th ICS, LSB	S_1 S_2	Holosystolic, continuous
Mitral stenosis	Diastole	Apical	S_2 S_1	Rumble sound that becomes louder toward the end, continuous

(continued)

TABLE 22–4 **Classifications of Heart Murmurs** **(continued)**

MURMUR	CARDIAC CYCLE TIMING	AUSCULTATION SITE	CONFIGURATION OF SOUND	CONTINUITY
Tricuspid stenosis	Diastole	Lower LSB	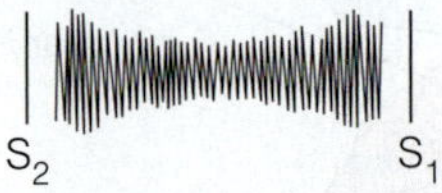 S_2 S_1	Rumble sound that becomes louder toward the end, continuous
Ventricular septal defect (left-to-right shunt)	Systole	3rd to 5th ICS, LSB	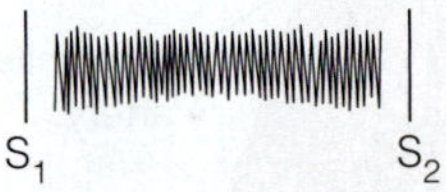 S_1 S_2	Holosystolic, continuous
Aortic regurgitation	Diastole (early)	3rd ICS, LSB	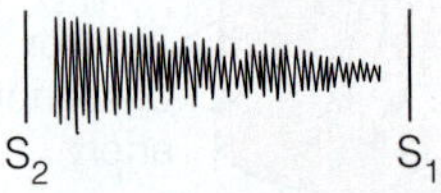 S_2 S_1	Decrescendo, continuous
Pulmonic regurgitation	Diastole (early)	3rd ICS, LSB	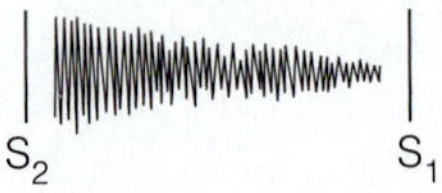 S_2 S_1	Decrescendo, continuous

MURMUR	QUALITY	PITCH	RADIATION	CHANGES WITH RESPIRATIONS
Aortic stenosis	Usually harsh, coarse	Medium	Most commonly into neck, into carotid area, and down left sternal border, possibly apex	Expiration may intensify the sound of the murmur
Pulmonary stenosis	Usually harsh	Medium	Toward the left upper neck and shoulder areas	Inspiration may intensify sound of the the murmur
Mitral regurgitation	Blowing, can be harsh in sound quality	High	Usually to left axilla, LSB, and base	Expiration may intensify the sound of the murmur
Tricuspid regurgitation	Blowing	High	May radiate to LSB and mid-clavicular line but not to axilla	Inspiration may intensify the sound of the murmur
Mitral stenosis	Rumbling	Low, best heard with bell	Rare	Expiration may intensify the sound of the murmur
Tricuspid stenosis	Rumbling	Low	Rare	Inspiration may intensify the sound of the murmur
Ventricular septal defect (left-to-right shunt)	Harsh	High	May radiate across precordium but not to axilla	Expiration may intensify the sound of the murmur
Aortic regurgitation	Blowing	High, best auscultated with diaphragm unless client is sitting up and leaning forward	May radiate to 2nd ICS, RSB, and may proceed to apex	Expiration may intensify the sound of the murmur if the client leans forward and sits up
Pulmonic regurgitation	Blowing	High, best auscultated with diaphragm	May radiate to 2nd ICS, RSB, and may proceed to apex	Inspiration may intensify the sound of the murmur

cyanotic heart disease appear relatively comfortable even when the arterial partial pressure of oxygen (PaO_2) is between 20 and 25 mmHg, in contrast to healthy newborns, who have a PaO_2 of between 83 and 108 mmHg. Older children and adults would rapidly develop acidosis and cerebral anoxia with such a low PaO_2. Figure 22–8 ■ compares fetal and postnatal circulation through the heart.

The Cardiac Cycle and Cardiac Output

The contraction and relaxation of the heart constitutes one heartbeat and is called the **cardiac cycle** (Figure 22–9 ■). As mentioned, ventricular filling is followed by ventricular systole, a phase during which the ventricles contract and eject blood into the pulmonary and systemic circuits. Systole is followed by a relaxation phase known as diastole, during which the ventricles

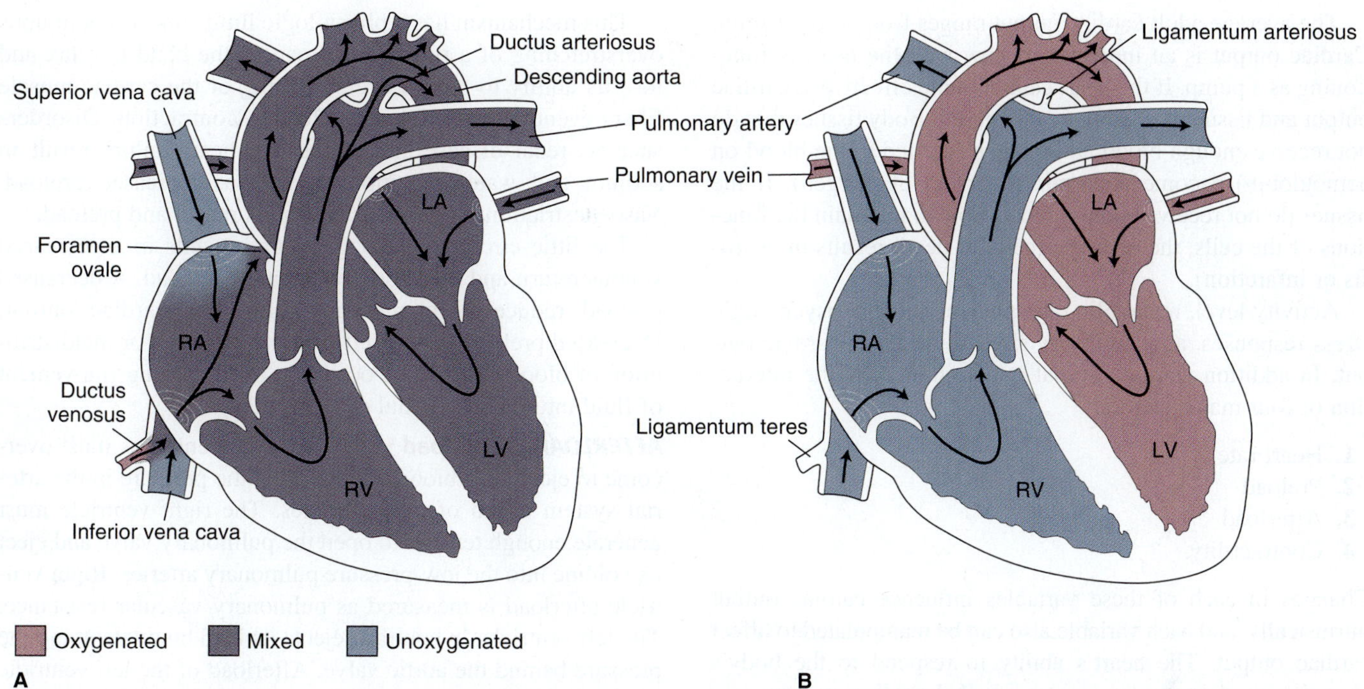

Figure 22–8 ■ The arrows indicate the flow of blood through the heart while the color indicates level of oxygen saturation in the blood. *A*, Fetal circulation. *B*, Pulmonary circulation. LA, left atrium; LV, left ventricle; RA, right atrium; RV, right ventricle.

refill, the atria contract, and the myocardium is perfused. Normally, the complete cardiac cycle occurs approximately 70–80 times per minute, measured as the heart rate (HR).

During diastole, the volume in the ventricles is increased to approximately 120 mL (the end-diastolic volume), and at the end of systole, approximately 50 mL of blood remains in the ventricles (the end-systolic volume). The difference between the end-diastolic volume and the end-systolic volume is called the **stroke volume (SV)**. Stroke volume ranges from 60 to 100 mL/beat and averages approximately 70 mL/beat in an adult. The **cardiac output (CO)** is the amount of blood pumped by the ventricles into the pulmonary and systemic circulations in 1 minute. Multiplying the stroke volume (SV) by the heart rate (HR) determines the cardiac output (CO):

$$SV \times HR = CO$$

The **ejection fraction** is the stroke volume divided by the end-diastolic volume and represents the fraction or percent of the diastolic volume that is ejected from the heart during systole (Porth, 2005). For example, an end-diastolic volume of 120 mL divided by a stroke volume of 80 mL equals an ejection fraction of 66%. The normal ejection fraction ranges from 50% to 70%.

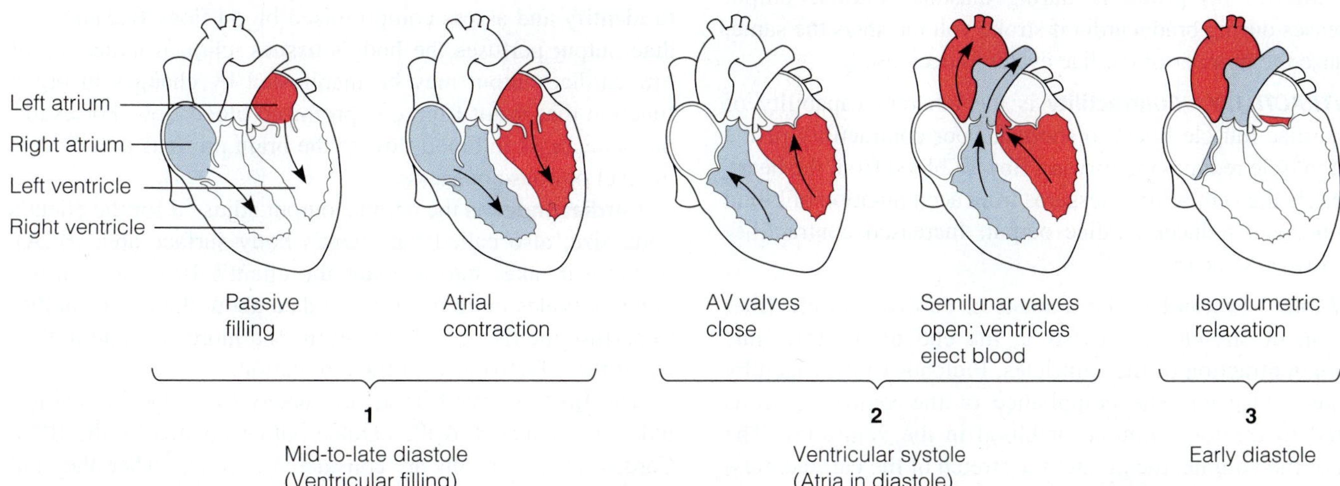

Figure 22–9 ■ The cardiac cycle has three events: (1) ventricular filling in mid-to-late diastole, (2) ventricular systole, and (3) isovolumetric relaxation in early diastole.

The average adult cardiac output ranges from 4 to 8 L/min. Cardiac output is an indicator of how well the heart is functioning as a pump. If the heart cannot pump effectively, cardiac output and tissue perfusion are decreased. Body tissues that do not receive enough blood and oxygen (carried in the blood on hemoglobin) become **ischemic** (deprived of oxygen). If the tissues do not receive enough blood flow to maintain the functions of the cells, the cells die (cellular death results in necrosis or infarction).

Activity level, metabolic rate, physiologic and psychologic stress responses, age, and body size all influence cardiac output. In addition, cardiac output is determined by the interaction of four major factors:

1. Heart rate
2. Preload
3. Afterload
4. Contractility.

Changes in each of these variables influence cardiac output intrinsically, and each variable also can be manipulated to affect cardiac output. The heart's ability to respond to the body's changing need for cardiac output is called **cardiac reserve**.

HEART RATE Heart rate is affected by both direct and indirect autonomic nervous system stimulation. Direct stimulation is accomplished through innervation of the heart muscle by sympathetic and parasympathetic nerves. The sympathetic nervous system increases the heart rate, whereas the parasympathetic vagal tone slows the heart rate. Reflex regulation of the heart rate in response to systemic blood pressure also occurs through activation of sensory receptors known as baroreceptors or pressure receptors located in the carotid sinus, aortic arch, venae cavae, and pulmonary veins.

If heart rate increases, cardiac output also increases (up to a point) even if there is no change in stroke volume. However, rapid heart rates decrease the amount of time available for ventricular filling during diastole. Cardiac output then falls, because decreased filling time decreases stroke volume. Coronary artery perfusion also decreases, because the coronary arteries fill primarily during diastole. Cardiac output decreases during bradycardia if stroke volume stays the same, because the number of cardiac cycles is decreased.

CONTRACTILITY **Contractility** is the inherent capability of the cardiac muscle fibers to shorten. Poor contractility of the heart muscle reduces the forward flow of blood from the heart, increases the ventricular pressures from accumulation of blood volume, and reduces cardiac output. Increased contractility may stress the heart.

PRELOAD **Preload** is the amount of cardiac muscle fiber tension, or stretch, that exists at the end of diastole, just before contraction of the ventricles. Preload is influenced by venous return and the compliance of the ventricles. It is related to the total volume of blood in the ventricles: The greater the volume, the greater the stretch of the cardiac muscle fibers, and the greater the force with which the fibers contract to accomplish emptying. (This principle is called Starling's law of the heart.)

This mechanism has a physiologic limit. Just as continuous overstretching of a rubber band causes the band to relax and lose its ability to recoil, overstretching of the cardiac muscle fibers eventually results in ineffective contraction. Disorders such as renal disease and congestive heart failure result in sodium and water retention as well as increased preload. Vasoconstriction also increases venous return and preload.

Too little circulating blood volume results in a decreased venous return and therefore a decreased preload. A decreased preload reduces stroke volume and thus cardiac output. Decreased preload may result from hemorrhage or maldistribution of blood volume, as occurs in third spacing (movement of fluid into the interstitial comaprtment).

AFTERLOAD **Afterload** is the force the ventricles must overcome to eject their blood volume. It is the pressure in the arterial system ahead of the ventricles. The right ventricle must generate enough tension to open the pulmonary valve and eject its volume into the low-pressure pulmonary arteries. Right ventricle afterload is measured as pulmonary vascular resistance. The left ventricle, in contrast, ejects its load by overcoming the pressure behind the aortic valve. Afterload of the left ventricle is measured as systemic vascular resistance. Arterial pressures are much higher than pulmonary pressures; thus, the left ventricle has to work much harder than the right ventricle.

Alterations in vascular tone affect afterload and ventricular work. As the pulmonary or arterial blood pressure increases (e.g., through vasoconstriction), pulmonary vascular resistance and/or systemic vascular resistance increases, and the work of the ventricles increases. As workload increases, consumption of myocardial oxygen also increases. A compromised heart cannot effectively meet this increased oxygen demand, and a vicious cycle ensues. By contrast, a very low afterload decreases the forward flow of blood into the systemic circulation and the coronary arteries.

CLINICAL INDICATORS OF CARDIAC OUTPUT For many clients who are critically ill, invasive hemodynamic monitoring catheters are used to measure cardiac output in quantifiable numbers. However, advanced technology is not the only way to identify and assess compromised blood flow. Because cardiac output perfuses the body's tissues, clinical indicators of low cardiac output may be manifested by changes in organ function that result from compromised blood flow. For example, a decrease in blood flow to the brain presents as a change in level of consciousness.

Cardiac index is the cardiac output adjusted for the client's body size, also called the client's body surface area (BSA). Because it takes into account the client's BSA, the cardiac index provides more meaningful data about the heart's ability to perfuse the tissues and therefore is a more accurate indicator of the effectiveness of the circulation.

The BSA is stated in square meters (m^2), and the cardiac index is calculated as the cardiac output divided by the BSA. Cardiac measurements are considered adequate when they fall within the range of 2.5–4.2 L/min/m^2. For example, two clients are determined to have a cardiac output of 4 L/min. This parameter is within normal limits. However, one client is 5 feet,

2 inches (157 cm) tall and weighs 120 lb (54.5 kg), with a BSA of 1.54 m^2. This client's cardiac index is 4 ÷ 1.54, or 2.6 L/min/m^2. The second client is 6 feet, 2 inches (188 cm) tall and weighs 280 lb (81.7 kg), with a BSA of 2.52 m^2. This client's cardiac index is 4 ÷ 2.52, or 1.6 L/min/m^2. The cardiac index results show that the same cardiac output of 4 L/min is adequate for the first client but is grossly inadequate for the second.

The Conduction System of the Heart

The cardiac cycle is perpetuated by a complex electrical circuit commonly known as the intrinsic conduction system of the heart. Cardiac muscle cells possess an inherent characteristic of self-excitation, which enables them to initiate and transmit impulses independent of a stimulus. However, specialized areas of myocardial cells typically exert a controlling influence in this electrical pathway.

One of these specialized areas is the sinoatrial (SA) node, located at the junction of the superior vena cava and right atrium (Figure 22–10 ■). The SA node acts as the normal "pacemaker" of the heart, usually generating an impulse 60–100 times per minute. This impulse travels across the atria via internodal pathways to the AV node, in the floor of the interatrial septum. The very small junctional fibers of the AV node slow the impulse, slightly delaying its transmission to the ventricles. It then passes through the bundle of His at the AV junction and continues down the interventricular septum through the right and left bundle branches and out to the Purkinje fibers in the ventricular muscle walls.

This path of electrical transmission produces a series of changes in ion concentration across the membrane of each cardiac muscle cell. The electrical stimulus increases the permeability of the cell membrane, creating an action potential (electrical potential). The result is an exchange of sodium, potassium, and calcium ions across the cell membrane, which changes the intracellular electrical charge to a positive state. This process of depolarization results in myocardial contraction. As the ion exchange reverses and the cell returns to its resting state of electronegativity, the cell is repolarized, and the cardiac muscle relaxes. The cellular action potential serves as the basis for **electrocardiography** (a diagnostic test of cardiac function).

THE ACTION POTENTIAL Movement of ions across cell membranes causes the electrical impulse that stimulates muscle contraction. This electrical activity, called the **action potential**, produces the waveforms represented on electrocardiogram (ECG) strips.

In the resting state, positive and negative ions align on either side of the cell membrane, producing a relatively negative charge within the cell and a positive extracellular charge (Figure 22–11 ■). The cell is said to be polarized. The negative resting membrane potential is maintained at approximately –90 mV by the sodium–potassium pump in the cell membrane.

Depolarization **Depolarization** is the phase when the heart contracts, resulting from ion channel functions. Two types of ion channels function to produce the electrical changes that occur during the depolarization phase: the fast sodium channels and the slow calcium channels. A fast action potential occurs in atrial and ventricular muscle cells and the Purkinje conduction system, and it uses the fast sodium channels. A slow action potential occurs in the SA and AV nodes, which use the slow calcium channels. The action potential for contraction of the heart is initiated in the SA node. When a resting cell is

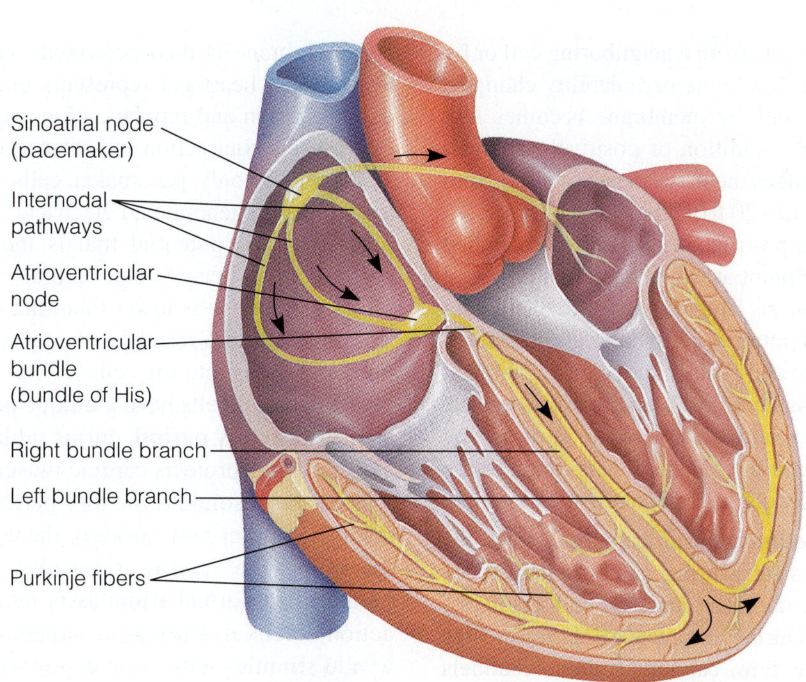

Figure 22–10 ■ The intrinsic conduction system of the heart.

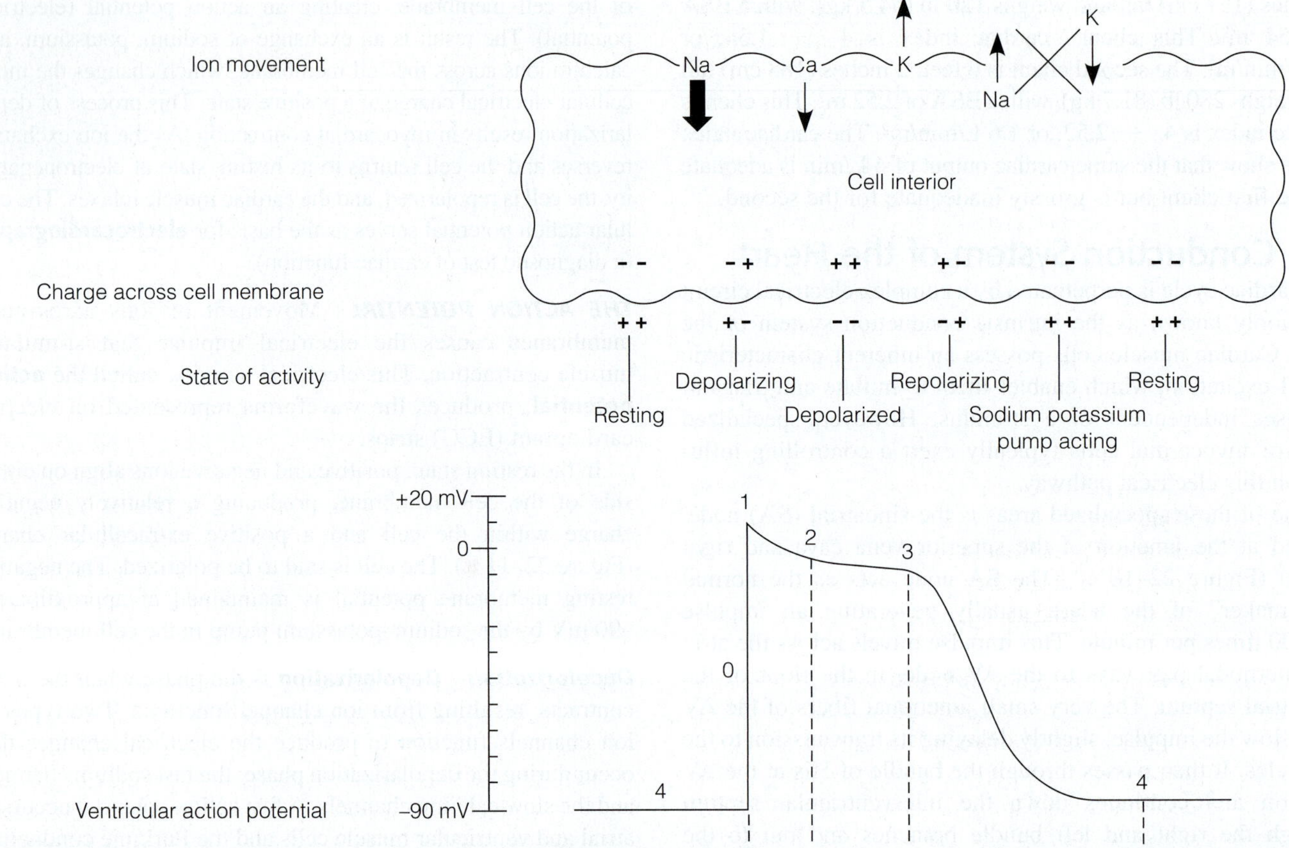

Figure 22–11 ■ Action potential of a cardiac muscle cell. In the resting state (phase 4), the cell membrane is polarized; the cell's interior has a negative charge compared to that of extracellular fluid. On depolarization (phase 0), sodium ions diffuse rapidly across the cell membrane into the cell, and calcium channels open. In the fully depolarized state (phase 1), the cell's interior has a net positive charge compared to its exterior. During the plateau period (phase 2), calcium moves into the cell and potassium diffusion slows, prolonging the action potential. In phase 3, calcium channels close, the sodium–potassium pump removes sodium from the cell, and the cell membrane again becomes polarized with a net negative charge.

stimulated by an electrical charge from a neighboring cell or by a spontaneous event, its cell membrane permeability changes. Sodium ions enter the cell, and the membrane becomes less permeable to potassium ions. Addition of positively charged ions to intracellular fluid changes the membrane potential from negative to slightly positive, at +20 to +30 mV.

As the cell becomes more positive, it reaches a point called the **threshold potential** (the point at which an action potential is capable of being generated). The response to the action potential in the myocardial muscle cells causes a chemical reaction of calcium within the cell. This in turn causes actin and myosin filaments to slide together, producing cardiac muscle contraction. The action potential then spreads to surrounding cells, causing a coordinated muscle contraction. As soon as the myocardium is completely depolarized, repolarization begins.

Repolarization **Repolarization** is the process that returns the cell to its resting, polarized state. During rapid repolarization, fast sodium channels close abruptly, and the cell begins to regain its negative charge. During the plateau phase, muscle contraction is prolonged as slow calcium–sodium channels remain open. When these channels close, the sodium–potassium pump restores ion concentration to normal resting levels. The cell membrane is then polarized, ready for the cycle to start again. Each heartbeat represents one cardiac cycle, with one depolarization and repolarization cycle and one complete cardiac muscle contraction and relaxation (systole and diastole).

Normally, only pacemaker cells demonstrate automaticity (capability to generate an electrical impulse). Pacemaker cells have a resting potential that is much less negative (–70 to –50 mV) than that of other cardiac muscle cells. Their threshold potential also is lower than that of other myocardial cells. These differences result from constant leakage of sodium and potassium ions into the cell.

Myocardial cells have a unique protective property, known as the **refractory period**, during which they resist stimulation. This property protects cardiac muscle from spasm and tetany. During the absolute refractory period, depolarization will not occur no matter how strongly the cell is stimulated. It is followed by the relative refractory period, during which a greater-than-normal stimulus is required to generate another action potential. During the supernormal period that follows, a mild stimulus will cause depolarization. Many cardiac dysrhythmias are triggered during the relative refractory and supernormal periods.

ANATOMIC LANDMARKS FOR CARDIOVASCULAR ASSESSMENT Anatomic landmarks for assessing the cardiovascular system include the sternum, clavicles, and ribs. By correlating assessment findings with the overlying body landmarks, the nurse may gain vital information concerning underlying pathologic mechanisms. Many landmarks identified during the respiratory assessment are also utilized when performing a cardiac assessment. These include, but are not limited to, the sternum and the second ICS through the fifth ICS.

The sternum is the flat, narrow center bone of the upper anterior chest (Figure 22–12 ■). There are three portions of the adult sternum. The upper sternum is called the manubrium, the middle part is called the body, and the inferior piece is called the xiphoid process. The average sternal length in an adult is 18 cm (7 in.). During cardiovascular assessment, the sternum is used as a vertical landmark, and the angle of Louis is used to locate the second ICS.

The clavicles are bones that attach at the top of the manubrium of the sternum above the first rib (see Figure 22–12). The midclavicular line is used as a landmark for cardiovascular assessment.

The ribs are flat, arched bones that form the thoracic cage. There are 12 pairs of ribs. Between each rib is an ICS. The first ICS lies between the first and the second rib, and each remaining ICS is numbered successively (see Figure 22–12). The intercostal spaces, horizontal landmarks for cardiac assessment, are used to locate the base of the heart and the apex of the heart and to auscultate the valvular sounds. The second ICS is located by feeling the angle of Louis, sliding the finger laterally to the second rib, and then sliding the finger down below the rib to the ICS. Each succeeding ICS is located by sliding the finger over the rib into the ICS.

Pulse

The **pulse** is a wave of blood created by contraction of the left ventricle of the heart. Generally the pulse wave represents the stroke volume output or the amount of blood that enters the arteries with each ventricular contraction. **Compliance** of the arteries refers to their ability to contract and expand. When a person's arteries lose their distensibility, as can happen in old age, greater pressure is required to pump the blood into the arteries.

In a healthy person, the pulse reflects the heartbeat; that is, the pulse rate is the same as the rate of the ventricular contractions of the heart. However, in some types of cardiovascular disease, the heartbeat and pulse rates can differ. For example, a client's heart may produce very weak or small pulse waves that are not detectable in a peripheral pulse far from the heart. In these instances, the nurse should assess the heartbeat and the peripheral pulse. A **peripheral pulse** is a pulse located away from the heart, for example, in the foot or wrist. The **apical pulse**, in contrast, is a central pulse; that is, it is located at the apex of the heart. It is also referred to as the **point of maximal impulse (PMI)**.

FACTORS AFFECTING THE PULSE The rate of the pulse is expressed in beats per minute (BPM). A pulse rate varies according to a number of factors. The nurse should consider each of the following factors when assessing a client's pulse:

- *Age.* As age increases, the pulse rate gradually decreases overall. See Table 22–5 for specific variations in pulse rates from birth to adulthood.
- *Gender.* After puberty, the average male's pulse rate is slightly lower than the female's.
- *Exercise.* The pulse rate normally increases with activity. The rate of increase in the professional athlete is often less

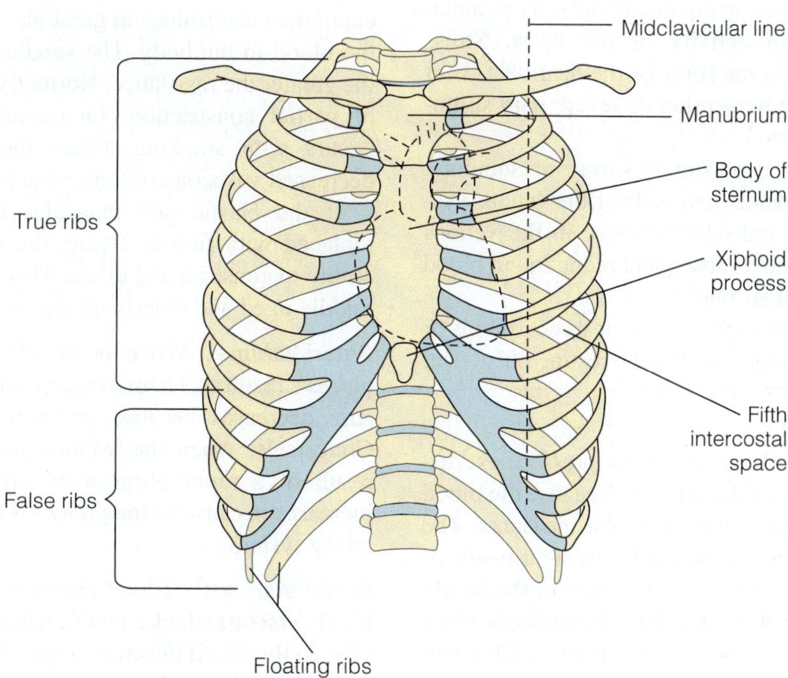

Figure 22–12 ■ Landmarks for cardiovascular assessment.

TABLE 22–5 Variations in Pulse and Respirations by Age

AGE	PULSE AVERAGE (AND RANGES)	RESPIRATIONS AVERAGE (AND RANGES)
Newborn	130 (80–180)	35 (30–80)
1 year	120 (80–140)	30 (20–40)
5–8 years	100 (75–120)	20 (15–25)
10 years	70 (50–90)	19 (15–25)
Teen	75 (50–90)	18 (15–20)
Adult	80 (60–100)	16 (12–20)
Older adult	70 (60–100)	16 (15–20)

than in the average person because of greater cardiac size, strength, and efficiency.

- *Fever.* The pulse rate increases (a) in response to the lowered blood pressure that results from peripheral vasodilatation associated with elevated body temperature and (b) because of the increased metabolic rate.
- *Medications.* Some medications decrease the pulse rate, and others increase it. For example, cardiotonics (e.g., digitalis preparations) decrease the heart rate, whereas epinephrine increases it.
- *Hypovolemia.* Loss of blood from the vascular system normally increases pulse rate. In adults the loss of circulating volume results in an adjustment of the heart rate to increase blood pressure as the body compensates for the lost blood volume. Adults can usually lose up to 10% of their normal circulating volume without adverse effects.
- *Stress.* In response to stress, sympathetic nervous stimulation increases the overall activity of the heart. Stress increases the rate as well as the force of the heartbeat. Fear and anxiety as well as the perception of severe pain stimulate the sympathetic system.
- *Position changes.* When a person is sitting or standing, blood usually pools in dependent vessels of the venous system. Pooling results in a transient decrease in the venous blood return to the heart and a subsequent reduction in blood pressure and increase in heart rate.
- *Pathology.* Certain diseases such as some heart conditions or those that impair oxygenation can alter the resting pulse rate.

Blood Pressure

Arterial blood pressure is a measure of the pressure exerted by the blood as it flows through the arteries. Because the blood moves in waves, there are two blood pressure measures. The **systolic pressure** is the pressure of the blood as a result of contraction of the ventricles, that is, the pressure of the height of the blood wave. The **diastolic pressure** is the pressure when the ventricles are at rest. Diastolic pressure, then, is the lower pressure, present at all times within the arteries. The difference between the diastolic and the systolic pressures is called the **pulse pressure**. A normal pulse pressure is about 40 mmHg but can be as high as 100 mmHg during exercise. A consistently elevated pulse pressure occurs in arteriosclerosis. A low pulse pressure (e.g., less than 25 mmHg) occurs in conditions such as severe heart failure.

Blood pressure is measured in millimeters of mercury (mmHg) and recorded as a fraction: systolic pressure over the diastolic pressure. A typical blood pressure for a healthy adult is 120/80 mmHg (pulse pressure of 40). A number of conditions are reflected by changes in blood pressure. Because blood pressure can vary considerably among individuals, it is important for the nurse to know a specific client's baseline blood pressure. For example, if a client's usual blood pressure is 180/100 mmHg, and it is assessed following surgery to be 120/80 mmHg, this significant drop in pressure may indicate complications and must be reported to the primary care provider.

DETERMINANTS OF BLOOD PRESSURE Arterial blood pressure is the result of several factors: the pumping action of the heart, the peripheral vascular resistance (the resistance supplied by the blood vessels through which the blood flows), and the blood volume and viscosity.

Pumping Action of the Heart When the pumping action of the heart is weak, less blood is pumped into arteries (lower cardiac output), and the blood pressure decreases. When the heart's pumping action is strong and the volume of blood pumped into the circulation increases (higher cardiac output), the blood pressure increases.

Peripheral Vascular Resistance Peripheral resistance can increase blood pressure. The diastolic pressure especially is affected. Some factors that create resistance in the arterial system are the capacity of the arterioles and capillaries, the compliance of the arteries, and the viscosity of the blood.

The internal diameter or capacity of the arterioles and the capillaries determines in great part the peripheral resistance to the blood in the body. The smaller the space within a vessel, the greater the resistance. Normally, the arterioles are in a state of partial constriction. Increased vasoconstriction, such as occurs with smoking, raises the blood pressure, whereas decreased vasoconstriction lowers the blood pressure.

If the elastic and muscular tissues of the arteries are replaced with fibrous tissue, the arteries lose much of their ability to constrict and dilate. This condition, most common in middle-aged and elderly adults, is known as **arteriosclerosis**.

Blood Volume When the blood volume decreases (for example, as a result of a hemorrhage or dehydration), the blood pressure decreases because of decreased fluid in the arteries. Conversely, when the volume increases (for example, as a result of a rapid intravenous infusion), the blood pressure increases because of the greater fluid volume within the circulatory system.

Blood Viscosity Blood pressure is higher when the blood is highly **viscous** (thick), that is, when the proportion of red blood cells to the blood plasma is high. This proportion is referred to as the **hematocrit**. The viscosity increases markedly when the hematocrit is more than 60–65%.

FACTORS AFFECTING BLOOD PRESSURE Among the factors influencing blood pressure are age, exercise, stress, race, obesity, sex, medications, diurnal variations, and disease processes.

- *Age.* Newborns have a mean systolic pressure of about 75 mmHg. The pressure rises with age, reaching a peak at the onset of puberty, and then tends to decline somewhat. In elders, elasticity of the arteries is decreased—the arteries are more rigid and less yielding to the pressure of the blood. This produces an elevated systolic pressure. Because the walls no longer retract as flexibly with decreased pressure, the diastolic pressure may also be high.
- *Exercise.* Physical activity increases the cardiac output and hence the blood pressure; thus 20–30 minutes of rest following exercise is indicated before the resting blood pressure can be reliably assessed.
- *Stress.* Stimulation of the sympathetic nervous system increases cardiac output and vasoconstriction of the arterioles, thus increasing the blood pressure reading; however, severe pain can decrease blood pressure greatly by inhibiting the vasomotor center and producing vasodilatation.
- *Race.* African American males over 35 years have higher blood pressures than European American males of the same age.
- *Gender.* After puberty, females usually have lower blood pressures than males of the same age; this difference is thought to be due to hormonal variations. After menopause, women generally have higher blood pressures than before.
- *Medications.* Many medications, including caffeine, may increase or decrease the blood pressure.
- *Obesity.* Both childhood and adult obesity predispose to hypertension.
- *Diurnal variations.* Pressure is usually lowest early in the morning, when the metabolic rate is lowest, then rises throughout the day and peaks in the late afternoon or early evening.
- *Disease process.* Any condition affecting the cardiac output, blood volume, blood viscosity, and/or compliance of the arteries has a direct effect on the blood pressure.

DEVELOPMENTAL ASPECTS

Cardiac function and perfusion differ as the fetus makes the required adaptation to extrauterine life. Fluid volume differences impact pediatric cardiology, while the aging heart affects perfusion in the older adult. This section discusses developmental aspects of normal cardiac function.

Pediatric Differences

It is important for nurses who care for children to understand the differences in pediatric cardiology. These differences impact not only how a child responds to cardiac alterations but also their response to therapy.

CARDIAC FUNCTIONING Infants have a greater risk of heart failure than older children do, because the immature heart is more sensitive to volume or pressure overload. During infancy, the heart's muscle fibers are less developed and less organized, resulting in limited functional capacity. Less compliance of the heart muscle means that the stroke volume cannot increase substantially until the heart muscle is fully developed at 5 years of age. The heart muscle fibers develop during early childhood; by 9 years of age, the weight of the heart has increased by six times (Connor, 2006). As the child's heart grows and develops, the systolic blood pressure rises, reaching adult levels by puberty.

The infant's metabolic rate and oxygen requirements double at birth, so the heart rate is high to maintain a high cardiac output and adequate oxygen transport. During stress, exercise, fever, or respiratory distress, infants and children have tachycardia, which increases their cardiac output. The infant has little cardiac output reserve capacity until oxygen requirements begin to decrease.

OXYGENATION Hematocrit and hemoglobin concentrations appropriate for the child's age are necessary for adequate oxygen transport. The oxygen arterial saturation is the amount of oxygen that can potentially be delivered to the tissues. **Desaturated blood** results when oxygenated and unoxygenated blood mix because of a congenital heart defect. Cyanosis, which indicates **hypoxemia** (lower-than-normal amounts of oxygen in the blood), results from a concentration of 5 or more grams of deoxygenated hemoglobin per 100 mL of blood or from arterial saturations of less than 85%.

The child's bone marrow responds to chronic hypoxemia by producing more red blood cells to increase the amount of hemoglobin available for oxygenation. This increase is known as **polycythemia**. A hematocrit value of 50% or higher is common in children with cyanotic heart defects.

Children respond to severe hypoxemia with bradycardia. Cardiac arrest in children generally results from prolonged hypoxemia related to respiratory failure or shock rather than from a primary cardiac insult (as in adults). Bradycardia is therefore a significant warning sign of cardiac arrest. Appropriate management of hypoxemia often reverses bradycardia and prevents cardiac arrest.

Alterations in cardiovascular function may be the result of a congenital defect, acquired infection, or injury. Congenital heart disease is the leading cause of death, excluding prematurity, during the first year of life. It is estimated that about one-third of children born with congenital heart disease die as a result of their cardiac disease, and about one-third of those deaths occur in the first year of life (Connor, 2006). Rapid advances in the treatment of congenital heart defects have allowed children to undergo surgery at younger ages. As a result, the nursing care required to identify and manage responses of infants and children with heart disease has become more challenging.

Cardiovascular Changes in Pregnancy

During pregnancy, blood flow increases to organ systems with an increased workload. Thus, blood flow increases to the uterus, placenta, and breasts, whereas blood flow to the liver and brain remains unchanged. Cardiac output begins to increase early in pregnancy, and at 25–30 weeks of gestation it peaks at 30–50% above prepregnant levels. During the third trimester, cardiac output becomes less predictable; it is likely that any changes are individually determined (Gordon, 2007).

The pulse may increase by as many as 10–15 bpm at term. The blood pressure decreases slightly, reaching its lowest point during the second trimester, then gradually increases to near prepregnant levels by the end of the third trimester.

The enlarging uterus puts pressure on pelvic and femoral vessels, interfering with returning blood flow and causing stasis of blood in the lower extremities. This condition may lead to dependent edema and varicosity of the veins in the legs, vulva, and rectum (hemorrhoids) during late pregnancy. This increased blood volume in the lower legs may also make the woman who is pregnant prone to postural hypotension.

When the woman lies supine, the enlarging uterus may press on the vena cava, thus reducing blood flow to the right atrium, lowering blood pressure, and causing dizziness, pallor, and clamminess. Research indicates that the enlarging uterus may also press on the aorta and its collateral circulation (Cunningham et al., 2005). This condition is called supine hypotensive syndrome; it may also be referred to as vena caval syndrome or aortocaval compression (Figure 22–13 ■). It can be corrected by having the woman lie on her left side or by placing a pillow or wedge under the woman's right hip as she lies in a supine position.

Blood volume progressively increases beginning in the first trimester, increases rapidly until about 30–34 weeks of gestation, and then plateaus until birth at approximately 40–50% above prepregnant levels. This increase occurs because of increases in both erythrocytes and plasma (Gordon, 2007).

The total erythrocyte (red blood cell) volume increases by approximately 30% in women who receive iron supplementation (but only by ~18% without iron supplementation). This increase in erythrocytes is necessary to transport the additional oxygen required during pregnancy. However, the increase in plasma volume during pregnancy averages approximately 50%. Because the plasma volume increase (50%) is greater than the erythrocyte increase (30%), the hematocrit, which measures the concentration of red blood cells in the plasma, decreases slightly (Gordon, 2007). This decrease is referred to as the **physiologic anemia of pregnancy** (pseudoanemia).

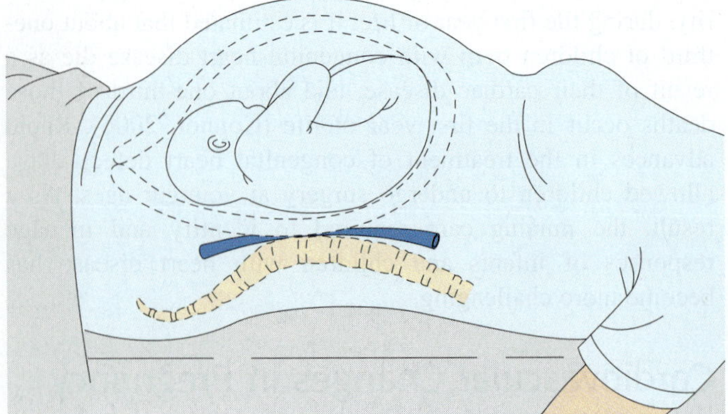

Figure 22–13 ■ Vena caval syndrome. The gravid uterus compresses the vena cava when the woman is supine. This reduces the blood flow returning to the heart and may cause maternal hypotension.

Iron is necessary for hemoglobin formation, and hemoglobin is the oxygen-carrying component of erythrocytes. Thus, the increase in erythrocyte levels results in an increased need for iron by the woman who is pregnant. Even though the gastrointestinal absorption of iron is moderately increased during pregnancy, it is usually necessary to add supplemental iron to the diet to meet the expanded red blood cell and fetal needs.

Leukocyte production increases slightly to an average of 8,500/mm^3, with a range of 5,600 to 12,200/mm^3. During labor and the early postpartum period, these levels may reach 20,000–30,000/mm^3. Because of this normal increase in white blood cells, the result should not be used clinically to diagnose the presence of infection (Gordon, 2007).

Both the fibrin and plasma fibrinogen levels increase during pregnancy. Although the blood-clotting time of the woman who is pregnant does not differ significantly from that of the woman who is not, clotting factors VII, VIII, IX, and X increase; thus, pregnancy is a somewhat hypercoagulable state. These changes, coupled with venous stasis in late pregnancy, increase the woman's risk of developing venous thrombosis during pregnancy.

Normal Changes of Aging

A wide range of changes can occur with aging, but it is often difficult to distinguish between disease processes and the natural consequences of aging. A decrease in cardiovascular reserve or in cardiac output may be the result of deconditioning or disease and not the result of natural aging processes. Differences in cardiovascular functioning also exist from one person to another. The very old person with a good family history and healthy lifestyle can enjoy much greater cardiac function than a middle-aged person with a family history of cardiovascular problems or a history of smoking. Older people should not expect to become debilitated from aging alone.

It is important to remember the concept of compensation in cardiovascular function. Changes such as decreased renal functioning may occur with aging, and this causes a change in other systems in order to try to improve functioning. Sometimes, these compensatory changes cause problems of their own. For example, kidneys that are poorly perfused as a result of decreased cardiac output produce renin, which eventually increases blood pressure and sodium retention. These gradual compensatory changes are initially benign but can lead to decreased cardiac and renal function and to fluid overload. See Figure 22–14 ■ for normal changes of aging in the cardiovascular system.

How an individual person ages is determined by genetic factors as well as by physical and social environments. Aging changes are gradual and may not be noticed by the individual or by members of the family. Different body systems age at different rates. One person might have orthopaedic problems but relatively few cardiovascular problems. Many cardiovascular functions also involve neurologic or endocrine systems, and these interrelated processes are vulnerable to aging in that a

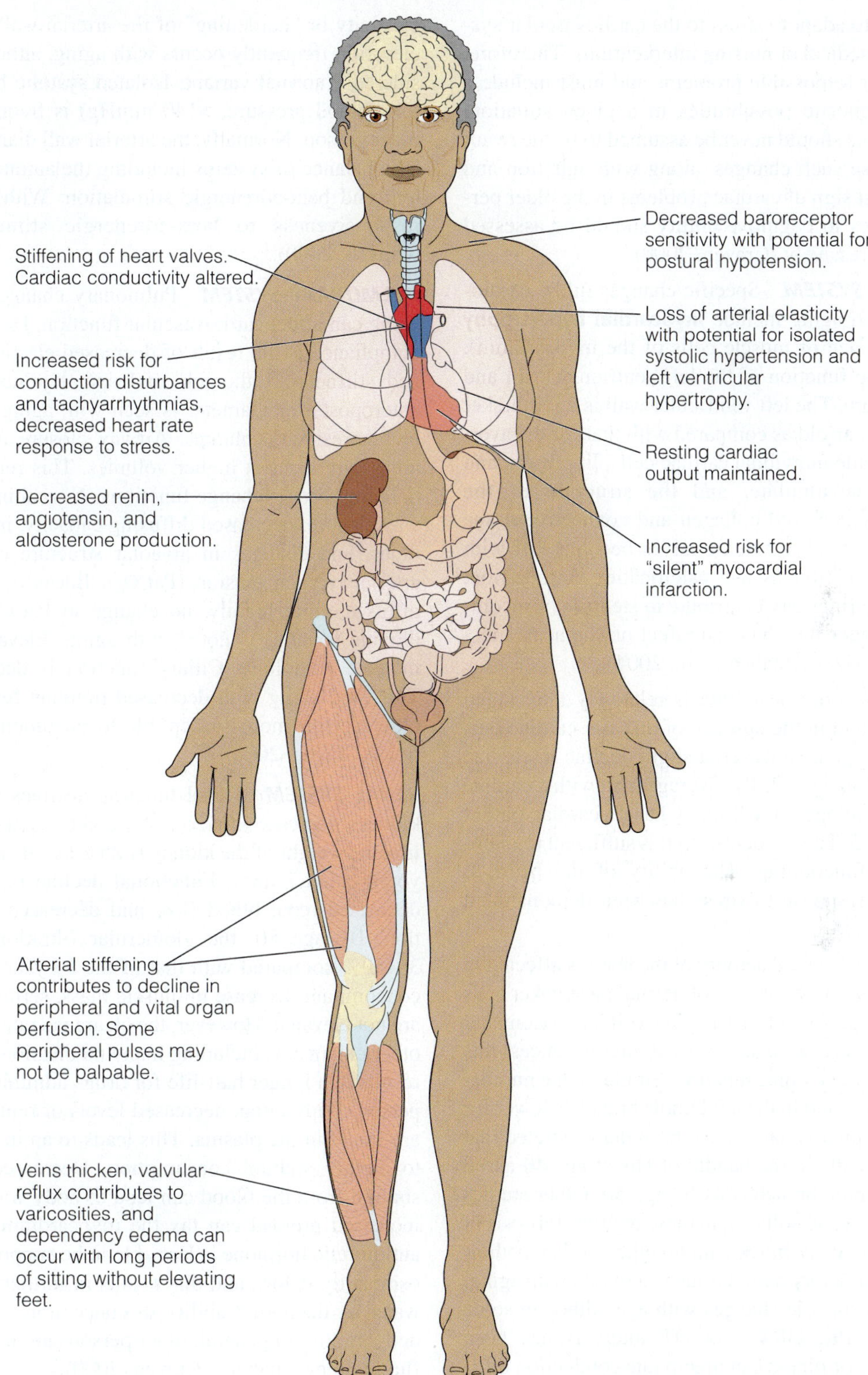
Decreased baroreceptor sensitivity with potential for postural hypotension.
Stiffening of heart valves. Cardiac conductivity altered.
Loss of arterial elasticity with potential for isolated systolic hypertension and left ventricular hypertrophy.
Increased risk for conduction disturbances and tachyarrhythmias, decreased heart rate response to stress.
Resting cardiac output maintained.
Decreased renin, angiotensin, and aldosterone production.
Increased risk for "silent" myocardial infarction.
Arterial stiffening contributes to decline in peripheral and vital organ perfusion. Some peripheral pulses may not be palpable.
Veins thicken, valvular reflux contributes to varicosities, and dependency edema can occur with long periods of sitting without elevating feet.

Figure 22–14 ■ Normal changes of aging in the cardiovascular system.

change in one system can affect the functioning of many others. Furthermore, physical or emotional stress can cause greater response and require a longer time for recovery. Taking a trip or getting the flu can cause much greater stress and negative changes for a frail older person.

Another feature of aging is the atypical presentation of disease in an older person. For example, a middle-aged person experiencing a myocardial infarction will most likely complain of the typical substernal chest pain with radiation down the left arm; however, the older person may complain of heartburn, nausea and vomiting, or excessive fatigue. Complaints of fatigue, decreased activity, sleep disturbance, or pain are not normal and should be investigated. The older person has a decreased capacity to adapt to stress to the cardiovascular system and may need medical or nursing interventions. Therefore, nurses must be alert to possible problems and must include a wide range of diagnostic possibilities in a given situation. Mental status changes should never be assumed to be the result of dementia, because such changes, along with agitation and falls, may be the first sign of cardiac problems in the older person. Sudden changes in cognitive ability should be assessed completely and aggressively (Craven, 2000).

CARDIOVASCULAR SYSTEM Specific changes in the cardiovascular system with aging include **myocardial hypertrophy** (an increase in the size of muscle cells of the myocardium). This will change the function of the left ventricular wall and the ventricular septum. The left ventricular wall is 25% thicker for the average 80-year-old as compared with that for the average 30-year-old. Inside individual cardiac cells, lipofuscin and amyloid deposits accumulate, and the structure of the myocardium shows increased collagen and connective tissue (McCance & Huether, 2001). Heart valves become stiff with aging as the result of fibrosis and calcification. In addition, changes in the valve rings can contribute to stenosis or incompetence. These changes then have an effect on the heart muscle and on chamber sizes (Reuben et al., 2004).

Cardiac Output Resting heart rate is relatively unchanged with normal aging, and in the absence of disease, cardiac output is not much changed. However, a slight decline in cardiac output does occur after age 20. The average man with a cardiac output of 5.0 L/min at age 20 will likely have a cardiac output of 3.5 L/min at age 75. This cardiac output is sufficient to maintain normal adult functioning. The ability of the heart to increase its rate in response to stress has been demonstrated (Craven, 2000).

Electrical Activity Electrical activity of the heart is affected in aging, with a decrease in the number of normal pacemaker cells in the SA node. By age 75, only 10% of the original pacemaker cells are still functional, but under normal circumstances, this number can still support cardiac function. Similarly, the number of cells in the AV node and in the left bundle branch is lower for the older person. Similar changes have been demonstrated that show a decrease in cells in the bundle of His at age 40 and a decrease in right bundle branch cells by age 50. Other studies show an increase in fat and collagen in these regions. Fibrosis of the AV node can lead to AV block with no other cardiac pathology. The AV node refractory period is also increased with aging. The ECG shows no specific changes with age, although some lengthening of the PR, QRS, and QT intervals has been described. The stress of illness can precipitate conduction difficulties for the older person (Craven, 2000).

VASCULAR SYSTEM The vascular system undergoes a range of changes with aging. The layers of the vascular system change, with a thickening of the intimal and medial layers. For arteries, the endothelial layer becomes irregular, with more connective tissue. Lipid deposits and calcification occur. Calcification can extend to the medial layer with increased collagen deposits. These changes can all lead to decreased elasticity or "hardening" of the arterial walls. Blood pressure elevation frequently occurs with aging, although it is not considered a normal variant. Isolated systolic hypertension (systolic blood pressure, >140 mmHg) is frequently seen in the older person. Normally, the arterial wall diameter is controlled by a balance of systems including the autonomic nervous system and beta-adrenergic stimulation. With aging, decreased responsiveness to beta-adrenergic stimulation is noted (Craven, 2000).

PULMONARY SYSTEM Pulmonary changes that occur with aging can affect cardiovascular function. Decreased chest wall compliance is the result of decreased elasticity of lung tissue and stiffness of thoracic and spinal joints. An increase in anteroposterior diameter is seen with aging. This can lead to higher residual volumes. Airway closure in dependent lung areas can occur at higher volumes. This removes portions of the lung from exchange functions. A combination of early airway closure, decreased diffusing capacity, increased lung volumes, and changes in alveolar structure can lead to lower arterial oxygen tension ($PaCO_2$). Because carbon dioxide is diffused more readily, no change in $PaCO_2$ (arterial carbon dioxide tension) is noted with aging. Elevated $PaCO_2$ would indicate pathology. Ciliary function is decreased with age. This fact, along with decreased immune function, makes the older person more susceptible to pneumonia or other infections (Craven, 2000).

RENAL SYSTEM Renal function declines with age, and the kidneys decrease in size and weight. By the ninth decade of life, the weight of the kidney is 25% less than the weight of the young adult kidney. Functional decline is also the result of decreased renal blood flow and decreased glomerular filtration. By age 80, the glomerular filtration rate is reduced 30–50% compared with that of the 30-year-old. Because of a concomitant decrease in muscle mass, serum creatinine levels are not elevated. However, the clearance rate for creatinine and other chemicals, including many medications, is reduced. This results in a longer half-life for drugs administered to the older person. With aging, decreased levels of renin and aldosterone are found in the plasma. This leads to an increased sensitivity to dietary sodium consumption. Decreased ability to clear sodium from the blood can lead to body water overload. This increased preload can tax the myocardium. Additionally, an antidiuretic hormone is less able to be suppressed when serum osmolality is low, and this results in further retention of body water. A decreased ability to concentrate urine can result in dehydration. In general, older persons are less able to adapt to fluid volume changes (Craven, 2000).

ALTERATIONS

Nurses care for many clients with alterations in cardiac function secondary to the prevalence of cardiac disease in the United States. Clients may present with cardiac disease as a primary diagnosis or they may be seen for a variety of other problems complicated by cardiac disease as a secondary diagnosis.

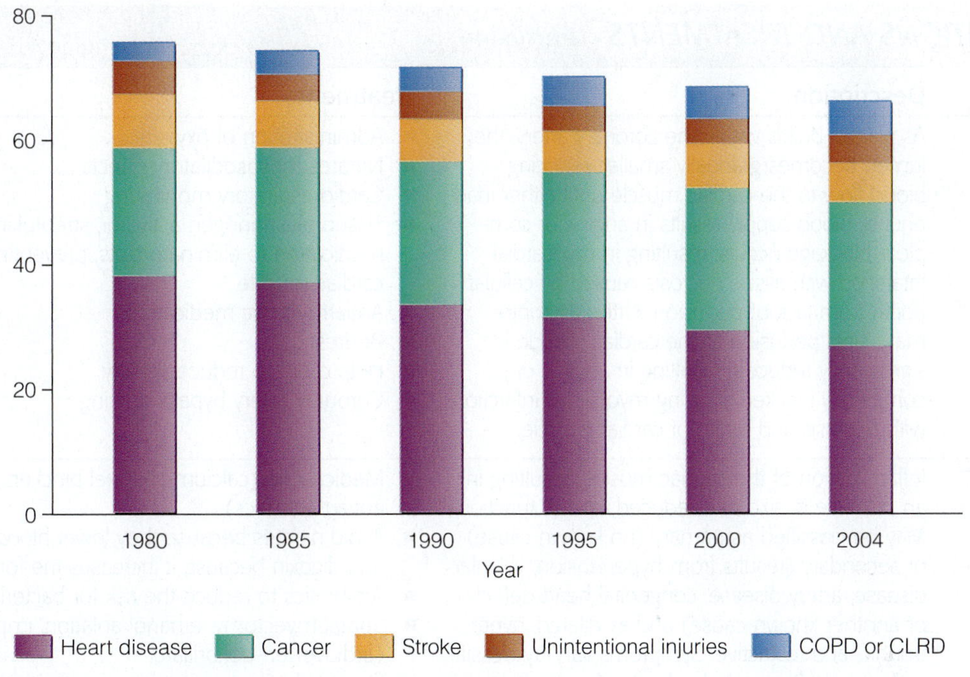

Figure 22–15 ■ Top five causes of death in the United States—1980–2004.

Source: Heron (2007). Courtesy of Scott M. Grundy, MD, PhD, Center for Human Nutrition, Departments of Clinical Nutrition and Internal Medicine, University of Texas, Southwestern Medical Center at Dallas.

Alterations in Pediatric Cardiology

Most pediatric disorders are related to congenital cardiac defects. With the advances in pediatric cardiology children who would not have survived to their first birthday are now entering adolescence. As a result, nurses may care for clients with profound alterations in cardiac anatomy requiring special considerations when planning care. Cardiac congenital anomalies are discussed in more detail in the exemplar.

Common Cardiovascular Illnesses of Aging

In the United States, it is difficult to determine the actual prevalence of cardiovascular disorders, because no national database tracks such things. Some recent surveys have failed to include clients older than 80 years or who live in nursing homes (Centers for Disease Control and Prevention, 2004). Heart disease is the number one cause of death for older people in the United States. Figure 22–15 ■ illustrates the most common causes of death in the United States for the years 1980–2004.

Cardiovascular disease develops slowly and can become more severe with the passage of time, impacting other organ systems such as the kidney and lung. Some common conditions, such as hypertension or hyperlipidemia, are risk factors for developing more serious conditions at any stage in life, and these conditions require ongoing assessment and treatment at any age (Table 22–6).

TABLE 22–6 **Age-Related Cardiac Changes**

AGE-RELATED CHANGE	SIGNIFICANCE
Myocardium: ↓ efficiency and contractibility. Sinoatrial node: ↑ in thickness of shell surrounding the node and ↓ in number of pacemaker cells.	■ Decreased cardiac output when under physiologic stress, with resulting tachycardia that lasts longer than in younger people. The person may require rest time between physical activities.
Left ventricle: Slight hypertrophy, prolonged isometric contraction phase and relaxation time; ↑ time for diastolic filling and systolic emptying cycle.	■ Stroke volume may increase to compensate for tachycardia, leading to increased blood pressure.
Valves and blood vessels: Aorta is elongated and dilated, valves are thicker and more rigid, and resistance to peripheral blood flow increases by 1% per year.	■ Blood pressure increases to compensate for increased peripheral resistance and decreased cardiac output.

ALTERATIONS AND TREATMENTS Perfusion

Alteration	Description	Treatment
Coronary artery disease	As plaque builds within the coronary artery, the lumen becomes gradually smaller, reducing blood flow to the cardiac muscle until either inadequate blood supply results in angina or complete blockage occurs, resulting in myocardial infarction with tissue necrosis caused by cellular death from lack of perfusion. Often asymptomatic until perfusion to the cardiac muscle is significantly reduced, resulting in angina, or is completely blocked, causing myocardial infarction with necrosis and death of cardiac muscle.	▪ Administration of oxygen ▪ Nitrates for vasodilatory effects ▪ Cardiorespiratory monitoring ▪ Tissue plasminogen activator, streptokinase, or other medication to eliminate clots, preventing perfusion of cardiac muscle ▪ Antiarrhythmic medications ▪ Bedrest ▪ Help client to reduce anxiety ▪ Coronary artery bypass grafting
Cardiomyopathy	Inflammation of the cardiac muscle, resulting in an increase in size and reduced cardiac function. May be classified as primary (no known cause) or secondary (results from hypertension, valvular disease, artery disease, congenital heart defects, or another known cause) and as dilated, hypertrophic, and restrictive. Symptoms vary by classification and often include chest pain, shortness of breath, syncope, and arrhythmias.	▪ Medications (calcium-channel blockers, beta-blockers, antiarrhythmics) ▪ Avoid nitrates because they lower blood pressure (BP), and digoxin because it increases the force of contractions ▪ Antibiotics to reduce the risk for bacterial endocarditis ▪ Septal myectomy, ethanol ablation, implantable cardioverter–defibrillator ▪ Heart failure management ▪ Fluid and sodium restriction ▪ Regular follow-up care
Dysrhythmia	Irregular electrical pattern seen on an electrocardiogram that may be the result of tissue damage (myocardial infarction), creating a new conduction path or a malfunction within the conduction system.	▪ Holter monitoring to capture appearance if arrhythmia occurs intermittently ▪ Antiarrhythmic medications ▪ Cardioversion or defibrillation ▪ Implanted cardioverter–defibrillator
Valve disease	May involve any valve and either stenosis (stiff, narrow opening, reducing blood flow) or insufficiency (incomplete closing of valves, allowing blood to regurgitate and reducing cardiac output). Symptoms depend on severity of the problem and may include shortness of breath, palpitations, edema of lower extremities, weakness, dizziness, weight gain, and chest pressure.	▪ Surgery may be indicated depending on severity of disorder, potentially requiring valve replacement ▪ Antibiotics to prevent bacterial endocarditis ▪ Medical management may include diuretics, antiarrhythmics, vasodilators, angiotensin-converting enzyme inhibitors, beta-blockers, and/or anticoagulants
Shock	Inadequate perfusion of the tissues as a result of blood loss, infection, destruction of or inadequate production of blood cells, reduced cardiac output caused by cardiac disease, or systemic vasodilation. Symptoms include pale, cool skin; hypotension; dizziness; light-headedness; confusion or change in level of consciousness; rapid pulse and respiration; and reduced urine output.	▪ Administer fluids and, depending on cause, blood transfusions or volume expanders ▪ Medications may include vasoconstrictors and those needed to treat the underlying cause ▪ Monitor and assess cardiorespiratory function and oxygen saturation ▪ Administer oxygen as indicated ▪ Assess level of consciousness, and report significant deviations from baseline ▪ Those in acute shock may require mechanical ventilation
Hypertension	Pressure in the arterial blood vessels is elevated, causing the heart to pump with much more force in order to overcome higher pressures. Causes may be primary (no known cause; most often diagnosed) or secondary (result of another disease process, e.g., diabetes mellitus, pheochromocytoma, or arteriosclerosis). Clients are often asymptomatic until hypertension becomes significant.	▪ Reduce weight ▪ Reduce salt intake ▪ Antihypertensive medications ▪ Exercise ▪ Client teaching needs to stress the importance of taking medications daily ▪ Teach client to monitor BP and to maintain a log

ALTERATIONS AND TREATMENTS Perfusion (continued)

Alteration	Description	Treatment
Pregnancy-induced hypertension	Blood pressure elevates, causing damage to nephrons with leakage of protein into the urine. As BP continues to rise, can result in fetal demise, seizures, stroke, and death. Signs and symptoms include proteinuria, headache, and edema of the face, hands, and lower extremities.	■ Reduce salt intake ■ Monitor BP ■ Elevate extremities ■ If BP exceeds acceptable limits, client will be admitted and intravenous magnesium sulfate administered ■ If unable to control BP with magnesium sulfate, the only option is to deliver the baby, which will resolve the problem and gradually return BP to normal limits
Stroke	Can result from a blood clot in a small vessel in the brain blocking blood flow to neurons or from rupture of a blood vessel with bleeding into the tissues, resulting in pressure and damage to nephrons. Symptoms include a sudden loss of motor and/or sensation.	■ Brain visualization in the form of computed tomography, magnetic resonance imagine, or positron-emission tomography ■ Antithrombotic medications may be used if bleeding can be eliminated as the cause ■ Supportive care to lower intracranial pressure ■ Rehabilitation to restore function ■ Monitor vital functions during the acute phase

ASSESSMENT

Physical assessment, including assessment of pulse and blood pressure, and the collection of subjective data are essential to designing the nursing plan of care. Symptoms such as pain, fatigue, and shortness of breath can only be truly assessed by careful questioning of the client.

Physical Assessment

Physical assessment of the cardiovascular system requires the use of inspection, palpation, percussion, and auscultation. During each of the procedures, the nurse is gathering objective data related to the function of the heart as determined by the heart rate and the quality and characteristics of the heart sounds. In addition, the nurse observes for signs of appropriate cardiac function in relation to oxygen perfusion by assessing skin color and temperature, abnormal pulsations, and the characteristics of the client's respiratory effort. Knowledge of normal parameters and expected findings is essential in determining the meaning of the data during a physical health assessment.

Adults normally have uniform skin color on the face, trunk, and extremities. The eyes are symmetric. The periorbital area is flat, and the eyes do not bulge. The sclera of the eye should be white, the cornea clear, and the conjunctiva pink. The lips should be smooth and noncyanotic. The head should be steady and the skull proportional to the face. The earlobe should be smooth and without creases. The jugular veins are not visible when the chest is upright. Furthermore, the jugular veins distend only 3 cm above the sternal angle when the client is at a 45° angle. Carotid pulsations are visible bilaterally. The fingers should be round and even, with flat, pink nails. The respiratory pattern is even, regular, and unlabored. Intercostal spaces and clavicles are visible; chest veins are evenly distributed and flat; no bulges or masses are visible. Pulsations over the pericardium are absent; however, aortic pulsations in the epigastric area are visible in clients who are thin. The lower extremities are of uniform color and temperature, with even hair distribution. The skeleton should be free of deformity, and the neck and extremities should be in proportion to the torso. Palpation over the pericardium reveals slight vibration at the apical area only. Carotid pulses are palpable and equal in intensity. Dullness to percussion should extend to the midclavicular line at the fifth ICS. S_1 and S_2 are heard equally at Erb's point (third left ICS). However, S_2 is louder than S_1 at the aortic and pulmonic auscultatory areas, and S_1 is louder than S_2 at the tricuspid and apical areas. Murmurs are absent. The carotid pulse is synchronous with the apical pulse.

Physical assessment of the cardiovascular system follows an organized pattern. It begins with inspection of the client's head and neck, including eyes, ears, lips, face, skull, and neck vessels. The upper extremities, chest, abdomen, and lower extremities are also inspected. Palpation includes the precordium and carotid pulses. Percussion of the chest is conducted to determine the cardiac borders. Auscultation includes the heart in five areas with the diaphragm and the bell of the stethoscope. The carotid arteries and the apical pulse are auscultated. Helpful hints for the physical assessment are listed in Box 22–1.

Box 22–1 Helpful Hints for Physical Assessment of the Cardiovascular System

- Provide specific instructions throughout the assessment. Explain what is expected of the client, and state that he or she will be able to breathe regularly throughout the examination.
- Assessment of the heart will require several position changes; the nurse should assist the client if necessary. Allow time for movement if the client is uncomfortable, and explain the purpose of the position change.
- The nurse's hands and the stethoscope should be warmed before beginning the examination.
- The room should be quiet so that subtle sounds may be heard.
- Provide adequate draping to prevent unnecessary exposure of the female breasts.
- Use Standard Precautions.

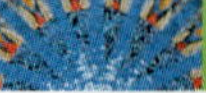

Perfusion Assessments

Technique/Normal Findings	Abnormal Findings
Apical Impulse Assessment	
First using the palmar surface and then repeating with finger pads, palpate the precordium for symmetry of movement and the apical impulse for location, size, amplitude, and duration. The sequence for palpation is shown in Figure 22–16 ■. To locate the apical impulse, ask the client to assume a left lateral recumbent position. Simultaneous palpation of the carotid pulse may also be helpful. *The apical impulse is not palpable in all clients. The apical impulse may be palpated in the mitral area and has only a brief, small amplitude.*	■ An enlarged or displaced heart is associated with an apical impulse lateral to the midclavicular line or below the fifth left intercostal space (ICS). ■ Increased size, amplitude, and duration of the apical impulse are associated with left ventricular volume overload (increased afterload) in conditions such as hypertension (HTN) and aortic stenosis and with pressure overload (increased preload) in conditions such as aortic or mitral regurgitation. ■ Increased amplitude alone may occur with hyperkinetic states, such as anxiety, hyperthyroidism, and anemia. ■ Decreased amplitude is associated with a dilated heart in cardiomyopathy. ■ Displacement alone may also occur with dextrocardia, diaphragmatic hernia, gastric distention, or chronic lung disease. ■ A **thrill** (a palpable vibration over the precordium or an artery) may accompany severe valve stenosis. ■ A marked increase in amplitude of the apical impulse at the right ventricular area occurs with right ventricular volume overload in atrial septal defect. ■ An increase in amplitude and duration occurs with right ventricular pressure overload in pulmonic stenosis and pulmonary hypertension. A lift or heave may also be seen in these conditions and in chronic lung disease. ■ A palpable thrill in this area occurs with ventricular septal defect.
Palpate the subxiphoid area with the index and middle finger. *No pulsations or vibrations should be palpated.*	■ Right ventricular enlargement may produce a downward pulsation against the fingertips. ■ An accentuated pulsation at the pulmonary area may be present in hyperkinetic states. ■ A prominent pulsation reflects increased flow or dilation of the pulmonary artery. ■ A thrill may be associated with aortic or pulmonary stenosis, aortic stenosis, pulmonary HTN, or atrial septal defect. ■ Increased pulsation at the aortic area may suggest aortic aneurysm. ■ A palpable S_2 may be noted with systemic HTN.
Cardiac Rate and Rhythm Assessment	
Auscultate heart rate. *The heart rate should be 60–100 bpm, with regular rhythm.*	■ A heart rate of >100 bpm is tachycardia. A heart rate of <60 bpm is bradycardia.
Simultaneously palpate the radial pulse while listening to the apical pulse. *The radial and apical pulses should be equal.*	■ If the radial pulse falls behind the apical rate, the client has a **pulse deficit**, indicating weak, ineffective contractions of the left ventricle.
Auscultate heart rhythm. *The heart rhythm should be regular.*	■ **Dysrhythmias** (abnormal heart rate or rhythm) may be regular or irregular in rhythm; their rates may be slow or fast. Irregular rhythms may occur in a pattern (e.g., an early beat every second beat, called bigeminy), sporadically, or with frequency and disorganization (e.g., atrial fibrillation). A pattern of gradual increase and decrease in heart rate that is within the normal range and that correlates with inspiration and expiration is called sinus arrhythmia.

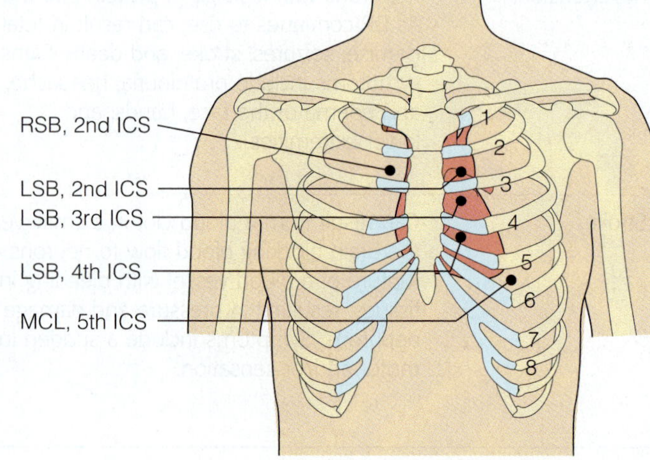

Figure 22–16 ■ Areas for inspection and palpation of the precordium, indicating the sequence for palpation.

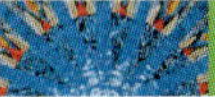

Perfusion Assessments (continued)

Technique/Normal Findings | **Abnormal Findings**

Heart Sounds Assessment

See guidelines for cardiac auscultation in Box 22–2.

Box 22–2 Guidelines for Cardiac Auscultation

1. Locate the major auscultatory areas on the precordium (see Figure 22–17 ■).
2. Choose a sequence of listening. Either begin from the apex and move upward along the sternal border to the base, or begin at the base and move downward to the apex. One suggested sequence is shown in Figure 22–17.
3. Listen first with the client in the sitting or supine position. Then, ask the client to lie on his or her left side, and focus on the apex. Lastly, ask the client to sit up and lean forward. These position changes bring the heart closer to the chest wall and enhance auscultation. Carry out the following steps when the client assumes each of these positions:
   a. First, auscultate each area with the diaphragm of the stethoscope to listen for high-pitched sounds (S_1, S_2, murmurs, and pericardial friction rubs).
   b. Next, auscultate each area with the bell of the stethoscope to listen for lower-pitched sounds (S_3, S_4, and murmurs).
   c. Listen for the effect of respirations on each sound. While the client is sitting up and leaning forward, ask the client to exhale and hold the breath while you listen to heart sounds.

Identify S_1, and note its intensity. At each auscultatory area, listen for several cardiac cycles. See Figure 22–17 for auscultation areas. *S_1 is loudest at the apex of the heart.*

- An accentuated S_1 occurs with tachycardia, states in which cardiac output is high (e.g., fever, anxiety, exercise, anemia, stress, and hyperthyroidism), complete heart block, and mitral stenosis.
- A diminished S_1 occurs with first-degree heart block, mitral regurgitation, congestive heart failure (CHF), coronary artery disease, and pulmonary or systemic HTN. The intensity is also decreased with obesity, emphysema, and pericardial effusion. Varying intensity of S_1 occurs with complete heart block and grossly irregular rhythms.

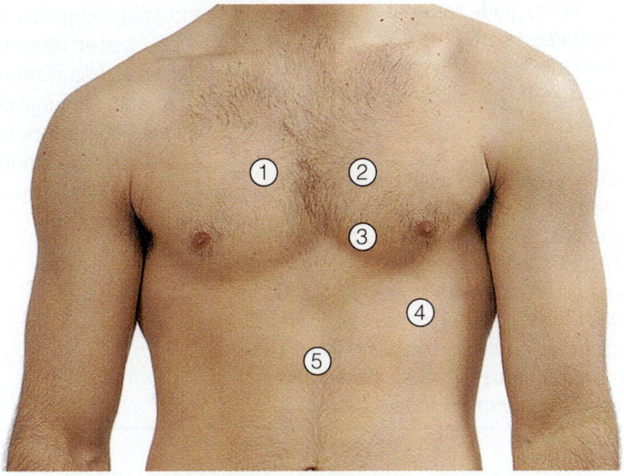

Figure 22–17 ■ Areas for auscultation of the heart.

Listen for splitting of S_1. *Splitting of S_1 may occur during inspiration.*

- Abnormal splitting of S_1 may be heard with right bundle branch block and premature ventricular contractions.

Identify S_2, and note its intensity. *S_2 immediately follows S_1 and is loudest at the base of the heart.*

- An accentuated S_2 may be heard with HTN, exercise, excitement, and conditions of pulmonary HTN, such as CHF and cor pulmonale.
- A diminished S_2 occurs with aortic stenosis, a fall in systolic blood pressure (shock), and increased anteroposterior chest diameter.

Listen for splitting of S_2. *No splitting of S_2 should be heard.*

- Wide splitting of S_2 is associated with delayed emptying of the right ventricle, resulting in delayed pulmonary valve closure (e.g., mitral regurgitation, pulmonary stenosis, and right bundle branch block).
- Fixed splitting occurs when right ventricular output is greater than left ventricular output and pulmonary valve closure is delayed (e.g., with atrial septal defect and right ventricular failure).
- Paradoxic splitting occurs when closure of the aortic valve is delayed (e.g., left bundle branch block).

Identify extra heart sounds in systole. *No extra heart sounds should be heard.*

- Ejection sounds (or clicks) result from the opening of deformed semilunar valves (e.g., aortic and pulmonary stenosis).
- A midsystolic click is heard with mitral valve prolapse.

(continued)

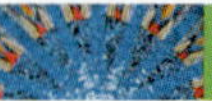

Perfusion Assessments (continued)

Technique/Normal Findings	Abnormal Findings
Identify the presence of extra heart sounds in diastole. *No extra heart sounds should be heard.*	■ An opening snap results from the opening sound of a stenotic mitral valve. ■ A pathologic S_3 (a third heart sound that immediately follows S_2, called a ventricular gallop) results from myocardial failure and ventricular volume overload (e.g., CHF and mitral or tricuspid regurgitation). ■ An S_4 (a fourth heart sound that immediately precedes S_1, called an atrial gallop) results from increased resistance to ventricular filling after atrial contraction (e.g., HTN, coronary artery disease, aortic stenosis, and cardiomyopathy). ■ A combined S_3 and S_4 is called a summation gallop and occurs with severe CHF.
Identify extra heart sounds in both systole and diastole. *No extra heart sounds should be heard during systole and diastole.*	■ A pericardial friction rub results from inflammation of the pericardial sac, as with pericarditis.
Murmur Assessment	
Identify any murmurs. Note location, timing, presence during systole or diastole, and intensity. Use the following scale to grade murmurs: I = Barely heard II = Quietly heard III = Clearly heard IV = Loud V = Very loud VI = Loudest; may be heard with stethoscope off the chest. (A thrill may accompany murmurs of grade IV to grade VI.) Note pitch (low, medium, or high), and quality (harsh, blowing, or musical). Note pattern/shape, crescendo, decrescendo, and radiation/transmission (to axilla or neck). *No murmurs should be heard.*	■ Midsystolic murmurs are heard with semilunar valve disease (e.g., aortic and pulmonary stenosis) and with hypertrophic cardiomyopathy. ■ Pansystolic (holosystolic) murmurs are heard with atrioventricular valve disease (e.g., mitral and tricuspid regurgitation, ventricular septal defect). ■ A late systolic murmur is heard with mitral valve prolapse. ■ Early diastolic murmurs occur with regurgitant flow across incompetent semilunar valves (e.g., aortic regurgitation). ■ Middiastolic and presystolic murmurs, such as with mitral stenosis, occur with turbulent flow across the atrioventricular valves. ■ Continuous murmurs throughout systole and all or part of diastole occur with patent ductus arteriosus.

Assessing the Pulse

A pulse is commonly assessed by palpation (feeling) or auscultation (hearing). The middle three fingertips are used for palpating all pulse sites except the apex of the heart. A stethoscope is used for assessing apical pulses. A Doppler ultrasound stethoscope (DUS; see Figure 22–18 ■) is used for pulses that are difficult to assess. The DUS headset has earpieces similar to standard stethoscope earpieces, but it has a long cord attached to a volume-controlled audio unit and an ultrasound transducer. The DUS detects movement of red blood cells through a blood vessel. In contrast to the conventional stethoscope, it excludes environmental sounds.

A pulse is normally palpated by applying moderate pressure with the three middle fingers of the hand. The pads on the most distal aspects of the finger are the most sensitive areas for detecting a pulse. With excessive pressure one can obliterate a pulse, whereas with too little pressure one may not be able to detect it. Before the nurse assesses the resting pulse, the client should assume a comfortable position. The nurse should also be aware of the following:

- Any medication that could affect the heart rate.
- Whether the client has been physically active. If so, wait 10–15 minutes until the client has rested and the pulse has slowed to its usual rate.
- Any baseline data about the normal heart rate for the client. For example, a physically fit athlete may have a heart rate below 60 BPM.

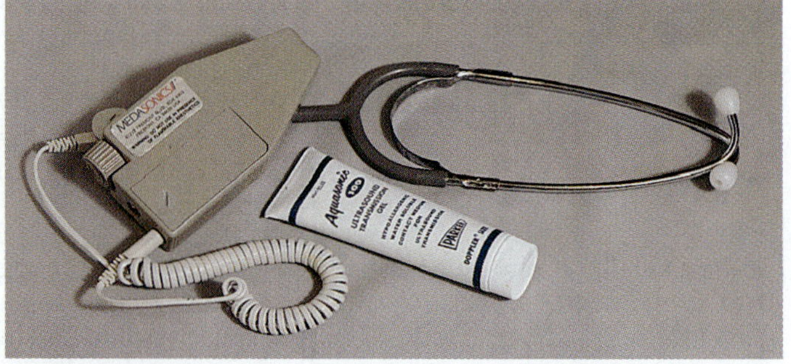

Figure 22–18 ■ A Doppler ultrasound stethoscope (DUS).

- Whether the client should assume a particular position (e.g., sitting). In some clients, the rate changes with the position because of changes in blood flow volume and autonomic nervous system activity.

When assessing the pulse, the nurse collects the following data: the rate, rhythm, volume, arterial wall elasticity, and presence or absence of bilateral equality. An excessively fast heart rate (e.g., over 100 BPM in an adult) is referred to as **tachycardia**. A heart rate in an adult of less than 60 BPM is called **bradycardia**. If a client has either tachycardia or bradycardia, the apical pulse should be assessed.

The **pulse rhythm** is the pattern of the beats and the intervals between the beats. Equal time elapses between beats of a normal pulse. A pulse with an irregular rhythm is referred to as a **dysrhythmia** or **arrhythmia**. It may consist of random, irregular beats or a predictable pattern of irregular beats (documented as "regularly irregular"). When a dysrhythmia is detected, the apical pulse should be assessed. An electrocardiogram (ECG or EKG) is necessary to define the dysrhythmia further.

Pulse volume, also called the pulse strength or amplitude, refers to the force of blood with each beat. Usually, the pulse volume is the same with each beat. It can range from absent to bounding. A normal pulse can be felt with moderate pressure of the fingers and can be obliterated with greater pressure. A forceful or full blood volume that is obliterated only with difficulty is called a full or bounding pulse. A pulse that is readily obliterated with pressure from the fingers is referred to as weak, feeble, or thready.

The **elasticity of the arterial wall** reflects its expansibility or its deformities. A healthy, normal artery feels straight, smooth, soft, and pliable. Elders often have inelastic arteries that feel twisted (tortuous) and irregular upon palpation.

When assessing a peripheral pulse to determine the adequacy of blood flow to a particular area of the body (perfusion), the nurse should also assess the corresponding pulse on the other side of the body. The second assessment gives the nurse data with which to compare the pulses. For example, when assessing the blood flow to the right foot, the nurse assesses the right dorsalis pedis pulse and then the left dorsalis pedis pulse. If the client's right and left pulses are the same, the client's dorsalis pedis pulses are bilaterally equal. The pulse rate does not need to be counted when assessing for perfusion and equality.

When a peripheral pulse is located, it indicates that pulses more proximal to that location will also be present. For example, if the dorsalis pedis, the most distal pulse of the lower extremity, cannot be felt, the nurse next palpates for the posterior tibial pulse. If it is not felt, the popliteal pulse must be assessed. If the popliteal pulse is found, it is not necessary to assess the femoral pulse since it must also be present in order for the more distal pulse to exist.

PULSE SITES A pulse may be measured in nine sites (see Figure 22–19 ■).

1. *Temporal*, where the temporal artery passes over the temporal bone of the head. The site is superior (above) and lateral to (away from the midline of) the eye.

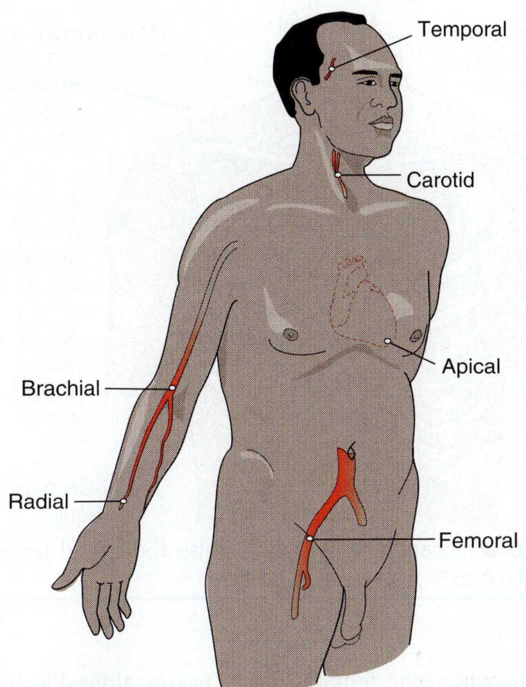

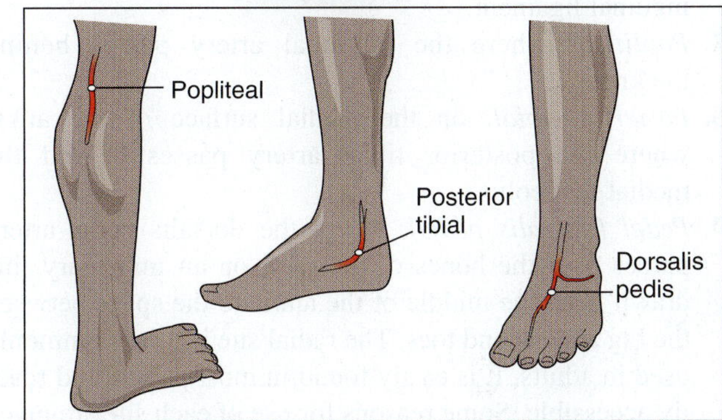

Figure 22–19 ■ Nine sites for assessing pulse.

2. Carotid, at the side of the neck where the carotid artery runs between the trachea and the sternocleidomastoid muscle.

PRACTICE ALERT

Never press both carotids at the same time because this can cause a reflex drop in blood pressure or pulse rate.

3. *Apical*, at the apex of the heart. In an adult this is located on the left side of the chest, about 8 cm (3 in.) to the left of the sternum (breastbone) and at the fourth, fifth, or sixth intercostal space (area between the ribs). In elders, the apex may be further left if there are conditions that have led to an enlarged heart. Before 4 years of age the apex is left of the midclavicular line (MCL); between 4 and 6 years, it is at the MCL (see Figure 22–20 ■). For a child 7 to 9 years of age, the apical pulse is located at the fourth or fifth intercostal space.
4. *Brachial*, at the inner aspect of the biceps muscle of the arm or medially in the antecubital space.
5. *Radial*, where the radial artery runs along the radial bone, on the thumb side of the inner aspect of the wrist.

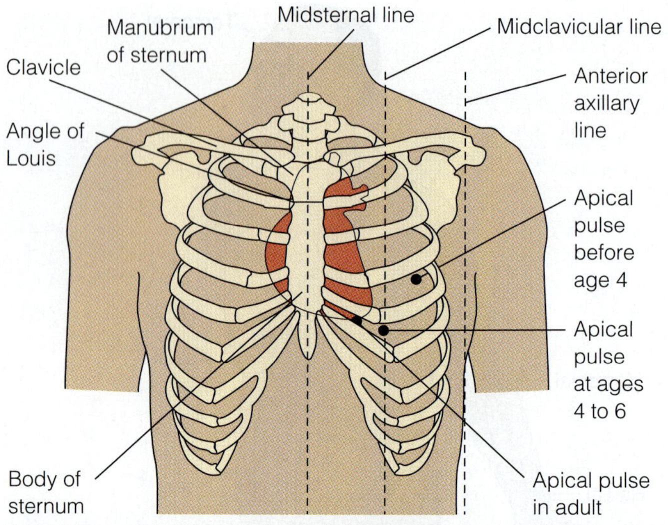

Figure 22–20 ■ Location of the apical pulse for a child under 4 years, a child 4 to 6 years, and an adult.

6. *Femoral*, where the femoral artery passes alongside the inguinal ligament.
7. *Popliteal*, where the popliteal artery passes behind the knee.
8. *Posterior tibial*, on the medial surface of the ankle where the posterior tibial artery passes behind the medial malleolus.
9. *Pedal (dorsalis pedis)*, where the dorsalis pedis artery passes over the bones of the foot, on an imaginary line drawn from the middle of the ankle to the space between the big and second toes. The radial site is most commonly used in adults. It is easily found in most people and readily accessible. Some reasons for use of each site are given in Table 22–7.

TABLE 22–7 **Reasons for Using Specific Pulse Site**

PULSE SITE	REASONS FOR USE
Radial	Readily accessible
Temporal	Used when radial pulse is not accessible
Carotid	Used during cardiac arrest/shock in adults Used to determine circulation to the brain
Apical	Routinely used for infants and children up to 3 years of age Used to determine discrepancies with radial pulse Used in conjunction with some medications
Brachial	Used to measure blood pressure Used during cardiac arrest for infants
Femoral	Used in cases of cardiac arrest/shock Used to determine circulation to a leg
Popliteal	Used to determine circulation to the lower leg
Posterior tibial	Used to determine circulation to the foot
Dorsal pedal	Used to determine circulation to the foot

CARE SETTINGS Monitoring Pulse in the Home

- Assist in obtaining and using an electronic pulse device if indicated.
- Teach the client to monitor the pulse prior to taking medications that affect the heart rate. Tell the client to report any notable changes in heart rate or rhythm (regularity) to the health care provider.

APICAL PULSE ASSESSMENT Assessment of the apical pulse is indicated for clients whose peripheral pulse is irregular or unavailable as well as for clients with known cardiovascular, pulmonary, and renal diseases. It is commonly assessed prior to administering medications that affect heart rate. The apical site is also used to assess the pulse for newborns, infants, and children up to 2 to 3 years old.

APICAL-RADIAL PULSE ASSESSMENT An **apical-radial pulse** may need to be assessed for clients with certain cardiovascular disorders. Normally, the apical and radial rates are identical. An apical pulse rate greater than a radial pulse rate can indicate that the thrust of the blood from the heart is too weak for the wave to be felt at the peripheral pulse site, or it can indicate that vascular disease is preventing impulses from being transmitted. Any discrepancy between the two pulse rates is called a **pulse deficit** and needs to be reported promptly. In no instance is the radial pulse greater than the apical pulse.

Assessing Blood Pressure

Blood pressure is measured with a blood pressure cuff, a sphygmomanometer, and a stethoscope. The blood pressure cuff consists of a rubber bag that can be inflated with air called the bladder (Figure 22–21 ■). It is covered with cloth and has

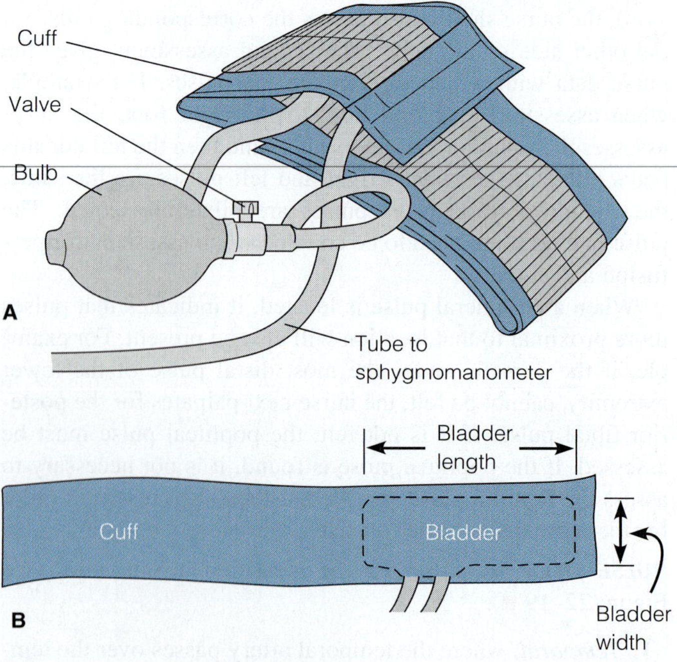

Figure 22–21 ■ *A*, A blood pressure cuff and bulb; *B*, the bladder inside the cuff.

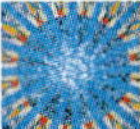

DEVELOPMENTAL CONSIDERATIONS Assessing the Pulse

INFANTS

- Use the apical pulse for the heart rate of newborns, infants, and children 2 to 3 years old to establish baseline data for subsequent evaluation, to determine whether the cardiac rate is within normal range, and to determine if the rhythm is regular.
- Place a baby in a supine position, and offer a pacifier if the baby is crying or restless. Crying and physical activity will increase the pulse rate. For this reason, take the apical pulse rate of infants and small children before assessing body temperatures.
- Locate the apical pulse in the fourth intercostal space, lateral to the midclavicular line during infancy.
- Brachial, popliteal, and femoral pulses may be palpated. Due to a normally low blood pressure and rapid heart rate, infants' other distal pulses may be hard to feel.
- Newborn infants may have heart murmurs that are not pathological, but reflect functional incomplete closure of fetal heart structures (ductus arteriosus or foramen ovale).

CHILDREN

- To take a peripheral pulse, position the child comfortably in the adult's arms, or have the adult remain close by. This may decrease anxiety and yield more accurate results.
- To assess the apical pulse, assist a young child to a comfortable supine or sitting position.
- Demonstrate the procedure to the child using a stuffed animal or doll, and allow the child to handle the stethoscope before beginning the procedure. This will decrease anxiety and promote cooperation.
- The apex of the heart is normally located in the fourth intercostal space in young children; fifth intercostal space in children 7 years of age and over.
- Locate the apical impulse along the fourth intercostal space, between the MCL and the anterior axillary line (see Figure 22–20 ■).
- Count the pulse prior to other uncomfortable procedures so that the rate is not artificially elevated by the discomfort.

ELDERS

- If the client has severe hand or arm tremors, the radial pulse may be difficult to count.
- Cardiac changes in elders, such as decrease in cardiac output, sclerotic changes to heart valves, and dysrhythmias often indicate that obtaining an apical pulse will be more accurate.
- Elders often have decreased peripheral circulation, so pedal pulses should also be checked for regularity, volume, and symmetry.
- The pulse returns to baseline after exercise more slowly than with other age groups.

two tubes attached to it. One tube connects to a rubber bulb that inflates the bladder. A small valve on the side of this bulb traps and releases the air in the bladder.

The other tube is attached to a sphygmomanometer. The sphygmomanometer indicates the pressure of the air within the bladder. There are two types of sphygmomanometers: aneroid and digital. The aneroid sphygmomanometer is a calibrated dial with a needle that points to the calibrations (Figure 22–22 ■).

Many agencies use digital (electronic) sphygmomanometers (Figure 22–23 ■), which eliminate the need to listen for the sounds of the client's systolic and diastolic blood pressures through a stethoscope. Electronic blood pressure devices should be calibrated periodically to check accuracy. All health care facilities should have manual blood pressure equipment available as backup.

Doppler ultrasound stethoscopes are also used to assess blood pressure (see Figure 22–18 earlier in the chapter). These are of particular value when blood pressure sounds are difficult to hear, such as in infants, obese clients, and clients in shock. Systolic pressure may be the only blood pressure obtainable with some ultrasound models.

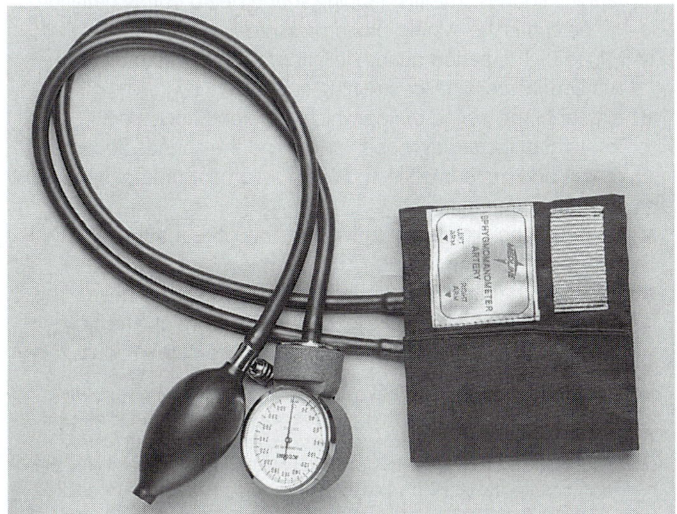

Figure 22–22 ■ An aneroid sphygmomanometer and cuff.

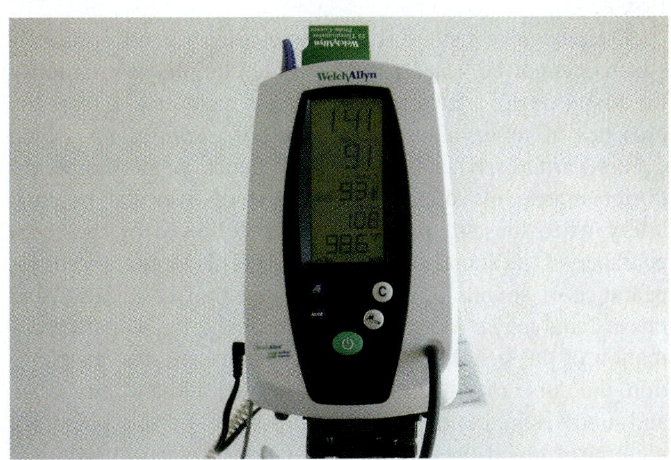

Figure 22–23 ■ Blood pressure monitors register systolic and diastolic blood pressures and often other vital signs.

BLOOD PRESSURE SITES The blood pressure is usually assessed in the client's upper arm using the brachial artery and a standard stethoscope. Assessing the blood pressure on a client's thigh is indicated in these situations:

- The blood pressure cannot be measured on either arm (e.g., because of burns or other trauma).
- The blood pressure in one thigh is to be compared with the blood pressure in the other thigh.

Blood pressure is not measured on a particular client's limb in the following situations:

- The shoulder, arm, or hand (or the hip, knee, or ankle) is injured or diseased.
- A cast or bulky bandage is on any part of the limb.
- The client has had surgical removal of axilla (or hip) lymph nodes on that side, such as for cancer.
- The client has an intravenous infusion in that limb.
- The client has an arteriovenous fistula (e.g., for renal dialysis) in that limb.

METHODS Blood pressure can be assessed directly or indirectly. Direct (invasive monitoring) measurement involves the insertion of a catheter into the brachial, radial, or femoral artery. Arterial pressure is represented as wavelike forms displayed on a monitor. With correct placement, this pressure reading is highly accurate.

Two noninvasive indirect methods of measuring blood pressure are the auscultatory and palpatory methods. The auscultatory method is most commonly used in hospitals, clinics, and homes. Required equipment is a sphygmomanometer, a cuff, and a stethoscope. When carried out correctly, the auscultatory method is relatively accurate.

When taking a blood pressure using a stethoscope, the nurse identifies phases in the series of sounds called *Korotkoff's sounds* (Figure 22–24 ■). First the nurse pumps the cuff up to about 30 mmHg above the point where the pulse is no longer felt; that is the point when the blood flow in the artery is stopped. Then the pressure is released slowly (2–3 mmHg per second) while the nurse observes the readings on the manometer and relates them to the sounds heard through the stethoscope. Five phases occur but may not always be audible (see Box 22–3).

The palpatory method is sometimes used when Korotkoff's sounds cannot be heard and electronic equipment to amplify the sounds is not available, or to prevent misdirection from the presence of an auscultatory gap. An *auscultatory gap*, which occurs particularly in hypertensive clients, is the temporary disappearance of sounds normally heard over the brachial artery when the cuff pressure is high followed by the reappearance of the sounds at a lower level. This temporary disappearance of sounds occurs in the latter part of phase 1 and phase 2 and may cover a range of 40 mmHg. If a palpated estimation of the systolic pressure is not made prior to auscultation, the nurse may begin listening in the middle of this range and underestimate the systolic pressure. In the palpatory method of blood pressure determination, instead of listening for the blood flow sounds, the nurse uses light to moderate pressure to palpate the pulsations of the artery as the pressure

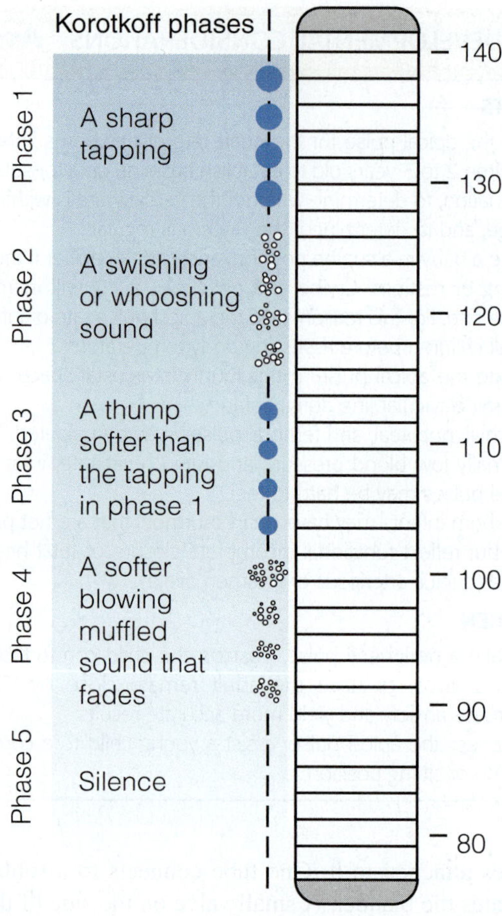

Figure 22–24 ■ Korotkoff's sounds can be differentiated into five phases. In the illustration, the blood pressure is 138/90 or 138/102/90.

Box 22–3 Korotkoff's Sounds

- *Phase 1:* The pressure level at which the first faint, clear tapping or thumping sounds are heard. These sounds gradually become more intense. To ensure that they are not extraneous sounds, the nurse should identify at least two consecutive tapping sounds. The first tapping sound heard during deflation of the cuff is the systolic blood pressure.
- *Phase 2:* The period during deflation when the sounds have a muffled, whooshing, or swishing quality.
- *Phase 3:* The period during which the blood flows freely through an increasingly open artery and the sounds become crisper and more intense and again assume a thumping quality but softer than in phase 1.
- *Phase 4:* The time when the sounds become muffled and have a soft, blowing quality.
- *Phase 5:* The pressure level when the last sound is heard. This is followed by a period of silence. The pressure at which the last sound is heard is the diastolic blood pressure in adults.*

*In agencies where the fourth phase is considered the diastolic pressure, three measures are recommended (systolic pressure, diastolic pressure, and phase 5). These may be referred to as systolic, first diastolic, and second diastolic pressures. The phase 5 (second diastolic pressure) reading may be zero; that is, the muffled sounds are heard even when there is no air pressure in the blood pressure cuff. In some instances, muffled sounds are never heard, in which case a dash is inserted where the reading would normally be recorded (e.g.,/–/110).

in the cuff is released. The pressure is read from the sphygmomanometer when the first pulsation is felt.

COMMON ERRORS IN ASSESSING BLOOD PRESSURE The importance of the accuracy of blood pressure assessments cannot be overemphasized. Many judgments about a client's health are made on the basis of blood pressure. It is an important indicator of the client's condition and is used extensively as a basis for nursing interventions. Two possible reasons for blood pressure errors are haste on the part of the nurse and subconscious bias. For example, a nurse may be influenced by the client's previous blood pressure measurements or diagnosis and "hear" a value consonant with the practitioner's expectations. Some reasons for erroneous blood pressure readings are given in Table 22–8.

PRACTICE ALERT

Electronic/automatic blood pressure cuffs can be left in place for many hours. Remove the cuff and check skin condition periodically.

HYPOTENSION **Hypotension** is a blood pressure that is below normal, that is, a systolic reading consistently between 85 and 110 mmHg in an adult whose normal pressure is higher than this. **Orthostatic hypotension** is a blood pressure that falls when the client sits or stands. It is usually the result of peripheral vasodilatation in which blood leaves the central body organs, especially the brain, and moves to the periphery, often causing the person to feel faint. Hypotension can also be caused by analgesics such as meperidine hydrochloride (Demerol), bleeding, severe burns, and dehydration. It is important to monitor hypotensive clients carefully to prevent falls. When assessing for orthostatic hypotension:

- Place the client in a supine position for 10 minutes.
- Record the client's pulse and blood pressure.
- Assist the client to slowly sit or stand. Support the client in case of faintness.
- Immediately recheck the pulse and blood pressure in the same sites as previously.
- Repeat the pulse and blood pressure after 3 minutes.

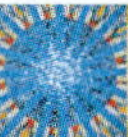

DEVELOPMENTAL CONSIDERATIONS Blood Pressure

INFANTS

- Use a pediatric stethoscope with a small diaphragm.
- The lower edge of the blood pressure cuff can be closer to the antecubital space of an infant.
- Use the palpation method if auscultation with a stethoscope or DUS is unsuccessful.
- Arm and thigh pressures are equivalent in children under 1 year of age.
- One quick way to determine the normal systolic blood pressure of a child is to use the following formula:
  Normal systolic BP = 80 + (2 × child's age in years)

CHILDREN

- Blood pressure should be measured in all children over 3 years of age and in children under 3 years of age with certain medical conditions (e.g., congenital heart disease, renal malformation, medications that affect blood pressure).
- Explain each step of the process and what it will feel like. Demonstrate on a doll.
- Use the palpation technique for children under 3 years old.
- Cuff bladder width should be 40% and length should be 80–100% of the arm circumference (Figure 22–25 ■).
- Take the blood pressure prior to other uncomfortable procedures so that the blood pressure is not artificially elevated by the discomfort.
- In children, the diastolic pressure is considered to be the onset of phase 4, where the sounds become muffled.
- In children, the thigh pressure is about 10 mmHg higher than the arm.

ELDERS

- Skin may be very fragile. Do not allow cuff pressure to remain high any longer than necessary.
- Determine if the client is taking antihypertensives and, if so, when the last dose was taken.
- Medications that cause vasodilation (antihypertensive medications) along with the loss of baroreceptor efficiency in the elderly place them at increased risk for having orthostatic hypotension. Measuring blood pressure while the client is in the lying, sitting, and standing positions, and noting any changes can determine this.
- If the client has arm contractures, assess the blood pressure by palpation, with the arm in a relaxed position. If this is not possible, take a thigh blood pressure.

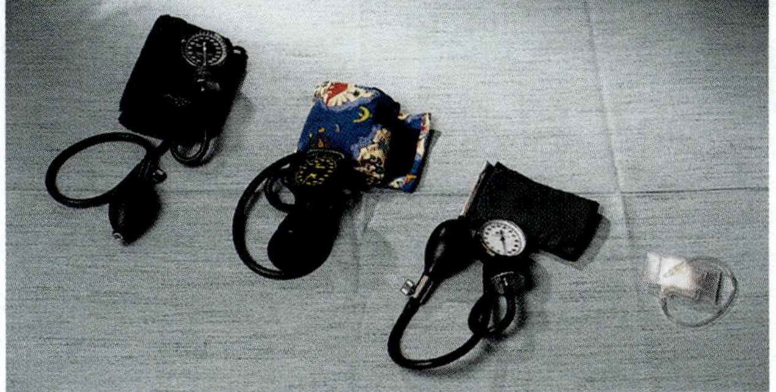

Figure 22–25 ■ Pediatric blood pressure cuffs (with manometers).

TABLE 22–8 Selected Sources of Error in Blood Pressure Assessment

ERROR	EFFECT
Bladder cuff too narrow	Erroneously high
Bladder cuff too wide	Erroneously low
Arm unsupported	Erroneously high
Insufficient rest before the assessment	Erroneously high
Repeating assessment too quickly	Erroneously high systolic or low diastolic readings
Cuff wrapped too loosely or unevenly	Erroneously high
Deflating cuff too quickly	Erroneously low systolic and high diastolic readings
Deflating cuff too slowly	Erroneously high diastolic reading
Failure to use the same arm consistently	Inconsistent measurements
Arm above level of the heart	Erroneously low
Assessing immediately after a meal or while client smokes or has pain	Erroneously high
Failure to identify auscultatory gap	Erroneously low systolic pressure and erroneously low diastolic pressure

- Record the results. A rise in pulse of 15–30 beats per minute or a drop in blood pressure of 20 mmHg systolic or 10 mmHg diastolic indicates orthostatic hypotension (Irvin & White, 2004).

Health Assessment Interview

A health assessment interview to determine problems with cardiac structure and function may be conducted during a health screening, may focus on a chief complaint (e.g., chest pain), or may be part of a total health assessment. If the client has a problem with cardiac function, analyze its onset, characteristics, course, severity, precipitating and relieving factors, and any associated symptoms, noting the timing and circumstances. For example, ask the client the following:

- What is the location of the chest pain you experienced? Did it move up to your jaw or into your left arm?
- Describe the type of activity that brings on your chest pain.
- Have you noticed any changes in your energy level?
- Have you felt light-headed during the times your heart is racing?

The interview begins by exploring the client's chief complaint (e.g., chest pain, palpitations, or shortness of breath). For the client with chest pain, assess in terms of location, quality or character, timing, setting or precipitating factors, severity, aggravating and relieving factors, and associated symptoms (Table 22–9).

Explore the client's history for heart disorders, such as angina, heart attack, congestive heart failure, hypertension, and valvular disease. Ask the client about previous heart surgery or illnesses, such as rheumatic fever, scarlet fever, or recurrent streptococcal throat infections. Also ask about the presence and treatment of other chronic illnesses, such as diabetes mellitus, bleeding disorders, or endocrine disorders. Review the client's family history

CARE SETTINGS Taking Blood Pressure Readings in the Home

- If the client takes blood pressure readings at home, use the same equipment or calibrate it against a system known to be accurate.
- Observe the client or family member taking the blood pressure and provide feedback if further instruction is needed.
- Home blood pressure measurement done by the client or family can detect elevated pressures not identified when the client is seen in a medical office (Bobrie et al., 2004).
- If the client is in a chair or low bed, position yourself so that you maintain the client's arm at heart level and you can read the sphygmomanometer at eye level.

TABLE 22–9 Assessing Chest Pain

CHARACTERISTIC	EXAMPLES
Location	Substernal, precordial, jaw, back Localized or diffuse Radiation to neck, jaw, shoulder, arm
Character/quality	Pressure; tightness; crushing, burning, or aching quality; heaviness; dullness; "heartburn" or indigestion
Timing	Onset: Sudden or gradual? Duration: How many minutes does the pain last? Frequency: Is the pain continuous or periodic?
Setting/precipitating factors	Awake, at rest, sleep interrupted? With activity? With eating, exertion, exercise, elimination, emotional upset?
Intensity/severity	Can range from 0 (no pain) to 10 (worst pain ever felt)
Aggravating factors	Activity, breathing, temperature
Relieving factors	Medication (nitroglycerin, antacid), rest; there may be no relieving factors
Associated symptoms	Fatigue, shortness of breath, palpitations, nausea and vomiting, sweating, anxiety, light-headedness or dizziness

Assessment Interview The Cardiac System

Interview Questions and Leading Statements

Current and Past Medical History

- Have you ever had any problems with your heart, such as angina (pain), heart attack, or disease of the valves? If so, describe. How were these problems treated?
- Have you been diagnosed with high blood pressure? If so, how is it treated?
- Do you have a history of rheumatic fever, scarlet fever, or strep throat infections? If so, describe them and their treatment.
- Have you had your cholesterol checked recently? If so, what is it? If you have high cholesterol, how is it treated?
- Have you ever had tests to check the function of your heart? If so, describe them.
- Do you take any medications to make your heart function more effectively, such as aspirin, those to control heart rate, anticoagulants, or diuretics? If so, how often do you take them?
- Do you have a pacemaker? If so, at what age did you receive it, and for what problem? How do you check the batteries?

Lifestyle

- Do you smoke, chew tobacco, or use snuff? If so, how often and how much?
- Do you drink alcohol? If so, what type, how much, and for how long?
- Are you able to manage your activities of daily living and work independently? Explain.
- Describe your food and liquid intake during a 24-hour period. How often do you eat fried foods, fast foods, or meat?
- How much salt do you use on food?
- Do you eat high-fiber foods? If so, what are they, and how often do you eat them?

Signs and Symptoms

- Have you had a recent weight gain or loss? Explain.
- Have you noticed any change in the color of your skin (e.g., pale or dusky or flushed)? If so, do you know what causes this?
- Have you had any swelling in your feet or legs? If so, where and how much? What do you do to relieve it?
- Describe any chest pain you have experienced. When did it occur? Where was it located? On a scale of 0–10, with 10 being the worst pain you have ever had, rate the pain and describe it (e.g., burning, crushing, stabbing, squeezing, heavy, or tight).
- What were you doing when the pain began (e.g., were you working or resting)? Did it begin suddenly or gradually? How long did it last?
- Did you have any other symptoms with the pain, such as nausea or vomiting, sweating, racing heart, pale skin, palpitations?
- What made the pain worse? What did you do to try to relieve the pain? Did that work?
- Describe any cough you have had. Was it dry or wet? Do you cough up mucus? If so, what color is it? How long have you had the cough?
- Have you experienced any numbness or tingling, dizziness or light-headedness, or palpitations? If so, describe.
- Have you ever used oxygen?

Sleep and Rest

- How long do you sleep each night? Do you feel rested after you sleep?
- Does your heart problem interfere with your ability to sleep and rest? Explain.
- How many pillows do you use at night?
- Where do you sleep at night (e.g., in a recliner to breathe more easily)?
- Do you ever feel short of breath while you are resting or sleeping? If so, does this wake you up? Explain.

Self

- How does having this condition make you feel about yourself?
- How does this condition affect your relationships with others?
- Has having this condition interfered with your ability to work? Explain.
- Has this condition interfered with your usual sexual activity?
- Have you ever had chest pain during sexual activity? What do you do for it?
- Do you use a slower pace or different positions that are less stressful for you during sexual activities? Does this help?

Stress and Coping

- Has having this condition created stress for you?
- Have you experienced any kind of stress that makes this condition worse? Explain.
- Describe what you do when you feel stressed.
- Describe how specific relationships or activities help you cope with this problem.
- Describe specific cultural beliefs or practices that affect how you care for and feel about this problem.
- Are there any specific treatments that you would not use to treat this problem?

for coronary artery disease, hypertension, stroke, hyperlipidemia, diabetes, congenital heart disease, or sudden death.

Ask the client about past or present occurrence of various cardiac symptoms, such as chest pain, shortness of breath, difficulty breathing, cough, palpitations, fatigue, light-headedness or dizziness, fainting, heart murmur, blood clots, or swelling. Because cardiac function affects all other body systems, a full history may need to explore other related systems, such as respiratory function and/or peripheral vascular function.

Review the client's personal habits and nutritional history, including body weight; eating patterns; dietary intake of fats, salt, and fluids; dietary restrictions; hypersensitivities or intolerances to food or medication; and use of caffeine and alcohol. If the client uses tobacco products, ask about type (e.g., cigarettes, pipe, cigars, or snuff), duration, amount, and efforts to quit. If the client uses street drugs, ask about type, method of intake (e.g., inhaled or injected), duration of use, and efforts to quit. Include questions about the client's activity level and tolerance, recreational activities, and relaxation habits. Assess the client's sleep patterns for interruptions in sleep caused by dyspnea, cough, discomfort, urination, or stress. Ask how many pillows the client uses when sleeping.

Also consider psychosocial factors that may affect the client's stress level: What is the client's marital status, family composition, and role within the family? Have there been any changes? What is the client's occupation, level of education, and socioeconomic level? Are resources for support available? What is the client's emotional disposition and personality type? How does the client perceive his or her state of health or illness, and how able is the client to comply with treatment?

Genetic Considerations

When conducting a health assessment interview and physical assessment, it is important for the nurse to consider genetic influences on the health of the adult. During the health assessment interview, ask about family members with health problems affecting cardiac function or a family history of high cholesterol levels or early onset coronary artery disease. During the physical assessment, assess for any manifestations that might indicate a genetic disorder (Box 22–4). If data are found to indicate genetic risk factors or alterations, ask about genetic testing and refer for appropriate genetic counseling and evaluation.

DIAGNOSTIC TESTS

The results of diagnostic tests of cardiac function are used to support the diagnosis of a specific disease, to provide information to identify or modify the appropriate medications or therapy used to treat the disease, and to help nurses monitor the client's responses to treatment and nursing care interventions. Diagnostic tests appropriate for determining cardiac function may include the following:

- Serum cholesterol, triglycerides, and lipids
- Stress/exercise tests
- X-ray, magnetic resonance imaging (MRI), computed tomography (CT), or positron-emission tomography test
- Echocardiogram
- A transesophageal echocardiogram
- Cardiac catheterization with either coronary angiography or coronary arteriography
- Pericardiocentesis
- Electrocardiography (see Boxes 22–5 and 22–6)
- Troponin, MB isoenzyme of creatine kinase.

Regardless of the type of diagnostic test, the nurse is responsible for explaining the procedure and any special preparation needed, assessing for medication use that may affect the outcome of the tests, supporting the client during the examination as necessary, documenting the procedures as appropriate, and monitoring the results of the tests.

Box 22–4 **Genetic Considerations for Cardiac Disorders**

- Familial hypercholesterolemia is a single-gene disorder that results in atherosclerosis and coronary artery disease, which may occur at an earlier age than in the general population (i.e., before age 55 in men and age 65 in women). However, increased cholesterol levels may also be inherited and are a risk factor for coronary artery disease in both men and women.
- Marfan syndrome is an autosomal-dominant inherited disorder that affects the skeleton, eyes, and cardiovascular system. The cardiovascular effects are a dilatation of the proximal aorta and aortic dissection associated with degeneration of the elastic fibers in the tunica media of the aorta. There may also be thoracic aortic aneurysms.
- Supraventricular aortic stenosis is a genetic vascular disorder resulting in an hourglass-shaped stenosis of the ascending aorta. It may also affect other major arteries, including the pulmonary, carotid, cerebral, renal, and coronary arteries.
- Hypertropic cardiomyopathy, a disease of sarcomere proteins, has a genetic transmission.
- Williams syndrome is a rare genetic disorder characterized by characteristic "elfin-like" features and heart and blood vessel problems (as well as other physical problems).
- Long QT syndrome is an inherited genetic disorder that results from structural abnormalities of the potassium channels in the heart, leading to dysrhythmias. This can result in unconsciousness and may cause sudden cardiac death in teenagers and young adults when exposed to stressors ranging from exercise to loud sounds.

CARING INTERVENTIONS

Nursing interventions are aimed at supporting, improving, and promoting perfusion adequate to meet the client's oxygenation needs and prevent tissue damage. Depending on the disease process involved, this may include caring interventions to reduce stress on the heart, decrease the cardiac workload, increase the efficacy of cardiac contractions, and meet fluid needs.

Nurses also provide teaching at a primary level to reduce the risk of cardiac disease in later life. Teaching the importance of reducing fat intake, aerobic exercise adequate to attain optimal heart rate, and eating a well-balanced diet can all reduce the risk of coronary artery disease.

Once an initial assessment of a client for alterations in circulation has been made, the nurse develops a plan of care and prioritizes interventions. Interventions for circulatory problems usually fall into three broad categories: inputs, outputs, and pressure supports. Inputs include arterial lines, venous lines, fluids, drug regimens, transfusions, and blood component therapies. Outputs include suctioning with specialized equipment such as hemovacs and chest tubes and procedures such as thoracentesis. Pressure supports include dressings, direct compression, tourniquets, and cardiopulmonary resuscitation. An evaluation of the planned actions, based on the client's response, should be continuous and modified as the client's condition dictates.

In coping with alterations in circulation, care should be directed toward promoting, maintaining, or regaining the best possible cardiopulmonary function. The design for nursing action is to assess the situation and client for stressors. The client should be interviewed if possible, observed, and examined to identify actual and/or potential circulatory problems. The client's responses are determined to be appropriate, deficient, or excessive, and interventions are planned accordingly. The nurse attempts to reduce client stress, supports adaptive behaviors, replaces deficiencies, modifies or removes excessive responses, and prevents injury and complications. The nurse should always assist in the evaluation of planned actions, report client responses, and assist in modifying the interventions as indicated.

Skills specific used to care for the client with perfusion related problems include the following:

- Assessing pulses
- Recording and interpreting an ECG
- Administering cardiopulmonary resuscitation
- Achieving defibrillation

(Text continues on page 1329.)

Box 22–5 The Electrocardiogram

The **electrocardiogram (ECG)** is a graphic record of the heart's activity. Electrodes applied to the body surface are used to obtain a graphic representation of cardiac electrical activity. These electrodes detect the magnitude and direction of electrical currents produced in the heart. They attach to the electrocardiograph by an insulated wire called a **lead**. The electrocardiograph converts the electrical impulses it receives into a series of waveforms that represent cardiac depolarization and repolarization. Placement of electrodes on different parts of the body allows different views of this electrical activity, much like turning the head while holding a camera provides different views of the scenery. ECG waveforms and patterns are examined to detect dysrhythmias as well as myocardial damage, effects of drugs, and electrolyte imbalances.

The ECG waveforms reflect the direction of electrical flow in relation to a positive electrode. Current flowing toward the positive electrode produces an upward (positive) waveform; current flowing away from the positive electrode produces a downward (negative) waveform. Current flowing perpendicular to the positive pole produces a biphasic (both positive and negative) waveform. Absence of electrical activity is represented by a straight line called the **isoelectric line**.

The ECG waveforms are recorded by a heated stylus on heat-sensitive paper. The paper is marked at standard intervals that represent time and voltage or amplitude (Figure 22–26 ■). Each small box is 1 mm^2. The recording speed of the standard ECG is 25 mm/second, so each small box represents 0.04 second. Five small boxes horizontally and vertically make one large box, equivalent to 0.20 second. Five large boxes represent 1 full second. Measured vertically, each small box represents 0.1 mV.

Both bipolar and unipolar leads are used in recording the ECG. A bipolar lead uses two electrodes of opposite polarity (negative and positive). A unipolar lead uses one positive electrode and a negative reference point at the center of the heart. The electrical potential between the two monitoring points is graphically recorded as the ECG waveform.

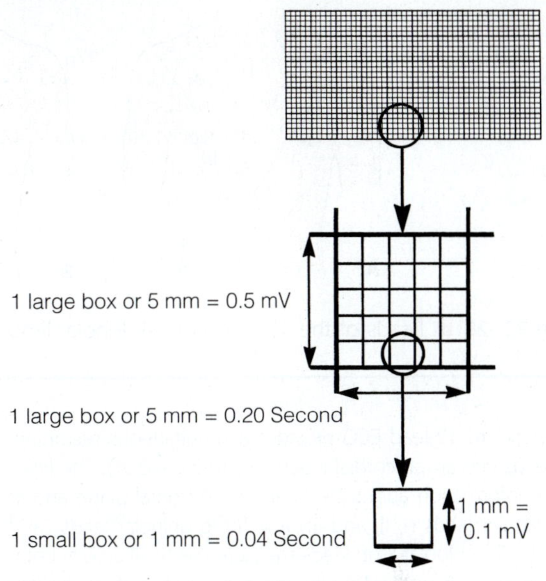

Figure 22–26 ■ Time and voltage measurements on ECG paper at a recording speed of 25 mm/second.

The heart can be viewed from both the frontal plane and the horizontal plane (Figure 22–27 ■). Each plane provides a unique perspective of the heart muscle. The frontal plane is an imaginary cut through the body that views the heart from top to bottom (superior to inferior) and side to side (right to left). This perspective of the heart is analogous to a paper doll cutout. It provides information about the inferior and lateral walls of the heart. The horizontal plane is a cross-sectional view of the heart from front to back (anterior to posterior) and side to side (right to left). Information regarding the anterior, septal, and lateral walls of the heart, as well as the posterior wall, are obtained from this view.

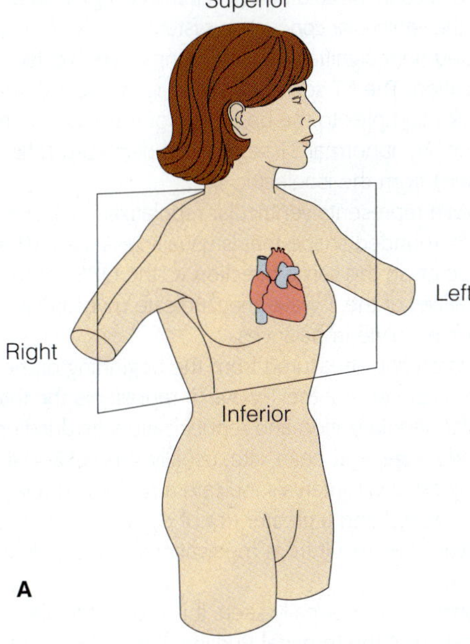

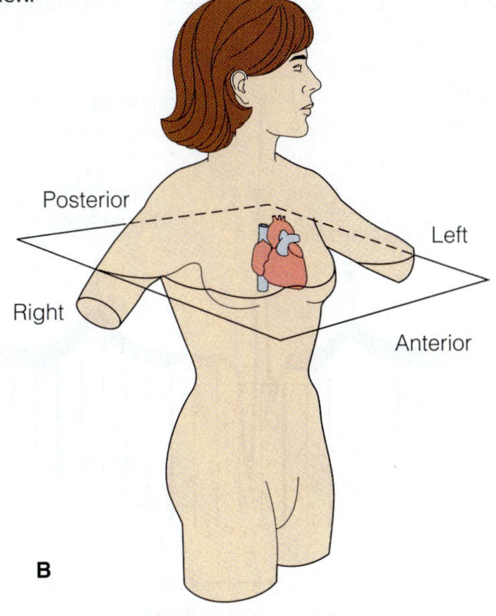

Figure 22–27 ■ Planes of the heart. *A,* Frontal plane; *B,* horizontal plane.

(continued)

Box 22–5 **The Electrocardiogram (continued)**

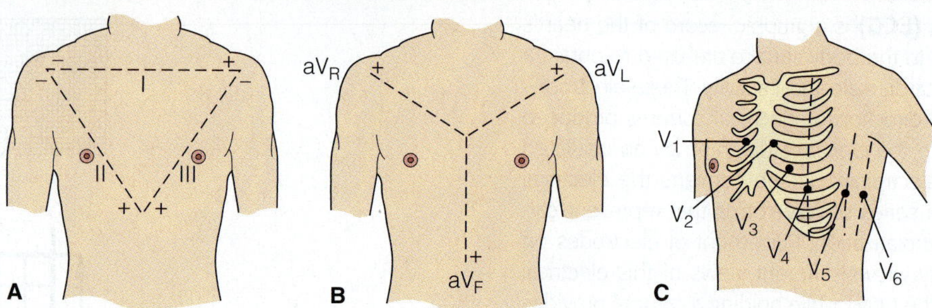

Figure 22–28 ■ Leads of the 12-lead ECG. *A,* Bipolar limb leads I, II, III; *B,* Unipolar limb leads aVR, aVL, aVF; *C,* Unipolar precordial leads V1 to V6.

A standard 12-lead ECG provides a simultaneous recording of six limb leads and six precordial leads (Figure 22–28 ■). The limb leads provide information about the heart in the frontal plane and include three bipolar leads (I, II, and III) and three unipolar leads (aVR, aVL, and aVF). The bipolar limb leads measure electrical activity between a negative lead on one extremity and a positive lead on another. The unipolar limb leads (called augmented leads) measure the electrical activity between a single positive electrode on a limb (right arm [R], left arm [L], or left leg [F for foot]), and the center of the heart.

The precordial leads, also known as chest leads or V leads, view the heart in the horizontal plane. They include six unipolar leads (V_1, V_2, V_3, V_4, V_5, and V_6), which measure electrical activity between the center of the heart and a positive electrode on the chest wall.

The cardiac cycle is depicted as a series of waveforms, the P, Q, R, S, T, and U waves (see Figure 22–29 ■):

- The *P wave* represents atrial depolarization and contraction. The impulse is from the sinoatrial node. The P wave precedes the QRS complex and is normally smooth, round, and upright. P waves may be absent when the SA node is not acting as the pacemaker. Atrial repolarization occurs during ventricular depolarization and usually is not seen on the ECG.
- The *PR interval* represents the time required for the sinus impulse to travel to the AV node and into the Purkinje fibers. This interval is measured from the beginning of the P wave to the beginning of the QRS complex. If no Q wave is seen, the beginning of the R wave is used. The PR interval is normally 0.12–0.20 second (up to 0.24 second is considered normal in clients over age 65). PR intervals greater than 0.20 second indicate a delay in conduction from the SA node to the ventricles.
- The *QRS complex* represents ventricular depolarization and contraction. The QRS complex includes three separate waves: The Q wave is the first negative deflection, the R wave is the positive or upright deflection, and the S wave is the first negative deflection after the R wave. All three waves may not be present in every QRS but the name remains unchanged. The normal duration of a QRS complex is from 0.06 to 0.10 second. QRS complexes of greater than 0.10 second indicate delays in transmitting the impulse through the ventricular conduction system.
- The *ST segment* signifies the beginning of ventricular repolarization. The ST segment, which is the period from the end of the QRS complex to the beginning of the T wave, should be isoelectric. An abnormal ST segment is displaced (elevated or depressed) from the isoelectric line.
- The *T wave* represents ventricular repolarization. It normally has a smooth, rounded shape that is usually less than 10 mm tall. It usually points in the same direction as the QRS complex. Abnormalities of the T wave may indicate myocardial ischemia or injury or electrolyte imbalances.
- The *QT interval* is measured from the beginning of the QRS complex to the end of the T wave. It represents the total time of ventricular depolarization and repolarization. Its duration varies with gender, age, and heart rate; usually, it is 0.32–0.44 second long. Prolonged QT intervals indicate a prolonged relative refractory period and a greater risk of dysrhythmias. Shortened QT intervals may result from medications or electrolyte imbalances.
- The *U wave* is not normally seen. It is thought to signify repolarization of the terminal Purkinje fibers. If present, the U wave follows the same direction as the T wave. It is most commonly seen in hypokalemia.

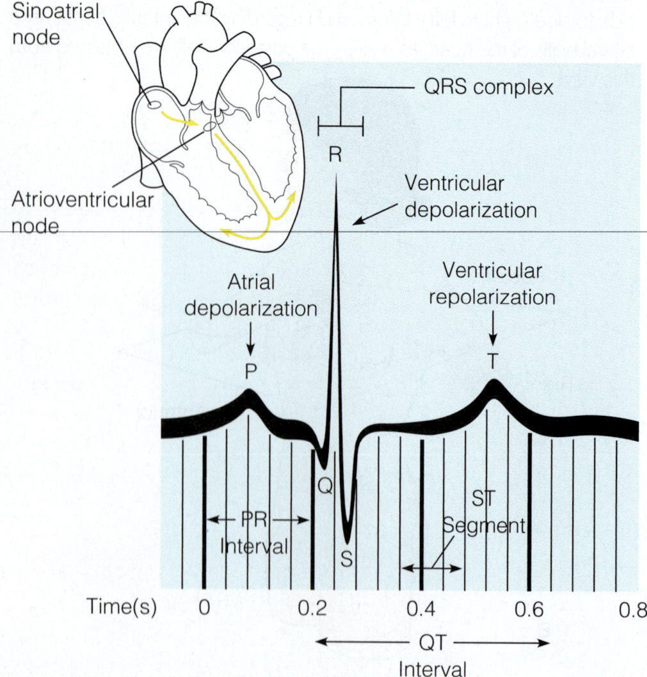

Figure 22–29 ■ Normal ECG waveform and intervals.

Box 22–6 **Interpreting an Electrocardiogram**

Interpreting an electrocardiogram (ECG) strip to determine the cardiac rhythm is a skill that takes practice to learn and master. Many methods are used to analyze ECGs, and it is important to use a consistent method for such analysis. Identifying and interpreting complex dysrhythmias requires advanced skills and knowledge obtained through further training. One method for analyzing an ECG strip is the following:

- *Step 1: Determine rate.* Assess heart rate. Use P waves to determine the atrial rate and R waves for the ventricular rate. Several approaches can determine the heart rate:
  a. Count the number of complexes in a 6-second rhythm strip (the top margin of ECG paper is marked at 3-second intervals), and multiply by 10. This provides an estimate of the rate and is particularly valuable if rhythms are irregular.
  b. Count the number of large boxes between two consecutive complexes, and divide 300 (the number of large boxes in 1 min) by this number. For example, there are 6 large boxes between two R waves; 300 divided by 6 equals a ventricular rate of 50 bpm. Memorize the following sequence for rapid rate determination: 300, 150, 100, 75, 60, 50, 43. One large box between complexes equals a rate of 300; two large boxes, a rate of 150; three, a rate of 100; and so on.
  c. Count the number of small boxes between two consecutive complexes, and divide 1,500 (the number of small boxes in 1 min) by this number. For example, there are 19 small boxes between two R waves; 1,500 divided by 19 equals a ventricular rate of 79 bpm. This is the most precise measurement of heart rate.
- *Step 2: Determine regularity.* Regularity is the consistency with which the P waves or QRS complexes occur. In a regular rhythm, all waves occur at a consistent rate. Rhythm regularity is determined by measuring the interval between consecutive waves. Place one point of an ECG caliper (a measuring device) on the peak of the P wave (for atrial rhythm) or the R wave (for ventricular rhythm). Adjust the other point to the peak of the next wave, P to P or R to R (Figure 22–30 ■). Keeping the calipers set at this distance, evaluate the intervals between consecutive waves. The rhythm is regular if all caliper points fall on succeeding wave peaks. Alternately, use a strip of blank paper on top of the ECG strip, and mark the peaks of two or three consecutive waves. Then, move the paper along the strip to consecutive waves. Wave peaks that vary by more than one to three small boxes (depending on the rate) are irregular. Irregular rhythms may be irregularly irregular (if the intervals have no pattern) or regularly irregular (if a consistent pattern to the irregularity can be identified).
- *Step 3: Assess P waves.* The presence or absence of P waves helps determine the origin of the rhythm. All the P waves should be alike in size and shape (morphology). If P waves are not seen or if they differ in shape, the rhythm may not originate in the sinoatrial node.

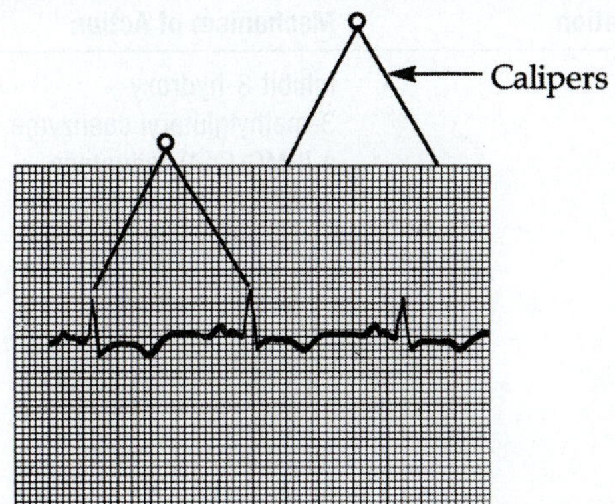

Figure 22–30 ■ Using calipers to evaluate intervals between consecutive waves.

- *Step 4: Assess the P to QRS relationship.* Determine the relationship between P waves and QRS complexes. There should be one—and only one—P wave for every QRS complex, because the normal stimulus for ventricular contraction originates in the sinoatrial node.
- *Step 5: Determine interval durations.* To evaluate impulse transmission through the cardiac conduction system, measure the PR interval, QRS duration, and QT interval. To measure, count the number of small boxes from the beginning of the interval to the end, and multiply by 0.04 second. Then, determine whether the interval duration is within its normal limits. For example, assume the PR interval is 3.5 small boxes wide, or 0.14 second. This is within the normal limits of 0.12–0.20 second. This interval should be consistent, not varying from beat to beat. A PR interval of greater than 0.20 second or one that varies from beat to beat is abnormal.

  The QRS complex duration is normally between 0.06 and 0.10 second. A QRS complex of greater than 0.12 second indicates delayed ventricular conduction.

  The QT interval is normally 0.32–0.44 second. It varies inversely with the heart rate: The faster the heart rate, the shorter the QT interval. As a general rule, the QT interval should be no more than half the previous R–R interval. A prolonged QT interval indicates a prolonged relative refractory period of the heart.
- *Step 6: Identify abnormalities.* Note the presence and frequency of **ectopic** (extra) beats, deviation of the ST segment above or below the baseline, and abnormalities in waveform shape and duration.

- Measuring for and application of elastic compression stockings
- Fetal monitoring
- Applying sequential compression devices
- Applying continuous cardiorespiratory monitoring
- Obtaining capillary wedge pressures
- Measuring cardiac output
- Reading central and peripheral blood pressures
- Caring for the client with arterial pressure monitor.

PHARMACOLOGIC THERAPIES

Many of the medications administered by nurses have an impact on perfusion. Beta blockers, antihypertensives, cardiac glycosides and even some narcotics, like morphine sulfate, have profound impact on cardiac functioning and perfusion. The Medications box on the next page describes some of the more commonly prescribed medications.

MEDICATIONS Perfusion

Classification	Mechanism of Action	Generic Drug	Nursing Considerations
Statins	Inhibit 3-hydroxy-3-methylglutaryl coenzyme, a (HMG-CoA) reductase, which results in less cholesterol biosynthesis.	atorvastatin, fluvastatin, lovastatin, pravastatin	■ Assess triglyceride, total cholesterol, low-density lipoprotein, and high-density lipoprotein levels. ■ Avoid in clients who are or may become pregnant or are nursing. ■ Monitor liver function tests. ■ Avoid in clients with liver disease or heavy alcohol consumption. ■ Teach client to avoid alcohol while taking. ■ Assess for muscle pain, tenderness, or weakness.
Antihypertensives			
Diuretics	Reduce fluid volume in the vessels.	furosemide, hydrochlorothiazide, bumetanide, triamterene, spironolactone, metolazone	■ Monitor serum electrolyte levels. ■ Obtain client's weight daily. ■ Teach client importance of compliance with the medication regimen. ■ Assess hydration status. ■ Monitor breath sounds for fluid volume excess.
Angiotensin-converting enzyme (ACE) inhibitors and angiotensin II receptor blockers	Angiotensin II is a potent natural vasoconstrictor; its actions are blocked by ACE inhibitors and angiotensin inhibitors.	benazepril, captopril, lisinopril, losartan, valsartan	■ Follow vital sign changes. ■ First dose may cause severe hypotension, so monitor blood pressure (BP) carefully. ■ It's best to administer first dose at bedtime. ■ Monitor BP carefully if given intravenously (IV), and with subsequent alteration in level of consciousness if this occurs. ■ Assess for angioedema, which can be life-threatening. ■ Monitor complete blood count for neutropenia or agranulocytosis.
Combination drugs	These contain a diuretic, usually a potassium-sparing diuretic, and another class of drugs, such as adrenergic agents or ACE inhibitors.	Combines hydrochlorothiazide with propranolol, metoprolol, timolol, or bisoprolol	■ Monitor serum electrolyte levels. ■ Obtain client's weight daily. ■ Teach client importance of compliance with the medication regimen. ■ Assess hydration status. ■ Monitor breath sounds for fluid volume excess.
Vasodilators	These cause dilation of blood vessels.	diazoxide, hydralazine, minoxidil, nitroprusside	■ These may produce reflex tachycardia. ■ These may produce angina in clients with coronary artery disease. ■ Monitor for sodium and water retention. ■ IV nitroprusside is the drug of choice for treating hypertensive emergency, but care must be taken not to drop BP too quickly. Metabolizes to cyanide, so careful monitoring is required.

MEDICATIONS **Perfusion** (continued)

Classification	Mechanism of Action	Generic Drug	Nursing Considerations
Adrenergic antagonists	These reduce autonomic nervous system effects by blocking $beta_1$-adrenergic receptor sites in the heart, blocking $alpha_1$-adrenergic receptors in arterioles, stimulating $alpha_2$ receptors in the brainstem, and/or blocking peripheral adrenergic neurons.	Beta blockers: atenolol, bisoprolol, metoprolol $Alpha_1$ antagonists: doxazosin, prazosin, terazosin $Alpha_2$ agonists: clonidine, guanabenz, methyldopa $Alpha_1$ and beta blockers: carteolol, labetalol Adrenergic neuron blockers: guanadrel, guanethidine, reserpine	■ Monitor vital signs. ■ Hold medication if heart rate is <60 bpm or if BP is <90/60 mmHg. ■ Use care when ambulating, monitoring for potential orthostatic hypotension. ■ Monitor clients with diabetes for hypoglycemia.
Calcium-channel blockers	Treats angina, dysrhythmias, and hypertension, reducing available calcium, muscular contractility, peripheral vascular resistance and BP.	nifedipine, verapamil, diltiazem, nicardipine	■ Obtain baseline electrocardiogram, heart rate, and BP before beginning therapy. ■ Teach client to maintain a daily BP log and about the need for compliance with the medication regimen. ■ Contraindicated in clients with third-degree block of sick sinus syndrome. ■ Monitor for tachycardia and hypotension if administered IV. ■ Teach client to avoid grapefruit juice.
Cardiac glycosides	Causes the heart to beat more forcefully and more slowly, improving cardiac output (positive inotropic affect).	digoxin	■ Monitor serum potassium. ■ Administer with caution to older adults and to those post-myocardial infarction or with incomplete heart block or renal insufficiency. ■ Side effects such as drowsiness, fatigue, dizziness, visual disturbances, anorexia, nausea, or vomiting may indicate toxic levels. ■ Follow serum drug levels in order to maintain therapeutic levels.
Phosphodiesterase inhibitors	Block the enzyme phosphodiesterase in cardiac and smooth muscle, increasing the amount of calcium available for myocardial contraction, which results in positive inotropic actions and vasodilation.	milrinone	■ Assess serum potassium levels. ■ Monitor for dysrhythmia. ■ During IV administration, monitor for ventricular dysrhythmias.
Nitrates	Potent vasodilators that dilate both arterial and venous smooth muscle. Dilation of veins reduces preload.	amyl nitrite, isosorbide dinitrate, nitroglycerine	■ Monitor BP frequently for hypotension. ■ To prevent falls and lessen dizziness, as well as to reduce the oxygen demands on the heart, have client lie down when taking this medication for chest pain. ■ Teach client how to take medication when having chest pain and how often it may be repeated before calling 911. ■ Contraindicated in clients with cardiac tamponade and pericarditis or clients with head injury, shock, and increased intracranial pressure. ■ Teach client to avoid alcohol consumption, which can lead to severe hypotension and cardiovascular collapse.

(continued)

MEDICATIONS **Perfusion** (continued)

Classification	Mechanism of Action	Generic Drug	Nursing Considerations
Thrombolytics	Administered to dissolve clots resulting in myocardial infarction or stroke, with quick restoration of circulation.	reteplase, tissue plasminogen activator (t-PA), alteplase, tenecteplase, anistreplase, streptokinase, urokinase	■ Must be administered within 12 hours of symptom onset; best if given within 4 hours. ■ Research suggests clients older than 75 years do not experience reduced mortality from these drugs. ■ Monitor clients carefully for bleeding, because all clots, even those formed as the result of venipuncture, are dissolved. ■ In clients who may be receiving thrombolytics, attempt to minimize invasive procedures in order to avoid future bleeding sites. ■ Do not administer to clients who have recently (within the past 2 weeks) fallen, been involved in an motor-vehicle accident, or experienced any form of trauma. ■ Closely monitor cardiac rhythm, because return of perfusion to the blocked vessel often results in reperfusion arrhythmias that may include ventricular tachycardia.

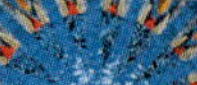

22.1 CARDIOMYOPATHY

KEY TERMS

Cardiomyopathy, *1332*
Dilated cardiomyopathy, *1333*
Hypertrophic cardiomyopathy, *1333*
Mural thrombi, *1334*
Peripartum cardiomyopathy, *1334*
Restrictive cardiomyopathy, *1333*
Syncope, *1334*

BASIS FOR SELECTION OF EXEMPLAR

Centers for Disease Control and Prevention
Institute of Medicine
Leading cause of death

LEARNING OUTCOMES

After reading about this exemplar, you will be able to:

1. Describe the pathophysiology, etiology, clinical manifestations, and direct and indirect causes of cardiomyopathy.
2. Identify risk factors associated with cardiomyopathy.
3. Illustrate the nursing process in providing culturally competent care across the life span for individuals with cardiomyopathy.
4. Formulate priority nursing diagnoses appropriate for an individual with cardiomyopathy.
5. Create a plan of care for individuals with cardiomyopathy and their family members.
6. Asses expected outcomes for an individual with cardiomyopathy.
7. Discuss therapies used in the collaborative care of an individual with cardiomyopathy.
8. Employ evidence-based caring interventions for an individual with cardiomyopathy.

OVERVIEW

The term **cardiomyopathy** describes a diverse group of disorders that affect both systolic and diastolic functions. Cardiomyopathies, which may be either primary or secondary in origin, affect the heart muscle itself. Primary cardiomyopathies are idiopathic: Their cause is unknown. Secondary cardiomyopathies occur as a result of other processes, such as ischemia, infectious disease, exposure to toxins, connective tissue disorders, metabolic disorders, or nutritional deficiencies. Close to 27,000 deaths annually are directly attributed to cardiomyopathy. Mortality associated with cardiomyopathy is higher in older adults, men, and African Americans (American Heart Association [AHA], 2005).

PATHOPHYSIOLOGY AND ETIOLOGY

Cardiomyopathies are categorized by their pathophysiology and presentation into three groups: dilated, hypertrophic, and restrictive. Table 22–10 compares the causes, pathophysiology, manifestations, and management of the cardiomyopathies.

TABLE 22–10 **Classifications of Cardiomyopathy**

	DILATED	HYPERTROPHIC	RESTRICTIVE
Causes	Usually idiopathic; may be secondary to chronic alcoholism or myocarditis	Hereditary; may be secondary to chronic hypertension	Usually secondary to amyloidosis, radiation, or myocardial fibrosis
Pathophysiology	Scarring and atrophy of myocardial cells Thickening of ventricular wall Dilation of heart chambers Impaired ventricular pumping Increased end-diastolic and end-systolic volumes Mural thrombi common	Hypertrophy of ventricular muscle mass Small left ventricular volume Septal hypertrophy may obstruct left ventricular outflow Left atrial dilation	Excess rigidity of ventricular walls restricts filling Myocardial contractility remains relatively normal
Manifestations	Heart failure Cardiomegaly Dysrhythmias S_3 and S_4 gallop; murmur of mitral regurgitation Dyspnea, anginal pain, syncope	Left ventricular hypertrophy Dysrhythmias Loud S_4 Sudden death	Dyspnea, fatigue Right-sided heart failure Mild to moderate cardiomegaly S_3 and S_4 Mitral regurgitation murmur
Management	Management of heart failure Implantable cardioverter–defibrillator (ICD) as needed Cardiac transplantation	Beta-blockers Antidysrhythmic agents Calcium-channel blockers ICD, dual-chamber pacing Surgical excision of part of the ventricular septum	Management of heart failure Exercise restriction

Dilated Cardiomyopathy

Dilated cardiomyopathy is the most common type of cardiomyopathy, accounting for 87% of cases (AHA, 2005). Dilated cardiomyopathy also is a common cause of heart failure, accounting for approximately one in three cases. It is primarily a disease of middle-aged males; African American males have a higher risk than whites (Kasper et al., 2005).

In dilated cardiomyopathy, heart chambers dilate and ventricular contraction is impaired. Both end-diastolic and end-systolic volumes increase, and the left ventricular ejection fraction is substantially reduced, decreasing cardiac output. Left ventricular dilation is prominent; left ventricular hypertrophy is usually minimal. The right ventricle also may be enlarged. Extensive interstitial fibrosis (scarring) is evident, and necrotic myocardial cells may be seen (Kasper et al., 2005).

The prognosis for dilated cardiomyopathy is grim. Most clients get progressively worse. Fifty percent die within 5 years after the diagnosis, and 75% die within 10 years (AHA, 2005).

Hypertrophic Cardiomyopathy

Hypertrophic cardiomyopathy is characterized by decreased compliance of the left ventricle and hypertrophy of the ventricular muscle mass. This impairs ventricular filling, leading to small end-diastolic volumes and low cardiac output.

The pattern of left ventricular hypertrophy is unique in that the muscle may not hypertrophy equally. In a majority of clients, the interventricular septal mass, especially the upper portion, increases to a greater extent than the free wall of the ventricle. The enlarged upper septum narrows the passageway of blood into the aorta, impairing ventricular outflow. For this reason, this disorder is also known as idiopathic hypertrophic subaortic stenosis or hypertrophic obstructive cardiomyopathy.

Restrictive Cardiomyopathy

The least common form of cardiomyopathy, **restrictive cardiomyopathy**, is characterized by rigid ventricular walls that impair diastolic filling. Decreased ventricular compliance impairs filling, with decreased ventricular size, elevated end-diastolic pressures, and decreased cardiac output. Contractility is unaffected, and the ejection fraction is normal.

Peripartum Cardiomyopathy

Peripartum cardiomyopathy is a relatively rare but serious dysfunction of the left ventricle that may occur in the last month of pregnancy or the first 5 months postpartum in a woman with no previous history of heart disease. Subsequent pregnancy is strongly discouraged, because the disease tends to recur. The mortality rate is as high as 18–56% (Klein & Galan, 2004).

Etiology

The cause of dilated cardiomyopathy is unknown, although it appears to result frequently from toxins, metabolic conditions, or infection. Reversible dilated cardiomyopathy may develop as a result of alcohol and cocaine abuse, chemotherapeutic drugs, pregnancy, and systemic hypertension. Up to 20% of cases of dilated cardiomyopathy may be genetic in origin, most commonly transmitted in an autosomal dominant pattern, although autosomal recessive, X-linked, and mitochondrial patterns of inheritance also are evident (Kasper et al., 2005; Porth, 2005).

Causes of restrictive cardiomyopathy include myocardial fibrosis and infiltrative processes, such as amyloidosis. Fibrosis of the myocardium and endocardium causes excessive stiffness and rigidity of the ventricles.

The cause of peripartum cardiomyopathy is unknown, but hypertrophic cardiomyopathy results from autosomal dominant transmission and is caused by mutations in any one of 10 genes (Maron, 2004). About half of all clients with hypertrophic cardiomyopathy have a family history of the disease.

Risk Factors

Clients with hypertension, excessive alcohol consumption, and valvular heart disease are at increased risk for developing a cardiomyopathy. However, many forms of cardiomyopathy are idiopathic, with no known cause or risk factors, and often result in death, because there is no known treatment other than supportive care.

CLINICAL MANIFESTATIONS

Each form of cardiomyopathy has subtle differences in symptoms. Manifestations of *dilated cardiomyopathy* develop gradually. Heart failure often presents years after the onset of dilation and pump failure. Both right- and left-sided failure occur, with dyspnea on exertion, orthopnea, paroxysmal nocturnal dyspnea, weakness, fatigue, peripheral edema, and ascites. Both S_3 and S_4 are commonly heard, as well as an AV regurgitation murmur. Dysrhythmias are common, including supraventricular tachycardias, atrial fibrillation, and complex ventricular tachycardias. Untreated dysrhythmias can lead to sudden death (Porth, 2005). **Mural thrombi** (blood clots in the heart wall) may form in the left ventricular apex and embolize to other parts of the body.

Hypertrophic cardiomyopathy may be asymptomatic for many years. Symptoms typically occur when increased oxygen demand causes increased ventricular contractility; they may develop suddenly during or after physical activity. In children and young adults, sudden cardiac death may be the first sign of the disorder. Hypertrophic cardiomyopathy is the probable or definite cause of death in 36% of young athletes who die suddenly (AHA, 2005). It is hypothesized that sudden cardiac death is the result of ventricular dysrhythmias or hemodynamic factors. Predictors of sudden cardiac death in clients with hypertrophic cardiomyopathy include family history of sudden death, age of less than 30 years, syncopal episodes, severe ventricular hypertrophy, and ventricular tachycardia seen on ambulatory ECG monitoring (Kasper et al., 2005).

The usual manifestations of hypertrophic cardiomyopathy are dyspnea, angina, and syncope. Angina may result from ischemia caused by overgrowth of the ventricular muscle, coronary artery abnormalities, or decreased coronary artery perfusion. **Syncope** (transient loss of consciousness and muscle tone after exercise or activity) may occur when the outflow tract obstruction severely decreases cardiac output and blood flow to the brain. Ventricular dysrhythmias are common; atrial fibrillation also may develop. Other manifestations of hypertrophic cardiomyopathy include fatigue, dizziness, and palpitations. A harsh, crescendo–decrescendo systolic murmur of variable intensity, heard best at the lower left sternal border and apex, is characteristic in hypertrophic cardiomyopathy. S_4 may also be noted on auscultation.

The manifestations of *restrictive cardiomyopathy* are those of heart failure and decreased tissue perfusion. Dyspnea on exertion and exercise intolerance are common. Jugular venous pressure is elevated, and S_3 and S_4 are common. The prognosis for restrictive cardiomyopathy is poor. Most clients die within 3 years, and the systemic nature of the underlying disease process precludes effective treatment.

Peripartum cardiomyopathy is a condition usually presents with anemia and infection. Consequently, treatment focuses on underlying abnormalities. Peripartum cardiomyopathy may resolve with bedrest as the heart gradually returns to normal size.

COLLABORATION

With the exception of therapy for an underlying cause, little can be done to treat either dilated or restrictive cardiomyopathies. For these disorders, treatment focuses on managing heart failure and treating dysrhythmias. Treatment of hypertrophic cardiomyopathy focuses on reducing contractility and preventing sudden cardiac death. Strenuous physical exertion is restricted, because it may precipitate dysrhythmias or sudden cardiac death. Dietary and sodium restrictions may help diminish the manifestations. Peripartum cardiomyopathy may resolve with bedrest as the heart gradually returns to normal size.

CLINICAL MANIFESTATIONS AND THERAPIES **Cardiomyoparthy**

ETIOLOGY	CLINICAL MANIFESTATION	CLINICAL THERAPIES
Heart failure (both left and right sided) often develops as the result of reduced cardiac output.	Dyspnea on exertion, orthopnea, paroxysmal nocturnal dyspnea, weakness, fatigue, peripheral edema, and ascites	■ Treatment of underlying cause ■ Medications to include diuretics, vasodilators, beta-blockers, and calcium-channel blockers ■ Monitor client's weight daily and client's intake and output ■ Elastic stockings to improve venous return ■ Abdominocentesis to reduce ascites ■ Sleeping in semi-Fowler's position ■ Periods of activity followed by periods of rest
Dysrhythmias are common because of dilation of the heart muscle that damages conduction pathways and leads to the formation of alternate paths.	Electrocardiogram may show supraventricular tachycardias, atrial fibrillation, and complex ventricular tachycardias	■ Treatment of underlying cause ■ Medications to include antiarrhythmics, nitrates, and beta-blockers ■ May potentially require implanted cardiac defibrillator ■ Client teaching regarding awareness of pulse rate and rhythm and when to interact with health care team
Mural thrombi (blood clots in the heart wall) may form in the left ventricular apex and embolize to other parts of the body.	Manifestations depend on where the clot lodges and may result in deep venous thrombosis, pulmonary emboli, myocardial infarction, or stroke	■ Treatment of underlying cause ■ Medications to include anticoagulants or thrombolytics if clot lodges in coronary arteries or brain
Angina may result from ischemia caused by overgrowth of the ventricular muscle, coronary artery abnormalities, or decreased coronary artery perfusion.	Chest pain radiating to the jaw, back, or left arm; shortness of breath; activity intolerance; intermittent claudication; and nausea or vomiting	■ Treatment of underlying cause ■ Medications to include nitrates and beta-blockers ■ Client teaching regarding how to respond to symptoms and when to call 911 ■ Surgery may be required to repair damaged coronary arteries
Syncope may occur when the outflow tract obstruction severely decreases cardiac output and blood flow to the brain.	Dizziness, light-headedness, fainting (sudden loss of consciousness), and nausea	■ Treatment of underlying cause ■ Medications to include beta-blockers ■ Teach client the importance of sitting down as soon as symptoms start in order to prevent injuries from falls

Diagnostic Tests

Diagnosis begins with a history and physical assessment to rule out known causes of heart failure. Other tests may include the following:

- Echocardiography
- Electrocardiography and ambulatory ECG monitoring
- Chest x-ray
- Hemodynamic studies
- Radionuclear scans
- Cardiac catheterization and coronary angiography
- Myocardial biopsy.

Pharmacologic Therapies

The same drug regimen used to treat heart failure is used for dilated or restrictive cardiomyopathy. This includes angiotensin-converting enzyme inhibitors, vasodilators, and digitalis. Beta-blockers also may be used with caution in clients who have dilated cardiomyopathy. Anticoagulants are given to reduce the risk of thrombus formation and embolization. Antidysrhythmic drugs are avoided if possible because of their tendency to precipitate further dysrhythmias (Kasper et al., 2005).

Beta-blockers are the drugs of choice to reduce anginal symptoms and syncopal episodes associated with hypertrophic cardiomyopathy. The negative inotropic effects of beta-blockers and calcium-channel blockers decrease the myocardial contractility, thus decreasing obstruction of the outflow tract. Beta-blockers also decrease heart rate and increase ventricular compliance, thus increasing diastolic filling time and cardiac output. Vasodilators, digitalis, nitrates, and diuretics are contraindicated. Amiodarone may be used to treat ventricular dysrhythmias (Kasper et al., 2005).

Surgery

Without definitive treatment, clients with cardiomyopathy develop end-stage heart failure. Cardiac transplant is the definitive treatment for dilated cardiomyopathy. Ventricular assist devices may be used to support cardiac output until a donor heart is available. Transplantation is not a viable option for restrictive cardiomyopathy, however. Transplantation does not eliminate the underlying process causing infiltration or fibrosis, and eventually, the transplanted organ is affected as well. (See Exemplar 22.6, Heart Failure, for more information about cardiac transplantation.)

In severely symptomatic clients with obstructive hypertrophic cardiomyopathy, excess muscle may be surgically resected from the aortic valve outflow tract. The septum is incised, and tissue is removed. This procedure provides lasting improvement in approximately 75% of clients (Kasper et al., 2005).

An implantable cardioverter–defibrillator often is inserted to treat potentially lethal dysrhythmias, reducing the need for antidysrhythmic medications. A dual-chamber pacemaker also may be used to treat hypertrophic cardiomyopathy.

NURSING PROCESS

Nursing assessment and care for clients with dilated or restrictive cardiomyopathy are similar to those for clients with heart failure. Teaching about the disease process and its management is vital. Some degree of activity restriction often is necessary; assist the client to conserve energy while encouraging self-care. Support coping skills and adaptation to required lifestyle changes. Provide information and support for decision making about cardiac transplantation if that is an option. Discuss the toxic and vasodilator effects of alcohol, and encourage abstinence.

The client with hypertrophic cardiomyopathy requires care similar to that provided for the client with myocardial ischemia; nitrates and other vasodilators, however, are avoided. If surgery is performed, nursing care is similar to that for any client undergoing open-heart surgery or cardiac transplant. Discuss the genetic transmission of hypertrophic cardiomyopathy, and suggest screening of close relatives (parents and siblings).

Provide pre- and postoperative care and teaching as appropriate for clients undergoing invasive procedures or surgery for cardiomyopathy.

Assessment

Obtain both subjective and objective data when assessing the client with cardiomyopathy:

- *Health history.* Complaints of increasing shortness of breath, dyspnea with exertion, decreasing activity tolerance, or paroxysmal nocturnal dyspnea; number of pillows used for sleeping; recent weight gain; presence of a cough; chest or abdominal pain; anorexia or nausea; history of cardiac disease, previous episodes of heart failure; other risk factors, such as hypertension or diabetes; current medications; and usual diet and activity, as well as any recent changes.
- *Physical examination.* General appearance; ease of breathing, conversing, changing positions; apparent anxiety; vital signs, including apical pulse; color of skin and mucous membranes; neck vein distention, peripheral pulses, capillary refill, presence and degree of edema; heart and breath sounds; abdominal contour, bowel sounds, tenderness; right upper abdominal tenderness, and liver enlargement.

Diagnosis

Nursing diagnoses that may be appropriate for clients with cardiomyopathy include the following:

- Decreased Cardiac Output related to impaired left ventricular filling, contractility, or outflow obstruction
- Fatigue related to decreased cardiac output
- Excess Fluid Volume related to compensatory mechanisms
- Activity Intolerance related to decreasing cardiac function
- Deficient Knowledge related to the importance of a low-sodium diet
- Anticipatory Grieving related to poor prognosis.

Plan

Goals of care will be determined based on the type and severity of cardiomyopathy as well as on the individual needs of the client. These goals may include the following:

- The client will maintain blood pressure within specified limits.
- The client will alter his or her lifestyle to demonstrate adjustment to alterations in activity level caused by the disease process.
- The client will modify his or her diet to support long-term management of the condition.

Implementation

When providing care for the client with alterations in perfusion, it is important to monitor for subtle changes in vital signs and other signs and symptoms. Alterations in peripheral capillary refill time, pulse rate or volume, and level of consciousness may be early warning signs of reduced perfusion.

Decreased Cardiac Output

As the heart fails as a pump, stroke volume and tissue perfusion decrease.

- Monitor vital signs and oxygen saturation as indicated. Decreased cardiac output stimulates the sympathetic nervous system to increase the heart rate in an attempt to restore cardiac output. Tachycardia at rest is common. Diastolic blood pressure may initially be elevated because of vasoconstriction. In late stages, however, compensatory mechanisms fail, and blood pressure falls. Oxygen saturation levels provide a measure of gas exchange and tissue perfusion.
- Monitor BNP (B-type natriuretic peptide) levels, and report trends. BNP levels indicate the severity of heart failure: As the cardiac index decreases and left ventricular pressures increase, BNP levels increase. Noting trends provides additional information about cardiac output and effectiveness of the cardiac pump.
- Auscultate heart and breath sounds regularly. S_1 and S_2 may be diminished if cardiac function is poor. A ventricular gallop (S_3) is an early sign of heart failure; an atrial gallop (S_4) may also be present. Crackles are often heard in the lung bases; increasing crackles, dyspnea, and shortness of breath indicate worsening failure.
- Administer supplemental oxygen as needed. This improves oxygenation of the blood, decreasing the effects of hypoxia and ischemia.
- Administer prescribed medications as ordered. Drugs are used to decrease the cardiac workload and increase the effectiveness of contractions.
- Encourage rest, and explain the rationale. Elevate the head of the bed to reduce the work of breathing. Provide a bedside commode, and assist with activities of daily living (ADLs). Instruct the client to avoid the Valsalva maneuver. These measures reduce cardiac workload.

Excess Fluid Volume

As cardiac output falls, compensatory mechanisms cause salt and water retention, increasing blood volume. This increased fluid volume places additional stress on the already failing ventricles, making them work harder to move the fluid load.

- Assess respiratory status and auscultate lung sounds at least every 4 hours. Notify the physician of significant changes in condition. Declining respiratory status indicates worsening left heart failure.
- Monitor intake and output. Notify the physician if urine output is less than 30 mL/hr. Weigh the client daily. Careful monitoring of fluid volume is important during treatment of heart failure. Diuretics may reduce circulating volume, producing hypovolemia despite persistent peripheral edema. A fall in urine output may indicate significantly reduced cardiac output and renal ischemia. Weight is an objective measure of fluid status: 1 L of fluid is equal to 2.2 lb of weight.
- Record abdominal girth every shift. Note complaints of a loss of appetite, abdominal discomfort, or nausea. Venous congestion can lead to ascites and may affect gastrointestinal function and nutritional status.
- Monitor and record hemodynamic measurements. Report significant changes and negative trends. Hemodynamic measurements provide a means of monitoring condition and response to treatment.
- Restrict fluids as ordered. Allow choices of fluid type and timing of intake, scheduling most fluid intake during morning and afternoon hours. Offer ice chips and frequent mouth care; provide hard candies if allowed. Providing choices increases the client's sense of control. Ice chips, hard candies, and mouth care relieve dry mouth and thirst and promote comfort.

Activity Intolerance

Clients with heart failure have little or no cardiac reserve to meet increased oxygen demands. As the disease progresses and cardiac function is further compromised, activity intolerance increases. The low cardiac output and inability to participate in activities may hinder self-care.

- Organize nursing care to allow rest periods. Grouping care activities together allows adequate time to "recharge."
- Assist with ADLs as needed. Encourage independence within prescribed limits. Assisting with ADLs helps ensure that care needs are met while reducing cardiac workload. Involving the client promotes a sense of control and reduces a sense of helplessness.
- Plan and implement progressive activities. Use passive and active range-of-motion (ROM) exercises as appropriate. Consult with a physical therapist on an activity plan. Progressive activity slowly increases exercise capacity by strengthening and improving cardiac function without strain. Activity also helps prevent skeletal muscle atrophy. ROM exercises prevent complications of immobility in severely compromised clients.

CLIENT TEACHING **Cardiomyopathy**

Cardiomyopathies are chronic, progressive disorders generally managed in home and community care settings unless surgery or transplant is planned or end-stage heart failure develops. When teaching the client and family about home care, include the following topics:

- Activity restrictions and dietary changes to reduce manifestations and prevent complications
- The prescribed drug regimen, its rationale, and its intended and possible adverse effects
- The disease process, its expected ultimate outcome, and treatment options
- Cardiac transplantation, including the procedure, the need for lifetime immunosuppression to prevent transplant rejection, and the risks of postoperative infection and long-term immunosuppression
- Symptoms to report to the physician or for which immediate care is needed
- Cardiopulmonary resuscitation procedures and available training sites.

Refer the client and family for home and social services and counseling as indicated. Provide community resources such as support groups or the AHA.

- Provide written and verbal information about activity after discharge. Written information provides a reference for important information. Verbal information allows clarification and validation of the material.

Deficient Knowledge: Low-Sodium Diet

Diet is an important part of long-term management of heart failure. It also contributes to reducing fluid retention.

- Discuss the rationale for sodium restrictions. Understanding fosters compliance with the prescribed diet.
- Consult with dietitian to plan and teach a low-sodium and, if necessary for weight control, low-kilocalorie diet. Provide a list of high-sodium, high-fat, high-cholesterol foods to avoid. Provide AHA materials. Dietary planning and teaching increase the client's sense of control and participation in disease management. Food lists are useful memory aids.

Evaluation

The effectiveness of nursing care, and changes in client needs based on response to nursing care and collaborative treatment, will be evaluated in light of the nursing diagnosis and may include the following expected outcomes:

- The client will list symptoms to report to provider immediately upon noting.
- The client will maintain blood pressure within acceptable range to demonstrate adequate tissue perfusion.
- The client suggests strategies for maintaining as normal a lifestyle as possible within the requirements of activity intolerance.
- The client articulates a change to a low-sodium diet.

REVIEW Cardiomyopathy

RELATE: LINK THE CONCEPTS

Linking the exemplar of Cardiomyopathy with the concept of Oxygenation:

1. What physical assessment findings related to oxygenation would you anticipate for the client with cardiomyopathy?
2. What are your priorities of care for the client with cardiomyopathy who comes to the emergency department with dyspnea?

Linking the exemplar of Cardiomyopathy with the concept of Comfort:

3. The client with cardiomyopathy reports fatigue that is interfering with ADLs. What strategies might you recommend to help this client improve independence in performing ADLs?
4. What techniques will you teach the client with cardiomyopathy to improve sleep and rest in the home setting?

READY: GO TO COMPANION SKILLS MANUAL

- Monitor intake and output
- Oxygen saturation (using a pulse oximeter)
- Using digital pressure
- Assessing the heart and central vessels
- Assessing an apical-radial pulse
- Assessing an apical pulse
- Assessing peripheral pulses
- Assessing respirations
- Assessing blood pressure
- Assessing pulse oximeter
- Measuring abdominal girth
- Assessing the heart rate
- Assessing the respiratory rate

REFER: GO TO MYNURSINGKIT

REFLECT: CASE STUDY

Deshawn Milby is a 28-year-old African-American male who plays professional basketball. He is 6 feet 2 inches tall and weighs 180 pounds. Deshawn's wife, Sylvia, owns a popular local restaurant. Sylvia and Deshawn have a 2-year-old son, Pete. Deshawn is away much of the winter when the team plays out of town. Deshawn and Sylvia's families live in town and often help with child care.

Deshawn's father died suddenly while running track at the age of 30. He was diagnosed on autopsy with hypertrophic cardiomyopathy. Deshawn's mother is alive and healthy and helps Sylvia at the restaurant as well as caring for Pete when needed. Deshawn's younger sister May is away at college.

Deshawn has had occasional twinges of chest pain when practicing basketball and has decided to see a family physician for a full physical.

1. What factors in Deshawn's history put him at risk for cardiomyopathy?
2. What assessment data will you gather when examining Deshawn?
3. How will you respond to Deshawn when he tells you that he is afraid that he will die the same way his father did?

22.2 CONGENITAL HEART DEFECTS

KEY TERMS

Aortic stenosis, *1347*
Atrial septal defect (ASD), *1340*
Atrioventricular (AV) canal, *1341*
Coarctation of the aorta, *1347*
Congenital heart defect, *1339*
Endocardial cushions, *1341*
Heaving, *1356*
Holosystolic, *1342*
Hypercyanotic episode, *1342*
Hypoplastic left heart syndrome, *1348*
Palliative procedure, *1351*
Patent ductus arteriosus, *1339*
Preload, *1343*

Pulmonary atresia, *1344*
Septal defect, *1339*
Shunt, *1349*
Stenosis, *1343*
Syncope, *1350*
Tetralogy of Fallot, *1342*
Total anomalous pulmonary venous return, *1346*
Transposition of the great arteries (TGA), *1345*
Tricuspid atresia, *1344*
Truncus arteriosus, *1345*
Ventricular septal defect (VSD), *1341*

BASIS FOR SELECTION OF EXEMPLAR

American Academy of Pediatrics
Centers for Disease Control and Prevention

LEARNING OUTCOMES

After reading about this exemplar, you will be able to:

1. Describe the pathophysiology, etiology, clinical manifestations, and direct and indirect causes of congenital heart defects.
2. Identify risk factors associated with congenital heart defects.
3. Illustrate the nursing process in providing culturally competent care across the life span for individuals with congenital heart defects.
4. Formulate priority nursing diagnoses appropriate for an individual with congenital heart defects.
5. Create a plan of care for individuals with congenital heart defects and their families.
6. Assess expected outcomes for an individual with congenital heart defects.
7. Discuss therapies used in the collaborative care of an individual with congenital heart defects.
8. Employ evidence-based caring interventions for an individual with congenital heart defects.

OVERVIEW

The term **congenital heart defect** refers to a defect in the heart or great vessels that results from an alteration in normal fetal development or persistence of a fetal structure that does not convert to extrauterine anatomy after birth. Congenital heart defects occur in an estimated 1% of all pregnancies and one in every 170 live births (Neilson & Robin, 2002). More than 35 types of heart defects have been documented. Deaths from heart defects have declined dramatically over the past 50 years, and now approximately 85% of newborns with congenital heart disease are expected to survive to adulthood (Green, 2004). This change is attributed to diagnostic advances, refinements in surgical technique, and increased sophistication of intensive care.

PHYSIOLOGY AND ETIOLOGY

Congenital heart defects were previously categorized as to whether the child had or did not have cyanosis—that is, as cyanotic or acyanotic. Defects are now categorized by pathophysiology and hemodynamics. These categories include the following:

- Defects increasing pulmonary blood flow
- Defects decreasing pulmonary blood flow
- Mixed defects
- Defects obstructing system blood flow.

Defects Increasing Pulmonary Blood Flow

The most common congenital heart defects result from a connection between the left and right side of the heart (**septal defect**) or between the great arteries (**patent ductus arteriosus**) that allows blood to flow between the left and right side of the heart. The pressures on the left side of the heart are higher than the pressures on the right side, so blood shunts from the left side of the heart to the right side and increases the amount of blood pumped to the lungs. The size of the connection and how much blood passes through it determine how quickly the child develops signs of congestive heart failure. The increased blood flow to the lungs causes increased pulmonary vascular resistance (constriction of the pulmonary vascular bed, in an effort to reduce the blood flow) as well as pulmonary artery hypertension. Right ventricular hypertrophy develops to overcome the increasing pulmonary vascular resistance and deliver the blood to the lungs.

Table 22–11 describes the pathophysiology, clinical manifestations, and clinical therapy for heart defects that increase pulmonary blood flow.

Defects Decreasing Pulmonary Blood Flow

Defects that obstruct the pulmonary blood flow result in little or no blood reaching the lungs to be oxygenated. If an atrial or ventricular septal opening exists between the left and right side of the heart, the right-sided pressures exceed those on the left, resulting in right-to-left shunting. In this case, cyanosis often results.

The bone marrow is stimulated to produce more red blood cells to increase the hemoglobin available to carry oxygen. Polycythemia may result and place the child at risk for thromboembolism. Over time, platelet survival is reduced and clotting factors are impaired, increasing the infant's risk of bleeding with surgery. Brain abscesses are also more common in children with cyanotic heart defects.

When infants and children with cyanosis rise in the morning, they may experience an abrupt decrease in systemic resistance and pulmonary blood flow. This physiologic change can

TABLE 22–11 Pathophysiology, Clinical Manifestations, and Clinical Therapy for Heart Defects That Increase Pulmonary Blood Flow

PATHOPHYSIOLOGY, CLINICAL MANIFESTATIONS, AND CLINICAL THERAPY

ANATOMY

PATENT DUCTUS ARTERIOSUS (PDA)

This is a common congenital defect caused by persistent fetal circulation that accounts for 10% of all congenital heart defects (Rome & Kreutzer, 2004). When pulmonary circulation is established and systemic vascular resistance increases at birth, pressures in the aorta become greater than pressures in the pulmonary arteries. Blood is then shunted from the aorta to the pulmonary arteries, increasing circulation to the pulmonary system. It is a common problem of preterm infants and is present in nearly all preterm infants delivered at less than 27 weeks of gestation (Tran, 2002). The ductus arteriosus in the preterm newborn is not as responsive to the increased oxygen content with the conversion to pulmonary circulation, and it is less likely to close.

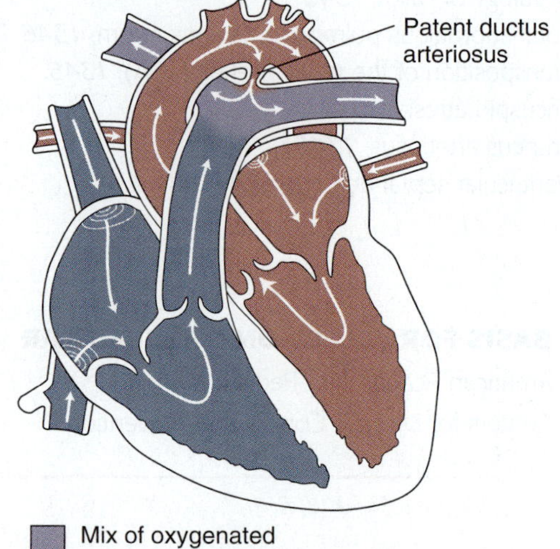

Clinical Manifestations

Dyspnea; tachypnea; tachycardia; full, bounding pulses; widened pulse pressure; hypotension may be noted when cardiac output is low.

Congestive heart failure (CHF), intercostal retractions, hepatomegaly, and growth failure when a large PDA exists.

A continuous "machinery" murmur during systole and diastole, and a thrill in the pulmonic area.

High risk for frequent respiratory infections, pneumonia, and infective endocarditis.

Diagnostic Procedures

Chest x-ray and electrocardiogram (ECG) show left ventricular hypertrophy.

The PDA can be visualized, and a left-to-right shunt can be measured on echocardiogram.

Clinical Therapy

Surgical ligation of PDA is the treatment of choice.

Intravenous indomethacin often stimulates closure of the ductus arteriosus in premature infants.

Transcatheter closure by obstructive device is sometimes attempted in children older than 18 months. Prophylaxis for infective endocarditis is required until the PDA is closed.

Prognosis

No long-term sequelae occur if treated before pulmonary vascular disease develops. If PDA is not treated, the child's life span is shortened, because pulmonary hypertension and pulmonary vascular obstructive disease develop.

ATRIAL SEPTAL DEFECT (ASD)

An **atrial septal defect (ASD)** is an opening in the atrial septum that permits left-to-right shunting of blood. Three types of ASDs occur: ostium secundum, which is a small septal opening in the fetus that normally closes at birth; ostium primum, which is an endocardial cushion defect with anomalies of one or both of the tricuspid and mitral valves; and sinus venosus, which is associated with partial anomalous pulmonary venous connection. The opening may be small, as when the foramen ovale fails to close, or large, as when the septum may be completely absent. Of children with congenital heart defects, 10% have an ASD (Rome & Kreutzer, 2004).

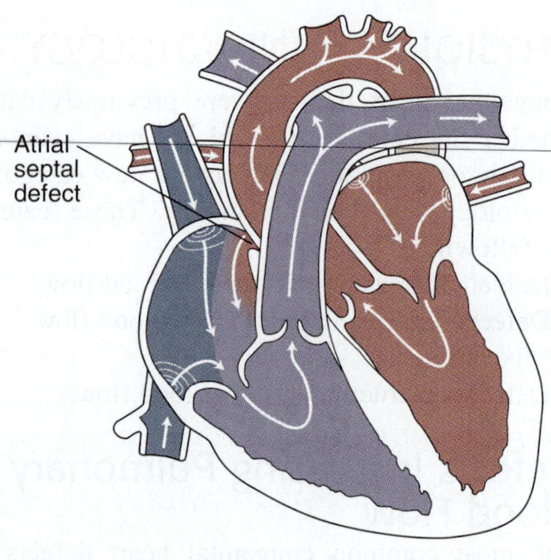

Clinical Manifestations

Infants and young children usually have no symptoms. Small and moderate-size ASDs may not be diagnosed until preschool years or later.

CHF, easy tiring, and poor growth occur with a large ASD.

A soft systolic ejection murmur occurs in the pulmonic area with wide splitting of the second heart sound (S_2). The split S_2 is fixed through all phases of respiration.

Diagnostic Procedures

Echocardiogram identifies a dilated right ventricle caused by blood overload and the shunt size.

Chest x-ray and ECG reveal little information unless the ASD is large, has excessive shunting, and right ventricular hypertrophy is present.

TABLE 22–11 **Pathophysiology, Clinical Manifestations, and Clinical Therapy for Heart Defects That Increase Pulmonary Blood Flow** **(continued)**

PATHOPHYSIOLOGY, CLINICAL MANIFESTATIONS, AND CLINICAL THERAPY	ANATOMY

Clinical Therapy

Spontaneous closure of some ASDs occurs within the first 4 years of life. No activity limitations are needed.

Surgery to close or patch the ASD is performed when significant increased pulmonary blood flow causes CHF or when spontaneous closure has not occurred by 4 years of age.

Secundum ASDs may be closed by a transcatheter device (septal occluder) during cardiac catheterization.

Prognosis

Many persons with uncorrected small and moderate-size ASDs have lived to middle age without symptoms, but CHF and pulmonary hypertension may develop in untreated adults. Atrial arrhythmias may also occur in adults.

VENTRICULAR SEPTAL DEFECT (VSD)

A **ventricular septal defect (VSD)** is an opening in the ventricular septum that causes increased pulmonary blood flow. Blood is shunted from the left ventricle directly across the open septum into the pulmonary artery. This is the most common congenital heart defect, accounting for 40% of all defects (Rome & Kreutzer, 2004).

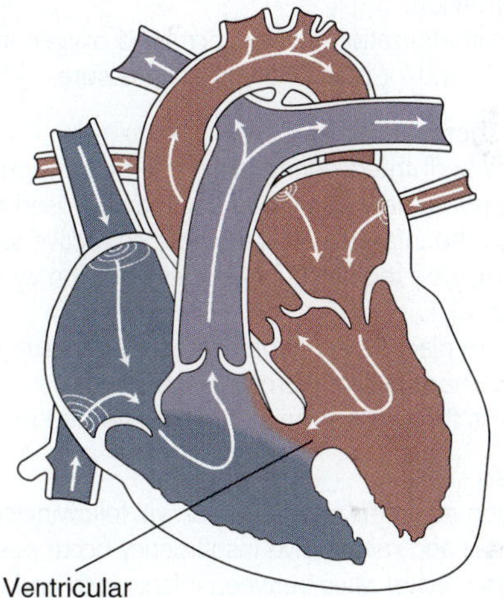

Clinical Manifestations

Only 15% of VSDs are large enough to cause CHF, an increased number of pulmonary infections, and pulmonary hypertension.

A systolic murmur is auscultated at the third or fourth left intercostal space at the sternal border.

Diagnostic Procedures

Chest x-ray and ECG reveal little when VSDs are small. An enlarged heart and pulmonary vascular markings may be seen on the chest x-ray when a large VSD causes shunting. Right and left ventricular hypertrophy may be seen on the ECG.

Echocardiogram establishes the diagnosis if shunting is present.

Cardiac catheterization is used only in preparation for surgery. Findings reveal increased oxygen in the right ventricle and increased systolic pressure in the right ventricle and pulmonary artery.

Clinical Therapy

Most small VSDs close spontaneously within the first 6 months of life. Treatment is conservative when no signs of CHF or pulmonary artery hypertension are present.

Surgical patching of VSD during infancy is performed when poor growth is evident.

Closure of VSD by transcatheter device (i.e., Rashkind device) during cardiac catheterization may be attempted for some defects.

Prophylaxis for infective endocarditis is required.

Prognosis

Highest risk associated with surgical repair is in the first few months of life. Children respond well to surgery and experience substantial catch-up growth.

Tachyarrhythmias and right bundle branch block are possible complications.

ATRIOVENTRICULAR (AV) CANAL (ENDOCARDIAL CUSHION DEFECT)

Atrioventricular (AV) canal refers to a combination of defects in the atrial and ventricular septa and portions of tricuspid and mitral valves. Approximately 2% of children with congenital heart defects have a total AV canal (Park, 2002). This defect is associated with Down syndrome. **Endocardial cushions** are fetal growth centers for mitral and tricuspid valves and AV septum. The most complex AV canal defect results in one AV valve and large septal defects between both atria and ventricles.

(continued)

TABLE 22–11 Pathophysiology, Clinical Manifestations, and Clinical Therapy for Heart Defects That Increase Pulmonary Blood Flow (continued)

PATHOPHYSIOLOGY, CLINICAL MANIFESTATIONS, AND CLINICAL THERAPY	ANATOMY
Clinical Manifestations Severity of symptoms depends on the amount of mitral regurgitation and the left-to-right shunting of blood across the septum. Infants have CHF, tachypnea, tachycardia, poor growth, recurrent respiratory infections, and repeated respiratory failure. A **holosystolic** (heard during the entire phase of systole) murmur is loudest at the left lower sternal border, and the intensity reflects the amount of mitral regurgitation. The first heart sound (S_1) is accentuated, and S2 is split. **Diagnostic Procedures** Chest x-ray shows cardiomegaly and pulmonary vascular markings. ECG reveals atrial enlargement, right ventricular hypertrophy, and an incomplete right bundle branch block. Echocardiogram reveals dilation of the ventricles, septal defects, and details of valve malformation. Cardiac catheterization reveals increased oxygen in the right atrium and increased right ventricle and/or pulmonary artery pressure. **Clinical Therapy** Surgery is performed during infancy to prevent pulmonary vascular disease. Palliative pulmonary artery banding may be used to reduce blood flow to the lungs and CHF so the infant can grow before corrective surgery. Oxygen may be required until surgery, but it may increase pulmonary blood flow and worsen CHF. Patches are placed over septal defects, and valve tissue is used to form functioning valves. The mitral valve may be replaced. Prophylaxis for infective endocarditis is required. **Prognosis** Information regarding long-term survival following successful surgery is lacking. Arrhythmias and mitral valve insufficiency occur postoperatively. There is no difference in short-term survival rates between infants with and without Down syndrome.	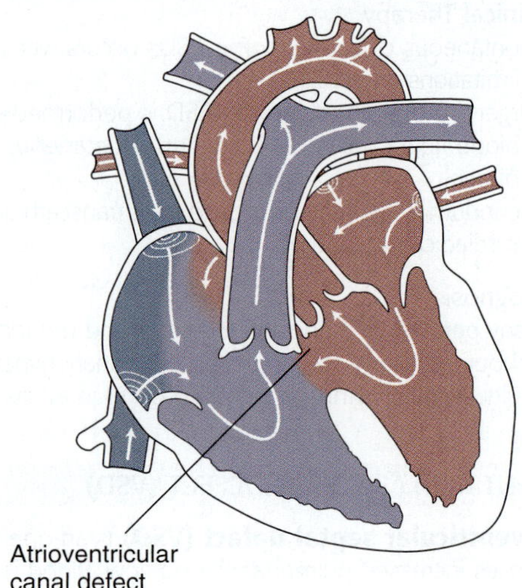 Atrioventricular canal defect

trigger a **hypercyanotic episode** (also known as a hypoxic or "tet" episode) when combined with a sudden increase in cardiac output and venous return associated with crying, feeding, exercise, a warm bath, and straining with defecation. The partial pressure of oxygen (PO_2) is lowered, and the partial pressure of carbon dioxide (PCO_2) rises. Hypoxemia becomes progressively worse as the respiratory center in the brain overreacts, increasing the respiratory effort. The extra respiratory effort further increases the cardiac output and contributes to a life-threatening decline unless rapid intervention is successful.

Table 22–12 describes the pathophysiology, clinical manifestations, and clinical therapy for defects with decreased pulmonary blood flow.

Mixed Defects

Many complex congenital heart defects involve a combination of defects that make the newborn dependent upon mixing pulmonary and systemic circulations for survival during the postnatal period. This mixing of oxygen-saturated and desaturated blood results in a general, desaturated systemic blood flow and cyanosis. Pulmonary congestion occurs because of increased pulmonary blood flow and obstruction of systemic flow.

The pathophysiology, clinical manifestations, and clinical therapy for mixed defects are shown in Table 22–13.

Defects Obstructing Systemic Blood Flow

An anatomic stenosis of the aorta causes obstruction of blood flow and results in a pressure load on the left ventricle and decreased cardiac output. The greater the narrowing, the more obstructed the blood flow to the circulation. This results in higher pressure in the ventricle and decreased cardiac output. Neonates with severe left outflow obstruction or left ventricular dysfunction may develop decreased cardiac output and shock.

The pathophysiology, clinical manifestations, and clinical therapy for defects that obstruct the systemic blood flow are shown in Table 22–14.

TABLE 22–12 **Pathophysiology, Clinical Manifestations, and Clinical Therapy for Defects With Decreased Pulmonary Blood Flow**

DEFECT PATHOPHYSIOLOGY, CLINICAL MANIFESTATIONS, AND CLINICAL THERAPY	ANATOMY
PULMONIC STENOSIS (PS)	
Stenosis (narrowing of the valve, valve area, or great artery above the valve) can be above valve, below valve, or at valve. Stenosis obstructs blood flow into the pulmonary artery, which increases **preload** (the volume of blood in the ventricle at the end of diastole that stretches the heart muscle before contraction) and results in right ventricular hypertrophy. This is the second most common congenital heart defect, accounting for 8–12% of all cases (Park, 2002). Stenosis may progress in the subvalvular area as the heart muscle grows and develops. **Clinical Manifestation** Children with mild stenosis may have no symptoms and grow normally. In moderate stenosis, dyspnea and fatigue occur on exertion. Signs of congestive heart failure (CHF) and hepatosplenomegaly are rare but may result from chronic pressure overload. Heart failure and chest pain on exertion occur in severe cases. A loud systolic ejection murmur with a widely split second heart sound (S_2), and thrill may be found in the pulmonic listening area. **Diagnostic Procedures** Chest x-ray may show an enlarged pulmonary artery with normal heart size and normal pulmonary vascularity. Electrocardiogram (ECG) may show right atrial enlargement and right ventricular hypertrophy. Echocardiogram provides information about the pressure gradient across the valve and size of valve ring. Cardiac catheterization findings include increased right ventricular pressure and a normal or slightly lowered pulmonary artery pressure. **Clinical Therapy** Dilation by balloon valvuloplasty, performed during cardiac catheterization, treats simple pulmonic stenosis. Surgical valvotomy may be used when other defects such as ventricular septal defect (VSD) are present. Surgical resection may be needed for narrowing above the valve area. Pulmonary regurgitation may result but is not a significant problem. **Prognosis** Pulmonic stenosis does not typically increase in severity. Lifelong infective endocarditis prophylaxis is necessary.	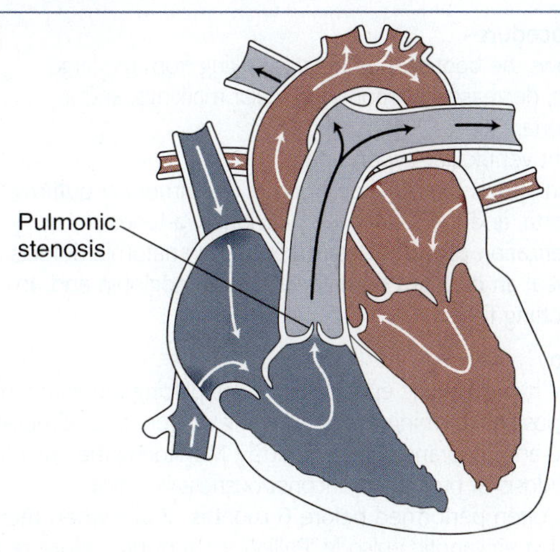 Decreased unoxygenated blood flow
TETRALOGY OF FALLOT (TOF)	
Tetralogy of Fallot consists of four defects—pulmonic stenosis, right ventricular hypertrophy, VSD, and an overriding aorta (aorta positioned directly over a VSD). Some children have a fifth defect, an open foramen ovale or atrial septal defect (ASD). Approximately 10% of children with congenital heart defects have TOF (Park, 2002). Elevated pressures in the right side of the heart cause a right-to-left shunt. **Clinical Manifestations** The infant becomes hypoxic and cyanotic as the ductus arteriosus closes. The degree of pulmonary stenosis determines the severity of symptoms. A systolic murmur is heard in the pulmonic area and is transmitted to the suprasternal notch. A thrill may be palpated in the pulmonic area. Polycythemia, hypoxic episodes, metabolic acidosis, poor growth, clubbing of the fingers, and exercise intolerance may develop. Toddlers with uncorrected defects instinctively squat (assume a knee–chest position) to decrease the return of systemic venous blood to the heart. See Figure 22–32 ■.	

(continued)

TABLE 22–12 Pathophysiology, Clinical Manifestations, and Clinical Therapy for Defects With Decreased Pulmonary Blood Flow (continued)

DEFECT PATHOPHYSIOLOGY, CLINICAL MANIFESTATIONS, AND CLINICAL THERAPY	ANATOMY

Diagnostic Procedures

Chest x-ray shows the boot-shaped heart, resulting from the large right ventricle, decreased pulmonary vascular markings, and a prominent aorta.

ECG shows right ventricular hypertrophy.

Echocardiogram shows the VSD, obstruction of pulmonary outflow, an overriding aorta, and the size of the pulmonary arteries.

Cardiac catheterization provides details about the anatomic defects.

Blood tests reveal an elevated hematocrit and hemoglobin and an increased clotting time.

Clinical Therapy

Management of hypercyanotic episodes includes placing the infant in the knee–chest position, calming the child, giving oxygen, and administering morphine and propranolol intravenously. Monitoring the child for metabolic acidosis or prolonged unconsciousness is critical.

A total repair is often performed before 6 months of age when the infant has a hypercyanotic episode. Palliative shunt procedure (e.g., Blalock–Taussig) may be performed to allow the child to grow and improve outcomes with corrective surgery.

Prognosis

Not all children are cured by surgery, but most have improved quality of life and improved longevity. Arrhythmias may be residual problems (Park, 2002). Lifelong infective endocarditis prophylaxis is required.

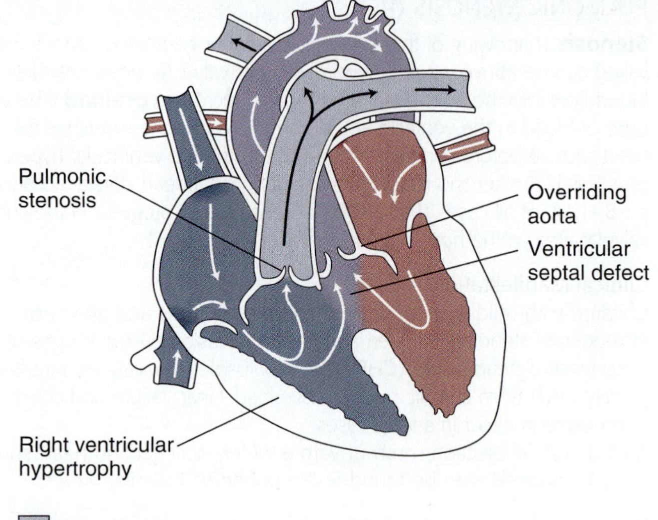

PULMONARY OR TRICUSPID ATRESIA

Pulmonary atresia is the absence of communication between the right ventricle and the pulmonary artery, either at the site of the pulmonary valve or in the main pulmonary artery. It occurs in less than 1% of children with congenital heart defects. In **tricuspid atresia**, the tricuspid valve is absent. It occurs in 1–3% of congenital heart defects (Park, 2002). Blood flows to the left side of the heart through the foramen ovale. The patent ductus arteriosus (PDA) provides the only flow of blood to the pulmonary arteries. A VSD or transposition of the great arteries is also often present.

Clinical Manifestations

Cyanosis is present at birth.

Tachypnea, CHF, pulmonary edema, hepatomegaly, acidosis, hypoxic episodes, clubbing, polycythemia, and growth delays occur.

A continuous murmur from the PDA is heard in the pulmonic area. A single S_2 is heard in the aortic area, and a harsh systolic murmur may be heard in the tricuspid area.

Diagnostic Procedures

Chest x-ray may reveal a normal size or slightly enlarged sized heart.

ECG may reveal right atrial hypertrophy.

Echocardiogram shows a small hypoplastic right ventricular cavity and tricuspid valve, an absent right ventricular outflow tract, a dilated right atrium, and right-to-left shunting across the atrial septum.

Clinical Therapy

Prostaglandin E_1 is given immediately to maintain a PDA. Digoxin and diuretics are also used.

Rastelli balloon atrial septostomy is performed to increase the atrial opening.

Rastelli or modified Fontan procedure results in improved survival.

Prognosis

Outcome depends upon the size of the pulmonary outflow tract developed by surgery and the fibrosis in the right ventricle. The child has increased risk for arrhythmia and right ventricular dysfunction.

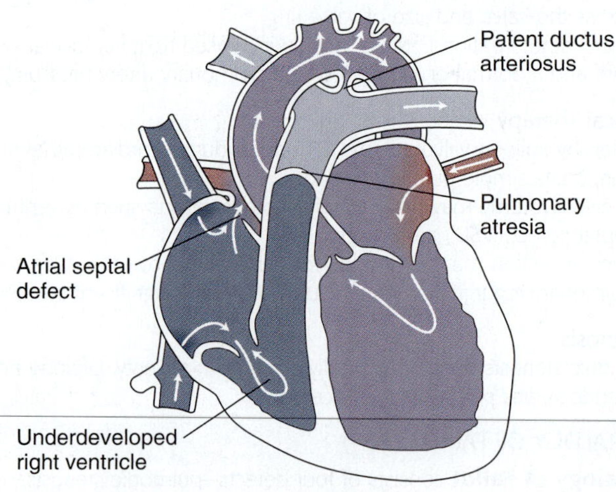

TABLE 22–13 **Pathophysiology, Clinical Manifestations, and Clinical Therapy for Mixed Defects**

DEFECT PATHOPHYSIOLOGY, CLINICAL MANIFESTATIONS, AND CLINICAL THERAPY	ANATOMY

TRANSPOSITION OF THE GREAT ARTERIES (TGA)

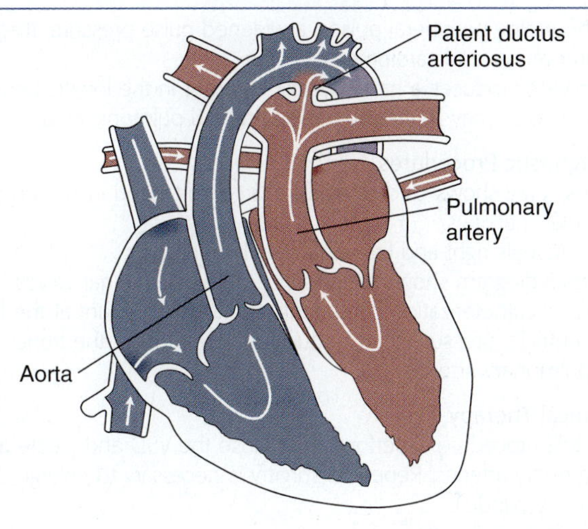

In **transposition of the great arteries (TGA)**, the pulmonary artery, which is the outflow tract for the left ventricle, and the aorta, which is the outflow tract for the right ventricle, are transposed. TGA is life-threatening at birth, and survival initially depends on an open ductus arteriosus and foramen ovale. This condition occurs in approximately 5% of children with congenital heart disease (Park, 2002). An atrial septal defect (ASD) or ventricular septal defect (VSD) may also be present with TGA.

Clinical Manifestations

Cyanosis, apparent soon after birth, progresses to hypoxia and acidosis. Cyanosis does not improve with oxygen administration. Cyanosis may be less apparent when a large VSD is present.

Congestive heart failure (CHF) may develop immediately or over days or weeks. Tachypnea (60 breaths/min) is often present without retractions or other signs of dyspnea.

A systolic murmur is present if a VSD is present; no other murmur is generally heard. The second heart sounds (S_2) is loud.

Infants take a long time to feed and need frequent rest periods because of rapid respiratory rate and fatigue.

Growth failure may be evident as early as 2 weeks of age if corrective surgery is not performed.

Diagnostic Procedures

Chest x-ray may reveal a classic egg-shaped heart on a string (narrow superior mediastinum) with enlarged ventricles and increased pulmonary vascular markings.

Electrocardiogram (ECG) reveals right ventricular hypertrophy.

Echocardiogram often shows the abnormal position of the great arteries rising from ventricles.

Hyperoxitest confirms a cyanotic congenital heart defect.

Cardiac catheterization shows increased right ventricular pressure, and the catheter can enter the aorta through the right ventricle.

Blood tests reveal an increased hematocrit and hemoglobin or polycythemia.

Clinical Therapy

Prostaglandin E_1 is ordered to maintain a patent ductus arteriosus until a palliative procedure can be performed. Oxygen is administered for severe hypoxemia.

Balloon atrial septostomy may be performed during cardiac catheterization in newborns as a first stage. The defect may also be corrected surgically. Other defects may be repaired in stages as the infant grows.

Corrective surgery (arterial switch) is usually performed before 1 week of age.

Prognosis

Survival without surgery is impossible. The 5-year survival rate following an arterial switch is greater than 80% (Park, 2002). Arrhythmias, decreased right ventricular function, pulmonary vascular disease, and sudden death are long-term complications after the Mustard and Senning procedures, so follow-up every 6–12 months as needed (Park, 2002). Other complications of surgical repair include pulmonary artery or aortic stenosis, coronary artery obstruction, and mitral regurgitation. Infective endocarditis prophylaxis may be necessary.

TRUNCUS ARTERIOSUS

In **truncus arteriosus**, a single large vessel empties both ventricles and provides circulation for the pulmonary, systemic, and coronary circulations. A VSD is usually present. This occurs in less than 1% of congenital heart defects (Park, 2002).

Clinical Manifestations

Cyanosis develops soon after birth; however, this is also a condition of increased pulmonary blood flow. Severe CHF, dyspnea, retractions, fatigue, poor feeding, poor growth, polycythemia, clubbing, increased pulse pressure,

(continued)

TABLE 22–13 Pathophysiology, Clinical Manifestations, and Clinical Therapy for Mixed Defects (continued)

DEFECT PATHOPHYSIOLOGY, CLINICAL MANIFESTATIONS, AND CLINICAL THERAPY	ANATOMY
bounding peripheral pulses, a widened pulse pressure, frequent respiratory infections, and cardiomegaly occur. The VSD produces a harsh systolic murmur in the lower sternal border. A systolic click may be heard in the apex and pulmonic area. **Diagnostic Procedures** Chest x-ray shows cardiomegaly, a large aorta, and increased pulmonary vascular markings. ECG reveals right and left ventricular hypertrophy. Echocardiogram shows the absence of two semilunar valves. Cardiac catheterization documents a left-to-right shunt at the level of the ventricle, pressure that is equal in the ventricles, the truncus, and pulmonary arteries. **Clinical Therapy** Rastelli procedure is performed to close the VSD and create a passage to pulmonary arteries. Repeated surgery is necessary to enlarge the pulmonary artery conduit. Digoxin and diuretics are given. **Prognosis** Survival is improved, but truncal valve stenosis and regurgitation result. The long-term prognosis is unknown. The child should not participate in competitive sports.	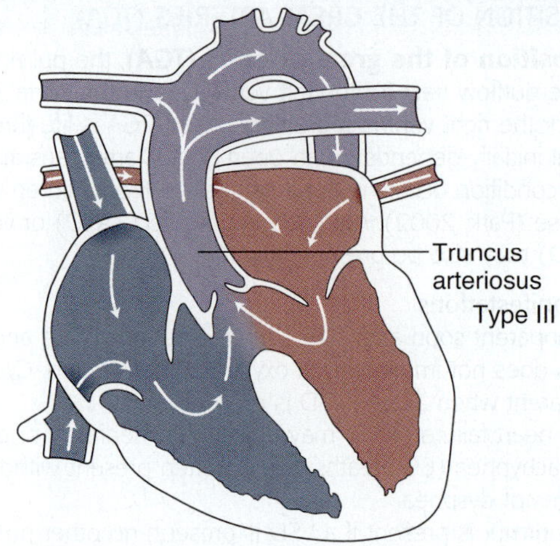
TOTAL ANOMALOUS PULMONARY VENOUS RETURN	
In **total anomalous pulmonary venous return**, the pulmonary veins empty into the right atrium, or into veins leading to the right atrium, rather than into the left atrium. The foramen ovale must remain patent for mixed blood from the right atrium to pass to the systemic circulation. Any obstruction of the pulmonary veins increases the condition's severity. It occurs in approximately 1% of children with a congenital heart defect (Park, 2002). **Clinical Manifestations** Mild cyanosis and frequent respiratory infections occur. Increased cyanosis may occur with feedings as the filled esophagus compresses the common pulmonary vein. If the pulmonary veins are obstructed in any way, cyanosis will be increased. Increased pulmonary blood flow will result in signs of CHF. A precordial bulge may be palpated. S_2 has a wide, fixed split when there is no pulmonary vein obstruction. An ejection murmur and gallop rhythm may be heard in the pulmonic area. **Diagnostic Procedures** Chest x-ray shows cardiac enlargement, a large pulmonary artery, and increased pulmonary blood flow. ECG reveals hypertrophy of the right atrium and ventricle. Echocardiogram shows enlargement of the right atrium, a patent foramen ovale, and lack of connection between the pulmonary veins and left atrium. Cardiac catheterization shows a higher oxygen level in the right atrium and the abnormal circulation. **Clinical Therapy** Prostaglandin E_1 is given to maintain a patent ductus arteriosus. Hypoxemia and CHF are treated. Balloon atrial septostomy may be performed to promote better mixing of blood so surgery can be delayed until the infant is stabilized. Surgery to reconnect or baffle the pulmonary veins to the left atrium is performed. **Prognosis** Survivors have lived more than 20 years after correction.	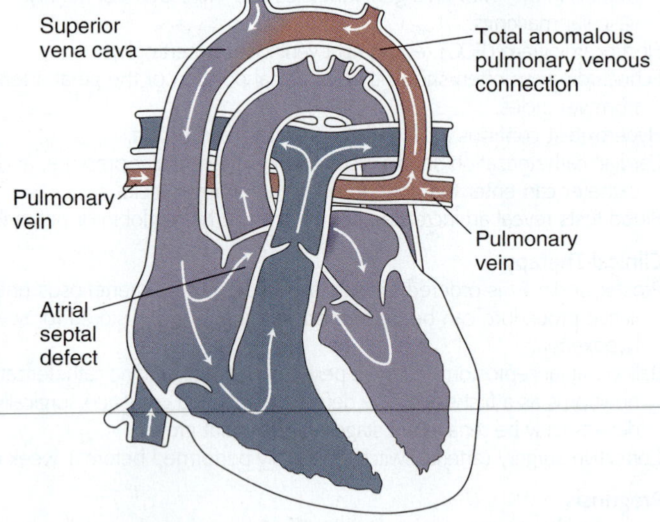

TABLE 22–14 **Pathophysiology, Clinical Manifestations, and Clinical Therapy for Defects That Obstruct the Systemic Blood Flow**

DEFECT PATHOPHYSIOLOGY, CLINICAL MANIFESTATIONS, AND CLINICAL THERAPY	ANATOMY
AORTIC STENOSIS (AS)	
In **aortic stenosis**, narrowing of the aortic valve obstructs blood flow to systemic circulation. The valve is often bicuspid rather than tricuspid. The pressure gradient across the valve usually increases as the child grows and cardiac output increases. Aortic stenosis accounts for 3–6% of all cases of congenital heart defects (Park, 2002). **Clinical Manifestations** Most infants and children are asymptomatic, with normal growth and development. Life-threatening aortic stenosis is detected in some newborns. Congestive heart failure (CHF) develops in infants with significant stenosis. Blood pressure is normal, but a narrow pulse pressure may be noted. Peripheral pulses may be weak. The child may complain of chest pain after exercise, but exercise intolerance is uncommon. Syncope and dizziness are serious signs that require intervention. A systolic heart murmur and thrill occur in the aortic or pulmonic areas with transmission to the neck. An ejection click may be heard. Splitting of the second heart sound (S_2) may be noted with severe aortic stenosis. **Diagnostic Procedures** Chest x-ray is usually normal but may reveal a slight prominence of the left ventricle and aorta with increased severity. Electrocardiogram (ECG) is usually normal in mild cases but may show mild left ventricular hypertrophy and inverted T waves with increased severity. Echocardiogram reveals the number of the valve cusps, pressure gradient across the valve, and size of the aorta. Stress testing may be used in asymptomatic children to determine the amount of obstruction present with exercise. **Clinical Therapy** Newborns with life-threatening aortic stenosis need prostaglandin E_1 to maintain a patent ductus arteriosus until the aortic valve can be dilated. The aortic valve may be successfully dilated by balloon valvuloplasty during cardiac catheterization. Surgical valvuloplasty may also be performed. Surgical treatment is palliative rather than curative. Aortic valve replacement is performed when stenosis is severe or if significant regurgitation results from other interventions. **Prognosis** Chest pain, syncope, and sudden death can occur in symptomatic children, particularly during vigorous exercise. Stenosis is usually progressive during childhood as the valve calcifies. Valve replacement may be necessary once the child reaches adulthood, requiring lifelong anticoagulant therapy. Lifelong infective endocarditis prophylaxis is required.	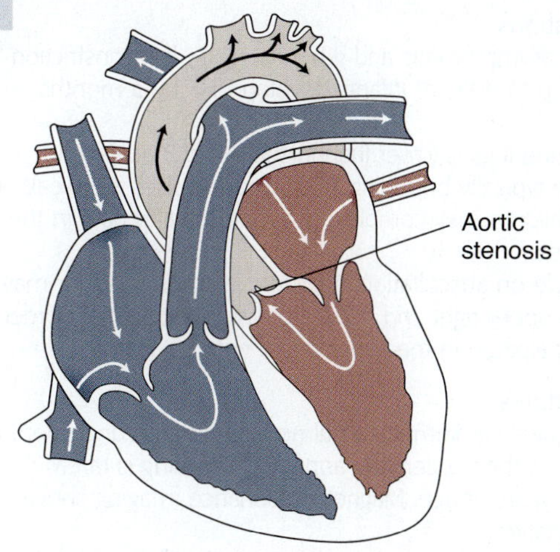
COARCTATION OF THE AORTA (COA)	
In **coarctation of the aorta**, narrowing or constriction in the descending aorta, often near the ductus arteriosus or left subclavian artery, obstructs the systemic blood outflow. This defect is common, occurring in 5% of all children with congenital heart disease (Rome & Kreutzer, 2004). Up to 30% of girls with Turner syndrome have COA (Park, 2002).	

(continued)

TABLE 22–14 **Pathophysiology, Clinical Manifestations, and Clinical Therapy for Defects That Obstruct the Systemic Blood Flow (continued)**

DEFECT PATHOPHYSIOLOGY, CLINICAL MANIFESTATIONS, AND CLINICAL THERAPY	ANATOMY
Clinical Manifestations Many children are asymptomatic and grow normally, but constriction is progressive. Up to 30% of infants develop CHF by 3 months of age. Blood pressure in the legs is lower than in the arms. Brachial and radial pulses are typically bounding, but femoral pulses are weak or absent. Older children may complain of weakness and pain in the legs after exercise. S_2 is loud and single on auscultation. A systolic ejection murmur may be heard at the upper right and middle or lower left sternal border. A thrill may be palpated in the suprasternal notch. **Diagnostic Procedures** Chest x-ray may reveal cardiomegaly, pulmonary venous congestion, and indentation of the descending aorta. Rib notching is rarely seen before 10 years of age. Magnetic resonance imaging shows the site of coarctation. ECG shows left ventricular hypertrophy; right ventricular hypertrophy may be seen in severe cases. Echocardiogram shows the size of the aorta, the actual coarctation, and the function of the aortic valve and left ventricle. **Clinical Therapy** Balloon dilation occurs during cardiac catheterization for initial relief and recoarctation. Balloon dilation on infants under 3 months of age may be performed through the umbilical artery to avoid injury to the femoral artery (Rao, Jureidini, Balfour et al., 2003). Surgical resection with end-to-end anastomosis or with patching using the subclavian artery may be performed. Repair in the first year of life is preferred to decrease exposure to hypertension. **Prognosis** If coarctation recurs, balloon valvuloplasty is usually performed. Persistent hypertension in adulthood is common. Infective endocarditis prophylaxis is needed.	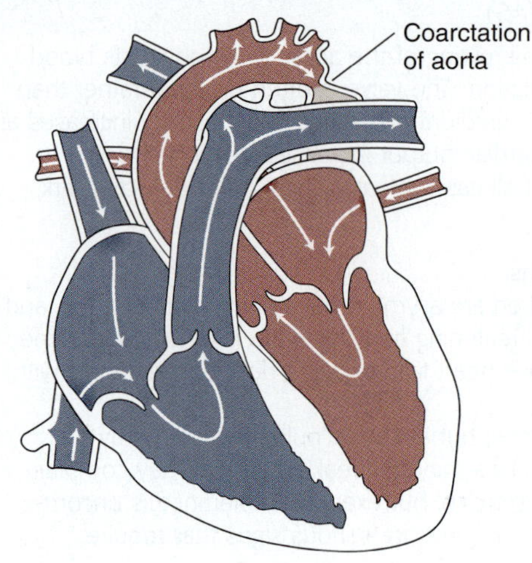
HYPOPLASTIC LEFT HEART SYNDROME (HLHS)	
Hypoplastic left heart syndrome (HLHS) is one of the most severe congenital heart defects, with absence or stenosis of mitral and aortic valves, an abnormally small left ventricle, a small aorta, and aortic or mitral stenosis or atresia. It occurs in 1% of all cases of congenital heart defects (Park, 2002). **Clinical Manifestations** With closure of the ductus arteriosus, the newborn has progressive cyanosis, tachycardia, tachypnea, dyspnea, retractions, and decreased peripheral pulses. A systolic murmur may be present or absent. Poor peripheral perfusion, pulmonary edema, and CHF lead to shock, acidosis, and death. **Diagnostic Procedures** Chest x-ray shows cardiomegaly and increased pulmonary vascularity. Echocardiogram shows the small left ventricle. This condition may be diagnosed prenatally. Cardiac catheterization may be performed in preparation of surgical intervention or to perform an atrial septostomy to promote blood mixing.	

TABLE 22–14 **Pathophysiology, Clinical Manifestations, and Clinical Therapy for Defects That Obstruct the Systemic Blood Flow (continued)**

DEFECT PATHOPHYSIOLOGY, CLINICAL MANIFESTATIONS, AND CLINICAL THERAPY	ANATOMY
Clinical Therapy Prostaglandin E1 is given to maintain a patent ductus arteriosus. Supplemental oxygen is avoided. Treatment options include comfort or palliative care, the Norwood procedure, and heart transplantation. Many infants waiting for a heart transplant die because of the scarcity of donor hearts. The Norwood procedure has become a more common intervention as outcomes have improved. Surgery is performed in three stages. The Norwood procedure is performed in the first week of life, followed by the Glenn procedure at approximately 3–8 months of age and then the Fontan procedure at between 18 months and 3 years of age. **Prognosis** Without surgery, the median survival time is 3 days. HLHS is the largest contributor of infant deaths resulting from congenital heart disease. Mortality rates in infants having a first-stage Norwood procedure are approximately 10–20% in the first year of life (Cook & Higgins, 2004). Some large centers have achieved a 5-year survival rate of 70% with the Norwood procedure (Chang, Chen, & Klitzner, 2002). The child will have some limitations in physical activity because of a single ventricle. Many children have significant neurocognitive and neurodevelopmental impairment whether treated with transplantation or staged Fontan procedure (Ikle, Hale, Fashaw et al., 2003; Mahle, Visconti, Freier et al., 2006; Shillingford & Wernovsky, 2004). Failure of the single ventricle occurs over time, and these children may require a heart transplant during adolescence or adulthood.	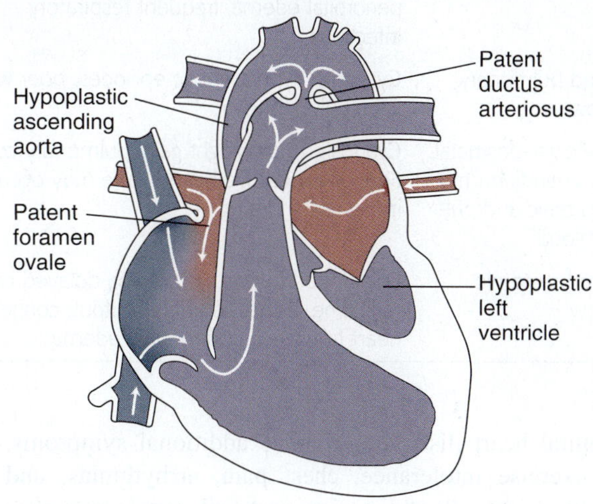

Etiology

Most congenital heart defects develop during the first 8 weeks of gestation. They are usually the result of a combined or interactive effect of genetic and environmental factors, such as the following:

- Fetal exposure to drugs (e.g., phenytoin, lithium, warfarin, and alcohol.)
- Maternal viral infections (e.g., rubella and coxsackie B5).
- Maternal metabolic disorders (e.g., phenylketonuria, diabetes mellitus, and hypercalcemia).
- Maternal complications of pregnancy (e.g., increased age and antepartal bleeding).
- Genetic factors (family recurrence patterns). T transmission is higher when the mother is the affected parent (Park, 2002).
- Chromosomal abnormalities (e.g., Turner syndrome, Noonan syndrome, Marfan syndrome, DiGeorge syndrome, cri du chat syndrome, Down syndrome, and trisomy syndromes 13, 15, 18, and 21). The prevalence of heart defects is approximately 50% in children with Down syndrome, and in children with trisomy 13 and 18, the incidence increases to 90% or more (Park, 2002).

Deletion of chromosome 22q11 is associated with development of several cardiovascular defects, such as interrupted aortic arch, truncus arteriosus, tetralogy of Fallot, and ventricular septal defects (Goldmuntz, 2004). Knowledge about other chromosome deletions or mutations associated with cardiovascular defects is emerging. Because of this genetic component, the incidence of congenital heart defects is expected to slowly rise as people with some of these defects survive and have children of their own. Depending on the type of defect, signs and symptoms may be present at birth or may develop later.

CLINICAL MANIFESTATIONS

The presence of a heart murmur is often the first indication of a congenital heart defect. A loud murmur indicates blood is flowing with higher-than-normal pressure to get through a narrowed valve or vessel, or through a **shunt** (movement of blood between the systemic and pulmonary circulation through an abnormal anatomic opening, such as through the right and left ventricles). Other clinical manifestations and the timing of their appearance vary by the pathophysiology and severity of the defect (see Table 22–15). Some infants and children, such as those with a small atrial septal defect, may be asymptomatic except for a heart murmur. Older children with the diagnosis

TABLE 22–15 **Clinical Manifestations of Heart Defects by Pathophysiology**

PATHOPHYSIOLOGY	CLINICAL MANIFESTATION	TYPES OF DEFECTS
Increased pulmonary blood flow	Tachypnea, tachycardia, murmur, congestive heart failure, poor weight gain, diaphoresis, periorbital edema, frequent respiratory infections	Patent ductus arteriosus, atrial septal defect, ventricular septal defect, atrioventricular canal defect (endocardial cushion defect), truncus arteriosus, total anomalous pulmonary venous return
Decreased pulmonary blood flow	Cyanosis, hypercyanotic episodes, poor weight gain, polycythemia	Pulmonic stenosis, tetralogy of Fallot, pulmonary atresia, tricuspid atresia, transposition of the great arteries
Mixed defects—postnatal survival depends on mixing of systemic and pulmonary blood	Cyanosis, poor weight gain, pulmonary congestion, or congestive heart failure may occur with increased shunting	Transposition of great arteries, total anomalous pulmonary venous connection, truncus arteriosus, double outlet right ventricle
Obstructed systemic blood flow	Diminished pulses, poor color, delayed capillary refill time, decreased urine output, congestive heart failure with pulmonary edema	Coarctation of aorta, aortic stenosis, hypoplastic left heart syndrome, mitral stenosis, interrupted aortic arch

of congenital heart disease may have additional symptoms, such as exercise intolerance, chest pain, arrhythmias, and **syncope** (transient loss of consciousness and muscle tone after exercise or activity).

Defects Increasing Pulmonary Blood Flow

The infant's heart rate, respiratory rate, and metabolic rate are increased because of the high pulmonary blood flow. Sucking breast milk or formula takes energy, and diaphoresis often occurs with feeding. The infant may be unable to take in enough calories to support the metabolic rate and growth, so poor weight gain is noted. If congestive heart failure develops, signs include dyspnea, tachypnea, intercostal retractions, and periorbital edema. Frequent respiratory infections occur as the wet environment in the lungs supports bacterial growth. See Table 22–8 for the pathophysiology, clinical manifestations, and clinical therapy for specific congenital heart defects with increased pulmonary blood flow.

Defects Decreasing Pulmonary Blood Flow

Initially, clinical manifestations in infants include cyanosis shortly after birth, dyspnea, and a loud murmur. The skin may be ruddy or mottled before cyanosis is observed. Cyanosis that does not respond as expected to oxygen is a classic sign (Figure 22–31 ■). Signs and symptoms of chronic hypoxemia include fatigue, clubbing of the fingers and toes, exertional dyspnea, and delayed developmental milestones. The infants may need to stop sucking periodically during feedings to breathe, and diaphoresis may be seen with the increased work of feeding. These infants have a higher metabolic rate, and inadequate calories may be consumed, resulting in poor weight gain. See Table 22–9 for the pathophysiology, clinical manifestations, and clinical therapy for these defects.

When the infant or child has severe obstruction to pulmonary blood flow, hypercyanotic episodes can occur suddenly. Toddlers with uncorrected cyanotic heart disease often squat to relieve dyspnea (Figure 22–32 ■). The knee–chest position reduces the cardiac output by decreasing the venous return from the lower extremities and by increasing the systemic vascular resistance. Hypercyanotic episodes usually appear between 2 months and 2 years of age. Signs include increased rate and depth of respirations; increased heart rate; increased cyanosis,

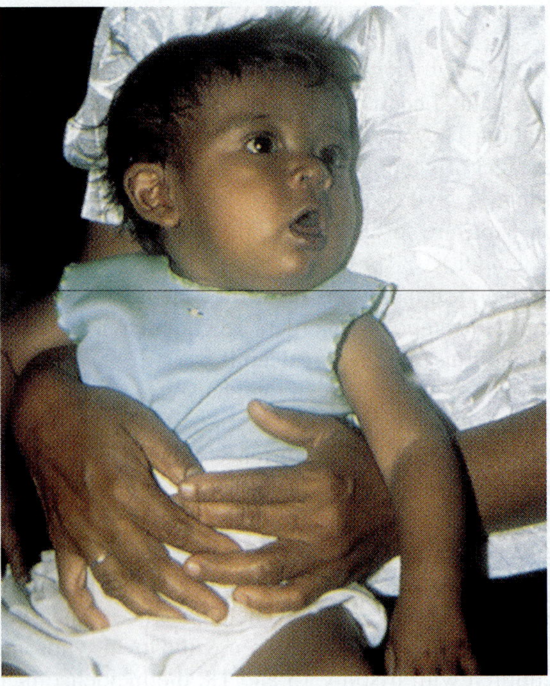

Figure 22–31 ■ The infant is cyanotic due to a heart defect that reduces pulmonary blood flow.

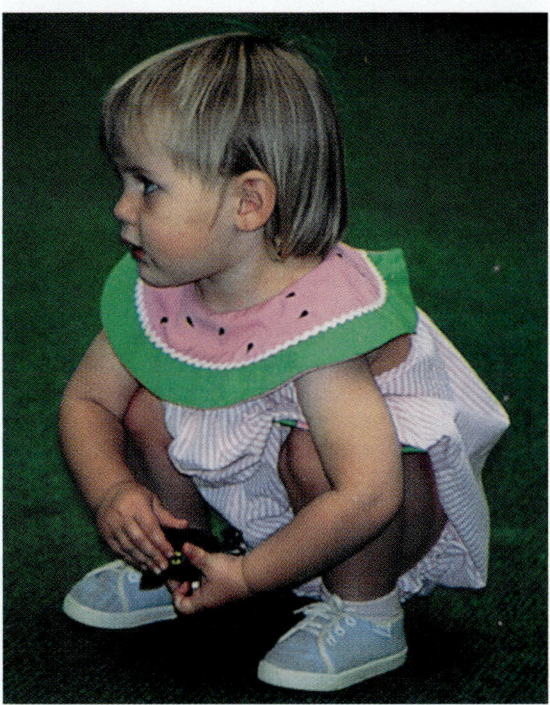

Figure 22–32 ■ A young child with an uncorrected or partially corrected defect that reduces pulmonary blood flow may squat (assumes a knee–chest position) to reduce systemic blood flow return to the heart.

pallor, and poor tissue perfusion; diaphoresis; irritability and crying; and seizures and loss of consciousness.

Older children may have additional symptoms, such as exercise-induced dizziness and syncope. These are serious signs indicating a need for medical evaluation.

Mixed Defects

These complex congenital heart defects cause varying degrees of cyanosis and congestive heart failure. When the pulmonary vascular resistance is lower than the systemic resistance, pulmonary congestion develops, followed by congestive heart failure. When the pulmonary blood flow is decreased, the infant will have more severe cyanosis and polycythemia (Suddaby, 2001). See Table 22–10 for the pathophysiology, clinical manifestations, and clinical therapy for the congenital heart defects that obstruct systemic blood flow.

Defects Obstructing Systemic Blood Flow

Low cardiac output is responsible for the following clinical manifestations: diminished pulses, poor color, delayed capillary refill time, and decreased urinary output. The blood cannot move past the obstruction, so it backs up into the left atrium and then the lungs, causing congestive heart failure and pulmonary edema. Children with mild obstruction may have leg cramps, cooler feet than hands, and stronger pulses and higher blood pressure in the upper extremities than in the lower extremities. Decreased blood supply to the gastrointestinal tract may lead to necrotizing enterocolitis. See Table 22–11 for the pathophysiology, clinical manifestations, and clinical therapy for the congenital heart defects that obstruct systemic blood flow.

COLLABORATION

Some children with mild congenital defects may only require monitoring until the defect resolves on its own. Other defects may be life-threatening and impact life for as long as the child lives. Care of these children requires collaboration between pediatricians, cardiac surgeons, teachers, nurses, occupational therapists, respiratory therapists, and physical therapists in order to help the client meet developmental, physical, and psychosocial milestones.

Diagnostic Tests

Diagnostic procedures and laboratory tests used to evaluate congenital cardiac conditions are described in Table 22–16.

Pharmacologic Therapies

Medications administered to children with congenital heart defects may include any of those discussed under Pharmacologic Therapies in the About section of this concept. In addition, prostaglandin may be administered to maintain fetal circulation, specifically to maintain a patent ductus arteriosus, which allows blood to pass through the ductus and perfuse the rest of the body. Prostaglandin is only used for defects that rely on the patent ductuc arteriosus.

Clinical Interventions

One-third of infants born with congenital heart defects develop life-threatening symptoms in the first few days of life. Treatment for congenital heart defects depends on the severity of symptoms and whether the condition is imminently life-threatening.

Interventional catheterization or surgical correction is the treatment of choice for many defects. Many heart defects can be completely repaired, with restoration of normal hemodynamics and physiology. For complex heart defects, however, treatment may only be a **palliative procedure**, a surgical or interventional cardiac catheterization procedure that does not create normal anatomic or hemodynamic results but allows adequate blood flow to oxygenate the tissues. A palliative procedure may be used for children with a potentially fatal or lethal condition or as an initial procedure while the infant is small and before definitive corrective surgery can be performed. Table 22–17 lists the types of interventions during cardiac catheterization and surgical procedures performed on children with congenital heart defects.

TABLE 22–16 **Diagnostic Procedures and Laboratory Tests Used to Evaluate Cardiac Conditions**

DIAGNOSTIC PROCEDURE	PURPOSE	NURSING IMPLICATIONS
Cardiac catheterization	An invasive procedure that passes a radiopaque catheter through a large vein or artery in an arm or leg to the heart. The catheter is threaded to the heart chambers, coronary arteries, or both and is guided by fluoroscopy, which enables precise measurement of oxygen saturation within the heart's chambers and great arteries and of pressure gradients in the pulmonary vessels or heart chambers. This helps identify congenital heart defects, cardiac valvular disease, and coronary artery disease. In some cases a biopsy of the heart muscle may be obtained to evaluate muscle function problems, inflammation, or heart transplant rejection. Also, cardiac catheterization can aid in evaluation of artificial valves and rhythm disturbances.	■ No food or fluid 6–8 hours before test. ■ Obtain history of hypersensitivity to iodine, seafood, or contrast dye. Antihistamines and/or steroids may be ordered before the procedure if allergy exists. Assess for allergic reaction during the procedure. ■ Oral anticoagulant therapy is discontinued. ■ An intravenous line may be started for administering sedation or emergency drugs, as needed. ■ Vital signs and heart rhythm are monitored during the procedure. ■ Once the catheter and guidewires are removed, apply direct pressure on the catheterization site for 15 minutes, and then apply a pressure dressing for 6 hours. ■ Monitor the site for bleeding, and assess the distal extremity for pulse, capillary refill, and temperature according to agency guidelines. ■ Maintain bed rest for 6 hours after the procedure, and then limit activities for 24 hours. ■ Monitor intake and output as the contrast dye causes diuresis.
Chest x-ray	As the most common form of imaging, radiographs use irradiation to obtain images and capture them on film for diagnostic and screening purposes. They reveal the size and contour of the heart and characteristics of pulmonary vascular markings.	■ Explain the procedure to parents and child. Inform them that several images may be taken from different angles. ■ Explain that modern equipment decreases radiation exposure. ■ Have the child practice holding still and holding a breath in preparation for the test.
Echocardiography	This is a noninvasive ultrasound study of the heart. An ultrasound probe (transducer) is held over the chest to produce an ultrasound beam to the tissues. The reflected sound waves or tissues are then transformed into scans, graphs, or sounds (Doppler). It identifies the heart size, structure, pattern of movement, hemodynamics, blood flow, and blood flow disturbances.	■ Explain the procedure to parents and child. Inform the child of the need to hold still for the procedure. ■ Inform the child that a gel will be applied to the skin and a transducer will move over the area, but that the test causes no pain.
Electrocardiography (ECG)	This records the electrical impulses of the heart via electrodes and a galvanometer (ECG machine). Electrodes with electropaste or pads are strapped to the four extremities, and chest electrodes are applied. The lead selector is turned to read the 12 standard leads. Purposes of this procedure include detection of cardiac dysrhythmias, identification of electrolyte imbalances, and monitoring ECG changes during the stress test.	■ Obtain a list of current medications and when the medications last taken. ■ When applying the chest and extremity leads, explain to the child that the procedure is not painful. ■ Tell the child about the need to hold still for a very short time. A pacifier or bottle may help the infant hold still. ■ Teach methods to relieve anxiety and remain relaxed.
Exercise testing	This is a test performed with a treadmill or stationary exercise bicycle that will evaluate exercise tolerance. ECG leads, a blood pressure cuff, and sometimes an oxygen consumption monitor are attached, and the adolescent begins the exercise. Acceleration and pitch of the treadmill or bicycle are increased at intervals until the adolescent is fatigued or a predetermined endpoint is reached. This enables ECG recording with controlled increase in activity to identify significant cardiac compensation or inadequate cardiac output.	■ Inform the adolescent about the test, what to expect, and that the test can be stopped at any time. ■ Instruct the adolescent to report vertigo, extreme shortness of breath, chest pain, and excessive fatigue. ■ Ensure that the adolescent understands the test is of greater value when the exercise continues to the predetermined stopping level. ■ Take baseline vital sign measurements before the exercise.

TABLE 22–16 Diagnostic Procedures and Laboratory Tests Used to Evaluate Cardiac Conditions (continued)

DIAGNOSTIC PROCEDURE	PURPOSE	NURSING IMPLICATIONS
Holter monitor (ambulatory ECG)	ECG leads are attached, and a portable recorder is used to enable continuous, 24- to 48-hour recording of the ECG on magnetic tape. It is used to detect rhythm disturbances, changes in heart rate with activity or during sleep, as well as responses to antiarrhythmic medications.	■ The child may not swim or bathe in a tub or shower until the electrodes are removed. ■ The child can engage in other usual activities. ■ A diary of any events or emotional stress that cause symptoms should be kept. A daily schedule of sleep, eating, exercise, and other activities may be requested.
Hyperoxitest	Arterial blood is collected before and at least 10 minutes after giving the child 100% oxygen. It measures differences in arterial blood gas level when an infant has central cyanosis to help distinguish between cardiac disease, pulmonary disease, or central nervous system depression (Park, 2002).	■ Administer oxygen through a plastic hood for at least 10 minutes to replace all alveolar air with oxygen.
Magnetic resonance imaging (MRI)	MRI produces results similar to those of a computed tomographic scan, but it does not use ionizing radiation. The MRI scanner is a large, doughnut-shaped cylinder. The child lies on a table and is guided into the cylinder until the body part to be imaged is within the magnetic field. It provides images of the heart's myocardium, structure, valve function, blood vessels, and other soft tissues.	■ Prepare the child for the sounds, size of equipment, and tunnel. ■ Ensure that the child has no metallic implants, and is not connected to metal equipment (e.g., oxygen tank). ■ Use sedation, if needed, to keep the infant or child still. ■ Monitor the child according to agency guidelines.

LABORATORY TEST	PURPOSE	NURSING IMPLICATIONS
Arterial blood gas	Blood is collected from an artery to monitor the adequacy of ventilation and oxygenation, the oxygen-carrying capacity of the blood, and acid–base levels. It enables a direct measurement of the arterial blood pH, partial pressures of oxygen and carbon dioxide, and bicarbonate.	■ Perform arterial puncture on the radial, brachial, and femoral arteries, if desired. ■ Use an anesthetizing agent to reduce pain associated with the arterial puncture. ■ Following blood collection, put pressure over the puncture site for 5–10 minutes to prevent hematoma formation.
Complete blood count	Blood is collected from a vein or capillary puncture. The hematocrit and hemoglobin levels are assessed to identify polycythemia or anemia. The white blood cell count provides evidence of infection.	■ Inform the child about what to expect and how to cooperate. ■ Use the approved skin preparation, and wipe the skin dry with gauze. ■ Warm the skin before blood collection to improve blood flow. ■ Apply pressure briefly, and cover with a bandage.
Serum digoxin level	Blood is collected from a vein to assess the drug level for therapeutic range or toxicity.	■ Collect 1 mL of blood. ■ Record the dosage, route, and time since last digoxin dose on the requisition.
Anti-streptolysin O antibody titer	This provides documentation of a recent group A beta-hemolytic streptococcal infection.	■ Collect venous blood.
Erythrocyte sedimentation rate (ESR)	ESR measures the speed with which red blood cells settle in a tube of anticoagulated blood. It provides evidence of inflammation or infection but does not reveal location. Changes in the ESR help evaluate the condition's acuteness.	■ Collect 5 mL of uncoagulated blood. ■ Follow guidelines for venous blood collection.
C-reactive protein	This nonspecific test provides evidence of inflammation but does not reveal the location. It is used to monitor rheumatic fever.	■ Collect 3 mL of venous blood. ■ Follow guidelines for venous blood collection.
Serum lipid panel	This detects dyslipidemias.	■ Fasting is not needed for total cholesterol screening. ■ Fasting for 12 hours is needed for a total lipid panel.

Source: Corbett, J. V. (2004). *Laboratory tests and diagnostic procedures with nursing diagnoses* (6th ed.). Upper Saddle River, NJ: Prentice Hall; and Park, M. (2002). *Pediatric cardiology for practitioners* (4th ed., pp. 374–375). St. Louis: Mosby.

TABLE 22–17 **Clinical Interventions for Congenital Heart Defects**

CARDIAC CATHETERIZATION PROCEDURE	INTERVENTION	THERAPEUTIC USE AND DEFECT TREATED
Angioplasty	Dilatation of coarctation of aorta (COA) or a stenotic vessel during cardiac catheterization	Palliative or corrective for COA
Balloon valvuloplasty	A deflated balloon is inserted into the opening of a narrowed valve and inflated to stretch the valve open during cardiac catheterization	Corrective or palliative for pulmonic stenosis (PS) and aortic stenosis (AS)
Patent ductus arteriosus (PDA) closure	Closure of ductus arteriosus by an umbrella or coil device during cardiac catheterization	Corrective for PDA
Rashkind–Balloon atrial septostomy	Creation of larger defect (at the foramen ovale) between atria to increase blood mixing, performed during cardiac catheterization	Palliative for transposition of the great arteries (TGA)
Transcatheter closure	Closure of a septal defect by a device such as a septal occluder during cardiac catheterization	Corrective for atrial septal defect and ventricular septal defect (VSD)

SURGICAL PROCEDURE	INTERVENTION	THERAPEUTIC USE AND DEFECT TREATED
Aorta end-to-end anastomosis	Resection of the narrowed section of the aorta and connection of the proximal and distal sections	Corrective for COA
Blalock–Taussig shunt, modified	Creation of aortopulmonary conduit (from the subclavian artery to pulmonary artery) to increase pulmonary blood flow	Palliative for tetralogy of Fallot (TOF) and other defects of decreased pulmonary blood flow
Brock	Blind incision of pulmonary valve	Corrective for PS
Damus–Kaye–Stansel	Pulmonary artery is cut in two, with the proximal section attached to the ascending aorta and the distal section to the right ventricle	Corrective for TGA and complex single-ventricle defects
Fontan	Creation of conduit between inferior vena cava and pulmonary artery to increase pulmonary blood flow—total right heart bypass. This permits the right ventricle to assume the responsibility for the systemic circulation and eject blood into the aorta.	Palliative for hypoplastic left heart syndrome (HLHS) and single-ventricle defects
Glenn	Superior vena cava connected to right pulmonary artery along with closure of aortopulmonary shunt; systemic venous blood from the head sent to the lungs directly without ventricular pumping	Palliative for HLHS and single-ventricle defects
Jatene (arterial switch)	Aorta and pulmonary arteries transected and reanastomosed to opposite stumps; coronary arteries moved to the new aorta area	Corrective for TGA
Mustard or Senning (venous switch or intra-atrial baffle)	Baffling blood in atria to reestablish a proper blood flow in transposition of great arteries	Palliative for TGA
Norwood	Atrial septectomy, anastomosis of the main pulmonary artery to the aorta, and an arterial–pulmonary shunt	Palliative for HLHS
Norwood with Sano modification	Creation of a right ventricle to pulmonary artery conduit so that both the direct pulmonary and aorta blood flow originate in the right ventricle	Palliative for HLHS
Patch aortoplasty	Insertion of a Dacron patch to expand the lumen of the aorta	Corrective for COA

TABLE 22–17 Clinical Interventions for Congenital Heart Defects (continued)

SURGICAL PROCEDURE	INTERVENTION	THERAPEUTIC USE AND DEFECT TREATED
Pulmonary artery banding	Placement of constricting band around pulmonary artery to reduce pulmonary blood flow	Palliative for VSD, atrioventricular canal, single-ventricle defects
Rastelli	Creation of a conduit between the right ventricle to pulmonary artery with closure of the VSD; in the case of truncus arteriosus, the pulmonary arteries are removed from the truncus	Corrective for TGA with PS, TOF, tricuspid atresia, and truncus arteriosus
Ross	The diseased aortic valve is replaced with the client's pulmonic valve (pulmonary autograft), and a homograft (valve from a human donor) replaces the pulmonic valve	Corrective for AS
Subclavian flap aortoplasty	Division of the distal subclavian artery and insertion of a flap into the aorta through the coarcted segment	Corrective for COA
Transplant	Replacement of diseased heart with donor heart	Corrective for HLHS, complex defects, and cardiomyopathies

NURSING PROCESS

Nursing care of clients with a congenital anomaly should address the family's needs as well as those of the infant. Parents and grandparents often are overwhelmed by the complexity of the neonate's medical condition, worried the infant will die, and confused by the decisions they are asked to make. Siblings are often frightened as a result of the anxiety they sense from the adults in their life and also need support.

Assessment

Frequently, the first assessment finding in a child with a congenital heart defect is a heart murmur. The location and sound of the murmur can provide significant detail regarding the type of defect the child has. Assessing heart murmurs is a very specialized skill that requires practice.

When caring for a child with a congenital heart defect, it is important to gather data regarding the mother's prenatal and antepartum experience. Family history of heart defects or other congenital anomalies should also be documented.

Performing a nursing assessment of the child with a potential or actual cardiac condition involves a careful review of the signs and symptoms in many body systems and an analysis of their relationship to cardiac functioning. Use the guidelines in Table 22–18 to perform a comprehensive nursing assessment of the cardiovascular system.

Physiologic Assessment

Before surgery, the infant or child is seen regularly to assess growth and to detect signs of worsening congestive heart failure. Many infants with a small defect will have no problems with growth. Failure to gain weight is an indication of an increased metabolic rate and an inability to consume adequate calories for both metabolic function and growth. Assessment of length and head circumference helps determine the full impact of the condition on growth.

Psychosocial Assessment

Assess the parents' ability to cope with the infant's diagnosis. Parents may initially be in shock and feel guilty or anxious. Parents need an opportunity to express their feelings and learn to cope with the child's illness. The initial period of diagnosis, hospitalization, and early care of the infant at home are very stressful. Parents need special support if their infant has a life-threatening heart defect.

Diagnosis

Potential nursing diagnoses for the child with a congenital heart defect that increases pulmonary blood flow include the following:

- Excess Fluid Volume related to heart failure and pulmonary vasculature overload
- Ineffective Infant Feeding Pattern related to shortness of breath and fatigue
- Risk for Infection related to pulmonary vascular congestion and chronic illness
- Interrupted Family Processes related to crisis of child's serious illness.

Examples of nursing diagnoses that may apply to a child with a congenital heart defect that decreases pulmonary blood flow include the following:

- Decreased Cardiac Output related to ventricular restriction and an obstructed outflow tract
- Risk for Infection related to unfiltered bacteria in the blood and sites of blood shunting that promote bacterial growth
- Caregiver Role Strain related to care of a child with chronic illness
- Activity Intolerance related to cyanosis and dyspnea on exertion
- Delayed Growth and Development related to congenital anomaly and hypoxemia.

TABLE 22–18 **Assessment Guidelines for the Child With a Cardiac Condition**

ASSESSMENT FOCUS	ASSESSMENT GUIDELINES
Respirations	■ Inspect the rate, depth, and respiratory effort. ■ Is a cough present? ■ Identify the signs of increased respiratory effort: tachypnea (rapid rate of respirations), dyspnea, retractions, nasal flaring, and expiratory grunting. ■ Auscultate breath sounds for adventitious sounds (wheezes, crackles).
Pulses	■ Assess the pulse rate, rhythm, and quality. ■ Compare the apical, brachial, and radial pulse rates. ■ Compare the brachial and femoral pulses for strength.
Blood pressure	■ Compare the blood pressure to expected value for age, sex, and height percentiles. ■ Compare blood pressure values between upper and lower extremities.
Color	■ Observe overall color; note pallor, dusky color, or cyanosis. ■ Contrast color in peripheral and central locations (e.g., nail beds to mucous membranes). Note whether crying improves or worsens color.
Heart	■ Inspect the anterior chest for bulging or **heaving** (lifting of the chest wall during contraction). ■ Palpate the chest wall for pulsations, heaves, or vibrations. ■ Locate the point of maximum intensity. ■ Auscultate the heart for the heart sounds and their quality (loud versus weak, distinct versus muffled). Muffled or indistinct sounds are associated with congestive heart failure or a heart defect. ■ Are extra heart sounds or murmurs present? Describe murmurs by intensity, location, radiation, timing, and quality. ■ Auscultate the heart with the child in sitting and reclining positions to detect differences in heart sounds.
Fluid status	■ Observe for signs of periorbital, facial, or peripheral edema. ■ Observe for abdominal distention. ■ Palpate the liver to detect hepatomegaly. ■ Observe for signs of dehydration with acute illnesses.
Activity and behavior	■ Is exercise intolerance present? ■ Does the child tire with feeding? ■ Identify changes in activity level or behavior.
General	■ Assess growth. ■ Note presence of diaphoresis and when it occurs.

Examples of nursing diagnoses for a child following cardiac surgery include the following:

- Ineffective Breathing Pattern related to respiratory muscle fatigue
- Acute Pain related to surgical incision and expansion of chest with coughing and deep breathing exercises
- Risk for Imbalanced Fluid Volume related to impact of surgery on heart's pumping action
- Risk for Infection related to surgery and chronic disease status.

Plan

The primary goal when caring for the child with a congenital heart defect is to support perfusion adequate to at least meet the minimum required to sustain life. Other goals of care include the following:

- The parents and family will verbalize concerns and fears related to the child's diagnosis.
- The parents and family will articulate resources available in the community, such as support groups and financial assistance agencies.
- The parents will articulate an understanding of the child's diagnosis and participate in the treatment plan.
- The child will maintain oxygenation and perfusion to meet needs of the tissues.
- The child will remain free of pain.

Implementation

Participate with members of the cardiology team to provide information to and educate the family about the child's condition. Information may include the following:

- General information about the congenital heart defect, including a description of the heart's anatomy and physiology and of the defect itself
- Information about genetic and environmental influences associated with the congenital heart defect
- Overview of the child's prognosis and timing of medical and surgical interventions
- Interventions for congestive heart failure if it develops.

Psychosocial Support

Parents often need support for anxiety about an uncertain surgical outcome. Determine if parents have a support system as they learn about the infant's diagnosis and make difficult decisions about the child's surgery. If the parents do not have adequate support systems, identify some resources for support, such as social services, pastoral services, or a parent of a child with a similar heart defect. Some parents may be concerned that signing consent for surgery places the child in even more danger of illness or even death.

Parents should be offered genetic counseling if planning a future pregnancy.

Presurgical Home Care

Children are often managed at home until surgery. Parents should encourage feeding to promote growth, and recognize the infant may take longer to eat. Breastfeeding is encouraged because of its beneficial effects for the infant. A high-calorie formula may be used if the infant does not gain enough weight. Feedings through a nasogastric or gastrostomy tube may also be given at night or 24 hours a day to ensure that adequate calories are ingested. Even when nasogastric or gastrostomy feedings are used, encourage the infant to take some formula orally to provide positive oral stimulation.

PRACTICE ALERT

Positioning the baby in an infant seat at a 45° angle decreases venous return to the heart and its metabolic demand. This is a favorable position for feeding and interacting with the infant to promote development (Cook & Higgins, 2004).

Efforts should be made to reduce the infant's exposure to infectious diseases. Nurses, parents, family members, and caregivers should wash their hands frequently. Respiratory infections make hypoxemia worse in children with cyanosis. Fever increases the metabolic rates and oxygen demands. Vomiting and diarrhea may cause an electrolyte disturbance and digoxin toxicity (Cook & Higgins, 2004). The physician should be notified about fever, poor feeding, vomiting, and diarrhea.

Health promotion visits are important. Provide all immunizations according to the recommended schedule. Monthly prophylaxis for respiratory syncytial virus with palivizumab should be provided during the peak season.

Preparation for Surgery

When the child is preschool age or older, prepare the child for the settings, equipment, and experiences to expect before and after surgery. If an infant or toddler is having surgery, provide parents with information about how the child will look, the equipment that will be used, and what care will be provided during the immediate postoperative period.

Postoperative Care

In the immediate postoperative period, the child will be cared for in the intensive care unit. When the child returns to the general nursing unit, assessment focuses on signs of surgical complications, such as infection, arrhythmias, and impaired tissue perfusion.

Monitor the vital signs, including blood pressure and the fifth vital sign–pain. The child may not be on a cardiac monitor, so auscultate the apical pulse to detect an irregular heart rate or bradycardia, which are both signs of reduced cardiac output that require immediate intervention. Assess the respiratory system for breath sounds, respiratory effort, and signs of distress that may indicate pneumonia or fluid in the pleural space. Check pulse oximetry, capillary refill, extremity warmth, pedal pulses, level of consciousness, and urine output to assess impaired tissue perfusion. Reduced urine output is another sign of decreased cardiac output.

Monitor the child's temperature, and inspect the surgical incision site. Fever, excessive incisional pain, spreading erythema around the incision, and wound drainage beginning 3–4 days postoperatively may be early signs of infection.

Pain Management

Pain management with 24-hour intravenous opioids should be provided for several days postoperatively until the child is taking fluids. Once the child is taking oral fluids and foods, oral analgesics may be given around the clock. Teach parents and caregivers to lift and move the child carefully and avoid stress on the incision to reduce potential pain.

PRACTICE ALERT

Holding a pillow or stuffed animal against the chest reduces the pain from coughing and deep breathing.

Promote Respiratory Function

Encourage the child to take deep breaths and cough or to perform spirometry exercises regularly to promote full lung expansion. Chest physiotherapy may be performed in children under 3 years of age.

Manage Fluids and Nutrition

Encourage the infant or child to begin oral fluids and nutrition when permitted. Although oral fluids are rarely limited, intake and output should be carefully assessed. Parents may be encouraged to bring in favorite foods for the child when they can be tolerated. Administer antibiotics as ordered. If intravenous antibiotics are continued after the child's oral intake is normal, the line can be converted to a heparin or saline lock.

Activity

Encourage the child to increase activity gradually, with longer periods out of bed every day, but ensure adequate rest periods to promote healing. Provide diversional activities and opportunities for therapeutic play so the child can better manage the stresses associated with pain and frightening procedures (Box 22–7).

Discharge Planning and Postsurgical Home Care

Infants and children may be discharged from the hospital within a few days of surgery. Parents need information spread over several days to prepare for care of the child at home. Encourage a nutritious diet and snacks so the infant or child has an opportunity to catch up for previous growth deficits. Acetaminophen or ibuprofen may be used for pain management after discharge.

Prepare parents for potential behavior problems of young children that may result from the stress of hospitalization, such as nightmares, separation anxiety, and overdependence

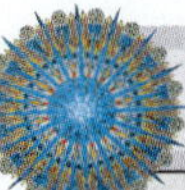

NURSING CARE PLAN A Client With Ventricular Septal Defect

Baby Girl Polasani is born to Theresa and Jason Polasani. She is their third child; they have a 4-year-old girl and 6-year-old boy at home.

ASSESSMENT

Upon admission to the newborn nursery, the baby is weighed (4,000 g), measured (chest, 33 cm; height, 53.34 cm), and found by exam to be at 39 weeks of gestation. Vital signs are as follows: T_{AX} 98.0°F, P 148, R 52, 68/44. When performing a complete assessment, the nurse finds nothing abnormal until assessing heart sounds, when a loud systolic murmur is heard. An echocardiogram is ordered, which demonstrates a large ventricular septal defect (VSD).

The pediatrician recommends monitoring her condition and allows her to remain in the normal nursery and spend time with her mother so long as she remains stable. Two days later, her weight has increased to 4,400 g, she is edematous, and she has course crackles throughout the lung fields. She is tachypneic, and her oxygen saturation is 88% on room air. She is lethargic, and vital signs are as follows: temperature, 98°F axillary; pulse, 188 bpm; respirations, 76/minute; and BP 54/36 mmHg. The pediatrician diagnoses her with congestive heart failure secondary to her VSD, and she is transferred to the neonatal intensive care unit.

DIAGNOSES

- Decreased Cardiac Output related to cardiac anomaly (VSD)
- Excess Fluid Volume related to heart failure
- Risk for Impaired Skin Integrity related to altered fluid status
- Imbalanced Nutrition: Less Than Body Requirements related to increased metabolic needs and rapid tiring during feedings
- Compromised Family Coping related to situational crisis with child's health problems

PLANNING

Goals of care include the following:

- The child's cardiac output will be sufficient to meet the body's metabolic demands.
- The child will manifest adequate oxygenation.
- The child's peripheral and central edema will decrease.
- Intake and output will be balanced once excess fluid is excreted.
- The infant will demonstrate normal weight gain for age.

IMPLEMENTATION

- Administer digoxin as ordered.
- Take apical pulse, and listen to heart sounds regularly, especially before each dose of digoxin. Record apical pulse with each recorded dose of digoxin.
- Place infant on a cardiorespiratory monitor.
- Prevent injury by monitoring for digoxin side effects and serum potassium level.
- Stagger care to provide for rest periods.
- Place child in semi-Fowler's position.
- Evaluate respiratory rate and sounds.
- Take pulse oximetry readings to determine oxygen saturation.
- Provide oxygen and humidification if ordered. Observe for diaphoresis, a sign of increased respiratory effort.
- Administer diuretics as ordered.
- Weigh daily. Measure abdominal girth daily. Observe for peripheral edema.
- Measure intake and output carefully by weighing diapers.
- Maintain fluid restrictions as ordered.
- Monitor electrolytes.
- Provide skin care for edematous body parts, and elevate extremities.
- Change child's position frequently.
- Inspect skin frequently for redness and skin breakdown over pressure points.
- Hold infant at a 45° angle for feeding.
- Give frequent small feedings with rest periods in between, or insert a feeding tube per order.
- Use high-calorie formula.
- Transition to supplemental nasogastric feeding if the infant is not able to gain weight.
- Encourage parents to room-in or visit infant frequently.
- Explain procedures and treatment.
- Involve parents in care as much as possible.
- Have parents hold the child often.
- At discharge, provide clear instructions and information about what to do in an emergency as well as whom and where to call with questions.
- Allow parents to verbalize questions, concerns, and feelings.
- Refer parents to support groups or other resources as needed.

EVALUATION

Expected outcomes used to evaluate the child's response to care include the following:

- The child's cardiac output is sufficient, as indicated by increased energy, adequate feeding intake, and decreased edema.
- The child maintains normal serum levels of potassium and therapeutic levels of digoxin.
- The child has adequate energy to eat.
- The child has normal respiratory rate for age, with no evidence of adventitious sounds or diaphoresis.
- The child's intake and output are proportional, and electrolyte levels remain within normal ranges.
- The child has no skin breakdown after edema resolves.
- The infant gains recommended weight according to growth grids, with all dietary requirements met.
- The parents participate in developing and implementing the treatment plan and in providing care to the child.

CRITICAL THINKING

1. How would you explain the child's congenital defect and rationale for why she developed congestive heart failure?
2. Why would this baby have an increased metabolic rate and need for increased calories?
3. How will this infant's care needs change as she grows if surgery is delayed until she is older?

Box 22–7 Post-Traumatic Stress Disorder and Heart Surgery

Children between 5 and 12 years of age were evaluated for symptoms of post-traumatic stress disorder (PTSD) 1–3 days before and 4–8 weeks after undergoing heart surgery. No children had PTSD at the preoperative assessment, even though 18 (42%) had had prior cardiac surgery. Results indicated that the number of PTSD symptoms increased in children who spent 48 hours or more in the intensive care unit. No significant relationship was found in PTSD scores for children with prior cardiac surgery or chronologic age. These findings are similar to those of other studies of PTSD in children after hospitalization for other serious medical illnesses and injuries such as cancer and liver transplantation (Connolly, McClowry, Hayman et al., 2004). See Concept 28, Stress and Coping, for more information about PTSD.

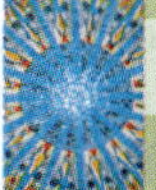

ALTERNATIVE THERAPIES Congenital Heart Defects

Caution parents of children with congenital heart defects to avoid using complementary therapies, such as herbal products, that may interfere with the medications prescribed to manage the child's heart condition. Products containing ginkgo are known to interact with warfarin, which is of particular concern for any child on anticoagulant therapy. Many of these herbal remedies have not been researched fully, so the potential side effects and interactions with prescribed medications are not known (Cook & Higgins, 2004).

on parents. Encourage parents to reassure children about their security and to promote play and other means to deal with their feelings. If the child's symptoms continue for several weeks, a referral for psychologic evaluation and care may be needed.

Reassure parents of children with a complete correction of the cardiac defect that there should be no further cardiovascular problems. Provide parents with full information about the child's defect and the surgery performed to share with the child's current and future health care providers. Encourage parents to allow the child to live a normal and active life.

Children are at risk for infective endocarditis, especially within the first 6 months after surgery. Prophylactic antibiotics are indicated for invasive procedures. Any unexplained fever or malaise seen in the 2 months following surgical repair or after dental work may be a sign of infection. The child should be examined for petechiae and splenomegaly and evaluated for infective endocarditis.

Evaluation

Examples of expected outcomes of nursing care include the following:

- The child's pain is managed effectively.
- Full lung expansion is maintained with incentive spirometry exercises or chest physiotherapy.
- The child's incision heals without infection.
- Catch-up growth occurs over the next few months to years.

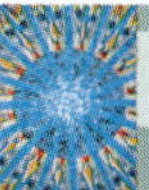

EVIDENCE-BASED PRACTICE Parental Stress Associated With Having a Child With a Congenital Heart Defect

Clinical Question

Do parents of a child with a congenital heart defect have any more or less stress than parents of children with other chronic conditions?

Evidence

Prior studies identified that parents of infants with congenital heart defects reported higher stress than parents of children with cystic fibrosis or with cleft lip and/or cleft palate (Goldberg, Morris, Simmons et al., 1990; Pelchat, Ricard, Bouchard et al., 1999). Recently, a 36-item self-report Parenting Stress Index (PSI) was used to measure the amount of stress experienced by parents of young children with congenital heart defects. The PSI has three subscales to help interpret findings: parental distress, parent–child dysfunctional interaction, and difficult child. The 80 parents of children with congenital heart disease reported significantly greater stress than the parent population in whom the PSI had been normalized, and 17.5% reported a total stress score at or above the 90th percentile. The parents also had significantly higher stress scores for the difficult child subscale. Parenting stress was not related to the severity of the child's heart disease (Uzark & Jones, 2003).

A second study compared the parents of 26 children with a complex heart defect requiring multiple surgeries to the parents of 32 children with a simple defect (ventricular septal defect) requiring a single surgery. No significant differences were found in parental stress (even when scores of mothers and fathers were analyzed separately) by the type of their child's congenital heart defect (Mörelius, Lundh, & Nelson, 2002). These findings were consistent with those of a study that included children with 11 different types of congenital heart defects (Davis, Brown, Bakeman, & Campbell, 1998).

Best Practice

The heart is known to be an organ essential for survival, so it is appropriate for parents to be fearful of their child's survival. However, these studies reveal that while most parents of children with congenital heart defects have significant stress, the stress is not related to the severity of the heart defect. An important nursing role therefore is to identify factors that could contribute to the parent's stress and help them find coping mechanisms. Families need information about the child's condition that is reinforced in future visits, especially when the child has a simple heart defect. Allow the parents to tell their stories of living with the child to help understand their stresses and strengths. A family assessment may help identify social supports, strengths, and resources available. Encourage the parents to raise the child as close to normal as possible. Help them by providing age-appropriate expectations regarding development and activity and by discussing strategies for discipline.

REVIEW Congenital Heart Defects

RELATE: LINK THE CONCEPTS

Linking the exemplar of Congenital Heart Defects with the concept of Family:

1. What is you priority of care for the family of a newborn diagnosed with a cyanotic heart defect?
2. How might you support the family of the newborn requiring extensive and numerous open heart surgeries?

Linking the exemplar of Congenital Heart Defects with the concept of Development:

3. Why might the child with a significant unrepaired congential defect fail to meet developmental milestones?
4. What interventions would you initate for the family whose infant is not meeting developmental milestones due to a congenital heart defect?

READY: GO TO COMPANION SKILLS MANUAL

- Monitoring intake and output
- Assessing vital signs
- Assessing the client in pain
- Using an incentive spirometer
- Preparing a client for chest physiotherapy
- Preparing a client for surgery

REFER: GO TO MYNURSINGKIT

REFLECT: CASE STUDY

Billy Secton is a few hours old; he was born at 32 weeks gestation to Randy and Barbara Sexton. Randy, age 26, is in law school and Barbara, age 25, teaches first grade at the local elementary school. Billy is their first child. Billy is taken to the neonatal ICU where he is examined and diagnosed with tetralogy of fallot following a cardac echocardiogram.

Randy and Barbara leave the NICU in a state of shock and don't even know what questions to ask the doctor. The doctor has told them that Billy will require open heart surgery when he is older and has gained weight. Until that time, Billy will be treated medically. The idea of taking him home with such a serious heart problem is truly frightening to Barbara. Randy finds himself wondering if his son will survive and, if he does, will he ever be able to act like a normal child.

1. How will you help Randy and Barbara understand the pathophysiology of Billy's heart defect?
2. What is your priority nursing diagnosis for Billy?
3. Create a teaching plan for the family to prepare them for Billy's discharge from the hospital.

22.3 CORONARY ARTERY DISEASE

KEY TERMS

Acute coronary syndrome (ACS), *1361*
Acute myocardial infarction (AMI), *1361*
Angina pectoris, *1361*
Arrhythmogenic, *1368*
Atherosclerosis, *1361*
Bradydysrhythmia, *1369*
Cardiac markers, *1371*
Cardiac rehabilitation, *1382*
Cardiac tamponade, *1380*
Cardiogenic shock, *1369*
CK-MB, *1371*
Collateral channels, *1361*
Coronary artery disease (CAD), *1360*
Dermatome, *1362*
Dysrhythmias, *1368*
Ischemia, *1362*
Homocysteine, *1366*
Metabolic syndrome, *1366*
Pericarditis, *1369*
Regurgitation, *1369*
Troponins, *1371*
Ventricular aneurysm, *1369*

BASIS FOR SELECTION OF EXEMPLAR

Healthy People 2010

LEARNING OUTCOMES

After reading about this exemplar, you will be able to:

1. Describe the pathophysiology, etiology, clinical manifestations, and direct and indirect causes of coronary artery disease.
2. Identify risk factors associated with coronary artery disease.
3. Illustrate the nursing process in providing culturally competent care across the life span for individuals with coronary artery disease.
4. Formulate priority nursing diagnoses appropriate for an individual with coronary artery disease.
5. Create a plan of care for individuals with coronary artery disease and their families.
6. Asses expected outcomes for an individual with coronary artery disease.
7. Discuss therapies used in the collaborative care of an individual with coronary artery disease.
8. Employ evidence-based caring interventions for an individual with coronary artery disease.

OVERVIEW

Coronary artery disease (CAD) affects 13.2 million people in the United States and causes more than 500,000 deaths annually (National Heart, Lung, and Blood Institute [NHLBI], 2004). CAD is caused by impaired blood flow to the myocardium. Accumulation of atherosclerotic plaque in the coronary arteries is the usual cause. CAD may be asymptomatic, or it may lead to angina pectoris, acute coronary syndrome, myocardial infarction (MI) or heart attack, dysrhythmias, heart failure, and even sudden death.

Angina pectoris (or angina) is chest pain resulting from reduced coronary blood flow, which causes a temporary imbalance between myocardial blood supply and demand. The imbalance may be caused by CAD, atherosclerosis, or vessel constriction that impairs the myocardial blood supply. Hypermetabolic conditions, such as exercise, thyrotoxicosis, stimulant abuse (e.g., cocaine), hyperthyroidism, and emotional stress, can increase myocardial oxygen demand, precipitating angina. Anemia, heart failure, ventricular hypertrophy, or pulmonary diseases may affect blood and oxygen supplies as well, causing angina.

Acute coronary syndrome (ACS) is a condition of unstable cardiac ischemia. ACS includes unstable angina and acute myocardial ischemia with or without significant injury of myocardial tissue. An estimated 1.4 million Americans are admitted to the hospital annually with ACS (Kasper et al., 2005).

An **acute myocardial infarction (AMI)**, which refers to necrosis (death) of myocardial cells, is a life-threatening event. It occurs when blood flow to a portion of the cardiac muscle is blocked. If circulation to the affected myocardium is not promptly restored, loss of functional myocardium affects the heart's ability to maintain an effective cardiac output. This may ultimately lead to cardiogenic shock and death.

Heart disease remains the leading cause of death in the United States. Of the major heart diseases, MI, or *heart attack*, as well as other forms of ischemic heart disease cause the majority of deaths. Annually, approximately 700,000 people in the United States experience their first MI; another 500,000 suffer an MI subsequent to the initial one. Nearly 492,000 people died of CAD in 2002, with most of these deaths related to MI (NHLBI, 2004).

The majority of deaths from MI occur during the initial period after symptoms begin: approximately 60% within the first hour, and 40% before hospitalization. Heightening public awareness of the manifestations of MI, the importance of seeking immediate medical assistance, and training in cardiopulmonary resuscitation (CPR) techniques are vital to decreasing the number of deaths caused by MI.

PATHOPHYSIOLOGY AND ETIOLOGY

The two main coronary arteries, the left and the right, supply blood, oxygen, and nutrients to the myocardium. They originate in the root of the aorta, just outside the aortic valve. The left main coronary artery divides to form the anterior descending and circumflex arteries. The anterior descending artery supplies the anterior interventricular septum and the left ventricle, including the apex of the heart. The circumflex branch supplies the lateral wall of the left ventricle. The right coronary artery supplies the right ventricle and forms the posterior descending artery. The posterior descending artery supplies the posterior portion of the heart (see Figure 22–7 in the About section).

Blood flow through the coronary arteries is regulated by several factors. Aortic pressure is the primary factor. Other factors include heart rate (most of the flow occurs during diastole, when the muscle is relaxed), metabolic activity of the heart, blood vessel tone (constriction), and collateral circulation. Although no connections occur between the large coronary arteries, small arteries are joined by **collateral channels** (sometimes called collateral circulation; these are small blood vessels that develop to connect small arteries). If large vessels are gradually occluded, these channels enlarge, providing alternative routes for blood flow (Porth, 2005).

Coronary atherosclerosis is the most common cause of reduced coronary blood flow. **Atherosclerosis** is a progressive disease characterized by atheroma (plaque) formation, which affects the intimal and medial layers of large and midsized arteries. Atherosclerosis is initiated by unknown precipitating factors that cause lipoproteins and fibrous tissue to accumulate in the arterial wall. Although the precise mechanisms are unknown, abnormal lipid metabolism and injury to, or inflammation of, endothelial cells lining the artery appear to be key to its development.

In the bloodstream, lipids are transported while attached to proteins called apoproteins. High levels of certain lipoproteins (a type of apoprotein) increase the risk of atherosclerosis. Low-density lipoproteins (LDLs), which are high in cholesterol, carry cholesterol to peripheral tissues, where some of it is released to be taken up and incorporated into cells for use in producing energy. Very-low-density lipoproteins (VLDLs), which are large molecules composed primarily of triglycerides and cholesterol, carry triglycerides to muscle and fat cells. When the triglycerides are released into these tissues, the remainder of the molecule is an LDL. High-density lipoproteins (HDLs), in contrast, attract cholesterol, returning it from peripheral tissues to the liver.

Hyperlipidemia itself may damage arterial endothelium. Other potential mechanisms of vessel injury include excessive pressures within the arterial system (hypertension), toxins found in cigarette smoke, infections, and inflammation (Copstead & Banasik, 2005). Endothelial damage promotes platelet adhesion and aggregation and attracts leukocytes to the area.

At the site of injury, atherogenic (atherosclerosis-promoting) lipoproteins collect in the intimal lining of the artery. These lipoproteins appear to actually bind with the extracellular portion of the vessel endothelium. Macrophages migrate to the injured site as part of the inflammatory process. Contact with platelets, cholesterol, and other blood components stimulates smooth muscle cells and connective tissue within the vessel wall to proliferate abnormally. Although blood flow is not affected at this stage, the early lesion appears as a yellowish, fatty streak on the inner lining of the artery. Fibrous plaque develops as smooth muscle cells enlarge, collagen fibers proliferate, and blood lipids accumulate. The lesion protrudes into the arterial lumen and is fixed to the inner wall of the intima. It may invade the muscular media layer of the vessel as well. The developing plaque not only gradually occludes the vessel lumen but also impairs the vessel's ability to dilate in response to increased oxygen demands. Fibrous plaque lesions often develop at arterial bifurcations or curves or in areas of narrowing. As the plaque expands, it can produce severe stenosis or total occlusion of the artery.

The final stage of the process is the development of atheromas, which are complex lesions consisting of lipids, fibrous tissue, collagen, calcium, cellular debris, and capillaries. These calcified lesions can ulcerate or rupture, stimulating thrombosis. The vessel lumen may be rapidly occluded by the thrombus (clot), or it may embolize to occlude a distal vessel.

Plaque formation may be eccentric (located in a specific, asymmetric region of the vessel wall) or concentric (involving the entire vessel circumference). Manifestations of the process usually do not appear until approximately 75% of the arterial lumen has been occluded.

Atherosclerosis tends to develop where arteries bifurcate or branch. Certain vessels have a higher likelihood of being affected, including the coronary arteries (the left anterior descending artery in particular), the renal arteries, the bifurcation of the carotid arteries, and the branching sections of peripheral arteries. In addition to obstructing or occluding blood flow, atherosclerosis weakens arterial walls and is a major cause of aneurysm in vessels such as the aorta and iliac arteries.

Ischemia

As a result of declining artery circumference, blood supply to the cardiac tissue is reduced, and the imbalance between myocardial blood supply and demand causes temporary and reversible myocardial ischemia. **Ischemia** results when the oxygen supply is inadequate to meet metabolic demands. The critical factors in meeting metabolic demands of cardiac cells are coronary perfusion and myocardial workload. Coronary perfusion can be affected by several different mechanisms:

- One or more vessels may be partially occluded by large, stable areas of plaque.
- Platelets can aggregate in narrowed vessels, forming a thrombus.
- Normal or already narrowed vessels may spasm.
- A drop in blood pressure may lead to inadequate flow through coronary vessels.
- Normal autoregulatory mechanisms that increase flow to working muscles may fail (Copstead & Banasik, 2005).

Workload is affected by heart rate, myocardial contractility, preload (the amount of blood in the ventricles just prior to systole), and afterload (the peripheral pressure that must be overcome to move blood out of the heart into the circulation). The oxygen content of the blood and hematocrit are contributing factors to myocardial ischemia. Table 22–19 lists factors that may lead to myocardial ischemia.

Cellular processes are compromised as adenosine triphosphate stores are depleted in ischemic tissue. Reduced oxygen causes cells to switch from aerobic metabolism to anaerobic metabolism. Anaerobic metabolism causes lactic acid to build up in the cells. It also affects cell membrane permeability, releasing substances such as histamine, kinins, and specific enzymes that stimulate terminal nerve fibers in the cardiac muscle and send pain impulses to the central nervous system. The pain radiates to the upper body because the heart shares the same **dermatome** (an area supplied with afferent nerve fibers by a single posterior spinal root) as this region. If blood flow is restored within 20 minutes, aerobic metabolism and contractility are restored, and cellular repair begins (McCance & Huether, 2006). Continued ischemia results in cell necrosis and death (infarction).

Angina results from ischemia and can be a one-time event or a chronic condition. Angina is categorized into three types:

1. *Stable angina* is the most common and predictable form of angina. It occurs with a predictable amount of activity or stress and is a common manifestation of CAD. Stable angina usually occurs when the work of the heart is increased by physical exertion, exposure to cold, or stress. Stable angina is relieved by rest and nitrates.
2. *Prinzmetal's (variant) angina* is atypical angina that occurs unpredictably (unrelated to activity) and often at night. It is caused by coronary artery spasm with or without an atherosclerotic lesion. The exact mechanism of coronary artery spasm is unknown. It may result from hyperactive sympathetic nervous system responses, altered calcium flow in smooth muscle, or reduced prostaglandins that promote vasodilation.
3. *Unstable angina* occurs with increasing frequency, severity, and duration. Pain is unpredictable, occurs with decreasing levels of activity or stress, and may occur at rest. Clients with unstable angina are at risk for MI. (Unstable angina is discussed further in under Acute Coronary Syndrome.)

Silent myocardial ischemia, or asymptomatic ischemia, is thought to be common in people with CAD. Silent ischemia may occur with either activity or with mental stress. Mental stress increases the heart rate and blood pressure, increasing myocardial oxygen demand (McCance & Huether, 2006). Like symptomatic angina, silent myocardial ischemia is associated with an increased chance of MI and death (Kasper et al., 2005).

Acute Coronary Syndrome

Acute coronary syndrome is a dynamic state in which coronary blood flow is acutely reduced but not fully occluded. Myocardial cells are injured by the acute ischemia that results.

TABLE 22–19 Factors Contributing to Myocardial Ischemia

CORONARY PERFUSION	MYOCARDIAL WORKLOAD	BLOOD OXYGEN CONTENT
■ Atherosclerosis	■ Rapid heart rate	■ Reduced atmospheric oxygen pressure
■ Thrombosis	■ Increased preload, afterload, or contractility	■ Impaired gas exchange
■ Vasospasm	■ Increased metabolic demands (e.g., hyperthyroidism)	■ Low red blood cell count and hemoglobin content
■ Poor perfusion pressure		

Most people affected by ACS have significant stenosis of one or more coronary arteries.

Acute coronary syndrome is precipitated by one or more of the following processes:

1. Rupture or erosion of atherosclerotic plaque, with formation of a blood clot that does not fully occlude the vessel
2. Coronary artery spasm (e.g., Prinzmetal's angina)
3. Progressive vessel obstruction by atherosclerotic plaque or restenosis following a percutaneous revascularization procedure
4. Inflammation of a coronary artery
5. Increased myocardial oxygen demand and/or decreased supply (e.g., acute blood loss or anemia) (Braunwald et al., 2002).

Of these, ruptured or eroded plaque is the predominant pathophysiology underlying ACS (AHA, 2005a). Plaque rupture often is triggered by hemodynamic factors, such as increased heart rate, blood flow, and blood pressure in response to a surge of sympathetic nervous system activity. Increased sympathetic nervous system activity also is thought to contribute to the higher incidence of plaque rupture within the first hour after arising from bed in the morning (Porth, 2005).

When atherosclerotic plaque ruptures or erodes, the exposed lipid core of the plaque stimulates platelet aggregation and the extrinsic clotting pathway. Thrombin is generated and fibrin is deposited, forming a clot that severely impairs or obstructs blood flow to tissue distal to the area of plaque rupture. As a result, these cells become ischemic.

Injured myocardial cells contract less effectively, potentially reducing cardiac output if a large area of myocardium is affected. Lactic acid released from ischemic cells stimulates pain receptors, causing chest pain. Ischemia and injury affect electrical impulse conduction, producing inversion of the T wave and possibly elevation of the ST segment on the ECG.

Acute Myocardial Infarction

Atherosclerotic plaque may form stable or unstable lesions. Stable lesions progress by gradually occluding the vessel lumen, whereas unstable (or complicated) lesions are prone to rupture and thrombus formation. Stable lesions often cause angina; unstable lesions often lead to ACS or acute ischemic heart diseases. ACS can include unstable angina, MI, and sudden cardiac death (Braunwald et al., 2002).

Myocardial infarction occurs when blood flow to a portion of cardiac muscle is completely blocked, resulting in prolonged tissue ischemia and irreversible cell damage. Coronary occlusion is usually caused by ulceration or rupture of a complicated atherosclerotic lesion. When an atherosclerotic lesion ruptures or ulcerates, substances are released that stimulate platelet aggregation, thrombin generation, and local vasomotor tone. As a result, the vessel constricts and a thrombus forms, occluding the vessel and interrupting blood flow to the myocardium distal to the obstruction.

Cellular injury occurs when the cells are denied adequate oxygen and nutrients. When ischemia is prolonged, lasting more than 20–45 minutes, irreversible hypoxemic damage causes cellular death and tissue necrosis. Oxygen, glycogen, and adenosine triphosphate stores of ischemic cells are rapidly depleted. Cellular metabolism shifts to an anaerobic process, producing hydrogen ions and lactic acid. Cellular acidosis increases the vulnerability of cells to further damage. Intracellular enzymes are released through damaged cell membranes into interstitial spaces.

Cellular acidosis, electrolyte imbalances, and hormones released in response to cellular ischemia affect impulse conduction and myocardial contractility. The risk for dysrhythmias increases, and myocardial contractility decreases, reducing stroke volume, cardiac output, blood pressure, and tissue perfusion.

The subendocardium suffers the initial damage, within 20 minutes of injury, because this area is the most susceptible to changes in coronary blood flow. If blood flow is restored at this point, the infarction is limited to subendocardial tissue (a subendocardial or non-Q-wave infarction). If blood flow is not restored, the damage progresses to the epicardium within 1–6 hours. When all layers of the myocardium are affected, it is known as a transmural infarction. A significant Q wave develops with a transmural infarction, so this also may be called a Q-wave MI. Complications such as heart failure are more frequently associated with Q-wave MIs; however, clients with non-Q-wave MIs frequently experience recurrent ischemia or subsequent MI within weeks or months of the event (Woods et al., 2004).

The necrotic, infarcted tissue is surrounded by regions of injured and ischemic tissues. Tissue in this ischemic area is potentially viable; restoration of blood flow minimizes the amount of tissue lost. This surrounding tissue also undergoes metabolic changes. It may be stunned (its contractility impaired for hours or days following reperfusion) or hibernating (a process that protects myocytes until perfusion is restored). Myocardial remodeling also may occur, with cellular hypertrophy and loss of contractility in regions distant from the infarction. Rapid restoration of blood flow limits these changes (McCance & Huether, 2006).

When a larger artery is compromised, collateral vessels connecting smaller arteries in the coronary system dilate to maintain blood flow to the cardiac muscle. The degree of collateral circulation helps determine the extent of myocardial damage from ischemia. Acute occlusion of a coronary artery without any collateral flow results in massive tissue damage and may result in death. Progressive narrowing of the larger coronary arteries allows collateral vessels to develop and enlarge, meeting the demand for blood flow. Good collateral circulation can limit the size of an MI.

Myocardial infarctions are described by the damaged area of the heart. The coronary artery that is occluded determines the area of damage. MI usually affects the left ventricle, because it is the major "workhorse" of the heart. Its muscle mass is greater, as are its oxygen demands. Occlusion of the left anterior descending artery affects blood flow to the anterior wall of the left ventricle (an *anterior* MI) and part of the interventricular septum. Occlusion of the left circumflex artery causes a *lateral* MI. Right ventricular, inferior, and posterior infarcts involve occlusions of the right coronary artery and posterior descending artery. Occlusion of the left main coronary artery is the most devastating, causing ischemia of the entire left ventricle and a grave prognosis. Identifying the infarct site helps predict possible complications and determine appropriate therapy.

Acute myocardial infarction may also develop as a result of cocaine intoxication. Cocaine increases sympathetic nervous system activity by both increasing the release of catecholamines from central and peripheral stores and interfering with the reuptake of catecholamines. This increased catecholamine concentration stimulates the heart rate and increases its contractility, increases the automaticity of cardiac tissues and the risk of dysrhythmias, and causes vasoconstriction and hypertension. The client with cocaine-induced MI may present with an altered level of consciousness, confusion and restlessness, seizure activity, tachycardia, hypotension, increased respiratory rate, and respiratory crackles. (Further information about the effects of cocaine may be found in Concept 2, Addiction Behaviors.)

Etiology

The underlying cause of atherosclerosis and related disease are unknown. A person's tendency to develop cardiovascular disease may be inherited. Lifestyle habits such as diet, smoking, and physical activity also play a role.

Risk Factors

The causes of atherosclerosis are not known, but certain risk factors have been linked with the development of atherosclerotic plaques. The Framingham Heart Study provided vital research into the relationship between risk factors and the development of heart disease (see the Evidence-Based Practice feature that follows). Research into CAD is ongoing, looking at causative factors, manifestations, and protective measures for many populations. Risk factors for CAD are frequently classified as nonmodifiable (factors that cannot be changed) and modifiable (factors that can be changed). Table 22–20 lists risk factors for coronary artery disease.

The development of CAD is the primary risk factor for angina and MI. While ischemic heart disease can result from trauma, stimulant drug use (cocaine, amphetamines), or other causes, these are not common.

NONMODIFIABLE RISK FACTORS Age is a nonmodifiable risk factor for CAD. More than 50% of those who experience a heart attack are age 65 or older; 80% of deaths caused by MI occur in this age group. Gender and genetic factors also are nonmodifiable risk factors for CAD. Men are affected by CAD at an earlier age than women. A family history of CAD in a male first-degree relative younger than age 55, or in a female first-degree relative younger than 65, also has been identified as a risk factor for CAD (National Cholesterol Education Program [NCEP], 2002).

MODIFIABLE RISK FACTORS Modifiable risk factors include lifestyle factors and pathologic conditions that predispose the client to developing CAD. Behavioral or lifestyle factors can be controlled or completely eliminated. Lifestyle changes require significant commitment by the client; ongoing support from the health care team is vital for success.

Disease conditions that contribute to CAD include hypertension, diabetes mellitus, and hyperlipidemia. Although these conditions are not a matter of choice; they are modifiable risk factors that can often be controlled through medication, weight control, diet, and exercise.

Hypertension Hypertension is consistent blood pressure readings of greater than 140 mmHg systolic or 90 mmHg diastolic. Hypertension is common, affecting more than one-third

TABLE 22–20 **Risk Factors for Coronary Artery Disease**

NONMODIFIABLE	MODIFIABLE	
	PATHOPHYSIOLOGIC	LIFESTYLE
Age	Hyperlipidemia	Cigarette smoking
Men ≥ 45 years	Elevated low-density lipoprotein cholesterol	Obesity
Women ≥ 55 years	Elevated triglycerides	Physical inactivity
Gender	Low high-density lipoprotein cholesterol	Atherogenic diet
Heredity	Hypertension	Use of oral contraceptives (women only)
	Diabetes mellitus	Hormone replacement therapy (women only)
	Premature menopause (women only)	
	Emerging risk factors:	
	Elevated homocysteine levels	
	Thrombogenic factors	
	Inflammatory factors	
	Impaired fasting glucose	

EVIDENCE-BASED PRACTICE The Framingham Heart Study

Evidence

The Framingham Heart Study (FHS) is an ongoing, significant clinical research study that has provided data about cardiovascular disease for more than 50 years. The study was initiated in 1948 with an original group of 5,209 participants in the town of Framingham, Massachusetts. Every 2 years, this original group is evaluated for cardiovascular "events" via their medical history, physical findings, and diagnostic testing. Children of the original group have also been studied as part of the Framingham Offspring Study. It was in reports of the Framingham study that the term "risk factor" first appeared.

Best Practice

The data collected from both the Framingham Heart Study and the Framingham Offspring Study provide a rich database from which to develop evidence-based approaches for clients with heart disease. A major application of these research findings to practice is in primary preventive education, for example, through community cardiovascular health programs. As noted in the text, research shows that increased public awareness of cardiovascular risk factors has lowered morbidity and mortality from heart disease, but heart disease remains the number-one killer in the United States. Education about the effects of lifestyle on the cardiovascular system must begin in the early school years and be reinforced throughout the formative years. When healthy choices become habit, cardiac disease will be reduced.

A second application of these findings is in interdisciplinary treatment. Nurses should keep up to date about the latest strategies for medical treatment so they can provide accurate rationales to clients and formulate effective nursing treatment plans that complement medical management strategies. The result is better communication, a sense of collegiality and teamwork, and positive client outcomes.

Critical Thinking

1. What kinds of strategies can be used in elementary school settings to teach cardiovascular health in a fun, informative manner?
2. Which health care providers should be included in a multidisciplinary effort to encourage clients to modify their lifestyles?
3. What changes do you need to make in your lifestyle to role model heart healthy living?

of people over age 50 in the United States. Its prevalence is higher in African Americans than in Hispanics and is higher in Hispanics than in White Americans. Hypertension damages the endothelial cells of arteries, possibly by excess pressure and altered characteristics of blood flow. This damage can stimulate the development of atherosclerotic plaque.

Diabetes Mellitus Diabetes mellitus contributes to CAD in several ways. Diabetes is associated with higher blood lipid levels, a higher incidence of hypertension, and obesity—all risk factors in their own right. In addition, diabetes affects the endothelium of blood vessels, contributing to the process of atherosclerosis. Hyperglycemia and hyperinsulinemia, altered platelet function, elevated fibrinogen levels, and inflammation also are thought to play a role in the development of atherosclerosis in people with diabetes.

Hyperlipidemia Hyperlipidemia is an abnormally high level of blood lipids and lipoproteins. Lipoproteins carry cholesterol in the blood. Low density lipids (LDLs) are the primary carriers of cholesterol. High levels of LDL (memory cue: LDLs = **l**ess **d**esirable **l**ipoproteins) promote atherosclerosis, because LDL deposits cholesterol on artery walls. Table 22–21 lists desirable and high-risk levels for total and LDL cholesterol. In contrast, high density lipids (HDLs) (memory cue: HDLs = **h**ighly **d**esirable **l**ipoproteins) help clear cholesterol from the arteries, transporting it to the liver for excretion. HDL levels of greater than 35 mg/dL have a protective effect, reducing the risk of CAD; in contrast, HDL levels of lower than 35 mg/dL are associated with an increased risk for CAD. Triglycerides (compounds of fatty acids bound to glycerol and used for fat storage by the body) are carried on VLDL molecules. Elevated triglycerides also contribute to the risk for CAD.

Cigarette Smoking Cigarette smoking, an independent risk factor for CAD, is responsible for more deaths from CAD than from lung cancer or pulmonary disease (Woods et al., 2004). The effects of smoking on the cardiovascular system are dose dependent (NCEP, 2002). The male cigarette smoker has two to three times the risk for developing heart disease compared with the nonsmoker; the female smoker has up to four times the risk. For both men and women who stop smoking, the risk of mortality from CAD is reduced by half. Second-hand (or environmental)

TABLE 22–21 **Classification of Serum Cholesterol and Triglyceride Values**

	TOTAL CHOLESTEROL (mg/dl)	LOW-DENSITY LIPOPROTEIN CHOLESTEROL (mg/dl)	TRIGLYCERIDE (mg/dl)
Optimal		<100	
Desirable	<200	100–129	<150
Borderline high	200–239	130–159	150–199
High	≥ 240 or higher	160–189	200–499
Very high		≥ 190	≥ 500

Note. As defined by the NHLBI's NCEP.

tobacco smoke also increases the risk of death from CAD, by as much as 30% (Woods et al., 2004).

Tobacco smoke promotes CAD in several ways. Carbon monoxide damages vascular endothelium, promoting cholesterol deposition. Nicotine stimulates catecholamine release, increasing blood pressure, heart rate, and myocardial oxygen use. Nicotine also constricts arteries, limiting tissue perfusion (blood flow and oxygen delivery). Furthermore, nicotine reduces HDL levels and increases platelet aggregation, increasing the risk of thrombus formation.

Obesity Obesity (excess adipose tissue) is generally defined as a body mass index of 30 kg/m^2 or greater and affects the risk for CAD. People who are obese have higher rates of hypertension, diabetes, and hyperlipidemia. In the Framingham study, obese men over age 50 had twice the incidence of CAD and AMI of those who were within 10% of their ideal weight.

Fat distribution also affects the risk for CAD. Central obesity, or intra-abdominal fat, is associated with an increased risk. The best indicator of central obesity is the waist circumference. A waist-to-hip ratio of greater than 0.8 (women) or 0.9 (men) increases the risk for CAD.

Physical Inactivity Physical inactivity is associated with a higher risk for CAD. Research data indicate that people who maintain a regular program of physical activity are less prone to developing CAD than sedentary people. Cardiovascular benefits of exercise include increased availability of oxygen to the heart muscle, decreased oxygen demand and cardiac workload, and increased myocardial function and electrical stability. Other positive effects of regular physical activity include decreased blood pressure, blood lipids, insulin levels, platelet aggregation, and weight.

Diet Diet is a risk factor for CAD, independent of fat and cholesterol intake. Diets high in fruits, vegetables, whole grains, and unsaturated fatty acids appear to have a protective effect. The underlying factors are not clear but probably relate to nutrients such as antioxidants, folic acid, other B vitamins, omega-3 fatty acids, and other unidentified micronutrients (NCEP, 2002).

EMERGING RISK FACTORS Recent research demonstrates a link between elevated serum levels of **homocysteine** (an amino acid that is a homologue of cysteine) and CAD. Until menopause, women have lower homocysteine levels than men, which may partially explain their lower risk for CAD. Homocysteine levels are negatively correlated with serum folate and dietary folate intake; that is, increasing folate intake lowers homocysteine levels.

Based on evidence that aspirin and antiplatelet therapies reduce the risk for MI, clot-promoting factors are identified as risk factors for CAD. Inflammation also has recently been identified as a risk factor. Inflammatory processes may increase the development of atherosclerotic plaque, and they are implicated in plaque rupture (NCEP, 2002). Inflammation also promotes clot formation at the site of ruptured plaque. It is not generally recommended that clients routinely be tested for these factors.

The **metabolic syndrome** is a group of metabolic risk factors occurring in an individual that create a highly elevated risk for CAD (Box 22–8). In fact, metabolic syndrome has emerged as a risk factor for premature CAD that is equal to cigarette smoking. Three underlying causes of metabolic syndrome have been identified: overweight/obesity, physical inactivity, and genetic factors. Metabolic syndrome is closely associated with insulin resistance (impaired tissue responses to insulin). Genetic factors play a role in insulin resistance, as do the acquired factors of abdominal obesity and physical inactivity (NCEP, 2002).

RISK FACTORS UNIQUE TO WOMEN Risk factors unique to women include premature menopause, oral contraceptive use, and hormone replacement therapy (HRT). At menopause, serum HDL levels drop and LDL levels rise, increasing the risk for CAD. Early menopause (natural or surgically induced) increases the risk for CAD and MI. Women who have bilateral oophorectomy without hormone replacement before age 35 are eight times more likely to have an MI than women experiencing natural menopause. Estrogen replacement therapy reduces the risk for CAD and MI in these women. Oral contraceptives, by contrast, increase the risk for MI, particularly in women who also smoke. This increased risk is caused by the tendency of oral contraceptives to promote clotting and their effects on blood pressure, serum lipids, and glucose tolerance (Woods et al., 2004). The Women's Health Initiative randomized trial of HRT showed an increased risk for CAD in previously healthy women taking a commonly prescribed combination of estrogen and progestin (Writing Group, 2002). This well-controlled research study was terminated early, however, when it showed a small but significant increased risk for CAD, stroke, pulmonary embolism, and invasive breast cancer in women taking HRT.

CLINICAL MANIFESTATIONS

While the clinical manifestations of angina and MI are similar initially, important differences exist. Differentiating between ischemic causes of chest pain and other causes can be subtle and complex; chest pain should always be assessed by experienced health care professionals.

Angina

The cardinal manifestation of angina is chest pain. The pain typically is precipitated by an identifiable event, such as physical activity, strong emotion, stress, eating a heavy meal, or exposure to cold. The classic sequence of angina is activity–pain, rest–relief. The client may describe the pain as a

Box 22–8 Characteristics of Metabolic Syndrome

- Abdominal obesity
- Abnormal blood lipids (low HDL, high triglycerides)
- Hypertension
- Elevated fasting blood glucose
- Clotting tendency
- Inflammatory factors

Box 22–9 Manifestations of Angina

- *Chest pain:* substernal or precordial (across the chest wall); may radiate to neck, arms, shoulders, or jaw
- *Quality:* Tight, squeezing, constricting, or heavy sensation; may also be described as burning, aching, choking, dull, or constant
- *Associated manifestations:* dyspnea, pallor, tachycardia, anxiety, and fear
- *Atypical manifestations:* indigestion, nausea, vomiting, upper back pain
- *Precipitating factors:* exercise or activity, strong emotion, stress, cold, heavy meal
- *Relieving factors:* rest, position change; nitroglycerin

tight, squeezing, heavy pressure or a constricting sensation. It characteristically begins beneath the sternum and may radiate to the jaw, neck, shoulder, or arm. Less characteristically, the pain may be felt in the jaw, epigastric region, or back. Anginal pain usually occurs in a crescendo–decrescendo pattern (increasing to a peak, then gradually decreasing) and typically lasts 2–5 minutes. It generally is relieved by rest. Additional manifestations of angina include dyspnea, pallor, tachycardia, and great anxiety and fear.

Women frequently present with atypical symptoms of angina, including indigestion or nausea, vomiting, fatigue, and upper back pain. The manifestations of angina are summarized in Box 22–9.

The severity of angina can be graded by the degree to which it limits the client's activities. Class I angina does not occur with ordinary physical activities. It is prompted by strenuous, rapid, or prolonged physical exertion. Class II angina may develop with rapid or prolonged walking or stair climbing, whereas Class III angina significantly limits ordinary physical activities. The client with Class IV angina may have angina at rest as well as with any physical activity (Kasper et al., 2005).

Acute Coronary Syndrome

The cardinal manifestation of ACS is chest pain, usually substernal or epigastric. The pain often radiates to the neck, left shoulder, and/or left arm. The pain may occur at rest, and it typically lasts longer than 10–20 minutes. In ACS, the chest pain is more severe and prolonged than that previously experienced by the client. It may be a new onset of pain, or it may represent a pattern of increasing frequency and severity of anginal pain. Dyspnea, diaphoresis, pallor, and cool skin may be present. Tachycardia and hypotension may occur. The client may be nauseated or feel light-headed. Table 22–22 compares the features of stable angina, ACS, and AMI.

Acute Myocardial Infarction

Pain is a classic manifestation of MI. Chest pain resulting from MI is more severe than anginal pain. However, it is not the intensity of the chest pain that distinguishes MI from angina or ACS but its duration and its continuous nature. The onset of pain is sudden and usually is not associated with activity. In

TABLE 22–22 Comparing Stable Angina, Acute Coronary Syndrome, and Acute Myocardial Infarction

	STABLE ANGINA	ACUTE CORONARY SYNDROME	ACUTE MYOCARDIAL INFARCTION
Pathophysiology	Myocardial ischemia occurs with increased workload (e.g., during exercise) as a result of stable atherosclerotic plaque narrowing the coronary arteries	Coronary artery spasm or partial occlusion results from unstable plaque and thrombus formation with increasing myocardial ischemia	Obstruction of a coronary artery by a thrombus blocks the blood supply to a portion of myocardium, resulting in necrosis
Chest pain	Stable and predictable, occurring with exertion or emotion	Occurs at rest; increasing frequency and severity	Begins abruptly, unrelated to rest or exercise
	Crescendo–decrescendo pattern	Lasts 10 minutes or longer	Severe, "crushing"
	May radiate to neck, shoulder, and arms	Radiates to neck, left shoulder, and arm	Unrelieved by rest or nitroglycerin
	Usually lasts 2–5 minutes, relieved by rest		Radiates to arms, neck, and jaw
Other manifestations	Indigestion, nausea	Epigastric pain	Epigastric pain, nausea
	Possible shortness of breath	Dyspnea	Dyspnea
	Anxiety	Tachycardia, hypotension	Pallor, diaphoresis
		Cool, pale skin	Tachycardia or bradycardia, hypertension or hypotension
Diagnosis			
Electrocardiogram	T-wave inversion during anginal episodes	ST-segment depression, T-wave inversion	ST-segment elevation, possible Q wave

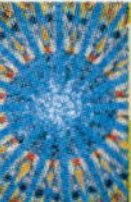

DEVELOPMENTAL CONSIDERATIONS Recognizing Acute Myocardial Infarction in Women and Older Adults

Women and older adults often present with atypical manifestations of myocardial infarction (MI). However, heart disease is the number-one cause of death in both groups, making early recognition and aggressive treatment vital.

Women are more likely than men to have a "silent" or unrecognized heart attack or to present in cardiac arrest or with cardiogenic shock. Women often experience epigastric pain and nausea, causing them to blame their discomfort on heartburn. Shortness of breath is common, as are fatigue and weakness of the shoulders and upper arms.

Older people often seek treatment for vague complaints of difficulty breathing, confusion, fainting, dizziness, abdominal pain, or cough. They often attribute their symptoms to a stroke. The prevalence of silent ischemia is greater in older adults.

Stress the importance of quickly seeking medical help for atypical manifestations of MI. Prompt diagnosis and intervention reduces the mortality and morbidity of MI in women and older adults, just as it does in men. Despite this fact, both women and older adults are more likely to delay seeking treatment and are less likely to be accurately diagnosed and aggressively treated for cardiac heart disease (CHD). Younger women are a particularly important group to reach; their mortality rate when MI occurs is twice that of men (Kasper et al., 2005).

fact, most MIs occur in the early morning. Clients with a history of angina may have more frequent anginal attacks in the days or weeks before an MI (unstable angina or ACS). Chest pain may be described as crushing and severe; as pressure, heaviness, or a squeezing sensation; or as chest tightness or burning. The pain often begins in the center of the chest (substernal) and may radiate to the shoulders, neck, jaw, or arms. It lasts more than 15–20 minutes and is not relieved by rest or nitroglycerin.

Women and older adults often experience atypical chest pain, presenting with complaints of indigestion, heartburn, nausea, and vomiting (see the Developmental Considerations feature that follows). Up to 25% of clients with acute MI deny chest discomfort (Woods et al., 2004).

Compensatory mechanisms cause many of the other symptoms of MI. Sympathetic nervous system stimulation causes anxiety, tachycardia, and vasoconstriction. This results in cool, clammy, mottled skin. Pain and blood chemistry changes stimulate the respiratory center, causing tachypnea. The client often has a sense of impending doom and death. Tissue necrosis causes an inflammatory reaction that increases the white blood cell count and elevates the temperature. Serum cardiac enzyme levels rise as enzymes are released from necrotic cardiac cells.

Other manifestations may vary, depending on the location and amount of infarcted tissue. Hypertension, hypotension, or signs of heart failure may develop. Vagal stimulation may cause nausea and vomiting, bradycardia, and hypotension. Hiccuping may develop as a result of diaphragmatic irritation. If a large vessel is occluded, the first sign of MI may be sudden death. Typical manifestations of MI are listed in Box 22–10.

It is not uncommon for the man experiencing chest pain for the first time to attribute it to indigestion. It is important to help the client overcome his denial in order to promote rapid notification of the emergency medical system, because the first hour following the beginning of chest pain is a time of increased risk for sudden death. If thrombolytics (also called fibrinolytics) are considered for treatment (discussed under Collaboration), it is vitally important to see the client in the emergency department as soon as possible after ischemia occurs.

Refer back to Table 22–22 for a comparison of the signs and symptoms of stable angina, ACS, and AMI.

COMPLICATIONS The risk for complications associated with MI is related to the size and location of the MI.

Dysrhythmias Infarcted tissue is **arrhythmogenic**—that is, it affects the generation and conduction of electrical impulses in the heart. This increases the risk for disturbances or irregularities of heart rhythm (**dysrhythmias**), which are the most frequent complication of MI.

Premature ventricular contractions are common following MI, developing in more than 90% of clients with an acute MI. While not dangerous in themselves, they may be predictive of more dangerous dysrhythmias, such as ventricular tachycardia or ventricular fibrillation (Woods et al., 2004). The risk of ventricular fibrillation is greatest the first hour after MI; it is a frequent cause of sudden cardiac death associated with acute myocardial infarction. Its incidence declines with time.

If the infarct affects a conduction pathway, electrical conduction may be affected. Any degree of AV block may occur following MI, especially when the anterior wall is infarcted.

Box 22–10 Manifestations of Acute Myocardial Infarction

- Chest pain: substernal or precordial (across the entire chest wall); may radiate to neck, jaw, shoulder(s), or left arm
- Tachycardia, tachypnea
- Dyspnea, shortness of breath
- Nausea and vomiting
- Anxiety, sense of impending doom
- Diaphoresis
- Cool, mottled skin; diminished peripheral pulses
- Hypotension or hypertension
- Palpitations, dysrhythmias
- Signs of left heart failure
- Decreased level of consciousness

CLINICAL MANIFESTATIONS AND THERAPIES Coronary Artery Disease

ETIOLOGY	CLINICAL MANIFESTATION	CLINICAL THERAPIES
Damage to cardiac cells as well as anaerobic metabolism, increasing the risk of dysrhythmias	Premature ventricular contractions, tachycardia, heart block, with increased risk for ventricular fibrillation Pulse rate irregularities, may be weak	■ Antiarrhythmic medications ■ Oxygen administration ■ Nitrates to restore cardiac perfusion ■ Placement of stent in coronary artery to restore cardiac perfusion ■ Continuous cardiac monitoring
Increased quantities of lactic acid, causing pain	Feeling of pressure or banding around the chest, with reports of acute and severe pain that may be stabbing or burning and with radiation to the left arm, jaw, back, or neck	■ Administration of an analgesic, often morphine sulfate, which causes coronary vasodilation in addition to pain control ■ Administration of nitrates and oxygen to reduce ischemia ■ Continuous cardiac monitoring
Reduced cardiac output and sympathetic nervous system stimulation, causing tachypnea	Color may be gray or pale, capillary refill time may be delayed if output is significantly reduced, hypotension, symptoms of shock, altered level of consciousness	■ Reduce cardiac workload ■ Administer oxygen ■ Administer vasoconstricting s to improve blood pressure as indicated

First-degree and Mobitz I (Wenckebach) blocks are most common, although complete heart block may develop. **Bradydysrhythmia** (abnormal slow rhythms) also may develop, particularly when the inferior wall of the ventricle is affected.

Pump Failure Myocardial infarction reduces myocardial contractility, ventricular wall motion, and compliance. Impaired contractility and filling may produce pump failure. The risk of heart failure is greatest when large portions of the left ventricle are infarcted. Heart failure may be more severe with an anterior infarction. Loss of 20–30% of the left ventricular muscle mass may cause manifestations of left-sided heart failure, including dyspnea, fatigue, weakness, and respiratory crackles on auscultation. Inferior or right ventricular MI may lead to right-sided heart failure, with manifestations such as neck vein distention and peripheral edema. Hemodynamic monitoring is often initiated for clients with evidence of heart failure.

Cardiogenic Shock **Cardiogenic shock** (impaired tissue perfusion resulting from pump failure), results when functioning myocardial muscle mass decreases by more than 40%. The heart is unable to pump enough blood to meet the needs of the body and maintain organ function. Low cardiac output resulting from cardiogenic shock also impairs perfusion of the coronary arteries and myocardium, further increasing tissue damage. Mortality from cardiogenic shock is greater than 70%, although this can be reduced by prompt intervention with revascularization procedures.

Infarct Extension Approximately 10% of clients experience extension or reinfarction in the area of the original infarction during the first 10–14 days after an MI. Extension of the MI is characterized by increased myocardial necrosis from continued impairment of blood flow and ongoing injury. Expansion of the MI is described as a permanent expansion of the infarcted area from thinning and dilation of the muscle. Infarct extension and expansion may cause manifestations such as continuing chest pain, hemodynamic compromise, and worsening heart failure.

Structural Defects Necrotic muscle is replaced by scar tissue that is thinner than the ventricular muscle mass. This can lead to such complications as ventricular aneurysm, rupture of the interventricular septum or papillary muscle, and myocardial rupture.

A **ventricular aneurysm** is an outpouching of the ventricular wall. It may develop when a large section of the ventricle is replaced by scar tissue. Because it does not contract during systole, stroke volume decreases. Blood may pool within the aneurysm, causing clots to form.

Ischemia of the papillary muscle or chordae tendineae may cause structural damage leading to papillary muscle dysfunction or rupture. This affects AV valve function (usually the mitral valve), causing **regurgitation** (backflow of blood into the atria during systole). The interventricular septum may perforate or rupture as a result of ischemia and infarction.

Myocardial rupture is a risk between days 4 and 7 after MI, when the injured tissue is soft and weak. This potential complication of MI is often fatal.

Pericarditis Tissue necrosis prompts an inflammatory response. **Pericarditis** (inflammation of the pericardial tissue surrounding the heart) may complicate AMI, usually within 2–3 days. Pericarditis causes chest pain that may be aching or sharp and stabbing, and aggravated by movement or deep breathing. A pericardial friction rub may be heard on auscultation of heart sounds.

Dressler syndrome, which is thought to be a hypersensitivity response to necrotic tissue or an autoimmune disorder, may develop days to weeks after AMI. It is a symptom complex characterized by fever, chest pain, and dyspnea. Dressler syndrome may spontaneously resolve or recur over several months, causing significant discomfort and distress.

COLLABORATION

Care of clients with CAD focuses on aggressive risk factor management to slow the atherosclerotic process and maintain myocardial perfusion. Until manifestations of chronic or acute ischemia are experienced, the diagnosis often is presumptive, based on history and the presence of risk factors.

The management of stable angina focuses on maintaining coronary blood flow and cardiac function. Stable angina often can be managed by medical therapy. As for CAD, risk factor management is a vital component of care for the client with angina.

Immediate treatment goals for the MI client are as follows:

- Relieve chest pain.
- Reduce the extent of myocardial damage.
- Maintain cardiovascular stability.
- Decrease cardiac workload.
- Prevent complications.

Slowing the process of CAD and reducing the risk of future MI is a major long-term management goal for the client.

Rapid assessment and early diagnosis is important in treating AMI. "Time is muscle" is a medical truism for the client with AMI. The evolution of an AMI is dynamic: The quicker the artery is reopened (medically, surgically, or spontaneously), the more myocardium can be salvaged. Survival and long-term outcomes following AMI are improved by rapidly restoring blood flow to the "stunned" myocardium surrounding the infracted tissue, reducing myocardial oxygen demand, and limiting the accumulation of toxic by-products of necrosis and reperfusion (Kasper et al., 2005). The AHA recommends initiation of definitive treatment within 1 hour of entry into the health care system. A recent study by De Luca et al. (2004) showed that every minute of delay in treating clients with AMI affects the mortality risk during the first year.

The major problem interfering with timely reperfusion is delay in seeking medical care following the onset of symptoms. Up to 44% of clients with symptoms of chest discomfort or pain wait more than 4 hours before seeking treatment. Many factors are cited as reasons for treatment delay, including advanced age, perception of the seriousness of symptoms, denial, access to medical care, availability of an emergency response system, and in-hospital delays. Immediate evaluation of the client presenting with manifestations of MI is essential to early diagnosis and treatment.

Diagnostic Tests

Laboratory testing is used to assess for risk factors such as an abnormal blood lipid profile (elevated triglyceride and LDL levels and decreased HDL levels). Total serum cholesterol is elevated in hyperlipidemia. A lipid profile also includes triglyceride, HDL, and LDL levels and enables calculation of the ratio of HDL to total cholesterol. The ratio should be at least 1:5, with 1:3 being the ideal ratio. Elevated lipid levels are associated with an increased risk of atherosclerosis (see Table 22–18). In clients with a strong family history of premature CAD or familial hypercholesterolemia, lipoprotein (a) also may be measured. Elevated levels of lipoprotein (a) may independently increase the risk of CAD. Other subsets of blood lipids may also be measured in selected clients.

Diagnostic tests to identify subclinical (asymptomatic) CAD may be indicated when multiple risk factors are present. Relevant diagnostic tests include the following:

- *C-reactive protein* is a serum protein associated with inflammatory processes. Recent evidence suggests that elevated blood levels of this protein may be predictive of CAD.
- *Ankle–brachial blood pressure index (ABI)* is an inexpensive, noninvasive test for peripheral vascular disease that may be predictive of CAD. The systolic blood pressure in the brachial, posterior tibial, and dorsalis pedis arteries is measured by Doppler. An ABI of less than 0.9 in either leg indicates the presence of peripheral arterial disease and a significant risk for CAD.
- *Exercise ECG testing* may be performed. ECGs are used to assess the response to increased cardiac workload induced by exercise. The test is considered "positive" for CAD if myocardial ischemia is detected on the ECG (depression of the ST segment by >3 mm; see Figure 22–33 ■), the client develops chest pain, or the test is stopped because of excess fatigue, dysrhythmias, or other symptoms before the predicted maximal heart rate is achieved.
- *Electron beam computed tomography* creates a three-dimensional image of the heart and coronary arteries that can reveal plaque and other abnormalities. This noninvasive test requires no special preparation and can identify clients at risk for developing myocardial ischemia.

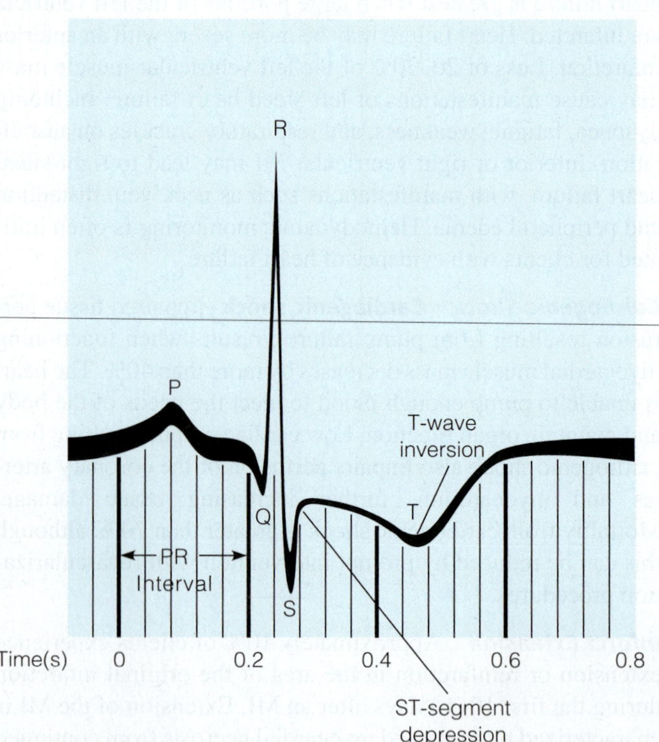

Figure 22–33 ■ ECG changes during an episode of angina. Note characteristic T-wave inversion and ST-segment depression of myocardial ischemia.

- *Myocardial perfusion imaging* may be used to evaluate myocardial blood flow and perfusion, both at rest and during stress testing (exercise or mental stress). Perfusion imaging studies are costly, however, and therefore are not recommended for routine CAD risk assessment.

Diagnostic testing to establish the diagnosis of AMI involves serum levels of **cardiac markers** (proteins released from necrotic heart muscle). These tests are ordered on admission and for 3 succeeding days. Serial blood levels help establish the diagnosis and determine the extent of myocardial damage. The proteins most specific for diagnosis of MI are creatine kinase (CK), or creatine phosphokinase, and cardiac-specific troponins (Table 22–23):

- *Creatine kinase (CK)* is an important enzyme for cellular function found principally in cardiac and skeletal muscle and the brain. CK levels rise rapidly with damage to these tissues, appearing in the serum 4–6 hours after AMI, peaking within 12–24 hours, and then declining over the next 48–72 hours. The CK level correlates with the size of the infarction: The greater the amount of infarcted tissue, the higher the serum CK level.
- **CK-MB** (also called MB-bands) is a subset of CK specific to cardiac muscle. This isoenzyme of CK is considered the most sensitive indicator of MI. Elevated CK alone is not specific for MI; however, elevated CK-MB of greater than 5% is considered a positive indicator of MI. CK-MB levels do not normally rise with chest pain from angina or causes other than MI.
- *Cardiac muscle* **troponins**, *cardiac-specific troponin T (cT_nT), and cardiac-specific troponin I (cT_nI)* are proteins released during MI that are sensitive indicators of myocardial damage. These proteins are part of the actin–myoclin unit in cardiac muscle and normally are not detectable in the blood. With necrosis of cardiac muscle, troponins are released and blood levels rise. The specificity of cT_nT and cT_nI to cardiac muscle necrosis makes these markers particularly useful when skeletal muscle trauma contributes to elevated CK levels (e.g., when CPR has been performed or traumatic injury occurred at the time of the MI). They are sensitive enough to detect very small infarctions that do not cause significant CK elevation. Both cT_nT and cT_nI remain in the blood for 10–14 days after an MI, making them useful to diagnose MI when medical treatment is delayed.

Other laboratory tests may include the following:

- *Myoglobin* is one of the first cardiac markers to be detectable in the blood after an MI. It is released within a few hours of symptom onset. However, its lack of specificity to cardiac muscle and rapid excretion (blood levels return to normal within 24 hours) limit its use (Kasper et al., 2005).
- *Complete blood count* shows an elevated white blood cell count resulting from inflammation of the injured myocardium. The erythrocyte sedimentation rate also rises because of inflammation.
- *Arterial blood gas* may be ordered to assess blood oxygen levels and acid–base balance.

Electrocardiography, echocardiography, and myocardial nuclear scans are the most common diagnostic tests performed when AMI is suspected. With the exception of the ECG, the timing of these tests depends on the client's immediate condition. Hemodynamic monitoring may be initiated in the unstable client following MI. Specifically consider the following:

- The ECG reflects changes in conduction resulting from myocardial ischemia and necrosis. Classic ECG changes seen in AMI include T-wave inversion, ST-segment elevation, and formation of a Q wave. Ischemic changes in the heart are seen as depression of the ST segment or inversion of the T wave (Figure 22–34 ■). With myocardial injury, elevation of the ST segment occurs (Figure 22–35A ■). Significant Q-wave development (Figure 22–27B) indicates a transmural, or full-thickness, infarction. Myocardial damage can be localized using the 12-lead ECG.
- For the client with CAD, diagnostic testing may include stress electrocardiography (exercise stress test), which uses ECGs to monitor the cardiac response to an increased workload during progressive exercise.
- *Echocardiography* is done to evaluate cardiac wall motion and left ventricular function. Stunned and infarcted tissue does not contract as effectively (if at all) as healthy myocardium.

TABLE 22–23 **Cardiac Markers**

				CHANGES OCCURRING WITH MI		
MARKER	NORMAL LEVEL	PRIMARY TISSUE LOCATION	SIGNIFICANCE OF ELEVATION	APPEARS	PEAKS	DURATION
CK (CPK)	Male: 12–80 unit/L Female: 10–70 unit/L	Cardiac muscle, skeletal muscle, brain	Injury to muscle cells	3–6 hr	12–24 hr	24–48 hr
CK-MB	0–3% of total CK	Cardiac muscle	MI, cardiac ischemia, myocarditis, cardiac contusion, defibrillation	4–8 hr	18–24 hr	72 hr
cT_nT	< 0.2 mcg/L	Cardiac muscle	Acute MI, unstable angina	2–4 hr	24–36 hr	10–14 days
cT_nI	< 3.1 mcg/L	Cardiac muscle	Acute MI, unstable angina	2–4 hr	24–36 hr	7–10 days

Note: CK = creatine kinase; CPK = creatine phosphokinase; CK-MB = MB isoenzyme of creatine kinase; cT_nI = cardiac-specific troponin I; cT_nT = cardiac-specific troponin T.

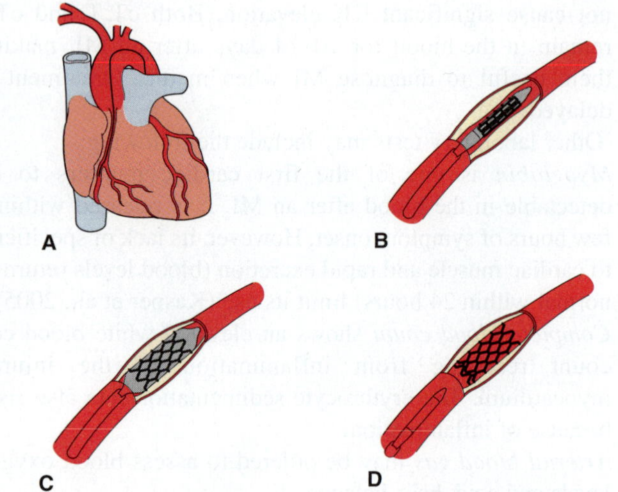

Figure 22–34 ■ Percutaneous coronary revascularization. *A,* The balloon catheter with the stent is threaded into the affected coronary artery. *B, C,* The stent is positioned across the blockage and expanded. The balloon is deflated and removed, leaving the stent in place.

- *Radionuclide imaging* may be done to evaluate myocardial perfusion. These studies cannot differentiate between an acute MI and old scar tissue but do help identify the specific area of myocardial ischemia and damage.
- *Hemodynamic monitoring* may be initiated when AMI significantly affects cardiac output and hemodynamic status.

Conservative Management

Conservative management of CAD focuses on risk factor modification, including smoking, diet, exercise, and management of contributing conditions, such as hypertension and diabetes.

SMOKING Smoking cessation reduces the risk for CAD within months after quitting and improves cardiovascular status. People who quit reduce their risk by 50%, regardless of how long they smoked before quitting. For women, the risk becomes equivalent to a nonsmoker within 3–5 years of smoking cessation (Woods et al., 2004). In addition, stopping smoking improves HDL levels, lowers LDL levels, and reduces blood viscosity. All smokers are advised to quit. Health promotion activities focus on preventing children, teenagers, and adults from starting to smoke.

DIET Dietary recommendations by the NCEP (2002) include reduced saturated fat and cholesterol intake as well as strategies to lower LDL levels (Table 22–24). Most fats are a mixture of saturated and unsaturated fatty acids. The highest proportions of saturated fat are found in whole-milk products, red meats, and coconut oil. Nonfat dairy products, fish, and poultry as primary protein sources are recommended. Solidified vegetable fats (e.g., margarine and shortening) contain *trans* fatty acids, which behave more like saturated fats. Soft margarines and vegetable oil spreads contain low levels of *trans* fatty acids and should be used instead of butter, stick margarine, and shortening. Monounsaturated fats, found in olive, canola, and peanut oils, actually lower LDL and cholesterol levels. Certain cold-water fish, such as tuna, salmon, and mackerel, contain high levels of omega-3 fatty acids, which

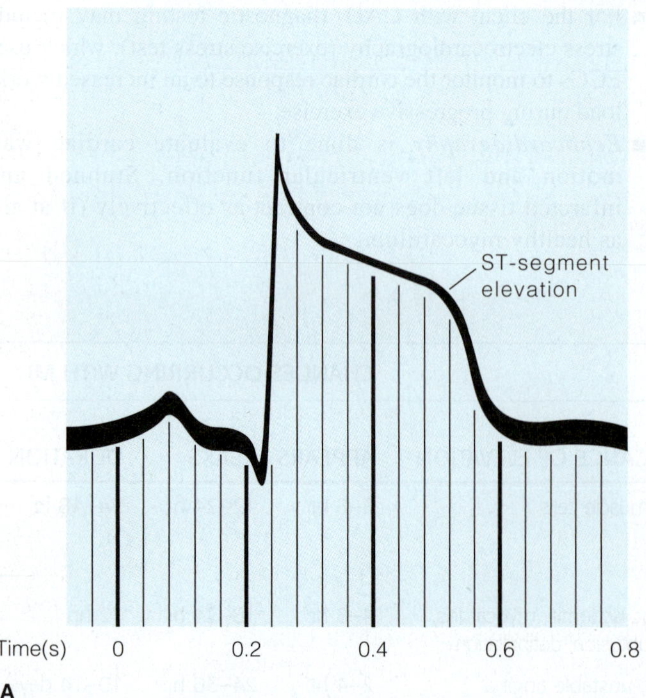

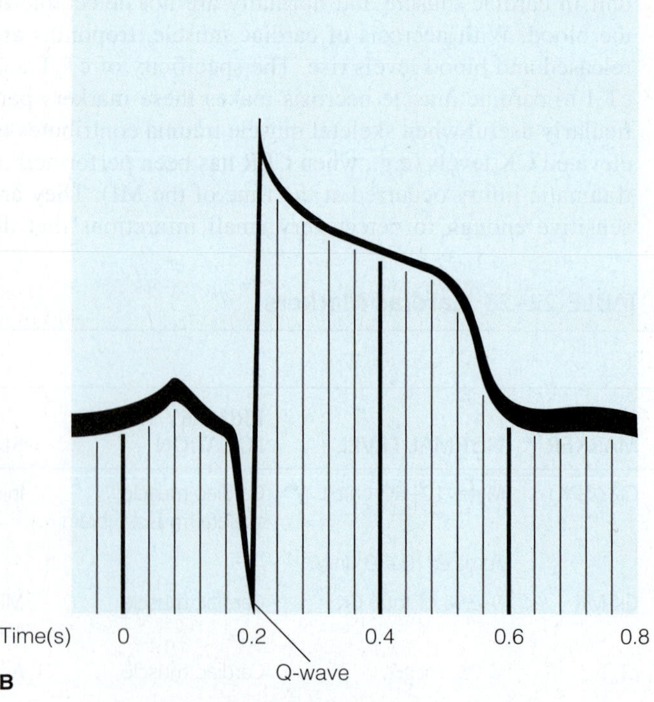

Figure 22–35 ■ ECG changes characteristic of MI. *A,* ST-segment elevation characteristic of myocardial injury. *B,* Clinically significant Q-wave characteristic of a transmural infarction.

TABLE 22–24 Dietary Recommendations From the National Cholesterol Education Program

NUTRIENT	RECOMMENDATION
Calories	Adjusted to attain/maintain desirable body weight
Total fat	25–35% of total calories
■ Saturated fats	■ < 7% of total calories
■ Polyunsaturated fat	■ ≤ 10% of total calories
■ Monounsaturated fat	■ 20% of total calories
■ Cholesterol	■ < 200 mg/day
Carbohydrate (primarily complex carbohydrates; e.g., whole grains, fruits, and vegetables)	50–60% of total calories
Dietary fiber	20–30 g/day
Protein	~15% of total calories

Source: Compiled from NCEP (2002).

help raise HDL levels and decrease serum triglycerides, total serum cholesterol, and blood pressure.

In addition, increased intake of soluble fiber (found in oats, psyllium, pectin-rich fruit, and beans) and insoluble fiber (found in whole grains, vegetables, and fruit) is recommended. Folic acid and vitamins B_6 and B_{12} affect homocysteine metabolism, reducing serum levels. Leafy green vegetables (e.g., spinach and broccoli) and legumes (e.g., black-eyed peas, dried beans, and lentils) are rich sources of folate. Meat, fish, and poultry are rich in vitamins B_6 and B_{12}. Vitamin B_6 also is found in soy products; vitamin B_{12} is in fortified cereals. Increased intake of antioxidant nutrients (vitamin E, in particular) and foods rich in antioxidants (fruits and vegetables) appears to increase HDL levels and have a protective effect against CAD.

In middle-aged and older adults, moderate alcohol intake may reduce the risk for CAD (NCEP, 2002). Consumption of no more than two drinks per day for men or one drink per day for women is recommended. A drink is 5 ounces of wine, 12 ounces of beer, or 1.5 ounces of whiskey. People who do not drink alcohol, however, should not be encouraged to start consuming it as a heart-protective measure.

People who are overweight or obese are encouraged to lose weight through a combination of reduced calorie intake (maintaining a nutritionally sound diet) and increased exercise. High-protein, high-fat weight loss programs are not recommended for weight reduction.

EXERCISE Regular physical exercise reduces the risk for CAD in several ways. It lowers VLDL, LDL, and triglyceride levels, and it raises HDL levels. Regular exercise reduces blood pressure and insulin resistance. Unless contraindicated, all clients are encouraged to participate in at least 30 minutes of moderate-intensity physical activity 5–6 days each week. To achieve weight loss and prevent weight gain, 60–90 minutes of moderate-intensity exercise daily is recommended (U.S. Department of Health and Human Services, 2005).

HYPERTENSION Although hypertension often cannot be prevented or cured, it can be controlled. Hypertension control (maintaining a blood pressure of <140/90 mmHg) is vital to reduce its atherosclerosis-promoting effects and the workload of the heart. Management strategies include reducing sodium intake, increasing calcium intake, regular exercise, stress management, and medications.

DIABETES Diabetes increases the risk of CAD by accelerating the atherosclerotic process. Weight loss (if appropriate), reduced fat intake, and exercise are particularly important for the client with diabetes. Because hyperglycemia apparently also contributes to atherosclerosis, consistent blood glucose management is vital.

Pharmacologic Therapies

Medications are used extensively, both in treatment of existing cardiac disease as well as in prevention. A number of drug groups are useful.

DRUGS USED TO LOWER CHOLESTEROL Drug therapy to lower total serum cholesterol and LDL levels and to raise HDL levels now is an integral part of CAD management (Box 22–11). This therapy is used in conjunction with diet and other lifestyle changes and is based on the client's overall risk for CAD.

Drugs used to treat hyperlipidemia act specifically by lowering LDL levels. The goal of treatment is to achieve an LDL level of less than 130 mg/dL (NCEP, 2002). Medications to treat hyperlipidemia are not inexpensive; the cost–benefit ratio needs to be considered, because long-term treatment may be required. The four major classes of cholesterol-lowering drugs are statins, bile acid sequestrants, nicotinic acid, and fibrates.

The statins, including lovastatin (Mevacor), pravastatin (Pravachol), simvastatin (Zocor), and others, are first-line drugs for treating hyperlipidemia. They effectively lower LDL levels and may also increase HDL levels. The statins can cause myopathy; all clients are instructed to report muscle pain and weakness or brown urine. Liver function tests are monitored during therapy, because these drugs may increase liver enzyme levels.

The other cholesterol-lowering drugs, such as the bile acid sequestrants, nicotinic acid, and fibrates, are primarily used

Box 22–11 Medication Administration: Cholesterol-Lowering Drugs

STATINS

Lovastatin (Mevacor)
Pravastatin (Pravachol)
Simvastatin (Zocor)
Fluvastatin (Lescol)
Atorvastatin (Lipitor)

Statins inhibit the enzyme 3-hydroxy-3-methylglutaryl coenzyme A reductase in the liver, lowering low-density lipoprotein (LDL) synthesis and serum levels. The statins are first-line treatment for elevated LDL and are used in conjunction with diet and lifestyle changes. Although their side effects are minimal, they may cause increased serum liver enzyme levels and myopathy.

Nursing Responsibilities

- Monitor serum cholesterol and liver enzyme levels before and during therapy. Report elevated liver enzyme levels.
- Assess for muscle pain and tenderness. Monitor creatine phosphokinase level if present.
- If taking digoxin concurrently, monitor for and report digoxin toxicity.

Health Education for the Client and Family

- Promptly report muscle pain, tenderness, or weakness; skin rash, hives, or changes in skin color; abdominal pain, nausea, or vomiting.
- Do not use these drugs if you are pregnant or plan to become pregnant.
- Inform your doctor if you are taking any other medications concurrently.

BILE ACID SEQUESTRANTS

Cholestyramine (Questran)
Colestipol (Colestid)
Colesevelam (Welchol)

Bile acid sequestrants lower LDL levels by binding bile acids in the intestine, reducing their reabsorption and cholesterol production in the liver. These medications are used in combination therapy regimens and for women who are considering pregnancy. Their primary disadvantages are inconvenience of administration (because of bulk) and gastrointestinal side effects (e.g., constipation).

Nursing Responsibilities

- Mix cholestyramine and colestipol powders with 4–6 oz of water or juice; administer once or twice a day as ordered with meals.
- Store in a tightly closed container.

Health Education for the Client and Family

- Promptly report constipation, severe gastric distress with nausea and vomiting, unexplained weight loss, black or bloody stools, or sudden back pain to your doctor.
- Drinking ample amounts of fluid while taking these drugs reduces problems of constipation and bloating.
- Do not omit doses, because this may affect the absorption of other drugs you are taking.

NICOTINIC ACID

Niacin (Nicobid, Nicolar, Niaspan, others)

Nicotinic acid in both prescription and nonprescription forms lowers total and LDL cholesterol and triglyceride levels. The crystalline form and Niaspan, a prescription extended-release tablet, also raise HDL levels. Because the doses required to achieve significant cholesterol-lowering effects are associated with multiple side effects, nicotinic acid generally is used in combination therapy, particularly with the statin drugs.

Nursing Responsibilities

- Give oral preparations with meals accompanied by a cold beverage to minimize gastrointestinal effects.
- Administer with caution to clients who have active liver disease, peptic ulcer disease, gout, or type 2 diabetes.
- Monitor blood glucose, uric acid levels, and liver function tests during treatment.

Health Education for the Client and Family

- Flushing of the face, neck, and ears may occur within 2 hours following dose; these effects generally subside as treatment continues. Alcohol use during nicotinic acid therapy may worsen this effect.
- Report weakness or dizziness with changes in posture (lying to sitting; sitting to standing) to your doctor. Change positions slowly to reduce the risk of injury.

FIBRIC ACID DERIVATIVES

Gemfibrozil (Lopid)
Fenofibrate (Tricor)
Clofibrate (Atromid-S)

The fibrates are used to lower serum triglyceride levels; they have only a slight to modest effect on LDL. They affect lipid regulation by blocking triglyceride synthesis. They are used to treat very high triglyceride levels and may be used in combination with statins.

Nursing Responsibilities

- Monitor serum LDL and VLDL levels, electrolytes, glucose, liver enzymes, renal function tests, and complete blood count during therapy. Report abnormal values.
- Up to 2 months of treatment may be required to achieve a therapeutic effect; rebound, with decreasing benefit, may occur in the second or third month of treatment.

Health Education for the Client and Family

- Take with meals if the drug causes gastric distress.
- Promptly report flulike symptoms (e.g., fatigue, muscle aching, soreness, or weakness) to your doctor.
- Do not use this drug if you are pregnant or plan to become pregnant. Use reliable birth control measures while taking this drug.
- Contact your doctor before stopping this drug and before taking any over-the-counter preparations.

when combination therapy is required to effectively lower serum cholesterol levels. They also may be used for selected clients, such as younger adults and women who wish to become pregnant, or to specifically lower triglyceride levels.

Clients at high risk for MI are often started on prophylactic low-dose aspirin therapy. The dose ranges from 80–325 mg/day (Tierney et al., 2005). In women, the benefit of low-dose aspirin in reducing the risk for CAD is not clear before age 65 (NHLBI, 2005). Aspirin is contraindicated for clients with a history of aspirin sensitivity, bleeding disorders, or active peptic ulcer disease. Angiotensin-converting enzyme inhibitors or angiotensin-receptor blockers also may be prescribed for high-risk clients, including those with diabetes or those with other CAD risk factors.

DRUGS USED TO TREAT ANGINA Drugs may be used for both acute and long-term relief of angina. The goal of drug treatment is to reduce oxygen demand and increase oxygen supply to the myocardium. Three main classes of drugs are used to treat angina: nitrates, beta-blockers, and calcium-channel blockers.

Nitrates Nitrates, including nitroglycerin and longer-acting nitrate preparations, are used to treat acute anginal attacks and prevent angina.

Sublingual nitroglycerin is the drug of choice to treat acute angina. It acts within 1–2 minutes, decreasing myocardial work and oxygen demand through venous and arterial dilation, which in turn reduce preload and afterload. It may also improve myocardial oxygen supply by dilating collateral blood vessels and reducing stenosis. Rapid-acting nitroglycerin is also available as a buccal spray in a metered system. For some clients, this may be easier to handle than small nitroglycerin tablets.

Longer-acting nitroglycerin preparations (oral tablets, ointment, or transdermal patches) are used to prevent attacks of angina, not to treat an acute attack. The primary problem with long-term nitrate use is the development of tolerance (a decreasing effect from the same dose of medication). Tolerance can be limited by a dosing schedule that allows a nitrate-free period of at least 8–10 hours daily. This is usually scheduled at night, when angina is less likely to occur.

Headache is a common side effect of nitrates and may limit their usefulness. Nausea, dizziness, and hypotension are also common effects of therapy.

Beta-Blockers Beta-blockers, including propranolol, metoprolol, nadolol, and atenolol, are considered first-line drugs to treat stable angina. They block the cardiac-stimulating effects of norepinephrine and epinephrine, preventing anginal attacks by reducing heart rate, myocardial contractility, and blood pressure, thus reducing myocardial oxygen demand. Beta-blockers may be used alone or with other medications to prevent angina.

Beta-blockers are contraindicated for clients with asthma or severe chronic obstructive pulmonary disease, because they may cause severe bronchospasm. They are not used in clients with significant bradycardia or AV conduction blocks, and they are used cautiously in clients with heart failure. Beta-blockers are not used to treat Prinzmetal's angina, because they may make it worse.

Calcium-Channel Blockers Calcium-channel blockers reduce myocardial oxygen demand and increase myocardial blood and oxygen supply. These drugs (which include verapamil, diltiazem, and nifedipine) lower blood pressure, reduce myocardial contractility, and in some cases, lower heart rate, decreasing myocardial oxygen demand. They are also potent coronary vasodilators, effectively increasing oxygen supply. Like beta-blockers, calcium-channel blockers act too slowly to effectively treat an acute attack of angina; they are used for long-term prophylaxis. Because they may actually increase ischemia and mortality in clients with heart failure or left ventricular dysfunction, however, these drugs are not usually prescribed in the initial treatment of angina. They are used cautiously in clients with dysrhythmias, heart failure, or hypotension.

Aspirin The client with angina, particularly unstable angina, is at risk for MI because of significant narrowing of the coronary arteries. Low-dose aspirin (80–325 mg/day) is often prescribed to reduce the risk of platelet aggregation and thrombus formation.

DRUGS USED TO TREAT MYOCARDIAL INFARCTION Fibrinolytic, analgesic, and antidysrhythmic agents are among the principal classes of drugs used in treating AMI. In addition, aspirin, a platelet inhibitor, is now considered an essential part of treating AMI. A 160- to 325-mg aspirin tablet is given by emergency personnel, with the instruction that it is to be chewed (for buccal absorption). This initial dose is followed by a daily oral dose of 160–325 mg.

Analgesics Pain relief is vital in treating the client with AMI. Pain stimulates the sympathetic nervous system, increasing the heart rate and blood pressure and, in turn, the myocardial workload. Sublingual nitroglycerin may be given (up to three 0.4-mg doses at 5-minute intervals). Intravenous nitroglycerin may be continued for the first 24– 48 hours to reduce myocardial work. In addition to pain relief, nitroglycerin decreases myocardial oxygen demand and may increase the supply of oxygen to the myocardium. Nitroglycerin is a peripheral and arterial vasodilator that reduces afterload. It dilates coronary arteries and collateral channels in the heart, increasing coronary blood flow to save myocardial tissue at risk. Nitrates may, however, cause reflex tachycardia or excessive hypotension, so close monitoring is necessary during administration. It also is important to ask the client about use of sildenafil (Viagra) within the 24 hours before administering nitroglycerin, because the combination can precipitate a significant drop in blood pressure.

Morphine sulfate is the drug of choice for pain unrelieved by nitroglycerin and for sedation. Following an initial intravenous dose of 4–8 mg, small doses (2–4 mg) may be repeated intravenously every 5 minutes until pain is relieved. It is important to assess frequently for pain relief and possible adverse effects of analgesia, such as excessive sedation. Pain unrelieved by expected or usual doses should be reported to the physician, because it may indicate a complication such as extension of the infarct. Antianxiety agents such as diazepam (Valium) may also be administered to promote rest.

Fibrinolytics Fibrinolytic agents, which are drugs that dissolve or break up blood clots, are first-line drugs used to treat acute MI when access to a cardiac catheterization lab for revascularization procedures is not immediately available. Fibrinolytic drugs activate the fibrinolytic system to lyse, or destroy, the clot, restoring blood flow to the obstructed artery. Early fibrinolytic administration (within the first 6 hours of MI onset) limits infarct size, reduces heart damage, and improves outcomes. Activation of the fibrinolytic system can cause multiple complications; approximately 0.5–5% of clients receiving fibrinolytic drugs experience serious bleeding complications. In addition, not every client is a candidate for fibrinolytic therapy; for example, it is contraindicated in clients with known bleeding disorders, history of cerebrovascular disease, uncontrolled hypertension, pregnancy, or recent trauma or surgery of the head or spine (Tierney et al., 2005).

Several fibrinolytic agents are commonly used today. Among these, little difference in effectiveness has been demonstrated; there are, however, big differences in cost. Streptokinase, a biologic agent derived from group C *Streptococcus* organisms, is the least expensive of the drugs. Its primary drawback is the risk for a severe hypersensitivity reaction, including anaphylaxis. Streptokinase is administered by intravenous infusion. Anisoylated plasminogen streptokinase activator complex, or APSAC, is a related drug that can be administered by bolus over 2–5 minutes. It has many of the same effects as streptokinase but is considerably more expensive. Tissue plasminogen activator, tenecteplase, and reteplase are more effective in reestablishing myocardial perfusion, especially when the pain developed more than 3 hours previously. These drugs, however, are the most expensive.

Antidysrhythmics Dysrhythmias are a common complication of AMI, particularly in the first 12–24 hours. Antidysrhythmic medications are used as needed to treat dysrhythmias. They also may be given prophylactically to prevent dysrhythmias. Ventricular dysrhythmias are treated with a class I or class III antidysrhythmic. Symptomatic bradycardia (bradycardia with associated hypotension and other signs of low cardiac output) is treated with intravenous atropine, 0.5–1 mg. Intravenous verapamil or the short-acting beta-blocker esmolol (Brevibloc) may be ordered to treat atrial fibrillation or other supraventricular tachydysrhythmias.

Other Medications Beta-blockers such as propranolol (Inderal), atenolol (Tenormin), and metoprolol (Lopressor) reduce pain, limit infarct size, and decrease the incidence of serious ventricular dysrhythmias in AMI. These drugs decrease the heart rate, reducing cardiac work and myocardial oxygen demand. Initial doses are given intravenously. Oral beta-blocker therapy is continued to reduce the risk of reinfarction and death related to cardiovascular causes (Kasper et al., 2005).

Angiotensin-converting enzyme inhibitors also reduce mortality associated with AMI. These drugs reduce ventricular remodeling following an MI, reducing the risk for subsequent heart failure. They also may reduce the risk of reinfarction (Kasper et al., 2002).

Anticoagulants and antiplatelet medications often are prescribed to maintain coronary artery patency following thrombolysis or a revascularization procedure. Abciximab (ReoPro) suppresses platelet aggregation and reduces the risk of reocclusion following angioplasty. It also improves vessel opening with fibrinolytic therapy, permitting lower doses of fibrinolytic drugs. Standard or low-molecular-weight heparin preparations often are given to clients with AMI. Heparin helps establish and maintain patency of the affected coronary artery. It also is used, along with long-term warfarin, to prevent systemic or pulmonary embolism in clients with significant left ventricular impairment or atrial fibrillation following AMI. See Box 22–12 for the nursing implications of antiplatelet drugs.

Clients with pump failure and hypotension may receive intravenous dopamine, a vasopressor. At low doses (< 5 mg • kg^{-1} • min^{-1}), it improves blood flow to the kidneys, preventing renal ischemia and possible acute renal failure. With increasing doses, dopamine increases myocardial contractility and causes vasoconstriction, improving blood pressure and cardiac output.

Antilipemic agents are used for the client with hyperlipidemia. A stool softener, such as docusate sodium, is prescribed to maintain normal bowel function and reduce straining.

Clinical Therapies

The client with a suspected or confirmed MI is monitored continuously. Care is provided in the intensive coronary care unit for the first 24–48 hours, after which time less intensive monitoring (e.g., telemetry) may be required. An intravenous line is established to allow rapid administration of emergency medications.

Bedrest is prescribed for the first 12 hours to reduce the cardiac workload. The bedside commode generally is allowed; studies have shown this to be less stressful than using a bedpan. If the client's condition is stable, sitting in a chair at the bedside is permitted after 12 hours. Activities are gradually increased as tolerated. A quiet, calm environment with limited outside stimuli is preferred. Visitors are limited to promote rest. Oxygen is administered by nasal cannula at 2–5 L/minute to improve oxygenation of the myocardium and other tissues.

A liquid diet may be prescribed for the first 4–12 hours to reduce gastric distention and myocardial work. Following that, a low-fat, low-cholesterol, reduced-sodium diet is allowed. Sodium restrictions may be lifted after 2–3 days if no evidence of heart failure is present. Small, frequent feedings are often recommended. Drinks containing caffeine, as well as very hot and cold foods, may also be limited.

Revascularization Procedures

Several procedures may be used to restore blood flow and oxygen to ischemic tissue. Nonsurgical techniques include transluminal coronary angioplasty, laser angioplasty, coronary atherectomy, and intracoronary stents. Coronary artery bypass grafting (CABG) is a surgical procedure that may be used.

PERCUTANEOUS CORONARY REVASCULARIZATION

Percutaneous coronary revascularization (PCR) procedures are used to restore blood flow to the ischemic myocardium in clients with CAD. Approximately 600,000 PCR procedures are done annually in the United States. PCR is used to treat clients with the following:

- Moderately severe, chronic stable angina unrelieved by medical therapy
- Unstable angina
- AMI
- Significant stenosis of the left anterior descending coronary artery
- Stenosis of a CABG (Kasper et al., 2005; Tierney et al., 2005).

Box 22–12 **Medication Administration: Antiplatelet Drugs**

ORAL ANTIPLATELET DRUGS

Aspirin
Clopidogrel (Plavix)

Antiplatelet drugs suppress platelet aggregation in arteries, preventing the development of an arterial thrombus. Aspirin and clopidogrel block different platelet activation pathways to inhibit platelet aggregation and clot formation. The dose of aspirin given to achieve antiplatelet effects is low, typically 80–25 mg/day.

Nursing Responsibilities

- Inquire about a history of intracranial hemorrhage, upper gastrointestinal bleeding, peptic ulcer disease, or known bleeding tendency.
- Observe for and report increased bruising, petechiae, purpura, and apparent or occult bleeding (e.g., melena and hematemesis).
- Do not administer concurrently with warfarin (Coumadin).

Health Education for the Client and Family

- Take as directed. Take aspirin with food or milk; clopidogrel may be taken at any time of day.
- Do not use nonsteroidal anti-inflammatory drugs (NSAIDs) or other over-the-counter drugs that may contain aspirin or an NSAID unless prescribed by your physician.
- Check with your physician before using any herbal remedies, such as evening primrose oil, feverfew, garlic, ginkgo biloba, or grapeseed extract, while taking these medications.
- Report unusual bruising or excessive bleeding.
- Inform all care providers (including dental professionals) about use of these drugs.

INTRAVENOUS ANTIPLATELET DRUGS

Abciximab (ReoPro)
Eptifibatide (Integrelin)
Tirofiban (Aggrastat)

The intravenously administered antiplatelet drugs abciximab, epifibatide, and tirofiban, block the final common pathway of platelet activation and thus are more effective than the orally administered antiplatelet drugs. However, the risk of bleeding is greater than with the orally administered antiplatelet drugs.

Nursing Responsibilities

- Determine history of bleeding disorders, intracranial hemorrhage, or recent trauma or surgery.
- Inquire about recent use of oral antiplatelet or anticoagulant drugs.
- Monitor complete blood count, including hemoglobin, hematocrit, and platelet count; clotting studies, including prothrombin time, International Normalized Ratio, partial thromboplastin time; vital signs; and electrocardiogram during therapy.
- Maintain separate intravenous lines for blood draws and for administration of other drugs during infusion.
- Closely observe for and immediately report anaphylaxis or bleeding uncontrolled by pressure. Keep resuscitation equipment readily available.
- Maintain bedrest during infusion.

Health Education for the Client and Family

- This drug is given to reduce the risk of clotting and myocardial infarction. It helps maintain blood flow through the affected vessel following angioplasty and stent placement.
- Immediately report any chest tightness, difficulty breathing, shortness of breath, or itching that develops during the infusion.
- Your risk of bleeding should return to normal within about 2 days following the infusion.
- Immediately report any unusual bruising or bleeding to your doctor.

The PCR procedures are similar to the procedure used for coronary angiography. A catheter introduced into the arterial circulation is guided into the opening of the narrowed coronary artery. A flexible guidewire is inserted through the catheter lumen into the affected vessel. The guidewire is then used to thread an angioplasty balloon, arterial stent, or other therapeutic device into the narrowed segment of the artery. The procedure is performed in the cardiac catheterization laboratory using local anesthesia. The hospital stay is short (1–2 days), minimizing costs.

In a percutaneous transluminal coronary angioplasty, a balloon-tipped catheter is threaded over the guidewire, with the balloon positioned across the area of narrowing (see Figure 22–34). The balloon is inflated in a step-by-step fashion for approximately 30 seconds to 2 minutes to compress the plaque against the arterial wall, with a goal of reducing the vessel obstruction to less than 50% of the arterial lumen. Percutaneous transluminal coronary angioplasty typically is accompanied by placement of a stent. Intracoronary stents are metallic scaffolds used to maintain an open arterial lumen. Stents reduce the rate of restenosis following angioplasty by about one-third and are now used in the majority of all PCR procedures (Kasper et al., 2005). The stent is placed over a balloon catheter, guided into position, and expanded as the balloon is inflated. It then remains in the artery as a prop after the balloon is removed. Endothelial cells will completely line the inner wall of the stent to produce a smooth inner lining. Antiplatelet medications (aspirin and ticlopidine) are given following stent insertion to reduce the risk of thrombus formation at the site. Nursing care of the client having a PCR is described in Box 22–13.

In contrast to stent procedures, which enlarge the artery by displacing plaque, atherectomy procedures remove plaque from the identified lesion. The directional atherectomy catheter shaves the plaque off vessel walls using a rotary cutting head, retaining the fragments in its housing and removing them from the vessel. Rotational atherectomy catheters pulverize plaque into particles small enough to pass through the coronary microcirculation. Laser atherectomy devices use laser energy to remove plaque.

Complications following PCR procedures include hematoma at the catheter insertion site, pseudoaneurysm, embolism, hypersensitivity to contrast dye, dysrhythmias,

Box 22–13 Nursing Care of the Client Having Percutaneous Coronary Revascularization

BEFORE THE PROCEDURE

- Assess the client's knowledge of the procedure and expectations of treatment. *This allows information to be tailored to the client's needs and provides an opportunity to clarify misconceptions.*
- Describe the cardiac catheterization laboratory and the planned PCR procedure. Include the following topics:
  a. Preoperative preparation
  b. Planned anesthesia or sedation to be used
  c. Drugs that may be given during the procedure, such as anticoagulants to reduce the risk of thrombus formation and intravenous nitroglycerin and a calcium-channel blocker to dilate coronary arteries and prevent anginal pain.
- Discuss possible sensations during the procedure, including flushing or warmth, a metallic taste in the mouth as the contrast dye is injected, and a feeling of pressure or chest pain during balloon inflation. *Advanced preparation for expected sensations reduces anxiety and improves outcomes.*
- Perform a comprehensive assessment, including hydration status (skin and mucous membrane moisture, turgor) and peripheral circulation (color, warmth, sensation, pulses, and capillary refill). *Hydration status may be impacted by medications or fluid restriction and both hydration and peripheral circulation is an indicator of perfusion.*

AFTER THE PROCEDURE

- Complete a head-to-toe assessment. Note any complaints of chest pain or evidence of decreased cardiac output or myocardial infarction. *Assessment provides a baseline for subsequent assessments and allows early identification of possible complications.*
- Monitor vital signs and cardiac rhythm continuously. Treat dysrhythmias as ordered. Obtain a 12-lead electrocardiogram if signs of ischemia develop, and notify the physician. *Vital signs reflect cardiac output. Dysrhythmias may develop with reperfusion of the ischemic myocardium. Electrocardiographic changes may indicate infarction or restenosis of the affected vessel.*
- Maintain intravenous nitroglycerin infusion. Administer anticoagulant and antiplatelet medications, nitrates, and calcium-channel blockers as ordered. *These drugs decrease oxygen demand and increase oxygen supply by dilating the coronary arteries and systemic vasculature. They also reduce the risk of thrombus formation.*
- Monitor for and treat or report chest pain as indicated. *Chest pain may indicate ischemia and possible myocardial infarction.*
- Maintain bedrest as ordered, with the head of the bed at an angle of 30° or less. Prevent flexion of the leg on the affected side. Following sheath removal, follow protocol for pressure dressing or device or sandbag placement. *A large puncture wound occurs at the insertion site. Immobilization allows the wound to seal; a pressure dressing helps prevent bleeding.*
- Monitor distal pulses, color, movement, sensation, and temperature of the affected leg and insertion site every 15 minutes for the first hour, every 30 minutes for the next hour, every hour for the next 8 hours, and then every 4 hours. *A clot may form at the site, reducing perfusion of the affected leg. The site and dressing are monitored for excessive bleeding, hematoma formation, or pseudoaneurysm. Pseudoaneurysm occurs as a result of inadequate hemostasis after catheter removal.*
- Monitor intake and output, serum electrolytes, blood urea nitrogen, creatinine, complete blood count, partial thromboplastin time, and cardiac enzymes. Report abnormal results to the physician. *Contrast dye causes osmotic diuresis and may cause renal damage or a hypersensitivity reaction. Electrolyte imbalances increase the risk of dysrhythmias. Cardiac enzymes are monitored for indications of possible myocardial damage during the procedure. The partial thromboplastin time monitors the effectiveness of heparin therapy.*
- Monitor for bradycardia, light-headedness, hypotension, diaphoresis, and loss of consciousness during sheath removal. Keep atropine at bedside during sheath removal. *Bradycardia and signs of decreased cardiac output may occur during sheath removal because of a vasovagal reaction. Atropine decreases vagal tone and increases heart rate.*

bleeding, vessel perforation, and restenosis or reocclusion of the treated vessel.

CORONARY ARTERY BYPASS GRAFTING Surgery for CAD involves using a section of a vein or an artery to create a connection, or bypass, between the aorta and the coronary artery beyond the obstruction (Figure 22–36 ■). This allows blood to perfuse the ischemic portion of the heart. The internal mammary artery (IMA) in the chest and the saphenous vein from the leg are the vessels most commonly used for CABG.

Bypass grafts are safe and effective. Angina is totally relieved or significantly reduced in 90% of clients who undergo complete revascularization. While anginal pain may recur within 3 years, it rarely is as severe as before surgery. CABG has a positive effect on mortality in many cases. It is recommended for clients who have multiple-vessel disease and impaired left ventricular function or diabetes and for clients who have significant obstruction of the left main coronary artery (Kasper et al., 2005).

A median sternotomy commonly is used to access the heart. The heart is usually stopped during surgery. A cardiopulmonary bypass (CPB) pump is used to maintain perfusion to the rest of the organs during open-heart surgery. Venous blood is removed from the body through a cannula placed in the right atrium or the superior and inferior venae cavae. Blood then circulates through the CPB pump, where it is oxygenated, has its temperature regulated, and is filtered. Oxygenated blood is returned to the body through a cannula in the ascending aorta (Figure 22–37 ■). CPB enables surgeons to operate on a quiet heart and a relatively bloodless field. Hypothermia can be maintained to reduce the metabolic rate and decrease oxygen demand during surgery.

Newer techniques have been developed that allow surgeons to perform CABG without cardioplegia (stopping the heart) and CPB. Off-pump coronary artery bypass (OPCAB) allows use of a smaller incision for access. Although CPB is employed for the majority of coronary artery bypass procedures, OPCAB

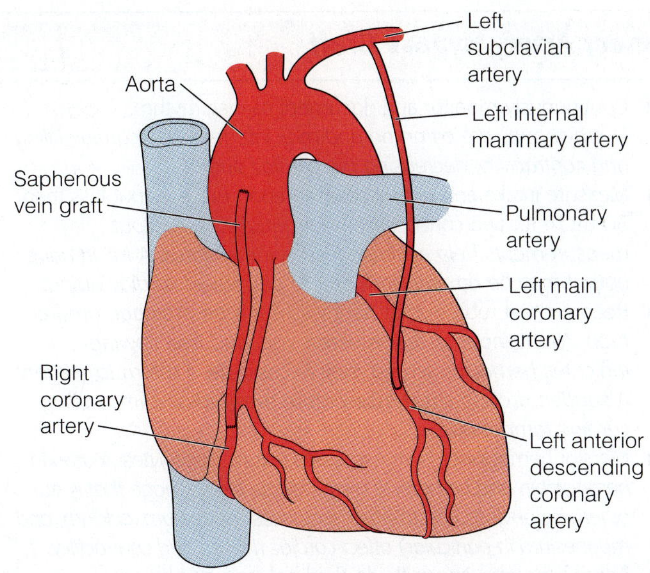

Figure 22–36 ■ Coronary artery bypass grafting using the internal mammary artery and a saphenous vein graft.

is a promising alternative. Controlled studies demonstrate lower mortality and morbidity rates as well as faster recovery for clients undergoing OPCAB as compared to CABG with CPB (Eagle et al., 2004).

When the saphenous vein is used for the graft, it is excised from its normal attachments in the leg, flushed with a cold heparinized saline solution, and then reversed so that its valves do not interfere with blood flow. When appropriate, a laparoscopic approach may be used to remove the vein. The vein is anastomosed (grafted) to the aorta and the coronary artery, distal to the occlusion (see Figure 22–36). This provides a bridge, or conduit, for blood flow past the obstruction. If the IMA is used, its distal end is excised and anastomosed to the coronary artery distal to the obstruction. The IMA often is used to revascularize the left coronary artery because of the greater oxygen demand of the left ventricle.

Once grafting is completed, CPB is discontinued and the client is rewarmed. Rewarming stimulates the heart to resume beating. Temporary pacing wires are sutured in place and passed through the chest wall in case temporary pacing is necessary. Chest tubes are placed in the pleural space and mediastinum to drain blood and reestablish negative pressure in the thoracic cavity. The sternum is closed using heavy wires and bone wax. The skin is closed with sutures or staples, and sterile dressings are applied over sternal and leg incisions. Nursing care of the client having a CABG is described in Box 22–14.

MINIMALLY INVASIVE CORONARY ARTERY SURGERY Minimally invasive coronary artery surgery is a potential future alternative to CABG. Two approaches may be used: Port-access coronary artery bypass uses several small holes, or

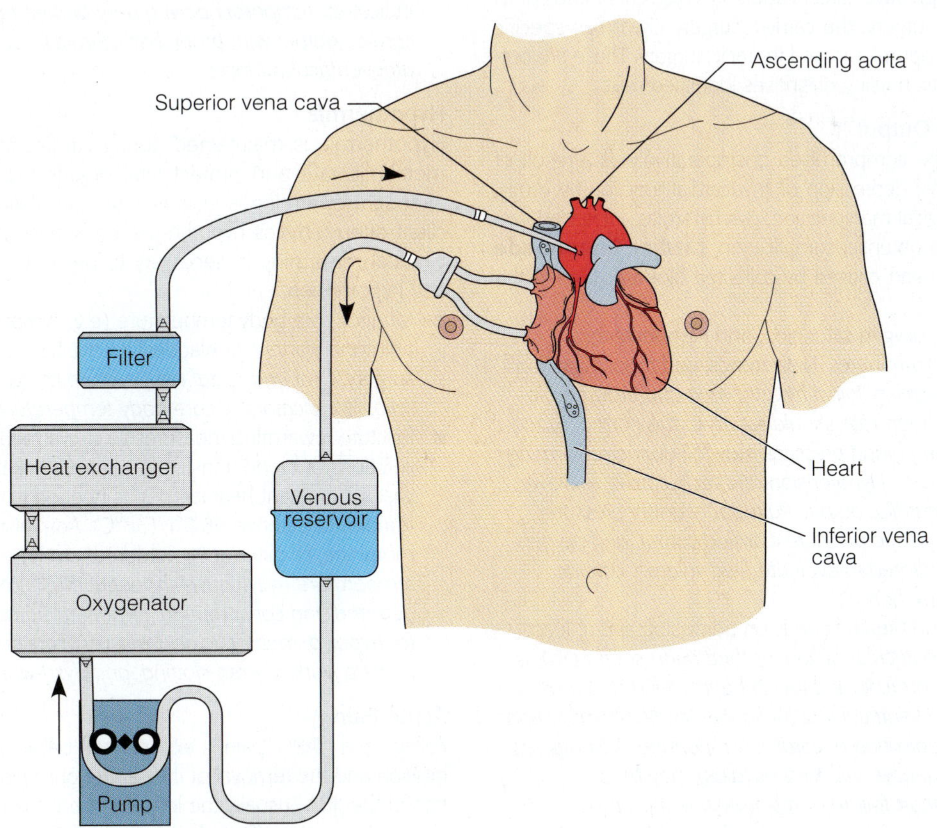

Figure 22–37 ■ A diagrammatic representation of cardiopulmonary bypass. A cannula in the superior and inferior venae cavae removes venous blood, which is then pumped through an oxygenator and heat exchanger. After filtering, oxygenated blood is returned to the ascending aorta.

Box 22–14 **Nursing Care of the Client Having a Coronary Artery Bypass Graft**

PREOPERATIVE CARE

- Provide routine preoperative care and teaching. *Teaching clients what to expect during and after surgery reduces anxiety and helps improve client outcomes if postoperative requrirements such as deep breathing, turning, and coughing are properly performed.*
- Verify presence of laboratory and diagnostic test results in the chart, including complete blood count, coagulation profile, urinalysis, chest x-ray, and coronary angiogram. *These baseline data are important for comparison of postoperative results and values.*
- Type and crossmatch four or more units of blood as ordered. *Blood is made available for use during and after surgery as needed.*
- Provide specific client and family teaching related to procedure and postoperative care. Include the following topics:
  a. Cardiac recovery unit; sensory stimuli, personnel; noise and alarms; visiting policies
  b. Tubes, drains, and general appearance
  c. Monitoring equipment, including cardiac and hemodynamic monitoring systems
  d. Respiratory support: ventilator, endotracheal tube, suctioning; communication while intubated
  e. Incisions and dressings
  f. Pain management.

  Preoperative teaching reduces anxiety and prepares the client and family for the postoperative environment and expected sensations.

POSTOPERATIVE CARE

Provide routine postoperative care. In addition to the care needs of all clients having major surgery, the cardiac surgery client has specific care needs related to open-heart and thoracic surgery. These are outlined under the specific nursing diagnoses identified next.

Decreased Cardiac Output

Cardiac output may be compromised postoperatively as a result of bleeding and fluid loss; depression of myocardial function by drugs, hypothermia, and surgical manipulation; dysrhythmias; increased vascular resistance; and a potential complication, **cardiac tamponade** (compression of the heart caused by collected blood or fluid in the pericardium).

- Monitor vital signs, oxygen saturation, and hemodynamic parameters every 15 minutes. Note trends, and report significant changes to the physician. *Initial hypothermia and bradycardia are expected; the heart rate should return to the normal range with rewarming. The blood pressure may fall during rewarming as vasodilation occurs. Hypotension and tachycardia, however, may indicate low cardiac output. Pulmonary artery pressure, pulmonary artery wedge pressure, cardiac output, and oxygen saturation are monitored to evaluate fluid volume, cardiac function, and gas exchange.*
- Auscultate heart and breath sounds on admission and at least every 4 hours. *A ventricular gallop, or third heart sound (S_3), is an early sign of heart failure; a fourth heart sound (S_4) may indicate decreased ventricular compliance. Muffled heart sounds may be an early indication of cardiac tamponade. Adventitious breath sounds (wheezes, crackles, or rales) may be a manifestation of heart failure or respiratory compromise.*
- Assess skin color and temperature, peripheral pulses, and level of consciousness with vital signs. *Pale, mottled, or cyanotic coloring; cool and clammy skin; and diminished pulse amplitude are indicators of decreased cardiac output.*
- Continuously monitor and document cardiac rhythm. *Dysrhythmias are common and may interfere with cardiac filling and contractility, decreasing the cardiac output.*
- Measure intake and output hourly. Report urine output less than 30 mL/h for two consecutive hours. *Intake and output measurements help evaluate fluid volume status. A fall in urine output may be an early indicator of decreased cardiac output.*
- Record chest tube output hourly. *Chest tube drainage greater than 70 mL/hour or that is warm, red, and free flowing indicates hemorrhage and may necessitate a return to surgery. A sudden drop in chest tube output may indicate impending cardiac tamponade.*
- Monitor hemoglobin, hematocrit, and serum electrolytes. *A drop in hemoglobin and hematocrit may indicate hemorrhage that is not otherwise obvious. Electrolyte imbalances (potassium, calcium, and magnesium in particular) affect cardiac rhythm and contractility.*
- Administer intravenous fluids, fluid boluses, and blood transfusions as ordered. *Fluid and blood replacement helps ensure adequate blood volume and oxygen-carrying capacity.*
- Administer medications as ordered. *Medications ordered in the early postoperative period to maintain the cardiac output include inotropic drugs (e.g., dopamine or dobutamine) to increase the force of myocardial contractions, vasodilators (e.g., nitroprusside or nitroglycerin) to decrease vascular resistance and afterload, and antidysrhythmics to correct dysrhythmias that affect cardiac output.*
- Keep a temporary pacemaker at the bedside; initiate pacing as indicated. *Temporary pacing may be needed to maintain the cardiac output with bradydysrhythmias, such as high-level atrioventricular blocks.*

Hypothermia

Hypothermia is maintained during cardiac surgery to reduce the metabolic rate and protect vital organs from ischemic damage. Although rewarming is instituted on completion of the surgery, the client often remains hypothermic on admission to cardiac recovery. Gradual rewarming is necessary to prevent peripheral vasodilation and hypotension.

- Monitor core body temperature (e.g., tympanic membrane, pulmonary artery, or bladder) for the first 8 hours following surgery. *Oral and rectal temperature measurements are not reliable indicators of core body temperature during this period.*
- Institute rewarming measures (e.g., warmed intravenous solutions or blood transfusion, warm blankets, warm inspired gases, or radiant heat lamps) as needed to maintain a temperature above 96.8°F (36°C). Administer chlorpromazine, morphine, or diltiazem as ordered to relieve shivering. *Low body temperature may cause shivering, thus increasing oxygen demand and consumption. Hypothermia also increases the risk for hypoxia, metabolic acidosis, vasoconstriction and increased cardiac work, altered clotting, and dysrhythmias.*

Acute Pain

Following a CABG, pain is experienced because of both the thoracic incision and the removal of the saphenous vein from the leg. Dissection of the IMA (usually the left IMA) from the chest wall also causes chest pain on the affected side. Chest tube sites are also uncomfortable. The leg from which the saphenous vein graft was obtained may be more painful than the chest incision.

Box 22–14 **Nursing Care of the Client Having a Coronary Artery Bypass Graft (continued)**

- Frequently assess for pain, including its location and character. Document its intensity using a standard pain scale. Assess for verbal and nonverbal indicators of pain. Validate pain cues with the client. *Pain is subjective and differs among individuals. Incisional pain is expected; however, anginal pain also may develop. It is important to differentiate the type of pain.*
- Administer analgesics on a scheduled basis, by PCA, or by continuous infusion for the first 24–48 hours. *Research demonstrates that adequate pain management in the immediate postoperative period reduces complications from sympathetic stimulation and allows faster recovery. Pain causes muscle tension and vasoconstriction, impairing circulation and tissue perfusion, slowing wound healing, and increasing cardiac work.*
- Premedicate 30 minutes before activities or planned procedures. *Premedication and the subsequent reduction of pain improves client participation and cooperation with care.*

Ineffective Airway Clearance/Impaired Gas Exchange

Atelectasis resulting from impaired ventilation and airway clearance is a common pulmonary complication of cardiac surgery. Gas exchange may also be affected by blood loss and decreased oxygen-carrying capacity following surgery. Phrenic nerve paralysis is a potential complication of cardiac surgery that may also contribute to impaired ventilation and gas exchange.

- Evaluate respiratory rate, depth, effort, symmetry of chest expansion, and breath sounds frequently. *Pain, anxiety, excess fluid volume, surgical injury, narcotics and anesthesia, and altered homeostasis can affect respiratory rate, depth, and effort postoperatively. Decreased chest expansion or asymmetrical movement may indicate impaired ventilation of one lung and needs further evaluation.*
- Note endotracheal tube (ETT) placement on chest x-ray. Mark tube position and secure in place. Insert an oral airway if an oral ETT is used. *The chest x-ray documents correct ETT placement above the bifurcation to the right and left mainstem bronchus. Marking its appropriate placement allows evaluation of potential tube movement. Secure the tube firmly in place to prevent slippage or inadvertent removal. An oral airway helps prevent obstruction of an oral ETT by biting.*
- Maintain ventilator settings as ordered. Monitor arterial blood gas levels as ordered. *Mechanical ventilation promotes optimal lung expansion and oxygenation postoperatively. Arterial blood gas levels are used to evaluate oxygenation and acid–base balance.*
- Suction as needed. *Suctioning is performed only as indicated to clear airway secretions.*
- Prepare for ventilator weaning and extubation as appropriate. *The client is removed from the ventilator and extubated as soon as possible to reduce complications associated with mechanical ventilation and intubation.*
- After extubation, teach use of the incentive spirometer, and encourage its use every 2 hours. Encourage deep breathing; advise against vigorous coughing. Teach use of a "cough pillow" to splint chest incision and decrease pain. Frequently turn and encourage movement. Dangle on postoperative day 1. *Deep breathing, controlled coughing, and position changes improve ventilation and airway clearance and help prevent complications. Vigorous coughing may excessively increase intrathoracic pressure and cause sternal instability.*

Risk for Infection

Following an open chest procedure, a sternal infection may develop that can progress to involve the mediastinum. Incisions for removal of the saphenous vein also may become infected. Clients with IMA grafts or who have diabetes, are older, or are malnourished are at high risk: Harvesting of the IMA disrupts blood supply to the sternum, and these clients have impaired immune responses and healing.

- Assess sternal incision and leg wounds every shift. Document redness, warmth, swelling, and/or drainage from the site. Note wound approximation. *These assessments provide indicators of inflammation and healing.*
- Maintain a sterile dressing for the first 48 hours, then leave the incision open to air. Use Steri-Strips as needed to maintain approximation of the wound edges. *The sterile dressing prevents early contamination of the wound, whereas exposing the incision after 48 hours promotes healing.*
- Report signs of wound infection: a swollen, reddened area that is hot and painful to the touch; drainage from the wound; impaired healing; or healed areas that reopen. *Evidence of infection or impaired healing requires further evaluation and treatment.*
- Culture wound drainage as indicated. *Identifying the infective organism facilitates appropriate antibiotic therapy.*
- Collaborate with the dietitian to promote nutrition and fluid intake. *Good nutritional status is vital to healing and immune function.*

Disturbed Thought Processes

Many factors affect neuropsychologic function after CABG, including length of the CPB, age, presurgery organic brain dysfunction, severity of illness, and decreased cardiac output. Sensory overload and deprivation, sleep disruption, and numerous drugs also affect thinking and mental clarity.

- Frequently reorient the client during the initial recovery period. State that surgery is over and that the client is in the recovery area. *Frequent reorientation provides emotional support and reality checks.*
- Explain all procedures before performing them. Speak in a clear, calm voice. Encourage questions, and give honest answers. *These measures provide information, decrease anxiety, and establish trust.*
- Secure all intravenous lines and invasive catheters/tubes (e.g., ETT, Foley catheter, or nasogastric tube). *Disoriented clients may tug or pull at invasive equipment, disrupting them and increasing the risk of injury.*
- Note verbal responses to questions. Correct misconceptions immediately (e.g., "Mr. Snow, look at all the special equipment in this room. Does this room look like your bedroom at home?"). *Helping the client recognize differences in the hospital environment offers a basis for continual reality checks.*
- Maintain a calendar and clock within the client's view. *This provides current information regarding day, date, and time.*
- Involve family members in providing reorientation. Place familiar objects and photographs within view. Encourage family presence. *The family provides reassurance and contact with the familiar, assisting with orientation.*
- Promote client participation in care and decision making as appropriate. *This allows the client to maintain a degree of power and control and enables the client to take an active role in recovery.*

(continued)

Box 22–14 Nursing Care of the Client Having a Coronary Artery Bypass Graft (continued)

- Report signs of hallucinations, delusions, depression, or agitation. *These may indicate progressive deterioration of mental status.*
- Administer sedatives cautiously. *Mild sedation may help prevent injury. Some sedatives may, however, have adverse effects, increasing confusion and disorientation.*
- Reevaluate neurologic status every shift. *These data allow evaluation of the effect of interventions.*

"ports," in the chest wall to access vessels for connection to the CPB pump and the surgical site. Alternatively, the femoral artery and femoral vein may be used for CPB (Eagle et al., 2004). CPB is avoided altogether using the minimally invasive direct coronary artery bypass (MIDCAB) approach. With MIDCAB, a small surgical incision and several chest wall ports are used to graft a chest wall artery to the affected coronary vessel while the heart continues to beat.

TRANSMYOCARDIAL LASER REVASCULARIZATION A new development in myocardial revascularization techniques is called transmyocardial laser revascularization. In this procedure, a laser is used to drill tiny holes into the myocardial muscle itself to provide collateral blood flow to ischemic muscle. Clients whose coronary artery obstructions are too diffuse to bypass are candidates for this new surgical treatment.

Other Invasive Procedures

For clients with large MIs and evidence of pump failure, invasive devices may be used to temporarily take over the function of the heart, allowing the injured myocardium to heal. The intra-aortic balloon pump is widely used to augment cardiac output. Ventricular assist devices are indicated for clients requiring more or longer-term artificial support than the intra-aortic balloon pump provides.

INTRA-AORTIC BALLOON PUMP The intra-aortic balloon pump (IABP), also called intra-aortic balloon counterpulsation, is a mechanical circulatory support device that may be used after cardiac surgery or to treat cardiogenic shock following AMI. The IABP temporarily supports cardiac function, allowing the heart to recover gradually by decreasing myocardial workload and oxygen demand and increasing perfusion of the coronary arteries.

A catheter with a 30–40-mL balloon is introduced into the aorta, usually via the femoral artery. The balloon catheter is connected to a console that regulates the inflation and deflation of the balloon. The IABP catheter inflates during diastole, increasing perfusion of the coronary and renal arteries, and deflates just before systole, decreasing afterload and cardiac workload (Figure 22–38 ■). The inflation–deflation sequence is triggered by the ECG pattern. During the most acute period, the balloon inflates and deflates with each heartbeat (1:1 ratio), providing maximal assistance to the heart. As the client's condition improves, the IABP is weaned to inflate–deflate at varying intervals (e.g., 1:2, 1:4, and 1:8). This provides a continually decreasing amount of support as the heart muscle recovers. When mechanical assistance is no longer required, the IABP catheter is removed.

VENTRICULAR ASSIST DEVICES Use of ventricular assist devices (VADs) to aid the failing heart is becoming more common as technology advances. Whereas the IABP can supplement cardiac output by approximately 10–15%, the VAD temporarily takes partial or complete control of cardiac function, depending on the type of device used. VADs may be used as temporarily or completely in AMI and cardiogenic shock when there is a chance for recovery of normal heart function after a period of cardiac rest. The device also may be used as a bridge to heart transplant. Nursing care for the client with a VAD is supportive and includes assessing hemodynamic status and for complications associated with the device. Clients with VAD are at considerable risk for infection; strict aseptic technique is used with all invasive catheters and dressing changes. Pneumonia also is a risk because of immobility and ventilatory support. Mechanical failure of the VAD is a life-threatening event that requires immediate intervention (Urden et al., 2006).

Cardiac Rehabilitation

Cardiac rehabilitation is a long-term program of medical evaluation, exercise, risk factor modification, education, and counseling designed to limit the physical and psychologic

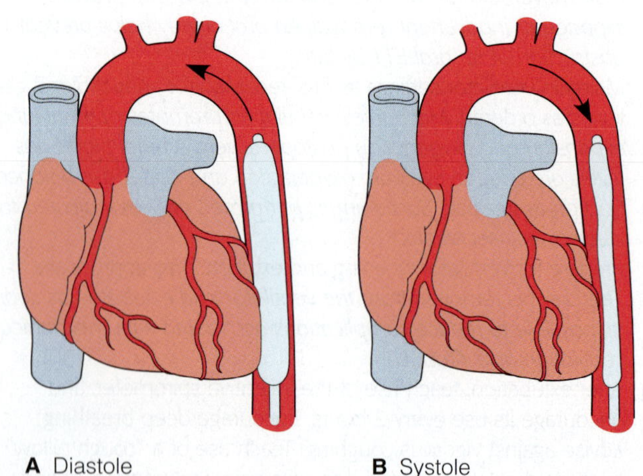

Figure 22–38 ■ The intra-aortic balloon pump. *A,* When inflated during diastole, the balloon supports cerebral, renal, and coronary artery perfusion. *B,* The balloon deflates during systole, so cardiac output is unimpeded.

effects of cardiac illness and improve the client's quality of life (Woods et al., 2004). Cardiac rehabilitation begins with admission for a cardiac event such as an AMI or a revascularization procedure. Phase 1 of the program is the inpatient phase. A thorough assessment of the client's history, current status, risk factors, and motivation is obtained. During this phase, activity progresses from bedrest to independent performance of ADLs and ambulation within the facility. Both subjective and objective responses to increasing activity levels are evaluated. Excess fatigue, shortness of breath, chest pain, tachypnea, tachycardia, or cool, clammy skin indicates activity intolerance. Phase 2, immediate outpatient cardiac rehabilitation, begins within 3 weeks of the cardiac event. The goals for the outpatient program are to increase activity level, participation, and capacity; improve psychosocial status and treat anxiety or depression; and provide education and support for risk factor reduction. Phase 3, continuation programs, are directed at providing a transition to independent exercise and exercise maintenance. During this final phase, the client may "check in" every 3 months to evaluate risk factors, quality of life, and exercise habits (Woods et al., 2004).

Complementary Therapies

Diet and exercise programs that emphasize physical conditioning and a low-fat diet rich in antioxidants have been shown to be effective in managing CAD (Box 22–15). Supplements of vitamins C, E, B_6, and B_{12}, as well as folic acid, may be beneficial. Other potentially helpful complementary therapies include herbals such as ginkgo biloba, garlic, curcumin, and green tea, and consumption of red wine, foods containing bioflavonoids, and nuts. Emphasize the need for clients to talk to their physicians before taking any herbal preparations, as interactions with prescribed drugs are common. Behavioral therapies of benefit for clients with CAD include relaxation and stress management, guided imagery, treatment of depression, anger/hostility management, meditation, tai chi, and yoga.

Box 22–15 Complementary Therapies: Diet for CHD

Two diet programs have been shown to have a beneficial effect on CHD. These are the Pritikin diet and the Ornish diet.

The Pritikin diet is basically vegetarian, high in complex carbohydrates and fiber, low in cholesterol, and extremely low in fat (<10% of daily calories). Egg whites and limited amounts of nonfat dairy or soy products are allowed. The Pritikin program requires 45 minutes of walking daily and recommends multivitamin supplements, including vitamins C and E and folate.

The Ornish diet also is vegetarian, although egg whites and a cup of nonfat milk or yogurt per day are allowed. No oil or fat is permitted, even for cooking. Two ounces of alcohol a day are permitted. The Ornish program also calls for stress reduction, emotional–social support systems, daily stretching, and walking for 1 hour three times a week.

NURSING PROCESS

The focus of nursing care for clients with angina is similar to the interdisciplinary care focus—that is, to reduce myocardial oxygen demand and improve the oxygen supply. Angina usually is treated in community settings; the primary nursing focus is education.

Nursing care of the client with an AMI focuses on reducing cardiac work, identifying and treating complications in a timely manner, and preparing the client for rehabilitation.

Nurses are instrumental in educating adults about their risk for CAD, promoting participation in screening programs to identify that risk, and teaching all clients measures to reduce their risk for CAD. Present information about healthy lifestyle habits to community and religious groups, school children (grades K–12), and through the print media. In promoting healthy lifestyle habits, nurses can positively affect the incidence, morbidity, and mortality from CAD.

Strongly encourage all clients to avoid smoking in the first place, and to stop all forms of tobacco use. Discuss the adverse effects of smoking and the benefits of quitting. Provide information about dietary recommendations to maintain a healthy weight and optimal cholesterol levels. Discuss the benefits and importance of regular exercise. Finally, encourage clients with cardiovascular risk factors to undergo regular screening for hypertension, diabetes, and abnormal blood lipids.

In addition to health promotion measures identified for CAD, emphasize the importance of actively managing CAD risk factors to slow progression of the disease. As mentioned, encourage clients to stop smoking. Discuss the use of cholesterol-lowering drug therapy with clients who have hypercholesterolemia. Encourage regular aerobic exercise and a diet based on AHA or NCEP guidelines.

Assessment

Nursing assessment for CAD focuses on identifying risk factors. Obtain the following data when assessing the client:

- *Health history.* Current manifestations, such as chest pain or heaviness, shortness of breath, and weakness; current diet, exercise patterns, and medications; smoking history and pattern of alcohol intake; history of heart disease, hypertension, or diabetes; and family history of CAD or other cardiac problems.
- *Physical examination.* Current weight and its appropriateness for height; body mass index; waist-to-hip ratio; blood pressure; and strength and equality of peripheral pulses.

Focused assessment data for the client with angina include the following:

- *Health history.* Chest pain, including type, intensity, duration, frequency, aggravating factors, and relief measures; associated symptoms; history of other cardiovascular disorders, peripheral vascular disease, or stroke; current medications and treatment; usual diet, exercise, and alcohol intake patterns; smoking history; and use of other recreational drugs.

- *Physical assessment.* Vital signs and heart sounds; strength and equality of peripheral pulses; skin color and temperature (central and peripheral); and physical appearance during pain episode (e.g., shortness of breath, apparent anxiety, color, and diaphoresis).

Nursing assessment for the client with AMI must be both timely and ongoing. Assessment data related to AMI include the following:

- *Health history.* Complaints of chest pain, including its location, intensity, character, radiation, and timing; associated symptoms, such as nausea, heartburn, shortness of breath, and anxiety; treatment measures taken since onset of pain; past medical history, especially cardiac related; chronic diseases; current medications and any known allergies to medications; and smoking history as well as use of recreational drugs and alcohol.
- *Physical examination.* General appearance, including obvious signs of distress; vital signs; peripheral pulses; skin color, temperature, and moisture; level of consciousness; heart and breath sounds; cardiac rhythm (on bedside monitor); and bowel sounds and abdominal tenderness.

Diagnosis

Nursing diagnoses that may apply to the client with CAD include the following:

- Imbalanced Nutrition: More Than Body Requirements
- Ineffective Health Maintenance.

Nursing diagnoses appropriate for a client with angina include the following:

- Ineffective Tissue Perfusion: Cardiac
- Risk for Ineffective Therapeutic Regimen Management.

Specific nursing diagnoses for a client with AMI include the following:

- Acute Pain
- Ineffective Tissue Perfusion
- Ineffective Coping
- Fear.

Plan

Planning care for the client at risk for CAD may include the following goals:

- The client will verbalize modifiable risk factors.
- The client will describe dietary changes to reduce the risk for CAD.
- The client will alter lifestyle to include increasing activity, quitting smoking, or changing diet.

Planning care for the client with symptomatic CAD may include the following goals:

- The client will describe lifestyle choices that may worsen CAD.
- The client will prevent cardiac muscle damage by complying with treatment regimen.
- The client will control blood pressure through the proper administration of medications, teaching dietary changes and promoting exercise as tolerated.

Planning care for the client with ineffective tissue perfusion may include the following:

- The client will understand how to take medications and what symptoms to report to health care provider.
- The client with reduce activity as needed to maintain optimal tissue perfusion.
- The client will describe emergency actions to take when experiencing chest pain.

Implementation

The focus of nursing care is on improving cardiac output, reducing cardiac workload, maximizing function, and teaching clients how to care for themselves at home while reducing the risk of further cardiac damage. It is important to treat the client holistically, dealing with the client's psychosocial, spiritual, and cultural needs as well as the client's physical needs. Learning of a diagnosis that impacts the heart is very frightening to clients, and they often require assistance in coping with fear and anxiety.

Imbalanced Nutrition: More Than Body Requirements

This nursing diagnosis may be appropriate for clients who are obese, have a waist-to-hip ratio of greater than 0.8 (female) or 0.9 (male), or whose diet history or serum cholesterol levels indicate a need to reduce fat and cholesterol intake.

- Encourage assessment of food intake and eating patterns to help identify areas that can be improved. Clients often are unaware of their fat and cholesterol intake, particularly when many meals are eaten away from home. Careful assessment increases awareness and allows the client to make conscious changes.
- Discuss AHA and therapeutic lifestyle change dietary recommendations, emphasizing the role of diet in heart disease. Provide guidance regarding specific food choices, with healthy alternatives. Specific diet information and suggestions help the client make better food choices.
- Refer to a clinical dietitian for diet planning and further teaching. Suggest cookbooks that offer low-fat recipes to encourage healthier eating, and provide AHA and American Cancer Society recipe pamphlets and information on low-fat eating. These resources provide tools for the client to use as eating patterns change.
- Encourage gradual but progressive dietary changes. Drastic changes in eating patterns may cause frustration and discourage the client from maintaining a healthy diet over the long term.
- Discourage use of high-fat, low-carbohydrate, or other fad diets for weight loss. These diets may adversely affect serum cholesterol and triglyceride levels, and they often are too drastic to maintain over the long term.
- Encourage reasonable goals for weight loss (e.g., 1.0–1.5 lb per week and a 10% weight loss over 6 months). Provide information about weight loss programs and support groups, such as Weight Watchers and Take Off Pounds Sensibly (TOPS). Gradual but steady weight loss is more likely to be sustained. Recognized programs that emphasize

healthy eating provide support and incentive for making lifetime dietary changes.

Ineffective Health Maintenance

Clients with risk factors for CAD may be unable to identify or independently manage their risk factors.

- Discuss risk factors for CAD, stressing how changing or managing those factors that can be modified reduces the client's overall risk for the disease. Clients with significant nonmodifiable risk factors may be discouraged, reducing their ability to eliminate or control modifiable risk factors.
- Discuss the immediate benefits of smoking cessation. Provide resource materials from the AHA, the American Lung Association, and the American Cancer Society. Refer to a structured smoking cessation program to increase the likelihood of success in quitting. Long-time smokers may assume that the damage from smoking has already been done and that quitting would not be "worth the price."
- Help the client identify specific sources of psychosocial and physical support for smoking cessation, dietary, and lifestyle changes. Support persons, groups, and aids such as nicotine patches help the client achieve success and provide encouragement during difficult times (e.g., during withdrawal symptoms).
- Discuss the benefits of regular exercise for cardiovascular health and weight loss. Help identify favorite forms of exercise or physical activity. Encourage planning for 30 minutes of continuous aerobic activity (e.g., walking, running, bicycling, or swimming) four to five times a week. Encourage identification of an "exercise buddy" to help maintain motivation. Engaging in preferred activities with a partner maintains motivation and increases the likelihood of maintaining an exercise program. Encourage continuation of the plan, even when days are missed. Exercise is cumulative, so increasing the duration of exercise on subsequent days can "make up" for a lost day.
- Provide information and teaching about prescribed medications, such as cholesterol-lowering drugs. Discuss the relationship between hypertension, diabetes, and CAD. Teaching is important to promote understanding of and compliance with the prescribed drug regimen.

Acute Pain

Chest pain occurs when the oxygen supply to the heart muscle does not meet the demand. Myocardial ischemia and infarction cause pain, as does reperfusion of an ischemic area following fibrinolytic therapy or emergent percutaneous transluminal coronary angioplasty. Pain stimulates the sympathetic nervous system, increasing cardiac work. Pain relief is a priority of care for the client with AMI.

- Assess for verbal and nonverbal signs of pain. Document the characteristics and intensity of the pain, using a standard pain scale. Verify nonverbal indicators of pain with the client. Frequent, careful pain assessment allows early intervention to reduce the risk of further damage. Pain is a subjective experience; its expression may vary with location and intensity, previous experiences, and cultural and social background. Pain scales provide an objective tool for measuring pain and a way to assess pain relief or reduction.
- Administer oxygen at 2–5 L/minute per nasal cannula. Supplemental oxygen increases oxygen supply to the myocardium, decreasing ischemia and pain.
- Promote physical and psychologic rest. Provide information and emotional support. Rest decreases cardiac workload and sympathetic nervous system stimulation, promoting comfort. Information and emotional support help decrease anxiety and provide psychologic rest.
- Titrate intravenous nitroglycerin as ordered to relieve chest pain, maintaining a systolic blood pressure of greater than 100 mmHg. Nitroglycerin decreases chest pain by dilating peripheral vessels, reducing cardiac work, and dilating coronary vessels, including collateral channels, thus improving blood flow to ischemic tissue.
- Administer 2–4 mg of morphine by intravenous push for chest pain as needed. Morphine is an effective narcotic analgesic for chest pain. It decreases pain and anxiety, acts as a venodilator, and decreases the respiratory rate. The resulting reduction in preload and sympathetic nervous system stimulation reduces cardiac work and oxygen consumption.

Ineffective Tissue Perfusion

Cardiac muscle damage affects compliance, contractility, and cardiac output. The extent of the effect on tissue perfusion depends on the location and amount of damage. Anterior wall infarcts have a greater effect on cardiac output than do right ventricular infarcts. Infarcted muscle also increases the risk for cardiac dysrhythmias, which can also affect the delivery of blood and oxygen to the tissues.

- Assess and document vital signs. Report increases in heart rate and changes in rhythm, blood pressure, and respiratory rate. Decreased cardiac output activates compensatory mechanisms that may cause tachycardia and vasoconstriction, increasing cardiac work.
- Assess for changes in level of consciousness; decreased urine output; moist, cool, pale, mottled, or cyanotic skin; dusky or cyanotic mucous membranes and nail beds; diminished to absent peripheral pulses; and delayed capillary refill. These are manifestations of impaired tissue perfusion. A change in level of consciousness is often the first manifestation of altered perfusion, because brain tissue and cerebral function depend on a continuous supply of oxygen.
- Auscultate heart and breath sounds. Note abnormal heart sounds (e.g., an S_3 or S_4 gallop or a murmur) or adventitious lung sounds. Abnormal heart sounds or adventitious lung sounds may indicate impaired cardiac filling or output, increasing the risk for decreased tissue perfusion.
- Monitor ECG rhythm continuously. Dysrhythmias can further impair cardiac output and tissue perfusion.
- Monitor oxygen saturation levels. Administer oxygen as ordered. Obtain and assess arterial blood gas levels as indicated. Oxygen saturation is an indicator of gas exchange, tissue perfusion, and the effectiveness of oxygen administration. Arterial blood gas levels provide a

more precise measurement of blood oxygen levels and allow assessment of acid–base balance.

- Administer antidysrhythmic medications as needed. Dysrhythmias affect tissue perfusion by altering cardiac output.
- Obtain serial CK, isoenzyme, and troponin levels as ordered. Levels of cardiac markers, CK isoenzymes in particular, correlate with the extent of myocardial damage.
- Plan for invasive hemodynamic monitoring. Hemodynamic monitoring facilitates AMI management and treatment evaluation by providing a means of assessing pressures in the systemic and pulmonary arteries, the relationship between oxygen supply and demand, cardiac output, and cardiac index.

Ineffective Coping

Coping mechanisms help a person deal with a life-threatening event or with acute changes in health. However, certain coping mechanisms may be detrimental to restoring health, particularly if the client relies on them for a prolonged period. Denial, for example, is a common coping mechanism among clients after an MI. During the initial stages, denial can reduce anxiety. Continued denial, however, can interfere with both learning and compliance with treatment.

- Establish an environment of caring and trust. Encourage the client to express feelings. Establishing a trusting nurse–client relationship provides a safe environment for the client to discuss feelings of helplessness, powerlessness, anxiety, and hopelessness. The nurse may then be able to provide additional resources to meet the client's needs.
- Accept denial as a coping mechanism, but do not reinforce it. Denial may initially help by diminishing the psychologic threat to health, decreasing anxiety. However, its prolonged use can interfere with acceptance of reality and cooperation, possibly delaying treatment and hindering recovery.
- Note aggressive behaviors, hostility, or anger. Document any failure to comply with treatments. These signs may indicate anxiety and denial.
- Help the client identify positive coping skills used in the past (e.g., problem-solving skills, verbalization of feelings, asking for help, or prayer). Reinforce use of positive coping behaviors. Coping behaviors that have been successful in the past can help the client deal with the current situation. These familiar methods can decrease feelings of powerlessness.
- Provide opportunities, as possible, for the client to make decisions about the plan of care. This promotes self-confidence and independence. Participating in care planning gives the client a sense of control and the opportunity to use positive coping skills.
- Provide privacy for the client and significant other to share their questions and concerns. Privacy provides an opportunity for the client and partner to share their feelings and fears, offer support and encouragement to one another, relieve anxiety, and establish effective coping methods.

Fear

The fear of death and disability can be a paralyzing emotion that adversely affects the client's recovery from AMI.

- Identify the client's level of fear, noting verbal and nonverbal signs. This information enables the nurse to plan appropriate interventions. Clients may not voice concerns; attention to nonverbal indicators is important. Controlling fear helps decrease sympathetic nervous system responses and catecholamine release that may increase feelings of fear and anxiety.
- Acknowledge the client's perception of the situation. Allow the client to verbalize concerns. A sudden change in health status causes anxiety and fear of the unknown. Verbalizing these fears may help the client cope with change and allow the health care team to provide information and correct misconceptions.
- Encourage questions, and provide consistent, factual answers. Repeat information as needed. Accurate and consistent information can reduce fear. Honest explanations help strengthen the client–nurse relationship and help the client develop realistic expectations. Anxiety and fear decrease the ability to concentrate and retain information; therefore, information may need to be repeated.
- Encourage self-care. Allow the client to make decisions regarding the plan of care. This promotes personal responsibility for health and allows some control over the situation. Clients' confidence increases as their dependence decreases.
- Administer antianxiety medications as ordered. These medications promote rest and relaxation and decrease feelings of anxiety, which may act as barriers to health restoration.
- Teach nonpharmacologic methods of stress reduction (e.g., relaxation techniques, mental imagery, music therapy, breathing exercises, meditation, and massage). Stress management techniques can help reduce tension and anxiety, provide a sense of control, and enhance coping skills.

Ineffective Tissue Perfusion: Cardiac

The pain of angina results from impaired blood flow and oxygen supply to the myocardium. Nursing interventions can both prevent ischemia and shorten the duration of pain.

- Keep prescribed nitroglycerin tablets at the client's side so one can be taken at the onset of pain. Anginal pain indicates myocardial ischemia. Nitroglycerin reduces cardiac work and may improve myocardial blood flow, relieving ischemia and pain.
- Start oxygen at 4–6 L/minute per nasal cannula or as prescribed. Supplemental oxygen reduces myocardial hypoxia.
- Space activities to allow rest between them. Activity increases cardiac work and may precipitate angina. Spacing of activities allows the heart to recover.
- Teach about prescribed medications to maintain myocardial perfusion and reduce cardiac work. Emphasize that long-acting nitrates, beta-blockers, and calcium-channel blockers are used to *prevent* anginal attacks, not to *treat* an acute attack. It is important for the client to understand the purpose and use of prescribed drugs to maintain optimal myocardial perfusion.

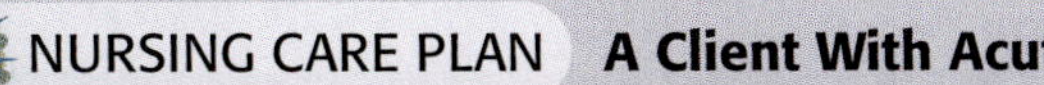

NURSING CARE PLAN A Client With Acute Myocardial Infarction

Betty Williams, a 62-year-old psychologist, is admitted to the emergency department with complaints of severe substernal chest pain. Mrs. Williams states that the pain began after lunch, about 4 hours ago. She initially attributed the pain to indigestion. She described the pain, which now radiates to her jaw and left arm, as "really severe heartburn." It is accompanied by a "choking feeling," severe shortness of breath, and diaphoresis. The pain is unrelieved by rest, antacids, or three sublingual nitroglycerin tablets (0.4 mg).

Oxygen is started per nasal cannula at 5 L/minute. Central and peripheral intravenous lines are inserted. A 12-lead electrocardiogram (ECG) and the following labwork are obtained: cardiac troponins, CK and CK isoenzymes, arterial blood gas levels, complete blood count, and a chemistry panel. Morphine sulfate relieves Mrs. Williams's pain.

Mrs. Williams's medical history includes type 2 diabetes, angina, and hypertension. She has a 45-year history of cigarette smoking, averaging 1.5–2 packs per day. Family history reveals that Mrs. Williams's father died at age 42 of acute myocardial infarction (AMI), and her paternal grandfather died at age 65 of AMI. Mrs. Williams is taking the following medications: tolbutamide (Orinase), hydrochlorothiazide, and isosorbide (Isordil).

Based on ECG changes and cardiac markers, an acute anterior MI is diagnosed. Mrs. Williams has no contraindications to fibrinolytic therapy and is deemed a good candidate. Intravenous alteplase (Activase) is given by bolus, followed by intravenous infusions of alteplase and heparin. She is transferred to the coronary care unit.

ASSESSMENT

Dan Morales, RN, is Mrs. Williams's primary care nurse. Mrs. Williams is alert and oriented to person, place, and time. Vital signs are as follows: temperature, 99.6°F (37.5°C); pulse, 118 bpm; respirations, 24/mind with adequate depth; and blood pressure, 172/92 mmHg. Auscultation reveals a fourth heard sound (S_4) and fine crackles in the bases of both lungs. The ECG shows sinus tachycardia with occasional premature ventricular contractions (PVCs). Her skin is cool and slightly diaphoretic. Capillary refill is less than 3 seconds, and peripheral pulses are strong and equal. Her nail beds are pink.

A triple-lumen central line is in place. Nitroglycerin is infusing at 200 mcg/min in the distal lumen. The alteplase infusion is in the middle lumen, and a heparin infusion is in the proximal lumen. The peripheral intravenous line has a saline lock. Mrs. Williams states, "The pain is better since the nurse in the ER gave me a shot. But it has been coming and going. I would rate it a 4 right now, but it was terrible before. The doctor told me that this drug I'm getting will quickly open up the artery that is blocked. I hope it works! Do many people get this drug?"

DIAGNOSES

- Acute Pain related to ischemic myocardial tissue
- Anxiety and Fear related to change in health status
- Ineffective Protection related to the risk of bleeding secondary to fibrinolytic therapy
- Risk for Decreased Cardiac Output related to altered cardiac rate and rhythm

PLANNING

Goals of care include the following:

- The client will rate chest pain as 2 or lower on a pain scale of 0–10.
- The client will verbalize reduced anxiety and fear.
- The client will demonstrate no signs of internal or external bleeding.
- The client will maintain an adequate cardiac output during and following reperfusion therapy.

IMPLEMENTATION

- Instruct to report all chest pain. Monitor and evaluate pain using a scale of 0–10. Titrate intravenous nitroglycerin infusion for chest pain; stop infusion if systolic blood pressure is below 100 mmHg. Administer 2–4 mg of morphine intravenously for chest pain unrelieved by nitroglycerin infusion.
- Encourage verbalization of fears and concerns. Respond honestly, and correct misconceptions about the disease, therapeutic interventions, or prognosis.
- Assess knowledge of CAD. Explain the purpose of fibrinolytic therapy to dissolve the fresh clot and reperfuse the heart muscle, limiting heart damage.
- Explain the need for frequent monitoring of vital signs and potential bleeding.
- Assess for manifestations of internal or intracranial bleeding: complaints of back or abdominal pain, headache, decreased level of consciousness, dizziness, bloody secretions or excretions, or pallor. Test all stools, urine, and vomitus for occult blood. Notify physician immediately of any abnormal findings.
- Monitor for signs of reperfusion: decreased chest pain, return of ST segment to baseline, and reperfusion dysrhythmias (e.g., PVCs, bradycardia, and heart block).
- Continuously monitor ECG for changes in cardiac rate, rhythm, and conduction. Assess vital signs.
- Treat dangerous dysrhythmias or other cardiac events per protocol. Notify the physician.
- Discuss continuing cardiac care and rehabilitation.

EVALUATION

The initial morphine dose reduces Mrs. Williams's chest pain from a rating of 8 to 4. The nitroglycerin infusion and fibrinolytic therapy further reduce her pain to 2. The nitroglycerin infusion is gradually discontinued after 24 hours. As her pain subsides, Mrs. Williams states that she feels "much better now that the pain is gone. I was afraid it would just get worse." She verbalizes an understanding of fibrinolytic therapy to limit myocardial damage. No indication of bleeding problems are noted. Reperfusion is indicated by relief of chest pain, return of the ST segment to baseline on the ECG, early peaking of CK levels, and increased frequency of PVCs but no significant dysrhythmias. Mrs. Williams remains in coronary care unit for 36 hours and is then transferred to the floor.

NURSING CARE PLAN A Client With Acute Myocardial Infarction *continued*

CRITICAL THINKING

1. How would the initial plan of care have changed if Mrs. Williams were not a candidate for fibrinolytic therapy?
2. Two days after her initial therapy, Mrs. Williams complains of palpitations. You notice frequent PVCs on the ECG monitor. What do you do?
3. What health promotion topics would you teach Mrs. Williams before discharge?
4. Mrs. Williams states, "I've been smoking for over 45 years, and I'm not going to stop now! Besides, it calms me down when I'm anxious." How would you respond to this statement?

- Instruct to take sublingual nitroglycerin before engaging in activities that precipitate angina (e.g., climbing stairs or sexual intercourse). This prophylactic dose of nitroglycerin helps maintain cardiac perfusion when increased work is anticipated, preventing ischemia and chest pain.
- Encourage to implement and maintain a progressive exercise program under the supervision of the primary care provider or a cardiac rehabilitation professional. Exercise slows the atherosclerotic process and helps develop collateral circulation to the heart muscle.
- Refer to a smoking cessation program as indicated. Nicotine causes vasoconstriction and increases the heart rate, decreasing myocardial perfusion and increasing cardiac workload.

Risk for Ineffective Therapeutic Regimen Management

Denial may be strong in the client with angina pectoris. Because many people think of the heart as the locus of life itself, problems such as angina remind people of their mortality, an uncomfortable fact. Denial may lead to "forgetting" to take prescribed medications or attempting activities that will precipitate angina. Some clients, by contrast, may become "cardiac cripples," afraid to engage in activities because of anticipated chest pain. Their inactivity may actually hasten the atherosclerotic process and inhibit collateral circulation development, worsening angina.

- Assess the client's knowledge and understanding of angina. Assessment allows tailoring of teaching and interventions to the needs of the client.
- Teach about angina and atherosclerosis as needed, building on current knowledge base. This can help the client understand that angina is a manageable disease and that pain can usually be controlled and progression of the disease slowed.
- Provide written and verbal instructions about prescribed medications and their use. Written instructions reinforce teaching and are available to the client for future reference.
- Stress the importance of taking chest pains seriously while maintaining a positive attitude. Although it is vital to recognize the significance of chest pain and deal with it appropriately, it is also important to maintain a positive outlook.
- Refer to a cardiac rehabilitation program or other organized activities and support groups for clients with CAD. Programs such as these help the client develop risk factor management strategies, maintain a program of supervised activity, and gain coping skills.

Evaluation

Client care is evaluated based on the client's progress toward goals and may be based on the following expected outcomes:

- The client demonstrates adequate circulation as evidenced by PaO_2 and $PaCO_2$ within normal limits.

CLIENT TEACHING Cardiac Rehabilitation

Cardiac rehabilitation begins with admission to the health care facility and continues through the inpatient stay and after discharge into the rehabilitative period. The emphasis is on realistic application of information to maintain lifestyle changes.

Assessing readiness to learn is an important first step in preparing for home care. The client in strong denial may not identify any relevance to the information being taught. Evaluate ability to learn, assessing physiologic and psychologic health, beliefs regarding personal responsibility for health, and expectations of the health care system. Also assess developmental level, ability to perform psychomotor skills, cognitive function, learning disabilities, existing knowledge base, and the influence of previous learning experiences. Provide written material to supplement teaching and encourage questions.

Include the following topics in teaching for home care:

- The normal anatomy and physiology of the heart, and the specific area of heart damage
- The process of CAD and implications of MI
- Purposes and side effects of prescribed medications
- The importance of complying with the medical regimen and cardiac rehabilitation program and of keeping follow-up appointments
- Information about community resources, such as the local chapter of the AHA.

After discharge, follow up by telephone within 1 week and periodically thereafter during the recovery period. Provide telephone numbers of resource personnel who are available to respond to questions and concerns after discharge. Research demonstrates the value of motivational and social support in adopting healthier behaviors after AMI.

Because the client who has had an MI is at high risk for sudden cardiac death, encourage family members to learn CPR and provide information about community resources for CPR training.

- The client maintains systolic blood pressure, pulse pressure, mean blood pressure, central venous pressure, and/or pulmonary wedge pressures within the normal range.
- The client reduces anginal events and demonstrates proper actions when angina begins.
- The client shows an absence of complications resulting from CAD.

REVIEW Coronary Artery Disease

RELATE: LINK THE CONCEPTS

Linking the exemplar of Coronary Artery Disease with the concept of Health, Wellness, and Illness:

1. What nutritional recommendations will you teachr the client with, or at risk for, CAD?
2. What will you teach the client about physical fitness and exercise in regards to reducing the risk of CAD?

Linking the exemplar of Coronary Artery Disease with the concept of Metabolism:

3. What role does obesity play in regards to risk for CAD? Explain the physiology of this impact.
4. What teaching would you provide the client with type 2 diabetes mellitus to reduce the risk of CAD?

READY: GO TO COMPANION SKILLS MANUAL

- Oxygen saturation (using a pulse oximeter)
- Administering oxygen by cannula, face mask, or face tent
- Interpreting an ECG strip
- Recording a 12-le ECG
- Assessing the client in pain
- Assessing appearance and mental status
- Assessing vital signs
- Assessing the heart and central vessels
- Administering oral medications

REFER: GO TO MYNURSINGKIT

REFLECT: CASE STUDY

Norma James is a 65-year-old widow who lives alone. Although she has lived in the neighborhood for years, she is somewhat socially isolated. She has two adult sons with whom she has limited contact; they live out of the state and rarely call. She has only a few individuals whom she considers friends; she does not particularly like people and prefers the company of her six cats.

Mrs. James has a long history of type 2 diabetes mellitus and hypertension. In more recent years, she has been diagnosed with atrial fibrillation. She has multiple physicians and takes multiple medications including:

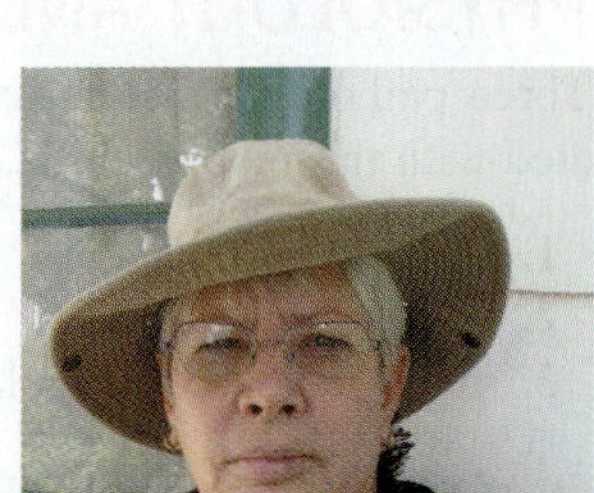

- Glucotrol: 10 mg, twice a day
- Captopril, 50 mg, twice a day
- Digoxin, 125 mcg, once a day
- Coumadin, 5 mg, once a day

Mrs. James has a known drug allergy to penicillin.

Mrs. James does not work; she has very limited savings and relies on Social Security benefits for income. She smokes about ½ pack of cigarettes a day and has been a smoker since she was in her 20s. She drinks alcohol "a couple times a year, usually a glass of wine at a special dinner."

She does not drive and relies on her friends, neighbors, or the city bus for transportation. She lives near a grocery store and prides herself in being able to get most things she needs without any assistance. She spends most of her time alone at home and occupies herself by watching television, reading, and doing crossword and jigsaw puzzles.

1. According to Mrs. James history, what are her risks for developing coronary artery disease?
2. What lifestyle changes would you discuss with Mrs. James to reduce this risk?
3. Create a teaching plan to help Mrs.James understand the risks associated with her lifestyle behaviors that are increasing her risk of CAD.

22.4 DEEP VENOUS THROMBOSIS

KEY TERMS

Homan's sign, *1391*
Venous thrombectomy, *1392*
Venous thrombosis, *1390*
Virchow's triad, *1390*

BASIS FOR SELECTION OF EXEMPLAR

Most common condition

LEARNING OUTCOMES

After reading about this exemplar, you will be able to:

1. Describe the pathophysiology, etiology, clinical manifestations, and direct and indirect causes of deep venous thrombosis.
2. Identify risk factors associated with deep venous thrombosis.
3. Illustrate the nursing process in providing culturally competent care across the life span for individuals with deep venous thrombosis.
4. Formulate priority nursing diagnoses appropriate for an individual with deep venous thrombosis.
5. Create a plan of care for individuals with deep venous thrombosis and their families.
6. Assess expected outcomes for an individual with deep venous thrombosis.
7. Discuss therapies used in the collaborative care of an individual with deep venous thrombosis.
8. Employ evidence-based caring interventions for an individual with deep venous thrombosis.

OVERVIEW

Venous thrombosis (also known as thrombophlebitis) is a condition in which a blood clot (thrombus) forms on the wall of a vein, accompanied by inflammation of the vein wall and some degree of obstructed venous blood flow. As the name implies, deep venous thrombosis (DVT) occurs when the thrombosis is located in a deep vein of the body. Prevention of venous thrombosis is an important nursing action when caring for the immobilized, postoperative, or postpartum client.

PHYSIOLOGY AND ETIOLOGY

Three pathologic factors, called **Virchow's triad**, are associated with thrombophlebitis. These pathologic factors are

1. stasis of blood,
2. vessel damage, and
3. increased blood coagulability.

Vessel trauma stimulates the clotting cascade. Platelets aggregate at the site, particularly when venous stasis is present. Platelets and fibrin form the initial clot. Red blood cells are trapped in the fibrin meshwork, and the thrombus propagates (grows) in the direction of blood flow. The inflammatory response is triggered, causing tenderness, swelling, and erythema in the area of the thrombus.

Initially, the thrombus floats within the vein. Pieces of the thrombus may break loose and travel through the circulation as emboli. Fibroblasts eventually invade the thrombus, scarring the vein wall and destroying venous valves. Although patency of the vein may be restored, valve damage is permanent, affecting directional flow (Tierney et al., 2005).

The deep veins of the legs, primarily in the calf, and of the pelvis provide the most hospitable environment for venous thrombosis. Approximately 80% of DVTs begin in the deep veins of the calf, often propagating into the popliteal and femoral veins (Figure 22–39 ■) (Tierney et al., 2005). DVT usually is asymptomatic; in some clients, a pulmonary embolism may be the first indication.

Etiology

Venous thrombi are more common than arterial thrombi because of lower pressures and flow within the venous system (McCance & Huether, 2006). Thrombi can form in either superficial or deep veins. DVT is a common complication of hospitalization, surgery, and immobilization. Obstetric and orthopaedic procedures carry a higher risk for venous thrombosis; it may develop in more than 50% of clients having orthopaedic surgery, particularly surgeries involving the hip or knee (Kasper et al., 2005). Other significant risk factors for venous thrombosis include abdominal or thoracic surgery,

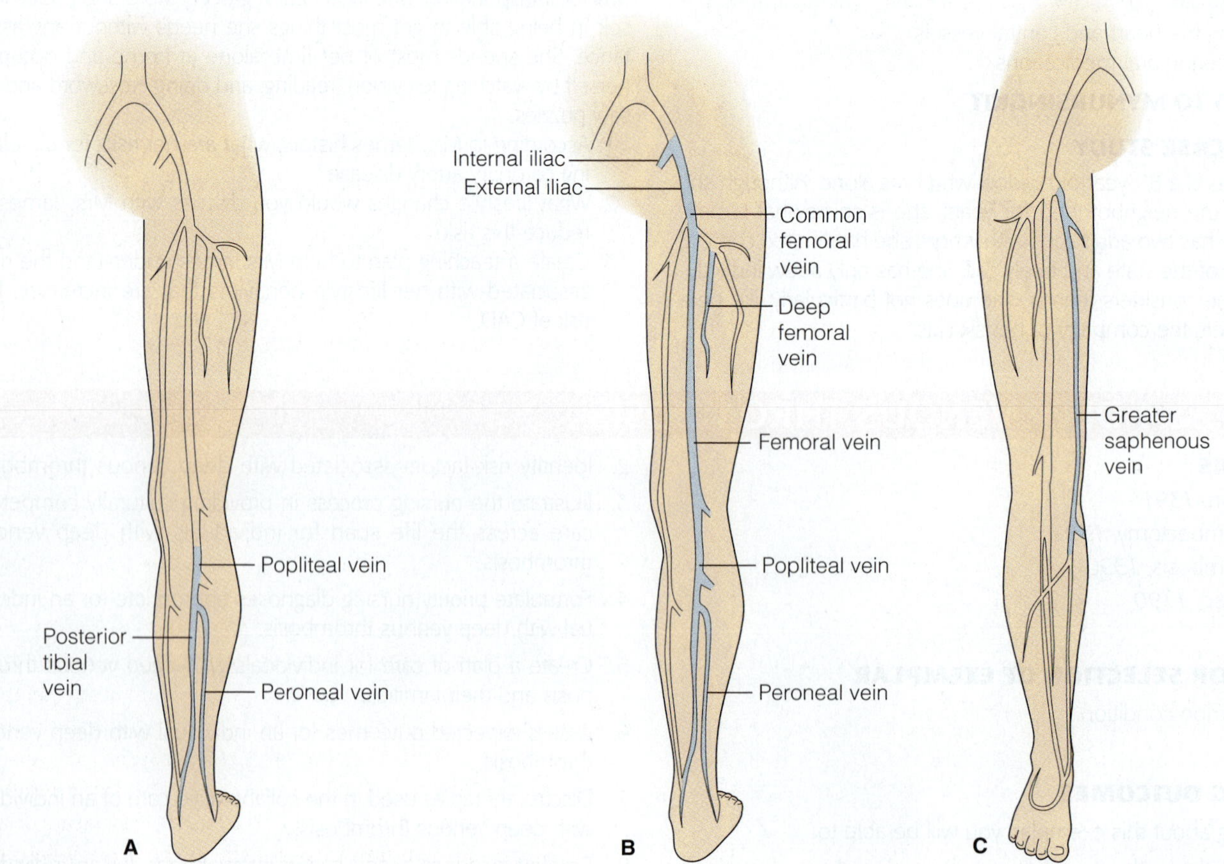

Figure 22–39 ■ Common locations of venous thrombosis. *A*, The most common sites of DVT. *B*, DVT extending from the calf to the iliac veins. *C*, Superficial venous thrombosis.

certain cancers, trauma, pregnancy, and use of oral contraceptives or hormone replacement therapy (Box 22–16).

Risk Factors

Preventive approaches are individualized to minimize the risk factors that can predispose to DVT. Specific conditions warranting prevention include the following:

- *Orthopaedic procedures.* Examples include total hip replacement, traumatic hip fracture, and total knee replacement. For total hip replacement, the incidence of DVT without prophylaxis is 25%; for traumatic hip fracture, approximately 50%; and for total knee replacement, as high as 60%.
- *Atrial fibrillation.* Persons with atrial fibrillation can form thrombi within the atria that can enter the general circulation and cause stroke. Transesophageal echocardiography identifies clients at risk for thromboembolism.
- *Acute myocardial infarction.* The risk of DVT in clients who have had an MI approaches 20%. Older clients with heart failure, recurrent angina, or ventricular arrhythmias are most at risk.
- *Ischemic stroke.* In clients with stroke and paralyzed lower extremities, the incidence of DVT is 40%.

Deep venous thrombosis is more frequently seen in women with a history of thrombosis. Certain obstetric complications, such as hydramnios, preeclampsia, and operative birth, are also associated with an increased incidence. After a clinical diagnosis of DVT, a woman's risk in a subsequent pregnancy increases.

CLINICAL MANIFESTATIONS

When present, the manifestations of DVT are primarily caused by the inflammatory process accompanying the thrombus. Calf pain, which may be described as tightness or a dull, aching pain in the affected extremity, particularly upon walking, is the most common symptom. Tenderness, swelling, warmth, and erythema may be noted along the course of involved veins. The affected extremity may be cyanotic and often is edematous. Rarely, a cord may be palpated over the affected vein. A positive **Homan's sign** (pain in the calf when the foot is dorsiflexed) is an unreliable indicator of DVT. See Box 22–17 for a summary of the manifestations of DVT.

Box 22–16 Factors Associated With Venous Thrombosis

- Immobilization: myocardial infarction, heart failure, stroke, postoperative
- Surgery: orthopaedic, thoracic, abdominal, genitourinary
- Cancer: pancreatic, lung, ovary, testes, urinary tract, breast, stomach
- Trauma: fractures of the spine, pelvis, femur, tibia; spinal cord injury
- Pregnancy and delivery
- Hormone therapy: oral contraceptives, hormone replacement therapy
- Coagulation disorders

Box 22–17 Manifestations of Deep Venous Thrombosis

- Usually asymptomatic
- Dull, aching pain in affected extremity, especially when walking
- Possible tenderness, warmth, erythema along affected vein
- Cyanosis of affected extremity
- Edema of affected extremity

The major complications of DVT are chronic venous and pulmonary embolism. Pulmonary embolism occurs when the clot fragments or breaks loose from the vein wall. As the clot travels, it moves through progressively larger veins and into the right side of the heart. From there, it enters the pulmonary circulation, where it eventually occludes arterial flow to a portion of the lungs. The result is a mismatch between ventilation (air flow) and perfusion (blood flow) in a portion of the lungs. The effect on gas exchange depends on the size of the embolism and the vessel it occludes.

COLLABORATION

It is important to differentiate venous thrombosis from other causes of extremity pain, such as cellulitis, muscle strain, contusion, and lymphedema. The history, physical examination, and diagnostic tests are used to establish the diagnosis. Treatment focuses on preventing further clotting or extension of the clot and addressing underlying causes.

Diagnostic Tests

Laboratory studies that may be ordered include D-dimer, prothrombin time, partial thromboplastin time, bleeding time, and platelet count may be ordered. Information about these studies can be found in Appendix B. Diagnostic tests for DVT include the following:

- *Duplex venous ultrasonography* is a noninvasive test used to visualize the vein and measure the velocity of blood flow in the veins. Although the clot often cannot be visualized directly, its presence can be inferred by an inability to compress the vein during the examination.
- *Plethysmography* is a noninvasive test that measures changes in blood flow through the veins. It is often used in conjunction with Doppler ultrasonography. Plethysmography is most valuable in diagnosing thromboses of larger or more superficial veins.
- *Magnetic resonance imaging (MRI)* is another noninvasive means of detecting DVT. It is particularly useful when thrombosis of the venae cavae or pelvic veins is suspected.
- *Ascending contrast venography* uses an injected contrast medium to assess the location and extent of venous thrombosis. Although invasive, expensive, and uncomfortable, contrast venography is the most accurate diagnostic tool for venous thrombosis. It is used when the results of less invasive tests leave the diagnosis unclear (Tierney et al., 2005).

Prophylaxis

Medications and other measures are used to prevent venous thrombosis when the risk is high. Low-molecular-weight heparins prevent DVT in clients who are undergoing general or orthopaedic surgery, experiencing acute medical illness, or on prolonged bedrest. Oral anticoagulation also may be used as a prophylactic measure in clients with fractures or who are undergoing orthopedic surgery.

Elevating the foot of the bed with the knees slightly flexed promotes venous return. Early mobilization and leg exercises such as ankle flexion and extension assist venous flow by muscle compression. Intermittent pneumatic compression devices applied to the legs are effective to prevent DVT and are used when anticoagulation is contraindicated because of the increased risk for bleeding (Kasper et al., 2005). Elastic stockings are also used to prevent venous thrombosis in clients who are at risk.

Pharmacologic Therapies

Anticoagulants to prevent clot propagation and enable the body's own lytic system to dissolve the clot are the mainstay of treatment for venous thrombosis. Fibrinolytic drugs such as streptokinase or t-PA may accelerate the process of clot lysis and prevent damage to venous valves. There is, however, no evidence that fibrinolytic therapy is more effective in preventing pulmonary embolism in clients with existing DVT than anticoagulants (Kasper et al., 2005). It also significantly increases the risk for bleeding and hemorrhage.

Nonsteroidal anti-inflammatory agents (NSAIDs) such as indomethacin (Indocin) or naproxen (Naprosyn) may be ordered to reduce inflammation in the veins and provide symptomatic relief, particularly for clients with superficial venous thrombosis.

ANTICOAGULANTS Anticoagulants are given to prevent clot extension and reduce the risk of subsequent pulmonary embolism. See Box 22–18 for the nursing implications for anticoagulant therapy.

Anticoagulation is initiated with unfractionated heparin or LMW heparin. Following an initial intravenous bolus of 7500–10,000 units of unfractionated heparin, a continuous heparin infusion of 1000 to 1500 international units per hour is started. The dosage is calculated to maintain the aPTT at approximately twice the control or normal value. An infusion pump is used to deliver the prescribed dosage. Frequent monitoring of the infusion is an important nursing responsibility. Subcutaneous heparin injections may be used as an alternative to intravenous infusion in some instances.

LMW heparins are increasingly used to prevent and treat venous thrombosis. They do not require the close laboratory monitoring of unfractionated heparins. LMW heparin is administered subcutaneously in fixed doses once or twice daily, allowing the option of outpatient treatment. LMW heparins have additional advantages, in that they are more effective and carry lower risks for bleeding and thrombocytopenia than conventional, unfractionated heparins.

Oral anticoagulation with warfarin may be initiated concurrently with heparin therapy. Overlapping heparin and warfarin therapy for 4–5 days is important because the full anticoagulant effect of warfarin is delayed, and it may actually promote clotting during the first few days of therapy (Tierney et al., 2005). Warfarin doses are adjusted to maintain the INR at 2.0–3.0 (Kasper et al., 2005).

Once this level is achieved, the heparin is discontinued and a maintenance dose of warfarin is prescribed to prevent recurrent thrombosis. Anticoagulation generally is continued for at least 3 months. When DVT is recurrent or risk factors such as altered coagulability or cancer are present, anticoagulant therapy may be prolonged. Regular follow-up is necessary to be sure prothrombin times (INR) remain within the desirable range for anticoagulation.

Surgery

Venous thrombosis usually is effectively treated with conservative measures and anticoagulation. In some cases, however, surgery is required to remove the thrombus, prevent its extension into deep veins, or prevent the effects of embolization.

Venous thrombectomy is done when thrombi lodge in the femoral vein and their removal is necessary to prevent pulmonary embolism or gangrene. Successful thrombus removal rapidly improves venous circulation. The duration of this effect varies.

When venous thrombosis is recurrent and anticoagulant therapy is contraindicated, a filter may be inserted into the vena cava to capture emboli from the pelvis and lower extremities, preventing pulmonary embolism. Several different filters are available (Figure 22–40 ■). The Greenfield filter is widely used for its ability to trap emboli within its apex while maintaining patency of the vena cava. The filter can be inserted under fluoroscopy with local anesthesia. Mortality and morbidity associated with the filter are very low.

Extensive thrombosis of the saphenous vein may necessitate ligation and division of the saphenous vein where it joins the femoral vein to prevent clot extension into the deep venous system. A vein affected by septic venous thrombosis is excised to control the infection. Antibiotic therapy also is initiated.

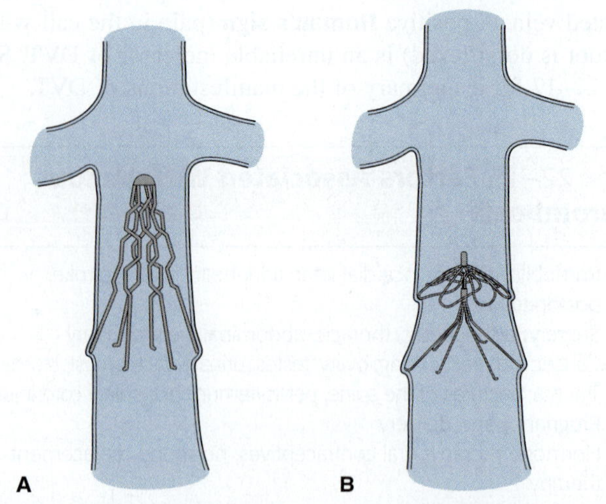

Figure 22–40 ■ Venal caval filters. *A*, Greenfield filter. *B*, Nitinol filter.

Box 22–18 **Medication Administration: Anticoagulant Therapy**

HEPARIN

Heparin interferes with the clotting cascade by inhibiting the effects of thrombin and preventing the conversion of fibrinogen to fibrin. This prevents the formation of a stable fibrin clot. At therapeutic levels, heparin prolongs the thrombin time, clotting time, and activated partial thromboplastin time. When given intravenously, its effect is immediate. Given subcutaneously, its onset of action is within 1 hour. When heparin is discontinued, clotting times return to normal within 2–6 hours (Spratto & Woods, 2003). *Heparin-induced thrombocytopenia (HIT)* is a potential complication of therapy with unfractionated heparin.

Nursing Responsibilities

- Assess for history of unexplained or active bleeding. Assess laboratory results for abnormal clotting profile or evidence of active bleeding.
- Give a test dose as indicated to clients with a history of multiple allergies or a history of asthma.
- Administer by deep subcutaneous injection; abdominal sites are preferred. Avoid injecting within 2 inches of the umbilicus. Rotate sites. Do not aspirate prior to injecting or massage after the injection.
- Intravenous solutions may be diluted with dextrose, normal saline, or Ringer's solution. Use an infusion pump.
- Keep protamine sulfate, a heparin antagonist, available to treat excessive bleeding.
- Monitor and report abnormal laboratory results and aPTT values outside the desired range.
- Promptly report evidence of bleeding such as hematemesis, hematuria, bleeding gums, or unexplained abdominal or back pain.

Health Education for the Client and Family

- Report unusual bleeding or excessive menstrual flow.
- Use an electric razor and a soft-bristle toothbrush; prevent injury by clearing pathways, using a night light, and other measures. Do not consume alcohol.
- Avoid contact sports while on anticoagulant therapy.
- Do not consume large amounts of food rich in vitamin K (yellow and dark green vegetables).
- Do not use aspirin or NSAIDs while on heparin therapy unless advised to do so by your physician.
- Wear a Medic-Alert tag and advise all health care providers (including dentists and podiatrists) of therapy.

LOW-MOLECULAR-WEIGHT HEPARINS

Ardeparin (Normiflo)
Dalteparin (Fragmin)
Enoxaparin (Lovenox)
Tinzaparin (Innohep)

LMW heparins are the most bioavailable fraction of heparin. They provide a more precise and predictable anticoagulant effect than unfractionated heparins. Like unfractionated heparin, LMW heparin prevents conversion of prothrombin to thrombin, liberation of thromboplastin from platelets, and formation of a stable clot. LMW heparins cannot be used interchangeably with each other or with unfractionated heparin. Although the risk of heparin-induced thrombocytopenia is significantly lower with LMW heparin, clients who were previously treated with unfractionated heparin may develop HIT when treated with LMW heparin.

Nursing Responsibilities

- Assess for evidence of active bleeding, a history of bleeding disorders or thrombocytopenia, or sensitivity to heparin, sulfites, or pork products.
- Monitor for unusual or masked bleeding. PT and aPTT levels may be within normal levels even in the presence of hemorrhage.
- Administer by deep subcutaneous injection into abdominal wall, thigh, or buttocks. Rotate sites. Do not aspirate or massage.

Health Education for the Client and Family

- Subcutaneous self-administration technique, timing of doses, and site rotation. Do not rub site after administering to minimize bruising.
- Do not take aspirin, NSAIDs, or other over-the-counter drugs unless recommended by your physician.
- Promptly report excessive bruising or bleeding, chest pain, difficulty breathing, itching, rash, or swelling to your health care provider.
- Keep follow-up appointments as scheduled.

ORAL ANTICOAGULANT

Warfarin (Coumadin)

Warfarin interferes with synthesis of vitamin K–dependent clotting factors by the liver, leading to depletion of these factors. It has no effect on already circulating clotting factors or on existing clots. Warfarin inhibits extension of existing thrombi and the formation of new clots. Its action is cumulative and more prolonged than that of heparin.

Nursing Responsibilities

- Assess laboratory results and history for evidence of abnormal bleeding.
- Multiple drugs affect the metabolism and protein binding of warfarin; note all medications and assess for interactions with warfarin.
- Do not give during pregnancy because warfarin may cause congenital malformations.
- Oral tablets may be crushed and given without regard to meals.
- Dilute intravenous warfarin with supplied diluent; administer within 4 hours by direct intravenous injection at a rate of 25 mg/min.
- Keep vitamin K available to reverse effects of warfarin in the event of excessive bleeding or hemorrhage.
- Monitor PT or INR; report values outside the desired range.

Health Education for the Client and Family

- If bleeding occurs (hematemesis, bright red or black tarry feces, hematuria, bleeding gums, excessive bruising, etc.), do not take your prescribed dose and notify your physician immediately. Report rash or manifestations of hepatitis (dark urine, malaise, yellow skin or sclera).
- Take your warfarin at the same time every day; do not change brands because their effects may differ.
- Menstrual bleeding may be slightly increased; contact your health care provider if it increases significantly. Use reliable birth control to prevent pregnancy while taking warfarin. Immediately contact your health care provider if you think you may be pregnant.
- Take precautions to prevent injury and bleeding: use a soft-bristle toothbrush and electric razor, wear shoes, and use a night light. Avoid participating in contact sports.
- Do not smoke, use alcohol, or take any over-the-counter drugs unless specifically recommended by your health care provider. Notify all health care providers, including dentists and podiatrists, of therapy. Wear a Medic-Alert tag.
- Obtain lab tests as scheduled and keep all scheduled follow-up appointments.

Clinical Therapies

Treatment of venous thrombosis also includes measures to relieve symptoms and reduce inflammation. With superficial venous thrombosis, applying warm, moist compresses over the affected vein, extremity rest, and anti-inflammatory agents usually provide relief of symptoms.

Bedrest may be ordered for DVT. The duration of bedrest typically is determined by the extent of leg edema. The legs are elevated 15–20°, with the knees slightly flexed, above the level of the heart to promote venous return and discourage venous pooling. Elastic antiembolism stockings (TEDS) or pneumatic compression devices are also frequently ordered to stimulate the muscle-pumping mechanism that promotes the return of blood to the heart. When permitted, walking is encouraged, as is avoiding prolonged standing or sitting. Crossing the legs also is avoided, as are tight-fitting garments or stockings that bind.

NURSING PROCESS

Prevention of venous thrombosis is an important component of nursing care for all at-risk clients. Position clients to promote venous blood flow from the lower extremities, with the feet elevated and the knees slightly bent. Avoid placing pillows under the knees and positions in which the hips and knees are sharply flexed. Use a recliner chair or footstool when sitting. Ambulate clients as soon as possible, and maintain a regular schedule of ambulation throughout the day. Teach ankle flexion and extension exercises, and frequently remind clients to perform them. Apply elastic hose and pneumatic compression devices when appropriate. Instruct clients to avoid crossing legs when in bed or sitting. Inquire about possible prophylactic heparin or warfarin therapy for clients undergoing orthopaedic surgery or other high-risk procedures. Frequently assess intravenous sites. Change the site and catheter as dictated by agency protocol and if evidence of local inflammation is noted.

Assessment

Assess clients at risk for venous thrombosis for manifestations and risk factors, and obtain the following information:

- *Health history.* Complaints of leg or calf pain, its duration and characteristics, and the effect of walking on the pain; history of venous thrombosis or other clotting disorders; current medications.
- *Physical examination.* Redness and edema of the affected extremity; tenderness, warmth, and cordlike structures on palpation; body temperature.

Diagnosis

Nursing diagnoses that apply to the client with DVT include the following:

- Pain
- Ineffective Tissue Perfusion: Peripheral
- Ineffective Protection
- Impaired Physical Mobility
- Risk for Ineffective Tissue Perfusion: Cardiopulmonary.

Plan

Goals of nursing care include the following:

- The client will have pain control sufficient to allow rest and comfort.
- The client will not experience complications resulting from embolization of thrombus.
- The client will have increased tissue perfusion to prevent cellular damage.

Implementation

In addition to preventive measures, priority nursing diagnoses for the client with venous thrombosis relate to pain, maintenance of tissue perfusion and integrity, and the potential adverse effects of prescribed treatments.

Pain

The pain associated with venous thrombosis results from inflammation of the involved vein. It may be aggravated by use of the involved extremity. Associated edema and swelling may contribute to discomfort. Measures to reduce the inflammation often help relieve the pain.

- Regularly assess pain location, characteristics, and level using a standardized pain scale. Report increasing pain or changes in its location or characteristics. Tissue substances released during the inflammatory process can stimulate pain receptors. In addition, localized swelling presses on pain-sensitive structures in the area of the inflammation, contributing to discomfort. As inflammation and swelling are reduced, pain should abate. Continued or increasing pain may indicate extension of the thrombosis. Sudden chest pain may indicate a pulmonary embolism, necessitating immediate intervention.
- Measure calf and thigh diameter of the affected extremity on admission and daily thereafter. Report increases promptly. The inflammatory process causes vasodilation and increases vessel permeability, in turn causing edema of the affected extremity. Baseline and subsequent measurements provide a measure of treatment effectiveness.
- Apply warm, moist heat to the affected extremity at least four times daily, using warm, moist compresses or an aqua-K pad. Moist heat penetrates tissues to a greater depth. Warmth promotes vasodilation, allowing reabsorption of excess fluid into the circulation. Vasodilation also reduces resistance within the affected vessel, reducing pain. As edema subsides, pressure on surrounding tissues is relieved, thereby reducing pain.
- Maintain bedrest as ordered. Using leg muscles during walking exacerbates the inflammatory process and increases edema. This, in turn, increases venous compression and pain.

Ineffective Tissue Perfusion: Peripheral

As thrombi develop, they occlude the lumen of the vein and obstruct blood flow. In addition, the accompanying inflammatory response may precipitate vessel spasms, further impairing arterial and venous blood flow as well as tissue perfusion. Impaired tissue perfusion in turn deprives tissues of nutrients and oxygen. As a result, distal tissues of the affected extremity are at risk for ulceration and infection.

- Assess the skin of the affected lower leg and foot at least every 8 hours, or more often as indicated. Frequent assessment is important to rapidly detect early signs of tissue breakdown and implementation of measures to protect vulnerable tissues. Early intervention allows healing and restoration of tissue integrity; if allowed to continue, the process can lead to necrosis and potential gangrene.
- Elevate extremities at all times, keeping knees slightly flexed and legs above the level of the heart. Elevation of the extremities promotes venous return and reduces peripheral edema. Knee flexion promotes muscle relaxation.
- Use mild soaps, solutions, and lotions to clean the affected leg and foot daily. Pat dry after washing, and apply a nonalcohol-based lotion or moisturizing cream. Daily hygiene with nondrying soaps and solutions removes potential pathogens from the skin surface and maintains skin integrity and the first line of defense against infection. Caustic or harsh soaps or solutions can dry and crack the skin. Dry, cracked skin permits bacteria and other microorganisms to enter and infect the tissue, potentially leading to ulceration and venous gangrene.
- Use an egg-crate mattress or sheepskin on the bed as needed. Egg-crate mattresses and sheepskins distribute weight more evenly, preventing excess pressure on affected tissues.
- Encourage frequent position changes (at least every 2 hours) while awake. Frequent position changes reduce pressure on bony prominences and edematous tissue, reducing the risk of tissue breakdown.

Ineffective Protection

Anticoagulant therapy interferes with the body's normal clotting mechanisms, increasing the risk for bleeding and hemorrhage.

- Monitor laboratory results, including the INR (prothrombin time), aPTT, hemoglobin, and hematocrit as indicated. Report values outside the normal or desired range. Coagulation studies are used to monitor the effect of anticoagulant medications. Values within the desired range prevent further clot development while carrying a low risk for bleeding and hemorrhage. A fall in the hemoglobin and hematocrit may indicate undetected bleeding.

Impaired Physical Mobility

Although prolonged bedrest rarely is required, it is associated with many problems, including constipation, joint contractures, muscle atrophy, and boredom. Nursing care goals include maintaining joint ROM, minimizing muscle atrophy, and reducing boredom.

- Encourage active ROM exercises at least every 8 hours. Provide passive ROM as needed. ROM exercises maintain joint mobility and prevent contractures. Active ROM (performed by the client) also helps prevent muscle atrophy and preserve function. While passive ROM exercises do not prevent muscle atrophy, they do maintain joint mobility.
- Encourage frequent position changes, deep breathing, and coughing. Prolonged immobility can lead to impaired airway clearance and respiratory complications, such as atelectasis or pneumonia. Turning, coughing, and deep breathing facilitate expulsion of secretions from the respiratory tract, airway clearance, and alveolar ventilation.
- Encourage increased fluid and dietary fiber intake. Constipation is a frequent complication of immobility that results from decreased gastrointestinal motility and loss of abdominal muscle strength. Increasing fluid and fiber intake helps maintain soft, easily expelled stools.
- Assist with and encourage ambulation as allowed. Ambulation promotes venous blood flow, helps maintain muscle tone and joint mobility, and increases the sense of well-being.
- Encourage diversional activities, such as reading, handiwork or other hobbies, television or video games, and socializing. Boredom may lead to dozing and inertia, with little physical movement or mental stimulation, increasing the risk for complications of immobility.

Risk for Ineffective Tissue Perfusion: Cardiopulmonary

A thrombus that forms in the deep veins of the legs or pelvis may break loose or fragment, becoming an embolism. Emboli that originate in the venous system usually become trapped in the pulmonary circulation (pulmonary embolism). Gas exchange in the affected area is impaired as blood flow ceases or is reduced to an area of the lungs that is well ventilated.

- Frequently assess respiratory status, including rate, depth, ease, and oxygen saturation levels. A mismatch of ventilation and perfusion can significantly affect gas exchange,

CLIENT TEACHING **Home Care for Deep Venous Thrombosis**

Treatment measures for venous thrombosis may be initiated and carried out on an outpatient basis or continued for an extended period of time following hospital discharge. Include the following topics when teaching for home care:

- Explanation of the disease process
- Treatment measures, including laboratory tests and their purposes as well as medications and adverse effects that should be reported
- Appropriate methods of heat application
- Prescribed activity restrictions
- Measures to prevent future episodes of venous thrombosis
- The importance of follow-up visits and laboratory tests as scheduled.

Refer clients for community nursing services for continued assessment and reinforcement of teaching. Provide referrals for assistance with activities of daily living and home maintenance services as indicated. Consider referral for physical therapy if needed.

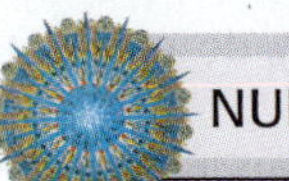

NURSING CARE PLAN A Client With Deep Venous Thrombosis

ASSESSMENT

Mrs. Opal Hipps, age 75, lives alone with her dog, Chester, in her family home in the suburbs. She retired from her job as a postal clerk 10 years ago and now spends a lot of time reading and watching television. Over the past week, she has developed a vague, aching pain in her right leg. She ignored the pain until last night, when it developed into a much more severe pain in her right calf. She noticed that her right lower leg seemed larger than the left, and it was very tender to the touch. After seeing her physician and undergoing Doppler ultrasound studies, Mrs. Hipps is admitted to the hospital with the diagnosis of deep venous thrombosis in the right leg. She is placed on bedrest and intravenous heparin. Michael Cookson, RN, is assigned to admit and care for Mrs. Hipps.

Mr. Cookson notices that Mrs. Hipps was admitted 14 months ago for repair of a fractured femur. Mrs. Hipps says, "This business about a blood clot really has me worried." She also tells Mr. Cookson that she is worried about who will care for her dog while she is in the hospital. Physical findings include the following: height, 62 in. (157 cm); weight, 149 lb (68 kg); temperature, 99.2°F (37.3°C); vital signs within normal limits otherwise. Her left leg is warm and pink, with strong peripheral pulses and good capillary refill. Her right calf is dark red, very warm, and dry to the touch. It is tender to palpation. The right femoral and popliteal pulses are strong, but the pedal and posterior tibial pulses are difficult to locate. The right calf diameter is 0.5 in. (1.27 cm) larger than the left.

DIAGNOSES

- Pain related to inflammatory response in affected vein
- Anxiety related to unexpected hospitalization and uncertainty about the seriousness of her illness
- Ineffective Tissue Perfusion: Peripheral related to decreased venous circulation in the right leg
- Risk for Impaired Skin Integrity related to pooling of venous blood in the right leg

PLANNING

Goals of care include the following:

- The client will verbalize relief of right leg pain by the day of discharge.
- The client will verbalize reduced anxiety by the second day of hospitalization.
- The client will demonstrate reduced right leg diameter by 0.25 in. (0.64 cm) by the fifth day of hospitalization.
- The client will maintain intact skin in the right foot throughout the hospital stay.

IMPLEMENTATION

- Elevate legs, maintaining slight knee flexion, while in bed.
- Apply warm, moist compresses to right leg using a 2-hours-on, 2-hours-off schedule around the clock.
- Administer prescribed analgesics, and evaluate their effectiveness.
- Spend time with Mrs. Hipps to explain venous thrombosis and its treatment.
- Arrange for a friend or neighbor to care for Mrs. Hipps's dog.
- Apply antiembolism stockings as ordered; remove for 30 minutes every 8 hours.
- Monitor laboratory values to assess effect of anticoagulant therapy; report values outside the desired range.
- Assist with progressive ambulation when allowed.
- Inspect legs and feet, and record findings, every 8 hours.

EVALUATION

Seven days after admission, the pain in Mrs. Hipps's right leg has subsided and the diameter of her right calf is equal to that of her left calf. Mrs. Hipps admits to Mr. Cookson that her fears really relate to a cousin who was hospitalized for a similar problem and had his leg amputated. After talking about her condition and the steps she can take to prevent its recurrence, she is much less anxious. Before discharge, Mr. Cookson reviews instructions for antiembolism stockings, daily walking, warfarin schedule, and scheduled follow-up appointment. Mrs. Hipps's neighbor, Kate, comes to pick her up. As Mr. Cookson is helping Mrs. Hipps into the car, Kate hands her a small brown dog and says, "I took good care of Chester for you, but he's missed you." Mrs. Hipps smiles, and assures Mr. Cookson that she will call the number he provided if she has any questions.

CRITICAL THINKING

1. Describe the pathophysiologic reasons for the pain in Mrs. Hipps's right leg.
2. How would you respond if Mrs. Hipps tells you she does not have the money to buy the prescribed anticoagulant when she goes home?
3. How would you change your teaching and discharge planning if Mrs. Hipps had difficulty caring for herself?
4. Design a plan of care for Mrs. Hipps for the nursing diagnosis activity intolerance.

leading to rapid and shallow respirations, dyspnea and air hunger, and a fall in oxygen saturation levels.

- Initiate oxygen therapy, elevate the head of the bed, and reassure the client who is experiencing manifestations of pulmonary embolism. Oxygen therapy and elevating the head of the bed promote ventilation and gas exchange in those alveoli that are well perfused, helping maintain tissue oxygenation. Reassurance helps reduce anxiety and slow the respiratory rate, promoting greater respiratory depth and alveolar ventilation.

Evaluation

Client outcomes are evaluated based on their progress in meeting goals and may include the following expected outcomes:

- The client reports pain control adequate to allow rest and comfort.
- The client experiences no complications related to reduced perfusion.
- The client experiences no complications secondary to immobility.
- The client describes strategies for preventing reoccurrence of DVT.

REVIEW Deep Venous Thrombosis

RELATE: LINK THE CONCEPTS

Linking the exemplar of Deep Venous Thrombosis with the concept of Mobility:

1. What strategies can you implement to reduce the risk of DVT in the client who is confined to bed?
2. Develop a teaching plan aimed at reducing the risk of DVT in an older client who has limited mobility.

Linking the exemplar of Deep Venous Thrombosis with the concept of Reproduction:

3. Why is the pregnant client at increased risk for DVT?
4. Explain the specific factors that increase risk fo DVT at each stage of pregnancy (prenatal, antenatal, and post partum)

READY: GO TO COMPANION SKILLS MANUAL

- Assessing the client in pain
- Assessing the skin
- Assessing respirations
- Oxygen saturation (using a pulse oximeter)
- Administering oxygen by cannula, face mask, or face tent
- Applying compresses and moist packs
- Performing passive range of motion exercises

REFER: GO TO MYNURSINGKIT

REFLECT: CASE STUDY

Jennifer Walker is a 20-year-old female college student majoring in business. She lives with her boyfriend, Sam age 21, in an off-campus apartment. Jennifer and Sam enjoy walking around the campus with their dog, Shelby, and playing tennis and golf. Sam's parents are both doctors and Jennifer's mother is a nurse.

At her examination several months ago, Jennifer obtained a prescription for oral contraceptives. Jennifer has been taking them daily. Recently, she began to notice pain in her left leg when she walks. She ignored it for several days thinking she just pulled a muscle while playing tennis but the pain gets worse. Today she is unable to put any pressure on the leg. She also notes a red area on the calf of her leg that is hot to touch and very tender. She calls the campus clinic and makes an appointment to be seen today.

1. What factors in Jennifer's history puts her at risk for developing a DVT?
2. What is you priority nursing diagnosis for Jennifer?
3. What teaching will you provide Jennifer during her visit to the campus clinic?

22.5 DISSEMINATED INTRAVASCULAR COAGULATION

KEY TERMS

Disseminated intravascular coagulation (DIC), *1398*
Fibrin degradation products, *1398*
Schistocytes, *1399*

BASIS FOR SELECTION OF EXEMPLAR

Centers for Disease Control and Prevention
Institute of Medicine

LEARNING OUTCOMES

After reading about this exemplar, you will be able to:

1. Describe the pathophysiology, etiology, clinical manifestations, and direct and indirect causes of disseminated intravascular coagulation.
2. Identify risk factors associated with disseminated intravascular coagulation.
3. Illustrate the nursing process in providing culturally competent care across the life span for individuals with disseminated intravascular coagulation.
4. Formulate priority nursing diagnoses appropriate for an individual with disseminated intravascular coagulation.
5. Create a plan of care for individuals with disseminated intravascular coagulation and their families.
6. Assess expected outcomes for an individual with disseminated intravascular coagulation.
7. Discuss therapies used in the collaborative care of an individual with disseminated intravascular coagulation.
8. Employ evidence-based caring interventions for an individual with disseminated intravascular coagulation.

OVERVIEW

Disseminated intravascular coagulation (DIC) is a disruption of hemostasis characterized by widespread intravascular clotting and bleeding. It may be acute and life-threatening, or it may be relatively mild.

PHYSIOLOGY AND ETIOLOGY

Disseminated intravascular coagulation is triggered by endothelial damage, release of tissue factors into the circulation, or inappropriate activation of the clotting cascade by an endotoxin. Both the intrinsic and the extrinsic clotting cascade may be activated, although the extrinsic cascade usually is the one activated. Extensive thrombin entering the systemic circulation overwhelms natural anticoagulants, leading to unrestricted clot formation (McCance & Huether, 2006). Clotting may be localized to an individual organ, or it may be widespread, with deposition of small thrombi and emboli throughout the microvasculature (Kasper et al., 2005). The widespread clotting consumes clotting factors (prothrombin, platelets, factor V, and factor VIII in particular) and activates fibrinolytic processes with anticoagulant production. As a result, hemorrhage occurs (Figure 22–41 ■).

The sequence of DIC is as follows:

1. Endothelial damage, tissue factors, or toxins stimulate the clotting cascade.
2. Excess thrombin within the circulation overwhelms naturally occurring anticoagulants.
3. Widespread clotting occurs within the microvasculature.
4. Thrombi and emboli impair tissue perfusion, leading to ischemia, infarction, and necrosis.
5. Clotting factors and platelets are consumed faster than they can be replaced.
6. Clotting activates fibrinolytic processes, which begin to break down clots.
7. **Fibrin degradation products** (potent anticoagulants) are released, contributing to bleeding.
8. Clotting factors are depleted, the ability to form clots is lost, and hemorrhage occurs.

Etiology

Disseminated intravascular coagulation is a clinical syndrome that develops as a complication of a wide variety of other disorders (Box 22–19). Sepsis is the most common cause of DIC. Gram-negative and gram-positive bacteria as well as viruses, fungi, and protozoal infections may lead to DIC (McCance & Huether, 2006).

Risk Factors

Disseminated intravascular coagulation occurs more often in pregnancies complicated by preeclampsia, abruptio placentae, intrauterine fetal demise, amniotic fluid embolism, maternal liver disease, and septic abortion. Although DIC is not considered a

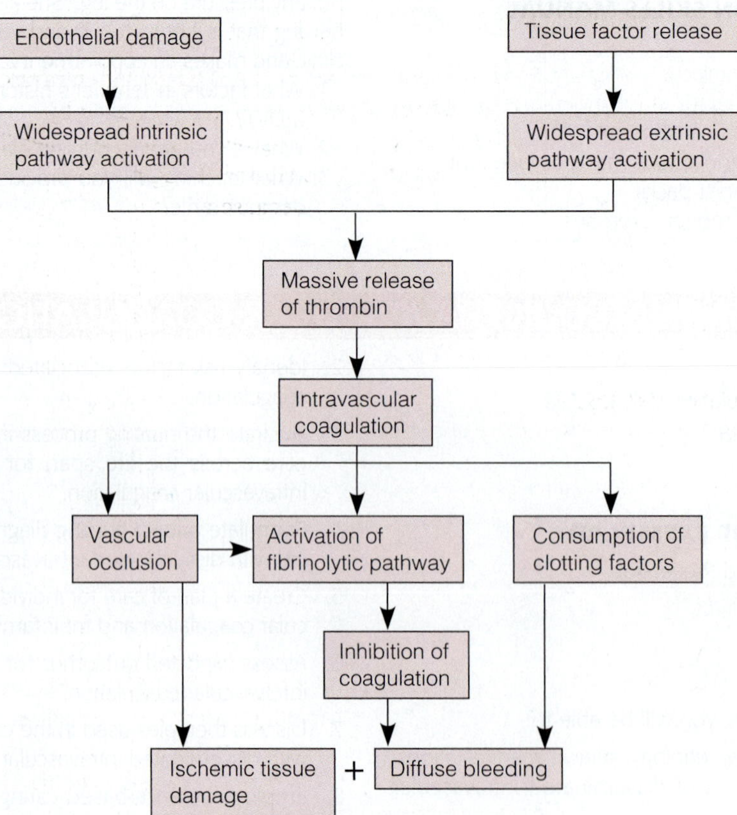

Figure 22–41 ■ Disseminated intravascular coagulation (DIC). Endothelial cell injury or release of tissue factors activate the intrinsic or extrinsic clotting pathway (or both). As a result, numerous microthrombi form throughout the vasculature, causing ischemic tissue damage. Simultaneously, rapid consumption of clotting factors and activation of fibrinolytic mechanisms trigger widespread bleeding.

component of severe preeclampsia, eclampsia, or HELLP syndrome (group of symptoms that occur in pregnancy including hemolysis, elevated liver enzymes, and low platelet count), it can occur as a complication when any of these conditions exist. The incidence of DIC occurring when HELLP is the only risk factor is approximately 5% (Sibai, 2007).

CLINICAL MANIFESTATIONS

The manifestations of DIC result from both clotting and bleeding, although bleeding is more obvious, especially in acute DIC. Bleeding ranges from oozing blood following an injection to frank hemorrhage from every body orifice. Chronic DIC may be asymptomatic, or it may present with peripheral cyanosis, thrombosis, and pregangrenous changes in the fingers and toes, nose, and genitalia (Kasper et al., 2005). See the Clinical Manifestations and Therapies feature on the following page.

COLLABORATION

Treatment of DIC is directed toward treating the underlying disorder and preventing further bleeding or massive thrombosis. Treatment stabilizes the client, reduces complications, and allows recovery to occur; it does not cure DIC (Kasper et al., 2005).

Diagnostic Tests

Diagnostic tests are used to confirm the diagnosis of DIC and evaluate the risk for hemorrhage. Relevant diagnostic tests include the following:

- *Complete blood count* and *platelet count* are used to evaluate the hemoglobin, hematocrit, and number of circulating platelets. **Schistocytes** (fragmented red blood cells) may be noted as a result of cell trapping and damage within fibrin thrombi. The platelet count is decreased.
- *Coagulation studies* show prolonged prothrombin time, partial thromboplastin time, and thrombin time as well as a low fibrinogen level caused by depletion of clotting factors. The fibrinogen level helps predict bleeding in DIC: As it falls, the risk of bleeding increases (Kasper et al., 2005).
- *Fibrin degradation products* or *fibrin split products* are increased as a result of the fibrinolysis that occurs with DIC.

Box 22–19 Conditions That May Precipitate Disseminated Intravascular Coagulation

TISSUE DAMAGE

- Trauma: burns, gunshot wounds, frostbite, head injury
- Obstetric complications: septic abortion, abruptio placentae, amniotic fluid embolus, retained dead fetus
- Neoplasms: acute leukemia, adenocarcinomas
- Hemolysis
- Fat embolism

VESSEL DAMAGE

- Aortic aneurysm
- Acute glomerulonephritis
- Hemolytic uremic syndrome

INFECTIONS

- Bacterial infection or sepsis
- Viral or mycotic infections
- Parasitic or rickettsial infection

Clinical Therapies

When bleeding is the major manifestation of DIC, fresh frozen plasma and platelet concentrates are given to restore clotting factors and platelets. Heparin, although controversial, may be administered. Heparin interferes with the clotting cascade and may prevent further clotting factor consumption as a result of uncontrolled thrombosis. It is used when bleeding is not controlled by plasma and platelets as well as when the client has manifestations of thrombotic problems, such as acrocyanosis (cyanotic, or blue, color in the hands and/or feet) and possible gangrene. Long-term heparin therapy (administered by injection or continuous infusion using a portable pump) may be necessary for clients with chronic DIC.

In severe cases of DIC, supportive care is essential to maintain life. Intracranial bleeding may result in altered levels of consciousness, damage to the respiratory center, and increased intracranial pressure. Supportive care may include mechanical ventilation and control of organ damage caused by reduced perfusion.

NURSING PROCESS

Disseminated intravascular coagulation is a complex disorder that is managed by a critical care team. Nursing care focuses on assessing the bleeding, preventing further injury, and administering prescribed therapies.

Because all body systems can be involved, careful assessment of all systems is needed on a continual basis. Observe for petechiae, ecchymoses, and oozing every 1–2 hours. Check dependent areas because blood will pool there. Intravenous sites are particularly prone to oozing and should be assessed every 15 minutes. Examine stool for the presence of blood, and measure blood loss as accurately as possible. Assess extremities for capillary refill, warmth, and pulses. Frequently assess vital signs and level of consciousness. Measure intake and output. Monitor urine for the presence of blood. Blood urea nitrogen and creatinine are monitored to assess renal function.

Institute bleeding-control precautions, monitor prescribed therapy (transfusion or anticoagulant therapy), and report any signs of complications. Monitor oxygen saturation and arterial blood gases. The child may require mechanical ventilation. Maintain patency of the airway, and ensure correct endotracheal tube position.

Implement measures to maintain skin integrity, such as gentle repositioning. Implement a nutritional plan of tube feedings or total parenteral nutrition. Identify the family members' coping strategies and support system to facilitate their ability to manage this life-threatening crisis.

CLINICAL MANIFESTATIONS AND THERAPIES Disseminated Intravascular Coagulation

ETIOLOGY	CLINICAL MANIFESTATION	CLINICAL THERAPIES
CARDIOVASCULAR SYSTEM		
Tachycardia	Decreased perfusion, shock	■ Administer fluids as ordered; monitor intake and output
Hypotension	Inappropriate clotting	
Circulatory collapse		■ Monitor vital signs
Major vessel thrombosis		
RESPIRATORY SYSTEM		
Tachypnea	Impaired gas exchange resulting from microclots in the pulmonary vasculature	■ Monitor respiratory status
Decreased breath sounds		■ Maintain ventilatory support if required
CENTRAL NERVOUS SYSTEM		
Confusion	Impaired cerebral perfusion	■ Conduct neurologic assessment every 2 hours during critical period, then every 4 hours until stabilized
Coma		
Seizures		
URINARY SYSTEM		
Oliguria	Impaired renal perfusion	■ Monitor urine output hourly
Anuria	Impaired clotting mechanisms lead to bleeding	■ Maintain patent urinary catheter
Renal failure		■ Monitor urine for blood
Hematuria		
GASTROINTESTINAL SYSTEM		
Gastrointestinal bleeding	Impaired clotting mechanisms lead to bleeding	■ Monitor for occult blood in stools and emesis
Abdominal distention		■ Monitor for overt signs of bleeding from gums
Bleeding from mucous membranes		■ Measure abdominal girth every 4 hours
Occult blood in stool or emesis		
INTEGUMENTARY SYSTEM		
Petechiae	Impaired clotting mechanism leads to bleeding	■ Monitor skin for evidence of bleeding
Purpura	Impaired tissue perfusion	■ Protect from injury
Ecchymosis		■ Monitor distal pulses, temperature, and capillary refill
Bleeding or oozing from wounds or intravenous access site		
Pallor		
Cool extremities		
Cyanosis of extremities		
GANGRENE		
General: weakness, malaise	Shock, decreased perfusion	■ Cluster care to allow for rest periods
Oozing from body orifices	Impaired clotting mechanism leads to bleeding	■ Maintain bedrest

Assessment

Focused nursing assessment for DIC includes obtaining the following information:

- *Health history.* Recent abortion (spontaneous or therapeutic) or current pregnancy; presence of a known malignant tumor; history of abnormal bleeding episodes or a hematologic disorder.
- *Physical examination.* Bleeding from puncture wounds (e.g., injections), intravenous sites, or incisions; hematuria, obvious or occult blood in emesis or stool, epistaxis, or other abnormal bleeding; vital signs; heart and breath sounds; abdominal assessment, including girth, contour, bowel sounds, tenderness, or guarding to palpation; color, temperature, and skin condition of hands, feet, and digits; petechiae or purpura of skin or mucous membranes.

Diagnosis

Clients with acute DIC often are critically ill, with multiple nursing care needs. As mentioned, septic shock may precipitate DIC; hemorrhagic shock may occur as a complication of DIC. Priority nursing diagnoses discussed in this section include the following:

- Ineffective Tissue Perfusion
- Impaired Gas Exchange
- Pain
- Fear.

Plan

Goals of nursing care may include the following:

- The client will demonstrate adequate tissue perfusion, as evidenced by capillary refill time, vital signs, and hemoglobin and hematocrit within acceptable limits.
- The client will demonstrate adequate gas exchange, as evidenced by arterial blood gas results, oxygen saturation monitoring, and respiratory status.
- The client will demonstrate adequate pain control, as evidenced by ability to rest and client's description of pain.
- The client will exhibit fear self-control, as evidenced by seeking information, using relaxation techniques, and ability to maintain role performance.

Implementation

Care of the client diagnosed with DIC often requires specialized nursing in critical care. Continuous monitoring for inadequate oxygenation, altered perfusion, and bleeding are priorities of nursing care.

Ineffective Tissue Perfusion

Thrombi and emboli forming throughout the microcirculation affect the perfusion of multiple organs and tissues. Additionally, bleeding as a result of clotting factor consumption affects cardiac output and blood flow to these tissues.

- Assess extremity pulses, warmth, and capillary refill. Monitor level of consciousness and mental status. Monitoring central and peripheral tissue perfusion facilitates early treatment of impaired perfusion.
- Carefully reposition at least every 2 hours. Position changes facilitate circulation and tissue perfusion and also provide an opportunity to assess for purpura, pallor, and bleeding.
- Discourage crossing the legs, and do not elevate the knees on the bed or with a pillow. These positions may impair arterial and venous flow to the lower legs and feet, increasing vascular stasis and the risk for thrombosis.
- Minimize use of tape on the skin, using binders, nonadhesive dressings, and other devices as needed. Preventing skin trauma reduces the risk for bleeding and potential infection.

Impaired Gas Exchange

Microclots in the pulmonary vasculature are likely to interfere with gas exchange in the client with DIC.

- Monitor oxygen saturation continuously. Administer oxygen as ordered. Oxygen saturation levels are a noninvasive means of assessing gas exchange. Supplemental oxygen promotes gas exchange and reduces cardiac work, relieving dyspnea.
- Place in Fowler's or high-Fowler's position as tolerated. Elevating the head of the bed improves diaphragmatic excursion and alveolar ventilation.
- Maintain bedrest. Bedrest reduces oxygen demands and cardiac work.
- Encourage deep breathing and effective coughing. Increased respiratory depth and clearance of secretions from airways improves alveolar ventilation and oxygenation.
- Cautious nasotracheal suctioning may be instituted if cough is ineffective or an endotracheal tube is in place. Removal of secretions facilitates ventilation and oxygenation. However, care must be used to minimize suction-induced hypoxia and airway trauma.
- Administer analgesics and antianxiety drugs as needed to control pain and anxiety. Provide reassurance and comfort measures. Pain and anxiety increase the respiratory rate and decrease the depth of respirations, reducing effective ventilation and gas exchange.

Pain

Both the underlying cause of DIC and the tissue ischemia from microvascular clots can cause pain. Identifying the etiology of pain is important to identify potential complications or harmful effects of DIC and institute effective treatment.

- Use a standard pain scale to evaluate and monitor pain and analgesic effectiveness. Monitoring pain and response to medication facilitates development of an appropriate and effective treatment plan.
- Handle extremities gently. Gentle handling reduces the risk of further injury to and pain in ischemic tissues.

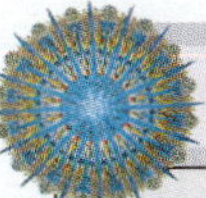

NURSING CARE PLAN A Client With Disseminated Intravascular Coagulation

Addy McMannis, 19 years old, is admitted to the hospital with toxic shock syndrome believed to have resulted from improper use of tampons. She has intravenous fluids infusing at 125 mL/hr and is receiving broad-spectrum antibiotics. She reports feeling very weak and fatigued and says all she wants to do is sleep. Two days later, she is diagnosed with disseminated intravascular coagulation.

ASSESSMENT	DIAGNOSES	PLANNING
Petechia and small bruises are noted over all of her extremities. Ms. McMannis also reports bleeding from the gums during oral care. Hematuria is noted. Laboratory studies are as follows: platelet count, 71,000; hematocrit, 28%; prolonged prothrombin time, partial thromboplastin time, and thrombin time; low fibrinogen level; elevated white blood cell count. Vital signs are as follows: temperature, 100.2°F oral; pulse, 108 bpm; respirations, 24 minutes; and blood pressure, 104/60 mmHg.	■ Ineffective Tissue Perfusion ■ Fatigue ■ Risk for Injury	Goals of care include the following: ■ Provide ongoing and continuous assessment of oxygenation, perfusion, and neurological status. ■ Promote rest for the client and minimize oxygen metabolism. ■ Provide support and education for the client and family related to the diagnosis, treatment, and diagnostic testing. ■ Monitor for and reduce bleeding to reduce risk of complications. ■ Promote tissue perfusion to reduce risk of complications.

IMPLEMENTATION

- Assess pulses, warmth, and capillary refill in extremities, and monitor level of consciousness.
- Teach client to use sponge for oral care to reduce risk of gum trauma and only an electric razor when shaving.
- Administer medications as indicated.
- Support oxygenation which may include mechanical ventilation.
- Monitor for bleeding (stools, venipunctures, open wounds, and emesis).
- Encourage gentle repositioning frequently to prevent loss of skin integrity.
- Discourage crossing of the legs or elevation of the knees to promote circulation to the feet.
- Minimize use of tape on the skin to prevent altered skin integrity.
- Schedule care to allow periods of uninterrupted sleep and prevent overtiring.
- Provide emotional support to client and family.
- Monitor respiratory pattern, breath sounds, and oxygenation.

EVALUATION

Ms. McMannis continues to receive antibiotics to treat toxic shock syndrome and is also given fresh frozen plasma and platelet concentrates, which controls bleeding. Her platelet count decreases initially but eventually returns to near normal, and she is discharged a week later with instructions to follow up with her primary care provider and immediately report any signs of bleeding or bruising.

CRITICAL THINKING

1. Why, if the disease is caused by small clots forming, do clients manifest this disease with bleeding?
2. What effect does the administration of platelet concentrate have on platelet production?
3. Was the diagnosis of toxic shock syndrome related to the occurrence of disseminated intravascular coagulation? Explain your answer.

- Apply cool compresses to painful joints. Application of cold decreases pain through the gate-control mechanism, inhibiting the dorsal horn of the spinal cord and reducing the sensation of pain.

Fear

The underlying serious illness and a complication such as DIC result in an uncertain prognosis, often accompanied by fear.

- Encourage the client and family to verbalize concerns. This helps the client and family identify their concerns and frame questions.
- Answer questions truthfully. Providing honest answers is vital to developing a therapeutic nurse–client relationship. Accurate responses allow the client and family to set priorities as they plan for an uncertain future.

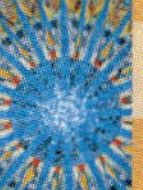

CLIENT TEACHING Disseminated Intravascular Coagulation

Although the immediate crisis of acute DIC is resolved before discharge, the client may have some continuing effects of the disorder, such as impaired tissue integrity of distal extremities. Teach the client and family about specific care needs, such as foot care or dressing changes. Provide instruction about any continuing medications and follow-up care.

Clients with chronic DIC may require continuing heparin therapy, using either intermittent subcutaneous injections or a portable infusion pump. Teach the client and family members how to administer the injection or manage the infusion pump. Provide a referral to home health care or home intravenous management service for assistance. Discuss the manifestations of excessive bleeding or recurrent clotting that need to be reported to the physician.

- Help the client and family identify coping strategies to manage this significant situational stressor. Implementing previously effective coping methods may provide the skills to manage the current crisis.
- Provide emotional support. The presence of a caring nurse helps reduce the fear and anxiety associated with a crisis.
- Maintain a calm environment. A calm environment provides reassurance that the situation is in control, reduces anxiety, and promotes rest.
- Respond promptly when the client calls for help. Prompt response to expressed needs helps develop a trusting relationship and a sense of security that assistance is readily available.
- Teach relaxation techniques. Relaxation techniques can reduce muscle tension and other signs of anxiety. Gaining control over physical responses can help the client gain a sense of control over the situation.

Evaluation

The client's response to nursing care may be evaluated using the following expected outcomes:

- Client experiences no complications from DIC
- Family demonstrates effective coping techniques to deal with severity of client's illness
- Client's bleeding is controlled
- Client's body systems are capable of meeting needs of oxygenation and perfusion to prevent tissue distruction.

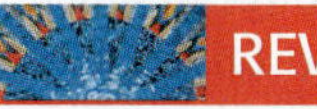

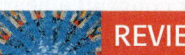

REVIEW Disseminated Intravascular Coagulation

RELATE: LINK THE CONCEPTS

Linking the exemplar of Disseminated Intravascular Coagulation with the concept of Elimination:

1. What pathophysiology places the client with DIC at increased risk for renal failure?
2. Prioritize care for the client diagnosed with DIC who experiences acute renal failure as a result.

Linking the exemplar of Disseminated Intravascular Coagulation with the concept of Intracranial Regulation:

3. What assessment findings would indicate possible increased intracranial pressure in the client diagnosed with DIC?
4. What is your priority nursing intervention if signs of increased intracranial pressure are found in the client with DIC?

READY: GO TO COMPANION SKILLS MANUAL

- Applying compresses and moist packs
- Supporting a client in Fowler's position
- Deep breathing and coughing
- Oxygen saturation using a pulse oximeter
- Administering oxygen by cannula, face mask, or face tent
- Assessing the client in pain
- Assessing respirations
- Assessing an apical pulse
- Assessing blood pressure

REFER: GO TO MYNURSINGKIT

REFLECT: CASE STUDY

Rhonda Fischer, 29 years old, has just delivered her fourth child by emergency cesarean section at 36 weeks' gestation secondary to beta strep sepsis. Rhonda lives with her husband Mark and their three other children, Lisa age 4, Robin age 5, and Fred age 7. Rhonda is a stay-at-home mother. Mark is 30 years old and is up for partner in the law firm where he works.

Rhonda tested positive for vaginal strep at 28 weeks and was given a course of antibiotics. However, she developed another infection after the antibiotics were finished. In order to protect the baby, the doctor opted for a cesarean section. Rhonda and Mark agreed. Rhonda was placed on IV antibiotics prior to surgery and is now on the postpartum unit. During a focused assessment, the nurse notes that Rhonda is having frank bleeding from her incision and she is oozing blood from around her IV site. Her vital signs include T_O 99.7, P 96, R 28, BP 100/65.

1. What are the first laboratory data you will want to review on Rhonda's medical record?
2. What nursing diagnosis will you add to Rhonda's plan of care based on these assessment findings?
3. What nursing interventions will you initiate for Rhonda?
4. What client teaching will you provide Rhonda and Mark to explain the diagnosis of DIC made by the obstetrician?

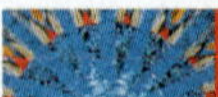

22.6 HEART FAILURE

KEY TERMS

Decompensation, *1404*
Exercise intolerance, *1416*
Frank–Starling mechanism, *1405*
Heart failure, *1404*
Hemodynamics, *1411*
Mean arterial pressure (MAP), *1411*
Nocturia, *1408*
Orthopnea, *1408*
Paroxysmal nocturnal dyspnea, *1408*
Pulmonary edema, *1404*

BASIS FOR SELECTION OF EXEMPLAR

Centers for Disease Control and Prevention
Healthy People 2010

LEARNING OUTCOMES

After reading about this exemplar, you will be able to:

1. Describe the pathophysiology, etiology, clinical manifestations, and direct and indirect causes of heart failure.
2. Identify risk factors associated with heart failure.
3. Illustrate the nursing process in providing culturally competent care across the life span for individuals with heart failure.
4. Formulate priority nursing diagnoses appropriate for an individual with heart failure.
5. Create a plan of care for individuals with heart failure and their families.
6. Asses expected outcomes for an individual with heart failure.
7. Discuss therapies used in the collaborative care of an individual with heart failure.
8. Employ evidence-based caring interventions for an individual with heart failure.

OVERVIEW

Heart failure is a complex syndrome resulting from cardiac disorders that impair the ability of the ventricles to fill with and effectively pump blood (Hunt et al., 2005). In heart failure, the heart is unable to pump enough blood to meet the metabolic demands of the body.

Heart failure is the end result of many conditions. Frequently, it is a long-term effect of coronary heart disease and MI when left ventricular damage is extensive enough to impair cardiac output. Other diseases of the heart, including structural and inflammatory disorders, also may cause heart failure. In normal hearts, failure can result from excessive demands placed on the heart. Heart failure may be acute or chronic.

Heart failure develops when the heart cannot effectively fill or contract with adequate strength to function as a pump to meet the needs of the body. As a result, cardiac output falls, leading to decreased tissue perfusion. The body initially adjusts to reduced cardiac output by activating inherent compensatory mechanisms to restore tissue perfusion. These normal mechanisms may result in vascular congestion—hence, the commonly used term *congestive heart failure*. As these mechanisms are exhausted, heart failure ensues, with increased morbidity and mortality.

Heart failure is a disorder of cardiac function. It frequently is the result of impaired myocardial contraction, which may result from coronary heart disease and myocardial ischemia or infarct or from a primary cardiac muscle disorder, such as cardiomyopathy or myocarditis. Structural cardiac disorders, such as valve disorders or congenital heart defects, and hypertension also can lead to heart failure when the heart muscle is damaged by the long-standing excessive workload associated with these conditions. Other clients without a primary abnormality of myocardial function may present with manifestations of heart failure as a result of acute excess demands placed on the myocardium, such as volume overload, hyperthyroidism, and massive pulmonary embolus (Table 22–25).

Pulmonary edema is an abnormal accumulation of fluid in the interstitial tissue and alveoli of the lung. Both cardiac and noncardiac disorders can cause pulmonary edema. Cardiac causes include AMI, acute heart failure, and valvular disease. Cardiogenic pulmonary edema, the focus of this section, is a sign of severe cardiac **decompensation** (the loss of effective compensation). Noncardiac causes of pulmonary edema include primary pulmonary disorders, such as acute respiratory distress syndrome, trauma, sepsis, drug overdose, or neurologic sequelae.

TABLE 22–25 **Selected Causes of Heart Failure**

IMPAIRED MYOCARDIAL FUNCTION	INCREASED CARDIAC WORKLOAD	ACUTE NONCARDIAC CONDITIONS
■ Coronary heart disease	■ Hypertension	■ Volume overload
■ Cardiomyopathies	■ Valve disorders	■ Hyperthyroidism
■ Rheumatic fever	■ Anemias	■ Fever, infection
■ Infective endocarditis	■ Congenital heart defects	■ Massive pulmonary embolus

Pulmonary edema is a medical emergency: The client is literally drowning in the fluid in the alveolar and interstitial pulmonary spaces. Its onset may be acute or gradual, progressing to severe respiratory distress. Immediate treatment is necessary.

PHYSIOLOGY AND ETIOLOGY

The mechanical pumping action of cardiac muscle propels the blood it receives to the pulmonary and systemic vascular systems for reoxygenation and delivery to the tissues. Cardiac output is the amount of blood pumped from the ventricles in 1 minute. Cardiac output is used to assess cardiac performance, especially left ventricular function. Effective cardiac output depends on adequate functional muscle mass and the ability of the ventricles to work together. Cardiac output normally is regulated by the oxygen needs of the body: As oxygen use increases, cardiac output increases to maintain cellular function. Cardiac reserve is the ability of the heart to increase cardiac output to meet metabolic demand. Ventricular damage reduces the cardiac reserve.

Cardiac output (CO) is a product of heart rate (HR) and stroke volume (SV). Heart rate affects cardiac output by controlling the number of ventricular contractions per minute. It is influenced by the autonomic nervous system, catecholamines, and thyroid hormones. Activation of a stress response (e.g., hypovolemia or fear) stimulates the sympathetic nervous system (SNS), increasing the heart rate and its contractility. Elevated heart rates increase cardiac output. Very rapid heart rates, however, shorten ventricular filling time (diastole), reducing stroke volume and cardiac output. On the other hand, a slow heart rate reduces cardiac output simply because of fewer cardiac cycles.

Stroke volume (the volume of blood ejected with each heartbeat) is determined by preload, afterload, and myocardial contractility. Preload is the volume of blood in the ventricles at end diastole (just before contraction). The blood in the ventricles exerts pressure on the ventricle walls, stretching muscle fibers. The greater the blood volume, the greater the force with which the ventricle contracts to expel the blood. End-diastolic volume depends on the amount of blood returning to the ventricles (venous return) and on the distensibility or stiffness of the ventricles (compliance).

Afterload is the force needed to eject blood into the circulation. This force must be great enough to overcome arterial pressures within the pulmonary and systemic vascular systems. The right ventricle must generate enough force to open the pulmonary valve and eject its blood into the pulmonary artery. The left ventricle ejects its blood into the systemic circulation by overcoming the arterial resistance behind the aortic valve. Increased systemic vascular resistance (e.g., hypertension) increases afterload, impairing stroke volume and increasing myocardial work.

Contractility is the natural ability of cardiac muscle fibers to shorten during systole. Contractility is necessary to overcome arterial pressures and eject blood during systole. Impaired contractility affects cardiac output by reducing stroke volume. The ejection fraction is the percentage of blood in the ventricle that is ejected during systole. A normal ejection fraction is 50–70%.

When the heart begins to fail, mechanisms are activated to compensate for the impaired function and maintain the cardiac output. The primary compensatory mechanisms are as follows:

1. The Frank–Starling mechanism
2. Neuroendocrine responses, including activation of the SNS and the renin–angiotensin system
3. Myocardial hypertrophy.

These mechanisms and their effects are summarized in Table 22–26.

Decreased cardiac output initially stimulates aortic baroreceptors, which in turn stimulate the SNS. Stimulation of the SNS produces both cardiac and vascular responses through the release of norepinephrine. Norepinephrine increases heart rate and contractility by stimulating cardiac beta-receptors. Cardiac output improves as both heart rate and stroke volume increase. Norepinephrine also causes arterial and venous vasoconstriction, increasing venous return to the heart. Increased venous return increases ventricular filling and myocardial stretch, increasing the force of contraction (the **Frank–Starling mechanism**). Overstretching the muscle fibers past their physiologic limit results in an ineffective contraction.

Blood flow is redistributed to the brain and the heart to maintain perfusion of these vital organs. Decreased renal perfusion causes renin to be released from the kidneys. Activation of the renin–angiotensin system produces additional vasoconstriction and stimulates the adrenal cortex to produce aldosterone and the posterior pituitary to release antidiuretic hormone (ADH). Aldosterone stimulates sodium reabsorption in renal tubules, promoting water retention. ADH acts on the distal tubule to inhibit water excretion, and it also causes vasoconstriction. The effect of these hormones is significant vasoconstriction as well as salt and water retention, with a resulting increase in vascular volume. Increased ventricular filling increases the force of contraction, improving cardiac output.

The effects of the renin–angiotensin–aldosterone system and ADH release are counterbalanced to a certain extent by two additional hormones. The increased vascular volume and venous return prompted by vasoconstriction and sodium and water retention increase the volume and pressures in the heart. Stimulation of stretch receptors in the atria and ventricles lead to the release of atrial natriuretic peptide (ANP) and brain natriuretic peptide (BNP) from stores in the atria (ANP and BNP) and ventricles (BNP). These hormones promote sodium and water excretion and inhibit the release of norepinephrine, renin, and ADH, with resulting vasodilation. Although beneficial, the effects of these hormones are too weak to completely counteract the vasoconstriction and the sodium and water retention that occurs in heart failure.

Ventricular remodeling occurs as the heart chambers and myocardium adapt to fluid volume and pressure increases. The chambers dilate to accommodate excess fluid resulting from increased vascular volume and incomplete emptying. Initially,

TABLE 22–26 **Compensatory Mechanisms Activated in Heart Failure**

MECHANISM	PHYSIOLOGY	EFFECT ON BODY SYSTEMS	COMPLICATIONS
Frank–Starling mechanism	The greater the stretch of cardiac muscle fibers, the greater the force of contraction.	■ Increased contractile force leading to increased CO	■ Increased myocardial oxygen demand ■ Limited by overstretching
Neuroendocrine response	Decreased CO stimulates the sympathetic nervous system and catecholamine release.	■ Increased heart rate, blood pressure, and contractility ■ Increased vascular resistance ■ Increased venous return	■ Increased vascular resistance ■ Tachycardia, with decreased filling time and decreased CO ■ Increased myocardial work and oxygen demand
	Decreased CO and decreased renal perfusion stimulate the renin–angiotensin system. Angiotensin stimulates aldosterone release from adrenal cortex. Antidiuretic hormone is released from posterior pituitary. Atrial natriuretic peptide and brain natriuretic peptide are released. Blood flow is redistributed to vital organs (heart and brain).	■ Vasoconstriction and increased blood pressure ■ Salt and water retention by the kidneys ■ Increased vascular volume ■ Water excretion inhibited ■ Increased sodium excretion ■ Diuresis ■ Vasodilation ■ Decreased perfusion of other organ systems ■ Decreased perfusion of skin and muscles	■ Increased myocardial work ■ Renal vasoconstriction and decreased renal perfusion ■ Increased preload and afterload ■ Pulmonary congestion ■ Fluid retention and increased preload and afterload ■ Pulmonary congestion ■ Renal failure ■ Anaerobic metabolism and lactic acidosis
Ventricular hypertrophy	Increased cardiac workload causes myocardial muscle to hypertrophy and ventricles to dilate.	■ Increased contractile force to maintain CO	■ Increased myocardial oxygen demand ■ Cellular enlargement

this additional stretch causes more effective contractions. Ventricular hypertrophy occurs as existing cardiac muscle cells enlarge, increasing their contractile elements (actin and myosin) and force of contraction.

Although these responses may help in the short-term regulation of cardiac output, it is now recognized that they also hasten the deterioration of cardiac function. The onset of heart failure is heralded by decompensation. Heart failure progresses as a result of the very mechanisms that initially maintained circulatory stability.

The rapid heart rate shortens diastolic filling time, compromises coronary artery perfusion, and increases myocardial oxygen demand. Resulting ischemia further impairs cardiac output. Beta-receptors in the heart become less sensitive to continued SNS stimulation, decreasing heart rate and contractility. As the beta-receptors become less sensitive, norepinephrine stores in the cardiac muscle become depleted. In contrast, alpha-receptors on peripheral blood vessels become increasingly sensitive to persistent stimulation, promoting vasoconstriction and increasing afterload and cardiac work.

As mentioned, ventricular hypertrophy and dilation initially increase cardiac output, but chronic distention eventually causes the ventricular wall to thin and degenerate. The purpose of hypertrophy is thus defeated. In addition, chronic overloading of the dilated ventricle eventually stretches the fibers beyond the optimal point for effective contraction. The ventricles continue to dilate to accommodate the excess fluid, but the heart loses the ability to contract forcefully. The heart muscle may eventually become so large that the coronary blood supply is inadequate, causing ischemia.

Chronic distention exhausts stores of ANP and BNP. The effects of norepinephrine, renin, and ADH prevail, and the renin–angiotensin pathway is continually stimulated. This mechanism ultimately raises the hemodynamic stress on the heart by increasing both preload and afterload. As heart function deteriorates, less blood is delivered to the tissues and to the heart itself. Ischemia and necrosis of the myocardium further weaken the already failing heart, and the cycle repeats.

In normal hearts, the cardiac reserve allows the heart to adjust its output to meet metabolic needs of the body, increasing the cardiac output by up to five times the basal level during exercise. Clients with heart failure have minimal to no cardiac reserve. At rest, they may be unaffected; however, any stressor (e.g., exercise, illness) taxes their ability to meet the demand for oxygen and nutrients. Manifestations of activity intolerance when the person is at rest indicate a critical level of cardiac decompensation.

Classifications

Heart failure is commonly classified in several different ways, depending on the underlying pathology. Classifications include systolic versus diastolic failure, left-sided versus right-sided failure, high-output versus low-output failure, or acute versus chronic failure.

SYSTOLIC VERSUS DIASTOLIC FAILURE Systolic failure occurs when the ventricle fails to contract adequately to eject a sufficient volume of blood into the arterial system. Systolic function is affected by loss of myocardial cells as a result of ischemia and infarction, cardiomyopathy, or inflammation.

Diastolic failure results when the heart cannot completely relax in diastole, disrupting normal filling. Passive diastolic filling decreases, increasing the importance of atrial contraction to preload. Diastolic dysfunction results from decreased ventricular compliance caused by hypertrophic and cellular changes and impaired relaxation of the heart muscle.

LEFT-SIDED VERSUS RIGHT-SIDED FAILURE Depending on the pathophysiology involved, either the left or the right ventricle may be primarily affected. In chronic heart failure, however, both ventricles typically are impaired to some degree.

Coronary heart disease and hypertension are common causes of left-sided heart failure, whereas right-sided heart failure often is caused by conditions that restrict blood flow to the lungs, such as acute or chronic pulmonary disease. Left-sided heart failure also can lead to right-sided failure as pressures in the pulmonary vascular system increase with congestion behind the failing left ventricle.

As left ventricular function fails, cardiac output falls. Pressures in the left ventricle and atrium increase as the amount of blood remaining in the ventricle after systole increases. These increased pressures impair filling, causing congestion and increased pressures in the pulmonary vascular system. Increased pressures in this normally low-pressure system increase fluid movement from the blood vessels into interstitial tissues and the alveoli (Figure 22–42 ■). The manifestations of left-sided heart failure result from pulmonary congestion (backward effects) and decreased cardiac output (forward effects).

In right-sided heart failure, increased pressures in the pulmonary vasculature or right ventricular muscle damage impair the right ventricle's ability to pump blood into the pulmonary circulation. The right ventricle and atrium become distended, and blood accumulates in the systemic venous system. Increased venous pressures cause abdominal organs to become congested and peripheral tissue edema to develop (Figure 22–43 ■).

Dependent tissues tend to be affected because of the effects of gravity.

LOW-OUTPUT VERSUS HIGH-OUTPUT FAILURE Clients with heart failure resulting from coronary heart disease, hypertension, cardiomyopathy, and other primary cardiac disorders develop low-output failure and manifestations such as those previously described. Clients in hypermetabolic states (e.g., hyperthyroidism, infection, anemia, or pregnancy) require increased cardiac output to maintain blood flow and oxygen to the tissues. If the increased blood flow cannot meet the oxygen demands of the tissues, compensatory mechanisms are activated to further increase cardiac output, which in turn further increases oxygen demand. Thus, even though cardiac output is high, the heart is unable to meet increased oxygen demands. This condition is known as high-output failure.

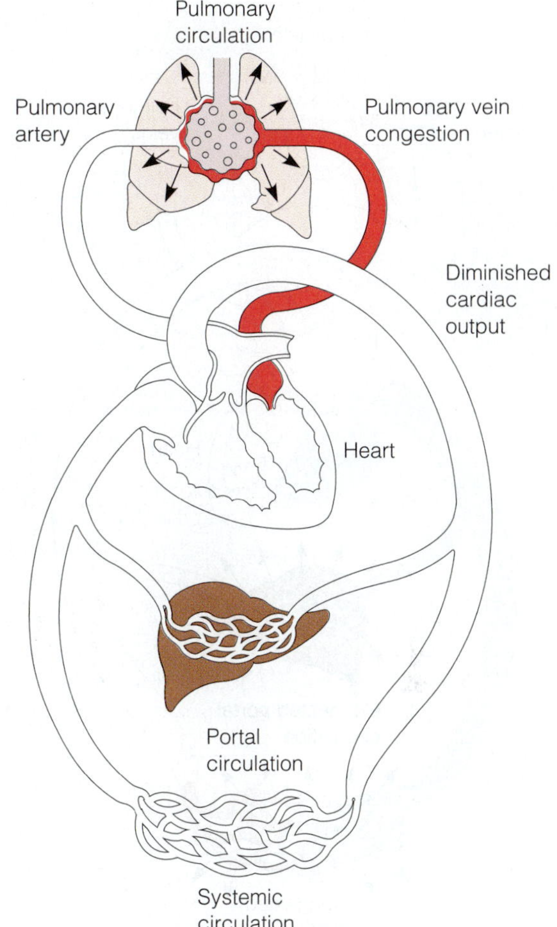

Figure 22–42 ■ The hemodynamic effects of left-sided heart failure.

ACUTE VERSUS CHRONIC FAILURE Acute failure is the abrupt onset of a myocardial injury (e.g., a massive MI) resulting in suddenly decreased cardiac function and signs of decreased cardiac output. Chronic failure is a progressive deterioration of the heart muscle as a result of cardiomyopathies, valvular disease, or coronary heart disease.

PULMONARY EDEMA In cardiogenic pulmonary edema, the contractility of the left ventricle is severely impaired. The ejection fraction falls because the ventricle is unable to eject the blood that enters it, causing a sharp rise in end-diastolic volume and pressure. Pulmonary hydrostatic pressures rise, ultimately exceeding the osmotic pressure of the blood. As a result, fluid leaking from the pulmonary capillaries congests interstitial tissues, decreasing lung compliance and interfering with gas exchange. As capillary and interstitial pressures increase further, the tight junctions of the alveolar walls are disrupted, and the fluid enters the alveoli, along with large red blood cells and protein molecules. Ventilation and gas exchange are severely disrupted, and hypoxia worsens.

Etiology

Ischemic heart disease (coronary heart disease) is the leading cause of heart failure. Cardiomyopathies are the second leading cause of heart failure. Other, less common causes of heart

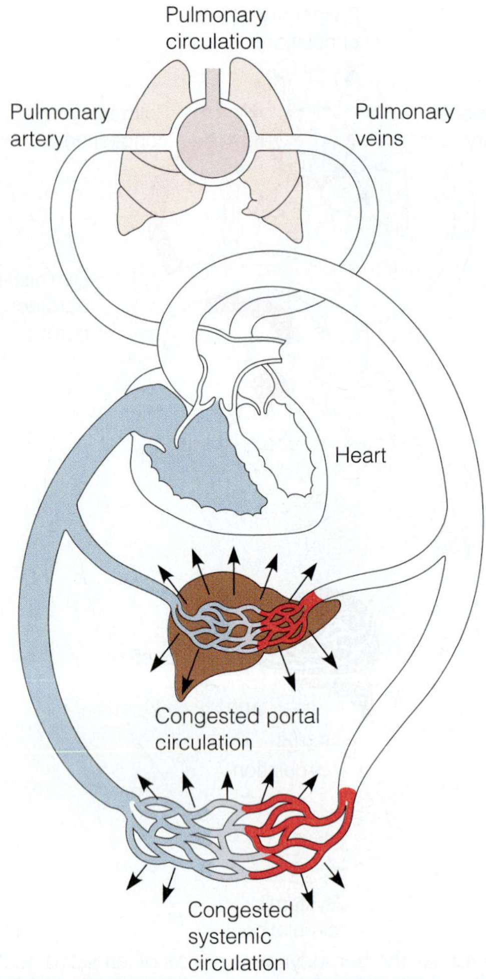

Figure 22–43 ■ The hemodynamic effects of right-sided heart failure.

failure are hypertension and congenital and valvular heart disease (Kasper et al., 2005).

Nearly 5 million people in the United States are currently living with heart failure; approximately 550,000 new cases of heart failure are diagnosed annually (AHA, 2005). Its incidence and prevalence increase with age: Less than 5% of people between the ages of 55 and 64 have heart failure, whereas 6–10% of people older than 65 are affected (AHA, 2005). The prevalence and mortality rate for heart failure is higher in African Americans than in whites.

The prognosis for a client with heart failure depends on its underlying cause and how effectively the precipitating factors can be treated. Most clients with heart failure die within 8 years of the diagnosis. Clients with heart failure have a dramatically increased risk for sudden cardiac death, which occurs at a rate six to nine times that of the general population (AHA, 2005).

Risk Factors

The most common risk factors for heart failure include coronary artery disease and hypertension. The high prevalence of these conditions makes many people susceptible to heart failure. Other risk factors include family history, cardiotoxic drugs (some cancer chemotherapy drugs), smoking, obesity, alcohol abuse, and diabetes mellitus. Reducing modifiable risk factors is important at all stages of heart failure, and the nurse can do much to support clients in making lifestyle changes.

CLINICAL MANIFESTATIONS

The manifestations of systolic failure are those of decreased cardiac output: weakness, fatigue, and decreased exercise tolerance. The manifestations of diastolic failure include shortness of breath, tachypnea, and respiratory crackles if the left ventricle is affected; distended neck veins, liver enlargement, anorexia, and nausea if the right ventricle is affected. Many clients have components of both systolic and diastolic failure. Multisystem effects of heart failure are shown in the following feature.

Left-Sided Failure

Fatigue and activity intolerance are common early manifestations of left-sided heart failure. Dizziness and syncope also may result from decreased cardiac output. Pulmonary congestion causes dyspnea, shortness of breath, and cough. The client may develop **orthopnea** (difficulty breathing when supine), prompting use of two or three pillows or a recliner for sleeping. Cyanosis from impaired gas exchange may be noted. On auscultation of the lungs, inspiratory crackles (rales) and wheezes may be heard in lung bases. An S_3 gallop may be present, reflecting the heart's attempts to fill an already distended ventricle.

Right-Sided Failure

In right-sided heart failure, edema develops in the feet and legs or, if the client is bedridden, in the sacrum. Congestion of gastrointestinal tract vessels causes anorexia and nausea. Right upper quadrant pain may result from liver engorgement. Neck veins distend and become visible, even when the client is upright, because of increased venous pressure.

Other Manifestations

In addition to the previous manifestations for the various classifications of heart failure, other signs and symptoms commonly are seen. A fall in cardiac output activates mechanisms that cause increased salt and water retention. This causes weight gain and further increases pressures in the capillaries, resulting in edema. **Nocturia** (voiding two or more times at night) develops as edema fluid from dependent tissues is reabsorbed while the client is supine. **Paroxysmal nocturnal dyspnea**, a frightening condition in which the client awakens at night acutely short of breath, also may develop. Paroxysmal nocturnal dyspnea occurs when edema fluid that has accumulated during the day is reabsorbed into the circulation at night, causing fluid overload and pulmonary congestion. Severe heart failure may cause dyspnea at rest as well as with activity, signifying little or no cardiac reserve. Both an S_3 and an S_4 gallop may be heard on auscultation.

MULTISYSTEM EFFECTS OF **Heart Failure**

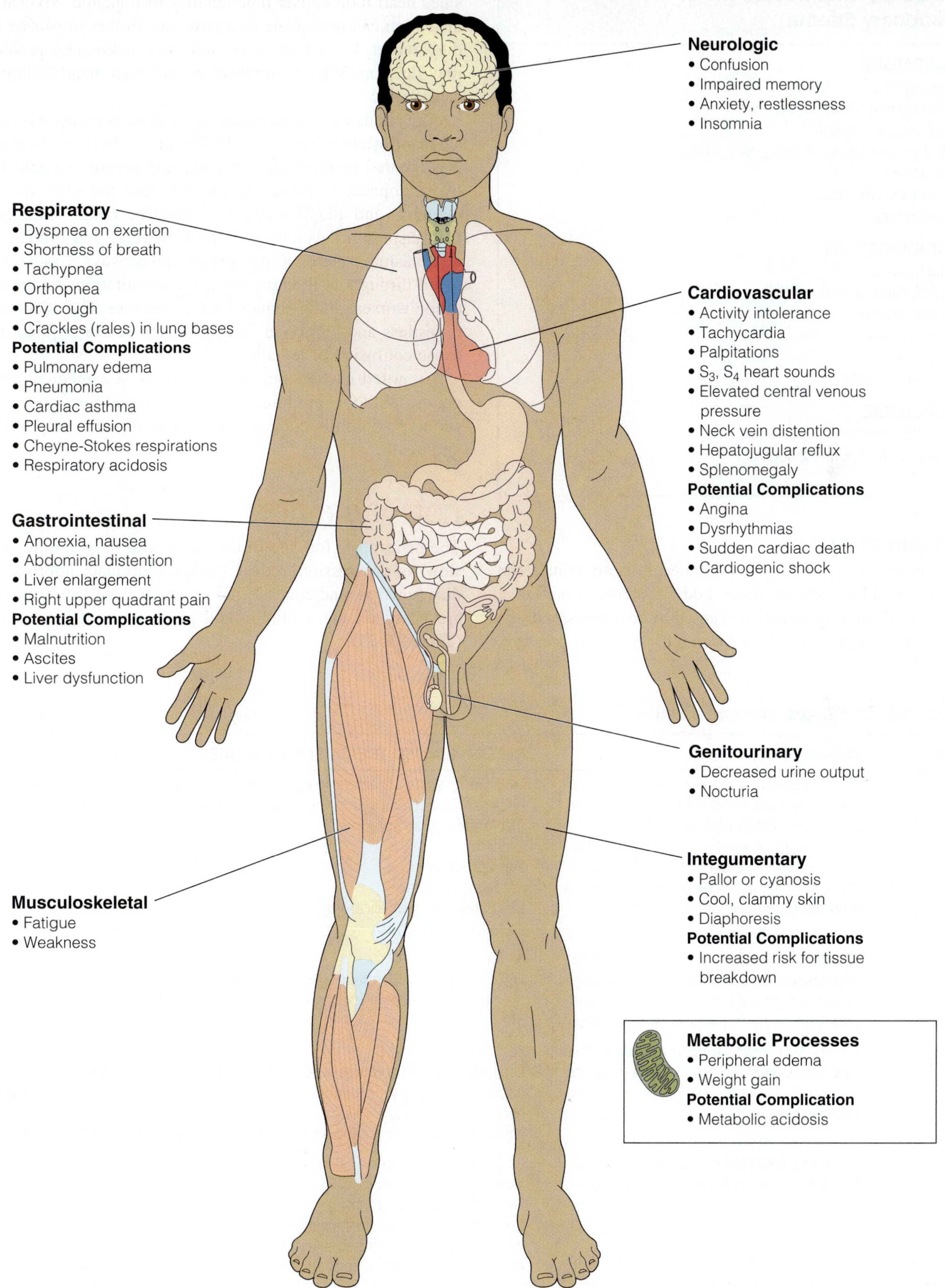

Neurologic
• Confusion
• Impaired memory
• Anxiety, restlessness
• Insomnia
Respiratory
• Dyspnea on exertion
• Shortness of breath
• Tachypnea
• Orthopnea
• Dry cough
• Crackles (rales) in lung bases
Potential Complications
• Pulmonary edema
• Pneumonia
• Cardiac asthma
• Pleural effusion
• Cheyne-Stokes respirations
• Respiratory acidosis
Cardiovascular
• Activity intolerance
• Tachycardia
• Palpitations
• S_3, S_4 heart sounds
• Elevated central venous pressure
• Neck vein distention
• Hepatojugular reflux
• Splenomegaly
Potential Complications
• Angina
• Dysrhythmias
• Sudden cardiac death
• Cardiogenic shock
Gastrointestinal
• Anorexia, nausea
• Abdominal distention
• Liver enlargement
• Right upper quadrant pain
Potential Complications
• Malnutrition
• Ascites
• Liver dysfunction
Genitourinary
• Decreased urine output
• Nocturia
Integumentary
• Pallor or cyanosis
• Cool, clammy skin
• Diaphoresis
Potential Complications
• Increased risk for tissue breakdown
Musculoskeletal
• Fatigue
• Weakness
Metabolic Processes
• Peripheral edema
• Weight gain
Potential Complication
• Metabolic acidosis

Box 22–20 Manifestations of Pulmonary Edema

RESPIRATORY
- Tachypnea
- Paroxysmal nocturnal dyspnea
- Labored respirations
- Cough productive of frothy, pink sputum
- Dyspnea
- Crackles, wheezes
- Orthopnea

CARDIOVASCULAR
- Tachycardia
- Cool, clammy skin
- Hypotension
- Hypoxemia
- Cyanosis
- Ventricular gallop

NEUROLOGIC
- Restlessness
- Feeling of impending doom
- Anxiety

Complications

The compensatory mechanisms initiated in heart failure can lead to complications in other body systems. Congestive hepatomegaly and splenomegaly caused by engorgement of the portal venous system result in increased abdominal pressure, ascites, and gastrointestinal problems. With prolonged right-sided heart failure, liver function may be impaired. Myocardial distention can precipitate dysrhythmias, further impairing cardiac output. Pleural effusions and other pulmonary problems may develop. Major complications of severe heart failure are cardiogenic

The client with acute pulmonary edema presents with classic manifestations (Box 22–20). Dyspnea, shortness of breath, and labored respirations are acute and severe, accompanied by orthopnea. Cyanosis is present, and the skin is cool, clammy, and diaphoretic. A productive cough with pink, frothy sputum develops as a result of fluid, red blood cells, and plasma proteins in the alveoli and airways. Crackles are heard throughout the lung fields on auscultation. As the condition worsens, lung sounds become harsher. The client often is restless and highly anxious, although severe hypoxia may cause confusion or lethargy.

As noted earlier, pulmonary edema is a medical emergency. Without rapid and effective intervention, severe tissue hypoxia and acidosis will lead to organ system failure and death.

COLLABORATION

The main goals for care of the client with heart failure are to slow its progression, reduce cardiac workload, improve cardiac function, and control fluid retention. Treatment strategies are based on the evolution and progression of heart failure (Table 22–27).

TABLE 22–27 Stages of Heart Failure

STAGE	DESCRIPTION	RECOMMENDED TREATMENT MEASURES
A	Clients at high risk for developing heart failure but without structural heart disease or symptoms of heart failure (clients with hypertension, coronary heart disease, diabetes, obesity, metabolic syndrome; who have a family history of cardiomyopathy; or who are taking cardiotoxic drugs)	Treat underlying risk factors (e.g., hypertension) including lipid disorders Angiotensin-converting enzyme (ACE) inhibitor or angiotensin-receptor blocker (ARB) therapy as appropriate Exercise Salt restriction Smoking cessation Discourage alcohol, illicit drug use Control blood glucose in clients with metabolic syndrome
B	Clients with structural heart disease but no manifestations of heart failure (clients with previous myocardial infarction, asymptomatic valve disease, or left ventricular dysfunction)	As for stage A ACE inhibitor or ARB therapy as appropriate Beta-blocker therapy if indicated
C	Clients with structural heart disease and current or previous symptoms of heart failure (shortness of breath, fatigue, or decreased exercise tolerance)	As for stages A and B Drug therapy with a diuretic, ACE inhibitor, and/or beta-blocker Additional drugs as indicated, such as an aldosterone antagonist, ARB, digitalis, hydralazine, nitrates Ventricular pacing or an implantable cardioverter–defibrillator (ICD) as indicated
D	Refractory heart failure (clients with manifestations of heart failure at rest despite aggressive treatment)	As for stages A, B, and C as appropriate Hospice care Hemodynamic monitoring Continual infusion of positive inotropic agents Valve replacement, cardiac transplant as indicated Permanent mechanical support; experimental surgery or drug therapy

Source: Adapted from Hunt et al. (2005).

Diagnostic Tests

Diagnosis of heart failure is based on the history, physical examination, and diagnostic findings. Relevant diagnostic tests include the following:

- *Atrial natriuretic peptide (ANP),* also called *atrial natriuretic hormone,* and *brain natriuretic peptide (BNP)* are hormones released by the heart muscle in response to changes in blood volume. Blood levels of these hormones increase in heart failure. BNP levels, in particular, have been shown to positively correlate with pressures in the left ventricle and the pulmonary vascular system. As the severity of left ventricular failure increases, BNP levels increase (White, 2005). It is important to remember, however, that BNP levels may be elevated in women and in people older than 60 years who do not have heart failure. Therefore, an elevated BNP cannot be used alone to diagnose heart failure (Hunt et al., 2005).
- *Serum electrolytes* are measured to evaluate fluid and electrolyte status. Serum osmolarity may be low because of fluid retention. Sodium, potassium, and chloride levels provide a baseline for evaluating the effects of treatment; serum calcium and magnesium are measured as well.
- *Urinalysis, blood urea nitrogen,* and *serum creatinine* are obtained to evaluate renal function.
- *Liver function tests,* including alanine aminotransferase, aspartate aminotransferase, lactate dehydrogenase, serum bilirubin, and total protein and albumin levels, are obtained to evaluate possible effects of heart failure on liver function.
- *Thyroid function tests,* including thyroid-stimulating hormone and thyroid hormone levels, are obtained because both hyperthyroidism and hypothyroidism can be either a primary or a contributing cause of heart failure (Hunt et al., 2005).
- *Arterial blood gas* levels are determined to evaluate gas exchange in the lungs and tissues in the client with acute heart failure.
- *Chest x-ray* may show pulmonary vascular congestion and cardiomegaly in heart failure.
- *Electrocardiography* is used to identify ECG changes associated with ventricular enlargement and to detect dysrhythmias, myocardial ischemia, or infarction.
- *Echocardiography with Doppler flow studies* is performed to evaluate left ventricular function. Either transthoracic echocardiography or transesophageal echocardiography may be used.

Hemodynamic Monitoring

Hemodynamics is the study of forces involved in blood circulation. Hemodynamic monitoring is used to assess cardiovascular function in the client who is critically ill or unstable. The main goals of invasive hemodynamic monitoring are to evaluate cardiac and circulatory function and the response to interventions.

Hemodynamic parameters include heart rate, arterial blood pressure, central venous or right atrial pressure, pulmonary pressures, and cardiac output. Direct hemodynamic parameters are obtained straight from the monitoring device (e.g., heart rate and arterial and venous pressures). Indirect or derived measurements are calculated using the direct data (e.g., the cardiac index, mean arterial blood pressure, and stroke volume). Invasive hemodynamic monitoring is routinely used in critical care units.

Hemodynamic monitoring systems measure the pressure within a vessel and convert this signal into an electrical waveform that is amplified and displayed. The electrical signal may be recorded on graph paper and displayed digitally on the monitor. System components include an invasive catheter threaded into an artery or vein connected to a transducer by stiff, high-pressure tubing. The pressure transducer translates pressures into an electrical signal that is relayed to the monitor. Additional components of the system include stopcocks and a continuous flush system with normal saline or heparinized saline and an infusion pressure bag to prevent clots from forming in the catheter. Figure 22–44 ■ illustrates a pressure transducer and typical hemodynamic monitoring system.

Hemodynamic pressure monitoring may be used to measure peripheral arterery pressures or central pressures, such as central venous pressure or right atrial pressure and pulmonary artery pressure. Although the information obtained from invasive monitoring is valuable, the procedure is not without risk. Box 22–21 lists potential complications of central pressure monitoring.

INTRA-ARTERIAL PRESSURE MONITORING Intra-arterial pressure monitoring is commonly used in intensive and coronary care units. An indwelling arterial line, commonly called an art line or an A line, allows direct and continuous monitoring of systolic, diastolic, and mean arterial blood pressure and provides easy access for arterial blood sampling. Arterial lines are used to assess blood volume, to monitor the effects of vasoactive drugs, and to obtain frequent arterial blood gas determinations. Because the invasive catheter is inserted directly into the artery, it offers immediate access for blood gas measurements and blood testing.

The arterial blood pressure reflects the cardiac output and the resistance to blood flow created by the elastic arterial walls (systemic vascular resistance [SVR]). Cardiac output is determined by the blood volume and the ability of the ventricles to fill and effectively pump that blood. Systemic vascular resistance is primarily determined by vessel diameter and distensibility (compliance). Factors such as SNS input, circulating hormones (e.g., epinephrine, norepinephrine, ANP, and vasopressin), and the renin–angiotensin system affect systemic vascular resistance.

The systolic blood pressure, normally approximately 120 mmHg in healthy adults, reflects the pressure generated during ventricular systole. During diastole, elastic arterial walls keep a minimum pressure within the vessel (diastolic blood pressure) to maintain blood flow through the capillary beds. The average diastolic pressure in a healthy adult is 80 mmHg. The **mean arterial pressure (MAP)** is the average pressure in the arterial circulation throughout the cardiac cycle. It reflects the driving pressure, or perfusion pressure, an indicator of tissue perfusion. The formula MAP = CO × SVR often is used to show the relationships between factors

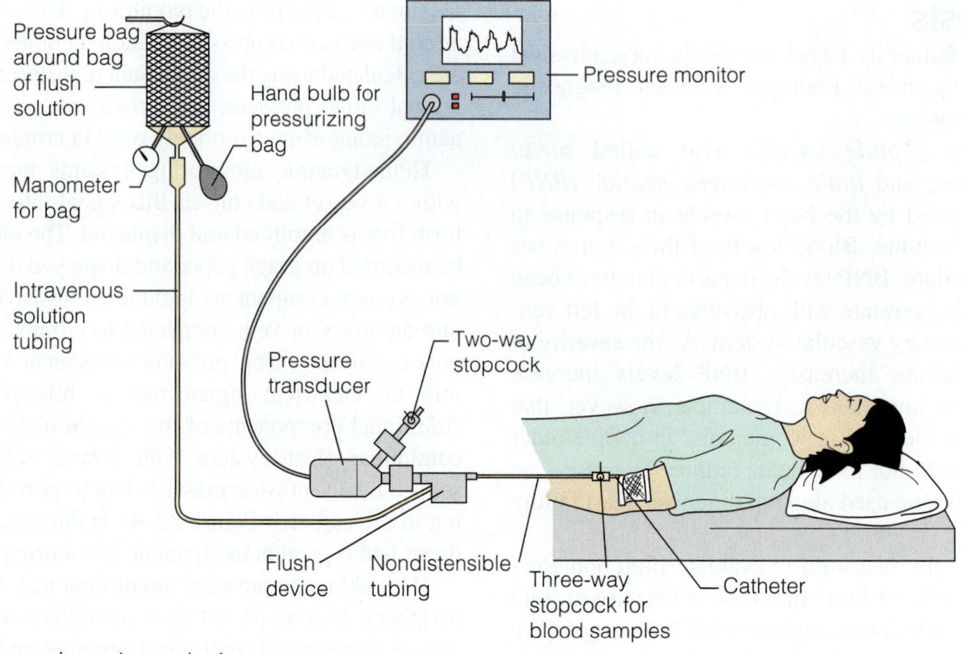

Figure 22–44 ■ A hemodynamic monitoring setup.

determining the blood pressure. MAP can be calculated by adding one-third of the pulse pressure (PP) to the diastolic blood pressure (DBP)—that is, MAP = DBP + PP/3. For example, a blood pressure of 120/80 results in a MAP of 93. MAPs of 70 to 90 mmHg are desirable. Perfusion to vital organs is severely jeopardized at MAPs of 50 or less; MAPs of greater than 105 mmHg may indicate hypertension or vasoconstriction.

VENOUS PRESSURE MONITORING Central venous pressure (CVP) and right atrial pressure are measures of blood volume and venous return. They also reflect right heart filling pressures. Pressures are elevated in right-sided heart failure. CVP and right atrial pressure are primarily used to monitor fluid volume status. To measure venous and atrial pressures, a catheter is inserted in the internal jugular or subclavian vein. The distal tip of the catheter is positioned in the superior vena cava just above or just inside the right atrium.

Box 22–21 Potential Complications of Central Catheters

- Bleeding
- Hematoma
- Pneumothorax
- Hemothorax
- Arterial puncture
- Dysrhythmias
- Venospasm
- Infection
- Air embolism
- Thromboembolism
- Brachial nerve injury
- Thoracic nerve injury

CVP may be measured in either centimeters of water (cm H_2O) or millimeters of mercury (mmHg). A water manometer is a clear tube with calibrated markings that is attached between a central catheter and the intravenous fluid bag. Pressure in the venous system causes fluid in the manometer to rise or fall. The CVP is recorded by noting the fluid level in the manometer. If the central line is connected to a pressure transducer, venous pressure is displayed digitally in millimeters of mercury.

The normal range for CVP is 2–8 cm H_2O or 2–6 mmHg, but CVP varies in individual clients. Hypovolemia and shock decrease the CVP; fluid overload, vasoconstriction, and cardiac tamponade increase CVP.

PULMONARY ARTERY PRESSURE MONITORING The pulmonary artery (PA) catheter is a flow-directed, balloon-tipped catheter first used in the early 1970s. The PA catheter is often called a Swan–Ganz catheter, after the physicians who developed it. The PA catheter is used to evaluate left ventricular and overall cardiac function. The PA catheter is inserted into a central vein, usually the internal jugular or subclavian vein, and threaded into the right atrium. A small balloon at the tip of the catheter allows the catheter to be drawn into the right ventricle and, from there, into the pulmonary artery (Figure 22–45 ■). The inflated balloon carries the catheter forward until the balloon wedges in a small branch of pulmonary vasculature. Once in place, the balloon is deflated, and multiple lumens of the catheter allow measurement of pressures in the right atrium, pulmonary artery, and left ventricle. The normal PA pressure is approximately 25/10 mmHg; normal mean pulmonary artery pressure is approximately 15 mmHg (Figure 22–46A ■). Pulmonary artery pressure is increased in left-sided heart failure.

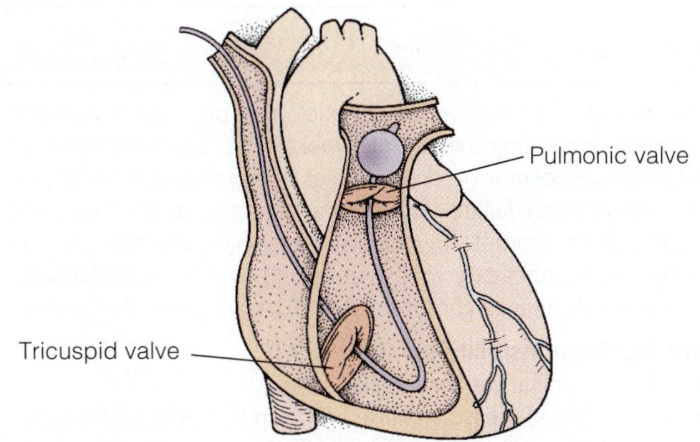

Figure 22–45 ■ Inflation of the balloon on the flow-directed catheter allows it to be carried through the pulmonic valve into the pulmonary artery.

Inflation of the balloon effectively blocks pressure from behind the balloon and allows measurement of pressures generated by the left ventricle. This is known as the pulmonary artery wedge pressure (PAWP) and is used to assess left ventricular function. The normal PAWP is 8–12 mmHg (Figure 22–46B). PAWP is increased in left ventricular failure and pericardial tamponade, and decreased in hypovolemia.

Cardiac output also can be measured with the PA catheter using a technique called thermodilution. Cardiac output and the cardiac index are used to assess the heart's ability to meet the body's oxygen demands. Because body size affects overall cardiac output, the cardiac index is a more precise measure of heart function. The cardiac index is a calculation of cardiac output per square meter of body surface area. The normal cardiac index is 2.8–4.2 L/min/m^2.

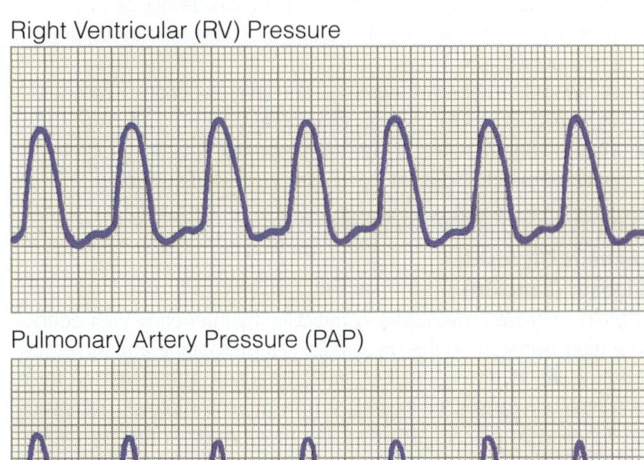

Figure 22–46 ■ Typical waveforms seen when measuring, *A*, pulmonary artery pressure and, *B*, pulmonary wedge pressure.

Pharmacologic Therapies

Clients with heart failure often receive multiple medications to reduce cardiac work and improve cardiac function. The main drug classes used to treat heart failure are the ACE inhibitors, ARBs, beta-blockers, diuretics, positive inotropic medications (including digitalis, sympathomimetic agents, and phosphodiesterase inhibitors), direct vasodilators, and antidysrhythmic drugs. Medication administration for heart failure is summarized in Box 22–22.

ANGIOTENSIN-CONVERTING ENZYME INHIBITORS Angiotensin-converting enzyme inhibitors interrupt the conversion of angiotensin I to angiotensin II by inhibiting the enzyme that mediates the conversion (i.e., ACE). Angiotensin II causes intense vasoconstriction, increasing afterload and ventricular wall stress and increasing preload and ventricular dilation. It also stimulates aldosterone and ADH production, causing fluid retention. ACE inhibitors block this renin–angiotensin system activity, decreasing cardiac work and increasing cardiac output. They reduce the progression and manifestations of heart failure, thus reducing the number and frequency of hospital admissions, decreasing mortality rates, and preventing cardiac complications (Kasper et al., 2005).

ANGIOTENSIN II–RECEPTOR BLOCKERS In contrast to ACE inhibitors, ARBs do not block the production of angiotensin II; instead, they block its action. The pharmacologic effect is similar, and they also are used in heart failure to slow its progression, reduce manifestations, and prevent cardiac complications.

BETA-BLOCKERS Beta-blockers improve cardiac function in heart failure by inhibiting SNS activity. This prevents the long-term deleterious effects of sympathetic stimulation. Because beta-blockers reduce the force of myocardial contraction and may actually worsen symptoms, they are used in low doses. The combination of ACE inhibitors and beta-blockers improves client outcomes.

DIURETICS Clients with symptomatic heart failure often are treated with diuretics, which relieve symptoms related to fluid retention. Diuretics may, however, cause significant electrolyte imbalances and rapid fluid loss. Clients with severe heart failure are often treated with a loop, or high-ceiling, diuretic, such as furosemide (Lasix), bumetanide (Bumex), torsemide (Demadex), or ethacrynic acid (Edecrin). These drugs have a rapid onset of action, inhibiting chloride reabsorption in the ascending loop of Henle and thus prompting sodium and water excretion. Their major drawback is their efficacy in promoting diuresis; loss of vascular volume can stimulate the SNS. Thiazide diuretics may be used for clients with less severe manifestations of heart failure. These agents promote fluid excretion by blocking sodium reabsorption in the terminal loop of Henle and the distal tubule.

VASODILATORS Vasodilators relax smooth muscle in blood vessels, causing dilation. Asrterial dilation reduces peripheral vascular resistance and afterload, reducing myocardial work. Venous dilation reduces venous return and preload. Pulmonary vascular relaxation reduces pulmonary capillary pressure,

Box 22–22 Medication Administration: Heart Failure

ANGIOTENSIN-CONVERTING ENZYME (ACE) INHIBITORS

Enalapril (Vasotec) **Lisinopril (Prinivil, Zestril)**
Captopril (Capoten) **Fosinopril (Monopril)**
Moexipril (Univasc) **Quinapril (Accupril)**
Ramipril (Altace) **Trandolapril (Mavik)**

ANGIOTENSIN II–RECEPTOR BLOCKERS (ARBS)

Candesartan (Atacand) **Irbesartan (Avapro)**
Losartan (Cozaar) **Telmisartan (Micardis)**
Valsartan (Diovan)

ACE inhibitors and ARBs prevent acute coronary events and reduce mortality in heart failure. ACE inhibitors interfere with production of angiotensin II, resulting in vasodilation, reduced blood volume, and prevention of its effects in the heart and blood vessels. In heart failure, ACE inhibitors reduce afterload and improve cardiac output and renal blood flow. They also reduce pulmonary congestion and peripheral edema. ACE inhibitors suppress myocyte growth and reduce ventricular remodeling in heart failure. While the pharmacologic effect of ARBs is similar, they block the action of angiotensin II at the receptor rather than interfering with its production.

Nursing Responsibilities

- Do not give these drugs to women in the second and third trimesters of pregnancy.
- Carefully monitor clients who are volume depleted or have impaired renal function.
- Use an infusion pump when administering ACE inhibitors intravenously.
- Monitor blood pressure closely for 2 hours following the first dose and as indicated thereafter.
- Monitor serum potassium levels; ACE inhibitors can cause hyperkalemia (this is less of a concern with ARBs).
- Monitor white blood cell count for potential neutropenia. Report to the physician.

Health Education for the Client and Family

- Take the drug at the same time every day to ensure a stable blood level.
- Monitor your blood pressure and weight weekly. Report significant changes to your doctor.
- Avoid making sudden position changes (e.g., rise from bed slowly). Lie down if you become dizzy or lightheaded, particularly after the first dose.
- Report any signs of easy bruising and bleeding, sore throat or fever, edema, or skin rash. Immediately report swelling of the face, lips, or eyelids and any itching or breathing problems.
- A persistent, dry cough may develop if you are taking an ACE inhibitor. Contact your doctor if this becomes a problem.
- Take captopril or moexipril 1 hour before meals.

DIURETICS

Chlorothiazide (Diuril) **Spironolactone (Aldactone)**
Furosemide (Lasix) **Triamterene (Dyrenium)**
Ethacrynic acid (Edecrin) **Amiloride (Midamor)**
Bumetanide (Bumex) **Acetazolamide (Diamox)**
Hydrochlorothiazide (HydroDIURIL)

Diuretics act on different portions of the kidney tubule to inhibit the reabsorption of sodium and water and promote their excretion. With the exception of the potassium-sparing diuretics—spironolactone, triamterene, and amiloride—diuretics also promote potassium excretion, increasing the risk of hypokalemia. Spironolactone, an aldosterone-receptor blocker, reduces symptoms and slows progression of heart failure. Aldosterone receptors in the heart and blood vessels promote myocardial remodeling and fibrosis, activate the sympathetic nervous system, and promote vascular fibrosis (which decreases compliance) and baroreceptor dysfunction.

Nursing Responsibilities

- Obtain baseline weight and vital signs.
- Monitor blood pressure, intake and output, weight, skin turgor, and edema as indicators of fluid volume status.
- Assess for volume depletion, particularly with loop diuretics (furosemide, ethacrynic acid, and bumetanide): dizziness, orthostatic hypotension, tachycardia, and muscle cramping.
- Report abnormal serum electrolyte levels to the physician. Replace electrolytes as indicated.
- Do not administer potassium replacements to clients receiving a potassium-sparing diuretic.
- Evaluate renal function by assessing urine output, blood urea nitrogen, and serum creatinine.
- Administer intravenous furosemide slowly, no faster than 20 mg/min. Evaluate for signs of ototoxicity. Do not administer this drug or ethacrynic acid concurrently with aminoglycoside antibiotics (e.g., gentamicin), which are also ototoxic.

Health Education for the Client and Family

- Drink at least six to eight glasses of water per day.
- Take your diuretic at times that will be least disruptive to your lifestyle, usually in the morning and early afternoon if a second dose is ordered. Take with meals to decrease gastric upset.
- Monitor your blood pressure, pulse, and weight weekly. Report significant weight changes to your doctor.
- Report any of the following to your doctor: severe abdominal pain; jaundice; dark urine; abnormal bleeding or bruising; flulike symptoms; and signs of hypokalemia, hyponatremia, or dehydration (e.g., thirst, salt craving, dizziness, weakness, and rapid pulse).
- Avoid sudden position changes. You may experience dizziness, lightheadedness, or feelings of faintness.
- Unless you are taking a potassium-sparing diuretic, integrate potassium-rich foods into your diet. Limit sodium use.

POSITIVE INOTROPIC AGENTS

Digitalis Glycosides
Digoxin (Lanoxin)

Digitalis improves myocardial contractility by interfering with adenosine triphosphatase in the myocardial cell membrane and increasing the amount of calcium available for contraction. The increased force of contraction causes the heart to empty more completely, increasing stroke volume and cardiac output. Improved cardiac output improves renal perfusion, decreasing renin secretion. This decreases preload and afterload, reducing cardiac work. Digitalis also has electrophysiologic effects, slowing conduction through the atrioventricular node. This decreases the heart rate and reduces oxygen consumption.

Nursing Responsibilities

- Assess apical pulse before administering. Withhold digitalis and notify the physician if heart rate is below 60 bpm and/or manifestations of decreased cardiac output are noted. Record apical rate on medication record.

Box 22–22 Medication Administration: Heart Failure (continued)

- Evaluate the electrocardiogram for scooped (spoon-shaped) ST segment, AV block, bradycardia, and other dysrhythmias (especially premature ventricular contractions and atrial tachycardias).
- Report manifestations of digitalis toxicity: anorexia, nausea and vomiting, abdominal pain, weakness, vision changes (e.g., diplopia, blurred vision, or yellow-green or white halos seen around objects), and new-onset dysrhythmias.
- Assess potassium, magnesium, calcium, and serum digoxin levels before giving digitalis. Hypokalemia can precipitate toxicity even when the serum digitalis level is in the "normal" range (*adult:* 0.5–2 ng/ml, 0.5–2 nmol/l (SI units); *infants:* 1–3 ng/ml).
- Monitor clients with renal insufficiency or renal failure and older adults carefully for digitalis toxicity.
- Prepare to administer digoxin immune fab (Digibind) for digoxin toxicity.

Health Education for the Client and Family

- Take your pulse daily before taking your digoxin. Do not take the digoxin if your pulse is below 60 bpm or if you are weak, fatigued, lightheaded, dizzy, short of breath, or having chest pain. Instead, notify your physician immediately.
- Contact your doctor if you develop manifestations of digitalis toxicity: palpitations, weakness, loss of appetite, nausea and vomiting, abdominal pain, blurred or colored vision, or double vision.
- Avoid using antacids and laxatives; they decrease digoxin absorption.
- Notify your physician immediately if you develop manifestations of potassium deficiency: weakness, lethargy, thirst, depression, muscle cramps, or vomiting.
- Incorporate potassium-rich foods into your diet: fresh orange or tomato juice, bananas, raisins, dates, figs, prunes, apricots, spinach, cauliflower, and potatoes.

SYMPATHOMIMETIC AGENTS

Dopamine (Intropin)
Dobutamine (Dobutrex)

Sympathomimetic agents stimulate the heart, improving the force of contraction. Dobutamine is preferred in managing heart failure because it does not increase the heart rate as much as dopamine and it has a mild vasodilatory effect. These drugs are given by intravenous infusion and may be titrated to obtain their optimal effects.

PHOSPHODIESTERASE INHIBITORS

Amrinone (Inocor)
Milrinone (Primacor)

Phosphodiesterase inhibitors are used in treating acute heart failure to increase myocardial contractility and cause vasodilation. The net effects are an increase in cardiac output and a decrease in afterload.

Nursing Responsibilities

- Use an infusion pump to administer these agents. Monitor hemodynamic parameters carefully.
- Avoid discontinuing these drugs abruptly.
- Change solutions and tubing every 24 hours.
- Amrinone is given as an intravenous bolus over 2–3 minutes, followed by an infusion of 5–10 mg • kg^{-1} • min^{-1}.
- Amrinone may be infused full strength or diluted in either normal or half-strength saline. Do not mix this drug with dextrose solutions. After dilution, amrinone can be piggybacked into a line containing a dextrose solution.
- Monitor liver function and platelet counts; amrinone may cause hepatotoxicity and thrombocytopenia.

Health Education for the Client and Family

- Notify the nursing staff if you experience abdominal pain or notice a skin rash or bruising.

allowing reabsorption of fluid from interstitial tissues and the alveoli. Vasodilators include nitrates, hydralazine, and prazosin, an alpha-adrenergic blocker.

Nitrates produce both arterial and venous vasodilation. They may be given by nasal spray or the sublingual, oral, or intravenous route. Sodium nitroprusside is a potent vasodilator that may be used to treat acute heart failure. It can cause excessive hypotension, however, so it is often given along with dopamine or dobutamine to maintain the blood pressure. Isosorbide or nitroglycerin ointment may be used in long-term management of heart failure.

In 2005, the U.S. Food and Drug Administration (FDA) approved a new drug for treatment of heart failure in African Americans. This drug, known as BiDil, is a combination of two vasodilators, hydralazine and isosorbide, in fixed doses. In a study of African Americans with severe heart failure, BiDil improved symptoms and significantly reduced the number of hospitalizations and deaths attributed to heart failure (U.S. FDA, 2005).

DIGITALIS Digitalis glycosides are used judiciously in symptomatic heart failure. Digitalis has a positive inotropic effect on the heart, increasing the strength of myocardial contraction by increasing the intracellular calcium concentrations. Digitalis also decreases SA node automaticity and slows conduction through the AV node, increasing ventricular filling time.

Digitalis has a narrow therapeutic index; in other words, therapeutic levels are very close to toxic levels. Early manifestations of digitalis toxicity include anorexia, nausea and vomiting, headache, altered vision, and confusion. A number of cardiac dysrhythmias are also associated with digitalis toxicity, including sinus arrest, supraventricular and ventricular tachycardias, and high levels of AV block. Low serum potassium levels increase the risk of digitalis toxicity, as do low magnesium and high calcium levels. Older adults are at particular risk for digitalis toxicity.

Digitalis levels may be affected by a number of other drugs. Check for potential interactions.

ANTIDYSRHYTHMICS Dysrhythmias are common in clients with heart failure. Although premature ventricular contractions may be frequent, they are often not associated with an increased risk of ventricular tachycardia and fibrillation. Because many antidysrhythmic medications depress left ventricular function, premature ventricular contractions are frequently left untreated in heart failure. Amiodarone is the drug of choice to treat nonsustained ventricular tachycardia, which is associated with a poor prognosis.

Nutrition and Activity

A sodium-restricted diet is recommended to minimize sodium and water retention. Intake is generally limited to 1.5–2 g of sodium per day, a moderate restriction. See Exemplar 11.3, Fluid and Electrolyte Imbalance, for a list of high-sodium foods to avoid (Box 11–13) and for client teaching regarding a sodium-restricted diet.

Exercise intolerance (decreased ability to participate in activities using large skeletal muscles because of fatigue or dyspnea) is a common early manifestation of heart failure. Activity may be restricted to bedrest during acute episodes of heart failure to reduce cardiac workload and allow the heart to recompensate. Prolonged bedrest and continued activity limitations, however, are not recommended. A moderate, progressive activity program is prescribed to improve myocardial function. Exercise should be performed 3–5 days per week, and each session should include a 10- to 15-minute warm-up period, 20–30 minutes of exercise at the recommended intensity, and a cool-down period. Walking is encouraged on nontraining days (Piña et al., 2003).

Surgery

In end-stage heart failure, devices to provide circulatory assistance or surgery may be required. Surgery may be used to treat the underlying cause of failure (e.g., replacement of diseased valves) or improve quality of life. Heart transplant is currently the only clearly effective surgical treatment for end-stage heart failure; however, its use is limited by the availability of donor hearts.

CIRCULATORY ASSISTANCE Devices such as the intra-aortic balloon pump or a left-ventricular assist device may be used when the client is expected to recover or as a bridge to transplant. Newer devices that will allow longer-term support outside the hospital are in the developmental stages. These devices will serve either as a bridge to transplant or allow the myocardium to heal over an extended period of time.

CARDIAC TRANSPLANTATION Heart transplant is the treatment of choice for end-stage heart disease. Survival rates are good: 83% at 1 year, and 76% at 3 years. More than 90% of clients return to normal, unrestricted functional abilities following transplant (Kasper et al., 2005).

The most frequently used transplant procedure leaves the posterior walls of the atria, the superior and inferior venae cavae, and the pulmonary veins of the recipient intact (Figure 22–47A ■). The atrial walls of the donor heart are then anastomosed to the recipient's atria (Figure 22–47B), and the donor pulmonary artery and aorta are anastomosed to the recipient vessels (Figure 22–47C). Care is taken to avoid damaging the sinus node of the donor heart and to ensure integrity of the suture line to prevent postoperative bleeding. Donor organs typically are obtained from young accident victims with no evidence of cardiac trauma.

Nursing care of the client with a heart transplant is similar to care of the client with any cardiac surgery. Bleeding is a major concern during the early postoperative period. Chest tube drainage is frequently monitored (initially every 15 minutes), as are the cardiac output, pulmonary artery pressures, and CVP. Cardiac tamponade (compression of the heart) can develop, presenting as either a sudden event or a gradual process. Chest tubes are gently milked (not stripped) as needed to maintain patency. Atrial dysrhythmias are relatively common following cardiac transplant. Temporary pacing wires are placed during surgery because the conduction system may be disrupted by surgical manipulation or postoperative swelling. Hypothermia is induced during surgery; postoperatively, the client is gradually rewarmed over a 1- to 2-hour period. Prevention of rapid rewarming and shivering are important to maintain hemodynamic stability and reduce

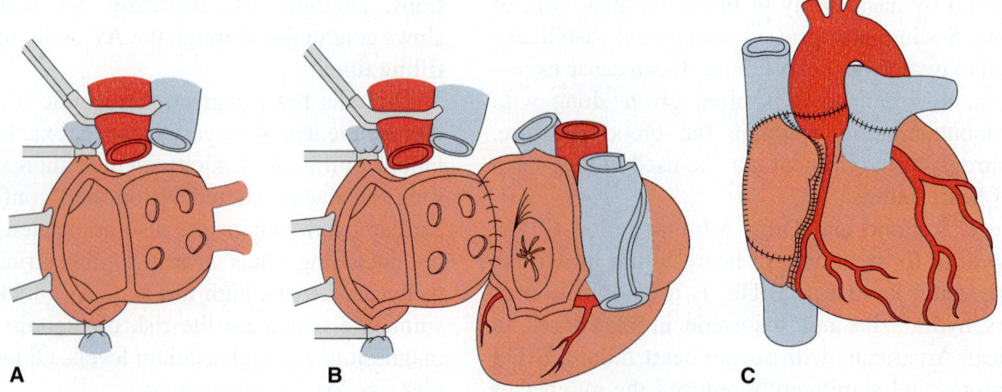

Figure 22–47 ■ Cardiac transplantation. *A*, The heart is removed, leaving the posterior walls of the atria intact. *B*, The donor heart is anastomosed to the atria, *C*, and the great vessels.

oxygen consumption. Cardiac function is impaired in up to 50% of transplanted hearts during the early postoperative period. Inotropic agents, such as low-dose dopamine, dobutamine, or milrinone, may be required to support cardiac function and circulation (Wade, Rieth, Sikora, & Augustine, 2004).

Infection and rejection are major postoperative concerns; these are the chief causes of mortality in clients with a transplant. Rejection may develop immediately after transplant (a rare occurrence), within weeks to months, or years after the transplant. Acute rejection usually presents within weeks of the transplant, developing when the transplanted organ is recognized by the immune system as foreign. Lymphocytes infiltrate the organ, and myocardial cell necrosis can be detected on biopsy. Acute rejection often can be treated using immunosuppressive drugs (Wade et al., 2004). These drugs also are given to prevent rejection of the transplanted organ, even when the tissue match is good. Although immunosuppressive medications help prevent organ rejection, they impair the client's defenses against infection. Early postoperative infections commonly are bacterial or fungal (*Candida* sp.). Multiple invasive lines, prolonged ventilator support, and immunosuppressive therapy contribute to the transplant recipient's risk for infection. Aggressive nursing care directed at prevention of infection is vital: limiting visitors with communicable diseases, pulmonary hygiene measures, early ambulation, and strict aseptic technique (Wade et al., 2004).

The donor heart is denervated during the transplant procedure. Lack of innervation by the autonomic nervous system affects the heart rate (usually 90–110 bpm in transplanted hearts), its response to position changes, stress, exercise, and certain drugs.

OTHER PROCEDURES Other surgical procedures, such as cardiomyoplasty and ventricular reduction surgery, do not improve the prognosis or quality of life in clients with end-stage heart failure. Cardiomyoplasty involves wrapping the latissimus dorsi muscle around the heart to support the failing myocardium. The muscle is stimulated in synchrony with the heart, providing a more forceful contraction and increasing cardiac output. In ventricular reduction surgery (or partial ventriculectomy), a portion of the anterolateral left ventricular wall is resected to improve cardiac function (Tierney et al., 2005).

Complementary Therapies

Strong evidence supports the use of several complementary therapies for heart failure. Hawthorn, a shrubby tree, contains natural cardiotonic ingredients in its blossoms, leaves, and fruit. It increases the force of myocardial contraction, dilates blood vessels, and has a natural ACE inhibitor. Hawthorn should never be used without consulting an experienced herb practitioner and advising the physician (Fontaine, 2005). Nutritional supplements of coenzyme Q10, magnesium, and thiamine may be used in conjunction with other treatments. Coenzyme Q10 improves mitochondria function and energy production.

End-of-Life Care

Unless a cardiac transplant is performed, chronic heart failure is ultimately a terminal disease. The client and family need honest discussions about the anticipated course of the disease and treatment options. It is important to discuss advance directives, such as the living will and medical power of attorney, differentiating potential acute events from which recovery would be anticipated (e.g., a reversible exacerbation of heart failure or a sudden cardiac arrest) from prolonged life support without reasonable expectation of functional recovery. Hospice services are available for clients with heart failure and should be offered when appropriate. Severe dyspnea is common in the final stages of the disease. It may be managed with narcotic analgesics or with frequent intravenous diuretics and continuous infusion of a positive inotropic agent (Hunt et al., 2005).

NURSING PROCESS

Health promotion activities to reduce the risk for and incidence of heart failure are directed at lifestyle changes. Teach clients about coronary heart disease, the primary underlying cause of heart failure. Discuss risk factors for coronary heart disease and ways to reduce those risk factors.

Hypertension also is a major cause of heart failure. Routinely screen clients for elevated blood pressure, and refer clients to a primary care provider as indicated. Discuss the importance of effectively managing hypertension to reduce the future risk for heart failure. Likewise, stress the relationship between effective diabetes management and reduced risk for heart failure.

Heart failure impacts quality of life, interfering with such daily activities as self-care and role performance. Reducing the oxygen demand of the heart is a major nursing care goal for the client in acute heart failure. This includes providing rest and carrying out prescribed treatment measures to reduce cardiac work, improve contractility, and manage symptoms.

Assessment

Obtain the following subjective and objective data when assessing the client with heart failure:

- *Health history.* Complaints of increasing shortness of breath, dyspnea with exertion, decreasing activity tolerance, or paroxysmal nocturnal dyspnea; number of pillows used for sleeping; recent weight gain; presence of a cough; chest or abdominal pain; anorexia or nausea; history of cardiac disease or previous episodes of heart failure; other risk factors, such as hypertension or diabetes; current medications; usual diet and activity as well as any recent changes.
- *Physical examination.* General appearance; ease of breathing, conversing, and changing positions; apparent anxiety; vital signs, including apical pulse; color of the skin and mucous membranes; neck vein distention, peripheral pulses, capillary refill, and presence and degree of edema; heart and breath sounds; abdominal contour, bowel sounds, and tenderness; right upper abdominal tenderness and liver enlargement.

Diagnosis

Nursing diagnoses appropriate for the client diagnosed with heart failure may include the following:

- Decreased Cardiac Output
- Excess Fluid Volume
- Activity Intolerance
- Deficient Knowledge: Low-Sodium Diet.

Plan

Goals of care for the client with heart failure often include the following:

- The client will describe the purpose of each medication prescribed and which symptoms to report.
- The client will maintain adequate oxygenation, as demonstrated by respiratory status, breath sounds, oxygen saturation, and vital signs.
- The client will maintain adequate tissue perfusion and myocardial function, as demonstrated by capillary refill, hemodynamic monitoring, assessment of pulses, and vital signs.
- The client will meet the body's energy needs through adequate and appropriate nutrition.

Implementation

Nursing care is focused on promoting perfusion, improving oxygenation, and reducing fear and anxiety. When the client is diagnosed with a disorder related to the heart it often produces great fear of death and disability because the heart is vital to life. Helping the client and family to cope with this fear is an important component of nursing care. Anxiety secondary to hypoxia is also anticipated and requires nursing intervention.

Decreased Cardiac Output

As the heart fails as a pump, stroke volume and tissue perfusion decrease.

- Monitor vital signs and oxygen saturation as indicated. Decreased cardiac output stimulates the SNS to increase the heart rate in an attempt to restore output. Tachycardia at rest is common. Diastolic blood pressure may initially be elevated because of vasoconstriction; in late stages, compensatory mechanisms fail and blood pressure falls. Oxygen saturation levels provide a measure of gas exchange and tissue perfusion.
- Monitor BNP levels, reporting trends. BNP levels indicate the severity of heart failure: As the cardiac index decreases and left ventricular pressures increase, BNP levels increase. Noting trends provides additional information about cardiac output and effectiveness of the cardiac pump.
- Auscultate heart and breath sounds regularly. S_1 and S_2 may be diminished if cardiac function is poor. A ventricular gallop (S_3) is an early sign of heart failure; an atrial gallop (S_4) may also be present. Crackles are often heard in the lung bases; increasing crackles, dyspnea, and shortness of breath indicate worsening failure.
- Administer supplemental oxygen as needed. This improves oxygenation of the blood, decreasing the effects of hypoxia and ischemia.
- Administer prescribed medications as ordered. Drugs are used to decrease the cardiac workload and increase the effectiveness of contractions.
- Encourage rest, explaining the rationale. Elevate the head of the bed to reduce the work of breathing. Provide a bedside commode, and assist with ADLs. Instruct to avoid the Valsalva maneuver. These measures reduce cardiac workload.

Excess Fluid Volume

As cardiac output falls, compensatory mechanisms cause salt and water retention, increasing blood volume. This increased fluid volume places additional stress on the already failing ventricles, making them work harder to move the fluid load.

- Assess respiratory status and auscultate lung sounds at least every 4 hours. Notify the physician of significant changes in condition. Declining respiratory status indicates worsening left heart failure.
- Monitor intake and output. Notify the physician if urine output is less than 30 mL/hr. Weigh the client daily. Careful monitoring of fluid volume is important during treatment of heart failure. Diuretics may reduce circulating volume, producing hypovolemia despite persistent peripheral edema. A fall in urine output may indicate significantly reduced cardiac output and renal ischemia. Weight is an objective measure of fluid status: 1 L of fluid is equal to 2.2 lb of weight.
- Record abdominal girth every shift. Note complaints of a loss of appetite, abdominal discomfort, or nausea. Venous congestion can lead to ascites and may affect gastrointestinal function and nutritional status.
- Monitor and record hemodynamic measurements. Report significant changes and negative trends. Hemodynamic measurements provide a means of monitoring condition and response to treatment.
- Restrict fluids as ordered. Allow choices of fluid type and timing of intake, scheduling most fluid intake during morning and afternoon hours. Offer ice chips and frequent mouth care; provide hard candies if allowed. Providing choices increases the client's sense of control. Ice chips, hard candies, and mouth care relieve dry mouth and thirst and promote comfort.

Activity Intolerance

Clients with heart failure have little or no cardiac reserve to meet increased oxygen demands. As the disease progresses and cardiac function is further compromised, activity intolerance increases. The low cardiac output and inability to participate in activities may hinder self-care.

- Organize nursing care to allow rest periods. Grouping activities together allows adequate time to "recharge."
- Assist with ADLs as needed. Encourage independence within prescribed limits. Assisting with ADLs helps ensure that care needs are met while reducing cardiac workload. Involving the client promotes a sense of control and reduces helplessness.

NURSING CARE PLAN A Client With Heart Failure

ASSESSMENT

One year ago, Arthur Jackson, 67 years old, had a large anterior wall MI and underwent subsequent coronary artery bypass surgery. On discharge, he was started on a regimen of enalapril (Vasotec), digoxin, furosemide (Lasix), warfarin (Coumadin), and a potassium chloride supplement. He is now in the cardiac unit complaining of severe shortness of breath, hemoptysis, and poor appetite for 1 week. He is diagnosed with acute heart failure.

Mr. Jackson refuses to settle in bed, preferring to sit in the bedside recliner in high Fowler's position. He states, "Lately, this is the only way I can breathe." Mr. Jackson states that he has not been able to work in his garden without getting short of breath. He complains of his shoes and belt being too tight.

When Ms. Takashi, RN, Mr. Jackson's nurse, obtains his nursing history, Mr. Jackson insists that he takes his medications regularly. He states that he normally works in his garden for light exercise. In his diet history, Mr. Jackson admits fondness for bacon and Chinese food and sheepishly admits to snacking between meals "even though I need to lose weight."

Mr. Jackson's vital signs are as follows: blood pressure, 95/72 mmHg; pulse, 124 bpm and irregular; respirations, 28/min and labored; and temperature 97.5°F (36.5°C). The cardiac monitor shows atrial fibrillation. An S_3 is noted on auscultation; the cardiac impulse is left of the midclavicular line. Mr. Jackson has crackles and diminished breath sounds in the bases of both lungs. Significant jugular venous distention, 3+ pitting edema of feet and ankles, and abdominal distention are noted. Liver size is within normal limits by percussion. Skin is cool and diaphoretic. Chest x-ray shows cardiomegaly and pulmonary infiltrates.

DIAGNOSES

- Excess Fluid Volume related to impaired cardiac pump and salt and water retention
- Activity Intolerance related to impaired cardiac output
- Impaired Health Maintenance related to lack of knowledge about diet restrictions

PLANNING

Goals of care include the following:

- The client will demonstrate loss of excess fluid by weight loss and decreases in edema, jugular venous distention, and abdominal distention.
- The client will demonstrate improved activity tolerance.
- The client will verbalize understanding of diet restrictions.

IMPLEMENTATION

- Take hourly vital signs and hemodynamic pressure measurements.
- Administer and monitor effects of prescribed diuretics and vasodilators.
- Weigh the client daily; strict intake and output.
- Monitor for edema
- Enforce fluid restriction of 1,500 mL/24 hr (600 mL day shift, 600 mL evening shift, and 300 mL at night).
- Auscultate heart and breath sounds every 4 hours and as indicated.
- Administer oxygen per nasal cannula at 2 L/min. Monitor oxygen saturation continuously; notify physician if less than 94%.
- Place in High Fowler's or position of comfort.
- Notify physician of significant changes in laboratory values.
- Teach about all medications and how to take and record pulse. Provide information about anticoagulant therapy and signs of bleeding.
- Design an activity plan that incorporates preferred activities and scheduled rest periods.
- Instruct about sodium-restricted diet. Allow meal choices within allowed limits.
- Consult dietitian for planning and teaching about a low-sodium diet.

EVALUATION

Mr. Jackson is discharged after 3 days in the cardiac unit. He has lost 8 lb during his stay, and he states that it is much easier to breathe and his shoes fit better. He is able to sleep in semi-Fowler's position with only one pillow. His peripheral edema has resolved. Mr. and Mrs. Jackson met with the dietitian, who helped them develop a realistic eating plan to limit sodium, sugar, and fats. The dietitian also provided a list of high-sodium foods to avoid. Mr. Jackson is relieved to know that he can still enjoy Chinese food prepared without monosodium glutamate (MSG) or added salt. Ms. Takashi and the physical therapist designed a progressive activity plan with Mr. Jackson that he will continue at home. He remains in atrial fibrillation, a chronic condition. His knowledge of digoxin and Coumadin has been assessed and reinforced. Ms. Takashi confirms that he is able to accurately check his pulse and can list signs of digoxin toxicity and excessive bleeding.

CRITICAL THINKING

1. Mr. Jackson's medication regimen remains the same after discharge. What specific teaching does he need related to potential interactions of these drugs?
2. Mr. Jackson tells you, "Talk to my wife about my medications—she's Tarzan and I'm Jane now." How would you respond?
3. Design an exercise plan for Mr. Jackson to prevent deconditioning and conserve energy.
4. Mr. Jackson tells you, "Sometimes I forget whether I have taken my aspirin, so I'll take another just to be sure. After all, they are only baby aspirin. One or two extra a day shouldn't hurt, right?" What is your response?
5. Mr. Jackson is admitted to the neuro unit 6 months later with a cerebral vascular accident. What is the probable cause of his stroke?

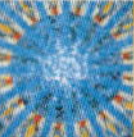

CLIENT TEACHING Home Care for a Client With Heart Failure

Heart failure is a chronic condition requiring active participation by the client and family for effective management. In teaching for home care, include the following topics:

- The disease process and its effects on the client's life
- Warning signals of cardiac decompensation that require treatment
- Desired and adverse effects of prescribed drugs, monitoring for effects, and importance of compliance with drug regimen to prevent acute and long-term complications of heart failure
- Prescribed diet and sodium restriction, practical suggestions for reducing salt intake, and AHA materials and recipes
- Exercise recommendations to strengthen the heart muscle and improve aerobic capacity (Box 22–23)
- The importance of keeping scheduled follow-up appointments to monitor disease progression and effects of therapy.

Provide referrals for home health care and household assistance (shopping, transportation, personal needs, and housekeeping) as indicated. Referrals to community agencies, such as local cardiac rehabilitation programs, heart support groups, or the AHA, can provide the client and family with additional materials and psychosocial support.

- Plan and implement progressive activities. Use passive and active ROM exercises as appropriate. Consult with the physical therapist on an activity plan. Progressive activity slowly increases exercise capacity by strengthening and improving cardiac function without strain. Activity also helps prevent skeletal muscle atrophy. ROM exercises prevent complications of immobility in severely compromised clients.
- Provide written and verbal information about activity after discharge. Written information provides a reference for important information. Verbal information allows clarification and validation of the material.

Deficient Knowledge: Low-Sodium Diet

Diet is an important part of long-term management of heart failure to manage fluid retention.

- Discuss the rationale for sodium restrictions. Understanding fosters compliance with the prescribed diet.
- Consult with a dietitian to plan and teach a low-sodium and, if necessary for weight control, low-kilocalorie diet. Provide a list of high-sodium, high-fat, high-cholesterol foods to avoid. Provide AHA materials. Dietary planning and teaching increase the client's sense of control and participation in disease management. Food lists are useful memory aids.

Evaluation

Client progress toward goals is evaluated based on the following suggested expected outcomes:

- The client describes each medication prescribed along with the symptoms that should be reported to provider immediately.
- The client explains the importance of daily weights and keeping a log along with the importance of reporting significant weight gain.
- The client chooses appropriate foods from a menu reflecting a low sodium diet.
- The client modifies daily routine to allow adequate periods of rest and activity.

Box 22–23 Home Activity Guidelines for the Client With Heart Failure

- Perform as many activities as independently as you can.
- Space your meals and activities.
  a. Eat six small meals a day.
  b. Allow time during the day for periods of rest and relaxation.
- Perform all activities at a comfortable pace.
  a. If you get tired during any activity, stop what you are doing and rest for 15 minutes.
  b. Resume activity only if you feel up to it.
- Stop any activity that causes chest pain, shortness of breath, dizziness, faintness, excessive weakness, or sweating. Rest. Notify your physician if your activity tolerance changes and if symptoms continue after rest.
- Avoid straining. Do not lift heavy objects. To prevent constipation, eat a high-fiber diet and drink plenty of water. Use laxatives or stool softeners, as approved by your physician, to avoid constipation and straining during bowel movements.
- Begin a graded exercise program. Walking is good exercise that does not require any special equipment (except a good pair of walking shoes). Plan to walk twice a day at a comfortable, slow pace for the first couple of weeks at home, and then gradually increase the distance and pace. Below is a suggested schedule—but progress at your own speed. Take your time. Aim for walking at least three times per week (every other day).

Week 1	200–400 feet	Twice a day, slow and leisurely pace
Week 2	1/4 mile	15 minutes, minimum of three times per week
Weeks 2–3	1/2 mile	30 minutes, minimum of three times per week
Weeks 3–4	1 mile	30 minutes, minimum of three times per week
Weeks 4–5	1 1/2 mile	30 minutes, minimum of three times per week
Weeks 5–6	2 miles	40 minutes, minimum of three times per week

REVIEW Heart Failure

RELATE: LINK THE CONCEPTS

Linking the exemplar of Heart Failure with the concept of Oxygenation:

1. What is the nursing priority of care when caring for a client with heart failure and pulmonary edema? Explain your answer.
2. What impact does heart failure have on the client's oxygenation status if pulmonary edema is not found?

Linking the exemplar of Heart Failure with the concept of Cognition:

3. Why might heart failure induce confusion in the older client?
4. What teaching would you provide the family of an older client diagnosed with heart failure who becomes suddenly confused and disoriented?

READY: GO TO COMPANION SKILLS MANUAL

- Supporting a client in Fowler's position
- Oxygen saturation using a pulse oximeter
- Administering oxygen via cannula
- Assessing respirations
- Assessing an apical pulse
- Assessing blood pressure
- Assessing vital signs
- Measuring abdominal girth
- Measuring weight
- Monitoring intake and output

REFER: GO TO MYNURSINGKIT

REFLECT: CASE STUDY

Dr. Danilo Ocampo is a 74-year-old retired pathologist. He lives in his home with Lydia, his wife of 51 years. Their only child, a son, was killed at age 22 in an automobile accident. Dr. Ocampo was born and raised in the Philippines and came to the United States when he was 23. He is the last living member of his immediate family. He has a few nephews and nieces in the Philippines, but no relatives live nearby.

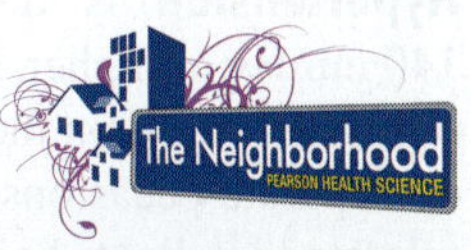

Dr. Ocampo's health has been declining for the past few years. He has a medical history that includes hypertension, myocardial infarction, angina, and class 2 heart failure. Because of these cardiovascular disorders, he takes multiple medications, including metoprolol, lisinopril, spironolactone, furosemide (intermittently as needed), potassium supplements (when taking furosemide), aspirin, isosorbide dinitrate, and nitroglycerin. He has a good understanding of the pharmaceutical properties of the medications. At times, he is not sure he gets good health care because of all the medications he takes. He often does not believe the medications are helpful because he experiences many side effects, and he has required multiple admissions to the hospital. He usually feels better after a few days in the hospital, but typically checks himself out of the hospital before his physicians are ready to discharge him.

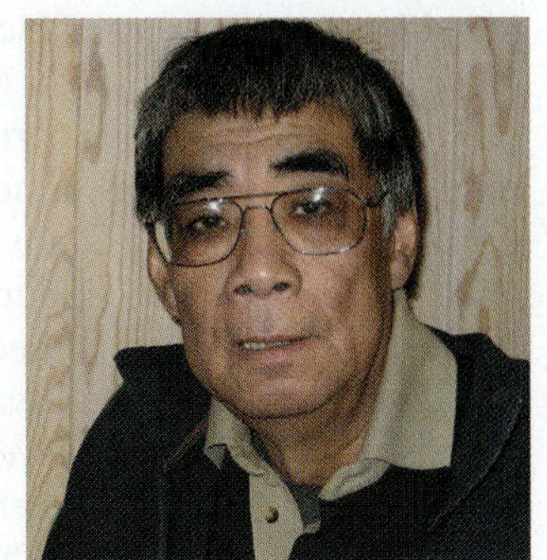

Because his wife Lydia has dementia, most of Dr. Ocampo's time and energy are spent managing their household and taking care of her. He has been resistant to outside help, believing he can care for her better than anyone else. He maintains a very consistent schedule, and they get along quite well. Although at one time in their lives they were very socially active, at this point, they rarely go out.

1. What interventions can you initiate to help Dr. Ocampo minimize the side effects of the multiple medications he is taking?
2. What nutritional assessment would be appropriate for Dr. Ocampo. Why?
3. Should you intervene to help Dr. Ocampo accept help with the care of Lydia to decrease his own stress and improve his health? Explain your answer.

22.7 HYPERTENSION

KEY TERMS

Blood flow, *1422*
Blood pressure, *1422*
Diastolic blood pressure, *1422*
Hypertension, *1422*
Hypertensive emergency, *1425*
Hypertensive encephalopathy, *1427*
Mean arterial pressure, 1422
Peripheral vascular resistance, *1422*
Primary hypertension, *1424*
Pulse pressure, *1422*
Secondary hypertension, *1424*
Step-down therapy, *1433*
Systolic blood pressure, *1422*

BASIS FOR SELECTION OF EXEMPLAR

Centers for Disease Control and Prevention
Institute of Medicine

LEARNING OUTCOMES

After reading about this exemplar, you will be able to:

1. Describe the pathophysiology, etiology, clinical manifestations, and direct and indirect causes of hypertension.
2. Identify risk factors associated with hypertension.
3. Illustrate the nursing process in providing culturally competent care across the life span for individuals with hypertension.
4. Formulate priority nursing diagnoses appropriate for an individual with hypertension.
5. Create a plan of care for individuals with hypertension and their family members.
6. Assess expected outcomes for an individual with hypertension.
7. Discuss therapies used in the collaborative care of an individual with hypertension.
8. Employ evidence-based caring interventions for an individual with hypertension.

OVERVIEW

Hypertension is defined as systolic blood pressure of 140 mmHg or higher, or a diastolic blood pressure of 90 mmHg or higher, based on the average of three or more readings taken on separate occasions (NHLBI, 2004b). Higher levels may be tolerated in clients being treated for hypertension. Table 22–28 identifies classifications of blood pressure for adults age 18 and older as defined by the Joint National Committee.

Hypertension is an important public health issue: While it rarely causes symptoms or noticeably limits the client's functional health, hypertension is a major risk factor for coronary heart disease, heart failure, stroke, and renal failure. Hypertension and its consequences are not unique to the United States. The World Health Organization identifies blood pressure above optimal levels (systolic, > 115 mmHg) as responsible for 62% of cerebrovascular disease and 49% of ischemic heart disease worldwide (NHLBI, 2004b).

While the identification and treatment of hypertension in the United States has improved significantly during the past 25 years, approximately 30% of adults with hypertension remain unaware of their condition. Although 59% of adults with hypertension adults are being treated for the disorder, effective blood pressure control is achieved only in approximately 34% (NHLBI, 2004b).

PATHOPHYSIOLOGY AND ETIOLOGY

The factors that affect arterial circulation are blood flow, peripheral vascular resistance, and blood pressure. **Blood pressure** is the force exerted against the walls of the arteries by the blood as it is pumped from the heart. It is most accurately referred to as **mean arterial pressure (MAP)**, which specifically denotes the average pressure in the arterial circulation throughout the cardiac cycle. The highest pressure exerted against the arterial walls at the peak of ventricular contraction (systole) is called the **systolic blood pressure.** The lowest pressure exerted during ventricular relaxation (diastole) is the **diastolic blood pressure**.

TABLE 22–28 Classification of Blood Pressure for Adults[a]

CATEGORY	SYSTOLIC (mmHG)		DIASTOLIC (mmHG)
Normal	< 120	*and*	< 80
Prehypertension	120–139	*or*	80–89
Hypertension[b]			
Stage 1	140–159	*or*	90–99
Stage 2	≥ 160	*or*	≥ 100

Source: Adapted from NHLBI. (2004b). *The Seventh Report of the Joint National Committee on Prevention, Detection, Education, and Treatment of High Blood Pressure,* NIH Publication No. 04-5250. Bethesda, MD: National Institutes of Health. Retrieved from http://www.nhlbi.nih.gov/guidelines/hypertension

[a]When systolic and diastolic blood pressures fall into different categories, the reading that is highest or most out of acceptable range is used to classify blood pressure status.

[b]Based on the average of two or more readings taken at each of two or more visits after an initial screening.

Mean arterial blood pressure is regulated mainly by cardiac output (CO) and peripheral vascular resistance (PVR), as represented in this formula: MAP = CO × PVR. For clinical use, the MAP may be estimated by calculating the diastolic blood pressure plus one third of the pulse pressure (the difference between the systolic and diastolic blood pressure).

Blood flow refers to the volume of blood transported in a vessel, in an organ, or throughout the entire circulation over a given period of time. It is commonly expressed as liters or milliliters per minute or as cubic centimeters per second. Blood flow through the circulatory system requires sufficient blood volume to fill the blood vessels and pressure differences within the system to allow blood to move forward.

The arterial, or supply, side of the circulation has relatively high pressures created by the thick elastic walls of the arteries and arterioles. The venous, or return, side of the system is a low-pressure system of thin-walled, distensible veins. Blood flows through the capillaries linking these two systems from the higher-pressure arterial side to the lower-pressure venous side.

The arterial blood pressure is created by the ejection of blood from the heart during systole (cardiac output) and the tension (resistance to blood flow) created by the elastic arterial walls (systemic vascular resistance). The blood pressure (the force exerted against the walls of the arteries by the blood as it is pumped from the heart) rises as the heart contracts during systole, ejecting its blood. This pressure wave, or systolic blood pressure, is felt as the peripheral pulse and is heard as the Korotkoff's sounds during blood pressure measurement. In healthy adults, the average systolic pressure is less than 120 mmHg. During diastole (cardiac relaxation and filling), elastic arterial walls maintain a minimum pressure, or diastolic blood pressure, to maintain blood flow through the capillary beds. The average diastolic pressure in a healthy adult is less than 80 mmHg. The difference between the systolic and diastolic pressure (normally ~40 mmHg) is known as the **pulse pressure**. The MAP is the average pressure in the arterial circulation throughout the cardiac cycle; it can be calculated using the formula [systolic blood pressure + 2(diastolic blood pressure)]/3.

Cardiac output is determined by the blood volume and the ability of the ventricles to fill and effectively pump that blood. A number of factors contribute to systemic vascular resistance, including vessel length, blood viscosity, and vessel diameter and distensibility (compliance). While vessel length and blood viscosity remain relatively constant, vessel diameter and compliance are subject to normal regulatory activities and disease. These factors also affect **peripheral vascular resistance**, which refers to the opposing forces or impedance to blood flow as the arterial channels become more and more distant from the heart.

Peripheral vascular resistance is determined by three factors:

1. *Blood viscosity:* The greater the viscosity, or thickness, of the blood, the greater its resistance to moving and flowing.

2. *Length of the vessel.* The longer the vessel, the greater the resistance to blood flow.
3. *Diameter of the vessel.* The smaller the diameter of a vessel, the greater the friction against the walls of the vessel and, thus, the greater the impedance to blood flow.

Factors Influencing Arterial Blood Pressure

The arterioles normally determine the systemic vascular resistance as their diameter changes in response to a variety of stimuli. These stimuli include the following:

Sympathetic nervous system (SNS) stimulation. Baroreceptors in the aortic arch and carotid sinus signal the SNS via the cardiovascular control center in the medulla when the MAP changes. A drop in MAP stimulates the SNS, increasing the heart rate and cardiac output and constricting arterioles (except in skeletal muscle). As a result, blood pressure rises. A rise in MAP has the opposite effect, decreasing the heart rate and cardiac output and causing arteriolar vasodilation.

- *Circulating epinephrine and norepinephrine* from the adrenal cortex (e.g., the fight-or-flight response) have the same effect as SNS stimulation.
- *Renin–angiotensin–aldosterone system* responds to renal perfusion. A drop in renal perfusion stimulates renin release. Renin converts angiotensinogen to angiotensin I, which is subsequently converted to angiotensin II in the lungs by ACE. Angiotensin II is a potent vasoconstrictor. It also promotes sodium and water retention, both directly and by stimulating the adrenal medulla to release aldosterone. Both systemic vascular resistance and cardiac output increase, raising blood pressure.
- *Atrial natriuretic peptide (ANP)* and *brain natriuretic peptide (BNP)* are released from atrial cells in response to stretching by excess blood volume. These hormones promote vasodilation and sodium and water excretion, lowering blood pressure.
- *Adrenomedullin* is a peptide synthesized and released by endothelial and smooth muscle cells in blood vessels. It is a potent vasodilator.
- *Vasopressin* or *antidiuretic hormone (ADH)*, from the posterior pituitary gland, promotes water retention and vasoconstriction, raising blood pressure.
- *Local factors*, such as inflammatory mediators and various metabolites, can promote vasodilation, affecting blood pressure.

Other factors that can affect vessel compliance is the extent of arteriosclerosis (hardening of the arteries) and atherosclerosis (plaque accumulation). Figure 22–48 ■ summarizes the interrelationships of major factors regulating blood pressure. The cardiovascular system adapts to increased blood volume by increasing cardiac output. Autoregulatory mechanisms in the systemic arteries react to the increased volume, causing vasoconstriction. The increased systemic vascular resistance causes hypertension.

Blood flow, peripheral vascular resistance, and blood pressure, which influence arterial circulation, are in turn influenced by various factors. These factors include the following:

- The sympathetic and parasympathetic nervous systems are the primary mechanisms that regulate blood pressure. Stimulation of the SNS exerts a major effect on peripheral resistance by causing vasoconstriction of the arterioles, thereby increasing

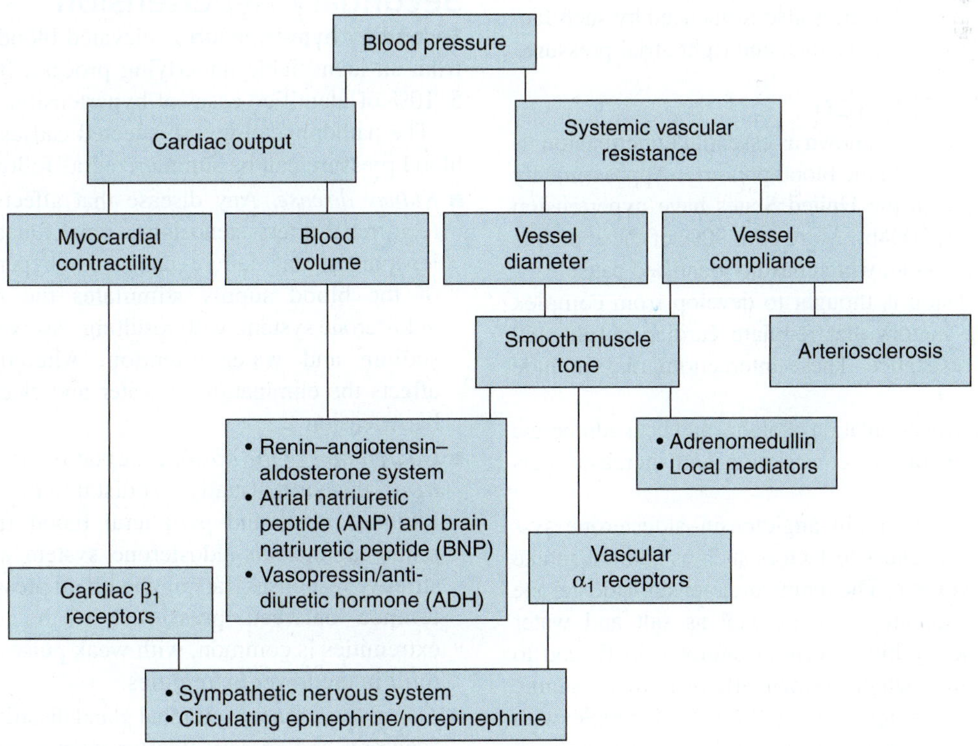

Figure 22–48 ■ Factors affecting blood pressure.

blood pressure. Parasympathetic stimulation causes vasodilation of the arterioles, lowering blood pressure.

- Baroreceptors and chemoreceptors in the aortic arch, carotid sinus, and other large vessels are sensitive to pressure and chemical changes and cause reflex sympathetic stimulation, resulting in vasoconstriction, increased heart rate, and increased blood pressure.
- The kidneys help maintain blood pressure by excreting or conserving sodium and water. When blood pressure decreases, the kidneys initiate the renin–angiotensin mechanism. This stimulates vasoconstriction, resulting in the release of the hormone aldosterone from the adrenal cortex, increasing sodium ion reabsorption and water retention. In addition, pituitary release of ADH promotes renal reabsorption of water. The net result is an increase in blood volume and a consequent increase in cardiac output and blood pressure.
- Temperatures may also affect peripheral resistance: Cold causes vasoconstriction, whereas warmth produces vasodilation. Many chemicals, hormones, and drugs influence blood pressure by affecting CO and/or peripheral vascular resistance. For example, epinephrine causes vasoconstriction and increased heart rate; prostaglandins dilate blood vessel diameter (by relaxing vascular smooth muscle); endothelin, a chemical released by the inner lining of vessels, is a potent vasoconstrictor; nicotine causes vasoconstriction; and alcohol and histamine cause vasodilation.
- Dietary factors, such as intake of salt, saturated fats, and cholesterol, elevate blood pressure by affecting blood volume and vessel diameter.
- Race, gender, age, weight, time of day, position, exercise, and emotional state may also affect blood pressure. These factors influence the arterial pressure. Systemic venous pressure, though it is much lower, is also influenced by such factors as blood volume, venous tone, and right atrial pressure.

Primary Hypertension

Primary hypertension, also known as essential hypertension, is a persistently elevated systemic blood pressure. Approximately 50–65 million people in the United States have hypertension (AHA, 2005; NHLBI, 2004b). More than 90% of these people have primary hypertension, which has no identified cause.

Primary hypertension is thought to develop from complex interactions among factors that regulate cardiac output and systemic vascular resistance. These interactions may include the following:

- Excess SNS with overstimulation of alpha- and beta-adrenergic receptors, resulting in vasoconstriction and increased cardiac output.
- Altered function of the renin–angiotensin–aldosterone system and its responsiveness to factors such as sodium intake and overall fluid volume. The renin–angiotensin–aldosterone system affects vasomotor tone as well as salt and water excretion. Chronically high levels of angiotensin II lead to arteriolar remodeling, which permanently increases systemic vascular resistance. In approximately 20% of people with primary hypertension, renin levels are lower than normal. Increased sodium intake increases the blood pressure in these clients. Low plasma renin levels are more commonly seen in African Americans than in whites. Another 15% of clients with hypertension have higher-than-normal plasma renin levels. For these clients, salt intake has less of an effect on blood pressure (Kasper et al., 2005). Most people with hypertension have normal levels of renin activity.
- Other chemical mediators of vasomotor tone and blood volume, such as ANP, also play a role by affecting vasomotor tone and sodium and water excretion. Vascular endothelium itself produces hormones (endothelins) that also affect vasomotor tone. Endothelin-1 is a potent vasoconstrictor (Copstead & Banasik, 2005).
- The interaction between insulin resistance, hyperinsulinemia, and endothelial function may be a primary cause of hypertension. Excess insulin has several effects that potentially contribute to hypertension: sodium retention by the kidneys, increased SNS activity, hypertrophy of vascular smooth muscle, and changes in ion transport across cell membranes (Kasper et al., 2005).

The result is sustained increases in blood volume and peripheral resistance. The cardiovascular system adapts to increased blood volume by increasing cardiac output. Autoregulatory mechanisms in the systemic arteries react to the increased volume, causing vasoconstriction. The increased systemic vascular resistance causes hypertension.

It appears unlikely that one single cause and pathologic process will be found to account for essential hypertension. Increasingly, evidence points to hypertension as a diverse group of pathophysiologic mechanisms resulting in the common manifestation of elevated blood pressure.

Secondary Hypertension

Secondary hypertension is elevated blood pressure resulting from an identifiable underlying process. It accounts for only 5–10% of identified cases of hypertension.

The pathophysiology of selected causes of secondary high blood pressure can be summarized as follows:

- *Kidney disease.* Any disease that affects renal blood flow (e.g., renal artery stenosis) or renal function (e.g., glomerulonephritis, renal failure) can lead to hypertension. Disruption of the blood supply stimulates the renin–angiotensin–aldosterone system, with resulting vasoconstriction as well as sodium and water retention. Altered kidney function affects the elimination of water and electrolytes, leading to hypertension.
- *Coarctation of the aorta.* Coarctation of the aorta is narrowing of the aorta, usually just distal to the subclavian arteries. Reduced renal and peripheral blood flow stimulates the renin–angiotensin–aldosterone system and local vasoconstrictive responses, raising the blood pressure. A marked difference between pressures in the upper and lower extremities is common, with weak pulses and poor capillary refill in the lower extremities.
- *Endocrine disorders.* Adrenal gland disorders, such as Cushing syndrome and primary aldosteronism, can cause hypertension. A rare tumor of the adrenal medulla, pheochromocytoma,

causes persistent or intermittent hypertension. Other endocrine disorders, such as hyperthyroidism and pituitary disorders, also can lead to hypertension.

- *Neurologic disorders.* Increased intracranial pressure causes an elevated blood pressure as the body attempts to maintain cerebral blood flow. Disorders that interfere with autonomic nervous system regulation (e.g., high spinal cord injury) may allow the SNS to predominate, increasing systemic vascular resistance and blood pressure.
- *Drug use.* Estrogen and oral contraceptive use may lead to hypertension, possibly by prompting sodium and water retention and affecting the renin–angiotensin–aldosterone system. Stimulant drugs, such as cocaine and methamphetamines, increase systemic vascular resistance and cardiac output, resulting in hypertension.
- *Pregnancy.* Approximately 10% of all pregnant women are hypertensive. Hypertension may predate pregnancy, or it may occur as a direct response to the pregnancy. The mechanism of pregnancy-induced hypertension is unclear. It is a significant cause of maternal and fetal morbidity and mortality, and it requires careful perinatal management. (See Exemplar 22.10, Pregnancy-Induced Hypertension, for more details.)

The pattern of secondary hypertension varies depending on its cause. Pheochromocytoma may cause attacks of hypertension that last for minutes to hours, accompanied by anxiety, palpitations, diaphoresis, pallor, and nausea and vomiting. Primary aldosteronism may cause hypertension, weakness, paresthesias, polyuria, and nocturia. Symptoms of kidney disease accompany hypertension when a renal disorder is the cause.

Hypertensive Emergency

Some clients with hypertension may, for reasons not clearly understood, develop rapid, significant elevations in systolic and/or diastolic pressures. In a **hypertensive emergency** (or malignant hypertension), the systolic pressure is greater than 180 mmHg and the diastolic pressure higher than 120 mmHg. Immediate treatment (within 1 hour) is vital to prevent cardiac, renal, and vascular damage and to reduce morbidity and mortality. Intense cerebral artery spasms help protect the brain from excess pressure; however, cerebral edema often develops. Prolonged severe hypertension damages walls of the arterioles and renal blood vessels and may lead to intravascular coagulation and acute renal failure.

Hypertension and Pregnancy

In women with chronic hypertension, the goals of care are to prevent the development of preeclampsia and ensure normal growth of the fetus. Preeclampsia develops in approximaetly 10–25% of women previously found to have chronic hypertension (Habli & Sibai, 2008).

Gestational hypertension occurs after 20 weeks, often during the last weeks of pregnancy. Its distinction from preeclampsia is the lack of proteinuria. Women in whom gestational hypertension occurs are at increased risk for developing chronic hypertension later in life.

Close monitoring and careful management of the client who is pregnant are indicated if the following signs develop:

- Elevations of systolic blood pressure 30 mmHg above the baseline, or diastolic blood pressure 15–20 mmHg above the baseline, on two occasions at least 6 hours apart
- Proteinuria
- Edema occurring in the upper half of the body.

A woman with chronic hypertension who develops superimposed preeclampsia often progresses quickly to eclampsia, sometimes before 30 weeks of pregnancy.

Etiology

Hypertension primarily affects middle-aged and older adults: More than 50% of people ages 60–69 and approximately 75% of those age 70 and older are hypertensive (NHLBI, 2004b). An age-related increase in the systolic blood pressure is the primary factor leading to the high incidence of hypertension in older adults. Unlike the diastolic blood pressure, which tends to rise until approximately age 50 and then level off, the systolic blood pressure continues to rise with aging (NHLBI, 2004b).

The prevalence of hypertension is significantly higher in blacks than in whites and Hispanics. Nearly 40% of black adults are hypertensive, whereas less than 30% of adult white and Hispanic people are affected. In whites and Hispanics, more males than females are hypertensive; in blacks, more women than men are affected (NHLBI, 2004a). Essential hypertension affects people of all income groups, having great financial effects because of its effects on other body systems.

The underlying causes of hypertension are not known in most cases. Only in a small number of cases can specific causes be determined. In general, several mechanisms may be involved, including the following:

1. Autonomic nervous system dysfunction, with an exaggerated response to autonomic triggers
2. Genetic differences in renal sodium reabsorption, which may be particularly prevalent among non-Hispanic blacks
3. Dysfunction of the renin–angiotensin aldosterone system, which results in increased body water
4. Impaired endovascular responsiveness
5. Insulin resistance, noted because hypertension and diabetes frequently occur together.

Primary hypertension is diagnosed when no specific cause is known.

Kidney disease is the most common identifiable cause of secondary high blood pressure in both adults and children (Copstead & Banasik, 2005). Other common identifiable causes of hypertension in adults include renovascular disease (reduced blood flow to the kidneys), disorders of the adrenal cortex, pheochromocytoma, coarctation of the aorta, and sleep apnea.

Risk Factors

A number of risk factors have been identified for primary hypertension (Box 22–24). Genetics plays a role, as do environmental factors.

Box 22–24 **Factors Contributing to Hypertension**

MODIFIABLE FACTORS

- High sodium intake
- Low potassium, calcium, and magnesium intake
- Obesity
- Excess alcohol consumption
- Insulin resistance

NONMODIFIABLE FACTORS

- Genetic factors
- Age
- Family history
- Race

Specific risk factors include the following:

- *Family history.* Studies show a genetic link in approximately 30% of people with primary hypertension (Kasper et al., 2005). Genes involved in the renin–angiotensin–aldosterone system and others that affect vascular tone, salt and water transportation in the kidney, obesity, and insulin resistance likely are involved in the development of hypertension, although no consistent genetic linkages have been found.
- *Age.* The incidence of hypertension rises with increasing age. Aging affects baroreceptors involved in blood pressure regulation as well as arterial compliance. As the arteries become less compliant, pressure within the vessels increases. This is often most apparent as a gradual increase in the systolic pressure with aging.
- *Race.* Essential hypertension is more common and more severe in blacks than in people of other ethnic backgrounds (see the Focus on Diversity and Culture feature that follows). It also tends to develop at an earlier age and is associated with more cardiovascular and renal damage. More African Americans with hypertension have low renin levels and altered renal excretion of sodium at normal blood pressure levels. This genetic tendency to conserve salt may have developed as an adaptation to working in a warm environment, where salt and water conservation are beneficial (Porth, 2005).
- *Mineral intake.* High sodium intake often is associated with fluid retention. Hypertension related to sodium intake involves a number of different physiologic mechanisms, including the renin–angiotensin–aldosterone system, nitric oxide, catecholamines, endothelin, and ANP (Copstead & Banasik, 2005). Low potassium, calcium, and magnesium intakes also contribute to hypertension by unknown mechanisms. The ratio of sodium to potassium intake appears to play a role, possibly through the effects of increased potassium intake on sodium excretion. Potassium also promotes vasodilation by reducing responses to catecholamines and angiotensin II. Calcium has a vasodilator effect as well. While magnesium has been shown to reduce the blood pressure, the mechanism of action is unclear.
- *Obesity.* Central obesity (fat cell deposits in the abdomen), as determined by an increased waist-to-hip ratio, has a stronger correlation with hypertension than body mass index or skinfold thickness. Although a clear correlation exists between obesity and hypertension, the relationship may be one of common cause: Genetic factors appear to play a role in the common triad of obesity, hypertension, and insulin resistance.
- *Insulin resistance.* Insulin resistance with resulting hyperinsulinemia is linked with hypertension by its effects of excess circulating insulin on the SNS, vascular smooth muscle, renal regulation of sodium and water, and ion transport across cell membranes. Insulin resistance may be a genetic or an acquired trait. Although it is more commonly seen in individuals who are obese, insulin resistance also has been found in people of normal weight.
- *Excess alcohol consumption.* Regular consumption of three or more drinks a day increases the risk of hypertension. Decreasing or discontinuing alcohol consumption reduces the blood pressure, particularly systolic readings. Lifestyle factors associated with excessive alcohol intake (obesity and lack of exercise) may contribute to hypertension as well.
- *Stress.* Physical and emotional stress cause transient elevations of blood pressure, but the role of stress in primary hypertension is less clear. Blood pressure normally fluctuates throughout the day, increasing with activity, discomfort, or emotional responses such as anger. Frequent or continued stress may cause vascular smooth muscle hypertrophy or affect central integrative pathways of the brain (Porth, 2005).

Most hypertensive emergencies occur when clients suddenly stop taking their medications or their hypertension is poorly controlled. Younger clients (30–50 years), African American men, pregnant women with preeclampsia, and people with collagen and/or renal disease also are at higher risk for a hypertensive emergency (Porth, 2005).

FOCUS ON DIVERSITY AND CULTURE
Hypertension in African Americans

- The prevalence of hypertension among African Americans living in the United States is among the highest in the world: In African American adults, 41.8% of males and 45.4% of females are hypertensive.
- African Americans with the highest risk for hypertension tend to be
  a. middle aged or older,
  b. less educated,
  c. overweight or obese,
  d. physically inactive, and
  e. affected by diabetes (AHA, 2005).

CLINICAL MANIFESTATIONS

The early stages of primary hypertension typically are asymptomatic, marked only by elevated blood pressure. Blood pressure elevations initially are transient but eventually become permanent. When symptoms do appear, they are usually vague. Headache, generally in the back of the head and neck, may be present on awakening, subsiding during the day. Other symptoms result from target organ damage and may include

CLINICAL MANIFESTATIONS AND THERAPIES **Hypertension**

ETIOLOGY	CLINICAL MANIFESTATION	CLINICAL THERAPIES
Hypertensive crisis	Rapid onset, blurred vision, papilledema, systolic pressure > 180 mmHg, diastolic pressure > 120 mmHg, headache, confusion, motor or sensory deficits	■ Medication administration: vasodilators, calcium-channel blockers, angiotensin-converting enzyme inhibitors, or adrenergic blockers ■ Blood pressure (BP) should be lowered gradually to prevent shock ■ Monitor BP continuously ■ Reduce client anxiety, which can cause BP to rise ■ Teach importance of maintaining treatment for hypertension
Stroke	Sudden onset of loss of sensation and/or movement: may be hemiplegia, hemiparesis, flaccidity, spasticity, or sensory loss of vision, hearing, taste, touch, proprioception, or smell	■ Monitor level of consciousness ■ Medication administration: anticoagulant, thrombolytic, corticosteroids, or antihypertensives ■ Surgery: carotid endarterectomy, extracranial–intracranial bypass, or carotid angioplasty ■ Reduce intracranial pressure to prevent further damage

nocturia, confusion, nausea and vomiting, and visual disturbances. Examination of the retina of the eye may reveal narrowed arterioles, hemorrhages, exudates, and papilledema (swelling of the optic nerve).

Sustained hypertension affects the cardiovascular, neurologic, and renal systems. The rate of atherosclerosis accelerates, increasing the risk for coronary heart disease and stroke. The workload of the left ventricle increases, leading to ventricular hypertrophy, which then increases the risk for coronary heart disease, dysrhythmias, and heart failure. The diastolic blood pressure is a significant cardiovascular risk factor until age 50; the systolic pressure then becomes the more important factor contributing to cardiovascular risk (NHLBI, 2004b). Most deaths caused by hypertension result from coronary heart disease and AMI or heart failure (Kasper et al., 2005).

Accelerated atherosclerosis associated with hypertension increases the risk for cerebral infarction (stroke). Increased pressure in the cerebral vessels can lead to development of microaneurysms and an increased risk for cerebral hemorrhage. **Hypertensive encephalopathy**, a syndrome characterized by extremely high blood pressure, altered level of consciousness, increased intracranial pressure, papilledema, and seizures, may develop. Its etiology is unclear.

Box 22–25 **Manifestations of Hypertensive Emergencies**

- Rapid onset
- Blurred vision, papilledema
- Systolic pressure > 180 mmHg
- Diastolic pressure > 120 mmHg
- Headache
- Confusion
- Motor and sensory deficits

Hypertension also can lead to nephrosclerosis and renal insufficiency. Proteinuria and microscopic hematuria develop, as do signs of chronic renal failure. African Americans experience hypertensive kidney disease more frequently than whites. Renal failure causes approximately 10% of deaths attributed to hypertension (Kasper et al., 2005).

Clients presenting with a hypertensive emergency may have manifestations such as headache, confusion, swelling of the optic nerve (papilledema), blurred vision, restlessness, and motor and sensory deficits. Manifestations of hypertensive emergencies are listed in Box 22–25.

COLLABORATION

Although there is no cure for hypertension, it can be controlled. Management of hypertension focuses on reducing the blood pressure to less than 140 mmHg systolic and 90 mmHg diastolic. The ultimate goal of hypertension management is to reduce cardiovascular and renal morbidity and mortality. The risk of cardiovascular complications (coronary heart disease, heart failure, and stroke) decreases when the average blood pressure is less than 140/90 mmHg; when the client also has diabetes or renal disease, the treatment goal is a blood pressure of less than 130/80 mmHg. It now is recognized that most people with hypertension will require a combination of two or more drugs along with lifestyle changes to achieve recommended blood pressure levels (NHLBI, 2004b). Figure 22–49 ■ shows the recommended algorithm for hypertension management.

Diagnostic Tests

The client with hypertension is evaluated for the presence of identifiable causes of hypertension, cardiovascular risk factors, and the presence or absence of target organ damage (heart, brain, kidneys, peripheral vascular systems, and retina

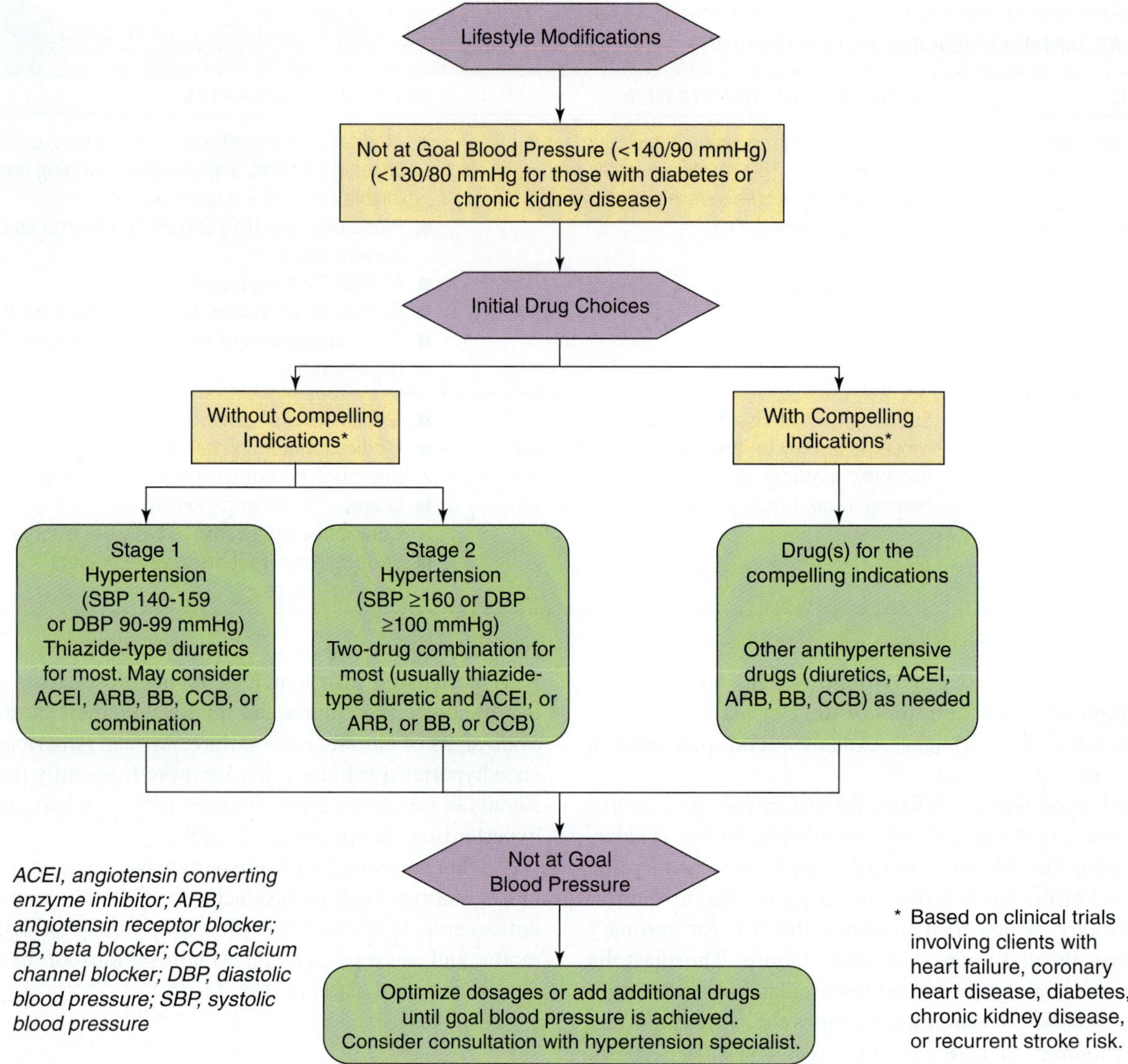

Figure 22–49 ■ Algorithm for treating hypertension.

Source: Adapted from NHLBI. (2004b). *The Seventh Report of the Joint National Committee on Prevention, Detection, Education, and Treatment of High Blood Pressure,* NIH Publication No. 04-5250. Bethesda, MD: National Institutes of Health.

of the eye). Before treatment is started, the following diagnostic tests are performed:

- ECG
- Urinalysis
- Blood glucose
- Hematocrit
- Serum potassium, creatinine, and calcium
- Cholesterol and lipoprotein profile, including HDL, LDL, and triglycerides.

Additional tests that may be done include urinary albumin excretion, evaluation of the glomerular filtration rate (e.g., creatinine clearance), and tests for emerging cardiovascular risk factors, such as C-reactive protein and homocystine levels.

The following diagnostic tests may be ordered to differentiate primary from secondary hypertension:

- *Renal function studies* and *urinalysis* to identify renal causes of hypertension. Elevated serum creatinine and blood urea nitrogen, reduced creatinine clearance, and hematuria, proteinuria, and casts often indicate kidney disease.
- *Serum potassium*, which is decreased in hyperaldosteronism.
- *Blood chemistries*, including serum electrolytes, glucose, and lipid studies, to detect abnormalities indicative of endocrine or cardiovascular disease.
- *Intravenous pyelography, renal ultrasonography, renal arteriography,* and *computed tomography (CT)* or *magnetic resonance imaging (MRI)* when secondary hypertension is suspected.

Lifestyle Modifications

Lifestyle modifications are recommended for all clients whose blood pressure falls within the prehypertension range (120–139/80–89 mm Hg) and for everyone with intermittent or sustained hypertension. These modifications include weight loss, dietary changes, restricted alcohol use and cigarette smoking, increased physical activity, and stress reduction (Box 22–26).

DIET Dietary approaches to managing hypertension focus on reducing sodium intake, maintaining adequate potassium and calcium intakes, and reducing total and saturated fat intake. A mild to moderate sodium restriction (no added salt) lowers blood pressure and potentiates the effect of antihypertensive drugs for most clients. The DASH (Dietary Approaches to Stop Hypertension) diet has proven beneficial in lowering blood pressure. This diet (Box 22–27) focuses on whole foods rather than individual nutrients. It is rich in fruits and vegetables (up to 10 servings per day) and is low in total and saturated fats.

Weight Loss

Weight loss is recommended for clients who are obese. Loss of as little as 10 lb (4.5 kg) reduces blood pressure in many people (NHLBI, 2004b). A balanced diet, such as the DASH diet, is recommended for weight loss.

PHYSICAL ACTIVITY Regular exercise (e.g., walking, cycling, jogging, or swimming) reduces blood pressure and contributes to weight loss, stress reduction, and feelings of overall well-being. Previously sedentary clients are encouraged to engage in aerobic exercise for 30–45 minutes per day most days of the week (5–6 days). Isometric exercise (e.g., weight training) may not be appropriate, because it can raise the systolic blood pressure.

ALCOHOL AND TOBACCO USE The recommended alcohol intake for clients with hypertension is no more than 1 oz of ethanol or two drinks per day. A drink is 12 oz of beer, 5 oz of wine, or 1.5 oz of 80-proof whiskey. Women and lighter-weight people should reduce this limit by half. Although alcohol withdrawal may increase blood pressure, this is usually temporary and diminishes as abstinence or restricted intake continues.

Although nicotine is a vasoconstrictor, substantial data linking smoking to hypertension are lacking. A definitive link exists between smoking and heart disease, however. Clients who smoke are strongly urged to quit. Smoking also reduces the effect of some antihypertensive medications, such as propranolol (Inderal). Smoking cessation aids, such as nicotine patches and gum, contain lower amounts of nicotine and usually do not raise blood pressure.

Box 22–26 **Lifestyle Modifications for Hypertension**

- Maintain normal body weight; lose weight if overweight.
- Dietary modifications:
  a. Eat a diet rich in fruits, vegetables, and low-fat dairy products.
  b. Reduce sodium intake.
  c. Reduce intake of cholesterol and of total and saturated fat.
- Limit alcohol intake to no more than 1 oz of ethanol (1/2 oz for women and lighter-weight people) per day.
- Engage in aerobic exercise for 30 minutes most days of the week (5–6 days/week).
- Stop smoking.
- Use stress management techniques, such as relaxation therapy.

Box 22–27 **DASH Diet Recommendations**

- Grains: 7–8 servings per day
- Vegetables: 4–5 servings per day
- Fruits: 4–5 servings per day
- Nonfat/low-fat dairy products: 2–3 servings per day
- Meats, poultry, and fish: £ 2 servings (3 oz each) per day
- Nuts, seeds, and dry beans: 4–5 servings per week
- Fats and oils: 2–3 servings per day
- Sweets: 5 servings per week (should be low in fat)

STRESS REDUCTION Stress stimulates the systemic nervous system, increasing vasoconstriction, systemic vascular resistance, cardiac output, and blood pressure. Regular, moderate exercise is the treatment of choice for reducing stress in clients with hypertension. Relaxation techniques, such as biofeedback, therapeutic touch, yoga, and meditation, to relax both mind and body may also lower blood pressure, although their effect has not been proven in hypertension management.

Pharmacologic Therapies

Current pharmacologic treatment of hypertension involves using one or more of the following drug classes: diuretics, alpha-adrenergic blockers, beta-adrenergic blockers, centrally acting sympatholytics, vasodilators, ACE inhibitors, angiotensin II receptor blockers, and calcium-channel blockers (Box 22–28). For most clients, two or more antihypertensive drugs selected from different drug classes are necessary to achieve effective control. These drug classes have different sites of action (see Figure 22–50 ■ on page 1432).

DRUG CLASSES Diuretics are the preferred treatment for systolic hypertension in older adults. Diuretics are relatively safe and well-tolerated drugs; in addition, most are relatively inexpensive. Thiazide diuretics, such as hydrochlorothiazide (HydroDIURIL), are widely used. In major clinical studies, treatment with a single diuretic controlled blood pressure in approximately 50% of clients and reduced hypertension-linked morbidity and mortality related to coronary heart disease. Diuretics control hypertension primarily by preventing tubular reabsorption of sodium, thus promoting sodium and water excretion and reducing blood volume. Thiazide diuretics also reduce systemic vascular resistance through an unknown mechanism. Diuretics are particularly effective in African Americans and in clients who are obese, older, or have increased plasma volume or low renin activity. The adverse effects of diuretics generally are dose-related. In addition to hypokalemia, diuretics may affect serum levels of glucose, triglycerides, uric acid, LDLs, and insulin.

Clients with heart failure, coronary heart disease, or diabetes may initially be treated with a beta-blocker. These drugs lower blood pressure, apparently by reducing peripheral vascular resistance. They may also reduce the amount of renin released by the kidneys by blocking beta$_1$-receptors in the kidney. Beta-blockers reduce the risk of complications such as heart failure and stroke. They are, however, relatively contraindicated for clients with asthma or chronic obstructive pulmonary disease because they promote bronchial constriction.

Box 22–28 **Medication Administration: Antihypertensive Drugs**

ALPHA-ADRENERGIC BLOCKERS

Doxazosin (Cardura)
Prazosin (Minipress)
Terazosin (Hytrin)

Alpha-adrenergic blocking agents block alpha-receptors in vascular smooth muscle, decreasing vasomotor tone and vasoconstriction. They also reduce serum levels of low-density lipoproteins and very-low-density lipoproteins. However, vasodilation may cause orthostatic hypotension and reflex stimulation of the heart, resulting in tachycardia and palpitations. A beta-blocker may be ordered to minimize this effect.

Nursing Responsibilities

- Give the first dose at bedtime to minimize risk of fainting (called "first-dose syncope"). If the first dose is given in the daytime (or if the dose is increased), instruct the client to remain in bed for 3–4 hours.
- Assess blood pressure and apical pulse before each dose and as indicated thereafter.

Health Education for the Client and Family

- There is a risk of fainting after taking the first dose of this drug. Take the drug at bedtime to reduce this risk, and do not drive or engage in other hazardous activities for 12–24 hours after the first dose.
- This drug may cause dizziness or lightheadedness. Change positions slowly, and sit down if you become dizzy or lightheaded.
- Notify your primary care provider if you develop nasal congestion or impotence while taking this drug.
- Notify your primary care provider before discontinuing this medication.

ANGIOTENSIN-CONVERTING ENZYME (ACE) INHIBITORS

Benazepril (Lotensin)	**Moexipril (Univasc)**
Captopril (Capoten)	**Perindopril (Aceon)**
Enalapril (Vasotec)	**Quinapril (Accupril)**
Fosinopril (Monopril)	**Ramipril (Altace)**
Lisinopril (Prinivil, Zestril)	**Trandolapril (Mavik)**

ANGIOTENSIN II–RECEPTOR BLOCKERS (ARBS)

Candesartan (Atacand)	**Olmesartan (Benicar)**
Eprosartan (Teveten)	**Telmisartan (Micardis)**
Irbesartan (Avapro)	**Valsartan (Diovan)**
Losartan (Cozaar)	

The ACE inhibitors lower blood pressure by preventing conversion of angiotensin I to angiotensin II. This in turn prevents vasoconstriction and sodium and water retention. ARBs have the same effect, but they act by blocking the effect of angiotensin II on receptors. Both ACE inhibitors and ARBs are less effective in clients who are black, and both are contraindicated in women who are pregnant (Lehne, 2004). Their primary adverse effects are persistent cough, first-dose hypotension, and hyperkalemia.

Nursing Responsibilities

- Assess blood pressure and white blood cell count before giving the first dose. Monitor blood pressure for 2 hours after the first dose and regularly thereafter.
- Administer orally 1 hour before meals; tablets may be crushed.
- Report changes in white blood cell count or differential, hyperkalemia, or changes in blood urea nitrogen or serum creatinine to the primary care provider.
- Do not administer to clients with renal artery stenosis or who are pregnant.
- Immediately report and treat manifestations of angioedema (giant wheals and edema of the tongue, glottis, and pharynx). Initiate resuscitation measures as needed. Discontinue drug immediately, and do not use in the future.

Health Education for the Client and Family

- Report peripheral edema, signs of infection, or difficulty breathing to your primary care provider.
- Change position (lying to sitting and sitting to standing) slowly to prevent dizziness; sit down if dizziness or lightheadedness develops.
- Do not take a potassium supplement or use a potassium-based salt substitute while taking this drug unless prescribed by your physician.
- Notify your physician if you become pregnant while taking this drug. Although it is safe early in pregnancy, taking the drug during the second and third trimesters may harm the fetus.

BETA-ADRENERGIC BLOCKING AGENTS

Acebutolol (Sectral)	**Nadolol (Corgard)**
Atenolol (Tenormin)	**Penbutolol (Levatol)**
Betaxolol (Kerlone)	**Pindolol (Visken)**
Bisoprolol (Zebeta)	**Propranolol (Inderal)**
Metoprolol tartrate (Lopressor)	**Timolol (Blocadren)**

Combined with an alpha-adrenergic blocking agent:

Carvedilol (Coreg)	**Labetalol (Normodyne)**

Beta-adrenergic blocking agents are commonly used to control hypertension. Beta-blockers reduce blood pressure by preventing beta-receptor stimulation in the heart, thereby decreasing heart rate and cardiac output. Beta-blockers also interfere with renin release by the kidneys, decreasing the effects of angiotensin and aldosterone. Potential adverse effects of beta-blockers include bronchospasm, fatigue, sleep disturbances, nightmares, bradycardia, heart block, worsening of heart failure, gastrointestinal disturbances, impotence, and increased triglyceride levels.

Nursing Responsibilities

- Before giving the initial dose, assess for contraindications to beta-blockers, such as asthma, chronic lung disease, bradycardia, or heart block.
- Assess blood pressure and apical pulse before giving; notify primary care provider if vital signs are outside established parameters.
- Report adverse effects, such as bradycardia, decreased cardiac output (fatigue, dyspnea with exertion, hypotension, or decreased level of consciousness), heart failure, heart block, bronchoconstriction (wheezing or dyspnea), or altered blood glucose levels (in clients with diabetes).
- Carefully monitor responses of the older client.

Health Education for the Client and Family

- Monitor blood pressure and pulse daily as instructed.
- Change position (lying to sitting and sitting to standing) slowly to prevent dizziness and possible falls.
- Report effects such as fatigue, lethargy, and impotence to your primary care provider.
- Notify your physician if you become short of breath or develop a cough or swelling of your extremities.

Box 22–28 **Medication Administration: Antihypertensive Drugs** (continued)

- If you have diabetes, check blood glucose levels more frequently, because hypoglycemia may develop with few symptoms.
- Talk to your primary care provider before taking any over-the-counter medications.
- Carry an adequate supply of the drug when traveling. Do not stop taking this drug without notifying your primary care provider.

CALCIUM-CHANNEL BLOCKERS

Amlodipine (Norvasc)
Diltiazem (Cardizem)
Felodipine (Plendil)
Isradipine (DynaCirc)
Nicardipine (Cardene)
Nifedipine (Procardia)
Nisoldipine (Sular)
Verapamil (Isoptin)

Calcium-channel blockers inhibit the flow of calcium ions across the cell membrane of vascular tissue and cardiac cells. In doing so, they relax arterial smooth muscle, lowering peripheral resistance through vasodilation. Calcium-channel blockers can cause reflex tachycardia, and some (e.g., verapamil and diltiazem) may impair cardiac function, worsening heart failure.

Nursing Responsibilities

- Assess blood pressure, apical pulse, and liver and renal function tests before giving these drugs.
- Calcium-channel blockers may be given orally or intravenously.
- Do not administer verapamil or diltiazem to clients with severe hypotension, sinus, or atrioventricular blocks. Administer with caution to clients also taking digoxin or a beta-blocker.
- Periodically monitor blood pressure and apical pulse during therapy. Promptly report signs of bradycardia, atrioventricular block, or heart failure to the physician.

Health Education for the Client and Family

- Take blood pressure and pulse daily as taught. Notify your physician if your pulse is less than 60 bpm or your blood pressure is not within the specified range.
- This drug may cause constipation. Drink six to eight glasses of water each day, and increase the amount of fiber in your diet.
- Report shortness of breath, weight gain, or swelling in feet or ankles to your primary care provider.

CENTRALLY ACTING SYMPATHOLYTICS

Clonidine (Catapres)
Guanfacine (Tenex)
Methyldopa (Aldomet)
Reserpine (generic)

The centrally acting sympatholytics stimulate the alpha$_2$-receptors in the central nervous system to suppress sympathetic outflow to the heart and blood vessels. A fall in cardiac output and in vasodilation results, reducing blood pressure. Dry mouth and sedation are common adverse effects. Severe reflex hypertension may occur if abruptly discontinued. Clonidine is contraindicated during pregnancy; methyldopa is contraindicated for clients with active liver disease.

Nursing Responsibilities

- Assess for contraindications to therapy. Obtain baseline blood pressure, complete blood count, Coombs' test, and liver function studies.
- Administer oral doses at bedtime to minimize effects of sedation.
- Methyldopa may be given intravenously for hypertensive emergencies.
- Apply transdermal clonidine patch to a dry, hairless area of intact skin on the chest or upper arm. Assess for rash, which indicates allergy, at area of application.
- Promptly report changes in laboratory values to the physician. Discontinue methyldopa if manifestations of liver dysfunction develop.

Health Education for the Client and Family

- Relieve dry mouth by sipping water or chewing sugarless gum.
- Take with meals if gastric upset or nausea develop.
- Change position (lying to sitting and sitting to standing) slowly to prevent dizziness and possible falls.
- Do not suddenly discontinue medication or skip doses; this could cause serious hypertension.
- Report mental depression or decreased mental acuity to your health care provider.
- Side effects (e.g., dry mouth, nausea, and dizziness) tend to diminish over time.
- Do not drive a car if the medications cause drowsiness.

VASODILATORS

Hydralazine (Apresoline)
Minoxidil (Loniten)

Vasodilators reduce blood pressure by relaxing vascular smooth muscle (especially in the arterioles) and decreasing peripheral vascular resistance. These drugs are often prescribed in combination with a diuretic or beta-blocker because they can cause reflex tachycardia and fluid retention. Because these drugs can have significant toxic effects, they are not routinely used to manage chronic hypertension.

Nursing Responsibilities

- Hydralazine may be given orally or intravenously; minoxidil is given orally.
- Assess blood pressure and pulse before giving the drug, and monitor during therapy as indicated. Report tachycardia or hypotension to the physician.
- Report peripheral edema and manifestations of volume overload and heart failure.
- Immediately report muffled heart sounds or paradoxic pulse, because pericardial effusion and possible cardiac tamponade may develop during minoxidil therapy.
- Discontinue hydralazine and report manifestations of a systemic lupus erythematosus–like syndrome: muscle or joint pain, fever, or symptoms of nephritis or pericarditis.

Health Education for the Client and Family

- Change position (lying to sitting and sitting to standing) slowly to prevent dizziness and possible falls.
- Report muscle, joint aches, and fever to your health care provider.
- Headache, palpitations, and rapid pulse may develop but should abate in about 10 days.
- Do not discontinue the medication without talking to your health care provider.
- Minoxidil may cause excessive hair growth. Contact your physician if this becomes troublesome.

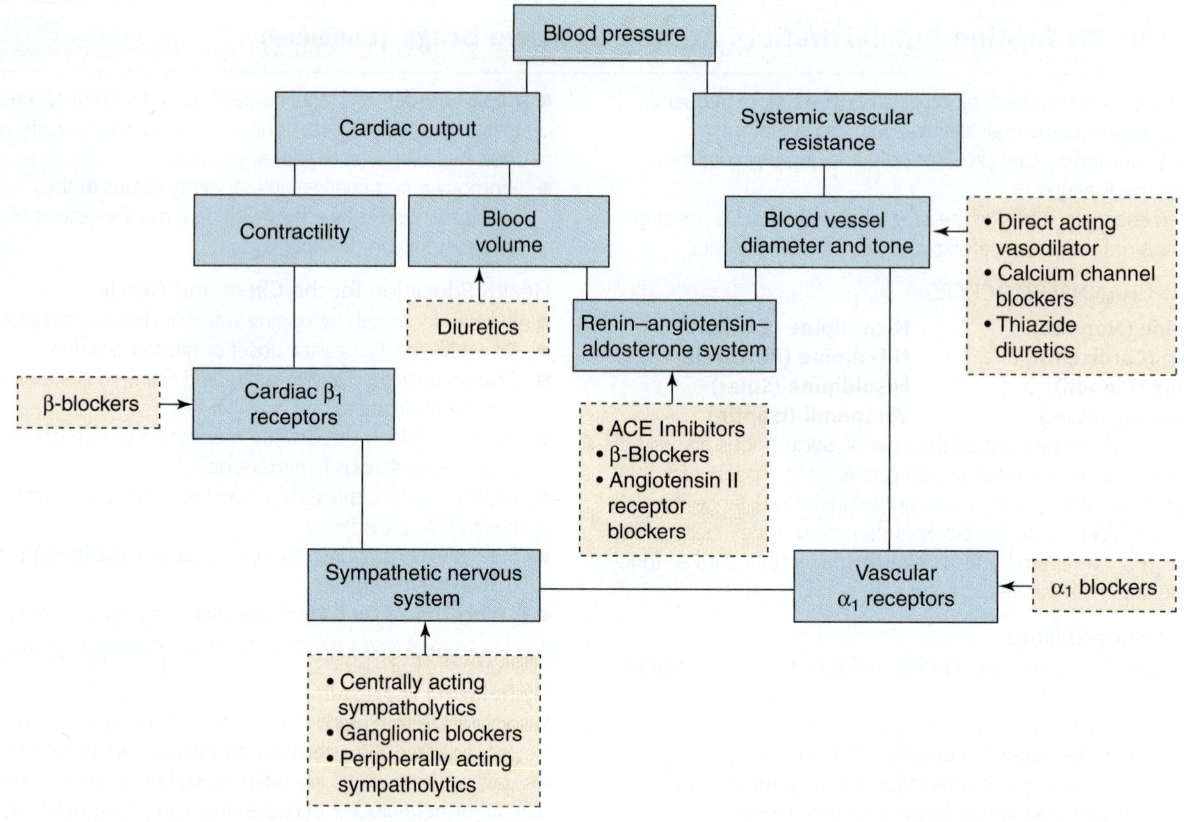

Figure 22–50 ■ Sites of antihypertensive drug action.

The ACE inhibitors and ARBs also are commonly used in the initial treatment of hypertension, particularly for clients with diabetes or heart failure, a history of MI, or chronic kidney disease. ACE inhibitors block formation of angiotensin II by inhibiting the action of ACE. Angiotensin II is a potent vasoconstrictor that also stimulates aldosterone release from the adrenal gland; blocking its action prevents vasoconstriction and sodium and water retention resulting from aldosterone release. ARBs have a very similar effect, although their action is to block angiotensin II receptors, thus preventing its vasoconstrictive and volume expansion effects.

Several drug classes work through their ability to promote vasodilation and reduce peripheral vascular resistance. Alpha-blockers, such as prazosin and terazosin, block stimulation of alpha$_1$-receptors on arterioles and veins, preventing vasoconstriction. Because of their ability to dilate both arterioles and veins, alpha-blockers can cause significant orthostatic hypotension, particularly following the initial dose. Calcium-channel blockers promote dilation of arterioles, the primary regulators of peripheral vascular resistance. These drugs can cause reflex tachycardia. Some calcium-channel blockers (verapamil and diltiazem in particular) also suppress heart function, reducing stroke volume and cardiac output. Reflex tachycardia is minimal with these calcium-channel blockers. Direct-acting vasodilators, such as hydralazine and minoxidil, also directly affect the arterioles, reducing peripheral vascular resistance. These drugs have little effect on veins, so the risk of orthostatic hypotension is minimal. They are, however, associated with reflex tachycardia and fluid retention, so they are rarely administered as in single-drug treatment regimens.

Other factors considered in selecting drugs for treating hypertension include demographic characteristics of the client, concurrent conditions, quality of life, cost, and possible interactions among prescribed drugs. In general, diuretics and calcium-channel blockers are more effective for treating hypertension in African Americans than beta-blockers or ACE inhibitors. Beta-blockers are preferred to treat hypertension with concurrent coronary heart disease and angina but are contraindicated for clients who have asthma or depression. Beta-blockers also reduce exercise tolerance and may adversely affect lifestyle for some clients.

DRUG REGIMENS Treatment usually is initiated using a single antihypertensive drug at a low dose. Unless otherwise indicated, a diuretic is recommended as the initial drug of choice. The dose is slowly increased until optimal blood pressure control is achieved. If the drug does not effectively lower the blood pressure or has troubling side effects, a different drug from another class of antihypertensive medications is substituted. If, on the other hand, the drug is tolerated well but does not lower blood pressure to the desired level, a second drug from another class may be added to the treatment regimen.

Treatment of clients with stage 2 hypertension generally is more aggressive in order to minimize the risk of MI, heart failure, or stroke. When the average blood pressure is greater

ALTERNATIVE THERAPIES Transcendental Meditation for Stress Management and Blood Pressure Control

The relationship between stress and cardiovascular reactivity and subsequent development of primary hypertension in adults has been documented. African American adolescents have been found to exhibit greater blood pressure reactivity to stress than white adolescents. A randomized clinical trial with 35 adolescents (aged 15–18 years) with high normal resting blood pressure (between the 85th and 95th percentiles) compared the impact of a 2-month transcendental meditation program with a control group that received lifestyle education sessions. Each group had similar numbers of males and females, but 34 of the participants were African American and only 1 was white. Participants in the transcendental meditation group practiced two 15-minute sessions while sitting comfortably with eyes closed to obtain a deeply restful state of wakefulness. Participants in the control group attended seven weekly 1-hour health education sessions. The study was conducted in collaboration with the public school system. Anthropometric measurements, heart rate, blood pressure, cardiac output, and total peripheral resistance were evaluated at the beginning of the study and during exposure to stressful experiences (a car driving simulation and a social situation interview). Study results revealed that the transcendental meditation group had greater decreases in resting systolic blood pressure and a trend toward greater decreases in diastolic blood pressure than the control group, particularly with the car driving simulation. Transcendental meditation shows promise as a potential complementary therapy to help control blood pressure in adolescents. Further study is needed to determine if the blood pressure reductions are sustained long term with this intervention (Barnes, Treiber, & Davis, 2001).

than 200/120 mmHg, immediate therapy (and possible hospitalization) is vital.

After a year of effective hypertension control, an effort may be made to reduce the dosage and number of drugs. This is known as **step-down therapy**. It is more successful in clients who have made lifestyle modifications. Careful blood pressure monitoring is necessary during and after step-down therapy because the blood pressure often rises again to hypertensive levels.

Complementary Therapies

Behavioral and mind–body therapies may be helpful for some clients in lowering blood pressure. Blood pressure increases in response to physiologic and psychologic stress and anxiety. Mind–body therapies, such as yoga and t'ai chi, meditation, and guided imagery, are designed to modify both physiologic and cognitive aspects of the stress response. In a study of older African American men and women with moderate hypertension, transcendental mediation was shown to reduce the blood pressure. Eastern exercises such as yoga and t'ai chi, which often combine imagery, meditation, and physical exercise, have been shown to reduce sympathetic nervous system activity, blood pressure, and heart and respiratory rates (Spencer & Jacobs, 2003). A nursing research study of clients with hypertension in Thailand demonstrated the effectiveness of yoga to reduce blood pressure, heart rate, and body mass index (McCaffrey, Ruknui, Hatthakit, & Kasetsomboon, 2005).

NURSING PROCESS

Health promotion teaching and activities focus on modifiable risk factors for hypertension. Advise all clients (as well as children and adolescents) to stop or never start smoking. Discuss the risks of obesity, excess alcohol intake, and a sedentary lifestyle with clients. Encourage all clients to eat a diet rich in fruits and vegetables and low in total and saturated fat. Discuss the potential benefits of following the DASH diet or a similar eating plan. Advise all clients to remain active and engage in aerobic exercise 5 days or more each week. Discuss the stress-reducing benefits of exercise. Offer blood pressure screening, and refer clients for follow up.

Assessment

Obtain the following information during focused assessment of the client with hypertension:

- *Health history.* Complaints of morning headache or cervical pain; cardiovascular or central nervous system manifestations; history of hypertension, renal disease, or diabetes; family history of high blood pressure, heart failure, or kidney disease; current medications.
- *Physical examination.* Vital signs, including blood pressure in both arms as well as apical and peripheral pulses; ophthalmologic exam of retinal fundus as appropriate.

Diagnosis

Nursing diagnoses that may apply to the client with primary hypertension include the following:

- Ineffective Health Maintenance
- Risk for Noncompliance
- Imbalanced Nutrition: More Than Body Requirements
- Excess Fluid Volume.

Plan

Goals of nursing care include the following:

- The client will describe lifestyle choices that can prevent, reduce, or resolve hypertension.
- The client's blood pressure will remain within the acceptable range for age and condition.
- The client will reduce sodium consumption.
- The client will maintain fluid balance.

Implementation

Primary nursing interventions are aimed at preventing hypertension through client teaching. Secondary interventions are aimed at controlling blood pressure to prevent complications.

Ineffective Health Maintenance

Unhealthy lifestyle and behaviors can contribute to health problems such as hypertension. When hypertension has been identified, knowledge regarding the disease and its management is vital for the client. Willingness to take responsibility for hypertension management is central to effective blood pressure control. Adopting healthy lifestyle changes enhances drug therapy; in some cases, the need for medications may be eliminated or reduced. Because hypertension is often an asymptomatic disease and many antihypertensive drugs have unpleasant side effects, it is vital that the client understand the chronic progressive nature of the disease and its long-term consequences.

- Assist with identifying current behaviors that contribute to hypertension. The client must first identify contributory behaviors before he or she can change them. Using knowledge of hypertension risk factors, the nurse can help identify behaviors and factors contributing to hypertension that can be changed. Including the family in this process is important to reduce potential sabotage of the client's efforts to adopt healthier behaviors.
- Assist in developing a realistic health maintenance plan. Preparing a health maintenance plan for the client does little to encourage personal responsibility for health. However, nurses can guide clients in developing realistic goals and expectations for the treatment plan and for modifying risk factors such as smoking, exercise, diet, and stress.
- Help the client and family identify strengths and weaknesses in maintaining health. Discussing areas of the health maintenance plan that are working well and those that present difficulties can help identify necessary changes in the plan and additional strategies for implementing it.

Risk for Noncompliance

Noncompliance, or failure to follow the identified treatment plan, is a continuing risk for any client with a chronic disease. Recommended lifestyle changes, such as diet, exercise, restricted alcohol intake, stress reduction, and smoking cessation, often are difficult to maintain on a continuing basis. In addition, prescribed medications may have undesirable effects, whereas hypertension itself often has no symptoms or noticeable effects.

- Inquire about reasons for noncompliance with the recommended treatment plan. Listen openly and without judging. Nonthreatening discussion of factors contributing to noncompliance validates the client's self-esteem and partnership in the treatment plan.
- Evaluate knowledge regarding hypertension, its long-term effects, and treatment. Provide additional information and reinforce teaching as needed. Knowledge increases the sense of control, which also increases the likelihood of compliance with treatment.
- Assist the client to develop realistic short-term goals for lifestyle changes. Attempting to lose weight, exercise daily, stop smoking, and dramatically change the diet all at the same time may be overwhelming, leading to a sense of failure. Smaller, gradual changes are more easily incorporated into lifestyle and daily activities, improving compliance.
- Help the client identify cues and develop reminders (e.g., written notes or a medication box filled weekly) to assist with maintaining a schedule for exercise and medications. Cues and other devices provide helpful reminders of activities and schedules until they are incorporated into habits.
- Reassure the client that relapse into old habits and behaviors is common. Encourage the client to avoid feelings of guilt associated with relapse and use the circumstance to renew efforts to comply with treatment. Guilt and feelings of failure can lead to further noncompliance unless the event is used to identify reasons for noncompliance and ways to prevent it from recurring in the future.

Imbalanced Nutrition: More Than Body Requirements

The relationship between obesity, excess alcohol intake, and hypertension is well documented. Hypertension is particularly associated with central obesity, identified by waist circumference greater than hip circumference. Although weight loss is difficult and takes commitment to changing both eating and exercise habits, it is possible for most clients to achieve.

- Assess usual daily food intake, and discuss possible contributing factors to excess weight, such as a sedentary lifestyle or using food as a reward or stress reliever. Inquire about diversional activities, exercise patterns, and previous weight reduction efforts (e.g., participation in weight reduction programs or using fad or crash diets). Assessment data provide clues about factors contributing to obesity and about the client's knowledge base about the relationship between eating and exercise habits and weight as well as safe weight-loss strategies. This provides direction for further teaching and for developing a realistic weight reduction plan.
- Mutually determine with the client a realistic target weight (e.g., loss of 10% of current body weight over a 6-month period). Regularly monitor weight. Encourage a system of nonfood rewards for achieving small, incremental goals. Setting weight loss goals helps formalize the process and provides motivation for continued progress. Developing realistic goals may be difficult; unrealistic goals, however, set the client up for failure. Continuous incremental weight loss provides reassurance that the goal can be achieved and promotes permanent weight reduction.
- Refer to a dietitian for information about low-fat, low-calorie foods and eating plans. Focus on changing eating habits as opposed to "following a diet." Focusing on changing eating habits promotes the sense that low-fat, low-calorie eating patterns should become a part of the client's lifestyle rather than a short-term measure to be endured until the weight loss goal is achieved.

CLIENT TEACHING Control of Hypertension

Effective control of hypertension requires the client not only to participate in the plan of care but also to take an active role in managing the disease. Include the following topics when teaching the client and family about hypertension:

- Specific lifestyle changes recommended for the client and suggestions for implementing them. For example:
  a. Increase activity gradually. Develop a realistic exercise program that is enjoyable and fits into the individual's lifestyle. Identify an exercise buddy for additional motivation. Activity and exercise, through a gradual conditioning of muscles and blood vessels, lower blood pressure by reducing peripheral vascular resistance. As the heart becomes conditioned and pumps more efficiently, kidney perfusion improves and intravascular volume falls, further reducing blood pressure. Exercise also reduces stress and contributes to weight loss and maintenance. Aerobic exercise, such as walking, jogging, swimming, and cycling, are appropriate; isometric activities (e.g., such as weight lifting) should be avoided without physician approval.
  b. Adopt healthy eating patterns, following a low-fat, low-cholesterol, moderate sodium diet that also is rich in fruits and vegetables and includes at least two servings of low-fat milk or milk products daily. Do not give up if you slip into old eating habits on occasion; use such occasions to identify ways to avoid future lapses.
  c. Stop smoking. Participating in organized smoking cessation programs or using aids such as nicotine patches can help.
  d. Use alcohol in moderation if at all, consuming no more than 1.5 oz of hard liquor, 5–10 oz of wine, or 12–20 oz of beer per day.
  e. Use stress-reducing techniques, such as meditation, relaxation, deep breathing, and exercise, to manage stress. Anger and hostility intensify vasoconstriction; channeling these emotions into more positive responses, such as using a change process to modify factors that provoke these emotions, can reduce their harmful effects on blood pressure.
- Prescribed medications, their intended effect, dose and timing, interactions, and possible adverse effects. Discuss effects that should be reported to the physician and those that can be managed by the client or that will diminish over time.
- The importance of monitoring blood pressure and regular visits to the primary care provider or hypertension clinic to monitor treatment. During follow-up visits, assess the blood pressure and specific laboratory work (e.g., serum creatinine, blood urea nitrogen, and/or serum electrolytes) to evaluate the disease and the effects of antihypertensive medications.

Refer the client to community blood pressure clinics and to home health services as needed for regular follow up and reinforcement of teaching. Refer to a dietitian or an organized weight loss program as indicated for further teaching and weight loss support.

- Recommend participating in an approved weight loss program such as Weight Watchers, Overeaters Anonymous, or Take off Pounds Sensibly (TOPS). Organized weight loss programs provide structure for a balanced weight reduction program as well as mutual support from others trying to lose weight.

Excess Fluid Volume

Excess fluid volume often contributes to hypertension by increasing cardiac output. A number of factors associated with hypertension can cause excess fluid volume, including sodium retention and disruption of the renin–angiotensin–aldosterone system. In addition, some antihypertensive drugs, such as calcium-channel blockers and vasodilators, can contribute to excess fluid in the interstitial spaces and peripheral edema.

- Monitor intake and output, and weigh the client daily (if in an acute or long-term care facility) or weekly (in the community). Rapid weight changes (over days) more accurately reflect fluid balance compared with intake and output records. One liter of fluid weighs 1 kg (2.2 lb). Weight changes and intake and output records help monitor the effects of therapy.
- Monitor for peripheral edema (sacral edema in the client who is bedridden). Drugs such as vasodilators can cause fluid accumulation in interstitial tissues, leading to peripheral or dependent edema. Adding a diuretic to the treatment plan may be necessary.
- Refer to a dietitian for teaching about a restricted sodium diet. Discuss the relationship between sodium intake and fluid retention. Provide opportunities to choose low-sodium foods from simulated menus. Support efforts, and reassure that lifestyle changes such as consuming less sodium take time. Knowledge provides the power to take control of sodium intake. Patience and perseverance are needed to succeed; positive reinforcement of efforts to change long-standing dietary patterns is important.
- Discuss the importance of adhering to treatment plans, such as dietary restrictions and medication schedules. Understanding the rationale for treatment measures promotes the client's sense of control and encourages compliance with the treatment regimen.

Evaluation

Evaluation of the effectiveness of client care may be based on the following expected outcomes:

- The client describes strategies for maintaining normal blood pressure, including exercise, quitting smoking, losing weight, and managing stress.
- The client describes expected actions of medications, side effects to report to the health care provider, and importance of taking medication every day.
- The client demonstrates accurate performance of blood pressure monitoring and maintains a log of readings to share with the health care provider.
- The client demonstrates ability to choose foods that are low in sodium.

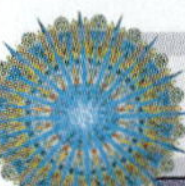

NURSING CARE PLAN A Client With Hypertension

ASSESSMENT

Margaret Spezia is a married, 49-year-old Italian American with eight children whose ages range from 3–18 years. For the past 2 months, Mrs. Spezia has had frequent morning headaches as well as occasional dizziness and blurred vision. At her annual physical examination 1 month ago, her blood pressure was 168/104 and 156/94 mmHg. She was instructed to reduce her fat and cholesterol intake, to avoid using salt at the table, and to start walking for 30–45 minutes daily. Mrs. Spezia returns to the clinic for follow up.

While escorting Mrs. Spezia to the exam room and obtaining her weight, blood pressure, and history, Lisa Christos, RN, notices that Mrs. Spezia seems restless and upset. Ms. Christos says, "You look upset about something. Is everything OK?" Mrs. Spezia responds, "Well, my head is throbbing, and I'm sort of dizzy. I think I'm just overdoing it and not getting enough rest. You know, raising eight children is a lot of work and expense. I just started working part-time so we wouldn't get behind in our bills. I thought the extra money might relieve some of my stress, but I'm not so sure that's really happening. I'm not getting any better and I'm worried that I'll lose my job or become disabled and that my husband won't be able to manage the children by himself. I really need to go home, but first, I want to get rid of this awful headache. Would you please get me a couple of aspirin or something?"

Mrs. Spezia's history shows a steady weight gain during the past 18 years. She has no known family history of hypertension. Physical findings include the following: height, 63 in. (160 cm); weight, 225 lb (102 kg); temperature, 99°F (37.2°C); pulse, 100 bpm and regular; respirations, 16/min; and blood pressure, 180/115 mmHg(lying), 170/110 mmHg (sitting), and 165/105 mmHg (standing), with an average 10-point difference in readings between right and left arm (lower on left). Her skin is cool and dry, with capillary refill of 4 seconds in the right hand and 3 seconds in the left hand. Mrs. Spezia's total serum cholesterol is 245 mg/dL (normal, < 200 mg/dL). All other blood and urine studies are within normal limits. Based on analysis of the data, Mrs. Spezia is started on enalapril, 5 mg, and hydrochlorothiazide, 12.5 mg, in a combination drug (Vaseretic) and is placed on a low-fat, low-cholesterol, no-added-salt diet.

DIAGNOSES

- Fatigue related to effects of hypertension and stresses of daily life
- Imbalanced Nutrition: More Than Body Requirements related to excessive food intake
- Ineffective Health Maintenance related to inability to modify lifestyle
- Deficient Knowledge related to effects of prescribed treatment

PLANNING

Goals of care include the following:

- The client will reduce her blood pressure readings to less than 150 mmHg systolic and 90 mmHg diastolic by the return visit next week.
- The client will incorporate into her diet low-sodium and low-fat foods from a list provided.
- The client will develop a plan for regular exercise.
- The client will verbalize understanding of the effects of the prescribed drug, dietary restrictions, exercise, and follow-up visits to help control hypertension.

IMPLEMENTATION

- Teach to take own blood pressure daily and record it, bringing the record to scheduled clinic visits.
- Teach name, dose, action, and side effects of her antihypertensive medication.
- Instruct to walk for 15 minutes each day this week and to investigate swimming classes at the local pool.
- Discuss strategies for achieving a realistic weight-loss goal.
- Refer to a dietary consultation for further teaching about fat and sodium restrictions.
- Discuss stress-reducing techniques, helping identify possible choices.

EVALUATION

Mrs. Spezia returns to the clinic 1 week later. Her average blood pressure is now 148/88 mmHg. She has lost 1.5 lb and states that her oldest daughter has suggested they join a weight reduction program together. Mrs. Spezia is walking for an average of 20 minutes at a local mall each day. She verbalizes an understanding of her medication and is taking it in the morning and before dinner each day. She met with the dietitian and discussed ways to reduce the sodium and fat in her diet. The dietitian provided a list of low-fat, low-sodium foods and recommended cookbooks to help Mrs. Spezia modify her cooking. Mrs. Spezia tells Ms. Christos, "I just can't believe how much better I feel already. My headaches are gone, and I've actually lost some weight—and I feel motivated to keep going. If I had only known how much better I could feel! I don't expect I'll ever go back to my old habits again; it's just not worth it!"

NURSING CARE PLAN A Client With Hypertension *continued*

CRITICAL THINKING

1. Identify the factors that contributed to Mrs. Spezia's hypertension. Which were modifiable, and which were not?
2. What is the rationale for reducing sodium and fat in Mrs. Spezia's diet?
3. Suppose your client with hypertension is homeless and has no source of income. How could you help ensure your client would follow the treatment plan? What would you do if the client did not follow it?
4. Discuss the role of stress in hypertension. What factors in Mrs. Spezia's life contribute to her stress level?
5. Develop a plan of care for the nursing diagnosis low-self esteem related to obesity.

HEALTH CARE

Evidence-Based Practice

Conduct a search of the peer-reviewed literature, and find an article addressing medications found to be more effective for clients from a specific race or culture. Based on your reading, why might one medication be more effective for one client over another? If a client from this race told you he or she had read that the "better medication" is being given to clients from other races, how would you respond in order to help the client understand the pharmacodynamics of the prescribed medication?

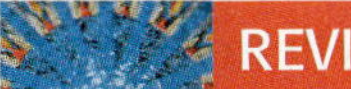

REVIEW Hypertension

RELATE: LINK THE CONCEPTS

Linking the exemplar of Hypertension with the concept of Metabolism:

1. Create a plan of care, including nutrition, for the client diagnosed with both hypertension and type 2 diabetes mellitus.
2. You receive a call from a client, diagnosed with hypertension and diabetes mellitus, asking what over-the-counter medications would be safe to take to treat a mild upper respiratory infection (a cold). How will you respond to this question?

Linking the exemplar of Hypertension with the concept of Fluid and Electrolytes:

3. Explain the impact hypertension has on urinary elimination.
4. What teaching will you provide the client diagnosed with hypertension to reduce this impact on the renal system?

READY: GO TO COMPANION SKILLS MANUAL

- Monitoring intake and output
- Measuring weights
- Assessing blood pressure
- Assessing vital signs

REFER: GO TO MYNURSINGKIT

REFLECT: CASE STUDY

Yvonne Genmar is a 42-year-old female with primary hypertension. She is married to Tom who has a 17-year-old son from a previous marriage. Yvonne and Tom have two children together, Sabrina 14 and Charlie 3. Tom runs his own business installing sprinkler systems and Yvonne is a real estate agent and home inspector. Yvonne spends a great deal of time in her car showing houses and taking the kids to their various after-school activities.

Yvonne's mother has type 2 diabetes and her father is fairly healthy. Yvonne has been prescribed several different antihypertensives but her blood pressure remains elevated. Most recently, she was placed on captopril 50 mg twice a day, which seems to be maintaining her blood pressure within acceptable limits.

1. What precautions would you teach Yvonne regarding captopril in conjunction with her lifestyle?
2. If you admitted Yvonne to the provider's office before captopril was prescribed, what interview questions would you want to explore in order to determine lifestyle factors that may be contributing to her continued hypertension?
3. What nutritional recommendations will you make to Yvonne to help her control her hypertension?

22.8 LIFE-THREATENING DYSRHYTHMIAS

KEY TERMS

Asystole, *1454*
Atrial kick, *1438*
Cardiac arrest, *1454*
Cardiopulmonary resuscitation (CPR), *1455*
Couplet, *1446*
Defibrillation, *1449*
Dysrhythmia, *1438*
Ectopic beats, *1440*
Heart block, *1440*
Multifocal, *1446*
Normal sinus rhythm, *1440*
Pacemaker, *1450*
Paroxysmal, *1444*
Premature junctional contractions, *1445*
Retrograde conduction, *1445*
Sudden cardiac death (SCD), *1454*
Synchronized cardioversion, *1449*
Torsades de pointes, *1446*
Triplet, *1446*
Unifocal, *1446*
Valsalva maneuver, *1454*
Ventricular bigeminy, *1446*
Ventricular trigeminy, *1446*

BASIS FOR SELECTION OF EXEMPLAR

Agency for Health Care Research and Quality

Common cause of death

Top 20 reasons to be admitted through the emergency department

LEARNING OUTCOMES

After reading about this exemplar, you will be able to:

1. Describe the pathophysiology, etiology, clinical manifestations, and direct and indirect causes of life-threatening dysrhythmias.
2. Identify risk factors associated with life-threatening dysrhythmias.
3. Illustrate the nursing process in providing culturally competent care across the life span for individuals with life-threatening dysrhythmias.
4. Formulate priority nursing diagnoses appropriate for an individual with life-threatening dysrhythmias.
5. Create a plan of care for individuals with life-threatening dysrhythmias and their families.
6. Assess expected outcomes for an individual with life-threatening dysrhythmias.
7. Discuss therapies used in the collaborative care of an individual with life-threatening dysrhythmias.
8. Employ evidence-based caring interventions for an individual with life-threatening dysrhythmias.

OVERVIEW

Heart muscle contracts in response to electrical stimulation. In the normal heart, electrical stimulation produces a synchronized, rhythmic heart muscle contraction that propels blood into the vascular system. Changes in cardiac rhythm affect this synchronized activity and the heart's ability to effectively pump blood to body tissues.

A cardiac **dysrhythmia** is an abnormal heart rate or rhythm; more specifically, a disturbance or irregularity in the electrical system of the heart. Cardiac dysrhythmias may be benign or have lethal consequences. Prompt recognition of a lethal dysrhythmia and quick action can truly be lifesaving.

Dysrhythmias develop for many reasons. Not all are pathologic; some alterations in cardiac rhythm occur in response to events such as exercise or fear. For example, a rapid heart rate as a result of exercise, fever, or excitement is a normal response to the body's demand for oxygen or to stimulation of the sympathetic nervous system (SNS). Slow heart rates also may be normal. Athletic heart syndrome, which results from long-term training of the heart muscle, allows the heart to beat more slowly and forcefully while maintaining cardiac output and tissue perfusion at a slower rate. Many athletes have a heart rate of less than 60 bpm, and heart rate may be as low as 44–48 beats per minute (bpm) in a very-well-conditioned athlete. Aging affects cardiac rhythm as well.

Regardless of cause, a dysrhythmia can significantly affect cardiac performance, depending on the health of the heart muscle. The client's response to the dysrhythmia is key in determining the urgency and type of treatment needed.

PATHOPHYSIOLOGY AND ETIOLOGY

Five unique properties of cardiac cells allow effective heart function. Four properties are electrical; the fifth is cardiac muscle's mechanical response to electrical stimulation. These five properties are as follows:

1. *Automaticity* is the ability of pacemaker cells to spontaneously initiate an electrical impulse (action potential). The SA node is the dominant pacemaker, generating impulses at 60–100 times a minute. Myocardial muscle cells do not possess this ability.
2. *Excitability* is the ability of myocardial cells to respond to stimuli generated by pacemaker cells.
3. *Conductivity* is the ability to transmit an impulse from cell to cell. When one cell is stimulated, the impulse rapidly spreads throughout the heart muscle.
4. *Refractoriness* is the inability of cardiac cells to respond to additional stimuli immediately following depolarization. In the absolute refractory period, depolarization will not occur in response to any stimulus. A stronger-than-normal stimulus is required to initiate depolarization during the relative refractory period. This is followed by the supernormal period, during which a mild stimulus will cause depolarization.
5. *Contractility* is the ability of myocardial fibers to shorten in response to a stimulus. Heart muscle responds in an all-or-nothing manner: Stimulation of one muscle fiber causes the entire muscle mass to contract to its fullest extent as one unit.

Electrical activity of the heart is normally controlled by the cardiac conduction system (see Figure 22–10 on page 1333). The SA node, which is the primary pacemaker of the heart, usually generates impulses at a regular rate of 60–100 bpm. The impulse spreads through the atria, is briefly delayed at the AV node, then spreads through conduction pathways of the ventricles and to ventricular muscle. The AV nodal delay allows the atria to contract, delivering an extra bolus of blood to the ventricles before they contract (the **atrial kick**). The AV node also controls the number of impulses that reach the ventricles, preventing extremely rapid heart rates.

Dysrhythmias arise through disruption of the very properties that stimulate and control the heartbeat: automaticity, excitability, conductivity, and refractoriness. Dysrhythmias that result from altered impulse formation include changes in rate and rhythm and the development of ectopic beats. This category includes tachydysrhythmia (rapid heart rates), bradydysrhythmia (slow heart rates), and ectopic rhythms. These

DEVELOPMENTAL CONSIDERATIONS Cardiac Dysrhythmias

CHILDREN

Cardiac arrhythmias (abnormal heart rhythms or dysrhythmias) occur frequently in children but less commonly than in adults. Arrhythmias can cause decreased cardiac output and congestive heart failure or further progress to an even more serious arrhythmia that could result in sudden death.

Tachyarrhythmias (e.g., sinus tachycardia) often occur with acute conditions, such as hypoxia, anemia, hypovolemia, shock, hyper- or hypokalemia, hyperthyroidism, catecholamine medications, and stimulant or illicit drug use. Acute conditions associated with bradyarrhythmias (e.g., sinus bradycardia) include hypoxemia, vagal stimulation, acidosis, severe sepsis, and acute increased intracranial pressure (Doniger & Sharieff, 2006). These types of arrhythmias generally resolve once the underlying condition is treated. Some arrhythmias result from genetic conditions, such as forms of supraventricular tachycardia (SVT) and long QT syndrome. Less common arrhythmias are often associated with congenital heart disease, especially as many more children are now surviving surgeries for complex defects.

Neonates and young children may be predisposed to SVT because of a congenital heart defect or Wolff–Parkinson–White syndrome. Short periods of arrhythmia (several seconds), which may be caused by paroxysmal atrial tachycardia, are rarely dangerous; however, prolonged episodes (>24 hours) of continuous SVT may be life-threatening and can progress to congestive heart failure or cardiogenic shock. Cardiac output is affected because blood returning during diastole cannot keep pace with such a rapid heart rate.

Nursing Assessment

- The child suspected of having an arrhythmia should be monitored for level of consciousness, heart rate, and other vital signs. A cardiorespiratory monitor and pulse oximetry should be used to identify deterioration of the child's condition.
- A change in the child's level of consciousness may indicate the beginning of cardiopulmonary compromise (Green, Kitchen, & Ray, 2005). Changes in color, weakness, irritability, and changes in feeding pattern may indicate the development of hypoxia.
- Any child in the community found to have an abnormal ECG finding, unusual heart rhythm, syncope (especially with exercise), or dizziness with palpitations should be referred to a pediatric cardiologist for evaluation.

Home Care Teaching

Episodes of arrhythmia are frightening for both the child and parents, as are the unpredictability of recurrent episodes and the risk for sudden cardiac death with some arrhythmias. Provide support, and encourage the parents to promote the child's normal development between episodes. Emphasize that medications help prevent or reduce episode frequency.

- Carefully explain the treatment plan and home care.
- Teach parents to take the child's apical pulse. Make sure parents are trained in CPR and use of Valsalva maneuvers.
- Provide telephone numbers of emergency medical facilities, and help parents plan how to seek emergency care.
- Make sure the parents and child with SVT understand the need to avoid using cardiac stimulant drugs, such as decongestants, because these drugs might trigger another episode.
- Describe and provide written instructions about the danger signs indicating a recurrence of the acute condition and how to seek emergency care.
- Provide preparation for the child and family for procedures such as radiofrequency ablation or implantation of a pacemaker or cardioverter–defibrillator.

OLDER ADULTS

Aging affects the heart and the cardiac conduction system, increasing the incidence of dysrhythmias and conduction defects. Older adults may experience dysrhythmias even when no evidence of heart disease is found.

Older adults have a higher incidence of both ventricular and supraventricular dysrhythmias without detrimental effects compared with younger people. Ectopic beats, including short runs of ventricular tachycardia, occur more commonly during exercise in older adults. These dysrhythmias do not affect cardiac morbidity or mortality. Fibrosis of the bundle branches can lead to atrioventricular blocks; a prolonged PR interval is common in clients over the age of 65. Older adults also have a higher incidence of diseases that may affect heart rhythm. An older client with hyperthyroidism, for example, may present with atrial fibrillation, syncope, and confusion instead of the usual manifestations of goiter, tremor, and exophthalmos.

Nursing Assessment

Assessment of the older adult for problems related to cardiac dysrhythmias focuses on the effect of the dysrhythmia on functional health status.

- Ask about a history of cardiovascular disease and current medications.
- Inquire about symptoms such as episodes of dizziness, lightheadedness, fainting, palpitations, chest pain, or shortness of breath.
- Ask about the relationship of symptoms such as palpitations to intake of certain foods and caffeine-containing beverages.
- Evaluate for other contributing factors, such as smoking or alcohol intake.
- Inquire about a history of falls, particularly those occurring without apparent reason.

Home Care Teaching

Teach measures to reduce the risk of cardiac dysrhythmias and potential adverse consequences of dysrhythmias.

- Emphasize the importance of taking medications as prescribed. Discuss possible effects of over-the-counter medications on the heart.
- Encourage reducing or eliminating caffeine intake. Caffeine increases the risk of ectopic beats and rapid heart rates.
- Encourage participation in a smoking cessation program and reduction or elimination of alcohol intake if appropriate.
- Encourage engaging in regular exercise. Discuss the beneficial effects of exercise to maintain muscle mass, including cardiac muscle, and cardiovascular health.
- Instruct to contact the primary care provider for evaluation of symptoms such as dizziness, fainting, frequent palpitations, shortness of breath, unexplained falls, or chest pain.

dysrhythmias result from a change in the automaticity of cardiac cells. The rate of impulse formation may abnormally increase or decrease. Aberrant (abnormal) impulses may originate outside normal conduction pathways, causing ectopic beats. **Ectopic beats** interrupt the normal conduction sequence and may not initiate a normal muscle contraction. Depending on the site and timing of abnormal impulses, they may have little effect on the client or pose a significant threat.

Ischemia, injury, and infarction of myocardial tissue affect its excitability and ability to conduct and respond to an electrical stimulus. Conduction abnormalities cause varying degrees of **heart block** (a block in the normal conduction pathways). Myocardial injury or infarction can obstruct or delay impulse conduction. Bundle branch blocks are common in acute MI.

The reentry phenomenon, a phenomenon of normal and slow conduction, is a major cause of tachydysrhythmia. A stimulus such as an ectopic beat triggers the reentry phenomenon. The impulse is delayed in one area of the heart (e.g., an area of ischemia or injury) but is conducted normally through the rest. Muscle that has been depolarized by the normally conducted impulse is repolarized by the time the impulse travelling through the area of slow conduction reaches it, thus initiating another cycle of depolarization (Porth, 2005). The result is a dysrhythmia that propagates itself.

Several forms of reentry may occur. The impulse may travel through a set pathway to reenter repolarized tissue. Many atrial dysrhythmias follow this pattern, including atrial flutter. In functional reentry, local differences in the conduction of an impulse interrupt the normal wave of depolarization, sending it back upon itself in a spiral pattern and setting up a permanent rotation. This type of pattern suppresses normal pacemaker activity and can lead to atrial fibrillation (Porth, 2005).

Cardiac rhythms are classified according to the site of impulse formation or the site and degree of conduction block. Supraventricular rhythms arise above the ventricles. These rhythms usually produce a QRS complex within the normal range. Sinus rhythms, atrial rhythms, and junctional (arising from the AV junction) rhythms are all supraventricular rhythms. Ventricular rhythms originate in the ventricles and may prove fatal if left untreated. AV conduction blocks result from a defect in impulse transmission from the atria to the ventricles. The major normal and abnormal cardiac rhythms are summarized in Table 22–29.

Supraventricular Rhythms

To improve understanding, rhythms are presented in sections based on the site of origination. Supraventricular rhythms are those that originate above the ventricle. Junctional rhythms originate at atrioventricular node. Ventricular rhythms originate below the AV node and are the most life threatening because of their impact on cardiac output.

NORMAL SINUS RHYTHM **Normal sinus rhythm** is the normal heart rhythm, in which impulses originate in the SA (sinus) node and travel through all normal conduction pathways without delay. All waveforms are of normal configuration, look alike, and have consistent (fixed) durations. The rate is between 60 and 100 bpm.

SINUS NODE DYSRHYTHMIAS Sinus node, also called sinoatrial node, dysrhythmias may occur as a normal compensatory response (e.g., to exercise) or because of altered automaticity. In these rhythms, as in normal sinus rhythm, the initiating impulse is from the SA node. They differ from normal sinus rhythms in rate or regularity of the rhythm. Sinus dysrhythmias include sinus arrhythmia, sinus tachycardia, and sinus bradycardia.

Sinus Arrhythmia *Sinus arrhythmia* is a sinus rhythm in which the rate varies with respirations, causing an irregular rhythm. The rate increases during inspiration and decreases with expiration. Sinus arrhythmia is common in the very young and the very old. It can be caused by an increase in vagal tone, by digitalis toxicity, or by morphine administration.

Sinus Tachycardia *Sinus tachycardia* has all of the characteristics of NSR, except that the rate is greater than 100 bpm. Tachycardia arises from enhanced automaticity in response to changes in the internal environment. Sympathetic nervous system stimulation or blocked vagal (parasympathetic) activity increases the heart rate. Tachycardia is a normal response to any condition or event that increases the body's demand for oxygen and nutrients, such as exercise or hypoxia. In the client on bed rest, tachycardia is an ominous sign. Sinus tachycardia may be an early sign of cardiac dysfunction, such as heart failure. Tachycardia is detrimental in clients with cardiac disease because it increases cardiac work and oxygen use.

Common causes of sinus tachycardia include exercise, excitement, anxiety, pain, fever, hypoxia, hypovolemia, anemia, hyperthyroidism, myocardial infarction, heart failure, cardiogenic shock, pulmonary embolism, caffeine intake, and certain drugs, such as atropine, epinephrine (Adrenalin), or isoproterenol (Isuprel).

Manifestations of sinus tachycardia include a rapid pulse rate. The client may complain of feeling that the heart is "racing," shortness of breath, and dizziness. In the presence of heart disease, sinus tachycardia may precipitate chest pain.

Sinus Bradycardia *Sinus bradycardia* has all of the characteristics of NSR, but the rate is less than 60 beats/minute. Sinus bradycardia may result from increased vagal (parasympathetic) activity or from depressed automaticity due to injury or ischemia to the sinus node. Sinus bradycardia may be normal (e.g., in clients with athletic heart syndrome). The heart rate also normally slows during sleep because the parasympathetic nervous system is dominant at this time. Other causes of sinus bradycardia include pain, increased intracranial pressure, sinus node disease, AMI (especially with inferior wall damage), hypothermia, acidosis, and certain drugs.

Sinus bradycardia may be asymptomatic; it is important to assess the client before treating the rhythm. Manifestations of decreased cardiac output, such as decreased level of consciousness, syncope (faintness), or hypotension, indicate a need for intervention.

TABLE 22–29 Characteristics of Selected Cardiac Rhythms and Dysrhythmias

RHYTHM/ECG APPEARANCE	ECG CHARACTERISTICS	MANAGEMENT
SUPRAVENTRICULAR RHYTHMS		
Normal sinus rhythm (NSR) 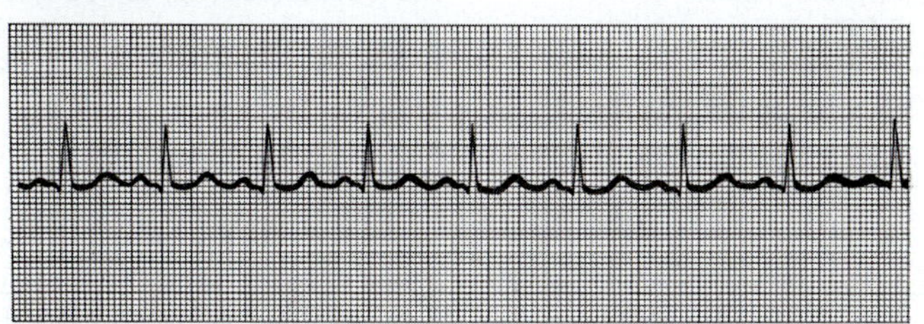	Rate: 60–100 bpm Rhythm: regular P:QRS: 1:1 PR interval: 0.12–0.20 sec QRS complex: 0.6–0.10 sec	None; normal heart rhythm
Sinus arrhythmia 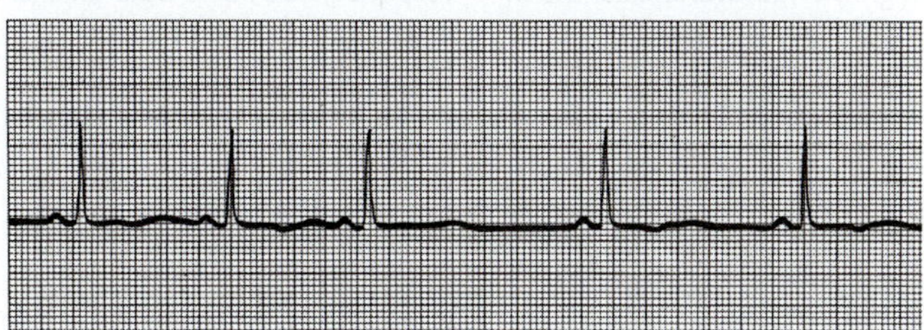	Rate: 60–100 bpm Rhythm: irregular, varying with respirations P:QRS: 1:1 PR interval: 0.12–0.20 sec QRS complex: 0.6–0.10 sec	Generally none; considered a normal rhythm in the very young and very old
Sinus tachycardia 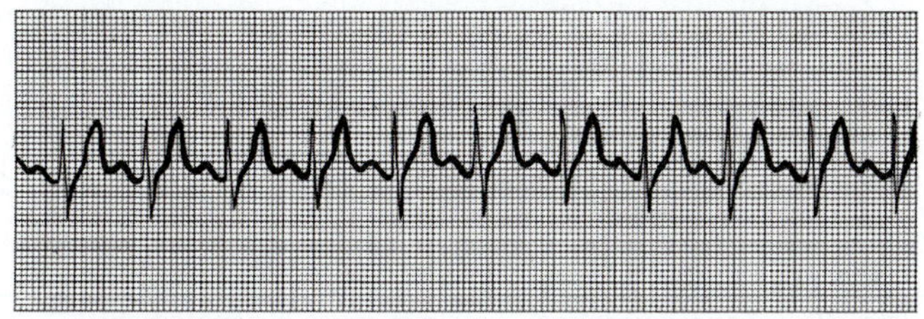	Rate: 101–150 bpm Rhythm: regular P:QRS: 1:1 (with very fast rates, P wave may be hidden in preceding T wave) PR interval: 0.12–0.20 sec QRS complex: 0.6–0.10 sec	Treated only if symptomatic or client is at risk for myocardial damage Treat underlying cause (e.g., hypovolemia, fever, pain) Beta-blockers or verapamil may be used
Sinus bradycardia 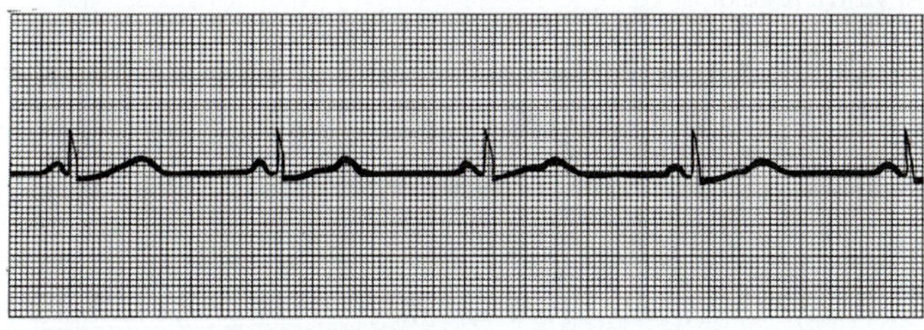	Rate: <60 bpm Rhythm: regular P:QRS: 1:1 PR interval: 0.12–0.20 sec QRS complex: 0.6–0.10 sec	Treated only if symptomatic Intravenous atropine or isoproterenol, and/or pacemaker therapy may be used
Premature atrial contractions (PAC) 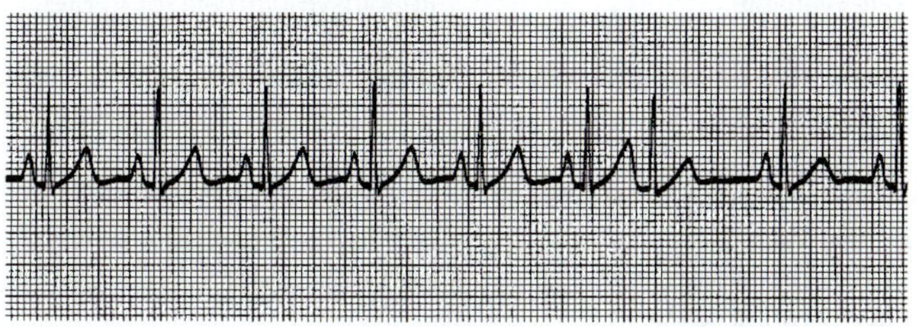	Rate: variable Rhythm: irregular, with normal rhythm interrupted by early beats arising in the atria P:QRS: 1:1 PR interval: 0.12–0.20 sec, but may be prolonged QRS complex: 0.6–0.10 sec	Usually require no treatment Advise to reduce alcohol and caffeine intake, to reduce stress, and to stop smoking Beta-blocker may be prescribed

(continued)

TABLE 22–29 **Characteristics of Selected Cardiac Rhythms and Dysrhythmias** **(continued)**

RHYTHM/ECG APPEARANCE	ECG CHARACTERISTICS	MANAGEMENT
Paroxysmal supraventricular tachycardia (PSVT) 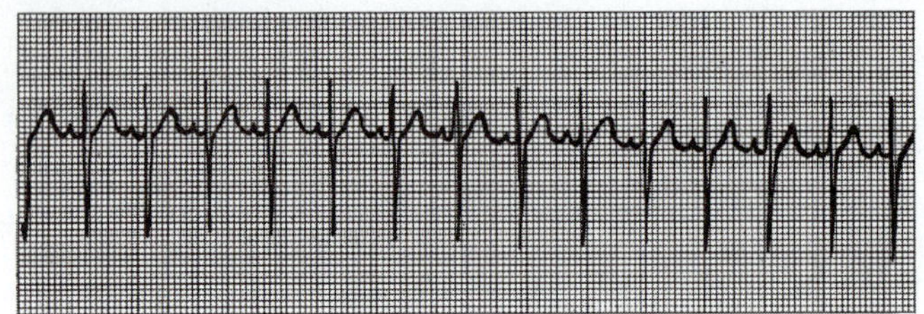	Rate: 100–280 bpm (usually 150–200 bpm) Rhythm: regular P:QRS: P waves often not identifiable PR interval: not measured QRS complex: 0.6–0.10 sec	Treat if symptomatic Treatment may include vagal maneuvers (Valsalva, carotid sinus massage), oxygen therapy, adenosine or a beta-blocker, temporary pacing, or synchronized cardioversion
Atrial flutter 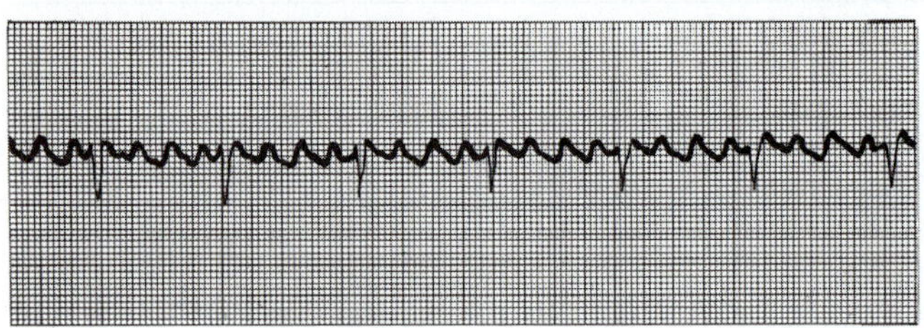	Rate: atrial, 240–360 bpm; ventricular rate depends on degree of atrioventricular block and usually is <150 bpm Rhythm: atrial, regular; ventricular, usually regular P:QRS: 2:1, 4:1, 6:1; may vary PR interval: not measured QRS complex: 0.6–0.10 sec	Synchronized cardioversion; medications to slow ventricular response, such as a beta-blocker or calcium-channel blocker, followed by a class I antidysrhythmic agent or amiodarone
Atrial fibrillation 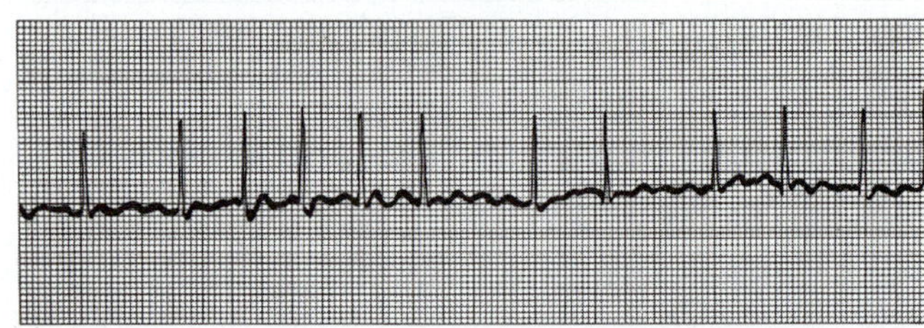	Rate: atrial, 300–600 bpm (too rapid to count); ventricular, 100–180 bpm in untreated clients Rhythm: irregularly irregular P:QRS: variable PR interval: not measured QRS complex: 0.06–0.10 sec	Synchronized cardioversion; medications to reduce ventricular response rate: metaprolol, diltiazem, or digoxin; anticoagulant therapy to reduce risk of clot formation and stroke
Junctional escape rhythm 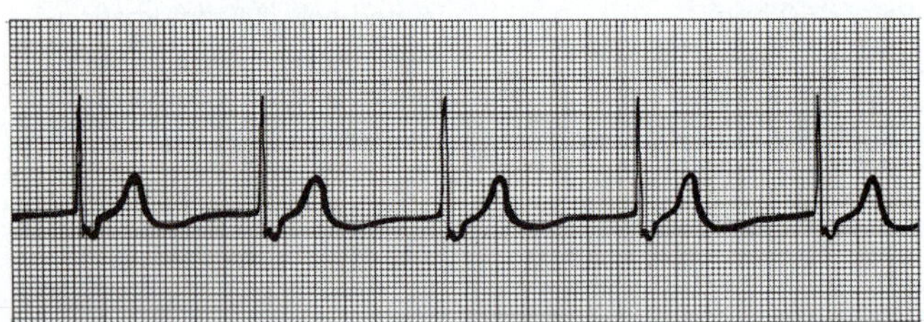	Rate: 40–60 bpm; junctional tachycardia, 60–140 bpm Rhythm: regular P:QRS: P waves may be absent, inverted and immediately preceding or succeeding QRS complex, or hidden in QRS complex PR interval: <0.10 sec QRS complex: 0.06–0.10 sec	Treat cause if symptomatic
VENTRICULAR RHYTHMS		
Premature ventricular contractions (PVC) 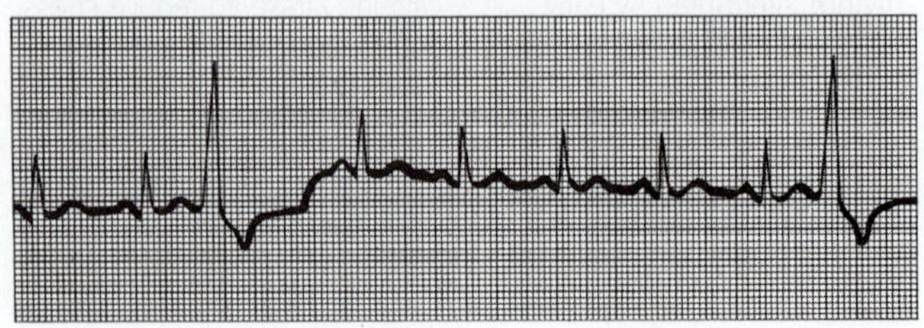	Rate: variable Rhythm: irregular, with PVC interrupting underlying rhythm and followed by a compensatory pause P:QRS: no P wave noted before PVC PR interval: absent with PVC QRS complex: wide (>0.12 sec) and bizarre in appearance; differs from normal QRS complex	Treat if symptomatic or in presence of severe heart disease; advise against stimulant use (caffeine, nicotine); beta-blockers, or class I or III antidysrhythmic agents may be used in clients with severe heart disease who are symptomatic

TABLE 22–29 Characteristics of Selected Cardiac Rhythms and Dysrhythmias (continued)

RHYTHM/ECG APPEARANCE	ECG CHARACTERISTICS	MANAGEMENT
Ventricular tachycardia (VT, V tach) 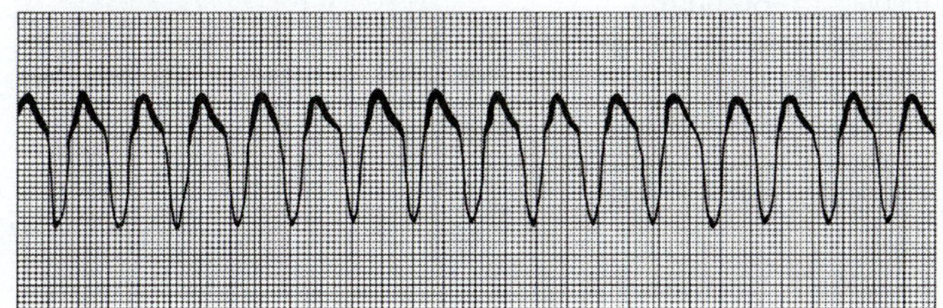	Rate: 100–250 bpm Rhythm: regular P:QRS: P waves usually not identifiable PR interval: not measured QRS complex: ≥ 0.12 sec; bizarre shape	Treat if VT is sustained, symptomatic, or associated with organic heart disease Treatment includes DC cardioversion or intravenous procainamide, lidocaine, or a class III antidysrhythmic agent if hemodynamic instability accompanies; surgical ablation or antitachycardia pacing with an implanted cardioverter–defibrillator for repeated episodes
Ventricular fibrillation (VF, V fib) 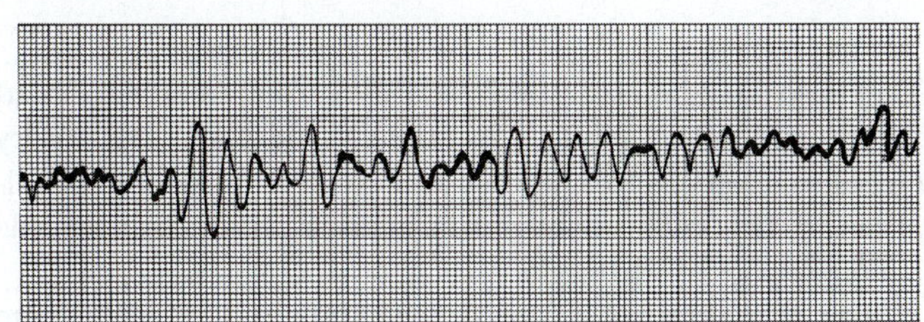	Rate: too rapid to count Rhythm: grossly irregular P:QRS: no identifiable P waves PR interval: none QRS: bizarre, varying in shape and direction	Immediate cardioversion/defibrillation
ATRIOVENTRICULAR (AV) CONDUCTION BLOCKS		
First-degree AV block 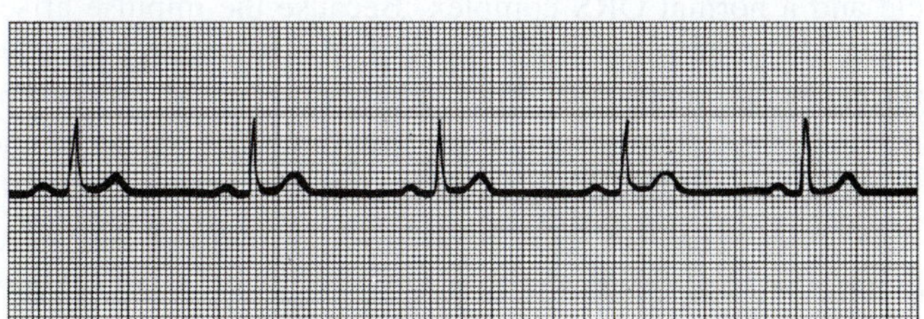	Rate: usually 60–100 bpm Rhythm: regular P:QRS: 1:1 PR interval: >0.21 sec QRS complex: 0.06–0.10 sec	None required
Second-degree AV block, type I (Mobitz I, Wenckebach) 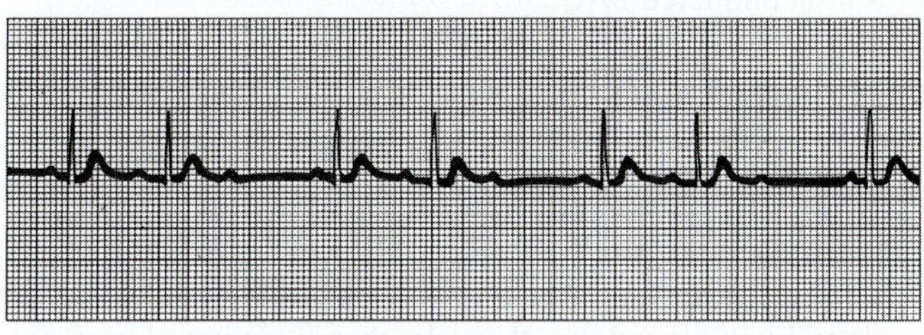	Rate: 60–100 bpm Rhythm: atrial, regular; ventricular, irregular P:QRS: 1:1 until P wave blocked with no subsequent QRS complex PR interval: progressively lengthens in a regular pattern QRS complex: 0.06–0.10 sec; sudden absence of QRS complex	Monitoring and observation; rarely progresses to a higher degree of block or requires treatment
Second-degree AV block, type II (Mobitz II) 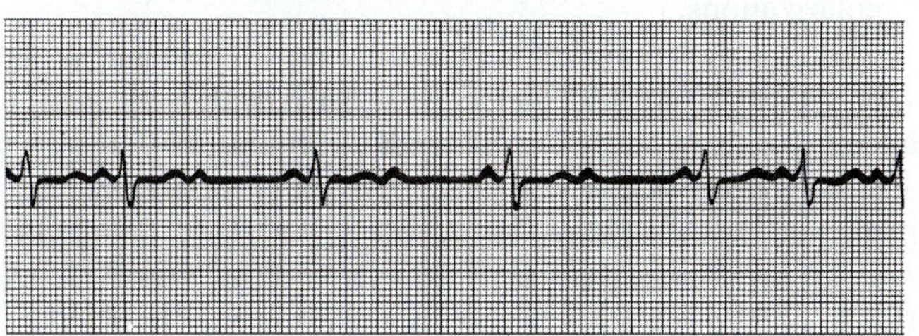	Rate: atrial, 60–100 bpm; ventricular, <60 bpm Rhythm: atrial, regular; ventricular, irregular P:QRS: typically 2:1, may vary PR interval: constant PR interval for each conducted QRS complex QRS complex: 0.06–0.10 sec	Atropine or isoproterenol; pacemaker therapy

(continued)

TABLE 22–29 Characteristics of Selected Cardiac Rhythms and Dysrhythmias (continued)

RHYTHM/ECG APPEARANCE	ECG CHARACTERISTICS	MANAGEMENT
Third-degree AV block (complete heart block) 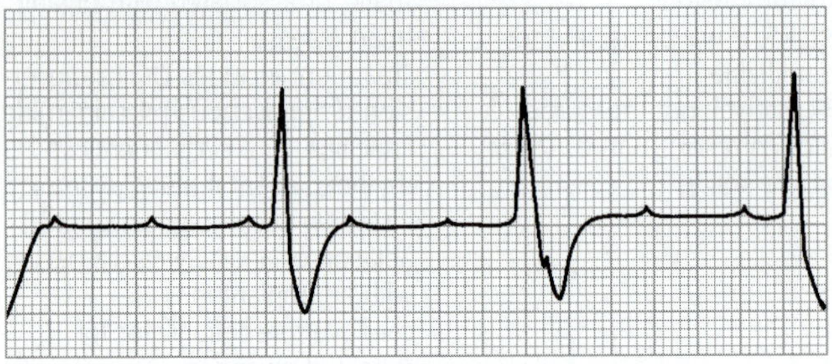	Rate: atrial, 60–100 bpm; ventricular, 15–60 bpm Rhythm: atrial, regular; ventricular, regular P:QRS: no relationship between P waves and QRS complexes; independent rhythms PR interval: not measured QRS complex: 0.06–0.10 sec if junctional escape rhythm; > 0.12 sec if ventricular escape rhythm	Immediate pacemaker therapy

Sick Sinus Syndrome *Sick sinus syndrome (SSS)* results from sinus node disease or dysfunction that causes problems with impulse formation, transmission, and conduction. Sick sinus syndrome is often found in older adults. It may be caused by direct injury to sinus tissue, fibrosis of conduction fibers associated with aging, and such drugs as digitalis, beta blockers, and calcium channel blockers.

ECG characteristics of SSS include sinus bradycardia, sinus arrhythmia, sinus pauses or arrest, and atrial tachydysrhythmias such as atrial fibrillation, atrial flutter, or atrial tachycardia. Bradycardia-tachycardia syndrome, characterized either by **paroxysmal** (abrupt onset and termination) atrial tachycardia followed by prolonged sinus pauses or alternating periods of bradycardia and tachycardia also may indicate sinus node dysfunction.

Manifestations of sinus node dysfunction often are intermittent, related to a drop in cardiac output caused by the irregular rhythm. Fatigue, dizziness, light-headedness, and syncope are common. The heart rate may not increase in response to stressors such as exercise or fever.

SUPRAVENTRICULAR DYSRHYTHMIAS When an action potential originates in atrial tissue outside the SA node, the resulting rhythm is classified as a supraventricular rhythm. In these dysrhythmias, an ectopic pacemaker takes over, or overrides, the SA node. They may also occur when the SA node fails; an escape rhythm develops as a fail-safe mechanism to maintain the heart rate. The most common supraventricular dysrhythmias are premature atrial contractions, paroxysmal supraventricular tachycardia, atrial flutter, and atrial fibrillation. These rhythms may be paroxysmal—that is, occur in bursts, with an abrupt beginning and end.

Premature Atrial Contractions A *premature atrial contraction (PAC)* is an ectopic atrial beat that occurs earlier than the next expected sinus beat. PACs can arise anywhere in the atria. They are usually asymptomatic and benign, but they may initiate paroxysmal supraventricular tachycardia in susceptible individuals. PACs are common in older adults, often occurring without an obvious cause. Strong emotions, excessive alcohol intake, tobacco, and stimulants such as caffeine can precipitate PACs. They also may be associated with myocardial infarction, heart failure and other cardiac disorders, hypoxemia, pulmonary embolism, digitalis toxicity, and electrolyte or acid–base imbalances. In clients with underlying heart disease, PACs may precede a more serious dysrhythmia.

The ECG tracing shows interruption of the underlying rhythm by a premature complex that looks similar to the underlying beats. The ectopic impulse of the PAC is usually conducted normally, leading to depolarization of cardiac muscle and a normal QRS complex. Because the impulse arises above the ventricles, it follows normal conduction pathways through the ventricles. The QRS complex is narrow or matches those of the underlying rhythm. The shape of the P wave of a PAC differs from normal P waves because its impulse arises outside the sinus node. A *non-compensatory pause* usually follows, as the PAC resets the SA node rhythm. Occasionally, the ectopic impulse may not be conducted through the heart, resulting in a lone P wave without a QRS, or a nonconducted PAC.

PACs cause few manifestations. If frequent, they may cause palpitations or a fluttering sensation in the chest. Early beats may be noted on auscultating or palpating the pulse.

Paroxysmal Supraventricular Tachycardia *Paroxysmal supra-ventricular tachycardia (PSVT)* is tachycardia of sudden onset and termination. PSVT is usually initiated by a reentry loop in or around the AV node; that is, an impulse reenters the same section of tissue over and over, causing repeated depolarizations.

PSVT occurs more frequently in women. Sympathetic nervous system stimulation and stressors such as fever, sepsis, and hyperthyroidism may precipitate PSVT. It also may be associated with heart diseases such as CHD, myocardial infarction, rheumatic heart disease, myocarditis, or acute pericarditis. Abnormal conduction pathways associated with Wolff-Parkinson-White (WPW) syndrome may account for PSVT.

PSVT affects ventricular filling and cardiac output, and decreases coronary artery perfusion. Its manifestations include complaints of palpitations and a "racing" heart, anxiety, dizziness, dyspnea, anginal pain, diaphoresis, extreme fatigue, and polyuria (urine output may reach up to 3 L in the first few hours after PSVT onset).

Atrial Flutter *Atrial flutter* is a rapid and regular atrial rhythm thought to result from an intra-atrial reentry mechanism. Causes include sympathetic nervous system stimulation due to anxiety or caffeine and alcohol intake; thyrotoxicosis; coronary heart disease or myocardial infarction; pulmonary embolism; and abnormal conduction syndromes, such as WPW syndrome. Older persons with rheumatic heart disease and/or valvular disease are especially vulnerable.

Two types of atrial flutter have been identified. Type I atrial flutter has an atrial rate of 240–340 beats per minute. It develops due to a reentry mechanism in the right atrium. The mechanism leading to type II atrial flutter has not been identified. In this type of flutter, the atrial rate is faster, to 350 beats per minute.

Clients with atrial flutter may complain of palpitations or a fluttering sensation in the chest or throat. If the ventricular rate is rapid, manifestations of decreased cardiac output, such as decreased level of consciousness, hypotension, decreased urinary output, and cool clammy skin, may be noted. The atrial kick (additional ventricular filling with atrial contraction) is lost because of inadequate atrial filling.

ECG characteristics include a "sawtooth" or "picket fence" appearance of P waves, which are labeled flutter (F) waves. The atrial rate is rapid, often around 300 beats/minute. As a protective mechanism, many impulses are blocked at the AV node, and the ventricular rate is rarely greater than 150–170 beats/minute. Usually, atrial impulses are evenly conducted through the AV node, for example, two impulses to one QRS complex (2:1), four impulses to one QRS complex (4:1), or six impulses to one QRS complex (6:1). A constant conduction ratio results in a regular ventricular rhythm; the ventricular rhythm is irregular if the conduction ratio varies. The ventricular rate usually ranges from 150–170 beats/minute in 2:1 conduction and 60–75 beats/minute for lower conduction ratios. The T wave is usually hidden by overriding F waves; some F waves may be hidden in the QRS complex.

Atrial Fibrillation *Atrial fibrillation* is a common dysrhythmia characterized by disorganized atrial activity without discrete atrial contractions. Multiple small reentry circuits develop in the atria. Atrial cells cannot repolarize in time to respond to the next stimulus (Porth, 2005). Extremely rapid atrial impulses bombard the AV node, resulting in an irregularly irregular ventricular response. Atrial fibrillation may occur suddenly and recur, or it may persist as a chronic dysrhythmia. Atrial fibrillation is commonly associated with heart failure, rheumatic heart disease, coronary heart disease, hypertension, and hyperthyroidism.

Manifestations of atrial fibrillation relate to the rate of the ventricular response. With rapid response rates, manifestations of decreased cardiac output such as hypotension, shortness of breath, fatigue, and angina may develop. Clients with extensive heart disease may develop syncope or heart failure. Peripheral pulses are irregular and of variable amplitude (strength).

The specific ECG characteristics of atrial fibrillation include an irregularly irregular rhythm and the absence of identifiable P waves. The atrial rate is so rapid that it is not measurable. The ventricular rate varies.

Atrial fibrillation increases the risk for formation of thromboemboli. Organ infarction may occur as a result; the incidence of stroke is high.

Junctional Dysrhythmias

Rhythms that originate in AV nodal tissue are termed *junctional.* The AV junction includes the AV node and the bundle of His, which branches into the right and left bundle branches. An impulse arising from the AV junction may occur in response to failure of higher pacemakers, as in a *junctional escape rhythm,* or it may result from an abnormal mechanism, such as altered automaticity. An impulse arising from the AV junction may or may not be conducted back up to the atria. This conduction against the normal flow or pattern is called **retrograde conduction**. The resulting atrial wave, called a P′ wave, may be found before, during, or after the QRS complex, depending on the speed of conduction. The P′ wave is inverted in some ECG leads because the impulse moves from the AV node up to the atria instead of from the SA node down toward the AV node. In addition, the P′R interval is shorter than normal (less than 0.12 sec). The QRS complex is typically narrow.

A junctional rhythm may be due to drug toxicity (e.g., digitalis, beta blockers, or calcium channel blockers) or other causes such as hypoxemia, hyperkalemia, increased vagal tone or damage to the AV node, myocardial infarction, and heart failure. Loss of synchronized atrial contraction and the atrial kick may affect cardiac output, leading to manifestations of decreased cardiac output and impaired myocardial tissue perfusion. Heart failure may develop.

Premature junctional contractions occur before the next expected beat of the underlying rhythm. Isolated premature junctional contractions may occur in healthy people and are insignificant. Junctional tachycardia is a junctional rhythm with a rate greater than 60 bpm. It is caused by increased automaticity of AV nodal tissue. The ventricular rate is usually less than 140 bpm. Both rhythms are most commonly associated with digitalis toxicity, hypoxia, ischemia, or electrolyte imbalances.

Ventricular Dysrhythmias

Ventricular dysrhythmias originate in the ventricles. Because the ventricles pump blood into the pulmonary and systemic vasculature, any disruption of their rhythm can affect cardiac output and tissue perfusion. A wide and bizarre QRS complex (>0.12 sec) is a characteristic feature of ventricular dysrhythmias. This occurs because ventricular ectopic impulses begin and travel outside normal conduction pathways. Other characteristics include no relationship of the QRS complex to a P wave, increased amplitude of the QRS complex, an abnormal ST segment, and a T wave deflected in the opposite direction from the QRS complex.

PREMATURE VENTRICULAR CONTRACTIONS Premature ventricular contractions (PVCs) are ectopic ventricular beats that occur before the next expected beat of the underlying rhythm. They usually do not reset the atrial rhythm and are followed by a full compensatory pause. PVCs often have no significance in people without heart disease. Frequent, recurrent, or multifocal PVCs may be associated with an increased risk for lethal dysrhythmias. PVCs result from either enhanced automaticity or a reentry phenomenon. They may be triggered by anxiety or stress; tobacco, alcohol, or caffeine use; hypoxia, acidosis, and electrolyte imbalances; sympathomimetic drugs; coronary heart disease; heart failure; and mechanical stimulation of the heart (e.g., the insertion of a cardiac catheter); or reperfusion after fibrinolytic therapy. The incidence and significance of PVCs is greatest after MI.

Premature ventricular contractions may be isolated or occur in a specific pattern. Two PVCs in a row are called a **couplet**, or paired PVCs. Three consecutive PVCs (a **triplet**, or salvo) is a short run of ventricular tachycardia. **Ventricular bigeminy** is characterized by a PVC following each normal beat; a PVC noted every third beat is called **ventricular trigeminy**. When the ventricular impulse arises from one ectopic site, all PVCs look the same (monomorphic) and are called **unifocal** PVCs. **Multifocal** PVCs arise from different ectopic sites and appear different from one another on the ECG (polymorphic).

The frequency and patterns of PVCs can be indicative of myocardial irritability and the risk for a lethal dysrhythmia. The following are considered warning signs in the client with acute heart disease (e.g., an acute MI):

- PVCs that develop within the first 4 hours of an MI
- Frequent PVCs (six or more per minute)
- Couplets or triplets
- Multifocal PVCs
- R-on-T phenomenon (PVCs falling on the T wave).

In people without heart disease, isolated PVCs usually are insignificant and do not require treatment. In clients with preexisting heart disease, PVCs may indicate a drug toxicity or an increased risk for lethal dysrhythmias and cardiac arrest. The risk is greatest following acute MI.

VENTRICULAR TACHYCARDIA Ventricular tachycardia is a rapid ventricular rhythm defined as three or more consecutive PVCs. Ventricular tachycardia may occur in short bursts, or "runs," or it may persist for more than 30 sec (sustained ventricular tachycardia). The rate is greater than 100 bpm, and the rhythm is usually regular. Reentry is the usual electrophysiologic mechanism responsible for ventricular tachycardia. Myocardial ischemia and infarction are the most common predisposing factors for ventricular tachycardia. VT also is associated with cardiac structural disorders such as valvular disease, rheumatic heart disease, or cardiomyopathy. It may occur in the absence of heart disease, and with anorexia nervosa, metabolic disorders, and drug toxicity.

Nonsustained ventricular tachycardia may occur paroxysmally and convert back to an effective rhythm spontaneously. The client may experience a fluttering sensation in the chest or complain of palpitations and brief shortness of breath. Clients in sustained VT generally develop signs and symptoms of decreased cardiac output and hemodynamic instability, including severe hypotension, a weak or nonpalpable pulse, and loss of consciousness. Allowed to continue, VT can deteriorate into ventricular fibrillation. Sustained ventricular tachycardia is a medical emergency that requires immediate intervention, particularly in clients with cardiac disease.

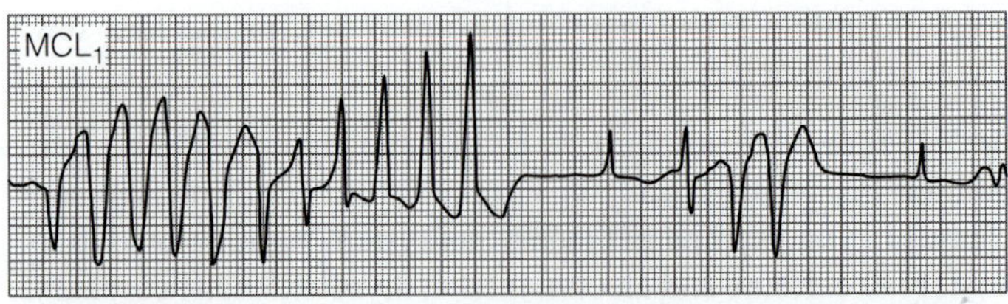

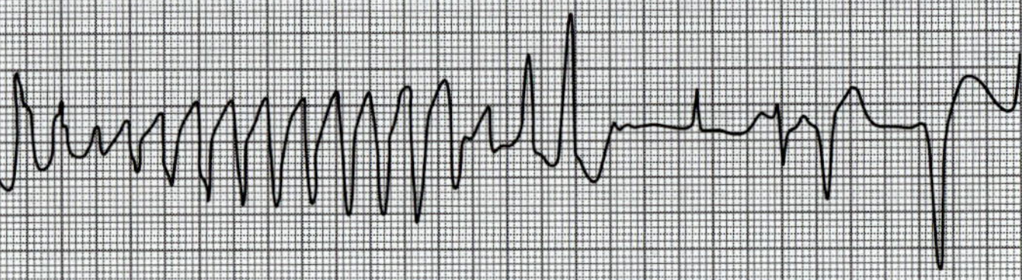

Figure 22–51 ■ Toursades de pointes. Note the wide and bizarre QRS complexes of varying size, shape (morphology), and amplitude.

Torsades de pointes is a type of ventricular tachycardia associated with long QT syndrome (a prolongation of the QT interval). Long QT syndrome may be genetic or acquired, occurring secondarily to electrolyte disruptions, MI, cocaine use, liquid protein diets, medications, or other conditions. In torsades de pointes, the QRS complexes vary in size, shape, and amplitude (Figure 22–51 ■). Clients with torsades de pointes may have multiple bursts or episodes of ventricular tachycardia or may develop ventricular fibrillation and sudden cardiac death (Kasper et al., 2005; Porth, 2005).

VENTRICULAR FIBRILLATION Ventricular fibrillation is extremely rapid, chaotic ventricular depolarization causing the ventricles to quiver and cease contracting; the heart does not pump. This is known as cardiac arrest; it is a medical emergency requiring immediate intervention with CPR. Death will follow the onset of ventricular fibrillation within 4 minutes if the rhythm is not recognized and terminated and an effective perfusing rhythm reestablished.

Ventricular fibrillation is usually triggered by severe myocardial ischemia or infarction. It occurs without warning 50% of the time. It is the terminal event in many disease processes or traumatic conditions. Ventricular fibrillation may be precipitated by a single PVC or may follow ventricular tachycardia. Other causes of ventricular fibrillation include digitalis toxicity, reperfusion therapy, antidysrhythmic drugs, hypokalemia and hyperkalemia, hypothermia, metabolic acidosis, mechanical stimulation (as with the insertion of cardiac catheters or pacing wires), and electric shock.

Clinically, loss of ventricular contractions results in absence of a palpable or audible pulse. The client loses consciousness and stops breathing as perfusion ceases. The ECG shows grossly irregular, bizarre complexes with no discernible rate or rhythm.

Atrioventricular Conduction Blocks

Conduction defects that delay or block transmission of the sinus impulse through the AV node are called AV conduction blocks. Impaired conduction may result from tissue injury or

CLINICAL MANIFESTATIONS AND THERAPIES Life-Threatening Dysrhythmias

ETIOLOGY	CLINICAL MANIFESTATION	CLINICAL THERAPIES
Decreased cardiac output	Changes in level of consciousness (LOC) ranging from dizziness to complete loss of consciousness; ischemia, reduced tissue perfusion, hypotension	■ Antiarrhythmic medications. ■ Defibrillation or cardioversion (external or implanted). ■ Pacemaker (external or implanted). ■ Reduce cardiac workload.
Alterations in oxygenation	Cyanosis, shortness of breath, hypoxemia, hypercapnia, altered LOC, death	■ Administration of oxygen. ■ Mechanical ventilation. ■ Reduce activity to decrease oxygen demands on the body.
Stasis of blood in the heart	Increased risk of emboli formation that manifests differently depending on where the thrombus occurs. May result in myocardial infarction, stroke, or deep venous thrombosis	■ Administration of anticoagulants. ■ Treat the underlying dysrhythmia to promote movement of blood through the chambers of the heart.
Sudden cardiac death	Pulselessness, absence of respirations, death	■ Cardiopulmonary resuscitation. ■ Antiarrhythmic medications. ■ Administration of oxygen. ■ Cardiorespiratory monitoring after successful resuscitation.

disease, increased vagal (parasympathetic) tone, drug effects, or a congenital defect. AV conduction blocks vary in severity from benign to severe.

FIRST-DEGREE AV BLOCK First-degree AV block is a benign conduction delay that generally poses no threat, has no symptoms, and requires no treatment. Impulse conduction through the AV node is slowed, but all atrial impulses are conducted to the ventricles. It may result from injury or infarct of the AV node, other cardiac diseases, or drug effects. The ECG shows all characteristics of normal sinus rhythm, except the PR interval is greater than 0.20 second.

SECOND-DEGREE AV BLOCK Second-degree AV block is characterized by failure to conduct one or more impulses from the atria to the ventricles. Two patterns of second-degree AV block are seen, identified as type I and type II.

Second-Degree AV Block–Type I Type I second-degree AV block (Mobitz type I or Wenckebach phenomenon) is characterized by a repeating pattern of increasing AV conduction delays until an impulse fails to conduct to the ventricles. On the ECG, PR intervals progressively lengthen until one QRS complex is not conducted (or dropped). The ventricular rate remains adequate to maintain cardiac output, and the client usually is asymptomatic. Mobitz type I AV block usually is transient, associated with acute MI or drug intoxication (e.g., digitalis, beta-blockers, or calcium-channel blockers). It rarely progresses to complete heart block.

Second-Degree AV Block–Type II Type II second-degree AV block (Mobitz type II) involves intermittent failure of the AV node to conduct an impulse to the ventricles without preceding delays in conduction. The PR interval remains constant, but not all P waves are followed by QRS complexes (e.g., there may be two P waves for every QRS). Conduction through the His–Purkinje system usually is delayed as well, causing a widened QRS complex (Braunwald et al., 2002). Mobitz type II block is frequently associated with acute anterior wall MI and a high rate of mortality (Porth, 2005). Manifestations of Mobitz type II block depend on the ventricular rate. Pacemaker therapy may be required to maintain the cardiac output.

THIRD-DEGREE AV BLOCK Third-degree AV block (complete heart block) occurs when atrial impulses are completely blocked at the AV node and fail to reach the ventricles. As a result, the atria and ventricles are controlled by different and independent pacemakers, with separate rates and rhythms. The ventricular impulse arises from either junctional fibers (with a rate of 40–60 bpm) or a ventricular pacemaker at a rate of less than 40 bpm. The width of the QRS complex depends on the location of the escape pacemaker. The QRS is wide and the rate is slow when the rhythm arises distal to the bundle of His.

Third-degree AV block is frequently associated with an inferior or anteroseptal MI. Other causes include congenital conditions, acute or degenerative cardiac disease or damage, drug effects, and electrolyte imbalances. The slow escape rhythm significantly affects cardiac output, causing manifestations such as syncope (known as a *Stokes-Adams attack*), dizziness, fatigue, exercise intolerance, and heart failure. Third-degree AV block is life threatening and requires immediate intervention to maintain adequate cardiac output.

ATRIOVENTRICULAR DISSOCIATION Complete dissociation of atrial and ventricular rhythms can occur in conditions other than third-degree AV block. The two primary factors leading to AV dissociation are severe sinus bradycardia and a lower pacemaker (junctional or ventricular) that competes with or exceeds the normal sinus rhythm (Braunwald et al., 2002). AV dissociation may result from acute myocardial ischemia or infarction, cardiac surgery, or drug effects. The ECG shows separate and competing atrial (P waves) and ventricular (QRS complexes) rhythms.

Intraventricular Conduction Blocks

Once the impulse enters the ventricles, its conduction through the right and left bundle branches may be impaired (bundle branch block). As a result, the impulse is conducted more slowly than normal through the ventricles. On the ECG, the QRS complex is prolonged. Its appearance varies, depending on the affected bundle (right or left). Typically, no clinical manifestations are associated with bundle branch block unless it occurs in conjunction with an AV block.

COLLABORATION

Cardiac dysrhythmias may be either benign or critical: Recognizing lethal dysrhythmias is a matter of life and death. Major goals of care include identifying the dysrhythmia, evaluating its effect on physical and psychosocial well-being, and treating the underlying causes. This may involve correcting fluid and electrolyte or acid–base imbalances; treating hypoxia, pain, or anxiety; administering antidysrhythmic medications; or performing mechanical and surgical interventions.

Diagnostic Tests

Diagnostic tests for dysrhythmias include ECG, cardiac monitoring, and electrophysiology studies. Laboratory tests, such as serum electrolytes, drug levels, and arterial blood gases, may be done to help identify the cause of the dysrhythmia.

ELECTROCARDIOGRAM The 12-lead ECG may be required to accurately diagnose a dysrhythmia. It also provides information about underlying disease processes, such as MI or other cardiac disease. The ECG may also be used to monitor the effects of treatment.

CARDIAC MONITORING Cardiac monitoring allows continuous observation of the cardiac rhythm. It is used in many different circumstances (Box 22–29). Different types of ECG monitoring are employed for different situations.

Box 22–29 Indications for Cardiac Monitoring

- Perioperative monitoring of heart rate and rhythm
- Detecting and identifying dysrhythmias
- Monitoring the effects of cardiac and noncardiac diseases on the heart
- Monitoring clients with potentially life-threatening conditions:
  a. Major trauma (especially cardiac trauma)
  b. Dissecting aneurysm
  c. Acute myocardial infarction
  d. Heart failure
  e. Shock
  f. Other emergency conditions.
- Evaluating responses to procedures and interventions:
  a. Drug therapies
  b. Diagnostic procedures
  c. Ablative techniques
  d. Angioplasty or cardiac catheterization
  e. Cardiac surgery
  f. Pacemaker function
  g. Automatic implantable cardioverter–defibrillator function.

Continuous Cardiac Monitoring Continuous monitoring of the cardiac rhythm is provided by bedside and central monitoring stations. Electrodes placed on the client's chest attach to cables connected to a monitor. The heart rate and rhythm is visually displayed on a bedside monitor connected to a central monitoring station. The central station allows simultaneous monitoring of multiple clients within a nursing unit. Alarms on both bedside and central monitors warn of potential problems, such as very rapid or very slow heart rates. Alarm limits are preset by the nurse for the individual client.

Telemetry may be used in acute care settings when the client is ambulatory. Chest electrodes are connected to a portable transmitter worn around the neck or waist, and the ECG is transmitted electronically to a central monitoring station for continuous monitoring.

Home Monitoring Clients often complain of palpitations or other heart symptoms but are asymptomatic during evaluation in a hospital or community-based setting. Ambulatory or Holter monitoring may be used to identify intermittent dysrhythmias, to detect silent ischemia, to monitor the effects of treatment, and to assess pacemaker or automatic cardioverter–defibrillator function. Electrodes are applied and the leads attached to the portable telemetry monitor that records and stores all electrical activity. Clients are instructed to leave the electrode pads in place during monitoring and record any cardiac symptoms or events (e.g., chest pain, palpitations, or syncope) in a journal. After the prescribed period, usually 48–72 hours, the client returns to the clinic, and the monitor is removed. Diary entries are compared to the recorded heart rhythms to identify the effects of dysrhythmias.

ELECTROPHYSIOLOGY STUDIES Diagnostic cardiac electrophysiology procedures are performed to identify dysrhythmias and their causes. Electrophysiology studies are used to analyze components of the conduction system, identify sites of ectopic stimulation, and evaluate the effectiveness of treatment. Electrophysiology procedures can be employed for both diagnosis and as a therapeutic intervention.

In the electrophysiology laboratory, electrode catheters are guided by fluoroscopy into the heart through the femoral or brachial vein. The timing and sequence of electrical activation during normal and abnormal (aberrant) rhythms is observed and measured. Electrical stimulation may be used to induce dysrhythmias similar to the client's clinical dysrhythmia (Woods et al., 2004). Following diagnosis, an electrophysiology procedure may be used to treat the dysrhythmia—for example, by overdrive pacing (stimulating the client's heart to a rate faster than that of the tachydysrhythmia) to break the dysrhythmia's cycle, or to perform ablative therapy to destroy the ectopic site. (See the discussion under Cardiac Mapping and Catheter Ablation for further information.)

Nursing care for the client undergoing an electrophysiology procedure is similar to that for the client undergoing percutaneous coronary revascularization. (See the discussion under Revascularization Procedures in Exemplar 22.3, Coronary Artery Disease, for more details.) The procedure and expected sensations are explained. The client remains awake during the procedure; antianxiety medications or sedatives are given to reduce apprehension. Intravenous heparin may be given during the procedure to reduce the risk of thromboembolism.

Pharmacologic Therapies

The goal of drug therapy is to suppress dysrhythmia formation. No drug has been found to be completely safe and effective. Antidysrhythmic drugs are primarily used for acute treatment of dysrhythmias, although they may also be used to manage chronic conditions. The overall goal of therapy is to maintain an effective cardiac output by stabilizing cardiac rhythm.

It is important to remember that virtually all antidysrhythmic drugs also have prodysrhythmic effects; that is, they can worsen existing dysrhythmias and precipitate new ones. Because of this tendency, studies that demonstrate higher mortality rates in clients receiving antidysrhythmic medications, and the increasing safety and availability of interventional techniques, antidysrhythmic medications are used sparingly.

Most antidysrhythmic drugs are classified by their effects on the cardiac action potential. Most are class I drugs, or fast sodium-channel blockers. By blocking sodium channels, these drugs slow impulse conduction in the atria and ventricles. This class is further divided into subclasses A, B, and C. Class II drugs are beta-blockers, which decrease SA node automaticity, AV conduction velocity, and myocardial contractility. Class III agents block potassium channels, delaying repolarization and prolonging the relative refractory period. Class IV drugs are calcium-channel blockers. Their effect is similar to that of beta-blockers. Adenosine and digoxin do not fit within the major classes. Both drugs reduce SA node automaticity and slow AV conduction. Ibutilide and magnesium also fall outside the major classes but are used to treat dysrhythmias. Box 22–30 identifies common antidysrhythmic drugs within each class and the nursing implications in caring for clients receiving these drugs.

Drugs that affect the autonomic nervous system may also be used to treat dysrhythmias. Sympathomimetics, such as epinephrine, stimulate the heart, increasing both heart rate and contractility. Anticholinergic agents, such as atropine, are used to decrease vagal tone and increase heart rate. Magnesium sulfate is an unclassified drug that has been shown to be safe and effective in treating ventricular tachycardias.

Countershock

Countershock is used to interrupt cardiac rhythms that compromise cardiac output and the client's welfare. Delivery of a direct current charge depolarizes all cardiac cells at the same time. This simultaneous depolarization may stop a tachydysrhythmia and allow the SA node to recover control of impulse formation. There are two types of countershock: synchronized cardioversion and defibrillation.

SYNCHRONIZED CARDIOVERSION **Synchronized cardioversion** delivers direct electrical current synchronized with the client's heart rhythm. Synchronization of the shock with the QRS complex prevents ventricular fibrillation by avoiding current delivery during the vulnerable period of repolarization. Cardioversion is usually done as an elective procedure to treat supraventricular tachycardia, atrial fibrillation, atrial flutter, or hemodynamically stable ventricular tachycardia.

The nurse assists with cardioversion by preparing the client before the procedure; obtaining any laboratory tests ordered; obtaining and documenting ECG strips before, during, and after treatment; setting up the equipment; and monitoring the client's response.

Clients in atrial fibrillation are at high risk for thromboembolism following cardioversion. Loss of atrial contractions with atrial fibrillation leads to blood pooling in the atria, increasing the risk of clot formation. When the atria begin to contract following successful cardioversion, clots may be dislodged, embolizing to the pulmonary or systemic circulation. If possible, anticoagulants are given for several weeks before cardioversion is attempted.

DEFIBRILLATION Unlike carefully synchronized cardioversion, **defibrillation** is an emergency procedure that delivers direct current without regard to the cardiac cycle. Ventricular fibrillation is immediately treated as soon as the dysrhythmia is recognized. Early defibrillation has been shown to improve survival in clients experiencing ventricular fibrillation.

Defibrillation can be delivered by external or internal paddles or pads. Conductive gel pads or paste is applied, and external paddles or pads are placed on the chest wall at the apex and base of the heart (Figure 22–52 ■). Internal paddles are applied directly on the heart and may be used in surgery, the emergency department, or critical care. Internal defibrillation is done only by a physician; external defibrillation may be performed by any health care provider who has been trained in the procedure. Automatic external defibrillators are available on most hospital units to allow early defibrillation for cardiac arrest.

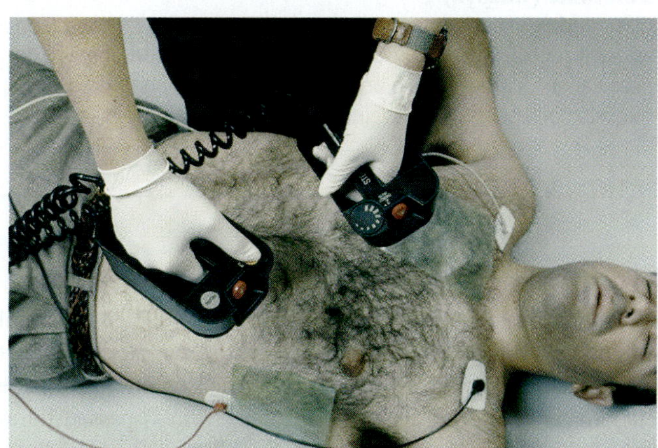

Figure 22–52 ■ Placement of paddles for defibrillation.

Source: Floyd Jackson.

Box 22–30 Medication Administration: Antidysrhythmic Drugs

CLASS I DRUGS: SODIUM-CHANNEL BLOCKERS

Class IA

Quinidine (Cardioquin, Quinidex, Quinaglute)
Procainamide (Pronestyl, Procan SR)
Disopyramide (Norpace, Norpace CR)
Moricizine (Ethmozine)

Class IA drugs decrease the flow of sodium into the cell and prolong the action potential. This decreases automaticity, slows the rate of impulse conduction, and prolongs refractoriness. They are used to treat both supraventricular and ventricular tachycardias.

Class IB

Lidocaine (Xylocaine) **Tocainide (Tonocard)**
Mexiletine (Mexitil) **Phenytoin (Dilantin)**

Class IB, or lidocaine-like, drugs decrease the refractory period but have little effect on automaticity. Drugs in this class are used primarily to treat ventricular dysrhythmias, including premature ventricular contractions and ventricular tachycardia.

Class IC

Flecainide (Tambocor) **Propafenone (Rythmol)**

Class IC drugs slow impulse conduction velocity but have little effect on refractoriness. They are used to reduce or eliminate tachydysrhythmias associated with reentry. Their significant prodysrhythmic effects limit their usefulness, but they may be used to treat supraventricular tachycardia.

CLASS II DRUGS: BETA-BLOCKERS

Esmolol (Brevibloc)
Propranolol (Inderal)
Metoprolol (Toprol)

Class II drugs are beta-blockers that decrease automaticity and conduction through the atrioventricular (AV) node. They also reduce the heart rate and myocardial contractility. They are used to treat supraventricular tachycardia and to slow the ventricular response rate to atrial fibrillation. These drugs may cause bronchospasm and are contraindicated for clients with asthma, chronic obstructive pulmonary disease, or other restrictive or obstructive lung diseases.

CLASS III DRUGS: POTASSIUM-CHANNEL BLOCKERS

Sotalol (Betapace) **Bretylium (Bretylol)**
Amiodarone (Cordarone) **Ibutilide (Corvert)**
Dofetilide (Tikosyn)

Class III drugs block potassium channels, prolonging repolarization and the refractory period. Drugs in this class are used primarily to treat ventricular tachycardia and ventricular fibrillation. Amiodarone may also be used for supraventricular tachycardias.

CLASS IV DRUGS: CALCIUM-CHANNEL BLOCKERS

Verapamil (Calan, Isoptin, Verelan)
Diltiazem (Cardizem, Dilacor XR)

Calcium-channel blockers decrease automaticity and AV nodal conduction. They are used to manage supraventricular tachycardias. Like the beta-blockers, calcium-channel blockers reduce myocardial contractility.

OTHER DRUGS

Adenosine (Adenocard) **Digoxin**

Adenosine and digoxin decrease conduction through the AV node and are used to treat supraventricular tachycardias.

Nursing Responsibilities

- Obtain baseline data, including vital signs, cardiac rhythm (including rate, PR and QT intervals, and QRS duration), and physical assessment (especially cardiac, neurologic, and respiratory status).
- Assess medication regimen to identify drugs that may interfere with antidysrhythmic therapy.
- Monitor electrocardiogram to evaluate the effectiveness of therapy and assess for possible dysrhythmias precipitated by treatment.
- Immediately report manifestations of drug toxicity:
  a. Procainamide: signs of heart failure; conduction delays or ventricular dysrhythmias; skin rash, myalgias or arthralgias, flu-like symptoms
  b. Disopyramide: urinary retention, heart failure, eye pain
  c. Lidocaine: changes in neurologic status, such as agitation, confusion, dizziness, nervousness
  d. Amiodarone: pulmonary fibrosis (increasing dyspnea, cough, hepatic dysfunction—changes in liver function tests, jaundice); vision changes, photosensitivity
  e. Digoxin: anorexia, nausea, vomiting; blurred or double vision; yellow-green halos; new-onset dysrhythmias.
- Use an infusion pump to administer intravenous infusions. Monitor the dose, and assess its appropriateness (in mg/min or mcg · kg^{-1} · min^{-1}).

Heath Education For The Client and Family

- Take the drug exactly as prescribed. Do not skip or double doses. Check with your physician if a dose is missed.
- Take your pulse and record the rate daily before rising. Count the pulse for a full minute. Bring the record with you to each office or clinic visit.
- Report the following to the physician: irregular pulse rate or rhythm, dizziness, eye pain, changes in vision, skin rashes or color changes, wheezing or other respiratory problems, and changes in behavior.

Pacemaker Therapy

A **pacemaker** is a pulse generator used to provide an electrical stimulus to the heart when the heart fails to generate or conduct its own at a rate that maintains the cardiac output. The pulse generator is connected to leads (insulated wires) passed intravenously into the heart or sutured directly to the epicardium. The leads sense intrinsic electrical activity of the heart and provide an electrical stimulus to the heart when necessary (pacing).

Pacemakers are used to treat both acute and chronic conduction defects, such as third-degree AV block. They also may be used to treat bradydysrhythmias and tachydysrhythmias.

Temporary pacemakers use an external pulse generator (Figure 22–53 ■) attached to a lead threaded intravenously into the right ventricle, to temporary pacing wires implanted during cardiac surgery, or to external conductive pads placed on the chest wall for emergency pacing. Permanent pacemakers use an

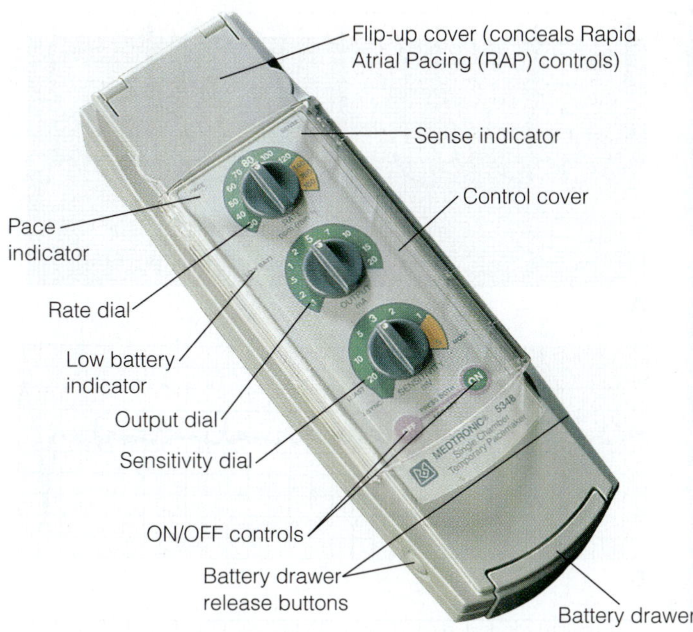

Figure 22–53 ■ Programmable settings on a temporary pacemaker.

Courtesy of Medtronics, Inc.

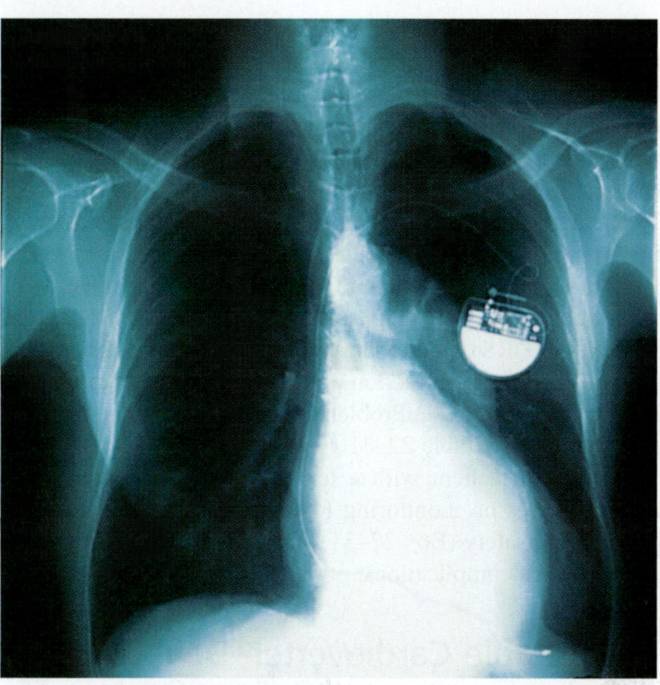

Figure 22–55 ■ A permanent transvenous (endocardial) pacemaker with the lead placed in the right ventricule via the subclavian vein.

Source: Phototake NYC.

internal pulse generator placed in a subcutaneous pocket in the subclavian space or abdominal wall. The generator connects to leads sewn directly onto the heart (epicardial) or passed transvenously into the heart (endocardial). Epicardial pacemakers (Figure 22–54 ■) require surgical exposure of the heart. Leads may be placed during cardiac surgery or using a small subxiphoid incision to expose on the heart. Transvenous pacemaker leads are positioned in the right heart via the cephalic, subclavian, or jugular vein (Figure 22–55 ■). Local anesthesia can be used for permanent pacemaker insertion.

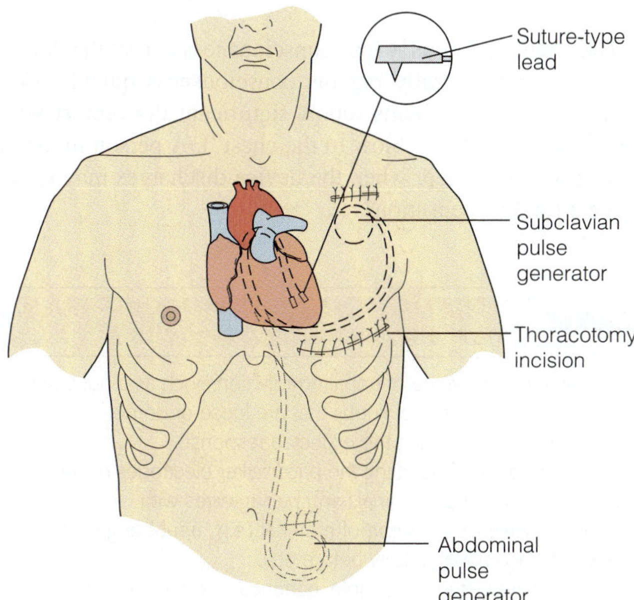

Figure 22–54 ■ A permanent epicardial pacemaker. The pulse generator may be placed in subcutaneous pockets in the subclavian or abdominal regions.

Pacemakers are programmed to stimulate the atria or the ventricles (single-chamber pacing) or both (dual-chamber pacing). Table 22–30 defines terms used to describe pacemaker modes and functions. The most commonly used pacemakers

TABLE 22–30 Terms Used to Describe Pacemaker Functions

TERM	DEFINITION
Asynchronous pacing	Pacemaker delivers a pacing stimulus at a set rate regardless of intrinsic cardiac activity.
Base rate	Rate at which the pacemaker paces when no cardiac activity is sensed.
Capture	The ability of the pacing stimulus to generate a cardiac depolarization.
Demand pacing	Pacemaker delivers a pacing stimulus only when the intrinsic rate falls below the pacemaker's base rate.
Dual-chamber pacing	Allows both the atria and the ventricles to be paced; most frequently used permanent pacing mode.
Lead	An insulated wire that senses intrinsic cardiac activity and delivers a pacing stimulus as programmed.
Output	The electrical stimulus delivered by the pulse generator.
Pacing spike	A small vertical spike noted on the electrocardiogram with every pacemaker stimulus.
Sensing	The pacemaker's ability to identify and respond to intrinsic cardiac activity.
Single-chamber pacing	Pacing of only the atria or the ventricles, not both; most commonly used temporary pacing mode.

Source: Adapted from S. L. Woods, E. S. Froelicher, S. A. Motzer, & E. Bridges. (2004). *Cardiac Nursing* (5th ed.) Philadelphia: Lippincott.

either sense activity in and pace the ventricles only or sense activity in and pace both the atria and the ventricles. Dual-chamber or atrioventricular sequential pacing stimulates both chambers of the heart in sequence. AV pacing imitates the normal sequence of atrial contraction followed by ventricular contraction, improving cardiac output.

Pacing is detected on the ECG strip by the presence of pacing artifact (Figure 22–56 ■). A sharp spike is noted before the P wave with atrial pacing and before the QRS complex with ventricular pacing. Pacing spikes are seen before both the P wave and QRS complex in AV sequential pacing. Capture is noted if there is a contraction of the chamber immediately following the pacer spike. Problems in sensing, pacing, and capture are noted in Table 22–31.

Care of the client with a temporary or permanent pacemaker focuses on monitoring for pacemaker malfunctioning, maintaining safety (Box 22–31), and preventing infection and postoperative complications.

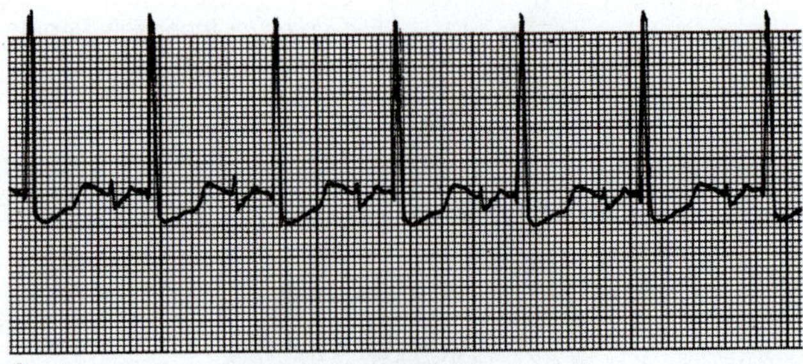
A

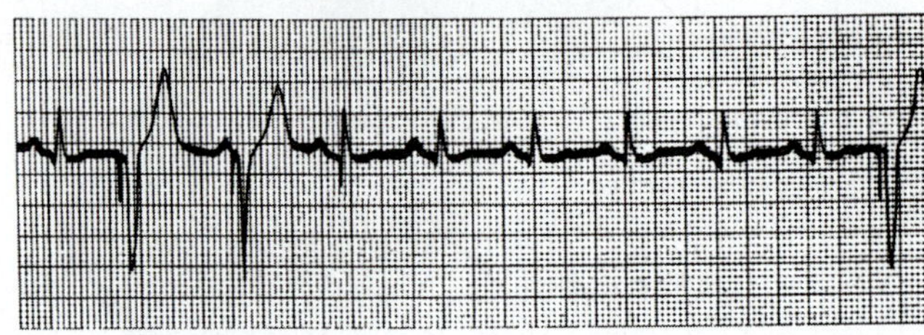
B

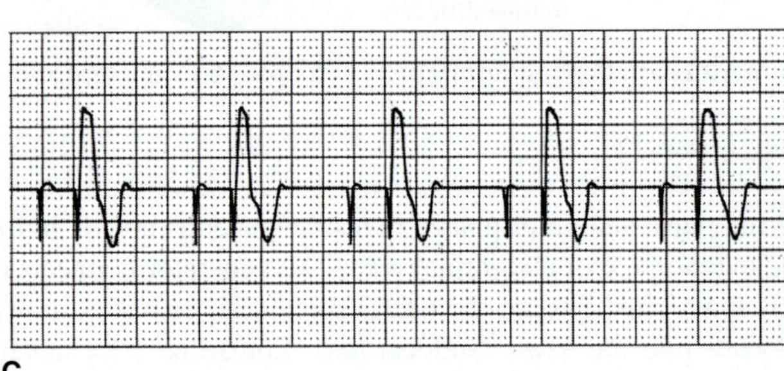
C

Figure 22–56 ■ Pacing artifacts. *A,* Atrial pacing and ventricular sensing. Note the pacer spike preceding the P wave. *B,* Ventricular demand pacing. Note the absence of pacer spikes when the client's natural rhythm predominates. *C,* Atrioventricular pacing. Note the pacer spikes preceding both P waves and QRS complexes.

Implantable Cardioverter–Defibrillator

The implantable cardioverter-defibrillator (ICD) detects life-threatening changes in the cardiac rhythm and automatically delivers an electric shock to convert the dysrhythmia back into a normal rhythm. ICDs are used for survivors of SCD, clients with recurrent ventricular tachycardia, and clients with demonstrated risk factors for SCD. ICDs can deliver a shock as needed, provide pacing on demand, and store ECG records of tachycardic episodes (Woods et al., 2004).

A pulse generator connected to lead electrodes for rhythm detection and current delivery is implanted in the left pectoral region. The lead is threaded transvenously to the apex of the right ventricle. The ICD is programmed to sense a change in heart rate or rhythm. When it detects a potentially lethal rhythm, it shocks the heart to convert the rhythm. The device can be programmed or reprogrammed at the bedside as necessary. The ICD may be tested before discharge.

Local or general anesthesia is used, and the client may be discharged within 24 hours. The lithium-powered battery must be surgically replaced every 5 years. Complications and nursing care are similar to those for a client having a permanent pacemaker implant.

The client may briefly lose consciousness before the device discharges but typically regains consciousness quickly after the episode. Some clients report significant discomfort with ICD discharge (like a "blow to the chest"). A person in direct contact with the client when the device discharges may experience a tingling sensation.

Box 22–31 **Safety for Clients With a Temporary Pacemaker**

- Ensure that all electrical equipment in use has a grounded plug; do not use adapters or extension cords.
- Encourage use of battery-powered equipment (e.g., electric razor).
- Remove any damaged electrical equipment from the unit, including equipment that
  a. has been abused (e.g., has been dropped or in which liquid has been spilled).
  b. has given anyone a shock.
  c. has frayed, worn, or otherwise damaged electrical cords or plugs.
  d. has other evidence of impaired function, such as a hot smell during use or control knobs that are loose or do not consistently produce the expected response.
- Wear gloves when handling the pacemaker electrodes or wires.
- Insulate pacemaker terminals and pacing wires with nonconductive, moistureproof material (e.g., a rubber glove).
- Test the pacemaker battery before use.
- Keep a spare pacemaker, cable, batteries, and battery tester available at all times.
- Immediately report any apparent deviation from expected pacemaker function.

TABLE 22–31 Potential Pacemaker Problems and Corrective Strategies

PROBLEM	POSSIBLE CAUSES	CORRECTIVE MEASURES
UNDERSENSING		
Device fails to detect existing cardiac depolarizations and therefore competes with the native rhythms. 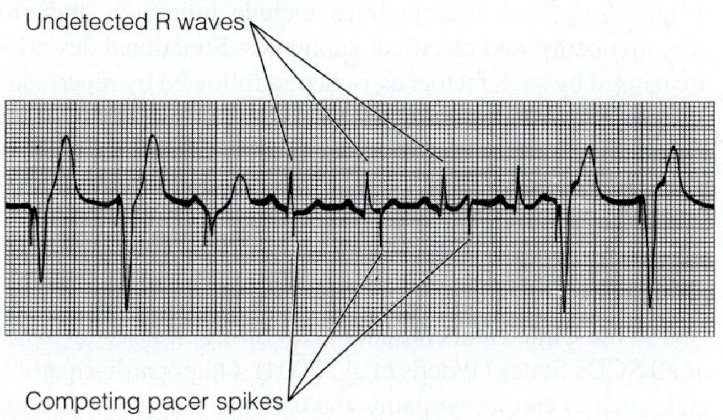	Lead disconnected from pacer or from viable myocardium. Sensitivity set too low. Lead fracture. Low battery.	Check connection of lead to pacer. Increase sensitivity. Reposition or change lead. Change battery.
OVERSENSING		
Device detects noncardiac electrical events, interprets them as cardiac depolarizations, and therefore is wrongly inhibited from pacing. 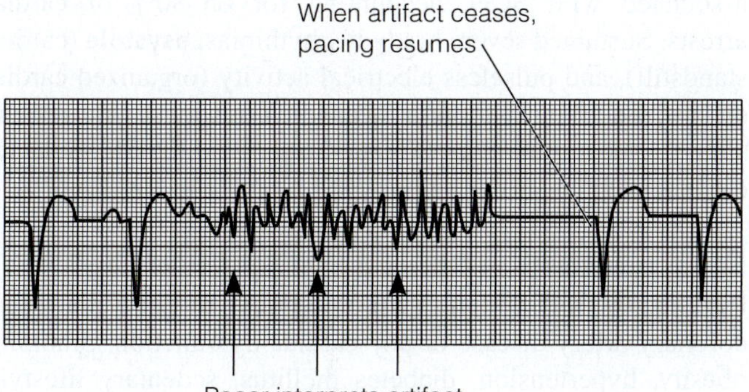	Sensitivity set too high. Interference from electrical sources (ungrounded equipment, short circuits) is detected and misinterpreted by the device. Lead disconnected from pacer or from viable myocardium.	Decrease sensitivity (turn sensing control to a LARGER number). Remove all ungrounded electrical equipment or have it evaluated by hospital engineers. Check connection of lead to pacer.
NONCAPTURE		
Device emits stimuli that fail to depolarize the myocardium. 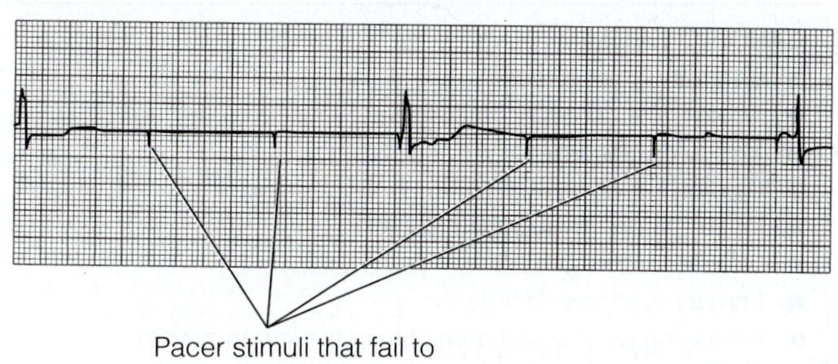	Output set too low in the noncaptured chamber. Lead fracture. High pacing threshold caused by medication or metabolic changes. Low battery.	Increase output in the noncaptured chamber. Reposition or change lead. Alter medication regimen, correct metabolic changes. Change battery.

Source: From C. L. Witherell. (1994). Cardiac rhythm control devices. *Critical Care Nursing Clinics of North America, 6*(1), 92.

Cardiac Mapping and Catheter Ablation

Cardiac mapping and catheter ablation are used to locate and destroy an ectopic focus. These diagnostic and therapeutic measures use electrophysiology techniques and can be performed in the cardiac catheterization laboratory. Cardiac mapping is used to identify the site of earliest impulse formation in the atria or ventricles. Intracardiac and extracardiac catheter electrodes and computer technology are used to pinpoint the ectopic site on a map of the heart. These same catheters can be used to deliver the ablative intervention.

Ablation destroys, removes, or isolates an ectopic focus. In most instances, radiofrequency energy produced by high-frequency alternating current is used to create heat as it passes through tissue. Catheter ablation is used to treat supraventricular tachycardias, atrial fibrillation and flutter, and in some cases, paroxysmal ventricular tachycardia (Woods et al., 2004). Anticoagulant therapy may be started after catheter ablation to reduce the risk of clot formation at the ablation site.

Other Therapies

In addition to medications and interventional techniques, other measures may be used to treat selected dysrhythmias. Vagal maneuvers that stimulate the parasympathetic nervous system may be used to slow the heart rate in supraventricular tachycardias. These maneuvers include carotid sinus massage and the Valsalva maneuver. Carotid sinus massage is performed only by a physician during continuous cardiac monitoring. Excessive slowing of the heart rate may result. The **Valsalva maneuver**, or forced exhalation against a closed glottis (e.g., bearing down), increases intrathoracic pressure and vagal tone, slowing the pulse rate.

Sudden Cardiac Death

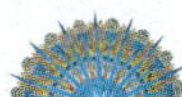

Sudden cardiac death (SCD) is defined as unexpected death occurring within 1 hour of the onset of cardiovascular symptoms. It usually is caused by ventricular fibrillation and cardiac arrest. **Cardiac arrest** is the cessation of heart function that precedes biologic death. Worldwide, less than 6% of out-of-hospital victims of cardiac arrest survive. In communities of North America that have organized lay rescuer and automated external defibrillator programs, the survival rate is significantly better, ranging from 49–74% when a witnessed arrest caused by ventricular fibrillation occurs (AHA, 2005a).

Almost 50% of all deaths from coronary heart disease are attributed to SCD. Risk factors for SCD are those associated with coronary heart disease. Advancing age and male gender are powerful risk factors. After age 65, the gap between male and female incidence of SCD narrows (Kasper et al., 2005). Clients with dysrhythmias such as recurrent ventricular tachycardia may have a higher risk of SCD. Women with acute MI, however, are more likely to present with cardiac arrest and cardiogenic shock than with ventricular tachycardia (Kasper et al., 2005).

Evidence of coronary heart disease with significant atherosclerosis and narrowing of two or more major coronary arteries is found in 75% of SCD victims. Although most have had previous MI, only 20–30% have recent acute MI. An acute change in cardiovascular status precedes cardiac arrest by up to 1 hour; however, the onset often is instantaneous or abrupt. Tachycardia develops, and the number of PVCs increases. This is followed by a run of ventricular tachycardia that deteriorates into ventricular fibrillation (Kasper et al., 2005).

Abnormalities of myocardial structure or function also contribute. Structural abnormalities include infarction, hypertrophy, myopathy, and electrical anomalies. Functional deviations are caused by such factors as ischemia followed by reperfusion, altered homeostasis, autonomic nervous system and hormone interactions, and toxic effects. The interactions of the two cause myocardial instability and may precipitate fatal dysrhythmias.

Etiology

In the United States, SCD claims more than 300,000 lives per year in the United and coronary heart disease causes up to 80% of all SCDs States (Woods et al., 2004). Other cardiac pathologies, such as cardiomyopathy and valvular disorders, also may lead to SCD. Noncardiac causes of sudden death include electrocution, pulmonary embolism, and rapid blood loss from a ruptured aortic aneurysm.

Ventricular fibrillation is the most common dysrhythmia associated with SCD, accounting for 65–80% of cardiac arrests. Sustained severe bradydysrhythmias, **asystole** (cardiac standstill), and pulseless electrical activity (organized cardiac electrical activity without a mechanical response) are responsible for most remaining SCDs (Kasper et al., 2005). Selected cardiac and noncardiac causes of SCD are listed in Box 22–32.

Risk Factors

Risk factors for sudden death are similar to those that cause coronary artery disease or any cardiac dysfunction. Smoking, obesity, hypertension, diabetes mellitus, sedentary lifestyle,

Box 22–32 **Selected Causes of Sudden Cardiac Death**

CARDIAC CAUSES

- Coronary heart disease
- Reperfusion following ischemia
- Myocardial hypertrophy
- Cardiomyopathy
- Inflammatory myocardial disorders
- Valve disorders
- Primary electrical disorders
- Dissecting or ruptured aortic or ventricular aneurysm
- Cardiac drug toxicity

NONCARDIAC CAUSES

- Pulmonary embolism
- Cerebral hemorrhage
- Autonomic dysfunction
- Choking
- Electrical shock
- Electrolyte and acid–base imbalances

and high-fat diets can result in cardiac disease. Alterations in cardiac function can impact the electrical activity resulting in dysrhythmias.

Manifestations

Sudden cardiac death may be preceded by typical manifestations of acute coronary syndrome or MI, including severe chest pain, dyspnea or orthopnea, and palpitations or lightheadedness. The event itself is abrupt, with complete loss of consciousness and death within minutes. If ventricular tachycardia precedes cardiac arrest, consciousness and mentation may be impaired prior to collapse and loss of consciousness.

Collaborative Care

The goal of care for the client with SCD is to restore cardiac output and tissue perfusion. Treatment measures are initiated as soon as clinical cardiac arrest is verified by the absence of respirations and carotid or femoral pulses. Basic and advanced cardiac life support measures must be instituted within 2–4 minutes of cardiac arrest to prevent permanent neurologic damage and ischemic injury to other organs.

BASIC LIFE SUPPORT Basic life support begins with identification of the cardiac arrest and initiation of an emergency response. Providers trained in use of the automated external defibrillator should immediately defibrillate the client in ventricular fibrillation. Self-adhesive conductive pads attached to connecting cables are positioned on the chest (Figure 22–57 ■). The automated external defibrillator analyzes the rhythm and advises the provider to charge the device if ventricular fibrillation is detected. After all personnel have been warned to stand clear, the shock button is depressed to deliver a shock. Following the shock, CPR is immediately initiated. After approximately 2 minutes, or five cycles of CPR, the rhythm is evaluated and circulation checked. The sequence of analysis, shock, CPR is continued, and advanced cardiac life support protocols are initiated (AHA, 2005a).

Cardiopulmonary resuscitation (CPR) is a mechanical attempt to maintain tissue perfusion and oxygenation using oral resuscitation and external cardiac compressions. All health care providers need to be proficient in CPR. The technique should be performed according to AHA guidelines and hospital protocol (Box 22–33) Research demonstrates clear benefit from sustained, effective chest compressions, yet compressions often are interrupted for ventilation, assessment of pulses, and other measures. Many clients are excessively ventilated and underperfused during CPR (Sanders & Ewy, 2005). The AHA 2005 guidelines for CPR reflect this research (AHA, 2005a). New guidelines are anticipated in 2010 and will be found at http://www.americanheart.org/presenter.jhtml?identifier=3011764

Cardiopulmonary resuscitation carries a high risk for both cardiac and noncardiac trauma. CPR-related complications include injuries to the skin, thorax, upper airway, abdomen, lungs, heart, and great vessels. These complications can be minimized by adhering to accepted CPR techniques.

ADVANCED LIFE SUPPORT Advanced life support, provided by specially trained health care personnel, includes advanced airway support (insertion of a laryngeal mask airway, esophageal–tracheal Combitube, or endotracheal intubation) to maintain the airway and oxygenation, use of intravenous drugs following specific protocols, and additional interventions, such as repeated defibrillation procedures and cardiac pacing. Epinephrine, vasopressin, sodium bicarbonate, and antidysrhythmic drugs, such as amiodarone, bretylium, lidocaine, procainamide, magnesium sulfate, and atropine are used to attempt to restore and maintain an effective cardiac rhythm.

POSTRESUSCITATION CARE Clients who experience SCD associated with ventricular fibrillation and acute MI have the best prognosis (Kasper et al., 2005). The client is transferred to a coronary care unit, and MI treatment measures are instituted. Antidysrhythmic drugs may be continued for 24–48 hours to reduce the risk of subsequent episodes of ventricular fibrillation.

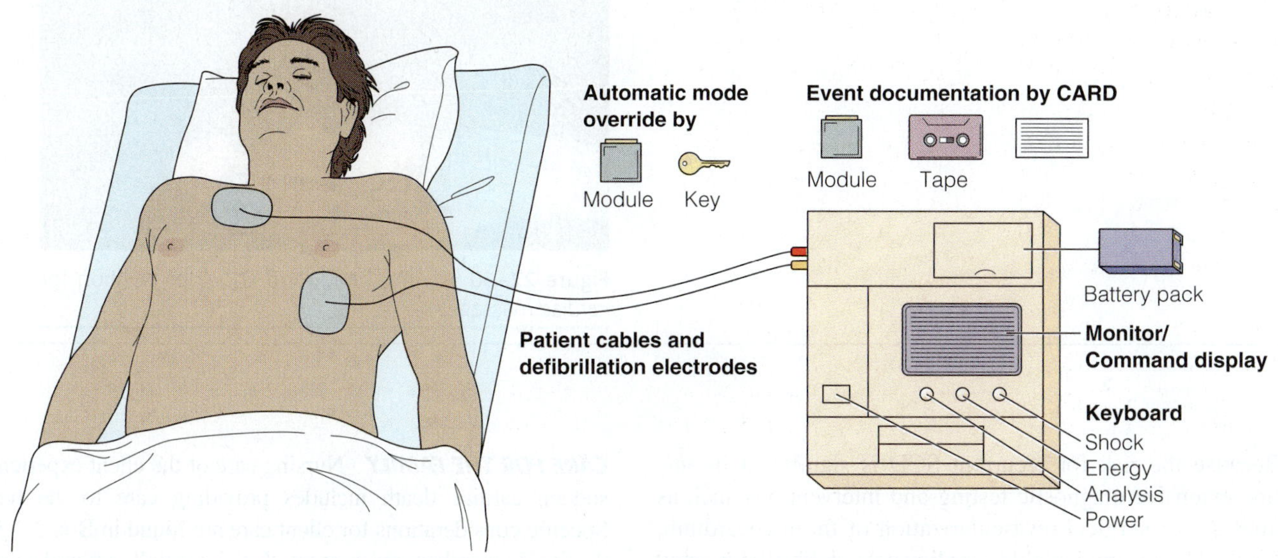

Figure 22–57 ■ Schematic of an automated external defrillator (AED) attached to a client.

Box 22–33 Cardiopulmonary Resuscitation

1. Assess for responsiveness; shake the client and shout.
2. Call for help. Dial 911 (if outside the health care facility) or initiate the institutional code or cardiac arrest procedure.
3. Open the airway using the head-tilt/chin-lift maneuver. Simultaneously press down on the forehead with one hand while lifting the chin upward with the other (Figure 22–58 ■).
4. Check for breathing; look and listen. Inspect the chest for rise and fall with respirations; listen and feel for air movement through the nose or mouth. This step should take no more than 10 seconds.
5. If not breathing, begin rescue breathing using a pocket mask, mouth shield, or bag-valve mask (see Figure 22–45). Administer two breaths (1 second per breath), observing for rise of the chest with each breath.
6. Check the carotid or femoral artery for a pulse (≤10 second).
7. If a pulse is present, continue rescue breathing, administering 8–10 breaths per minute, until help arrives or spontaneous respirations resume. Recheck the carotid pulse every 2 minutes.
8. If no pulse is present, analyze rhythm and defibrillate or, if the arrest was not witnessed or an automated external defibrillator is not available, initiate external cardiac compressions. Place on a firm surface. Position the heel of one hand in the center of the chest between the nipples (child and adult), with the other hand on top and the fingers either interlocked or extended (Figure 22–59 ■).
9. Initiate hard and fast cardiac compressions, pressing straight down to depress the sternum 1.5–2 in., keeping the elbows locked and positioning the shoulders directly over the hands (Figure 22–60 ■). Release pressure completely between compressions, but do not lift the hands from the chest.
10. Compress the chest at a rate of approximately 100 times per minute. With one- or two-rescuer CPR, provide two breaths after every 30 compressions. Assess the pulse after five complete cycles of 30 compressions and two breaths; continue CPR until help arrives.

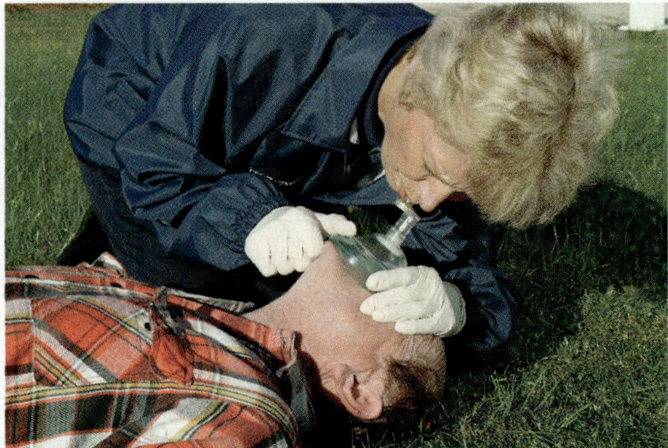

Figure 22–58 ■ Head-tilt/chin-lift maneuver using a bag-mask.

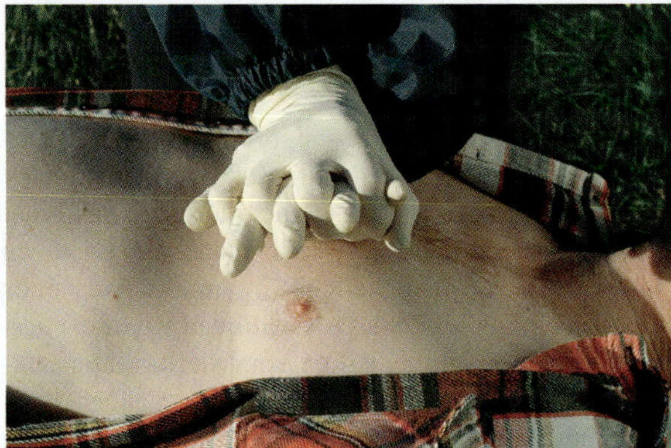

Figure 22–59 ■ Placement of hands on the sternum between the nipples.

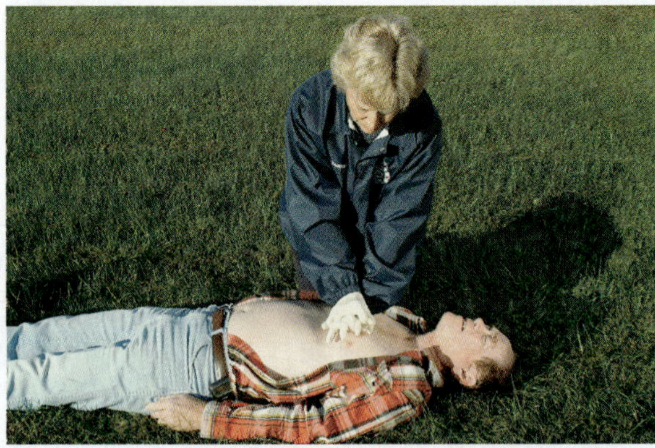

Figure 22–60 ■ Arm, hand, and shoulder position for cardiac massage.

Because the risk for recurrent SCD is significant in survivors, extensive diagnostic testing and interventions such as angioplasty or surgical revascularization of the myocardium, ablation, or an implantable cardioverter–defibrillator may be indicated.

CARE FOR THE FAMILY Nursing care of the client experiencing sudden cardiac death includes providing care to the family. Specific considerations for client care are found in Box 22–34. If the family members are present, they are usually offered a private consultation room in which to await the outcome. If the family

Box 22–34 Nursing Care of Clients Experiencing Sudden Cardiac Death

Nursing care of the client experiencing sudden cardiac death requires prompt recognition of the event and immediate initiation of basic and advanced life support protocols. Fast and effective cardiac compressions and early defibrillation of unstable ventricular tachycardia and fibrillation are the most important keys to survival of cardiac arrest victims. Important concepts of emergency cardiac care include the following:

- Treat the client, not the monitor. Recognize signs and symptoms of cardiac compromise early.
- Activate the emergency medical services system (call a code or 911).
- Begin and continue basic cardiac life support principles throughout the resuscitation effort.
- Continually assess the effectiveness of emergency interventions.
- Defibrillate pulseless ventricular tachycardia or fibrillation as soon as possible.
- Initiate advance life support protocols early.

members are not present, they are notified that their family member is not doing well and asked to come to the hospital as soon as possible. The situation is presented in a careful manner to prevent the family from racing to the hospital, precipitating an automobile crash. The nurse offers pastoral care or the family's choice of spiritual support to help during this difficult time. Attendance of family members during resuscitation efforts is controversial and depends on institutional protocols and family desires.

After successful resuscitation, the nurse provides care specific to the client's underlying disease processes and needs. Intravenous infusions, such as lidocaine, bretylium, or dopamine, may be ordered to prevent further dysrhythmias and maintain hemodynamic stability. The nurse provides honest information about the client's condition to the family in a supportive manner, and assesses the family's coping abilities and resources.

If the client does not survive the arrest, the nurse provides postmortem care to the client and emotional and spiritual support to the family.

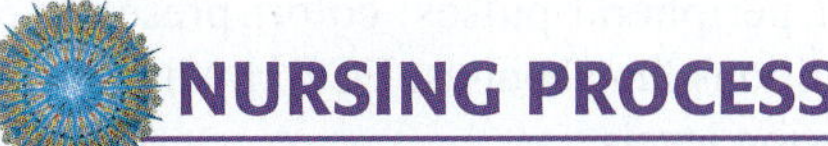

NURSING PROCESS

Caring for the client with cardiac dysrhythmias requires the ability to recognize, identify, and in some cases, promptly treat the dysrhythmia. The urgency of intervention is determined by the effects of the dysrhythmia on the client. Nursing care focuses on maintaining cardiac output, monitoring the response to therapy, and teaching. Nurses working in critical care areas are likely to care for clients with dysrhythmias on a regular basis and should be certified in advanced cardiac life support.

Health promotion measures to prevent coronary heart disease also reduce the risk for dysrhythmias. In most cases, dysrhythmias develop as a result of ischemic or structural changes in the heart rather than develop in isolation. Advise clients who are at risk or who complain of occasional palpitations or "flutters" in their chest to reduce their intake of caffeine and other SNS stimulants, such as excess chocolate.

Assessment

Assessment is vital before treating any suspected dysrhythmia. What appears to be ventricular tachycardia on the monitor may be the client scratching or even brushing teeth. Apparent asystole on the monitor may be the result of a loose electrode patch. Similarly, a heart rate of 52 bpm may not affect the overall cardiac output in some clients.

Obtain the following data when assessing the client with a dysrhythmia:

- *Health history.* Complaints of palpitations (ask for further definition of palpitations), "fluttering" sensations, or a sensation of the heart racing; episodes of dizziness, light-headedness, or syncope (fainting); timing (duration, time of day); correlation with food or beverage intake or activity; presence of chest pain, shortness of breath, or other associated symptoms; history of heart or endocrine disease (e.g., hyperthyroidism); current medications.
- *Physical examination.* Level of consciousness; vital signs, including apical pulse for a full minute; regularity

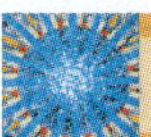

CLIENT TEACHING Home Care for Clients With Dysrhythmias

Dysrhythmias have a significant physical and psychological impact on the client and all family members. Many of these clients and their families are under a great deal of stress from frequent hospitalizations, experimentation with therapies, frustration, and the fear of sudden cardiac death. A major teaching effort focuses on coping strategies and lifestyle changes, as well as on specific management of prescribed therapies. Include the following topics as appropriate when teaching the client and family for home care:

- Function, maintenance, precautions, and signs of malfunction or complications of any implanted device, such as a pacemaker or implantable cardioverter–defibrillator
- Monitoring pulse rate and rhythm
- Activity or dietary restrictions, and any potential effects of the dysrhythmia or its treatment on lifestyle
- Medication management to reduce the risk of dysrhythmias, including the desired and potential adverse effects of antidysrhythmic drugs
- Specific instructions related to planned diagnostic tests or procedures
- The importance of follow-up visits with the cardiologist
- The importance of and where to obtain training in cardiopulmonary resuscitation for the client and family members.

In addition, discuss fears related to treatment or implanted devices, such as that of shocking a significant other during close contact or sexual activity. Explain that if a shock occurs, the partner may feel a slight buzz or tingling but should not be harmed. Refer to, and encourage the client and family to attend, a peer support group for the specific condition.

and amplitude of peripheral pulses; color; presence of dyspnea or adventitious lung sounds; ECG rhythm analysis; oxygen saturation levels.

Diagnosis

Potential diagnoses for the client experiencing SCD include the following:

- Ineffective Tissue Perfusion: Cerebral related to ineffective cardiac output
- Decreased Cardiac Output
- Activity Intolerance
- Impaired Spontaneous Ventilation related to cardiac arrest
- Spiritual Distress related to unexplained sudden cardiac death
- Disturbed Thought Processes related to compromised cerebral circulation
- Fear related to risk for future episodes of sudden cardiac death.

Plan

Goals for client care may include the following:

- The client will have adequate oxygenation, as evidenced by arterial blood gas analysis, respiratory status, and client condition.
- The client will have cardiac output adequate to meet the body's perfusion requirements.
- The client will provide self-care after discharge.
- The client will comply with the medical treatment regimen.
- The client will perform proper medication self-administration and care of implanted devices.
- The client will verbalize symptoms to be reported to provider if they occur.

Implementation

The effect of the dysrhythmia on cardiac output is the priority of nursing care.

Decreased Cardiac Output

Dysrhythmias can affect cardiac output. Bradycardias decrease cardiac output if the stroke volume does not increase to compensate for the slow heart rate. Tachycardia reduces diastolic filling time, affecting stroke volume and coronary artery perfusion. Loss of the atrial kick in junctional rhythms, atrial fibrillation, and AV blocks also decreases ventricular filling and cardiac output. In ventricular fibrillation, loss of ventricular contractions causes cardiac arrest and no cardiac output.

PRACTICE ALERT

Before treating any dysrhythmia, assess the client, not just the monitor! Loose electrode pads, disconnected leads or cables, and muscle movement can simulate critical dysrhythmias. The client's condition is the best indicator of the need for treatment.

- Assess for decreased cardiac output: decreased level of consciousness; tachycardia; tachypnea; hypotension; low oxygen saturation; diaphoresis; low urine output; cool, clammy, mottled skin; pallor or cyanosis; and diminished peripheral pulses. Initial signs of decreased cardiac output may be subtle, such as decreased level of consciousness. Early recognition of the dysrhythmia's effect on cardiac output facilitates appropriate treatment and may prevent further adverse effects.
- Monitor ECG; post the ECG strip every shift and when rhythm changes occur. Documenting cardiac rhythm provides a record of disease progression and treatment effectiveness.

PRACTICE ALERT

Assess vital signs, ECG, and oxygen saturation every 5–15 minutes during acute dysrhythmic episodes and during antidysrhythmic drug infusions. These data provide a record of cardiac output during the dysrhythmia. Antidysrhythmic drugs can adversely affect heart rate, rhythm, and blood pressure, further decreasing cardiac output.

- Assess for underlying causes of dysrhythmias, such as hypovolemia, hypoxia, anemia, vagal stimulation, or medications. Sinus tachycardia often develops in response to tissue hypoxia. Vagal stimulation (e.g., the Valsalva maneuver) can precipitate bradycardia.
- Assess serum electrolytes (especially potassium, calcium, and magnesium) and digitalis and antidysrhythmic drug levels as indicated. Report abnormal values. Electrolyte imbalances affect cardiac depolarization and repolarization and may cause dysrhythmias. Toxic levels of digitalis and antidysrhythmic drugs can precipitate further dysrhythmias. Impaired renal or hepatic function increases the risk for toxicity, as does aging.

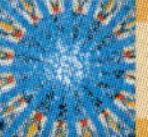

CLIENT TEACHING Home Care for Clients at Risk for Sudden Cardiac Death

The risk for a future episode of sudden cardiac death requires careful and effective teaching for home care before discharge. Discuss the following topics with the client and family:

- Risk factor reduction for coronary heart disease
- Planned diagnostic studies to identify the cause of sudden cardiac death and possible interventions
- The risks and benefits of an implantable cardioverter–defibrillator if appropriate
- The importance of carrying a card at all times listing all current medications and the health care provider
- Early manifestations or warning signs of cardiac arrest
- The importance of training and maintaining proficiency in performing cardiopulmonary resuscitation (provide referral to local training providers or scheduled classes through the American Heart Association or American Red Cross).

Box 22–35 **Nursing Care for the Client Having a Permanent Pacemaker Implant**

PREOPERATIVE CARE

- Provide routine preoperative care and teaching.
- Assess knowledge and understanding of the procedure, clarifying and expanding on existing knowledge as needed. *Clarifying knowledge, providing information, and conveying emotional support reduces anxiety and fear and allows the client to develop a realistic outlook regarding pacer therapy.*
- Place electrocardiographic monitor electrodes away from potential incision sites. *This helps preserve skin integrity.*
- Teach range-of-motion (ROM) exercises for the affected side. *ROM exercises of the affected arm and shoulder prevent stiffness and impaired function following pacemaker insertion.*

POSTOPERATIVE CARE

- Provide postoperative monitoring, analgesia, and care.
- Obtain a chest x-ray as ordered. *A postoperative chest x-ray is used to identify lead location and detect possible complications, such as pneumothorax or pleural effusion.*
- Position for comfort. Minimize movement of the affected arm and shoulder during the initial postoperative period. *Restricting movement minimizes discomfort on the operative side and allows the leads to become anchored, reducing the risk of dislodging.*
- Assist with gentle ROM exercises at least three times daily, beginning 24 hours after pacemaker implantation. *ROM exercises help restore normal shoulder movement and prevent contractures on the affected side.*
- Monitor pacemaker function with cardiac monitoring or intermittent ECGs. Report pacemaker problems to the physician:
    a. Failure to pace: *This may indicate battery depletion, damage or dislodgement of pacer wires, or inappropriate sensing.*
    b. Failure to capture (the pacemaker stimulus is not followed by ventricular depolarization): *The electrical output of the pacemaker may not be adequate, or the lead may be dislodged.*
    c. Improper sensing (the pacemaker is firing, or not firing, regardless of the intrinsic rate): *This increases the risk for decreased cardiac output and dysrhythmias.*
    d. Runaway pacemaker (a pacemaker firing at a rapid rate): *This may be the result of a generator malfunction or problems with sensing.*
    e. Hiccups: *A lead positioned near the diaphragm can stimulate it, causing hiccups. Hiccups may occur in extremely thin clients or may indicate a medical emergency with perforation of the right ventricle by the pacing electrode tip.*
- Assess for dysrhythmias, and treat as indicated. *Until the catheter is "seated" or adheres to the myocardium, its movement may cause myocardial irritability and dysrhythmias. Fibrotic tissue develops within 2–3 days.*
- Document the date of pacemaker insertion, the model and type, and settings. *This information is important for future reference.*
- Immediately report signs of potential complications, including myocardial perforation, cardiac tamponade, pneumothorax or hemothorax, emboli, skin breakdown, bleeding, infection, endocarditis, or poor wound healing. *Early identification of complications allows for aggressive intervention.*
- Provide a pacemaker identification card, including the manufacturer's name, model number, mode of operation, rate parameters, and expected battery life. *This card provides a reference for the client and future health care providers.*

HOME CARE

Provide appropriate teaching for the client and family about the following:

- Placement of the pacemaker generator and leads in relation to the heart.
- How the pacemaker works and the rate at which it is set.
- Battery replacement. Most pacemaker batteries last 6–12 years. Replacement requires an outpatient surgery to open the subcutaneous pocket and replace the battery.
- How to take and record the pulse rate. Instruct to assess pulse daily before arising and to notify the physician if 5 or more bpm slower than the preset pacemaker rate.
- Incision care and signs of infection. Bruising may be present following surgery.
- Signs of pacemaker malfunction to report, including dizziness, fainting, fatigue, weakness, chest pain, or palpitations.
- Activity restrictions as ordered. This usually is limited to contact sports, which may damage the generator, and to avoiding heavy lifting for 2 months after surgery.
- Resume sexual activity as recommended by the physician. Avoid positions that cause pressure on the site.
- Avoid tight-fitting clothing over the pacemaker site to reduce irritation and avoid skin breakdown.
- Carry the pacemaker identification card at all times, and wear a Medic-Alert bracelet or tag.
- Notify all care providers of the pacemaker.
- Do not hold or use certain electrical devices over the pacemaker site, including household appliances or tools, garage door openers, antitheft devices, or burglar alarms. The pacemaker will set off airport security detectors; notify security officials of its presence.
- Maintain follow-up care with the physician as recommended.

- Be prepared to administer antidysrhythmic medications as indicated. Implement advanced cardiac life support protocols as needed. Emergency drugs should be readily available, especially on units with high-risk clients. See Box 22–30 for drugs used to treat common dysrhythmias that may affect cardiac output.
- If appropriate, instruct to perform the Valsalva maneuver (bear down as if straining or coughing) for supraventricular tachycardia or ventricular tachycardia without angina. Vagal maneuvers stimulate the parasympathetic system and may terminate some dysrhythmias. The Valsalva maneuver is contraindicated if chest pain occurs with the dysrhythmia.
- Prepare to assist with cardioversion. Prepare the client per orders or hospital protocol. Explain the procedure to reduce anxiety. Have emergency equipment readily available. Elective or emergency cardioversion is a treatment of choice for certain dysrhythmias.

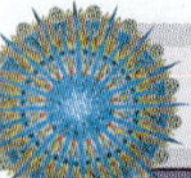

NURSING CARE PLAN A Client With Supraventricular Tachycardia

ASSESSMENT

Elisa Vasquez, 53 years old, is admitted to the cardiac unit with complaints of palpitations, light-headedness, and shortness of breath. Her history reveals rheumatic fever at age 12, with subsequent rheumatic heart disease and mitral stenosis. An intravenous line is in place, and she is receiving oxygen. Marcia Lewin, RN, is assigned to Ms. Vasquez.

Ms. Lewin's assessment reveals that Ms. Vasquez is moderately anxious. Her electrocardiogram (ECG) shows supraventricular tachycardia with a rate of 154 bpm. Vital signs are as follows: temperature, 98.8°F (37.1°C); respirations, 26/minute; and blood pressure, 95/60 mmHg. Peripheral pulses are weak but equal. Mucous membranes are pale pink, and skin is cool and dry. Fine crackles are noted in both lung bases. A loud S_3 gallop and a diastolic murmur are noted. Ms. Vasquez is still complaining of palpitations and tells Ms. Lewin, "I feel so nervous and weak and dizzy." Ms. Vasquez's cardiologist orders 2.5 mg of verapamil to be given slowly via intravenous push and tells Ms. Lewin to prepare to assist with synchronized cardioversion if drug therapy does not control the ventricular rate.

DIAGNOSES

- Decreased Cardiac Output related to inadequate ventricular filling associated with rapid tachycardia
- Ineffective Tissue Perfusion: Cerebral/Cardiopulmonary/Peripheral related to decreased cardiac output
- Anxiety related to unknown outcome of altered health state

PLANNING

Goals of care include the following:

- The client will maintain adequate cardiac output and tissue perfusion.
- The client will demonstrate a ventricular rate within normal limits and stable vital signs.
- The client will verbalize reduced anxiety.
- The client will verbalize an understanding of the rationale for the treatment measures to control the heart rate.

IMPLEMENTATION

- Provide oxygen per nasal cannula at 4 L/min.
- Continuously monitor ECG for rate, rhythm, and conduction. Assess vital signs and associated symptoms with changes in ECG. Report findings to physician.
- Explain the importance of rapidly reducing the heart rate. Explain the cardioversion procedure, and encourage questions.
- Encourage verbalization of fears and concerns. Answer questions honestly, correcting misconceptions about the disease process, treatment, or prognosis.
- Administer intravenous diazepam as ordered before cardioversion.
- Document pretreatment vital signs, level of consciousness, and peripheral pulses.
- Place emergency cart with drugs and airway management supplies in client unit.
- Assist with cardioversion as indicated.
- Assess level of consciousness, level of sedation, cardiovascular and respiratory status, and skin condition following cardioversion.
- Document procedure and postcardioversion rhythm and also response to intervention.

EVALUATION

Intravenous verapamil lowers Ms. Vasquez's heart rate to 138 bpm for a short time, after which it increases to 164 bpm, with a blood pressure of 82/64 mmHg. Her cardiologist, Dr. Mullins, performs carotid sinus massage. The ventricular rate slows to 126 bpm for 2 minutes, revealing atrial flutter waves, and then returns to a rate of 150 bpm. Dr. Mullins explains the treatment options, including synchronized cardioversion. Ms. Vasquez agrees to the procedure.

Ms. Vasquez is lightly sedated, and synchronized cardioversion is performed. One countershock converts Ms. Vasquez to regular sinus rhythm at 96 bpm, with a blood pressure of 112/60 mmHg.

Ms. Vasquez is sleepy from the sedation but recovers without incident. She states that she feels "much better," and her vital signs return to her normal levels. She remains in normal sinus rhythm, with a rate of 86–92 bpm for the remainder of her hospital stay. Dr. Mullins places Ms. Vasquez on furosemide to treat manifestations of mild heart failure.

CRITICAL THINKING

1. What is the scientific basis for using carotid massage to treat supraventricular tachycardias? Was this an appropriate maneuver in the case of Ms. Vasquez?
2. What other treatment options might the physician have used to treat Ms. Vasquez's supraventricular tachycardia if she had been asymptomatic with stable vital signs?
3. Develop a teaching plan for Ms. Vasquez related to her prescription for furosemide.

PRACTICE ALERT

On recognizing ventricular fibrillation and cardiac arrest, begin emergency procedures. Call for help. Obtain defibrillator and immediately defibrillate. If the defibrillator will be brought by another health care provider, begin CPR. Initiate ACLS protocols and assist with resuscitation measures as directed. Cardiac output ceases with ventricular fibrillation. Immediate or early defibrillation has been shown to have the greatest impact on survival following cardiac arrest.

- After cardiac arrest, transfer to critical care. Perform and document head-to-toe assessment; obtain laboratory tests, 12-lead ECG, and chest x-ray as ordered. Monitor and maintain oxygenation and intravenous infusions, and monitor vital signs and cardiac rhythm. The period following resuscitation is critical, necessitating careful monitoring. Postarrest assessment allows comparison of the client's condition with prearrest status and may identify CPR-related injuries. Correcting electrolyte disturbances, hypoxia, and acid–base imbalances is important to prevent further dysrhythmias and potential adverse effects on cardiac output. Intravenous access is crucial to maintain drug infusions. Hemodynamic monitoring may be instituted. The 12-lead ECG documents myocardial status, and the chest x-ray provides information about pulmonary status and possible thoracic injury resulting from CPR.
- Notify the family of significant changes in the client's condition or cardiac arrest, providing up-to-date information. Prepare family members before visits by explaining interventions (e.g., invasive tubes, a ventilator, or additional equipment) implemented since the last visit. Concern for the family and significant others is part of holistic nursing. Clients and families need and appreciate honest communication, information about their loved one's condition, and compassionate care. Preparing the family for critical changes in the client's condition and plan of care helps them to cope with a situational crisis.

Evaluation

Expected outcomes of nursing care include the following:

- The client will experience reduced frequency of dysrhythmic episodes through adherence to medication regimen.
- The client and family will respond appropriately to an episode of dysrhythmia.

REVIEW Life-Threatening Dysrhythmias

RELATE: LINK THE CONCEPTS

Linking the exemplar of Life-Threatening Dysrhythmias with the concept of Safety:

1. What safety teaching will you provide the client with atrial fibrillation?
2. Your client has an internal pacemaker in place secondary to 3rd degree heart block. When providing safety instructions the client asks why battery powered equipment is used rather than electrically powered equipment. How will you respond?

Linking the exemplar of Life-Threatening Dysrhythmias with the concept of Addiction Behaviors:

3. What information will you provide the client with supraventricular tachycardia who plans to continue smoking cigarettes ?
4. What alterations will you make to your plan of care for the client with a dysrhythmia who also abuses cocaine ?

READY: GO TO COMPANION SKILLS MANUAL

- Assessing an apical pulse
- Assessing vital signs
- Assessing respirations
- Assessing blood pressure
- Assessing the heart rate
- Assessing the respiratory rate
- Glasgow Coma Scale
- Neurovascular assessment
- Administering intravenous medications using IV push
- Administering cardiac compressions
- Administering automated external defibrillator
- Interpreting an ECG strip
- Recording a 12-lead ECG

REFER: GO TO MYNURSINGKIT

REFLECT: CASE STUDY

Regina Moss, a 24-year-old female, is 6 weeks postpartum after delivering her first baby, Mickey. The delivery was uncomplicated; Mickey weighed 8 pounds at birth. Mickey has adapted well to the home environment, eating and sleeping well. Regina lives with Greg, a foreman for a construction crew. Regina has taken 3 months leave from her job as a legal secretary. Regina is enjoying her time at home with Mickey and is not sure she wants to return to work full time when her leave is up. Both her parents and Greg's live in town, and they have all offered to care for Mickey when Regina goes back to work.

This morning Mickey is pale and seems to be lethargic and is having trouble eating. Regina calls Greg and they go to the hospital where they are told that Mickey has supraventricular tachycardia. The emergency room physicians have given Mickey propranolol (Inderal) and are planning to admit Mickey to the pediatric ICU.

1. What is your priority nursing diagnosis for Mickey?
2. What teaching will you provide Regina and Greg?
3. How will you respond to Regina when she states that she must have done something wrong because Mickey had been so healthy?

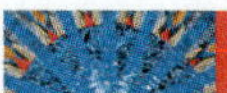

22.9 PERIPHERAL VASCULAR DISEASE

KEY TERMS

Arteriosclerosis, *1462*
Atherosclerosis, *1462*
Chronic venous insufficiency, *1462*
Intermittent claudication, *1463*
Peripheral vascular disease (PVD), *1462*
Rest pain, *1463*
Venous stasis, *1462*

BASIS FOR SELECTION OF EXEMPLAR

Most common condition

LEARNING OUTCOMES

After reading this exemplar, you will be able to:

1. Describe the pathophysiology, etiology, clinical manifestations, and direct and indirect causes of peripheral vascular disease.
2. Identify risk factors associated with peripheral vascular disease.
3. Illustrate the nursing process in providing culturally competent care across the life span for individuals with peripheral vascular disease.
4. Formulate priority nursing diagnoses appropriate for an individual with peripheral vascular disease.
5. Create a plan of care for individuals with peripheral vascular disease and their families.
6. Assess expected outcomes for an individual with peripheral vascular disease.
7. Discuss therapies used in the collaborative care of an individual with peripheral vascular disease.
8. Employ evidence-based caring interventions for an individual with peripheral vascular disease.

OVERVIEW

Peripheral vascular diseases are conditions affecting the peripheral arteries and veins. **Arteriosclerosis**, which is characterized by thickening, loss of elasticity, and calcification of arterial walls, is the most common chronic arterial disorder. **Atherosclerosis** is a form of arteriosclerosis in which deposits of fat and fibrin obstruct and harden the arteries. In the peripheral circulation, these pathologic changes impair the blood supply to peripheral tissues, particularly the lower extremities. This is known as **peripheral vascular disease (PVD)** or peripheral artery disease.

Chronic venous insufficiency is a disorder of inadequate venous return over a prolonged period. DVT is the most frequent cause of chronic venous insufficiency. Other conditions, such as varicose veins or leg trauma, may contribute; in some instances, it develops without an identified precipitating cause (Kasper et al., 2005; Tierney et al., 2005).

PATHOPHYSIOLOGY AND ETIOLOGY

Atherosclerotic lesions involve both the intima and the media of the involved arteries. Lesions typically develop in large and mid-sized arteries, particularly the abdominal aorta and iliac arteries (30% of symptomatic clients), the femoral and popliteal arteries (80–90% of clients), and more distal arteries (40–50% of clients) (Kasper et al., 2005). Arteriosclerosis in the abdominal aorta leads to the development of aneurysms as plaque erodes the vessel wall.

Plaque tends to form at arterial bifurcations. The vessel lumen is progressively obstructed, decreasing blood flow to the lower extremities. Tissue hypoxia or anoxia results. With gradual obstruction of the vessel, collateral circulation often develops. However, the collateral circulation is usually not adequate to supply tissue needs, especially when metabolic demand increases (e.g., during exercise). Manifestations typically develop only when the vessel is occluded by 60% or more.

Chronic venous insufficiency results when venous blood collects and stagnates in the lower leg (**venous stasis**). Venous pressures in the calf and lower leg increase, particularly during ambulation. This increased pressure impairs arterial circulation to the lower extremities as well. The body's ability to provide sufficient oxygen and nutrients to the cells and remove metabolic waste products diminishes. Eventually, there is so little oxygen and nutrients that cells begin to die. The skin atrophies, and subcutaneous fat deposits necrose. Breakdown of red blood cells in the congested tissues causes brown skin pigmentation (Porth, 2005). Venous stasis ulcers develop. Congested tissues impair the body's ability to increase the supply of oxygen, nutrients, and metabolic energy to heal the ulcer. As a result, the condition worsens and, over time, the ulcers enlarge. The congested venous circulation also prevents the blood from mounting effective inflammatory and immune responses, significantly increasing the risk for infection in the ulcerated tissue (McCance & Huether, 2006).

Etiology

Peripheral vascular disease usually affects people in their 60s and 70s; men are more often affected than women. Deaths attributed to peripheral arterial disease are about the same for black and white males but are higher among black women than white women (NHLBI, 2004).

Risk Factors

Risk factors for PVD are similar to those for atherosclerosis and coronary heart disease. Diabetes mellitus, hypercholesterolemia, hypertension, cigarette smoking, and high homocystine levels are risk factors for PVD (Kasper et al., 2005).

Several risk factors predispose a client to the development of venous insufficiency. Thrombophlebitis sometimes results in damage to the valves of the deep veins. Obesity and occupations that require prolonged standing or sitting can also lead to venous insufficiency.

CLINICAL MANIFESTATIONS

Pain is the primary symptom of peripheral atherosclerosis. **Intermittent claudication** (a cramping or aching pain in the calves of the legs, the thighs, and the buttocks that occurs with a predictable level of activity) is characteristic of PVD. The pain is often accompanied by weakness and is relieved by rest.

Rest pain, in contrast, occurs during periods of inactivity. It is often described as a burning sensation in the lower legs. Rest pain increases when the legs are elevated and decreases when the legs are dependent (e.g., hanging over the side of the bed). The legs also may feel cold or numb along with the pain. Sensation is diminished, and the muscles may atrophy.

Peripheral pulses may be decreased or absent. A bruit (unusual sound made by blood rushing past an obstruction) may be heard over large affected arteries, such as the femoral artery and the abdominal aorta. The legs are pale when elevated but often are dark red (dependent rubor) when dependent. The skin often is thin, shiny, and hairless, with discolored areas. Toenails may be thickened. Areas of skin breakdown and ulceration may be evident. Edema may develop with severe PVD.

Box 22–36 lists the manifestations of peripheral atherosclerosis. Complications of peripheral atherosclerosis include gangrene and extremity amputation, rupture of abdominal aortic aneurysms, and possible infection and sepsis.

Manifestations of chronic venous insufficiency include lower leg edema, itching, and discomfort of the affected extremity that increase with prolonged standing (Box 22–37). The extremity is cyanotic. Recurrent stasis ulcers develop (Figure 22–61 ■), usually forming just above the ankle, on the medial or anterior aspect of the leg. They heal poorly, forming scar tissue that breaks down easily. Tissue surrounding the ulcer is shiny, atrophic, and cyanotic, and there is a brownish pigmentation to the skin. Other skin changes, such as eczema or stasis dermatitis, also may develop. Necrosis and fibrosis of subcutaneous tissue causes the affected area of the leg to feel hard and somewhat leathery to the touch, but even the slightest trauma to the area can produce serious tissue breakdown. Table 22–32 compares venous and arterial ulcers.

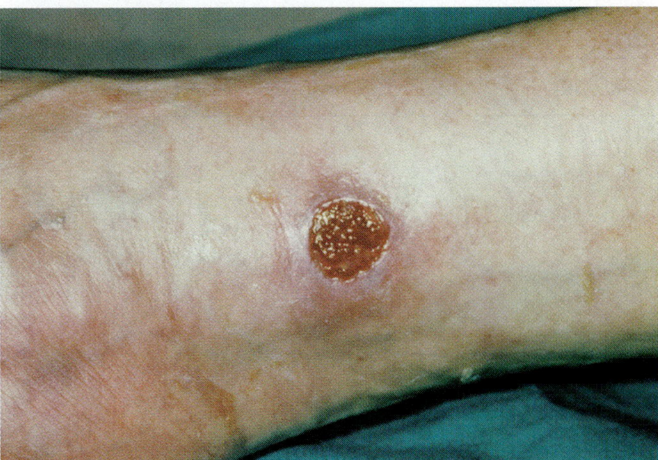

Figure 22–61 ■ Chronic venous insufficiency. Note the discoloration of the ankle and the stasis ulcer.

Source: Dr. P. Marazzi, Photo Researchers, Inc.

COLLABORATION

Management of PVD focuses on slowing the atherosclerotic process and maintaining tissue perfusion. Collaborative care for the client with venous insufficiency focuses on relieving symptoms, promoting adequate circulation, and healing and preventing tissue damage.

The history and physical examination often establish the diagnosis of chronic venous insufficiency. Because a history of DVT is a major risk factor, careful evaluation of the past medical history and questioning of the client is important. There are no specific diagnostic tests to confirm the diagnosis of chronic venous insufficiency.

Conservative management of venous insufficiency focuses on reducing edema and treating ulcerations. Prolonged standing or sitting is discouraged. Graduated compression hosiery is ordered for daytime use, and frequent elevation of the legs and feet during the day is recommended. At night, the legs and feet should be elevated above the level of the heart by raising the foot of the mattress.

Box 22–36 Manifestations of Peripheral Atherosclerosis

- Intermittent claudication
- Rest pain
- Paresthesias (numbness, decreased sensation)
- Diminished or absent peripheral pulses
- Pallor with extremity elevation, dependent rubor when dependent
- Thin, shiny, hairless skin; thickened toenails
- Areas of discoloration or skin breakdown

Box 22–37 Manifestations of Chronic Venous Insufficiency

- Lower extremity edema that worsens with standing
- Itching, dull leg discomfort or pain that increases with standing
- Thin, shiny, atrophic skin
- Cyanosis and brown skin pigmentation of lower leg and foot
- Possible weeping dermatitis
- Thick, fibrous (hard) subcutaneous tissue
- Recurrent ulcerations of medial or anterior ankle

TABLE 22–32 **Comparison of Arterial and Venous Leg Ulcers**

FACTOR	ARTERIAL ULCERS	VENOUS ULCERS
Location	Toes, feet, shin	Over medial or anterior ankle
Ulcer appearance	Deep, pale	Superficial, pink
Skin appearance	Normal to atrophic	Brown discoloration
	Pallor on elevation	Stasis dermatitis
	Rubor on dependency	Cyanosis on dependency
Skin temperature	Cool	Normal
Edema	Absent or mild	May be significant
Pain	Usually severe	Usually mild
	Intermittent claudication	Aching pain
	Rest pain	
Gangrene	May occur	Does not occur
Pulses	Decreased or absent	Normal

Treatment of associated stasis dermatitis varies, based on the duration of the condition. Wet compresses of boric acid, buffered aluminum acetate (Burow's solution), or isotonic saline solution are applied to acute weeping dermatitis four times a day for 1-hour periods. Following the compress, a topical corticosteroid (e.g., 0.5% hydrocortisone cream) is applied. Bed rest is prescribed during the acute period. Stasis dermatitis that is subsiding or chronic may be treated with a topical corticosteroid, zinc oxide ointment, or a topical, broad-spectrum antifungal cream, such as clotrimazole (Lotrimin) cream or miconazole (Monistat) cream (Tierney et al., 2005).

Isotonic saline compresses or wet-to-dry dressings are applied to stasis ulcers to promote healing. A dilute topical antibiotic solution also may be used (Kasper et al., 2005). The ulcer may be treated by using a semirigid boot applied to the foot and lower leg. This device may be made of Unna's paste or Gauzetex bandage. Bony prominences must be well padded. The boot must be changed every 1–2 weeks, depending on the amount of drainage from the ulcer. This device often allows ambulatory treatment.

A very large, chronic ulcer may require surgery. In this case, the incompetent veins are ligated, the ulcer is excised, and the area is covered with a skin graft.

Diagnostic Tests

Although PVD often can be diagnosed based on the history and physical examination, diagnostic tests may be ordered to evaluate its extent. Noninvasive studies often are sufficient. Diagnostic tests for PVD include the following:

- *Segmental pressure measurements* use sphygmomanometer cuffs and a Doppler device to compare blood pressures between the upper and lower extremities (normally similar) and within different segments of the affected extremity. In PVD, the blood pressure may be lower in the legs than in the arms.
- *Stress testing* using a treadmill provides functional assessment of limitations. In PVD, pressure at the ankle may decline even further with exercise, confirming the diagnosis. Evaluation for coronary heart disease may be done simultaneously during exercise testing (Kasper et al., 2005).

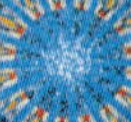

CLIENT TEACHING **Foot Care for the Client With Peripheral Atherosclerosis**

1. Keep legs and feet clean, dry, and comfortable.
   - Wash legs and feet daily in warm water, using mild soap.
   - Pat dry using a soft towel; be sure to dry between the toes.
   - Apply moisturizing cream to prevent drying.
   - Use powder on the feet and between the toes.
   - Buy shoes in the afternoon (when feet are largest); never buy shoes that are uncomfortable. Be sure toes have adequate room.
   - Wear a clean pair of cotton socks each day.
2. Prevent accidents and injuries to the feet.
   - Always wear shoes or slippers when getting out of bed.
   - Walk on level ground and avoid crowds, if possible.
   - Do not go barefoot.
   - Inspect legs and feet daily; use a mirror to examine backs of legs and bottoms of feet.
   - Have a professional foot care provider trim toenails and care for corns, calluses, ingrown toenails, or athlete's foot.
   - Always check the temperature of the water before stepping into the tub.
   - Do not get the legs or tops of the feet sunburned.
   - Report leg or foot problems (increased pain, cuts, bruises, blistering, redness, or open areas) to your health care provider.
3. Improve blood supply to the legs and feet.
   - Do not cross legs.
   - Do not wear garters or knee stockings.
   - Do not swim or wade in cold water.

- *Doppler ultrasound* uses sound waves reflected off moving red blood cells within a vessel to evaluate blood flow. The impulses may be translated into an audible signal or a graphic waveform. With significant PVD, the waveform becomes progressively flatter as the transducer is moved distally along the affected vessel. Segmental pressures may be used to locate the site of obstruction.
- *Duplex Doppler ultrasound* combines the audible or graphic Doppler ultrasound with ultrasound imaging to identify arterial or venous abnormalities. Ultrasonic imaging provides views of the affected vessel while Doppler ultrasound evaluates blood flow. *Color-flow Doppler ultrasound* provides color images of the vessel and blood flow.
- *Transcutaneous oximetry* evaluates oxygenation of tissues.
- *Angiography* or *magnetic resonance angiography* is done before revascularization procedures to locate and evaluate the extent of arterial obstruction. For angiography, a contrast medium is injected and vessels are visualized using fluoroscopy and x-rays. Magnetic resonance angiography does not require injection of a contrast medium and may replace angiography.

Pharmacologic Therapies

Drug treatment of peripheral atherosclerosis is less effective than that for coronary heart disease. Medications to inhibit platelet aggregation, such as aspirin or clopidogrel (Plavix), are ordered to reduce the risk of arterial thrombosis. Cilostazol (Pletal), a platelet inhibitor with vasodilator properties, improves claudication. Pentoxifylline (Trental) decreases blood viscosity and increases red blood cell flexibility, increasing blood flow to the microcirculation and tissues of the extremities. Parenteral vasodilator prostaglandins may be given on a long-term basis to decrease pain and facilitate healing in clients with severe limb ischemia (Kasper et al., 2005).

Clinical Therapies

Smoking cessation is vital for the treatment of PVD. Nicotine not only promotes atherosclerosis, it also causes vasospasm, further reducing blood flow to the extremities.

Meticulous foot care is vital to prevent ulceration and infection. Elastic support hose, which reduce circulation to the skin, are avoided. Elevating the head of the bed on blocks may help relieve rest pain. Regular, progressively strenuous exercise, such as 30–45 minutes of walking daily, is important. The client is taught to rest at the onset of claudication, resuming activity when the pain resolves.

Other measures to slow the process of atherosclerosis, such as controlling diabetes and hypertension, lowering cholesterol levels, and weight loss, also are recommended.

Surgery

Revascularization may be performed if symptoms are progressive, severe, or disabling. Other indications for surgery include symptoms that significantly interfere with ADLs, rest pain, and pregangrenous or gangrenous lesions. Either nonsurgical revascularization procedures or surgery may be performed.

Nonsurgical procedures include percutaneous transluminal angioplasty, stent placement, or atherectomy. Techniques may include balloon angioplasty to dilate the narrowed lumen, mechanical atherectomy to remove plaque, or laser or thermal angioplasty to vaporize the occluding material. In either case, a stent typically is placed at the time of angioplasty to maintain vessel patency. Iliac and femoral–popliteal percutaneous transluminal angioplasty initially reestablish good blood flow and relieve symptoms in more than 80% of clients. While the 3-year success rate is lower, stent placement improves the duration of symptom relief (Kasper et al., 2005).

Surgical options include endarterectomy (to remove occlusive plaque from the artery) and bypass grafts. Knitted Dacron bypass grafts are commonly used. Both immediate and long-term graft patency is better with bypass grafting than with nonsurgical revascularization procedures, but the risk for operative complications, such as MI, stroke, infection, and peripheral embolization, is higher (Kasper et al., 2005).

Complementary Therapies

Complementary therapies for PVD include interventions to improve circulation and reduce stress. A number of complementary therapies may improve peripheral circulation: aromatherapy with rosemary or vetiver; biofeedback; healing or therapeutic touch and massage; herbals, such as ginkgo, garlic, cayenne, hawthorn, and bilberry; and exercise including yoga. Aromatherapy and yoga also may reduce stress, as can breathing exercises, meditation, and counseling. In addition, complementary therapies to reduce atherosclerosis and lower cholesterol levels may slow the progress of PVD. Measures such as a very low-fat or vegetarian diet, including antioxidant nutrients or using vitamin C, vitamin E, or garlic supplements, and traditional Chinese medicine may be useful.

NURSING PROCESS

Discuss healthy lifestyle habits with community and religious groups, with schoolchildren (grades K–12), and through the print media to reduce the incidence and slow the progression of atherosclerosis. Strongly encourage all clients to avoid smoking in the first place and to stop all forms of tobacco use. Discuss the adverse effects of smoking and the benefits of quitting. Provide information about dietary recommendations to maintain a healthy weight and optimal cholesterol levels. Discuss the benefits and importance of regular exercise. Finally, encourage clients with cardiovascular risk factors to undergo regular screening for hypertension, diabetes, and hyperlipidemia.

Nursing care for the client with chronic venous insufficiency is primarily educative and supportive. Client teaching includes the following recommendations:

- Elevate the legs while resting and during sleep.
- Walk as much as possible, but avoid sitting or standing for long periods of time.

- When sitting, do not cross your legs or allow pressure on the back of the knees (e.g., sitting on the side of the bed).
- Do not wear anything that pinches your legs (e.g., knee-high hose, garters, or girdles).
- Wear elastic hose as prescribed. The elastic hose should be tighter over the feet than at the top of the leg. Be sure the tops of the elastic hose do not cut into your legs. Put on the hose after you have had your legs elevated.
- Keep the skin on your feet and legs clean, soft, and dry.
- Follow guidelines in the Client Teaching feature on page 1464 for care of the legs and feet.

Assessment

Focused assessment related to peripheral atherosclerosis includes the following:

- *Health history*. Complaints of pain, its relationship to exercise or rest, timing, associated symptoms, and relief measures; history of coronary heart disease, PVD, hyperlipidemia, hypertension, or diabetes; current medications; smoking history; usual diet and activity patterns.
- *Physical examination*. Vital signs; strength and equality of peripheral pulses of all extremities; capillary refill; skin color, temperature, hair distribution, and presence of any discolorations or lesions; movement and sensation of lower extremities.

Diagnosis

Nursing diagnoses that may be useful for the client with PVD include the following:

- Ineffective Tissue Perfusion: Peripheral
- Pain
- Impaired Skin Integrity
- Activity Intolerance.

Nursing diagnoses that may apply to the client with chronic venous insufficiency include the following:

- Disturbed Body Image related to edema and stasis ulcers on lower leg
- Ineffective Health Maintenance related to lack of knowledge about disorder and prescribed treatments
- Risk for Infection related to ulcerations
- Impaired Physical Mobility related to pain and edema in lower legs
- Impaired Skin Integrity related to presence of stasis ulcers
- Ineffective Tissue Perfusion: Peripheral related to incompetent venous valves.

Plan

Goals of nursing care may include the following:

- Promote wound healing
- Manage pain to allow for client comfort and rest
- Promote tissue perfusion
- Optimize activity tolerance.

Implementation

Nursing care is focused on improving tissue perfusion and preventing tissue damage. Any time tissues receive inadequate blood supply, the client will experience very severe pain. As a result, pain management until perfusion can be improved is also a primary nursing focus.

Ineffective Tissue Perfusion: Peripheral

Impaired blood flow to the lower extremities affects gas, nutrient, and waste product exchange between the capillaries and cells. Oxygen and nutrient deprivation impairs cell function and tissue integrity, causing pain and impaired healing. Pain develops with exercise and when extremities are elevated.

- Assess peripheral pulses, pain, color, temperature, and capillary refill every 4 hours and as needed. Use a Doppler device if pulses are not palpable. Mark pulse locations with an indelible marker. Assessment data provide a baseline for evaluating the effectiveness of interventions and identifies changes in arterial blood flow.
- Position the client with extremities dependent. Gravity promotes arterial flow to the dependent extremity, increasing tissue perfusion and relieving pain.
- Discuss the benefits of regular exercise. Exercise promotes development of collateral circulation to ischemic tissues and slows the process of atherosclerosis.
- Use a foot cradle and lightweight blankets, socks, and slippers to keep extremities warm. Avoid electric heating pads or hot water bottles. Keeping extremities warm conserves heat, prevents vasospasm, and promotes arterial flow. External heating devices are avoided to reduce the

CLIENT TEACHING **Home Care for Clients With Peripheral Vascular Disease**

Discuss the following topics when preparing the client and family for home and community-based care:

- Smoking cessation strategies and ways to avoid second-hand smoke
- Prescribed medications and anticoagulants, their purpose, doses, and desired and adverse effects
- Signs of excess bleeding to report to the physician
- Skin surveillance and foot care (see Client Teaching feature on page 1464)
- Recommended diet and exercise
- Weight loss strategies if appropriate

If revascularization or surgery has been performed, include the following topics as appropriate:

- Incision care
- Manifestations of complications (e.g., infection, graft leakage, or thrombosis) to be reported to the physician
- Activity limitations

Provide referrals to home health services, physical or occupational therapy, and home maintenance assistance services as indicated. Consider resources such as Meals-on-Wheels for clients who are severely limited by their disease.

risk of burns in the client with impaired sensation. The foot cradle protects tissues from compression by linens.

- Encourage frequent position changes. Instruct to avoid crossing legs or using a pillow under the knees. Position changes promote blood flow and reduce damage caused by pressure. Leg crossing and excessive flexion of the hip or knee joints can compress partially obstructed arteries and impair blood flow to distal tissues.

Pain

Impaired blood flow results in tissue ischemia. Metabolism shifts from an efficient aerobic process to an anaerobic process. Lactic acid and metabolic waste products accumulate in tissues, causing pain. Severe and cramping pain generally occurs with exercise early in the disease. Rest initially produces relief, similar to the process of angina. As the disease progresses, pain develops with less exercise and often occurs even at rest. Rest pain disrupts sleep, the sense of well-being, and has significant disruptive effects on life roles.

- Assess pain at least every 4 hours using a standard pain scale. Pain is a subjective experience. Using a standard pain scale allows evaluation of treatment measures in relieving pain and restoring blood flow. Examples of pain scales may be found in Exemplar 5.1, Acute Pain, and in the Companion Skills Manual.
- Keep extremities warm. Cooling leads to vasoconstriction, increasing pain. Warming the extremities promotes vasodilation and improves arterial flow, reducing pain.
- Teach pain relief and stress reduction techniques, such as relaxation, meditation, and guided imagery. Pain increases stress. The stress response leads to vasoconstriction, increasing pain. Stress reduction techniques, when combined with other measures to promote blood flow, can help reduce pain.

Impaired Skin Integrity

Clients with PVD are at risk for impaired skin integrity as a result of oxygen and nutrient deprivation. Chronic tissue ischemia leads to dry, scaly, and atrophied skin. Pruritus can lead to scratching; minor injuries may go unnoticed because of impaired sensation. Impaired tissue healing can lead to ulceration, infection, and potential gangrene.

- Provide meticulous daily skin care, keeping the skin clean and dry. Apply a moisturizing cream to dry or scaly areas. Intact skin is the body's first defense against bacterial invasion. Ischemic tissues of the injured extremity provide an excellent medium for microorganism growth. Clean, dry, supple skin decreases the risk of breakdown.
- Apply a bed cradle. The bed cradle suspends bed linens over the legs, preventing them from placing pressure on extremities and injured tissues. Minimizing pressure on the tissues promotes capillary blood flow.
- Provide an egg-crate mattress, flotation pad, sheepskin, or heel protectors. Ischemic tissues may be damaged by minor trauma, such as that created by the shearing forces of skin against bed linens.

Activity Intolerance

Pain and impaired perfusion of peripheral tissues may limit the client's ability to engage in desired activities, even impairing self-care.

- Assist with care activities as needed. Severe claudication or rest pain may limit activities. Muscle atrophy of affected extremities is common, leading to fatigue and weakness.
- Unless contraindicated, encourage gradual increases in duration and intensity of exercise. Teach to rest with extremities dependent when claudication develops, resuming activity after pain has abated. Gradual increases in the duration and intensity of exercise promote development of collateral circulation, improve exercise tolerance, provide a sense of well-being, and support self-esteem.
- Provide diversional activities during periods of prescribed bed rest. Encourage relaxation techniques to reduce muscle tension. Diversional activities help prevent boredom and stress associated with enforced rest. Relaxation techniques reduce vasoconstriction induced by stress, improving peripheral circulation.
- Encourage frequent position changes and active range-of-motion exercises. Encourage self-care to the extent possible. Position changes relieve pressure on tissues, improving capillary circulation and reducing tissue ischemia. ROM exercises help prevent muscle atrophy and joint contractures. Self-care supports self-esteem.

Evaluation

Client progress toward goals may be evaluated based on the following expected outcomes:

- The client demonstrates proper positioning to promote perfusion to extremities.
- The client abstains from use of tobacco products.
- The client demonstrates appropriate wound care.
- The client reports symptoms to report to provider if they occur.

REVIEW Peripheral Vascular Disease

RELATE: LINK THE CONCEPTS

Linking the exemplar of Peripheral Vascular Disease with the concept of Infection:

1. What factors related to PVD would increase the risk for infection in wounds to the lower extremities?
2. What client teaching will you provide the client with PVD to reduce the risk of infection?

Linking the exemplar of Peripheral Vascular Disease with the concept of Comfort:

3. Explain the relationship between physical exercise and pain in the client with PVD.
4. Compare the pain experienced during exercise for client with PVD to that of the client with angina.

READY: GO TO COMPANION SKILLS MANUAL

- Assessing the client in pain
- Assessing the skin
- Assessing vital signs
- Administering oral medications

REFER: GO TO MYNURSINGKIT

REFLECT: CASE STUDY

Vincent D'Angelo is a 69-year-old male who retired recently from Ford Motor Company where he worked on the assembly line in one of its truck factories. Vincent and his wife Pat are enjoying retirement and spending time together. Pat and Vincent own their own home. Their children, Laurie and Peter, live nearby. Vincent has not had any major health issues until recently, when he started experiencing pain during evening walks with Pat.

Vincent drinks an occasional glass of wine at special functions. Ten years ago, he quit a two-pack-a-day smoking habit. Pat and Vincent eat relatively healthy meals, mostly cooked by Pat. Pat has finally convinced Vincent to see his primary care provider to find out why he's having leg pain.

1. Describe the noninvasive diagnostic tests that the doctor might order to confirm Vincent's diagnosis of PVD.
2. What nursing assessments will you perform to support the diagnosis of PVD?
3. Create a teaching plan to reduce the risk of complications associated with PVD for this client.

22.10 PREGNANCY-INDUCED HYPERTENSION

KEY TERMS

Eclampsia, *1468*
HELPP syndrome, *1469*
Preeclampsia, *1468*

BASIS FOR SELECTION OF EXEMPLAR

Healthy People 2010

LEARNING OUTCOMES

After reading about this exemplar, you will be able to:

1. Describe the pathophysiology, etiology, clinical manifestations, and direct and indirect causes of pregnancy-induced hypertension.
2. Identify risk factors associated with pregnancy-induced hypertension.
3. Illustrate the nursing process in providing culturally competent care for individuals with pregnancy-induced hypertension.
4. Formulate priority nursing diagnoses appropriate for an individual with pregnancy-induced hypertension.
5. Create a plan of care for individuals with pregnancy-induced hypertension and their families.
6. Assess expected outcomes for an individual with pregnancy-induced hypertension.
7. Discuss therapies used in the collaborative care of an individual with pregnancy-induced hypertension.
8. Employ evidence-based caring interventions for an individual with pregnancy-induced hypertension.

OVERVIEW

Hypertensive disorders, which affect 5–10% of pregnant women, are the most common medical complications in pregnancies (Habli & Sibai, 2008). Various attempts have been made to classify these disorders. For clinical purposes, the following classification (Sibai, 2007) may be used:

- Pregnancy-induced hypertension
- Preeclampsia–eclampsia
- Chronic hypertension
- Chronic hypertension with superimposed preeclampsia or eclampsia.

Preeclampsia, the most common hypertensive disorder in pregnancy, occurs in 2–7% of pregnancies, although the incidence is significantly higher (14%) in women with a twin pregnancy (Habli & Sibai, 2008). In the United States, it is the second-leading cause of maternal death (Baxter & Weinstein, 2004). **Preeclampsia** is defined as an increase in blood pressure after 20 weeks of gestation accompanied by proteinuria. Previously, edema was included in the definition but was removed because it is such a common finding in pregnancy. However, sudden onset of severe edema warrants close evaluation to rule out preeclampsia or other pathologic processes, such as renal disease.

Preeclampsia, typically categorized as mild or severe, is a progressive disorder. In its most severe form, **eclampsia**, generalized seizures or coma develop. Most often, preeclampsia is seen in the last 10 weeks of gestation, during labor, or in the first 48 hours after childbirth. Although birth of the fetus and removal of the placenta is the only known cure for preeclampsia, it can be controlled with early diagnosis and careful management.

PATHOPHYSIOLOGY AND ETIOLOGY

In normal pregnancy, the lowered peripheral vascular resistance and increased maternal resistance to the pressor effects of angiotensin II result in lowered blood pressure. In preeclampsia, blood pressure begins to rise after 20 weeks of gestation, probably in response to a gradual loss of resistance to angiotensin II. This response has been linked to the ratio between the prostaglandins prostacyclin and thromboxane. Prostacyclin is a potent vasodilator. It is decreased in preeclampsia, often several weeks before symptoms develop. This changes the ratio between the two prostaglandins, allowing the potent vasoconstriction and platelet-aggregating effects of thromboxane to dominate. These hormones are produced partially by the placenta, which would help explain the reversal of the condition when the placenta is removed and why the incidence is increased when there is a larger-than-normal placental mass.

In addition, nitric oxide, a potent vasodilator, plays a role in the pregnant woman's resistance to vasopressors. Decreased nitric oxide production in women with preeclampsia may contribute to the development of hypertension.

The loss of normal vasodilation of uterine arterioles and the concurrent maternal vasospasm result in decreased placental perfusion. The effect on the fetus may be growth restriction, decrease in fetal movement, and chronic hypoxia or nonreassuring fetal status.

In preeclampsia, normal renal perfusion is decreased. With a reduction of the glomerular filtration rate, serum levels of creatinine, blood urea nitrogen, and uric acid begin to rise from normal pregnant levels, whereas urine output decreases. Sodium is retained in increased amounts, which results in increased extracellular volume, increased sensitivity to angiotensin II, and edema. Stretching of the capillary walls of the glomerular endothelial cells allows the large protein molecules, primarily albumin, to escape in the urine, decreasing serum albumin levels. The decreased serum albumin concentration causes decreased plasma colloid osmotic pressure. This lowered pressure results in a further movement of fluid to the extracellular spaces, which also contributes to the development of edema. The decreased intravascular volume causes increased viscosity of the blood and a corresponding rise in hematocrit.

HELLP Syndrome

HELLP syndrome (***h***emolysis, ***e***levated ***l***iver enzymes, and ***l***ow ***p***latelet count) is sometimes associated with severe preeclampsia. Women who experience this multiple-organ-failure syndrome have high morbidity and mortality rates, as do their offspring.

The hemolysis that occurs in HELLP syndrome is termed microangiopathic hemolytic anemia. It is thought that red blood cells are distorted or fragmented during passage through small, damaged blood vessels. Vascular damage is associated with vasospasm, and platelets aggregate at sites of damage, resulting in low platelet count (<100,000/mm^3) (Baxter & Weinstein, 2004). Elevated liver enzymes occur from blood flow that is obstructed by fibrin deposits. Hyperbilirubinemia and jaundice may also be seen. Liver distention causes epigastric pain and may ultimately result in liver rupture. Symptoms may include nausea, vomiting, flulike symptoms, or epigastric pain. HELLP syndrome is sometimes complicated by disseminated intravascular coagulation.

Women with HELLP syndrome are best cared for in a tertiary care center. Initially the mother's condition should be assessed and stabilized, especially if her platelet counts are very low. The fetus is also assessed, using a nonstress test and biophysical profile. Once HELLP syndrome is diagnosed and the woman's condition is stable, expeditious birth of the child is indicated regardless of gestational age.

Etiology

Preeclampsia is seen more often in teenagers and in women over age 35, especially if they are primigravidas. The exact cause of pregnancy-induced hypertension remains unknown, despite decades of research.

Risk Factors

Women with a history of preeclampsia are at increased risk, as are women with a large placental mass associated with multiple gestation, gestational trophoblastic disease (GTD), Rh incompatibility, and diabetes mellitus.

CLINICAL MANIFESTATIONS

Central nervous system changes associated with preeclampsia are hyperreflexia, headache, and seizures. Hyperreflexia may be caused by increased intracellular sodium and decreased intracellular potassium levels. Cerebral vasospasm causes headaches, and cerebral edema and vasoconstriction are responsible for seizures. Thrombocytopenia (platelet count, <100,000/mm^3) is a frequent finding in preeclampsia. It occurs when platelets aggregate at the sites of vascular damage associated with vasospasm.

Women with severe preeclampsia or eclampsia are at increased risk for renal failure, abruptio placentae, disseminated intravascular coagulation, ruptured liver, and pulmonary embolism.

Infants of women with preeclampsia tend to be small for gestational age. The cause is related specifically to maternal vasospasm and hypovolemia, which result in fetal hypoxia and malnutrition. In addition, the newborn may be premature because of the necessity for early birth.

At birth, the newborn may be oversedated because of medications administered to the mother. The newborn may also have hypermagnesemia caused by treatment of the woman with large doses of magnesium sulfate.

Mild Preeclampsia

Women with mild preeclampsia may exhibit few if any symptoms. The blood pressure is elevated to 140/90 mmHg or higher, and the proteinuria is 1 g or less in 24 hours (2+ dipstick).

Although edema is no longer considered a diagnostic criterion, generalized edema (seen as puffy face or hands) and edema in dependent areas, such as the ankles, may be present. Edema is identified by a weight gain of more than 1.5 kg (3.3 lb) per month in the second trimester or more than 0.5 kg (1.1 lb) per week in the third trimester. Edema is assessed on a 1+ to 4+ scale.

Severe Preeclampsia

Severe preeclampsia may develop suddenly. In this form of preeclampsia, blood pressure is 160/110 mm Hg or higher on two occasions at least 6 hours apart while the woman is on bed rest. Proteinuria of 5 g or more is found in a 24-hour urine collection, while a dipstick urine protein measurement is 3+ to 4+ on two random samples obtained at least 4 hours apart. Oliguria

CLINICAL MANIFESTATIONS AND THERAPIES **Pregnancy-Induced Hypertension**

ETIOLOGY	CLINICAL MANIFESTATION	CLINICAL THERAPIES
Central nervous system changes	Hyperreflexia, headache, seizures	■ Reduce stimuli ■ Bed rest ■ Anticonvulsant: magnesium sulfate ■ If a seizure occurs, fetus must be delivered to prevent further seizure activity
Decreased nitric oxide production	Hypertension; edema of the face, hands, and lower extremities	■ Frequent monitoring of blood pressure ■ Elevate extremities to reduce edema ■ Complete bed rest ■ High-protein, low-sodium diet
Loss of normal vasodilation of uterine arterioles	Decreased placental perfusion, fetal growth restriction, decreased fetal movement, chronic fetal hypoxia	■ Frequent fetal monitoring ■ Teach pregnant woman to report absence of movement ■ Fetal distress may require emergent delivery
Decreased renal perfusion	Elevated serum creatinine, blood urea nitrogen, uric acid Sodium retained, increasing extracellular fluid retention and resulting in edema, hypertension Stretching of capillary walls in glomeruli results in proteinuria and decreasing serum albumin levels, further contributing to edema	■ Frequent monitoring of blood pressure ■ Elevate extremities to reduce edema ■ Complete bed rest ■ High-protein, low-sodium diet ■ Monitor intake and output

is present, with urine output of 500 mL or less in 24 hours. Other characteristic symptoms include visual or cerebral disturbances (frontal headaches, blurred vision, or scotomata [spots before the eyes]); cyanosis or pulmonary edema; epigastric or right upper quadrant pain; impaired liver function; thrombocytopenia, evidence of hemolysis, or both; and intrauterine fetal growth restriction. Other signs or symptoms that may be present include nausea, vomiting, irritability, hyperreflexia, and retinal edema (retinas appear wet and glistening), with narrowed segments on the retinal arterioles when examined with an ophthalmoscope. Epigastric pain is often the sign of impending convulsion and is thought to be caused by increased vascular engorgement of the liver.

Eclampsia

Eclampsia, characterized by a grand mal convulsion or coma, may occur before the onset of labor, during labor, or early in the postpartal period. Some women experience only one seizure; others have several. Unless seizures occur quite frequently, the woman often regains consciousness between them.

COLLABORATION

The goals of medical management are prompt diagnosis of the disease; prevention of cerebral hemorrhage, seizures, hematologic complications, and renal and hepatic diseases; and birth of an uncompromised newborn as close to term as possible. Reduction of elevated blood pressure is essential in accomplishing these goals.

Antepartal Management

The clinical therapy for preeclampsia depends on the severity of the disease. In general, women with preeclampsia are admitted to the hospital. However, for some women with mild preeclampsia, home care is now an option. The woman assesses her blood pressure, weight, and urine protein daily and does daily fetal movement monitoring. Weight gains of 1.4 kg (3 lb) in 24 hours or 1.8 kg (4 lb) in a 3-day period are generally cause for concern. Remote nonstress tests (NSTs) are performed twice per week, or biophysical profiles are done weekly. Nursing contact varies from daily to weekly, depending on physician request. It is extremely important to advise the woman to report to the doctor any signs of worsening preeclampsia.

The woman is placed on bed rest, primarily on her left side, to decrease pressure on the vena cava, thereby increasing venous return, circulatory volume, and placental and renal perfusion. Improved renal blood flow helps decrease angiotensin II levels, promotes diuresis, and lowers blood pressure.

The woman is weighed daily and evaluated for worsening edema, persistent headache, visual changes, or epigastric pain. Urine dipstick is done daily to assess for protein; blood pressure is checked at least four times per day. Diet should be well balanced and moderate to high in protein (80–100 g/day, or 1.5 $g \cdot kg^{-1} \cdot day^{-1}$) to replace protein lost in the urine. Sodium intake should be moderate, not to exceed 6 g/day. Excessively salty foods should be avoided, but sodium restriction and diuretics are no longer used in treating preeclampsia.

To achieve a safe outcome for the fetus, tests to evaluate fetal status are done more frequently as preeclampsia progresses. The following tests are used:

- Fetal movement record
- Nonstress test
- Ultrasonography every 3 or 4 weeks for serial determination of growth
- Biophysical profile
- Amniocentesis to determine fetal lung maturity
- Doppler velocimetry beginning at 30–32 weeks of gestation to screen for fetal compromise.

SEVERE PREECLAMPSIA If the uterine environment is considered detrimental to fetal well-being, birth may be the treatment of choice for both mother and fetus, even if the fetus is immature. Other medical therapies for severe preeclampsia include the following:

- *Bed rest.* Bed rest must be complete. Stimuli that may bring on a seizure should be reduced.
- *Diet.* A high-protein, moderate-sodium diet is given as long as the woman is alert and has no nausea or indication of impending seizure.
- *Anticonvulsants.* Magnesium sulfate is the treatment of choice for convulsions. Its depressant action on the central nervous system reduces the possibility of seizure.
- *Fluid and electrolyte replacement.* The goal of fluid intake is to achieve a balance between correcting hypovolemia and preventing circulatory overload. Fluid intake may be oral or supplemented with intravenous therapy. Intravenous fluids may be started "to keep lines open" in case they are needed for drug therapy even when oral intake is adequate. Electrolytes are replaced as indicated by daily serum electrolyte levels.
- *Corticosteroids.* Betamethasone or dexamethasone is often administered to the woman whose fetus has an immature lung profile. Corticosteroids may also have a beneficial effect in women with HELLP syndrome.
- *Antihypertensives.* Antihypertensive therapy is generally given for sustained systolic blood pressure of at least 160–180 mmHg or diastolic blood pressures of 105–110 mmHg or higher. Hydralazine (Apresoline) is the antihypertensive medication most commonly used. It is generally administered in as an intravenous bolus. Methyldopa is often used for long-term control of mild to moderate hypertension in pregnancy, because it is effective and has a well-documented safety record. Recent studies indicate that intravenous labetalol and oral nifedipine are as effective as intravenous hydralazine and have fewer side effects (Sibai, 2007).

ECLAMPSIA An eclamptic seizure requires immediate, effective treatment. A bolus of 4–6 g of magnesium sulfate is given intravenously over 5 minutes to control convulsions. Antihypertensive agents are used to keep the diastolic blood pressure between 90 and 100 mmHg, thus avoiding a potential reduction in uteroplacental blood flow or cerebral perfusion. A sedative, such as diazepam or amobarbital, is used only if the seizures are not controlled by magnesium sulfate. Dilantin may be used for seizure prevention. The lungs are auscultated for pulmonary edema. The woman is observed for circulatory and renal failure and for signs of cerebral hemorrhage. Furosemide (Lasix) may be given for pulmonary edema; digitalis may be given for circulatory failure. Intake and output are monitored hourly.

The woman is assessed for signs of labor. She is also checked every 15 minutes for evidence of vaginal bleeding and abdominal rigidity, which might indicate abruptio placentae. While she is comatose, she is positioned on her side with the side rails up.

Because of the severity of her condition, the woman is often cared for in an intensive care unit. Invasive hemodynamic monitoring of either central venous pressure or pulmonary artery wedge pressure may be started using a Swan–Ganz catheter. Both procedures carry risk to the woman, and the decision to use either of them should be made judiciously. When the condition of the woman and the fetus are stabilized, induction of labor is considered, because birth is the only known cure for preeclampsia. The woman and her partner should be given a careful explanation about her status and that of her unborn child and about the treatment they are receiving. Plans for further treatment and for birth must be discussed with them.

Intrapartal Management

Labor may be induced by intravenous oxytocin when there is evidence of fetal maturity and cervical readiness. In severe cases, cesarean birth may be necessary even if the fetus is immature.

Assessment for signs of worsening preeclampsia continues. The woman may receive intravenous oxytocin and magnesium sulfate simultaneously. Infusion pumps should be used, and bags and tubing must be carefully labeled. Magnesium levels are assessed regularly.

Meperidine (Demerol) or fentanyl may be given intravenously for pain relief in labor. A pudendal block is often used for vaginal birth. An epidural block may be used if it is administered by a skilled anesthesiologist who is knowledgeable about preeclampsia. However, spinal or epidural anesthesia is contraindicated in the presence of coagulopathy or a platelet count of 50,000/mm^3 (Sibai, 2005).

Electronic fetal monitoring is used to assess fetal status continuously. Birth in the Sims' or semi-sitting position should be considered. If the lithotomy position is used, a wedge should be placed under the right buttock to displace the uterus. The wedge should also be used if birth is by cesarean. Oxygen is administered to the woman during labor if the need is indicated by fetal response to the contractions.

A pediatrician or neonatal nurse practitioner must be available to care for the newborn at birth. This caregiver must be informed of all amounts and times of any medication the woman has received during labor.

Postpartal Management

The woman with preeclampsia usually improves rapidly after giving birth, although seizures can still occur during the first 48 hours postpartum. When the hypertension is severe, the woman may continue to receive hydralazine or magnesium sulfate postpartally.

In general, the recurrence rate of preeclampsia is 18–25% in subsequent pregnancies. The rate is substantially higher in women with multiple gestations, early onset preeclampsia–eclampsia, previous HELLP syndrome, or underlying vascular disease (Sibai, 2005). Women who have had a normotensive previous pregnancy are at increased risk when they conceive with a new partner. Also, in vitro fertilization using donor eggs and/or donor sperm has a higher incidence of preeclampsia (Wiggins & Elliott, 2005).

NURSING PROCESS

When caring for the pregnant woman with pregnancy-induced hypertension, it is important to always remember there are two clients involved. In addition to meeting the needs of the woman, the fetus's needs must also be met in order to promote a good outcome following delivery.

Assessment

Blood pressure is taken and recorded during each antepartal visit. If the blood pressure rises, or if the normal slight decrease in blood pressure expected between 8 and 28 weeks of pregnancy does not occur, the woman should be followed closely. The woman's urine is checked for proteinuria at each visit.

If hospitalization becomes necessary, the nurse assesses the following:

- *Blood pressure.* Blood pressure should be assessed every 1–4 hours, or more frequently if indicated by medication or other changes in the woman's status.
- *Temperature.* Temperature should be taken every 4 hours, or every 2 hours if elevated.
- *Pulse and respirations.* Pulse rate and respirations should be determined along with blood pressure.
- *Fetal heart rate.* The fetal heart rate should be checked with the blood pressure or monitored continuously with the electronic fetal monitor if the situation indicates.
- *Urinary output.* Every voiding should be measured. The woman frequently has an indwelling catheter. In this case, urine output can be assessed hourly. Output should be 700 mL or greater in 24 hours, or at least 30 mL/hr.
- *Urine protein.* Urinary protein is evaluated hourly if an indwelling catheter is in place or with each voiding. Readings of 3+ or 4+ indicate loss of 5 g or more of protein in 24 hours.
- *Urine specific gravity.* Specific gravity of the urine should be checked hourly or with each voiding. Readings over 1.040 correlate with oliguria and proteinuria.
- *Edema.* The face (especially the eyelids and cheekbone area), fingers, hands, arms (ulnar surface and wrist), legs (tibial surface), ankles, feet, and sacral area are inspected and palpated for edema. The degree of pitting is determined by pressing over bony areas.
- *Weight.* The woman is weighed daily at the same time, wearing the same robe or gown and slippers. Weighing may be omitted if the woman is to maintain strict bed rest.
- *Pulmonary edema.* The woman is observed for coughing. The lungs are auscultated for moist respirations.
- *Deep tendon reflexes.* The woman is assessed for evidence of hyperreflexia in the brachial, wrist, patellar, or Achilles tendons. The patellar reflex is the easiest to assess. Clonus should also be assessed by vigorously dorsiflexing the foot while the knee is held in a fixed position. Normally no clonus is present. If it is present, it is measured as beats and recorded as such.
- *Placental separation.* The woman should be assessed hourly for vaginal bleeding and/or uterine rigidity.
- *Headache.* The woman should be questioned about the existence and location of any headache.
- *Visual disturbance.* The woman should be questioned about any visual blurring or changes or scotomata. The results of the daily funduscopic exam should be recorded on the chart.
- *Epigastric pain.* The woman should be asked about any epigastric pain. It is important to differentiate it from simple heartburn, which tends to be familiar and less intense.
- *Laboratory blood tests.* Daily tests of hematocrit to measure hemoconcentration; blood urea nitrogen, creatinine, and uric acid levels to assess kidney function; clotting studies for any indication of thrombocytopenia or disseminated intravascular coagulation; liver enzymes; and electrolyte levels for deficiencies are all indicated. Magnesium levels are monitored regularly in women receiving magnesium sulfate.
- *Level of consciousness.* The woman is observed for alertness, mood changes, and any signs of impending convulsion or coma.
- *Emotional response and level of understanding.* The woman's emotional response should be carefully assessed so that support and teaching can be planned accordingly.

In addition, the nurse continues to assess the effects of any medications administered. Because the administration of prescribed medications is an important aspect of care, the nurse is, of course, familiar with the more commonly used medications and their purpose, implications, and associated untoward or toxic effects.

Diagnosis

Nursing diagnoses that might apply to the woman with preeclampsia include the following:

- Deficient Fluid Volume related to fluid shift from intravascular to extravascular space secondary to vasospasm
- Risk for Injury related to the possibility of seizure secondary to cerebral vasospasm or edema.

Plan

Goals of nursing care may include the following:

- Fetal perfusion will remain adequate to sustain normal growth, as demonstrated by fetal heart rate, fetal monitoring, and fetal movement.
- Maternal blood pressure will remain within the acceptable range.

- The woman will maintain nutritional status.
- Safety of the client and fetus will be maintained.
- The woman will maintain fluid status.

Implementation

When caring for a client with PIH, the focus of nursing care is to reduce blood pressure while supporting the pregnancy. However, if blood pressure continues to rise or remains elevated, delivery of the premature fetus may be unavoidable. In that case, nursing care is focused on optimizing outcomes for both the client and the newborn.

Community-Based Nursing Care

A woman with preeclampsia has several major concerns. She may fear losing her fetus, she may worry about her personal relationship with her other children and her personal and sexual relationship with her partner, she may be concerned about finances, and she may also feel bored and a little resentful if she faces prolonged bed rest. If she has small children, she may have trouble providing for their care. The nurse should help the couple identify and discuss these concerns. The nurse can offer information and explanations if certain aspects of therapy cause difficulty. The nurse can also refer the woman and her family to community resources, such as support groups or homemaker services, as appropriate.

The woman needs to know which symptoms are significant and should be reported at once. Usually, the woman with mild preeclampsia is seen once or twice a week, but she may need to come in earlier than her next scheduled appointment if symptoms indicate that her condition is progressing. She must understand her diet plan, which should reflect her culture, finances, and lifestyle (Figure 22–62 ■).

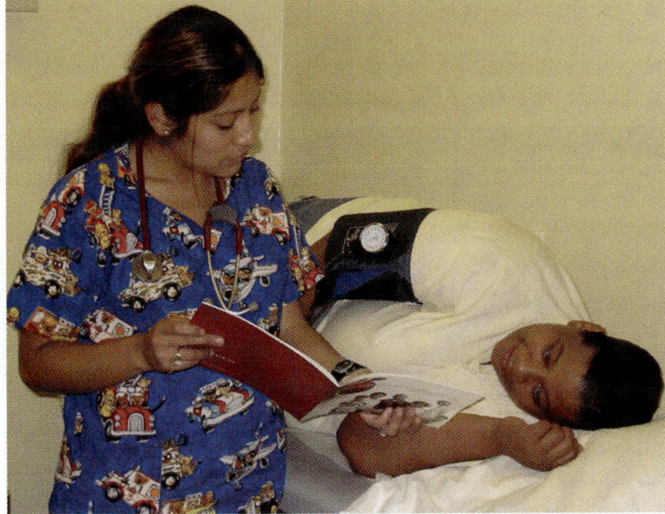

Figure 22–62 ■ The nurse ensures that the client with preeclampsia clearly understands her plan of care, especially with regard to the significance of her symptoms, her diet plan, and the importance of the side-lying position.

Hospital-Based Nursing Care

The development of severe preeclampsia is a cause for increased concern for the woman and her family. The most immediate concerns usually are about the prognosis for the woman and her fetus. The nurse can explain medical therapy and its purpose and offer honest, hopeful information. The nurse keeps the couple informed of fetal status and discusses other concerns the couple may express. The nurse provides as much information as possible and seeks other sources of information or aid for the family as needed. The nurse can also offer to contact a member of the clergy or hospital chaplain for additional support if the couple so chooses.

The nurse maintains a quiet, low-stimulus environment for the woman. The woman is generally placed in a private room in a quiet location where she can be watched closely. Visitors are limited to close family members or main support persons. The woman should maintain the left lateral recumbent position most of the time, with side rails up for her protection. Unlimited phone calls are avoided because the phone ringing unexpectedly may be too jarring. To avoid a sense of isolation, however, some women find it preferable to allow calls during a certain time of day. Bright lights and sudden loud noises may precipitate seizures in the woman with severe preeclampsia.

The occurrence of a convulsion is frightening to any family members who may be present, although the woman will not be able to recall it when she becomes conscious. Therefore, it is essential to offer explanations to the family members and the woman herself later.

A grand mal seizure has both a tonic phase, marked by pronounced muscular contraction and rigidity, and a clonic phase, marked by alternate contraction and relaxation of the muscles, which causes the woman to thrash about wildly. When the tonic phase of the contraction begins, the woman should be turned to her side (if she is not already in that position) to aid circulation to the placenta. Her head should be turned face down to allow saliva to drain from her mouth. The side rails should be padded or a pillow put between the woman and each side rail.

After 15–20 seconds, the clonic phase starts. When the thrashing subsides, intensive monitoring and therapy begin. An oral airway is inserted, the woman's nasopharynx is suctioned, and oxygen is administered by nasal catheter. Fetal heart tones are monitored continuously. Maternal vital signs are monitored every 5 minutes until they are stable, and then every 15 minutes thereafter.

Nursing Management During Labor and Birth

During labor, the woman with preeclampsia must receive all the care and precautions necessary for normal labor, as well as those required for managing preeclampsia. The woman is kept positioned on her left side as much as possible. Both the woman and the fetus are monitored carefully throughout labor. The nurse notes the progress of labor and is alert to signs of worsening preeclampsia or its complications.

During the second stage of labor, the woman is encouraged to push in the side-lying position if possible. If she is unable to do so comfortably or effectively, she can be helped to a semi-sitting position for pushing and can then resume the lateral

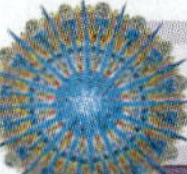

NURSING CARE PLAN A Client With Pregnancy-Induced Hypertension

ASSESSMENT

Ingrid Fruehauf, a 36-year-old primigravida, is 34 weeks pregnant. Four days ago, during a routine prenatal visit, the nurse discovered that her blood pressure was elevated slightly, to 130/84 mmHg. Normally, Ms. Fruehauf's blood pressure readings had been 118/74 mmHg. She had gained 4 lb since her previous monthly visit. A trace level of protein was found with a dipstick urine. In addition, Ms. Fruehauf reported experiencing some headaches over the previous few days that had not been relieved by acetaminophen. The nurse explained the signs and symptoms of preeclampsia and encouraged her to call the clinic if her condition worsened over the next few days. Ms. Fruehauf was sent home on bed rest and scheduled for a recheck in 4 days.

When Ms. Fruehauf returns to the clinic today, she is admitted to the hospital with worsening preeclampsia. She is placed on complete bed rest. The nurse monitors her closely for signs of severe preeclampsia, which include hypertension, proteinuria, oliguria, cerebral or visual disturbances, pulmonary edema, epigastric pain, and sudden onset of severe edema. She is also observed for eclamptic seizure. Tests for fetal status, such as documentation of fetal movement, nonstress tests, serial ultrasounds, biophysical profile, amniocentesis, and Doppler flow studies, are performed. The nurse reassures Ms. Fruehauf that everything will be done to make her comfortable and ensure the well-being of her baby.

Ms. Fruehauf reports headache and irritability. Scotomata are noted. Other findings are as follows: blood pressure, 148/90 mmHg; deep tendon reflexes are 3+; 600 mL of urine collected over the last 24 hours with a protein level of 5 g/L; weight gain of 3 lb over last 4 days; and 2+ pitting edema on lower extremities.

DIAGNOSES

- Deficient Fluid Volume related to fluid shift from intravascular to extravascular space secondary to vasospasm
- Risk for Injury to Fetus related to uteroplacental insufficiency secondary to vasospasm

PLANNING

Goals of care include the following:

- The client's signs and symptoms of preeclampsia will decrease, as evidenced by decreased blood pressure, decreased levels of protein in urine, and deep tendon reflexes return to normal (2+).
- The fetus will have adequate supply of oxygen and nutrients, as evidenced by no signs of fetal distress and fetal diagnostic tests within normal limits.

IMPLEMENTATION

- Encourage the woman to lie in the left lateral recumbent position.
- Assess blood pressure every 1–4 hours as necessary.
- Monitor urine for volume and proteinuria every shift or every hour per agency protocol.
- Assess deep tendon reflexes and clonus.
- Assess for edema.
- Administer magnesium sulfate per infusion pump as ordered.
- Assess for magnesium sulfate toxicity.
- Provide a balanced diet that includes 80 to 100 g/day or 1.5 $g \cdot kg^{-1} \cdot day^{-1}$ of protein.
- Instruct the woman to count fetal movements three times a day for 20–30 minutes, maintain a record of movement, and share the record with the nurse.
- Encourage the woman to rest in the left lateral recumbent position.
- Assist with serial ultrasounds.
- Perform nonstress tests as ordered.
- Describe for the woman the purposes of a biophysical profile.
- Assist with amniocentesis to obtain lecithin/sphingomyelin ratio.
- Explain the purpose of Doppler flow studies.

EVALUATION

Ms. Fruehauf's blood pressure returns to her normal level. Her urine protein levels decrease to zero. Her deep tendon reflexes remain at 2+ with no beats of clonus. All diagnostic tests are within normal limits, which indicates that uteroplacental sufficiency is maintained. No signs of fetal distress are documented during testing.

CRITICAL THINKING

1. A woman gives birth at 39 weeks of gestation. The prenatal record reveals a history of preeclampsia with this pregnancy. Even though the newborn was full term, the birth weight falls below the 10th percentile. Describe how preeclampsia in the prenatal period can affect the growth of the fetus.
2. The nurse is assisting a woman with preeclampsia to select a dinner menu. The choices include the following:
   a. Menu #1: grilled chicken, broccoli with peanut sauce, brown rice, an oatmeal cookie, and a milkshake
   b. Menu #2: pasta with tomato sauce, fresh green salad, garlic bread, chocolate cake, and iced tea
   Which menu plan is best for a woman with preeclampsia? Why?

NURSING CARE PLAN A Client With Pregnancy-Induced Hypertension *continued*

3. The nurse is admitting three women to the antepartum unit. Two rooms are available: one private room and one double occupancy room. One woman being admitted is in preterm labor, the second has preeclampsia, and the third has third-trimester bleeding. Which room assignment would be most appropriate for the woman with preeclampsia? Why?
4. Your assessment of a client receiving magnesium sulfate for severe preeclampsia includes nausea and vomiting, blurred vision, absent deep tendon reflexes (previously deep tendon reflexes were 3+), and 70 mL of total urine output over 4 hours. Are these findings normal? What, if any, actions would you take?

position between contractions. Birth is in the side-lying position or in the lithotomy position with a wedge placed under the woman's right hip.

A family member or other support person is encouraged to stay with the woman as much as possible. The woman in labor and the support person are kept informed of the progress and plan of care. In addition, their wishes concerning the birth experience are respected when possible. Preferably, the woman should be cared for by the same nurses throughout her stay.

Nursing Management During the Postpartal Period

Because the woman with preeclampsia is hypovolemic, even normal blood loss can be serious. The amount of vaginal bleeding must be assessed and the woman observed for signs of shock. Blood pressure and pulse are monitored every 4 hours for 48 hours. Hematocrit is checked daily. The woman is assessed for any further signs of preeclampsia. Intake and output are measured. Normal postpartum diuresis helps eliminate edema and is a favorable sign.

Postpartal depression can develop after such a difficult pregnancy. To help prevent it, the nurse provides opportunities for frequent maternal–infant contact and encourages family members to visit. The couple may have many questions, and the nurse should be available for discussion. The couple should be given family-planning information. Oral contraceptives may be used if the woman's blood pressure has returned to normal by the time they are prescribed (usually 4–6 weeks after birth).

Evaluation

Expected outcomes of nursing care include the following:

- The woman is able to explain preeclampsia, its implications for her pregnancy, the treatment regimen, and possible complications.
- The woman suffers no eclamptic seizures.
- The woman and her caregivers detect early evidence for increasing severity of the preeclampsia or possible complications so that appropriate treatment measures can be instituted.
- The woman gives birth to a healthy newborn.

REVIEW Pregnancy-Induced Hypertension

RELATE: LINK THE CONCEPTS

Linking the exemplar of Pregnancy-Induced Hypertension with the concept of Intracranial Regulation:

1. What independent nursing intervetions might you initiate to reduce the risk of seizures in the client with PIH who is 28 weeks pregnant?
2. When caring for a pregnant female in the early stages of PIH what teaching would you provide to reduce disease advancement?

Linking the exemplar of Pregnancy-Induced Hypertension with the concept of Oxygenation:

3. What impact will PIH have on fetal oxygenation?
4. List short- and long-term goals for the client with PIH aimed at optimizing client and fetal oxygenation.

READY: GO TO COMPANION SKILLS MANUAL

- Assessing the skin
- Monitoring input and output
- Assessing blood pressure
- Assessment of fetal well-being: nonstress test
- Auscultating fetal heart rate

REFER: GO TO MYNURSINGKIT

REFLECT: CASE STUDY

Ginny Sims is a 36-year-old primigravida who is 34 weeks gestation. Ginny is married to Paul, whose job as a buyer for a major department store chain requires a great deal of travel. Ginny and Paul had plans to have children when they first married, but they had trouble conceiving. Ginny is the manager of a Starbuck's. When she began feeling very tired and nauseated in the mornings, she decided she was in early menopause because her period was late. As fatigue continued to hurt her ability to concentrate at work, Ginny finally made an appointment with her OB/GYN and found out she was pregnant. She and Paul are thrilled and can't wait to greet their newborn. Paul is investigating the possibility of taking a job closer to home so he can spend more time with his family.

Ginny is seeing the nurse practitioner today for her routine prenatal examination. The nurse takes Ginny's blood pressure and it is 130/85, increased from her baseline of 110/70. Ginny's ankles are slightly swollen and Ginny admits to an occasional recurrent nagging headache. Ginny's urine was slightly positive for protein.

1. What further physical assessments would you perform to support the diagnosis of early PIH?
2. What teaching will you provide before sending Ginny home from the office?
3. What assessment findings would indicate worsening PIH in this client?

22.11 PULMONARY EMBOLISM

KEY TERMS

Dead space, *1477*
Embolus, *1476*
Lyse, *1479*
Pulmonary embolism, *1476*
Thromboemboli, *1476*

BASIS FOR SELECTION OF EXEMPLAR

Leading cause of death

LEARNING OUTCOMES

After reading about this exemplar, you will be able to:

1. Describe the pathophysiology, etiology, clinical manifestations, and direct and indirect causes of pulmonary embolism.
2. Identify risk factors associated with pulmonary embolism.
3. Illustrate the nursing process in providing culturally competent care across the life span for individuals with pulmonary embolism.
4. Formulate priority nursing diagnoses appropriate for an individual with pulmonary embolism.
5. Create a plan of care for individuals with pulmonary embolism and their family members.
6. Assess expected outcomes for an individual with pulmonary embolism.
7. Discuss therapies used in the collaborative care of an individual with pulmonary embolism.
8. Employ evidence-based caring interventions for an individual with pulmonary embolism.

OVERVIEW

Pulmonary embolism, or pulmonary thromboembolism, is the obstruction of blood flow in part of the pulmonary vascular system by an **embolus** (debris blocking a blood vessel; may be a particle or aggregate of a substance that may be blood, fat, or clump of pathogens). **Thromboemboli** (emboli created by a blood clots) that develop in the venous system (DVT) or right side of the heart are the most frequent cause of pulmonary embolism. Other sources of emboli include tumors that have invaded the venous circulation, fat or bone marrow entering the circulation as a result of fracture or other trauma, amniotic fluid released into the circulation during childbirth, and intravenous injection of air or other foreign substances.

Pulmonary embolism is a medical emergency. Fifty percent of deaths from pulmonary embolism occur within the first 2 hours following embolization. In many cases, DVT has not been recognized or treated; often, embolization also goes undetected. Prevention is the most effective treatment strategy. Pulmonary embolism causes an estimated 200,000 deaths annually, making it the third-leading cause of death in hospitalized clients (Tierney et al., 2005).

PHYSIOLOGY AND ETIOLOGY

The right heart receives deoxygenated blood from the systemic venous circulation. The entire output of the right ventricle enters the pulmonary circulation via the pulmonary artery. This artery branches into successively smaller arteries, arterioles, and capillaries of the pulmonary vascular system. Each alveolus of the lungs is surrounded by a meshwork of capillaries. Oxygen and carbon dioxide readily diffuse across the alveolar–capillary membrane, driven by a concentration gradient. The partial pressure of oxygen in the alveolus is greater than that in the capillary; therefore, oxygen diffuses into the blood. Carbon dioxide diffuses from the capillaries into the alveoli, driven by the higher pressure of dissolved carbon dioxide in venous blood.

A match between blood flow through the pulmonary vascular system (perfusion) and lung ventilation is necessary for effective respiration (gas exchange) (Figure 22–63 ■). Local factors regulate ventilation and perfusion to maintain this match. A low alveolar PO_2 constricts alveolar capillaries, directing blood flow to better-ventilated areas of the lung. A high alveolar PCO_2 causes local bronchodilation, increasing airflow and eliminating excess carbon dioxide.

Thrombi affecting only the deep veins of the calf rarely embolize to the pulmonary circulation. However, thrombi often propagate proximally to the popliteal and ileofemoral veins, and from there, they may break loose to become an embolus. As vessels of the venous system become progressively larger, the embolus moves freely until it enters the pulmonary arterial system, with its progressively smaller vessels leading to the pulmonary capillary beds (Figure 22–64 ■).

The impact of a pulmonary embolus depends on the extent to which pulmonary blood flow is obstructed, the size of the embolus, its nature, and any secondary effects of the obstruction. The effects can range widely:

- Occlusion of a large pulmonary artery with sudden death. Gas exchange is significantly reduced or prevented, and cardiac output falls dramatically as blood fails to move through the pulmonary vascular system and return to the left heart.
- Lung tissue infarction caused by occlusion of a significant portion of pulmonary blood flow. Fewer than 10% of pulmonary emboli result in pulmonary infarction.
- Obstruction of a small segment of the pulmonary circulation with no permanent lung injury.
- Chronic or recurrent, possibly multiple, small emboli with recurring symptoms.

Obstruction of pulmonary blood flow by an embolus affects both perfusion and ventilation. Neurohumoral reflexes triggered by obstruction cause vasoconstriction, increasing pulmonary vascular resistance. In severe cases, this can lead to pulmonary hypertension and right ventricular heart failure. Systemically, hypotension and a drop in cardiac output may

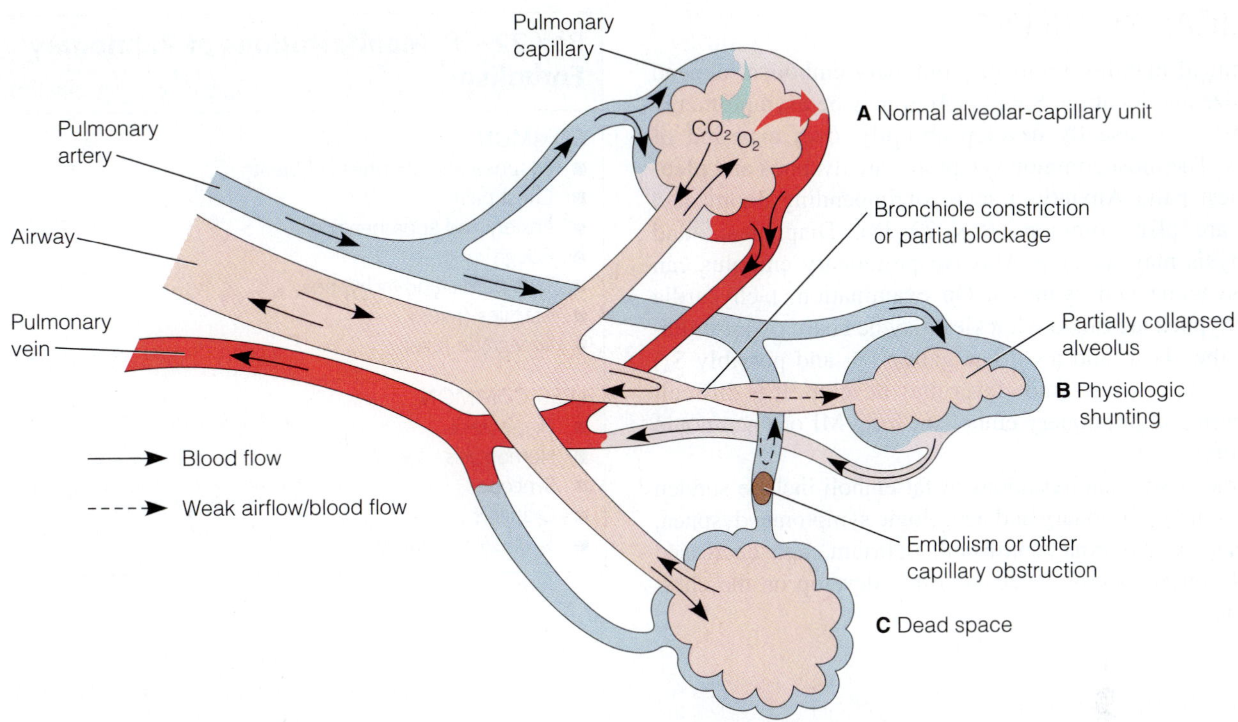

Figure 22–63 ■ Ventilation-perfusion relationships. *A,* Normal alveolar-capillary unit with an ideal match of ventilation and blood flow. Maximum gas exchange occurs between alveolus and blood. *B,* Physiologic shunting: A unit with adequate perfusion but inadequate ventilation. *C,* Dead space: A unit with adequate ventilation but inadequate perfusion. In the latter two cases, gas exchange is impaired.

develop. Bronchoconstriction occurs in the affected area of lung. **Dead space** (areas of the lung that are ventilated but not perfused) increases. Alveolar surfactant decreases, increasing the risk for atelectasis.

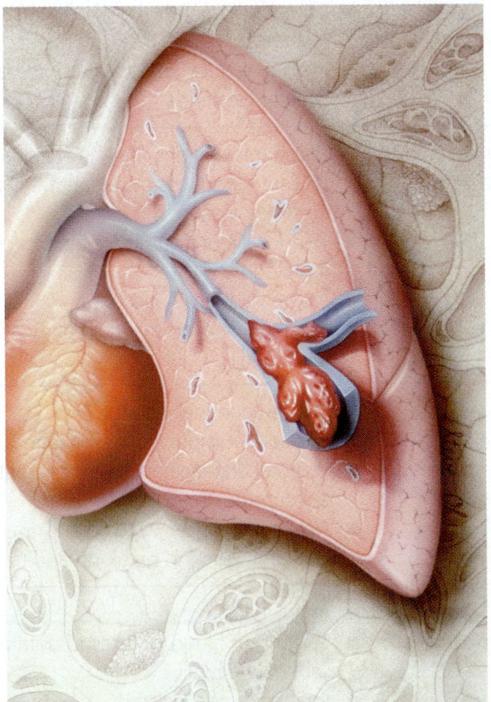

Figure 22–64 ■ A thromboembolism lodged in a pulmonary vessel.

Source: Steve Oh, M. S., Phototake NYC.

If infarction does not occur, the fibrinolytic system ultimately dissolves the clot, and pulmonary function returns to normal. If infarction does occur, the infarcted tissue becomes scarred and fibrotic.

Fat emboli are the most common nonthrombotic pulmonary emboli. A fat embolism usually occurs after fracture of long bone (typically the femur) releases bone marrow fat into the circulation. Adipose tissue or liver trauma may also lead to fat emboli.

Etiology

Thrombus arising from the deep veins of the legs is the leading cause of pulmonary embolism. Another less common source of emboli is fatty tissue that enters the circulatory systems as the result of surgery or trauma. This is most commonly seen when fatty marrow enters the circulation after a fracture to a large bone, most often the femur or pelvis.

Risk Factors

The risk factors for pulmonary embolus are similar to those for DVT, including stasis of venous blood flow, vessel wall damage, and altered blood coagulation. Risk factors for DVT include prolonged immobility; trauma, including hip and femur fractures; surgery (orthopaedic, pelvic, and gynecologic surgery in particular); MI and heart failure; obesity; and advanced age. Women who use oral contraceptives or estrogen therapy are at risk, as are women during pregnancy and childbirth. Smoking cigarettes also increases the risk of pulmonary emboli.

CLINICAL MANIFESTATIONS

The clinical manifestations of pulmonary embolism depend on its size and location. Small emboli may be asymptomatic. Manifestations usually develop abruptly, over a period of minutes. The most common symptoms are dyspnea and pleuritic chest pain. Anxiety, a sense of impending doom, and cough are also common (Box 22–38). Diaphoresis and hemoptysis may develop. Massive pulmonary embolus can cause syncope and cyanosis. On examination, tachycardia and tachypnea are noted. Crackles may be heard on auscultation of the chest, and a cardiac gallop (S_3 and possibly S_4) may be noted. A low-grade fever may develop. It is difficult to differentiate pulmonary embolism from MI or pneumonia by manifestations.

Characteristic manifestations of fat emboli include sudden onset of cardiopulmonary and neurologic symptoms: dyspnea, tachypnea, tachycardia, confusion, delirium, and decreased level of consciousness. Petechiae often develop on the chest and arms.

Box 22–38 **Manifestations of Pulmonary Embolism**

COMMON

- Dyspnea and shortness of breath
- Chest pain
- Anxiety and apprehension
- Cough
- Tachycardia and tachypnea
- Crackles (rales)
- Low-grade fever

LESS COMMON

- Diaphoresis
- Hemoptysis
- Syncope
- Cyanosis
- S_3 and/or S_4 gallop

CLINICAL MANIFESTATIONS AND THERAPIES **Pulmonary Embolism**

ETIOLOGY	CLINICAL MANIFESTATION	CLINICAL THERAPIES
Hypoxia may result if blood flow to a significant number of alveoli is blocked as a result of a thrombus blocking blood flow in a larger arteriole.	Anxiety, chest pain, shortness of breath, dyspnea, cyanosis, use of accessory muscles of respiration, respiratory acidosis, tachycardia, and tachypnea	■ Administration of oxygen ■ Position to facilitate breathing ■ Mechanical ventilation if unable to meet oxygen demands ■ Anticoagulants ■ Thrombolytics may be considered as a last resort ■ Help to reduce anxiety, which increases oxygen demands
Arterial congestion may increase pressure in distal arterioles as a result of impeded blood flow, resulting in rupture of small arterioles.	Hemoptysis, course crackles in the affected lung lobe, cough, shortness of breath, and dyspnea	■ Blood transfusions may be required if significant blood loss occurs, but this is not commonly seen ■ Reduce client's anxiety related to coughing blood ■ Oxygen administration ■ Suction airway to maintain patency if needed
Alveoli may collapse as a result of tissue necrosis and initiation of inflammatory process.	Absence of breath sounds in involved area, hypoxia, dyspnea, productive cough, and chest pain	■ Oxygen administration ■ Position to improve air exchange ■ Postural drainage and use of incentive spirometer ■ Avoid percussion, which can cause section of thrombi to break off and travel
Fever may result secondary to inflammation or infection	Elevated temperature, tachycardia, tachypnea, fluid volume deficiency, and cough	■ Antipyretics ■ Sputum or blood cultures to determine causative agent ■ Antibiotics as indicated

COLLABORATION

Because DVT may not be identified until pulmonary embolism occurs, prevention is the primary goal in treating pulmonary embolism. Early ambulation of medical and surgical clients is an effective means of preventing venous stasis and reducing the incidence of pulmonary embolism. External pneumatic compression of the legs is also effective for clients undergoing neurosurgery, urologic surgery, or major surgery of the hip or knee, or when anticoagulant therapy is contraindicated. Other preventive measures include elevating the legs and active and passive leg exercises.

When pulmonary embolism occurs, treatment is supportive. Oxygen therapy is initiated, and analgesics may be ordered to relieve severe pleuritic pain and anxiety. Pulmonary artery and wedge pressures are monitored with a balloon (Swan-Ganz) catheter. Cardiac outputs also may be assessed. Cardiac rhythm is monitored to detect dysrhythmias.

Diagnostic Tests

The studies performed to identify DVT differ from those used to diagnose a pulmonary embolism and include the following:

- *Plasma D-dimer levels* are highly specific to the presence of a thrombus. *D-Dimer* is a fragment of fibrin formed during lysis of a blood clot; elevated blood levels indicate thrombus formation and lysis (e.g., DVT and pulmonary embolism).
- *Chest CT with contrast* is the principal test used to diagnose pulmonary embolism. Chest CT effectively shows large, central pulmonary emboli; newer-generation scanners also can detect peripheral emboli.
- *Lung scans,* including perfusion and ventilation scans, may be used. In a perfusion lung scan, radiotagged albumin is injected intravenously and distributed in the lungs by the pulmonary blood flow. The lungs are then scanned for distribution of the isotope. An area of lung in which the isotope cannot be detected is suggestive of occluded blood flow and pulmonary embolism. For a ventilation scan, a radiotagged gas is inhaled and the lungs are scanned for gas distribution. Combined perfusion and ventilation scans allow identification of areas of the lungs that are ventilated but not perfused, a characteristic of pulmonary embolism.
- *Pulmonary angiography* is the definitive test for pulmonary embolism when other, less invasive tests are inconclusive. It is possible to detect very small emboli with angiography. A contrast medium injected into the pulmonary arteries illustrates the pulmonary vascular system on x-ray.
- *Chest x-ray* often shows pulmonary infiltration and occasionally pleural effusion.
- *Electrocardiography* is ordered to rule out acute MI as the cause of symptoms. Electrocardiographic findings commonly associated with pulmonary embolism include tachycardia and nonspecific T-wave changes.
- *Arterial blood gas* measurements usually show hypoxemia ($PaO_2 < 80$ mmHg) and often respiratory alkalosis (pH > 7.45, $PaCO_2 < 38$ mmHg) caused by tachypnea and hyperventilation.
- *$ETCO_2$ (end-tidal carbon dioxide*, a measurement of carbon dioxide exhaled) may be measured to evaluate alveolar perfusion. The normal $ETCO_2$ reading is 35–45 mmHg; it is decreased when pulmonary perfusion is impaired.
- *Coagulation studies* are ordered to monitor the response to therapy. The activated partial thromboplastin time (aPTT also called PTT) is used to assess the intrinsic clotting pathway and the response to heparin therapy. Desired levels with anticoagulant therapy are 1.5–2 times the control value. The risk of recurrent thromboembolism is high at lower levels; the risk of bleeding increases at higher levels. The International Normalized Ratio (INR) is used to assess the extrinsic clotting system and oral anticoagulation with warfarin (Coumadin). The goal of anticoagulant therapy is to achieve a therapeutic INR range of 2.0–3.0.

Pharmacologic Therapies

Anticoagulant therapy is the standard treatment to prevent pulmonary emboli. It is often instituted in high-risk clients who have no evidence of pulmonary embolism in order to prevent possible devastating effects. In the client with DVT or a pulmonary embolus, anticoagulants are administered to prevent further clotting and embolization.

For the client with a pulmonary embolus, heparin therapy is initiated with an intravenous bolus of 5,000–10,000 U, followed by continuous infusion at the rate of 1,000–1,500 U/hr. The aPTT or PTT is monitored frequently until stabilized. Heparin therapy is typically continued for approximately 5 days, or until oral anticoagulant therapy has become fully effective.

Oral anticoagulant therapy with warfarin sodium (Coumadin) is initiated at the same time as heparin. Warfarin sodium alters the synthesis of vitamin K–dependent clotting factors and requires 5–7 days to be fully effective. Anticoagulant therapy is continued for 2–3 months when few risk factors for thromboemboli exist; long-term therapy is used when chronic disorders that increase the risk of thromboemboli are present.

Bleeding is a risk associated with anticoagulant therapy. Although major hemorrhage is uncommon, it occurs in approximately 5% of clients receiving intravenous heparin. Cardiac, hepatic, and renal disease all increase the risk of significant bleeding, as does age over 60 years. Protamine, a protein that combines with heparin to inactivate it, is used to stop its anticoagulant effect if major bleeding occurs. Vitamin K is given to treat bleeding associated with Coumadin therapy.

Fibrinolytic therapy may be used to treat a massive pulmonary embolus and hypotension. Streptokinase, urokinase, or tissue plasminogen activators are used to **lyse** (disintegrate) the embolus, restore pulmonary blood flow, and reduce pulmonary artery and right heart pressures. Although fibrinolytic therapy may not reduce the mortality associated with pulmonary embolus, it may reduce the incidence of pulmonary hypertension, which develops 3–5 years after an embolism. Fibrinolysis significantly increases the risk of bleeding, particularly cerebral bleeding. Contraindications to fibrinolysis include intracranial disease, recent stroke, active bleeding or a bleeding disorder, pregnancy, severe hypertension, and recent surgery or trauma. Because of the increased risk of hemorrhage, invasive procedures are avoided after fibrinolysis.

Surgery

When anticoagulant therapy fails to prevent recurrent emboli or is contraindicated, an umbrella-like filter may be inserted into the inferior vena cava to trap large emboli while allowing continued blood flow (see Figure 22–40 on page 1392). The filter usually is inserted percutaneously, via either the femoral or jugular vein.

NURSING PROCESS

Nurses play a primary role in preventing pulmonary embolism. Encouraging clients to ambulate after surgery or illness, applying compression stockings or pneumatic compression devices, teaching and encouraging leg exercises, and discouraging the use of pillows under the knees, all help prevent DVT and subsequent pulmonary emboli.

Teach clients to reduce the risks associated with long periods of immobility, stopping every 1–2 hours during long automobile trips for a brief stretch and walk, getting up every hour or so and doing leg exercises while seated during long flights, and avoiding crossing the legs to prevent venous stasis and pooling. Regular exercise, such as walking, also reduces the risk for DVT. Instruct clients who stand for long periods to use well-fitted elastic stockings, being careful to avoid hose that bind around the knee or thigh.

Assessment

Because pulmonary embolism can be a medical emergency, assessment may be very focused. In other instances, when emboli are small and not life-threatening, a more extensive nursing assessment may be done. Obtain the following data when assessing the client with, or at risk for, a pulmonary embolus:

- *Health history.* Chest pain, shortness of breath, and other symptoms, including onset, severity, and precipitating factors; history of recent surgery, venous thrombosis, or other risk factor, such as childbirth or malignancy; current medications
- *Physical examination.* Level of consciousness, presence of respirations and pulse; skin color, temperature, and moisture; vital signs, including apical pulse and temperature; breath sounds and heart sounds; oxygen saturation level; neck vein distention and peripheral edema.

Diagnosis

Nursing diagnoses appropriate for a client with pulmonary embolism may include the following:

- Impaired Gas Exchange
- Decreased Cardiac Output
- Ineffective Protection
- Anxiety.

Plan

Goals of nursing care are individualized based on the client's specific needs and may include the following:

- The client will demonstrate an oxygen saturation that remains greater than 94%.
- The client will verbalize fears resulting from respiratory distress.
- The client will obtain relief from pain to allow for adequate rest and comfort.
- The client will demonstrate adequate tissue perfusion.

Implementation

The primary and most emergent focus of nursing care is to promote oxygenation and gas exchange. Other considerations include pain management and reduction of anxiety that often results from hypoxia.

Impaired Gas Exchange

Pulmonary embolism results in areas of the lung that are ventilated but not perfused; these areas receive no capillary blood flow. If the embolus is large and a major segment of the lung is not perfused, gas exchange is significantly affected. Nursing interventions are directed toward compensating for impaired gas exchange.

- Frequently assess respiratory status, including rate, depth, effort, lung sounds, and oxygen saturation. Impaired ventilation will further compromise gas exchange and worsen hypoxemia. Oxygen saturation can be monitored continuously and noninvasively to evaluate gas exchange.
- Place the client in Fowler's or high-Fowler's position, with the lower extremities dependent (e.g., hanging over the side of the bed). This position facilitates maximal lung expansion and reduces venous return to the right side of the heart, lowering pressures in the pulmonary vascular system.
- Monitor arterial blood gas results, reporting abnormal findings as indicated. Arterial blood gas results are used to assess gas exchange and tissue oxygenation. An arterial line may be inserted for monitoring arterial pressure and arterial blood sampling.

CLIENT TEACHING Pulmonary Embolism

Discuss the following topics when preparing the client with pulmonary embolism and family members for home care:

- Use of prescribed anticoagulant, including drug interactions, scheduled laboratory testing, and manifestations of bleeding to report to the primary care provider
- Using a soft toothbrush and electric razor to reduce the risk of bleeding
- Avoiding aspirin (unless prescribed) and other over-the-counter medications unless approved by the physician
- Importance of wearing a Medic-Alert tag for anticoagulant use
- Health promotion measures to reduce the risk of recurrent pulmonary embolism
- Symptoms of recurrent pulmonary embolism, such as sudden chest pain, shortness of breath, and possibly bloody sputum.

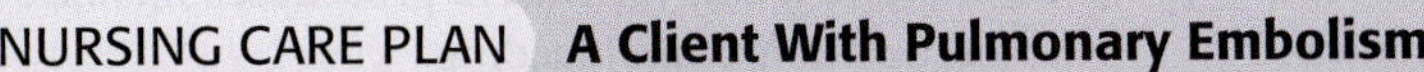

NURSING CARE PLAN A Client With Pulmonary Embolism

Frank Marlin, 52 years old, is traveling home with his wife from their 3-week vacation in Australia. The flight is 14½ hours long. As they approach their destination, Frank experiences a sharp, stabbing pain in his right chest, which he assumes is a pulled muscle that resulted from a sudden cough he developed a few hours ago. When the plane lands, he gathers their carry-on luggage, walks with his wife through the concourse toward the baggage area, and he notices he feels short of breath. He tells his wife he needs to sit down for a minute, secretly worried that he might be having a heart attack, but the pain remains on the right side of his chest. He begins to feel increasingly more anxious, and his wife notices he is breathing rapidly and perspiring. She asks for help from a customer service clerk, who calls the paramedics, who transport him to the local emergency room.

ASSESSMENT

On admission to the emergency department, the nurse collects the following data: temperature, 99.2°F tympanic; pulse, 98 bpm; respirations, 26/min; BP, 142/84 mmHg. Mr. Marlin's oxygen saturation is 87%. His breath sounds clear and equal, with fine rales in the upper right base. His lips and fingernails are mildly cyanotic. Mr. Marlin is alert, oriented, and anxious, asking the nurses "Am I going to die?" His chest x-ray is normal; however, computed tomography (CT) with contrast shows obstructed pulmonary circulation in the right upper lobe. His D-dimer level is elevated. Mr. Marlin is diagnosed with right upper lobe pulmonary emboli.

DIAGNOSES

- Impaired Gas Exchange
- Pain
- Anxiety

PLANNING

Goals of care include the following:

- Improve gas exchange, as evidenced by an oxygen saturation of greater than 90%.
- Obtain pain control sufficient to improve comfort, as evidenced by a reported pain level of 3 or less.
- Reduced anxiety, as evidenced by client's ability to sleep and express less fear.

IMPLEMENTATION

- Apply oxygen via face mask.
- Place cardiorespiratory monitor and oxygen saturation monitor on the client to allow for continuous monitoring of vital signs and oxygen saturation.
- Administer analgesics, per orders, and evaluate client's response to medication.
- Teach the client and family about risk factors contributing to development of pulmonary emboli.
- Answer client and family questions about the diagnosis of pulmonary emboli.
- Promote deep breathing.
- Position the client in semi-Fowler's position, lying on the right side to maximize expansion of healthy lungs.
- Remain with the client until vital signs normalize and oxygen saturation improves.
- Administer anticoagulants, and teach the client how to reduce bleeding risk.

EVALUATION

Mr. Marlin remains hospitalized for 5 days and is discharged on oral warfarin. Follow-up CT with contrast shows resolution of the emboli without permanent scarring or damage to lung tissue.

CRITICAL THINKING

1. Based on Mr. Marlin's symptoms, rate the severity of his pulmonary emboli.
2. What measures might you implement to reduce the client's anxiety?
3. Could Mr. Marlin's vital signs have been monitored manually instead of placement of a cardiorespiratory monitor? Why is the monitor placed?

- Maintain bed rest. Bed rest reduces metabolic demands and tissue needs for oxygen.

Decreased Cardiac Output

The impact of a large pulmonary embolus on hemodynamic status can be significant. Pressures in the pulmonary vascular system and right heart increase; blood return to the left heart and cardiac output may significantly decrease. Nursing interventions focus on preserving adequate blood pressure and organ function until cardiopulmonary status stabilizes. A central line for hemodynamic monitoring may be instituted.

- Auscultate heart sounds every 2–4 hours, and report any abnormalities. Sounds such as an S_3 or S_4 gallop may indicate cardiac compromise.
- Assess skin color and temperature. These assessments monitor tissue perfusion.
- Monitor cardiac rhythm. A drop in cardiac output and other hemodynamic alterations resulting from pulmonary embolism can precipitate dysrhythmias, which in turn can further impair cardiac output.
- Administer vasopressors and other medications as ordered. Carefully monitor the response to prescribed medications. Drugs may be prescribed to maintain adequate arterial

pressure and tissue perfusion. Potent drugs, such as vasopressors, require careful monitoring for desired and adverse effects.

- Monitor pulmonary arterial pressures, neck vein distention, and peripheral edema. Report findings as indicated. Right-sided heart failure is a potential complication of pulmonary embolism because of increased pulmonary arterial pressures.
- Maintain intravenous and arterial access sites as well as central lines. The client may be in unstable and critical condition, potentially needing immediate interventions to maintain life.
- Instruct to report chest pain or other symptoms. Decreased cardiac output and an increased workload resulting from pulmonary hypertension may cause anginal pain.

Ineffective Protection

Fibrinolytics and anticoagulant therapy impair normal clotting mechanisms, increasing the risk for bleeding and hemorrhage. This risk is particularly acute during the first 24–48 hours following fibrinolytic drug administration.

- Assess frequently for overt and covert signs of bleeding: bleeding gums; hematuria; obvious or occult blood in stool or vomitus; incisional bleeding, bleeding or bruising of injection sites or with minor trauma; joint pain or immobility; and abdominal or flank pain. Careful monitoring is necessary to identify early signs of abnormal bleeding and prevent potential hemorrhage.
- Report coagulation study results outside the desired range for anticoagulant therapy. Levels less than the target range may indicate an increased risk for further clot development and pulmonary emboli; levels above the target range indicate an increased risk for bleeding.
- Keep protamine sulfate available for heparin therapy and vitamin K available for warfarin (Coumadin) therapy. Bleeding or hemorrhage resulting from excess anticoagulant may require antidote administration to rapidly reverse the anticoagulant effects.
- Assess the medication regimen for possible drug interactions that could potentiate or inhibit anticoagulant effects. Drug interactions can increase the risk for hemorrhage or further embolus formation.
- Avoid invasive procedures, injections, and venous punctures when possible, particularly during and following fibrinolytic therapy. Invasive procedures increase the risk of tissue trauma and bleeding.
- Maintain firm pressure on injection and venipuncture sites. Maintain pressure for 30 minutes following arterial puncture. Firm pressure reduces the risk for bleeding into the tissues.
- Maintain adequate fluid intake. Administer stool softeners as ordered. These measures help prevent constipation and straining, which may precipitate bleeding of hemorrhoids.

Anxiety

Pulmonary embolism is a physiologic and psychologic threat to safety and integrity. It is a major physiologic stressor, eliciting a strong neuroendocrine stress response. The feeling of suffocation and inability to catch one's breath that accompanies a pulmonary embolus is also a strong psychologic stressor. Fear, anxiety, and apprehension are common responses.

- Assess the client's anxiety level. Appropriate interventions are determined by the level of anxiety.
- Remain with the client as much as possible. The presence of a caring nurse helps reduce fear.
- Explain procedures and treatments, using short, simple sentences. Providing clearly understood, simple instructions reduces fear of the unknown.
- Reduce environmental stimuli, and use a calm, reassuring manner. These measures help reduce anxiety for both the nurse and the client.
- Allow supportive family members to remain with the client as much as possible. Calm, supportive family members provide further reassurance.
- Administer morphine sulfate as ordered. Morphine is given to reduce pain and anxiety.

Evaluation

Client progress toward meeting goals set during the planning stage of care is evaluated based on the following expected outcomes:

- The client maintains adequate tissue perfusion to prevent complications or tissue necrosis.
- The client obtains pain relief to allow for adequate rest.
- The client maintains adequate oxygenation to meet the body's oxygen demands.

REVIEW Pulmonary Embolism

RELATE: LINK THE CONCEPTS

Linking the exemplar of Pulmonary Embolism with the concept of Acid–Base Balance:

1. What impact on acid–base balance would you anticipate finding when reviewing the results of an arterial blood gas drawn from a client with a significant pulmonary emboli?
2. What assessment findings would you anticipate when examining the client described in question 1?

Linking the exemplar of Pulmonary Embolism with the concept of Comfort:

3. Contrast the effectiveness of pharmacological versus nonpharmacological therapies to control the pain associated with pulmonary embolism.
4. What risk is associated with administration of narcotics to a client with pulmonary emboli? How would you reduce these risks?

READY: GO TO COMPANION SKILLS MANUAL

- Assisting with arterial line insertion
- Monitoring arterial blood pressure
- Supporting a client in Fowler's position
- Assessing the client in pain
- Assessing the skin
- Assessing the heart and central vessels
- Assessing an apical-radial pulse
- Assessing respirations
- Assessing the heart rate
- Assessing the respiratory rate

REFER: GO TO MYNURSINGKIT

REFLECT: CASE STUDY

Jennifer Walker is a 20-year-old female who is attending college in the Midwest. She is majoring in business and lives with her boyfriend, Sam age 21, in an off-campus apartment. Jennifer had an annual physical with a physician on campus and obtained a prescription for oral contraceptives. Jennifer and Sam enjoy walking around the campus with their dog, Shelby, and are very active playing tennis and golf. Sam's parents are both doctors and Jennifer's mother is a nurse.

Jennifer begins to notice that she has pain in her left leg when she walks Shelby and when she is playing tennis. Sam suggests that she return to the physician for a check-up.

Jennifer's doctor admits her to the hospital and places her on Heparin and bedrest for her thrombophlebitis. Jennifer is on her third day in the hospital and she and Sam are studying together in her room. She develops dyspnea and chest pain and becomes very apprehensive. Sam goes to the nurse's station to inform the staff of Jennifer's new symptoms.

1. What is the priority intervention for Jennifer at this time?
2. What is the physiological rationale for pain control for Jennifer?
3. Create a plan of care for Jennifer and Sam regarding teaching interventions needed for discharge.

22.12 SHOCK

KEY TERMS

Anaphylactic shock, *1489*
Cardiac output (CO), *1484*
Cardiogenic shock, *1488*
Distributive shock, *1489*
Hypovolemic shock, *1488*
Mean arterial pressure (MAP), *1484*
Neurogenic shock, *1489*
Obstructive shock, *1489*
Septic shock, *1489*
Shock, *1483*
Stroke volume (SV), *1483*
Sympathetic tone, *1484*
Tone, *1483*
Vasogenic shock, *1489*

LEARNING OUTCOMES

After reading about this exemplar, you will be able to:

1. Describe the pathophysiology, etiology, clinical manifestations, and direct and indirect causes of shock.
2. Identify risk factors associated with shock.
3. Illustrate the nursing process in providing culturally competent care across the life span for individuals with shock.
4. Formulate priority nursing diagnoses appropriate for an individual with shock.
5. Create a plan of care for individuals with shock and their families.
6. Assess expected outcomes for an individual with shock.
7. Discuss therapies used in the collaborative care of an individual with shock.
8. Employ evidence-based caring interventions for an individual with shock.

BASIS FOR SELECTION OF EXEMPLAR

Standards of Nursing Practice

OVERVIEW

Shock is a clinical syndrome characterized by a systemic imbalance between oxygen supply and demand. This imbalance results in a state of inadequate blood flow to body organs and tissues, causing life-threatening cellular dysfunction.

To maintain cellular metabolism, cells of all body organs and tissues require a regular and consistent supply of oxygen and the removal of metabolic wastes. This homeostatic regulation is maintained primarily by the cardiovascular system and depends on four physiologic components:

1. A cardiac output sufficient to meet bodily requirements
2. An uncompromised vascular system, in which the vessels have a diameter sufficient to allow unimpeded blood flow and have good **tone** (the ability to constrict or dilate to maintain normal pressure)
3. A volume of blood sufficient to fill the circulatory system, and a blood pressure adequate to maintain blood flow
4. Tissues that are able to extract and use the oxygen delivered through the capillaries.

In a healthy person, these components function as a system to maintain tissue perfusion. During shock, however, one or more of these components are disrupted. An understanding of basic hemodynamics is necessary to understand the pathophysiology of shock:

- **Stroke volume (SV)** is the amount of blood pumped into the aorta with each contraction of the left ventricle.

- **Cardiac output (CO)** is the amount of blood pumped per minute into the aorta by the left ventricle. It is determined by multiplying SV by the heart rate (HR): CO = SV × HR.
- **Mean arterial pressure (MAP)** is the average pressure in the arterial circulation throughout the cardiac cycle. It is the product of CO and systemic vascular resistance (SVR): MAP = CO × SVR. When CO, SVR, or total blood volume rises, MAP and tissue perfusion increase. Conversely, when CO, SVR, or total blood volume falls, MAP and tissue perfusion decrease.
- The *sympathetic nervous system (SNS)* maintains the smooth muscle surrounding the arteries and arterioles in a state of partial contraction called **sympathetic tone**. Increased sympathetic stimulation increases vasoconstriction and systemic vascular resistance; decreased sympathetic stimulation allows vasodilatation, which decreases systemic vascular resistance.
- *Pulse pressure* (the difference between systolic and diastolic blood pressure) is often an early indicator of shock. Narrowing pulse pressure is consistent with hypovolemic and cardiogenic shock as a result of reduced cardiac output while septic shock causes a widening pulse pressure.

PATHOPHYSIOLOGY AND ETIOLOGY

When one or more cardiovascular components do not function properly, the body's hemodynamic properties are altered. Consequently, tissue perfusion may be inadequate to sustain normal cellular metabolism. The result is the clinical syndrome known as shock.

The manifestations of shock result from the body's attempts to maintain vital organs (heart and brain) and to preserve life following a drop in cellular perfusion. However, if the injury or condition triggering shock is severe enough or of long enough duration, then cellular hypoxia and cellular death occur.

Shock is triggered by a sustained drop in MAP. This drop can occur after a decrease in cardiac output, a decrease in the circulating blood volume, or an increase in the size of the vascular bed as a result of peripheral vasodilatation. If intervention is timely and effective, the physiologic events that characterize shock may be stopped; if not, shock may lead to death. See Table 22–33 for classifications of shock.

Stage I: Early, Reversible, and Compensatory Shock

The initial stage of shock begins when baroreceptors in the aortic arch and the carotid sinus detect a sustained drop in MAP of less than 10 mmHg from normal levels. The circulating blood volume may decrease (usually to < 500 mL), but not enough to cause serious effects.

The body reacts to the decrease in arterial pressure as it would to any physical stressor. The cerebral integration center initiates the body's response systems, causing the SNS to increase the heart rate and the force of cardiac contraction, thus increasing cardiac output. Sympathetic stimulation also causes peripheral vasoconstriction, resulting in increased systemic vascular resistance and a rise in arterial pressure. The net result is that the perfusion of cells, tissues, and organs is maintained.

Symptoms are almost imperceptible during the early stage of shock. The pulse rate may be slightly elevated. If the injury is minor or of short duration, arterial pressure is usually maintained, and no further symptoms occur.

Compensatory shock begins after the MAP falls 10–15 mmHg below normal levels. The circulating blood volume is reduced by 25–35% (1,000 mL or more), but compensatory mechanisms are able to maintain blood pressure and tissue perfusion to vital organs, thereby preventing cell damage. These compensatory mechanisms include the following:

- Stimulation of the SNS results in the release of epinephrine from the adrenal medulla and the release of norepinephrine from the adrenal medulla and the sympathetic fibers. Both hormones rapidly stimulate the alpha- and beta-adrenergic fibers. Stimulated alpha-adrenergic fibers cause vasoconstriction in the blood vessels supplying the skin and most of the abdominal viscera. Perfusion of these areas decreases. Stimulated beta-adrenergic fibers cause vasodilatation in vessels supplying the heart and skeletal muscles ($beta_1$ response) and increase the heart rate and force of cardiac contraction ($beta_2$ response). Furthermore, blood vessels in the respiratory

TABLE 22–33 **Classification of Hemorrhagic Shock and Client Presentation**

	COMPENSATED/CLASS I	MILD/CLASS II	MODERATE/CLASS III	SEVERE/CLASS IV
Blood loss	< 750 mL	750–1,500 mL	1,500–2,000 mL	> 2,000 mL
% of blood volume loss	< 15%	15–30%	30–40%	> 40%
Heart rate	< 100	> 100	> 120	> 140
Blood pressure	Normal or increased	Normal	Decreased	Markedly decreased
Pulse pressure	Normal or increased	Decreased	Decreased	Decreased
Capillary refill	Normal	Mild increase	Usually delayed	Delayed
Respiratory rate	Normal	Mild increase	Moderate tachypnea	Markedly tachypnea
Urine output (mL/hr)	> 30 mL	20–30 mL	5–15 mL	Anuria
Mental status	Normal–slightly anxious	Mildly anxious–agitated	Anxious–confused	Lethargic–obtunded

system dilate, and the respiratory rate increases (beta$_2$ response). Thus, stimulation of the SNS results in increased cardiac output and oxygenation of these tissues.

- The renin–angiotensin response occurs as the blood flow to the kidneys decreases. Renin released from the kidneys converts a plasma protein to angiotensin II, which causes vasoconstriction and stimulates the adrenal cortex to release aldosterone. Aldosterone causes the kidneys to reabsorb water and sodium and to lose potassium. The absorption of water maintains circulating blood volume while increased vasoconstriction increases systemic vascular resistance, maintaining central vascular volume and raising blood pressure.
- The hypothalamus releases adrenocorticotropic hormone, causing the adrenal glands to secrete aldosterone. Aldosterone promotes the reabsorption of water and sodium by the kidneys, preserving blood volume and pressure.
- The posterior pituitary gland releases antidiuretic hormone, which increases renal reabsorption of water to increase intravascular volume. The combined effects of hormones released by the hypothalamus and posterior pituitary glands work to conserve central vascular volume.
- As MAP falls in the compensatory stage of shock, decreased capillary hydrostatic pressure causes a fluid shift from the interstitial space into the capillaries. The net gain of fluid raises the blood volume.

Working together, these compensatory mechanisms can maintain MAP for only a short period of time. During this period, the perfusion and oxygenation of the heart and brain are adequate. If effective treatment is provided, the process is arrested, and no permanent damage occurs. However, unless the underlying cause of shock is reversed, these compensatory mechanisms soon become harmful, and shock perpetuates shock.

Stage II: Intermediate or Progressive Shock

The progressive stage of shock occurs after a sustained decrease in MAP of 20 mmHg or more below normal levels and a fluid loss of 35–50% (1,800–2,500 mL). Although the compensatory mechanisms in the previous state remain activated, they are no longer able to maintain MAP at a level sufficient to ensure perfusion of vital organs.

The vasoconstriction response that first helped sustain MAP eventually limits blood flow to the point that cells become oxygen deficient. To remain alive, the affected cells switch from aerobic to anaerobic metabolism. The lactic acid formed as a by-product of anaerobic metabolism contributes to an acidotic state at the cellular level. As a result, adenosine triphosphate, the source of cellular energy, is produced inefficiently. Lacking energy, the sodium–potassium pump fails. Potassium moves out of the cell, while sodium and water move inward. As this process continues, the cell swells, cell membrane integrity is lost, and cell organelles are damaged. Lysosomes within the cell spill out their digestive enzymes, which disintegrate any remaining organelles. Some enzymes spread to adjacent cells, where they erode and rupture cell membranes.

The acid by-products of anaerobic metabolism dilate the precapillary arterioles and constrict the postcapillary venules. This causes increased hydrostatic pressure within the capillary, and fluid shifts back into the interstitial space. The capillaries also become increasingly permeable, allowing serum proteins to shift from the vascular space into the interstitium. The buildup of plasma proteins increases the osmotic pressure in the interstitium, further accelerating the fluid shift out of the capillaries.

Throughout this period, the heart rate and vasoconstriction increase; however, perfusion of the skin, skeletal muscles, kidneys, and gastrointestinal organs is greatly diminished. Cells in the heart and brain become hypoxic, while other body cells and tissues become ischemic and anoxic. A generalized state of acidosis and hyperkalemia ensues. Unless this stage of shock is treated rapidly, the client's chances of survival are poor.

Stage III: Refractory or Irreversible Shock

If shock progresses to the irreversible stage, tissue anoxia becomes so generalized and cellular death so widespread that no treatment can reverse the damage. Even if MAP is temporarily restored, too much cellular damage has occurred to maintain life. Death of cells is followed by death of tissues, which results in death of organs. Death of vital organs contributes to subsequent death of the body.

Effects of Shock on Body Systems

Whatever its causes, shock produces predictable effects on the body's organ systems.

CARDIOVASCULAR SYSTEM The perfusion and oxygenation of the heart are adequate in the early stages of shock. As shock progresses, myocardial cells become hypoxic, and myocardial muscle function diminishes. Initially, the blood pressure may be normal or even slightly elevated (as a result of compensatory mechanisms) and the heart rate only slightly increased. Sympathetic stimulation increases the heart rate (a sinus tachycardia of 120 bpm is common) in an effort to increase cardiac output. As a result of vasoconstriction and decreased blood volume, the palpated pulse is rapid, weak, and thready; as shock progresses, peripheral pulses are usually nonpalpable.

Tachycardia reduces the time available for left ventricular filling and coronary artery perfusion, further reducing cardiac output. With progressive shock, altered acid–base balance, hypoxia, and hyperkalemia damage the heart's electrical systems and contractility. Consequently, cardiac dysrhythmias may develop. Decreased blood volume with decreased venous return also decreases cardiac output, and blood pressure falls.

The blood pressure changes produced by shock are characterized by a progressive decrease in both systolic and diastolic pressures and a narrowing pulse pressure. Auscultation of blood pressure is often difficult or impossible and is an inaccurate reflection of blood pressure status. For this reason, hemodynamic monitoring is usually instituted to follow the client's cardiovascular status accurately.

MULTISYSTEM EFFECTS OF **Shock**

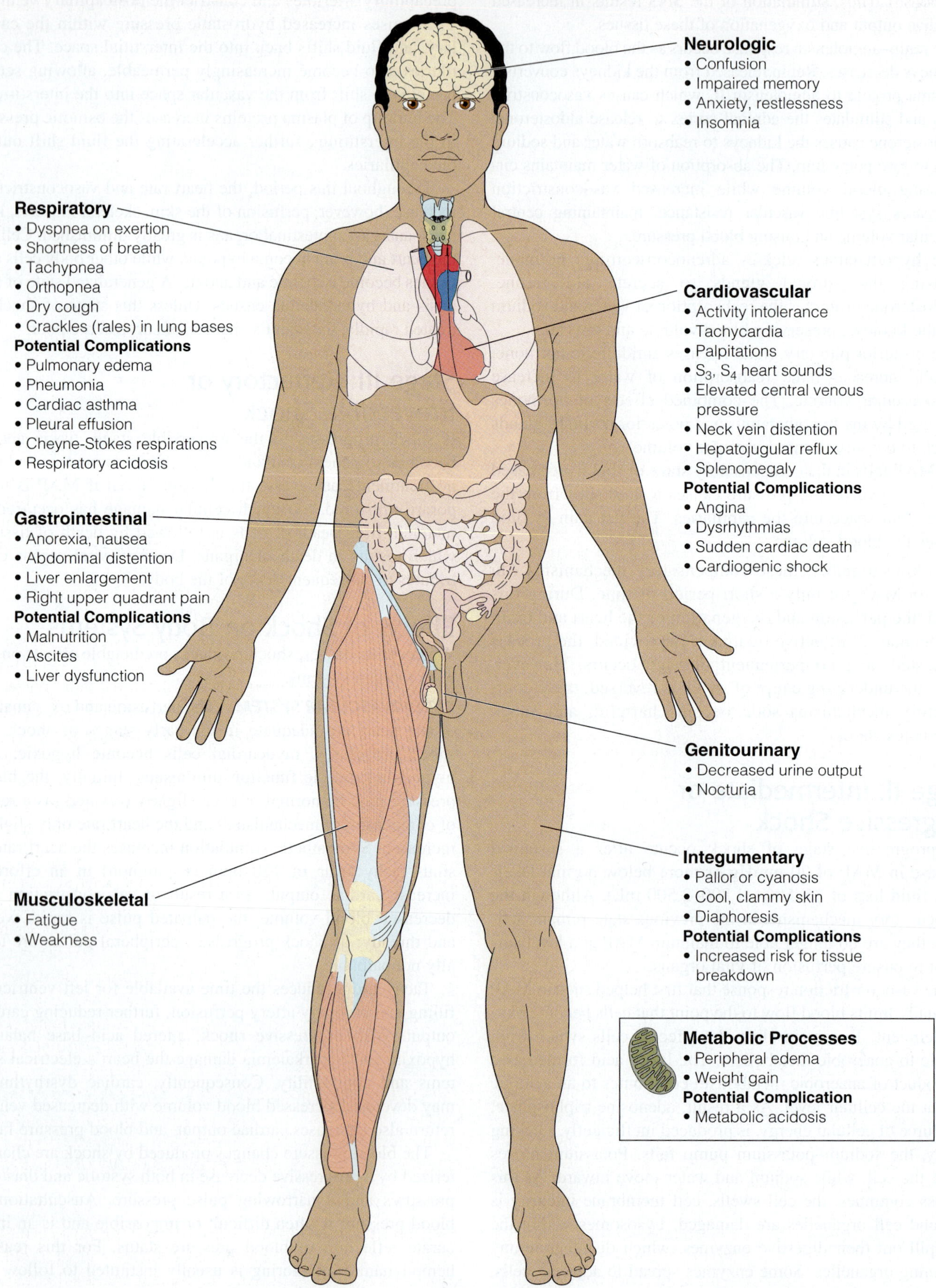

RESPIRATORY SYSTEM During shock, oxygen delivery to cells may be impaired by a drop in circulating blood volume or, in the case of blood loss, by an insufficient number of red blood cells that carry oxygen. Although the respiratory rate increases because of compensatory mechanisms that promote oxygenation, the number of alveoli that are perfused decreases, and gas exchange is impaired. As a result, oxygen levels in the blood decrease, and carbon dioxide levels increase. As perfusion of the lungs diminishes, carbon dioxide is retained, and respiratory acidosis occurs.

A complication of decreased perfusion of the lungs is acute respiratory distress syndrome, or "shock lung." The exact mechanism that produces acute respiratory distress syndrome is unknown, but some contributing factors have been identified. The pulmonary capillaries become increasingly permeable to proteins and water, resulting in noncardiogenic pulmonary edema. Production of surfactant, which controls surface tension within alveoli, is impaired, and the alveoli collapse or fill with fluid. This potentially lethal form of respiratory failure may result from any condition that causes hypoperfusion of the lungs, but it is more common in shock caused by hemorrhage, severe allergic responses, trauma, and infection.

GASTROINTESTINAL SYSTEMS The gastrointestinal organs normally receive 25% of the cardiac output through the splanchnic circulation. Shock constricts the splanchnic arterioles and redirects arterial blood flow to the heart and brain. Consequently, gastrointestinal organs become ischemic and may be irreversibly damaged.

Gastric mucosa tends to ulcerate when it becomes ischemic. Lesions of the gastric and duodenal mucosa (stress ulcers) can develop within hours of severe trauma, sepsis, or burns (Porth, 2005). Gastrointestinal ulcers may hemorrhage within 2–10 days following the original cause of shock. In addition, the permeability of damaged mucosa increases, allowing enteric bacteria or their toxins to enter the abdominal cavity and then progress to the circulation, resulting in sepsis.

Gastric and intestinal motility is impaired during shock, and paralytic ileus may result. If the episode of shock is prolonged, necrosis of the bowel may occur. In many cases, alterations in the structure and function of the gastrointestinal tract impair absorption of nutrients, such as protein and glucose.

Shock also alters the metabolic functions of the liver. Initially, gluconeogenesis (the process of forming glucose from noncarbohydrate sources) and glycogenolysis (the breakdown of glycogen into glucose) increase. This process allows blood glucose levels to increase as the body attempts to respond to the stressor; however, as shock progresses, liver functions are impaired and hypoglycemia develops. Metabolism of fats and protein is impaired, and the liver can no longer effectively remove lactic acid, contributing to the development of metabolic acidosis.

The destruction of the liver's reticuloendothelial Kupffer cells (phagocytes that destroy bacteria) causes a further problem. Bacteria may proliferate within the circulatory system, causing overwhelming bacterial infection and toxicity.

NEUROLOGIC SYSTEM The primary effects of shock on the neurologic system involve changes in mental status and orientation. Cerebral hypoxia produces altered levels of consciousness, beginning with apathy and lethargy and progressing to coma. A common early symptom of cerebral hypoxia is restlessness. Continued ischemia of brain cells eventually causes swelling, resulting in cerebral edema, neurotransmitter failure, and irreversible brain cell damage.

As cerebral ischemia worsens, the sympathetic activity and vasomotor centers are depressed. This leads to a loss of sympathetic tone, causing systemic vasodilatation and pooling of blood in the periphery. As a result, venous return and cardiac output further decrease.

PRACTICE ALERT

An early sign of shock is a change in level of consciousness. Late signs of shock include mental status changes, hypotension, and marked tachycardia.

RENAL SYSTEM Blood that normally perfuses the kidneys is shunted to the heart and brain during the progressive stage of shock, resulting in renal hypoperfusion. The drop in renal perfusion is reflected in a corresponding decrease in the glomerular filtration rate. Urine output is reduced, and the urine that is produced is highly concentrated. Oliguria of less than 20 mL/hr indicates progressive shock.

Healthy kidneys can tolerate a drop in perfusion only for approximately 20 minutes; thereafter, acute tubular necrosis develops (Porth, 2005). As tubular necrosis occurs, epithelial cells slough off and block the tubules, disrupting nephron function. The accumulating loss of functional nephrons eventually causes renal failure. Without normal renal function, metabolic waste products are retained in the plasma.

If treatment restores renal perfusion, the kidneys can regenerate the lost epithelial cells in the tubules, and renal function usually returns to normal. However, in a client who is older, chronically ill, or in sustained shock, loss of renal function may become permanent.

EFFECTS ON SKIN, TEMPERATURE, AND THIRST In most types of shock, blood vessels supplying the skin are vasoconstricted, and the sweat glands are activated. As a result, changes in skin color occur. The skin of white clients becomes pale. In people with darker skin (e.g., those of African, Hispanic, or Mediterranean descent), shock-related skin color changes may be assessed as paleness of the lips, oral mucous membranes, nail beds, and conjunctiva. The skin is usually cool and moist and, in the later stages of shock, often edematous.

The body temperature decreases as shock progresses, the result of a decrease in overall body metabolism. Some people with shock become thirsty, probably a response to decreased blood volume and increased serum osmolality (Porth, 2005).

Etiology

Shock is identified according to its underlying cause. All types of shock progress through the same stages and exert similar effects on body systems. Any differences are noted in the following discussion.

HYPOVOLEMIC SHOCK **Hypovolemic shock** is caused by a decrease in intravascular volume of 15% or more (Porth, 2005). In hypovolemic shock, the venous blood returning to the heart decreases, and ventricular filling drops. As a result, stroke volume, cardiac output, and blood pressure decrease. Hypovolemic shock is the most common type of shock, and it often occurs simultaneously with other types.

The decrease in circulating blood volume that triggers hypovolemic shock may result from the following:

- Loss of blood volume from hemorrhage (from surgery, trauma, gastrointestinal bleeding, blood coagulation disorders, or ruptured esophageal varices)
- Loss of intravascular fluid from the skin because of injuries such as burns
- Loss of blood volume from severe dehydration
- Loss of body fluid from the gastrointestinal system because of persistent and severe vomiting or diarrhea or continuous nasogastric suctioning
- Renal losses of fluid because of diuretic use or endocrine disorders, such as diabetes insipidus
- Conditions causing fluid shifts from the intravascular compartment to the interstitial space
- Third spacing because of such disorders as liver diseases with ascites, pleural effusion, or intestinal obstruction.

Hypovolemic shock affects all body systems. Its effects vary depending on the client's age, general state of health, extent of injury or severity of illness, length of time before treatment is provided, and rate of volume loss.

The manifestations of hypovolemic shock result directly from the decrease in circulating blood volume and the initiation of compensatory mechanisms (Figure 22–65 ■). The loss of circulating blood volume reduces cardiac output by decreasing venous return to the heart. As a result, blood pressure drops. The carotid and cardiac baroreceptors sense the decrease in blood pressure and communicate it to the vasomotor centers in the brainstem. The vasomotor centers then induce the sympathetic compensatory responses. If the fluid loss is less than 500 mL, activation of the sympathetic response is generally adequate to restore cardiac output and blood pressure to near normal, although the heart rate may remain elevated.

With a sustained loss of blood volume (1,000 mL or more), the shock stage progresses. Heart rate and vasoconstriction increase, and blood flow to the skin, skeletal muscles, kidneys, and abdominal organs decreases. Several renal mechanisms and a decline in capillary pressure help conserve blood volume. Eventually, the amount of blood flowing to cells is too low to oxygenate them and sustain production of cellular energy. Anaerobic metabolism begins, producing an acidotic environment for cells. As a result, cells lose their physical integrity. If untreated, shock causes multiple organ failure, and death results.

With aging comes a relative decrease in sympathetic activity in relation to the cardiovascular system. Cardiac compliance also decreases with age. Atherosclerosis affects many vital organs' sensitivity to even the slightest reduction in blood flow. Many older adults experience secondary volume depletion because of chronic diuretic use or malnutrition. Also, clients prescribed beta-blockers may not present with tachycardia as an early indicator of shock. This important sign can be masked because of beta-adrenergic blockade. These clients will require early invasive monitoring in order to avoid excessive or inadequate volume restoration. This should be considered early in the treatment phase.

CARDIOGENIC SHOCK **Cardiogenic shock** occurs when the heart's pumping ability is compromised to the point that it cannot maintain cardiac output and adequate tissue perfusion. The

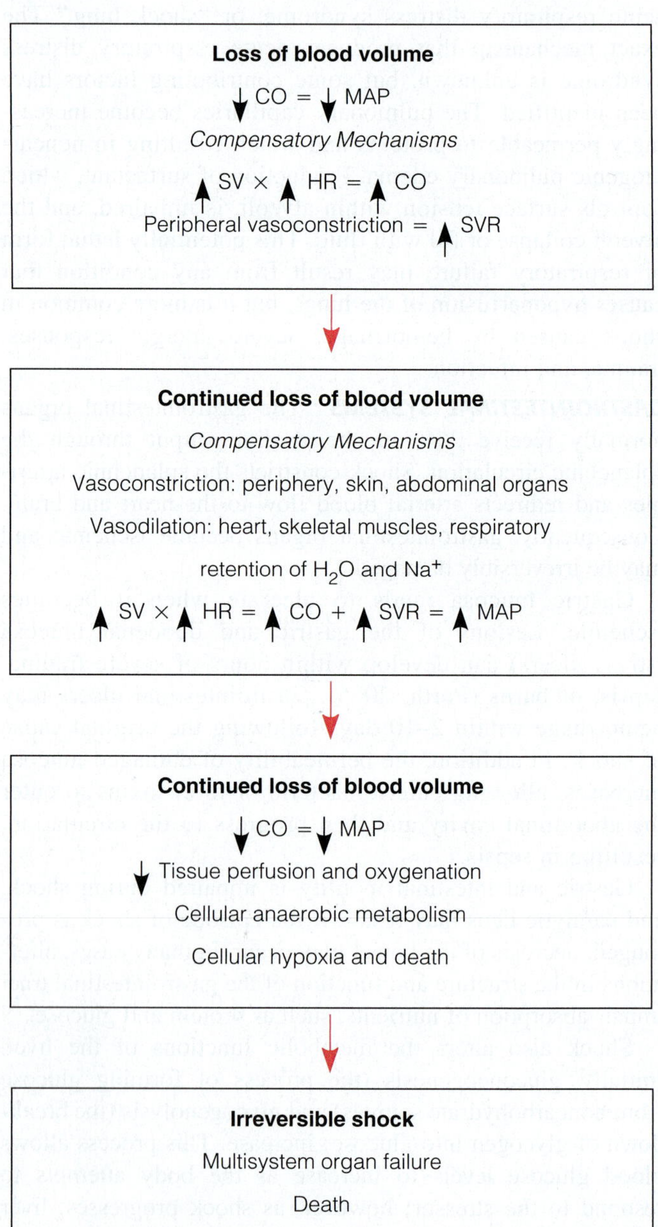

Figure 22–65 ■ Stages of hypovolemic shock.

loss of the pumping action of the heart may be caused by the following conditions:

- MI
- Cardiac tamponade
- Restrictive pericarditis
- Cardiac arrest
- Dysrhythmias, such as fibrillation or ventricular tachycardia
- Pathologic changes in the valves
- Cardiomyopathies from hypertension, alcohol, bacterial or viral infections, or ischemia
- Complications of cardiac surgery
- Electrolyte imbalances, especially changes in normal potassium and calcium levels
- Drugs affecting cardiac muscle contractility
- Head injuries causing damage to the cardioregulatory center.

Myocardial infarction is the most common cause of cardiogenic shock. Clients admitted to the hospital for treatment of MI or cardiac surgery are at risk for cardiogenic shock. The severity and progression of shock are related to the amount of myocardial damage.

Whatever the cardiogenic cause, the decrease in cardiac output causes a decrease in MAP. Heart rate may increase in response to compensatory mechanisms. However, tachycardia, increases myocardial oxygen consumption, and decreases coronary perfusion. The myocardium becomes progressively depleted of oxygen, causing further myocardial ischemia and necrosis. The typical sequence of shock is essentially unchanged in cardiogenic shock.

Cyanosis, however, is more common in cardiogenic shock, because stagnating blood increases extraction of oxygen from the hemoglobin at the capillary beds. As a result, the skin, lips, and nail beds may appear cyanotic. As cardiac failure and cardiogenic shock progress, left ventricular end-diastolic pressure increases. The increase is transmitted to the pulmonary capillary bed, and pulmonary edema may occur. Retention of blood in the right side of the heart increases right atrial pressure, which leads to jugular venous distention as a result of backflow through the vena cava.

OBSTRUCTIVE SHOCK **Obstructive shock** is caused by an obstruction in the heart or great vessels that either impedes venous return or prevents effective cardiac pumping action. The causes of obstructive shock are impaired diastolic filling (e.g., pericardial tamponade or pneumothorax), increased right ventricular afterload (e.g., pulmonary emboli), and increased left ventricular afterload (e.g., aortic stenosis or abdominal distention). The manifestations are the result of decreased cardiac output and blood pressure, with reduced tissue perfusion and cellular metabolism.

DISTRIBUTIVE SHOCK **Distributive shock**, also called **vasogenic shock**, includes several types of shock that result from widespread vasodilatation and decreased peripheral resistance. Because the blood volume does not change, relative hypovolemia results.

SEPTIC SHOCK **Septic shock**, also known as septicemia, is the leading cause of death for clients in intensive care units. It is one part of a progressive syndrome called systemic inflammatory response syndrome. This condition is most often the result of gram-negative bacterial infections (i.e., *Pseudomonas, Escherichia coli,* or *Klebsiella*) but may also follow gram-positive infections from *Staphylococcus* and *Streptococcus* bacteria. Septic shock is discussed in more detail in Concept 15, Exemplar 15.6, Sepsis.

NEUROGENIC SHOCK **Neurogenic shock** is the result of an imbalance between parasympathetic and sympathetic stimulation of vascular smooth muscle. If parasympathetic overstimulation or sympathetic understimulation persists, sustained vasodilatation occurs, and blood pools in the venous and capillary beds.

Neurogenic shock causes dramatic reduction in systemic vascular resistance as the size of the vascular compartment increases. As systemic vascular resistance decreases, pressure in the blood vessels becomes too low to drive nutrients across capillary membranes, and cellular metabolism is impaired.

The following conditions can cause neurogenic shock by increasing parasympathetic stimulation or inhibiting sympathetic stimulation of the smooth muscle of blood vessels:

- Head injury
- Trauma to the spinal cord
- Insulin reactions (which cause hypoglycemia, decreasing glucose to the medulla)
- Central nervous system depressant drugs (e.g., sedatives, barbiturates, or narcotics)
- Anesthesia (spinal and general)
- Severe pain
- Prolonged exposure to heat.

Bradycardia occurs early, but tachycardia begins as compensatory mechanisms are initiated. CVP drops as veins dilate, venous return to the heart decreases, stroke volume decreases, and MAP falls. In early stages, the extremities are warm and pink (from the pooling of blood), but as shock progresses, the skin becomes pale and cool.

ANAPHYLACTIC SHOCK **Anaphylactic shock** is the result of a widespread hypersensitivity reaction (called anaphylaxis). The pathophysiology in this type of shock includes vasodilation, pooling of blood in the periphery, and hypovolemia with altered cellular metabolism. These physiologic alterations occur when a sensitized person has contact with an allergen (a foreign substance to which an individual is hypersensitive). Many different allergens can cause anaphylactic shock, including medications, blood administration, latex, foods, snake

DEVELOPMENTAL CONSIDERATIONS

Blood Volume in Children

The child's total blood volume varies by weight. The child has approximately 80 mL of blood for every kilogram of body weight.

- Newborn: 3 kg × 80 mL = 240 mL (1 cup)
- 5 year old: 25 kg × 80 mL = 2,000 mL (2 quarts)
- 13 year old: 50 kg × 80 mL = 4,000 mL (1 gallon)

venom, and insect stings. Anaphylactic shock is discussed in more detail in Concept 14, Exemplar 14.2, Hypersensitivity.

Risk Factors

Advancing cardiac disease increases the risk for cardiogenic shock. Those who practice high-risk behaviors, ranging from driving while under the influence of a mind-altering substance to those who participate in dangerous sports, are at increased risk for trauma and shock that results from bleeding or multisystem injury. Clients with diseases that slow the body's ability to clot, such as hemophilia, are also at increased risk for hemorrhagic shock.

CLINICAL MANIFESTATIONS

Specific manifestations for different forms of shock are included in the descriptions under Pathophysiology and Etiology. The onset of shock may be rapid or slow, depending on its cause and severity. Signs of early shock may be nonspecific. As the body compensates for hypotension or decreased blood volume, signs of shock include tachycardia, increased respiratory effort, and decreased urine output. The client may also be diaphoretic or perspire excessively.

If treatment is not begun in the early stages of shock, the condition progresses until the client can no longer compensate. At that time, the systolic blood pressure drops, and the pulse pressure narrows. Reduced cerebral blood flow ultimately results in a decreased level of consciousness. If shock is not reversed, the condition progresses to cardiopulmonary failure.

COLLABORATION

Medical care for the client with shock focuses on treating the underlying cause, increasing arterial oxygenation, and improving tissue perfusion. Depending on the cause and type of shock, interventions include emergency care measures, oxygen therapy, fluid replacement, and medications. Emergency care is often the first course of collaborative action taken to arrest shock.

Diagnostic Tests

The following diagnostic tests can help identify the type of shock and assess the client's physical status:

- *Blood hemoglobin* and *hematocrit.* Changes in hemoglobin and hematocrit concentrations usually occur in hypovolemic shock. These changes reflect the underlying etiology. In hypovolemic shock resulting from hemorrhage, the hemoglobin and hematocrit concentrations are lower than normal. In hypovolemic shock resulting from intravascular fluid loss, the hemoglobin and hematocrit concentrations are higher than normal.
- *Arterial blood gases* to determine oxygen and carbon dioxide levels and pH. The effects of shock and of the body's compensatory mechanisms cause a decrease in pH (indicating acidosis), a decrease in the PaO_2 and in total oxygen saturation, and an increase in $PaCO_2$.
- *Serum electrolytes* to monitor the severity and progression of shock. As shock progresses, glucose levels decrease, sodium levels decrease, and potassium levels increase.
- *Blood urea nitrogen, serum creatinine levels, urine specific gravity,* and *osmolality* to check renal function. As perfusion of the kidneys is decreased and renal function is reduced, the blood urea nitrogen and creatinine levels increase, as does urine specific gravity and osmolality.
- *Blood cultures* to identify the causative organism in septic shock.
- *White blood cell count* and *differential* in the client with septic or anaphylactic shock. The total white blood cell count is increased in septic shock. Elevated neutrophils indicate acute infection, increased monocytes indicate a bacterial infection, and increased eosinophils indicate an allergic response.
- *Serum cardiac enzymes,* which are elevated in cardiogenic shock: lactate dehydrogenase, creatine phosphokinase, and serum glutamic-oxaloacetic transaminase.
- *Central venous catheterization* to aid in the differential diagnosis of shock and provide information about the preload of the heart. A pulmonary artery catheter may be inserted to monitor cardiac dynamics, fluid balance, and the effects of vasoactive medications.

Other diagnostic tests may be ordered to determine the extent of injury or damage or to locate the site of internal hemorrhage. These tests might include x-ray studies, CT scans, MRI, endoscopic examinations, and echocardiograms. Newer diagnostic methods for hypoperfusion include gastric tonometry and sublingual $PaCO_2$. Gastric tonometry measures $PaCO_2$ in the gastric lumen. The measurement of sublingual carbon dioxide correlates well with decreased MAP (Sole et al., 2001).

Pharmacologic Therapies

When fluid replacement alone is not sufficient to reverse shock, vasoactive drugs (drugs causing vasoconstriction or vasodilatation) and inotropic drugs (drugs improving cardiac contractility) may be administered. When used to treat shock, these drugs increase venous return through vasoconstriction of peripheral vessels; they also improve the pumping ability of the heart by facilitating myocardial contractility and by dilating coronary arteries to increase perfusion of the myocardium.

Drugs used to treat shock are discussed in Box 22–39. Other drugs that may be administered to the client with shock include the following:

- Diuretics to increase urine output after fluid replacement has been initiated
- Sodium bicarbonate to treat acidosis
- Calcium to replace calcium lost as a result of blood transfusions
- Antiarrhythmic agents to stabilize heart rhythm
- Broad-spectrum antibiotics to suppress organisms responsible for septic shock
- A cardiotonic glycoside (e.g., digitalis) to treat cardiac failure
- Corticosteroids to treat anaphylactic shock
- Morphine to dilate veins and decrease anxiety.

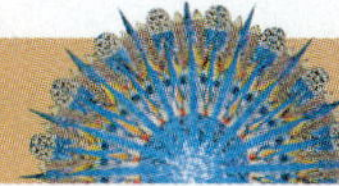

CLINICAL MANIFESTATIONS AND THERAPIES **Shock**

ETIOLOGY	CLINICAL MANIFESTATION	CLINICAL THERAPIES
Hypovolemic shock	**Initial Stage** ■ Blood pressure: normal to slightly decreased ■ Pulse: slightly increased from baseline ■ Respirations: normal (baseline) ■ Skin: cool, pale (in periphery), moist ■ Mental status: alert and oriented ■ Urine output: slight decrease ■ Other: thirst, decreased capillary refill time **Compensatory and Progressive Stages** ■ Blood pressure: hypotension ■ Pulse: rapid, thready ■ Respirations: increased ■ Skin: cool, pale (includes trunk); poor turgor with fluid loss, edematous with fluid shift ■ Mental status: restless, anxious, confused, or agitated ■ Urine output: oliguria (< 30 mL/hr) ■ Other: marked thirst, acidosis, hyperkalemia, decreased capillary refill time, decreased or absent peripheral pulses **Irreversible Stage** ■ Blood pressure: severe hypotension (systolic pressure often is < 80 mmHg) ■ Pulse: very rapid, weak ■ Respirations: rapid, shallow; crackles and wheezes ■ Skin: cool, pale, mottled with cyanosis ■ Mental status: disoriented, lethargic, comatose ■ Urine output: anuria ■ Other: loss of reflexes, decreased or absent peripheral pulses	■ Administer blood ■ Administer intravenous (IV) fluid and volume expanders ■ NPO until gastrointestinal (GI) function returns to normal ■ Administer oxygen ■ Support vital functions until perfusion is restored ■ Assess level of consciousness (LOC) ■ Monitor effectiveness of respiratory effort—may require mechanical ventilation to meet the body's oxygen demands ■ Monitor lab data, including hemoglobin and hematocrit, arterial blood gases (ABG), serum electrolytes, blood urea nitrogen (BUN) ■ Medications may include sodium bicarbonate to treat acidosis, calcium to replace loss from transfusions, antiarrhythmic
Cardiogenic shock	■ Blood pressure: hypotension ■ Pulse: rapid, thready; distention of veins of hands and neck ■ Respirations: increased, labored; crackles and wheezes; pulmonary edema ■ Skin: pale, cyanotic, cold, moist ■ Mental status: restless, anxious, lethargic progressing to comatose ■ Urine output: oliguria to anuria ■ Other: dependent edema; elevated central venous pressure (CVP); elevated pulmonary capillary wedge pressure; arrhythmias	■ Administer IV fluid cautiously to avoid fluid overload placing more stress on the heart ■ NPO until GI function returns to normal ■ Treat underlying cause ■ Medications may include diuretics, sodium bicarbonate, antiarrhythmic agents, cardiotonic glycoside ■ Administer oxygen ■ Support vital functions until perfusion is restored ■ Assess LOC ■ Monitor effectiveness of respiratory effort—may require mechanical ventilation to meet the body's oxygen demands ■ Monitor lab data including ABG, serum electrolytes, BUN, creatinine, cardiac enzymes, CVP, pulmonary wedge pressure, cardiac output

(continued)

CLINICAL MANIFESTATIONS AND THERAPIES Shock (continued)

ETIOLOGY	CLINICAL MANIFESTATION	CLINICAL THERAPIES
Obstructive shock	■ Tachycardia ■ Tachypnea ■ Hypotension ■ Delayed capillary refill in extremities ■ Decreased urine output ■ Peripheral edema	■ Treat underlying cause ■ Reduce cardiac workload ■ Administer oxygen ■ Support vital functions until perfusion is restored ■ Assess LOC ■ Monitor effectiveness of respiratory effort—may require mechanical ventilation to meet the body's oxygen demands
Distributive (vasogenic) shock	■ Tachycardia ■ Tachypnea ■ Hypotension ■ Delayed capillary refill in extremities ■ Decreased urine output ■ Peripheral edema ■ Absent or weak peripheral pulses	■ Treat underlying cause ■ Administer vasoconstricting medications to increase peripheral vascular resistance and restore perfusion
Septic shock	**Early (Warm) Septic Shock** ■ Blood pressure: normal to hypotension ■ Pulse: increased, thready ■ Respirations: rapid and deep ■ Skin: warm, flushed ■ Mental status: alert, oriented, anxious ■ Urine output: normal ■ Other: increased body temperature; chills; weakness; nausea, vomiting, diarrhea; decreased CVP **Late (Cold) Septic Shock** ■ Blood pressure: hypotension ■ Pulse: tachycardia, arrhythmias ■ Respirations: rapid, shallow, dyspneic ■ Skin: cool, pale, edematous ■ Mental status: lethargic to comatose ■ Urine output: oliguria to anuria ■ Other: normal to decreased body temperature; decreased CVP	■ Treat underlying cause ■ Administer antibiotics and IV fluids ■ Assess for potential disseminated intravascular coagulation ■ Support vital functions until perfusion is restored ■ Assess LOC ■ Monitor effectiveness of respiratory effort—may require mechanical ventilation to meet the body's oxygen demands ■ Obtain cultures prior to administration of antibiotics to determine source of infection and pathogen involved
Neurogenic shock	■ Blood pressure: hypotension ■ Pulse: slow and bounding ■ Respirations: vary ■ Skin: warm, dry ■ Mental status: anxious, restless, lethargic progressing to comatose ■ Urine output: oliguria to anuria ■ Other: lowered body temperature	■ Treat underlying injury ■ Reduce parasympathetic stimulation or sympathetic understimulation ■ Medications may include corticosteroids and vasoactive agents
Anaphylactic shock	■ Blood pressure: hypotension ■ Pulse: increased, dysrhythmias ■ Respirations: dyspnea, stridor, wheezes, laryngospasm, bronchospasm, pulmonary edema ■ Skin: warm, edematous (lips, eyelids, tongue, hands, feet, genitals) ■ Mental status: restless, anxious, lethargic to comatose ■ Urine output: oliguria to anuria ■ Other: paresthesias; pruritus; abdominal cramps, vomiting, diarrhea	■ Treat underlying cause ■ Medications may include corticosteroids and albuterol to treat histamine induced bronchospasm ■ Remove allergen ■ Monitor blood pressure and respirations ■ Insertion of an artificial airway may be required to maintain a functional airway if tracheal edema occurs ■ Administer oxygen

Box 22–39 Medication Administration: The Client With Shock

ADRENERGICS (SYMPATHOMIMETICS)

Vasoconstrictors

Norepinephrine (Levophed)
Metaraminol (Aramine)

Inotropes

Dopamine (Inotropin)*
Dobutamine (Dobutrex)
Isoproterenol (Isuprel)

Adrenergic drugs (also called sympathomimetics) mimic the fight-or-flight response of the SNS, selectively stimulating alpha-adrenergic and beta-adrenergic receptors. Many of these drugs have both vasopressor (vasoconstricting) effects and positive inotropic effects (Table 22–34). Stimulation of alpha-adrenergic receptors results in vasoconstriction and increased systemic blood pressure. Stimulation of beta-adrenergic receptors increases the force and rate of myocardial contraction.

The physiologic effect of these drugs includes improved perfusion and oxygenation of the heart, with increased stroke volume and heart rate, and increased cardiac output. In turn, increased cardiac output increases tissue perfusion and oxygenation. The major disadvantage is that increases in stroke volume and heart rate also increase the oxygen requirements of the myocardium. These drugs may be used during the early stages of shock, especially in types of shock characterized by vasodilation.

Nursing Responsibilities

- Carefully monitor responses in the older adult, who may be especially sensitive to sympathomimetics and require lower doses.
- When administering these drugs by the subcutaneous route, carefully aspirate the injection site to avoid injecting the drug directly into a blood vessel.
- Use the intravenous route only with continuous-infusion pumps. Carefully adjust the dose to accommodate the client's cardiovascular status (as ordered by the physician or by written protocol).
- Document lung sounds, vital signs, and hemodynamic parameters before starting the medication and then according to institutional policy (usually every 5–15 minutes).
- Record and monitor urine output. Report output of less than 30 mL/hr.
- Be aware that the sympathomimetics are incompatible with sodium bicarbonate or alkaline solutions.
- When administering drugs that cause vasoconstriction, such as norepinephrine (Levophed) and metaraminol (Aramine), monitor the intravenous insertion site for infiltration. If infiltration does occur, stop the infusion and notify the physician immediately. (Infiltration may cause ischemia and necrosis of tissue.)

Health Education for the Client and Family

- Because these drugs mimic a physiologic reaction to stress, they may cause feelings of anxiety.
- Close monitoring to adjust the dose will be carried out by qualified nurses using written protocols.
- Report heart palpitations or chest pain immediately.

VASODILATORS

Nitroglycerin (Tridil) **Nitroprusside (Nipride)**

Drugs that cause vasodilation act directly on smooth muscle, affecting both arterioles and veins. Peripheral resistance, cardiac output, and pulmonary wedge pressure are all reduced as a result of the vasodilation. These effects decrease the oxygen need of the heart and decrease pulmonary congestion. Vasodilators are used primarily in the treatment of cardiogenic shock and may be combined with a sympathomimetic (e.g., dopamine).

Nursing Responsibilities

- Protect these drugs from light by wrapping the intravenous bag in the package that is provided.
- Mix only with 5% dextrose in water.
- Infuse with an infusion pump, and use within 4 hours of reconstitution.
- Do not add other medications to the solution.
- Assess mental status, blood pressure, and pulse before initiating medication. Thereafter, assess blood pressure and pulse according to institutional policy (usually every 5 minutes initially, then every 15 minutes until stable, and then every hour).
- Monitor for confusion, dizziness, tachycardia, arrhythmias, hypotension, and adventitious breath sounds. If they occur, report immediately, and slow the infusion to a keep-open rate.
- Monitor for signs of thiocyanate poisoning (nausea, disorientation, muscle spasms, and decreased or absent reflexes) if infusion lasts longer than 72 hours.
- Keep client in bed with side rails up.

Health Education for the Client and Family

- It is important to stay in bed and change positions slowly to avoid dizziness.
- The blood pressure and pulse are taken frequently to adjust the dose of medication.
- Headache is a common side effect.

TABLE 22–34 Adrenergic Drugs Used to Treat Shock

ACTION	DRUG	RECEPTOR
Vasoconstrictors	Norepinephrine (Levophed)	A
	Metaraminol (Aramine)	A
Inotropes	Dopamine (Inotropin)*	A, B^1
	Dobutamine (Dobutrex)	B^1
	Isoproterenol (Isuprel)	B^1, B^2

Note: *Receptors are dose dependent.

Oxygen Therapy

Establishing and maintaining a patent airway and ensuring adequate oxygenation are critical interventions in reversing shock. All clients with shock (even those with adequate respirations) should receive oxygen therapy (usually by mask or nasal cannula) to maintain the PaO_2 at greater than 80 mmHg during the first 4–6 hours of care. If the client's unassisted respiration cannot maintain PaO_2 at this level, ventilatory assistance may be necessary.

Fluid Replacement Therapy

The most effective treatment for the client with hypovolemic shock is the administration of intravenous fluids or blood. Fluids also treat septic and neurogenic shock. However, the client with cardiogenic shock may require either fluid replacement or restriction, depending on pulmonary artery pressure.

Various fluids may be administered alone or in combination as part of fluid replacement therapy in treating shock. Whole blood or blood products increase the oxygen-carrying capacity of the blood and thus increase oxygenation of cells. Fluid replacements, such as crystalloid and colloid solutions, increase circulating blood volume and tissue perfusion. Fluid replacements are administered in massive amounts through two large-bore peripheral lines or through a central line.

CRYSTALLOID SOLUTIONS Crystalloid solutions contain dextrose or electrolytes dissolved in water; they are either isotonic or hypotonic. Isotonic solutions include normal saline (0.9%), lactated Ringer's solution, and Ringer's solution. Hypotonic solutions include one-half normal saline (0.45%) and 5% dextrose in water.

All crystalloid solutions increase fluid volume in both the intravascular and the interstitial space. Of the total amount infused, only approximately 25% remains in the intravascular system; the remaining 75% moves into the interstitial space. Consequently, fluid volume is only minimally expanded, and the potential for peripheral edema is increased when crystalloid solutions are used. However, Ringer's lactate (an electrolyte solution) and 0.9% saline are the fluids of choice in treating hypovolemic shock, especially during the emergency phase of care while blood is being typed and crossmatched. Large amounts of these solutions may be infused rapidly, increasing blood volume and tissue perfusion.

COLLOID SOLUTIONS Colloid solutions contain substances (colloids) that should not diffuse through capillary walls. Hence, colloids tend to remain in the vascular system and increase the osmotic pressure of the serum, causing fluid to move into the vascular compartment from the interstitial space. As a result, plasma volume expands. Colloid solutions used to treat shock include 5% albumin, 25% albumin, hetastarch, plasma protein fraction, and dextran (Box 22–40).

Colloid products reduce platelet adhesiveness and have been associated with reductions in blood coagulation. Consequently, the client's prothrombin time (PT), INR, platelet count, and aPTT should be monitored when these solutions are administered. Normal values are as follows:

PT	10–15 s
INR	1–1.2 s
Platelets	150,000–400,000/mm^3
aPTT	< 35 s

Box 22–40 **Medication Administration: Colloid Solutions**

COLLOID SOLUTIONS (PLASMA EXPANDERS)

Albumin 5% (Albuminar-5, Buminate 5%)
Albumin 25% (Albuminar-25, Buminate 25%)
Dextran 40 (Gentran 40)
Dextran 70 (Gentran 70, Macrodex)
Dextran 75 (Gentran 75)
Hetastarch (Hespan [HES])
Plasma protein fraction (Plasmanate, Plasma-Plex, Plasmatein, Protenate)

These solutions are blood volume expanders and are used to treat hypovolemic shock caused by surgery, hemorrhage, burns, or other trauma. Albumin and plasma protein fraction are prepared from healthy blood donors. Dextran and hetastarch are synthetically prepared large molecules. The solutions promote circulatory volume and tissue perfusion by rapidly expanding plasma volume. Dextran solutions are infrequently used.

Nursing Responsibilities

- Before infusion begins, establish a baseline of vital signs, lung sounds, heart sounds, and (if possible) CVP and pulmonary artery wedge pressure.
- Start administration of ordered intravenous fluids, using a large-gauge (18- or 19-gauge) infusion needle.
- Take and record vital signs as required by institutional policy (usually every 15–60 minutes) and client status.
- Take and record intake and output every 1–2 hours.
- Monitor for manifestations of congestive heart failure or pulmonary edema (dyspnea, cyanosis, cough, crackles, or wheezes). If these manifestations appear, stop the fluids, and notify the physician immediately.
- Monitor for bleeding from new sites; an increase in blood pressure may cause bleeding in severed vessels that did not bleed with decreased blood pressure.
- Monitor for manifestations of dehydration (dry lips; scant, dark-colored urine; or loss of skin turgor). Increased intravenous fluids are usually ordered if the client becomes dehydrated.
- Monitor for manifestations of circulatory overload (jugular vein distention, increase in central venous pressure, or increase in pulmonary artery wedge pressure). If these manifestations occur, slow the rate of infusion and notify the physician.
- Monitor prothrombin time, partial thromboplastin time, and platelet counts.
- If administering dextran or plasma protein fraction, have epinephrine and antihistamines readily available for any manifestations of a hypersensitivity reaction (fever, chills, rash, headache, wheezing, or flushing).
- Maintain client on bedrest with side rails elevated.

Health Education for the Client and Family

- The solutions are given to replace lost serum protein, which helps maintain the volume of blood.
- The vital signs are taken frequently to ensure the safety of the client.

BLOOD AND BLOOD PRODUCTS If hypovolemic shock is caused by hemorrhage, the infusion of blood and blood products may be indicated. The goal of blood administration is to keep the hematocrit at 30–35% and the hemoglobin level between 12.5 and 14.5 g/100 mL. Available blood and blood products include fresh whole blood, stored whole blood, packed red blood cells, platelet concentrate, fresh-frozen plasma, and cryoprecipitate. Often, packed red blood cells are given to provide hemoglobin concentration and are supplemented with crystalloids to maintain an adequate circulatory volume.

NURSING PROCESS

The priority of nursing care for the client with shock often requires rapid assessment and reaction to subtle symptoms in order to prevent a downward cascade of events. Anticipating the potential for shock to occur can promote rapid intervention when symptoms are caught early.

Assessment

Nursing assessments are critical in preventing shock. Identifying clients at risk and making focused assessments are essential. Although shock may occur at any age, physiologic changes with aging make the older adult a high-risk population.

- *Hypovolemic shock:* Clients who have undergone surgery, have sustained multiple traumatic injuries, or have been seriously burned are most likely to develop hypovolemic shock. Monitoring fluid status is essential to prevent shock and includes daily assessments of weight, fluid intake by all routes, measurable fluid loss (e.g., urine, vomitus, wound drainage, gastric drainage, and chest tube drainage), and fluid loss that must be estimated, such as fluid lost via profuse perspiration and wound drainage. Assessments for the critically ill client are ongoing and include fluid balance, hemodynamic values, and vital signs.
- *Cardiogenic shock:* Clients with left anterior wall MIs are at risk for developing cardiogenic shock. Nursing care to prevent the development of cardiogenic shock focuses on maintaining or improving myocardial oxygen supply by providing immediate pain relief, maintaining rest, and administering supplemental oxygen.
- *Neurogenic shock:* The risk of neurogenic shock is increased in clients who have spinal cord injuries and those who have received spinal anesthesia. Preventive nursing care includes maintaining immobility of clients with spinal cord trauma and elevating the head of the bed 15–20° following spinal anesthesia. Elevations of more than 20°, however, can potentiate headaches following spinal anesthesia and should be avoided.
- *Anaphylactic shock:* Prevent anaphylactic shock by collecting information about allergies and drug reactions during the health history. Note these allergies clearly on all documents, and place a special armband on the client. Careful and frequent assessments during blood administration may prevent serious reactions to blood or blood products.
- *Septic shock:* Clients who are hospitalized, are debilitated, are chronically ill, or have undergone invasive procedures or tube insertions are at high risk for septic shock. Nursing care to prevent septic shock includes careful and consistent hand washing, the use of aseptic techniques for procedures (e.g., catheterizations, suctioning, changing dressings, starting and maintaining intravenous fluids or medications), and monitoring for local and systemic manifestations (e.g., white blood cell and differential counts) of infection.

Diagnosis

Different types and causes of shock will determine which nursing diagnoses are most appropriate. Priority nursing diagnoses that may be appropriate for the client with any type of shock include the following:

- Decreased Cardiac Output
- Ineffective Tissue Perfusion
- Anxiety.

Plan

Goals for nursing care may include the following:

- Maintain airway, breathing, and circulation.
- Maintain perfusion adequate to meet the body's needs.
- Explain all procedures.
- Encourage client to verbalize feelings to reduce anxiety.
- Reduced cardiac workload.

Implementation

Nurses in the emergency department and intensive care unit participate in the resuscitation of the client in hypovolemic shock and often have guidelines or protocols for nursing actions. Assist with the client's assessment and the establishment of intravenous access. Calculate and prepare the amount of intravenous fluid needed for administration. Ensure rapid fluid administration by intravenous push or pressure bag. Monitor the client's physiologic response to the fluid bolus within 5 minutes. Prepare a second and third fluid bolus. Warmed intravenous fluids are used for resuscitation, because hypothermia may interfere with the client's response to treatment.

When packed red blood cells are administered, verify that the correct blood has been obtained for the client. Change the intravenous fluid to normal saline solution to prevent clotting during blood administration. Assess the client carefully for a transfusion reaction. Monitor the client's physiologic circulatory responses for improvement or deterioration in status. Notify the physician of any deterioration.

Decreased Cardiac Output

Decreased cardiac output is the primary problem for the client with shock. Although much of the care related to this diagnosis is collaborative, many independent nursing interventions are critical to the care of the client with shock.

- Assess and monitor cardiovascular function via the following:
  a. Blood pressure
  b. Heart rate and rhythm
  c. Pulse oximetry
  d. Peripheral pulses
  e. Hemodynamic monitoring of arterial pressures, pulmonary artery pressures, and CVPs.

A baseline assessment is necessary to establish the stage of shock. If palpable peripheral pulses and audible (to auscultation) blood pressure are lost, inserting central arterial, venous, and pulmonary artery catheters is essential to establish progression of shock accurately and to evaluate the client's response to therapy.

- Measure and record intake and output (total output and urinary output) hourly. A decrease in circulating blood volume with hypotension and the effect of the compensatory mechanisms associated with shock can cause renal failure. Urinary output of less than 30 mL/hr in an acutely ill adult indicates reduced renal blood flow.
- Monitor bowel sounds, abdominal distention, and abdominal pain. Decreased splanchnic blood flow reduces bowel motility and peristalsis; paralytic ileus may result.
- Monitor for sudden, sharp chest pain and for dyspnea, cyanosis, anxiety, and restlessness. Hemoconcentration and increased platelet aggregation may result in pulmonary emboli.
- Maintain bedrest, and provide (to the extent possible) a calm, quiet environment. Place in a supine position with the legs elevated to approximately 20°, trunk flat, and head and shoulders elevated higher than the chest (≈10°) (Figure 22–66 ■). Limiting activity and ensuring rest decreases the workload of the heart. The supine position with legs elevated increases venous return; however, this position should not be used for clients with cardiogenic shock. The Trendelenburg position is no longer recommended, because it causes the abdominal organs to press against the diaphragm (limiting respirations), decreases filling of the coronary arteries, and initiates aortic and carotid sinus reflexes.

Ineffective Tissue Perfusion

As shock progresses, diminished tissue perfusion causes ischemia and hypoxia of major organ systems. As shock worsens, blood flow and oxygenation of the lungs, heart, and brain are also impaired. Hypoxia and ischemia result from decreased tissue perfusion in the kidneys, brain, heart, lungs, gastrointestinal tract, and the periphery.

- Monitor skin color, temperature, turgor, and moisture. Decreased tissue perfusion is evidenced by the skin becoming pale, cool, and moist; as hemoglobin concentrations decrease, cyanosis occurs.

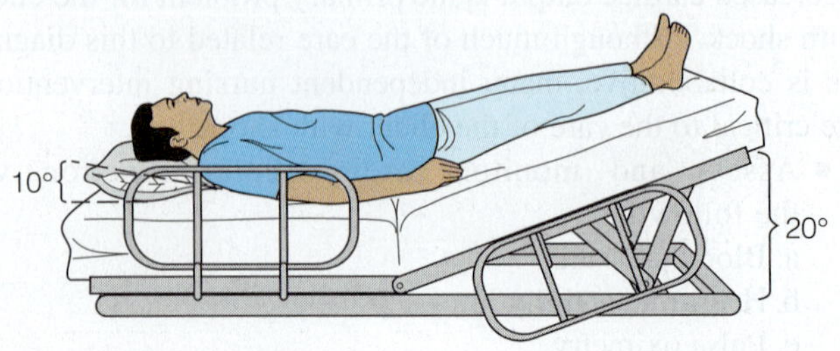

Figure 22–66 ■ The client in shock should be positioned with the lower extremities elevated approximately 20 degrees (knees straight), and the head elevated about 10 degrees.

- Monitor cardiopulmonary function by assessing/monitoring the following:
  a. Blood pressure (by auscultation or by hemodynamic monitoring)
  b. Rate and depth of respirations
  c. Lung sounds
  d. Pulse oximetry
  e. Peripheral pulses (brachial, radial, dorsalis pedis, and posterior tibial); include presence, equality, rate, rhythm, and quality (if unable to palpate pulses, use a device such as a Doppler ultrasound flowmeter to assess peripheral arterial blood flow)
  f. Jugular vein distention
  g. CVP measurements.

Baseline vital signs are necessary to determine trends in subsequent findings. As shock progresses, the blood pressure decreases, and the pulse becomes rapid, weak, and thready. As perfusion of the lungs decreases, crackles, wheezes, and dyspnea are commonly assessed. Capillary refill is prolonged, and peripheral pulses are weak or nonpalpable. Neck veins that cannot be seen when the client is in the supine position indicate decreased intravascular volume. CVP is an accurate means of determining fluid status in the client with shock; the findings will be low (5–15 cm H_2O is normal) in hypovolemic shock because of the decreased blood volume.

- Monitor body temperature. An elevated body temperature increases metabolic demands, depleting energy reserves. It also increases myocardial oxygen demand and may place the client with previous cardiac problems at even greater risk for hypoperfusion.
- Monitor urinary output per Foley catheter hourly, using a urometer. Urine output is a reliable indicator of renal perfusion.
- Assess mental status and level of consciousness. The appropriateness of the client's behavior and responses reflects the adequacy of cerebral circulation. Restlessness and anxiety are common early in shock; during later stages, the client may become lethargic and progress to a comatose state. Altered levels of consciousness are the result of both cerebral hypoxia and the effects of acidosis on brain cells.

Anxiety

Many clients with hypovolemic shock have experienced some form of major trauma and may have life-threatening, multiple injuries. Following on-the-scene treatment, the client is usually admitted to the health care setting through the emergency department. Surgery may be required to treat injuries, followed by care in a critical care unit. Throughout this sequence of crisis events, treatment is invasive, and contact with family is minimal. Client and family responses to these situations of uncertainty, instability, and change include anxiety, fear, and powerlessness. These responses are affected by age, developmental level, cultural and ethnic group, experience with illness and the health care system, and support systems.

- Assess the cause(s) of the anxiety, and manipulate the environment to provide periods of rest. Reducing stimuli that cause anxiety is calming and facilitates rest, which is necessary in the client at risk for bleeding.

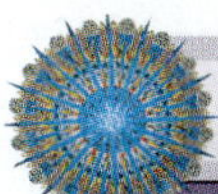

NURSING CARE PLAN A Client With Septic Shock

ASSESSMENT

Huang Mei Lan is a 43-year-old, unmarried female who lives alone in a major West Coast city. Ms. Huang came to America 15 years ago from China; she speaks English well. Her family still lives in China. She worked in a neighborhood sewing shop until 3 years ago, when she was diagnosed with breast cancer. Her treatment included mastectomy of the affected breast and follow-up chemotherapy.

Last month, Ms. Huang experienced a recurrence of cancer in the liver. Surgery to remove the tumor and a lobe of the liver was performed and chemotherapy is planned. Ms. Huang has a central line, a urinary catheter, and a midline abdominal surgical incision. She is underweight, weak, and depressed.

Ms. Huang's primary nurse enters her room early in the morning to make an initial assessment and finds Ms. Huang huddled in the middle of the bed. Ms. Huang reports that she feels cold. The nurse finds Ms. Huang's dressing saturated with bright red blood. She rolls Ms. Huang onto her side and finds the bed filled with blood. The nurse measures the size of the blood stain and records it is 18 X 38 inches. Her vital signs are T_O 99.2$_O$°F , P 110, R 30, BP 106/66. Pulse is weak and regular. Her skin is cool, dry, and pale with poor turgor. She is alert and oriented but restless and appears anxious. Ms. Huang states she is nauseated and suddenly begins vomiting and is incontinent of liquid stool. Laboratory data indicate leukocytosis, respiratory alkalosis, and reduced red blood cell, hemoglobin and hematocrit.

Plasma expanders in the form of albumin are administered while a type and crossmatch for four units of blood can be performed. IV fluid rate is increased and the client's vital signs are monitored. Ms. Huang is taken back to surgery to repair the source of the bleeding and loses an additional 2 pints of blood. She receives 3 units of blood in the operative suite and returns to the unit with the fourth unit running. The physician's orders indicate dopamine is to be started if her blood pressure falls below 90/60 following administration of the fourth unit of blood. Despite treatment, Ms. Huang's condition worsens. Her blood pressure continues to drop, her skin becomes cool and cyanotic, and she begins to have periods of disorientation. She is transferred to the critical care unit. As she is being prepared for the transfer, she begins to cry and asks, "Am I going to die?"

DIAGNOSES

- Deficient Fluid Volume related to bleeding, vomiting, diarrhea, and shift of intravascular volume to interstitial spaces
- Ineffective Breathing Pattern related to rapid respirations and progression of hypovolemic shock
- Ineffective Tissue Perfusion related to progression of hypovolemic shock with decreased cardiac output, hypotension, and massive vasodilatation
- Anxiety related to hypoxia, serious health status, and transfer to critical care unit

PLANNING

Goals of care include the following:

- Maintain adequate oxygenation.
- Maintain adequate circulating blood volume.
- Promote breathing to maintain acid–base within acceptable parameters.
- Promote stable hemodynamic status.
- Assist client to verbalize increased ability to cope with stressors.

IMPLEMENTATION

- Continuously monitor oxygenation status to include pulse oximetry, skin color, and breathing pattern
- Monitor neurologic status, including mental status and level of consciousness.
- Continuously monitor cardiovascular status, including arterial blood pressure; rate, rhythm, and quality of pulses; central venous pressure; pulmonary artery pressure; and cardiac output.
- Monitor color and character of skin, wound dressing for further bleeding.
- Monitor results of arterial blood gases, blood counts, clotting times, and platelet counts.
- Monitor respiratory status, including respiratory rate, rhythm, and breath sounds.
- Monitor urinary output hourly, reporting any output of less than 30 mL/hr.
- Administer blood and IV fluids as ordered.
- Explain procedures, and provide comfort measures (e.g., oral care, skin care, turning, and positioning).

EVALUATION

After administration of the fourth unit of blood, Ms. Huang's blood pressure remains stable and dopamine is not required. Urine output is less than 30 mL/hr for 3 hours and fluid administration is increased until her urine output improves and hemodynamic status stabilizes. She remains in the critical care area for two days and is then transferred back to the oncology unit.

(continued)

NURSING CARE PLAN A Client With Septic Shock *continued*

CRITICAL THINKING

1. Vasopressors may be used in the treatment of shock. Explain the rationale for their use.
2. While monitoring Ms. Huang's arterial blood gases, the nurse notes that her PaO_2 is less than 60 mmHg and her $PaCO_2$ is greater than 50 mmHg. What do these findings indicate, and why have they occurred?
3. Ms. Huang has been given large amounts of colloids intravenously. Hemodynamic monitoring indicates higher-than-normal central venous pressure and pulmonary artery pressure. What do these findings indicate? What physical assessments would you make to confirm the changes?

- Administer prescribed pain medications on a regular basis. Pain precipitates and/or aggravates anxiety.
- Provide interventions to increase comfort and reduce restlessness:
  a. Maintain a clean environment.
  b. Provide skin and oral care.
  c. Monitor the effectiveness of ventilation or oxygen therapy.
  d. Eliminate all nonessential activities.
  e. Remain with the client during procedures.
  f. Speak slowly and calmly, using short sentences.
  g. Use touch to provide support.

Unfamiliar sounds, sights, and odors can increase anxiety. Damp skin or a dry mouth increases discomfort. Inadequate gas exchange with a decrease in oxygen or an increase in carbon dioxide in the blood may cause the client to experience a "feeling of doom." Activity increases the body's need for oxygen. Listening and touch provide support in an environment in which the client often feels alone and abandoned. Severe anxiety interferes with the ability to understand others and to respond appropriately.

- Provide support for the client and family:
  a. Provide time, space, and privacy for family members.
  b. Allow family members access to the client when feasible.
  c. Encourage the expression of feelings and concerns. Provide anticipatory guidance to prepare for recovery or death and to support realistic hope.
  d. Acknowledge the beliefs, values, and expectations of the client and family.

Allowing the family access to the client reduces anxiety and gives both the client and the family some feeling of control. If prognosis is poor, access and involvement allow the family to begin the grieving process. If recovery is expected, contact provides the client and family with a feeling of hope. Supporting the client and family facilitates concrete problem solving, promotes acceptance of the illness and its implications, and helps them begin to establish ways of managing the illness experience.

- Provide information about the current setting to both the client and family; give the family information about available resources (e.g., pastoral care, social services, temporary housing, and meals). Knowing what to expect and how to control the environment to meet basic needs reduces anxiety.

Evaluation

Examples of expected nursing care outcomes include the following:

- Prevention of progression to uncompensated shock by fluid resuscitation
- Family coping with the stress of the client's injury.

REVIEW Shock

RELATE: LINK THE CONCEPTS

Linking the exemplar of Shock with the concept of Religion:

1. While caring for a pediatric client in hypovolemic shock following a bicycle accident, the family members refuse blood, explaining that it is against their religious beliefs. How will you respond?
2. What options for treatment might be considered for this child without conflicting with the family's religious beliefs?

Linking the exemplar of Shock with the concept of Fluids and Electrolytes:

3. Contrast the administration of IV fluids for the client in hypovolemic shock versus the client in cardiogenic shock.
4. Contrast the administration of colloids versus crystalloids in treating the client with hypovolemic shock.

READY: GO TO COMPANION SKILLS MANUAL

- Monitoring intake and output
- Establishing intravenous infusions
- Maintaining infusions
- Infusing IV fluids through a central line
- Infusing IV lipids
- Administering blood components
- Managing central lines
- Administering intravenous medications using IV push
- Assessing the skin
- Assessing blood pressure
- Assessing apical-radial pulse
- Assessing peripheral pulses
- Assessing pulse oximeter
- Assessing heart rate
- Intracranial pressure monitoring and daily care

REFER: GO TO MYNURSINGKIT

REFLECT: CASE STUDY

Stacie Horton is a 15-year-old client who required a heart transplant 5 years ago to repair damage done by a viral illness. She is compliant with her medication regimen and adheres to the prescribed diet.

Stacie is captain of the cheerleading squad at her school where she is also an honor student. Stacie lives with her parents and her older brother. While she appreciates the watchfulness of her parents, Stacie sometimes wishes that her family wouldn't hover over her as much as they do.

Stacie is in class and begins to feel faint and nauseated. Her skin is cold and clammy and her color is slightly cyanotic. Her respirations are 30 breathes per minute and her pulse is weak and thready at a rate of 124 beats per minute. Knowing her history, the teacher alerts the school nurse who immediately calls 911 and Stacie's family.

1. What interventions will you initiate for Stacie until the paramedics arrive?
2. If you were the nurse admitting Stacie in the emergency department what would your priority assessment include?
3. When Stacie's parents arrive what family teaching will you initiate?

22.13 STROKE

KEY TERMS

Agnosia, *1502*
Aphasia, *1504*
Apraxia, *1502*
Contralateral deficit, *1500*
Dysphagia, *1512*
Flaccidity, *1505*
Hemianopia, *1502*
Hemiparesis, *1505*
Hemiplegia, *1505*
Neglect syndrome, *1502*
Penumbra, *1500*
Proprioception, *1502*
Spasticity, *1505*
Stroke, *1499*
Transient ischemic attack (TIA), *1500*

BASIS FOR SELECTION OF EXEMPLAR

Centers for Disease Control and Prevention
Healthy People 2010
Institute of Medicine

LEARNING OUTCOMES

After reading about this exemplar, you will be able to:

1. Describe the pathophysiology, etiology, clinical manifestations, and direct and indirect causes of stroke.
2. Identify risk factors associated with stroke.
3. Illustrate the nursing process in providing culturally competent care across the life span for individuals with stroke.
4. Formulate priority nursing diagnoses appropriate for an individual with stroke.
5. Create a plan of care for individuals with stroke and their families.
6. Assess expected outcomes for an individual with stroke.
7. Discuss therapies used in the collaborative care of an individual with stroke.
8. Employ evidence-based caring interventions for an individual with stroke.

OVERVIEW

A **stroke** (also known as cerebrovascular accident, or brain attack) is a condition in which neurologic deficits result from a sudden decrease in blood flow to a localized area of the brain. Strokes may be ischemic (when the blood supply to a part of the brain is suddenly interrupted by a thrombus [blood clot], embolus [foreign matter traveling through the circulation], stenosis [narrowing]) or hemorrhagic [when a blood vessel breaks open, spilling blood into spaces surrounding neurons]. The neurologic deficits caused by ischemia and the resultant necrosis of cells in the brain vary according to the area of the brain involved, the size of the affected area, and the length of time blood flow is decreased or stopped. A major loss of blood supply to the brain can cause severe disability or death. When the duration of decreased blood flow is short and the anatomic area involved is small, the person may not be aware that damage has been done.

On average, someone in the United States has a stroke every 45 seconds and dies of a stroke every 3 minutes. Stroke is the third leading cause of death and disability in North America, where approximately 700,000 people suffer a stroke each year. Of those, 160,000 die, and many clients who survive are left with some type of functional impairment. Although strokes occur in every age group, the highest incidence occurs in people over 65 years of age; 28% of strokes occur in people under the age of 65. Strokes occur more frequently in men than women, although the risk of stroke may be greater in women during pregnancy and for the 6 weeks following birth (American Heart Association [AHA], 2005a).

PATHOPHYSIOLOGY AND ETIOLOGY

The brain, which makes up only 2% of total body weight, receives approximately 20% of the cardiac output each minute (≈750 mL) and accounts for 20% of the body's oxygen consumption. Cerebral blood flow, especially in the deep cerebral vessels, is largely self-regulated by the brain to meet metabolic needs. This self-regulation (also called autoregulation) allows the brain to maintain a constant blood flow despite changes in systemic blood pressure. However, autoregulation is not effective when systemic blood pressure falls below 50 mmHg or rises above 160 mmHg. In the latter case, the increased systemic pressure (as in hypertension) causes an increase in cerebral blood flow with resultant overdistention of cerebral vessels. Cerebral blood flow also increases in response to increased carbon dioxide concentrations, increased hydrogen ion concentrations, and decreased oxygen concentrations.

When blood flow to and oxygenation of cerebral neurons are decreased or interrupted, pathophysiologic changes at the cellular level take place in 4 to 5 minutes. Cellular metabolism ceases as glucose, glycogen, and adenosine triphosphate are depleted and the sodium–potassium pump fails. Cells swell as sodium draws water into the cell. Cerebral blood vessel walls also swell, further decreasing blood flow. Even if circulation is restored, vasospasm and increased blood viscosity can continue to impede blood flow. Severe or prolonged ischemia leads to cellular death. A central core of dead or dying cells is surrounded by a band of minimally perfused cells, called the **penumbra**. Although cells in the penumbra have impaired metabolic activities, their structural integrity is maintained. The survival of these cells depends on a timely return of adequate circulation, the volume of toxic products released by adjacent dying cells, the degree of cerebral edema, and alterations in local blood flow. The potential survival of cells in the penumbra has led to the use of fibrinolytic agents in the early treatment of ischemic stroke (Porth, 2005).

The neurologic deficits that occur as a result of a stroke can often be used to identify its location. Because the motor pathways cross at the junction of the medulla and spinal cord (decussation), strokes lead to loss or impairment of sensorimotor functions on the side of the body opposite the side of the brain that is damaged. This effect, known as a **contralateral deficit**, causes a stroke in the right hemisphere of the brain to be manifested by deficits in the left side of the body (and vice versa).

A stroke is characterized by a gradual or rapid onset of neurologic deficits resulting from compromised cerebral blood flow. Strokes may result from a variety of problems, including cerebral thrombosis, cerebral embolism, and cerebral hemorrhage.

Ischemic Strokes

Ischemic strokes result from blockage and/or stenosis of a cerebral artery, decreasing or stopping blood flow and ultimately causing a brain infarction. This type of stroke accounts for approximately 80% of all strokes (National Institute of Neurologic Disorders and Stroke [NINDS], 2005a). The blockage may result from a blood clot (either as a thrombus or an emboli) or from stenosis of a vessel resulting from a buildup of plaque. Plaque may cause stenosis in large blood vessels (called large vessel disease) or small blood vessels (called small vessel disease). Large vessel disease usually is the result of thrombi. Small vessel strokes, called lacunar infarcts, are small to very small infarcts in the deep, noncortical areas of the brain or the brainstem. Ischemic strokes are classified as transient, thrombotic, or embolic.

TRANSIENT ISCHEMIC ATTACK A **transient ischemic attack (TIA)**, sometimes called a mini-stroke, is a brief period of localized cerebral ischemia that causes neurologic deficits lasting for less than 24 hours (usually < 1–2 hours) (Porth, 2005). The deficits may be present for only minutes or may last for hours. TIAs are often warning signals of an ischemic thrombotic stroke. One or many TIAs may precede a stroke, with the time between the TIA and a stroke ranging from hours to months. Of the 50,000 Americans who have a TIA each year, approximately one-third will have an acute stroke some time in the future (NINDS, 2005).

The etiology of TIA includes inflammatory artery disorders, sickle cell anemia, atherosclerotic changes in cerebral blood vessels, thrombosis, and emboli. Neurologic manifestations of a TIA vary according to the location and size of the cerebral vessel involved. Manifestations have a sudden onset and often disappear within minutes or hours. Commonly occurring deficits include contralateral numbness or weakness of the leg, hand, forearm, and corner of the mouth (because of middle cerebral artery involvement); aphasia (because of ischemia of the left hemisphere); and visual disturbances, such as blurring (because of involvement of the posterior cerebral artery) (Porth, 2005). The client may also experience a visual disturbance called amaurosis fugax (a fleeting blindness of one eye, described as a shade coming down over vision with the affected eye).

THROMBOTIC STROKE A thrombotic stroke is caused by occlusion of a large cerebral vessel by a thrombus (blood clot). Thrombotic cerebrovascular accidents most often occur in older people who are resting or sleeping. The blood pressure is lower during sleep, so there is less pressure to push the blood through an already narrowed arterial lumen and ischemia may result.

Thrombi tend to form in large arteries that bifurcate and have narrowed lumens as a result of deposits of atherosclerotic plaque. The plaque involves the intima of the arteries, causing the internal elastic lamina to become thin and frayed with exposure of underlying connective tissue. This structural change causes platelets to adhere to the rough surface and release the enzyme adenosine diphosphate. This enzyme initiates the clotting sequence, and the thrombus forms. A thrombus may remain in place and continue to enlarge, completely occluding the lumen of the vessel, or a part of it may break off and become an embolus.

The most common locations of thrombi are the internal carotid artery, the vertebral arteries, and the junction of the vertebral and basilar arteries. Thrombotic strokes affecting the smaller cerebral vessels are called lacunar strokes, because the infarcted areas slough off, leaving a small cavity or "lake" in the brain tissue. A thrombotic stroke usually affects only one region of the brain, supplied by a single cerebral artery.

A thrombotic stroke occurs rapidly but progresses slowly. It often begins with a TIA and continues to worsen over 1–2 days; the condition is called a stroke-in-evolution. When maximum neurologic deficit has been reached, usually in 3 days, the condition is called a completed stroke. At that time, the damaged area of brain tissue is edematous and necrotic.

EMBOLIC STROKE An embolic stroke occurs when a blood clot or clump of matter traveling through the cerebral blood vessels becomes lodged in a vessel that is too narrow to permit further movement. The area of the brain supplied by the blocked vessel becomes ischemic. The most frequent sites of cerebral emboli are at bifurcations of vessels, particularly those of the carotid and middle cerebral arteries. This type of stroke is typically seen in clients who are younger than those experiencing thrombotic strokes, and it occurs when the client is awake and active.

Many embolic strokes originate from a thrombus in the left chambers of the heart, formed during atrial fibrillation. These are referred to as cardiogenic embolic strokes. Emboli result when parts of the thrombus break off and are carried through the arterial system to the brain. Cerebral emboli may also be the result of carotid artery atherosclerotic plaque, bacterial endocarditis, recent MI, rheumatic heart disease, and ventricular aneurysm.

An embolic stroke has a sudden onset and causes immediate deficits. If the embolus breaks up into smaller fragments and is absorbed by the body, manifestations will disappear in a few hours to a few days. If the embolus is not absorbed, manifestations will persist. Even if the embolus is absorbed, the vessel wall where the embolus lodges may be weakened, increasing the potential for cerebral hemorrhage.

Hemorrhagic Stroke

A hemorrhagic stroke, or intracranial hemorrhage, occurs when a cerebral blood vessel ruptures. It occurs most often in people with sustained increase in systolic–diastolic blood pressure. Intracranial hemorrhage usually occurs suddenly, often when the affected person is engaged in some activity. Although hypertension is the most common cause, a variety of factors may contribute to a hemorrhagic stroke, including rupture of a brittle, plaque-encrusted artery wall; ruptured intracranial aneurysms; trauma; erosion of blood vessels by tumors; arteriovenous malformations; anticoagulant therapy; and blood disorders. Of all forms of stroke, this form is most often fatal and accounts for approximately 20% of all strokes (NINDS, 2005). There are two types of hemorrhagic strokes: intracerebral hemorrhage and subarachnoid hemorrhage.

As a result of the blood vessel rupture, blood enters the brain tissue, the cerebral ventricles, or the subarachnoid space, compressing adjacent tissues and causing blood vessel spasm and cerebral edema. Blood in the ventricles or subarachnoid space irritates the meninges and brain tissue, causing an inflammatory reaction and impairing absorption and circulation of cerebrospinal fluid (CSF).

The onset of manifestations from a hemorrhagic stroke is rapid. Manifestations depend on the location of the hemorrhage but may include vomiting, headache, seizures, hemiplegia, and loss of consciousness. Pressure on the brain tissue from increased intracranial pressure may cause coma and death.

Risk Factors

Certain diseases, lifestyle habits, and ethnic backgrounds increase the risk of a stroke. Specific risk factors include the following (NINDS, 2005):

- *Hypertension.* Hypertension is the greatest risk factor for a stroke. Increased systolic and diastolic blood pressure is associated with damage to all blood vessels, including the cerebral vessels. People with hypertension have a four to six times greater risk for stroke than do those without hypertension. One third of the adult American population has hypertension.
- *Heart disease.* Atrial fibrillation is the second greatest risk factor for stroke. Affecting as many as 2.2 million people, fibrillation increases the risk for stroke by 4–6% (AHA, 2005a). Other cardiovascular problems that increase the risk for a stroke are mitral valve stenosis, patent foramen ovale, and cardiac surgery.
- *Diabetes mellitus.* Diabetes leads to vascular changes in both the systemic and cerebral circulation and increases the risk of hypertension (the prevalence of hypertension is 40% higher in people with diabetes). People with diabetes are three times more likely to have a stroke compared to those without diabetes.
- *Sleep apnea.* Considered a major risk for stroke, sleep apnea increases blood pressure and causes decreased oxygen and increased carbon dioxide in the blood.
- *Blood cholesterol levels.* Increased blood cholesterol levels contribute to the risk of atherosclerosis, including arteries in the cerebral circulation.
- *Smoking.* Cigarette smoking doubles a person's risk for ischemic stroke and increases the risk for cerebral hemorrhage by up to 3.5%. Smoking is directly responsible for more strokes in young adults.

FOCUS ON DIVERSITY AND CULTURE Risk Factors for Stroke

AFRICAN AMERICAN

- African Americans have almost twice the number of first-ever strokes compared to whites.
- The prevalence of hypertension in African Americans is the highest in the world.
- Among African Americans age 20 and older, 62.9% of men and 77.2% of women are overweight or obese.

HISPANICS

- Mexican Americans have an increased incidence of intracerebral hemorrhage, subarachnoid hemorrhage, ischemic stroke, transient ischemic attack, and transient ischemic attack at a younger age when compared to non-Hispanic whites.
- Diabetes is more common among Hispanics, with estimates that 30% or more of Hispanic adults have the disease.
- Hispanics have a greater proportion of hypertension.
- Obesity is more prevalent among Hispanics than among non-Hispanic whites.
- As a result of language barriers and lack of transportation, Hispanics are more likely to delay or drop out of care.

Source: American Stroke Association (2003).

- *Sickle cell disease.* Changes in the shape of the red blood cells increase blood viscosity and produce erythrocyte clumps that may occlude small cerebral vessels.
- *Substance abuse.* The injection of unpurified substances increases the risk for a stroke, and abuse of certain drugs can decrease cerebral blood flow and increase the risk for intracranial hemorrhage. Substances associated with strokes include marijuana, anabolic steroids, heroin, amphetamines, and cocaine.
- *Living in the stroke belt.* People living in the southeastern United States have the highest stroke mortality rate in the country. The cause has not been identified.

Other risk factors include a family history of stroke, obesity, a sedentary lifestyle, recent viral and bacterial infections, and previous TIAs. Risk factors specific to women are oral contraceptive use, pregnancy, childbirth, menopause, migraine headaches with aura, autoimmune disorders (e.g., diabetes and lupus), and clotting disorders.

In addition, having a stroke is a major risk factor for having another stroke (called recurrent stroke); approximately 5–14% of people who have a stroke and recover have another stroke within 1 year (AHA, 2005a). The risk is highest immediately after a stroke, then decreases with time. Approximately 3% of clients with a stroke have another stroke within 30 days, and one third of recurrent strokes occur within 2 years of the first stroke (NINDS, 2005).

CLINICAL MANIFESTATIONS

Manifestations of a stroke vary according to the cerebral artery involved and the area of the brain affected. Manifestations are always sudden in onset, focal, and usually one sided. The most common manifestation is weakness involving the face and arm, and sometimes the leg. Other common manifestations are numbness on one side, loss of vision, speech difficulties, a sudden severe headache, and difficulties with balance. The various deficits associated with involvement of a specific cerebral artery are collectively referred to as stroke syndromes, although the deficits often overlap, as shown in Box 22–41. Specific manifestations of individual types of stroke are discussed in the subsections under Pathophysiology and Etiology.

Complications

Typical complications include sensory–perceptual deficits, cognitive and behavioral changes, communication disorders, motor deficits, and elimination disorders. These may be transient or permanent, depending on the degree of ischemia and necrosis as well as time of treatment. As a result of the neurologic deficits, the client with a stroke has complications that involve many different body systems. The disabilities resulting from a stroke often cause serious alterations in functional health status (Box 22–42).

SENSORY–PERCEPTUAL DEFICITS A stroke may involve pathologic changes in neurologic pathways that alter the ability to integrate, interpret, and attend to sensory data. The client may experience deficits in vision, hearing, equilibrium, taste, and sense of smell. The ability to perceive vibration, pain, warmth, cold, and pressure may be impaired, as may **proprioception** (the body's sense of its position). The loss of these sensory abilities increases the risk for injury.

Sensory–perceptual deficits may include the following:

- **Hemianopia,** the loss of half of the visual field of one or both eyes; when the same half is missing in each eye, the condition is called homonymous hemianopia (Figure 22–67 ■).
- **Agnosia,** the inability to recognize one or more subjects that were previously familiar; agnosia may be visual, tactile, or auditory.
- **Apraxia,** the inability to carry out some motor pattern (e.g., drawing a figure or getting dressed) even when strength and coordination are adequate.

Another form of sensory–perceptual deficit is the **neglect syndrome** (or unilateral neglect), in which the client has a disorder of attention. In this syndrome, the person cannot integrate

Box 22–41 Manifestations of a Stroke by Involved Cerebral Vessel

INTERNAL CAROTID ARTERY
- Contralateral paralysis of the arm, leg, and face
- Contralateral sensory deficits of the arm, leg, and face
- If the dominant hemisphere is involved: aphasia
- If the nondominant hemisphere is involved: apraxia, agnosia, unilateral neglect
- Homonymous hemianopia

MIDDLE CEREBRAL ARTERY
- Drowsiness, stupor, coma
- Contralateral hemiplegia of the arm and face
- Contralateral sensory deficits of the arm and face
- Global aphasia (if dominant hemisphere involved)
- Homonymous hemianopia

ANTERIOR CEREBRAL ARTERY
- Contralateral weakness or paralysis of the foot and leg
- Contralateral sensory loss of the toes, foot, and leg
- Loss of ability to make decisions or act voluntarily
- Urinary incontinence

VERTEBRAL ARTERY
- Pain in face, nose, or eye
- Numbness and weakness of the face on involved side
- Problems with gait
- Dysphagia

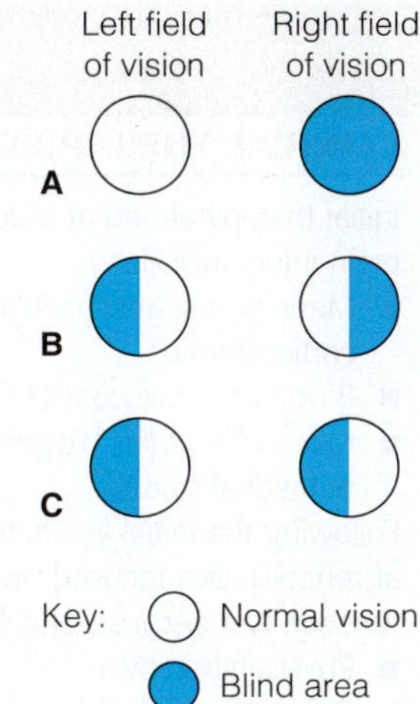

Figure 22–67 ■ Abnormal visual fields. *A*, Normal left field of vision with loss of vision in right field. *B*, Loss of vision in temporal half of both fields (bitemporal hemianopia). *C*, Loss of vision in nasal field of right eye and temporal field of left eye (homonymous hemianopia).

and use perceptions from the affected side of the body or from the environment on the affected side and therefore ignores that part. In severe cases, the client may even deny the paralysis. This deficit is more common following a stroke of the right hemisphere, where damage to the parietal lobe (a center for mediation of directed attention) results in perceptual deficits.

Pain and discomfort may accompany a stroke, with the client experiencing acute pain, numbness, or strange sensations. Although not common, damage to the thalamus may cause central stroke pain or central pain syndrome. The pain in this syndrome includes hot and cold, burning, tingling, and sharp, stabbing pain, most often in the extremities. It is worsened by movement and temperature changes. The painful sensations are not relieved by pain medications, nor are there any specific treatments.

COGNITIVE AND BEHAVIORAL CHANGES A change in consciousness, ranging from mild confusion to coma, is a common manifestation of a stroke. This change may result from tissue damage following ischemia or hemorrhage involving either the carotid or vertebral arteries. Altered consciousness may also be the result of cerebral edema or increased intracranial pressure.

Behavioral changes include emotional lability (in which the client may laugh or cry inappropriately), loss of self-control (manifested by behavior such as swearing or refusing to wear clothing), and decreased tolerance for stress (resulting in anger or depression). Intellectual changes may include memory loss, decreased attention span, poor judgment, and an inability to think abstractly.

COMMUNICATION DISORDERS Communication is a complex process involving motor functions, speech, language, memory, reasoning, and emotions. Communication disorders are usually the result of a stroke affecting the dominant hemisphere.

Box 22–42 **Complications of Stroke**

INTEGUMENT
- Decubitus (pressure) ulcers

NEUROLOGIC
- Hyperthermia
- Neglect syndrome
- Seizures
- Agnosias
- Communication deficits
  - a. Expressive aphasia
  - b. Receptive aphasia
  - c. Global aphasia
  - d. Agraphia
- Visual deficits
  - a. Homonymous hemianopia
  - b. Diplopia
  - c. Decreased acuity
- Cognitive changes
  - a. Memory loss
  - b. Short attention span
  - c. Distractibility
  - d. Poor judgment
  - e. Poor problem-solving ability
  - f. Disorientation
- Behavioral changes
  - a. Emotional lability
  - b. Loss of social inhibitions
  - c. Fear
  - d. Hostility
  - e. Anger
  - f. Depression
- Increased intracranial pressure
- Alterations in consciousness
- Sensory loss (touch, pain, heat, cold, pressure)

RESPIRATORY
- Respiratory center damage
- Airway obstruction
- Decreased ability to cough

GASTROINTESTINAL
- Dysphagia
- Constipation
- Stool impaction

GENITOURINARY
- Incontinence
- Frequency
- Urgency
- Urinary retention
- Renal calculi

MUSCULOSKELETAL
- Hemiplegia
- Contractures
- Bony ankylosis
- Disuse atrophy
- Dysarthria

CLINICAL MANIFESTATIONS AND THERAPIES **Stroke**

ETIOLOGY	CLINICAL MANIFESTATION	CLINICAL THERAPIES
Damage to neurons, depending on number and location, often results in loss of sensory and/or motor function.	Hemiplegia, hemiparesis, flaccidity, paresthesias, spasticity, weakness, or paralysis	Initial therapy aimed at reducing amount of brain injury includes: ■ Medications: anticoagulant, thrombolytic, corticosteroids ■ Blood pressure control ■ Maintaining fluid, oxygen, and nutritional status. Following the initial insult, therapy is aimed at rehabilitation focused on restoring any function lost because of cellular damage: ■ Physical therapy ■ Occupational therapy ■ Home health assessment.
Alterations in ability to communicate often results if the cellular damage occurs on the dominant side of the brain.	Aphasia, expressive aphasia, receptive aphasia, mixed or global aphasia, dysarthria	Develop alternate means of communicating: ■ Use of hand signals ■ Speech therapy ■ Allow client time to express thoughts.
Sensory perceptual deficits may occur if the neurologic pathways are involved.	Vision, hearing, equilibrium, taste, or sense of smell deficits Ability to perceive vibration, pain, warmth, cold, and pressure Altered proprioception Hemianopia, agnosia, apraxia, neglect syndrome	■ Provide reassurance and support ■ Physical and occupational therapy when condition stabilizes ■ Maintain client safety
Pain or strange sensations may result with damage to the thalamus.	Pain that may be hot, cold, burning, tingling, or sharp and stabbing in the extremities, worsened by movement or temperature changes, and not relieved by analgesics	No treatment has been found
Cognitive and behavioral changes resulting from ischemia or hemorrhage involving either the carotid or vertebral arteries, cerebral edema, or increased intracranial pressure.	Emotional lability, loss of self-control, decreased tolerance for stress, memory loss, decreased attention span, poor judgment, lack of ability for abstract thought	Behavioral and cognitive therapy

The left hemisphere is dominant in approximately 95% of people who are right-handed and 70% of people who are left-handed (Porth, 2005).

Many different impairments may occur, and most are partial. Disorders of communication affect both speech (the mechanical act of articulating language through the spoken word) and language (the vocal or written formulation of ideas to communicate thoughts and feelings). Language involves oral and written expression as well as auditory and reading comprehension. Among these disorders are the following:

- **Aphasia:** the inability to use or understand language; aphasia may be expressive, receptive, or mixed (global).
- *Expressive aphasia:* a motor speech problem in which one can understand what is being said but can respond verbally only in short phrases; also called Broca's aphasia.
- *Receptive aphasia:* a sensory speech problem in which one cannot understand the spoken (and often written) word. Speech may be fluent but with inappropriate content; also called Wernicke's aphasia.
- *Mixed or global aphasia:* language dysfunction in both understanding and expression.
- *Dysarthria:* any disturbance in muscular control of speech.

MOTOR DEFICITS Body movement results from a complex interaction between the brain, spinal cord, and peripheral nerves. The motor areas of the cerebral cortex, the basal ganglia, and the cerebellum initiate voluntary movement by sending messages to the spinal cord, which then transmits the messages to the peripheral nerves. A stroke may interrupt the central nervous system component of this relay system and produce effects in the contralateral side ranging from mild weakness to severe limitation of any kind of movement.

Depending on the area of the brain involved, strokes may cause weakness, paralysis, and/or spasticity. Specific motor deficits include the following:

- **Hemiplegia:** paralysis of the left or right half of the body (Figure 22–68 ■).
- **Hemiparesis:** weakness of the left or right half of the body.
- **Flaccidity:** absence of muscle tone (hypotonia).
- **Spasticity:** increased muscle tone (hypertonia), usually with some degree of weakness. The flexor muscles are usually more strongly affected in the upper extremities, and the extensor muscles are more strongly affected in the lower extremities.

When the corticospinal tract is involved, the affected arm and leg almost always are initially flaccid and then become spastic within 6–8 weeks. Spasticity often causes characteristic body positioning: adduction of the shoulder, pronation of the forearm, flexion of the fingers, and extension of the hip and knee. There is often foot drop, outward rotation of the leg, and dependent edema in the involved extremities.

The motor deficits may result in altered mobility, further impairing body function. The complications of immobility involve multiple body systems and include orthostatic hypotension, increased thrombus formation, decreased cardiac output, impaired respiratory function, osteoporosis, formation of renal calculi, contractures, and decubitus ulcer formation.

ELIMINATION DISORDERS Disorders of bladder and bowel elimination are common. A stroke may cause partial loss of the sensations that trigger bladder elimination, resulting in urinary frequency, urgency, or incontinence. Control of urination may be altered as a result of cognitive deficits. Changes in bowel elimination are common, resulting from changes in level of consciousness, immobility, and dehydration (Hickey, 2003).

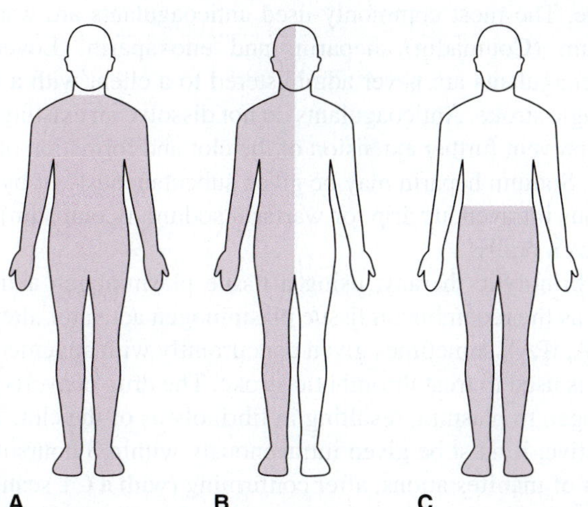

Figure 22–68 ■ Types of paralysis. *A*, Quadriplegia is complete or partial paralysis of the upper extremities and complete paralysis of the lower part of the body. *B*, Hemiplegia is paralysis of one-half of the body when it is divided along the median sagittal plane. *C*, Paraplegia is paralysis of the lower part of the body.

COLLABORATION

The type of treatment a client with a stroke receives depends on the stage of the disease. In general, there are three treatment stages:

1. Stroke prevention
2. Acute care immediately after a stroke
3. Rehabilitation after a stroke.

The client with an acute stroke may receive medical and/or surgical treatment. The focus in the acute care phase is on diagnosing the type and cause of the stroke, supporting cerebral circulation, and controlling or preventing further deficits. The goals of stroke care, defined by the AHA (2005), are to minimize brain injury and maximize client recovery by the following:

- Rapid recognition and reaction to stroke warning signs
- Rapid emergency medical services (EMS) dispatch
- Rapid EMS system transport and hospital prenotification
- Rapid diagnosis and treatment in the hospital.

Diagnostic Tests

Diagnosis begins with a complete history and careful physical assessment, including a thorough neurologic examination. The time of the onset of stroke manifestations is a critical part of assessment. The National Institutes of Health Stroke Scale is a clinical evaluation tool widely used to assess neurologic outcome and degree of recovery. Part of the scale is illustrated in Table 22–35. The tool measures level of consciousness, vision, facial paralysis, motor abilities, ataxia, sensation, language, and attention.

Imaging tests are used to identify an increased risk for a stroke or to identify pathophysiologic changes after a stroke has occurred. CT is the first imaging technique used to demonstrate the presence of hemorrhage, tumors, aneurysm, ischemia, edema, and tissue necrosis. A CT scan can also demonstrate a shift in intracranial contents and is useful in distinguishing the type of stroke (e.g., a hemorrhagic stroke results in an increase in density). Cerebral infarctions usually are visible with a CT scan 6–8 hours poststroke; hemorrhage is visible immediately. Other imaging tests that may be used for diagnosis include cerebral arteriography, transcranial Doppler ultrasound, MRI, magnetic resonance angiography, position emission tomography, and single photon emission CT.

In addition to imaging tests, a blood test has recently been approved to screen for recurrent stroke risk. The PLAC test scans the blood for high levels of lipoprotein-associated phospholipase A2, which is more common in people who have had strokes. A lumbar puncture may be performed to obtain CSF for examination if there is no danger of increased intracranial pressure. (Removal of CSF when intracranial pressure is increased can result in herniation of the brainstem.) A thrombotic stroke may elevate CSF pressure; after a hemorrhagic stroke, frank blood may be seen in the CSF.

TABLE 22–35 National Institutes of Health Stroke Scale: Assessment of Level of Consciousness

INSTRUCTIONS	SCALE DEFINITION	SCORE
1a. *Level of Consciousness (LOC):* The investigator must choose a response, even if a full evaluation is prevented by such obstacles as an endotracheal tube, language barrier, orotracheal trauma/bandages. A 3 is scored only if the client makes no movement (other than reflexive posturing) in response to noxious stimulation.	0 = Alert, keenly responsive 1 = Not alert, but arousable by minor stimulation to obey, answer, or respond 2 = Not alert, requires repeated stimulation to attend, or is obtunded and requires strong or painful stimulation to make movements (not stereotyped) 3 = Responds only with reflex motor or autonomic effects or totally unresponsive, flaccid, areflexic	______
1b. *LOC Questions:* The client is asked the month and his or her age. The answer must be correct. There is no partial credit for being close. Aphasic and stuporous clients who do not comprehend the questions will score a 2. Clients unable to speak because of endotracheal intubation, orotracheal trauma, severe dysarthria from any cause, language barrier, or any other problem not secondary to aphasia are given a 1. It is important that only the initial answer be graded and that the examiner not "help" the client with verbal or nonverbal cues.	0 = Answers both questions correctly. 1 = Answers one question correctly. 2 = Answers neither question correctly.	______
1c. *LOC Commands:* The client is asked to open and close the eyes and then to grip and release the nonparetic hand. Substitute another one-step command if the hands cannot be used. Credit is given if an unequivocal attempt is made but not completed because of weakness. If the client does not respond to the command, the task should be demonstrated (pantomime) and the results scored (i.e., follows none, one, or two commands). Clients with trauma, amputation, or other physical impediments should be given suitable one-step commands. Only the first attempt is scored.	0 = Performs both tasks correctly. 1 = Performs one task correctly. 2 = Performs neither task correctly.	______

Note: This is a sample of only one part of the National Institutes of Health Stroke Scale. The entire scale may be viewed as a PDF file at http://www.ninds.nih.gov/doctors/NIH_Stroke_Scale.pdf

Pharmacologic Therapies

Medications are administered to prevent a stroke in clients with TIAs or a previous stroke and to treat the client during the acute phase of a stroke.

PREVENTION Antiplatelet agents are often used to treat clients with TIAs or who have had a previous stroke. Platelets are concentrated in high-blood-flow arteries, where they adhere to endothelial tissue damaged by atherosclerosis and occlude the vessel. The drugs used to prevent clot formation and blood vessel occlusion include aspirin, clopidogrel (Plavix), dipyridamole (Persantine), and ticlopidine (Ticlid).

Daily low-dose aspirin reduces TIA occurrence and stroke risk by interfering with platelet aggregation. Ticlopidine (Ticlid) is a platelet-aggregation inhibitor that reduces thrombotic stroke risk.

ACUTE STROKE Medications are used to treat the client during the acute phase of an ischemic stroke to prevent further thrombosis formation, increase cerebral blood flow, and protect cerebral neurons. The type of medication used varies according to the type of stroke.

Anticoagulant drug therapy is often ordered for an ischemic stroke. The most commonly used anticoagulants are warfarin sodium (Coumadin), heparin, and enoxaparin (Lovenox). Anticoagulants are never administered to a client with a hemorrhagic stroke. Anticoagulants do not dissolve an existing clot; they prevent further extension of the clot and formation of new clots. Sodium heparin may be given subcutaneously or by continuous intravenous drip, or warfarin sodium (Coumadin) may be given orally.

Fibrinolytic therapy, using a tissue plasminogen activator such as the recombinant tissue plasminogen activator alteplase (rt-PA, tPA), sometimes given concurrently with an anticoagulant, is used to treat thrombotic stroke. The drug converts plasminogen to plasmin, resulting in fibrinolysis of the clot. To be effective, it must be given intravenously within 3 hours of the onset of manifestations, after confirming (with a CT scan) that the client has had an ischemic stroke (Tierney et al., 2005). Antithrombotic drugs, which inhibit the platelet phase of clot formation, have been used as a preventive measure for clients at risk for embolic and thrombotic cerebrovascular accident. Both aspirin and dipyridamole have been used for this purpose. These drugs are sometimes also used in combination with other drugs during acute treatment. Antiplatelet agents are contraindicated in clients with a hemorrhagic stroke.

Management of hypertension during the acute phase of stroke is controversial, but if the client is eligible for fibrinolytic therapy, blood pressure control is essential to decrease the risk for bleeding. If the blood pressure is sustained at levels of greater than 185 mmHg systolic or greater than 110 mmHg diastolic, the client cannot be treated with intravenous tPA (AHA, 2005b).

Corticosteroids, such as prednisone or dexamethasone, have been used to treat cerebral edema, but the results are not always positive. If the client has increased intracranial pressure, hyperosmolar solutions (e.g., mannitol) or diuretics (e.g., furosemide) may be administered. Anticonvulsants, such as phenytoin (Dilantin), and barbiturates may be prescribed if increased intracranial pressure causes seizures.

Surgery

Surgery may be performed to prevent the occurrence of a stroke, to restore blood flow when a stroke has already occurred, or to repair vascular damage or malformations. In people who have had TIAs or are in danger of having another stroke, a carotid endarterectomy at the carotid artery bifurcation may be performed to remove atherosclerotic plaque (Figure 22–69 ■).

When an occluded or stenotic vessel is not directly accessible, an extracranial–intracranial bypass may be performed. Bypass of the internal carotid, middle cerebral, or vertebral arteries may be required. The indications for the bypass are manifestations of ischemia caused by TIAs or a mild completed stroke. The procedure reestablishes blood flow to the affected area of the brain.

A carotid angioplasty with stenting is a newer option for treating cerebral stenosis. During the procedure, an angioplasty balloon catheter is inserted through an artery in the client's arm or leg. Under fluoroscopy, the catheter is advanced to the area of carotid artery stenosis, and a small filter is inserted to catch any clots or pieces of debris that might break loose. The balloon is then inflated to widen the artery, followed by insertion of a permanent stent in the area of the angioplasty (Palmieri, 2006).

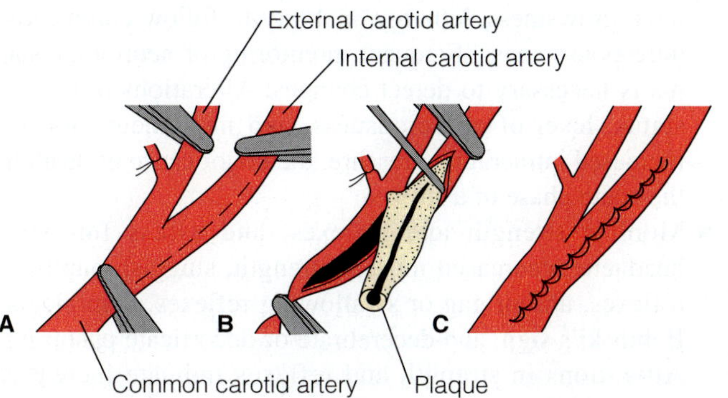

Figure 22–69 ■ Carotid endarterectomy. *A*, The occluded area is clamped off and an incision is made in the artery. *B*, Plaque is removed from the inner layer of the artery. *C*, To restore blood flow through the artery, the artery is sutured, or a graft is completed.

Rehabilitation

Various types of therapy are necessary for poststroke rehabilitation. The types and goals of the therapies used are as follows:

- *Physical therapy* may help prevent contractures and improve muscle strength and coordination. Physical therapists teach exercises to enable the client to relearn how to walk, sit, lie down, and change from one type of movement to another.
- *Occupational therapy* provides assistive devices and a plan for regaining lost motor skills that greatly improve quality of life after a stroke. These skills include eating, drinking, bathing, cooking, reading, writing, and toileting.
- *Speech therapy* is provided to help the client relearn language and communication skills as well as improve swallowing.

NURSING PROCESS

Even though many people who have a stroke experience full recovery, a substantial number are left with disabilities that affect their physical, emotional, interpersonal, and family status. The required nursing care is often complex and multidimensional, requiring consideration of continuity of care for clients in acute care settings, long-term care settings, rehabilitation centers, and the home.

Nurses caring for clients who have had a stroke require knowledge and skill to meet client needs during both the acute and rehabilitative phases of care. The client may have losses in multiple areas: mobility, ability to provide self-care, communications, concept of self, and interpersonal or intimate relationships with others. Holistic, individualized nursing care is essential in all settings and focuses on promoting the achievement of maximum potential and quality of life.

The client's family is often faced with many changes. The young to middle-aged adult with a family member who has had a stroke may be faced with economic difficulties and social isolation. The middle-aged adult family member may become the caretaker for an older parent, in essence switching roles with the parent. An older adult may not be able to care for a spouse and may have to accept nursing home placement. In addition, the older adult who has no family may have to struggle alone to regain the ability to function independently. Although not all of these problems are amenable to nursing solutions, the nurse is most often the health care provider who assesses and identifies the needs of each individual and who provides information and referrals to clients and families to help meet those needs.

Because a stroke has the potential to cause many different health problems, a wide variety of nursing diagnoses may be appropriate. It is important to remember that each person will be affected differently, depending on the degree of ischemia and the area of the brain involved. Nursing diagnoses discussed in this section focus on problems with cerebral tissue perfusion (specific to nursing care during the acute phase), physical mobility, self-care, communication, sensory-perceptual deficits, bowel and urine elimination, and swallowing (specific to prevention of complications and rehabilitation).

Health promotion activities focus on stroke prevention, especially for those people with known risk factors. It is important to discuss, as appropriate, the importance of stopping smoking and drug use with clients of all ages. Maintaining a normal weight through diet and exercise can help reduce obesity, which increases the risk of hypertension and type 2 diabetes mellitus (both in turn increase the risk for stroke). Cholesterol levels should be screened regularly to monitor for hyperlipidemia. Regular health care to monitor for and treat cardiovascular disorders and to detect and treat infections such as infective endocarditis is important. It is also important to increase public awareness of the signs of a TIA or stroke and of the need to call 911 or seek care immediately if the following warning signs or symptoms occur:

- Sudden weakness or numbness of the face, arm, or leg, especially on one side of the body
- Sudden confusion, difficulty speaking, or difficulty understanding speech
- Sudden trouble walking, dizziness, loss of coordination
- Sudden difficulty with vision in one or both eyes
- Sudden severe headache without a cause.

Assessment

The following data are collected through the health history and physical examination:

- *Health history*. Risk factors, previous stroke, drug use (prescribed, over-the-counter, street drugs), smoking history, when manifestations began, severity of manifestations, presence of incontinence, level of consciousness, family support system.
- *Physical assessment*. Level of consciousness, motor strength, coordination, communication, cranial nerves, sensory function.

If the client is a woman, she has risks for stroke different than from a man and should be asked questions specific to her gender.

Diagnosis

Nursing diagnoses that may apply to the client with stroke include the following:

- Ineffective Tissue Perfusion: Cerebral
- Impaired Physical Mobility
- Self-Care Deficit
- Impaired Verbal Communication
- Impaired Urinary Elimination and Risk for Constipation
- Impaired Swallowing.

Plan

Goals of care for the client who has had a stroke include the following:

- The client's blood pressure will remain within the normal range.
- The client will participate in rehabilitation to improve function and ability to perform ADLs autonomously.
- The client will not experience complications as a result of immobility.
- The client will be assisted to communicate needs effectively.
- The client's nutritional needs will be met without risk of aspiration.

Implementation

The focus of care will be determined by the severity of the stroke, the neurologic deficits that result, and on whether the client is in the acute stages or rehabilitative stages of the event. In the acute phase, assuring airway, breathing, and circulation will be the priority focus. Once the ABCs of care are met, the nurse's priority shifts to reducing loss of neurological function. Psychosocial support for the client and family also is an important role of the nurse.

Ineffective Tissue Perfusion: Cerebral

The initial assessment and care of the client admitted for intensive care focuses on identifying changes that may indicate altered cerebral perfusion. The client's airway, breathing, circulation, and neurologic status are monitored, and interventions are provided to maintain cerebral perfusion.

- Monitor respiratory status and airway patency. Auscultate pulmonary sounds and monitor respiratory rate and results of studies of arterial blood gases. The client is often unconscious, and breathing may be impaired. Respiratory complications develop rapidly, as manifested by crackles and wheezes, rapid respirations, and respiratory acidosis.
- Suction as necessary, using care to suction no longer than 10 seconds at any one time and using sterile technique. Suctioning removes secretions that not only obstruct airflow but also poses the risk for aspiration and pneumonia. Suctioning for longer than 10 seconds at a time may increase intracranial pressure (Hickey, 2003).
- Place in a side-lying position.
- Administer oxygen as prescribed. Administration of oxygen decreases the risk for hypoxia and hypercapnia, which can increase cerebral ischemia and intracranial pressure.
- Monitor mental status and level of consciousness: restlessness, drowsiness, lethargy, inability to follow commands, unresponsiveness. Frequent monitoring of neurologic status is necessary to detect changes. Alterations in mental status, level of consciousness, and movement indicate increased intracranial pressure, the major cause of death in the acute phase of a stroke.
- Monitor strength and reflexes, and assess for pain, headache, decreased muscle strength, sluggish pupillary reflexes, absent gag or swallowing reflexes, hemiplegia, Babinski's sign, and decerebrate or decorticate posturing. Alterations in strength and reflexes indicate increased intracranial pressure, the major cause of death in the acute phase of a stroke.
- Continuously monitor cardiac status, observing for dysrhythmias. A stroke may cause cardiac dysrhythmias, including bradycardia, PVCs, tachycardia, and AV block.

Characteristic ECG changes include a shortened PR interval, peaked T waves, and a depressed ST segment.

- Monitor body temperature. Hyperthermia may develop if the hypothalamus is affected.
- Maintain accurate intake and output records; measure urinary output via a Foley catheter. A stroke may damage the pituitary gland, resulting in diabetes insipidus and the possibility of dehydration from greatly increased urinary output.
- Monitor for seizures. Pad the side rails, and administer prescribed anticonvulsants. Seizures may be the result of cerebral tissue damage or increased intracranial pressure. Padded side rails prevent injury if a seizure occurs. Anticonvulsants prevent or treat seizures.

Impaired Physical Mobility

The goals of care for clients with impaired mobility are to maintain and improve functional abilities (by maintaining normal function and alignment, preventing edema of extremities, and reducing spasticity) and to prevent complications.

- Encourage active ROM exercises for unaffected extremities, and perform passive ROM exercises for affected extremities every 4 hours during day and evening shifts and once during the night shift. Support the joint during passive ROM exercises. Active ROM exercises maintain or improve muscle strength and endurance and help maintain cardiopulmonary function. Passive ROM exercises do not strengthen muscles but do help maintain joint flexibility.
- Turn the client every 2 hours around the clock, following a posted schedule for side-to-side and supine-to-prone position changes (verify prone positioning with the physician). Maintain body alignment, and support extremities in proper position with pillows. Elevate the head of the bed 30 degrees. Turning on a regular basis, accompanied by proper positioning, maintains joint function, alleviates pressure on bony prominences that can lead to skin breakdown, decreases dependent edema in hands and feet, reduces intracranial pressure, and lessens the risk of complications resulting from immobility (Figure 22–70 ■).
- Monitor the lower extremities each shift for symptoms of thrombophlebitis. Assess for increased warmth and redness in calves; measure the circumference of the calves and thighs. Clients on bedrest (especially those with loss of muscle strength and tone) are particularly prone to the development of deep venous thrombosis. Promptly report manifestations of thrombophlebitis.
- Collaborate with the physical therapist as the client gains mobility, using consistent techniques to move the client from the bed to the wheelchair and to help the client ambulate. The use of consistent techniques facilitates rehabilitation.

Self-Care Deficit

The client who has had a stroke may have a self-care deficit as a result of impaired mobility or mental confusion. It is important for clients to perform as much of their own physical care and grooming as possible to promote functional ability, increase independence, decrease feelings of powerlessness, and improve self-esteem.

Before establishing a plan to increase self-care, determine which hand was dominant before the stroke. If the client's dominant side is affected, self-care will be more difficult.

- Encourage use of the unaffected arm to bathe, brush teeth, comb hair, dress, and eat. Use of the unaffected arm promotes functional ability and independence.
- Teach the client to put on clothing by first dressing the affected extremities and then dressing the unaffected extremities. This technique facilitates self-dressing with minimal assistance.
- Collaborate with the occupational therapist in scheduling times for training for upper extremity functioning necessary for ADLs. Encourage the use of assistive devices (if required) for eating, physical hygiene, and dressing. Following a regular schedule in daily routines promotes learning. Use of assistive devices promotes independence and decreases feelings of powerlessness. Optimal grooming facilitates positive self-concept.

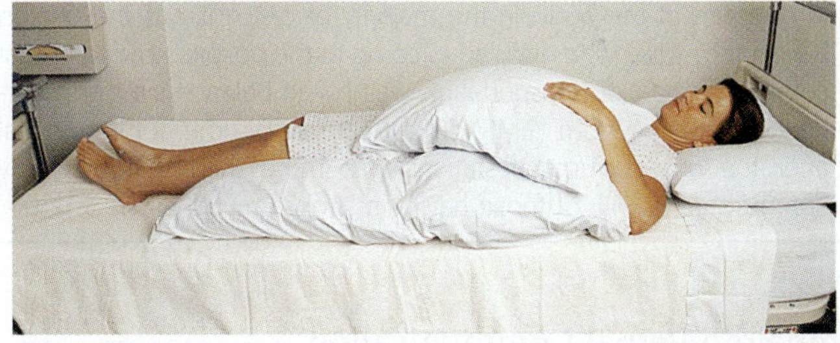

A

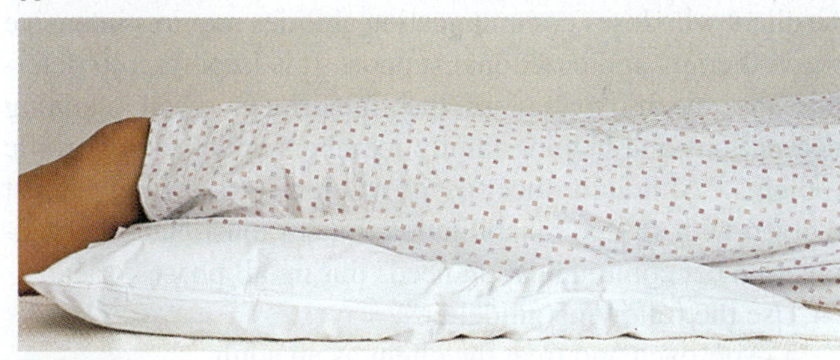

B

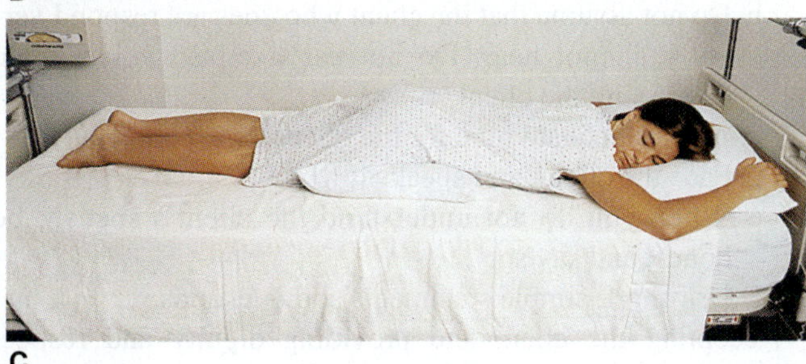

C

Figure 22–70 ■ Positioning the client with hemiplegia is important in preventing deformity of the affected extremities. *A*, With the client in a supine position, place a pillow in the axilla (to prevent adduction) and under the hand and arm, with the hand higher than the elbow (to prevent flexion and edema). *B*, When the client is lying supine, use a pillow from the iliac crest to the middle of the thigh to prevent external rotation of the hip. *C*, When the client is in the prone position, place a pillow under the pelvis to promote hip hyperextension.

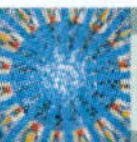

EVIDENCE-BASED PRACTICE Treating Stroke With tPA

Clinical Question

Stroke is the third-leading cause of death in the United States and is also a leading cause of severe, long-term disability. The risk of disability and death can be reduced in people who experience a sudden ischemic stroke by the administration of tissue plasminogen activator (tPA). To be effective, tPA must be administered within 3 hours of the warning signs of a stroke, but the public's awareness of stroke manifestations and the need for immediate treatment remain poor. This is especially true for those most at risk: people older than 75 years of age, African Americans, and men.

Evidence

Maze and Bakas (2004) conducted a study to determine (1) the most common manifestations leading to the decision to seek medical care, (2) who makes the decision, (3) the most common mode of transportation, (4) hospital arrival time in relation to onset of warning signs, and (5) factors most associated with hospital arrival time. They found that the most common warning sign leading people to come to the hospital was sudden confusion or trouble speaking or understanding speech, followed by sudden numbness or weakness in one part of the body. In the majority of cases, it was the person having the stroke who decided to come to the hospital, and the most common mode of transportation was by ambulance via the emergency medical system (EMS). The mean arrival time at the hospital after the onset of manifestations was more than 5 hours; only approximately 29% of those having a stroke arrived within 3 hours. Those that arrived by EMS and reported their incomes as adequate had the shortest arrival times.

Best Practice

Nurses provide information to the public in a wide variety of health promotion activities, including stroke awareness and the need for immediate treatment to ensure the best outcomes of care. It is important that the programs be geared toward the specific population most at risk and target people from all socioeconomic and cultural backgrounds. Although not measured in this study, factors that affect behavior, such as perceived risk, benefits and barriers of care, readiness to change, and self-efficacy, are areas that may be effective in designing educational programs to increase stroke awareness.

Critical Thinking

1. If you were planning a stroke awareness educational program, where would you have it in order to reach the largest number of the population? How would you advertise stroke warning manifestations to reach the most people?
2. How would you change the design of your program for the following groups?
   a. Long-term care or assisted living residents
   b. A men's study group in an African American church
   c. A group of Mexican American women.
3. Think of a slogan for the public that increases awareness of the 3-hour time limit for treatment with tPA.

Impaired Verbal Communication

The client who loses communication abilities requires intensive speech therapy and emotional support. It is important to determine the specific nature of the impairment when planning interventions and helping family members understand specific problems. Although the speech therapist is usually most involved with speech rehabilitation, nurses must plan interventions to meet communication needs during all phases of care.

- Use the following guidelines:
  a. Approach and treat the client as an adult.
  b. Do not assume that the client who does not respond verbally cannot hear. Do not use a raised voice when addressing the client.
  c. Allow adequate time for the client to respond.
  d. Face the client, and speak slowly.
  e. When you do not understand the client's speech, be honest and say so.
  f. Use short, simple statements and questions.

Accepting the client and providing dignity and respect enhances the nurse–client relationship. Allowing adequate response time and using short verbal statements or questions while facing the client motivates the client to communicate and decreases frustration.

- Accept frustration and anger as a normal reaction to the loss of function. Anger represents the client's frustration at the inability to control the loss of function.
- Try alternate methods of communication, including writing tablets, flash cards, and computerized talking boards.

Clients unable to communicate verbally may use other methods effectively.

Impaired Urinary Elimination and Risk for Constipation

Both urinary and bowel elimination may be altered because of neurologic deficits, impaired mobility, cognitive impairment, communication deficits, or preexisting problems (especially if the client is an older adult). Other causes can include changes in food and fluid intake and side effects of medications. Urinary incontinence or retention and constipation and fecal impaction are the usual manifestations.

- Assess for urinary frequency, urgency, incontinence, nocturia, and voiding in small amounts. In addition, assess the client's ability to respond to the need to void, the ability to use the call light, and the ability to use toileting equipment.
- Encourage bladder training by having client void on schedule, such as every 2 hours, rather than in response to the urge to void. Voiding every 2 hours or on schedule promotes bladder tone and urine storage.
- Teach Kegel exercises. To perform Kegel exercises, the client contracts the perineal muscles as though stopping urination, holds the contraction for 5 seconds, and then releases. Kegel exercises increase pubococcygeal muscle tone and bladder control, decreasing incontinence.
- Use positive reinforcement (verbal praise) for successful management of urinary elimination. Positive reinforcement can be a useful part of the teaching program.

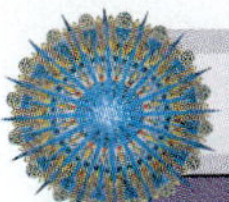

NURSING CARE PLAN A Client With a Stroke

ASSESSMENT

Orville Boren is a 63-year-old African American male who had a stroke caused by right cerebral thrombosis 1 week ago. He is a history instructor at the local community college. His hobbies are wood carving and gardening. Mr. Boren is also an active member of his church. For the past 2 years, Mr. Boren has been taking medication for hypertension, but his wife Emily reports that he often forgets to take it and that his blood pressure was high at his last physical examination. Mrs. Boren tells the staff that she has never had to worry about her husband's health before and that she wants to learn everything she can to care for him at home. However, she says that her husband was always the one to make the decisions and pay the bills. Mrs. Boren adds that all the children, grandchildren, neighbors, and family pastor want to see Mr. Boren back at home as soon as possible.

Carol Merck, RN, the nurse assigned to Mr. Boren, completes a health history and physical assessment, with Mrs. Boren providing information for the history. Mrs. Boren reports that her husband did have several spells of dizziness and blurred vision the week before his stroke, but they lasted only a few minutes and he believed them to be caused by "old age and working out in the sun." On the morning of admission, Mr. Boren woke up and could not move his left arm or leg; he also could not speak sensibly. Mrs. Boren called 911, and an ambulance took her husband to the hospital.

Physical assessment findings include the following: Mr. Boren is drowsy but responds to verbal stimuli. Although he does not respond verbally, he can nod his head to indicate "yes" when asked questions. Flaccid paralysis is present in his left arm and left leg, with no response noted to touch in those extremities (he is left-handed). Visual fields are decreased in a pattern consistent with homonymous hemianopia. A computed tomographic scan, negative on admission, is repeated on the day after admission and confirms the medical diagnosis of a right-brain stroke caused by a thrombus of the middle cerebral artery.

Mr. Boren's medical treatment includes heparin sodium administered by continuous intravenous drip, with clotting studies to be performed every 4 hours and the dose adjusted accordingly.

DIAGNOSES

- Feeding Self-Care Deficit related to loss of the ability to use the left hand and arm
- Impaired Physical Mobility related to neurologic deficits causing left hemiplegia
- Risk for Impaired Skin Integrity related to inability to change position
- Sensory Perception Disturbed: Visual related to changes in visual fields
- Impaired Verbal Communication related to cerebral injury

PLANNING

Goals of care include the following:

- The client will learn to use his right hand to feed himself.
- The client will participate in exercises necessary to maintain muscle strength and tone.
- The client will maintain skin integrity.
- The client will indicate an understanding that visual fields may improve in a few weeks.
- The client will practice and implement speech therapy activities while at the same time using alternative methods of communication.

IMPLEMENTATION

- Arrange mealtimes so that Mr. Boren is sitting up by the window in a clean and private environment.
- Provide adaptive devices (silverware with thick handles and nonslip plates).
- Encourage Mrs. Boren to visit at mealtimes, to assist with meals, and periodically to bring a favorite food from home.
- Provide passive ROM exercises for the left arm and leg; schedule active ROM exercises for the right extremities as well as quadriceps and gluteal sets every 4 hours during waking hours.
- Keep the skin clean and dry at all times.
- Establish and maintain a regular schedule for turning when Mr. Boren is in bed.
- Place objects (e.g., call bell and tissues) on the unaffected side, and approach Mr. Boren from that side.
- Support attempts to communicate verbally; when Mr. Boren is not understood, he prefers to use a large marker and tablet.

EVALUATION

Mr. Boren is discharged to his home after being in the hospital for 10 days. During the first 2 months after discharge, Martha Grimes, RN, the home health nurse, visits Mr. and Mrs. Boren at home. At the end of 2 months, Mr. Boren is using his right hand to feed himself. He has regained partial use of his left arm and leg and is using a walker to move around the house and yard; he is even able to work in his flower garden. His skin has remained intact, and his vision is back to normal. He is slowly relearning speech; this has been the most difficult change for him to accept. Once he writes on his tablet, "I think God has forgotten me."

(continued)

NURSING CARE PLAN A Client With a Stroke *continued*

CRITICAL THINKING

1. Hypertension is sometimes referred to as "the silent killer." Provide justifications for this statement.
2. The functional changes Mr. Boren has experienced may make a return to teaching difficult. What other uses of his knowledge and abilities might you suggest?
3. What would be your reply if, after you had completed passive ROM on Mr. Boren's left arm, he wrote: "I just ignore that part of my body—it doesn't work anyway"?

- Discuss prestroke bowel habits as well as the pattern of bowel elimination since the stroke.
- If the client is able to swallow without difficulty, encourage fluids (up to 2,000 mL/day) and a high-fiber diet. Increased fluids and fiber stimulate intestinal motility.
- Increase physical activity as tolerated. Increased activity stimulates intestinal motility.
- Assist in using the toilet facilities at the same time each day (based on usual patterns of bowel elimination), ensuring privacy and having the client sit in an upright position if at all possible. Establishing a regular daily time for bowel movements in the upright position and in privacy promotes normal bowel elimination.
- Administer prescribed stool softeners if the client is following a bowel elimination routine or is not drinking sufficient fluids. Stool softeners help prevent the formation of hard stool that is more difficult to expel.

Impaired Swallowing

A stroke may impair the ability to swallow. Weakness or lack of coordination of the tongue, attention deficits, and deficits involving the swallowing reflex all play a role. **Dysphagia** (difficulty swallowing) may result in choking, drooling, aspiration, or regurgitation. Nursing care focuses on maintaining safety by preventing aspiration and on ensuring adequate nutrition.

- Monitor results of swallowing studies before providing oral food and fluids.
- Ensure safety when eating.
  a. Position in upright sitting position with neck slightly flexed.
  b. Order puréed or soft food. Liquids should be of the same consistency as honey.
  c. Feed or teach client to eat by putting food behind the front teeth on the unaffected side of mouth and tilting the head slightly backward. Teach to swallow one bite at a time.
  d. Assess for coughing with eating or drinking.
  e. Have suction equipment available at the bedside in case of choking or aspiration.

Sitting upright with the head and neck first slightly flexed and then tilted back helps the client swallow. The client can usually swallow puréed or soft foods more easily than liquid or solid foods. Using the unaffected side of the mouth helps prevent food from collecting in the mouth and makes swallowing safer; in addition, food is less likely to fall out of the mouth. Coughing may be indicative of dysphagia.

- Monitor lung sounds. Coarse lung sounds heard in the right upper and/or lower lobes may indicate aspiration as the right bronchus is the first division of the bronchi and where the majority of aspirations occur.
- Minimize distractions and, if necessary, give step-by-step instructions for eating. Distractions increase the risk of aspiration. Complex activities are easier to perform when broken down into small steps.

Evaluation

Client outcomes may be evaluated based on the following expected outcomes:

- The client participates in rehabilitation.
- The client communicates needs effectively.
- The client receives adequate family and/or community support upon discharge from the facility.
- The client experiences no complications resulting from immobility, dysphagia, or reduced motor or sensory function.

REVIEW Stroke

RELATE: LINK THE CONCEPTS

Linking the exemplar of Stroke with the concept of Thermoregulation:

1. What impact related to thermoregulation might be seen in the client who has had a massive stroke?
2. You are caring for a client who had a stroke. The client requires mechanical ventilation due to inadequate breathing patterns. The client's temperature is 106.2 axillary. What are your priorities of care? Will over-the-counter antipyretics be effective? Explain your answer.

Linking the exemplar of Stroke with the concept of Safety:

3. You are caring for a 56-year-old male client in the rehabilitation facility who experienced a stroke 6 months ago resulting in hemiplegia of the left side. What risks to safety do you anticipate for this client?
4. What interventions, including client teaching, will you provide to reduce this client's risk of injury?

READY: GO TO COMPANION SKILLS MANUAL

- Monitoring intake and output
- Assessing the skin
- Assessing blood pressure
- Assessing apical-radial pulse
- Assessing peripheral pulses
- Assessing pulse oximeter
- Assessing heart rate
- Assessing respirations
- Oropharyngeal, nasopharyngeal, and nasotracheal suctioning
- Assisting the client to the commode
- Developing a regular bowel routine

REFER: GO TO MYNURSINGKIT

REFLECT: CASE STUDY

Ted Marist is a 68-year-old man who lives with his wife Maggie in a condominium on the sixth floor of a high-rise building. Ted is recently retired from the police force. Ted smoked two packs a day until 1 year ago when his doctor discovered a bruit in his right carotid artery. The doctor placed Ted on Coumadin (1.5 mg. a day) and Maggie insisted Ted quit smoking. He still smokes an occasional cigarette when he's out with friends, but he no longer smokes regularly. Ted and Maggie have three grown children and five grandchildren.

Maggie attempts to regulate Ted's diet and encourages him to take a walk with her every night after dinner. Ted comes to the doctor's office today to have his clotting times checked. Maggie says she is very concerned because Ted has had two episodes of staring off into space and not responding to her questions. She says his eyes were open but he looked like "there was nobody home behind his eyes" and even when she screamed he did not respond. When the episode stopped he complained of a headache and insisted on taking a nap, saying he felt much better when he awoke.

1. What do you suspect is causing Ted's symptoms?
2. How will you respond to Maggie's concerns when she tells you about these events?
3. What orders do you anticipate receiving from the provider related to these symptoms?
4. Considering Ted's history, what type of stroke is Ted most at risk for?

EXPLORE PEARSON **mynursingkit**™

MyNursingKit is your one stop for online chapter review materials and resources. Prepare for success with additional NCLEX®-style practice questions, interactive assignments and activities, web links, animations and videos, and more!

Register your access code from the front of your book at **www.mynursingkit.com**.

REFERENCES

American Heart Association. (2005). *Heart disease and stroke statistics—2005 update.* Dallas, TX: Author.

American Heart Association. (2005a). 2005 Guidelines for CPR and ECC. *Circulation, 112,* IV1–IV205. Retrieved from http://www.circulationaha.org

American Heart Association. (2005b). *Part 9: Adult stroke.* Supplement to Circulation. (2005). 112: IV-111-IV-120.

American Stroke Association. (2003). *Stroke among Hispanics.* Retrieved from http://www.strokeassociation.org/presenter.jhtml?identifier=3030389

Barnes, V. A., Treiber, F. A., & Davis, H. (2001). Impact of transcendental meditation on cardiovascular function at rest and during acute stress in adolescents with high normal blood pressure. *Journal of Psychosomatic Research, 51,* 597–605.

Baxter, J. K., & Weinstein, L. (2004). HELLP syndrome: The state of the art. *Obstetrical & Gynecological Survey, 59*(12), 838–845

Bobrie, G., Chatellier, G., Genes, N., Clerson, P., Vaur, L., Vaisse, B., et al. (2004). Cardiovascular prognosis of "masked hypertension" detected by blood pressure self-measurement in elderly treated hypertensive patients. *Journal of the American Medical Association, 291,* 1342–1349.

Braunwald, E., Antman, E. M., Beasley, J. W., Califf, R. M., Cheitlin, M. D., Hochman, J. S., et al. (2002). *ACC/AHA 2002 guideline update for the management of patients with unstable angina and non-ST-segment elevation myocardial infarction: A report of the American College of Cardiology/American Heart Association Task Force on Practice Guidelines (Committee on the Management of Patients with Unstable Angina).* Retrieved from http://www.acc.org/clinical/guidelines/unstable/unstable.pdf

Centers for Disease Control and Prevention. (2004). *Chronic disease overview.* Retrieved October 15, 2004, from http://www.cdc.gov/nccdphp/overview.htm

Chang, R. R., Chen, A.Y., & Klitzner, T. S. (2002). Clinical management of infants with hypoplastic left heart syndrome in the United States, 1988–1997. *Pediatrics, 110*(2), 292–298.

Connolly, C., McClowry, S., Hayman, L., Mahony, L., & Artman, M. (2004). Posttraumatic stress disorder in children after cardiac surgery. *Journal of Pediatrics, 144*(4), 480–484.

Connor, J. A. (2006). Alterations in cardiovascular function in children. In K. L. McCance & S. E. Huether (Eds.), *Pathophysiology: The biologic basis for disease in adults and children.* (5th ed., pp. 1147–1180). St. Louis: Mosby.

Cook, E. H., & Higgins, S. S. (2004). Congenital heart disease. In P. Jackson Allen & J. A. Vessey, *Primary care of the child with a chronic condition* (4th ed., 382–403). St. Louis, MO: Mosby.

Copstead, L. C., & Banasik, J. L. (2005). *Pathophysiology* (3rd ed.). St. Louis, MO: Saunders.

Corbett, J. V. (2004). *Laboratory tests and diagnostic procedures with nursing diagnoses* (6th ed.). Upper Saddle River, NJ: Prentice Hall.

Craven, R. F. (2000). Physiologic adaptation with aging. In S. L. Woods, E. S. S. Froelicher, & S. A. Motzer (Eds.), *Cardiac nursing* (4th ed., pp. 180–185). Philadelphia: Lippincott.

Cunningham, F. G., Leveno, K. J., Bloom, S. L., Hauth, J. C., Gilstrap III, L. C., & Wenstrom, K. D. (2005.) *Williams obstetrics* (22nd ed.). New York: McGraw-Hill.

Davis, C. C., Brown, R. T., Bakeman, R., & Campbell, R. (1998). Psychological adaptation and adjustment of mothers of children with congenital heart disease: Stress, coping, and family functioning. *Journal of Pediatric Psychology, 23*(4), 219–228.

De Luca, G., Suryapranata, H., Ottervanger, J. P., & Antman, E. M. (2004). Time delay to treatment and mortality in primary angioplasty for acute myocardial infarction: Every minute of delay counts. *Circulation,* March 16, 2004. Retrieved October 26, 2009, from http://www.circulationaha.org

Doniger, S. J., & Sharieff, G. Q. (2006). Pediatric dysrhythmias. *Pediatric Clinics of North America, 53,* 85–105.

Eagle, K. A., Guyton, R. A., Davidoff, R., Edwards, F. H., Ewy, G. A., Gardner, T. J., et al. (2004). *ACC/AHA 2004 guideline update for coronary artery bypass graft surgery: A report of the American College of Cardiology/American Heart Association Task Force on Practice Guidelines.* Retrieved October 26, 2009, from http://www.acc.org/qualityandscience/clinical/guidelines/cabg/index_rev.pdf

Fontaine, K. L. (2005). *Healing practices: Alternative therapies for nursing* (2nd ed.). Upper Saddle River, NJ: Prentice Hall Health.

Goldberg, S., Morris, P., Simmons, R. J., Fowler, R. S., & Levinson, H. (1990). Chronic illness in infancy and parenting stress: A comparison of three groups of parents. *Journal of Pediatric Psychology, 15,* 347–358.

Goldmuntz, E. (2004). The genetic contribution to congenital heart disease. *Pediatric Clinics of North America, 51,* 1721–1737.

Gordon, M. C. (2007). Maternal physiology. In S. G. Gabbe, J. R. Niebyl, & J. L. Simpson (Eds.), *Obstetrics: Normal and problem pregnancies* (5th ed.). New York: Churchill-Livingstone.

Green, A. (2004). Outcomes of congenital heart disease: A review. *Pediatric Nursing, 30*(4), 280–284.

Green, A., Kitchen, B., & Ray, T. (2005). Supraventricular tachycardia in children: Symptoms distinguish from sinus tachycardia. *Journal of Emergency Nursing, 31*(1), 105–108.

Habli, M., & Sibai, B. M. (2008). Hypertensive disorders of pregnancy. In R. S. Gibbs, B. Y. Karlan, A. F. Haney, & I. E. Nygaard (Eds.), *Danforth's obstetrics and gynecology* (10th ed.). Philadelphia: Wolters Kluwer/Lippincott Williams & Wilkins.

Hickey, J. (2003). *The clinical practice of neurological and neurosurgical nursing* (4th ed.). Philadelphia: Lippincott

Hunt, S. A., Abraham, W. T., Chin, M. H., Feldman, A. M., Francis, G. S., Ganiats, T. G., et al. (2005). *ACC/AHA 2005 guideline update for the diagnosis and management of chronic heart failure in the adult: A report of the American College of Cardiology/American Heart Association Task Force on Practice Guidelines (Writing Committee to Update the 2001 Guidelines for the Evaluation and Management of Heart Failure).* Retrieved from http://www.acc.org/clinical/guidelines/ failure/index/pdf

Ikle, L., Hale, K., Fashaw, L., Boucek, M., & Rosenberg, A. A. (2003). Developmental outcome of patients with hypoplastic left heart syndrome treated with heart transplantation. *Journal of Pediatrics, 142*(1), 20–25.

Irvin, D. J., & White, M. (2004). The importance of accurately assessing orthostatic hypotension. *Geriatric Nursing, 25,* 99–101.

Kasper, D. L., Braunwald, E., Fauci, A. S., Hauser, S. L., Longo, D. L., & Jameson, J. L. (Eds.). (2005). *Harrison's principles of internal medicine* (16th ed.). New York: McGraw-Hill.

Klein, L. L., & Galan, H. L. (2004). Cardiac disease in pregnancy. *Obstetrics & Gynecology Clinics of North America, 31*(2), viii, 429–459.

Lehne, R. A. (2004). *Pharmacology for nursing care* (5th ed). St. Louis: Saunders.

Mahle, W. T., Visconti, K. J., Freier, M. C., Kanne, S. M., Hamilton, W. G., et al. (2006). Relationship of surgical approach to neurodevelopmental outcomes in hypoplastic left heart syndrome. *Pediatrics, 117*(1), e90–e97.

Maron, B. J. (2004). Hypertrophic cardiomyopathy in childhood. *Pediatric Clinics of North America, 51,* 1305–1346.

Maze, L., & Bakas, T. (2004). Factors associated with hospital arrival time for stroke patients. *Journal of Neuroscience Nursing, 36*(3), 136–141, 155.

McCaffrey, R., Ruknui, P., Hatthakit, U., & Kasetsomboon, P. (2005). The effects of yoga on hypertensive persons in Thailand. *Holistic Nursing Practice, 19*(4), 173–180.

McCance, K., & Huether, S. (2001). *Pathophysiology: The biologic basis for disease in adults and children.* St. Louis, MO: Mosby.

McCance, K., & Huether, S. (2006). *Pathophysiology: The biologic basis for disease in adults and children.* St. Louis, MO: Mosby.

Mörelius, E., Lundh, U., & Nelson, N. (2002). Parental stress in relation to the severity of congenital heart disease in the offspring. *Pediatric Nursing, 28*(1), 28–32.

National Cholesterol Education Program. (2002). *Third report of the National Cholesterol Education Program (NCEP) Expert Panel on detection, evaluation, and treatment of high blood cholesterol in adults (Adult Treatment Panel III). Final report.* Bethesda, MD: National Institutes of Health.

National Heart, Lung, and Blood Institute. (2004). *Morbidity & mortality: 2004 chart book of cardiovascular, lung, and blood diseases.* Bethesda, MD: National Institutes of Health.

National Heart, Lung, and Blood Institute (2004a). *Morbidity & mortality: 2004 chart book of cardiovascular, lung, and blood diseases.* Bethesda, MD: National Institutes of Health.

National Heart, Lung, and Blood Institute. (2004b). *The seventh report of the Joint National Committee on prevention, detection, evaluation, and treatment of high blood pressure.* Bethesda, MD: National High Blood Pressure Education Program, National Institutes of Health.

National Heart, Lung, and Blood Institute. (2005). Statement from Elizabeth G. Nabel, M.D., director of the National Heart, Lung, and Blood Institute of the National Institutes of Health on the findings of the Women's Health Study, *NIH News,* March 7. Retrieved from www.nhlbi.nih.gov

National Institute of Neurological Disorders and Stroke. (2005). *Stroke: Hope through research.* Retrieved 10/26/2009 from http://www.ninds.nih.gov/disorders/stroke/detail_stroke.htm

National Institute of Neurological Disorders and Stroke [NINDS]. (2005a). *Low back pain fact sheet.* Available http://www.ninds.nih.gov/disorders/backpain/detail_backpain.htm

Neilson, D. E., & Robin, N. H. (2002). Advances in the genetics of pediatric heart disease. *Contemporary Pediatrics, 19*(1), 85–100.

Palmieri, R. (2006). Cerebral artery stenosis paves the way for a stroke. *Nursing, 36*(6), 36–42.

Park, M. K. (2002). *Pediatric cardiology for practitioners* (4th ed.). St. Louis: Mosby.

Pelchat, D., Ricard, N., Bouchard, J. M., Perreault, M., Saucier, J. F., Berrthiaume, M., et al. (1999). Adaptation of parents in relation to their 6-month-old infant's type of disability. *Child: Care, Health and Development, 25,* 377–397.

Piña, I. L., Apstein, C. S., Balady, G. J., Belardinelli, R., Chaitman, B. R., Duscha, B. D., et al. (2003). *AHA scientific statement: Exercise and heart failure.* Retrieved October 25, 2009, from http://www.circulationaha.org

Porth, C. M. (2005). *Pathophysiology: Concepts of altered health states* (7th ed.). Philadelphia: Lippincott.

Rao, P. S., Jureidini, S. B., Balfour, I. C., Singh, G. K., & Chen, S. (2003). Severe aortic coarctation in infants less than three months: Successful palliation by balloon angioplasty. *Journal of Invasive Cardiology, 15*(4), 202–208.

Reuben, D., Herr, K., Pacala, J., Pollock, B., Potter, J., & Semla, T. (2004). *Geriatrics at your fingertips.* Malden, MA: American Geriatrics Society, Blackwell.

Rome, J. J., & Kreutzer, J. (2004). Pediatric interventional catheterization: Reasonable expectations and outcomes. *Pediatric Clinics of North America, 51,* 1589–1610.

Sanders, A. B., & Ewy, G. A. (2005). Cardiopulmonary resuscitation in the real world: When will the guidelines get the message? *JAMA, 293*(3), 363–365.

Shillingford, A. J., & Wernovsky, G. (2004). Academic performance and behavioral difficulties after neonatal and infant heart surgery. *Pediatric Clinics of North America, 51,* 1625–1639.

Sibai, B. M. (2005). Diagnosis, prevention, and management of eclampsia. *Obstetrics and Gynecology, 105*(2), 402–410.

Sibai, B. M. (2007). Hypertension. In S. G. Gabbe, J. R. Niebyl, & J. L. Simpson (Eds.), *Obstetrics: Normal and problem pregnancies* (5th ed.). Philadelphia: Churchill Livingstone.

Sole, M. L., Lamborn, M. L., & Hartshorn, J. C. (Eds.). (2001). *Introduction to critical care nursing* (3rd ed.). Philadelphia: Saunders.

Spencer, J. W., & Jacobs, J. J. (2003). *Complementary and alternative medicine: An evidence-based approach* (2nd ed.). St. Louis, MO: Mosby.

Suddaby, E. C. (2001). Contemporary thinking for congenital heart disease. *Pediatric Nursing, 27*(3), 233–238, 270.

Tierney, L. M., McPhee, S. J., & Papadakis, M. A. (2005). *Current medical diagnosis & treatment* (44th ed.). New York: Lange Medical Books/McGraw-Hill.

Tran, J. T. (2002). Current treatment strategies of symptomatic patent ductus arteriosis. *Journal of Pediatric Health Care, 16*(6), 306–310.

Urden, L. D., Stacy, K. M., & Lough, M. E. (2006). *Thelan's critical care nursing: Diagnosis and management* (5th ed.). St. Louis, MO: Mosby.

U.S. Department of Health & Human Services. (2005). *Dietary guidelines for Americans 2005.* Washington, DC: U.S. Department of Agriculture. Retrieved from http://www.healthierus.gov/dietaryguidelines

U.S. FDA. (2005). *FDA Approves BiDil Heart Failure Drug for Black Patients.* Retrieved October 25, 2009, from http://www.fda.gov/NewsEvents/Newsroom/PressAnnouncements/2005/ucm108445.htm

Uzark, K., & Jones, K. (2003). Parenting stress and children with heart disease. *Journal of Pediatric Health Care, 17*(4), 163–168.

Wade, C. R., Reith, K. K., Sikora, J. H., & Augustine, S. M. (2004). Postoperative nursing care of the cardiac transplant recipient. *Critical Care Nursing Quarterly, 27*(1), 17–28.

White, R. M. (2005). The role of brain natriuretic peptide in systolic heart failure. *Dimensions of Critical Care Nursing, 24*(4), 171–174.

Wiggens, D. A., & Elliott, M. (2005). Outcomes of pregnancies achieved by donor egg in vitro fertilization—A comparison with standard in vitro fertilization pregnancies. *American Journal of Obstetrics and Gynecology, 192*(6), 2002–2008.

Woods, S. L., Froelicher, E. S., Motzer, S. A., & Bridges, E. (2004). *Cardiac nursing* (5th ed.). Philadelphia: Lippincott.

Writing Group for the Women's Health Initiative Investigators. (2002). Risks and benefits of estrogen plus progestin in healthy postmenopausal women. (On-line). *JAMA, 288*(3). Retrieved from http://jama.ama-assn.org/issues/v288n3/fffull/joc21036.html

Reproduction 23

Concept at-a-Glance

Concept Learning Outcomes

After reading about this concept, you will be able to:

1. Summarize the structure and physiology of the reproductive system related to childbearing.
2. List factors affecting reproduction.
3. Identify commonly occurring alterations in reproduction and their related treatments.
4. Explain common physical assessment procedures used to examine reproductive health across the life span.
5. Outline diagnostic and laboratory tests used to determine the individual's reproductive status.
6. Explain the management of reproductive health and prevention of reproductive illness.
7. Demonstrate the nursing process in providing culturally competent care across the life span for pregnant individuals and their families.
8. Identify pharmacologic interventions used in caring for individuals with alterations in reproduction.

Concept Key Terms

Acrosomal reaction, *1525*
Amnion, *1527*
Amniotic fluid, *1527*
Aortocaval compression, *1542*
Ballottement, *1548*
Blastocyst, *1527*
Braxton Hicks contractions, *1533*
Capacitation, *1525*
Chadwick's sign, *1542*
Chloasma, *1543*
Chorion, *1527*
Conjugate vera, *1517*
Corpus luteum, *1522*
Cotyledons, *1531*
Diagonal conjugate, *1517*
Diastasis recti, *1544*
Ductus arteriosus, *1534*
Ductus venosus, *1534*
Embryo, *1538*
Embryonic membranes, *1527*
False pelvis, *1517*
Female reproductive cycle (FRC), *1519*
Fertilization, *1524*
Fetus, *1539*
Foramen ovale, *1534*
Gametes, *1516*
Gametogenesis, *1524*
Goodell's sign, *1542*
Graafian follicle, *1522*
Hegar's sign, *1547*
McDonald's sign, *1547*
Meiosis, *1523*
Melasma gravidarum, *1543*
Mitosis, *1523*
Morning sickness, *1546*
Morula, *1527*
Obstetric conjugate, *1517*
Oogenesis, *1524*
Ovulation, *1522*
Pelvic inlet, *1517*
Pelvic outlet, *1518*
Physiologic anemia of pregnancy, *1543*
Placenta, *1530*
Postconception age periods, *1538*
Prenatal education, *1571*
Quickening, *1546*
Risk factors, *1561*
Spermatogenesis, *1524*
Striae, *1542*
Supine hypotensive syndrome, *1542*
Transverse diameter, *1517*
Trophoblast, *1527*
True pelvis, *1517*
Umbilical cord, *1530*
Vena caval syndrome, *1542*
Vernix caseosa, *1541*
Wharton's jelly, *1530*
Zygote, *1524*

See also Box 23–1 on page 1559 for additional key terms.

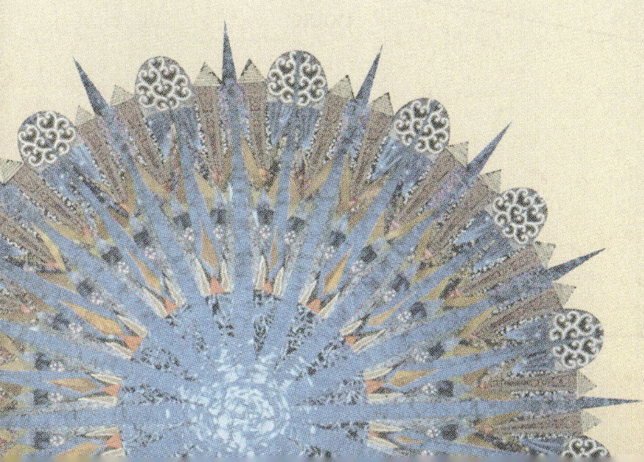

About Reproduction

Understanding reproduction requires more than understanding sexual intercourse or the process by which the female and male sex cells unite. The nurse also must be familiar with the structures and functions that make childbearing possible and the phenomena that initiate it. The primary functions of both female and male reproductive systems are to produce sex cells and transport them to locations where their union can occur. The sex cells, called **gametes**, are produced by specialized organs called gonads. A series of ducts and glands in both the male and female reproductive system contributes to the production and transport of the gametes. •

KEY COMPONENTS OF THE FEMALE REPRODUCTIVE SYSTEM

The female reproductive system is described in detail in Concept 26, Sexuality. Two key components discussed here in relation to their importance in conception and childbearing are the bony pelvis and the female reproductive cycle (FRC).

Bony Pelvis

The female bony pelvis has two unique functions:

- To support and protect the pelvic contents
- To form the relatively fixed axis of the birth passage

Because the pelvis is so important to childbearing, its structure must be understood clearly.

BONY STRUCTURE The pelvis is made up of four bones: two innominate bones, the sacrum, and the coccyx. The pelvis resembles a bowl or basin; its sides are the innominate bones, and its back is the sacrum and coccyx. Lined with fibrocartilage and held tightly together by ligaments (Figure 23–1 ■), the four bones join at the symphysis pubis, the two sacroiliac joints, and the sacrococcygeal joints.

The innominate bones, also known as the hip bones, are made up of three separate bones: the ilium, ischium, and pubis. These bones fuse to form a circular cavity, the acetabulum, which articulates with the femur.

The ilium is the broad, upper prominence of the hip. The iliac crest is the margin of the ilium. The ischial spines, the foremost projections nearest the groin, are the site of attachment for ligaments and muscles.

The ischium, the strongest bone, is under the ilium and below the acetabulum. The L-shaped ischium ends in a marked protuberance, the ischial tuberosity, on which the weight of a seated body rests. The ischial spines arise near the junction of the ilium and ischium and jut into the pelvic cavity. The shortest diameter of the pelvic cavity is between the ischial spines. The ischial spines serve as reference points during labor to evaluate the descent of the fetal head into the birth canal.

The pubis forms the slightly bowed front portion of the innominate bone. Extending medially from the acetabulum to the midpoint of the bony pelvis, each pubis meets the other to form a joint called the symphysis pubis. The triangular space below this junction is known as the pubic arch. The fetal head passes under this arch during birth. The symphysis pubis is formed by heavy fibrocartilage and the superior and inferior pubic ligaments. The mobility of the inferior ligament increases during a first pregnancy and to a greater extent in subsequent pregnancies.

The sacroiliac joints also have a degree of mobility that increases near the end of pregnancy as the result of an upward gliding movement. The pelvic outlet may be increased by 1.5–2 cm in the squatting, sitting, and dorsal

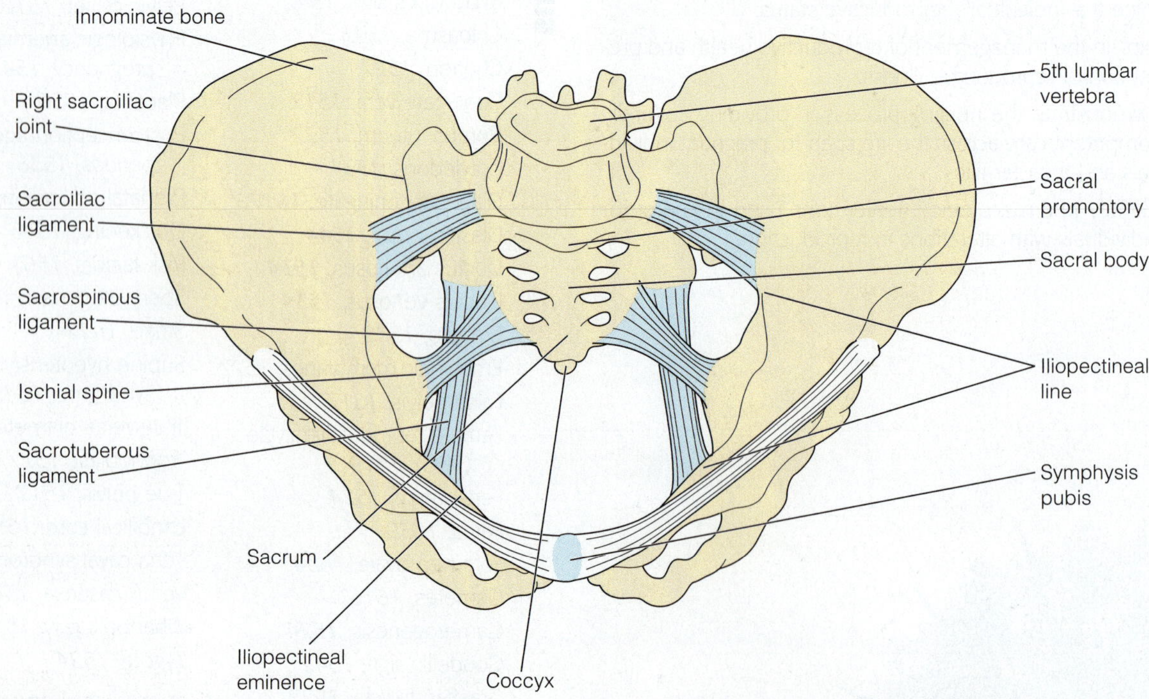

Figure 23–1 ■ Pelvic bones with supporting ligaments.

lithotomy positions. These relaxations of the joints are induced by the hormones of pregnancy.

The sacrum is a wedge-shaped bone formed by the fusion of five vertebrae. The anterior upper portion of the sacrum has a projection into the pelvic cavity known as the sacral promontory. This projection is another obstetric guide in determining pelvic measurements.

The small triangular bone last on the vertebral column is the coccyx. It articulates with the sacrum at the sacrococcygeal joint. The coccyx usually moves backward during labor to provide more room for the fetus.

PELVIC FLOOR The muscular floor of the bony pelvis is designed to overcome the force of gravity exerted on the pelvic organs. It acts as a buttress to the irregularly shaped pelvic outlet, thereby providing stability and support for surrounding structures.

Deep fascia, the levator ani, and coccygeal muscles form the part of the pelvic floor known as the pelvic diaphragm. The components of the pelvic diaphragm function as a whole, yet they are able to move over one another. This feature provides an exceptional capacity for dilatation during birth and return to prepregnancy condition following birth. Above the pelvic diaphragm is the pelvic cavity; below and behind it is the perineum. The sacrum is located posteriorly.

The levator ani muscle makes up the major portion of the pelvic diaphragm and consists of four muscles: the iliococcygeus, pubococcygeus, puborectalis, and pubovaginalis. The iliococcygeal muscle, a thin muscular sheet underlying the sacrospinous ligament, helps the levator ani support the pelvic organs. Muscles of the pelvic floor are shown in Figure 23–2 ■ and are discussed in Table 23–1.

PELVIC DIVISION The pelvic cavity is divided into the false pelvis and the true pelvis (Figure 23–3A ■). The **false pelvis**, the portion above the pelvic brim, or linea terminalis, supports the weight of the enlarged pregnant uterus and directs the presenting fetal part into the true pelvis below.

The **true pelvis** is the portion that lies below the linea terminalis. The bony circumference of the true pelvis is made up of the sacrum, coccyx, and innominate bones and represents the bony limits of the birth canal. The relationship between the true pelvis and the fetal head is of paramount importance: The size and shape of the true pelvis must be adequate for normal fetal passage during labor and at birth. The true pelvis consists of three parts: the inlet, the pelvic cavity, and the outlet (Figure 23–3B). Each part has distinct measurements that aid in evaluating the adequacy of the pelvis for childbirth.

The **pelvic inlet** is the upper border of the true pelvis and is typically rounded. Its size and shape are determined by assessing three anteroposterior diameters. The **diagonal conjugate** extends from the subpubic angle to the middle of the sacral promontory and is typically 11.5 cm in diameter. The diagonal conjugate can be measured manually during a pelvic examination. The **obstetric conjugate** extends from the middle of the sacral promontory to an area approximately 1 cm below the pubic crest. Its length is estimated by subtracting 1.5 cm from the length of the diagonal conjugate (Figure 23–4 ■). The fetus passes through the obstetric conjugate, whose diameter determines whether the fetus can move down into the birth canal for engagement to occur. The true (anatomic) conjugate, or **conjugate vera**, extends from the middle of the sacral promontory to the middle of the pubic crest (superior surface of the symphysis). One additional measurement, the transverse diameter, helps determine the shape of the inlet. The **transverse diameter** is the largest diameter of the inlet and is measured by using the linea terminalis as the point of reference.

The pelvic cavity (canal) is a curved canal with a longer posterior than anterior wall. A change in the lumbar curve can increase or decrease the tilt of the pelvis and influence the progress of labor because the fetus has to adjust itself to this curved path as well as to the different diameters of the true pelvis (Figure 23–3B).

TABLE 23–1 **Muscles of the Pelvic Floor**

MUSCLE	ORIGIN	INSERTION	INNERVATION	ACTION
Levator ani	Pubis, lateral pelvic wall, and ischial spine	Blends with organs in pelvic cavity	Inferior rectal, 2nd, and 3rd sacral nerves in addition to anterior rami of 3rd and 4th sacral nerves	Supports pelvic viscera; helps form pelvic diaphragm
Iliococcygeus	Pelvic surface of ischial spine and pelvic fascia	Central point of perineum, coccygeal raphe, and coccyx		Assists in supporting abdominal and pelvic viscera
Pubococcygeus	Pubis and pelvic fascia	Coccyx		
Puborectalis	Pubis	Blends with rectum; meets similar fibers from opposite side		Forms sling for rectum, just posterior to it; raises anus
Pubovaginalis	Pubis	Blends into vagina		Supports vagina
Coccygeus	Ischial spine and sacrospinous ligament	Lateral border of lower sacrum and upper coccyx	3rd and 4th sacral nerves	Supports pelvic viscera; helps form pelvic diaphragm; flexes and abducts coccyx

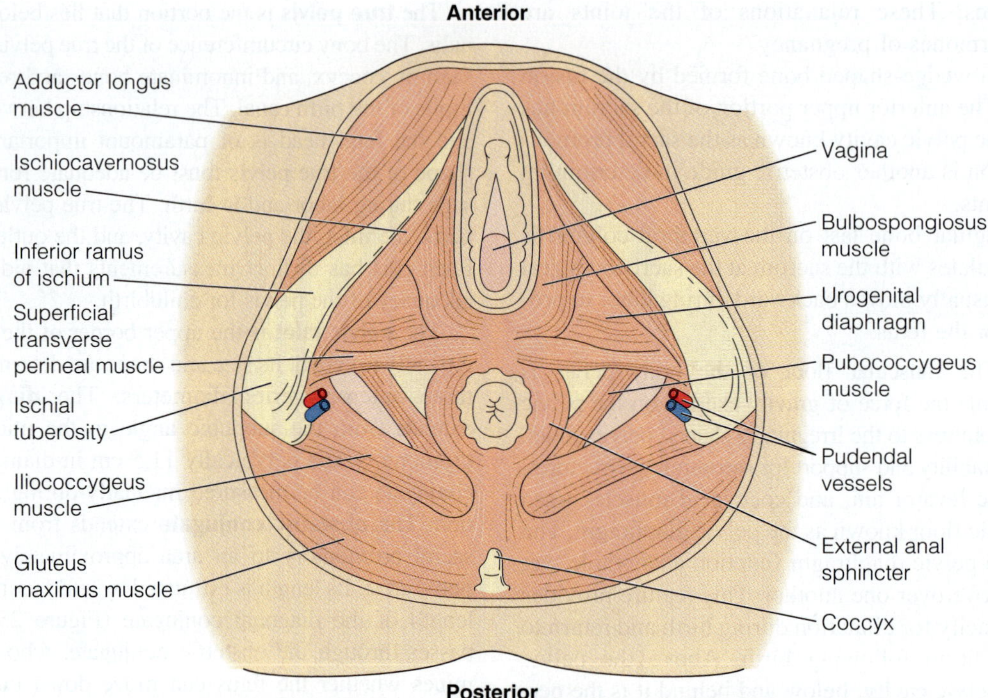

Figure 23–2 ■ Muscles of the pelvic floor. (The puborectalis, pubovaginalis, and coccygeal muscles cannot be seen from this view.)

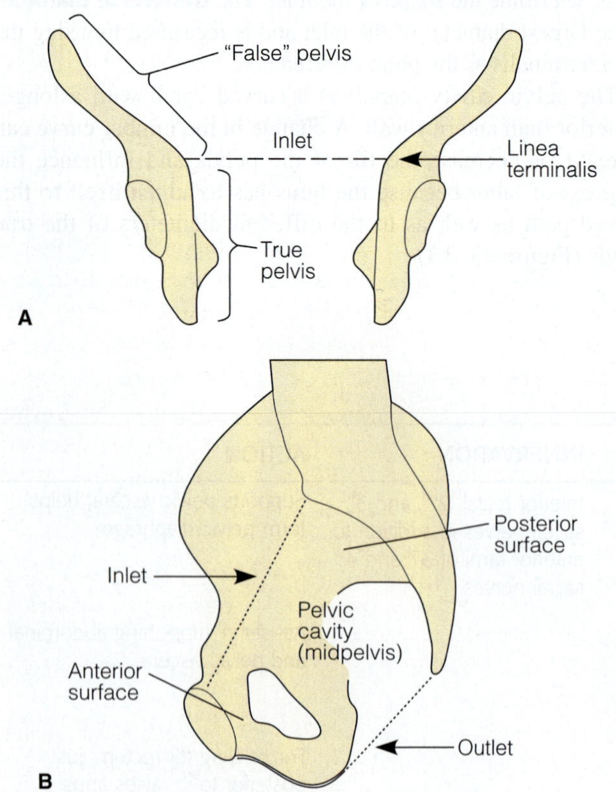

Figure 23–3 ■ Female pelvis. *A,* False pelvis is a shallow cavity above the inlet; true pelvis is the deeper portion of the cavity below the inlet. *B,* True pelvis consists of inlet, cavity (midpelvis), and outlet.

The **pelvic outlet** is at the lower border of the true pelvis. The size of the pelvic outlet can be determined by assessing the transverse diameter. The anteroposterior diameter of the pelvic outlet increases during birth as the presenting part pushes the coccyx posteriorly at the mobile sacrococcygeal joint. Decreased mobility, a large head, and/or a forceful birth can cause the coccyx to break. As the infant's head emerges, the long diameter of the head (occipital frontal) parallels the long diameter of the outlet (anteroposterior).

The transverse diameter (bi-ischial or intertuberous) extends from the inner surface of one ischial tuberosity to the other. It is the shortest diameter of the pelvic outlet and becomes even shorter when the woman has a narrowed pubic arch. The pubic arch is of great importance because the fetus must pass under it during birth. If it is narrow, the baby's head may be pushed backward toward the coccyx, making extension of the head difficult. This situation, known as outlet dystocia, may require the use of forceps or a cesarean birth. The shoulders of a large baby also may become wedged under the pubic arch, making birth more difficult.

PELVIC TYPES The Caldwell–Moloy classification of pelves is widely used to differentiate bony pelvic types (Caldwell & Moloy, 1933). The four basic types are gynecoid, android, anthropoid, and platypelloid (Figure 23–5 ■). However, variations in the female pelvis are so great that classic types are not usual. Each type has a characteristic shape, and each shape has implications for labor and birth.

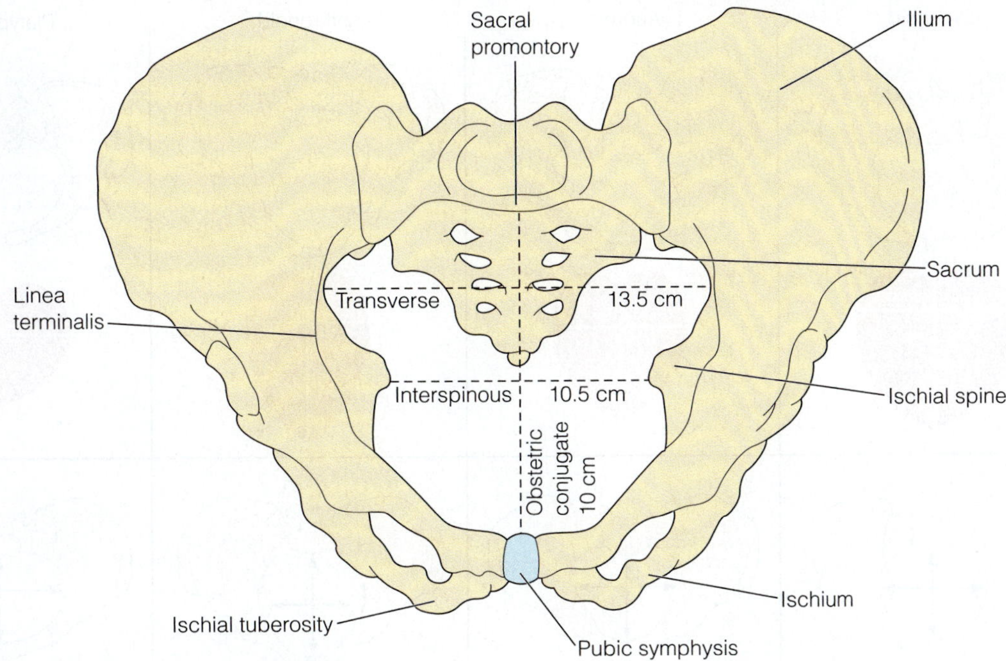

Figure 23–4 ■ Pelvic planes: coronal section and diameters of the bony pelvis.

The Female Reproductive Cycle

The **female reproductive cycle (FRC)** is composed of the ovarian cycle, during which ovulation occurs, and the uterine cycle, during which menstruation occurs. These two cycles take place simultaneously (Figure 23–6 ■).

EFFECTS OF FEMALE HORMONES After menarche, a female undergoes a cyclic pattern of ovulation and menstruation, which is disrupted only by pregnancy, for a period of 30–40 years. This cycle is an orderly process under neurohormonal control. Each month one oocyte matures, ruptures from the ovary, and enters the fallopian tube. The ovary, vagina, uterus, and fallopian tubes are major target organs for female hormones.

The ovaries produce mature gametes and secrete hormones. Ovarian hormones include the estrogens, progesterone, and testosterone. The ovary is sensitive to follicle-stimulating hormone (FSH) and luteinizing hormone (LH). The uterus is sensitive to estrogen and progesterone. The relative proportion of these hormones to each other controls the events of both ovarian and menstrual cycles.

Estrogens Estrogens are hormones associated with characteristics contributing to "femaleness." The major estrogenic effects are due primarily to three classical estrogens: estrone, β-estradiol, and estriol. The major estrogen is β-estradiol.

Estrogens control the development of the female secondary sex characteristics: breast development, growth of body hair, widening of the hips, and deposits of tissue (fat) in the buttocks and mons pubis. Estrogens also assist in the maturation of the ovarian follicles and cause the endometrial mucosa to proliferate following menstruation. The amount of estrogens is greatest during the proliferative (follicular or estrogenic) phase of the menstrual cycle. Estrogens also cause the uterus to increase in size and weight because of increased glycogen, amino acids, electrolytes, and water. Blood supply is expanded as well. Under the influence of estrogens, myometrial contractility increases in both the uterus and fallopian tubes and uterine sensitivity to oxytocin increases. Estrogens inhibit FSH production and stimulate LH production.

Estrogens have effects on many hormones and other carrier proteins. For example, they contribute to the increased amount of protein-bound iodine in pregnant women and in women who use oral contraceptives containing estrogen. Estrogens also may increase libidinal feelings in humans. They decrease the excitability of the hypothalamus, which may cause an increase in sexual desire.

Progesterone Progesterone is secreted by the corpus luteum and is found in greatest amounts during the secretory (luteal or progestational) phase of the menstrual cycle. Progesterone decreases uterine motility and contractility caused by estrogens, thereby preparing the uterus for implantation after the ovum is fertilized. The endometrial mucosa is in a ready state as a result of estrogenic influence. Progesterone causes the uterine endometrium to further increase its supply of glycogen, arterial blood, secretory glands, amino acids, and water.

This hormone is often called the hormone of pregnancy because its effects on the uterus allow pregnancy to be maintained. Under the influence of progesterone, the vaginal epithelium proliferates and the cervix secretes thick, viscous mucus. Breast glandular tissue increases in size and complexity. Progesterone also prepares the breasts for lactation.

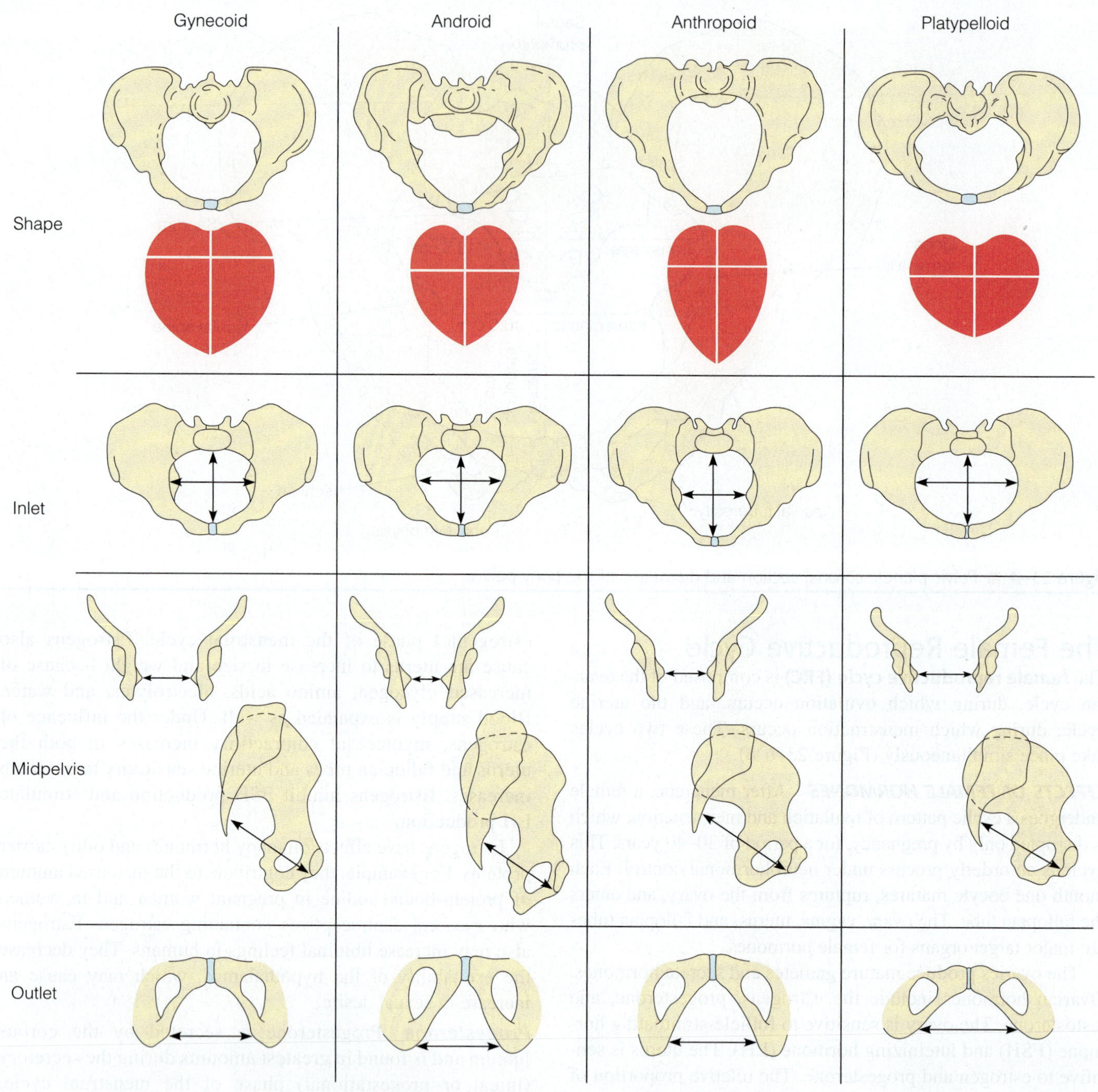

Figure 23–5 ■ Comparison of Caldwell–Moloy pelvic types.

The temperature rise of about 0.3–0.6°C (0.5–1.0°F) that accompanies ovulation and persists throughout the secretory phase of the menstrual cycle is due to progesterone.

Prostaglandins (PGs) Prostaglandins (PGs), oxygenated fatty acids, are produced by the cells of the endometrium. They are classified as hormones. Prostaglandins have varied action in the body. The two primary types of PGs are group E and F. Generally, PGE relaxes smooth muscles and is a potent vasodilator; PGF is a potent vasoconstrictor and increases the contractility of muscles and arteries. Although the primary actions of PGE and PGF seem antagonistic, their basic regulatory functions in cells are achieved through an intricate pattern of reciprocal events.

Prostaglandin production increases during follicular maturation, is dependent on gonadotropins, and seems to be critical to follicular rupture (Cunningham, Leveno, Bloom, Hauth, & Wenstrom, 2005). Extrusion of the ovum, resulting from follicular swelling and increased contractility of the smooth muscle in the theca externa layer of the mature follicle, is thought to be caused in part by $PGF_{2\alpha}$. Significant amounts of PGs are found in and around the follicle at the time of ovulation.

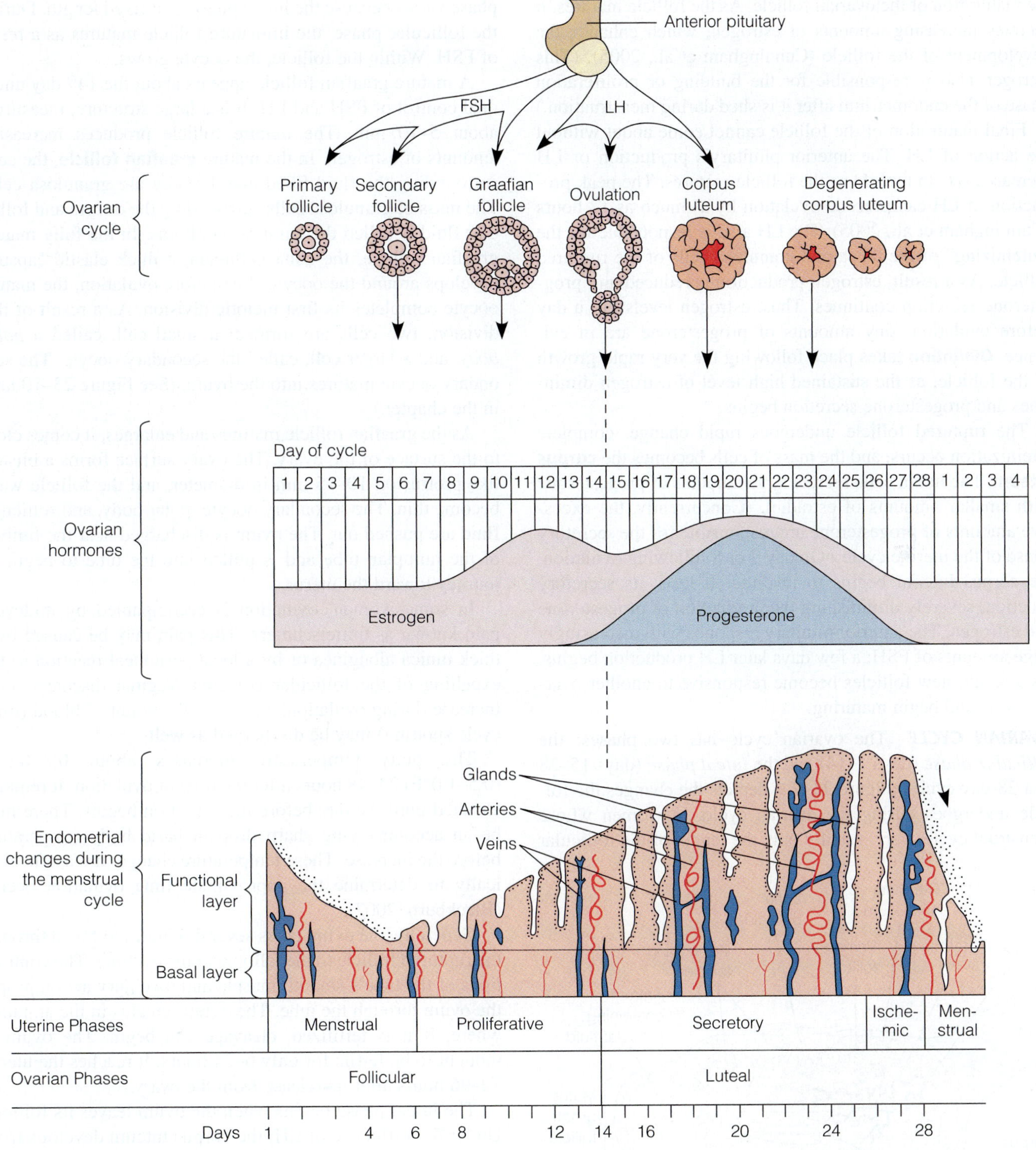

Figure 23–6 ■ Female reproductive cycle: interrelationships of hormones with the four phases of the uterine cycle and the two phases of the ovarian cycle in an ideal 28-day cycle.

NEUROHUMORAL BASIS OF THE FEMALE REPRODUCTIVE CYCLE The FRC is controlled by complex interactions between the nervous and endocrine systems and their target tissues. These interactions involve the hypothalamus, anterior pituitary, and ovaries.

The hypothalamus secretes gonadotropin-releasing hormone (GnRH) to the pituitary gland in response to signals received from the central nervous system (CNS). This releasing hormone is often called luteinizing hormone-releasing hormone (LHRH) and follicle-stimulating hormone-releasing hormone (FSHRH) (Blackburn, 2007).

In response to GnRH, the anterior pituitary secretes the gonadotropic hormones follicle-stimulating hormone (FSH) and luteinizing hormone (LH). FSH is primarily responsible for the maturation of the ovarian follicle. As the follicle matures, it secretes increasing amounts of estrogen, which enhance the development of the follicle (Cunningham et al., 2005). (This estrogen also is responsible for the building or proliferation phase of the endometrium after it is shed during menstruation.)

Final maturation of the follicle cannot come about without the action of LH. The anterior pituitary's production of LH increases six- to tenfold as the follicle matures. The peak production of LH can precede ovulation by as much as 12 hours (Cunningham et al., 2005). The LH also is responsible for the "luteinizing" of the theca and granulosa cells of the ruptured follicle. As a result, estrogen production is reduced and progesterone secretion continues. Thus, estrogen levels fall a day before ovulation; tiny amounts of progesterone are in evidence. **Ovulation** takes place following the very rapid growth of the follicle, as the sustained high level of estrogen diminishes and progesterone secretion begins.

The ruptured follicle undergoes rapid change, complete luteinization occurs, and the mass of cells becomes the **corpus luteum**. The lutein cells secrete large amounts of progesterone with smaller amounts of estradiol. (Concurrently, the excessive amounts of progesterone are responsible for the secretory phase of the uterine cycle.) On day 7 or 8 following ovulation, the corpus luteum begins to involute. It loses its secretory function, severely diminishing the production of progesterone and estrogen. The anterior pituitary responds with increasingly large amounts of FSH; a few days later LH production begins. As a result, new follicles become responsive to another ovarian cycle and begin maturing.

OVARIAN CYCLE The ovarian cycle has two phases: the *follicular phase* (days 1–14) and the *luteal phase* (days 15–28 in a 28-day cycle). Figure 23–7 ■ depicts the changes the follicle undergoes during the ovarian cycle. In women whose menstrual cycles vary, usually only the length of the follicular

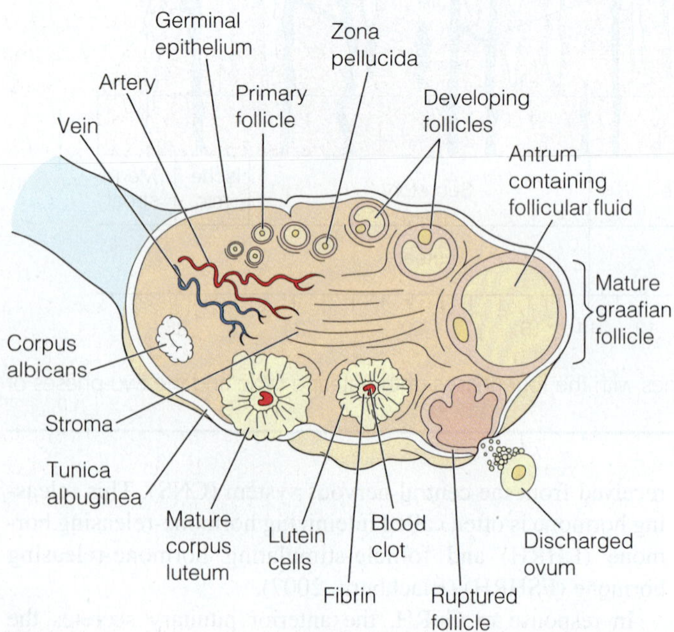

Figure 23–7 ■ Various stages of development of the ovarian follicles.

phase varies because the luteal phase is of fixed length. During the follicular phase, the immature follicle matures as a result of FSH. Within the follicle, the oocyte grows.

A mature graafian follicle appears about the 14th day under dual control of FSH and LH. It is a large structure, measuring about 5–10 mm. The mature follicle produces increasing amounts of estrogen. In the mature **graafian follicle**, the cells surrounding the fluid-filled antral cavity are granulosa cells. The mass of granulosa cells surrounding the oocyte and follicular fluid is called the cumulus oophorus. In the fully mature graafian follicle, the zona pellucida, a thick elastic capsule, develops around the oocyte. Just before ovulation, the mature oocyte completes its first meiotic division. As a result of this division, two cells are formed: a small cell, called a *polar body,* and a larger cell, called the secondary oocyte. The secondary oocyte matures into the ovum. (See Figure 23–10 later in the chapter.)

As the graafian follicle matures and enlarges, it comes close to the surface of the ovary. The ovary surface forms a blister-like protrusion 10–15 mm in diameter, and the follicle walls become thin. The secondary oocyte, polar body, and follicular fluid are pushed out. The ovum is discharged near the fimbria of the fallopian tube and is pulled into the tube to begin its journey toward the uterus.

In some women, ovulation is accompanied by midcycle pain known as mittelschmerz. This pain may be caused by a thick tunica albuginea or by a local peritoneal reaction to the expelling of the follicular contents. Vaginal discharge may increase during ovulation, and a small amount of blood (midcycle spotting) may be discharged as well.

The body temperature increases about 0.3–0.6°C (0.5–1.0°F) 24–48 hours after the time of ovulation. It remains elevated until the day before menstruation begins. There may be an accompanying sharp drop in basal body temperature before the increase. These temperature changes are useful clinically to determine the approximate time ovulation occurs (Blackburn, 2007).

Generally, the ovum takes several minutes to travel through the ruptured follicle to the fallopian tube opening. The contractions of the tube's smooth muscle and its ciliary action propel the ovum through the tube. The ovum remains in the ampulla, where, if it is fertilized, cleavage can begin. The ovum is thought to be fertile for only 6–24 hours. It reaches the uterus 72–96 hours after its release from the ovary.

The luteal phase begins when the ovum leaves its follicle. Under the influence of LH, the corpus luteum develops from the ruptured follicle. Within 2 or 3 days, the corpus luteum becomes yellowish and spherical and increases in vascularity. If the ovum is fertilized and implants in the endometrium, the fertilized egg begins to secrete human chorionic gonadotropin (hCG), which is needed to maintain the corpus luteum. If fertilization does not occur, within about a week after ovulation, the corpus luteum begins to degenerate, eventually becoming a connective tissue scar called the corpus albicans. With degeneration comes a decrease in estrogen and progesterone. This allows for an increase in LH and FSH, which trigger the hypothalamus.

MENSTRUAL CYCLE *Menstruation* is cyclic uterine bleeding in response to cyclic hormonal changes. Menstruation occurs when the ovum is not fertilized and begins about 14 days after ovulation in an ideal 28-day cycle. The menstrual discharge, also referred to as the menses or menstrual flow, is composed of blood mixed with fluid, cervical and vaginal secretions, bacteria, mucus, leukocytes, and other cellular debris. The menstrual discharge is dark red and has a distinctive odor.

Menstrual parameters vary greatly among individuals. Generally, menstruation occurs every 29 days, but varies from 21–35 days. Some women have longer cycles, which can skew standard calculations of the estimated date of birth (EDB). Emotional and physical factors such as illness, excessive fatigue, stress or anxiety, and vigorous exercise programs can alter the cycle interval. Certain environmental factors such as temperature and altitude also may affect the cycle.

The duration of menses is from 2–8 days, with the blood loss averaging 25–60 mL, and the loss of iron averaging 0.5–1 mg daily.

The uterine (menstrual) cycle has four phases: menstrual, proliferative, secretory, and ischemic. Menstruation occurs during the menstrual phase. Some endometrial areas are shed, although others remain. Some of the remaining tips of the endometrial glands begin to regenerate. The endometrium is in a resting state following menstruation. Estrogen levels are low, and the endometrium is 1–2 mm deep. During this part of the cycle, the cervical mucosa is scanty, viscous, and opaque.

The *proliferative phase* begins when the endometrial glands enlarge, becoming twisted and longer in response to increasing amounts of estrogen. The blood vessels become prominent and dilated, and the endometrium increases in thickness six- to eight-fold. This gradual process reaches its peak just before ovulation. The cervical mucosa becomes thin, clear, watery, and more alkaline, making the mucosa more favorable to spermatozoa. As ovulation nears, the cervical mucosa shows increased elasticity, called spinnbarkeit. At ovulation, the mucus will stretch more than 5 cm. The pH of the cervical mucosa increases from below 7.0 to 7.5 at the time of ovulation. On microscopic examination, the mucosa shows a characteristic ferning pattern (Figure 23–8 ■). This fern pattern is useful in assessing ovulation time.

The *secretory phase* follows ovulation. The endometrium, under estrogenic influence, undergoes slight cellular growth. Progesterone, however, causes such marked swelling and growth that the epithelium is warped into folds. The amount of tissue glycogen increases. The glandular epithelial cells begin to fill with cellular debris, become twisted, and dilate. The glands secrete small quantities of endometrial fluid in preparation for a fertilized ovum. The vascularity of the entire uterus increases greatly, providing a nourishing bed for implantation. If implantation occurs, the endometrium, under the influence of progesterone, continues to develop and become even.

If fertilization does not occur, the *ischemic phase* begins. The corpus luteum begins to degenerate, and as a result, both estrogen and progesterone levels fall. Areas of necrosis appear under the epithelial lining. Extensive vascular changes also occur. Small blood vessels rupture, and the spiral arteries constrict and retract, causing a deficiency of blood in the endometrium, which becomes pale. This ischemic phase is characterized by the escape of blood into the stromal cells of the uterus. The menstrual flow begins, thus beginning the menstrual cycle again. After menstruation, the basal layer remains so that the tips of the glands can regenerate the new functional endometrial layer.

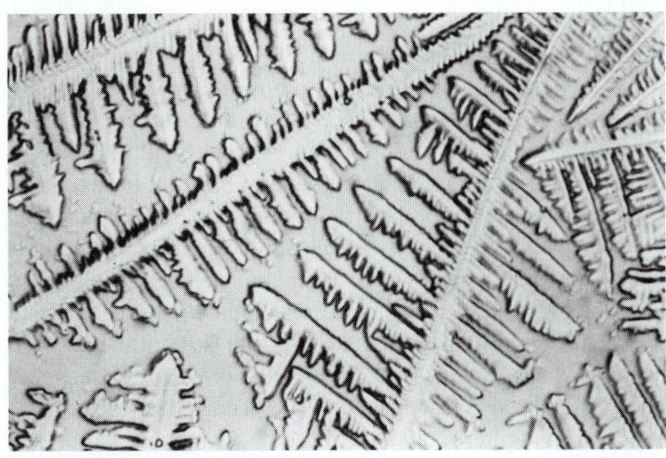

Figure 23–8 ■ Ferning pattern.

Source: Courtesy of Lavena Porter, OB/GYN.

CONCEPTION AND FETAL DEVELOPMENT

Each human begins life as a single cell called a fertilized ovum, or zygote. This single cell reproduces itself, and in turn, each resulting cell reproduces itself in a continuing process. The new cells are similar to the cells from which they came. Cells are reproduced by mitosis or meiosis, two different but related processes.

Mitosis results in the production of diploid body (somatic) cells, which are exact copies of the original cell. Mitosis makes growth and development possible, and in mature individuals, it is the process by which the body cells continue to divide and replace themselves. **Meiosis** is a process of cell division leading to the development of eggs and sperm needed to produce a new organism. Unlike cells produced during mitosis, the cells produced during meiosis contain only half the genetic material or number of chromosomes (the haploid number).

Mitosis

During mitosis, the cell undergoes several changes, ending in cell division. As the last phase of cell division nears completion, a furrow develops in the cell cytoplasm, which divides it into two daughter cells, each with its own nucleus. Daughter cells have the same diploid number of chromosomes (46) and same genetic makeup as the cell from which they came. After a cell with 46 chromosomes goes through mitosis, the result is two identical cells, each with 46 chromosomes.

Meiosis

Meiosis is a special type of cell division by which diploid cells in the testes and ovaries give rise to gametes (sperm and ova) with the haploid number of chromosomes, which is 23.

Meiosis consists of two successive cell divisions. In the first division, the chromosomes replicate. Next, a pairing takes place between homologous chromosomes (Sadler, 2006). Instead of separating immediately, as in mitosis, the chromosomes become closely intertwined. At each point of contact, there is a physical exchange of genetic material between the chromatids (the arms of the chromosomes). New combinations are provided by the newly formed chromosomes; these combinations account for the wide variation of traits in people (e.g., hair and eye color). The chromosome pairs then separate, and the members of the pair move to opposite sides of the cell. (In contrast, during mitosis, the chromatids of each chromosome separate and move to opposite poles.) The cell divides, forming two daughter cells, each with 23 double-structured chromosomes—the same amount of deoxyribonucleic acid (DNA) as a normal somatic cell. In the second division, the chromatids of each chromosome separate and move to opposite poles of each of the daughter cells. Cell division occurs, resulting in the formation of four cells, each containing 23 single chromosomes (the haploid number of chromosomes). These daughter cells contain only half the DNA of a normal somatic cell (Sadler, 2006).

Mutations may occur during the second meiotic division if two of the chromatids do not move apart rapidly enough when the cell divides. The still-paired chromatids are carried into one of the daughter cells and eventually form an extra chromosome. This condition, autosomal nondisjunction (chromosomal mutation), is harmful to the offspring that may result should fertilization occur. Another type of chromosomal mutation can occur if chromosomes break during meiosis. If the broken segment is lost, the result is a shorter chromosome—a situation known as deletion. If the broken segment becomes attached to another chromosome, a harmful mutation called a translocation results.

Meiosis occurs during **gametogenesis**, the process by which germ cells, or gametes *(ovum and sperm)*, are produced. These cells contain only half the genetic material of a typical body cell. The gametes must have a haploid number (23) of chromosomes so that when the female gamete (egg or ovum) and the male gamete (sperm or spermatozoon) unite to form the **zygote** (fertilized ovum), the normal human diploid number of chromosomes (46) is reestablished.

Oogenesis

Oogenesis is the process that produces the female gamete, called an ovum (egg). The ovaries begin to develop early in the fetal life of the female. All of the ova that the female will produce in her lifetime are present at birth. The ovary gives rise to oogonial cells, which develop into oocytes. Meiosis begins in all oocytes before the female fetus is born, but stops before the first division is complete and remains in this arrested phase until puberty. During puberty, the mature primary oocyte proceeds (by oogenesis) through the first meiotic division in the graafian follicle of the ovary.

The first meiotic division produces two cells of unequal size with different amounts of cytoplasm but with the same number of chromosomes. These two cells are the secondary oocyte and a minute polar body. Both the secondary oocyte and the polar body contain 22 double-structured autosomal chromosomes and one double-structured sex chromosome (X).

At ovulation, a second meiotic division begins immediately and proceeds as the oocyte moves down the fallopian tube. Division is again not equal, and the secondary oocyte moves into the metaphase stage of cell division, where its meiotic division is arrested until and unless the oocyte is fertilized.

When the secondary oocyte completes the second meiotic division after fertilization, the result is a mature ovum with the haploid number of chromosomes and virtually all of the cytoplasm. In addition, the second polar body (also haploid) forms at this time. The first polar body now has also divided, producing two additional polar bodies. Thus, at the completion of meiosis, four haploid cells have been produced: the three polar bodies, which eventually disintegrate, and one ovum (Sadler, 2006) (Figure 23–9 ■).

Spermatogenesis

During puberty, the germinal epithelium in the seminiferous tubules of the testes begins the process of **spermatogenesis**, which produces the male gamete (sperm). The diploid spermatogonium replicates before it enters the first meiotic division, during which it is called the primary spermatocyte. During this first meiotic division, the spermatogonium replicates and forms two cells called secondary spermatocytes, each of which contains 22 double-structured autosomal chromosomes and either a double-structured X sex chromosome or a double-structured Y sex chromosome. During the second meiotic division, they divide to form four spermatids, each with the haploid number of chromosomes. The spermatids undergo a series of changes during which they lose most of their cytoplasm and become sperm (spermatozoa) (Figure 23–9). The nucleus becomes compacted into the head of the sperm, which is covered by a cap called an acrosome that is, in turn, covered by a plasma membrane. A long tail is produced from one of the centrioles.

Fertilization

Fertilization is the process by which a sperm fuses with an ovum to form a new diploid cell, or zygote. The zygote begins life as a single cell with a complete set of genetic material, 23 chromosomes from the mother's ovum and 23 chromosomes from the father's sperm for a total of 46 chromosomes. The following events lead to fertilization.

PREPARATION FOR FERTILIZATION The mature ovum and spermatozoa have only a brief time to unite. Ova are considered fertile for about 12–24 hours after ovulation. Sperm can survive in the female reproductive tract for 48–72 hours, but are believed to be healthy and highly fertile for only about 24 hours.

The ovum's cell membrane is surrounded by two layers of tissue. The layer closest to the cell membrane is called the zona pellucida. It is a clear, noncellular layer whose thickness influences the fertilization rate. Surrounding the zona pellucida is a ring of elongated cells, called the corona radiata because they radiate from the ovum like the gaseous corona around the sun. These cells are held together by hyaluronic

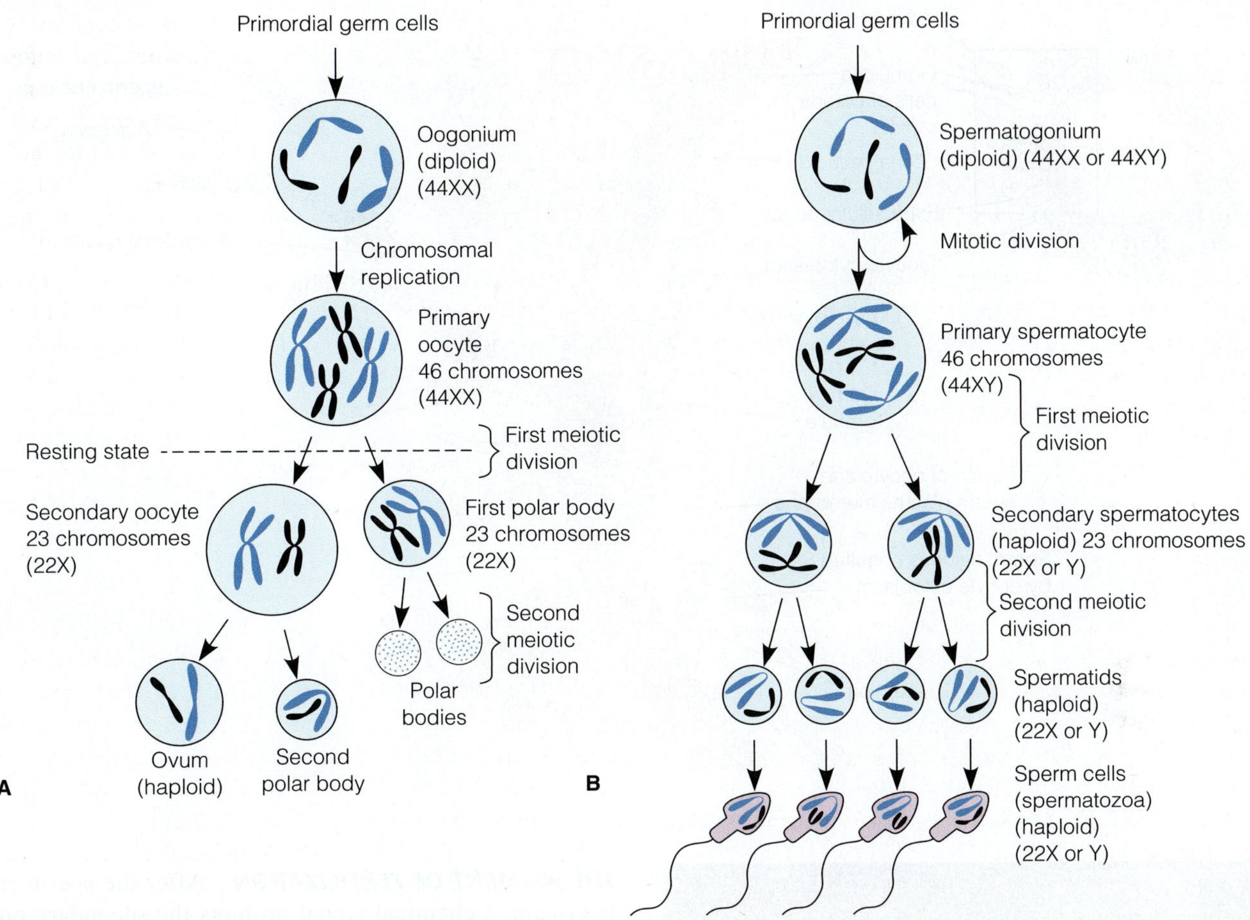

Figure 23–9 ■ Gametogenesis involves meiosis within the ovary and testis. *A,* During meiosis, each oogonium produces a single haploid ovum once some cytoplasm moves into the polar bodies. *B,* Each spermatogonium produces four haploid spermatozoa.

acid. The ovum has no inherent power of movement. During ovulation, high estrogen levels increase peristalsis in the fallopian tubes, which helps move the ovum through the tube toward the uterus. The high estrogen levels also cause a thinning of the cervical mucus, facilitating movement of the sperm through the cervix, into the uterus, and up the fallopian tube.

The process of fertilization takes place in the ampulla (outer third) of the fallopian tube. In a single ejaculation, the male deposits approximately 200–300 million spermatozoa into the vagina, of which only hundreds of sperm actually reach the ampulla (Sadler, 2006). Fructose in the semen, secreted by the seminal vesicles, is the energy source for the sperm. The spermatozoa propel themselves up the female tract by the flagellar movement of their tails. Transit time from the cervix into the fallopian tube can be as short as 5 minutes but usually takes an average of 2–7 hours after ejaculation (Sadler, 2006). Prostaglandins in the semen may increase uterine smooth muscle contractions, which help transport the sperm. The fallopian tubes have a dual ciliary action that facilitates movement of the ovum toward the uterus and movement of the sperm from the uterus toward the ovary.

The sperm must undergo two processes before fertilization can occur: capacitation and the acrosomal reaction. **Capacitation** is the removal of the plasma membrane overlying the spermatozoa's acrosomal area and the loss of seminal plasma proteins. If the glycoprotein coat is not removed, the sperm will not be able to fertilize the ovum (Sadler, 2006). Capacitation occurs in the female reproductive tract (aided by uterine enzymes) and is thought to take about 7 hours. Sperm that undergo capacitation take on three characteristics: (1) the ability to undergo the acrosomal reaction, (2) the ability to bind to the zona pellucida, and (3) the acquisition of hypermotility.

The **acrosomal reaction** follows capacitation, whereby the acrosomes of the sperm surrounding the ovum release their enzymes (hyaluronidase, a protease called acrosin, and trypsinlike substances) and thus break down the hyaluronic acid in the ovum's corona radiata (Sadler, 2006). Hundreds of acrosomes must rupture before enough hyaluronic acid is cleared for a single sperm to penetrate the ovum's zona pellucida successfully.

At the moment of penetration by a fertilizing sperm, the zona pellucida undergoes a reaction that prevents additional sperm from entering a single ovum. This is known as the block to polyspermy. This cellular change is mediated by release of materials from the cortical granules, organelles found just below the ovum's surface, and is called the cortical reaction (Figure 23–10 ■).

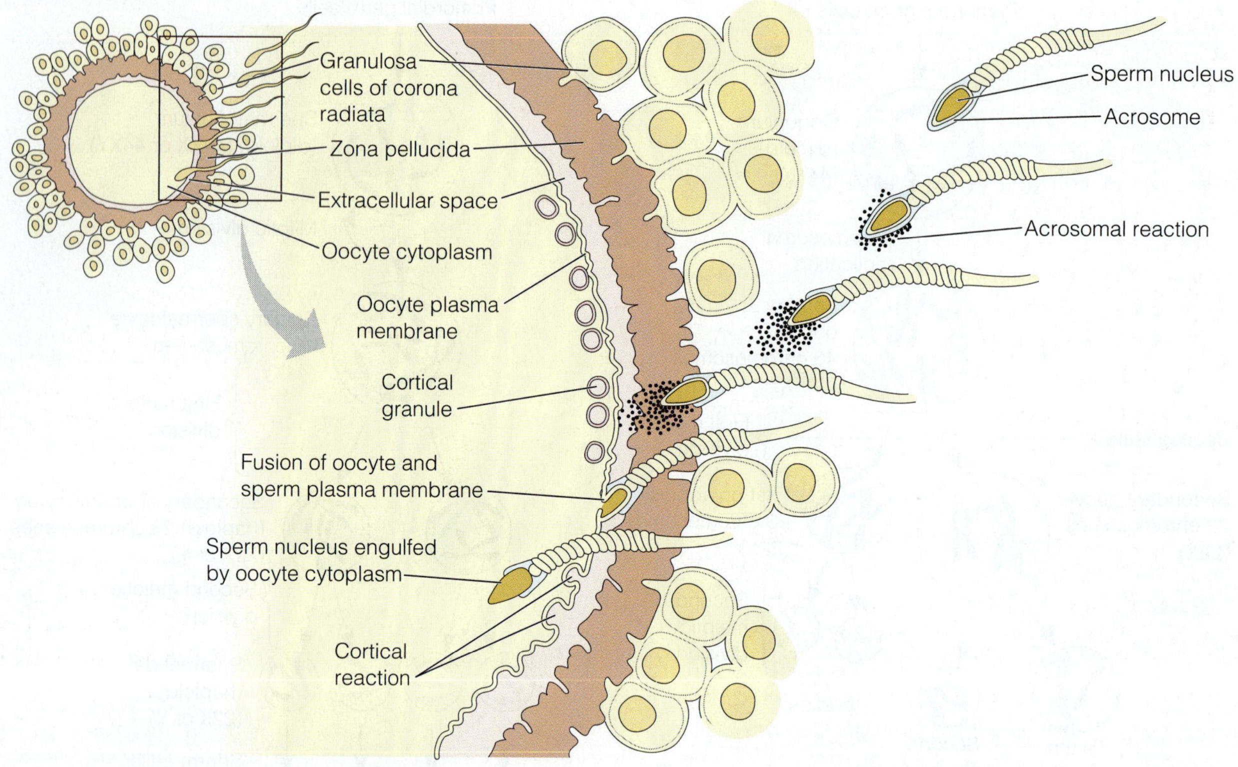

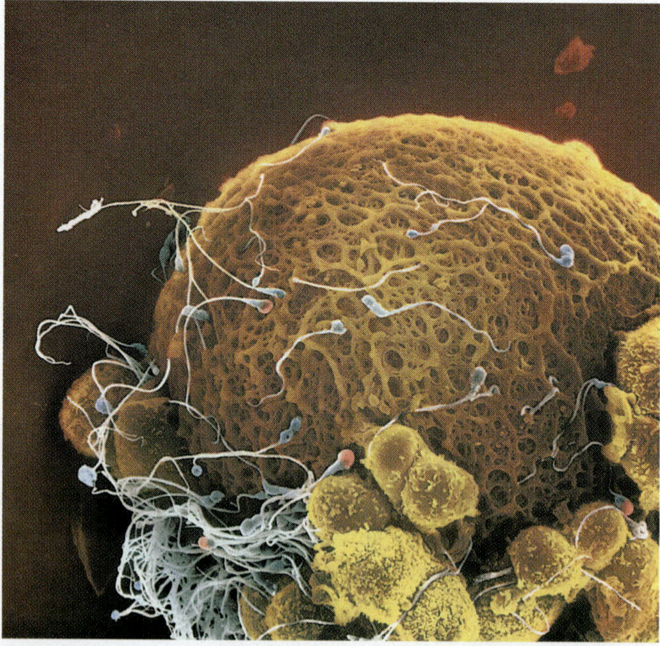

Figure 23–10 ■ Sperm penetration of an ovum. *A*, The sequential steps of oocyte penetration by a sperm are depicted moving from top to bottom. *B*, Scanning electron micrograph of a human sperm surrounding a human ovum (750X). The smaller spherical cells are granulosa cells of the corona radiata.

Source: (B) Scanning electron micrograph from Nilsson, L. (1990). *A child is born.* New York: Dell Publishing.

THE MOMENT OF FERTILIZATION After the sperm enters the ovum, a chemical signal prompts the secondary oocyte to complete the second meiotic division, forming the nucleus of the ovum and ejecting the second polar body. Then the nuclei of the ovum and sperm swell and approach each other. The true moment of fertilization occurs as the nuclei unite. Their individual nuclear membranes disappear, and their chromosomes pair up to produce the diploid zygote. Because each nucleus contains a haploid number of chromosomes (23), this union restores the diploid number (46). The zygote contains a new combination of genetic material that results in an individual different from either parent and from anyone else.

The moment of fertilization is when the sex of the zygote is determined. The two chromosomes (the sex chromosomes) of the 23rd pair—either XX or XY—determine the sex of an individual. The X chromosome is larger and bears more genes than the Y chromosome. Females have two X chromosomes, and males have an X and a Y chromosome. Whereas the mature ovum produced by oogenesis can have only one type of sex chromosome—an X—spermatogenesis produces two sperm with an X chromosome and two sperm with a Y chromosome. When each gamete contributes an X chromosome, the resulting zygote is female. When the ovum contributes an X and the sperm contributes a Y chromosome, the resulting zygote is male. Certain traits are termed *sex-linked* because they are controlled by the genes on the X sex chromosome. Two examples of sex-linked traits are color blindness and hemophilia.

Preembryonic Development

The first 14 days of development, starting the day the ovum is fertilized (conception), are called the preembryonic stage, or the stage of the ovum. Development after fertilization can be divided into two phases: cellular multiplication and cellular differentiation. These phases are characterized by rapid cellular multiplication and differentiation and establishment of the primary germ layers and embryonic membranes. Synchronized development of both the endometrium and embryo is a prerequisite for implantation to succeed (Moore & Persaud, 2008). These phases and the process of implantation (nidation), which occurs between them, are discussed next.

CELLULAR MULTIPLICATION Cellular multiplication begins as the zygote moves through the fallopian tube toward the cavity of the uterus. This transport takes 3 days or more and is accomplished mainly by a weak fluid current in the fallopian tube resulting from the beating action of the ciliated epithelium that lines the tube.

The zygote now enters a period of rapid mitotic divisions called cleavage, during which it divides into two cells, four cells, eight cells, etc. These cells, called blastomeres, are so small that the developing cell mass is only slightly larger than the original zygote. The blastomeres are held together by the zona pellucida, which is under the corona radiata. The blastomeres eventually form a solid ball of 12–16 cells called the **morula**.

As the morula enters the uterus, two things happen: The intracellular fluid in the morula increases, and a central cavity forms within the cell mass. Inside this cavity is an inner solid mass of cells called the **blastocyst**. The outer layer of cells that surrounds the cavity and replaces the zona pellucida is the **trophoblast**. Eventually, the trophoblast develops into one of the two embryonic membranes, the chorion. The blastocyst develops into a double layer of cells called the embryonic disc, from which the embryo and the amnion (embryonic membrane) develop. The journey of the fertilized ovum to its destination in the uterus is illustrated in Figure 23–11 ■.

Early pregnancy factor (EPF), an immunosuppressant protein, is secreted by the trophoblastic cells. This factor appears in the maternal serum within 24–48 hours after fertilization and forms the basis of a pregnancy test during the first 10 days of development (Moore & Persaud, 2008).

IMPLANTATION (NIDATION) While floating in the uterine cavity, the blastocyst is nourished by the uterine glands, which secrete a mixture of lipids, mucopolysaccharides, and glycogen. The trophoblast attaches to the surface of the endometrium for further nourishment. The most frequent site of attachment is the upper part of the posterior uterine wall. Between 7 and 10 days after fertilization, the zona pellucida disappears and the blastocyst implants itself by burrowing into the uterine lining and penetrating down toward the maternal capillaries until it is

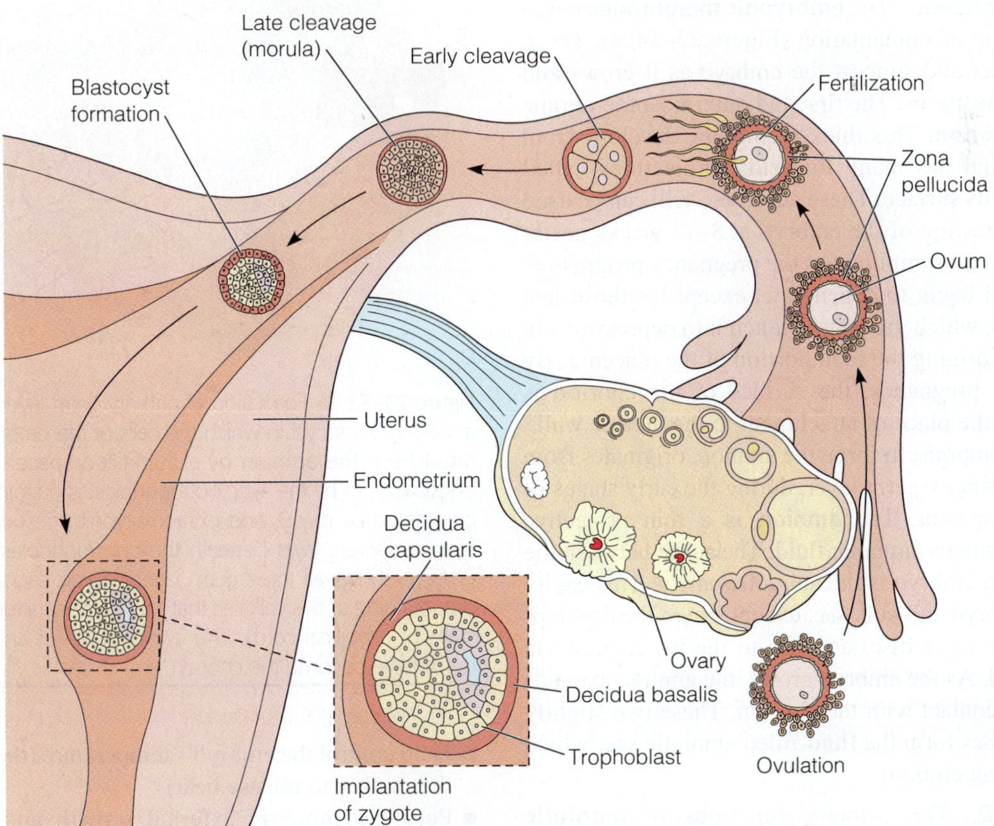

Figure 23–11 ■ During ovulation, the ovum leaves the ovary and enters the fallopian tube. Fertilization generally occurs in the outer third of the fallopian tube. The figure depicts subsequent changes in the fertilized ovum from conception to implantation.

completely covered (Moore & Persaud, 2008). The lining of the uterus thickens below the implanted blastocyst, and the cells of the trophoblast grow down into the thickened lining, forming processes that will be called chorionic villi.

Under the influence of progesterone, the endometrium increases in thickness and vascularity in preparation for implantation and nutrition of the ovum. After implantation, the endometrium is called the decidua. The portion of the decidua that covers the blastocyst is called the decidua capsularis, the portion directly under the implanted blastocyst is the decidua basalis, and the portion that lines the rest of the uterine cavity is the decidua vera (parietalis). The maternal part of the placenta develops from the decidua basalis, which contains large numbers of blood vessels (magnified inset in Figure 23–11) (Moore & Persaud, 2008). The chorionic villi (discussed shortly) in contact with the decidua basalis will form the fetal portion of the placenta.

CELLULAR DIFFERENTIATION

Primary Germ Layers About the 10th–14th day after conception, the homogeneous mass of blastocyst cells differentiates into the primary germ layers (Figure 23–12 ■). These three layers—the ectoderm, mesoderm, and endoderm—are formed at the same time as the embryonic membranes. All tissues, organs, and organ systems will develop from these primary germ cell layers (Table 23–2). For example, differentiation of the endoderm results in the formation of epithelium lining the respiratory and digestive tracts (Figure 23–13 ■).

Embryonic Membranes The **embryonic membranes** begin to form at the time of implantation (Figure 23–14 ■). These membranes protect and support the embryo as it grows and develops inside the uterus. The first and outermost membrane to form is the **chorion**. This thick membrane develops from the trophoblast and has many fingerlike projections called chorionic villi on its surface. These chorionic villi can be used for early genetic testing of the embryo at 8–11 weeks gestation by chorionic villi sampling. As the pregnancy progresses, the chorionic villi begin to degenerate, except for those just under the embryo, which grow and branch into depressions in the uterine wall, forming the fetal portion of the placenta. By the 4th month of pregnancy, the surface of the chorion is smooth except at the place of attachment to the uterine wall.

The second membrane to form, the amnion, originates from the ectoderm, a primary germ layer, during the early stages of embryonic development. The **amnion** is a thin protective membrane that contains amniotic fluid. The space between the membrane and the embryo is the amniotic cavity. This cavity surrounds the embryo and yolk sac, except where the developing embryo (germ-layer disc) attaches to the trophoblast via the umbilical cord. As the embryo grows, the amnion expands until it comes in contact with the chorion. These two slightly adherent membranes form the fluid-filled amniotic sac, which protects the floating embryo.

AMNIOTIC FLUID The primary functions of **amniotic fluid** are to:

- Act as a cushion to protect the embryo against mechanical injury

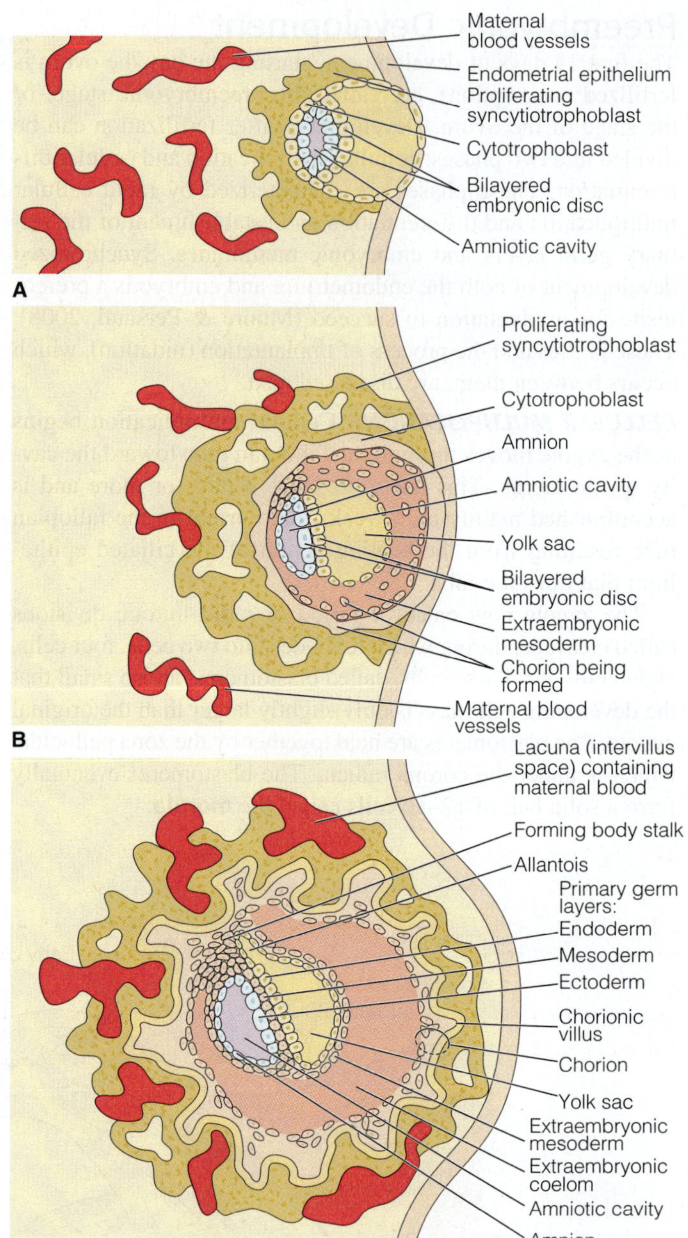

Figure 23–12 ■ Formation of primary germ layers. *A*, Implantation of a 7½-day blastocyst in which the cells of the embryonic disc are separated from the amnion by a fluid-filled space. The erosion of the endometrium by the syncytiotrophoblast is ongoing. *B*, Implantation is completed by day 9, and extraembryonic mesoderm is beginning to form a discrete layer beneath the cytotrophoblast. *C*, By day 16, the embryo shows all three germ layers, a yolk sac, and an allantois (an outpouching of the yolk sac that forms the structural basis of the body stalk, or umbilical cord). The cytotrophoblast and associated mesoderm have become the chorion, and chorionic villi are developing.

- Help control the embryo's temperature (the embryo relies on the mother to release heat)
- Permit symmetric external growth and development of the embryo
- Prevent adherence of the embryo–fetus to the amnion (decreases chance of amniotic band syndrome) to allow

TABLE 23–2 Derivation of Body Structures from Primary Cell Layers

ECTODERM	MESODERM	ENDODERM
Epidermis	Dermis	Respiratory tract epithelium
Sweat glands	Wall of digestive tract	Epithelium (except nasal), including pharynx, tongue, tonsils, thyroid, parathyroid, thymus, tympanic cavity
Sebaceous glands	Kidneys and ureter (suprarenal cortex)	
Nails	Reproductive organs (gonads, genital ducts)	Lining of digestive tract
Hair follicles	Connective tissue (cartilage, bone, joint cavities)	Primary tissue of liver and pancreas
Lens of eye	Skeleton	Urethra and associated glands
Sensory epithelium of internal and external ear, nasal cavity, sinuses, mouth, anal canal	Muscles (all types)	Urinary bladder (except trigone)
	Cardiovascular system (heart, arteries, veins, blood, bone marrow)	Vagina (parts)
Central and peripheral nervous systems	Pleura	
Nasal cavity	Lymphatic tissue and cells	
Oral glands and tooth enamel	Spleen	
Pituitary gland		
Mammary glands		

freedom of movement so that the embryo–fetus can change position (flexion and extension), thus aiding in musculoskeletal development

- Allow the umbilical cord to be relatively free of compression
- Act as an extension of fetal extracellular space (hydropic infants have increased amniotic fluid)
- Act as a wedge during labor
- Provide fluid for analysis to determine fetal health and maturity.

Amniotic fluid is slightly alkaline and contains albumin, uric acid, creatinine, lecithin, sphingomyelin, bilirubin, vernix, leukocytes, epithelial cells, enzymes, and fine hair called lanugo. The amount of amniotic fluid at 10 weeks is about 30 mL, and it increases to 350 mL at 20 weeks. After 20 weeks, the volume ranges from 700–1000 mL. The amniotic fluid volume is constantly changing as the fluid moves back and forth across the placental membrane. Water and solutes must pass between the amniotic fluid and fetus. As the pregnancy continues, the fetus

Figure 23–13 ■ Endoderm differentiates to form the epithelial lining of the digestive and respiratory tracts and associated glands.

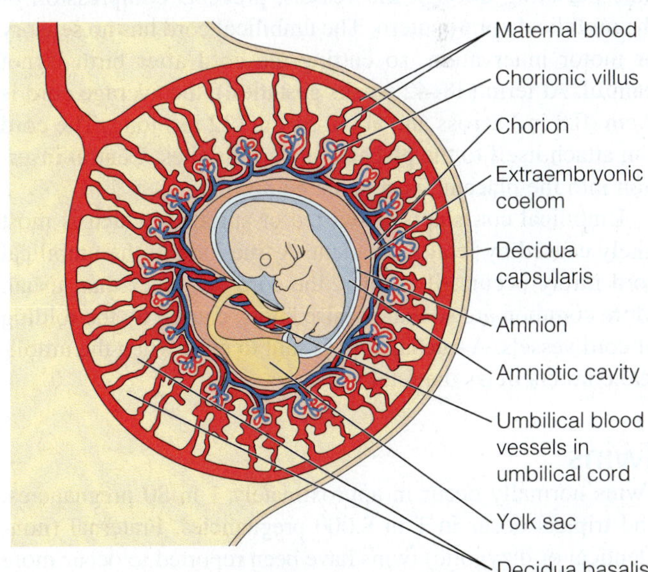

Figure 23–14 ■ Early development of primary embryonic membranes. At 4½ weeks, the decidua capsularis (placental portion enclosing the embryo on the uterine surface) and decidua basalis (placental portion encompassing the elaborate chorionic villi and maternal endometrium) are well formed. The chorionic villi lie in blood-filled intervillous spaces within the endometrium. The amnion and yolk sac are well developed.

contributes to the volume of amniotic fluid by excreting urine. The fetus also swallows up to 262 mL/kg/day. About 400 mL of lung fluid flows out of the fetal lungs each day (Gilbert, 2007). Abnormal variations in amniotic fluid volume are oligohydramnios (less than 400 mL of amniotic fluid) and hydramnios (more than 2000 mL of amniotic fluid or an amniotic fluid index greater than the 97.5 percentile for the corresponding gestational age). Hydramnios is also called polyhydramnios.

YOLK SAC In humans, the yolk sac is small and functions early in embryonic life. It develops as a second cavity in the blastocyst on about day 8 or 9 after conception. It forms primitive red blood cells (RBCs) during the first 6 weeks of development, until the embryo's liver takes over the process. As the embryo develops, the yolk sac is incorporated into the umbilical cord, where it can be seen as a degenerated structure after birth.

UMBILICAL CORD As the placenta develops, the **umbilical cord** is being formed from the amnion. The body stalk, which attaches the embryo to the yolk sac, contains blood vessels that extend into the chorionic villi. The body stalk fuses with the embryonic portion of the placenta to provide a circulatory pathway from the chorionic villi to the embryo. As the body stalk elongates to become the umbilical cord, the vessels in the cord decrease to one large vein and two smaller arteries. About 1% of umbilical cords have only two vessels: an artery and a vein; this condition may be associated with congenital malformations primarily of the renal, gastrointestinal, and cardiovascular systems. A specialized connective tissue known as **Wharton's jelly** surrounds the blood vessels in the umbilical cord. This tissue, in addition to the high blood volume pulsating through the vessels, prevents compression of the umbilical cord in utero. The umbilical cord has no sensory or motor innervation, so cutting the cord after birth is not painful. At term (38–42 weeks gestation), the average cord is 2 cm (0.8 in.) across and about 55 cm (22 in.) long. The cord can attach itself to the placenta at various sites. Central insertion into the placenta is considered normal.

Umbilical cords appear twisted or spiraled, which is most likely caused by fetal movement. A true knot in the umbilical cord rarely occurs; if it does, the cord is longer than usual. More common are so-called false knots, caused by the folding of cord vessels. A nuchal cord is said to exist when the umbilical cord encircles the fetal neck.

Twins

Twins normally occur in approximately 1 in 80 pregnancies, and triplets occur in 1 in 8,000 pregnancies. Fraternal (nonidentical or dizygotic) twins have been reported to occur more often among black than white women and more often among white women than women of Asian origin (Moore & Persaud, 2008). Among all groups, as parity (having given birth to a viable infant) increases, so does the chance for multiple births.

Twins may be fraternal or identical (Figure 23–15 ■). If twins are fraternal, they are dizygotic, which means that they arise from two separate ova fertilized by two separate spermatozoa. There are two placentas, two chorions, and two amnions; however, the placentas sometimes fuse and look as if they are one. Despite their birth relationship, fraternal twins are no more similar to each other than they would be to siblings born singly. They may be of the same or different sex.

Dizygotic twinning increases with maternal age up to about age 35 and then decreases abruptly. The chance of dizygotic twins increases with parity, in conceptions that occur in the first 3 months of marriage, and also with coital frequency. The chance of dizygotic twinning decreases during periods of malnutrition and during winter and spring for women living in the Northern Hemisphere. Studies indicate that dizygotic twins occur in certain families, perhaps because of genotype (genetic constitution) of the mother that results in elevated serum gonadotropin levels leading to double ovulation (Moore & Persaud, 2008). The incidence of dizygotic twinning varies greatly from approximately 1 in 500 in Asians, 1 in 125 in whites, and as high as 1 in 20 in some African populations, whereas the incidence of monozygotic twins is approximately the same in all populations (Moore & Persaud, 2008).

Identical, or monozygotic, twins develop from a single fertilized ovum. They are of the same sex and have the same phenotype (appearance). Identical twins usually have a common placenta. Monozygosity is not affected by environment, race, physical characteristics, or fertility.

Monozygotic twins originate from division of the fertilized ovum at different stages of early development, after the zygote consists of thousands of cells. Complete separation of the cellular mass into two parts is necessary for twin formation. The number of amnions and chorions present depends on the timing of the division.

- If division occurs within 3 days of fertilization (before the inner cell mass and chorion are formed), two embryos, two amnions, and two chorions will develop. This dichorionic–diamniotic situation occurs about 20–30% of the time, and there may be two distinct placentas or a single fused placenta.
- If division occurs about 5 days after fertilization (when the inner cell mass is formed and the chorion cells have differentiated but those of the amnion have not), two embryos develop with separate amnion sacs. These sacs will eventually be covered by a common chorion; thus, there will be a monochorionic–diamniotic placenta (Figure 23–15B).
- If the amnion has already developed, approximately 7–13 days after fertilization, division results in two embryos with a common amnion sac and a common chorion (a monochorionic–monoamniotic placenta). This type rarely occurs.

Monozygotic twinning is considered a random event and occurs in approximately 3–4 per 1,000 live births (Sadler, 2006). The survival rate of monozygotic twins is lower than that of dizygotic twins, and congenital anomalies are more prevalent. Both twins may have the same malformation.

Development and Functions of the Placenta

The **placenta** is the means of metabolic and nutrient exchange between the embryonic and maternal circulations. Placental development and circulation do not begin until the 3rd week of

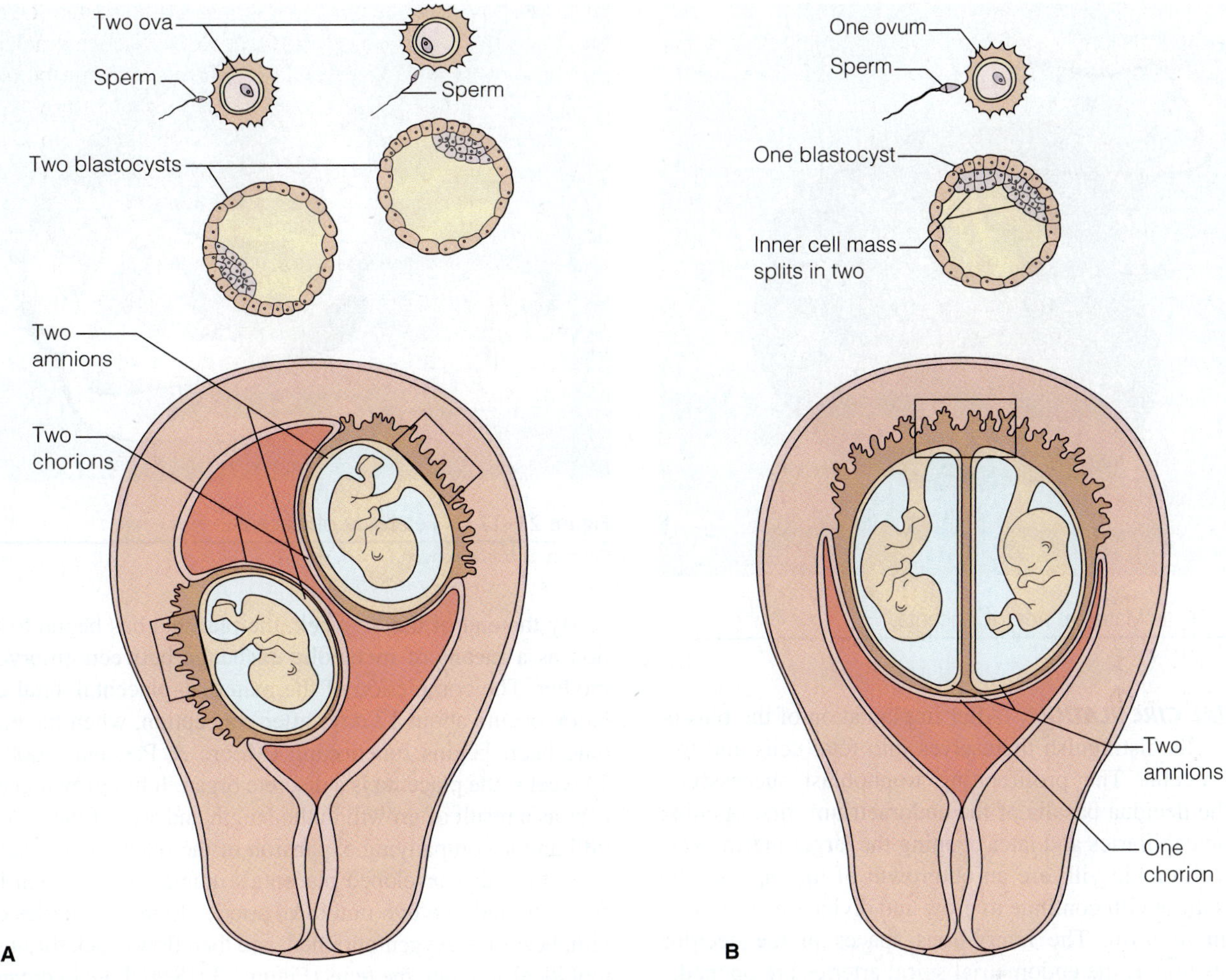

Figure 23–15 ■ *A*, Formation of fraternal twins. (Note separate placentas.) *B*, Formation of identical twins.

embryonic development. The placenta develops at the site where the embryo attaches to the uterine wall. Expansion of the placenta continues until about 20 weeks, when it covers approximately one half of the internal surface of the uterus. After 20 weeks gestation, the placenta becomes thicker but not wider. At 40 weeks gestation, the placenta is about 15–20 cm (5.9–7.9 in.) in diameter and 2.5–3.0 cm (1.0–1.2 in.) in thickness. At that time, it weighs about 400–600 g (14–21 oz).

The placenta has two parts: the maternal and fetal portions. The maternal portion consists of the decidua basalis and its circulation. Its surface is red and fleshlike. The fetal portion consists of the chorionic villi and their circulation. The fetal surface of the placenta is covered by the amnion, which gives it a shiny gray appearance (Figures 23–16 ■ and 23–17 ■).

Development of the placenta begins with the chorionic villi. The trophoblastic cells of the chorionic villi form spaces in the tissue of the decidua basalis. These spaces fill with maternal blood, and the chorionic villi grow into them. As the chorionic villi differentiate, two trophoblastic layers appear: an outer layer, called the syncytium (consisting of syncytiotrophoblasts), and an inner layer, known as the cytotrophoblast (Figure 23–12). The cytotrophoblast thins out and disappears about the 5th month, leaving only a single layer of syncytium covering the chorionic villi. The syncytium is in direct contact with the maternal blood in the intervillous spaces. It is the functional layer of the placenta, and it secretes the placental hormones of pregnancy.

A third inner layer of connective mesoderm develops in the chorionic villi, forming anchoring villi. These anchoring villi eventually form the septa (partitions) of the placenta. The septa divide the mature placenta into 15–20 segments called **cotyledons** (subdivisions of the placenta made up of anchoring villi and decidual tissue). In each cotyledon, the branching villi form a highly complex vascular system that allows compartmentalization of the uteroplacental circulation. The exchange of gases and nutrients takes place across these vascular systems.

Exchange of substances across the placenta is minimal during the first 3–5 months of development because the villous membrane is initially too thick, which limits its permeability. As the villous membrane thins, placental permeability increases until about the last month of pregnancy, when permeability begins to decrease as the placenta ages. In the fully developed placenta, fetal blood in the villi and maternal blood in the intervillous spaces are separated by three or four thin layers of tissue.

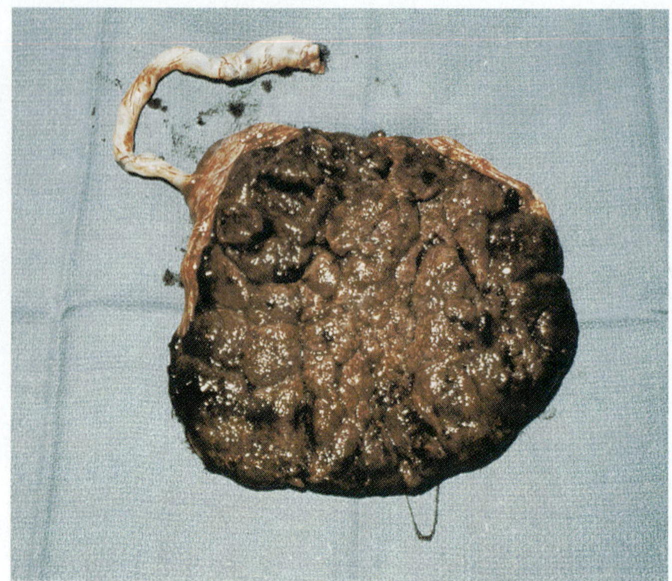

Figure 23–16 ■ Maternal side of placenta.

Courtesy of Marcia London.

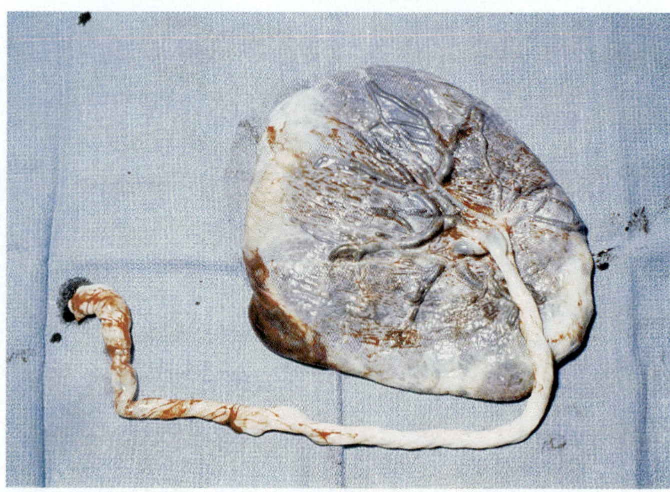

Figure 23–17 ■ Fetal side of placenta.

Courtesy of Marcia London.

PLACENTAL CIRCULATION After implantation of the blastocyst, the cells distinguish themselves into fetal cells and trophoblastic cells. The proliferating trophoblast successfully invades the decidua basalis of the endometrium, first opening the uterine capillaries and later opening the larger uterine vessels. The chorionic villi are an outgrowth of the blastocystic tissue. As these villi continue to grow and divide, the fetal vessels begin to form. The intervillous spaces in the decidua basalis develop as the endometrial spiral arteries are opened.

By the end of the 4th week, the placenta has begun to function as a means of metabolic exchange between embryo and mother. The completion of the maternal–placental–fetal circulation occurs about 17 days after conception, when the embryonic heart begins functioning (Moore & Persaud, 2008). By 14 weeks, the placenta is a discrete organ. It has grown in thickness as a result of growth in the length and size of the chorionic villi and accompanying expansion of the intervillous space.

In the fully developed placenta's umbilical cord, fetal blood flows through the two umbilical arteries to the capillaries of the villi, becomes oxygen-enriched, and then flows back through the umbilical vein into the fetus (Figure 23–18 ■). Late in pregnancy

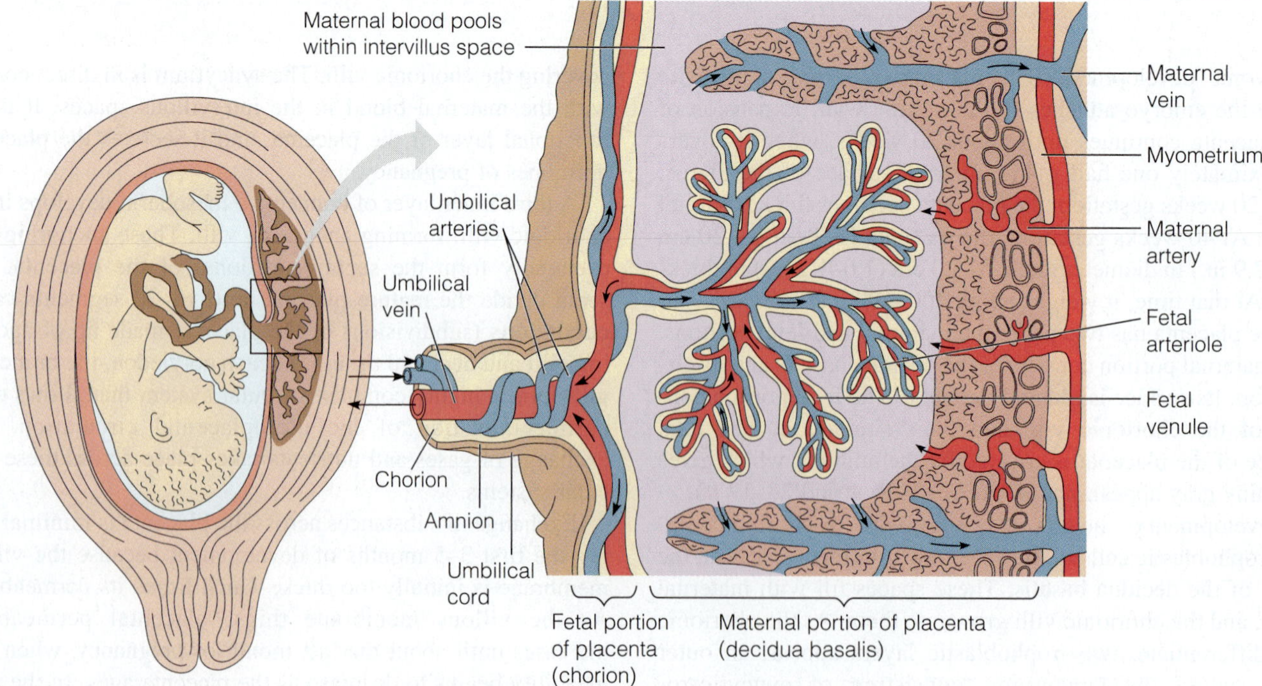

Figure 23–18 ■ Vascular arrangement of the placenta. Arrows indicate the direction of blood flow. Maternal blood flows through the uterine arteries to the intervillous spaces of the placenta and returns through the uterine veins to maternal circulation. Fetal blood flows through the umbilical arteries into the villous capillaries of the placenta and returns through the umbilical vein to the fetal circulation.

a soft blowing sound (funic souffle) can be heard over the area of the umbilical cord. The sound is synchronous with the fetal heartbeat and fetal blood flow through the umbilical arteries.

Maternal blood, rich in oxygen and nutrients, spurts from the spiral uterine arteries into the intervillous spaces. These spurts are produced by the maternal blood pressure. The spurt of blood is directed toward the chorionic plate, and as the blood loses pressure, it becomes lateral (spreads out). Fresh blood enters continuously and exerts pressure on the contents of the intervillous spaces, pushing blood toward the exits in the basal plate. The blood then drains through the uterine and other pelvic veins. A uterine souffle, timed precisely with the mother's pulse, also is heard just above the mother's symphysis pubis during the last months of pregnancy. This souffle is caused by the augmented blood flow entering the dilated uterine arteries.

Braxton Hicks contractions are intermittent painless uterine contractions that may occur every 10–20 minutes and occur more frequently near the end of pregnancy. These contractions are believed to facilitate placental circulation by enhancing the movement of blood from the center of the cotyledon through the intervillous space. Placental blood flow is enhanced when the woman is lying on her side because venous return from the lower extremities is not compromised (Blackburn, 2007).

PLACENTAL FUNCTIONS Placental exchange functions occur only in those fetal vessels that are in intimate contact with the covering syncytial membrane. The syncytium villi have brush borders containing many microvilli, which greatly increase the exchange rate between maternal and fetal circulation (Sadler, 2006).

The placental functions, many of which begin soon after implantation, include fetal respiration, nutrition, and excretion. To carry out these functions, the placenta is involved in metabolic and transfer activities. In addition, it has endocrine functions and special immunologic properties. (See the discussion later in this section.)

METABOLIC ACTIVITIES The placenta continuously produces glycogen, cholesterol, and fatty acids for fetal use and hormone production. The placenta also produces numerous enzymes (such as sulfatase, which enhances excretion of fetal estrogen precursors, and insulinase, which increases the barrier to insulin) required for fetoplacental transfer and breaks down certain substances such as epinephrine and histamine (Blackburn, 2007). In addition, it stores glycogen and iron.

TRANSPORT FUNCTION The placental membranes actively control the transfer of a wide range of substances by a variety of transport mechanisms.

- *Simple diffusion* moves substances from an area of higher concentration to an area of lower concentration. Substances that move across the placenta by simple diffusion include water, oxygen, carbon dioxide, electrolytes (sodium and chloride), anesthetic gases, and drugs. Insulin and steroid hormones originating from the adrenals, as well as thyroid hormones, also cross the placenta. However, this happens at a very slow rate. The rate of oxygen transfer across the placental membrane is greater than that allowed by simple diffusion, indicating that oxygen also is transferred by some type of facilitated diffusion transport. Unfortunately, many substances of abuse, such as cocaine and heroin, cross the placenta via simple diffusion.
- *Facilitated transport* involves a carrier system to move molecules from an area of greater concentration to an area of lower concentration. Molecules such as glucose, galactose, and some oxygen are transported by this method. Ordinarily, the glucose level in the fetal blood is approximately 20–30% lower than the glucose level in the maternal blood because the fetus is metabolizing glucose rapidly. This, in turn, causes rapid transport of additional glucose from the maternal blood to the fetal blood.
- *Active transport* can work against a concentration gradient and allows molecules to move from areas of lower concentration to areas of higher concentration. Amino acids, calcium, iron, iodine, water-soluble vitamins, and glucose are transferred across the placenta this way. The measured amino acid content of fetal blood is greater than that of maternal blood, and calcium and inorganic phosphate occur in greater concentration in fetal blood than in maternal blood (Blackburn, 2007).

Other modes of transfer also exist. Pinocytosis is important for transferring large molecules such as albumin and gamma globulin. Materials are engulfed by amoeba-like cells, forming plasma droplets. Hydrostatic and osmotic pressures allow the bulk flow of water and some solutes. Also, fetal RBCs can pass into the maternal circulation through breaks in the capillaries and placental membrane, particularly during labor and birth. Certain cells (e.g., maternal leukocytes) and microorganisms such as viruses (e.g., HIV, which causes AIDS), rubella, cytomegalovirus, polio, and the bacterium Treponema pallidum (which causes syphilis), also can cross the placental membrane under their own power (Moore & Persaud, 2008). Some bacteria and protozoa infect the placenta by causing lesions and then entering the fetal blood system.

Reduction of the placental surface area, as with abruptio placentae (partial or complete premature separation of an abnormally implanted placenta), lessens the area that is functional for exchange. Placental diffusion distance also affects exchange. In conditions such as diabetes and placental infection, edema of the villi increases the diffusion distance, thus increasing the distance the substance must be transferred.

Blood flow alteration changes the transfer rate of substances. Decreased blood flow in the intervillous space is seen in labor and with certain maternal diseases such as hypertension. Mild fetal hypoxia increases the umbilical blood flow, but severe hypoxia results in decreased blood flow.

As the maternal blood picks up fetal waste products and carbon dioxide, it drains back into the maternal circulation through the veins in the basal plate. Fetal blood is hypoxic by comparison; therefore, it attracts oxygen from the mother's blood. Affinity for oxygen increases as the fetal blood gives up its carbon dioxide, which also decreases its acidity.

ENDOCRINE FUNCTIONS The placenta produces hormones that are vital to the survival of the fetus. These include hCG; human placental lactogen (hPL); and two steroid hormones, estrogen and progesterone.

The hormone hCG is similar to LH and prevents the normal involution of the corpus luteum at the end of the menstrual cycle. If the corpus luteum stops functioning before the 11th week of pregnancy, spontaneous abortion occurs. The hCG also causes the corpus luteum to secrete increased amounts of estrogen and progesterone.

After the 11th week, the placenta produces enough progesterone and estrogen to maintain pregnancy. In the male fetus, hCG also exerts an interstitial cell-stimulating effect on the testes, resulting in the production of testosterone. This small secretion of testosterone during embryonic development is the factor that causes male sex organs to grow. Human chorionic gonadotropin may play a role in the trophoblast's immunologic capabilities (ability to exempt the placenta and embryo from rejection by the mother's system). This hormone is used as a basis for pregnancy tests.

Human chorionic gonadotropin is present in maternal blood serum 8–10 days after fertilization, just as soon as implantation has occurred, and is detectable in maternal urine at the time of missed menses. After reaching its maximum level at 50–70 days gestation, hCG begins to decrease as placental hormone production increases.

Progesterone is an essential hormone for pregnancy. It increases the secretions of the fallopian tubes and uterus to provide appropriate nutritive matter for the developing morula and blastocyst. It also appears to aid in ovum transport through the fallopian tube. Progesterone causes decidual cells to develop in the uterine endometrium, and it must be present in high levels for implantation to occur. Progesterone also decreases the contractility of the uterus, thus preventing uterine contractions from causing spontaneous abortion.

Before stimulation by hCG occurs, the production of progesterone by the corpus luteum reaches a peak about 7–10 days after ovulation. Implantation occurs at about the same time as this peak. Sixteen days after ovulation, progesterone reaches a level between 25 and 50 mg per day and continues to rise slowly in subsequent weeks. After 11 weeks, the placenta (specifically, the syncytiotrophoblast) takes over the production of progesterone and secretes it in tremendous quantities, reaching levels of more than 250 mg per day late in pregnancy.

By 7 weeks, the placenta produces more than 50% of the estrogens in the maternal circulation. Estrogens serve mainly a proliferative function, causing enlargement of the uterus, breasts, and breast glandular tissue. Estrogens also have a significant role in increasing vascularity and vasodilation, particularly in the villous capillaries toward the end of pregnancy. Placental estrogens increase markedly toward the end of pregnancy, to as much as 30 times the daily production in the middle of a normal monthly menstrual cycle. The primary estrogen secreted by the placenta is different from that secreted by the ovaries. The placenta secretes mainly estriol, whereas the ovaries secrete primarily estradiol. The placenta cannot synthesize estriol by itself. Essential precursors such as dehydroepiandrosterone sulfate (DHEA-S) is provided by the fetal adrenal glands; is processed by fetal liver; and is transported to the placenta for the final conversion to estrone, estradiol, and estriol (Blackburn, 2007; Knuppel, 2007).

The hormone hPL, also referred to as human chorionic somatomammotropin (hCS), is similar to human pituitary growth hormone; hPL stimulates certain changes in the mother's metabolic processes. These changes ensure that more protein, glucose, and minerals are available for the fetus. Secretion of hPL can be detected by about 4 weeks after conception.

IMMUNOLOGIC PROPERTIES The placenta and embryo are transplants of living tissue within the same species and therefore are considered homografts. Unlike other homografts, the placenta and embryo appear exempt from immunologic reaction by the host. Most recent data suggest that there is a suppression of cellular immunity by the placental hormones (progesterone and hCG) during pregnancy (Knuppel, 2007). One theory suggests that chorionic villi syncytiotrophoblastic tissue is immunologically inert. The chorionic villi may lack major histocompatibility (MHC) antigens and thus do not evoke rejection responses. It does, however, protect against antibody formation. Extravillous trophoblast (EVT) cells, which invade the uterine deciduas, have HLA-G, which is not readily recognized by sensitized T lymphocytes and natural killer cells (Moore & Persaud, 2008).

Development of the Fetal Circulatory System

The circulatory system of the fetus has several unique features that, by maintaining the blood flow to the placenta, provide the fetus with oxygen and nutrients while removing carbon dioxide and other waste products.

Most of the blood supply bypasses the fetal lungs because they do not carry out respiratory gas exchange. The placenta assumes the function of the fetal lungs by supplying oxygen and allowing the fetus to excrete carbon dioxide into the maternal bloodstream. Figure 23–19 ■ shows the fetal circulatory system. The blood from the placenta flows through the umbilical vein, which enters the abdominal wall of the fetus at the site that, after birth, is the umbilicus (belly button). As umbilical venous blood approaches the liver, a small portion of the blood enters the liver sinusoids, mixes with blood from the portal circulation, and then enters the inferior vena cava via hepatic veins. Most of the umbilical vein's blood flows through the **ductus venosus** directly into the fetal inferior vena cava, bypassing the liver. This blood then enters the right atrium; passes through the **foramen ovale** into the left atrium; and pours into the left ventricle, which pumps blood into the aorta. Some blood returning from the head and upper extremities by way of the superior vena cava is emptied into the right atrium and passes through the tricuspid valve into the right ventricle. This blood is pumped into the pulmonary artery, and a small amount passes to the lungs for nourishment only. The larger portion of blood passes from the pulmonary artery through the **ductus arteriosus** into the descending aorta, bypassing the lungs. Finally, blood returns to the placenta through the two umbilical arteries, and the process is repeated.

The fetus obtains oxygen via diffusion from the maternal circulation because of the gradient difference of PO_2 of 50 mmHg in maternal blood in the placenta to 30 mmHg PO_2

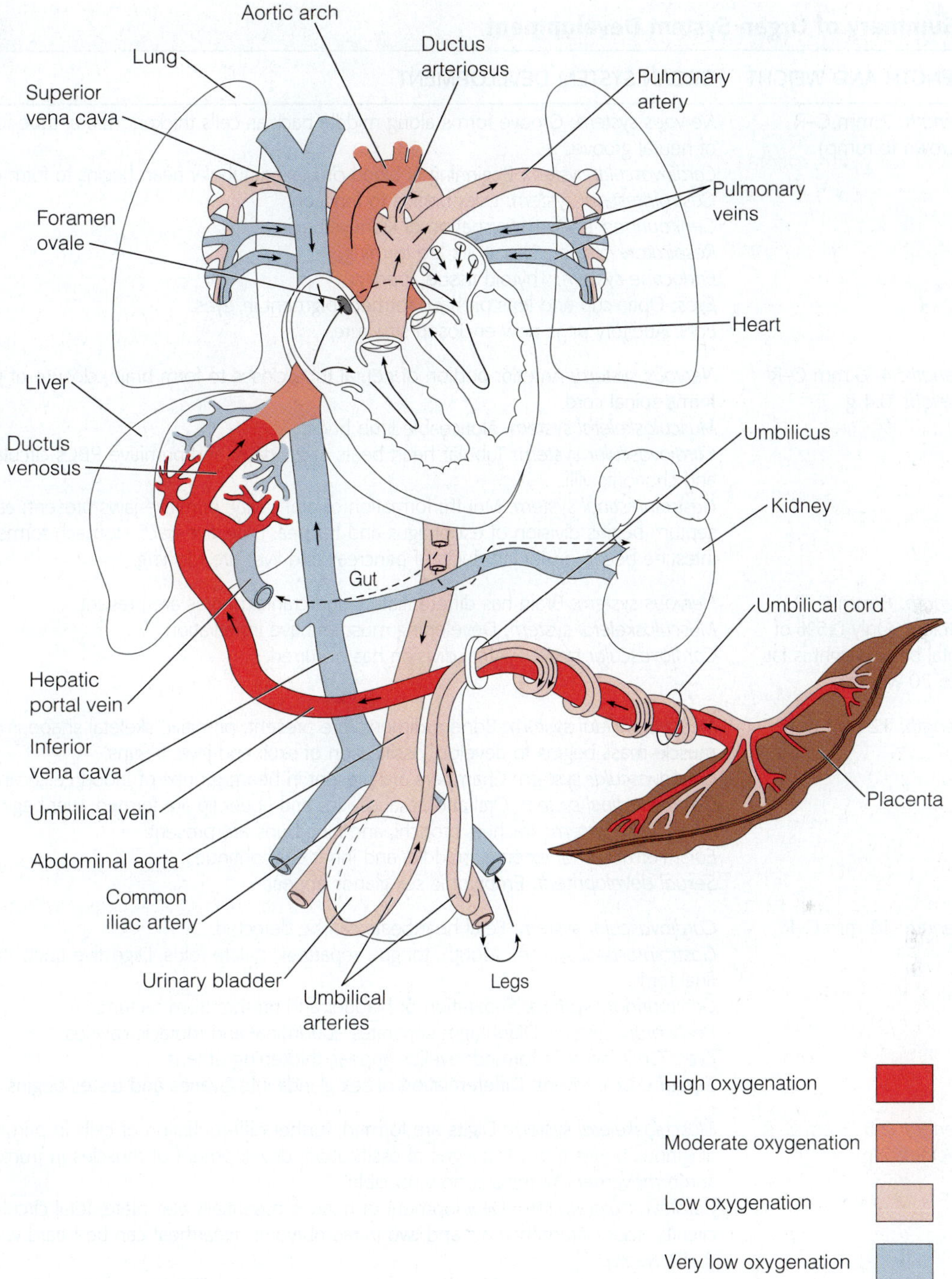

Figure 23–19 ■ Fetal circulation. Blood leaves the placenta and enters the fetus through the umbilical vein. After circulating through the fetus, the blood returns to the placenta through the umbilical arteries. The ductus venosus, the foramen ovale, and the ductus arteriosus allow the blood to bypass the fetal liver and lungs.

in the fetus. At term, the fetus receives oxygen from the mother's circulation at a rate of 20–30 mL per minute (Sadler, 2006). Fetal hemoglobin facilitates obtaining oxygen from the maternal circulation because it carries as much as 20–30% more oxygen than adult hemoglobin.

Fetal circulation delivers the highest available oxygen concentration to the head, neck, brain, and heart (coronary circulation) and a lesser amount of oxygenated blood to the abdominal organs and the lower body. This circulatory pattern leads to cephalocaudal (head-to-tail) development in the fetus.

Embryonic and Fetal Development

Pregnancy is calculated to last an average of 10 lunar months: 40 weeks, or 280 days. This period of 280 days is calculated from the onset of the last normal menstrual period to the time of birth. Estimated date of birth, sometimes referred to as the

TABLE 23–3 **Summary of Organ System Development**

AGE	LENGTH AND WEIGHT	ORGAN SYSTEM DEVELOPMENT
2–3 weeks	*Length*: 2 mm C–R (crown to rump)	*Nervous system:* Groove forms along middle back as cells thicken; neural tube forms from closure of neural groove. *Cardiovascular system:* Beginning of blood circulation; tubular heart begins to form during 3rd week. *Gastrointestinal system:* Liver begins to function. *Genitourinary system:* Formation of kidneys begins. *Respiratory system:* Nasal pits are forming. *Endocrine system:* Thyroid tissue appears. *Eyes:* Optic cup and lens pit have formed; pigment in eyes. *Ears:* Auditory pit is now enclosed structure.
4 weeks	*Length:* 4–6 mm C–R *Weight:* 0.4 g	*Nervous system:* Anterior portion of neural tube closes to form brain; closure of posterior end forms spinal cord. *Musculoskeletal system:* Noticeable limb buds. *Cardiovascular system:* Tubular heart beats at 28 days, and primitive RBCs circulate through fetus and chorionic villi. *Gastrointestinal system:* Mouth: formation of oral cavity; primitive jaws present; esophagotracheal septum begins division of esophagus and trachea. Digestive tract: stomach forms; esophagus and intestine become tubular; ducts of pancreas and liver are forming.
5 weeks	*Length:* 8 mm C–R *Weight:* Only 0.5% of total body weight is fat (to 20 weeks)	*Nervous system:* Brain has differentiated, and cranial nerves are present. *Musculoskeletal system:* Developing muscles have innervation. *Cardiovascular system:* Atrial division has occurred.
6 weeks	*Length:* 12 mm C–R	*Musculoskeletal system:* Bone rudiments are present; primitive skeletal shape is forming; muscle mass begins to develop; ossification of skull and jaws begins. *Cardiovascular system:* Chambers are present in heart; groups of blood cells can be identified. *Gastrointestinal system:* Oral and nasal cavities and upper lip are formed; liver begins to form RBCs. *Respiratory system:* Trachea, bronchi, and lung buds are present. *Ears:* Formation of external, middle, and inner ear continues. *Sexual development:* Embryonic sex glands appear.
7 weeks	*Length:* 18 mm C–R	*Cardiovascular system:* Fetal heartbeats can be detected. *Gastrointestinal system:* Mouth: tongue separates; palate folds. Digestive tract: stomach attains final form. *Genitourinary system:* Separation of bladder and urethra from rectum. *Respiratory system:* Diaphragm separates abdominal and thoracic cavities. *Eyes:* Optic nerve is formed; eyelids appear, thickening of lens. *Sexual development:* Differentiation of sex glands into ovaries and testes begins.
8 weeks	*Length:* 2.5–3 cm C–R *Weight:* 2 g	*Musculoskeletal system:* Digits are formed; further differentiation of cells in primitive skeleton; cartilaginous bones show first signs of ossification; development of muscles in trunk, limbs, and head; some movement of fetus is now possible. *Cardiovascular system:* Development of heart is essentially complete; fetal circulation follows two circuits—four extraembryonic and two intraembryonic. Heartbeat can be heard with Doppler at 8–12 weeks. *Gastrointestinal system:* Mouth: completion of lip fusion. Digestive tract: rotation in midgut; anal membrane has perforated. *Ears:* External, middle, and inner ear are assuming final form. *Sexual development:* Male and female external genitals appear similar until end of 9th week.
10 weeks	*Length:* 5–6 cm C–H (crown to heel) *Weight:* 14 g	*Nervous system:* Neurons appear at caudal end of spinal cord; basic divisions of brain are present. *Musculoskeletal system:* Fingers and toes begin nail growth. *Gastrointestinal system:* Mouth: separation of lips from jaw; fusion of palate folds. Digestive tract: developing intestines are enclosed in abdomen. *Genitourinary system:* Bladder sac is formed. *Endocrine system:* Islets of Langerhans are differentiated. *Eyes:* Eyelids are fused closed; development of lacrimal duct. *Sexual development:* Males: production of testosterone and physical characteristics between 8 and 12 weeks.

TABLE 23–3 **Summary of Organ System Development** **(continued)**

AGE	LENGTH AND WEIGHT	ORGAN SYSTEM DEVELOPMENT
12 weeks	*Length:* 8 cm C–R; 11.5 cm C–H *Weight:* 45 g	*Musculoskeletal system:* Clear outlining of miniature bones (12–20 weeks); process of ossification is established throughout fetal body; appearance of involuntary muscles in viscera. *Gastrointestinal system:* Mouth: completion of palate. Digestive tract: appearance of muscles in gut; bile secretion begins; liver is major producer of RBCs. *Respiratory system:* Lungs acquire definitive shape. *Skin:* Pink and delicate. *Endocrine system:* Hormonal secretion from thyroid; insulin is present in pancreas. *Immunologic system:* Appearance of lymphoid tissue in fetal thymus gland.
16 weeks	*Length:* 13.5 cm C–R; 15 cm C–H *Weight:* 100 g	*Musculoskeletal system:* Teeth beginning to form hard tissue that will become central incisors. *Gastrointestinal system:* Mouth: differentiation of hard and soft palate. Digestive tract: development of gastric and intestinal glands; intestines begin to collect meconium. *Genitourinary system:* Kidneys assume typical shape and organization. *Skin:* Appearance of scalp hair; lanugo present on body; transparent skin with visible blood vessels; sweat glands are developing. *Eyes, ears, and nose:* Formed. *Sexual development:* Sex determination is possible.
18 weeks	*Length:* 14.2 cm C-R; *Weight* 140 g	*Musculoskeletal system:* Teeth beginning to form hard tissue (enamel and dentine) that will become lateral incisors. *Cardiovascular system:* Fetal heart tones audible with fetoscope at 16–20 weeks.
20 weeks	*Length:* 19 cm C–R; 25 cm C–H *Weight:* 435 g (6% of total body weight is fat)	*Nervous system:* Myelination of spinal cord begins. *Musculoskeletal system:* Teeth beginning to form hard tissue that will become canine and first molar. Lower limbs are of final relative proportions. *Gastrointestinal system:* Fetus actively sucks and swallows amniotic fluid; peristaltic movements begin. *Skin:* Lanugo covers entire body; brown fat begins to form; vernix caseosa begins to form. *Immunologic system:* Detectable levels of fetal antibodies (IgG type). *Blood formation:* Iron is stored, and bone marrow is increasingly important.
24 weeks	*Length:* 23 cm C–R; 28 cm C–H *Weight:* 780 g	*Nervous system:* Brain looks like mature brain. *Musculoskeletal system:* Teeth are beginning to form hard tissue that will become the second molars. *Respiratory system:* Respiratory movements may occur (24–40 weeks). Nostrils reopen. Alveoli appear in lungs and begin production of surfactant; gas exchange is possible. *Skin:* Reddish and wrinkled; vernix caseosa is present. *Immunologic system:* IgG levels reach maternal levels.
28 weeks	*Length:* 27 cm C–R; 35 cm C–H *Weight:* 1200–1250 g	*Nervous system:* Begins regulation of some body functions. *Skin:* Adipose tissue accumulates rapidly; nails appear; eyebrows and eyelashes are present. *Eyes:* Eyelids are open (26–29 weeks). *Sexual development:* Males: testes descend into inguinal canal and upper scrotum.
32 weeks	*Length:* 31 cm C–R; 38–43 cm C–H *Weight:* 2000 g	*Nervous system:* More reflexes are present.
36 weeks	*Length:* 35 cm C–R; 42–48 cm C–H *Weight:* 2500–2750 g	*Musculoskeletal system:* Distal femoral ossification centers are present. *Skin:* Pale; body is rounded, lanugo is disappearing, hair is fuzzy or woolly; few sole creases; sebaceous glands are active and helping to produce vernix caseosa (36–40 weeks). *Ears:* Earlobes are soft with little cartilage. *Sexual development:* Males: scrotum is small and few rugae are present; descent of testes into upper scrotum to stay (36–40 weeks). Females: labia majora and minora are equally prominent.
38–40 weeks	*Length:* 40 cm C–R; 48–52 cm C–H *Weight:* 3200+ g (16% of total body weight is fat)	*Respiratory system:* At 38 weeks, lecithin/sphingomyelin (L/S) ratio approaches 2:1 (indicates decreased risk of respiratory distress from inadequate surfactant production if born now). *Skin:* Smooth and pink; vernix is present in skin folds; moderate to profuse silky hair; lanugo on shoulders and upper back; nails extend over tips of digits; creases cover sole. *Ears:* Earlobes are firmer because of increased cartilage. *Sexual development:* Males: rugous scrotum. Females: labia majora is well developed, and minora is small or completely covered.

Source: Data from Sadler, T. W. (2006). *Langman's medical embryology* (10th ed.). Baltimore: Lippincott Williams & Wilkins.

Note: Age refers to postfertilization or postconception age.

estimated date of delivery (EDD), is usually calculated by this method. Most fetuses are born within 10–14 days of the calculated date of birth. The fertilization age (or postconception age) of the fetus is calculated to be *about* 2 weeks less, or 266 days (38 weeks), or 9.5 calendar months. The latter measurement is more accurate because it measures time from the fertilization of the ovum, or conception.

The basic events of organ development in the embryo and fetus are outlined in Table 23–3. The time periods in the table are **postconception age periods**. During the period from fertilization to the end of the embryonic period (8 weeks), age is often expressed in days but can be given in weeks. During the fetal period (9th week until birth), age is given in weeks (Moore & Persaud, 2008).

In review, human development follows three stages. The preembryonic stage, as discussed earlier in the chapter, consists of the first 14 days of development after the ovum is fertilized. The embryonic stage covers the period from day 15 until approximately the end of the 8th week, and the fetal stage extends from the end of the 8th week until birth. (See the detailed discussion of the embryonic and fetal stages next.)

EMBRYONIC STAGE The stage of the **embryo** starts on day 15 (the beginning of the 3rd week after conception) and continues until approximately the 8th week, or until the embryo reaches a crown-to-rump (C–R) length of 3 cm (1.2 in.). This length is usually reached about 56 days after fertilization (the end of the 8th gestational week). During the embryonic stage, tissues differentiate into essential organs and the main external features develop (Figure 23–20 ■). The embryo is most vulnerable to *teratogens* during this period.

Three Weeks In the third week, the embryonic disk becomes elongated and pear-shaped, with a broad cephalic end and a narrow caudal end. The ectoderm has formed a long cylindrical tube for brain and spinal cord development. The gastrointestinal tract, created from the endoderm, appears as another tube-like structure communicating with the yolk sac. The most advanced organ is the heart. At 3 weeks, a single tubular heart forms just outside the body cavity of the embryo.

Four to Five Weeks During days 21–32, somites (a series of mesodermal blocks) form on either side of the embryo's midline. The vertebrae that form the spinal column will develop from these somites. Before 28 days, arm and leg buds are not visible, but the tail bud is present. The pharyngeal arches—which will form the lower jaw, hyoid bone, and larynx—develop at this time. The pharyngeal pouches appear now; these pouches will form the eustachian tube and cavity of the middle ear, the tonsils, and the parathyroid and thymus glands. The primordia of the ear and eye also are present. By the end of 28 days, the tubular heart is beating at

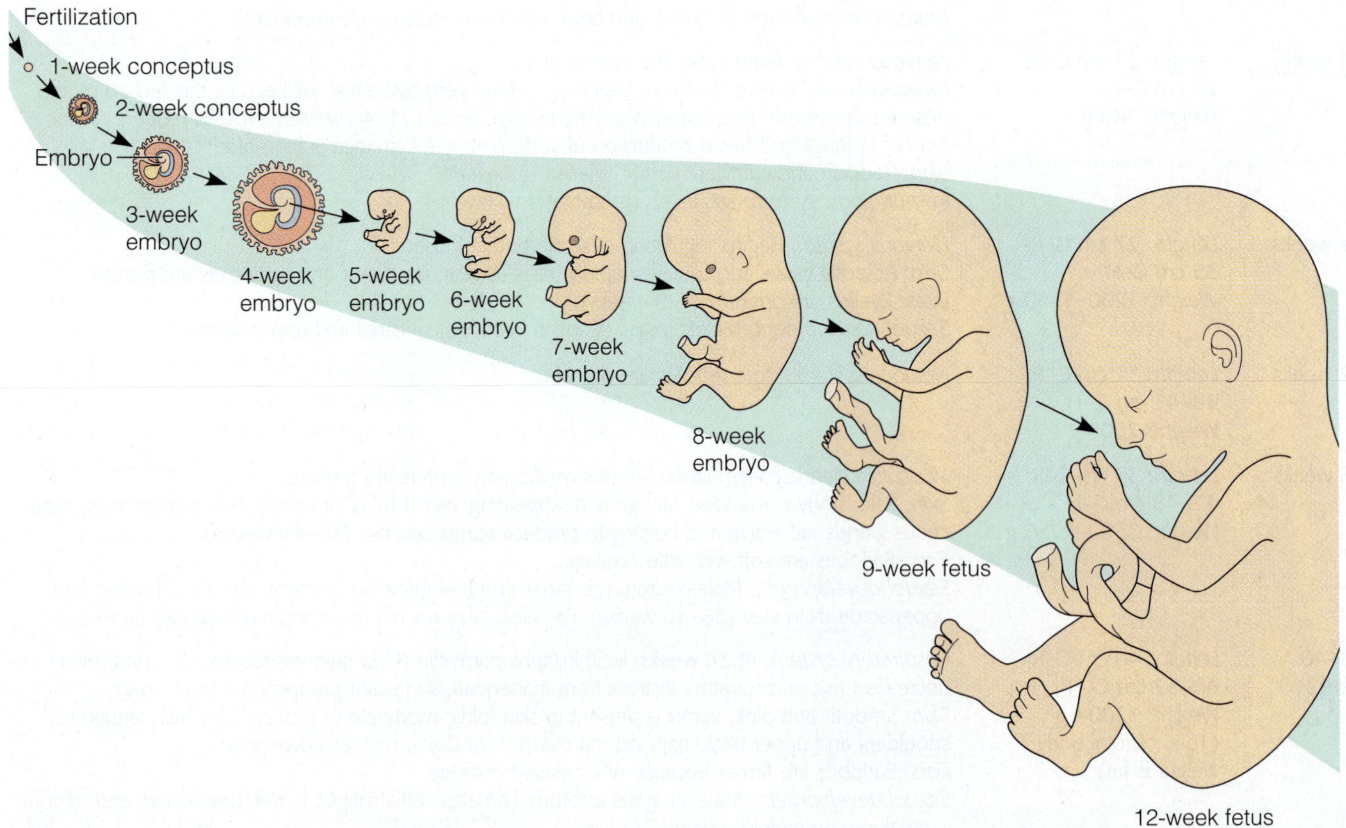

Figure 23–20 ■ The actual size of a human conceptus from fertilization to the early fetal stage. The embryonic stage begins in the third week after fertilization; the fetal stage begins in the ninth week.

a regular rhythm and pushing its own primitive blood cells through the main blood vessels.

During the fifth week, the optic cups and lens vessels of the eye form and the nasal pits develop. Partitioning in the heart occurs with division of the atrium. The embryo has a marked C-shaped body, accentuated by the rudimentary tail and the large head folded over a protuberant trunk (Figure 23–21 ■). By day 35, the arm and leg buds are well developed, with paddle-shaped hand and foot plates. The heart, circulatory system, and brain show the most advanced development. The brain has differentiated into five areas, and 10 pairs of cranial nerves are recognizable.

Six Weeks At 6 weeks, the head structures are more highly developed and the trunk is straighter than in earlier stages. The upper and lower jaws are recognizable, and the external nares are well formed. The trachea has developed, and its caudal end is bifurcated for beginning lung formation. The upper lip has formed, and the palate is developing. The ears are developing rapidly. The arms have begun to extend ventrally across the chest, and both arms and legs have digits, although they may still be webbed. There is a slight elbow bend in the arms, which are more advanced in development than the legs. Beginning at this stage, the prominent tail will recede. The heart now has most of its definitive characteristics, and fetal circulation begins to be established. The liver starts to produce blood cells.

Seven Weeks At 7 weeks, the head of the embryo is rounded and nearly erect (Figure 23–22 ■). The eyes have shifted and are closer together, and the eyelids are beginning to form. The palate is near completion, and the tongue is developing in the formed mouth. The gastrointestinal and genitourinary tracts undergo significant changes during the 7th week. Before this time, the rectal and urogenital passages formed one tube that ended in a blind pouch; they now separate into two tubular structures. The intestines enter the extraembryonic coelom in the area of the umbilical cord (called umbilical herniation) (Moore & Persaud, 2008). The beginning of all essential external and internal structures are present.

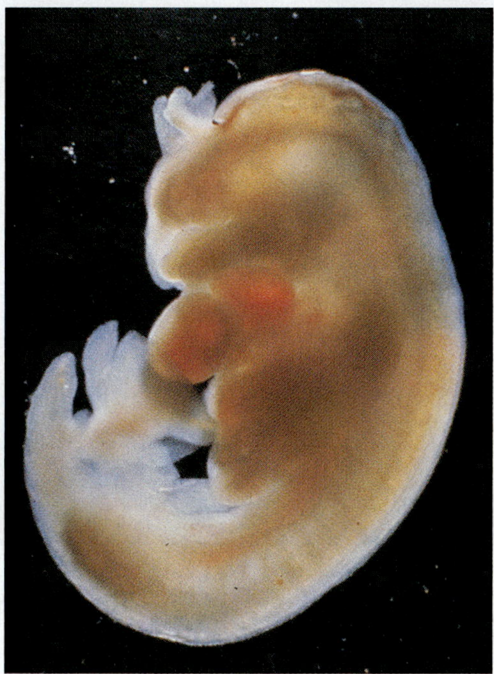

Figure 23–21 ■ The embryo at 5 weeks. The embryo has a marked C-shaped body and a rudimentary tail.

Source: © Petit Format/Nestle/Science Source/Photo Researchers, Inc.

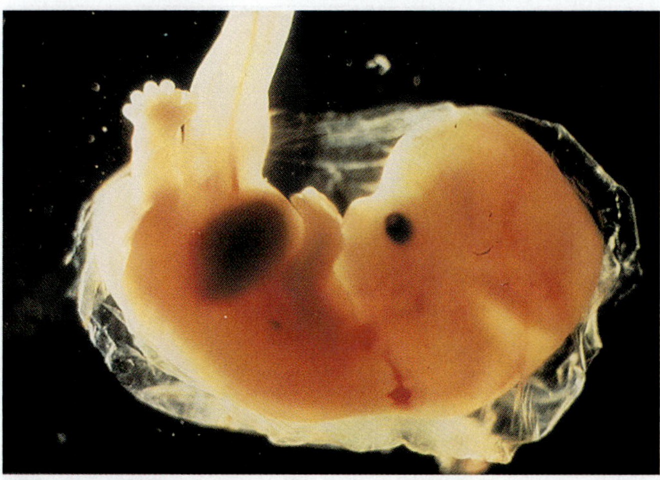

Figure 23–22 ■ The embryo at 7 weeks. The head is rounded and nearly erect. The eyes have shifted forward and closer together, and the eyelids begin to form.

Source: © Petit Format/Nestle/Science Source/Photo Researchers, Inc.

Eight Weeks At 8 weeks, the embryo is approximately 3 cm (1.2 in.) C–R length and clearly resembles a human being. Facial features continue to develop. The eyelids begin to fuse. Auricles of the external ears begin to assume their final shape, but they are still set low (Moore & Persaud, 2008). External genitals appear, but the embryo's sex is not clearly identifiable. The rectal passage opens with the perforation of the anal membrane. The circulatory system through the umbilical cord is well established. Long bones are beginning to form, and the large muscles are now capable of contracting.

FETAL STAGE By the end of the eighth week, the embryo is sufficiently developed to be called a **fetus**. Every organ system and external structure that will be found in the full-term newborn is present. The remainder of gestation is devoted to refining structures and perfecting function.

Nine to Twelve Weeks By the end of the ninth week, the fetus reaches a C–R length of 5 cm (2 in.) and weighs about 14 g (0.5 oz). The head is large and comprises almost half of the fetus's entire size (Figure 23–23 ■). At 12 weeks, the fetus reaches 8 cm (3.2 in.) C–R length and weighs about 45 g (1.6 oz). The face is well formed, with the nose protruding, the chin small and receding, and the ears acquiring a more adult shape. The eyelids close at about the 10th week and do not reopen until about the 26- to 29-week period. Some movement of the lips suggestive of the sucking reflex has been observed at 3 months. Tooth buds now appear for all 20 of the child's first teeth (baby teeth). The limbs are long and slender with well-formed digits. The fetus can curl the fingers toward the palm and begins to make a tiny fist.

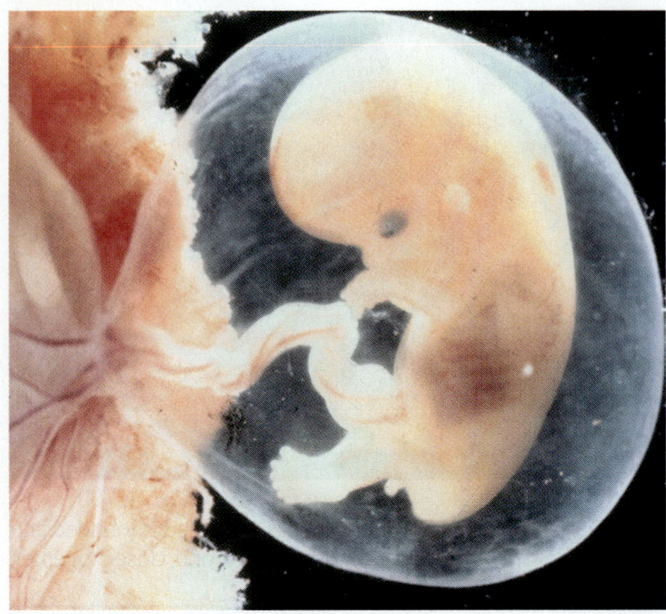

Figure 23–23 ■ The fetus at 9 weeks. Every organ system and external structure is present.

Source: Nilsson, L. (1990). *A child is born.* New York: Dell Publishing.

The legs are still shorter and less developed than the arms. The urogenital tract completes its development, well-differentiated genitals appear, and the kidneys begin to produce urine. Red blood cells are produced primarily by the liver. Spontaneous movements of the fetus now occur. Fetal heart rates (FHRs) can be ascertained by electronic devices between 8 and 12 weeks. The rate is 120–160 beats per minute.

Thirteen to Sixteen Weeks This is a period of rapid growth. At 13 weeks, the fetus weighs 55–60 g (1.9–2.1 oz) and is about 9 cm (3.6 in.) in C–R length. Lanugo, or fine hair, begins to develop, especially on the head. The skin is so transparent that blood vessels are clearly visible beneath it. More muscle tissue and body skeleton have developed and hold the fetus more erect (Figure 23–24 ■). Active movements are present; the fetus stretches and exercises its arms and legs. It makes sucking motions, swallows amniotic fluid, and produces meconium in the intestinal tract. Bronchial tubes are branching out in the primitive lungs, and sweat glands are developing. The liver and pancreas now begin production of their appropriate secretions. By the beginning of week 16, skeletal ossification is clearly identifiable.

Twenty Weeks The fetus doubles its C–R length and now measures 19 cm (8 in.) long. Fetal weight is between 435 and 465 g (15.2 and 16.3 oz). Lanugo covers the entire body and is especially prominent on the shoulders. Subcutaneous deposits of brown fat, which has a rich blood supply, make the skin less transparent. Nipples now appear over the mammary glands. The head is covered with fine "woolly" hair, and the eyebrows and eyelashes are beginning to form. Nails are present on both fingers and toes. Muscles are well developed, and the fetus is active (Figure 23–25 ■). The mother feels fetal movement, known as

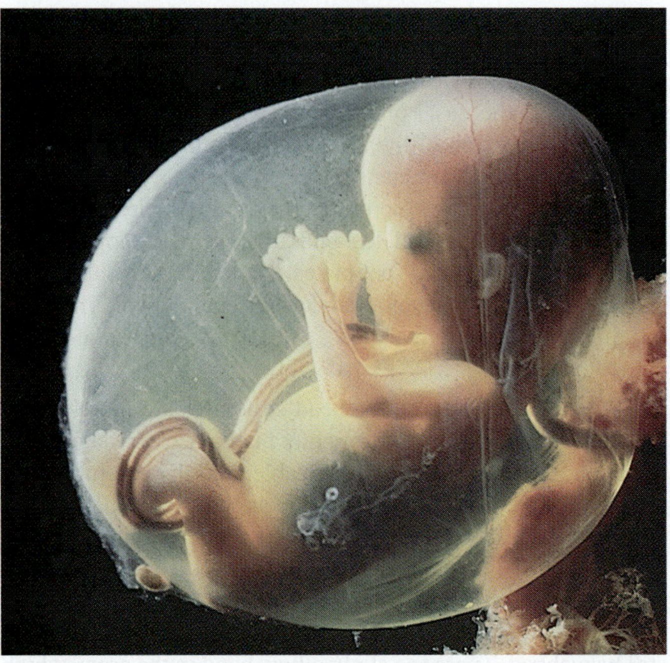

Figure 23–24 ■ The fetus at 14 weeks. During this period of rapid growth, the skin is so transparent that blood vessels are visible beneath it. More muscle tissue and body skeleton have developed, and they hold the fetus more erect.

Source: Nilsson, L. (1990). *A child is born.* New York: Dell Publishing.

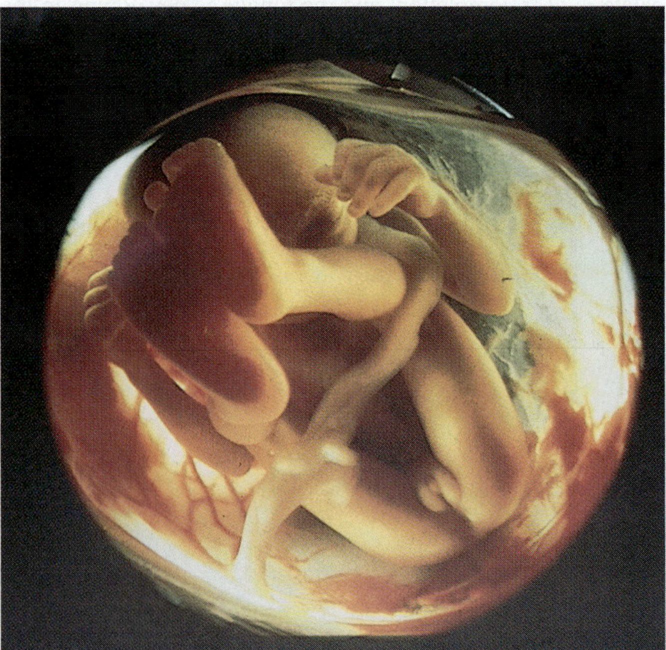

Figure 23–25 ■ The fetus at 20 weeks. The fetus now weighs 435–465 g (15.2–16.3 oz) and measures about 19 cm (7.5 in.). Subcutaneous deposits of brown fat make the skin a little less transparent. "Woolly" hair covers the head, and nails have developed on the fingers and toes.

Source: Nilsson, L. (1990). *A child is born.* New York: Dell Publishing.

quickening. The fetal heartbeat is audible through a fetoscope. Quickening and fetal heartbeat can help validate the EDB.

Twenty-Four Weeks At 24 weeks, the fetus reaches a crown-to-heel (C–H) length of 28 cm (11.2 in.). It weighs about 780 g (1 lb 10 oz). The hair on the head is growing long, and eyebrows and eyelashes have formed. The eye is structurally complete and will soon open. The fetus has a reflex hand grip (grasp reflex) and, by the end of 6 months, a startle reflex. Skin covering the body is reddish and wrinkled with little subcutaneous fat. Skin on the hands and feet has thickened, with skin ridges on palms and soles forming distinct foot- and fingerprints. The skin over the entire body is covered with **vernix caseosa**, a protective cheeselike, fatty substance secreted by the sebaceous glands. The alveoli in the lungs are just beginning to form.

Twenty-Five to Twenty-Eight Weeks At 6 calendar months, the fetal skin is still red, wrinkled, and covered with vernix caseosa. The brain is developing rapidly, and the nervous system is complete enough to provide some degree of regulation of body functions. The eyelids, under neural control, open and close. The fetus has nails on both fingers and toes. In the male fetus, the testes begin to descend into the scrotal sac. Even though the lungs are still physiologically immature, they are sufficiently developed to provide gas exchange. A fetus born at this time requires immediate and prolonged intensive care to survive and then to decrease the risk of major handicap. The fetus at 28 weeks is about 35–38 cm (14–15 in.) long C–H and weighs 1200–1250 g (2 lb 10.5 oz–2 lb 12 oz).

Twenty-Nine to Thirty-Two Weeks At 30 weeks, the pupillary light reflex is present (Moore & Persaud, 2008). The fetus is gaining weight from an increase in body muscle and fat and weighs about 2000 g (4 lb 6.5 oz), with a C–H length of about 38–43 cm (15–17 in.) by 32 weeks of age. The CNS has matured enough to direct rhythmic breathing movements and to partially control body temperature; however, the lungs are not yet fully mature. Bones are fully developed but soft and flexible. The fetus begins storing iron, calcium, and phosphorus. In males, the testicles may be located in the scrotal sac but are often still high in the inguinal canals.

Thirty-Five to Thirty-Six Weeks The fetus begins to get plump, and less wrinkled skin covers the deposits of subcutaneous fat. Lanugo begins to disappear, and the nails reach the edge of the fingertips. By 35 weeks of age, the fetus has a firm grasp and exhibits spontaneous orientation to light. By 36 weeks of age, the weight is usually 2500–2750 g (5 lb 12 oz–6 lb 11.5 oz) and the C–H length of the fetus is about 42–48 cm (16–19 in.). An infant born at this time has a good chance of surviving but may require special care, especially if there is intrauterine growth restriction (IUGR).

Thirty-Eight to Forty Weeks The fetus is considered full term at 38 weeks and up to 40 weeks after conception. The C–H length varies from 48–52 cm (19–21 in.), with males usually longer than females. Males also usually weigh more than females. The weight at term is about 3000–3600 g (6 lb 10 oz–7 lb 15 oz) and varies in different ethnic groups. The skin is pink and has a smooth, polished look. The only lanugo left is on the upper arms and shoulders. The hair on the head is no longer woolly, but is coarse and about 1 in. long. Vernix caseosa is present, with heavier deposits remaining in the creases and folds of the skin. The body and extremities are plump, with good skin turgor, and the fingernails extend beyond the fingertips. The chest is prominent but still a little smaller than the head, and mammary glands protrude in both sexes. In males, the testes are in the scrotum or are palpable in the inguinal canals.

As the fetus enlarges, amniotic fluid diminishes to about 500 mL or less and the fetal body mass fills the uterine cavity. The fetus assumes what is called its position of comfort, or lie. The head is generally pointed downward, following the shape of the uterus (and possibly because the head is heavier than the feet). The extremities, and often the head, are well flexed. After 5 months, patterns in feeding, sleeping, and activity become established; so at term, the fetus has its own body rhythms and individual style of response.

PHYSICAL AND PSYCHOLOGIC CHANGES OF PREGNANCY

The growth of the developing fetus and the physical and psychologic changes that occur in the pregnant mother continue to inspire feelings of awe and amazement, not to mention curiosity. First, it is nothing short of a miracle that the union of two microscopic entities—an ovum and a sperm—can produce a living being. Second, the woman's body must undergo extraordinary physical changes to maintain a pregnancy.

Pregnancy is divided into three trimesters, each approximately a 3-month period. Each trimester brings predictable changes for both mother and fetus. This section describes these physical and psychologic changes. It also presents the various cultural factors that can affect a pregnant woman's well-being.

Anatomy and Physiology of Pregnancy

The changes that occur in the pregnant woman's body may result from hormonal influences, the growth of the fetus, or the mother's physiologic adaptation to the pregnancy. Virtually every system must adapt to support the growing fetus and maintain the pregnant woman's body functions.

REPRODUCTIVE SYSTEM Some of the most dramatic changes of pregnancy occur in the reproductive organs.

Uterus The changes in the uterus during pregnancy are amazing. Before pregnancy, the uterus is a small, semisolid, pear-shaped organ measuring approximately 7.5 × 5 × 2.5 cm and weighing about 60 g (2 oz). At the end of pregnancy, it measures about 28 × 24 × 21 cm and weighs approximately 1100 g (2.5 lb); its capacity also has increased from about 10 mL to 5000 mL (5 L) or more (Cunningham et al., 2005).

The enlargement of the uterus is primarily because of the enlargement (hypertrophy) of the preexisting myometrial cells as a result of the stimulating influence of estrogen and the distention caused by the growing fetus. Only a limited increase in cell number (hyperplasia) occurs. The fibrous tissue between the muscle bands increases markedly, which adds to the strength and elasticity of the muscle wall. The enlarging uterus, developing placenta, and growing fetus require additional blood flow to the uterus. By the end of pregnancy, one sixth of the total maternal blood volume is contained in the vascular system of the uterus.

Braxton Hicks contractions, which are irregular, generally painless contractions of the uterus, occur intermittently throughout pregnancy. They may be felt through the abdominal wall beginning about the fourth month of pregnancy. In later months, these contractions become uncomfortable and may be confused with true labor contractions.

Cervix Estrogen stimulates the glandular tissue of the cervix, which increases in cell number and becomes hyperactive. The endocervical glands secrete a thick, sticky mucus that accumulates and forms a mucous plug, which seals the endocervical canal and prevents the ascent of microorganisms into the uterus. This plug is expelled when cervical dilatation begins. The hyperactivity of the glandular tissue also increases the normal physiologic mucorrhea, at times resulting in profuse discharge. Increased cervical vascularity also causes both the softening of the cervix (**Goodell's sign**) and its bluish discoloration (**Chadwick's sign**).

Ovaries The ovaries stop producing ova during pregnancy, but the corpus luteum continues to produce hormones until about weeks 6–8. It secretes progesterone until about the 7th week of pregnancy to maintain the endometrium until the placenta assumes the task. The corpus luteum then begins to disintegrate slowly.

Vagina Estrogen causes a thickening of the vaginal mucosa, a loosening of the connective tissue, and an increase in vaginal secretions. These secretions are thick, white, and acidic (pH 3.5–6.0). The acid pH helps prevent bacterial infection but favors the growth of yeast organisms. Thus, the pregnant woman is more susceptible to *Candida* infection than usual.

The supportive connective tissue of the vagina loosens throughout pregnancy. By the end of pregnancy, the vagina and perineal body are sufficiently relaxed to permit passage of the infant. Because blood flow to the vagina is increased, the vagina may show the same blue-purple color (Chadwick's sign) as the cervix.

BREASTS Estrogen and progesterone cause many changes in the mammary glands. The breasts enlarge and become more nodular as the glands increase in size and number in preparation for lactation. Superficial veins become more prominent, the nipples become more erectile, and the areolas darken. Montgomery's follicles (sebaceous glands) enlarge, and **striae** (reddish stretch marks that slowly turn silver after childbirth) may develop.

Colostrum, an antibody-rich yellow secretion, may leak or be expressed from the breasts during the last trimester. Colostrum gradually converts to mature milk during the first few days after childbirth.

RESPIRATORY SYSTEM Many respiratory changes occur to meet the increased oxygen requirements of a pregnant woman. The volume of air breathed each minute increases 30–40%. In addition, progesterone decreases airway resistance, permitting a 15–20% increase in oxygen consumption as well as increases in carbon dioxide production and in the respiratory functional reserve.

As the uterus enlarges, it presses upward and elevates the diaphragm. The subcostal angle increases, so that the rib cage flares. The anteroposterior diameter increases, and the chest circumference expands by as much as 6 cm; as a result, there is no significant loss of intrathoracic volume. Breathing changes from abdominal to thoracic as pregnancy progresses, and descent of the diaphragm on inspiration becomes less possible. Some hyperventilation and difficulty in breathing may occur.

Nasal stuffiness and epistaxis (nosebleeds) also may occur because of estrogen-induced edema and vascular congestion of the nasal mucosa.

CARDIOVASCULAR SYSTEM During pregnancy, blood flow increases to organ systems with an increased workload. Thus, blood flow increases to the uterus, placenta, and breasts, whereas hepatic and cerebral flow remains unchanged. Cardiac output begins to increase early in pregnancy and peaks at 25–30 weeks gestation at 30–50% above prepregnant levels. In the 3rd trimester, cardiac output becomes less predictable; it is likely that any changes are individually determined (Gordon, 2007).

The pulse may increase by as many as 10–15 beats per minute at term. The blood pressure decreases slightly, reaching its lowest point during the 2nd trimester. It gradually increases to near prepregnant levels by the end of the 3rd trimester.

The enlarging uterus puts pressure on pelvic and femoral vessels, interfering with returning blood flow and causing stasis of blood in the lower extremities. This condition may lead to dependent edema and varicosity of the veins in the legs, vulva, and rectum (hemorrhoids) in late pregnancy. This increased blood volume in the lower legs also may make the pregnant woman prone to postural hypotension.

When the pregnant woman lies supine, the enlarging uterus may press on the vena cava. This reduces blood flow to the right atrium; lowers blood pressure; and causes dizziness, pallor, and clamminess. Research indicates that the enlarging uterus also may press on the aorta and its collateral circulation (Cunningham et al., 2005). This condition is called **supine hypotensive syndrome**. It also may be referred to as **vena caval syndrome** or **aortocaval compression** (Figure 23–26 ■).

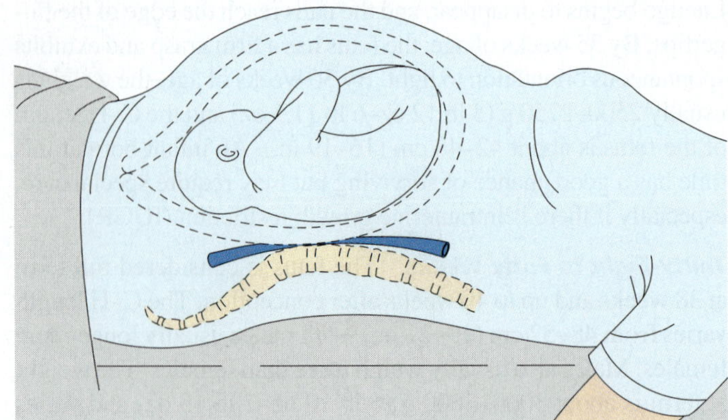

Figure 23–26 ■ Vena caval syndrome. The gravid uterus compresses the vena cava when the woman is supine. This reduces the blood flow returning to the heart and may cause maternal hypotension.

It can be corrected by having the woman lie on her left side or by placing a pillow or wedge under her right hip as she lies in a supine position.

Blood volume progressively increases beginning in the first trimester, increases rapidly until about 30–34 weeks, and then plateaus until birth at about 40–50% above nonpregnant levels. This increase occurs because of increases in both erythrocytes and plasma (Gordon, 2007).

The total erythrocyte (RBC) volume increases by about 30% in women who receive iron supplementation (but only about 18% without iron supplementation). This increase in erythrocytes is necessary to transport the additional oxygen required during pregnancy. However, the increase in plasma volume during pregnancy averages about 50%. Because the plasma volume increase (50%) is greater than the erythrocyte increase (30%), the hematocrit, which measures the concentration of RBCs in the plasma, decreases slightly (Gordon, 2007). This decrease is referred to as the **physiologic anemia of pregnancy** (pseudoanemia).

Iron is necessary for hemoglobin formation, and hemoglobin is the oxygen-carrying component of erythrocytes. Thus, the increase in erythrocyte levels results in the pregnant woman's increased need for iron. Even though the gastrointestinal absorption of iron is moderately increased during pregnancy, it is usually necessary to add supplemental iron to the diet to meet the expanded RBC and fetal needs.

Leukocyte production increases slightly to an average of 8500 mm^3, with a range of 5600–12,200 mm^3. During labor and the early postpartum period, these levels may reach 20,000–30,000 mm^3. Because of this normal increase in WBCs, the result should not be used clinically to diagnose the presence of infection (Gordon, 2007).

Both the fibrin and plasma fibrinogen levels increase during pregnancy. Although the blood-clotting time of the pregnant woman does not differ significantly from that of the nonpregnant woman, clotting factors VII, VIII, IX, and X increase; thus, pregnancy is a somewhat hypercoagulable state. These changes, coupled with venous stasis in late pregnancy, increase the pregnant woman's risk of developing venous thrombosis.

GASTROINTESTINAL SYSTEM Nausea and vomiting are common during the first trimester because of elevated hCG levels and changed carbohydrate metabolism. Gum tissue may soften and bleed easily. The secretion of saliva may increase and even become excessive (ptyalism).

Elevated progesterone levels cause smooth muscle relaxation, resulting in delayed gastric emptying and decreased peristalsis. As a result, the pregnant woman may complain of bloating and constipation. These symptoms are aggravated as the enlarging uterus displaces the stomach upward and the intestines are moved laterally and posteriorly. The cardiac sphincter also relaxes, and heartburn (pyrosis) may occur because of reflux of acidic secretions into the lower esophagus. Hemorrhoids frequently develop in late pregnancy from constipation and from pressure on vessels below the level of the uterus.

Only minor liver changes occur with pregnancy. Plasma albumin concentrations and serum cholinesterase activity decrease with normal pregnancy, as with certain liver diseases.

The emptying time of the gallbladder is prolonged during pregnancy as a result of smooth muscle relaxation from progesterone. This, coupled with the elevated levels of cholesterol in the bile, can predispose the woman to gallstone formation.

URINARY TRACT During the first trimester, the enlarging uterus is still a pelvic organ and presses against the bladder, producing urinary frequency. This symptom decreases during the 2nd trimester, when the uterus becomes an abdominal organ and pressure against the bladder lessens. Frequency reappears during the third trimester, when the presenting part descends into the pelvis and again presses on the bladder, reducing bladder capacity, contributing to hyperemia, and irritating the bladder.

The ureters (especially the right ureter) elongate and dilate above the pelvic brim. The glomerular filtration rate (GFR) rises by as much as 50% beginning in the 2nd trimester and remains elevated until birth. To compensate for this increase, renal tubular reabsorption also increases. However, glycosuria sometimes is seen during pregnancy because of the kidneys' inability to reabsorb all of the glucose filtered by the glomeruli. Glycosuria may be normal or may indicate gestational diabetes, so it always warrants further testing.

SKIN AND HAIR Changes in skin pigmentation commonly occur during pregnancy. Increased estrogen, progesterone, and α-melanocyte-stimulating hormone levels are thought to stimulate these changes. Pigmentation of the skin increases primarily in areas that are already hyperpigmented: the areola, the nipples, the vulva, and the perianal area. The skin in the middle of the abdomen may develop a pigmented line, the linea nigra, which usually extends from the umbilicus or above to the pubic area (Figure 23–27 ■). Facial **chloasma**, or **melasma gravidarum** (also known as the "mask of pregnancy"), a darkening of the

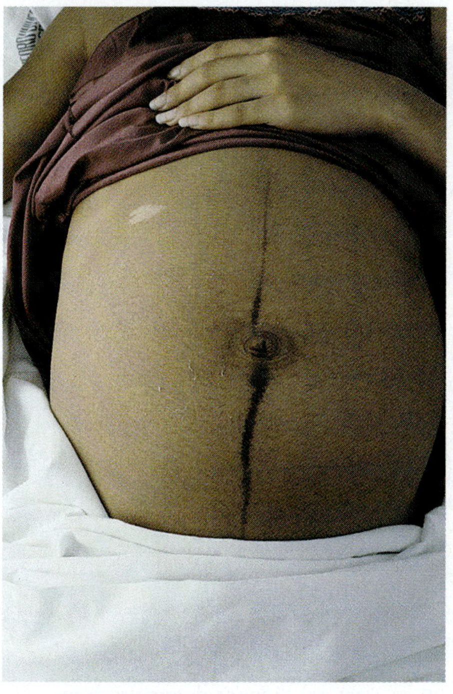

Figure 23–27 ■ Linea nigra.

skin over the cheeks, nose, and forehead, may develop. Chloasma or melasma is more prominent in dark-haired women and is aggravated by exposure to the sun. Fortunately, the condition fades or becomes less prominent soon after childbirth, when the hormonal influence of pregnancy subsides.

In addition, the sweat and sebaceous glands are often hyperactive during pregnancy.

Striae, or stretch marks, may appear on the abdomen, thighs, buttocks, and breasts. They result from reduced connective tissue strength because of elevated adrenal steroid levels.

Vascular spider nevi—small, bright red elevations of the skin radiating from a central body—may develop on the chest, neck, face, arms, and legs. They may be caused by increased subcutaneous blood flow in response to elevated estrogen levels.

The rate of hair growth may decrease during pregnancy; the number of hair follicles in the resting or dormant phase also decreases. After birth, the number of hair follicles in the resting phase increases sharply and the woman may notice increased hair shedding for 1–4 months. Practically all hair is replaced within 6–12 months, however (Cunningham et al., 2005).

MUSCULOSKELETAL SYSTEM No demonstrable changes occur in the teeth of pregnant women. The dental caries that sometimes accompany pregnancy are probably caused by inadequate oral hygiene and dental care, especially if the woman has problems with bleeding gums or nausea and vomiting.

The joints of the pelvis relax somewhat because of hormonal influences. The result is often a waddling gait. As the pregnant woman's center of gravity gradually changes, the lumbar spinal curve becomes accentuated and her posture changes (Figure 23–28 ■). This posture change compensates for the increased weight of the uterus anteriorly and frequently results in low backache.

Pressure of the enlarging uterus on the abdominal muscles may cause the rectus abdominis muscle to separate, producing **diastasis recti**. If the separation is severe and muscle tone is not regained postpartally, subsequent pregnancies will not have adequate support and the woman's abdomen may appear pendulous.

CENTRAL NERVOUS SYSTEM (CNS) Pregnant women frequently describe decreased attention, concentration, and memory during and shortly after pregnancy, but few studies have explored this phenomenon. One study did compare a group of pregnant women against a control group, finding a decline in memory that could not be attributed to depression, anxiety, sleep deprivation, or other physical changes of pregnancy. This memory loss disappears soon after childbirth (Cunningham et al., 2005).

EYES During pregnancy, intraocular pressure decreases, probably because of increased vitreous outflow, and the cornea thickens slightly because of fluid retention. As a result, some pregnant women experience difficulty wearing previously comfortable contact lenses (Cunningham et al., 2005). These changes usually disappear by 6 weeks postpartum.

METABOLISM Most metabolic functions increase during pregnancy because of the increased demands of the growing fetus and its support system. The expectant mother must meet both her own tissue replacement needs and those of her unborn child. Her body also must anticipate the needs of labor and lactation.

Weight Gain Adequate nutrition and weight gain are important during pregnancy. The recommended weight gain for women of normal weight before pregnancy is 11.4–15.9 kg (25–35 lb), whereas women who are overweight should limit their gain to 6.8 kg (15 lb). Underweight women may gain up to 18.1 kg (40 lb) (Johnson, Gregory, & Niebyl, 2007). The average pattern of

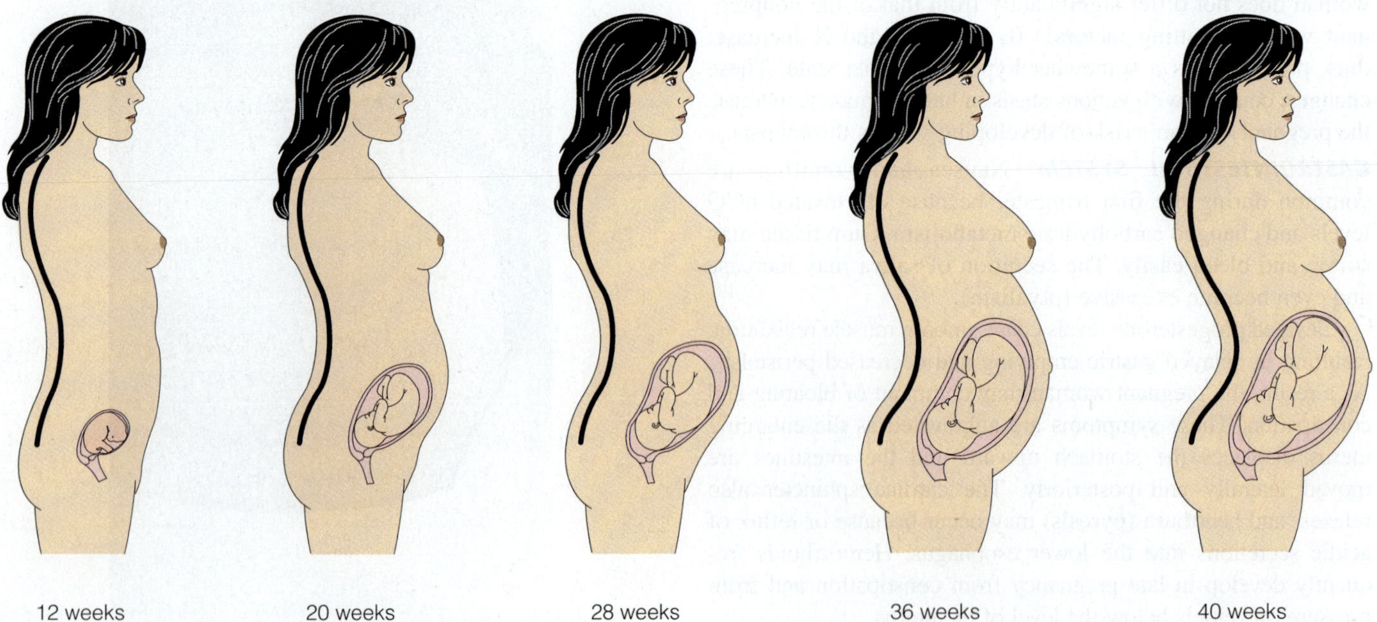

Figure 23–28 ■ Postural changes during pregnancy. Note the increasing lordosis of the lumbosacral spine and the increasing curvature of the thoracic area.

weight gain is 1.6–2.3 kg (3.5– to 5.0 lb) during the first trimester and 5.5–6.8 kg (12–15 lb) during each of the last two trimesters.

Water Metabolism Increased water retention, a basic alteration of pregnancy, is caused by several interrelated factors. The increased level of steroid sex hormones affects sodium and fluid retention. The lowered serum protein also influences fluid balance, as do increased intracapillary pressure and permeability. The extra water is needed for the fetus, placenta, and amniotic fluid and the mother's increased blood volume, interstitial fluids, and enlarged organs.

Nutrient Metabolism The fetus makes its greatest protein and fat demands during the second half of pregnancy, doubling in weight during the last 6–8 weeks. Protein (contributing nitrogen) must be stored during pregnancy to maintain a constant level in the breast milk and to avoid depletion of maternal tissues. Carbohydrate needs also increase, especially during the 2nd and 3rd trimesters.

Fats are more completely absorbed during pregnancy, and the level of free fatty acids increases in response to hPL. The levels of lipoproteins and cholesterol also increase. Because of these changes, increased levels of dietary fat or reduced carbohydrate production may lead to ketonuria in the pregnant woman.

ENDOCRINE SYSTEM

Thyroid The thyroid gland often enlarges slightly during pregnancy because of increased vascularity and hyperplasia of glandular tissue. Its capacity to bind thyroxine is greater, resulting in an increase in serum protein-bound iodine. These changes are because of higher blood levels of estrogen during pregnancy.

The basal metabolic rate increases by as much as 20–25% during pregnancy. The increased oxygen consumption is primarily because of fetal metabolic activity. Within a few weeks after birth, all thyroid function returns to normal limits.

Pituitary Pregnancy is made possible by the hypothalamic stimulation of the anterior pituitary gland. The anterior pituitary produces FSH, which stimulates ovum growth, and LH, which brings about ovulation. Stimulation of the pituitary also prolongs the ovary's corpus luteal phase, which maintains the endometrium in case conception occurs. Prolactin, another anterior pituitary hormone, is responsible for lactation.

The posterior pituitary secretes vasopressin (antidiuretic hormone) and oxytocin. Vasopressin causes vasoconstriction, which results in increased blood pressure; it also helps regulate water balance. Oxytocin promotes uterine contractility and stimulates ejection of milk from the breasts (the letdown reflex) in the postpartum period.

Adrenals No significant increase in the weight of the adrenal glands occurs during pregnancy. Circulating cortisol, which regulates carbohydrate and protein metabolism, increases in response to increased estrogen levels. Cortisol blood levels return to normal within 1–6 weeks postpartum.

The adrenals secrete increased levels of aldosterone by the early part of the 2nd trimester. This increase in aldosterone in a normal pregnancy may be the body's protective response to the increased sodium excretion associated with progesterone (Cunningham et al., 2005).

Pancreas The pregnant woman has increased insulin needs, and the pancreatic islets of Langerhans, which secrete insulin, are stressed to meet this increased demand. Any marginal pancreatic function quickly becomes apparent, and the woman may show signs of gestational diabetes.

Hormones in Pregnancy Several hormones are required to maintain pregnancy. Most of them are initially produced by the corpus luteum; then the placenta takes over production.

Human Chorionic Gonadotropin (hCG) The trophoblast secretes hCG in early pregnancy. This hormone stimulates progesterone and estrogen production by the corpus luteum to maintain the pregnancy until the placenta is developed sufficiently to assume that function. Human chorionic gonadotropin can be detected in maternal blood and urine as early as 8 days post-fertilization and peaks at 9–10 weeks (Burton, Sibley, & Jauniaux, 2007).

Human Placental Lactogen (hPL) Also called human chorionic somatomammotropin, hPL is produced by the syncytiotrophoblast. Human placental lactogen is an antagonist of insulin; it increases the amount of circulating free fatty acids for maternal metabolic needs and decreases maternal metabolism of glucose to favor fetal growth.

Estrogen, secreted originally by the corpus luteum, is produced primarily by the placenta as early as the 7th week of pregnancy. Estrogen stimulates uterine development to provide a suitable environment for the fetus. It also helps develop the ductal system of the breasts in preparation for lactation.

Progesterone Progesterone, also produced initially by the corpus luteum and then by the placenta, plays the greatest role in maintaining pregnancy. It maintains the endometrium and inhibits spontaneous uterine contractility, thus preventing early spontaneous abortion. Progesterone also helps develop the acini and lobules of the breasts in preparation for lactation.

Relaxin Relaxin is detectable in the serum of a pregnant woman by the time of the first missed menstrual period. Relaxin inhibits uterine activity, diminishes the strength of uterine contractions, aids in the softening of the cervix, and has the long-term effect of remodeling collagen. Its primary source is the corpus luteum, but small amounts are believed to be produced by the placenta and uterine decidua.

Prostaglandins in Pregnancy Prostaglandins are lipid substances that can arise from most body tissues but occur in high concentrations in the female reproductive tract and are present in the decidua during pregnancy. The exact functions of PGs during pregnancy are still unknown, although it has been proposed that they are responsible for maintaining reduced placental vascular resistance. Decreased PG levels may contribute to hypertension and preeclampsia. Prostaglandins also are believed to play a role in the complex biochemistry that initiates labor.

Signs of Pregnancy

Many of the changes women experience during pregnancy are used to diagnose the pregnancy itself. They are called the subjective, or presumptive, changes; the objective, or probable, changes; and the diagnostic, or positive, changes of pregnancy.

SUBJECTIVE (PRESUMPTIVE) CHANGES The subjective changes of pregnancy are the symptoms the woman experiences and reports. Because they can be caused by other conditions, they cannot be considered proof of pregnancy (Table 23–4). The following subjective signs can be diagnostic clues when other signs and symptoms of pregnancy are also present.

Amenorrhea, or the absence of menses, is the earliest symptom of pregnancy. The missing of more than one menstrual period, especially in a woman whose cycle is ordinarily regular, is an especially useful diagnostic clue. Excessive fatigue may be noted within a few weeks after the first missed menstrual period and may persist throughout the first trimester. Urinary frequency is experienced during the first trimester as the enlarging uterus presses on the bladder. This improves during the second trimester when the enlarging uterus escapes the pelvis and then recurs in the third trimester when the growing fetus presses on the bladder.

Nausea and vomiting in pregnancy (NVP) occur frequently during the first trimester and may be the result of elevated hCG levels and changed carbohydrate metabolism. Because these symptoms often occur in the early part of the day, they are commonly referred to as **morning sickness**. In reality, the symptoms may occur at any time and can range from a mere distaste for food to severe vomiting. Research indicates that women who experience NVP often have a more favorable pregnancy outcome than those who do not (Gordon, 2007).

Changes in the breasts are frequently noted in early pregnancy. These changes include tenderness and tingling sensations, increased pigmentation of the areola and nipple, and changes in Montgomery's glands. The veins also become more visible and form a bluish pattern beneath the skin.

Quickening, or the mother's perception of fetal movement, occurs about 18–20 weeks after the last menstrual period (LMP) in a woman pregnant for the first time but may occur as early as 16 weeks in a woman who has been pregnant before. Quickening is a fluttering sensation in the abdomen that gradually increases in intensity and frequency.

OBJECTIVE (PROBABLE) CHANGES An examiner can perceive the objective changes that occur in pregnancy. Because these changes also have other causes, they do not confirm pregnancy (Table 23–5).

TABLE 23–4 **Differential Diagnosis of Pregnancy—Subjective Changes**

SUBJECTIVE CHANGES	POSSIBLE ALTERNATIVE CAUSES
Amenorrhea	Endocrine factors: early menopause; lactation; thyroid, pituitary, adrenal, ovarian dysfunction
	Metabolic factors: malnutrition, anemia, climatic changes, diabetes mellitus, degenerative disorders, long-distance running
	Psychologic factors: emotional shock, fear of pregnancy or sexually transmitted infection (STI), intense desire for pregnancy (pseudocyesis), stress
	Obliteration of endometrial cavity by infection or curettage
	Systemic disease (acute or chronic) such as tuberculosis or malignancy
Nausea and vomiting	Gastrointestinal disorders
	Acute infections such as encephalitis
	Emotional disorders such as pseudocyesis or anorexia nervosa
Urinary frequency	Urinary tract infection
	Cystocele
	Pelvic tumors
	Urethral diverticula
	Emotional tension
Breast tenderness	Premenstrual tension
	Chronic cystic mastitis
	Pseudocyesis
	Hyperestrogenism
Quickening	Increased peristalsis
	Flatus (gas)
	Abdominal muscle contractions
	Shifting of abdominal contents

TABLE 23–5 **Differential Diagnosis of Pregnancy—Objective Changes**

OBJECTIVE CHANGES	POSSIBLE ALTERNATIVE CAUSES
Changes in pelvic organs	Increased vascular congestion
Goodell's sign	Estrogen–progestin oral contraceptives
Chadwick's sign	Vulvar, vaginal, cervical hyperemia
Hegar's sign	Excessively soft walls of nonpregnant uterus
Uterine enlargement	Uterine tumors
Von Braun-Fernwald's sign	Uterine tumors
Enlargement of abdomen	Obesity, ascites, pelvic tumors
Braxton Hicks contractions	Hematometra; pedunculated, submucous, and soft myomas
Uterine souffle	Large uterine myomas, large ovarian tumors, or any condition with greatly increased uterine blood flow
Pigmentation of skin	Estrogen–progestin oral contraceptives
Chloasma (Melasma)	Melanocyte hormonal stimulation
Linea nigra	
Nipples/areola	
Abdominal striae	Obesity, pelvic tumor
Ballottement	Uterine tumors/polyps, ascites
Pregnancy tests	Increased pituitary gonadotropins at menopause, choriocarcinoma, hydatidiform mole
Palpation for fetal outline	Uterine myomas

Changes in the pelvic organs—the only physical changes detectable during the first 3 months of pregnancy—are caused by increased vascular congestion. These changes are noted on pelvic examination. As noted earlier, there is a softening of the cervix called Goodell's sign. Chadwick's sign is a bluish, purple, or deep red discoloration of the mucous membranes of the cervix, vagina, and vulva. (Some sources consider this a presumptive sign.) **Hegar's sign** is a softening of the isthmus of the uterus, the area between the cervix and the body of the uterus (Figure 23–29 ■). **McDonald's sign** is an ease in flexing the body of the uterus against the cervix.

General enlargement and softening of the body of the uterus can be noted after the 8th week of pregnancy. The fundus of the uterus is palpable just above the symphysis pubis at about 10–12 weeks gestation and at the level of the umbilicus at 20–22 weeks gestation (Figure 23–30 ■).

Enlargement of the abdomen during the childbearing years is usually regarded as evidence of pregnancy, especially if it is continuous and accompanied by amenorrhea.

Braxton Hicks contractions can be palpated most commonly after 28 weeks. As the woman approaches the end of pregnancy, these contractions may become uncomfortable. They are then often called false labor.

Uterine souffle may be heard when the examiner auscultates the abdomen over the uterus. It is a soft blowing sound that occurs at the same rate as the maternal pulse and is caused by

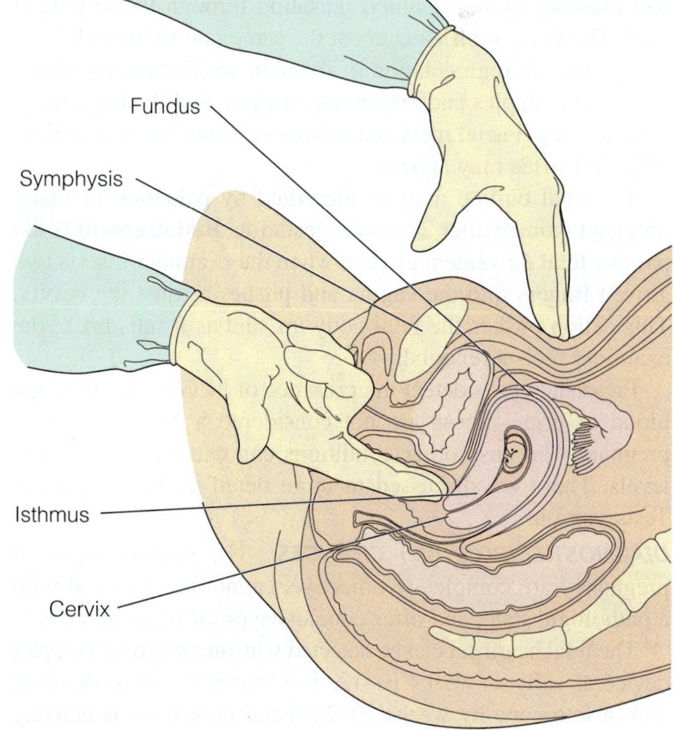

Figure 23–29 ■ Hegar's sign, a softening of the isthmus of the uterus, can be determined by the examiner during a vaginal examination.

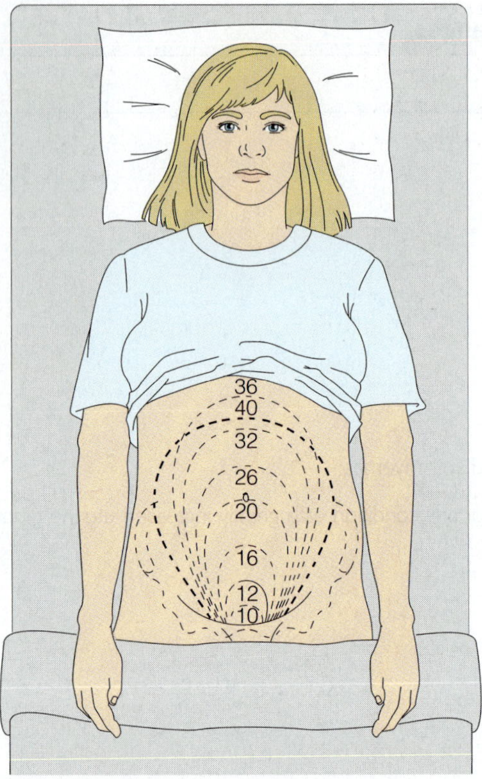

Figure 23–30 ■ Approximate height of the fundus at various weeks of pregnancy.

the increased uterine blood flow and blood pulsating through the placenta. It is sometimes confused with the funic souffle, a soft blowing sound of blood pulsating through the umbilical cord. The funic souffle occurs at the same rate as the FHR.

Changes in pigmentation of the skin are common in pregnancy. The nipples and areola may darken, and the linea nigra may develop. Facial melasma (chloasma) may become noticeable, and striae may appear.

The fetal outline may be identified by palpation in many pregnant women after 24 weeks gestation. **Ballottement** is the passive fetal movement elicited when the examiner inserts two gloved fingers into the vagina and pushes against the cervix. This action pushes the fetal body up, and as it falls back, the examiner feels a rebound.

Pregnancy tests detect the presence of hCG in the maternal blood or urine. These are not considered a positive sign of pregnancy because other conditions can cause elevated hCG levels. These are discussed in more detail in the Diagnostic Tests section.

DIAGNOSTIC (POSITIVE) CHANGES The positive signs of pregnancy are completely objective, cannot be confused with a pathologic state, and offer conclusive proof of pregnancy.

The fetal heartbeat can be detected with an electronic Doppler device as early as weeks 10–12. The heartbeat can be detected with a fetoscope by weeks 17–20. Fetal movement is actively palpable by a trained examiner after about week 20 of pregnancy.

Visualization of the fetus by ultrasound examination confirms a pregnancy. The gestational sac can be observed by 4–5 weeks gestation (2–3 weeks after conception). Fetal parts and fetal heart movement can be seen as early as 8 weeks gestation. More recently ultrasound using a vaginal probe has been used to detect a gestational sac as early as 10 days after implantation (Cunningham et al., 2005).

Psychologic Response of the Expectant Family to Pregnancy

Pregnancy is a turning point in a family's life, accompanied by stress and anxiety, whether the pregnancy is desired or not. Especially when this is their first child, the expectant parents may be unaware of the physical, emotional, and cognitive changes of pregnancy and may anticipate no problems from such a normal event. Thus, they may be confused and distressed by new feelings and behaviors that are essentially normal.

For beginning families, pregnancy is the transition period from childlessness to parenthood. If the expectant woman is married or has a stable partner, she is no longer only a mate, but also must assume the role of mother. Her partner, whether male or female, will become a parent too. The anticipation of parenthood brings significant role changes for them. Career goals and mobility may be affected, and the couple's relationship takes on a different meaning to them and their families and community. If the pregnancy results in the birth of a child, the couple enters a new, irreversible stage of their life together. With each subsequent pregnancy, routines and family dynamics are again altered, requiring readjustment and realignment.

In most pregnancies, finances are an important consideration. Traditional lore relegates to the father the role of primary breadwinner, and finances are often a very real concern for fathers. In today's society, however, there are many types of families and even pregnant women with stable partners recognize the financial impact of a child and may be concerned about financial issues. Decisions about financial matters need to be made at this time. Will the woman work during her pregnancy and return to work after her child is born? If so, who will provide child care? Couples also may need to decide about the division of domestic tasks. Any differences of opinion must be discussed openly and resolved so that the family can meet the needs of its members.

If the pregnant woman has no stable partner, she must deal with the role changes, fears, and adjustments of pregnancy alone or seek support from family or friends. She also faces the reality of planning for the future as a single parent. Finances may be a major source of concern. Even if the pregnant woman plans to relinquish her infant, she still must deal with the adjustments of pregnancy. This adjustment can be especially difficult without a good support system.

DEVELOPMENTAL TASKS OF THE EXPECTANT COUPLE Pregnancy can be viewed as a developmental stage with its own distinct developmental tasks. For a couple, it can be a time of support or conflict depending on the amount of adjustment each is willing to make to maintain the family's equilibrium.

During a first pregnancy, the couple plans together for the child's arrival, collecting information on how to be parents. At the same time, each continues to participate in some separate activities with friends or family members. The availability of social support is an important factor in psychosocial well-being during pregnancy. The social network is often a major source of advice for the pregnant woman; however, both sound and unsound information may be conveyed.

During pregnancy, the expectant parents face significant changes and must deal with major psychosocial adjustments (Table 23–6). Other family members, especially other children of the woman or couple and the grandparents-to-be, also must adjust to the pregnancy.

For some, pregnancy is more than a developmental stage; it is a crisis. *Crisis* can be defined as "a disturbance or conflict in which the individual cannot maintain a state of equilibrium." Pregnancy can be considered a *maturational crisis,* as it is a common event in the normal growth and development of the family. During such a crisis, the individual or family is in disequilibrium. Egos weaken, usual defense mechanisms are not effective, unresolved material from the past reappears, and relationships shift. The period of disequilibrium and disorganization is marked by unsuccessful attempts to solve the perceived problems. If the crisis is not resolved, it will result in maladaptive behaviors in one or more family members and possible disintegration of the family. Families that are able to resolve a maturational crisis will return successfully to normal functioning and can even strengthen the bonds in the family relationship.

THE MOTHER Pregnancy is a condition that alters body image and necessitates a reordering of social relationships and changes in roles of family members. The way each woman meets the stresses of pregnancy is influenced by her emotional makeup, her sociologic and cultural background, and her acceptance or rejection of the pregnancy. However, many women manifest similar psychologic and emotional responses during pregnancy, including ambivalence, acceptance, introversion, mood swings, and changes in body image.

TABLE 23–6 **Parental Reactions to Pregnancy**

FIRST TRIMESTER	SECOND TRIMESTER	THIRD TRIMESTER
Mother's Reactions	**Mother's Reactions**	**Mother's Reactions**
Informs father secretively or openly. Feels ambivalent toward pregnancy, anxious about labor and responsibility of child. Is aware of physical changes, daydreams of possible miscarriage. Develops special feelings for and renewed interest in her own mother, with formation of a personal identity.	Remains regressive and introspective, projects all problems with authority figures onto partner, may become angry as if lack of interest is sign of weakness in him. Continues to deal with feelings as a mother and looks for furniture as something concrete. May have other extreme of anxiety and wait until 9th month to look for furniture and clothes for baby. Feels movement and is aware of fetus and incorporates it into herself. Dreams that partner will be killed, telephones him often for reassurance. Experiences more distinct physical changes; sexual desires may increase or decrease.	Experiences more anxiety and tension, with physical awkwardness. Feels much discomfort and insomnia from physical condition. Prepares for birth, assembles layette, picks out names. Dreams often about misplacing baby or not being able to give birth, fears birth of deformed baby. Feels ecstasy and excitement, has spurt of energy during last month.
Father's Reactions	**Father's Reactions**	**Father's Reactions**
Differ according to age, parity, desire for child, economic stability. Acceptance of pregnant woman's attitude or complete rejection and lack of communication. Is aware of his own sexual feelings, may develop more or less sexual arousal. Accepts, rejects, or resents mother-in-law. May develop new hobby outside of family as sign of stress.	If he can cope, will give partner extra attention she needs; if he cannot cope, will develop a new time-consuming interest outside the home. May develop a creative feeling and a "closeness to nature." May become involved in pregnancy and buy or make furniture. Feels for movement of baby, listens to heartbeat, or remains aloof, with no physical contact. May have fears and fantasies about himself being pregnant, may become uneasy with this feminine aspect in himself. May react negatively if partner is too demanding, may become jealous of physician and of physician's importance to partner and her pregnancy.	Adapts to alternative methods of sexual contact. Becomes concerned over financial responsibility. May show new sense of tenderness and concern, treats partner like a doll. Daydreams about child as if older and not newborn, dreams of losing partner. Renewed sexual attraction to partner. Feels responsible for whatever happens.

A woman's attitude toward her pregnancy can be a significant factor in its outcome. Even if the pregnancy is planned, there is an element of surprise at first. Many women commonly experience feelings of ambivalence during early pregnancy. This ambivalence may be related to feelings that the timing is somehow wrong; worries about the need to modify existing relationships or career plans; fears about assuming a new role; unresolved emotional conflicts with the woman's own mother; and fears about pregnancy, labor, and birth. These feelings may be more pronounced if the pregnancy is unplanned or unwanted. Indirect expressions of ambivalence include complaints about considerable physical discomfort, prolonged or frequent depression, significant dissatisfaction with changing body shape, excessive mood swings, and difficulty in accepting the life changes resulting from the pregnancy.

Many pregnancies are unintended, but not all unintended pregnancies are unwanted. A pregnancy can be unintended and wanted at the same time. For some women, an unintended pregnancy has more psychologic and social advantages than disadvantages. It provides purpose and direction to life and allows a woman to test the devotion and love of her partner and family. However, an unintended pregnancy can be a risk factor for depression. Women with an unintended pregnancy also may perceive life events as being more stressful than women with an intended pregnancy—another contributor to depression. Depression, in turn, can negatively impact a woman's health choices and behaviors (Messer, Dole, Kaufman, & Savitz, 2005).

Conflicts about adapting to pregnancy are no more pronounced for older pregnant women (aged 35 and over) than for younger ones. Moreover, older pregnant women tend to be less concerned about the normal physical changes of pregnancy and are confident about handling issues that arise during pregnancy and parenting. This difference may result because mature pregnant women have more experience with problem solving. However, mature pregnant women may have fewer pregnant peers and thus may have fewer people with whom to share concerns and expectations.

Pregnancy produces marked changes in a woman's body within a relatively short period of time. Pregnant women experience changes in body image because of physical alterations and may feel a loss of control over their bodies during pregnancy and later during childbirth. These perceptions are related to a certain extent to personality factors, social network responses, and attitudes toward pregnancy. Although changes in body image are normal, they can be very stressful for the woman. Explanation and discussion of the changes may help both the woman and her partner deal with the stress associated with this aspect of pregnancy.

Fantasies about the unborn child are common among pregnant women. The themes of the fantasies (baby's appearance, gender, traits, impact on parents, etc.) vary by trimester and differ between women who are pregnant for the first time and women who already have children.

First Trimester During the first trimester, feelings of disbelief and ambivalence are paramount. The woman's baby does not seem real, and she focuses on herself and her pregnancy. She may experience one or more of the early symptoms of pregnancy, such as breast tenderness or morning sickness, which are unsettling and at times unpleasant.

At this time, the expectant mother also begins to exhibit some characteristic behavioral changes. She may become increasingly introspective and passive. She may be emotionally labile, with characteristic mood swings from joy to despair. She may fantasize about a miscarriage and feel guilt because of these fantasies. She may worry that these thoughts will harm the baby in some way.

Second Trimester During the second trimester, quickening occurs. This perception of fetal movement helps the woman think of her baby as a separate person, and she generally becomes excited about the pregnancy even if she had not been looking forward to the pregnancy earlier. The woman becomes increasingly introspective as she evaluates her life, her plans, and her child's future. This introspection helps the woman prepare for her new mothering role. Emotional lability, which may be unsettling to her partner, persists. In some instances, the partner may react by withdrawing. This withdrawal is especially distressing to the woman because she needs increased love and affection. Once the couple understands that these behaviors are characteristic of pregnancy, it is easier for the couple to deal with them effectively, although to some extent they may be sources of stress throughout pregnancy.

As pregnancy becomes more noticeable, the woman's body image changes. She may feel great pride, embarrassment, or concern. Generally, women feel best during the second trimester, which is a relatively tranquil time.

Third Trimester In the third trimester, the woman feels both pride about her pregnancy and anxiety about labor and birth. Physical discomforts increase, and the woman is eager for the pregnancy to end. She experiences increased fatigue, her body movements are more awkward, and her interest in sexual activity may decrease. During this time, the woman tends to be concerned about the health and safety of her unborn child and may worry that she will not cope well during childbirth. Toward the end of this period, the woman often experiences a surge of energy as she prepares a "nest" for the infant. Many women report bursts of energy, during which they vigorously clean and organize the home.

Psychologic Tasks of the Mother Rubin (1984) identified four major tasks that the pregnant woman undertakes to maintain her intactness and that of her family and at the same time to incorporate her new child into the family system. These tasks form the foundation for a mutually gratifying relationship with her infant.

1. *Ensuring safe passage through pregnancy, labor, and birth.* The pregnant woman feels concern for her unborn child and for herself. She looks for competent maternity care to provide a sense of control. She may seek information from literature, observation of other pregnant women and new mothers, and discussion with others. She also attempts to ensure safe passage by engaging in self-care activities related to diet, exercise, alcohol consumption,

etc. In the 3rd trimester, she becomes more aware of external threats in the environment—a toy on the stairs, the awkwardness of an escalator—that pose a threat to her well-being. She may worry if her partner is late or if she is home alone. Sleep becomes more difficult, and she longs for birth even though it, too, is frightening.

2. *Seeking acceptance of this child by others.* The birth of a child alters a woman's primary support group (her family) and her secondary affiliative groups. The woman slowly and subtly alters her network to meet the needs of her pregnancy. In this adjustment, the woman's partner is the most important figure. The partner's support and acceptance help form a maternal identity. If there are other children in the home, the mother also works to ensure their acceptance of the coming child. Acceptance of the anticipated change is sometimes stressful, and the woman may work to maintain special time with her partner or older children. The woman without a partner looks to others, such as a family member or friend, for this support.
3. *Seeking commitment and acceptance of herself as mother to the infant (binding in).* During the first trimester, the child remains a rather abstract concept. With quickening, however, the child begins to become a real person and the mother begins to develop bonds of attachment. The mother experiences the movement of the child within her in an intimate, exclusive way, and out of this experience, bonds of love form. This binding-in process, characterized by its strong emotional component, motivates the pregnant woman to become competent in her role and provides satisfaction for her in the role of mother. This possessive love increases her maternal commitment to protect her fetus now and her child after he or she is born.
4. *Learning to give of oneself on behalf of one's child.* Childbirth involves many acts of giving. The man "gives" a child to the woman; she in turn "gives" a child to him. Life is given to an infant; a sibling is given to older children of the family. The woman begins to develop a capacity for self-denial and learns to delay immediate personal gratification to meet the needs of another. Baby showers and gifts are acts of giving that increase the mother's self-esteem and help her recognize the separateness and needs of the coming baby.

Accomplishment of these tasks helps the expectant woman develop her self-concept as mother. The expectant woman who was well nurtured by her own mother may view her mother as a role model and emulate her; the woman who views her mother as a "poor mother" may worry that she will make similar mistakes. A woman's self-concept as a mother expands with experience and continues to grow through subsequent childbearing and childrearing. Occasionally, a woman fails to accept the mother role, instead playing the role of babysitter or older sister to her child.

THE FATHER For the expectant father, pregnancy is a psychologically stressful time because he, too, must make the transition from nonparent to parent or from parent of one or more to parent of two or more. Research indicates that most men handle the transition to fatherhood well and that in general, any anxieties they feel resolve over time. However, the anxieties they have are sometimes missed prenatally because most attention is devoted to the expectant mother (Buist, Morse, & Durkin, 2003).

Initially, expectant fathers may feel pride in their virility, which pregnancy confirms, but also have many of the same ambivalent feelings as expectant mothers. The extent of ambivalence depends on many factors, including the father's relationship with his partner, his previous experience with pregnancy, his age, and his economic stability and whether the pregnancy was planned.

In adjusting to his role, the expectant father must first deal with the reality of the pregnancy and then struggle to gain recognition as a parent from his partner, family, friends, coworkers, and society—and from his baby. The expectant mother can help her partner be a participant and not merely a helpmate to her if she has a definite sense of the experience as *their* pregnancy and *their* infant and not *her* pregnancy and *her* infant.

The expectant father must establish a fatherhood role, just as the woman develops a motherhood role. Fathers who are most successful at this task generally like children, are excited about the prospect of fatherhood, are eager to nurture a child, and have confidence in their ability to be a parent. They also share the experiences of pregnancy and birth with their partner (Table 23–6).

First Trimester After the initial excitement attending the announcement of the pregnancy, an expectant father may begin to feel left out. He may be confused by his partner's mood changes. He might resent the attention she receives and her need to modify their relationship as she experiences fatigue and possibly a decreased interest in sex. In addition, he might be concerned about what kind of father he will be. During this time, his child is a "potential" baby. Fathers often picture themselves interacting with a child of 5 or 6 years, not a newborn. The pregnancy itself may seem unreal until the woman shows more physical signs.

Second Trimester The father's role in the pregnancy is still vague in the 2nd trimester, but his involvement may increase as he watches and feels fetal movement and listens to the fetal heartbeat during a prenatal visit. For many men, seeing their infant on ultrasound is an important experience in accepting the reality of pregnancy. Like expectant mothers, expectant fathers need to confront and resolve some of their conflicts about the fathering they received. A father needs to sort out which behaviors of his own father he wants to imitate and which he wants to avoid.

Evidence suggests that the father-to-be's anxiety is lessened when both parents agree on the paternal role the man is to assume. For example, if both of them see his role as that of breadwinner, the man's stress is low. However, if the man views his role as that of breadwinner and the woman expects him to be actively involved in child care, his stress increases. An open, honest discussion about the expectations the parents have about their roles will help the father-to-be in his transition to fatherhood (Goodman, 2005).

As the woman's appearance begins to change, her partner may have several reactions. Her changed appearance may decrease his sexual interest, or it may have the opposite effect. Because of the variety of emotions both partners may feel, continued communication and acceptance are important.

Third Trimester If the couple's relationship has grown through effective communication of their concerns and feelings, the 3rd trimester is often a rewarding time. They may attend childbirth classes and make concrete preparations for the arrival of the baby. If the father has developed a detached attitude about the pregnancy, however, it is unlikely he will become a willing participant, even though his role becomes more obvious.

Concerns and fears may recur. The father may worry about hurting the unborn baby during intercourse or become concerned about labor and birth. Also, he may wonder what kind of parents he and his partner will be.

SIBLINGS Bringing a new baby home often marks the beginning of sibling rivalry. The siblings view the baby as a threat to the security of their relationships with their parents. Parents who recognize this potential problem early in pregnancy and begin constructive actions can minimize the problem of sibling rivalry.

Preparation of the young child begins several weeks before the anticipated birth. Because they do not have a clear concept of time, young children should not be told too early about the pregnancy. From the toddler's point of view, several weeks is an extremely long time. The mother may let the child feel the baby moving in her uterus, explaining that the uterus is "a special place where babies grow." The child can help the parents put the baby clothes in drawers and prepare the nursery.

The concept of consistency is important in dealing with young children. They need reassurance that certain people, special things, and familiar places will continue to exist after the new baby arrives. The crib is often an important although transient object in a child's life. If it is to be given to the new baby, the parents should thoughtfully help the older child adjust to this change. Any move from crib to bed or from one room to another should precede the baby's birth by at least several weeks. If the new baby is to share a room with siblings, the parents also must discuss this situation with the older child or children.

FOCUS ON DIVERSITY AND CULTURE
Couvade

Traditionally, couvade has referred to the male's observance of certain rituals and taboos to signify the transition to fatherhood. This observance affirms his psychosocial and biophysical relationship to the woman and child. Some taboos restrict his actions. For example, in some cultures, the man may be forbidden to eat certain foods or carry certain weapons before and immediately after the birth. More recently, the term has been used to describe the unintentional development of physical symptoms such as fatigue, increased appetite, difficulty sleeping, depression, headache, or backache by the partner of a pregnant woman. Men who demonstrate couvade syndrome tend to have a higher degree of paternal role preparation and be involved in more activities related to this preparation.

Some parents advocate cosleeping (one or both parents sleeping with the baby or young child), in which case the crib is less of an issue. Cosleeping, common in many non-Western cultures, is on the increase in the United States. Opinion varies sharply about the advantages and risks of the practice, especially in light of an American Academy of Pediatrics (AAP) policy statement (2005) that recommends against cosleeping because of the increased risk of sudden infant death syndrome (SIDS). The AAP stresses that the infant can be brought to the bed to be comforted or to be breastfed, but should be placed supine in a separate bed ("back to bed") to sleep. Parents who choose to cosleep must make decisions about the sleeping arrangements of other siblings following the birth of the baby.

If the child is ready, toilet training is most effective several months before or after the baby's arrival. It is not unusual for an older toilet-trained child to regress to wetting or soiling because of the attention given to the newborn for such behavior. The older weaned child may want to nurse or drink from the bottle again after the baby arrives. If the new mother anticipates these behaviors, they will be less frustrating during her early postpartum days.

Pregnant women may find it helpful to bring their children on a prenatal visit to the certified nurse-midwife (CNM) or physician to give them an opportunity to listen to the fetal heartbeat. This visit helps make the baby more real to the children; they also may become involved in the prenatal care.

If siblings are school-age children, pregnancy should be viewed as a family affair. Teaching should be suitable to the child's level of understanding and may be supplemented with appropriate books. Taking part in family discussions, attending sibling preparation classes, feeling fetal movement, and listening to the fetal heartbeat help the school-age child take part in the experience of pregnancy and not feel like an outsider.

Older children and adolescents may appear to have sophisticated knowledge but may have many misconceptions about pregnancy and birth. The parents should discuss their concerns and involve the children in preparations for the new baby.

Even after birth, siblings need to feel that they are taking part. Having siblings visit their mother and the new baby at the hospital or birthing center will help. After the baby comes home, siblings can share in showing off the new baby.

Sibling preparation is essential, but other factors are equally important. These factors include how much parental attention the new arrival receives, how much attention the older child receives after the baby comes home, and how well the parents handle regressive or aggressive behavior.

GRANDPARENTS The first relatives told about a pregnancy are usually the grandparents. Often the expectant grandparents become increasingly supportive of the couple even if conflicts existed previously. But even sensitive grandparents may have difficulty knowing how deeply to become involved in the childrearing process.

Because grandparenting can occur over a wide expanse of years, people's response to this role varies considerably. Younger grandparents leading active lives may not demonstrate as much interest as the young couple would like. In other cases, expectant grandparents may give advice and gifts unsparingly. For grandparents, conflict may be related to the expectant couple's need to feel in control of their lives or it may stem from events signaling changing roles in the grandparents' lives (e.g., retirement, financial concerns, menopause, or death of a friend). Some parents of expectant couples may already be grandparents with a developed style of grandparenting. This influences their response to the pregnancy.

Because childbearing and childrearing practices have changed, family cohesiveness is promoted by effective communication and frank discussion between young couples and interested grandparents about the changes and the reasons for those changes. Clarifying the role of the helping grandparent ensures a comfortable situation for all.

Classes for grandparents may provide information about changes in birth and parenting practices. These classes help familiarize grandparents with new parents' needs and may offer suggestions for ways in which the grandparents can support the childbearing couple.

Cultural Values and Pregnancy

A universal tendency exists to create ceremonial rituals or rites around important life events. Thus, pregnancy, childbirth, marriage, and death are often tied to ritual. The rituals and customs of a group are a reflection of the group's values. Therefore, the identification of cultural values is useful in predicting reactions to pregnancy. An understanding of male and female roles, family lifestyles, religious values, or the meaning of children in a culture may explain reactions of joy or shame.

Generalization about cultural characteristics or values is difficult because not every individual in a culture may display these characteristics. Just as variations are seen between cultures, variations are also seen within cultures. For example, because of their exposure to the American culture, a third-generation Chinese American family might have different values and beliefs from those of a Chinese family that has recently immigrated to America. For this reason, the nurse needs to supplement a general knowledge of cultural values and practices with a complete assessment of the individual's values and practices. The following Focus on Diversity and Culture feature summarizes the key actions a nurse can take to become more culturally aware.

Cultural assessment is an important aspect of prenatal care. Increasingly, health care professionals know that they must address cultural needs in the prenatal assessment to provide culturally sensitive health care during pregnancy. The nurse needs to identify the prospective parents' main beliefs, values, and behaviors related to pregnancy and childbearing. This includes information about ethnic background, degree of affiliation with the ethnic group, patterns of decision making, religious preference, language, communication style, and common etiquette practices. The nurse also can explore the woman's (or family's) expectations of the health care system. Once this information is gathered, the nurse can plan and provide care that is appropriate and responsive to family needs.

FOCUS ON DIVERSITY AND CULTURE
Providing Culturally Sensitive Care

Nurses who are interacting with expectant families from a different culture or ethnic group can provide more effective, culturally sensitive nursing care by

- Critically examining their own cultural beliefs
- Identifying personal biases, attitudes, stereotypes, and prejudices
- Making a conscious commitment to respect and study the values and beliefs of others
- Using sensitive, current language when describing others' cultures
- Learning the rituals, customs, and practices of the major cultural and ethnic groups with whom they have contact
- Including cultural assessment and assessment of the family's expectations of the health care system as a routine part of prenatal nursing care
- Incorporating the family's cultural and spiritual practices into prenatal care as much as possible
- Fostering an attitude of respect for and cooperation with alternative healers and caregivers when possible
- Providing for the services of an interpreter when language barriers exist
- Learning the language (or at least several key phrases) of at least one of the cultural groups with whom they interact
- Recognizing that ultimately it is the woman's right to make her own health care choices
- Evaluating whether the client's health care beliefs have any potential negative consequences for her health

ADOLESCENT PREGNANCY

Factors Contributing to Adolescent Pregnancy

SOCIOECONOMIC AND CULTURAL FACTORS Poverty is a major risk factor for adolescent pregnancy. Adolescents who do not have access to middle-class opportunities tend to maintain their pregnancies because they see pregnancy as their only option for adult status; 85% of births to unmarried teens occur among those adolescents from poor or low-income families (Alan Guttmacher Institute, 2006). Not surprisingly, research indicates that the more time high school students spend without adult supervision, the greater their level of sexual activity.

In the United States, the adolescent birth rate is higher among African American teens (63.7 births per 1,000) and Hispanic teens (83 births per 1,000) than among white teens (26.6 births per 1,000). However, until 2006, these pregnancy rates had been declining (Hamilton, Martin, & Ventura, 2007). To some degree, the higher teenage pregnancy rate in these groups reflects the impact of poverty, as a disproportionately higher number of African American and Hispanic youths live in poverty.

Low educational achievement is another major risk factor for adolescent pregnancy. Teenage girls who participate in after-school activities are less likely to be sexually experienced than girls who do not participate (Cohen, Farley, Taylor, Martin, & Schuster, 2002). Similarly, compared with other teens, teens with future goals (i.e., college or work) tend to use birth control more consistently; if they do become pregnant, they are more likely to have abortions.

The younger the teen when she first gets pregnant, the more likely she is to have another pregnancy in her teens. Moreover, the likelihood of repeat pregnancies increases when the teen is living with a sexual partner and has dropped out of school. Daughters and sisters of women who had a baby in their early teens tend to have intercourse earlier and are at higher risk for teen pregnancy (Short & Rosenthal, 2003).

Internationally, adolescent women are more likely to welcome a pregnancy in a country (1) in which Islam is the predominant religion, (2) where large families are desired, (3) where social change is slow in coming, and (4) where most childbearing occurs within marriage. Early pregnancy is less desired in countries in which the reverse is true.

HIGH-RISK BEHAVIORS Developmentally, adolescents, especially younger ones, are not yet able to foresee the consequences of their actions. As a result, they may have a sense of invulnerability that leads to the mistaken idea that harm will not befall them. This sense of invulnerability also may result in an overly optimistic view of the risks associated with their actions (King-Jones, 2008).

Among American adolescents, there is tremendous peer pressure to become sexually active during the teen years. Premarital sexual activity is commonplace, and teenage pregnancy is more socially acceptable today than it was in the past. In fact, nearly half (46%) of all teens aged 15–19 have had sex at least once (Alan Guttmacher Institute , 2006). Sexual innuendo permeates every aspect of the popular media, including music, music videos, television, and movies, but issues of sexual responsibility are commonly ignored.

High-risk sexual behaviors, including, for example, multiple partners and lack of contraceptive use, are of concern. Research indicates that young people aged 15–24 comprise 25% of the sexually experienced population in the United States; however, they account for 48% of the new cases of STIs. This is particularly worrisome because many STIs, including HIV, are asymptomatic. Thus, apparently healthy young people who are infected may not have a reason to seek health care (Weinstock, Berman, & Cates, 2004).

Worldwide, people younger than 25 account for the greatest proportion of STIs. Moreover, estimates suggest that 6,000 young people are infected with HIV *daily* (Bearinger, Sieving, Ferguson, & Sharma, 2007).

Statistics have demonstrated an increased use of condoms among the adolescent population, probably because of the tremendous educational efforts related to HIV. Among currently sexually active students, 62.8% report using a condom during their last sexual intercourse (Eaton et al., 2006). Nevertheless, adolescents remain inconsistent contraceptive users. Contraceptive use is more consistent when teens discuss contraception before having sex, when they have waited a longer time after starting a relationship to have sex with that person, and when they use dual methods of contraception (Manlove, Ryan, & Franzetta, 2003).

Many teens lack accurate and adequate knowledge about contraceptive options. This is a common topic of sex education programs; however, debate continues about the appropriateness of such programs in schools. Proponents advocate early sex education to provide teens with the knowledge they need to avoid unwanted pregnancy and the risk of STIs. Opponents believe that sex education is the responsibility of parents and worry that sex education in the schools will promote sexual activity. However, a review of research on sex education reveals that it does not increase initiation of sexual activity at an earlier age (Doniger, Adams, Utter, & Riley, 2001). Other factors affecting the use of contraception include access or availability, cost of supplies, and concern about confidentiality.

PSYCHOSOCIAL FACTORS Family dysfunction and poor self-esteem are also major risk factors for adolescent pregnancy. Some young teenagers deliberately plan to get pregnant. The adolescent girl may use pregnancy for various subconscious or conscious reasons: to punish her father and/or mother, to escape from an undesirable home situation, to gain attention, or to feel that she has someone to love and to love her. Pregnancy also may be a young woman's form of acting out. In some circumstances, pregnancy may represent an important milestone that leads to positive lifestyle changes and healthier behaviors (Klima, 2003).

Teenage pregnancy can result from an incestuous relationship. In the very young adolescent, incest or sexual abuse should be suspected as a possible cause of pregnancy. More teens who become pregnant, compared with teens who have not been pregnant, have been physically, emotionally, or sexually abused. In fact, maltreatment of any kind is a high-risk contributor to early teen pregnancy (Montgomery, 2003). Teenage pregnancy also may be the result of other nonvoluntary sexual experiences such as acquaintance rape.

Risks to the Adolescent Mother

Adolescent pregnancy carries a number of risks, especially for those who become pregnant before age 15. It carries greater risk when the mother does not receive timely prenatal care, regardless of her age at conception. This section discusses the risks associated with adolescent pregnancy.

PHYSIOLOGIC RISKS Adolescents over age 15 who receive early, thorough prenatal care are at no greater risk during pregnancy than women over age 20. Unfortunately, adolescents typically begin prenatal care later in pregnancy than any other age group. Thus, risks for pregnant adolescents include preterm births, low-birth-weight infants, cephalopelvic disproportion (CPD), iron deficiency anemia, and preeclampsia–eclampsia and its sequelae. In the adolescent age group, prenatal care is the critical factor that most influences pregnancy outcome.

Teenagers ages 15–19 have a high incidence of sexually transmitted infections, including genital herpes, syphilis, and gonorrhea. The incidence of chlamydial infection also increases in this age group. The presence of such infections during a pregnancy greatly increases the risk to the fetus. (Refer to Concept 26, Sexuality.) Other problems seen in adolescents are cigarette smoking and drug use. By the time pregnancy is confirmed in a young woman, these substances may have already harmed the fetus.

PSYCHOLOGIC RISKS The major psychologic risk to the pregnant adolescent is the interruption of her developmental tasks. Adding the tasks of pregnancy to her other developmental tasks creates an overwhelming amount of psychologic work, the completion of which will affect the adolescent's future and that of her newborn. Table 23–7 suggests typical behaviors of the early, middle, and late adolescent when she becomes aware of her pregnancy. In reviewing these behaviors, the nurse should realize that other factors may influence individual response.

SOCIOLOGIC RISKS Being forced into adult roles before completing adolescent developmental tasks causes a series of events that affects the adolescent's entire life. These events may result in a prolonged dependence on parents, a lack of stable relationships with the opposite sex, and a lack of economic and social stability.

Many teenage mothers drop out of school during their pregnancy and then are less likely to complete their schooling. Similarly, they are less likely to go to college, more likely to have big families, and more likely to be single. Lack of education, in turn, reduces the quality of jobs available. Childbearing at an early age is a strong predictor that the adolescent mother's children will live in poverty (Kirby, 2007).

Adolescent mothers frequently fail to establish a stable family, especially when they have a second child while still in their teens. Their family structure tends to be a single-parent, matriarchal structure—often the same type in which the adolescents themselves were raised.

Some pregnant adolescents choose to marry the father of the baby, who also may be a teenager. Unfortunately, the majority of adolescent marriages end in divorce. This fact should not be surprising because pregnancy and marriage interrupt the adolescents' childhood and basic education. Lack of maturity in dealing with an intimate relationship also contributes to marital breakdown in this age group.

Studies suggest that 16–37% of pregnant teens experience domestic violence. This rate is higher than that estimated for pregnant adults and suggests that teens are more susceptible to such victimization than are pregnant adults (Scheiman & Zeoli, 2003). Dating violence is often an issue for teens, especially for younger girls dating older boys. These younger teens may interpret such actions as hitting, pushing, and making verbal threats as signs of love and caring and a deep commitment to the relationship that will ultimately produce long-term positive results (Glass, Fredland, Campbell, Yonas, Sharps, & Kub, 2003).

TABLE 23–7 **Initial Reaction to Awareness of Pregnancy**

AGE	ADOLESCENT BEHAVIOR	NURSING IMPLICATIONS
Early adolescent (14 and under)	Fears rejection by family and peers. Enters health care system with an adult, most likely mother (parents still seen as locus of control). Value system still closely reflects that of parents, so still turns to parents for decision or approval of decision. Pregnancy probably is not the result of intimate relationship. Is self-conscious about normal adolescent changes in body. Self-consciousness and low self-esteem likely to increase with rapid breast enlargement and abdominal enlargement of pregnancy.	Be nonjudgmental in approach to care. Focus on needs and concerns of adolescent, but if parent accompanies daughter, include parent in plan of care. Encourage both to express concerns and feelings regarding pregnancy and options: having an abortion, maintaining pregnancy, giving baby up for adoption. Be realistic and concrete in discussing implications of each option. During physical exam of adolescent, respect increased sense of modesty. Explain in simple and concrete terms physical changes that are produced by pregnancy versus puberty. Explain each step of physical exam in simple and concrete terms.
Middle adolescent (15–17 years)	Fears rejection by peers and parents. Unsure in whom to confide. May seek confirmation of pregnancy on own with increased awareness of options and services such as over-the-counter pregnancy kits, Planned Parenthood, and Birthright. If in an ongoing, caring relationship with partner (peer), adolescent may choose him as confidant. Economic dependence on parents may determine if and when parents are told. Future educational plans and perception of parental support or lack of support are significant factors in decision regarding termination or maintenance of the pregnancy. Possible conflict in parental and own developing value system.	Be nonjudgmental in approach to care. Reassure the adolescent that confidentiality will be maintained. Help adolescent identify significant individuals in whom she can confide to help make a decision about the pregnancy. Be aware of state laws regarding requirement of parental notification if abortion is intended. Also be aware of state laws regarding requirements for marriage: minimum age for both parties is usually18; in most states, 16- and 17-year-olds are allowed to marry only with consent of parents. Encourage adolescent to be realistic about parental response to pregnancy.
Late adolescent (18–19 years)	Most likely to confirm pregnancy on own and at an earlier date because of increased acceptance and awareness of consequences of behavior. Likely to use pregnancy kit for confirmation. Relationship with father of baby, future educational plans, and own value system are among significant determinants of decision about pregnancy.	Be nonjudgmental in approach to care. Reassure the adolescent that confidentiality will be maintained. Encourage adolescent to identify significant individuals in whom she can confide. Refer to counseling as appropriate. Encourage adolescent to be realistic about parental response to pregnancy.

The increased incidence of maternal complications, premature birth, and low-birth-weight babies among adolescent mothers also has an impact on society because many of these mothers receive government support. The need for increased financial support for good prenatal care and nutritional programs remains critical.

Table 23–8 identifies the early adolescent's response to the developmental tasks of pregnancy. Middle and older adolescents respond differently, reflecting their progression through the developmental tasks. In addition to her maturational level, the amount of nurturing the pregnant adolescent receives is a critical factor in the way she handles pregnancy and motherhood.

Risks to the Child

Children of adolescent parents are at a disadvantage in many ways because teens are not developmentally or economically prepared to be parents. In general, children of teenage mothers are found to be at a developmental disadvantage compared with children whose mothers were older at the time of their birth. Many factors contribute to these differences, especially the adverse social and economic conditions that many teenage mothers face. These factors result in high rates of family instability, disadvantaged neighborhoods, and high rates of behavior problems. In addition, these children do not do as well in school and are less likely to complete high school. Children born to adolescent mothers also have higher rates of abuse and neglect (National Campaign to Prevent Teen Pregnancy, 2004).

Partners of Adolescent Mothers

Approximately two thirds of the fathers of infants born to adolescent mothers are not teens, but are 20 years of age and older. In particular, teens in poorer, recently immigrated populations have considerably older partners (Males, 2004).

TABLE 23–8 **The Early Adolescent's Response to the Developmental Tasks of Pregnancy**

STAGE	DEVELOPMENTAL TASKS OF PREGNANCY	EARLY ADOLESCENT'S RESPONSE TO PREGNANCY	NURSING IMPLICATIONS
First trimester	Pregnancy confirmation. Seeking early prenatal care as a confirmation tool. Begins to evaluate her diet and general health habits. Initial ambivalence is common. Usually a supportive partner.	May delay confirmation of pregnancy until late in first trimester or later. Reasons for delay may include lack of awareness that she is pregnant, fear of confiding in anyone, or denial. Rapid enlargement and sensitivity of breasts are embarrassing and frightening to early adolescent—may be perceived as changes of puberty. If confiding in mother, may be experiencing family turmoil in response to pregnancy.	Emphasize need for good nutrition as important for her well-being as much as infant's (prevention of preeclampsia and anemia). Use simple explanations and many audiovisuals. Have adolescent listen to FHR with Doppler.
Second trimester	Changes in physical appearance begin, and fetal movement is experienced, causing pregnancy to be experienced as a reality. Begins wearing maternity clothes to accommodate the physical changes. As a result of quickening, perceives her fetus as a real baby and begins preparing for the maternal role and new relationships with her partner and members of her family.	Some teenagers may delay validation of pregnancy until now, with family turmoil occurring at this time. Abdominal enlargement and quickening may be perceived as loss of control over body image. May try to maintain prepregnant weight and wear restrictive clothing to control and conceal changing body. Becomes dependent on her own mother for support. Egocentric; unable to develop a maternal role at this time.	Continue to discuss importance of good nutrition and adequate weight gain as previously noted. Discuss ways of utilizing common teenage clothing (large sweatshirts, blouses) to promote comfort but preserve adolescent image to some degree. Discuss plans being made for baby, continued educational plans, and role of teen's parents.
Third trimester	At end of second trimester, begins to view fetus as separate from self. Buys baby clothes and supplies. Prepares a place for the baby. Realistic about what baby is like. Prepares to give birth to infant. Anxiety increases as labor and birth approach; adolescent has concerns about well-being of fetus.	May focus on "wanting it to be over." May have trouble individuating fetus. May have fantasies, dreams, or nightmares about childbirth. Natural fears of labor and birth are greater than with older primigravida. Probably has not been in a hospital and may associate this with negative experiences. Explain physiologic changes of pregnancy versus those associated with puberty. Explain that ambivalence is normal with any pregnancy, but recognize it as a much greater concern with adolescent pregnancy.	Assess whether adolescent is preparing for baby by buying supplies and preparing a place in the home. Childbirth education is important. Provide hospital tour. Assess for discomforts of pregnancy, such as heartburn and constipation. Adolescent may be uncomfortable mentioning these and other problems.

Adolescent males tend to become sexually active at an earlier age than females, and they have more sexual partners in their teenage years (Marcell, Raine, & Eyre, 2003). When the father is an adolescent, he, too, has uncompleted developmental tasks for his age group and is no better prepared psychologically than his female counterpart to deal with the consequences of pregnancy. Consequently, the adolescent who attempts to assume his responsibility as a father faces many of the same psychologic and sociologic risks as the adolescent mother. The mother and father are generally from similar socioeconomic backgrounds and have similar educational levels.

Although not married, many adolescent couples are involved in meaningful relationships. Adolescent fathers may be involved in the pregnancy and be present for the birth. In situations in which the adolescent father wants to assume some responsibility, health care providers should support him in his decision. It is important, however, that the pregnant adolescent have the opportunity to decide whether she wants the father to participate in her health care.

The lack of responsibility shown by some unwed fathers has caused a shift in cultural and community attitudes. Fathers are being included on birth certificates far more frequently today than in the past. Legal paternity gives children access to military and Social Security benefits and to medical information about their fathers. In addition, this inclusion helps ensure the fathers' rights and encourages fathers to meet their responsibilities to their children.

In some situations, the pregnant adolescent female may not want to identify or contact the baby's father and the male may not readily acknowledge paternity. Those situations include rape, exploitative sexual relations, incest, and casual sexual relations. If health care providers suspect any of the first three causes, further investigation into the situation is important for the well-being of the pregnant adolescent and referral to other resources should be made as appropriate. If the adolescents perceive that they have a caring relationship, the adolescent father may want to be supportive and protective but may not understand the physical and psychologic changes that his partner is experiencing. The young man will need education about pregnancy, childbirth, child care, and parenting.

Even if the adolescent father has been included in the health care of the young woman throughout the pregnancy, it is not unusual for her to want her mother as her primary support person during labor and birth. Younger adolescents are especially likely to choose their mothers for this role. It is important to support the pregnant adolescent's wishes and to acknowledge and support the adolescent father's wishes as appropriate.

As a part of counseling, the nurse should assess the young man's stressors, his support systems, his plans for involvement in the pregnancy and childbearing, and his future plans. He should be referred to social services for an opportunity for counseling regarding his educational and vocational future. When the father is involved in the pregnancy, the young mother feels less alone, more confident in her decision making, and better able to discuss her future. Relationships between fathers, teenage mothers, and their infants appear prone to deterioration over time. Research suggests, however, that many young fathers genuinely want to be involved with their children and would have more contact and input if they could. Issues such as conflicts with the teen mother or maternal grandparents and a lack of financial resources may act as barriers for the young father (Bunting & McAuley, 2004).

Reactions of Family and Social Network to Adolescent Pregnancy

The reactions of family members and support groups to adolescent pregnancy are as varied as the motivation and cause of the pregnancy. In families that foster their children's educational and career goals, adolescent pregnancy is often a shock. Anger, shame, and sorrow are common reactions. The majority of pregnant adolescents from these families are likely to use contraception or choose abortion, with the exception of teens whose cultural and religious beliefs prevent them from seeking abortions.

Some adolescent fathers also face negative reactions from people, including their own families and the families of their young partners. They may experience others' anger, shame, and disappointment. Relationships with their peers may be altered as well.

In populations in which adolescent pregnancy is more prevalent and more socially acceptable, family and friends may be more supportive of the adolescent parents. In many cases, the teen's friends and mother are present at the birth. The expectant couple also may have friends who are already teen parents. Some male partners of these adolescent mothers see pregnancy and the birth of a baby as signs of adult status and increased sexual prowess—a source of pride.

The mother of the pregnant adolescent is usually among the first to be told about the pregnancy. She typically becomes involved with decision making, especially with the young adolescent, about issues such as maintaining the pregnancy, deciding whether to seek an abortion, and dealing with the father-to-be and his family.

Once the pregnant adolescent decides how to proceed, it is often the mother who helps the teen access health care and accompanies her to her first prenatal visit. If the pregnancy is maintained, the mother may participate in prenatal care and classes and can be an excellent source of support for her daughter. She should be encouraged to participate if the mother–daughter relationship is positive. If the baby's father is involved in the pregnancy, he and the pregnant adolescent's mother may be able to work together to support the teenage mother. The nurse can update the pregnant adolescent's mother on childbearing practices to clarify any misconceptions she might have. During labor and birth, the mother may be a key figure for her daughter, offering her reassurance and instilling confidence. The younger the adolescent is when she gives birth, the more she needs her mother's support. Children of adolescent parents experience more negative outcomes, including more aggressive behavior at a younger age, when the adolescent is in constant conflict with her mother and becomes less involved in parenting.

OVERVIEW OF EXEMPLARS FOR NURSING CARE OF PREGNANT WOMEN

This concept includes five exemplars for nursing care of pregnant women and their related priorities for care: care for the mother during the antepartum, intrapartum, and postpartum stages of pregnancy; newborn care; and prematurity. The following sections and Table 23–9 provide an overview of the material. The complete exemplars can be found at www.mynursingkit.com.

Exemplar 23.1: Antepartum Care

This exemplar reviews the care required by the pregnant client until the time labor begins. While the focus of the exemplar is the normal pregnancy, some discussion is directed toward pregnancy-induced complications and complications of pregnancy resulting from preexisting health alterations such as diabetes, systemic lupus erythematosus, and cardiac disorders.

Exemplar 23.2: Intrapartum Care

The exemplar on intrapartum care begins with the woman in labor and ends with delivery and the immediate postpartum period. As with the antepartum exemplar, the approach is focused on the normal labor and delivery process with some discussion of common complications and nursing care required.

Exemplar 23.3: Postpartum Care

Postpartum care is discussed with a focus on meeting the care needs of the family immediately following delivery until approximately 6 weeks later. Common alterations in the postpartum client are also discussed.

Exemplar 23.4: Newborn Care

This exemplar takes a family-centered approach and focuses on the normal adaptations of the newborn and the nursing care required to support health and promote family. Assessment of the newborn with discussion of normal and abnormal findings

TABLE 23–9 **Overview of Reproduction Exemplars**

EXEMPLAR	DESCRIPTION	PRIORITIES FOR NURSING CARE
Antepartum care	Care of the pregnant client throughout the pregnancy from the first prenatal contact to the time when the woman begins to labor.	■ Teaching self-care to promote health and safety including avoidance of teratogens ■ Assessing client for potential or existing alterations ■ Assessing both maternal and fetal response to required adaptations ■ Preparing client for labor and delivery ■ Minimizing symptoms of common discomforts experienced during pregnancy
Intrapartum care	The period of labor and delivery.	■ Assessing maternal and fetal response to labor ■ Supporting the laboring client to reduce anxiety and fear ■ Managing pain throughout the labor and delivery process ■ Caring for the client during labor ■ Caring for the newborn immediately after birth ■ Potential complications of labor and delivery
Postpartum care	The period immediately following pregnancy, including the physical changes following pregnancy. (Postpartum depression is covered in Concept 20, Mood and Affect.)	■ Caring for the woman following delivery ■ Promoting incorporation of the newborn into the family ■ Preventing complications during the postpartum period ■ Teaching the client newborn and self-care to promote health and safety ■ Assessing maternal adaptation following delivery
Newborn care	Care of the newborn immediately upon birth.	■ Characteristics of the normal newborn ■ Assessing and supporting adaptation of the newborn to extrauterine life ■ Assessing normal and abnormal findings ■ Teaching parents to care for the newborn and meet routine needs of the neonate ■ Common alterations found in the newborn
Prematurity	Care of the infant born prematurely.	■ Assessing gestational age ■ Anticipated alterations in the premature neonate ■ Promoting growth in the premature neonate ■ Promoting bonding in the parents of a neonate ■ Reducing the risk of complications in the premature neonate

is included. While the focus of the exemplar is on the normal newborn, common alterations are also included.

Exemplar 23.5: Prematurity

This exemplar discusses the unique needs of the neonate born prematurely. A broad overview of physiological differences found in the premature infant are explained along with basic nursing care needs.

ASSESSMENT

The nurse caring for a woman who is pregnant establishes an environment of comfort and open communication with each antepartal visit. The nurse conveys interest in the woman as an individual and discusses the woman's concerns and desires. Typically, the registered nurse may complete many areas of prenatal assessment. Advanced practice nurses such as certified nurse-midwives (CNM) and certified women's health nurse practitioners have the education and skill to perform full and complete antepartal assessments.

This section focuses on the initial prenatal assessment.

Initial Client History

The course of a pregnancy depends on a number of factors, including the woman's prepregnancy health, the presence of disease states, the woman's emotional status, and her past health care. A thorough history is useful in determining the status of a woman's prepregnancy health. Terms useful for recording history of maternity clients are listed in Box 23–1.

CLIENT PROFILE The history is essentially a screening tool that identifies factors that may place the mother or fetus at risk during the pregnancy. The following information is obtained for each pregnant woman at the first prenatal assessment.

1. *Current pregnancy*
   - First day of last normal menstrual period. Is she sure or unsure of the date? Do her cycles normally occur every 28 days, or do her cycles tend to be longer?
   - Presence of cramping, bleeding, or spotting since LMP
   - Woman's opinion about the time when conception occurred and when infant is due
   - Woman's attitude toward pregnancy (Is this pregnancy planned? Wanted?)
   - Results of pregnancy tests, if completed
   - Any discomforts since LMP (e.g., nausea, vomiting, urinary frequency, fatigue, or breast tenderness)
2. *Past pregnancies*
   - Number of pregnancies
   - Number of abortions, spontaneous or induced
   - Number of living children
   - History of previous pregnancies, length of pregnancy, length of labor and birth, type of birth (vaginal, forceps or vacuum-assisted birth, or cesarean), type of anesthesia used (if any), woman's perception of the experience, and complications (antepartal, intrapartal, and postpartal)
   - Neonatal status of previous children: Apgar scores, birth weights, general development, complications, and feeding patterns (breast milk or formula)
   - Loss of a child (miscarriage, elective or medically indicated abortion, stillbirth, neonatal death, relinquishment, or death after the neonatal period). What was the experience like for her? What coping skills helped? How did her partner, if involved, respond?
   - If Rh-negative, was medication received after birth to prevent sensitization?
   - Prenatal education classes and resources (books)

Box 23–1 **Definition of Terms**

The following terms are used in recording the history of maternity clients:

Abortion: Birth that occurs before the end of 20 weeks' gestation or the birth of a fetus–newborn who weighs less than 500 g (Cunningham, Leveno, Bloom et al., 2005)

Antepartum: Time between conception and the onset of labor; often used to describe the period during which a woman is pregnant; used interchangeably with *prenatal*

Gestation: The number of weeks since the first day of the last menstrual period

Gravida*: Any pregnancy, regardless of duration, including present pregnancy

Intrapartum: Time from the onset of true labor until the birth of the infant and placenta

Multigravida: A woman who is in her second or any subsequent pregnancy

Multipara: A woman who has had two or more births at more than 20 weeks' gestation

Nulligravida: A woman who has never been pregnant

Nullipara: A woman who has had no births at more than 20 weeks' gestation

Para*: Birth after 20 weeks' gestation regardless of whether the infant is born alive or dead

Postpartum: Time from birth until the woman's body returns to an essentially prepregnant condition

Postterm labor: Labor that occurs after 42 weeks' gestation

Preterm or premature labor: Labor that occurs after 20 weeks' but before completion of 37 weeks' gestation

Primigravida: A woman who is pregnant for the first time

Primipara: A woman who has had one birth at more than 20 weeks' gestation, regardless of whether the infant was born alive or dead

Stillbirth: An infant born dead after 20 weeks' gestation

Term: The normal duration of pregnancy (38– to 42 weeks' gestation)

*The terms *gravida* and *para* are used in relation to pregnancies, not the number of fetuses. Thus, twins, triplets, etc., count as one pregnancy and one birth.

3. *Gynecologic history*
   - Date of last Pap smear; any history of abnormal Pap smear; any follow-up therapy completed
   - Previous infections: vaginal, cervical, tubal, sexually transmitted
   - Previous surgery
   - Age at menarche
   - Regularity, frequency, and duration of menstrual flow
   - History of dysmenorrhea
   - Sexual history
   - Contraceptive history (If birth control pills were used, did pregnancy occur immediately following cessation of pills? If not, how long after?)
   - Any issues related to infertility or fertility treatments

4. *Current medical history*
   - Weight
   - Blood type and Rh factor if known
   - General health, including nutrition (dietary practices such as vegetarianism) and regular exercise program (type, frequency, and duration)
   - Any medications presently being taken (including non-prescription, homeopathic, or herbal medications) or taken since the onset of pregnancy
   - Previous or present use of alcohol, tobacco, or caffeine (Ask specifically about the amount of alcohol, cigarettes, and caffeine (specify coffee, tea, cola, and chocolate) consumed each day.)
   - Illicit drug use or abuse (Ask about specific drugs such as cocaine, crack, methamphetamines, and marijuana.)
   - Drug allergies and other allergies (Ask about latex allergies or sensitivities.)
   - Potential teratogenic insults to this pregnancy, such as viral infections, medications, x-ray examinations, surgery, or cats in the home (possible source of toxoplasmosis)
   - Presence of disease conditions such as diabetes, hypertension, cardiovascular disease, renal problems, or thyroid disorder
   - Record of immunizations (especially rubella)
   - Presence of any abnormal symptoms

5. *Past medical history*
   - Childhood diseases
   - Past treatment for any disease condition (Any hospitalizations? History of hepatitis? Rheumatic fever? Pyelonephritis? Cancer?)
   - Surgical procedures
   - Presence of bleeding disorders or tendencies (Has she received blood transfusions?)

6. *Family medical history*
   - Presence of diabetes, cardiovascular disease, cancer, hypertension, hematologic disorders, tuberculosis, or preeclampsia–eclampsia
   - Occurrence of multiple births
   - History of congenital diseases or deformities
   - History of mental illness
   - Causes of death of deceased parents or siblings
   - Occurrence of cesarean births and cause if known

7. *Religious, spiritual, and cultural history*
   - Does the woman want to specify a religious preference on her chart? Does she have any spiritual beliefs or practices that might influence her health care or that of her child, such as prohibition against receiving blood products, dietary considerations, or circumcision rites?
   - What practices are important to maintaining her spiritual well-being?
   - Might practices in her culture or that of her partner influence her care or that of her child?

8. *Occupational history*
   - Occupation
   - Physical demands (Does she stand all day, or are there opportunities to sit and elevate her legs? Any heavy lifting?)
   - Exposure to chemicals or other harmful substances
   - Opportunity for regular meals and breaks for nutritious snacks
   - Provision for maternity or family leave

9. Partner's history
   - Presence of genetic conditions or diseases in him or in his family history
   - Age
   - Significant health problems
   - Previous or present alcohol intake, drug use, or tobacco use
   - Blood type and Rh factor
   - Occupation
   - Educational level; methods by which he learns best
   - Attitude toward the pregnancy

10. *Personal information about the woman (Social history)*
    - Age
    - Educational level; methods by which she learns best
    - Race or ethnic group (to identify need for prenatal genetic screening and racially or ethnically related risk factors)
    - Housing; stability of living conditions
    - Economic level
    - Acceptance of pregnancy, whether intended or unintended
    - Any history of emotional or physical deprivation or abuse of herself or children or any abuse in her current relationship (Ask specifically whether she has been hit, slapped, kicked, or hurt within the past year or since she has become pregnant. Ask whether she is afraid of her partner or anyone else. If yes, of whom is she afraid? Note: Ask these questions when the woman is alone.)
    - History of emotional problems
    - Support systems
    - Personal preferences about the birth (expectations of both the woman and her partner, presence of others, etc.)
    - Plans for care of child following birth
    - Feeding preference for the baby (breast milk or formula?)

OBTAINING DATA In many instances, a questionnaire is used to obtain information. The woman should complete the questionnaire in a quiet place with a minimum of distractions. The nurse can obtain further information in an interview, which allows the pregnant woman to clarify her responses to questions and gives the nurse and client the opportunity to begin developing rapport.

The expectant father or partner can be encouraged to attend the prenatal examinations, often able to contribute to the history. Encourage partners to use the opportunity to ask questions or express concerns that are important to them.

PRENATAL HIGH-RISK SCREENING **Risk factors** are any findings that suggest that the pregnancy may have a negative outcome, for either the woman or her unborn child. Screening for risk factors is an important part of the prenatal assessment. Many risk factors can be identified during the initial assessment; others may be detected during subsequent prenatal visits. It is important to identify high-risk pregnancies early so that appropriate interventions can be started promptly. Not all risk factors threaten a pregnancy equally; thus, many agencies use a scoring sheet to determine the degree of risk. Information must be updated throughout pregnancy as necessary. Any pregnancy may begin as low-risk and change to high-risk because of complications.

Physical Examination

The physical examination begins with assessment of vital signs; then the woman's body is examined. The pelvic examination is performed last.

Before the examination, the woman should provide a clean urine specimen. When her bladder is empty, the woman is more comfortable during the pelvic examination and the examiner can palpate the pelvic organs more easily. After the woman has emptied her bladder, the nurse asks her to disrobe and gives her a gown and sheet or some other protective covering.

Increasing numbers of nurses (e.g., CNMs and other nurses in advanced practice) are prepared to perform complete physical examinations. The nurse who does not yet possess advanced assessment skills assesses the woman's vital signs, explains the procedures to allay apprehension, positions her for examination, and assists the examiner as necessary. Each nurse is responsible for operating at the expected standard for his or her skill and knowledge base.

Thoroughness and a systematic procedure are the most important considerations when performing the physical portion of an antepartal examination. To promote completeness, the Assessment Guide: Initial Prenatal Assessment, starting on page 1562, is organized in three columns that address the areas to be assessed (and normal findings), the variations or alterations that may be observed, and nursing responses to the data. The nurse should be aware that certain organs and systems are assessed concurrently with others during the physical portion of the examination.

A gestation calculator or wheel permits the caregiver to calculate the EDB even more quickly (Figure 23–31 ■).

If a woman with a history of menses every 28 days remembers her LMP and was not taking oral contraceptives before becoming pregnant, Nägele's rule may be a fairly accurate determiner of the EDB. However, *ovulation usually occurs 14 days before the onset of the next menses, not 14 days after the previous menses.* Consequently, if her cycle is irregular, or more than 28 days long, the time of ovulation may be delayed. If she has been using oral contraceptives, ovulation may be delayed several weeks following her last menses. Then, too, a postpartum woman who is breastfeeding may resume ovulating but be amenorrheic for a time, making calculation impossible. Thus, Nägele's rule, although helpful, is not foolproof.

UTERINE ASSESSMENT

Physical Examination When a woman is examined in the first 10–12 weeks of pregnancy and her uterine size is compatible with her menstrual history, uterine size may be the single most important clinical method for dating her pregnancy. In many cases, however, women do not seek maternity care until well into their second trimester, when it becomes more difficult to evaluate specific uterine size. In obese women, it is difficult to determine uterine size early in a pregnancy because the uterus is more difficult to palpate.

Fundal Height Fundal height may be used as an indicator of uterine size, although this method is less accurate late in pregnancy. A centimeter tape measure is used to measure the distance abdominally from the top of the symphysis pubis to the top of the

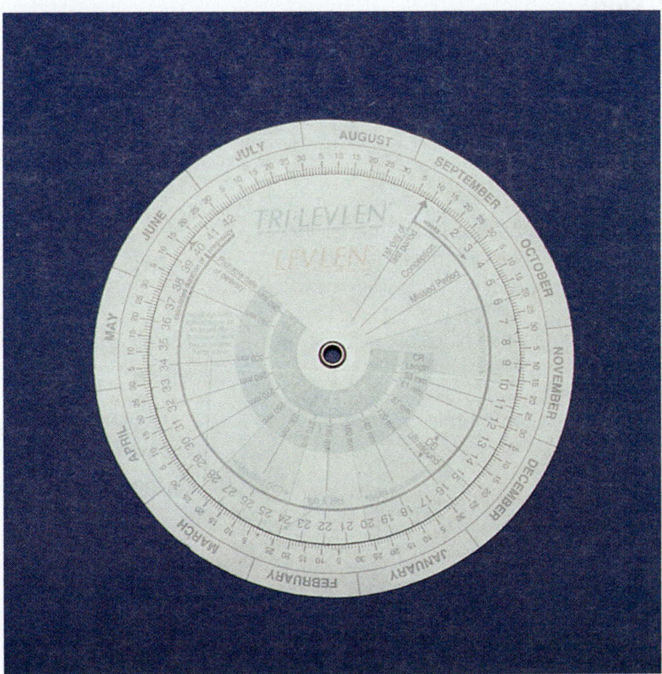

Figure 23–31 ■ The EDB wheel can be used to calculate the due date. To use it, place the arrow labeled "1st day of last period" on the date of the woman's LMP. Then read the EDB at the arrow labeled 40. In this case, the LMP is September 8 and the EDB is June 17.

Initial Prenatal Assessment

Physical Assessment/Normal Findings	Alterations and Possible Causes	Nursing Responses to Data
Vital Signs		
Blood Pressure (BP): Less than or equal to 135/85 mmHg	High BP (essential hypertension; renal disease; pregestational hypertension, apprehension or anxiety associated with pregnancy diagnosis, exam, or other crises; preeclampsia if initial assessment not done until after 20 weeks gestation)	BP greater than 140/90 requires immediate consideration; establish woman's BP; refer to health care provider if necessary. Assess woman's knowledge about high BP; counsel on self-care and medical management.
Pulse: 60–90 beats/minute; rate may increase 10 beats/minute during pregnancy	Increased pulse rate (excitement or anxiety, cardiac disorders)	Count for 1 full minute; note irregularities.
Respirations: 12–22 breaths/minute (or pulse rate divided by 4); pregnancy may induce a degree of hyperventilation; thoracic breathing predominant	Marked tachypnea or abnormal patterns	Assess for respiratory disease.
Temperature: 36.2–37.6°C (97.0–99.6°F)	Elevated temperature (infection)	Assess for infection process of disease state if temperature is elevated; refer to health care provider.
Weight		
Depends on body build	Weight less than 45 kg (100 lb) or greater than 91 kg (200 lb); rapid, sudden weight gain (preeclampsia)	Evaluate need for nutritional counseling; obtain information on eating habits, cooking practices, food regularly eaten, income limitations, need for food supplements, pica and other abnormal food habits. Note initial weight to establish baseline for weight gain throughout pregnancy.
Skin		
Color: Consistent with racial background; pink nail beds	Pallor (anemia); bronze, yellow (hepatic disease; other causes of jaundice)	The following tests should be performed: complete blood count (CBC), bilirubin level, urinalysis, and blood urea nitrogen (BUN).
	Bluish, reddish, mottled; dusky appearance or pallor of palms and nail beds in dark-skinned women (anemia)	If abnormal, refer to health care provider.
Condition: Absence of edema (slight edema of lower extremities is normal during pregnancy)	Edema (preeclampsia); rashes, dermatitis (allergic response)	Counsel on relief measures for slight edema. Initiate preeclampsia assessment; refer to health care provider.
Lesions: Absence of lesions	Ulceration (varicose veins, decreased circulation)	Further assess circulatory status; refer to health care provider if lesion is severe.
Spider nevi common in pregnancy	Petechiae, multiple bruises, ecchymosis (hemorrhagic disorders; abuse)	Evaluate for bleeding or clotting disorder. Provide opportunities to discuss abuse if suspected.
	Change in size or color (carcinoma)	Refer to health care provider.
Moles		
Pigmentation: Pigmentation changes of pregnancy include linea nigra, striae gravidarum, melasma		Assure woman that these are normal manifestations of pregnancy and explain the physiologic basis for the changes.
Café-au-lait spots	Six or more (Albright syndrome or neurofibromatosis)	Consult with health care provider.

Initial Prenatal Assessment (continued)

Physical Assessment/Normal Findings	Alterations and Possible Causes	Nursing Responses to Data
Nose		
Character of mucosa: Redder than oral mucosa; in pregnancy, nasal mucosa is edematous in response to increased estrogen, resulting in nasal stuffiness (rhinitis of pregnancy) and nosebleeds	Olfactory loss (first cranial nerve deficit)	Counsel woman about possible relief measures for nasal stuffiness and nosebleeds (epistaxis); refer to health care provider for olfactory loss.
Mouth		
May note hypertrophy of gingival tissue because of estrogen	Edema, inflammation (infection); pale in color (anemia)	Assess hematocrit for anemia; counsel regarding dental hygiene habits. Refer to health care provider or dentist if necessary. Routine dental care is appropriate during pregnancy (no x-ray studies, no nitrous anesthesia).
Neck		
Nodes: Small, mobile, nontender nodes	Tender, hard, fixed, or prominent nodes (infection, carcinoma)	Examine for local infection; refer to health care provider.
Thyroid: Small, smooth, lateral lobes palpable on either side of trachea; slight hyperplasia by third month of pregnancy	Enlargement or nodule tenderness (hyperthyroidism)	Listen over thyroid for bruits, which may indicate hyperthyroidism. Question woman about dietary habits (iodine intake). Ascertain history of thyroid problems; refer to health care provider.
Chest and Lungs		
Chest: Symmetric, elliptic, smaller AP than transverse diameter	Increased AP diameter, funnel chest, pigeon chest (emphysema, asthma, chronic obstructive pulmonary disease (COPD))	Evaluate for emphysema, asthma, pulmonary disease (COPD).
Ribs: Slope downward from nipple line	More horizontal (COPD) angular bumps (rachitic rosary) (vitamin C deficiency)	Evaluate for COPD. Evaluate for fractures. Consult health care provider. Consult nutritionist.
Inspection and palpation: No retraction or bulging of intercostal spaces (ICS) during inspiration or expiration; symmetric expansion	ICS retractions with inspirations, bulging with expiration; unequal expansion (respiratory disease)	Do thorough initial assessment. Refer to health care provider.
Tactile fremitus	Tachypnea, hyperpnea, Cheyne-Stokes respirations (respiratory disease)	Refer to health care provider.
Percussion: Bilateral symmetry in tone	Flatness of percussion, which may be affected by chest wall thickness	Evaluate for pleural effusions, consolidations, or tumor.
Low-pitched resonance of moderate intensity	High diaphragm (atelectasis or paralysis), pleural effusion	Refer to health care provider.
Auscultation: Upper lobes: bronchovesicular sounds above sternum and scapulas; equal expiratory and inspiratory phases	Abnormal if heard over any other area of chest	Refer to health care provider.
Remainder of chest: Vesicular breath sounds heard; inspiratory phase longer (3:1)	Rales, rhonchi, wheezes; pleural friction rub; absence of breath sounds; bronchophony, egophony, whispered pectoriloquy	Refer to health care provider.
Breasts		
Supple: Symmetric in size and contour; darker pigmentation of nipple and areola; may have supernumerary nipples, usually 5–6 cm below normal nipple line Axillary nodes unpalpable or pellet-sized	"Pigskin" or orange-peel appearance, nipple retractions, swelling, hardness (carcinoma); redness, heat, tenderness, cracked or fissured nipple (infection) Tenderness, enlargement, hard node (carcinoma); may be visible bump (infection)	Encourage monthly self-examination; instruct woman how to examine her breasts. Refer to health care provider if evidence of inflammation.

(continued)

Initial Prenatal Assessment (continued)

Physical Assessment/Normal Findings	Alterations and Possible Causes	Nursing Responses to Data
Pregnancy changes: 1. Size increase noted primarily in first 20 weeks. 2. Become nodular. 3. Tingling sensation may be felt during first and third trimester; woman may report feeling of heaviness. 4. Pigmentation of nipples and areolae darkens. 5. Superficial veins dilate and become more prominent. 6. Striae seen in multiparas. 7. Tubercles of Montgomery enlarge. 8. Colostrum may be present after 12th week. 9. Secondary areola appears at 20 weeks, characterized by series of washed-out spots surrounding primary areola. 10. Breasts less firm, old striae may be present in multiparas.		Discuss normalcy of changes and their meaning. Teach and/or institute appropriate relief measures. Encourage use of supportive, well-fitting brassiere.
Heart		
Normal rate, rhythm, and heart sounds	Enlargement, thrills, thrusts, gross irregularity or skipped beats, gallop rhythm or extra sounds (cardiac disease)	Complete an initial assessment. Explain normal pregnancy-induced changes. Refer to health care provider if indicated.
Pregnancy changes: 1. Palpitations may occur due to sympathetic nervous system disturbance. 2. Short systolic murmurs that increase in held expiration are normal due to increased volume.		
Abdomen		
Normal appearance, skin texture, and hair distribution; liver nonpalpable; abdomen nontender	Muscle guarding (anxiety, acute tenderness); tenderness, mass (ectopic pregnancy, inflammation, carcinoma)	Assure woman of normalcy of diastasis. Provide initial information about appropriate prenatal and postpartum exercises. Evaluate woman's anxiety level. Refer to health care provider if indicated.
Pregnancy changes: 1. Purple striae may be present (or silver striae on a multipara) as well as linea nigra. 2. Diastasis of the rectus muscles late in pregnancy.		
3. Size: Flat or rotund abdomen; progressive enlargement of uterus due to pregnancy. 10–12 weeks: Fundus slightly above symphysis pubis. 16 weeks: Fundus halfway between symphysis and umbilicus. 20–22 weeks: Fundus at umbilicus. 28 weeks: Fundus three finger breadths above umbilicus. 36 weeks: Fundus just below ensiform cartilage.	Size of uterus inconsistent with length of gestation (IUGR, multiple pregnancy, fetal demise, hydatidiform mole)	Reassess menstrual history regarding pregnancy dating. Evaluate increase in size using McDonald's method. Use ultrasound to establish diagnosis.
4. Fetal heart rate: 110–160 beats/minute may be heard with Doppler at 10–12 weeks gestation; may be heard with fetoscope at 17–20 weeks.	Failure to hear fetal heartbeat with Doppler (fetal demise, hydatidiform mole)	Refer to health care provider. Administer pregnancy tests. Use ultrasound to establish diagnosis.
5. Fetal movement palpable by a trained examiner after 18th week.	Failure to feel fetal movements after 20 weeks gestation (fetal demise, hydatidiform mole)	Refer to health care provider for evaluation of fetal status.

Initial Prenatal Assessment (continued)

Physical Assessment/Normal Findings	Alterations and Possible Causes	Nursing Responses to Data
Pregnancy changes: (continued) 6. Ballottement: During fourth to fifth month, fetus rises and then rebounds to original position when uterus is tapped sharply.	No ballottement (oligohydramnios)	Refer to health care provider for evaluation of fetal status.
Extremities		
Skin warm, pulses palpable, full range of motion; may be some edema of hands and ankles in late pregnancy; varicose veins may become more pronounced; palmar erythema may be present	Unpalpable or diminished pulses (arterial insufficiency); marked edema (preeclampsia)	Evaluate for other symptoms of heart disease; initiate follow-up if woman mentions that her rings feel tight. Discuss prevention and self-treatment measures for varicose veins; refer to health care provider if indicated.
Spine		
Normal spinal curves: Concave cervical, convex thoracic, concave lumbar	Abnormal spinal curves; flatness, kyphosis, lordosis	Refer to health care provider for assessment of cephalopelvic disproportion.
In pregnancy, lumbar spinal curve may be accentuated	Backache	May have implications for administration of spinal anesthetics.
Shoulders and iliac crests should be even	Uneven shoulders and iliac crests (scoliosis)	Refer very young women to health care provider; discuss back-stretching exercise with older women.
Reflexes		
Normal and symmetric	Hyperactivity, clonus (preeclampsia)	Evaluate for other symptoms of preeclampsia.
Pelvic Area		
External female genitals: Normally formed with female hair distribution; in multiparas, labia majora loose and pigmented; urinary and vaginal orifices visible and appropriately located	Lesions, hematomas, varicosities, inflammation of Bartholin's glands; clitoral hypertrophy (masculinization)	Explain pelvic examination procedure. Encourage woman to minimize her discomfort by relaxing her hips. Provide privacy.
Vagina: Pink or dark pink, vaginal discharge odorless, nonirritating; in multiparas, vaginal folds smooth and flattened; may have episiotomy scar	Abnormal discharge associated with vaginal infections	Obtain vaginal smear. Provide understandable verbal and written instructions about treatment for woman and partner if indicated.
Cervix: Pink color; os closed except in multiparas, in whom os admits fingertip	Eversion, reddish erosion, nabothian or retention cysts, cervical polyp; granular area that bleeds (carcinoma of cervix); lesions (herpes, human papilloma virus [HPV]); presence of string or plastic tip from cervix (intrauterine device [IUD] in uterus)	Provide woman with a hand mirror and identify genital structures for her; encourage her to view her cervix if she wishes. Refer to health care provider if indicated. Advise woman of potential serious risks of leaving an IUD in place during pregnancy; refer to health care provider for removal.
Pregnancy changes: 1–4 weeks gestation: Enlargement in AP diameter		
4–6 weeks gestation: Softening of cervix (Goodell's sign); softening of isthmus of uterus (Hegar's sign); cervix takes on bluish coloring (Chadwick's sign)	Absence of Goodell's sign (inflammatory conditions, carcinoma)	Refer to health care provider.
8–12 weeks gestation: Vagina and cervix appear bluish violet in color (Chadwick's sign)	Fixed (pelvic inflammatory disease [PID]); nodular surface (fibromas)	Refer to health care provider.

(continued)

Initial Prenatal Assessment (continued)

Physical Assessment/Normal Findings	Alterations and Possible Causes	Nursing Responses to Data
Uterus: Pear-shaped, mobile; smooth surface		
Ovaries: Small, walnut-shaped, nontender (ovaries and fallopian tubes are located in adnexal areas)	Pain on movement of cervix (PID); enlarged or nodular ovaries (cyst, tumor, tubal pregnancy, corpus luteum of pregnancy)	Evaluate adnexal areas; refer to health care provider.
Pelvic Measurements		
Internal measurements:	Measurement below normal	Vaginal birth may not be possible if deviations are present.
1. Diagonal conjugate is at least 11.5 cm.		
2. Obstetric conjugate is estimated by subtracting 1.5–2.0 cm from diagonal conjugate.	Disproportion of pubic arch	
3. Inclination of sacrum.	Abnormal curvature of sacrum	
4. Motility of coccyx; external intertubular diameter is greater than 8 cm.	Fixed or malposition of coccyx	
Anus and Rectum		
No lumps, rashes, excoriation, tenderness; cervix may be felt through rectal wall	Hemorrhoids, rectal prolapse; nodular lesion (carcinoma)	Counsel about appropriate prevention and relief measures; refer to health care provider for further evaluation.
Laboratory Evaluation		
Hemoglobin: 12–16 g/dL; women residing in areas of high altitude may have higher levels of hemoglobin	Less than 11 g/dL (anemia)	Note: Wear nonlatex gloves when drawing blood. Hemoglobin less than 12 g/dL requires nutritional counseling; less than 11 g/dL requires iron supplementation.
ABO and Rh typing: Normal distribution of blood types	Rh negative	If Rh-negative, check for presence of anti-Rh antibodies. Check partner's blood type; if partner is Rh-positive, discuss with woman the need for antibody titers during pregnancy, management during the intrapartal period, and possible need for Rh immune globulin.
CBC		
Hematocrit: 38–47% physiologic anemia (pseudoanemia) may occur	Marked anemia or blood dyscrasias	Perform CBC and Schilling differential cell count.
RBCs: 4.2–5.4 million/microliter		
White blood cells (WBCs): 5,000–12,000/microliter	Presence of infection; may be elevated in pregnancy and with labor	Evaluate for other signs of infection.
Differential Neutrophils: 40–60% Bands: up to 5% Eosinophils: 1–3% Basophils: up to 1% Lymphocytes: 20–40% Monocytes: 4–8%		
First trimester aneuploidy screening (testing to detect conditions related to abnormal chromosome number): if nuchal translucency (NT) testing is available, offer first-trimester screening for Down syndrome using NT and serum markers (PAPP-A and free b-hCG). Normal range.	Increased NT, elevated β-hCG, and reduced PAPP-A (Down syndrome, trisomy 18, trisomy 13, Turner syndrome)	If findings are positive, genetic counseling and diagnostic testing using chorionic villus sampling (CVS) or second-trimester amniocentesis is offered (ACOG, 2007).

Initial Prenatal Assessment (continued)

Physical Assessment/Normal Findings	Alterations and Possible Causes	Nursing Responses to Data
Integrated screening: combines first-trimester aneuploidy screening results with second-trimester quad screen to detect aneuploidy and neural tube defects; may be used in areas in which NT testing is not available		
Syphilis tests: Serologic tests for syphilis (STS), complement fixation test, venereal disease research laboratory (VDRL) test—nonreactive	Positive reaction STS—tests may have 25–45% incidence of biologic false-positive results; false results may occur in individuals who have acute viral or bacterial infections, hypersensitivity reactions, recent vaccinations, collagen disease, malaria, or tuberculosis	Positive results may be confirmed with the fluorescent treponemal antibody-absorption (FTA-ABS) test; all tests for syphilis give positive results in the secondary stage of the disease; antibiotic tests may cause negative test results.
Gonorrhea culture: Negative	Positive	Refer for treatment.
Urinalysis: Normal color, specific gravity; pH 4.6–8.0	Abnormal color (porphyria, hemoglobinuria, bilirubinemia): alkaline urine (metabolic alkalemia, *Proteus* infection, old specimen)	Repeat u/a; refer to health care provider.
Negative for protein, RBCs, WBCs, casts	Positive findings (contaminated specimen, kidney disease)	Repeat u/a; refer to health care provider.
Glucose: Negative (small degree of glycosuria may occur in pregnancy)	Glycosuria (low renal threshold for glucose, diabetes mellitus)	Assess blood glucose level; test urine for ketones.
Rubella titer: Hemagglutination-inhibition (HAI) test—1:10 or above indicates woman is immune	HAI titer less than 1:10	Immunization will be given postpartum or within 6 weeks after childbirth. Instruct woman whose titers are less than 1:10 to avoid children who have rubella.
Hepatitis B screen for hepatitis B surface antigen (HbsAg): negative	Positive	If negative, consider referral for hepatitis B vaccine. If positive, refer to physician. Infants born to women who test positive are given hepatitis B immune globulin soon after birth, followed by first dose of hepatitis B vaccine.
HIV screen: Offered to all women; encouraged for those at risk; negative	Positive	Refer to health care provider.
Illicit drug screen: Offered to all women; negative	Positive	Refer to health care provider.
Sickle-cell screen for clients of African descent: Negative	Positive; test results would include a description of cells	Refer to health care provider.
Pap smear: Negative	Test results that show atypical cells	Refer to health care provider. Discuss with the woman the meaning of the findings and the importance of follow-up.

Cultural Assessment	Variations to Consider*	Nursing Responses to Data[†]
Determine the woman's fluency in written and oral English.	Woman may be fluent in language other than English.	Work with a knowledgeable translator to provide information and answer questions.
Ask the woman how she prefers to be addressed.	Some women prefer informality; others prefer to use titles.	Address the woman according to her preference. Maintain formality in introducing oneself if that seems preferred.
Determine customs and practices regarding prenatal care:	Practices are influenced by individual preference, cultural expectations, or religious beliefs.	Honor a woman's practices and provide for specific preferences unless they are contraindicated because of safety.

(continued)

Initial Prenatal Assessment (continued)

Physical Assessment/Normal Findings	Alterations and Possible Causes	Nursing Responses to Data
■ Ask the woman if there are certain practices she expects to follow when she is pregnant.	Some women believe they should perform certain acts related to sleep, activity, or clothing.	Have information printed in the language of different cultural groups that live in the area.
■ Ask the woman if there are any activities she cannot do while she is pregnant.	Some women have restrictions or taboos they follow related to work, activity, sexual, environmental, or emotional factors.	
■ Ask the woman whether there are certain foods she is expected to eat or avoid while she is pregnant. Determine whether she has lactose intolerance.	Foods are an important cultural factor. Some women may have certain foods they must eat or avoid; many women have lactose intolerance and have difficulty consuming sufficient calcium.	Respect the woman's food preferences, help her plan an adequate prenatal diet within the framework of her preferences, and refer to a dietitian if necessary.
■ Ask the woman whether the gender of her caregiver is of concern.	Some women are comfortable only with a female caregiver.	Arrange for a female caregiver if it is the woman's preference.
■ Ask the woman about the degree of involvement in her pregnancy that she expects or wants from her support person, mother, and other significant people.	A woman may not want her partner involved in the pregnancy. The role may fall to the woman's mother or a female relative or friend.	Respect the woman's preferences about her partner or husband's involvement; avoid imposing personal values or expectations.
■ Ask the woman about her sources of support and counseling during pregnancy.	Some women seek advice from a family member, *curandera*, or tribal healer.	Respect and honor the woman's sources of support.
Psychologic Status		
Excitement and/or apprehension, ambivalence	Marked anxiety (fear of pregnancy diagnosis, fear of medical facility)	Establish lines of communication. Active listening is useful. Establish trusting relationship. Encourage woman to take active part in her care.
	Apathy; display of anger with pregnancy diagnosis	Establish communication and begin counseling. Use active listening techniques.
Educational Needs		
May have questions about pregnancy or may need time to adjust to reality of pregnancy		Establish educational, supporting environment that can be expanded throughout pregnancy.
Support System		
Can identify at least two or three individuals with whom she is emotionally intimate (partner, parent, sibling, friend)	Isolated (no telephone, unlisted number); cannot name a neighbor or friend whom she can call upon in an emergency; does not perceive parents as part of her support system	Institute support system through community groups. Help woman to develop trusting relationship with health care professionals.
Family Functioning		
Emotionally supportive Adequate communication Mutually satisfying Cohesiveness in times of trouble	Long-term problems or specific problems related to this pregnancy, potential stressors within the family, pessimistic attitudes, unilateral decision making, unrealistic expectations of this pregnancy or child	Help identify the problems and stressors, encourage communication, and discuss role changes and adaptations.
Economic Status		
Source of income is stable and sufficient to meet basic needs of daily living and medical needs	Limited prenatal care; poor physical health; limited use of health care system; unstable economic status	Discuss available resources for health maintenance and the birth. Institute appropriate referral for meeting expanding family's needs (e.g., food stamps).

Initial Prenatal Assessment (continued)

Cultural Assessment	Variations to Consider	Nursing Responses to Data
Stability of Living Conditions		
Adequate, stable housing for expanding family's needs	Crowded living conditions; questionable supportive environment for newborn	Refer to appropriate community agency. Work with family on self-help ways to improve situation.

uterine fundus (McDonald's method) (Figure 23–32 ■). Fundal height in centimeters correlates well with weeks of gestation between 22–24 weeks and 34 weeks. Thus, at 26 weeks gestation, fundal height is probably about 26 cm. If the woman is very tall or very short, fundal height will differ. To ensure accuracy, fundal height should be measured by the same examiner each time. The woman should have voided within 30 minutes of the exam and should lie in the same position each time. In the third trimester, variations in fetal weight decrease the accuracy of fundal height measurements.

A lag in progression of measurements of fundal height from month to month and week to week may signal IUGR. A sudden increase in fundal height may indicate twins or hydramnios (excessive amount of amniotic fluid).

ASSESSMENT OF FETAL DEVELOPMENT

Quickening Fetal movements felt by the mother, called *quickening,* may indicate that the fetus is nearing 20 weeks gestation. However, quickening may be experienced between 16 and 22 weeks gestation, so this method is not completely accurate.

Fetal Heartbeat The ultrasonic Doppler device (Figure 23–33 ■) is the primary tool for assessing fetal heartbeat. It can detect fetal heartbeat, on average, at 8–12 weeks gestation. If an ultrasonic Doppler is not available, a fetoscope may be used, although in current practice, it is seldom necessary. The fetal heartbeat can be detected by fetoscope as early as week 16 and usually by 19 or 20 weeks gestation.

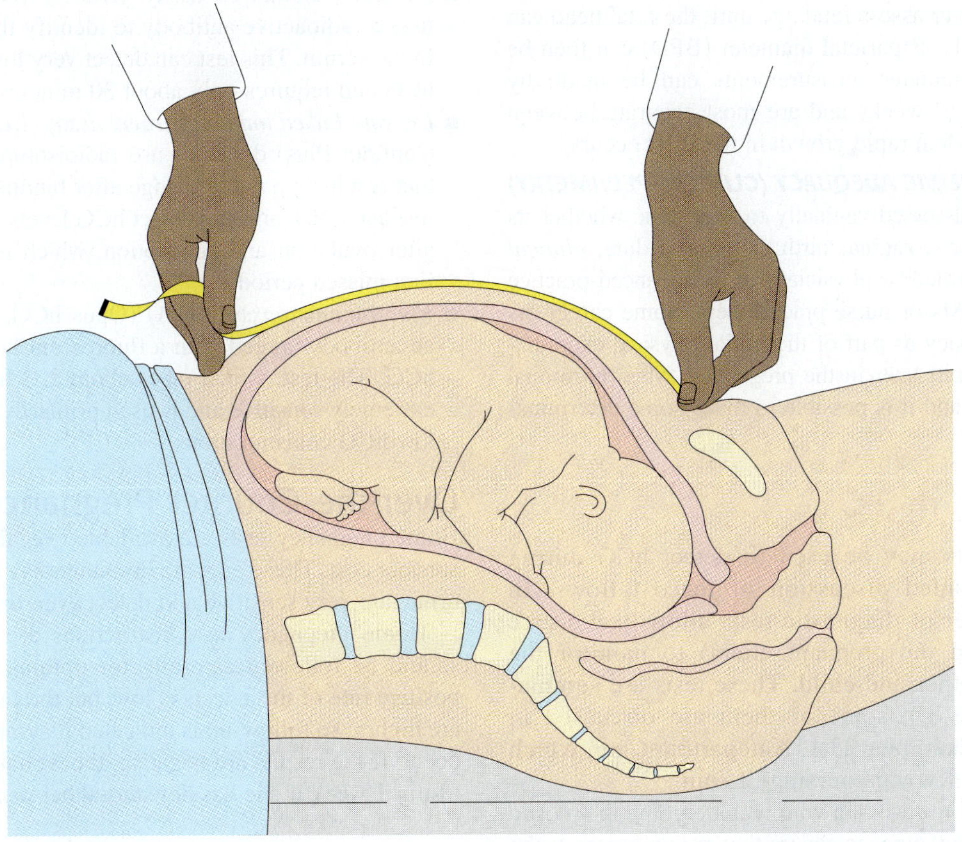

Figure 23–32 ■ A cross-sectional view of fetal position when McDonald's method is used to assess the fundal height.

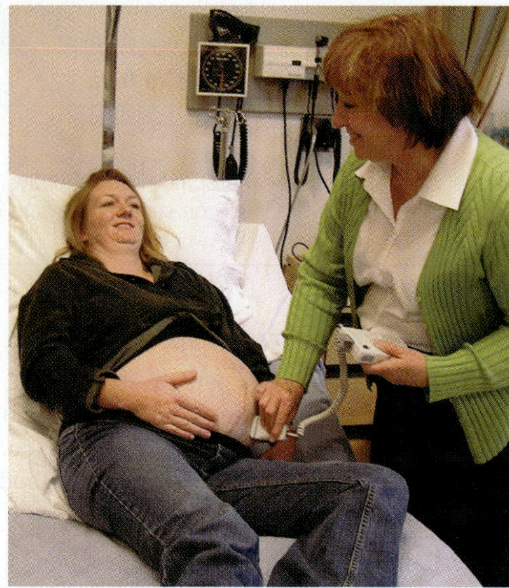

Figure 23–33 ■ Listening to the fetal heartbeat with a Doppler device.

Ultrasound In the first trimester, ultrasound scanning can detect a gestational sac as early as 5–6 weeks after the LMP, fetal heart activity by 6–7 weeks, and fetal breathing movement by 10–11 weeks of pregnancy. Crown-to-rump measurements can be made to assess fetal age until the fetal head can be visualized clearly. Biparietal diameter (BPD) can then be used. Biparietal diameter measurements can be made by approximately 12–13 weeks and are most accurate between 20 and 30 weeks, when rapid growth in the BPD occurs.

ASSESSMENT OF PELVIC ADEQUACY (CLINICAL PELVIMETRY) The pelvis can be assessed vaginally to determine whether its size is adequate for a vaginal birth. This procedure, *clinical pelvimetry,* is performed by physicians or by advanced-practice nurses such as CNMs or nurse practitioners. Some caregivers assess pelvic adequacy as part of the initial physical examination. Others wait until later in the pregnancy, when hormonal effects are greatest and it is possible to make some determination of fetal size.

DIAGNOSTIC TESTS

A number of tests may be used to detect hCG during pregnancy; a detailed discussion of these follows. In addition, a number of diagnostic tests allow health care professionals (and the pregnant client) to monitor the safety of both mother and child. These tests are summarized in Table 23–10; some of them are discussed in greater detail in Exemplar 23.1, Antepartum Care, which you can access at www.mynursingkit.com.

Nursing care for the woman who is undergoing diagnostic testing focuses on outcomes to ensure that she understands the reasons for the test, understands the test results, and has support during the test. In addition, other objectives include completing the tests without complication and ensuring that the safety of the mother and her unborn child has been maintained.

Clinical Pregnancy Tests

A variety of assay techniques are available to detect hCG during early pregnancy. Historically, the following two tests were commonly performed on the first morning urine specimen. These tests become positive within 10–14 days after the first missed period.

- *Hemagglutination inhibition test* (Pregnosticon R test), an immunoassay, is based on the fact that no clumping of cells occurs when the urine of a pregnant woman is added to the hCG-sensitized RBCs of sheep.
- *Latex agglutination test* (Gravindex and Pregnosticon Slide tests), also an immunoassay, is based on the fact that latex particle agglutination is inhibited in the presence of urine containing hCG.

Several newer pregnancy tests are available, including the following:

- *β-subunit radioimmunoassay (RIA)* uses an antiserum with specificity for the β-subunit of hCG in maternal blood. This accurate pregnancy test becomes positive a few days after presumed implantation, thereby permitting early diagnosis of pregnancy. This test also is used in the diagnosis of ectopic pregnancy or trophoblastic disease. However, because it requires several hours to perform and has only limited sensitivity, it is being replaced by other, technically simpler tests such as the immunoradiometric assay (IRMA).
- *Immunoradiometric assay (IRMA)* (Neocept, Pregnosis) uses a radioactive antibody to identify the presence of hCG in the serum. This test can detect very low concentrations of hCG and requires only about 30 minutes to perform.
- *Enzyme-linked immunosorbent assay (ELISA)* (Sensichrome, Confidot Plus) does not use radioisotopes, but a substance that results in a color change after binding. The test is sensitive and quick and can detect hCG levels as early as 7–9 days after ovulation and conception, which is 5 days before the first missed period.
- *Fluoroimmunoassay (FIA)* (Opus hCG, Stratus hCG) uses an antibody tagged with a fluorescent label to detect serum hCG. The test, which takes about 2–3 hours to perform, is extremely sensitive and is used primarily to identify and follow hCG concentrations.

Over-the-Counter Pregnancy Tests

Home pregnancy tests are available over the counter at a reasonable cost. These enzyme immunoassay tests, performed on urine, are very sensitive and detect even low levels of hCG.

Home pregnancy test instructions are quite explicit and should be followed carefully for optimal results. The false-positive rate of these tests is low, but the false-negative results are higher; so follow-up is indicated if symptoms of pregnancy occur. If the results are negative, the woman should repeat the test in 1 week if she has not started her period.

CARING INTERVENTIONS

Caring interventions for the pregnant woman are focused on teaching the client appropriate self-care techniques, especially with regard to protecting the fetus and relieving discomfort.

TABLE 23–10 **Summary of Screening and Diagnostic Tests**

GOAL	TEST	TIMING
To validate the pregnancy	Ultrasound: gestational sac volume	5 and 6 weeks after last menstrual period (LMP) by transvaginal ultrasound
To determine how advanced the pregnancy is	Ultrasound: crown–rump length	6–10 weeks gestation
	Ultrasound: BPD, femur length, abdomen circumference	13–40 weeks gestation
To identify normal growth of the fetus	Ultrasound: biparietal diameter	
	Most useful from 20–30 weeks gestation	
	Ultrasound: head/abdomen ratio	13–40 weeks gestation
	Ultrasound: estimated fetal weight	About 24–40 weeks gestation
To detect congenital anomalies and problems	Nuchal translucency testing	9–13 weeks gestation
	Ultrasound	18–40 weeks gestation
	Chorionic villus sampling	10–12 weeks gestation
	Amniocentesis	15–20 weeks gestation
	Fetoscopy	18 weeks gestation
	First-trimester combination screening test or quadruple test	Generally 15–20 weeks gestation
To localize the placenta	Ultrasound	Usually in third trimester or before amniocentesis
To assess fetal status	Biophysical profile	Approximately 28 weeks to birth
	Maternal assessment of fetal activity	Approximately 28 weeks to birth
	Nonstress test	Approximately 28 weeks to birth
	Contraction stress test	After 28 weeks
To diagnose cardiac problems	Fetal echocardiography	Second and third trimesters
To assess fetal lung maturity	Amniocentesis	33–40 weeks
	L/S ratio	33 weeks to birth
	Phosphatidylglycerol	33 weeks to birth
	Phosphatidylcholine	33 weeks to birth
	Lamellar body counts	33 weeks to birth
To obtain more information about breech presentation	Ultrasound	Just before labor is anticipated or during labor

Many of these interventions are discussed in the exemplars on antepartum and intrapartum care. Those that are covered here are related to fetal safety and to some of the most common discomforts experienced by the pregnant woman.

Prenatal Education

Prenatal education programs provide important opportunities to share information about pregnancy and childbirth and to enhance the parents' decision-making skills. The content of each class is generally directed by the overall goals of the program. For example, in classes that aim to provide preconceptual information, preparations for becoming pregnant and optimizing the woman's health status are the major topics. Other classes may be directed toward childbirth choices available today, preparation of the mother and her partner for pregnancy and birth, preparation for a vaginal birth after a (previous) cesarean (VBAC) birth, and preparation for the birth by specific people such as grandparents or siblings. The nurse who knows the types of prenatal programs available in the community can direct expectant parents to programs that meet their special needs and learning goals.

From the expectant parents' point of view, class content is best presented in chronology with the pregnancy. It is important to begin the classes by finding out what each parent wants to learn and including a discussion of related choices. Whereas both parents may expect to learn breathing and relaxation techniques and infant care, fathers usually expect facts and mothers expect coping strategies. Classes for partners provide a forum for expectant fathers or partners to ask questions and interact with others who are sharing similar circumstances and have the same types of concerns (Premburg & Lundgren, 2006).

A family's culture may influence its beliefs about and practices surrounding many aspects of childbearing and childrearing. The accompanying Focus on Diversity and Culture describes some cultural beliefs and attitudes about pregnancy.

TERATOGENIC SUBSTANCES Prenatal education must include teaching the parents about teratogenic substances and the use of medications during pregnancy. Substances that adversely affect the normal growth and development of the fetus are called *teratogens*. Many substances are known or suspected teratogens, including, for example, certain medications, psychotropic drugs, and alcohol. The harmful effects of other teratogens, such as some pesticides and exposure to x-rays in the first trimester of pregnancy, also have been documented. It is essential that pregnant women receive information about recognized teratogens and

FOCUS ON DIVERSITY AND CULTURE Beliefs and Attitudes About Pregnancy

Children are generally valued all over the world, not only for the joy they bring, but also because they ensure continuation of the family and cultural values. This valuing of children may manifest itself in different ways, however. Families in the United States and many Western countries commonly have only one or two children out of a desire to provide the children with the best home and education they can afford and to spend as much free time with them as possible. In contrast, in many cultures throughout the world, it is common to have as many children as possible.

In some cultures, a woman who gives birth achieves a higher status, especially when the child is male (Safadi, 2005). This is especially true in the traditional Chinese culture and in some Middle Eastern cultures (Do, 2005). Similarly, in the western United States, people of the Mormon faith view motherhood as the most important aspect of a woman's life, comparable with the male role of priesthood (Faust, 2005). In Mexican American society and among many other Latino groups, having children is evidence of the male's virility and is a sign of manliness or *machismo,* a desired trait.

Culture also may influence attitudes and beliefs about contraception. For example, Muslims from the Middle East may use birth control but do not believe in sterilization because it is a permanent method (Hammond, White, & Fetters, 2005). Other Muslims may not practice contraception because children are highly valued and it is believed that the traditional role of women is to bear children. In Chinese society, in contrast, where state policy limits the number of children a couple can have, contraception is common.

Health values and beliefs are also important in understanding reactions and behavior. Certain behaviors can be expected if a culture views pregnancy as a sickness, whereas other behaviors can be expected if the culture views pregnancy as a natural occurrence. For example, because Native Americans, African Americans, and Mexican Americans generally view pregnancy as a natural and desirable condition, prenatal care may not be a priority. In other cultures, pregnancy may be seen as a time of increased vulnerability. In Orthodox Judaism, for example, it is a man's responsibility to procreate, but it is a woman's right, not her obligation, to do so. This is because, according to Orthodox Jewish law, the health of the mother, both physically and mentally, is of primary concern and she should never be obliged to do something that threatens her life (Semenic, Callister, & Feldman, 2004).

Individuals of many cultures take certain protective precautions based on their beliefs. For example, many Southeast Asian women fear they will have a complicated labor and birth if they sit in a doorway or on a step. Thus, they tend to avoid areas near doors in waiting rooms and examining rooms. In the Mexican American culture, a common belief is that *mal aire,* or bad air, may enter the body and cause harm. Preventive measures such as keeping the windows closed or covering the head are used. Some Latinos place a raisin on the cord stump of newborns to prevent drafts from entering their bodies. A *taboo* is a behavior or thing to be avoided. Many cultures, including those in the United States, have taboos centered on the unborn baby and/or newborn that are meant to ensure that the baby will survive. For example, it is common among Muslims to avoid naming the baby until after birth; similarly, many Orthodox Jewish women wait to set up the nursery until after the baby is born.

In developing countries, mortality rates among infants and young children are extremely high; thus, certain traditions focus on protecting the baby from evil spirits. For example, many Muslim parents pin an amulet to the newborn's clothes as protection. This may be a palm, an eye, a blue stone, or a verse from the Quaran. Following birth, it is common for a male family member to whisper prayers in the newborn baby's ear to declare faith and protect the baby (Cassar, 2006).

Some cultures subscribe to the *equilibrium model of health,* based on the concept of balance between light and dark, heat and cold. This model affects the treatment of pregnant women. Some Eastern philosophies focus on the notion of *yin* and *yang.* Yin represents the female (passive) principle—darkness, cold, wetness; yang is the masculine (active) principle—light, heat, and dryness. When the two are combined, they are all that can be. The hot–cold classification is seen in cultures in Latin America, the Near East, and Asia.

Some Mexican Americans consider illness to be an excess of either hot or cold. To restore health, imbalances are often corrected by the proper use of foods, medications, or herbs. These substances also are classified as hot or cold. For example, an illness attributed to an excess of cold is treated only with hot foods or medications. The classification of foods is not always consistent, but it conforms to a general structure of traditional knowledge. Certain foods, spices, herbs, and medications are perceived to cool or heat the body. These perceptions do not necessarily correspond to the actual temperature; some hot dishes are said to have a cooling quality.

Southeast Asians believe it is important to keep the woman "warm" after birth because blood, which is considered "hot," has been lost and the woman is at risk of becoming "cold." Therefore, they avoid cold drinks and foods following birth. In contrast, many women in India consider pregnancy a "hot" period and eat "cool" foods to balance the hot state (Holroyd, Twinn, & Yim, 2004).

The concepts of hot and cold are not as important in Native American or African American beliefs. Similarities exist in all of these groups, however, because of their emphasis on a balance in nature.

environmental risks. An overview of the risks associated with medications and tobacco is provided here. For a more thorough discussion of the risks of substance abuse during pregnancy, please see Exemplar 2.3, Prenatal Substance Exposure.

Medications The use of medications during pregnancy, including prescriptions, over-the-counter drugs, and herbal remedies, is of great concern because maternal drug exposure is thought to account for at least 10% of birth defects (Black & Hill, 2003). Many pregnant women need medication for therapeutic purposes, such as the treatment of infections, allergies, or other pathologic processes. In these situations, the problem can be complex. Known teratogenic agents are not prescribed and usually can be replaced with medications that are considered safe. Even when a woman is highly motivated to avoid taking any medications, she may have taken potentially teratogenic medications before her pregnancy was confirmed, especially if she has an irregular menstrual cycle.

The greatest potential for gross abnormalities in the fetus occurs during the first trimester of pregnancy, when fetal organs are first developing. The classic period of teratogenesis in a woman with a 28-day cycle extends from day 31 after the LMP (17 days after fertilization) to day 71 (54 days after fertilization) (Niebyl & Simpson, 2007). Many factors influence teratogenic effects, including the specific type of teratogen and the dose, the stage of embryonic development, and the genetic sensitivity of the mother and fetus. For example, the commonly prescribed acne medication isotretinoin (Accutane) is associated with a high incidence of spontaneous abortion and congenital malformations if taken early in pregnancy.

To provide information for caregivers and clients, the U.S. Food and Drug Administration (FDA) has developed the following classification system for medications administered during pregnancy:

- Category A*:* Controlled studies in women have demonstrated no associated fetal risk. Few drugs fall into this category.
- Category B*:* Animal studies show no risk but there are no controlled studies in women, or animal studies indicate a risk but controlled human studies fail to demonstrate a risk. The penicillins fall into this category.
- Category C*:* Either (1) no adequate animal or human studies are available or (2) animal studies show teratogenic effects but no controlled studies in women are available. Many drugs fall into this category, which, because of the lack of information, is a problematic one for caregivers. Epinephrine, beta-blockers, and zidovudine (a drug used to decrease perinatal transmission of HIV) fall into this category.
- Category D*:* Evidence of human fetal risk exists, but the benefits of the drug in certain situations are thought to outweigh the risks. Examples of drugs in this category include tetracycline, vincristine, lithium, and hydrochlorothiazide.
- Category X: The demonstrated fetal risks clearly outweigh any possible benefit. Examples of drugs in this category include isotretinoin (Accutane), the acne medication, which can cause multiple CNS, facial, and cardiovascular anomalies.

If a woman has taken a drug in category D or X, she should be informed of the risks associated with that drug and of her alternatives. Similarly, a woman who has taken a drug in the safer categories can be reassured (Cunningham et al., 2005).

This system, although useful, has been criticized because the use of letters suggests a risk grading that is not necessarily accurate. More importantly, not all drugs in a category have the same risk level. Currently, the FDA is working to develop a new labeling system (Cunningham et al., 2005).

Although the first trimester is the critical period for teratogenesis, some medications are known to have a teratogenic effect when taken in the second and third trimesters. For example, tetracycline taken in late pregnancy is commonly associated with staining of teeth in children and has been shown to depress skeletal growth, especially in premature infants. Sulfonamides taken in the last few weeks of pregnancy are known to compete with bilirubin attachment of protein-binding sites, increasing the risk of jaundice in the newborn (Niebyl & Simpson, 2007).

Pregnant women need to avoid all medication—prescribed, homeopathic, or over-the-counter—if possible. If no alternative exists, they should select a well-known medication rather than a newer drug whose potential teratogenic effects may not be known. When possible, the oral form of a drug should be used and it should be prescribed in the lowest possible therapeutic dose for the shortest time possible. Finally, the caregiver needs to consider the multiple components of the medication. Caution is the watchword for nurses caring for pregnant women who have been taking medications. It is essential that pregnant women check with their CNMs or physicians about any herbs or medications they were taking when pregnancy occurred and about any nonprescription drugs they are thinking of using. The advantage of using a particular medication must outweigh the risks. Any medication with possible teratogenic effects is best avoided.

Tobacco In the United States, smoking during pregnancy is one of the most significant, modifiable causes of poor pregnancy outcomes. Smoking during pregnancy has a strong association with low-birth-weight infants. In addition, mothers who smoke have an increased risk of preterm birth, premature rupture of the membranes, fetal demise, placentae previa, abruptio placentae, premature rupture of membranes, and preterm birth (Hartmann et al., 2007). Pregnant women who smoke and participate in other unhealthy behaviors, such as alcohol use, further increase their risk for low-birth-weight infants (Okah, Cai, & Hoff, 2005). Research also links maternal smoking, both during and after pregnancy, with an increased risk of SIDS. Maternal smoking exposes young children to other risks of secondhand smoke, including middle ear infections, acute and chronic respiratory tract illnesses, and behavioral and learning disabilities (Albrecht et al., 2004).

Relief of the Common Discomforts of Pregnancy

The common discomforts of pregnancy result from physiologic and anatomic changes and are fairly specific to each of the three trimesters. Health professionals often refer to these discomforts as minor, but they are not minor to the pregnant woman. They can make her quite uncomfortable and, if they are unexpected, anxious. Table 23–11 identifies the common

TABLE 23–11 Self-Care Measures for Common Discomforts of Pregnancy

DISCOMFORT	INFLUENCING FACTORS	SELF-CARE MEASURES
First Trimester		
Nausea and vomiting	Increased levels of hCG Changes in carbohydrate metabolism Emotional factors Fatigue	Avoid odors or causative factors. Eat dry crackers or toast before arising in morning. Have small but frequent meals. Avoid greasy or highly seasoned foods. Take dry meals with fluids between meals. Drink carbonated beverages.
Urinary frequency	Pressure of uterus on bladder in both first and third trimesters	Void when urge is felt. Increase fluid intake during the day. Decrease fluid intake *only* in the evening to decrease nocturia.
Fatigue	Unknown specific causative factors May be aggravated by nocturia due to urinary frequency	Plan time for a nap or rest period daily. Go to bed early. Seek family support and assistance with responsibilities so that more time is available to rest.
Breast tenderness	Increased levels of estrogen and progesterone	Wear well-fitting, supportive bra.
Increased vaginal discharge	Hyperplasia of vaginal mucosa and increased production of mucus by the endocervical glands due to the increase in estrogen levels	Promote cleanliness by daily bathing. Avoid douching, nylon underpants, and pantyhose; cotton underpants are more absorbent; powder can be used to maintain dryness if not allowed to cake.
Nasal stuffiness and nosebleed (epistaxis)	Elevated estrogen levels	May be unresponsive, but cool-air vaporizer may help; avoid use of nasal sprays and decongestants.
Ptyalism (excessive, often bitter salivation)	Unknown specific causative factors	Use astringent mouthwashes, chew gum, or suck hard candy.
Second and Third Trimesters		
Heartburn (pyrosis)	Increased production of progesterone, decreasing gastrointestinal motility and increasing relaxation of cardiac sphincter, displacement of stomach by enlarging uterus, thus regurgitation of acidic gastric contents into the esophagus	Eat small and more frequent meals. Use low-sodium antacids. Avoid overeating, eating fatty and fried foods, lying down after eating, and taking sodium bicarbonate.
Ankle edema	Prolonged standing or sitting Increased levels of sodium due to hormonal influences Circulatory congestion of lower extremities Increased capillary permeability Varicose veins	Practice frequent dorsiflexion of feet when prolonged sitting or standing is necessary. Elevate legs when sitting or resting. Avoid tight garters or restrictive bands around legs.
Varicose veins	Venous congestion in the lower veins that increases with pregnancy Hereditary factors (weakening of walls of veins, faulty valves) Increased age and weight gain	Elevate legs frequently. Wear supportive hose. Avoid crossing legs at the knees, standing for long periods, wearing garters, and wearing hosiery with constrictive bands.
Hemorrhoids	Constipation (see following discussion) Increased pressure from gravid uterus on hemorrhoidal veins	Avoid constipation. Apply ice packs, topical ointments, anesthetic agents, warm soaks, or sitz baths; gently reinsert hemorrhoid into rectum as necessary.
Constipation	Increased levels of progesterone, which cause general bowel sluggishness Pressure of enlarging uterus on intestine Iron supplements Diet, lack of exercise, and decreased fluids	Increase fluid intake, fiber in the diet, and exercise. Develop regular bowel habits. Use stool softeners as recommended by physician.

TABLE 23–11 Self-Care Measures for Common Discomforts of Pregnancy (continued)

DISCOMFORT	INFLUENCING FACTORS	SELF-CARE MEASURES
Backache	Increased curvature of the lumbosacral vertebrae as the uterus enlarges Increased levels of hormones, which cause softening of cartilage in body joints Fatigue Poor body mechanics	Use proper body mechanics. Practice the pelvic-tilt exercise. Avoid uncomfortable working heights, high-heeled shoes, lifting of heavy loads, and fatigue.
Leg cramps	Imbalance of calcium/phosphorus ratio Increased pressure of uterus on nerves Fatigue Poor circulation to lower extremities Pointing the toes	Practice dorsiflexion of feet to stretch affected muscle. Evaluate diet. Apply heat to affected muscles. Arise slowly from resting position.
Faintness	Postural hypotension Sudden change of position causing venous pooling in dependent veins Standing for long periods in warm area Anemia	Avoid prolonged standing in warm or stuffy environments. Evaluate hematocrit and hemoglobin.
Dyspnea	Decreased vital capacity from pressure of enlarging uterus on the diaphragm	Use proper posture when sitting and standing. Sleep propped up with pillows for relief if problem occurs at night.
Flatulence	Decreased gastrointestinal motility leading to delayed emptying time Pressure of growing uterus on large intestine Air swallowing	Avoid gas-forming foods. Chew food thoroughly. Get regular daily exercise. Maintain normal bowel habits.
Carpal tunnel syndrome	Compression of median nerve in carpal tunnel of wrist Aggravated by repetitive hand movements	Use splint as prescribed. Elevate affected arm. Avoid aggravating hand movements.

discomforts of pregnancy, their possible causes, and the self-care measures that might relieve discomfort.

PRACTICE ALERT

At each prenatal visit, provide client teaching on changes or possible discomforts the woman might encounter during the coming month and the next trimester. If the pregnancy is progressing normally, spend a few minutes describing her baby at that particular stage of development.

NAUSEA AND VOMITING Nausea and vomiting of pregnancy (NVP) are early, very common symptoms occurring in 70–85% of pregnant women (ACOG, 2004). These symptoms appear sometime after the first missed menstrual period and usually cease by the fourth missed menstrual period. Some women develop an aversion to specific foods, many experience nausea upon arising in the morning, and others experience nausea throughout the day or in the evening.

The exact cause of NVP is unknown, but it is thought to be multifactorial. An elevated hCG level is believed to be a major factor, but changes in carbohydrate metabolism, fatigue, and emotional factors also may play a role. Research suggests that pregnant women should start taking a multivitamin before reaching 6 weeks gestation to reduce the effects of NVP (ACOG, 2004).

In addition to the self-care measures identified in Table 23–11, certain complementary therapies may be useful. For example, many women find that acupressure applied to pressure points in the wrists is helpful (Figure 23–34 ■). Ginger also may relieve

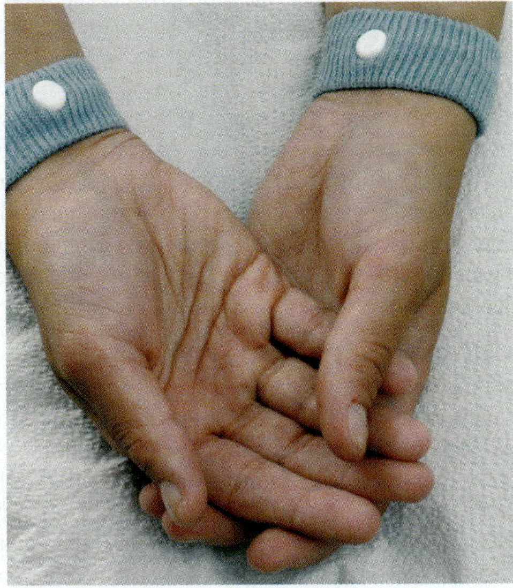

Figure 23–34 ■ Acupressure wristbands are sometimes used to help relieve nausea during early pregnancy.

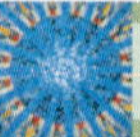

ALTERNATIVE THERAPIES Ginger for Morning Sickness

Women who experience NVP often try alternative approaches to relieve their symptoms because they are reluctant to take medication for fear of harming their fetus. Ginger, long used in traditional Chinese medicine for a variety of maladies ranging from gastrointestinal problems to headaches, is becoming an increasingly popular treatment for NVP, and its safety has been demonstrated in clinical trials (White, 2007). Ginger is available in a variety of forms, including the fresh root, capsules, tea, candy, cookies, crystals, inhaled powdered ginger, and sugared ginger (Lie, 2004). In the first trimester, the daily dosage should not exceed 2 g of dried ginger or 1 g of ginger syrup (Born & Barron, 2005).

NVP. (See Alternative Therapies: Ginger for Morning Sickness.) Pyridoxine (vitamin B_6) or vitamin B_6 plus doxylamine (Unisom), an over-the-counter antihistamine, is considered a first-line treatment. Antihistamine H_1 receptor blockers, benzamines, and phenothiazines are considered safe and effective for treating refractory cases. In severe cases, methylprednisolone, a steroid, may be used, but as a last resort because it poses a potential risk to the fetus (ACOG, 2004).

A woman should be advised to contact her health care provider if she vomits more than once a day or shows signs of dehydration such as dry mouth and concentrated urine. In such cases, the physician/CNM might order an antiemetic such as promethazine (Phenergan). However, if possible, antiemetics should be avoided during this time because of possible harmful effects on embryonic development.

URINARY FREQUENCY Urinary frequency, a common discomfort of pregnancy, occurs early in pregnancy and again during the third trimester because of pressure of the enlarging uterus on the bladder. Although frequency is considered normal during the first and third trimesters, the woman is advised to report to her health care provider signs of bladder infection such as pain, burning with voiding, or blood in the urine. Fluid intake should never be decreased to prevent frequency. The woman needs to maintain an adequate fluid intake—at least 2000 mL (eight to ten 8 oz glasses) per day. She also should be encouraged to empty her bladder frequently (about every 2 hours while awake).

BACKACHE Over 50% of women experience backache during pregnancy (Johnson, Gregory, & Niebyl, 2007). Backache is due primarily to exaggeration of the lumbosacral curve that occurs as the uterus enlarges and becomes heavier. Maintaining good posture and using proper body mechanics throughout pregnancy can help prevent backache. The pregnant woman is advised to avoid bending over at the waist to pick up objects and should bend from the knees instead. (See Figure 19–36 in Concept 19, Mobility.) She should place her feet 12–18 inches apart to maintain body balance. If the

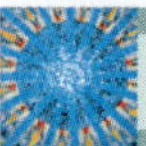

EVIDENCE-BASED PRACTICE Preventing and Treating Back Pain in Pregnancy

Clinical Question

What interventions can prevent back pain in pregnancy? How can back pain be safely treated during the prenatal period?

The Evidence

A descriptive study of the prevalence of prenatal back pain revealed that more than two thirds of pregnant women report back pain during pregnancy. Of these women, 21% described the pain as "severe," 80% reported that it interfered with sleep, and 75% took pain medication for relief. Unfortunately, 85% of these women reported that they had not been offered any treatment for their pain. A systematic review of randomized trials revealed very little research dealing specifically with prevention of back pain. Eight studies examined the effects of exercise, physical therapy, acupuncture, and the use of sleep pillows to treat the pain. This aggregation of randomized trials comparing pain interventions to standard prenatal care represents the strongest level of evidence for practice.

What Is Effective?

Exercises to strengthen the lower back, including pelvic tilt exercises, reduced pain intensity. Water aerobics reduced pain severity and decreased the number of missed work days because of pain. Acupuncture reduced pain intensity and provided relief from evening pain, thereby helping with sleep. Supporting the back with standard bed pillows did not demonstrate any therapeutic effect. Mothers who received standard prenatal care with no back pain interventions reported more use of analgesics than mothers who used these treatments.

What Is Inconclusive?

How much pain relief is achieved by these methods and how long the pain relief is sustained is unclear. Aside from strengthening exercises, the benefits of physical therapy for back pain in pregnancy were inconclusive. It is not known if any of these interventions can prevent back pain from starting in the first place.

Best Practice

The nurse should ask clients if they are experiencing back pain during pregnancy, as most women do. Offer treatments that have been shown to be effective, such as strengthening exercises and water aerobics. The latter may help women miss less work and enable them to continue normal daily activities. Women who are considering acupuncture can be encouraged to pursue this option, as it has been shown to provide relief from pain, particularly in the evening. Helping mothers use these interventions may reduce their reliance on pharmacologic pain relievers.

References

Granath, A., Hellgren, M., & Gunnarsson, R. (2006). Water aerobics reduces sick leave due to low back pain during pregnancy. *JOGNN: Journal of Obstetric, Gynecologic, & Neonatal Nursing, 35*(4), 465–471.

Pennick, R., & Young, G. (2007). Interventions for preventing and treating pelvic and back pain in pregnancy. *Cochrane Database of Systematic Reviews,* 4.

Skaggs, C., Prather, H., Gross, G., George, J., Thompson, P., & Nelson, D. (2007). Back and pelvic pain in an underserved United States pregnant population: A preliminary descriptive survey. *Journal of Manipulative & Physiological Therapeutics, 30*(2), 130–134.

woman uses work surfaces that require her to bend, the nurse can advise her to adjust the height of the surfaces.

PHARMACOLOGIC THERAPIES

A number of pharmacologic therapies may be used safely to protect the health and safety of the mother and fetus. Some of these are listed in the Medications: Pregnancy and Birth feature box.

A pregnant woman who lives with chronic illness or disease needs to discuss the treatment of her illness during her pregnancy with both her obstetrician and treating physician. The nurse's responsibility is to elicit information about any preexisting illness when obtaining the client's health history. Particular consideration should be given to clients with existing respiratory or cardiac disease, diabetes mellitus, and HIV. Pregnant clients living with a chronic disease require additional teaching regarding management of their disease during pregnancy. Collaboration among all of the health care professionals working with these clients is essential to promoting client self-care and fetal development.

It is important to recognize that pregnancy is usually a normal process that ends with the delivery of a healthy newborn. The nurse's role in these cases is health promotion and client teaching. However, alterations can result in injury to either the fetus or the client or both. The nurse assesses clients at each encounter in order to rapidly intervene to minimize complications and promote expected outcomes. Holistic, culturally appropriate care is important to make the experience as positive as possible for the client and her family.

MEDICATIONS Pregnancy and Birth

Classification	Action	Drug Examples	Nursing Considerations
Uterine stimulants (oxytocics)	Stimulates uterus to contract as levels increase, thus promoting labor and the delivery of the baby and the placenta. It also promotes the letdown reflex to promote milk production for breastfeeding mothers.	oxytocin, ergonovine maleate, methylergonovine maleate, carboprost tromethamine, dinoprostone, misoprostol	■ Monitor mother's condition and FHR frequently. ■ In order to administer these medications, fetus must be viable and vaginal delivery must be possible. ■ Do not administer if mother has a history of invasive cervical cancer, active herpes genitalia, or cord prolapse. ■ Contraindicated when client has had prior uterine or cervical surgery, including cesarean section, client is a grand multipara, or client is older than 35 years of age. ■ Discontinue if fetal distress occurs or uterine hyperstimulation results.
Uterine relaxants (tocolytics, $beta_2$ adrenergic agonists)	Relaxes smooth muscles of the uterus and diminishes premature contractions.	ritodrine hydrochloride, terbutaline sulfate, magnesium sulfate, nifedipine	■ Prepare mother for potential premature birth. ■ Monitor for possible tachycardia in the mother or fetus. ■ Asses magnesium levels and potential signs of magnesium toxicity.
Vitamin and mineral supplement	Administered to provide all essential vitamins and minerals required for both the growing fetus and the pregnant female.	multivitamin, multivitamin with iron	■ Vitamins without iron are given during the first trimester to reduce complication of nausea and vomiting.

PEARSON

EXPLORE mynursingkit™

MyNursingKit is your one stop for online chapter review materials and resources. Prepare for success with additional NCLEX®-style practice questions, interactive assignments and activities, web links, animations and videos, and more!

Register your access code from the front of your book at **www.mynursingkit.com**.

REFERENCES

Alan Guttmacher Institute. (2006a). *Facts on American teens' sexual and reproductive health.* Retrieved January 11, 2008, from http://www.guttmacher.org

Albrecht, S. A., Maloni, J. A., Thomas, K. K., Jones, R., Halleran, J., & Osborne, J. (2004). Smoking cessation for pregnant women who smoke: Scientific basis for practice: 'AWHONN's SUCCESS Project. *Journal of Obstetric, Gynecologic, and Neonatal Nursing, 33*(3), 298–305.

American Academy of Pediatrics (AAP). (2005). Policy statement: The changing concept of sudden infant death syndrome: Diagnostic coding shifts, controversies regarding the sleeping environment, and new variables to consider in reducing risk. *Pediatrics, 116*(5), 1245–1255.

American College of Obstetricians and Gynecologists (ACOG). (2004). *Diagnosis and treatment of nausea and vomiting in pregnancy* (ACOG Practice Bulletin No. 52). Washington, DC: Author.

American College of Obstetricians and Gynecologists (ACOG). (2007). Intrauterine device and adolescents (Committee Opinion No. 392). Washington, DC: Author.

Bearinger, L. H., Sieving, R. E., Ferguson, J., & Sharma, V. (2007). Global perspectives on the sexual and reproductive health of adolescents: Patterns, prevention, and potential. *The Lancet, 369*, 1220–1229.

Black, R. A., & Hill, D. A. (2003). Over-the-counter medications in pregnancy. *American Family Physician, 67*(12), 2517–2524.

Blackburn, S. T. (2007). *Maternal, fetal, & neonatal physiology: A clinical perspective* (2nd ed.). St. Louis, MO: Saunders.

Born, D., & Barron, M. L. (2005). Herb use in pregnancy. *American Journal of Maternal Child Nursing, 30*(3), 201–206.

Buist, A., Morse, C. A., & Durkin, S. (2003). Men's adjustment to fatherhood: Implications for obstetric health care. *Journal of Obstetric, Gynecologic, and Neonatal Nursing, 32*(2), 172–180.

Bunting, L., & McAuley, C. (2004). Research review: Teenage pregnancy and parenthood: The role of fathers. *Child and Family Social Work, (9)*, 295–303.

Burton, G. J., Sibley, C. P., & Jauniaux, E. R. M. (2007). Placental anatomy and physiology. In S. G. Gabbe, J. R. Niebyl, & J. L. Simpson (Eds.), *Obstetrics: Normal and problem pregnancies* (5th ed.). New York: Churchill-Livingstone.

Caldwell, W. E., & Moloy, H. C. (1933). Anatomical variations in the female pelvis and their effect on labor with a suggested classification [Historical article]. *American Journal of Obstetrics and Gynecology, 26*, 479–505.

Cassar, L. (2006). Cultural expectations of Muslims and Orthodox Jews in regard to pregnancy and the postpartum period: A study in comparison and contrast. *International Journal of Childbirth Education, 21*(2), 27–30.

Cohen, D. A., Farley, T. A., Taylor, S. N., Martin, D. H., & Schuster, M. A. (2002). When and where do youths have sex? The potential role of adult supervision. *Pediatrics, 110*(6), 66–69.

Cunningham, F. G., Leveno, K. J., Bloom, S. L., Hauth, J. C., & Wenstrom, K. D. (2005). *William's obstetrics* (22nd ed.). New York: McGraw-Hill.

Do, H. (2005). Chinese culture. *Ethnomed.* Retrieved November 29, 2005, from http://ethnomed.org

Doniger, A., Adams, E., Utter, C., & Riley, J. (2001). Impact evaluation of the "not me, not now" abstinence-oriented adolescent pregnancy prevention communication program, Monroe County, New York. *Journal of Health Communication, 6*(1), 45–60.

Eaton, D. K., Kann, L., Kinchen, S., Ross, L., Hawkins, J., Harris, W. A., et al. (2006, June 9). Youth risk behavior surveillance—United States, 2005. *Morbidity and Mortality Weekly Reports, 55*(SS05), 1–108.

Faust, J. E. (2005). Instruments in the hands of God. *Liahona Archives.* Retrieved January 4, 2008, from www.lds.org

Gilbert, W. M. (2007). Amniotic fluid disorders. In S. G. Gabbe, J. R. Niebyl, & J. L. Simpson (Eds.), *Obstetrics: Normal and problem pregnancies.* (5th ed., pp. 834–845). Philadelphia: Churchill Livingstone Elsevier.

Glass, N., Fredland, N., Campbell, J., Yonas, M., Sharps, P., & Kub, J. (2003). Adolescent dating violence: Prevalence, risk factors, health outcomes, and implications for clinical practice. *Journal of Obstetric, Gynecologic, and Neonatal Nursing, 32*(2), 227–238.

Goodman, J. H. (2005). Becoming an involved father of an infant. *Journal of Obstetric, Gynecologic, and Neonatal Nursing, 34*(2), 190–200.

Gordon, M. C. (2007). Maternal physiology. In S. G. Gabbe, J. R. Niebyl, & J. L. Simpson (Eds.), *Obstetrics: Normal and problem pregnancies* (5th ed.). New York: Churchill-Livingstone.

Hamilton, B. E., Martin, J., & Ventura, S. J. (2007). Births: Preliminary data for 2006. *National Vital Statistics Reports, 56*(7), 1–18.

Hammond, M. M., White, C. B., & Fetters, M. D. (2005). Opening cultural doors: Providing culturally sensitive healthcare to Arab American and American Muslim patients. *American Journal of Obstetrics & Gynecology, 193*(4), 1307–1311.

Hartmann, K. E., Wechter, M. E., Payne, P., Salisbury, K., Jackson, R. D., & Melvin, C. L. (2007). Best practice smoking cessation and resource needs of prenatal care providers. *Obstetrics & Gynecology, 110*(4), 765–770.

Holroyd, E., Twinn, S., & Yim, I. W. (2004). Exploring Chinese women's cultural beliefs and behaviors regarding the practice of "doing the month." *Women's Health, 40*(3), 109–123.

Johnson, T. R. B., Gregory, K. D., & Niebyl, J., R. (2007). Preconception and prenatal care: Part of the continuum. In S. G. Gabbe, J. R. Niebyl, & J. L. Simpson (Eds.), *Obstetrics: Normal and problem pregnancies* (5th ed.). New York: Churchill-Livingstone.

King-Jones, T. C. (2008). Pregnant adolescents: Perils and pearls of communication. *Nursing for Women's Health, 12*(2), 114–119.

Kirby, D. (2007). Emerging answers: Research findings on programs to reduce teen pregnancy and sexually transmitted diseases. The National Campaign to Prevent Teen and Unplanned Pregnancy. Retrieved April 17, 2008, from http://www.thenationalcampaign.org/EA2007/EA2007_sum.pdf

Klima, C. S. (2003). Centering pregnancy: A model for pregnant adolescents. *Journal of Midwifery & Women's Health, 48*(3), 220–225.

Knuppel, R. A. (2007). Maternal–placental–fetal unit: Fetal & early neonatal physiology. In A. H. Decherney, L. Nathan, T. M Goodwin, & N. Laufer (Eds.), *Current diagnosis and treatment: Obstetrics & gynecology* (10th ed.). Boston: McGraw-Hill.

Lie, D. (2004). Ginger helpful for nausea and vomiting of pregnancy. Medscape CME offering. Retrieved January 13, 2004, from www.medscape.com/viewarticle/466746_print

Males, M. (2004). Teens and older partners. *Resource Center for Adolescent Pregnancy Prevention (ReCAPP)* Retrieved January 15, 2008, from www.etr.org/recap/research/AuthoredPapOlderPrtnrs0504.htm

Manlove, J., Ryan, S., & Franzetta, K. (2003). Patterns of contraceptive use within teenagers' first sexual relationships. *Perspectives on Sexual and Reproductive Health, 35*(6), 246–255.

Marcell, A. V., Raine, T., & Eyre, S. L. (2003). Where does reproductive health fit into the lives of adolescent males? *Perspectives on Sexual and Reproductive Health, 35*(4), 180–186.

Messer, L. C., Dole, N., Kaufman, J. S., & Savitz, D. A. (2005). Pregnancy intendedness, maternal psychosocial factors and preterm birth. *Maternal and Child Health Journal, 9*(4), 403–412.

Montgomery, K. S. (2003). Nursing care for pregnant adolescents. *Journal of Obstetric, Gynecologic, and Neonatal Nursing, 32*(2), 249–257.

Moore, K. L., & Persaud, T. V. N. (2008). *The developing human: Clinical oriented embryology* (8th ed.). Philadelphia: Saunders.

National Campaign to Prevent Teen Pregnancy. (2004). Survey slices: Highlights from the National Campaign's 2003 Annual Survey. Retrieved January 22, 2004, from www.teenpregnancy.org

Niebyl, J. R., & Simpson, J. L. (2007). Drugs and environmental agents in pregnancy and lactation: Embryology, teratology, epidemiology. In S. G. Gabbe, J. R. Niebyl, & J. L. Simpson (Eds.), *Obstetrics: Normal and problem pregnancies* (5th ed.). New York: Churchill-Livingstone.

Okah, F. A., Cai, J., & Hoff, G. L. (2005). Term gestation low birth weight and health compromising behaviors during pregnancy. *Obstetrics and Gynecology, 105*(3), 543–550.

Premburg, A., & Lundgren, I. (2006). Fathers' experiences of childbirth education. *Journal of Perinatal Education, 15*(2), 21–28.

Rubin, R. (1984). *Maternal identity and the maternal experience.* New York: Springer.

Sadler, T. W. (2006). *Langman's medical embryology* (10th ed.). Philadelphia: Lippincott Williams & Wilkins.

Safadi, R. (2005). Jordanian women: Perceptions and practices of first-time pregnancy. *International Journal of Nursing Practice, 11*(6), 269–276.

Scheiman, L., & Zeoli, A. M. (2003). Adolescents' experiences of dating and intimate partner violence: "Once is not enough." *Journal of Midwifery and Women's Health, 48*(3), 226–228.

Semenic, S. E., Callister, L. C., & Feldman, P. (2004). Giving birth: The voices of Orthodox Jewish women living in Canada. *Journal of Obstetric, Gynecologic, and Neonatal Nursing, 33*(1), 80–87.

Short, M. B., & Rosenthal, S. L. (2003). Helping teenaged girls make wise sexual decisions. *Contemporary OB/GYN, 48*(5), 84–95.

Weinstock, H., Berman, S., & Cates, W. (2004). Sexually transmitted diseases among American youth: Incidence and prevalence estimates, 2000. *Perspectives on Sexual and Reproductive Health, 36*(1), 6–10.

White, B. (2007). Ginger: An overview. *American Family Physician, 75*, 1689–1691.

Self 24

Concept at-a-Glance

Concept Learning Outcomes

After reading about this concept, you will be able to:

1. Summarize the characteristics and psychosocial processes related to self-concept.
2. List factors affecting self-concept.
3. Identify commonly occurring alterations in self-concept and their related treatments.
4. Relate methods of assessing the client's self-concept.
5. Explore strategies to promote a healthy self-concept.
6. Demonstrate the nursing process in providing culturally competent and caring interventions across the life span for clients with alterations in self-concept.
7. Identify pharmacological interventions for the individual with alterations in self-concept.

Concept Key Terms

Anorexia nervosa, *1584*
Body image, *1582*
Bulimia nervosa, *1584*
Eating disorder, *1584*
Global self, *1580*
Global self-esteem, *1583*
Ideal self, *1581*
Introspection, *1580*
Personal identity, *1582*
Personality disorder, *1587*
Prader–Willi syndrome, *1585*
Purging, *1584*
Role, *1582*
Role ambiguity, *1583*
Role conflicts, *1583*
Role development, *1583*
Role mastery, *1582*
Role performance, *1582*
Role strain, *1583*
Self-awareness, *1580*
Self-concept, *1579*
Self-esteem, *1583*
Specific self-esteem, *1583*

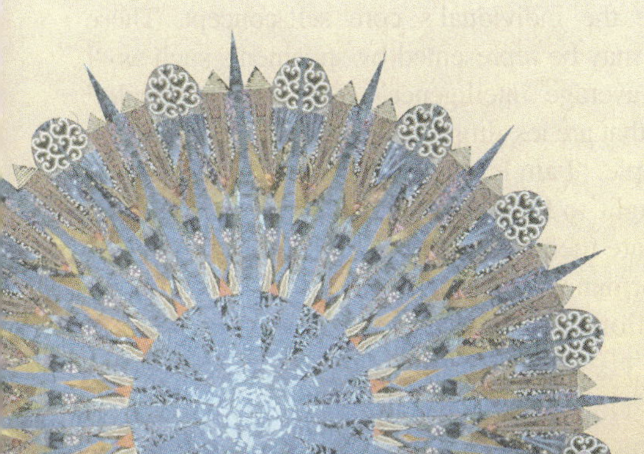

About Self-Concept

Self-concept is one's mental image of oneself. A positive self-concept is essential to a person's mental and physical health. Individuals with a positive self-concept are better able to develop and maintain interpersonal relationships and resist psychological and physical illness. An individual possessing a strong self-concept should be better able to accept or adapt to changes that may occur over the life span. How one views oneself affects one's interaction with others.

Nurses have a responsibility to assess clients for a negative self-concept and to identify the possible causes in order to help them develop a more positive view of themselves. Individuals who have a poor self-concept may express feelings of worthlessness, self-dislike, or even self-hatred. They may feel sad or hopeless, and may state they lack energy to perform even the simplest of tasks. ●

NORMAL PRESENTATION

Self-concept involves all of the self-perceptions—appearance, values, and beliefs—that influence behavior and are referred to when using the words *I* or *me*. Self-concept is a complex idea that influences the following:

- How one thinks, talks, and acts
- How one sees and treats another person
- Choices one makes
- Ability to give and receive love
- Ability to take action and to change things.

There are four dimensions of self-concept:

- Self-knowledge: the knowledge that one has about oneself, including insights into one's abilities, nature, and limitations
- Self-expectation: what one expects of oneself; may be a realistic or unrealistic expectation
- Social self: how a person is perceived by others and society
- Social evaluation: the appraisal of oneself in relationship to others, events, or situations.

Individuals who value "how I perceive me" above "how others perceive me" can be termed *me-centered*. They try hard to live up to their own expectations and compete only with themselves, not others. In contrast, strongly *other-centered* people have a high need for approval from others; they try hard to live up to the expectations of others, comparing, competing, and evaluating themselves in relation to others. Other-centered people tend not to deal with their personal shortcomings, are unable to assert themselves, and fear disapproval. The positive self-concept, therefore, is me-centered and is formed with minimal reference to others' opinions.

Assessing and promoting a positive self-concept is not limited to the nurse acting on the client. A nurse's own self-concept is also important. Nurses who understand the different dimensions of themselves are better able to understand the needs, desires, feelings, and conflicts of their clients. Nurses who feel positive about themselves are more likely to help clients meet their needs.

Self-awareness refers to the relationship between an individual's perception of himself or herself and others' perceptions of him or her. Thus, a nurse who is very self-aware has perceptions that are very congruent. Becoming more self-aware is a process that requires time and energy and is never complete. One important component of the process is **introspection**, which involves the individual considering his or her own beliefs, attitudes, motivations, strengths, and limitations (Donnelly, 2004). By using individual reflective exercises such as introspection, the nurse may increase his or her insight into the self. Working with other nurses who serve as mentors and talking seriously and acting on the feedback obtained during regular performance reviews also helps the nurse gain self-awareness.

Once the nurse has developed a clear understanding and awareness of self, the nurse can respect and avoid projecting his or her own beliefs onto others. While in the caregiver role, the self-aware nurse is able to suspend judgment and focus on the needs of the client, even if they differ from those of the nurse. When conflicts arise, the nurse can analyze his or her own reactions through introspection and by asking,

- "What is there in me that produces this kind of reaction in the client?"
- "Why do I react this way (fear, anger, anxiety, annoyance, worry)?"
- "Can I change the way I respond to this situation to affect the client's reaction in a helpful way?"

Formation of Self-Concept

A person is not born with a self-concept; rather, it develops as a result of social interactions with others. Concept 7 discusses the development of self-concept, including Erikson's stages of development, Piaget's cognitive developmental stages, and Havighurst's developmental tasks.

According to Erikson (1963), throughout life people face developmental tasks associated with eight psychosocial stages that provide a theoretical framework. The success with which a person copes with these developmental tasks largely determines the development of self-concept. Difficulty in coping results in self-concept problems at the time and, often, later in life. Table 24–1 lists examples of behaviors indicating successful and unsuccessful resolution of these developmental tasks.

There are three broad steps in the development of one's self-concept:

- The infant learns that the physical self is separate and different from the environment.
- The child internalizes others' attitudes toward self.
- The child and adult internalize the standards of society.

The term **global self** refers to the collective beliefs and images one holds about oneself. It is the most complete description that individuals can give of themselves at any one time. It is also a person's frame of reference for experiencing and viewing the world. Some of these beliefs and images represent statements of fact, for example, "I am a woman"; "I am a father"; "I am short." Others refer to less tangible aspects of self, for instance, "I am competent"; "I am shy."

Each separate image and belief one holds about oneself has a bearing on self-concept. However, self-concept is not simply the sum of its parts. The various images and beliefs people hold about themselves are not given equal weight and prominence. Each person's self-concept is like a piece of art. At the center of the art are the beliefs and images that are most vital to the individual's identity, that constitute the individual's core self-concept. These beliefs and images may be represented by statements such as "I am very smart/of average intelligence"; "I am male/female." Images and beliefs that are less important to the person are on the periphery, for example, "I am left-/right-handed."

People are thought to base their self-concept on how they perceive and evaluate themselves in these areas:

- Vocational performance
- Intellectual functioning

TABLE 24–1 **Examples of Behaviors Associated with Erikson's Stages of Psychosocial Development**

STAGE: DEVELOPMENTAL TASKS	BEHAVIORS INDICATING POSITIVE RESOLUTION	BEHAVIORS INDICATING NEGATIVE RESOLUTION
Infancy: trust vs. mistrust	Requesting assistance and expecting to receive it Expressing belief of another person Sharing time, opinions, and experiences	Restricting conversation to superficialities Refusing to provide a person with personal information Being unable to accept assistance
Toddlerhood: autonomy vs. shame and doubt	Accepting the rules of a group but also expressing disagreement when it is felt Expressing one's own opinion Easily accepting deferment of a wish fulfillment	Failing to express needs Not expressing one's own opinion when opposed Overconcern about being clean
Early childhood: initiative vs. guilt	Starting projects eagerly Expressing curiosity about many things Demonstrating original thought	Imitating others rather than developing independent ideas Apologizing and being very embarrassed over small mistakes Verbalizing fear about starting a new project
Early school years: industry vs. inferiority	Completing a task once it has been started Working well with others Using time effectively Not completing tasks started	Not assisting with the work of others Not organizing work
Adolescence: identity vs. role confusion	Asserting independence Planning realistically for future roles Establishing close interpersonal relationships	Failing to assume responsibility for directing one's own behavior Accepting the values of others without question Failing to set goals in life
Early adulthood: intimacy vs. isolation	Establishing a close, intimate relationship with another person Making a commitment to that relationship, even in times of stress and sacrifice Accepting sexual behavior as desirable	Remaining alone Avoiding close interpersonal relationships
Middle-aged adults: generativity vs. stagnation	Being willing to share with another person Guiding others Establishing a priority of needs, recognizing both self and others	Talking about oneself instead of listening to others Showing concern for oneself in spite of the needs of others Being unable to accept interdependence
Older adults: integrity vs. despair	Using past experience to assist others Maintaining productivity in some areas Accepting limitations	Crying and being apathetic Not accepting changes Demanding unnecessary assistance and attention from others

- Personal appearance and physical attractiveness
- Sexual attractiveness and performance
- Being liked by others
- Ability to cope with and resolve problems
- Independence
- Particular talents.

Self-concept in these areas also extends to the choices people make and perceptions they have about their health. Persons with strong positive self-concept about appearance are likely to value healthy behaviors and take action to maintain the health of their skin, hair, and body tone. Individuals with negative self-concepts may be less proactive about health promotion and illness prevention activities.

Maintaining and evaluating one's self-concept is an ongoing process. Events or situations may change the level of self-concept over time. Having a basic self-concept includes how we see ourselves and how we are seen by others. There is also the **ideal self**, which is how we should be or would prefer to be. The ideal self is the individual's perception of how one should behave based on certain personal standards, aspirations, goals, and values. Sometimes this ideal self is realistic; sometimes it is not. When perceived self is close to ideal self, people do not wish to be much different from what they believe they already are. A discrepancy between ideal self and perceived self can be an incentive to self-improvement. When the discrepancy is great, however, low self-esteem may result.

Nurses, like other adults, view themselves based on both internal and external inputs acquired over many years. The ability to appraise one's own strengths, the desire to follow in the steps of role models, and the feedback received from colleagues and clients are some of the influences on the nurse's self-concept.

Components of Self-Concept

There are four components of self-concept: personal identity, body image, role performance, and self-esteem.

PERSONAL IDENTITY **Personal identity** is the conscious sense of individuality and uniqueness that is continually evolving throughout life. People often view their identity in terms of name, sex, age, race, ethnic origin or culture, occupation or roles, talents, and other situational characteristics (e.g., marital status and education).

Personal identity also includes beliefs and values, personality, and character. For instance, is the individual outgoing, friendly, reserved, generous, selfish? Personal identity thus encompasses both the tangible and factual, such as name and sex, and the intangible, such as values and beliefs. Identity is what distinguishes self from others.

A person with a strong sense of identity has integrated body image, role performance, and self-esteem into a complete self-concept. This sense of identity provides the individual with a feeling of continuity and a unity of personality. Furthermore, the individual sees himself or herself as a unique person.

BODY IMAGE The image of physical self, or **body image**, is how an individual perceives the size, appearance, and functioning of his or her body and its parts. Body image has both cognitive and affective aspects. The cognitive is the knowledge of the material body; the affective includes the sensations of the body, such as pain, pleasure, fatigue, and physical movement. Body image is the sum of these attitudes, conscious and unconscious, that a person has toward his or her body.

Body image includes clothing, makeup, hairstyle, jewelry, and other things intimately connected to the person (Figure 24–1 ■). It also includes body prostheses, such as artificial limbs, dentures, and hairpieces, as well as devices required for functioning, such as wheelchairs, canes, and eyeglasses. Past as well as present perceptions and how the body has evolved over time are part of one's body image.

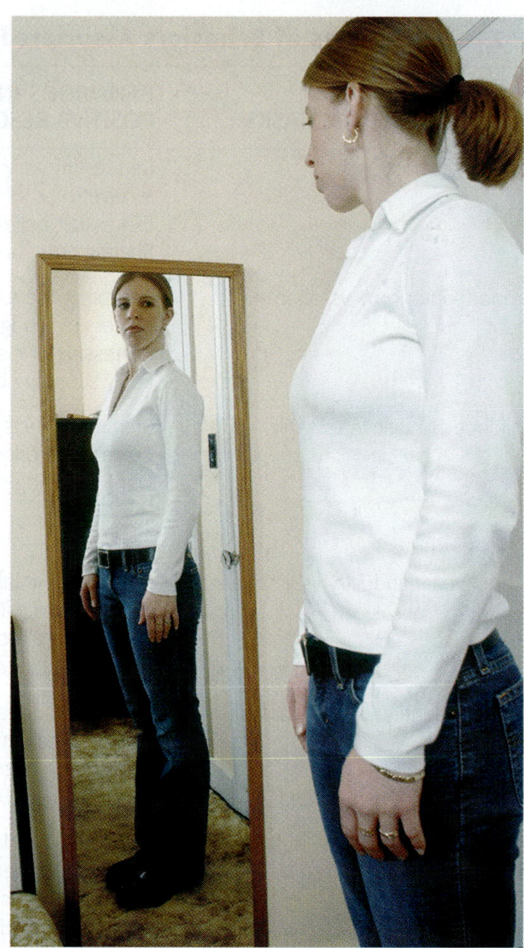

Figure 24–1 ■ Body image is the sum of a person's conscious and unconscious attitudes about his or her body.

An individual's body image develops partly from others' attitudes and responses to that person's body and partly from the individual's own exploration of the body. For example, body image develops in infancy as the parents or caregivers respond to the child with smiles, holding, and touching, and as the child explores its own body sensations during breastfeeding, thumb sucking, and the bath. Cultural and societal values also influence the individual's body image.

The various information and entertainment media have played a part over the years in how individuals view themselves and others. During adolescence, concerns related to body image are of paramount interest. The "ideal" person portrayed by the media is really an unrealistic goal for many.

If a person's body image closely resembles one's body ideal, the individual is more likely to think positively about the physical and nonphysical components of the self. The body ideal is greatly influenced by cultural standards. For example, currently in North America the fit, well-toned body is admired.

Another aspect of body image is the understanding that different parts of the body have different values for different people. For example, large breasts may be highly important to one woman and unimportant to another, or the occurrence of gray hair may be traumatic to one individual and barely noticed by another.

The individual with a healthy body image will normally show concern for both health and appearance. This person will seek help if ill and will include health-promoting practices in daily activities. The individual who has an unhealthy body image is likely to be overly concerned about minor illness and to neglect activities like sleep and a healthy diet that are important to health.

The individual who has a body image disturbance may hide, not look at, or not touch a body part that is significantly changed in structure by illness or trauma. Some individuals may also express feelings of helplessness, hopelessness, powerlessness, and vulnerability, and may exhibit self-destructive behavior such as under- or overeating or attempting suicide.

ROLE PERFORMANCE Throughout life, people undergo numerous role changes. A **role** is a set of expectations about how the person occupying one position behaves. **Role performance** relates what a person in a particular role does to the behaviors expected of that role. **Role mastery** means that the individual's behaviors meet social expectations. Expectations, or standards of behavior of a role, are set by society; a cultural or religious group, such as a tribe or a congregation; or a smaller group to which the individual belongs. Each individual usually has several roles, such as husband, parent, brother, son, employee, friend, nurse, and church member. Some roles are assumed for only limited periods, such as client, student, and ill person. **Role development** involves socialization into a particular role. For example, nursing students are socialized into nursing through exposure to their instructors, clinical experience, classes, laboratory simulations, and seminars.

To act appropriately, people need to know who they are in relation to others and what society expects for the positions they hold. **Role ambiguity** occurs when expectations are unclear, and when people do not know how to perform their roles and are unable to predict the reactions of others to their behavior. Failure to master a role creates frustration and feelings of inadequacy, often resulting in lower self-esteem.

Self-concept is also affected by role strain and role conflicts. People undergoing **role strain** are frustrated because they feel or are made to feel inadequate or unsuited to a role. Role strain is often associated with sex role stereotypes. For example, women in occupations traditionally held by men might be treated as having less knowledge and competence than men in the same roles.

Role conflicts arise from opposing or incompatible expectations. In an interpersonal conflict, people have different expectations about a particular role. For example, a grandparent may have different expectations than the mother about how she should care for her children. In an inter-role conflict, one person's or group's role expectations differ from the expectations of another person or group. For example, a woman who has little flexibility in her full-time job schedule has a role conflict if her husband expects her to handle all child care problems. In a person-role conflict, role expectations violate the beliefs or values of the role occupant. For example, a nurse in a family planning clinic may be expected to advise couples about birth control methods that are not consistent with the nurse's belief system regarding prevention or management of unwanted pregnancy. Role conflict can lead to tension, decrease in self-esteem, and embarrassment if needs for achievement, independence, and recognition are unmet.

SELF-ESTEEM **Self-esteem** refers to one's judgment of one's own worth; that is, how the individual's standards and performances compare to others and to the individual's ideal self. If a person's self-esteem does not match with the ideal self, then poor self-concept results.

There are two types of self-esteem: global and specific. **Global self-esteem** is how much one likes oneself as a whole. **Specific self-esteem** is how much one approves of a certain part of oneself. Global self-esteem is influenced by specific self-esteem. For example, if a man values his looks, then how he looks will strongly affect his global self-esteem. By contrast, if a man places little value on his cooking skills, then how well or badly he cooks will have little influence on his global self-esteem.

Self-esteem is derived from self and others. In infancy, self-esteem is related to the caregiver's evaluations and acceptances. Later the child's self-esteem is affected by competition with others. As an adult, an individual who has high self-esteem has feelings of significance, of competence, of the ability to cope with life, and of control over his or her destiny.

The individual establishes a foundation for self-esteem during early life experiences, usually within the family structure. However, an adult's level of overall self-esteem may change markedly from day to day and moment to moment. Severe stress—for example, stress related to prolonged illness or unemployment—can substantially lower a person's self-esteem. In health care, clients who believe that their condition is viewed negatively by society may have lower self-esteem (Berge & Ranney, 2005). People frequently focus on their negative aspects and spend less time on their positive aspects. It is important that nurses assist clients to identify both strengths and weaknesses in order to promote self-esteem and health-promoting behaviors.

Factors That Affect Self-Concept

Many factors affect a person's self-concept. Major factors are stage of development, family and culture, stressors, resources, history of success and failure, and illness.

EVIDENCE-BASED PRACTICE Can Assertiveness Training Improve Nursing Students' Self-Esteem?

A study reported in a 2004 issue of *Nurse Education Today* attempted to evaluate a training program on nursing and medical students' assertiveness, self-esteem, and interpersonal communication satisfaction. The researchers followed 69 participants who had been identified as having low assertiveness that were assigned to either an experimental or comparison group. Participants in the experimental group received assertiveness training once a week. Data were collected before and after training and again one month after the end of the training. The assertiveness and self-esteem of the experimental group were significantly improved in nursing and medical students after assertiveness training, although interpersonal communication satisfaction of the experimental group was not significantly improved after the training program.

Implications

This study shows that it is possible to improve both self-esteem and assertiveness through educational intervention if the initial level of assertiveness is low. It is unknown for how long the improvement might last. The details regarding the training, and the meaning of the failure to improve satisfaction with communication, need to be evaluated for influence of culture. Communication styles differ significantly among ethnic groups and it is important to determine whether the ethnicity of health care providers is similar to or different from that of the dominant society.

Note: From Lin, Y., Shiah, I., Lai, T., Wang, K., & Chou, K. (2004). Evaluation of an assertiveness training program on nursing and medical students' assertiveness, self esteem, and interpersonal communication satisfaction. *Nurse Education Today, 24*(8), 656–665.

STAGE OF DEVELOPMENT As an individual develops, the conditions that affect self-concept change. For example, an infant requires a supportive, caring environment, while a child requires freedom to explore and learn. Older adults' self-concept is based on their experiences in progressing through life's stages.

FAMILY AND CULTURE A young child's values are largely influenced by family and culture. As the client grows, peer influence becomes more important and has a greater affect on the sense of self. When the child is confronted by differing expectations from family, culture, and peers, the child's sense of self is often confused (Figure 24–2 ■). For example, a child's parents may expect him to abstain from alcohol and to attend religious services each Saturday evening, while his peers drink beer and encourage him to spend Saturday evenings with them.

STRESSORS Stressors can strengthen the self-concept as an individual copes successfully with problems or cause maladaptive responses, such as substance abuse, withdrawal, and anxiety, in the individual who is unable to cope successfully with them. The ability of a person to handle stressors largely depends on personal resources.

RESOURCES An individual's resources are internal and external. Examples of internal resources include confidence and values, whereas external resources include a support network, sufficient finances, and organizations. Generally the greater the number of resources a person has and uses, the more positive the effect on the self-concept. Stress, coping, and resources are discussed in further detail in Concept 28.

HISTORY OF SUCCESS AND FAILURE People who have a history of failures come to see themselves as failures, whereas people with a history of successes develop a more positive self-concept. Likewise, persons with a positive self-concept tend to find contentment in their level of success, while those with a negative self-concept may come to view their life situation as negative.

ILLNESS Illness and trauma can also affect the self-concept. A woman who has a mastectomy may see herself as less attractive, and the loss may affect how she acts and values herself.

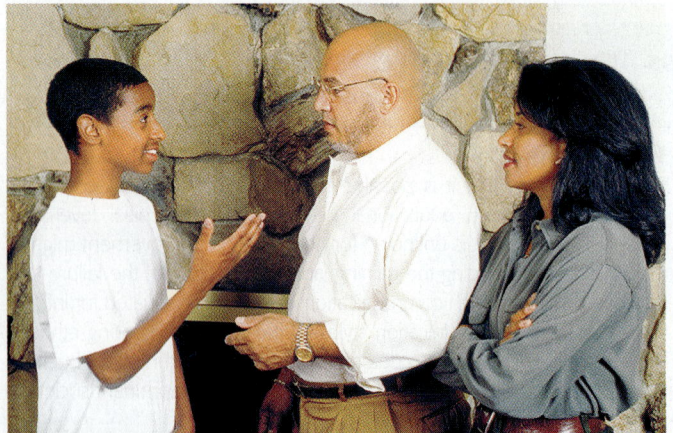

Figure 24–2 ■ A child is often pulled in opposite directions by family and peer expectations.

Source: Jonathan Nourak/Photoedit.

People respond to stressors such as illness and alterations in function related to aging in a variety of ways. Acceptance, denial, withdrawal, and depression are common reactions.

It is sometimes difficult to determine the direction of the relationship between self-concept and health. Some research has shown that persons with a positive self-concept may enhance their health because they are more likely to follow the health care plan (Burkhart & Rayens, 2005). Other research shows that health conditions, including psychosocial situations such as loss and grieving, have an impact on self-concept (see Montpetit, Bisconti, & Bergeman, 2004). Thus, self-concept and health-related behavior are intertwined.

ALTERATIONS

People exhibit alterations of self-concept in a variety of ways. Individuals with a more positive sense of self may experience temporary alterations when confronted with a difficult but time-limited event, such as a move across the country or the transition from college to employment. These individuals normally exhibit or develop the behaviors they need to master new situations or roles without assistance from health care professionals. Those with lower self-esteem may develop a set of maladaptive behaviors that continue over time and require intervention and treatment. Eating disorders and personality disorders are two categories of alterations of self that require interaction with the health care system.

Eating Disorders

An **eating disorder** is a set of maladaptive responses to stress or anxiety characterized by obsessions with food and weight to the extent that daily functioning is impaired and physical and psychological health are threatened. Individuals who have eating disorders suffer deeply both emotionally and physically. These disorders cause low self-esteem, self-hatred, fear, and hopelessness and put the individual at risk for a variety of physiological problems (see Multisystem Effects of Malnutrition on page 1586). Those with eating disorders often also have other mental disorders such as anxiety disorder (Concept 28, Stress and Coping), substance abuse (Concept 2, Addictive Behaviors), and depression (Concept 20, Mood and Affect) (Spearing, 2001). Eating disorders can be fatal. Nurses should not underestimate the significance of these disorders.

ANOREXIA NERVOSA AND BULIMIA NERVOSA Anorexia nervosa and bulimia nervosa are often thought of as separate diseases, because their primary symptoms are different: **Anorexia nervosa** is a potentially life-threatening disorder characterized by extreme perfectionism; weight fear; significant weight loss; body image disturbances; strenuous exercising; peculiar food-handling patterns; and reductions in heart rate, blood pressure, metabolic rate, and the production of estrogen or testosterone. Individuals with **bulimia nervosa** develop cycles of binge eating followed by **purging** (self-induced vomiting or the misuse of laxitives, diuretics, or enemas). The severity of the disorder is determined by the frequency of the binge–purge cycles. Despite these very different manifestations, anorexia nervosa and bulimia nervosa

ALTERATIONS AND TREATMENTS Self-Concept

Alteration	Description	Treatment
Eating disorders	Maladaptive responses to stress or anxiety characterized by obsessions with food and weight to the extent that daily functioning is impaired and physical and psychological health are threatened	■ Pharmacologic therapy for comorbid disorders or to manage acute symptoms ■ Medical treatment as appropriate for manifestations related to malnutrition ■ Psychotherapy
Personality disorders	An enduring pattern of inner experience and behavior that occurs over time and deviates markedly from the expectations of the individual's culture	■ Pharmacologic therapy for comorbid disorders or to manage acute symptoms ■ Long-term psychotherapy

are not single diseases but syndromes with multiple predisposing factors and a variety of characteristics. Although the most obvious symptom is the eating problem, these disorders are not simply a matter of eating too much or too little. It is because of the complex interaction of biological, psychological, developmental, familial, and sociocultural factors that certain individuals develop eating disorders.

There is no clear-cut distinction between the two disorders, and they have many features in common. The traditional division of anorexia and bulimia is still appropriate until more is known about them. Body weight may be a significant distinguishing characteristic; individuals with anorexia are severely underweight and people with bulimia are at normal or near-normal weight. About 30% of people with bulimia have a history of anorexia. As many as 62% of people with anorexia exhibit bulimic behaviors. Conversion from anorexia to bulimia may be a way of moving from a "visible" to an "invisible" eating disorder to deceive family, friends, and health care providers. Thus, the two disorders can occur in the same person, or the person can go from one disorder to the other. There are far more similarities than differences between anorexia and bulimia (Finfgeld, 2002; Tozzi et al., 2005). However, to help explain the differences, the disorders have been separated in this chapter (see Box 24–3, the *DSM-IV-TR* Classifications feature, later in this chapter).

BINGE-EATING DISORDER The bulimic pattern is different from binge-eating disorder, which is often associated with obesity. This is a proposed new category that needs further study before inclusion into the *Diagnostic and Statistical Manual of Mental Disorders* (4th ed., Text Revision) (*DSM-IV-TR*) (APA, 2000). The prevalence in the general population is 1–3% and as high as 25% in those people seeking help for weight loss (Pull, 2004).

Obese individuals who overeat tend to follow one of two patterns, neither of which includes purging the body after excessive food intake. The first pattern is overeating and feeling out of control in response to a number of feelings such as anxiety or depression. The diagnosis of binge-eating disorder is given when binging occurs at least twice a week for 6 months. Some binge in response to losing control over a weight-loss diet. Although these individuals lose weight in weight-control programs, they regain it after going off the diet. People with this eating pattern say that their eating or weight interferes with their relationships and their self-esteem. Women are more likely to have this eating pattern than men. There is evidence that several drugs are effective for this disorder including sibutramine (Meridia), an appetite suppressant; citalopram (Celexa), a selective serotonin reuptake inhibitor (SSRI) antidepressant; and topiramate (Topamax), an anticonvulsant and mood stabilizer (Appolinario et al., 2003; Neumark-Sztainer, 2005; Pull, 2004).

The second pattern is overeating because of the enjoyment of food. Seldom attempting to diet, these individuals have no sense of loss of control. They are more accepting of their body size and understand it to be the result of their enjoyment of eating.

OTHER DISORDERS The exemplar on eating disorders will discuss anorexia nervosa, bulimia nervosa, and binge-eating disorder in detail. Other eating disorders of which the nurse should be aware are purging disorder, nocturnal sleep-related eating disorder, and Prader–Willi syndrome.

Purging Disorder Purging disorder is a separate clinical disorder from bulimia. Individuals with purging disorder do not binge eat but do purge frequently. Screening tests may miss this group of individuals because they are of normal weight and respond negatively to the binge-eating questions. Given that purging itself has serious medical consequences, it is important to identify these clients (Keel, Haedt, & Edler, 2005).

Nocturnal Sleep-Related Eating Disorder Nocturnal sleep-related eating disorder is a newly recognized form of binge eating. It is characterized by sleepwalking and sleep eating. Safety becomes a problem when individuals actually prepare meals while asleep, resulting in burns or even a fire. Some sufferers discover bruises and lacerations from bumping into walls or furniture while sleepwalking. Upon awakening, the individual may have no recall or may have vague recall of the nighttime behavior. This eating disorder is found in those individuals of normal weight and those who are overweight. Some may also experience a daytime eating disorder such as anorexia or bulimia (Pull, 2004).

Prader–Willi Syndrome **Prader–Willi syndrome (PWS)** is a congenital disorder of the 15th chromosome. Estimated prevalence is 1 in 10,000 to 15,000 live births. PWS not only causes an unrelenting feeling of hunger, but also low muscle tone, short stature, incomplete sexual development, mild to severe

MULTISYSTEM EFFECTS OF **Malnutrition**

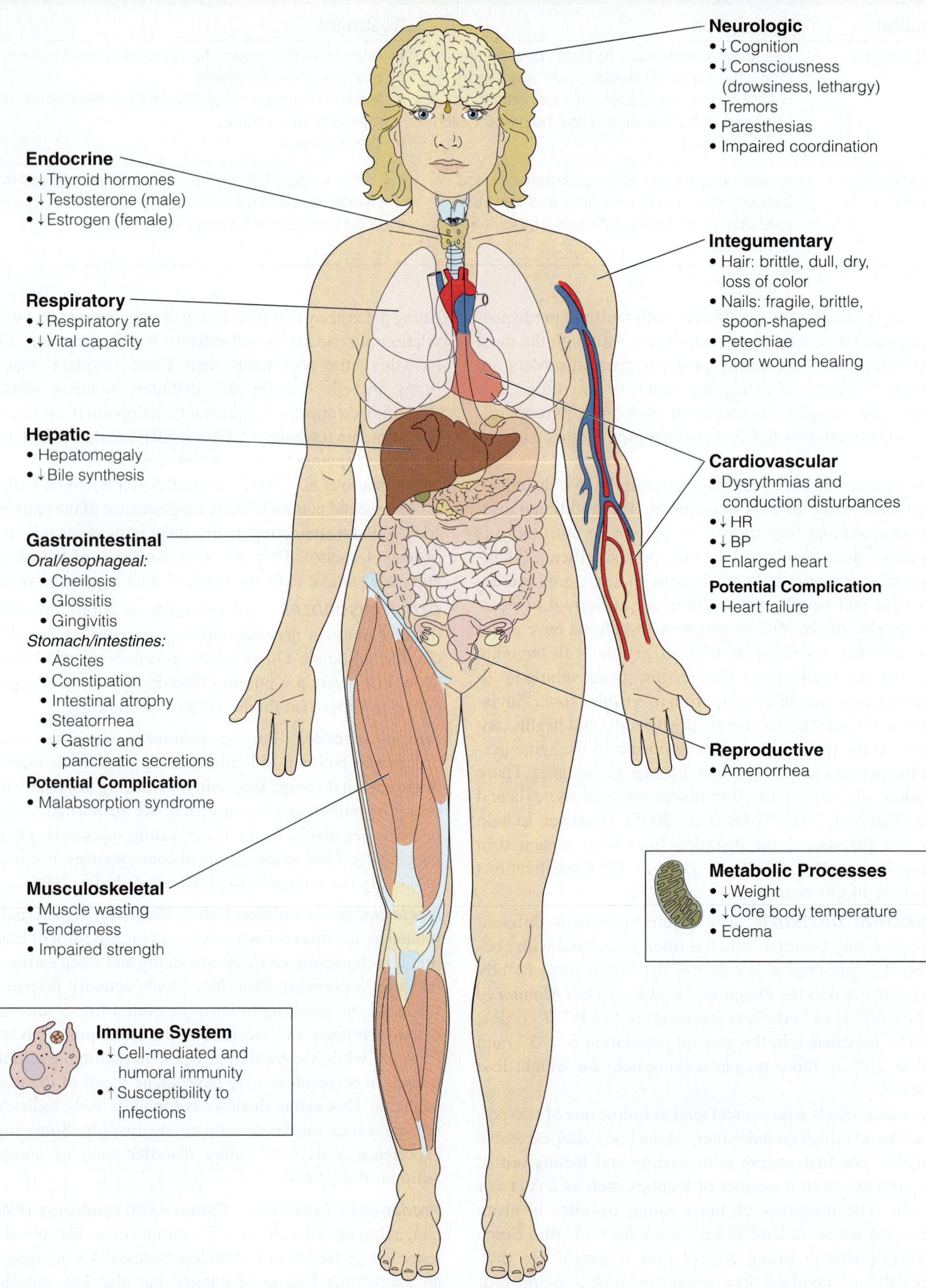
Neurologic
• ↓ Cognition
• ↓ Consciousness (drowsiness, lethargy)
• Tremors
• Paresthesias
• Impaired coordination
Endocrine
• ↓ Thyroid hormones
• ↓ Testosterone (male)
• ↓ Estrogen (female)
Integumentary
• Hair: brittle, dull, dry, loss of color
• Nails: fragile, brittle, spoon-shaped
• Petechiae
• Poor wound healing
Respiratory
• ↓ Respiratory rate
• ↓ Vital capacity
Hepatic
• Hepatomegaly
• ↓ Bile synthesis
Cardiovascular
• Dysrythmias and conduction disturbances
• ↓ HR
• ↓ BP
• Enlarged heart
Potential Complication
• Heart failure
Gastrointestinal
Oral/esophageal:
• Cheilosis
• Glossitis
• Gingivitis
Stomach/intestines:
• Ascites
• Constipation
• Intestinal atrophy
• Steatorrhea
• ↓ Gastric and pancreatic secretions
Potential Complication
• Malabsorption syndrome
Reproductive
• Amenorrhea
Metabolic Processes
• ↓ Weight
• ↓ Core body temperature
• Edema
Musculoskeletal
• Muscle wasting
• Tenderness
• Impaired strength
Immune System
• ↓ Cell-mediated and humoral immunity
• ↑ Susceptibility to infections

mental retardation, and behavioral problems. By age 2 or 3 years, the child's appetite becomes insatiable and there is a rapid and excessive weight gain. The physiologically driven eating behavior is not under the individual's cognitive control. The person cannot decide "not to eat." Compounding the excessive appetite is decreased calorie utilization in those with PWS due to low muscle mass and inactivity. Their calorie needs are about 60% of other persons. Access to food must be rigidly enforced if they are not to become morbidly obese. Restricting food intake must extend from the home and into school, work, and community settings. Hoarding food and stealing money to buy food are very common problems for this group of individuals. Morbid obesity may lead to serious medical consequences, including cardiovascular diseases, diabetes mellitus, sleep disturbances, and respiratory compromise. These are the most common causes of premature death among those suffering from PWS (Nolan, 2003).

Behavioral problems can lead to curtailed psychosocial development and poor social functioning. Symptoms may include temper tantrums, oppositional behavior and stubbornness, labile emotions, and obsessive thinking or compulsive behaviors, such as skin picking. Some individuals compulsively engage in rectal digging, which often causes embarrassment to them and their families. Rectal digging has potential risks, ranging from fecal contamination to rectal bleeding and sphincter problems. Treatment of PWS is growth hormone that increases muscle tone and enhances growth. For those who are depressed or anxious, antidepressants are often prescribed (Nolan, 2003).

Personality Disorders

Although the normal range of human behavior, feelings, and thought is broad, it is possible for personality to be outside the normal range. A **personality disorder (PD)** is an enduring pattern of inner experience and behavior that has the following characteristics (American Psychiatric Association, 2000):

- It deviates markedly from the expectations of the individual's culture.
- It is pervasive and inflexible.
- It begins in adolescence or young adulthood.

FOCUS ON DIVERSITY AND CULTURE
Personality and Culture

Any judgment about a client's personality must take into account that individual's ethnic, cultural, and social background. People who are immigrants from other cultures are especially at risk of being diagnosed with disorders of mental function and personality when they are acting or thinking in a way that is accepted in their culture of origin but not in their new home. For example, a Cuban immigrant stated to the nurse that her dead father talked to her and told her to be careful when talking to strangers. In the Cuban culture, "talking" with deceased people may mean the same as "This is what my father would have wanted me to do" in the European American culture. The nurse can become more culturally sensitive to this client by talking with other Cuban people or learning more about the client's culture in other ways.

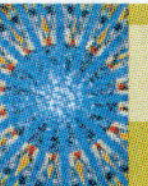

DEVELOPMENTAL CONSIDERATIONS
Personality Disorders in Children

Whether there are early signs of personality disorders in children is a current research question. Studies have found that both personality traits and environmental experiences in childhood appear to contribute to the development of personality disorders in adulthood. There is not a direct correlation, but children who have a conduct disorder are statistically more likely to develop antisocial personality disorder as adults. Children with self-mutilating behavior and impulse control problems are more likely to develop borderline personality disorder. Obsessive–compulsive personality disorder appears to have a more clearly genetic basis. Adults with obsessive–compulsive personality disorder often had a history of symptoms beginning in childhood (De Clercq & De Fruyt, 2007).

- It is stable over time.
- It leads to distress for the individual or impairment of functioning.

An individual's personality significantly affects how he or she responds to life events, including illnesses. The response a client has to a mental disorder will be affected by that client's personality as well. A client's culture also affects the client's behavior and personality. The Focus on Culture and Diversity feature shows the importance of considering a client's cultural background when interpreting behavior.

The American Psychiatric Association (2000) describes 11 types of personality disorders. Ten of these disorders are grouped into three clusters by their similarities. The clusters are based on similar observed behaviors:

1. Odd and eccentric
2. Dramatic and emotional
3. Anxiety and fear-based personality disorders.

Table 24–2 provides an outline of the categories.

The 11th disorder does not meet the diagnostic criteria for any of the others and is designated as *personality disorder not otherwise specified*. In some clients, there will be features of more than one disorder of personality. Such a client may have a diagnosis of "mixed" personality disorder.

TABLE 24–2 **Personality Disorders by Cluster**

CLUSTER	PERSONALITY DISORDER
A: Odd-eccentric	Paranoid Personality Disorder Schizoid Personality Disorder Schizotypal Personality Disorder
B: Dramatic-emotional	Antisocial Personality Disorder Borderline Personality Disorder Histrionic Personality Disorder Narcissistic Personality Disorder
C: Anxious-fearful	Avoidant Personality Disorder Dependent Personality Disorder Obsessive-Compulsive Personality Disorder

Source: American Psychiatric Association. (2000). *Diagnostic and statistical manual of mental disorders* (4th ed., Text Revision). Washington, DC: Author.

COMMON CLINICAL FEATURES ***Impaired Sense of Self*** Impaired sense of self is a central problem in disorders of personality. The sense of identity often is not adequately formed in people with personality disorders. Sense of self, or identity, is necessary for goal-directed behavior and for satisfying interpersonal relationships (Limandri & Boyd, 2005).

Thinking Patterns Thinking patterns are distorted in individuals with personality disorders. The individual's ability to decode stimuli and to interpret environmental events is impaired. Maladaptive thinking patterns cause individuals to misinterpret the actions of others. The misinterpretations result in maladaptive responses by the affected individual.

Emotions Emotions, in their intensity and quality, appear to be affected by disorders of personality. Individuals affected by personality disorders have blunted or distorted emotional experiences. They tend to have more negative emotional experiences. Their ability to function in daily life and even to learn new things is affected.

Behavior Behavior is a part of personality. First, personality disorders cause *impulsive behavior*. These disorders appear to make it more difficult for individuals to foresee the consequences of their actions or to control their impulses despite probable negative consequences.

Second, these disorders cause *inflexibility* of behavior. Affected clients tend to be rigid. They are unable to change their usual behavior when circumstances suggest that a change is indicated. Usually, people learn to change their behavior when they try new actions and receive positive reinforcement from the new approach. The inflexibility in personality disorders makes it difficult for affected individuals to learn new ways to behave or cope.

This inflexibility traps these clients in a vicious cycle of behaviors that are self-defeating. They become rigid and inflexible in role functions and personal interactions. The inflexibility provokes predicaments and problems. The more inflexible they are, the more problems they have. The more problems they have, the more inflexible they become. This vicious circle reduces learning opportunities and alienates other people (Millon & Davis, 1999). Figure 24–3 ■ illustrates this vicious cycle.

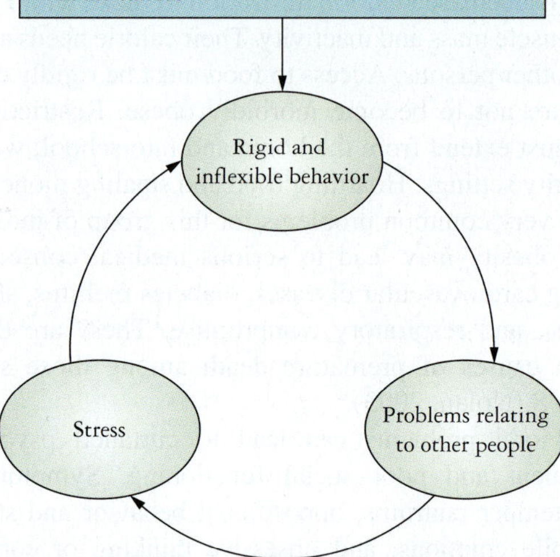

Figure 24–3 ■ Vicious Cycle of Personality Disorders.

ASSESSMENT

A thorough assessment of self-concept includes a psychosocial assessment of the client. Including the family, significant other, or close friends may provide clues to actual or potential problems. The nurse assessing self-concept focuses on the four components: (1) personal identity, (2) body image, (3) role performance, and (4) self-esteem.

Before conducting a psychosocial assessment, the nurse must establish trust and a working relationship with the client. Guidelines for conducting a psychosocial assessment include the following:

- Be aware of your own biases and discomforts that could influence the assessment.
- Minimize interruptions if possible.
- Maintain appropriate eye contact.
- Sit at eye level with the client.
- Demonstrate an interest in the client's concerns.
- Indicate acceptance of the client by not criticizing, frowning, or demonstrating shock.
- Ask open-ended questions to encourage the client to talk rather than close-ended questions that tend to block free sharing.
- Avoid asking more personal questions than are actually needed.
- Minimize writing detailed notes during the interview because this can create client concern that confidential material is being "recorded" as well as interfere with your ability to focus on what the client is saying.
- Determine whether the family can provide additional information.
- Maintain confidentiality.
- Create a quiet, private environment.
- Consider how the client's behavior is influenced by culture.

It is also important that the nurse identify any stressors that may affect aspects of the self-concept. See Box 24–1 for

FOCUS ON CULTURE AND DIVERSITY

Assessing Self-Concept

It is the nurse's responsibility to use therapeutic communication and to remain sensitive to the effect that cultural influences will have on the client's behaviors and needs. Cultural background is assessed directly and considered as a factor in the areas of self-perception, role relationships, major stressors, and coping strategies. In the area of behaviors that may suggest low self-esteem, nurses need to ask themselves the following question: Is this really a behavior that would suggest a low self-esteem or is it part of the cultural behavior(s) of the client? In addition, might the client be experiencing cultural dissonance, a situation in which there are conflicting beliefs and attitudes between the client's culture and the one in which the client is living?

Box 24–1 Stressors Affecting Self-Concept

IDENTITY STRESSORS

- Change in physical appearance (e.g., facial wrinkles)
- Declining physical, mental, or sensory abilities
- Inability to achieve goals
- Relationship concerns
- Sexuality concerns
- Unrealistic ideal self

BODY IMAGE STRESSORS

- Loss of body parts (e.g., amputation, mastectomy, hysterectomy)
- Loss of body functions (e.g., from stroke, spinal cord injury, neuromuscular disease, arthritis, declining mental or sensory abilities)
- Disfigurement (e.g., through pregnancy, severe burns, facial blemishes, colostomy, tracheostomy)
- Unrealistic body ideal (e.g., a muscular configuration that cannot be achieved)

SELF-ESTEEM STRESSORS

- Lack of positive feedback from significant others
- Repeated failures
- Unrealistic expectations
- Abusive relationship
- Loss of financial security

ROLE STRESSORS

- Loss of parent, spouse, child, or close friend
- Change or loss of job or other significant role
- Divorce
- Illness
- Ambiguous or conflicting role expectations
- Inability to meet role expectations

examples of stressors that may place a client at risk for problems with self-concept.

When stressors are identified, the nurse needs to determine how the client perceives the stressor. A positive, growth-oriented perception of stressful events reinforces self-worth; a negative, hopeless, defeatist perception leads to decreased self-esteem. The nurse should also identify the client's coping style and determine whether this style is effective by asking the client such questions as these:

- When you have a problem or face a stressful situation, how do you usually deal with it?
- Do these methods work?

PRACTICE ALERT

The degree to which a stressor is perceived to affect self-concept varies from person to person. For example, whereas some people may respond to repeated failures by trying harder, others may give up.

Personal Identity

When assessing self-concept, the information the nurse first needs is about the client's personal identity. This involves who the client believes he or she is. See the accompanying Assessment Interview for examples of questions to ask.

Body Image

If there are indications of a body image disturbance, the nurse should assess the client carefully for possible functional or physical problems. The disturbance may be a result of an anticipated or present deformity or malfunction. In addition to the stated responses about the problem, it is important to

Assessment Interview Self-esteem

PERSONAL IDENTITY

- How would you describe your personal characteristics? Or, how do you see yourself as a person?
- How do others describe you as a person?
- What do you like about yourself?
- What do you do well?
- What are your personal strengths, talents, and abilities?
- What would you change about yourself if you could?
- Does it bother you a great deal if you think someone doesn't like you?

BODY IMAGE

- Is there any part of your body you would like to change?
- Are you comfortable discussing your surgery?
- Do you feel different or inferior to others?
- How do you feel about your appearance?
- What changes in your body do you expect following your surgery?
- How have significant others in your life reacted to changes in your body?

SELF-ESTEEM

- Are you satisfied with your life?
- How do you feel about yourself?
- Are you accomplishing what you want?
- What goals in life are important to you?

ROLE PERFORMANCE

Family Relationships

- Tell me about your family.
- What is home like?
- How is your relationship with your spouse/partner/significant other? (if appropriate)
- What are your relationships like with your other relatives?
- How are important decisions made in your family?
- What are your responsibilities in the family?
- What about your role or responsibilities would you like changed?
- Do you feel your family members are proud of you?

Work Roles and Social Roles

- Do you like your work?
- How do you get along at work?
- What about your work would you like to change if you could?
- How do you spend your free time?
- Are you most comfortable alone, with one other person, or in a group?
- Who is most important to you?
- Who do you go to when you need help?

assess related behavior, such as wearing clothes in such a way as to hide a deformity. See the accompanying Assessment Interview for examples of questions to ask about body image.

Role Performance

The nurse assesses the client's satisfactions and dissatisfactions associated with role responsibilities and relationships: family roles, work roles, student roles, and social roles. Family roles are especially important to people because family relationships are particularly close. Relationships can be supportive and growth producing or, at the opposite extreme, highly stressful if there is violence or abuse. Assessment of family role relationships may begin with structural aspects such as the number in the family group, ages, residence location, and how often members of the family see each other or interact. To obtain data related to the client's family relationships and satisfaction or dissatisfaction with work roles and social roles, the nurse might ask some of the questions shown in the accompanying Assessment Interview. Keep in mind, however, that questions need to be tailored to the individual and his or her culture, age, and situation.

Self-Esteem

A nurse can ask questions to determine a client's self-esteem. See the accompanying Assessment Interview for examples of such questions.

It is important for the nurse to determine the client's cultural background in order not to misinterpret specific behaviors. The following behaviors might reflect low self-esteem or may be misinterpreted due to the client's cultural background:

- Avoids eye contact
- Stoops in posture and moves slowly
- Is poorly groomed and has an unkempt appearance
- Is hesitant or halting in speech
- Is overly critical of self (e.g., "I'm no good," "I'm ugly," or "People don't like me.")
- May be overly critical of others
- Is unable to accept positive remarks about self
- Apologizes frequently
- Verbalizes feelings of hopelessness, helplessness, and powerlessness, such as "I really don't care what happens," "I'll do whatever anyone wants," "Whatever is destined will happen."

CARING INTERVENTIONS

Nursing interventions to promote a positive self-concept include helping a client to identify areas of strength. In addition, for clients who have an altered self-concept, nurses should establish therapeutic relationships and assist clients to evaluate themselves and make behavioral changes.

Identifying Areas of Strength

Healthy people often perceive their problems and weaknesses more easily than their assets and strengths. Individuals with low self-esteem tend to focus even more on their limitations and to be aware of fewer strengths and many more problems. When a client has difficulty identifying personality strengths and assets, the nurse provides the client with a set of guidelines or a framework for identifying personality strengths (Box 24–2).

Box 24–2 **Framework for Identifying Personality Strengths**

Note past, present, and anticipated future participation in the following:

- Hobbies and crafts
- Expressive arts such as writing, painting, sketching, or music appreciation
- Sports and outdoor activities, including spectator sports
- Education, training, and related areas (including self-education)
- Work, vocation, job, or position.

In addition, determine the following:

- Sense of humor and the ability to laugh at oneself and take kidding
- Health status including healthy aspects of body function and good health maintenance practices
- Special aptitudes such as sales or mechanical ability; a "green thumb"; ability to recognize and enjoy beauty; ability to solve problems; a liking for adventure or pioneering; having perseverance and the drive needed to get things done
- Relationship strengths including the ability to make people feel comfortable, the capacity to enjoy being with people, being aware of people's needs and feelings, and being able to listen
- Emotional strengths including the capacity to give and receive warmth, affection, and love; the ability to "take" anger and to feel and express a wide range of emotions; and the capacity for empathy
- Spiritual strengths such as religious faith or love of God, membership and participation in church and related activities.

Nurses can employ the following specific strategies to reinforce strengths:

- Stress positive thinking rather than self-negation.
- Notice and verbally reinforce client strengths.
- Encourage the setting of attainable goals.
- Acknowledge goals that have been attained.
- Provide honest, positive feedback.

Enhancing Self-Esteem

Nurses assisting clients who have an altered self-concept must establish a therapeutic relationship. To do this nurses must have self-awareness and effective communication skills. The following nursing techniques may help clients analyze the problem and enhance the self-concept:

- Encourage clients to appraise the situation and express their feelings.
- Encourage clients to ask questions.
- Provide accurate information.
- Become aware of distortions, inappropriate or unrealistic standards, and faulty labels in clients' speech.
- Explore clients' positive qualities and strengths.
- Encourage clients to express positive self-evaluation more than negative self-evaluation.
- Avoid criticism.
- Teach clients to substitute negative self-talk ("I can't walk to the store anymore") with positive self-talk ("I can walk half a block each morning"). Negative self-talk reinforces a negative self-concept.

Certain strategies vary depending on the age of the client (see the Developmental Considerations box on page 1591).

DEVELOPMENTAL CONSIDERATIONS **Enhancing Self-Esteem**

CHILDREN

- Children build strong self-esteem if they develop five basic attitudes: (1) security and trust, (2) identity, (3) belonging, (4) purpose, and (5) personal competence.
- Security and trust are developed early in life; infants should not be left "to cry it out," for example, but should learn that they can rely on their parents to meet their needs promptly and consistently. With older children, trust and security are strengthened when adults spend time with them: listening, playing, reading, or just being there. Both emotional and physical contact, such as a hug, convey warmth and caring.
- Identity is developed when children are allowed to explore and experiment with the world around them and to express themselves as unique individuals in that world. They should be given opportunities to "practice" who they are. Preschoolers, for example, love to dress themselves and should be allowed to wear outlandish outfits (within limits of weather and safety) if they choose. Teenagers who try new hair colors and styles, some of which may "offend" their parents, are engaging in a crucial developmental step.
- Belonging is essential for all humans, and having a sense that others in the child's social network care about the child, want him or her there, and that the child's contribution is important to healthy self-esteem. Children gain this sense of belonging by being included in activities; by being praised for their efforts and achievements; and by being valued by parents, siblings, caregivers, and other adults. Parents should make an effort to "catch their children doing well" and praise them for it (e.g., "I like the way you share with your brother"). Children should also hear that they are valued just for being themselves (e.g., "I like doing things with you. Remember when we went to the park? Wasn't that fun?").
- Purpose and belonging are closely related. Children need opportunities to participate in the family and their community in order to discover what they can best contribute based on their strengths and skills. One mother, for example, stated "Leo (age 4) is our actor. He is wonderful with costumes and can make any of us smile when he starts his routine." Leo may never become an actor, but he knows he makes a significant contribution to his family's well-being. He brings them joy.
- Personal competence grows as children identify and refine their skill sets. Children develop competence as they confront and solve problems, face challenges, expand their thinking, and are asked to do more than they think they can do. Adults must, however, provide children with support, guidance, appropriate assistance, and constructive feedback (including praise) in order to prevent the child from being overwhelmed. Too much frustration or uncertainty can lead to giving up, avoidance, lying, bullying, and other antisocial behaviors. If adults help children to accomplish goals that are important to them, children are more likely to develop a sense of personal competence and independence.
- Key ingredients for helping children develop high self-esteem are love, acceptance, firmness, consistency, and the establishment of expectations. Such qualities provide children with a safe, loving, supportive, and predictable world in which to live.

ADOLESCENTS

- Provide increasing levels of responsibility. Adolescents need to experience successes and failures and the consequences of their own behavior.
- Encourage discussion about issues including problems and mistakes.
- Show appreciation for effort and contributions. Emphasize the process, not just the result.
- Ask for their opinions and suggestions.
- Encourage participation in decision making in areas that affect the adolescent. Show confidence in the teen's judgments.
- Avoid comparison with or ridicule or punishment in front of others.
- Assist in the creation of realistic goals and standards.
- Adolescents often engage in volunteer activities in their schools or communities, helping them to identify their strengths and find meaning in their activities. Knowing that they have a purpose and make a difference gives children strong self-esteem.

ADULTS

- Explore the meaning of self-esteem and how his or her self-esteem has influenced past behaviors and actions (and can influence present and future plans and decisions).
- Assist the client in assessing the internal and external forces contributing to or retarding his or her self-esteem.
- Act in ways that demonstrate belief that the person can cope with the realities and demands of life and is worthy of experiencing joy and happiness.
- Avoid comparisons with other people.
- Discourage statements about the self that are negative.
- Encourage the use of affirmations to enhance self-esteem: statements such as "I like myself" or "I am a valuable person."
- Encourage associations with positive, supportive people.
- Make positive statements about the person's past successes (major or minor).
- Assist the person to make a list of his or her positive qualities and to review this list often.
- Suggest the person do things for others. Making a positive contribution enhances positive feelings of self-worth.

OLDER ADULTS

Older adults who become increasingly dependent can develop low self-esteem. Old age is frequently accompanied by changes such as reduced income, decline in physical health, loss of friends and family, and retirement. In addition to those actions listed previously for use with adults, nurses can use the following techniques to help older adults enhance their self-esteem:

- Encourage clients to participate in planning their own care.
- Listen carefully to their concerns.
- Assist clients to identify and use their own strengths.
- Encourage them to participate in activities in which they can be successful.
- Communicate that the client is valued. Use the client's name and ask for advice.
- Encourage older adults to stay connected with their memories. Reminiscing by writing or recording an autobiography or storytelling are excellent ways to do this.
- For older clients who are in hospitals or nursing homes, make sure that they are always shown respect and dignity and are provided privacy.

(continued)

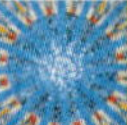

DEVELOPMENTAL CONSIDERATIONS **Enhancing Self-Esteem (continued)**

- Encourage creative activities to tap their resources. Examples are music, art, storytelling, quilting, and photography.
- Work with clients to establish goals in small steps that are achievable—this, in itself, can bolster self-esteem.

WEAVING THE TAPESTRY OF LIFE

The mainstays of the tapestry of life are the powers in one's life—self-esteem, love of life and humanity, and closeness to and recognition of the spirituality in oneself and others.

The weavings that form the patterns in one's life are experiences, knowledge, and dreams. Beauty can be seen throughout, but strength of the fabric increases with age as the tapestry displays interweavings and integration of these special qualities.

As time goes on, aging is often accompanied by a fragileness of the physical body and an increased number of inevitable losses—emotional and social, as well as physical. This is when the integration of those special fibers—strengthening qualities—becomes so crucial to the overall quality of life of the individual.

When these strengths are displayed in the tapestry of life, the individual is not only given a feeling of self-worth and self-love, but the tapestry is a beautiful gift for all who behold it and are somehow touched by it. —Grace Miller

PHARMACOLOGIC THERAPIES

Pharmacologic therapy may benefit clients with alterations of self-concept, particularly when used in conjunction with psychotherapy. Because different medications work better for some clients than others, several prescriptions may be tried before the best treatment is found.

Eating Disorders

Medications, primarily antidepressants, are used to reduce the frequency of disturbed eating behaviors such as binge eating and vomiting. In addition, medications are used to ease symptoms that may accompany eating disorders such as depression, anxiety, obsessions, or impulse control problems.

For people with anorexia, drug trials have been disappointing, although there is some interest in exploring the use of second-generation antipsychotic medication. Fluoxetine (Prozac), an SSRI, is effective for clients with bulimia when given at the higher dose of 50–60 mg per day. Typically, the medication is continued until 6 months following the disappearance of symptoms. In the past, tricyclic antidepressants have been used but the dropout rate is higher than with the SSRIs (Bacaltchuk & Hay, 2003).

Personality Disorders

Studies are being conducted on the effectiveness of medications in treating personality disorders. Medications are used to target specific symptoms. Psychotic symptoms appear to respond to low doses of the antipsychotic agents. These medications are best used for relief of acute symptoms and are typically discontinued when the psychotic features disappear. A number of medications are being tried to decrease the impulsive, aggressive, and self-destructive behavior patterns of borderline personality disorders (BPD). SSRIs, clonidine (Catapres), and guanfacine (Tenex) diminish rage and rapid mood swings as well as decrease aggression and impulsive and self-destructive behavior. SSRIs are also used to treat obsessive ruminations in people with personality disorders. SSRIs include fluoxetine (Prozac), paroxetine (Paxil), and sertraline (Zoloft). Medications should be viewed as a means of controlling symptoms that are disabling. The overall treatment plan includes individual, group, family, and behavioral therapy. As more is learned about these disorders, improved techniques can be designed to better meet individual client needs (Keshavan, Shad, Soloff, & Schooler, 2004; Soler et al., 2005).

24.1 EATING DISORDERS

KEY TERMS

Anorexia nervosa, *1599*
Binge eating, *1600*
Binge-eating disorder, *1601*
Bulimia nervosa, *1600*
Metabolism, *1597*
Nutrients, *1593*
Nutrition, *1593*
Purging, *1600*

BASIS FOR SELECTION OF EXEMPLAR

Healthy People 2010
National Institute of Mental Health
Institute of Medicine
Centers for Disease Control and Prevention

LEARNING OUTCOMES

After reading about this exemplar, you will be able to:

1. Describe the pathophysiology, etiology, clinical manifestations, and direct and indirect causes of eating disorders.
2. Identify risk factors associated with eating disorders.
3. Illustrate the nursing process in providing culturally competent care across the life span for individuals with eating disorders.
4. Formulate priority nursing diagnoses for an individual with an eating disorder.
5. Create a plan of care for individuals with eating disorders and their family members.
6. Assess expected outcomes for an individual with an eating disorder.
7. Discuss therapies used in the collaborative care of an individual with an eating disorder.
8. Employ evidence-based caring interventions for an individual with an eating disorder.

OVERVIEW

The body relies on an adequate supply of nutrients to meet energy needs such as metabolism, cellular regulation, and thermoregulation. When inadequate nutrients are supplied, the body finds other sources to meet its needs, often metabolizing muscles to produce energy. Eating disorders disrupt the supply of nutrients to the body, resulting in biochemical and physiological changes that can endanger bodily systems.

For many, eating symbolizes parental nurturing—the love and care that are the prototype of, and basis for, all future intimate relationships. For some, however, eating creates anxiety because of its association with unsatisfactory and unpleasant parent–child interactions. Clearly, food and eating have greater individual and cultural meaning and importance than merely sustaining life. Disturbed eating patterns also may develop as a means of coping with stress.

The three major eating disorders discussed in this chapter—anorexia nervosa, bulimia nervosa, and binge-eating disorder—create biologic, psychologic, and social imbalances that interfere with the individual's normal functioning. In addition to interfering with the supply of nutrients to the body, eating disorders create depression, isolation, and sometimes self-destructive behavior.

NORMAL NUTRITION

Nutrition is the process by which the body ingests, absorbs, transports, uses, and eliminates nutrients in food. **Nutrients** are substances found in food that are used by the body to promote growth, maintenance, and repair. The categories of nutrients are carbohydrates, proteins, fats, vitamins, minerals, and water. Dietary guidelines for Americans specific to nutrients are summarized in Table 24–3.

Carbohydrates

The primary sources of carbohydrates (which include sugars and starches) are plant foods. Monosaccharides and disaccharides come from milk, sugar cane, sugar beets, honey, and fruits. Polysaccharide starch is found in grains, legumes, and root vegetables. Following ingestion, digestion, and metabolism, carbohydrates are converted primarily to glucose, the molecule body cells use to make adenosine triphosphate (ATP). Excess glucose in the healthy person is converted to glycogen or fat. Glycogen is stored in the liver and muscles; fat is stored as adipose tissue. Carbohydrate use by the body is shown in Figure 24–4A ■.

Regardless of the source, all carbohydrates supply 4 kcal per gram. The minimum necessary daily carbohydrate intake

TABLE 24–3 **Recommended Dietary Guidelines for Americans, 2005**

CATEGORY	RECOMMENDATION
General dietary guidelines	■ Consume a variety of nutrient-dense foods and beverages within and among the basic food groups while choosing foods that limit the intake of saturated and *trans* fats, cholesterol, added sugars, salt, and alcohol. ■ Meet recommended intakes by adopting a balanced eating pattern, such as that provided by the USDA Food Guide Pyramid. ■ Balance calories from foods and beverages with calories expended to maintain body weight. ■ Over time, make small decreases in food and beverage calories and increase physical activity to prevent gradual weight gain.
Food groups	■ For a 2000-calorie diet, consume 2 cups of fruit and 2 1/2 cups of vegetables per day (increase or decrease amounts depending on calorie level). ■ Select from all five vegetable subgroups (dark green, orange, legumes, starchy vegetables, other vegetables) several times a week. ■ Consume 3 or more ounce equivalents of whole-grain products each day, with the rest of recommended grains coming from enriched or whole-grain products. In general, at least half of the grains should be from whole grains. ■ Consume 3 cups per day of fat-free or low-fat milk or equivalent milk products.
Carbohydrates	■ Choose fiber-rich foods, vegetables, and whole grains often. ■ Choose and prepare foods with little added sugars or caloric sweeteners.
Fats	■ Consume less than 10% of calories from saturated fatty acids and less than 300 mg/day of cholesterol; keep *trans* fatty acid consumption as low as possible. ■ Keep total fat intake between 20% and 35% of calories, with most fats coming from sources of polyunsaturated and monounsaturated fatty acids, such as fish, nuts, and vegetable oil. ■ When selecting and preparing meats, poultry, dry beans, and milk or milk products, make choices that are lean, low fat, or fat free.
Sodium and potassium	■ Consume less than 2300 mg (about 1 teaspoon of salt) of sodium each day. ■ Choose and prepare foods with little salt. ■ Consume potassium-rich foods, such as fruits and vegetables.

Source: United States Department of Agriculture. (2005). *Dietary guidelines for Americans 2005. Key recommendations for the general population*. Available at http://www.health.gov/dietaryguidelines/dga2005/recommendations.htm

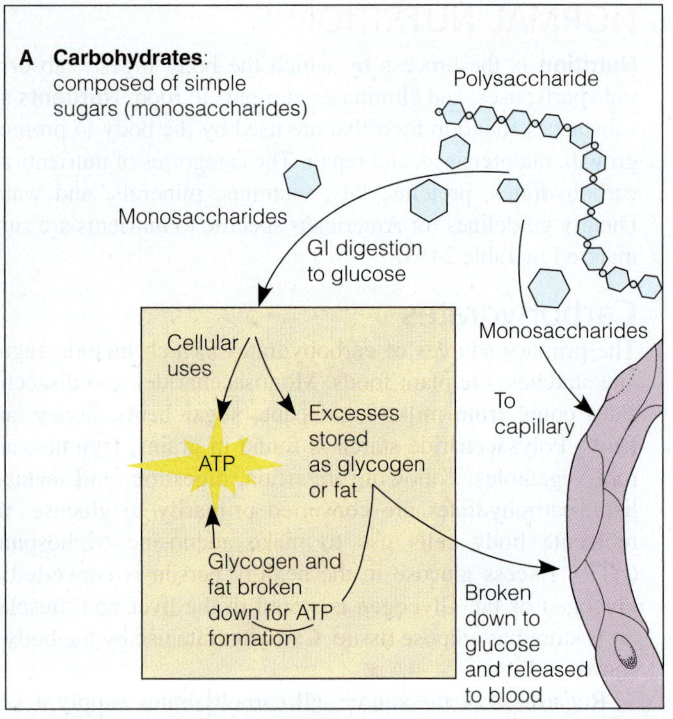

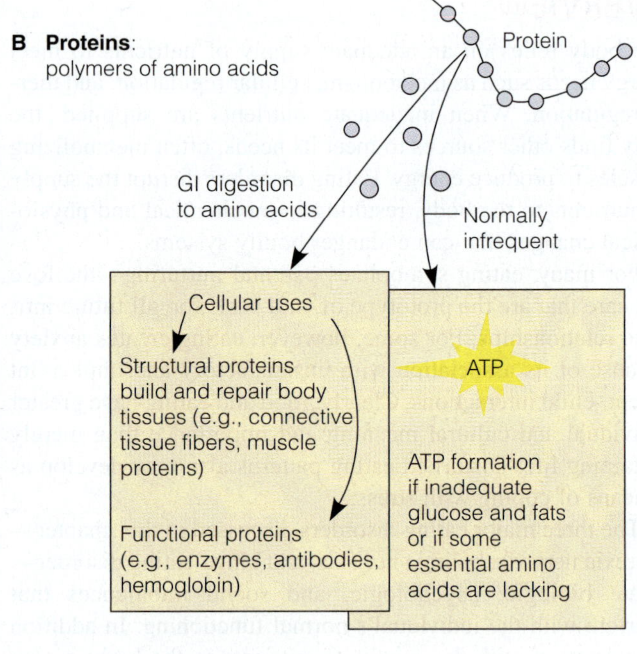

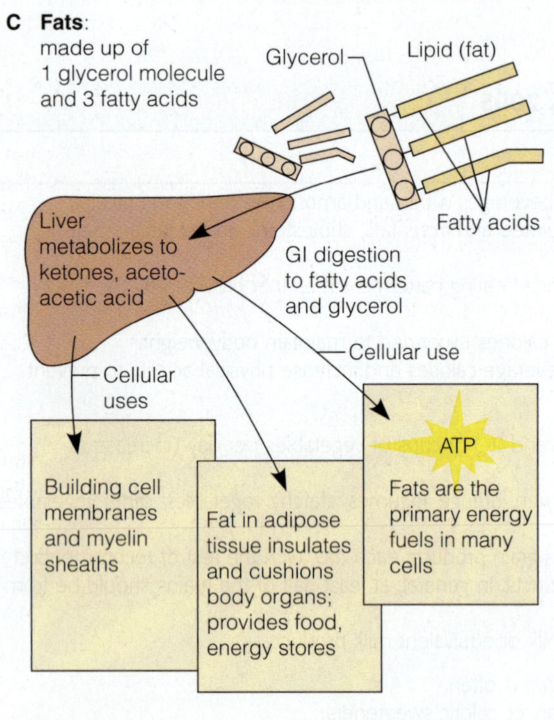

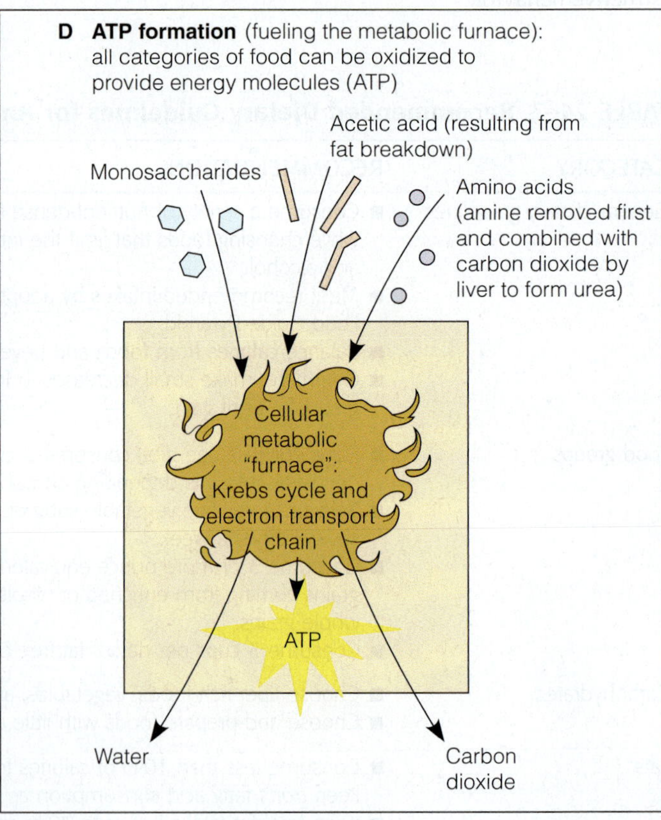

Figure 24–4 ■ A schematic overview of nutrient use by body cells, including *A*, carbohydrates; *B*, proteins; *C*, fats; and *D*, ATP formation.

is unknown, but the recommended daily intake is 125 to 175 g, most of which should be complex carbohydrates (such as milk, potatoes, and whole grains). Excess intake of carbohydrates over time can result in obesity, dental caries, and elevated plasma triglycerides. Over extended periods of time, carbohydrate deficiencies lead to tissue wasting from protein breakdown and metabolic acidosis from an excess of ketones as a by-product of fat breakdown.

Proteins

Proteins are classified as either complete or incomplete. Complete proteins are found in animal products such as eggs, milk, milk products, and meat. They contain the greatest amount of amino acids and meet the body's amino acid requirements for tissue growth and maintenance. Incomplete proteins are found in legumes, nuts, grains, cereals, and vegetables. These sources are low in or lack one or more of the amino acids essential for building complete proteins.

The body uses proteins to build many different structures, including skin keratin, the collagen and elastin in connective tissues, and muscles. They also are used to make enzymes, hemoglobin, plasma proteins, and some hormones. Protein use by the body is shown in Figure 24–4B.

Proteins provide 4 kcal per gram. The recommended daily intake of protein is 56 g for men and 45 g for women. Healthy people with adequate caloric intake have an equal rate of protein synthesis and protein breakdown and loss, reflected as nitrogen balance. If the breakdown and loss of proteins exceed intake, a negative nitrogen balance results. This may occur from starvation, altered physical states (e.g., from injury or illness), or altered emotional states (such as depression or anxiety). Protein deficits can cause weight loss, tissue wasting, edema, and anemia. When protein intake exceeds breakdown, a positive nitrogen balance occurs. This is normal during growth, tissue repair, and pregnancy. Abnormal rates of protein use may result during times of stress, when the body releases adrenal corticosteroids to increase protein breakdown and conversion of amino acids to glucose. Anabolic steroids may affect the rate of protein use, as may excessive intake of proteins. Excessive intake of proteins may lead to obesity, impacting a number of bodily systems.

Fats (Lipids)

Fats, or lipids, include phospholipids; sterols, such as cholesterol; and neutral fats, more commonly known as triglycerides. Neutral fats are the most abundant fats in the diet. They may be either saturated or unsaturated. Saturated fats are found in animal products (milk and meats) and in some plant products (such as coconut). Unsaturated fats are found in seeds, nuts, and most vegetable oils. Sources of cholesterol include meats, milk products, and egg yolks. Fat use by the body is shown in Figure 24–4C.

Fats supply 9 kcal per gram. When a person consumes more than the body requires, the excess is stored as adipose tissue, increasing the risk of obesity and heart disease. A deficit of fats may cause excessive weight loss and skin lesions.

Fats are a necessary part of the structure and function of the body. For example,

- phospholipids are a part of all cell membranes.
- triglycerides are the major energy source for hepatocytes and skeletal muscle cells.
- dietary fats facilitate absorption of fat-soluble vitamins.
- linoleic acid, an essential fatty acid, helps form prostaglandins, regulatory molecules that assist in smooth muscle contraction, maintenance of blood pressure, and control of inflammatory responses.
- cholesterol is the essential component of bile salts, steroid hormones, and vitamin D.
- adipose tissue serves as a protection around body organs, as a layer of insulation under the skin, and as a concentrated source of fuel for cellular energy.

Vitamins

Vitamins are organic compounds that facilitate the body's use of carbohydrates, proteins, and fats. All of the vitamins except vitamins D and K must be ingested in foods or taken as supplements. Vitamin D is made by ultraviolet irradiation of cholesterol molecules in the skin, and vitamin K is synthesized by bacteria in the intestine.

Vitamins are categorized as either fat soluble or water soluble. The fat-soluble vitamins (A, D, E, and K) bind to ingested fats and are absorbed as the fats are absorbed. Water-soluble vitamins (the B complex and C) are absorbed with water in the GI tract (however, vitamin B_{12} must become attached to intrinsic factor to be absorbed). Fat-soluble vitamins are stored in the body, and excesses may cause toxicity; water-soluble vitamins in excess of body requirements are excreted in the urine.

The recommended amounts of vitamins, previously labeled recommended daily allowances (RDAs), are now labeled by the National Academy of Sciences as dietary reference intakes (DRIs) per day. The source, function, and minimum daily recommended intake levels are provided for each vitamin in Table 24–4 and Table 24–5. Since these DRIs were established, a number of new studies on the importance of vitamin D have been released. As a result, the Food and Nutrition Board (FNB) at the Institute of Medicine has established a committee to review the recommendations regarding DRIs for vitamin D. Research suggests that current recommended levels may be insufficient, especially for individuals who do not get adequate sunlight, infants who are breastfed, and older adults (NIH, 2009).

Minerals

Minerals work with other nutrients to maintain the structure and function of the body. An adequate supply of calcium, phosphorus, potassium, sulfur, sodium, chloride, and magnesium—as well as other trace elements such as iron, iodine, copper,

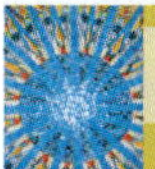

DEVELOPMENTAL CONSIDERATIONS

Nutrition and the Older Adult

The older adult has some unique nutritional requirements due to the physical and functional changes that occur with aging. While many older adults experience a decline in physical activity level and have lower calorie needs, there is not a decreased need for most vitamins and minerals with age. In fact, the dietary requirement for some nutrients increases with age. For example, the daily recommended intake for the general adult population and the older adult population is the same with the exception of vitamin D, calcium, vitamin B_{12}, vitamin B_6, and energy. Obtaining a well-balanced diet while consuming fewer calories overall can present a challenge to many older adults.

TABLE 24–4 Recommended Daily Intake of Fat-Soluble Vitamins

NAME	SOURCE	FUNCTION	MINIMUM RECOMMENDED DAILY INTAKE (M = MEN, W = WOMEN)
Vitamin A (retinol)	■ Fish liver oils ■ Egg yolk ■ Liver ■ Fortified milk ■ Margarine	Necessary for vision, integrity of skin and mucous membranes, cell membrane function, and reproductive function	M = 900 mcg W = 700 mcg
Vitamin D	■ The action of sunshine on cholesterol in the skin	Necessary for blood calcium homeostasis (in turn necessary for blood clotting), bone formation, and neuromuscular function	M and W = 5 mcg (10 mcg for those over 50)
Vitamin E	■ Vegetable oils ■ Margarine ■ Whole grains ■ Dark green leafy vegetables	As an antioxidant, helps prevent the oxidation of vitamins A and C in the intestines and decreases the oxidation of unsaturated fatty acids to facilitate cell membrane integrity	M and W = 15 mcg
Vitamin K	■ Synthesized by coliform teria in the large intestine ■ Green, leafy vegetables ■ Cabbage ■ Cauliflower ■ Pork	Essential for the formation of clotting proteins in the liver	M = 120 mcg W = 90 mcg

TABLE 24–5 Recommended Daily Intake of Water-Soluble Vitamins

NAME	SOURCE	FUNCTION	MINIMUM RECOMMENDED DAILY INTAKE (M = MEN, W = WOMEN)
Vitamin B_1 (thiamin)	■ Lean meats ■ Liver ■ Eggs ■ Green leafy vegetables ■ Legumes ■ Whole grains	An essential coenzyme for carbohydrate metabolism and use; also for healthy function of nerves, muscles, and the heart	M = 1.2 mg W = 1.1 mg
Vitamin B_2 (riboflavin)	■ Liver ■ Egg white ■ Whole grains ■ Meat ■ Poultry ■ Fish ■ Milk	Involved in the catabolism and use of carbohydrates, fats, and proteins; the use of other B vitamins; and is important for the production of adrenal hormones	M = 1.3 mg W = 1.1 mg
Vitamin B_6 (pyridoxine)	■ Meat ■ Poultry ■ Fish ■ Potatoes ■ Tomatoes ■ Sweet potatoes ■ Spinach	Necessary for amino acid metabolism, formation of antibodies, and formation of hemoglobin	M and W < age 51 = 1.3 M > age 51 = 1.7 mg W > age 51 = 1.5 mg
Vitamin B_{12} (cyanocobalamin)	■ Liver ■ Meat ■ Poultry ■ Dairy foods (except butter) ■ Eggs	Essential for the production of nucleic acids and red blood cells in the bone marrow; also plays an important role in the use of folic acid and carbohydrates, and in healthy function of the nervous system	M and W = 2.4 mcg
Vitamin C (ascorbic acid)	■ Citrus fruits ■ Potatoes ■ Tomatoes ■ Green leafy vegetables	Acts as an antioxidant and vasoconstrictor; also serves in the formation of connective tissue, conversion for cholesterol to bile salts, iron absorption and use, and conversion of folic acid to an active form	M = 90 mg W = 75 mg

TABLE 24–5 Recommended Daily Intake of Water-Soluble Vitamins (continued)

NAME	SOURCE	FUNCTION	MINIMUM RECOMMENDED DAILY INTAKE (M = MEN, W = WOMEN)
Vitamin B_3 niacin (nicotinamide)	■ Meat ■ Poultry ■ Fish ■ Liver ■ Peanuts ■ Green leafy vegetables	Plays an important role in the metabolism of carbohydrates and fats; inhibits cholesterol synthesis; important for integumentary, nervous, and digestive system health; assists in the manufacture of reproductive hormones	M and W = 35 mg
Biotin	■ Liver ■ Eggs ■ Nuts ■ Legumes	Essential for the catabolism of fatty acids and carbohydrates, and helps dispose of the waste products of protein catabolism	M and W = 30 mcg
Pantothenic acid	■ Meats ■ Whole grains ■ Egg yolk ■ Liver ■ Yeast ■ Legumes	Assists in the synthesis of steroids and of the heme in hemoglobin; is essential for the metabolism of carbohydrates and fats, and for the manufacture of reproductive hormones	M and W = 5 mg
Folic acid (folate)	■ Liver ■ Dark green vegetables ■ Lean beef ■ Eggs ■ Veal ■ Whole grains ■ Synthesized by bacteria in the intestine	The basis of a coenzyme necessary for the manufacture of nucleic acids and so is essential for the formation of red blood cells, growth and development, and nervous system health	M and W = 400 mcg

and zinc—is necessary to health. Most minerals in the body are found in body fluids or are bound to organic compounds. The best sources of minerals are vegetables, legumes, milk, and some meats. The recommended daily intake for minerals is outlined in Table 24–6.

TABLE 24–6 Recommended Daily Intake of Minerals

NAME	MINIMUM RECOMMENDED DAILY INTAKE (M = MEN, W = WOMEN)
Calcium	M and W = 1000 mg W > menopause = 1200 mg
Phosphorus	M and W = 1000 mg
Iron	M and W = 18 mg
Zinc	M and W = 15 mg
Manganese	M = 2.3 mg W = 1.8 mg
Molybdenum	M and W = 75 mcg
Chromium	M and W = 120 mcg
Iodine	M and W = 150 mcg
Selenium	M and W = 70 mcg
Magnesium	M and W = 400 mg
Copper	M and W = 2.0 mg
Chloride	M and W = 3400 mg

Metabolism

After nutrients (carbohydrates, fats, and proteins) are ingested, digested, absorbed, and transported across cell membranes, they must be metabolized to produce and provide energy to maintain life. **Metabolism** is the process of biochemical reactions occurring in the body's cells that are necessary to sustain life. Metabolic processes are either catabolic or anabolic. Catabolism involves the breakdown of complex structures into simpler forms, for example, the breakdown of carbohydrates to produce ATP, an energy molecule that fuels cellular activity. In the process of anabolism, simpler molecules combine to build more complex structures; for example, amino acids bond to form proteins.

The biochemical reactions of metabolism produce water, carbon dioxide, and ATP (see Figure 24–4D on page 1594). The energy value of foods is measured in kilocalories (kcal). A kilocalorie is defined as the amount of heat energy needed to raise the temperature of 1 kilogram (kg) of water 1 degree centigrade.

PATHOPHYSIOLOGY AND ETIOLOGY OF EATING DISORDERS

The causes of eating disorders are multiple in individuals and across a variety of people. Fatness and thinness are outcomes of biological, psychological, and social processes. The balance between energy intake and expenditure determines weight, and this balance is the product of many influences. Although family and culture may provide a trigger, it seems increasingly likely that hormones and brain chemicals prime a certain group of people to push themselves to starvation. Having a knowledge base about the major theories will help the nurse understand individual clients from a composite perspective.

Genetics

Family risk studies show that relatives of clients with eating disorders are five to ten times more likely to develop an eating disorder. It appears that in anorexia, the more severe the disorder, the more likely a strong genetic predisposition. Twin studies for anorexia show that the concordance rate for monozygotic twins is 55–71% and for dizygotic twins it is 0–32%. These data suggest that there may be a *genetic predisposition* to anorexia. Concordance rates for bulimia range from 23–83% for monozygotic twins and 0–27% for dizygotic twins (Slof-O't Landt et al., 2005).

Genetic research focuses on behavioral, neurobiological, and temperamental variables that may represent core features of these disorders. These features include perfectionism, orderliness, low tolerance for new situations, low self-esteem, and overall high anxiety. Even if an individual has a high genetic risk, however, he or she might develop an eating disorder even if he or she did not live in a culture that stresses dieting and thinness (Bulik, 2005).

Neurobiology

Recent studies indicate that *neurotransmitter dysregulation* may be involved in eating disorders, particularly serotonin (5-HT). Being full of food to the point of satisfaction is referred to as *satiety*. Normally, a low level of 5-HT decreases a person's satiety and thereby increases food intake. In contrast, a high level of 5-HT increases satiety and thereby decreases food intake. Carbohydrates are involved in the synthesis of 5-HT by increasing tryptophan, the precursor of 5-HT. The neurotransmitter hypothesis of bulimia is that the recurrent binge episodes may result from a deficiency in 5-HT and low satiety levels. Since people with bulimia tend to binge on high-carbohydrate foods, this may be a reflection of the body's adaptive attempt to increase 5-HT levels. The neurotransmitter hypothesis of anorexia is that decreased food intake is related to excess 5-HT and increased satiety (Romano, Halmi, Sarkar, Koke, & Lee, 2002).

The level of spontaneous physical activity appears to be related to energy expenditure and thus to body weight. Orexin neurons in the lateral hypothalamus appear to integrate this activity with feeding behavior (Kotz, 2006).

Other neurotransmitters affect eating behavior. Norepinephrine (NE) and neuropeptide Y (NPY) increase eating behavior while dopamine suppresses food intake. Dopamine agonists such as amphetamines and cocaine are appetite suppressants (Frank et al., 2005).

Endogenous opioids, such as endorphins, are associated with food intake and mood. Opioids increase food intake and enhance positive mood states; therefore, insufficient levels cause decreased food intake and depressed mood. It has been found that underweight people have significantly lower levels of endorphins compared to healthy volunteers. When the person's weight is returned to normal levels, the endorphin level is also within normal limits.

Neuroimaging studies have shown a low level of functioning in the frontal lobes, parietal lobes, and the anterior cingulate of individuals with anorexia and bulimia. When these individuals viewed high-calorie foods, they experienced abnormally increased activity in those same brain regions (Uher et al., 2004).

Intrapersonal Factors

Intrapersonal theorists believe that people at higher risk for eating disorders have low self-esteem, experience significant adolescent turmoil, and have difficulty with identity formation. Personality characteristics of people with anorexia are perfectionism, low tolerance for new situations, low self-esteem, and difficulty achieving the maturational tasks of adolescence. People with bulimia are described in terms of perfectionism, affective instability, and poor impulse control. Feelings of incompetence and fear of losing control contribute to a tenuous self-definition, which is masked by the eating disorder (Stein & Corte, 2003).

Impulsive personality traits are characteristic of many people suffering from bulimia. The loss of control and the inability to stop binging once started is the typical bulimic pattern. This impulsivity resembles other addictive disorders.

Cognitive Theory

Cognitive theorists believe that cognitive distortions and dysfunctional thoughts such as dichotomous thinking and catastrophizing (exaggerating failures in one's life) contribute to disordered eating patterns. The extreme belief is "It is absolutely essential that I be thin." This belief leads to dieting, avoidant behavior, and increased isolation, which in turn cause a lack of responsiveness to alternative cognitive input. Given the cultural emphasis on thinness, there is a sense of gratification, self-control, mastery, and approval of or concern from others.

Behavioral Theory

Behavioral theorists are concerned with what the disordered behavior accomplishes rather than why the behavior occurs. Eating disorders are considered phobias. In this context, anxiety increases with eating and decreases with fasting or purging. Anxiety reduction is the reinforcer for both anorexia and bulimia.

Family Factors

Most family theorists believe family issues are not specific to eating disorders. The family is viewed more as an enabler of the disorder than as a primary causative factor. Some people with eating disorders are survivors of childhood or adolescent sexual abuse, which may or may not have occurred within the family or extended family system. (Sexual abuse is discussed further in Concept 31, Violence.)

As the result of anorexia, some families become enmeshed; that is, the boundaries between the members are weak, interactions are intense, dependency on one another is high, and autonomy is minimal. Everybody is involved in each member's concerns, and there is minimal privacy. The enmeshed family system becomes overprotective of the child, and the entire family system becomes preoccupied with food, eating, and rituals involving meals. In contrast, current research indicates that families of people with bulimia are less enmeshed than those of anorexic people. Family members tend to be isolated from one another, and eating behavior may be an attempt to decrease feelings of loneliness and boredom.

Many families of individuals with eating disorders have difficulty with conflict resolution. When problems are denied for the sake of family harmony, they cannot be resolved, and growth of the family system is inhibited. The anorexic child may protect and maintain the family unit. In some family systems, the parents avoid conflict with each other by uniting in a common concern for the child's welfare. In other family systems, the issues of marital conflict are converted into disagreements over how the anorexic child should be managed. In both systems, the marital problems are camouflaged to prevent the disruption of the family unit.

Many families of clients with eating disorders are achievement and performance oriented, with high ambition for the success of all members. In these families, body shape is related to success, and priorities are established for physical appearance and fitness. The family's focus on professional achievement as well as on food, diet, exercise, and weight control may become obsessional.

Gender

Cultural stereotypes contribute to women's preoccupation with their bodies. Attractiveness is determined by how closely a woman's appearance matches the cultural ideal of thinness. Thus, identity and self-esteem are dependent on physical appearance. Being disgusted with one's flesh is the same as having an adversarial relationship with the body—a relationship that often results in eating disorders.

Etiology

Determining the incidence of anorexia and bulimia is difficult because of the variety of definitions that exist. Certainly the frequency of these disorders has been increasing, but the increase may be due partly to increased reporting. Ninety percent of women and 25% of men diet at some time in their lives. Over half of teenage girls and one-third of teenage boys use unhealthy weight control behaviors such as skipping meals, fasting, vomiting, using laxatives, and smoking cigarettes. It is estimated that clinical eating disorders affect 8–20% of the population. They are more commonly seen among females, with estimates of the male–female ratio ranging from 1:6 to 1:10, although 19–30% of younger people with anorexia are male. The estimate may be low, as primary health care providers are less likely to diagnose an eating disorder in a male than in a female (Tozzi et al., 2005).

Risk Factors

Risk factors for eating disorders include the following:

- Female gender
- Age (eating disorders tend to develop in the teens and 20s)
- Emotional disorders
- Dieting
- Sports and artistic endeavors
- Family influences (including sexual abuse)
- Societal influences (e.g., media stereotypes).

CLINICAL MANIFESTATIONS

Clinical manifestations of eating disorders vary, but there are some similarities including body image disturbances, presence of anxiety, and ineffective coping skills.

Anorexia Nervosa

Anorexia nervosa is a potentially life-threatening disorder characterized by extreme perfectionism, weight fear; significant weight loss; body image disturbances; strenuous exercising; peculiar food-handling patterns; and reductions in heart rate, blood pressure, metabolic rate, and the production of estrogen or testosterone. The *DSM-IV-TR* diagnostic criteria for anorexia nervosa are shown in Box 24–3. A well-known pioneer in the treatment of eating-disordered clients, Hilde Bruch (1978), called anorexia nervosa "the relentless pursuit of thinness."

Rigidity and overcontrol are the hallmarks of anorexia. To control themselves and their environment, anorexics develop rigid rules. Such rigidity often develops into *obsessive rituals*, particularly concerning eating and exercise. Cutting all food

Box 24–3 *DSM-IV-TR:* Diagnostic Criteria for Anorexia Nervosa

A. Refusal to maintain body weight at or above a minimally normal weight for age and height (e.g., weight loss leading to maintenance of body weight less than 85% of that expected; or failure to make expected weight gain during period of growth, leading to body weight less than 85% of that expected).
B. Intense fear of gaining weight or becoming fat, even though underweight.
C. Disturbance in the way in which one's body image or shape is experienced, undue influence of body weight or shape on self-evaluation, or denial of the seriousness of the current low body weight.
D. In postmenarcheal females, amenorrhea, i.e., the absence of at least three consecutive menstrual cycles. (A woman is considered to have amenorrhea if her periods occur only following hormone–e.g., estrogen–administration.)

RESTRICTING TYPE

During the current episode of Anorexia Nervosa, the person has not regularly engaged in binge-eating or purging behavior (i.e., self-induced vomiting or the misuse of laxatives, diuretics, or enemas).

BINGE-EATING/PURGING TYPE

During the current episode of Anorexia Nervosa, the person has regularly engaged in binge eating or purging behavior (i.e., self-induced vomiting or the misuse of laxatives, diuretics, or enemas).

Source: Reprinted with permission from the American Psychiatric Association. (2000). *Diagnostic and statistical manual of mental disorders* (4th ed., Text Revision). Washington, DC: Author.

into a predetermined size or number of pieces, chewing all food a certain number of times, allowing only certain combinations of foods in a meal, accomplishing a fixed number of exercise routines, and having an inflexible pattern of exercises are rituals common to anorexic people. These rules and rituals help keep anxiety beyond conscious awareness. If the rituals are disrupted, the anxiety becomes intolerable. Paradoxically, all these efforts to stay in control lead to out-of-control behaviors (Tozzi et al., 2005).

Many people with anorexia are hyperactive and discover that overexercise is a way to increase their weight loss. Solitary running tends to be the exercise of choice. Anorexics who overexercise often develop obsessive behaviors about the exercise itself. For example, they believe that before they can eat, they have to earn calories by exercising. Conversely, if they overeat, they believe they must punish themselves with excessive exercise. Excessive exercise signifies the triumph of will over the body and is a possible indication of poor prognosis in recovery (Neumark-Sztainer, 2005).

Anorexic young women have a desperate need to please others. Their self-worth depends on responses from others rather than on their own self-approval. Thus, their behavior is often overcompliant; they always try to meet the expectations of others in order to be accepted. They may overachieve in academic and extracurricular activities, but these accomplishments are usually an attempt to please parents rather than a source of self-satisfaction.

People with anorexia often feel hopeless, helpless, and ineffective. Because of being overcompliant with their parents, they believe they have always been controlled by others. Their refusal to eat may be an attempt to assert themselves and gain some control within the family. As weight is lost, they are rewarded with praise, admiration, and envy from their peers, which reinforces the restricted eating pattern.

PRACTICE ALERT

Health care providers often use language unfamiliar to clients and their families. Explain *amenorrhea in postmenarcheal females* in a way that would help a family understand the characteristics of anorexia nervosa.

Bulimia Nervosa

There is a cyclic behavioral pattern in **bulimia nervosa**. It begins with skipping meals sporadically and overstrict dieting or fasting. In an effort to refrain from eating, the person may use amphetamines, which can lead to extreme hunger, fatigue, and low blood glucose levels. The next part of the cycle is a period of **binge eating**, in which the person ingests huge amounts of food (about 3,500 kcal) within a short time (about 1 hour). Binges can last up to 8 hours, with consumption of 12,000 kcal. Binge eating usually occurs when the person is alone and at home, and most frequently during the evening. The cycle may occur once or twice a month for some and as often as five or ten times a day for others. The binge part of the cycle may be triggered by the ingestion of certain foods, but this is not consistent for everyone. Although eating binges may involve any kind of food, they usually consist of junk foods, fast foods, and high-calorie foods.

The final part of the cycle is **purging** the body of the ingested food. After excessive eating, people with bulimia force themselves to vomit. They often abuse laxatives and diuretics in order to purge their bodies of the food. Some use as many as 50 to 100 laxatives per day. In rare cases, bulimics may resort to Syrup of Ipecac to induce vomiting. Purging becomes a purification rite and a means of regaining self-control. Some describe it as feeling "completely fresh and clean again." The *DSM-IV-TR* diagnostic criteria for bulimia nervosa are shown in Box 24–4.

After the purging, the cycle begins all over again, with a return to strict dieting or fasting. Some people with bulimia eat highly nutritious meals when not binge eating/purging to repair harm done to the body.

Binge eating and purging begin as a way to eat and stay slim. Before long, the behavior becomes a response to stress and a way to cope with negative feelings such as anger, anxiety, and depression. For some it is poor impulse control, and for others it is an expression of rebellion against family members.

People with bulimia may engage in sporadic excessive exercise, but they usually do not develop compulsive exercise

Box 24–4 *DSM-IV-TR:* Diagnostic Criteria for Bulimia Nervosa

A. Recurrent episodes of binge eating. An episode of binge eating is characterized by both of the following:
  1. Eating, in a discrete period of time (e.g., within any 2-hour period), an amount of food that is definitely larger than most people would eat during a similar period of time and under similar circumstances
  2. A sense of lack of control over eating during the episode (e.g., a feeling that one cannot stop eating or control what or how much one is eating).

B. Recurrent inappropriate compensatory behavior in order to prevent weight gain, such as self-induced vomiting; misuse of laxatives, diuretics, enemas, or other medications; fasting; or excessive exercise.

C. The binge eating and inappropriate compensatory behaviors both occur, on average, at least twice a week for 3 months.

D. Self-evaluation is unduly influenced by body shape and weight.

E. The disturbance does not occur exclusively during episodes of Anorexia Nervosa.

PURGING TYPE

During the current episode of bulimia nervosa, the person has regularly engaged in self-induced vomiting or the misuse of laxatives, diuretics, or enemas.

NONPURGING TYPE

During the current episode of bulimia nervosa, the person has used other inappropriate compensatory behaviors, such as fasting or excessive exercise, but has not regularly engaged in self-induced vomiting or the misuse of laxatives, diuretics, or enemas.

Source: Reprinted with permission from the American Psychiatric Association. (2000). *Diagnostic and statistical manual of mental disorders* (4th ed., Text Revision). Washington, DC: Author.

CLINICAL MANIFESTATIONS AND THERAPIES Eating Disorders

ETIOLOGY	CLINICAL MANIFESTATIONS	CLINICAL THERAPIES
Anorexia nervosa	■ Withholding of food, obsessive behaviors regarding food ■ Extreme perfectionism ■ Rigidity, overcontrol, obsessive rituals ■ Significant weight loss ■ Body disturbances ■ Strenuous exercises ■ Reductions in heart rate, blood pressure, metabolic rate, and production of estrogen or testosterone ■ Feelings of hopelessness, helplessness	■ Antidepressants ■ Cognitive-behavior therapy ■ Family therapy
Bulimia nervosa	■ Cycle of binging and purging food ■ Body image disturbances ■ Abuse of laxatives ■ Hoarding food ■ Secretive behaviors	■ Antidepressants ■ Cognitive-behavioral therapy ■ Family therapy
Binge-eating disorder	■ Binging twice or more a week for at least 6 months ■ Absence of purging ■ Sense of loss of control ■ Allow eating and weight to interfere with personal relationships ■ Sense of embarrassment, disgust after overeating	■ Antidepressants ■ Cognitive-behavior therapy

routines. They are more likely to abuse street drugs to decrease their appetite and alcohol to reduce their anxiety. Since their binges are often expensive, costing as much as $100 per day, they may resort to stealing food or money to buy the food. The binge–purge cycle can become so consuming that it disrupts activities and relationships. To keep the behavior secret, the bulimic often resorts to excuses and lies.

Binge-Eating Disorder

The bulimic pattern is different from **binge-eating disorder**, which is often associated with obesity. This disorder is a proposed new category that needs further study before inclusion in the *Diagnostic and Statistical Manual of Mental Disorders* (4th ed., text revision) (*DSM-IV-TR*) (APA, 2000). The research criteria for binge-eating disorder are in Box 24–5. The prevalence in the general population is 1–3% and as high as 25% among people seeking help for weight loss (Pull, 2004).

Obese individuals who overeat tend to follow one of two patterns, neither of which includes purging the body after excessive food intake. The first pattern is overeating and feeling out of control in response to a number of feelings such as anxiety or depression. The diagnosis of binge-eating disorder is given when bingeing occurs at least twice a week for 6 months. Some individuals binge in response to losing control over a weight-loss diet. Although these people lose weight in weight-control programs, they regain it after going off the diet. People

Box 24–5 *DSM-IV-TR:* Research Criteria for Binge-Eating Disorder

A. Recurrent episodes of binge eating. An episode of binge eating is characterized by both of the following:
  1. Eating, in a discrete period of time (e.g., within any 2-hour period), an amount of food that is definitely larger than most people would eat in a similar period of time under similar circumstances.
  2. A sense of lack of control over eating during the episode (e.g., a feeling that one cannot stop eating or control what or how much one is eating).

B. The binge-eating episodes are associated with three (or more) of the following:
  1. Eating much more rapidly than normal
  2. Eating until feeling uncomfortably full
  3. Eating large amounts of food when not feeling physically hungry
  4. Eating alone because of being embarrassed by how much one is eating
  5. Feeling disgusted with oneself, depressed, or very guilty after overeating

C. Marked distress regarding binge eating is present.

D. The binge eating occurs, on average, at least 2 days a week for 6 months.

Note: The method of determining frequency differs from that used for bulimia nervosa; future research should address whether the preferred method of setting a frequency threshold is counting the number of days on which binges occur or counting the number of episodes of binge eating.

E. The binge eating is not associated with the regular use of inappropriate compensatory behaviors (e.g., purging, fasting, excessive exercise) and does not occur exclusively during the course of anorexia nervosa or bulimia nervosa.

Source: Reprinted with permission from the American Psychiatric Association. (2000). *Diagnostic and statistical manual of mental disorders* (4th ed., Text Revision). Washington, DC: Author.

with this eating pattern say that their eating or weight interferes with their relationships and their self-esteem. Women are more likely to have this eating pattern than men. There is evidence that several medications are effective for this disorder including sibutramine (Meridia), an appetite suppressant; citalopram (Celexa), a selective serotonin reuptake inhibitor (SSRI) antidepressant; and topiramate (Topamax), an anticonvulsant and mood stabilizer (Appolinario et al., 2003; Pull, 2004). The following clinical example discusses overeating in response to emotional distress.

PRACTICE ALERT

Health care providers often use language unfamiliar to clients and their families. Explain *inappropriate compensatory behavior* in a way that would help a family better understand the characteristics of binge-eating disorder.

COLLABORATION

Individual treatment and family therapy are used to address dysfunctional family patterns and assist the family to accept and deal with the client as an independent and less than perfect individual. Family involvement is crucial to effect a lasting change in the client and is most successful with young teens. Nurses, psychologists, family therapists, and dietitians commonly partner to plan and implement therapy. The nurse's role as a member of the health care team is detailed in the Nursing Process section.

Diagnostic Tests

Laboratory tests may reveal electrolyte abnormalities, particularly low serum potassium. Potentially fatal cardiac arrhythmias may result. The overuse of Syrup of Ipecac, an emetic agent, can create cumulative systemic toxicity affecting the gastrointestinal, neuromuscular, and cardiovascular systems, potentially leading to death from cardiotoxicity. Because the frequency of bulimia in diabetics is increasing, particularly among young women, bulimic clients should be tested for diabetes. Diabetes as a comorbid disorder carries the potential for lethality, because binge eating and purging increase the risk for both hypoglycemic episodes and diabetic ketoacidosis (DKA). Close monitoring of blood glucose levels is indicated for these clients.

Clinical Therapy

Long-term outpatient treatment, in either an individual or a group setting, is frequently necessary. Counseling that applies cognitive behavioral therapy may be continued for 2–3 years to ensure that weight gain and self-image are maintained.

Indications for hospitalization include loss of 25–30% of body weight, fluid and electrolyte imbalances or arrhythmias, or the need to provide a more intense period of therapy if outpatient treatment fails to produce improvement. Behavior modification techniques are used extensively in combination with counseling and other methods in care of the hospitalized anorectic client.

Antidepressants are the pharmalogic therapy of choice, with SSRIs being the first choice of treatment. It is generally recognized, however, that pharmacologic therapy is not effective in all clients and is less effective when not used in conjunction with psychotherapy.

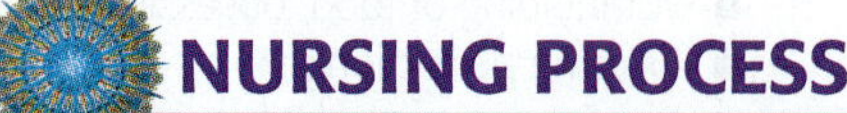

NURSING PROCESS

This section discusses the specific steps of the nursing process for clients with eating disorders. While pieces of the process will vary according to the nature of the eating disorder, the steps presented here may apply to any of the disorders, depending on the specific symptomology of the client.

Nurses must be aware of their own potential reactions to clients with eating disorders. Self-aware nurses recognize their own emotional reactions to clients and view clients' self-absorption and manipulativeness as symptoms of the disorder.

Assessment

When assessing clients with dramatic weight loss or gain, the nurse must not lose sight of the fact that both can be caused by physical conditions. Certain illnesses must be ruled out before an eating disorder diagnosis can be made. Wasting conditions such as advanced cancer, tuberculosis, AIDS, hyperthyroidism, pyloric obstruction, and drug abuse must be considered when weight loss is a feature. Rapid weight gain can result from a brain tumor, from an endocrine disorder, or as a side effect of medications. A good history and physical examination are often needed to provide information to eliminate the possibility of a physical basis for sudden weight loss or gain. After the presence of an eating disorder is established, the nurse will assess the client using the following subjective and objective data. Nutritional status is assessed by findings from diagnostic tests, a health assessment interview to collect subjective data, and a physical assessment to collect objective data. See Box 24–6 for sample documentation of a nutritional status assessment.

Nursing History

In addition to collecting data about the client's medical history and eating patterns, the nurse conducting the assessment should ask questions about the client's self-esteem and perception of self. This is critical to confirming the presence of an eating disorder. Clients with anorexia nervosa, for example, perceive themselves as overweight, no matter how thin they

Box 24–6 Sample Documentation

ASSESSMENT OF NUTRITIONAL STATUS

Twenty-two-year-old female visiting health clinic for regular checkup. Height 5 feet, 5 inches (165 cm); Weight 128 pounds (58 kg). BMI: 24. MAC: 28 cm. Waist-to-hip ratio: 0.6. Skin is warm, moist, and smooth without lesions other than well-healed scar on RLQ of abdomen from appendectomy, age 15. Oral mucosa and tongue pink and moist. No breath odor. All teeth present with evidence of dental care. Abdomen slightly concave when lying on back, bowel sounds present in all four quadrants, liver nonpalpable, tympany over lower abdomen on percussion.

may be. However emaciated their bodies, they can always find some body part they believe is fat.

Nurses should keep in mind that anorexics frequently deny that they have a weight problem. They insist they have never felt better and simply wish to be left alone about food while at the same time reporting feeling strong, powerful, and good as a result of self-denial. They report feeling guilty, self-indulgent, and weak when they eat. They therefore resist treatment, although they may admit to feeling isolated and lonely and may even describe themselves as exhausted with the effort it takes to achieve the perfection they seek. They tend to have difficulty accepting nurturing behavior from others and therefore have difficulty forming therapeutic alliances. They report a loss of interest in sex but do not perceive this as a problem.

Unlike anorexics, clients with bulimia nervosa recognize that their eating behaviors are abnormal and bizarre. Clients with bulimia nervosa have feelings of low self-esteem, worthlessness, inadequacy, and guilt. They experience shame and embarrassment over their secret binges (eating several quarts of ice cream, buckets of popcorn, or eight or more candy bars is not unusual) and subsequent purging activities. This shame may be manifested in self-deprecating remarks. Clients report feeling out of control, but at the same time they feel an excessive need to control. Anxiety and unsatisfactory interpersonal relationships are features of this disorder. Anxiety is intensified when others see the bulimic as successful and in control, and they often appear so to others. They are impulsive and cannot delay gratification. Preoccupation with food, weight, and dieting is a prominent feature. Bulimic clients may report feeling weak and lethargic.

PRACTICE ALERT

When interviewing the anorexic client, be sure to ask about amenorrhea; it is extremely common and is thought to be related to the degree of stress the woman is experiencing, the percentage of body fat lost, and altered hypothalamic function. With low estrogen levels, these young women are at higher risk for osteopenia leading to osteoporosis. This is a serious medical complication with no known effective treatment.

Physical Examination

The anorexic client is emaciated, with sunken eyes and a skeletal appearence. In very young clients, growth failure may be present. Lanugo growth (babylike, fine hair) on the face, extremities, and trunk may occur. Other physical symptoms include bradycardia, hypotension, arrhythmias, delayed gastric motility, and a hypothyroid-like state manifested by dry skin, listlessness, and dry hair that falls out at a higher-than-normal rate. Peripheral edema may be a feature in advanced starvation. Clients will likely have lost 25% of their weight, but a loss as high as 50% is possible. Laboratory tests may reveal leukopenia, anemia, low serum potassium, and elevated blood urea nitrogen (BUN). There may also be low thyroid levels and elevated serum cortisol.

Physical signs of bulimia nervosa include hoarseness and esophagitis, dental enamel erosion, enlarged parotid glands, abrasions or calluses on knuckles from inducing vomiting, and amenorrhea in about 40% of cases. The client may also have symptoms of fluid volume deficit: concentrated urine, decreased urine output, hypotension, elevated temperature, poor skin turgor, and weakness. The bulimic client's weight is usually normal or slightly above, unless anorexia is a co-occurring disorder.

Diagnosis

Once the assessment process is completed, determine appropriate nursing diagnoses. Any of the following may be appropriate for the client with an eating disorder:

- Imbalanced Nutrition related to self-starvation, binging, or purging (exacerbated if laxatives or emetics are used to promote vomiting)
- Ineffective Coping related to impaired adaptive behaviors, such as impulse control
- Disturbed Body Image related to an inability to see oneself realistically and underestimating one's own bodily needs, even in the face of overwhelming malnutrition
- Chronic Low Self-Esteem manifested by the client's lack of confidence in self, feelings of inferiority, unrealistic expectations of self and others, and unmet dependency needs
- Anxiety related to preoccupation with body image
- Deficient Fluid Volume related to purging.

PRACTICE ALERT

By the time clients with eating disorders are seen in treatment, their physical condition is often so deteriorated from self-imposed starvation, purging, or binge eating that nutritional status becomes the priority for nursing care. Life-threatening malnourishment is seen in 5–20% of anorexic clients. Death may occur from malnutrition, infection, or cardiac abnormalities related to electrolyte imbalances. For the anorexic client, intravenous therapy, tube feedings, and total parenteral hyperalimentation (TPH) are required in cases of medical emergency.

Plan

In order for the client to be successful, the client must participate in the planning process and take ownership of the care plan. Appropriate goals include the following:

- The client will return to and maintain at least 90% of normal weight for height and age.
- The client will demonstrate an understanding of nutrition as evidenced by a healthy change in eating patterns.
- The client will achieve and maintain normal elimination patterns, vital signs, and muscle tone.
- The female client will experience normal menstrual cycles.
- The client will identify adaptive coping behaviors and integrate them into daily routines.
- The client will express less anxiety about weight and appearance and verbalize other means of feeling in control.
- The bulimic client will refrain from purging following meals.

Implementation

Implementing care for the client with an eating disorder can be difficult when clients are submerged in the pathology of their illness to the extent that they cannot focus on anything else. Nurses must be patient with these clients, and must acknowledge small gains as well as large ones.

Facilitating Coping

The best way to promote individual coping is by involving clients in their own treatment planning. Self-determination fosters adaptive coping mechanisms in clients' day-to-day experiences.

Although trust is difficult to establish with clients with eating disorders, it is the basis for all therapeutic relationships. Being honest, available, and matter-of-fact helps establish trust and encourages clients to express their feelings. If necessary, allow clients to assume a dependent role at first, but as trust is developed and physical condition improves, encourage them to take more responsibility for themselves. Involving clients in care planning ensures autonomy and gives clients opportunities to practice making decisions. Letting clients have input into their treatment plans also fosters adherence. Provide flexibility in activities of daily living, type and timing of exercise, and choice of occupational and recreational therapy activities. This autonomy increases clients' sense of responsibility for themselves.

Giving clients the opportunity to practice problem solving may lead to power struggles if the nurse disagrees with clients' choices. Demonstrate positive belief in clients' ability to regain healthy functioning and a willingness to tolerate "mistakes." The treatment team must set firm and clear limits, however, to provide the secure environment clients need to learn more effective coping behaviors. Also help clients identify ways to feel in control other than by abusing food or relying on manipulative behaviors.

Clients need to explore their obsessive feelings about weight before they can relinquish maladaptive behaviors. It is helpful to explore with clients their feelings about their family, their role in the family, and their autonomy within the family system.

Enhancing Body Image

To help clients regain an accurate perception of their body size and nutritional needs, first encourage them to express feelings about body size. Reframe clients' misperceptions by using language that emphasizes health, strength, and evaluation. For example, if the client says "My thighs are huge," reply "Your thighs are becoming stronger now that you're gaining weight. Healthy muscles are rounded and firm, like yours." With practice, clients can replace negative thinking with positive self-talk. Teach and reinforce this skill, and help them practice it. For example, ask clients to make three positive statements (positive affirmations) about their bodies each day.

If clients are unable or unwilling to discuss their feelings about body size, ask them to draw themselves as they are now and as they desire to be. These drawings not only focus the discussion of body size and nutritional needs but also help the

FAMILY TEACHING **Teaching About Eating Disorders**

Friends and family members of people with eating disorders are often at a loss as to how to help. Heather L. Howard, former administrator for the National Association of Anorexia Nervosa and Associated Disorders (ANAD), recommends the following guidelines:

- Accept that there are no quick and easy solutions. Attitudes and behaviors must change.
- Change takes time and requires the cooperation of the person with the disorder.
- Family and friends must also change to accommodate the person's growth.
- Cooperate fully with the person's therapist.
- Avoid arguments about weight and food.
- Express love and affection both verbally and physically.
- Admit your anger, frustration, helplessness, and powerlessness and help the person see that these feelings do not mean you don't love him or her.
- Do things with the person that do not involve food.
- Don't diet yourself or talk about food, calories, fat grams, and the like.
- Avoid power struggles.
- Recognize that the person will make progress, then retreat into rituals for a time.
- Learn all you can about the disorder (see resource list).
- If the person will not seek help, CONFRONT in the following way:

  Concern—The reason you are confronting is that you care about the person.

  Organize—Decide who will be involved, when and where the confrontation will occur, and what to say.

  Needs—What resources will be needed after the confrontation? Therapist or support group; other resources.

  Face—Face the actual confrontation. Be direct; do not back down if the person angrily denies having a problem.

  Respond—Respond after listening carefully.

  Offer—Offer help and suggestions; offer yourself as a sounding-board.

  Negotiate—Negotiate another time to talk and set a time frame for the person to seek professional help.

  Time—Time to begin work. Remember to stress that recovery takes time and patience but that it is time to begin the process. There is much to be gained by seeking help and much to lose if the behaviors continue.

RESOURCES

National Association of Anorexia Nervosa and Associated Disorders, Inc
P.O. Box 640
Naperville, IL 60566
Helpline: 630-577-1330 Business Line: 630-577-1333
http://www.anad.org/

National Eating Disorders Association
603 Steward St., Suite 803
Seattle, WA 98101
206–382–3587
www.nationaleatingdisorders.org

Office on Women's Health
200 Independence Avenue SW, Room 730B
Washington, DC 20201
202–690–7650
http://www.womenshealth.gov/bodyimage/

Weight-Control Information Network (WIN)
1 Win Way
Bethesda, MD 20892–3665
877–946–4627
http://win.niddk.nih.gov/index.htm

Source: Heather L. Howard, former administrator. National Association of Anorexia Nervosa and Associated Disorders (ANAD). Retrieved September 11, 2007, from www.anad.org

NURSING CARE PLAN **A Client With Bulimia Nervosa**

ASSESSMENT

Lauren Franklin, a 28-year-old married woman, was admitted to the psychiatric unit from the emergency department where she was taken after collapsing during a marathon. She is a social worker with a master's degree who works in a drug abuse prevention program.

Lauren reports that she has been training for the marathon for about a year, running at least 35 miles a week. She believes that she had to be hospitalized because she did not ingest sufficient carbohydrates and fluids before the race.

Lauren states that she has been binge eating and purging for about 3 years. On a typical day she arises at 5:00 a.m., runs at least 5 miles, and then gets ready for work. On the way to work she buys and consumes a dozen doughnuts. She arrives at work before anyone else and vomits in the employees' bathroom. She eats no lunch unless she can be sure of access to a "good" bathroom, which she describes as one with a single toilet and an outside door that locks. In the evening, while preparing dinner, she consumes a can of salted peanuts and four or five glasses of wine. She denies ever getting "high." After a large dinner she showers, vomiting while the shower is running. Her husband of 4 years is unaware of her "problem" but worries about her drinking and wonders how she can eat so much and never gain weight.

Ms. Franklin has no prior psychiatric history, is the oldest of three children, and the only female. Her parents, both retired schoolteachers, live in a nearby town. She sees them infrequently because "they still treat me like I'm a little girl." She rarely sees her younger brothers and feels closer to her husband's family. There is no family history of eating disorders or substance abuse.

As the daughter of two schoolteachers, Ms. Franklin was expected to be the top student in her school. She had few friends because she was "the class geek." In college she excelled academically but was a "social failure." She states that she can drink an entire bottle of wine, vomit, and "sober up instantly." She has few friends or interests except running. She describes her job as "not fulfilling."

Ms. Franklin has no significant health problems. Vital signs: T_O 98.2; P 68; R 14; Ht 5′ 7″; Wt 110 lb; BP 108/68. She reports that she has not had a menstrual period in over 1 year. She takes no medications.

DIAGNOSES

- Anxiety related to low self-esteem
- Deficient Fluid Volume related to self-induced vomiting and excessive exercising
- Ineffective Individual Coping related to feelings of helplessness and lack of control

PLANNING

- The client will identify at least three sources of anxiety.
- The client will demonstrate the use of relaxation techniques to manage anxiety.
- The client will drink a minimum of 2 ounces of fluid every hour.
- The client will not vomit following meals.
- The client will eat regularly within one week.
- The client will refrain from discussing body image dissatisfaction for one week.

IMPLEMENTATION

- Adopt a calm, reassuring attitude when caring for Ms. Franklin.
- Help client recognize situations and events that create anxiety.
- Encourage client to identify health responses to anxiety.
- Teach relaxation techniques.
- Negotiate client contract to limit hoarding food, vomiting, and other compulsive behaviors.
- Teach client the importance of adequate fluid and nutritional intake.
- Teach client to weigh daily to evaluate rehydration and to keep accurate intake and output records while preparing her for the weight gain that will result from adequate hydration.
- Observe client for at least 1 hour after meals to prevention purging (or if outpatient, have the client ask a friend or relative).
- Encourage client to identify ways of nurturing herself without using alcohol or food.

EVALUATION

Ms. Franklin enters an inpatient rehabilitation facility that specializes in treatment of eating disorders. She attends daily cognitive-behavioral therapy sessions and begins to recognize how her parents' expectations and her own desire to please them has impacted her thought processes and behavior. She is initially repulsed by the weight gain that results from attaining a normal fluid balance but admits she has more energy and feels better when she eats properly. She attends nutrition classes and learns how to meet her body's nutritional needs while maintaining her desired level of fitness. Upon discharge both she and her husband continue to attend ongoing therapy sessions and report they are much happier.

CRITICAL THINKING

1. What factors may have contributed to bulimia for Ms. Franklin?
2. Based on her assessment information, design an appropriate diet for Ms. Franklin to meet her nutritional and fluid needs.
3. Early in her inpatient treatment regimen she turns to the nurse and says, "No one in this place will be happy until I'm so fat I waddle." How would you respond to this statement?

nurse understand how clients view their bodies. Because clients with eating disorders have distorted body images, this activity can be incorporated into their plans of care as well.

When clients share feelings honestly, show improvement in accurate perception of body image, or demonstrate healthier eating behaviors, reinforce their efforts through verbal recognition.

Improving Self-Esteem

Help clients reexamine negative feelings about themselves and identify their positive attributes. Encourage clients to record in a diary those thoughts that are difficult to share directly. Be nonjudgmental in your acceptance of negative feelings and positively reinforce the honest expression of all feelings. Encouragement is particularly important when clients experiment with independently made decisions, even when outcomes are not entirely positive. The client needs to interpret each experience as worthwhile. Emphasize the feeling of control gained through independent decision making.

Together, the nurse and the client explore the client's attempt to achieve perfection by controlling weight. The idea is for the client to realize that perfection is an unrealistic goal. The nurse is a role model for the person who accepts imperfection yet retains self-esteem. One way to model strong self-esteem is to admit errors willingly. Also model appropriate expressions of anger and teach clients the destructive effects of unexpressed anger.

Managing Fluids and Electrolytes

The importance of accurate intake and output records cannot be overstated, especially for the client who requires inpatient treatment. Daily consumption of 2,000–3,000 mL of liquid promotes rehydration. Accurate daily weights are needed. Always weigh the client at the same time of day (immediately upon arising is preferred) and on the same scale. Assess and document the condition of the skin and oral mucous membranes as well as pulses and blood pressure daily, and monitor laboratory values, particularly urine specific gravity, reporting significant alterations to the physician. Observe clients for at least an hour after meals to prevent purging. To promote comfort in the dehydrated client, give frequent mouth care.

Evaluation

Evaluation of the effectiveness of nursing interventions with these disorders is an ongoing part of the nursing process. Answers to the following questions will help determine if the client has met treatment objectives:

- Has the client regained and is the client maintaining at least 90% of normal weight for height and age?
- Is the client following an eating pattern that demonstrates an understanding of nutrition?
- Is the client maintaining normal elimination patterns, vital signs, and muscle tone?
- Is the female client experiencing normal menstrual cycles?
- Does the client demonstrate interest and competence in self-care activities?
- Does the client accurately identify both maladaptive coping behaviors and adaptive coping behaviors that can be integrated into daily routines?
- Does the client express less anxiety about weight and verbalize other means of feeling in control?
- Does the client verbalize positive statements about his or her body?
- Does the client accept compliments and positive feedback and show greater interest in activities?
- Does the client demonstrate interpersonal relationships that are substantially free of manipulation?

REVIEW Eating Disorders

RELATE: LINK THE CONCEPTS

Linking the exemplar of Eating Disorders with the concept of Sexuality:

1. A girl develops anorexia at the age of 13, which continues untreated for several years. How might this affect her sexual development?
2. How would anorexia affect the sexual development of a boy who developed anorexia at the same age?

Linking the exemplar of Eating Disorders with the concept of Fluids and Electrolytes:

3. What effect does bulimia nervosa have on fluid and electrolyte balance?
4. At what point would bulimia nervosa become life threatening related to fluid, electrolytes, and acid–base?

READY: GO TO COMPANION SKILLS MANUAL

- Monitoring intake and output
- Collecting routine urine specimen
- Establishing intravenous infusions
- Maintaining infusions
- Discontinuing infusion devices
- Measuring height
- Measuring weight
- Measuring body mass index

REFER: GO TO MYNURSINGKIT

REFLECT: CASE STUDY

Anisha Robinson is an 18-year-old college student. She is on the college's gymnastics team. A tiny little thing, Anisha is a bundle of energy and regularly complains about her weight. Sometimes she is so wound up at night that she can't sleep. In order not to keep her roommate up, she'll go out and run 2–3 miles in the middle of the night. Her friends worry about her because they don't know how she can keep her strength up when she eats so little, despite the fact that she'll go exercise for an hour or more after every meal. Her roommate becomes worried when they return from Thanksgiving break and she hears the gymnastics coach complaining that Anisha has gained 3 pounds over the holiday.

1. What are the priority nursing diagnoses for Anisha?
2. What caring interventions would you design for Anisha?
3. What symptoms would indicate that Anisha's health is deteriorating?

24.2 PERSONALITY DISORDERS

KEY TERMS

Antisocial personality disorder (ASPD), *1617*
Avoidant personality disorder (APD), *1618*
Borderline personality disorder (BPD), *1614*
Dependent personality disorder (DPD), *1619*
Depersonalization, *1613*
Derealization, *1613*
Ego-syntonic, *1607*
Histrionic personality disorder (HPD), *1616*
Impulsiveness, *1610*
Manipulation, *1610*
Narcissism, *1610*
Narcissistic personality disorder (NPD), *1616*
Obsessive–compulsive personality disorder (OCPD), *1619*
Paranoid personality disorder, *1611*
Personality, *1607*
Personality disorder (PD), *1607*
Personality traits, *1607*
Schizoid personality disorder, *1613*
Schizotypal personality disorder, *1613*
Splitting, *1615*

BASIS FOR SELECTION OF EXEMPLAR

National Institute of Mental Health

LEARNING OUTCOMES

After reading about this exemplar, you will be able to:

1. Describe the pathophysiology, etiology, clinical manifestations, and direct and indirect causes of personality disorders.
2. Identify risk factors associated with personality disorders.
3. Illustrate the nursing process in providing culturally competent care across the life span for individuals with personality disorders.
4. Formulate priority nursing diagnoses for an individual with a personality disorder.
5. Create a plan of care for individuals with personality disorders and their family members.
6. Assess expected outcomes for an individual with a personality disorder.
7. Discuss therapies used in the collaborative care of an individual with a personality disorder.
8. Employ evidence-based caring interventions for an individual with a personality disorder.

OVERVIEW

What distinguishes an individual from others is referred to as **personality**, which is defined as the individual qualities, including habitual behavior patterns, that make a person unique. **Personality traits** are persistent behavioral patterns. Even though the behaviors may be annoying or frustrating to others, they do not significantly interfere with the person's life. Both personality and personality traits tend to be stable over time. On the other hand, a **personality disorder (PD)** is a rigid, stereotyped behavioral pattern that deviates markedly from the norm of an individual's culture and persists throughout the person's life. A PD is a lifelong maladaptive pattern of perceiving, thinking, and relating that impairs social or occupational functioning and can be traced back to at least adolescence or early adulthood.

Individuals who have a PD have unique ways of perceiving themselves, other people, and the events in their lives. The range, intensity, and appropriateness of their emotional responses are often out of order. They lack insight; that is, they have no understanding of the impact of their behavior on the environment. They fail to accept the consequences of their own behavior and, when feeling threatened, attempt to ease the stress by changing the environment rather than changing their own behavior. Personality-disordered individuals' relationships are usually characterized by superficiality.

This exemplar discusses the various types of PDs and the major characteristics of each. Note that the goal of therapeutic approaches is not to restructure the client's basic personality, which is likely to be an impossible task. It is a well-known psychiatric axiom that one's basic personality is fixed by the age of 6. Instead, interventions are implemented to help those with PDs learn to deal with others in more productive, less stressful ways.

PATHOPHYSIOLOGY AND ETIOLOGY

A personality becomes *disordered* when the patterns are exaggerated, inflexible, and maladaptive. Personality disorders represent the extremes of normal variation of personality. The dysfunction may be a failure to establish personal identity, an inability to initiate or maintain intimate relationships, or a lack of social skills that interfere with cooperative relationships. Some people with personality disorders have intense emotional pain, whereas others seem invulnerable to painful feelings. Some are able to maintain relationships and careers, whereas others become functionally impaired.

Clients with personality disorders are among the most difficult to treat. Most will never enter a psychiatric hospital, seek or receive outpatient treatment, or undergo a diagnostic evaluation. Some will enter the mental health system through family pressure or because of a court order. With those who do come into the system, mental health professionals find their expertise tested. In most cases, the personality problems are **ego-syntonic**, that is clients perceive their difficulties in dealing with other people to be external to them. Incapable of considering that their problems have anything to do with them personally, they will describe being victimized by specific others or by "the system." Some may develop an awareness of their self-defeating behavior but remain at a loss as to how they got that way or how to begin to change.

Personality disorders are diagnosed or coded on Axis II of the *Diagnostic and Statistical Manual of Mental Disorders* (4th ed., Text Revision) (*DSM-IV-TR*) (American Psychiatric Association, 2000) (See Box 24–7). The personality disorders have a high degree of overlap, and many individuals exhibit traits of several disorders. Thus, individuals who receive any personality disorder diagnosis typically receive several. This lack of precision continues to be a criticism of the *DSM-IV-TR*. Some clinicians prefer to conceptualize personality disorders on a continuum from mild to moderate to severe.

Typically, personality disorders become apparent before or during adolescence and persist throughout life. In some cases, the symptoms become less obvious by middle or old age. Studies show that personality disorders have an impact on an individual's quality of life (Chen et al. 2006).

Etiology

It is extremely difficult to estimate the incidence of personality disorders. Many people with personality disorders never come to the attention of the mental health system. Personality disorders are frequently diagnosed among the psychiatric client population.

As with other psychiatric disorders, a number of theories have been offered to identify the causes of personality disorders. With continuing refinement of diagnostic criteria for each cluster of disorders, it will become possible to conduct useful research on specific populations that have been accurately diagnosed. In the past, wide differences in the application of specific diagnostic labels precluded the gathering of reliable data. Since there was so little agreement about whether a person should be included in the category at the outset, it is easy to understand why the search for any common factors—in genetics, early experiences, family patterns, or any other variable—failed to yield results from which general conclusions could be drawn.

Remaining obstacles are the refusal to seek treatment on the part of the client and the relatively infrequent need for psychiatric hospitalization. Thus, research has usually focused on those individuals who seek therapy or those who are referred through the criminal system (most often with antisocial personality disorder).

There is no single cause of the personality disorders. Most likely, they arise from an interaction between biological factors and the environment. Just as one's biology or constitution can alter experiences in life, so too can experiences alter one's basic biology. The brain constantly changes to absorb new experiences.

Box 24–7 *DSM-IV-TR:* Diagnostic Criteria for a Personality Disorder

A. An enduring pattern of inner experience and behavior that deviates markedly from the expectations of the individual's culture. This pattern is manifested in two (or more) of the following areas:
  1. Cognition (i.e., ways of perceiving and interpreting self, other people, and events)
  2. Affectivity (i.e., the range, intensity, lability, and appropriateness of emotional response)
  3. Interpersonal functioning
  4. Impulse control.

B. The enduring pattern is inflexible and pervasive across a broad range of personal and social situations.

C. The enduring pattern leads to clinically significant distress or impairment in social, occupational, or other important areas of functioning.

D. The pattern is stable and of long duration and its onset can be traced back at least to adolescence or early adulthood.

E. The enduring pattern is not better accounted for as a manifestation or consequence of another mental disorder.

F. The enduring pattern is not due to the direct physiological effects of a substance (e.g., a drug of abuse, a medication) or a general medical condition (e.g., head trauma).

Source: Reprinted with permission from the American Psychiatric Association. (2000). *Diagnostic and statistical manual of mental disorders,* (4th ed., p. 689, Text Revision). Washington, DC: Author.

Genetics

Studies suggest a common genetic factor in schizotypal personality disorder and schizophrenia. Individuals in both groups have an equal probability of having a sibling with schizophrenia. This shared genetic vulnerability has led many people to consider schizotypal personality disorder as one of the schizophrenia spectrum disorders (Keshavan et al., 2005).

Extreme shyness beginning in infancy may be associated with Cluster C disorders. Overanxious children are more likely to be overprotected and vulnerable to developing dependent traits. It is critical, however, that labels not be attached to behavior that is developmentally appropriate (American Psychiatric Association, 2000).

A strong predictor of the development of antisocial behavior is antisocial personality disorder in one or both parents. This seems to be due to both genetic and environmental factors. There also appears to be a genetic link between antisocial and borderline personality disorders. It is believed that people with both disorders are born with an innate biological tendency to react intensely to low levels of stress (Paris, 2001).

Neurobiology

Some of the personality disorders are primarily disorders of impulse control. There may be problems with limbic system regulation. Brain imaging studies report reduced glucose utilization in the limbic system and the prefrontal cortex of people who exhibit impulsive aggression when compared to normal controls. People diagnosed with borderline personality disorder and antisocial personality disorder appears to have lower serotonin (5-HT) activity than control groups. The lower the 5-HT levels, the more likely the client is to self-mutilate, experience intense rage, and behave aggressively toward others. A concurrent high level of norepinephrine (NE) creates hypersensitivity to the environment and is related to aggressive behavior. Abnormalities in levels of dopamine (DA) may explain the psychotic episodes experienced by some clients with borderline personality disorder (BPD) and schizotypal personality disorder (MacFarlane, 2004; Ni et al., 2006).

Many people with personality disorders have a history of traumatic childhood events such as physical or sexual abuse. Trauma increases activity in the hypothalamic–pituitary–adrenocortical axis, which, with long-term stimulation, increases anxiety and self-destructive behavior. Childhood trauma may also reduce the volume of the hippocampus (Brambilla et al., 2004; Lee, Geracioti, Kasckow, & Coccaro, 2005).

Recent research has found that there may be a relationship between criminal behavior and physiological under arousal to stimulation. Heart rate, skin conductance, and electroencephalogram (EEG) readings are lower in people with antisocial personality disorder (ASPD) than in those without the disorder. This underarousal can be interpreted in two ways: Either the person seeks inappropriate stimulation to counteract the underaroused state or it is a marker of low fear levels, which interfere with the anticipation of danger (Ratey, 2001).

Intrapersonal Factors

The idea that most children are *resilient* to adversity is critical for understanding the impact of negative events in childhood. Some aspects of resilience are biological. Children with positive personality traits and higher levels of intelligence are more adept at finding ways to cope with adversity. In contrast, children with negative personality traits and lower levels of intelligence experience more stress as they attempt to cope with adversity. Psychosocial aspects of resiliency are positive relationships, which buffer negative experiences. Thus, growing up in a dysfunctional family can be offset by attachments to competent extended family members.

People with Cluster A personality disorders have been studied minimally because they seldom request or are forced into treatment. Intrapersonal theory suggests that the primary defense mechanism is one of projection; that is, they project their own hostility on others and respond to them in a fearful and distrustful manner. It is also thought that they defensively withdraw from others for fear they will be hurt.

Intrapersonal theory explains ASPD as a developmental delay or failure. It is believed that people with ASPD have an underdeveloped superego, in that authority and cultural mores have not been internalized. Conformity to cultural expectations is situational and superficial, and there is an inability to experience guilt when rules are violated.

Individuals with BPD often think, feel, and behave more like toddlers than adults. When young children experience inadequate parenting, their basic needs and desires remain unsatisfied. Unmet needs lead to hostility toward those on whom their lives depend. At the same time, these children are terrified by the destructiveness of their anger. They begin to believe that they have been, or will be, abandoned, and the parents are unable to provide good experiences to balance the intense feelings of neglect. All of this contributes to adults who feel so utterly empty inside that they can never get enough attention and nurturing. At the same time, they are terrified of intimacy because of their fears of abandonment. This constant tension between need and fear leads to acting out feelings of rage and self-destructive behavior to manage the guilt.

Sociocultural Factors

Negative childhood experiences do not necessarily lead to mental disorders in adulthood. Risk factors may, however, increase the likelihood of negative outcomes. In community populations, psychosocial stressors contribute to pathology in only a minority of those who are exposed. In clinical populations, people with a variety of mental disorders report more psychosocial stressors during childhood than do those without mental disorders. In other words, most people are resilient to adversity but those who develop mental disorders have an underlying vulnerability to stress.

A variety of social conditions lead to low self-esteem, negative self-concept, and even self-hatred. When one is on the receiving end of social oppression, it is more difficult to develop self-esteem and a healthy identity.

Social expectations encourage some kinds of behavior and suppress others. Traditional societies are more tolerant of dependence, and people are expected to conform to family and group norms. Some believe that industrialization has contributed to a changing value system and that Cluster B personality disorders may be a response to society's increasing complexity. We have come to recognize current values such as these: Personal needs are more important than group needs, expediency is more important than morality, and appearance is more important than inner worth. Believing that survival depends solely on themselves, those with Cluster B personality disorders develop a value system of "Every person for herself or himself" and "Take care of number one first."

Family Theory

Many individuals diagnosed with personality disorders report dysfunctional families of origin. This may reflect some reality but may also reflect how distressed adults account for their present difficulties by blaming their parents. Abnormal parenting (abuse, neglect, overcontrol) may be a risk factor for personality disorder. However, multiple negative experiences in childhood are more likely to cause problems.

The diathesis–stress model states that biology and social environment of the family interact in such a way as to produce personality disorders (Orth, Robins, & Meier, 2009). For example, children who are born with a temperament of impulsivity and mood instability may be badly treated by family members. Other children who are born with an anxious temperament and who have problems with peer relationships may be overprotected or rejected by parental caregivers. Children with difficult temperaments come into conflict with peers and parents, increasing the likelihood of either social rejection or physical abuse.

People with ASPD are thought to come from families with inconsistent parenting that resulted in emotional deprivation in the children. Because of their own personality or substance abuse problems, parents may be unable to supervise and discipline their children, or they may even model antisocial behavior for the children. Others seem to come from healthy families and had good childhood experiences.

Family theorists view BPD as a dysfunction of the entire family system across several generations, with similar dynamics of blurred generational boundaries of the incestuous family. BPD usually occurs in an enmeshed family system. With a high family value on children's loyalty to parents, adult children cling to their parents even after marriage. As a result, the marital couple is unable to bond with each other. When children are born, they are encouraged to cling, and normal separation behavior is discouraged. Often, the children end up in a caretaking role with parents and must assume a high level of family responsibility. During late adolescence, they are unable to separate from their parents because of an incorporated family theme that separation and loss are intolerable. It is within the third or fourth generation of enmeshed families that borderline traits develop into the personality disorder. Male children with BPD tend not to marry and remain connected with their families of origin. Female children with BPD often marry but tend to pick passive and distant partners who are enmeshed with their own families (Livesley, 2003; Magnavita & MacFarlane, 2004).

It is believed that a chaotic, depriving, abusive, or brutalizing environment is a major factor in the development of BPD. Research shows that 50–70% of clients diagnosed with BPD have a history of abuse. Tentative findings at this point indicate that the abuse began at an early age, that the child was neglected as well as abused, that sexual abuse was often combined with physical abuse, and that there was usually more than one perpetrator. It must be noted that abuse within the family is not a single incident but rather part of a dysfunctional family behavior pattern that is either chaotic or coercively controlling. Dysfunctional families distort all interactions and relationships (Livesley, 2003).

Gender-Bias Theory

Girls and boys are socialized very differently in America. Boys are encouraged to be independent, self-sufficient, active, and thinking rather than feeling individuals. Girls are taught to be dependent, submissive, passive, and feeling individuals who are more concerned with the needs of others than with their own needs. Such rigid role expectations can lead to identity difficulties. The same behaviors that may be considered acceptable in men (impulsiveness, expressing anger, argumentativeness, making demands) are labeled pathological in women. It is more likely that men are diagnosed as having antisocial personality disorder and women are diagnosed as having BPD when exhibiting similar behaviors. These differences in diagnoses reflect the real and unfortunate consequences of gender-role stereotyping in American culture (Sperry, 2004).

Risk Factors

As discussed in the preceding sections, risk factors for personality disorders include genetic and environmental factors:

- Family history of mental illness
- History of child abuse, neglect, or other victimization (e.g., rape)
- Instability in family life during childhood (parental loss, homelessness, etc.)
- Client history of other mental illness or conduct disorder.

CLINICAL MANIFESTATIONS

There are 11 personality disorders. Three major categories, or *clusters,* of PDs have been established by the American Psychiatric Association (APA). Each cluster is discussed separately in this section. Even though there are some differences among the three clusters, three traits are common to people with all types of PDs:

- Lack of insight—individuals lack understanding of the impact of their behavior on others.
- External response to stress—when feeling threatened, individuals try to change the environment instead of changing themselves.
- Failure to accept the consequences of their own behavior.

The essential characteristics of personality disorders are chronicity, pervasiveness, and maladaptation. The individual with a PD often goes through life repeating the same dysfunctional patterns. The PD affects every dimension of life and seriously impairs interpersonal and functional abilities.

Other problematic behaviors that are characteristic of people with PDs include manipulation, narcissism, and impulsiveness. **Manipulation** refers to controlling behavior which the individual uses to exploit others for personal gain. **Narcissism** is self-centered behavior in which the individual feels entitled to special favors due to a mistaken perception of oneself as the "center of the universe." **Impulsiveness** refers to acting without considering the consequences of one's behavior.

The *DSM-IV-TR* delineates diagnostic criteria for PDs on Axis II. Essential features of these disorders include significant distress or impairment in at least two of the following areas of functioning:

- Cognition
- Affect
- Interpersonal relationships
- Impulse control.

These behavior patterns must be evident by early adulthood and not be a result of other mental disorders or substance abuse (APA, 2000). It is important to distinguish the behaviors that define personality disorders from responses that may emerge as a result of specific situational stressors or transient mental states. Therefore, it is often necessary and important to conduct more than one interview with the client over a period of time. While personality-disordered people display enduring, inflexible, and pervasive maladaptive behaviors in a broad variety of personal, occupational, and social situations, they may not view their lifestyles as abnormal. Typically, they do not seek professional help unless they are very stressed.

Personality disorders may coexist with extreme psychopathology, such as the disorders included in *DSM-IV-TR* Axis I groupings. In addition, when under stress, the individual with a personality disorder may progressively deteriorate even to the point of psychosis.

What follows is a description of each cluster and its specific disorders. Table 24–7 outlines the major features of each cluster and some of the characteristics of specific disorders.

TABLE 24–7 **Clinical Manifestations of Personality Disorders**

ETIOLOGY	MAJOR FEATURES	SPECIFIC CHARACTERISTICS
Cluster A (Odd–Eccentric)	■ Pervasive distrust ■ Social detachment ■ Subsequent impairment of social and occupational functioning ■ Cognitive impairments ■ Peculiar behaviors ■ Maladaptive defense mechanisms	**Paranoid Personality Disorder** ■ Suspicious and mistrustful ■ Persistently bears grudges ■ Reads hidden or threatening meanings into benign comments **Schizoid Personality Disorder** ■ Neither desires nor enjoys close relationships ■ Chooses solitary activities ■ Rarely takes pleasure in activities ■ Emotional coldness, detachment, or flattened affect **Schizotypal Personality Disorder** ■ Odd beliefs or magical thinking that influence behaviors ■ Odd thinking or speech ■ Inappropriate or constructed affect ■ Paranoid ideation
Cluster B (Dramatic–Emotional)	■ Impulsive behavior ■ Live in the present moment ■ Act without evaluating potential consequences ■ Inability to delay gratification	**Borderline Personality Disorder** ■ Frantic efforts to avoid real or imagined abandonment ■ Impulsive, self-damaging behavior ■ Disturbed sense of personal identity ■ Marked reactivity of mood ■ Chronic feelings of emptiness **Histrionic Personality Disorder** ■ Inappropriate sexually provocative behavior ■ Rapidly shifting and shallow expressions of emotion ■ Speech is excessively impressionistic and lacking in detail ■ Theatrical; exaggerated expressions of emotion **Narcissistic Personality Disorder** ■ Grandiose sense of self-importance ■ Preoccupied fantasies of success, power, beauty, etc. ■ Requires excessive admiration ■ Lacks empathy **Antisocial Personality Disorder** ■ Failure to conform to social norms; unlawful behaviors ■ Deceitful, impulsive ■ Irritable, aggressive ■ Reckless disregard for safety of self and others
Cluster C (Anxious–Fearful)	■ Restricted affect ■ Problems expressing feelings ■ Unrealistic expectations of others ■ Impaired decision making and problem solving ■ Intense emotional repression ■ Behaviors that are socially isolating and self-defeating	**Avoidant Personality Disorder** ■ Social withdrawal ■ Overly serious, painfully shy ■ Hypersensitive to potential rejection or shame **Dependent Personality Disorder** ■ Difficulty making decisions without excessive advice and reassurance ■ Goes to excessive lengths to obtain support from others ■ Needs others to assume responsibility in most areas of his or her life **Obsessive–Compulsive Personality Disorder** ■ Preoccupation with details, rules, lists ■ Perfectionism interferes with task completion ■ Excessive devotion to work and productivity ■ Rigid, stubborn

Cluster A Personality Disorders: Odd–Eccentric

Cluster A consists of the paranoid, schizoid, and schizotypal personality disorders. The major features of these disorders are pervasive distrust, social detachment, and subsequent impairment in social and occupational functioning. People with odd–eccentric personality disorders have the most cognitive impairments as well as the most peculiar behaviors and maladaptive defensive styles of people with PDs. Box 24–8, the *DSM-IV-TR* Diagnostic Criteria feature, describes the characteristics of persons with odd–eccentric personality disorders.

PARANOID PERSONALITY DISORDER Clients with **paranoid personality disorder** engage in a pattern of pervasive mistrust of others, misinterpreting benign comments and actions as

Box 24–8 *DSM-IV-TR:* Diagnostic Criteria for Personality Disorders: Cluster A (Odd–Eccentric)

PARANOID PERSONALITY DISORDER

A pervasive distrust and suspiciousness of others such that their motives are interpreted as malevolent, beginning by early adulthood and present in a variety of contexts, as indicated by four (or more) of the following:

1. Suspects, without sufficient basis, that others are exploiting, harming, or deceiving him or her
2. Is preoccupied with unjustified doubts about the loyalty or trustworthiness of friends or associates
3. Is reluctant to confide in others because of unwarranted fear that the information will be used maliciously against him or her
4. Reads hidden demeaning or threatening meanings into benign remarks or events
5. Persistently bears grudges (i.e., is unforgiving of insults, injuries, or slights)
6. Perceives attacks on his or her character or reputation that are not apparent to others and is quick to react angrily or to counterattack
7. Has recurrent suspicions, without justification, regarding fidelity of spouse or sexual partner.

SCHIZOID PERSONALITY DISORDER

A pervasive pattern of detachment from social relationships and a restricted range of expression of emotions in interpersonal settings, beginning by early adulthood and present in a variety of contexts, as indicated by four (or more) of the following:

1. Neither desires nor enjoys close relationships, including being part of a family
2. Almost always chooses solitary activities
3. Has little, if any, interest in having sexual experiences with another person
4. Takes pleasure in few, if any, activities
5. Lacks close friends or confidants other than first-degree relatives
6. Appears indifferent to the praise or criticism of others
7. Shows emotional coldness, detachment, or flattened affect
8. Considers relationships to be more intimate than they actually are.

SCHIZOTYPAL PERSONALITY DISORDER

A pervasive pattern of social and interpersonal deficits marked by acute discomfort with, and reduced capacity for, close relationships as well as by cognitive or perceptual distortions and eccentricities of behavior, beginning by early adulthood and present in a variety of contexts, as indicated by five (or more) of the following:

1. Ideas of reference (excluding delusions of reference)
2. Odd beliefs or magical thinking that influences behavior and is inconsistent with subcultural norms (e.g., superstitiousness, belief in clairvoyance, telepathy, or "sixth sense"; in children and adolescents, bizarre fantasies or preoccupations)
3. Unusual perceptual experiences, including bodily illusions
4. Odd thinking and speech (e.g., vague, circumstantial, metaphorical, overelaborate, or stereotyped)
5. Suspiciousness or paranoid ideation
6. Inappropriate or constricted affect
7. Behavior or appearance that is odd, eccentric, or peculiar
8. Lack of close friends or confidants other than first-degree relatives
9. Excessive social anxiety that does not diminish with familiarity and tends to be associated with paranoid fears rather than negative judgments about self.

Source: Reprinted with permission from the American Psychiatric Association. (2000). *Diagnostic and statistical manual of mental disorders* (4th ed., Text Revision). Washington, DC: Author.

threatening. These clients often report that others plot against them or attempt to use or deceive them. They talk about disloyal friends and coworkers and the irreversible harm others' actions have caused. They may be surprised by, but mistrustful of, loyalty shown to them; they often refuse to answer questions, saying, "That is no one's business." A frequent theme of clients with a paranoid personality disorder is pathologic suspicion of spousal or partner infidelity. Unrealistic grandiose fantasies often emerge; clients may discuss activities with others who share their beliefs, such as special interest groups or cults. Client affect may be labile, with hostile, stubborn sarcasm being predominant.

Suspiciousness and Mistrust Suspiciousness and mistrust reflect an attitude of doubt toward the trustworthiness of objects or people. Suspiciousness is also a way of thinking and includes such manifestations as expectations of trickery or harm, guardedness, secretiveness, pathologic jealousy, and excessive concern with hidden motives and special meanings. For example, the suspicious person may perceive a birthday gift as a trick to create an obligation. Legal disputes may arise from the client's response to perceived threats.

Projection People who are paranoid attribute their own ego-alien (intolerable) motivations, drives, or feelings to others. Projection is used to attribute to others the harmful intentions that they themselves feel. In this way, the idea that one may be harmed really reflects one's own wish to harm others.

Restricted Affect Labile emotional expressiveness and a lack of spontaneity characterize people with paranoid personality disorder. They often appear cold, humorless, and devoid of tender, sensitive feelings. Although they may demonstrate temper outbursts, they pride themselves on remaining objective and reasonable and frequently use intellectualization and rationalization to avoid affective experiences. Some paranoid people may appear friendly, but in fact this friendliness is a "script" that helps them adapt to social situations or achieve their goals.

Exclusion Because of the paranoid person's antagonism and suspiciousness, tension develops between the person and significant others. The persistent strain on relationships causes others to define the paranoid person as more than simply "different." Instead, they see the individual as unreliable or untrustworthy, and others begin to interact according to their perceptions. These behaviors reinforce the suspicions and beliefs of the paranoid person. The effects of this process include the following:

- Blocked communication, which increases the process of exclusion
- Emergence of a crisis, which formally excludes the paranoid person
- Reinforcement of the paranoid person's beliefs, interpretations, or ideas of reference.

Because paranoid people are generally intelligent, persuasive, and creative in justifying their beliefs, they often try to adapt by one of two ways. They may join quasi-political groups, esoteric religions, cults, or quasi-scientific organizations that reinforce their interpretations of reality. Or they may join organizations that challenge societal norms and trends in an effort to direct and thus control their hostile feelings.

The nurse may encounter clients with paranoid personality disorder in any health care setting.

SCHIZOID PERSONALITY DISORDER People with **schizoid personality disorder** generally have a detached and aloof social style and display a range of adjustment. Some are fairly well-adjusted individuals who are loners; others live out their lives in protective environments, such as group homes, mental hospitals, and prisons.

Schizoid personality disorder is found in about 3% of the population (APA, 2000). Individuals who are diagnosed with schizoid personality disorder are rarely seen in clinical settings, but when they are it is usually for treatment of symptoms associated with anxiety, depression, or dysphoric affect. They may experience transient psychotic episodes, which may last a few minutes to several hours.

Individuals with schizoid personality disorder show a preference for solitary interests—they claim to enjoy being alone—and occupations that require minimal social interaction. They tend to choose solitary hobbies such as solitaire and computer games, and jobs such as night security guard or bridge tender. They may decline job promotions because social demands (meetings, supervisory responsibilities) accompany the promotion. When questioned about sexual activity, clients with schizoid PD usually deny interest or involvement in intimate relationships. They may appear cool, aloof, or bored, and may seem to be cognitively impaired. When asked if they think their loner-type behavior is unusual, a typical response is, "I never thought about it much…it doesn't much matter to me." Schizoid clients acknowledge that they rarely become excited, angry, upset, or joyful. Indifference and humorlessness are hallmarks of the individual with schizoid personality disorder.

SCHIZOTYPAL PERSONALITY DISORDER Suspicion, including paranoid ideation, is usually noted in the schizotypal client. Maintaining eye contact may be difficult, and communication strategies such as humor to defuse anxiety may be met with a stare and questions about the meaning or purpose of the joking. Be careful about using humor with mentally disordered people. Their interpretation of humor or joking will not always match that of others.

Clients with **schizotypal personality disorder** report a great deal of subjective anxiety in social situations, have cognitive or perceptual distortions, and display eccentric behavior. They often report bizarre fantasies, especially of paranormal events. During an interview, they may remark, "I know what you're going to ask me before you say it," believing they are endowed with special powers or have the ability to control others' behavior by simply "willing it to happen." Often, these clients have speech patterns that are loose, digressive, or vague; this often makes them difficult to interview. The client may acknowledge this behavior by stating, "I was never talkative" (APA, 2000). Clients with schizotypal PD appear absent-minded; they daydream, are vague about goals, are indecisive, and lack social skills. Often, they act as if they are "in a fog." They fail to respond in a usual manner to social cues and seem like social misfits.

The schizotypal-personality-disordered client demonstrates eccentricities in communication and behavior not seen in a person with schizoid personality. Examples include such oddities of thought as magical thinking and ideas of reference; altered perceptions, such as illusions, **depersonalization** (a feeling of strangeness or unreality about the self), and **derealization** (a feeling of disconnection from the environment); speech alterations, including circumstantiality (giving detailed, factual but nonessential information), digression, metaphoric speech patterns, and overly concrete or abstract responses; and an odd or unkempt manner of dress, which includes ill-fitting, stained, and mismatched clothing.

They have a history of being loners and neither desire nor enjoy close relationships. They are indifferent to feedback and insensitive to others. The detachment from social relationships is also noted in the client's lack of interest in having intimate or sexual relationships.

Onset of schizotypal PD is believed to be in childhood or early adolescence. Clients report poor academic achievement and poor peer relationships as well as social anxiety, even as children. Clients with schizotypal personality disorders may experience psychotic episodes of very short duration, lasting from a few minutes to several hours (APA, 2000).

Cluster B Personality Disorders: Dramatic–Emotional

The *DSM-IV-TR* identifies the borderline, histrionic, narcissistic, and antisocial personality disorders as dramatic, emotional, and erratic dysfunctions. Individuals with these disorders are often in conflict with society because of their impulsive behavior. Impulsive people view the world as a discontinuous, fragmented collection of opportunities, frustrations, and affective experiences. They live only in the present moment and, therefore, lack the ability to formulate long-range plans. They act decisively without critical evaluation of consequences. The focus of their intellectual and emotional goals is to achieve immediate satisfaction. This lack of impulse control and inability to delay gratification often result in both verbal and nonverbal outbursts of anger, which may be self-directed or other-directed. Indeed, clients with dramatic–emotional personality disorders may experience rapid escalation of anxiety when their own angry impulses are not controlled by others. A description of the Cluster B personality disorders is shown in Box 24–9.

BORDERLINE PERSONALITY DISORDER Individuals with **borderline personality disorder (BPD)** have unstable interpersonal relationships, self-image, and affect, and are impulsive. It is common for such clients to experience psychotic breaks from reality whenever they experience severe stress. Prevalence of this disorder is about 2% (APA, 2000).

Approximately 50% of individuals with BPD also have other coexisting mental disorders, such as major depression, bipolar disorder, eating disorders, and substance abuse (National Alliance on Mental Illness, 2007). Individuals with BPD may also have coexisting physical problems. Medical–surgical nurses may meet them as clients in general hospital settings.

Impulsivity Impulsiveness may be expressed in self-damaging ways, demonstrating a lack of responsibility and disregard for the consequences of one's behavior. The responses of individuals with BPD fluctuate in situations that are subjectively interpreted and often distorted. These individuals do not learn from their mistakes and, therefore, do not change their behavior, which reinforces their impulsive responses (de Bruijn et al., 2006). Impulsiveness is manifested in spending habits, sexual

Box 24–9 *DSM-IV-TR:* Diagnostic Criteria for Personality Disorders: Cluster B (Dramatic–Emotional)

BORDERLINE PERSONALITY DISORDER

A pervasive pattern of instability of interpersonal relationships, self-image, and affects, and marked impulsivity beginning by early adulthood and present in a variety of contexts, as indicated by five (or more) of the following:

1. Frantic efforts to avoid real or imagined abandonment

Note: Do not include suicidal or self-mutilating behavior covered in Criterion 5.

2. A pattern of unstable and intense interpersonal relationships characterized by alternating between extremes of idealization and devaluation
3. Identity disturbance: markedly and persistently unstable self-image or sense of self
4. Impulsivity in at least two areas that are potentially self-damaging (e.g., spending, sex, substance abuse, reckless driving, binge eating)
5. Recurrent suicidal behavior, gestures, or threats, or self-mutilating behavior
6. Affective instability due to a marked reactivity of mood (e.g., intense episodic dysphoria, irritability, or anxiety usually lasting a few hours and only rarely more than a few days)
7. Chronic feelings of emptiness
8. Inappropriate, intense anger or difficulty controlling anger (e.g., frequent displays of temper, constant anger, recurrent physical fights)
9. Transient, stress-related paranoid ideation or severe dissociative symptoms.

HISTRIONIC PERSONALITY DISORDER

A pervasive pattern of excessive emotionality and attention seeking, beginning by early adulthood and present in a variety of contexts, as indicated by five (or more) of the following:

1. Is uncomfortable in situations in which he or she is not the center of attention
2. Interaction with others is often characterized by inappropriate sexually seductive or provocative behavior
3. Displays rapidly shifting and shallow expression of emotions
4. Consistently uses physical appearance to draw attention to self
5. Has a style of speech that is excessively impressionistic and lacking in detail
6. Shows self-dramatization, theatricality, and exaggerated expression of emotion
7. Is suggestible (i.e., easily influenced by others or circumstances).

NARCISSISTIC PERSONALITY DISORDER

A pervasive pattern of grandiosity (in fantasy or behavior), need for admiration, and lack of empathy, beginning by early adulthood and present in a variety of contexts, as indicated by five (or more) of the following:

1. Has a grandiose sense of self-importance (e.g., exaggerates achievements and talents, expects to be recognized as superior without commensurate achievements)
2. Is preoccupied with fantasies of unlimited success, power, brilliance, beauty, or ideal love
3. Believes that he or she is "special" and unique and can only be understood by, or should associate with, other special or high-status people (or institutions)
4. Requires excessive admiration
5. Has a sense of entitlement (i.e., unreasonable expectations of especially favorable treatment or automatic compliance with his or her expectations)
6. Is interpersonally exploitative (i.e., takes advantage of others to achieve his or her own ends)
7. Lacks empathy: is unwilling to recognize or identify with the feelings and needs of others
8. Is often envious of others or believes that others are envious of him or her
9. Shows arrogant, haughty behaviors or attitudes.

ANTISOCIAL PERSONALITY DISORDER

There is a pervasive pattern of disregard for and violation of the rights of others occurring since age 15 years, as indicated by three (or more) of the following:

1. Failure to conform to social norms with respect to lawful behaviors as indicated by repeatedly performing acts that are grounds for arrest
2. Deceitfulness, as indicated by repeated lying, use of aliases, or conning others for personal profit or pleasure
3. Impulsivity or failure to plan ahead
4. Irritability and aggressiveness, as indicated by repeated physical fights or assaults
5. Reckless disregard for safety of self or others
6. Consistent irresponsibility, as indicated by repeated failure to sustain consistent work behavior or honor financial obligations
7. Lack of remorse, as indicated by being indifferent to or rationalizing having hurt, mistreated, or stolen from another.

Source: Reprinted with permission from the American Psychiatric Association. (2000). *Diagnostic and statistical manual of mental disorders* (4th ed., Text Revision). Washington, DC: Author.

promiscuity, substance use, abnormal eating habits, shoplifting, and frequent job changes. "I just told my boss to take this job and shove it" may be the response to a work situation that is perceived as intolerable. "I just got another credit card with a $5,000 limit, so I don't have to worry about going over the limit on my other three cards." "I only drink wine when I'm driving, so I don't worry about DUIs." "I don't worry about AIDS; all my partners come from high-rent districts, so they are clean and safe." Responses such as "I don't know why I did it, I just did" are common when clients are questioned about the reasons for particular actions.

Intense Anger Clients with BPD tend to instigate problems as they become involved in therapeutic relationships. The anger may manifest itself in accusations, frequent displays of temper, inability to control anger (acting out), irritability, sarcasm, argumentativeness, devaluing others, and overreaction to minor irritants. Such behaviors usually sabotage their treatment.

These clients are unable to tolerate their own "bad" image and therefore project it onto others, often raging at the perceived attributes of the other. Anger tends to be greatest toward those people who remind them of a nurturing/frustrating parent.

Identity Diffusion Clients with BPD display behaviors that show confusion about values and goals in life. These clients are described as chameleon-like because they are constantly changing their behavior to match the behavior of those around them. An intense fear of rejection causes borderline individuals to say what they think others want to hear and to behave in a manner that they believe will win them popularity or special favors. It is difficult to determine what borderline individuals really think or feel. They cannot genuinely experience feelings and emotions; their core personality is hollow. They do not assume responsibility for their actions but project blame and credit onto others.

Unstable Interpersonal Relationships Clients relate stories of "one-night stands" in search of the perfect partner. Any real or perceived threat of abandonment results in the client's "switching" to another partner. "He's never there when I need him" may be used in conjunction with "I always see to it that his shirts are ironed and his dinner is ready when he gets home from work." These clients need a payback in return for any giving they do. The failure to resolve the separation–individuation process described by Mahler, Pine, and Bergman (1975) in their classic work is reflected in the person's attitudes toward self and others.

Unstable interpersonal relationships may include such behaviors as the following:

- Manipulation of others
- Pitting individuals against one another
- Intense attachment
- Explosive separations
- Sudden shifts in attitude toward others perceived as good or bad
- Clinging, demanding
- Controlling, exploiting
- Sadism or masochism in close relationships
- Relationships motivated by a need to avoid being alone rather than a need to be with others
- Lack of empathy
- Diminished capacity to evaluate others realistically
- Transient, superficial relationships.

Problems of identity diffusion are also apparent in the areas of sexual intimacy and gender identity. Sexual intimacy is disturbed as a result of the person's fears of being either engulfed and destroyed or else abandoned by another. An approach–avoidance conflict emerges as a consequence of the parent or caretaker having thwarted independence and rewarded dependent behavior. As a result, the borderline client develops two major fears: the fear of abandonment, which leads to clinging behavior, and fear of engulfment, which leads to distancing from others. The client desperately wants intimate relationships but is terrified of losing the self. These fears are reminiscent of the early choice between parent's love and autonomy, which is the core of the borderline conflict.

This conflict is managed by using the primitive dissociation defense, also called **splitting**, which can best be described as the inability to integrate contradictory experiences. Splitting is based on dichotomous thinking, a cognitive distortion in which the person has an "all-or-none" mentality about others; people are viewed as either all "good" or all "bad."

Gender identity disturbance may be manifested by the selection of rejecting or abusive partners, the preference for homosexual relationships while maintaining a heterosexual lifestyle, and bizarre fantasies.

Another area of identity diffusion is temporal discontinuity, which is manifested by a searching for one's origins or keeping detailed chronologic journals. Borderline individuals seem unable to integrate past, present, and future into a continuum. They may frantically plan for the future while reminiscing about past events. These behaviors often lead to difficulty in choosing long-term goals, making career choices, and reassessing personal values. "I can't make up my mind if I should stay in nursing or try interior design" (after completing 1 year in a 2-year nursing program).

Affective Instability The failure to resolve the issues described previously is also related to the inability of the person with BPD to maintain a consistent, satisfying, affective state. Characteristics of this disorder include intense fluctuations of mood, normally of short duration (a few hours or a few days); intense, discrete episodes of depression with accompanying suicidal ideation and gestures; and hypomanic or elated episodes. "Of course I knew I wouldn't kill myself when I took those pills—do you think I'm stupid or something?" "I only told him [partner] I was HIV positive to see if he really cared for me as much as he said."

Feelings of Emptiness and Aloneness Individuals with borderline personality disorder report hollow, empty feelings, lack of peaceful solitude, a sense of being disconnected, and anhedonia (absence of pleasure in performing ordinarily pleasurable acts). The person may attempt to combat these feelings by compulsive eating, drinking, drug abuse, sexual encounters, and self-mutilation. "I get depressed and I think about taking some pills, but then my boyfriend calls and we'll go out and I won't be depressed anymore," or, "I feel so totally empty inside. I burned my wrist with the cigarette just to see if I could still feel."

Self-Damaging Acts Impulsiveness, together with identity disturbances, often leads to self-destructive behaviors. People with BPD are often depressed, but they may make self-destructive gestures in an attempt to affirm their reality and relieve tension rather than to express a wish to die. Self-damaging behaviors include self-mutilation (cigarette burns, cutting, taking drug overdoses), recurrent accidents, and physical fights. Individuals who engage in self-mutilating behaviors often experience boundary disturbances and lack insight. "I don't see what's the big deal, so I tried to cut my wrists a couple of times—doesn't everybody?" "Yeah, I vomit after I eat; it keeps my weight down and I still get to have all the desserts I want."

Distortions of Reality When identity diffusion reaches panic proportions, the borderline individual may experience both depersonalization and derealization.

HISTRIONIC PERSONALITY DISORDER People with **histrionic personality disorder (HPD)** show a lifelong tendency for dramatic, egocentric, attention-seeking response patterns. Their seeming lack of sincerity and emotional commitment contributes to disturbances in interpersonal relationships. These people appear to be continually "on stage" and acting out a role. Their coping patterns are based on repression, denial, and dissociation.

As with other personality disorders, it is important to consider the client's cultural and ethnic background before assuming that the diagnosis of HPD is correct because norms for interpersonal behavior, dress and appearance, and emotional expression vary widely among cultures, genders (sex-role stereotyping), and age groups. Approximately 3% of the general population are diagnosed with this disorder. More females than males are diagnosed with this condition (APA, 2000).

Dramatic, Exhibitionistic, and Egocentric Responses The behaviors of individuals with HPD are characterized by exaggerated emotional expression. They demonstrate an excessive craving for attention, activity, and excitement. Often, these individuals behave frivolously, acting silly and making nuisances of themselves.

When confronted with minor stressors, the individual with HPD overreacts with irrational emotional outbursts and temper tantrums.

Dysfunctional Interpersonal Relationships People with HPD constantly need love, reassurance, and validation of their existence because of their feelings of dependence and helplessness. For this reason, they have problems with significant relationships. They are likely to manipulate others in order to hold on to them while at the same time being highly inconsiderate and lacking empathy.

Impaired Sexual Expression People with HPD are generally provocative and seductive and use sexual expression to manipulate and control others in relationships. Clients are often unaware of this flamboyance and how others perceive it. They are often competitive with those of the same sex and seductive with members of the opposite sex. A potential problem is promiscuous sexual activity and the risk of developing and spreading sexually transmitted diseases. Disregard for the welfare and safety of others may be noted in sexual acting-out, including intimate relationships with other clients in the healthcare facility, if the client is hospitalized. When confronted, the client may say, "I've been talking to the social worker about the need for conjugal visits; maybe now you'll understand how important it is for us to get sex as well as therapy."

Dysphoric Mood Clients may express dysphoria as a sense of disquiet or restlessness. Histrionic clients may experience dysphoria when their demands for attention and affection are not met. They may act out in a suicidal fashion to manipulate or coerce others.

Cognitive Alterations Clients with HPD are much more interested in creative or imaginative pursuits than in analytic or academic achievements. They tend to be impressionable and highly suggestible and tend to look to authority figures for magical solutions to problems.

Impaired Health Patterns Regression and the development of somatic and/or dissociative symptoms are frequent among histrionic people. These disabling symptoms may serve the purpose of calling attention to themselves. Generally, the symptoms occur when an audience is present or when an unpleasant situation is anticipated. Substance use, depression, seizure-like activity, blackouts, falling, dizziness, or reactive psychoses may lead to hospitalization.

NARCISSISTIC PERSONALITY DISORDER People with **narcissistic personality disorder (NPD)** engage in a pattern of grandiosity, have difficulty regulating self-esteem, and need admiration and attention from others. Their self-evaluation is dependent on admiration and devotion from others. The constant desire to be the center of attention is based on a strong sense of entitlement; narcissistic people feel they deserve to be treated in a special manner. When their need for constant attention is not met, the narcissistic person feels rejected and may retaliate through acting-out behavior. Characteristics most frequently observed include a sense of entitlement, lack of empathy, indifference toward others, and interpersonal manipulation.

About 1% of the general population has NPD, and the incidence is increasing steadily. Of those diagnosed, 50–75% are male (APA, 2000). There may be a higher than usual risk in children of narcissistic parents who impart to them an unrealistic sense of omnipotence, grandiosity, beauty, and talent (Sadock & Sadock, 2005). While narcissistic traits are quite common (and developmentally appropriate) in adolescents, the majority of teens who exhibit narcissism do not necessarily develop NPD as adults (APA, 2000).

Grandiosity Grandiosity is evidenced by expressions of exaggerated self-importance, self-absorption, and egocentricity. This inflated self-concept may be a compensation for feelings of diminished self-worth. Isolating a child from the feedback of others and the parents' failing to mirror the child's behavior may contribute to the development of grandiosity. Mirroring, or mirror images, reflect what the parents think of and how they treat the child. When coming in contact with people outside the home, the child may discover a discrepancy between treatment from others and the mirror images developed at home. Excessive boasting may result from the inconsistency in self-concept.

Exhibitionism Exhibitionistic behavior is demonstrated by the constant seeking of support and admiration from others. Because of their limited interests, these clients boast about themselves to the point of boring others. Concern over declining physical attractiveness and occupational limitations may lead them to seek cosmetic surgery.

Labile Affective Respons Despite the narcissistic individual's extensive use of rationalization for failures, there is an underlying sense of rage, shame, and diminished self-esteem. The perceptive nurse may observe cool indifference, emptiness, humiliation, uncontrolled anger, or desire for revenge. The following clinical example illustrates this lack of empathy.

Dysfunctional Interpersonal Relationships Clients with NPD feel entitled to special favors and attention. Further, they refuse to assume mutual responsibilities in relationships and tend to exploit and disregard the rights of others. They lack empathy, especially toward those whom they perceive to be of lower status.

In his classic work on narcissism that remains the standard for understanding this disorder, Kernberg (1975) emphasizes that chronic, intense envy and defenses against envy lead to idealization or devaluation of others. Responses to others may include lack of concern, mistrust, lack of intimacy, accusations of incompetence, and demand for unattainable perfection. Clients with NPD see interpersonal relationships as a means of enhancing their own self-esteem. A narcissistic person often selects a spouse or partner who will be dutiful and subservient in return for assurances of security and faithfulness. More recently, Kernberg has identified what he calls the "almost untreatable" narcissistic client (Kernberg, 2007). This is a client who combines the characteristics of NPD and BPD, and possibly antisocial personality disorder as well, representing the most severe cases of pathological narcissism.

Impaired Sexual Expression Perverse sexual fantasies and promiscuity may be associated with NPD. There may be confusion regarding sex-role behavior. Sexual favors may be used as bartering tools with partners.

ANTISOCIAL PERSONALITY DISORDER **Antisocial personality disorder (ASPD)**, a pattern of disregard for and violation of the rights of others, was one of the earliest personality disorders to be identified. It has been labeled *psychopathy*, *sociopathy*, *dyssocial disorder*, and *moral insanity*. Most people with ASPD do not seek medical help but often come to the attention of authorities because of criminal activity that leads to judicial commitment to psychiatric facilities or incarceration in correctional facilities. In clinical settings, 3–30% of the population may have this disorder. Higher prevalence rates are found in substance abuse treatment centers and forensic settings (APA, 2000).

Manipulation, which is a hallmark of the antisocial client's behavior, can be a normal, nondestructive mode of meeting one's needs. However, when used to control others, manipulation interferes with interpersonal relationships. In antisocial clients, the drive to manipulate others is paramount, because these clients feel a need to be "number one" at all times. Manipulation may be evident in the client's attempt to form alliances with the staff at the mental health or forensic facility.

In making contact with antisocial people, the nurse may find them initially charming. They are often intellectually bright, conversationally glib, and they tell you what you want to hear. Because they are so astute in identifying others' vulnerabilities, nurses are frequently amazed at the "empathy" they show for others. These behaviors are manipulative and are used to create a situation that the person with ASPD can control.

During the initial assessment interview, it is common for the person diagnosed with ASPD to refuse responsibility for admission to the mental health or forensic facility. In fact, this individual will probably claim that the victim of his or her actions is at fault and fail to show any remorse.

Antisocial clients exhibit impulsiveness by making quick decisions without regard for the consequences. "I'm going to leave the facility for a little while right now; it doesn't matter if you discharge me AMA [against medical advice]." The client may exhibit agression by fighting with other clients, particularly when the client feels a need for excitement or has not received sufficient attention from the staff. The client's explanation might be, "Hey, if you guys would get more sports going for us here, we wouldn't be getting on each other's nerves so much."

Lack of anxiety is notable with antisocial individuals, unless there is extreme external stress, in which case they may act out in ways that put them at high risk for accidents, physical injury, or suicidal acts. History of violence toward others is very common, including sex offenses (i.e., rape, child pornography, child molestation) and murder. These clients often have histories of drug dealing and substance abuse, prostitution, homelessness, erratic job histories, and exploitive sexual relationships. While these individuals can identify what is correct and appropriate behavior, they do not believe the rules apply to them.

People with ASPD need immediate gratification in most situations but can delay rewards to the extent that they need planning time to achieve what they want. They are often admitted to mental health facilities for depressive symptoms, suicidal attempts, substance abuse, somatic disorders, and/or anxiety disorders.

Cluster C Personality Disorders: Anxious–Fearful

According to the *DSM-IV-TR*, personality-disordered individuals who are primarily anxious or fearful may be diagnosed with avoidant, dependent, or obsessive–compulsive personality disorder. Anxious–fearful people generally experience both social and occupational impairments as a result of their restricted affect, nonassertiveness, problems expressing feelings, unrealistic expectations of others, and impaired decision making and problem solving. The lifestyle of the anxious–fearful person is characterized by intense emotional repression and behaviors that are socially isolating and self-defeating. The behaviors of anxious–fearful personalities tend to overlap, and common diagnostic features are described in Box 24–10.

PRACTICE ALERT

It is often difficult for nurses to relate to these clients because of the clients' poor social skills. To work with clients with personality disorders, nurses must understand themselves first. Nurses must have the insight to know what type of behavior is stressful to them so they can manage their own stress without giving it back to the client. Direct communication with clear expectations for client behavior and clear and consistent limits is important for these clients.

AVOIDANT PERSONALITY DISORDER The essential feature of people with **avoidant personality disorder (APD)** is a pattern of social withdrawal along with a sense of inadequacy, fear, and hypersensitivity to potential rejection or shame. These people withdraw socially even though they deeply desire affection and acceptance. Their avoidant behavior results in visiting public places (movies, museums, and ballparks) simply to experience the presence of other people because they do not enjoy being alone. When in public places, however, they maintain a safe distance from others. For example, in a movie theater, one can be physically close to people without feeling that one's personal space is being invaded.

Avoidant people devalue their own achievements. They appear overly serious, humorless, and painfully shy. Speech is often slow, and they do not readily express their feelings. Thought content is generally serious.

Box 24–10 *DSM-IV-TR:* Diagnostic Criteria for Personality Disorders: Cluster C (Fearful–Anxious)

AVOIDANT PERSONALITY DISORDER

A pervasive pattern of social inhibition, feelings of inadequacy, and hypersensitivity to negative evaluation, beginning by early adulthood and present in a variety of contexts, as indicated by four (or more) of the following:

1. Avoids occupational activities that involve significant interpersonal contact, because of fears of criticism, disapproval, or rejection
2. Is unwilling to get involved with people unless certain of being liked
3. Shows restraint within intimate relationships because of the fear of being shamed or ridiculed
4. Is preoccupied with being criticized or rejected in social situations

Note: Do not include suicidal or self-mutilating behavior covered in Criterion 5.

5. Is inhibited in new interpersonal situations because of feelings of inadequacy
6. Views self as socially inept, personally unappealing, or inferior to others
7. Is unusually reluctant to take personal risks or to engage in any new activities because they may prove embarrassing.

DEPENDENT PERSONALITY DISORDER

A pervasive and excessive need to be taken care of that leads to submissive and clinging behavior and fears of separation, beginning by early adulthood and present in a variety of contexts, as indicated by five (or more) of the following:

1. Has difficulty making everyday decisions without an excessive amount of advice and reassurance from others
2. Needs others to assume responsibility for most major areas of his or her life
3. Has difficulty expressing disagreement with others because of fear of loss of support or approval

Note: Do not include realistic fears of retribution.

4. Has difficulty initiating projects or doing things on his or her own (because of a lack of self-confidence in judgment or abilities rather than a lack of motivation or energy)
5. Goes to excessive lengths to obtain nurturance and support from others, to the point of volunteering to do things that are unpleasant
6. Feels uncomfortable or helpless when alone because of exaggerated fears of being unable to care for himself or herself
7. Urgently seeks another relationship as a source of care and support when a close relationship ends
8. Is unrealistically preoccupied with fears of being left to take care of himself or herself.

OBSESSIVE–COMPULSIVE PERSONALITY DISORDER

A pervasive pattern of preoccupation with orderliness, perfectionism, and mental and interpersonal control—at the expense of flexibility, openness, and efficiency—beginning by early adulthood and present in a variety of contexts, as indicated by four (or more) of the following:

1. Is preoccupied with details, rules, lists, order, organization, or schedules to the extent that the major point of the activity is lost
2. Shows perfectionism that interferes with task completion (e.g., is unable to complete a project because his or her own overly strict standards are not met)
3. Is excessively devoted to work and productivity to the exclusion of leisure activities and friendships (not accounted for by obvious economic necessity)
4. Is overconscientious, scrupulous, and inflexible about matters of morality, ethics, or values (not accounted for by cultural or religious identification)
5. Is unable to discard worn-out or worthless objects even when they have no sentimental value
6. Is reluctant to delegate tasks or to work with others unless they submit to exactly his or her way of doing things
7. Adopts a miserly spending style toward both self and others; money is viewed as something to be hoarded for future catastrophes
8. Shows rigidity and stubbornness.

Source: Reprinted with permission from the American Psychiatric Association. (2000). *Diagnostic and statistical manual of mental disorders* (4th ed., Text Revision). Washington, DC: Author.

DEPENDENT PERSONALITY DISORDER The essential features of **dependent personality disorder (DPD)** include a pervasive, excessive, and unrealistic need to be cared for; fear of separation; lack of self-confidence; an inability to make decisions; and an inability to function independently. In sharp contrast to the avoidant person, dependent people cling to others and passively accept their dictates and leadership. Dependent people view themselves as "helpless" or "stupid" and seek out dominant others to rely on for guidance, control, and support as well as for "permission" to behave. These individuals have difficulty initiating projects and function adequately only when assured of approval and supervision.

In dependent people, the normal symbiotic parent–child relationship has been excessively prolonged, impairing their capacity for thinking, feeling, and responding on their own. They believe they must be taken care of and consequently rely on others to mirror their feelings to them.

Dependent people subordinate their desires and needs to the wishes of others in order to maintain relationships. They often appear friendly, helpful, and indispensable. Indeed, they will volunteer for unpleasant tasks if they think they will be reciprocated with nurturing. When the dominant other is unavailable, or perceived as unavailable, dependent people experience intense anxiety. This may lead to feelings of unhappiness, anger, resentment, or depression. It is also noteworthy that significant others may eventually respond to dependent people with anger and resentment because of their continuous clinging and ingratiating behaviors.

OBSESSIVE–COMPULSIVE PERSONALITY DISORDER People with **obsessive–compulsive personality disorder (OCPD)** demonstrate fear and anxiety concerning loss of control over situations, objects, or people. They demonstrate perfectionism, preoccupation with details, and hoarding behavior. The person with OCPD strives at all times to keep the world predictable and organized. The major features of this disorder are an excessive need for order, extreme dedication to work and productivity, and perfectionism to the exclusion of feelings and pleasure. A person with OCPD may be likened to a drill sergeant in the military who is rigid, serious, detail-oriented, and stingy with emotions.

People with OCPD tend to focus on trivial details. Although they may be highly praised for their organizational skills and work ethic, eventually their rigidity causes them to fear making mistakes. Because they repeatedly check their work, they are not good time managers; thus, projects may not get completed. They are self-critical and adhere strictly and concretely to rules. Consequently, they postpone making decisions. They tend to resent authority but rarely express this resentment openly. Instead, they may engage in passive–aggressive behavior, such as procrastination and stubbornness.

People who are excessively conscientious and rigid often exhibit a contradictory pattern of slovenliness, which is also compulsive. Thus, a compulsive housewife may scrub her kitchen floor daily but allow bags of garbage to accumulate and become infested. When clients with OCPD describe their lifestyle, the nurse will quickly become aware of their rigidity, concreteness, and need for order and perfection.

People with OCPD are also keenly aware of other people's expectations; of the threat of possible criticism; of the weight and direction of authority; of rules, regulations, and conventions; and of a great collection of moral principles. They feel required to fulfill unending duties, responsibilities, and tasks. Obsessive–compulsive people do not view taking work home and working long hours as an imposition, since work organizes their lives and binds their anxiety. Indeed, they will manage to make work out of pleasurable activities.

COLLABORATION

Treatment of clients with personality disorders can be challenging, often requiring significant collaboration among health care professionals, the client, and family members. The nurse performs a variety of roles in such a collaboration, including tracking and following up on information and referrals, client teaching, and even acting as "cheerleader" by providing positive reinforcement to clients and families as they successfully begin to change behaviors. The priority of care is the safety of the client and others. Beyond that, helping the client develop adaptive behaviors and social skills are key components of treating any personality disorder.

Pharmacologic Therapies

Currently no medications exist to treat personality disorders. Antidepressants and antipsychotics may be used to target specific symptoms or to treat comorbid Axis I disorders. Medications should be viewed as a means of controlling symptoms that are disabling. The overall treatment plan includes individual, group, family, and behavioral therapy, with long-term therapy seen as being the most effective treatment.

Cognitive-Behavioral Therapy

Cognitive-behavioral therapy (CBT) can help clients learn to reframe negative thinking patterns and learn adaptive coping mechanisms and relaxation techniques. CBT provides a supportive setting in which a client can role-play adaptive behaviors and talk through the consequences of maladaptive behaviors.

DIALECTICAL BEHAVIOR THERAPY *Dialectical behavior therapy* is a cognitive and behavioral therapy used specifically for borderline personality disorder. Dialectical behavior therapy (DBT) has been shown to decrease suicidal behavior, hospitalization, and treatment dropout while improving interpersonal functioning and anger management. DBT theory begins with a validating treatment environment. Treatment focuses on client education and prioritizing treatment goals. Treatment techniques include behavior analysis, skills training and coaching, and management of responses to behavior (Swenson, Sanderson, Dulit, & Linehan, 2001).

Alternative Therapies

There are no specific alternative therapies for individuals with personality disorders. Those who experience anxiety may find chamomile tea to be helpful. Yoga and meditation may also decrease levels of anxiety. People who have a concomitant

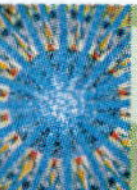

ALTERNATIVE THERAPIES **Relaxation Techniques**

Throughout the day the client may find hundreds of opportunities to integrate some deep breathing, relaxation, self-massage, and gentle movement techniques into usual activities. Teach some of these techniques to the client:

- You are sitting at a stoplight. Take a deep breath.
- You are just about to fall asleep or have just awakened. Breathe deeply and allow your whole body to become completely relaxed.
- You are in the shower washing your hair. As you apply shampoo, massage your scalp vigorously; rub your ears, relax, and take several deep breaths.
- As you apply lotion or oil to your body following your bath, do so with the intent of relaxing each muscle group as you gently massage your entire body.
- You are watching television. During each commercial break, massage your hands, feet, and ears. Breathe deeply and relax.
- You are vacuuming the house. Relax your shoulders, breathe deeply, and coordinate your movements with your breathing.

Source: Adapted from Jahnke, R. (1997). *The healer within*. San Francisco: Harper San Francisco.

mild or moderate depression may find St. John's wort or SAMe helpful. Vitamin B_{12} is necessary for the production of dopamine and serotonin, which may be lowered in depressive states. Omega-3 fatty acids are helpful in decreasing depression, which may be comorbid with the personality disorders.

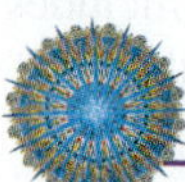

NURSING PROCESS

Although the symptomatology of clients with personality disorders varies, the commonalities allow nurses and other professionals to identify treatment priorities. Priorities of care for clients with personality disorders are as follows:

- Safety
- Managing crises
- Setting limits
- Improving socialization.

Nurses working with clients with personality disorders should remember that some of the symptoms (e.g., labile affect and impairments in social skills) make it difficult to develop the nurse–client relationship, especially when the client denies the presence of symptoms or problems.

Assessment

As with other psychiatric disorders, data collection serves as the starting point for the nursing process for clients with personality disorders. The main obstacle to assessment is the probability that the client will not perceive that a problem exists. If possible, interview family members for their perceptions of the problem. Exercise professional judgment in seeking information from others about their relationships with the client. Although the objective is to obtain a description of the client's functioning within various family and social contexts, the nurse must be certain that the client's rights are protected. By remaining alert to the potential for a breach of confidentiality, the nurse can ensure that neither the legal nor the ethical limits of the professional domain are exceeded. Table 24–8 provides examples of how thoughts, behavior, and feelings relate to one another in the various personality disorders.

Nursing History

Assess work history; history of behavior problems, including violence directed at self or others; history of suicidal ideation; methods of resolving conflicts; alcohol and drug use; and nature of relationships with family members, coworkers, and friends. Ask questions that encourage the client to describe aspects of self:

- When was the last time you were upset? What upset you? How did you handle it?
- How do others describe you?
- How would you describe yourself?
- What do you like about yourself? What would you like to change?
- How do you usually relate to others?

Physical Examination: Assess for signs of self-directed violence, such as cutting (Figure 24–5 ■); assess for evidence of alcohol or drug use.

Diagnosis

A number of nursing diagnoses may be appropriate for the client with a personality disorder. In synthesizing the assessment data, consider how well the client functions in daily life, the stability of the client's affect, how the client gets along with others, and what the client's skills and talents are (North American Nursing Diagnosis Association, 2007). Some appropriate nursing diagnoses include the following:

- Risk for Violence, Self-directed, related to poor impulse control
- Self-mutilation related to poor impulse control
- Ineffective Coping related to intense, labile affect
- Anxiety related to fear of rejection, fear of separation, fear of embarrassment
- Deficient Knowledge related to diagnosis, outcomes, commitment to treatment

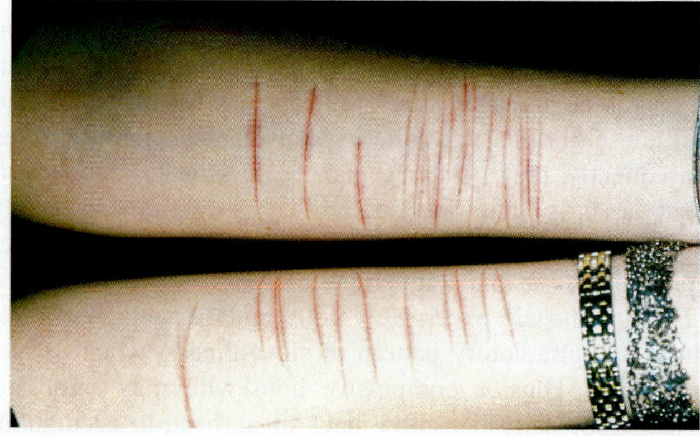

Figure 24–5 ■ Some people with borderline personality disorders engage in recurrent suicidal gestures or self-mutilating behavior.

TABLE 24–8 **Characteristics Related to Types of Disorders**

Behavioral Characteristics	
Impulsive	ASPD—difficulty delaying gratification; criminal behavior
	BPD—behavior unpredictable; self-destructive
Rigid	OCPD—perfectionism interferes with task completion
	AVPD—doesn't want to be embarrassed by trying new activities
Affective Characteristics	
Intense, unstable, inappropriate affect	BPD—affect instability; difficulty moderating strong feelings
	HPD—rapidly shifting and shallow expression of emotions; overly dramatic
	ASPD—irritable, aggressive
	PPD—quick expression of anger; bears grudges; pathological jealousy
Restricted, flat affect	SZPD—cold and detached
	STPD—inappropriate or constricted
	OCPD—unable to express emotions; fearful
	AVPD—fearful; shy
Cognitive Characteristics	
Hostile, paranoid world view	STPD, BPD—transient paranoid ideation
	PPD—hyperalert to danger; secretive
Negative sense of self	NPD—envious of others or believes others are envious of them
	AVPD—views self as socially inept or inferior
	DPD—can't do things on own; lack of self-confidence in judgment or abilities
Lack of sense of self	BPD—unstable self-image or sense of self
Exaggerated sense of self	HPD—needs to be the center of attention
	NPD—grandiose sense of self-importance
	ASPD—egocentric and grandiose
Peculiar thought processes	Odd beliefs, magical thinking
	Poverty of thoughts (schizoid)
Social Characteristics	
Overly close relationships	BPD—unstable and intense; alternate between idealization and devaluation
	HPD—considers relationships to be more intimate than they actually are
	DPD—goes to excessive lengths to obtain nurturance and support from others
Distant/avoidant relationships	OCPD—excessively devoted to work to exclusion of friendships; unable to compromise
	PPD—argumentative; fear information and relationships will be used against them
	SZPD—doesn't want relationships
	STPD—only maintains contact with family
	AVPD—fears criticism, disapproval, or rejection from others
Lack of concern for other's needs	ASPD—indifferent to others' feelings; no remorse for hurting others
	NPD—unreasonable expectations of others; exploits others

Sources: Geiger, T. C., & Crick, N. R. (2001). A developmental psychopathology perspective on vulnerability to personality disorders. In R. E. Ingram & J. M. Price (Eds.), *Vulnerability to psychopathology* (pp. 57–102). New York: Guilford Press; Livesley, W. J. (2001). Conceptual and taxonomic issues. In W. J. Livesley (Ed.), *Handbook of personality disorders* (pp. 3–38). New York: Guilford Press; and Paris, J. (1999). *Nature and nurture in psychiatry*. Washington, DC: American Psychiatric Press.

PPD, paranoid; SZPD, schizoid; STPD, schizotypal; ASPD, antisocial; BPD, borderline; HPD, histrionic; NPD, narcissistic; AVPD, avoidant; DPD, dependent; OCPD, obsessive–compulsive

- Social Isolation related to inability to trust, odd behavior, fear of relationships
- Impaired Social Interaction related to manipulation, egocentricity, quick anger
- Ineffective Role Performance related to inappropriate affect, manipulation, inflexibility, highly dependent
- Disturbed Personal Identity related to vague self-descriptions, grandiosity, deprecation
- Interrupted Family Processes related to extreme dependency, fear of abandonment, exploitation of family members.

Plan

Client goals are specific behavioral prescriptions that the nurse, the client, and significant others identify as realistic and attainable. Be aware that many of these clients have a tendency

FOCUS ON DIVERSITY AND CULTURE

Personality Disorders Around the World

Personality disorders can be diagnosed in clinical populations all over the world. Social expectations of any given culture encourage some kinds of behavior and suppress others. Thus, if culture has some influence in shaping personality, these disorders should have different prevalence rates. For example, antisocial personality disorder is rapidly increasing in North America and has very low rates in certain East Asian societies such as Taiwan. It is thought that North American families increase risk factors by failing to discipline their children effectively. In contrast, the Taiwanese have a strong belief in discipline and suppress most of the impulsive behaviors in children and adolescents (Paris, 2001).

to set broad, vague goals, such as "feel better," and may need assistance in being specific. The following are examples of appropriate goals:

- The client will refrain from violent behaviors.
- The client will use the problem-solving process.
- The client will interact socially with others.
- The client will verbalize decreased anxiety.

Implementation

Individuals with personality disorders do not respond to therapy very easily and treatment tends to be prolonged—years rather than months. Building a therapeutic relationship is critically important to any success. When clients are in acute distress they are more motivated to attempt changes. In the chronic phase, it is often very difficult for them to envision anything changing. The nurse's role is to provide support, respect, empathy, and validation. Over the course of time, ideally you become a role model for the client (Perseius, Ekdahl, Asberg, & Samuelsson, 2005).

Approach clients with *Cluster A* personality disorders in a gentle, interested, and nonintrusive manner that is respectful of the client's need for distance, privacy, and respites from interpersonal interactions. Demands for trust or self-disclosure may heighten anxiety and even precipitate a transient psychotic state. Nurses must understand that clients' social withdrawal and lack of feeling or responses are self-protective rather than unappreciative. Nurses should demonstrate their trustworthiness through their actions. Nurses should only make offers that they are willing and able to follow through on. Try to be clear and consistent.

Clients with *Cluster B* personality disorders require much more patience and structure from nurses. The approach must be one of consistency and limit setting. It is critically important that staff members keep open and clear lines of communication with one another. Nurses working with these clients must know how to deal with problems of anger and dishonesty. Since some clients alternate between criticism and flattery, nurses should avoid personalizing clients' behavior.

Clients with *Cluster C* diagnoses will find it helpful when the nurse points out their avoidance behavior and secondary gains. Assertiveness training helps these clients manage their dependency and anger. Anxiety may lessen when they learn to modify their perfectionistic standards.

Three fundamental beliefs should guide the nurse's approach in working with persons experiencing personality disorders. The first is *self-determination*. Clients are partners in treatment and have the right to choose their own course in life. Second, the focus is on *role functioning* while recognizing that not all symptoms will disappear. Third is *maintaining hope*. These clients are particularly susceptible to loss of hope for change and giving up on treatment.

Maintaining Boundaries

The boundaries between people are those edges that maintain a clear distinction between individuals. In terms of the nurse–client relationship, clear boundaries are designed to create an atmosphere of safety and predictability within which the nursing process can be implemented. Individuals experiencing identity confusion may be unclear about the norms of social and professional interaction. Teach them about physical, social, emotional, and sexual boundaries. Help them understand when they inadvertently or purposefully cross those boundaries.

Some individuals cannot separate their own experiences from those of others. Their self-image changes according to the reactions of others. Talk about how they adopt other's thoughts and feelings as their own. Teach them that when someone makes a personal comment to them, they have a choice of what they do with this comment. Ask them to imagine the comment as a brick. They can choose to accept the brick and build it into their wall of self-image. Alternatively, they can set the brick down, they can give it back, or they can throw it away. Point out the choices they have, for example, if someone says, "You are an ugly person." They can take that opinion and build it into their self-image and believe that they indeed are ugly. They can simply ignore the comment or tell themselves that the person must have a hidden agenda to say such a mean thing. Or, alternatively, they can give the "brick" back by saying, "I'm sorry you see me that way. I don't believe I am ugly."

Help clients establish and maintain their own boundaries. Begin with simply asking them to list their likes and preferences. Move on to goals they would like to achieve and decisions they need to make. Role-play situations in which their boundaries may be violated and how they may respond to this situation.

Teaching

Individuals with personality disorders are often puzzled by their problems and their inability to manage their lives. Telling clients the diagnosis is essential to establishing a relationship and validating their sense that their suffering is real. Many are relieved to learn that they have an identifiable disorder and that there is hope for change. It is helpful to teach them the nature and origin of personality and personality difficulties. Explore the way in which past events influence the way they think about themselves and others. Connect their patterns of thinking to their mood and emotions. Provide information on the treatment process including goal setting, commitment to change, and evaluation. Explain that changes occur slowly and the process will take time.

Modifying Cognitive Distortions

Clients with personality disorders have a number of cognitive distortions such as dichotomous thinking, overgeneralization, magnification, and suspiciousness. Help clients understand how these cognitive distortions relate to behavioral and social problems. Do not try to talk them out of their beliefs but rather suggest that each thought is just one of a number of possibilities. For clients who believe that others are especially looking at them, assign them to go to a shopping mall and sit and watch people. Ask them to analyze when individuals look at others and under what conditions. This exercise may help them recognize that they are not the focus of other people's attention (McLean & McLean, 2004). Box 24–11 contains some helpful statements for correcting the distorted thoughts of clients with personality disorders.

NURSING CARE PLAN A Client With Borderline Personality Disorder

Brenda Bacon is a 23-year-old Bulgarian American female client admitted to the short-stay unit for multiple lacerations she received when she ran through a glass door. She seems to be a very passionate person who expresses her concerns loudly and with emotion. She told the admitting nurse that she ran through the door because her boyfriend was planning to leave her and she could not stand it. The client was seeing a psychiatrist and a therapist regularly for borderline personality disorder but stopped treatment because "It wasn't helping."

ASSESSMENT	DIAGNOSES	PLANNING
Brenda's lacerations on her head, shoulders, and right knee are sutured and the dressings are clean and dry. On admission the chart says that she was loud and emotional. Now she is quiet and expressing remorse for her impulsive behavior. She states that she is worthless and that her boyfriend is too good to deserve such a terrible person. She is right-handed and has multiple healed laceration scars on her left arm. When the nurse asked about them, Brenda stated, "Sometimes I have to cut myself to know that I'm alive. Sometimes I do it to stop the stress." When it was time for the nurse's shift to end, Brenda cried and begged the nurse not to leave her like everyone else has.	■ Risk for Self-Directed Violence ■ Ineffective Coping ■ Impaired Skin Integrity	■ The client will not harm herself. ■ The client will notify the nurse when she feels stressed or feels like cutting herself. ■ The client will verbalize her feelings to the nurse. ■ The client will verbalize adaptive coping mechanisms that she could use instead of hurting herself. ■ The client will keep lacerations clean and dry.

IMPLEMENTATION

- Assign consistent staff to the client and provide consistent expectations for behavior.
- Show the client how to contact the nurse.
- Teach the client to call the nurse when she is stressed, so that she can share her feelings with the nurse and the nurse can teach her adaptive coping mechanisms to use.
- Actively listen to the client's concerns.
- Help the client list adaptive coping mechanisms when she is feeling anxious or stressed.
- Teach basic wound care.

EVALUATION

Brenda was hospitalized for 2 days. During that time she had several angry outbursts at staff members when she perceived that her needs were not being met. She had long discussions with the nurse about her feelings and abuse history. She did not injure herself while she was in the hospital. Her boyfriend decided to stay with her, because she needs him so badly. Her lacerations healed well.

CRITICAL THINKING

1. What other interventions might be appropriate for Brenda?
2. The nurse believes that Brenda should return to therapy for her personality disorder. What can the nurse do to ensure that this happens?
3. When Brenda said, "You won't give me more medication! I hate you! Give me another nurse!" What response from the nurse is best for Brenda?

Box 24–11 Corrective Statements for Distorted Thoughts

Thought Distortion: "This is the worst thing that has ever happened."
Corrective Statement: "True, this is a bad thing, but it is not the worst thing that ever happened." (*Giving perspective allows the client to see the real placement of this stressful event as it relates to life priorities.*)

Thought Distortion: "I could NEVER do anything like you are suggesting."
Corrective Statement: "You have already done things like this before, such as…" (*Giving examples makes the implied generalization specific.*)

Thought Distortion: "If only I hadn't made him mad, he wouldn't have beat me up."
Corrective Statement: "He is an adult and responsible for his own behavior. You are responsible for your own behavior, not his." (*Stating the mature reality of the situation helps the client see it from another point of view.*)

Thought Distortion: "My boyfriend left me. This will kill me. I can't go on."
Corrective Statement: "You have survived disappointments before. You are strong enough to handle this. Let's talk about how you feel." (*Allowing the client to discuss and examine feelings increases insight and promotes the ability to learn from past experiences and to apply current learning to future situations.*)

Thought Distortion: "Nobody understands me."
Corrective Statement: "Let's talk about how you feel, so I can understand." (*Suggesting a problem-solving approach promotes adaptive coping.*)

As specific cognitive distortions are identified, ask clients to write these in a journal along with evidence against the thought. The client's thought may be that "People want to tease me and bully me." Evidence against that thought might be, "This happened when I was young but has not happened recently" or "These people do not tease or bully other individuals, so why would they want to do that to me?" The journal writing will help clients develop a range of alternative interpretations for core beliefs.

Improving Family Communication

Personality disorders often have a negative impact on the family and friends surrounding the individual. It is important to include families in the treatment process. Families need information about the nature of the disorder, its course, and the available treatments. See Box 24–12 for topics to include in family education.

Teach friends and family members how to set limits with individuals who are manipulative. Family members tend to get drawn into dysfunctional interactions. Support them in setting limits and establishing consequences for manipulative behavior. Explain that they need to be consistent in what they will and will not tolerate. Teach friends and family how to set limits with individuals who are passive–aggressive. To avoid the "misunderstandings," the nurse should have the person repeat back the instructions given before the person sets out to perform the task. Family members and friends should never take it for granted that the person has understood. To deal with a person who procrastinates, they should set a precise, never vague, deadline and establish a penalty for delays. The same is true for latecomers—a clearly set consequence is established for late behavior. Family and friends must consistently enforce all consequences in order to lessen the passive–aggressive behavior. Teach families how to solve problems and negotiate conflict. When family conflict arises, ask all members to identify specific behavior that triggers the conflict and to tell one another how they felt as a result of the conflict. Discourage the use of "you" language since that assigns blame and leads to further arguing. An example of a "you" statement is "You drive me crazy by wanting me by your side all the time." Teach the use of "I" language, in which all individuals assume responsibility for themselves. An example of an "I" statement is "I feel overloaded with your requests that I be with you so much of the time." Encourage each person involved in the conflict to explain what specific behavior change he or she would like to see and would be willing to make. Throughout this process provide clear direction and coaching to reduce emotional overreaction. Teach *empathic listening* and *responding* since most people with personality disorders have difficulty with this. The person who is listening concentrates on the other person's statements and tries to understand what the speaker is saying. The listener then restates what the other person has said, ensuring that the communication was clear and understood. The roles are then reversed and the process begins again.

Box 24–12 Family Education

- Personality disorders are long-standing and inflexible patterns of relating to the world and other people.
- Affected people usually have little insight into their behavior.
- Their loved one is handicapped but not disabled.
- There are frequent comorbid conditions such as depression, anxiety disorders, psychotic episodes, and substance abuse.
- Life stresses make clients more vulnerable to relapse.
- Go slowly. Recovery takes time.
- Maintain family routines as much as possible.
- Do not ignore threats of self-harm.

Evaluation

To complete the nursing process, the nurse should evaluate clients' responses to nursing interventions based on the selected outcomes. Personality traits are almost always too ingrained for radical change through therapy. Because the problems associated with personality disorders have been with most clients for their entire lives, clients respond to intervention strategies very slowly. The nurse must help the client define small steps toward the achievement of therapeutic goals. The nurse can assist them most by helping them see how their behavior affects their lives so that they can learn to modify patterns enough to develop a more adaptive lifestyle.

Expected outcomes may include:

- Client identifies impact of behavior on their life and the lives of those close to them.
- Client voices interest in changing their patterns of behavior.
- Client attends regular therapy sessions.
- Client sets short term and long term goals.

REVIEW Personality Disorders

RELATE: LINK THE CONCEPTS

Linking the exemplar of Personality Disorders with the concept of Reproduction:

1. What nursing considerations would be appropriate for an expectant mother with narcissistic personality disorder?
2. What client teaching would be appropriate for this mother?

Linking the exemplar of Personality Disorder with the concept of Violence:

3. Which personality disorders carry the greatest risk for spousal or child abuse?
4. What is the priority of care for the client with a personality disorder who is abusing his or her spouse or child? What short- and long-term interventions would be appropriate?

REFER: GO TO MYNURSINGKIT

REFLECT: CASE STUDY

David is a 23-year-old Nigerian American male client admitted to the hospital for peritonitis following an appendectomy for a ruptured appendix. He sees a therapist weekly to work on his dependent personality disorder. The nurse asks David during the nursing admission history if he is going to school or working. He states that his mother wants him to attend Portland Community College to study computer technology. He has been an ideal client: he drinks, eats, and ambulates when he is told, even if he is not hungry or thirsty or has too much pain to want to ambulate. He is anxious when his mother leaves the hospital to buy some school clothes for him.

David will have a wound drain with a simple dressing change that must be done daily when he goes home. When the nurse wants to teach him how to do the dressing change, he says, "My mother will do it. Please wait to teach her. She'll be back in 15 minutes."

1. How can the nurse promote David's independence?
2. What other client teaching would be appropriate for David? For his mother?
3. What cultural beliefs or practices should the nurse consider?

PEARSON

EXPLORE mynursingkit™

MyNursingKit is your one stop for online chapter review materials and resources. Prepare for success with additional NCLEX®-style practice questions, interactive assignments and activities, web links, animations and videos, and more!

Register your access code from the front of your book at **www.mynursingkit.com**.

REFERENCES

American Psychiatric Association. (2000). *Diagnostic and statistical manual of mental disorders* (4th ed., Text Revision). Washington, DC: Author.

Appolinario, J. C., Bacaltchuk, J., Sichieri, R., Claudino, A. M., Godoy-Matos, A., Morgan, C., et al. (2003). A randomized, double-blind, placebo-controlled study of sibutramine in the treatment of binge-eating disorder. *Archives of General Psychiatry, 60*(11), 1109–1116.

Bacaltchuk, J., & Hay, P. (2003). Antidepressants versus placebo for people with bulimia nervosa. *Cochrane Database of Systematic Reviews* (4): CD003391.

Berge, M., & Ranney, M. (2005). Self esteem and stigma among persons with schizophrenia: Implications for mental health. *Journal of Long Term Home Health Care, 6,* 139–144.

Brambilla, P., Soloff, P. H., Sala, M., Nicoletti, M. A., Keshavan, M. S., & Soares, J. C. (2004). Anatomical MRI study of borderline personality disorder patients. *Psychiatry Research, 131*(2), 125–133.

Bruch, H. (1978). *The golden cage: The enigma of anorexia nervosa.* Cambridge, MA: Harvard University Press.

Bulik, C. M. (2005). Exploring the gene-environment nexus in eating disorders. *Journal of Psychiatry & Neuroscience, 30*(5), 335–339.

Burkhart, P. V., & Rayens, M. K. (2005). Self-concept and health locus of control: Factors related to children's adherence to recommended asthma regimen. *Pediatric Nursing, 31,* 404–409.

Chen, H., Cohen, P., Crawford, T. N., Kasen, S., Johnson, J. G., & Berenson, K. (2006). Relative impact of young adult personality disorders on subsequent quality of life. *Journal of Personality Disorders, 20*(5), 510–523.

de Bruijn, E. R., Grooten, K. P., Verkes, R. J., Buchholz, V., Hummelen, J. W., & Hulstijn, W. (2006). Neural correlates of impulsive responding in borderline personality disorder: EFP evidence for reduced action monitoring. *Journal of Psychiatric Research, 40,* 428–437.

De Clercq, B., & De Fruyt, F. (2007). Childhood antecedents of personality disorder. *Current Opinion in Psychiatry, 20*(1), 57–61.

Donnelly, G. (2004). Thinking about feeling: The value of introspection. *Holistic Nursing Practice, 18,* 275.

Erikson, E. H. (1963). *Childhood and society* (2nd ed.). New York: Norton.

Finfgeld, D. L. (2002). Anorexia nervosa: Analysis of long-term outcomes and clinical implications. *Archives of Psychiatric Nursing, 16*(4), 176–186.

Frank, G. K., Bailer, U. F., Henry, S. E., Drevets, W., Meltzer, C. C., Price, J. C., et al. (2005). Increased dopamine D2/D3 receptor binding after recovery from anorexia nervosa. *Biological Psychiatry, 58*(11), 908–12. Published ahead of print June 29, 2005.

Keel, P. K., Haedt, A., & Edler, C. (2005). Purging disorder. *International Journal of Eating Disorders, 38*(3), 191–199.

Kernberg, O. (1975). *Borderline conditions and pathological narcissism*. New York: Aronson.

Keshavan, M. S., Duggal, H. S., Veeragandham, G., McLaughlin, N. M., Montrose, D. M., Haas, G. L., et al. (2005). Personality dimensions in first-episode psychoses. *American Journal of Psychiatry, 162*(1), 102–109.

Keshavan, M. S., Shad, M., Soloff, P., & Schooler, N. (2004). Efficacy and tolerability of olanzapine in the treatment of schizotypal personality disorder. *Schizophrenia Research, 71*(1), 97–101.

Kernberg, O. F. (1975). The almost untreatable narcissistic patient. *Journal of the American Psychoanalytic Association, 55*(2), 503–539.

Kotz, C. M. (2006). Integration of feeding and spontaneous physical activity. *Physiology & Behavior, 88*(3), 294–301.

Lee, R., Geracioti, T. D., Kasckow, J. W., & Coccaro, E. F. (2005). Childhood trauma and personality disorder. *American Journal of Psychiatry, 162*(5), 995–997.

Limandri, B., & Boyd, M. A. (2005). Personality and impulse control disorders. In M. A. Boyd (Ed.), *Psychiatric nursing: Contemporary practice* (3rd ed.). Philadelphia: Lippincott.

Lin, Y., Shiah, I., Chang, Y., Lai, T., Wang, K., & Chou, K. (2004). Evaluation of an assertiveness training program on nursing and medical students' assertiveness, self esteem, and interpersonal communication satisfaction. *Nurse Education Today, 24*(8), 656–665.

Livesley, W. J. (2003). *Practical management of personality disorder*. New York: Guilford Press.

MacFarlane, M. M. (2004). Systemic treatment of borderline personality disorder. In M. M. MacFarlane (Ed.), *Family treatment of personality disorders* (pp. 205–240). New York: Haworth Clinical Practice Press.

Magnavita, J. J., & MacFarlane, M. M. (2004). Family treatment of personality disorder: Historical overview and current perspectives. In M. M. MacFarlane (Ed.), *Family treatment of personality disorders* (pp. 3–39). New York: Haworth Clinical Practice Press.

Mahler, M. S., Pine, F., & Bergman, A. (1975). *The psychological birth of the human infant: Symbiosis and individuation*. New York: Basic Books.

McLean, P. D., & McLean, C. P. (2004). Family therapy of avoidant personality disorder. In M. M. MacFarlane (Ed.), *Family treatment of personality disorders* (pp. 273–303). New York: Haworth Clinical Practice Press.

Millon, T., & Davis, R. (1999). *Personality disorders in modern life*. New York: John Wiley & Sons.

Montpetit, M., Bisconti, T., & Bergeman, C. (2004). Self-concept in bereavement: Evidence for structural change. *Gerontologist, 44,* 572–573.

NANDA International. (2007). *NANDA nursing diagnoses: Definitions and classification 2007–2008.* Philadelphia: Author.

National Alliance on Mental Illness. (2007). *Borderline personality disorder.* Retrieved January 2007, from www.nami.org/PrinterTemplate.cfm?Section=By_Illness&Template=TaggedPage[&|mu|&]

National Institutes of Health, Office of Dietary Supplements. (2009). *Dietary supplement fact sheet: Vitamin D.* Retrieved September 18, 2009 from http://dietary-supplements.info.nih.gov/factsheets/vitamind.asp

Neumark-Sztainer, D. (2005). *"I'm, like, SO fat!"* New York: Guilford Press.

Ni, X., Chan, K., Bulgin, N., Sicard, T., Bismil, R., McMain, S., & Kennedy, J. L. (2006). Association between serotonin transporter gene and borderline personality disorder. *Journal of Psychiatric Research, 40*(5), 448–453.

Nolan, M. E. (2003). Anticipatory guidance for parents of Prader–Willi children. *Pediatric Nursing, 29*(6), 427–430.

North American Nursing Diagnosis Association. (2007). *Nursing diagnoses: Definitions and classification, 2007* to *2008*. Philadelphia: Author.

Orth, U., Robins, R. W., & Meier, L. L. (2009). Disentangling the effects of low self-esteem and stressful events on depression: Findings from three longitudinal studies. *Journal of Personality and Social Psychology, 97*(2), 307–321.

Paris, J. (2001). Psychosocial adversity. In W. J. Livesley (Ed.), *Handbook of personality disorders* (pp. 231–241). New York: Guilford Press.

Perseius, K. I., Ekdahl, S., Asberg, M., & Samuelsson, M. (2005). To tame a volcano: Patients with borderline personality disorder and their perceptions of suffering. *Archives of Psychiatric Nursing, 19*(4), 160–168.

Pull, C. B. (2004). Binge eating disorder. *Current Opinions in Psychiatry, 17*(1), 43–48.

Ratey, J. J. (2001). *A user's guide to the brain*. New York: Pantheon Books.

Romano, S. J., Halmi, K. A., Sarkar, N. P., Koke, S. C., & Lee, J. S. (2002). A placebo-controlled study of fluoxetine in continued treatment of bulimia nervosa after successful acute fluoxetine treatment. *American Journal of Psychiatry, 159*(1), 96–102.

Sadock, B. J., & Sadock, V. A. (2005). *Kaplan & Sadock's pocket handbook of clinical psychiatry* (4th ed.). Philadelphia: Lippincott Williams & Wilkins.

Slof-O't Landt, M. C., van Furth, E. F., Meulenbelt, I., Slagboom, P. E., Bartels, M., Boomsma, D. I., et al. (2005). Eating disorders: From twin studies to candidate genes and beyond. *Twin Research and Human Genetics, 8*(5), 467–482.

Soler, J., Pascual, J. C., Campins, J., Barrachina, J., Puigdemont, D., Alvarez, E., et al. (2005). Double-blind, placebo-controlled study of dialectical behavior therapy plus olanzapine for borderline personality disorder. *American Journal of Psychiatry, 162*(6), 1221–1224.

Spearing, M. (2001). *Eating disorders: Facts about eating disorders and the search for solutions* [NIH Publication No. 01-4901]. National Institute of Mental Health.

Sperry, L. (2004). Family therapy with a histrionic-obsessive couple. In M. M. MacFarlane (Ed.), *Family treatment of personality disorders* (pp. 149–172). New York: Haworth Clinical Practice Press.

Stein, K. F., & Corte, C. (2003). Reconceptualizing causative factors and intervention strategies in the eating disorders: A shift from body image to self-concept impairments. *Archives of Psychiatric Nursing, 17*(2), 57–66.

Swenson, C. R., Sanderson, C., Dulit, R. A., & Linehan, M. M. (2001). The application of dialectical behavior therapy for patients with borderline personality disorder on inpatient units. *Psychiatric Quarterly, 72*(4), 307–324.

Tozzi, F., Thornton, L. M., Klump, K. L., Fichter, M. M., Halmi, K. A., Kaplan, A. S., et al. (2005). Symptom fluctuation in eating disorders. *American Journal of Psychiatry, 162*(4), 732–740.

Uher, R., Murphy, T., Brammer, M. J., Dalgleish, T., Phillips, M. L., Ng, V. W., et al. (2004). Medial prefrontal cortex activity associated with symptom provocation in eating disorders. *American Journal of Psychiatry*, 161(7), 1238–1246.

Sensory Perception 25

Concept at-a-Glance

Concept Learning Outcomes

After reading about this concept, you will be able to:

1. Summarize the structure and physiologic processes of the sensory organs related to sensory perception.
2. List factors affecting sensory perception.
3. Identify commonly occurring alterations in sensory perception and their related treatments.
4. Explain common physical assessment procedures used to examine sensory perception functioning of clients across the life span.
5. Outline diagnostic and laboratory tests to determine the individual's sensory perception status.
6. Explain management of altered sensory perception and prevention of illness.
7. Demonstrate the nursing process in providing culturally competent and caring interventions across the life span for individuals with common alterations in sensory perception.
8. Identify pharmacologic interventions in caring for the individual with alterations in sensory perception.

Concept Key Terms

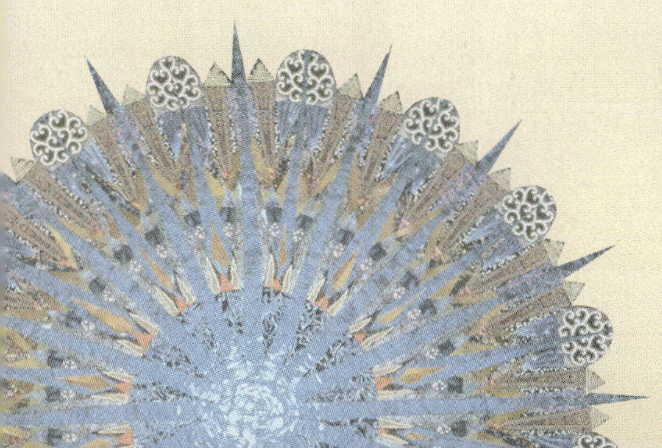

About Sensory Perception

An individual's senses are essential for growth, development, and survival. Sensory stimuli give meaning to events in the environment. Any alteration in sensory functions can affect one's ability to operate within the environment. For example, many clients have impaired sensory functions that put them at risk in an institutional setting such as a school or assisted living facility; nurses can help these clients find ways to function safely in these often confusing environments. ●

The sensory process involves two components: reception and perception. **Sensory reception** is the process of receiving stimuli or data. These stimuli are either external or internal to the body. External stimuli are **visual** (sight), **auditory** (hearing), **olfactory** (smell), **tactile** (touch), and **gustatory** (taste). Gustatory stimuli can be internal as well. Other types of internal stimuli are kinesthetic and visceral. **Kinesthetic** refers to awareness of the position and movement of body parts. For example, a person walking is aware of which leg is forward. A related sense is **stereognosis**, the ability to perceive and understand an object through touch by its size, shape, and texture. A person holding a tennis ball is aware of its size, round shape, and soft surface without seeing it. **Visceral** means of or relating to any large organ within the body. Visceral organs may produce stimuli that make a person aware of them (e.g., a full stomach). **Sensory perception** involves the conscious organization and translation of the data or stimuli into meaningful information.

For an individual to be aware of his or her surroundings, four aspects of the sensory process must be present: a stimulus, a receptor, impulse conduction, and perception.

- **Stimulus.** This is an agent or act that stimulates a nerve receptor.
- **Receptor.** A nerve cell acts as a receptor by converting the stimulus to a nerve impulse. Most receptors are specific, that is, sensitive to only one type of stimulus, such as visual, auditory, or touch.
- **Impulse conduction.** The impulse travels along nerve pathways to the spinal cord or directly to the brain. The cranial nerves (listed in Table 25–1 along with their functions) are important nerves controlling many actions required for

TABLE 25–1 **Cranial Nerves and Their Functions**

NAME	FUNCTION
I Olfactory	Sense of smell
II Optic	Vision
III Oculomotor	Eyeball movement Raising of upper eyelid Constriction of pupil Proprioception
IV Trochlear	Eyeball movement
V Trigeminal	Sensation of the upper scalp, upper eyelid, nose, nasal cavity, cornea, and lacrimal gland Sensation of the palate, upper teeth, cheek, top lip, lower eyelid, and scalp; sensation of the tongue, lower teeth, chin, and temporal scalp Chewing
VI Abducens	Lateral movement of the eyeball
VII Facial	Movement of facial muscles Secretions of lacrimal, nasal, submandibular, and sublingual glands Sensation of taste
VIII Acoustic	Sense of equilibrium Sense of hearing
IX Glossopharyngeal	Swallowing Gag reflex Secretions of parotid salivary gland Sense of taste Touch, pressure, and pain from pharynx and posterior tongue Pressure from carotid arteries Receptors to regulate blood pressure
X Vagus	Swallowing Regulation of cardiac rate Regulation of respirations Digestion Sensation from thoracic and abdominal organs Proprioception Sense of taste
XI Accessory	Movement of head and neck Proprioception
XII Hypoglossal	Movement of tongue for speech and swallowing

sensory perception (Figure 25–1 ■). For example, auditory impulses travel to the organ of Corti in the inner ear. From there, the impulses travel along the eighth cranial nerve to the temporal lobe of the brain.

- **Perception.** Perception, or awareness and interpretation of stimuli, takes place in the brain. Specialized brain cells interpret the nature and the quality of the sensory stimuli. The level of consciousness affects the perception of the stimuli.

The brain has the capacity to adapt to sensory stimuli. For example, a person living in a city may not notice traffic noise that someone from a rural area finds loud and disturbing. Not all sensory stimuli are acted on; some are stored in the memory to be used at a later date. Sensory processing is not the same as cognition or awareness. Cognition is the process by which an individual learns, stores, retrieves, and uses information. **Awareness** is the ability to perceive environmental stimuli and body reactions and to respond appropriately through thought and action. The normal, alert person can assimilate many kinds of information at one time.

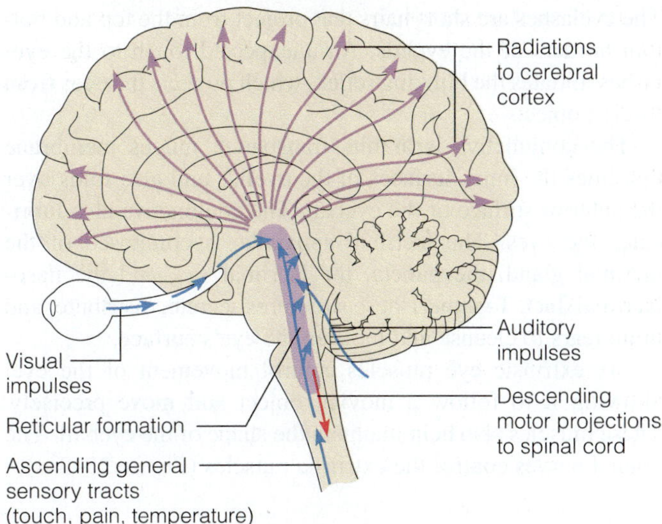

Figure 25–1 ■ The nerve impulses run along the ascending sensory tracts to reach the reticular activating system (RAS); then certain impulses reach the cerebral cortex where they are preceived.

Source: From Marieb, E. N., & Hoehn, K. (2007). *Human Anatomy & Physiology*, (7th ed., p.455). Benjamin Cummings Publishing Company. Reprinted by permission of Pearson Education, Inc.

NORMAL PRESENTATION

Our sensory organs provide pathways for stimuli to reach the brain, allowing us to experience the world in which we live. Deficits in sensory perception may limit self-care, mobility, safety, independence, communication, and relationships with others.

Eyes

The eyes are complex structures, containing 70% of the body's sensory receptors. Both extraocular and intraocular structures are considered parts of the eye. Each eye is a sphere measuring about 1 in. (2.5 cm) in diameter, surrounded and protected by a bony orbit and cushions of fat. The primary functions of the eye are to encode the patterns of light from the environment through photoreceptors and to carry the coded information from the eyes to the brain. The brain gives meaning to the coded information, allowing us to make sense of what we see.

EXTRAOCULAR STRUCTURES Although the extraocular structures of the eye are outside the eyeball, they are vital to its protection. These structures are the eyebrows, eyelids, eyelashes, conjunctiva, lacrimal apparatus, and extrinsic eye muscles (Figure 25–2 ■).

The eyebrows shade the eyes and keep perspiration away from them. The eyelids are thin, loose folds of skin covering the anterior eye. They protect the eye from foreign bodies, regulate the entry of light into the eye, and distribute tears by blinking.

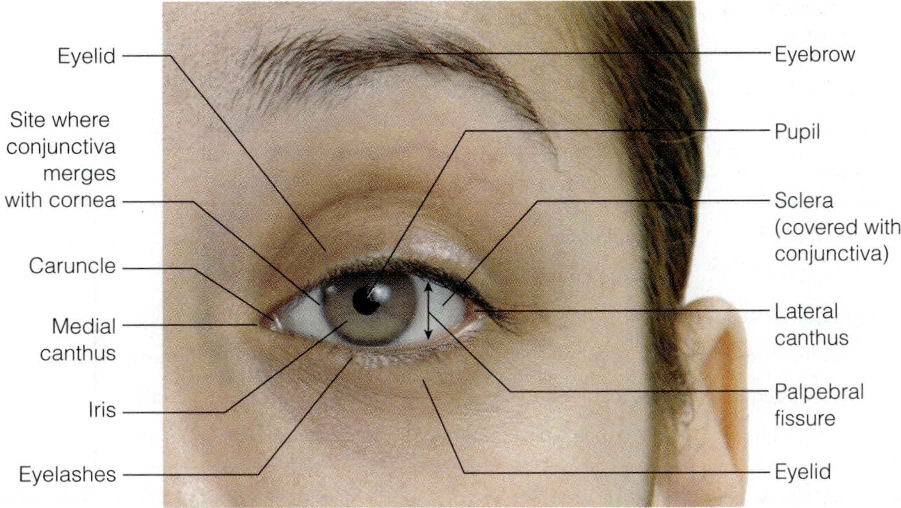

Figure 25–2 ■ Structures of the external eye.

The eyelashes are short hairs that project from the top and bottom borders of the eyelids. An unexpected touch to the eyelashes initiates the blinking reflex, which protects the eyes from foreign objects.

The conjunctiva is a thin, transparent mucus membrane that lines the inner surfaces of the eyelids and also folds over the anterior surface of the eyeball. The conjunctiva also lubricates the eyes. The lacrimal apparatus is composed of the lacrimal gland, the puncta, the lacrimal sac, and the nasolacrimal duct. Together, these structures secrete, distribute, and drain tears to cleanse and moisten the eye's surface.

Six extrinsic eye muscles control movement of the eye, allowing it to follow a moving object and move precisely. These muscles also help maintain the shape of the eyeball. The cranial nerves control the extrinsic muscles (Figure 25–3 ■).

INTRAOCULAR STRUCTURES The intraocular structures transmit visual images and maintain homeostasis of the inner eye. Those in the anterior portion of each eyeball are the sclera and the cornea, the iris, the pupil, and the anterior cavity (Figure 25–4 ■).

Sclera and Cornea The white sclera lines the outside of the eyeball, protecting it and giving it shape. The sclera gives way to the cornea over the iris and pupil. The cornea is transparent, avascular, and sensitive to touch. It forms a window that allows light to enter the eye and is a part of its light-bending apparatus. When the cornea is touched, the eyelids blink (**corneal reflex**) and tears are secreted.

Iris and Pupil The iris is a disc of muscle surrounding the pupil and lying between the cornea and the lens. The iris gives the eye its color and regulates light entry by controlling the size

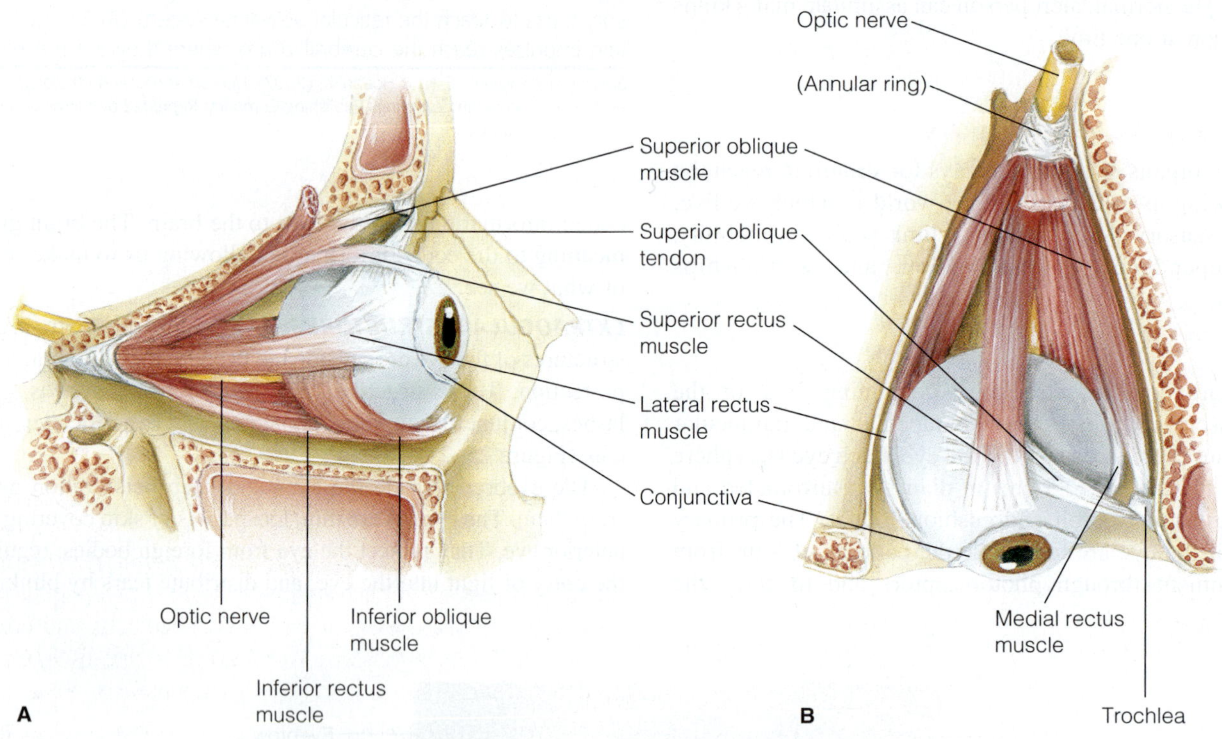

Name	Controlling cranial nerve	Action
Lateral rectus	VI (abducens)	Moves eye laterally
Medial rectus	III (oculomotor)	Moves eye medially
Superior rectus	III (oculomotor)	Elevates eye or rolls it superiorly
Inferior rectus	III (oculomotor)	Depresses eye or rolls it inferiorly
Inferior oblique	III (oculomotor)	Elevates eye and turns it laterally
Superior oblique	IV (trochlear)	Depresses eye and turns it laterally

C

Figure 25–3 ■ Extraocular muscles. *A*, Lateral view of the right eye. *B*, Superior view to the right eye. *C*, Innervation of the extraocular by the cranial nerves.

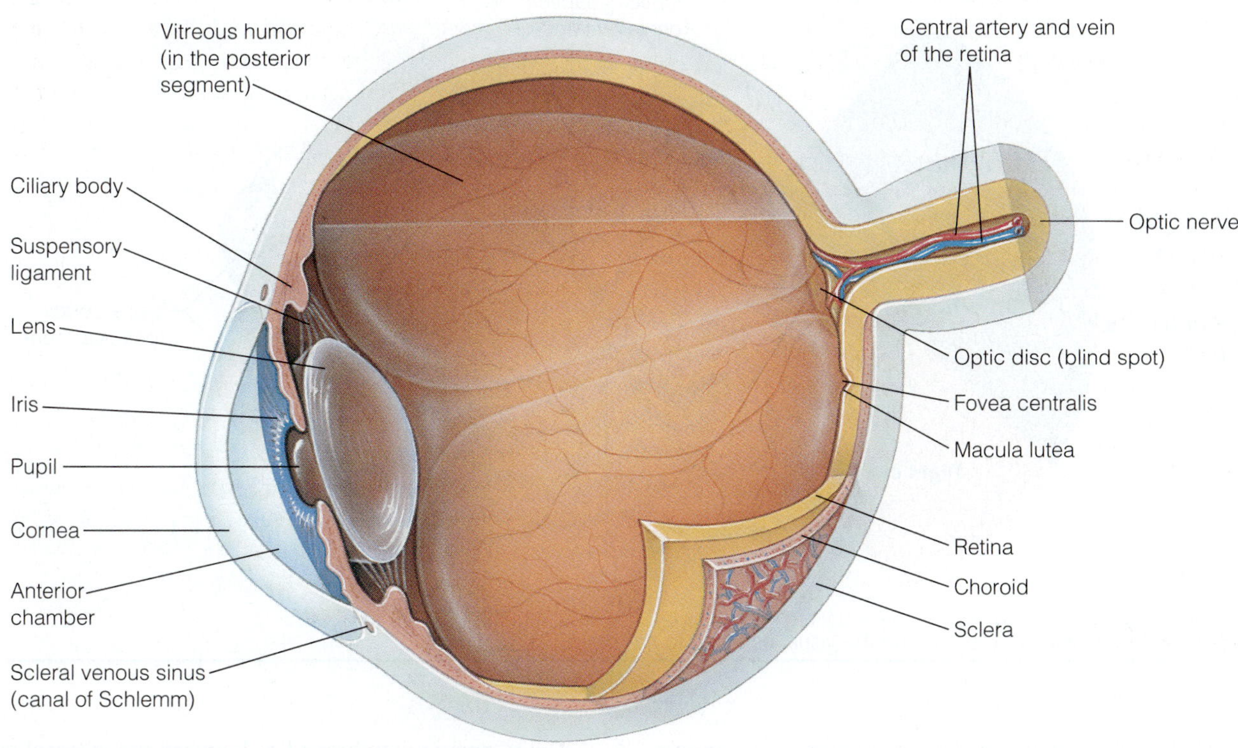

Figure 25–4 ■ Interior of the eye.

of the pupil. The pupil is the dark center of the eye through which light enters. It constricts when bright light enters the eye and when it is used for near vision; it dilates when light conditions are dim and when the eye is used for far vision. In response to intense light, the pupil constricts rapidly in the **pupillary light reflex**.

Anterior Cavity The anterior cavity is made of the anterior chamber (the space between the cornea and the iris) and the posterior chamber (the space between the iris and the lens). The anterior cavity is filled with aqueous humor. Aqueous humor, a clear fluid, is constantly formed and drained to maintain a relatively constant pressure in the eye of from 15 to 20 mmHg. The canal of Schlemm, provides the drainage system for fluid moving between the anterior and posterior chambers. Aqueous humor provides nutrients and oxygen for the cornea and the lens.

Internal Chamber The intraocular structures that lie in the internal chamber of the eye are the lens, the posterior cavity and vitreous humor, the ciliary body, the uvea, and the retina.

- The lens is a biconvex, avascular, transparent structure located directly behind the pupil. It can change shape to focus and refract light onto the retina.
- The posterior cavity lies behind the lens. It supports the posterior surface of the lens, maintains the position of the retina, and transmits light.
- The uvea is the middle layer of the eyeball. This pigmented layer has three components: the iris, ciliary body, and choroid.
- The ciliary body encircles the lens and, along with the iris, regulates the amount of light reaching the retina by controlling the shape of the lens. Blood vessels of the choroid nourish the layers of the eyeball. Its pigmented areas absorb light, preventing it from scattering within the eyeball.
- The retina is the innermost lining of the eyeball. It has an outer pigmented layer and an inner neural layer. The outer layer, next to the choroid, serves as the link between visual stimuli and the brain. The transparent inner layer is made up of millions of light receptors in structures called rods and cones. Rods enable peripheral vision and vision in dim light. Cones enable vision in bright light and the perception of color.

REFRACTION **Refraction** is the bending of light rays as they pass from one medium to another medium of different optical density. As light rays pass through the eye, they are refracted at several points: as they enter the cornea, as they leave the cornea and enter the aqueous humor, as they enter the lens, and as they leave the lens and enter the vitreous humor. At the lens, light is bent so that it converges at a single point on the retina. This focusing of the image is called **accommodation**. Because the lens is convex, the image projected onto the retina (the real image) is upside down and reversed from left to right. This real image is coded as electric signals that are sent to the brain. The brain decodes the image so that the person perceives it as it occurs in space (Figure 25–5 ■).

The eyes are best adapted to see distant objects. Both eyes fix on the same distant image and do not require any change in accommodation. For people with normal vision, the distance

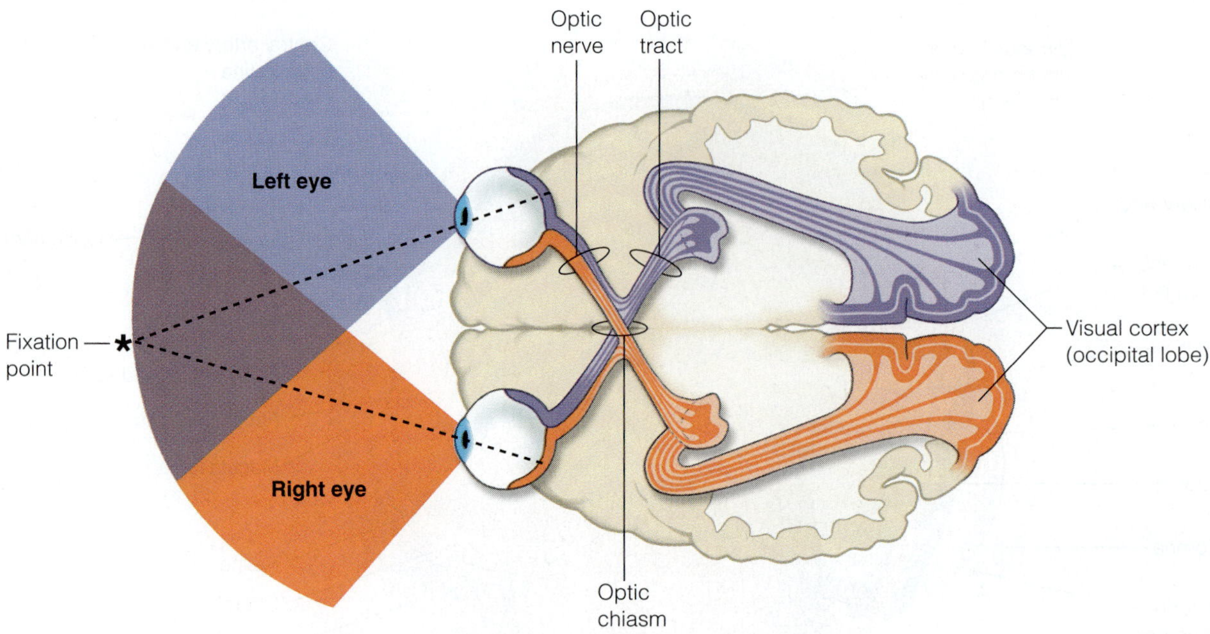

Figure 25–5 ■ Visual fields of the eye and the visual pathway to the brain.

from the viewed object at which the eyes require no accommodation is 20 ft (6 m). This point is called the far point of vision. To focus for near vision, the eyes must instantly accommodate the lens, constrict the pupils, and converge the eyeballs. The closest point on which a person can focus is called the near point of vision; in young adults with normal vision this is usually 8–10 in. (20–25 cm). Pupillary constriction helps eliminate most of the divergent light rays and sharpens focus. **Convergence** (the medial rotation of the eyeballs so that each is directed toward the viewed object) allows the image to be focused on the retinal fovea of each eye.

Ears

As a sensory organ, the ears have two primary functions, hearing and maintaining equilibrium. Anatomically, each ear is divided into three areas: the external ear, the middle ear, and the inner ear (Figure 25–6 ■). Each area has a unique function. All three are involved in hearing, but only the inner ear is involved in equilibrium.

EXTERNAL EAR The external ear consists of the auricles (or pinna), the external auditory canal, and the tympanic membrane.

The auricles are elastic cartilage covered with thin skin. They contain sebaceous and sweat glands and sometimes hair. Each auricle has a rim (the helix) and a lobe. The auricle serves to direct sound waves into the ear.

The external auditory canal serves as a resonator for the range of sound waves typical of human speech and increases the pressure that sound waves in this frequency range place on the tympanic membrane. The canal's ceruminous glands (modified apocrine glands) secrete a yellow to brown waxy substance called **cerumen** (earwax). Cerumen traps foreign bodies; it also has bacteriostatic properties, protecting the tympanic membrane and the middle ear from infections.

The tympanic membrane lies between the external ear and the middle ear. It is a thin, semitransparent, fibrous structure covered with skin on the external side and mucosa on the inner side. The membrane vibrates as sound waves strike it; these vibrations are transferred as sound waves to the middle ear.

MIDDLE EAR The middle ear is an air-filled cavity in the temporal bone. The posterior wall of the middle ear contains the mastoid antrum. This cavity communicates with the mastoid sinuses, which help the middle ear adjust to changes in pressure. The mastoid antrum also opens into the eustachian tube, which connects with the nasopharynx. The eustachian tube helps to equalize the air pressure in the middle ear by opening briefly in response to differences between middle ear pressure and atmospheric pressure. This action also ensures that vibrations of the tympanic membrane remain adequate. The mucous membrane lining the middle ear is continuous with the mucous membranes lining the throat.

The middle ear contains three auditory ossicles: the malleus, the incus, and the stapes. The malleus attaches to the tympanic membrane and articulates with the incus, which in turn articulates with the stapes. The stapes fits into the oval window. Vibrations of the tympanic membrane are conducted across the middle ear to the oval window by the ossicles. The vibrations then set in motion the fluids of the inner ear, which in turn stimulate the hearing receptors. Two small muscles attached to the ossicles contract reflexively in response to sudden loud noises, decreasing the vibrations and protecting the inner ear.

INNER EAR The inner ear is a maze of bony chambers located deep within the temporal bone just behind the eye socket. Within the inner ear the cochlea houses the organ of Corti, the receptor organ for hearing. The organ of Corti is a series of sensory hair cells, arranged in a single row of inner hair cells and three rows of outer hair cells. The hair cells are

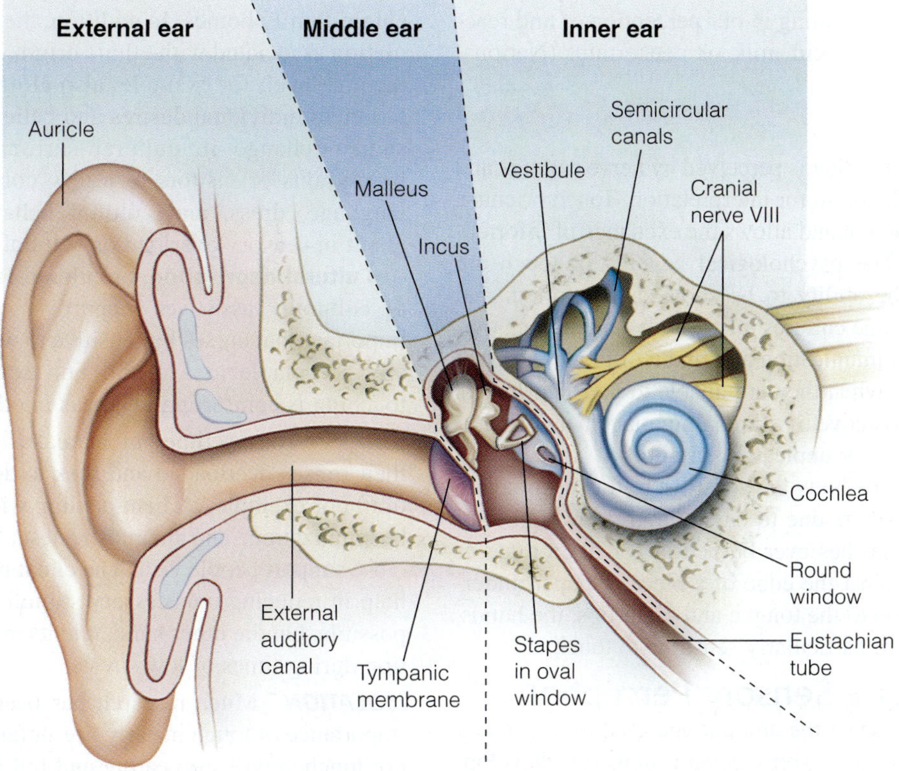

Figure 25–6 ■ The three parts of the ear.

innervated by sensory fibers from cranial nerve VIII. The organ of Corti is supported in the cochlea by the flexible basilar membrane, which has fibers of varying lengths that respond to different sound wave frequencies.

SOUND CONDUCTION Hearing is the perception and interpretation of sound. Sound is produced when the molecules of a medium are compressed, resulting in a pressure disturbance evidenced as a sound wave. The intensity or loudness of sound is determined by the amplitude (height) of the sound wave, with greater amplitudes causing louder sounds. The frequency of the sound wave in vibrations per second determines the pitch or tone of the sound, with higher frequencies resulting in higher sounds.

Sound waves enter the external auditory canal and cause the tympanic membrane to vibrate at the same frequency. The ossicles not only transmit the motion of the tympanic membrane to the oval window, but also amplify the energy of the sound wave.

Several brainstem auditory nuclei transmit impulses to the cerebral cortex. Fibers from each ear cross, with each auditory cortex receiving impulses from both ears. Auditory processing is so finely tuned that a wide variety of sounds of different pitch and loudness can be heard at any one time. In addition, the sources of the sounds can be localized.

EQUILIBRIUM The inner ear also provides information about the position of the head. This information is used to coordinate body movements so that equilibrium and balance are maintained. The types of equilibrium are static balance (affected by changes in the position of the head) and dynamic balance (affected by the movement of the head).

Receptors called maculae detect changes in the position of the head. Maculae are groups of hair cells in the inner ear that have protrusions covered with a gelatinous substance. Embedded in this gelatinous substance are tiny particles of calcium carbonate called otoliths (ear stones) which sense gravity and movement.

Taste and Smell

The sense of taste is mediated by taste buds located on the dorsal surface of the tongue, in the lateral folds on the side of the tongue, on the epiglottis, on the larynx, and even on the first third of the esophagus. Many nerves are responsible for transmitting taste information to the brain, including cranial nerves VII, IX, and X. Taste buds are continually bathed in secretions from the salivary glands.

Taste is not the same thing as flavor. Traditionally five tastes have been identified: sour, sweet, bitter, salty, and umami. Taste combines with texture, temperature, and the perception of odor from the olfactory senses to produce the perception of flavor. Flavor is greatly regulated by sense of smell. Someone with a bad head cold, for example, may repeatedly complain that he or she cannot taste anything (National Institutes of Health, 2009).

The olfactory cells, located in the roof of the nasal cavity, form filaments that connect to the olfactory nerve (cranial nerve I) and are primarily responsible for the sense of smell. Nerve endings in the ear, throat, and mouth also play a part in the sense of smell, participating in our perception of and reaction to smells such as rancid milk or peppermint (National Institutes of Health, 2009).

Touch

Touch is the tactile sense that is perceived by nerve endings and transmits signals to the brain for interpretation. Touch orients a person to the environment and allows the exchange of information and sensation. The psychological benefits of touch are many and include the ability to be soothed, comforted, and held. Individuals in some cultures rely heavily on touching others during routine communication and find it difficult to refrain from touching others when they are unable to use their hands. Touch can also be protective by stimulating movement or withdrawal from hot, sharp, or unpleasant stimuli.

While all areas of the body are sensitive to touch, some are more sensitive than others due to having a greater number of receptors. Anyone who has ever burned his or her tongue or sliced a finger tip against the edge of a piece of paper understands this. In addition to the tongue and fingertips, the hands, feet, face and neck are particularly sensitive to touch.

Factors Affecting Sensory Perception

A number of factors affect the amount and quality of sensory stimulation, including a person's genetic make-up, developmental stage, culture, level of stress, isolation, medications and illness, and lifestyle.

CONGENITAL AND HEREDITARY CONDITIONS Many conditions lead to temporary or permanent impairment of sensory perception. Infants who are premature; whose mothers were infected prenatally with rubella, toxoplasmosis, or other viruses; or who have certain congenital and hereditary conditions are at a high risk for visual problems. Fetal alcohol syndrome (FAS) is a major cause of prenatal visual disturbance. Auditory Processing Disorder, a condition in which the individual has difficulty differentiating individual sounds in words, is one of several hearing disorders with which a child may be born. It creates difficulty for individuals in some environments, especially school. Its cause is unknown. Some people are born with impairment of the senses of smell and taste, but these can also be acquired from exposure to insecticides or radiation and through other means.

CULTURE An individual's culture often determines the amount of stimulation the person considers usual or "normal." For example, a child reared in a big-city Latino neighborhood, where extended families share responsibilities for all the children, may be accustomed to more stimulation than a child reared in a European-American suburb of scattered single-family homes. In addition, the normal amount of stimulation associated with ethnic origin, religious affiliation, and income level, for example, also affects the amount of stimulation an individual desires and believes to be meaningful. A sudden change in cultural surroundings experienced by immigrants or visitors to a new country—especially where language, dress, and cultural behaviors differ—may also result in sensory overload or cultural shock.

Cultural deprivation, or cultural care deprivation, is a lack of culturally assistive, supportive, or facilitative acts. It is important that nurses be sensitive to what stimulation is culturally acceptable to a client. For example, in some cultures touching is comforting, whereas in others it is offensive.

STRESS During times of increased stress, people may find their senses overloaded and seek to decrease sensory stimulation. For example, a client dealing with physical illness, pain, hospitalization, and diagnostic tests may wish to have only close support people visit. The client may also need the nurse's help in reducing unnecessary stimuli (e.g., noise) as much as possible. On the other hand, clients may seek sensory stimulation during times of low stress.

ISOLATION Much research has been done to document the importance of touch in early life. Infants in incubators who are not touched will stop eating and fail to thrive. The same may be true for older people, especially those with cognitive or sensory impairments. Institutionalized older persons deprived of caring touch and nurturing physical contact experience a diminishing quality of life, a lessening of their desire to relate to others, and a weakening of what may already be a fragile relationship with physical reality (Nelson, 2001).

MEDICATION AND ILLNESS Certain medications can alter an individual's awareness of environmental stimuli. Narcotics and sedatives, for example, can decrease awareness of stimuli. Some antidepressants can alter perceptions of stimuli. Anyone taking several medications concurrently may show alterations in sensory function. Elders are especially at risk and need to be monitored carefully, particularly if they are simultaneously taking multiple medications for a variety of conditions. Certain medications, if taken over a long period of time, become ototoxic, injuring the auditory nerve and causing hearing loss that may be irreversible. (See Exemplar 25.1, the exemplar on hearing impairment.)

Diseases such as atherosclerosis restrict blood flow to the receptor organs and the brain, thereby decreasing awareness and slowing responses. Uncontrolled diabetes mellitus can

FOCUS ON DIVERSITY AND CULTURE Otitis Media

Native American and Alaska Native (NA/AN) children have a very high rate of otitis media, perhaps related to culture-specific bony structure of the ear, nose, and mouth. One study found that NA/AN children are seen about three times more frequently in outpatient clinics for otitis media than are other children in the United States (Curns et al., 2002). Nurses should be alert for the high incidence in these population groups, plan prevention programs, and ensure prompt care and teaching about treatments for families of children affected. What prevention measures would you emphasize with these families?

impair vision and is a leading cause of blindness in the United States. Some central nervous system diseases cause varying degrees of paralysis and sensory loss.

LIFESTYLE AND PERSONALITY Lifestyle influences the quality and quantity of stimulation to which an individual is accustomed. A client who is employed in a large company may be accustomed to diverse stimuli, whereas a client who is self-employed and works in the home is exposed to fewer, less diverse stimuli. People's personalities also differ in terms of the quantity and quality of stimuli with which they are comfortable. Some people delight in constantly changing stimuli and excitement, whereas others prefer a more structured life with few changes.

Age-Related Changes in Sensory Perception

The eyes of neonates differ from the eyes of adults in several ways. Visual acuity in neonates ranges between 20/100 and 20/400. Because the optic nerve is not yet completely myelinated, the ability to distinguish color and other details is decreased. The rectus muscles that control binocular vision may be somewhat uncoordinated at birth. By the age of 3 months, the eyes should be aligned and movement coordinated. Transient **nystagmus** (involuntary rapid eye movement) and **esotropia** (momentary turning inward of eyes) are common in neonates, but decrease in incidence during the first few months of life.

The cornea occupies a larger portion of the orbit in the infant and young child than in the adult; the infant's eyeball is about three-fourths of its adult size (Chamley, Carson, Randall, & Sandwell, 2005). Because the infant's eyeball is relatively unprotected laterally, it is more easily injured. The sclera of the neonate is thin and translucent with a bluish tinge, and the iris is blue or gray. Eye color changes during the first 6 months of life. By the age of 2 or 3 years, most children have a visual acuity of 20/50, and by the age of 6 or 7 years, visual acuity reaches 20/20.

Why do infants and young children have more ear problems than adults? The eustachian tube, which connects the nasopharynx to the middle ear, is proportionately shorter, wider, and more horizontal in infants than in older children or adults (see Figure 25–6). During sucking, yawning, and other movements, the tube opens for milliseconds, allowing free passage of air between the nasopharynx and the middle ear. These factors predispose young children to development of otitis media or middle ear infection.

Although auditory nerve function is not fully mature until about 5 months of age, the fetus begins to hear at about 20 weeks' gestation. Before 34 weeks' gestation, the external ear is soft, with little cartilage apparent. The external ear canal is small at birth, although the internal ear and middle ear are relatively large. As a result, the tympanic membrane is close to the surface and can be easily injured.

Newborns should be screened for hearing loss prior to hospital discharge. Universal screening of all newborns is mandated in at least 30 states, and in all states screening is done for children who are at high risk (e.g., have a history of infection during gestation, or are born with anomalies of the head or face). If hearing loss is detected early, treatment can begin early and complications such as speech impairment or loss can be prevented. If an infant is found to have hearing loss, it is recommended that treatment begin before 6 months of age (Joint Committee on Infant Hearing, 2000).

Changes in vision, hearing, smell, taste, and touch occur naturally throughout the aging process (Tables 25–2 and 25–3). The greatest declines in accommodation occur between 45 and 55 years of age, making this more a problem for middle-aged adults than for older adults. There is usually no change in accommodation after 60 years of age (Burke, 2002). However, normal physiologic changes in older adults put them at higher risk for altered sensory function, particularly hearing loss. Hearing loss is the third most common condition reported by the elderly. Approximately 40–45% of people over the age of 65 and more than 83% over the age of 70 have a hearing impairment (Gordon-Salant, 2005).

Although normal age-related changes in vision occur gradually, over time these changes can limit the functional ability of the older adult. Approximately 1.8 million community-dwelling older people report some difficulty with basic activities such as bathing, dressing, and walking around the house, in part because they are visually impaired. Unfortunately, visual impairment increases with age. Visual impairment is defined as visual acuity of 20/40 or worse while wearing corrective lenses, and legal blindness or severe visual impairment is 20/200 or more as measured by a Snellen wall chart at 20 ft.

The prevalence of blindness also increases with age, reaching its peak at about the age of 85. Fortunately, the prevalence of blindness in both eyes in the United States is low, about 1% among persons 70–74 years of age and 2.4% in persons 85 and older (Centers for Disease Control and Prevention, 2002). Visual impairment and blindness in the older person has four main causes: cataracts, age-related macular degeneration (ARMD), glaucoma, and diabetic retinopathy.

A diminished sense of taste, **hypogeusia**, is a normal sensory change usually occurring after the age of 70. The exact pathophysiology behind age-related gustatory changes remains unclear. However, studies have shown that both taste discrimination and sensitivity significantly change with age.

Olfactory dysfunction is more common than taste dysfunction. The three most common causes of loss of smell are nasal and sinus disease, upper respiratory infection, and head trauma (Bromley, 2000). Normal age-related changes influencing olfactory function are attributed to injury of the olfactory mucosa and reduction in both the number of sensory cells and neurotransmitters. Structural alterations of the upper airway, olfactory tract and bulb, hippocampus, amygdaloid complex, and hypothalamus have also been observed as contributing factors for diminished sense of smell, or **hyposmia**, in older adults (Schiffman, 1997).

Older persons with one or more sensory impairments are at risk for injury, weight loss, falls, malnutrition, and social isolation. Intact senses allow the older person to accurately

TABLE 25–2 **Age-Related Changes in the Eye**

AGE-RELATED CHANGE	SIGNIFICANCE
The lens:	
■ ↓ elasticity, decreasing focus and accommodation for near vision (presbyopia) ■ ↑ density and size, making lens more stiff and opaque ■ Yellowing of the lens and changes in the retina affecting color perception	Most older adults require corrective lenses to accommodate close and detailed work. Increased opacity leads to the development of cataracts. As cataracts develop, they increase sensitivity to glare and interfere with night vision.
The cornea:	
■ Fat deposits around the periphery and throughout the cornea	A partial or complete white circle may form around the cornea (*arcus senilis*). Lipid deposits in the cornea cause vision to be blurred.
■ ↓ corneal sensitivity	Decreased sensitivity increases the risk of injury to the eye.
The pupil:	
■ ↓ size and responsiveness to light pupil; sphincter hardening	Increased light perception threshold and difficulty seeing in dim light or at night means increased light is needed to see adequately.
The retina and visual pathways:	
■ Visual fields narrow ■ Photoreceptor cells lost ■ Rods working less effectively ■ Macular degeneration ■ Depth perception distortion ■ Adaptation to dark and light taking longer	Peripheral vision is decreased and central vision may be lost due to macular degeneration. Increased risk of falls results from changes in depth perception and adaptation to changes in light. Vision progressively declines with age.
The lacrimal apparatus:	
■ ↓ reabsorption of intraocular fluid	Increased risk of developing glaucoma; eyes feel and look dry.
■ ↓ production of tears	
The posterior cavity:	
■ Debris and condensation becoming visible ■ Vitreous body maybe pulling away from the retina	Vision is blurred and distorted. "Floaters" are often seen by the older person.

TABLE 25–3 **Age-Related Changes in the Ear**

AGE-RELATED CHANGE	SIGNIFICANCE
Inner ear:	
■ Loss of hair cells, ↓ blood supply, less flexible basilar membrane, degeneration of spiral ganglion cells, and ↓ production of endolymph resulting in progressive hearing loss with age (**presbycusis**) ■ High-frequency sounds lost; middle- and low-frequency sounds maybe also lost or decreased ■ Vestibular structures degenerating, organ of Corti and cochlea	Older adults may require hearing aids to hear well. With loss of high-frequency sounds, speech may be distorted, contributing to a risk for problems with communication. Degeneration of inner ear structures concerned with balance and equilibrium increase the risk for falls, atrophy.
Middle ear:	
■ Muscles and ligaments weakening and stiffening, decreasing the acoustic reflex	Sounds made from one's own body and speech are louder and may further interfere with hearing, speech, and communications.
External ear:	
■ Higher keratin content of cerumen, contributing to increased cerumen in the ear canal	Accumulated cerumen may impair hearing.

perceive the environment and remain appropriately involved with other people, places, and objects. Safety is compromised when the older person cannot see fall hazards on the floor, cannot smell a natural gas leak from a stove, cannot recognize the taste of spoiled milk, cannot hear a signaling fire alarm, and cannot feel a pebble in the shoe that could lead to a blister or foot ulcer. Older persons with sensory dysfunction may suffer functional impairment, injury, social isolation, and depression.

ALTERATIONS

Common problems related to sensory impairment include injury, cataracts, glaucoma, and macular degeneration. Chronic use of certain medications and chronic diseases such as Alzheimer's can cause impairment of smell. Hearing impairment is discussed later in this concept.

Injuries

Children are particularly at risk for eye injury. In the United States, eye injuries are common in boys 11–15 years of age and in all children ages 9–11 years. Boys from 11 to 15 years have four times more eye injuries than girls. Approximately half of the 42,000 sports injuries that occur annually involve children (Committee on Sports Medicine and Fitness, 2004). Sports, darts, fireworks, air-powered BB guns, blunt and sharp objects, chemical and thermal burns, physical irritants, and abuse all may cause eye trauma (Behrman, Kliegman, & Jenson, 2004). Older children may be injured by chemicals in school science laboratories. Athletes, particularly those involved in sports that do not require use of a helmet, are at risk for eye injuries, whether they play professionally or recreationally. Use of projectile toys of any kind increases the risk of eye injury. Professionals such as contractors, woodworkers, welders, and electricians are also at risk of eye injury and should wear protective goggles at all times.

Many eye injuries are minor, but without timely and appropriate intervention even a minor injury can threaten vision. For this reason, all eye injuries should be considered medical emergencies requiring immediate evaluation and intervention.

PRACTICE ALERT

Linking the Concepts—Sensory Perception, Family, Violence
External eye injuries are very common in children and by themselves will rarely indicate some form of abuse or nonaccidental trauma. Two black eyes, however, rarely occur by accident and raccoon eyes accompanied by swelling and skin injury are more likely to accompany nonaccidental fracture at the base of the skull (National Criminal Justice Reference Service, 2009). Ruptured tympanic membranes in combination with conjunctival and retinal hemorrhage are indicative of shaken baby syndrome. Retinal hemorrhage rarely occurs with any other type of injury. A nurse who suspects child abuse should follow his or her agency's protocol for reporting to Child Protective Services.

Ear injuries of many types are common in children. Lacerations, infections, and hematomas may occur in the external ear structures, especially the pinna. Children may place foreign objects in the ear, and insects may enter the ear canal.

Rupture of the tympanic membrane may result from head injuries, blows to the ear, or insertion of objects into the ear canal. Serous drainage from the ear can indicate a basilar skull fracture. Any injury resulting in earache, decreased hearing, persistent bleeding, or other discharge should be evaluated by a physician.

ALTERATIONS AND TREATMENTS Sensory Perception

ALTERATION	DESCRIPTION	TREATMENTS
Eye Injury	Damage to the structure of the eye; a common cause of vision loss in children. Often caused by sports injury or chemicals.	■ All eye injuries should be considered medical emergencies requiring immediate evaluation and intervention ■ Treatment varies due to type and severity of injury; treatments may include irrigation, foreign body removal and surgery
Cataracts	Opacification of eye that prevents refraction of light rays onto the retina; may be congenital or acquired.	■ Surgical removal of lens; lens may be implanted
Glaucoma	Optic neuropathy with gradual loss of peripheral vision; there are two main types, open-angle and angle-closure glaucoma.	■ Medications to control intraocular pressure and preserve vision in open-angle glaucoma ■ Surgery ■ Laser trabeculoplasty ■ Trabulectomy ■ Photocoagulation ■ Gionioplasty ■ Laser iridotomy
Macular degeneration (AMD)	Progressive disorder involving loss of central vision due to damage to the retina; there are two types, nonexudative andexudative.	■ High-dose antioxidants and zinc (early-to-intermediate dry AMD) ■ Laser surgery or photodynamic therapy (wet AMD)

> **PRACTICE ALERT**
> Often referred to simply as *vertigo,* benign positional vertigo is an inner ear condition usually caused by head injury, viral infection, or inflammation. Typical symptoms are dizziness, especially when readjusting the body's position (e.g., sitting up to get out of bed), and nausea. Temporary benign positional vertigo may be seen in athletes who have experienced a minor head injury because these injuries can dislodge one or more otoliths. In most cases, this type of vertigo resolves on its own within a few weeks as the otoliths return to their normal positions.

Cataracts

A **cataract** is an opacification (clouding) of the lens of the eye. This opacification can significantly interfere with light transmission to the retina and the ability to perceive images clearly. Cataracts are a common and significant cause of visual deficits, affecting nearly 20.5 million people over age 40 in the United States. By age 80, nearly half of the population is affected.

Glaucoma

Glaucoma is a condition characterized by optic neuropathy with gradual loss of peripheral vision and, usually, increased intraocular pressure of the eye. Glaucoma is a silent thief of vision. The client typically experiences no manifestations other than narrowing of the visual field, which occurs so gradually that it often goes unnoticed until late in the disease process.

Macular Degeneration

The leading cause of legal blindness and impaired vision in people over the age of 65 is age-related **macular degeneration** (AMD) (Prevent Blindness America, 2002).

SENSORY ASSESSMENT

Nursing assessment of sensory-perceptual functioning includes six components: (a) nursing history, (b) mental status examination, (c) identification of clients at risk, (d) the client's environment, (e) social support network, and (f) physical assessment.

Nursing History

During the nursing history, the nurse assesses present sensory perceptions, usual functioning, sensory deficits, and potential problems. In some instances, significant others or family members can provide data the client cannot. For example, family members may reveal signs of recent changes in the client's hearing ability, such as inattention to others, recent mood swings, difficulty following clear instructions, frequent requests to have something repeated, and unusually loud radio or television volumes. Assessment should include questions to obtain information related to noise exposure—loud, constant sounds from any type of equipment, for example—as well as hobbies or work that can cause burns or injuries. The nurse should always assess for chronic diseases or illness as well as medications taken by the client, regardless of the type of impairment suspected. The following Assessment Interview provides examples of interview questions to elicit data about the client's sensory-perceptual functioning.

Mental Status and Cognition

Mental status is critical to any evaluation of the sensory-perceptual process. The nurse should assess for any recent history of mood swings or delirium. The nurse should also assess for any problems with cognitive function, including level of consciousness, orientation, memory, and attention span. It is important to note that sensory alterations can cause changes in mental status and cognitive functioning (adapted from Wahl & Heyl, 2003).

Assessment Interview Sensory-Perceptual Functioning

VISUAL

- How would you rate your vision (excellent, good, fair, or poor)?
- Do you wear eyeglasses or contact lenses?
- Describe any recent changes in your vision.
- Do you have any difficulty seeing near or far objects?
- Do you have any difficulty seeing at night? Have you ever experienced blurred vision, double vision, spots moving in front of your eyes, blind spots, light sensitivity, flashing lights, or halos around objects?
- When did you last visit an eye doctor?

AUDITORY

- How would you rate your hearing (excellent, good, fair, or poor)?
- Do you wear a hearing aid?
- Describe any recent changes in your hearing.
- Can you locate the direction of sounds and distinguish various voices?
- Are you having any trouble with balance?
- Do you experience any dizziness or vertigo? Do you experience any ringing, buzzing, humming, crackling noises, or fullness in the ears?
- Do you listen to loud music on a regular basis?
- Are you exposed to any loud noises at work? If so, what are they? How much or how often?

GUSTATORY

- Have you experienced any changes in taste (e.g., difficulty in differentiating sweet, sour, salty, and bitter tastes)?
- Do you enjoy the taste of foods as you did previously?

OLFACTORY

- Have you experienced any changes in smell?
- Do things (foods, flowers, perfumes, and so on) smell the same as previously?
- Can you distinguish foods by their odors and tell when something is burning?
- Have you experienced any changes in appetite? (Changes in appetite may be related to an impaired sense of smell.)

TACTILE

- Are you experiencing any pain or discomfort?
- Have you experienced any decrease in your ability to perceive heat, cold, or pain in your limbs?
- Do you have any numbness or tingling in your extremities?

KINESTHETIC

- Have you noticed any difficulty in perceiving the position of parts of your body?
- Do you need any assistance standing or sitting down?

Client Environment

The nurse assesses the client's environment for quantity, quality, and type of stimuli. The client's environment may produce insufficient stimuli, placing the client at risk for sensory deprivation, or excessive stimuli, placing the client at risk for sensory overload. Nonstimulating environments include those that (a) severely restrict physical activity and (b) limit social contact with family and friends. Because appropriate or meaningful stimuli decrease the incidence of sensory deprivation, the nurse must consider the client's health care environment for the presence of the following stimuli:

- Radio or other auditory device (e.g., cassette or CD player), including television and use of earphones with portable devices
- Clock or calendar
- Reading material (or toys for children)
- Number and compatibility of roommates (which may affect number of auditory devices used at one time, level of overall noise in the environment)
- Number of visitors.

In the client's home, the nurse may also note the presence of a video/DVD recorder, pets, bright colors, and adequate lighting.

To assess a health care environment that produces excessive stimuli, the nurse considers, for example, bright lights, noise, therapeutic measures, and frequency of assessments and procedures.

Social Support Network

The degree of isolation a person feels is significantly influenced by the quality and quantity of support from family members and friends. The nurse assesses (a) whether the client lives

Eye and Vision Assessment

Vision Assessment

Visual acuity is assessed with an eye chart such as the Snellen chart or the E chart for testing distance vision and the Rosenbaum chart for testing near vision. The Snellen chart contains rows of letters in various sizes, with standardized numbers at the end of each row. The number at the end of the row indicates the visual acuity of a client who can read the row at a distance of 20 feet. (If the client is unable to read or does not read English, you can use the E chart to test visual acuity.) The top number at the end of the row is always 20, representing the distance between the client and the chart. The bottom number is the distance (in feet) at which a person with normal vision can read the line. A person with normal vision can read the row marked 20/20. To conduct the assessment, ask the person to stand 20 feet from the chart in a well-lit area. Ask the client to cover one eye with an opaque cover (Figure 25–7 ■). Then ask the client to read each row of letters, moving from largest letters to the smallest ones that the client can see. Measure visual acuity in the other eye in the same way, and then assess visual acuity while the client has both eyes uncovered. You may test the client who wears corrective lenses with and without the lenses.

The Rosenbaum chart is held at a distance of from 12 to 14 inches from the eyes, with visual acuity measured in the same manner as with the Snellen chart (Figure 25–8 ■). A gross estimate of near vision may also be assessed by asking the person to read from a magazine or newspaper.

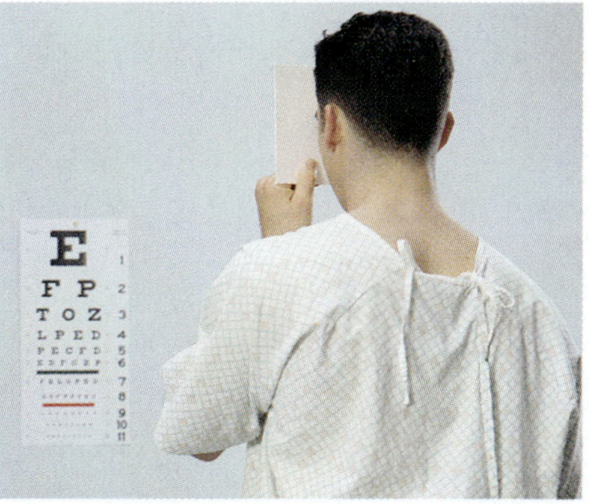

Figure 25–7 ■ Testing distant vision using the Snellen eye chart.

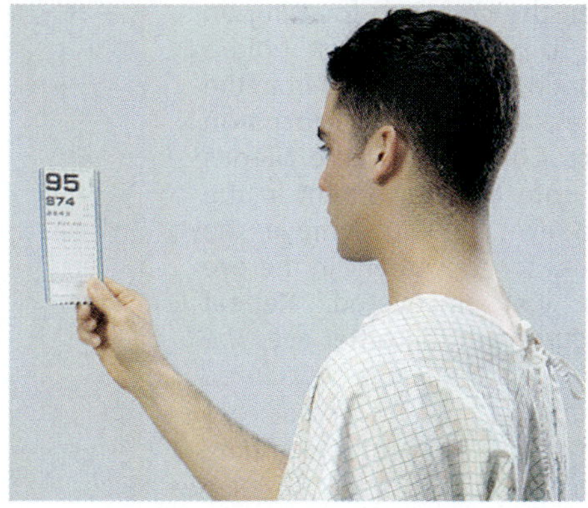

Figure 25–8 ■ Testing near vision using Rosenbaum eye chart.

Technique/Normal Findings	Abnormal Findings
Assess distant vision, using the Snellen or E chart. *When standing 20 feet from the chart, the client can read the smallest line of letters with or without corrective lenses (recorded as 20/20).*	■ Changes in distant vision are most commonly the result of **myopia** (nearsightedness). For example, a reading of 20/100 indicates impaired distance vision. A person has to stand 20 feet from the chart to read a line that a person with normal vision could read 100 feet from the chart.
Assess near vision, using a Rosenbaum chart or a card with newsprint held 12–14 inches from the client's eyes. *Normal near visual acuity is 14/14 with or without corrective lenses.*	■ Changes in near vision, especially in clients over age 45, can indicate **presbyopia**, impaired near vision resulting from a loss of elasticity of the lens related to aging. In younger clients, this condition is referred to as **hyperopia** (farsightedness).

(continued)

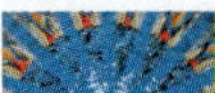

Eye and Vision Assessment (continued)

Technique/Normal Findings	Abnormal Findings

Eye Movement Assessment

Assess the cardinal fields of vision to gain information about extraocular eye movements. Ask the client to follow a pen or your finger while keeping the head stationary. Move the pen or your finger through the six fields one at a time, returning to the central starting point before proceeding to the next field (Figure 25–9 ■). *The eyes should move through each field without involuntary movements.*

- Failure of one or both eyes to follow the object in any given direction may indicate extraocular muscle weakness or cranial nerve dysfunction.
- An involuntary rhythmic movement of the eyes, nystagmus, is associated with neurologic disorders and the use of some medications.

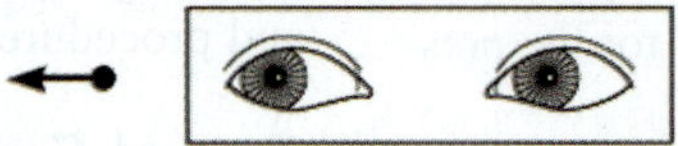

1 Penlight is to nurse's extreme left.

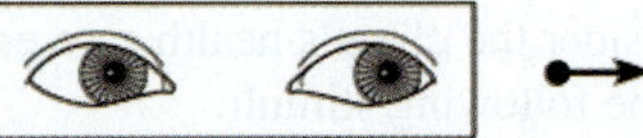

4 Penlight is to nurse's extreme right.

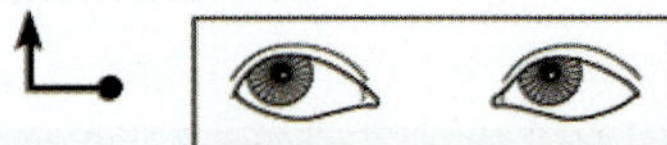

2 Penlight is left and up.

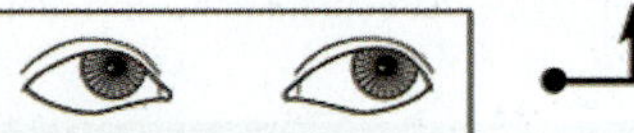

5 Penlight is right and up.

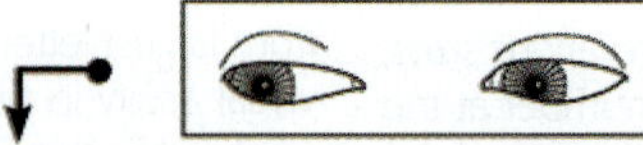

3 Penlight is left and down.

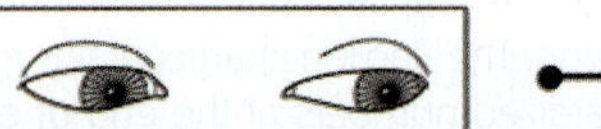

6 Penlight is right and down.

Figure 25–9 ■ The six cardinal fields of vision.

The cover–uncover test is a test for strabismus, a weakening of a muscle that causes one eye to deviate from the other when the person is focusing on an object. To conduct the test, hold a pen or your finger about 1 foot from the eyes and ask the person to focus on that object. Cover one of the client's eyes and note any movement in the uncovered eye; as you remove the cover, assess for movement in the eye that was just uncovered. Repeat the procedure with the other eye. *The uncovered eye should remain fixed straight ahead. The covered eye should remain fixed straight ahead after being uncovered.*

Assess convergence. *Ask the client to follow an object as you move it toward the client's eyes. Normally both eyes converge toward the center.*

- Failure of the eyes to converge equally on an approaching object may indicate a neuromuscular disorder or improper eye alignment.

Assess the corneal light reflex. *Direct a light source onto the bridge of the nose from 12 to 15 inches. Observe for equal reflection of the light from each eye.*

- Reflections of the light from different sites on the eyes reveal improper alignment.

Pupillary Assessment

Observe pupil size and equality. *Pupils should be of equal size, 3–5 mm.*

- Pupils that are unequal in size may indicate a severe neurologic problem, such as increased intracranial pressure.

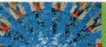

Eye and Vision Assessment (continued)

Technique/Normal Findings	Abnormal Findings
Assess direct and consensual pupil response. *Ask the client to look straight ahead. Shine a light obliquely into one eye at a time. Observe for constriction of the pupil in the illuminated eye. Test both eyes. To test consensual pupil response, again shine a light obliquely into one eye at a time as the client looks straight ahead. Observe constriction of the pupil in the opposite eye. The normal direct and consensual pupillary response is constriction.*	■ Failure of the pupils to respond to light may indicate degeneration of the retina or destruction of the optic nerve. ■ A client who has one dilated and unresponsive pupil may have paralysis of the oculomotor nerve. ■ Some eye medications may cause unequal dilation, constriction, or inequality of pupil size. Morphine and narcotic drugs may cause small, unresponsive pupils, and anticholinergic drugs such as atropine may cause dilated, unresponsive pupils.
Test for accommodation. *Hold an object at a distance of a few feet from the client. The pupils should dilate. Ask the client to follow the object as you bring it to within a few inches of the client's nose. The pupils should constrict and converge as they change focus to follow the object.*	■ Failure of accommodation along with lack of pupil response to light may signal a neurologic problem. ■ Lack of response to light with appropriate response to accommodation is often seen in clients with diabetes.

External Eye Assessment

Technique/Normal Findings	Abnormal Findings
Inspect the eyelids. *Eyelids should be the color of the client's facial skin, without redness, discharge, or drooping. The sclera should not be visible.*	■ Unusual redness or discharge may indicate an inflammatory state due to trauma, allergies, or infection. ■ Drooping of one eyelid, called **ptosis**, may be the result of a stroke, indicate a neuromuscular disorder, or be congenital (Figure 25–10 ■). ■ Unusual widening of the lids may be due to exophthalmos, protrusion of the eyeball. Exophthalmos is often associated with hyperthyroid conditions. ■ Yellow plaques noted on or near the lid margins are referred to as xanthelasma and may indicate high lipid levels. ■ An acute localized inflammation of a hair follicle is known as a hordeolum (sty) and is generally caused by staphylococcal organisms. ■ A chalazion is an infection or retention cyst of the meibomian glands.
Inspect the puncta. *The puncta should be free of redness or discharge.*	■ Unusual redness or discharge from the puncta may indicate an inflammation due to trauma, infection, or allergies.
Inspect the bulbar and palpebral conjunctiva. *The conjunctiva should be clear, moist, and smooth. The upper and lower palpebral conjunctiva should be clear, without redness or swelling.*	■ Increased erythema or the presence of exudate may indicate acute conjunctivitis. ■ A cobblestone appearance is often associated with allergies. ■ A fold in the conjunctiva, called a pterygium, may be seen as a clouded area that extends over the cornea. This is an abnormal growth of the bulbar conjunctiva, usually seen on the nasal side of the cornea. It may interfere with vision if it covers the pupil.
Inspect the sclera. *The sclera is white in Caucasians; people with darker skin normally have yellow sclera.*	■ Unusual redness may indicate an inflammatory state as a result of trauma, allergies, or infection. ■ Yellow discoloration of the sclera in clients with fair skin may be seen in conditions involving the liver, such as hepatitis. ■ Bright red areas in the sclera are often subconjunctival hemorrhages and may indicate trauma or bleeding disorders. They may also occur spontaneously.

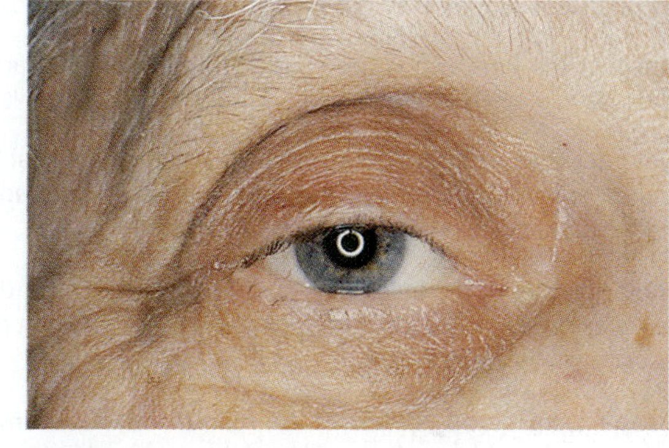

Figure 25–10 ■ Ptosis.

Source: Leonard Lessen/Peter Arnold, Inc. Custom Medical Stock Photo, Inc.

(continued)

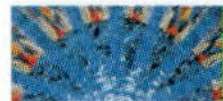

Eye and Vision Assessment (continued)

Technique/Normal Findings	Abnormal Findings
Inspect the cornea. *The cornea is normally transparent.*	■ Dullness, opacities, or irregularities of the cornea may be abnormal. ■ Corneal arcus is a thin, grayish-white arc seen toward the edge of the cornea. It is normal in older clients.
Assess corneal sensitivity. *Lightly touch a wisp of cotton to the client's cornea. This action should cause a corneal reflex (blinking the eye).*	■ Failure of the corneal reflex may indicate a neurologic disorder.
Inspect the iris. *The iris is normally round, flat, and evenly colored.*	■ Lack of clarity of the iris may indicate a cloudiness of the cornea. ■ Constriction of the pupil accompanied by pain and circumcorneal redness indicates acute iritis.
Internal Eye Assessment	
Assess internal structures of the eye by using the ophthalmoscope, an instrument that allows visualization of the lens, the vitreous humor, and the retina. Box 25–1 provides guidelines for using the ophthalmoscope.	
Inspect for the red reflex. *The red reflex should be clearly visible.*	■ Absence of a red reflex often indicates improper position of the ophthalmoscope, but also may indicate total opacity of the pupil by a cataract or a hemorrhage into the vitreous humor.
Inspect the lens and vitreous body. *The lens should be clear.*	■ A cataract is an opacity of the lens, often seen as a dark shadow on ophthalmoscopic examination. It may be due to aging, trauma, diabetes, or a congenital defect.
Inspect the retina. *There should be no visible hemorrhages, exudate, or white patches.*	■ Areas of hemorrhage, exudate, and white patches may be a result of diabetes or long-standing hypertension.
Inspect the optic disc. *The optic disc should be round to oval in shape with clear, well-defined borders.*	■ Loss of definition of the optic disc, as well as an increase in the size of the physiologic cup, is seen in papilledema from increased intracranial pressure.
Inspect the blood vessels of the retina. *The retinal blood vessels should be distinct.*	■ Glaucoma often results in displacement of blood vessels from the center of the optic disc due to increased intraocular pressure. ■ Hypertension may cause a narrowing of the vein where an arteriole crosses over. ■ Engorged veins may occur with diabetes, atherosclerosis, and blood disorders.
Inspect the retinal background. *The retina should be a consistent red-orange color, becoming lighter around the optic disc.*	■ Variations in color or a pale color overall may indicate disease.
Inspect the macula. *The macula should be visible on the temporal side of the optic disc.*	■ Absence of the fovea centralis is common in older clients. It may indicate macular degeneration, a cause of loss of central vision.
Palpate over the lacrimal glands, puncta, and nasolacrimal duct. *There should be no tenderness, drainage, or excessive tearing.*	■ Tenderness over any of these areas or drainage from the puncta may indicate an infectious process. (Wear gloves if you see any drainage.) ■ Excessive tearing may indicate a blockage of the nasolacrimal duct.

alone, (b) who visits and when, and (c) any signs indicating social deprivation. Signs of social deprivation may include withdrawal from contact with others to avoid embarrassment or dependence on others; negative self-image; reports of lack of meaningful communication with others; and absence of opportunities to discuss fears or concerns that facilitate coping mechanisms.

Physical Assessment

Physical assessment determines whether the senses are impaired. During the physical examination, the nurse assesses vision (including color vision) and hearing, and the olfactory, gustatory, tactile, and kinesthetic senses. The examination should reveal the client's specific visual and hearing abilities; perception of heat, cold, light touch, using pain in the limbs; and awareness of the position of the body parts. Specific sensory tests include the following:

- Visual acuity, using a Snellen chart or other reading material such as a newspaper, and visual fields, using picture charts for those with limited reading or language proficiency
- Hearing acuity, by observing the client's conversation with others and by performing the whisper test and the Weber and Rinne tuning fork tests

- Olfactory sense, by identifying specific aromas
- Gustatory sense, by identifying three tastes such as lemon, salt, and sugar
- Tactile sense, by testing light touch, sharp and dull sensation, two-point discrimination, hot and cold sensation, vibration sense, position sense, and stereognosis

If the client uses sensory adaptive devices such as eyeglasses or a hearing aid, the nurse should determine whether or not these function properly and if the client is compliant in using them.

Taste and Smell Assessment

One reason decreased sense of smell fails to be detected is that it is not adequately tested. Most physical examination records state "cranial nerves II–XII intact," completely omitting cranial nerve I. The nurse can examine the mucous

Ear and Hearing Assessment

Hearing Assessment

Tuning forks are used to determine whether a hearing loss is conductive or perceptive (sensorineural). Hold the tuning fork at the base and make it ring softly by stroking the prongs or by lightly tapping them on the heel of the opposite hand. The vibrating tuning fork emits sound waves of a particular frequency, measured in hertz (Hz). Tuning forks with a frequency of 512–1024 Hz are preferred for auditory evaluation, because that range corresponds to the range of normal speech.

Technique/Normal Findings	Abnormal Findings
Perform the Weber test. Place the base of a vibrating tuning fork on the midline vertex of the client's head (Figure 25–11 ■). Ask whether the client hears the sound equally in both ears or better in one than the other. *Sound is normally heard equally in both ears.*	■ Sound heard in, or lateralized to, one ear indicates either a conductive loss in that ear or a sensorineural loss in the other ear. The sound will be louder on the impaired side with a conductive hearing loss. The sound will be softer on the impaired side with a sensorineural hearing loss. Conductive losses may be due to a buildup of cerumen, an infection such as otitis media, or perforation of the eardrum.
Perform the Rinne test. Place the base of a vibrating tuning fork on the client's mastoid bone. Ask the client to indicate when the sound is no longer heard. When the client does so, quickly reposition the tuning fork in front of the client's ear close to the ear canal. Ask whether the client can hear the sound. If the client says yes, ask the client to indicate when the sound is no longer heard. Repeat over the opposite mastoid bone (Figure 25–12 ■). *The client with no conductive hearing loss will hear the sound twice as long by air conduction as by bone conduction.*	■ Bone conduction is greater than air conduction in the ear with a conductive loss. The normal pattern is AC > BC (air conduction greater than bone conduction).

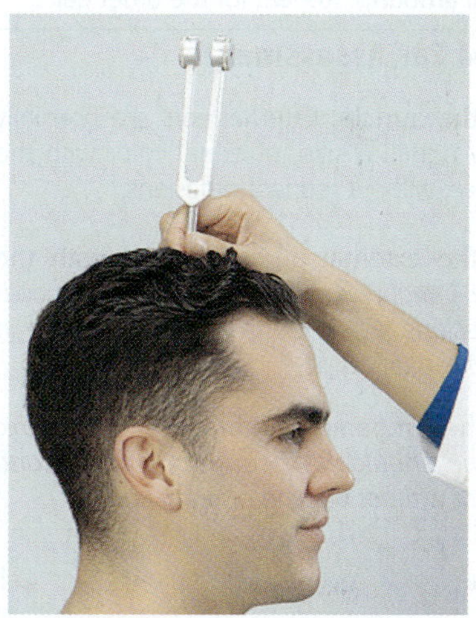

Figure 25–11 ■ Performing the Weber test with a tuning fork.

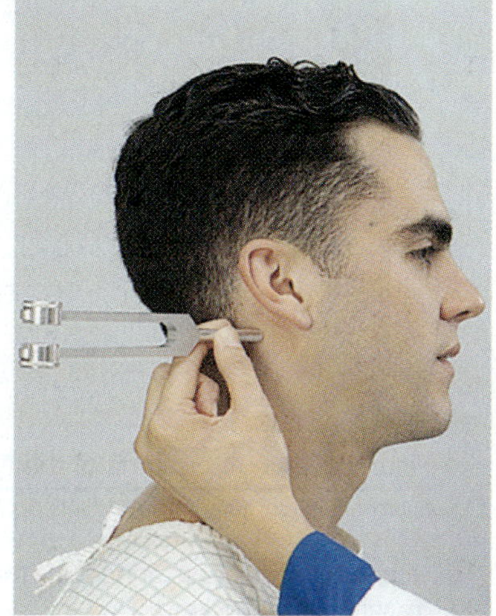

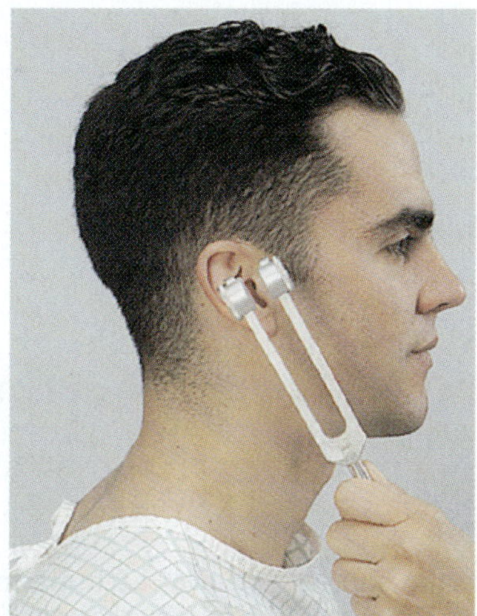

Figure 25–12 ■ Performing the Rinne test with a tuning fork.

(continued)

Ear and Hearing Assessment (continued)

Technique/Normal Findings	Abnormal Findings
Perform the whisper test. Ask the client to occlude one ear with a finger. Stand 1–2 feet away from the client, on the side of the unoccluded ear. Softly whisper numbers and ask the client to repeat them. Repeat the procedure, having the client occlude the other ear. Note whether you need to raise your voice or to stand closer to make the client hear you.	■ This test provides a rough estimate of hearing loss.
Use a tympanogram to measure the pressure of the middle ear and observe the tympanic membrane's response to waves of pressure. Insert the device into the ear canal. Ask the client not to speak, move, swallow, or jump when hearing a sound. Tell the client he or she will hear a loud tone as the measurements are taken. The normal pressure inside the middle ear is a 100 daPa (a very small amount). Repeat for the other ear.	■ Abnormal findings may include fluid in the middle ear, a perforated eardrum, impacted earwax, or a tumor of the middle ear.

External Ear Assessment

Inspect the auricle. External ears are normally bilaterally equal in size, of equal color with the client's face, without redness or lesions.

- Unusual redness or drainage may indicate an inflammatory response to infection or trauma.
- Scales or skin lesions around the rim of the auricle may indicate skin cancer.
- Small, raised lesions on the rim of the ear are known as tophi and indicate gout.

Inspect the external auditory canal with the otoscope. *Canal walls should be pink and smooth without lesions. Cerumen is normally present in small, odorless amounts.*

- Unusual redness, lesions, or purulent drainage may indicate an infection.
- Cerumen varies in color and texture, but hardened, dry, or foul-smelling cerumen may indicate an infection or an impaction of cerumen that requires removal. People with darker skin tend to have darker cerumen.

Inspect the tympanic membrane. *The tympanic membrane should be pearly gray, shiny, and translucent without bulging or retraction.*

- White, opaque areas on the tympanic membrane are often scars from previous perforations (Figure 25–13 ■).
- Inconsistent texture and color may be due to scarring from previous perforations caused by infection, allergies, or trauma.
- Bulging membranes are indicated by a loss of bony landmarks and a distorted light reflex. Such bulges may be the result of otitis media or malfunctioning auditory tubes.
- Retracted tympanic membranes are indicated by accentuated bony landmarks and a distorted light reflex. Such retraction is often due to an obstructed auditory tube.

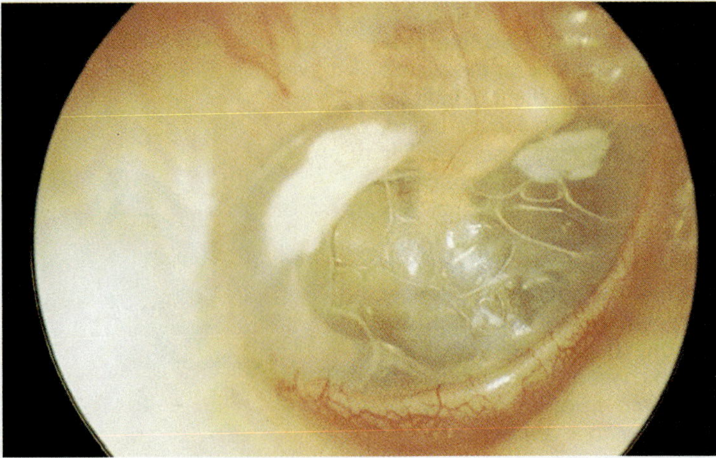

Figure 25–13 ■ Scarring of the tympanic membrane.

Source: Professor Tony Wright, Institute of Laryngology and Otology/SPL/Photo Researchers, Inc.

Palpate the auricles and over each mastoid process. *There should be no pain or swelling on palpation.*

- Tenderness, swelling, or nodules may indicate inflammation of the external auditory canal or mastoiditis.

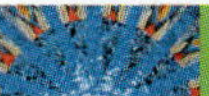

Cranial Nerve Assessment

Assessment	Findings
Test CN I (olfactory). Note client's ability to smell scents (e.g., soap, coffee) with each nostril. This test is usually done only if a problem with the ability to smell is reported. Sense of smell should be equal in both nostrils.	■ Anosmia (an inability to smell) may be seen with lesions of the frontal lobe and may also occur with impaired blood flow to the middle cerebral artery.
Assess ability to perceive various sensations. Touch both sides of various parts of the body (the chest, abdomen, arms, and legs) with one or more of the following: ■ Cotton wisp ■ Sharp object ■ Dull object ■ Vibrating tuning fork placed on bony prominences. Client should be able to differentiate between soft and sharp, and feel vibrations appropriately.	■ Decreased sensation of pain occurs with injury to the spinothalamic tract. ■ Decreased vibratory sensations are seen with injuries to the posterior column tract. ■ Transient numbness of face, arm, or hand is seen with TIAs. ■ Sensory loss on one side of the body is seen with lesions of higher pathways to the spinal cord. ■ Bilateral sensory loss is seen in polyneuropathy (a disease in which multiple peripheral nerves are affected, such as Guillain-Barré syndrome or diabetes mellitus). Sensations are impaired with strokes, brain tumors, and spinal cord trauma or compression.
Assess sense of position (kinesthesia). Move the client's finger or big toe up or down. Ask the client to describe the movement. Client should be able to accurately describe position of finger or toe when moved up or down.	■ Lesions of the posterior column of the spinal cord may affect sense of position.
Assess ability to discriminate fine touch. Ask the client to identify the following: 1. Object in hand, such as a coin or key (tests stereognosis) 2. Number written on hand (tests graphesthesia) 3. Two points of simultaneous pinpricks on the hand (tests two-point discrimination) 4. Where he or she is being touched (tests localization) 5. How many sensations are felt when touched simultaneously on both sides of the body (tests extinction). Client should be able to identify and discriminate fine touch.	■ Inability to discriminate fine touch (stereognosis, graphesthesia, two points, point localization, and extinction) may occur with injury to the posterior columns or sensory cortex.

membranes of the nares using a penlight or an otoscope and speculum, taking care not to touch the septum. The mucous membranes of the nares should be free from polyps, slightly red in color, and without ulceration or copious exudates. The nurse can then ask the patient to occlude one side of the nose, close the eyes, and identify a familiar smell such as vanilla, coffee, or an alcohol swab. This maneuver is repeated on the opposite side using a different odor. Using familiar odors enhances the validity of the test. Commercially prepared scratch-and-sniff tests are available in some smell assessment clinics. These tests contain over 40 odorants and provide more complete information regarding deficits in smell. Patients with obvious deficits in smell should be referred to their primary care provider, an otolaryngologist, and a neurologist.

DIAGNOSTIC TESTS

Diagnostic tests of the structure and functions of the eyes are used to diagnose a specific injury, disease, or vision problem; to provide information to identify or modify the appropriate medications or assistive devices used to treat the disease or problem; and to help nurses monitor the client's responses to treatment and nursing care interventions. Diagnostic tests of the eye,

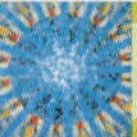

DEVELOPMENTAL CONSIDERATIONS Assessing Sensory Function in Children

INFANT SENSORY FUNCTION

An infant's sensory function is not routinely assessed. Withdrawal responses to painful stimuli indicate normal sensory function.

SUPERFICIAL TACTILE SENSATION

Stroke the skin on the lower leg or arm with a cotton ball or a finger while the child's eyes are closed. Cooperative children over 2 years of age can normally point to the location touched.

SUPERFICIAL PAIN SENSATION

Break a tongue blade to get a sharp point. After asking the child to close the eyes, touch the child in various places on each arm and leg, alternating the sharp and dull ends of the tongue blade. A paper clip may also be used. Children over 4 years of age can normally distinguish between a sharp and dull sensation each time. To improve the child's accuracy with the test, let the child practice telling you the difference between the sharp and dull stimulation.

An inability to identify superficial touch and pain sensation may indicate sensory loss. Identify the extent of sensory loss, such as all areas below the knee. Other sensory function tests (temperature, vibratory, deep pressure pain, and position sense) are performed when sensory loss is found.

especially for vision testing, are most often conducted in a health care provider's office. Diagnostic tests to assess the structure and functions of the eyes are described and summarized in the following bulleted list.

- Refractive errors (with prescription for corrective lenses) are evaluated by retinoscopy and/or refractometry. Pupils must be dilated for accurate diagnosis.
- Tonometry is used to identify and evaluate increased intraocular pressure, characteristic of glaucoma.
- A CT scan may be used to identify foreign objects or tumors of the eye.
- Scratches or injuries from foreign matter may be assessed by staining the sclera and examining the eye with an ultraviolet light.

Hearing evaluation includes gross tests of hearing (such as the whisper test), the Rinne and Weber tests, and audiometry. Diagnostic tests of the structure and functions of the ears are used to diagnose a specific injury, disease, or hearing problems; to provide information to identify or modify the appropriate medications or assistive devices used to treat the disease or problem; and to help nurses monitor the client's responses to treatment and nursing care interventions. Diagnostic tests of the ear, especially for hearing, are most often conducted in a health care provider's office. Sometimes, however, a speech therapist or audiologist may perform diagnostic tests of the ear in a school or educational setting. Diagnostic tests to assess the structure and functions of the ears are described and summarized in the following bulleted list:

- Rinne and Weber tests compare air and bone sound conduction. When bone conduction of sound is better than air conduction, the hearing deficit is a conductive loss. The Rinne test can identify even mild conductive hearing losses. If both air and bone conduction are impaired, a sensorineural loss is indicated.
- Audiometry identifies the type and pattern of hearing loss. Specific sound frequencies are presented to each ear by either air or bone conduction.
- Speech audiometry identifies the intensity at which speech can be recognized and interpreted. Speech discrimination evaluates the ability to discriminate among various speech sounds.
- Tympanometry is an indirect measurement of the compliance and impedance of the middle ear to sound transmission. The external auditory meatus is subjected to neutral, positive, and negative air pressure while the resultant sound energy flow is monitored.
- Acoustic reflex testing uses a tone presented at various intensities to evaluate movement of the structures of the middle ear.

Regardless of the type of diagnostic test, the nurse is responsible for explaining the procedure and any special preparation needed, for assessing for any medication use that might affect the outcome of the tests, for supporting the client during the examination as necessary, for documenting the procedures as appropriate, and for monitoring the results of the tests.

CARING INTERVENTIONS

Medical management of altered sensory perception is based on the cause and severity of the problem. The physician will prescribe medications or assistive devices such as eyeglasses and hearing aids. The nurse will teach the client appropriate use of any medication prescribed, and ensure that the client understands the importance of regular use of both medications and assistive devices. The nurse will employ caring interventions to assist the patient in meeting outcomes as defined in the client's care plan.

Common outcomes for clients with sensory-perception alterations include the following:

- Preventing injury
- Maintaining the function of existing senses
- Developing an effective method of communication
- Preventing sensory overload or deprivation
- Reducing social isolation
- Performing activities of daily living independently and safely.

Nurses can assist clients with sensory alterations by promoting healthy sensory function, adjusting environmental stimuli, and helping clients to manage acute sensory deficits. This includes helping clients access the resources necessary to obtain any assistive communication devices. Nurses also teach clients and families how to find freedom within the limitations imposed by the client's sensory loss. Clients with visual impairments, for example, may find comfort and joy in attending live music performances and in downloading reading material that has been converted into spoken word via the Internet. Clients with hearing impairments may experience frustration when talking on the phone, even if they have a hearing aid that works well. These clients may increase use of communication via e-mail and text messages in order to minimize frustration with audio communications.

Promoting Healthy Sensory Function

Children with chronic ear infections and people who live or work in an environment where the noise level is high should receive routine auditory testing. Women who are considering pregnancy should be advised of the importance of testing for syphilis and rubella, both of which can cause hearing impairments in newborns. Periodic vision screening of all newborns and children is recommended to detect congenital blindness, strabismus, and refractive errors (Ball & Bindler, 2006, p. 251).

Healthy sensory function can be promoted with environmental stimuli that provide appropriate sensory input. This input should vary and be neither excessive nor too limited. As many senses as possible should be stimulated. Various colors, sounds, textures, smells, and body positions can provide various sensations. Nurses can teach parents to stimulate infants and children, and teach family members to stimulate an elderly person and others in the home with sensory deficits. Nurses should explain that initially there may be some trial and error as parents and caregivers learn what materials and activities stimulate the family member as well as what the family member enjoys. Exercise and social activities often help stimulate the mind and the senses.

Nurses should also teach clients at risk of sensory loss how to prevent or reduce the loss. They should teach clients general health measures, such as getting regular eye examinations and controlling chronic diseases such as diabetes. Avoidance of risk factors, such as hot temperatures for the touch-impaired individual, is also critical.

Adjusting Environmental Stimuli

The client functions best when the environment is somewhat similar to that of the individual's ordinary daily life. Sometimes nurses need to take steps to adjust the client's environment to prevent either sensory overload or sensory deprivation.

Preventing Sensory Overload

For clients who are at risk of overstimulation, nurses should assist with reducing the number and type of environmental stimuli. The nurse can counteract sensory overload by blocking stimuli and by helping the client organize the stimuli and alter responses to the stimuli.

Dark glasses with ultraviolet (UV) light protection can partially block light rays, and a window shade or drape can reduce visual stimulation. Earplugs reduce auditory stimuli, as do soft background music and earphones. The odor from a draining wound can be minimized by keeping the dressing dry and clean and applying a liquid deodorant with gauze near the wound.

Another method of blocking stimuli is to reduce novelty and surprise and provide rest intervals free of interruptions. Sometimes the number of visitors and the length of visits must be restricted. Also, if the nurse carries out several nursing measures together, the client may need to have a scheduled quiet period before the next activity.

By explaining sounds in the environment, the nurse can help the client organize them mentally: A bell signals a change of shift; a beep, an IV alarm. When clients understand the meaning of environmental sounds, these stimuli become less confusing and more easily ignored. People can also learn through practice and feedback to alter their responses to the stimuli. Clients can employ relaxation techniques to reduce anxiety and stress despite continual sensory stimulation.

Preventing Sensory Deprivation

For clients who are at risk for sensory deprivation, nurses can increase environmental stimuli in a number of ways. For example, newspapers, books, music, and television can stimulate the visual and auditory senses. Providing objects that are pleasant to touch, such as a pet to stroke, can provide tactile and interactive stimulation. Clocks that differentiate night from day by color can help orient a client to time. The olfactory sense can be stimulated by the presence of fresh flowers or plants.

Arrangements should also be made for people to visit and talk with the client regularly. Many church and community groups provide visitors to "shut-ins," that is, people who are confined to their homes or who reside in nursing homes.

Managing Acute Sensory Deficits

When assisting clients who have a sensory deficit, the nurse needs to (a) encourage the use of sensory aids to support residual sensory function, (b) promote the use of other senses, (c) communicate effectively, and (d) ensure client safety.

SENSORY AIDS Many sensory aids are available for clients who have visual and hearing deficits. Examples are listed in Box 25–1. A popular, but expensive example, are service dogs. Service dogs both protect sensory impaired individuals from risk as well as assist them with activities of daily living, such as opening doors and fetching object. Raising and training service dogs can cost upwards of $40,000 before the dog is ready to go into active service. The cost along with the shortage of trainers sometimes results in long waiting lists for service dogs. Some training programs provide dogs to sensory-impaired individuals free of charge, but some do charge fees.

Sensory aids can be used in the health care setting as well as in the home. In all situations, the assistance of support people needs to be enlisted whenever possible to help the client deal with the deficit.

PROMOTING THE USE OF OTHER SENSES When one sense is lost, the nurse can teach the client to use other senses to supplement the loss. This stimulation is similar to that provided to prevent sensory deprivation, discussed earlier. However, the type of stimulation needs to be adapted in accordance with the client's specific deficit. For example, for the visually impaired client, stimulation of hearing, taste, smell, and touch can be encouraged. A radio, audiotapes of

Box 25–1 Sensory Aids for Visual and Hearing Deficits

VISUAL
- Eyeglasses of the correct prescription, clean and in good repair
- Adequate room lighting, including night-lights
- Sunglasses or shades on windows to reduce glare
- Bright contrasting colors in the environment
- Magnifying glass
- Phone dialer with large numbers
- Clock and wristwatch with large numbers
- Color code or texture code on stoves, washer, medicine containers, and so on
- Colored or raised rims on dishes
- Reading material with large print
- Braille or recorded books
- Seeing-eye dog

HEARING
- Hearing aid in good order
- Lip reading
- Sign language
- Amplified telephones
- Telecommunication device for the deaf (TDD)
- Amplified telephone ringers and doorbells
- Flashing alarm clocks
- Flashing smoke detectors

music or books, clocks that chime, music boxes, and wind chimes can be used for auditory stimulation. Diets that include a variety of flavors, temperatures, and textures can be planned to stimulate the taste buds. Taking sips of water between foods and eating foods separately can enhance the taste sensation. Fresh flowers, scented candles (safely used), room fragrances, brewing coffee, and baking can stimulate the sense of smell. Clients can also be encouraged to remember pleasant or familiar odors such as the perfume of sweet peas. Measures such as providing a hug, massage, hair brushing, grooming, different textures in clothing and upholstery fabrics, and pets can be taken to stimulate touch receptors.

COMMUNICATING EFFECTIVELY Communication with clients who have sensory deficits should convey respect, enhance the person's self-esteem, and ensure the exchange of correct information. A person with a hearing impairment has to concentrate more than other people and therefore tires more readily. Fatigue compounded by an illness can further reduce the person's ability to hear. A person with impaired vision is unable to observe most nonverbal cues during communication and relies largely on the spoken word and tone of voice. Guidelines for communicating with people who are visually or hearing impaired are shown in Box 25–2.

SAFETY CONSIDERATIONS Client teaching regarding safety for the sensory impaired client is a critical intervention for the nurse. Safety prevention techniques and devices vary depending on the nature of the impairment.

Impaired Vision For clients with visual impairments, nurses should provide (in a health care setting) and teach clients and families the importance of (for use at home) the following:
- An uncluttered environment with plenty of lighting
- Clear pathways (chairs pushed under tables, things put away); furniture should not be arranged without orienting the client
- Organizing self-care articles within the client's reach

Box 25–2 Communicating With Clients Who Have a Visual or Hearing Deficit

VISUAL DEFICIT
- Always announce your presence when entering the client's room and identify yourself by name.
- Stay in the client's field of vision if the client has a partial vision loss.
- Speak in a warm and pleasant tone of voice. Some people tend to speak louder than necessary when talking to a blind person.
- Always explain what you are about to do before touching the person.
- Explain the sounds in the environment.
- Indicate when the conversation has ended and when you are leaving the room.

HEARING DEFICIT
- Before initiating conversation, convey your presence by moving to a position where you can be seen or by gently touching the person.
- Decrease background noises (e.g., television) before speaking.
- Talk at a moderate rate and in a normal tone of voice. Shouting does not make your voice more distinct and in some instances makes understanding more difficult.
- Address the person directly. Do not turn away in the middle of a remark or story. Make sure the person can see your face easily and that it is well lighted.
- Avoid talking when you have something in your mouth, such as chewing gum. Avoid covering your mouth with your hand.
- Keep your voice at about the same volume throughout each sentence without dropping the voice at the end of each sentence.
- Always speak as clearly and accurately as possible. Articulate consonants with particular care.
- Do not "overarticulate"; mouthing or overdoing articulation is just as troublesome as mumbling. Pantomime or write ideas, or use sign language or finger spelling as appropriate.
- Use longer phrases, which tend to be easier to understand than short ones. For example, "Would you like a drink of water?" presents much less difficulty than "Would you like a drink?" Word choice is important: "Fifteen cents" and "fifty cents" may be confused, but "half a dollar" is clear.
- Pronounce every name with care. Make a reference to the name for easier understanding, for example, "Joan, the girl from the office" or "Sears, the big downtown store."
- Change to a new subject at a slower rate, making sure that the person follows the change to the new subject. A key word or two at the beginning of a new topic is a good indicator.

FOCUS ON DIVERSITY AND CULTURE Vision Impairment and Older Adults

The most common vision diseases affecting older adults are macular degeneration, glaucoma, cataract, and diabetic retinopathy.

- Age-related macular degeneration (ARMD) is the most common cause of new cases of vision impairment in people older than 65. It is the leading cause of vision impairment in adults 75 and older. The prevalence of ARMD is the same for African Americans and Caucasians up to age 75, with rates higher for Caucasians after 75.
- African Americans are three to four times more likely to have open-angle glaucoma.
- People of Asian descent and Eskimos are more likely to have closed-angle glaucoma.
- Diabetic retinopathy is more prevalent among African Americans, Hispanics, and Native Americans than Caucasians.

Source: From Horowitz, A. (2004). The prevalence and consequences of vision impairment in later life. *Topics in Geriatric Rehabilitation, 20*(3), pp. 185–195. Reprinted with permission.

- Orienting the client to a new location when traveling or running errands
- Keeping call lights and assistive devices within easy reach
- Assisting with ambulation (as necessary) by standing at the client's side, walking about one foot ahead, and allowing the person to grasp your arm. Confirm whether the client prefers grasping your arm with the dominant or nondominant hand.

Research has established an association between vision impairment and greater disability in activities of daily living (e.g., bathing, dressing, eating) and instrumental tasks (e.g., shopping, housekeeping) (Horowitz, 2004). Studies have also shown that visual impairment increases the risk of depression among older adults living in the community (Horowitz, 2003, 2004). Explanations for this relationship vary. One explanation is that vision loss leads to increased disability, which leads to depression. Another explanation is that loss of vision causes fear—a fear of losing one's autonomy and becoming dependent on another or others. Visual loss also affects how a person obtains information (e.g., reading the newspaper). In addition, reading is often a leisure activity and its loss can affect a person's quality of life. It is important for the nurse to be aware of and assess for signs of depression and intervene as appropriate if an older adult is experiencing depression as a result of a visual impairment.

Impaired Hearing Clients with hearing impairments who are unable to hear the alarms of IV pumps and cardiac monitors need to be assessed frequently. They can be taught to use their visual sense to identify kinks in the IV tubing or a loose electrocardiogram (ECG) lead, and so on. For home safety, clients with impaired hearing need to obtain devices that either amplify sounds or respond with flashing lights to sounds such as a doorbell or smoke detector, a baby crying, or a burglar alarm. The sounds of doorbells and alarm clocks may be amplified or changed to a lower frequency or buzzerlike sound. These devices can be obtained from hearing aid dealers, telephone companies, and appliance stores.

Impaired Olfactory Sense Clients with an impaired sense of smell should be taught about the dangers of cleaning with chemicals such as ammonia. Because a gas leak can go undetected, clients should keep gas stoves and heaters in good working order. Strong chemicals such as ammonia used in confined spaces such as a bathroom may affect the client before they are smelled. Food poisoning is a concern with clients who have difficulty detecting spoiled meat or dairy products. Clients need to carefully inspect food for freshness (check its color and texture) and check expiration dates on food packages.

Impaired Tactile Sense Clients with an impaired sense of touch may not be aware of hot temperatures, which can cause burns, or pressure on bony prominences, which can produce pressure ulcers. Clients with decreased sensation to temperature should have the temperature adjusted on their hot water heater and test water temperature with a thermometer before bathing. Clients with decreased sensation to pressure must change their position frequently.

PHARMACOLOGIC THERAPIES

The eye is vulnerable to a variety of conditions, many of which can be prevented, controlled, or reversed with proper treatment. A simple scratch can cause the client almost unbearable discomfort as well as concern about the effect the damage may have on vision. Other eye disorders may be more bearable, but extremely dangerous—including glaucoma, one of the leading causes of preventable blindness in the world. Although medications cannot cure glaucoma, many clients with open-angle glaucoma can control intraocular pressure and preserve vision indefinitely with medications. Medications are used alone or in combination with the timing and dosage individually determined by pressure measurements. The primary pharmacologic agents used to treat glaucoma are topical beta-adrenergic blocking agents, adrenergics (mydriatics), prostaglandin analogs, or carbonic anhydrase inhibitors. An oral carbonic anhydrase inhibitor also may be used.

Clients suffering from macular degeneration may benefit from medications that slow the formation of new blood vessels. Photodynamic therapy, in which a light-activated drug is injected in the body, may be used. When macular degeneration does not improve with medications, laser surgery to destroy affected blood vessels may be indicated.

Treatment of olfactory impairment generally may be resolved by treating the underlying cause of the impairment. However, olfactory impairment sometimes presents with the onset of serious illnesses, such as diabetes, hypertension, and Parkinson's disease. Treatment of the underlying disease does not always restore olfactory function.

MEDICATIONS Antiglaucoma Drugs

Drug Classifications	Mechanism of Action	Commonly Prescribed Drugs	Nursing Considerations
■ Prostaglandins	Drugs for glaucoma work by one of two mechanisms: increasing the outflow of aqueous humor at the canal of Schlemm or decreasing the formation of aqueous humor at the ciliary body. Many agents for glaucoma act by affecting the autonomic nervous system	■ bimatoprost (Lumigan) ■ latanoprost (Xalatan) ■ travoprost (Travatan) ■ unoprostone isopropyl (Rescula)	■ Assess and note eye color, presence of inflammation, exudates, or pain. ■ Note vital signs and most recent liver function test results because these may be altered by the drug.
■ Beta-adrenergic blockers		■ betaxolol (Betoptic) ■ carteolol (Ocupress) ■ levobunolol (Betagan) ■ metipranolol (OptiPranolol) ■ timolol (Betimol, Timoptic, and others)	■ Assess the client for allergies or contraindications to beta-blocker therapy, including asthma, chronic obstructive pulmonary disease (COPD), heart block, and heart failure. ■ Maintain pressure over the lacrimal sac after administration to prevent systemic absorption. ■ Assess for side effects such as bradycardia, hypotension, and depression. ■ Teach about the drug, its dose, administration, and desired and side effects.
■ $Alpha_2$-adrenergic agonists		■ apraclonidine (Iopidine) ■ brimonidine tartrate (Alphagan)	■ Assess the client for contraindications and adverse reactions to adrenergic agonists, including acute angle-closure glaucoma, hypertension, cardiac dysrhythmias, and coronary heart disease. ■ Assess for central nervous system side effects of anxiety, nervousness, and muscle tremors. If these side effects are severe, notify the physician. ■ Assess for a hypersensitivity reaction, including itching, lid edema, and discharge from the eyes. Notify the physician if you notice these signs.
■ Carbonic anhydrase inhibitors		■ acetazolamide (Diamox) ■ brinzolamide (Azopt) ■ methazolamide (Neptazane)	■ Assess for allergies or other contraindications to the use of carbonic anhydrase inhibitors, including known allergy to sulfa, or severe renal or hepatic disease. ■ Monitor for increased drug interactions of amphetamines, procainamide, quinidine, tricyclic antidepressants, and ephedrine and pseudoephedrine. ■ Assess daily weight, intake and output, serum electrolytes, and vital signs in clients taking oral or parenteral carbonic anhydrase inhibitors. ■ Administer PO in the morning to prevent sleep disruption because of the diuretic effect. ■ If used with another topical ophthalmic, administer 10 minutes apart. ■ Teach the client about the drug, its dose, administration, and desired and side effects.

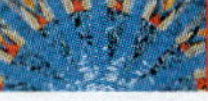

25.1 HEARING IMPAIRMENT

KEY TERMS

Decibels, *1651*

Tinnitus, *1652*

BASIS FOR SELECTION OF EXEMPLAR

Healthy People 2010

LEARNING OUTCOMES

After reading about this exemplar, you will be able to:

1. Describe the pathophysiology, etiology, clinical manifestations, and direct and indirect causes of hearing impairment.
2. Identify risk factors associated with hearing impairment.
3. Illustrate the nursing process in providing culturally competent care across the life span for individuals with hearing impairment.
4. Formulate priority nursing diagnoses appropriate for an individual with hearing impairment.
5. Create a plan of care for an individual with hearing impairment and their family members.
6. Assess expected outcomes for an individual with hearing impairment.
7. Discuss therapies used in the collaborative care of an individual with hearing impairment.
8. Employ evidence-based caring interventions for an individual with hearing impairment.

OVERVIEW

Approximately one million children in the United States have some form of hearing impairment. Hearing loss is present in 2 out of every 1,000 births (Moore, 2006; Yaeger et al., 2006). These hearing impairments are expressed in terms of **decibels** (dB), which are units of loudness, and rated according to severity (Table 25–4). Children who have only a mild hearing loss (35–40 dB) may miss as much as 50% of everyday conversation and are considered at high risk for difficulty in school. Anyone with a hearing loss of more than 90 dB is considered legally deaf.

Hearing loss is a significant problem for adults as well, affecting an estimated 10% of adults in the United States (Kasper et al., 2005). The problem of hearing loss is particularly significant in older adults, affecting about 30–35% of people between the ages of 65 and 74, and more than 40% of those over age 75 (National Institute on Deafness and Other Communication Disorders, 2005d). As many as 70% of nursing home residents have impaired hearing.

Hearing loss impairs the ability to communicate in a world filled with sound and hearing individuals. A hearing deficit can be partial or total, congenital or acquired. It may affect one or both ears. In some types of hearing loss, the ability to perceive sound at specific frequencies is lost. In others, hearing is diminished across all frequencies.

PATHOPHYSIOLOGY AND ETIOLOGY

Etiology

Lesions in the outer ear, middle ear, inner ear, or central auditory pathways can result in hearing loss. The process of aging also can affect the structures of the ear and hearing. Hearing loss is classified as conductive, sensorineural, or mixed, depending on what portion of the auditory system is affected. Profound deafness is often a congenital condition.

CONDUCTIVE HEARING LOSS Anything that disrupts the transmission of sound from the external auditory meatus to the inner ear results in a conductive hearing loss. The most common cause of conductive hearing loss is obstruction of the external ear canal. Impacted cerumen, edema of the canal lining, stenosis, and neoplasms all may lead to canal obstruction. Other causes of conductive loss include a perforated tympanic membrane, disruption or fixation of the ossicles of the middle ear, fluid, scarring, and tumors of the middle ear. Conductive loss also occurs if the tympanic membrane does not fully vibrate, as in otitis media. In these cases, loss may be restored after the infection clears. Chronic and untreated ear infections may lead to ear structural changes and permanent hearing impairment. The loss of acuity may be gradual or rapid and results in diminished hearing in all ranges.

TABLE 25–4 **Severity of Hearing Loss**

TYPE OF LOSS	DECIBEL LEVEL (DB)	HEARING ABILITY
Slight/mild	26–40	Some speech sounds are difficult to perceive, particularly unvoiced consonant sounds
Moderate	41–60	Most normal conversational speech sounds are missed
Severe	61–80	Speech sounds cannot be heard at a normal conversational level
Profound	81–90	No speech sounds can be heard
Deaf	>90	No sound at all can be heard

SENSORINEURAL HEARING LOSS Disorders that affect the inner ear, the auditory nerve, or the auditory pathways of the brain may lead to a sensorineural hearing loss. In this type of hearing loss, sound waves are effectively transmitted to the inner ear. In the inner ear, however, lost or damaged receptor cells, changes in the cochlear apparatus, or auditory nerve abnormalities decrease or distort the ability to receive and interpret stimuli. Conditions leading to sensorineural hearing loss may be congenital, genetic, or acquired. In sensorineural hearing loss, high-frequency sounds are most affected.

A significant cause of sensorineural hearing deficit is damage to the hair cells of the organ of Corti. In the United States, noise exposure is the major cause. Damage may result from either loud impulse noise (e.g., an explosion) or loud continuous noise (e.g., machinery). Exposure to a high level of noise (e.g., standing close to the stage or speakers at a rock concert) on an intermittent or continuing basis damages the hair and supporting cells of the organ of Corti. Ototoxic drugs also damage the hair cells; when combined with high noise levels, the damage is greater and resultant hearing loss more profound.

PRACTICE ALERT

Ototoxic drugs include aspirin, furosemide (Lasix), aminoglycosides, streptomycin, vancomycin (Vancocin), antimalarial drugs, and chemotherapy such as cisplatin (Platinol). Other potential causes of sensory hearing loss include prenatal exposure to rubella, viral infections, meningitis, trauma, Ménière's disease, and aging.

Tumors such as acoustic neuromas, vascular disorders, demyelinating or degenerative diseases, infections (bacterial meningitis in particular), or trauma may affect the central auditory pathways and produce a neural hearing loss

PRESBYCUSIS With aging, the hair cells of the cochlea degenerate, producing a progressive sensorineural hearing loss. In presbycusis, hearing acuity begins to decrease in early adulthood and progresses as long as the individual lives. Higher-pitched tones and conversational speech are lost initially.

Risk Factors

About 50% of hearing loss in children is genetically caused, usually with a recessive inheritance pattern with GJB2 gene abnormalities (Yaeger et al., 2006). Another 25% is due to environmental causes around the time of birth; the remainder is due to unknown causes. Although many infants with hearing loss have no known risk factors, identified risks include the following:

- Family history of congenital hearing loss*
- Positive titer for TORCH infections (toxoplasmosis, rubella, cytomegalovirus, syphilis, herpes)
- Craniofacial abnormalities
- Very low birth weight (<1500 g)*
- Bilirubin greater than 16 mg/dL
- Aminoglycoside medication administration for more than 5 days
- Low Apgar score at 1 or 5 min*
- Bacterial meningitis
- Mechanical ventilation for over 5 days
- Presence of syndromes associated with hearing loss (Down syndrome, Pierre Robin syndrome, Arnold-Chiari malformation)*

*Primary risk factors (Chu et al., 2003).

CLINICAL MANIFESTATIONS

Conductive hearing loss involves an equal loss of hearing at all sound frequencies. If the level of sound is greater than the threshold for hearing, speech discrimination is good. Because of this, the client with a conductive hearing loss benefits from amplification by a hearing aid.

Sensorineural hearing losses typically affect the ability to hear high-frequency tones more than low-frequency tones. This loss makes speech discrimination difficult, especially in a noisy environment. Hearing aids are often not useful, because they amplify both speech and background noise. The increased sound intensity may actually cause discomfort for the client.

Because the hearing loss of presbycusis is gradual, the client and family may not realize the extent of the deficit. The individual with a hearing impairment may be described as unsociable or paranoid. The family may worry that the person is becoming increasingly forgetful, absentminded, or perhaps "senile." Depression, confusion, inattentiveness, tension, and negativism have been noted in older adults with hearing impairments. Functional problems such as poor general health, reduced mobility, and impaired interpersonal communication are also associated with hearing loss. Caregivers need to be alert for signs of impaired hearing such as cupping an ear, difficulty understanding verbal communication when the person cannot see the speaker's face, difficulty following conversation in a large group, and withdrawal from social activities. Hearing aids and other amplification devices are useful for most clients with presbycusis.

Tinnitus

Tinnitus is the perception of sound or noise in the ears without stimulus from the environment. The sound may be steady, intermittent, or pulsatile and is often described as a buzzing, roaring, or ringing.

Tinnitus usually associated with hearing loss (conductive or sensorineural); however, the mechanism producing the sound is poorly understood. It is often an early symptom of noise-induced hearing damage and drug-related ototoxicity. Tinnitus is especially associated with salicylate, quinine, or quinidine toxicity. Other etiologies include obstruction of the auditory meatus, presbycusis, middle or inner ear inflammations and infections, otosclerosis, and Ménière's disease. Most tinnitus, however, is chronic and has no pathologic importance.

Early identification of hearing loss is a key element in successful treatment. Detection of hearing loss in infants is important to ensure optimal development. Clients need to know the risk for hearing damage and how to prevent it. Awareness of the effects of noise exposure, especially when combined with the ototoxic effects of aspirin or other drugs, is important in preventing sensorineural hearing loss.

CLINICAL MANIFESTATIONS AND THERAPIES Hearing Impairment

ETIOLOGY	CLINICAL MANIFESTATIONS	CLINICAL THERAPIES
Conductive hearing loss	■ Equal loss of hearing at all sound frequencies	■ Hearing aid ■ Treat underlying condition, such as infection in otitis media ■ Surgery
Sensorineural hearing loss	■ Lesser ability to hear high-frequency tones more than low-frequency tones ■ Difficulty discriminating speech	■ Cochlear implant
Presbycusis	■ Personality manifestations, such as depression, confusion, forgetfulness, not being sociable; poor health, reduced mobility, withdrawal; signs of impaired hearing, such as cupping an ear	■ Hearing aid
Tinnitus Mechanism not fully understood, etiology varies to include noise, ototoxicity; infection or inflammation, underlying conditions such as Ménière's disease	■ Buzzing, roaring, or ringing in the ears	■ Treat underlying cause ■ Tinnitus maskers such as ambient noise

COLLABORATION

If hearing loss in a client is uncorrectable, a multidisciplinary team should be formed to assist the client and family with adaptation to the disability. Team members may include any of the following: physician, nurse, a speech/language, occupational or physical therapist, an audiologist, a teacher, a social worker, and family members and caregivers. The team may provide strategies and accommodations for a client whose loss is correctable until surgery is completed or other treatments take effect. Therapists and social workers can often assist clients in accessing assistive technology devices at relatively low cost, especially if they are not covered by insurance, as well as help the client learn how to use these tools.

Amplification

A hearing aid or other amplification device can help many clients with hearing deficits. These assistive devices do nothing to prevent, minimize, or treat the hearing loss itself. They amplify the sound presented to the hearing apparatus of the ear, which may bring the level of sound above the hearing threshold, allowing more accurate perception and interpretation of its meaning. When sound perception is distorted, a hearing aid may be less helpful, because it simply amplifies the distorted sound.

Unfortunately, less than one-fifth of older clients with a hearing deficit have or use a hearing aid. Denial of the deficit, other health problems, poor visual acuity, decreased manual dexterity, and cost all contribute to this low usage. Cost is another factor. Typically health insurance and will cover only one pair of hearing aids within a certain time frame, and in most states Medicare does not pay for hearing aids at all. Some clients choose not to pay for hearing aids. Hearing aids must be individually prescribed by an audiologist. Proper design, proper fit, and regular maintenance are necessary for their effectiveness.

All hearing aids include a microphone, amplifier, speaker, earpiece, and volume control. Many include an option to turn off the microphone when using the telephone; others can be adjusted for the client's pattern of hearing loss. Hearing aids are available in a variety of styles, each with advantages and disadvantages:

- Canal hearing aids (in-the-canal and completely-in-canal) are the least noticeable style, fitting in the ear canal. They are appropriate for mild to moderately severe hearing loss. These small and unobtrusive devices allow use of the telephone and can be worn during exercise. Because of their small size, the client must have good manual dexterity to insert, clean, and change the batteries in canal hearing aids. For this reason, older clients or clients with impaired dexterity may be unable to use them.
- The in-ear style of hearing aid fits into the external ear and is used for mild to severe hearing loss (Figure 25–14 ■). Its larger size makes manipulation somewhat easier, although it

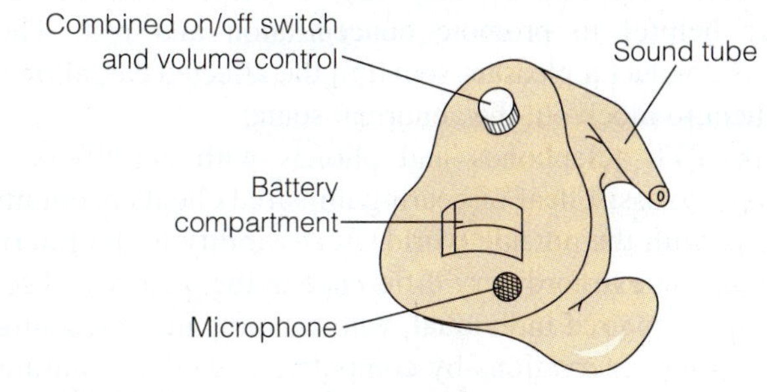

Figure 25–14 ■ An in-ear hearing aid.

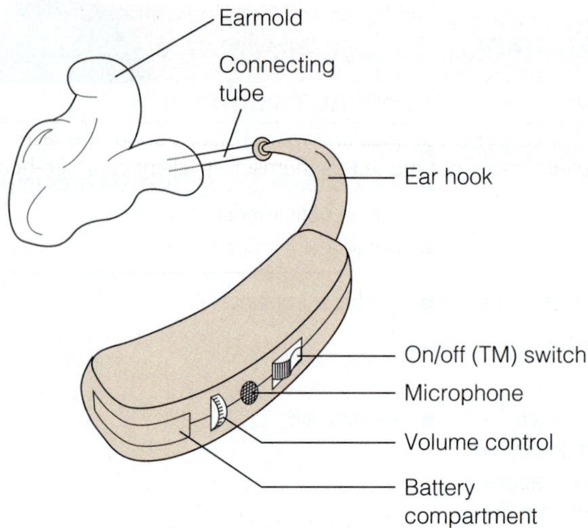

Figure 25–15 ■ A behind-ear hearing aid.

still may be difficult for less dexterous individuals. A greater degree of amplification is possible with the in-ear aid. Many have a toggle switch for telephone usage.

- The behind-ear hearing aid allows finer adjustment of the level of amplification and is easier for the client to manipulate (Figure 25–15 ■). The device can be used by clients with mild to profound hearing loss. For the client who wears glasses, this style can be modified, with all components fitting into the temple of the eyeglasses.
- Clients with profound hearing loss may require a body hearing aid. The microphone and amplifier of this aid are contained in a pocket-sized case that the client clips on to clothing, slips into a pocket, or carries in a harness. The receiver is attached by a cord to the case and clips onto the ear mold, which delivers the sound to the ear canal.

With both the in-canal and in-ear style, cleaning is important. Small portals may become plugged with cerumen, interfering with sound transmission.

For the client who does not have a hearing aid, an *assistive listening device*, or "pocket talker," with a microphone and "Walkman"-type earpieces, is useful. Pocket talkers are available over-the-counter or through an audiologist and are relatively inexpensive. The earpiece requires no special fitting, and the external microphone allows the client to focus on the desired sound rather than simply amplifying all sounds. Assistive listening devices may also be used in conjunction with a hearing aid.

Clients with tinnitus may find a white noise–masking device helpful to promote concentration and rest. These devices conduct a pleasant sound to the affected ear, allowing the client to block out the abnormal sound.

TTD/TTY telephones and phones with amplifiers are available to assist deaf or hearing impaired clients in communicating with the outside world. Accessibility to the Internet can make an extraordinary difference in the quality of life to a hearing impaired individual, who can now make restaurant and airplane reservations by computer, as well as communicate by e-mail.

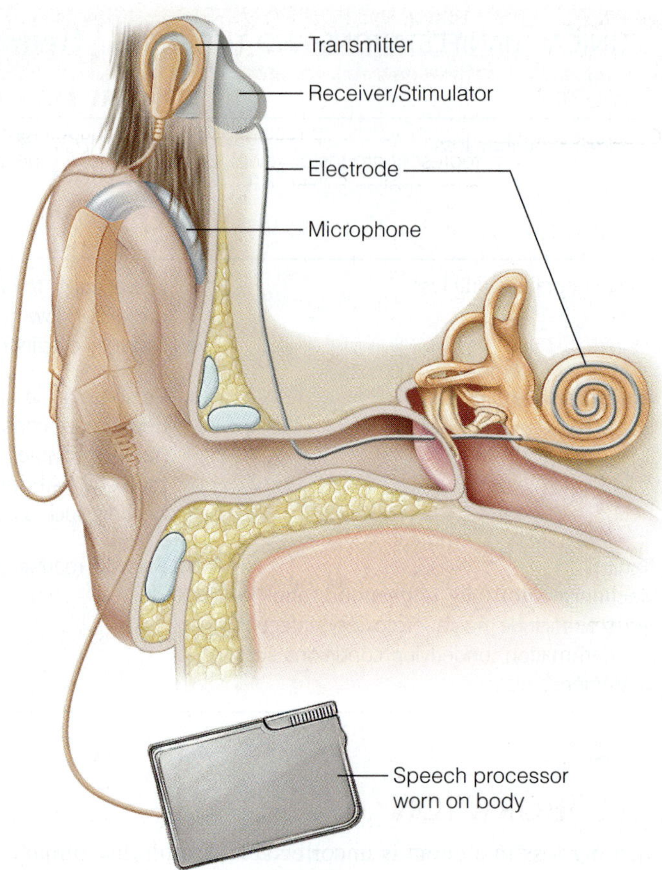

Figure 25–16 ■ A cochlear implant for sensorineural hearing loss.

Surgery

Reconstructive surgeries of the middle ear, such as a stapedectomy or tympanoplasty, may help restore hearing with a conductive hearing loss. Stapedectomy is the removal and replacement of the stapes. This procedure is used to treat hearing loss related to otosclerosis.

In a tympanoplasty, the structures of the middle ear are reconstructed to improve conductive hearing deficits. Chronic otitis media with necrosis and scarring of the middle ear is a common indication for this type of surgery.

For the client with a sensorineural hearing loss, a *cochlear implant* may be the only hope for restoring sound perception. The cochlear implant consists of a microphone, speech processor, transmitter and receiver/stimulator, and electrodes (Figure 25–16 ■). Its function is more similar to the way the ear normally receives and processes sounds than it is to that of a hearing aid. The microphone picks up sounds, sending them to the speech processor, which selects and processes those that are useful. The transmitter and receiver/stimulator receive signals from the speech processor, convert them to electrical impulses, and send these impulses to the electrodes for transmission to the brain.

Cochlear implants provide sound perception but not normal hearing. The client is able to recognize warning sounds such as automobiles, sirens, telephones, and doors opening or closing. Clients also receive stimuli to alert them to incoming communication so they can focus on the person speaking. Many

TABLE 25–5 **Communication Techniques for Clients Who Are Hearing Impaired**

TECHNIQUE	DESCRIPTION
Cued speech	Supplement to lip-reading; eight hand shapes represent groups of consonant sounds and four positions about the face represent groups of vowel sounds; based on the sounds the letters make, not the letters themselves; client can "see-hear" every spoken syllable a hearing person hears.
Oral approach	Uses only spoken language for face-to-face communication; avoids use of formal signs; uses hearing aids and residual hearing.
Total communication	Uses speech and sign, finger-spelling, lip-reading, and residual hearing simultaneously; client selects communication technique depending on the situation.
Sign language	A separate or foreign language that allows the user to communicate quickly and accurately with others who understand signs. The signs or hand movements represent words or concepts. When a sign is not available, the word can be spelled out using signs. American Sign Language (ASL) is most often used; British Sign Language (BSL) is common in Europe.

clients learn to interpret perceived sounds as words, especially when the hearing loss is acquired as an adult.

For uncorrectable hearing loss, several approaches are used to enhance communication (Table 25–5). Clients with hearing impairment may receive speech therapy and instructions in lip-reading, signing, cuing, and finger-spelling.

NURSING PROCESS

In planning and implementing nursing care for the client with a hearing deficit, the type and extent of hearing loss, the client's adaptation to the loss, and the availability of assistive hearing devices are considered, as well as the client's ability and willingness to use assistive devices.

Assessment

- *Health history.* Perceived ability to hear; effect of hearing loss on function and lifestyle; risk factors such as use of ototoxic medications; upper respiratory tract or frequent ear infection; noise exposure; presence of vertigo, tinnitus, unsteadiness, or imbalance
- *Physical examination.* Apparent perception of normal speech; inspection of external ear, tympanic membrane; whisper, Rinne, and Weber tests; tests of balance and cranial nerve function

Diagnoses

Possible nursing diagnosis for the client with hearing impairment may include the following:

- Disturbed Sensory Perception: Auditory
- Impaired Verbal Communication
- Social Isolation.

Planning and Implementation

Disturbed Sensory Perception: Auditory

Whether the client's hearing deficit is partial or total, impaired sound perception is the primary problem. The client needs to understand what causes the deficit and what to expect for the future. Nursing interventions focus on maximizing available hearing and preventing further deterioration to the extent possible.

- Encourage the client to talk about the hearing loss and its effect on activities of daily living. Hearing loss affects each individual in a different way. The client may be denying the extent of the deficit or grieving the loss. Listening and providing support encourage the client to develop coping strategies.
- Provide information about the type of hearing loss. Refer to an audiologist for evaluation of the hearing loss and possible exploration of amplification devices. With improved understanding of the deficit, the client can plan ways to compensate.
- Replace batteries in hearing aids regularly and as needed. Hearing aid batteries last approximately 1 week. If a battery is old or has been improperly stored, the life may be reduced further.
- If the hearing aid has a toggle switch for microphone/telephone, be sure it is in the appropriate position. This ensures proper amplification with the hearing aid.
- Talk with the family members about techniques they can use to make communication with the client easier. The same techniques the nurse employs, as listed in Box 25–2, can be used by family members.

PRACTICE ALERT

Check hearing aids for patency, cleaning out cerumen as necessary.

Impaired Verbal Communication

A hearing deficit impairs the client's ability to receive and interpret verbal communication. A hearing loss affects the client's ability to follow conversations, use the telephone, and enjoy television or other forms of entertainment.

- Use the following techniques to improve communication:
  a. Wave the hand or tap the shoulder before beginning to speak.
  b. If the client wears corrective lenses, ensure that they are clean, and encourage the client to wear them.
  c. When speaking, face the client and keep your hands away from your face.
  d. Keep your face in full light.
  e. Reduce the noise in the environment before speaking.
  f. Use a low voice pitch with normal loudness.
  g. Use short sentences and pause at the end of each sentence.
  h. Speak at a normal rate, and do not overarticulate.
  i. Use facial expressions or gestures.
  j. Provide a magic slate for written communication.

Individuals with hearing impairments often lip-read, making good visibility of the speaker's face necessary. Excessive environmental noise interferes with the ability to perceive the message. Higher tones are typically lost with presbycusis and other types of hearing loss. Using short sentences and pausing give the client time to interpret the message. Overarticulating makes it more difficult to follow the flow and to lip-read. Nonverbal cues and written messages enhance the client's understanding.

- Be sure hearing aid is properly placed, is turned on, and has fresh batteries. The client may not be aware that the hearing aid is not functioning well.
- Do not place intravenous catheters in the dominant hand. The client may need to use that hand to write.
- Rephrase sentences when the client has difficulty understanding. Hearing losses may affect different sound tones, making some words more difficult to comprehend. Using alternative words and phrases may increase the client's ability to perceive the message.
- Repeat important information. The nurse must make sure that the client understands the information.
- Inform other staff about the client's hearing deficit and effective strategies for communication. Consistent use of effective strategies for communication decreases the client's frustration.

Social Isolation

The client with impaired hearing often becomes socially isolated. This isolation may be self-imposed because of difficulty communicating, especially in a group. Often, however, the isolation comes about gradually and without intention. The client finds social settings such as family dinners or community gatherings increasingly difficult. Friends and family become frustrated trying to communicate with someone who has a hearing impairment, and invitations to participate in social activities dwindle.

- Identify the extent and cause of the social isolation. Help to differentiate the reality of the isolation and its cause from the client's perception of isolation. Clients with impaired hearing may be unaware that they are isolated. Identifying factors that contribute to isolation may provide the needed impetus to remedy the hearing loss. Clients may also experience paranoid thinking as a result of impaired communication and believe that friends and family have purposely begun to avoid interactions.
- Encourage client to interact with friends and family on a one-to-one basis in quiet settings. Clients with impaired hearing are more successful in understanding conversations that take place in small groups and quiet settings.
- Treat client with dignity and remind friends and family that a hearing deficit does not indicate loss of mental faculties. Inappropriate responses due to a hearing deficit can cause others to perceive the client as "stupid" or demented.
- Involve client in activities that do not require acute hearing, such as checkers and chess. The client has an opportunity to interact socially without the stress of straining to hear.
- Obtain a pocket talker or encourage the client and family to do so.
- Refer the client to an audiologist for evaluation and possible hearing-aid fitting.
- Refer to resources such as support groups and senior citizen centers. These groups provide new social outlets.

Community-Based Care

Teaching for home and community-based care for the client with hearing loss focuses on managing the deficit and developing coping strategies. Referral to an audiologist for evaluation of the deficit and the usefulness of a hearing aid may be appropriate. In addition, discuss the following topics as appropriate for each client:

Evaluation

Expected outcomes of nursing care for a client with hearing impairment include the following:

- The client will demonstrate successful establishment of a communication method.
- The client will manifest growth and developmental milestones to maximum potential.
- The client and family will demonstrate positive methods of coping.

REVIEW Hearing Impairment

RELATE: LINK THE CONCEPTS

Linking the exemplar of Sensory Perception with the concept of Development:

1. When caring for a young child who receives a cochlear implant after being deaf from birth to age 5, how will the child's speech patterns differ from the normal 5 year old?
2. What strategies can the nurse employ to help this 5-year-old client improve speech patterns?

Linking the exemplar of Hearing Impairment with the concept of Cognition:

3. How might hearing loss impact an older client's cognition?
4. What can the nurse implement to promote cognition in the hearing impaired older adult?

READY: GO TO COMPANION SKILLS MANUAL

- Assessing the ears and hearing

REFLECT: CASE STUDY

Mrs. Smith is an 87-year-old woman who recently moved into an assisted living home after hospitalization for uncontrolled diabetes. She enjoyed reading, but for a long time she has not been able to read due to poor vision acuity. During the admission assessment, the nurse also documents a hearing loss.

1. Discuss the importance of a thorough sensory assessment in this client.
2. Describe the benefits of improving Mrs. Smith's sensory deficits.
3. What recommendations will the nurse make to Mrs. Smith to improve her hearing?
4. How does diabetes mellitus impact her sense of hearing?

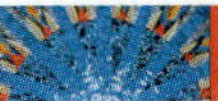

25.2 CATARACTS

KEY TERMS

Cataract, *1657*
Congenital cataracts, *1657*
Extracapsular extraction, *1658*
Radiation cataracts, *1657*
Secondary cataracts, *1657*
Traumatic cataracts, *1657*

BASIS FOR SELECTION OF EXEMPLAR

Healthy People 2010

LEARNING OUTCOMES

After reading about this exemplar, you will be able to:

1. Describe the pathophysiology, etiology, clinical manifestations, and direct and indirect causes of cataracts.
2. Identify risk factors associated with cataracts.
3. Illustrate the nursing process in providing culturally competent care across the life span for individuals with cataracts.
4. Formulate priority nursing diagnoses appropriate for an individual with cataracts.
5. Create a plan of care for individuals with cataracts and their family members.
6. Assess expected outcomes for an individual with cataracts.
7. Discuss therapies used in the collaborative care of an individual with cataracts.
8. Employ evidence-based caring interventions for an individual with cataracts.

OVERVIEW

A **cataract** is an opacification (clouding) of the lens of the eye; it can significantly interfere with light transmission to the retina and the ability to perceive images clearly. Cataracts are a common cause of visual deficits, and by age 80, nearly half of the population is affected. In many cases, however, cataracts do not significantly impair vision.

PATHOPHYSIOLOGY AND ETIOLOGY

Pathophysiology

The majority of cataracts are senile cataracts, formed as a result of the aging process. As the lens ages, its fibers and proteins change and degenerate. The proteins clump, clouding the lens and reducing light transmission to the retina. This process generally begins at the periphery of the lens, gradually spreading to involve the central portion. As the cataract continues to develop, the entire lens may become opaque. When only a portion of the lens is affected, the cataract is called immature. A mature cataract is opacity of the entire lens. In addition to clouding, the lens may discolor over time, affecting the ability to accurately discriminate colors.

Four types of cataracts occur independent of the aging process. **Secondary cataracts** can form after surgery to treat another eye disorder, such as glaucoma, or as an effect of medication or another primary disorder. Clients who require regular or recurring doses of corticosteroids, for example, are at risk for secondary cataracts. **Traumatic cataracts** may result from an injury to the eye. **Radiation cataracts** may result from long-term exposure to radiation. **Congenital cataracts** may appear in a child at birth or in childhood, usually in both eyes (National Eye Institute, 2009a).

Etiology

The prevalence of cataracts in the United States increases rapidly with aging.

- 2.5% (just over 1 million) of adults ages 40–49 are affected.
- This increases to more than 2 million (or 6.8%) of those ages 50–59 and nearly doubles to over 4 million (or 20%) of adults ages 60–69.
- 68.3% of adults ages 80 and older (over 6 million) are affected by cataracts (National Eye Institute, 2004).

Risk Factors

Age is the greatest single risk factor for cataracts. Genetics may contribute to the risk, although the link is unclear. Environmental and lifestyle factors play a role. Long-term exposure to sunlight (UVB rays) increases the risk for cataracts; cigarette smoking and heavy alcohol consumption are associated with earlier cataract development. Eye trauma, including injury to the lens capsule by a foreign body, blunt trauma, or exposure to heat or radiation, can precipitate cataract formation. Diabetes mellitus is associated with earlier development of cataracts, especially when the blood glucose

DEVELOPMENTAL CONSIDERATIONS Cataracts in Children

- Some cataracts are present at birth, whereas others are acquired during childhood.
- Some of the causes of acquired cataracts include retinopathy of prematurity, metabolic diseases such as galactosemia, and long-term use of corticosteroids.
- A major cause of congenital cataracts in the past was congenital rubella syndrome, the mother's infection with rubella during gestation. Now that children and women receive the rubella vaccine, there are very few cases of cataracts due to congenital rubella syndrome.

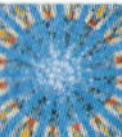

FOCUS ON DIVERSITY AND CULTURE Blindness

Blindness affects African Americans more often than white Americans and Hispanics. Cataracts and glaucoma are responsible for more than 50% of cases of blindness in African Americans. Beginning at age 40, African Americans should have a comprehensive dilated eye exam at least every 2 years (National Women's Health Center, 2008). Unfortunately, due to disparities in access to health services, this population is less likely to seek preventive eye care. Nurses working with these clients should inquire about the frequency of eye examinations at each health care interaction.

level is not carefully controlled at or near normal levels. Certain drugs, such as systemic or inhaled corticosteroids, chlorpromazine (Thorazine), and busulfan (Myleran) also prompt the formation of cataracts.

CLINICAL MANIFESTATIONS

Cataracts tend to occur bilaterally unless related to eye trauma. Fortunately, they tend to develop at different rates, and one cataract generally matures more rapidly than the other. As a cataract interferes with light transmission through the lens, visual acuity decreases, affecting both close and distance vision (Figure 25–17 ■). Light rays are scattered as they pass through the lens, causing complaints of glare. Glare affects the ability to adjust between light and dark environments. Color discrimination is impaired, particularly in the blue to purple range. When the cataract is mature, the pupil may appear cloudy gray or white rather than black.

The diagnosis of a cataract is made based on the history and eye examination. Ophthalmoscopic examination confirms the diagnosis by identifying the location and extent of a cataract. As the cataract matures, ophthalmoscopy reveals a dark area instead of the red reflex.

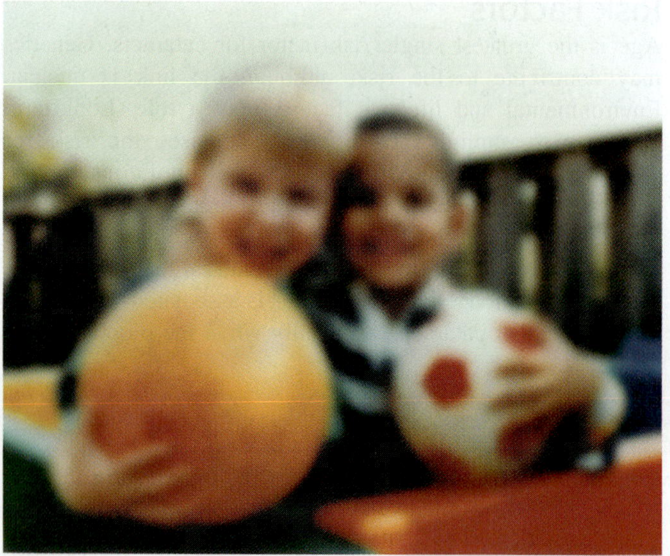

Figure 25–17 ■ A scene as viewed by a client with cataracts.

Source: Courtesy of National Eye Institute, National Institutes of Health.

COLLABORATION

Surgery

Surgical removal is the only treatment used at this time for cataracts; no medical treatment is available to prevent or treat them. If the client presents with bilateral cataracts, surgery is performed on only one eye at a time. If an intraocular lens (an artificial lens to replace the diseased lens of the eye) is to be implanted during surgery, the corneal curvature and anteroposterior diameter of the eye are measured prior to surgery. This allows the health care team to determine the lens power needed for the intraocular lens implant.

Surgical removal of the cataract and lens is indicated when the cataract has developed to the point that vision and activities of daily living are affected. A mature cataract also may be removed when it causes a secondary condition such as glaucoma or uveitis.

Cataract surgery typically is done on an outpatient basis using local anesthesia. If general anesthesia is required, the client may be hospitalized overnight. The entire lens and its surrounding capsule may be removed in a procedure called *intracapsular extraction*. Intracapsular extraction is rarely used today (Way & Doherty, 2003). **Extracapsular extraction**, in which the anterior capsule, nucleus, and cortex of the lens are removed leaving the posterior capsule intact, is the procedure of choice (Figure 25–18 ■). Using an operating microscope, the surgeon makes a small incision at the edge of the cornea and extracts the lens intact or via emulsification and aspiration. In the latter technique, ultrasound vibrations are used to break the lens material into fragments (phacoemulsification), which are then suctioned out of the eye. Phacoemulsification lens removal requires a smaller incision and usually is preferred over extracting the lens intact. (Way & Doherty, 2003). The remaining capsule supports the lens implant and protects the retina.

After removal of the lens, the eye can no longer focus light on the retina and vision is seriously affected. Usually a polymethylmethacrylate (PMMA or Plexiglas) intraocular lens is implanted at the time of surgery. This implant rapidly restores binocular vision and depth perception. Following extracapsular lens removal, the intraocular lens is positioned in the posterior capsule behind the iris (Figure 25–18).

If an intraocular lens cannot be implanted, convex corrective glasses or contact lenses may be used to correct vision after cataract removal. Although contact lenses can provide excellent vision correction following cataract surgery, they

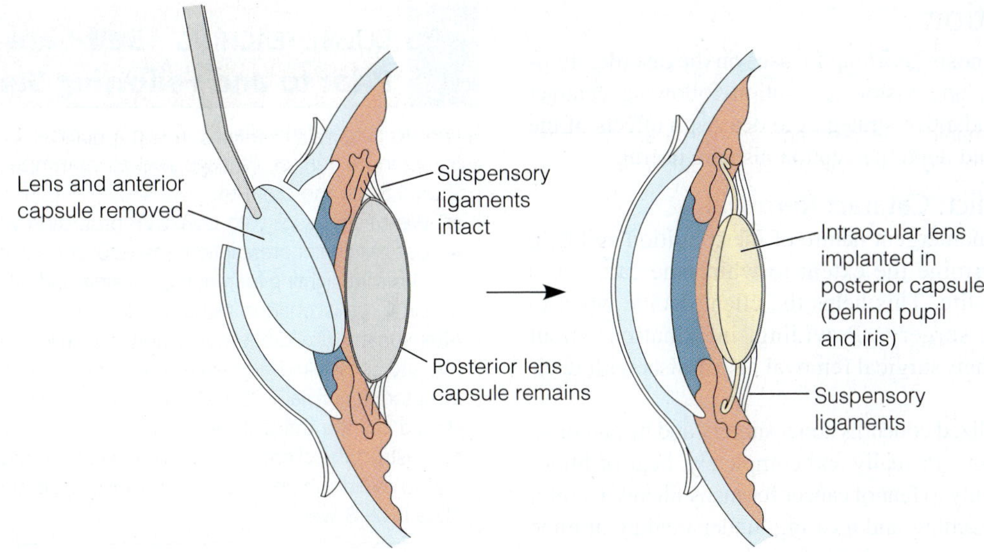

Figure 25–18 ■ Extracapsular cataract extraction with removal of the lens and anterior capsule, leaving the posterior capsule intact. The intraocular lens is implanted within the posterior capsule.

may be difficult for some clients to adapt to or manipulate. The client with a preexisting refractive error may continue to require corrective lenses and often needs a prescriptive change after surgery.

Complications of cataract surgery are unusual and occur in less than 1% of the surgeries. Potential complications include loss of vitreous humor, corneal edema, increased intraocular pressure, hemorrhage, inflammation or infection, retinal detachment, and displacement of the implanted lens. Up to 35% of clients who undergo extracapsular extraction may develop opacification of the remaining posterior capsule. Vision can be restored using laser capsulotomy (creation of an opening for light to pass through the opacified capsule) or surgical incision into the posterior capsule to allow light to reach the retina (Kasper et al., 2005; Way & Doherty, 2003).

Complementary and Alternative Therapies

Insufficient data exists to support the treatment of cataracts with alternative therapies. Some clients may find that acupuncture relieves perceived symptoms of discomfort, but there is no sufficient evidence to support the use of acupuncture to treat cataracts. Some complementary and alternative medicine (CAM) practitioners believe that antioxidants improve cataracts because they reduce the amount of free radicals that can cause damage to the eyes. It is thought that there may be a link between lactose and cataracts formation, but more studies in this area need to be conducted.

NURSING PROCESS

Advise all clients about the importance of protecting their eyes by wearing eye protection during activities, such as welding, and by wearing sunglasses with UVA/UVB protection when out of doors. Discuss the link between heavy smoking and cataract development. Provide education about anti-tobacco use for young people and resources for smokers to help them stop smoking.

Assessment

- *Health history.* Effect of vision changes on lifestyle and activities (e.g., ability to read, watch television, participate in work and recreational activities); history of smoking, diabetes, use of prescription drugs associated with increased risk of cataract.
- *Physical examination.* General health; visual acuity (using corrective lenses and Snellen chart) in each eye; presence of red reflex, cloudy gray or white pupil.

Diagnosis

The client with cataracts has few physical care nursing needs. Patient advocacy, psychologic and emotional support, and teaching/learning needs are typically of higher priority for these clients.

Nursing diagnoses for the client with cataracts may include the following:

- Decisional Conflict: Cataract Removal
- Risk for Ineffective Therapeutic Regimen Management
- Disturbed Sensory Perception: Visual.

Plan

Appropriate outcomes for the client diagnosed with cataracts include the following:

- Client will be able to articulate an understanding of the reasons for and risks involved with surgery.
- Client will participate in self-care activities to protect eyes from further damage and to maximize safety.
- Client will follow self-care instructions following surgery to ensure healing and to maximize benefits of surgery.

Implementation

With the initial diagnosis, teaching focuses on the disorder, indications for surgery, and vision restoration following cataract removal. Teaching adaptive strategies to deal with effects of the cataract on vision and depth perception also are useful.

Decisional Conflict: Cataract Removal

- Explain the nonemergent nature of the condition and help the client determine the extent to which the cataract is affecting daily life. This helps the client decide when to proceed with surgery. Providing information about cataracts and their surgical removal also assists with decision making.
- Attend to verbalized concerns about surgery and its outcome. Address questions factually and completely. Fear of blindness is second only to fear of cancer for many clients. Careful listening and teaching and a caring, understanding attitude can help the client deal with this fear prior to surgery.

Risk for Ineffective Therapeutic Regimen Management

- Assess for factors that may interfere with the client's ability to provide self-care postoperatively. A chronic condition that may affect the ability to administer eyedrops, such as arthritis, may indicate the need to include a family member in teaching.
- Assess for other care needs that may be impacted by vision changes in the early postoperative period. Other care needs, such as insulin injections, may suggest the need for home health or nursing care postoperatively.

When surgery is scheduled, provide pre- and postoperative teaching. Include a significant other in teaching sessions. Reinforce the following information with written instructions:

- Limitations such as avoiding reading, lifting, bending to pick up objects, strenuous activity, and sleeping on operative side
- Importance of not disturbing the eye dressing
- Prescribed medications and side effects
- Importance of follow-up appointments
- Manifestations of postoperative complications such as eye pain, decreased visual acuity or other change in vision, headache, nausea, or itching and redness of the affected eye
- Administration of eyedrops and application of eye patch or shield
- Care, insertion, and removal of contact lenses as appropriate
- Visual changes associated with thick-lensed eyeglasses as appropriate.

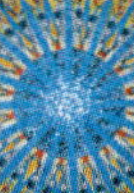

CLIENT TEACHING Self-Care Activities Prior to and Following Surgery

Prior to surgery, the client can use a number of self-care activities to minimize further damage and to maximize safety. The nurse should teach the client to:

- Wear sunglasses with UVA/UVB protection when outdoors.
- Use reading or prescription glasses or contact lenses as necessary.
- Maximize lighting for reading, cooking, and other indoor activities.
- Limit or discontinue nighttime driving.

After surgery, the client may experience mild to moderate discomfort and some fluid discharge. The nurse should explain that these symptoms normally subside in 1 or 2 days but that the client should call the office if the symptoms persist or become intolerable. Instruct the client to continue to wear eye protection as ordered and to avoid rubbing the eye. In most cases, healing will be complete in 7–8 weeks.

For more information about perioperative nursing care, please see the Appendicitis exemplar in Concept 16, Inflammation.

Care in the Community

Care of the client in the community revolves around prevention.

- Encourage clients with diabetes, previous history of visual problems, or disorders that require frequent use of corticosteroids to see an ophthalmologist at least every 2 years.
- Encourage clients who smoke to enroll in a smoking cessation program.
- Encourage all clients to use appropriate eye protection when using tools and when spending time outside.
- Conduct an eye and vision assessment at each health care interaction with clients ages 65 years and older; inquire about any problems with vision and date of last appointment with an ophthalmologist or optometrist.

Evaluation

Expected outcomes for the client with cataracts include the following:

- The client will make an informed decision regarding cataract surgery.
- The client will verbalize concerns about home care.
- The client will verbalize appropriate home care activities.
- The client will demonstrate correct medication administration.

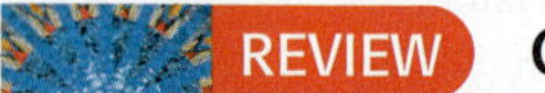

REVIEW Cataracts

RELATE: LINK THE CONCEPTS

The nurse is caring for a client undergoing surgery for cataracts. The client is 78-years-old and lives alone on a third-floor walk-up with no elevator.

Linking the exemplar of Cataracts with the concept of Safety:

1. What safety issues will the nurse address when teaching this client?
2. What issues place this client at increased risk for injury?

Linking the exemplar of Cataracts with the concept of Development:

3. How might the development of cataracts interfere with the older adult's ability to meet developmental milestones?
4. Prior to cataract repair, what interventions might the nurse initiate to help the older adult meet his or her developmental needs?

READY: GO TO COMPANION SKILLS MANUAL

- Assessing the eyes and vision

REFER: GO TO MYNURSINGKIT

REFLECT: CASE STUDY

Mary Martin, a 75-year-old widow with osteoporosis, has an appointment with her ophthalmologist this week. The ophthalmologist notes that Mary's cataracts continue to worsen and recommends that she consider surgery. Mary does not admit the fact that she is afraid to have surgery on her eyes. She tells the doctor that she might have the surgery at some point but that she is too busy to do it right now. The physician gives Mary a new prescription for her eyeglasses, knowing that this will help her vision at least for a little while. Mary is told to increase the amount of light and to use reading glasses or a magnifying glass for reading.

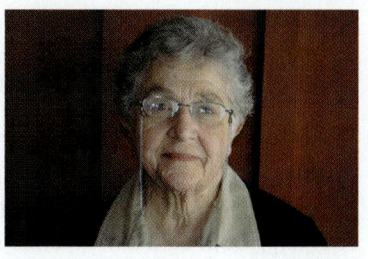

1. What nursing diagnosis would be appropriate for this client?
2. How will the nurse address the client's concerns regarding surgery?
3. What factors may impact Mary's home care?

25.3 EYE INJURIES

KEY TERMS

Aphakia, *1662*
Blepharism, *1665*
Corneal abrasion, *1661*
Enophthalmos, *1662*
Hyphema, *1662*
Penetrating injury, *1662*
Perforating injury, *1662*
Pneumatic retinopexy, *1664*
Retinal detachment, *1664*
Scleral buckling, *1664*

BASIS FOR SELECTION OF EXEMPLAR

Emergency department visits

LEARNING OUTCOMES

After reading about this exemplar, you will be able to:

1. Describe the pathophysiology, etiology, clinical manifestations, and direct and indirect causes of eye injuries.
2. Identify risk factors associated with eye injuries.
3. Illustrate the nursing process in providing culturally competent care across the life span for individuals with eye injuries.
4. Formulate priority nursing diagnoses appropriate for an individual with an eye injury.
5. Create a plan of care for individuals with an eye injury and their family members.
6. Assess expected outcomes for an individual with an eye injury.
7. Discuss therapies used in the collaborative care of an individual with an eye injury.
8. Employ evidence-based caring interventions for an individual with an eye injury.

OVERVIEW

Any part of the eye, especially the exposed parts, may be affected by trauma. Foreign bodies, abrasions, and lacerations are the most common types of eye injury. Traumatic injury also may be due to a burn, penetrating object, or blunt force.

PATHOPHYSIOLOGY AND ETIOLOGY

Etiology

As discussed in the About section, eye injuries are fairly common in children, especially in children ages 9–11 years. Boys from 11–15 years have 4 times more eye injuries than girls. Eye injuries from playing sports are so common among children that the American Society for Testing and Materials has developed standards for protective eyewear for various sports. While it is recommended that children and adolescents wear eye goggles particular to their sport, it is most important that they wear protective gear made with polycarbonate lenses (Wu, 2005).

Eye injuries result in more than $300 million each year in medical expenses, loss of production time, and workers' compensation. A number of Occupational Safety and Health Administration (OSHA) regulations exist to protect employees who work in environments that are hazardous to the eyes (Occupational Safety and Health Administration, 2008).

Risk Factors

Sports, darts, fireworks, air-powered BB guns, blunt and sharp objects, chemical and thermal burns, physical irritants, and abuse may cause eye trauma (Behrman, Kliegman, & Jenson, 2004). Recreational activities, such as sports and projectile toys, are common causes of eye injuries. The most common injuries occur in baseball, basketball, swimming, bicycling, and football (Center for Health and Health Care in Schools, 2004).

Older children may be injured by chemicals in school science laboratories. Adults who fail to wear protective eyewear while working outside or using tools also risk injury to the eyes.

CLINICAL MANIFESTATIONS

Corneal Abrasion

Corneal abrasion is disruption of the superficial epithelium of the cornea. Objects commonly causing corneal abrasion include contact lenses, eyelashes, small foreign bodies such as dust and dirt, and fingernails. Drying of the eye surface and chemical irritants also may result in a corneal abrasion.

Superficial abrasions of the cornea are extremely painful but generally heal rapidly without complication or scarring.

Photophobia and tearing are commonly present. When the stroma is damaged by a deep abrasion or laceration, there is an increased risk of infection, slowed healing, and scar formation.

Burns

The outer surface of the eye may be subjected to burns caused by heat, radiation, or explosion, but chemical burns are most common. Both acid and alkaline substances can burn the eye. Ammonia, products that contain lye (such as oven and drain cleaners), acids from car batteries, and other sources are often implicated in eye injuries. Burns caused by alkaline substances are particularly serious because tiny particles of the chemical may remain in the conjunctival sac, causing progressive damage. Acid causes rapid damage to the eye, but generally causes less serious burns than alkaline substances.

Explosions and flash burn injuries pose the greatest risk for thermal burns of the eye. Ultraviolet rays also can cause corneal damage ranging in severity from mild to extensive. Depending on the source of the ultraviolet light, these burns may be referred to as snowblindness, welder's arc burn, or flash burn.

The client who experiences a burn to the eye will give a history of face and eye contact with a caustic substance or another burning agent and will complain of eye pain and decreased vision. The client's eyelids may be swollen; his or her face and lips may be affected. The appearance of the client's eye may vary depending on the type of burn. Typically, the conjunctiva is reddened and edematous. Sloughing may be seen, particularly with chemical burns. The cornea often appears cloudy or hazy, and ulcerations may be evident.

Penetrating Trauma

Perforation of the eye occurs from a variety of causes. Metal flakes or other particles produced by high-speed drilling or grinding, glass shards, or other substances may penetrate the eye. Gunshots (including BBs), arrows, and knives can penetrate the eye. In a **penetrating injury**, the layers of the eye spontaneously reapproximate after entry of a sharp-pointed object or small missile (e.g., a BB) into the globe. These injuries may not be readily apparent when the eye is inspected. In a **perforating injury**, the layers of the eye do not spontaneously reapproximate, resulting in rupture of the globe and potential loss of ocular contents (Way & Doherty, 2003).

Penetrating injuries may be hidden because of tissue swelling. They may be missed when the client has other significant injuries that command attention. When the eyelid is lacerated or has a puncture wound, it is vital to inspect the underlying eye tissue for possible damage. Eye perforations cause pain, partial or complete loss of vision, and possibly bleeding or extrusion of eye contents.

Blunt Trauma

Sports injuries are a common cause of blunt trauma to the eye, which may be struck with a ball (a baseball, tennis ball, racquetball, and handball are frequently implicated) or injured during contact sports such as basketball, football, boxing, and wrestling. Motor vehicle crashes, falls, and physical assault are examples of other causes of blunt eye trauma.

Blunt trauma may lead to a minor eye injury such as lid ecchymosis (black eye) or subconjunctival hemorrhage, which is caused by rupture of a blood vessel in the conjunctiva. With subconjunctival hemorrhage, a well-defined bright area of erythema appears under the conjunctiva. No pain or discomfort is associated with the hemorrhage, and no treatment is necessary. The blood typically reabsorbs within 2–3 weeks.

Hyphema, bleeding into the anterior chamber of the eye, is a potential result of blunt eye trauma. When the highly vascular uveal tract of the eye is disrupted by blunt force, hemorrhage may result, filling the anterior chamber. The client complains of feeling eye pain, experiencing decreased visual acuity, and seeing a reddish tint. Blood is visible in the anterior chamber.

An orbital blowout fracture is another potential result of blunt eye trauma. Although any part of the eye orbit may be fractured, the ethmoid bone on the orbital floor is the most likely site. Orbital contents, including fat, muscles, and the eye itself, may herniate through the fracture into the underlying maxillary sinus. The client complains of diplopia (double vision), pain with upward movement of the affected eye, and decreased sensation on the affected cheek. The eye appears sunken (**enophthalmos**) and has limited movement on examination.

Detached Retina

Separation of the retina, or sensory portion of the eye, from the choroid, the pigmented vascular layer, is known as a **retinal detachment**. Although retinal detachment may be precipitated by trauma, it usually occurs spontaneously. The vitreous humor normally adheres to the retina at the optic disc, the macula, and the periphery of the eye. With aging, the vitreous humor shrinks and may pull the retina away from the choroid. Therefore, aging is a common risk factor, as are myopia and **aphakia**, absence of the lens (e.g., following lens removal for cataracts) (Porth, 2005; Tierney, McPhee, & Papadakis, 2005).

The retina may actually tear and fold back on itself, or the retina may remain intact but no longer adhere to the choroid. A break or tear in the retina allows fluid from the vitreous cavity to enter the defect. This, along with fluid that escapes from choroid vessels, the pull of gravity, and traction exerted by the vitreous humor, separates the retina from the choroid. The detached area may rapidly increase in size, increasing loss of vision. Unless contact between the retina and choroid is reestablished, the neurons of the retina become ischemic and die, causing permanent vision loss. For that reason, retinal detachment is a true medical emergency, requiring prompt ophthalmologic referral and treatment.

When the retina detaches, the client experiences floaters, or spots, and lines or flashes of light in the visual field. Often the client describes the sensation of having a curtain drawn across the vision, much like a curtain being drawn over a window. The area of the visual field affected is directly related to the area of detachment. For example, because light rays cross as they pass through the lens, a retinal tear in the superior portion of the eye results in a deficit in the lower part of the visual field. The client feels no pain, and the eye appears normal to visual inspection.

CLINICAL MANIFESTATIONS AND THERAPIES Eye Injuries

CONDITION AND ETIOLOGY	CLINICAL MANIFESTATIONS	CLINICAL THERAPIES
Corneal abrasion	■ Intense pain and redness ■ Photophobia ■ Tearing	■ Superficial corneal abrasions are diagnosed by touching a sterile fluorescein strip to lower conjunctiva; dye remains where corneal epithelial cells are disrupted. ■ Most corneal abrasions heal spontaneously. Antibiotic ointment may be prescribed and eyes patched in some clients.
Burns (Alkaline burns readily penetrate the cornea and are more serious than acid burns.)	■ Pain and/or complaints of "blindness" or vision loss ■ Swollen eyelids ■ Red, edematous conjunctiva ■ Cloudy or hazy conjunctiva ■ Possible presence of ulcerations	■ For chemical burns, eyes are irrigated, preferably with normal saline. ■ Pupils are dilated to reduce pain and prevent adhesions; after irrigation is complete, eyes are patched and antibiotics are prescribed. ■ Topical anesthetic is applied.
Penetrating and perforating injuries	■ Pain ■ Partial or complete vision loss ■ Possible bleeding or extrusion of eye contents	■ *Note: If foreign object is embedded in or sticking out of eye, do not remove. Immobilize object and protect eye until ophthalmologist arrives. Manage pain.* ■ Irrigation ■ Removal of object using a sterile cotton-tipped applicator or a sterile needle or other equipment ■ Application of antibiotic ointment after removal ■ Application of eye patch ■ Surgery
Blunt trauma	■ Pain and redness ■ Ecchymosis ■ Subconjunctival hemorrhage ■ Hyphema ■ Possible diplopia, enophthalmos ■ Personnel should be aware that retinal hemorrhage is a common presentation of the type of child abuse called shaken-baby syndrome.	■ Client is placed in semi-Fowler's position. ■ Eye is protected with eye shield; also, unaffected eye is patched to minimize eye movement. ■ A carbonic anhydrase inhibitor may be prescribed.
Subconjunctival hemorrhage (caused by coughing, mild trauma, or increased physical activity)	■ Reddened area in conjunctiva	■ Usually heals spontaneously; client should see ophthalmologist if most of sclera is covered or if condition does not clear up in 1–2 weeks.
Periorbital ecchymosis	■ Black eye or bruising of the skin around the eye	■ Ice is applied to eye area (both eyes) for 5–15 minutes every hour for the first 1–2 days after injury (even if only one eye is affected, both eyes may discolor); then warm compresses are applied beginning the second day after injury.
Foreign body on conjunctiva	■ Intense pain or feeling of something in the eye	■ Client must not rub eye; material on surface of eye is removed by closing upper lid over lower lid, irrigating or everting upper lid, visualizing material, and removing it with a slightly damp handkerchief; eye is patched and client transported to emergency department if foreign body cannot be removed.
Detached retina	■ Floaters: irregular dark lines or spots in the field of vision ■ Flashes of light ■ Blurred vision ■ Progressive deterioration of vision ■ Sensation of a curtain or veil being drawn across the field of vision ■ If macula is involved, loss of central vision	■ Prompt treatment to preserve vision ■ Proper positioning ■ Cryotherapy ■ Laser photocoagulation ■ Scleral buckling ■ Laser therapy

COLLABORATION

Diagnostic Tests

Facial x-rays and CT scans are used to identify orbital fractures or foreign bodies in the globe. Ultrasonography may be employed to detect a detached retina or vitreous hemorrhage.

Clinical Therapies

Foreign bodies are removed using irrigation, a sterile cotton-tipped applicator, or a sterile needle or other instrument. Antibiotic ointment—erythromycin or sulfacetamide sodium—is applied after the foreign bodies are removed. In clients with corneal abrasions and large foreign bodies in the eye, an eye patch is applied firmly after application of the antibiotic to keep the eye closed for approximately 24 hours.

The immediate priority of care for clients with chemical burns is flushing the affected eye with copious amounts of fluid. Normal saline is preferred; however, water may be used if saline is not available. A special contact lens irrigating unit (Morgan Lens) or a bottle of irrigant with intravenous tubing held to flush all eye surfaces may be useful. The eyelid is everted to identify and remove material from the conjunctival sac. A topical anesthetic, such as tetracaine drops, helps relieve pain, making inspection and irrigation easier. During irrigation, fluid is directed from the inner to the outer canthus of the eye. Slightly tipping the client's head to the affected side prevents contamination of the unaffected eye. Irrigation is continued until the pH of the eye is normal (in the range of 7.2–7.4). Following irrigation, a topical antibiotic ointment, such as gentamicin ophthalmic, is applied.

Penetrating wounds of the eye generally require surgical intervention by an ophthalmic surgeon. Immediate care focuses on relieving pain and protecting the eye from further injury. To prevent loss of intraocular contents, do not place pressure on the eye itself, but gently cover it with sterile gauze or an eye pad. If a foreign body is embedded in or sticking out of the eye, no attempt should be made to remove it. The object should be immobilized and the eye protected with a metal eye shield until an ophthalmologist can see the client. A paper cup or another protective device may be used if the object is too large for an eye shield. Patching the unaffected eye will help decrease ocular movement. Pain is managed using narcotic analgesics (e.g., morphine). The client also may require sedation (e.g., diazepam) and antiemetic medications to prevent vomiting. Antibiotics such as intravenous cefazolin (Ancef) and gentamicin (Garamycin) are prescribed to prevent infection.

Interventions for the client with blunt trauma to the eye include placing the client on bed rest in semi-Fowler's position and protecting the eye from further injury with an eye shield. The unaffected eye should be patched to minimize eye movement. A carbonic anhydrase inhibitor, such as acetazolamide (Diamox) or dichlorphenamide (Daranide), may be prescribed to reduce intraocular pressure.

Treatment of Retinal Detachment

Retinal detachment is a medical emergency; prompt treatment is necessary to preserve vision. The manifestations and examination of the ocular fundus by ophthalmoscopy establish the diagnosis of retinal detachment. Early diagnosis and intervention are vital. If the condition is left untreated, the detached portion will become necrotic because of separation from the vascular supply of the choroid. Permanent blindness in that portion of the eye results.

If an ophthalmologist is not readily available, the client's head is positioned so that gravity pulls the detached portion of the retina into closer contact with the choroid. The client should lay flat in bed with the head midline. This position may not be tolerated by clients with certain cardiorespiratory diseases.

Interventions are directed toward bringing the retina and choroid back into contact and reestablishing the blood and nutrient supply to the retina. Either cryotherapy, using a supercooled probe, or laser photocoagulation may be used to create an area of inflammation and adhesion to "weld" the layers together.

A surgical procedure called **scleral buckling** also may be used. In this procedure, an indentation or fold is created in the sclera, bringing the choroid into contact with the retina. Contact is maintained with a local implant on the sclera or an encircling strap or "buckle." In a procedure called **pneumatic retinopexy**, air is injected into the vitreous cavity. The client is positioned so that the air bubble pushes the detached portion of the retina into contact with the choroid.

NURSING PROCESS

The nursing role involves educating people about the prevention of eye injuries and providing direct care to clients with eye injuries.

Assessment

Ocular injuries require immediate interventions simultaneously with assessment and collection of accurate history. Determine the time, type, and extent of injury and the circumstances under which it occurred. In addition, ask about preexisting visual problems.

If the client normally wears corrective lenses, perform a vision assessment while the client is wearing lenses. Evaluate eye movement unless a penetrating object is present, and inspect the lid and eye for lacerations. Perform inspection using strong light and magnification with a headband loupe or slit lamp. Topical anesthesia may be used prior to inspection if eye pain and photophobia make opening the eye difficult. Fluorescein staining can help identify foreign bodies and abrasions. Note any conjunctival or anterior chamber hemorrhage as well as the presence or absence of the red reflex.

For the client with a detached retina, the nursing focus is on early identification and treatment. Because early intervention is vital to preserve the client's sight, nurses must recognize early manifestations of retinal detachment and intervene appropriately to obtain definitive treatment for the client. Retinal detachment can be successfully treated on an outpatient basis, often in an ophthalmologist's office.

PRACTICE ALERT

Check the immunization status of the child with an eye injury. If the child has not had a tetanus booster within 5 years, this immunization should be given. A tetanus-diphtheria (Td) or tetanus-diphtheria-pertussis (Tdap) booster should be administered in most cases.

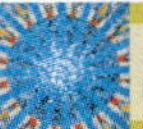

DEVELOPMENTAL CONSIDERATIONS **Eye Injuries**

CHILDREN

- Visual impairment caused by trauma is largely preventable. Scissors, knives, and other sharp objects should be out of the reach of young children. Young children should be supervised when using scissors, pencils, and other sharp objects.
- Parents should be aware of sharp and exploding parts of toys and purchase only those intended for the age of the child.
- Household products containing harmful chemicals and solutions should be kept out of the reach of young children. One example of such a risk is packets of liquid detergent that can break open and spray into the eyes of children (Horgan, McLoone, Lannigan, & Flitcroft, 2005).
- All children should be encouraged to wear protective eyewear during sports that commonly lead to eye injury. School nurses can ensure that students use protective eye gear in chemistry classes and that emergency treatment for injury is posted in classrooms.
- When eye injury does occur, the nurse may care for the child at home and in the community. The permanent loss of vision from an injury can cause feelings of guilt and anger in the child and family, in which case the nurse may need to provide emotional support.

Diagnosis

Nursing diagnoses for the client with an eye injury may include the following:

- Impaired Tissue Integrity: Ocular
- Pain, Acute
- Anxiety
- Ineffective Tissue Perfusion: Retinal.

Plan

Planning with the client is based on the nature and extent of the injury. Typical outcomes may include the following:

- Client will be free of pain associated with the injury.
- Client will articulate and follow instructions regarding eye protection and the healing process.
- Client will describe when to call the primary care provider in the event of worsening symptoms or condition.
- Client will experience healing and restoration of vision to the maximum extent possible.

Implementation

All types of eye trauma pose the risk of violating the integrity of the eye, threatening vision. Therefore, the goals of nursing care are preserving vision and the integrity of the eye and preventing further damage.

Impaired Tissue Integrity: Ocular

- Assess vision in each eye and both eyes, with and without corrective lenses, upon client's entry to the emergency department or primary care setting. An initial assessment provides valuable information about the effect of the injury on the client's vision and a baseline for future comparisons.
- Inspect eye(s) carefully for evidence of foreign bodies, burns, penetrating injury, or blunt trauma. Note whether lacerations, burns, or other trauma are evident in tissues surrounding the eye. Eye trauma may be hidden by other injuries and thus remain untreated.
- If a burn or foreign body is present, consider administering anesthetic drops and irrigating the eye before or after the physician evaluates the client. **Blepharism** (spasms that cause the eye to blink continuously) and eye pain may prevent assessment of the injured eye. Irrigation to remove the chemical is of higher priority than assessment of the eye.
- Remove any loose foreign bodies using a moist, sterile cotton-tipped applicator. Prompt removal of foreign bodies may prevent corneal abrasion.
- For a severe or penetrating injury, promote rest and stabilize the injured eye by applying an eye pad or gauze dressing loosely over both the affected and unaffected eye. Stabilize any penetrating object if possible. These measures reduce eye movement and can help preserve the client's vision.
- Following treatment, apply eyedrops or ointment as prescribed and apply an eye pad or shield if ordered. Apply an eyepad to the affected eye to reduce pain and photophobia and to promote healing.
- Following an injury, discuss the following topics with the client and family:
  a. Prescribed medications and possible adverse effects
  b. Strategies to prevent further trauma
  c. Application of the eye pad or shield
  d. Avoidance of activities that increase intraocular pressure
  e. Importance of activity restrictions.

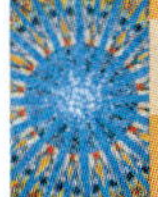

CLIENT TEACHING **Eye Injuries: Prevention and First Aid**

Teaching related to eye injuries focuses on prevention and first-aid measures. Teaching individuals and groups how to prevent eye injuries is an important nursing role, especially for people involved in hazardous occupations and activities. Children in particular are at risk for eye injuries. Whenever the extent of injury is not clear, recommend that the child be evaluated in an emergency care facility. Protective eyewear should be used by participants in all sports with a risk of eye injury. Stress the importance of using seat belts and air bags to prevent eye injury in automobile crashes.

Instruct clients and their families about steps to take for a variety of eye injuries. If a chemical splash occurs, they should immediately flush the eye with copious amounts of water. They can remove loose, visible foreign bodies using a clean, moistened cotton-tipped swab. If an abrasion, penetrating, or blunt injury is suspected, they should cover the eye loosely with sterile gauze and seek immediate medical attention. Instruct clients and their families *not* to remove objects that penetrate the eye.

Interventions for Retinal Detachment

Restoring contact between the retina and choroid is a priority of nursing and medical care for the client with retinal detachment. Vitreous humor may leak through a retinal tear, and fluid exudate may collect behind the tear, causing further detachment. If the macula is detached, central vision is lost, and the likelihood of restoring full vision decreases.

- Notify physician and ophthalmologist immediately. To preserve vision, immediate medical intervention is required in clients with retinal detachment.
- Position the client so the area of detachment is inferior. For instance, for a superior temporal retinal detachment of the right eye (with corresponding vision loss in the inferior medial visual field of that eye), place the client supine with head turned to the right. Correct positioning allows the contents of the posterior portion of the eye to place pressure on the detached area, bringing the retina in closer contact with the choroid.
- Maintain a calm, confident attitude while carrying out priority interventions. Administering care in a calm, although urgent, manner helps reassure the client that the problem is treatable and that appropriate measures are being taken.
- Reassure the client that most retinal detachments are successfully treated, usually on an outpatient basis. Reassurance can help allay the client's fear of permanent vision loss.
- Explain all procedures fully, including the reason for positioning. Explanations facilitate understanding and help relieve anxiety in unfamiliar settings.
- Allow supportive family members or friends to remain with the client as much as possible. Additional support helps lower the client's anxiety level.

Teaching for the client undergoing surgical repair of retinal detachment is similar to that for clients experiencing other types of eye surgery (Box 25–3). If the retina remains detached, provide instructions about the change in peripheral vision or other visual fields and changes in depth perception.

Discuss the following topics with the client and family to prepare for home care:

- Limitations on positioning the head before or following repair
- Activity restrictions such as no bending or straining at stool
- Use of eye shield
- Early manifestations and importance of seeking immediate treatment
- Follow-up treatment with the ophthalmologist.

Box 25–3 Nursing Care of the Client Having Eye Surgery

PREOPERATIVE CARE

- Assess visual acuity of the nonoperative eye prior to surgery. The client with limited vision in the nonoperative eye may need additional postoperative attention and assistance with activities of daily living to ensure safety.
- Assess the client's support systems and the possible effect of impaired vision on lifestyle and ability to perform activities of daily living in the postoperative period. Safety measures, such as installing handrails and removing throw rugs from the home, can help promote mobility and safety, especially if the client has limited vision in the unaffected eye.
- Teach measures to prevent eye injury postoperatively: avoid vomiting, straining at stool, coughing, sneezing, lifting more than 5 pounds, and bending over at the waist. These activities temporarily increase intraocular pressure and may lead to postoperative complications.
- Remove all eye makeup and contact lenses or glasses prior to surgery. Store corrective lenses in a safe place and make them readily available to the client upon return from surgery. Maintaining visual acuity in the unaffected eye helps reduce fear and maintain safety.
- Administer preoperative medications and eyedrops or ointments as prescribed. Mydriatic (pupil-dilating) or cycloplegic (ciliary paralytic) drops and drops to lower intraocular pressure may be prescribed preoperatively.

POSTOPERATIVE CARE

- Assess eye dressing for bleeding or drainage following surgery. Bleeding or drainage may indicate a surgical complication.
- Maintain the eye patch or shield in place. The eye patch or shield helps prevent inadvertent injury to the operative site.
- Place in semi-Fowler's or Fowler's position on the unaffected side. Lying with the head of the bed elevated and lying on the unaffected side reduce intraocular pressure in the affected eye.
- Remind the client to avoid coughing, sneezing, or straining as needed. These activities increase intraocular pressure.
- Assess and medicate as necessary for complaints of pain, aching, or a scratchy sensation in affected eye. Immediately report complaints of sudden, sharp eye pain to the physician. An abrupt increase in or onset of eye pain may indicate hemorrhage or other ocular emergency requiring immediate intervention to preserve sight.
- Assess for the following potential complications:
  a. Pain in or drainage from the affected eye
  b. Hemorrhage with blood in the anterior chamber of the eye
  c. Flashes of light, floaters, or the sensation of a curtain being drawn over the eye (indicators of retinal detachment)
  d. Cloudy appearance to the cornea (corneal edema).

Evidence of complications or unusual complaints should be reported to the physician at once. Early intervention is often necessary to preserve sight.

- Approach the client on the unaffected side. This approach facilitates eye contact and communication.
- Place personal articles and the call light within easy reach. These measures prevent the client from stretching and straining.
- Administer antibiotic, anti-inflammatory, and other systemic and topical eye medications as prescribed. Medications are prescribed to prevent infection or inflammation of the operative site, maintain pupil constriction, and control intraocular pressure.
- Administer antiemetic medication as needed. It is important to prevent vomiting to maintain normal intraocular pressures.

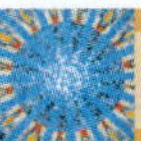

CLIENT TEACHING Home Care Post Eye Surgery

- Teach the client and family about home care:
  a. How to instill eyedrops
  b. What the name, dosage, schedule, duration, purpose, and side effects of medications are
  c. How and when to use the eye patch and eye shield
  d. Why it is important to avoid scratching, rubbing, touching, or squeezing the affected eye
  e. What measures should be used to avoid constipation and straining
  f. What, if any, limitations in activities have been ordered
  g. What symptoms should be reported, including eye pain or pressure, redness or cloudiness, drainage, decreased vision, floaters or flashes of light, or halos around bright objects
  h. Why it is important to wear sunglasses with side shields when outdoors to reduce photophobia.
- Remind the client that vision may not stabilize for several weeks following eye surgery. New corrective lenses, if necessary, are not prescribed until vision has stabilized. The client may be alarmed that vision seems worse after surgery than it did before surgery; reassure the client that visual acuity usually improves with time and healing of the affected eye.
- Emphasize the importance of keeping recommended follow-up appointments. Provide referral as needed to a community home health agency for assistance with home care after discharge.

Evaluation

The client's progress and response to the nursing plan of care may be evaluated using the following expected outcomes:

- Client maintains optimal vision following injury.
- Client experiences no loss of vision as the result of preventable complications.
- Client reports pain management to acceptable levels.

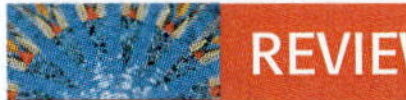

REVIEW Eye Injuries

RELATE: LINK THE CONCEPTS

Mr. Callahan was admitted to the medical surgical unit with a retinal detachment and is scheduled for a scleral buckling procedure in the morning.

Linking the exemplar of Eye Injuries with the concept of Safety:

1. What is Mr. Callahan's priority nursing diagnosis?
2. What post-op teaching does the nurse include for Mr. Callahan and his wife prior to discharge to reduce his risk of injury?

Linking the exemplar of Eye Injuries with the concept of Cognition:

3. When caring for a older adult client with an eye injury, how might his or her cognition be impacted?
4. What nursing interventions might the nurse initiate to reduce the impact of reduced vision on the adult client's cognition?

READY: GO TO COMPANION SKILLS MANUAL

- Assessing the eyes and vision
- Administering ophthalmic medications

REFER: GO TO MYNURSINGKIT

REFLECT: CASE STUDY

Seth Moore, aged 17, presents to the emergency room with his parents after he was hit in the eye with a paintball. Seth was running through an outdoor course with his friends when his right eye was struck. At the time of his injury, Seth was not wearing the eye protection provided to him at the course.

Seth reports eye pain and decreased visual acuity. Examination reveals visible blood in the right eye.

1. What are the potential nursing diagnoses?
2. What are the immediate nursing interventions?
3. What teaching might help Seth avoid injury in the future?

25.4 GLAUCOMA

KEY TERMS

Angle-closure glaucoma, *1669*
Glaucoma, *1668*
Intraocular Pressure, *1668*
Mydriasis, *1669*
Open-angle glaucoma, *1668*
Photophobia, *1669*

BASIS FOR SELECTION OF EXEMPLAR

Most common condition

LEARNING OUTCOMES

After reading about this exemplar, you will be able to:

1. Describe the pathophysiology, etiology, clinical manifestations, and direct and indirect causes of glaucoma.
2. Identify risk factors associated with glaucoma.
3. Illustrate the nursing process in providing culturally competent care across the life span for individuals with glaucoma.
4. Formulate priority nursing diagnoses appropriate for an individual with glaucoma.
5. Create a plan of care for individuals with glaucoma and their family members.
6. Assess expected outcomes for an individual with glaucoma.
7. Discuss therapies used in the collaborative care of an individual with glaucoma.
8. Employ evidence-based caring interventions for an individual with glaucoma.

OVERVIEW

Glaucoma is a condition characterized by optic neuropathy with gradual loss of peripheral vision and (usually) increased **intraocular pressure** of the eye (force within the eye causing tissue damage). Glaucoma is a silent thief of vision. The client typically experiences no manifestations other than narrowing of the visual field, which occurs so gradually that it often goes unnoticed until late in the disease process. In the United States, glaucoma affects about 2.2 million people over the age of 40; it remains undetected in approximately 25% of these cases.

PATHOPHYSIOLOGY AND ETIOLOGY

Aqueous humor, a thick fluid, occupies the anterior and posterior chambers of the eye. The normal intraocular pressure of approximately 12–15 mmHg is maintained by a balance between the production of aqueous humor in the ciliary body, its flow through the pupil from the posterior to the anterior chamber of the eye, and its outflow or absorption through the trabecular meshwork and canal of Schlemm. When this balance is disrupted, usually because of a decrease in the outflow or absorption of aqueous humor, intraocular pressure increases. Although the exact relationship is unclear, it appears that increased intraocular pressure injures the optic nerve. Axons in the periphery of the optic disc are damaged first. As optic fibers are destroyed, the rim of the optic disc shrinks and the normal depression in its center (the *optic cup*) becomes larger and deeper (called optic "cupping"). These changes to the optic disc are visible before changes in the visual field can be detected (Porth, 2005). As the disease progresses, there is a painless, progressive narrowing of the visual field (Figure 25–19 ■) and eventual blindness. Vision loss is often significant before the client seeks treatment and glaucoma is diagnosed.

Primary glaucoma in adults has two major forms: open-angle glaucoma and angle-closure glaucoma. Both terms refer to the angle formed at the point where the iris meets the cornea in the eye's anterior chamber (Figure 25–20 ■).

Some infants have congenital glaucoma present at birth, and other children manifest a genetically caused glaucoma sometime during childhood. Secondary or acquired glaucoma can result from eye injury or prolonged steroid use. The pressure can alter structures of the eye when left untreated, leading to permanent visual impairment.

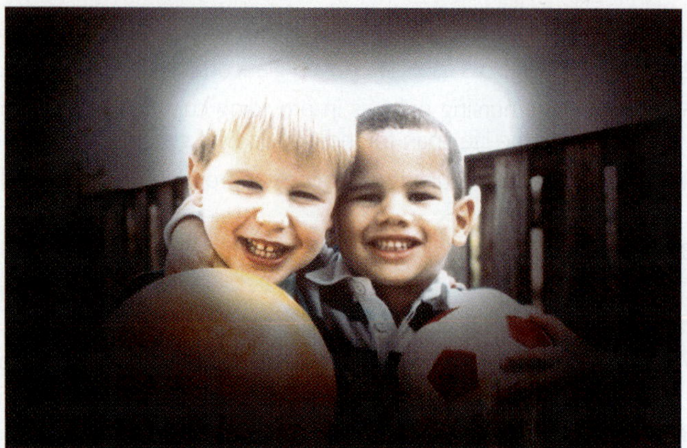

Figure 25–19 ■ Narrowing of visual fields typical of untreated glaucoma.

Source: Courtesy of National Eye Institute, National Institutes of Health.

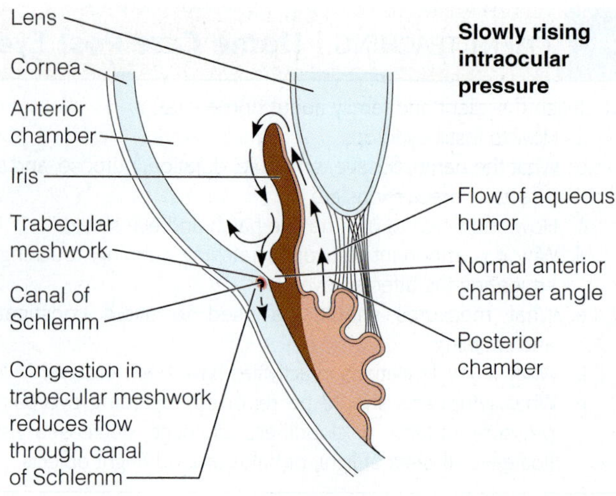

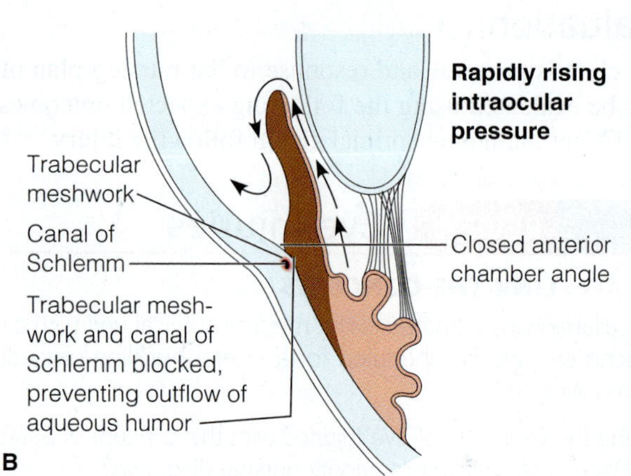

Figure 25–20 ■ Forms of primary adult glaucoma. *A*, In chronic open-angle glaucoma, the anterior chamber angle remains open, but drainage of aqueous humor through the canal of Schlemm is impaired. *B*, In acute angle-closure glaucoma, the angle of the iris and anterior chamber narrows, obstructing the outflow of aqueous humor.

Open-Angle Glaucoma

Glaucoma is usually a primary condition without an identified cause. **Open-angle glaucoma**, often called chronic simple glaucoma, is the most common form in adults, accounting for approximately 90% of all glaucomas. Its cause is unknown; it is thought to have a hereditary component, but no clear inheritance pattern can be identified. Open-angle glaucoma occurs more frequently and at an earlier age in African Americans than in whites (Tierney et al., 2005).

Open-angle glaucoma tends to be a chronic, gradually progressive disease. It typically affects both eyes, although the pressures and progression may not be symmetric. In open-angle glaucoma, the anterior chamber angle between the iris and cornea is normal (thus the term *open angle*). However, the flow of aqueous humor through the trabecular meshwork and into the

FOCUS ON DIVERSITY AND CULTURE Asians and Glaucoma

Narrow-angle glaucoma is more prevalent among Asians than whites. In general, the Asian population has a shorter anteroposterior distance between the lens and the cornea. This may result in the iris obstructing the egress of aqueous fluid, as it can potentially obstruct the trabecular meshwork. While narrow-angle glaucoma is typically free of symptoms, it can cause intermittent pain or **photophobia** (sensitivity to light). The incidence of narrow-angle glaucoma increases with age as the lens swells related to the aging process (Chang, 2009).

canal of Schlemm is relatively obstructed; the cause of this obstruction is unknown. The trabecular meshwork increasingly inhibits the outflow of aqueous humor, and the intraocular pressure gradually increases. The result is neuronal ischemia and optic nerve degeneration, leading to gradual loss of vision.

Angle-Closure Glaucoma

Acute angle-closure (also called narrow-angle or closed-angle) glaucoma is the other, less common form of primary glaucoma in adults. It accounts for approximately 5–10% of all cases of glaucoma (Porth, 2005). Approximately 1% of people over the age of 35 have narrowed anterior chamber angles; the incidence is higher in older adults and in people of Far Eastern, Asian, or Inuit (Alaskan native) ancestry (Porth, 2005).

Narrowing of the anterior chamber angle (see Figure 25–20A for an illustration of the normal anterior chamber angle) occurs because of corneal flattening or bulging of the iris into the anterior chamber. When the lens thickens during accommodation or the iris thickens during pupil dilation, this angle can close completely. Closure of the angle blocks the outflow of aqueous humor through the trabecular meshwork and canal of Schlemm, and the intraocular pressure rises abruptly (Figure 25–20B). This increase in intraocular pressure damages the neurons of the retina and the optic nerve, leading to a rapid and permanent loss of vision if not treated promptly.

Episodes of angle-closure glaucoma are typically unilateral. However, a history of angle-closure glaucoma of one eye increases the risk that it will occur in the other eye.

Because of the effect of pupil dilation on aqueous outflow in angle-closure glaucoma, episodes often occur in association with darkness, emotional upset, or other factors that cause the pupil to dilate. Clients may have intermittent episodes lasting several hours before they have a more typical prolonged attack of angle-closure glaucoma. Clients with a history of the condition must avoid medications, such as atropine and other anticholinergics, which may cause **mydriasis**, or dilation of the pupil.

Risk Factors

Glaucoma is a leading cause of blindness worldwide. Age and race are the primary identified risk factors. Glaucoma is five times more likely to occur in African Americans than in whites, and it is about four times more likely to cause blindness in African American than in whites. The prevalence of glaucoma rises rapidly in Mexican Americans over age 60 (National Eye Institute, 2009b).

CLINICAL MANIFESTATIONS

Open-angle glaucoma is painless, with gradual loss of visual fields. This loss of peripheral vision generally occurs so gradually that the client is often unaware of it until it is detected through a comprehensive vision examination Intraocular pressure is usually, but not always, elevated (Kasper et al., 2005).

Symptoms such as experiencing severe eye and face pain, general malaise, nausea and vomiting, seeing colored halos around lights, and experiencing an abrupt decrease in visual

CLINICAL MANIFESTATIONS AND THERAPIES Glaucoma

GLAUCOMA TYPE	CLINICAL MANIFESTATIONS	CLINICAL THERAPIES
Open-angle glaucoma	■ No initial manifestations ■ Frequent lens changes in glasses ■ Impaired dark adaptation ■ Halos around lights ■ Gradual reduction of visual fields with preservation of central vision until late in the disease ■ Mild to severe increased intraocular pressure	■ Topical medications such as miotics, beta blockers, prostaglandin analogs ■ Carbonic anhydrase inhibitors ■ Laser trabeculoplasty, trabeculectomy
Angle-closure glaucoma	■ Abrupt onset of eye pain, headache ■ Decreased visual acuity ■ Nausea and vomiting ■ Reddened conjunctiva ■ Cloudy cornea ■ Fixed pupil ■ Rapid, significant increase in intraocular pressure	■ Topical miotics or beta blockers ■ Systemic osmotic agents, carbonic anhydrase inhibitors ■ Laser iridotomy or peripheral iridectomy

acuity are associated with acute episodes of angle-closure glaucoma. The conjunctiva of the affected eye may be reddened and the cornea clouded with corneal edema. The pupil may be fixed (nonreactive to light) at midpoint.

Symptoms of juvenile glaucoma include the child constantly bumping into objects in the periphery (painless visual field loss) and seeing halos around objects.

COLLABORATION

Although glaucoma cannot be predicted, prevented, or cured, in most cases, it can be controlled and vision preserved if diagnosed early. Because the most prevalent type of glaucoma, open-angle glaucoma, has few symptoms, routine eye examinations are recommended for early detection. Measurement of intraocular pressure, fundoscopy to assess the optic disc, and visual field testing are used to diagnose glaucoma and monitor the effectiveness of treatment.

Diagnostic Tests

The following diagnostic studies are used to detect and evaluate the presence, severity, type, and effects of glaucoma.

- *Tonometry* indirectly measures intraocular pressure. Contact or noncontact tonometry may be used. Routine tonometry screening is recommended for everyone over the age of 60. A single elevated pressure reading does not warrant a diagnosis of glaucoma; variations in intraocular pressure occur throughout the day.
- *Fundoscopy* (visual inspection of the optic fundus using an ophthalmoscope) identifies pallor and an increase in the size and depth of the optic cup on the optic disc. These changes are significant for a diagnosis of glaucoma.
- *Gonioscopy* uses a gonioscope to measure the depth of the anterior chamber. This test differentiates open-angle from angle-closure glaucoma.
- *Visual field testing* identifies the degree of central visual field narrowing and peripheral vision loss. The client with glaucoma may retain 20/20 central vision even when there is severe peripheral vision loss.

Pharmacologic Therapies

Topical beta-adrenergic blocking agents reduce intraocular pressure by decreasing the production of aqueous humor in the ciliary body. Beta-adrenergic blockers may be prescribed for use once or twice a day depending on the specific drug and dosage form. When administering beta blockers or teaching about their use, it is important to remember that they can produce systemic effects, including bronchospasm, bradycardia, and heart failure.

Prostaglandin analogs such as latanoprost (Xalatan) are a newer class of ophthalmics used to increase aqueous outflow. They are similar to beta blockers in that their longer duration of action means they require only a daily dose. Although they have fewer systemic effects, these drugs may cause conjunctival hyperemia and permanent changes in the color of the iris and eyebrows.

The adrenergic agonist brimonidine may be prescribed along with a beta blocker or in cases when beta blockers are contraindicated (e.g., in a client with heart failure, asthma, or COPD). Another adrenergic agonist, apraclonidine, may be prescribed when other drugs do not sufficiently reduce intraocular pressure, but adverse effects make it inappropriate for long-term use (Tierney et al., 2005).

Dorzolamide (Trusopt), a carbonic anhydrase inhibitor, decreases the production of aqueous humor and reduces intraocular pressure. It is used with other drugs to control pressures and in clients for whom beta blockers are contraindicated because of heart failure or reactive airway disease. Acetazolamide (Diamox), a systemic carbonic anhydrase inhibitor, also may be used for some clients.

Nursing implications for medications used to control chronic glaucoma are outlined in Box 25–4.

In acute angle-closure glaucoma, diuretics may be administered intravenously to achieve a rapid decrease in intraocular pressure prior to surgical intervention. Both the carbonic anhydrase inhibitor acetazolamide and osmotic diuretics, such as mannitol, are used. Fast-acting miotic drops, such as acetylcholine, also are administered to constrict the pupil and draw the iris away from the angle and from the canal of Schlemm.

Surgery

Surgical management of chronic open-angle glaucoma involves improving the drainage of aqueous humor from the anterior chamber of the eye. Trabeculoplasty and trabeculectomy filtration surgery are the most commonly used procedures.

In a *laser trabeculoplasty,* an argon laser is aimed through a gonioscope to create multiple laser burns spaced evenly around the trabecular meshwork. As the burns heal, the scars they create cause tension, stretching and opening the meshwork. This noninvasive technique requires no incision and can be performed as an outpatient procedure, making it the treatment of choice.

Trabeculectomy is a type of filtration surgery in which a permanent fistula is created to drain aqueous humor from the

DEVELOPMENTAL CONSIDERATIONS **Glaucoma in Children**

- Surgery to reduce intraocular pressure is the treatment of choice because medications used to combat glaucoma in adults are not as effective in children.
- Treatment is not always successful, especially if the child has congenital glaucoma. So parents' feelings regarding care of a visually handicapped child should be explored.
- If treatment is not successful, the nurse should refer the family to resources for families with visually impaired children and, when appropriate, for counseling. School-age children are eligible for services from the public school system. Young children may receive early intervention services through agencies such as preschool developmental day centers.

Box 25–4 **Medication Administration for the Client With Glaucoma**

ADRENERGIC AGONISTS (MYDRIATICS)
Brimonidine (Alphagan)
Apraclonidine

Adrenergic agonists dilate the pupil, reduce the production of aqueous humor, and increase its absorption, effectively reducing intraocular pressure in open-angle glaucoma.

Nursing Responsibilities

- Assess the client for contraindications and adverse reactions to adrenergic agonists, including acute angle-closure glaucoma, hypertension, cardiac dysrhythmias, and coronary heart disease.
- Assess for central nervous system (CNS) side effects of anxiety, nervousness, and muscle tremors. If they are severe, notify the physician.
- Assess for a hypersensitivity reaction, including itching, lid edema, and discharge from the eyes. Notify the physician if you notice these signs.

Health Education for the Client and Family

- Report any change in visual acuity or eye pain. (Eye pain may indicate an attack of angle-closure glaucoma and must be reported to the physician immediately.)
- Avoid over-the-counter sinus and cold medications containing pseudoephedrine and phenylephrine. They may accentuate the side effects of this drug.

BETA-ADRENERGIC BLOCKERS
Betaxolol (Betoptic)
Carteolol (Cartrol, Ocupress)
Levobunolol (Betagan)
Metipranolol (OptiPranolol)
Timolol (Timoptic)

Selected beta-adrenergic blockers reduce intraocular pressure by decreasing the production of aqueous humor. Because beta blockers do not affect pupil size and lens accommodation, they do not have the adverse effects on visual acuity that adrenergic agonists do. Their systemic effects, however, may limit their usefulness for certain clients.

Nursing Responsibilities

- Assess the client for allergies or contraindications to beta blocker therapy, including asthma, COPD, heart block, and heart failure.
- Maintain pressure over the lacrimal sac after administration to prevent systemic absorption.
- Assess for side effects such as bradycardia, hypotension, and depression.
- Teach the client about the drug and its dose, administration, desired effects, and side effects.

Health Education for the Client and Family

- Put pressure on the lacrimal sac, at the corner of the eye near the bridge of the nose, to keep the drug from entering client's system.
- Remember that vision may be blurred during the initial period of therapy, but it will improve with continued use of the drug.
- Report adverse effects, including worsening vision, difficulty breathing, reduced exercise tolerance, and sweating or flushing, to the physician.

CARBONIC ANHYDRASE INHIBITORS
Dorzolamide (Trusopt)
Brinzolamide (Azopt)
Acetazolamide (Diamox)

The carbonic anhydrate inhibitors lower intraocular pressure and are used primarily as adjunctive therapy. Dorzolamide and brinzolamide are administered as eyedrops, whereas acetazolamide may be given orally, intramuscularly, or intravenously.

Nursing Responsibilities

- Assess for allergies or other contraindications to the use of carbonic anhydrase inhibitors, including known allergy to sulfa, or severe renal or hepatic disease.
- Monitor for increased drug interactions of amphetamines, procainamide, quinidine, tricyclic antidepressants, and ephedrine and pseudoephedrine.
- Assess daily weight, intake and output, serum electrolytes, and vital signs in clients taking oral or parenteral carbonic anhydrase inhibitors.
- Administer orally in the morning to prevent sleep disruption because of the diuretic effect.
- If used with another topical ophthalmic, administer 10 minutes apart.
- Teach the client about the drug and its dose, administration, desired effects, and side effects.

Health Education for the Client and Family

- For oral medications, maintain a fluid intake of 2–3 L per day and rise slowly from lying or sitting to prevent dizziness when first standing (orthostatic hypotension).
- For topical medications, notify the physician if there is prolonged eye irritation.

PROSTAGLANDIN ANALOGS
Bimatoprost (Lumigan)
Latanoprost (Xalatan)
Travoprost (Travatan)

The prostaglandin analog drugs relax the ciliary muscle, improving the outflow of aqueous humor and reducing intraocular pressure. These drugs have the advantage of requiring only a single daily dose. However, they do have some adverse effects, such as blurred vision and stinging, and when used long-term, they cause permanent darkening of the iris of the eye and eyebrows, increased growth of eyelashes, and conjunctival hyperemia (redness).

Nursing Responsibilities

- Assess and note eye color, presence of inflammation, exudates, or pain.
- Note vital signs and most recent liver function test results because these may be altered by the drug.

Health Education for the Client and Family

- Use once daily at bedtime as directed. Because this drug may blur vision, use at bedtime minimizes associated safety risks.
- Remove contact lenses before administering this drug.
- Remember that minor eye discomfort, including burning and tearing, may occur with this drug. Notify your doctor if adverse effects are severe or intolerable.
- Remember that this drug may cause darkening of the iris, the skin around the eyes, and the eyebrows, as well as increased growth of the eyelashes. These color changes are permanent but will not progress if your doctor discontinues the drug.

anterior chamber of the eye. A portion of trabecular meshwork is removed, and a flap of sclera is left unsutured to create a channel, or fistula, between the anterior chamber and the subconjunctival space. Aqueous humor drains into the space under the conjunctiva, where it can be absorbed into the systemic circulation. A trabeculectomy is usually performed under general anesthesia and requires hospitalization.

If these procedures are not effective, photocoagulation using an argon laser (heat) or cyclocryotherapy using a probe to freeze tissue may be employed to destroy portions of the ciliary body. This destruction of tissue reduces the production of aqueous humor, subsequently reducing intraocular pressure. Another surgical procedure involves inserting a glaucoma drainage device that regulates the outflow of aqueous humor.

Surgical procedures used in the treatment of acute angle-closure glaucoma include gonioplasty, laser iridotomy, and peripheral iridectomy. Because of the high risk for a future attack of angle-closure glaucoma in the unaffected eye, these procedures are often performed prophylactically.

In *gonioplasty,* the healing and scarring of microscopic lesions created at the periphery of the iris draw the iris away from the cornea, widening the anterior chamber. This widening of the chamber increases the angle and opens drainage channels for aqueous humor.

Laser iridotomy is a noninvasive procedure using a laser to create multiple small perforations in the iris of the eye. These perforations allow aqueous humor to drain from the posterior chamber to the anterior chamber and out through the trabecular meshwork and the canal of Schlemm. During an *iridectomy,* a small segment of the iris is removed to facilitate the flow of aqueous humor between the posterior and anterior chambers and to open the anterior chamber angle.

Exercise

There is some evidence that regular exercise lowers intraocular pressure by increasing blood flow to the retina and the optic nerve. Studies indicate that walking three or more times a week is sufficient exercise to slow progression of glaucoma, but the benefit only lasts as long as the individual continues to exercise. Yoga participants should take care to avoid inverted poses, as studies have shown that these can increase intraocular pressure (Johns Hopkins Medicine, 2007).

NURSING PROCESS

When planning and providing nursing care for the client with glaucoma, nurses must consider the specific form of the disease and its actual or potential effects on the client's vision, lifestyle, safety, and psychosocial well-being. In the hospitalized client, glaucoma is typically a concurrent diagnosis rather than the primary reason for seeking care, unless the diagnosis is acute angle-closure glaucoma.

Although glaucoma cannot be prevented, its severity and potentially deleterious permanent effects can be limited with early visual screening. The nurse assumes an important role in educating the public about the risk factors for glaucoma. These include increased age and the higher incidence in African Americans and Asians. Everyone over the age of 40 should be encouraged to receive an eye examination every 2–4 years that includes tonometry screening. Those with a predominant family history or another risk factor, such as frequent use of corticosteroids, should be evaluated more frequently, every 1–2 years. After the age of 65, yearly ophthalmologic examinations are recommended.

Assessment

Collect the following data through a health history and physical examination:

- *Health history.* Family history; presence of altered vision, halos, and excessive tearing; sudden, severe eye pain; use of corrective lenses; most recent eye examination; history of chronic illness; medication history.
- *Physical examination.* Distant and near vision, peripheral fields, retina for optic nerve cupping.

Diagnosis

Nursing care planning focuses on problems associated with the temporary or permanent visual impairment, the resultant increased risk for injury, and the psychosocial problems of anxiety and coping. Potential diagnoses include the following:

- Disturbed Sensory Perception: Visual
- Risk for Injury
- Anxiety.

Plan

Appropriate outcomes for the client with glaucoma include the following:

- The client will follow glaucoma care guidelines and have no further vision loss.
- The client will remain free from injury.
- The client will report control over environment and reduced anxiety.

Implementation

Whether glaucoma and resulting impaired vision is the client's primary problem or a preexisting condition in a client with another disorder, it must be a primary consideration in nursing care planning.

Disturbed Sensory Perception: Visual

- Address the client by name and identify yourself with each interaction. Orient to time, place, person, and situation as indicated. State the purpose of your visit. The client with impaired vision must rely on input from the other senses. A lack of visual cues increases the importance of verbal ones. For example, the client with impaired vision cannot see the nurse checking an intravenous infusion and needs a verbal explanation of who is in the room and why. When the client's normal daily routine is disrupted by illness or hospitalization, additional sensory input such as a radio, a television, and explanations of the routine and activities are useful to maintain the client's orientation.
- Provide any visual aids that are routinely used. Keep them close to the client, making sure the client knows where

they are and can reach them easily. Easy access encourages the client to use these items and enhances the ability to provide self-care.

- Orient the client to the environment. Explain the location of the call bell, personal items, and furniture in the room. If the client is able, provide a tour of client's room, including the bathroom and sink. Clients with visual impairments are usually capable of providing self-care in a known environment.
- Provide other tools or items that can help compensate for diminished vision, as follows:
  a. Bright, nonglare lighting
  b. Books, magazines, and instructions in large print
  c. Books on tape
  d. Telephones with oversize push buttons
  e. A clock with numbers and hands that can be felt.
- Assist with meals by:
  a. Reading menu selections and marking choices.
  b. Describing the position of foods on a meal tray according to the clock system. For example, On the plate, the peas are at 9 o'clock, the mashed potatoes are at 1 o'clock, and the chicken breast is at 6 o'clock. The milk glass is at 2 o'clock on the tray above the plate, and coffee is at 11 o'clock.
  c. Placing the utensils in a readily accessible position.
  d. Removing lids from containers, buttering the bread, and cutting meat as needed.
  e. Feeding the client or providing continued assistance as needed during the meal if the client's visual impairment is new or temporary.

Providing assistance during eating is important to maintain the client's nutritional status. The client may be ashamed of needing help or embarrassed to request it and may respond by not eating or by claiming not to be hungry.

- As needed, assist with mobility and ambulation as follows:
  a. Have the client hold your arm or elbow and walk slightly ahead as a guide. Do not hold the client's arm or elbow.
  b. Describe the surroundings and progress as you proceed. Warn in advance of potential hazards, turns, and steps.
  c. Teach the client to feel the chair, bed, or commode with the hands and the back of the legs before sitting.

These measures help ensure the client's safety while providing mobility and helping prevent complications associated with immobility.

- If the client's vision loss is unilateral and recent, provide instructions related to unilateral vision loss and change in depth perception as follows:
  a. Caution the client about the loss of depth perception and teach safety precautions such as reaching slowly for objects and using visual cues as to distance, especially when driving.
  b. Teach the client to scan, turning the head fully toward the affected side to identify potential hazards and looking up and down to compensate for the loss of depth perception.

  The client with a unilateral vision loss is often unaware of its effect on peripheral vision and depth perception.

Clients who are experiencing a sudden loss of vision due to acute angle-closure glaucoma or are experiencing significant visual impairment due to inadequately managed chronic glaucoma face increased risk for injury. Clients who have had surgical interventions for glaucoma are at even greater risk.

- Assess the client's ability to perform activities of daily living. Clients may be reluctant to request assistance, believing that they should be able to perform these familiar tasks. Carefully assessing and providing needed assistance helps prevent injury and maintain the client's self-esteem.
- Notify housekeeping and place a sign on the client's door to alert all personnel not to change the arrangement of the client's room. The client with impaired vision is at high risk for falling in an unfamiliar environment. It is important to maintain a safe, familiar room when the client is hospitalized.
- Raise two or three side rails on the client's bed. Raised rails remind clients to ask for assistance before ambulating in an unfamiliar environment.
- Discuss possible adaptations in the home to help the client remain as independent as possible and to prevent falls or other injuries. Often minor changes in the home environment, such as removing scatter rugs and small items of furniture, allow the client to navigate safely in this already familiar environment.

Anxiety

The actual or potential loss of sight threatens the client's self-concept, role functioning, patterns of interaction, and, potentially, environment. The client with impaired vision who functions well in a familiar environment will feel anxious in the unfamiliar setting of a hospital or care facility.

- Assess for verbal and nonverbal indications of anxiety level and for normal coping mechanisms. Repeated

CLIENT TEACHING **Managing Glaucoma at Home**

Clients with glaucoma must be provided with strategies for managing the disease at home. They need to understand the importance of lifetime therapy to control the disease and prevent blindness. If a permanent visual impairment has resulted, the client needs information on achieving maximum independence while maintaining safety. The following topics should be discussed with the client and family:

- Importance of not taking certain prescription and over-the-counter medications without consulting a physician
- Prescribed medications, including proper way to administer eyedrops
- Periodic eye examinations with measurement of intraocular pressure
- Risks, warning signs, and management of acute angle-closure glaucoma
- Possible surgical options
- Community resources such as the National Association for Local Societies of Visually Impaired People, local libraries, and transportation services
- Helpful resources such as The Glaucoma Foundation,Young and Under Pressure, the Glaucoma Research Foundation, and Prevent Blindness America.

NURSING CARE PLAN A Client With Glaucoma and Cataracts

Lila Rainey is an 80-year-old widow who lives alone in the house she and her late husband built 50 years ago. She has worn glasses for nearsightedness since she was a young girl; she now wears bifocals to correct her near vision as well. She was diagnosed 4 years ago with chronic open-angle glaucoma, for which she takes timolol maleate (Timoptic) 0.5%. Recently she has noticed difficulty reading and watching television despite a new lens prescription. She has stopped driving at night because the glare of oncoming headlights makes it difficult for her to see. Mrs. Rainey's ophthalmologist has told her that she has cataracts but that they do not need to come out until they bother her. Although her glaucoma is still controlled with timolol maleate 0.5%, one drop in each eye twice a day, her intraocular pressure measurements have been gradually increasing. Mrs. Rainey has taken 325 mg of aspirin daily since a transient ischemic attack 8 years ago. She is being admitted to the outpatient surgery unit for cataract removal and intraocular lens implant in her right eye.

ASSESSMENT

Mrs. Rainey is admitted to the eye surgery unit by Susan Schafer, RN. In her assessment, Ms. Schafer finds Mrs. Rainey to be alert and oriented, although apprehensive about her upcoming surgery. Assessment findings include P 86, R 18, BP 134/72 . Mrs. Rainey's neurologic, respiratory, cardiovascular, and abdominal assessments are essentially normal. Her pupils are round and equal and react briskly to light and accommodation. Her conjunctivae are pink; sclera and corneas, clear. Using the ophthalmoscope, Ms. Schafer notes that the red reflex in Mrs. Rainey's right eye is diminished. Ophthalmic examination shows visual acuity of 20/150 OD (right eye) and 20/50 OS (left eye) with corrective lenses. Her intraocular pressures are 21 mmHg OD and 17 mmHg OS. On fundoscopic exam, no disease of the blood vessels, retina, macula, or disc is found. Ms. Schafer reviews the operative procedure with Mrs. Rainey, answering her questions and telling her what to expect after surgery. Following preoperative protocols, Mrs. Rainey is prepared and transported to surgery.

DIAGNOSES

- Disturbed Sensory Perception: Visual related to myopia and lens extraction
- Anxiety related to anticipated surgery
- Deficient Knowledge related to lack of information regarding postoperative care
- Impaired Home Maintenance related to activity restrictions and impaired vision

PLANNING

Goals of nursing care may include:

- Regain sufficient visual acuity to maintain activities of daily living, including reading and watching television for enjoyment.
- Demonstrate a reduced level of anxiety.
- Demonstrate the procedure for instilling eyedrops postoperatively.
- Demonstrate knowledge of the home care she will require after surgery, signs of complications, and actions to take if complications occur.
- Use appropriate resources to assist with home maintenance until vision stabilizes and activity restrictions are lifted.

IMPLEMENTATION

- Provide a safe environment, placing the call light and personal care items within easy reach.
- Encourage Mrs. Rainey to express her fears about surgery and its potential effect on vision.
- Explain all procedures related to surgery and recovery.
- Instruct Mrs. Rainey to avoid shutting the eyelids tightly, sneezing, coughing, laughing, bending over, lifting, or straining to have a bowel movement. Teach her to wear glasses during the day and an eye shield at night to prevent injury to the surgical site.
- Explain and demonstrate the procedure for administering eyedrops.
- Provide verbal and written instructions about postoperative care, including a schedule of follow-up examinations, potential complications, and actions to take in response.
- Refer Mrs. Rainey to a discharge planner or social worker to help establish a plan for home maintenance.

EVALUATION

Mrs. Rainey is discharged the morning after her surgery. She is visibly relieved when the eye patch is removed because her vision in the operated eye is better than before surgery, even without her glasses. She is able to relate the recommended activity restrictions. Mrs. Rainey administers her own eyedrops before discharge and relates an understanding of the prescribed postoperative care and safety precautions. Mrs. Rainey's daughter plans to visit her mother two or three times a week to help with laundry and vacuuming until Mrs. Rainey can resume all of her household activities. Mrs. Rainey says that she won't "be so scared when I need my other eye done." She understands the chronic nature of her glaucoma and says that her vision is too important for her to neglect her timolol drops and routine eye exams.

expressions of concern or denial that the vision change will affect the client's life indicate anxiety. Nonverbal indicators include tension, difficulty concentrating or thinking, restlessness, poor eye contact, and changes in vocalization (rapid speech, quivering voice). Physical indicators include tachycardia, dilated pupils, cool and clammy skin, and tremors. The client may not recognize this feeling as anxiety. Identifying and acknowledging the anxiety can help the client recognize and deal with it.

- Encourage the client to verbalize fears, anger, and feelings of anxiety. Verbalizing helps externalize the anxiety and allows fears to be addressed.

- Discuss the client's perception of the eye condition and its effects on lifestyle and roles. Discussion provides an opportunity to correct misperceptions and introduce alternative activities and assistive devices for clients with visual impairments.
- Introduce yourself when entering the room. Explain all procedures fully before they are performed and while they are being performed. Use touch to convey proximity and caring. The client with impaired vision must rely on the other senses to make up for the loss of sight. Because the client cannot see what you are doing, complete explanations of such simple tasks as refilling a water glass help to relieve anxiety.
- Identify coping strategies that have been useful in the past and adapt these strategies to the present situation. Previously successful coping strategies may be employed to increase the client's sense of control.

Evaluation

Expected outcomes for the client with glaucoma may include:

- Client demonstrates proper self-administration of eye drops.
- Client describes need for compliance with plan of care and follow up care to avoid complications or vision loss.
- Client lists resources available within the community.

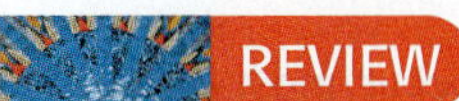

REVIEW Glaucoma

RELATE: LINK THE CONCEPTS

Linking the exemplar of Glaucoma with the concept of Safety:

1. What interventions are appropriate for the nurse to initiate to ensure safety for the client with glaucoma?
2. Why would it be important for the nurse to give anticipatory guidance to the client with glaucoma?

Susan Parkerson is a 40-year-old woman with severe, persistent asthma. In addition to receiving bimonthly immunotherapy, she takes an inhaled corticosteroid with a long-acting beta-agonist and an antihistamine daily. Each year she has four or five acute exacerbations of asthma that usually require a taper of oral prednisone.

Linking the exemplar of Glaucoma with the concept of Oxygenation:

3. What are Ms. Parkerson's risk factors for glaucoma?
4. What client teaching should the nurse provide Ms. Parkerson to reduce her risk of developing glaucoma?

READY: GO TO COMPANION SKILLS MANUAL

- Assessing the eyes and vision
- Administering ophthalmic medications

REFER: GO TO MYNURSINGKIT

REFLECT: CASE STUDY

Jane Baker is a 75-year-old female who was recently widowed. She and her husband were married 40 years when he died from cancer. She has limited income because her husband's pension terminated when he died. She receives $652 a month in Social Security benefits.

Mrs. Baker does not see particularly well. She is in excellent health; the only health-related problems she is aware of are osteoporosis and glaucoma, for which she sees an ophthalmologist on a regular basis. The only prescription drugs and over-the-counter supplements she uses are Fosamax, calcium, and latanoprost ophthalmic solution (Xalatan) eyedrops to manage her glaucoma (her dose is 1 drop in each eye once a day); her only complaint about the eyedrops is the cost. Although Mrs. Baker has a car and a driver's license, she does not drive very often due to problems with vision. She prefers that friends and family members take her places she needs to go.

At her latest visit to the ophthalmologist, the doctor notes increased intraocular pressure.

1. Based on the information provided, what might be the cause of Mrs. Baker's increased intraocular pressure?
2. What is the priority nursing diagnosis?
3. What resources might be available to help Mrs. Baker meet her needs?

25.5 MACULAR DEGENERATION

KEY TERMS

Age-related macular degeneration, *1676*
Exudative macular degeneration, *1676*
Macular degeneration, *1675*
Nonexudative macular degeneration, *1676*

BASIS FOR SELECTION OF EXEMPLAR

Chronic Disease Management

LEARNING OUTCOMES

After reading about this exemplar, you will be able to:

1. Describe the pathophysiology, etiology, clinical manifestations, and direct and indirect causes of macular degeneration.
2. Identify risk factors associated with macular degeneration.
3. Illustrate the nursing process in providing culturally competent care across the life span for individuals with macular degeneration.
4. Formulate priority nursing diagnoses appropriate for an individual with macular degeneration.
5. Create a plan of care for individuals with macular degeneration and their family members.
6. Assess expected outcomes for an individual with macular degeneration.
7. Discuss therapies used in the collaborative care of an individual with macular degeneration.
8. Employ evidence-based caring interventions for an individual with macular degeneration.

OVERVIEW

The leading cause of legal blindness and impaired vision in people over the age of 65 is **age-related macular degeneration** (AMD), a gradual process of degeneration in the macular area of the retina. Only 2.1% of people ages 40–49 have intermediate or advanced AMD. The incidence and prevalence of AMD increases rapidly with aging, affecting over 7% of people ages 60–69, more than 14% of people ages 70–79, and 35% of people ages 80 and older (National Eye Institute, 2004).

PATHOPHYSIOLOGY AND ETIOLOGY

The macula is the area of the retina that provides sharp central vision, which it does by receiving light from the center of the visual field. Two forms of AMD are identified, a nonexudative (dry) form and an exudative (wet) form. Although both are progressive disorders, their manifestations and management differ.

Nonexudative, or dry, **macular degeneration** is the more common form of AMD. It is a gradual process that begins with the accumulation of deposits called *drusen* beneath the pigment epithelium of the retina. Over time, these deposits enlarge and increase in number. The pigment epithelium detaches in small areas and becomes atrophic, interfering with sensory function of the macula. Typically, vision loss is not significant, and the disorder progresses slowly. However, there is a risk that the disorder will progress to an exudative stage of the disease.

Exudative macular degeneration (wet) is characterized by the formation of new, weak blood vessels in the potential space between the choroid (vascular layer of the eye) and the retina (neurosensory layer). These new vessels are prone to leak, elevating the retina from the choroid and distorting vision. Although exudative macular degeneration typically is a gradual process, bleeding can lead to acute vision loss in some cases. With significant or repeated bleeding episodes, scar tissue forms, and central vision is permanently lost (Kasper et al., 2005).

Etiology

Approximately 15 million Americans have AMD, with approximately 200,000 new diagnoses occurring each year. AMD is the number one cause of severe vision loss and legal blindness in Americans over the age of 60 (Macular Degeneration Partnership, n.d.). There are indications that the risk for AMD is much lower for Asians, leading credence to the theory that diet and sun exposure may play a role, as Asians typically have an aversion to sun exposure and have diets high in dark leafy greens (Chang, 2009). Darker pigmentation also may play a part, as those with darker skin are less likely to develop AMD.

Risk Factors

Although the exact cause of AMD is unknown, factors associated with it include aging, smoking, race, cardiovascular health, and possibly genetic factors. Whites have a significantly higher risk of developing AMD than do African Americans, Hispanics, and people of Asian ancestry. However,

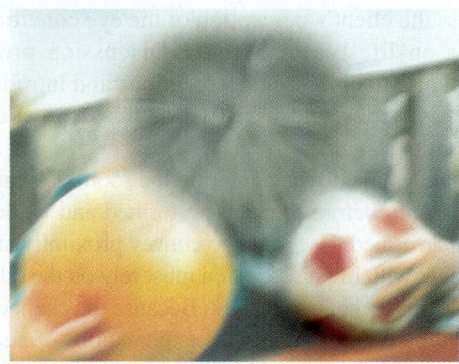

Figure 25–21 ■ Loss of central vision with advanced age-related macular degeneration.

Source: Courtesy of National Eye Institute, National Institutes of Health.

the destructive changes in the macula occur most often as a response to the aging process. AMD affects males and females equally. Evidence suggests that the risk for developing AMD may be reduced by consumption of certain antioxidant nutrients, including vitamin C, vitamin E, beta-carotene, and zinc (National Eye Institute, 2009c).

CLINICAL MANIFESTATIONS

When the macula is damaged, central vision becomes blurred and distorted, but peripheral vision remains intact. With the loss of central vision, activities that require close central vision, such as reading and sewing, are particularly affected (Figure 25–21 ■).

Clients with AMD often experience blurry vision, central scotomas (blind spots within the visual field), and metamorphopsia in which images are distorted to look smaller (micropsia) or larger (macropsia) than they actually are.

Another symptom typical of wet AMD is that straight lines appear crooked or wavy. The Amsler grid was developed as a screening tool to assess for AMD (Figure 25–22 ■). Clients with AMD experience visual distortions of the lines and central scotomas.

AMD typically affects central vision and peripheral vision remains intact. A client with macular degeneration will experience a dark spot in the center of the field of vision and must learn to rely on and interpret peripheral vision in order to function (see Figure 25–21).

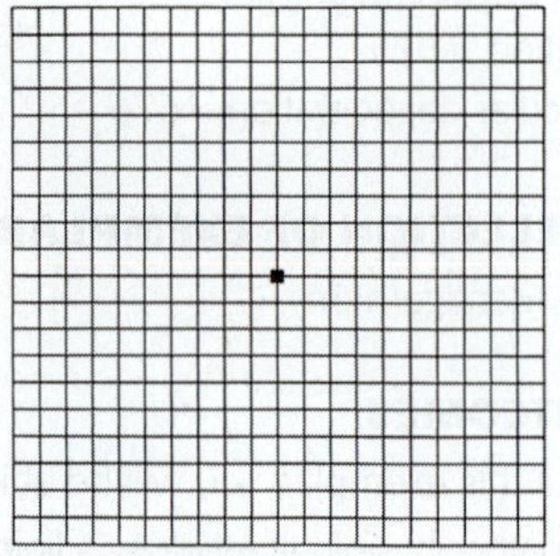

Figure 25–22 ■ The Amsler grid.

CLINICAL MANIFESTATIONS AND THERAPIES Macular Degeneration

TYPE OF MACULAR DEGENERATION	CLINICAL MANIFESTATIONS	CLINICAL THERAPIES
Nonexudative macular degeneration (dry)	■ Slow progression ■ Need for increasingly brighter light when reading ■ Possible blurriness of printed words ■ Difficulty recognizing faces ■ Overall haziness in vision ■ Blurred or blind spot in the center of visual field; activities, such as reading and sewing, are affected.	■ High-dose antioxidants and zinc
Exudative macular degeneration (wet)	■ Possible abrupt onset ■ Visual distortions ■ Visual hallucinations ■ Impaired color vision ■ Blurred spot in the center of visual field	■ Laser surgery ■ Photodynamic therapy

COLLABORATION

Diagnostic Tests

AMD is diagnosed through vision and retinal examination. The Amsler grid may be used to identify distortion of central vision caused by AMD. If treatment for wet AMD is planned, a *fluorescein angiogram* may be done. Pictures are taken as the dye passes through the blood vessels of the retina, allowing detection of leaks.

Pharmacologic Therapies

In photodynamic therapy, verteporfin, a drug that tends to adhere to the surface of new blood vessels, is injected systemically. Shining a light into the affected eye activates the drug and destroys new blood vessels. This treatment is relatively fast and painless, but it does require avoiding exposure to direct sunlight or bright indoor light for 5 days following treatment (National Eye Institute, 2003a).

Surgery

Wet AMD is treated with laser surgery or photodynamic therapy. Although these treatments do not cure the disease, they may slow the rate of vision loss. In laser surgery, fragile blood vessels are destroyed, preventing bleeding. Risks include damage to surrounding healthy tissue, some vision loss, and continued growth of new vessels.

Nonpharmacologic Therapies

In its early or intermediate stages, the progress of dry AMD can be slowed through the use of high-dose antioxidants and zinc. Research demonstrated a benefit when vitamin C, vitamin E, beta-carotene (vitamin A), zinc, and copper were administered daily.

Large-print books and magazines, the use of a magnifying glass, and high-intensity lighting can help the client cope with the reduced vision of macular degeneration.

NURSING PROCESS

Nurses should be alert for clients demonstrating new and rapid onset of macular degeneration and promptly refer these clients for ophthalmologic evaluation. Early intervention may preserve a greater degree of vision and slow the progress of the disease.

Assessment

- *Health history.* Effect of vision changes on lifestyle and activities (e.g., ability to read, watch television, participate in work and recreational activities); family history of macular degeneration, nutrient intake, history of cigarette smoking
- *Physical examination.* General health; visual acuity, including Amsler grid

Diagnosis

For clients with slowly progressive manifestations, the nursing focus is on helping the client and family members adapt to the gradual decline in vision by recommending visual aids and other coping strategies. Client education materials should be in a large-print format. Patient advocacy, psychologic and emotional support, and teaching/learning needs are typically of higher priority for these clients.

Nursing diagnoses for the client with macular degeneration may include the following:

- Disturbed Sensory Perception: Visual
- Risk for injury
- Fear.

Plan

Goals for nursing care may include:

- Promote client safety
- Encourage client to express feelings related to diagnosis and reduced vision
- Assist client to identify strategies to promote client's self-care and daily routine.

Implementation

Due to the severity of vision loss as a result of AMD, nurses can play an important role in patient education. Routine ophthalmic examinations are important to detect early signs of the disease. Nurses should encourage preventive measures such as wearing ultraviolet protective lenses in the sun, stopping smoking, and exercising. In addition, nurses should encourage a healthy diet consisting of fruits and vegetables. These may be helpful not only in increasing consumption of antioxidants, but also in reducing the risk of cardiovascular disease. When working with the client who is experiencing severe vision loss due to AMD, nurses should assess the client for grief or fear related to the client's loss of vision and anxiety related to the disease and treatment options.

- Explain the nature of the condition and help the client determine the extent to which it is affecting daily life.
- Attend to verbalized concerns. Address questions factually and completely. For many clients, fear of blindness is second only to fear of cancer. Careful listening and teaching and a caring, understanding attitude can help the client deal with this fear.
- Assess for factors that may interfere with the client's ability to provide self-care, such as environmental barriers that compromise safety.
- Recommend visual aids when appropriate (e.g., magnifying glass and large-type books).
- Teach client and caregiver about the benefits of a diet high in antioxidants, such as leafy green vegetables and fish; also offer information about supplements.
- Offer resources on smoking cessation.
- Explain the need for regular eye exams.
- Assess for other care needs that may be impacted by vision changes. Some health care needs, such as insulin injections, may suggest the need for home health or nursing care postoperatively.
- Encourage use of other senses, such as touch. Touch allows the client to become familiar with objects.
- Encourage use of radios, compact discs (CDs), and audio books. Radio and television can help the client remain aware of day and time.
- If needed, consult with occupational therapy for assistive devices.
- Make referrals to appropriate home health agency.
- Educate family and caregivers and provide resources.

Evaluation

Expected outcomes for the client with macular degeneration may include the following:

- The client will verbalize concerns and identify appropriate resources.
- The client will demonstrate the ability to safely compensate for visual deficits.
- Client will describe strategies to promote self-care.

REVIEW Macular Degeneration

RELATE: LINK THE CONCEPTS

Linking the exemplar of Macular Degeneration with the concept of Health, Wellness, and Illness:

1. What challenges might the client with late-stage AMD experience at the dinner table?

Linking the exemplar of Macular Degeneration with the concept of Cognition:

2. What effect might advancing macular degeneration have on the client's cognition?
3. What strategies can the nurse implement to promote cognitive functioning?

READY: GO TO COMPANION SKILLS MANUAL

- Assessing the eyes and vision

REFER: GO TO MYNURSINGKIT

REFLECT: CASE STUDY

Margaret Marlborough, 58 years old, is a librarian in good health. She has never smoked and has no history of heart disease. She has made an appointment with her ophthalmologist because she has noticed pages getting blurry and she sometimes can't see her coworkers' faces clearly. At first, she thought her glasses might be dirty, but cleaning them didn't seem to help.

1. Based on the information above, what visual examinations will be performed?
2. What type of AMD is Margaret likely to have?
3. What is the priority nursing diagnosis?
4. What interventions will be of most benefit to Margaret?

25.6 PERIPHERAL NEUROPATHY

KEY TERMS

BASIS FOR SELECTION OF EXEMPLAR

Chronic Disease Management

LEARNING OUTCOMES

After reading about this exemplar, you will be able to:

1. Describe the pathophysiology, etiology, clinical manifestations, and direct and indirect causes of peripheral neuropathy.
2. Identify risk factors associated with peripheral neuropathy.
3. Illustrate the nursing process in providing culturally competent care across the life span for individuals with peripheral neuropathy.
4. Formulate priority nursing diagnoses appropriate for an individual with peripheral neuropathy.
5. Create a plan of care for individuals with peripheral neuropathy and their family members.
6. Assess expected outcomes for an individual with peripheral neuropathy.
7. Discuss therapies used in the collaborative care of an individual with peripheral neuropathy.
8. Employ evidence-based caring interventions for an individual with peripheral neuropathy.

OVERVIEW

Peripheral neuropathy results when trauma or disease process interferes with innervation of peripheral nerves. The overall effectiveness of blood vessels decreases, and superficial blood vessels constrict to divert blood to larger vessels. With the constriction of peripheral blood vessels, peripheral nerve endings in the constricted area suffer effects of decreased blood flow, and neuropathy develops. Although most peripheral neuropathies progress slowly over time, the symptoms, including pain and muscle weakness, can significantly affect quality of life.

PATHOPHYSIOLOGY AND ETIOLOGY

The peripheral nervous system (PNS) links the central nervous system (CNS) with the rest of the body. The PNS is responsible for receiving and transmitting information from and about the external environment. It consists of nerves, ganglia (groups of nerve cells), and sensory receptors located outside—or peripheral to—the brain and spinal cord. The PNS is divided into a sensory (afferent) division and a motor (efferent) division. Most nerves of the PNS contain fibers for both divisions, and all nerves are classified regionally as either spinal nerves or cranial nerves. Damage to these nerves can interrupt communication between the brain and the body, affecting normal muscle movement and sensory perception and causing pain.

The main components of peripheral nerves are the axon and myelin. Peripheral neuropathy can be classified according to the predominant pathology: axonal degeneration or segmental demyelination.

The peripheral neuropathies (also called *somatic neuropathies*) include polyneuropathies and mononeuropathies. **Polyneuropathies**, the most common types of neuropathy associated with diabetes, are bilateral sensory disorders. The manifestations appear first in the toes and feet and progress upward. The fingers and hands also may be involved, but usually only in later stages of diabetes. The manifestations of polyneuropathies depend on the nerve fibers involved.

Mononeuropathies are isolated peripheral neuropathies that affect a single nerve. Injury or trauma is the most common cause, although repetitive motions, such as those resulting in carpal tunnel syndrome, also can cause mononeuropathy.

Neuropathies are classified by one of three causes: acquired, hereditary, or idiopathic. Acquired neuropathies include those caused by disease or illness, nutritional deficits, infection, trauma, and toxins. Hereditary, or inherited, neuropathies include Charcot-Marie-Tooth disease. Idiopathic neuropathies are from an unknown cause and account for up to 30% of neuropathies.

The etiology of polyneuropathy is varied; it often is caused by complications of diseases such as diabetes, exposure to toxins, and poor nutrition (in particular, vitamin B deficiency). One of the most serious polyneuropathies is **Guillain-Barré syndrome (GBS)**, an acute inflammatory demyelinating disorder of the peripheral nervous system characterized by an acute onset of motor paralysis (usually ascending). The classification of Guillain-Barré subtypes includes acute inflammatory demyelinating polyradiculoneuropathy, acute axonal motor neuropathy, and acute motor and sensory axonal neuropathy.

Guillain-Barré syndrome is one of the most common peripheral nervous system disorders, affecting about 3,500 people in the United States and Canada each year (Porth, 2005). The cause is unknown, but precipitating events include a respiratory or gastrointestinal viral or bacterial infection 1–3 weeks prior to the onset of manifestations, surgery, viral immunizations, and other viral illnesses. In 60% of cases, *Campylobacter jejuni* is identified as the cause of the preceding infection. Approximately 80–90% of clients with GBS have a spontaneous recovery with little or no residual disabilities.

The disease is characterized by progressive ascending flaccid paralysis, accompanied by **paresthesias** (a subjective feeling of a change in sensation, such as numbness or tingling) and numbness. About 20% of clients have respiratory involvement to the point that ventilatory assistance is required. GBS is often a medical emergency.

The primary pathophysiologic process in GBS is the destruction of myelin sheaths covering the axons of peripheral nerves. The demyelination is thought to be the result of both a humoral- and cell-mediated immunologic response. The loss of myelin results in poor conduction of nerve impulses, causing sudden muscle weakness and loss of reflex response. Other manifestations occur when nerve conduction to various muscles is interrupted.

Systemic diseases are often the cause of peripheral neuropathy. Damage from disease processes such as metabolic and endocrine disorders affects the body's ability to process waste products and utilize nutrients. At least half of all people with diabetes develop some type of neuropathy (Mayo Clinic,

2008). Conditions that decrease oxygen supply may cause a thickening of the walls of blood vessels that supply nerves, resulting in a reduced blood flow.

Autoimmune disorders and infections also can cause peripheral neuropathy. Viruses and bacteria can attack nerve tissues (or cause the body to attack nerve tissues), resulting in the destruction of nerve axons or myelin sheath. Sensory neuropathies with manifestations of numbness, tingling, and pain in the lower extremities affect about 30% of clients with AIDS. A Guillain-Barré type of inflammatory demyelinating polyneuropathy also can occur, resulting in progressive weakness and paralysis. In addition, untreated Lyme disease can cause extensive peripheral nerve damage.

Alcoholic neuropathy is damage to the nerves that results from long-term excessive use of alcohol. Malnutrition is a serious complication of chronic alcoholism; thiamine (B_1) deficiency that may be associated with chronic alcoholism is characterized by progressive cognitive deterioration, confabulation, myopathy, and peripheral neuropathy.

Inflammation, cancer, and toxins, including some types of chemotherapy, other medications, and environmental chemicals, such as lead, can damage nerve tissue and fibers, resulting in peripheral neuropathy.

Inflammation and swelling in tendon sheaths can lead to peripheral neuropathy. The carpal tunnel is a canal through which flexor tendons and the median nerve pass from the wrist to the hand. Carpal tunnel syndrome develops from narrowing of the tunnel and compression of the median nerve as a result of inflammation and swelling of the synovial lining of the tendon sheaths.

Charcot-Marie-Tooth syndrome, the most common inherited peripheral neuropathy in the world, is characterized by a slowly progressive degeneration of the muscles of the foot, lower leg, hand, and forearm. Symptoms usually present between adolescence and young adulthood.

The prognosis for clients with peripheral neuropathy ranges from the neuropathy resolving (e.g., the underlying cause is successfully treated) to cases in which the client does not respond to treatment or the cause is not identifed and the condition persists indefinitely.

Risk Factors

Risk factors for acquired peripheral neuropathies include the following:

- Diabetes
- Alcohol abuse
- Vitamin deficiencies, particularly B vitamins
- Immune system suppression
- Autoimmune diseases
- Kidney, liver, or thyroid disorders
- Exposure to toxins, including some medications.

Age also appears to have a role in risk for peripheral neuropathy. Studies show that the incidence of peripheral neuropathy increases significantly in older adults (Centers for Disease Control and Prevention, 2004; Mold, Vesely, Keyl, Schenk, & Roberts, 2004). Although some changes in the peripheral system are due to the normal aging process, they are not usually associated with changes in functional status.

CLINICAL MANIFESTATIONS

Clinical manifestations of peripheral neuropathy depend upon the affected nerve or nerves and the amount of damage. The primary goal of treatment is to correct or manage the underlying cause so that symptoms are controlled and further nerve damage is minimized.

The client with polyneuropathy commonly has distal paresthesias; pain described as aching, burning, or shooting; and feelings of cold feet. Other manifestations may include impaired sensations of pain, temperature, light touch, two-point discrimination, and vibration. With GBS, there is frequently a "stocking–glove" pattern—feeling as though stockings and gloves are being worn when they are not—with pain in the hands, feet, and legs.

Weakness in the arm or legs is often caused by damage to motor nerves; clients may report difficulty walking or running, stumbling, dropping things, and tiring easily. A general feeling of lack of coordination or clumsiness may be reported, and the client may compensate by changing the walking pattern to maintain balance.

CLINICAL MANIFESTATIONS AND THERAPIES Peripheral Neuropathy

ETIOLOGY	CLINICAL MANIFESTATIONS	CLINICAL THERAPIES
Motor nerve damage	■ Muscle weakness ■ Cramps ■ Fasciculations ■ Muscle loss	■ Treatment of underlying cause ■ Physical therapy ■ Necessity for surgery (e.g., to remove tumor causing compression)
Sensory nerve damage	■ Numbness ■ Pain ■ Burning or shooting pain ■ Impaired touch, temperature, and pain sensation	■ Treatment of underlying cause ■ Medication ■ Physical therapy

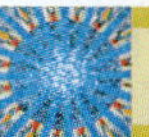

DEVELOPMENTAL CONSIDERATIONS **Manifestations of GBS in Children**

INFANTS

- Infants have an onset of rapidly progressive severe hypotonia, possible respiratory distress, irritability, and feeding difficulties.

CHILDREN

- Older children exhibit rapidly progressive symmetric weakness and muscle pain with varying degrees of distal paresthesia and numbness in the legs. This ascending weakness spreads to the upper extremities, trunk, chest, neck, face, and head. Deep tendon reflexes may be diminished or absent. The child may develop acute ataxia or an inability to walk.
- Difficulty swallowing and facial weakness are signs of impending respiratory failure. Respiratory effort may be inadequate for proper ventilation.
- Cranial nerves may be affected, causing Bell's palsy, for example. A dysfunctional autonomic nervous system may cause such symptoms as a labile blood pressure and cardiac rate, postural hypotension, or profound bradycardia (Sarnat, 2004).

COLLABORATION

Because peripheral neuropathy can involve multiple systems, collaboration is likely to include specialists (e.g., a neurologist or an endocrinologist, physical or occupational therapists, and pain specialists).

Diagnostic Tests

In addition to a medical history and neurologic exam, diagnostics for peripheral neuropathy may include the following:

- Electromyography
- Complete blood count (CBC)
- Thyroid function tests
- Serum levels for B_{12} and thiamin
- Metabolic panel
- Urine screening
- Nerve biopsy.

Lyme disease and HIV tests also may be indicated.

Treatment

There is no specific treatment for polyneuropathy, as it is a symptom with many potential causes. The primary goals of treatment are to care for and manage the underlying cause. However, a combination of medication, lifestyle modifications, and physical therapy can be effective in treating symptoms and increasing quality of life.

There is no catch-all drug to treat pain resulting from peripheral neuropathy, as drug therapy is individualized and based on comorbidities, extent of nerve damage, and nerve affected. Medications used include pain relievers, anticonvulsants, antidepressants, and a lidocaine patch.

Physical or occupational therapy may help the client maintain mobility and avoid further changes in functional status.

Complementary Therapies

Complementary and alternative therapies include acupuncture, biofeedback, transcutaneous electrical nerve stimulation (TENS), and massage.

Changes in daily life may be required to maintain or restore health. These include:

- Compliance with therapeutic regimen for primary condition (e.g., maintain blood glucose control)
- A healthy, well-balanced diet (vitamin supplements may be necessary)
- Maintenance of optimal weight
- Regular exercise to increase/maintain muscle strength
- Smoking cessation
- Limits on alcohol intake
- Daily foot care.

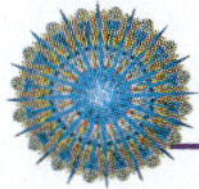

NURSING PROCESS

Assessment

A health assessment to determine problems with the peripheral nervous system may be conducted during a health screening, may focus on a chief complaint (such as tingling), or may be part of a total health assessment. Analyze onset, characteristics, course, severity, precipitating and relieving factors, and any associated symptoms, noting the time and circumstances. For example, ask the client the following questions:

- Describe the location and intensity of the pain you have been experiencing in your left leg. Is it made worse by coughing, sneezing, or walking?
- When did you first notice that you were having numbness in your fingers?

Questions about present health status include information about numbness, tingling sensations, tremors, problems with coordination or balance, and loss of movement in any part of the body. In older adults, impaired balance or falls should be carefully assessed. Ask the client about difficulty speaking, seeing, hearing, tasting, or detecting odors. In addition, elicit information about memory, feeling state (such as anxiety or depression), recent changes in sleep patterns, ability to perform self-care and activities of daily living, sexual activity, and weight. If the client is taking prescribed medications, over-the-counter medications, or herbal supplements, ask about the type and purpose as well as the frequency and duration of use.

Ask about past history of seizures; fainting; dizziness; headaches; infection and any trauma; tumors; and surgery of the brain, spinal cord, or nerves. Discuss illnesses that may cause neurologic manifestations, including cardiac disease, strokes, pernicious anemia, sinus infections, liver disease, and/or renal failure. Also ask the client about family history of neurologic health problems, diabetes mellitus, hypertension, seizures, or mental health problems.

Question the client about occupational hazards, such as exposure to toxic chemicals or materials, and the amount of time spent performing repetitive motions (e.g., data entry and assembly). Ask questions about self-care to assess the client's diet and use of tobacco, drugs, or alcohol. Ask whether the client wears a helmet when riding a bike or motorcycle or participating in contact sports or uses seat belts when driving a vehicle.

A physical exam should include cranial nerve and sensory/motor assessments.

Diagnosis

Nursing diagnoses for the client with peripheral neuropathy will differ based on the type of neuropathy and comorbidities. They may include the following:

- Pain
- Disturbed sensory perception
- Anxiety.

Plan

Goals of nursing care may include:

- Promote client safety and prevent injury related to reduced sensation
- Assess client pain and promote nonpharmacological interventions to reduce pain before initiating pharmacological management
- Encourage client to voice feelings and concerns related to sensory loss.

Implementation

Nursing care is focused on promoting client comfort and safety. Thorough assessment of sensory loss should be conducted before beginning implementation of nursing care.

Pain

Pain experienced with peripheral neuropathy varies. Pain and tenderness in muscles can be severe; interventions must be individualized to client needs. The intense pain combined with altered sensations leads to anxiety. Nursing interventions can make a difference in breaking the cycle of increasing pain that leads to increased anxiety, which, can cause more pain.

- Listen to the description of pain; determine presence of triggers or a pattern. Acknowledging the client's perception of pain is a basis for treatment; listening establishes trust.
- Use a pain scale for determining extent of pain. Consistent measurement is essential to evaluate degree of pain and effectiveness of intervention.
- Use the following complementary therapies to help manage pain:
  a. Application of heat/cold
  b. Guided imagery
  c. Relaxation techniques
  d. Massage.

Presenting options for managing pain gives the client control over the situation and helps reduce anxiety. Noninvasive interventions may augment the therapeutic benefit of medications.

- Provide analgesics as indicated; administer on a regular schedule rather than waiting until pain becomes severe. Anticipating and managing pain before it becomes severe decreases anxiety and averts the cycle of increased anxiety leading to increased pain.
- For clients with GBS, monitor for side effects of analgesics, particularly respiratory depression; assess respirations and lung sounds. Perform routine pulmonary care measures and monitor for aspiration. Frequent respiratory monitoring is indicated.

Disturbed Sensory Perception

Ensure client safety. Those with compromised feeling in extremities may be unaware that they have sustained injury.

- Teach clients and their families preventive and comfort measures. Clients with GBS may require frequent teaching if anxiety interferes with ability to understand. When possible, include the client and family in decision making; for example, seek their input when planning a daily schedule of care that incorporates various therapies.

Teaching topics, depending on the type of peripheral neuropathic and the extent of nerve damage, may include:

- Foot care, as the client may not feel injuries to the feet—especially important for clients with diabetes
- Exercise
- Smoking cessation
- Avoidance of toxic chemicals
- Nutrition, stressing the importance and identifying sources of B_{12}
- Avoidance of repetitive motion and/or prolonged pressure
- Massage to improve circulation, stimulate nerves, and reduce pain
- Referrals as appropriate.

Evaluation

Nursing care is evaluated based on client progress in meeting expected outcomes, which may include:

- Client experiences pain control to allow for rest and comfort
- Client lists strategies to reduce the risk of injury and promote safety
- Client describes treatment plan to reduce further deterioration of sensation.

of nursing care relate to treatment of underling condition, prevention of further nerve damage, and relief from symptoms.

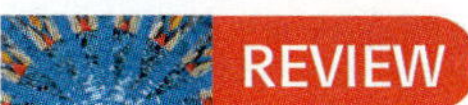

REVIEW Peripheral Neuropathy

RELATE: LINK THE CONCEPTS

Linking the exemplar of Peripheral Neuropathy with the concept of Comfort:

1. How would nursing interventions for pain differ for a client with GBS and a client with carpal tunnel syndrome?
2. What client teaching would you provide each client to prevent and/or manage pain?

Linking the exemplar of Peripheral Neuropathy with the concept of Cellular Metabolism:

3. What client teaching would you provide the newly diagnosed diabetic client to reduce the risk of later development of peripheral neuropathy?
4. Describe the pathophysiology of diabetes that contributes to the development of peripheral neuropathy.

READY: GO TO COMPANION SKILLS MANUAL

- Assessing the eyes and vision
- Assessing the client in pain

REFER: GO TO MYNURSINGKIT

REFLECT: CASE STUDY

Bob Bendy is an assembly line worker who started to feel numbness in his feet at work, where he stands 8–10 hours a day. Lately, he has noticed that he tires more easily, but he has been ignoring it "for a while" because he fears losing his job if he complains. He called in sick today because "I feel like my feet are freezing and on fire at the same time." Bob is 55 years old and lives alone on the second floor of an apartment complex. Client is 6′ and 195 pounds. He eats "mostly junk," drinks four or five beers a night, and has smoked a pack of cigarettes a day for 30 years. Despite this, he reports "good health." Bob was adopted and has no knowledge of his family's health history. His vital signs are T_O 98.9°F, P 80, R 20, BP 130/80.

1. What laboratory and diagnostic tests would you expect to be preformed?
2. What nursing diagnosis would be appropriate for this client?
3. What interventions would you initiate for this client?
4. What teaching will this client need prior to discharge?

PEARSON

EXPLORE mynursingkit™

MyNursingKit is your one stop for online chapter review materials and resources. Prepare for success with additional NCLEX®-style practice questions, interactive assignments and activities, web links, animations and videos, and more!

Register your access code from the front of your book at **www.mynursingkit.com**.

REFERENCES

Behrman, R. E., Kliegman, R. M., & Jenson, H. B. (2004). *Nelson textbook of pediatrics* (17th ed.). Philadelphia: Saunders.

Center for Health and Health Care in Schools. (2004). *Childhood vision: What the research tells us.* Retrieved June 15, 2004, from http://www.healthinschools.org

Centers for Disease Control and Prevention. (2004). National Center for Health Statistics (NCHS). *National Health and Nutrition Examination Survey Data.* http://www.cdc.gov/nchs/data/nhanes/survey_content_99_10.pdf

Chang, T. (2009). Eye diseases in Asians. *Federation of Chinese American and Chinese Canadian medical studies 9th annual conference on health care of the Chinese in North America.* Retrieved August 7, 2009, from http://www.fcmsdocs.org/HealthResources/FCMSConferences/1998/Document/TChang.php

Horgan, N., McLoone, E., Lannigan, B., & Flitcroft, I. (2005). Eye injuries in children: A new household risk. *Lancet, 366,* 547–548.

Johns Hopkins Medicine. (2007). Exercise and glaucoma: Staying fit benefits your eyes. Retrieved August 7, 2009, from http://www.johnshopkinshealthalerts.com/alerts/vision/JohnsHopkinsVisionEyeCareHealthAlert_738-1.html

Kasper, D. L., Braunwald, E., Fauci, A. S., Hauser, S. L., Longo, D. L., & Jameson, J. L. (Eds.). (2005). *Harrison's principles of internal medicine* (16th ed.). New York: McGraw-Hill.

Mayo Clinic. (2008, January 16). *Diabetic neuropathy.* Retrieved October 16, 2009, from http://www.mayoclinic.com/health/diabetic-neuropathy/DS01045/DSECTION=symptoms

Mold, J. W., Vesely, S. K., Keyl, B. A., Schenk, J. B., & Roberts, M. (2004). The prevalence, predictors, and consequences of peripheral sensory neuropathy in older patients. *The Journal of the American Board of Family Practice, 173,* 309–318.

Macular Degeneration Partnership. (n.d.). *Macular degeneration.* Retrieved August 8, 2009, from http://www.amd.org

National Eye Institute, National Institutes of Health. (2003). *Glaucoma: What you should know* (NIH Publication No. 03-651). Bethesda, MD: Author.

National Eye Institute, National Institutes of Health. (2004). *Statistics and data.* Retrieved from http://www.nei.nih.gov/eyedata/pbd_tables.asp

National Eye Institute, National Institutes of Health. (2009a). *Facts about cataract.* Retrieved August 7, 2009, from http://www.nei.nih.gov/health/cataract/cataract_facts.asp

National Eye Institute, National Institutes of Health. (2009b). *Glaucoma.* Retrieved October 9, 2009, from http://www.nei.nih.gov/health/glaucoma/glaucoma_facts.asp

National Eye Institute, National Institutes of Health. (2009c). *Age-related macular degeneration.* Retrieved October 9, 2009, from http://www.nei.nih.gov/health/maculardegen/armd_facts.asp

National Women's Health Center, Office of Womens Health, U.S. Department of Health and Human Services. (2008).

Cataracts. Retrieved August 8, 2009, from http://www.womenshealth.gov/minority/africanamerican/cataracts.cfm

Occupational Safety and Health Administration. (2008). *Safety and health topics: Eye and face protection.* Retrieved August 7, 2009, from http://www.osha.gov/SLTC/eyefaceprotection/index.html

Porth, C. M. (2005). *Pathophysiology: Concepts of altered health states* (7th ed.). Philadelphia: Lippincott.

Prevent Blindness America & National Eye Institute, National Institutes of Health. (2002). *Vision problems in the U.S. Prevalence of adult vision impairment and age-related eye disease in America.* Retrieved from http://www.usvisionproblems.org

Sarnat, H. B. (2004). Guillaine-Barre syndrome. In R. E. Behrman, R. M. Kliegman, & H. B. Jepson, *Nelson textbook of pediatrics* (17th ed., pp. 2080–2081). Philadelphia: Saunders.

Tierney, L. M., McPhee, S. J., & Papadakis, M. A. (Eds.). (2005). *Current medical diagnosis & treatment* (44th ed.). Stamford, CT: Appleton & Lange.

Way, L. W., & Doherty, G. M. (2003). *Current surgical diagnosis & treatment* (11th ed.). New York: McGraw-Hill.

Wu, C. (2005). Sports-related eye injuries. Retrieved August 8, 2009, from http://www.childrenshospital.org/patientsfamilies/Site1393/mainpageS1393P201sublevel154Flevel164.html

Sexuality 26

Concept at-a-Glance

Concept Learning Outcomes

After reading about this concept, you will be able to:

1. Summarize the structure and physiology of the reproductive system related to sexuality.
2. List factors affecting sexuality.
3. Identify commonly occurring alterations in sexuality and their related treatments.
4. Explain common physical assessment procedures used to examine sexual health across the life span.
5. Outline diagnostic and laboratory tests to determine the individual's reproductive system status.
6. Explain management of sexual health and prevention of alterations in sexuality.
7. Demonstrate the nursing process in providing culturally competent and caring interventions across the life span for individuals with common alterations in sexuality.
8. Identify pharmacologic interventions in caring for the individual with alterations in sexuality.

Concept Key Terms

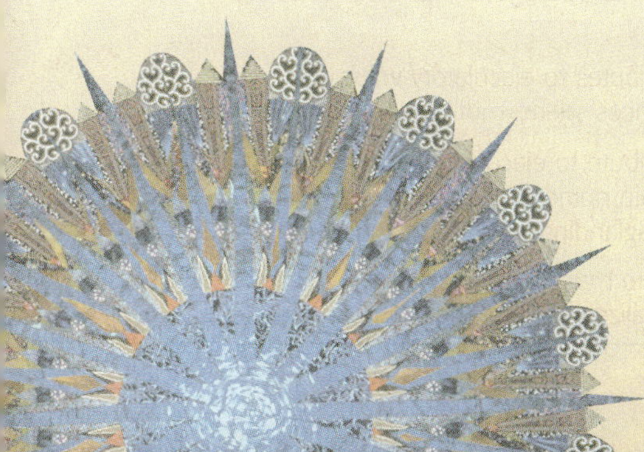

About Sexuality

Sexuality is an individually expressed and highly personal phenomenon whose meaning evolves from life experiences. Physiological, psychosocial, and cultural factors influence a person's sexuality and lead to the wide range of attitudes and behaviors seen in humans. There are no normal, universal sexual behaviors. Satisfying or "normal" sexual expression can generally be described as whatever behaviors give pleasure and satisfaction to those adults involved, without threat of coercion or injury to self or others. What constitutes "normal" sexual expression, however, varies among cultures and religions. •

REPRODUCTIVE ANATOMY AND PHYSIOLOGY

Sexuality involves more than just the anatomy and physiology of the reproductive system. Many psychological components influence sexuality, some of which will be discussed later in this section.

Male Anatomy and Physiology

The male reproductive system consists of the paired testes, scrotum, ducts, glands, and penis (Figure 26–1 ■). The breasts are part of the male reproductive system and are also assessed. The location and functions of the male reproductive organs are summarized in Table 26–1.

THE PENIS The penis is the genital organ that encloses the urethra (see Figure 26–1). It is homologous to the clitoris of the female. The penis is composed of a shaft and a tip called the glans, which is covered in the uncircumcised man by the foreskin (or prepuce). The shaft contains three columns of erectile tissue: The two lateral columns are called the corpora cavernosa, and the central mass is called the corpus spongiosum.

Erection occurs when the penile masses become filled with blood in response to a reflex that triggers the parasympathetic nervous system to stimulate arteriolar vasodilation. The erection reflex may be initiated by touch, pressure, sights, sounds, smells, or thoughts of a sexual encounter. After ejaculation, the arterioles vasoconstrict, and the penis becomes flaccid.

THE SCROTUM The scrotum is a sac or pouch made of two layers. The outer layer is continuous with the skin of the perineum and thighs. The inner layer is made of muscle and fascia.

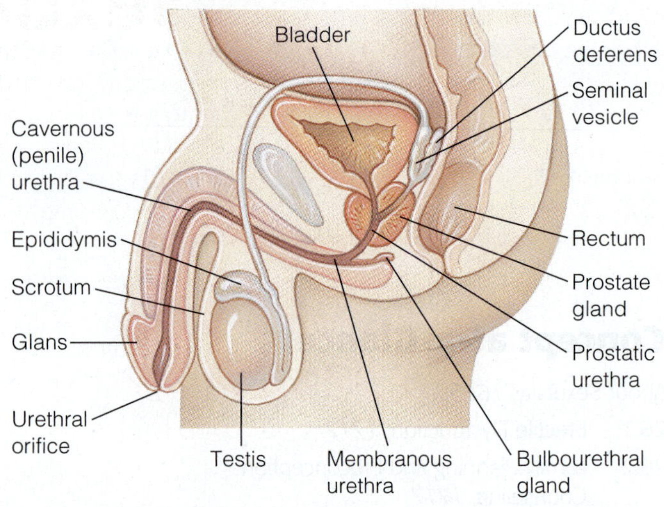

Figure 26–1 ■ The male reproductive system.

The scrotum hangs at the base of the penis, anterior to the anus, and regulates the temperature of the testes. The optimum temperature for sperm production is about 2 to 3 degrees below body temperature. When the testicular temperature is too low, the scrotum contracts to bring the testes up against the body. When the testicular temperature is too high, the scrotum relaxes to allow the testes to lie farther away from the body.

THE TESTES The testes develop in the abdominal cavity of the fetus and then descend through the inguinal canal into the scrotum. They are homologous to the female's ovaries. The testes produce sperm and testosterone. These paired organs are each about 1.5 inches (4 cm) long and 1 inch (2.5 cm) in

TABLE 26–1 **Location and Function of the Male Reproductive Organs**

MALE REPRODUCTIVE ORGAN	LOCATION	FUNCTION
Penis	Attached to front and sides of the pubic arch Proximal, ventral surface is directly continuous with the scrotum	Excretes semen and urine Deposits sperm in female reproductive tract
Scrotum	Hangs from body at root of penis	Contains testes, epididymis, and portions of the vas (ductus) deferens
Testes	In the scrotal sac	Produce sperm and testosterone
Epididymis	Posterolateral to upper aspect of each testis	Stores sperm Promotes sperm maturation Transports sperm to vas deferens
Vas deferens (ductus deferens)	Between the epididymis and the seminal vesicle forming the ejaculatory duct	Stores sperm Transports sperm
Urethra	Begins at bladder and passes through prostate and penis	Serves as passageway for urine or semen
Prostate gland	Encircles the urethra at the neck of the bladder	Contributes to ejaculatory volume Enhances sperm motility and fertility
Seminal vesicles	Lie on posterior bladder wall.	Contribute to ejaculatory volume Contain nutrients to sustain sperm and prostaglandins to facilitate sperm motility
Bulbourethral (Cowper's) glands	Inferior to the prostate	Secrete mucus into urethra Neutralize traces of acidic urine in the urethra

diameter. They are suspended in the scrotum by the spermatic cord. Each is surrounded by two coverings: an outer tunica vaginalis and an inner tunica albuginea. Each testis is divided into 250 to 300 lobules, with each lobule containing one to four seminiferous tubules. The seminiferous tubules are responsible for sperm production. Leydig's cells (or interstitial cells) lie in the connective tissue surrounding the seminiferous tubules and produce testosterone.

THE DUCTS AND SEMEN The seminiferous tubules lead into the efferent ducts and become the rete testis. From the rete testis, 10,000 to 20,000 efferent ducts join the epididymis, a long coiled tube that lies over the outer surface of each testis. The epididymis is the final area for the storage and maturation of sperm. When a man is sexually excited, the epididymis contracts to propel the sperm through the vas deferens to the ampulla, where the sperm are stored until ejaculation.

The seminal vesicles at the base of the bladder produce about 60% of the volume of seminal fluid. Seminal fluid is also made of secretions from the accessory sex organs, the epididymis, the prostate gland, and Cowper's glands. Seminal fluid nourishes the sperm, provides bulk, and increases its alkalinity. (An alkaline pH is essential to mobilize the sperm and ensure fertilization of the ova.) Sperm mixed with this fluid is called **semen**. Each seminal vesicle joins its corresponding vas deferens to form an ejaculatory duct, which enters the prostatic urethra. During ejaculation, seminal fluid mixes with sperm at the ejaculatory duct and enters the urethra for expulsion.

The total amount of semen ejaculated is 2 to 4 mL, although the amount varies. The total ejaculate of a healthy male contains from 100 million to 400 million sperm.

THE PROSTATE GLAND The prostate gland is about the size of a walnut. It encircles the urethra just below the urinary bladder (see Figure 26–1). It is made of 20 to 30 tubuloalveolar glands surrounded by smooth muscle. Secretions of the prostate gland make up about one-third of the volume of the semen. These secretions enter the urethra through several ducts during ejaculation.

SPERMATOGENESIS Spermatogenesis is the series of physiologic events that generate sperm in the seminiferous tubules. This process begins with puberty and continues throughout a man's life, with several hundred million sperm produced each day.

The inner layer of the seminiferous tubules consists of sustentacular cells (or Sertoli's cells), which contain the spermatocytes and sperm in different stages of development. Sertoli's cells secrete a nourishing fluid for the developing sperm, as well as enzymes that help convert spermatocytes to sperm. The events in spermatogenesis, which takes 64 to 72 days, are as follows:

1. The spermatogonia (sperm stem cells) undergo rapid mitotic division. As these cells multiply, the more mature spermatogonia divide into two daughter cells. These daughter cells grow and become the primary spermatocytes (and eventually become sperm).
2. Primary spermatocytes divide by meiosis to form two smaller secondary spermatocytes, which in turn divide to form two spermatids. This process occurs over several weeks.
3. The spermatids elongate into a mature sperm cell with a head and a tail. The head contains enzymes essential to the penetration and fertilization of the ova. The flagellar motion of the tail allows the sperm to move. The sperm cells then move to the epididymis to mature further and develop motility.

MALE SEX HORMONES The male sex hormones are called **androgens**. Most androgens are produced in the testes, although the adrenal cortex also produces a small amount. **Testosterone**, the primary androgen produced by the testes, is essential for the development and maintenance of sexual organs and secondary sex characteristics, and for spermatogenesis. It also promotes metabolism, growth of muscles and bone, and libido (sexual desire).

THE BREASTS The male breast is comprised primarily of an areola (circular pigmented area) and a small nipple. These lie over a thin disk of undeveloped breast tissue that may not be overtly different from surrounding tissue. Approximately one in three men have a firm area of breast tissue 2 cm or larger; the limits of normal size of this area have not been established (Bickley & Szilagyi, 2007).

Female Anatomy and Physiology

The female reproductive system consists of the external genitalia (mons pubis, labia, clitoris, vaginal and urethral openings, and glands) and the internal organs (vagina, cervix, uterus, fallopian tubes, and ovaries). The breasts are also a part of women's reproductive organs. In women, the urethra and urinary meatus are separated from the reproductive organs; however, they are so close to each other that a health problem with one often affects the other. The location and function of the female reproductive organs are summarized in Table 26–2.

THE EXTERNAL GENITALIA The external genitalia collectively are called the vulva. They include the mons pubis, the labia, the clitoris, the vaginal and urethral openings, and glands (Figure 26–2 ■).

The mons pubis is a pad of adipose (fat) tissue covered with skin. It lies anterior to the symphysis pubis. After puberty, the mons is covered with hair.

The labia are divided into two structures. The labia majora, folds of skin and adipose tissue covered with hair, are outermost; they begin at the base of the mons pubis and end at the anus. The labia minora, located between the clitoris and the base of the vagina, are enclosed by the labia majora. They are made of skin, adipose tissue, and some erectile tissues. They are usually light pink and hairless.

The area between the labia is called the vestibule and contains the openings for the vagina and the urethra as well as the Bartholin's glands. Skene's glands open onto the vestibule on each side of the urethra. Prior to menopause, Bartholin's and Skene's glands secrete lubricating fluid during the sexual response cycle.

TABLE 26–2 **Location and Function of the Female Reproductive Organs**

FEMALE REPRODUCTIVE ORGAN	LOCATION	FUNCTION
Mons pubis (mons veneris)	Anterior and superior to the pubis	Enhances sexual sensations Protects and cushions pubic symphysis during intercourse
Labia majora	Extend from mons pubis to perineum	Protect labia minora, urethral and vaginal openings Enhance sexual arousal
Labia minora	Enclosed by the labia majora	Protect clitoris Inferiorly, merge to form posterior ring of vaginal introitus (fourchette) Lubricate vulva Enhance sexual arousal
Vestibule	Area enclosed by labia minora	Contains openings for urethra, vagina, Bartholin's glands, and Skene's glands
Bartholin's (greater vestibular) glands	Posterior on each side of the vaginal orifice Open onto the sides of the vestibule in the groove between the labia minora and hymen	Secrete clear, viscid mucus during intercourse
Skene's (lesser vestibular, paraurethral) glands	Open onto the vestibule on each side of the urethra	Drain urethral glands Produce lubricating mucus
Clitoris	Small bud of erectile tissue just below the superior joining of the labia minora	Stimulates and elevates levels of sexual arousal
Perineum	Skin-covered muscular area between vaginal opening and anus	Provides support for pelvic organs
Mammary glands	Contained within breasts anterior to pectoral muscles of thorax	Produce human milk Play a role in sexual arousal
Ovaries	Lie on each side of the uterus below and behind the uterine tubes	Produce and secrete ova Produce the hormones estrogen and progesterone
Fallopian tubes (uterine tubes, oviducts)	One tube extends medially from the area of each ovary and empties into the upper portion (fundus) of the uterus.	Transport ova
Uterus (adnexa of the uterus are composed of the uterine tubes and ovaries)	Anterior to the rectum and posterior/superior to the bladder	Receives, retains, and nourishes the fertilized ovum Contracts rhythmically to expel infant Cyclically sheds lining when ovum is not fertilized
Cervix	Lower portion of uterus extending into the vagina	Connects uterine cavity with vagina Opens to allow passage of menstrual flow and infant
Vagina	Extends from the external orifice in the vestibule to the cervix	Receives penis and semen during intercourse Passageway for menstrual flow and expulsion of infant at birth.

The clitoris is an erectile organ analogous to the penis in the male. It is formed by the joining of the labia minora. Like the penis, it is highly sensitive and distends during sexual arousal.

The vaginal opening, called the introitus, is the opening between the internal and the external genitals. Prior to first intercourse or trauma, the introitus is surrounded by a connective tissue membrane called the hymen.

THE INTERNAL ORGANS The vagina and cervix, uterus, fallopian tubes, and ovaries are the internal organs of the female reproductive system (Figure 26–3 ■). The ovaries are the primary reproductive organs in women and also produce female sex hormones. The vagina, uterus, and fallopian tubes serve as accessory ducts for the ovaries and a developing fetus.

The Vagina and Cervix The vagina is a fibromuscular tube about 3 to 4 inches (8 to 10 cm) in length located posterior to the bladder and urethra and anterior to the rectum. The upper end contains the uterine cervix in an area called the fornix. The walls of the vagina are membranes that form folds, called rugae. These membranes are composed of mucous-secreting, squamous, stratified epithelial cells. The vagina serves as a

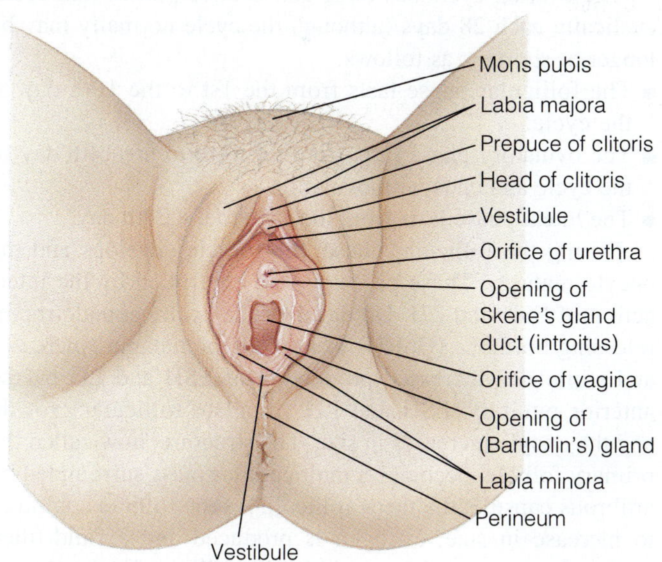

Figure 26–2 ■ The external organs of the female reproductive system.

route for the excretion of secretions, including menstrual fluid, as an organ of sexual response, and as a passageway for the birth of an infant.

The walls of the vagina are usually moist and maintain a pH ranging from 3.8 to 4.2. This pH is bacteriostatic and is maintained by the action of estrogen and normal vaginal flora. **Estrogen** stimulates the growth of vaginal mucosal cells so that they thicken and have increased glycogen content. The glycogen is fermented to lactic acid by Döderlein's bacilli (lactobacilli that normally inhabit the vagina), slightly acidifying the vaginal fluid.

The cervix projects into the vagina and forms a pathway between the uterus and the vagina. The uterine opening of the cervix is called the internal os; the vaginal opening is called the external os. The space between these openings, the endocervical canal, serves as a route for the discharge of menstrual fluid, the entrance for sperm, and the expulsion of the infant during birth. The cervix is a firm structure, protected by mucus that changes consistency and quantity during the menstrual cycle and during pregnancy.

The Uterus The uterus is a hollow, pear-shaped muscular organ with thick walls located between the bladder and the rectum. It has three parts: the fundus, the body, and the cervix. It is supported in the abdominal cavity by the broad ligaments, the round ligaments, the uterosacral ligaments, and the transverse cervical ligaments. The uterus receives the fertilized ovum and provides a site for growth and development of the fetus.

The uterine wall has three layers. The perimetrium is the outer serous layer that merges with the peritoneum. The myometrium is the middle layer and makes up most of the uterine wall. This layer has muscle fibers that run in various directions, allowing contractions during **menstruation** (the periodic shedding of the uterine lining in a woman of childbearing age who is not pregnant) or childbirth, and expansion as the fetus grows. The endometrium lines the uterus; its outermost layer is shed during menstruation.

The Fallopian Tubes The fallopian tubes are thin, cylindrical structures about 4 inches (10 cm) long and 2.5 inches (1 cm) in diameter. They are attached to the uterus on one end and are supported by the broad ligaments. The lateral ends of the fallopian tubes are open and made of projections called fimbriae that drape over the ovary. The fimbriae pick up the ovum after it is discharged from the ovary.

The fallopian tubes are made of smooth muscle and are lined with ciliated, mucous-producing epithelial cells. The movement of the cilia and contractions of the smooth muscle move the ovum through the tubes toward the uterus. Fertilization of the ovum by the sperm usually occurs in the outer portion of a fallopian tube.

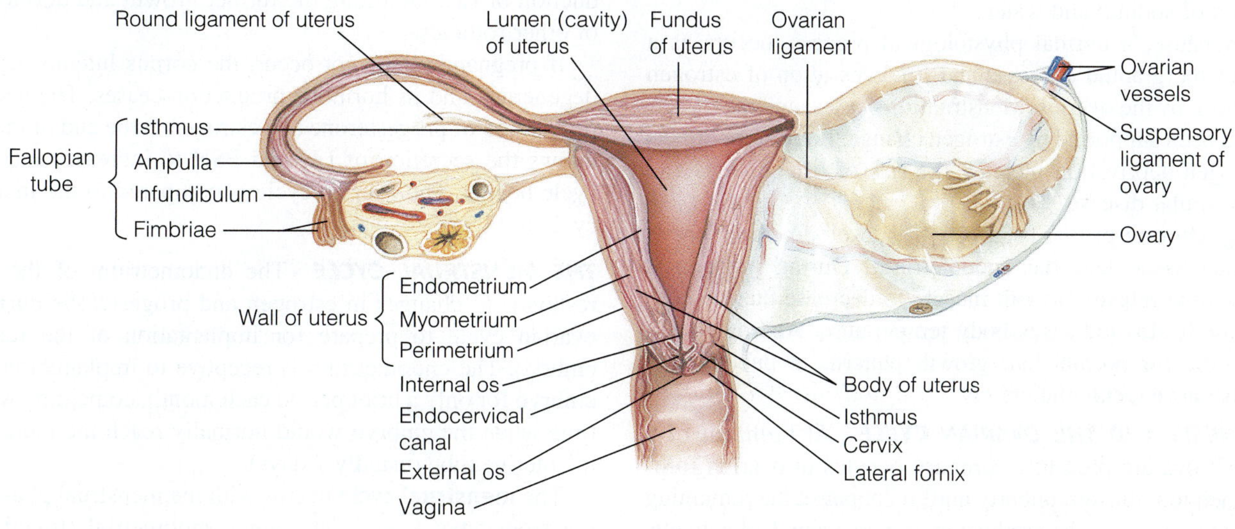

Figure 26–3 ■ The internal organs of the female reproductive system.

The Ovaries The ovaries in the adult woman are flat, almond-shaped structures located on either side of the uterus below the ends of the fallopian tubes. They are homologous to the male's testes. They are attached to the uterus by a ligament and are also attached to the broad ligament. The ovaries store the female germ cells and produce the female hormones estrogen and progesterone. A woman's total number of ova is present at birth.

Each ovary contains many small structures called ovarian follicles. Each follicle contains an immature ovum, called an oocyte. Each month, several follicles are stimulated by follicle-stimulating hormone (FSH) and luteinizing hormone (LH) to mature. The developing follicles are surrounded by layers of follicle cells, with the mature follicles called graafian follicles. The graafian follicles produce estrogen, which stimulates the development of endometrium. Each month in the menstruating woman, one or two of the mature follicles eject an oocyte in a process called ovulation. The ruptured follicle then becomes a structure called the corpus luteum. The corpus luteum produces both estrogen and progesterone to support the endometrium until conception occurs or the cycle begins again. The corpus luteum slowly degenerates, leaving a scar on the surface of the ovary.

FEMALE SEX HORMONES The ovaries produce estrogens, progesterone, and androgens in a cyclic pattern. Estrogens are steroid hormones that occur naturally in three forms: estrone (E_1), estradiol (E_2), and estriol (E_3). Estradiol is the most potent and is the form secreted in greatest amount by the ovaries. Although estrogens are secreted throughout the menstrual cycle, they are at a higher level during certain phases of the cycle, as discussed shortly.

Estrogens are essential for the development and maintenance of secondary sex characteristics, and in conjunction with other hormones, they stimulate the female reproductive organs to prepare for growth of a fetus. Estrogens are responsible for the normal structure of skin and blood vessels. They also decrease the rate of bone resorption, promote increased high-density lipoproteins, reduce cholesterol levels, and enhance the clotting of blood. Estrogens also promote the retention of sodium and water.

Menopause, a normal physiological process, occurs as a result of the gradual decrease and final cessation of estrogen production by the ovaries. Menstruation ceases, and the tissues that had been supported by estrogen change. Long-term effects of estrogen deprivation increase the risk of osteoporosis and cardiovascular disease.

Progesterone primarily affects the development of breast glandular tissue and the endometrium. During pregnancy, progesterone relaxes smooth muscle to decrease uterine contractions. It also increases body temperature. Androgens are responsible for normal hair growth patterns at puberty and may also have metabolic effects.

OOGENESIS AND THE OVARIAN CYCLE At birth, all of a woman's ova are present as primary oocytes in ovarian follicles. Each month from puberty until menopause the remaining events of oogenesis (the production of ova) occur. Collectively, these events are known as the **ovarian cycle**.

The ovarian cycle has three consecutive phases that occur cyclically each 28 days (although the cycle normally may be longer or shorter), as follows:

- The follicular phase lasts from the 1st to the 10th day of the cycle.
- The ovulatory phase lasts from the 11th to the 14th day of the cycle and ends with ovulation.
- The luteal phase lasts from the 14th to the 28th day.

During the follicular phase, the follicle develops and the oocyte matures. These processes are controlled by the interaction of FSH and LH. On day 1 of the cycle, gonadotropin-releasing hormone (GnRH) from the hypothalamus increases and stimulates increased production of FSH and LH by the anterior pituitary. FSH and LH stimulate follicular growth, and the oocyte increases in size. The structure, now called the primary follicle, becomes a multicellular mass surrounded by a fibrous capsule, the theca folliculi. As the follicle continues to increase in size, estrogen is produced and a fluid-filled space (the antrum) forms within the follicle. The oocyte is enclosed by a membrane, the zona pellucida. By about day 10, the follicle is a mature graafian follicle and bulges out from the surface of the ovary. There are always follicles at different stages of development in each ovary, but usually only one follicle becomes dominant and matures to ovulation, while the others degenerate.

The ovulatory phase begins when estrogen levels reach a level high enough to stimulate the anterior pituitary, and a surge of LH is produced. The LH stimulates meiosis in the developing oocyte, and its first meiotic division occurs. The LH also stimulates enzymes that act on the bulging ovarian wall, causing it to rupture and discharge the antrum fluid and the oocyte. The oocyte is expelled from the mature ovarian follicle in the process called ovulation.

During the luteal phase, the surge in LH also stimulates the ruptured follicle to change into a corpus luteum and then stimulates the corpus luteum to begin immediately producing progesterone and estrogen. The increase of progesterone and estrogen in the blood has a negative feedback effect on the production of LH, inhibiting the further growth and development of other follicles.

If pregnancy does not occur, the corpus luteum begins to degenerate, and its hormone production ceases. The declining production of progesterone and estrogen at the end of the cycle allows the secretion of LH and FSH to increase, and a new cycle begins. The ovarian cycle is compared to the menstrual cycle in Figure 26–4 ■.

THE MENSTRUAL CYCLE The endometrium of the uterus responds to changes in estrogen and progesterone during the ovarian cycle to prepare for implantation of the fertilized embryo. The endometrium is receptive to implantation of the embryo for only a brief period each month, coinciding with the time when the embryo would normally reach the uterus from the uterine tube (usually 7 days).

The **menstrual cycle** begins with the menstrual phase, lasting from days 1 to 5. The inner endometrial (functionalis) layer detaches and is expelled as menstrual fluid (fluid and blood) for 3 to 5 days. As the maturing follicle begins to produce estrogen (days 6 to 14), the proliferative phase begins. In response, the functionalis layer is repaired and thickens, while spiral arteries increase in number and tubular glands form. Cervical mucus changes to a thin, crystalline substance, forming channels to help the sperm move up into the uterus.

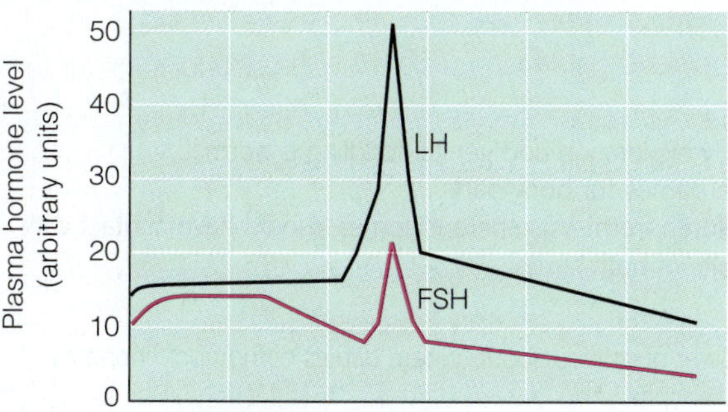

A Fluctuation of gonadotropin levels

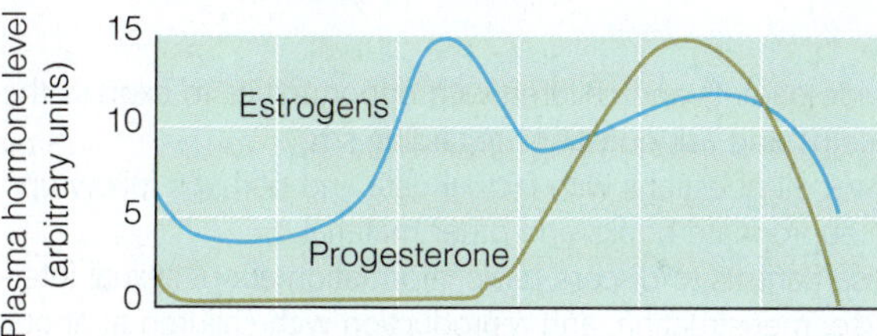

B Fluctuation of ovarian hormone levels

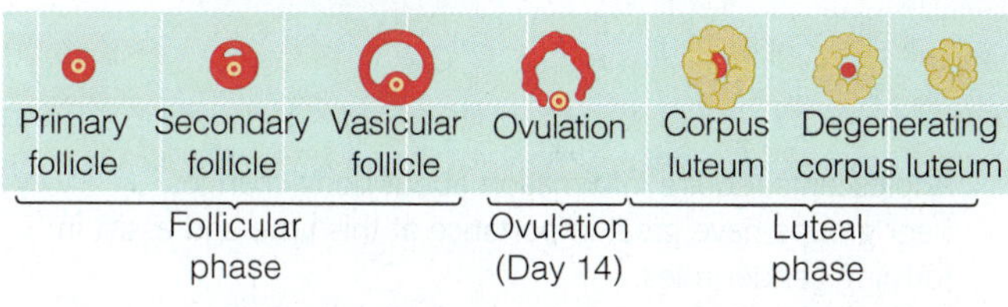

C Ovarian cycle

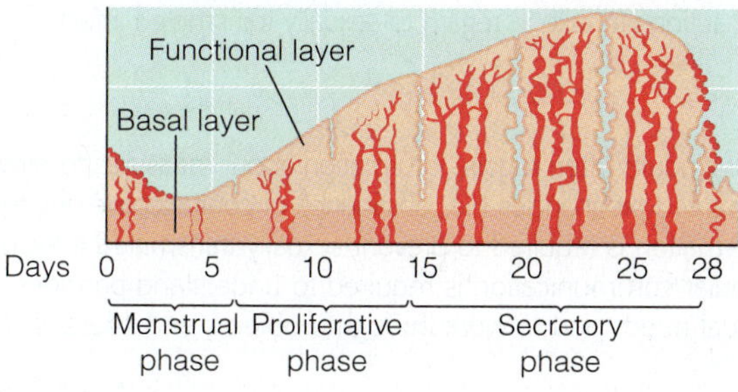

D Menstrual cycle

Figure 26–4 ■ Comparison of the ovarian and menstrual cycles. *A*, Fluctuating levels of follicle-stimulating hormone (FSH) and luteinizing hormone (LH), the pituitary gonadotropins regulating the ovarian cycle. *B*, Fluctuating levels of ovarian hormones that cause endometrial changes during the menstrual cycle. *C*, Changes in the ovarian follicles during the 28-day menstrual cycle. *D*, Corresponding changes in the endometrium during the menstrual cycle.

The final phase, lasting from days 14 to 28, is the secretory phase. As the corpus luteum produces progesterone, the rising levels act on the endometrium, causing increased vascularity, changing the inner layer to secretory mucosa, stimulating the secretion of glycogen into the uterine cavity, and causing the cervical mucus again to become thick and block the internal os. If fertilization does not occur, hormone levels fall. Spasm of the spiral arteries causes hypoxia of the endometrial cells, which begin to degenerate and slough off. As with the ovarian cycle, the process begins again with the sloughing of the functionalis layer.

THE BREASTS The breasts (or mammary glands) are located between the third and seventh ribs on the anterior chest wall. They are supported by the pectoral muscles and are richly supplied with nerves, blood, and lymph (Figure 26–5 ■). A pigmented area called the areola is located slightly below the center of each breast and contains sebaceous glands and a nipple. The nipple is usually protrusive and becomes erect in response to cold and stimulation.

The breasts are made of adipose tissue, fibrous connective tissue, and glandular tissue. Cooper's ligaments support the breast and extend from the outer breast tissue to the nipple, dividing the breast into 15 to 25 lobes. Each lobe is made of alveolar glands connected by ducts that open to the nipple.

DEVELOPMENT AND SEXUALITY

The development of sexuality begins with conception and continues throughout the life span. While this concept discusses development in terms of sexuality, it is important that nurses

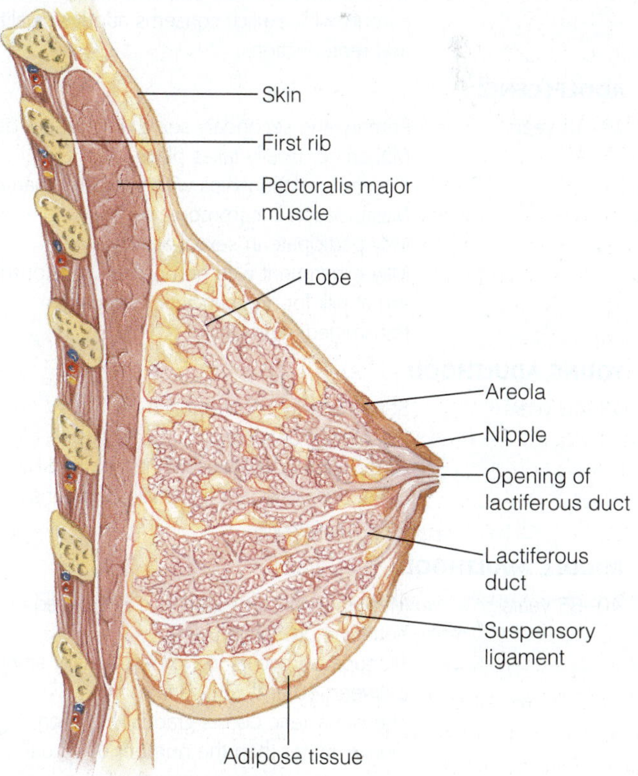

Figure 26–5 ■ Structure of the female breast.

DEVELOPMENTAL CONSIDERATIONS Sexual Development Throughout the Life Span

STAGE	CHARACTERISTICS	NURSING INTERVENTIONS AND TEACHING GUIDELINES
INFANCY		
Birth to 18 months	Given gender assignment of male or female. Differentiates self from others gradually. External genitals are sensitive to touch. Male infants have penile erections; females, vaginal lubrication.	Self-manipulation of the genitals is normal. Caregivers need to recognize these behaviors as common in children.
TODDLER		
1–3 years	Continues to develop gender identity. Able to identify own gender.	Body exploration and genital fondling is normal. Use names for body parts. Children from single-parent homes should have contact with adults of both sexes.
PRESCHOOLER		
4–5 years	Becomes increasingly aware of self. Explores own and playmates' body parts. Learns correct names for body parts. Learns to control feelings and behavior. Focuses love on parent of the other sex.	Answer questions about "where babies come from" honestly and simply. Parental overreaction to exploration of genitals and masturbation can lead to feelings that sex is "bad."
SCHOOL AGE		
6–12 years	Has strong identification with parent of same gender. Tends to have friends of the same gender. Has increasing awareness of self. Increased modesty, desire for privacy. Continues self-stimulating behavior. Learns the role and concepts of own gender as part of the total self-concept. At about 8 or 9 years becomes concerned about specific sex behaviors and often approaches parents with explicit concerns about sexuality and reproduction.	Provide parents and children with opportunities to express their concerns and ask questions regarding sex. Answer all questions with factual data and perhaps follow up with appropriate books and other material. Advise parents to discuss basic information about sexual intercourse, menstruation, and reproduction with children at about 10 years of age. Give children reading material and then discuss it with them.
ADOLESCENCE		
12–18 years	Primary and secondary sex characteristics develop. Menarche usually takes place. Develops relationships with interested partners. Masturbation is common. May participate in sexual activity. May experiment with homosexual relationships. Are at risk for pregnancy and sexually transmitted infections.	Adolescents require information about body changes. Peer groups have great importance at this time and assist in forming gender roles. Dating helps adolescents prepare for adult roles. Parents influence values and beliefs regarding behavior. Teenagers require information about contraceptive measures and precautions to take in regard to sexually transmitted infections.
YOUNG ADULTHOOD		
18–40 years	Sexual activity is common. Establishes own lifestyle and values. Homosexual identity usually established by mid-20s. Many couples share financial obligations and household tasks.	Young adults often require information about measures to prevent unwanted pregnancies (i.e., abstinence or contraceptive devices). Information is required to prevent sexually transmitted infections. Regular communication is required to understand partner's sexual needs and to work through problems and stresses.
MIDDLE ADULTHOOD		
40–65 years	Men and women experience decreased hormone production. Menopause occurs in women, usually anywhere between 40 and 55 years. The climacteric occurs gradually in men. Quality rather than the number of sexual experiences becomes important. Individuals establish independent moral and ethical standards.	Women and men may need help adjusting to new roles. People may require counseling to help them reevaluate and direct their energies. Encourage couples to look at the positive aspects of this time of life.

DEVELOPMENTAL CONSIDERATIONS **Sexual Development Throughout the Life Span (continued)**

STAGE	CHARACTERISTICS	NURSING INTERVENTIONS AND TEACHING GUIDELINES
LATE ADULTHOOD		
65 years and over	Interest in sexual activity often continues. Sexual activity may be less frequent. Women's vaginal secretions diminish, and breasts atrophy. Men produce fewer sperm and need more time to achieve an erection and to ejaculate.	Older adults often continue to be sexually active. Couples may require counseling about adapting their affection and sexual needs to physical limitations.

consider this in the larger context of the development of the individual. The concept on Development, discusses the various stages of individual development. Sexual development throughout the life span is discussed in the Developmental Considerations feature.

Birth to 12 Years

The ability of the human body to experience a sexual response is present before birth. As evidenced by ultrasound, males have erections several months before birth. They continue to experience erections after birth. Since females have vaginal lubrication at birth, it is assumed that lubrication also occurs prior to birth. When babies find their fingers and toes, they also find their genitals. They seem to experience a pleasurable sensation from the touch but one would not call this a sexual experience. By the age of 3, more purposeful masturbation begins, and the orgasmic response is quite common, although males do not ejaculate until after puberty. By age 2 1/2 or 3, children know what gender they are and have beginning awareness of genital differences between males and females.

Around age 9 or 10, the first physical changes of puberty begin—the development of breast buds in girls and the growth of pubic hair. As the adrenal glands mature they produce more testosterone and estradiol, which contribute to the first experiences of sexual attraction to another person. Girls need to be taught about menstruation (monthly uterine bleeding) and related self-care.

Adolescence

During early adolescence (12 to 13 years), primary and secondary sex characteristics continue to develop, necessitating more information about body changes. For boys, the testes and scrotum increase in size, the skin over the scrotum becomes darker, pubic hair grows, and axillary sweating begins. Development of the genitals to adult size takes about 5 to 6 years. For girls, the pelvis and hips broaden, the breast tissue develops, pubic hair grows, axillary sweating begins, and vaginal secretions become milky and change from an alkaline to an acid pH.

Teenage girls may have irregular menstruation initially, which can lead to embarrassment because of stained clothing. They can be taught to be aware of subtle signs of impending menstruation, such as tender breasts, water retention or bloating, or the appearance of skin eruptions or pimples. Girls should also be counseled regarding the variety of feminine hygiene products available (e.g., sanitary pads and tampons) so that they can make intelligent choices. Parents and nurses should advise teenage girls to wash their hands thoroughly before inserting a tampon, to change tampons frequently, to alternate tampons with sanitary pads, and to use pads at night. These measures will help to decrease the risk of infection, including the risk of "toxic shock," a particular type of *Staphylococcus aureus* infection. Thorough cleaning of the genital area and wiping from front to back will also decrease infection and prevent odors.

Dysmenorrhea (painful menstruation) is prevalent among adolescent females. Cramping, lower abdominal pain radiating to the back and upper thighs, nausea, vomiting, diarrhea, and headaches may occur for a few hours up to 3 days. Dysmenorrhea results from powerful uterine contractions, which cause ischemia and, in turn, cramping pain. The symptoms of dysmenorrhea are treated with bed rest, administration of analgesics such as aspirin, application of heat to the abdomen, certain exercises such as abdominal muscle strengthening, biofeedback, and nonsteroidal anti-inflammatory medications, such as ibuprofen. Masturbation to orgasm also eases cramping through the associated uterine contractions and increased blood flow.

Although it is difficult to apply statistical data on large populations to local populations, it is generally accepted that sexual experimentation is currently occurring at ages younger than in previous decades. One study showed first sexual experience reported occurring within ages 10 to 16 for one-third of the sample of almost 10,000 young adults (Kaestle, Halpern, Miller, & Ford, 2005). Sexually transmitted infections (STIs) are the most common bacterial infections among adolescents.

All adolescents want to know about sexual behaviors but are often uneasy about discussing these concerns with their parents. Nurses, the schools, and the family need to provide accurate information. During the nursing assessment, teenagers should be asked directly what they know about sex, contraception, and reproduction. Sometimes a lot of the teenager's information is based on popular myths and little, if any, fact. The nurse should discuss factual information about sex, sexual actions and their consequences, the individual's right to make a decision regarding ways to express oneself sexually, and the responsibilities of each person with respect to sexual activity.

Young and Middle Adulthood

In young adulthood, many people begin to form intimate relationships with long-term implications. These relationships may take the form of dating, cohabitation, or marriage. Note, however, that some people do not form intimate relationships until late adulthood and that some never form these types of relationships.

Young adult men and women are often concerned about normal sexual response, for both themselves and their partners. In heterosexual relationships, problems may arise because of basic differences in male and female expectations and responses. Gay and lesbian couples often fare better in this respect. Couples need to communicate their needs to one another early in their courtship so that a successful intimate relationship can develop and grow. Young adults should also be aware that because sexual needs and responses may change, each partner should listen and respond to the needs of the other.

During middle adulthood, both men and women experience decreased hormone production, causing the climacteric, usually called menopause in women. These events often affect the individual's sexual self-concept, body image, and sexual identity.

Sexuality and Older Adults

Interest in sexual activity is not lost as people age. For men, however, more time is needed to achieve an erection and to ejaculate (the erection may last longer than at a younger age), more direct genital stimulation is required to achieve an erection, the volume of ejaculated fluid decreases, and the intensity of contractions with orgasm may decrease. The refractory period after orgasm is longer.

Older women remain capable of multiple orgasms and may, in fact, experience an increase in sexual desire after menopause; vaginal lubrication and elasticity decrease with menopause and decreased estrogen, and phases of the sexual response cycle may take longer to occur.

Many products are available to assist older adults with enhancing their sexual experiences. These range from simple lubricants to surgically implanted devices that enable penile erections. Although older adults' technique may require modification, the nurse should never assume that they are less interested or motivated to have an active sex life.

Older adults may define sexuality far more broadly and include in their definition such things as touching, hugging, romantic gestures (e.g., giving or receiving roses), comfort, warmth, dressing up, joy, spirituality, and beauty.

Older adults continue to need **intimacy**, chosen emotional interconnectedness between two people that includes mutual caring and responsibility, although there may be fewer opportunities and strong social sanctions against this. Intimacy entails five important aspects: commitment, affective intimacy, cognitive intimacy, physical intimacy, and mutuality (Blieszner & de Vries, 2001). Close friendships, sexual relationships, strong ties to family members, and beloved pets can all contribute to meeting the older adult's need for intimacy but are not always available. Nursing care may include touching intimate areas of an older person's body, but in a detached and clinical fashion. This may leave the older adult feeling bereft. Awareness on the part of the nurse can be an asset to older adults and their quest for intimacy.

The age-related changes in sexual response in both men and women do not preclude a satisfying sex life. Because arousal takes longer in both sexes, foreplay is even more important than in younger adults. Hugging, kissing, and caressing are sexual activities that both men and women enjoy. They can be preludes to sexual intercourse or satisfying activities in themselves (Johnson, 1996). The older adults Johnson studied were generally open-minded and knowledgeable about sexual matters, but health status was a barrier to sexual expression.

Chronic pain and osteoarthritis are two common problems that have deleterious effects on sexual activity in older adults. Arthritis in the hip joint presents the greatest challenge to satisfying sexual activity (Butler & Lewis, 2003), but it can be ameliorated by changes in coital position, use of heat applications, and timing during the day when joints are less painful. The "spoon" position, in which partners lie on their sides with the woman in front, allows for penile penetration of the vagina without undue strain to either partner (Monga et al., 1999). Warm baths can also help relieve pain and can be incorporated as foreplay.

Many older adults who suffer from cardiovascular disease are concerned about the safety of sex. In general, if an older adult can climb two flights of stairs or walk at a rate of 2 miles per hour without chest pain or shortness of breath, he or she should have no cardiac problems during sexual intercourse (Butler & Lewis, 2003). Consideration should be given to the partner with the less stable vital signs, particularly blood pressure, and that person should not be positioned on top. Sexual intercourse with one partner in a chair and the other directly in front of the chair is another variation that may help some older couples (Monga et al., 1999).

Dyspareunia, painful intercourse for the older woman, may be related to decreased vaginal lubrication as well as lack of elevation of the labia during sexual arousal (Monga et al., 1999). Penetration is difficult as the vaginal opening may be partially obscured by the labia, and the lack of lubrication further inhibits entrance of the penis. The older couple might be advised to use a vaginal lubricant as part of their sexual activity and to have the woman use her hand to guide her partner's penis into the vagina.

Diabetes mellitus can have negative effects on the sexual expression of both men and women. It is correlated with erectile dysfunction in the man and even greater reduction of lubrication in the woman (Monga et al., 1999). Alternative expressions of sexuality, such as body caressing, manipulation of the partner's genitals with the hand, or mutual masturbation, may be suggested.

DISCUSSING SEXUALITY WITH OLDER ADULTS The PLISSIT model of intervention for sexual concerns, developed over 30 years ago, is still a valid method for nurses to use with older adults (Annon, 1974; Hartford Institute for Geriatric Nursing, 2001). **P** stands for permission, in which the nurse validates the older adult's desire for sexual activity. The nurse may start the conversation with a neutral phrase such as "Many people think older adults aren't interested in sex any more, but that's not true. I wonder if you have questions that I might answer for you." The permission phase is concerned with normalizing the older adult's feelings and concerns.

LI is limited information, and the nurse offers specific, factual information pertinent to the older client. For example, an older man may appreciate knowing that although his erection is not as firm as it once was, he can still satisfy himself and his partner. **SS** stands for specific suggestions, such as coital positions or timing of pain medication. **IT** is intensive therapy, which requires a referral to an advanced practice nurse or other expert.

SEXUALITY IN LONG-TERM CARE Meeting the intimacy needs of older adults in long-term care settings can be a challenge to the nurse. A poignant description of the negative view nurses hold of sexuality and older adults in institutions was written by Nay (1992), who concluded, "It is not possible to provide care that aims at maximizing potential, independence, and control, while denying or ridiculing a 'core' aspect of identity. It is not enough to care for the body; recognition of the whole person, including sexuality, must be reflected in nursing care" (p. 314). That being said, there are both legal and ethical concerns when it comes to sexual activity among residents of long-term care facilities.

Nursing homes have a lack of privacy for residents, and safety is a concern when there are no beds large enough to accommodate two people and sexual activity. Pushing two beds together is not a safe option unless they are securely fastened together. The attitudes of staff and adult children, however, may be the biggest hurdle sexually active older adults have to face (Lichtenberg, 1997; Nay, 1992). Many parties may have concerns related to physical intimacy between nursing home residents, including the adult children of the involved residents, the unit staff, governmental agencies, and the administrative team of the nursing home. In fact, adult children may collude with staff members to keep their parent away from a romantic interest.

If one or both of the older adults involved in physical intimacy is cognitively impaired, both legal and ethical responsibilities arise. The nurse must intervene to ensure that both parties are making an informed decision to participate in sexual activity or at least that there is no exploitation involved (Lichtenberg, 1997). A person with dementia who is unable to make an informed decision should be protected from exploitation. There is no generally accepted standard for when a person with cognitive changes is no longer able to give informed consent, and the nurse will have to assess each situation.

Some older adults with dementias will engage in sexual activity that is inappropriate, for example, masturbation in public. One nursing intervention is to redirect the older adult to a private area or provide distraction (Monga et al., 1999). It is important to consider the motive that may be driving the sexual behavior and attempt to meet those needs (Duffy, 1998). For example, fondling the genitals may be an indication that the older person needs to urinate. At no time should a punitive approach be taken.

SEXUAL HEALTH

Sexual health is an individual and constantly changing phenomenon falling within the wide range of human sexual thoughts, feelings, needs, and desires. For most people, sexual health is not considered until its absence or an impairment is noticed. A person's degree of sexual health is best determined by that individual, sometimes with the assistance of a qualified professional. The World Health Organization defined **sexual health** in 1975 as "the integration of the somatic, emotional, intellectual, and social aspects of sexual being, in ways that are positively enriching and that enhance personality, communication, and love" (p. 6). This definition recognizes the biological, psychological, and sociocultural dimensions of sexuality. Characteristics of sexual health are listed in Box 26–1.

Components of Sexual Health

Five critical components of sexual health are sexual self-concept, body image, gender identity, gender-role behavior, and freedoms and responsibilities.

One's **sexual self-concept** (how one values oneself as a sexual being) determines with whom one will have sex; the gender and kinds of people one is attracted to; and the values about when, where, with whom, and how one expresses sexuality. A positive sexual self-concept enables people to form intimate relationships throughout life. A negative sexual self-concept may impede the formation of relationships.

Body image, a central part of the sense of self, is constantly changing. Pregnancy, aging, trauma, disease, and therapies can alter an individual's appearance and function, which can affect body image. How a person feels about his or her body is related to his or her sexuality. People who feel good about their bodies are likely to be comfortable with and enjoy sexual activity. People who have a poor body image may respond negatively to sexual arousal. A major influence on body image for women is the media focus on physical attractiveness and large breasts. Likewise, many men worry about penis size. The myth that "larger is better," particularly if it is erect and has staying power,

Box 26–1 **Characteristics of Sexual Health**

- Knowledge about sexuality and sexual behavior
- Ability to express one's full sexual potential, excluding all forms of sexual coercion, exploitation, and abuse
- Ability to make autonomous decisions about one's sexual life within a context of personal and social ethics
- Experience of sexual pleasure as a source of physical, psychological, cognitive, and spiritual well-being
- Capability to express sexuality through communication, touch, emotional expression, and love
- Right to make free and responsible reproductive choices
- Ability to access sexual health care for the prevention and treatment of all sexual concerns, problems, and disorders

Note: From *Declaration of Sexual Rights*, by the World Association of Sexology, 1999, Adopted at the 14th World Congress of Sexology, Hong Kong and People's Republic of China. Reprinted with permission from the World Association for Sexual Health (WAS). All rights reserved.

is pervasive in North America. A person's body image can suffer when the person is unable to achieve these expectations.

Gender identity is one's self-image as a female or male. More than just the biological component, it also includes social and cultural norms. Gender identity is the result of a long series of developmental events that may or may not conform to one's apparent biological sex. Once gender identity is established, it cannot be easily changed.

Gender-role behavior is the outward expression of a person's sense of maleness or femaleness as well as the expression of what is perceived as gender-appropriate behavior. Each society defines its roles for males and females; boys are given reinforcement for behaving in a "masculine" way, and girls receive reinforcement for exhibiting "feminine" behaviors.

Physical structure, variations in the internal sense of what is male or female, family values, and cultural values all influence gender-role behavior. In North America, expected adult male roles include breadwinner, heterosexual lover, father, and athlete. Expected male behaviors include wearing trousers, demonstrating physical strength, and expressing feelings in a controlled fashion. Women are expected to express their emotions more freely and to be gentler in their physical responses; they also have a broader choice of clothing than men do.

Androgyny, or flexibility in gender roles, is the belief that most characteristics and behaviors are human qualities that should not be limited to one specific gender or the other. Being androgynous does not mean being sexually neutral or imply anything about one's sexual orientation. Rather, it describes the degree of flexibility a person has regarding gender-stereotypic behaviors. Adults who can behave flexibly regarding their sexual roles may be able to adapt better than those who adopt rigid stereotyped gender roles.

Sexual health includes both *freedoms* and *responsibilities*. Sexually healthy people engage in activities that are freely chosen, including both self-pleasuring and shared-pleasuring activities. Individuals also have freedom of their sexual thoughts, feelings, and fantasies. Sexually healthy people are ethically motivated to exercise behavioral, emotional, economic, and social responsibility for themselves ("Vision of Sexual Health," 2004).

Varieties of Sexuality

There are many varieties of sexuality. There is a tremendous range of variation in how people experience and express their sexuality. There are also many differences in the priority people place on sexuality in their lives. Sexual varieties include sexual orientation, gender identity, erotic preferences, and sexual lifestyles.

SEXUAL ORIENTATION One's attraction to people of the same sex, the other sex, or both sexes is referred to as **sexual orientation**. Sexual orientation lies along a continuum with a wide range between the two extremes of exclusively heterosexual attraction and exclusively homosexual attraction. Individuals who are attracted to people of both genders are referred to as *bisexuals*.

The origins of sexual orientation are still not well understood. Some biological theories describe sexual orientation in terms of the genetic composition of the individual. Psychological theories stress the role of early learning experiences and cognitive processes. Other theories acknowledge the confluence of genetics and the environment in the development of sexual orientation.

Estimates of the percentage of the population with a homosexual orientation vary, although the usual figure is 5% to 10% of men and 2% to 4% of women (McCammon, Knox, & Schacht, 2004). Because these individuals grow up acutely aware of the discrimination they face in North America, many do not disclose their sexual orientation; therefore, actual figures are not available.

GENDER IDENTITY Western culture is deeply committed to the idea that there are only two sexes. Biologically speaking, however, there are many gradations running from female to male; this is known as **transgenderism**. In some cases, gender is clear; in other cases, there is a blending of both genders within the same individual; and in some cases, it is unclear.

Intersex About 1 in every 2,000 babies is born with an intersex condition, in which there are contradictions among chromosomal gender, gonadal gender, internal organs, and external genital appearance. The gender of such an infant is ambiguous. What this means is that an intersexed person has some parts usually associated with males and some parts usually associated with females. Intersex anatomy may not be apparent at birth. Sometimes it is undetected until puberty, until the person is identified as an infertile adult, or until the person dies and is autopsied. For more information, see the Intersex Society of North America.

Transsexuals The medical profession considers **transsexuals** to have a condition called *gender dysphoria* (strong and persistent feelings of discomfort with one's assigned gender) or *gender identity disorder*. For the transsexual person, sexual anatomy is not consistent with gender identity. Those who are born physically male but are emotionally and psychologically female are called male-to-female (MTF) transsexuals. Those who are born female but are emotionally and psychologically male are called female-to-male (FTM) transsexuals.

Most transsexuals report that they have felt gender dysphoria since early childhood. They often suffer for many years and try to hide the situation from family and friends for fear of being considered "crazy." Being transgendered puts women and men at extreme risk of the following:

- Ridicule and humiliation
- Discrimination in hiring and employment practices
- Eviction without cause from restaurants and stores
- Discrimination in housing
- Being refused medical treatment, even to save a life (Lips, 2005).

As self-understanding and acceptance increase, many transsexuals live part or full time as members of the other sex. Cross-dressing (dressing in the clothing of the other sex) not only makes their outward appearance consistent with their inner identity and gender role, but also increases their comfort with themselves. Their sexual orientation may be heterosexual, homosexual, or bisexual.

Cross-Dressers **Cross-dressers** are typically males who cross-dress to express the feminine side of their personality. In most instances, cross-dressers are not interested in permanently altering their bodies through surgical means, especially since the majority of them are comfortable with their original birth identity and behavior in their public and professional lives.

Cross-dressing is a conscious choice and may occur at home or in public settings. The frequency of the activity ranges from rarely to often. It is not unusual for cross-dressers to have a female name to go with the female personality and wardrobe. Cross-dressing occurs more frequently in cultures where males are expected to be strong, independent, and unemotional protectors. If the social climate is considered to be one with rigid gender roles, some men may need to express their gentleness and dependence by creating a separate world and female persona within that social climate (Barnett & Rivers, 2004).

EROTIC PREFERENCES Over a lifetime, sexual fantasies and single-partner sex are the most common sexual outlets for women and men, single and coupled persons, and heterosexual, gay/lesbian, and bisexual persons. **Masturbation** is the self-stimulation of one's genitals for sexual pleasure. It may be an expression of the ongoing love affair that each of us has with ourselves throughout our lifetime. It is the way we discover our erotic feelings and learn about our sexual response. Mutual masturbation can provide sexual pleasuring and intimacy without hurrying to genital interaction before both partners are ready. Masturbation shared with a partner is a safe alternative to unprotected genital sex.

Male-to-female or female-to-female **oral–genital sex** is known as *cunnilingus.* This involves kissing, licking, or sucking of the female genitals, including the mons pubis, vulva, clitoris, labia, and vagina. *Fellatio* is oral stimulation of the penis by licking and sucking. *Sixty-nine* is simultaneous oral–genital stimulation by two people. Preconceptions and myths are a major deterrent for those who have not tried oral sex. However, like most sexual practices, oral–genital sex is not completely free of the potential for transmission of infection, and safe sex practices must be used.

Anal stimulation can be a source of sexual pleasure because the anus has a rich nerve supply. Stimulation may be applied with fingers, mouth, or sex toys such as vibrators. The anus is surrounded by strong muscles, and the rectum contains no natural lubrication. Therefore, inserting a finger or penis into the rectum requires relaxation and water-soluble lubricant.

A common form of sexual activity for heterosexual couples is **genital intercourse**. Penile–vaginal intercourse (coitus) can be both physically and emotionally satisfying. There are varieties of positions for this kind of intercourse; the most common is lying face to face (with the female or male on top). Side-lying, standing, sitting, and rear-entry positions are also used. Side-lying, female-on-top, and rear-entry positions facilitate clitoral stimulation, by either penile or manual contact. The choice of intercourse positions and activities depends on physical comfort and beliefs, values, and attitudes about different practices.

During intercourse, the man moves the penis back and forth along the vaginal walls by rhythmic thrusting movements of his hips. At the same time, the woman may move her own body to match the partner's hip movements. Movements usually continue until orgasm is achieved by one or both partners. Simultaneous orgasm can be difficult to achieve. After coitus, caressing, hugging, and kissing can increase the shared intimacy and should be encouraged.

The other form of genital intercourse is *anal intercourse,* during which the penis is inserted into the anus and rectum of the partner. Anal intercourse is commonly practiced by gay men, but a number of heterosexual couples engage in it as well. Positions for anal intercourse are similar to those for penile–vaginal intercourse, with minor differences due to the position of the anus.

Current practice dictates the use of a condom in both forms of intercourse to prevent the transmission of disease. Because anorectal tissue is not self-lubricating, a lubricant must be used on the condom. Also, since normal bacterial flora from the bowel can produce infection in other parts of the body, the used condom should be removed and another applied before inserting the penis into other body orifices.

There are many other varieties of sexuality that are beyond the scope of this chapter. These include several or many partners, nudism, swinging, group sex, fetishism, sexual sadism, and sexual masochism.

Sexual Response Cycle

Commonly occurring phases of the human sexual response follow a similar sequence in females and males regardless of sexual orientation. It does not matter whether the motive for being sexually active is true love or passionate lust. Table 26–3 provides a summary of the physiological changes associated with each of the phases of the cycle.

The response cycle starts in the brain, with conscious sexual desires called the **desire phase**. Sexually arousing stimuli, often called *erotic stimuli,* may be real or symbolic. Sight, hearing, smell, touch, and imagination (sexual fantasy) can all invoke sexual arousal. Sexual desire fluctuates within each person and varies from person to person. If people suppress or block out conscious sexual desires, they may not experience any physiological response. Although psychological issues are the more common causes of lack of sexual desire, medications, drugs, and hormone imbalances can also interfere.

The **excitement phase** involves two primary physiological changes (see Figure 26–6 ■). *Vasocongestion* is an increase in the blood flow to various body parts resulting in erection of the penis and clitoris and swelling of the labia, testes, and breasts. Vasocongestion stimulates sensory receptors within these body parts, which in turn transmit messages to the conscious brain, where they are usually interpreted as pleasurable sensations. When stimulation is continued, vasocongestion increases until it either is released by orgasm or fades away. Likewise, *myotonia,* an increase of tension in muscles, may increase until released by orgasm, or it may also simply fade away.

The **orgasmic phase** is the involuntary climax of sexual tension, accompanied by physiological and psychological release. This phase is considered the measurable peak of the sexual experience. Although the entire body is involved, the major focus of the orgasm is felt in the pelvic region. Male

TABLE 26–3 **Physiological Changes Associated With the Sexual Response Cycle**

PHASE OF THE SEXUAL RESPONSE CYCLE	SIGNS PRESENT IN BOTH SEXES	SIGNS PRESENT IN MALES ONLY	SIGNS PRESENT IN FEMALES ONLY
Excitement/Plateau	Muscle tension increases as excitement increases.	Penile erection; glans size increases as excitement increases.	Erection of the clitoris.
	Sex flush, usually on chest.	Appearance of a few drops of lubricant, which may contain sperm.	Vaginal lubrication.
	Nipple erection.		Labia may increase 2 to 3 times in size.
			Breasts enlarge.
			Inner two-thirds of vagina widens and lengthens; outer third swells and narrows.
			Uterus elevates.
Orgasmic	Respirations may increase to 40 breaths per minute.	Rhythmic, expulsive contractions of the penis at 0.8-second intervals.	Approximately 5–12 contractions in the orgasmic platform at 0.8-second intervals.
	Involuntary spasms of muscle groups throughout the body.	Emission of seminal fluid into the prostatic urethra from contraction of the vas deferens and accessory organs (stage 1 of the expulsive process).	Contraction of the muscles of the pelvic floor and the uterine muscles.
	Diminished sensory awareness.	Closing of the internal bladder sphincter just before ejaculation to prevent retrograde ejaculation into bladder.	Varied pattern of orgasms, including minor surges and contractions, multiple orgasms, or a simple intense orgasm similar to that of the male.
	Involuntary contractions of the anal sphincter.	Orgasm may occur without ejaculation.	
	Peak heart rate (110–180 BPM), respiratory rate (40/min or greater), and blood pressure (systolic 30–80 mm Hg and diastolic 20–50 mm Hg above normal).	Ejaculation of semen through the penile urethra and expulsion from the urethral meatus.	
		The force of ejaculation varies from man to man and at different times but diminishes after the first two to three contractions (stage 2 of the expulsive process).	
Resolution	Reversal of vasocongestion in 10–30 minutes; disappearance of all signs of myotonia within 5 minutes.	A refractory period during which the body will not respond to sexual stimulation; varies, depending on age and other factors, from a few moments to hours or days.	
	Genitals and breasts return to their preexcitement states.		
	Sex flush disappears in reverse order of appearance.		
	Heart rate, respiratory rate, and blood pressure return to normal.		
	Other reactions include sleepiness, relaxation, and emotional outbursts such as crying or laughing.		

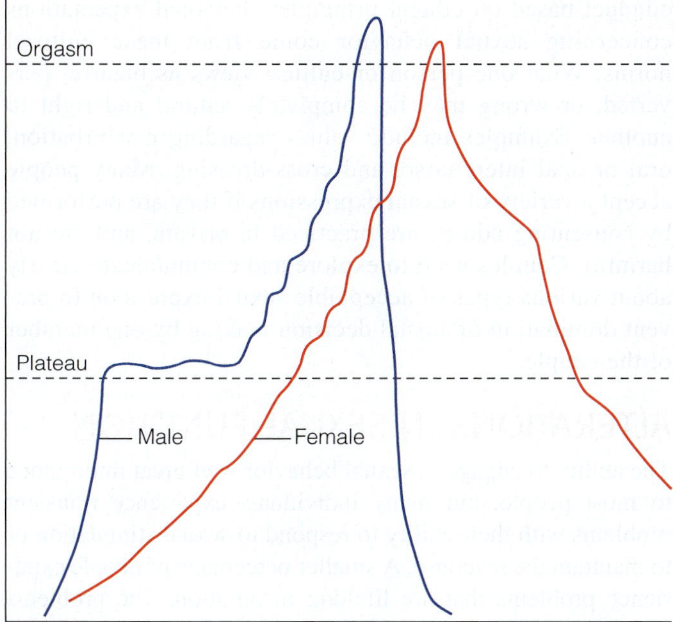

Figure 26–6 ■ Phases of the sexual response cycle.

orgasms usually last 10 to 30 seconds, while female orgasms last 10 to 50 seconds. Men usually have an *ejaculation* and expel semen as part of their orgasm. Before puberty and in later years, males experience orgasms without ejaculation.

The **resolution phase**, the period of return to the unaroused state, may last 10 to 15 minutes after orgasm or longer if there is no orgasm. This phase in females is quite varied; some women experience multiple successive orgasms followed by a longer period of resolution.

Factors Influencing Sexuality

Many factors influence a person's sexuality. Discussed here are family, culture, religion, and personal expectations and ethics.

FAMILY For the majority of us, the family is the earliest and most enduring social relationship. Families are the fabric of our day-to-day lives and shape the quality of our lives by influencing our outlooks on life, our motivations, our strategies for achievement, and our styles for coping with adversity. It is within our families that we develop our gender identity, body image, sexual self-concept, and capacity for intimacy. Through family interactions, we learn about relationships and gender roles and our expectations of others and ourselves.

From earliest beginnings, children observe their parents and model themselves after these adults. If parents are able to share affection with one another and other family members, children will most likely become adults who are able to give and receive affection. If parents seldom hug, hold hands, or kiss each other, their children may become adults who are very uncomfortable with romantic touch. If family gender role behavior is very rigid, arguments and hurt feelings will abound if a person from this system is partnered with a person who grew up in an androgynous family system. Family messages about sex range from "sex is so shameful it shouldn't be talked about" to "sex is a joyful part of adult relationships." The following are some common sexual messages children get from their families:

- Sex is dirty.
- Premarital sex is sinful.
- Good girls don't do it.
- Masturbation is disgusting.
- Men should be the sexual experts.
- Sex is mainly for procreating.
- Bodies, including genitals, are beautiful.
- Sex should be fun for both women and men.
- Sexual thoughts and feelings are natural.
- Masturbation is a common, pleasurable activity.
- There is great variety in sexual behaviors.

CULTURE Sexuality is regulated by the individual's culture. For example, culture influences the sexual nature of dress, rules about marriage, expectations of role behavior and social responsibilities, and specific sex practices. Societal attitudes vary widely. Attitudes about childhood sexual play with self or with children of the same gender or other gender may be restrictive or permissive. Premarital and extramarital sex and homosexuality may be unacceptable or tolerated. Polygamy (several marriage partners) or monogamy (one marriage partner) may be the norm. Gender role behavior also varies from culture to culture. Culture is so much a part of everyday life that it is taken for granted. We tend to assume that others share our own perspective, including those for whom we provide care. It is impossible to provide sensitive nursing care if we believe that our own culture is more important than, and preferable to, any other culture.

Cultures differ with regard to which body parts they find to be erotic. In some cultures, legs are erotic and breasts are not. Body weight may also be a determinant of sexual attractiveness. There is a great deal of pressure in American culture to be very thin. Women who would be considered obese in America are found highly attractive in other cultures. The degree of public nudity ranges from women's entire bodies and faces being covered in Islamic societies to complete nudity in some cultures in New Guinea and Australia.

Female circumcision, also known as female genital mutilation (FGM) or female ritual cutting (FRC), is a dangerous practice that is common in parts of Africa. Some of the cultural beliefs behind the practice include the following: female genitals are offensive to men, if not removed the clitoris will become the size of a penis, the labia get in the way of intercourse, the cutting enhances fertility, and the procedure prepares the woman for childbirth. Removal of the clitoris may or may not be accompanied by removal of the labia and closure of the vaginal entrance except for a small opening. Long-term medical complications include urinary incontinence, chronic urinary tract infections, vaginal scarring, pain syndromes, infertility, and sexual dysfunctions. FGM is illegal in several African and European countries and in Canada and the United States. In 1980, the World Health Organization and the United Nations Children's Fund (UNICEF) unanimously recommended that all forms of female circumcision be abolished (Elwood, 2005).

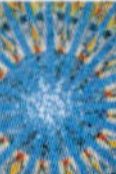

FOCUS ON DIVERSITY AND CULTURE

Selected Facts on Sexual Health

- Female circumcision or female genital mutilation (FGM) is a traditional or cultural practice in Africa, Asia, and Middle Eastern countries.
- FGM is increasingly found in the United States and Canada among immigrants from Africa, Asia, and the Middle East.
- The death rate from cervical cancer is higher than average in African Americans, Hispanics, and Native Americans.
- Leiomyosarcoma, one form of uterine cancer, occurs with greater frequency in African Americans than in other groups.
- In many cultures and religions, physical examination by a health care provider of the opposite sex is prohibited.
- Discussion of sexual activity and reproductive function is unacceptable in many cultures.
- Language barriers often prevent females from seeking or obtaining information or actual care associated with female reproductive issues.

Male circumcision is controversial. The American Academy of Pediatrics Committee on the Fetus and Newborn stated in 1971 that there were no valid medical indications for circumcision for newborns. The academy's current policy is that "Existing scientific evidence demonstrates potential medical benefits of newborn male circumcision; however, these data are not sufficient to recommend routine neonatal circumcision" (American Academy of Pediatrics Task Force on Circumcision, 1999). It supports informed decision making on the part of parents. The change of rate of circumcisions is variably reported. Some studies show an increase (Nelson, Dunn, Wan, & Wei, 2005), while the U.S. National Center for Health Statistics (2005) indicates little change in the overall rate of about 65% in the past 20 years. All studies show the highest rates in the Midwest segment of the country (81%) and the lowest rates in the West (37%).

RELIGION Religion influences sexual expression. It provides guidelines for sexual behavior and acceptable circumstances for the behavior, as well as prohibited sexual behavior and the consequences of breaking the sexual rules. The guidelines or rules may be detailed and rigid or broad and flexible. For example, some religions view forms of sexual expression other than male–female intercourse as unnatural and hold virginity before marriage to be the rule.

Many religious values conflict with the more flexible values of society that have developed during the last few decades (often labeled the "sexual revolution"), such as the acceptance of premarital sex, unwed parenthood, homosexuality, and abortion. These conflicts create marked anxiety and potential sexual dysfunctions in some individuals.

PERSONAL EXPECTATIONS AND ETHICS Although ethics is integral to religion, ethical thought and ethical approaches to sexuality can be viewed separately from religion. Cultures have developed written or unwritten codes of conduct based on ethical principles. Personal expectations concerning sexual behavior come from these cultural norms. What one person or culture views as bizarre, perverted, or wrong may be completely natural and right to another. Examples include values regarding masturbation, oral or anal intercourse, and cross-dressing. Many people accept a variety of sexual expressions if they are performed by consenting adults, are practiced in private, and are not harmful. Couples need to explore and communicate clearly about various types of acceptable sexual expression to prevent domination of sexual decision making by one member of the couple.

ALTERATIONS IN SEXUAL FUNCTION

The ability to engage in sexual behavior is of great importance to most people, but many individuals experience transient problems with their ability to respond to sexual stimulation or to maintain the response. A smaller percentage of people experience problems that are lifelong in duration. The problems may be generalized to all sexual interactions and settings, or they may be situational, occurring in a specific setting or with specific types of sexual activity. It is often difficult to sort out the multiple factors contributing to an individual's or a couple's sexual problems. Generally a number of past and current factors are involved.

Past and Current Factors

Sociocultural factors interfering in sexual function include a very restrictive upbringing accompanied by inadequate sex education. Rigid gender role socialization may inhibit exploration of sexual activities, positions, toys, and other lovemaking behaviors. If the religion to which a person is affiliated believes that sex is only for procreation, there may be great difficulty in celebrating the pleasure and fun of a loving sexual relationship. Another factor may be parental punishment for normally exploring one's genitals or for normal childhood sex play. In our current culture, the pressures of family and work often leave couples with too little time and not enough energy to enjoy sex.

Psychological factors may include negative feelings, such as guilt, anxiety, or fear, that interfere with the ability to experience pleasure and joy. Some people experience guilt when they simply enjoy sex or when they participate in what they label "unusual" sexual activities, or guilt regarding the choice of the partner. Adults who have been sexually abused at any time of their lives may experience overwhelming anxiety when faced with the decision to engage in sex. Fears may include pregnancy, sexually transmitted infections, or pain. Because vulnerability and intimacy are inherent in most sexual relationships, fear of these may lead to an avoidance of sex. Fear of failure in sexual performance often becomes a vicious cycle; that is, fear of failure creates actual failure, which in turn produces more fear. Spectatoring is the detached appraisal of sexual performance or the body during a sexual act: "Am I going to lose my erection?" "Am I going to have an orgasm this time?" "My stomach is too flabby." "When did his thighs get that fat?"

Depressed people lose interest in sexual activity and often experience a complete loss of sexual desire and fulfillment.

Cognitive factors include the internalization of negative expectations and beliefs. Those with low self-esteem may not understand how another person could value and love them and also find them sexually attractive. For those who have not yet accepted their sexual orientation or gender identity, this cognitive conflict may interfere with sexual relationships.

Sexual problems may also be symptomatic of *relationship* problems. Conflict and anger with one's partner are not conducive to positive sexual interaction. Some people lose the physical attraction to their partner or feel more attracted to someone else.

Lack of intimacy and feeling like a sex object inhibit the feeling of communion and connection that is an important part of making love. Another factor is expecting one's partner to read one's mind about sexual needs. Failure to communicate may result in one or both partners not knowing how to please the other. Unless the partners experiment, sex may, in time, become boring. Disagreements in sexual frequency and/or sexual activities may lead to further relationship conflict.

Health factors can interfere with people's expression of sexuality. Physical changes brought on by illness, injury, or surgery may inhibit full sexual expression. Throughout your program of nursing education, you will learn about the sexual side effects of a number of diseases such as heart disease, diabetes mellitus, joint disease, cancer, and mental disorders. You will also study the impact of surgeries such as hysterectomy, prostate surgery, and radical surgeries that alter a person's body image. Spinal cord injuries, traumatic amputations, or disfiguring accidents negatively affect sexual functioning. The presence of an STI in one partner induces fear of transmission in the other, often resulting in abstinence of sexual contact. In some situations, the presence of an STI is unknown and transmission occurs.

Many prescription medications beyond those intended to impact sexual functioning have side effects that affect such functioning. Most frequently, the impact is negative, but sometimes there is a positive impact. Table 26–4 provides an overview of the effects of medications on sexual function. For example, antidepressants may slow ejaculation. This may be a problem for the man who finds himself suddenly feeling unable to ejaculate. If the man is suffering from rapid ejaculation, however, the antidepressant may "cure" this problem. Some street drugs, such as marijuana, amphetamines, and cocaine, enhance sexual functioning. Others, such as opioids and anabolic steroids, interfere with sexual functioning.

TABLE 26–4 **Effects of Medications on Sexual Function**

MEDICATION	POSSIBLE EFFECTS*
Alcohol	Moderate amounts: increased sexual functioning; chronic use: decreased sexual desire, orgasmic dysfunction, and erectile dysfunction
Alpha-blockers	Inability to ejaculate
Amphetamines	Increased sex drive, delayed orgasm
Amyl nitrate	Reported enhanced orgasm; vasodilation, fainting
Anabolic steroids	Decreased sex drive, shrinking of testicles and infertility in men
Antianxiety agents	Decreased sexual desire; orgasmic dysfunction in women; delayed ejaculation
Anticonvulsants	Decreased sexual desire; reduced sexual response
Antidepressants	Decreased sexual desire; orgasmic delay or dysfunction in women; delayed or failed ejaculation; painful erection
Antihistamines	Decreased vaginal lubrication; decreased desire
Antihypertensives	Decreased sexual desire; erectile failure; ejaculation dysfunction
Antipsychotics	Decreased sexual desire; orgasmic dysfunction in women; delayed ejaculation; ejaculatory failure
Barbiturates	In low doses, increased sexual pleasure; in large doses, decreased sexual desire, orgasmic dysfunction, and erectile dysfunction
Beta-blockers	Decreased sexual desire
Cardiotonics	Decreased sexual desire
Cocaine	Increased intensity of sexual experience; with chronic use, decreased sexual desire and sexual dysfunction
Diuretics	Decreased vaginal lubrication; decreased sexual desire; erectile dysfunction
Marijuana	As above for cocaine, but prolonged use reduces testosterone levels and reduces sperm production
Narcotics	Inhibited sexual desire and response; erectile and ejaculatory dysfunctions

**Nurses and clients must familiarize themselves with the specific medication prescribed or used, because effects vary in each category of drug.*

ALTERATIONS AND TREATMENTS Alterations in Sexuality

Alteration	Description	Treatment
Priapism	Tightening of the foreskin causing tears and scarring when the penis becomes erect	Circumcision
Orgasmic disorder	Inability to reach a satisfactory conclusion or orgasm from sexual activity	Assess for possible physical cause Psychotherapy
Sexual arousal disorder	Lack of lubrication in the female; failure to attain or maintain an erection, lack of subjective sexual excitement	Medications – phosphodiesterase type 5 Artificial lubrication
Sexual pain disorders	Pain during or immediately after intercourse	Screen for STI Alternative forms of contraception Insertion of dilators that gradually increase in size Psychological counseling if no physical alteration is found
Menstrual dysfunction	Abnormal vaginal bleeding or pain during or immediately before menstruation	Oral contraceptives Dilation and curettage Hysterectomy
Sexually transmitted infections	May be no manifestations Abnormal drainage from vagina or urethra; chancre sores	If bacterial, treated with antibiotics If viral, treated with antivirals If fungal, treated with antifungals Surgery may be required to remove genital warts

Sexual Desire Disorders

For most people, sexual desire varies from day to day as well as over the years. Some people, however, report a deficiency in or absence of sexual fantasies and persistently low interest or a total lack of interest in sexual activity; these clients suffer from **hypoactive sexual desire disorder**. If both individuals in a relationship are similarly uninterested in sex, there really is no problem. More typically, there is a disparity of sexual needs, and the person with the greater desire becomes dissatisfied with the sexual relationship. The key issue in the relationship is not frequency but rather the negotiating of both partners' needs.

Sexual aversion disorder is a severe distaste for sexual activity or the thought of sexual activity, which then leads to a phobic avoidance of sex. It occurs in both women and men. Intense emotional dread of an impending sexual interaction also can trigger the physiological symptoms of anxiety: sweating, increased heart rate, and extreme muscle tension. The person then stops the sexual interaction or prevents it from even beginning. The most common cause of sexual aversion disorder is childhood sexual abuse or adult rape. The severe trauma can lead to a phobic response to sexual activity (McCammon et al., 2004).

Sexual Arousal Disorders

Sexual arousal refers to the physiological responses and subjective sense of excitement experienced during sexual activity. Lack of lubrication and failure to attain or maintain an erection are the major disorders of the arousal phase. In **female sexual arousal disorder**, the lack of vaginal lubrication causes discomfort or pain during sexual intercourse. The diagnosis of **male erectile disorder** is usually made when the man has erection problems during 25% or more of his sexual interactions. Arousal disorder may also be diagnosed even when lubrication and erection are adequate if individuals report a persistent or recurring lack of subjective sexual excitement or pleasure.

Orgasmic Disorders

The term commonly applied in the past to women who did not experience orgasm, *frigid*, implied that the woman was totally incapable of responding sexually. The more accurate and objective term is **female orgasmic disorder**, which simply means that the sexual response stops before orgasm occurs. *Preorgasmic* women have never experienced an orgasm. Studies indicate that 10–15% of women are preorgasmic, and another 20–22% report irregular orgasms. Compounding the orgasmic difficulty is the associated anxiety. In the preoccupation with orgasm, the real goal of being sexual—mutual pleasuring and intimacy—is lost, and the interchange becomes one of anxiety, frustration, and anger (McCammon et al., 2004).

Some men suffer from **male orgasmic disorder**. Men with this disorder can maintain an erection for long periods (an hour or more) but have extreme difficulty ejaculating, referred to as *retarded ejaculation.* In heterosexual intercourse, the difficulty may be limited to ejaculation in the vagina. Some men ejaculate after self-stimulation or manual or oral stimulation by the partner; others have great difficulty ejaculating with any type of stimulation. This disorder is much less common than rapid ejaculation.

Rapid ejaculation is one of the most common sexual dysfunctions among men. There are many definitions, with descriptions including ejaculating before being touched, ejaculating before penetration, ejaculating with one internal thrust, and ejaculating within a minute or two of penetration. A more helpful description is the absence of voluntary control of ejaculation. The problem is best self-defined, as when a man is concerned about his ejaculatory control or the couple agrees that ejaculation is too rapid for mutual satisfaction.

Sexual Pain Disorders

Both women and men can experience dyspareunia. It is associated with many physiological causes, especially those that inhibit lubrication. Thus, skin irritations, vaginal infections, estrogen deficiencies, and use of medications that dry vaginal secretions can cause women to experience discomfort with intercourse.

Pelvic disorders, such as infections, lesions, endometriosis, scar tissue, or tumors, can result in painful intercourse. In males, infection or inflammation of the glans penis or other genitourinary organs can cause pain with intercourse. Also, some contraceptive foams, creams, sponges, or latex products can irritate either the vagina or penis.

Vaginismus is the involuntary spasm of the outer one-third of the vaginal muscles, making penetration of the vagina painful and sometimes impossible. The woman often experiences desire, excitement, and orgasm with stimulation of the external sexual structures. Attempts at intercourse, however, elicit the involuntary spasm. The woman may have similar difficulty undergoing pelvic exams and inserting tampons or a diaphragm.

Vulvodynia is constant, unremitting burning that is localized to the vulva with an acute onset. The girl or woman has problems in sitting, standing, and sleeping related to the intensity of pain. **Vestibulitis** causes severe pain only on touch or attempted vaginal entry. Half of the women with vestibulitis report lifelong dyspareunia. Women with either of these disorders report a negative impact on their sexual functioning and partner relationships, as well as their self-esteem and mental health (Metzger, 2004).

Problems with Satisfaction

Some people experience sexual desire, arousal, and orgasm yet feel dissatisfied with their sexual relationships. These sexual problems are more commonly related to the emotional tone of the relationship than to the physiological response. Since giving and receiving pleasure in a mutually intimate relationship are the primary goals of sex for most people, **dissatisfaction problems** may be more disturbing than other types of sexual dysfunctions.

At times, satisfaction problems may be situational. For example, one partner may choose an inconvenient time, or a partner may feel anxious and therefore cannot experience much pleasure or joy. Some people describe their problems as being related to lack of extragenital satisfaction. These people describe how much they miss and continue to need all the touching and caressing of their earlier lovemaking experiences. Unfortunately, people who have been relating sexually for a long time often become genitally focused and neglect the rest of the body. One or both partners may feel touch starved, long for more extragenital loving, and become dissatisfied with sex.

Satisfaction problems are often related to relationship difficulties. The inability to communicate effectively in other relationship areas frequently results in sexual frustration. Partners who are angry with each other and make love without resolving the conflict may feel unhappy about the relationship despite having experienced arousal and orgasm. Couples who define their relationship in terms of rigid, unequal power and gender roles may have difficulty negotiating and compromising about sexual issues. Not infrequently, the person with the least amount of power feels helpless and dissatisfied with the sexual interchanges.

Lack of intimacy or a feeling of connectedness is understandably related to satisfaction problems. If one has sex with a stranger, the body may function well, but there is often a sense of something missing after the sexual experience. Making love to one person while feeling more attracted to or in love with another person can result in feelings of emptiness or disconnection. Even couples in a committed relationship may complain of lack of intimacy. Dissatisfaction issues include lack of romance, love, tenderness, and nurturance. Fulfillment of sexuality, then, depends on the ability to relate to a partner in an intimate and mutually pleasing manner that is compatible with one's values and chosen lifestyle.

Clients at risk for altered sexual patterns include those experiencing the following:

- Altered body structure or function due to trauma, pregnancy, recent childbirth, anatomical abnormalities of the genitals, or a variety of diseases
- Physical, psychosocial, emotional, or sexual abuse; sexual assault
- Disfiguring conditions, such as burns, skin conditions, birthmarks, scars (e.g., mastectomy), and ostomies
- Specific medication therapy that causes sexual problems (see Table 26–4)
- Temporary or long-term impaired physical ability to perform grooming and maintain sexual attractiveness
- Value conflicts between personal beliefs and religious doctrine
- Loss of a partner
- Lack of knowledge or misinformation about sexual functioning and expression.

PHYSICAL ASSESSMENT

In performing a physical assessment involving the genitalia, it is important for the nurse to be very professional in approach in order to reduce the client's anxiety. The nurse must also use caution to avoid misperception by the client of sexual harassment or sexual abuse by touching in a nonintimate fashion, obtaining consent from the client before performing any assessment or procedure, and explaining what will happen before proceeding. It is always best to have another health care provider in the room during physical examination of the genitalia.

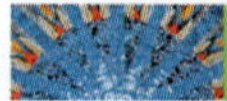

Male Reproductive System Assessments

Technique/Normal Findings	Abnormal Findings
Breast and Lymph Node Assessment	
Inspect and palpate both breasts, including areola and nipple. *Breast tissue should not be swollen, tender, or enlarged (although soft, fatty, and enlarged breast tissue does occur with obesity in men).*	■ A smooth, firm, mobile, tender disk of breast tissue behind the areola indicates **gynecomastia**, abnormal enlargement of the breast(s) in men. Gynecomastia requires additional investigation to determine cause. ■ A hard, irregular nodule in the nipple area suggests carcinoma.
Palpate the axillary and supraclavicular lymph nodes. *Lymph nodes should not be palpable.*	■ Enlarged axillary nodes are common with infections of the hand or arm but may be caused by cancer. ■ Enlarged supraclavicular nodes may indicate metastasis.
External Genitalia Assessment	
Inspect and palpate the inguinal and femoral area for bulges. Ask the man to bear down or cough as you palpate (Figure 26–7 ■). *There should be no bulging with coughing or bearing down.*	■ A bulge that increases with coughing or straining suggests a hernia.
Inspect the penis. If the man is uncircumcised, retract the foreskin or ask him to do so. *When nonerect, the penis is normally soft, flaccid, and nontender. The foreskin should be without lesions, of color equal with the penis, and should retract easily. The glans is normally free of lesions.*	■ **Phimosis** (tightness of prepuce that prevents retraction of foreskin) may be congenital or due to recurrent balanoposthitis (generalized infection of glans penis and prepuce). ■ Narrow or inflamed foreskin can cause paraphimosis, retraction of the foreskin that causes painful swelling of the glans. ■ Balanitis (inflammation of the glans) is associated with bacterial or fungal infections. ■ Ulcers, vesicles, or warts suggest a sexually transmitted infection. ■ Nodules or sores seen in uncircumcised men may be cancer.
Inspect the external urinary meatus. Press the glans between the thumb and forefinger (Figure 26–8 ■). Replace the foreskin if appropriate. *The external urinary meatus is normally in the center of the glans, without redness or discharge.*	■ Erythema or discharge indicates inflammatory disease. Further assessment is required.

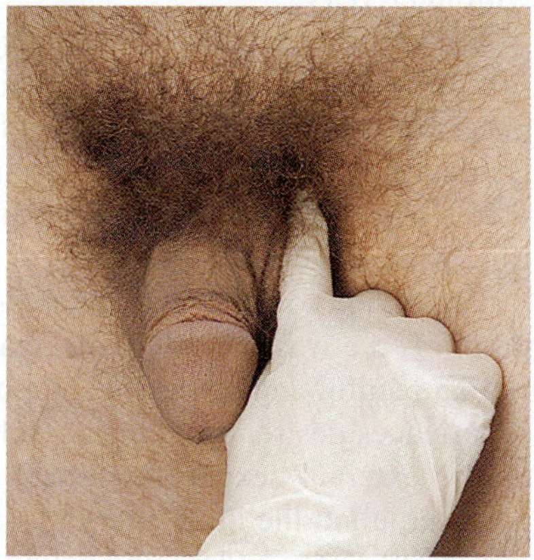

Figure 26–7 ■ Palpating the male inguinal area for bulges.

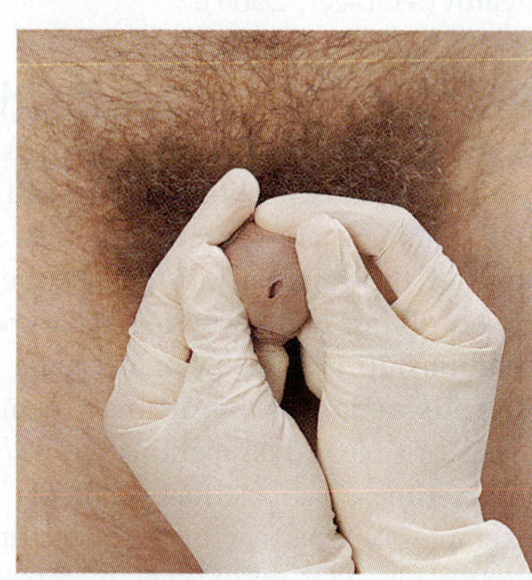

Figure 26–8 ■ Inspecting the external urinary meatus of the male.

Male Reproductive System Assessments (continued)

Technique/Normal Findings	Abnormal Findings
Inspect the skin on the shaft of the penis. *The skin on the shaft of the penis should be free of redness or lesions.*	■ Excoriation or inflammation suggests lice or scabies.
Palpate the shaft of the penis. *The shaft of the penis should not be tender.*	■ Induration with tenderness along the ventral surface suggests urethral stricture with inflammation.
Inspect the scrotum. Further assess any swelling in the scrotum using transillumination: Darken the room, and place a lighted flashlight against the skin of the scrotum. *The normal scrotum and epididymis appear as dark masses with regular borders.*	■ A unilateral or bilateral poorly developed scrotum suggests cryptorchidism (failure of one or both testes to descend into the scrotum). ■ Swelling of the scrotum may indicate indirect inguinal hernia, hydrocele (accumulation of fluid in the scrotum), or scrotal edema. Swellings containing serous fluid will transilluminate. Swellings containing blood or tissue will not transilluminate.
Palpate each testis and epididymis. *The testes should not be tender or swollen.*	■ Tender, painful scrotal swelling occurs in acute epididymitis, acute orchitis, torsion of the spermatic cord, and strangulated hernia. ■ A painless nodule in the testis is associated with testicular cancer.
Prostate Assessment	
The prostate gland is assessed by digital rectal examination (DRE). With a gloved index finger, palpate the posterior rectal wall for the rounded, two-lobed structure of the posterior prostate. *The prostate is normally nontender, with two lateral lobes that are divided, smooth, and about 2.5 cm long.*	■ Enlargement (1 cm protrusion into the rectum) with obliteration of the median sulcus suggests benign prostatic hypertrophy. ■ Enlargement with asymmetry and tenderness suggests prostatitis. ■ A hard, irregular nodule is suspicious of carcinoma.

Female Reproductive System Assessments

Technique/Normal Findings	Abnormal Findings
Breast Assessment	
Inspect both breasts simultaneously with the woman seated in the following positions: arms at sides, arms overhead, hands pressed on hips, leaning forward. Inspect breast size, symmetry, contour, skin color, texture, venous patterns, and lesions. Lift the breasts, and inspect the lower and lateral aspects. *Breasts normally vary in size and shape, and one breast may normally be larger than the other. Color should be consistent with the skin tone and texture smooth. There should be no redness, swelling, prominent veins, or lesions.*	■ Retractions, dimpling, and abnormal contours suggest benign lesions, but may also suggest malignancy. ■ Thickened, dimpled skin with enlarged pores (called *peau d'orange*, *orange peel*, or *pig skin*) and unilateral venous patterns are also associated with malignancy. ■ Redness may be seen with infection or carcinoma.
Inspect the areolae and nipples. *The color of the areolae should be consistent with the woman's skin color (ranging from dark pink to dark brown), and Montgomery tubercles may be present. The nipples should be equal bilaterally in size, centrally located in each breast, and free of lesions or discharge. Nipples are usually everted, but may normally be inverted or flat.*	■ Peau d'orange may be noted first in the areola. ■ Recent unilateral inversion of the nipple or asymmetry in the directions in which the nipples point suggests cancer.

(continued)

Female Reproductive System Assessments (continued)

Technique/Normal Findings	Abnormal Findings
Palpate both breasts, axillae, and supraclavicular areas. Figure 26–9 ■ illustrates a possible pattern for breast palpation. Various palpation patterns may be used as long as every part of each breast is palpated, including the axillary tail (also called tail of Spence), which is the breast tissue that extends from the upper outer quadrant toward and into the axillae. Ask the woman to assume a supine position with a small pillow under the shoulder and the arm over the head, and repeat the systematic palpation sequence. Describe identified masses by location, size, shape, consistency, tenderness, mobility, and delineation of borders. *Breasts should feel smooth, firm, and elastic, without palpable masses. Prior to the menstrual cycle, there may be increased nodularity and tenderness.*	■ Tenderness may be related to premenstrual fullness, fibrocystic disease, or inflammation. Tenderness may also indicate cancer. ■ Nodules in the tail of the breast may be enlarged lymph nodes. ■ Hard, irregular, fixed unilateral masses that are poorly delineated suggest carcinoma. ■ Bilateral, single or multiple, round, mobile, well-delineated masses are consistent with fibrocystic breast disease or fibroadenoma. ■ Swelling, tenderness, erythema, and heat may be seen with mastitis.
Palpate the nipple then compress it between the thumb and index finger. Note the color of any discharge. *Nipples should be firm and elastic, normally without discharge (although some women normally have a clear discharge, and a milky substance may be expressed during pregnancy and lactation).*	■ Loss of nipple elasticity is seen in cancer. ■ Bloody or serous discharge is associated with intraductal papilloma. ■ Milky discharge not due to prior pregnancy and found on both sides suggests galactorrhea (lactation not associated with pregnancy or nursing), which is sometimes associated with a pituitary tumor. ■ Unilateral discharge from one or two ducts can be seen in fibrocystic breast disease, intraductal papilloma, or carcinoma.

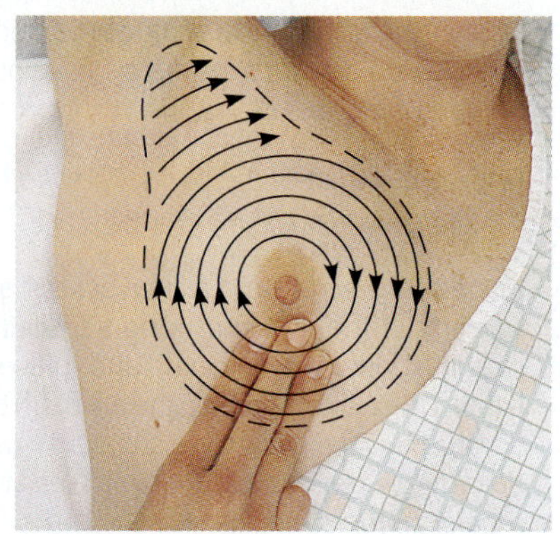

Figure 26–9 ■ Possible pattern for palpation of the breast.

Axillary Assessment

Technique/Normal Findings	Abnormal Findings
Inspect the skin of the axillae. *There should be no redness, irritation, lesions, or enlarged lymph nodes on palpation.*	■ Rash may be due to allergy or other causes. ■ Signs of inflammation and infection may be due to infection of the sweat glands. ■ Palpate all sections of both axillae for palpable nodes (Figure 26–10 ■). ■ Enlarged axillary nodes are most often due to infection of the hand or arm but can be caused by malignancy. ■ Enlarged supraclavicular nodes are associated with lymphatic metastases from abdominal or thoracic carcinoma.

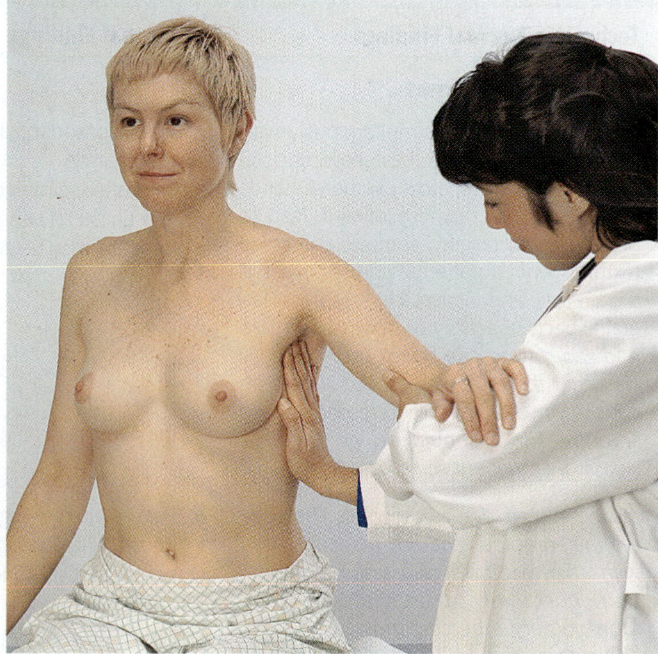

Figure 26–10 ■ Palpating the axillary lymph nodes.

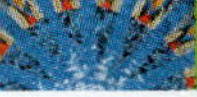

Female Reproductive System Assessments (continued)

Technique/Normal Findings	Abnormal Findings
External Genitalia Assessment	
Help the woman to the lithotomy position with the knees flexed and separated.	
Inspect and palpate the labia majora. *The labia majora should be equal in size and free of lesions or bulging.*	■ Excoriation, rashes, or lesions suggest inflammatory or infective processes. ■ Bulging of the labia that increases with straining suggests a hernia. ■ Varicosities may be present on the labia.
Inspect the labia minora. Separate the labia majora for better visualization. *The labia minora should be symmetrical, dark pink and moist, without redness or lesions.*	■ Inflammation, irritation, excoriation, or caking of discharge in tissue folds suggests vaginal infection or poor hygiene. ■ Ulcers or vesicles may be symptoms of sexually transmitted infection.
Palpate the inside of the labia minora between thumb and forefinger. *There should be no nodules, ulcers, or lesions.*	■ Small, firm, round cystic nodules in labia suggest sebaceous cysts. ■ Wartlike lesions suggest condylomata acuminata (genital warts). ■ Firm, painless ulcers suggest chancre of primary syphilis. ■ Shallow, painful ulcers suggest herpes infection. ■ Ulcerated or red raised lesions in older women suggest vulvar carcinoma.
Inspect the clitoris. *The clitoris is normally not enlarged.*	■ Enlargement may be a symptom of a masculinizing condition.
Inspect the vaginal opening. *There should be no swelling, discoloration, lacerations, discharge, or lesions visible in the vaginal opening.*	■ Swelling, discoloration, or lacerations may be caused by trauma. ■ Discharge or lesions may be symptoms of infection. ■ Fissures or fistulas may be related to injury, infection, spreading of a malignancy, or trauma.
Palpate Skene's glands. Using the index finger, "milk" Skene's glands on both sides and over the urethra and inspect for possible discharge (Figure 26–11 ■). *There should be no discharge or tenderness present.*	■ Discharge from Skene's glands and/or tenderness suggests infection.

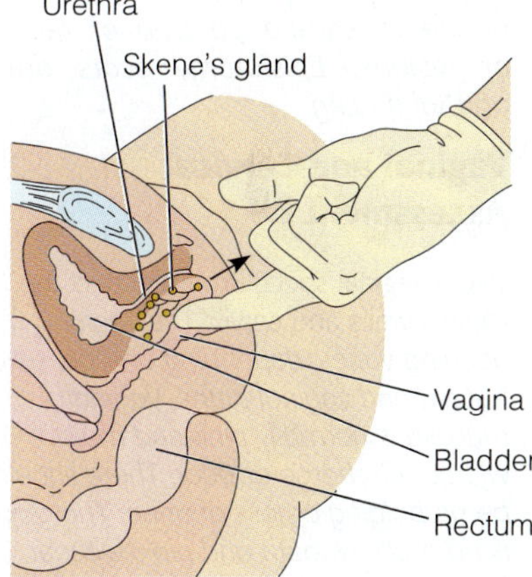

Figure 26–11 ■ Palpating Skene's glands.

(continued)

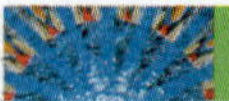

Female Reproductive System Assessments (continued)

Technique/Normal Findings	Abnormal Findings
Palpate Bartholin's glands at the posterior labia majora (Figure 26–12 ■). *There should be no masses, redness, swelling, or tenderness on palpation.*	■ A nontender mass in the posterolateral portion of the labia majora is indicative of a Bartholin's cyst. ■ Swelling, redness, or tenderness, especially if unilateral, may indicate abscess of Bartholin's glands.

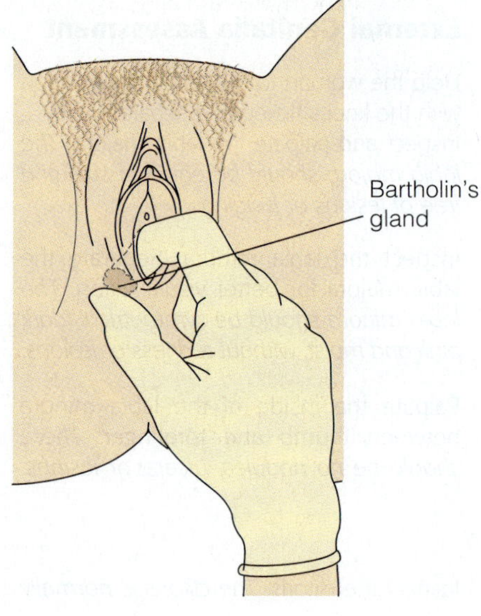

Figure 26–12 ■ Palpating Bartholin's glands.

Technique/Normal Findings	Abnormal Findings
Inspect the vaginal orifice for bulging and urinary incontinence. Ask the woman to strain or "bear down." *No bulging should be visible with straining.*	■ Bulging of the anterior vaginal wall and urinary incontinence suggest a cystocele. ■ Bulging of the posterior wall suggests a rectocele. ■ Protrusion of the cervix or uterus into the vagina indicates uterine prolapse.
Inspect and palpate the perineum. *The perineum should be free of redness or lesions. Episiotomy scars are a normal finding.*	■ Inflammation, lesions, and growths may be seen in infections or cancer. ■ Fistulas may be the result of injury, trauma, infection, or spreading of a malignancy.
Vaginal and Cervical Assessment	
Use a vaginal speculum to inspect the vaginal walls and cervix. *The vaginal opening varies, depending on age, sexual history, and vaginal births. Vaginal mucosa is normally pink and moist, without discharge or odor. There should be no bulging or loss of urine. The cervix is normally smooth and pink, without lesions and has a consistency similar to the tip of the nose.*	■ Bluish color of the cervix and vaginal mucosa may be a sign of pregnancy. ■ A pale cervix is associated with anemia. ■ A cervix to the right or left of the midline may indicate a pelvic mass, uterine adhesions, or pregnancy. ■ Projection of the cervix more than 3 cm into the vaginal canal may indicate a pelvic or uterine mass. ■ Transverse or star-shaped cervical lacerations reflect trauma causing tearing of the cervix. ■ An enlarged cervix is associated with infection. ■ Nabothian cysts (small, white, or yellow raised, round areas on the cervix) are considered normal but may become infected.
■ Cervical polyps may be cervical or endometrial in origin. Palpate the cervix, uterus, and ovaries. *The cervix can be moved slightly without discomfort. The uterus is normally at the level of the pubis, moves freely, and is nontender. The ovaries (about the size of a walnut) are firm, smooth, mobile, and slightly tender on palpation. The ovaries are not usually palpable 3 to 5 years after menopause. A small amount of clear drainage is normal.*	■ The uterus may be retroverted (tilted backward) or retroflexed (angled backward). ■ Pain on movement of the cervix during manual examination suggests pelvic inflammatory disease (PID). ■ Softening of the uterine isthmus (Hegar's sign), softening of the cervix (Goodell's sign), and uterine enlargement may be objective signs of pregnancy. ■ Firm, irregular nodules that vary greatly with size and are continuous with the uterine surface are likely to be myomas (fibroids). ■ Unilateral or bilateral smooth, compressible adnexal masses are found in ovarian tumors. ■ Profuse menstrual bleeding is seen with endometrial polyps, dysfunctional uterine bleeding (DUB), and use of an intrauterine device. ■ Irregular bleeding may be associated with endometrial polyps, DUB, uterine or cervical carcinoma, or oral contraceptives. ■ Postmenopausal bleeding is seen with endometrial hyperplasia, estrogen therapy, and endometrial cancer.

Assessment Interview Sexuality

ASSESSING MEN

A health assessment interview to determine problems with the male reproductive system may be conducted during a health screening, may focus on a chief complaint (such as a discharge from the penis), or may be part of a total health assessment. The man may perceive the interview as less threatening if the discussion begins with more general questions and then progresses to specific questions and if questions are asked in a way that gives him permission to describe behaviors and manifestations. For example, rather than asking a man if he has difficulty achieving or maintaining an erection, ask him to describe any changes he has noticed in his erections.

Men may be embarrassed to discuss health problems or concerns involving their reproductive organs; it is important for the nurse to ask questions in a nonthreatening, matter-of-fact manner. Consider the psychological, social, and cultural factors that affect sexuality and sexual activity. Use words that the man can understand, and do not be embarrassed or offended by the words he uses.

If the man has a health problem, analyze its onset, characteristics and course, severity, precipitating and relieving factors, and any associated symptoms, noting the timing and circumstances. For example, the nurse may ask the man the following:

- When did you first notice that you were having difficulty urinating?
- Did you use a different brand of condoms before you noticed the rash on your penis?
- Describe the changes that occurred in your ability to have an erection after you started taking medicine for high blood pressure.

In questioning the man about past medical history, ask about chronic illnesses such as diabetes, chronic renal failure, cardiovascular disease, multiple sclerosis, spinal cord tumors or trauma, or thyroid disease. The effects of these illnesses as well as the treatment of the illnesses may cause **impotence** (inability to achieve or maintain an erection). The following drugs may cause sexual function problems: antihypertensives, antidepressants, antispasmodics, tranquilizers, sedatives, and histamine$_2$-receptor antagonists. Psychosocial stressors also may contribute to impotence.

If the man was born to a woman who was treated during pregnancy with diethylstilbestrol (DES), a drug used in the 1940s and 1950s to prevent miscarriage, he may have congenital deformities of the urinary tract as well as decreased semen levels. If the man had mumps as a child, sterility is possible. The risk for testicular cancer is greatest in men who have a history of an undescended testicle, an inguinal hernia, testicular swelling with mumps, a history of maternal use of DES or oral contraceptives, and a family history of testicular cancer.

Explore the man's lifestyle and social history; the use of alcohol, cigarettes, or street drugs may affect sexual function. Frequent sexual intercourse, especially if unprotected, increases the potential for sexually transmitted infections, including HIV infection. Ask about sexual preference. Sexual intercourse with same-sex partners further increases the risk for HIV infection. Other questions about sexuality may include number of sexual partners; history of premature ejaculation, impotence, or other sexual problems; any history of sexual trauma; use of condoms or other contraceptives; and current level of sexual satisfaction.

ASSESSING WOMEN

A health assessment interview to determine problems with the female reproductive system may be conducted during a health screening, may focus on a chief complaint (such as severe menstrual cramping), or may be part of a total health assessment. The woman may perceive the interview as less threatening if the discussion begins with more general questions and then progresses to specific questions and if questions are asked in a way that gives the woman permission to describe behaviors and manifestations. For example, first ask a female client about menstrual and childbirth histories before asking questions about sexually transmitted infections.

Women may be embarrassed to discuss health problems or concerns involving their reproductive organs; it is important for the nurse to ask questions in a nonthreatening, matter-of-fact manner. Consider the psychological, social, and cultural factors that affect sexuality and sexual activity. Use words that the woman can understand, and do not be embarrassed or offended by the words she uses.

The focused interview for the female reproductive system is usually extensive. However, the questions may in many instances be tailored to the specific health problem of the woman. As with the assessment of other body systems, analyze and document the onset of the problem, its duration, frequency, precipitating and relieving factors, any associated symptoms, treatment, self-care, and outcomes. For example, the nurse may ask the woman the following:

- Have you noticed vaginal bleeding after intercourse?
- Does over-the-counter medication relieve the vaginal itching and discharge?
- Have you had any fever or abdominal pain with this vaginal infection?

Ask about menstrual history, obstetric history, use of contraceptives, sexual history, use of medications, and reproductive system examinations. Also assess the use of condoms during intercourse; unprotected sexual intercourse increases the risk of sexually transmitted infections, including HIV infection. Also ask about smoking; a history of smoking increases the risk of circulatory problems in the woman taking oral contraceptives. Smoking also increases the risk for cancer of the cervix.

Chronic illnesses may affect the function of the female reproductive system. Diabetes mellitus increases the risk of vaginal infections and vaginal dryness, both of which interfere with sexual pleasure. Chronic heavy menstrual flow may result in anemia. Thyroid and adrenal disorders may affect secondary sex characteristics, the menstrual cycle, and the ability to become pregnant.

Obtaining any family history of cancer is important. The risk for endometrial cancer is higher in women with a family history of endometrial, breast or colon cancer, the risk for ovarian cancer is higher in women with a family history of ovarian or breast cancer, and the risk for breast cancer is higher in women with a family history of breast cancer. Exposure to DES in utero increases the risk of cancer of the cervix and vagina. Exposure to asbestos poses a risk of cancer of the ovary. The risk for breast cancer is also greater if the woman has a history of fibrocystic disease.

Carefully explore any history of vaginal bleeding and vaginal discharge. Ask about the onset of vaginal bleeding, any related factors, the color (pink, red, dark red, brown), the character (thin, watery, presence of mucus, size and number of clots), the amount (spotting, how many pads or tampons in a specific amount of time), and relationship to the woman's menstrual cycle. Regarding vaginal discharge, ask about the onset, color (white, green, gray), character (thin, thick, curdlike), odor, itching, and rash.

Questions about sexuality may include sexual preference, number of sexual partners; history of **anorgasmia** (absence of orgasm), dyspareunia (painful intercourse), or other problems with intercourse; history of sexual trauma; use of condoms or other contraceptives; and current level of sexual satisfaction.

DIAGNOSTIC TESTS

Diagnostic tests related to sexuality may include the following:

- Culture and sensitivity to determine causative agent of STI or other infections
- Serum hormone levels
- Urinalysis
- Papanicolaou smear (Pap smear)
- Colposcopy
- Biopsy
- Complete blood count with differential.

CARING INTERVENTIONS

Caring interventions for the client with an alteration related to sexuality may include the following:

- Assisting with a pelvic examination
- Assisting with collection of a Pap smear
- Teaching the client to perform breast or testicular self-examination
- Teaching related to prevention of STIs or prevention of transmission of STIs
- Providing sexual health teaching
- Counseling for altered sexual function.

Dealing With Inappropriate Sexual Behavior

Nurses, both male and female, may encounter a variety of sexually inappropriate behaviors for a number of reasons. The behavior may be either aggressive or nonaggressive. Clients may act out sexually by doing the following:

- Exposing themselves
- Asking the nurse to provide intimate physical care, such as bathing genital areas, when they are capable of doing this themselves
- Touching or grabbing the nurse's genitals or buttocks
- Making blatant sexual statements to the nurse
- Offering the nurse sex
- Whistling and/or making comments about the nurse's attractiveness or desirability
- Making sexual comments to another client in the same room or to visitors about the "sexy" nurse or what they would like to do sexually with the nurse.

Following are some possible reasons for this inappropriate behavior:

- Fear or anxiety over future ability to function sexually
- Unmet needs for intimacy and sexual closeness because of hospitalization, injury, illness, treatment, lack of a partner, or lack of privacy
- Misinterpretation of the nurse's behavior as sexual or provocative
- Need for reassurance that they are still sexual beings and still sexually attractive
- Need for attention
- Confusion: Neurological impairment or trauma can lead clients to use profane sexual language, engage in masturbation, expose themselves, or inappropriately touch or grab at the nurse
- Need to control: Clients may be experiencing loss of control over their lives because of hospitalization, injury, or illness
- Need for power
- Belief that flirtatious behavior is expected because of media portrayals of nurses as sexy, available, and experienced.

Before implementing any nursing interventions, the nurse should first determine whether the behavior is inappropriate or an attempt to communicate a physical need. For example, clients may expose themselves if they are febrile, pull at the penis if a catheter is uncomfortable or irritating, or reach for the nurse if unable to communicate verbally. Nursing strategies to deal with inappropriate sexual behavior are listed in Box 26–2.

PHARMACOLOGIC THERAPIES

Several different types of medications may be used to help clients maintain sexual health and ability. Oral contraceptives and female infertility medications impact the woman's reproductive system in decidedly different ways. Hormone replacement and hormone replacement therapy may help maintain hormone levels and are sometimes used in the treatment of certain cancers. Refer to the Medications feature for examples and nursing considerations.

Box 26–2 Nursing Strategies for Inappropriate Sexual Behavior

- Communicate that the behavior is not acceptable by saying, for example, "I really do not like the things you are saying," or "I see you are not dressed. I will be back in 10 minutes and will help you with breakfast when you get your clothes on."
- Tell the client how the behavior makes you feel: "When you act like that toward me, I am very uncomfortable. It embarrasses me and makes it hard for me to give you the kind of nursing care you need."
- Identify the behavior you expect: "Please call me by my name, not 'honey,'" or "I expect you to keep yourself covered when I am in the room."
- Set firm limits: Take the client's hand and move it away, use direct eye contact, and say, "Don't do that!"
- Try to refocus clients from the inappropriate behavior to their real concerns and fears; offer to discuss sexuality concerns: "All morning you have been making very personal sexual comments about yourself. Sometimes people talk like that when they are concerned about the sexual part of their life and how their illness will affect them. Are there things that you have questions about or would like to talk about?"
- Report the incident to your nursing instructor, charge nurse, or clinical nurse specialist. Discuss the incident, your feelings, and possible interventions.
- Assign a nurse who will confront the behavior and relate to the client in a consistent manner.
- Clarify the consequences of continued inappropriate behavior (avoidance, withdrawal of services, no chance to help resolve the client's underlying concerns).

MEDICATIONS Sexuality

Classification	Action	Drug Examples	Nursing Considerations
Oral contraceptives	If taken appropriately prevents pregnancy with almost 100% effectiveness by providing negative feedback to the pituitary to shut down the secretion of LH and FSH	Depo-Provera, Lunelle, Norplant, Ortho Evra, NuvaRing, Mirena	■ Effectiveness declines when taking antibiotics so alternate method of birth control is required ■ Teach client how to take the medication and how to respond if a dose is missed ■ Avoid use in women over 35 or those who smoke due to risk of DVT ■ While no risk has been found if taken while pregnant, client should be screened for pregnancy prior to use ■ Monitor blood pressure and screen for hypertension as possible side effect ■ Use with caution in clients with hypertension, DVT, cardiac or renal disease, liver dysfunction, diabetes, gallbladder disease, and a history of depression
Hormone replacement therapy (estrogen and progestin)	Replaces hormones that are produced in declining amounts post-menopause. May also be used to treat hormone-dependent cancers (male hormones given if dependent on female hormones or female hormones for male-hormone-dependent cancers	Estrogen/progestin conjugated estrogens and conjugated estrogens with medroxyprogesterone	■ Contraindicated if client has or has a history of breast cancer or any suspected estrogen-dependent cancer ■ Contraindicated in pregnancy ■ Assess for thrombohemolytic disease ■ Teach importance of regular screening exams due to increased risk of cancer ■ When using female hormones to treat male clients teach about potential secondary sex characteristics that may occur with use ■ Teach client to immediately report calf tenderness, chest pain, dyspnea and to take with food if gastrointestinal upset occurs
Hormone replacement (androgens)	Used to treat hypogonadism resulting from insufficient testosterone. May also be used to treat estrogen dependent cancers	danazol, fluoxymesterone, methyltestosterone, nandrolone phenpropionate	■ Monitor liver enzymes and serum electrolytes ■ Secondary male sexual characteristics (deepening voice, facial hair, enlarged clitoris) may occur in women taking these medications ■ Monitor weight ■ Diabetic clients should carefully monitor glucose owing to risk of hypoglycemia ■ Teach client to report soreness at injection site, prolonged or painful erections
Female Infertility Medications	Acting as an antiestrogen, they stimulate release of LH to promote conception. May also be used to treat endometriosis	bromocriptine mesylate, clomiphene, danazol, urofollitropin, follitropin alfa, cetrorelix acetate, leuprolide acetate, nafarelin acetate	■ Warn client of increased risk of multiple birth ■ Teach client to report abdominal pain, unusual vaginal bleeding, uterine contractions, or calf tenderness

refractory period (time to next erection) is lengthened to several hours or, in some cases, as long as 24 hours (McCance & Huether, 2001).

The decreased levels of testosterone in the older man change the vascular responses that are part of arousal. Arousal occurs more in response to direct penile stimulation than to psychic factors (Masters, 1986; Schiavi & Rehman, 1995). In general, the older man's libido may decrease but does not disappear. If an older man reports a loss in sexual interest, the nurse should be as concerned as when a younger man reports a loss of interest in sexual activity. Older men achieve an erection that is less firm than that in younger men but is still capable of penetration. Ejaculation may take longer to occur, and the older man may have difficulty anticipating or delaying ejaculation.

COLLABORATION

The management of men with ED is growing in importance and scale, because the population as a whole is aging, so the incidence is increasing proportionately. Another factor is the gradual change in the willingness of men and their partners to discuss sexual concerns. Although sexuality is still a very sensitive and private area for most people, the knowledge that help is available is causing men to seek answers. Many older men are coming to believe that loss of erectile function is not an inevitable part of aging.

Diagnostic Tests

The diagnostic tests that may be ordered include blood studies, penile monitoring, and penile blood flow.

Blood chemistry, testosterone, prolactin, thyroxin, and prostate specific antigen (PSA) levels are measured to identify metabolic and endocrine problems that may be causing the dysfunction. Nocturnal penile tumescence and rigidity (NPTR) monitoring helps differentiate between psychogenic and organic causes. These tests can be performed in a sleep laboratory, although home testing with portable devices is an alternative. The number and quality of erections occurring during REM sleep can be determined. Cavernosometry and cavernosography of the corpora are used to evaluate arterial inflow and venous outflow of blood in the penis.

Pharmacologic Therapies

Erectile dysfunction can be treated with medications taken orally, injected directly into the penis, or inserted into the urethra at the tip of the penis.

ORAL MEDICATIONS The oral medications used to treat erectile dysfunction include sildenafil citrate (Viagra), vardenafil hydrochloride (Levitra), or tadalafil (Cialis). Viagra and Levitra are taken an hour before sexual activity and enhance the effects of nitrous oxide to facilitate relaxation of the smooth muscle in the penis during sexual stimulation to increase blood flow. These drugs should be taken no more than once a day and should not be taken by men who are also taking nitrate-based drugs (for health problems) or alpha-blockers (used to treat hypertension and prostate enlargement). Cialis is a selective phosphodiesterase type 5 inhibitor that allows smooth muscle relaxation to facilitate inflow of blood into the penis. Its action lasts for 36 hours, but an erection only occurs with sexual stimulation. Cialis should not be taken if the man is also taking nitrates, alpha-blockers, erythromycin or rifampicin (antibiotics), ketoconazole or itraconazole (antifungals), or protease inhibitors (for HIV).

INJECTABLE MEDICATIONS Hormone replacement therapy with testosterone injections (200 mg IM every 3 weeks) or topical patches may be used for men who have documented androgen deficiency and do not have prostate cancer. Injectable medications, including papaverine and prostaglandin E injections, may be used. When injected directly into the penis, papaverine relaxes the arterioles and smooth muscles of the cavernosum, thus inducing tumescence (swelling). An erection usually develops that lasts from 30 minutes to 4 hours. Prostaglandin E functions much as papaverine does, but has fewer side effects. One problem with this treatment is its mode of delivery. There is a high attrition rate, and clients report dissatisfaction with lack of spontaneity, loss of interest in sex, physical limitations, cost, and, occasionally, pain. Alprostadil (Caverject) is another injectable medication that may be used to treat ED. It may be injected into the penis or placed in the urethra as a minisuppository

Mechanical Devices

A frequently prescribed mechanical device for ED is the vacuum constriction device (VCD). The VCD draws blood into the penis with a vacuum, trapping it there with a constricting band at the base of the penis. After the device is removed for intercourse, a single small band, often called an O-ring, is left at the base of the penis to maintain the erection. If the man can attain an erection but cannot maintain it, then an O-ring alone can be used.

Surgery

Surgical treatment for ED involves either revascularization procedures or implantation of prosthetic devices. Venous or arterial procedures are generally not successful. The result is often temporary, because the underlying cause of the vascular insufficiency is usually not corrected. Implantation of penile prostheses is now common (Figure 26–13 ■). Men are generally satisfied with their prostheses, and they rank the inflatable type highest. Partners are also more likely to report satisfaction with the penile implant, although not to the same degree as clients. Some partners report that the implanted penis is harder than a normal erect penis and therefore causes pain. Also, the man can have intercourse for a prolonged period of time, and some partners do not find prolonged penetration enjoyable. Client and partner teaching is mandatory. Counseling by a sex therapist may be needed to facilitate adaptation to the implant.

TABLE 26–5 Causes of Erectile Dysfunction

MAJOR PATHOLOGICAL CAUSES		MAJOR IATROGENIC CAUSES	
		Medications	**Procedures and Infections**
Neurogenic	*Arterial*	*Antihypertensives*	*Surgery*
Spinal cord injury	Atherosclerosis	Hydrochlorothiazide	Coronary artery bypass
Stroke	Hypertension	Spironolactone	Pelvic lymphadenectomy
Parkinson's disease	Aortic aneurysm	Methyldopa	Radical prostatectomy
Multiple sclerosis	Sickle cell anemia	Clonidine	Radical cystectomy
Endocrinological	*Mechanical*	Prazosin	Abdominal perineal resection
Diabetes mellitus	Decreased penile distensibility	Propranolol	Sympathectomy
Hypogonadism	Congenital disorders	Reserpine	Aortic aneurysm repair
Hypothyroidism	Morbid obesity	*Psychotropic Agents*	Transplant surgeries
Inflammatory	Hydrocele	Phenothiazines	*Other*
Prostatitis	Hip or pelvic fractures	Butyrophenones	Severe nosocomial infection
Cystitis	*Psychogenic*	Tricyclic antidepressants	Radiation therapy to pelvis
Activity Intolerance	Depression	MAO inhibitors	
Pulmonary problems	Stress	Diazepam	
Anemias	Fatigue	Chlorodiazepoxide	
Myocardial infarction	Fear of failure	*Endocrinological Agents*	
Congestive heart failure	*Compulsive Food Disorders*	Lutenizing hormone releasing hormone agonists	
Hepatic diseases	Compulsive overeating	Estrogen compounds	
Renal failure	Anorexia nervosa	Progesterone	
Substance Dependency	Bulimia	*Other*	
Alcohol		Antiparkinsonian agents	
Marijuana		Anticholinergic agents	
Narcotics		Immunosuppressive agents	
Sedatives		Antihistamines	
Tobacco			

illnesses, it is not surprising that many older men have problems with ED.

Risk Factors

The risk factors for ED are numerous; they include advancing age, diseases such as heart disease and diabetes, trauma, and the use of prescription or illicit drugs. Excessive use of alcohol can also result in ED.

CLINICAL MANIFESTATIONS

Erectile dysfunction can manifest as either the complete inability to attain an erection or the inability to sustain an erection. A man may achieve erection but be unable to sustain it, or the penis may become semi-erect but lack rigidity sufficient for intercourse. Erectile dysfunction can occur in men of any age and can be chronic, intermittent, or episodic.

The older man will notice several age-related changes in his sexual response and performance, but it is important for both the client and nurse to know that sexual response and performance should be present in the older adult. For both men and women, the major age-related change in sexual response is timing. It takes longer to become sexually aroused, longer to complete intercourse, and longer before sexual arousal can occur again (Butler & Lewis, 2003).

The orgasm of older men differs from that of younger men in that there are fewer contractions of the urethra, the amount of seminal fluid decreases, and the force of ejaculation lessens. The nipples may not engorge to firm erections, and the rectal sphincter contractions that accompany climax are less frequent. After orgasm, the erection is rapidly lost. The refractory period (time to next erection) is lengthened to several hours or, in some cases, as long as 24 hours (McCance & Huether, 2001).

The decreased levels of testosterone in the older man change the vascular responses that are part of arousal. Arousal occurs more in response to direct penile stimulation than to psychic factors (Masters, 1986; Schiavi & Rehman, 1995). In general, the older man's libido may decrease but does not disappear. If an older man reports a loss in sexual interest, the nurse should be as concerned as when a younger man reports a loss of interest in sexual activity. Older men achieve an erection that is less firm than that in younger men but is still capable of penetration. Ejaculation may take longer to occur, and the older man may have difficulty anticipating or delaying ejaculation.

COLLABORATION

The management of men with ED is growing in importance and scale, because the population as a whole is aging, so the incidence is increasing proportionately. Another factor is the gradual change in the willingness of men and their partners to discuss sexual concerns. Although sexuality is still a very sensitive and private area for most people, the knowledge that help is available is causing men to seek answers. Many older men are coming to believe that loss of erectile function is not an inevitable part of aging.

Diagnostic Tests

The diagnostic tests that may be ordered include blood studies, penile monitoring, and penile blood flow.

Blood chemistry, testosterone, prolactin, thyroxin, and prostate specific antigen (PSA) levels are measured to identify metabolic and endocrine problems that may be causing the dysfunction. Nocturnal penile tumescence and rigidity (NPTR) monitoring helps differentiate between psychogenic and organic causes. These tests can be performed in a sleep laboratory, although home testing with portable devices is an alternative. The number and quality of erections occurring during REM sleep can be determined. Cavernosometry and cavernosography of the corpora are used to evaluate arterial inflow and venous outflow of blood in the penis.

Pharmacologic Therapies

Erectile dysfunction can be treated with medications taken orally, injected directly into the penis, or inserted into the urethra at the tip of the penis.

ORAL MEDICATIONS The oral medications used to treat erectile dysfunction include sildenafil citrate (Viagra), vardenafil hydrochloride (Levitra), or tadalafil (Cialis). Viagra and Levitra are taken an hour before sexual activity and enhance the effects of nitrous oxide to facilitate relaxation of the smooth muscle in the penis during sexual stimulation to increase blood flow. These drugs should be taken no more than once a day and should not be taken by men who are also taking nitrate-based drugs (for health problems) or alpha-blockers (used to treat hypertension and prostate enlargement). Cialis is a selective phosphodiesterase type 5 inhibitor that allows smooth muscle relaxation to facilitate inflow of blood into the penis. Its action lasts for 36 hours, but an erection only occurs with sexual stimulation. Cialis should not be taken if the man is also taking nitrates, alpha-blockers, erythromycin or rifampicin (antibiotics), ketoconazole or itraconazole (antifungals), or protease inhibitors (for HIV).

INJECTABLE MEDICATIONS Hormone replacement therapy with testosterone injections (200 mg IM every 3 weeks) or topical patches may be used for men who have documented androgen deficiency and do not have prostate cancer. Injectable medications, including papaverine and prostaglandin E injections, may be used. When injected directly into the penis, papaverine relaxes the arterioles and smooth muscles of the cavernosum, thus inducing tumescence (swelling). An erection usually develops that lasts from 30 minutes to 4 hours. Prostaglandin E functions much as papaverine does, but has fewer side effects. One problem with this treatment is its mode of delivery. There is a high attrition rate, and clients report dissatisfaction with lack of spontaneity, loss of interest in sex, physical limitations, cost, and, occasionally, pain. Alprostadil (Caverject) is another injectable medication that may be used to treat ED. It may be injected into the penis or placed in the urethra as a minisuppository

Mechanical Devices

A frequently prescribed mechanical device for ED is the vacuum constriction device (VCD). The VCD draws blood into the penis with a vacuum, trapping it there with a constricting band at the base of the penis. After the device is removed for intercourse, a single small band, often called an O-ring, is left at the base of the penis to maintain the erection. If the man can attain an erection but cannot maintain it, then an O-ring alone can be used.

Surgery

Surgical treatment for ED involves either revascularization procedures or implantation of prosthetic devices. Venous or arterial procedures are generally not successful. The result is often temporary, because the underlying cause of the vascular insufficiency is usually not corrected. Implantation of penile prostheses is now common (Figure 26–13 ■). Men are generally satisfied with their prostheses, and they rank the inflatable type highest. Partners are also more likely to report satisfaction with the penile implant, although not to the same degree as clients. Some partners report that the implanted penis is harder than a normal erect penis and therefore causes pain. Also, the man can have intercourse for a prolonged period of time, and some partners do not find prolonged penetration enjoyable. Client and partner teaching is mandatory. Counseling by a sex therapist may be needed to facilitate adaptation to the implant.

MEDICATIONS Sexuality

Classification	Action	Drug Examples	Nursing Considerations
Oral contraceptives	If taken appropriately prevents pregnancy with almost 100% effectiveness by providing negative feedback to the pituitary to shut down the secretion of LH and FSH	Depo-Provera, Lunelle, Norplant, Ortho Evra, NuvaRing, Mirena	■ Effectiveness declines when taking antibiotics so alternate method of birth control is required ■ Teach client how to take the medication and how to respond if a dose is missed ■ Avoid use in women over 35 or those who smoke due to risk of DVT ■ While no risk has been found if taken while pregnant, client should be screened for pregnancy prior to use ■ Monitor blood pressure and screen for hypertension as possible side effect ■ Use with caution in clients with hypertension, DVT, cardiac or renal disease, liver dysfunction, diabetes, gallbladder disease, and a history of depression
Hormone replacement therapy (estrogen and progestin)	Replaces hormones that are produced in declining amounts post-menopause. May also be used to treat hormone-dependent cancers (male hormones given if dependent on female hormones or female hormones for male-hormone-dependent cancers	Estrogen/progestin conjugated estrogens and conjugated estrogens with medroxyprogesterone	■ Contraindicated if client has or has a history of breast cancer or any suspected estrogen-dependent cancer ■ Contraindicated in pregnancy ■ Assess for thrombohemolytic disease ■ Teach importance of regular screening exams due to increased risk of cancer ■ When using female hormones to treat male clients teach about potential secondary sex characteristics that may occur with use ■ Teach client to immediately report calf tenderness, chest pain, dyspnea and to take with food if gastrointestinal upset occurs
Hormone replacement (androgens)	Used to treat hypogonadism resulting from insufficient testosterone. May also be used to treat estrogen dependent cancers	danazol, fluoxymesterone, methyltestosterone, nandrolone phenpropionate	■ Monitor liver enzymes and serum electrolytes ■ Secondary male sexual characteristics (deepening voice, facial hair, enlarged clitoris) may occur in women taking these medications ■ Monitor weight ■ Diabetic clients should carefully monitor glucose owing to risk of hypoglycemia ■ Teach client to report soreness at injection site, prolonged or painful erections
Female Infertility Medications	Acting as an antiestrogen, they stimulate release of LH to promote conception. May also be used to treat endometriosis	bromocriptine mesylate, clomiphene, danazol, urofollitropin, follitropin alfa, cetrorelix acetate, leuprolide acetate, nafarelin acetate	■ Warn client of increased risk of multiple birth ■ Teach client to report abdominal pain, unusual vaginal bleeding, uterine contractions, or calf tenderness

Maintaining sexual health is important for both sexual pleasure and physical health. A number of issues in sexual health can cause anxiety, embarrassment, and physical discomfort. Some issues, such as sexually transmitted diseases, can present a physical danger to the client. The exemplars that follow offer guidelines for the provision of culturally competent nursing care in a range of issues impacting individual sexuality.

26.1 ERECTILE DYSFUNCTION

KEY TERMS

Erectile dysfunction, *1712*
Impotence, *1712*
Libido, *1712*

BASIS FOR SELECTION OF EXEMPLAR

Common condition

LEARNING OUTCOMES

After reading about this exemplar, you will be able to:

1. Describe the pathophysiology, etiology, clinical manifestations, and direct and indirect causes of erectile dysfunction.
2. Identify risk factors associated with erectile dysfunction.
3. Illustrate the nursing process in providing culturally competent care across the life span for individuals with erectile dysfunction.
4. Formulate priority nursing diagnoses appropriate for an individual with erectile dysfunction.
5. Create a plan of care for individuals with erectile dysfunction and their family members.
6. Assess expected outcomes for an individual with erectile dysfunction.
7. Discuss therapies used in the collaborative care of an individual with erectile dysfunction.
8. Employ evidence-based caring interventions for an individual with erectile dysfunction.

OVERVIEW

Erectile dysfunction (often abbreviated as ED) is the inability of the male to attain and maintain an erection sufficient to permit satisfactory sexual intercourse. **Impotence**, a term often used synonymously with *erectile dysfunction*, may involve a total inability to achieve erection, an inconsistent ability to achieve erection, or the ability to sustain only brief erections. Erectile dysfunction has many possible causes (Table 26–5), and may or may not be associated with a loss of **libido** (sexual desire).

The incidence of ED is difficult to estimate because many affected men may not report the disorder. An estimated 15 to 30 million men in the United States have ED, and most are older than age 65 (National Kidney and Urologic Disease Information Clearinghouse [NKUDIC], 2003a). The incidence of the problem increases with age.

PATHOPHYSIOLOGY AND ETIOLOGY

The weight of the testes does not decrease in old age, although they become less firm. Approximately half of all men continue to produce viable sperm up to the age of 90 years (McCance & Huether, 2001). The number of seminiferous tubules that contain sperm decreases dramatically with age, but the adage "it only takes one" seems to apply here.

The testes gradually produce less testosterone, starting at approximately age 50 (Tan, 1999). Concomitantly, FSH and LH levels increase, probably in response to a decrease in circulating testosterone. The secondary sex characteristics supported by testosterone, such as muscle mass and body and facial hair growth, tend to diminish.

Other age-related changes in sexual function involve cellular and tissue changes in the penis, decreased sensory activity, hypogonadism, and the effects of chronic illness. In the penis, a change from elastic collagen to a more rigid collagen results in decreased distensibility (a less rigid erection). This, in turn, interferes with the veno-occlusive mechanism, which prevents blood from "leaking" out of the penis into the general vasculature prematurely. Problems with this mechanism result in incomplete erections. Vibrotactile sensation over the skin of the penis declines with age. This decline may explain why some older men require longer stimulation to achieve an erection. Hypogonadism, common in aging men, results in decreased testosterone levels. There may be a relationship between lower androgen levels and erectile function.

Etiology

Most problems with erection are the result of a disease, injury, or chemical substance (such as prescribed medications, alcohol, nicotine, cocaine, or marijuana) that decreases blood flow in the penis (Cleveland Clinic, 2004). Damage to arteries, smooth muscles, and fibrous tissues are the most common causes of impotence. Diseases such as diabetes, kidney disease, chronic alcoholism, atherosclerosis, and vascular disease are responsible for organic ED. Iatrogenic causes, that is, problems that result from treatment and therapy, must always be considered. For example, innervation and blood flow to the penis may be damaged during surgery, prostate surgery in particular. Given the effects of aging on the vasculature of the penis, the increased incidence of chronic illness, and the multiple medications and treatments required to manage those

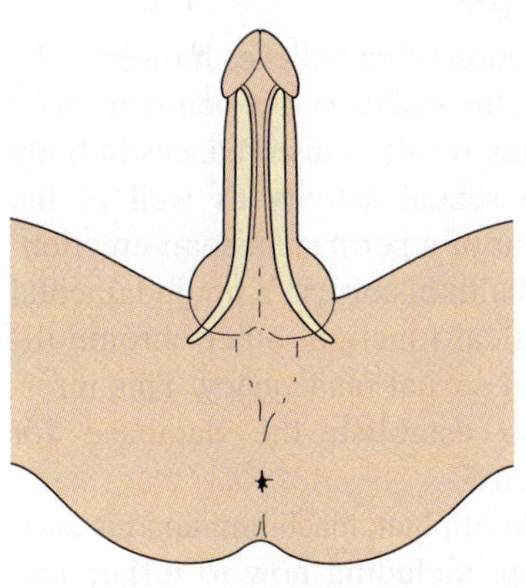
A Semirigid

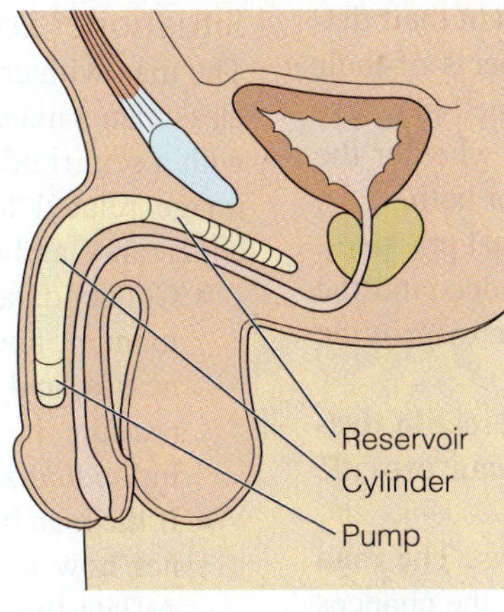

B Self-contained

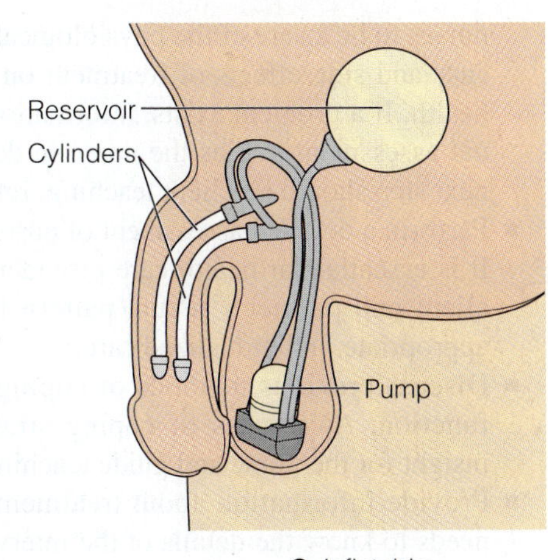

C Inflatable

Figure 26–13 ■ Types of penile implants. *A*, With semirigid rods implanted in the corpora cavernosa, the penis is always in a state of semi-erection, which may not be acceptable to the man. *B*, With a self-contained penile implant, the penis remains flaccid until the man compresses a pump at the head of the penis, which transfers fluid from a reservoir to a cylinder within the penis to achieve an erection. The man presses a release valve to return the fluid to the reservoir. *C*, With an inflatable penile implant, the penis remains flaccid until the man compresses a pump in the scrotum, which transfers fluid from an abdominal reservoir to cylinders in the corpora cavernosa to achieve an erection. Pressing a release valve returns the fluid to the reservoir.

NURSING PROCESS

Nurses in any health care setting may encounter men with erectile dysfunction, either through routine examinations or through careful assessment of clients' conditions and treatments that may incidentally cause ED. Nurses employed in clinics, operating rooms, and surgical units with urological services commonly encounter men being treated for ED. Nurses in a variety of settings, including long-term care, encounter men who have had surgical interventions, such as penile implants.

Because nurses often complete a client's health history, they are most likely to discover problems of erectile dysfunction. Once a problem is known, nurses are involved in giving information, providing emotional support, and referring clients to physicians or counselors.

Assessment

Whether the client presents with reports of erectile dysfunction or it is discovered during the nursing interview, it is important to perform a complete physical examination to reveal data that may contribute to the problem. Question the client to determine all medications, social habits, surgical history, and procedures that may be contributing factors.

PRACTICE ALERT

Many men will not volunteer information about sexual function unless asked, but then will be open about concerns and appreciate being asked.

Diagnosis

Appropriate nursing diagnoses for clients with erectile dysfunction often include the following:

- Sexual Dysfunction
- Situational Low Self-Esteem.

Plan

Goals of nursing care include the following:

- Client will discuss concerns without embarrassment or anxiety.
- Client will understand medication teaching aimed at preventing client from discontinuing necessary medications.
- Client will understand treatment options and make an informed decision.

Implementation

While some interventions will vary based on the inidividualized client needs, the nurse typically will provide ongoing assessment and client teaching regarding the nature of erectile dysfunction and its treatments. It is important the nurse maintain a very professional affect when discussing sensitive sexual dysfunction issues with the client, recognizing that the client may find it difficult to discuss sexual performance with a young nurse of either sex.

Sexual Dysfunction

Many men who lose erectile function are not aware of the cause. Often the man blames the loss on unrelated factors, such as age, a medication for an illness, a dangerous illness, or his sexual partner. Not knowing causes anxiety, which may disrupt the relationship with his partner or lead him to discontinue an important medication.

- Assess for risk factors for erectile dysfunction. Be especially alert to men who have recently begun medications or had recent surgeries that could cause ED. Awareness of risk factors helps the nurse to prioritize care, although nurses must remember that almost all aging clients have at least one risk factor for ED.
- Assess for sexual dysfunction. Men have shown increasing willingness to discuss sexual concerns and expect

nurses to be aware of the physiological effects of their disease and side effects of treatment on all aspects of their health. If a problem exists, information obtained in a sexual assessment guides the nurse in deciding whether the next step should be client teaching, referral, or both.

- Perform a detailed assessment of current sexual practices. It is essential for health care providers to understand the client and partner's sexual pattern in order to provide appropriate, individualized care.
- Discuss previous methods of coping with erectile dysfunction. Awareness of coping strategies can provide insight for the nurse and guide teaching.
- Provide information about treatment options. The man needs to know the details of the intervention, the chances for success, and the possible complications.

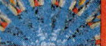

CLIENT TEACHING Erectile Dysfunction

Many nurses find that men with ED and their partners have lived in isolation with the problem for many years. The partner may even be unaware of the problem. The partner may believe that the man is seeing someone else or that the man has lost his attraction to the partner. The man may have kept his problem a secret because an intense feeling of shame makes him unable to admit that he cannot perform sexually. Many men greet the information about the high incidence of ED with a sense of relief that they are not alone in having this problem. All men and their partners need to be aware of support services available to them. Referral sources include the following:

- Sexual Function Health Council
- American Urological Association
- American Association of Sex Educators, Counselors, and Therapists.

Situational Low Self-Esteem

The man with erectile dysfunction often believes himself to be "less than a man." In addition, the insertion of a penile implant with a semirigid prosthesis may result in disturbances in body image related to changes in sexual activity as well as the appearance and embarrassment of a permanent semi-erection.

- Collect data during the health history, in a nonjudgmental manner, about physiological function, other chronic illnesses, and feelings about sexual inadequacy. This information is necessary to establish the database for individualized interventions.
- If the man has had a penile implant, teach him and his partner how to use the pump, including how to inflate and deflate the device. Suggest that he practice inflation and deflation during the postoperative period. Suggest wearing snug-fitting underwear with the penis placed in an upright position on the abdomen and loose trousers. Provide information about length of healing, and inform the client that sexual activity may resume within 6–8 weeks following surgery. Practice using the pump will maintain the pump position and promote tissue growth around the implant. The type of clothing worn can improve the ability to conceal a semirigid prosthesis and decrease embarrassment. Recovery from surgery is necessary before resuming sexual activity.

Evaluation

Client outcomes may be evaluated based on the following expected outcomes:

- Client makes informed decision regarding treatment options.
- Client understands that the problem is not related to his masculinity.

REVIEW Erectile Dysfunction

RELATE: LINK THE CONCEPTS

Linking the exemplar of Erectile Dysfunction with the concept of Self:

1. Why might the client's self-concept be negatively affected by ED?
2. What can the nurse do to help reduce this negative impact?

Linking the exemplar of Erectile Dysfunction with the concept of Perfusion:

3. What effect does arteriosclerosis have on the man's ability to attain an erection?
4. What preventive teaching can the nurse provide to younger men to prevent ED as the result of altered perfusion?

READY: GO TO COMPANION SKILLS MANUAL

- Assessing the male genital and inguinal area

REFER: GO TO MYNURSINGKIT

REFLECT: CASE STUDY

Steve Young is a 41-year-old African-American male in excellent health. He has been married to his wife Angie for 8 years. They have two children, Kelsey and Marcus. Angie and Steve met in college and were married shortly after Steve graduated with a degree in accounting. Following graduation, he took the CPA exam and has worked for a large corporate accounting firm ever since. He has been extremely successful in his firm and has an income that easily supports his family. He is pleased that his wife is able to be a stay-at-home mother, but his success requires long working hours. Steve has few outside interests and rarely exercises. His world revolves around work and home. He recognizes his inactivity has led to weight gain over the last few years, but is not concerned about it.

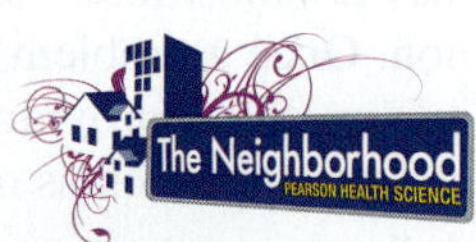

Steve began smoking at age 17 and, at this time, has a 10 pack/year smoking history. He knows he should quit, but he likes it and figures he can probably get away with it for a little while longer without complications. Because he knows it is a source of irritation with his wife, he plans to quit smoking eventually.

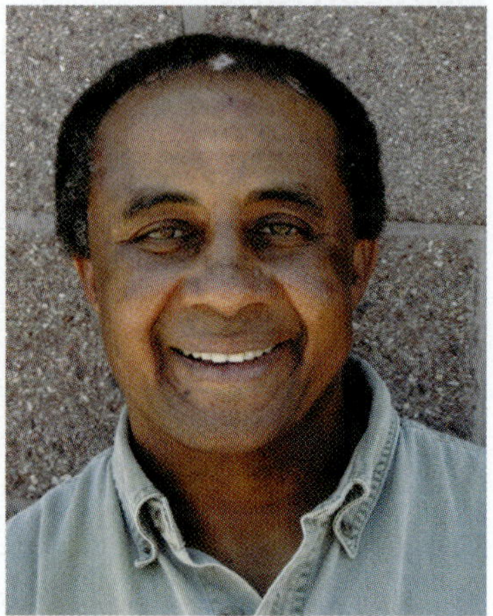

1. What risk factors does Steve have for developing erectile dysfunction?
2. What client teaching can you provide to reduce Steve's risk for erectile dysfunction?
3. How might you approach Steve to discuss any sexual function issues he may have experienced?

26.2 FAMILY PLANNING AND PRECONCEPTION COUNSELING

KEY TERMS

Autosomes, *1720*
Cervical cap, *1729*
Chromosomes, *1720*
Coitus interruptus, *1726*
Combined oral contraceptives (COCs), *1731*
Condom, *1727*
Depo-Provera, *1733*
Diaphragm, *1728*
Fertility awareness–based methods, *1725*
Genotype, *1723*
Infertility, *1718*
In vitro fertilization (IVF), *1736*
Intrauterine device (IUD), *1730*
Karyotype, *1720*
Mendelian (single-gene) inheritance, *1723*
Monosomies, *1721*
Mosaicism, *1721*
Non-Mendelian (multifactorial) inheritance, *1723*
Pedigree, *1723*
Phenotype, *1723*
Postcoital contraception, *1733*
Secondary infertility, *1718*
Spermicide, *1727*
Sterilization, *1733*
Subdermal implant, *1732*
Subfertility, *1718*
Therapeutic insemination, *1735*
Trisomies, *1720*
Tubal ligation, *1733*
Vasectomy, *1733*

BASIS FOR SELECTION OF EXEMPLAR

Healthy People 2010

LEARNING OUTCOMES

After reading about this exemplar, you will be able to:

1. Describe decisions to be made by couples prior to beginning preconception counseling.
2. Identify factors associated with family planning.
3. Illustrate the nursing process in providing culturally competent care across the life span for individuals requiring preconception counseling.
4. Formulate priority nursing diagnoses appropriate for a family requiring preconception counseling.
5. Create a plan of care for individuals seeking preconception counseling.
6. Assess expected outcomes for an individual receiving preconception counseling.
7. Discuss therapies used in the collaborative care of a couple dealing with infertility.
8. Employ evidence-based caring interventions for a couple who seek preconception or infertility counseling.

OVERVIEW

Some of the most serious decisions couples must make relate to family planning and reproduction—whether and when to have children as well as how many children they want. Information provided by nurses and other health professionals can help clients make informed decisions about contraception and childbearing. Some couples are unable to fulfill their dream of having the desired baby because of infertility or genetic problems. Developments in medicine can help growing numbers of couples overcome infertility issues.

Contraception

The decision to use a method of contraception may be made individually by a woman (or, in the case of vasectomy, by a man) or jointly by a couple. The decision may be motivated by a desire to avoid pregnancy, to gain control over the number of children conceived, or to determine the spacing of future children. In choosing a specific method, consistency of use outweighs the absolute reliability of the given method.

Decisions about contraception should be made voluntarily, with full knowledge of advantages, disadvantages, effectiveness, side effects, contraindications, and long-term effects. Many outside factors influence this choice, including cultural practices, religious beliefs, attitudes and personal preferences, cost, effectiveness, misinformation, practicality of method, and self-esteem. Different methods of contraception may be appropriate at different times for couples.

Preconception Counseling

Making the decision to have children is the first step a couple makes in the process of conception. For some couples, this decision is part of discussions during the dating process. Others do not make the decision to have children until after marriage or later in their relationship. This decision involves consideration of each person's goals, expectations of the relationship, and desire to be a parent. Sometimes one individual wishes to have a child, but the other does not. In such situations, an open discussion is essential to reach a mutually acceptable decision.

Couples who wish to have children face a decision about the timing of pregnancy. At what point in their lives do they believe it would be best to become parents? Pregnancy is a life-changing event and never proceeds just as the couple anticipates, even when the pregnancy is planned and the timing is convenient.

For couples who have religious beliefs that do not support contraception or who feel that fertility planning is unnatural, planning the timing of the pregnancy is unacceptable and irrelevant. These couples can still take steps to ensure that they are in the best possible physical and mental health if and when pregnancy occurs.

PRECONCEPTION HEALTH MEASURES Most preconception recommendations focus on helping the couple attain their best possible health state so that they do not enter pregnancy with unnecessary risks. The nurse begins by teaching the couple about known or suspected health risks.

The nurse advises the woman to stop smoking or at least to limit her cigarette intake as much as possible. Because of the hazards of secondhand smoke, it is helpful for the woman to avoid environments where secondhand smoke is common and to ask her partner to refrain from smoking around her. Although the effects of caffeine are less clearly understood, the woman is advised to avoid or limit her intake of caffeine. Alcohol, social drugs, and street drugs pose a real threat to the fetus. A woman who uses any prescription or over-the-counter medications needs to discuss the implications of their use with her health care provider.

Women with chronic health problems, such as thyroid disorders, seizures, hypertension, and diabetes, should have a preconception visit with the appropriate specialist to determine whether pregnancy is advised and medication changes or treatment plan changes are warranted. Because of the possible teratogenic effects of environmental hazards, the nurse urges the couple contemplating pregnancy to determine possible exposure to any environmental hazards, such as radiation or chemical exposure, at work or in their community.

PHYSICAL EXAMINATION It is advisable for both partners to have a physical examination to identify any health problems so that these can be corrected if possible. These problems might include medical conditions, such as high blood pressure, diabetes, or obesity; problems that pose a threat to fertility, such as certain sexually transmitted infections; or conditions that keep the individual from achieving optimal health, such as anemia or colitis. If the family history indicates previous genetic disorders or if the couple is planning pregnancy when the woman is over age 35, the health care provider may suggest that the couple consider genetic counseling. In addition to the history and physical exam, the woman may have a variety of laboratory tests. Before conception, the woman is also advised to have a dental examination and any necessary dental work to avoid exposure to x-rays, local anesthetics, and the risk of infection while pregnant.

NUTRITION Before conception, it is advisable for the woman to be at an average weight for her body build and height. Women who are underweight should be advised to gain weight, whereas women who are overweight should try to get their weight down because maternal obesity is a risk factor for multiple pregnancy complications. The woman is advised to follow a nutritious diet that contains ample quantities of all the essential nutrients. Some nutritionists advocate emphasizing the following nutrients: calcium, protein, iron, B complex vitamins, vitamin C, and magnesium. Folic acid supplementation before conception is recommended, as these supplements decrease the risk of neural tube defects. Intake of vitamins in greater than the recommended dietary allowance (RDA) can cause severe fetal problems and should be avoided. An assessment that includes unique dietary practices that can affect nutrition should also be explored. Cultural norms that affect nutritional intake should also be reviewed.

EXERCISE A woman is advised to continue her present pattern of exercise or to establish a regular exercise plan beginning at least 3 months before she attempts to become pregnant. An exercise routine that she enjoys and maintains will provide the best results. Exercise that includes some aerobic conditioning and some general muscle toning will improve the woman's circulation and general health. Once an exercise program is well established, the woman is generally encouraged to continue it during pregnancy. During pregnancy, at least 30 minutes of moderate exercise daily or at least most days is recommended (Penney, 2008).

Infertility Counseling

Infertility, a lack of conception despite unprotected sexual intercourse for at least 12 months (Kumar, Ghadir, Eskandari, & DeCherney, 2007), has a profound emotional, psychological, and economic impact on affected couples and society. The term *sterility* is applied when there is an absolute factor preventing reproduction. **Subfertility** is used to describe a couple who has difficulty conceiving because both partners have reduced fertility. The term **secondary infertility** is applied to couples who have been unable to conceive after one or more successful pregnancies or who cannot sustain a pregnancy.

Approximately 10–15% of couples in their reproductive years in the United States are infertile (Wright & Johnson, 2008). Public perception is that the incidence of infertility is increasing, but in fact there has been no significant change in the proportion of infertile couples in the United States. What has changed is the composition of the infertile population; the infertility diagnosis has increased in the age group 25 to 44 because of delayed childbearing and the entry of the baby boom cohort into this age range in Western society.

Understanding the elements that are essential for normal fertility can help the nurse identify the many factors that may cause infertility. The following components must be present for normal fertility:

Female partner

- The cervical mucus must be favorable to ensure survival of spermatozoa and facilitate passage to the upper genital tract.
- The fallopian tubes must be patent and have normal fimbriae with peristaltic movements toward the uterus to facilitate transport and interaction of ovum and sperm.

- The ovaries must produce and release normal ova in a regular, cyclic fashion.
- There must be no obstruction between the ovaries and the uterus.
- The endometrium must be in a physiological state to allow implantation of the blastocyst and to sustain normal growth.
- Adequate reproductive hormones must be present.

Male partner

- The testes must produce spermatozoa of normal quality, quantity, and motility.
- The male genital tract must not be obstructed.
- The male genital tract secretions must be normal.
- Ejaculated spermatozoa must be deposited in the female vaginal tract in such a manner that they reach the cervix.

These normal findings are correlated with possible causes of deviation in Table 26–6. With timing and environment playing such a crucial role, it is an impressive natural phenomenon that the majority of couples in the United States are able to conceive. The remaining couples suffer infertility because of a male factor (40%), a female factor (40%), or either an unknown cause (unexplained infertility) or a problem with both partners (20%) (American Society of Reproductive Medicine, 2006b). Professional intervention can help approximately 65% of infertile couples achieve pregnancy.

Young couples with no history that is suggestive of reproductive disorders should be referred for infertility evaluation if they have been unable to conceive after at least 1 year of attempting to achieve pregnancy. An earlier workup is indicated in couples with positive history for fertility-lowering disease or advancing maternal age (Wright & Johnson, 2008). If the woman is over age 35, it may be appropriate to refer the couple after only 6–9 months of unprotected intercourse without conception. At age 25, when couples are the most fertile, conception occurs within the first month of unprotected intercourse in about 25% of cases (Wright & Johnson, 2008).

GENETICS

Even when conception has been achieved, families can have special reproductive concerns. The desired and expected outcome of any pregnancy is the birth of a healthy, "perfect" baby.

TABLE 26–6 **Possible Causes of Infertility**

NECESSARY NORMS	DEVIATIONS FROM NORMAL
Female	
Favorable cervical mucus	Cervicitis, cervical stenosis, use of coital lubricants, antisperm antibodies (immunological response)
Clear passage between cervix and tubes	Myomas, adhesions, adenomyosis, polyps, endometritis, cervical stenosis, endometriosis, congenital anomalies (e.g., septate uterus, diethylstilbestrol [DES] exposure)
Patent tubes with normal motility	Pelvic inflammatory disease, peritubal adhesions, endometriosis, intrauterine device (IUD), salpingitis (e.g., chlamydia, recurrent sexually transmitted infections [STIs]), neoplasm, ectopic pregnancy, tubal ligation
Ovulation and release of ova	Primary ovarian failure, polycystic ovarian disease, hypothyroidism, pituitary tumor, lactation, periovarian adhesions, endometriosis, premature ovarian failure, hyperprolactinemia, Turner syndrome
No obstruction between ovary and tubes	Adhesions, endometriosis, pelvic inflammatory disease
Endometrial preparation	Anovulation, luteal phase defect, malformation, uterine infection, Asherman syndrome
Male	
Normal semen analysis	Abnormalities of sperm or semen, polyspermia, congenital defect in testicular development, mumps after adolescence, cryptorchidism, infections, gonadal exposure to x-rays, chemotherapy, smoking, alcohol abuse, malnutrition, chronic or acute metabolic disease, medications (e.g., morphine, aspirin [ASA], ibuprofen), cocaine, marijuana use, constrictive underclothing, heat
Unobstructed genital tract	Infections, tumors, congenital anomalies, vasectomy, strictures, trauma, varicocele
Normal genital tract secretions	Infections, autoimmunity to semen, tumors
Ejaculate deposited at the cervix	Premature ejaculation, impotence, hypospadias, retrograde ejaculation (e.g., diabetic), neurological cord lesions, obesity (inhibiting adequate penetration)

Parents experience grief, fear, and anger when they discover that their baby has been born with a defect or a genetic disease. Such an abnormality may be evident at birth or may not appear for some time. The baby may have inherited a disorder from one parent or both, creating guilt and strife within the family.

Regardless of the type or scope of the problem, parents will have many questions: "What did I do?" "What caused it?" "How do I cope with it?" "Will it happen again?" The nurse must anticipate the couple's questions and concerns and guide, direct, and support the family. To do so, the nurse must have a basic knowledge of genetics and genetic counseling. Professional nurses can help expedite this process if they understand the principles involved and can direct the family to the appropriate resources.

Genetic Disorders

All hereditary material is carried on tightly coiled strands of DNA known as **chromosomes**. The chromosomes carry the *genes*, the smallest units of inheritance. The Human Genome Project has made remarkable advances toward determining the exact DNA sequence of human genes and the precise genes that are associated with certain abnormalities such as fragile X syndrome and cystic fibrosis (Ward, 2008).

All *somatic (body) cells* contain 46 chromosomes, which is the *diploid* number; the sperm and egg contain half as many (23) chromosomes, or *the haploid* number. There are 23 pairs of homologous chromosomes (a matched pair of chromosomes, one inherited from each parent). Twenty-two of the pairs are **autosomes** (nonsex chromosomes), and one pair is made up of the sex chromosomes, X and Y. A normal female has a 46, XX chromosome constitution (Figure 26–14 ■); a normal male has a 46, XY chromosome constitution (Figure 26–15 ■).

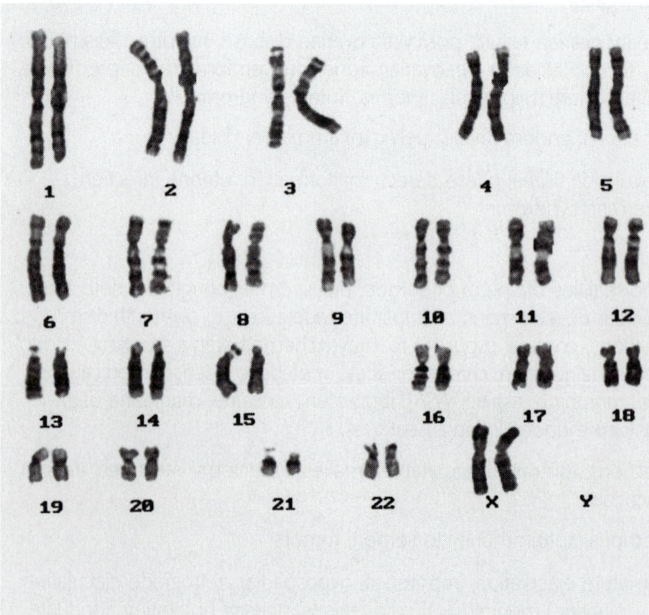

Figure 26–14 ■ Normal female karyotype.

Source: Courtesy of David Peakman, Reproductive Genetic Center, Denver, CO.

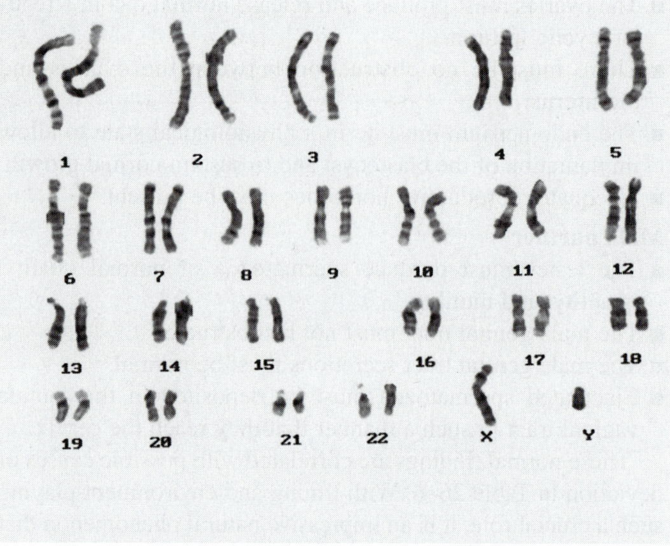

Figure 26–15 ■ Normal male karyotype.

Source: Courtesy of David Peakman, Reproductive Genetic Center, Denver, CO.

The **karyotype**, or pictorial analysis of these chromosomes, is usually obtained from specially treated and stained peripheral blood lymphocytes. Placental tissue taken from a site near the insertion of the cord and deep enough to include chorion can also be sent for karyotyping of the fetus.

Chromosome abnormalities can occur in either the autosomes or the sex chromosomes and can be divided into two categories: abnormalities of number and abnormalities of structure. Even small alterations in chromosomes can cause problems, especially those associated with delayed growth and development. Some of these abnormalities can be passed on to other offspring. Thus, in some cases, chromosomal analysis is appropriate even if clinical manifestations are mild.

ABNORMALITIES OF CHROMOSOMAL NUMBER

Abnormalities of chromosomal number are most often caused by nondisjunction, a failure of paired chromosomes to separate during cell division. If nondisjunction occurs in either the sperm or the egg before fertilization, the resulting zygote (fertilized egg) will have an abnormal chromosome makeup in all of the cells (trisomy or monosomy). If nondisjunction occurs after fertilization, the developing zygote will have cells with two or more different chromosome makeups, evolving into two or more different cell lines (mosaicism). These abnormalities are most commonly seen as trisomies, monosomies, and mosaicism.

Trisomies are the product of the union of a normal gamete (egg or sperm) with a gamete that contains an extra chromosome. The individual will have 47 chromosomes and be trisomic (has three copies of the same chromosome) for whichever chromosome is extra (Table 26–7). Down syndrome (formerly called mongolism) is the most common trisomy abnormality seen in children (see Figure 26–16 ■). The presence of the extra chromosome 21 produces distinctive clinical features (Figure 26–17 ■). Although children born with Down syndrome have a variety of physical ailments, advances in medical science have extended their life expectancy.

Two other common trisomies are trisomy 18 and trisomy 13 (refer to Table 26–7). The prognosis for both trisomies 13 and 18 is extremely poor. Most children with these trisomies (70%) die within the first 3 months of life secondary to complications related to respiratory and cardiac abnormalities. However, 10% survive the first year of life; therefore, the family needs to plan for the possibility of long-term care of a severely affected infant and for family support.

Monosomies occur when a normal gamete unites with a gamete that is missing a chromosome. In this case, the individual has only 45 chromosomes and is said to be monosomic. Monosomy of an entire autosomal chromosome is incompatible with life.

Mosaicism occurs after fertilization and results in an individual who has two different cell lines, each with a different chromosomal number. Mosaicism tends to be more common in the sex chromosomes than in the autosomes; when it occurs in the autosomes, it is most common in Down syndrome. An individual with many classic signs of Down syndrome but with normal or near-normal intelligence should be investigated for the possibility of mosaicism.

TABLE 26–7 **Chromosomal Syndromes**

ALTERED CHROMOSOME	GENETIC DEFECT AND INCIDENCE	CHARACTERISTICS
21	*Genetic defect:* trisomy 21 (Down syndrome) (secondary nondisjunction or 14/21 unbalanced translocation) *Incidence:* average 1 in 700 live births, incidence variable with age of woman	*CNS:* mental retardation; hypotonia at birth *Head:* flattened occiput; depressed nasal bridge; mongoloid slant of eyes; epicanthal folds; white specking of the iris (Brushfield spots); protrusion of the tongue; high, arched palate; low-set ears *Hands:* broad, short fingers; abnormalities of finger and foot; dermal ridge patterns (dermatoglyphics); transverse palmar crease *Other:* congenital heart disease
18	*Genetic defect:* trisomy 18 *Incidence:* 1 in 3,000 live births	*CNS:* mental retardation; severe hypotonia *Head:* prominent occiput; low-set ears; corneal opacities; ptosis (drooping eyelids) *Hands:* third and fourth fingers overlapped by second and fifth fingers; abnormal dermatoglyphics; syndactyly (webbing of fingers) *Other:* congenital heart defects; renal abnormalities; single umbilical artery; gastrointestinal tract abnormalities; rocker-bottom feet; cryptorchidism; various malformations of other organs
13	*Genetic defect:* trisomy 13 *Incidence:* 1 in 5,000 live births	*CNS:* mental retardation; severe hypotonia; seizures *Head:* microcephaly; microphthalmia, and/or coloboma (keyhole-shaped pupil); malformed ears; aplasia of external auditory canal; micrognathia (abnormally small lower jaw); cleft lip and palate *Hands:* polydactyly (extra digits); abnormal posturing of fingers; abnormal dermatoglyphics *Other:* congenital heart defects; hemangiomas; gastrointestinal tract defects; various malformations of other organs
5P	*Genetic defect:* deletion of short arm of chromosome 5 (cri du chat, or cat-cry syndrome) *Incidence:* 1 in 20,000 live births	*CNS:* severe mental retardation; a catlike cry in infancy *Head:* microcephaly; hypertelorism (widely spaced eyes); epicanthal folds; low-set ears *Other:* failure to thrive; various organ malformations
XO (sex chromosome)	*Genetic defect:* only one X chromosome or partially missing second X chromosome in female (Turner syndrome) *Incidence:* 1 in 300 to 7,000 live female births	*CNS:* no intellectual impairment; some perceptual difficulties *Head:* low hairline; webbed neck *Trunk:* short stature; cubitus valgus (increased carrying angle of arm); excessive nevi (congenital discoloration of skin because of pigmentation); broad, shieldlike chest with widely spaced nipples; puffy feet; no toenails *Other:* fibrous streaks in ovaries; underdeveloped secondary sex characteristics; primary amenorrhea; usually infertile; renal anomalies; coarctation of the aorta
XXY (sex chromosome)	*Genetic defect:* extra X chromosome in male (Klinefelter syndrome) *Incidence:* 1 in 1,000 live male births, approximately 1% to 2% of institutionalized males	*CNS:* mild mental retardation *Trunk:* occasional gynecomastia (abnormally large male breasts); eunuchoid body proportions (lack of male muscular and sexual development) *Other:* small, soft testes; underdeveloped secondary sex characteristics; usually sterile

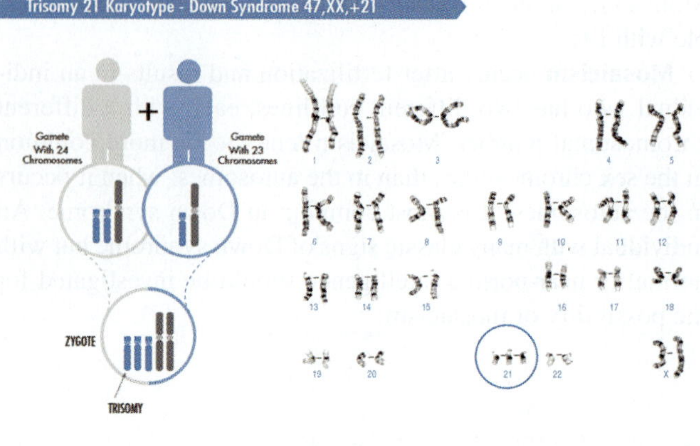

Figure 26–16 ■ Karyotype of a female who has trisomy 21, Down syndrome. Note the extra 21 chromosome.

Source: Courtesy of Greenwood Genetics Center. (2007). *Genetic counseling aids*, 5th ed.

ABNORMALITIES OF CHROMOSOME STRUCTURE Abnormalities of chromosome structure involve only parts of the chromosome and occur in two forms: translocation and deletions or additions. Some children born with Down syndrome have an abnormal rearrangement of chromosomal material known as a *translocation*. Clinically, the two types of Down syndrome are indistinguishable; the only way to distinguish them is to do a chromosome analysis.

The translocation occurs when the carrier parent has 45 chromosomes, usually with one chromosome fused to another. For example, a common translocation is one in which a particle of chromosome 14 breaks and fuses to chromosome 21. The parent has one normal 14, one normal 21, and one 14/21 chromosome. Because all the chromosomal material is present and functioning normally, the parent is clinically normal. This individual is known as a *balanced translocation carrier*. When a person who is a balanced translocation carrier has a child with a partner who has a structurally normal chromosome constitution, the child can have a normal number of chromosomes, be a carrier, or have an extra chromosome 21. Such a child has an *unbalanced translocation* and has Down syndrome.

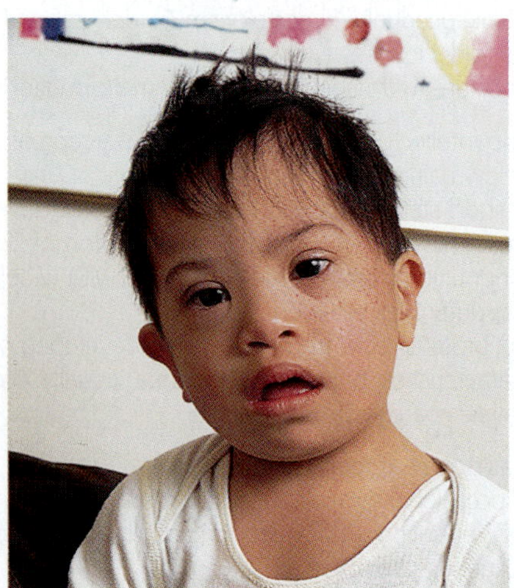

Figure 26–17 ■ A boy with Down syndrome.

Structure abnormality is also caused by additions or deletions of chromosomal material. Any portion of a chromosome may be lost or added, generally leading to some adverse effect. Depending on how much chromosomal material is involved, the clinical effects may be mild or severe. Many types of additions and deletions have been described, such as the deletion of the short arm of chromosome 5 (*cri du chat*, or cat-cry syndrome) or the deletion of the long arm of chromosome 18 (Edwards syndrome). Table 26–7 lists other chromosomal syndromes.

SEX CHROMOSOME ABNORMALITIES To better understand abnormalities of the sex chromosomes, the nurse should know that in a female, at an early embryonic stage, one of the two normal X chromosomes becomes inactive. The inactive X chromosome forms a dark staining area known as the *Barr body*. The normal female has one Barr body, because one of her two X chromosomes has been inactivated. The normal male has no Barr bodies because he has only one X chromosome.

The most common sex chromosome abnormalities are Turner syndrome in females (45, XO with no Barr bodies present; see Figure 26–18 ■) and Klinefelter syndrome in males

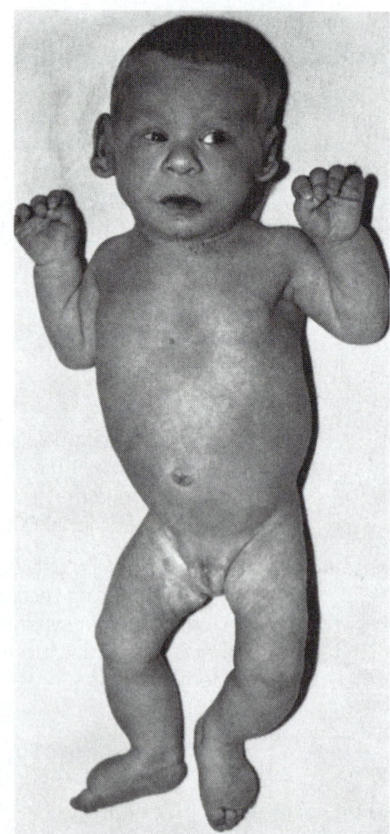

Figure 26–18 ■ Infant with Turner syndrome at 1 month of age. Note prominent ears.

Source: Lemli, L., & Smith, D. W. (1963). The XO syndrome: A study of the differentiated phenotype in 25 patients. *Journal of Pediatrics, 63*, 577, with permission from Elsevier Science.

(47, XXY with one Barr body present). See Table 26–7 for clinical descriptions of these abnormalities.

The mosaic form of the XO chromosome is associated with daughters of women who took the drug diethylstil-bestrol (DES) during pregnancy. The fertility of women with the mosaic form of the XO chromosome may not be impaired; however, there is a higher percentage of uterine malformation and hormonal difficulty associated with it and therefore a high degree of miscarriage.

There is a concern that children born as a result of intracytoplasmic sperm injection (ICSI) might be at increased risk for chromosomal and other major congenital anomalies, cancer, or infertility, because ICSI may override natural safeguards that serve to prevent fertilization. Therefore, it is strongly recommended that karyotyping and Y chromosome deletion analysis be offered to all men with severe male factor infertility who are candidates for in vitro fertilization and ICSI (Speroff & Fritz, 2005).

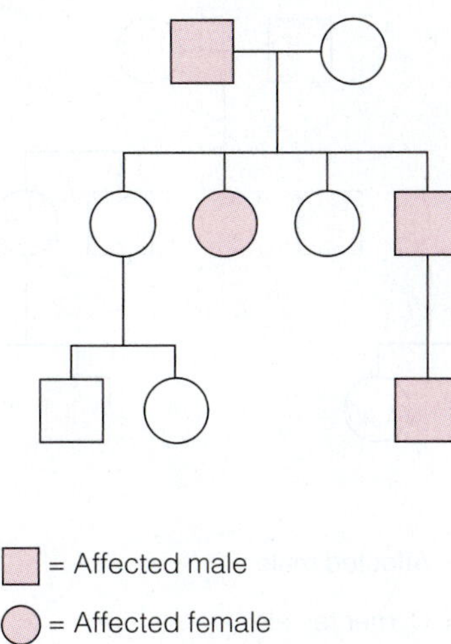

Figure 26–19 ■ Autosomal dominant pedigree. One parent is affected. Statistically, 50% of offspring will be affected regardless of gender.

Modes of Inheritance

Many inherited diseases are produced by an abnormality in a single gene or pair of genes. In such instances, the chromosomes are normal on the gross level. The defect is at the gene level. Some of these gene defects can be detected by technologies such as DNA and other biochemical assays.

The two major categories of inheritance are **Mendelian (single-gene) inheritance** and **non-Mendelian (multifactorial) inheritance**. Each single-gene trait is determined by a pair of genes working together. These genes are responsible for the observable expression of the traits (e.g., brown eyes, dark skin), referred to as the **phenotype**. The total genetic makeup of an individual is referred to as the **genotype** (pattern of the genes on the chromosomes).

One of the genes for a trait is inherited from the mother, the other from the father. An individual who has two identical genes at a given locus is considered to be *homozygous* for that trait. Individuals are considered to be *heterozygous* for a particular trait when they have two different alleles (alternative forms of the same gene) at a given locus on a pair of homologous chromosomes.

The best known modes of single-gene inheritance are autosomal dominant, autosomal recessive, and X-linked (sex-linked) recessive. There is also an X-linked dominant mode of inheritance, which is less common, and the new identified mode of inheritance, fragile X syndrome.

AUTOSOMAL DOMINANT INHERITANCE A person is said to have an autosomal dominant inherited disorder if the disease trait is heterozygous—that is, the abnormal gene overshadows the normal gene of the pair to produce the trait. It is essential to remember that in autosomal dominant inheritance the following occurs:

- An affected individual generally has an affected parent. Thus the family **pedigree** (graphic representation of a family tree) usually shows multiple generations with the disorder.
- Affected individuals have a 50% chance of passing on the abnormal gene to each of their children (Figure 26–19 ■).
- Males and females are equally affected, and a father can pass the abnormal gene on to his son. This is an important principle when distinguishing autosomal dominant disorders from X-linked disorders.
- Autosomal dominant inherited disorders have varying degrees of presentation. This is an important factor when counseling families concerning autosomal dominant disorders. Although a parent may have a mild form of the disease, the child may have a more severe form.

Autosomal dominant conditions such as phocomelia (a developmental anomaly characterized by the absence of the upper portion of the limbs) can have minimal expression in a parent but severe effects in a child. Other common autosomal dominant inherited disorders are Huntington disease, polycystic kidney disease, neurofibromatosis (von Recklinghausen disease), and achondroplastic dwarfism.

AUTOSOMAL RECESSIVE INHERITANCE In an autosomal recessive inherited disorder, the individual must have two abnormal genes to be affected. The notion of a carrier state is appropriate here. A *carrier* is an individual who is heterozygous for the abnormal gene and clinically normal. It is not until two individuals mate and pass on the same abnormal gene that affected children may appear. It is essential to remember that in autosomal recessive inheritance, the following occurs:

- An affected individual may have clinically normal parents, but both parents are carriers of the abnormal gene (Figure 26–20 ■).
- In the case in which both parents are carriers, there is a 25% chance that the abnormal gene will be passed on to any of their offspring. Each pregnancy has a 25% chance of resulting in an affected child.
- If a child of two carrier parents is clinically normal, there is a 50% chance that the child is a carrier of the gene.
- Both males and females are equally affected.
- There is an increased history of consanguineous matings (mating of close relatives).

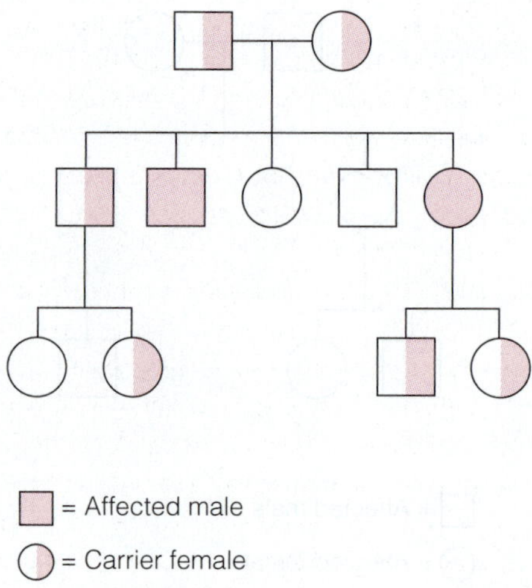

Figure 26–20 ■ Autosomal recessive pedigree. Both parents are carriers. Statistically, 25% of offspring are affected regardless of gender.

Some common autosomal recessive inherited disorders are cystic fibrosis, phenylketonuria (PKU), galactosemia, sickle cell anemia, Tay–Sachs disease, and most metabolic disorders.

X-LINKED RECESSIVE INHERITANCE X-linked, or sex-linked, disorders are those for which the abnormal gene is carried on the X chromosome. Thus an X-linked disorder is manifested in a male who carries the abnormal gene on his X chromosome. His mother is considered to be a carrier when the normal gene on one X chromosome overshadows the abnormal gene on the other X chromosome. It is essential to remember that in X-linked recessive inheritance the following occurs:

- There is no male-to-male transmission. Affected males are related through the female line (see Figure 26–21 ■).
- There is a 50% chance that a carrier mother will pass the abnormal gene to each of her sons, who will thus be affected.
- There is a 50% chance that a carrier mother will pass the normal gene to each of her sons, who will thus be unaffected.

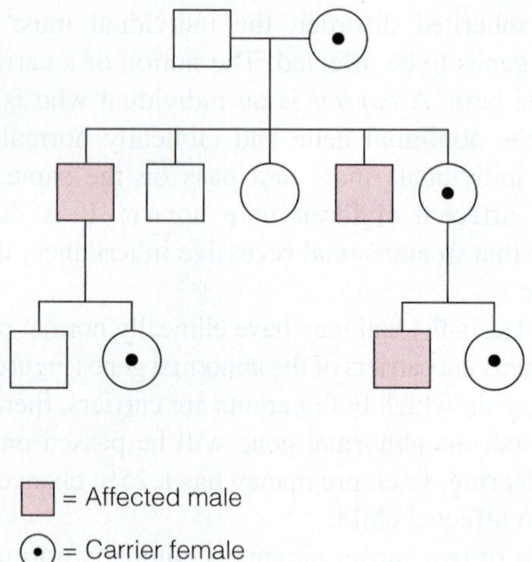

Figure 26–21 ■ X-linked recessive pedigree. The mother is the carrier. Statistically, 50% of male offspring are affected, and 50% of female offspring are carriers.

- There is a 50% chance that a carrier mother will pass the abnormal gene to each of her daughters, who become carriers.
- Fathers affected with an X-linked disorder cannot pass the disorder to their sons, but all their daughters become carriers of the disorder.

Common X-linked recessive disorders are hemophilia, Duchenne muscular dystrophy, and color blindness.

X-LINKED DOMINANT INHERITANCE The X-linked dominant disorders are rare, with the most common being vitamin D-resistant rickets and fragile X syndrome. When X-linked dominance does occur, the pattern is similar to that of X-linked recessive inheritance except that heterozygous females are affected. It is essential to remember that in X-linked dominant inheritance there is no male-to-male transmission. Affected fathers will have affected daughters; however, because they pass only the Y chromosome to male offspring, any sons will not be affected.

Fragile X Syndrome Fragile X syndrome is an inherited form of mental retardation; it is second only to Down syndrome among all causes of moderate mental retardation in males. Fragile X syndrome is a central nervous system disorder linked to a "fragile" site on the X chromosome. It is characterized by moderate mental retardation, large protuberant ears, and large testes after puberty. The carrier females do not have the abnormal features, but about one-third are mildly retarded.

MULTIFACTORIAL INHERITANCE Many common congenital malformations such as cleft palate, heart defects, spina bifida, dislocated hips, clubfoot, and pyloric stenosis are caused by an interaction of many genes and environmental factors. They are, therefore, multifactorial in origin. It is essential to remember that in multifactorial inheritance the following occurs:

- The malformations may vary from mild to severe. For example, spina bifida may range in severity from mild (spina bifida occulta) to more severe (myelomeningocele). It is believed that the more severe the defect, the greater the number of genes present for that defect.
- There is often a sex bias. For example, pyloric stenosis is more common in males, whereas cleft palate is more common in females. When a member of the less commonly affected sex shows the condition, a greater number of genes must usually be present to cause the defect.
- In the presence of environmental influences (such as seasonal changes, altitude, radiation exposure, chemicals in the environment, or exposure to toxic substances), fewer genes are needed to manifest the disease in the offspring.
- In contrast to single-gene disorders, there is an additive effect in multifactorial inheritance. The more family members who have the defect, the greater the risk that the next pregnancy will also be affected (Ward, 2008).

Although most congenital malformations are multifactorial, a careful family history should always be taken, because cleft lip and palate, certain congenital heart defects, and other malformations occasionally can be inherited as autosomal dominant or recessive traits. Other disorders thought to be within the multifactorial inheritance group are diabetes, hypertension, some heart diseases, and mental illness.

CONTRACEPTION

Many couples use contraception to allow them to plan pregnancy and/or avoid conception. It is important to understand the client's cultural and religious beliefs regarding the use of contraceptives in order to provide information on the best contraceptive choices for the client or couple.

Fertility Awareness Methods

Fertility awareness–based methods, also known as *natural family planning*, are based on an understanding of the changes that occur throughout a woman's ovulatory cycle. Fertility awareness methods take into account the life span of sperm (2–7 days) and the ovum (1–3 days) in the female reproductive tract. Maximum fertility for the woman occurs approximately 5 days before ovulation and decreases rapidly the day after (Speroff & Darney, 2005). All these methods require periods of abstinence and recording of certain events throughout the cycle; cooperation of the partner is important.

Fertility awareness methods are free, safe, and acceptable to many whose religious beliefs prohibit other methods. They provide increased awareness of the body, involve no artificial substances or devices, encourage a couple to communicate about sexual activity and family planning, and are useful in helping a couple plan a pregnancy.

However, these methods require extensive initial counseling to be used effectively. They may interfere with sexual spontaneity; they require careful maintenance of records for several cycles before beginning to use them; they may be difficult or impossible for women with irregular cycles to use; and although theoretically they should be very reliable, in practice they may not be as reliable in preventing pregnancy as other methods.

The *calendar rhythm method* is based on the assumptions that ovulation tends to occur about 14 days before the start of the next menstrual period, sperm are viable for up to 7 days, and the ovum is viable for up to 3 days. To use this method, the woman must record her menstrual cycles for 6 months to identify the shortest and longest cycles. The first day of menstruation is the first day of the cycle. The fertile phase is calculated from 18 days before the end of the shortest recorded cycle through 11 days from the end of the longest recorded cycle. For example, if a woman's cycle lasts from 24–28 days, the fertile phase would be calculated as day 6 through day 17. Once this information is obtained, the woman can identify the fertile and infertile phases of her cycle. For effective use of this method, she must abstain from intercourse during the fertile phase. The calendar method is the least reliable of the fertility awareness methods and has largely been replaced by other, more scientific approaches.

The *basal body temperature (BBT) method* to detect ovulation requires that a woman take her BBT every morning upon awakening (before any activity) and record the readings on a temperature graph. To do this, she uses a basal body temperature thermometer, which shows tenths of a degree rather than the two-tenths shown on standard thermometers. She may also use tympanic thermometry (an "ear thermometer"). After 3–4 months of recording temperatures, a woman with regular cycles should be able to predict when ovulation will occur. The method is based on the fact that the temperature sometimes drops just before ovulation and almost always rises and remains elevated for several days afterward. The temperature rise occurs in response to the increased progesterone levels that occur in the second half of the cycle. Figure 26–22 ■ shows a sample BBT chart. To avoid conception, the couple abstains from intercourse on the day of the temperature rise and for 3 days afterward. Because the temperature rise does not occur until after ovulation, a woman who had intercourse just before the rise is at risk of pregnancy. To decrease this risk, some couples abstain from intercourse for several days before the anticipated time of ovulation and then for 3 days afterward.

The *ovulation method*, sometimes called the *cervical mucus method* or the *Billings method*, involves the assessment of cervical mucus changes that occur during the menstrual cycle. The amount and character of cervical mucus change because of the influence of estrogen and progesterone. At the time of ovulation, the mucus (estrogen-dominant mucus) is clearer, more stretchable (a quality called *spinnbarkeit*) and more permeable to sperm. It also shows a characteristic fern pattern when placed on a glass slide and allowed to dry. During the

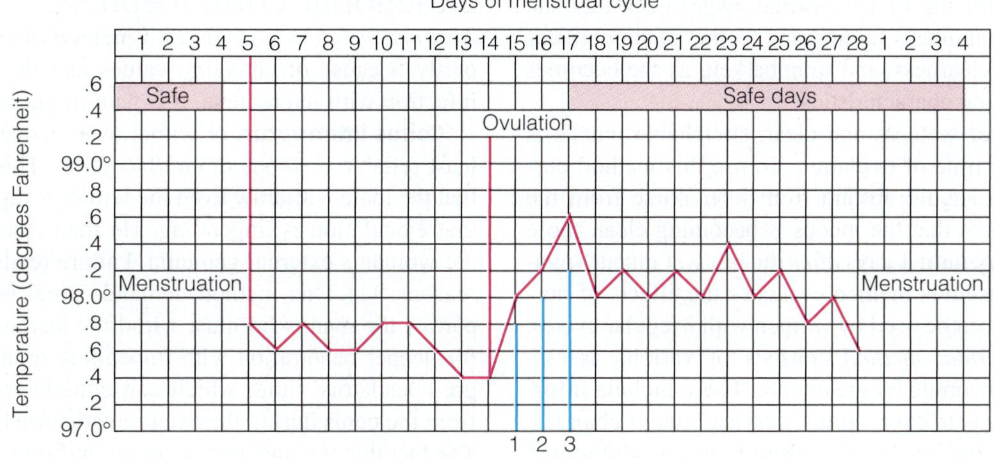

Figure 26–22 ■ Sample basal body temperature chart.

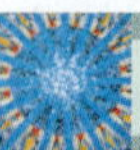

EVIDENCE-BASED PRACTICE **Natural Family Planning**

Clinical Question

What is the effectiveness of natural family planning methods for determining times of fertility?

The Evidence

The most common natural methods for estimating the fertile phase of the menstrual cycle are calendar-based formulas, daily measurement of basal body temperature (BBT), and observation of the characteristics of cervical mucus. A technology-based approach to fertility monitoring is a handheld, home-use device that measures urinary luteinizing hormones. Data about the effectiveness of each method when used singly or in combination have been generated through meta-analysis, a multisite prospective clinical efficacy trial, and a longitudinal study of more than 900 women. The data from these sources are the strongest evidence for practice.

What Is Effective?

Identifying the peak fertility period and avoiding unprotected sex during this time are essential for natural family planning methods to work. Calendar-based methods are the least accurate and require the longest periods of abstinence; when used alone, 15–18% of women became pregnant in 1 year. Two methods—BBT and urine hormone detection—identify ovulation at its peak. Because fertilization is most common in the 2 days before ovulation, these methods do not present a long enough warning period. Cervical mucus observation alone had a much lower pregnancy rate (1–3.4%), but women often found it confusing to use correctly. When used incorrectly, the cervical mucus method resulted in 15.2–22.5 pregnancies per 100 women. The best results were achieved when two methods were used in tandem. The cervical mucus method combined with BBT detection had an associated pregnancy rate of 1.8%. Combining urine hormone detection with cervical mucus had a correct use pregnancy rate of 2.1%. One of the studies found that nearly 10% of women discontinue mixed methods of natural family planning because they found them difficult to use consistently.

What Is Inconclusive?

Efficacy is usually reported as two rates: one for couples who used the methods correctly and one for couples who either used the methods incorrectly or who had unprotected intercourse during the fertile period. Most of these studies did not require the participants to report sexual activity, so incorrect application of the method may not be because of incorrect usage but rather because of unprotected sex during an identified fertile period.

Best Practice

Professional nurses are often in a position to recommend natural family planning methods to women who desire nonpharmacological methods of protection against unintended pregnancy. Teaching focused on the correct use of any natural family planning method is essential. Focus on both the use of the method and the need to avoid unprotected intercourse during times of peak fertility. Encourage women to use multiple methods, specifically cervical mucus observation along with BBT monitoring or a home urine hormone detection device, to get maximum effectiveness from these methods.

References

Colombo, B., Mion, A., Passarin, K., & Scarpa, B. (2006). Cervical mucus symptom and daily fecundability: First results from a new database. *Statistical Methods in Medical Research, 15*, 161–180.

Fehring, R., Schneider, M., Raviele, K., & Barron, K. (2007). Efficacy of cervical mucus observations plus electronic hormonal fertility monitoring as a method of natural family planning. *JOGNN: The Journal of Obstetric, Gynecological & Neonatal Nursing, 36*, 152–160.

Frank-Herrmann, P., et al. (2007). The effectiveness of a fertility awareness based method to avoid pregnancy in relation to a couple's sexual behaviour during the fertile time: A prospective longitudinal study. *Human Reproduction, 22*(5), 1310–1319.

luteal phase, the cervical mucus is thick and sticky (progesterone-dominant mucus) and forms a network that traps sperm, making their passage more difficult.

To use the cervical mucus method, the woman abstains from intercourse for the first menstrual cycle. Each day she assesses her cervical mucus for amount, feeling of slipperiness or wetness, color, clearness, and spinnbarkeit, as she becomes familiar with varying characteristics.

The peak day of wetness and clear, stretchable mucus is assumed to be the time of ovulation. To use this method correctly, the woman should abstain from intercourse from the time she *first* notices that the mucus is becoming clear, more elastic, and slippery until 4 days *after* the last wet mucus (ovulation) day. Because this method evaluates the effects of hormonal changes, it can be used by women with irregular cycles.

The *symptothermal method* consists of various assessments made and recorded by the couple. These include information regarding cycle days, coitus, cervical mucus changes, and secondary signs such as increased libido, abdominal bloating, *mittelschmerz* (midcycle abdominal pain), and basal body temperature. Through the various assessments, the couple learns to recognize signs that indicate ovulation. This combined approach tends to improve the effectiveness of fertility awareness as a method of birth control.

Situational Contraceptives

Abstinence can be considered a method of contraception, and, partly because of changing values and the increased risk of infection with intercourse, it is gaining increased acceptance.

Coitus interruptus, or withdrawal, is one of the oldest and least reliable methods of contraception. This method requires that the male withdraw from the female's vagina when he feels that ejaculation is impending. He then ejaculates away from the woman's external genitalia. Failure tends to occur for two reasons: (1) This method demands great self-control on the part of the man, who must withdraw just as he feels the urge for deeper penetration with impending orgasm, and (2) some pre-ejaculatory fluid, which can contain sperm, may escape from the penis during the excitement phase before ejaculation. The fact that the quantity of sperm in this pre-ejaculatory fluid is increased after a recent ejaculation is especially significant for couples who engage in repeated episodes of intercourse within a short period of time. Couples who use this method should be aware of postcoital contraceptive options in case the man fails to withdraw in time.

Douching after intercourse is an ineffective method of contraception and is not recommended. It may actually facilitate conception by pushing sperm farther up the birth canal.

Spermicides

The **spermicide** nonoxynol-9 (N-9), which is approved for use in the United States, is available as a cream, jelly, foam, vaginal film, and suppository. A spermicide is inserted into the vagina before intercourse. It destroys sperm by disrupting the cell membrane. A spermicide that effervesces in a moist environment offers more rapid protection, and coitus may take place immediately after it is inserted. A suppository may require up to 30 minutes to dissolve and will not offer protection until it has done so. The nurse instructs the woman to insert any of these spermicide preparations high in the vagina and to maintain a supine position.

N-9 is minimally effective when used alone. Its effectiveness increases in conjunction with a diaphragm or condom. The major advantages of spermicides are their wide availability and low toxicity. Skin irritation and allergic reactions to spermicides are the primary disadvantages. In 2007 the Food and Drug Administration (FDA) issued a ruling requiring that a warning and label information be added for all over-the-counter vaginal contraceptives containing N-9. The ruling states that N-9 does not offer protection against infection from the human immunodeficiency virus, which causes HIV/AIDS, or against any other sexually transmitted infection. Moreover, N-9 may actually increase a woman's risk of HIV infection because it irritates vaginal tissue, making them more susceptible to invasion by organisms such as HIV (FDA, 2007).

Barrier Methods of Contraception

Barrier methods of contraception prevent the transport of sperm to the ovum, immobilize sperm, or are lethal against sperm.

MALE AND FEMALE CONDOMS The male **condom** offers a viable means of contraception when used consistently and properly (Figure 26–23 ■). Acceptance has been increasing as a growing number of men are assuming responsibility for regulation of fertility. The condom is applied to the erect penis, rolled from the tip to the end of the shaft, before vulvar or vaginal contact. A small space must be left at the end of the condom to allow for collection of the ejaculate, so that the condom will not break at the time of ejaculation. If the condom or vagina is dry, water-soluble lubricants such as K-Y jelly should be used to prevent irritation and possible condom breakage.

Care must be taken in removing the condom after intercourse. For optimal effectiveness, the man should withdraw his penis from the vagina while it is still erect and hold the condom rim to prevent spillage. If after ejaculation the penis becomes flaccid while still in the vagina, the male should hold onto the edge of the condom while withdrawing to avoid spilling the semen and to prevent the condom from slipping off.

The effectiveness of male condoms is largely determined by their use. The condom is small, disposable, and inexpensive; it has no side effects (if neither partner is allergic to latex), requires no medical examination or supervision, and offers visual evidence of effectiveness. Most condoms are made of latex, although polyurethane and silicone rubber condoms are available for individuals allergic to latex. All condoms except natural "skin" condoms, made from lamb's intestines, offer protection against both pregnancy and STIs. Breakage, displacement, perineal or vaginal irritation, and dulled sensation are possible disadvantages. Condoms should not be stored in hot conditions because heat accelerates their deterioration, making them more susceptible to breaking.

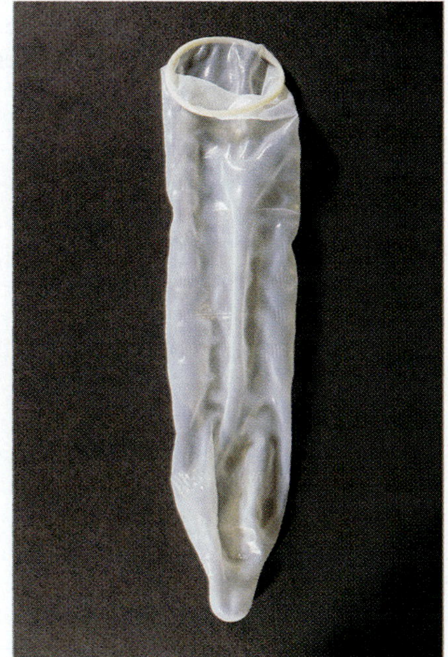

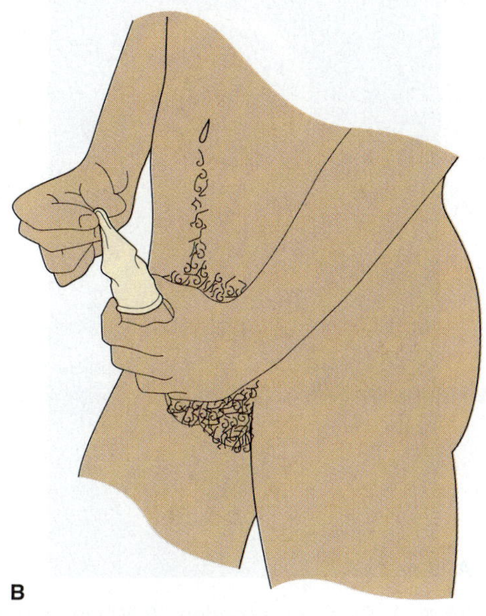

Figure 26–23 ■ *A*, An unrolled condom with reservoir tip. *B*, Correct use.

Thus, men should avoid placing them in their car glove box or in their wallets in a rear pants pocket.

The male condom is becoming increasingly popular because of the protection it offers from infections. For women, sexually transmitted infection increases the risk of pelvic inflammatory disease and resultant infertility. Many women are beginning to insist that their sexual partners use condoms, and many women carry condoms with them.

The *Reality female condom* (Figure 26–24 ■) is a thin polyurethane sheath with a flexible ring at each end. The inner ring, at the closed end of the condom, serves as the means of insertion and fits over the cervix like a diaphragm. The second ring remains outside the vagina and covers a portion of the woman's perineum. It also covers the base of the man's penis during intercourse. Available over the counter and designed for one-time use, the condom may be inserted up to 8 hours before intercourse. The inner sheath is prelubricated but does not contain spermicide and is not designed to be used with a male condom. Because it also covers a portion of the vulva, it probably provides better protection than other contraceptive methods against some pathogens. High cost, noisiness during intercourse, and the cumbersome feel of the device make acceptability a problem for some couples.

DIAPHRAGM AND CERVICAL CAP The **diaphragm** (Figure 26–25 ■) is used with spermicidal cream or jelly and offers a good level of protection from conception. The woman must be fitted with a diaphragm and instructed in its use by trained personnel. The diaphragm should be rechecked for correct size after each childbirth and whenever a woman has gained or lost 10–15 pounds or more.

The diaphragm must be inserted before intercourse, with approximately 1 teaspoonful (or 1.5 inches as squeezed from the tube) of spermicidal jelly placed around its rim and in the cup. This chemical barrier supplements the mechanical barrier of the diaphragm. The diaphragm is inserted through the vagina and covers the cervix. The last step in insertion is to push the edge of the diaphragm under the symphysis pubis, which may result in a "popping" sensation. When fitted properly and correctly in place, the diaphragm should not cause discomfort to the woman or her partner. Correct placement of the diaphragm can be checked by touching the cervix with a fingertip through the cup. The cervix feels like a small, firm, rounded structure and has a consistency similar to that of the tip of the nose. The center of the diaphragm should be over the cervix. If more than 6 hours elapse between insertion of the diaphragm and intercourse, additional spermicidal cream should be used. It is necessary to leave the diaphragm in place for at least 6 hours after coitus. If intercourse is desired again within the 6 hours, another type of contraception must be used or additional spermicidal jelly placed in the vagina with an applicator, taking care not to disturb the placement of the diaphragm. The diaphragm should not remain in the vagina for more than 24 hours. Periodically, the diaphragm should be held up to the light and inspected for tears or holes.

Some couples feel that the use of a diaphragm interferes with the spontaneity of intercourse. The nurse can suggest that the partner insert the diaphragm as part of foreplay. The woman can then easily verify the placement herself.

Diaphragms are an excellent contraceptive method for women who are lactating, who cannot or do not wish to use the pill (oral contraceptives), who are smokers over age 35, or who wish to avoid the increased risk of pelvic inflammatory disease associated with intrauterine devices. A silicone diaphragm is available for women with a latex allergy.

Women who object to touching their genitals to insert the diaphragm, check its placement, and remove it may find this method unsatisfactory. Women who are very obese or who have short fingers may find the diaphragm difficult to insert. The diaphragm is not recommended for women with a history of urinary tract infection (UTI), because pressure from the diaphragm on the urethra may interfere with complete bladder emptying

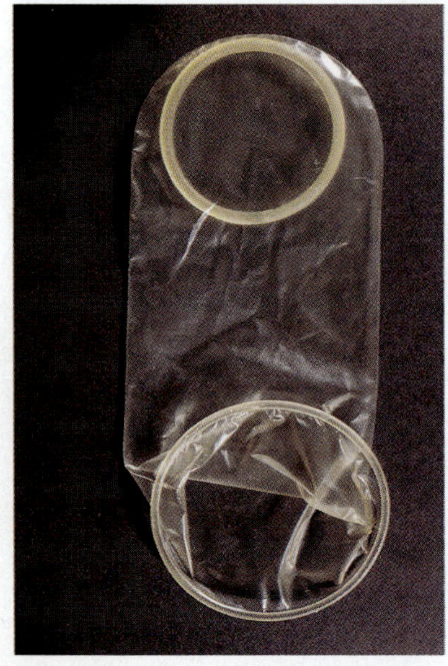

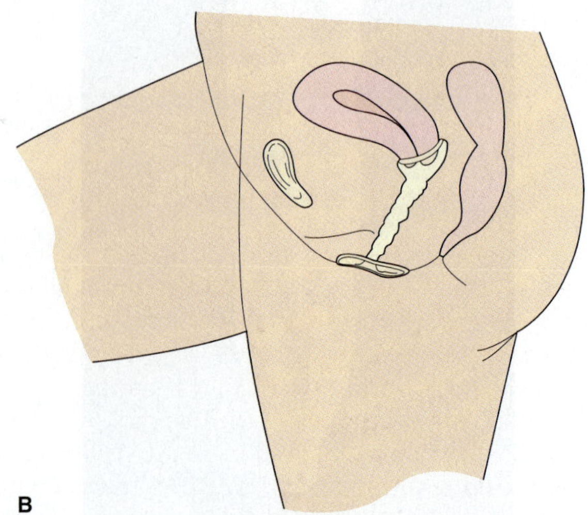

Figure 26–24 ■ *A*, The female condom. *B*, When properly inserted, the outer ring should rest on the folds of the skin around the vaginal opening, and the inner ring (closed end) should fit loosely against the cervix.

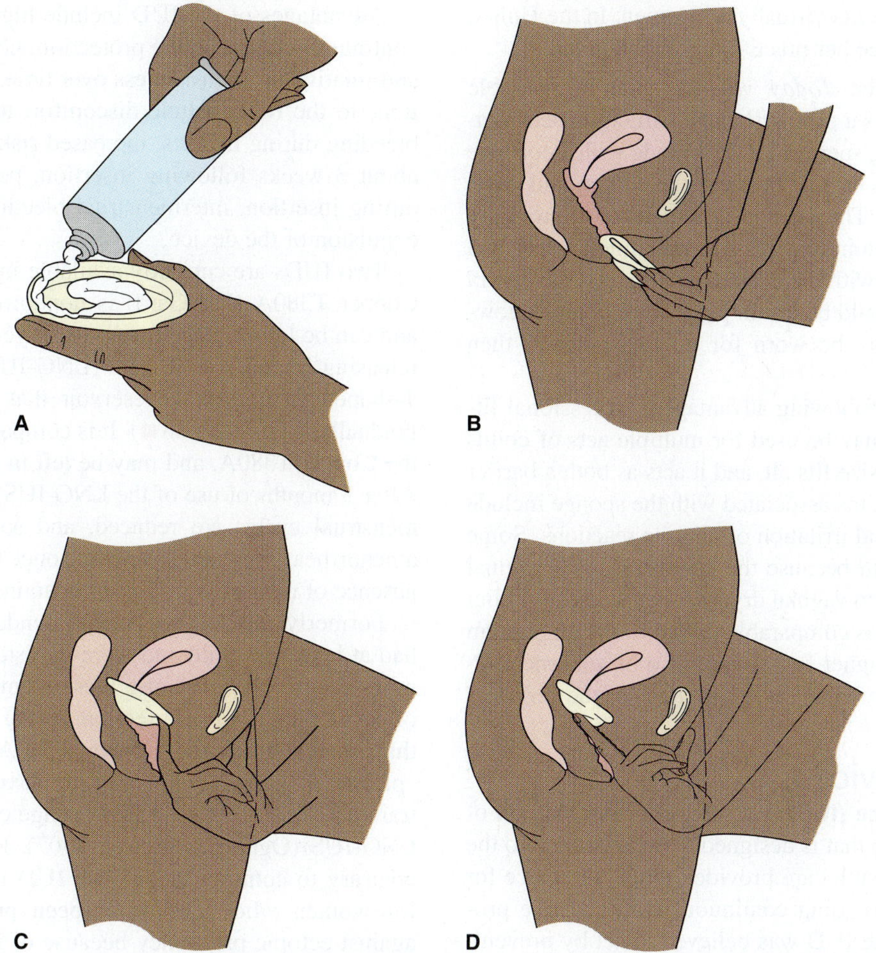

Figure 26–25 ■ Inserting the diaphragm. *A*, Apply jelly to the rim and center of the diaphragm. *B*, Insert the diaphragm. *C*, Push the rim of the diaphragm under the pubic symphysis. *D*, Check placement of the diaphragm. The cervix should be felt through the diaphragm.

and lead to recurrent UTIs. Women with a history of toxic shock syndrome should not use diaphragms or any of the barrier methods because they are left in place for prolonged periods. For the same reason, the diaphragm should not be used during a menstrual period or if a woman has abnormal vaginal discharge.

The Prentiff Cavity Rim **cervical cap** (Figure 26–26 ■) is a latex cup-shaped device, used with spermicidal cream or jelly, that fits snugly over the cervix and is held in place by suction. Effectiveness rates and method of insertion are similar to those for the diaphragm. The cap may be left in place for up to 48 hours, and repeated acts of intercourse do not require additional spermicide. Advantages, disadvantages, and contraindications are similar to those associated with the diaphragm. The cervical cap may be more difficult to fit because of limited size options. It also tends to be more difficult for women to insert and remove. A newer form of cervical cap—the FemCap—is also available. It looks like a small sailor's cap and has a strap placed over the dome that allows easier removal.

A systematic research review indicates that the Prentiff cervical cap is comparable to the diaphragm in preventing pregnancy; however, the FemCap is not as effective as a diaphragm. Both forms of cap are medically safe to use (Gallo, Grimes, & Schulz, 2006).

Lea's shield is a reusable silicone vaginal barrier method that completely covers the cervix. It is similar to the cervical cap but contains a centrally located valve that permits the passage of cervical secretions and air. A spermicide should be used with it, and it should not be worn for more than 48 hours with a single application of spermicide. The device has been available over the counter in several European countries for over a

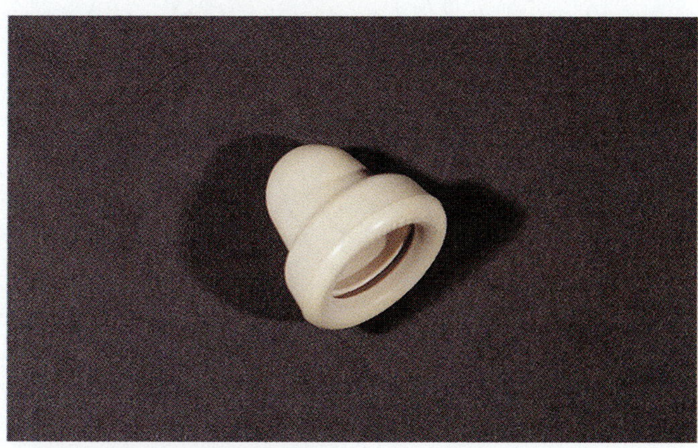

Figure 26–26 ■ A cervical cap.

decade because one size fits virtually all women. In the United States, a woman must see her practitioner to obtain one.

VAGINAL SPONGE The *Today vaginal sponge,* available without a prescription, is a pillow-shaped, soft, absorbent synthetic sponge containing spermicide. It is made with a concave or cupped area on one side that fits over the cervix, and has a loop for easy removal. The sponge is moistened thoroughly with water before insertion to activate the spermicide and then inserted into the vagina with the cupped side against the cervix (Figure 26–27 ■). It should be left in place for 6 hours following intercourse and may be worn for up to 24 hours, then removed and discarded.

The sponge has the following advantages: Professional fitting is not required, it may be used for multiple acts of coitus for up to 24 hours, one size fits all, and it acts as both a barrier and a spermicide. Problems associated with the sponge include difficulty removing it and irritation or allergic reactions. Some women report a problem because the sponge absorbs vaginal secretions, contributing to vaginal dryness. For women without children the failure rate is comparable to that of the diaphragm and cervical cap. It is higher for women who have borne children, possibly because of changes in the shape of the cervix.

Intrauterine Devices

The **intrauterine device (IUD)** is a safe, effective method of reversible contraception that is designed to be inserted into the uterus by a qualified health care provider and left in place for an extended period, providing continuous contraceptive protection. Traditionally the IUD was believed to act by preventing the implantation of a fertilized ovum. Therefore, the IUD was considered an abortifacient (abortion-causing) method. This belief is not accurate. IUDs truly are contraceptives; they trigger a spermicidal type reaction in the body, thereby preventing fertilization. The IUD is also known to have local inflammatory effects on the endometrium.

Advantages of the IUD include high rate of effectiveness, continuous contraceptive protection, no coitus-related activity, and relative inexpensiveness over time. Possible adverse reactions to the IUD include discomfort to the wearer, increased bleeding during menses, increased risk of pelvic infection for about 3 weeks following insertion, perforation of the uterus during insertion, intermenstrual bleeding, dysmenorrhea, and expulsion of the device.

Two IUDs are currently available in the United States. The Copper T380A (ParaGard) is nonhormonal, highly effective, and can be left in place for up to 10 years. The levonorgestrel-releasing intrauterine system (LNG-IUS) (Mirena) is a small, T-shaped frame with a reservoir that releases levonorgestrel gradually (Figure 26–28 ■). It is comparable in effectiveness to the Copper T380A, and may be left in place for up to 5 years. After 3 months of use of the LNG-IUS, bleeding and length of menstrual cycles are reduced, and some women experience amenorrhea, which they welcome once they are advised that the absence of menses is safe and not an indication of pregnancy.

Formerly, the IUD was recommended only for women who had at least one child and were in a stable, mutually monogamous relationship, because these women have the lowest risk of developing a pelvic infection. At the request of the company that manufactures the Copper T380A, the FDA removed a "patient or partner with multiple sexual partners" as a contraindication for its use. This change can apply as well to the LNG-IUS (Ogburn & Espey, 2007). Research indicates that, contrary to common belief, the IUD is reliable and effective for women who have never been pregnant; it is effective against ectopic pregnancy because of its overall effectiveness in preventing any pregnancy. Moreover, the copper IUD is a good choice for women who cannot use hormonal forms of contraception (Jacobstein, 2007).

The IUD is inserted into the uterus with its string or tail protruding through the cervix into the vagina. It may be inserted at any time during a woman's cycle, provided that she

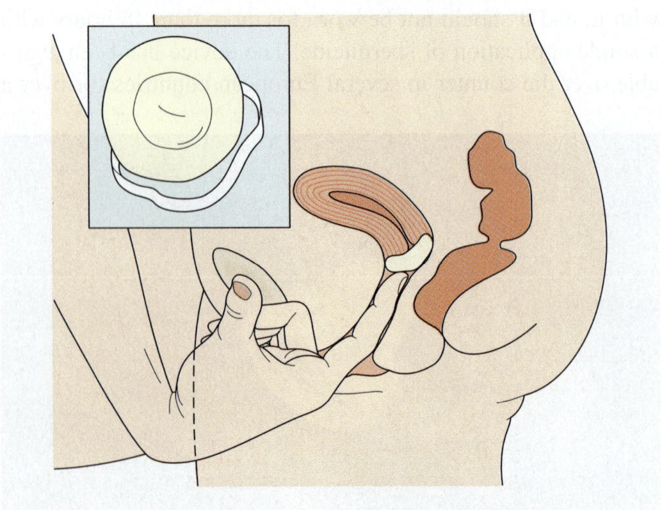

Figure 26–27 ■ The contraceptive sponge is moistened well with water and inserted into the vagina with the concave portion positioned over the cervix.

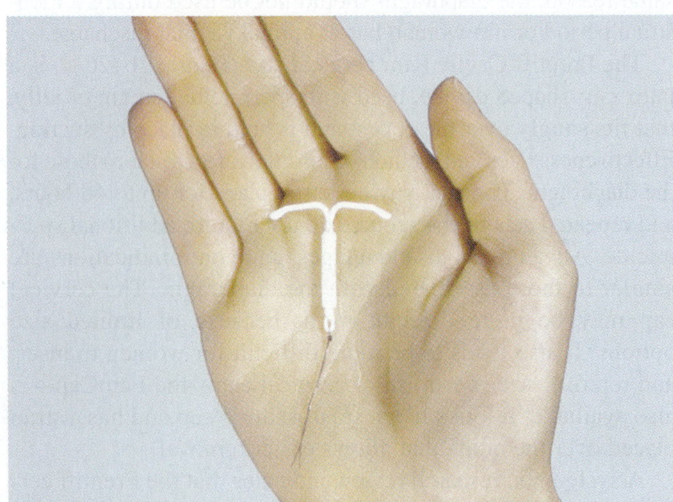

Figure 26–28 ■ The Mirena Intrauterine Contraceptive, which releases levonorgestrel gradually, may be left in place for up to 5 years.

Source: Courtesy of Berlex, Inc.

is not pregnant, or during the 4- to 6-week postpartum check. The Copper IUD may be inserted up to 5 days after unprotected intercourse as a method of emergency contraception. After insertion, the clinician instructs the woman to check for the presence of the string once a week for the first month and then after each menses. She is told that she may have some cramping or bleeding intermittently for 2–6 weeks and that her first few menses may be irregular. Follow-up examination is suggested 4–8 weeks after insertion.

Women with IUDs should contact their health care providers if they are exposed to an STI or if they develop the following warning signs: late period, abnormal spotting or bleeding, pain with intercourse, abdominal pain, abnormal discharge, signs of infection (fever, chills, and malaise), or missing string. If the woman becomes pregnant with an IUD in place, the device should be removed as soon as possible to prevent infection.

Hormonal Contraceptives

Hormonal contraceptives are available in a variety of forms. They may be progestin-only hormones, most often using a synthetic form of progesterone called progestin, or a combination of estrogen and a progestin.

COMBINED ESTROGEN–PROGESTIN APPROACHES Combined hormonal approaches work by inhibiting the release of an ovum, by creating an atrophic endometrium, and by maintaining a thick cervical mucus that slows sperm transport and inhibits the process that allows sperm to penetrate the ovum.

Combined Oral Contraceptives **Combined oral contraceptives (COCs)**, also called *birth control pills*, are a combination of estrogen and progestin. COCs are safe, highly effective, and rapidly reversible. COCs are generally taken daily for 21 days, typically beginning on the Sunday after the first day of the menstrual cycle although the woman can also start on day 1 of her menstrual cycle. In most cases, menses occurs 1–4 days after the last pill is taken. Seven days after taking her last pill, the woman restarts the pill. Thus, the woman always begins the pill on the same day. Some companies offer a 28-day pack with seven "blank" pills so that the woman never stops taking a pill. The pill should be taken at approximately the same time each day—usually upon arising or before retiring in the evening.

Research suggests that traditional 21/7 approaches may need to be modified. With today's low-dose COCs, the 7 hormone-free days may result in failure to completely suppress ovarian function, resulting in the development of an ovarian follicle and possible ovulation (Sulak, 2008). Consequently there is growing interest in extended oral contraceptives. Seasonale and Seasonique are the first FDA-approved extended cycle COCs. They both are 91-day regimens in which a woman takes an active pill daily for 84 consecutive days followed by 7 days of inactive tablets, during which the woman has a period. Thus, a woman has only four periods a year. Extended use reduces the side effects of COCs, such as bloating, headache, breast tenderness, and cramping (Abboud, 2006). Another COC, Lybrel, has been approved by the FDA for continuous 365-day use with no scheduled hormone-free periods.

Although they are highly effective when taken correctly, COCs may produce a variety of side effects, which may be either progesterone or estrogen related (Table 26–8). The use of low-dose (35 mcg or less estrogen) preparations has reduced many of the side effects. The newer 20- or 25-mcg pills have even fewer side effects, but they may result in less contraceptive effectiveness and in weaker cycle control.

Absolute contraindications to the use of oral contraceptives include pregnancy, previous history of thrombophlebitis or thromboembolic disease, acute or chronic liver disease of cholestatic type with abnormal function, presence of estrogen-dependent carcinomas, undiagnosed uterine bleeding, heavy smoking, gallbladder disease, hypertension, diabetes, and hyperlipidemia. In addition, women with the following relative contraindications need to be monitored frequently: migraine headaches, epilepsy, depression, oligomenorrhea, and amenorrhea. Women who choose this method of contraception should be fully advised of its potential side effects.

TABLE 26–8 **Side Effects Associated With Oral Contraceptives**

ESTROGEN EFFECTS	PROGESTIN EFFECTS
Alterations in lipid metabolism	Acne, oily skin
Breast tenderness; engorgement; increased breast size	Breast tenderness; increased breast size
Cerebrovascular accident	Decreased libido
Changes in carbohydrate metabolism	Decreased high-density lipoprotein (HDL) cholesterol levels
Chloasma	Depression
Fluid retention; cyclic weight gain	Fatigue
Headache	Hirsutism
Hepatic adenomas	Increased appetite; weight gain
Hypertension	Increased low-density lipoprotein (LDL) cholesterol levels
Leukorrhea, cervical erosion, ectopia	Oligomenorrhea, amenorrhea
Nausea	Pruritus
Nervousness, irritability	Sebaceous cysts
Telangiectasia	
Thromboembolic complications: thrombophlebitis, pulmonary embolism	

COCs also have some important noncontraceptive benefits. Many women experience relief of uncomfortable menstrual symptoms. Cramps are lessened, flow is decreased, and cycle regularity is increased. Mittelschmerz is eliminated, and the incidence of functional ovarian cysts is decreased. There is also a substantial reduction in the incidence of ectopic pregnancy, ovarian cancer, endometrial cancer, iron deficiency anemia, and benign breast disease. COCs are considered a good solution to the physiological problems some women experience during the perimenopause. However, because of the increased risk of myocardial infarction (heart attack), women over age 35 who smoke should not take COCs. The woman using oral contraceptives should contact her health care provider if she becomes depressed, becomes jaundiced, develops a breast lump, or experiences any of the following warning signs: severe abdominal pain, severe chest pain or shortness of breath, severe headaches, dizziness, changes in vision (vision loss or blurring), speech problems, or severe leg pain.

Another COC is the progestin-only pill, also called the *minipill*. It is used primarily by nursing mothers because it does not interfere with breast milk production. It is also used by women who have a contraindication to the estrogen component of the combination preparation, such as history of thrombophlebitis, but are strongly motivated to use this form of contraception. The major problems with this preparation are amenorrhea or irregular spotting and bleeding patterns.

Other Combined Hormonal Methods Hormones can now be administered transdermally using a *contraceptive skin patch* called Ortho Evra, which is roughly the size of a silver dollar but square. The woman applies the patch weekly for 3 weeks to one of four sites: her abdomen, buttocks, upper outer arm, or trunk (excluding the breasts). During the fourth week, no patch is worn and menses occurs. The patch is highly effective in women who weigh less than 198 pounds. The patch is as safe and reliable as COCs and has a better rate of compliance.

Because skin absorption of transdermal estrogen is 60% greater than oral absorption of a 35-mcg COC, questions have arisen as to whether this increases a woman's risk of serious side effects or complications. It has been noted that women using the patch still have about a 25% lower peak blood level of estrogen than women taking typical COCs (U.S. Food and Drug Administration, 2006). Preliminary research suggests that the incidence of stroke and acute MI is no higher in women using the patch than in women using 35-mcg COCs (Jick & Jick, 2007). Research is ongoing. In the meantime, this method is considered a safe birth control option.

NuvaRing vaginal contraceptive ring (manufactured by Orgonon), another form of low-dose, sustained release hormonal contraceptive, is a flexible, soft ring that the woman inserts into her vagina (Figure 26–29 ■). The ring is left in place for 3 weeks and then removed for 1 week to allow for withdrawal bleeding. One size fits virtually all women. The ring is highly effective and has minimal side effects. The ring can be worn during intercourse and is comfortable for both the woman and her partner. Replacement rings should be kept in the refrigerator to maintain integrity.

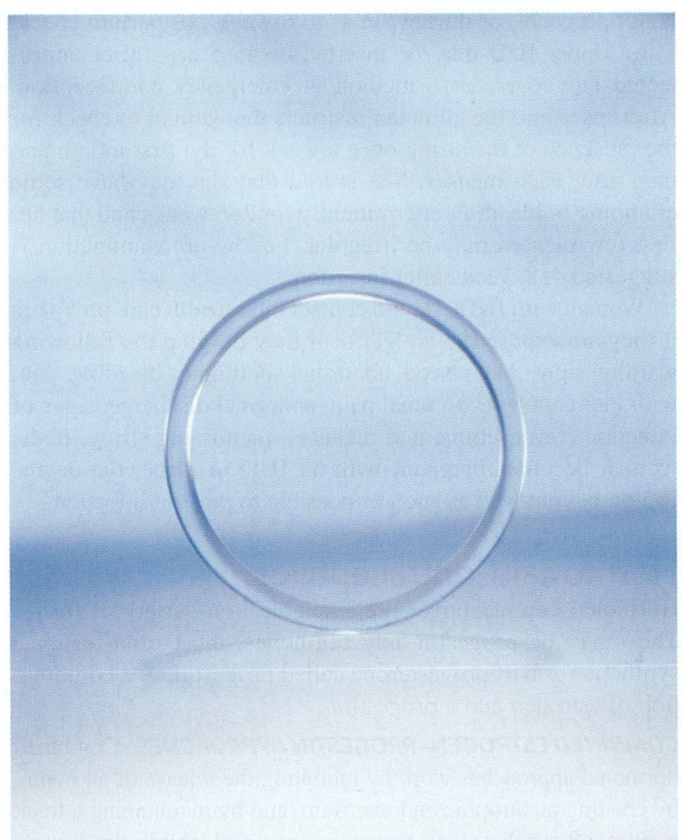

Figure 26–29 ■ The NuvaRing vaginal contraceptive ring.

Source: Courtesy of Orgonon, Inc.

Lunelle, an injectable combination of medroxyprogesterone acetate (MPA) and estradiol cypionate (E_2C), is now off the market in the United States and Canada but is available in many countries worldwide under the name Cyclofem. Administered every 28 to 30 days (not to exceed 33 days) intramuscularly, it is a highly effective contraceptive that has a side effect pattern similar to that of COCs.

LONG-ACTING PROGESTIN CONTRACEPTIVES Norplant, a system consisting of six silastic capsules containing levonorgestrel (a progestin) that are implanted in a woman's arm, was the original **subdermal implant**. It is now off the market in the United States. Norplant II, which consists of a two-rod system that is effective for up to 5 years, was never introduced in the United States, although it is marketed elsewhere as Jadelle.

Implanon, a single-capsule implant also inserted under the skin of the arm, is effective for up to 3 years. It is impregnated with etonogestrel, another progestin. Its release in the United States has been postponed but remains anticipated.

Subdermal implants prevent ovulation in most women. They also stimulate the production of thick cervical mucus, which inhibits sperm penetration. Norplant provides effective continuous contraception removed from the act of coitus. Possible side effects include spotting, irregular bleeding or amenorrhea, an increased incidence of ovarian cysts, weight gain, headaches, fluid retention, acne, mood changes, and depression.

Implants are mentioned in this chapter because some women may not have had their six Norplant rods removed or the nurse may care for women from foreign countries who use Jadelle or Implanon. A minor surgical procedure is required to insert and remove the implants.

Depot-medroxyprogesterone acetate (DMPA) (**Depo-Provera**), another long-acting progesterone, provides highly effective birth control for 3 months when given as a single injection of 150 mg. DMPA, which acts primarily by suppressing ovulation, is safe, convenient, private, and relatively inexpensive. It also separates birth control from the act of coitus. It can safely be given to nursing mothers because it contains no estrogen. DMPA provides levels of progesterone high enough to block the LH surge, thereby suppressing ovulation. It also thickens the cervical mucus to block sperm penetration. Side effects include menstrual irregularities, headache, weight gain, breast tenderness, and depression. Return of fertility may be delayed for an average of 9 months.

Depo-Provera is not recommended for use longer than 2 years without specific informed consent by the woman. It has been associated with calcium loss from the bones that may not resolve after discontinuing use. Women who remain on DMPA longer than 2 years must be educated about this serious side effect and need to exercise and take 1,200 mg of calcium daily.

Depo-Provera 104 mg subcutaneously is an alternative to Depo-Provera 150 mg. Originally approved by the FDA for the treatment of endometriosis, it subsequently was approved as a contraceptive. Because there is 30% less drug available compared with the 150-mg preparation, it may result in less bone density loss for long-term users. It is administered subcutaneously every 10–13 weeks.

EMERGENCY POSTCOITAL CONTRACEPTION Emergency **postcoital contraception** is indicated when a woman is worried about pregnancy because of unprotected intercourse, rape, or possible contraceptive failure (e.g., broken condom, slipped diaphragm, missed COCs, or too long a time between DMPA injections). Plan B, a progestin-only (levonorgestrel) approach, is the only emergency contraceptive currently available in the United States.

The phrase "morning-after pill" is misleading. The woman actually takes her first dose as soon after intercourse as possible (but not longer than 72 hours) and a second dose 12 hours later. Emergency contraception taken within 72 hours can reduce the risk of pregnancy after a single act of intercourse by 89% (Office of Population Research & Association of Reproductive Health Professionals, 2007). In 2006, the FDA approved Plan B for over-the-counter sale to women 18 years and older. A prescription for this pill is still required for teens under age 18.

A combined hormonal approach (levonorgestrel and ethinyl estradiol) called Preven is no longer available in the United States. However, a woman can use COCs for emergency contraception if necessary. She is advised to consult her health care provider about specifics.

Placement of the Copper IUD within 5 days of unprotected intercourse may reduce pregnancy risk by as much as 99% (Hatcher et al., 2004).

PRACTICE ALERT

Emergency contraceptives are controversial and may be declined by some women with strong beliefs about right to life. The emergency contraceptive does not prevent conception but instead prevents implantation of the fertilized ova. Some people view this as similar to abortion and may prefer not to take the medication.

Operative Sterilization

Operative **sterilization** is an inclusive term that refers to surgical procedures that permanently prevent pregnancy. Before sterilization is performed on either partner, the physician provides a thorough explanation of the procedure to both. Each needs to understand that sterilization is not a decision to be taken lightly or entered into when psychological stresses, such as separation or divorce, exist. Even though both male and female procedures are theoretically reversible, the permanence of the procedure should be stressed and understood.

PRACTICE ALERT

The decision to have a sterilization procedure is the client's. The nurse's responsibility is to provide client teaching about the procedure, its permanence, and side effects (if any). The nurse should not impose his or her beliefs about sterilization on the client, and should accept the client's decision. In addition, the nurse should not provide information in a way that makes the procedure sound intimidating or conveys any implication about the morality of the procedure. The nurse must support the client in his or her decision, regardless of the nurse's personal beliefs about the procedure.

Male sterilization is achieved through a relatively minor procedure called a **vasectomy**. This procedure involves surgically severing the vas deferens in both sides of the scrotum. It takes about 4–6 weeks and 6–36 ejaculations to clear the remaining sperm from the vas deferens. During that period, the couple is advised to use another method of birth control and to bring in two or three semen samples for a sperm count. The man is rechecked at 6 and 12 months to ensure that fertility has not been restored by recanalization. Possible side effects of a vasectomy include pain, infection, hematoma, sperm granulomas, and spontaneous reanastomosis (reconnecting).

Vasectomies can sometimes be reversed by using microsurgery techniques. Restored fertility, as measured by subsequent pregnancy, ranges from 38% to 82% (Hatcher et al., 2004).

Female sterilization is most frequently accomplished by **tubal ligation**. The tubes are located through a small subumbilical incision or by minilaparotomy techniques and are clipped, ligated, electrocoagulated, banded, or plugged. Tubal ligation may be done at any time; however, the postpartal period is an ideal time to perform the procedure because the tubes are somewhat enlarged and easily located.

Complications of female sterilization procedures include coagulation burns on the bowel, perforation of the bowel, pain, infection, hemorrhage, and adverse anesthesia effects. Reversal of a tubal ligation depends on the type of procedure performed.

The *Essure* method of permanent sterilization requires no surgical incision. Under hysteroscopy, stainless steel microinserts are placed in the tubes, stimulating the growth of local tissue, which then results in tubal blockage—by 3 months for 96% of women and 6 months postprocedure for 100% (Memmel & Gilliam, 2008). Essure eliminates the need for transabdominal surgery, but it does require some specialized training and a hysterosalpingogram (HSG) 3 months following the procedure to confirm that the tubes are occluded. The woman should use a backup contraceptive method until the HSG confirms that the tubes are occluded.

Male Contraception

The vasectomy and the condom, discussed previously, are currently the only forms of male contraception available in the United States. Hormonal contraception for men has yet to be developed, although studies are underway. Developing safe, effective, and reversible male contraceptives is challenging: It is easier to interrupt a woman's cyclic process than to interrupt a man's continuous fertility.

Discontinuing Contraception

A woman who uses hormonal contraception—such as COCs, mini-pills, the NuvaRing, Ortho Evra patch, or Depo-Provera—is advised to stop using the hormonal birth control method and have two or three normal menstrual cycles before attempting to conceive. This waiting period allows the natural hormonal cycle to return and facilitates dating the subsequent pregnancy. A woman using an intrauterine device is advised to have it removed and wait 1 month before attempting to conceive. During the waiting period she can use barrier methods of contraception (condoms, diaphragm, or cervical cap with spermicides). Women who have used Depo-Provera should be advised that it could take up to 12 months to conceive after discontinuation.

COLLABORATION

Care of the client or couple seeking family, infertility, genetic, or contraceptive care often involves several members of the health care team. Geneticists, psychologists, and infertility experts may be included in the client's health care team.

Diagnostic Tests

Diagnostic testing that may be used in the care for a client with infertility includes the following:

- Basal body temperature recording
- Hormonal assessments of ovulatory function
- Endometrial biopsy
- Transvaginal ultrasound
- Hysterosalpingography
- Hysteroscopy
- Laparoscopy.

Diagnostic tests that may be used for potential genetic issues include the following:

- Genetic screening
- Genetic ultrasound
- Genetic amniocentesis
- Percutaneous umbilical cord sampling and chorionic villus sampling
- Alpha-fetoprotein
- Preimplantation genetic testing.

Fertility Medications

Pharmacological agents are commonly used for ovarian stimulation in the follicular phase, control of midcycle release, and support of the luteal phase. The pharmacological treatment chosen depends on the specific cause of infertility. Table 26–9 lists some of the drugs commonly used and indications for use.

Clinical Interruption of Pregnancy

Although abortion was legalized in the United States in 1973, the associated controversy over moral and legal issues continues. This controversy is as readily apparent in the medical and nursing professions as in other groups.

Some people are strongly opposed to abortion for religious, ethical, or personal reasons. Some people feel that access to a safe, legal abortion is every woman's right. A number of physical and psychosocial factors influence a woman's decision to seek an abortion. The presence of a disease or health state that jeopardizes the mother's life and serious, life-threatening fetal problems are frequently suggested as indications for abortion. In other instances, the timing or circumstance of the pregnancy creates an inordinate stress on the woman and she chooses an abortion. Some of these situations may involve contraceptive failure, sexual assault, or incest.

Medical abortion, now available in the United States, provides an effective alternative to surgical abortion for many women with unintended pregnancy. *Mifepristone* (Mifeprex), originally called RU 486, may be used to induce abortion medically during the first 7 weeks of pregnancy (up to 49 days following conception). (*Note:* Some clinicians support the use of a slightly modified dosage regimen through 63 days' gestation [Creinin, Blumenthal, & Shulman, 2006].)

Mifepristone blocks the action of progesterone, thereby altering the endometrium. After the length of the woman's gestation is confirmed, she takes a dose of mifepristone. Between 1–3 days later (depending upon gestation), she returns to her caregiver and takes a dose of the prostaglandin misoprostol, which induces contractions that expel the embryo/fetus. About 14 days after taking the misoprostol, the woman is seen a third time to confirm that the abortion was successful.

Since 2001, seven deaths that may possibly have been related to the oral mifepristone/vaginal misoprostol regimen have been reported. Four of these deaths were related to an infection caused by a rare organism, *Clostridium sordelli* (Creinin et al., 2006). Therefore, *any* woman who has taken the oral mifepristone/vaginal misoprostol regimen within the last 24 hours who develops stomach pain, weakness, nausea, vomiting or diarrhea, with or without fever, should contact her health care provider *immediately* (U.S. FDA, 2007). Currently, mifepristone is still considered safe and use of routine prophylactic antibiotics is not recommended.

In the first trimester, surgical abortion may be performed by dilation and curettage (D&C), minisuction, or vacuum curettage. The major risks include perforation of the uterus, laceration of the cervix, systemic reaction to the anesthetic

TABLE 26–9 **Drugs Commonly Used to Treat Infertility**

DRUGS	WOMEN	MEN
Clomiphene citrate (Clomid, Serophene)	■ PCOS ■ Hyper-androgenemia ■ Premature follicle rupture	■ Low levels of gonadotrophins ■ Hypothalamic hypogonadism
Human menopausal gonadotropin (hMG), (Repronex, Bravelle)	■ Hypothalamic ovulatory dysfunction (after failure of clomiphene) ■ Hypopituitarism ■ PCOS (rarely) ■ Luteinized unruptured follicle syndrome (after failure of hCG alone) ■ Inadequate cervical mucus ■ In vitro fertilization, GIFT, ZIFT ■ Controlled super-ovulation	■ Hypothalamic pituitary failure due to Kallmann syndrome or delayed puberty ■ Hypogonadotrophic hypogonadism (deficiency of FSH and LH)
Recombinant follicle-stimulating hormone (rFSH) (Follistim, Gonal-F)	■ PCOS ■ Too-long cycles ■ In vitro fertilization, GIFT, ZIFT	
Human chorionic gonadotropin (hCG) (Pregnyl, Novarel, A.P.L)	■ Induces dominant follicle to release egg ■ Luteinized unruptured follicle syndrome	
Bromocriptine (Parlodel)	■ Pituitary adenoma	■ Hyperprolactinemia (functional or pituitary adenoma)
Cabergoline (Dostinex)	■ Hyperpituitarism	
Gonadotropin releasing hormone (GnRh) (Factral, Lutre-pulse)	■ Hypothalamic ovulatory dysfunction—to ensure a pulsatile release of GnRH by a small pump	■ Hypothalamic pituitary failure due to Kallmann syndrome or delayed puberty (pulsed infusion)
GnRh analogs	■ Premature follicular rupture	
■ Leuprolide acetate (Lupron)	■ In vitro fertilization, GIFT, ZIFT	■ Hypogonadotrophic hypogonadism
■ Nafarelin acetate (Synarel)	■ Endometriosis	
■ Goserelin acetate (Zoladex)		
GnRH antagonists	■ Same as GnRH analogs	
■ Ganirelix acetate (Antagon)		
■ Progesterone (Crinone, Prometrium, progesterone in oil)	■ Luteal phase dysfunction ■ Luteal phase support	

Source: Adapted from American Society for Reproductive Medicine Booklet. (2006). *Medications for inducing ovulation—A guide for patients.* Retrieved from http://www.org/patientbooklets/ovulation_drugs.pdf; Shane, J. (1993). Evaluation and treatment of infertility. *Clinical Symposia, 45*(2); Wilson, B. A., Shannon, M. T., Shields, K. M., & Stang, C. L. (2009). *Prentice Hall nurse's drug guide 2009.* Upper Saddle River, NJ: Pearson Education.

agent, hemorrhage, and infection. Second trimester abortion may be done using dilatation and extraction (D&E), hypertonic saline, systemic prostaglandins, and intrauterine prostaglandins. Surgical abortion in the first trimester is technically easier and safer than abortion in the second trimester.

PRACTICE ALERT

Important aspects of nursing care for a woman who chooses to have an abortion include providing information about the methods of abortion and associated risks; counseling regarding available alternatives to abortion and their implications; encouraging verbalization by the woman; providing support before, during, and after the procedure; monitoring vital signs, intake, and output; providing for physical comfort and privacy throughout the procedure; and health teaching about self-care, the importance of the postabortion checkup, and contraception review.

Therapeutic Insemination

Therapeutic insemination has replaced the previously used term *artificial insemination* and involves the depositing of semen at the cervical os or in the uterus by mechanical means. *Therapeutic donor insemination (TDI)* is the current term for use of donor semen, and *therapeutic husband insemination (THI)* is the current term for use of the husband's semen.

THI is generally indicated for such seminal deficiencies as oligospermia (low sperm count), asthenospermia (decreased motility), and teratospermia (low percentage, abnormal morphology); for anatomical defects accompanied by inadequate deposition of semen such as hypospadia (a congenital abnormal male urethral opening on the underside of the penis); and for ejaculatory dysfunction (such as retrograde ejaculation). THI is also indicated in cases of unexplained infertility and some cases of female factor infertility, such as scant or inhospitable mucus, persistent cervicitis, or cervical stenosis. In some cases, intrauterine insemination (IUI) would be indicated to bypass the cervical factor. Seminal fluid contains high levels of prostaglandins, which can cause nausea, severe cramps, abdominal pain, and diarrhea when absorbed by the uterine lining. Therefore, sperm preparation for IUI involves washing sperm from the seminal plasma. IUI, with or without ovulation induction therapy, is an option for many couples before more aggressive treatments such as in vitro fertilization are employed.

TDI is considered in cases of azoospermia (absence of sperm), severe oligospermia or asthenospermia, inherited male sex-linked disorders, and autosomal dominant disorders. In the past several years, indications for donor insemination have expanded to include single women or lesbians desirous of pregnancy. Some states have specified the parental rights of single women and donors, but most are silent on this issue.

TDI has become more complicated and expensive in the past decade because of the need for strict screening and processing procedures to prevent transmission of a genetic defect or sexually transmitted infection to the offspring or recipient. Guidelines have been established that include mandatory medical (genetic) and infectious disease screening of both donor and recipient, the need for informed consent from all parties, the need to limit the number of pregnancies per donor, and the need for accurate means of record keeping. Finally, because of the risk of transmitting infectious diseases, donated sperm must be frozen and quarantined for 6 months from the time of acquisition, and the donor must be retested before sperm can be released for use.

Numerous factors need to be evaluated before TDI is performed. Has every possible effort been made to diagnose and treat the cause of the male infertility? Do tests indicate normal fertility and sperm–ovum transport in the woman? Has the couple had an opportunity to discuss this option with an infertility counselor to explore the issues of secrecy, disclosure, and potential feelings of loss the couple (particularly the male partner) may feel about not having a genetic child? Are there any religious constraints? After making the decision, the couple should allow themselves time to further assess their concerns and explore their feelings individually and together to ensure that this option is acceptable to both.

In Vitro Fertilization

In vitro fertilization (IVF) is selectively used in cases when infertility has resulted from tubal factors, mucous abnormalities, male infertility, unexplained infertility, male and female immunological infertility, and cervical factors. In IVF, a woman's eggs are collected from her ovaries, fertilized in the laboratory, and placed into her uterus after normal embryo development has begun. If the procedure is successful, the embryo continues to develop in the uterus, and pregnancy proceeds naturally (Figure 26–30 ■).

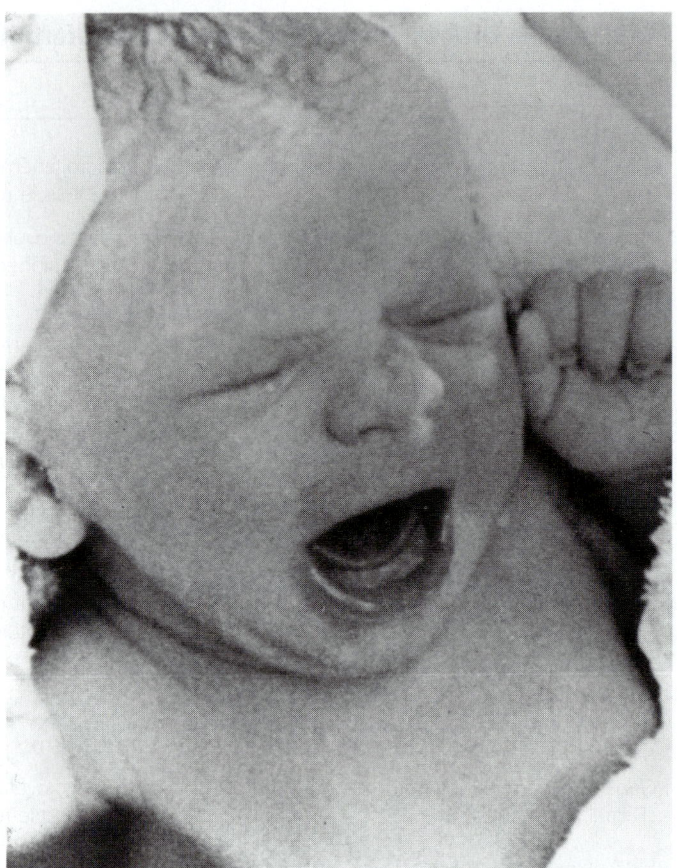

Figure 26–30 ■ Louis Joy Brown, the world's first "test tube baby" shown shortly after her birth by cesarean section on July 25, 1978. IVF was pioneered by Drs. Bob Edwards and Patrick Steptoe.

The potential for a successful pregnancy with IVF is maximized when three to four embryos (rather than one) are placed into the uterus. For this reason, fertility drugs are used to induce ovulation before the process. Follicular development and oocyte maturity are monitored frequently with ultrasound and hormonal assays. Monitoring usually begins around cycle day 5, and medications are titrated according to individual response. When follicles appear mature, hCG is given to stimulate final egg maturation and control the induction of ovulation. Egg retrieval is performed approximately 35 hours later, before ovulation occurs.

In the majority of cases, egg retrieval is performed by a transvaginal approach under ultrasound guidance (Figure 26–31 ■). It

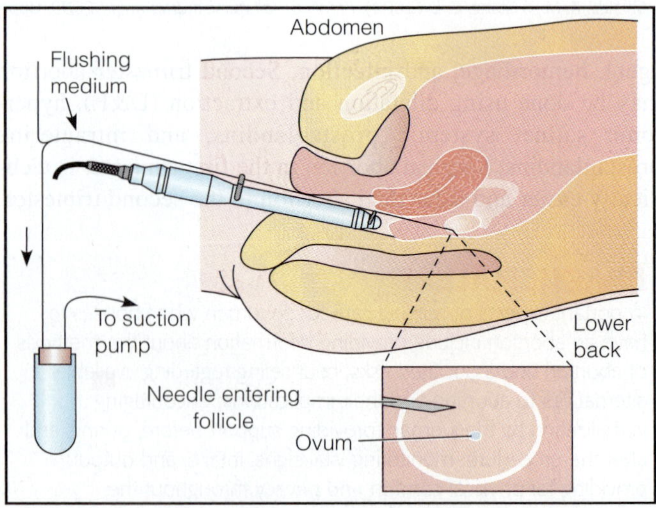

Figure 26–31 ■ Transvaginal ultrasound-guided oocyte retrieval.
Source: Courtesy of Serono, Inc., Rockland, MA.

is an outpatient procedure performed with intravenous sedation and a cervical block for anesthesia. Many follicles can be aspirated with only one puncture, and the procedure generally lasts no more than 30 minutes. Once the eggs are fertilized and progress to the embryo stage, the embryos are placed in the uterus. This occurs 1–2 days after conception. After the procedure, the woman is advised to engage in only minimal activity for 12–24 hours, and progesterone supplementation is prescribed. The progesterone supplementation is given to promote implantation and support the early pregnancy; therefore, the woman will not have a period even if she is not pregnant. (The pregnancy is usually determined by transvaginal ultrasound.)

Sperm used to fertilize the eggs in vitro can be obtained naturally or via microsurgical epididymal sperm aspiration (MESA) or testicular sperm aspiration (TESA). These are procedures that address severe male factor infertility. MESA and TESA involve the retrieval of sperm from the gonadal tissue of men who have azoospermia or an ejaculatory disorder (Figure 26–32 ■). Percutaneous epididymal sperm aspiration (PESA) and TESA are replacing MESA as the preferred techniques for retrieval of sperm because they are not surgical procedures. ICSI is a microscopic procedure to inject a single sperm into the outer layer of an ovum so that fertilization will occur (Devine, 2008).

Success with IVF depends on many factors, especially the woman's age and the specific indication. Women have a good chance of achieving pregnancy with an average of three cycles of IVF. Many couples find the emotional, physical, and financial costs of going beyond three cycles too great. Costs vary by treatment and by region of the country; one cycle of IVF-ET averages $12,400 (American Society of Reproductive Medicine, 2006a). Clinical birth rates reported by the Society of Assisted Reproductive Technology (SART) were 40–45% per egg donation for women regardless of age or indication in the United States (American Society of Reproductive Medicine, 2007). The increase in maternal and neonatal morbidity associated with IVF because of the rates of multiple fetuses remains an issue.

Other Assisted Reproduction Techniques

Other assisted reproductive techniques include procedures for transfer of gametes, zygotes, or embryos; cryopreservation of embryos; IVF using donor oocytes; micromanipulation techniques; and use of a gestational carrier.

Preimplantation Genetic Diagnosis

Other recent advances in micromanipulation allow a single cell to be removed from the embryo for genetic study. Couples at risk for having a detectable single gene or chromosomal anomaly may wish to undergo such preimplantation genetic testing, called *blastomere analysis* or, more recently, *preimplantation*

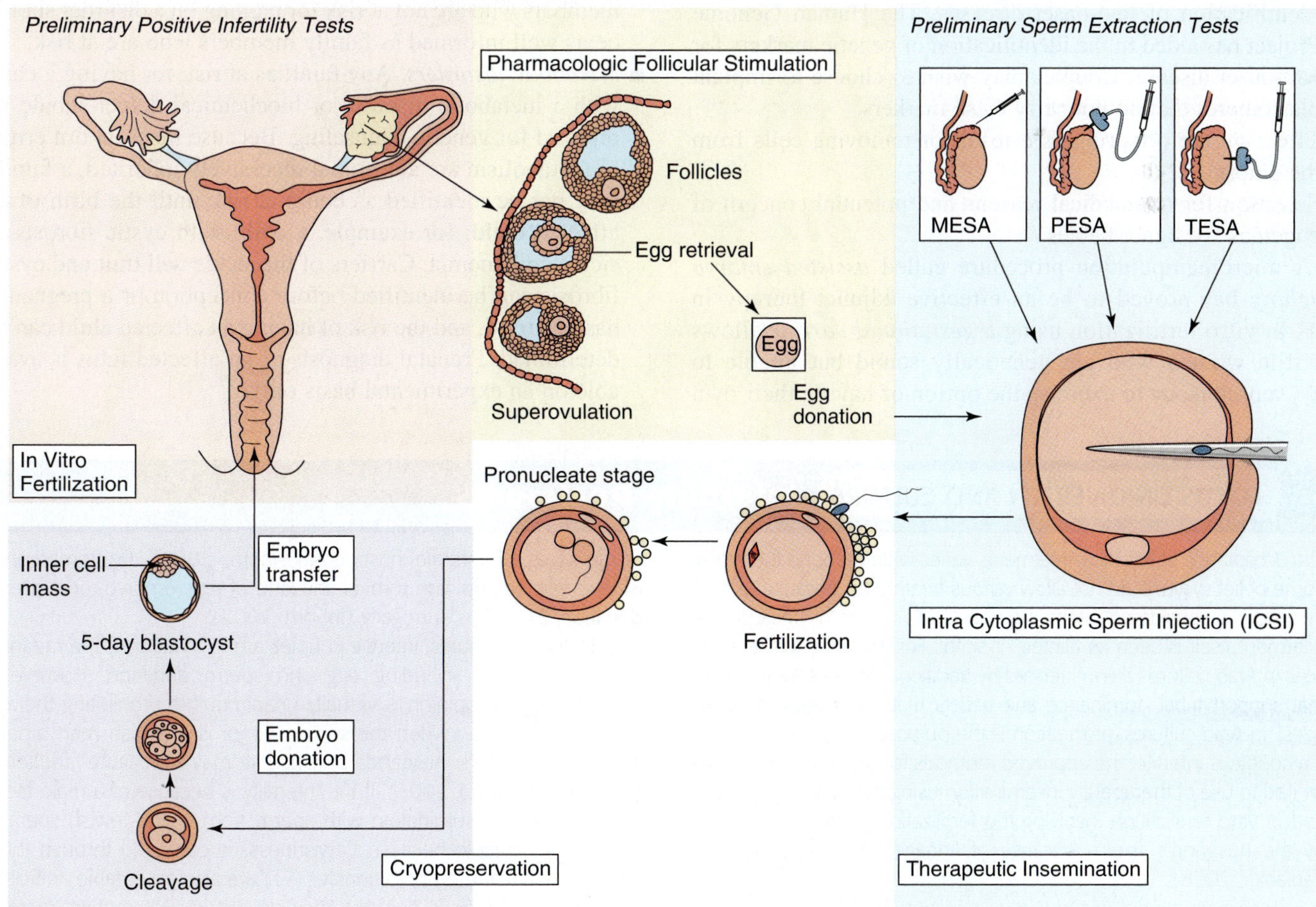

Figure 26–32 ■ Assisted reproductive techniques.

genetic diagnosis (PGD). The single cell is obtained from a six- to eight-cell embryo by a process known as *blastomere biopsy*. The genetic content of the cell is examined using polymerase chain reaction (PCR) technique or fluorescence in situ (FISH). Results of genetic testing on the preimplantation embryos are available in 4–24 hours, so unaffected embryos may still be transferred during the required biological window of time without the need for cryopreservation.

The diagnosis of genetic disorders before implantation provides couples with the option of forgoing the attempt to establish a pregnancy and thereby avoiding a difficult decision about terminating an affected pregnancy (Simpson & Holzgreve, 2007). This technology also raises several ethical issues, including the following:

- Identification of couples at risk. There is a need for criteria that identify couples at risk for diseases that constitute significant hardship and suffering so that "wrongful birth" cases can be avoided.
- Availability of and access to centers providing PGD. Should society provide access for those at risk for genetic transfer of disease but without the financial resources to pay for the services?
- Analysis of blastomeres for sex chromosome testing when a genetic disorder carried on the sex chromosomes is suspected. In X-linked diseases, the only way to prevent the disorder is to select against the blastomere with the Y chromosome.
- Identification of late-onset diseases. The Human Genome Project has aided in the identification of genetic markers for late-onset disease. Couples may wish to choose to implant blastomeres that do not carry these markers.
- Effect on the offspring as a result of removing cells from the embryo
- Selection for nonmedical reasons and potential concern of eugenics "designer babies."

A micromanipulation procedure called *assisted embryo hatching* has proved to be an effective adjunct therapy in IVF. In vitro fertilization using a *gestational carrier* allows infertile women who are genetically sound but unable to carry a pregnancy to exercise the option of having their own biological child. Other technologies involve oocyte donation and cryopreservation of the embryo.

Genetic Counseling Referral

Genetic counseling is a communication process in which a genetic counselor, physician, or specially trained and certified nurse tries to provide a family with the most complete and accurate information about the occurrence or the risk of recurrence of a genetic disease in that family. Genetic counseling is thus an appropriate course of action for any family wondering, "Will it happen again?"

A genetic counseling referral is advised for any of the following categories:

- *Congenital abnormalities, including mental retardation.* Any couple who has a child or a relative with a congenital malformation may be at increased risk and should be so informed. If mental retardation of unidentified cause has occurred in a family, there may be an increased risk of recurrence.
- *Familial disorders.* Families should be told that certain diseases may have a genetic component and that the risk of their occurrence in a particular family may be higher than that in the general population. Such disorders as diabetes, heart disease, cancer, and mental illness fall into this category.
- *Known inherited diseases.* Families may know that a disease is inherited but not know the mechanism or the specific risk for them. An important point to remember is that family members who are not at risk for passing on a disorder should be as well informed as family members who are at risk.
- *Metabolic disorders.* Any families at risk for having a child with a metabolic disorder or biochemical defect should be referred for genetic counseling. Because most inborn errors of metabolism are autosomal recessively inherited, a family may not be identified as being at risk until the birth of an affected child; for example, a child with cystic fibrosis or sickle cell anemia. Carriers of the sickle cell trait and cystic fibrosis can be identified before conception or a pregnancy has occurred, and the risk of having an affected child can be determined. Prenatal diagnosis of an affected fetus is available on an experimental basis only.

FOCUS ON DIVERSITY AND CULTURE Infertility Treatments

The acceptance of infertility treatments varies widely around the world. Some belief systems do not allow various treatments, because using a treatment is considered interfering with God's design or because the treatment itself is seen as tainted or sinful. For example, fertility practices in Arab cultures are influenced by traditional Arab Bedouin values that support tribal dominance and beliefs that "God decides family sizes." In Arab cultures, procreation is the purpose of marriage.

If a couple is infertile, the approved methods for treating infertility are limited to use of therapeutic insemination using the husband's sperm and in vitro fertilization involving the fertilization of the wife's ovum by the husband's sperm because of lineage concerns (Purnell & Paulanka, 2008).

Sterility in a woman can lead to rejection and divorce. Also with the use of ICSI, male-initiated divorce is becoming more common for aging wives of infertile husbands (Inhorn, 2002). Contemporary Islamic religious opinion forbids any kind of egg, embryo, or semen donation, as well as surrogacy (Inhorn, 2002).

In Jewish cultures, infertile couples are to try all possible means to have children, including egg and sperm donation. However, Orthodox Jewish opinion is virtually unanimous in prohibiting therapeutic insemination when the semen donor is a Jewish man other than the woman's husband, because it may constitute adultery (Purnell & Paulanka, 2008). If the infertility is because of a male factor, therapeutic insemination with sperm from a non-Jewish sperm donor is acceptable because "Jewishness" is conferred through the matrilineal. IVF and embryo transfer (ET) are also acceptable artificial insemination methods because they do not involve putting sperm into another's wife (Kahn, 2002).

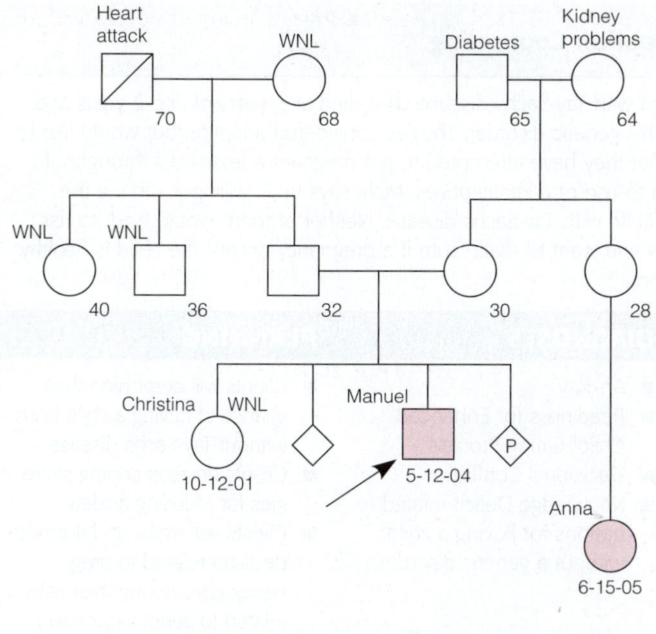

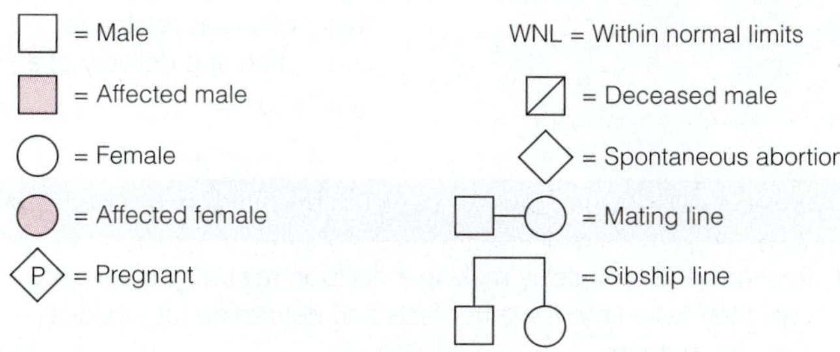

Figure 26–33 ■ Screening pedigree. Arrow indicates the nearest family member affected with the disorder being investigated. Basic data have been recorded. Numbers refer to the ages of the family.

- *Chromosomal abnormalities.* As discussed previously, any couple who has had a child with a chromosomal abnormality may be at increased risk of having another child similarly affected. This group includes families in which there is concern about a possible translocation.

After a couple has been referred to the genetics clinic, they are sent a form requesting information on the health status of various family members. This information assists the genetic counselor in creating the family's pedigree.

Together, the pedigree and history facilitate identification of other family members who might also be at risk for the same disorder (Figure 26–33 ■). The family being counseled may wish to notify relatives at risk so that they, too, can begin genetic counseling. When done correctly, the family history and pedigree can be powerful tools for determining a family's risk.

NURSING PROCESS

The priority of nursing care for the client with family planning considerations is to identify specific needs, provide emotional support, and teach the client about options so he or she can make the best informed decision.

Assessment

When assessing men and women for reproductive issues, the nurse must use a nonjudgmental attitude and open communication. Many clients are uncomfortable discussing their sexuality and sexual activity. The nurse must approach the topic in a matter-of-fact manner, with reassurance of confidentiality within the law. Some questions are the same for both genders:

- Ask about history of sexual activity, including the age at first sexual intercourse.
- Ask about the number of sexual partners, currently and in the past.
- Ask about the use of contraceptives.
- Ask about the use of barriers to prevent STIs.
- Ask about a history of sexual trauma, including abuse, rape, or incest.

Women

- Ask about risk factors for breast cancer, including family history.
- Ask about breast self-exam, how often she does it, and any abnormal findings.
- Perform a breast examination, palpating the breast for masses, irregularities in contour, and drainage, if warranted.
- Ask about menstrual history, including onset of menstruation, the date of the last menses, and any irregularities.

Men

- Ask about testicular self-examination, how often he does it, and any abnormal findings.
- Perform a testicular examination, palpating for masses and inspecting the genitals for lesions and drainage, if warranted.
- Ask about difficulty voiding, including difficulty starting or stopping and the size of the stream. Include symptoms of burning, frequency, urgency, or nocturia.
- Ask about sexual functioning, including premature ejaculation, impotence, or other sexual problems.

Diagnosis

Possible nursing diagnoses that may be appropriate for clients with family planning needs include the following:

- Risk for Disturbed Body Image
- Sexual Dysfunction
- Deficient Knowledge related to family planning, infertility, contraception, or genetics.

Plan

Goals of nursing care include the following:

- Client describes options available for treatment and chooses the option that best fits his or her needs, beliefs, and values.
- Client acknowledges the impact of the situation on existing personal relationships and lifestyle.
- Client describes actual change in body function.
- Client maintains close social interactions and personal relationships.

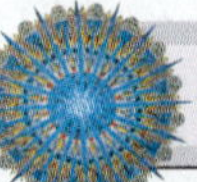

NURSING CARE PLAN A Client Requesting Preconception Counseling

Donner Everson and her significant other, Mola Langerson, had a child born with Tay-Sachs disease who died at 3 years of age 2 years ago. They would love to have another child but fear having another child with this genetic disorder. They've considered adoption but would like to know whether there is any chance of having a normal child. They report that they have attempted to get pregnant a few times throughout the last year, but when it didn't happen immediately, they decide to return to use of contraceptives. Mola says he is willing to "throw the dice," but Donner says she would rather be childless than deliver another child with Tay-Sachs disease. Neither of them would want to risk having to make a decision about aborting a child conceived with Tay-Sachs and want to make sure if a pregnancy occurs, the child is healthy. They have come to talk with their family provider to learn about their options.

ASSESSMENT	DIAGNOSES	PLANNING
Both Donner and Mola are healthy with no significant current, chronic, or past medical or surgical history. Vital signs are within normal limits, their weights are appropriate for their heights, and they are both physically active. Neither client has a substance abuse issue or history, and they report an occasional glass of wine, perhaps twice a week. They are both orthodox Jews whose grandparents lived in Germany prior to World War II. Donner's family history includes two children born with Tay-Sachs disease, one born to her maternal aunt and one to her paternal aunt. She has no siblings. Mola had a brother who died who was born with Tay-Sachs disease, but there is no other family history of congenital or genetic anomalies. Their family provider collects blood for genetic testing and refers them to a genetic counselor.	■ Anxiety ■ Readiness for Enhanced Childbearing Process ■ Decisional Conflict ■ Knowledge Deficit related to options for having a child without a genetic disorder	■ Clients will determine their chance of having a child born without Tay-Sachs disease. ■ Clients develop coping strategies for reducing anxiety. ■ Clients will make an informed decision related to pregnancy, considering their risks related to genetic disorders. ■ Clients will understand their options as related to conception and delivery of a healthy child.

IMPLEMENTATION

The nurse's role in caring for these clients is largely supportive, as well as providing the necessary teaching to help them understand what they are told as well as any options that they are provided.

- Encourage clients to verbalize their feelings.
- Suggest coping strategies to reduce anxiety.
- Recommend they delay making a decision regarding pregnancy until they have time to gather facts and determine the options available to them.
- Describe the role of the genetic counselor and the type of information the geneticist can provide based on the blood test that was collected.

EVALUATION

Donner and Mola spoke with the genetic counselor and learned there was a 50% chance that a baby conceived naturally would be born with Tay-Sachs disease. The genetic counselor told them about in vitro fertilization that could be performed, allowing the doctor to choose only the sperm and ova that were free of the genetic mutation and, once conception took place, could be implanted into Donner's uterus, allowing the couple a 100% likelihood of conceiving a child without Tay-Sachs disease. However, the genetic counselor cautioned that this method would not eliminate risks related to other congenital or pregnancy-induced disorders. They opted to try this procedure, and Donner became pregnant and delivered a healthy baby girl.

CRITICAL THINKING

1. One of the implementations for this couple is to encourage them to delay conception until they receive information related to their options. Is this an appropriate nursing implementation? Explain your answer.
2. Define the role of the genetic counselor and explain what information genetic counseling can provide this couple.
3. Describe the in vitro process and explain how this process can reduce the risk of having a child born with Tay-Sachs disease.

Implementation

Family planning considerations can cause a great deal of stress for the couple or client. By providing a nonjudgmental, accepting atmosphere and thorough client teaching, nurses can help clients resolve difficult decision making in a way that suits the client best. This facilitates both the nurse-client relationship as well as the client's ability to learn and act on information.

Risk for Disturbed Body Image

- Encourage verbalization of feelings.
- Provide resources (pamphlets, books, tapes, referrals to support groups and counselors) as appropriate.
- Teach client (and significant other if appropriate) about reproductive physiology as it applies to use of contraceptive, infertility issue, or genetic issue.

Sexual Dysfunction

- Encourage discussion of sexual function among client, partner, and health care provider.
- Provide information given by the health care provider regarding treatment options.
- Encourage the client to discuss concerns of sexuality with a therapist or counselor.

Deficient Knowledge Related to Risk Factors, Disease Prevention, and Treatment, Including Medications

- Teach clients about risk factors for reproductive dysfunction. For example, STIs increase the risk of infertility.
- Teach clients about disease prevention. For example, teach about use of contraceptives and application of condoms. By understanding disease prevention, clients can take measures to protect themselves.
- Teach clients (and significant others if appropriate) about their specific disease and prescribed treatment.

Evaluation

Clients may be evaluated using the following expected outcomes:

- Client makes informed decisions about treatment based on the disorder and individual choice.
- Client verbalizes understanding of information presented.
- Client expresses feelings openly.

REVIEW Family Planning and Preconception Counseling

RELATE: LINK THE CONCEPTS

Linking the exemplar of Family Planning and Preconception Counseling with the concept Addiction Behaviors:

1. You are working with a young couple who are planning to have a baby. The potential father smokes cigarettes. What teaching regarding the effects of paternal smoking on planned children will you provide?
2. What information about risks associated with alcohol consumption would you provide the woman who plans to become pregnant and drinks an average of 4 alcoholic drinks a week?

Linking the exemplar of Family Planning and Preconception Counseling with the concept Immunity:

3. What client teaching will you provide a client diagnosed with systemic lupus erythematosus who plans to become pregnant?
4. What is your priority of care for the woman, diagnosed with rheumatoid arthritis, who is anticipating pregnancy?

READY: GO TO COMPANION SKILLS MANUAL

- Assessing the Female Genitals and Inguinal Area
- Assessing the Male Genitalias and Inguinal Area

REFER: GO TO MYNURSINGKIT

REFLECT: CASE STUDY

Lisa Daniels is an 18-year-old woman recently married to her high school sweetheart, Dan. Lisa is planning to begin college in the fall to study interior decorating. Dan is 24 and working as the manager of a local food chain store. Lisa's family lives a few towns away and is thrilled with her marriage to Dan. Her younger brother, Tom, enjoys playing basketball with Dan. Dan's family lives across the country, but are very fond of Lisa and excited about the marriage.

Lisa and Dan have come to the OB/GYN clinic to talk about planning for a family. Neither Lisa nor Dan has any health issues that would put them or a child at risk. Lisa feels that she can handle going to school part time and also care for a baby. Both Lisa and Dan are very excited about the prospect of starting their family. Lisa and Dan just bought a house and have furnished it with hand-me-downs from family and friends. They both laugh when they talk about living paycheck to paycheck.

1. What topics will you raise with Lisa and Dan as they consider starting a family?
2. What nutritional teaching will you provide Lisa to help her optimize her status before becoming pregnant?
3. If Dan and Lisa decide to begin attempting to become pregnant, what teaching will you provide this couple?

26.3 MENOPAUSE

KEY TERMS

Hormone replacement therapy (HRT), *1743*
Menopause, *1742*

BASIS FOR SELECTION OF EXEMPLAR

Standards of Nursing Practice
Common condition

LEARNING OUTCOMES

After reading about this exemplar, you will be able to:

1. Describe the physiology, etiology, and clinical manifestations, of menopause.
2. Identify risk factors associated with menopause.
3. Illustrate the nursing process in providing culturally competent care for menopausal individuals.
4. Formulate priority nursing diagnoses appropriate for a menopausal individual.
5. Create a plan of care for menopausal individuals and their families.
6. Assess expected outcomes for a menopausal individual.
7. Discuss therapies used in the collaborative care of an individual with alterations related to menopause.
8. Employ evidence-based caring interventions for a menopausal individual.

OVERVIEW

Menopause is the permanent cessation of menses. The *climacteric*, or *perimenopausal*, period denotes the time during which reproductive function gradually ceases. For most women, the perimenopausal period lasts several years. It begins with a decline in the production of the hormone estrogen, includes the permanent cessation of menstruation due to loss of ovarian function, and extends for 1 year after the final menstrual period, at which time a woman is said to be *postmenopausal*. The average woman will live one-third of her life after menopause.

Menopause is neither a disease nor a disorder, but a normal physiological process. It is included here because it does increase the risk of physical disorders as well as affect various aspects of women's health. Many women welcome the freedom from monthly menstrual periods and have relatively minor physical effects from the estrogen depletion. However, the hormonal changes that occur can be accompanied by side effects. There is wide variation in how individual women experience these side effects. In the United States, most women stop menstruating between 48 and 55 years of age. Earlier menopause is associated with genetics, smoking, higher altitude, and obesity (Association of Reproductive Health Professionals [ARHP], 2005b). Certain health risks increase after menopause, including heart disease, osteoporosis, macular degeneration, cognitive changes, and breast cancer.

PHYSIOLOGY AND ETIOLOGY

The menopausal period marks the natural biological end of reproductive ability. *Surgical menopause* occurs when the ovaries are removed in premenopausal women, dramatically reducing the production of estrogen and progestins. *Chemical menopause* often occurs during cancer chemotherapy, when cytotoxic drugs arrest ovarian function.

As ovarian function decreases, the production of estradiol (E_2), the most biologically active estrogen, decreases and is ultimately replaced by estrone as the major ovarian estrogen. Estrone is produced in small amounts and has only about one-tenth the biological activity of estradiol. With decreased ovarian function, the second ovarian hormone, progesterone, which is produced during the luteal phase of the menstrual cycle, also is markedly reduced.

CLINICAL MANIFESTATIONS

Although menopause is an age-related process, not pathology, some women have troublesome health experiences after the cessation of menses. As estrogen decreases, various tissues are affected. The breast tissue, body hair, skin elasticity, and subcutaneous fat decrease. The ovaries and uterus become smaller, and the cervix and vagina also decrease in size and become pale in color. These changes may result in problems with vaginal dryness, dyspareunia, urinary stress incontinence, urinary tract infections (UTIs), and vaginitis. Atrophic vaginitis may lead to urogenital infection, ulceration, and uncomfortable sexual intercourse. Vasomotor instability often results in hot flashes, palpitations, dizziness, and headaches. Other problems resulting from vasomotor instability include insomnia, frequent awakening, perspiration (night sweats), osteoporosis, and increased cardiovascular disease (Welner, 1999). The woman may experience irritability, anxiety, and depression as a result of these events.

Hoerger et al. (1999) have estimated that annual medical costs for postmenopausal health problems are $186 billion, with the majority spent on cardiovascular disease. Menopause is an emotionally laden subject with many cultural implications. Different societies view aging women differently, and the older woman may internalize some of these views. Women may experience negative changes in their body image, or a feeling that they are no longer sexually viable people (Daniluk, 1998). Some women may celebrate menopause; others attach no significance to it.

Long-term estrogen deprivation results in an imbalance in bone remodeling and osteoporosis, leading to fractures and kyphosis. The risk for cardiovascular diseases increases in response to an increase in atherosclerosis (from an increase in the LDL-to-HDL cholesterol ratio).

CLINICAL MANIFESTATIONS AND THERAPIES **Menopause**

ETIOLOGY	CLINICAL MANIFESTATIONS	CLINICAL THERAPIES
Increase in vaginal pH	Risk of urinary tract infection (burning, frequency, hesitancy, and urgency to urinate) and vaginal infection (vaginitis, vaginal drainage)	■ Medications, antibiotics or antifungal ■ Encourage adequate fluid intake ■ Teach importance of wiping from front to back ■ Teach symptoms to report
Reduced vaginal lubrication	Dyspareunia, injury, and fungal infections	■ Teach use of artificial water-based lubricant to reduce symptoms
Vasomotor instability	Hot flashes, diaphoresis, increased risk of heart disease	■ If severe, hormone supplements may be prescribed
Osteoporosis	Fractures, kyphosis, increased bone fragility	■ Teach importance of calcium, vitamin D, and phosphorus intake

Box 26–3 Manifestations of the Perimenopausal Period

- Menstrual cycles become erratic. Menstrual flow varies widely in amount and duration and eventually ceases.
- Vaginal, vulval, and urethral tissues begin to atrophy.
- Vaginal pH rises, predisposing the woman to bacterial infections.
- Vaginal lubrication decreases, and vaginal rugae decrease in number. This may result in dyspareunia, injury, and fungal infections.
- Vasomotor instability due to a decrease in estrogen may result in hot flashes and night sweats. A hot flash starts in the chest and moves upward toward the face and may last from seconds to several minutes.
- Psychological symptoms may include moodiness, nervousness, insomnia, headaches, irritability, anxiety, inability to concentrate, and depression.

Manifestations of the perimenopausal period are listed in Box 26–3. These manifestations vary widely. Some women experience severe symptoms, others experience moderate symptoms, and some women experience few or no symptoms.

COLLABORATION

Care of the woman experiencing menopausal symptoms focuses on relieving symptoms and minimizing postmenopausal health risks.

Diagnostic Tests

As estrogen secretion diminishes, levels of follicle-stimulating hormone (FSH) and luteinizing hormone (LH) rise and remain elevated. A woman who has not menstruated for 1 full year or who has an increased FSH blood level is considered menopausal (Porth, 2005).

Pharmacologic Therapies

Although controversial, **hormone replacement therapy (HRT)** may be prescribed to alleviate severe manifestations of menopause, but only for a limited amount of time and only after a woman has been provided with known risks. HRT may include estrogen alone for women who have had a hysterectomy or a combination of estrogen and progestin. The addition of progestin stimulates monthly shedding of the intrauterine lining, decreasing the risk of uterine cancer. HRT relieves hot flashes and night sweats and decreases problems of vaginal dryness and urogenital tissue atrophy, which can lead to painful intercourse and urinary incontinence. Long-term HRT may increase the risk for breast cancer, ovarian cancer, stroke, heart attacks, and venous thrombosis (Tierney et al., 2004). However, women who have had a hysterectomy and take estrogen alone do not have an increased risk of breast cancer (Health & Science, 2006).

Selective estrogen receptor modulators (SERMs) such as raloxifene (Evista) and triphenylethylene (tamoxifen) bind to estrogen receptors and exert site-specific effects in different target tissues. Tamoxifen and toremifene (a derivative of tamoxifen) have a beneficial effect on bone mineral density and serum lipids and decrease the risk of invasive breast cancer in women at high risk. They also provide an alternative to HRT for preventing osteoporosis.

Until recently, HRT was commonplace to relieve the problematic effects of menopause. In 2001, however, the American Heart Association strongly advised health care providers to stop prescribing HRT to postmenopausal women for cardioprotection ("AHA Cautions," 2001). The recommendation was based on a number of clinical research trials that demonstrated that HRT was not cardioprotective and could be deleterious to women with concomitant cardiovascular disease (Manson et al., 2003). In this large clinical investigation, women on HRT had demonstrated higher rates of myocardial infarction, stroke, breast cancer, pulmonary embolism, and deep vein thrombosis. In 2003, the U.S. Food and Drug Administration went even further, requiring explicit labeling of HRT products to caution potential users of a number of serious risks related to use ("FDA Orders Estrogen Safety Warnings," 2003). Current recommendations are that HRT be used only for the relief of vasomotor symptoms related to menopause, for women at high risk of osteoporosis, and for prevention of colorectal cancer (Nelson, Humphrey, Nygren, Teutsch, & Allan, 2002). The potential for harm from HRT should be thoroughly discussed with the woman before she initiates the therapy.

Menopausal women may be anxious about using estrogen-containing preparations, even if their vasomotor symptoms are severe. The hot flashes of menopause range from mild feelings of being overly warm to intense feelings of uncomfortable heat over the upper body (Noblett & Ostergard, 1999). Some women find that dressing in layers allows them to remove and replace clothing as the hot flashes come and go. If the hot flashes occur frequently, the older woman should discuss her concerns with her primary care provider. Soy products and black cohosh have been shown to relieve hot flashes without serious side effects and may be acceptable to older women (Morelli & Naquin, 2002).

Alternative and Complementary Therapies

As a result of the controversy surrounding the use of HRT, nontraditional or alternative therapies have become more popular. The following complementary therapies are examples of those used by menopausal women to reduce associated discomforts (ARHP, 2005b; Mayo Clinic, 2004):

- Acupuncture
- Biofeedback
- Massage
- Herbs and botanicals (see Alternative Therapies on page 1744)
- Supplements: vitamin E, soy protein (soy is high in plant estrogens)
- Bioidentical hormones
- Meditation and yoga.

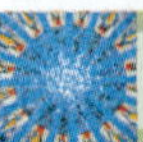

ALTERNATIVE THERAPIES Use of Botanicals for Menopausal Symptoms

The following botanicals were reviewed during a 2005 National Institutes of Health (NIH) State-of-the-Science conference on the management of menopausal symptoms. The panel found the following:

- *Black cohosh.* This substance has received the most attention of all the botanicals. It does not act as an estrogen, as was once believed. Studies of its effectiveness in relieving hot flashes have had mixed results, but it has a good safety record over many years.
- *Red clover.* Five controlled studies found no conclusive or consistent evidence that hot flashes were reduced in women using red clover leaf extract. Few side effects have been reported, and no serious health problems have been cited in the literature. Animal studies have raised a concern as to whether red clover might be harmful to estrogen-sensitive tissue such as the uterus and breasts.
- *Dong quai.* In the only randomized controlled study reported, dong quai was not found to be effective in reducing hot flashes. Because dong quai is known to interact with and increase the activity of warfarin (Coumadin), its use by women on warfarin can lead to bleeding problems.
- *Ginseng.* Although it has not been found to be effective in relieving hot flashes, ginseng may help with other menopausal symptoms, such as sleep disturbances and mood swings.
- *Kava.* No evidence supports its effectiveness in relieving hot flashes, although it may decrease anxiety. The FDA has issued a warning about kava because it has been associated with liver disease.
- *Soy.* Results about the use of soy to relieve hot flashes are mixed. Its use as a dietary supplement for short periods of time is not associated with any serious side effects, although long-term use has been associated with a thickening of the uterine lining.

Source: National Center for Complementary and Alternative Medicine (NCCAM). (2006). Do CAM therapies help menopausal symptoms? Retrieved March 8, 2006, from http://nccam.nih.gov/health/menopauseandcam/

NURSING PROCESS

Nursing care during and after the menopausal period focuses on minimizing the symptoms associated with hormonal changes; reducing the risk of cardiovascular disease, cancer, and osteoporosis; and educating the woman about lifestyle changes important to health and well-being.

The American Cancer Society recommends a cancer-related checkup every year after the age of 40. This checkup includes examination for cancers of the thyroid, ovaries, lymph nodes, oral cavity, and skin. Other important checkups include screening for cervical, breast, and colorectal cancer. Health counseling should also include information about alcohol and tobacco use, sun exposure, diet and nutrition, exercise, risk factors, sexual practices, and environmental and occupational exposures. It is important to discuss the benefits of rest and exercise, as well as a diet that includes fruits, vegetables, and fiber. In addition, suggest the following resources for further information:

- National Institute on Aging
- Centers for Disease Control and Prevention
- North American Menopause Society
- Association of Reproductive Health Professionals
- Women's Health Initiative
- National Women's Health Information Center.

Assessment

Collect the following data through the health history and physical examination. When assessing the older woman, be aware of normal changes with aging.

- *Health history.* Problems with urinary frequency, urgency, or incontinence; menstrual history; sexual history; dyspareunia; use of alcohol, nicotine, and drugs; medications, sleep patterns, hot flashes, night sweats, changes in emotional responses.
- *Physical assessment.* Height and weight, posture, vital signs, breast examination, pelvic examination, abdominal assessment.

Diagnosis

The nursing diagnoses that may apply to the client with menopause include the following:

- Deficient Knowledge
- Ineffective Sexuality Pattern
- Situational Low Self-Esteem
- Disturbed Body Image.

Plan

Goals of client care may include the following:

- Promoting self-esteem
- Teaching strategies to reduce and cope with symptoms
- Informing client of potential symptoms to reduce anxiety.

Implementation

Menopause is viewed differently by different women and it is important to determine what it means to each client before beginning implementation. While some women may view it as a relief, others may see it as the end of their youth and the beginning of old age. Implementations should be aimed at helping the woman understand the processs of menopause, cope with symptoms as they arise, and make healthy lifestyle choices.

Deficient Knowledge

Because menopausal manifestations vary widely, it is difficult to predict their effect on an individual woman. However, the well-informed woman is better prepared to deal with whatever symptoms she experiences.

- Discuss physiological manifestations, such as hot flashes and night sweats. The underlying cause of hot flashes is not known (Porth, 2005). Many physiological effects of menopause are amenable to nonpharmacological methods of relief, such as lifestyle changes.

PRACTICE ALERT

When hot flashes occur at night and are accompanied by perspiration, they are called night sweats. Night sweats often interfere with normal sleep patterns, leading to increased fatigue and irritability.

- Provide information about dietary recommendations. The recommended daily intake of calcium for women over 50 is 1,200 mg. Some women need to use calcium supplements or calcium-containing antacid tablets to meet this requirement.
- Emphasize the importance of weight-bearing exercise. Weight-bearing exercise reduces the rate of bone loss, helps maintain optimum weight, and reduces cardiovascular risk.
- Provide information about the benefits and risks of HRT. Not every woman will need or want it. Every woman needs to understand both the risks and the benefits before deciding whether to use HRT.
- Encourage the woman to obtain yearly mammograms, clinical breast examinations, and Pap smears, and to perform monthly breast self-examination on the same day each month. The increased risk for cancer of the breast and pelvic reproductive organs makes self-examination and health care provider screening during and after menopause even more important.

Ineffective Sexuality Pattern

Vaginal dryness and atrophy, together with the emotional effect of menopause, can interfere with sexual expression and satisfaction. Suggesting measures to help the woman and her partner cope with these changes can enable them to continue or resume a mutually satisfying sexual relationship.

- Encourage expression of feelings and concerns about how menopause is changing her sex life. Midlife and older women may not be comfortable in discussing their intimate sexual behavior.
- Suggest ways to increase vaginal lubrication, such as spending more time in foreplay and/or using water-soluble gels (e.g., Replens) for vaginal lubrication. A more leisurely approach to sexual activity can be mutually gratifying for the woman and her partner. Use of water-soluble gels can prevent vaginal pain and irritation and improve the quality of the sexual experience.

PRACTICE ALERT

Plant estrogens, found in food such as brown rice, corn, green beans, lemon and orange peels, and tofu, are mildly estrogenic and may improve vaginal dryness.

- Explain that as women age, it may take longer for vaginal lubrication and orgasm to occur. This information is important to prevent the woman from believing something is wrong with her or her partner believing he or she is no longer interesting or sexually exciting.

Situational Low Self-Esteem

Each woman responds to the aging process in her own way, and most women have coping skills that adequately equip them to deal with the gradual changes associated with aging. Among the factors that may provoke a self-esteem disturbance are the loss of youth, a sense of emptiness as children leave home, and the need to redefine one's self-concept and roles as parenting becomes less important. Women who place a high value on their physical attractiveness may experience a painful psychological response to the physical changes of menopause.

- Encourage expression of fears and concerns related to changes in interpersonal and family functions. Many women associate aging with "uselessness" and unattractiveness.
- Suggest volunteer activities or employment for the woman who has extra time. This enables the woman to feel that she is still a contributing member of society. Volunteering for activities involving young people can help reduce anxiety about the loss of reproductive ability or any late regrets about not having had children.
- Discuss the importance of a healthy lifestyle in maintaining physical attractiveness. Identify risk factors and high-risk behaviors. Lifestyle habits and behaviors affect many body systems and physical appearance. For example, cigarette smoking and overexposure to the sun make the skin age faster, contributing to wrinkles. Active women who exercise and eat a well-balanced diet look and feel better.

Disturbed Body Image

As women progress through the perimenopausal period, changes in appearance and the loss of childbearing ability may combine to make the woman feel "old," "ugly," and "useless." Although this is far from the truth, with women living at least one-third of their lives after menopause in productive careers and activities, it nevertheless is the perception of women as well as society. The physical changes the woman often experiences include growth of facial hair, excessive perspiration and flushing of the face, and weight gain.

- Encourage the woman to describe her perceptions of her own body. This information is necessary to obtain data to establish an individualized plan of care.
- Encourage verbalization of feelings of concern, anger, anxiety, loss, and fear over body changes. Expressing these emotions can facilitate the grieving process and acceptance of change.
- Stress that certain physical characteristics of a person cannot be changed; emphasize the importance of learning to recognize and appreciate one's own special strengths. These help the woman gain acceptance and a realistic appraisal of self.
- Refer, as appropriate, for dietary management, exercise, stress management, and cosmetic assistance (e.g., for aggravating facial hair). These actions increase wellness and a positive sense of self.

Evaluation

Expected outcomes to evaluate the client's progress toward goals may include the following:

- Client demonstrates a positive sense of self as evidenced by stable weight, participation in a regular exercise program, and ability to manage stress.
- Client verbalizes feelings related to changes that have occurred.
- Client describes strategies for maintaining health.

REVIEW Menopause

RELATE: LINK THE CONCEPTS

Linking the exemplar of Menopause with the concept Self:

1. What interventions will you initiate for the woman entering menopause who feels she is no longer attractive and has lost her feminity?
2. What is your priority of care for the woman experiencing menopause that has low self-esteem?

Linking the exemplar of Menopause with the concept Health Wellness, and Illness:

3. What health promotion interventions will be a priority for the client entering menopause?
4. What nutritional and exercise behaviors would you promote for the woman in menopause. Explain your answer.

READY: GO TO COMPANION SKILLS MANUAL

- Assessing the female genitals and inguinal area

REFER: GO TO MYNURSINGKIT

REFLECT: CASE STUDY

Marly Cutler is a 51-year old woman who is married to Fred. They live in a small rural community and own their farm. Marly and Fred have two adult children who live in the city. Fred has hypertension that is being treated with lisinopril, 10 mg/day and high cholesterol for which he takes simvastatin 20 mg/day. Marly has no real health issues and is compliant with yearly screening examinations. Last year her physician told her to take calcium 1200 mg/day to reduce the risk of osteoporosis.

Marly has come to the OB/GYN clinic today because she has missed some periods, is having night sweats, and is experiencing mood swings that are affecting her relationship with Fred. She wonders if she has caught the flu.

1. What client teaching will you provide Marly?
2. What strategies might you suggest to reduce the severity of the symptoms she reports?
3. How will you assess Marly's mental stuatus?

26.4 MENSTRUAL DYSFUNCTION

KEY TERMS

Amenorrhea, *1748*
Dysfunctional uterine bleeding (DUB), *1748*
Dysmenorrhea, *1748*
Menorrhagia, *1748*
Metrorrhagia, *1748*
Premenstrual syndrome (PMS), *1746*

BASIS FOR SELECTION OF EXEMPLAR

Standards of Nursing Practice
Common disorder

LEARNING OUTCOMES

After reading about this exemplar, you will be able to:

1. Describe the pathophysiology, etiology, clinical manifestations, and direct and indirect causes of menstrual dysfunction.
2. Identify risk factors associated with menstrual dysfunction.
3. Illustrate the nursing process in providing culturally competent care across the life span for individuals with menstrual dysfunction.
4. Formulate priority nursing diagnoses appropriate for an individual with menstrual dysfunction.
5. Create a plan of care for individuals with menstrual dysfunction and their family members.
6. Assess expected outcomes for an individual with menstrual dysfunction.
7. Discuss therapies used in the collaborative care of an individual with menstrual dysfunction.
8. Employ evidence-based caring interventions for an individual with menstrual dysfunction.

OVERVIEW

Monthly menstruation normally involves some minor discomfort, including breast tenderness, a feeling of heaviness and congestion in the pelvic area, uterine cramping, and lower backache. Many women, however, experience more serious effects, both physiological and psychological.

Premenstrual syndrome (PMS) is a complex of manifestations (e.g., mood swings, breast tenderness, fatigue, irritability, food cravings, and depression) that are limited to 3–14 days before menstruation and relieved by the onset of menses. Premenstrual syndrome can be a factor in absenteeism at school or work, decreased productivity, interpersonal relationship difficulties, and lifestyle disruption. It is estimated that 25–40% of all adult women experience mild to moderate symptoms and 2–5% have severe symptoms (Porth, 2005). For a small number of women, PMS is so disabling that it is called by the psychiatric label *premenstrual dysphoric disorder (PMDD)*.

MULTISYSTEM EFFECTS OF PREMENSTRUAL SYNDROME

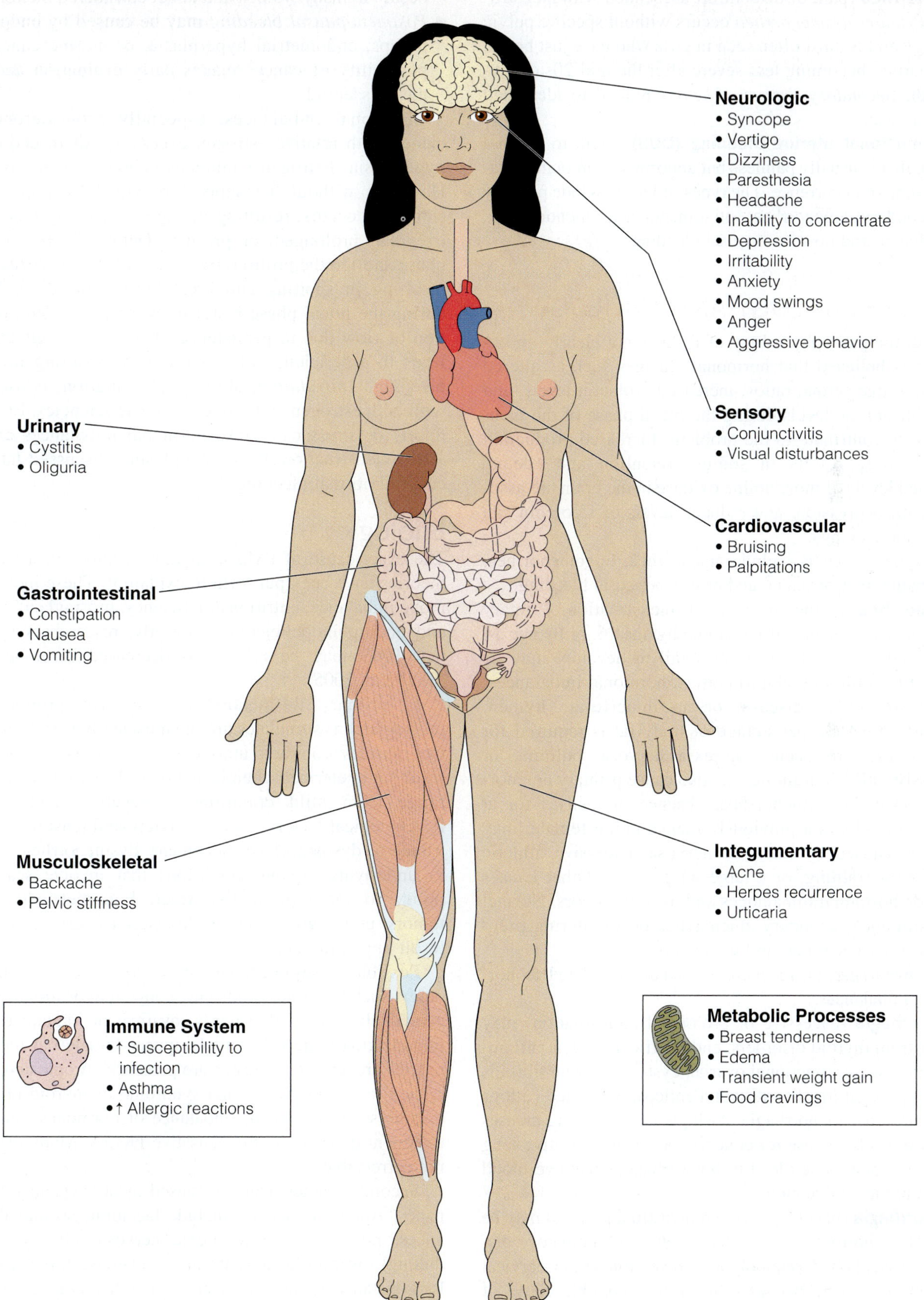
Neurologic
• Syncope
• Vertigo
• Dizziness
• Paresthesia
• Headache
• Inability to concentrate
• Depression
• Irritability
• Anxiety
• Mood swings
• Anger
• Aggressive behavior
Urinary
• Cystitis
• Oliguria
Sensory
• Conjunctivitis
• Visual disturbances
Cardiovascular
• Bruising
• Palpitations
Gastrointestinal
• Constipation
• Nausea
• Vomiting
Musculoskeletal
• Backache
• Pelvic stiffness
Integumentary
• Acne
• Herpes recurrence
• Urticaria
Immune System
• ↑ Susceptibility to infection
• Asthma
• ↑ Allergic reactions
Metabolic Processes
• Breast tenderness
• Edema
• Transient weight gain
• Food cravings

A significant number of menstruating women experience **dysmenorrhea** (pain or discomfort associated with menstruation). *Primary dysmenorrhea* occurs without specific pelvic pathology and is most often seen in girls who have just begun menstruating, becoming less severe after the mid-20s or giving birth. *Secondary dysmenorrhea* is related to identified pelvic disease.

Dysfunctional uterine bleeding (DUB) refers to vaginal bleeding that is usually painless but abnormal in amount, duration, or time of occurrence. The types of DUB include primary and secondary amenorrhea, oligomenorrhea, menorrhagia, metrorrhagia, and postmenopausal bleeding.

PATHOPHYSIOLOGY AND ETIOLOGY

Although the pathophysiology of PMS is not clearly understood, it is believed that hormonal changes such as altered estrogen–progesterone ratios, increased prolactin levels, and rising aldosterone levels during the luteal phase of the menstrual cycle contribute to the problem. Increased production of aldosterone results in sodium retention and edema. Decreased levels of monoamine oxidase in the brain are associated with depression, and reduced levels of serotonin can lead to mood swings.

The types of DUB include amenorrhea, oligomenorrhea, menorrhagia, metrorrhagia, and postmenopausal bleeding.

- **Amenorrhea** is the absence of menstruation. Primary amenorrhea, absence of menarche by age 16, or by age 14 if secondary sex characteristics fail to develop, may be caused by structural abnormalities, hormonal imbalances, polycystic ovary disease, or an imperforate hymen. Because a certain percentage of body fat is required for menstruation to occur, anorexia nervosa, bulimia, or excessive athletic training can also cause primary amenorrhea. Secondary amenorrhea, absence of menses for at least 6 months in a previously menstruating female, may also be caused by anorexia nervosa, excessive athletic activity or training, or a large weight loss. Other causes include hormonal imbalances and ovarian tumors. Normal (physiologic) secondary amenorrhea occurs during pregnancy, breast-feeding, and menopause.
- *Oligomenorrhea* (scant menses) usually is related to hormonal imbalances.
- **Menorrhagia** (excessive or prolonged menstruation) may result from thyroid disorders, endometriosis, pelvic inflammatory disease, functional ovarian cysts, or uterine fibroids or polyps. Clotting disorders and anticoagulant medications also can cause menorrhagia. A single heavy or long menses is not in itself a cause for concern; however, repetitive long or heavy menses can lead to hemorrhage, excessive blood loss, fatigue, and anemia.
- **Metrorrhagia** (bleeding between menstrual periods) may be caused by hormonal imbalances, pelvic inflammatory disease, cervical or uterine polyps, uterine fibroids, or cervical or uterine cancer. Because cancer is a possible cause of metrorrhagia, early evaluation and treatment are extremely important. Midcycle spotting associated with ovulation occurs in many women and is not considered metrorrhagia.
- *Postmenopausal bleeding* may be caused by endometrial polyps, endometrial hyperplasia, or uterine cancer. The possibility of cancer makes early evaluation and treatment essential.

Hormonal imbalances, especially progesterone deficiency with relative estrogen excess, result in endometrial hyperplasia. Estrogen stimulates endometrial proliferation. However, without the support provided by progesterone, sloughing occurs, resulting in vaginal bleeding that may be irregular, prolonged, or profuse. Defects in the follicular phase shorten the proliferative phase of the menstrual cycle, resulting in spotting and breakthrough bleeding. Defects during the luteal phase result in excessive amount or duration of flow due to persistence of the corpus luteum. This leads to a deficiency of progesterone, resulting in vaginal bleeding. *Anovulation*, absence of ovulation, is associated with both estrogen and progesterone deficiencies. Emotional upsets or stress can cause hormonal imbalances and thus affect menstruation. Pelvic neoplasms, discussed later, also cause abnormal bleeding.

Etiology

The exact cause of PMS is unknown, although a variety of theories have been put forth to explain it. These include hormone imbalance, nutritional deficiency, prostaglandin excess, and endorphin deficiency. Currently, researchers speculate that PMS may be related to decreased serotonin levels (Shulman, 2005).

In primary dysmenorrhea, excessive production of prostaglandins stimulates uterine muscle fibers to contract. As the muscles contract, uterine circulation is compromised, resulting in uterine ischemia and pain. These contractions can range from mild cramping to severe muscle spasms. Psychological factors, such as anxiety and tension, may contribute to dysmenorrhea. Secondary dysmenorrhea is related to underlying organic conditions that involve scarring or injury to the reproductive tract. Endometriosis, fibroid tumors, pelvic inflammatory disease, or ovarian cancer may result in painful menses.

Possible causes of primary amenorrhea include genetic disorders such as Turner syndrome; congenital obstructions; congenital absence of the uterus, ovaries, or vagina; testicular feminization (external genitals appear female but uterus and ovaries are absent and testes are present); chronic anovulation related to polycystic ovarian syndrome or thyroid or adrenal disorders; or absence or imbalance of hormones. Success of treatment depends on the causative factors. Many causes are not correctable.

Secondary amenorrhea is caused most frequently by pregnancy. Additional causes include lactation, hormonal imbalances, poor nutrition (anorexia nervosa, obesity, and fad dieting), ovarian lesions, strenuous exercise (associated with long-distance runners, dancers, and other athletes with low body fat ratios), debilitating systemic diseases, stress of high

Box 26–4 Manifestations of Primary Dysmenorrhea

- Abdominal pain beginning with onset of menses and lasting 12–48 hours
- Pain radiating to lower back and thighs
- Headache
- Nausea
- Vomiting
- Diarrhea
- Fatigue
- Breast tenderness

intensity and/or long duration, stressful life events, a change in season or climate, use of oral contraceptives, use of the phenothiazine and chlorpromazine group of tranquilizers, exposure to radiation or chemotherapy, viral infection, and syndromes such as Cushing and Sheehan syndromes.

Risk Factors

PMS is seen less frequently during the teens and 20s, reaching a peak in women in their mid-30s. Major life stressors, age greater than 30, and depression are risk factors associated with PMS.

A number of factors may predispose a woman to DUB. These factors include stress, extreme weight changes, use of oral contraceptive agents or intrauterine devices (IUDs), and postmenopausal status. Dysfunctional uterine bleeding is usually related to hormonal imbalances or pelvic neoplasms, either benign or malignant.

CLINICAL MANIFESTATIONS

Manifestations of PMS occur during the luteal phase of the menstrual cycle (7–10 days prior to the onset of the menstrual flow), abating when the menstrual flow begins (Box 26–4). Although PMS may produce a variety of physiological and psychological manifestations, the exact nature of these manifestations and their intensity are individualized for each woman with this disorder. The manifestations may even differ from month to month in the same woman.

Manifestations of primary dysmenorrhea may be severe enough to disrupt activities of daily living, sexual function, and even fertility.

COLLABORATION

If no organic cause for the signs and symptoms of PMS can be identified, the goals of care are to relieve manifestations and to help develop self-care patterns that will help the woman anticipate and cope more effectively with future episodes of PMS. There are no definitive diagnostic tests for PMS. The regular recurrence of manifestations preceding the onset of menses for at least 3 months leads to a diagnosis of PMS. The treatment of PMS integrates this self-monitored record of manifestations, regular exercise, avoiding caffeine, and a diet low in simple sugars and high in lean proteins (Porth, 2005).

Although many different medications, vitamins, and herbal supplements have been used to treat the manifestations of PMS, the most promising appears to be the use of selective serotonin reuptake inhibitors (SSRIs).

Care of the woman with menstrual pain focuses on identifying the underlying cause, reestablishing functional capacity, and managing pain.

A careful history and physical assessment are performed to rule out any underlying organic cause of dysmenorrhea. If no organic cause can be found, the diagnosis is primary dysmenorrhea. In addition, attitudes and expectations about menstruation and lifestyle disruption are identified and explored.

The care of the woman with DUB focuses on identifying and treating the underlying disease. A careful history and physical examination are performed. Abdominal and pelvic examinations are performed to rule out abdominal masses. The woman may need to keep a menstrual history and basal body temperature chart for several months to determine whether ovulation is occurring.

Diagnostic Tests

Various diagnostic tests are performed to identify structural abnormalities, hormonal imbalances, and pathological conditions that could cause menstrual pain.

CLINICAL MANIFESTATIONS AND THERAPIES Menstrual Dysfunction

ETIOLOGY	CLINICAL MANIFESTATIONS	CLINICAL THERAPIES
Shock	Hypotension, delayed capillary refill, cyanosis, hypoxia, dizziness, change in LOC, low urine output, diminished bowel motility, pale skin, activity intolerance, tachycardia, tachypnea	■ Blood transfusions ■ IV fluid administration ■ Monitor ABCs ■ Administer oxygen ■ Measure intake and output
Anemia	Pale skin, activity intolerance, fatigue,	■ Administer iron supplements ■ Promote diet high in iron ■ Encourage fluid intake

Diagnosis is made based on findings from a pelvic examination and diagnostic procedures, including a Pap smear and cervical and vaginal cultures; ultrasound of the pelvis and vagina; and CT scan or MRI to detect structural abnormalities, malignancy, or infections. Laboratory tests used to assess possible causes of dysmenorrhea are as follows:

- FSH and LH levels to assess the function of the pituitary gland. The results are correlated with the time of the menstrual cycle
- Progesterone and estradiol levels to assess ovarian function
- Thyroid function tests (T_3 and T_4) to assess thyroid function.

Laparoscopy is used to diagnose structural defects and blockages caused by scarring, endometriosis, tumors, and cysts (Figure 26–34 ■). A dilation and curettage (D&C) of the uterus may be performed to obtain tissue for evaluation or to relieve dysmenorrhea and heavy menstrual bleeding.

A variety of diagnostic tests are used to diagnose the cause of DUB. Diagnostic tests include a Pap smear to rule out or identify cervical carcinoma, a pelvic ultrasound to identify luteal cysts, a hysteroscopy to detect abnormalities of the uterine cavity, or an endometrial biopsy to obtain endometrial tissue for histological examination.

Laboratory studies may include the following:

- A complete blood count (CBC) to rule out systemic disease as a contributing factor to DUB and to evaluate its effects
- Thyroid function studies, including measurement of triiodothyronine (T_3), thyroxine (T_4), and thyroid-stimulating hormone (TSH) levels, to rule out hyper- or hypothyroidism as a cause of DUB
- Endocrine studies to evaluate pituitary and adrenal function. Pituitary dysfunction may first be manifested by menstrual irregularities
- Serum progesterone levels to determine the level of progesterone deficiency.

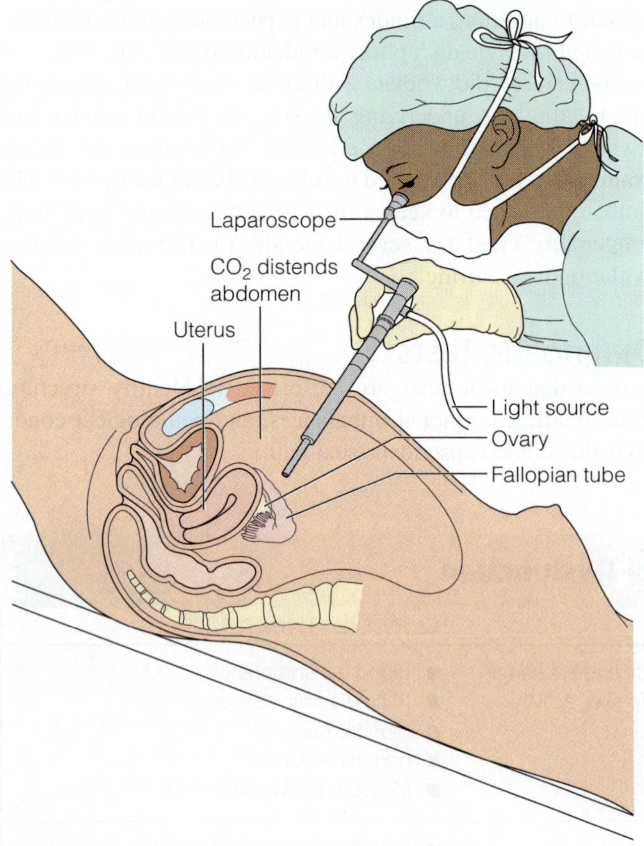

Figure 26–34 ■ Laparoscopy. In this surgical procedure, a flexible, lighted instrument (laparoscope) is inserted through a periumbilical incision. Laparoscopy allows visualization of the pelvic cavity.

Pharmacologic Therapies

If the manifestations of PMS are severe or incapacitating, ovulation may be suppressed by the use of gonadotropin-releasing hormone (GnRH) agonists, oral contraceptives, or danazol. Progesterone and antiprostaglandin agents such as nonsteroidal anti-inflammatory drugs (NSAIDs) may help relieve cramping. Diuretics may be prescribed to relieve bloating. SSRIs such as fluoxetine (Prozac), sertraline (Zoloft), and paroxetine (Paxil) may be used to manage mood and some physical manifestations of PMS.

Dysmenorrhea may be treated with analgesics, prostaglandin inhibitors such as NSAIDs, or oral contraceptives.

For many women with DUB, hormonal agents can correct menstrual irregularities. For anovulatory DUB, oral contraceptives may be prescribed for 3 to 6 months. Progesterone or medroxyprogesterone also may be prescribed to regulate uterine bleeding.

Ovulatory DUB may be treated with progestins during the luteal phase. Oral iron supplements may be prescribed to replace iron lost through menstrual bleeding.

Surgery

Surgical intervention emphasizes the least invasive method that proves effective relief, beginning with a therapeutic D&C, then endometrial ablation, and, finally, hysterectomy.

THERAPEUTIC D&C In a therapeutic D&C, the cervical canal is dilated and the uterine wall is scraped. D&C, the most frequently performed minor gynecological surgical procedure, is used to diagnose and treat DUB and other disorders of the female reproductive system. It may be performed to correct excessive or prolonged bleeding. D&C is contraindicated in any woman who has been taking anticoagulant drugs or whose condition precludes the use of regional or general anesthesia.

ENDOMETRIAL ABLATION In an endometrial ablation, the endometrial layer of the uterus is permanently destroyed using laser surgery or electrosurgical resection. It is performed in women who do not respond to pharmacological management or D&C. The woman needs to understand that this procedure ends menstruation and reproduction.

HYSTERECTOMY Hysterectomy, or removal of the uterus, may be performed when medical management of bleeding disorders is unsuccessful or malignancy is present, particularly if the woman no longer wishes to bear children. In premenopausal women, the ovaries are usually left in place; in postmenopausal women, a total hysterectomy, or panhysterectomy, may be performed; this procedure involves removal of the uterus, fallopian tubes, and ovaries.

Hysterectomy may involve either an abdominal or a vaginal approach. The choice depends on the underlying disorder, the need to explore the abdominal cavity, and the preference of the surgeon and woman. Nursing care of the woman undergoing a hysterectomy is described in Box 26–5.

Abdominal hysterectomy is performed when a preexisting abdominal scar is present, when adhesions are thought to be present, or when a large operating field is necessary. For example, the woman with endometriosis is more likely to have an abdominal hysterectomy because endometrial tissue implants that may be present on other abdominal organs need to be removed. The surgical incision may be either longitudinal, made in the midline from umbilicus to pubis, or a Pfannenstiel incision, also known as the bikini cut.

Vaginal hysterectomy, removal of the uterus through the vagina, is desirable when the uterus has descended into the vagina or if the urinary bladder or rectum have prolapsed into the vagina. Vaginal hysterectomy leaves no visible abdominal scar. Laparoscopy-assisted vaginal hysterectomy (LAVH) is most often performed.

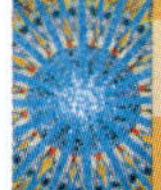

CLIENT TEACHING **Dysfunctional Uterine Bleeding**

Provide support, appropriate reassurance, and information to help the woman and her family better understand her disorder and the therapeutic interventions indicated. Teaching also includes self-care measures that help minimize the effects of DUB on the daily functioning of the woman. The following topics should be included:

- Administration and side effects of prescribed medications, including iron
- The need to maintain a balanced diet, increasing iron-rich foods such as eggs, beans, liver, beef, and shrimp. (Inform the woman that while orange juice may improve the absorption of iron, foods high in calcium and oxalic acid, such as spinach, may reduce its absorption.)
- Importance of maintaining a fluid intake of 2,000 to 3,000 mL a day
- The need to immediately report recurring episodes of DUB, particularly in postmenopausal women, to the health care provider.

Box 26–5 **Nursing Care of the Client Having a Hysterectomy**

PREOPERATIVE CARE

- Assess the woman's understanding of the procedure. Provide explanation, clarification, and emotional support as needed. Reassure that the anesthesia will eliminate any pain during surgery and that medication will be administered postoperatively to minimize discomfort. *The woman who understands the procedure to be performed and what to expect after surgery will be less anxious.*
- Cleanse the abdominal and perineal area, and, if ordered, shave the perineal area.
- If ordered, administer a small cleansing enema and ask the woman to empty her bladder. *This precaution helps prevent contamination from the bowel or bladder during surgery.*
- Administer preoperative medications as ordered.
- Check the chart to ensure that the consent form has been signed.

POSTOPERATIVE CARE

- Assess for signs of hemorrhage. *Hemorrhage is more common after vaginal hysterectomy than after abdominal hysterectomy.*
- Monitor vital signs every 4 hours, auscultate lungs every shift, and measure intake and output. *These data are important indicators of hemodynamic status and complications.*
- Once the catheter has been removed, measure the amount of urine voided.
- Assess for complications, including infection, ileus, shock or hemorrhage, thrombophlebitis, and pulmonary embolus.
- Assess vaginal discharge; instruct the woman in perineal care.
- Assess incision and bowel sounds every shift.
- Encourage turning, coughing, deep breathing, and early ambulation.
- Encourage fluid intake.
- Teach the woman to splint the abdomen and cough deeply. Teach the use of the incentive spirometer.
- Instruct the woman to restrict physical activity for 4–6 weeks. Heavy lifting, stair climbing, douching, tampons, and sexual intercourse should be avoided. The woman should shower, avoiding tub baths, until bleeding has ceased. *Infection and hemorrhage are the greatest postoperative risks; restricting activities and preventing the introduction of any foreign material into the vagina helps reduce these risks.*
- Explain to the woman that she may feel tired for several days after surgery and needs to rest periodically.
- Explain that appetite may be depressed and bowel elimination may be sluggish. *These are after effects of general anesthesia, handling of the bowel during surgery, and loss of muscle tone in the bowel while empty.*
- Teach the woman to recognize signs of complications that should be reported to the physician or nurse:
  a. Temperature greater than 37.7°C (100°F)
  b. Vaginal bleeding that is greater than a typical menstrual period or is bright red
  c. Urinary incontinence, urgency, burning, or frequency
  d. Severe pain.
- Encourage the woman to express feelings that may signal a negative self-concept. Correct any misconceptions. *Some women believe that hysterectomy means weight gain, the end of sexual activity, and the growth of facial hair.*
- Provide information on risks and benefits of hormone replacement therapy, if indicated. *If the ovaries have also been removed, the woman is immediately thrust into menopause and may want or need hormone replacement therapy.*
- Reinforce the need to obtain gynecological examinations regularly even after hysterectomy.

Alternative and Complementary Therapies

Alternative and complementary therapies the woman with PMS may find helpful focus on diet, exercise, relaxation, and stress management:

- A diet high in complex carbohydrates with limited simple sugars and alcohol is recommended to minimize reactive hypoglycemia, which can contribute to the manifestations of PMS.
- Reduced sodium intake helps minimize fluid retention. Increased intake of calcium (1,200 mg per day), magnesium (200 mg per day), vitamin B_6 (50 to 100 mg per day), and vitamin E (400 international units per day) may be helpful (Mayo Clinic, 2004).
- Caffeine is restricted to reduce irritability.
- Herbal remedies include black cohosh, ginger, chaste tree berry, and evening primrose oil. Natural progesterone creams, derived from wild yams and soybeans, relieve manifestations in some women (Mayo Clinic, 2004). These alternative therapies should be discussed with the health care provider.
- Exercise is beneficial, but adequate rest also is necessary.
- Techniques for relaxation and stress management include deep abdominal breathing, meditation, muscle relaxation, and guided imagery.

The complementary therapies listed for the woman with PMS may also be useful for the woman with dysmenorrhea. Other helpful activities are regular physical exercise, supplementing the diet with zinc and calcium, and using herbal remedies such as *Viburnum prunifolium*, black cohosh, evening primrose oil, and blue cohosh (About Women's Health, 2005). Using a heating pad on the abdomen or taking a warm bath also helps reduce pain.

NURSING PROCESS

Nursing care for the woman with PMS focuses on relieving manifestations. Most women experiencing PMS require interventions to manage pain and enhance coping.

Nursing care for the woman with primary dysmenorrhea focuses on controlling manifestations and providing education about the normal physiology of the menstrual cycle and self-care measures. Care of the woman with secondary dysmenorrhea varies according to the underlying cause. Nursing interventions previously described for the woman with PMS are also appropriate for the woman with dysmenorrhea.

DUB usually causes the woman anxiety. Her self-image, sexuality, or reproductive capacity may be threatened, and she may fear the possibility of cancer. She may be embarrassed to discuss her menstrual history and hygiene practices.

Assessment

Menstrual habits of the client should be assessed whenever the woman seeks health care. Determination of last menstrual period, normal length of menstruation and time between periods, as well as any symptoms associated with menstruation should be assessed. Cultural influences often play a role in how the women views and responds to menstruation and should also be assessed

It is essential to create an atmosphere that facilitates open communication and comfort for the client. Clients commonly experience anxiety, fear, and embarrassment when questioned about a topic that, in most clients' minds, is very personal. These emotions may be expressed either verbally or nonverbally. The nurse should approach the client in as nonthreatening a manner as possible and assure the client that the information provided and the results of the physical examination will remain confidential.

Throughout the assessment process, the nurse gathers subjective and objective data reflecting the client's state of health.

- *Objective Data:* Results of Papanicolaou smear, examination of genitalia, hemaglobin and hematocrit levels.
- *Subjective Data:* Date of last menstrual period and length of cycle; age at which menses began; date of last OB-GYN exam; date of last sexual encounter and typical sexual practices, including types of birth control used; medications; preexisting conditions, obstetric history.

Diagnosis

The nursing diagnoses for a client with PMS include the following:

- Acute Pain
- Ineffective Coping.

Nursing diagnoses that may be appropriate for the client with DUB include the following:

- Anxiety
- Sexual Dysfunction.

Plan

Goals of nursing care include the following:

- Reduce pain and discomfort to an acceptable level for the client.
- Promote comfort in discussing sexual dysfunction.
- Help client to identify coping strategies to reduce anxiety.
- Teach client to maintain a journal of symptoms.

Implementation

Nursing interventions focus on relieving symptoms and providing client teaching to decrease anxiety and increase coping skills, Assisting the client to identify lifestyle choices that may be contributing to menstrual disorders such as heavy lifting, nutrition, and substance abuse can help the nurse implement the most effective plan of care.

Acute Pain

The woman with PMS may have pain from headache (including migraine), menstrual cramps, excessive fluid retention, breast swelling, joint and muscle pain, and backache.

- Teach effective pharmacological and nonpharmacological self-care measures to relieve pain: application of heat, relaxation techniques (such as breathing exercises, imagery techniques, or meditation), and exercise. Heat relieves muscle spasms and dilates blood vessels, increasing blood supply to the pelvis and uterine muscles. Relaxation and exercise aid the release of naturally produced pain relievers called endorphins.

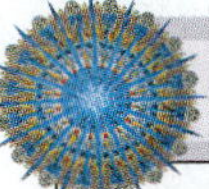

NURSING CARE PLAN **A Client With Menstrual Dysfunction**

Angela Hall is a 31-year-old married accountant, who relates a history of severe dysmenorrhea and menorrhagia, a feeling of pelvic heaviness and pain that radiates down her thighs. Because of her discomfort, her husband has complained about the quality of their sex life and has expressed concerns about their plans for having children. Mrs. Hall reports being so tired she doesn't care whether she has sex or not and, in fact, would really prefer not to: "Sex hurts so much, I just can't stand it." Endometriosis is suspected, and a diagnostic laparoscopy has been scheduled.

ASSESSMENT	DIAGNOSES	PLANNING
Christine Brigham, RN, NP, interviews Mrs. Hall and makes the following assessments: T_O 36.7°C (98.2°F), P 68, R 18, BP 110/70. Mrs. Hall's weight is 59 kg (130 lb) and within normal limits for her height. Review of laboratory findings indicate a hemoglobin level of 9.8 g/dL (normal range: 12 to 16 g/dL) and a hematocrit of 33.1% (normal range: 35% to 45%). Physical examination reveals pelvic tenderness on manipulation of the cervix and small masses that are palpable on abdominal/pelvic examination.	▪ Chronic Pain related to endometrial pelvic implants ▪ Anxiety related to effect of endometriosis on fertility ▪ Deficient Knowledge related to diagnosis and treatment options ▪ Ineffective Sexuality Pattern related to the manifestations of endometriosis	▪ The client will use effective self-care measures to deal with the pain and discomfort. ▪ The client will verbalize decreased anxiety. ▪ The client will demonstrate understanding of the disease and treatment options. ▪ The client will articulate an improvement in sexual functioning and a decrease in interpersonal stress between herself and her husband.

IMPLEMENTATION

- Identify the location, type, duration, and history of the pain.
- Recommend analgesics and heat therapy.
- Provide information on biofeedback, relaxation, and imagery to lessen pain.
- Discuss with Mr. and Mrs. Hall the causes of endometriosis and its manifestations.
- Encourage the Halls to discuss their feelings about the effect of the disease on their sex life, lifestyle, and fertility.
- Refer the couple to the local mental health center if appropriate.

EVALUATION

Two years after the initiation of treatment, Mr. and Mrs. Hall have become parents of a baby girl. Mrs. Hall states that the discomfort and other manifestations of endometriosis have eased. Relaxation and imagery have effectively minimized her pain and brought about improvement in her function as wife, mother, and sexual partner. Counseling has improved the interpersonal and sexual relations between the Halls. Dietary management has improved her anemia, although the menorrhagia persists. The Halls are trying to have a second child, understanding the advantages of rapid succession of pregnancies. They will be followed in the nursing clinic and referred to an infertility clinic if conception does not occur within 1 year.

CRITICAL THINKING

1. Explain the pathophysiological basis for Mrs. Hall's anemia.
2. How would you handle the situation if Mr. and Mrs. Hall were extremely uncomfortable and embarrassed about discussing their sexual problems?
3. Develop a plan of care for Mrs. Hall for the nursing diagnosis *Situational Low Self-Esteem* related to the manifestations of endometriosis.

- Review daily activities and suggest ways to balance rest periods and activity. During rest periods, energy and oxygen requirements decrease, increasing the amount of energy and oxygen available to muscles.
- Review manifestations and, if possible, correlate these with dietary patterns and activity levels. Encourage the woman to keep a diary of PMS manifestations. Maintaining a diary of PMS manifestations, activity, and foods eaten can provide data to identify modifiable causes of discomfort.
- If appropriate, suggest sexual activity (including masturbation) as a way to lessen menstrual cramps. Orgasm may help relieve dysmenorrhea.

Ineffective Coping

Many women experience wide mood swings during episodes of PMS, sometimes exhibiting self-destructive or aggressive behaviors toward others. These mood swings can interfere with a woman's ability to manage her responsibilities at home or at work.

- Encourage the woman to keep a journal of her menstrual cycle and to document her mood changes in the 7–10 days prior to menstruation. Recognizing the signs and timing of PMS is the first step in developing methods to cope with the problem.

- Explore possible ways to rearrange or reschedule activities when experiencing PMS. Planning ahead enables the woman to assume more control and promotes coping methods.
- Explore what, if any, self-care measures have helped cope with mood alterations in the past. Encourage healthful coping mechanisms, such as relaxation techniques and exercise. Some women may rely on alcohol or other drugs during PMS, which only exacerbate the manifestations.

Anxiety

The anxiety associated with abnormal uterine bleeding can be intense. Until the cause of the bleeding is identified and has been addressed, the woman may fear cancer or other life-threatening conditions.

- Discuss the results of tests and examinations with the woman. This allows for open exchange of information.
- Provide information about the causes, treatments, risks, long-term effects of treatments, and prognosis. This allows the woman to assume responsibility for her own health and become involved in her own treatment plan.
- Evaluate coping strategies and psychosocial support systems. Teach coping strategies if indicated. The possibility of surgery or cancer represents a crisis for the woman and her support system. Support groups can provide assistance for the woman through crisis intervention.

Sexual Dysfunction

The woman with DUB may be unwilling to express herself sexually, particularly if bleeding is frequent or heavy. Additionally, fatigue may prevent her from participating in sexual activity.

- Offer information about engaging in sexual activity during menstruation. Explain that conception is possible during this time and that orgasm may help relieve symptoms. Some women mistakenly believe that birth control measures are unnecessary during menstruation. Orgasm causes a release of tension and vascular congestion and frequently provides at least temporary relief of symptoms.
- Provide an opportunity for the expression of concerns related to alterations in lifestyle and sexual functioning. Some women have had a prolonged period of sexual abstinence related to DUB. Allowing women to verbalize concerns can assist them in working collaboratively with the health care provider to minimize the impact of illness and optimize function.
- Encourage frequent rest periods. This conserves energy and may allow sexual activities to resume.
- Provide information about alternative methods of sexual expression. Methods of sexual expression other than vaginal intercourse may satisfy the needs of both partners.

Evaluation

Client progress toward goals is evaluated on the basis of appropriate learning outcomes which may include the following:

- Client experiences less pain, allowing her to perform activities of daily living.
- Client reports reduced anxiety.
- Client reports return to baseline menstruation.
- Client is able to participate in sexual activity without symptoms.

REVIEW Menstrual Dysfunction

RELATE: LINK THE CONCEPTS

Linking the exemplar of Menstrual Dysfunction with the concept of Elimination:

1. What teaching will you initiate for the client with premenstrual syndrome regarding urinary health?
2. What nutritional counseling will you offer the client with premenstrual syndrome to prevent constipation?

Linking the exemplar of Menstrual Dysfunction with the concept of Stress and Coping:

3. What assessment data would alert you that the client with dysfunctional uterine bleeding is experiencing anxiety?
4. What priority interventions will you implement to help the woman with dysfunctional uterine bleeding to cope with fears?

READY: GO TO COMPANION SKILLS MANUAL

- Assessing the female genital and inguinal area
- Assessing the client in pain

REFER: GO TO MYNURSINGKIT

REFLECT: CASE STUDY

Angie Able is a 35-year-old woman married to Joe. Angie and Joe have four children, Ted 12, Abel 10, Susie 8, and Linda 4. Joe is a chef who owns a very successful restaurant in town. Angie is an administrative assistant to the CEO of the largest bank in the area. She is a well-organized, detail person with high energy. She manages the children, her home, her husband, and her job with aplomb. Angie has enjoyed good health with only mild seasonal colds.

Angie has been having heavier than usual menstrual periods over the past 6 months, and it is beginning to interfere with her work. She has needed to leave work to change clothes several times and has begun carrying extra clothes with her during her menstrual period. Besides being very embarrassed, Angie is afraid that there is something seriously wrong with her. She feels tired all the time and is always thirsty. Angie decides to visit her gynecologist before her next menstrual period begins.

1. What could explain Angie's symptoms of fatigue and thirst?
2. What diagnostic tests do you anticipate will be ordered?
3. What teaching will you provide Angie to reduce her current symptoms?

26.5 SEXUALLY TRANSMITTED INFECTIONS

KEY TERMS

Chancre, *1761*
Chlamydia, *1759*
Genital herpes, *1757*
Genital warts, *1758*
Gonorrhea, *1760*
Sexually transmitted infections (STIs), *1755*
Syphilis, *1760*

BASIS FOR SELECTION OF EXEMPLAR

Standards of Nursing Practice
Common disorder

LEARNING OUTCOMES

After reading about this exemplar, you will be able to:

1. Describe the pathophysiology, etiology, clinical manifestations, and direct and indirect causes of sexually transmitted infection.
2. Identify risk factors associated with sexually transmitted infections.
3. Illustrate the nursing process in providing culturally competent care across the life span for individuals with sexually transmitted infections.
4. Formulate priority nursing diagnoses appropriate for an individual with sexually transmitted infections.
5. Create a plan of care for individuals with sexually transmitted infections and their significant other.
6. Assess expected outcomes for an individual with a sexually transmitted infection.
7. Discuss therapies used in the collaborative care of an individual with a sexually transmitted infection.
8. Employ evidence-based caring interventions for an individual with a sexually transmitted infection.

OVERVIEW

Infections transmitted by vaginal, oral, and anal intimate contact and intercourse are referred to as **sexually transmitted infections (STIs)**. Infections transmitted by sexual intercourse are also labeled as *sexually transmitted diseases (STDs)* or *venereal diseases*. STIs also include systemic diseases (such as tuberculosis, hepatitis, and HIV/AIDS) that can be transmitted from an infected person to a partner. This chapter discusses STIs that involve the urogenital system. Vaginal infections are included in this chapter because they are also included in the Centers for Disease Control and Prevention (CDC) 2006 treatment guidelines.

Sexually transmitted infections include those caused by bacteria, *Chlamydiae*, viruses, fungi, protozoa, and parasites. Portals of entry for these agents of transmission include the mouth, genitalia, urinary meatus, anus, rectum, and skin. STIs have many consequences, and nurses have the responsibility of teaching sexually active clients how to prevent STIs, regardless of their gender, age, or sexual orientation. Nurses have a critical role in the prevention of STIs by teaching clients about these diseases, their prevention, treatment, and potential complications.

Incidence and Prevalence

STIs have reached epidemic proportions in the United States and are on the increase worldwide (Box 26–6). They are the most frequent infections encountered by professionals in the field of reproductive health and occur in more than half of all people at some point in their life (American Social Health Association [ASHA], 2005).

Women and infants are disproportionately affected by STIs. Many STIs are more easily transmitted from a man to a woman than from a woman to a man. Women often experience few early manifestations of the infection, delaying diagnosis and treatment. Furthermore, women are at greater risk for complications of STIs such as pelvic inflammatory disease (PID) and genital cancers.

Several factors help explain the escalating incidence of STIs. The so-called sexual revolution of the 1960s and 1970s, fueled by "the pill" and the freedom from unplanned pregnancy, led to a more permissive attitude about sexuality and increases in sexual activity and the number of sexual partners. In addition, since oral contraceptives were introduced to American women in 1961, they have replaced the condom as a birth control method for many couples. However, oral contraceptives do not protect against STIs, a fact of increasing importance.

STIs affect men and women of all ages, backgrounds, and socioeconomic levels. Of the 15 million new STI cases each year, approximately 25% occur in adolescents. Female adolescents have the highest reported rates of STIs, and they have the

Box 26–6 Selected Facts About Sexually Transmitted Infections

- The CDC estimates that approximately 19 million new sexually transmitted infections occur each year, almost half of them among young people 15–24 years of age.
- Biological factors place women at greater risk than men for the severe health consequences of STIs. Chlamydia and gonorrhea can both result in infertility if left untreated.
- Chlamydia, gonorrhea, syphilis, and herpes are also associated with increased HIV transmission, which is of particular concern among men who have sex with men of all races and African American men and women, where the HIV burden is now greatest.

Source: Sexually Transmitted Diseases Surveillance. (2007). Centers for Disease Control and Prevention. Retrieved September 25, 2009, from http://www.cdc.gov/std/stats07/trends.htm

potential for more complications, such as pelvic inflammatory disease (Shafii & Burstein, 2004). Results from the CDC National 2007 Youth Risk Behavior Survey revealed that 47.8% of high school students had engaged in sexual intercourse and 38.5% of sexually active adolescents had not used a condom at last sexual intercourse (CDC, 2008). Adolescents are considered an at-risk population related to their inexperience and lack of knowledge about STIs. Studies have determined that adolescents possess minimal knowledge about non-HIV sexually transmitted infections, their treatments, and curability (Clark, Jackson, & Allen-Taylor, 2002). Factors contributing to the risk to the child and adolescent include the avoidance of protective barriers, multiple sexual partners, engaging in sex frequently, and failure to seek medical treatment until symptoms are well advanced.

The incidence of STIs is highest in young adults ages 15–24 and in minorities. Drug abuse, unprotected sexual activity, and sexual activity with multiple partners also are associated with increased incidence of STIs (Blair, 2004). A further factor in the increasing incidence is that young people are becoming sexually active at an earlier age, marrying later, and divorce is more common. As a result, sexually active people today are more likely to have multiple sex partners in their lifetime and are potentially at risk for STIs (National Institute of Allergy and Infectious Diseases, 2003).

PRACTICE ALERT

When a child younger than 10 years is found to have gonorrhea or other sexually transmitted infection, consider the possibility of sexual abuse. When anorectal symptoms or disease or trauma are found, suspect molestation (see Concept 31, Violence, for a discussion of child abuse).

The emergence of HIV/AIDS has created a kind of "epidemiological synergy" among all STIs. Other STIs, such as syphilis, herpes simplex virus (HSV), and chancroid, facilitate the transmission of HIV/AIDS, and the immune suppression caused by HIV potentiates the infectious process of other STIs. In fact, individuals who are infected with STIs are at greater risk of acquiring HIV if they are exposed to the virus. This is the result of several factors: Genital ulcers create a portal of entry for HIV, nonulcerative STIs increase the concentration of cells in genital secretions that can be targets for HIV, and infection with both an STI and HIV results in an increased likelihood of having HIV in genital secretions and semen.

Characteristics

Although STIs are caused by various organisms, they have several characteristics in common:

- Most can be prevented by the use of latex condoms.
- They can be transmitted during both heterosexual and homosexual activities, including nonpenetrating intimate exposure.
- For treatment to be effective, sexual partners of the infected person must also be treated.
- Two or more STIs frequently coexist in the same client.

The complications of STIs in women include PID, ectopic pregnancy, infertility, chronic pelvic pain, neonatal illness and death, and genital cancer. Some bacterial STIs can be cured through appropriate early treatment with antibiotics. Others, such as genital herpes, are chronic conditions that can be managed but not cured because they are caused by viruses. The most serious STI is AIDS, which at this time is incurable. Treatment guidelines for STIs are updated regularly and are available from the CDC.

Prevention and Control

The prevention and control of STIs are based on the principles of education, detection, effective diagnosis, and treatment of infected persons and the evaluation, treatment, and counseling of sex partners of people who are infected. The ability of the health care provider to obtain an accurate sexual history is essential to prevention and control efforts. One approach to collecting accurate information about key areas of interest has been summarized by the CDC (2006). This approach includes the Five Ps: Partners, Prevention of Pregnancy, Protection from STIs, Practice, and Past History of STIs. Suggested questions to use are found on the CDC website.

The most effective way to prevent sexual transmission of HIV and other STIs is to avoid sexual intercourse with an infected partner. It is recommended that both partners be tested for STIs, including HIV, before beginning to have sexual intercourse. If a person chooses to have intercourse with an infected partner or one whose infection status is unknown, a new condom should be used for each act of intercourse. See Meeting Individualized Needs below for recommended STI barrier guidelines (CDC, 2006).

Prevention teaching for the person who is an injecting-drug user includes the following:

- Enroll or continue in a drug treatment program.
- Do not use injection equipment that has been used by another person. If equipment is shared, first clean the syringe and needle with bleach and water (to reduce the rate of HIV transmission).
- If needles can legally be obtained in the community, obtain and use clean needles.

PRACTICE ALERT

Eliminating further transmission and reinfection of STIs is critical to control. For treatable STIs, this means that referral of sex partners for diagnosis, treatment, and counseling is essential. Gonorrhea, syphilis, and AIDS are reportable diseases in every state, and chlamydial infections are reportable in most states. When a health care professional refers infected clients to a local or state department of health, every effort is made to identify and contact sex partners. Reports of STI and HIV infections are maintained in strictest confidence, and are protected by law from subpoena.

Suggested resources for people with STIs are listed in Box 26–7.

Common Sexually Transmitted Infections

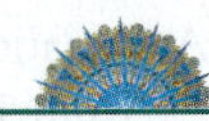

Sexually transmitted infection is a general term used to describe many different infections. Each infection has distinct pathophysiology, etiology, risk factors, and clinical manifestations, so each will be addressed separately.

Box 26–7 **Resources for Clients with Sexually Transmitted Infections**

- CDC National STD Hotline
- CDC National Prevention Information Network
- National Center for HIV, STD, and TB Prevention
- National HPV and Cervical Cancer Resource Center and Hotline
- National Herpes Hotline
- American Social Health Association

GENITAL HERPES

Genital herpes are caused by the herpes simplex viruses HSV-1 and HSV-2. Like most STIs, genital herpes are most commonly found in young, sexually active adults and are associated with early onset of sexual activity and multiple sexual partners. Approximately 50 million people ages 12 and older, or 1 out of every 5 teens and adults, have had genital HSV infections (CDC, 2006). There is no cure, and the treatments are primarily symptomatic.

Pathophysiology

One hundred types of HSV viruses have been identified, with more than 30 affecting the urogenital area. HSV-1 is associated with cold sores but may be transmitted to the genital area by oral intercourse or by self-inoculation through poor handwashing practices. HSV-2 is transmitted by sexual activity or during childbirth from an infected woman and is the virus that causes genital herpes. HSV infections begin with an exposure to the virus by contact with infectious lesions or secretions. The virus then moves into the stratified squamous epithelium, stimulating the replication of the epithelium and infecting the neurons that innervate the area. HSV viruses are neurotropic viruses, meaning that they grow in neurons and can maintain their disease potential even when there are no manifestations. The virus ascends through the peripheral nerves to the dorsal root ganglia, where it can remain dormant. For unknown reasons, the virus may reactivate and return to the nerve root of the skin, causing lesions. During dormancy, the virus is impervious to treatment. The incubation period ranges from 6 weeks to 8 months (Porth, 2005). Genital HSV-2 infection is more common in women (approximately one in four women) than it is in men (almost one of five) (CDC, 2004).

Manifestations

Within 2–10 days after exposure to the herpes virus, painful red papules appear in the genital area. In men, the lesions generally occur on the glans or shaft of the penis. In women, the lesions commonly occur on the labia, vagina, and cervix. Anal intercourse or oral–anal sexual contact may result in lesions in and around the anus.

Soon after the papules appear, they form small painful blisters filled with clear fluid containing virus particles (Figure 26–35 ■). The blisters break, shedding the highly infectious virus and creating patches of painful ulcers that last 6 weeks (or longer if they become infected). Touching these blisters and then rubbing or scratching in another place can spread the infection to other areas of the body (*autoinoculation*).

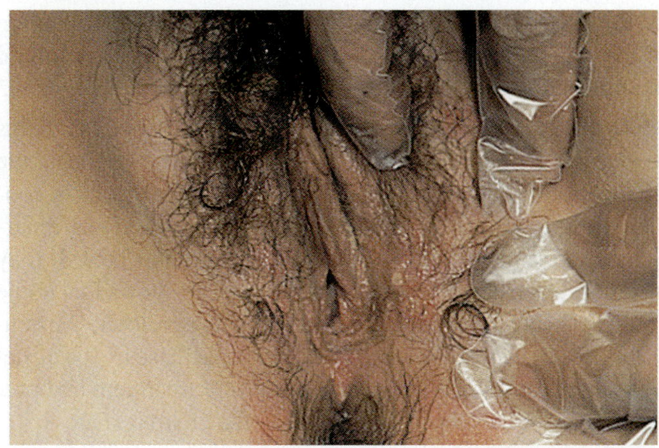

Figure 26–35 ■ Genital herpes blisters as they appear on the labia.

The first outbreak of herpes lesions is called *first episode infection*, with an average duration of 12 days. Subsequent occurrences, usually less severe, are termed *recurrent infections* (average duration of 4–5 days). The period between episodes is called *latency*, during which time the person remains infectious even though no symptoms are present. During latency, the virus withdraws into the nerve fibers that lead from the infected site to the lower spine, remaining dormant until recurrence, at which time it retraces its path to the genital area.

The manifestations of genital herpes are listed in Box 26–8. Prodromal symptoms of recurrent outbreaks of genital herpes can include burning, itching, tingling, or throbbing at the sites where lesions commonly appear. These sensations may be accompanied by pain in the legs, groin, or buttocks. Some authorities believe that prodromal symptoms signal increased levels of infectiousness, during which sexual contact should be avoided.

Collaboration

Presumptive diagnosis of genital herpes is based on history and physical examination of the client, including lesions and patterns of recurrence. Because there is no cure for genital herpes, treatment focuses on relieving symptoms and preventing spread of the infection. Client education is essential to prevent further transmission of the disease and to help clients integrate management of a chronic disease into their lifestyles.

Box 26–8 **Manifestations of Genital Herpes**

- Herpetic lesions
- Regional lymphadenopathy
- Headache
- Fever
- General malaise
- Dysuria
- Urinary retention
- Vaginal discharge
- Urethral discharge (men)

DIAGNOSTIC TESTS Definitive diagnosis requires isolation of the virus in tissue culture. Ideally, tissue specimens should be obtained within 48 hours of the appearance of the blisters.

PHARMACOLOGIC THERAPIES Acyclovir (Zovirax) helps reduce the length and severity of the first episode and is the treatment of choice for genital herpes. The oral form is considered most effective for the first episode as well as recurrences and is given for 7–10 days or until lesions heal. It may also be administered intravenously. Evidence shows that some strains of HSV are becoming resistant to acyclovir, particularly in HIV-positive people. In those cases, foscarnet (Foscavir) is used. Other antivirals used for treatment and prevention are valacyclovir (Valtrex) and famciclovir (Famvir).

GENITAL WARTS

Genital warts (*condylomata acuminata*), caused by the human papillomavirus (HPV), are the most common infectious genital infections in the United States and are considered epidemic. Genital warts are chronic and, in many people, largely asymptomatic. Currently, they are incurable.

Women are at greater risk for HPV genital infections because they have a larger mucosal surface area exposed in the genital area. Most HPV infections are asymptomatic or unrecognized. An estimated 20 million Americans are infected with the virus, and up to 6.2 million new cases are diagnosed annually (CDC, 2006) (Box 26–9).

Although the majority of people infected with genital warts are asymptomatic, others experience frequent recurrences. Other than recurrences, men are not likely to experience serious physical complications of genital warts. Women, however, face concerns about the increased risk of cervical cancer, with HPV DNA having been identified in almost all cervical cancers worldwide and in approximately 50–80% of vaginal, vulvar, and anogenital cancers (Porth, 2005).

Pathophysiology

Genital warts are caused by HPV and are transmitted by vaginal, anal, or oral–genital contact. The incubation period is 6 weeks to 8 months (Porth, 2005).

Box 26–9 Selected Facts About Genital HPV Infection

- At least 50% of sexually active men and women acquire genital HPV infection at some point in their lives.
- By age 50, at least 80% of women will have acquired genital HPV infection.
- Most people with a genital HPV infection do not know they are infected; most women are diagnosed by abnormal Pap smears.

Source: CDC (2004).

Manifestations

Although some people with HPV may not have manifestations, others exhibit characteristic lesions: single or multiple painless, soft, moist, pink or flesh-colored swellings in the vulvovaginal area, perineum, penis, urethra, anus, groin, or thigh (Figure 26–36 ■). In women, the growths may be in the vagina or on the cervix and may be apparent only during a pelvic examination.

The four types of genital warts are as follows:

- *Condyloma acuminata:* cauliflower-shaped lesions that appear on moist skin surfaces such as the vagina or anus
- *Keratotic warts:* thick, hard lesions that develop on keratinized skin such as the labia major, penis, or scrotum
- *Papular warts:* smooth lesions that also develop on keratinized skin
- *Flat warts:* slightly raised lesions, often invisible to the naked eye, that also develop on keratinized skin.

Collaboration

Treatment is directed at removal of the warts, relief of symptoms, and health teaching to reduce the risk of recurrence and future transmission. Infection with HPV is considered chronic; however, research has shown that for about 90% of women, cervical HPV becomes undetectable within 2 years (CDC, 2004).

Genital and anal warts are diagnosed primarily by clinical appearance. An HPV DNA test is specific for diagnosis in women. There are no HPV tests for men.

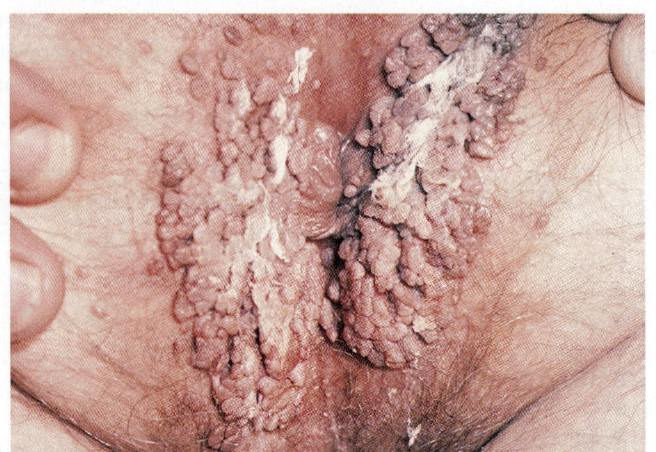

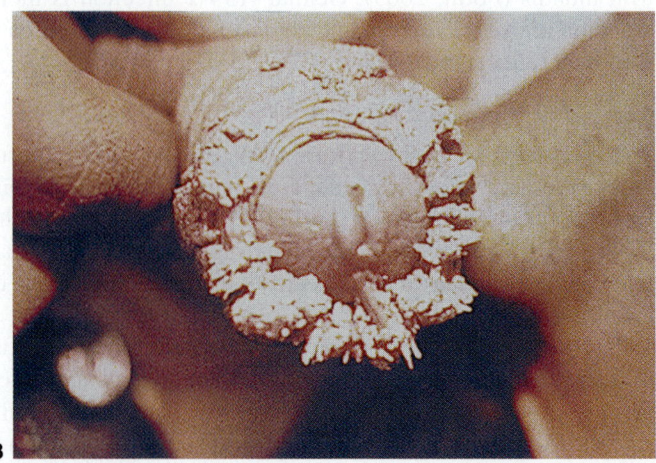

Figure 26–36 ■ Genital warts (condyloma acuminatum) on the *A*, vulva and *B*, penis.

PHARMACOLOGIC THERAPIES Topical agents used to treat genital warts include podofilox and imiquimod (both can be applied by the client) or podophyllin and trichloroacetic acid (provider-administered treatments). Podophyllin (Condylox, Podofin) is contraindicated during pregnancy and can have side effects in any client, ranging from nausea, diarrhea, and lethargy to paralysis and coma (see Box 26–10). Gardasil is a vaccine developed to prevent genital warts, precancerous genital lesions, and cervical cancer due to HPV. It is administered by 3 intramuscular injections given over a 6-month period. As HPV is so closely associated with cervical cancer, a federal advisory panel has recommended that the vaccine be targeted for females, aged 9–26. The vaccine does not protect against the effects of an existing HPV infection.

OTHER TREATMENTS Genital warts may also be removed by cryotherapy, electrocautery, laser vaporization, or surgical excision. Carbon dioxide laser surgery is becoming increasingly common for removal of extensive warts.

CHLAMYDIA

Chlamydias are a group of STIs, caused by *Chlamydia trachomatis*, a bacterium that behaves like a virus, reproducing only within the host cell. The bacterium is spread by any sexual contact and to the neonate by passage through the birth canal of an infected mother. The infections caused by *Chlamydia* include acute urethral syndrome, nongonococcal urethritis, mucopurulent cervicitis, and PID.

Chlamydia is the most commonly reported bacterial STI in the United States, affecting an estimated 2–3 million people each year (CDC, 2004). Of that number, three of every four reported cases occurred in people under age 25. Risk factors for chlamydia are listed in Box 26–11.

Because chlamydia is asymptomatic in most women until the uterus and fallopian tubes have been invaded, treatment may be delayed, resulting in devastating long-term complications. Nearly a third of men with urethral chlamydia are also asymptomatic. Chlamydia is a leading cause of preventable blindness in the newborn.

Box 26–11 **Risk Factors for Chlamydial Infection**

- Personal or partner history of STI
- Pregnancy
- Adolescent sexual activity
- Oral contraceptive use
- Unprotected sexual activity
- Multiple sexual partners

Pathophysiology

C. trachomatis is an intracellular bacterial pathogen that resembles both a virus and a bacterium. The organism enters the body as an elementary body, a form in which it is capable of entering uninfected cells. The infection begins when the organism enters a cell and changes into a reticulate body. The reticulate body divides within the cell, bursting the cell and infecting adjoining cells.

Manifestations

The incubation period is from 1–3 weeks; however, chlamydia may be present for months or years without producing noticeable symptoms in women. Chlamydia typically invades the same target organs as gonorrhea (cervix and male urethra) and results in similar manifestations (dysuria, urinary frequency, and discharge). Clients may be asymptomatic; however, they are still potentially infectious.

Complications

If a chlamydial infection in a woman is not treated, it ascends into the upper reproductive tract, causing such complications as PID, which includes endometritis and salpingitis. Chronic pelvic pain may result. These infections are a major cause of

Box 26–10 **Medication Administration for the Client With Genital Warts**

TOPICAL APPLICATIONS

Podophyllin

Trichloroacetic Acid

Although cryotherapy using liquid nitrogen or a cryoprobe is more commonly used to treat genital warts, podophyllum preparations are sometimes used. Podophyllin is applied topically to the warts by the physician once weekly for 3–5 weeks.

Podophyllin is contraindicated during pregnancy; the alternative is cryotherapy. Podophyllin is also contraindicated in cervical, urethral, oral, or anorectal warts. It is important to avoid contact of podophyllin resin with the eyes.

Adverse effects of podophyllin include local irritation, severe ulceration of surrounding tissue, nausea, diarrhea, lethargy, paralysis, and coma.

Nursing Responsibilities

- Establish baseline data, including mental status, vital signs, and weight.
- Document and report any existing lesions (genital, anal, or oral).
- Cover the tissue surrounding the warts with petrolatum or a paste of baking soda and water to protect the tissue from the caustic treatment solution.

Health Education for the Client and Family

- Wash the treated area thoroughly within 1–4 hours after the first application; gradually increase this period to 6–8 hours after the second and subsequent applications.
- Return for regular treatment until warts are gone.
- Refer partners for examination and any necessary treatment.
- Report any adverse effects (nausea, diarrhea, local irritation, lethargy, numbness).
- Avoid sexual activity until you and your partners have been free of disease for 1 month.
- Use condoms to prevent future infections.
- Return for an annual Pap smear.

infertility and ectopic pregnancy, a potentially life-threatening disorder in women. Complications of chlamydial infections in men include epididymitis, prostatitis, sterility, and Reiter's syndrome. Routine screening for sexually active adolescents and young adults has been suggested by the CDC to minimize these serious complications in asymptomatic people (Porth, 2005).

Collaboration

C. trachomatis is treated with medications to eradicate the infection. Its prevalence, particularly in younger populations, makes widespread screening necessary if the disease is to be controlled. Because chlamydia is often asymptomatic, treatment is often begun on a presumptive basis.

DIAGNOSTIC TESTS The diagnostic tests that may be ordered include a Gram stain of discharge from the female endocervix and urethra or from the male urethra to look for polymorphonuclear leukocytes (considered evidence of infection).

Tests for antibodies to chlamydia such as the direct fluorescent antibody (DFA) test and an enzyme-linked immunosorbent assay (ELISA), as well as polymerase chain reaction (PCR) or ligase chain reaction (LCR) tests, are highly sensitive and specific tests performed on cervical and urethral swab specimens. However, nucleic acid amplification tests (NAATs), also performed on cervical and urethral swab specimens, have become the diagnostic method of choice (Porth, 2005).

PHARMACOLOGIC THERAPIES The antibiotic recommended by the CDC for chlamydial infections in men and nonpregnant women is azithromycin (Zithromax), orally in a single dose, or doxycycline (Adoxa, Apo-Doxy), orally for 7 days. Both sexual partners must be treated at the same time or prior to resuming sexual intercourse.

GONORRHEA

Gonorrhea, also known as "GC" or "the clap," is caused by *Neisseria gonorrhoeae*, a Gram-negative diplococcus. Gonorrhea is the most common reportable communicable disease in the United States. The CDC (2004) estimates that approximately 700,000 new cases occur annually, with the rate of reported gonorrhea increasing.

Gonorrhea rates for African Americans are 30% higher than rates for non-Hispanic whites. Other risk factors include residence in large urban areas, being transient, early onset of sexual activity, multiple serial or consecutive sex partners, drug use, prostitution, and previous gonorrheal or concurrent STI infection.

Pathophysiology

The causative organism of gonorrhea is a pyogenic (pus-forming) bacteria that causes inflammation characterized by purulent exudate. Humans are the only host for the organism. Gonorrhea is transmitted by direct hetero-and homosexual intercourse and during delivery as the neonate passes through the birth canal. The portal of entry can be the genitourinary tract, eyes, oropharynx, anorectum, or skin. The incubation period is 2–7 days after exposure. The organism initially targets the female cervix and the male urethra. Without treatment, the disease ultimately disseminates (spreads widely) to other organs. In men, gonorrhea can cause acute, painful inflammation of the prostate, epididymis, and periurethral glands and can lead to sterility. In women, it can cause PID, endometritis, salpingitis, and pelvic peritonitis.

Manifestations

Manifestations of gonorrhea in men include dysuria and serous, milky, or purulent discharge from the penis. Some men also experience regional lymphadenopathy. About 20% of men and 80% of women remain asymptomatic until the disease is advanced. Women with symptoms experience dysuria, urinary frequency, abnormal menses (increased flow or dysmenorrhea), increased vaginal discharge, and dyspareunia.

Anorectal gonorrhea is seen most often in homosexual men. The manifestations include pruritus, mucopurulent rectal discharge, rectal bleeding and pain, and constipation. Gonococcal pharyngitis occurs primarily in homosexual or bisexual men or heterosexual women after oral sexual contact (fellatio) with an infected partner. The manifestations include fever, sore throat, and enlarged lymph glands.

Complications

The complications of untreated gonorrhea in both men and women may be permanent and serious. They include the following:

- PID in women, leading to internal abscesses, chronic pain, ectopic pregnancy, and infertility
- Blindness, infection of joints, and potentially lethal infections of the blood in the newborn, contracted during delivery
- Epididymitis and prostatitis in men, resulting in infertility and dysuria
- Spread of the infection to the blood and joints
- Increased susceptibility to and transmission of HIV.

Collaboration

The goals of treatment for the client with gonorrhea include eradication of the organism and any coexisting disease and prevention of reinfection or transmission. It is important to emphasize the importance of taking all medications as prescribed and abstaining from sexual contact until the infection is cured in both client and partners. Condom use to prevent future infections is essential, particularly for pregnant women whose partners may be infected.

DIAGNOSTIC TESTS Diagnosis of gonorrhea is based on cultures from the infected mucous membranes (cervix, urethra, rectum, or throat), examination of urine from an infected person, and a Gram stain to visualize the bacteria under the microscope. Testing for other STIs (especially chlamydia and syphilis) at the same time is recommended. Pregnant women are routinely screened during their first prenatal visit.

SYPHILIS

Syphilis is a complex systemic STI caused by the spirochete *Treponema pallidum*, and it can infect almost any body tissue or organ. It is transmitted from open lesions during any sexual contact (genital, oral–genital, or anal–genital). The organism is highly susceptible to heat and drying but can survive for days in fluids; thus, it may also be transmitted by infected blood or other body fluid such as saliva. The incubation period ranges from 10–90 days, averaging 21 days. If not treated appropriately, syphilis can lead to blindness, paralysis, mental illness, cardiovascular damage, and death. Syphilis often occurs with one or more other STIs, such as HIV/AIDS or chlamydial infection.

Although in 1996 the rate of syphilis infection reached its lowest level in many years, it has risen since then and remains a significant problem in certain geographic regions and among specific populations such as African Americans. Rates also remain high in many urban centers, with higher infection rates found in drug users, transients, and the homeless. The incidence of primary and secondary syphilis is highest in people 20–39 years of age, with the incidence in women decreasing. However, the rate of syphilis among men having sex with men (MSM) is increasing (CDC, 2004).

Pathophysiology

Any break in the skin or mucous membrane is vulnerable to invasion by the spirochete. Once it has entered the system, the spirochete is spread through the blood and lymphatic system. Congenital syphilis is transferred to the fetus through the placental circulation.

Manifestations

Syphilis is generally characterized by three clinical stages: primary, secondary, and tertiary. Each stage has characteristic manifestations (Box 26–12). The client with syphilis also may experience a latency period when no signs of the disease are evident.

PRIMARY SYPHILIS The primary stage of syphilis is characterized by the appearance of a **chancre** (Figure 26–37 ■) and by regional enlargement of lymph nodes; little or no pain accompanies these warning signs. The chancre appears at the site of inoculation (such as the genitals, anus, mouth, breast, fingers) 3–4 weeks after the infectious contact. In women, a genital chancre may go unnoticed, disappearing within 4–6 weeks. In both primary and secondary stages, syphilis remains highly infectious, even if no symptoms are evident.

SECONDARY SYPHILIS Manifestations of secondary syphilis may appear any time from 2 weeks to 6 months after the initial chancre disappears. These symptoms can include a skin rash, especially on the palms of the hands or soles of the feet, mucous patches in the oral cavity; sore throat; generalized

Box 26–12 **Manifestations of Syphilis**

REPRODUCTIVE

Primary
- Genital chancre (may be internal in female)

Secondary
- Condyloma lata

INTEGUMENTARY SYSTEM

Secondary
- Rash on palms of hands and soles of feet

Tertiary
- Granulomatous lesions involving mucous membranes and skin

GASTROINTESTINAL SYSTEM

Secondary
- Anorexia
- Oral mucous patches

NEUROLOGICAL SYSTEM

Secondary
- Asymptomatic
- Meningitis
- Headache
- Cranial neuropathies

Tertiary
- Asymptomatic
- Tabes dorsalis
- Neurosyphilis
- Seizures, hemiparesis, hemiplegia
- Personality changes, hyperactive reflexes, Argyll Robertson pupil, decreased memory, slurred speech, optic atrophy

MUSCULOSKELETAL SYSTEM

Secondary
- Arthralgia
- Myalgia
- Bone and joint arthritis
- Periostitis

Tertiary
- Gummas

CARDIOVASCULAR SYSTEM

Tertiary
- Aortic insufficiency
- Aortic aneurysm
- Stenosis of openings to coronary arteries

RENAL SYSTEM

Secondary
- Glomerulonephritis
- Nephrotic syndrome

OTHER

Primary
- Regional lymphadenopathy

Secondary
- Generalized lymphadenopathy
- Fever
- Hepatitis
- Malaise
- Alopecia

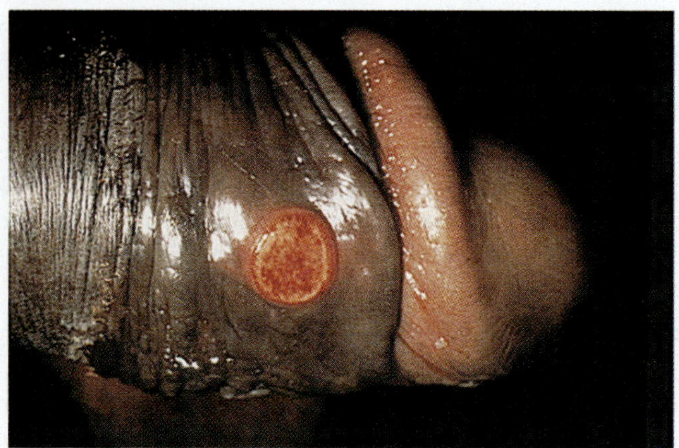

Figure 26–37 ■ Chancre of primary syphilis on the penis.

lymphadenopathy; condyloma lata (flat, broad-based papules, unlike the pedunculated structure of genital warts) on the labia, anus, or corner of the mouth; flulike symptoms; and alopecia. These manifestations generally disappear within 2–6 weeks, and an asymptomatic latency period begins.

LATENT AND TERTIARY SYPHILIS The latent stage of syphilis begins 2 or more years after the initial infection and can last up to 50 years. During this stage, no symptoms of syphilis are apparent, and the disease is not transmissible by sexual contact. It can be transmitted by infected blood, however; therefore, all prospective blood donors must be screened for syphilis. In two-thirds of all cases, the latent stage persists without further complications. Unless treated, the remaining one-third of infected people progress to late-stage or tertiary syphilis. In the presence of HIV infection, disease progression seems to be more rapid.

Two types of late-stage syphilis occur. Benign late syphilis, of rapid onset, is characterized by localized development of infiltrating tumors (*gummas*) in skin, bones, and liver, generally responding promptly to treatment. Of more insidious onset is a diffuse inflammatory response that involves the central nervous system and the cardiovascular system. Though the disease can still be treated at this stage, much of the cardiovascular and central nervous system damage is irreversible.

Collaboration

The goals of treatment are to inactivate the spirochete and educate the client about how to prevent reinfection or further transmission. Treatment includes antibiotic therapy and identification and referral of partners for testing and treatment if necessary, follow-up testing, and education about condom use to prevent reinfection of self and transmission of disease to partners. In addition, clients should be screened for chlamydial infection and advised to have an HIV test.

DIAGNOSTIC TESTS Diagnosis of syphilis is complex because it mimics many other diseases. A careful history and physical examination are obtained, as well as laboratory evaluations of lesions and blood.

The VDRL (Venereal Disease Research Laboratory) and RPR (rapid plasma reagin) blood tests measure antibody production. People with syphilis become positive about 4–6 weeks after infection. However, these tests are not specific for syphilis, and other diseases may also cause positive results. Additional tests are required for definitive diagnosis.

The FTA-ABS (fluorescent treponemal antibody absorption) test is specific for *T. pallidum* and can be used to confirm VDRL and RPR findings. It may be used for clients whose clinical picture indicates syphilis but who have negative VDRL results. In immunofluorescent staining a specimen is obtained from early lesions or aspiration of lymph nodes and is specially treated and examined microscopically for the presence of *T. pallidum.* Darkfield microscopy involves examining a specimen from the chancre for the presence of *T. pallidum* using a darkfield microscope.

PHARMACOLOGIC THERAPIES The treatment of choice for all stages of syphilis in adults is penicillin G, given intramuscularly (IM) in a single dose. Clients allergic to penicillin are given oral doxycycline or tetracycline for 28 days.

Treatment of syphilis may result in a severe reaction called the *Jarisch-Herxheimer reaction*, which involves fever, musculoskeletal pain, tachycardia, and sometimes hypotension. This is not a reaction to the penicillin itself, but to the sudden and massive destruction of spirochetes by the penicillin and the resulting release of toxins into the bloodstream. The Jarisch-Herxheimer reaction generally begins within 24 hours of treatment and subsides in another 24 hours. Treatment should not be discontinued unless symptoms become life threatening.

NURSING PROCESS

In providing nursing care for the client with a sexually transmitted infection, the nurse needs to consider both short-term and long-term implications. Although the immediate priority is symptom relief, treatment, and prevention of further transmission, the client may need assistance to deal with the diagnosis if the STI is a chronic disease or may require repeated screening for potential complications. Although this nursing process focuses on the client with genital herpes, the principles addressed may be applied to clients with any STI.

Assessment

The focused interview of the female concerns data related to the client's sexual practices and health history, including menstrual cycle, forms of birth control used, number of partners, frequency of sexual encounters, medication use, and preexisting conditions. Open-ended or closed questions are used to obtain information. Often a number of follow-up questions or requests for descriptions are required to clarify data or gather missing information. Follow-up questions are aimed at identifying the source of problems, duration of difficulties, measures to alleviate problems, and clues about the client's knowledge of her own health.

Information about the genital areas, reproduction, and sexual activity is generally considered very private. The nurse must be sensitive to the client's need for privacy and carefully explain that all information is confidential. A conversational approach with the use of open-ended statements

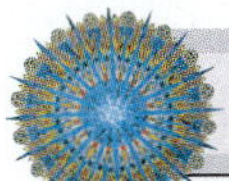

NURSING CARE PLAN A Client With Gonorrhea

Janet Cirit, a 33-year-old legal secretary, lives in a suburban midwestern community. She is unmarried but dating a man named Jim Adkins, who lives in an adjacent suburb. Ms. Cirit visits her gynecologist because her periods have become irregular and she is experiencing pelvic pain and an abnormal amount of vaginal discharge. Recently she has developed a sore throat. The pelvic pain has begun to disrupt her sleeping pattern, and she is concerned that she might have cancer because her mother recently died of ovarian cancer.

ASSESSMENT

When Ms. Cirit arrives for her appointment at the gynecologist's office, Marsha Davidson, the nurse practitioner, interviews her. Ms. Davidson completes a thorough medical and sexual history, including questions about her menstrual periods, pain associated with urination or sexual intercourse, urinary frequency, most recent Pap smear, birth control method, history of STI and drug use, and types of sexual activity. Ms. Cirit reports her symptoms and her concern about ovarian cancer. She also indicates that she is taking oral contraceptives and therefore sees no need for her boyfriend to use a condom because she believes their relationship is monogamous.

Physical examination reveals both pharyngeal and cervical inflammation and lower abdominal tenderness. Her temperature is 37.0°C (98.5°F). There are no signs or symptoms of pregnancy.

The gynecologist orders a Pap smear and cultures of the cervix, urethra, and pharynx to evaluate for gonorrhea and chlamydial infection. Blood is drawn for a white blood cell count (WBC). Test results are positive for gonorrhea and negative for chlamydia. The WBC is slightly elevated, indicating possible salpingitis. Because Mr. Adkins has been Ms. Cirit's only sexual partner, it is clear that he is the source of infection and needs to be treated as well.

DIAGNOSES

- Acute Pain related to the infectious process
- Anxiety related to fear about possible cancer
- Situational Low Self-Esteem related to shame and guilt because of having an STI
- Ineffective Sexuality Patterns related to the impaired relationship and fear of reinfection

PLANNING

- The client will experience relief of pain, indicating that the infection has been eradicated.
- The client will articulate that she has nothing to be ashamed of and that she has been wise to seek treatment as soon as symptoms occurred.
- The client will verbalize that she will insist her partner use condoms during future sexual activity.

IMPLEMENTATION

- Administer ceftriaxone IM as ordered.
- Emphasize the need for regular Pap smears and pelvic examinations because of the family history of ovarian cancer.
- Discuss feelings and concerns about the diagnosis of gonorrhea. Stress that such a diagnosis does not reflect on one's worth as a person.
- Teach the client how to talk with a future sexual partner about condom use.

EVALUATION

A week later during her follow-up visit. Ms. Cirit states that she is feeling much better and sleeping well at night since the pain has ended. She has terminated her relationship with Mr. Adkins and is considering joining a health club in the hope of increasing her level of fitness and perhaps meeting someone new.

CRITICAL THINKING

1. How are Ms. Cirit's manifestations related to the infectious process of gonorrhea?
2. Should the nurse have suggested that Ms. Cirit also be tested for HIV? Why or why not?
3. Develop a care plan for Ms. Cirit for the nursing diagnosis impaired social interaction.

is often helpful in a situation that promotes anxiety and embarrassment. The client's terminology about body parts and functions should guide the nurse's questions.

The focused interview guides the physical assessment. The information is always considered in relation to normal parameters and expectations about the health of the system. Therefore, the nurse must consider age, gender, race, culture, environment, health practices, past and concurrent problems, and therapies when framing questions and using techniques to elicit information.

The nurse must consider the client's ability to participate in the focused interview and physical assessment of the reproductive system. If a client is experiencing pain or anxiety, attention must focus on relief of these symptoms. Because of the close proximity of some of the female reproductive structures to the urethra, data gathered during the focused interview will relate to the status of the urinary system as well.

Abnormal vaginal discharge, pelvic pain, inflammation, infection, and suspicion of contracting an STI are some of the more frequent problems that the female reports. Examination

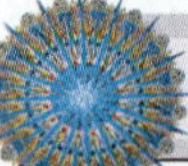

NURSING CARE PLAN A Client With Syphilis

Eddie Kratz, age 22, works as bellman at a large hotel. For the past year, he has shared a small apartment with Maria Jones, who is 5 months pregnant with his child. Although he intends to marry Ms. Jones before the baby is born, he has continued a previous relationship with a woman named Justine Simpson. His sexual activities with Ms. Simpson have increased in frequency as Ms. Jones's pregnancy has advanced. Recently Mr. Kratz has noticed a swelling in his groin and a sore on his penis.

ASSESSMENT

When Mr. Kratz comes to the community clinic, he is interviewed by the nurse practitioner, Sally Morovitz. She takes a thorough medical and sexual history, including questions about drug use, allergies, difficulty with urination, urinary frequency, itching or discharge from the penis, recent sexual activities, precautions taken against infection, history of STIs, and sexual function. She determines that Mr. Kratz has been having unprotected sex with both Ms. Jones and Ms. Simpson. He believes that Ms. Jones is not having sex with anyone except him, but he is not sure.

Physical assessment reveals a classic syphilitic chancre on the shaft of the penis and regional lymphadenopathy. A specimen of exudates from the chancre is sent for darkfield examination. Ms. Morovitz discusses with Mr. Kratz the likelihood that he has syphilis and the need to tell both Ms. Jones and Ms. Simpson so that they can be tested and, if necessary, treated. Ms. Morovitz also suggests that Mr. Kratz be tested for HIV, since he has been having unprotected sex with two women, at least one of whom may be sexually active with other partners. He agrees, and blood is drawn for an ELISA test. Darkfield analysis of the chancre exudate confirms the diagnosis of syphilis; the ELISA results are negative for HIV.

DIAGNOSES

- Risk for Injury to the client, his partners, and the infant, related to the disease process
- Ineffective Health Maintenance related to a lack of knowledge about the disease process, its transmission, and the need for treatment
- Interrupted Family Processes related to the effects of the diagnosis of syphilis on the couple's relationship
- Anxiety related to the effects of the infection on the unborn child

PLANNING

- The client will receive prompt treatment to cure the syphilis.
- The client will articulate understanding for the need to abstain from sexual contact during treatment, complete all medications, return for follow-up visits, and use condoms to prevent reinfection.
- The client will verbalize an ability to cope with the effect of diagnosis and treatment on the relationship.
- The client will verbalize decreased anxiety following education and treatment.

IMPLEMENTATION

- Administer IM injection of penicillin G as ordered.
- Discuss the importance of abstaining from sexual activity until he and his partners are cured and of using condoms to prevent reinfection.
- Explain the need to return for follow-up testing in 3 months and again at 6 months. Provide a copy of the STI prevention checklist, and document that reminders need to be sent at 3- and 6-month intervals.
- Notify sexual partners that they need to come to the clinic for testing.
- Refer to a social worker for counseling about the effect of the disease on the couple's relationship.
- Teach the couple about the importance of treatment to the health of their infant.

EVALUATION

At the 3-month follow-up visit, the chancre on Mr. Kratz's penis has healed, and he reports that he is using a condom any time he has sex. Ms. Jones has also tested positive for syphilis and negative for HIV, so she, too, is given penicillin G, and verbal and written follow-up instructions, including follow-up until the infant is born. The couple is meeting every other week with the social worker and say that their relationship is improving. Ms. Simpson has received similar test results and is given a prescription for doxycycline because she is allergic to penicillin.

CRITICAL THINKING

1. What manifestations might a client with early syphilis experience?
2. List some appropriate questions for taking a sexual history when you suspect the presence of one or more STIs.
3. How might you counsel Mr. Kratz to help him break the news of the diagnosis to Ms. Jones?

of the perianal area is included in assessment of the female reproductive system. Related problems include hemorrhoids, fissures, and infectious processes.

Diagnosis

Nursing diagnoses that may be appropriate for clients diagnosed with a sexually transmitted infection may include the following:

- Acute Pain
- Sexual Dysfunction
- Knowledge Deficit.

Plan

When planning care of the client with a diagnosed or suspected STI, the following goals may be appropriate:

- Client describes strategies for reducing the risk of contracting an STI.
- Client develops a plan to contact anyone who may have been exposed to the diagnosed STI through sexual contact.
- Client abstains from sexual activity until the STI is resolved or takes appropriate actions to avoid infecting others.

- Pain is controlled to reduce severity of pain to a tolerable level.

Implementation

Nursing diagnoses discussed in this section focus on pain and sexual dysfunction.

Acute Pain

For the client with genital herpes, herpetic lesions are very painful and can become infected. Because the virus resides in the nerve ganglia, pain may also occur in the legs, thighs, groin, or buttocks. Although acyclovir diminishes the pain of herpes and accelerates the healing process, additional measures can relieve the discomfort further.

- Teach the client how to keep herpes blisters clean and dry. A solution of warm water, soap, and hydrogen peroxide (if lesions are not open) can be used to cleanse the lesions two or three times daily. Burrow's solution (a liquid containing aluminum sulfate, acetic acid, precipitated calcium carbonate, and water) can also be used. Lesions should be dried using a hair dryer turned to a cool setting. It is important to wear loose cotton clothing that will not trap moisture and to avoid wearing panty hose and tight jeans. Keeping the lesions clean and dry reduces the possibility of secondary infection and speeds the healing process.
- For dysuria, suggest pouring water over the genitals while urinating. Drinking additional fluids also helps dilute the acidity of the urine; however, fluids that increase acidity, such as cranberry juice, should be avoided. These measures dilute the acid content of urine and thereby reduce the burning sensation.
- Suggest the use of sitz baths (with tepid water) for 15–30 minutes several times a day. The warm water is soothing and decreases pain from ulcers and an irritated urethral meatus. It also facilitates wound healing.

Sexual Dysfunction

Clients who learn that they are infected with an incurable STI may believe they can no longer have a normal sex life. Fortunately, many people have learned to live with and manage genital herpes without infecting their partners or their children.

- Provide a supportive, nonjudgmental environment for the client to discuss feelings and ask questions about what this diagnosis means to future sexual relationships. Feelings of guilt, shame, and anger are natural responses to such a diagnosis and can lead to a total avoidance of sexual intimacy.
- Offer information about support groups and other resources for people with herpes such as the National Herpes Information Hotline. Information about how others cope with this disease can offset feelings of shame and hopelessness.

Deficient Knowledge

Health teaching for clients with genital herpes involves helping them manage this chronic disease with the least possible disruption in lifestyle and relationships. Understanding the disease process and factors that affect it helps the client regain a sense of control and see the potential for future sexual intimacy without transmission of infection. The following topics should be addressed:

- How to recognize prodromal symptoms of recurrence and factors that seem to trigger recurrences (such as emotional stress, acidic food, sun exposure)
- The need for abstinence from sexual contact from the time prodromal symptoms appear until 10 days after all lesions have healed
- If lesions become infected, use of topical acyclovir (Painful lesions can be protected with sterile petroleum jelly or aloe vera gel.)
- Use of latex condoms due to viral shedding at any time and careful hygiene practices (such as not sharing towels or other personal items) even during latency periods
- The need for prompt treatment and the necessity for sexual abstinence until lesions have healed, or using a condom while lesions are present
- The increased risk of cervical cancer and the importance of an annual Pap smear when diagnosed with HPV
- The importance of thorough handwashing.

Evaluation

Client care may be evaluated on the basis of the following expected outcomes:

- Resolution of the STI (for those STIs that can be treated and cured by antibiotics)
- Client explains strategies to prevent infection of others
- Client abstains from sexual activity until STI is treated
- Client describes barrier methods to reduce risk of contracting an STI.

REVIEW Sexually Transmitted Infections

RELATE: LINK THE CONCEPTS

Linking the exemplar of Sexually Transmitted Infection with the concept of Reproduction:

1. How will care of the pregnant client with genital herpes differ from the care provided to a pregnant client who does not have this infection?
2. What is your priority nursing diagnosis for the young couple contemplating pregnancy who are both diagnosed with genital warts?

Linking the exemplar of Sexually Transmitted Infection with the concept of Comfort:

3. Create a plan of care addressing pain management for the client diagnosed with candidiasis.
4. What teaching will you provide the client using sitz baths for pain relief resulting from genital warts?

READY: GO TO COMPANION SKILLS MANUAL

- Assessing the female genital and inguinal area
- Assessing the male genital and inguinal area

REFER: GO TO MYNURSINGKIT

REFLECT: CASE STUDY

Maggie Lynch is a 14-year-old who has a 6-month old daughter named Amy. Maggie lives with her single mother, Marcia, who has become very controlling of Maggie since she became pregnant. Marcia has forced Maggie to go back to school, which Maggie was very much against. Maggie participates very little in Amy's care. Marcia treats Amy as if she were her own child. There is a great deal of friction between Marcia and Maggie.

Maggie has been skipping class occasionally to be with her 16-year-old boyfriend, Brett, who is Amy's father. Brett has no interest in Amy but his parents make the effort to see Amy often. Maggie and Brett have resumed their physical relationship despite objections from both families.

Marcia accidentally interrupts Maggie in the bathroom and notices a foul odor in the room. Marcia questions Maggie and learns she has noticed a frothy yellow vaginal discharge in addition to the foul odor. Marcia arranges for Maggie to be seen by her gynecologist.

1. The nurse calls Maggie from the waiting room. Should she allow Maggie's mother to accompany them to the exam room? Explain your answer.
2. What teaching will you initiate for Maggie once diagnosis is made and treatment ordered?
3. How will you respond to Marcia when she demands that you tell her what is wrong with Maggie?

PEARSON

EXPLORE mynursingkit™

MyNursingKit is your one stop for online chapter review materials and resources. Prepare for success with additional NCLEX®-style practice questions, interactive assignments and activities, web links, animations and videos, and more!

Register your access code from the front of your book at **www.mynursingkit.com.**

REFERENCES

About Women's Health. (2005). *Causes and treatments for menstrual cramps.* Retrieved from http://womenshealth.about.com/cs/crampsmenstrual/a/cramps.htm

AHA cautions against using HRT to prevent CVD. (2001). *Geriatrics, 56*(9), 15–16.

American Academy of Pediatrics Task Force on Circumcision. (1999). Circumcision policy statement. *Pediatrics, 103,* 686–693.

American Social Health Association. (2005). *Facts & answers about STDs: Statistics.* Retrieved from http://www.ashastd.org/stdfaqs/statistics.html

American Society of Reproductive Medicine (ASRM). (2006a). *Frequently asked questions about infertility.* Retrieved March 24, 2008, from www.asrm.org/patients/faqs.htm

American Society of Reproductive Medicine (ASRM). (2006b). *Frequently asked questions. The psychological component of infertility.* Retrieved March 24, 2008, from www.asrm.org/patients/faqs.htm

American Society of Reproductive Medicine (ASRM). (2007). *Assisted reproductive technologies: A guide for parents.* Retrieved March 24, 2008, from www.asrm.org/patientbooklets/assisted

Annon, J. (1974). *The behavioral treatment of sexual problems: Volume I, Brief therapy.* Honolulu, HI: Enabling Systems.

Association of Reproductive Health Professionals. (2005b). *Physiology of the perimenopause: Treatment options.* Retrieved from http://www.arhp.org/healthcareproviders/onlinepublications/ clinicalproceedings.cfm?ID=177

Bickley, L., & Szilagyi, P. (2007). *Bates' guide to physical examination and history taking* (9th ed.). Philadelphia: Lippincott.

Blair, M. (2004). Sexually transmitted diseases: An update. *Urology Nursing, 24*(6), 467–473.

Blieszner, R., & deVries, B. (2001). Perspectives on intimacy. *Generations, 25*(2), 7–8.

Butler, R. N., & Lewis, M. I. (2003). Sexuality and aging. In W. R. Hazzard, J. P. Blass, J. B. Halter, J. G. Ouslander, & M. E. Tinetti (Eds.), *Principles of geriatric medicine and gerontology* (5th ed., pp. 1277–1282). New York: McGraw-Hill.

Centers for Disease Control and Prevention (CDC). (2004). *STD general information (PID, syphilis, trichomoniasis, human papillomavirus, genital herpes, HPV, chlamydia).* Retrieved from http://www.cdc.gov/std.htm

Centers for Disease Control and Prevention (CDC). (2006). Treatment guidelines for sexually transmitted diseases. Retrieved from http://www.cdc. gov/std/treatment.htm

CenterS for Disease Control and Prevention (CDC). (2007). Unintended pregnancy prevention. Retrieved on February 11, 2008, from http://www.cdc.gov/reproductivehealth/UnintendedPregnancy/index.htm

Centers for Disease Control and Prevention (CDC). (2008). Youth risk behavioral surveillance—United States 2007. *Morbidity and Mortality Weekly Report, 57*(SS-4).

Clark, L. R., Jackson, M., & Allen-Taylor, L. (2002). Adolescent knowledge about sexually transmitted diseases. *Sexually Transmitted Diseases, 29*(8), 436–443.

Cleveland Clinic. (2004). *Erectile dysfunction: Drugs linked to erectile dysfunction.* Retrieved from http://my.webmd.com/content/article/57/66229

Daniluk, J. C. (1998). *Women's sexuality across the life span: Challenging myths, creating meanings.* New York: Guilford Press.

Devine, K. S. (2008). *Challenges and management of infertility, including assisted reproductive technologies.* White Plains, NY: March of Dimes Foundation.

Elwood, A. (2005). Female genital cutting, 'circumcision' and mutilation. *Contemporary Sexuality, 39*(1), i–vii.

FDA orders estrogen safety warnings: Agency offers guidance for HRT use. (2003). *Journal of the American Medical Association, 289,* 537–538.

Food and Drug Administration (FDA). (2007). Over-the-counter vaginal contraceptive and spermicide drug products containing nonoxynol 9; required labeling. Final rule. *Federal Register, 72*(243), 71769–71785.

Hatcher, R. A., Trussell, J., Stewart, F., Nelson, A., Cates, W., Guest, F., & Kowal, D. (2004). *Contraceptive technology* (18th ed.). New York: Ardent Media, Inc.

Hartford Institute for Geriatric Nursing. (2001). *Incorporating essential gerontologic content into baccalaureate nursing education and staff development* (3rd ed.). New York: Author.

Health & Science. (2006). *Study: Estrogen protects some from breast cancer.* Retrieved from http://cis.nci.nih.gov/fact/5_29.htm

Inhorn, M. C. (2002). "Local" confronts the "Global": Infertile bodies and the new reproductive technology in Egypt. In M. C. Inhorn & F. Van Balen (Eds.), *Infertility around the globe: New thinking on childness, gender, and reproductive technologies.* Berkeley and Los Angeles: University of California Press.

Jick, S. S., & Jick, H. (2007). The *contraceptive patch* in relation to ischemic stroke and acute myocardial infarction. *Pharmacotherapy, 27*(2), 218–220.

Johnson, B. K. (1996). Older adults and sexuality: A multidimensional perspective. *Journal of Gerontological Nursing, 22*(2), 6–15.

Kaestle, C. E., Halpern, C. T., Miller, W. C., & Ford, C. A. (2005). Young age at first sexual intercourse and sexually transmitted infections in adolescents and young adults. *American Journal of Epidemiology, 161,* 774–780.

Kahn, S. M. (2002). Rabbis and reproduction: The uses of new reproductive technologies among Ultraorthodox Jews in Israel. In M. C. Inhorn & F. Van Balen (Eds.), *Infertility around the globe: New thinking on childness, gender, and reproductive technologies.* Berkeley and Los Angeles: University of California Press.

Kumar, A., Ghadir, S., Eskandari, N., & DeCherney, A. H. (2007). Infertility. In A. H. DeCherney, L. Nathan, T. M. Goodwin, & N. Laufer (Eds.), *Current diagnosis and treatment: Obstetrics & gynecology* (10th ed.). Boston: McGraw Hill.

Lichtenberg, P. A. (1997). Clinical perspectives on sexual issues in nursing homes. *Topics in Geriatric Rehabilitation, 12*(4), 1–10.

Masters, W. H. (1986). Sex and aging: Expectations and reality. *Hospital Practice, 21*(8), 177.

Mayo Clinic. (2004). *Premenstrual syndrome: Complementary and alternative medicines*. Retrieved from http://www.mayoclinic.com/invoke.cfm?objectid=95C74A46-ACOA-405D-AEC831A8CF4&dsect

McCance, K., & Huether, S. (2001). *Pathophysiology: The biologic basis of disease in adults and children.* St. Louis, MO: Mosby.

McCammon, S. L., Knox, D., & Schacht, C. (2004). *Choices in sexuality* (2nd ed.). Cincinnati, OH: Atomic Dog Publishing.

Memmel, L., & Gilliam, M. (2008). Contraception. In R. S. Gibbs, B. Y. Karlan, A. F. Haney, & I. E. Nygaard, (Eds.), *Danforth's Obstetrics and Gynecology* (10th ed.). Philadelphia: Wolters Kluwer/Lippincott Williams & Wilkins.

Metzger, D. A. (2004). New advances in the diagnosis and treatment of vulvar/vestibular pain disorders. *Conference proceedings: Women's Sexual Health.* The Berman Center and Northwestern University, Feinberg School of Medicine, Department of Obstetrics and Gynecology, Chicago.

Monga, T. N., Monga, U., Tan, G., & Grabois, M. (1999). Coital positions and sexual functioning in patients with chronic pain. *Sexuality and Disability, 17,* 287–297.

Morelli, V., & Naquin, C. (2002). Alternative therapies for traditional disease states: Menopause. *American Family Physician, 66,* 129–134.

National Kidney and Urologic Diseases Information Clearinghouse (NKUDIC). (2003a). Erectile dysfunction. Available http://kidney.niddk.nih.gov/kudiseases/pubs/impotence/

Nelson, H. D., Humphrey, L. L., Nygren, P., Teutsch, S. M., & Allan, J. D. (2002). Postmenopausal hormone replacement therapy: Scientific review. *Journal of the American Medical Association, 288,* 872–881.

Noblett, K. L., & Ostergard, D. R. (1999). Gynecologic disorders. In W. R. Hazzard, J. P. Blass, W. H. Ettinger, J. B. Halter, & J. G. Ouslander (Eds.), *Principles of geriatric medicine and gerontology* (4th ed., 797–807). New York: McGraw-Hill.

Office of Population Research & Association of Reproductive Health Professionals. (2007). Emergency contraception pills ("Morning after pills"). Retrieved September 9, 2007, from http://ec.princeton.edu/info/ecp.html

Penney, D. S. (2008). The effects of vigorous exercise during pregnancy. (2008). *Journal of Midwifery and Women's Health, 53*(2), 155–159.

Porth, C. M. (2005). *Pathophysiology: Concepts of altered health states* (7th ed.). Philadelphia: Lippincott.

Purnell, L. D., & Paulanka, B. J. (2008). *Transcultural health care: A culturally competent approach*. Philadelphia: F. A. Davis.

Schiavi, R. C., & Rehman, J. (1995). Sexuality and aging. *Urological Clinics of North America, 22,* 711–726.

Shafii, T., & Burstein, G. R. (2004). An overview of sexually transmitted infections among adolescents. *Adolescent Medicine Clinics, 15*(2), 201–214.

Shulman, L. P. (2005). Unique progestational impact on PMS/PMDD. Innovative options for patient care, a new way of thinking. CE Monograph. Released February 2005.

Simpson, J. L., & Holzgreve, W. (2007). Genetic counseling and genetic screening. In S. G. Gabbe, J. R. Niebyl, & J. L. Simpson (Eds.), *Obstetrics: Normal and problem pregnancies* (5th ed., pp. 138–151). Philadelphia, PA: Churchill Livingstone.

Speroff, L., & Darney, P. (2005). *A clinical guide for contraception* (4th ed.). Philadelphia: Lippincott Williams & Wilkins.

Nay, R. (1992). Sexuality and aged women in nursing homes. *Geriatric Nursing, 13*(6), 312–314.

Nelson, C. P., Dunn, R., Wan, J., & Wei, J. T. (2005). The increasing incidence of newborn circumcision: Data from the nationwide inpatient sample. *Journal of Urology, 173,* 978–981.

Speroff, L., & Fritz, M. (2005). *Clinical gynecologic endocrinology and infertility*. Philadelphia, PA: Lippincott Williams & Wilkins.

Ward, K. (2008). Genetics in obstetrics and gynecology. In R. S. Gibbs, B. Y. Karlan, A. F. Haney, & I. Nygaard (Eds.), *Danforth's obstetrics and gynecology* (10th ed., pp. 88–110). Philadelphia, PA: Lippincott Williams & Wilkins.

Welner, S. L. (1999). Menopausal issues. *Sexuality and Disability, 17*(3), 259–267.

World Health Organization. (1975). *Education and treatment in human sexuality: The training of health professionals*. Geneva: Author.

Wright, K. P., & Johnson, J. (2008). Infertility. In R. S. Gibbs, B. Y. Karlan, A. F. Haney, & I. Nygaard (Eds.), *Danforth's obstetrics and gynecology* (10th ed., pp. 705–715). Philadelphia, PA: Lippincott Williams & Wilkins.

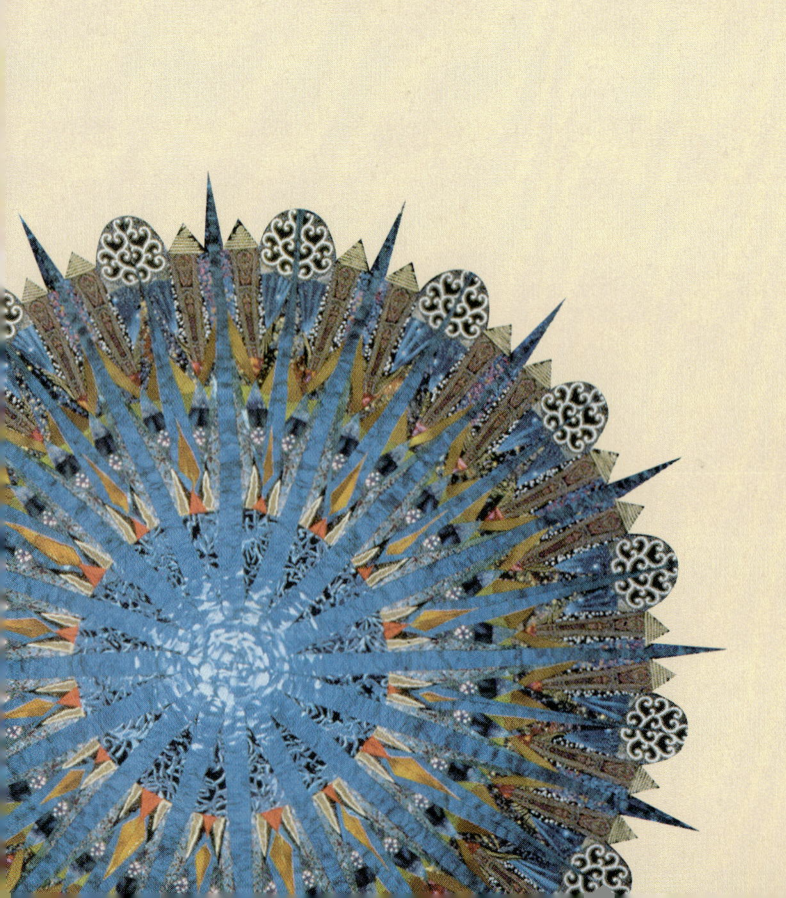

Spirituality 27

Concept at-a-Glance

Concept Learning Outcomes

After reading about this concept, you will be able to:

1. Define the concept of spirituality as it relates to nursing and health care.
2. Identify characteristics of spiritual health.
3. Identify factors associated with, and manifestations of, spiritual distress.
4. Describe the spiritual development of the individual across the life span.
5. Describe the influence of spiritual beliefs on diet, dress, meditation, prayer, birth, and death as they impact health care.
6. Demonstrate common assessments to determine the spiritual needs of clients.
7. Describe evidenced-based nursing interventions to support clients' spiritual beliefs and meet spiritual needs.
8. Identify desired outcomes for evaluating the client's spiritual health.

Concept Key Terms

Agnostic, *1771*
Atheist, *1771*
Faith, *1771*
Hope, *1772*
Kosher, *1773*
Monotheism, *1771*
Polytheism, *1771*
Religion, *1771*
Spiritual distress, *1771*
Spiritual health, *1770*
Spiritual well-being, *1770*
Spirituality, *1769*
Transcendence, *1772*

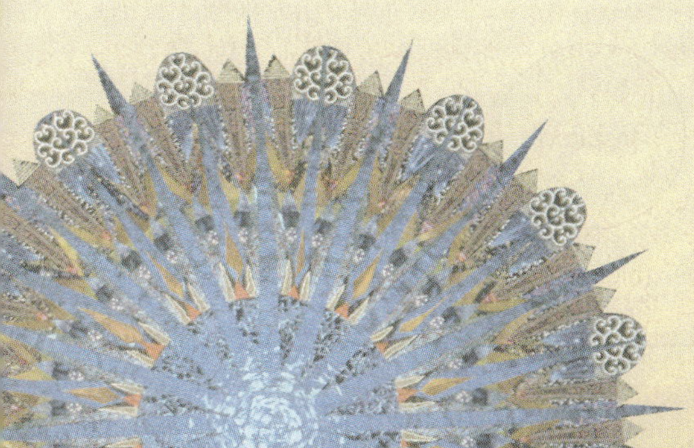

About Spirituality

Spirituality, faith, and religion are separate entities, yet the words are often used interchangeably. The word *spiritual* derives from the Latin word *spirare*, which means "to blow" or "to breathe," and has come to connote that which gives life or essence to being human. **Spirituality** refers to the part of being human that seeks meaningfulness through intrapersonal, interpersonal, and transpersonal connection (Reed, 1992). Spirituality generally involves a belief in a relationship with some higher power, creative force, divine being, or infinite source of energy. For example, a person may believe in *God*, *Allah*, the *Great Spirit*, or a *Higher Power*. Spirituality includes the following aspects (Martsolf & Mickley, 1998):

- Meaning (having purpose, making sense of life)
- Value (having cherished beliefs and standards)
- Transcendence (appreciating a dimension that is beyond the self)
- Connecting (relating to others, nature, Ultimate Other)
- Becoming (involves reflection, allowing life to unfold, and knowing who one is).

Words or concepts that are reflective of spirituality, such as faith, courage, cheer, and hope, may be used in ordinary speech in discussing spirituality.

Spirituality can be described by measuring it, so to speak, on a "spirit titer" (Jourard, 1971). One's spirit titer is influenced by numerous factors, such as life experiences, coping skills, social supports, and individual belief systems. Individuals experience multiple changes and losses over their life span, and if their spirit titer is low, they may become dispirited, or depressed. If they have a high spirit titer, they will lean toward being inspired and becoming an inspiration to others in spite of hardships they experience (Figure 27–1 ■). Nurses need to direct their goals and planning to assist clients in attaining and maintaining a high spirit titer. •

COMPONENTS OF SPIRITUALITY

Spirituality incorporates a number of components including spiritual needs, spiritual health and well being, spiritual distress, and core aspects of spirituality such as religion, faith, and hope. It is important for nurses to have a solid understanding of spirituality itself, how spirituality influences a client's decision making, and how spirituality can be impacted by illness.

Spiritual Needs

Just as everybody has a spiritual dimension, all clients have needs that reflect their spirituality. These needs are often accentuated by an illness or other health crisis. Clients who have well-defined spiritual beliefs may find that their beliefs are challenged by their health situation or may cling to their beliefs more firmly and appreciatively. Clients who have no defined beliefs may suddenly come face to face with challenging questions such as "Why me?" and others related to the meaning and purpose of life. Nurses need to be sensitive to indications of the client's spiritual needs and respond appropriately, as will be discussed later. Examples of spiritual needs are listed in Box 27–1.

Box 27–1 Examples of Spiritual Needs

NEEDS RELATED TO THE SELF:

- Need for meaning and purpose
- Need to express creativity
- Need for hope
- Need to transcend life challenges
- Need for personal dignity
- Need for gratitude
- Need for vision
- Need to prepare for and accept death.

NEEDS RELATED TO OTHERS:

- Need to forgive others
- Need to cope with loss of loved ones.

NEEDS RELATED TO THE ULTIMATE OTHER:

- Need to be certain there is a God or Ultimate Power in the universe
- Need to believe that God is loving and personally present
- Need to worship.

NEEDS AMONG AND WITHIN GROUPS:

- Need to contribute or improve one's community
- Need to be respected and valued
- Need to know what and when to give and take.

Note: From Taylor, E. J. (2002). *Spiritual care: Nursing theory, research, and practice.* Upper Saddle River, NJ: Prentice Hall. Reprinted by permission of Pearson Education, Inc., Upper Saddle River, New Jersey.

Spiritual Health and Well-Being

Spiritual health, or **spiritual well-being**, is manifested by a feeling of being "generally alive, purposeful, and fulfilled" (Ellison, 1983, p. 332). According to Pilch (1998), spiritual wellness is "a way of living, a lifestyle that views and lives life as purposeful and pleasurable, that seeks out life-sustaining and life-enriching options to be chosen freely at every opportunity, and that sinks its roots deeply into spiritual values and/or specific religious beliefs" (p. 31). Spiritual health, as defined by the Nursing Outcomes Classification project (Moorhead, Johnson, & Maas, 2004, p. 519) is the "connectedness with self, others, higher power, all life, nature and the universe that transcends and empowers the self." Indicators of spiritual health are shown in Box 27–2.

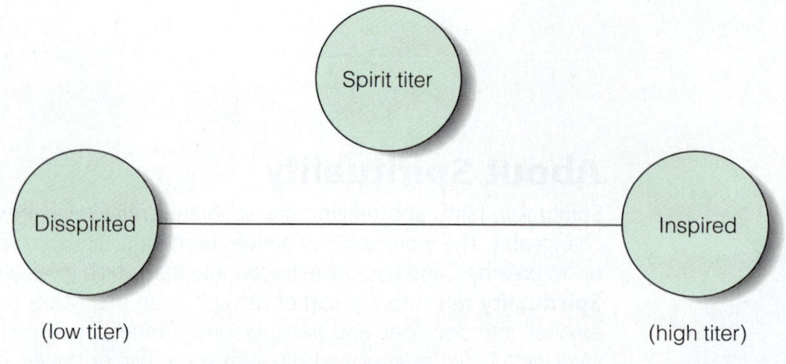

Figure 27–1 ■ Spirit titer.

Box 27–2 Indicators of Spiritual Health

UNCOMPROMISED. . .
Faith
Hope
Meaning and purpose in life
Achievement of spiritual world
Feelings of peacefulness
Ability to love
Ability to forgive
Ability to pray
Ability to worship
Spiritual experiences
Participation in spiritual rites and passages
Participation in meditation
Participation in spiritual reading
Interaction with spiritual leaders
Expression through song/music
Expression through art
Expression through writing
Connectedness with inner self
Connectedness with others
Interaction with others to share thoughts, feelings, and beliefs

Note: Reprinted from Moorhead, S., Johnson, M., & Mass, M. (2004). *Iowa intervention project: Nursing outcome classification*. With permission from Elsevier.

People nurture or enhance their spirituality in many ways. Some focus on development of the inner self; others focus on the expression of their spiritual energy with others or the outer world. Relating to one's inner self or soul may be achieved by conducting an inner dialogue with a higher power or with oneself through prayer or meditation, by analyzing dreams, by communing with nature, or by experiencing the inspiration of art (e.g., drama, music, dance). The expression of a person's spiritual energy to others is manifested in loving relationships with and service to others, joy and laughter, participation in religious services and associated fellowship gatherings and activities, and expression of compassion, empathy, forgiveness, and hope. Nurses who attend to their own spirituality are better able to work with clients who have spiritual needs (Taylor, 2005). Therefore, it is important to be comfortable with one's own spirituality.

Spiritual Distress

Spiritual distress refers to a challenge to one's spiritual well-being or to the belief system that provides strength, hope, and meaning to life. Some factors that may be associated with or contribute to a person's spiritual distress include physiological problems, treatment-related concerns, and situational concerns. Physiological problems include having a medical diagnosis of a terminal or debilitating disease, experiencing pain, experiencing the loss of a body part or function, or experiencing a miscarriage or stillbirth. Treatment-related factors include recommendation for blood transfusions, abortion, surgery, dietary restrictions, amputation of a body part, or isolation. Situational factors include the death or illness of a significant other, inability to practice one's spiritual rituals, or feelings of embarrassment when practicing them (Carpenito-Moyet, 2006).

Core Aspects of Spirituality

Because spirituality is a reflection of an inner experience that is expressed individually, it includes as many representations as there are human beings. Core aspects of spirituality include religion, faith, hope, transcendence, and forgiveness.

RELIGION **Religion** is an organized system of beliefs and practices. It offers a way of spiritual expression that provides guidance for believers in responding to life's questions and challenges. According to Vardey (1996, p. xv), organized religions offer the following:

- A sense of community bound by common beliefs
- The collective study of scripture (the Torah, Bible, Koran, or others)
- The performance of ritual
- The use of disciplines and practices, commandments, and sacraments
- Ways of taking care of the person's spirit (such as fasting, prayer, and meditation).

Many traditional religious practices and rituals are related to such life events as birth, transition from childhood to adulthood, marriage, illness, and death. Religious rules of conduct, typically influenced concurrently by culture, may also apply to matters of daily life such as dress, food, social interaction, menstruation, and sexual relationships.

Religious development of an individual refers to the acceptance of specific beliefs, values, rules of conduct, and rituals. Religious development may or may not parallel spiritual development. For example, a person may follow certain religious practices and yet not internalize the symbolic meaning behind the practices. Often religious development strengthens and enhances spirituality by providing a system of belief that can suggest areas of growth to the believer. For example, the daily prayers of the Muslims bring the believers into direct relationship with the profound questions of life several times per day.

An **agnostic** is a person who doubts the existence of God or a supreme being or who believes that the existence of God has not been proved. An **atheist** is a person who does not believe in a God. **Monotheism** is the belief in the existence of one god, while **polytheism** is the belief in more than one god.

FAITH **Faith** is to believe in or be committed to something or someone. Fowler (1981) described faith as being present in both religious and nonreligious people. Faith gives life meaning, providing the individual with strength in times of difficulty. For the client who is ill, faith—whether in a higher authority (e.g., God, Allah, Jehovah), in oneself, in the health care team, or in a combination of all of these—provides strength and hope. The term *faith* may be used in a way that is interchangeable with the term *religion*. For example, the term *faith-based organization* is often used to refer to an organization or agency that is affiliated with a particular religion or religious faith.

HOPE **Hope** is a concept that incorporates spirituality. Stephenson (1991) suggested this definition: "a process of anticipation that involves the interaction of thinking, acting, feeling, and relating, and is directed toward a future fulfillment that is personally meaningful" (p. 1459). In the absence of hope, the client gives up, losing spirit. In the client who has lost hope, illness is likely to progress more rapidly.

TRANSCENDENCE The term **transcendence** is often used interchangeably with self-transcendence, which Coward (1990) defined as "the capacity to reach out beyond oneself, to extend oneself beyond personal concerns and to take on broader life perspectives, activities, and purposes" (p. 162). Transcendence is also thought to involve a person's recognition that there is something other or greater than the self and a seeking and valuing of that greater other, whether it is an ultimate being, force, or value.

FORGIVENESS The concept of forgiveness is receiving increased attention among health care professionals. For many clients, illness or disability brings a sense of shame or guilt. The health problem is interpreted as a punishment for past sins (e.g., "Having sex before I got married is why I have breast cancer"). Clients facing imminent death may seek forgiveness from others as well as from God. Mickley and Cowles's (2001) research suggested that nurses can play a pivotal role in assisting clients to understand the process of forgiveness and to persevere through it.

Spiritual Development

Just as individuals develop physically, cognitively, and morally, they also develop spiritually. Several theologians have identified specific linear stages through which individuals may progress while maturing spiritually. Westerhoff (1976), for example, described faith as a way of behaving that evolves from a faith guided by parents and others during infancy and childhood to an owned faith that is internalized in adulthood and serves as a directive for action. Table 27–1 describes some of the aspects of spiritual development and healthful religious behaviors during different life stages.

SPIRITUAL PRACTICES AFFECTING NURSING CARE

Clients frequently identify religious practices such as prayer as important strategies for coping with illness (Mauk & Schmidt, 2004; Taylor, 2003b). The most common practices affecting the nursing care of clients include practices associated with diet, nutrition, healing, dress, birth, and death.

It is possible for nurses to unethically impose personal spiritual beliefs on clients, whose circumstances inherently leave them vulnerable. Observing guidelines for ethical conduct in spiritual caregiving is essential. The following

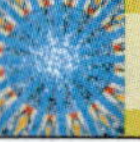

DEVELOPMENTAL CONSIDERATIONS Spiritual Development

CHILDREN

The development of spirituality in children parallels their cognitive and psychosocial development. As children mature, they are increasingly capable of understanding spiritual matters, stating spiritual beliefs, and incorporating spirituality into their lives.

A developing spirituality includes the following:

- A sense of wholeness, having internal resources and identity
- Being attached to others, and being a part of a greater, even transcendent, world
- Having a sense of meaning and purpose in one's life
- Being able to express hope, even in the face of fear, uncertainty, and serious illness (Howden, 1992).

Nurses should help ill or injured children and their parents identify and express these qualities. This can be done by actively listening, by offering opportunities to practice religious rituals, and by providing materials for nonverbal expression (e.g., painting, play, music).

OLDER ADULTS

Many older adults frequently use and highly value religious coping strategies such as prayer. Evidence shows spiritual well-being to be directly correlated with mental health and less medical illness among older adults (Koenig, 2002). It is, therefore, important to address the spiritual issues of this population. Older adults may be especially concerned about living a purposeful life, about maintaining loving relationships to avoid social isolation, and about preparing for a good death. Nursing care for older adults that attends to such spiritual issues includes

- supporting meaning-making activities (e.g., conducting a life review or reminiscence therapy; allowing the client to weave together the strands of lived life; encouraging the client to become dedicated to some social, political, religious, or artistic cause; supporting the client to leave a legacy or do an altruistic deed). Such activities provide older adults with a sense of purpose for their life and assist them to make sense of the life that they have lived.
- allowing open discussions about suffering and dying, encouraging client disclosure by asking open-ended questions, and providing responses that are respectful and compassionate. Do not avoid discomforting topics and questions that older adults raise by imposing positivity, giving pat answers, or otherwise minimizing or avoiding their spiritual pain.
- as appropriate, supporting older adults to reframe the "losses" of aging as "liberations." For example, older adults possess great wisdom and are in a season of life that promotes spiritual growth.

Clients with dementia present special circumstances for spiritual caregiving. Nurses can help those with early stages of dementia to focus on the positives, the "haves" rather than the losses. Allowing older adults with dementia to tell their stories helps them to maintain some identity (amidst a disease that threatens the very sense of self) and gives the nurse a window into their world. Clients with dementia can also worship and express their hope and creativity through various art forms (e.g., movement, painting, music). It is also possible for them to experience the compassion of others when they feel their caring touch or hear their soothing voice.

TABLE 27–1 Stages of Spiritual Development

DEVELOPMENTAL STAGE	CHARACTERISTICS
0–3 years	Neonates and toddlers acquire fundamental spiritual qualities of trust, mutuality, courage, hope, and love. Transition to the next stage of faith begins when the child's language and thought begin to allow use of symbolism.
3–7 years	Fantasy-filled, imitative phase when child can be influenced by examples, moods, actions. Child relates intuitively to ultimate conditions of existence through stories and images, the fusion of facts and feelings. Make-believe is experienced as reality (Santa Claus, God as grandfather in the sky).
7–12 years, even into adulthood	Child attempts to sort fantasy from fact by demanding proofs or demonstrations of reality. Stories are important for finding meaning and organizing experiences. Child accepts stories and beliefs literally. Child has the ability to learn the beliefs and practices of the culture, religion.
Adolescence	Experience of the world beyond the family unit and spiritual beliefs can aid understanding of extended environment. Adolescents generally conform to the beliefs of those around them; they begin to examine beliefs objectively, especially in late adolescence.
Young adulthood	The young adult develops a self-identity and worldview differentiated from those of others. The individual forms independent commitments, lifestyle, beliefs, and attitudes, and begins to develop personal meaning for symbols of religion and faith.
Mid-adulthood	The person finds newfound appreciation for the past; increased respect for inner voice; and more awareness of myths, prejudices, and images that exist because of social background. Individual attempts to reconcile contradictions in mind and experience and to remain open to others' truths.
Mid- to late adulthood	Individual is able to believe in, and live with a sense of participation in, a nonexclusive community. May work to resolve social, political, economic, or ideological problems in society. Able to embrace life, yet hold it loosely. (Martin Luther King, Jr., Mahatma Gandhi, and Mother Teresa illustrate this stage.)

Note: Adapted from content from Fowler, J. W. (1981). *Stages of faith development: The psychology of human development and the quest for meaning.* Reprinted with permission of HarperCollins Publishers.

guidelines for nurses were offered by Winslow and Winslow (2003):

- First seek a basic understanding of clients' spiritual needs, resources, and preferences (i.e., assess).
- Follow the client's expressed wishes regarding spiritual care.
- Do not prescribe or urge clients to adopt certain spiritual beliefs or practices, and do not pressure them to relinquish any of their beliefs or practices.
- Strive to understand personal spirituality and how it influences caregiving.
- Provide spiritual care in a way that is consonant with personal beliefs.

PRACTICE ALERT

While some clients are eager for nurses' overt offers of "spiritual care," others may be uncertain or opposed to such offers (Taylor, 2003a). Clients often confuse religiosity with spirituality; this may contribute to their uncertainty about receiving spiritual care from nurses. Observing and using the client's language for spirituality (e.g., "being at peace" or "faith"), as well as large measures of sensitivity and respect, will help nurses to converse therapeutically with clients to provide spiritual care.

Beliefs Affecting Diet and Nutrition

Many religions have proscriptions regarding diet. There may be rules about which foods and beverages are allowed and which are prohibited. For example, Orthodox Jews are not to eat shellfish or pork, and Muslims are not to drink alcoholic beverages or eat pork. Members of the Church of Jesus Christ of Latter-Day Saints (Mormons) are not to drink caffeinated or alcoholic beverages. Older Catholics may choose not to eat meat on Fridays because it was proscribed in years past, and abstinence from meat is still required on some days during Lent. Buddhists and Hindus are generally vegetarian, not wanting to take life to support life. Religious law may also dictate how food is prepared; for example, many Jewish people require **kosher** food, which is food prepared according to Jewish law.

Some solemn religious observances are marked by fasting, which is the abstinence from food for a specified period of time. Some religions also restrict beverages; others allow drinking of water or other sustaining beverages on fast days. Examples of religions that observe fasting include Islam, Judaism, and Catholicism. During the month of Ramadan, devout Muslims eat no food and avoid beverages during daylight hours; the fast is broken after sunset. Members of Jewish synagogues fast on Yom Kippur, and devout Catholics may fast on Ash Wednesday and Good Friday. Most religions lift the fasting requirements for seriously ill believers for whom fasting may be a detriment to health (e.g., diabetic clients). Some religions may exempt nursing mothers or menstruating women from fasting requirements.

It is important that health care providers prescribe diet plans with an awareness of the client's dietary and fasting beliefs.

Beliefs Related to Healing

Clients may have religious beliefs that attribute illness to a spiritual disruption. Healing for such clients may appear to be unrelated to current treatment practices. The nurse needs to assess the client's beliefs and, if possible, include some aspects of healing that are part of the client's belief system in the planning of care.

Beliefs Related to Dress

Many religions have laws or traditions that dictate dress. For example, Orthodox and Conservative Jewish men believe that it is important to have their heads covered at all times and therefore wear yarmulkes. Orthodox Jewish women cover their hair with a wig or scarf as a sign of respect to God. Many Muslim women also cover their hair in accordance with their particular ethnic or national background. Mormons may wear temple undergarments in compliance with religious law.

Some religions require that women dress in a conservative manner, which may include wearing sleeves and modestly cut tops, and skirts that cover the knees. Some religions, such as Islam, may require that the body (torso, arms, and legs) be covered. Hindu women accustomed to wearing saris prefer to cover all of the body except arms and feet (Figure 27–2 ■). Hospital gowns may make women who wish to comply with religious dress codes uneasy and uncomfortable. Clients may be especially disconcerted when undergoing diagnostic tests or treatments, such as mammography, that require body parts to be bared.

Beliefs Related to Birth

For all religions, the birth of a child is an important event giving cause for celebration. Many religions have specific ritual ceremonies that consecrate the new child to God. When a Muslim child is born, "someone recites the call to prayer in the infant's ear." On the seventh day after birth, the child is named, and a tuft of hair is shaved from the head (Denny, 1993, p. 682).

In the Christian faith, baptism and christening ceremonies may take place after the birth of a child to confirm that the "infant [was] born into a Christian family as part of the organism of the church" (Frankiel, 1993, p. 556). Christian parents of seriously ill infants may want baptism performed at birth by the nurse or primary care provider if a chaplain or clergy person is not present.

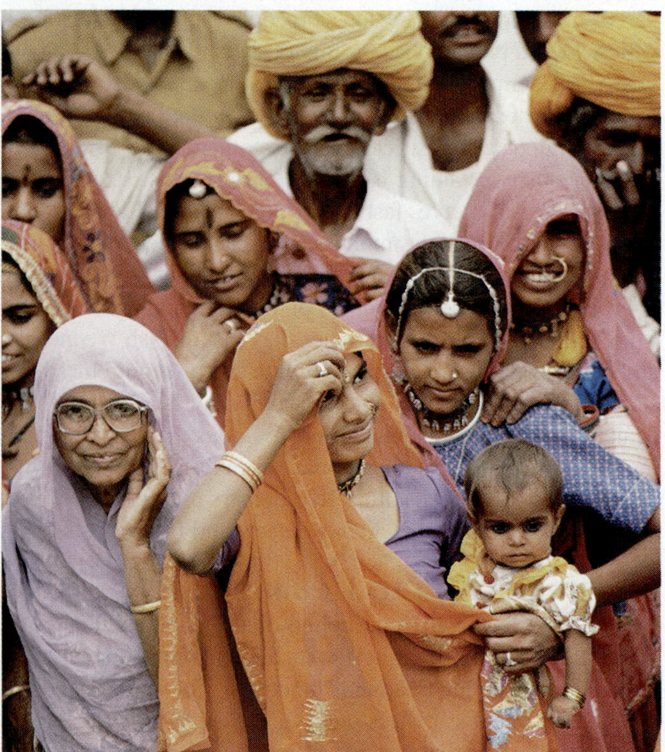
Figure 27–2 ■ Hindu women dressed in saris.

In the Jewish religion, the ritual circumcision conducted on male children on the eighth day after birth is an expression of the religious bond between the prophet Abraham, his descendants, and their God. Following the ritual circumcision by the trained person, called a *mohel*, the child is named. Girls are named in the synagogue on the Sabbath after the birth (Fishbane, 1993).

When nurses are aware of the religious needs of families and their infants, they can assist families in fulfilling their religious obligations. This is especially important when the newborn infant is seriously ill or in danger of dying, because some people believe that if religious obligations are not fulfilled the infant will not be accepted into the community of the faithful after death.

Beliefs Related to Death

Spiritual and religious beliefs play a significant role in the believer's approach to death just as they do in other major life events. Many believe that the person who dies transcends this life for a better place or state of being.

Some religions have special rituals surrounding dying and death that must be observed by the faithful. Observance of these rituals provides comfort to the dying person and his or her loved ones. Some rituals are carried out while the person is still alive, and can include special prayers, singing or chants, and reading of sacred scriptures. Roman Catholic priests perform the sacrament of Anointing of the Sick (previously referred to as the Last Rites or Extreme Unction) when clients are very ill or near death. Muslims who are dying want their body or head turned toward Mecca (Denny, 1993).

Jews have a tradition of burial within 24 hours following death, except on the Sabbath, and they sit Shiva (gather to pay respects), draping any mirrors in black to ensure that guests are focused on memory of the deceased rather than on themselves. Tibetan Buddhists read the *Tibetan Book of the Dead* within 7 days of the death to release the soul of the deceased from the Bardos, or nether worlds. Hindus cremate the body within 24 hours to release the soul from any earthly attachment.

Griffith (1996) suggested that during a terminal illness the client and family should be queried about observances or rituals that follow death. Some religions require that the body of the deceased be touched only by members of that faith. In both the Muslim (Denny, 1993) and Jewish (Fishbane, 1993) religions, believers may require that a ritual bath be given after death by a family member or by a ritual burial society. Religious symbols or objects should be treated with respect and kept with the body (Griffith, 1996). The nurse can support the family of the deceased by providing an environment conducive to the performance of its traditional death rituals.

PRACTICE ALERT

Before sharing personal beliefs or practices, a nurse must consider questions such as the following:

- For what purpose am I sharing my beliefs or practices? By doing so, am I meeting my needs or my client's?
- Is my spiritual care reflecting a spiritual assessment?
- Am I preying on a vulnerable client?
- Am I offering my beliefs or practices in a manner that allows my client to comfortably refuse?
- Does my spiritual care hurt or contribute to a therapeutic relationship with the client?

ASSESSMENT

Data about a client's spiritual beliefs are obtained from the client's general history (religious preferences or orientation); through a nursing history; and by clinical observations of the client's behavior, verbalizations, mood, and interactions with others. Nurses should never assume that a client follows all the practices of the client's stated religion.

Nursing History

The Joint Commission on Accreditation of Healthcare Organizations (2000) mandates that each client admitted to an institution's care must be assessed for spiritual beliefs and practices. Several experts (Cole, Benore, & Pargament, 2004; Koenig, 2002; Massey, Fitchett, & Roberts, 2004; Taylor, 2002) recommend a two-tiered approach to spiritual assessment. All clients can be asked a general question or two (e.g., "What spiritual beliefs or practices are important to you now while you live with illness?" "How would you like your health care team to support you spiritually?"). Only clients who manifest some type of unhealthful spiritual need or are at risk for spiritual distress need be subjected to a more thorough spiritual assessment. Even this assessment can be streamlined to hone in on the particular spiritual concern present.

Although the nurse will continually be assessing, the initial spiritual assessment is best taken at the end of the assessment process or following the psychosocial assessment, after the nurse has developed a relationship with the client and/or support person. A nurse who has demonstrated sensitivity and personal warmth, earning some rapport, will be more successful during a spiritual assessment.

Remembering an acronym such as FICA can also help the nurse to ask appropriate questions:

F (faith or beliefs)—for example, "What spiritual beliefs are most important to you?"

I (implications or influence)—for example, "How is your faith affecting the way you cope now?"

C (community)—for example, "Is there a group of like-minded believers with which you regularly meet?"

A (address)—for example, "How would you like your health care team to support you spiritually?" (Dameron, 2005; Massey et al., 2004).

Clinical Assessment

Cues to spiritual and religious preferences, strengths, concerns, or distress may be revealed by one or more of the following (Taylor, 2002):

- *Environment.* Does the client have a Bible, Torah, Koran, other prayer book, devotional literature, religious medals, rosary, cross, Star of David, or religious get-well cards in the room? Does a church send altar flowers or Sunday bulletins?
- *Behavior.* Does the client appear to pray before meals or at other times or read religious literature? Does the client have nightmares and sleep disturbances or express anger at religious representatives or at a deity?
- *Verbalization.* Does the client mention God or a higher power, prayer, faith, a church, a synagogue, a temple, a spiritual or religious leader, or religious topics? Does the client ask about a visit from the clergy? Does the client express fear of death, concern with the meaning of life, inner conflict about religious beliefs, concern about a relationship with a deity, questions about the meaning of existence or the meaning of suffering, or questions about the moral or ethical implications of therapy?
- *Affect and attitude.* Does the client appear lonely, depressed, angry, anxious, agitated, apathetic, or preoccupied?
- *Interpersonal relationships.* Who visits? How does the client respond to visitors? Does a minister or other spiritual mentor come? How does the client relate to other clients and nursing personnel?

In order to provide holistic care, it is important for the nurse to understand the spiritual needs and beliefs of the client. Understanding and support of a client's spiritual beliefs and practices builds trust in the nurse-client relationship, makes the client feel more comfortable in strange environments, and individualizes the nursing plan of care to meet each person's unique needs. Specific considerations and appropriate interventions are detailed in the exemplars that follow.

Assessment Interview Spirituality

- Are any particular religious practices important to you? If so, could you please tell me about them?
- How will being sick interfere with your religious practices?
- How is your faith helpful to you? In what ways is it important to you right now?
- In what ways can I support your spirit? For example, would you like me to read your prayer book to you?
- Would you like a visit from your spiritual counselor or the hospital chaplain?
- What are your hopes and your sources of strength right now? What comforts you during hard times?

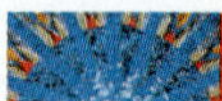

27.1 MORALITY

KEY TERMS

Accountability, *1778*
Autonomy, *1777*
Beneficence, *1777*
Bioethics, *1776*
Consequence-based (teleological) theories, *1777*
Ethics, *1776*
Fidelity, *1778*
Justice, *1778*
Moral development, *1776*
Moral rules, *1777*
Morality, *1776*
Nonmaleficence, *1777*
Nursing ethics, *1776*
Principles-based (deontological) theories, *1777*
Relationship-based (caring) theories, *1777*
Responsibility, *1778*
Utilitarianism, *1777*
Utility, *1777*
Veracity, *1778*

BASIS FOR SELECTION OF EXEMPLAR

NLN Competency

LEARNING OUTCOMES

After reading about this exemplar, you will be able to:

1. Define the concepts of morality as it relates to nursing and health care.
2. Identify factors associated with conflicts in, or alterations of, morality.
3. Describe theories, frameworks, and principles of moral development.
4. Describe nursing interventions to support clients experiencing moral dilemmas or distress.
5. Identify desired outcomes for clients experiencing moral dilemmas or distress.

OVERVIEW OF MORALITY AND ETHICS

The term **ethics** has several meanings in common use. It refers to (a) a method of inquiry that helps people to understand the morality of human behavior (i.e., it is the study of morality), (b) the practices or beliefs of a certain group (e.g., medical ethics, nursing ethics), and (c) the expected standards of moral behavior of a particular group as described in the group's formal code of ethics. The term **bioethics** describes the application of ethics to issues of human life or health (e.g., to decisions about abortion or euthanasia). The term **nursing ethics** refers to ethical issues that occur in nursing practice. The revised *Scope and Standards of Practice* (2003) of the American Nurses Association (ANA) holds nurses accountable for their ethical conduct. Nurses are repeatedly named as among the most ethical of professionals in various surveys (Gallup, 2005; Medical News Today, 2009).

Morality (or morals) is similar to ethics, and many people use the terms interchangeably. **Morality** usually refers to private, personal standards of what is right and wrong in conduct, character, and attitude. Sometimes the first clue to the moral nature of a situation is an aroused conscience or an awareness of feelings such as guilt, hope, or shame. Another indicator is the tendency to respond to the situation with words such as *ought*, *should*, *right*, *wrong*, *good*, and *bad*. Moral issues are concerned with important social values and norms; they are not about trivial things.

Nurses must be able to distinguish between morality and law. Laws reflect the moral values of a society, and they offer guidance in determining what is moral. However, an action can be legal but not moral. For example, an order for full resuscitation of a dying client is legal, but one could still question whether the act is moral. Conversely, an action can be moral but illegal. For example, if a child at home stops breathing, it is moral but not legal to exceed the speed limit when driving to the hospital. Legal aspects of nursing practice are covered in Concept 47, Legal Issues.

Nurses should also distinguish between morality and religion as they relate to health practices, although the two concepts are related. For example, according to some religious beliefs, women should undergo procedures such as female circumcision that may cause physical mutilation. Other religions or groups may consider this practice to be an ethical violation of the human right to self-determination (Hellsten, 2004) and an action that discriminates against women. Other common instances of differences in moral perspectives on health involving religious beliefs include blood transfusions, abortion, sterilization, and contraceptive and safer sex counseling.

Moral Development

Ethical decisions require persons to think and reason. Reasoning is a cognitive function and is, therefore, developmental. **Moral development** is the process of learning to tell

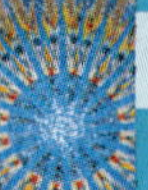

FOCUS ON DIVERSITY AND CULTURE
Confucian and Buddhist Religions

Many Chinese people are members of either the Confucian or the Buddhist religion. Confucian religious beliefs do not consider a fetus a human being. However, Buddhists believe the fetus is a form of human life. As a result, Chinese people may vary from each other in their views on abortion, depending on their religious affiliation.

the difference between right and wrong and of learning what ought and ought not to be done. It is a complex process that begins in childhood and continues throughout life.

Theories of moral development attempt to answer questions such as these: How does a person become moral? What factors influence the way a person behaves in a situation involving a question of morals? Two well-known theorists of moral development are Lawrence Kohlberg (1969) and Carol Gilligan (1982). Kohlberg's theory emphasizes rights and formal reasoning; Gilligan's theory emphasizes care and responsibility, although it points out that people use the concepts of both theorists in their moral reasoning. For a full discussion of these two theories, see Concept 7, Development.

Moral Frameworks

Moral theories provide different frameworks through which nurses can view and clarify client care situations. Nurses can use moral theories in developing explanations for their ethical decisions and actions and in discussing problem situations with others. Three types of moral theories are widely used, and they can be differentiated by their emphasis on (1) consequences, (2) principles and duties, or (3) relationships.

Consequence-based (teleological) theories look to the outcomes (consequences) of an action in judging whether that action is right or wrong. **Utilitarianism**, one form of consequentialist theory, views a good act as one that brings the most good and the least harm for the greatest number of people. This is called the principle of **utility**. This approach is often used in making decisions about the funding and delivery of health care. Teleological theories focus on issues of fairness.

Principles-based (deontological) theories involve logical and formal processes and emphasize individual rights, duties, and obligations. The morality of an action is determined not by its consequences, but by whether it is done according to an impartial, objective principle. For example, following the rule "Do not lie," a nurse might believe he or she should tell the truth to a dying client, even though the physician has given instruction not to do so. There are many deontological theories; each justifies the rules of acceptable behavior differently.

Relationship-based (caring) theories stress courage, generosity, commitment, and the need to nurture and maintain relationships. Unlike the two preceding types of theories, which frame problems in terms of justice (fairness) and formal reasoning, caring theories judge actions according to a perspective of caring and responsibility. Principles-based theories stress individual rights, but caring theories promote the common good or the welfare of the group.

A moral framework guides moral decisions, but it does not determine the outcome. Imagine a situation in which a frail, elderly client has made it clear that he does not want further surgery but the family and surgeon insist. Three nurses have each decided that they will not help with preparations for surgery and that they will work through proper channels to try to prevent it. Using consequence-based reasoning, Nurse A thinks, "Surgery will cause him more suffering; he probably will not survive it anyway, and the family may even feel guilty later." Using principles-based reasoning, Nurse B thinks, "This violates the principle of autonomy. This man has a right to decide what happens to his body." Using caring-based reasoning, Nurse C thinks, "My relationship to this client commits me to protecting him and meeting his needs, and I feel such compassion for him. I must try to help the family understand that he needs their support." Each of these different perspectives is based on the nurse's moral framework.

Moral Principles

Moral principles are statements about broad, general, philosophical concepts such as autonomy and justice. They provide the foundation for **moral rules**, which are specific prescriptions for actions. For example, the rule "People should not lie" is based on the moral principle of respect for persons (autonomy). Principles are useful in ethical discussions because even if people disagree about which action is right in a situation, they may be able to agree on the principles that apply. Such an agreement can serve as the basis for a solution that is acceptable to all parties. For example, most people would agree to the principle that nurses are obligated to respect their clients, even if they disagree as to whether the nurse should deceive a particular client about his or her prognosis.

Autonomy refers to the right to make one's own decisions. Nurses who follow this principle recognize that each client is unique, has the right to be who or what he or she is, and has the right to choose personal goals. People have "inward autonomy" if they have the ability to make choices; they have "outward autonomy" if their choices are not limited or imposed by others.

Honoring the principle of autonomy means that the nurse respects a client's right to make decisions even when those choices seem to the nurse not to be in the client's best interest. It also means treating others with consideration. In a health care setting, this principle is violated, for example, when a nurse disregards clients' subjective accounts of their symptoms (e.g., pain). Finally, respect for autonomy means that people should not be treated as an impersonal source of knowledge or training. This principle comes into play, for example, in the requirement that clients provide informed consent before tests, procedures, or involvement as a research participant can be carried out.

Nonmaleficence is the duty to "do no harm." Although this would seem to be a simple principle to follow, in reality it is complex. Harm can mean intentionally causing harm, placing someone at risk of harm, and unintentionally causing harm. In nursing, intentional harm is never acceptable. However, placing a person at risk of harm has many facets. A client may be at risk of harm as a known consequence of a nursing intervention that is intended to be helpful. For example, a client may react adversely to a medication. Unintentional harm occurs when the risk could not have been anticipated. For example, while catching a client who is falling, a nurse might grip the client tightly enough to cause bruises to the client's arm. Caregivers do not always agree on the degree of risk that is morally permissible in order to attempt the beneficial result.

Beneficence means "doing good." Nurses are obligated to do good, that is, to implement actions that benefit clients and their support persons. However, doing good can also pose a risk of doing harm. For example, a nurse may advise a client about a strenuous exercise program to improve general health but should not do so if the client is at risk of a heart attack.

Justice is often referred to as *fairness*. Nurses often face decisions in which a sense of justice should prevail. For example, a nurse making home visits finds one client tearful and depressed and knows that she could help by staying for 30 more minutes to talk. However, that would take time from her next client, who is a diabetic who needs a great deal of teaching and observation. The nurse will need to weigh the facts carefully in order to divide her time justly among her clients.

Fidelity means to be faithful to agreements and promises. By virtue of their standing as professional caregivers, nurses have responsibilities to clients, employers, government, and society, as well as to themselves. Nurses often make promises such as "I'll be right back with your pain medication" or "I'll find out for you." Clients take such promises seriously, and so should nurses.

Veracity refers to telling the truth. Although this seems straightforward, in practice choices are not always clear. Should a nurse tell the truth when it is known that it will cause harm? Does a nurse tell a lie when it is known that the lie will relieve anxiety and fear? Lying to sick or dying people is rarely justified. The loss of trust in the nurse and the anxiety caused by not knowing the truth, for example, usually outweigh any benefits derived from lying.

Nurses must also have professional accountability and responsibility. According to the *Code of Ethics for Nurses* (ANA, 2001), **accountability** means "answerable to oneself and others for one's own actions," while **responsibility** refers to "the specific accountability or liability associated with the performance of duties of a particular role." Thus, the ethical nurse is able to explain the rationale behind every action and recognizes the standards to which he or she will be held.

MORALITY AND THE PRACTICE OF NURSING

The Stanford Encyclopedia of Philosophy states that morality can be used to "normatively refer to a code of conduct that, given specified conditions, would be put forward by all rational persons." Given that nurses are seen as among the most ethical of professionals, it is difficult to accept that there are nurses who abuse their clients and nurses who witness abuse or are cognizant of it and say nothing. Unfortunately, such unethical or immoral behavior occurs. Certainly, it is exhibited by only a very few in the nursing profession, but it is behavior that all nurses must be able to identify, discourage, and report. Every nurse must understand that to know about the abuse of a client by a nurse or other health care professional and not report it is a violation of the *Code of Ethics for Nurses*; condoning or ignoring abuse is a violation of the nurse–client relationship.

In a series of articles in the fall of 2008, *Nursing Standard* explored the reasons why some nurses abuse, and sometimes kill, clients in their care (Wright, 2008). In a survey conducted by *Nursing Standard* and *Nursing Elder People*, 58% of 848 nurses surveyed said they would not report abuse of an older client or other client in their care for fear of "misinterpreting" the situation. Some respondents also cited fear of becoming a target of the abuser as a reason for not making a report (Doughty, 2007). The idea of a nurse willfully harming a client or allowing a client to be harmed is unthinkable, yet it happens.

Another "unthinkable" situation is described in a 2007 report of the American Red Cross, which found that nurses, physicians, and other health care professionals at Guantanamo Bay witnessed and condoned the torture of prisoners. Some detainees even reported that health care professionals had, at times, given interrogators instructions "to continue, to adjust, or to stop particular methods" of interrogation (Shane, 2009).

To rise above questionable and unethical practices, nurses must have a thorough understanding of their own morality and what constitutes right and wrong for them as individuals. They must also have a thorough understanding of their professional code of ethics and be able to identify when the ethics of another professional or another agency are contrary to the *Code of Ethics for Nurses.*

NURSING PROCESS

Just as the nurse will encounter clients of various cultural and religious backgrounds, he or she will encounter clients at various stages of moral development, clients with questionable or confusing morals, and even clients who are immoral. Nursing ethics and professional codes of conduct require nurses to deliver high-quality, professional care to all clients, regardless of client morality. This can challenge even the most professional, experienced nurse. Examples of these challenges include the following scenarios:

1. A client with HIV is transferred to the critical care unit (CCU) of a hospital from the prison infirmary. In addition to HIV, the client is paraplegic with no ability to move his legs. He is in prison on a life sentence for repeated child molestation and rape.
2. A young woman comes to the local free health clinic with her boyfriend to get a pregnancy test. The test is positive. The boyfriend immediately starts talking to her about how she'll have to get an abortion.
3. An older woman is brought to the emergency room by a friend who came to visit and found her lying in her own feces. She is weak and dehydrated. The friend says that the older woman lives with her son and his wife.
4. The nurse on the day shift at an inpatient rehabilitation center makes her morning rounds. She finds a young female client awake in her bed, crying. The woman has bruises on her wrists and forearms that were not there when the nurse last visited with the client the previous afternoon. When the nurse asks the client what happened, she responds only by shaking her head, and she pulls away when the nurse reaches out to comfort her. The nurse checks the visitor logs and confirms that the client had no visitors the night before.

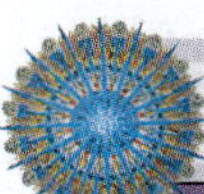

NURSING CARE PLAN **A Client Presenting Morality Issues**

ASSESSMENT

Michael Dunham is a 50-year-old white male with HIV who is also paraplegic. Mr. Dunham is admitted to the critical care unit of the local hospital from the prison infirmary, where he has been for more than a month. He is on oxygen by cannula. He is restrained to his bed. Almost every time the nursing staff works with him, he tries to spit on them in an effort to "give" them his disease. Upon arrival, the prison transport unit informs the head nurse that Mr. Dunham is serving a life sentence for molesting children and that he used his disability to trick the children into coming close enough for him to handcuff them to his wheelchair so they could not escape his sexual abuse. Before releasing them he would threaten to kill their parents if the children told anyone what happened.

Upon physical examination, the nurses working with this client find the following:

- T_O 37.9°C (100.2°F), P 104, R 32, BP 102/60
- Oxygen saturation 84%; breath sounds reveal course crackles in the left lower base
- Mild cyanosis of nail beds and mucous membranes
- Use of accessory muscles to breath with intercostal and suprasternal retractions
- Flaccid paralysis of lower extremities since he was 8 years old
- ECG shows 2–3 premature ventricular contractions per minute
- HIV positive with CD 4 T cell count of 64, CBC showed WBC of 9.8, elevated lymphocyte and low segs
- Chest x-ray shows characteristic appearance of *Pneumocystis carinii.*

DIAGNOSES

- Moral Distress
- Impaired Social Interaction
- Social Isolation
- Impaired Gas Exchange
- Risk-Prone Health Behavior

PLANNING

- The client will participate appropriately as able in the therapeutic regimen.
- The client will refrain from causing disruptions that affect other clients and staff.
- The client will be appropriately supervised during caring interventions, diagnostic procedures, and other activities.
- Nursing staff will take appropriate precautions to prevent spread of HIV.

IMPLEMENTATION

- A correctional officer or member of the hospital security staff will be present during any intervention in which removing the restraints is necessary.
- Nurses will provide care in groups of two or more.
- The client will be offered counseling and a referral to the hospital chaplain.
- The nurses caring for the client will share their concerns with their supervisor or mentor.
- The client will be consulted and give permission for all treatments and therapies.
- Additional interventions as warranted for medical condition and ordered by the attending physician.

EVALUATION

Mr. Dunham's condition continued to deteriorate and he was placed on the mechanical ventilator. As it became increasingly difficult to meet his oxygenation needs, he was given paralytics and ultimately died of cardiorespiratory failure.

CRITICAL THINKING

1. Does a nurse, assigned to care for this client, have the option of requesting a different assignment based on his or her feelings of revulsion, disgust, or anger at the client's past history and behavior? Why or why not?
2. What interventions would be the most difficult for you to provide this client? Explain your answer.
3. How would your conflicting moral beliefs with this client impact your nursing care? Is it appropriate to reduce the quality of care you provide as a result? Explain your answer.

To care for clients such as these, nurses must have an awareness of their own ethics, a thorough understanding of the requirements they must follow under the professional code of ethics, and an understanding of the reporting requirements in their own state and the procedures they must follow in their place of employment. The nurse's own personal beliefs, morality, and bias will influence how he or she manages each situation. It is important that every nurse remember his or her moral duty to provide the best possible care, no matter what the client's morality or immorality may be. It is never appropriate for the nurse to allow his or her feelings about the client to affect care.

Assessment

As with any client, the assessment of the client who is immoral or who is exposed to immorality leading to abuse or mistreatment includes a nursing history and physical examination.

Clients who are immoral may not be able to participate in a trusting nurse–client relationship and may not respond to attempts at therapeutic communication. The nurse attempting to interview these clients should maintain a calm, nonjudgmental manner and should ask open-ended questions in a matter-of-fact tone.

Diagnosis

Nursing diagnoses for an immoral client or a client with a family member or significant other with questionable morals will vary. Diagnoses in the scenarios mentioned earlier may include the following:

- The prisoner transferred to the CCU will have a number of diagnoses appropriate to his medical condition. In addition, the following may be appropriate:
  a. Risk Prone Health Behavior
  b. Moral Distress
  c. Noncompliance
  d. Social Isolation.
- The young woman who has just found out she's pregnant may be diagnosed with the following:
  a. Risk for Situational Low Self-Esteem
  b. Impaired Individual Resilience.

Plan

Immoral clients may exhibit difficulty in participating in the planning process; in fact, they may even show disdain for it. The nurse may try to obtain cooperation by capitalizing on needs presented during the assessment. "I remember that you said you didn't want to be in pain any more. We need to run these tests to find out what is causing your pain, so that we can treat it." "I know you don't like the food here, but remember we discussed that to feel better, you have to get appropriate nutrition." While goals for these clients will vary widely, a few appropriate goals include the following:

- The client will participate appropriately as able in the therapeutic regimen.
- The client will refrain from causing disruptions that affect other clients and staff.
- The client will be appropriately supervised during caring interventions, diagnostic procedures, and other activities. For example, a security staff member or member of law enforcement will be present during caring interventions for a client with a history of assault.

Implementation

Caring for clients who lack morality consistent with what society deems normal can be challenging, unpleasant, and time consuming. Interventions that may be appropriate in working with these clients may include any of the following:

- Following procedures that ensure the safety of staff working with the client. For example, the nurse working with a client who is potentially dangerous should stay between the client and the door and should notify security to be present as necessary.
- Adding precautions or procedures as necessary to ensure safety of other clients and staff. This may include restraining the client, providing additional staff for interventions and procedures, and transporting the client for procedures when hallways and other areas have the fewest people around.
- Encouraging clients to make informed decisions without pressure from others. In the earlier example of the young woman who learned she was pregnant, her boyfriend was attempting to influence her decision. While clients are free to seek advice from whomever they wish, the nurse must ensure that the client makes a treatment decision free from coercion.
- Refer clients to spiritual leaders or mental health professionals as necessary to help the clients in the decision-making process.

Evaluation

Treatment decisions that challenge individual morality and ethics, such as abortion and organ transplantation, are often the decisions that most leave clients and family members second guessing the decision after it is made. Evaluation of the client making a decision that poses a challenge to the client's morality or evaluation of the client who is without morality is based on the question "Is the client comfortable that the best possible decision was made?" Nurses working with clients in these situations should support autonomy; provide a listening, nonjudgmental ear; and continue to support the client's decision following the conclusion of treatment.

REVIEW Morality

RELATE: LINK THE CONCEPTS

A mother brings her 13-year-old daughter to her gynecologist's office for the daughter's first pelvic examination. The daughter is autistic and has a spoken vocabulary of less than 500 words. The mother tells the nurse she wants to talk to the physician about getting her daughter's tubes tied "or some other" procedure that will keep her daughter from getting pregnant if anyone molests her.

Linking the exemplar of Morality with the concept of Ethics:

1. How would you respond to this mother's request?
2. What ethical responsibilities do you have to the daughter in this situation?

Linking the exemplar of Morality with the concept of Comfort:

3. What moral or ethical issues are involved in clients' advance directives and do-not-resuscitate orders?
4. What are your feelings about the morality of do-not-resuscitate orders? How would you keep these feelings from influencing your discussions with a client about do-not-resuscitate orders? Would your feelings change if the client were a child or adolescent?

READY: GO TO COMPANION SKILLS MANUAL

- Managing clients in restraints
- Using a bed or chair exit safety monitoring device
- Applying wrist or ankle restraint

- Maintaining nurses' safety
- Assessing home for safe environment
- Evaluating client's safety
- Assessing caregiver's safety
- Assessing for elder abuse

REFER: GO TO MYNURSINGKIT

REFLECT: CASE STUDY

The nurse on the day shift at an inpatient rehabilitation center makes her morning rounds. She finds a young female client awake in her bed, crying. The woman has bruises on her wrists and forearms that were not there when the nurse last visited with the client the previous afternoon. When the nurse asks the client what happened, she responds only by shaking her head, and she pulls away when the nurse reaches out to comfort her. The nurse checks the visitor logs and confirms the client had no visitors the night before.

1. What are the priorities of care for the client at this moment?
2. What steps should the nurse take to try to determine what happened to this client?
3. How should the nurse document her findings, and with whom should the nurse share them?
4. Does the nurse have an obligation to report these findings and to whom?

27.2 RELIGION

KEY TERMS

Denomination, *1783*
Holy day, *1781*
Meditation, *1783*
Prayer, *1782*

BASIS FOR SELECTION OF EXEMPLAR

NLN Competency

LEARNING OUTCOMES

After reading about this exemplar, you will be able to:

1. Define the concept of religion as it relates to nursing and health care.
2. Identify components of different religious practices.
3. Describe how religious practices may impact nursing care.
4. Describe culturally competent nursing interventions to support religious needs of clients.
5. Identify desired outcomes for clients and their families at risk for impaired religiosity.

OVERVIEW OF RELIGION AND RELIGIOUS PRACTICES

Religion is an organized, communal approach to human spirituality. In its simplest terms, a religion provides its members with the constructs of beliefs, moral values, and spiritual practices that guide its members' expressions of their spirituality. While religion is typically practiced in a community setting, such as a church, synagogue, or mosque, most religious individuals also practice their religion alone in various ways, and those who are separated from their religious community will often continue their observations of holy days and rituals in private.

Religions have more differences than they have similarities, but all religions share some common characteristics. These include the following:

- Belief in a god or higher power. A few religions, including Hinduism and Buddhism, worship multiple gods.
- Belief that the god or higher power has influence over humanity.
- Forms of communication with the higher power, usually in the form of prayer or rituals.
- Community. Religions are typically practiced in a communal setting, such as a church, synagogue, or mosque.
- Rituals to honor the god or gods or to incorporate the community into the religious faith. Baptism is an example of a ritual that brings the newly baptized into the Christian faith.
- Ethical or moral codes. Probably the single best-known example of a religious moral code is the Ten Commandments.

Beyond these shared characteristics, religions have various similarities and differences, including how they approach medicine and certain aspects of health care. The very brief descriptions included later in this exemplar are mere snapshots intended to raise the nurse's awareness of some important areas of health care that an individual's religion can impact. Nurses working with clients of faith should ask appropriate questions to learn how the client's religion affects the client's own specific health care decision-making processes. Nurses should ask questions to gain information necessary about religious holy days, sacred writings and symbols, and times and needs regarding prayer and meditation.

Holy Days

A **holy day** is a day set aside for special religious observance; all the world religions observe certain holy days. For example, Christians observe Easter and Christmas, Jews observe Yom Kippur and Passover, Buddhists observe the birthday of the Buddha, Muslims observe the month-long holy period of Ramadan, and Hindus observe Mahashivarathri, a celebration of Lord Shiva. Many religions require fasting, extended prayer, and reflection or ritual observances on sacred (or high holy) days. Believers who are seriously ill are often exempted from such requirements.

The concept of the Sabbath is common to both Christians and Jews, in response to the biblical commandment "Remember the Sabbath day to keep it holy." Most Christians observe the Sabbath on Sunday, whereas Jews and sabbatarian

Christians (e.g., Seventh-Day Adventists) observe Saturday as their Sabbath. Clients who are devout in their religious practices may want to avoid any special treatments or other intrusions on their day of rest and reflection.

Muslims follow the practice of prayer fives times a day, and the Muslim client may need assistance to maintain this commitment (Figure 27–3 ■). In addition, Muslims traditionally gather on Friday at noon to worship and learn about their faith. Both Hindus and Buddhists practice meditation, and the nurse may create a quiet time for them to meditate.

Solemn religious observances throughout the year may be referred to as *high holy days* and may include fasting, reflection, and prayer. Examples of such holy days are Rosh Hashanah and Yom Kippur (Jewish), Good Friday (Christian), and the month-long Ramadan (Islam). Many hospitals and health organizations facilitate ritual observances for clients and staff on holy days. Because many religions follow calendars other than the Gregorian calendar, a multifaith calendar can be used to identify the holy days of the various religious groups (Griffith, 1996).

Sacred Writings

Each religion has sacred and authoritative scriptures that provide guidance for its adherents' beliefs and behaviors; in addition, sacred writings frequently tell instructive stories of the religion's leaders, kings, and heroes. In most religions, these scriptures are thought to be the word of the Supreme Being as written down by prophets or other human representatives. Christians rely on the Bible, Jews on the Torah and Talmud, and Muslims on the Koran; Hindus have several holy texts, or Vedas, and Buddhists value the teachings of the Tripitakas. Scriptures generally set forth religious law in the form of admonitions and rules for living (e.g., the Ten Commandments). This religious law may be interpreted in various ways by subgroups of a religion's adherents and may affect a client's willingness to accept treatment suggestions. For example, blood transfusions are in conflict with the religious admonitions of Jehovah's Witnesses.

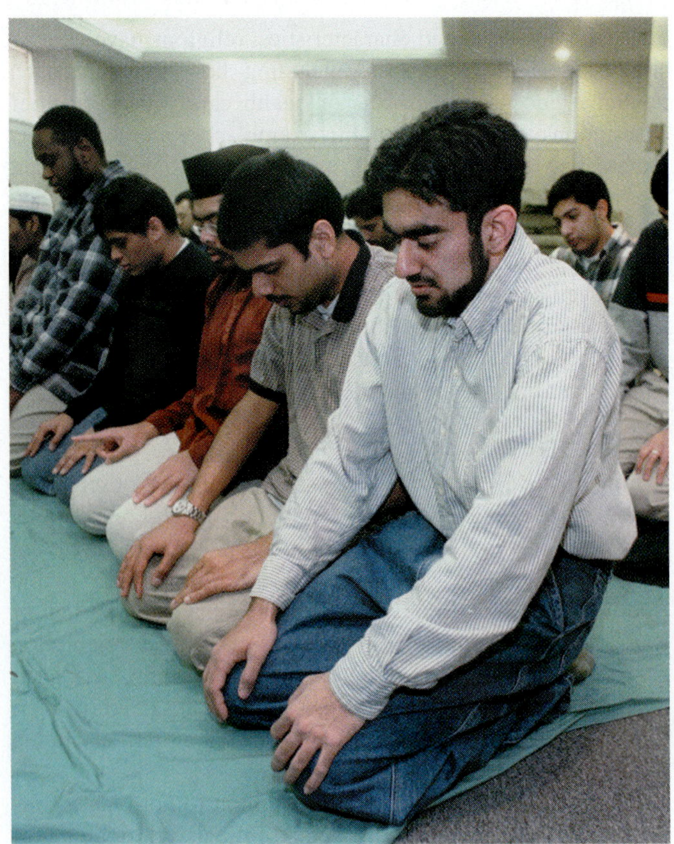
Figure 27–3 ■ Muslim students at Johns Hopkins University at their weekly prayer meeting.

People often gain strength and hope from reading religious writings when they are ill or in crisis. Examples of scriptural stories that may give comfort to clients are Job's suffering, in both the Jewish and Christian scriptures, and Jesus' healing of people who were physically or mentally ill, in the New Testament.

Sacred Symbols

Sacred symbols include jewelry, medals, amulets, icons, totems, or body ornamentation (e.g., tattoos) that carry religious or spiritual significance. They may be worn to pronounce one's faith, to remind the practitioner of the faith, to provide spiritual protection, or to be a source of comfort or strength. People may wear religious medals at all times, and they may wish to wear them when they are undergoing diagnostic studies, medical treatment, or surgery. People who are Roman Catholic may carry a rosary for prayer; a person who is Muslim may carry a mala, or string of prayer beads (Figure 27–4 ■).

People may have religious icons or statues in their home, car, or place of work as a personal reminder of their faith or as part of a personal place of worship or meditation. Hospitalized clients or long-term care residents may wish to have their spiritual icons or statues with them as a source of comfort.

Prayer and Meditation

Prayer is a spiritual practice; for many, it is also a religious practice. An encyclopedia of religion defines **prayer** simply as "human communication with divine and spiritual entities" (Gill, 1987, p. 489). Some argue that because prayer requires a belief in a divine or spiritual entity not all people pray, while others consider prayer a universal phenomenon that does not require such belief. Ulanov and Ulanov (1983), for example, proposed that everyone prays: "People pray whether or not they call it prayer. We pray every time we ask for help, understanding, or strength, in or out of religion . . . who and what we are speak out of us. . . . To pray is to listen to and hear this self who is speaking" (p. 1). Prayer is intention plus love, often communicated with "the Absolute," according to Dossey (1999); that is, prayer is a loving wish or thought for oneself or another and not an invocation of positive or negative forms of magic.

There are different types of prayer experience. Poloma and Gallup (1991) categorized prayer experiences as follows:

- Ritual (e.g., the Lord's Prayer, memorized prayers that can be repeated)
- Petitionary (e.g., "God, cure me!" or intercessory prayers when one is requesting something of the divine)
- Colloquial (i.e., conversational prayers)
- Meditational (e.g., moments of silence focused on nothing, a meaningful phrase, or a certain aspect of the divine).

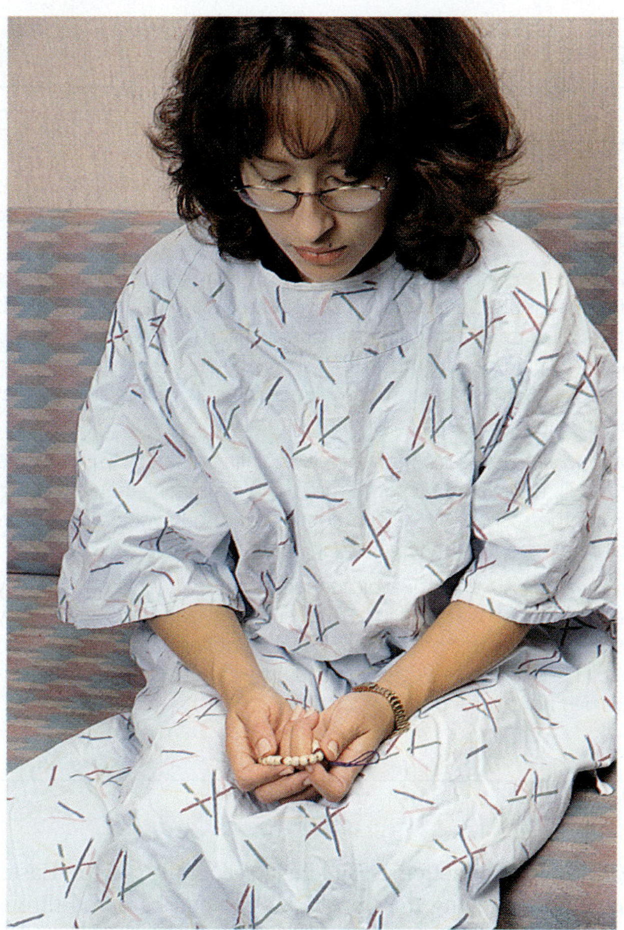

Figure 27–4 ■ Clients may bring objects to the hospital to use in prayer or other religious rituals. Caregivers should respect such objects, because they usually have great significance for clients.

While meditational and colloquial prayer experiences have been found to be associated with spiritual well-being and quality of life in healthy adults, ritual and petitionary prayer experiences may be most comforting and appropriate for those who are ill.

Some religions have prescribed prayers that are printed in a prayer book, such as the Anglican/Episcopal *Book of Common Prayer* or the Catholic missal. Some religious prayers are attributed to the source of faith; for example, the Lord's Prayer for Christians is attributed to Jesus, and the first sutra for Muslims is attributed to Mohammed.

Some religions require daily prayers or dictate specific times for prayer and worship: the five daily prayers, or Salat, of the Muslims (performed while facing east toward Mecca at dawn, noon, midafternoon, sunset, and evening), the daily Kaddish of the Jews, or the seven canonical prayers of the Roman Catholics. People who are ill may want to continue or increase their prayer practices (Moschella, Pressman, Pressman, & Weissman, 1997). They may need uninterrupted quiet time during which they have their prayer books, rosaries, malas, or other icons available to them.

Meditation is the act of focusing one's thoughts or engaging in self-reflection or contemplation. Some people believe that, through deep meditation, one can influence or control physical and psychological functioning and the course of illness.

Religion and Medical Care

There are many broad forms, or categories, of religions. Within each category, there are any number of **denominations**, groups of members that adhere to the same practices and beliefs. Even within a specific denomination, such as the Baptist faith, there may be further sects or denominations within the larger group. For example, the Southern Baptist Church has a number of different groups, including traditionalists, fundamentalists, and revivalists (Wax, 2008). Because of the great number of different groups that may be affiliated with a particular religion, nurses must be careful not to make assumptions about the client's beliefs and practices based on what religion the client professes. The client may belong to a group that practices the religion somewhat differently or may have belonged to the religion as a child and has since modified his or her practices to suit evolving beliefs. In addition to the following information, see Box 27–3 for health-related information about specific religions.

JUDAISM Typically, Jewish people participate actively in their medical care and seek treatment from modern Western doctors. Some Jews keep to the traditional kosher diet. This is a complex dietary code laid out in the Torah, the first five books of the Old Testament. Some of its rules are not eating meat and dairy foods together and not eating meat from animals that do not both chew their cud and have cleft feet; this includes pork.

Traditionally Jews will use all medical care necessary to extend life. Because there are prescribed Jewish rituals for individuals who are near death and for the time of and after death, Jewish families will often request a rabbi, a Jewish spiritual leader, when they know a loved one is near death. Jewish burial customs require the dead to be buried as soon as possible, preferably within 24 hours.

ISLAM Islam is the second largest religion in the world, with most of its members living outside Arab countries. Those who practice Islam are called Muslims. Many Muslims view events in their lives as a direct result of God's will, may view illness or death as the will of God, and therefore believe that healing can take place only through God's will. Muslims pray five times a day, so nurses working with Muslim clients should take their prayer times into consideration, especially those in a hospital or institutional setting. Cleanliness and modesty are of great importance; ideally, the Muslim client should have a nurse of the same gender. During the holy period of Ramadan, Muslims fast. If a client wishes to fast and doing so may endanger his or her health, a nurse or physician may want to consult a Muslim elder, or Imam, to speak with the client, as there are some allowable exceptions to the fasting laws. Practicing Muslims follow dietary codes similar to those of Judaism, particularly regarding pork and pork-based products (al-Shahri & al-Khenaizan, 2005).

Box 27–3 Health-Related Information About Specific Religions

A SAMPLER

Amish, Mennonites—Likely will not have insurance coverage; rely on religious community for support.

Anglicans, Episcopalians, Roman Catholics—Appreciate receiving Eucharist (Holy Communion), a ritual of ingesting bread and wine (or grape juice) led by clergy or lay leaders to commemorate the death of Jesus. Lenten season (Ash Wednesday to Easter) may involve some degree of abstention from food.

Buddhists—May be vegetarian. Facilitate meditation (may desire incense, visual focal point, use breathing or chanting, etc.).

Christian Scientists—Typically oppose Western medical interventions, relying instead on lay and professional Christian Science practitioners.

Hindus—Most eat no beef; many are vegetarian. Cleanliness highly valued. Many food preferences (e.g., foods fresh or cooked in oil).

Jehovah's Witnesses—Abstain from most blood products; need to discuss alternative treatments such as blood conservation strategies, autologous techniques, hematopoietic agents, nonblood volume expanders, and so on; contact local Jehovah's Witness hospital liaison committee.

Jews—Some observe kosher diet to varying degrees (e.g., avoid pork and shellfish, do not mix dairy and meat). Sabbath observance varies (e.g., Orthodox Jews avoid traveling in vehicles, writing, turning on electric appliances and lights, etc.).

Latter-Day Saints (LDS or Mormons)—Avoid alcohol, caffeine, smoking. Prefer to wear temple undergarments. Arrange for priestly blessing if requested.

Muslims—Respect modesty, avoid nakedness. Provide same-gender nurse if possible. Support prayers five times daily (may need to assist with ritual washing and positioning beforehand). Allow for family and imam (religious leader) to follow Islamic guidelines for burial when client dies. Eat no pork. Children, pregnant, elderly, and sick exempt from daytime fast during month of Ramadan.

Roman Catholics—Sacrament of the Anointing of the Sick appropriate for the ill. Be aware that some may think rite means they are dying, though the sacrament may be administered to anyone who is seriously ill or about to undergo a major operation.

Seventh-Day Adventists—Avoid unnecessary treatments on Saturday (Sabbath). Sabbath begins at Friday sundown and ends at Saturday sundown. Adventists prefer restful, spirit-nurturing, family activities on Sabbaths. Likely to be vegetarian and abstain from caffeinated beverages. Do not smoke or drink alcohol.

ROMAN CATHOLICISM Roman Catholics generally participate in Western medicine. Catholics typically have a great respect for life, so a Catholic's religious beliefs will most likely inform decisions about childbearing and end-of-life care for him- or herself or other family members. This is not always true, however. Many Roman Catholics use birth control despite religious laws against it. Roman Catholics have a great deal of respect for the rituals of the sacrament of Anointing of the Sick (formerly known as Last Rites or Extreme Unction). Nurses working with a very sick or dying member of the Roman Catholic faith will want to make sure that the family has the opportunity to call for a priest to administer rituals important to their faith.

PROTESTANT CHRISTIANITY The umbrella of Protestant Christianity covers many religions. Episcopalians, Methodists, Southern Baptists, African Methodist Episcopalians, and Lutherans are just a few of them. Protestants generally embrace Western medicine, although they may differ in their views about birth control and end-of-life care.

HINDUISM Hinduism is a religion practiced by people from India and other parts of Asia. Typically, Hindus embrace Western medicine, but they will also employ alternative therapies from their culture such as yoga and various homeopathic remedies. Hindus generally do not eat meat and may prefer not to use medications that are derived from animals. Hindus generally believe that they have more than one life, and as a result may choose not to participate in organ donation. As with many other religions, Hindus have ceremonial rites that are practiced at the time of dying and immediately after death.

BUDDHISM Practicing Buddhists generally prefer Eastern medicine, believing that most illnesses can be cured through the mind and the use of herbs. Many also use acupuncture. This does not mean, however, that Buddhists will refuse Western medicine. In fact, Buddhists see giving blood as a great gift. However, a Buddhist client or client of Asian origin may use traditional therapies in addition to those prescribed by a physician or nurse practitioner.

JEHOVAH'S WITNESSES Although Jehovah's Witnesses are not one of the larger populations of faith, it is important to note that traditionally they have prohibited blood transfusions, to the extent of shunning members who received certain types of transfusions. This can have important consequences for care in emergency and labor and delivery departments. Organ donation and organ transplants, however, are seen as personal decisions.

ALTERATIONS

Any number of situations can threaten an individual's or community's ability to express or practice religion. Globally, many countries do not guarantee their citizens the kind of freedom of religion that is guaranteed in the United States. In some countries, certain religious faiths are prohibited. For example, the Communist Party in China does not permit its members to hold religious beliefs and has a history of persecuting Christians who worship in public. Although the persecution of Christians by the Chinese government is not as frequent as it once was, most Christians living in China meet in "house churches" in groups of fewer than 25 (*Economist*, 2008). Within the United

States, there are active, passionate discussions about the separation of church and state, with many Christians feeling that the Christian religion should be practiced in public schools, on public property, and at public events, despite knowing that the United States has no official religion and guarantees the freedom of religion for all of its people.

Any number of medical situations can threaten an individual's ability to practice his or her religion. NANDA International has recently accepted three new nursing diagnoses that reflect client religious issues including Impaired Religiousity, Risk for Impaired Religiousity, and Readiness for Enhanced Religiousity (Burkhardt, 2005, p. 10).

Impaired religiosity is the "impaired ability to exercise reliance on religious beliefs and/or participate in rituals of a particular faith tradition." Illness or injury that disrupts religious practice can impair the client's religiosity and result in emotional distress. An example of impaired religiousity might be the Roman Catholic cleint who attends daily Mass or the Muslim client who says evening prayers daily at the local mosque who is on enforced bedrest or requires an extended hospitalization.

Similarly, there are times when a medical condition may require a decision that is in conflict with a client's or family's religious practice. For example, a pregnant client who believes that life begins at conception discovers at 20–22 weeks gestation learns that she will not be able to carry the fetus to term and attempting to do so will most likely result in her death. How will she decide what to do? If she had been trying for years to get pregnant without success, how would that influence her decision? How would her decision be affected if she had two small children at home? In such a situation in which a medical condition presents a complication that is at odds with a client's faith, the client may be at *risk for impaired religiosity*.

The relationship between the individual and his or her religion and religious practices is complex. Sometimes events that might threaten one person's faith strengthen the faith of another. *Readiness for enhanced religiosity* is defined as the "ability to increase reliance on religious beliefs and/or participate in rituals of a particular faith tradition." *Spiritual Distress,* an existing nursing diagnosis, is discussed in detail in the exemplar that follows.

NURSING PROCESS

It is important to determine the client's religious practices during the admissions process. If the client denies a formal religious affiliation, the nurse must determine any practices the client may not identify as religious that are spiritual in nature and would affect the delivery of care. Meditating at regular intervals is one example of such a practice.

Assessment

As discussed in the About Spirituality section of this concept, assessment of the client's religious faith, practices, and spirituality occurs as part of the nursing history. Certainly the nurse should assess the religious and spiritual needs of any client who is going to be receiving care in an institution for more than a few hours. The longer the client's hospitalization or institutionalization, the more important this assessment becomes. In addition, any client with an illness or injury that may result in a threat to life should be assessed for religious practices and spiritual needs. Nurses should inquire about religious practices related to all of the following:

- Diet and nutrition, including types of foods prohibited and any required meals or meal times
- Prayers observed, including any requirements regarding the times that prayers must be observed
- Use of sacred objects or texts during prayers
- Prohibitions regarding medical procedures (if any)
- Other medical-related requirements or prohibitions.

Diagnosis

The nursing diagnoses appropriate to religious practices are the following:

- Risk for Impaired Religiosity
- Impaired Religiosity
- Readiness for Enhanced Religiosity.

The religious client and family may practice a number of observations of their faith at home, and these may be an essential part in each day in the life of the family. Interrupted family processes and readiness for enhanced family coping may also be appropriate if these normal daily practices are disturbed by hospitalization. Because the individual's sense of self may be closely tied to his or her religious practices, risk for compromised human dignity and risk for powerlessness may also be appropriate.

Plan

When planning care, the nurse attempts to preserve the client's and family's observance of religious practices to every extent possible and may include the following goals of care:

- The client will be able to participate in religious observances if he or she desires.
- The client will be able to participate in prayer at prescribed times without interruption.
- The client will receive meals in keeping with religious dietary restrictions or requirements.
- The client will have access to religious resources, including ministers, prayer partners, sacred texts, and sacred objects.

Implementation

Providing care related to the client's religious needs must be done with great tact and sensitivity. The nurse's own religious beliefs may influence the approach to implementing care, but it is important to remember it is never the nurse's place to preach or proselytize his or her own beliefs and practices; rather, the nurse should focus on supporting the needs of the client.

Supporting Religious Practices

During the assessment of the client, the nurse obtains specific information about the client's religious preference and practices. Nurses need to consider specific religious practices that

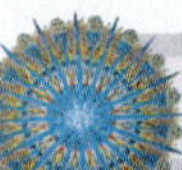

NURSING CARE PLAN A Client at Risk for Impaired Religiosity

ASSESSMENT

Mohammed Al-Hussein is a 45-year-old husband and father of four who was badly hurt in a motor vehicle accident. Upon admission to the rehabilitation center, where he is expected to stay for several weeks, he informs the nurse that he is Muslim and a strict follower of prayer rituals and dietary restrictions. He and his wife are both science professors at the nearby university. His wife teaches an early class and has to leave for work before the school bus arrives. His oldest child, a daughter, is 16, and he says that she has been helping her mother with the younger children since the accident, almost a week ago. He admits that he is concerned that the extra burden on his daughter may affect her school work but says that she does not complain. He says he can deal with the pain and discomfort but that he misses the company of his wife and children greatly. Currently confined to a wheelchair because of a hip fracture, Dr. Al-Hussein has orders for daily physical and occupational therapy.

DIAGNOSES

- Risk for Impaired Religiosity
- Impaired Physical Mobility
- Impaired Transfer Ability
- Risk for Caregiver Role Strain
- Interrupted Family Processes

PLANNING

Together with Mr. Al-Hussein and his wife, the nurse develops a plan of care that includes the following:

- The client will observe all five prayer times daily.
- The client's diet will follow Islamic restrictions.
- The client will talk with the imam at his mosque about the possibilities of additional help around the house while the client is in rehab.
- The entire family will visit regularly to pray together and to talk about what is happening at home and school while the client is in the rehabilitation center.

IMPLEMENTATION

- The nurse will talk with the occupational and physical therapists about scheduling therapy sessions around the client's prayer schedule.
- The nurse will talk with his or her supervisor about moving the client's bed to face east so that even though he cannot kneel, he can pray in the appropriate direction.
- The nurse will facilitate the client contacting his imam.
- The nurse will notify the registered dietitian of the client's needs for dietary considerations and follow up with the client after the first meal.

EVALUATION

Evaluation of Mr. Al-Hussein's plan of care should include checking with him to make sure that his meals meet his requirements and that staff are not interrupting him during prayer times. The nurse should also follow-up with his wife to make sure that there are not any additional considerations that need to be made for the family.

CRITICAL THINKING

1. What are the prescribed times for daily Islamic prayers? Which times might be most difficult for nursing staff to accommodate?
2. What other interventions can the nurse make to support Mr. Al-Hussein as he tries to maintain his religious observes while in the rehab unit?
3. Where can the nurse go for more information about the Islamic faith?

will affect nursing care, such as the client's beliefs about birth, death, dress, diet, prayer, sacred symbols, sacred writings, and holy days as discussed earlier in this chapter. See Box 27–4 for ways the nurse can help clients to continue their usual spiritual practices.

Assisting Clients with Prayer

Prayer involves a sense of love and connection, as well as a reaching out. It has many health benefits and healing properties (Dossey, 1996). It offers a means for someone to talk to a greater power, a mechanism for expressing care, and a sense of serenity and connection with something greater.

Clients may choose to participate in private prayer or want group prayer with family, friends, or clergy. In such situations the nurse's major responsibility is to ensure a quiet environment and privacy. Nursing care may need to be adjusted to accommodate periods for prayer.

Illness can interfere with some clients' ability to pray (Taylor, 2003a). Feelings such as anxiety, fear, guilt, grief, despair, and isolation can produce barriers to relationships in general and to the relationship the person has with the Divine. In these instances, the client may ask the nurse to pray with him or her. Prayers with clients should be done only when there is mutual agreement between the clients and those praying with them. Nurses who are unaccustomed to praying aloud or in public may find it helpful to have a formal prayer or a scriptural passage readily available. Because prayer can evoke deep feelings, the nurse needs to spend time with the client following a prayer to enable the client to express these feelings.

Box 27–4 **Supporting Religious Practices**

- Create a trusting relationship with the client so that any religious concerns or practices can be openly discussed and addressed.
- If unsure of the client's religious needs, ask how nurses can assist in having these needs met. Avoid relying on personal assumptions when caring for clients.
- Do not discuss personal spiritual beliefs with a client unless the client requests it. Be sure to assess whether such self-disclosure contributes to a therapeutic nurse–client relationship.
- Inform clients and family caregivers about spiritual support available at your institution (e.g., chapel or meditation room, chaplain services).
- Allow time and privacy for, and provide comfort measures prior to, private worship, prayer, meditation, reading, or other spiritual activities.
- Respect and ensure safety of the client's religious articles (e.g., icons, amulets, clothing, jewelry).
- If desired by the client, facilitate clergy or spiritual care specialist visitation. Collaborate with the chaplain (if available).
- Prepare the client's environment for spiritual rituals or clergy visitations as needed (e.g., have a chair near the bedside for clergy, create private space).
- Make arrangements with the dietitian so that dietary needs can be met. If the institution cannot accommodate the client's needs, ask the family to bring food. (Most religions have some recommendations about diet, such as espousing vegetarianism, rejecting alcohol.)
- Acquaint yourself with the religions, spiritual practices, and cultures of the area in which you are working.
- Remember the difference between facilitating/supporting a client's religious practice and participating in it yourself.
- Ask another nurse to assist you if a particular religious practice makes you uncomfortable.
- All spiritual interventions must be done within agency guidelines.

Clients' preferences for prayer reflect their personalities. That is, introverts may prefer being alone to pray, and their prayers will reflect their capacity for introspection. In contrast, extroverts' prayers may revolve around their relationships with others and be expressed in creative, verbal ways. Similarly, a prayer of a feeling-type client may be emotion filled, whereas the prayer of a thinking-type client may be based on ideas and logic. Structure prayer interventions accordingly (Box 27–5).

Evaluation

Evaluation will be based on answers to the following questions:

- Has the client been provided the opportunity to practice religious rituals, including prayers?
- Did the nursing and dietary staff make appropriate considerations regarding dietary restrictions?
- Has the client successfully maintained connection with his or her religious practices and community of faith?

Box 27–5 **Praying with Clients**

- When assessing whether a client would like you to pray, ask to pray in a way that allows both of you to feel comfortable if the answer is no. ("Some people tell me prayer helps them to cope with rough times like this. Would you feel comfortable if I prayed with you?")
- Assess how the client approaches the addressee of prayer. For example, a Baptist may pray to Jesus, whereas a Jew would pray directly to God, or Yahweh. This assessment can usually be made while listening to a client talk about religious beliefs.
- Before praying, assess what the client would like you to pray. Listen carefully. The answer may provide greater insight into his or her fears and concerns.
- Personalize the prayer. Present your client's name and personal concerns to the Divine.
- Prayer can be used to summarize a conversation. This lets the client know you have heard what was said. It may also help the client to view circumstances more objectively.
- Prayer may be the springboard to further discussion or catharsis. Stay with the client after a prayer until there has been time for conversation.
- Follow a prayer with nonverbal communication (e.g., eye contact or touch) to convey "See, I am me, a person, and you are you, and we have returned from our brief journey inward."
- Remember that some clients would like to pray aloud with you, just as you may with them. This can be a beautiful experience that nurtures both the client and nurse. It allows the client to reciprocate caring.
- Be mindful of one difference between magic and prayer. Magic invokes a greater power for personal gain. Prayer allows the greater power to do the greater good ("Thy will be done").
- Praying with a client may not involve verbalization. You may feel it will be more comfortable or appropriate if you remain quiet and fully present, praying silently.
- Facilitate the clients' prayer practices. Schedule time when he or she will be undisturbed, palliate distressing symptoms that interfere with praying, help with articles that accompany prayers (e.g., rosaries, prayer garments, books of prayers), and so on.
- In times of distress, a client or loved one may not be able to construct a prayer spontaneously. You may want to teach a centering prayer that is very brief (e.g., "Lord, have mercy/healing"). Nurses can discuss with care recipients what prayer would benefit them most and encourage them to use it while alone. These prayers may be more beneficial when they are framed in a positive sense. To illustrate, "Jesus loves me" or "The Lord has mercy."
- Encourage clients to think (privately or with you) about what prayer means to them. Offer questions like these: Why do you pray? What do you expect from your praying? Are these expectations appropriate? How content are you with your prayer experiences? Is there a yearning for something more in your prayer experience?

Note: From Taylor, E. J. (1998). Caring for the sprit. In C. C. Burke (Ed.), *Psychosocial dimensions of oncology nursing care* (pp. 55–75). Pittsburgh, PA: Oncology Nursing Press. Adapted with permission.

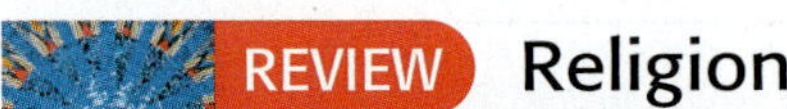

REVIEW Religion

RELATE: LINK THE CONCEPTS

Linking the exemplar of Religion with the concept of Stress and Coping:

1. How might the client's inability to perform customary religious rituals during times of illness result in anxiety?
2. How does helping the client meet his or her religious needs, thus reducing anxiety, help the client to recover more quickly?

Linking the exemplar of Religion with the concept of Development:

3. How do a person's religious beliefs change as they age?
4. In assisting the client to meet his or her needs related to religion, how might the nurse's interventions differ based on the developmental stage of the client?

REFER: GO TO MYNURSINGKIT

REFLECT: CASE STUDY

Olivia Rossi is an 80-year-old woman who attends Mass at her church every day. She enjoys shopping at the Italian market that is within walking distance of her home. A couple of years ago she was diagnosed with Parkinson's disease. At first she did well, thanks to medication and therapy, but in the last few months her symptoms have become worse, and she is afraid to continue to live on her own. After going to visit several assisted living centers, she and her adult children chose one that is very nice, with a very well-qualified staff, but is a fifteen-minute drive from the nearest Catholic church. After a few weeks, the nurse working on Mrs. Rossi's floor notices that Mrs. Rossi has become depressed. The nurse approaches Mrs. Rossi and begins to talk with her about the changes she's experienced since moving to the center. Mrs. Rossi expresses her sadness at not being able to attend Mass and says that she misses her church community.

1. What are the priority diagnoses for Mrs. Rossi?
2. What caring interventions could the nurse implement to help Mrs. Rossi?
3. What are the possible outcomes if Mrs. Rossi does not receive any nursing interventions?

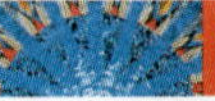

27.3 SPIRITUAL DISTRESS

KEY TERMS

Presencing, *1789*

BASIS FOR SELECTION OF EXEMPLAR

NLN Competency

LEARNING OUTCOMES

After reading about this exemplar you should be able to:

1. Define the concept of spiritual distress as it relates to nursing and health care.
2. Identify components of spiritual health and well-being.
3. Describe nursing interventions to support clients with spiritual distress.
4. Identify desired outcomes for clients with spiritual distress.

OVERVIEW

When working with clients and their families, it is essential that the nurse assess them for spiritual health. Faith, a firm connection with others, and a belief in the future and in a higher power can be a strongly sustaining influence for critically or chronically ill clients and their families. In diagnosing spiritual health, the nurse may find that spiritual problems provide the diagnostic label or that spiritual distress is the etiology of the problem.

NANDA International (2007) offers the following as defining characteristics of spiritual distress:

- Expresses lack of hope, meaning and purpose in life, forgiveness of self
- Expresses being abandoned by or having anger toward God
- Refuses interaction with friends, family
- Undergoes sudden changes in spiritual practices
- Requests to see a religious leader
- Lacks interest in nature, reading spiritual literature.

No list could be complete, however, considering the complexity and variability of people and their spiritual dimensions.

SPIRITUAL OR RELIGIOUS DISTRESS AS THE ETIOLOGY

Spiritual distress may affect other areas of functioning and indicate other diagnoses. In these instances, spiritual distress becomes the etiology. Examples include the following:

- Fear related to apprehension about the soul's future after death and unpreparedness for death
- Chronic or Situational Low Self-Esteem related to failure to live within the precepts of one's faith
- Disturbed Sleep Pattern related to spiritual distress
- Ineffective Coping related to feelings of abandonment by God and loss of religious faith
- Decisional Conflict related to conflict between treatment plan and religious beliefs.

NURSING PROCESS

Clients in spiritual distress require the nurse's thoughtful interventions. While the nurse may not be able to provide the spiritual guidance clients require, it is possible to help clients explore their feelings and work through their distress, as well as help them talk with those who can provide the necessary spiritual guidance such as a religious leader, spiritual guide, or elder in their community. Sensitivity and tact are important skills for the nurse to employ.

Assessment

As part of the assessment of the client, the nurse should ask questions to determine the client's spiritual beliefs and practices, and how they affect or are affected by the client's health condition. Asking open-ended questions such as "How did you feel when the doctor told you about the risks associated with the surgery?" serve to build the nurse–client relationship as well as eliciting information the nurse will need to inform the plan of care. Client statements such as "Why is God doing this to me?" "I don't care anymore," and "I wish I were dead" indicate that the client is in spiritual distress.

Diagnosis

NANDA International (2007) recognizes three diagnoses related to spirituality:

- Spiritual Distress is "impaired ability to experience and integrate meaning and purpose in life through a person's connectedness with self, others, art, music, literature, nature, or a power greater than oneself" (p. 186).
- Readiness for Enhanced Spiritual Well-Being recognizes that spiritual well-being is the "ability to experience and integrate meaning and purpose in life through a person's connectedness with self, others, art, music, literature, nature, or a power greater than oneself" (p. 189). This wellness diagnosis describing spiritual health acknowledges that some people respond to adversity with an increased sensitivity to spirituality or spiritual maturation.
- Risk for Spiritual Distress is defined by NANDA (2005) as being "at risk for an impaired ability to experience and integrate meaning and purpose in life through a person's connectedness with self, other persons, art, music, literature, nature, and/or a power greater than oneself" (p. 188). This diagnosis may be appropriate for a client who currently shows no indication of this disruption of spirit yet may if a nurse fails to intervene.

Plan

In the planning phase, the nurse identifies interventions to help the client achieve the overall goal of maintaining or restoring spiritual well-being so that the client may realize spiritual strength, serenity, and satisfaction. Goals of care may include the following:

- The client will fulfill religious obligations.
- The client will draw on and use inner resources more effectively to meet the present situation.
- The client will maintain or establish a dynamic, personal relationship with a supreme being in the face of unpleasant circumstances.
- The client will find meaning in existence and the present situation.
- The client will feel a sense of hope.
- The client will have access to spiritual resources as needed.

Implementation

Numerous nursing actions are available to help clients meet their spiritual needs (Cole et al., 2004; Mauk & Schmidt, 2004; Taylor, 2002). Spiritual care may include any of the following diverse actions:

- Recognizing and validating inner resources of an individual, such as coping methods, humor, motivation, self-determination, positive attitude, and optimism.
- Assisting the client to leave a legacy by storytelling and/or recording life stories for family and friends, and encouraging creative expression through art, music, and writing. (This keeps the imagination alive and serves to regenerate the body, mind, and spirit.)
- Fostering ways for clients to keep in touch with nature and maintain a sense of wonder are also forms of spiritual care.
- Recognizing that the seasons, the emergence of flowers in spring, the phases of the moon, the migrations of birds, and the unchanging stars provide examples of orderliness in the universe, even in the midst of chaos and loss.

A client with a good measure of spiritual health will find hope, meaning, purpose, and value in existence. Although nursing therapeutics that enhance spiritual health are diverse, some of the most common and most desired include (a) providing presence, (b) supporting religious practices, (c) assisting clients with prayer, and (d) referring clients for spiritual counseling (Taylor & Mamier, 2005).

Providing Presence

Presencing, which is defined as being present, being there, or just being with a client, is a term that identifies one of the competencies incorporated by expert nurses (Zerwekh, 1997). Pettigrew (1990) identified four distinguishing features of presencing:

1. Giving of self in the present moment
2. Being available with all of the self
3. Listening, with full awareness of the privilege of doing so
4. Being there in a way that is meaningful to another person.

Fredriksson (1999) noted that presencing is a "gift of self" given by the nurse who maintains an attitude of attentiveness toward the client. Thus, nurses who listen attentively to clients yet fail to give of self (i.e., inwardly "make room") diminish their effectiveness.

There are multiple levels of presencing. Osterman and Schwartz-Barcott (1996) identified four ways of being present for clients:

1. Presence (when a nurse is physically present but not focused on the client)
2. Partial presence (when a nurse is physically present and attending to some task on the client's behalf but not relating to the client on any but the most superficial level)
3. Full presence (when a nurse is mentally, emotionally, and physically present; intentionally focusing on the client)
4. Transcendent presence (when a nurse is physically, mentally, emotionally, and spiritually present for a client; involves a transpersonal and transforming experience).

Presencing is often the best and sometimes the only intervention to support a client who suffers under circumstances that medical interventions cannot address. When a client is helpless, powerless, and vulnerable, a nurse's presencing can be most beneficial. Rather than worrying about saying or doing "the right thing," nurses should focus on being fully present (Taylor, 2002).

Referring Clients for Spiritual Counseling

There are times when spiritual care is best referred to other members of the health care team. Referrals can be made for hospitalized clients and their families through the hospital chaplain's office if one is available (Figure 27–5 ■). Nurses in home and community health settings can identify spiritual resources by checking directories of community service agencies, telephone directories, or religious directories that describe available spiritual counselors and the services provided through the religious community. Many religious counselors will provide assistance to members of their faith who are not members of their specific religious community. For example, a priest may attend a client in the hospital or at home even though the person is not a member of the priest's parish.

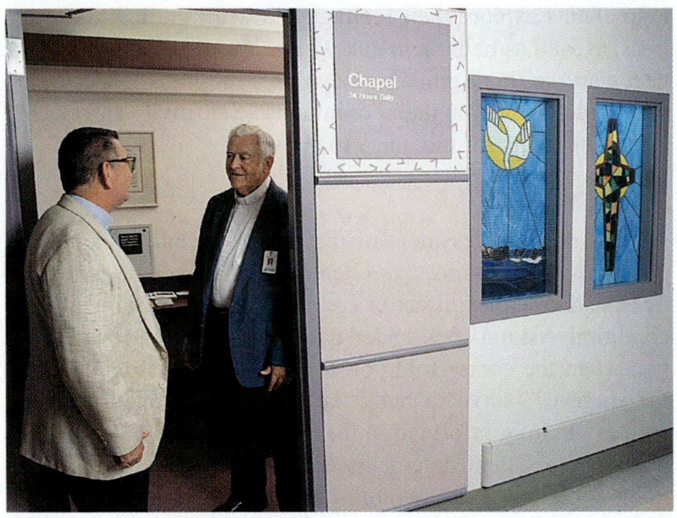

Figure 27–5 ■ Hospital chaplains minister to clients and their families.

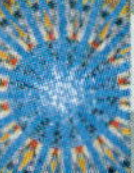

PRACTICE ALERT

When the nurse's spiritual beliefs conflict with the client's, the nurse must remember his or her role is as a health care provider and not a spiritual counselor. If the conflict is minor, the nurse may be able support the client's beliefs and help the client to resolve issues of concern. However, if the conflict is great and the nurse cannot support the client in an objective manner, it is most appropriate for the nurse to find a spiritual counselor who shares the client's beliefs. The client's permission is needed before seeking an outside counselor in order to protect the client's right to confidentiality.

Referrals may be necessary when the nurse makes a diagnosis of spiritual distress. In this situation, the nurse and religious counselor can work together to meet the client's needs. One situation the nurse may encounter is client refusal of necessary medical intervention because of religious tenets. In this case, the nurse encourages the client, primary care provider, and spiritual adviser to discuss the conflict and consider alternative methods of therapy. The nurse's major roles are to provide information the client needs to make an informed decision and to support the client's decision.

Evaluation

Using the measurable desired outcomes developed during the planning stage, the nurse collects data needed to judge whether client goals and outcomes have been achieved. Appropriate

EVIDENCE-BASED PRACTICE Spiritual Care Nursing: What Do Cancer Clients and Family Caregivers Want?

A convenience sample of 156 adult cancer clients and 68 family caregivers self-completed the Nurse Spiritual Therapeutics Scale, which measured how much these clients would want a nurse to provide different spiritual care therapeutics—for example, how much they would want a nurse to help them have quiet time or space, listen to them talk about spiritual concerns, ask them about religious practices, arrange for a minister or chaplain to visit, pray, and so forth.

Findings from these data indicated that while some cancer clients and family members are eager for a nurse to provide some spiritual care "therapeutics," others do not want it. Therapeutics that did not involve much intimacy, are traditional, and are not overtly religious are those most desired by clients. To illustrate, these participants *most wanted* the nurse to provide

- humor,
- private prayer,
- and help to find quiet time or space.

Least wanted therapeutics included instruction about writing or drawing their spirituality, discussion about the difficulties of praying when sick, and help with understanding dreams. No differences were observed between client and family member preferences. A modest, positive correlation was also found between frequency of attending religious services and greater desire for nurse-provided spiritual care.

Implications

The researchers concluded that nurses must be sensitive to providing spiritual care in ways that are welcomed by clients.

Note: From Taylor, E. J. & Mamier, I. (2005). Spiritual care nursing: What cancer patients and family caregivers want. *Journal of advanced nursing, 49*(3) 260–267. Blackwell Publishing. Reprinted with permission.

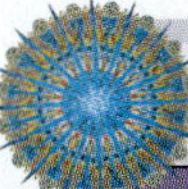

NURSING CARE PLAN A Client With Spiritual Distress

ASSESSMENT	DIAGNOSIS	PLANNING
Mrs. Sally Horton is a 60-year-old hospitalized homemaker who is recovering from a right radical mastectomy. Her primary care provider told her yesterday that due to metastases of the cancer, her prognosis is poor. This morning her nurse finds her tearful, stating that she slept poorly and has no appetite. She asks the nurse, "Why has God done this to me? Perhaps it's because I have sinned in my life. I've not gone to church or spoken to a minister in several years. Is there a chapel in the hospital where I could go and pray? I'm terribly afraid of dying and what awaits me." **Physical Examination** Height: 165.1 cm (5'5")	■ Spiritual Distress related to feelings of guilt and alienation from God as evidenced by questioning why "God has done this"; inquiries about praying in a chapel; insomnia; no appetite	■ The client will interact with a spiritual leader from her faith. ■ The client will observe a spiritual practice that provides her comfort. ■ The client will connect with others to share thoughts, feelings, beliefs.

IMPLEMENTATION

- Create an accepting, nonjudgmental atmosphere.
- Be open to Mrs. Horton's feelings about illness and death.
- Assist her to express and relieve anger in appropriate ways.
- Encourage the use of spiritual resources, if desired by the client.
- Encourage her to list values that guide behavior in times of tragedy.
- Encourage verbalization of feelings, perceptions, and fears. Allow time for grieving.

EVALUATION

Outcome met. Mrs. Horton has been visited on several occasions by her minister. She reads scripture each day and has found consolation in reading the book of Psalms. She states, "God is merciful and will help me bear my suffering."

CRITICAL THINKING

1. What spiritual resources might you recommend for this client?
2. If Mrs. Horton's spiritual leader supports the concept that disease is a result of sins committed throughout life, how can the nurse help this client?
3. If your religious beliefs would help this client obtain spiritual well-being what actions could you take to help this client?

outcomes for the client who needs to maintain or be restored to spiritual health include the following:

- The client will participate in religious observances; e.g., the client will observe prayer times.
- The client will articulate a sense of hopefulness about the future.
- The client will articulate faith in a higher power.
- The client will articulate how to access spiritual resources.
- The client will find meaning and existence in the present situation.

REVIEW Spiritual Distress

RELATE: LINK THE CONCEPTS

Linking the exemplar of Spiritual Distress with the concept of Oxygenation:

1. Describe the risk for spiritual distress faced by the parents of a child who has just died from sudden infant death syndrome.
2. What caring interventions would you offer to the child's parents?

Linking the exemplar of Spiritual Distress with the concept of Development:

3. What signals or words might indicate that an 8-year-old child from a Protestant Christian family is in spiritual distress? What caring interventions would be appropriate for a child this age?
4. How might a teenager communicate spiritual distress differently? What interventions would be appropriate for a teenager that would not be appropriate for a younger child?

REFER: GO TO MYNURSINGKIT

REFLECT: CASE STUDY

Terry is a 32-year-old male who received several pints of blood following an automobile crash 10 years ago. Five years ago he was diagnosed with acquired immune deficiency syndrome (AIDS), and he is now in the hospital with pneumonia and severe diarrhea. He is very ill and very discouraged. While you are caring for Terry, he comments, "I might as well die right now because I'm not going to get well. My folks were Methodist, but I guess I'm being punished because I'm not very religious."

1. Terry stated that he was "not very religious." Does that mean that he is not spiritual? Explain.
2. What data suggest that Terry may be experiencing spiritual distress?
3. How might illness affect one's spiritual beliefs? Religious beliefs?
4. How might a spiritual assessment be of benefit to both you and Terry?

PEARSON

EXPLORE mynursingkit™

MyNursingKit is your one stop for online chapter review materials and resources. Prepare for success with additional NCLEX®-style practice questions, interactive assignments and activities, web links, animations and videos, and more!

Register your access code from the front of your book at **www.mynursingkit.com**.

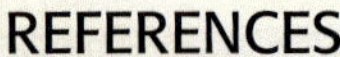

REFERENCES

Burkhardt, M. A. (1989). Spirituality: An analysis of the concept. *Holistic Nursing Practice, 3*(3), 69–77.

Burkhart, L. (2005). A click away: Documenting spiritual care. *Journal of Christian Nursing, 22*(1), 6–12.

Carpenito-Moyet, L. J. (2006). *Nursing diagnosis: Application to clinical practice* (11th ed.). Philadelphia: Lippincott.

Cole, B., Benore, E., & Pargament, K. I. (2004). Spirituality and coping with trauma. In S. Sorajjakool & H. Lamberton (Eds.), *Spirituality, health, and wholeness* (pp. 49–76). New York: Haworth Press.

Coward, D. D. (1990). The lived experience of self-transcendence in women with advanced breast cancer. *Nursing Science Quarterly, 3*(4), 162–169.

Dameron, C. M. (2005). Spiritual assessment made easy. . . with acronyms! *Journal of Christian Nursing, 22*(1), 14–16.

Denny, F. M. (1993). Islam and the Muslim community. In H. Byron Earhart (Ed.), *Religious traditions of the world* (pp. 603–713). New York: HarperSanFrancisco.

Dochterman, J. M., & Bulechek, G. M. (Eds.). (2004). *Nursing interventions classification (NIC)* (4th ed.). St. Louis, MO: Mosby.

Dossey, L. (1996). *Prayer is good medicine. How to reap the benefits of prayer.* New York: HarperCollins.

Dossey, L. (1999). Healing and the nonlocal mind: Interview by Bonnie Horrigan. *Alternative Therapies in Health and Medicine, 5*(6), 85–93.

Doughty, S. (2007). Six in ten nurses would turn "blind eye" to the abuse of the elderly. *The Daily Mail Online.* Retrieved September 14, 2009 from http://www.dailymail.co.uk/health/article-478352/Six-10-nurses-turn-blind-eye-abuse-elderly.html

Economist (2008). Sons of heaven: Christianity in China. Retrieved September 13, 2009, from http://www.economist.com/world/asia/displaystory.cfm?story_id=12342509

Ellison, C. W. (1983, April). Spiritual well-being: Conceptualization and measurement. *Journal of Psychology and Theology, 11*, 330–340.

Fishbane, M. (1993). Judaism: Revelation and traditions. In H. Byron Earhart (Ed.), *Religious traditions of the world* (pp. 373–484). New York: HarperSanFrancisco.

Fowler, J. W. (1981). *Stages of faith development: The psychology of human development and the quest for meaning.* San Francisco: Harper & Row.

Frankiel, S. S. (1993). Christianity: A way of salvation. In H. Byron Earhart (Ed.), *Religious traditions of the world* (pp. 484–601). New York: HarperSanFrancisco.

Fredriksson, L. (1999). Modes of relating in a caring conversation: A research synthesis on presence, touch, and listening. *Journal of Advanced Nursing, 30*, 1167–1176.

Gill, S. D. (1987). Prayer. In M. Eliade (Ed.), *The encyclopedia of religion* (pp. 489–492). New York: Macmillan.

Griffith, J. K. (1996). *The religious aspects of nursing care.* Vancouver, BC: Author.

Howden, J. W. (1992). *Development and psychometric characteristics of the Spirituality Assessment Scale.* Unpublished doctoral dissertation, Texas Women's University, Denton.

Joint Commission on Accreditation of Healthcare Organizations. (2000). *Hospital accreditation standards.* Oakbrook, IL: Author.

Jourard, S. (1971). *The transparent self.* London: D. Van Nostrand.

Koenig, H. G. (2002). *Spirituality in patient care: Why, how, when, and what.* Radnor, PA: Templeton Press.

Martsolf, D. S., & Mickley, J. R. (1998). The concept of spirituality in nursing theories: Differing world-views and extent of focus. *Journal of Advanced Nursing, 27*, 294–303.

Massey, K., Fitchett, G., & Roberts, P. A. (2004). In K. L. Mauk & N. K. Schmidt (Eds.), *Spiritual care in nursing practice. Assessment and diagnosis in spiritual care* (Chapter 14, pp. 209–242). Philadelphia: Lippincott Williams & Wilkins.

Mauk, K. L., & Schmidt, N. K. (2004). *Spiritual care in nursing practice.* Philadelphia: Lippincott Williams & Wilkins.

Medical News Today. (2009). The Australian community continues to value nurses: Nurses voted the most 'ethical and honest' profession for the 15th year running. Retrieved September 14, 2009, from http://www.medicalnewstoday.com/articles/154046.php

Mickley, J. R., & Cowles, K. (2001). Ameliorating the tension: Use of forgiveness for healing. *Oncology Nursing Forum, 28*, 31–38.

Moorhead, S., Johnson, M., & Maas, M. (2004). *Iowa intervention project: Nursing outcome classification.* St. Louis, MO: Mosby.

Moschella, V. D., Pressman, K. R., Pressman, P., & Weissman, D. E. (1997). The problem of theodicy and religious responses to cancer. *Journal of Religion & Health, 36*(1), 17–20.

NANDA International. (2007). *NANDA nursing diagnoses: Definitions and classification 2007–2008.* Philadelphia: Author.

Osterman, P., & Schwartz-Barcott, D. (1996). Presence: Four ways of being there. *Nursing Forum, 31*(2), 23–30.

Pettigrew, J. (1990). Intensive nursing care: The ministry of presence. *Critical Care Nursing Clinics of North America, 2*, 503–508.

Pilch, J. J. (1998, May/June). Wellness spirituality. *Health Values, 12*, 28–31.

Poloma, M. M., & Gallup, G. H., Jr. (1991). *Varieties of prayer: A survey report.* Philadelphia: Trinity Press International.

Reed, P. G. (1992). An emerging paradigm for the investigation of spirituality in nursing. *Research in Nursing and Health, 15*, 349–357.

al-Shahri, M.Z, & al-Khenaiza, A. (2005) Palliative care for Muslim paitents. *Journal of Supportive Oncology, 3*(6), 432–436. Retrieved September 13, 2009, from http://www.supportiveoncology.net/journal/articles/0306432.pdf

Shane, S. (2009). Report outlines medical workers' role in torture. *New York Times.* Retrieved September 14, 2009, from http://www.nytimes.com/2009/04/07/world/07detain.html

Stephenson, C. (1991). The concept of hope revisited for nursing. *Journal of Advances in Nursing, 16*, 1456–1461.

Taylor, E. J. (1998). Caring for the spirit. In C. C. Burke (Ed.), *Psychosocial dimensions of oncology nursing care.* Pittsburgh: Oncology Nursing Press.

Taylor, E. J. (2001). Spirituality, culture, and cancer care. *Seminars in Oncology Nursing, 17*(3), 197–205.

Taylor, E. J. (2002). *Spiritual care: Nursing theory, research, and practice.* Upper Saddle River, NJ: Prentice Hall.

Taylor, E. J. (2003a). Nurses caring for the spirit: Patients with cancer and family caregiver expectations. *Oncology Nursing Forum, 30*, 585–594.

Taylor, E. J. (2003b). Prayer's clinical issues and implications. *Holistic Nursing Practice, 17*(4), 179–188.

Taylor, E. J. (2005). What have we learned from spiritual care research? *Journal of Christian Nursing, 22*(1), 22–28.

Taylor, E. J., & Mamier, I. (2005). Spiritual care nursing: what cancer patients and family caregivers want. *Journal of Advanced Nursing, 49*(3), 260–267.

Ulanov, A., & Ulanov, B. (1983). *Primary speech: A psychology of prayer.* Atlanta, GA: John Knox Press. (Classic.)

Vardey, L. (1996). *God in all worlds.* Toronto: Vintage Canada.

Wax, Trevin. (2008). Seven Types of Southern Baptists. Retrieved September 13, 2009, from http://trevinwax.com/2008/06/10/7-types-of-southern-baptists/

Westerhoff, J. (1976). *Will our children have faith?* New York: Seabury Press.

Winslow, G. R., & Winslow, B. W. (2003). Examining the ethics of praying with patients. *Holistic Nursing Practice, 17*(4), 170–177.

Wright, S. (2008). When nurses do. *Nursing Standard, 23*(6), 18–20.

Zerwekh, J. V. (1997). The practice of presencing. *Seminars in Oncology Nursing, 13*, 260–262.

Stress and Coping 28

Concept at-a-Glance

Concept Learning Outcomes

After reading about this concept, you will be able to:

1. Summarize the dynamics of stress, appraisal, coping, and adaptation.
2. List factors affecting stress and coping.
3. Identify commonly occurring alterations in stress and coping and their related treatments.
4. Explain common assessment procedures used to examine the stress response of clients across the life span.
5. Outline diagnostic and laboratory tests to determine the individual's stress and coping status.
6. Explain the management of stress to facilitate healthy coping and the prevention of illness.
7. Demonstrate the nursing process in providing culturally competent and caring interventions across the life span for individuals with common alterations in stress and coping.
8. Identify pharmacological interventions in caring for individuals with alterations in stress response, coping, and adaptation.

Concept Key Terms

Adaptation, *1794*
Anger, *1800*
Anxiety, *1800*
Appraisal-focused coping, *1799*
Approach-coping, *1799*
Avoidance-coping, *1799*
Basic needs, *1798*
Burnout, *1807*
Cognitive appraisal, *1796*
Cognitive-behavioral therapy (CBT), *1806*
Coping, *1794*
Countershock phase, *1794*
Depression, *1801*
Ego defense mechanisms, *1802*
Emotion-focused coping, *1799*
Eustress, *1797*
External environmental stressors, *1797*
Fear, *1800*
General adaptation syndrome (GAS), *1794*
Hassles, *1797*
Hildegard Peplau, *1796*
Homeostasis, *1793*
Internal environment, *1797*
Local adaptation syndrome (LAS), *1794*
Meta-needs, *1798*
Nursing transactional model, *1796*
Primary appraisal, *1796*
Problem-focused coping, *1799*
Reappraisal, *1796*
Secondary appraisal, *1796*
Shock phase, *1794*
Stage of exhaustion, *1795*
Stage of resistance, *1794*
Stimulus-based stress model, *1794*
Stress, *1793*
Stress response, *1794*
Stressor, *1794*

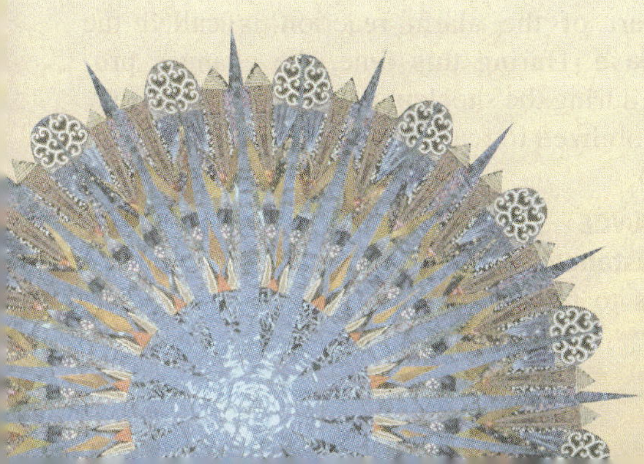

About Stress and Coping

The study of stress begins with the concept of homeostasis. In relation to stress and coping, **homeostasis** is the state of dynamic balance of the human body's internal environment, which is always adjusting in response to internal and external changes. This stable internal environment is necessary for survival. The ability of the body to maintain homeostasis depends on thousands of physiological control systems. These include the systems within the body that maintain fluid and electrolyte balance, oxygen levels, and even the neuroendocrine systems that influence behavior (Porth, 2007). **Stress** is the body's reaction to any stimulus in the environment that demands change or disrupts homeostasis.

The stimulus provoking the demand for change is commonly referred to as a **stressor**. The **stress response**, commonly referred to as **coping**, refers to the individual's response to one or more stressors and his or her attempt to restore homeostasis. In cases in which the individual cannot return to homeostasis, the individual may achieve **adaptation**, that is, he or she finds a way to function normally despite the fact that homeostasis is not or cannot be restored. For example, the individual who loses a limb will not get that limb back. However, through use of a prosthetic or other accommodations, the individual may achieve adaptation and return to a normal, healthy life.

The experience of stress is a multidimensional phenomenon. Not fully understood, it encompasses a variety of biological, psychological, cognitive, and neurological factors. Numerous behavioral, nursing, and medical scientists and scholars have labored to understand, define, and describe the stress response. The fact that every individual experiences and responds differently to stress makes it such a compelling issue. A modern day conversation rarely takes place without including one or more references to stressful occurrences.

The term *stress* has been in use since as far back as the fourteenth century, when it was used to describe hardship and adversity (Lazarus & Folkman, 1984). In the nineteenth century, the term became associated with an imbalance in homeostasis between an individual's internal and external forces. This definition was developed further by the scientific community to include ill health (Lazarus & Folkman, 1984). Historically, the medical model of care by Descartes was based on the philosophy and the belief that the human body operates as a machine separating the mind, body, and spirit (Carson & Arnold, 1996). Progressing further from this simplistic model, theorists began to focus on homeostatic mechanisms, physiological stress, and the effect of stress on the body. Our scientific understanding has progressed to the level that we understand that the individual is dynamic and in constant interaction with the environment (Lazarus & Folkman, 1984).

A number of theories and models exist to explain the phenomenon of stress. The importance and contribution of each of the models cannot be understated. This concept will discuss stimulus-based and response-based models briefly, before presenting the transactional model in more detail. •

Stimulus-Based Models

In **stimulus-based stress models**, stress is defined as a stimulus, a life event, or a set of circumstances that arouses physiological and/or psychological reactions that may increase the individual's vulnerability to illness. In their classic work, Holmes and Rahe (1967) assigned a numerical value to 43 life changes or events. The most recent version of that scale includes 77 items (Miller & Rahe, 1997), and a shortened version (54 items, full stress and coping inventory competed in 15 minutes) was created more recently (Rahe & Tolles, 2002). The scale of stressful life events is used to document a person's relatively recent experiences, such as marriage, divorce, pregnancy, and retirement. In this view, both positive and negative events are considered stressful.

Similar scales have since been developed, but all scales should be used with caution: The degree of stress one individual experiences related to an event may be very different from the amount of stress another individual feels. For example, a divorce may be highly traumatic to one person and cause relatively little anxiety to another. In addition, many scales have not been tested for age, socioeconomic status, or cultural sensitivity.

Response-Based Models

Stress may also be considered as a response. This definition was developed and described by Selye (1956, 1976) as "the nonspecific response of the body to any kind of demand made upon it" (1976, p. 1).

Selye's stress response is characterized by a chain or pattern of physiological events called **general adaptation syndrome (GAS)** or *stress syndrome*. To differentiate the cause of stress from the response to stress, Selye (1976) used the term *stressor* to denote any factor that produces stress and disturbs the body's equilibrium. Because stress is a state of the body, it can be observed only by the changes it produces in the body. This response of the body, the general adaptation syndrome, occurs with the release of certain adaptive hormones and subsequent changes in the structure and chemical composition of the body. Parts of the body particularly affected by stress are the gastrointestinal tract, the adrenal glands, and the lymphatic structures. With prolonged stress, the adrenal glands enlarge considerably; the lymphatic structures, such as the thymus, spleen, and lymph nodes, atrophy (shrink); and deep ulcers appear in the lining of the stomach.

In addition to adapting globally, the body can also react locally; that is, one organ or a part of the body reacts alone. This is referred to as **local adaptation syndrome (LAS)**. Local inflammation is one example of LAS. Selye (1976) proposed that both GAS and LAS have three stages: alarm reaction, resistance, and exhaustion (see Figure 28–1 ■).

ALARM REACTION The body's initial reaction is the alarm reaction, commonly referred to as the **shock phase**, which sets the stage for the cascade of physiological reactions to the stressor. This triggers the body's defenses by stimulating the sympathetic nervous system, which in turn stimulates the hypothalamus. The hypothalamus releases corticotrophin-releasing hormone (CRH), which stimulates the anterior pituitary gland to release adrenocorticotropic hormone (ACTH). This sympathetic stimulation results in secretion of epinephrine and norepinephrine. Significant body responses to epinephrine include increased myocardial activity, bronchial dilation, and increased fat mobilization. This adrenal hormonal activity prepares the individual for *fight or flight*. This primary response is short lived, lasting from 1 minute to 24 hours.

The second part of the alarm reaction is called the **countershock phase**. During this time, the changes produced in the body during the shock phase are reversed. Thus, a person is best mobilized to react during the shock phase of the alarm reaction.

STAGE OF RESISTANCE The second stage of GAS syndrome is the **stage of resistance**, in which the body begins to initiate adaptive responses to return to homeostasis and reduce the

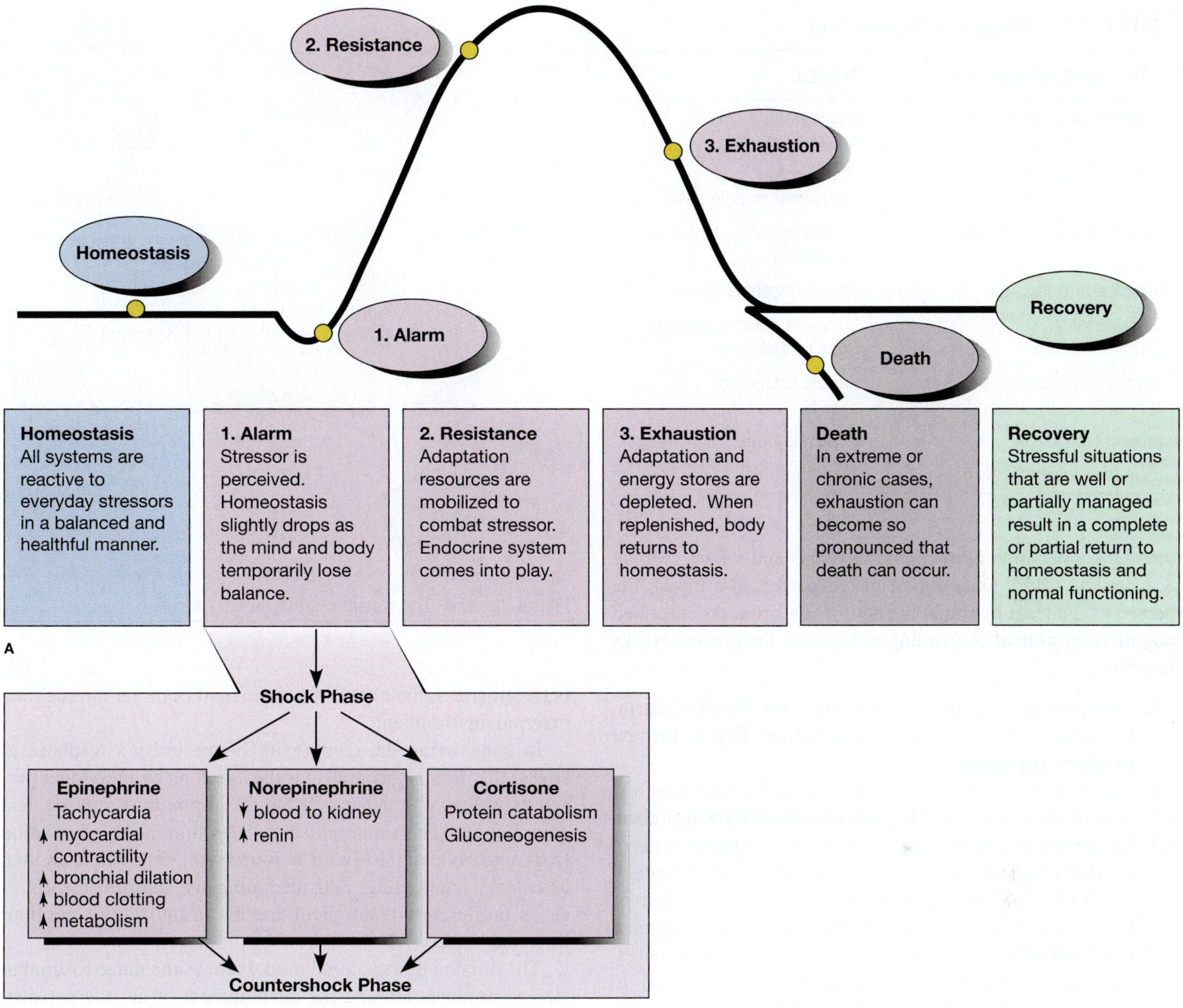

2. Resistance
3. Exhaustion
Homeostasis
1. Alarm
Recovery
Death
Homeostasis
All systems are reactive to everyday stressors in a balanced and healthful manner.
1. Alarm
Stressor is perceived. Homeostasis slightly drops as the mind and body temporarily lose balance.
2. Resistance
Adaptation resources are mobilized to combat stressor. Endocrine system comes into play.
3. Exhaustion
Adaptation and energy stores are depleted. When replenished, body returns to homeostasis.
Death
In extreme or chronic cases, exhaustion can become so pronounced that death can occur.
Recovery
Stressful situations that are well or partially managed result in a complete or partial return to homeostasis and normal functioning.
A
Shock Phase
Epinephrine
Tachycardia
↑ myocardial contractility
↑ bronchial dilation
↑ blood clotting
↑ metabolism
Norepinephrine
↓ blood to kidney
↑ renin
Cortisone
Protein catabolism
Gluconeogenesis
Countershock Phase
B

Figure 28–1 ■ The three stages of adaptation to stress: the alarm reaction, the stage of resistance, and the stage of exhaustion.

Source: Part A is from *Wellness: Concepts and application*, 6th ed. (p. 298) by D.J. Anspaugh, M. Hamrick, and F.D. Rosato, 2005, New York; McGraw-Hill. Reprinted with permission.

impact of the stressor on the individual. In other words, the body attempts to cope with the stressor and to limit the stressor to the smallest area of the body that can deal with it.

STAGE OF EXHAUSTION During the third stage, the **stage of exhaustion**, if the body cannot maintain its adaptation to the stressor, the stressor overwhelms the individual's ability to cope or mount a continued defense, resulting in the depletion of energy and resources. The body may rebound from the stressor after a period of rest or death may ensue. Table 28–1 summarizes this stage of the general adaptation syndrome. The end of this stage depends largely on the adaptive energy resources of the individual, the severity of the stressor, and the external adaptive resources that are provided. An example of this can be seen in the client who lives with chronic pain. The client may be able to tolerate the pain during the day, but at night finds the pain far more stressful because their energy resources are diminished to the point that the pain is intolerable.

TRANSACTIONAL MODEL OF STRESS AND COPING

The transactional model of stress and coping, originally presented in Lazarus and Folkman's work *Stress, Appraisal and Coping* (1984), differs from the stimulus-based and response-based models in that it accounts for individual differences in perceptions of and responses to stress. In the Lazarus model, perceived threat—what the person appraises as taxing or exceeding his or her resources or endangering his or her well-being—is the central characteristic of stressful situations because it

TABLE 28–1 Stages of Exhaustion

PARADOXICAL REACTION	SHOCK
Excretion of epinephrine	Depression of central nervous system
Elevated blood pressure	Hypotension Decreased muscle tone
Increased pulse pressure	Decreased white blood cell production
Increase in pulse rate	Hemoconcentration
Glycogenolysis Gluconeogenesis	Decrease plasma glucose Protein catabolism
Increase in cholesterol and free fatty acids in the blood for energy	Protein catabolism
Protein catabolism Increased respirations	Hypochloremia Hypothermia

threatens a person's most important goals and values (Monat & Lazarus, 1991). Once a person has perceived a threat, the person evaluates it by thinking about it. This process is termed **cognitive appraisal**. According to Lazarus, the process works like this:

1. The person assesses the potential for benefit, harm, loss, threat, or challenge in a situation. This is termed **primary appraisal**.
2. The person then evaluates his or her coping resources and options in the situation. This is termed **secondary appraisal**.
3. The person applies the coping resources and options at his or her disposal. This response to the stressor is termed *coping*.
4. The individual engages in ongoing reinterpretation of the situation based on new information. This is termed **reappraisal**. Reappraisal allows the individual to determine if the coping mechanisms he or she applied in response to the stressor worked, and helps the person appraise the next *transaction* or stress experience that comes along.

Cognitive appraisal and coping style are influenced by the culture of the individual. Providing culturally competent care requires understanding the client's perspective and recognizing that a client's cognitive appraisal of a situation may, and probably will, differ from one's own.

Lazarus believes that stress depends not only on external conditions but also on the person's physical vulnerability and the adequacy of that person's coping styles.

The nursing transactional model is an adaptation of Lazarus and Folkman's work. The **nursing transactional model** is defined as the relationship between the nurse, the client, and the environment in which they interact (Figure 28–2 ■). This interaction, or relationship, is dynamic, as with each transaction the individual and the stressor engage to form a new transaction with a particular meaning. This model has numerous implications for the profession of nursing and care of the individual experiencing stress. The emphasis is on the relationship

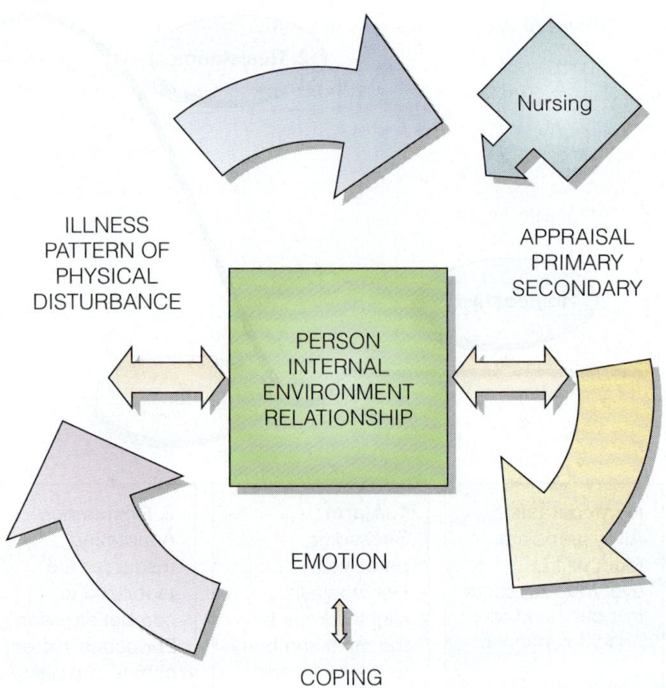

Figure 28–2 ■ The nursing transactional model.

between stress, the client, the nurse, and both the internal and external environment.

In considering the complexity of the client's response to stress, the nurse must consider the client as an individual person as well as a member of a family, community, culture, and environment. The astute nurse collects important information from each context to build a foundation for understanding, assessing, intervening, and mediating the harmful effects of stress on the individual client and his or her family, community, and society.

The nursing transactional model allows the nurse to emphasize communication and the development of an interpersonal relationship with the client with the intent of decreasing the client's anxiety and increasing or improving the client's coping resources. This approach owes much to **Hildegard Peplau**, who is known as the mother of psychiatric nursing. She was one of the first nurses to analyze nursing action using an interpersonal theoretical model and published this theory in her 1952 book *Interpersonal Relations in Nursing*. She defined nursing as a "significant therapeutic interpersonal process that makes health possible for individuals and groups." The major concepts of her theory include growth, development, communication, and roles.

Communication, described in detail in Concept 36, is a problem-solving process that takes place within the nurse–client relationship. Problem solving is a collaborative process in which the nurse may assume many roles in helping clients meet needs and continue their growth and development. As client conflicts and anxieties are resolved, personalities are strengthened. Peplau noted that both nurses' and clients' culture, religion, ethnicity, education, experiences, and preconceived ideas influence interpersonal relationships.

Peplau believed that psychodynamic nursing liberated nurses from a tradition of being task-oriented and gave them permission to focus on their excellent interpersonal skills. Peplau's perspective is humane and compassionate, encouraging nurses to listen carefully and develop the empathy essential for the therapeutic relationship. Peplau's work continues to be the essence of psychiatric nursing.

Stressors

Stress occurs when the individual appraises the stressor and determines whether or not the stressor is within the individual's coping range. Stressors are classified into four categories:

1. Acute and time limited
2. Sequential events following an initial stressor
3. Chronic intermittent
4. Chronic permanent.

See Table 28–2 for examples of each classification.

To understand the reciprocal and dynamic relationship between the individual and the environment, it is important to broaden the discussion of stressors to include sources of stress and types of stressors. The degree of the stressors range from benign (nonthreatening) daily hassles to catastrophic events within a person, family, and society such as the scenario at the beginning of this concept and natural disasters such as Hurricane Katrina in 2005. Box 28–1 lists some common stressors.

STRESSORS FROM THE INTERNAL ENVIRONMENT The **internal environment** includes the physical, spiritual, cognitive, emotional, and psychological well-being of the individual and is dependent upon the satisfaction of these basic human needs. According to Lazarus and Folkman (1984), the drive to fulfill human needs internally sparks the stimulus to produce the energy to seek gratification. This individual day-to-day tension is commonly referred to in stress and coping research as daily **hassles**. The holistic health and balance of individuals experiencing stressors affects their ability to cope with daily hassles. Consider the following examples of daily hassles: completing a day at school or work when experiencing a simple stress like the common cold, waking up feeling tired and having to care for a small child, or overdrawing one's bank account. Physical, emotional, and spiritual health affects whether or not the individual appraises a hassle as a minor inconvenience or a major strain. Alterations of health in any of these areas may overwhelm an individual's ability to cope with a specific stimulus or event, no matter how mild.

Dossey, Keegan, and Guzzetta (2005) address the spiritual dimension of the human condition as part of the individual's internal environment. The authors define *spirituality* as the essence of who we are and how we relate to the world. They incorporate elements of spirituality that include individual values, our place or fit in the world, and a sense of peace. Recent research has identified interconnectedness with the self, individuals, and the world around as important components of spirituality. For more information about spirituality, please see Concept 27.

STRESSORS FROM THE EXTERNAL ENVIRONMENT **External environmental stressors** include triggers outside of the individual that demand change or disrupt homeostasis. The change can be positive, known as **eustress**, such as graduation from college, or negative, such as lack of employment. It may be simultaneously positive and negative, as with the combination of pending college graduation and imminent lack of employment. The

TABLE 28–2 Classifications and Examples of Stressors

CLASSIFICATION OF STRESSORS	EXAMPLES
1. Acute and time limited	Roller coaster ride Nursing licensure exam
2. Sequential events following an initial stressor	Losing a job and subsequently filing for bankruptcy
3. Chronic intermittent	Strained relationship with in-laws Shared caretaking for an elderly parent
4. Chronic permanent	Paralysis Disability (e.g., blindness, deafness)

Box 28–1 Types of Stressors

DEVELOPMENTAL STRESSORS
Starting school
Playing and working with peers
Puberty
Education
Changes
Marriage
Birth of children
Aging

ENVIRONMENTAL STRESSORS
Major cataclysmic changes affecting a large number of people (natural disasters, war, floods, hurricanes)
Major changes affecting one or a few people (divorce, bereavement)

DAILY HASSLES
Roles of living
Caring for children
Pets
Work responsibility
Paying bills
Traffic
Neighbors

INTERNAL STRESSORS
Cognition (thoughts)
Spirituality
Emotions

TABLE 28–3 Factors Affecting Individual Stress Response

INDIVIDUAL FACTORS	ENVIRONMENTAL FACTORS
Genetic predisposition Past experience coping with stressors Ability to meet own basic human needs	Family support and connectedness Community support Financial resources Community resources Cultural beliefs and customs
Holistic health and well-being	Access to health care and education
Personal worldview and appraisal Coping mechanisms and history of coping successes	Family appraisal Social support

transactional model emphasizes that an event is a stressor if it creates a change in the individual or the individual's circumstances. Table 28–3 outlines specific individual and environmental factors that affect the individual's response to a stressor.

Appraisal

Appraisal is a key factor in the client's ability to cope with stressors. As the individual experiences exposure to a stressor, he or she appraises the stressor; that is, the individual mentally sorts, assesses, categorizes, evaluates and frames the significance of an event or stressor with respect to his or her well-being. The *primary appraisal* is the "first impression," occurring immediately upon exposure to a stressor. Based on the transactional model there are three ways in which a person categorizes a stimulus or demand: (1) irrelevant, (2) benign-positive, and (3) stressful. Irrelevant stressors are appraised as having no meaningful effect on the individual or his or her circumstance, and are disregarded. Benign-positive stressors are demands for change that are perceived as preserving or enhancing well-being, such as taking a driver's education class. Stressors or stimuli categorized as stressful include those viewed as harmful, threatening, or disturbing, such as the death of a family member or a threat to life or safety.

During the secondary appraisal, the individual attempts to predict the impact, intensity, and duration of the coping behavior necessary to respond to the stressor. At this time the individual selects a coping response.

MASLOW'S HIERARCHY OF BASIC HUMAN NEEDS When an individual appraises a stressor, he or she uses a number of factors to decide how to respond to the stressor. Included in these factors is the individual's perception of or state of need. How does the stressor affect the individual's need for food and shelter? For love? Are there other stressors that are of greater priority?

Abraham Maslow devised a hierarchy of needs to explain how human beings prioritize need and what levels of need must be met for the individual to *self-actualize*, that is, to reach peak capacity for fulfilling his or her potential (see Figure 28–3 ■).

- **Basic needs** are physiological, such as the need for food, water, and sleep.
- **Meta-needs** are growth-related and include such things as love and belonging, esteem, and self-actualization.

Under most circumstances, basic needs take precedence over meta-needs. A person who is hungry is less concerned with truth and justice than a person who is not hungry and whose basic needs have been met. Maslow felt that fulfilling meta-needs enables a person to rise above an animal level of existence. People who are unable to meet their growth needs, Maslow postulated, can become psychologically disturbed (Maslow, 1968).

Maslow looked primarily at the healthy, strong side of human nature. His is a *humanistic theory*, in which people are defined holistically as dynamic combinations of physical, emotional, cognitive, and spiritual processes. Maslow emphasized health rather than illness, success rather than failure. He even viewed basic drives, such as the sex drive, as natural rather than as unhealthy urges to be controlled. Maslow believed that people have an inborn nature that is essentially good or, at worst, neutral.

Coping

Coping is a process, not a trait. It includes all efforts mobilized by the individual to manage stressors. Coping involves constant change by the individual and includes spiritual, emotional, cognitive, and behavioral efforts to manage the demand. A stressor is appraised in terms of its effects or

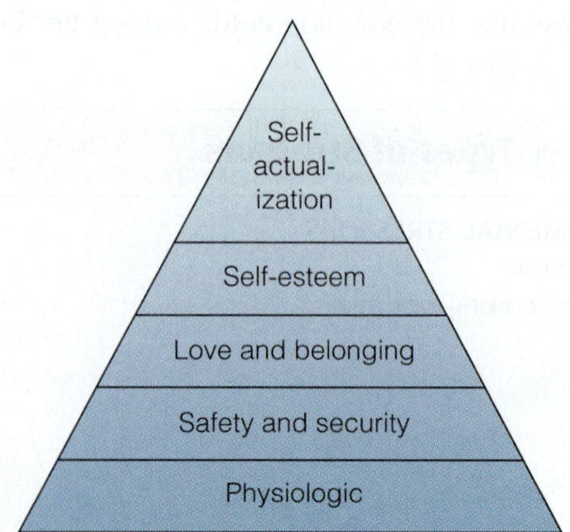

Figure 28–3 ■ Maslow's hierarchy of needs.

Source: From *Psychology of Human Behaviour*, 5th ed. by Kalish, copyright 1983. Reprinted with permission of Wadsworth, a division of Thomson Learning: www.thomsonrights.com. Fax 800-730-2215.

alterations on the physical, emotional, and spiritual conditions of the individual and/or on the individual's unmet needs or drives. Lazarus and Folkman's (1984) transactional model describes *coping* as a means to manage or alter the problem causing the distress. The appraisal process allows the individual to inform the coping response by incorporating the person's own spiritual, cognitive, affective, and inherent vulnerability. In essence, every person responds to a stressor according to his or her unique world view and condition.

There are two forms of coping: (1) **problem-focused coping**, which is aimed at managing or altering the stressor, event, or circumstance, and (2) **emotion-focused coping**, which is directed at regulating the emotional response to the distress. Emotion-focused coping is used most when the stressor is perceived to be beyond the individual's control. In problem-focused coping, the perception is generally that the stressor can be changed (Lazarus and Folkman, 1984). Additional subcategories of coping were added to the original model: **avoidance-coping** (using both behaviors and cognitive processes to avoid the stressor) and **approach-coping** (confronting and trying to change the stressor by taking direct action). Finally, there is also **appraisal-focused coping**, which involves revaluation to reduce the appraisal of a threat (Nicholls & Polman, 2007).

It is crucial for nurses to understand that any form of coping is an individual process influenced by the number of stressors; their source, type, intensity, and duration; and the individual's support, experience, and vulnerability. Critical to the nurse's ability to work with clients are an awareness of the nurse's own coping style and a nonjudgmental attitude about the coping mechanisms of individuals experiencing stressors. Table 28–4 depicts the various forms and examples of coping with stressors.

The importance of the individual's ability to respond to stress cannot be underestimated. Health care professionals and researchers have clearly established the strong and complex relationship between stress, coping, and physical and psychological illness (Sinah & Watson, 2007). It is estimated that the relationship between stress and coping accounts for almost 50% of psychological symptoms. A more global view includes cultural demands and the stress of the environment. A recent study by Sinah and Watson (2007) explored the social and cultural effects of stress on health and illness. Aldwin (1994) researched the impact of culture not only on the experience of stress, but also on the coping strategies that are used to deal with perceived stress. Lazarus and Folkman (1984) note that it is the reaction to the demand, not the stimulus itself, that causes the stressor. The nursing transactional model allows the nurse to consider individual client preferences, resources, culture, and environment in the assessment of the client's abilities to respond to stress and in the design of a care plan to assist the client in returning to homeostasis.

Reappraisal and Adaptation

Following attempts to cope with the stressor, the individual engages in a reappraisal process. During this time, the individual evaluates what coping mechanisms were successful and what were not and, ideally, begins another attempt to respond to the stressor and return to homeostasis. The individual who copes with the stressor successfully may reach a stage of adaptation. Adaptation refers to the quality of life experienced by the individual related to work and social activities, morale and life satisfaction, and holistic health. Stress is not viewed as "good" or "bad" but merely according to how much, what kinds, and under what conditions is it harmful or helpful (Lazarus & Folkman, 1984). Adaptation and or alterations in health are influenced by personal variables (Sinah & Watson, 2005). Variables that have been identified include ways of coping, the individual's perception of control, and quality of the individual's social support.

INDICATORS OF STRESS

Selye (1956) depicted stress as the reaction of an organism to continual bombardment from noxious agents in the environment. Selye presented this dynamic, complex, physiological cascade of events as GAS. This work stimulated increased interest in the concept of stress and helped to link the biology of the

TABLE 28–4 **Examples of Types of Coping**

TYPES	EMOTION-FOCUSED COPING (DEFENSIVE)	PROBLEM-FOCUSED COPING	AVOIDANCE	APPROACH	APPRAISAL
Cognitive	Minimizing the event. "Oh it's not that bad!"	Information gathering. "What are my odds of surviving?"	Denial of a situation or limiting information about stressful situations. "This is a bad dream!"	Confronting the situation	Primary control—attempting to change the environment
Behavioral	Performing physical activity to avoid thinking about a stressful situation	Adhering to a health care plan	Refusing to get a mammogram when a history of breast cancer runs in the family	Seeking means to exercise control	Attempting to fit into the environment. "I'll just go with the flow!"
Affective	Hoping for a miracle	Keeping feelings from interfering	Dealing with feelings later	Using feelings to motivate change	Seeking control of environment; regulating the emotional response to stress

stress response to the psychology and social sciences. Stress is further explained not as a stimulus, but as a dynamic state that occurs within the organism as a result of constant exposure to the environment. The environment holistically includes not only the physical environment, but also the psychological, emotional, spiritual, and cultural or external environment (Videbeck, 2004). To provide competent nursing care to individuals, the nurse needs a thorough understanding of the physiological, psychological, and cognitive events that occur within the individual as a result of an interaction with a stressor.

Physiological Indicators of Stress

Responses to stress vary depending on the individual's perception of events. The physiological signs and symptoms of stress result from activation of the sympathetic and neuroendocrine systems of the body. Box 28–2 lists physiological indicators of stress.

The harmful effects of stress on health emphasizing the mind–body connection are depicted in the Multisystem Effects of Stress feature on page 1801.

In the nursing transactional model, it is important to remain aware of the biological effects of stress on the individual. The person is considered a part of the environment, inseparable from it and in constant dynamic interaction with it. Stress occurs when the resources of the individual or the system become overwhelmed and tax the individual's ability to adapt.

Psychoemotional Indicators of Stress

Psychological manifestations of stress include anxiety, fear, anger, depression, and unconscious ego defense mechanisms. Some of these coping patterns are helpful; others may be detrimental, depending on the situation and the length of time they are used or experienced.

Box 28–2 **Physiological Indicators of Stress**

- Pupils dilate to increase visual perception when serious threats to the body arise.
- Sweat production (diaphoresis) increases to control elevated body heat due to increased metabolism.
- Heart rate and cardiac output increase to transport nutrients and by-products of metabolism more efficiently.
- Skin is pallid because of constriction of peripheral blood vessels, an effect of norepinephrine.
- Sodium and water retention increase due to release of mineralocorticoids, which increases blood volume.
- Rate and depth of respirations increase because of dilation of the bronchioles, promoting hyperventilation.
- Urinary output decreases.
- Mouth may be dry.
- Peristalsis of the intestines decreases, resulting in possible constipation and flatus.
- For serious threats, mental alertness improves.
- Muscle tension increases to prepare for rapid motor activity or defense.
- Blood sugar increases because of release of glucocorticoids and gluconeogenesis.

ANXIETY A common reaction to stress is **anxiety**, a state of mental uneasiness, apprehension, dread, or foreboding or a feeling of helplessness related to an impending or actual threat to self or significant relationships. Anxiety can be experienced at the conscious, subconscious, or unconscious level. As many as one-fourth of Americans experience an anxiety disorder sometime in their lifetime; over half of these are debilitating (Antai-Otong, 2003).

FEAR **Fear** is an emotion or feeling of apprehension aroused by impending or seeming danger, pain, or another perceived threat. The fear may be in response to something that has already occurred, to an immediate or current threat, or to something the person believes will happen. The object of fear may or may not be based in reality. For example, the beginning nursing student may be fearful in anticipation of the first experience in a client care setting. The student may fear that the client will not want to be cared for by the student or that the student might inadvertently harm the client.

Anxiety and fear differ in four ways:

1. The source of anxiety may not be identifiable; the source of fear is identifiable.
2. Anxiety is related to the future, that is, to an anticipated event. Fear is related to the present.
3. Anxiety is vague, whereas fear is definite.
4. Anxiety is the result of psychological or emotional conflict; fear is the result of a discrete physical or psychological entity.

PRACTICE ALERT

Mild or moderate anxiety motivates goal-directed behavior. In this sense, anxiety can be an effective coping strategy. For example, mild anxiety motivates students to study. Excessive anxiety, however, often has destructive effects.

ANGER **Anger** is an emotional state consisting of a subjective feeling of animosity or strong displeasure. People may feel guilty when they feel anger because they have been taught that to feel angry is wrong. However, anger can be expressed in a nonalienating manner; it is then considered a positive emotion and a sign of emotional maturity because growth and beneficial interactions result from it.

A verbal expression of anger can be considered a signal to others of one's internal psychological discomfort and a call for assistance to deal with perceived stress. In contrast, hostility is usually marked by overt antagonism and harmful or destructive behavior; aggression is an unprovoked attack or a hostile, injurious, or destructive action or outlook; and violence is the exertion of physical force to injure or abuse. Verbally expressed anger differs from hostility, aggression, and violence, but it can lead to destructiveness and violence if the anger persists unabated.

A clearly expressed verbal communication of anger, in which the angry person tells the other person about the anger and carefully identifies the source, is constructive. This clarity of communication gets the anger out into the open so that the other person can deal with it and help to alleviate it. The angry person "gets it off the chest" and prevents an emotional buildup.

MULTISYSTEM EFFECTS OF **Stress**

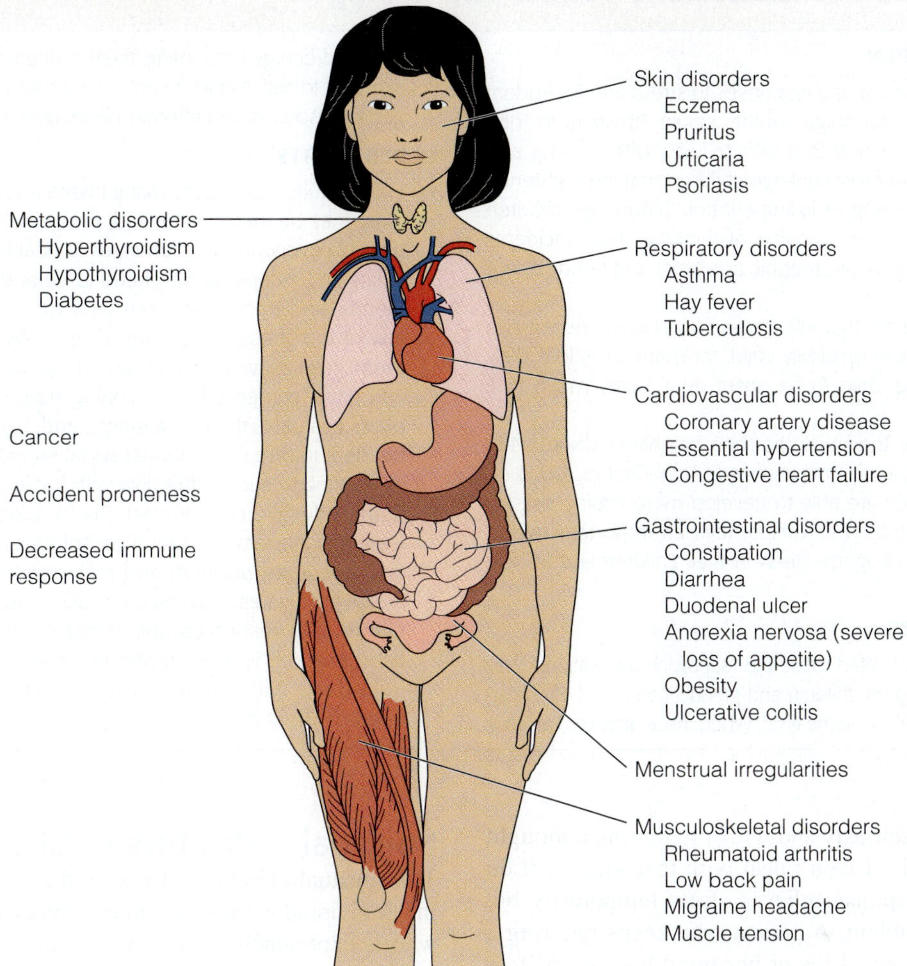

DEPRESSION Depression is a common reaction to events that seem overwhelming or negative. **Depression**, an extreme feeling of sadness, despair, dejection, lack of worth, or emptiness, affects millions of Americans every year. The signs and symptoms of depression and the severity of the problem vary with the client and the significance of the precipitating event. Emotional symptoms can include feelings of tiredness, sadness, emptiness, or numbness. Behavioral signs of depression include irritability, inability to concentrate, difficulty making decisions, loss of sexual desire, crying, sleep disturbance, and social withdrawal. Physical signs of depression may include loss of appetite, weight loss, constipation, headache, and dizziness. Many people experience short periods of depression in response to overwhelming stressful events, such as the death of a loved one or loss of a job; prolonged depression, however, is a cause for concern and may require treatment.

Cognitive Indicators of Stress

Cognitive indicators of stress are thinking responses that include problem solving, structuring, self-control or self-discipline, suppression, and fantasy.

Problem solving involves thinking through the threatening situation and using specific steps to arrive at a solution. The person assesses the situation or problem, analyzes or defines it, chooses alternatives, carries out the selected alternative, and evaluates whether the solution was successful.

Structuring is the arrangement or manipulation of a situation so that threatening events do not occur. For example, a nurse can structure or control an interview with a client by asking only direct, closed questions. Structuring can be productive in certain situations. A person who schedules a dental examination semiannually to prevent severe dental disease is using productive structuring.

Self-control (*discipline*) is assuming a manner and facial expression that convey a sense of being in control or in charge. When self-control prevents panic and harmful or nonproductive actions in a threatening situation, it is a helpful response that conveys strength. Self-control carried to an extreme, however, can delay problem solving and prevent a person from receiving the support of others, who may perceive the person as being unconcerned or as not needing support or assistance.

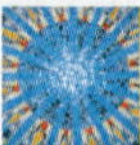

DEVELOPMENTAL CONSIDERATIONS Stress and Coping

INFANTS AND CHILDREN

- Children's perceptions of and responses to stress are dependent on their developmental stage. Infants sense stressors in their environment and respond in a diffuse way, often crying and clinging. Toddlers and preschool-age children may be frightened and react by withdrawing or losing control. School-age children and adolescents are more capable of thinking about incidents that cause stress (e.g., a catastrophic accident) and talking about it with adults.
- Temperament is a factor that influences how children respond to stress. An outgoing, low-sensitivity child, for example, is less likely than a timid, intense child to be upset by a family move to a different state.
- Anxiety disorders are the most common psychiatric disorders in children but are frequently unrecognized (Antai-Otong, 2003).
- As children grow, they are able to develop more coping skills to manage stressful situations. Nurses have an important role in teaching parents to recognize stress in their children and to help their children cope.

MIDDLE-AGED ADULTS

- Middle-aged adults are often called the "sandwich generation." They find themselves caring for children and grandchildren and often caring for aging parents at the same time. When these activities become time and energy consuming, there is often not enough time left for attention to self. Nurses need to be aware of this and assist in suggesting resources and effective planning to ease the strain.

OLDER ADULTS

- Older adults experience many losses and changes in their lives. They may be incremental and, over time, become stressful and possibly overwhelming. Changes in health, decreased functional ability and independence, need for relocation, loss of family and friends, and becoming a caregiver for a spouse or friend are a few of the stresses often experienced by older adults. Many of them have survived significant challenges in their earlier lives and have learned effective coping skills. Nurses can help them plan, evaluate their strategies, and learn new strategies, if needed. Informal and formal social supports are very important in learning to successfully live with these changes and stress.
- Some effective coping methods for older adults are exercise, learning different relaxation techniques, participation in activities, adequate nutrition and rest, and engaging in expressive creative activities, such as art, music, and journaling. Referral to community resources and supports should be done when appropriate. It is most important to see older adults as unique individuals with unique past experiences and very specific needs as they age.

Suppression is consciously and willfully putting a thought or feeling out of mind: "I won't deal with that today. I'll do it tomorrow." This response relieves stress temporarily but does not solve the problem. A person who keeps ignoring a toothache, pushing it out of his or her mind because of fear of the pain of having a filling, will not obtain relief of his or her symptoms.

Fantasy or *daydreaming* is likened to make-believe. Unfulfilled wishes and desires are imagined as fulfilled, or a threatening experience is reworked or replayed so that it ends differently from reality. Experiences can be relived, everyday problems solved, and plans for the future made. The outcome of current problems may also be fantasized. For example, a client who is awaiting the results of a breast biopsy may fantasize the surgeon as saying, "You do not have cancer." Fantasy responses can be helpful if they lead to problem solving. For example, the client awaiting breast biopsy results might say to herself, "Even if the doctor says, 'You have cancer,' as long as he also says it can be treated, I can accept that." Fantasies can be destructive and nonproductive if a person uses them to excess and retreats from reality.

Cognitive coping activities refer to the ability to think through stressors and problems. In addition to the cognitive appraisal processes previously discussed, behaviors intended to reduce the impact of the stressor on the individual are a part of the process of cognitive coping. These processes involve problem solving, identifying resources, planning resolution, and reevaluating our internal and external environment; they are necessary and protective responses that mediate the effects of stressors (Lazarus & Folkman, 1984).

Spiritual Indicators of Stress

The spiritual effects of stress on the individual are related to the individual's sense of interconnectedness. An individual who is experiencing great anxiety may become disconnected from his or her spiritual foundation and may question the meaning and purpose of life. Questions such as "Why is God doing this to me?" are not uncommon when stress and anxiety overwhelm an individual's spirituality. Dossey, Keegan, and Guzzetta (2005) summarize research related to spirituality, reporting higher scores on spirituality as significantly positively correlated with health-promoting behavior.

Ego Defense Mechanisms

Ego defense mechanisms (often referred to simply as *defense mechanisms*) are unconscious psychological adaptive mechanisms or, according to Sigmund Freud (1946), mental mechanisms that develop as the personality attempts to defend itself, establish compromises among conflicting impulses, and calm inner tensions. Defense mechanisms are the unconscious mind working to protect the person from anxiety. They can be considered precursors to conscious cognitive coping mechanisms that will ultimately solve the problem. Like some verbal and motor responses, defense mechanisms release tension. Table 28–5 describes these mechanisms and lists examples of their adaptive and maladaptive uses.

The importance of ego defense mechanisms cannot be overstated. Defenses mechanisms are essential to psychological survival. Just as the "fight or flight" response supports individual physical survival, the defense mechanisms protect our psychological state. Nurses must not only identify the

TABLE 28–5 **Ego Defense Mechanisms**

DEFENSE MECHANISM	EXAMPLE(S)	USE/PURPOSE
Compensation Covering up weaknesses by emphasizing a more desirable trait or by over-achievement in a more comfortable area	A high school student too small to play football becomes the star long distance runner for the track team.	Allows a person to overcome weakness and achieve success
Denial An attempt to screen or ignore unacceptable realities by refusing to acknowledge them	A woman, though told her father has metastatic cancer, continues to plan a family reunion 18 months in advance.	Temporarily isolates a person from the full impact of a traumatic situation
Displacement The transferring or discharging of emotional reactions from one object or person to another object or person	A husband and wife are fighting, and the husband becomes so angry he hits a door instead of his wife. A student gets a C on a paper she worked hard on and goes home and yells at her family.	Allows for feelings to be expressed through or to less dangerous objects or people
Identification An attempt to manage anxiety by imitating the behavior of someone feared or respected	A student nurse imitates the nurturing behavior she observes one of her instructors using with clients.	Helps a person avoid self-devaluation
Intellectualization A mechanism by which an emotional response that normally would accompany an uncomfortable or painful incident is evaded by the use of rational explanations that remove from the incident any personal significance and feelings	The pain over a parent's sudden death is reduced by saying, "He wouldn't have wanted to live disabled."	Protects a person from pain and traumatic events
Introjection A form of identification that allows for the acceptance of others' norms and values into oneself, even when contrary to one's previous assumptions	A 7-year-old tells his little sister, "Don't talk to strangers." He has introjected this value from the instructions of parents and teachers.	Helps a person avoid social retaliation and punishment; particularly important for the child's development of superego
Minimization Not acknowledging the significance of one's behavior	A person says, "Don't believe everything my wife tells you. I wasn't so drunk I couldn't drive."	Allows a person to decrease responsibility for own behavior
Projection A process in which blame is attached to others or the environment for unacceptable desires, thoughts, short-comings, and mistakes	A mother is told her child must repeat a grade in school, and she blames this on the teacher's poor instruction. A husband forgets to pay a bill and blames his wife for not giving it to him earlier.	Allows a person to deny the existence of shortcomings and mistakes; protects self-image
Rationalization justification of certain behaviors by faulty logic and ascription of motives that are socially acceptable but did not in fact inspire the behavior	A mother spanks her toddler too hard and says it was all right because he couldn't feel it through the diapers anyway.	Helps a person cope with the inability to meet goals or certain standards
Reaction formation A mechanism that causes people to act exactly opposite to the way they feel	An executive resents his bosses for calling in a consulting firm to make recommendations for change in his department but verbalizes complete support of the idea and is exceedingly polite and cooperative.	Aids in reinforcing repression by allowing feelings to be acted out in a more acceptable way
Regression Resorting to an earlier, more comfortable level of functioning that is characteristically less demanding and responsible	An adult throws a temper tantrum when he does not get his own way. A critically ill client allows the nurse to bathe and feed him.	Allows a person to return to a point in development when nurturing and dependency were needed and accepted with comfort
Repression An unconscious mechanism by which threatening thoughts, feelings, and desires are kept from becoming conscious; the repressed material is denied entry into consciousness	A teenager, seeing his best friend killed in a car accident, becomes amnesic about the circumstances surrounding the accident.	Protects a person from a traumatic experience until he or she has the resources to cope
Sublimation Displacement of energy associated with more primitive sexual or aggressive drives into socially acceptable activities	A person with excessive, primitive sexual drives invests psychic energy into a well-defined religious value system.	Protects a person from behaving in irrational, impulsive ways

(continued)

TABLE 28–5 **Ego Defense Mechanisms (continued)**

DEFENSE MECHANISM	EXAMPLE(S)	USE/PURPOSE
Substitution The replacement of a highly valued, unacceptable, or unavailable object by a less valuable, acceptable, or available object	A woman wants to marry a man exactly like her dead father and settles for someone who looks a little bit like him.	Helps a person achieve goals and minimizes frustration and disappointment
Undoing An action or words designed to cancel some disapproved thoughts, impulses, or acts in which the person relieves guilt by making reparation	A father spanks his child and the next evening brings home a present for him. A teacher writes an examination that is far too easy, then constructs a grading curve that makes it difficult to earn a high grade.	Allows a person to appease guilty feelings and atone for mistakes

defense mechanisms utilized by individuals entrusted to their care, but also use them to gain insight into their own defensive coping patterns. It is important to remember that defenses protect the individual and the ego. Providing a safe and nonjudgmental environment, both internal and external to the person, facilitates the letting go of some protective defenses and supports the client in coping with reality.

ALTERATIONS FROM NORMAL COPING RESPONSES

When an individual experiences anxiety so disabling that his or her functioning is adversely affected, the individual likely has developed an anxiety or dissociative disorder. According to Townsend (2006), anxiety disorders are the most common of all psychiatric disorders and produce distress that can be incapacitating and impair daily functioning. Anxiety disorders are more common/or reported more in women, at least twice as frequently as in men. The overall prevalence of anxiety disorders is approximately 15% of all adults in the United States over their life span (Videbeck, 2004). Some of the anxiety disorders include generalized anxiety disorder, phobias, panic disorder, obsessive compulsive disorder (OCD), and post-traumatic stress disorder (PTSD). Although crisis is not necessarily a disorder, this exemplar will be presented within the context of this concept as individuals in the course of daily living will experience a crisis at some point in their daily lives.

ASSESSMENT

Appraisal is to the transactional model of stress and coping what assessment is to the nursing process. Just as the nurse assesses and prioritizes client health concerns, individuals evaluate (appraise) and prioritize stressors. It is critical that the nurse, in making this transaction that is called assessment, support and affirm the client's anxiety and not do anything that might inadvertently cause anxiety for the client. Box 28–3 describes how nursing interactions can be used successfully with the anxious client.

ALTERATIONS AND TREATMENTS **Stress and Coping**

Alteration	Description	Treatments
Generalized anxiety disorder	Excessive worry about a number of everyday problems for at least 6 months, with anxiety that is more intense than the situation warrants	Counseling/Nursing /Therapy ▪ Cognitive-behavioral therapy (CBT) ▪ Stress management teaching ▪ Cognitive restructuring replacing maladaptive thoughts to more adaptive thought processes Medications are individualized and generally selected from the following classifications: ▪ Antidepressants ▪ Beta-blockers ▪ Antianxiety agents. Alternative Therapies ▪ Dietary (e.g., reduce caffeine intake) ▪ Eye movement desensitization (EMDR) ▪ Progressive relaxation ▪ Family counseling
Phobias	An intense, persistent, irrational fear of something dreaded; may be an object, situation, or activity that elicits panic and automatic avoidance of or repelling urge to stay away	
Panic disorder	A sudden attack of terror, accompanied by a pounding heart, sweatiness, weakness, faintness, or dizziness; can produce a sense of unreality, impending doom, or a fear of losing control	
Post-traumatic stress disorder (PTSD)	An anxiety disorder that can evolve after exposure to a traumatic or overwhelming event in which an individual's physical health was endangered (e.g., violent personal assaults, natural or human-caused disasters, accidents, military combat, dismemberment, incest and child abuse, traumatic childbirth, or invasive medical procedures) characterized by exaggerated stress responses to the event.	
Obsessive-compulsive disorder (OCD)	Characterized by obsessive thoughts and compulsive repetitive behaviors formed in response to the obsessive thoughts to lower the level of anxiety experienced	

Box 28–3 **Successful Nursing Interactions With the Anxious Client**

In the nursing transactional model, the nurse is part of the anxious client's environment and can influence changes in the client with both verbal and nonverbal cues. From the very first interaction with the client, the nurse's demeanor conveys a great deal of information to the client about how the client can expect to be treated. Initial nursing actions that inspire client confidence and that may help calm anxious clients include the following:

- Make eye contact, focusing on the person.
- Take a nonthreatening stance.
- Validate the client's feelings: "I know you are very uncomfortable; we will do everything we can to help you feel better."
- Determine and address the client's immediate concerns: "What can I do right away to help you?"
- Remember to address the client by name. Some clients find terms of endearment such as "honey" or "sweetie" impersonal or demeaning. Using the client's first name may be seen as patronizing if the client is expected to use the nurse's last name. On the other hand, some clients respond positively to the informality of first name use. Ask clients how they would prefer to be addressed and never use the first name of anyone over age 25 without permission.

Mrs. Betts is a 35-year-old woman who has come to her primary care physician's office with a number of complaints. The receptionist informs the nurse that Mrs. Betts is obviously anxious and is rambling a lot. As the nurse walks into the examination room, Mrs. Betts immediately begins talking about a number of issues. Wide-eyed, she complains of tingling in her arms, lack of sleep, and feeling like her heart is racing. She bombards the nurse with so many issues that he becomes confused. Sitting down, the nurse asks Mrs. Betts, "Tell me, which of those issues are you most concerned about?" Sitting down conveys that the nurse has time for Mrs. Betts. Asking her to prioritize or scale her concerns helps the nurse prioritize them as well.

Mrs. Betts replies, "I am having a heart attack and no one believes me." The nurse responds, "We know you're uncomfortable right now, and you must be worried. We're definitely going to check out your cardiac status. It will take a little time. What can I do to make you feel more comfortable right now?" By providing assurance and information, the nurse both empowers Mrs. Betts and assists her in making a secondary appraisal, deciding which concern is the next most important. This secondary appraisal is an important tool in helping Mrs. Betts learn the steps needed to lower her anxiety level. It also helps the nurse learn more about Mrs. Betts within a very short period of time.

The anxious client requires a holistic assessment process. A complete nursing history and a physical examination are the tools that will best help the nurse determine how to help the client.

Nursing History and Assessment Interview

The nurse should conduct a thorough nursing history with an assessment interview, asking about current and past illness, specific physical complaints, general health history, client-perceived stressors or stressful incidents, manifestations of stress, and past and present coping strategies. In addition to an assessment interview, the nurse may use a simple checklist while talking with and observing the client to note indications of stress. Box 28–4 provides a checklist to identify symptoms of stress. As was mentioned earlier, stress and stressors are a part of everyday life. The first step in mediating the effect of the stressor is conscious awareness of the manifestations of stress. Review the symptom checklist to increase your awareness of and assess your own stress reactions and behaviors.

The checklist in Box 28–4 is not meant to be all-encompassing; it is intended to provide points of reference to improve your conscious awareness of your own stress reactions and those of individuals with whom nurses interact. The experience of stress is an individual process; therefore, experiences that you have had or those of other individuals you know may not be listed in Box 28–4.

Physical Examination and Observation

The nurse should observe the client for verbal, motor, cognitive, or other physical manifestations of stress. Remember, however, that clinical signs and symptoms may not occur when cognitive coping is effective. The nurse will conduct a

Assessment Interview Stress and Coping Patterns

- On a scale of 1–10, where 1 is "very minor" and 10 is "extreme," how would you rate the stress you are experiencing in the following areas?
  a. Home
  b. Work or school
  c. Finance
  d. Recent illness or loss of loved one
  e. Your health
  f. Family responsibilities
  g. Relationships with friends
  h. Relationship with parents or children
  i. Relationship with partner
  j. Recent hospitalization
  k. Other (specify)
- How long have you been dealing with these stressors?
- How do you usually handle stressful situations? If the client does not adequately describe, prompt with the following:
  a. Cry
  b. Get angry
  c. Talk to someone (Who?)
  d. Withdraw from the situation
  e. Control others or situation
  f. Go for a walk or perform physical exercise
  g. Try to arrive at a solution
  h. Pray
  i. Laugh, joke, or use some other expression of humor
  j. Meditate or use some other relaxation technique such as yoga or guided imagery
- How well does your usual coping strategy work?

Box 28–4 **Stress Assessment Checklist**

BEHAVIORAL

Argumentativeness

Increase in compulsive behaviors (eating, drinking, nail biting, sexual activity, smoking)

Grinding teeth during sleep

Loud voice

Pacing

Vigilance

Withdrawal

COGNITIVE

Difficulty concentrating or listening

Short attention span

Trouble thinking

Forgetfulness

Lack of initiative

Lack of creativity

Memory lapses/loss

Ambivalence

Fear of the unknown

Worrying

Wanting to run away

Lacking a sense of humor

EMOTIONAL

Fear

Agitation/anger

Defensiveness

Hostility

Anxiety and feeling pressured

Crying

Irritability

Feeling overwhelmed

Feeling powerless

Easily annoyed

Jumpiness and nervousness

Sadness

Isolation

Suspiciousness

PHYSICAL

Diaphoresis

Restless

Fatigue Gastrointestinal upsets or butterflies

Headaches

Muscular stiffness and tension

Racing or pounding heart

Shakiness

Sweaty palms

Increase in blood sugar levels

Dry mouth

Pallor

Increase respiration rate

Urinary frequency

Source: Adapted from Benson, H. & Stuart, E. M. (1992). *The wellness book and holistic nursing* (p. 245).

physical examination, including assessing vital signs and urine (to determine alterations from normal, such as drug use).

Laboratory tests are not routinely done to evaluate anxiety because observation is faster and more accurate. However, tests may be necessary to rule out medical conditions that can cause or be exacerbated by anxiety. A complete blood count may show increased adrenal function, elevated levels of glucose and lactic acid, and decreased parathyroid function and oxygen and calcium levels. See Box 28–5 for a list of medical conditions associated with anxiety.

Box 28–5 **General Medical Conditions Associated With Anxiety**

- Hypoglycemia
- Hyperthyroidism
- Asthma
- Pneumonia
- Chronic obstructive pulmonary disease
- Pulmonary embolism
- Encephalitis
- Cardiac dysrhythmias
- Vitamin B12 deficiency
- Pheochromocytoma (adrenal tumor)
- Vestibular dysfunction
- Neoplasms

CARING INTERVENTIONS

A number of caring interventions may be appropriate for the client who is having difficulty coping with stressors. In addition to being well informed about various interventions and treatment options, such as psychotherapy, it is important that nurses be able to recognize and manage their own responses to stress.

Psychotherapy

Psychotherapy is a preferred method of treating anxiety disorders. Psychotherapy involves talking with a mental health professional, such as a psychiatrist, mental health nurse, advanced practice psychiatric nurse, psychologist, social worker, or counselor, to explore the nature and symptom management of the anxiety disorder (NIMH, 2008). The severity of symptoms may warrant hospitalization in a safe therapeutic *milieu,* or social setting, for the individual. Such an intervention provides needed protection from environmental stressors and the support of group therapy. The impact of overwhelming and disabling anxiety can create vulnerability to depression, suicidal thoughts, or self-harm.

Cognitive-behavioral therapy (CBT) is a form of psychotherapy that focuses on the role of the individual's thoughts and attitudes and their effect on feelings and behaviors. CBT is aimed at the reappraisal process. Referring back to Maslow, alterations in coping can occur when individuals do not feel a sense of safety or belonging. Most individuals suffering from anxiety feel isolated in their plight. In CBT, the nurse or other trained professional assists clients in learning to reframe the situation differently, empowering the clients to make choices, trust in themselves, and reappraise their stressors and responses in a safe environment.

CBT has yielded very positive results in treating anxiety disorders, primarily because it addresses both cognitive responses to stress, such as negative thought processes, and behavioral responses, such as the repetitive hand washing that sometimes occurs with obsessive-compulsive disorder. Techniques utilized involve providing stress management teaching, cognitive restructuring, and replacing maladaptive cognitions to more adaptive thoughts (Kopala & Keitel, 2003). Other techniques include exposure techniques to desensitize individuals from the specific stressor, which are repeated a number of times until the anxiety is extinguished. CBT therapists also use deep breathing, relaxation, and exercise to help clients relieve anxiety through relaxation (NIMH, 2008).

Interventions that the nurse may provide directly or by referral include administration of pharmacological therapy as ordered; therapeutic communication; psychosocial cognitive-behavioral interventions, such as teaching relaxation techniques; and supportive groups for the individual and family. Supporting an individual's feelings and validating them is of utmost importance to the building of self-esteem and fostering adaptive coping. Advice is not recommended other than in a crisis to protect individuals. Telling others what to do, which can feel demeaning to the client, is to be avoided. Reinforcing positive coping efforts, offering hope and reassurance to the individual about his or her ability to cope, and helping the person to identify successes in his or her life provides a sense of personal power and hope. Spiritual distress occurs when an individual loses hope of ever resolving or coping more adaptively. The chronic nature of anxiety disorders can be devastating and can erode an individual's sense of power and self-worth.

STRESS MANAGEMENT FOR NURSES

Nurses, like clients, are susceptible to experiencing anxiety and stress. Nursing practice involves many stressors related to both clients and the work environment: understaffing, increasing severity of client illnesses, adjusting to various work shifts, being expected to assume responsibilities for which one is not prepared, inadequate support from supervisors and peers, visiting homes that are depressing, caring for dying clients, and so on. Although most nurses cope effectively with the physical and emotional demands of nursing, in some situations nurses become overwhelmed and develop **burnout**, a complex syndrome of behaviors that can be likened to the exhaustion stage of the general adaptation syndrome. The nurse with burnout manifests physical and emotional depletion, a negative attitude and self-concept, and feelings of helplessness and hopelessness.

Nurses can prevent burnout by using the techniques to manage stress discussed for clients. Nurses must first recognize their stress and become attuned to such responses as feelings of being overwhelmed, fatigue, angry outbursts, physical illness, and increases in coffee drinking, smoking, or substance abuse. Once attuned to stress and personal reactions, it is necessary to identify which situations produce the most pronounced reactions so that steps may be taken to reduce the stress. Suggestions include the following:

- Plan a daily relaxation program with meaningful quiet times to reduce tension (e.g., read, listen to music, soak in a tub, meditate).
- Establish a regular exercise program to direct energy outward.
- Study assertiveness techniques to overcome feelings of powerlessness in relationships with others. Learn to say no.
- Learn to accept failures—your own and others—and make it a constructive learning experience. Recognize that most people do the best they can. Learn to ask for help, to discuss your feelings with colleagues, and to support your colleagues in times of need.
- Accept what cannot be changed. There are certain limitations in every situation. Get involved in constructive change efforts if organizational policies and procedures cause stress.
- Develop collegial support groups to deal with feelings and anxieties generated in the work setting.
- Participate in professional organizations to address workplace issues.
- Seek counseling if indicated to help clarify concerns.

PHARMACOLOGIC THERAPIES

The therapeutic goal of psychopharmacology is to manage symptoms and alleviate distress. Generally speaking, pharmacologic therapies are most successful when used in combination with psychotherapy. Many clients require medication for only short periods of time. Some treatment-resistant clients, however, may require longer courses of medication. Principal medications used to manage the physical symptoms of anxiety disorders are antianxiety, antidepressant, and beta-blocking medications. With proper treatment, many people with anxiety disorders can lead normal, fulfilling lives (NIMH, 2008).

Antianxiety medications (anxiolytic agents) are also known as minor tranquilizers. They are used to treat anxiety and

TABLE 28–6 **Frequently Prescribed Antianxiety Medications**

CLASSIFICATION	COMMON DRUGS
Benzodiazepines	Alprazolam (Xanax) Chlordiazepoxide HCL (Librium) Clorazepate dipotassium (Tranxene) Diazepam (Valium) Lorazepam (Ativan)
Antihistamine	Diphenhydramine (Benadryl)
Azapirone	Buspirone HCL (BuSpar)
Antidepressants	Selective serotonin reuptake inhibitors (SSRIs) (Paxil) Selective norepinephrine serotonin reuptake inhibitors (SNRIs) (Cymbalta)

insomnia (Table 28–6). Sedatives and hypnotics are no longer recommended for treatment of anxiety owing to potential for dependency and possible overdosage (Kee, Hayes, & McCuistion, 2006). They have properties similar to those of the anxiolytics (Antai-Otong, 2008). Benzodiazepines may be used for short-term treatment during an acute phase of an anxiety disorder. They may be effective in quickly lowering the severity of a client's anxiety, but they are generally not recommended for use beyond a few weeks because of their addictive properties. Clients experiencing anxiety secondary to short-term medical therapies, such as mechanical ventilation, may find benzodiazepines helpful.

28.1 ANXIETY DISORDERS

KEY TERMS

Acute stress disorder, *1814*
Anxiety, *1808*
Free-floating anxiety, *1808*
Generalized anxiety disorder (GAD), *1811*
Panic disorder, *1813*
Vulnerability, *1808*

BASIS FOR SELECTION OF EXEMPLAR

Healthy People 2010
National Institute of Mental Health
National Safety Council
United States Department of Health and Human Services
National Mental Health Information Center
World Health Organization

LEARNING OUTCOMES

After reading about this exemplar, you will be able to:

1. Describe the pathophysiology, psychopathology, etiology, clinical manifestations, and direct and indirect causes of anxiety disorders.
2. Identify risk factors associated with anxiety disorders.
3. Illustrate the nursing process in providing culturally competent care across the life span for individuals with anxiety disorders.
4. Formulate priority nursing diagnoses appropriate for an individual with anxiety disorders.
5. Create a plan of care for individuals with anxiety disorders and their family members.
6. Assess expected outcomes for an individual with anxiety disorders.
7. Discuss therapies used in the collaborative care of an individual with anxiety disorders.
8. Employ evidence-based caring interventions for an individual with anxiety disorders.

OVERVIEW

Anxiety is a stress response characterized by feelings of mental uneasiness, apprehension, dread, or foreboding or a feeling of helplessness related to an impending or actual threat to self or significant relationships. Generally anxiety helps the individual cope; it is an individual reaction to a stressor and is part of daily living. The energy exuded by anxiety can be a productive and necessary force in the life of every living individual. It is multidimensional and affects the entire realm of the individual. The experience is influenced by the individual's genetic makeup as well as emotional, developmental, physical, cognitive, socio-cultural, and spiritual factors.

Anxiety is also a feeling of dread accompanied by physical reactions such as elevated pulse, respirations, and blood pressure without a specific stimulus or threat (Frisch & Frisch, 2006) that occur when the autonomic nervous system is on overdrive. Anxiety can be experienced internally or externally to the individual. Internally, we experience the biological effects of the general adaptation syndrome; externally, we feel and experience environmental energy from the earth, groups, the family, the community, or global society.

An essential psychosocial competency for all nurses is the ability to differentiate healthy and expected stress responses from those that are harmful or threaten the person's well-being. Every individual experiences anxiety at times. The individual's anxiety is no longer healthy when the anxiety level reaches the point at which it prevents the individual from returning to homestasis through healthy coping and adaptation.

PATHOPHYSIOLOGY AND ETIOLOGY

Anxiety disorders affect individuals of all ages, from childhood to senescence, and are one of the most common forms of mental disorders affecting adolescents (Farrugia & Hudson, 2006). Each anxiety disorder has its own distinct characteristics, but they all have the common theme of excessive, irrational fear and dread.

In anxiety disorders, anxiety either is the predominant disturbance, as in generalized anxiety disorder, or is experienced as a defense mechanism when the person attempts to master the symptoms, as in confronting the dreaded object or situation in a phobic disorder. When anxiety is not related to a specific stimulus, it may be called **free-floating anxiety**.

Examples of anxiety disorders are listed in the About Stress and Coping section of this concept. This exemplar discusses generalized anxiety disorder, separation anxiety, and panic disorder.

Anxiety Theories

Vulnerability refers to the individual's susceptibility to react to a specific stressor. Vulnerability factors reported by Kneisl, Wilson, and Trigoboff (2004) include the neurobiology of the central nervous system. A number of models attempt to explain the alterations in the individual's ability to adapt successfully to stressors. A brief presentation of these theories provides a synopsis of the current assumptions.

NEUROBIOLOGICAL THEORIES Dysregulation of neurotransmitters has also been implicated in the development of anxiety. The neurotransmitters that are presumed to contribute to anxiety and the inability to adaptively cope are serotonin, norepinephrine, and gamma-aminobutyric acid (GABA).

Several areas of the brain orchestrate the experience of anxiety and the expression of the symptoms (Figure 28–4 ■). The amygdala is known as the "emotional brain" and is the focus of much research related to feelings of anxiety, fear, and anger, which are elicited in this area. The hippocampus stores memory related to fear. The locus coeruleus stimulates our arousal. Heart rate and respirations are regulated by the brain stem, and the hypothalamus activates the entire response. The frontal cortex assists with appraisal of a threat and is the center of cognitive processes. The thalamus integrates all sensory stimuli, and the basal ganglia are responsible for the tremors associated with anxiety (Townsend, 2004). Individual differences in the structure of the brain or injury to the brain will also alter the anxiety response.

NEUROCHEMICAL THEORIES Communication within the brain occurs between neurons through the transmission of electrical stimuli (Figures 28–5 ■ and 28–6 ■). To transmit a signal, a neuron releases chemicals called neurotransmitters. These chemicals deliver messages by binding to the receptors on the surface of another neuron, causing the neuron to fire and transmit the electrical impulse. Once the message is delivered, the neurotransmitter is taken back to a vesicle in

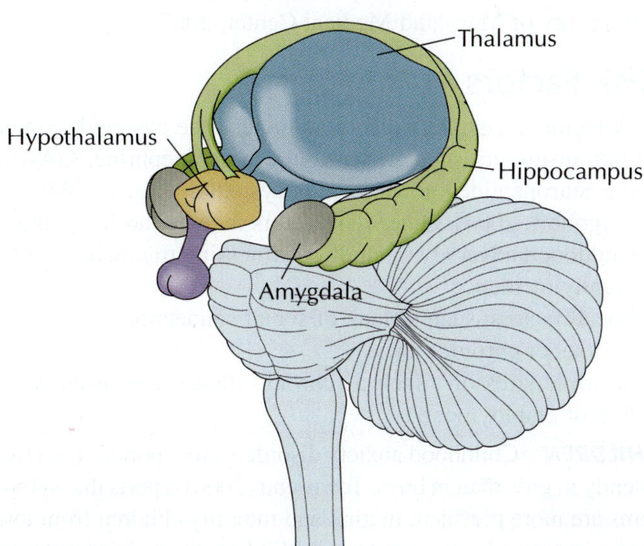

Figure 28–4 ■ The limbic system. Just above the inner core, yet surrounded by the cerebral cortex, the limbic system plays a role in motivation, emotion, and memory. The system is composed of many structures, including the thalamus, amygdale, hippocampus, and hypothalamus.

Source: Kassin, S. (2001). *Psychology* (3rd ed.). Upper Saddle River, NJ: Prentice Hall. Used with permission.

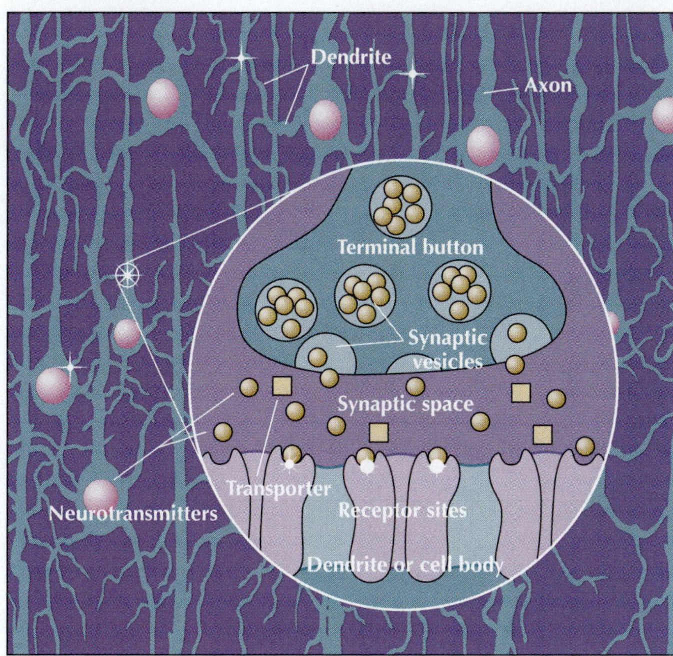

Figure 28–5 ■ Neurotransmission: How neurons communicate.

Source: Morris, C. G. & Maisto, A. A. (2001). *Understanding psychology* (3rd ed.). Upper Saddle River, NJ: Prentice Hall. Used with permission.

the presynaptic cell (NIMH, 2008). Any disruption in these transporters, binding sites, or cell structure can cause an alteration in cell functioning, leading to misfiring.

Structural anatomical differences, dysregulation of neurotransmitters, sensitivity of neuronal receptor sites, and the balance of neurotransmitters in the synaptic cleft all have an effect on the anxiety reaction. GABA is thought to be dysregulated with anxiety. GABA is an inhibitory neurotransmitter that "shuts down" or slows excitability in the cell. It is present in the locus coeruleus where norepinephrine is produced. Norepinephrine is an excitatory neurotransmitter that signals arousal and hyperarousal. Researchers believe that an imbalance in the regulation of these two neurotransmitters produces anxiety disorders (Videback, 2004). It is believed that GABA is decreased and norepinephrine is increased, creating anxiety. Serotonin is also implicated in the pathology of anxiety. It is thought to produce a feeling of well-being and is believed to be decreased in anxiety (Townsend, 2006).

PSYCHODYNAMIC THEORIES Antai-Otong (2008) describes the psychodynamic theories developed by Sigmund Freud based on the belief that anxiety occurs when the ego attempts to deal with conflict or tension. Anxiety is defined as a reaction to danger. In response to that reaction, the individual applies ego defense mechanisms. Defense mechanisms and the degree to which they are utilized reflect the individual's capacity to cope with the stressors of life.

COGNITIVE-BEHAVIORAL THEORIES Cognitive theorists attribute anxiety responses to faulty or distorted thinking that leads to a pattern of maladaptive behaviors. Distorted thinking creates feelings of powerlessness, fear, and a dysfunctional appraisal of the stressor or the situation. There is a lack of

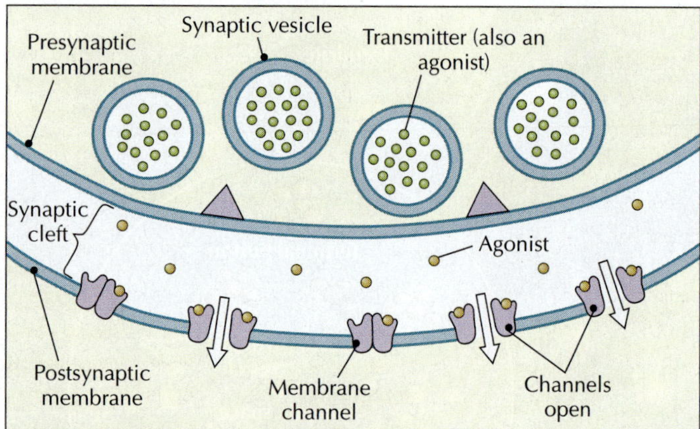

(A) Strong agonist activates receptors without transmission.

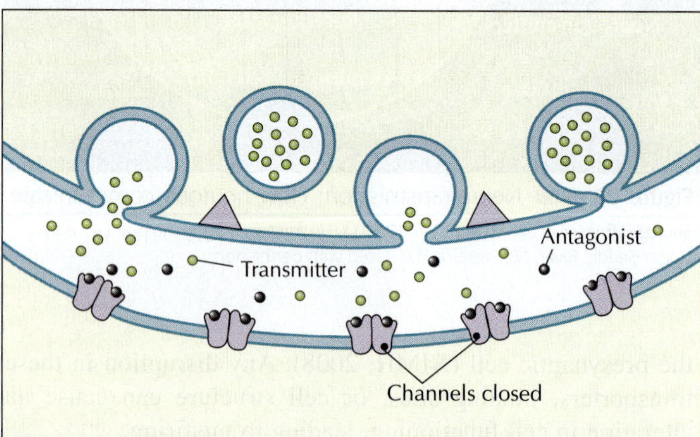

(B) Antagonist blocks receptors. Agonist cannot act.

Figure 28–6 ■ Ligands: Agonists and antagonists. Agonists and antagonists bind to the same binding site as transmitters. An agonist has potency, so it activates the cell biologically *A*, while antagonists bind and have no potency *B*, An antagonist produces its effect by blocking the binding site, preventing a transmitter from binding, and producing its biological effect.

Source: Smock, T. K. (1999). *Psysiological psychology: A Neuroscience approach.* Upper Saddle River, NJ: Prentice Hall. Used with permission.

rationality and ability to reason with the individual (Townsend, 2006) so anxious people often exaggerate the threat. Faulty thinking is described by Antai-Otong (2008) as overgeneralizations: "all or nothing" thinking.

Behaviorists believe that the faulty thinking and behavior is a learned dysfunctional response to stressors. They believe individuals can unlearn unhealthy behaviors by replacing them with new learned behaviors that are adaptive and reduce anxiety (Antai-Otong, 2008).

DEVELOPMENTAL THEORIES Attachment theory purports that the experience of anxiety begins with separation from the primary caregiver. The anxiety is expressed in stages beginning with protest, despair, and eventual detachment (Bowlby, 1969). Children who develop with inadequate attachment or bonding will experience impaired socialization and problem-solving skills. The ability to form normal social attachments provides the ability to moderate anxiety and cope with separation (Antai-Otong, 2008).

TRANSACTIONAL MODEL As described in the About Stress and Coping section of this concept, the transactional model views the individual within the system as a part of the system and in constant, dynamic interaction with the person, family, local and global communities, and universe. All internal and external environments are integral components of the model and are dynamic and interactive. Nurses interact with the individual in the appraisal process to facilitate adaptive coping. Nursing interventions are aimed at providing information and support. The nurse helps the individual to make the secondary appraisal and plan and implement appropriate coping responses.

Etiology

According to the National Institute of Mental Health (NIMH), the incidence of generalized anxiety disorder (GAD) in the United States is 6.8 million adults per year and therefore has been identified as a priority for health care providers. The World Health Organization (WHO) emphasizes the importance of differentiating anxiety disorder that causes suffering from the everyday lived experience of anxiety. Collectively, the prevalence reported in data from Western countries is estimated at 10–15% of the population. Current data available from the NIMH (2008) website reports that 28.8% of adults in the United States have had an anxiety disorder at some point in their lives. Anxiety disorders also affect youth and children in the United States. Researchers examined the psychiatric histories, from ages 11 through 32, of 1,037 adults; of the 232 adults with anxiety disorders, one third had suffered from anxiety or depression as a child.

Children and older adults are more vulnerable to physical reactions to anxiety and may not be able to adapt physically to overwhelming stressors and thus suffer exhaustion. GAD is the most common anxiety disorder among older adults (University of Maryland Medical Center, 2007).

Risk Factors

Risk factors for anxiety disorders include the dysregulation of neurotransmitters such as serotonin, norepinephrine, GABA, and a neuropeptide known as cholecystokinin (Kneisl, Wilson, & Trigoboff, 2004). Other risk factors include the following:

- Childhood adversity, including witnessing traumatic events
- Family incidence
- Social factors, such as lack of social connection
- Serious or chronic illness
- Multiple stressors, such as chronic illness concurrent with loss of employment.

CHILDREN Childhood anxiety disorders are reported more frequently in girls than in boys. Townsend (2006) reports that symptoms are more prevalent in girls and minority children from low socioeconomic backgrounds. All children from disadvantaged socioeconomic backgrounds are more vulnerable to emotional illness than their more advantaged peers. Familial predisposition is also a contributing vulnerability factor (Townsend, 2006).

OLDER ADULTS Older adults with cognitive impairments or one or more chronic physical impairments are at increased risk for developing anxiety. Significant emotional loss, such

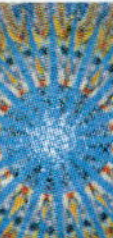

FOCUS ON DIVERSITY AND CULTURE

Anxiety Disorders in Immigrant Populations

There is some evidence to indicate that Mexican American immigrants born in the United States experience anxiety and other psychiatric disorders at higher rates than do those who recently immigrated. It is thought that new immigrants maintain closer ties to their home culture through greater contact with others who were born in their home country and with family members and friends who have not immigrated. More studies must be done to confirm this and to determine whether it is true for all immigrant populations. Studies also suggest that Mexican Americans born in the United States are at a lower risk for psychiatric disorder than U.S.-born non-Hispanic whites (Grant, Stinson, Hason, et al., 2004).

as the death of a spouse, also increases the older adult's risk for anxiety. Research on anxiety disorders among older adults is limited in comparison to research on depression and Alzheimer's disease (Anxiety Disorders Association of America, 2009).

CLINICAL MANIFESTATIONS

Anxiety states and clinical manifestations may range from mild or moderate to severe or panic. Mild anxiety is considered within the norm of human experiences. The harmful effects of anxiety are amplified with the severity of symptoms. Anxiety disorders range from mildly uncomfortable to diminishing the quality of a person's life. The Clinical Manifestations and Therapies feature discusses the levels of anxiety, associated symptoms, and appropriate therapies.

Generalized Anxiety Disorder

To differentiate between normal anxiety and generalized anxiety disorder, the diagnostic manual used by mental health professionals, the *DSM-IV-TR*, is the standard for diagnosis. The diagnostic criteria are outlined in Box 28–6. The fundamental characteristic of **generalized anxiety disorder (GAD)** is pervasive apprehension and worry. Additional symptoms of GAD include irritability, agitation, tachycardia, shortness of breath, and sleep disturbances. Depression may occur concurrently with an anxiety disorder. The diagnosis of GAD is determined by the advanced practice nurse, nurse practitioner, physician, or other health care practitioner.

CHILDREN AND GENERALIZED ANXIETY DISORDER GAD is often manifested in children with restlessness, excessive fatigue, poor concentration, irritability, muscle tension, and sleep disturbance. Anxiety is second only to substance abuse in incidence for mental disorders and is a common mental disorder of childhood. From 3 to 12% of children experience generalized anxiety disorder, with 8–19 years of age a common time for its emergence (Hudson, Deveney, & Taylor, 2005). Although all children experience anxiety at certain times, children with anxiety disorder are excessively worried about many things and are difficult to reassure. They worry about their health, the safety of the family, their performance in school, and the events in the world. They are not able to distract themselves from the worry. Many youth have accompanying physical complaints, such as headache or stomachache.

Anxiety disorders are strongly linked to familial and genetic factors. They may coexist with other mental health disorders, and children sometimes have more than one type of anxiety (Shear, Jin, Ruscio, et al., 2006). Diagnosis is performed by a mental health specialist. Treatment is usually cognitive-behavior therapy (CBT) and may involve medication. CBT can include child or family interventions

Box 28–6 ***DSM-IV-TR*** Diagnostic Criteria for Generalized Anxiety Disorder

A. Excessive anxiety and worry (apprehensive expectation), occurring more days than not for at least six months, about a number of events or activities (such as work or school performance).
B. The person finds it difficult to control the worry.
C. The anxiety and worry are associated with three (or more) of the following six symptoms (with at least some symptoms present for more days than not for the past 6 months). Note: Only one item is required in children.
   1. Restlessness or feeling keyed up or on edge
   2. Being easily fatigued
   3. Difficulty concentrating or mind going blank
   4. Irritability
   5. Muscle tension
   6. Sleep Disturbance (Difficulty falling or staying asleep, or restless unsatisfying sleep)
D. The focus of the anxiety and worry is not confined to features of an Axis I disorder, e.g., the anxiety or worry is not about having a panic attack (as in panic disorder), being embarrassed in public (as in social phobia), being contaminated (as in Obsessive-Compulsive Disorder), being away from home or close relatives (as in Separation Anxiety Disorder), gaining weight (as in Anorexia Nervosa), having multiple physical complaints (as in Somatization Disorder), or having a serious illness (as in Hypochondriasis), and the anxiety and worry do not occur exclusively during Post-Traumatic Stress Disorder.
E. The anxiety, worry, or physical symptoms cause clinically significant distress or impairment in social, occupational, or other important areas of functioning.
F. The disturbance is not due to the direct physiological effects of a substance (e.g., a drug of abuse, a medication) or a general medical condition (e.g., hyperthyroidism) and does not occur exclusively during a Mood Disorder, a Psychotic Disorder, or a Pervasive Developmental Disorder.

Source: Reprinted with permission from the American Psychiatric Association. (2000). *Diagnostic and statistical manual of mental disorders* (4th ed., Text Revision).

CLINICAL MANIFESTATIONS AND THERAPIES **Anxiety Disorders**

LEVEL OF SEVERITY OF ANXIETY	CLINICAL MANIFESTATIONS	CLINICAL THERAPIES
Mild	■ Increase in senses, perception, and arousal ■ Increase in alertness ■ Sleeplessness ■ Increase in motivation ■ Restlessness and irritability	Mild anxiety typically is resolved by an individual's coping mechanisms. Mild anxiety may be helpful to the client to accentuate focus and concentration. Clients who are distressed by mild anxiety may benefit from ■ improved sleep hygiene, ■ relaxation techniques, ■ behavior therapy, or ■ massage and aromatherapy.
Moderate	■ Narrowing of perceptual field and attention span ■ Reduction in alertness and awareness of surroundings ■ Feeling of discomfort and irritability with others ■ Self-absorption ■ Increased restlessness ■ Increase in respirations, heart rate, and muscle tension ■ Increase in perspiration ■ Rapid speech, louder tone, and higher pitch	■ Cognitive and behavior therapy to identify triggers and learn improved coping techniques ■ Relaxation techniques ■ Complementary and Alternative Medicine (CAM) therapies such as yoga, acupuncture, massage ■ Low-dose antianxiety medications if symptoms do not improve with other therapies or exacerbate chronic conditions
Severe	■ Perceptual field greatly reduced ■ Difficulty following directions ■ Feelings of dread, horror ■ Need to relieve anxiety ■ Headache ■ Dizziness ■ Nausea, trembling, insomnia ■ Palpitations, tachycardia, hyperventilating, diarrhea	■ Cognitive and behavior therapy to learn to identify triggers and to learn better coping techniques ■ Antianxiety medications which may include benzodiazepines ■ Relaxation techniques ■ CAM therapies such as yoga, acupuncture, massage ■ Hospitalization may be required initially to manage severe anxiety until improved coping mechanisms are developed
Panic	■ Inability to focus ■ Perception distorted ■ Terror ■ Feelings of doom ■ Bizarre behavior ■ Dilated pupils ■ Trembling, sleeplessness, palpitations pallor diaphoresis, muscular incoordination ■ Immobility or hyperactivity, incoherence	Immediate, structured intervention required. Immediate therapies include the following: ■ Placing client in a quiet, less stimulating environment ■ Use of repetitive or physical task to diffuse energy ■ Administration of antianxiety medications Long-term therapies include the following: ■ Cognitive and behavioral therapy ■ Pharmacological therapy ■ Relaxation techniques ■ Improved sleep hygiene ■ CAM therapies such as massage, acupuncture, yoga, hydrotherapy ■ Nutrition consultation ■ Mental health counseling.

that focus on relaxation, recognition of feelings, and self-talking. Medications that have been reported to be successful in children include sertraline and fluvoxamine

Separation Anxiety Disorder

Separation anxiety disorder is the most common type of anxiety disorder manifested by children. It is characterized by an extreme state of uneasiness when in unfamiliar surroundings and often by refusal to visit friends' homes or attend school for at least 2 weeks (Cartwright-Hatton, McNicol, & Doubleday, 2006). Approximately 75% of children with separation anxiety disorder refuse to attend school. This disorder occurs in approximately 4–5% of children and in twice as many girls as boys (Shear et al., 2006; Wren, Bridge, & Birmaher, 2004). The peak age for occurrence is 7–9 years. It may be recurrent and become worse at certain times. The condition may be acute in onset (often preceded by a traumatic event) or slow in developing over time (Hanna, Fischer, & Fluent, 2006).

Children with separation anxiety disorder tend to be perfectionistic, overly compliant, and eager to please. They appear to

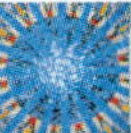

EVIDENCE-BASED PRACTICE The Effects of Psychosocial Stress on Cardiovascular Health

Das and O'Keefe (2008) studied the effects of psychosocial stress on cardiovascular health. They found that psychosocial stress exerts adverse effects on cardiovascular health. Psychosocial stress accounted for approximately 30% of the attributable risk of acute myocardial infarction. Hostility, depression, and anxiety are related to increased risk of coronary heart disease and death. Feelings of hopelessness, in particular, are strongly correlated with adverse cardiovascular outcomes. Psychosocial stress appears to adversely affect autonomic and hormonal homeostasis, resulting in metabolic abnormalities, inflammation, insulin resistance, and endothelial dysfunction. Many factors have been shown to be protective. These factors include social support, regular exercise, stress reduction, having a sense of humor, optimism, altruism, faith, and pet ownership. Simple screening questions are available to reliably indicate a client at risk for psychosocial-stress-related health problems.

cling to the parent or caretaker. They may use physical complaints such as headaches, abdominal pain, nausea, and vomiting in an attempt to avoid being away from the parent. Depression frequently accompanies separation anxiety disorder. The resulting avoidance behaviors can interfere with personal growth and development, academic achievement, and social functioning.

PRACTICE ALERT

The separation anxiety experienced by a toddler differs from psychiatric separation anxiety disorder in age appropriateness, duration, and severity. Separation anxiety disorder affects children of preschool age or older, lasts for at least 2 weeks, and is characterized by excessive anxiety. In contrast, the separation anxiety experienced by the toddler directly follows a separation from a familiar caretaker, lasts only for a short time after the separation, and is a normal developmental response in toddlers.

Diagnosis is made by a mental health specialist. Treatment includes cognitive-behavioral therapy (CBT) involving both the child and the parents. The parents learn about the disorder and how to structure the setting so that the child is expected to attend school. Consistency in expectations is necessary; if the child is permitted to stay home some days or has missed school and other activities for longer periods, treatment is more difficult. The child learns what situations cause anxiety and how to manage those situations and feelings. Both parents and child work out the expectations for behavior for the child with the mental health therapist. School personnel and those from other settings where the child spends time need to be included in the treatment plan. Medication may be used, but typically not until a child fails to improve through use of CBT (Jurbergs & Ledley, 2005). The SSRI fluoxetine has been used with a dose of 10–20 mg/day for children and adolescents; the dose may be increased as needed at weekly intervals to a maximum of 60 mg/day (Bindler & Howry, 2005).

Panic Disorder

A common disorder, **panic disorder** is characterized by recurrent attacks of severe anxiety lasting a few moments to an hour. These attacks typically are not associated with a stimulus, but seem to occur suddenly and spontaneously. These attacks may, however, become associated with certain situations, such as going to a shopping mall or driving a car. The individual usually experiences physical symptoms such as palpitations, nausea, diarrhea, dyspnea, rapid pulse, and a feeling of choking or suffocation. The individual's pupils become dilated and the face flushed. The inidividual may feel dizzy or faint and have a sense of impending doom or death. Restlessness is acute, and the person may make pleading, apprehensive appeals for help.

In its most advanced state, panic may create a group of symptoms that mimic myocardial infarction and mitral valve prolapse. This often contributes to a delay in proper diagnosis until after other medical diagnoses have been ruled out.

A rating scale for the severity of the symptoms provides direction for the multidisciplinary team working with clients with panic disorders (see Table 28–7).

Nocturnal panic disorder is a variation in which the client awakens with panic attacks within 1–4 hours after falling asleep, usually during non-REM sleep. No one knows the cause of nocturnal panic, although some believe it may be related to sleep apnea. Panic is further discussed in Exemplar 28.4.

CHILDREN AND PANIC DISORDER Panic disorder is the presence of recurrent, unexpected panic attacks. These attacks are periods of intense fear and discomfort in the absence of real danger. The risk of panic disorder ranges from 0.4% in adolescent boys to 0.7% in adolescent girls. Predictive factors for panic attacks in adolescence include a history of separation

TABLE 28–7 **Psychiatric Rating Scale: Levels of Severity for Panic Disorders**

LEVEL	DESCRIPTION
6	At least one panic episode per day
5	At least one panic episode per week but less than one per day
4	Persistent fear of panic
3	Limited-symptom panic
2	Sometimes feels on the verge of an attack but is able to control it
1	None of the above

Source: Adapted with permission from Yonkers, K. A., Zlotnick, C., Allsworth, J., Warshaw, M., Shea, T., & Keller, M. B. (1998). Is the course of panic disorder the same in women and men? *American Journal of Psychiatry, 155*(5), 596–602. Reprinted with permission from *American Journal of Psychiatry*, Copyright © (1998).

anxiety disorder earlier in life, history of parental panic attacks, and history of parental chronic illness (Hayward, Wilson, Lagle, et al., 2004).

Examples of the physical symptoms experienced are palpitations, sweating, chills, hot flashes, shaking, shortness of breath, choking, chest pain, nausea, and dizziness. The client describes feelings of danger or doom. As with anxiety disorder, treatment may involve child and family interventions using CBT and the use of SSRIs in some cases.

Acute Stress Disorder

Many people who experience or witness an extreme traumatic stressor develop **acute stress disorder**. During or shortly after the trauma, these individuals may feel numb and emotionally nonresponsive, may have a decreased awareness of their environment, and may experience amnesia for part, or all, of the event. Clients with acute stress disorder often experience recurrent images and flashbacks, which contribute to their tendency to avoid stimuli that remind them of the trauma. These behaviors cause significant distress and impair activities of daily living. Acute stress disorder begins within a month of the traumatic event, lasts at least 2 days, and goes away within 4 weeks. If symptoms persist beyond 4 weeks, the person is given the diagnosis of *post-traumatic stress disorder*.

COLLABORATION

The treatment of anxiety disorders is more apt to occur in the home and community than in the hospital, with the exception of acute anxiety or panic disorders (NIMH, 2008). Considering the level of distress that accompanies anxiety disorders, it is not difficult to understand the vulnerability of individuals with anxiety and the correlating increased incidence of substance abuse and/or depression. This combination is a threat to treatment success and positive outcomes for the individual. Because the individual is a part of a family and a larger community it is important for nurses to support positive outcomes for individuals by involving both the individual and his or her family in the treatment process. Such treatment is multimodal and involves the assessment of age, education, health and health practices, spirituality, and culturally specific needs (Antai-Otong, 2008).

Diagnostic Tests

Diagnosis of anxiety disorders is generally based on observation and client and family reports of clinical manifestations. Diagnostic tests such as urinalysis may be used to rule out the presence of other primary disorders, such as substance abuse. Complete blood count, thyroid function tests, and electrocardiograms may be used to detect alterations in biological functioning that may affect the individual's health status.

While magnetic resonance imagery and other similar tests are not currently used to diagnose anxiety disorders with any frequency, they are providing researchers with some new information that may, with more research and as the costs of these technologies decrease, become useful in the future.

Computer tomography (CT) scans and magnetic resonance imaging (MRI) provide a visual image of the structure of the brain (Videbeck, 2004). For example, Kneisl, Wilson, and Trigoboff (2004) note that researchers using MRI discovered that when individuals with panic disorder were compared with individuals who did not have panic, subjects with panic had smaller temporal lobes. Positron emission tomography (PET) scans use a radioactive tracer injected into the blood to follow the flow in the brain to monitor the brain while the person performs cognitive activities. Diminished blood flow and decreases in glucose metabolism have been detected in individuals with panic disorder (Videbeck, 2004).

Recent studies have found an association between panic and cholecystokinin, which can induce panic. The research suggests a variant gene that produces the cholecystokinin. Structural brain imaging studies have implicated abnormalities in the temporal lobes, especially the hippocampus (NIMH, 2008). Elevated levels of thyroid hormones and prolactin have been found in individuals with anxiety, and increased blood lactate levels have been found in individuals with panic (Townsend, 2006). A poor diet and low levels of vitamin B12 can also contribute to stress or anxiety. Vitamin B12 and the other B vitamins are important in the maintenance of the central nervous system. A rare tumor of the adrenal gland called a pheochromocytoma may also be the cause of anxiety. The symptoms are caused by an overproduction of hormones. Additional medical conditions that may cause anxiety are acute myocardial infarction, hypoglycemia, mitral valve prolapse, and seizure disorders (Goldman, 2004).

The most recent and convincing evidence points to the neurochemical studies conducted through the NIMH (2008) on chemical transporters and neurotransmitters like dopamine and serotonin. A technique called x-ray diffraction is used to visualize the structure of the "pocket" of the transporter that binds to the neurotransmitter. Based on this new three-dimensional imaging, researchers hypothesize that the pocket of the transporter acts to open a gate and facilitate the neurotransmitter into the cell (NIMH, 2008).

Pharmacologic Therapies

Antianxiety medication should be used cautiously and sparingly. Certain antianxiety medications (diazepam, for one) are among the most overprescribed and abused drugs in the United States and Canada.

Benzodiazepines (BZDs) have proved effective and relatively safe in controlling situational anxiety for periods of 4–8 weeks. Antianxiety agents such as diazepam and alprazolam (Xanax) or adrenergic blocking agents such as propranolol

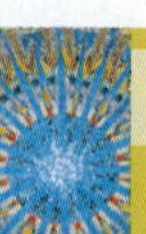

DEVELOPMENTAL CONSIDERATIONS

Treating Anxiety Disorders in Older Adults

Selective serotonin reuptake inhibitors are relatively tolerated and fairly effective in older adults. Therefore, they should be considered early as a treatment option. Cognitive-behavioral therapy has also been shown to be effective in the treatment of older adults with anxiety disorders (Lauderdale & Sheikh, 2003).

(Inderal) are sometimes used. Older adults are particularly sensitive to the effects of central nervous system depression associated with diazepam. If a benzodiazepine is necessary for an older person, lorazepam (Ativan) and oxazepam (Serax) are safer because the risk of toxicity is lower than with longer-acting benzodiazepines such as diazepam (Valium). The toxicity risk is lower due to the short elimination half-life and because they are not active metabolites and are not metabolized actively in the liver (Flint, 2005).

SSRIs are the class of medications of choice for treating anxiety disorders (Davidson, 2006), primarily because they cause fewer side effects than other medications. Other types of medications that can be used effectively in treating anxiety disorders include tricyclic antidepressants (TCAs), BZDs, beta-blockers, atypical antipsychotic agents, and buspirone (BuSpar), which often helps clients cope with a moderate level of anxiety.

Note that some antipsychotic medications may have a paradoxical effect and trigger the development of anxiety disorders. This is especially true of clozapine (Clozaril) as a precipitant to OCD in some individuals. When used to treat anxiety disorders, medications are started at a low dosage level and gradually increased until a therapeutic level is achieved. Inform clients that it may take up to 2–4 weeks before they begin to feel better. This information is crucial in helping clients continue to take the medication. In addition, many of these medications require that clients taper the dosage over a period of time, rather than quitting "cold turkey," when clients decide to stop taking the medication.

Although medications may alleviate the symptoms of anxiety, they do nothing to help clients understand the source of their anxiety. Ideally, these medications should be used for the short-term treatment of anxiety—days, weeks, or months instead of years. However, some clients may require longer-term treatment, depending on the degree of anxiety relief they need.

Cognitive Behavior Therapy

The ways in which a person thinks, feels, and acts all interact to predict how the individual adapts to stressors. Cognitive behavior therapy (CBT) is an important tool in the treatment of anxiety disorders and one in which the nurse can participate by modeling and teaching clients how to change thought patterns and behaviors.

The first step in teaching the management of stress is to teach the client to focus and develop an internal locus of control over thoughts and behaviors. *Locus of control* refers to the extent the client believes that he or she has influence over his or her own life. Sometimes referred to as *thought blocking*, this technique teaches the client to stop the train of obsessive thoughts that lead to increasing fear and anxiety. Clients with anxiety disorders frequently obsess over one or more specific stressors. Breaking the circle of obsessive thought frees the client for a myriad of other, healthy activities such as rest or reappraisal. It may free the client to consider alternative ways of thinking about a situation, and time and energy to engage in self-care. This is a critical tool, as it is difficult for clients to retain new information or develop new habits when they are engaged in obsessive thought processes. Additional cognitive techniques are listed in Box 28–7.

It is essential for the nurse to establish a trusting relationship with the client in order to know what to suggest that might facilitate relaxation. Teaching behavioral techniques to individuals suffering from anxiety supports an internal locus of control. Working out large muscle groups, writing in a journal, and seeking a supportive person to vent to can facilitate coping. Alternative therapies that may be helpful in reducing stress include aromatherapy such as lavender, progressive relaxation, yoga, and meditation. Nurses can provide several behavioral options to help individuals decrease their anxiety levels and build new coping mechanisms:

- Encouraging meditation in which the client repeats a word or phrase (Bormann et al, 2005). This technique activates the relaxation response.
- Developing goal-oriented contracts may help reduce a client's sense of inner chaos by providing structure and direction. The use of contracts also actively involves clients in their own healing process. This involvement increases their sense of control, thereby alleviating feelings of powerlessness.
- Helping clients test reality. This may help them realize that their sense of danger is often out of proportion to actual danger.

Box 28–7 **Coping Toolkit**

COGNITIVE COPING TOOLS

Thought stopping
Reflecting (distinguishing a thought from a feeling)
"Rethinking" or reframing
Retraining the brain (positive thoughts)
Distraction
Encouraging choice
Acceptance ("letting go")

BEHAVIORAL TOOLS

Reading self-help literature
Seeking social support (comforting person)
Journaling stressor and emotional responses and alternatives
Physical exertion
Talking and sharing with friends, therapist
Physical rest and leisure
Relaxation techniques (yoga, meditation, massage, aromatherapy, progressive relaxation, hypnosis)

EMOTIONAL TOOLS

Allowing oneself to emote feelings
Identifing and claiming feelings
Exploring emotional "hooks" attached to stress response

SPIRITUAL TOOLS

Expression of spirit through the arts
Symbols
Meditation
Prayer
Fellowship
Specific religious or cultural practices

Defensive clients may require assistance in identifying feelings and needs. Journaling assists individuals to explore and describe feelings. Helping clients find an outlet for expression of thoughts and feelings while offering nonjudgmental support empowers them to explore what it is they need to do to help themselves resolve the stressor.

Incorporating a person's cultural and spiritual beliefs is an important resource for some individuals coping with life stressors. Symbols and rituals can provide a source of strength and comfort for those dealing with overwhelming life stressors. Spiritual beliefs important to the person are a source of comfort during stressful times.

CHILDREN AND GROUP THERAPY Mental health nurses and other licensed professionals may conduct group therapy sessions with children both in inpatient and community settings. Group sessions for children often provide a forum for discussion of fears, an opportunity to enhance skills of working together, and an opportunity to learn coping skills. Being a member of a group with other children experiencing anxiety or trauma can remove the stigma and allow the child the freedom to explore feelings, behaviors, and their causes. Drawing and discussing pictures and telling stories are just some of the techniques used by mental health nurses and other professionals who lead child therapy groups.

Complementary and Alternative Therapies

A number of complementary and alternative therapies may be used to decrease feelings of stress and anxiety and promote relaxation. These include herbal or aromatherapy, massage and touch therapy, and yoga and meditation.

HERBS Several *herbs* are used for the treatment of anxiety disorders. Chamomile can be infused by pouring hot water over the herb, steeping it for 3–5 minutes, and straining before drinking. Honey or lemon may be added to taste. Chamomile can also be purchased as a tincture for a dosage of 1 teaspoon three times a day. Chamomile, a member of the ragweed family, should not be used by people who have ragweed allergy (Fontaine, 2005).

Kava, a South Pacific herb, contains alpha-pyrones, a recently discovered class of potent skeletal muscle relaxants. It is unknown whether kava affects the GABA (benzodiazepine) receptors. Kava should not be taken with St. John's wort, antianxiety medications, antidepressants, or alcohol because its effects may be increased. Reports of liver damage have led many countries to remove kava from their shelves. Currently, in the United States the FDA recommends caution in the use of kava (Basch & Ulbricht, 2005).

Many people find lavender relaxing, and some find it helpful in reducing anxiety. Lavender may be made into a tea, inhaled, added to bath water, or used with massage oil. Likewise, passion flower has a long history for use in agitation or anxiety.

MASSAGE AND TOUCH THERAPY Massage has been used with people having anxiety disorders as an adjunct to conventional psychiatric interventions. Clients are given an "executive massage," which is a massage done with the client fully dressed and seated on a massage chair. The head, neck, back, arms, and legs are massaged for 10–20 minutes per session.

> **EVIDENCE-BASED PRACTICE Acupuncture**
>
> Pilkington et al. (2007) reviewed the empirical evidence on the efficacy of acupuncture in the treatment of anxiety. Although positive findings were reported in the treatment of anxiety and situational anxiety such as preoperative anxiety, further studies are suggested.

Therapeutic touch (TT) works in conjunction with other medical or therapeutic techniques to alleviate anxiety and irritability. It also significantly reduces "state anxiety" in some clients and reduces stress in children and adults. TT also reduces anxiety levels for people who are hospitalized for medical–surgical problems (Newshan & Schuller-Civitella, 2003).

YOGA AND MEDITATION Yoga is tailored to the individual and can be done with great benefit at the beginner level as well as at the most advanced level. Attention is paid to how the body feels and what it is doing. Every movement is made gently and slowly. Every yoga session ends with a few minutes of complete relaxation. The psychiatric benefits of yoga include increasing brain endorphins, enkephalins, and serotonin; promoting relaxation; and managing stress.

If practiced regularly, even 15 minutes twice a day, meditation produces widespread positive effects on physical and psychological functioning. The autonomic nervous system responds with a decrease in heart rate, lower blood pressure, decreased respiratory rate and oxygen consumption, and a lower arousal threshold. All of this is helpful in reducing levels of general anxiety and worry. There are as many ways to meditate as there are people. When people say they have tried meditation and cannot do it, they just have not found the right practice for them. There is a variety of ways that one can meditate, including sitting, through repetitive prayers, swimming or running, walking, or through yoga or t'ai chi. Encourage clients to explore a variety of techniques and develop the habit of meditation on a daily basis.

NURSING PROCESS

Nursing interventions are focused on reducing the severity of the symptoms of anxiety. Specific interventions include establishing a rapport, communicating therapeutically, supporting and enhancing coping skills, assessing and identifying maladaptive coping, fostering mental health, maintaining a therapeutic milieu, minimizing the deleterious effects of anxiety, and promoting health of the individual. The generalist nurse provides case management, home health care, psychoeducation, and medication administration.

Assessment

The domain of nursing encompasses the professional role, competencies, practice, and process of providing safe individual care for the person and his or her family or community. The nurse begins with a complete nursing assessment based on

NURSING CARE PLAN A Client With Generalized Anxiety Disorder

ASSESSMENT	DIAGNOSES	PLANNING
Helen Martin comes to the community clinic complaining of indigestion and a feeling of soreness in her neck and shoulders. The nurse developing her health history learns that Ms. Martin has not slept well in some time. She has a hard time falling asleep because she worries about everything—the kids, money, problems at work, and recent problems on the national level affecting the country. Oftentimes, she gets up and paces about the house, trying to turn her mind off. Ms. Martin says the worrying and the sleeping problems have been going on for several months. ■ Dark circles under the eyes ■ Pulse rate elevated from baseline of 76 to current reading of 88 ■ Blood pressure 144/88 ■ Ms. Martin yawns several times during the examination	■ Anxiety ■ Disturbed Sleep Pattern ■ Ineffective Coping	The nurse, in collaboration with Ms. Martin, develops the following goals for care: ■ Client will obtain 8 hours of sleep per night ■ Explore source of anxiety ■ Attend cognitive-behavioral therapy to improve coping and reduce anxiety.

IMPLEMENTATION

- Teach Ms. Martin relaxation and meditation techniques to perform prior to going to bed in order to reduce anxiety at bedtime.
- Encourage Ms. Martin to keep a journal, writing her worries down each day before bedtime, and suggest that she "keep" her worries in the journal, and free herself to sleep.
- Encourage Ms. Martin to reduce caffeine intake, which can interfere with ability to sleep
- Suggest daily exercise to be performed at least 3 hours prior to bedtime to improve ability to sleep
- Provide a referral to a mental health provider specializing in treatment of anxiety
- Promote sleep hygiene.

EVALUATION

- Ms. Martin meets with mental health provider and attends regular sessions to improve coping skills and reduce anxiety.
- Upon next visitng the clinic Ms. Martin reports she is sleeping better and has more energy.

CRITICAL THINKING

1. Why might Ms. Martin find herself worrying at bedtime more than during the day?
2. When promoting sleep hygiene what specific strategies would you recommend?
3. Why is it important for Ms. Martin to exercise at least three hours prior to going to sleep? What impact would exercise immediately before bedtime have on her ability to sleep?

data collected from the individual and designs a plan of action to meet the needs of the individual.

- *Health History.* Including physical history, current medications, identifying current and past stressors
- *Physical Exam.* Including respiratory rate, oxygenation status, heart rate and rhythm, pupil dilation, cognitive and neurological status, pain level

Diagnosis

A number of diagnoses may be appropriate, depending on the extent of the client's anxiety, its etiology, and to what extent it is impacted or influenced by the client's family. Some appropriate diagnoses include the following:

- Anxiety
- Defensive Coping
- Disabled Family Coping
- Fear
- Impaired Adjustment
- Ineffective Coping
- Ineffective Denial.

Plan

The nursing plan of care, designed in collaboration with the client, may include the following goals:

- The client will report a decrease in level of and frequency of anxiety.
- The client will articulate successful coping mechanisms.
- The client will report increasing use of successful coping mechanisms.
- The client will participate in psychotherapy.

Implementation

Nursing interventions for individuals experiencing mild anxiety focus on appraisal. To gain understanding about the individual, the nurse acquires information about how the person appraises and prioritizes stressors. To facilitate the adaptive coping process, the nurse critically evaluates thoughts that may be increasing the person's anxiety.

Clients experiencing mild anxiety are often able to learn information and acquire new behaviors easily. The nurse is able to provide valuable information to these clients, teaching them ways to manage stress and modify thinking processes and behaviors.

Both mild and moderate anxiety need appropriate intervention to prevent the client from progressing to severe anxiety and panic. Due to the increase in physical autonomic responses described earlier, appropriate caring interventions for a person with moderate anxiety include both cognitive reframing and physical exertion to expend the client's excess energy due to excessive catecholamines. Walking briskly, running, or working out large muscle groups assists the individual to manage his or her own physical body.

Severe anxiety and panic require immediate intervention. The safety of the individual is at risk due to the narrowing of perception and inability to process information and think rationally. It is imperative to isolate the severely anxious or panicked client to prevent the client's distress from impacting, disturbing, or threatening others. Provide the individual with a safe, quiet, protective environment, do not leave the person unattended, and administer medications or other interventions as ordered by the health care provider. Benzodiazepines typically are used to treat severe anxiety and panic.

Encouraging Health Promotion Strategies

Several health promotion strategies are appropriate when caring for clients with stress-related nursing diagnoses including physical exercise, optimal nutrition, adequate rest and sleep, and time management. It is important to perform an assessment of each client to determine what strategies would be most helpful because all strategies do not apply to all clients.

- *Exercise.* Regular exercise promotes both physical and emotional health. Physiological benefits include improved muscle tone, increased cardiopulmonary function, and weight control. Psychological benefits include relief of tension, a feeling of well-being, and relaxation.
- *Nutrition.* Optimal nutrition is essential for health and increases the body's resistance to stress. Teach clients that, to minimize the negative effects of stress (e.g., irritability, hyperactivity, anxiety), they need to avoid excesses of caffeine, salt, sugar, and fat and deficiencies in vitamins.
- *Sleep.* Sleep restores the body's energy levels and is an essential aspect of stress management. Teach clients good sleep hygiene and relaxation techniques to help them restore good sleeping habits.
- *Time Management.* People who manage their time effectively usually experience less stress because they feel more in control of their circumstances. Clients who feel overwhelmed often need help to prioritize tasks and to consider whether modifications can be made to decrease role demands. Determining what time stressors the client is dealing with is an important first step for the nurse to assess. The nurse can then assist the client to develop a schedule to improve time management but should not create the schedule for them. The goal of teaching time management is for the client to learn to adapt their schedule as stressors and time constraints change. Parents who are employed full time, for example, may need to consider delegating tasks to other family members or hiring part-time help. Controlling the demands of others is also an important aspect of effective time management because requests made by others cannot always be met. Clients may need to learn to develop an awareness of which requests they can meet without undue stress, which ones can be negotiated, and which ones need to be declined. Feelings of control can be enhanced when clients schedule a daily or weekly period of time to deal with specific tasks.

PRACTICE ALERT

After encouraging the client to express feelings, be sure to listen attentively. Clients may express fear, anger, sadness, disappointment, or alienation, and it may be difficult for the nurse to hear about the client's pain. Some nurses feel helpless in the face of their client's catharsis and think they should be able to provide ready answers. In fact, ready answers are more likely to interfere with and thwart the client's communication. Genuine, concerned listening without judgment or giving advice is an effective intervention in itself.

Evaluation

Evaluation of the client experiencing anxiety is based on the symptoms with which they presented and their strengths and weaknesses. Suggested expected outcomes may include:

- Client anxiety diminishes as reflected by vital signs returning to baseline and client's self-report of anxiety level.
- Client demonstrates new or improved coping measures to reduce anxiety.
- Client self-moderates anxiety response when stressors occur.

REVIEW Anxiety Disorders

RELATE: LINK THE CONCEPTS

Linking the exemplar of Anxiety Disorders with the concept of Perfusion:

1. What impact does anxiety have on perfusion?
2. What medications normally prescribed for anxiety would be contraindicated for an individual with a history of heart disease?

Linking the exemplar of Anxiety Disorders with the concept of Acid–Base Balance:

3. How might anxiety impact acid–base balance?
4. What nursing interventions might the nurse recommend for the client with anxiety that is altering acid–base balance?

READY: GO TO COMPANION SKILLS MANUAL

- Assessing appearance and mental status

REFER: GO TO MYNURSINGKIT

REFLECT: CASE STUDY

Heather is a 34-year-old woman who is newly separated from her husband. She has been a stay-at-home mother of four children ages 7, 5, and 4, along with a 3-month-old infant. Her days are very busy caring for her young children, and she wonders how she will manage on her own, especially because she will need to find a job in order to provide for the financial needs of the household now that her husband has moved out. He has agreed to pay the mortgage on the house and provide a small stipend for other essentials for three months until Heather is able to become self-supporting. Heather had worked as a nurse before quitting when the oldest child was born. She looks into taking a refresher course so she can return to nursing and learns that several hospitals provide the course free of charge if she agrees to work for them after successful completion. She applies to one of these hospitals and is called for an interview. She wakes up early on the morning of the interview, feeds the older children and sends them to school, then takes the youngest child to a neighbor's house who has agreed to babysit. She returns home to dress for her interview, thinking about how she will find good childcare if she takes a full-time job and trying to figure out what salary she will need to meet her financial obligations if they are to stay in their home. After finishing dressing, she grabs copies of her resume that she typed last night after the children went to bed, takes one last look in the mirror, gets her purse, and heads out the door. As she is starting the car she suddenly finds she can't catch her breath, she feels lightheaded and dizzy, and she has acute chest pressure. She sits in the car concentrating on her breathing until the feeling subsides and then returns to the house to cancel her interview. She reschedules twice and each time the same physical symptoms begin before she can get to the interview. When she calls to reschedule a third time the hospital declines to set up another interview.

1. What is causing Heather's symptoms?
2. If Heather came to the clinic and you were admitting her to the office, what assessment questions would you ask?
3. What factors might be causing these events?
4. List specific interventions for this client.

28.2 CRISIS

KEY TERMS

Anticipatory guidance, *1826*
Crisis, *1819*
Crisis counseling, *1822*
Crisis intervention, *1821*
Maturational crisis, *1820*
Resilience, *1820*
Scaling, *1824*
Situational crisis, *1820*

BASIS FOR SELECTION OF EXEMPLAR

Healthy People 2010
Institute of Medicine
National Institute of Mental Health

LEARNING OUTCOMES

After reading about this exemplar, you will be able to:

1. Describe the pathophysiological response to crisis and the clinical manifestations of this response.
2. Identify risk factors associated with crisis.
3. Illustrate the nursing process in providing culturally competent care across the life span for individuals in crisis.
4. Formulate priority nursing diagnoses appropriate for an individual in crisis.
5. Create a plan of care for individuals in crisis and their family members.
6. Assess expected outcomes for an individual in crisis.
7. Discuss therapies used in the collaborative care of an individual in crisis.
8. Employ evidence-based caring interventions for an individual in crisis.

OVERVIEW

A part of life and the human condition is the experience of crisis. A **crisis** occurs when an event or circumstance overwhelms the individual's ability to resolve, manage, or process the event. A crisis refers to any acute incident that can evolve from a situation or event and which overwhelms the individual's normal coping process. Such an event may be a developmental, biological, psychosocial, environmental, or spiritual stressor. Crises occur when the typical or normal means a person utilizes to cope with stressful situations no longer reduces the anxiety or resolves the situation, producing an acute state of disequilibrium and turmoil. Adaptation and successful resolution of a crisis may involve a number of adjustments and may result in a change in the individual's coping process. A crisis also affords the individual an opportunity to grow and change as a result of successful adaptation to the crisis.

One of the many gifts of the profession of nursing is the privilege to work with individuals in crisis. The role of the nurse is to shine light and hope on the most abysmal of life circumstances. The most critical intervention begins with the question "What do you need from me right now?" The nurse's responsibility becomes that of facilitator in the acquisition of that need.

PATHOPHYSIOLOGY AND ETIOLOGY

A crisis is, by definition, an acute situation and is precipitated by an event that creates disequilibrium. Crises occur in the lives of all individuals. The characteristics of a crisis are listed in Box 28–8. The experience of crisis is an individual event. What is a crisis for one person may not constitute a crisis for someone else.

All crises afford opportunities for growth or deterioration (Townsend, 2006). There are typically three possible resolutions to a crisis. Generally, an individual will either (1) adapt to the crisis and return to the previous level of functioning,

Box 28–8 **Characteristics of Crisis**

- Something all individuals will experience as a part of living
- Presence of a specific stimulus or event
- Defined individually
- Acute event that will resolve (usually 4–6 weeks)
- Affords the opportunity for growth or deterioration

(2) utilize the opportunity to improve as an individual and cope with life more effectively, or (3) deteriorate to a lower level of functioning.

The contributions of Caplan (1964) to the prevention of mental illness have long provided the groundwork upon which to build what we know today as *crisis theory*. Individuals interact constantly with the environment; internally, they struggle to meet Maslow's hierarchy of needs (see Figure 28–3). These holistic needs, which include physical, psychological, social, and spiritual needs, are different as a person progresses through the life span. The individual's ability to fulfill needs, maintain homeostasis, regulate affect, mobilize resources, and maintain reality testing impacts whether or not the individual is able to achieve adaptation. The individual's perception of the crisis, resources, support, and ego strength all impact his or her capacity to return to prior levels of functioning after crisis. The intensity of the stressor and crisis can induce a range of symptoms from severe emotional pain and anxiety to the loss of reality testing.

Types of crisis involve both situational and maturational crisis. A **situational crisis** involves an unexpected stressor or circumstance that occurs in the course of daily living (Figure 28–7 ■). People experience acute stressors from the external environment, such as tornadoes or earthquakes; the internal environment, such as critical illness or disfigurement; and relational or interpersonal sources, such as the death of a loved one or a lost relationship. **Maturational crisis** occurs normally as people progress through the life cycle. Everyone experiences predictable stages of human growth and development as outlined by Erickson (1968). During each stage, the individual is subject to unique stressors. A failure at any one stage compromises the next stage of development.

Holistically, individual adaptation during the milestones of growth and development expends a tremendous amount of energy. Unexpected life events may alter the person's ability to adapt successfully to either maturational or situational crisis. This increases individual's vulnerability, often requiring supportive interventions from health care providers.

Resilience, Risk Factors, and Balancing Factors

Why do some people effectively manage disequilibrium while others go into crisis? The capacity to respond to stressors successfully is called **resilience**. Resilience is the ability not only to survive and bounce back from difficult and traumatic experiences, but also to continue to grow and develop emotionally

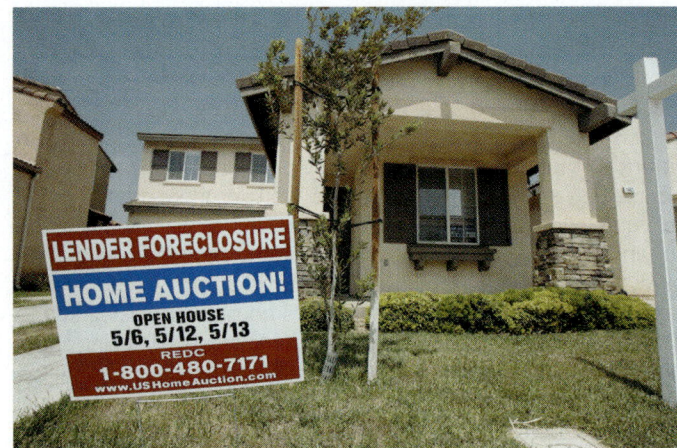

Figure 28–7 ■ The economic turmoil in the United States in 2008 and 2009 created crises for many families as they lost jobs and homes.

and psychologically. The notion of resilience encompasses the biological and psychological characteristics intrinsic to an individual, such as personality style and quality of interpersonal relationships, that confer protection against the development of psychopathology (Hoge, Austin, & Pollack, 2007). Resilience probably explains why not all maltreated children experience mental health problems as adults (Collishaw et al., 2007). Researchers and clinicians alike have been surprised by the prevalence of the capacity for resilience (Mancini & Bonanno, 2006), and clinicians are beginning to focus on uncovering and energizing pathways to resilience in their clients.

Several risk factors place individuals at high risk for crisis, the most obvious being the nature of the trauma or experience. Additional risk factors are identified in Box 28–9.

In addition to these risk factors, Aguilera (1998) indicates that the following three balancing factors are important to the successful resolution of disequilibrium:

1. *Perception of the event:* How individuals perceive and understand the event/crisis in their lives. Are they being punished? Is this happening only to them and never to anyone else? How will the event affect their future? Do they see the situation realistically, or is their view of it distorted?

Box 28–9 **Risk Factors for Crisis**

- Intensity of exposure to the situation
- Preexisting psychiatric symptoms and diagnoses
- Prior history of traumatic exposure
- Family history of psychiatric problems, anxiety, and/or antisocial behavior
- Early separation from parents
- Childhood abuse
- Poverty
- Cultural expectations that prohibit asking others for help
- Degree of threat to life (being on a plane that crashes versus watching a plane crash from a distance)

2. *Situational supports:* The availability of people who can help individuals in crisis solve the problem. Meaningful relationships with others give support and assistance during the crisis. Individuals with inadequate support are likely to experience a decrease in self-esteem. In turn, lowered self-esteem may make an event appear more threatening.
3. *Coping mechanisms:* All people use mechanisms to cope with anxiety and tension. Because the individual has used these coping mechanisms with success in the past, they become part of the coping repertoire. These tension-relieving mechanisms can be obvious or subtle.

If all these balancing factors—a realistic perception of the event, adequate situational support, adequate coping mechanisms—are present when an individual experiences a threat to homeostasis, the problem will be resolved and equilibrium will be regained, making it unlikely that a crisis will result. If, however, one or more balancing factors are absent, the problem is likely to be unresolved, disequilibrium is likely to continue, and a state of crisis will result.

CLINICAL MANIFESTATIONS

People in crisis need immediate assistance and support. Box 28–10 outlines the common clinical symptoms and manifestations of individuals in crisis.

The impact of a crisis may elicit intense emotions. To facilitate adaptive coping, it is essential that people be supported in expressing their feelings and that the nurse who is providing the support listen attentively. The nurse encourages and facilitates individuals to vent and emote. The goal in crisis is to stabilize the reactions of the individuals, thereby initiating the process of adaptation by reducing the disruption created by the crisis. Active participation from the nurse in the intervention process is required. The generalist nurse serves as communicator, facilitator, and resource expert for the individual.

Box 28–10 Clinical Manifestations of Crisis

- Difficulty problem solving
- Disorganized thought processes with difficulty processing information
- Disorientation
- Vulnerability
- Increased tension and helplessness
- Fearfulness and sense of being overwhelmed
- Intense emotional reactions
- Increased sensory input and bombardment
- Hypervigilance
- Intense physical reactions depicted in the fight or flight response
- Event is time limited by definition and resolves usually in 6 weeks

Caring Interventions

The nurse working with the client in crisis provides caring intervention at a time when the client needs it most. Times of crisis can be as challenging for the nurse as for the client. During these times the nurse should rely upon the essential element of nursing—caring intervention—to guide the care provided to the client.

Communicating with individuals in crisis requires frequent, brief, simple, and often directive communication. Biologically speaking, the brain of the individual in crisis is in the process of being bombarded with electrochemical reactions. Concentration and the ability to remember and retain information can be impaired. The nurse must continually reassess what the individual has heard or interpreted. In applying the transactional model, it is important to remember primary appraisal. What does the individual believe is happening? How can the nurse add resources and information to the reappraisal process to facilitate adaptive coping? Continual observation of patterns of communication within the family and/or group is essential. Due to the hyperarousal that occurs during the crisis, the nurse must be cognizant of nonverbal communication, tone, inflection, and mannerisms while communicating.

Concepts of caring in mental health nursing may seem somewhat abstract to the novice nurse. Frequently, nurses are more comfortable providing concrete care involving physical tasks such as dressing changes and medication administration. Exactly what skills are involved in dealing with crisis? The circumstances may seem quite overwhelming to the nurse as well. How can we administer care in desperate and distressing situations? The answer lies within the gentle spirit of each and every person. Caring is emitted not only in words but in deeds. Loving, caring energy is literally transmitted from one individual to another in need. The eyes are a reflection of what we hold inside. Eye contact is imperative. It is important to remain centered and know that words, energy, deeds and actions all carry a message to suffering individuals. Nurses cannot fix the life drama that they are frequently exposed to. Through supportive words, small acts of kindness, therapeutic touch, and a smile, nurses can provide individuals who are in emotional pain a blanket of loving support and energy, surrounding them with the assurance that they are not alone in their pain (Box 28–11).

Best practice for working with clients in crisis involves making contact by establishing a therapeutic relationship; ensuring client safety from the first moment of contact; mobilizing support through the significant other, family, relatives, friends, church support groups, and health care institutions; and collaborating with mental health professionals. Directive suggestion may be helpful, such as gently advising the mother of a critically sick child to go home and sleep while assuring her that she will be called immediately if her child's condition changes. Offering time, attention, and direction is most critical during a crisis. An arrangement for a follow-up care appointment suggests concern for the individual's well-being. The astute nurse looks for the opportunity to nurture vulnerable individuals in crisis. The opportunities to offer care in crisis are endless and may involve only a moment of time.

Crisis Intervention

Crisis intervention is a short-term helping process of assisting clients to work through a crisis to its resolution and restore their precrisis level of functioning. It is a process that includes

Box 28–11 Communicating Painful Information

One of the uncomfortable roles of the nurse is to communicate painful information to individuals. This task can be unnerving. A few simple guidelines convey a professional attitude of concern and care for those receiving dire news:

1. Greet the individuals with warmth, a kind smile, and an introduction.
2. Inform them that you are there and will assist during this difficult time.
3. Provide privacy, tissues, a drink, and a place to sit down to discuss the information.
4. Inquire about what they know, answer questions, and provide support.
5. Apprise them of the current circumstances in terms that they can understand.
6. Respond to their feelings and offer support.
7. Ask what they need from you and what has helped in the past to cope with difficult situations.
8. Incorporate cultural and religious practices of the individual in crisis to provide comfort.
9. Inform them you will facilitate communication and provide direction about the best means of accessing information.
10. Focus on the immediate reaction and needs of the individuals in crisis.
11. Write down specific contact numbers and instructions.
12. Inform them and check back with them as needed to see how they are doing.

not only the client in crisis, but also various members of the client's support network. Crisis intervention is not the specialty of any one professional group. People who intervene in crises come from the fields of nursing, medicine, psychology, social work, and theology (Figure 28–8 ■). Police officers, teachers, school guidance counselors, and rescue workers, among others, are often on the spot in moments of crisis (Figure 28–9 ■).

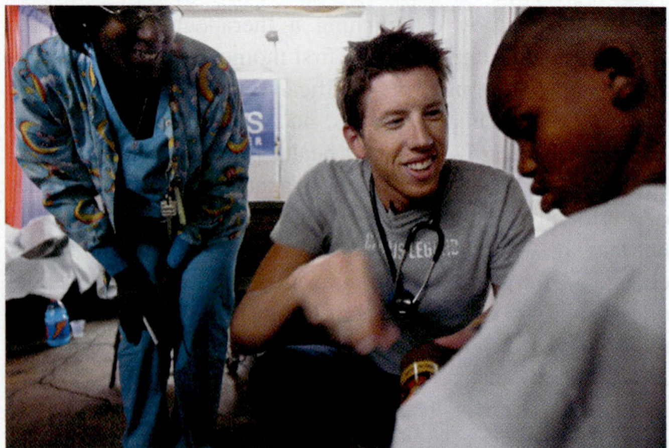

Figure 28–8 ■ Nurse Myeshia Westbrooks and Orthopedic Specialist Jarod Root talk with a 5-year-old evacuee from Hurricane Katrina as he receives medical attention at a newly erected medical clinic at the Dallas Convention Center in Dallas, Texas.

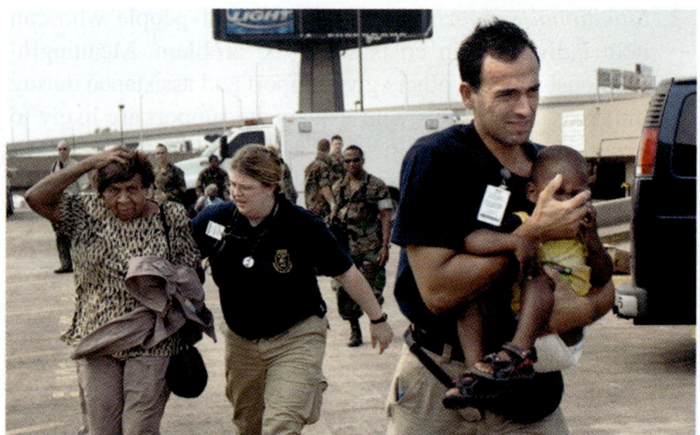

Figure 28–9 ■ A firefighter and a volunteer help evacuate a family from the New Orleans Superdome in the aftermath of Hurricane Katrina.

A person experiencing a crisis alone is more vulnerable to unsuccessful resolution of the crisis than is a person working through a crisis with help. Working with another person increases the likelihood that the person in crisis will resolve it in a positive way. Often a state of crisis offers the individual or family great potential for growth and change.

The traditional steps of the nursing process correspond closely to the steps of crisis intervention. In assessment, the nurse must focus on the client and the problem, collecting data about the client, the client's coping style, the precipitating event, the situational supports, the client's perception of the crisis, and the client's ability to handle the problem.

Effective planning for crisis intervention must be based on careful assessment and must be developed in active collaboration with the person in crisis and the significant people in that person's life.

Implementation involves crisis counseling and home crisis visits. **Crisis counseling** focuses on solving immediate problems, and it involves individuals, groups, or families. Crisis intervention centers rely heavily on telephone counseling by volunteers who have professional consultation available to them. Also known as hotlines and often available around the clock, these services allow callers to remain anonymous. The volunteers usually work within a protocol that indicates what information they need from the client to assess the crisis. Their goal is to plan steps to provide immediate relief and then long-term follow-up if necessary.

Crisis home visits are made when telephone counseling does not suffice or when the crisis workers need to obtain additional information by direct observation or to reach a client who is unobtainable by telephone. Home visits are appropriate when crisis workers need to initiate contacts rather than waiting for clients to come to them, for example, when a telephone caller is assessed to be highly suicidal or when a concerned neighbor, primary care provider, or clergy member informs the agency of clients in potential crisis.

A step-by-step intervention is outlined in Box 28–12. A crisis connection provides a lifeline for the client in crisis and allows the nurse to determine immediate needs.

Box 28–12 Crisis Connection

1. Make contact and connect with the individual.
2. Assess immediate safety needs.
3. Determine thought processes.
4. Scan for physical distress.
5. Listen intently, supporting emotional reactions.
6. Explore perceptions of the crisis.
7. Identify coping strengths.
8. Develop a support plan and a follow up plan.

COLLABORATION

Crisis counseling is focused on brief solution, focused interventions, and supportive care. During the course of a crisis it is important to consider the individual's physical vulnerability and stability (DeJong & Berg, 2008). The perception of the crisis, feelings of hopelessness, safety issues, and basic needs of the individual must be met. The alarm reaction, anxiety, and fear may prevent the person from resting, sleeping, or eating. Important members of the health care team during a crisis may include the hospital chaplain or family minister, a grief counselor, a social worker, a child and family therapist, and a teacher.

Pharmacologic Therapies

Pharmacologic therapies may be prescribed to address immediate medical needs, which vary widely depending on the nature of the crisis. Immediate needs that may require pharmacological treatment include:

- Pain following injury (e.g., associated with a motor vehicle accident)
- Threat of infection following injury or exposure to a bacterial infection (e.g., prophylactic treatment for tuberculosis following a lengthy stay in a hurricane shelter)
- Sleep disturbance
- Anxiety or depression.

Prayer and Faith

Many individuals find support during times of crisis from faith in a higher power. The relaxation response can be evoked with meditation and prayer (Matthews & Clark, 1998). The relaxation response buffers stress by clearing the mind and freeing the body from everyday tension. Practiced regularly, the relaxation response decreases heart rate, lowers metabolic rate, decreases respirations, and slows brain waves. In addition, it enhances measures of immunity. Benson (1997) found that when religious beliefs were added to relaxation response activities, worries and fears were significantly reduced when compared to the relaxation response alone.

Art Therapy

Art therapy can be a powerful tool in helping people process and manage crisis, especially children. Small children may not have the language skills they need to process crisis. Older children may be afraid or resistant to talk about crisis or afraid that adults may not believe them or may not respond to them in a supportive manner. This is particularly true for children who have experienced abuse (American Art Therapy Association, 2008). Art therapy helps clients express anger and fear or express frustrations about various types of crisis, from physical illness to disasters (Brinkman, 2004).

NURSING PROCESS

Ideally, the task of crisis intervention is to help the client in crisis understand the combination of events that led to the crisis and to guide the client, prior to a maladaptive response, toward a resolution that will meet the client's unique needs and foster future growth and strength. Especially during the acute phase, the goal of crisis intervention is to restore the client to the pretrauma level of functioning as quickly as possible.

Assessment

The nurse systematically assesses the client in crisis, beginning with making contact and connecting with the client. The first part of the assessment is focused on the individual client and should include assessing the safety of the self or others (explore suicidal and homicidal intent, feelings of hopelessness or threat to self or others, and/or potential for violence). During the assessment process, the nurse must also determine the client's thought processes, orientation, and ability to process information. Assessment of the client's physical condition includes any physical complaints and determining if the client is able to fulfill basic needs such as eating, rest, sleeping, and self care. Due to the intensity of the fight or flight reaction, vulnerable individuals may be at risk for physical illness during a crisis.

Assessment takes place on three levels: individual, family, and sociocultural.

Individual Assessment

Assessment of the individual is the first phase of crisis intervention. The nurse must focus on assessing the following elements that relate to the person and the problem. Collect data about the following:

- The client's resilience
- The client's coping style
- The precipitating event
- The situational supports
- The client's perception of the crisis
- Any guilt a disaster survivor may feel about having survived or about actions taken in order to survive
- The client's ability to handle the problem.

Assessment is an essential and critical step of crisis intervention and the basis for later decisions about how and when to intervene, and whom to call.

Safety is a key factor for individuals in crisis. During this time, the client may need to be hospitalized to ensure safety, and a referral to a therapist or an emergency room in a general hospital or a psychiatric emergency room may be necessary. Part of the overall assessment is to determine what is necessary to return this client to a homeostasis; this may be different from what is necessary to solve the problem.

Scaling assessment questions involve asking the client to rate the severity of symptoms or problems. This allows the nurse to determine the perceptions of the client. For example, the nurse may ask, "Mr. Smith, on a scale of 1–10, with 10 being absolutely intolerable, how would you score your distress right now?" Assessment information is prioritized on the basis of input from the individual. It is essential that the nurse be attune to caring for individuals' basic needs in a crisis, such as eating, sleeping, resting, self-care, and physical stability.

During a crisis situation, the nurse is more participative and directive than when working with a client who is experiencing anxiety but is not in crisis. The continued reassessment and monitoring by the nurse of individuals' responses to caring interventions is imperative. It is important to remember that the expression of feelings and interpretation of the event is culturally influenced and must be considered within the context of the individual's life.

Family Assessment

Family assessment is important when a client has experienced trauma, because trauma reverberates through an entire family (Wells, 2006), and when a crisis involves all or several members within a family. Meet with as many family members as possible to assess family resilience, family resources, coping skills, and interpersonal styles. Crises often accompany role changes in families or increased stresses in families that do not have the resources to meet the challenge.

Some common family crises are the death of a family member, the terminal illness of a family member, single parenting, divorce, drug/alcohol dependence, family violence, infidelity, remarriage, mental illness, incest, and "empty nest syndrome" (when all the children have grown and moved out of the family home).

Sociocultural Assessment

A critically important source of the meaning of an individual's response to stress or trauma is the broader sociocultural context in which the person lives. A client's culture influences the sources of distress a client experiences, as well as the client's symptomatology, interpretation of symptoms, and methods of coping.

How one is raised influences how one experiences distress, whether or not one seeks help, and whether or not one allows oneself to be disabled by a mental health problem. For example, in some cultures, anxiety is considered a sign of weakness rather than a mental health problem. This is particularly true for Asian American and Pacific Islander women, who are unlikely to seek help for mental illness until they reach a crisis stage (Office of Minority Women's Health, n.d.).

Cultural competence requires knowledge about other cultures and sensitivity to the culture of your clients in order to select the interventions that will likely be most helpful. Cultural sensitivity involves much more than simply identifying a family's ethnic origins or health practices.

To be effective in sociocultural assessment, you must also become aware of the influences and beliefs from your own experiences. If you are not familiar with a client's culture, ask respectful questions to help the client fully express his or her distress. For example, "I want to understand how all of this might affect you. Can you tell me more about how you feel about this situation? Tell me how your neighbors (your friends/your family) might feel about it."

Assessment Interview Crisis

INDIVIDUAL ASSESSMENT

1. What is the most significant stress/problem occurring in your life right now?
2. For whom is this a problem? You? Family members? Employer? Community?
3. How long has this been a problem?
4. Is this a temporary or permanent problem?
5. What does this problem mean to you?
6. What are the factors that cause this problem to continue?
7. Have you had similar stresses/problems in the past?
8. What other stresses do you have in your life?
9. How are you managing your usual life roles (partner, parent, homemaker, worker, student, etc.)?
10. In what way has your life changed as a result of this problem?
11. Are you feeling like you want to harm yourself or others?
12. Describe how you have managed problems in the past.
13. What have you done to try to solve the problem so far?
14. What happened when you tried this?
15. Describe possible resources (e.g., family, friends, employer, teacher, financial, spiritual).
16. What are your expectations and hopes concerning this problem?
17. What is the most you hope for when this problem is resolved?
18. What is the least you will settle for to resolve this problem?
19. What part of the overall problem is most important to deal with first?

FAMILY ASSESSMENT

1. How do you perceive the current problem?
2. In what way has the problem affected your roles in the family?
3. How has your lifestyle changed since this problem began?
4. Describe communication within the family before this current problem.
5. Describe communication within the family since the problem began.
6. How does the family typically manage problems?
7. What has the family done to try to solve the problem so far?
8. What happened when you tried this?
9. How well do you believe the family is coping at this time?
10. Describe possible resources (e.g., extended family, friends, finances).
11. What are your expectations and hopes concerning this problem?
12. Which part of the overall problem is most important to deal with first?

COMMUNITY ASSESSMENT

1. What are the special demands of the client's community?
2. What are the living conditions of the neighborhood?
3. Are recreational centers available?
4. Are there affordable child care services available?
5. Is there a community mental health center?
6. What support groups are available in the community?
7. What are the possible funding resources?

Disaster Assessment

Nurses as citizens are often at the scene of natural disasters or may be called on to help. Nurses can be particularly helpful during the initial stage of a disaster because, in addition to having the ability to provide care to the injured, they have the skills needed to perform physical assessments and assess psychological distress. The Red Cross trains health care professionals as responders in disasters. Go to www.redcross.org for more information.

Diagnosis

People in crisis may have a variety of problems and symptoms. The most common nursing diagnoses for people in crisis are as follows:

- Ineffective Coping
- Interrupted Family Processes
- Risk for Self-Directed Violence
- Anxiety
- Acute Confusion
- Spiritual Distress
- Sleep Deprivation
- Risk for Post-Trauma Syndrome.

Plan

The nursing care plan should be determined in collaboration with the client to avoid irrelevant goals and unworkable solutions. Consider the following as possible outcome criteria for a client in crisis:

- The client will be able to identify effective, as well as ineffective, coping patterns.
- The client will be able to employ effective coping strategies.
- The client will ask for help when necessary.
- The client will use available social support.
- The client will report an increase in psychological comfort and a decrease in negative feelings.

Implementation

Effective intervention is based on the ability to make interpersonal contact, establish rapport, and rapidly establish the relationship (conveying genuine regard and respect for the client, acceptance, reassurance, and a nonjudgmental attitude). One-to-one interventions to make interpersonal contact, establish rapport, and establish the relationship are important to an individual in crisis. However, nurses who work with people in crisis often need to use many nontraditional interventions, which can be as important as any verbal interventions. Working successfully with people in crisis is based on having a flexible, open view of what may be therapeutic with different individuals. You must have a full repertoire of skills and interventions that can be individualized to help all types of clients in crisis, including the ability to assist with spiritual needs.

Communication Strategies

- Use silence—this gives the person time to reflect and become more aware of feelings. Silence can prompt elaboration. Simply being with the person is supportive.
- Use nonverbal communication—maintaining, but not forcing, eye contact; head nodding; caring facial expressions; and occasional "uh-huhs" lets the person know that you are in tune.
- Paraphrase—understanding, empathy, and interest are conveyed by repeating portions of what the person said. Paraphrasing also checks for accuracy, clarifies misunderstandings, and lets people know they have been heard. You could say, "So, you are saying that …" or "I have heard you say that …."
- Reflect feelings—this helps the person identify and articulate emotions. You could say, "You sound angry [scared, etc.]. Does that fit for you?" See Box 28–13 for more help with what to say—and what not to say—to families in crisis.
- Allow the expression of emotions—this is an important part of healing. Venting often helps the person work through feelings in order to better engage in constructive problem solving.

FOCUS ON DIVERSITY AND CULTURE

How Cultural Differences Affect Crisis Intervention

Culture affects how and when clients seek help when they are in crisis, the considerations they make when appraising a crisis, and their coping mechanisms and resources. Cultural issues and factors that influence crisis intervention include the following:

- Language barriers
- Misunderstandings of expressions of distress
- Discrimination, mistrust
- Lack of representation of minorities and cultural groups in the research bases that support mental health services
- Disparities that impose a greater burden on minority populations (New York State Office of Mental Health, 2007).

Box 28–13 **Some Do's and Don'ts of Crisis Communication**

DO SAY:

- "These are normal reactions to an abnormal situation."
- "It is understandable that you feel this way."
- "It wasn't your fault; you did the best you could."
- "I am sorry that this happened."
- "Things will get better, and you will feel better, although they may never be the same again."

DON'T SAY:

- "It could have been worse."
- "You can always get another pet/car/house [or have another child, get married again, etc.]."
- "It's best if you just stay busy."
- "I know just how you feel."
- "You need to get on with your life."
- "If I were you I would…"

Source: Adapted from USDHHS Substance Abuse and Mental Health Services Administration. *Disaster counseling*. Retrieved November 27, 2007, from http://www.samhsa.gov

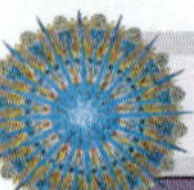

NURSING CARE PLAN **A Client in Crisis**

ASSESSMENT	DIAGNOSES	PLANNING
Deborah Smith is a 30-year-old African American woman who comes to the emergency department following a fall down the stairs outside her apartment. She breaks down in tears during the assessment. Not only is her ankle painful and swollen, but the father of her two small children has recently been arrested for nearly killing his girlfriend. She has no idea when he will be able to pay child support again, and she is afraid she will not be able to return work at her job as a waitress if her ankle is sprained. The physical assessment reveals the following: ■ VS: 98.0_0 – 96 – 18 138/86 ■ Hands are trembling, client is tearful and crying ■ Circular scars noted on both forearms the size of pencil erasers ■ Left ankle is edematous and painful to touch, unable to perform range of motion in ankle ■ Abrasions on the palm of the right hand, left elbow, and both knees.	The nurse diagnoses Ms. Smith with the following: ■ Acute Pain ■ Anxiety ■ Risk for Caregiver Role Strain ■ Risk for Compromised Resilience.	Nursing goals for Ms. Smith's care include: ■ Identify community resources that can provide assistance until Ms. Smith can return to work. ■ Identify Ms. Smith's strengths in terms of available resources and family support. ■ Manage pain to allow Ms. Smith to maintain comfort. ■ Teach client crutch walking and self-care for injured ankle.

IMPLEMENTATION

- Encourage Ms. Smith to express her feelings.
- Ask Ms. Smith whom she can look to for help. Are the children's grandparents supportive? Does she have a supportive spiritual community? Does her workplace have a sick leave policy? Are there resources within the community that can provide support and assistance?
- Provide referral to the hospital's department of social services to determine potential community resources.
- Encourage Ms. Smith to identify her strengths that can help her resolve her current crisis.
- Establish a follow up plan for both Ms. Smith's physical as well as psychosocial needs.
- Provide teaching on care of ankle injury, symptoms to report to provider immediately, crutch walking, and wound care.

EVALUATION

Social services assisted Ms. Smith in obtaining unemployment insurance during her medical leave of absence and provided anticipatory guidance to help her retain her job when she was able to return. Ms. Smith developed a stronger relationship with her church community who assisted in picking up the children from school, delivered meals, and helped to perform tasks such as laundry that Ms. Smith could not perform with limited mobility.

CRITICAL THINKING

1. If you were the nurse caring for Ms. Smith and lived in the same community would it be appropriate for you to offer to provide home care for her and the children when you had time available? Why or why not?
2. Is it appropriate for you, as the nurse caring for Ms. Smith, to solve problems for her? Explain your answer.
3. What functions can social service provide to help clients in crisis like Ms. Smith?

Assisting With Environmental Changes

Working with an individual or a family in crisis may require taking steps to provide shelter (Box 28–14). It may be necessary to find shelter for a homeless person, to obtain shelter in a safe house for an abused woman and her children, or to arrange for in-home health care. Nurses should be aware of the resources that are available in their communities.

Anticipatory Guidance

Anticipatory guidance is providing assistance in anticipation of the potential for crisis, thus averting it. These are some examples of anticipatory guidance: discussing methods of contraception with adolescents or young adults, preparing a child and the family for a tonsillectomy, arranging for a volunteer from the Reach for Recovery Program to visit a woman who has had a mastectomy, and preparing a list of helpful phone numbers for the newly discharged schizophrenic client.

Helping to Develop Social Supports

Immediate and tangible social support is crucial for clients in crisis because it may counteract or negate long-term adverse effects (Glass, Perrin, Campbell, & Soeken, 2007). Many people in crisis have limited social supports and are not always sure about how to access supports or develop them. Nurses can help a client develop tangible social supports by doing the following:

- Introducing someone whose spouse is an alcoholic to Al-Anon groups in his or her community

Box 28–14 ABCs of Crisis Counseling

ACHIEVE CONTACT (SAFETY AND SECURITY)

- Introduce yourself, your name, role, and purpose.
- Ensure the physical and emotional safety of the victim.
- Ask the victim how he or she would like to be addressed.
- As appropriate, collect information regarding residency and health conditions for contacting family members, any support systems, or friends.
- Assess whether the victim takes or needs medication.
- Identify the victim's feelings, reactions, and perceptions of the event.

BOIL DOWN THE PROBLEM (VENTILATE AND VALIDATE)

- Ask the victim to briefly describe what has just happened.
- Encourage the victim to talk about the present.
- Ask what is the most pressing problem (one at a time).
- Review and clarify what you heard as the primary and most immediate problem.
- Ask whether the victim has ever experienced a similar situation or crisis in the past.
- How was it handled? Consider how the victim can regain control.

COPE WITH THE PROBLEM (PREDICT AND PREPARE)

- What does the victim want to happen? (Give additional options that may be more realistic.)
- What is the most important need?
- Explore what the victim feels is the best solution.
- Help the victim formulate a plan of action with resources, activities, and a timeline for accomplishing the plan.
- Reaffirm the future and talk in hopeful terms of a "new normal" or a "new reality."
- Arrange for follow-up contact or visit with the victim.
- Connect the victim to resources that offer longer-term support.

Source: ABCD tip card was developed by the Association of Traumatic Stress Specialists, *"Recognizing Standards of Excellence in Response, Treatment & Service,"* PO Box 2747, Georgetown, TX, 78627, 512-868-3677, 512-868-3678 fax, admin//www.atss.com

- Referring a family with a terminally ill member to a local hospice
- Giving a rape victim the telephone number of the rape crisis hotline
- Informing the newly discharged client with bipolar disorder and the client's family about the National Alliance on Mental Illness (NAMI) local group or national website (www.nami.org).

Evaluation

Expected outcomes that may be appropriate for the client experiencing a crisis include:

- Client determines strengths and resources available to assist with crisis management.
- Client accurately perceives and describes events occurring as a result of crisis.
- Client creates a plan of action to cope with the crisis.
- Client verbalizes a feeling of control over managing the crisis.

REVIEW Crisis

RELATE: LINK THE CONCEPTS

Linking the exemplar of Crisis with the concept of Addiction Behavior:

1. When a crisis results from addiction behavior, what is the nurse's priority intervention? Explain your answer.
2. When a client's spouse is demonstrating addiction behavior that has caused the client's crisis, what community referrals might you consider suggesting to help the client?

Linking the exemplar of Crisis with the concept of Diversity:

3. Why might one series of events trigger a crisis for one client but not another?
4. How do coping strategies differ during times of crisis for clients from vulnerable populations versus those who are less vulnerable? How would your nursing interventions differ for each client?

READY: GO TO COMPANION SKILLS MANUAL

- Evaluating client safety
- Assessing appearance and mental status

REFER: GO TO MYNURSINGKIT

REFLECT: CASE STUDY

Carol is a 51-year-old mother of three. She is a nurse educator and works full time at a community college. Her son Paul recently moved back to live with her to attend college full time. Carol lives with her husband Tom and sons Paul and Mike. Her oldest and only daughter Angela lives in an apartment nearby. Arriving at the trauma unit at 3:00 a.m. after the dreaded call, all three enter the satellite unit. Carol is terrified her son is dead. Instantaneously, she detects what resembles her son. Gasping an audible breath, she slowly approaches the bedside. Tethered to a ventilator, his head seeps life's blood, the pillow is saturated. Scrupulously, Carol scans Mike's motionless body for signs of independent life. Splinters of glass are intermingled with hair, mud, and clotted blood. What appears to be a blue cable cord holds together a laceration that encompasses most of his head. Moving to his extremities, Carol inspects her son, recalling as she did, the day he was born. His left arm is swollen three times its size, and is blue and seeping from lacerations. Siblings Paul and Angela collapse into their mother's arms weeping. The nurse quietly gathers vital information from Carol. All three are directed to the lounge to await the insertion of the ventricular shunt. The neurosurgeon is unsure Mike will survive the night. Tom joins the group in the lounge after finding his way from the parking lot.

1. What type of crisis is this family experiencing?
2. Given the information presented thus far, which nursing diagnoses might be applicable?
3. List possible psychosocial interventions.
4. List specific interventions for this family.
5. What basic needs might this family require throughout the night?

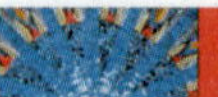

28.3 OBSESSIVE-COMPULSIVE DISORDER (OCD)

KEY TERMS

Compulsion, *1828*
Hoarding compulsions, *1830*
Obsession, *1828*
Obsessive-compulsive disorder (OCD), *1828*

BASIS FOR SELECTION OF EXEMPLAR

National Institute of Mental Health
Healthy People 2010

LEARNING OUTCOMES

After reading about this exemplar, you will be able to:

1. Describe the pathophysiology, psychopathology, etiology, clinical manifestations, and direct and indirect causes of obsessive-compulsive disorder.
2. Identify risk factors associated with obsessive-compulsive disorder.
3. Illustrate the nursing process in providing culturally competent care across the life span for individuals with obsessive-compulsive disorder.
4. Formulate priority nursing diagnoses appropriate for an individual with obsessive-compulsive disorder.
5. Create a plan of care for individuals with obsessive-compulsive disorder and their family members.
6. Assess expected outcomes for an individual with obsessive-compulsive disorder.
7. Discuss therapies used in the collaborative care of an individual with obsessive-compulsive disorder.
8. Employ evidence-based caring interventions for an individual with obsessive-compulsive disorder.

OVERVIEW

Obsessive-compulsive disorder (OCD) is a disabling anxiety disorder characterized by obsessive thoughts and compulsive, repetitive behaviors that dominate a person's life. An **obsession** is a recurrent, unwanted, and often distressing thought or image that leads to feelings of fear and anxiety. A **compulsion** is a repetitive behavior or mental activity (such as counting) used in response to the obsessive thoughts to help the individual lower his or her anxiety level (Gava et al., 2007). In order to be diagnosed with OCD, the individual must experience distress and lose time (more than one hour a day) due to the consuming rituals and repetitive behaviors associated with the disorder (APA, 2000).

PATHOPHYSIOLOGY AND ETIOLOGY

Conducting a review of recent research on OCD, Grados and Wilcox (2007) report significant gains made in the last decade. A specific gene has not yet been isolated, but epidemiological studies with families and twins strongly support a genetic linkage. The neurobiology of OCD also suggests the fronto-subcortical regions are affected. Abnormal neuroimaging in the basal ganglia and the orbito-frontal cortex has been found in individuals with OCD. Biochemical studies implicate dysregulation of serotonin in the etiology of OCD (Townsend, 2008), and a recent study conducted by German scientists suggests that both environmental and genetic factors strongly influence the disorder (Walitza, Renner, Wewetzer, & Warnke, 2008).

Recent research reported by the surgeon general (2008) discusses the development of OCD in children. Evidence suggests that a streptococcal infection may be the cause.

Diagnosis of obsessive-compulsive disorder may be challenging for those who are untrained or are uninformed about the disease. It is also made difficult by the variances that occur in the disorder, which are explained in detail in the Clinical Manifestations section. Contamination obsessions combined with washing and cleaning compulsions are probably the best-known variance of the disorder, in part due to the popularity of the television show *Monk*. Diagnosis of OCD is made by using the *DSM-IV-TR* criteria, provided in Box 28–15.

PRACTICE ALERT

Health care providers often use language that is unfamiliar to clients and their families. Explain obsession and compulsion in such a way that clients and family members can understand the difference.

Etiology

Approximately 2.2 million Americans have obsessive-compulsive disorder (National Institute of Mental Health, 2009). Obsessive-compulsive disorder typically begins in

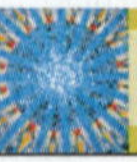

DEVELOPMENTAL CONSIDERATIONS OCD in Childhood and Adolescence

Recent research suggests that some children with OCD develop the condition after experiencing one type of streptococcal infection (Swedo et al., 1995). This condition is referred to by the acronym PANDAS, which stands for Pediatric Autoimmune Neuropsychiatric Disorders Associated with Streptococcal infections. Its hallmark is a sudden and abrupt exacerbation of OCD symptoms after a strep infection. The cause of this form of OCD appears to be antibodies mistakenly attacking a region of the brain. The selective serotonin reuptake inhibitors appear effective in alleviating symptoms of OCD in children. Several randomized, controlled trials revealed SSRIs to be effective in treating children and adolescents with OCD. CBT has been used to treat OCD but the evidence is not conclusive.

Box 28–15 *DSM-IV-TR* Diagnostic Criteria for Obsessive-Compulsive Disorder

A. Either obsessions or compulsions:

Obsessions as defined by 1, 2, 3, and 4:

1. recurrent and persistent thoughts, impulses, or images that are experienced, at some time during the disturbance, as intrusive and inappropriate and that cause marked anxiety or distress
2. the thoughts, impulses, or images are not simply excessive worries about real-life problems
3. the person attempts to ignore or suppress such thoughts, impulses, or images, or to neutralize them with some other thought or action
4. the person recognizes that the obsessional thoughts, impulses, or images are a product of his or her own mind (not imposed from without as in thought insertion)

Compulsions as defined by 1 and 2:

1. repetitive behaviors (e.g., hand washing, ordering, checking) or mental acts (e.g., praying, counting, repeating words silently) that the person feels driven to perform in response to an obsession, or according to rules that must be applied rigidly
2. the behaviors or mental acts are aimed at preventing or reducing distress or preventing some dreaded event or situation; however, these behaviors or mental acts either are not connected in a realistic way with what they are designed to neutralize or prevent or are clearly excessive

B. At some point during the course of the disorder, the person has recognized that the obsessions or compulsions are excessive or unreasonable.

Note: This does not apply to children.

C. The obsessions or compulsions cause marked distress, are time consuming (take more than 1 hour a day); or significantly interfere with the person's normal routine, occupational (or academic) functioning, or usual social activities or relationships.

D. If another Axis I disorder is present, the content of the obsessions or compulsions is not restricted to it (e.g., preoccupation with food in the presence of an Eating Disorder; hair pulling in the presence of Trichotillomania; concern with appearance in the presence of Body Dysmorphic Disorder; preoccupation with drugs in the presence of a Substance Use Disorder; preoccupation with having a serious illness in the presence of Hypochondriasis; preoccupation with sexual urges or fantasies in the presence of a Paraphilia; or guilty ruminations in the presence of Major Depressive Disorder).

E. The disturbance is not due to the direct physiological effects of a substance (e.g., a drug of abuse, a medication) or a general medical condition.

Specify if:

With Poor Insight: if, for most of the time during the current episode, the person does not recognize that the obsessions and compulsions are excessive or unreasonable

Source: Reprinted with permission from the American Psychiatric Association. (2000). *Diagnostic and statistical manual of mental disorders* (4th ed., Text Revision).

adolescence or early adulthood, although some cases do begin in childhood. It affects men and women equally, but men develop the disorder earlier: at ages 6–15 years for men and 20–29 years for women. One-third of adults with OCD developed it as children (NIMH, 2009). Stress can exacerbate the symptoms. About 15% of OCD clients show progressive deterioration in occupational and social functioning. Approximately 5% have an episodic course with minimal or no symptoms between episodes (APA, 2000).

Risk Factors

Risk factors for obsessive-compulsive disorder include family history and a major life stressor. Remember that OCD is an anxiety disorder and, as such, is a response to an underlying stressor.

CLINICAL MANIFESTATIONS

Obsessive-compulsive disorder is not to be confused with *obsessive-compulsive personality disorder*. The clinical manifestations of the personality disorder involve more of a preoccupation with perfection and are characterized by inflexibility.

The most frequently reported obsessions in OCD are repeated thoughts about contamination by shaking hands, repeated doubts with fear of having hurt someone or leaving a door unlocked, and a need to have things in a certain order. Aggressive impulses are often of a sexual nature or obscene. The obsessions are not rational or real-life problems. The client with OCD is, at some point, aware that the obsessions are not real (APA, 2000).

Compulsions are also part of OCD. The most commonly reported repetitive behaviors are hand washing, ordering, checking, and locking; mental activity such as praying, counting, and repeating words silently; and requesting or demanding assurances (APA, 2000). The person feels driven to perform the compulsion to reduce the anxiety produced by the obsession. Comments such as "I have to. I don't want to, but I have to" are common among OCD clients.

Of women with OCD, 90% are compulsive cleaners who have an unreasonable fear of contamination and avoid contact with anything thought to be unclean. They may spend many hours each day washing themselves and cleaning their environment. Cleaning rituals and avoidance of contamination decrease their anxiety and reestablish some sense of safety and control. Men with OCD are more likely to experience compulsive checking behavior, which is often associated with "magical" thinking, (irrational belief related to cause and effect). They hope to prevent an imagined future disaster by compulsive checking, even though they may recognize it to be irrational.

Other examples of obsessive behavior are arranging and rearranging objects, counting, hoarding, seeking order and precision, and repeating activities such as going in and out of a doorway. The *ritualistic behavior* may become so severe that the person may not be able to work or socialize. Professional help may not be sought until the individual is unable to meet basic needs or the family can no longer tolerate the symptoms (Clark, 2003).

The most common *preoccupations* involve dirt; safety; and violent, sexual, or blasphemous thoughts. There may be magical thinking, false beliefs, superstitions, or religious ideation, the content of which is culturally determined. These individuals say things like "No matter how hard I try, I cannot get these thoughts out of my mind."

Box 28–16 lists the most common types of obsessions and compulsions.

About 10% to 20% of individuals with OCD have **hoarding compulsions**, defined as the acquisition of and inability to discard worthless items. Underlying this behavior are obsessional fears that important items that might be needed at a later time may get lost, extreme beliefs about the importance of possessions, or an excessive emotional attachment to possessions. Individuals with hoarding compulsions, often called *hoarders*, are unable to decide what to keep and what to discard, so they save everything, including newspapers, magazines, old clothing, and junk mail. Living spaces become so cluttered that there may be only paths through the rooms. Since the disorder is egosyntonic (consistent with the individual's sense of self), the behavior can be especially troublesome for family members. As living space rapidly decreases, family members are forced to modify their daily activities. Some families acquire additional storage facilities, but these too are soon overrun with clutter. Family members are ashamed of the clutter but have little control over it. Embarrassment over the appearance of the home often leads to social isolation of the family. Hoarders often have little insight into their symptoms, making them less likely to seek treatment and more likely to divorce or never marry (Saxena et al., 2004).

Box 28–16 Types of Obsessions and Compulsions

AGGRESSIVE, SEXUAL, AND RELIGIOUS OBSESSIONS WITH CHECKING COMPULSIONS

- Checking, such as doors, locks, appliances, written work
- Frequent confession (of anything)
- The need to ask others repeatedly for reassurance

SYMMETRY OBSESSIONS WITH ORDERING, ARRANGING, AND REPEATING COMPULSIONS

- The need to have objects in fixed and symmetrical positions
- Repeating movements, such as going in and out of doorways, getting in and out of chairs, touching objects
- Counting or spelling silently or out loud

CONTAMINATION OBSESSIONS WITH WASHING AND CLEANING COMPULSIONS

- Grooming, such as washing hands, showering, bathing, brushing teeth
- Cleaning personal space

HOARDING, SAVING, AND COLLECTING SYMPTOMS

- Compulsive acquisition of items
- Difficulty discarding items
- Extreme clutter

The degree of interference in the lives of OCD sufferers can range from slight to incapacitating. Often, there is significant interference with home, school, work, and interpersonal functioning. Once begun, OCD usually runs a lifelong course, waxing and waning in severity but seldom stopping spontaneously. About 10% of people with OCD are disabled by this

CLINICAL MANIFESTATIONS AND THERAPIES Obsessive-Compulsive Disorder

ETIOLOGY	CLINICAL MANIFESTATIONS	CLINICAL THERAPIES
Aggressive, sexual, and religious obsessions with checking compulsions	■ Checks doors, locks, appliances, written work ■ Confesses frequently (to anything) ■ Needs to ask others repeatedly for assurance	**Pharmacological Therapies** include SSRIs: ■ Fluoxetine (Prozac) ■ Sertaline (Zoloft) ■ Fluvoxamine (Luvox) ■ Paroxetine (Paxil). Antipsychotic medications such as risperidone (Risperdal) may be helpful for those who do not respond to SSRIs. **Cognitive behavior therapy** may include *desensitization therapy* in which the person is carefully exposed over a period of time to an object that promotes fear. For example, the therapist and client may, at an appropriate time, agree that the client will touch the door knob. **Other therapies** *Deep brain stimulation* may be helpful to those who are treatment resistant.
Symmetry obsessions with ordering, arranging, and repeating compulsions	■ Needs to have objects in fixed and symmetrical positions ■ Repeats movements, such as going in and out of doorways, getting in and out of chairs, touching objects ■ Counts or spells silently or aloud	
Contamination obsessions with washing and cleaning compulsions	■ Repeatedly washes hands, showers, bathes, brushes teeth ■ Cleans personal space frequently	
Hoarding, saving, and collecting symptoms	■ Compulsively acquires items ■ Has difficulty discarding items ■ Extreme clutter	

illness. Rapoport (1989) describes the severity in terms of time involved in the compulsive behavior:

- *Mild:* Less than 1 hour a day
- *Moderate:* 1–3 hours a day
- *Severe:* 3–8 hours a day
- *Extreme:* Nearly constant

From 1 to 4% of children are affected with OCD. Affected children have recurrent obsessive thoughts, commonly about contamination, harm, sex, or moral concerns. Children with OCD differ from adults in several ways. Children have more aggressive obsessions, such as fears of catastrophe; more commonly hoard objects; and are more likely to have additional mental health disorders (Lewin et al., 2005).

The Importance of Early Intervention

Some evidence suggests that OCD clients who wait to seek intervention until late in the course of their illness when their symptoms are at the most extreme have poorer outcomes. The fact that one-third of OCD clients are treatment-resistant only compounds the difficulty in trying to find a combination of therapies that will work for the long-term OCD client with severe manifestations (Catapano, Perris, Masella, et al, 2006).

Social Isolation and OCD

Obsessive-compulsive behaviors frequently result in social isolation of the client with OCD. As was mentioned earlier, hoarders and their families are particularly affected by this. Other OCD clients are often isolated because of the time they devote to the compulsive activities in response to their obsessive thoughts. This social isolation is one of the many features of OCD that, for a long time, resulted in a negative stigma and stereotyping of individuals with OCD. Recently, however, society has begun to view OCD in a more compassionate light. Television shows such as *Monk* have brought warmth, humor, and understanding of individuals with OCD to the mainstream. Celebrities such as Mark Summers, a host on Nickelodeon and the Food Network, and Howie Mandel, the host of the NBC television show *Deal or No Deal*, have talked openly about their OCD and how they manage their obsessions and compulsions. All this contributes to a great communal understanding of OCD, increasing the possibility that individuals with the disorder will seek help.

COLLABORATION

It is important to coordinate individual care with the health care providers or physicians, clinicians, and community and social agencies such as schools and vocational rehabilitation programs. When OCD is disabling, the psychiatrist may need to assist the person with disability benefits from government agencies, financed health care, or government-supported housing or communicate with tax authorities, courts, schools, or employers. OCD clients who are parents of young children may want advice regarding the genetic risk of OCD. It is important for nurses to explain that there is a moderate risk of OCD in the children of affected individuals. Genetic counseling is available. OCD symptoms can interfere with the individual's parenting skills, and the nurse may need to elicit support from the nonaffected parent.

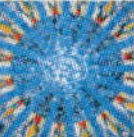

ALTERNATIVE THERAPIES Yoga and OCD

While it is thought that yoga may provide substantial benefit to clients with OCD, clinical evidence to prove or disprove its efficacy is lacking and further research is needed. However, experiential reports indicate the meditation involved in yoga may interrupt obsessive thinking patterns, while the postures and exercises may replace compulsive behaviors. Yoga may, therefore, help clients decrease their anxiety and give them a rest from compulsive behaviors. It may be particularly helpful for OCD clients to participate in yoga with a teacher, as the teacher's instructions and meditative talking may successfully interrupt the negative thought patterns of the client with OCD. Clients with obsessions about contamination should be encouraged to purchase their own mats, blankets, and other supplies, as they will not want to use those provided in class.

Diagnostic Tests

No definitive laboratory findings have been identified for diagnosing OCD. Abnormal laboratory findings have been noted in groups of individuals with OCD in comparison to control groups. There is some evidence that some serotonin agonists can cause increased symptoms in some individuals with the disorder.

Therapeutic Management

Conducting a review of current research, Gava and colleagues (2007) report that the most common therapy for OCD is pharmacological, followed by psychotherapies. They describe CBT as reporting the most evidence of effectiveness based on eight randomized controlled studies. These researchers assert there were no other trials of other forms of therapies and recommend further research on the long-term effectiveness of psychological therapies. The National Clearing House Guidelines for treatment of OCD are summarized in Box 28–17.

Pharmacologic Therapies

The first line of pharmacological agents for the treatment of obsessive-compulsive disorder is the SSRIs, such as fluvoximine (Luvox) and paroxitine (Paxil). Clomipramine (Anafranil) is also effective in the treatment of OCD. The nurse's role in the administration of medication is to provide

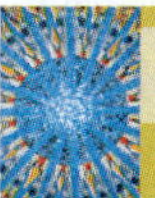

DEVELOPMENTAL CONSIDERATIONS Antidepressant Use in Young Adults

According to the National Guideline Clearinghouse, revised regulatory and/or warning information has been released. All antidepressant medications must include on the prescribing information a warning about the increased risks of suicidal thinking and behavior in young adults ages 18–24 years old during the first one to two months of treatment.

Source: http://www.guideline.gov/summary/summary.aspx?doc_id=5293&nbr=003616&string=ocd

Box 28–17 Guideline Summary for the Treatment of Individuals With Obsessive-Compulsive Disorder

PSYCHIATRIC MANAGEMENT

OCD is usually a chronic illness. Treatment is necessary when the symptoms interfere with functioning or cause significant distress. Therapeutic management consists of a variety of therapeutic interventions throughout the course of the illness.

PSYCHIATRIC ASSESSMENT

The psychiatrist will usually consider a medical evaluation and assessment of common comorbid conditions, such as depression, bipolar symptoms, other anxiety disorders, tics, impulse-control disorders, anorexia nervosa, bulimia nervosa, alcohol use, attention-deficit/hyperactivity disorder, and a history of panic attacks.

PHARMACOLOGICAL TREATMENT

- Clomipramine, fluoxetine, fluvoxamine, paroxetine, and sertraline, are approved by the U.S. Food and Drug Administration (FDA) for treatment of OCD. The SSRIs have fewer side effects than clomipramine and are recommended for the first medication trial.
- Successful medication treatment should be continued for 1–2 years before gradually tapering and while observing for symptom exacerbation.

PSYCHOTHERAPY

CBT that relies primarily on behavioral techniques such as exposure and response prevention (ERP) is recommended because it has the best evidentiary support. Family therapy may reduce interfamily tensions due to the individual's OCD symptoms.

Sources: Adapted from the National Clearing House Guidelines (2008); and American Psychiatric Association. (2007, p. 570). *Practice guideline for the treatment of patients with obsessive compulsive disorder*. Arlington (VA): Author.

client teaching regarding the safe administration of these medications and to work with the client to evaluate their effectiveness and resulting changes in behaviors.

The nurse also observes and evaluates factors contributing to failures to adhere to medication treatment. Due to the various unpleasant side effects and the chronic nature of anxiety disorders and OCD, it is important to teach and empower individuals to manage their own medications and provide strategies to increase compliance with their therapeutic regimen.

NURSING PROCESS

The primary nursing goals for the client with OCD are to ensure client safety and to alleviate anxiety and distress. Care must be taken not to prevent the performance of rituals which the client uses to reduce anxiety, but rather to promote new behavioral patterns and coping mechanism to make the rituals unnecessary while maintaining the safety of the client.

Assessment

The nursing assessment interviews of clients with OCD share many similarities for those used with clients who have other anxiety disorders. A thorough physical examination may determine physical problems resulting from manifestations of OCD. For example, excessive hand washing or the use of irritating cleansing agents may result in loss of tissue integrity.

Diagnosis

Appropriate nursing diagnoses for OCD may vary depending on the nature of the obsessive thoughts and compulsive behaviors and the severity of the illness. The presence of comorbid or co-occurring disorders must also be taken into consideration. For example, a hoarder who has allergic asthma may be at risk

Assessment Interview Obsessive Compulsive Disorder

CURRENT AND PAST MEDICAL HISTORY

- Does anyone in your family suffer from an anxiety disorders?
- Have you experienced intrusive or unwanted thoughts? Please describe the nature of the unwarranted thoughts.
- Do you find yourself performing repetitive actions and behaviors to alleviate your anxiety? Please describe.
- Describe how these compulsions have interfered with your life.
- How old where you when you first experienced these obsessive-compulsive thoughts and behaviors? Age of diagnosis?
- Approximately how much time out of your day is interrupted by dealing with these obsessions and compulsions?
- On a scale of 0–10, please rate your current level of distress (0 = no distress, 10 = intolerable anxiety).
- What have you tried in the past to alleviate the anxiety? What do you think was successful?
- Describe any repetitive or ritualistic behaviors.
- Do you use counting when feeling anxious?
- Have you experienced depression? Have you considered suicide? If yes, please rate on a scale from 0 to 10 how likely you are to act on these thoughts or impulses (0 = not at all, 10 = I will kill myself).
- Do you drink or use illicit drugs to manage your anxiety? If so please list name, frequency, and amount.

ACTIVITIES OF DAILY LIVING

- Is your health at risk as a result of the obsessions and compulsions?
- Describe a typical day (sleep, eating, activities, employment).
- How has this disorder affected your relationships?
- How has this disorder affected your spirituality?
- How has this disorder affected you emotional well-being and mental health?

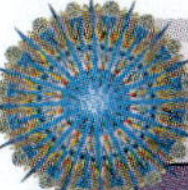

NURSING CARE PLAN A Client With Obsessive-Compulsive Disorder

ASSESSMENT

Margarita Hernandez is a 30-year-old Latino woman who comes to the local mental health clinic for help. As she sits in the waiting room, the receptionist notices that she keeps rearranging the magazines and counting aloud. The receptionist notifies Julie Watson, the intake nurse, prior to Ms. Hernandez's being called to an examination room.

Julie finds an exam room that has enough room for both her and Ms. Hernandez to sit down in chairs. She begins the interview by greeting Ms. Hernandez and introducing herself by name and asking, "How can we help you?" It takes a little while, and some client questioning, before Ms. Hernandez reveals that she feels "funny" all the time and can't stop touching objects and moving them around. She says her family keeps asking her to stop counting, which she says she does not notice doing. Her physical examination notes the following:

- Ms. Hernandez appears anxious and her eyes frequently dart about the room.
- She is unable to concentrate or follow a conversation and requires frequent restatement of questions before she is able to answer appropriately.
- When Ms. Hernandez is not talking to the nurse she mouths numbers, counting ceiling tiles and floor tiles.

DIAGNOSES

The nurse makes the following diagnoses for Ms. Hernandez:

- Anxiety
- Deficient Knowledge
- Ineffective Coping.

PLANNING

Goals of nursing care for the client with OCD often include:

- Assist Ms. Hernandez in recognizing the triggers for her obsessive-compulsive behaviors.
- Promote counseling as a means of returning control over hercondition to Ms. Hernandez.
- Encourage the family's support as Ms. Hernandez begins counseling.
- Emphasize the progress made by the client as symptoms of OCD begin to decline.

IMPLEMENTATION

- Use active listening when talking with Ms. Hernandez.
- Ask Ms. Hernandez whether there are times she feels worse or better. When she does feel better, can she say why?
- Confirm that Ms. Hernandez wants help feeling better more often.
- Teach Ms. Hernandez some relaxation techniques that she can do instead of counting, practicing them with her during her appointment.
- Refer Ms. Hernandez to a mental health provider at the clinic.
- Ask Ms. Hernandez to identify people who she can rely on for help when needed.
- Determine when Ms. Hernandez's behavior first started and whether there were any triggers proceeding the first performance of behaviors.
- Question Ms. Hernandez regarding family history of OCD.
- Allow Ms. Hernandez to perform ritualistic behaviors to avoid undue anxiety until treatment is initiated.
- Follow up with Ms. Hernandez by telephone in a couple of days to find out how she is doing.

EVALUATION

Ms Hernandez agrees that she would like help, saying she doesn't like feeling like a "freak" and would like to be able to live a normal life. She is reassured by the high success rate in treating OCD and begins seeing the mental health provider regularly. Six months later she proudly informs the nurse that all of her repetitive behavior has stopped and she feels so proud of her ability to help herself get better.

CRITICAL THINKING

1. What would you anticipate the outcome might be if the nurse did not allow Ms. Hernandez to perform her compulsive ritualistic behavior during the first visit?
2. Would it be acceptable to try to divert the client's attention away from performance of ritualistic behaviors?
3. What type of therapy would you anticipate the provider will initiate to help this client? Explain your answer.

for ineffective airway clearance and ineffective breathing pattern due to the presence of dust and debris in the house. Possible diagnoses for OCD clients include the following:

- Anxiety
- Fear
- Ineffective Coping
- Stress Overload
- Disturbed Sleep Pattern
- Insomnia
- Fatigue
- Deficient Knowledge
- Risk for Caregiver Role Strain.

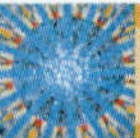

CLIENT TEACHING Adaptive Coping

Establishing a therapeutic relationship provides the nurse the opportunity to promote healthy adaptive coping. Client teaching about the nature of obsessive thinking is critical to lowering the client's feelings of shame and anxiety. The nurse can help the client realize that fears of hurting or killing family members arise from the *disease*, not from any actual desire of the client to harm others. Nurses can help clients reframe how they think about their disease and help them reframe thought processes in order to reduce ritual performance, such as helping the client meditate versus performing a ritual and then recognizing that nothing bad happened as a result of the absence of the ritual. The nurse has an essential role in helping the OCD client understand that he or she can decrease anxiety and gain control over the disease through pharmacological and behavior therapies.

Plan

Planning in collaboration with the client should be prioritized according to what the client identifies as most important and may include the following goals:

- Assist client in identifying triggers for obsessive compulsive behaviors.
- Promote a quiet restful environment for the client.
- Encourage client to identify strengths that can be used to reorder thinking in order to reduce obsessive compulsive behaviors.
- Reassure client that continued obsessive compulsive behaviors is not an indication of treatment failure and to identify reductions in behavior as positive progress.

Implementation

A supportive and nonjudgmental demeanor is essential in working with clients with OCD. Often the person is aware that the compulsive behaviors are unreasonable and feels embarrassed. Compulsive behaviors are designed to lower the level of anxiety or defensively "undo" the obsessive thoughts. Interrupting an individual during a ritual or compulsive behavior creates more anxiety and frequently leads to redoing or repeating the behavior to reduce anxiety. Working with the client to fit the ritual into the routine of the hospital may be necessary until relief is experienced from the pharmacological agents or cognitive-behavioral therapy. Administration of medications to lower anxiety and reevaluation of the client's response to the medication is the responsibility of the nurse in collaboration with the health care provider and the client.

Evaluation

Client response to nursing care may be evaluated by using the following expected outcomes:

- Client reports reduction in performance of ritualistic compulsive behaviors.
- Client demonstrates adequate coping skills to control anxiety related to absence of ritualistic compulsive behaviors.

HEALTH CARE

Advocacy

The covert discrimination of individuals with mental illness exists today in society and the health care system. The National Alliance for the Mentally Ill (NAMI, 2008) reports that one third of the homeless population suffers from mental illness and that people with mental illness suffer more and have more difficulty retaining employment. To learn more about advocating for individuals with mental illnesses, visit NAMI's website, www.nami.org. NAMI is the nation's largest organization for individuals suffering from mental illness and their families. NAMI has affiliates in every state and in more than 1,100 local communities across the country.

Every individual and nurse who cares enough about the plight of individuals living with mental illnesses has the ability to impact public policy. Organizations such as NAMI provide a platform for individuals to work collaboratively. Turning our conscience to the side as we pass homeless individuals with mental illness on the street does not make them disappear.

The Internet offers a wealth of information on issues that affect individuals living with mental illnesses in our global society. Ethical nursing practice involves developing expertise in accessing relevant current data and resources for the individual, hospital, and community.

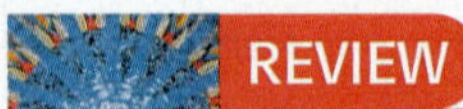

REVIEW Obsessive-Compulsive Disorder

RELATE: LINK THE CONCEPTS

Linking the exemplar of Obsessive-Compulsive Disorder with the concept of Mood and Affect:

1. How might mood be impacted in the client who is unable to control their ritualistic compulsive disorders?.
2. Is assessment for suicidal ideation important when admitting a new client with OCD? Why or why not?

Linking the exemplar of Obsessive-Compulsive Disorder with the concept of Advocacy:

3. If a client's rituals involve an act that places him or her in danger, what actions can the nurse take to advocate for the client while not causing increased anxiety that can result from not being able to perform the ritual?

4. While working on a medical unit in a local hospital you admit an adult client for surgery. While collecting the admission assessment you note what you suspect is ritualistic compulsive behavior. How can you best advocate for this client?

REFER: GO TO MYNURSINGKIT

REFLECT: CASE STUDY

A nurse is admitting a new client to the acute care psychiatric unit. Cheryl Franciotti is a married 46-year-old mother of two children. She was previously employed as a nurse but has not been able to work for the last 10 years. She complains of difficulty sleeping; exhaustion; weight loss; distressing and frightening obsessions; and feelings of guilt, shame, and self-incrimination. Her rituals involve hand washing, cleaning, and scrubbing handles and door knobs. Mrs. Franciotti is aware that her behavior is irrational but cannot interrupt her rituals. She expresses feeling hopeless, anxious, and guilty about the "burden I am on my husband and children." Mrs. Franciotti claims that she wishes she were dead, but because she is Catholic she is not sure she could kill herself. She has thought about driving her car off a bridge. "That way no one would know." Her history reveals panic attacks in college, and she claims, "I have always been the nervous type. My mother is the same way." Mrs. Franciotti's physical history is unremarkable with the exception of the excoriations on both hands. She says, "Sometimes I have to use bleach to kill the germs on my hand." She also reveals having used bleach on her genital area in order to be clean before going to a gynecology appointment. "See how crazy I am!" Mrs. Franciotti expresses doubt about her treatment, sighing, "I have been through this so many times. I just don't know."

1. Assessment: What objective and subjective data are available in this scenario?
2. Prioritize: Rank Mrs. Franciotti's individual needs in order to plan care.

28.4 PHOBIAS

KEY TERMS

Agoraphobia, *1836*
External locus of control, *1836*
Internal locus of control, *1836*
Locus of control, *1836*
Phobia, *1835*
Social phobia, *1837*
Specific phobia, *1838*

BASIS FOR SELECTION OF EXEMPLAR

Healthy People 2010
National Institute of Mental Health
National Mental Health Information Center
National Safety Council
United States Department of Health and Human Services
World Health Organization

LEARNING OUTCOMES

After reading about this exemplar, you will be able to:

1. Describe the pathophysiology, psychopathology, etiology, clinical manifestations, and direct and indirect causes of phobias.
2. Identify risk factors associated with phobias.
3. Illustrate the nursing process in providing culturally competent care across the life span for individuals with phobias.
4. Formulate priority nursing diagnoses appropriate for an individual with phobias.
5. Create a plan of care for individuals with phobias and their family members.
6. Assess expected outcomes for an individual with phobias..
7. Discuss therapies used in the collaborative care of an individual with phobias.
8. Employ evidence-based caring interventions for an individual with phobias.

OVERVIEW

A **phobia** is defined as an intense, persistent, irrational fear of a simple thing or social situation that compels the individual to avoid the stressor that elicits the fear. The stressor can be anything; needles and syringes, performance, airplanes, spiders, dogs, closed areas, and social activities are a few examples (Figure 28–10 ■). The individual with a phobic disorder will experience severe panic upon contact with the stressor. The intensity of the fear drives the individual to avoid the situation at all costs. Adults suffering from a phobic disorder are aware that the fear is irrational; children are not always able to make that distinction.

The maladaptive coping mechanism associated with phobias is the defensive mechanism known as displacement. The individual's unconscious, unresolved emotional issues are symbolically placed on the external object or situation. The individual moderates his or her anxiety by avoiding the object of fear. To be classified as a disorder, the phobia must be severe enough to interfere with the individual's daily functioning.

PATHOPHYSIOLOGY AND ETIOLOGY

The complex neurochemical and neuroendocrine systems are the focus of recent research studies linking dysregulation of neurotransmitters to anxiety disorders such as phobias. According to Antai-Otang (2008), recent data suggest that the dysregulation of three major neurotransmitters, norepinephrine (NE), serotonin (5-HT), and gamma-aminobutyricacid (GABA), are implicated in the origin of anxiety disorders.

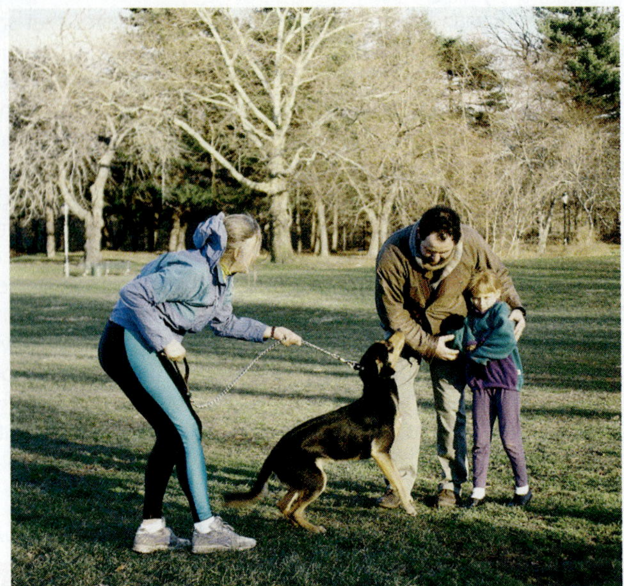

Figure 28–10 ■ People with specific phobias experience high levels of anxiety when confronted with the feared situation or object.

Source: Innervisions. Used with permission.

Etiology

According to the NIMH (2008), nearly 19.2 million Americans suffer from phobias. The incidence is twice as common in women as in men, and the onset usually begins in childhood or adolescence but can appear at any age and persist into adulthood. The causes of specific phobias have not yet been determined. The NIMH (2008) reports some evidence that there may be familial tendencies in the development of phobias. Often if the feared situation can be avoided, people with specific phobias do not seek treatment. It is when daily functioning is jeopardized that individuals most often seek help.

Risk Factors

According to the Mayo Clinic (2009), risk factors for developing phobias include the following:

- *Age:* Social phobia typically develops between the ages of 11 and 15 and almost never after the age of 25. Situational phobias generally develop by the mid-twenties.
- *Gender:* Girls and women are twice as likely to develop phobias as men, although this figure may be slightly skewed because men are less likely to seek help for anxiety disorders.
- *Family:* Individuals are at higher risk of developing a phobia if an immediate family member has the phobia.

An additional factor predisposing individuals to anxiety and phobias is an external locus of control. Lazarus and Folkman (1984) describe **locus of control** as the extent one believes he or she has control over the events in his or her life. Individuals with an **internal locus of control** believe their actions, choices and behaviors impact life events. Those with an **external locus of control** believe that powers outside of themselves, such as luck or fate, determine life events.

Factors that predispose people to develop phobias include the following (American Psychiatric Association, 2000):

- Traumatic events (e.g., being trapped in a closet or attacked by an animal)
- Unexpected panic attacks in the feared situation
- Observing others in the feared situation (e.g., seeing someone fall from a height)
- Seeing others demonstrate fear in the situation (e.g., the child's mother is afraid of going to the dentist)
- Informational transmission (e.g., media coverage of bombing, natural disasters, plane crashes, or repeated parental warnings about dangers of some situation).

CLINICAL MANIFESTATIONS

There are three general categories of phobias:

1. Agoraphobia
2. Social phobias
3. Specific phobias.

Agoraphobia

Agoraphobia is characterized by anxiety about being in places or situations where escape may be difficult (or embarrassing) or when help might not be available in the case of a panic attack. Agoraphobic fears typically include situations that involve being alone; away from home; in a crowd; standing in line; on a bridge; or traveling in a plane, train, bus, or automobile. The person avoids fear-producing situations, endures them with much anxiety and distress, or requires the presence of a companion (American Psychiatric Association, 2000). Agoraphobia is commonly associated with panic disorder. People who seek treatment for the disorder almost always also have panic disorder. Agoraphobia is more likely to occur in females than in males. It can severely impair social and occupational functioning when the individual avoids multiple anxiety-producing situations (APA, 2000). Figure 28–11 ■ shows a woman who is afraid to leave her home.

It is important to remember that not everyone who stays in the home all the time has agoraphobia. In some cultures,

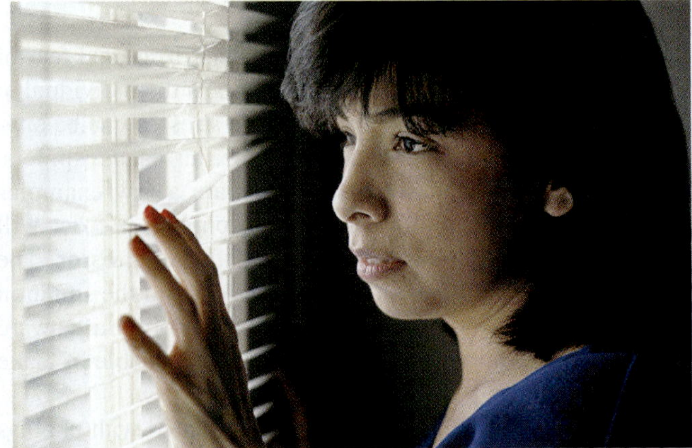

Figure 28–11 ■ People with agoraphobia do not feel safe outside their own homes.

Source: The Image Works.

CLINICAL MANIFESTATIONS AND THERAPIES **Phobias**

TYPES OF PHOBIAS	CLINICAL MANIFESTATIONS	CLINICAL THERAPIES
Agoraphobia	Fear of places or situations where the person feels unable to readily escape.	The short-term use of antianxiety agents, such as the benzodiazepines, may be indicated in severe cases (should not be used more than 2–4 weeks). SSRIs may be used for longer periods. Tricyclic antidepressants are also recommended. **Psychological therapies** ■ CBT ■ Supportive therapy ■ Desensitization and implosion therapy for specific phobias ■ Self-help groups and bibliotherapy (therapy that incorporates written forms of expression) based on CBT Discuss exercise and healthy nutrition. Phobic clients should decrease caffeine and nicotine intake. Assess alcohol intake.
Social phobias	Fear of being criticized or ridiculed by others.	
Specific phobias	Unreasonable fear triggered by the presence of an object or dreaded situation (e.g., animals, insects, thunder)	

Source: Data from National Institute for Clinical Excellence (2004), NIMH (2008), NGC (2008).

women are expected to remain at home, and their public activities are greatly limited. If a woman from such a culture stays at home, she is acting in accordance with cultural expectations and does not have a diagnosis of agoraphobia.

Social Phobia

Social phobia (also called *social anxiety disorder*) is characterized by a marked and persistent fear of social or performance situations in which embarrassment may occur. Exposure to the social or performance situation (such as public speaking or speaking to a supervisor) almost always results in an immediate anxiety reaction. Adults and adolescents with social phobia recognize that their fear is excessive. Affected children may not.

People with social phobia usually avoid the risky situations but may endure them with dread. Social phobia is diagnosed only if the fear, avoidance, or anxiety about encountering the social situation interferes significantly with daily routine or social, academic, or occupational life, or if the person is markedly distressed by the disorder. Anticipatory anxiety may begin weeks before an anticipated social event (American Psychiatric Association, 2000). In order for individuals younger than age 18 to be diagnosed, the symptoms must have lasted for more than 6 months. Temporary social anxiety in childhood or adolescence is quite common and does not constitute social phobia. Neither does fear of speaking in situations in which the fear may be justified, such as when the teacher calls on a student who has not done the homework.

Physical symptoms often go along with the anxiety in social phobia. These include blushing, excessive sweating, nausea, gastrointestinal distress, tremors, and difficulty talking. Although many realize that their fears are irrational, people with this disorder are unable to control it. Even after they have done the dreaded deed, people with this disorder continue to feel anxious about how they were perceived and judged by others. Making or keeping friends may be difficult. People with social phobia may medicate themselves with alcohol or drugs to make it possible for them to endure social situations.

DEVELOPMENTAL CONSIDERATIONS **Phobias**

CHILDREN

- Anxiety disorders and specific phobias are not uncommon in children.
- Children of parents who have been diagnosed with anxiety disorders have a higher incidence of separation anxiety and phobias. According to the *DSM-IV-TR* (APA, 2000), families that are close tend to exhibit a higher incidence of separation anxiety.
- Behaviors exhibited by children include clinging, crying, refusing to go to school, and difficulty staying away from home.
- Therapy for children involves the family and behavioral therapy and may involve school counselors or peer support groups.

OLDER ADULTS

- Anxiety disorders may occur later in life. They may be attributed to the fragility of the central nervous system or to a significant stressor, usually a loss such as the death of a spouse or loss of personal independence.
- According to Antai-Otong (2008), anxiety disorders are the most common psychiatric condition of older adults, yet research of anxiety disorders in the older adults lags behind that for dementias, such as Alzheimer's disease, and depression.
- Anxiety and depression tend to accompany each other in the older adult population.

Specific Phobias

A **specific phobia** is an excessive fear of a specific object or situation. It might be triggered by the presence or even the anticipation of the stressor. Affected people have an immediate anxiety reaction in response to the stressor, which may take the form of a panic attack. Some examples of specific phobias are fears of animals, flying, heights, or needles. Table 28–8 gives examples of specific phobias and their clinical names.

Adults with phobias generally recognize that their fears are unreasonable. They usually avoid the phobic stimulus but may endure it with intense anxiety or dread. A phobia seriously affects the person's daily routine, occupational or academic functioning, social life, or quality of life (American Psychiatric Association, 2000). When phobias involve situations or objects that are easy to avoid, people may not feel the need to seek treatment. However, phobias involving everyday experiences can be disabling. Fears of specific objects or situations are very common. Specific phobia is not diagnosed unless the phobia significantly interferes with the individual's functioning or causes severe distress.

Specific phobias often occur in people who also have other anxiety disorders, mood disorders, and substance-related disorders. Approximately 75% of people who have a blood-injection-injury–type phobia have a history of fainting from a vasovagal response. A vasovagal response is indicated by an initial rise in the heart rate and blood pressure, followed by a drop in heart rate and blood pressure that often causes fainting (American Psychiatric Association, 2000).

TABLE 28–8 **Common, Uncommon, and Curious Phobias**

NAME OF PHOBIA	SPECIFIC FEAR
Acrophobia	Heights
Agoraphobia	Open spaces or crowds
Algophobia	Pain
Androphobia	Men
Arachnophobia	Spiders
Astraphobia	Thunder and lightning
Astrophobia	Stars and celestial space
Aviophobia	Flying
Claustrophobia	Enclosed places
Coprophobia	Excrement
Cynophobia	Dogs
Entomophobia	Insects
Erythrophobia	Blushing
Hematophobia	Blood
Hydrophobia	Water
Iatrophobia	Doctors
Lalophobia	Speaking
Necrophobia	Dead bodies
Nyctophobia	Darkness, night
Odynophobia	Pain
Ophidiphobia	Snakes
Pathophobia	Disease
Peccatophobia	Committing a sin
Phonophobia	Speaking aloud
Pyrophobia	Fire
Sitophobia	Food, eating
Taphophobia	Being buried alive
Thanatophobia	Death
Toxophobia	Being poisoned
Xenophobia	Strangers
Zoophobia	Animals

COLLABORATION

It is the responsibility of nurses to collaborate and refer individuals with phobias and anxiety disorders to mental health professionals. These include advanced practice mental health nurses, counselors, therapists, and psychologists. Mental health professionals can help phobic clients develop more successful, healthier coping methods, decreasing their fear and improving their quality of life. Additional therapeutic professionals that support adaptive coping include exercise physiologists, dieticians, yoga instructors, massage therapists, and support groups.

Pharmacologic Therapy

Pharmacologic therapy options for the phobic client include benzodiazepines, SSRIs, and some antipsychotics. Because of their addictive qualities, benzodiazepines should be used for only a short period of time. Benzodiazepines work rapidly to alleviate emotional distress and induce relaxation. The level of distress with phobias and panic is severe and readily alters the quality of life for the individual. A short course of benzodiazepines may sufficiently reduce anxiety to allow the client to begin participation in psychotherapy where the client can learn new ways of coping with anxieties. Clients who need pharmacological support for a longer period of time may benefit from the use of SSRIs, which have fewer side effects than antipsychotics.

American culture has become a culture of immediate gratification. Pharmaceutical advertisements promoting chemicals for everything from headaches to anxiety, pain, and constipation are everywhere. The suggestion that human discomfort should be obliterated by chemicals and medication is epidemic and contributes to the addictive nature of contemporary society. Healthier coping mechanisms have taken a back seat to immediate gratification through chemistry. It is critical that the nurse working with the phobic client explain the importance of CBT as a treatment for the client's phobia and that any medication used as treatment will be less effective if not used in combination with cognitive-behavioral therapy.

TABLE 28–9 Cognitive-Behavioral Techniques for Treating Phobias

TECHNIQUE	DESCRIPTION	EXAMPLE
Systematic desensitization (exposure therapy)	A client is exposed to a series of increasingly anxiety-provoking situations, beginning with the least threatening. The client gradually becomes desensitized to each stimulus in the series until the stimulus that induced the most anxiety is no longer threatening.	A man who is terrified of earthworms might first talk about earthworms until the topic no longer evokes the same level of anxiety. Then he might be shown pictures of earthworms until he masters that level of closeness. Over time, he will progress to holding a live earthworm in his hand without experiencing severe or panic-level anxiety.
Reciprocal inhibition	The anxiety-provoking stimulus is paired with another stimulus associated with an opposite feeling strong enough to suppress the anxiety.	Through the use of meditation, yoga, biofeedback training, hypnosis, or antianxiety medications, a client learns how to induce a calm state.
Cognitive restructuring	This intervention is based on the belief that anxiety stems from erroneous interpretations of situations. The client learns to reframe (or relabel) a frightening situation, object, activity, or event so that it becomes less threatening.	A woman who fears she is going to die if she leaves her apartment learns to change her perception to one that is more reality based by saying, "I may feel uncomfortable but I will not die. I can do this."

Cognitive-Behavioral Therapy

As was discussed previously, CBT has shown great success in treatment of anxiety disorders. CBT techniques for clients with phobias include desensitization, reciprocal inhibition, and cognitive restructuring. See Table 28–9 for a description and example of each of these techniques.

Journal Writing

Journaling assists individuals to become consciously aware of unresolved issues and stressors. Stressors and issues that are undiscovered or denied cannot be consciously resolved. By discovering and acknowledging stressors, the phobic client can mobilize adaptive coping skills.

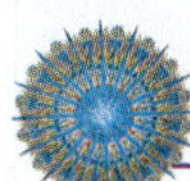

NURSING PROCESS

The role of the professional nurse in caring for clients with phobic disorders is to provide comfort to the client and family and alleviate emotional distress. This supports adaptive coping while empowering the client by providing information, accessing resources, and communicating therapeutically.

Assessment

Accurate assessment of the client experiencing a phobic disorder is essential. Although the treatment regimen is similar for the different types of phobias, it is important to obtain an accurate history from the individual about the attempts the individual has made to moderate his or her anxiety. Explore the possibility of comorbidity of depression and/or substance abuse, as the incidence for individuals suffering from anxiety disorders is high. Assess for any indication of suicidal ideation or past history of dangerous behavior.

Physical examination of the client should include assessment for symptoms related to substance abuse. Physical findings may be otherwise normal during the examination unless the client is currently experiencing anxiety related to the phobia.

Assessment Interview Individual Suffering From Phobias

CURRENT AND PAST MEDICAL HISTORY

- Do you have anxiety or avoid circumstances such as exposure to snakes or spiders?
- Do you avoid flying or are you afraid of heights?
- Do you avoid social situations where you might be evaluated by others such as eating or speaking in public?
- How often and in what circumstances do you leave home?
- Do you experience anxiety when anticipating or receiving criticism from others?
- Have you experienced feelings of irritability, guilt, depression, worthlessness, poor concentration, sleeplessness, suicidal intent?
- Have you sought treatment previously? What type of treatment have you tried? How helpful or effective was it?
- Do you have any history of substance abuse, alcohol abuse, or use of over the counter medication for anxiety? Do you use any herbs or supplements? Have you tried any alternative therapies, such as acupuncture or yoga?
- Whom can you rely on to understand and support you when you are distressed?
- Describe the qualities you like about yourself. What qualities do you dislike about yourself?
- Describe how family living patterns have changed around your fears.

SCALING QUESTIONS

- Ask the client to rank his or her anxiety on a scale of 0 (absence of symptoms) to 10 (completely disabling). Begin with current anxiety during the interview and progress to describe the 10 or worst experience of anxiety.
- Ask the client to rank how much the phobia interferes with daily routines or functioning.

RISK FACTORS

- Family history of anxiety disorders
- Family history of depression or substance abuse

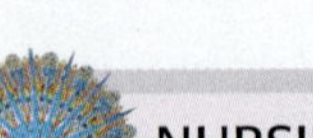

NURSING CARE PLAN A Client With Panic Disorder With Agoraphobia

ASSESSMENT

Mrs. Randolph is 43 years old, married, and the mother of four daughters in their late teens and early twenties. She is referred to the psychiatric outpatient clinic from the local ED following an acute panic attack with symptoms of racing heartbeat, sweating, feeling faint, and the belief that she was dying. She could not identify any events, thoughts, or feelings that precipitated the incident; it seemed to her to occur "out of the blue." She felt unable to cope with the severity of the symptoms of the attack: "I tried to talk myself out of it; to tell myself it would go away, but it only got worse." Mrs. Randolph reported she had had similar attacks lasting from 2 minutes to 2 hours in the past with no physical cause found by her family doctor. Her daily routine has become restricted, and she will not leave the house without a family member. She is not comfortable alone in her home and can't sleep if any family member is still out. She is ashamed and angry about her growing disability and often tries to cover up her fears to friends and family. Recent life events include a hysterectomy 4 weeks ago, loss of employment resulted from hospitalization, and the second anniversary of her father's sudden death is upcoming. She has no other history of mental health issues. She first saw a therapist for her panic disorder when they first started, "about the time I left home to marry" but did not follow up because she felt ashamed ("I've always been a strong and effective person!"), that the episodes were not so severe then, and that she found relief from panic attacks after she had the children. Her mother rarely left the house, never participating in social events unless they were in the home. She described her relationship with her husband as emotionally warm and supportive. She dreads seeing her daughters move from home.

Assessment findings:

- Attractive, carefully groomed woman who looks her stated age.
- Appears somewhat tense.
- Answers questions cooperatively, but at times with some hesitation, as if expecting criticism or judgment from the interviewer.
- Oriented to time, place, and person.
- Memory intact, good recall, no difficulty with calculations.
- Affect appears normal, with occasional evidence of anger in the form of irritability or sarcasm. Mood is within normal limits.
- Speech normal in flow and volume, pressured at times when she correct an impression
- Posture rigid at times, but she relaxes as she becomes more comfortable with the interview.

DIAGNOSES

- Ineffective Role Performance related to fear and anxiety level
- Disturbed Thought Processes related to high level of anxiety
- Ineffective Coping related to overwhelming fears

PLANNING

Goals of care include:

- Describe specific changes in role function.
- Demonstrate appropriate decision making.
- Demonstrate effective coping as evidenced by employing behaviors to reduce stress and reporting decreased negative feelings.

IMPLEMENTATION

- Maintain a calm manner.
- Stay with the client.
- Use short, simple sentences.
- Direct client's attention to repetitive or physical task.
- Administer antianxiety medication.
- Teach relaxation exercises.
- Encourage client to identify previous coping skills.
- Help client identify coping resources (including social supports).
- Teach client relaxation techniques.
- Encourage client to verbalize feelings.

EVALUATION

Expected outcomes to evaluate the client's response to care include:

- Client will demonstrate role performance as evidenced by the ability to meet role expectations, knowledge of role transition periods, and reported strategies for role changes.
- Client will demonstrate ability to choose between two or more alternatives.
- Client uses actions to manage stressors that tax personal resources.

NURSING CARE PLAN **A Client With Panic Disorder With Agoraphobia** *continued*

CRITICAL THINKING

1. What factors may be contributing to Mrs. Randolph's agoraphobia?
2. What interview questions would you like to ask Mrs. Randolph's family?
3. What strategies would you recommend to help Mrs. Randolph overcome her fear of leaving her house alone?

Diagnosis

The capacity of the client to manage his or her anxiety, reactions, behaviors, and judgments will inform the diagnoses. While the diagnoses may vary, some appropriate diagnoses may include the following:

- Anxiety
- Fear
- Ineffective Health Maintenance
- Deficient Knowledge
- Ineffective Coping.

Plan

The nursing plan of care, designed in collaboration with the client, may include any of the following goals:

- The client will report a decrease in the frequency and severity of phobic episodes.
- The client will verbalize healthy ways of responding to fear.
- The client will demonstrate relaxation techniques.
- The client will participate in the therapeutic regimen.

Implementation

Phobias with panic and severe anxiety must be treated immediately. As the level of a person's anxiety increases, his or her judgment and ability to listen, remember, and learn is impaired. This is not the time to teach or present new information. The professional nurse does not argue with the individual regarding his or her perception of reality or reaction to the object of the phobia. Empathic nurses offer understanding, support, and direction to ensure safety. The nurse validates concerns and fears; offers a quiet, safe environment; and provides the following:

- *One to one supervision.* This helps alleviate the client's anxiety by providing assurance to the client that he or she is in no danger. One-to-one supervision should be provided until the antianxiety medications have begun to take affect and the nurse has assessed that the client can be safely left alone.
- *Structure and direction for the individual.* This includes informing the client about the next step in the treatment process (e.g., "We're waiting to the doctor to finish with another client; then he will see you"). It may include gentle reminders to the client such as "You're safe here. Let's practice deep breathing again."
- *Antianxiety agents as prescribed.*

Once the person is stabilized, the nurse can effectively facilitate adaptive coping skills. The nurse encourages the client to vent feelings and describe his or her perception of the episode. As always, the nurse provides emotional support in a nonjudgmental manner. Specific interventions for the client experiencing phobia may include the following:

- Assisting the person to rethink or reframe the ability to manage his or her anxiety.
- Assisting the client to reappraise the level of the threat as less damaging. The first opportunity to do this will likely occur after the antianxiety medication has begun to take effect and the client's immediate anxiety level has decreased.
- Teaching the client relaxation techniques, such as deep breathing.
- Assisting the client to gain insight into his or her reactions.

Nurses working with the client over a period of time will have the opportunity to teach knowledge of defense mechanisms, to help the client work through unresolved issues and anxiety, and to help the client develop more adaptive coping mechanisms.

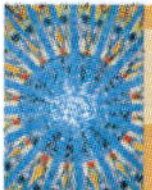

CLIENT TEACHING **Deep Breathing and Progressive Relaxation**

Essential teaching for individuals suffering from anxiety and phobias includes deep breathing and progressive relaxation techniques to lower anxiety responses. Avoidance of stimulants, caffeine, and nicotine is essential. Instructing individuals on the use of cognitive techniques can be helpful in lowering the individual's response to the threat. Strategies such as thought blocking, self-talk, and conversation with a support person all assist the person to manage and empower more adaptive coping skills. Physical exercise that makes use of large muscle groups, such as walking, running, weight lifting, hiking, and various sport activities, can dissipate pent-up energy. Exercising also releases natural chemicals such as endorphins, improving mood and natural pain relief.

Evaluation

Evaluation of nursing care is largely based upon the client's desire to overcome the phobia and willingness to follow the treatment regimen that requires confronting the phobia while controlling anxiety. When the client is able to encounter the phobia and not experience intolerable anxiety they have met the goal of care. However, the ability to face the phobia and control the anxiety using improved coping strategies is an indication of a measure of success.

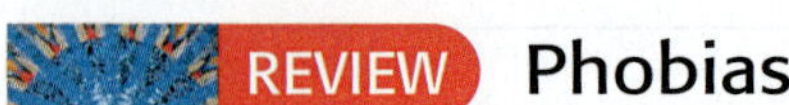

REVIEW Phobias

RELATE: LINK THE CONCEPTS

"My son Peter is scared to death to open his mouth! My friends come over to the house and he goes to his room or stands there like a fool and clams up. I tell him to say hello and he refuses. I think he does it to infuriate me."

Linking the exemplar of Phobias with the concept of Communication:

1. How could you respond therapeutically to this father's lack of empathy during the assessment process in an effort to educate the father about his son's phobia?
2. What strategies might you suggest to this father to improve communication between him and his son as well as reduce his son's anxiety related to talking with his father's friends?

Linking the exemplar of Phobias with the concept of Perfusion:

3. What impact on perfusion could be triggered by forcing someone to face a phobia prematurely?
4. What impact does acute anxiety have on perfusion?

READY: GO TO COMPANION SKILLS MANUAL

- Assessing appearance and mental status
- Evaluating client safety

REFER: GO TO MYNURSINGKIT

REFLECT: CASE STUDY

Providing further details about Peter—introduced in the previous Relate section—upon assessment the nurse collects the following data: Peter is an 8-year-old male who has a history of difficulty in school and refusal to go to school. Peter's mother recently caught Peter drinking pepper to induce vomiting in an attempt to fain illness in the hopes of staying home from school. Peter's mother is present during the initial nursing assessment. Peter barely responds during the assessment; he looks at the floor, shrugs his shoulders, and verbally responds in a barely audible voice "I don't know."

Objective data:

- Peter is having difficulty in school
- Poor attendance in school
- Peter is avoiding school
- Poor eye contact during the interview.

Subjective data:

- Peter responds "I don't know."

1. What further information would you want to collect about Peter from his mother?
2. What nursing diagnosis would be appropriate for Peter?
3. What do you suspect may be causing the described behaviors Peter is displaying?

28.5 POST-TRAUMATIC STRESS DISORDER

KEY TERMS

Depersonalization, *1843*
Eye movement desensitization and reprocessing (EMDR), *1845*
Flashbacks, *1842*
Post-traumatic stress disorder (PTSD), *1842*

BASIS FOR SELECTION OF EXEMPLAR

Healthy People 2010
National Institute of Mental Health

LEARNING OUTCOMES

After reading about this exemplar, you will be able to:

1. Describe the pathophysiology, psychopathology, etiology, clinical manifestations, and direct and indirect causes of post-traumatic stress disorder.
2. Identify risk factors associated with post-traumatic stress disorder.
3. Illustrate the nursing process in providing culturally competent care across the life span for individuals with post-traumatic stress disorder.
4. Formulate priority nursing diagnoses appropriate for an individual with post-traumatic stress disorder.
5. Create a plan of care for individuals with post-traumatic stress disorder and their family members.
6. Assess expected outcomes for an individual with post-traumatic stress disorder.
7. Discuss therapies used in the collaborative care of an individual with post-traumatic stress disorder.
8. Employ evidence-based caring interventions for an individual with post-traumatic stress disorder.

OVERVIEW

The NIMH (2008) defines **post-traumatic stress disorder (PTSD)** as an anxiety disorder that evolves after exposure to a traumatic or overwhelming event in which an individual's physical health was endangered. Extraordinary events that may trigger PTSD include violent personal assaults, natural or human-caused disasters, motor vehicle accidents, military combat, being taken hostage or tortured, imprisonment, dismemberment, incest and child abuse, traumatic childbirth, life-threatening illnesses, and invasive medical procedures (NIMH, 2008).

PATHOPHYSIOLOGY AND ETIOLOGY

Figure 28–12 ■ shows some survivors of the World Trade Center attacks. Many of them suffer from PTSD. Children may develop PTSD as a result of sexual abuse even if there is no actual or threatened injury. The disorder is more likely to occur and to be longer lasting when the stressor is of intentional human action, such as rape or torture (American Psychiatric Association, 2000).

People with PTSD can reexperience the traumatic event in various ways. The individual suffering from PTSD may experience **flashbacks**, the recurrence of images, sounds, smells, or

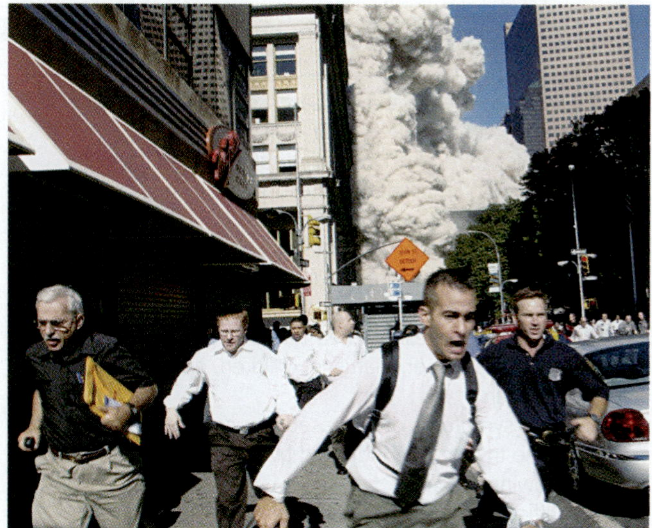

Figure 28–12 ■ Many people who survived the World Trade Center Attack on 9-11-01 are now experiencing PTSD.

Source: AP Wide World Photos.

feelings from the traumatic event, which are often triggered by daily events, such as a car backfiring on the street, the smell of a perpetrator's cologne. Commonly, the person has repeated intrusive memories or dreams of the event. Some people experience flashbacks in which they relive the event, believing that it is actually happening.

After extreme trauma, people often have some of the same symptoms as those of PTSD. The disorder is diagnosed only if symptoms persist for longer than a month. If a person is going to develop PTSD, it usually occurs within 3 months of the traumatic experience. The complete *DSM-IV-TR* criteria for PTSD are found in Box 28–18.

PRACTICE ALERT

Health care providers often use language that is unfamiliar to clients and their families. When discussing the diagnosis of PTSD, use terms that make it easier for clients and family members to understand, not phrases such as "recurrent and intrusive distressing recollections of the event."

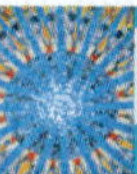

FOCUS ON DIVERSITY AND CULTURE
Post-Traumatic Stress Disorder

As a nurse in the United States, you will care for clients from all over the world. Refugees who immigrate from areas of war and unrest probably have increased rates of PTSD. Because of the nature of the disorder and the individual circumstances, affected people may be reluctant to discuss their experiences of torture and trauma. Refugees should be asked specifically about traumatic experiences and symptoms of PTSD. The nurse might ask, "Do you have nightmares about things that happened in your country?" or "Do you have recurring thoughts about bad things that happened to you?" Clients should be referred for treatment when indicated.

Etiology

Exposure to an overwhelming stressor can occur at any time or age in life. Childhood trauma, abuse, and molestation can create enduring effects and clinical symptoms that can last into adulthood. Additional factors that contribute to the development of PTSD are an individual history of a psychiatric disorder or a lack of emotional support or resources during the trauma. The incidence of PTSD is about 7.7 million, with women being more susceptible; some evidence suggests familial tendencies as reported by the NIMH (2008).

PTSD can occur at any age. Approximately half of affected people experience complete resolution of symptoms within 3 months. The most important factors affecting the likelihood of developing this disorder are severity of the traumatic event, duration of the trauma, and proximity of the individual's exposure.

Risk Factors

Why do some people who experience a traumatic event develop PTSD and others do not? Risk factors for PTSD include the following:

- The severity of the event itself, including whether or not the individual was harmed or watched others be harmed or killed
- Little or no social or psychological support following the trauma
- Additional stressors immediately following the event, such as loss of a spouse or family member or loss of employment
- Presence of preexisting mental illness.

CLINICAL MANIFESTATIONS

Clients who experience flashbacks may lose touch with reality emotionally and may cognitively return to the traumatic incident as if it is happening all over again. Some may experience **depersonalization**, an emotional numbing and a loss of their sense of reality, feelings, and sense of self in relation to others. Clients who experience depersonalization may have difficulty in interpersonal relationships. They may have difficulty trusting or being affectionate. Things they formerly enjoyed may not provide pleasure for them anymore. Irritability, aggression, and even violence may be expressed when these would be out of character for the person before the incident.

Depression sometimes occurs in people with PTSD. As with people affected by other anxiety disorders, people with PTSD may use alcohol and other substances to medicate their anxiety symptoms.

A common manifestation in individuals with PTSD is hyperarousal when reexperiencing the traumatic event. As a result, the person is unable to relax, hypervigilance occurs, and the person is always "on edge." Another common feature of PTSD is dissociation, in which emotions about the traumatic event are blocked. The individual becomes emotionally numb and experiences impaired social relationships.

People with PTSD avoid the stimuli associated with the traumatic event. For example, a woman who is raped in an

Box 28–18 *DSM-IV-TR* Diagnostic Criteria for Post-Traumatic Stress Disorder

A. The person has been exposed to a traumatic event in which both the following were present:
   1. the person experienced, witnessed, or was confronted with an event or events that involved actual or threatened death or serious injury, or a threat to the physical integrity of self or other
   2. the person's response involved intense fear, helplessness, or horror

Note: In children, this may be expressed instead by disorganized or agitated behavior.

B. The traumatic event is persistently reexperienced in one (or more) of the following ways:
   1. recurrent and intrusive distressing recollections of the event, including images, thoughts, or perceptions

Note: In young children, repetitive play may occur in which themes or aspects of the trauma are expressed.

   2. recurrent distressing dreams of the event

Note: In children, there may be frightening dreams without recognizable content.

   3. acting or feeling as if the traumatic event were recurring (includes a sense of reliving the experience, illusions, hallucinations, and dissociative flashback episodes, including those that occur on awakening or when intoxicated)

Note: In young children, trauma-specific reenactment may occur.

   4. intense psychological distress at exposure to internal or external cues that symbolize or resemble an aspect of the traumatic event
   5. physiological reactivity on exposure to internal or external cues that symbolize or resemble an aspect of the traumatic event

C. Persistent avoidance of stimuli associated with the trauma and numbing of general responsiveness (not present before the trauma), as indicated by three (or more) of the following:
   1. Efforts to avoid thoughts, feelings, or conversations associated with the trauma
   2. Efforts to avoid activities, places, or people that arouse recollections of the trauma
   3. Inability to recall an important aspect of the trauma
   4. Markedly diminished interest or participation in significant activities
   5. Feeling of detachment or estrangement from others
   6. Restricted range of affect (e.g., unable to have loving feelings)
   7. Sense of a foreshortened future (e.g., does not expect to have a career, marriage, children, or a normal life span)

D. Persistent symptoms of increased arousal (not present before the trauma), as indicated by two (or more) of the following:
   1. Difficulty falling or staying asleep
   2. Irritability or outbursts of anger
   3. Difficulty concentrating
   4. Hypervigilance
   5. Exaggerated startle response.

E. Duration of the disturbance (symptoms in Criteria B, C, and D) is more than 1 month.

F. The disturbance causes clinically significant distress or impairment in social, occupational, or other important areas of functioning.

Specify if:
Acute: if duration of symptoms is less than 3 months
Chronic: if duration of symptoms is 3 months or more

Specify if:
With Delayed Onset: if onset of symptoms is at least 6 months after the stressor.

Source: Reprinted with permission from the American Psychiatric Association. (2000). *Diagnostic and statistical manual of mental disorders,* (4th ed., Text Revision).

elevator may avoid using any elevator—an example of how PTSD can restrict daily functioning. A significant complicating problem occurs when the person uses alcohol or other substances in an attempt to maintain control and soothe emotions. See the *DSM-IV-TR* diagnostic criteria for PTSD in Box 28–18.

The course of PTSD is variable. Most people who have suffered a significant stressor tend to have an acute reaction from which they recover spontaneously. In others, however, the reaction may be delayed or prolonged and eventually become chronic. PTSD is characterized by high rates of chronicity and comorbidity. PTSD is divided into categories according to onset and duration of symptoms:

- Acute: Symptoms last less than 3 months
- Chronic: Symptoms last 3 months or more
- Delayed onset: At least 6 months have elapsed between the trauma and the occurrence of symptoms.

Manifestations in Children

Children approximately 8 years old and older exhibit symptoms fairly similar to those of adults. In young children, however, diagnosis may be more difficult. Relying on parental reports of a very young child's condition can be complicated, as children's responses to extreme stressors are often influenced by their parents' responses. In addition, there is some evidence to indicate that parents tend to underestimate the degree of their children's responses to stress. Incidence of multiple traumas, such as repeated episodes of child sexual abuse, increases the likelihood that a child will develop PTSD. This and direct exposure to one or more traumatic events are the two strongest risk factors for children. Regardless of the stressor, the mother's response is likely to modify (for better or for worse) the child's response (National Collaborative Centre for Mental Health, 2005).

CLINICAL MANIFESTATIONS AND THERAPIES Post-Traumatic Stress Disorder

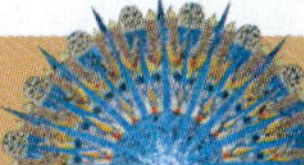

PTSD	CLINICAL MANIFESTATIONS	CLINICAL THERAPIES
Anxiety disorder that evolves from exposure to trauma or threat of physical harm. Recovery varies from one month to several years. Comorbidity may include depression, substance abuse, or other anxiety disorders.	■ Persistent frightening thoughts and memories or flashbacks of the event: images, sounds, smells, or feelings ■ Emotional numbing ■ Sleep disorders ■ Hypervigilance and exaggerated startle response ■ Re-experiencing the event ■ Trouble with affection ■ Irritability, aggressiveness, or violence ■ Avoidance of trauma-related situations or general social contacts ■ Drug and alcohol abuse ■ Depression ■ Suicidal thoughts or violence	■ Holistic approach to treatment includes CBT ■ EMDR ■ Supportive therapy ■ Group therapy

COLLABORATION

Trauma requires the skillful ability to assess, mobilize, communicate, and facilitate care of clients, families, and communities. As an advocate for clients, the nurse must acquire a strong information, referral, and resource base to network and connect individuals with the resources they need to recover successfully from trauma. These resources may include financial resources, such as local departments of social services; medical resources, such as free clinics and mental health providers who treat uninsured clients on a sliding scale basis; and agencies that provide food and shelter.

Because of the all-encompassing impact of trauma on a person's life, a holistic approach to treatment may be most effective, combining pharmacological and alternative therapies, such as relaxation techniques, cognitive-behavioral therapy, eye movement desensitization and response therapy (explained in the following section), and support from a multiagency team of providers.

Best practices and guidelines are posted on the National Guideline Clearing House website. Excellent guidelines for the treatment of PTSD are also available from the National Collaborating Centre for Mental Health in the United Kingdom and the Veterans Health Administration in the U.S. Department of Defense. A number of recommendations from these sources have been included in this exemplar.

Pharmacologic Therapies

Recent advances in psychopharmacology have led to the use of medication as an adjunct to the psychological treatment of PTSD. As is true for the other anxiety disorders, however, the nurse must be aware of the heightened potential for chemical abuse among extremely anxious clients. The desire for immediate, total relief is powerful and may foster chemical abuse and dependence.

Benzodiazepines, tricyclic antidepressants, selective serotonin reuptake inhibitors, lithium, beta blockers, alpha-adrenergic antagonists, and neuroleptics have all been reported to relieve PTSD symptoms. During the initial stage (4–8 weeks), the use of benzodiazepines may be helpful in the treatment of anxiety, insomnia, and nightmares.

Sleeplessness, another common feature of PTSD, is best treated with a behavioral approach such as relaxation techniques, guided imagery, muscle relaxation, and exclusion of daytime naps. Sedatives are discouraged except for very brief use. The goal is to help the client reestablish the ability to sleep naturally and cope more effectively without relying on the use of drugs.

EMDR Therapy

Eye movement desensitization and reprocessing (EMDR) is a form of psychotherapy that contains elements of a number of types of therapy, including cognitive-behavioral therapy and body-centered therapy. EMDR has been found effective in treating clients with PTSD. It is so named because one of the elements involves dual stimulation using eye movements, taps, or tones. *Dual stimulation* allows the client to reprocess or reappraise the trauma by focusing internally on the traumatic event or another stressor while simultaneously focusing on a different external stimulus (EMDR Institute, Inc., 2004).

Acupuncture

Preliminary research indicates that acupuncture may be effective in treating clients with PTSD. This research indicates the need for the client to participate in acupuncture on a regular period for a period of 3 months or more (NCCAM, n.d.). Nurses working with clients who are interested in trying acupuncture as a treatment for PTSD should encourage the clients to add acupuncture as an adjunctive therapy and not to abandon cognitive-behavioral and more traditional therapies.

NURSING PROCESS

PTSD clients experiencing hyperarousal and vigilance may exhibit unpredictable, aggressive, or bizarre behavior. The nursing priorities for these clients are ensuring the safety of the client and others while quickly lowering client anxiety levels. The PTSD client exhibiting extreme anxiety needs immediate pharmacological intervention, a quiet and calm environment, and reassurance of his or her safety. Once anxiety levels are reduce, the client can be helped to learn a new process of appraisal and coping mechanisms.

Due to the complexity of trauma, families may also suffer from PTSD and require the nurse's assistance and support. Evaluation of the impact on the family must also be included in the assessment, evaluation, and decision-making process. Families play a key role in the support of the individual. In the case of national disasters, entire communities may be involved in the trauma.

Assessment

According to the 2008 National Guideline Clearinghouse (NGC), recommendations for the assessment of PTSD sufferers include assessing physical, psychological, social, and risk factors. The assessment tool utilized for anxiety and phobias is adapted to the individual suffering from a traumatic event. Specific interview questions to ascertain the diagnosis of PTSD are aimed at the following clinical manifestations: re-experiencing or flashbacks, hyperarousal and vigilance, an exaggerated startle response, and sleep disturbances. In addition, the NGC (2008) suggests that identification of PTSD in children is improved when they are questioned directly about their experiences. Assessment of younger children involves questioning the child and/or the parents about significant changes in behavior and sleeping patterns.

Diagnosis

Evaluating assessment data for a person suffering PTSD can be challenging, due to the incidence of substance abuse, depression, and insomnia. Appropriate diagnoses for the client with PTSD may include any of the following:

- Post-Trauma Syndrome
- Anxiety
- Fear
- Ineffective Coping
- Compromised Family Coping
- Disturbed Sleep Patterns
- Risk for Self-Directed Violence
- Risk for Other-Directed Violence.

The nurse must explore the specific assessment questions directed at PTSD in order not to overlook the possibility of this diagnosis. It is important for the health care provider to involve the individual in the decision-making process and to facilitate the person's preferences.

Plan

Based on the assessment data, create a plan of care appropriate to the nursing diagnosis. Goals may include:

- Reduce high levls of anxiety
- Improve quality of life
- Verbalize feeling less anxious
- Develop effective coping behaviors
- Utilize support system when anxious
- Describe a state of spiritual well-being.

Implementation

The presence of PTSD is not an inevitable outcome of a traumatic event. Some individuals may require only limited interventions. It is important to remember that without early support or effective treatment, people may develop this chronic condition (NICE, 2008). Important indicators are the severity of the event itself and the severity of the individual's initial response.

In the United Kingdom, the National Collaborating Centre for Mental Health, with the assistance of the British Psychological Society, has outlined recommendations for caring interventions for clients with PTSD:

- *Mild symptoms present for 4 weeks or less:* Because not everyone who experiences trauma develops PTSD, interventions within the first 4 weeks of the event will involve ensuring or confirming the client's safety, shelter, and access to food and water. A nurse encountering a child who is a victim of abuse should follow agency requirements regarding child abuse and neglect reporting and ensuring the safety of the child following discharge (see Concept 31, Violence, Exemplar 31.1, Abuse). The nurse encountering the client within the first 4 weeks after the event should note

Assessment Interview Post-Traumatic Stress Disorder

- Under what circumstances do you experience outbursts of aggressive behavior?
- When was the last time you struck out in anger? How do you usually express anger?
- In what ways have you been reexperiencing the original trauma?
- In what ways do you attempt to avoid situations that may remind you of the original trauma?
- Are you able to laugh and cry at appropriate times/situations?
- How would you describe your mood right now? Happy? Sad? Depressed?
- Are you able to relax?
- How frequently do you participate in social activities?
- What types of activities do you enjoy doing?
- Have you had any employment difficulties since the original trauma?
- How much time during the day do you feel tense or irritable?
- When was the last time you lost your temper? Or said something without thinking first?
- How do you sleep at night? Any nightmares or repetitive dreams?
- Describe any difficulties you have had with your memory or with concentration.
- Are you able to finish tasks?
- Describe the qualities you like about yourself. Describe those qualities you do not like about yourself.

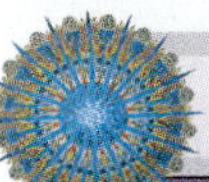

NURSING CARE PLAN A Client With Post-Traumatic Stress Disorder

ASSESSMENT

Sarah Green is a 44-year-old nurse whose teenage son was badly hurt in a car accident just over 3 months ago. She has been having flashbacks about the night of the accident and can barely control herself when she knows one of her children is driving or riding in a car Usually, when one of the children asks to borrow the car she just says "No" to avoid having to worry about them. Ms. Green knows she needs to see someone. She talks to a friend who is also a coworker, who recommends that she talk with an occupational health counselor at work. Ms. Green does not want anyone at work to know she is having trouble, but she agrees to see a mental health nurse that her friend recommends.

At her initial appointment, Ms. Green freely shares the flashbacks, which happen 2 or 3 times a week, usually at night. She says that when she knows her children are going anywhere, she can feel her heart racing, her breathing speeding up, and her palms getting sweaty. She tells the mental health nurse that she gets through these episodes by lying down and saying the Lord's Prayer out loud.

DIAGNOSES

The mental health nurse develops the following nursing diagnoses:

- Post-Trauma Stress Syndrome
- Anxiety
- Fear.

PLANNING

Goals for Ms Green's care include:

- Utilize deep breathing to control escalating anxiety.
- Express fears clearly.
- Describe the symptoms associated with the various levels of anxiety.
- Demonstrate breathing exercises to reduce anxiety.

IMPLEMENTATION

- Teach Ms. Green how to monitor physiological level of arousal.
- Teach use of abdmonial breathing at first sign of anxiety.
- Help client to express fears that interfere with her life.
- Encourage client to search for, confront, and relieve the source of the orginal anxiety.
- Teach distraction techniques that can control moderate levels of anxiety.
- Teach the use of positive imagery.
- Teach calming techniques such as muscle relaxation.
- Teach positive affirmations such as "I am calm and happy" or "I am very relaxed."
- Identify safe physical outlets for negative feelings such as exercise.

EVALUATION

- Client expresses feelings appropriately.
- Client spends less time thinking about the accident turning thoughts to more positive memories.
- Client allows adolescent to borrow the car setting reasonable limits to reduce her anxiety.

CRITICAL THINKING

1. What impact does Ms. Green's PTSD have on her children's development?
2. How would you teach Ms. Green relaxation techniques?

all information necessary to make a follow-up call a month after the event to reassess the client and determine whether further intervention is necessary.

- *When PTSD symptoms present within the first 3 months following the trauma:* Refer the client for psychological therapy. Be aware that therapies that do not focus directly on the trauma should not routinely be offered within the first 3 months of trauma; cognitive-behavioral therapy or EMDR is most appropriate for the client during this time. Relaxation techniques and alternative therapies may be used if the client finds comfort in them but should not take the place of proven psychological therapies.
- *Symptoms have been present for 3 or 4 months:* Refer the client for trauma-focused therapy (cognitive-behavioral therapy or EMDR). Clients who have experienced multiple traumas, have become disabled as a result of the traumatic event, or have comorbid social disorders will likely require more extensive therapy for longer periods of time. Help the client understand that continuous (weekly) therapy with the same experienced professional is the best way to ensure maximum benefit from therapy.

The National Collaborative Centre for Mental Health recommends pharmacologic therapy if the client is nonresponsive to trauma-focused therapy, refuses psychological therapy, or is likely to continue to experience trauma (e.g., abuse) (NCCMH, 2005).

CLIENT TEACHING Typical Human Responses to Traumatic Events

Clients suffering from PTSD should be given ample information about the typical human responses to traumatic events. Education about the process helps clients normalize the experience and gain information for reappraisal. Information and resources provide the hope for adaptive coping; conversely, a lack of resources may induce maladaptive coping. It is the responsibility of the nurse to provide information about the treatments available for PTSD to facilitate the individual and family to make informed choices.

Evaluation

The nurse evaluates the client's response to treatment using these suggested expected outcomes:

- Client utilizes self-calming techniques.
- Clients experience less cognitive distortions and decreased numinations or obsessions.
- Client will decrease time spent ruminating over worries, verbalizing more accurate predictions of future events.

HEALTH CARE

It is the ethical responsibility of the nurse to be knowledgeable about the resources within and outside of the health care system and the community, including state and local resources, such as city or county departments of social services. Many nonprofit agencies provide additional resources, especially during times of natural disasters. These include the American Red Cross, the Salvation Army, and faith organizations. Being able to navigate technology to access information for clients is an essential skill.

REVIEW Post-Traumatic Stress Disorder

RELATE: LINK THE CONCEPTS

Linking the exemplar of Post-Traumatic Stress Disorder with the concept of Development:

Explore the incidence of childhood abuse, molestation, and incest in the Unites States.

1. What impact does childhood abuse, molestation, and incest have on the growth and development of a child?
2. Childhood abuse, molestation, and incest can negatively affect the physical, emotional, spiritual, and cognitive processes of individuals What alterations in health are associated with abuse later in life?

Linking the exemplar of Post-Traumatic Stress Disorder with the concept of Violence:

3. How might PTSD cause a previously nonviolent individual to become more violent in their interactions with others?
4. What anticipatory guidance can you provide the client with PTSD to reduce the risk of future violence?

READY: GO TO COMPANION SKILLS MANUEL

- Assessing appearance and mental status

REFER: GO TO MYNURSINGKIT

REFLECT: CASE STUDY

Melinda Burns, 20 years old, lives in Manhattan. She is engaged to be married to a man she says she loves very much and while this should be the happiest time of her life, she is feeling very anxious and stressed.

She was 12 years old on 9/11/2001 and was in school when the planes hit the World Trade Center. They had to evacuate the school after the collapse of the buildings because the ash was so thick it made breathing difficult. Her father picked her up and they went to a hotel room in New Jersey because their apartment was also covered in ash and they weren't allowed to go home until several weeks later. Melinda's grandmother stayed with her in the hotel room while her father tried to find her mother, who worked on the 92nd floor of the North tower. Her Dad never found her mother and she never came home. Melinda says the worst part is her body was never identified from the wreckage so they she feels like she has no closure or confirmation that her mother is really dead. One of the New York fireman came to their home almost a year later to return a necklace that was found and the engraving helped them identify it as her mom's. Melinda treasures the necklace even though it is badly damaged and burned.

Melinda is seeking care because she is having trouble functioning normally. She reports severe anxiety whenever she hears a siren, has been waking from nightmares related to the World Trade Center several times a week, and she can't bring herself to watch any television programs or movies about the terrorist attack because they always make her cry. She has turned down a number of jobs because she can't bring herself to work on the upper levels of tall buildings. She says lately she has been having trouble concentrating, even on planning her wedding because she can't seem to think about anything other than the World Trade Center and what her mother's final minutes must have been like.

1. What nursing diagnosis is appropriate for Melinda?
2. What collaborative actions can the health care team take to help Melinda?
3. What independent nursing interventions would you initiate if Melinda was your client?

PEARSON

EXPLORE mynursingkit™

MyNursingKit is your one stop for online chapter review materials and resources. Prepare for success with additional NCLEX®-style practice questions, interactive assignments and activities, web links, animations and videos, and more!

Register your access code from the front of your book at **www.mynursingkit.com**.

REFERENCES

Agency for Health Care Research and Quality. (2008). Retrieved September 8, 2008, from http://effectivehealthcare.ahrq.gov/healthInfo.cfm?infotype=all#8

Aguilera, D. C. (1998). *Crisis intervention: Theory and methodology*. St. Louis, MO: Mosby.

Aldwin, C. M. (1994). *Stress, coping and development: An integrative perspective*. New York: Guilford.

American Art Therapy Association. (2008). Art therapy changes lives of abused children. Retrieved August 23, 2009, from http://www.arttherapy.org/news.htm?id=9

American Psychiatric Association. (2000). *Diagnostic and statistical manual of mental disorders* (4th ed.). Washington, DC: Author.

American Psychiatric Nurses Association (APNA). (2008). Curricular Guidelines for Undergraduate Education in Psychiatric Mental Health Nursing. Retrieved September 8, 2008, from http://www.apna.org/files/public/revmay08finalCurricular_Guidelines_for_Undergraduate_Education_in_Psychiatric_Mental_Health_Nursing.pdf

Antai-Otong, D. (2003). Anxiety disorders: Helping your patient conquer her fears. *Nursing, 33*(12), 36–41.

Antai-Otong, D. (2008). *Psychiatric nursing: Biological & behavioral concepts*. Canada: Delmar.

Anxiety Disorders Association of America. (2009) Anxiety disorders in older adults. Retrieved August 22, 2009, from http://www.adaa.org/GettingHelp/AnxietyDisordersinOlderAdults.asp

Basch, E. M., & Ulbricht, C. E. (2005). Natural standard. *Herb and supplement handbook*. St. Louis, MO: Elsevier/Mosby.

Benson, H. (1997). *Timeless healing*. New York: Fireside Book.

Berman, A., Snyder, S., Kozier, B., & Erb, G. (2008). *Kozier & Erb's fundamentals of nursing: Concepts, process and practice*. (8th ed.). New Jersey: Pearson Education, Inc.

Bindler, R., & Howry, L. (2005). *Pediatric drug guide*. Upper Saddle River, NJ: Prentice Hall Health.

Brinkman, J. (2004). Art therapy with children – a window to their world. Retrieved August 23, 2009, from http://www.uchsc.edu/news/bridge/2004/April/arttherapy.html

Clark, D. A. (2003). *Cognitive-behavioral therapy for OCD*. New York: Guilford Press.

Caplan, G. (1964). *Principles of preventive psychiatry*. New York: Basic Books.

Carrieri-Kohlman, V., Lindsey, A., & West. C. (2003). (3rd ed.). *Pathophysiological phenomena in nursing: Human responses to illness*. Missouri: Saunders.

Carson, V. & Arnold, E. (1996). *Mental health nursing: The nurse-patient journey*. Philadelphia: W.B. Saunders Company.

Cartwright-Hatton, S., McNicol, K., & Doubleday, E. (2006). Anxiety in a neglected population: Prevalence of anxiety disorders in pre-adolescent children. *Clinical Psychology Review, 26*, 817–833.

Catapano, F., Perris, F., Massella, M., et al. (2006). Obsessive-compulsive disorder: A 3-year prospective follow-up study of patients treated with serotonin reuptake inhibitors OCD follow-up study. *J Psychiatr Res 40*(6), 502–10. Retrieved August 24, 2009, from http://biopsychiatry.com/ocd-ssris.htm

Collishaw, S., Pickles, A., Messer, J., Rutter, M., Shearer, C., & Maugham, B. (2007). Resilience to adult psychopathology following childhood maltreatment: Evidence from a community sample. *Child Abuse and Neglect, 31*(3), 211–229.

Connolly, S. D., Bernstein, G. A., Work Group on Quality Issues. (2007). Practice parameter for the assessment and treatment of children and adolescents with anxiety disorders. *J Am Acad Child Adolesc Psychiatry, 46*(2), 267–83.

Das, S., O'Keefe, J. H., (2008). Behavioral cardiology: recognizing and addressing the profound impact of psychosocial stress on cardiovascular health. *Current Hypertension Reports, 10*(5), 374–378.

Davidson, J. R. (2006). Pharmacologic treatment of acute and chronic stress following trauma: 2006. *Journal of Clinical Psychiatry, 67*(Suppl 2), 34–39.

DeJong, P. & Berg, K. (2008). *Interviewing for Solutions*. CA: Thompson Brooks/Cole.

Dell Healthcare and Life Science Solutions. (2008). PACS medical imaging. Retrieved from http://www.dell.com/content/topics/global.aspx/sitelets/solutions/industry_application/pub_solutions/dell_healthcare_medical_imaging?c=us&cs=RC968571&l=en&s=hea&redirect=1

EMDR Institute, Inc. (2004). A brief description of EMDR. Retrieved August 26, 2009, from http://www.emdr.com/briefdes.htm

Erickson, E. H. (1963). *Childhood and society* (2nd ed.), New York: Norton.

Farrugia, S., & Hudson, J. (2006). Anxiety in adolescents with Asperger Syndrome: Negative thoughts, behavioral problems, and life interference. *Focus on Autism and Other Developmental Disabilities, 21*(1), 25–35.

Flint, A. J. (2005). Generalised anxiety disorder in elderly patients: Epidemiology, diagnosis and treatment options. *Drugs in Aging: 2005, 22*(2), 101–114.

Fontaine, K. L. (2005) *Complementary and alternative therapies for nursing practice* (2nd ed.). Upper Saddle River, NJ: Prentice Hall.

Frisch, N. & Frisch, L. (2006). *Psychiatric mental health nursing*. (3rd ed.) Canada: Thompson Delmar Learning.

Gava, I., Barbui, C., Aguglia, E., Carlino, D., Churchill, R., De Vanna, M., & McGuire, H.F. (2007). Psychological treatments versus treatment as usual for obsessive-compulsive disorder (OCD). *Cochrane Database of Systematic Reviews, 2*: CD005333.

Glass, N., Perrin, N., Campbell, J. C., & Soeken, K. (2007). The protective role of tangible support on post-traumatic stress disorder symptoms in urban women survivors of violence. *Research in Nursing and Health, 30*(5), 558–568.

Glynn, L., Hobel, C., Schetter, C., & Sndman, C. (2008). Pattern of perceived stress and anxiety in pregnancy predicts preterm birth. *Health* Psychology, *27*(1), 43–51.

Grados, M. & Wilcox, H. C. (2007). Genetics of obsessive-compulsive disorder: A research update. *Expert Review of Neurotherapeutics, 7*(8), 967–80. Retrieved June 30, 2008, from http://www.ncbi.nlm.nih.gov/pubmed/18386211?ordinalpos=1&itool=EntrezSystem2.PEntrez.Pubmed.Pubmed_ResultsPanel.Pubmed_DefaultReportPanel.Pubmed_RVDocSum

Grant, B. F., Frederick, S. S., Hasin, D. S., Dawson, D. A., Chou, S. P., & Anderson, K. (2004). Psychiatric disorders among Mexican Americans and Non-Hispanic Whites in the United States: Results from the National Epidemiologic Survey on alcohol and related conditions. *Archive of General Psychiatry, 61*, 1226–1233. Retrieved August 22, 2009, from www.archgenpsychiatry.com

Hanna, G. L., Fischer, D. J., & Fluent, T. E. (2006). Separation anxiety disorder and school refusal in children and adolescents. *Pediatrics in Review, 27*, 56–62.

Hayward, C., Wilson, K. A., Lagle, K., Killen, J. D., & Taylor, B. (2004). Parent-reported predictors of adolescent panic attacks. *Journal of the American Academy of Child and Adolescent Psychiatry, 43*, 613–620.

Hodge, D. (2006). Spiritually modified cognitive therapy: A review of the literature. *Social Work, 51*(2), 157–166.

Hoge, E. A., Austin, E. D., & Pollack, M. H. (2007). Resilience: Research evidence and conceptual considerations for posttraumatic stress disorder. *Depression and Anxiety, 24*(2), 139–152.

Holmes, T. H., & Rahe, R. H. (1967). The social readjustment rating scale. *Journal of Psychosomatic Research, 11*, 213–218.

Hudson, J. L., Deveney, C., & Taylor, L. (2005). Nature, assessment, and treatment of generalized anxiety disorder in children. *Pediatric Annals, 34*, 97–106.

Jurbergs, N., & Ledley, D. R. (2005). Separation anxiety disorder. *Pediatric Annals, 34*, 108–115.

Kee, J., Hayes, E., & McCuistion, L. (2006). *Pharmacology: A nursing process approach*. (5th ed.) MO: Mosby, Inc.

Kneisl, C., Wilson, H., & Trigoboff, E. (2004). *Contemporary psychiatric-mental health nursing*. New Jersey: Pearson, Education, Inc.

Lauderdale, S. A. & Sheikh, J. I. (2003). Anxiety disorders in older adults. *Clinics in Geriatric Medicine 19*(4), 721–741. Retrieved August 22, 2009, from http://www.ncbi.nlm.nih.gov/pubmed/15024809

Lazarus, R. S. (1991). *Emotion and adaptation*. New York: Oxford University Press.

Lazarus, R. S., & Folkman, S. (1984). *Stress, appraisal, and coping*. New York: Springer.

Lazarus, R. S., & Folkman, S. (1987). Transactional theory and research on emotion and coping. *European Journal of Personality, 1*, 141–169.

Lazarus, R. S., & Folkman, S. (1989). *Manual for the hassles and uplifts: Research edition*. Palo Alto, CA: Consulting Psychologists Press.

Lewin, A. B., Storch, E. A., Adkins, J., Murphy, T. K., & Geffken, G. R. (2005). Current directions in pediatric obsessive-compulsive disorder. *Pediatric Annals, 34*, 128–134.

Mancini, A. D., & Bonanno, G. A. (2006). Resilience in the face of potential trauma: Clinical practices and illustrations. *Journal of Clinical Psychology, 62*(8), 971–985.

Matthews, D. A., & Clark, C. (1998). *The Faith Factor: Proof of the Healing Power of Prayer*. New York: Viking.

Mayo Clinic. (2007). General anxiety disorder: risk factors. Retrieved August 20, 2009, from http://www.mayoclinic.com/health/generalized-anxiety-disorder/DS00502/DSECTION=risk-factors

Mayo Clinic. (2009). Phobias: risk factors. Retrieved August 24, 2009, from http://www.mayoclinic.com/health/phobias/DS00272/DSECTION=risk-factors

McGuire, H. F. Psychological treatments versus treatment as usual for obsessive compulsive disorder (OCD). *Cochrane Database of Systematic Reviews* 2007, Issue 2. Art. No.: CD005333. DOI: 10.1002/14651858.CD005333.pub2

Miller, M. A., & Rahe, R. H. (1997). Life changes scaling for the 1990s. *Journal of Psychosomatic Research, 43*, 279–292.

Monat, A., & Lazarus, R. S. (1991). *Stress and coping* (3rd ed.). New York: Columbia University Press.

National Center for Complimentary and Alternative Medicine. (n.d.) Acupuncture may help symptoms of post-traumatic stress disorder. Retrieved August 24, 2009, from http://nccam.nih.gov/research/results/spotlight/092107.htm

National Collaborating Centre for Mental Health. (2005). Post-traumatic stress disorder: The management of PTSD in adults and children in primary and secondary care. Retrieved August 26, 2009, from http://www.nccmh.org.uk/downloads/PTSD/CG026fullguideline.pdf

National Guideline Clearing House. (2008). Retrieved September 4, 2008, from http://www.guideline.gov/summary/summary.aspx?doc_id=5293&nbr=003616&string=ocd

National Guideline Clearing House. (2008). Retrieved September 4, 2008, from http://www.guideline.gov/summary/summary.aspx?doc_id=6850&nbr=004204&string=PTSD

National Institute for Clinical Excellence (NICE). (2004). Post-traumatic stress disorder (PTSD): The management of PTSD in adults and children in primary and secondary care. Retrieved September 20, 2008, from http://www.nice.org.uk/nicemedia/pdf/CG026NICEguideline.pdf

National Institute of Mental Health (NIMH). (2008). Anxiety disorders. Retrieved June 8, 2008, from http://www.nimh.nih.gov/health/topics/anxiety-disorders/index.shtml.

National Institute of Mental Health (NIMH). (2008). National institute of mental health: Fiscal year 2007 budget. Retrieved July 30, 2008, from http://www.nimh.nih.gov/health/topics/index.shtml

National Institute of Mental Health. (n.d.) Obsessive-compulsive disorder. Retrieved August 23, 2009, from http://www.nimh.nih.gov/health/topics/obsessive-compulsive-disorder-ocd/index.shtml

National Safety Council. (2005). Driving defensively. *National Safety Council*. Retrieved June 11, 2008, from http://www2.nsc.org/library/facts/defdriv.htm

New York State Office of Mental Health. (n.d.) Fact sheet: cultural competence, evidence-based practices, and planning. Retrieved August 22, 2009, from http://www.omh.state.ny.us/omhweb/EBP/culturalcompetence.htm

Newshan, G., & Schuller-Civitella, D. (2003). Large clinical study shows value of Therapeutic Touch program. *Holistic Nursing Practice, 17*(4), 189–192.

Nicholls, A. R. & Polman, R. C. J. (2007). *Coping in sport*: A systematic review. Journal of Sports Sciences, *25*, 11–31.

Office on Women's Health. (n.d.) Minority women's health: Suicide. Retrieved August 23, 2009, from http://www.womenshealth.gov/minority/asianamerican/suicide.cfm

Pilkington, K., Kirkwood, G., Rampes, H., Cummings, M. & Richardson, J. (2007). Acupuncture for anxiety and anxiety disorders – a systematic literature review. *Acupuncture in Medicine, 25*(1–2), 1–10.

Purnell, L. & Paulanka, B. (2005). *Guide to culturally competent health care*. Philadelphia: F. A. Davis Company.

Rahe, R. H., & Tolles, R. L. (2002). The brief stress and coping inventory: A useful stress management instrument. *International Journal of Stress Management, 9*, 61–70.

Rakel, D., & Faass, N. (2006). *Complementary medicine in clinical practice*. Boston: Jones Bartlett Publishers.

Rapoport, J. L. (1989). *The boy who couldn't stop washing*. Washington, DC: Dutton.

Saladin K. (2007). *Anatomy and physiology: The unity of form and function* (4th ed.). New York: McGraw-Hill Companies, Inc.

Sarason, I. G., Johnson, J. H., & Siegel, J. M. (1978). Assessing the impact of life changes: Development of the life experiences survey. *Journal of Consulting and Clinical Psychology, 46*, 932–946.

Saxena, S., Brody, A. L., Maidment, K. M., Smith, E. C., Zohrabi, N., Katz, E., et al. (2004). Cerebral glucose metabolism in obsessive–compulsive hoarding. *American Journal of Psychiatry, 61*(6), 1038–1048.

Selye, H. (1956). *The stress of life.* New York: McGraw-Hill.

Selye, H. (1976). *The stress of life* (revised ed.). New York: McGraw-Hill.

Shear, K., Jin, R., Ruscio, A. M., Walters, E. E., & Kessler, R. C. (2006). Prevalence and correlates of estimated *DSM-IV* child and adult separation anxiety disorder in the National Comorbidity Survey Replication. *American Journal of Psychiatry, 163*, 1074–1083.

Shoshani, A. & Slone, M. (2008). Efficacy of clinical interventions for indirect exposure to terrorism. *International Journal of Stress Management, 15*(1), 53–75.

Sinha, B. K. & Watson, D. C. (2007). Stress, coping and psychological illness: A cross-cultural study. *International Journal of Stress Management, 14*, (Issue 4), 1072–5245.

Surgeon General. (2008). Evidence based mental health: A report of the surgeon general. Children and Mental Health. Retrieved September 8, 2008, from http://mentalhealth .samhsa.gov/features/surgeongeneralreport/chapter3/ sec6.asp

Tamparo, C., & Lindh, W. (2000). *Therapeutic communications for health professionals.* (2nd ed.). Canada: Delmar.

Townsend, M. (2006). *Psychiatric mental health nursing: Concepts of care in evidence based practice* (5th ed.). Philadelphia: F. A. Davis.

University of Maryland Medical Center. (2007). Anxiety disorders: Risk factors. Retrieved August 20, 2009, from http://www.umm.edu/patiented/ articles/who_gets_anxiety_disorders_000028_3.htm

Van Voorhees, Benjamin W. (2007). Stress and anxiety. *Medline Plus.* Retrieved June 30, 2008, from http:// www.nlm.nih.gov/medlineplus/ency/article/003211.htm

Videbeck, S. (2004). *Psychiatric mental health nursing.* (2nd ed.) Philadelphia: Lippincott, Williams & Wilkins.

Walitza, S., Renner, T. J., Wewetzer, C. & Warnke, A. (2008). Klinik für Kinder- und Jugendpsychiatrie und Psychotherapie der Universität Würzburg. [Genetic findings in obsessive-compulsive disorder in childhood and adolescence and in adulthood]. [Article in German], 36(1), 45–52. walitza 18476602 [PubMed - indexed for MEDLINE]

Wells, M. E. (2006). Psychotherapy for families in the aftermath of a disaster. *Journal of Clinical Psychology, 62*(8), 1017–1027.

Wren, F. J., Bridge, J. A., & Birmaher, B. (2004). Screening for childhood anxiety symptoms in primary care: Integrating child and parent reports. *Journal of the American Academy of Child and Adolescent Psychiatry, 43*, 1364–1371.

Thermoregulation 29

Concept at-a-Glance

Concept Learning Outcomes

After reading about this concept, you will be able to:

1. Summarize the physiological processes of the thermoregulation.
2. List factors affecting thermoregulation.
3. Identify commonly occurring alterations in thermoregulation and their related treatments.
4. Explain common physical assessment procedures used to determine the temperature of clients across the life span.
5. Outline diagnostic and laboratory tests to determine causes of alterations in thermoregulation.
6. Explain management of clients with alterations in temperature.
7. Demonstrate the nursing process in providing culturally competent and caring interventions across the life span for individuals with common alterations in thermoregulation.
8. Identify pharmacological interventions in caring for the individual with alterations in thermoregulation.

Concept Key Terms

Afebrile, *1854*
Basal metabolic rate, *1852*
Body temperature, *1851*
Chemical thermogenesis, *1852*
Conduction, *1852*
Convection, *1853*
Febrile, *1854*
Fever, *1852*
Heat balance, *1852*
Hyperpyrexia, *1854*
Hyperthermia, *1852*
Hypothermia, *1852*
Insensible heat loss, *1853*
Insensible water loss, *1853*
Neutral thermal environment, *1854*
Pyrexia, *1854*
Radiation, *1852*
Surface temperature, *1851*
Thermoregulation, *1852*
Vaporization, *1853*

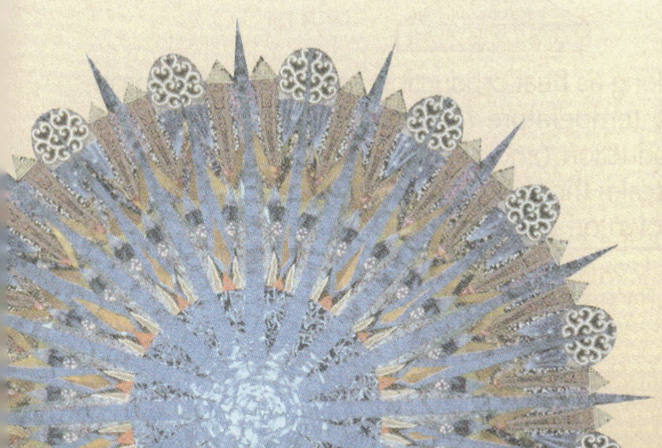

About Thermoregulation

Body temperature reflects the balance between the heat produced and the heat lost from the body, and is measured in heat units called degrees. The body's **surface temperature**—the temperature of the skin, subcutaneous tissues, and fat—fluctuates in response to environmental factors and is therefore unreliable for monitoring a client's health status. The nurse should monitor core body temperatures (or the deep tissues of the body) for a more reliable assessment. This temperature remains relatively constant at about 37°C, or 98.6°F.

Sensors in the hypothalamus regulate the body's core temperature. When these hypothalamic sensors detect heat, they signal the body to decrease heat production and increase heat loss by vasodilation and sweating. When sensors in the hypothalamus detect cold, they signal the body to increase heat production and decrease heat loss by shivering, vasoconstriction, and inhibition of sweating.

Much of the care nurses deliver is mysterious and new to clients who do not fully understand what is being done or why unless the nurse explains it. Thermoregulation is different in that most, if not all, adult clients understand what a temperature is; many can tell you exactly how they felt when their temperature began to change. Almost everyone has experienced shivering when cold or perspiring when hot. Most people want to know what the results are when their temperature is measured, especially if they are not feeling well or suspect they have a **fever** (temperature elevation). Have you ever heard someone say, "My temperature is normally low, so if I measure my temperature and it's 98.6 it means I have a fever"? Do you think this is true? If the person saying this was your client, would you feel like you needed to treat this temperature of 98.6°? •

NORMAL PRESENTATION

Thermoregulation is the body process that balances heat production and heat loss to maintain the body's temperature. There are two kinds of body temperature: core temperature and surface temperature. Core temperature remains relatively constant. The normal core body temperature is a range (Figure 29–1 ■). The surface temperature rises and falls in response to the environment. The body continually produces heat as a byproduct of metabolism. When the amount of heat produced by the body equals the amount of heat lost, the person is in **heat balance** (Figure 29–2 ■). If the body produces more heat than is lost, the client displays **hyperthermia**. If more heat is lost than produced, the client displays **hypothermia**.

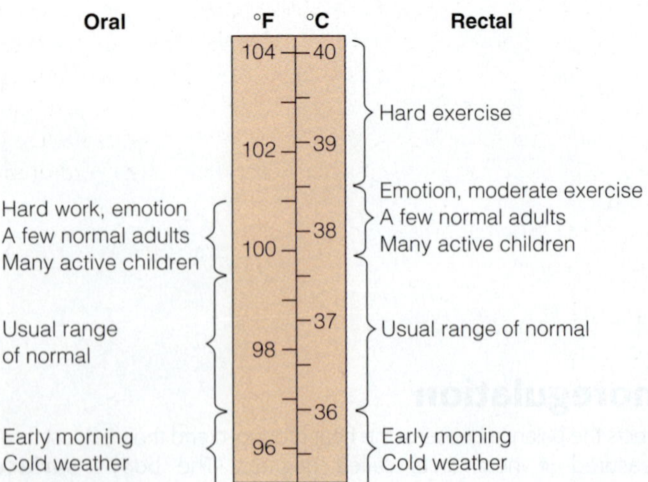

Figure 29–1 ■ Estimated ranges of body temperature in normal persons.

Source: From *Fever and the Regulation of Body Temperature*, by E.F. DuBois, 1948, Springfield, IL: Charles C. Thomas. Reprinted with permission.

A number of factors affect the body's heat production. The most important are these five:

1. *Basal metabolic rate (BMR).* The **basal metabolic rate (BMR)** is the rate of energy utilization the body requires to maintain essential activities such as breathing. Metabolic rates decrease with age. In general, the younger the person, the higher the BMR.
2. *Muscle activity.* Muscle activity, including shivering, increases the metabolic rate. All muscle activity produces heat.
3. *Thyroxine output.* Increased thyroxine output increases the rate of cellular metabolism throughout the body. This effect is called **chemical thermogenesis**, the stimulation of heat production in the body through increased cellular metabolism.
4. *Epinephrine, norepinephrine, and sympathetic stimulation/stress response.* These hormones are neurotransmitters that mount a sympathetic nervous system response that can immediately increase the rate of cellular metabolism in many body tissues. Epinephrine and norepinephrine directly affect liver and muscle cells, thereby increasing cellular metabolism.
5. *Fever.* Fever is a protective immune response to foreign antigens within the body that increases the cellular metabolic rate thus increasing the body's temperature.

Heat is lost from the body through radiation, conduction, convection, and vaporization. **Radiation** is the transfer of heat from the surface of one object to the surface of another without contact between the two objects, usually in the form of infrared rays. **Conduction** is transfer of heat from one molecule to a molecule of lower temperature. Because conductive

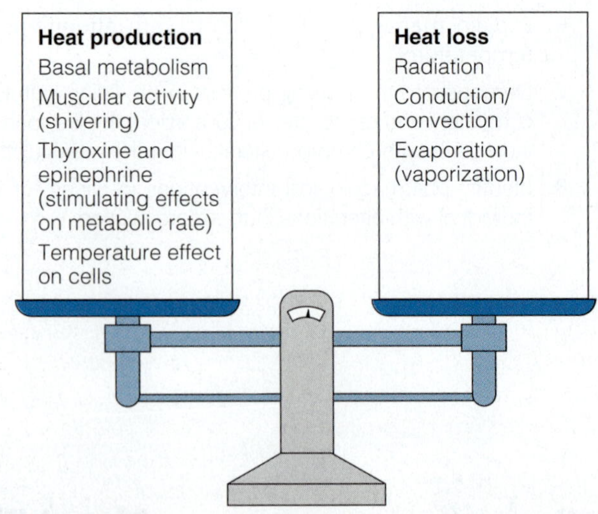

Figure 29–2 ■ As long as heat production and heat loss are properly balanced, body temperature remains constant. Factors contributing to heat production (and temperature rise) are shown on the left side of the scale; those contributing to heat loss (and temperature fall) are shown on the right side of the scale.

Source: From *Human Anatomy and Physiology*, 7th ed. (p. 985), by E. N. Marieb and K. Hoehn, 2007, San Francisco: Pearson Benjamin Cummings. Adapted with permission.

transfer cannot take place without contact between the molecules, it normally accounts for minimal heat loss except, for example, when a body is immersed in cold water. The amount of heat transferred depends on the temperature difference and the amount and duration of the contact.

Convection is the dispersion of heat by air currents. The body usually has a small amount of warm air adjacent to it. Because this warm air rises and is replaced by cooler air, people always lose a small amount of heat through convection. **Vaporization** is continuous evaporation of moisture from the respiratory tract, the mucosa of the mouth, and the skin. This continuous and unnoticed water loss is called **insensible water loss**; the accompanying heat loss is called **insensible heat loss**. Insensible heat loss accounts for about 10% of basal heat loss. When the body temperature increases, vaporization accounts for greater heat loss. Perspiration also results in vaporation of water and a cooling of body temperature.

Regulation of Body Temperature

The system that regulates body temperature has three main parts: sensors in the shell and in the core, an integrator in the hypothalamus, and an effector system that adjusts the production and loss of heat. Most sensors or sensory receptors are in the skin. The skin has more receptors for cold than warmth; therefore, skin sensors detect cold more efficiently than warmth.

When the skin becomes chilled over the entire body, three physiologic processes occur as the body attempts to regulate its temperature:

1. Shivering increases heat production.
2. Sweating is inhibited to decrease heat loss.
3. Vasoconstriction decreases heat loss.

The hypothalamic integrator, the center that controls the core temperature, is located in the preoptic area of the hypothalamus. When the sensors in the hypothalamus detect heat, they send out signals intended to reduce the temperature, that is, to decrease heat production and increase heat loss. In contrast, when the cold sensors are stimulated, they send out signals to increase heat production and decrease heat loss.

The signals from the cold-sensitive receptors of the hypothalamus initiate effectors such as vasoconstriction, shivering, and the release of epinephrine. Epinephrine increases cellular metabolism and, therefore, heat production. When the warmth-sensitive receptors in the hypothalamus are stimulated, the effector system sends out signals that initiate sweating and peripheral vasodilation. In addition to the body's thermoregulation responses, individuals consciously make appropriate adjustments, such as putting on additional clothing in response to cold or turning on a fan in response to heat.

Factors Affecting Body Temperature

Nurses should be aware of the factors that can affect a client's body temperature. They should also be able to recognize normal temperature variations as well as understand the significance of body temperature measurements that deviate from normal. The following are some factors that affect body temperature:

1. *Age.* Infants are greatly influenced by the temperature of the environment and must be protected from extreme changes. Until they reach puberty, children's temperatures continue to be more variable than those of adults. Many older people, particularly those over 75 years, are at risk of hypothermia (temperatures below 36°C, or 96.8°F) for a variety of reasons, including inadequate diet, loss of subcutaneous fat, lack of activity, and reduced thermoregulatory efficiency. Older adults are particularly sensitive to extremes in the environmental temperature due to decreased thermoregulatory controls.
2. *Diurnal variations (circadian rhythms).* Body temperatures normally change throughout the day, varying as much as 1.0°C (1.8°F) between the early morning and the late afternoon. The point of highest body temperature is usually reached between 4:00 and 6:00 p.m.) (Mackowiak, Wasserman, & Levine, 1992), and the lowest point is reached during sleep between 4:00 and 6:00 a.m.). (See Figure 29–3 ■).
3. *Exercise.* Hard work or strenuous exercise can increase body temperature to as high as 38.3–40°C (101–104°F), measured rectally, secondary to the heat produced by muscle action and increased metabolic rate.
4. *Hormones.* Women usually experience more fluctuations in hormone levels than men. In women, progesterone secretion at the time of ovulation raises body temperature by approximately 0.3–0.6°C (0.5–1.0°F) above basal temperature.
5. *Stress.* Stimulation of the sympathetic nervous system can increase the production of epinephrine and norepinephrine, thereby increasing metabolic activity and heat production. Nurses may anticipate that a highly stressed or anxious client could have a mildly elevated body temperature due to stress.
6. *Environment.* Extremes in environmental temperatures can affect a person's thermoregulation. In a very warm room, if a person's body temperature cannot be modified by convection, conduction, or radiation, his or her temperature will be elevated. Similarly, if a client has been outside in cold weather without suitable clothing, or if there is a medical condition preventing the client from controlling

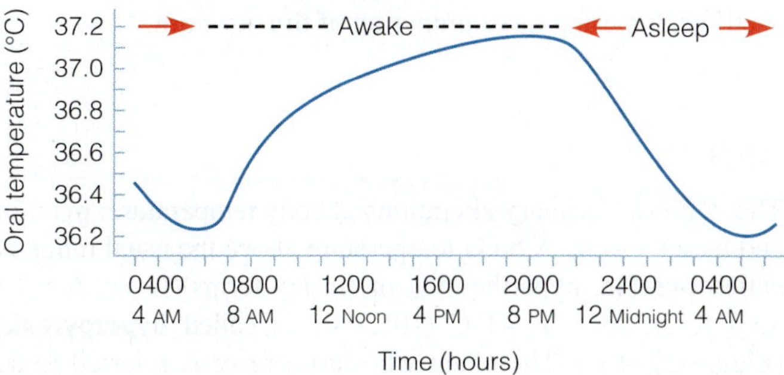

Figure 29–3 ■ Range of oral temperatures during 24 hours for a healthy young adult.

the temperature in the environment (e.g. the client has altered mental status or cannot dress self), her body temperature may be low.

Newborns are *homeothermic*; they attempt to stabilize their internal (core) body temperatures within a narrow range in spite of significant temperature variations in their environment. Thermoregulation in the newborn is closely related to the rate of metabolism and oxygen consumption. Within a specific environmental temperature range, called the **neutral thermal environment (NTE)** zone, the rates of oxygen consumption and metabolism are minimal, and internal body temperature is maintained because of thermal balance. For an unclothed, full-term newborn, the NTE is an ambient environmental temperature range of 32–34°C (89.6–93.2°F) within 50% relative humidity. The limits for an adult are 26–28°C (78.8–82.4°F) (Polin, Fox, & Abman, 2004). Thus, the normal newborn requires higher environmental temperatures to maintain a thermoneutral environment. Several newborn characteristics affect the establishment of thermal stability:

- The newborn has less subcutaneous fat than an adult and a thin epidermis.
- Blood vessels in the newborn are closer to the skin than those of an adult. Therefore, the newborn's circulating blood is more influenced by changes in environmental temperature and in turn influences the hypothalamic temperature-regulating center.
- The flexed posture of the term newborn decreases the surface area exposed to the environment, reducing heat loss. Size and age may also affect the establishment of an NTE. For example, the preterm or small-for-gestational-age (SGA) newborn has less adipose tissue and is hypoflexed, therefore requiring higher environmental temperatures to achieve an NTE. Larger, well-insulated newborns may be able to cope with lower environmental temperatures. If the environmental temperature falls below the lower limits of the NTE, the newborn responds with increased oxygen consumption and metabolism, which results in greater heat production. Prolonged exposure to the cold may result in depleted glycogen stores and acidosis. Oxygen consumption also increases if the environmental temperature is above the NTE.

Because neonates are adversely affected by heat loss through convection, be sure to place padding on any surface used for diapering or examination of the newborn.

ALTERATIONS

There are two primary alterations in body temperature: pyrexia and hypothermia. A body temperature above the usual range is called **pyrexia**, hyperthermia, or (in lay terms) fever. A very high fever, such as 41°C (105.8°F), is called **hyperpyrexia** (Figure 29–4 ■). The client who has a fever is referred to as **febrile**; one who does not is **afebrile**. Hypothermia is a core body temperature below the lower limit of normal. The three

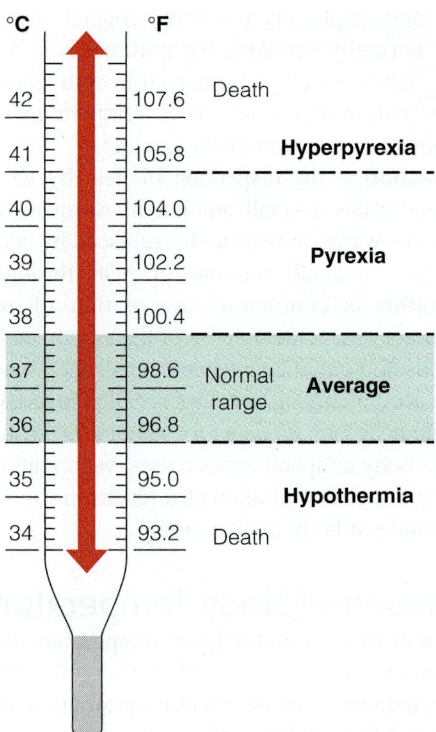

Figure 29–4 ■ Terms used to describe alterations in body temperature (oral measurements) and ranges in Celsius (centigrade) and Fahrenheit scales.

physiologic mechanisms of hypothermia are (a) excessive heat loss, (b) inadequate heat production to counteract heat loss, and (c) impaired hypothalamic thermoregulation.

PHYSICAL ASSESSMENT

Thermoregulation is assessed primarily by measuring body temperature. The body temperature is measured in degrees on two scales: Celsius (centigrade) and Fahrenheit. Sometimes a nurse needs to convert a Celsius reading to Fahrenheit, or vice versa. Although the conversion can be accomplished using several formulas, the most common is described here. To convert from Fahrenheit to Celsius, deduct 32 from the Fahrenheit reading and then multiply by the fraction 5/9:

$$C = (\text{Fahrenheit temperature} - 32) \times 5/9$$

For example, when the Fahrenheit reading is 100,

$$C = (100 - 32) \times 5/9 = (68) \times 5/9 = 37.8$$

To convert from Celsius to Fahrenheit, multiply the Celsius reading by the fraction 9/5 and then add 32:

$$F = (\text{Celsius temperature} \times 9/5) + 32$$

For example, when the Celsius reading is 40,

$$F = (40 \times 9/5) + 32 = (72 + 32) = 104$$

If using a calculator, the simplest way to convert Fahrenheit to Celsius will be to subtract 32 from the Fahrenheit temperature,

ALTERATIONS AND TREATMENTS Thermoregulation

Alteration	Description	Treatment
Hyperthermia	Increase in temperature as a result of more heat produced than lost	■ Monitor vital signs. ■ Assess skin color and temperature. ■ Monitor white blood cell count, hematocrit value, and other pertinent laboratory reports for indication of infection or dehydration. ■ Reduce covering (clothing, blankets, etc) to allow heat loss. ■ Lower room temperature. ■ Administer antipyretic medications. ■ Increase fluid intake and provide adequate nutrition. ■ Measure intake and output. ■ Reduce physical activity to limit heat production. ■ Provide oral hygiene to keep mucous membranes moist. ■ Administer tepid sponge bath to increase heat loss through conduction. ■ Provide dry clothing and bed linens if client is perspiring. ■ Use hypothermia blanket.
Hypothermia	Decrease in body temperature as a result of more heat lost than produced	■ Monitor vital signs. ■ Assess skin color and temperature. ■ Apply warm blankets or warm clothing. ■ Provide warm environment. ■ Provide dry clothing if heat loss is due to conduction. ■ Keep limbs close to body. ■ Cover scalp with cap or turban. ■ Use hyperthermia blanket. ■ Administer warmed oral or IV fluids. ■ Use heat lamps, hot water bottles, or heating pad.

divide the result by 9, and then multiply by 5. To convert Celsius to Fahrenheit, do exactly the opposite: Multiply by 9, divide by 5, and then add 32.

The most common sites for measuring body temperature are oral, rectal, axillary, tympanic membrane, and skin/temporal artery. Each of the sites has advantages and disadvantages (see Table 29–1).

The body temperature may be measured *orally*. If a client has been smoking or taking cold or hot food or fluids, the nurse should wait 30 minutes before taking the temperature orally. This ensures that the temperature of the mouth is not affected by the temperature of the warm smoke, food, or fluid.

Rectal temperature readings are considered to be very accurate. In some agencies, taking temperatures rectally is contraindicated for clients with myocardial infarction. It is believed that inserting a rectal thermometer can produce vagal stimulation, which can cause abnormal heart rhythms. However, not all authorities share this belief. Rectal temperatures are contraindicated for clients who are undergoing rectal surgery, have diarrhea or diseases of the rectum, are immunosuppressed, have a clotting disorder, or have significant hemorrhoids.

The *axilla* is the preferred site for measuring temperature in newborns because it is accessible and safe. However, some research indicates that the axillary method is inaccurate when assessing a fever (Bindler & Ball, 2003). Nurses should check agency protocol before they take the temperature of newborns, infants, toddlers, and children. Adult clients for whom the axillary method of temperature assessment is appropriate include those for whom other temperature sites are contraindicated.

The *tympanic membrane*, or nearby tissue in the ear canal, is a frequent site for estimating core body temperature. Like the sublingual oral site, the tympanic membrane has an abundant arterial blood supply, primarily from branches of the external carotid artery. Because temperature sensors applied directly to the tympanic membrane can be uncomfortable and involve risk of membrane injury or perforation, noninvasive infrared thermometers are used. Electronic tympanic thermometers are found extensively in both inpatient and ambulatory care settings.

The temperature may also be measured on the forehead using a chemical thermometer or a temporal artery thermometer. Forehead temperature measurements are most useful for infants and children for whom a more invasive measurement is not necessary.

Types of Thermometers

Traditionally, body temperatures were measured using mercury-in-glass thermometers. Glass thermometers can be hazardous if they crack or break because of the risk for exposure to mercury,

TABLE 29–1 Advantages and Disadvantages of Sites for Body Temperature Measurement

SITE	ADVANTAGES	DISADVANTAGES
Oral	Accessible and convenient	Thermometers can break if bitten. Inaccurate if client has just ingested hot or cold food or fluid or smoked. Could injure the mouth following oral surgery.
Rectal	Reliable measurement	Inconvenient and more unpleasant for clients; difficult for client who cannot turn to the side. Could injure the rectum following rectal surgery. Presence of stool may interfere with thermometer placement. If the stool is soft, the thermometer may be embedded in stool rather than against the wall of the rectum.
Axillary	Safe and noninvasive	The thermometer must be left in place a long time to obtain an accurate measurement.
Tympanic membrane	Readily accessible; reflects the core temperature Very fast	Can be uncomfortable and involves risk of injuring the membrane if the probe is inserted too far. Repeated measurements may vary. Right and left measurements can differ. Presence of cerumen can affect the reading.
Temporal artery	Safe and noninvasive; very fast	Requires electronic equipment that may be expensive or unavailable; variation in technique needed if the client has perspiration on the forehead.

which is toxic to humans, and the broken glass. In 1998, the U.S. Environmental Protection Agency and the American Hospital Association agreed on the goal of eliminating mercury from health care environments. Hospitals no longer use mercury-in-glass thermometers, and several cities have banned their sale and manufacture. Some modern versions of the thermometer have replaced glass with plastics and mercury with safer chemicals. However, the nurse may still encounter this type of thermometer.

The amount of mercury in a thermometer is minimal, but cleanup, should it break, involves several "dos and don'ts." Unsealed mercury slowly vaporizes into the air. The nurse should keep children and pets away from the area. Wearing rubber gloves, the nurse can wipe mercury beads off clothing, skin, or disposable items with a paper towel, and immediately place it into a plastic bag and discard. If the spill is on a porous material that cannot be discarded (e.g., carpet), a contractor trained in mercury disposal may be needed. If the mercury is on a hard surface, the nurse should use folded stiff cardboard to slowly gather the beads and pour them into a wide-mouthed container. The nurse should use a flashlight to search for the beads, since the light reflects off mercury, and then dispose of all items used in the cleanup in a plastic bag, which should then be sealed with tape. The nurse should shower or wash well after cleaning up, and keep the area well ventilated for several days. Vacuum cleaners or brooms should not be used since these will disperse the mercury and become contaminated. The mercury should not be poured down a toilet or drain; any contaminated materials should not be washed or reused.

PRACTICE ALERT

Whenever mercury-in-glass thermometers are encountered, the nurse should recommend their immediate replacement with less hazardous thermometers and their safe disposal.

Depending on the model, an electronic thermometer can provide a reading in only 2–60 seconds. The equipment consists of a battery-operated portable electronic unit, a probe that the nurse attaches to the unit, and a probe cover, which is usually disposable (Figure 29–5 ■). Some models have a different circuits and probes for oral and rectal measurement.

Basal and hypothermia thermometers are two specific types of oral thermometers that can be glass or electronic. A basal thermometer is calibrated with 0.1°F intervals and is used for fertility purposes, as it indicates the temperature rise associated with ovulation. Hypothermia thermometers have a greater low range than everyday thermometers, usually measuring temperatures from 81 to 108°F.

Chemical disposable thermometers are also used to measure body temperatures. Chemical thermometers using liquid crystal dots or bars or heat-sensitive tape or patches applied to the forehead change color to indicate temperature. Some of these are for single use; others may be reused several times. One type that has small chemical dots at one end is shown in Figure 29–6 ■. To read the temperature, the nurse notes the highest reading among the dots that have changed color.

Temperature-sensitive tape may also be used to obtain a general indication of body surface temperature. It does not indicate the core temperature. When the tape is applied to the skin, usually on the forehead or abdomen, the temperature digits respond by changing color (Figure 29–7 ■). The skin area should be dry. After the length of time specified by the manufacturer (e.g., 15 seconds), a color appears on the tape. This method is particularly useful at home and for use with infants.

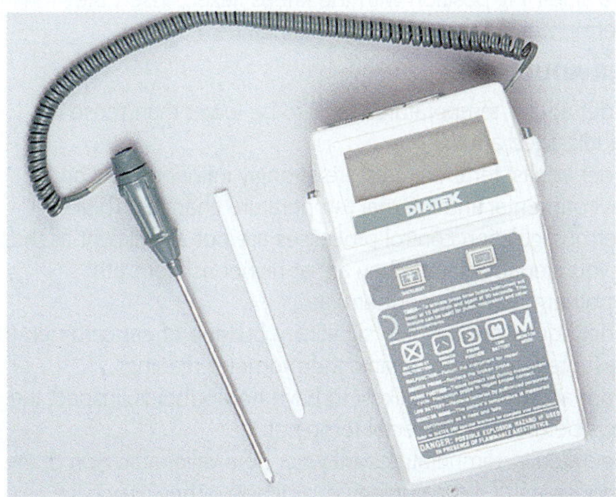

Figure 29–5 ■ An electronic thermometer. Note the probe and probe cover.

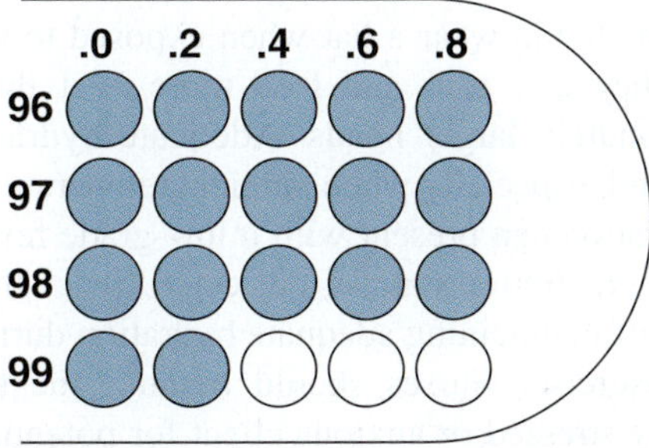

Figure 29–6 ■ A chemical thermometer showing a reading of 99.2°F.

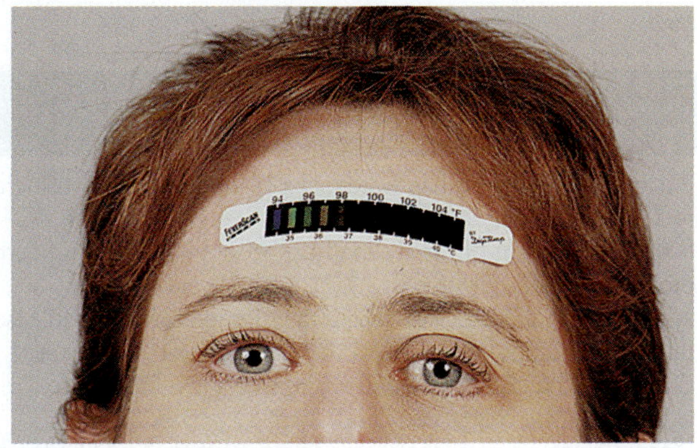

Figure 29–7 ■ A temperature-sensitive skin tape.

Infrared thermometers sense body heat in the form of infrared energy produced by a heat source. In the ear canal, this source is the tympanic membrane (Figure 29–8 ■). The infrared thermometer makes no contact with the tympanic membrane.

Temporal artery thermometers determine temperature using a scanning infrared thermometer that compares temperature in the temporal artery of the forehead to the temperature in the room and then calculates the heat balance to approximate the core temperature of the blood in the pulmonary artery (Roy, Powell, & Gerson, 2003). The probe is placed in the middle of the forehead and then drawn laterally to the hairline. If the client has perspiration on the forehead, the probe is also touched behind the earlobe so the thermometer can compensate for evaporative cooling (Figure 29–9 ■).

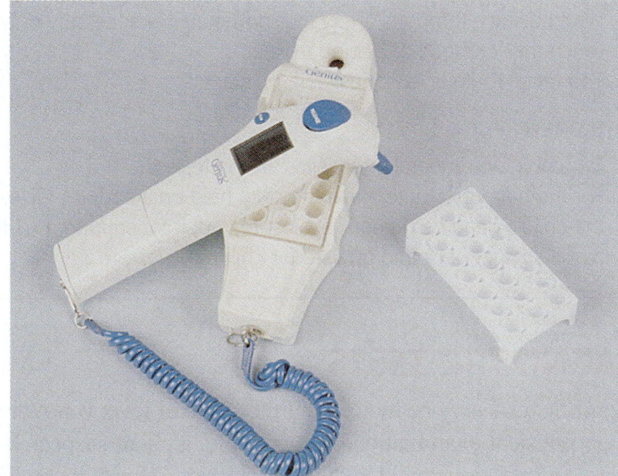

Figure 29–8 ■ An infrared (tympanic) thermometer used to measure the tympanic membrane temperature.

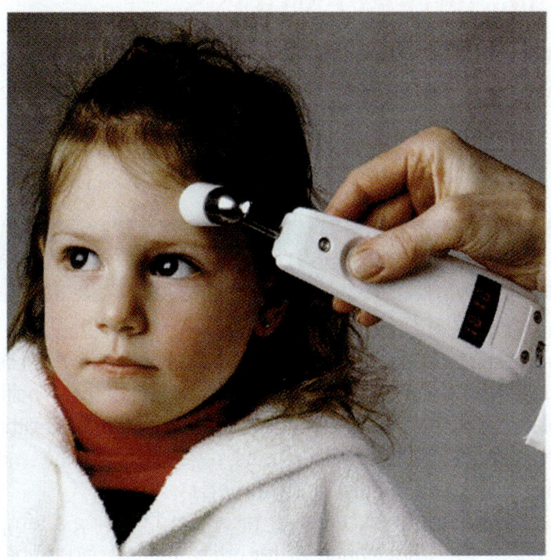

Figure 29–9 ■ A temporal artery thermometer.

Copyright © Exergen Corporation. All rights reserved.

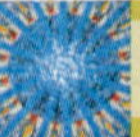

DEVELOPMENTAL CONSIDERATIONS Temperature

INFANTS

- The body temperature of newborns is extremely labile; newborns must be kept warm and dry to prevent hypothermia.
- Using the axillary site, you need to hold the infant's arm against the chest.
- The axillary route may not be as accurate as other routes for detecting fevers in children (Bindler & Ball, 2003).
- The tympanic route is fast and convenient. Place the infant supine and stabilize the head. Pull the pinna straight back and slightly downward. Direct the probe tip anteriorly and insert it far enough to seal the canal. The tip will not touch the tympanic membrane.
- Avoid the tympanic route in a child with active ear infections or tympanic membrane drainage tubes.
- The tympanic membrane route may be more accurate in determining temperature in febrile infants (Liu, Chang, & Chang, 2004; Nimah, Bshesh, Callahan, & Jacobs, 2006).
- When using a temporal artery thermometer, it is necessary only to touch the forehead or behind the ear.
- The rectal route is least desirable in infants.

CHILDREN

- Tympanic or temporal artery sites are preferred.
- For the tympanic route, have the child held on an adult's lap with the child's head held gently against the adult for support. Pull the pinna straight back and upward for children over age 3.
- Avoid the tympanic route in a child with active ear infections or tympanic membrane drainage tubes.
- The oral route may be used for children over age 3, but nonbreakable, electronic thermometers are recommended.
- For a rectal temperature, place the child prone across your lap or in a side-lying position with the knees flexed. Insert the thermometer 1 inch into the rectum.

OLDER ADULTS

- Older adults' temperatures tend to be lower than those of middle-aged adults.
- Older adults' temperatures are strongly influenced by both environmental and internal temperature changes. Their thermoregulation control processes are not as efficient as those of younger adults, and they are at higher risk for both hypothermia and hyperthermia.
- Older adults can develop significant buildup of ear cerumen that may interfere with tympanic thermometer readings.
- Older adults are more likely to have hemorrhoids. Inspect the anus before taking a rectal temperature.
- Older adults' temperatures may not be a valid indication of the seriousness of the pathology of a disease. They may have pneumonia or a urinary tract infection and exhibit only a slight temperature elevation. Other symptoms, such as confusion and restlessness, may be presented and need follow-up to determine if there is an underlying process.

DIAGNOSTIC TESTS

Diagnostic tests may be indicated if the cause of fever is not obvious on physical examination. For example, a client suspected of having an infection might require a complete blood count with differential to diagnose the type of infection, or a client whose fever is believed to be related to head trauma may require imaging studies to determine degree and location of trauma.

CARING INTERVENTIONS

Support the client's environment to maintain thermoregulatory mechanisms. Elderly clients and young infants may require a warmer environmental temperature than other clients. Infants and children should wear a hat when exposed to temperature extremes; they can gain and lose more heat through their disproportionately larger heads. Adequate hydration should be maintained, especially when ambient temperatures are very hot. Dehydration can present with a low-grade fever that will resolve when hydration status is corrected. Teach the client the importance of maintaining adequate hydration during times of strenuous exercise. Nurses should monitor the temperature of the highly stressed or anxious client for potential temperature elevation.

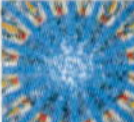

CARE SETTINGS Temperature

- Teach the client accurate use and reading of the type of thermometer to be used. Examine the thermometer the client uses in the home for safety and proper functioning. Facilitate the replacement of mercury-in-glass thermometers with other types. See page 1856 for instructions regarding management of a broken mercury-in-glass thermometer.
- Observe the client or caregiver taking and reading a temperature. Reinforce the importance of reporting the site and type of thermometer used and the value of using these consistently.
- Discuss means of keeping the thermometer clean, such as warm water and soap, and avoiding cross-contamination.
- Ensure that the client has water-soluble lubricant when using a rectal thermometer.
- Instruct the client or family member to notify the health care provider if the temperature is 37.7°C (100°F) or higher.
- When making a home visit, take a thermometer with you in case the clients do not have a functional thermometer of their own.
- Check that the client knows how to record the temperature. Provide a recording chart/table if indicated.
- Discuss environmental control modifications that should be taken during illness or extreme climate conditions (e.g., heating, air conditioning, appropriate clothing and bedding).

29.1 HYPERTHERMIA

KEY TERMS

CHCT, *1860*
Constant fever, *1859*
Endogenous pyrogens, *1860*
Febrile seizure, *1861*
Fever spike, *1859*
Heat exhaustion, *1859*
Heat stroke, *1859*
Intermittent fever, *1859*
Malignant hyperthermia, *1860*
Relapsing fever, *1859*
Remittent fever, *1859*

Basis for Selection of Exemplar
Nursing Skills B & I

LEARNING OUTCOMES

After reading about this exemplar, you will be able to:

1. Describe the pathophysiology, etiology, clinical manifestations, and direct and indirect causes of hyperthermia.
2. Identify risk factors associated with hyperthermia.
3. Illustrate the nursing process in providing culturally competent care across the life span for individuals with hyperthermia.
4. Formulate priority nursing diagnoses appropriate for an individual with hyperthermia.
5. Create a plan of care for individuals with hyperthermia and their family members.
6. Assess expected outcomes for an individual with hyperthermia.
7. Discuss therapies used in the collaborative care of an individual with hyperthermia.
8. Employ evidence-based caring interventions for an individual with hyperthermia.

OVERVIEW

To review, a body temperature above the usual range is called pyrexia, hyperthermia, or (in lay terms) fever. A very high fever, such as 41°C (105.8°F), is called hyperpyrexia (Figure 29–10 ■). The client who has a fever is referred to as febrile; the one who does not is afebrile.

Four common types of fevers are intermittent, remittent, relapsing, and constant. During an **intermittent fever**, the body temperature alternates at regular intervals between periods of fever and periods of normal or subnormal temperatures. Intermittent fever is common with some illnesses, such as malaria. During a **remittent fever**, such as with a cold or influenza, a wide range of temperature fluctuations (more than 2°C [3.6°F]) occurs over the 24-hour period, all of which are above normal. In a **relapsing fever**, short febrile periods of a few days are interspersed with periods of 1 or 2 days of normal temperature. During a **constant fever**, the body temperature fluctuates minimally but always remains above normal. This can occur with typhoid fever. A temperature that rises to fever level rapidly following a normal temperature and then returns to normal within a few hours is called a **fever spike**. Bacterial blood infections often cause fever spikes.

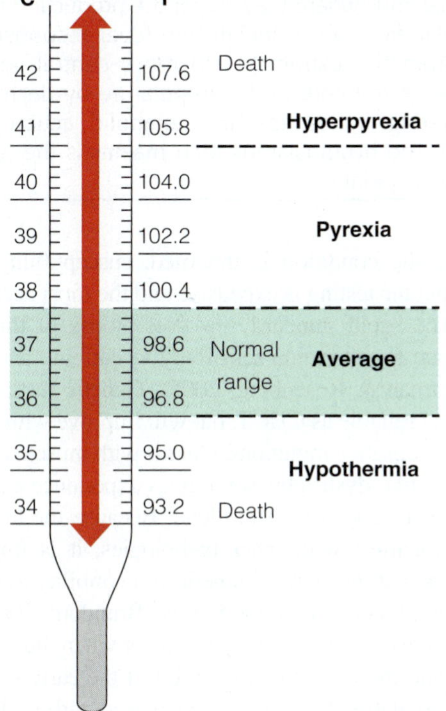

Figure 29–10 ■ Terms used to describe alterations in body temperature (oral measurements) and ranges in Celsius (centigrade) and Fahrenheit scales.

In some conditions, an elevated temperature is not a true fever. Two examples are heat exhaustion and heat stroke. **Heat exhaustion** is a result of excessive heat exposure and dehydration. Signs of heat exhaustion include paleness, dizziness, nausea, vomiting, fainting, and a moderately increased temperature (101–102°F). Persons experiencing **heat stroke**, a more serious form of heat exhaustion which can be life-threatening, generally have been exercising in hot weather, have warm, flushed skin, and often do not sweat. They usually have a temperature of 106°F or higher, and may be delirious, unconscious, or having seizures.

PATHOPHYSIOLOGY AND ETIOLOGY

The clinical signs of fever vary with the onset, course, and abatement stages. These signs occur as a result of changes in the set-point of the temperature control mechanism regulated by the hypothalamus. Under normal conditions, whenever the core temperature rises, the rate of heat loss increases, resulting in a decrease in temperature toward the set-point level. Conversely, when the core temperature falls, the rate of heat production is increased, resulting in a rise in temperature toward the set-point.

In a fever, however, the set-point of the hypothalamic thermostat changes suddenly from the normal level to a higher than normal value (e.g., 39.5°C [103.1°F]). This results from the effects on the hypothalamus of tissue destruction, pyrogenic substances, or dehydration. Although the set-point changes rapidly, the core body temperature (i.e., the blood temperature) reaches this new set-point only after several hours. During this interval, the usual heat production responses that elevate the body temperature occur: chills, feeling of coldness, cold skin due to vasoconstriction, and shivering. This is referred to as the chill phase.

When the core temperature reaches the new set-point, the client feels neither cold nor hot and no longer experiences chills (the plateau phase). Depending on the degree of temperature elevation, other signs may occur during the course of the fever. Very high temperatures, such as 41–42°C (106–108°F), damage the parenchyma of cells throughout the body, particularly in the brain where destruction of neuronal cells is irreversible. Damage to the liver, kidneys, and other body organs can also be great enough to disrupt functioning and eventually cause death.

When the cause of the high temperature is suddenly removed, the set-point of the hypothalamic thermostat is suddenly reduced to a lower value, perhaps even back to the original normal level. In this instance, the hypothalamus now attempts to lower the temperature, and the usual heat loss responses causing a reduction of the body temperature occur: excessive sweating and a hot, flushed skin due to sudden vasodilaation. This is referred to as the flush phase.

In response to an infection, macrophages release **endogenous pyrogens** (interleukins, interferons, and tumor necrosis factor). These pyrogens travel through the circulatory system to the hypothalamus, the control center for body temperature regulation. In the hypothalamus, the pyrogens trigger the production of prostaglandins, which are believed to raise the body's thermoregulatory set-point, thus causing the fever to occur (Crocetti & Serwint, 2005). See Figure 29–11 ■.

Heat loss from the body is reduced and the body temperature rises to the new temperature set-point. When the temperature is elevated, the heart rate increases. One degree of temperature elevation causes an increase in respiratory rate by four breaths per minute and increases the metabolic need for oxygen by 7%. Vasodilation occurs and the skin flushes, becoming warm to the touch.

Malignant hyperthermia (MH) is frequently inherited, and is a rare but serious reaction to volatile inhalational anesthetic gases and succinylcholine, a depolarizing neuromuscular blocker. The client manifests the following signs and symptoms: unexplained rise in end-tidal carbon dioxide that does not respond to ventilation, hyperthermia, tachypnea, tachycardia, and sustained skeletal muscle contraction (Carter-Templeton, 2005). If unchecked, the condition will progress to hyperkalemia, myoglobinuria, disseminated intravascular coagulation, congestive heart failure, bowel ischemia, and compartment syndrome in the limbs. Dantrolene sodium is the drug that inhibits the muscular pathology and prevents death.

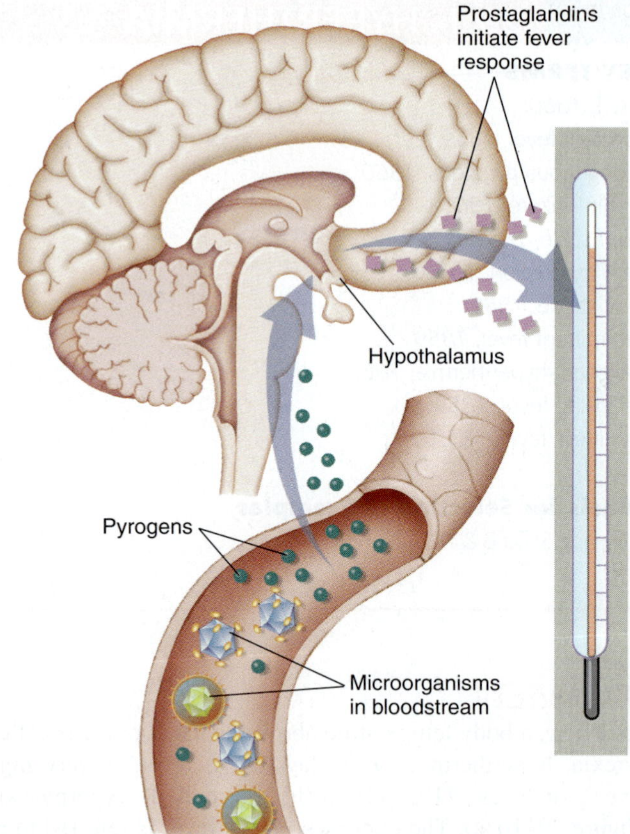

Figure 29–11 ■ The hypothalamus functions as the body's thermostat, directing the body to conserve or dissapate heat. When microorganisms invade the body, endogenous pyrogens are released into the bloodstream. These substances travel to the hypothalamus where they trigger the production and release of prostaglandins, which initiate the fever response. Blood is diverted from the extremities to more central vessels. This helps increase the core body temperature by decreasing heat loss. Shivering increases the metabolic action and heat production. The hypothalamus then maintains the temperature at the new set-point.

Because the condition is inherited, susceptibility testing is available, but the testing is expensive and the most accurate test is invasive. The "gold standard" involves biopsy of thigh skeletal muscle tissue to determine sensitivity to caffeine and halothane (**CHCT**) (Litman & Rosenberg, 2005). Genetic testing is not as sensitive and reliable as CHCT, but will improve with the discovery of more causative mutations. Clients with muscle myopathies, such as muscular dystrophy, sometimes experience early signs of MH and respond well to dantrolene. Because the symptoms of MH may manifest with other pathologies, it is important for clients to know if they have a genetic susceptibility to MH, which could affect all members of the family (Brandom, 2005).

MH can develop during an operation or when the client returns to the postanesthetic care unit (PACU). If the early symptoms of MH (e.g., escalating temperature, increased carbon dioxide production) are suspected, the nurse should immediately administer 100% oxygen with a nonrebreather mask, stay with the patient, ensure good intravenous (IV) access, and summon the anesthesia provider. The anesthesia provider will order 2.5 mg/kg of dantrolene, which can be given via IV push. The dantrolene can be repeated up to 10 mg/kg until the signs and symptoms of MH diminish. Measures to decrease core body temperature should be started at once and continued until core temperature is 36.0°C. A urinary catheter should be placed to monitor urine output, and blood drawn for testing. Blood gases should be drawn to measure pH; sodium bicarbonate is given to correct metabolic acidosis. Insulin may be ordered to decrease serum potassium. Expect this client to be transferred to the ICU for continued monitoring and doses of dantrolene every 4–6 hours.

Etiology

Hyperthermia may occur in response to viral or bacterial infections, or from tissue breakdown following myocardial infarction, malignancy, surgery, or trauma.

Risk Factors

Clients at risk for fever are those at risk for conditions resulting in fever. Diminished immune response increases the risk of infection, which increase the risk for fever. The very young and very old have diminished immunity, placing them at risk for fever. Adolescents who practice risky behavior resulting in infections or neurological trauma are also at risk for resulting fevers.

Fevers are most frequently seen in children, especially those in day care or exposed to many other children, because they have not developed immunity to common contagious diseases of childhood. Infections such as otitis media, upper respiratory infections, chickenpox, and other common diseases of childhood frequently result in fevers.

CLINICAL MANIFESTATIONS

The clinical manifestations of fever are frequently due, at least in part, to the cause of the fever. Signs and symptoms common to all fevers include flushing, skin that is warm or hot to the touch, increased metabolic rate resulting in an increased need for fluids, tachycardia, and tachypnea. Fatigue, malaise, weakness, decreased responsiveness, difficulty concentrating, skin rash, poor appetite, malaise, vomiting and/or diarrhea, and body aches are some common signs and symptoms that may accompany a fever.

Treatment for fever is not always indicated. A fever can be a beneficial physiologic response, helping to slow the growth of organisms that thrive at lower body temperatures. A fever helps mobilize the immune response by increasing neutrophil production and T-cell proliferation (Crocetti & Serwint, 2005). Fever is not inherently harmful until it reaches 41°C (105.9°F). For this reason, medical management may include postponing treatment of low-grade fevers under 38.9°C (102°F) in otherwise healthy children (101°F in adults) to promote the body's natural defenses against an infection. Fevers are more likely to be treated if associated with discomfort.

Acetaminophen and ibuprofen are the preferred antipyretics for children. Aspirin is no longer recommended for children because of its association with Reye's syndrome. Antipyretics reduce fever by inhibiting prostaglandin synthesis, which results in lowering of the body's temperature set-point.

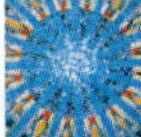

ALTERNATIVE THERAPIES Hot and Cold Theory

Many cultures subscribe to the hot and cold theory of disease causation. "Hot" and "cold" do not refer to temperature, but to categories. Fever, a hot condition, is treated by giving the patient cold substances (foods or medicines). Cold foods include vegetables, fruits, and fish. Cold medicines include orange flower water, linden, and sage.

Antibiotics may also be administered for infectious diseases. Antibiotics have been responsible for decreases in morbidity and mortality from infections among children. However, some strains of bacteria have developed resistance to many antibiotics. Children with chronic illnesses such as cystic fibrosis, sickle-cell disease, and AIDS are particularly susceptible to infection by drug-resistant pathogens.

PRACTICE ALERT

The practice of alternating acetaminophen with ibuprofen in the care of children with fever is not based on scientific evidence. Both medications are effective in managing fever. However, because they have different durations of action (4 hours for acetaminophen and 6 hours for ibuprofen) and many preparations, there is risk for overdosing the child if the administration schedule is not strictly adhered to. In addition, combining the two medications in an alternating schedule has a potentially synergistic effect on the kidneys that can cause renal tubular toxicity. An important patient safety initiative is to use only one antipyretic to manage fever, especially in children (Carson, 2003).

Febrile seizures are generalized seizures that usually occur in children as the result of rapid temperature rise above 39°C (102°F) in association with an acute illness. No evidence of intracranial infection or other defined cause is found. These seizures are usually seen in children between the ages of 3 months and 5 years, with a peak incidence between 17 and 24 months of age. There is often a family history of febrile seizures. In addition, children who have one febrile seizure have a 30–50% greater chance of having future seizures (Gill & Gieron-Korthals, 2002). The lower convulsive threshold of infants may explain this type of seizure.

COLLABORATION

Collaboration related to hyperthermia or fever will generally revolve around the underlying cause of the fever. For a child with a history of febrile seizures, the nurse from the child's pediatrician's office should collaborate with the child's preschool or classroom teacher, to ensure that any staff working with the child know what to do in the event the child has a seizure, and how to prevent the onset of a febrile seizure. Adequate hydration, shortened periods outside during hot weather, and shade are just some of the measures school staff can use to help prevent febrile seizures in children.

CLINICAL MANIFESTATIONS AND THERAPIES Hyperthermia

CLINICAL MANIFESTATION	CLINICAL THERAPY	RATIONALE
Flushing	Correction of temperature elevation	As body temperature rises the blood vessels vasodilate to bring more blood flow to the surface of the body. This allows cooler environmental temperatures to reduce the temperature of the blood flow as heat dissipates through convection.
Warm skin	Correction of temperature elevation	As body temperature raises, the blood vessels vasodilate to bring more blood flow to the surface of the body. This causes the skin to feel warm secondary to the warmth of the blood flow.
Tachycardia	Correction of temperature elevation	With the increase in temperature, there is an increased metabolic rate resulting in increased pulse rate and respiratory rate.
Tachypnea	Correction of temperature elevation	With the increase in temperature, there is an increased metabolic rate resulting in increased pulse rate and respiratory rate.
Increased fluid requirement	Increasing oral fluid intake or provide intravenous fluids; monitoring hydration status	Insensible water loss increases as the result of perspiration, tachypnea, and increased metabolic rate. Dehydration can occur quickly, especially in young children and older adults, if extra fluid intake is not provided.
Elevated body temperature	Ranges from no treatment for a low-grade fever (>102°F in children, >101°F in adults) to the following for higher temperatures: ■ Antipyretic ■ Tepid bath ■ Reducing clothing and skin covering ■ Increasing fluid intake (at least 2000 mL per day with additional fluids in hot weather or during strenuous exercise) ■ Applying cool washcloths or ice bags to axilla, groin, forehead, and nape of neck ■ Cooling blanket ■ For malignant hyperthermia, keeping emergency equipment nearby ■ Using a circulating fan in client's room	

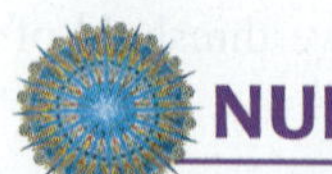

NURSING PROCESS

Assessment

The nurse assesses the client's hydration status and fluid intake, vital signs, comfort level, and appetite, and observes for seizures and a toxic appearance (lethargy, poor perfusion, hypoventilation or hyperventilation, and cyanosis), especially in the pediatric client. The client with a fever may be irritable and restless, sleep fitfully, and have nonspecific muscular pain. The nurse should identify those clients who may be at higher risk for a serious illness in association with a fever, the following in particular:

- Infants and children with a toxic appearance
- Neonates under 28 days of age with a temperature over 38°C (100.4°F)
- Children under 4 years of age with a temperature over 41°C (105.8°F)
- Children with conditions such as a ventriculoperitoneal shunt, congenital heart disease, asplenia, and sickle-cell disease
- Clients with immunosuppression, such as those receiving chemotherapy, undergoing organ transplantation, or diagnosed with HIV/AIDS
- Clients with chronic conditions such as diabetes mellitus, congestive heart failure, or pulmonary diseases.

The client should be observed for other signs of infection, such as a rash, nausea and vomiting, and/or diarrhea, as well as generalized symptoms of a poor appetite and malaise.

Diagnosis

Examples of nursing diagnoses that may be appropriate for clients with febrile illnesses include the following:

- Hyperthermia related to infectious disease process
- Risk for Deficient Fluid Volume related to hypermetabolic state
- Impaired Skin Integrity related to hyperthermia and self-mutilation of skin lesions
- Impaired Oral Mucous Membrane related to infectious disease process
- Deficient Fluid Volume related to repeated episodes of vomiting and diarrhea.

Plan

Care is planned for the client with hyperthermia based on the specific needs of the client and the cause of the temperature elevation. Goals specific to fever may include the following:

- Temperature will approach normal limits within 60 minutes of administration of antipyretic.
- Temperature will remain within normal limits within 48–72 hours of beginning antibiotic therapy.
- Temperature will be maintained within acceptable limits within 4 hours of application of hypothermia blanket.
- Client or parent will describe temperature elevations to be reported to the provider immediately.

Client or parent will recognize symptoms requiring consultation with health care provider.

Implementation

Nursing interventions for a client who has a fever are designed to support the body's normal physiologic processes, provide comfort, and prevent complications. During the course of fever, the nurse needs to monitor the client's vital signs closely.

Nursing measures during the chill phase are designed to help the client decrease heat loss. At this time, the body's physiologic processes are attempting to raise the core temperature to the new set-point temperature. During the flush or crisis phase, the body processes are attempting to lower the core temperature to the reduced or normal set-point temperature. At this time, the nurse takes measures to increase heat loss and decrease heat production. Nursing interventions for a client with fever are shown in Table 29–2 and Box 29–1.

Nursing care for treatment of fever includes administering antipyretics, removing unnecessary clothing, and careful continued monitoring of temperature progression. Identify clear fluids the client prefers to drink, and encourage the intake of extra fluids.

Care in the Community

The nurse teaches parents to care for their child at home, including how and when to give antipyretics. Parents often fear a fever, believing it is a disease rather than a symptom of an illness. Their greatest fears about the harmful effects of fever include seizure, brain damage, and death (Nativio, 2005). The nurse should provide information and reassurance, helping parents to recognize signs of the child's worsening condition in association with the child's specific disease (see Families Want to Know: Evaluating and Treating Fever in Children).

Evaluation

Expected outcomes of nursing care include the following:

- The client's fever is effectively managed with antipyretics.
- The client maintains adequate hydration as evidenced by skin turgor, moist mucous membranes, and hematocrit within normal range.

TABLE 29–2 **Identifying Nursing Diagnoses, Outcomes, and Interventions: Imbalanced Body Temperature**

NURSING DIAGNOSIS: DEFINITION	SAMPLE DESIRED OUTCOMES: DEFINITION	INDICATORS*	SELECTED INTERVENTIONS: DEFINITION†	SAMPLE ACTIVITIES (ALSO SEE BOX 29–1)
Risk for Imbalanced Body Temperature/At risk for failure to maintain body temperature within normal range	Hydration [0602]/ Adequate water in the intracellular and extracellular compartments of the body	■ Moist mucous membranes ■ Urine output	Temperature Regulation [3900]/Attaining and/or maintaining body temperature within a normal range	Monitor temperature every 2 hours, as appropriate. Promote adequate fluid and nutritional intake.
Hyperthermia/Body temperature elevated above normal range	Thermoregulation [0800]/*Balance among heat production, heat gain, and heat loss*	■ Skin temperature in expected range ■ Body temperature in expected range ■ Sweating when hot	Fever Treatment [3740]/ *Management of a patient with hyperpyrexia caused by nonenvironmental factors*	Monitor intake and output. Apply ice bag covered with a towel to groin. Cover the patient with only a sheet.

*The NOC # for desired outcomes and the NIC # for nursing interventions are listed in brackets following the appropriate outcome or intervention. Outcomes, indicators, interventions, and activities selected are only a sample of those suggested by NOC and NIC and should be further individualized for each client.

†The measurement scale for these indicators ranges from *extremely compromised* to *not compromised*.

Box 29–1 Evaluating and Treating Fever in Children

ABOUT FEVERS

- A fever is not a disease; it is the body's response to an infection. It means the child's body is using natural defenses to fight an infection.
- If the child has a fever and does not look sick, it may be better to let the child use the body's natural defenses to fight off the virus or bacteria causing the fever. Follow guidelines about when to contact the child's health care provider.

TREATING THE FEVER

- Use a thermometer to check the child's temperature every 4–6 hours.
- Administer either acetaminophen or ibuprofen to lower a fever. Check the label to make sure the correct dosage is given—drops and syrups do not have the same concentration. Do not alternate medications.
- Remove all but a light layer of the child's clothing.
- Monitor the child's behavior and response to fever medication. The fever medication will reduce the child's temperature, but the temperature may not return to normal until the child is recovering from the illness.
- If sponging the child, give fever medication first, and then use tepid water to sponge the child. Cool water may increase shivering and discomfort. Alcohol should not be used.
- The temperature may rise again 4 hours after acetaminophen or 6 hours after ibuprofen is given. Check the temperature and give another dose of fever medicine. Follow the recommendations on the bottle for the maximum number of doses allowed per day.

CALL YOUR HEALTH CARE PROVIDER IMMEDIATELY IF ANY OF THE FOLLOWING OCCUR

- The infant is under 2 months old and has a fever over 38.0°C (100.4°F).
- The child has a fever over 40.1°C (104.2°F) and any of the symptoms below are present:
- The child is crying inconsolably or whimpering. The child cries when moved or otherwise touched by the parent or other family members.
  - The child is difficult to awaken.
  - The child's neck is stiff.
  - There are purple spots present on the skin.
  - Breathing is difficult and no better after the nose is cleared.
  - The child is drooling saliva and is unable to swallow anything.
  - The child has a convulsion or seizure.
  - The child acts or looks very sick.

CALL YOUR HEALTH CARE PROVIDER WITHIN 24 HOURS IF ANY OF THE FOLLOWING OCCUR

- The child is 2–4 months old (unless fever occurs within 48 hours of a DTaP shot and the infant has no other serious symptoms).
- The fever is higher than 40.1°C (104.2°F) (especially if the child is under 3 years old).
- The child complains of burning or pain with urination.
- The fever has been present for more than 24 hours without an obvious cause or location of infection.
- The fever went away for more than 24 hours and then returned.

REVIEW Hyperthermia

RELATE: LINK THE CONCEPTS

Linking the exemplar of Hyperthermia with the concept of Infection:

1. Do all infections result in fevers? Explain your answer.
2. When treating a 4-year-old client with a viral infection and a temperature of 103.8 degrees Fahrenheit measured axillary, what independent nursing actions would you initiate? What collaborative interventions would you anticipate?

Linking the exemplar of Hyperthermia with the concept of Fluids and Electrolytes:

3. Explain the physiology that would cause a client to run a fever when dehydrated.
4. How does a client's fluid requirement change when he has a fever? Explain the physiology behind your answer.

READY: GO TO COMPANION SKILLS MANUAL

- Use of a hypothermia blanket
- Assessing body temperature

REFER: GO TO MYNURSINGKIT

REFLECT: CASE STUDY

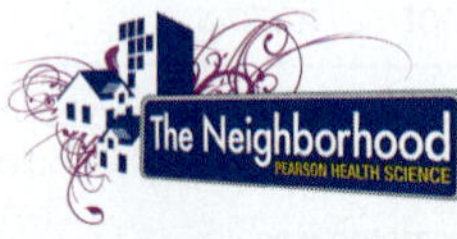

Carrie Holmes is six weeks old, born at 38 weeks' gestation by vaginal delivery secondary to a small placental abruptio attributed to her father, Casey Holmes, hitting her mother, Jessica Riley, in the abdomen. When she and her mother come home from the hospital they move into her grandmother's house with her big brother Ryan who is 3 years old. By six weeks of age Carrie is starting to become accustomed to the daily routine. Her grandmother Evelyn cares for her when her mother goes to work at the restaurant, feeding her a bottle and letting her sit in her infant seat to watch her big brother play with his toys.

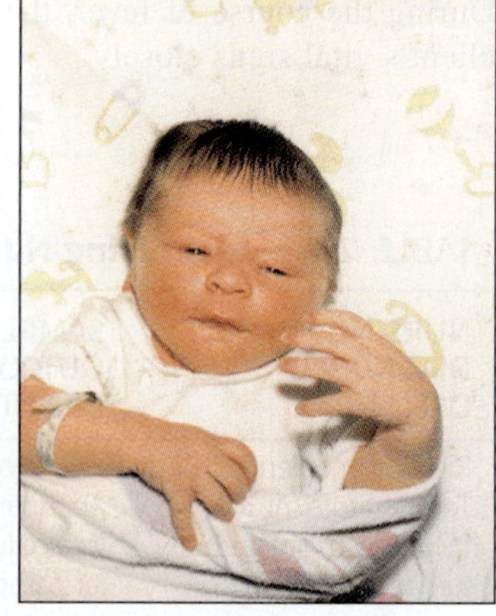

1. What factors would increase Carrie's risk of developing a fever?
2. If Jessica called the pediatrician's office to report that Carrie had a fever of 101.4°F, taken rectally what directions would you provide for her care? Explain the rationale for your answer.
3. If Ryan developed a fever of 101.4°F taken via the axillary route what instructions would you provide his mother for his care?

29.2 HYPOTHERMIA

KEY TERMS

Brown adipose tissue, *1866*
Chemical thermogenesis, *1866*
Frostbite, *1866*
Hyperthermia blanket, *1868*
Nonshivering thermogenesis, *1866*
Piloerection, *1868*

Basis for Selection of Exemplar

Nursing Skills B & I

LEARNING OUTCOMES

After reading about this exemplar, you will be able to:

1. Describe the pathophysiology, etiology, clinical manifestations, and direct and indirect causes of hypothermia.
2. Identify risk factors associated with hypothermia.
3. Illustrate the nursing process in providing culturally competent care across the life span for individuals with hypothermia.
4. Formulate priority nursing diagnoses appropriate for an individual with hypothermia.
5. Create a plan of care for individuals with hypothermia and their family members.
6. Assess expected outcomes for an individual with hypothermia.
7. Discuss therapies used in the collaborative care of an individual with hypothermia.
8. Employ evidence-based caring interventions for an individual with hypothermia.

OVERVIEW

Hypothermia is a condition in which the core body temperature falls below 35°C (95°F). This occurs when the heat the body produces is less than the heat lost. Hypothermia can be a life-threatening emergency, and can occur in any season and any geographic location.

PATHOPHYSIOLOGY AND ETIOLOGY

Hypothermia may be induced or accidental. Induced hypothermia is the deliberate lowering of the body temperature to decrease metabolic rate, reducing the body's need for oxygen. Accidental hypothermia may occur as the result of immersion in cold water, exposure to cold environments, or damage to the body's thermoregulatory processes.

As the body's core temperature falls, the body tries to conserve the core temperature at the expense of the extremities. Two major routes of heat loss are from the internal core of the body to the body surface and from the external surface to the environment. The core temperature is usually higher than the skin temperature, resulting in continuous transfer or conduction of heat to the surface. The greater the difference in temperature between core and skin, the more rapidly heat transfers. The transfer is accomplished through an increase in oxygen consumption, depletion of glycogen stores, and, in the newborn, metabolization of brown fat.

Induced Hypothermia

Hypothermia may be induced for a variety of reasons, but the most frequent reason for this treatment is to reduce metabolic rates and lower the cellular demand for oxygen in the tissues, particularly in the brain. Historically, induced hypothermia has been used to reduce neurological damage following head trauma, strokes, or during cardiac surgery. Kozik (2007) reports that elevated body temperatures following cardiac arrest increase the risk and amount of neurological damage from anoxia during the event. This study found that the lower the body temperature, the greater the neurological recovery will be. Based on this and other study results, the American Heart Association now recommends induced hypothermia in clients post–cardiac arrest. Research is being conducted to determine if there are benefits to emergency responders initiating hypothermia in the field (Clumpner & Mobley, 2008).

Cooling is initiated with iced saline gastric lavage and ice packs in the axilla and groin until the cooling blanket is started at 5°C. The goal is a client temperature of 33°C. After 24 hours, the temperature is gradually increased by one degree every 2–4 hours. It is important to stop all potassium administration during the rewarming phase: Potassium released by damaged cells will be circulated and serum potassium levels will rise. Clients are sedated and paralytic medications are administered to prevent the body's natural response to cold (shivering), which produces heat and reduces the effectiveness of the induced hypothermia (Kozik, 2007).

Etiology

Accidental hypothermia can result from (a) exposure to a cold environment, (b) immersion in cold water, or (c) lack of adequate clothing, shelter, or heat. Hypothermia is associated with near-drowning episodes because body heat is lost more quickly in water than in air. Other causes of hypothermia include ingestion of alcohol or barbiturates, trauma or a brain disorder that interferes with temperature regulation, and overwhelming sepsis. If skin and underlying tissues are damaged by freezing cold, frostbite results.

A newborn is at a distinct disadvantage in maintaining a normal temperature. With a large body surface in relation to mass and a limited amount of insulating subcutaneous fat, the full-term newborn loses about four times more heat than an adult. The newborn's poor thermal stability is primarily due to excessive heat loss rather than impaired heat production. Because of the risk of hypothermia and possible cold stress, minimizing heat loss in the newborn after birth is essential. Once the infant has been dried after birth, the highest losses of heat generally result from radiation and convection because of the newborn's large body surface compared with weight. Thermal conduction is also a risk because of the marked difference between the newborn's core temperature and skin temperature. The newborn can respond to the cooler environmental temperature with adequate peripheral vasoconstriction, but this mechanism is not entirely effective because of the minimal amount of fat insulation present, the large body surface, and ongoing thermal conduction. Minimizing the baby's heat loss and preventing hypothermia are imperative.

The newborn has several physiologic mechanisms that increase heat production, or thermogenesis. These mechanisms include increased basal metabolic rate, muscular activity, and **chemical thermogenesis** (also called **nonshivering thermogenesis** or NST) (Rosenberg, 2007). NST is an important mechanism of heat production unique to the newborn. It occurs when skin receptors perceive a drop in the environmental temperature and, in response, transmit sensations to stimulate the sympathetic nervous system. NST uses the newborn's stores of **brown adipose tissue (BAT)** (also called brown fat) to provide heat. Brown fat receives its name from its dark color, which is caused by its enriched blood supply, dense cellular content, and abundant nerve endings. These characteristics of brown fat cells promote rapid metabolism, heat generation, and heat transfer to the peripheral circulation. The large numbers of brown fat cells increase the speed with which triglycerides are metabolized to produce heat.

NST from BAT is the primary source of heat in the hypothermic newborn. It first appears in the fetus at about 26–30 weeks' gestation and continues to increase until 2–5 weeks after the birth of a term infant, unless the fat is depleted by cold stress. Brown fat is deposited in the midscapular area, around the neck, and in the axillas, with deeper placement around the trachea, esophagus, abdominal aorta, kidneys, and adrenal glands (Figure 29–12 ■). BAT constitutes 2–6% of the newborn's total body weight.

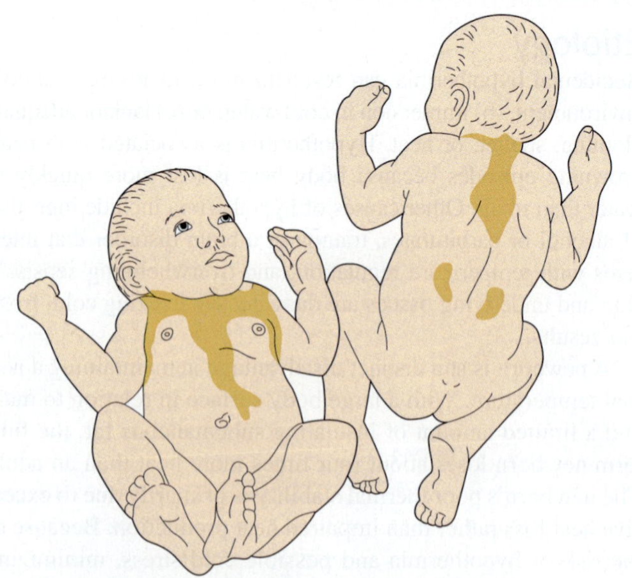

Figure 29–12 ■ The distribution of brown adipose tissue (brown fat) in the newborn.

Source: Adapted from Davis, V. (1980, November–December). Structure and function of brown adipose tissue in the neonate. *Journal of Obstetric, Gynecologic, and Neonatal Nursing, 9*, p.364.

Shivering, a form of muscular activity common in the cold adult, is rarely seen in the newborn, although it has been observed at ambient temperatures of 15°C (59°F) or less (Polin et al., 2004). If the newborn shivers, it means the newborn's metabolic rate has already doubled. The extra muscular activity does little to produce needed heat. Thermographic studies of newborns exposed to cold show an increase in the skin heat produced over the newborn's brown fat deposits between 1 and 14 days of age (Polin et al., 2004). However, if the brown fat supply has been depleted, the metabolic response to cold is limited or lacking. An increase in basal metabolism as a result of hypothermia results in an increase in oxygen consumption. A decrease in the environmental temperature of 2°C, from 33 to 31°C, is sufficient to double the oxygen consumption of a term newborn. Keeping the normal newborn warm promotes normal oxygen requirements, whereas chilling can cause signs of respiratory distress in the newborn.

When exposed to cold, the normal term newborn is usually able to cope with the increase in oxygen requirements. The preterm newborn, however, may be unable to increase ventilation to the necessary level of oxygen consumption. Because oxidation of fatty acids depends on the availability of oxygen, glucose, and adenosine triphosphate (ATP), the newborn's ability to generate heat can be altered by pathologic events. Such events include hypoxia, acidosis, and hypoglycemia or by medications that block the release of norepinephrine.

Meperidine (Demerol) given to a laboring woman or as a newborn analgesic can slow or prevent metabolism of newborn brown fat and lead to a greater decrease in the newborn's body temperature during the neonatal period. This effect of meperidine on brown fat is lessened if the mother and the newborn are well hydrated and in a neutral thermal environment. Newborn hypothermia prolongs as well as potentiates the effects of many analgesic and anesthetic drugs in the newborn.

The core temperature of infants is highly responsive to changes in the external environment; therefore, infants need extra protection from even mild variations in temperature. The core body temperature of children is more stable than that of infants but less so than that of adolescents or adults. However, older adults are more sensitive than middle adults to variations in environmental temperature. This increased sensitivity may be due to the decreased thermoregulatory control and loss of subcutaneous fat common in older adults, or it may be due to environmental factors such as lack of activity, inadequate diet, or lack of central heating. Illness or a central nervous system disorder may impair the thermostatic function of the hypothalamus.

FROSTBITE **Frostbite** is an injury of the skin resulting from freezing. If the exposure to freezing temperatures is limited, only the skin and subcutaneous tissues become involved. However, as exposure increases, deeper structures freeze. The skin freezes when the temperature drops to 14–24.8°F (21°–24°C). Frostbite is most common on exposed or peripheral areas of the body, such as the nose, ears, feet, and hands.

As human tissues freeze, ice crystals form, increasing intracellular sodium content. Small blood vessels initially vasoconstrict but then vasodilate and become more permeable, causing cells and tissues to swell. With continued exposure, vasoconstriction and increased viscosity of the blood cause infarction and necrosis of the affected tissue.

Superficial frostbite causes numbness, itching, and prickling. The skin appears cyanotic, reddened, or white. Deeper frostbite causes stiffness and paresthesias. As the skin and tissues thaw, the skin becomes white or yellow and loses its elasticity. The client experiences burning pain. Edema, blisters, necrosis, and gangrene may appear.

Rapid thawing may significantly decrease tissue necrosis. The following are general guidelines for rewarming areas of frostbite:

- Outdoors, treat superficial frostbite by applying firm pressure with a warm hand or by placing frostbitten hands in the axillae. If the feet are frostbitten, remove wet footwear, dry the feet, and put on dry footwear. Do not rub the areas with snow.
- In the hospital, rapidly rewarm affected areas in circulating warm water, 104–105°F (40–40.5°C) for 20–30 minutes. Do not rub or massage the areas.

Following rewarming, the client should kept on bedrest, with the affected parts elevated. Administer pain medications and anti-inflammatory agents and debride any blisters. Whirlpool therapy may be used to clean the skin and debride necrotic tissue. Recovery from frostbite is usually complete if the involved area has not become necrotic. Necrotic tissue may require amputation.

PRACTICE ALERT

Frostbite can also occur if a chemical ice pack (found in many first aid kits) is left in contact with the skin for too long. Avoid using these chemical packs in children if possible. When using a chemical ice pack, cover it with a few layers of clothing or towel and monitor the skin under the pack frequently. Remove the chemical ice pack if the skin starts to looks white or has decreased sensation. Remove the ice pack periodically to allow the skin to rewarm.

Risk Factors

Certain clients are at greater risk for accidental hypothermia. As people age, metabolic rate slows, placing the older adult at risk of hypothermia. This can be complicated further by reduced sensory perception, use of medications such as sedatives, and financial issues resulting in the inability to adequately heat their homes. Many suffer and die each year from hypothermia. A lowered metabolism and loss of normal insulation from thinning subcutaneous tissue decrease the older client's ability to retain heat. Older clients frequently prefer a warmer environment than younger adults. The older adult who spends time outdoors in cold weather or does not turn on the heat in the home is at significant risk for hypothermia.

Infants and young children are at risk because of immature temperature regulatory mechanisms, thinner skin, limited subcutaneous fat, and high ratios of skin surface area to body mass. Adolescents are at risk due to risk-taking behaviors including drug and alcohol use and engaging in remote outdoor activities without proper equipment or clothing. Alcohol causes peripheral vasodilation, which exposes the circulating bloodstream to more rapid cooling, resulting in a faster decrease in temperature. Drug and alcohol use may reduce the ability to sense cold, further exacerbating risk.

Other risk factors include damage to the hypothalamus, decreased ability to shiver, decreased metabolic rate, evaporation from skin in cool environments, exposure to a cool environment, illness, inactivity, inadequate clothing, malnutrition, medications, and trauma (NANDA, 2009). Hypothyroidism, immaturity of a newborn's temperature regulatory system, and ineffective thermoregulation can all contribute to hypothermia.

CLINICAL MANIFESTATIONS

Symptoms of mild hypothermia (32–35°C [90–95°F]) include fatigue, slurred speech, poor coordination and clumsiness, confusion and poor judgment, inappropriate behavior, shivering, tachycardia, and tachypnea. Symptoms of moderate hypothermia (28–32°C [82–90°F]) include depressed mental status, no shivering, depressed respirations, slow pulse or irregular heartbeat, low blood pressure, pale or cyanotic color, hallucinations, and coma. Profound hypothermia (body temperature below 28°C [82°F]) results in absence of respirations and pulse, ventricular fibrillation, dilated and unresponsive pupils, and coma.

PRACTICE ALERT

It is important to note that a client who is hypothermic should not be declared dead. Hypothermia reduces oxygen demands, and clients with hypothermia can survive cardiac arrest for far longer than those at normal temperature. As a result, clients in cardiac arrest who are hypothermic should be warmed and resuscitated. Only if resuscitation fails after warming should the client be declared dead.

COLLABORATION

Clients with severe hypothermia may require hemodialysis, peritoneal dialysis, or colonic irrigation in order to increase core body temperature. These interventions are typically used when hypothermia is the result of damage to the hypothalamus, usually due to trauma or cerebrovascular accidents (CVA). Such damage to the hypothalamus may make return of thermoregulation physiologically impossible.

Social service referrals may be indicated to assess the parents' ability to meet newborn or infant home care needs as well as for the client who experiences hypothermia because he or she is unable to provide a comfortable environmental temperature due to financial constraints or homelessness.

Free clinics and manufacturer prescription programs may be able to assist patients with limited incomes in getting some of their medications free or at reduced cost.

CLINICAL MANIFESTATIONS AND THERAPIES Hypothermia

ETIOLOGY	CLINICAL MANIFESTATION	CLINICAL THERAPIES
Reduction in temperature results in decreased metabolic rate and reduced oxygen demands, slowing respirations and pulse rate.	Decreased body temperature, pulse, and respirations	■ Provide a warm environment. ■ Provide dry clothing. ■ Apply warm blankets. ■ Keep limbs close to body. ■ Cover the client's scalp with a cap or turban. ■ Supply warm oral or intravenous fluids. ■ Apply warming pads.
The body's compensatory mechanism initiates shivering to produce heat from muscle activity.	Severe shivering (initially)	
	Feelings of cold and chills	
Hypothermia causes vasoconstriction to reduce exposure of the circulating bloodstream to the cold environment.	Pale, cool, waxy skin	
Vasoconstriction caused by hypothermia reduces peripheral circulation.	Frostbite (nose, fingers, toes)	■ Rapidly rewarm affected areas in circulating warm water, 104–105°F (40–40.5°C) for 20–30 minutes. ■ Do not rub or massage the areas. ■ Following rewarming, keep on bedrest with the affected parts elevated. ■ Administer analgesics and anti-inflammatory agents. ■ Debride blisters. ■ Administer whirlpool therapy to clean skin and debride necrotic tissue. ■ Necrotic tissue may require amputation. ■ Support respiratory and cardiac function. ■ Place on cardiorespiratory monitor. ■ Reduce handling as this increases the risk of cardiac fibrillation.
Reduced heart rate reduces cardiac output.	Hypotension	
Blood flow to the kidneys is reduced.	Decreased urinary output	
Blood flow to the brain is reduced secondary to slowed metabolic rate and reduced cardiac output.	Lack of muscle coordination	
	Disorientation	
	Drowsiness progressing to coma	

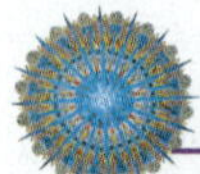

NURSING PROCESS

Assessment

The nurse assesses the client for defining characteristics of hypothermia, including the following:

- Lowered body temperature below normal range
- Cool skin
- Cyanotic nail beds due to vasoconstriction, resulting from the body's attempt to raise temperature and prevent further heat loss
- Hypertension
- Pallor
- **Piloerection** (goosebumps)
- Shivering
- Slowed capillary refill
- Tachycardia.

Diagnosis

Potential NANDA nursing diagnoses (NANDA, 2009) for the client with hypothermia include the following:

- Imbalanced Body Temperature
- Hypothermia.

Plan

Prevention is a primary nursing goal. Suggested Nursing Outcome Classifications recommends the following outcomes:

- Thermoregulation: balance among heat production, heat gain, and heat loss
- Thermoregulation in Neonate: balance among heat production, heat gain, and heat loss during the first 28 days of life
- Vital signs: extent to which temperature is within normal range.

Implementation

Managing hypothermia involves removing the client from the cold and rewarming the client's body. For mild hypothermia, warm the client by applying blankets; for severe hypothermia, apply a **hyperthermia blanket** (an electronically controlled blanket that provides a specified temperature) and give warm intravenous fluids. Wet clothing, which increases heat loss because of the high conductivity of water, should be replaced with dry clothing. See the Clinical Manifestations and Therapies box for nursing interventions used to treat clients with hypothermia. Monitor vital signs and urine output during active rewarming and assess the client for cold-related injuries.

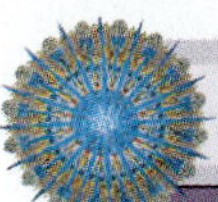

NURSING CARE PLAN **Hypothermia**

ASSESSMENT	DIAGNOSIS	PLANNING
Jerry Karpinski, an 87-year-old Caucasian male, is brought to the emergency room after his son found him unresponsive. The son reports that the client has lived alone in a single family home in Minnesota since his wife died 3 years ago. Mr. Karpinski depends on his Social Security income as his sole means of financial support and has been trying to keep his utility bills low by setting his thermostat to 15.6°C (60°F). His son checks on him every day and found him lying on the kitchen floor near the stove. Mr. Karpinski has a history of hypothyroidism and hypertension. He recently began taking sedatives to help him sleep at night. Vital signs: 29°C rectal – 52-6, BP 82/36. Height: 183 cm (6'). Weight: 72.7 kg (160 lb). Skin pale, cool to touch; nail beds cyanotic; breath sounds diminished throughout; pulse weak and thready. Nonresponsive to voice or stimulation. (Deep pain response not evaluated secondary to hypothermia.)	Hypothermia as evidenced by rectal temperature of 29°C	Mr. Karpinski will demonstrate thermoregulation as evidenced by the following indicators: ■ Increased skin temperature ■ Skin color becoming pink and less pale ■ Presence of piloerection when cold ■ Shivering when cold ■ Reported thermal comfort

IMPLEMENTATION

- Gradually rewarm Mr. Karpinski using a heating blanket until his temperature reaches 36°C.
- Administer warm IV solutions to maintain hydration.
- Utilize continuous core temperature monitoring device.
- Monitor continuously and record vital signs and cardiac rhythm on cardiorespiratory monitor.
- Make a referral to social services.
- Teach client and family how to prevent hypothermia.
- Teach client and family indications of hypothermia and appropriate emergency treatment.
- Reduce manual stimulation.

EVALUATION

As Mr. Karpinski's core temperature approaches normal range, he becomes increasingly more alert and vital signs return to normal ranges. Mr. Karpinski was at increased risk for hypothermia due to his age and poorly controlled hypothyroidism. Prior to discharge, Mr. Karpinski and his son were able to explain signs of early hypothermia, strategies for preventing hypothermia, and the importance of taking his thyroid hormone supplement every day. Social services contacted a local agency that can help the client pay for his prescription medications, freeing him to pay his utility bills to maintain an acceptable environmental temperature.

CRITICAL THINKING

1. What factors contributed to Mr. Karpinski's development of hypothermia?
2. The care plan focuses on the acute care of Mr. Karpinski's hypothermia. Once the client's temperature returns to normal range, what nursing care will this client require? Why will that care be required?
3. What client teaching (other than that mentioned in the plan of care) would the nurse initiate? Why?
4. Does this event indicate that the client is no longer able to care for himself? Explain the assessments you would perform to reach a decision about the client's competence for self-care.

Newborns

The amount of heat an infant loses depends to a large extent on the actions of the nurse or caregiver. During the transfer of a newborn in the neonatal intensive care unit (NICU) from one bed to another, a transient (although not significant) decrease in temperature may be noted for up to 1 hour. Prevention of heat loss is especially critical in the very-low-birth-weight (VLBW) infant. Placing the VLBW newborn in a polyethylene wrapping immediately following birth can decrease the postnatal drop in temperature that normally occurs. Using head coverings made of insulated fabrics, wool, polyolefin, or lined with Gamgee can significantly decrease heat loss after childbirth (Blackburn, 2007). Convective, radiant, and evaporative heat losses can all be reduced (Blackburn, 2007). Swaddling and nesting maintain flexion, which reduces exposed surface area and thus convective and radiant losses. The nurse observes all newborns for signs of cold stress, including increased movement and respirations, decreased skin temperature and peripheral perfusion, development of hypoglycemia, and possible development of metabolic acidosis. Vasoconstriction is the initial response to cold stress; because it initially decreases skin temperature, the nurse should monitor and assess skin temperature instead of rectal temperature. A decrease in rectal temperature means that the infant has longstanding cold stress. By monitoring skin temperature, a possible decrease will become apparent before the infant's core temperature is affected. If a decrease in skin temperature is noted, the nurse determines whether hypoglycemia is present. Hypoglycemia is a result of the metabolic effects of cold stress and is suggested by glucometer values below 40 mg/dL, tremors, irritability or lethargy, apnea, or seizure activity.

If hypothermia occurs with a newborn, the following nursing interventions should be initiated (Blackburn, 2007; Cloherty, Eichenwald, & Stark, 2008):

- Maintain a neutral thermal environment (NTE); adjust based on the gestational age and postnatal age.
- Warm the newborn slowly because rapid temperature elevation may cause hypotension and apnea.
- Increase the air temperature in hourly increments of 1°C (33.8°F) until the infant's temperature is stable.
- Monitor skin temperature every 15–30 minutes to determine if the newborn's temperature is increasing.
- Remove plastic wrap, caps, and heat shields while rewarming the infant so that cool air as well as warm air is not trapped.
- Warm intravenous fluids before infusion.
- Initiate efforts to block heat loss by evaporation, radiation, convection, and conduction; maintain the newborn in NTE such as a heated incubator for transport and radiant heater for procedures.

The nurse assesses for the presence of anaerobic metabolism and initiates interventions for the resulting metabolic acidosis. Attempts to burn brown fat increase oxygen consumption, lactic acid levels, and metabolic acidosis. Hypoglycemia may be reversed by adequate glucose intake.

Children

Parents should be educated to layer children's clothing and use hats in cold climates, recognize signs of hypothermia, decrease time of exposure to cold, and know how to treat mild hypothermia. The nurse teaches school-age children and adolescents who go on camping and hunting trips how to recognize and manage hypothermia in themselves and others. Teach preventive techniques, such as avoiding riding snow mobiles or walking on ice that may not be deep enough to support the child's weight. First aid for hypothermia includes moving the child to a dry area, removing any wet clothing, and protecting the child from further environmental exposure. The nurse should wrap the child in dry blankets or dress the child in warm, dry clothing, and encourage the child to drink a warm, high-calorie liquid, if able.

Older Adults

Older adults are at increased risk for hypothermia because their bodies are less able to maintain a constant internal temperature. Chronic conditions (problems with the circulatory or neurological systems, hypothyroidism, etc), medication use, reduced sensory perception, and cognitive disorders can all increase risk still further. Initial treatment is similar to treatment for hypothermia at any age, including removing wet clothing, increasing environmental temperatures, applying more clothing or blankets, and providing warm liquids. However, once the initial hypothermia is resolved, the nurse should assess for other issues that may place the geriatric client at increased risk for recurrent hypothermia. These may include nutritional status, financial concerns limiting their ability to heat their homes, and self-care deficits.

Evaluation

Evaluation criteria include determining that the client will:

- not exhibit piloerection or shivering,
- maintain core temperature within normal ranges,
- report thermal comfort,
- describe adaptive measures to minimize fluctuations in body temperature, and
- report early signs and symptoms of hypothermia (Wilkinson & Ahern, 2009).

HEALTH CARE

Further information regarding disparity in availability of health care may be found in Concept 8, Diversity; Concept 13, Health, Wellness, and Illness; and Concept 49, Safety.

REVIEW Hypothermia

RELATE: LINK THE CONCEPTS

Linking the exemplar of Hypothermia with the concept of Safety:

1. When teaching a class on safety at a long-term care facility, what teaching points would the nurse discuss regarding prevention of hypothermia in the geriatric client?
2. What safety measures should the nurse teach the new mother of a baby born prematurely to avoid hypothermia?

Linking the exemplar of Hypothermia with the concept of Safety:

1. Why is the client who abuses alcohol at increased risk for hypothermia?
2. A client is brought to the emergency department with no pulse, an elevated blood alcohol level, and a core temperature of 88.4 degrees Fahrenheit. What is the priority nursing action? Explain the rationale for your answer.

READY: GO TO COMPANION SKILLS MANUAL

- Assess body temperature

REFER: GO TO MYNURSINGKIT

REFLECT: CASE STUDY

Baby girl Cho is born at 34 weeks' gestation to Mr. and Mrs. Cho. This is their first child. They attended Lamaze classes because they wanted to deliver the baby using natural childbirth methods and avoided all medications during labor. The baby has made a successful transition to extrauterine life and is breathing independently and maintaining oxygenation without assistance. After spending 30 minutes bonding with her parents, the baby is brought to the newborn nursery. The baby's axillary temperature is 34.2°C and she begins to demonstrate mild substernal and intercostal retractions and nasal flaring. Respiratory rate is 52 and apical pulse is 148.

1. What factors may contribute to the baby's development of respiratory distress?
2. What are the priority nursing interventions for this newborn?
3. What nursing interventions would be appropriate to warm the newborn?

PEARSON
EXPLORE mynursingkit™

MyNursingKit is your one stop for online chapter review materials and resources. Prepare for success with additional NCLEX®-style practice questions, interactive assignments and activities, web links, animations and videos, and more!

Register your access code from the front of your book at **www.mynursingkit.com**.

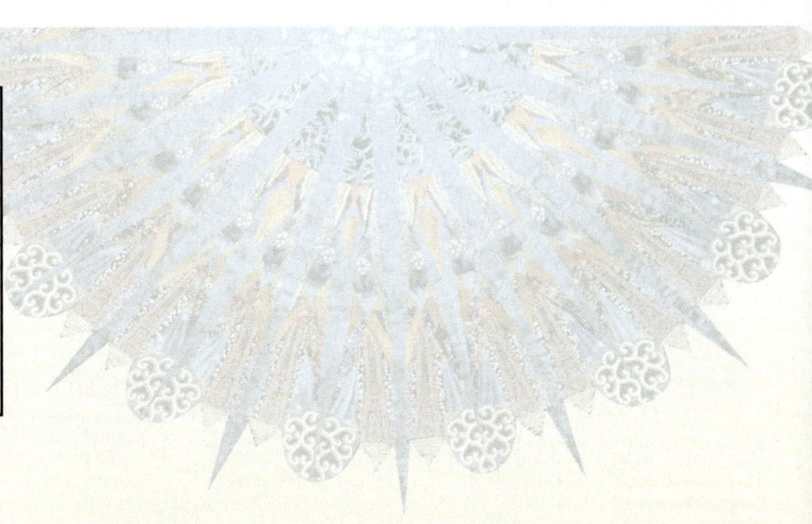

REFERENCES

Ball, J.W., & Bindler, R.C.(2008). *Pediatric nursing: Caring for children* (4th ed.). Upper Saddle River, NJ: Pearson, Inc.

Berman, A., Snyder, S.J., Kozier, B., & Erb, G. (2008). *Kozier & Erb's fundamentals of nursing: Concepts, process, and practice* (8th ed.). Upper Saddle River, NJ: Pearson, Inc.

Bindler, R. C., & Ball, J. W. (2003). *Clinical skills manual for pediatric nursing: Caring for children* (3rd ed.). Upper Saddle River, NJ: Prentice Hall Health.

Blackburn, S. T. (2007). *Maternal, fetal, & neonatal physiology: A clinical perspective* (3rd ed.). St. Louis: W.B. Saunders.

Brandom, B. W. (2005). The genetics of malignant hyperthermia. *Anesthesiology Clinics of North America, 23*, 615–619.

Carson, S. M. (2003). Alternating acetaminophen and ibuprofen in the febrile child: Examining the evidence regarding efficacy and safety. *Pediatric Nursing, 29*(5), 379–382.

Carter-Templeton, H. (2005). Malignant hyperthermia. *Nursing, 35*(6), 88.

Cloherty, J. P., Eichenwald, E. C., & Stark, A. R.(2008). *Manual of neonatal care* (6th ed.). Philadelphia: Lippincott Williams & Wilkins.

Clumpner, M., & Mobley, J. (2008). Raising the dead: Prehospital hypothermia for cardiac arrest victims may improve neurological outcome and survival to discharge. *EMS Magazine, 37*(9), 52–60.

Crocetti, M. T., & Serwint, J. R. (2005). Fever: Separating fact from fiction. *Contemporary Pediatrics, 22*(1), 34–41.

DuBois, E. F. (1948). *Fever and the regulation of body temperature*. Springfield, IL: Charles C. Thomas.

Gieron-Korthals, M., & Gill, J. K. (2002). Febrile convulsions: An ever changing story. What every pediatrician should know about it. *Contemporary Pediatrics, 19*(5):139-144.

Kozik, T. M. (2007). Induced hypothermia for patients with cardiac arrest: Role of a clinical nurse specialist. *Critical Care Nurse, 27*(5), 41–42.

Ladewig, P. W., London, M. L., & Davidson, M. R. (2010). *Contemporary maternal-newborn nursing care* (7th ed.). Upper Saddle River, NJ: Pearson, Inc.

LeMone, P., & Burke, K. (2008). *Medical-surgical nursing: Critical thinking in client care* (4th ed.). Upper Saddle River, NJ: Pearson, Inc.

Litman, R. S., & Rosenberg, H. (2005). Malignant hyperthermia: Update on susceptibility testing. *Journal of the American Medical Association, 293*(23), 2918–2924.

Liu, C. C., Chang, R. E., & Chang, W. C. (2004). Limitations of forehead infrared body temperature detection for fever screening for severe acute respiratory syndrome. *Infection Control Hospital Epidemiology, 25*, 1109–1111.

Mackowiak, P. A., Wasserman, S. S., & Levine, M. M. (1992). A critical appraisal of 98.6 degrees F, the upper limit of the normal body temperature, and other legacies of Carl Reinhold August Wunderlich. *Journal of the American Medical Association, 268*, 1578–1580.

Marieb, E. N. & Hoehn, K. (2007). *Human anatomy and physiology* (7th ed.). San Francisco: Benjamin Cummings.

NANDA International. (2009). *Nursing diagnoses: Definitions and classification 2009-2011*. Chichester, West Susex, UK: Wiley-Blackwell.

Nativio, D. G. (2005). Understanding fever in children. *American Journal for Nurse Practitioners, 9*(11/12), 47–52.

Nimah, M. M., Bshesh, K., Callahan, J., & Jacobs, B. R. (2006). Infrared tympanic thermometry in comparison with other temperature measurement techniques in febrile children. *Pediatric Critical Care Medicine, 7*, 48–55.

Polin, R. A., Fox, W.W., & Abman, S. H. (2004). *Fetal and neonatal physiology* (3rd ed.). Philadelphia: W.B. Saunders.

Rosenberg, A. A. (2007). The neonate. In S. G. Gabbe, J. R. Niebyl, & J. L. Simpson (Eds.). *Obstetrics: Normal and problem pregnancies* (5th ed., pp. 523–565). Philadelphia: Churchill Livingstone/Elsevier.

Roy, S., Powell, K., & Gerson, L. W. (2003). Temporal artery temperature measurements in healthy infants, children, and adolescents. *Clinical Pediatrics, 42*, 433–437.

Smith, L. S. (2004). Temperature measurement in critical care adults: A comparison of thermometry and measurement routes. *Biological Research for Nursing, 6*(2), 117–125.

Smith, L. S. (2004). Temperature monitoring in newborns, a comparison of thermometry and measurement sites. *Journal of Neonatal Nursing, 10*, 157–165.

Sund Levander, M., Grodzinsky, E., Loyd, D., & Wahren, L. K. (2004). Errors in body temperature assessment related to individual variation, measuring technique and equipment. *International Journal of Nursing Practice, 10*, 216–223.

Wilkinson, J. M., & Ahern, N. R. (2009). *Nursing diagnosis handbook* (9th ed.). Upper Saddle River, NJ: Prentice Hall.

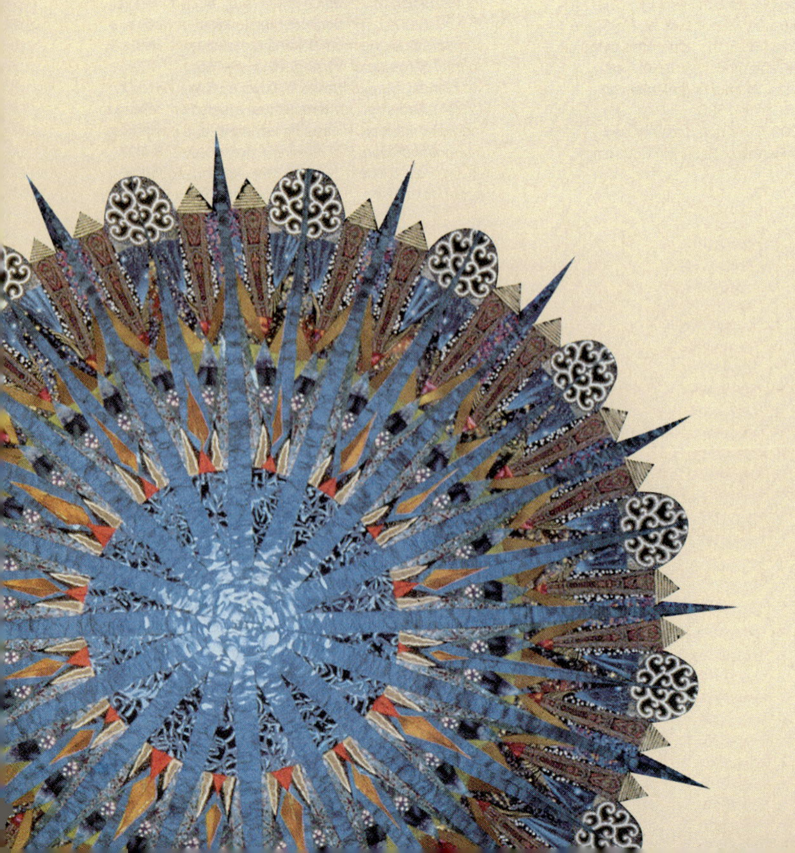

Tissue Integrity 30

Concept at-a-Glance

Concept Learning Outcomes

After reading about this concept, you will be able to:

1. Summarize the structure and physiological processes of the integumentary system related to skin and tissue integrity.
2. List factors affecting skin and tissue integrity.
3. Identify commonly occurring alterations in skin and tissue integrity and their related treatments.
4. Explain common physical assessment procedures used to examine skin and tissue health of clients across the life span.
5. Outline diagnostic and laboratory tests to determine the individual's skin and tissue health.
6. Explain management of skin and tissue health and prevention of alterations in skin and tissue integrity.
7. Demonstrate the nursing processes in providing culturally competent care across the life span for individuals with common alterations in skin and tissue integrity.
8. Identify pharmacologic interventions in caring for the individual with alterations in skin and tissue integrity.

Concept Key Terms

Alopecia, *1883*
Dermis, *1875*
Ecchymosis, *1882*
Edema, *1880*
Epidermis, *1874*
Erythema, *1876*
Hirsutism, *1883*
Hypodermis, *1875*
Integumentary system, *1873*
Keratin, *1874*
Lesion, *1876*
Lichenification, *1876*
Melanin, *1874*
Pruritus, *1876*
Senile purpura, *1875*
Subcutaneous, *1875*
Urticaria, *1882*
Vitiligo, *1882*

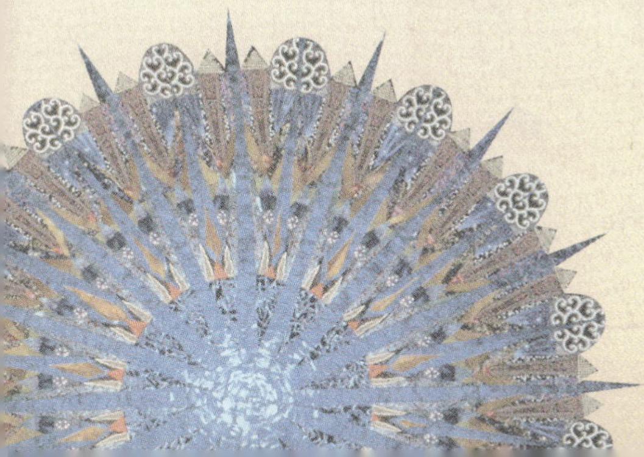

About Tissue Integrity

The largest organ in the body, the skin serves a variety of important functions in maintaining health and protecting the individual from injury. The skin is part of the body's **integumentary system**, which includes the skin, hair, and nails and the sebaceous, sweat, and mammary glands. Important nursing functions are maintaining skin integrity and promoting wound healing. Impaired skin integrity, that is, alterations to the dermis and epidermis, is not a serious problem for most healthy people but is a threat to older adults; to clients with restricted mobility, chronic illnesses, or trauma; and to those undergoing invasive health care procedures. To protect the skin and manage wounds effectively, the nurse must understand the factors that affect skin integrity, the physiology of wound healing, and specific measures that promote optimal conditions for the skin.

Tissue integrity includes integumentary, mucous membrane, corneal, or subcutaneous tissues uninterrupted by wounds. Tissue integrity is influenced by internal factors such as genetics, age, and the underlying health of the individual, as well as by external factors such as activity and injury. •

NORMAL PRESENTATION OF THE SKIN

The skin performs several essential functions. It protects underlying tissues from invasion by microorganisms and from trauma. The nerves in the skin enable the perception of touch, pain, pressure, heat, and cold. The skin also assists the body in regulating its temperature. Dilation of blood vessels and the secretion of sweat by the eccrine sweat glands, functioning under the control of the central nervous system, enable the body to release excess heat. The sweat glands, secreting a solution of water, electrolytes, and urea, also help rid the body of toxins. The skin supplements the body's intake of vitamin D by synthesizing this vitamin from ultraviolet light.

The skin has three distinct layers: the epidermis, the dermis, and the subcutaneous fatty layer that separates the skin from the underlying tissue (Figure 30–1 ■).

Epidermis

The **epidermis**, which is the surface or outermost part of the skin, consists of epithelial cells. The epidermis has either four or five layers, depending on its location. There are five layers over the palms of the hands and the soles of the feet, and there are four layers over the rest of the body.

The stratum basale is the deepest layer of the epidermis. It contains cells known as melanocytes, which produce the pigment melanin, and keratinocytes, which produce keratin. **Melanin** forms a protective shield to protect the keratinocytes and the nerve endings in the dermis from the damaging effects of ultraviolet light. Melanocyte activity probably accounts for the difference in skin color in humans. **Keratin** is a fibrous, water-repellent protein that gives the epidermis its tough, protective quality. As keratinocytes mature, they move upward through the epidermal layers, eventually becoming dead cells at the surface of the skin. Millions of these cells are worn off by abrasion each day, but millions more are simultaneously produced in the stratum basale. The next layer of the epidermis is the stratum spinosum. Several cells thick, this layer contains abundant cells that arise from the bone marrow and migrate to the epidermis. Mitosis occurs at this layer, although not as abundantly as in the stratum basale.

The stratum granulosum is only two to three cells thick. The cells of the stratum granulosum contain a glycolipid that slows water loss across the epidermis. Keratinization, a thickening of

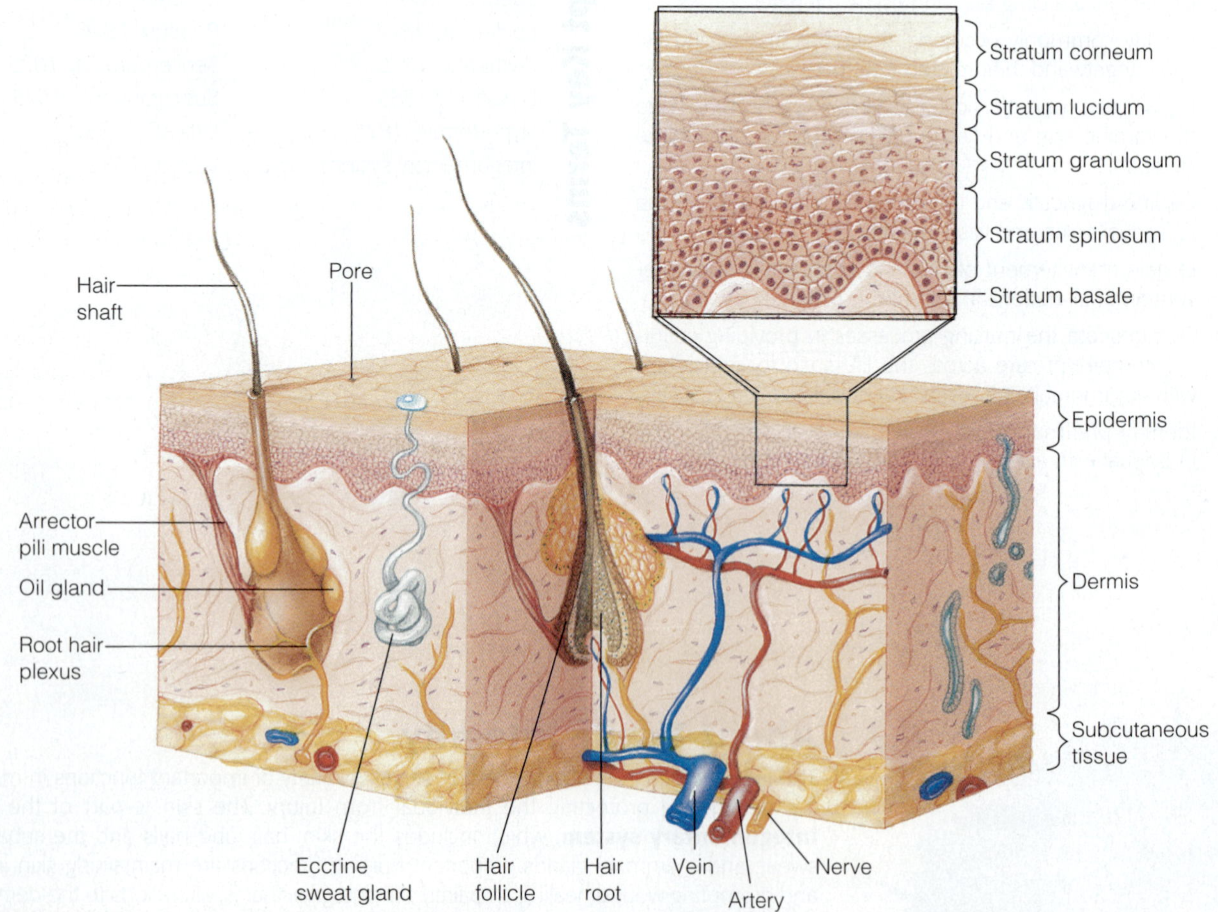

Figure 30–1 ■ Three-dimensional view of the skin, subcutaneous tissue, glands, and hairs.

the cells' plasma membranes, begins in the stratum granulosum. The stratum lucidum is present only in areas of thick skin. It is made up of flattened, dead keratinocytes.

The outermost layer of the epidermis, the stratum corneum, is also the thickest, making up about 75% of the total thickness of the epidermis. It consists of about 20–30 sheets of dead cells filled with keratin fragments arranged in "shingles" that flake off as dry skin.

Dermis

The **dermis** is the second, deeper layer of skin. Made of a flexible connective tissue, this layer is richly supplied with blood cells, nerve fibers, and lymphatic vessels. Most of the hair follicles, sebaceous glands, and sweat glands are located in the dermis. The dermis consists of a papillary and a reticular layer. The papillary layer contains ridges that indent the overlying epidermis. It also contains capillaries and receptors for pain and touch. The deeper, reticular layer contains blood vessels, sweat and sebaceous glands, deep pressure receptors, and dense bundles of collagen fibers. The regions between these bundles form lines of cleavage in the skin. Surgical incisions parallel to these lines of cleavage heal more easily and with less scarring than do incisions or traumatic wounds across cleavage lines.

Subcutaneous Tissue

The **subcutaneous** tissue (or **hypodermis**) is a loose connective tissue that stores approximately half of the body's fat cells. It cushions the body against trauma, insulates the body from heat loss, and stores fat for energy.

AGE-RELATED FACTORS

The newborn's skin is covered by vernix caseosa in utero, a greasy substance containing shed cells that cover and protect the fetal skin from amniotic fluid and urine (Chamley, 2005). It has many important properties, including anti-infective, antioxidant, moisturizing, and wound-healing agents (Stokowski, 2006).

The newborn's skin accounts for about 4% of body weight (Chamley, 2005). The infant's skin is thin, about 1 mm thick at birth, with little underlying subcutaneous fat. The skin grows to 2 mm thickness by adulthood. With thinner skin and less subcutaneous fat, the infant loses heat more rapidly, has greater difficulty regulating body temperature, and becomes chilled more quickly than an older child or an adult. The infant's thinner skin also allows increased absorption of harmful chemical substances and topical medications. The infant's skin contains more water than an adult's and has loosely attached cells. As the infant grows, the skin toughens and becomes less hydrated, making it less susceptible to bacteria.

Although changes occur in all of the body systems throughout life, skin and hair changes are the most visible and therefore greatly contribute to a person's self-perception and self-esteem. With normal aging, the thickness and elasticity of the skin decrease. These changes occur slowly, but by the seventh and eighth decades of life, they contribute to the appearance of wrinkled and sagging skin in the face, neck, and upper arms. The age-related changes in the skin's appearance correlate with changes in function (Table 30–1). To reduce risk factors and minimize negative consequences, it is important to understand normal changes, as well as environmentally induced damage. The normal changes of aging in the integumentary system are illustrated in the Developmental Considerations feature on page 1888.

Epidermis

The epidermal cells of the older person contain less moisture. This contributes to a dry, rough skin appearance. After 50 years of age, epidermal mitosis slows by 30%, resulting in a longer healing time for the older person. This increased healing time also may contribute to infection. Rete ridges, which connect the dermis and epidermis, flatten, resulting in fewer contact areas between these two layers. This increases the risk for skin tears in response to seemingly slight friction against the skin. The number and activity of melanocytes decrease with age, contributing to a paler complexion and an increased risk of damage from ultraviolet radiation for the light-skinned older person. Remaining cells may not function normally, resulting in scattered pigmented areas such as nevi, age spots, or liver spots and an increase in the number and size of freckles.

Dermis

The dermis decreases in thickness and functionality beginning in the third decade. Elastin decreases in quality but increases in quantity, resulting in wrinkling and sagging of the skin. Collagen becomes less organized, causing a loss of turgor. Men have a thicker dermal layer than women do, which explains the more rapid age-associated changes in the female facial appearance. The vascularity of the dermis decreases with age, contributing to a paler complexion in the light-skinned older person. The capillaries become thinner and more easily damaged, leading to bruised and discolored areas known as **senile purpura**. Both touch and pressure sensations gradually decline, putting the older person at risk for injuries such as burns and pressure ulcers.

Subcutaneous Tissue

With increasing age, gradual atrophy of subcutaneous tissue occurs in some areas of the body, and a gradual increase occurs in others. Subcutaneous tissue becomes thinner in the face, neck, hands, and lower legs, resulting in more visible veins in the exposed areas and skin that is more prone to damage. A gradual hypertrophy of subcutaneous tissue in some other areas of the body leads to an overall increase in the proportion of body fat for the older person. Overall, with aging, fat distribution is more pronounced in the abdomen and thighs in women and in the abdomen in men.

ALTERATIONS IN TISSUE INTEGRITY

Intact skin refers to the presence of normal skin and skin layers uninterrupted by wounds. The appearance of the skin and skin integrity are influenced by internal factors such as genetics, age, and the underlying health of the individual, as well as by external factors such as activity.

Many chronic illnesses and their treatments affect skin integrity. People with impaired peripheral arterial circulation

TABLE 30–1 Age-Related Skin Changes

AGE-RELATED CHANGE	SIGNIFICANCE
Epidermis: ↓ thickness and miotic activity	■ Skin more fragile and at greater risk for tears or injury ■ Delayed wound healing ■ Hyperkeratoses and skin cancers in sun-exposed areas more evident
Epidermis: ↑ permeability, ↓ Langerhans cells	■ Increased risk of reactions to irritants ■ Decreased inflammatory response ■ Increased susceptibility to sun exposure
Epidermis: hyperplasia of melanocytes, especially in sun-exposed areas	■ Small areas of hyperpigmentation (liver spots) and hypopigmentation (age spots), especially on the hands
Epidermis: ↓ vitamin D production	■ Increased risk of osteomalacia and osteoporosis ■ Increased risk of skin tears, purpura, and pressure ulcers
Dermis: ↓ perfusion	■ Greater susceptibility to dry skin ■ Decreased sensation (pain, touch, temperature, and peripheral vibration) ■ Increased risk of injury
Dermis: ↓ vasomotor response	■ Greater risk of hyperthermia and hypothermia
Dermis: elastic fiber degeneration	■ Decreased tone and elasticity, with wrinkle formation
Dermis: proliferation of capillaries	■ Cherry hemangiomas common
Subcutaneous skin layer: thinning	■ Greater risk of hypothermia ■ Increased risk of pressure ulcers
Subcutaneous skin layer: redistribution of adipose tissue	■ Cellulite formation ■ Bags over and under the eyes ■ Double chin formation ■ Increase in abdominal fat ■ Sagging of breasts ■ Skin slower to return to normal when pinched (tenting)
Glands: ↓ eccrine and apocrine activity	■ Dry skin common ■ Absent perspiration

may have skin on their legs that appears shiny, has lost its hair distribution, and damages easily. Some medications, such as corticosteroids, cause thinning of the skin, making it much more easily harmed. Many medications increase sensitivity to sunlight and can predispose one to severe sunburns. Some of the most common medications that cause this kind of damage are certain antibiotics, chemotherapy drugs for cancer, and some psychotherapeutic drugs. Poor nutrition alone can interfere with the appearance and function of normal skin.

Some skin disorders have vague, generalized signs and symptoms, and others have specific and easily identifiable causes. **Pruritus**, or itching, is a general condition associated with dry, scaly skin; it may also be a symptom of mite or lice infestation. Inflammation, a characteristic of burns and other traumatic disorders, occurs when damage to the skin is extensive. Local **erythema**, or redness, accompanies inflammation and many other skin disorders. Trauma to deeper tissues may cause additional symptoms, such as bleeding, bruising, and infections.

Skin disorders are diverse and difficult to classify. These disorders are summarized in Table 30–2. One simple classification method is to group them into the following general categories:

- *Infectious.* Bacterial, fungal, viral, and parasitic infections of the skin and mucous membranes are relatively common and are frequently indications for anti-infective pharmacotherapy.
- *Inflammatory.* Inflammatory disorders encompass a broad range of pathologies that includes acne, burns, eczema, dermatitis, and psoriasis.
- *Neoplastic.* Neoplastic disease includes malignant melanoma and basal cell carcinoma.

Dermatologic signs and symptoms may reflect disease processes occurring elsewhere in the body. Skin abnormalities, including surface lesions of various colors, sizes, types, and character, and abnormal skin turgor and moisture may have systemic causes. These can include liver or renal impairment, cardiovascular insufficiency, metastatic tumors, recent injury, and poor nutritional status.

Skin **lesions** (observable changes from normal skin structure) vary in size, shape, color, and texture characteristics. Primary lesions arise from previously healthy skin and include macules, patches, papules, nodules, tumors, vesicles, pustules, bullae, and wheals. Secondary lesions result from changes in primary lesions. They include crusts, scales, **lichenification** (thickening of the skin), scars, keloids, excoriation, fissures, erosion, and ulcers. It is

Normal Changes of Aging in the Integumentary System

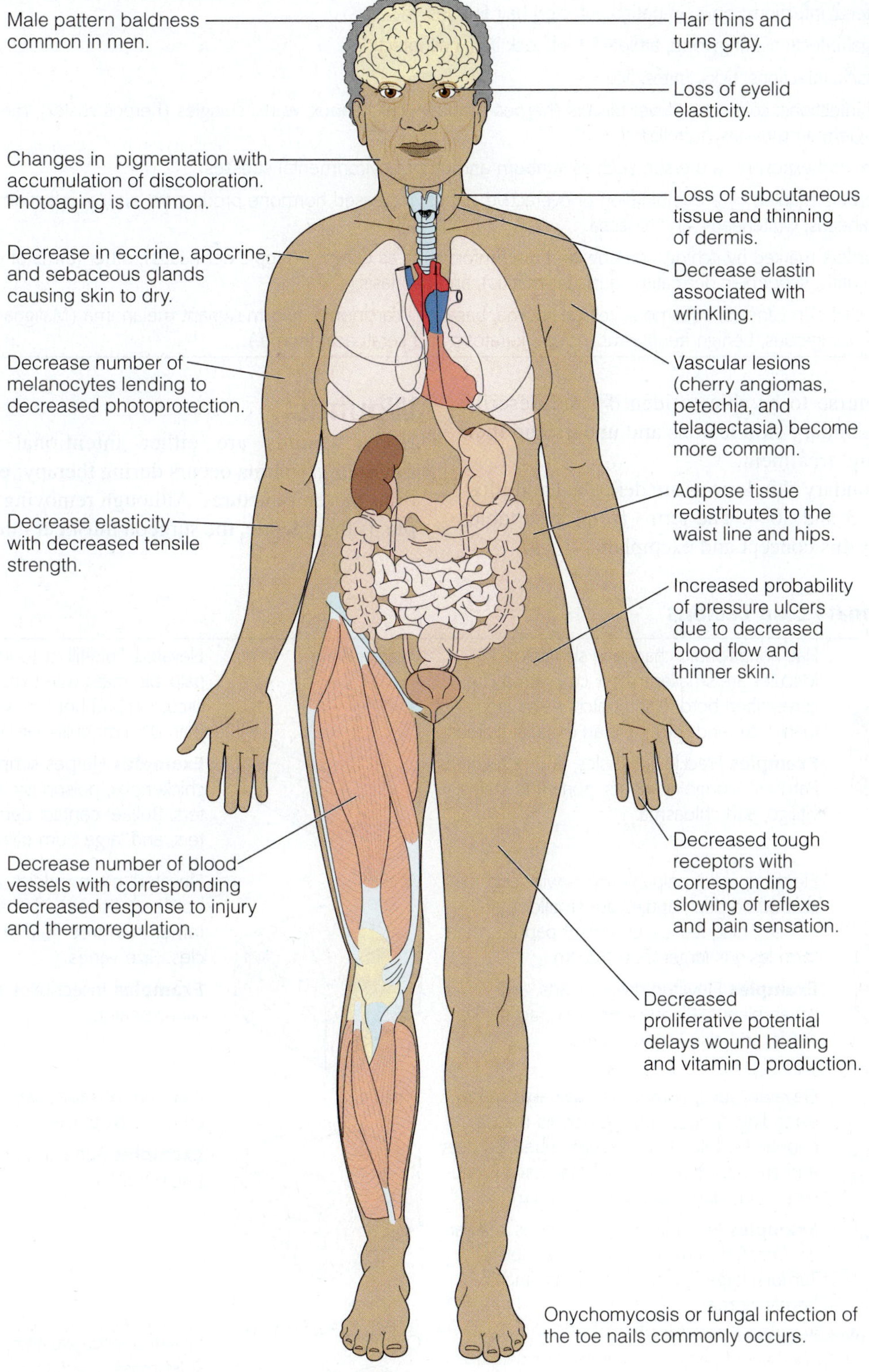
Male pattern baldness common in men.
Hair thins and turns gray.
Loss of eyelid elasticity.
Changes in pigmentation with accumulation of discoloration. Photoaging is common.
Loss of subcutaneous tissue and thinning of dermis.
Decrease in eccrine, apocrine, and sebaceous glands causing skin to dry.
Decrease elastin associated with wrinkling.
Decrease number of melanocytes lending to decreased photoprotection.
Vascular lesions (cherry angiomas, petechia, and telagectasia) become more common.
Adipose tissue redistributes to the waist line and hips.
Decrease elasticity with decreased tensile strength.
Increased probability of pressure ulcers due to decreased blood flow and thinner skin.
Decreased tough receptors with corresponding slowing of reflexes and pain sensation.
Decrease number of blood vessels with corresponding decreased response to injury and thermoregulation.
Decreased proliferative potential delays wound healing and vitamin D production.
Onychomycosis or fungal infection of the toe nails commonly occurs.

TABLE 30–2 **Classification of Skin Disorders**

TYPE	EXAMPLES
Infectious	Bacterial infections: boils, impetigo, infected hair follicles
	Fungal infections: ringworm, athlete's foot, jock itch, nail infection
	Parasitic infections: ticks, mites, lice
	Viral infections: cold sores, fever blisters (herpes simplex), chickenpox, warts, shingles (herpes zoster), measles (rubeola), and German measles (rubella)
Inflammatory	Injury and exposure to the sun such as sunburn and other environmental stresses
	Disorders marked by a combination of overactive glands, increased hormone production, and/or infection such as acne, blackheads, whiteheads, and rosacea
	Disorders marked by itching, cracking, and discomfort such as eczema (atopic dermatitis), other forms of dermatitis (contact dermatitis, seborrheic dermatitis, stasis dermatitis), and psoriasis
Neoplastic	Types of skin cancers: squamous cell carcinoma, basal cell carcinoma, and malignant melanoma (Malignant melanoma is the most dangerous; benign neoplasms include keratosis and keratoacanthoma.)

important for the nurse to be able to identify and describe the primary and secondary skin lesions and understand their underlying cause and treatment.

Primary and secondary skin lesions are described and illustrated in Tables 30–3 and 30–4. The terms from these tables are used throughout this concept and exemplars.

Wounds

Body wounds are either intentional or unintentional. *Intentional* trauma occurs during therapy; examples are operations or venipunctures. Although removing a tumor, for example, is therapeutic, the surgeon must cut into body tissues, thus

TABLE 30–3 **Primary Skin Lesions**

Macule, Patch

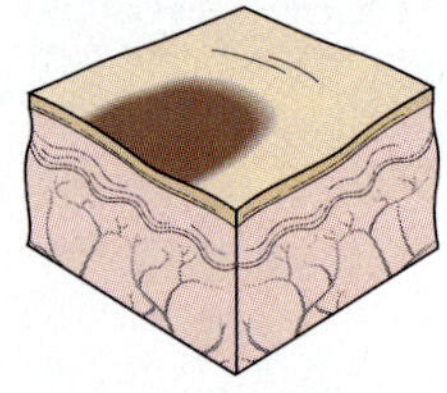

Flat, nonpalpable change in skin color. Macules are smaller than 1 cm, with a circumscribed border, and patches are larger than 1 cm and may have an irregular border.

Examples Freckles, measles, and petechiae. Patches: Mongolian spots, port-wine stains, vitiligo, and chloasma.

Papule, Plaque

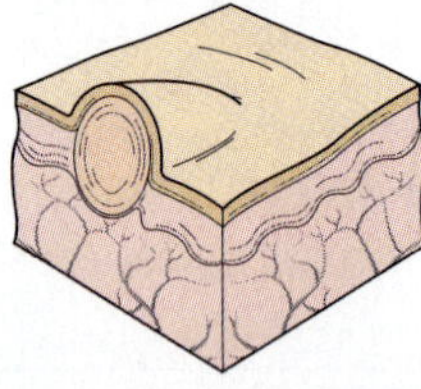

Elevated, solid, palpable mass with circumscribed border. Papules are smaller than 0.5 cm; plaques are groups of papules that form lesions larger than 0.5 cm.

Examples Elevated moles, warts, and lichen planus. Plaques: psoriasis, actinic keratosis, and also lichen planus.

Nodule, Tumor

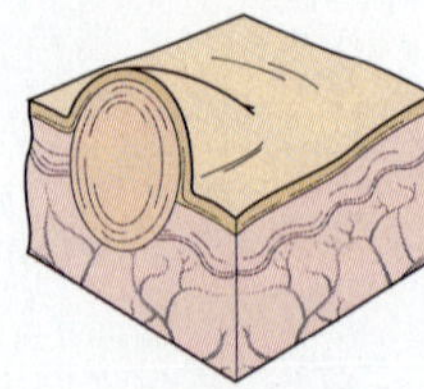

Elevated, solid, hard or soft palpable mass extending deeper into the dermis than a papule. Nodules have circumscribed borders and are 0.5–2 cm; tumors may have irregular borders and are larger than 2 cm.

Examples Small lipoma, squamous cell carcinoma, fibroma, and intradermal nevi. Tumors: large lipoma, carcinoma, and hemangioma.

Vesicle, Bulla

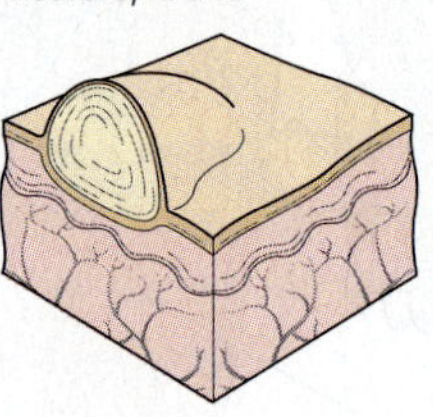

Elevated, fluid-filled, round or oval-shaped, palpable mass with thin, translucent walls and circumscribed borders. Vesicles are smaller than 0.5 cm; bullae are larger than 0.5 cm.

Examples Herpes simplex/zoster, early chickenpox, poison ivy, and small burn blisters. Bullae: contact dermatitis, friction blisters, and large burn blisters.

Wheal

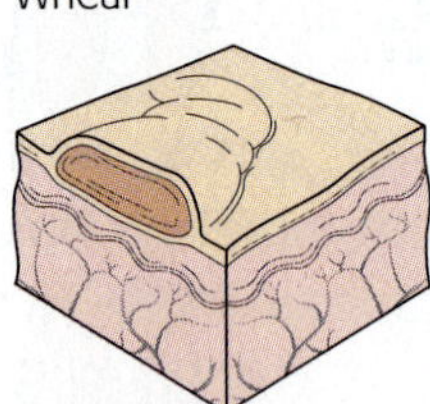

Elevated, often reddish area with irregular border caused by diffuse fluid in tissues rather than free fluid in a cavity, as in vesicles. Size varies.

Examples Insect bites and hives (extensive wheals).

Pustule

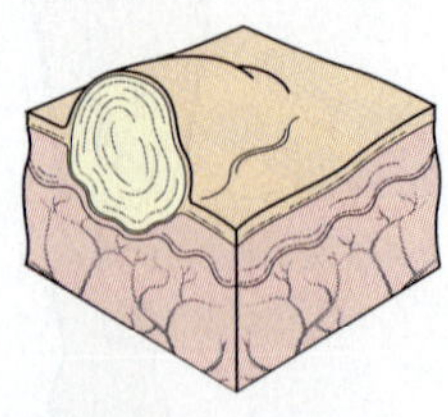

Elevated, pus-filled vesicle or bulla with circumscribed border. Size varies.

Examples Acne, impetigo, and carbuncles (large boils).

Cyst

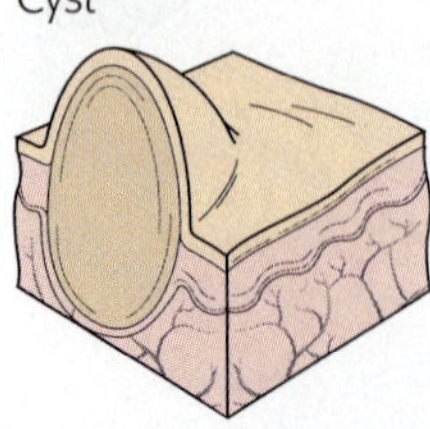

Elevated, encapsulated, fluid-filled or semisolid mass originating in the subcutaneous tissue or dermis, usually 1 cm or larger.

Examples Varieties include sebaceous cysts and epidermoid cysts.

TABLE 30–4 Secondary Skin Lesions

Lesion	Description	Lesion	Description
Atrophy 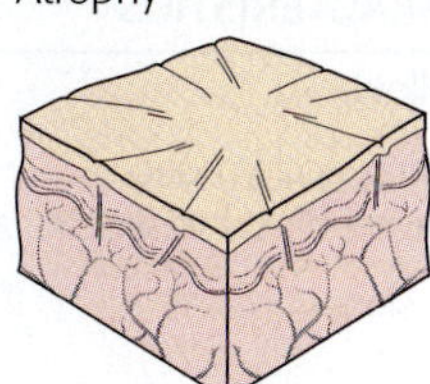	A translucent, dry, paper-like, sometimes wrinkled skin surface resulting from thinning or wasting of the skin due to loss of collagen and elastin. **Examples** Striae, aged skin.	Ulcer 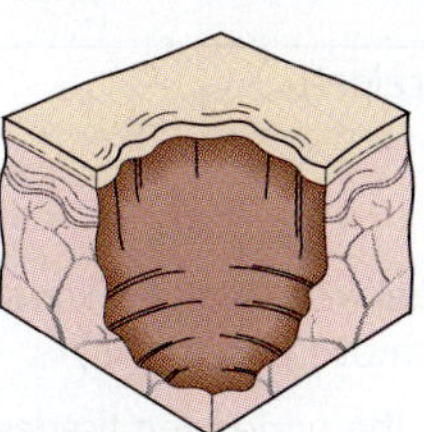	Deep, irregularly shaped area of skin loss extending into the dermis or sub cutaneous tissue. May bleed. May leave scar. **Examples** Decubitus ulcers (pressure sores), stasis ulcers, chancres.
Erosion 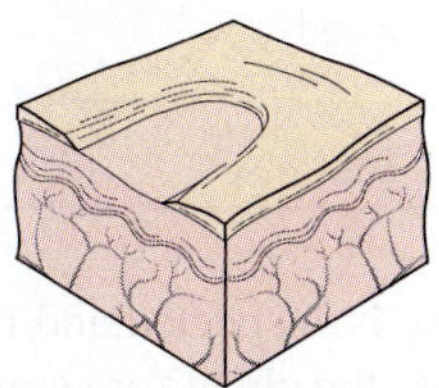	Wearing away of the superficial epidermis causing a moist, shallow depression. Because erosions do not extend into the dermis, they heal without scarring. **Examples** Scratch marks, ruptured vesicles.	Fissure 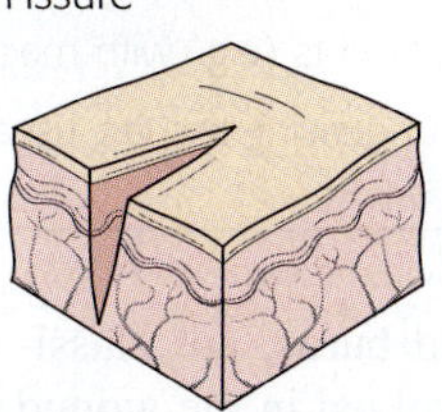	Linear crack with sharp edges, extending into the dermis. **Examples** Cracks at the corners of the mouth or in the hands, athlete's foot.
Lichenification 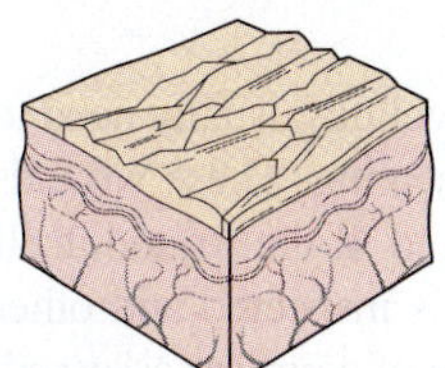	Rough, thickened, hardened area of epidermis resulting from chronic irritation such as scratching or rubbing. **Example** Chronic dermatitis.	Scar 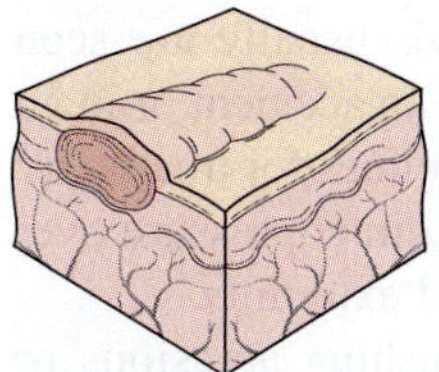	Flat, irregular area of connective tissue left after a lesion or wound has healed. New scars may be red or purple; older scars may be silvery or white. **Examples** Healed surgical wound or injury, healed acne.
Scales 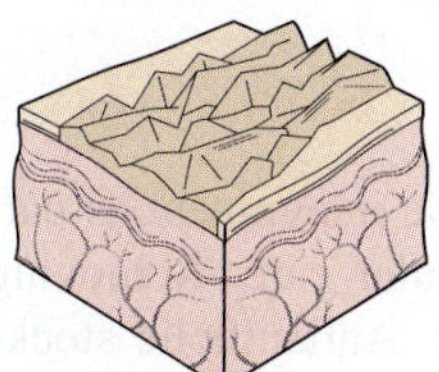	Shedding flakes of greasy, keratinized skin tissue. Color may be white, gray, or silver. Texture may vary from fine to thick. **Examples** Dry skin, dandruff, psoriasis, and eczema.	Keloid 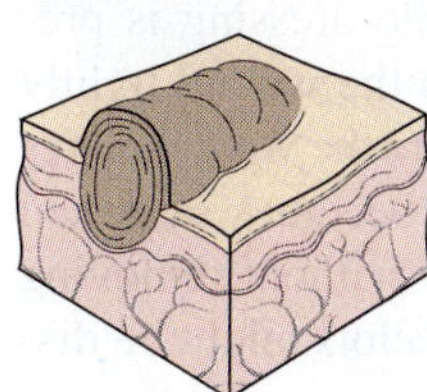	Elevated, irregular, darkened area of excess scar tissue caused by excessive collagen formation during healing. Extends beyond the site of the original injury. Higher incidence in people of African descent. **Examples** Keloid from ear piercing or surgery.
Crust 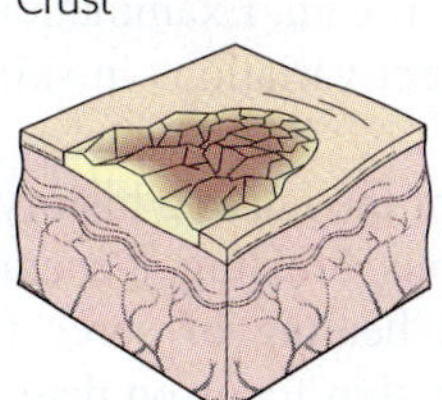	Dry blood, serum, or pus left on the skin surface when vesicles or pustules burst. Can be red-brown, orange, or yellow. Large crusts that adhere to the skin surface are called scabs. **Examples** Eczema, impetigo, herpes, or scabs following abrasion.		

traumatizing them. *Unintentional* wounds are accidental: For example, a person may fracture an arm in an automobile collision or a bicycle accident. If the tissues are traumatized without a break in the skin, the wound is closed. The wound is open when the skin or mucous membrane surface is broken.

Wounds may be described according to how they are acquired (Table 30–5). They also can be described according to the likelihood and degree of wound contamination.

- *Clean wounds* are uninfected wounds in which minimal inflammation is encountered and the respiratory, alimentary, genital, and urinary tracts are not entered. Clean wounds are primarily closed wounds.
- *Clean-contaminated wounds* are surgical wounds in which the respiratory, alimentary, genital, or urinary tract has been entered. Such wounds show no evidence of infection.
- *Contaminated wounds* include open, fresh, accidental wounds and surgical wounds that involve a major break in sterile technique or a large amount of spillage from the gastrointestinal tract. Contaminated wounds show evidence of inflammation.
- *Dirty* or *infected wounds* include wounds containing dead tissue and wounds with evidence of a clinical infection, such as purulent drainage.

TABLE 30–5 Types of Wounds

TYPE	CAUSE	DESCRIPTION AND CHARACTERISTICS
Incision	Sharp instrument (e.g., knife or scalpel)	Open wound; deep or shallow
Contusion	Blow from a blunt instrument	Closed wound; skin appearing ecchymotic (bruised) because of damaged blood vessels
Abrasion	Surface scrape, either unintentional (e.g., scraped knee from a fall) or intentional (e.g., dermal abrasion to remove pockmarks)	Open wound involving the skin
Puncture	Penetration of the skin and often the underlying tissues by a sharp instrument, either intentional or unintentional	Open wound
Laceration	Tissues torn apart, often from accidents (e.g., with machinery)	Open wound; edges often jagged
Penetrating Wound	Penetration of the skin and the underlying tissues, usually unintentional (e.g., from a bullet or metal fragments)	Open wound

Wounds, excluding pressure, ulcers and burns, are classified by depth, that is, the tissue layers involved in the wound (Box 30–1).

UNTREATED WOUNDS Untreated wounds usually are seen shortly after an injury (e.g., at the scene of an accident or in an emergency center). The following are guidelines for treatment:

- Control severe bleeding by (a) applying direct pressure over the wound and (b) elevating the involved extremity.
- Prevent infection by (a) cleaning or flushing abrasions or lacerations with normal saline and (b) covering the wound with a clean dressing if possible (a sterile dressing is preferred). When applying a dressing, wrap the wound tightly enough to apply pressure, and approximate the wound edges if possible. If the first layer of dressing becomes saturated with blood, apply a second layer. Do so without removing the first layer of dressing, because blood clots might be disturbed, resulting in more bleeding.
- Control swelling and pain by applying ice over the wound and surrounding tissues.
- If bleeding is severe or internal bleeding is suspected and if emergency equipment is available, assess the client for signs of shock (rapid, thready pulse; cold, clammy skin; pallor; lowered blood pressure).

Box 30–1 Classifying Wounds by Depth

- *Partial thickness:* Confined to the skin, that is, the dermis and epidermis; heal by regeneration
- *Full thickness:* Involving the dermis, epidermis, subcutaneous tissue, and possibly muscle and bone; require connective tissue repair

TREATED WOUNDS Treated or sutured wounds usually need to be observed to determine the progress of healing. These wounds may be inspected when a dressing is changed. If the wound itself cannot be directly inspected, the dressing is inspected and other data regarding the wound (e.g., the presence of pain) are assessed. See Exemplar 12.3, Wound Healing, for more information.

PHYSICAL ASSESSMENT

The nurse conducts an examination of the integument as part of a routine assessment and during regular care. Removing barriers to assessment is very important. Antiembolic stockings, braces, or other medical or assistive devices must be removed to assess the skin condition underneath. Examination of the skin requires good lighting to detect variations in skin color and to identify lesions.

During the review of systems as part of the nursing history, information about skin diseases, previous bruising, general skin condition, skin lesions, and usual healing of sores is obtained. Inspection and palpation of the skin focus on determining skin color distribution, skin turgor, presence of **edema** (swelling caused by excess fluid trapped in bodily tissue), and characteristics of any lesions that are present. Particular attention is paid to skin condition in areas that are most likely to break down: in skin folds such as under the breasts; in areas

Assessment Interview Skin and Tissue Integrity

SKIN CONDITIONS

- Have you ever had a skin problem?
- When were you diagnosed with the problem?
- What treatment was prescribed for the problem?
- Was the treatment helpful?
- What kinds of things do you do to help with the problem?
- Has the problem ever recurred (acute)?
- How are you managing the disease now (chronic)?
- Have you had an illness recently? If so, please describe it.
- Do you have or have you had a skin infection?
- When were you diagnosed with the infection?
- What treatment was prescribed for the problem?
- Was the treatment helpful? What kinds of things do you do to help with the problem?
- Has the problem ever recurred (acute)?
- How are you managing the infection now (chronic)?

Assessment Interview Skin and Tissue Integrity (continued)

SKIN CONDITION SYMPTOMS

- Do you have any sores or ulcers on your body that are slow in healing?
- Where are these?
- Do you have frequent boils or skin infections?
- Does your skin itch? If so, where?
- How severe is it?
- When does it occur?
- Have you noticed any rashes on your body? If so, please describe.
- Where on your body did the rash start? Where did it spread?
- When did you first notice it?
- Does the rash happen at the same time as any other symptoms, such as fever or chills?
- If you have a rash, do you notice it more after wearing certain clothes or jewelry? After using certain skin products?
- Did it occur soon after starting a new medication?
- Does the rash happen during or after any other activities such as gardening or washing dishes?
- Have you noticed any other lesions, lumps, bumps, tender spots, or painful areas on your body?
- If so, when did you first notice them? Where?
- Describe how they have spread and where they are located now.
- Have you noticed any drainage from any skin region?
- If so, where does the drainage come from? What does it look like? Does it have an odor?
- Is the drainage accompanied by any other symptoms? If so, please describe.
- Please describe anything you have done to treat your skin condition.
- When did you begin this treatment? How has your skin responded to the treatment?

PAIN

- Please describe any skin pain or discomfort.
- Have you experienced any pain or discomfort in any body folds, for example, between the toes, under the breasts, between the buttocks, or in the perianal area?
- Where is the pain?
- How often do you experience the pain?
- How long does the pain last?
- How long have you had the pain?
- How would you rate the pain on a scale of 1 to 10?
- Is there a trigger for the pain?
- What do you do to relieve the pain?
- Is this treatment effective?

BEHAVIORS

- Do you sunbathe?
- Have you ever sunbathed?
- Do you spend time in the sun exercising or playing sports?
- Do you work outdoors?
- How does your skin react to sun exposure?
- Do you use a lotion with sun protection factor (SPF) when spending time in the sun?
- What SPF lotion do you use? Do you reapply the lotion after several hours or after swimming?
- Do you remember having a sunburn that left blisters?
- How do you care for your skin?
- What kind of soap, cleansers, toners, or other treatments do you use?
- How do you clean your clothes?
- What kind of detergent do you use?
- How often do you bathe or shower?
- Do you now have or have you ever had a tattoo(s)?
- Have you had any problems with that area of the skin?
- Do you now have or have you ever had piercing of any part of your body?
- Where are the sites of piercing?
- How long have you had the piercing?
- Have any piercing sites closed?
- Have you ever had a problem at the piercing site?
- What was the problem?
- Did you seek treatment for the problem?
- What was the outcome of the treatment?
- What is the current condition of piercing sites?

INFANTS AND CHILDREN

- Does the child have any birthmarks? If so, where are they?
- Has the infant developed an orange hue in the skin?
- Does the child have a rash? If so, what seems to cause it?
- Have you introduced any new foods into your child's diet?
- How do you clean the child's diaper area?
- How do you wash the child's diapers?

OLDER ADULT

- What changes have you noticed in your skin in the past few years?
- Does your skin itch?
- Do you experience frequent falls?

INTERNAL ENVIRONMENT

- How would you describe your level of stress? Has it changed in the past few weeks? Few months? Describe.
- Are you now experiencing, or have you ever experienced, intermittent or prolonged anxiety or emotional upset?
- Describe the situation.
- Can you determine precipitating factors?
- Have you sought care or treatment for the problem?
- What do you do when the problem arises?
- Are you taking any prescription or over-the-counter medications?
- Have you changed your diet recently?
- Has the condition of your skin affected your social relationships in any way? Has it limited you in any way? If so, how?
- Female clients: Are you pregnant? If not, are you menstruating regularly? Describe your menstrual periods.

EXTERNAL ENVIRONMENT

- Have you been exposed recently to extremes in temperature?
- If so, when? How long was the exposure? Where did this occur?
- Describe the temperature of your home environment. Of your work environment.
- Do you work in an environment where radioisotopes or x-rays are used?
- If so, are you vigilant about following precautions and using protective gear?
- Do you wear gloves for work? If so, what types of gloves?
- How often do you travel?
- Have you traveled recently?
- If so, where?
- Have you come into contact with anyone who has a similar rash?
- Does your job or hobby require you to perform repetitive tasks? To work with any chemicals?
- Does your job or hobby require you to wear a specific type of helmet, hat, goggles, gloves, or shoes?

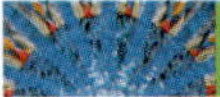

Integumentary Assessment

Technique/Normal Findings	Abnormal Findings
Inspect skin color and note any odors coming from the skin. *Skin color should be even, appropriate to the age and race of the client, without foul odors.*	■ A strong odor of perspiration may indicate poor hygiene and a need for client teaching. A foul odor may indicate a disorder of the sweat glands. ■ Pallor and/or cyanosis are seen with exposure to cold and with decreased perfusion and oxygenation. In cyanotic dark-skinned clients, skin loses glow and appears dull. Cyanosis may be more visible in the mucous membranes and nail beds of these clients. ■ In dark-skinned clients, jaundice may be most apparent in the sclerae of the eyes. ■ Redness, swelling, and pain are seen with various rashes, inflammations, infections, and burns. First-degree burns cause areas of painful erythema and swelling. Red, painful blisters appear in second-degree burns, whereas white or blackened areas are common in third-degree burns. ■ **Vitiligo**, an abnormal loss of melanin in patches, typically occurs over the face, hands, or groin. Vitiligo is thought to be an autoimmune disorder.
Inspect the skin for lesions and alterations, including calluses, scars, tattoos, and piercings. Include inspection of skin creases and folds. *Skin should be intact without abnormal lesions.*	■ Primary, secondary, and vascular lesions are described and shown in Tables 30–3 and 30–4. ■ Pearly edged nodules with a central ulcer are seen in basal cell carcinoma. ■ Scaly, red, fast-growing papules are seen in squamous cell carcinoma. ■ Dark, asymmetric, multicolored patches (sometimes moles) with irregular edges appear in malignant melanoma. ■ Circular lesions are usually present in ringworm and tinea versicolor. ■ Grouped vesicles may be seen in contact dermatitis. ■ Linear lesions appear in poison ivy and herpes zoster. ■ **Urticaria** (hives) appears as patches of pale, itchy wheals in an erythematous area. ■ In psoriasis, scaly red patches appear on the scalp, knees, back, and genitals. ■ In herpes zoster, vesicles appear along sensory nerve paths, turn into pustules, and then crust over. ■ Bruises (**ecchymosis**) are raised bluish or yellowish vascular lesions. Multiple bruises in various stages of healing suggest trauma or abuse.
Palpate skin temperature. *Skin should be warm.*	■ Skin is warm and red in inflammation and is generally warm with elevated body temperature. ■ Decreased blood flow decreases the skin temperature; this may be generalized, as in shock, or localized, as in arteriosclerosis.
Palpate skin texture. *Skin should be smooth.*	■ Changes in the texture of the skin may indicate irritation or trauma. ■ The skin is soft and smooth in hyperthyroidism and coarse in hypothyroidism.
Palpate skin moisture. *Skin should be dry.*	■ Excessively dry skin often is present in the older adult and in clients with hypothyroidism. ■ Oily skin is common in adolescents and young adults. Oily skin may be a normal finding, or it may accompany a skin disorder such as acne vulgaris. ■ Excessive perspiration may be associated with shock, fever, increased activity, or anxiety.
Palpate skin turgor. *Skin fold should return rapidly to normal position.*	■ Pinch the client's skin gently over the sternum or collarbone. Tenting, in which the skin remains pinched for a few moments before resuming its normal position, is common in older clients who are thin. ■ Skin turgor is decreased in dehydration. It is increased in edema and scleroderma.
Assess for edema. *No edema should be present.*	■ Assess edema (accumulation of fluid in the body's tissues) by depressing the client's skin (Figure 30–2 ■). Record findings as follows: 1+: Slight pitting, no obvious distortion 2+: Deeper pit, no obvious distortion 3+: Pit is obvious; extremities are swollen 4+: Pit remains with obvious distortion ■ Edema is common in cardiovascular disorders, renal failure, and cirrhosis of the liver. It also may be a side effect of certain drugs.

Integumentary Assessment (continued)

Technique/Normal Findings | **Abnormal Findings**

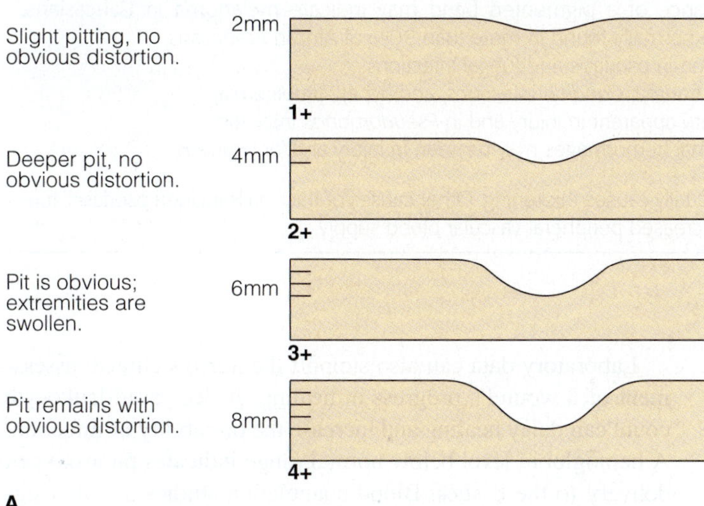

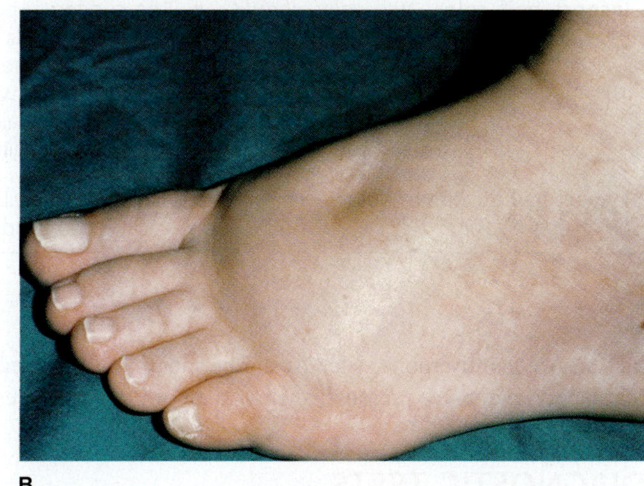

Figure 30–2 ■ *A*, Degrees of pitting in edema. *B*, 4+ pitting.
Source: Dr. P. Marazzi/Science Photo Library/Photo Researchers, Inc.

Inspect distribution and quality of hair. *Hair should be evenly distributed for client's gender.*

- A deviation in the normal hair distribution in the male or female genital area may indicate an endocrine disorder. **Hirsutism** (increased growth of coarse hair, usually on the face and trunk) is seen in Cushing's syndrome, acromegaly, and ovarian dysfunction. **Alopecia** (hair loss) may be related to changes in hormones, chemical or drug treatment, or radiation. In adult males whose hair loss follows the normal male pattern, the cause is usually genetic.

Palpate hair texture. *Hair should be of even texture.*

- Some systemic diseases change the texture of the hair. For instance, hypothyroidism causes the hair to coarsen, whereas hyperthyroidism causes the hair to become fine.

Inspect the scalp for lesions. *There should be no lesions on the scalp.*

- Mild dandruff is normal, but excessive, greasy flakes indicate seborrhea requiring treatment.
- Hair loss, pustules, and scales appear on the scalp in tinea capitis (scalp ringworm).
- Red, swollen pustules appear around infected hair follicles and are called folliculitis.
- Head lice may be seen as oval nits (eggs) adhering to the base of the hair shaft. Head lice are usually accompanied by itching.

Inspect nail curvature. *Nails should not be excessively curved.*

- Clubbing, in which the angle of the nail base is greater than 180 degrees, is seen in respiratory disorders, cardiovascular disorders, cirrhosis of the liver, colitis, and thyroid disease. The nail becomes thick, hard, shiny, and curved at the free end.
- The nail folds become inflamed and swollen and the nail loosens in paronychia an infection of the nails.

Inspect the surface of the nails. *Nail surfaces should be smooth and nail folds firm, without redness.*

- Inflammation and transverse rippling of the nail are associated with chronic paronychia and/or eczema.
- The nail plate may separate from the nail bed in trauma, psoriasis, and *Pseudomonas* and *Candida* infections. This separation is called oncolysis.
- Nail grooves may be caused by inflammation, by planus, or by nail biting.
- Nail pitting may be seen with psoriasis.
- A transverse groove (Beau's line) may be seen in trachoma and/or acute diseases.
- Thin spoon-shaped nails may be seen in anemia.

(continued)

Integumentary Assessment (continued)

Technique/Normal Findings	Abnormal Findings
Inspect nail color. *Nail color should be even.*	■ The sudden appearance of a pigmented band may indicate melanoma in Caucasians. Pigmented bands are normally found in more than 90% of African Americans. ■ Yellowish nails are seen in psoriasis and fungal infections. ■ Dark nails occur with trauma, *Candida* infections, and hyperbilirubinemia. ■ Blackish-green nails are apparent in injury and in *Pseudomonas* infection. ■ Red splinter longitudinal hemorrhages may be seen in injury and/or psoriasis.
Inspect nail thickness. *Nails should not be excessively thick.*	■ Trauma to the nails usually causes thickening. Other causes of thick nails include psoriasis, fungal infections, and decreased peripheral vascular blood supply.

that are frequently moist, such as the perineum; and in areas that receive extensive pressure, such as the bony prominences.

DIAGNOSTIC TESTS

The results of diagnostic tests of the structure and function of the integumentary system are used to support the diagnosis of a specific injury or disease. Diagnostic tests also provide information to identify or modify the appropriate medication or treatments used for the disease, and help nurses monitor the clients' responses to nursing care interventions. Diagnostic tests to assess the integumentary system are described in Diagnostic Tests: Integumentary System and are summarized in the following bulleted list.

- One of the most common diagnostic tests is a skin biopsy, which is used to differentiate a benign skin lesion from a skin cancer. Skin biopsies can be obtained by using a punch technique, incision, excision, or shaving.
- Cultures to identify infections may be conducted on tissue samples, on drainage and exudate (material, such as fluid and cells, that has escaped from blood vessels during the inflammatory process and is deposited in tissue or on tissue surfaces) from lesions, and (if an illness is generalized) on serum.
- Tests that are used to identify infections include immunofluorescent studies, Wood's lamp, potassium hydroxide, and the Tzanck test.
- Patch tests or scratch tests may be used to determine allergies.

Some studies are conducted to identify bacterial carriers. For example, if clients have repeated bacterial skin infections or if a health care unit or agency experiences numerous bacterial infections of clients, nasal cultures may be performed to determine whether the clients or health care workers are carriers of the bacteria. Regardless of the type of diagnostic test, the nurse is responsible for explaining the procedure to the client; explaining any special preparation needed, including fasting or avoiding allergy medications prior to testing; assessing for medication use that may affect the outcome of the tests; supporting the client during the examination as necessary; documenting the procedures as appropriate; and monitoring the results of the tests.

Laboratory data can also support the nurse's clinical assessment of a wound's progress in healing. A decreased leukocyte count can delay healing and increase the possibility of infection. A hemoglobin level below normal range indicates poor oxygen delivery to the tissues. Blood coagulation studies are also significant. Prolonged coagulation times can result in excessive blood loss and prolonged clot absorption. Hypercoagulability can lead to intravascular clotting. Intra-arterial clotting can result in a deficient blood supply to the wound area. Serum protein analysis provides an indication of the body's nutritional reserves for rebuilding cells. Albumin is an important indicator of nutritional status. A value below 3.5 g/dL indicates poor nutrition and may increase the risk of poor healing and infection. Wound cultures can either confirm or rule out the presence of infection. Sensitivity studies are helpful in the selection of appropriate antibiotic therapy. The nurse obtains a wound culture whenever an infection is suspected.

CARING INTERVENTIONS

Medical management of alterations in tissue integrity is based on the cause and severity of the condition. The goals of treatment are to control the severity of the disease, prevent infection, and promote healing. Palliative care may also be necessary, depending on the severity of the problem and the level of discomfort it presents for the client. The nurse should ask questions to determine whether the client is doing anything at home to relieve discomfort that could unintentionally inhibit healing, The nurse should also provide information about what home remedies will provide comfort while promoting healing.

PHARMACOLOGIC THERAPIES

There are many skin disorders; some warrant only localized or short-term pharmacotherapy. Examples include lice infestation, sunburn with minor irritation, and acne. Eczema, dermatitis, and psoriasis are more serious disorders that require extensive and sometimes prolonged therapy. Table 30–6 identifies some topical agents that are used to treat skin disorders, listed according to their level of potency. Some clients may use complementary therapies to treat skin lesions, as listed in the Alternative Therapies: Skin Lesions feature.

TABLE 30–6 **Topical Glucocorticoids for Dermatitis and Related Symptoms**

GENERIC NAME	TRADE NAMES
Highest Level of Potency	
Betamethasone	Benisone, Diprosone, Valisone
Clobetasol	Dermovate, Temovate
Diflorasone	Florone, Maxiflor, Psorcon
Middle Level of Potency	
Amcinonide	Cyclocort
Desoximetasone	Topicort, Topicort LP
Fluocinonide	Lidex, Lidex-E, others
Halcinonide	Halog
Mometasone	Elocon
Triamcinolone	Aristocort, Kenalog, others
Lower Level of Potency	
Clocortolone	Cloderm
Fluocinolone	Fluolar, Synalar, others
Flurandrenolide	Cordran, Cordran SP
Fluticasone	Flonase
Hydrocortisone	Hytone, Locoid, Westcort, others
Lowest Level of Potency	
Alclometasone	Aclovate
Desonide	DesOwen, Tridesilon
Dexamethasone	Decaderm, Decadron, others

ALTERNATIVE THERAPIES **Skin Lesions**

SKIN CONDITION	COMPLEMENTARY THERAPY
Atopic eczema	Evening primrose oil (oral)
Wound healing, superficial burns, and abrasions	Aloe vera gel (topical)
Skin inflammation	Chamomile (topical cream or ointment)

Source: Data from National Center for Complementary and Alternative Medicine. (2006). *Herbs at a glance.* Retrieved December 2, 2007, from http://nccam.nih.gov/health.

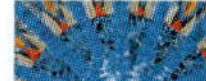

30.1 BURNS

KEY TERMS

BASIS OF SELECTION FOR EXEMPLAR

Emergency room admissions

LEARNING OUTCOMES

After reading about this exemplar, you will be able to:

1. Describe the pathophysiology, etiology, clinical manifestations, and direct and indirect causes of burns.
2. Identify risk factors associated with burns.
3. Illustrate the nursing process in providing culturally competent care across life span for individuals with burns.
4. Formulate priority nursing diagnoses appropriate for an individual with burns.
5. Create a plan of care for individuals with burns and their family members.
6. Assess expected outcomes for an individual with burns.
7. Discuss therapies used in the collaborative care of an individual with burns.
8. Employ evidence-based caring interventions for an individual with burns.

OVERVIEW

A **burn** is an injury resulting from exposure to heat, chemicals, radiation, or electric current. A transfer of energy from a source of heat to the human body initiates a sequence of physiologic events that, in the most severe cases, leads to irreversible tissue destruction. Burns range in severity from a minor loss of small segments of the outermost layer of the skin to a complex multisystem injury. Treatments vary from simple to an invasive, multisystem, interdisciplinary team approach in the aseptic environment of a burn center.

PATHOPHYSIOLOGY AND ETIOLOGY

The four types of burn injury are thermal, chemical, electrical, and radiation. Although all four types can lead to generalized tissue damage and multisystem involvement, the causative agents and priority treatment measures are unique to each.

Thermal Burns

Thermal burns result from exposure to dry heat (flames) or moist heat (steam and hot liquids). Thermal burns are the most common burn injuries and occur most often in children and older adults (Figure 30–3 ■). Direct exposure to the source of heat causes cellular destruction that can result in charring of vascular, bony, muscle, and nervous tissue.

Chemical Burns

Chemical burns are caused by direct skin contact with acids, alkaline agents, or organic compounds. More than 25,000 products found in the home or workplace can cause chemical burns. The chemical destroys tissue protein, leading to necrosis. Burns caused by alkalis (such as lye) are more difficult to neutralize than are burns caused by acids. Compared to acid burns, burns from alkalis tend to have deeper penetration, with a correspondingly more severe burn. Organic compound burns, such as those from petroleum distillates, cause cutaneous damage through fat solvent action and may cause renal and liver failure if absorbed.

Chemical agents are further classified according to the manner by which they structurally alter proteins. Oxidizing agents such as household bleach alter protein configuration through the chemical process of reduction. Corrosives such as lye cause extensive protein denaturation. Protoplasmic poisons such as organic compounds form salts with proteins, inhibiting calcium and other ions needed for cell viability. The severity of the chemical burn is related to the type of agent, the concentration of the agent, the mechanism of action, the duration of contact, and the amount of body surface area exposed. Box 30–2 lists household cleaning agents that may cause burns.

Electrical Burns

The severity of electrical burns depends on the type and duration of current and the amount of voltage. It is particularly difficult to assess the extent and depth of electrical burn injuries. Electricity follows the path of least resistance, which in the human body tends to lie along muscles, bone, blood vessels, and nerves. This can conceal the electrical insult, which may persist for weeks beyond the time of the initial injury. Further, entry and exit wounds tend to be small, masking widespread tissue damage underneath the wound. Tissue necrosis results from impaired blood flow secondary to blood coagulation at the site of the electrical injury. Because electrical burn wounds of the extremities often cause severe tissue necrosis, they frequently develop gangrene that necessitates amputation (Bishop, 2004).

Alternating current (AC), like that found in conventional households, produces repeated electrical surges that lead to

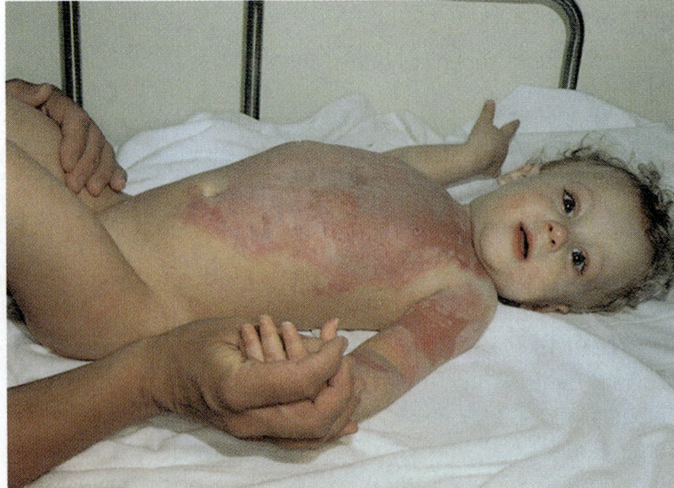

Figure 30–3 ■ Thermal (scald) burns are the most common burn injury in infants. Notice the distribution of the burned skin, a wide area on the upper chest and arm where the hottest liquid fell, with a narrower area near the umbilicus, indicating that the liquid cooled as it traveled down the chest.

Box 30–2 **Household Cleaning Agents That May Cause Burns**

- Drain cleaners
- Lye
- Industrial-strength ammonia
- Household ammonia
- Oven cleaners
- Toilet bowl cleaners
- Dishwasher detergents
- Bleach

tetanic muscle contractions. Such sustained muscle contractions inhibit respiratory efforts for the duration of contact and may result in respiratory arrest. The contractions also cause the person to clamp down on the power source (such as an electrical cord) which may increase the duration of contact with the source (Figure 30–4 ■).

Direct current, as in injury from a lightning bolt, exposes the body to very high voltage for an instantaneous period of time. High-voltage (lightning) injury usually results in entry and exit wounds. The flashover effect is a phenomenon unique to lightning injury. In a flashover, the lightning bolt flashes over the individual, the current traveling over the moist surface of the skin rather than through deeper structures, saving them from death. The individual suffering a lightning strike may experience instantaneous cardiopulmonary arrest. Other possible outcomes include brain injury resulting in loss of consciousness or even coma; injuries to the eyes and ears; temporary paralysis; and nerve damage. Many who survive have no memory of the event (Cooper, M., 2009).

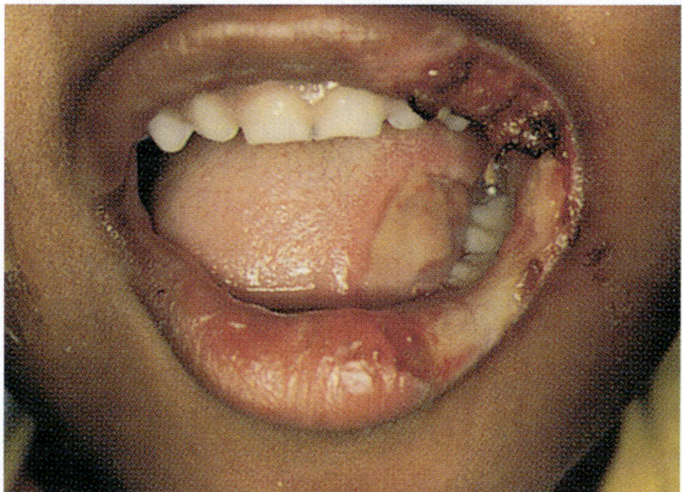

Figure 30–4 ■ Electrical burn caused by biting an electrical cord. The burn is caused when the current arcs through the lips, often causing a full-thickness injury through the mucosa, submucosa, muscle, nerves, and blood vessels. The labial artery may be injured and cause significant bleeding once the eschar falls off after 2–3 weeks.

Courtesy of Dr. Lezley McIlveen, Department of Dentistry, Children's National Medical Center, Washington, DC.

Radiation Burns

Radiation burns are usually associated with sunburn or radiation treatment for cancer. These kinds of burns tend to be superficial, involving only the outermost layers of the epidermis. All functions of the skin remain intact. Symptoms are limited to mild systemic reactions: headache, chills, local discomfort, nausea, and vomiting.

More extensive exposure to radiation or radioactive substances, as in nuclear power accidents, leads to the same degree of tissue damage and multisystem involvement associated with other types of burns.

Etiology

It is estimated that 1.1 million burn injuries require medical intervention each year in the United States and that approximately 45,000 of those require hospitalization. Each year, approximately 4,500 burn injuries result in death (National Institute of General Medical Sciences, 2005).

Burns are one of the top five leading causes of injury deaths in children between 1 and 14 years of age (National Center for Health Statistics, National Vital Statistics System, 2007). In 2003, approximately 83,300 children 14 years and under were treated in emergency departments for burn injuries (Duffy, McLaughlin, & Eichelberger, 2006). Males are at greater risk for burn injury and mortality (Klein & Herndon, 2004). About 10–25% of all burns in children are due to child abuse and are most commonly seen in children under 3 years of age (Horner, 2005).

The home is the most common site for fire-related burns. Home fires cause 80% of all fire-related deaths, with approximately eight people dying in home fires each day. Smoking materials, including cigarettes, cigars, and pipes, are the leading cause of home fire deaths, although unattended cooking also is responsible for many residential fires.

Risk Factors

Factors associated with deaths from burns are age (especially children under 5 and adults 65 and older), careless smoking, alcohol or drug intoxication, and physical and mental disabilities.

A common source of burns in young children is tap water scalds, whereas older children receive most burns from flame injuries. Fire injuries and deaths that occur among college-age students usually are due to alcohol use that impairs judgment and hampers escape (National Fire Protection Association, 2004). Occupations involving work with chemicals, gasoline, or electricity pose a risk for those who work with those elements.

Like young children, older adults are at high risk for tap water scalding. Older adults are more susceptible to deep burns from scalds because of their thinner skin. They generally are more vulnerable to fire and burn injury because of decreased visual acuity, depth perception, sense of smell, hearing, and impaired mobility. Alterations in cognition, such as dementia, are also risk factors. All of these factors increase the risk of accidentally starting a fire and diminish the ability to survive it.

Morbidity increases in clients with preexisting cardiac, pulmonary, or renal disorders and diabetes mellitus. Clients who are alcoholics have lower survival rates of a major burn injury due to the development of complications.

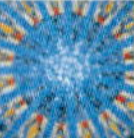

DEVELOPMENTAL CONSIDERATIONS Burns

CHILDREN

Children at different developmental stages are at risk for different types of burns, as follows:

- Infants are most often injured by thermal burns (scalding liquids, excessively hot bathwater, house fires)
- Toddlers are at risk for thermal burns (pulling hot liquids or grease onto themselves), electrical burns (biting electrical cords or chewing through insulation of electrical cords), contact burns, and chemical burns (ingesting cleaning agents and other substances) associated with exploring the environment.
- Preschool-age children are most often injured by scalding or contact with hot appliances (curling irons, ovens).
- School-age children are at risk for thermal burns (playing with matches and fireworks), electrical burns (climbing high-voltage towers, climbing trees, and making contact with electrical wires), and chemical burns (conducting combustion experiments) associated with their curiosity and interest in experimentation.
- Adolescents also experience thermal, chemical, and electrical burns, as well as radiation burns associated with sunbathing.

Infants and older adults have a greater risk of mortality from burn injuries.

OLDER ADULTS

- More than 1,200 deaths in adults 65 and older occur each year.
- Leading causes of fire-related deaths are smoking, heating, and cooking.
- One fifth of the deaths occur in physically challenged older adults.

Abuse is suspected when scald burns show a clear line of demarcation, indicating deliberate immersion. The presence of small, circular burns may be from cigarette burns inflicted by an abuser.

FACTORS AFFECTING BURN CLASSIFICATION

Tissue damage following a burn is determined primarily by two factors: depth of the burn (the layers of underlying tissue affected) and extent of the burn (the percentage of body surface area involved).

Depth of the Burn

The depth of a burn injury is determined by the elements of the skin that have been damaged or destroyed. Burn depth results from a combination of the temperature of the burning agent and the length of contact. Burns are classified as superficial, partial thickness, or full thickness (Figure 30–5 ■).

SUPERFICIAL BURNS **Superficial burns** involve only the epidermal layer of the skin. They most often result from damage from sunburn, ultraviolet light, minor flash injury (from a sudden ignition or explosion), or mild radiation associated with cancer treatment. Because the skin remains

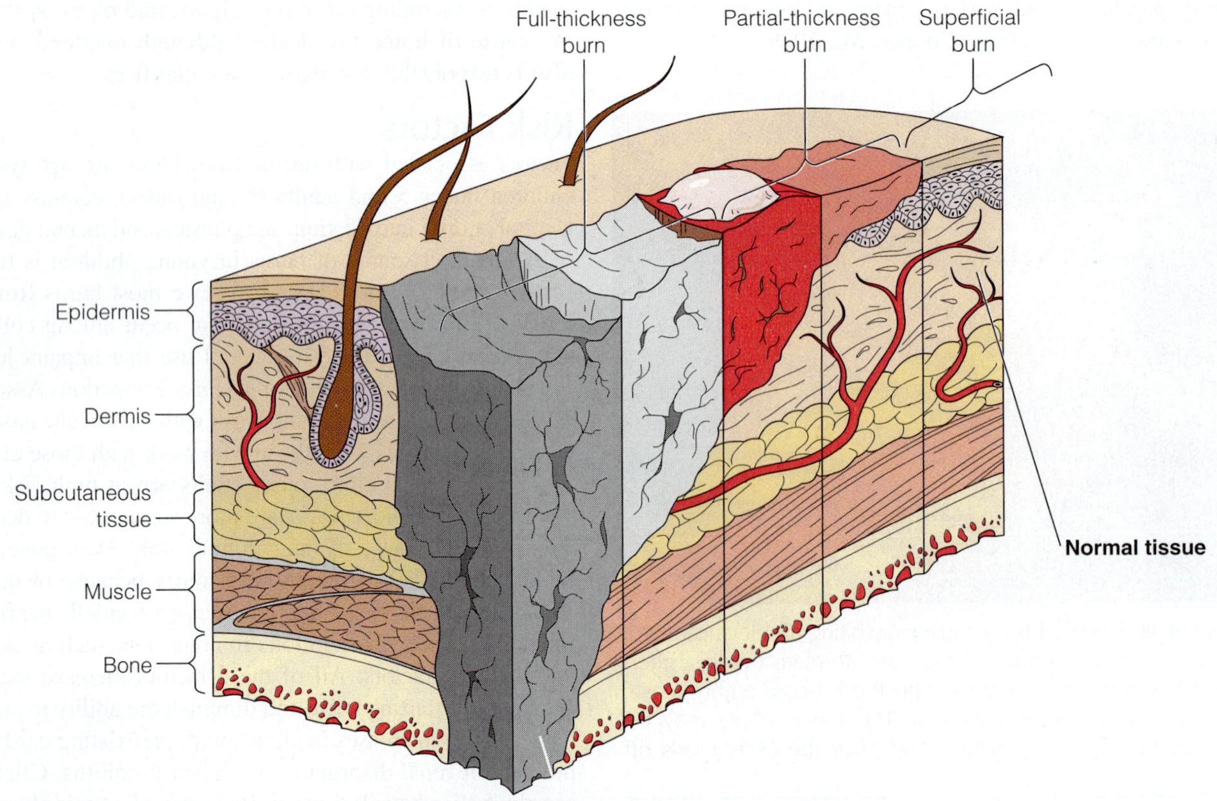

Figure 30–5 ■ Characteristics of burns by depth of thermal injury.

intact, this degree of burn is not calculated into the estimates of burn injury. The skin color ranges from pink to bright red, and there may be slight edema over the burned area. Superficial burns involving large body surface areas may be manifested by chills, headache, nausea, and vomiting. Superficial burns usually heal in 3–6 days, with dryness and peeling of the outer layer of skin and with no scar formation. Superficial burns are treated with mild analgesics and the application of water-soluble lotions. Extensive superficial burns, especially in older adults, may require intravenous (IV) fluid treatment.

PARTIAL-THICKNESS BURNS **Partial-thickness burns** involve the entire dermis and the papillae of the dermis (superficial partial-thickness burn) or extends into the hair follicles (deep partial-thickness burn). The classification depends on the depth of the burn.

A *superficial partial-thickness burn* (Figure 30–6 ■) may result from brief exposure to a flash flame or dilute chemical agents or contact with a hot surface. This burn is often bright red but has a moist, glistening appearance with blister formation. The burned area will blanch on pressure, and touch and pain sensation remain intact. Pain in response to temperature and air is usually severe. These burns typically heal within 21 days with minimal or no scarring, but pigment changes are common. Analgesics are administered, and if large blistered areas are disrupted, skin substitutes may be used.

A *deep partial-thickness burn* also involves the entire dermis but extends further into the dermis than a superficial partial-thickness burn. Hair follicles, sebaceous glands, and epidermal sweat glands remain intact (Porth, 2005). Hot liquids or solids, flash flame, direct flame, intense radiant energy, or chemical agents may cause this level of burn wound. The surface of the burn wound appears pale and waxy and may be moist or dry. Large, easily ruptured blisters may be present, or the blisters may look like flat, dry tissue paper. Capillary refill is decreased, and sensation to deep pressure is present. The burn wound is less painful than a superficial partial-thickness burn, but areas of pain and areas of decreased sensation may be present. Deep partial-thickness burn wounds often require more than 21 days for healing and may convert to a full-thickness injury if necrosis extends the depth of the wound. **Contractures**, permanent shortening of connective tissue, are possible, as are hypertrophic scarring and functional impairment (Figure 30–7 ■). Excision of the wound and skin grafting may be necessary to decrease scarring and loss of function.

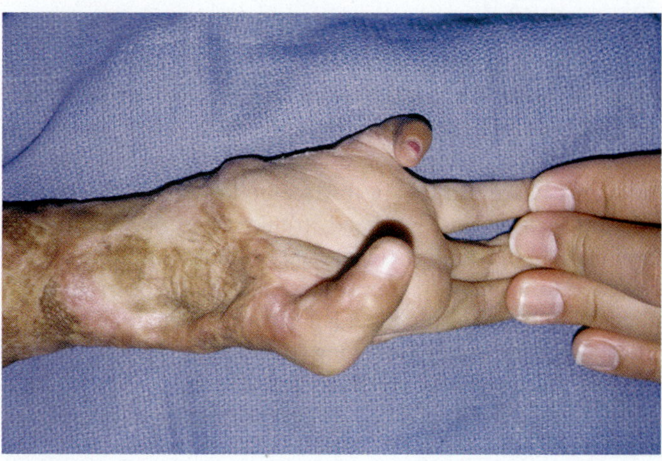

Figure 30–7 ■ Burn contracture.

Courtesy of JPD/Custom Medical Stock Photo, Inc.

FULL-THICKNESS BURNS A **full-thickness burn** involves all layers of the skin, including the epidermis, the dermis, and the epidermal appendages (Figure 30–8 ■). The burn wound may extend into the subcutaneous fat, connective tissue, muscle, and bone. Full-thickness burns are caused by prolonged contact with flames, steam, chemicals, or high-voltage electric current.

Depending on the cause of injury, the full-thickness burn wound may appear pale, waxy, yellow, brown, mottled, charred, or nonblanching red. The wound surface is dry, leathery, and firm to the touch. Thrombosed blood vessels may be visible under the surface of the wound. There is no sensation of pain or light touch because pain and touch receptors have been destroyed. Full-thickness burns require skin grafting to heal.

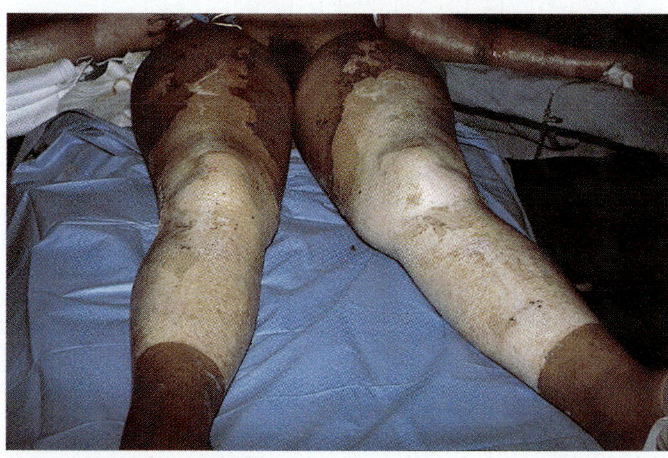

Figure 30–6 ■ Partial-thickness burn injury.

Courtesy of Dr. William Dominic, Valley Medical Center.

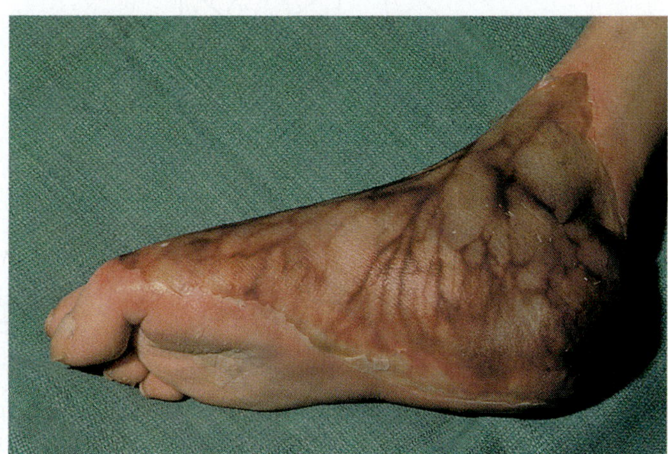

Figure 30–8 ■ Full-thickness burn injury.

Courtesy of Dr. William Dominic, Valley Medical Center.

Extent of the Burn

The extent of the burn injury is expressed as a percentage of the total body surface area (TBSA). Several methods are used to determine the extent of injury. The *rule of nines* is a rapid method of estimation used during the prehospital and emergency care phases. In this method, the body is divided into five surface areas—head, trunk, arms, legs, and perineum—and percentages that equal or total a sum of nine are assigned to each body area (Figure 30–9 ■). For example, a client with burns of the face, anterior right arm, and anterior trunk has burn injury involving 27% of the TBSA. (In this example, face = 4.5%, arm = 4.5%, and trunk = 18% to total 27%.) Only partial- and full-thickness burns are included in the estimation.

On the client's admission to the hospital, critical care unit, or burn center, more accurate methods for estimating the extent of injury are employed. For example, the Lund and Browder method (Figure 30–10 ■) determines surface area measurements for each body part according to the age of the client.

A recognized system for describing a burn injury, developed by the American Burn Association, uses both the extent and depth of burn to classify burns as minor, moderate, or major (Table 30–7).

BURN WOUND HEALING

Burns heal using the same processes as other wounds, but the wound healing phases occur more slowly and last longer. The healing process involves three phases: inflammation, proliferation, and remodeling (Carrougher, 1998; Porth, 2005).

Inflammation

Immediately following the injury, platelets coming into contact with the damaged tissue aggregate. Fibrin is deposited, trapping further platelets, and a thrombus forms. The thrombus, combined with local vasoconstriction, causes hemostasis, which walls off the wound from the systemic circulation.

Local vasodilation and an increase in capillary permeability follow hemostasis. Neutrophils infiltrate the wound and peak in about 24 hours, at which point monocytes predominate. The monocytes are converted into macrophages, which consume pathogens and dead tissue and secrete various growth factors. These growth factors stimulate the proliferation of fibroblasts and a deposit of a provisional wound matrix.

Proliferation

Within 2–3 days postburn, fibroblasts are the major cell in the wound. Their number peaks about 14 days after the injury. Granulation tissue begins to form, with complete

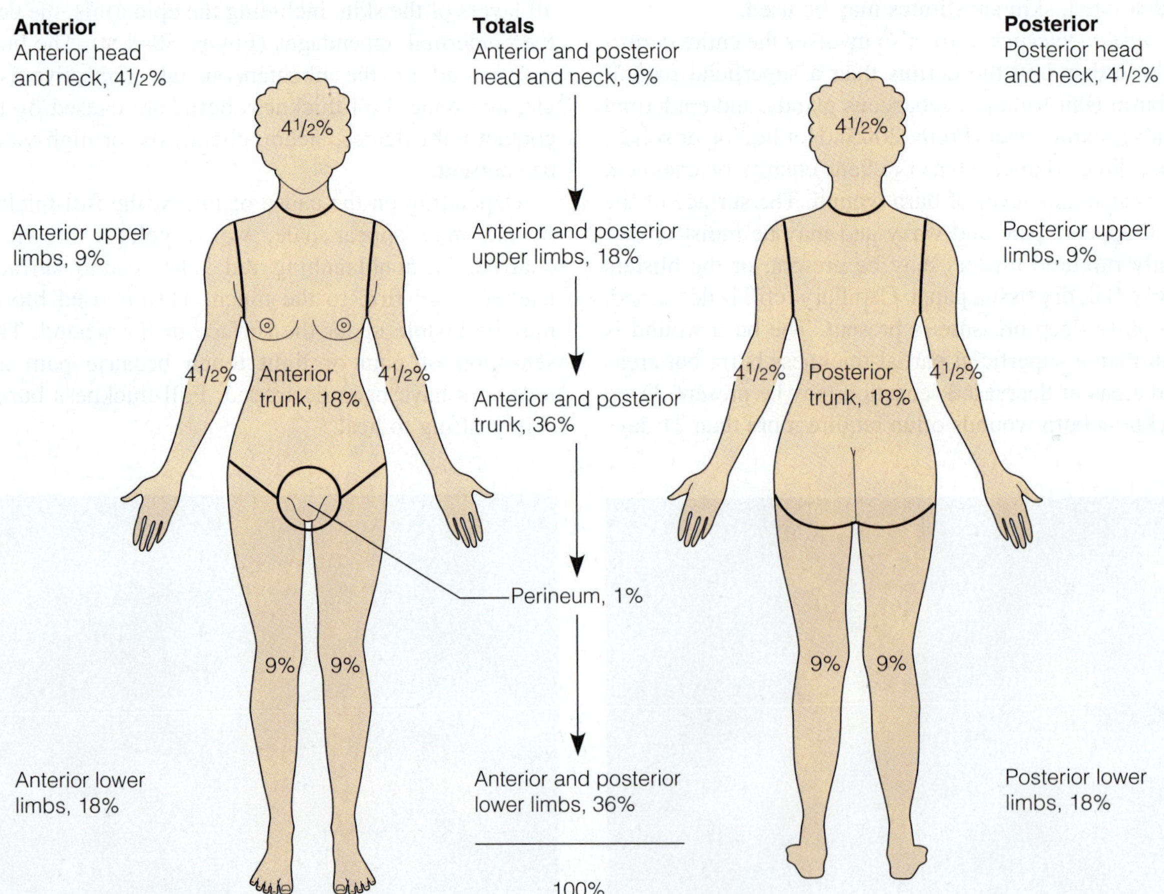

Figure 30–9 ■ The rule of nines is one method for quickly estimating the percentage of TBSA affected by a burn injury. Although useful in emergency care situations, the rule of nines is not accurate for estimating TBSA for adults who are short, obese, or very thin.

Area	Age (years)					% 1°	% 2°	% 3°	% Total
	0–1	1–4	5–9	10–15	Adult				
Head	19	17	13	10	7				
Neck	2	2	2	2	2				
Ant. trunk	13	13	13	13	13				
Post. trunk	13	13	13	13	13				
R. buttock	$2\frac{1}{2}$	$2\frac{1}{2}$	$2\frac{1}{2}$	$2\frac{1}{2}$	$2\frac{1}{2}$				
L. buttock	$2\frac{1}{2}$	$2\frac{1}{2}$	$2\frac{1}{2}$	$2\frac{1}{2}$	$2\frac{1}{2}$				
Genitalia	1	1	1	1	1				
R.U. arm	4	4	4	4	4				
L.U. arm	4	4	4	4	4				
R.L. arm	3	3	3	3	3				
L.L. arm	3	3	3	3	3				
R. hand	$2\frac{1}{2}$	$2\frac{1}{2}$	$2\frac{1}{2}$	$2\frac{1}{2}$	$2\frac{1}{2}$				
L. hand	$2\frac{1}{2}$	$2\frac{1}{2}$	$2\frac{1}{2}$	$2\frac{1}{2}$	$2\frac{1}{2}$				
R. thigh	$5\frac{1}{2}$	$6\frac{1}{2}$	$8\frac{1}{2}$	$8\frac{1}{2}$	$9\frac{1}{2}$				
L. thigh	$5\frac{1}{2}$	$6\frac{1}{2}$	$8\frac{1}{2}$	$8\frac{1}{2}$	$9\frac{1}{2}$				
R. leg	5	5	$5\frac{1}{2}$	6	7				
L. leg	5	5	$5\frac{1}{2}$	6	7				
R. foot	$3\frac{1}{2}$	$3\frac{1}{2}$	$3\frac{1}{2}$	$3\frac{1}{2}$	$3\frac{1}{2}$				
L. foot	$3\frac{1}{2}$	$3\frac{1}{2}$	$3\frac{1}{2}$	$3\frac{1}{2}$	$3\frac{1}{2}$				
					Total				

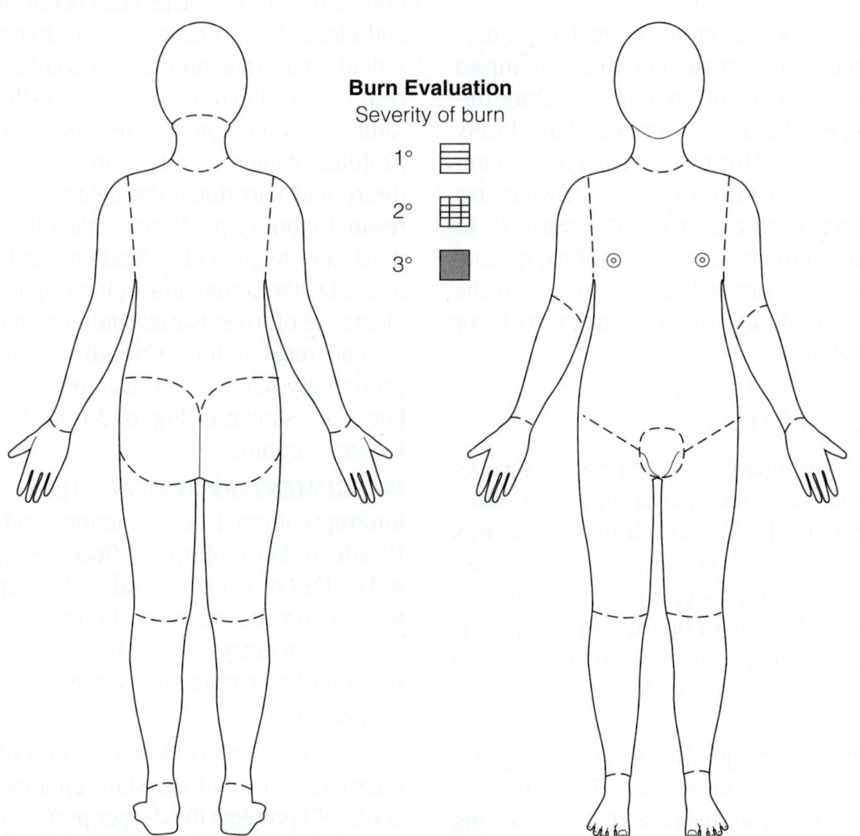

Figure 30–10 ■ The Lund and Browder burn assessment chart. This method of estimating TBSA affected by a burn injury is more accurate than the rule of nines because it accounts for changes in body surface area across the life span.

TABLE 30–7 **American Burn Association Classification of Burn Injury**

MINOR BURN INJURY	MODERATE BURN INJURY	MAJOR BURN INJURY
Excludes electrical injury, inhalation injury, complicated injuries (such as multiple trauma), and all clients who are considered to be at high risk (such as older adults and those with chronic illnesses)	Excludes electrical injury, inhalation injury, complicated injuries (such as multiple trauma), and all clients who are considered to be at high risk (such as older adults and those with chronic illnesses)	Includes all burns of the hands, face, eyes, ears, feet, and perineum; all electrical injuries, inhalation injuries, multiple-trauma injuries, and all clients who are considered to be at high risk
Partial-thickness burns of less than 15% of the TBSA in adults	Partial-thickness burns of 15–25% of the TBSA in adults	Partial-thickness burns of greater than 25% of the TBSA in adults
Full-thickness burns of less than 2% of the TBSA not involving special care areas (eyes, ears, face, hands, feet, joints, perineum)	Full-thickness burns of less than 10% of the TBSA not involving special care areas (eyes, ears, face, hands, feet, joints, perineum)	All full-thickness burns of 10% or greater of the TBSA

Note: Burn injuries described in this table (except minor burns) should be treated in a specialized burn center. These criteria have been established by the American Burn Association.

reepithelialization occurring during this stage. Epithelial cells cover the wound as each cell stretches across the wound surface to join with other epithelial cell sheets on the other side of the wound. The proliferation phase lasts until complete reepithelialization occurs by epithelial cell migration, surgical intervention, or a combination of the two.

Remodeling

This phase may last for years. Collagen fibers, laid down during the proliferative phase, reorganize into more compact areas. Scars contract and fade in color. In normal healing following a minor burn injury, the newly formed skin closely resembles its neighboring tissue. However, when a burn injury extends into the dermal layer of skin, two types of excessive scar may develop. A **hypertrophic scar** is an overgrowth of dermal tissue that remains within the boundaries of the wound. A **keloid** is a scar that extends beyond the boundaries of the original wound. Clients with dark skin are at greater risk for hypertrophic scars and keloids.

CLINICAL MANIFESTATIONS

Minor burn injuries consist of superficial burns that are involve only a small area of tissue; superficial partial-thickness burns that involve less than 15% of TBSA; and full-thickness burns that involve less than 2% of TBSA, excluding the special care areas are classified as minor burns (eyes, ears, face, hands, feet, perineum, and joints). Minor burn injuries are not associated with immunosuppression, hypermetabolism, or increased susceptibility to infection. Examples include sunburn and minor scald burns.

A major burn involves serious injury to the underlying layers of skin and covers a large body surface area. The American Burn Association defines a major burn as one that involves the following:

- >25% TBSA in adults less than 40 years of age
- >20% TBSA in adults more than 40 years of age
- >10% TBSA full-thickness burn
- Injuries to the face, eyes, ears, hands, feet, joints, or perineum
- High-voltage electrical injuries
- All burn injuries with inhalation injury or major trauma.

An overview of the classifications of burns and appropriate therapies is provided in the Clinical Manifestations and Therapies feature box. More detailed information follows.

Multisystem Effects

The pathophysiologic changes that result from major burn injuries involve all body systems. Extensive loss of skin (the body's protective barrier) can result in massive infection, fluid and electrolyte imbalances, and hypothermia. Often the individual inhales the products of combustion, thus compromising respiratory function. Cardiac dysrhythmias and circulatory failure are common manifestations of serious burn injuries. A profound catabolic state dramatically increases caloric expenditure and nutritional deficiencies. An alteration in gastrointestinal motility predisposes the client to developing paralytic ileus, and hyperacidity leads to gastric and duodenal ulcerations. Dehydration slows glomerular filtration rates and renal clearance of toxic wastes and may lead to acute tubular necrosis and renal failure. Overall, a significant burn injury may profoundly alter body metabolism. Systemic responses to burns are shown in Figure 30–11 ■ and discussed in the following sections.

INTEGUMENTARY SYSTEM The loss of skin in burn injuries interrupts normal skin functions and protective mechanisms. Results of burn injuries include the following:

- The loss of water secondary to evaporation
- Infection secondary to the loss of skin integrity to prevent pathogen entry into the body
- Difficulty maintaining temperature due to heat loss from open wounds.

Heat transfer to skin is a complex phenomenon. If the microcirculation of the skin remains intact during burning, it cools and protects the deeper portions of the skin and cools the outer surface once the heat source is removed. With extensive burn injury, the integrity of the microcirculation is lost and the burning process continues even after the heat source is removed. For this reason, stopping the burning process is important in extensive burn injuries.

Burns have a characteristic skin surface appearance that resembles a bull's-eye, with the most severe burn located

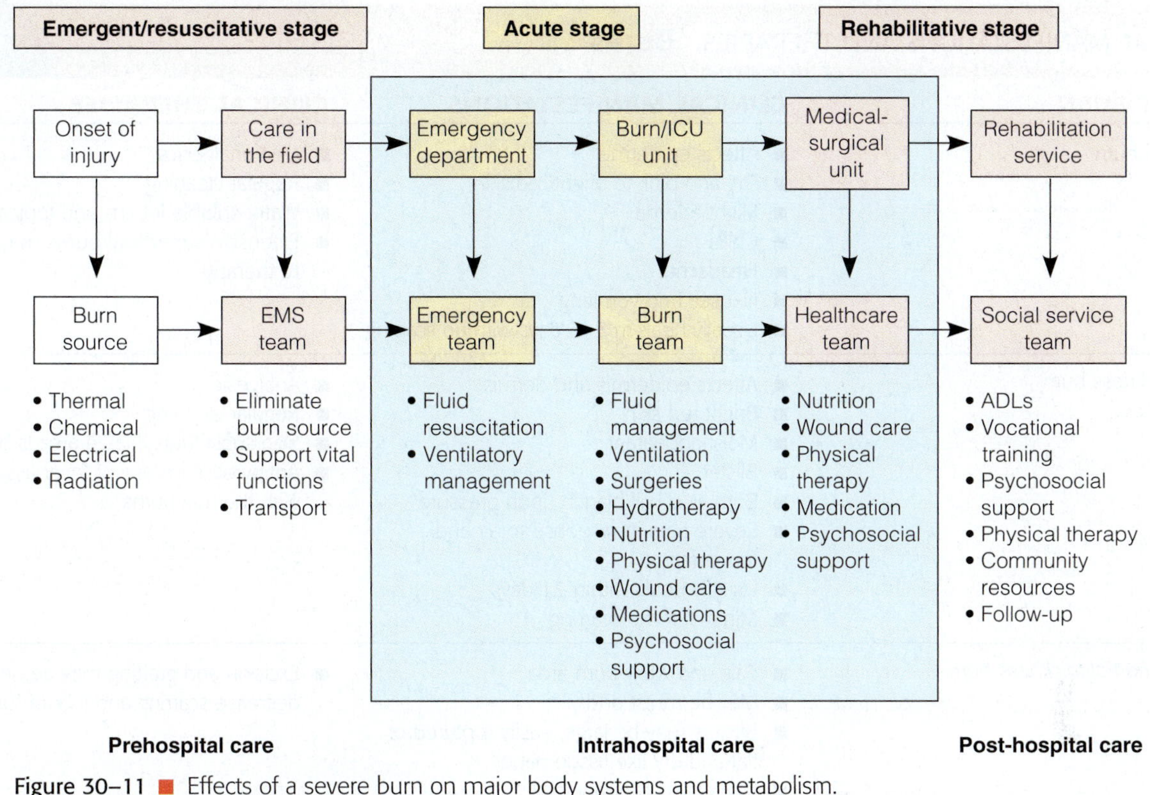

Figure 30–11 ■ Effects of a severe burn on major body systems and metabolism.

centrally and the lesser burns located along the peripheral wound edges. Depending on their intensity, burns consist of one, two, or three concentric three-dimensional zones closely corresponding on the skin surface to the depth of the burn (Figure 30–12 ■).

- The outer zone of hyperemia is unburned tissue, blanches on pressure, and heals in 2–7 days postburn.
- The medial zone of stasis is initially moist, red, and blistered, and blanches on pressure. It may recover or become pale and necrotic on days 3–7 postburn due to decreased perfusion or infection.
- The inner zone of coagulation immediately appears leathery and coagulated. It may merge with the zone of stasis in 3–7 days postburn.

The overall thickness of the dermis and epidermis varies considerably from one area of the body to another. As a result, similar temperatures produce different depths of injury in different body parts. For example, in the adult, skin covering the medial aspect of the forearm is thinner and more easily damaged than the skin covering the back of the same adult. Skin dissipates heat maximally in areas of greatest vascularization. When heat absorption exceeds the rate of dissipation, cellular temperatures rise and skin tissue is destroyed.

The burn injury results in the formation of necrotic skin and subcutaneous tissue. During the acute stage of the injury, a hard crust (**eschar**) forms, which covers the wound and harbors necrotic tissue. The eschar is characteristically leathery and rigid. Removal of the eschar facilitates healing.

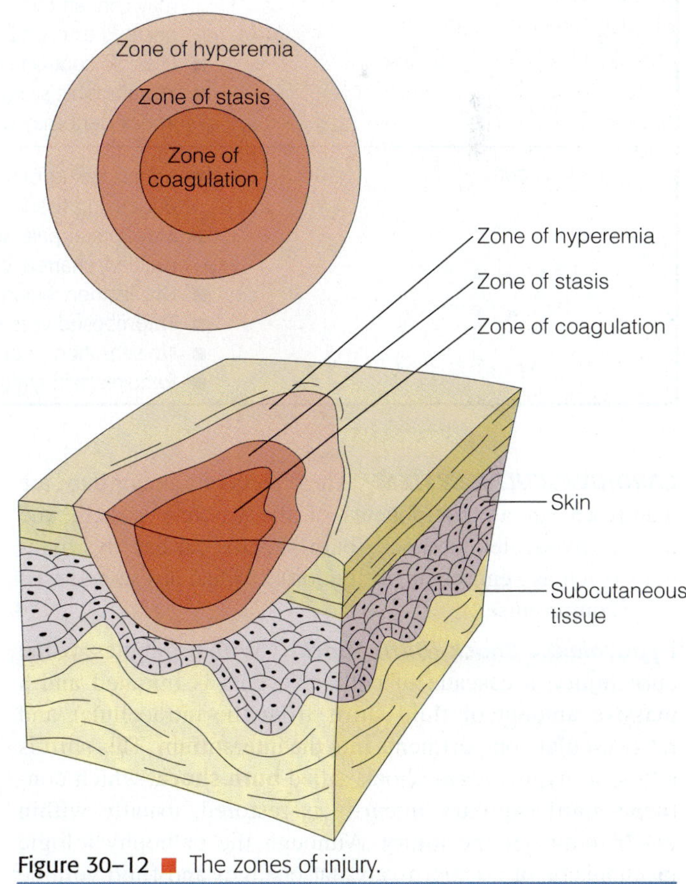

Figure 30–12 ■ The zones of injury.

CLINICAL MANIFESTATIONS AND THERAPIES **Burns**

TYPE OF BURN	CLINICAL MANIFESTATIONS	CLINICAL THERAPIES
Superficial burn	■ Affects epidermis ■ Dry and pink to bright red skin ■ Slight edema ■ Chills ■ Headache ■ Nausea and vomiting ■ Usually heals in 3–6 days with no scarring	■ Mild analgesics ■ Regular cleaning ■ Water-soluble lotions and topical agents ■ Extensive superficial burns may require IV therapy
Partial-thickness burn *Superficial*	■ Affects epidermis and dermis ■ Bright red skin ■ Moist appearance ■ Blister ■ Burn area will blanch upon pressure ■ Severe pain in response to air and temperature ■ Usually heals within 21 days ■ Minimal to no scarring	■ Analgesics ■ Regular cleaning ■ Skin substitutes if large area is burned ■ Antipyretics in case of fever associated with thermal burns
Deep partial-thickness burn	■ Pale and waxy burn area ■ May be moist or dry ■ Blisters may be large, easily ruptured or flat and dry like tissue paper ■ Decreased capillary refill ■ Sensation to deep pressure ■ Less painful than superficial partial-thickness burn ■ May require more than 21 days to heal; may convert to full-thickness injury if necrosis extends to depth of wound ■ Possible contractures ■ Hypertrophic scarring and functional impairment may occur	■ Excision and grafting may be necessary to decrease scarring and lack of function
Full-thickness burn	■ Affects epidermis, dermis, and underlying tissues ■ May appear pale, waxy, yellow, brown, mottled, charred, or non-blanching red ■ Dry, leathery wound surface ■ Thrombosed vessels visible ■ No sensation to pain or light touch ■ Requires skin grafting to heal	■ Regular cleaning ■ Topical agents ■ Skin substitutes ■ Excision of eschar ■ Skin grafting

CARDIOVASCULAR SYSTEM The effects of a major burn are manifested in all components of the vascular system and include hypovolemic shock (burn shock), cardiac dysrhythmias (such as ventricular fibrillation), cardiac arrest, and vascular compromise.

Hypovolemic Shock (Burn Shock) Within minutes of the burn injury, a cascade of cellular events is initiated and a massive amount of fluid shifts from the intracellular and intravascular compartments into the interstitium. This shift is a type of hypovolemic shock called **burn shock**, which continues until capillary integrity is restored, usually within 24–36 hours of the injury. Although the pathophysiologic mechanisms of postburn vascular changes and fluid volume shifts are not clearly understood, three processes occur early in the postburn phase in clients with burns involving 40% or more of the TBSA.

- Increase in microvascular permeability at the burn wound site
- Generalized impairment of cell wall function, resulting in intracellular edema
- Increase in osmotic pressure of the burned tissue, leading to extensive fluid accumulation

During burn shock, the shifting of fluid directly results from a loss of cell wall integrity at the site of injury and in the capillary bed. Fluid leaks from the capillaries into interstitial compartments located at the burn wound site and throughout the body, resulting in a decrease in fluid volume within the intravascular space. Plasma proteins and sodium escape into the interstitium, enhancing edema formation. Blood pressure falls as cardiac output diminishes.

Vasoconstriction results as the vascular system attempts to compensate for fluid loss. Abnormal platelet aggregation and white blood cell (WBC) accumulation result in ischemia (insufficient blood supply) in the deeper tissue below the burn, leading to eventual thrombosis. Red blood cells (RBCs) and WBCs remain in the circulation, producing an elevation in erythrocyte and leukocyte counts secondary to hemoconcentration.

The leakage of fluid into the interstitium compromises the lymphatic system, resulting in intravascular hypovolemia and edema at the burn wound site. Edematous body surfaces impair peripheral circulation and result in necrosis of the underlying tissue. During burn shock, potassium ions leave the intracellular compartment, putting the client at risk for cardiac dysrhythmia due to hypokalemia. The process of burn shock continues until capillary integrity is restored, usually within 24 hours of the injury.

Burn shock reverses when fluid is reabsorbed from the interstitium into the intravascular compartment. The blood pressure rises as cardiac output increases, and urinary output improves. Diuresis continues from several days to 2 weeks postburn. During this phase, the extra cardiac workload may predispose the older client or the client with cardiovascular disease to fluid volume overload.

Cardiac Rhythm Alterations Burns of more than 40% of the TBSA cause significant myocardial dysfunction, with a decrease in myocardial contractibility and cardiac output. These changes, which occur prior to a decrease in plasma volume, are believed to be due to the release of substances and oxygen-free radicals from the burn wound and from ischemic myocardial cells. Electrical burns often result in cardiac dysrhythmias or cardiopulmonary arrest caused by heat damage to the myocardium or electrical interference with cardiac electrical activity.

Peripheral Vascular Compromise Circumferential burns are those that result from injury that encircles an extremity. As scar tissue develops, the circumferential burn tightens, much like a rubber band, reducing or eliminating blood supply below the burn. Circulation to extremities may be further impaired by edema and by peripheral vasoconstriction that occurs during burn shock. In addition, **compartment syndrome** (in which the tissue pressure in a muscle compartment exceeds microvascular pressure, interrupting cellular perfusion) may result.

RESPIRATORY SYSTEM Breathing in hot gases and smoke may cause direct damage to the pulmonary tissues. Pulmonary damage also may result from the systemic response to the injury. Inhalation injury is a frequent and often lethal complication of burns. The injury may range from mild respiratory inflammation to massive pulmonary failure such as acute respiratory distress syndrome (ARDS). Exposure to heat, asphyxiants, and smoke initiates the pathophysiologic process associated with inhalation injury.

Inflammation occurs at localized sites in the airway and is manifested as hyperemia (increased blood supply). As a result, cells are destroyed and the bronchial cilia are rendered inactive. Because the mucociliary transport mechanism no longer functions, the client may develop bronchial congestion and infection.

Interstitial pulmonary edema develops secondary to the escape of fluid from the pulmonary vasculature into the interstitial compartment of the lung tissue. Surfactant is inactivated, resulting in atelectasis (collapse of lung tissue) and alveolar collapse. Sloughing of the damaged and dead lung tissue occasionally produces debris that may lead to complete airway obstruction.

Upper airway (above the level of the glottis) thermal injury results from the inhalation of heated air or chemicals dissolved in water. Inhalation injury should be suspected when the client has singed facial, scalp, or nasal hair. Physical findings include the presence of soot, charring, edema, blisters, and ulcerations along the mucosal lining of the oropharynx and larynx. The resulting edema in the airway peaks within the first 24–48 hours of injury. Ominous signs of hoarseness, labored breathing, or stridor indicate possible airway obstruction due to edema. Lower airway thermal injury is a rare occurrence. Because the lower airway is protected by laryngeal reflexes, thermal injury below the vocal cords is rare. However, when it does occur, it is typically associated with the inhalation of steam or explosive gases or the aspiration of hot liquids. Sputum containing soot or carbon particles is a classic manifestation of lower airway thermal injury (Sole, Klein, & Moseley, 2005).

Smoke poisoning results when toxic gases and particulate matter, the products of incomplete combustion, deposit directly on the pulmonary mucosa. The composition of the products of combustion depends on the combustible material, the rate at which the temperature increases, and the amount of ambient oxygen present. Irritant gases and particulate matter have a direct cytotoxic effect. The degree of injury is determined by their solubility in water, the duration of exposure, and the size of the particulate or aerosol droplet.

Carbon monoxide, a common asphyxiant, is a colorless, tasteless, odorless gas that has a 200 times greater affinity for hemoglobin than does oxygen. It displaces oxygen to bind with hemoglobin, forming carboxyhemoglobin. As a result, the decrease in arterial oxyhemoglobin produces tissue hypoxia. Carbon monoxide impairs both oxygen delivery and cellular oxygen use. The clinical manifestations of carbon monoxide poisoning range from headache, nausea, and dizziness to coma and death.

Cyanide gas is released when plastics, polyurethane, nylon, or silk is burned. The resultant production of cyanide gas affects cellular respiration. The brain and heart are most vulnerable to cyanide poisoning; manifestations include headache, dizziness, seizures, tachycardia, and lethal dysrhythmias.

GASTROINTESTINAL SYSTEM Dysfunction of the gastrointestinal system is directly related to the size of the burn wound. Clients with burns involving 20% or more of the TBSA experience decreased peristalsis with resultant gastric distention and increased risk of aspiration. A decrease in or absence of bowel sounds is a manifestation of paralytic ileus (adynamic bowel) secondary to burn trauma. The resulting cessation of intestinal motility leads to gastric distention, nausea, vomiting, and hematemesis.

Stress ulcers (**Curling's ulcers**) are acute ulcerations of the stomach or duodenum that form following the burn injury. Abdominal pain, acidic gastric pH levels, hematemesis, and blood in the stool may indicate a gastric ulcer.

URINARY SYSTEM During the early stages of the burn injury, renal blood flow and glomerular filtration rates are greatly reduced from the decreased intravascular blood volume and the release of antidiuretic hormone by the posterior pituitary. Urine output decreases, and serum creatinine and blood urea nitrogen increase.

Dark brown concentrated urine may indicate myoglobinuria or hemoglobinuria, the result of underlying muscle damage or the release of large amounts of dead or damaged erythrocytes after a major burn injury. When large amounts of these pigments are released, the liver cannot keep pace with conjugation and the pigments pass through the glomeruli. The pigments can occlude the renal tubules and cause renal failure, especially when dehydration, acidosis, or shock also is present.

IMMUNE SYSTEM The function of the immune system is to protect the human body from invasion by foreign microorganisms. The capillary leak that occurs in the early stages of the burn injury continues throughout the burn shock phase and impairs the active components of both the cell-mediated and humoral immune systems.

The humoral immune system relies on B cells to produce antibodies or immunoglobulins. In the burn client, the serum levels of all immunoglobulins are significantly diminished. Serum protein levels remain persistently low throughout the clinical course until wound closure is effected. A marked decrease in T-cell counts results in a reduction of cytotoxic activity and suppression of the cell-mediated immune system.

The compromise in the humoral and cell-mediated immune systems constitutes a state of acquired immunodeficiency, which places the burn client at risk for infection. The period of vulnerability is transient and may last from 1–4 weeks following the onset of the burn injury. During this time frame, opportunistic infections may be fatal despite aggressive antimicrobial therapy.

METABOLISM Two distinct phases characterize the body's metabolic response to the burn injury. The *ebb phase*, occurring during the first 3 days of the injury, is manifested by decreased oxygen consumption, fluid imbalance, shock, and inadequate circulating volume. These responses protect the body from the initial impact of the injury.

A second phase, *the flow phase*, occurs when adequate burn resuscitation has been accomplished. This phase is characterized by increases in cellular activity and protein catabolism, lipolysis, and gluconeogenesis. The basal metabolic rate (BMR) significantly increases, reaching twice the normal rate. Body weight and heat drop dramatically. Total energy expenditure may exceed 100% of normal BMR. Hypermetabolism persists until after wound closure has been accomplished and may reappear if complications occur.

COLLABORATION

The burn team is composed of an interdisciplinary group of health care professionals who plan the care and treatment of the burn-injured client during the acute and rehabilitative stages. The burn team typically consists of the nurse, physician, physical therapist, dietitian, and social worker. The team members meet regularly to discuss client progress and to determine collaboratively the most effective regimen of care and psychosocial support.

Clinical Therapies

Treatment for burns depends on the body surface area involved, the depth of skin damage, and the location of the burn. Burns that involve the airway require more careful monitoring than those involving extremities. Treatment often begins on scene, provided by family members, emergency services personnel, or specially trained personnel in occupational settings.

MINOR BURNS A minor burn injury is usually treated in an outpatient facility. The goal of therapy is to promote wound healing, eliminate discomfort, maintain mobility, and prevent infection.

Treatment for sunburn generally consists of applying mild lotions, increasing liquid intake, administering mild analgesics, and maintaining warmth. Older adults and young children should be monitored for evidence of dehydration. Using sunscreen properly and limiting sun exposure to the less hazardous hours of the day (before 10 a.m. and after 3 p.m.) can prevent sunburn.

For minor burns, the nurse provides client teaching regarding the application of antibiotic solutions and light dressings and the need to maintain adequate nutritional intake. Mild analgesics may be used to help the client carry out activities of daily living.

FOCUS ON DIVERSITY AND CULTURE *Litargirio* Use

When taking a history about methods used to treat minor burns in children, inquire about the use of *litargirio*. This traditional remedy is used as a treatment for burns and wounds and as a deodorant and foot fungicide in the Dominican Republic. The powder is sold in small packets at specialty stores that serve Spanish-speaking populations. The high lead content places the client at risk for lead poisoning. If a nurse determines a client has been using *litargirio*, the nurse should provide client teaching regarding the use of this medication and the client's lead levels should be checked. If the blood test determines treatment is necessary, the physician may prescribe DMSA (dimercaptosuccinic acid), an oral medicine that binds to lead and mercury.

CARE SETTINGS Burn Centers

Although many burn injuries are treated in local tertiary care facilities, the American Burn Association has developed guidelines for determining whether the client should be transported to a burn center for interdisciplinary approaches to treatment and rehabilitation. Adult clients who should be treated at burn centers include those with

- second- or third-degree burns >10% TBSA and older than 50 years of age.
- second- or third-degree burns >20% TBSA in adults younger than 50.
- third-degree burns >5% TBSA in adults of any age.
- burns involving the hands, feet, face, eyes, ears, joints, or perineum.
- electrical (including lightning), chemical, and inhalation injuries.
- circumferential burns of the extremities and/or chest.
- any burn associated with extenuating problems, preexisting illness, fractures, or other trauma.

Minor burns with blisters may be left intact or debrided. **Debridement** is the process of removing necrotic material, including all loose tissue, wound debris, and eschar (dead tissue), from the wound. Follow-up care for the minor burn injury includes twice daily wound cleansing with application of a topical ointment, range-of-motion (ROM) exercises to affected joints, and weekly clinic appointments until the wound heals completely.

MAJOR BURNS The clinical course of treatment for the client with a major burn is divided into three stages: the emergent/resuscitative stage, the acute stage, and the rehabilitative stage. Although these stages are useful predictors of the clinical needs of the client, it is important to recognize that the process of burn injury is dynamic and that, in many cases, the clinical stage may not be clearly delineated. This is one of the many reasons that ongoing assessment is necessary throughout the course of treatment. Figure 30–13 ■ shows the burn client's progression through the health care system. During each stage of care, different groups of nurses, physicians, and other health care specialists collaborate to manage the client's recovery.

Emergent/Resuscitative Stage The emergent/resuscitative stage lasts from the onset of injury through successful fluid resuscitation. During this stage, health care workers estimate the extent of burn injury, institute first-aid measures, and implement fluid resuscitation therapies. The client is assessed for shock and evidence of respiratory distress. If indicated, IV lines are inserted, and the client may be prophylactically intubated. During this stage, health care workers determine whether the client is to be transported to a burn center for the complex intervention strategies of the professional interdisciplinary burn team.

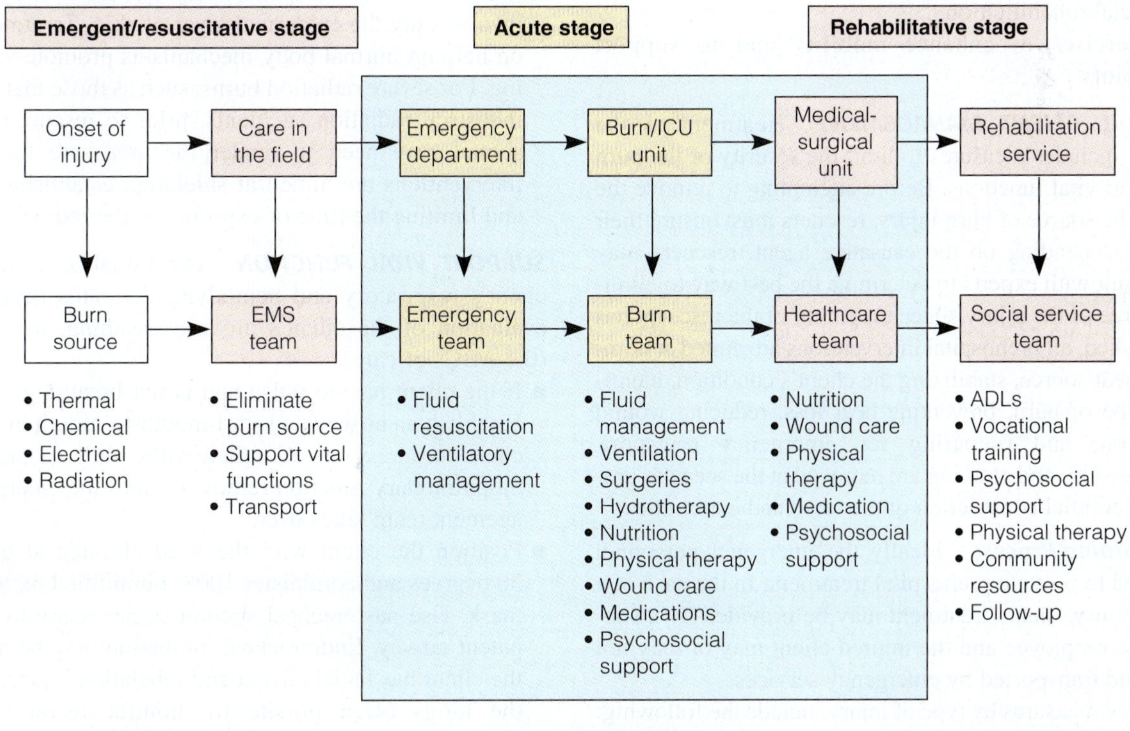

Figure 30–13 ■ The client's progression through the health care system during the emergent, acute, and rehabilitative stages of burn injury.

Acute Stage The acute stage begins with the start of diuresis and ends with closure of the burn wound (either by natural healing or by use of skin grafts). During this stage, the following therapies are implemented: wound care management, nutritional therapies, and measures to control infectious processes are initiated.

- *Wound care.* Hydrotherapy and excision and grafting of full-thickness wounds are performed as soon as possible after injury.
- *Nutrition therapy.* Enteral and parenteral nutritional interventions are started early in the treatment plan to address caloric needs resulting from extensive energy expenditure.
- *Infection prevention.* Measures to combat infection are implemented during this stage, including the administration of topical and systemic antimicrobial agents.
- *Pain management.* Pain management constitutes a significant segment of the nursing care plan throughout the clinical course of the burn-injured client. The administration of narcotic pharmaceutical agents must precede all invasive procedures to maximize client comfort and to reduce the anxieties associated with wound debridement and intensive physical therapy.

Rehabilitative Stage The rehabilitative stage begins with wound closure and ends when the client returns to the highest level of health restoration, which may take years. During this stage, the primary focus is the biopsychosocial adjustment of the client, which may include the following:

- The prevention of contractures and scars
- The client's successful resumption of work, family, and social roles through physical, vocational, occupational, and psychosocial rehabilitation
- ROM exercises to enhance mobility and to support injured joints.

PREHOSPITAL CLIENT MANAGEMENT Treatment at the injury scene includes measures to limit the severity of the burn and to support vital functions. Before attempting to remove the client from the source of burn injury, rescuers must ensure their own safety. Depending on the causative agent, rescuers may need to consult with experts to determine the best way to eliminate the source of the injury. Once the safety of the rescuers has been established, all prehospital interventions are aimed at eliminating the heat source, stabilizing the client's condition, identifying the type of burn, preventing heat loss, reducing wound contamination, and preparing for emergency transport. Restrictive jewelry and clothing are removed at the scene to prevent circumferential constriction of the torso and extremities.

Stop the Burning Process Ideally, the emergency personnel will be called to provide prehospital treatment. In the case of a workplace injury, onsite treatment may be provided by a specially trained employee and the injured client may or may not be treated and transported by emergency services.

Emergency measures by type of injury include the following:

- *Thermal Burns.* If the thermal injury has been caused by dry heat, smother inflamed clothing or lavage with water. Help the person "stop, drop, and roll" to extinguish the flame and limit the extent of burn. Once the flame has been extinguished, cover the body to prevent hypothermia. If the thermal injury has been caused by moist heat, lavage the area with cool water. Ice is not used for cooling because it causes vasoconstriction and may result in further injury. Tar and asphalt can be removed with mineral oil, petroleum ointments, Medisol (a citrus and petroleum distillate with hydrocarbon structure), or Crisco.
- *Chemical Burns.* For chemical burns, immediately remove the clothing and use a hose or shower to lavage the involved area thoroughly for a minimum of 20 minutes. Many chemicals are in powder form, and as much dry chemical as possible needs to be removed before the surface is flushed with water. Unusual chemicals may require consultation with a Poison Control Center about appropriate treatment. The rescuer should wear protective clothing during this process for protection from chemical exposure. Chemical splashes in or near the eye require immediate eye irrigation with clean, cool water or saline.
- *Electrical Burns.* Electrical injuries pose the potential of serious harm to both rescuer and burn victim. Ensure that the source of electrical current has been disconnected or move the person to safety away from the energy source using a nonconductive device such as an unpainted broomstick. If the person is unresponsive, assess for the presence of cardiac and respiratory function. If indicated, begin cardiopulmonary resuscitation (CPR). A spinal cord injury may be present secondary to the forceful contraction of the muscles of the neck and back during exposure to the current. If possible, place the person in a cervical collar and transport on a spinal board.
- *Radiation Burns.* Radiation injuries are usually minor and involve only the epidermal layer of skin. Treatment focuses on helping normal body mechanisms promote wound healing. For severe radiation burns, such as those that result from industrial radiation accidents, prior to rescue, trained personnel may need to render the area safe for entry. All interventions are aimed at shielding, establishing distance, and limiting the time of exposure to the radioactive source.

SUPPORT VITAL FUNCTION The initial assessment of the client's respiratory and hemodynamic status begins with an evaluation of the client's airway, breathing, and circulation (the ABCs of care).

- If the client has no pulse and is not breathing, begin CPR. Establish an airway and start mouth-to-mouth breathing and chest compressions. Continue CPR until spontaneous cardiopulmonary function returns or until the emergency management team takes over.
- Position the client with the head elevated at greater than 30 degrees and administer 100% humidified oxygen by face mask. Use nasotracheal suction as necessary to maintain a patent airway. Endotracheal intubation may be necessary if the client has facial edema and inhalation injury. Auscultate the lungs often on-site to monitor respiratory status. Continuous pulse oximetry provides ongoing assessment of the client's oxygen saturation levels.
- Monitor for cardiac dysrhythmias or arrest. When one is available, connect the client to a cardiac monitor and observe

for dysrhythmias. Elevate burned extremities above the level of the heart to facilitate circulation.

- Initiate fluid replacement therapy for burn wounds that involve more than 20% of the TBSA. Continuously assess heart and lung sounds and observe level of consciousness, cardiac rate and rhythm, blood pressure, and urine output.
- Cover the client to maintain body temperature and to prevent further wound contamination and tissue damage.

Emergency and Acute Care

Immediately upon arrival, the nurse obtains a history of the injury (including any medical interventions already implemented), estimates the depth and extent of the burn, begins fluid resuscitation, and maintains ventilation according to protocol.

FLUID RESUSCITATION **Fluid resuscitation** is the administration of intravenous (IV) fluids to restore the circulating blood volume during the acute period of increasing capillary permeability. To counteract the effects of burn shock, fluid resuscitation guidelines are used to replace the extensive fluid and electrolyte losses associated with major burn injuries. Fluid replacement is necessary in all burn wounds that involve 20% or more of the TBSA.

Crystalloid fluids are administered through two large-bore (14- to 16-gauge) catheters, preferably inserted through unburned skin. Because it most closely approximates the body's extracellular fluid composition, warmed lactated Ringer's solution is the IV fluid most widely used during the first 24 hours after burn injury. Several formulas may be used to replace fluid loss, including Parkland formula and ABLS Consensus formula.

These formulas specify the volume of fluid to be infused the first 24 hours from the time of the burn injury, with 50% of the fluid to be infused during the first 8 hours, followed by the remaining 50% during the next 16 hours (25% per 8 hours). During the second 24 hours, fluids for clients with larger burns (such as more than 30% TBSA) are changed to a crystalloid solution of 5% dextrose in water titrated to maintain urine output (Sole et al., 2005).

Hourly urine output is often used as the indicator of effective fluid resuscitation, with 30–50 mL for an adult considered adequate. (With electrical burns, a urine output of 75–100 mL should be maintained.) Another indicator is heart rate; if fluid resuscitation is adequate, the rate should be less than 120 beats per minute or in the upper limits of normal for age. However, underlying conditions and the fear, anxiety, and pain that accompany burn injuries often increase heart rate (Ahrns, 2004). Blood pressure changes are less reliable because significant hypotension does not develop until volume losses exceed 30% due to the body's compensatory mechanisms. Assessment for narrowed pulse pressure, which indicates shock earlier, should be considered along with urine output to monitor adequate fluid resuscitation (Sole et al., 2005).

During the fluid resuscitation stage, the client may require invasive hemodynamic monitoring. A pulmonary artery catheter may be used to monitor cardiac output, cardiac index, and pulmonary artery wedge pressures (PAWPs). All measurements must be maintained within normal limits to effect adequate fluid resuscitation.

RESPIRATORY MANAGEMENT Upon the client's admission to the emergency department, several baseline assessments of respiratory status must be obtained: a chest x-ray study, arterial blood gases (ABGs), vital signs, and carboxyhemoglobin levels. Intubation is indicated for all clients with burns of the chest, face, or neck. The primary treatment plan is oriented toward preventing atelectasis and maintaining alveolar oxygen exchange. The following interventions should be initiated:

- Maintain the head of the bed at 30 degrees or greater to maximize the client's ventilatory efforts. Turn the client side to side every 2 hours to prevent hypostatic pneumonia.
- To keep airway passages clear, suction the client frequently, encourage the client to use incentive spirometry hourly, and help the client perform coughing and deep-breathing exercises every 2 hours.
- In the face of impending airway obstruction, the client will require immediate intubation. Nasotracheal tube placement is the preferred route because it seems to be better tolerated and can be more effectively secured. If the client has suffered nasolabial burns, however, the orotracheal route is preferred. Nasotracheal and orotracheal intubation are reserved for short-term ventilatory management. For long-term ventilatory management (i.e., greater than 3 weeks), a tracheostomy is performed.
- Humidification of either room air or oxygen helps prevent the drying of tracheal secretions. Ambient air or oxygen flow is based on ABG results. The client may be placed on a face mask, steam collar, T-piece, mechanical ventilation with positive end-expiratory pressure, pressure support ventilation, or high-frequency jet ventilation. The goal of all therapies is to maintain adequate tissue oxygenation with the least amount of inspired oxygen flow necessary.
- Medications to dilate constricted bronchial passages are administered intravenously and as inhalants to control bronchospasms and wheezing. Mucolytic agents liquefy tenacious sputum and aid in expectoration.
- An arterial line is placed in the client with major burn injury for continuous assessment of ABGs. Pulmonary artery pressure (PAP) catheters may be inserted to measure pulmonary vascular resistance (PVR), PAP, PAWP, and mixed venous oxygen saturation (SvO_2). The PVR and PAP rise in the presence of hypoxia. The SvO_2 is the average percentage of hemoglobin bound with oxygen in the venous blood and reflects overall tissue utilization of oxygen. Pulse oximetry monitors arterial oxygen saturation levels.
- In the presence of carbon monoxide (CO) poisoning, monitor carboxyhemoglobin (COHgb) levels. Pulse oximetry cannot distinguish between oxyhemoglobin and COHgb, thus a false normal or high pulse oximetry reading is seen. High-flow 100% oxygen is given immediately by nonrebreather mask. Clients with COHgb greater than 15% may require hyperbaric oxygen therapy to replace the CO.
- Pain medications are administered if the client is not in shock.

After stabilization in the emergency department, the client is transferred to the critical care unit or a specialized burn center (a facility that has a burn physician as director of a specialized nursing unit with dedicated burn beds). In both settings, continuous monitoring of diagnostic tests, administration of medications, pain control, wound management, and nutrition support therapies constitute the initial plan of care.

Diagnostic Tests

The following diagnostic tests are used to evaluate the client's progress and to modify intervention strategies.

- *Urinalysis* indicates the adequacy of renal perfusion and the client's nutritional status. In catabolic states, nitrogen is excreted in large amounts into the urine. Nitrogen loss is measured through 24-hour urine collections for total nitrogen, urea nitrogen, and amino acid nitrogen. *Myoglobinuria,* which manifests as a dark brown, wine-colored urine, signals the development of acute tubular necrosis. Loss of plasma protein and dehydration lead to proteinuria and elevated urine specific gravity. Glycosuria is a transient development following major burn injury; it indicates a need to adjust the nutritional program.
- The *complete blood count* (CBC) is monitored regularly. Hematocrit is elevated secondary to hemoconcentration and fluid shifts from the intravascular compartment. Hemoglobin is decreased secondary to hemolysis. WBCs are elevated if infection is present.
- *Serum electrolytes* are monitored regularly. Sodium levels are decreased secondary to massive fluid shifts into the interstitium. Potassium levels initially are elevated during burn shock, as a result of cell lysis and fluid shifts into the extracellular space. Potassium levels decrease after burn shock resolves, as fluid shifts back to intracellular and intravascular compartments.
- *Renal function* test results are closely monitored. Blood urea nitrogen (BUN) is elevated secondary to dehydration. Creatinine is elevated in the presence of renal insufficiency.
- *Total protein, albumin, transferrin, prealbumin, retinol binding protein, alpha one-acid glycoprotein,* and *C-reactive protein* indicate protein synthesis and nutritional status. Because of the fluid shifts that occur during the early stages of the burn injury, they are more useful markers during the rehabilitative phase of care.
- *Creatine phosphokinase (CPK)* is elevated following an electrical burn, secondary to extensive muscle damage. Blood glucose is transiently elevated after major burn injury.
- *Serial ABGs* indicate the presence of hypoxia and acid–base disturbances and indicate client responses to changes in oxygen therapies. The burn-injured client may demonstrate elevated or lowered pH, decreased PCO_2, decreased PO_2, and low-normal bicarbonate levels.
- *Pulse oximetry* allows continuous assessment of oxygen saturation levels. The burn-injured client may have saturation levels below 95%.
- *Serial chest x-ray studies* document changes within the first 24–48 hours that may reflect the presence of atelectasis, pulmonary edema, or ARDS.
- *Serial 12-lead electrocardiograms (EKGs)* are necessary to monitor the development of dysrhythmias, especially those associated with hypokalemic and hyperkalemic states.

Pharmacologic Therapies

Medications are required to control pain, prevent infection, and reduce the risk of peptic ulcer disease. IV fluids and other medications to support vital functions also may be indicated in clients with severe burns.

PAIN CONTROL Burns often cause excruciating pain. In the emergent stages of care, intravenously administered narcotics such as morphine, hydromorphone, or fentanyl are the best means of managing pain. Morphine is the drug of choice in a typical dosage of 3–5 mg intravenously every 5–10 minutes for an adult. Avoid meperidine because of potential normeperidine accumulation, which can produce tremors and anxiety. Once the client has been stabilized, it is appropriate to administer narcotics, especially IV fentanyl, prior to initiating hydrotherapy or intensive exercising routines.

During the acute stage, opioids may be administered around the clock to decrease pain that occurs at rest. Patient-controlled analgesia (PCA) enhances the client's ability to cope with pain. Avoid the oral, subcutaneous, and intramuscular routes of administration until hemodynamic stability and unimpaired tissue perfusion return.

Burn treatments and the trauma associated with experiencing a major burn can produce high levels of anxiety. Antianxiety agents such as midazolam and lorazepam may be helpful, especially when administered 1 hour before wound care (Montgomery, 2004).

INFECTION CONTROL Systemic infection is a leading cause of death in clients with major burns. Gram-positive organisms such as *Staphylococcus* and *Streptococcus* colonize the burn surface during the first week postburn; gram-negative enteric organisms become more common with longer periods of hospitalization. Diagnosing infection is best done through a burn wound biopsy (DeSanti, 2005). Depending on protocol, topical antimicrobial therapy may be used to eliminate infection on the surface of the burn wound. Generally, topical antimicrobials are not applied until the client is admitted to a burn unit. Of the many antimicrobial agents available, the three most widely used are mafenide acetate (Sulfamylon) cream, silver nitrate 0.5% soaks, and sulfadiazine (Silvadene) cream. All three are broad-spectrum antibiotics. The choice of topical antibiotic is based on the extent of the burn wound; the presence of identified bacterial organisms; the method of treatment used, that is, whether open (exposing the wound to the air) or closed (using bulky dressings); and client response. Despite

> **ALTERNATIVE THERAPIES Pain Control**
>
> As the client enters the rehabilitative stage of care, alternative therapies for pain control may be added to the plan of care. Distraction, self-hypnosis, guided imagery, and relaxation techniques are helpful adjuncts in managing pain and coping with loss.

antimicrobial therapy, clients with major burn assault have a greater risk for sepsis and septic shock.

Clients with major burns are usually given prophylactic antibiotics. Systemic antimicrobial therapy is indicated in the immediate preoperative and postoperative periods associated with excision and autografting. Postoperatively, the therapy is discontinued as soon as the client's hemodynamic status returns to normal, usually within the first 24 hours. In the long-term treatment of identified infectious processes, drug administration is limited to the least amount of time required to eradicate the infection.

TETANUS PROPHYLAXIS If the client's immunization status is in doubt, administer tetanus toxoid intramuscularly early in the acute phase of care to prevent *Clostridium tetani* infection. If tetanus immunization is older than 5 years, a booster should be administered.

PREVENTION OF GASTRIC HYPERACIDITY Hyperacidity must be controlled to prevent Curling's ulcer. A nasogastric tube is placed during the emergent phase of care, and gastric aspirant is obtained hourly. The gastric pH should be assessed and maintained at levels above 5. To control gastric acid secretion during the acute phase of care, histamine H_2 blockers (e.g., famotidine (Pepcid)) or proton pump inhibitors (e.g., pantoprazole (Protonix)) can be administered intravenously, either intermittently or as continuous infusions. As soon as bowel sounds become audible, the client is placed on an antacid regimen.

Surgery

Three surgical interventions are commonly employed to manage the burn wound: escharotomy, surgical debridement, and autografting.

ESCHAROTOMY When the burn eschar forms circumferentially around the torso or extremities, it acts as a tourniquet, impairing circulation. Left unchecked, the affected body part becomes gangrenous. To prevent circumferential constriction of the torso or extremity, the physician performs an **escharotomy**, removing the eschar with a scalpel or by electrocautery (Figure 30–14 ■). A sterile surgical incision is made longitudinally along the extremity or the trunk to release taut skin and allow for expansion caused by edema formation. In the first 24 hours following the procedure, the incision should be gently packed with fine-mesh gauze. After 24 hours, the site may be treated with direct application of a topical antimicrobial agent.

SURGICAL DEBRIDEMENT **Surgical debridement** refers to the process of excising the wound to the level of fascia (**fascial excision**) or sequentially removing thin slices of the burn wound to the level of viable tissue (**tangential excision**). Because fascial excision, or **fasciectomy**, sacrifices potentially viable fat and lymphatic tissue, its use is reserved for clients with extensive or full-thickness burns. The most common technique is electrocautery with cutting and coagulating current capabilities. Tangential excision is performed with the use of a dermatome. Shallow burns and some burns of moderate depth bleed briskly after one slice. If bleeding does not occur, the procedure is repeated until a viable bed of dermis or subcutaneous fat is reached. Following surgical debridement, the client is returned to the burn unit.

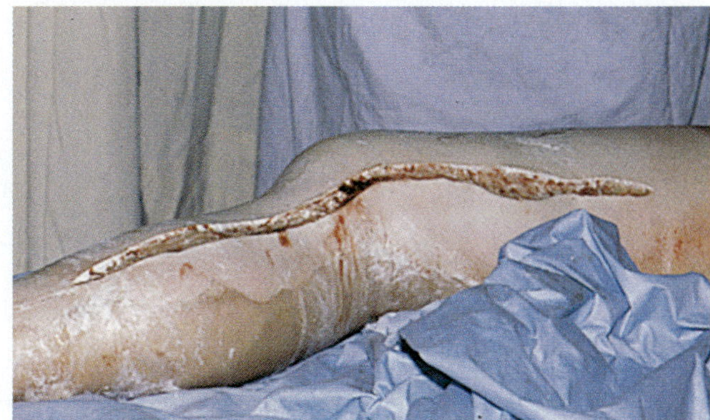

Figure 30–14 ■ Escharotomy, the surgical procedure that incises the eschar formed on the skin and underlying tissue following severe burns. The procedure is particularly helpful in restoring circulation to the extremities of clients when scar tissue forms a tight, constrictive band around the circumference of a limb.

Courtesy of Dr. William Dominic, Valley Medical Center.

AUTOGRAFTING **Autografting** is a procedure performed in the surgical suite in which part of the client's healthy skin is removed and used to effect permanent skin coverage over the wound area. Early burn wound excision and skin grafting decrease the hospital stay and enhance rehabilitation. Skin is removed from healthy tissue (donor site) of the burn-injured client and applied to the burn wound (Figures 30–15 ■ and 30–16 ■). After the autograft is applied, the grafted area is immobilized. The site is assessed daily for evidence of adherence. The client resumes ROM exercises 5 days postgraft. As the wound heals, the client may complain of itching, which can be treated with mild lotions.

Cultured epithelial autografting is a technique in which skin cells are removed from unburned sites on the client's body, then minced and placed in a culture medium for growth. Over a 5- to 7-day period, the cells expand 50–70 times the size of the initial biopsies. The cells are again separated out and placed in a new culture medium for continued growth. With this technique,

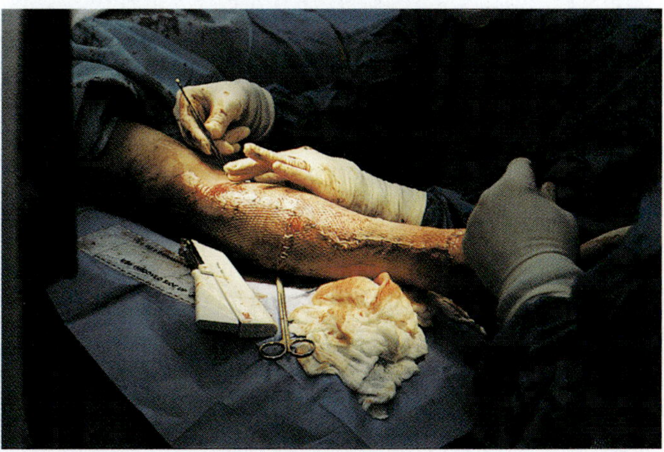

Figure 30–15 ■ Skin grafting procedure.

Courtesy of Dr. William Dominic, Valley Medical Center.

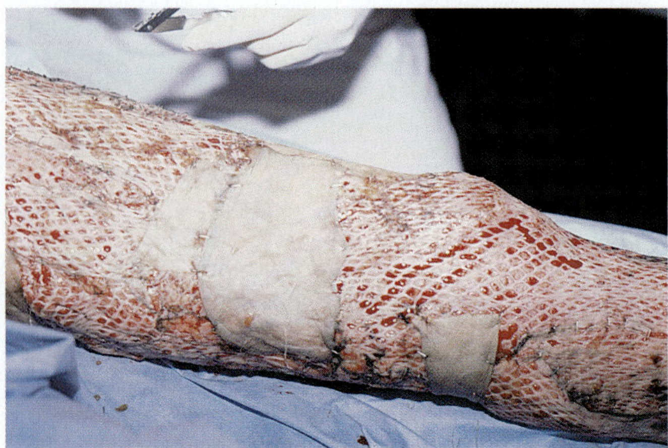

Figure 30–16 ■

Courtesy of Dr. William Dominic, Valley Medical Center.

enough skin can be grown over a period of 3–4 weeks to cover an entire human body. The cells are prepared in sheets and attached to petroleum jelly gauze backing, which is applied to the burn wound site. Problems with infection and lack of attachment have occurred.

Wound Management

The outcomes of care for the client with a major burn depend on the prevention and treatment of infection through daily topical wound care, wound monitoring, and wound excision and closure. The goals of wound management are as follows (Honari, 2004):

- Control microbial colonization and prevent wound infection.
- Prevent wound progression.
- Achieve wound coverage as early as possible.
- Promote function of healing skin.

Burned tissue releases chemical mediators that stimulate phagocytosis in an attempt to digest debris left by decaying necrotic tissue. Necrotic tissue that remains despite phagocytic action retards healing and prolongs inflammation. When this occurs, the necrotic tissue is removed by one of three ways: mechanical, enzymatic, or surgical debridement. Surgical debridement was discussed previously.

A nurse may perform mechanical debridement by applying and removing gauze dressings (wet-to-dry or wet-to-moist), or using hydrotherapy, irrigation, or scissors and tweezers. However, removal of gauze dressings can cause pain and possibly damage granulation tissue (Honari, 2004). During hydrotherapy (in an immersion tank, in a shower, or on a spray table), the burn injury may be gently washed with a mild, nonperfumed antimicrobial soap or wound cleanser solution to remove dead skin and separate eschar. The solution is then rinsed off with warm saline or tap water. Within the burn, body hair (except for eyebrows) should be shaved to within 2.5 cm of the wound edges. Blistered skin is grasped with dry gauze and gently removed. The edges of blisters or eschar are trimmed with blunt scissors. The wound is then covered with a topical antimicrobial agent.

Enzymatic debridement involves the use of a topical agent to dissolve and remove necrotic tissue as well as lift eschar. An enzyme such as Accuzyme, collagenase (Santyl), or fibrinolysis-deoxyribonuclease (Elase) is applied in a thin layer only within the wound area and covered with one layer of fine-mesh gauze. A topical antimicrobial agent is then applied and covered with a bulky wet dressing; the wound is immobilized with expandable mesh gauze. Enzymatic agents are discontinued once the eschar is removed and granulation tissue appears (Honari, 2004).

DRESSING THE WOUND Once the wound has been cleaned and debrided, it may be dressed using one of two methods. In the open method, the burn wound remains open to air, covered only by a topical antimicrobial agent. This method allows the wound to be easily assessed. Topical agents must be reapplied frequently because they tend to rub off onto the bedding. The open method also increases the risk for hypothermia (Sole et al., 2005).

In the closed method, a topical antimicrobial agent is applied to the wound site, which is covered with gauze or a nonadherent dressing and then gently wrapped with a gauze roll bandage (Figure 30–17 ■). With the closed method, burn wounds are usually dressed twice daily and as needed. Dressings are applied circumferentially in a distal-to-proximal manner. All fingers and toes are wrapped separately. Dressings are held in place with stockinettes rather than tape to prevent further skin injury. The closed method decreases heat loss but may impair ROM.

Contractures are a common problem for clients with burn injuries. During therapy, the client must be maintained in positions that prevent contractures from forming. Because flexion is the natural resting position of joints and extremities, early physical therapy includes maintaining antideformity positions. Splints immobilize body parts and prevent contractures of the joints. The splints are applied as soon as possible after the

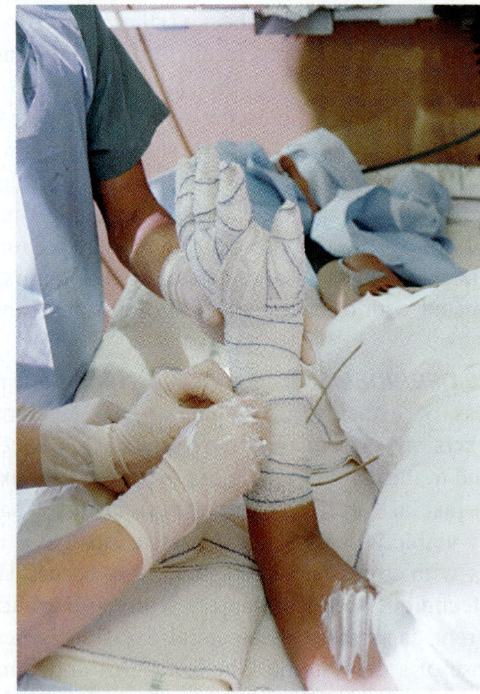

Figure 30–17 ■ Closed method of dressing a burn.

Courtesy of BSIP/Phototake NYC.

injury and removed according to schedules established by the physical therapist.

Early in the acute phase of care, the physical therapist prescribes active and passive ROM exercises, which are performed every 2 hours at the bedside, most often by physical therapy. Ideally, an exercise program is initiated on admission and continued until wounds are healed. Early ambulation also is part of the plan of care once the client's condition becomes stable.

Applying uniform pressure can prevent or reduce hypertrophic scarring. Tubular support bandages are applied 5–7 days postgraft to maintain tension ranging from 10–20 mmHg to control scarring. The client may wear custom-made elastic pressure garments (e.g., Jobst garments) for 6 months to a year postgraft (Figure 30–18 ■).

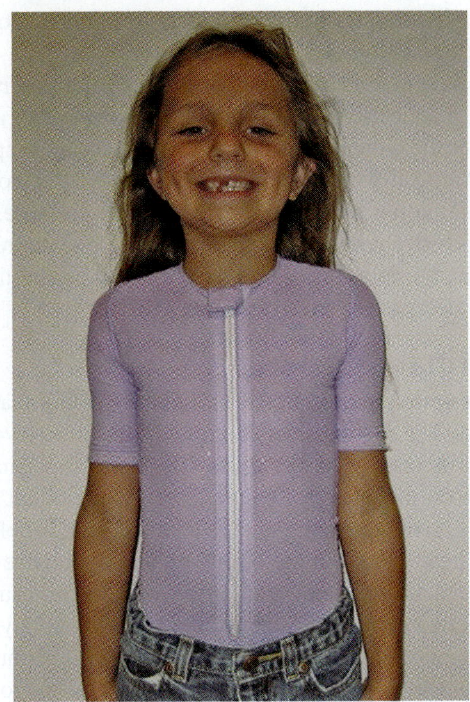

Figure 30–18 ■ Pressure garment used to reduce hypertrophic scarring from a burn to the chest and upper arms.

Courtesy of Martin R. Eichelberger, MD.

BIOLOGIC AND BIOSYNTHETIC DRESSINGS The terms *biological dressing* and *biosynthetic dressing* refer to any temporary material that rapidly adheres to the wound bed, promotes healing, and/or prepares the burn wound for permanent autograft coverage. Ideally, these kinds of dressings should be easy to apply and remove, inexpensive, nonantigenic, and elastic and should reduce pain, serve as a bacterial barrier, and enhance the natural healing process. The dressings are applied to the burn wound as soon as possible. Covering the wound eliminates the loss of water through evaporation, reduces infection, and promotes wound healing. Biological and biosynthetic dressings currently in use include homograft (allograft), heterograft (xenograft), amnionic membranes, and synthetic materials.

Homograft, or **allograft**, is human skin that has been harvested from cadavers. It is stored in skin banks located throughout the nation. The development of methods to achieve prolonged storage of viable frozen skin has increased the use of this dressing; however, its short supply and expense still pose problems. Homograft is cut to match the pattern of the burn and applied using sterile technique. As with any transplanted tissue, rejection is always a concern. Under normal circumstances, a homograft will demonstrate rejection within 14–21 days following application if it is not accepted However, even with rejection, the homograft acts as a covering to reduce infection and promote healing for as long as it remains in place.

Heterograft, or **xenograft**, is skin obtained from an animal, usually a pig. Although fresh porcine heterograft is available at some centers, frozen heterograft is more commonly used. Once applied, heterograft appears to undergo early softening and lysis from enzymatic action from the wound. As a result, frequent changes of the heterograft dressing are necessary. Because of the high infection rates associated with this dressing, silver nitrate-treated porcine heterograft has been developed to retard microbial growth.

The multiple problems associated with the use of biological dressings have driven the development of synthetic materials. One such material is Biobrane, a composite material consisting of nylon mesh bonded to silicone that has been successful in the temporary coverage of second- and third-degree burns. Whereas Biobrane adheres well to moderately clean wounds, it cannot adhere to or lower bacterial counts in grossly contaminated wounds. Biobrane dressing is supplied in various sizes, cut to fit the wound site, and secured with tape or Steri-Strips. It spontaneously separates from the wound when the underlying tissue heals. Hydrocolloid dressings are another type of biosynthetic material, which are occlusive wafers of gumlike materials that provide a water-resistant outer layer for coverage of the donor site. Hydrocolloid dressings protect healing tissue from excessive drying, liquefy necrotic tissue, and absorb wound drainage.

If dermal thickness is lost in deep partial-thickness or full-thickness burns, several products can serve as a dermal replacement. Integra is a synthetic dermal substitute, and AlloDerm is human cadaver allograft dermis that is nonimmunogenic. These products are placed in the wound, and split-thickness autografts are then placed over the dermal replacement. They provide temporary wound coverage, reduce pain, and facilitate healing.

Two recent temporary skin substitutes are TransCyte and Apligraf. TransCyte is a bioengineered substance derived from human fibroblast cells grown within mesh. As the cells grow, they secrete human dermal collagen, matrix proteins, and growth factors. The product is produced, extensively tested for infectious agents, and then frozen. It is used as a temporary covering for surgically debrided full-thickness and deep partial-thickness burn wounds and is an alternative to silver sulfadiazine and cadaver skin. TransCyte forms a transparent protective barrier over the wound surface and is typically applied only once. The best results have been obtained when it was applied within 24 hours of injury. Apligraf is a bilayered skin substitute cultured from neonatal foreskin.

The newest treatment method uses the vacuum-assisted closure (VAC) device (Figure 30–19 ■). VAC consists of a sponge placed over the wound with tubing that connects the sponge to a pump. An occlusive adhesive dressing covers the wound and tubing, sealing the wound to create negative pressure. VAC is showing positive results in reducing wound edema, removing exudate, and improving wound healing in partial-thickness burns and deep hand burns (DeSanti, 2005).

Nutritional Support

The client with a major burn is in a hypermetabolic and catabolic state. The resting energy expenditure after severe burn injury can increase by as much as 100% above normal levels depending on the extent of catabolism and the client's physical activity, size, age, and gender. This increase is believed to be due to heat loss from the burn wound, an increase in beta-adrenergic activity, pain, and infection. As a result, total caloric needs may be as great as 4000–6000 kcal/day.

Traditional dietary management based on oral intake seldom meets the kilocalorie requirements necessary to reverse negative nitrogen balance and begin the healing process. Therefore, enteral feedings with a nasointestinal feeding tube are instituted within 24–48 hours of the burn injury to offset hypermetabolism, improve nitrogen balance, decrease sepsis, and decrease length of hospital stay. A nasointestinal feeding tube is placed under fluoroscopy, with the tip extending past the pylorus to prevent reflux and aspiration.

Although enteral feeding is the preferred nutritional therapy, it is contraindicated in Curling's ulcer, bowel obstruction, feeding intolerance, pancreatitis, and septic ileus. When the enteral route cannot be used, a central venous catheter is inserted via the subclavian or jugular vein for the administration of total parenteral nutrition.

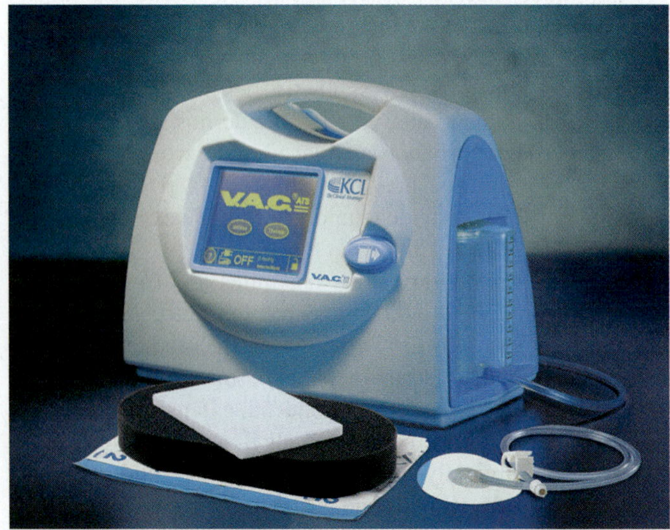

Figure 30–19 ■ Wound vacuum.

Courtesy of KCI Licensing, Inc.

NURSING PROCESS

The client with a major burn has complex multisystem needs. During the acute phase, life support and monitoring take priority. As the client begins to heal, the client begins to cope with scarring, hair loss, and powerlessness. Altered body image and loss of independence for a significant period of time, sometimes lifelong, must be considered when planning care.

Assessment

Nursing assessment is continuous from the initial contact with the client with a burn injury. This section describes the survey that is conducted when the client arrives at the emergency department. Once the client arrives, the staff must act quickly to obtain the history of the burn injury, including the time of injury, causative agents, early treatment, medical history, and client's age and body weight. In most cases, the client is awake and oriented and can relate the information during the emergent phase of care. Because changes in sensory abilities become evident within the first few hours following a major burn injury, the nurse obtains as much information as possible immediately upon the client's arrival.

- *Time of injury.* In many cases, the client is admitted to the emergency department an hour or more after the injury occurred. The time of the burn injury must be documented as precisely as possible at the scene because all fluid resuscitation calculations are based on the time of the burn injury, not on the client's time of arrival at the ER.
- *Cause of the injury.* Because the type of burn injury determines which nursing measures take priority, identify the specific causative agent to establish the appropriate plan of care.
- *First-aid treatment.* Prior to the arrival of medical personnel, the client or family may have applied home remedies to treat the burn wound. It is important for the nurse to ascertain and document the nature of all home treatment interventions, including the application of neutralizing agents, liquids, and immobilizing devices used to splint associated injuries.
- *Past medical history.* Clients with histories of respiratory, cardiac, renal, metabolic, neurologic, gastrointestinal, or skin diseases; alcohol abuse; or altered immune states require more intense observation. The nurse must obtain information about known allergies.
- *Age.* Children and older adults tend to require more supportive care.
- *Medications.* Drugs, either prescribed or recreational, taken by the client prior to the burn injury may further complicate the treatment regimen. Drugs that affect any of the major body systems or cause mood alterations need to be factored into the treatment plan. As part of the early assessment, the nurse must obtain and document blood levels of therapeutic pharmaceutical agents and mood-altering substances.

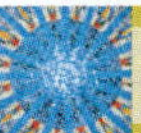

DEVELOPMENTAL CONSIDERATIONS Assessing a Child With a Burn Injury

Interviewing a parent about a child's burn injury can be difficult. If the injury was preventable, the parent may be emotionally stressed by feelings of guilt. The nurse must use caution to avoid sounding accusatory when questioning the parent about the injury.

The nurse should be alert to signs of child abuse when the history does not match the burn injury (e.g., glove and stocking burns; burns that spare flexor surfaces; contact burns from objects such as a curling iron, cigarettes, and irons; and zebra burn lines from contact with a hot grate) (Figure 30–20 ■). Photographs may be taken to document these burn injuries. Child neglect can be a factor in the burn of a child who was not adequately supervised.

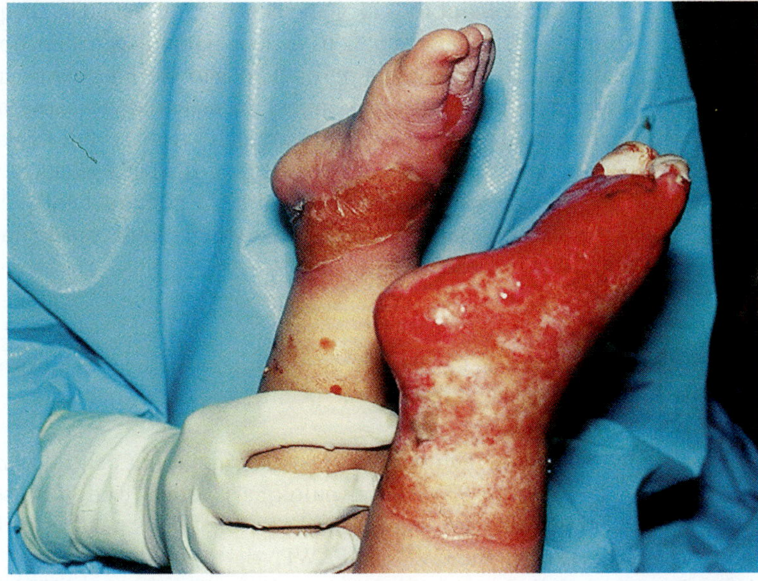

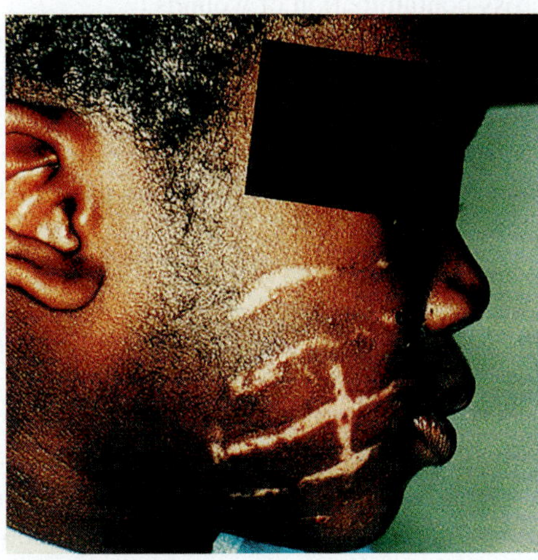

Figure 30–20 ■ Burn injuries associated with child abuse: *A,* Burns of the hands or feet that are distributed like gloves or stockings with a clear demarcation matching the depth of hot water and few splash marks are seen. *B,* Zebra burns from holding the face to a hot grate.

Courtesy of the American Academy of Pediatrics, Elk Grove, IL, and the Kempe Children's Center, Denver, CO.

- *Body weight.* During the acute and rehabilitative phases of the burn injury, the client will lose as much as 20% of preburn weight. This fact has significant implications for all clients, especially those who are underweight at the time of the injury.

Diagnosis

Each client's condition warrants individualized nursing diagnoses. Common diagnoses appropriate to care of the client with burns may include the following:

- Impaired Skin Integrity
- Deficient Fluid Volume
- Acute Pain
- Risk for Infection
- Impaired Physical Mobility
- Imbalanced Nutrition: Less Than Body Requirements
- Powerlessness.

Plan

A major burn affects virtually every body system, as well as social, cultural, economic, psychologic, and spiritual well-being. The plan of care changes as the client moves from stage to stage and requires frequent updating as different needs arise. Potential goals of nursing care are individualized and designed in collaboration with the client and family. These goals often include the following:

- The client will maintain adequate fluid volume.
- The client will receive adequate nutrition to meet the body's needs.
- The client will maintain adequate pain control reporting pain as a 3 or less.
- The client will not develop a nosocomial infection.
- The client will maintain full ROM following recovery.

Implementation

The first priority of care is to maintain life support by assuring the client has a functional airway, is breathing, and circulation is not impaired.and to stop the burning process. Once this is achieved, wound care, fluid volume, infection prevention, and pain management must be addressed. Continuous assessment is necessary until well into the healing process and should include assessment of client and family feelings regarding the injury and long-term effects.

Impaired Skin Integrity

The burn injury significantly impairs skin integrity. The severity of wounds varies according to the depth and extent of the burn. General treatment measures are designed to restore normal skin function as quickly as possible. Nursing care focuses on assessing and cleaning the wound and controlling infection.

- Estimate the extent and depth of the burn wound and recalculate extent of unhealed burns weekly. The severity of the burn injury is the basis for determining which types of interventions are appropriate. Reassessment on a regular basis is necessary to monitor the healing process.
- Provide daily wound care (including debridement method, dressing method, and medication administration) as prescribed to remove dead tissue, control infection, and promote reepithelialization as soon as possible. Avoid cross-contamination of wounds.
- Elevate burned or newly skin-grafted extremities at or above heart level to increase venous return and to prevent edema formation.
- Immobilize skin graft sites for 3–5 days or as ordered to promote graft adherence and to prevent loss of newly grafted skin.

PRACTICE ALERT
Move clients slowly and carefully across bed sheets to prevent shearing or dislodging new skin grafts.

- Provide special skin care to sensitive body areas as follows:
  a. Clean burns involving the eyes using normal saline or sterile water to prevent corneal and conjunctival drying and adherence. If contracture of the eyelid develops, apply drops or ointment to the eye to prevent corneal abrasion.
  b. Gently wipe burns of the lips with saline-soaked pads. Apply an antibiotic ointment as prescribed. Assess the mouth frequently and perform mouth care routinely. If an oral endotracheal tube is in place, reposition it often to prevent pressure ulcer formation.
  c. Gently debride burns of the nose and apply mafenide acetate (Sulfamylon) cream. Position nasogastric and nasotracheal tubes to prevent excessive pressure.
  d. Apply mafenide acetate (Sulfamylon) cream to burns of the ear. Gently debride and thoroughly clean the wound with a water spray. Do not cover ears with dressings. Do not use pillows; to reduce pressure to the area, use a foam doughnut instead. Burns of the ears are prone to infection; special positioning devices are necessary to decrease pressure ulcer formation.

Deficient Fluid Volume

Fluid resuscitation rates are adjusted periodically throughout the emergent stage of care. The nurse should be particularly aware of several situations that may warrant the administration of fluids at rates in excess of the calculations needed to maintain adequate urine output. Those situations include initial underestimation of the burn size, sequestration of fluid into the lung tissue in an inhalation injury, electrical injury (which tends to cause more extensive damage than is immediately visible), full-thickness burns, and inordinately delayed starts of fluid resuscitation.

- Assess blood pressure and heart rate frequently. Vital signs rapidly deteriorate when fluid resuscitation is inadequate.

PRACTICE ALERT
Tachycardia in the burn client is not a consideration until the heart rate is greater than 120 beats per minute.

- Monitor hemodynamic status, including central venous pressure (CVP) and pulmonary artery wedge pressure (PAWP). Inadequate fluid resuscitation is manifested by a drop in the CVP and PAWP.
- Follow prescribed protocols for intravenous (IV) fluid resuscitation. Therapy for burn shock is aimed at supporting the client through the period of hypovolemic instability.
- Monitor intake and output hourly. Report urine outputs of less than 50 mL/h. Intake and output measurements indicate the adequacy of fluid resuscitation and should range from 30–50 mL/h in an adult.
- Weigh daily. Body weight is used to calculate fluid requirements.
- Test all stools and emesis for the presence of blood. Occult blood in emesis or stool indicates gastrointestinal bleeding.
- Maintain a warm environment. Hypothermia leads to shivering and further loss of body fluid through increased energy expenditure and catabolism.

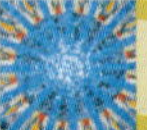

DEVELOPMENTAL CONSIDERATIONS **Burns in the Older Adult**

Older adults are at greater risk for burns of all degrees of severity, with burns and fires being a major cause of death. Most burns are accidental, resulting from slower reaction times, decreased mobility, visual deficits, a decreased sense of smell, forgetfulness, and impaired sensation. Many older adults are burned by stoves, hot water, hot food, irons, cookware, and heating pads. Older adults with cognitive impairment or dementia may start fires by leaving foods cooking unattended. The most common burns in this age group result from clothing catching on fire and scalding from tap water that is too hot.

The care of the older adult with burns often presents unique challenges. Older adults may delay seeking treatment, thus increasing the risk of infection. Their care is often complicated by the presence of other chronic illnesses. They may live alone and have no one to care for them during rehabilitation. Even small burns have the potential to become lethal in older adults.

Burn prevention topics for older adults include the following:

- Have a relative or neighbor routinely check for the odor of gas.
- Check the smoke detector battery once a month.
- Wear close-fitting clothing when cooking.
- Use a cooking timer with a loud alarm.
- Do not lay anything over a heating device.
- Set the temperature of the hot water heater no higher than 120°F.
- Install anti-scald devices in bathroom plumbing.
- Encourage no smoking in the house.

- Monitor for fluid volume overload. Older clients and those with underlying cardiac disease may demonstrate symptoms of heart failure during the fluid resuscitation stage.

PRACTICE ALERT

Major burn clients receive 10 or more liters of fluid and will gain weight with the fluid shifts. When capillary membrane integrity resumes, clients have a high CVP and urine output that necessitates monitoring of urine electrolytes.

Acute Pain

Extensive superficial and all partial-thickness burns can cause excrutiating pain, as can wound care and physical therapy. Increased levels of anxiety about treatments and outcomes may increase the perception of pain.

- Measure the client's level of pain using a consistent measurement tool. Pain tolerance is the duration and intensity of pain that the client is able to endure. Pain tolerance differs from one client to the next and may vary in the same client in different situations. A description of pain management tools can be found in Concept 5 in the exemplar on acute and chronic pain.
- Medicate before painful procedures and determine when PCA is appropriate. The inability to manage pain results in feelings of despair and frustration for the client.
- Administer IV narcotic analgesics as prescribed. Nurses' fears of precipitating addiction often make them reluctant to administer narcotics. During the acute stage of burn injury, however, invasive procedures and exposed neurosensory nerve endings dictate the need for narcotic pharmaceutical agents.
- Explain all procedures and expected levels of discomfort. Clients experience less stress when they are prepared for painful procedures and know beforehand the actual sensations they will feel.
- Use methods of nonnarcotic pain control in combination with medications for pain. Noninvasive pain relief measures (e.g., relaxation, massage, distraction) can enhance the therapeutic effects of pain relief medications.
- Allow the client to verbalize the pain experience. Each person experiences and expresses pain in his or her own manner using various sociocultural adaptation techniques.

PRACTICE ALERT

Narcotics are always administered intravenously (rather than orally, subcutaneously, or intramuscularly) in the emergent or acute stage of a burn due to decreased circulation and absorption of medications.

Risk for Infection

From the onset of the burn injury, loss of the body's natural barrier to the external environment increases the risk of infection. Nursing interventions focus on controlling infectious processes. Monitor the results of diagnostic tests; maintain nutritional therapies; and apply antimicrobial agents to monitor and prevent the spread of infection, a major complication of the burn injury.

- Monitor daily for manifestations of wound infection. Remove topical medications and wound exudate and examine the entire wound. Early manifestations of wound infection include swelling and inflammation in intact skin surrounding the wound; a change in the color, odor, or amount of exudate; increased pain; and loss of previously healed skin grafts.

PRACTICE ALERT

An increase in body temperature without other manifestations of infection is not indicative of infection in clients with large burn wounds (in which the hypermetabolic response resets the core temperature to a higher level).

- Monitor for positive blood cultures, which indicate bacteremia.
- Monitor for hyperemia, cough, chest pain, wheezing, rhonchi, decreased oxygen saturation, and purulent sputum, which are manifestations of pneumonia.
- Monitor for the presence of bacteria in the urine, fever, urgency, frequency, dysuria, and superpubic pain, which are manifestations of urinary tract infections.

PRACTICE ALERT

If the client has an indwelling catheter, assess the urine for cloudiness and a foul odor and obtain a urine culture and sensitivity at least weekly.

- Obtain daily WBC counts. Leukocyte counts are indicators of immune system function and increase in the presence of infection.
- Determine tetanus immunization status. Burn clients are at risk for anaerobic infection caused by *Clostridium tetani.*
- Maintain a high-kilocalorie intake. Nutritional support provides the nutrients needed to maintain the body's defense mechanisms.
- Maintain an aseptic environment using standard precautions (including gloving, gowning, and sterile procedures). Strict isolation technique deters the development of nosocomial infections.
- Culture all wounds and body secretions per protocol. Culture and sensitivity reports identify the presence of infectious microbes and indicate appropriate antimicrobial therapies.
- Administer prescribed antimicrobial medications to decrease invasive wound infections.

Impaired Physical Mobility

As the burn wound heals and new skin tissue forms, the involved area tends to shrink. Contractures form at the site and significantly limit mobility, especially when a joint is involved. Physical therapy is important beginning in the early stages of treatment. The nurse institutes ambulation and planned exercise regimens as soon as the client's condition stabilizes.

- Perform active or passive ROM exercises to all joints every 2 hours. Ambulate when stable. Regular exercise prevents further loss of motion, restores movement, and improves functional status.
- Apply splints as prescribed. Maintain antideformity positions and reposition the client hourly. Splinting and positioning retard the formation of contractures.

- Maintain limbs in functional alignment to preserve joint mobility.
- Anticipate the need for analgesia. Administering analgesics promotes the client's comfort during exercising sessions.

PRACTICE ALERT

Assess all clients, especially older adults, for indications of pressure ulcer formation under a splint.

Imbalanced Nutrition: Less Than Body Requirements

The burn injury initiates a complex series of events that have a profound effect on the body's use of nutrients and expenditure of energy. The dietitian determines daily kilocalorie requirements, and as soon as possible, enteral feedings are initiated. Nasointestinal tubes are placed to enhance intestinal absorption and retard gastric reflux. Parenteral nutrition is reserved for instances in which enteral feedings are contraindicated. Nursing measures focus on assessing feeding tolerance and use of nutrients.

- Maintain nasogastric/nasointestinal tube placement. Correct tube placement ensures appropriate absorption of nutrients and prevents aspiration.
- Maintain enteral/parenteral nutritional support as prescribed. Observe and report any evidence of feeding intolerance: diarrhea, vomiting, excessive gastric residual, abdominal distention, absent bowel sounds, and constipation. The dietitian, in collaboration with the physician, selects and individualizes the feeding formula according to the client's daily energy expenditure requirements and feeding tolerance. Failure to maintain rates of infusion predisposes the client to continued catabolism and negative nitrogen balance.
- Weigh the client daily. Weight indicates the adequacy of nutritional support therapies.
- Obtain daily laboratory values for protein, iron, CBC, glucose, and albumin. Decreased serum values indicate inadequate nutritional intake.

Powerlessness

Usually, the client with a major burn injury endures a lengthy hospital stay involving many treatments and care protocols that are beyond his or her control. During the early stages, much of the care regimen involves excruciating pain. Further, the foreign environment of the burn unit makes it difficult for the client to relate to the immediate surroundings. For example, the need to control infection in the burn unit requires hospital personnel and family members to don sterile clothing prior to coming to the client's bedside. Family members and nursing personnel appear radically different when they are masked and gowned, and their odd appearance can add to the burn-injured client's sense of alienation. The client's body image is often altered depending on the extent and location of the burn injury.

- Allow the client as much control over the surroundings and daily routine as possible. For example, allow the client to choose times of dressing changes. Powerlessness derives from the belief that one is unable to influence the outcome of a situation.
- Keep needed items (e.g., call bell, urinal, water pitcher, and tissues) within the client's reach to reinforce the client's feelings of control.
- Encourage the client to express feelings. The nurse can help the client cope by therapeutically listening, displaying a caring presence, clarifying misconceptions, and providing positive feedback.
- Set short-term, realistic goals for the client (e.g., to ambulate from bedside to chair twice daily). Small incremental gains are easier to achieve and allow for frequent positive reinforcement.

Table 30–8 lists overall nursing interventions for the emergent, acute, and rehabilitative stages of burn injury.

Evaluation

The client with a severe burn must be constantly evaluated and the plan of care changed to meet emerging or diminishing needs. It is not unusual for a client with a severe burn to be hospitalized for extended periods of time, requiring new care plan modifications as the client moves through the recovery

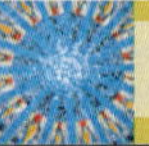

DEVELOPMENTAL CONSIDERATIONS Recovery From Burns

CHILDREN

Play therapy is encouraged for children even if they can only observe initially. Play therapy serves the following purposes for the child with a major burn:

- Provides an outlet for frustration, independence, and creativity
- Promotes activities that challenge ROM
- Normalizes the child's daily routine
- Encourages the child, who sees the progress that other children make day by day.

FAMILY

Families of children with major burns are at risk for emotional stress. They should be forewarned to expect edema and changes in the child's body with the injury response. Fear usually results from lack of knowledge about the severity of the burn and the child's status, especially in the early stages of burn care and admission to the hospital's intensive care unit (ICU). Include the family in the child's care when possible. The family must be given information and frequent updates to promote the development of trust between the family and the health care team. Parents often feel guilty and responsible for the child's injury. It is important to help parents focus on recovery rather than past actions.

TABLE 30–8 Interventions in Various Stages of Burn Injury

STAGE OF BURN INJURY	ONSET	END POINT	INTERVENTIONS
Emergent/resuscitative	Occurrence of burn injury	Successful fluid resuscitation	Remove client from heat source. Initiate first aid. Assess extent of burn injury. Prevent hypothermia. Assess for shock. Determine need for intubation. Determine need for IV therapy. Follow protocol for fluid resuscitation. Obtain history. Transport to tertiary care facility.
Acute	Diuresis	Wound closure	Begin hydrotherapy. Determine need for excision of burn wound. Control spread of infection. Institute wound care. Start nutrition support. Graft burn wound. Initiate physical therapy. Manage pain.
Rehabilitative	Wound closure	Return to highest level of health restoration	Prevent scar formation. Continue physical therapy. Address psychosocial, cultural, and spiritual needs. Consider occupational therapy. Consider vocational training. Assess home maintenance management.

process. Expected outcomes used to evaluate client progress may include the following:

- The client maintains stable vital signs as evidenced by values within normal limits.
- The client receives adequate pain management to allow for comfort as evidenced by being able to rest and reporting pain level as a 3 or less.
- The client's nutritional needs are met as evidenced by stable weight, balanced intake and output, and laboratory values within normal range.
- The client is infection-free as evidenced by CBC within normal range and wound healing.

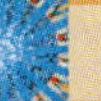

CLIENT TEACHING **Burn Care**

Client and family teaching is an important component of all phases of burn care. As treatment progresses, the nurse encourages family members to assume more responsibility in providing care. However, many burn centers perform burn dressing changes in a burn clinic because parents find it difficult to perform procedures they know will inflict pain on their child. If parents provide dressing changes, the nurse should provide client teaching regarding how to change the dressing(s) and how soon before the dressing change to give the pain medication. Specific guidelines for dressing changes should be outlined so that parents and health care team members have the same focus.

From admission to discharge, the nurse teaches the client and family to assess all findings, implement therapies, and evaluate progress. The nurse should address the following topics when preparing the client and family for home care:

- Long-term goals of rehabilitation care: to prevent soft tissue deformity, protect skin grafts, maintain physiologic function, manage scars, and return the client to an optimal level of independence
- Necessity of avoiding exposure to people with colds or infections and following aseptic technique meticulously when caring for the wound
- Need for progressive physical activity
- Procedures for applying splints, pressure support garments, and other assistive devices
- Dietary requirements with required kilocalories
- Alternative pain control therapies such as guided imagery, relaxation techniques, and diversional activities
- Care of the graft and donor sites
- Referral for occupational therapy, social service, clergy, and/or psychiatric services as appropriate
- Recommend resources as needed, including the following:
- American Burn Association
- International Society for Burn Injuries
- American Academy of Facial Plastic and Reconstructive Surgery
- The Phoenix Society for Burn Survivors, Inc.

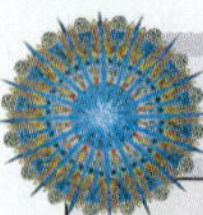

NURSING CARE PLAN A Client With a Major Burn

Craig Howard, a 39-year-old truck driver, is admitted to the hospital following an accident in which the cab of his truck caught on fire. He was freed from the truck by a passing motorist, who stayed with him until the rescue team arrived to transport him to a local emergency department. Mr. Howard's wife, Mary, and twin daughters, Jessica and Jane, age 10, have been notified.

ASSESSMENT

On his admission to the emergency department, Mr. Howard is diagnosed with deep partial-thickness and full-thickness burns of the anterior chest, arms, and hands. A quick assessment based on the rule of nines estimates the extent of his burn injury at 36% of TBSA. His vital signs are as follows: T 35.6°C rectal (96.2°F), P 140, R 40, BP 98/60. In the field, the paramedics had inserted a large-bore central line into Mr. Howard's right subclavian vein and started the rapid infusion of lactated Ringer's solution. Mr. Howard is receiving 40% humidified oxygen via face mask. Initial ABGs are pH 7.49, Po_2 60 mmHg, Pco_2 32 mmHg, and bicarbonate 22 mEq/L. Lung sounds indicate inspiratory and expiratory wheezing, and a persistent cough reveals sooty sputum production. A Foley catheter is inserted and initially drains a moderate amount of dark concentrated urine. A nasogastric tube is connected to low intermittent suction. Mr. Howard is alert and oriented and complains of severe pain associated with the burn injuries. The burn unit is notified, and Mr. Howard is transferred there.

DIAGNOSES

- Risk for Ineffective Airway Clearance related to increasing lung congestion secondary to smoke inhalation
- Deficient Fluid Volume related to abnormal fluid loss secondary to burn injury
- Risk for Ineffective Tissue Perfusion (peripheral) related to peripheral constriction secondary to circumferential burn wounds of the arms

PLANNING

Goals of nursing care include the following:

- Demonstrate a patent airway as evidenced by clear breath sounds; absence of cyanosis; and vital signs, chest x-ray findings, and ABGs within normal limits.
- Demonstrate adequate fluid volume and electrolyte balance as evidenced by urine output, vital signs, mental status, and laboratory findings within normal limits.
- Demonstrate adequate tissue perfusion as evidenced by palpable pulses, warm extremities, normal capillary refill, and absence of paresthesia.

IMPLEMENTATION

- Prepare for prophylactic nasotracheal intubation to maintain airway patency.
- Initiate fluid resuscitation therapy using the Parkland formula to calculate IV fluid rate for the first 24 hours postburn.
- Assist the physician to perform escharotomies of both upper extremities.

EVALUATION

The nurse anesthetist inserted a nasotracheal tube and connected Mr. Howard to a T-piece delivering 40% oxygen. Vigorous respiratory toileting has significantly improved his ABGs. Bronchodilators have been parenterally administered and mucolytic agents added to his respiratory treatments. His tracheal secretions have begun to show evidence of clearing. Hourly urine outputs indicate adequate fluid resuscitation. Urine output has been maintained at 50 mL/h, and color and concentration have improved. CVP readings have been maintained at 6 cm H_2O, and blood pressure has increased to 100/64. The pulse rate has decreased to 100.

To improve tissue perfusion of both arms, the physician has performed bilateral escharotomies, and the wounds have been dressed using sterile procedure. The extremities have demonstrated improved circulation.

CRITICAL THINKING

1. Explain the rationale for the immediate insertion of a Foley catheter and nasogastric tube.
2. An escharotomy was performed on both arms. Why was this procedure necessary in Mr. Howard's case?
3. What is the rationale supporting the IV administration of narcotics to control Mr. Howard's pain?
4. Explain the sequence of events that led to a fluid and electrolyte shift during the first 24–48 hours after Mr. Howard sustained his injury.

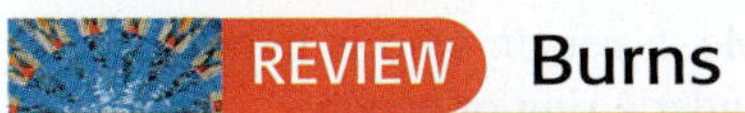

REVIEW Burns

RELATE: LINK THE CONCEPTS

Linking the exemplar of Burns with the concept of Comfort:

1. When providing care to the client with deep full thickness burns involving the entire right arm, will the nurse need to administer analgesics? Explain your answer.
2. The client is brought to the emergency department with partial-thickness burns of the chest and neck. The client is crying in pain. What nursing considerations will impact the plan for pain management for this client?

Linking the exemplar of Burns with the concept of Development:

3. When caring for a 12-year-old client admitted following a major burn, what pain scale is most appropriate for assessing pain? Explain your choice.
4. When caring for this 12-year-old client, and her physical condition stabilizes, how will the nurse address the client's developmental issues?

READY: GO TO COMPANION SKILLS MANUAL

- Monitoring intake and output
- Establishing intravenous infusions
- Regulating infusion flow rates
- Maintaining infusions
- Maintaining intermittent infusion devices
- Preparing for dressing change using individual supplies
- Changing a sterile dressing
- Adding medications to intravenous fluid containers
- Administering intravenous medications using IV push
- Managing pain with a PCA pump

REFER: GO TO MYNURSINGKIT

REFLECT: CASE STUDY

David Newton, aged 54, was smoking a cigarette and fell asleep, dropping the cigarette and igniting the bed linens. A neighbor discovered the fire and called 911. As a result, Mr. Newton was rescued by the fire department. He sustained full-thickness burns over the upper half of his chest and back and the posterior aspects of both upper arms. He also sustained superficial partial-thickness burns to his anterior and posterior head and neck. He was initially treated in the local emergency department and then transported via life flight to the specialized burn unit located 150 miles from his home. Upon his arrival in the burn unit, 5 hours after injury, the nurse notes the presence of a Foley catheter that is draining burgundy-colored urine. Mr. Newton also has a nasogastric tube that is draining dark yellow-green liquid. He was intubated in the emergency department and is now placed on a ventilator in the burn unit. Upon admission to the burn unit, his vital signs are: T_O 37.8°C (100°F), P 100, R 24, BP 96/56. His pain level is reported as a 9 on a 1–10 scale, and he is medicated with morphine sulfate 10 mg IV as per the physician's order.

1. The initial assessment in the emergency room (ER) is that Mr. Newton has sustained burns over 36% of his body. Using the rule of nines, how does the nurse analyze this total percentage?
2. Mr. Newton is in the phase of burn shock. His temperature is 37.8°C (100°F), pulse 100, respirations 24, and blood pressure 96/56. His urinary output for the past 5 hours has been 150 ml. What is the nurse's explanation for the physiology of shock related to a major burn injury?
3. Mr. Newton's diagnosis is impaired gas exchange related to swelling secondary to inhalation injury manifested by need for intubation and mechanical ventilation. Why was intubation necessary for Mr. Newton? What important nursing interventions are related to this?
4. Why was Mr. Newton's Foley catheter draining burgundy-colored urine at the time of admission to the burn unit?
5. Mr. Newton is put on enteral feeding during the recovery phase of the burn injury, and the nursing diagnosis established is imbalanced nutrition: less than body requirements related to hypermetabolic and catabolic stage secondary to a major burn. What is the rationale for this diagnosis?

30.2 CONTACT DERMATITIS

KEY TERMS

Allergic contact dermatitis, *1912*
Contact dermatitis, *1912*
Irritant contact dermatitis, *1912*
Patch testing, *1913*

BASIS FOR SELECTION OF EXEMPLAR

Frequency of office-based visits

LEARNING OUTCOMES

After reading about this exemplar, you will be able to:

1. Describe the pathophysiology, etiology, clinical manifestations, and direct and indirect causes of contact dermatitis.
2. Identify risk factors associated with contact dermatitis.
3. Illustrate the nursing process in providing culturally competent and caring interventions across the life span for individuals with contact dermatitis.
4. Formulate priority nursing diagnoses appropriate for an individual with contact dermatitis.
5. Create a plan of care for individuals with contact dermatitis and their family members.
6. Assess expected outcomes for an individual with contact dermatitis.
7. Discuss therapies used in the collaborative care of an individual with contact dermatitis.
8. Employ evidence-based caring interventions for an individual with contact dermatitis.

OVERVIEW

Contact dermatitis is an inflammation of the skin that occurs in response to direct contact with an allergen or irritant. The major sources known to cause contact dermatitis are dyes, perfumes, poison plants (ivy, oak, sumac), chemicals, and metals (Box 30–3). Latex (glove) dermatitis is a contact dermatitis that is common in the health care field.

> **PRACTICE ALERT**
>
> - The increased use of latex gloves among health care providers has resulted in increased reporting of latex allergies. It is estimated that 10–17% of health care providers are allergic to latex (Porth, 2005).
> - The most common type of allergic response to latex gloves is type IV, T cell-mediated contact dermatitis.
> - Type I, IgE-mediated hypersensitivity, manifested by urticaria, rhinoconjunctivitis, asthma, or anaphylaxis, is far more serious than the T cell-mediated type.
> - All clients with a latex allergy should be treated in a latex-free environment.
> - Health care providers with severe allergic responses to latex may have to seek a different type of employment.

PATHOPHYSIOLOGY AND ETIOLOGY

Allergic contact dermatitis is a cell-mediated or delayed hypersensitivity to a wide variety of allergens. Sensitizing antigens include microorganisms, plants, chemicals, drugs, metals, and foreign proteins. On initial contact with the skin, the allergen binds to a carrier protein, forming a sensitizing antigen. The antigen is processed and carried to the T cells, which in turn become sensitized to the antigen. The first exposure is the sensitizing contact: the individual does not experience manifestations until subsequent exposures. Manifestations include erythema, swelling, and pruritic vesicles in the area of allergen contact. For example, a person who is hypersensitive to metal may have lesions under a ring or watch.

Irritant contact dermatitis is an inflammation of the skin from irritants; it is not a hypersensitivity response. Common sources of irritant contact dermatitis include chemicals (such as acids), soaps, and detergents. The skin lesions are similar to those seen in allergic contact dermatitis.

> **Box 30–3 Common Causes of Contact Dermatitis**
>
> - Acids
> - Alkalis: soaps, detergents, household ammonia, lye, cleaners
> - Bromide
> - Chlorine
> - Cosmetics: perfumes, dyes, oils
> - Dusts of lime, arsenic, wood
> - Hydrocarbons: crude petroleum, lubricating oil, mineral oil, paraffin, asphalt, tar
> - Iodine
> - Insecticides
> - Fabrics: wool, polyester, dyes, sizing
> - Metal salts: calcium chloride, zinc chloride, copper, mercury, nickel, silver
> - Plants: ragweed, poison oak, poison sumac, poison ivy, pine
> - Coloring agents
> - Rubber products
> - Soot

Risk Factors

Risk factors for contact dermatitis include allergies, family history of eczema, regular exposure to a moist environment, burns, exposure to plants, chemicals, and metals, occupations that require frequent hand washing. The elderly are also at greater risk for contact dermatitis.

CLINICAL MANIFESTATIONS

Allergic contact dermatitis is characterized by erythema, edema, pruritus, vesicles, or bullae that rupture, ooze, and crust (Figure 30–21 ■). The rash is usually limited to the area of contact; for example, the rash may be linear where a poison ivy leaf brushed against the skin. Symptoms of allergic contact dermatitis can develop several hours to 3 days after exposure, when the immunologic response has been activated. The rash takes 2–4 weeks to resolve naturally without treatment (Amer & Fischer, 2006).

In contrast, irritant contact dermatitis is a discrete area of redness that corresponds to the exposure location. The rash usually develops within a few hours of contact, peaks within 24 hours, and quickly resolves with removal of the irritant. Reactions to irritants include painful erythema, edema, vesiculation, dryness of the skin, scaling, fissuring, and necrosis.

The distribution of the lesions provides clues about the source and identity of the allergen or irritant (Table 30–9). The diagnosis is often based on the manifestations of the disorder and a history of exposure to a known allergen. Scratch tests and intradermal tests are used to identify a specific allergen.

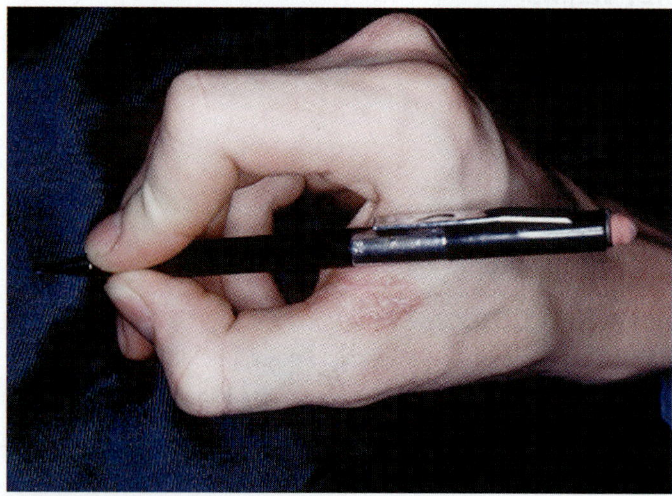

Figure 30–21 ■ Contact dermatitis.

Source: Copyright-protected material used with permission of Jane Ball and the University of Iowa's Virtual Hospital, http://www.vh.org.

TABLE 30-9 Distribution of Lesions by Type of Allergen

DISTRIBUTION OF LESION	ALLERGEN
Face, eyelids	Cosmetics, skin care products, nail cosmetics
Earlobes, neck	Nickel, fragrances
Lips, mouth	Oral hygiene products, gum, lipstick
Dorsal aspects of toes and feet	Rubber or leather chemical in shoes
Trunk	Snaps on pants, moisturizers, cleansers, sunscreens

Source: Adapted from Timm-Knudson, V. L., Johnson, J. S., Ortiz, K. J., & Yiannias, J. A. (2006). Allergic contact dermatitis to preservatives. *Dermatology Nursing, 18*(2), 130–136.

Patch testing, in which an adhesive patch with common allergens is placed on the back between the scapulae, may be used to identify the allergen.

PRACTICE ALERT

The patch for allergy testing stays on for 48–72 hours, and the client is not permitted to shower or exercise to the point of perspiring while the patch is in place. If severe pruritus develops, the health care provider should be contacted to remove the patch early to prevent skin sloughing (Mark & Slavin, 2006).

Treatment involves removing the offending agent (e.g., clothes, plant, soap). Calamine lotion can be applied to the affected skin. Cool compresses with aluminum acetate (Burow's solution) promote drying. Wet dressings or colloidal oatmeal soaks relieve itching. Antihistamines may be given to reduce itching or for a sedative effect when the itching makes the client too uncomfortable to sleep.

Acute allergic contact dermatitis is managed with medium-potency topical corticosteroids when less than 10% of the body surface area is affected; however, this topical medication should not be applied to open lesions. The topical corticosteroids limit the production of cytokines, stop lymphocyte proliferation, and limit the inflammatory response to the allergens. The topical corticosteroid is applied to the affected area twice a day for 2–3 weeks. Stopping the treatment too soon can cause rebound dermatitis. Reactions to poison ivy or other allergens covering more than 10% of the body surface area require treatment with oral corticosteroids for 7–10 days and a tapered dose over another 7–10 days. An antibiotic may be required if the area becomes infected (Table 30–10).

COLLABORATION

Collaborative care may be required for the client who experiences repeated episodes of contact dermatitis. For example, if a client is exposed to irritants at work, the nurse may need to encourage the client to speak with his or her employer or to contact an organization that provides training in OSHA regulations. A client who has repeated episodes due to allergy may need to be referred to an allergist for further testing and evaluation. A nurse working with a school-age child might want to speak with the school nurse or the child's classroom teacher to ensure that follow-up care is maintained at school and that the child is adequately hydrated.

TABLE 30–10 Medications Used to Treat Skin Disorders

TYPE	USE	EXAMPLES
Creams	Moisturize the skin	Aquacare Curel Nutraderm
Ointments	Lubricate the skin Retard water loss	Aquaphor Vaseline
Lotions	Moisturize the skin Lubricate the skin	Alpha-Keri Dermassage Lubriderm
Anesthetics	Relieve itching	Xylocaine
Antibiotics	Treat infection	Bacitracin Polysporin Gentamicin Silvadene
Corticosteroids	Suppress inflammation Relieve i tching	Dexamethasone Hydrocortisone Clocortolone Desonide

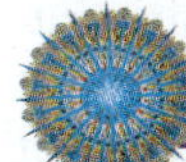

NURSING PROCESS

Assessment

A health assessment interview for a condition such as contact dermatitis focuses on a chief complaint (e.g., itching or a rash). If the client has a skin problem, the nurse analyzes its onset, characteristics and course, severity, and precipitating and relieving factors; the nurse also notes the timing and circumstances of any associated symptoms. The following are specific questions to ask the client:

- What type of itching have you experienced? When did it begin?
- Have you changed any household products lately? Have you changed any personal products lately, such as soap?
- Have you been anywhere unusual, for example, hiking in a new place?
- Do you have any allergies? Have you been in contact with anything to which you are allergic?

Ask about any change in health, rashes, itching, color changes, and the presence of lesions. Possible precipitating causes, such as medications, the use of new soaps and detergents, skin care agents, cosmetics, pets, travel, stress, or dietary changes should be explored.

The examination should be conducted in a warm, private room. The client removes all clothing and puts on a gown or drape. Fully expose the area to be examined, but protect the client's modesty by keeping other areas covered. The client may be standing, sitting, or lying down at various times in the examination. Wear disposable gloves when palpating open lesions, skin surfaces that are suggestive of infections or infestations, or discharge from lesions of the skin and mucous membranes. Adhere to standard precautions when conducting a skin assessment. Use a ruler to measure the size of the lesions and a flashlight to help examine them.

Diagnosis

Possible nursing diagnoses for the client with contact dermatitis may include the following:

- Impaired Skin Integrity related to contact dermatitis as evidenced by pruritus and rash
- Deficient Knowledge.

Plan

Appropriate goals for the client with contact dermatitis may include the following:

- The client's triggers will be identified and eliminated.
- The client will remain free of infection.

Implementation

Nursing care of the client with contact dermatitis focuses primarily on providing information for self-care at home. The client is responsible for managing skin problems and requires education and support. The nurse should address the following topics:

- Medications and treatments do not cure the disease; they only relieve the symptoms. Caution clients that using oatmeal soaks will make the tub slippery. Advise them to pat themselves dry to leave the oatmeal film in place. Wet dressings may be soothing and can help to loosen crusts. Applying Burow's or Domeboro solution to blistered or oozing lesions for 20 minutes daily helps dry lesions (Allen, 2004). Familiarize clients with the symptoms of infection in the affected area (e.g., increased redness, oozing, fever), and tell them when to return for follow-up care.
- Dry skin increases pruritus, which stimulates scratching. Scratching may in turn cause excoriation, which increases the risk of infection.
- It may be necessary to change the diet or environment to avoid contact with allergens. If a nickel allergy exists, make sure nickel jewelry and belt buckles are not used.
- Remove clothing worn after outside activities where suspected allergens may be present, and shower immediately after those activities.
- Wash all clothes before the first wearing, and rinse clothes an extra time to remove all soap. Mild soap should be used to clean the skin.
- Place a barrier between the allergen and the skin. For example, cover all metal snaps on clothing with cloth, and wear socks to avoid exposure to tanning chemicals left on shoe leather. If barriers do not reduce the dermatitis, then it may be necessary to try to find clothing without nickel or shoes with specific tanning chemicals.
- Apply topical corticosteroids, and keep using the ointment for 2–3 weeks, even when the skin shows signs of healing. When using steroid preparations, apply only a thin layer to slightly damp skin (e.g., after taking a bath). If using oral corticosteroids, never stop taking the medication abruptly. Follow instructions to taper the dosage gradually.
- If occlusive dressings are necessary, a plastic suit may be used.
- Antihistamines cause drowsiness. When using these medications, avoid alcohol and use caution when driving or working around machinery.

See Client Teaching: How to Relieve Reduce Dry Skin and Relieve Pruritus for suggestions on how to avoid drying of skin and how to relieve pruritus.

Evaluation

Expected outcomes of nursing care include the following:

- Control of the dermatitis is maintained, and no infection occurs.
- Triggers are identified and eliminated.
- The client's sleep is minimally disturbed by itching.

CLIENT TEACHING How to Reduce Dry Skin and Relieve Pruritus

- Wash clothing in a mild detergent and rinse twice; do not use fabric softeners.
- Avoid using perfumes and lotions containing alcohol.
- Apply skin lubricants after a bath to help retain moisture.
- Because soaps and hot water are drying, clean the skin with tepid water and either a mild soap or cleansing creams. If soap is used, rinse it off carefully.
- It is not necessary to take a bath every day.
- If bath oils are used, add them to the bath water at the end of the bath (the moist skin is more likely to retain the oil). Bath oils make the tub surface slippery, so they may be contraindicated for use by clients with poor balance or who are already at risk for falls.
- Use a humidifier to humidify the air.
- Apply creams and lotions when the skin is slightly damp after bathing.
- Increase fluid intake.
- Keep nails trimmed short, wear loose clothing, and keep the environment cool.
- A brief application of pressure or cold may relieve pruritus.
- Cotton gloves may be worn at night if scratching during sleep causes skin excoriation.
- Distraction or relaxation techniques may prove helpful.

REVIEW Contact Dermatitis

RELATE: LINK THE CONCEPTS

Linking the exemplar of Dermatitis with the concept of Immunity:

1. What is your priority nursing diagnosis for a client with contact dermatitis related to hypersensitivity?
2. How would your priority of care differ for this client if the contact dermatitis is located on or around the head and neck? Why?

Linking the exemplar of Dermatitis with the concept of Infection:

3. How will you respond to the client who insists on antibiotics for contact dermatitis?
4. When would a client with contact dermatitis need to be placed on antibiotic? What physical assessment findings would support the need for antibiotic therapy?

READY: GO TO COMPANION SKILLS MANUAL

- Aseptic technique
- Applying dressings
- Administering topical medication

REFER: GO TO MYNURSINGKIT

REFLECT: CASE STUDY

A 21-year-old female college student reported "an itchy rash" on the right side of her face. Examination revealed erythema, vesicles, and pruritus below her ear. Testing revealed a reaction to nickel. However, the client wore no nickel items. During the course of the assessment, the client took three calls on a cell phone; placement of the phone covered the rash.

1. Is it possible that the cell phone cause the reaction? Explain.
2. What kind of testing would determine a nickel allergy?
3. What can the client do to to reduce the risk of future reactions?

30.3 PRESSURE ULCERS

KEY TERMS

Debridement, *1924*
Eschar, *1918*
Excoriation, *1916*
Immobility, *1916*
Maceration, *1916*
Necrosis, *1915*
Pressure ulcers, *1915*
Shearing forces, *1916*

BASIS FOR SELECTION OF EXEMPLAR

Institute of Medicine (IOM)

LEARNING OUTCOMES

After reading about this exemplar, you will be able to:

1. Describe the pathophysiology, etiology, clinical manifestations, and direct and indirect causes of pressure ulcers.
2. Identify risk factors associated with pressure ulcers.
3. Illustrate the nursing process in providing culturally competent care across the life span for individuals with pressure ulcers.
4. Formulate priority nursing diagnoses appropriate for an individual with pressure ulcers.
5. Create a plan of care for individuals with pressure ulcers and their family members.
6. Assess expected outcomes for an individual with pressure ulcers.
7. Discuss therapies used in the collaborative care of an individual with pressure ulcers.
8. Use evidence-based caring interventions for an individual with pressure ulcers.

OVERVIEW

Pressure ulcers are ischemic lesions of the skin and underlying tissue caused by external pressure that impairs the flow of blood and lymph (Porth, 2005). The ischemia causes tissue **necrosis** (dead tissue) and eventual ulceration. These ulcers, also called bedsores or decubitus ulcers, tend to develop over a bony prominence (such as the heels, greater trochanter, sacrum, and ischia), but they may appear on the skin of any part of the body that is subjected to external pressure, friction, or shearing forces.

The incidence of pressure ulcers in hospitals, long-term care facilities, and home settings is high enough to warrant concern among health care providers. The incidence in hospitals has been reported to be as high as 8%, whereas the incidence in long-term care facilities is reported to range from 2.4–23% (Porth, 2005). Little research has been done to determine the extent of the problem in the home setting. However, with increasing numbers of clients (and especially older adult clients) being cared for in the home, it is probable that the incidence is great enough to warrant plans of care to prevent their occurrence.

PATHOPHYSIOLOGY AND ETIOLOGY

Pressure ulcers develop from external pressure that compresses blood vessels or from friction and shearing forces that tear and injure vessels. Both types of pressure cause traumatic injury and initiate the process of pressure ulcer development.

External pressure that is greater than capillary pressure and arteriolar pressure interrupts blood flow in capillary beds. When pressure is applied to skin over a bony prominence for

2 hours, tissue ischemia and hypoxia from external pressure cause irreversible tissue damage. For example, when the body is in the supine position, the body's weight applies pressure to the sacrum. A given amount of pressure causes more damage when it is applied to a small area than when it is distributed over a large surface.

Shearing forces result when one tissue layer slides over another. The stretching and bending of blood vessels cause injury and thrombosis. Clients in hospital beds are subject to shearing forces when the head of the bed is elevated and the torso slides down toward the foot of the bed. Pulling the client up in bed also subjects the client to shearing forces. (For this reason, always lift clients up in bed instead of pulling.) In both cases, friction and moisture cause the skin and superficial fascia to remain fixed to the bedsheet, while the deep fascia and bony skeleton slides in the direction of body movement.

When a person lies or sits in one position for an extended length of time without moving, pressure on the tissue between a bony prominence and the external surface of the body distorts capillaries and interferes with normal blood flow. If the pressure is relieved, blood flow to the area increases, and a brief period of reactive hyperemia occurs without permanent damage. If the pressure continues, platelets aggregate in the endothelial cells surrounding the capillaries and form microthrombi. These microthrombi impede blood flow, resulting in ischemia and hypoxia of tissues. Eventually, the cells and tissues of the immediate area of pressure and of the surrounding area die and become necrotic.

Alterations in the involved tissue depend on the depth of the injury. Injury to superficial layers of skin results in blister formation; injury to deeper structures causes the pressure ulcer area to appear dark reddish-blue. As the tissues die, the ulcer becomes an open wound that may be deep enough to expose the bone. The necrotic tissue elicits an inflammatory response, and the client experiences increases in temperature, pain, and white blood cell count. Secondary bacterial invasion is common. Enzymes from bacteria and macrophages dissolve necrotic tissue, resulting in a foul-smelling drainage.

Risk Factors

Although a pressure ulcer may develop in any adult who has impaired mobility, those who are most at risk are older adults with limited mobility, people with quadriplegia, and clients in the critical care setting (Porth, 2005).

Several factors contribute to the formation of pressure ulcers: immobility and inactivity, inadequate nutrition, fecal and urinary incontinence, decreased mental status, diminished sensation, excessive body heat, advanced age, and the presence of certain chronic conditions.

IMMOBILITY **Immobility** refers to a reduction in the amount and control of a person's movement. Normally, people move when they experience discomfort from pressure on an area of the body. Healthy people rarely exceed their tolerance to pressure. However, paralysis, extreme weakness, pain, or any cause of decreased activity can hinder a person's ability to change positions independently and relieve the pressure, even if the person can perceive the pressure.

INADEQUATE NUTRITION Prolonged inadequate nutrition causes weight loss, muscle atrophy, and the loss of subcutaneous tissue. These reduce the amount of padding between the skin and the bones, thus increasing the risk of pressure ulcer development. More specifically, inadequate intake of protein, carbohydrates, fluids, zinc, and vitamin C contributes to pressure ulcer formation.

Hypoproteinemia (abnormally low protein content in the blood), due to either inadequate intake or abnormal loss, predisposes the client to dependent edema. Edema (swelling caused by excess fluid trapped in bodily tissue) makes skin more prone to injury by decreasing its elasticity, resilience, and vitality. Edema increases the distance between the capillaries and the cells, thereby slowing the diffusion of oxygen to the tissue cells and of metabolites away from the cells.

FECAL AND URINARY INCONTINENCE Moisture from incontinence promotes skin **maceration** (tissues softened by prolonged wetting or soaking) and makes the epidermis more easily eroded and susceptible to injury. Digestive enzymes in feces, gastric tube drainage, and urea in urine also contribute to skin **excoriation** (area of loss of the superficial layers of the skin also known as *denuded* area). Any accumulation of secretions or excretions is irritating to the skin, harbors microorganisms, and makes the skin prone to breakdown and infection.

DECREASED MENTAL STATUS Individuals with a reduced level of awareness, including those who are unconscious, heavily sedated, or have dementia, are at risk for pressure ulcers because they are less able to recognize and respond to pain associated with prolonged pressure.

DIMINISHED SENSATION Paralysis, stroke, or other neurologic disease may cause loss of sensation in a body area. Loss of sensation reduces a person's ability to respond to trauma, to injurious heat and cold, and to the tingling ("pins and needles") that signals loss of circulation. Sensory loss also impairs the body's ability to recognize and provide healing mechanisms for a wound.

EXCESSIVE BODY HEAT Body heat is another factor in the development of pressure ulcers. An elevated body temperature increases the metabolic rate, thus increasing the cells' need for oxygen. This increased need is particularly severe in the cells of an area under pressure, which are already oxygen deficient. Severe infections with accompanying elevated body temperatures may affect the body's ability to deal with the effects of tissue compression.

ADVANCED AGE The aging process brings about several changes in the skin and its supporting structures, making the older person more prone to impaired skin integrity. These changes include the following:

- Loss of lean body mass
- Generalized thinning of the epidermis
- Decreased strength and elasticity of the skin due to changes in the collagen fibers of the dermis

- Increased dryness due to a decrease in the amount of oil produced by the sebaceous glands
- Diminished pain perception due to a reduction in the number of cutaneous end organs responsible for the sensation of pressure and light touch
- Diminished venous and arterial flow due to aging vascular walls.

CHRONIC MEDICAL CONDITIONS Certain chronic conditions such as diabetes and cardiovascular disease are risk factors for skin breakdown and delayed healing. These conditions compromise oxygen delivery to tissues, resulting in poor and delayed healing and increase risk of pressure sores.

OTHER FACTORS Other factors contributing to the formation of pressure ulcers are poor lifting and transferring techniques, incorrect positioning, hard support surfaces, and incorrect application of pressure-relieving devices.

CLINICAL MANIFESTATIONS

Pressure ulcers are graded or staged to classify the degree of damage. The stages are listed in Box 30–4. Diagnostic tests are conducted to determine the presence of a secondary infection and to differentiate the cause of the ulcer. If the ulcer is deep or appears infected, drainage or biopsied tissue is cultured to determine the causative organism.

Box 30–4 **Pressure Ulcer Staging**

STAGE I

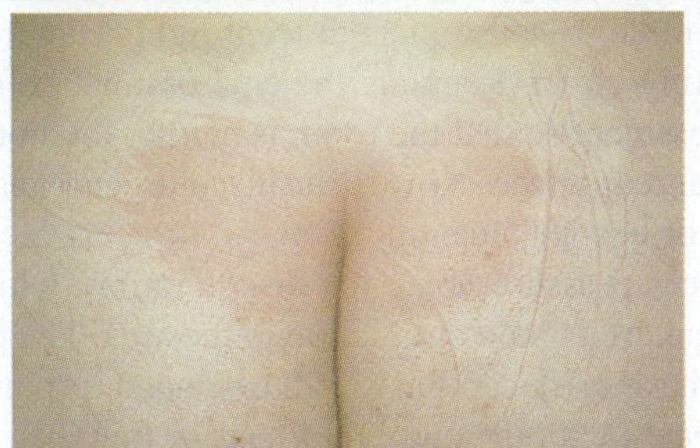

Nonblanchable erythema of intact skin; the heralding lesion of skin ulceration. Identification of stage I pressure ulcers may be difficult in clients with darkly pigmented skin.

Note: Reactive hyperemia can normally be expected to be present for one-half to three-fourths as long as the pressure occluded blood flow to the area. This should not be confused with stage I pressure ulcer.

STAGE II

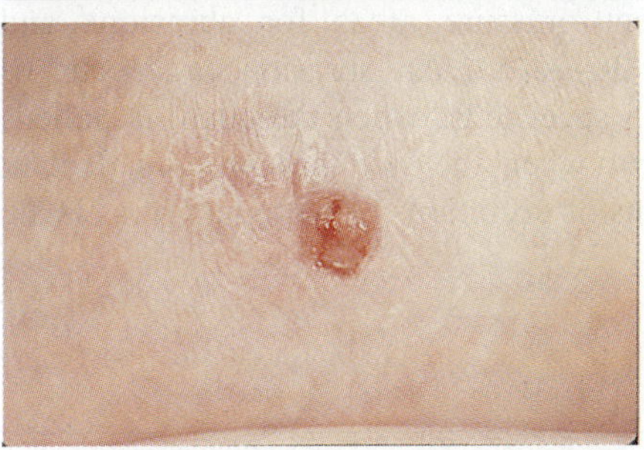

Partial-thickness skin loss involving epidermis and/or dermis. The ulcer is superficial and presents clinically as an abrasion, blister, or shallow crater.

STAGE III

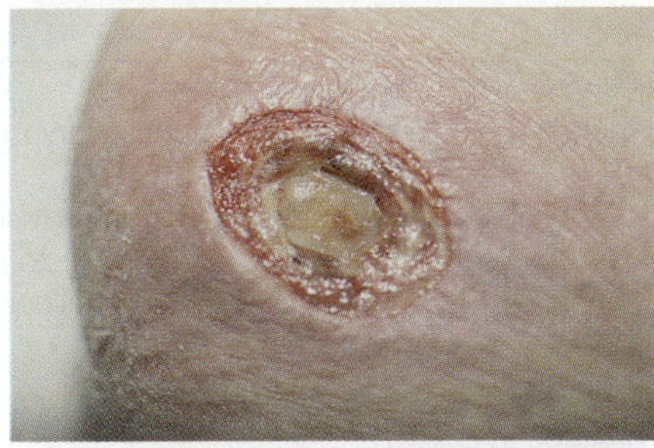

Full-thickness skin loss involving damage or necrosis of subcutaneous tissue that may extend down to, but not through, underlying fascia. The ulcer presents clinically as a deep crater with or without undermining of adjacent tissue.

STAGE IV

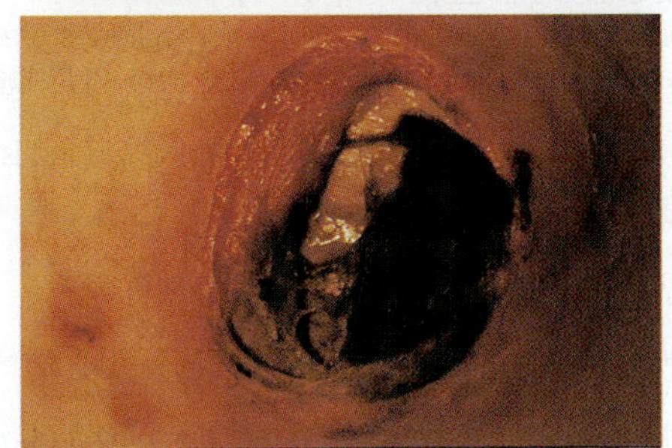

Full-thickness skin loss with extensive destruction, tissue necrosis, or damage to muscle, bone, or supporting structures (for example, tendon or joint capsule). Sinus tracts may also be associated with stage IV ulcers.

Note: When eschar is present, accurate staging of the pressure ulcer is not possible until the eschar has sloughed or the wound has been debrided.

Source: Text is from *Pressure Ulcers in Adults: Prediction and Prevention* by the Agency for Health Care Policy and Research, 1992 Rockville, MD: U.S. Department of Health and Human Services. Photos courtesy of Karen Lou Kennedy, RN, FPN, www.kennedyterminalulcer.com.

Topical and systemic antibiotics specific to the infectious organism eradicate any infection present. Additionally, a variety of topical products promote healing. Examples are listed in Table 30–11.

Surgical debridement may be necessary if the pressure ulcer is deep, if subcutaneous tissues are involved, or if an **eschar** (a scab or dry crust consisting of dried plasma proteins and dead cells that forms over skin damaged by burns, infections, or excoriations) has formed over the ulcer, preventing healing by granulation. Large wounds may require skin grafting for complete closure.

COLLABORATION

Nurses may find themselves collaborating with a number of individuals when providing care for a client who has or is at risk for pressure ulcers. Nurses frequently collaborate with physical therapists, especially in hospitals, rehabilitation centers, and nursing homes. When caring for a client who is living at home, the nurse will often collaborate with the individual's primary caregiver, be that a family member or a hired professional. Because many clients with pressure ulcers are older or have other serious illnesses, a caregiver may require teaching on such topics as the following:

- Definition and description of pressure ulcers
- Common locations of pressure ulcers
- Risk factors for the development of pressure ulcers
- Skin care
- Ways to avoid injury
- Diet.

Depending on the stage of the pressure ulcer, the nurse teaches the client or caregiver how to care for ulcers that are already present: how to change dressings, apply skin barriers, and avoid injury and infection. Referrals to a home health agency or community health department can help the family through the lengthy healing process.

NURSING PROCESS

Prevention is the goal for the client at risk for pressure ulcers. The client with one or more pressure ulcers not only has impaired skin integrity, but also is at increased risk for infection, pain, and decreased mobility. Pressure ulcers prolong treatment for other health problems, increase health care costs, and diminish the client's quality of life.

Assessment

Ensure that the lighting is good; natural or fluorescent lighting is preferable, because incandescent lights can create a transilluminating effect. Regulate the environment before beginning the assessment so that the room is neither too hot nor too cold. Heat can cause the skin to flush; cold can cause the skin to blanch or become cyanotic.

Inspect pressure areas for discoloration, which can result from impaired blood circulation to the area. The pressure areas should have brisk capillary refill or blanch response when gently palpated with the end of a finger or thumb.

Inspect pressure areas for abrasions and excoriations (Figure 30–22 ■). An abrasion can occur when skin rubs against a sheet (e.g., when the client is pulled). Excoriations can occur when the skin has prolonged contact with body secretions or excretions or with dampness in skin folds.

TABLE 30–11 **Products Used to Treat Pressure Ulcers**

STAGE	PRODUCT	PURPOSE
I	Skin Prep	Toughens intact skin and preserves skin integrity.
	Granulex	Prevents skin breakdown, increases blood supply, adds moisture, contains trypsin to aid in removal of necrotic tissue.
	Hydrocolloid dressing (e.g., DuoDerm)	Prevents skin breakdown and promotes healing without the formation of a crust over the ulcer; is permeable to air and water vapor; prevents the growth of anaerobic organisms.
	Transparent dressing (e.g., Tegaderm)	Prevents skin breakdown; prevents entrance of moisture and bacteria but allows oxygen and moisture vapor permeability.
II	Transparent dressing	Enhances healing (see transparent dressing in stage I).
	Hydrocolloid dressing	Enhances healing (see hydrocolloid dressing in stage I). (*Note:* If infection is present, these types of dressings are contraindicated. A sterile dressing should be applied instead.)
III	Wet-to-dry gauze dressing with sterile normal saline	Allows necrotic material to soften and adhere to the gauze, so that the wound is debrided.
	Hydrocolloid dressing	Enhances healing (see above).
	Proteolytic enzymes (such as Elase)	Serve as debriding agents in inflamed and infected lesions.
IV	Wet-to-dry gauze dressing with sterile normal saline	Enhances healing (see above). (*Note:* Transparent or hydrocolloid dressings or skin barriers are contraindicated.
	Vacuum-assisted closure (V.A.C.)	Creates a negative pressure to help reduce edema, increase blood supply and oxygenation, and decrease bacterial colonization; it also helps promote moist wound healing and the formation of granulation tissue.

CARE SETTINGS Assessing Common Pressure Sites

- Ensure the lighting is good, preferably natural or fluorescent, because incandescent lights can create a transilluminating effect.
- Regulate the environment before beginning the assessment so that the room is neither too hot nor too cold. Heat can cause the skin to flush; cold can cause the skin to blanch or become cyanotic.
- Inspect pressure areas (see Figure 30–22) for discoloration. This can be caused by impaired blood circulation to the area. The pressure areas should have brisk capillary refill or blanch response when gently palpated with the end of a finger or thumb.
- Inspect pressure areas for abrasions and excoriations. An abrasion can occur when skin rubs against a sheet (e.g., when the client is pulled). Excoriations can occur when the skin has prolonged contact with body secretions or excretions or with dampness in skin folds.
- Palpate the surface temperature of the skin over the pressure areas (warm your hands first). Normally, the temperature is the same as that of the surrounding skin. Increased temperature is abnormal and may be due to inflammation or blood trapped in the area.
- Palpate over bony prominences and dependent body areas for the presence of edema, which feels spongy or boggy.

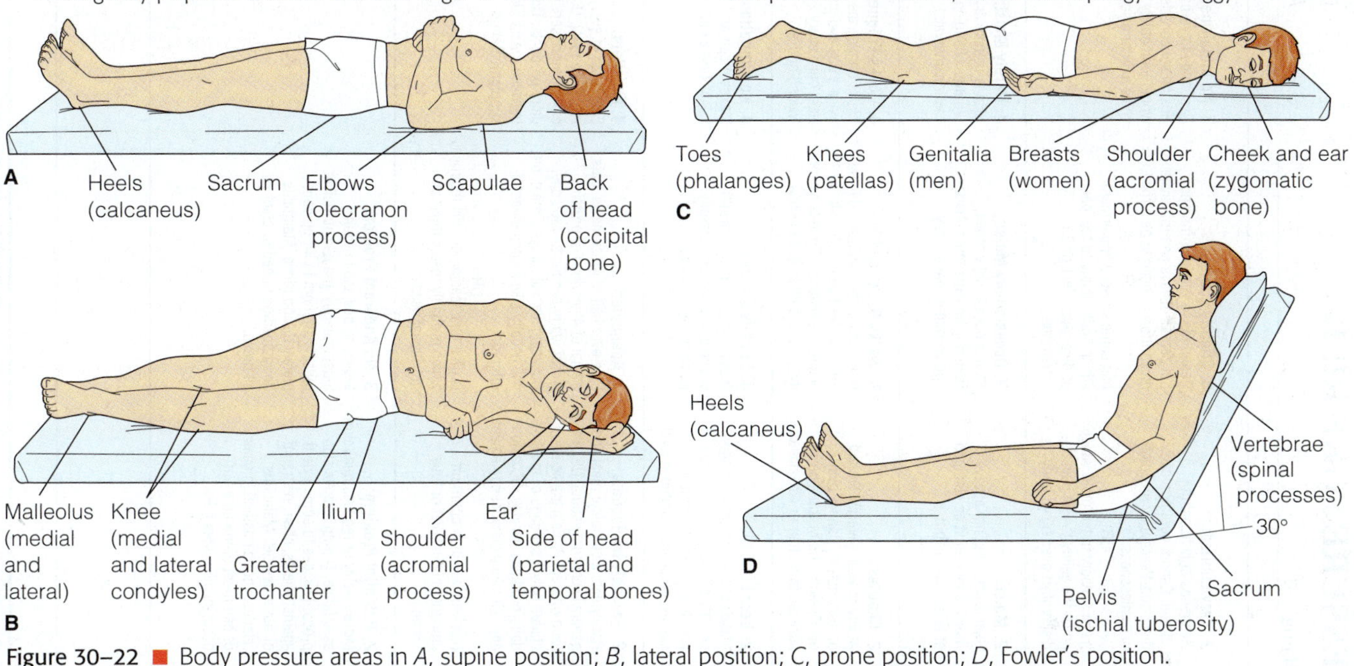

Figure 30–22 ■ Body pressure areas in *A*, supine position; *B*, lateral position; *C*, prone position; *D*, Fowler's position.

Palpate the surface temperature of the skin over the pressure areas (warm hands first). Normally, the temperature is the same as that of the surrounding skin. Increased temperature is abnormal and may be due to inflammation or blood trapped in the area. Palpate over bony prominences and dependent body areas for the presence of edema, which feels spongy or boggy. If a pressure ulcer is open or visibly infected, wear gloves during the examination.

If a pressure ulcer is present, the nurse notes the following:

- Location of the ulcer, related to a bony prominence
- Size of ulcer in centimeters (Measure length, width, and depth, beginning with length [head to toe] and then width [side to side]. To measure depth, insert a sterile applicator swab at the deepest part of the wound, and then measure it against a measuring guide.)
- Presence of undermining or sinus tracts, assessed as face on a clock, where 12 o'clock is the client's head
- Stage of the ulcer (see Box 30–4)
- Color of the wound bed and location of necrosis or eschar
- Condition of the wound margins
- Integrity of surrounding skin
- Clinical signs of infection, such as redness, warmth, swelling, pain, odor, and exudate (note color of exudate)
- Client complaints of pain or discomfort at the wound site
- Signs of infection such as fever, chills, or elevated white blood cell count (WBC).

Document the status of the client's skin and wounds on the standard agency form. It is important to be able to determine how these change over time.

Several risk assessment tools are available that provide the nurse with systematic means of identifying clients at high risk for pressure ulcer development. The Panel for the Prediction and Prevention of Pressure Ulcers in Adults (PPPPUA, 1992a) has recommended that the tools include data collection in the areas of immobility, incontinence, nutrition, and level of consciousness.

In 1987, Bergstrom, Braden, Laguzza, and Holman published the Braden Scale for Predicting Pressure Sore Risk. Their scale consists of six subscales: sensory perception, moisture, activity, mobility, nutrition, and friction and shear (Figure 30–23 ■). A total of 23 points is possible. An adult who scores below 18 points is considered at risk (Folkedahl & Frantz, 2002b). For best results, nurses should be trained in proper use of the scale.

BRADEN SCALE FOR PREDICTING PRESSURE SORE RISK

Patient's Name ________________ Evaluator's Name ________________

					Date of Assessment			
SENSORY PERCEPTION Ability to respond meaningfully to pressure-related discomfort	**1. Completely Limited:** Unresponsive (does not moan, flinch, or grasp) to painful stimuli, due to diminished level of consciousness or sedation, OR limited ability to feel pain over most of body surface.	**2. Very Limited:** Responds only to painful stimuli. Cannot communicate discomfort except by moaning or restlessness, OR has a sensory impairment which limits the ability to feel pain or discomfort over 1/2 of body.	**3. Slightly Limited:** Responds to verbal commands but cannot always communicate discomfort or need to be turned, OR has some sensory impairment which limits ability to feel pain or discomfort in 1 or 2 extremities.	**4. No Impairment:** Responds to verbal commands. Has no sensory deficit which would limit ability to feel or voice pain or discomfort.				
MOISTURE Degree to which skin is exposed to moisture	**1. Constantly Moist:** Skin is kept moist almost constantly by perspiration, urine, etc. Dampness is detected every time patient is moved or turned.	**2. Moist:** Skin is often but not always moist. Linen must be changed at least once a shift.	**3. Occasionally Moist:** Skin is occasionally moist, requiring an extra linen change approximately once a day.	**4. Rarely Moist:** Skin is usually dry; linen requires changing only at routine intervals.				
ACTIVITY Degree of physical activity	**1. Bedfast:** Confined to bed.	**2. Chairfast:** Ability to walk severely limited or nonexistent. Cannot bear own weight and/or must be assisted into chair or wheelchair.	**3. Walks Occasionally:** Walks occasionally during day but for very short distances, with or without assistance. Spends majority of each shift in bed or chair.	**4. Walks Frequently:** Walks outside the room at least twice a day and inside room at least once every 2 hours during waking hours.				
MOBILITY Ability to change and control body position	**1. Completely Immobile:** Does not make even slight changes in body or extremity position without assistance.	**2. Very Limited:** Makes occasional slight changes in body or extremity position but unable to make frequent or significant changes independently.	**3. Slightly Limited:** Makes frequent though slight changes in body or extremity position independently.	**4. No Limitations:** Makes major and frequent changes in position without assistance.				
NUTRITION Usual food intake pattern	**1. Very Poor:** Never eats a complete meal. Rarely eats more than 1/3 of any food offered. Eats 2 servings or less of protein (meat or dairy products) per day. Takes fluids poorly. Does not take a liquid dietary supplement, OR is NPO and/or maintained on clear liquids or IV's for more than 5 days.	**2. Probably Inadequate:** Rarely eats a complete meal and generally eats only about 1/2 of any food offered. Protein intake includes only 3 servings of meat or dairy products per day. Occasionally will take a dietary supplement, OR receives less than optimum amount of liquid diet or tube feeding.	**3. Adequate:** Eats over half of most meals. Eats a total of 4 servings of protein (meat, dairy products) each day. Occasionally will refuse a meal, but will usually take a supplement if offered, OR is on a tube feeding or TPN regimen, which probably meets most of nutritional needs.	**4. Excellent:** Eats most of every meal. Never refuses a meal. Usually eats a total of 4 or more servings of meat and dairy products. Occasionally eats between meals. Does not require supplementation.				
FRICTION AND SHEAR	**1. Problem:** Requires moderate to maximum assistance in moving. Complete lifting without sliding against sheets is impossible. Frequently slides down in bed or chair, requiring frequent repositioning with maximum assistance. Spasticity, contractures, or agitation leads to almost constant friction.	**2. Potential Problem:** Moves feebly or requires minimum assistance. During a move skin probably slides to some extent against sheets, chair, restraints, or other devices. Maintains relatively good position in chair or bed most of the time but occasionally slides down.	**3. No Apparent Problem:** Moves in bed and in chair independently and has sufficient muscle strength to lift up completely during move. Maintains good position in bed or chair at all times.					
				Total Score				

Figure 30–23 ■ Braden Scale for Predicting Pressure Sore Risk.

Source: Clinical Practice Guideline, Pressure Ulcers in Adults: Prediction and Prevention, by U.S. Department of Health and Human Services, PPPPUA Pub No. 92-0047, pp. 16–17, 1992, Rockville, MD: Public Health Service. Copyright © Barbara Braden and Nancy Bergstrom, 1988. Reprinted with permission.

Norton's Pressure Area Risk Assessment Form Scale includes the categories of general physical condition, mental state, activity, mobility, and incontinence. A category of medications was added in 1987, resulting in a possible score of 24. Scores of 15 or 16 should be viewed as indicators, not predictors, of risk. The Braden and Norton tools should be used when the client first enters the health care agency and whenever the client's condition changes. In some long-term care facilities, a risk assessment scale such as the Braden or Norton scale is used on admission and then on a regular basis, usually weekly. This increases awareness of specific risk factors and provides assessment data to use in planning goals and interventions to either maintain or improve skin integrity.

Diagnoses

The following NANDA diagnoses may be appropriate for the client with a pressure ulcer:

- Risk for Impaired Skin Integrity
- Impaired Skin Integrity
- Risk for Infection
- Imbalanced Nutrition: Less Than Body Requirements
- Risk for Compromised Human Dignity
- Situational Low Self-Esteem.

Plan

Outcomes to be developed in collaboration with the client and caregivers include the following:

- Client who is immobile or on bed rest will be repositioned every two hours. Appropriate positioning devices may be used.
- Client who is mobile will maintain or improve activity levels.
- Client will report any alterations such as changes in pain level, redness, numbness, tingling, or increased drainage.
- Client will articulate the importance of maintaining adequate nutrition and hydration.
- Client will describe measures to protect and heal tissue.

Implementation

Risk for Impaired Skin Integrity / Impaired Skin Integrity

In order to assist the client at risk for or with Impaired Skin Integrity, the nurse should consider the following:

- Conduct a systematic skin inspection at least once a day, paying particular attention to the bony prominences. Systematic, comprehensive, and routine skin care may decrease pressure ulcer incidence (although the exact role is unknown). Skin inspection provides data the nurse uses in designing interventions to reduce risk and in evaluating outcomes of those interventions.
- Clean the skin at the time of soiling and at routine intervals, as frequently as the client's need or preference dictates. Avoid hot water, use a mild cleansing agent, and clean the skin gently, applying as little force and friction as possible. Metabolic wastes and environmental contaminants accumulate on the skin; these potentially irritating substances should be removed frequently. Feces and urine cause chemical irritation and should be removed as soon as possible. Hot water may cause skin injury. Mild cleansing agents are less likely to remove the skin's natural barrier.
- Minimize environmental factors leading to skin drying, such as low humidity and exposure to cold. Treat dry skin with moisturizers. Well-hydrated skin resists mechanical trauma. Hydration decreases as the ambient air temperature decreases, especially when the air humidity is low. Poorly hydrated skin is less pliable, and severe dryness is associated with fissuring and cracking of the stratum corneum. Moisturizers reduce dry skin.
- Avoid massage over bony prominences. Although massage has been practiced for years, evidence now suggests that massage over bony prominences may lead to deep tissue trauma in clients at risk for, or with beginning, skin manifestations of a pressure ulcer.
- Minimize skin exposure to moisture due to incontinence, perspiration, or wound drainage. When these sources of moisture cannot be controlled, use underpads or briefs made of materials that absorb moisture and present a quick-drying surface to the skin. Change underpads and briefs frequently. Do not place plastic directly against the skin. Moisture from incontinence, perspiration, or wound drainage may contain factors that irritate the skin; moisture alone can increase the susceptibility of the skin to injury.
- To minimize skin injury due to friction and shearing forces, use proper positioning, transferring, and turning techniques. Lubricants (such as cornstarch or creams), protective films (such as transparent dressings and skin sealants), protective dressings (such as hydrocolloids), and protective padding may also reduce friction injuries. Shear injury occurs when skin remains stationary and the underlying tissue shifts. This shift diminishes the blood supply to the skin, resulting in ischemia and tissue damage. Proper positioning, however, can eliminate most shear injuries. Friction injuries occur when the skin moves across a coarse surface, such as bed linens. Most friction injuries can be avoided by using appropriate techniques to move clients so that their skin is never dragged across the linens. Any agent that eliminates contact or decreases the friction between the skin and the linens reduces the potential for injury.
- For the client who is immobile or on bedrest, provide interventions against the adverse effects of external mechanical forces of pressure, friction, and shear:
  a. Reposition all at-risk clients at least every 2 hours, using a written schedule for systematic turning and repositioning.
  b. For clients on bedrest, use positioning devices, such as pillows or foam wedges, to protect bony prominences.
- For completely immobile clients, use devices to totally relieve pressure on the heels (the most common method is to raise the heels off the bed). Do not use doughnut-type devices.

- Avoid placing clients in the side-lying position directly on the trochanter.
- Maintain the head of the bed at the lowest degree of elevation consistent with the client's medical condition and other restrictions. Limit the amount of time the head of the bed is elevated.
- Use assistive devices, such as a trapeze or bed linen, to move clients in bed who cannot assist during transfers and position changes.
- Place any at-risk client on a pressure-reducing device, such as foam, static air, alternating air, gel, or water mattress. Data indicate that the more spontaneous movements that bedridden, older adult clients make, the lower the incidence of pressure ulcers. Studies reveal that fewer pressure ulcers develop in at-risk clients who are turned every 2–3 hours. Proper positioning can reduce pressure on bony prominences. It is difficult to redistribute pressure under heels; suspending the heels is the best method. Do not use doughnut cushions, which are more likely to cause than to prevent pressure ulcers. Shearing forces are exerted on the body when the head of the bed is elevated. Lifting (rather than dragging) is less likely to cause injury from friction. Pressure-reducing devices and beds can reduce the incidence of pressure ulcers.
- For chair-bound clients, use pressure-reducing devices. Consider postural alignment, distribution of weight, balance and stability, and pressure relief when positioning these clients. Avoid uninterrupted sitting in a chair or wheelchair. Reposition the client every hour. Teach clients who can do so to shift their weight every 15 minutes. Use a written plan for positioning, movement, and the use of positioning devices. Do not use doughnut devices. Prolonged, uninterrupted mechanical pressure results in tissue breakdown. The client's weight should be shifted at least every hour.

Risk for Infection

Untreated pressure ulcers can become infected quickly. The nurse working with a client who is at risk for pressure ulcers should teach the client to guard against infection by doing the following:

- Maintaining skin hygiene
- Maintaining appropriate nutrition and hydration
- Recognizing the early stages of a pressure ulcer
- Contacting the officer at the earliest appearance of a pressure ulcer or change in skin integrity
- Maintaining or improving current activity levels.

Imbalanced Nutrition: Less than Body Requirements

Although the role nutrition plays in the development of (and to a lesser degree, the healing of) pressure ulcers is not understood, poor dietary intake of kilocalories, protein, and iron has been associated with the development of pressure ulcers. The nurse should do the following:

- Assess factors involved in inadequate dietary intake of protein or kilocalories.
- Offer nutritional supplements, and support the client during mealtimes as necessary to insure adequate dietary intake.
- If dietary intake remains inadequate, consult with a dietitian about other dietary interventions.

EVIDENCE-BASED PRACTICE Treating Pressure Ulcers

Despite advances in health care to extend life and improve functional status, older adults with chronic illnesses are at increased risk of developing pressure ulcers. The older adult, with age-related compromised cellular activity, is especially vulnerable to impaired healing of injured tissue, including pressure ulcers. Frantz (2004) describes an evidence-based protocol designed to enhance the healing of pressure ulcers in older clients by using evidence-based interventions. The following interventions are recommended:

- Assess all individuals admitted to a health care facility with a pressure ulcer for the risk of developing additional pressure ulcers by using a standardized risk assessment scale.
- Perform a complete history and physical examination, combined with a detailed assessment of the ulcer characteristics (location, stage, type of tissue, presence of tunneling or tracts, exudate, odor, and condition of skin around the ulcer).
- Remove necrotic tissue and debris from the ulcer to decrease the growth of bacteria. Remove foreign materials, such as exudates and metabolic wastes.
- Provide a moist wound environment to promote reepithelialization and healing.
- Control bacterial levels in the wound by using cleansing and debridement, as well as systemic and topical antibiotics.
- Supply essential substrates for tissue repair, including protein, calories, vitamins, and minerals. Maintain a positive nitrogen balance.
- Manage tissue loads by positioning to avoid external force on the ulcer.

Implications for Nursing

The design and implementation of a pressure ulcer prevention and treatment plan is essential for any person at risk, including older adults, those with debilitating or multiple illnesses, and those with health problems limiting mobility. To implement a plan effectively, it is important to prepare providers to use a standard protocol, and to monitor indicators of improvement or deterioration in the ulcer and presence or absence of new ulcers. These outcomes should be assessed and recorded on a weekly basis.

Critical Thinking in Client Care

1. Consider the activities to treat pressure ulcers. What would you do about the following:
   a. What level of health care provider would you delegate to care for the client?
   b. How much time in an 8-hour period would be needed for nursing care?
   c. What would you teach family caregivers about providing care at home?

Source: Franz, R. (2004). Treatment of pressure ulcers. *Journal of Gerontological Nursing, 30*(5), 4–10. Used with permission.

Risk for Compromised Human Dignity / Situational Low Self-Esteem

The immobile or nearly immobile client is at the mercy of those caring for him or her. If family members or caregivers do not effect interventions necessary to inhibit the growth of pressure ulcers and maintain client hygiene, the client is at risk for compromised human dignity. This can effect a client's moods and perception of self, in turn putting the client at risk for situational low self-esteem. Depression can follow quickly. The nurse can assist the client in these areas by doing the following:

- Conducting a physical examination at each health care interaction that includes examining the client for indicators of abuse or neglect.
- Develop a caring, trusting relationship with the client so that you will be able to get him or her to discuss issues related to human dignity and self-esteem. Refer for counseling as appropriate.
- Teaching family members and caregivers the importance of repositioning the client every two hours and teaching them about skin hygiene and how to position the client properly.
- Assisting family members and caregivers with obtaining supportive devices to assist in maintaining appropriate positioning of the client.

Preventing Pressure Ulcers

To reduce the likelihood of pressure ulcers developing in all clients, the nurse employs a variety of preventive measures (i.e., skin hygiene and pressure relief devices) to maintain the skin integrity and instructs the client, support people, and caregivers in how to prevent pressure ulcers.

PROVIDING NUTRITION Because an inadequate intake of calories, protein, vitamins, and iron is believed to be a risk factor for pressure ulcer development, nutritional supplements should be considered for nutritionally compromised clients. The diet should be similar to that which supports wound healing, as discussed earlier. The nurse should monitor weight regularly to help assess nutritional status. Pertinent lab work should also be monitored, including lymphocyte count, protein (especially albumin), and hemoglobin.

MAINTAINING SKIN HYGIENE The nurse should obtain baseline data using the established tool and then reassess the skin at least daily in the hospital and weekly at home. When bathing the client, the nurse should minimize the force and friction applied to the skin, using mild cleansing agents that minimize irritation and dryness and that do not disrupt the skin's "natural barriers." Also, the nurse should avoid using hot water, which increases skin dryness and irritation. Nurses can minimize dryness by avoiding exposure to cold and low humidity. Dry skin is best treated with moisturizing lotions applied while the skin is moist after bathing. The client's skin should be kept clean and dry and free of irritation and maceration by urine, feces, sweat, or incomplete drying after a bath. The nurse applies skin protection if indicated. Dimethicone-based creams or alcohol-free barrier films, which are available in liquid, spray, and moist wipe format, are very effective in preventing moisture or drainage from collecting on the skin. In most cases, the nurse can apply these without a primary care provider's order. Petroleum-based creams and ointments are no longer advised because of poor overall skin protection and interference with diaper/incontinence product absorption.

AVOIDING SKIN TRAUMA Providing the client with a smooth, firm, and wrinkle-free foundation on which to sit or lie helps prevent skin trauma. To prevent injury due to friction and shearing forces, clients must be positioned, transferred, and turned correctly. For bedridden clients, shearing force can be reduced by elevating the head of the bed to no more than 30 degrees, if this position is not contraindicated by the client's condition. (For example, clients with respiratory disorders may find it easier to breathe in Fowler's position.) When the head of the bed is raised, the skin and superficial fascia stick to the bed linen while the deep fascia and skeleton slide down toward the bottom of the bed. As a result, blood vessels in the sacral area become twisted, and the tissues in the area can become ischemic and necrotic. Baby powder and cornstarch are never used as friction or moisture prevention. These powders create harmful abrasive grit that is damaging to tissues and are considered a respiratory hazard when airborne. Instead, use moisturizing creams and protective films, such as transparent dressings and alcohol-free barrier films.

Frequent shifts in position, even if only slight, effectively change pressure points. The client who is able should shift weight 10–15 degrees every 15–30 minutes and, whenever possible, exercise or ambulate to stimulate blood circulation.

When lifting a client to change position, nurses should use a lifting device such as a trapeze rather than dragging the client across or up in bed. The friction that results from dragging the skin against a sheet can cause blisters and abrasions, which may contribute to more extensive tissue damage. Therefore, using devices that lift the client's weight off the bed surface is the method of choice. To deter shearing forces, the nurse should place a draw sheet that covers the bed from an individual's chest to buttocks and is folded to be wide enough to tuck under the mattress on either side when not in use.

Any at-risk client who is confined to bed—even when a special support mattress is used—should be repositioned at least every 2 hours, depending on the client's need, to allow another body surface to bear the weight. Six body positions can usually be used: prone, supine, right and left lateral (side-lying), and right and left Sims' positions. When a lateral position is used, the nurse should avoid positioning the client directly on the trochanter and should instead position the client on a 30-degree angle. A written schedule should be established for turning and repositioning.

PROVIDING SUPPORTIVE DEVICES For circulation to remain uncompromised, pressure on the bony prominences should remain below capillary pressure for as much time as possible through a combination of turning, positioning, and use of pressure-relieving surfaces. Mean capillary pressure can be estimated at 20 mmHg, although this varies. Some research has evaluated the effectiveness of pressure-reducing support surfaces in preventing pressure ulcers in clients at low, intermediate, or high risk; however, the results have been inconclusive (Cullum, McInnes, Bell-Syer, & Legood, 2005). The nurse should review the manufacturer's product descriptions that report the amount of time that the pressure between the surface and the bony prominence is above or below specified levels and determine whether this is adequate to protect a particular client.

For clients who are confined to bed, three types of support surfaces can be used to relieve pressure:

1. The overlay mattress is applied on top of the standard bed mattress. Use a replacement mattress instead of the standard mattress; most are made of foam and gel combinations.
2. Specialty beds replace hospital beds. They provide pressure relief, eliminate shearing and friction, and reduce moisture. Examples are high-air-loss beds, low-air-loss beds, and beds that provide kinetic therapy.
3. Kinetic beds provide continuous passive motion or oscillation therapy, both of which are intended to counteract the effects of a client's immobility.

When a client is confined to bed or to a chair, pressure-reducing devices, such as pillows made of foam, gel, air, or a combination of these, can be used. When the client is sitting, weight should be distributed over the entire seating surface so that pressure does not center on just one area. To protect a client's heels in bed, supports such as wedges or pillows can be used to raise the heels completely off the bed. Doughnut-type devices should not be used, since they limit blood flow and can cause tissue damage to the areas in direct contact with the device. Table 30–12 lists mechanical devices for reducing pressure on body parts.

Treating Pressure Ulcers

Pressure ulcers are a challenge for nurses because of the number of variables involved (e.g., risk factors, types of ulcers, and degrees of impairment) and the numerous treatment measures advocated. Existing and potential infections are the most serious complications of pressure ulcers. In treating pressure ulcers, nurses should follow the agency protocols and the primary care provider's orders, if any. Prompt treatment can prevent further tissue damage and pain and facilitate wound healing. See Box 30–5 regarding treating pressure ulcers.

Some wounds are covered with thick necrotic tissue, or eschar. These wounds require **debridement** (removal of the necrotic material). Nonviable tissue must be removed from a wound before the wound can be staged or heal. There are four types of debridement: sharp, mechanical, chemical, and autolytic. In *sharp debridement,* a scalpel or scissors are used to separate and remove dead tissue. In many settings, specially trained nurses (wound ostomy continence nurses, or WOCNs), physical therapists, and physician's assistants are permitted to perform sharp debridement. *Mechanical debridement* is accomplished through scrubbing force or moist-to-moist dressings. *Chemical debridement* is more selective than sharp or mechanical techniques. Collagenase enzyme agents such as

TABLE 30–12 **Mechanical Devices for Reducing Pressure on Body Parts**

DEVICE	DESCRIPTION/COMMENTS
Gel flotation pads	Polyvinyl, silicone, or Silastic™ pads filled with a gelatinous substance similar to fat
Pillows and wedges (foam, gel, air, fluid)	Support positioning and offloads bone on bone contact
Heel protectors (sheepskin boots, padded splints, off-loading inflatable boots, foam blocks)	Can raise or "float" a body part (e.g., heels) off the or surface; prevent shearing and limit pressure on heel area
Memory foam mattress/chair pad	Distributes weight over bony areas evenly; molds to the body
Alternating pressure mattress	Composed of a number of cells in which the pressure alternately increases and decreases; uses a pump
Water bed	Support surface filled with water; water temperature controllable
Static low-air-loss (LAL) bed	Consists of many air-filled cushions divided into four or five sections (Separate controls permit each section to be inflated to a different level of firmness; thus pressure can be reduced on bony prominences but increased under other body areas for support.)
Active or second-generation LAL bed	Like the static LAL but in addition gently pulsates or rotates from side to side, thus stimulating capillary blood flow and facilitating movement of pulmonary secretions
Air-fluidized (AF) bed (static high-air-loss bed)	Forced temperature-controlled air circulated around millions of tiny silicone-coated beads, producing a fluidlike movement; provides uniform support to body contours; decreases skin maceration by its drying effect (Moisture from the client penetrates the linens and soaks the beads. Air flow forces the beads away from the client and rapidly dries the sheet. A major disadvantage is that the head of the bed cannot be elevated. Some beds are a unique combination of air fluidized therapy and low-air-loss therapy on an articulating frame. These are used with clients who require head elevation.)

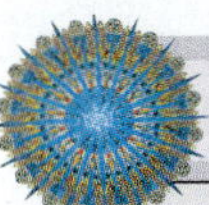

NURSING CARE PLAN **The Client With a Pressure Ulcer**

A registered nurse who works for a home health agency has been assigned to Mrs. Krebs, a 75-year-old client with a chronic stage III ulcer on her heel that has shown no progress in the last 3 months. The nurse notes that Mrs. Krebs has a smoking history of 40 pack years and has not followed her diet instruction. The supervisor of the home health agency has warned the nurse that if Mrs. Krebs does not improve, the insurance company will not continue to pay for the visits and treatment. Mrs. Krebs has refused to be admitted to the hospital for ulcer care and feels that the nurses and physician do not understand her situation.

ASSESSMENT

On the first visit, the nurse did a complete assessment and discussed the client's history, which includes peripheral vascular disease and hypertension. Mrs. Krebs's physical examination showed blood pressure 140/82 mmHg, pulse 76 beats/min, respirations 20 breaths/min, and temperature 98°F. On examination of the heel ulcer, the nurse noted a 4-cm by 6-cm stage III ulcer with a minimal amount of serous drainage and no local signs of inflammation.

Mrs. Krebs is eating poorly, mostly freezer and canned foods with little protein and high sodium. She admits that she is smoking and not following her diet. She states, "I lost my husband 6 months ago and have not been able to take care of things. I tried to quit smoking but it only lasted 5 days. I have been smoking for 40 years, and it is just too hard to stop. I'm doing the best I can."

DIAGNOSES

The current nursing diagnoses for Mrs. Krebs include the following:

- Impaired Skin Integrity: Stage III Ulcer related to prolonged pressure, inadequate nutrition, decreased vascular perfusion
- Ineffective Management of Therapeutic Regimen related to complex regimen: limited resources and impaired adjustment as manifested by client self-assessment of poor dietary intake, inability to rest and elevate foot, and smoking behavior
- Risk for Altered Nutrition: Less Than Body Requirements related to lack of physical and economic resources, and increased nutritional requirements related to ulcer.

EXPECTED OUTCOMES

The expected outcomes for the plan specify that Mrs. Krebs will do the following:

- Describe measures to protect and heal the tissue, including wound care.
- Report any additional symptoms, such as pain, redness, numbness, tingling, or increased drainage.
- Demonstrate an understanding of nutritional needs, including the need for supplemental protein drink and vitamins.
- Collaborate with the nurse to develop a therapeutic plan that is congruent with her goals and present lifestyle.

PLANNING AND IMPLEMENTATION

The following nursing interventions may be appropriate for Mrs. Krebs:

- Establish a trusting relationship with Mrs. Krebs.
- Begin to explore what the client's goals are in relation to her health care.
- Determine her daily habits and schedule, and find some small measures that can be started for health improvement.
- Begin to determine ways to work with Mrs. Krebs's family to motivate her toward a healthier lifestyle (i.e., nutrition, smoking cessation, foot care).
- Set priorities of care that Mrs. Krebs will agree to, such as (1) ulcer improvement, (2) diet adjustments, and (3) smoking reductions.

EVALUATION

The nurse hopes to develop a long-term relationship with Mrs. Krebs and make an impact on her health and well-being. The nurse will consider the plan a success on the basis of the following criteria:

- Mrs. Krebs will develop a trusting relationship and develop a plan with the nurse to improve her health.
- A family member will agree to assist Mrs. Krebs with her wound care and shopping issues.
- Mrs. Krebs will begin a smoking reduction effort.
- Mrs. Krebs will agree that if the ulcer is not healing in 4 weeks, she will seek inpatient treatment.

CRITICAL THINKING

1. What are the intrinsic and extrinsic factors that can cause skin problems in older adults? Make a list with two columns, and see how many factors you can identify.
2. How important is nutrition to the dermatologic health of your skin?
3. What type of dressings do you see used in your clinical rotations with older people? Are they consistent with current guidelines and recommendations?
4. What positioning techniques have you seen used in your clinical rotations?

Box 30–5 Treating Pressure Ulcers

- Minimize direct pressure on the ulcer. Reposition the client at least every 2 hours. Make a schedule, and record position changes on the client's chart. Provide devices to minimize or float pressure areas.
- Clean the pressure ulcer with every dressing change. The method of cleaning depends on the stage of the ulcer, products available, and agency protocol.
- Clean and dress the ulcer using surgical asepsis. Never use alcohol or hydrogen peroxide, as they are cytotoxic to tissue beds.
- If the pressure ulcer is infected, obtain a sample of the drainage to culture and test for sensitivity to antibiotic agents.
- Teach the client to move, even if only slightly, to relieve pressure.
- Provide range-of-motion (ROM) exercises and mobility out of bed as the client's condition permits.

papain-urea are currently most often recommended for this use. In *autolytic debridement,* dressings that contain wound moisture, such as hydrocolloid and clear absorbent acrylic dressings, trap the wound drainage against the eschar. The body's own enzymes in the drainage break down the necrotic tissue. Although this method takes longer than the other three, it is the most selective and therefore causes the least damage to healthy surrounding and healing tissues. Recently, the use of fly larvae (maggots, *Phaenicia sericata*) has received increased attention. Larval therapy can be extremely effective in cleansing chronic wounds because the maggots secrete enzymes that break down necrotic tissue (while leaving healthy tissue untouched), eat bacteria, and reduce bacterial growth by increasing surface pH that results from their presence (Sosin, 2005).

Evaluation

For clients who are immobile or on bed rest, the treatment plan may need to be evaluated and modified as often as daily, depending on the assessment of the client's skin integrity, client comfort and pain level, and whether or not the written repositioning plan has been followed. Clients who are in bed for long periods of time can experienced diminished appetites. If a client is not maintaining adequate dietary intake even if changes to the nutrition plan have been made, the nurse may need to arrange to consult with a nutritionist or dietician. For clients who are mobile, the nurse should provide instructions when to call the office if there is another appearance of a potential pressure ulcer or change in skin integrity.

REVIEW Pressure Ulcers

RELATE: LINK THE CONCEPTS

Linking the exemplar of Pressure Ulcers with the concept of Infection:

1. What assessment findings would cause you to believe a pressure ulcer is infected?
2. What nursing interventions can be implemented to reduce the risk of infection of a pressure ulcer?

Linking the exemplar of Pressure Ulcers with the concept of Mobility:

3. Contrast appropriate nursing interventions to prevent pressure ulcers in the clients aged 6, 30, and 80 years of age with limited mobility.
4. You are caring for a child who was involved in a bicycle accident resulting in below-the-waist paraplegia. How will you teach these parents to reduce the risk of pressure ulcers?

READY: GO TO COMPANION SKILLS MANUAL

- Moving and positioning clients in bed
- Performing safe and effective lifting and transfer techniques
- Maintaining body alignment
- Applying body mechanics
- Moving a client up in bed
- Using a turn or lift sheet

REFER: GO TO MYNURSINGKIT

REFLECT: CASE STUDY

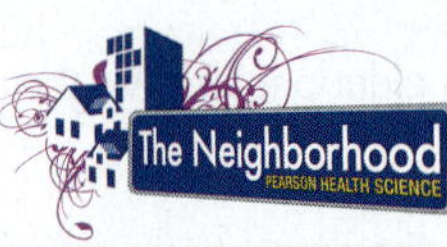

Lydia Ocampo is a 69-year-old widow who has recently been moved from a rehabilitation center to the skilled nursing wing of a nursing facility. She is still receiving care related to surgery on a broken hip a couple of months before. Before that, she had lived in the home that she shared with her husband of 50 years. Her husband died a few weeks ago. Lydia has Alzheimer's disease. At the nursing home, she exhibits intermittent confusion and is alternately passive and uncooperative with the staff. Over the course of the next month, her condition deteriorates. She eats very little and is fairly unresponsive to caregivers. She sleeps often.

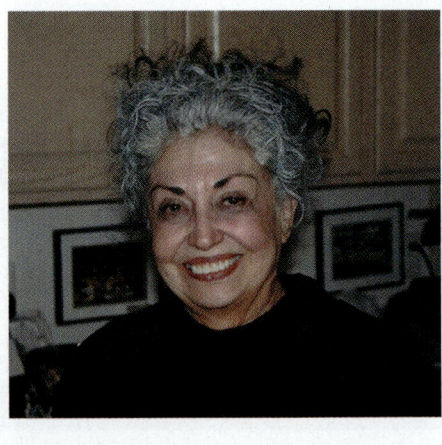

1. What data suggest that Lydia is particularly vulnerable to pressure ulcer development?
2. What additional information do you need in order to use the Braden scale to determine Lydia's potential for pressure ulcer development?
3. What independent measures can you take to protect Lydia's skin from further breakdown?
4. Considering that Lydia does not have any areas of skin breakdown, why is it important to institute treatment for pressure ulcers at this time?

30.4 WOUND HEALING

KEY TERMS

Approximated, *1927*
Collagen, *1928*
Dehiscence, *1929*
Evisceration, *1929*
Exudate, *1930*
Fibrin, *1927*
Granulation tissue, *1928*
Hematoma, *1929*
Hemorrhage, *1929*
Hemostasis, *1927*
Keloid, *1929*
Macrophages, *1928*
Phagocytosis, *1928*
Primary intention healing, *1927*
Purulent exudate, *1930*
Pus, *1930*
Pyogenic bacteria, *1930*
Regeneration, *1927*
Sanguineous (hemorrhagic) exudate, *1930*
Secondary intention healing, *1927*
Serosanguineous exudate, *1930*
Serous exudate, *1930*
Suppuration, *1930*
Tertiary intention healing, *1927*

BASIS FOR SELECTION OF EXEMPLAR

Institute of Medicine (IOM)

LEARNING OUTCOMES

After reading about this exemplar, you will be able to:

1. Describe the pathophysiology and clinical manifestations of wound healing along with etiology and factors that can impair wound healing.
2. Identify risk factors associated with open wounds.
3. Illustrate the nursing process in providing culturally competent care across the life span that promote wound healing for individuals with a wound.
4. Formulate priority nursing diagnoses appropriate for an individual with a wound or alterations in wound healing.
5. Create a plan of care for individuals with a wound or alterations in wound healing and their family members.
6. Assess expected outcomes for an individual with a wound or delayed wound healing.
7. Discuss therapies used in the collaborative care of an individual to promote wound healing.
8. Employ evidence-based caring interventions for an individual with a wound or delayed wound healing.

OVERVIEW

Healing is a quality of living tissue; it is also referred to as **regeneration** (renewal) of tissues. Healing can be considered in terms of *types of healing,* having to do with the caregiver's decision on whether to allow the wound to seal itself or to purposefully close the wound, and *phases of healing,* which refer to the steps in the body's natural processes of tissue repair. The phases are the same for all wounds, but the rate of healing depends on factors such as the type of healing, the location and size of the wound, and the client's health.

Types of Wound Healing

There are two types of healing, each influenced by the amount of tissue loss. **Primary intention healing** occurs where the tissue surfaces have been **approximated** (closed) and there is minimal or no tissue loss; it is characterized by the formation of minimal granulation tissue and scarring. It is also called *primary union* or *first intention healing.* An example of wound healing by primary intention is a closed surgical incision. Another example would be the use of tissue adhesive, a liquid "glue," to seal clean lacerations or incisions, which may result in better appearing scars (Coulthard, Worthington, Esposito, van der Elst, & van Waes, 2005).

A wound that is extensive and involves considerable tissue loss and in which the edges cannot or should not be approximated, heals by **secondary intention healing**. An example of wound healing by secondary intention is a pressure ulcer. Secondary intention healing differs from primary intention healing in three ways: (a) The repair time is longer, (b) the scarring is greater, and (c) the susceptibility to infection is greater.

Those wounds that are left open for 3–5 days to allow edema or infection to resolve or to permit exudate to drain and then are closed with sutures, staples, or adhesive skin closures, **tertiary intention healing**. This is also called delayed primary intention.

PATHOPHYSIOLOGY AND ETIOLOGY

Wound healing can be broken down into three phases: inflammatory, proliferative, and maturation or remodeling (Figure 30–24 ■).

Phases of Wound Healing

INFLAMMATORY PHASE The *inflammatory phase* is initiated immediately after injury and lasts 3–6 days. Two major processes occur during this phase: hemostasis and phagocytosis.

Hemostasis (the cessation of bleeding) results from vasoconstriction of the larger blood vessels in the affected area, retraction (drawing back) of injured blood vessels, the deposition of **fibrin** (connective tissue), and the formation of blood clots in the area. The blood clots, formed from blood platelets, provide a matrix of fibrin that becomes the framework for cell repair. A scab also forms on the surface of the wound. Consisting of clots and dead and dying tissue, the scab aids hemostasis and inhibits contamination of the wound by microorganisms. Below the scab, epithelial cells migrate into the wound from the edges. The epithelial cells serve as a barrier between the body and the environment, preventing the entry of microorganisms.

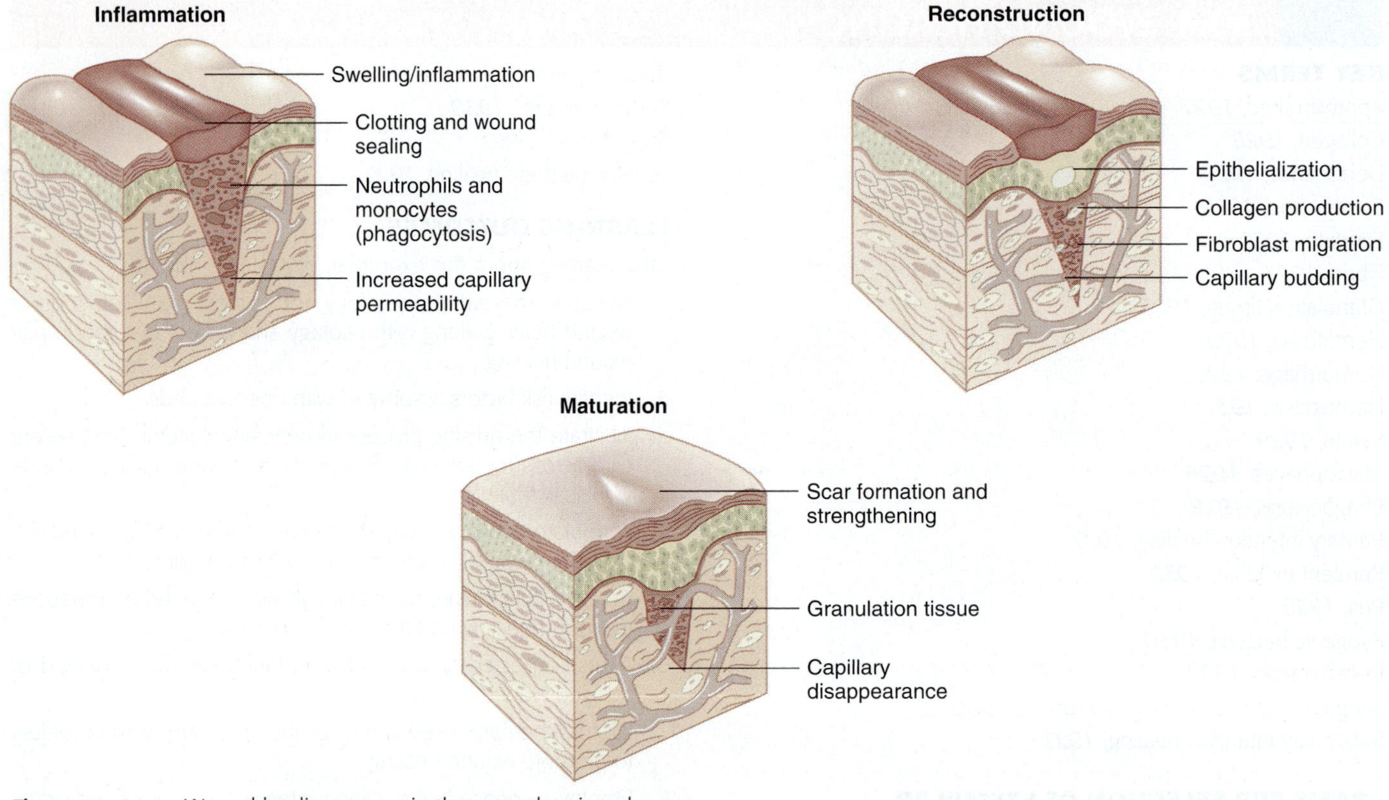

Figure 30–24 ■ Wound healing occurs in three overlapping phases.

Source: Data from Nicol, N. H., Heuther, S. E., & Weber, R. (2006). Structure, function, and disorders of the integument. In K. L. McCance & S. E. Huether, *Pathophysiology: The biologic basis for disease in adults and children* (5th ed., pp. 1573–1607). St. Louis: Elsevier Mosby.

The inflammatory phase also involves vascular and cellular responses intended to remove any foreign substances as well as dead and dying tissues. The blood supply to the wound increases, bringing with it oxygen and nutrients needed in the healing process. As a result, the area appears reddened and edematous. Exudate of fluid and cell debris is a normal accumulation and helps cleanse the wound. Overproduction of this exudate and other factors can impair wound healing, especially in chronic wounds (Hanson, Langemo, Thompson, Anderson, & Hunter, 2005).

During cell migration, leukocytes (specifically, neutrophils) move into the interstitial space. These are replaced about 24 hours after injury by **macrophages** (large cells of the immune system that remove waste and harmful microorganisms), which arise from the blood monocytes. These macrophages engulf microorganisms and cellular debris by a process known as **phagocytosis**. The macrophages also secrete an angiogenesis factor, which stimulates the formation of epithelial buds at the end of injured blood vessels. The microcirculatory network that results sustains the healing process and the wound during its life. This inflammatory response is essential to healing. Measures that impair inflammation, such as steroid medications, can place the healing process at risk.

PROLIFERATIVE PHASE The *proliferative phase,* the second phase in healing, extends from day 3 or 4 to about day 21 postinjury. Fibroblasts (connective tissue cells), which migrate into the wound starting about 24 hours after injury, begin to synthesize collagen. **Collagen** is a whitish protein substance that adds tensile strength to the wound. As the amount of collagen increases, so does the strength of the wound; thus the chance that the wound will remain closed increases progressively. If the wound is sutured, a raised "healing ridge" appears under the intact suture line. In a wound that is not sutured, the new collagen is often visible.

Capillaries grow across the wound, increasing the blood supply. Fibroblasts move from the bloodstream into the wound, depositing fibrin. As the capillary network develops, the tissue becomes a translucent red. This tissue, called **granulation tissue**, is fragile and bleeds easily.

When the skin edges of a wound are not sutured, the area must be filled in with granulation tissue. When the granulation tissue matures, marginal epithelial cells migrate to it, proliferating over this connective tissue base to fill the wound. If the wound does not close by epithelialization the area becomes covered by a scab or dry crust formed by dried plasma proteins and dead cells. This is called *eschar.* Initially, wounds healing by secondary intention seep blood-tinged (serosanguineous) drainage. Later, if they are not covered by epithelial cells, they become covered with thick, gray, fibrinous tissue that is eventually converted into dense scar tissue.

MATURATION PHASE The *maturation phase* begins about day 21 and can extend 1 or 2 years after the injury. Fibroblasts continue to synthesize collagen. The collagen fibers themselves, which were initially laid in a haphazard fashion, reorganize into a more orderly structure. During maturation, the wound is remodeled and contracted. The scar becomes stronger, but the repaired

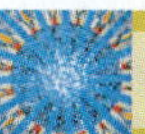

DEVELOPMENTAL CONSIDERATIONS Wound Care

INFANTS

- The skin of infants is more fragile than that of older children and adults and is more susceptible to infection, shearing from friction, and burns.

CHILDREN

- *Staphylococcus* and fungus are two major infectious agents affecting the skin of children. Abrasions or small lacerations, commonly experienced by children, provide an entry in the skin for these organisms. Clean minor wounds with warm, soapy water, and covered with a sterile bandage. Instruct children not to touch the wound.
- With more serious skin lesions, remind the child not to touch the wound, drains, or dressing. Cover with an appropriate bandage that will remain intact during the child's usual activities. Cover a transparent dressing with opaque material if viewing the site is distressing to the child. Restrain the child only when all alternatives have been tried and when absolutely necessary.
- For younger children, demonstrate wound care on a doll. Reassure the child that the wound will not be permanent and that nothing will fall out of the body.

OLDER ADULTS

- Hold wrinkled skin taut during application of a transparent dressing. Obtain assistance if needed.
- Skin is more fragile and can easily tear with removal of tape (especially adhesive tape). Use paper tape and tape remover as indicated, keeping tape use to the minimum required. Use extreme caution during tape removal.
- Older adults in long-term care facilities often have the following factors: immobility, malnutrition, and incontinence–all of which increase the risk for development of skin breakdown.
- Skin breakdown can occur as quickly as within 2 hours, so assessments should be done with each repositioning of the client.
- A thorough assessment of a client's heels should be done every shift. The skin can break down quickly from friction of movement in bed.

area is never as strong as the original tissue. In some individuals, particularly dark-skinned persons, an abnormal amount of collagen appears. This can result in a hypertrophic scar, or **keloid**.

Complications of Wound Healing

Several untoward events can interfere with the healing of a wound. These include hemorrhage, infection, and dehiscence and evisceration.

HEMORRHAGE Some escape of blood from a wound is normal. **Hemorrhage** (massive bleeding), however, is abnormal. A dislodged clot, a slipped stitch, or erosion of a blood vessel may cause severe bleeding.

Internal hemorrhage may be detected by swelling or distention in the area of the wound and, possibly, by sanguineous drainage from a surgical drain. Some clients will have a **hematoma**, a localized collection of blood underneath the skin that may appear as a reddish blue swelling (bruise). A large hematoma may be dangerous because it can place pressure on blood vessels, thereby obstructing blood flow.

The risk of hemorrhage is greatest during the first 48 hours after surgery. Hemorrhage is an emergency; the nurse applies pressure dressings to the area and monitors the client's vital signs. In many instances, the client must be taken to the operating room for surgical intervention.

INFECTION Contamination of a wound surface with microorganisms (colonization) is an inevitable result. Because the colonizing organisms compete with new cells for oxygen and nutrition and because their byproducts can interfere with a healthy surface condition, the presence of contamination can impair wound healing and lead to infection. When the microorganisms colonizing the wound multiply excessively or invade tissues, infection occurs. Infection suggested by the presence of a change in wound color, pain, or drainage is confirmed by performing a culture of the wound. Severe infection causes fever and elevated white blood cell count. Clients who are immunosuppressed, such as those with HIV or those receiving myelosuppressive treatment for cancer, are especially susceptible to wound infections.

A wound can be infected with microorganisms at the time of injury, during surgery, or postoperatively. Wounds that occur as a result of injury (e.g., bullet and knife wounds) are most likely to be contaminated at the time of injury. Surgery involving the intestines can also result in infection from the microorganisms inside the intestine. Surgical infection is most likely to become apparent 2–11 days postoperatively.

DEHISCENCE WITH POSSIBLE EVISCERATION **Dehiscence** is the partial or total rupturing of a sutured wound. Dehiscence usually involves an abdominal wound in which the layers below the skin also separate. **Evisceration** is the protrusion of the internal viscera through an incision. A number of factors, including obesity, poor nutrition, multiple trauma, failure of suturing, excessive coughing, vomiting, and dehydration heighten a client's risk of wound dehiscence. Wound dehiscence is more likely to occur 4–5 days postoperatively, before extensive collagen is deposited in the wound.

Sudden straining, such as coughing or sneezing, may precede dehiscence. It is not unusual for a client to feel that "something has given way." When dehiscence or evisceration occurs, the wound should be supported quickly by large sterile dressings soaked in sterile normal saline. The nurse should place the client in bed with knees bent to decrease pull on the incision. The surgeon must be notified because immediate surgical repair of the area may be necessary.

Factors Affecting Wound Healing

Characteristics of the individual such as age, nutritional status, lifestyle, and medications influence the speed of wound healing.

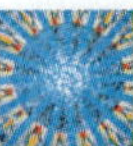

DEVELOPMENTAL CONSIDERATIONS Factors Inhibiting Wound Healing

OLDER ADULTS

- Vascular changes associated with aging, such as atherosclerosis and atrophy of capillaries in the skin, can impair blood flow to the wound.
- Collagen tissue is less flexible, which increases the risk of damage from pressure, friction, and shearing.
- Scar tissue is less elastic.
- Changes in the immune system may reduce the formation of the antibodies and monocytes necessary for wound healing.
- Nutritional deficiencies may reduce the numbers of red blood cells and leukocytes, thus impeding the delivery of oxygen and the inflammatory response essential for wound healing. Oxygen is needed for the synthesis of collagen and the formation of new epithelial cells.
- Having diabetes, chronic lung disease, or cardiovascular disease increases the risk of delayed healing due to impaired oxygen delivery to these tissues.
- Cell renewal is slower, resulting in delayed healing.

DEVELOPMENTAL CONSIDERATIONS Healthy children and adults often heal more quickly than do older adults, who are more likely to have chronic diseases that hinder healing. For example, reduced liver function can impair the synthesis of blood clotting factors. See Developmental Considerations: Wound Care for factors specific to children and to older adults and Developmental Considerations: Factors Inhibiting Wound Healing for factors inhibiting wound healing in older adults.

NUTRITION Wound healing places additional demands on the body. Clients require a diet rich in protein, carbohydrates, lipids, vitamins A and C, and minerals such as iron, zinc, and copper. Malnourished clients may require time to improve their nutritional status before surgery, if possible. Obese clients are at increased risk of wound infection and slower healing because adipose tissue usually has a minimal blood supply.

LIFESTYLE People who exercise regularly tend to have good circulation. Because blood brings oxygen and nourishment to the wound, clients who exercise regularly are more likely to heal quickly. Smoking reduces the amount of functional hemoglobin in the blood, thus limiting the oxygen-carrying capacity of the blood, and constricts arterioles. As a result, smokers are at risk for delayed healing.

MEDICATIONS Anti-inflammatory drugs (e.g., steroids and aspirin) and antineoplastic agents interfere with healing. Prolonged use of antibiotics may make a person susceptible to wound infection by resistant organisms.

CLINICAL MANIFESTATIONS

Exudate is material, such as fluid and dead phagocytic cells, that has escaped from blood vessels during the inflammatory process and is deposited in tissue or on tissue surfaces. The nature and amount of exudate vary according to the tissue involved, the intensity and duration of the inflammation, and the presence of microorganisms.

There are three major types of exudate: serous, purulent, and sanguineous (hemorrhagic). A **serous exudate** typically accompanies mild inflammation and presents as clear or straw colored. It is thin and watery and has few cells. An example is the fluid in a blister from a burn.

A **purulent exudate** is thicker than serous exudate and consists of a large quantity of cells and necrotic debris; it is usually opaque or milky in appearance. The formation of purulent exudate, commonly referred to as **pus**, is referred to as **suppuration**, and the bacteria that produce pus are called **pyogenic bacteria**. Not all microorganisms are pyogenic. Purulent exudates can vary in color, some acquiring tinges of blue, green, or yellow. The color may depend on the causative organism.

A **sanguineous (hemorrhagic) exudate** consists of large amounts of red blood cells, indicating damage to capillaries that is severe enough to allow the escape of red blood cells from plasma. This type of exudate is frequently seen in open wounds. Mixed types of exudates are often observed. A **serosanguineous exudate** (consisting of clear and blood-tinged drainage) is commonly seen in surgical incisions. A *purosanguineous* discharge (consisting of pus and blood) is often seen in a new wound that is infected.

PRACTICE ALERT

A bright sanguineous exudate indicates fresh bleeding, whereas dark sanguineous exudate denotes older bleeding.

COLLABORATION

The client with a wound receives care from a number of health care providers. Surgeons, nurses, scrub persons, anesthetists, phlebotomists, x-ray technicians, registration clerks, and emergency transporters are often involved in securing the safety and health of clients. Case managers and social workers are available based on client needs postdischarge. This interdisciplinary approach focuses on placing the client in the best possible health status to achieve successful wound healing.

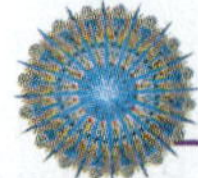

NURSING PROCESS

Assessment

Nurses commonly assess both untreated and treated wounds. Untreated wounds usually are seen shortly after an injury (e.g., at the scene of an accident or in an emergency center). Assessment for these wounds is as follows:

- Assess the location and extent of tissue damage (e.g., partial thickness or full thickness). Measure the length, width, and depth of the wound.

- Inspect the wound for bleeding. The amount of bleeding varies according to the type of wound and location. Penetrating wounds may cause internal bleeding.
- Inspect the wound for foreign bodies (soil, broken glass, shreds of cloth, or other foreign substances).
- Assess associated injuries such as fractures, internal bleeding, spinal cord injuries, or head trauma.
- If the wound is contaminated with foreign material, determine when the client last had a tetanus toxoid injection. A tetanus immunization or booster may be necessary.

Assessment of a treated (sutured) wound involves observation of its appearance, size, drainage, and the presence of swelling, pain, and status of drains or tubes. In some long-term facilities, home care situations, and outpatient clinics, photographs are taken weekly for a visual record of the progress of pressure ulcers and wounds. Other assessments are documented and dated along with the photograph.

Estimating the amount of wound drainage can be difficult. One recommendation is to describe the degree to which the dressing is saturated. Minimal drainage only stains the dressing; moderate drainage saturates the dressing without leakage prior to scheduled dressing changes; and heavy drainage overflows the dressing prior to scheduled changes (Brown, 2006). These terms, plus the description of the drainage and the amount and type of dressing material used, should be well understood by all care providers.

Sometimes the wound reaches under the skin surface (called *undermining*). The edges of the wound around an open center may be raw or appear healed, but the undermining can result in a sinus tract or tunnel that extends the wound many centimeters beyond the main wound surface. To assess the size of the wound, gently explore the undermined area with a thin, flexible probe. Do not use a cotton-tipped swab, since it can leave fibers in the wound. Once the end of the tract is reached, gently raise the probe so that the bulge created by the end can be seen and its length can be measured on the skin surface. Sinus tracts are often caused by infection and have significant drainage. They may be treated by using antibiotics, irrigation, surgical incision to open and drain the tract, or vacuum therapy for large tracts.

Diagnosis

The following nursing diagnoses relate to clients who have skin wounds or who are at risk for skin breakdown:

- Risk for Impaired Skin Integrity
- Impaired Skin Integrity
- Impaired Tissue Integrity.

Impaired Skin Integrity commonly applies to pressure ulcers and wounds that extend through the epidermis but not through the dermis. Impaired Tissue Integrity applies to pressure ulcers and wounds that extend into subcutaneous tissue, muscle, or bone. Additional nursing diagnoses may be appropriate for clients with existing impaired skin or tissue integrity, including the following examples:

- Risk for Infection if the skin impairment is severe, the client is immunosuppressed, or the wound is caused by trauma
- Pain related to nerve involvement within the tissue impairment or as a consequence of procedures used to treat the wound.

Plan

The major goals for clients at Risk for Impaired Skin Integrity are to maintain skin integrity and avoid potential associated risks. Clients with Impaired Skin Integrity need goals to demonstrate progressive wound healing and regain intact skin within a specified time. Client education for home care management focuses on maintaining skin integrity.

Implementation

The four major areas in which nurses can help clients develop optimal conditions for wound healing are maintaining moist wound healing, providing sufficient nutrition and hydration, preventing wound infections, and proper positioning.

Moist Wound Healing

The dressing and frequency of change should support moist wound bed conditions. Wound beds that are too dry or disturbed too often fail to heal.

CARE SETTINGS **Home Care for Wounds and Prevention of Pressure Ulcers**

CLIENT AND ENVIRONMENT

- Current level of knowledge: Understanding of the cause of the wound or risk for developing a pressure ulcer; prevention or treatment strategies
- Self-care abilities for mobility: Physical ability to change position, ambulate, and transfer including the use of assistive devices
- Self-care abilities for wound care: Manual dexterity and visual acuity necessary to perform skin assessments and wound treatments
- Facilities: Presence of running water, garbage container, bathroom needed to perform wound care and contain potentially infectious materials
- Current level of nutrition: Eating habits and preferences, laboratory values indicating need for teaching or other intervention

FAMILY

- Caregiver availability, skills, and responses: Understanding of the cause of the wound or risk for developing a pressure ulcer, prevention or treatment strategies, willingness to assist with wound care, and actions to prevent pressure ulcers
- Family role changes and coping: Effect on financial status, parenting and spousal roles, sexuality, and social roles
- Alternative potential primary or respite caregivers: For example, other family members, volunteers, church members, paid caregivers, or housekeeping services; available community respite care (adult day care, senior centers, etc.)

COMMUNITY

- Resources: Availability and familiarity with possible sources of assistance such as equipment and supply companies, organizations that offer medical supplies or financial assistance, home health agencies, and transportation to and from medical appointments, if needed

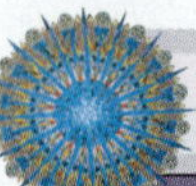

NURSING CARE PLAN **A Client With a Postoperative Wound**

ASSESSMENT

Mrs. Overbeck, 44 years old, underwent bariatric surgery 4 days ago. She says she knew it was time to do something dramatic when her doctor diagnosed both hypertension and type 2 diabetes mellitus on the same day. She has an 8 inch midline abdominal incision that appeared slightly red and began to ooze purulent drainage yesterday. The incision is stapled and has dissolvable sutures internally. She is NPO due to absent bowel sounds with an intravenous solution of dextrose and water infusing at 100 mL/h per infusion pump. The antibiotic ciprofloxacin hydrochloride (Cipro) is to be administered every 6 hours IV. Other medications include Regular Humulin insulin administered on a sliding scale based on finger-stick glucose levels, clevidipine butyrate administered PRN for hypertension, acetaminophen suppository PRN for fever greater than 100 degrees Fahrenheit, and morphine sulfate PRN for pain.

Assessment findings include:

- Drowsy but arousable and oriented X4
- Skin is pale and slightly cool
- Mrs. Overbeck states that she is cold and requests additional covers
- Mrs. Overbeck states that she is in no pain and would like to sleep
- Respirations unlabored
- Vital signs: T_O 101.2ºF, P 96, R 18, BP 128/86
- Large abdominal dressing over midline abdominal incision with purulent drainage the size of a silver dollar and a Jackson Pratt suction device connected to a drain with 10 mL dark red serosanguineous drainage coming from the distal part of the wound.
- Indwelling catheter in place with 210 mL clear amber urine
- This morning's lab results include: Fasting blood sugar–110, hemaglobin within normal limits, WBC–12, 400, serum albumin 2.6 g/dl.

DIAGNOSES

- Ineffective Thermoregulation
- Risk for Fluid Volume Deficit
- Impaired Skin Integrity
- Delayed Surgical Recovery

PLANNING

Goals for Mrs. Overbeck's plan of care include:

- Promote wound healing
- Maintain adequate hydration
- Control temperature within acceptable limits until fever subsides
- Reduce complications secondary to wound infection.

IMPLEMENTATION

- Use aseptic technique while changing dressing.
- Monitor temperature every 4 hours, with repeat measurement in 1 hour following administration of antipyretic if elevated higher than 100 degrees Fahrenheit.
- Assess wound every 4 hours for purulent drainage, odor, edges of wound for approximation, edema, redness, inflammation.
- Teach Mrs. Overbeck how to use aseptic technique when providing wound care.
- Promote comfort through use of appropriate pain management – both pharmacological and nonpharmacological.
- Monitor intake and output, daily weight, and hydration status
- Assess blood glucose four times per day and administer insulin on a sliding scale as ordered.
- Empty Jackson Pratt wound drain every 4 hours and notify provider if drainage increases beyond acceptable limits based on baseline drainage to date.
- Assist client to change positions at least every 2 hours.
- Teach proper nutrition to promote wound healing in keeping with postop bariatric surgical requirements.

EVALUATION

Expected outcomes for Mrs. Overbeck include:

- Client attains skin integrity of the abdominal incision
- Client demonstrates proper aseptic technique while performing dressing changes.
- Client reports control of pain at incision site
- Client's temperature will return to acceptable limits within 1 hour of receiving antipyretic.

CRITICAL THINKING

1. In addition to the nursing diagnosis identified in this plan of care, what other nursing diagnoses would be appropriate for her care?
2. Assess Mrs. Overbeck's nutritional status based on the data provided. Is it adequate to promote wound healing? Explain your answer and provide interventions as needed based on your response.
3. What impact will the client's preexisting conditions of hypertension and type 2 diabetes mellitus have on wound healing?
4. Other than the implementations listed in the plan of care, what else could you do to promote wound healing?
5. What discharge teaching will you provide this client to promote wound healing?

Nutrition and Fluids

Clients should be assisted to take in at least 2,500 mL of fluids a day unless other health conditions contraindicate this amount. Although there is no evidence that excessive doses of vitamins or minerals enhance wound healing, adequate amounts are extremely important. The nurse should ensure that clients receive sufficient protein, vitamins C, A, B, and B5, and zinc. Obtaining a consultation with a registered dietitian helps to ensure that correct supplementation needs are met. Nurses and those planning the client's meals should take into account both the client's personal and religious food preferences.

Preventing Infection

There are two main aspects to controlling wound infection: preventing microorganisms from entering the wound and preventing the transmission of bloodborne pathogens to or from the client to others.

Positioning

To promote wound healing, clients must be positioned to keep pressure off the wound (sometimes referred to as *off-loading*). Changes of position and transfers can be accomplished without shear or friction damage. In addition to proper positioning, the client should be assisted to be as mobile as possible because activity enhances circulation. If the client cannot move independently, range-of-motion exercises and a turning schedule are implemented. See the accompanying Nursing Care Plan and Care Settings: Home Care Assessment.

Evaluation

The major goals for clients at Risk for Impaired Skin Integrity are to maintain skin integrity and to avoid potential associated risks. Clients with Impaired Skin Integrity need goals to demonstrate progressive wound healing and regain intact skin within a specified time.

Expected outcomes of nursing care include the following:

- Skin and tissue integrity is maintained.
- Wound decreases in size.
- Client demonstrates understanding of preventive care measures.

REVIEW Wound Healing

RELATE: LINK THE CONCEPTS

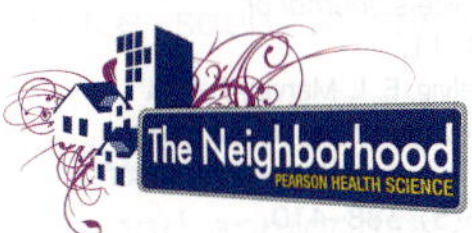

Mrs. James, a 65-year-old widow who lives alone, presents at the geriatric nursing clinic at the local senior center with a wound on her ankle about the size of a quarter. The wound is sore, with yellowish drainage. The skin around the wound is red and inflamed. Mrs. James says that she's had the sore about three weeks and that she treated it with butter for a while but that that seemed to make it worse. Mrs. James says that her foot hurts when she walks on it. The nurse at the clinic smells the cigarette smoke on Mrs. James clothing. When asked, Mrs. James reports that she smokes about a pack a day. In response to a question from the nurse, Mrs. James says that she has diabetes and high blood pressure. Mrs. James is not able to say what medicines she takes but estimates that she takes "about four different ones."

Linking the exemplar of Wound Healing with the concept of Metabolism:

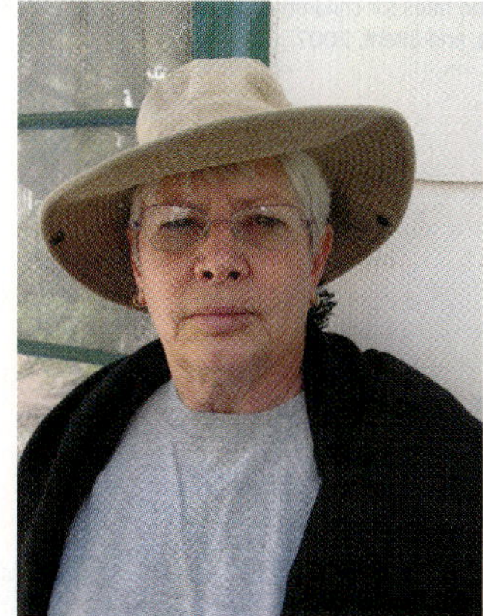

1. What metabolic factors will increase the risk of delayed wound healing?
2. What teaching can the nurse provide Mrs. James to promote wound healing in relation to metabolic concerns?

Linking the exemplar of Wound Healing with the concept of Perfusion:

3. What factors related to perfusion will increase the risk of delayed wound healing for Mrs. James?
4. What teaching will you provide Mrs. James to reduce these risks related to perfusion?

READY: GO TO COMPANION SKILLS MANUAL

- Obtaining a wound drainage specimen
- Irrigating a wound
- Maintaining closed wound drainage

REFER: GO TO MYNURSINGKIT

REFLECT: CASE STUDY

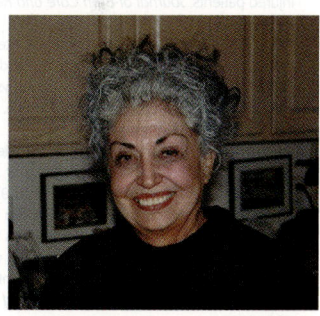

Lydia Ocampo, 69, wakes during the night to urinate but falls on the way to the bathroom. An ambulance takes her to the emergency department, where she is diagnosed with a left hip fracture. She is sent to the operating room for an open reduction internal fixation of the left hip. She is admitted to the medical-surgical floor following surgery.

Mrs. Ocampo remains at the hospital because she has developed an infection in her incision and needs intravenous antibiotics and dressing changes. Her oral intake has been inadequate, but she has been well hydrated by the intravenous fluids. She has been incontinent ever since the Foley catheter was removed. Attempts at physical therapy have been unproductive. The physical therapists are successful at transferring her from the bed to a chair, but this requires nearly full assistance.

1. Identify priority nursing diagnosis for Mrs. Ocampo.
2. List factors that put Mrs. Ocampo at risk for impaired tissue integrity.

- In 2007, U.S. child protective services investigated over 3 million reports of child abuse or neglect (U.S. Department of Health and Human Services, 2009a).
- Elder abuse in domestic settings affects hundreds of thousands of elderly across the United States; the problem is likely underreported, and the reported incidents may be only the tip of the iceberg (National Center on Elder Abuse, 2004).
- In 2006, 1.8 million emergency department visits were related to assault (CDC, 2006).
- In 2006, sexual assaults represented 10% of assault-related injury visits to emergency departments by females (CDC, 2007).
- In 2006, 5,958 young people ages 10–24 were murdered—an average of 16 each day (CDC, 2009a).
- Homicide victimization is 14 times higher in African American youth than in their white counterparts (CDC, n.d.)
- In 2007, over 631,000 violence-related injuries in young people ages 10–24 were treated in U.S. emergency rooms (CDC, 2009a).
- In a 2007 nationwide survey, 36% of high school students reported being in a physical fight during the past 12 months (CDC, 2007).
- In the same survey, nearly 6% of high school students reported taking a gun, knife, or club to school in the 30 days prior to the survey (CDC, 2007).
- Over 32,000 people in the U.S. commit suicide each year; suicide is the 11th leading cause of death among Americans.
- In 2006, there were 43,664 motor vehicle traffic deaths.

Societal violence and injury cost millions of dollars in hospital care alone and result in millions of days of lost work productivity. Add to this the personal costs of victimization as well as the mounting cost of police and other protective services and related court costs, and it becomes apparent that the United States cannot afford the current level of violence and must do something to contain it.

A major emphasis of *Healthy People 2010* is on violence reduction and prevention. The objectives are focused on reducing injury, disability, and death due to unintentional injury and violence (Centers for Disease Prevention and Control [CDC], 2005a). Selected objectives with baseline and target data are listed in Table 31–1. ●

TABLE 31–1 ***Healthy People 2010* Selected Objectives Related to Violence and Injury**

OBJECTIVE	BASELINE	TARGET
■ 15-3. Reduce firearm-related deaths to 4.9 per 1,000,000 population		
■ 15-4. Reduce the proportion of people living in homes with firearms that are loaded and unlocked	19%	16%
■ 15-5. Reduce nonfatal firearm-related injuries to 10.9 injuries per 100,000 population	23.5 per 100,000	9.1 per 100,00
■ 15-12. Reduce hospital emergency department visits caused by injuries to 112 hospital emergency department visits per 1,000 population	131 per 1,000	126 per 1,000
■ 15-15. Reduce deaths caused by motor vehicle crashes to 9.0 deaths per 100,000 population and 1 death per 100 million vehicle miles traveled (VMT)	8.0 per 100,000	126 per 1,000
■ 15-17. Reduce nonfatal injuries caused by motor vehicle crashes to 1,000 nonfatal injuries per 100,000 population.	1,181 per 100,000	933 per 100,000
■ 15-32. Reduce homicides (per 100,000 population)	6.0	3.0†
■ 15-33. Reduce		
a. Maltreatment of children (per 1,000 children)	12.6	10.3
b. Child maltreatment fatalities (per 100,000 children)	1.6	1.4†
■ 15-34. Reduce the rate of physical assault by current or former intimate partners (per 1,000 population)	4.4	3.3*
■ 15-35. Reduce the annual rate of rape or attempted rape (per 1,000 population)	0.8	0.7*
■ 15-36. Reduce sexual assault other than rape (per 1,000 population)	0.6	0.4
■ 15-37. Reduce physical assaults (per 1,000 population)	31.1	13.6
■ 15-39. Reduce weapon carrying by adolescents on school property	6.9%	4.9%
■ 18-1. Reduce the suicide rate (per 100,000 population)	10.5	5.0†
■ 16-2. Reduce the rate of suicide attempts by adolescents requiring medical attention (12-month average)	2.6%	1%†

* *Objective has been met*

† *Objective moving away from target*

Source: Centers for Disease Control and Prevention. (2005). *Healthy people data.* Retrieved August 23, 2009, from http://wonder.cdc.gov/data2010

Violence 31

Concept at-a-Glance

Concept Learning Outcomes

After reading about this concept, you will be able to:

1. Contrast prevalent types of violence seen in the United States.
2. Differentiate factors related to violent events.
3. Identify potential effects of violence and appropriate nursing considerations.
4. Explain common developmentally appropriate assessment procedures used to examine both risk of violence and related trauma.
5. Predict effective strategies to prevent violence.
6. Formulate a culturally appropriate plan of care for victims of violence.

Concept Key Terms

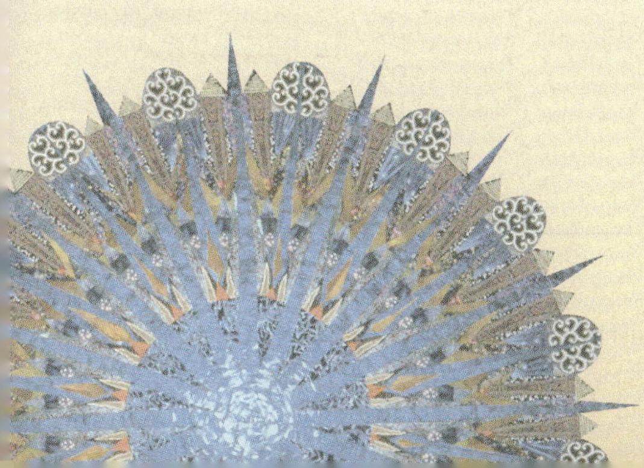

About Violence

Violence is a major health problem in the United States. Acts of violence can affect people of all ages, and may cause permanent physical or psychological scars. Violence can occur within any context: the family, the community, or the workplace.

- In 2007, 1,760 children died from maltreatment, including abuse and neglect; 76% of these children were younger than 4 years old (U.S. Department of Health and Human Services, 2009a).

- In 2007, U.S. child protective services investigated over 3 million reports of child abuse or neglect (U.S. Department of Health and Human Services, 2009a).
- Elder abuse in domestic settings affects hundreds of thousands of elderly across the United States; the problem is likely underreported, and the reported incidents may be only the tip of the iceberg (National Center on Elder Abuse, 2004).
- In 2006, 1.8 million emergency department visits were related to assault (CDC, 2006).
- In 2006, sexual assaults represented 10% of assault-related injury visits to emergency departments by females (CDC, 2007).
- In 2006, 5,958 young people ages 10–24 were murdered—an average of 16 each day (CDC, 2009a).
- Homicide victimization is 14 times higher in African American youth than in their white counterparts (CDC, n.d.)
- In 2007, over 631,000 violence-related injuries in young people ages 10–24 were treated in U.S. emergency rooms (CDC, 2009a).
- In a 2007 nationwide survey, 36% of high school students reported being in a physical fight during the past 12 months (CDC, 2007).
- In the same survey, nearly 6% of high school students reported taking a gun, knife, or club to school in the 30 days prior to the survey (CDC, 2007).
- Over 32,000 people in the U.S. commit suicide each year; suicide is the 11th leading cause of death among Americans.
- In 2006, there were 43,664 motor vehicle traffic deaths.

Societal violence and injury cost millions of dollars in hospital care alone and result in millions of days of lost work productivity. Add to this the personal costs of victimization as well as the mounting cost of police and other protective services and related court costs, and it becomes apparent that the United States cannot afford the current level of violence and must do something to contain it.

A major emphasis of *Healthy People 2010* is on violence reduction and prevention. The objectives are focused on reducing injury, disability, and death due to unintentional injury and violence (Centers for Disease Prevention and Control [CDC], 2005a). Selected objectives with baseline and target data are listed in Table 31–1. ●

TABLE 31–1 ***Healthy People 2010* Selected Objectives Related to Violence and Injury**

OBJECTIVE	BASELINE	TARGET
■ 15-3. Reduce firearm-related deaths to 4.9 per 1,000,000 population		
■ 15-4. Reduce the proportion of people living in homes with firearms that are loaded and unlocked	19%	16%
■ 15-5. Reduce nonfatal firearm-related injuries to 10.9 injuries per 100,000 population	23.5 per 100,000	9.1 per 100,00
■ 15-12. Reduce hospital emergency department visits caused by injuries to 112 hospital emergency department visits per 1,000 population	131 per 1,000	126 per 1,000
■ 15-15. Reduce deaths caused by motor vehicle crashes to 9.0 deaths per 100,000 population and 1 death per 100 million vehicle miles traveled (VMT)	8.0 per 100,000	126 per 1,000
■ 15-17. Reduce nonfatal injuries caused by motor vehicle crashes to 1,000 nonfatal injuries per 100,000 population.	1,181 per 100,000	933 per 100,000
■ 15-32. Reduce homicides (per 100,000 population)	6.0	3.0†
■ 15-33. Reduce		
a. Maltreatment of children (per 1,000 children)	12.6	10.3
b. Child maltreatment fatalities (per 100,000 children)	1.6	1.4†
■ 15-34. Reduce the rate of physical assault by current or former intimate partners (per 1,000 population)	4.4	3.3*
■ 15-35. Reduce the annual rate of rape or attempted rape (per 1,000 population)	0.8	0.7*
■ 15-36. Reduce sexual assault other than rape (per 1,000 population)	0.6	0.4
■ 15-37. Reduce physical assaults (per 1,000 population)	31.1	13.6
■ 15-39. Reduce weapon carrying by adolescents on school property	6.9%	4.9%
■ 18-1. Reduce the suicide rate (per 100,000 population)	10.5	5.0†
■ 16-2. Reduce the rate of suicide attempts by adolescents requiring medical attention (12-month average)	2.6%	1%†

** Objective has been met*

† Objective moving away from target

Source: Centers for Disease Control and Prevention. (2005). *Healthy people data*. Retrieved August 23, 2009, from http://wonder.cdc.gov/data2010

Nutrition and Fluids

Clients should be assisted to take in at least 2,500 mL of fluids a day unless other health conditions contraindicate this amount. Although there is no evidence that excessive doses of vitamins or minerals enhance wound healing, adequate amounts are extremely important. The nurse should ensure that clients receive sufficient protein, vitamins C, A, B, and B5, and zinc. Obtaining a consultation with a registered dietitian helps to ensure that correct supplementation needs are met. Nurses and those planning the client's meals should take into account both the client's personal and religious food preferences.

Preventing Infection

There are two main aspects to controlling wound infection: preventing microorganisms from entering the wound and preventing the transmission of bloodborne pathogens to or from the client to others.

Positioning

To promote wound healing, clients must be positioned to keep pressure off the wound (sometimes referred to as *off-loading*). Changes of position and transfers can be accomplished without shear or friction damage. In addition to proper positioning, the client should be assisted to be as mobile as possible because activity enhances circulation. If the client cannot move independently, range-of-motion exercises and a turning schedule are implemented. See the accompanying Nursing Care Plan and Care Settings: Home Care Assessment.

Evaluation

The major goals for clients at Risk for Impaired Skin Integrity are to maintain skin integrity and to avoid potential associated risks. Clients with Impaired Skin Integrity need goals to demonstrate progressive wound healing and regain intact skin within a specified time.

Expected outcomes of nursing care include the following:

- Skin and tissue integrity is maintained.
- Wound decreases in size.
- Client demonstrates understanding of preventive care measures.

REVIEW Wound Healing

RELATE: LINK THE CONCEPTS

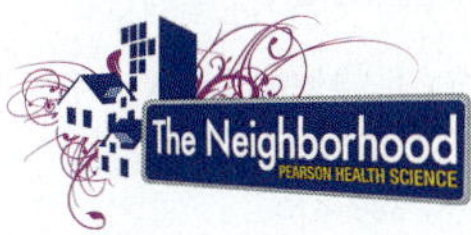

Mrs. James, a 65-year-old widow who lives alone, presents at the geriatric nursing clinic at the local senior center with a wound on her ankle about the size of a quarter. The wound is sore, with yellowish drainage. The skin around the wound is red and inflamed. Mrs. James says that she's had the sore about three weeks and that she treated it with butter for a while but that that seemed to make it worse. Mrs. James says that her foot hurts when she walks on it. The nurse at the clinic smells the cigarette smoke on Mrs. James clothing. When asked, Mrs. James reports that she smokes about a pack a day. In response to a question from the nurse, Mrs. James says that she has diabetes and high blood pressure. Mrs. James is not able to say what medicines she takes but estimates that she takes "about four different ones."

Linking the exemplar of Wound Healing with the concept of Metabolism:

1. What metabolic factors will increase the risk of delayed wound healing?
2. What teaching can the nurse provide Mrs. James to promote wound healing in relation to metabolic concerns?

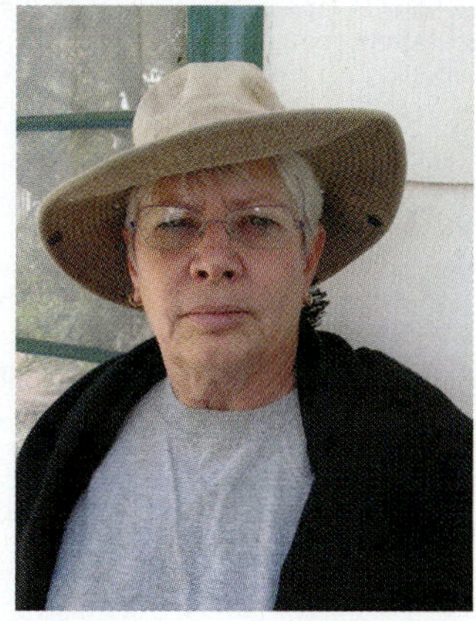

Linking the exemplar of Wound Healing with the concept of Perfusion:

3. What factors related to perfusion will increase the risk of delayed wound healing for Mrs. James?
4. What teaching will you provide Mrs. James to reduce these risks related to perfusion?

READY: GO TO COMPANION SKILLS MANUAL

- Obtaining a wound drainage specimen
- Irrigating a wound
- Maintaining closed wound drainage

REFER: GO TO MYNURSINGKIT

REFLECT: CASE STUDY

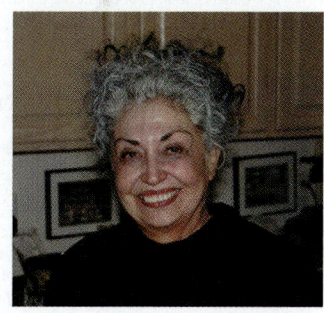

Lydia Ocampo, 69, wakes during the night to urinate but falls on the way to the bathroom. An ambulance takes her to the emergency department, where she is diagnosed with a left hip fracture. She is sent to the operating room for an open reduction internal fixation of the left hip. She is admitted to the medical-surgical floor following surgery.

Mrs. Ocampo remains at the hospital because she has developed an infection in her incision and needs intravenous antibiotics and dressing changes. Her oral intake has been inadequate, but she has been well hydrated by the intravenous fluids. She has been incontinent ever since the Foley catheter was removed. Attempts at physical therapy have been unproductive. The physical therapists are successful at transferring her from the bed to a chair, but this requires nearly full assistance.

1. Identify priority nursing diagnosis for Mrs. Ocampo.
2. List factors that put Mrs. Ocampo at risk for impaired tissue integrity.

PEARSON

EXPLORE mynursingkit™

MyNursingKit is your one stop for online chapter review materials and resources. Prepare for success with additional NCLEX®-style practice questions, interactive assignments and activities, web links, animations and videos, and more!

Register your access code from the front of your book at **www.mynursingkit.com**.

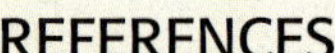

REFERENCES

Agency for Health Care Policy and Research. (1992). *Pressure ulcers in adults: Prediction and prevention.* Rockville, MD: U.S. Department of Health and Human Services.

__________. (1994). *Treatment of pressure ulcers.* Rockville, MD: U.S. Department of Health and Human Services.

Ahrns, K. S. (2004). Trends in burn resuscitation: Shifting the focus from fluids to adequate endpoint monitoring, edema control, and adjuvant therapies. *Critical Care Nursing Clinics of North America, 16,* 75–98.

Allen, P. L. J. (2004). Leaves of three, let them be: If it were only that easy! *Pediatric Nursing, 30*(2), 129–135.

Amer, A., & Fischer, H. (2006). Linear rash leaves your patient itching. *Contemporary Pediatrics, 23*(10), 20, 23.

Bishop, J. F. (2004). Burn wound assessment and surgical management. *Critical Care Nursing Clinics of North America, 16,* 145–177.

The Braden Scale for Predicting Pressure Sore Risk. *Nursing Research, 36*(4), 205–210.

Brown, G. (2006). Wound documentation: Managing risk. *Advances in Skin and Wound Care, 19,* 155–165.

Carrougher, G. (1998). *Burn care and therapy,* St. Louis: Mosby.

Carrougher, G. J., Ptacek, J. T., Sharar, S. R., Wiechman, S., Honari, S., Patterson, D. R., et al. (2003). Comparison of patient satisfaction and self-reports of pain in adult burn-injured patients. *Journal of Burn Care and Rehabilitation, 24*(1), 1–8.

Chamley, C. A. (2005). Development of the integumentary system. In C. A. Chamley, P. Carson, D. Randall, & M. Sandwell, *Developmental anatomy and physiology of children: A practical approach* (pp. 37–58). Edinburgh, UK: Elsevier Churchill Livingston.

Cooper, M. A. (2009). Lightning injuries. The Merck manuals online medical library. Retrieved September 21, 2009, from http://www.merck.com/mmhe/sec24/ch293/ch293c.html

Coulthard, P., Worthington, H., Esposito, M., van der Elst, M., & van Waes, O. J. F. (2005). Tissue adhesives for closure of surgical incisions. *The Cochrane Library* (ID #CD004287).

DeSanti, L. (2005). Pathophysiology and current management of burn injury. *Advances in Skin and Wound Care, 18*(6), 323–332.

Duffy, B. J., McLaughlin, P. M., & Eichelberger, M. R. (2006). Assessment, triage, and early management of burns in children. *Clinical Pediatric Emergency Medicine, 7,* 82–93.

Folkedahl, B. A., & Frantz, R. (2002b). *Treatment of pressure ulcers.* Iowa City: University of Iowa Gerontological Nursing Interventions Research Center, Research Dissemination Core. Retrieved June 9, 2006, from http://www.guideline.gov/summary/summary.aspx?view_id=1&doc_id=3457&nbr=2683

Frantz, R. (2004). Treatment of pressure ulcers. *Journal of Gerontological Nursing, 30*(5), 4–10.

Frantz, R. A., Tang, J. H., & Titler, M. G. (2004). Evidence-based protocol: Prevention of pressure ulcers. *Journal of Gerontological Nursing, 30*(5), 4–11.

Gordon, M. D., Gottschlich, M. M., Helvig, E. I., Marvin, J. A., & Richard, R. L. (2004). Review of evidence-based practice for the prevention of pressure sores in burn patients. *Journal of Burn Care and Rehabilitation, 25*(5), 388–410.

Hanson, D., Langemo, D., Thompson, P., Anderson, J., & Hunter, S. (2005). Understanding wound fluid and the phases of healing. *Advances in Skin & Wound Care, 18,* 360–362.

Honari, S. (2004). Topical therapies and antimicrobials in the management of burn wounds. *Critical Care Nursing Clinics of North America, 16,* 1–11.

Horner, G. (2005). Physical abuse: Recognition and reporting. *Journal of Pediatric Health Care, 19*(1), 4–11.

Klein, G. L., & Herndon, D. N. (2004). Burns. *Pediatrics in Review, 25*(12), 411–416.

Mark, B. J., & Slavin, R. G. (2006). Allergic contact dermatitis. *Medical Clinics of North America, 90,* 169–185.

Montgomery, R. K. (2004). Pain management in burn injury. *Critical Care Nursing Clinics of North America, 16,* 39–49.

National Center for Complementary and Alternative Medicine. (2006). *Herbs at a glance.* Retrieved December 2, 2007, from http://nccam.nih.gov/health

National Center for Health Statistics, National Vital Statistics System. (2007). Injury deaths and rates for children and teenagers by age, external cause, and intent, 2007. Retrieved July 21, 2007, from http://webapppa.cdc.gov/sasweb/ncicp/leadcause10.htm

National Fire Protection Association. (2004). *Leaving home: College fire safety and burn prevention campaign.* Quincy, MA: Author.

__________. (2005). *Smoking material-related fires.* Retrieved from http://www.nfpa.org/itemDetail.asp?categoryID=294&itemID19303&URL=Research%20&%20Reports/Fact%20sheets/Home%20safety/Smoking%20material-related%20fires

National Institute of General Medical Sciences. (2005). *Trauma, burn, shock, and injury: Facts and figures.* Retrieved from http://www.nigms.nih.gov/news/facts/traumaburnfactsfigures.html

Panel for the Prediction and Prevention of Pressure Ulcers in Adults. (1992a). *Clinical practice guideline, pressure ulcers in adults: Prediction and prevention* (Publication No. 92–0047). Rockville, MD: Agency for Health Care Policy and Research, Public Health Service, U.S. Department of Health and Human Services.

Porth, C. M. (2005). *Pathophysiology: Concepts of altered health states* (7th ed.). Philadelphia: Lippincott Williams & Wilkins.

Sole, M. L., Klein, D. G., & Moseley, M. J. (2005). *Introduction to critical care nursing* (4th ed.). St. Louis, MO: Elsevier.

Sosin, J. (2005). Ancient remedy heals today's wounds. *Nursing Spectrum, 14*(6), 32–33.

Stokowski, L. A. (2006). Neonatal skin: Back to nature? *Medscape Pediatrics.* Retrieved January 3, 2006, from http://www.medscape.com/viewarticle/519767?src=mp

Timm-Knudson, V. L., Johnson, J. S., Ortiz, K. J., & Yiannias, J. A. (2006). Allergic contact dermatitis to preservatives. *Dermatologic Nursing, 18*(2), 130–136.

U.S. Department of Health and Human Services. (2000). *Healthy people 2010: Understanding and improving health* (2nd ed.). Washington, DC: U.S. Government Printing Office.

NORMAL PRESENTATION

Generally speaking, violence results from a combination of predisposing, precipitating, and protective factors in several areas (Pirkis, Goldney, & Burgess, 2003). **Predisposing factors** are those that increase one's risk of violent victimization or perpetration of violence. Predisposing factors may be categorized as vulnerability factors or risk factors. In the context of violence, **vulnerability factors** increase one's risk of being a victim of violence; **risk factors** increase the potential that one will perpetrate violence on others. **Precipitating factors** are those that give rise to a specific incident of violence. **Protective factors**, on the other hand, decrease the risk of violence perpetration and victimization. For example, connectedness to school has been found to be a protective factor for youth violence (NCIPC, 2006d). Areas to be addressed in examining factors contributing to societal violence include biophysical, psychological, physical environmental, sociocultural, behavioral, and health care system considerations.

ALTERATIONS

Violence takes many forms. Perpetrators come in all guises. Almost anyone can be a victim. Within these statements can be found a number of patterns and alterations. The alterations that are covered in this concept are those related to abuse, including elder abuse, partner abuse, and the various forms of child abuse; assault and homicide; rape; suicide; and unintentional injury resulting from motor vehicle accidents.

Abuse

Interpersonal violence is the deliberate and systematic pattern of abuse used to establish power and control over a victim through fear and intimidation; see exemplars for a detailed discussion of specific types of violence. Abusive behavior is always intentional. Perpetrators choose to be violent and give themselves permission to be violent. Perpetrators are not out of control, as is commonly assumed. They may be enraged or cool and calculating, but in either case they choose to inflict violence. The victim cannot and does not "make them do it."

To the victim, violence often happens without warning and without a buildup of tension. A pattern of violence usually develops. Frustration or stress may precipitate the first incident. If the victim immediately refuses to accept the violence and seeks outside help, there are often no further episodes. If the victim submits to the violence, then physical force, without the stimulus of frustration or stress, becomes a way of relating, and the pattern becomes resistant to change. A typical **cycle of violence** occurs when conflict escalates into a violent episode, after which the perpetrator begs for the victim's forgiveness. The victim allows the cycle to continue because of promises to reform. With the next episode of conflict, the cycle of violence begins again and becomes part of the family dynamics. Table 31–2 outlines the cycle of violence.

Trauma

Trauma is defined as injury to human tissues and organs resulting from the transfer of energy from an external environmental source, such as a motor vehicle, a fire, or a sharp object. In the past the term *trauma* has been associated with the word *accident*. **Accident** means that the injury occurred without intent, regardless of whether or not the injury could have been prevented (e.g., by wearing a seat belt). Rather than using the term *accident*, trauma professionals generally define trauma as either *intentional* or *unintentional*. Intentional and unintentional trauma encompass a variety of injuries resulting from motor vehicle crashes, pedestrian injuries, gunshot wounds, falls, violence toward others, or self-inflicted violence. The injuries, disabilities, and deaths resulting from these incidents constitute a major health care challenge.

COMPONENTS OF TRAUMA Trauma results from an abnormal exchange of energy between a host and a mechanism in a predisposing environment. The *host* is the person or group at risk of injury. Multiple factors influence the host's potential for injury: age, sex, race, economic status, preexisting illnesses, and use of substances such as street drugs and alcohol.

The *mechanism* is the source of the energy transmitted to the host. The energy exchanged can be mechanical, gravitational, thermal, electrical, physical, or chemical. Table 31–3 lists the most common mechanisms for each type of energy. Mechanical energy is the most common type of energy transferred to a host that results in trauma. The most common mechanical source of injury in all adult age groups is the motor vehicle.

TABLE 31–2 **The Cycle of Violence**

PHASE	PERPETRATOR	VICTIM
Tension-building phase	Moody, withdraws affection, isolates victim, name-calling, verbally abusive, destroys property	Attempts to calm partner, nurturing, stays away from support systems, passive, feels as if walking on eggshells
Battering phase	Pushing, shoving, hitting, other acts of violence	Protects self any way possible; someone else calls police; victim leaves
Contrition phase	Says sorry, begs for forgiveness, promises never again	Agrees to stay or return; attempts to stop legal proceedings; hopeful

Source: Adapted with permission from Dutton, D. G. (1998). *The abusive personality*. New York: Guilford Press.

TABLE 31–3 Common Mechanisms of Injury by Energy Source

ENERGY SOURCE	COMMON MECHANISMS OF INJURY
Mechanical	Motor vehicles Firearms Machines
Gravitational	Falls
Thermal	Heating appliances Fire Freezing temperatures
Electrical	Wires, sockets, and other electrical objects Lightning
Physical	Fists, feet, and other body parts (as in physical assault) Sharp objects, such as knives Blunt objects, such as hammers or iron skillets Ultraviolet radiation Ionizing radiation Water (drowning) Submersion or entrapment (e.g., grain, falling debris) Explosions
Chemical	Drugs Poisons Industrial chemicals

Guns are another common mechanical source of injury. Trauma from gunshot wounds has steadily increased during the past 20 years and remains a major reason for emergency department and trauma center admissions, especially in large cities.

When describing a traumatic injury, *intention* is included as a component. Most gunshot and stab wounds are examples of intentional injuries. It is important to remember, however, that some gunshot wounds are unintentional, such as those that occur when children play with their parents' guns. Other common unintentional injuries result from motor vehicle crashes, falls, drownings, and fires. Although hunting accidents are rare in comparison to the number of people participating in the sport, hunting-related deaths and injuries have decreased with the implementation of mandatory "hunting safety" courses in some states.

The final component of trauma is the *environment.* For example, a road that has become slippery after a snowstorm is a physical environment that may contribute to an injury. Occupation is an important environmental factor to consider. Those in certain occupations face a high risk of trauma; examples include police officers, fire fighters, professional athletes, race car drivers, and taxi cab drivers. One's social environment also influences risk for injury.

TYPES OF TRAUMA **Minor trauma** causes injury to a single part or system of the body and is usually treated in a physician's office or in the hospital emergency department. A fracture of the clavicle, a small second-degree burn, and a laceration requiring sutures are examples of minor trauma. Major or **multiple trauma** involves serious single-system injury (such as the traumatic amputation of a leg) or multiple-system injuries. Multiple trauma is most often the result of a motor vehicle crash.

Trauma is further classified as either blunt or penetrating. **Blunt trauma** occurs when there is no communication between the damaged tissues and the outside environment; for example, a baseball batter being hit by a pitch. Blunt trauma is caused by various forces including *deceleration* (a decrease in the speed of a moving object), *acceleration* (an increase in the speed of a moving object), *shearing* (forces occurring across a plane, with structures slipping across each other), *compression*, and *crushing*. Blunt forces often cause multiple injuries that can affect the head, spinal cord, bones, thorax, and abdomen. Blunt trauma is frequently caused by motor vehicle crashes, falls, assaults, and sports activities.

Penetrating trauma occurs when a foreign object enters the body, causing damage to body structures. Structures commonly affected include the brain, lungs, heart, liver, spleen, intestines, and the vascular system. Examples of penetrating trauma are gunshot or stab wounds and impalement.

Other types of trauma include inhalation injuries from gases, smoke, or steam; burn or freezing injuries; and blast injuries from explosions. Blast injuries result from the temperature and velocity of air movement and the force of projectiles from the explosion. Blast injuries are more severe in water than in air because blast waves travel farther and faster in water. Trauma from blast injuries includes pulmonary edema and hemorrhage, damage to abdominal organs, burns, penetrating injuries, and ruptured tympanic membranes.

Prevention

Prevention efforts can reduce the incidence and severity of abuse and trauma related to violence and injury. Assessing for inadequate coping mechanisms, signs of inadequate anger

ALTERATIONS AND TREATMENTS **Violence**

Alteration	Description	Treatment/Prevention
Abuse	A pattern of behavior that dominates, controls, lowers self-esteem, or takes away freedom of choice. Can include elder abuse, child abuse, intimate partner abuse, and sexual abuse.	■ Medical interventions for trauma ■ Legal interventions ■ Community response and resources ■ Behavioral therapy ■ Family therapy ■ Support groups
Assault/Homicide	Injury from an act of violence where physical force is used with intent to harm, injure, or kill; in homicide, the injury is fatal.	■ Medical interventions for trauma ■ Legal intervention ■ Behavioral therapy ■ Family therapy ■ Support groups
Rape-Trauma Syndrome	The victim's response to the act of rape. Responses vary but can include flashbacks, fear, depression, and sexual dysfunction.	■ Medical interventions for trauma ■ Behavior therapy ■ Family therapy ■ Support groups ■ Medication ■ Legal intervention
Suicide	Suicide is the taking of one's own life.	■ Prevention ■ Intervention if the attempt was not fatal; intervention may include pharmacotherapy and psychotherapy in combination ■ Hospitalization may be necessary immediately following the attempt ■ Support groups and other therapies for surviving family members
Motor vehicle crashes		■ Medical interventions for trauma ■ Compliance with safety measures ■ Legislation

management, or inappropriate behavior can help to identify potentially violent tendencies and implement behavior therapy before someone is victimized. It is important for the nurse to remain current with new, evidence-based practice initiatives to help protect individuals, clients, facilities, and the community from violence.

ABUSE PREVENTION Nurses in all areas of practice (e.g., maternal/child health, school, community and occupational health, mental health, primary and acute care, and academic settings) need to take a proactive role to prevent family violence. Early screening of vulnerable individuals and efforts to promote a change in attitudes and beliefs about family violence are essential.

If they are to assist victims effectively, nurses must be aware of their own feelings about family violence. Nurses who are unclear about their own feelings about family violence may deny its existence, blame the victim in crisis, or minimize the effects of the violence (CNA, 1992, p. 8).

Nurses also can be instrumental as advocates in developing policies and programs, and providing in-service training and education to health care professionals and the public. Comprehensive violence prevention programs require a variety of disciplines and organizations working together, such as state or provincial and local health care agencies, criminal justice agencies, and social service agencies.

TRAUMA PREVENTION Areas of health promotion and trauma prevention interventions for individuals and communities include the following:

- *Motor vehicle safety:* seat belts, air bags, helmets, driving under the influence of alcohol or drugs, reckless driving, visual or cognitive deficits in the older adult, cell phone use (dialing, talking, texting), driver fatigue
- *Relationships:* domestic violence, child abuse, elder abuse, or neglect
- *Communities:* gun control, gangs, condition of streets, neighborhood safety.

In providing information about trauma prevention to members of the community, the nurse serves as a health care educator, political activist, and safety advocate.

Many city and county governments have multidisciplinary child abuse and prevention teams or child fatality prevention teams. These teams meet monthly to review child abuse or child fatality cases to determine whether any recommendations need to be made at the state level. Typically, teams do not review cases until any legal actions have been taken and resolved. For example, a child fatality team will not review a child homicide until after the perpetrator has been to trial. All team members must sign confidentiality statements. Examples of recommendations that may result from the efforts of these multidisciplinary teams include recommendations regarding requirements for car seat or bicycle helmet use. Team members are usually mandated by law and frequently include community health nurses, school nurses, preschool directors and school principles, members of law enforcement, and representatives of the district attorney's office.

ASSESSMENT

The priority when assessing any client always begins with the ABCs: airway, breathing, and circulation. Only when these priority needs have been met will the nurse go on to conduct a more complete physical survey. The focused assessment will vary depending on the type, severity, and location of injury.

Abuse

Often the nurse is the first person to discover that the client has been abused. Some victims may not disclose the abuse, may deny it despite obvious symptoms, or they may minimize its impact. However, it is the nurse's responsibility to be alert for symptoms of abuse. Because any client can be the victim of abuse, it is important for the nurse to not allow personal biases to impact who is assessed for these symptoms, but rather be alert for them in all client interactions. If the nurse acts on a bias that only certain types of individuals are abused, many abuse victims will not receive the care they need.

THE ASSESSMENT INTERVIEW During the assessment interview, the nurse must ensure privacy. The victim must feel safe from the perpetrator. It may be difficult for the client to admit to the reality of family violence until a trusting nurse–client relationship evolves. The nurse should assure the client of a genuine desire to help the entire family system. The nurse should also approach this topic as if it were any other health risk with a professional and calm demeanor. In addition, the nurse can offer the option of answering questions about incidents of abuse with "sometimes" instead of "yes" or "no"; this may encourage the client to make a first step to acknowledge the abuse.

Victims of violence enter the health care system for a variety of conditions associated with abuse. For example, common physical complaints include chronic pelvic pain, headache, irritable bowel syndrome, arthritis, pelvic inflammatory disease, and neurological damage. Psychiatric illness (e.g., alcoholism) may also be the result of a history of sexual or physical abuse. Depression is also common. The assessment interview should include a detailed nursing history as well as a description of current symptoms.

THE PHYSICAL EXAMINATION Victims of physical abuse may suffer a variety of injuries. During a head-to-toe assessment, the nurse may observe for indications of abuse, such as the following:

- *Head:* Bald patches on the scalp where hair has been pulled out; evidence of trauma from blows to the head, such as hematoma, facial bruises, facial fractures, bruised or swollen eyes, hemorrhages into the eyes; petechiae around the eyes from attempted strangulation
- *Skin:* Swelling or tenderness, bruises, burns, or scars of past injuries on the skin, genitals, and rectal areas
- *Musculoskeletal system:* Fractures or evidence of previous fractures, particularly of the face, arms/legs, and ribs; dislocated joints, especially in the shoulder when the victim is grabbed or pulled by the arm
- *Abdomen:* Bruises, wounds, or intra-abdominal injuries, especially if the person is pregnant
- *Neurological system:* Hyperactive reflexes due to neurological damage; paresthesias, numbness, or pain from old injuries.

If the nursing assessment reveals possible domestic violence, a team assessment needs to take place. The victim's medical condition and emotional state must be assessed. The severity and potential fatality of the situation must be considered, as well as the needs of dependent children and the legal ramifications.

The American Academy of Pediatrics has published guidelines for the evaluation of sexual abuse of children. These were developed by the committee on child abuse and neglect and are available from the AAP. Special considerations regarding the assessment of child victims of sexual abuse are discussed in Exemplar 31.1.

A collaborative team of nurse administrators and clinical nurses at Harris County Health Department in Houston, Texas, developed a screening and intervention triage tool for abuse. The triage structure facilitates appropriate intervention according to screening data. Each of the triage levels includes related interventions and essential documentation (Table 31–4).

It should be noted that research shows that screening for family violence as a routine part of health care results in reduction of abuse (Nelson et al., 2004). Therefore, nurses must detect signs of abuse when clients come to a health care facility and know what to do when family violence is detected. Nurses should carefully document the abuse and provide appropriate treatment to the client for both physical and psychological injuries. Nurses should also give abused clients information about protective services and how to access them. If the client returns for further treatment, nurses should follow-up with the client regarding the abuse (United States Preventive Services Task Force, 2004).

Several guidelines for the screening and management of intimate partner violence have been published. One method of assessment, developed with funding from the Agency for Healthcare Research and Quality, uses a critical pathway that is organized into the categories of physical assessment and treatment, psychiatric/mental health assessment and treatment, and social assessment and treatment (Dienemann & Wiederhorn, 2003). This type of assessment can provide guidance across all health care settings.

Trauma

Violence results in traumatic injury that may involve multiple systems. Because of the serious consequences of trauma, it is important to identify the client's injuries and institute appropriate

TABLE 31–4 **Screening and Intervention Triage for Abuse**

	TRIAGE		
STEPS	LEVEL I	LEVEL II	LEVEL III
SCREEN	No history or present threat of abuse	Recent or present abuse	Client presents with injuries
INTERVENE	Group or individual education about domestic violence; give handouts and pamphlets of community resources to client	Crisis intervention; individual counseling; assist client with escape plan; identify shelter and other emergency resources; assist client in contacting shelter	Crisis intervention; notify police; refer client to hospital for treatment (call ambulance); notify shelter; transport client to shelter
DOCUMENT	Statement of no abuse or threat of abuse; give handouts/education materials to client	Statement of present or recent abuse; counsel client; give numbers to shelter and police; plan escape route; note if client declines shelter assistance at this time, or if shelter should be contacted per client's request	Give statement of medical care given; notify emergency services; note where client was transported and in what condition

Source: Reprinted with permission from Lazzaro, M. V., & McFarlane, J. (October 1991). Establishing a Screening Program for Abused Women. *Journal of Nursing Administration, 21*, 10.

interventions immediately. When caring for the trauma victim the nurse must always prioritize assessments with airway, breathing, and circulation (ABC) as the highest priority concerns. Only after assessing the ABCs can the nurse go on to perform a detailed assessment of other systems or a focused assessment of the involved area of trauma.

Trauma usually occurs suddenly, leaving the client and family with little time to prepare for its consequences. Nurses provide a vital link in both the physical and psychosocial care for the injured client and family. In caring for the client who has experienced trauma, nurses must consider not only the initial physical injury, but also its long-term consequences, including rehabilitation and (in cases of accidents, abuse, or assault) prevention. Trauma may alter the client's previous way of life, potentially affecting independence, mobility, cognitive thinking, and appearance.

Death is a common result of serious traumatic injury, and may be immediate, early, or late. Immediate death happens at the scene from such injuries as a torn thoracic aorta or decapitation. Early death occurs within several hours of the injury from, for example, shock or delay in recognizing injuries. Late death generally occurs 1 or more days after the injury and results from multiple organ failure, sepsis, and blood loss.

EFFECTS ON THE FAMILY Trauma may result in death or cause injury serious enough to alter both the client's and the family's lives. The suddenness and seriousness of the event are precipitating factors in the development of a psychological crisis. Nurses working with the client who has experienced trauma should assess the family for a variety of needs, including immediate social and spiritual support. For clients who will require long-term rehabilitation, nurses may provide referrals to family members for counseling or financial support services.

Most hospitals employ a variety of professionals who can provide support to families of trauma victims. Nurses may call on the hospital chaplain, foreign language interpreter, social worker, victim's advocate, or other professional to provide assistance to a client who is the victim of violence or trauma and/or the client's family.

METHODS OF ASSESSMENT Many methods help health care providers determine the seriousness of the client's injuries and the potential for survival when violence results in serious trauma. Scoring systems such as the Champion Revised Trauma Scoring System can be helpful. A rapid but comprehensive trauma assessment, completed on the scene, includes the following:

- *Airway and breathing assessments* to determine if the airway is patent, maintainable, or nonmaintainable, and if ventilations are impeded in any way, such as by rib fractures or a collapsed lung
- *Circulation assessment* to palpate peripheral and central pulses; to assess capillary refill, skin color, and temperature; and to identify any external sources of bleeding
- *Level of consciousness* and *pupillary function assessments*
- Assessment for any obvious injuries.

The Glasgow Coma Scale is another scoring system that is used to quantify the level of consciousness following traumatic brain injury. For more information on the Glasgow Coma Scale, see Concept 17, Intracranial Regulation.

DIAGNOSTIC TESTS

The diagnostic tests ordered once the client reaches the hospital depend on the type of injury the client has sustained. Tests that may be ordered for victims of violence include the following:

- *Blood type and crossmatch* involves typing the client's blood for ABO antigens and Rh factor, screening the blood for antibodies, and crossmatching the client's serum and donor red blood cells.

- *Blood alcohol level* measures the amount of alcohol in a client's blood. Studies have found that between 20% and 50% of people who are injured may be intoxicated. Alcohol alters the client's level of consciousness and response to pain (NHTSA, 2006).
- *Urine drug screen* may also be ordered. Like alcohol, such drugs as cocaine alter the client's level of consciousness and overall response to the primary survey.
- *Pregnancy test* for any woman of childbearing age rules out the potential for pregnancy and fetal injury.
- The primary goal of the *focused assessment by sonography in trauma (FAST)* exam is to evaluate the unwelcome presence of blood in body cavities. Primary focus is on the peritoneum. It is also helpful in identification of blood in the pleura and pericardium.
- *Diagnostic peritoneal lavage* determines the presence of blood in the peritoneal cavity, which may indicate abdominal injury. This test is generally done in the emergency department. A local anesthetic (such as lidocaine) is injected subcutaneously, and a small incision is made in the lower abdomen. A catheter is placed into the peritoneal cavity, and any free blood is aspirated. If 10 mL of blood is found, the client is taken to the operating room for exploratory surgery. If no free blood is aspirated, 1 L of a warm isotonic solution (Ringer's solution or normal saline) is rapidly infused into the peritoneal cavity and then allowed to drain by gravity. If the solution returns pink and is found to have a red blood cell count of 100,000 mm^3, a white blood cell count of >500, or bile, food, or feces, the test is considered positive and the client is taken to the operating room for exploratory surgery. This procedure has been used less since the inception of the FAST exam.
- *Computerized tomography (CT) scans* can discover injuries to the brain, skull, spine, spinal cord, chest, and abdomen.
- *Magnetic resonance imaging (MRI) scans* can discover injuries to the brain and spinal cord.

CARING INTERVENTIONS

The nurse may be called upon to care for the victim of violence, the perpetrator of violence, or both. Nurses must provide quality care to both the perpetrator and the victim. Personal biases, judgments, and retribution have no place in nursing care. While caring for a victim of violence can arouse the nurse's sympathies, it is important to maintain objectivity to optimize care.

Abuse

The goals of treating abuse are (1) to empower the client to take control, (2) to support the client, and (3) to maximize the client's safety (CNA, 1992, p. 10).

Most people involved in intrafamily violence are disturbed by this behavior and would like it to end. Even though they want help to stop the abuse, they may not know how to seek the assistance they need. It is extremely important for nurses to be nonjudgmental in their interactions with all family members. The abusers may be distrustful of the motives of the nurse. Initially, the victims may be unwilling to trust because of family shame, fear of being blamed for remaining in the violent situation, and fear that the abuser will find out that they have revealed the abuse and the abuse will become worse. The nurse should avoid blaming the victim or the abuser or looking for pathological elements in anyone's behavior. It is vital not to impose personal values on the family by offering quick and easy solutions to intrafamily violence.

SHORT-TERM INTERVENTIONS Because the nurse may be the only professional to have the only contact with the client, it is essential that the nurse (1) determine the immediacy of danger, (2) convey that the person is not to blame and has the right to be safe, (3) explore options for help, and (4) provide information regarding available services.

It is important that the nurse avoid a judgmental attitude and support the person's choice about whether to leave the unsafe situation or return to the abusive relationship. Because severely battered women are at risk for homicide, the nurse needs to inform the client about associated risk factors and determine the immediacy of danger.

Nurses must familiarize themselves with agency protocols and resources available for victims of domestic violence. Most municipalities have crisis helplines and hotlines to provide assistance to victims of abuse. The nurse should also keep a record of telephone numbers for transition houses and rape crisis centers, alcohol and drug abuse information, support groups, religious organizations, and legal services. There are also several national organizations that offer toll-free contacts, such as the National Organization for Victim Assistance, the National Coalition Against Domestic Violence (in the United States), and the National Clearinghouse on Family Violence (in Canada).

Abused Children The priority nursing consideration regarding the abused child is to ensure safety. Once the child's safety is assured, developing a trusting relationship will allow the child to discuss his or her feelings and describe the abusive event. It is important that the child not be required to repeat the story for multiple reports because each retelling carries the possibility of creating trauma for the child. All hospitals and agencies working with abused children have standard protocols that support the child and ensure adequate information needed by law enforcement is obtained without further victimizing the child through a repetitive or unfriendly process.

The nurse working with the abused child needs to say that he or she believes the child's story; the nurse also must reassure the child that he or she has done nothing wrong. The nurse should avoid making negative comments about the abuser and must follow established protocols for mandatory reporting, documentation, and use of available support services (e.g., the police department, social service agencies, and child welfare agency).

Abused Older Adults Short-term interventions for abused older adults include developing a positive relationship with both the victim and the abuser, exploring ways for the older person to maximize independence, and exploring the need for additional home care services or alternative living arrangements.

LONG-TERM INTERVENTIONS Long-term goals for ongoing counseling and care may include (1) helping the client continue to choose to be safe from violence, (2) helping the client explore options for self-development, and (3) helping the client improve quality of life through increasing self-esteem (CNA, 1992, p. 14).

Usually, the best treatment for families experiencing violence is through a multidisciplinary approach involving nurses, physicians, social workers, police, protective services personnel, and, often, lawyers. Most families are more open to accepting help during a time of crisis than at other times. They most likely will be willing to develop new behavior patterns for a short time following a crisis. If they are not helped during that time, they will most likely return to previous behavior patterns, including violence.

Nurses should know the laws associated with reporting abuse. In the United States and Canada, nurses are required to report any suspected child abuse. The courts and child protective agencies make decisions in the child's interest. They may allow a child to remain in the home but under court supervision; they may remove the child from the home; and, in instances of very severe abuse or repeated abuse despite intervention, they may terminate parental rights.

State and provincial laws about reporting adult and elder abuse vary. Domestic violence is considered a violent crime; the victim has a right to be protected, and the perpetrator of the violence can be prosecuted.

The nurse plays a critical role on a multidisciplinary team, working with families involved in abuse. The nurse often spends the most time with clients and forms a trusting nurse–client relationship. As a result, the client feels most comfortable when talking with the nurse and is more likely to relate details of the abusive situation. The nurse's role may include teaching, support, or role modeling behavior. For example, if a child is transferred to foster care, the nurse may provide client teaching to the foster family to provide for the child's health care needs. Violence may be prevented through anticipatory teaching, such as teaching the new mother normal developmental milestones and best ways of providing care for the infant to reduce frustration that can lead to violence.

Trauma

Victims of violence often present in the emergency department with life-threatening injuries including hypovolemia due to blood loss, organ damage, and multisystem complications. The client will often be in both physical and psychological shock. Medical care for the client in shock focuses on treating the underlying cause, increasing arterial oxygenation, and improving tissue perfusion. Depending on the cause and type of shock, interventions include emergency care measures, oxygen therapy, fluid replacement, and medications.

Care of the trauma client depends on a team approach. Providing trauma care with a team focus helps each team member know his or her role. Prompt delegation of tasks and responsibilities improves the client's chances for survival and decreases the morbidity that may result from traumatic injuries.

The nurse's role in trauma care begins with **triage**, determining which client needs the most urgent medical intervention. Triage is based on the ABCs of trauma care—airway, breathing, and circulation. The nurse begins the triage process by performing a rapid general assessment including vital signs, level of consciousness, and a head-to-toe review looking for obvious physical alterations.

When caring for the client who experienced trauma, maintaining a patent airway and monitoring breathing and circulation is an ongoing responsibility. If the client has experienced blood loss, is in shock, or is in unstable condition, the initiation of an IV line is often a high priority allowing for administration of medications, fluid, and blood products. Changes in the client's condition are often marked by subtle alterations, so the nurse's primary role is in performing ongoing assessments in order to correct problems before they become more acute.

PHARMACOLOGIC THERAPIES

Medications used to treat the victim of violence can include virtually any drug, depending on the injury and system involved. The following general categories of medications may be used.

- Blood components and crystalloids may be administered intravenously in the initial treatment of traumatic shock to replace intravascular volume.
- Inotropic drugs (drugs that increase myocardial contractility) may be given to increase cardiac output and improve tissue perfusion. These drugs, administered only after fluid volume restoration, include dopamine (Dopastat, Intropin), dobutamine (Dobutrex), and isoproterenol (Isuprel).
- Vasopressors may be administered in conjunction with fluid replacement to treat neurogenic, septic, or anaphylactic shock. Examples of vasopressors include dopamine, epinephrine, norepinephrine, and phenylephrine.
- Opioids, administered by bolus or continuous infusion, are used to treat pain as soon as possible. However, the effects of the pain medications may alter client responses to injury and mask potential injuries. If pain medications are administered, they must be carefully regulated, and the client must be closely monitored.
- If the client has penetrating and open wounds, tetanus immunization status must be determined. If the client is unable to remember when the last tetanus immunization was given or is unable to answer, tetanus prophylaxis is given.

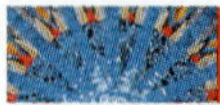

31.1 ABUSE

KEY TERMS

Abuse, *1944*
Battering, *1949*
Child abuse, *1946*
Child sexual abuse, *1947*
Elder abuse, *1945*
Emotional abuse, *1946*
Emotional neglect, *1947*
Female genital mutilation (FGM), *1949*
Incest, *1947*
Interpersonal violence, *1944*
Intimate partner violence, *1949*
Neglect, *1945*
Pedophile, *1947*
Physical abuse, *1945*
Physical neglect, *1946*
Psychological battering, *1949*
Self-neglect, *1945*
Shaken baby syndrome, *1951*

BASIS FOR SELECTION OF EXEMPLAR

Healthy People 2010

LEARNING OUTCOMES

After reading about this exemplar, you will be able to:

1. Describe the psychopathology, etiology, and clinical manifestations of abuse.
2. Identify risk factors associated with abuse.
3. Illustrate the nursing process in providing culturally competent care across the life span for individuals who have been abused or are at increased risk for abuse.
4. Formulate priority nursing diagnoses appropriate for an individual who has been abused or is at risk for abuse.
5. Create a plan of care for individuals who have been abused or are at risk for abuse and their family members.
6. Assess expected outcomes for an individual who have been abused or is at risk for abuse.
7. Discuss therapies used in the collaborative care of an individual who has been abused or are at risk for abuse.
8. Employ evidence-based caring interventions for an individual who has been abused.

OVERVIEW

Abuse refers to a pattern of behavior that dominates, controls, lowers self-esteem, or takes away freedom of choice. It is the systematic persecution of another individual, ranging from subtle words or actions to violent battering—acts of commission. Abuse also includes various types of neglect—acts of omission.

Healthy People 2010, published by the U.S. Department of Health and Human Services (2000), describes interpersonal violence as a significant problem in the United States. **Interpersonal violence**—violence between family members or friends—occurs at all levels in society. The myth is that violence occurs only among the poor and undereducated, but the reality is that violence occurs among the middle and upper classes and professional elite as well.

Unfortunately, family violence accounts for 11% of all violence in the United States. As many as 3.5 million incidents of family violence occur each year: 49% directed at spouses, 11% at children, with the remaining acts committed against other family members. Most of this violence involves simple assault, with less than 0.5% of cases resulting in homicide (Durose et al., 2005).

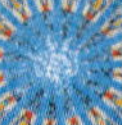

FOCUS ON DIVERSITY AND CULTURE Gender-based Family Violence

Women in many cultural groups adhere to cultural norms that permit men to control their lives even when this control may be harmful to themselves and to their children. Among many Chinese women, for example, family rules and values may promote intimate partner violence. Chinese women are expected to display "three obediences" to men: first to their fathers, then to their husbands, and later to their sons. Some authors report that because of traditional Asian cultural beliefs, many women do not perceive themselves as victims of violence. Even when they do see themselves as being victimized, they may be reluctant to report abuse because of feelings of shame, embarrassment, or loss of face. Others may also feel guilt, believing themselves to be at fault for the abuse (Magnussen et al., 2004).

Women's rights have not always been supported in the dominant U.S. culture either. In 1877, for example, all states had passed legislation that prohibited women from voting, and the 14th amendment to the Constitution specifically defined "citizens" and "voters" as male. It was not until 1920 that the 19th amendment granted women the right to vote, but the amendment was not actually ratified by Mississippi until 1984. In 1839, Mississippi became the first state to allow women to own property in their own name (with their husband's permission), and in 1855, the Missouri court ruled that a Black woman was considered property and did not have the right to defend herself from rape by her master. Similarly, in 1873, the U.S. Supreme Court ruled that states could prohibit married women from practicing law (National Women's History Project, n.d.), and the Equal Pay Act was not passed until 1963 (Imbornoni, 2006). It was not until 1976 that individual states slowly began to overturn laws which legalized marital rape. Based on the history of cultural attitudes to and legal and social restrictions on women, of which these are only a few examples, it is not surprising that many women may have internalized these perceptions.

Most victims of reported family violence are women and most perpetrators are men, although, as we will see later, these figures may be a function of willingness to report violence rather than representing the actual incidence of gender-based family violence (see Focus on Culture and Diversity).

Interpersonal violence encompasses child and elder maltreatment and intimate partner violence (IPV). In many families, these forms of abuse are intertwined, creating an intergenerational pattern of violence in which children who are subjected to or witness violence in the family internalize violence as a mode of family interaction (Abrahams & Jewkes, 2005). These children may then become abusive or enter abusive relationships in adulthood. These abusive relationships may also carry over into care of aging parents, particularly if the parents were abusive themselves. (See Table 31–2 in the About section for more on the cycle of violence.)

TYPES OF ABUSE

Nurses working in any professional environment may encounter a wide array of forms of abuse and neglect. This concept discusses elder abuse, including self-neglect; the abuse of children, including child sexual abuse; and interpersonal violence, including the abuse of pregnant women.

Elder Abuse

Elder abuse or maltreatment is purposeful physical or psychological harm or exploitation of elderly persons (Jech, 2002). Abuse of older adults can occur within families or in institutional settings, such as nursing homes and other residential facilities for the elderly. The focus of this section, however, is on the abuse of older adults by family members.

An estimated 700,000 to 1.2 million older adults are abused each year in the United States (Fulmer, 2002). U.S. reports of elder maltreatment increased by 150% from 1986 to 1996, due in part to better recognition of the problem (Jech, 2002). Several forms of elder abuse occur, many of them similar to the types of abuse found among children and couples. Types of abuse that may be encountered by nurses working with older clients are outlined in Table 31–5. These include **physical abuse**, the deliberate maltreatment of another individual that inflicts pain or injury and may result in permanent or temporary disfigurement or even death, and **neglect**, the deliberate withholding of or failure to provide the necessary and available resources to the older adult.

Older clients may also be financially exploited when their funds or material goods are appropriated by others rather than used to meet their needs. Older clients' personal rights may be violated if they are not allowed to participate in decisions regarding their lives when they are capable of making such decisions. Some older clients may be abandoned or deserted by those responsible for their care (Fulmer, 2002). Additional forms of elder abuse identified by the United Nations Economic and Social Council (2002) include loss of respect, systemic abuse, economic violence, and HIV/AIDS-related violence. In addition, community violence and political violence disproportionately affect the elderly as well as children.

TABLE 31–5 **Types of Elder Abuse**

TYPE OF ABUSE	DESCRIPTION
Physical Abuse	■ Injury ■ Inappropriate restraint ■ Improper medication
Sexual abuse	Forced participation in sexual acts
Neglect	■ Failure to meet physical or emotional needs ■ Failure to attend to medical needs ■ Self-neglect
Emotional abuse	■ Verbal abuse or disrespect ■ Social isolation

Perpetrators of elder maltreatment are usually family members or acquaintances (NCIPC, 2003), but older clients may also engage in self-neglect. **Self-neglect** has been defined as "behavior of an elderly person that threatens his or her safety" (Jech, 2002, p. 22); as many as 100,000 cases may occur each year (Mouton et al., 2004). *Institutional abuse* of the elderly may also occur and is defined as "abuse and neglect that occurs in residential facilities that care for the elderly" (Jech, 2002, p. 23). Others may also take advantage of older persons by defrauding them in financial scams (United Nations Economic and Social Council, 2002).

Older people who are physically or cognitively impaired or who have functional disabilities are at greater risk for abuse than those with better functional abilities. Women constitute 60% of abused elderly persons and 75% of those subjected to psychological abuse. Women are also more likely than older men to experience financial abuse (92% vs. 8%) (Jech, 2002). Consequences of abuse of older adults include injury, medication and substance abuse, decreased immune response, malnutrition or eating disorders, depression, fear and anxiety, and suicide (United Nations Economic and Social Council, 2002). As is the case with child maltreatment and intimate partner violence (IPV), elder maltreatment may end in death. In 2002 and 2003, the U.S. homicide rate for people over age 65 was 2.82 per 100,000 men and 1.38 for women (NCIPC, 2005).

CULTURAL PERCEPTIONS OF ELDER MISTREATMENT Definitions of the different subtypes of elder mistreatment need to be examined in the context of cultural considerations. Researchers and clinicians have documented differences in the way that people from different cultural groups define elder mistreatment as well as in the behaviors that they perceive as abusive or neglectful (SAMHSA, 2001; Moon & Benton, 2000). For example, in elder mistreatment studies involving older Chinese adults, researchers have found that loneliness (Dong, Simon, Gorbien, Percak, & Golden, 2007) and disrespect (Tam & Neysmith, 2006) are risk factors for elder mistreatment or abuse that perhaps are not assessed directly by instruments developed by Western researchers. Furthermore, other researchers have found that members of minority groups may not define abusive behavior the same way that professionals do and that when cultural norms and laws and regulations are in conflict, there is a need to educate and intervene to protect the vulnerable older person (Hudson, Armachain, Beasley, & Carlson, 1998; Hudson et al., 2000; National Center on Elder Abuse, 2006). Elder abuse or mistreatment cannot be tolerated, despite differing cultural perceptions.

These discrepancies across cultural and ethnic subgroups may be linked to the fact that these subgroups have different expectations about the responsibility that grown children and other relatives have for caring for older adults (Tam & Neysmith, 2006; Tomita, 1999). Some researchers speculate that cultural-specific approaches to interventions based on these differences in perception would be more effective than a general approach (Moon & Benton, 2000). However, the findings from research studies on elder mistreatment and culture are less than conclusive, with virtually no information to support or suggest different interventions for different cultural subgroups. At the very least, nurses and other clinicians should be aware of the possibility of differences in perceptions about what constitutes mistreatment based on culture, and should take this into account during assessment and care planning. The Institute of Medicine stresses the importance of clinicians understanding the physical, cultural, and community environments of their clients in order to adequately address family violence. Cultural and linguistic competences are important for successful intervention in cases of elder mistreatment (Institute of Medicine, 2002).

Child Abuse

Child abuse involves intentional physical or mental harm to a child by someone responsible for the child's welfare. Several different types of child abuse occur in the context of family–child interactions. These include physical abuse, emotional abuse, sexual abuse, and physical or emotional neglect (Massey-Stokes & Lanning, 2004).

As discussed earlier, physical abuse is the deliberate maltreatment of another individual that inflicts pain or injury and may result in permanent or temporary disfigurement or even death. Common methods of physical abuse in children are listed in Table 31–6.

Physical neglect is the deliberate withholding of or failure to provide the necessary and available resources to the child. Behaviors constituting physical neglect include failure to provide for the following basic needs: supervision appropriate for child's age, adequate nutrition and hydration, hygiene (e.g., clean diapers and clothes, bathing and toileting facilities), shelter (e.g., warmth in winter), and appropriate health care (e.g., immunizations, dental care, medications, eyeglasses). Neglect is the most common type of abuse, especially in infancy when it is responsible for 68.5% of maltreatment (Brodowski et al., 2008).

Emotional abuse usually involves shaming, ridiculing, embarrassing, or insulting the child. It can also include the destruction of a child's personal property, such as tearing up the child's favorite family photographs or letters, or harming, killing, or giving away the child's pet. These actions are frequently used as a means of frightening or controlling the child.

Box 31–1 **Methods of Physical Abuse in Children**

- Hitting, slapping, kicking, or punching
- Whipping with belts, shoes, or electrical cords (Figure 31–1 ■)

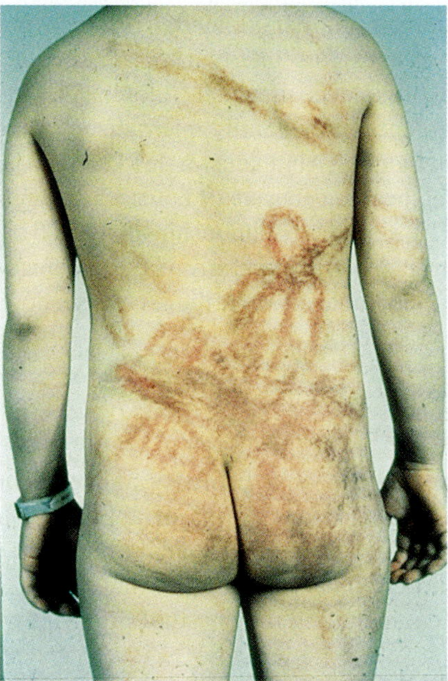

Figure 31–1 ■ Child who has been whipped.

- Inflicting burns with a lit cigarette or lighter (Figure 31–2 ■)

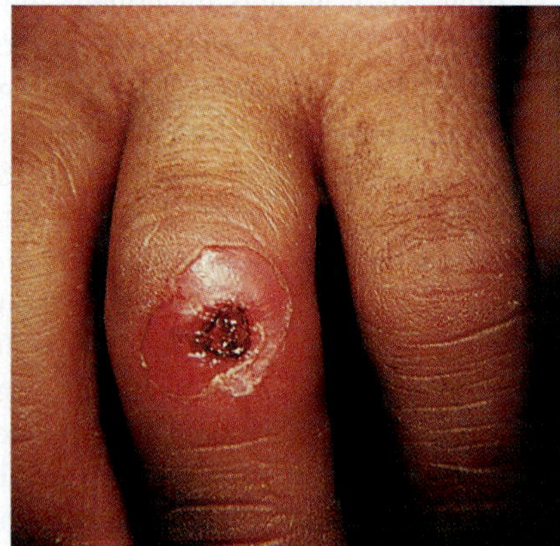

Figure 31–2 ■ Child burned with a cigarette.

- Immersing child or body part in scalding water (commonly legs, perineal area, hands, or feet: see Figure 30–20 ■ in Exemplar 30.1, Burns)
- Shaking the child violently ("shaken child" syndrome)
- Tying the child to a fence, bed, tree, or other object
- Throwing the child against a wall, down stairs, or against a window
- Choking or gagging the child
- Fracturing the legs, arms, ribs, or skull
- Deliberately administering excessive doses of prescribed or nonprescribed drugs
- Deliberately withholding prescribed medication

Source: Used with permission of the American Academy of Pediatrics, Visual Diagnosis of Child Physical Abuse Slide Kit. Photographs Copyright © AAP/Kempe.

Emotional neglect is characterized by the caretaker's emotional unavailability to the child. The usual style of interaction is cold and lacking in sensitive personal attention. The child suffers from a lack of nurturance and failure of the parent or caretaker to meet basic dependency needs. Another common example of emotional neglect occurs when the parent is mentally ill or abusing alcohol or other substances and cannot respond adequately to the child's developmental needs.

In 2007, more than 3.2 million reports of child maltreatment were made in the United States. Of the 794,000 classified as victims, 59% involved neglect, 11% involved physical abuse, 10% involved sexual abuse, and 4% involved emotional abuse; 1,760 children died from abuse and neglect, with 76% under 4 years of age (U.S. Department of Health and Human Services, 2009).

Perpetrators of child abuse tend to be family members, typically parents. Other perpetrators include mothers' boyfriends, stepfathers, and baby-sitters. A very small percentage of children are abused by older siblings; however, approximately 10% of family homicides are perpetrated by siblings (Hoffman & Edwards, 2004). More women than men are perpetrators of child abuse (U.S. Department of Health and Human Services, 2009).

Societal costs for child abuse are extensive. For example, direct judicial, law enforcement, and medical costs related to child abuse amount to more than $24 billion each year with another $69 billion in indirect costs (NCIPC, 2006a). In addition, abused children usually have longer hospital stays and charges (averaging $19,266 per child) twice those of children who are not abused. These additional charges are most often paid by Medicaid, further increasing the societal burden of child maltreatment (Rovi, Chen, & Johnson, 2004).

SEXUAL ABUSE **Child sexual abuse** is the exploitation of a child for the sexual gratification of an adult. About 1.2 per 1,000 children (almost 100,000) in the United States are sexually abused each year. Approximately 10% of schoolchildren report that they have been sexually abused. Many children who are sexually abused are under the age of 5 years; some are as young as 3 months old. The average age for sexual molestation is 4 years. The perpetrator is usually the parent (80% of the time) or another person legally responsible who does the following:

- Inflicts or allows another to inflict physical or emotional pain or injury
- Creates or allows another to create a significant risk of serious physical or emotional pain or injury
- Commits or allows another to commit an act of sexual abuse, as defined by law, against the child.

(U.S. Department of Health and Human Services, 2005)

The word *child* in sexual abuse and molestation refers to anyone who has not reached the age of consent, even if a teenager. **Incest** is sexual activity between close family members, so that marriage would be legally or culturally prohibited. Abusers often threaten to harm or kill the child or another family member if the child discloses the abuse; a variety of methods of sexual abuse occur.

Some abusers are **pedophiles**, people who have sexual impulses toward preadolescent children. The pedophile is at least 16 years of age and is at least 5 years older than the victim, and the victim is 13 years of age or younger. Another form of sexual abuse is exhibitionism, or obtaining sexual arousal by exposing one's genitals to a stranger. Some children are also victims of prostitution, forced to offer themselves for money or the pleasures of others, either in person or through videotapes and Internet sources. Common forms of sexual abuse are listed in Box 31–2.

Childhood sexual abuse does not discriminate. It occurs in all ethnic, religious, economic, and cultural subgroups. Affinity systems—immediate family, relatives, friends, neighbors, clergy members, scout leaders, coaches—account for 75% to 80% of the abuse. Heterosexual male perpetrators account for most of the reported cases. Children with mental retardation or physical disability are 4–10 times more vulnerable to sexual victimization than nondisabled children because disabled children may have difficulty asserting their rights or informing an adult protector. Although father–daughter incest is reported most, it is believed that sibling incest is the most widespread. Some siblings turn to each other for emotional nurturance and acceptance. In other instances, a sibling uses coercion or violence to perpetrate (National Center for Victims of Crime, 2004; Valente, 2005).

Having suffered sexual abuse in childhood is often a hidden feature of adult mental disorders. As much as 60–70% of psychiatric clients have a history of abuse. Repeated trauma in childhood distorts the personality. Since child victims cannot protect themselves, they must adapt to the trauma as well as they can. Behaviors that were originally adaptive become symptoms in adulthood. These people have a bewildering combination of symptoms, including anger, depression, anxiety, insomnia, suspicion, eating disorders, substance abuse, self-mutilation, and sexual dysfunction. Adult survivors often collect many different diagnoses before the underlying problem of post-traumatic stress disorder is correctly identified (Kaplow, Dodge, Amaya-Jackson, & Saxe, 2005; Kreidler, 2005).

Sexual abuse of children is an international public health problem; rates are similar for both industrialized and nonindustrialized countries. Any consideration of sexual abuse must take into account cultural views of appropriate and inappropriate sexual behavior. The aspects of culture relating to child sexual abuse include family structures, moral and religious principles, and child rearing practices. Other aspects include the relative value of interdependence, treatment of sexuality,

Box 31–2 **Common Forms of Child Sexual Abuse**

- Oral–genital contact
- Fondling and caressing the genitals
- Anal intercourse
- Sexual intercourse
- Rape
- Sodomy
- Prostitution
- Forcing viewing of or participation in pornography such as sexually explicit or nude photographs
- Encouraging nude photos or sexual activity via Internet or videotape

gender roles, and interpersonal boundaries. The ways in which communities view violence and sexual assault, and the action that is taken when these occur, reflect cultural values. It is only when we understand cultural diversity that we are able to develop effective prevention programs (Fontes, 2005; Warne & McAndrew, 2005).

Perpetrators Typically, adult perpetrators initiate sexual behavior in a manipulative or coercive manner. Often, the adult misrepresents the abuse as a game or "fun" activity. The behavior usually follows a progression of sexual activity, from exposure and fondling to oral, vaginal, or anal sex. The perpetrator imposes secrecy on the child by persuasion or threat. The abuser may say such things as, "If you tell, you'll be sent away," "If you tell, I won't love you anymore," "If you tell, I will kill you," and "If you tell, I'll do the same thing to your baby brother." Children know adults have absolute power over them, so they obey. When they have been threatened with abandonment or harm, they frequently choose to protect others. When asked, "Why didn't you tell sooner?" the answers are, "I didn't know who to tell," "I was scared," or "I did tell and no one believed me."

Sometimes, adult perpetrators use grooming behaviors to prepare or persuade victims to comply with the abuse. Grooming behaviors are used to gain the trust of children or family members before the abuse begins. These behaviors include hanging out with and participating in activities with the children, babysitting for the parents, or buying gifts for the children or other family members.

The Child's Response Some children who have been sexually abused form a clinging attachment to one or both parents. Some become extremely affectionate inside and outside the family system, while others have problems with impulse control and aggression toward others. Some children isolate themselves at school or in the neighborhood and limit most of their interactions to family members. They may act out sexually, by initiating oral or genital sex with other children or adults, for example. Some children, in an effort to master their trauma and regain a sense of personal control, victimize others as they were victimized. In addition, sexually abused children often engage in self-destructive behaviors such as head banging, self-mutilation, and suicide (Salter et al., 2003).

Adolescent victims may run away from home to escape an intolerable situation. Because they have learned, at home, that sexual behavior is rewarded by affection, love, and attention, some turn to prostitution. Others are forced into prostitution as a way to support themselves while living on the streets. Adolescents may unconsciously seek to repeat the trauma as a way of mastering it. This repetition may take the form of revictimization or perpetrating against others.

Children often feel responsible for the adult's behavior and ashamed that they have not been able to stop the abuse. Secrecy and guilt keep these children isolated, causing them to feel alienated from their peers. The feeling of powerlessness is extremely prevalent because what the victim says and does makes no difference. Children often will suppress their anger about the abuse until adolescence. When the suppressed rage comes to the surface, it may be directed against the self in self-defeating and self-destructive ways.

Some child victims use denial to cope with the trauma. Acknowledging the abuse would mean acknowledging that the world is dangerous and that those who are supposed to protect and nurture failed and caused harm. Other victims minimize the impact and say it was not important, saying things like, "It's not so bad; it only happens once a month" and "It's all right because it stopped when I was 11 years old."

Frequently, dissociation is the victim's major defense mechanism. The mind is "separated" from the body, so the victim is not emotionally present during the sexual attack. Dissociation prevents the feelings attached to the trauma from reaching conscious awareness in order to survive the trauma. Dissociation is evidenced by such statements as, "I put myself in the wall, where he couldn't reach all of me" and "When he would come into my room, I would close my eyes and go to my favorite place. Only my body stayed on the bed; the rest of me wasn't there." When sexual abuse is severe and sadistic, the victim may develop dissociative identity disorder (DID).

The Victim's Response in Adulthood Sexual behaviors are a trigger for some abuse survivors who only develop symptoms once they become sexually active. Some have a very strong aversion to sex and are filled with terror in sexual situations. Some are sexually inhibited and experience discomfort with sexual thoughts, feelings, and behaviors. Some engage in compulsive sexual behavior, perhaps as an unconscious way to validate their shame and guilt or a way to feel powerful. Other sexual symptoms include anger or disgust associated with touch, feeling emotionally distant during sex, experiencing intrusive sexual thoughts or images, and experiencing orgasmic, erectile, or ejaculatory difficulties. Many adult survivors go through a period of celibacy as they try to manage fear, anger, and distrust.

Many adult survivors continue to believe they were to blame for the abuse and should have been able to resist the adult. This self-blame often contributes to depression and anxiety and to panic attacks. For some, anger is the only emotion they experience or express, because they have repressed all other feelings.

It is not unusual for adult survivors to have total amnesia for the childhood sexual abuse. In such a case, amnesia is considered a defense mechanism in response to the trauma; amnesia is more likely to occur if the abuse began at a very young age. Recall of the abuse may be triggered by a significant life event, such as marriage or pregnancy, or during the process of psychotherapy.

Self-blame contributes to low self-esteem in adult survivors. They feel worthless and different from other people. Survivors often feel alienated from or even hate their bodies. They may believe they are only sex objects to be used and abused by others. They may suffer from flashbacks and nightmares. Many adult survivors have very little sense of self since their boundaries were violated so profoundly when they were children. This makes them more vulnerable to revictimization as adults.

Many adult survivors have difficulties with relationships. Superficial relationships are usually much easier than intimate relationships. As children, these adults learned that those who love you are the ones who hurt you, and that living in a family is not safe. There is a sense of betrayal by those they are dependent upon, a sense of powerlessness since they could do nothing to stop the abuse, and finally, a sense of stigmatization when they incorporate the shame and guilt that has been communicated to them.

Protective Services Intervention Nurses are among the professionals who are considered "mandatory reporters" of child abuse. Other professionals who are required to report abuse include teachers and school personnel and physicians. A nurse who suspects a child is being abused should follow his or her employment agency's policies and procedures for reporting abuse.

Abuse is reported to the local Child Protective Service (CPS) agency, typically in the county or local government's Department of Social Services. Upon receiving a report, CPS will conduct an investigation. In the event Child Protective Services determines that a child has been sexually abused by a family member, it will implement one of four plans:

1. The most frequent option is one in which the abuser is removed from the family. For this to occur, the nonabusing parent must be able to protect the child from any contact with the abuser.
2. When the nonabusing parent is unable to protect the child, both the child and the abuser are removed from the home. This option maximizes the safety of the child and decreases the child's feelings of responsibility.
3. In cases in which families have not used physical violence, where there is no substance abuse, and someone can ensure the child's safety, the family may be allowed to remain intact while participating in intensive therapy.
4. In a few instances, the child may be removed from the family when that appears to be the safest option. Unfortunately, this decision may place additional guilt on the child.

Intimate Partner Violence

Traditionally the term *domestic abuse* has been thought of as violence against a woman by a spouse or boyfriend. The Centers for Disease Control now use the term **intimate partner violence (IPV)**, which is defined as "the intentional emotional and/or physical abuse by a spouse, ex-spouse, boyfriend/girlfriend, ex-boyfriend/ex-girlfriend, or date" (CDC, 2000). Risk of severe violence may actually be higher once a relationship has been terminated than during the relationship (NCIPC, 2006b).

Nearly 4.8 million U.S. women and 2.9 million men experience IPV in a given year, although most incidents involve relatively minor actions such as pushing or slapping (NCIPC, 2006b). Each year, however, 1.5 million U.S. women and more than 835,000 men are raped or physically assaulted by an intimate partner (CDC, 2003a; Hahn et al., 2003a). Approximately 70% of rapes or sexual assaults of women are perpetrated by a family member or intimate partner (BJS, 2005a). Worldwide estimates of IPV range from 10–66% of women (Silverman, Mesh, Cuthbert, Slote, & Bancroft, 2004). These figures may vastly underrepresent the true incidence and prevalence of IPV since only about 20% of sexual assaults, 25% of physical assaults, and 50% of stalkings are reported to authorities (NCIPC, 2006b).

Intimate partners include spouses, ex-spouses, boyfriends or girlfriends, or former boyfriends or girlfriends. Risk of severe violence may actually be higher once a relationship has been terminated than during the relationship (NCIPC, 2006b). Intimate partner violence includes battering. **Battering** is chronic and continuing violence of one partner against another, resulting in the vulnerability, entrapment, and loss of control of one's life on the part of the abused partner. **Psychological battering** exists when there is no current physical or sexual abuse being perpetrated, but fear of potential abuse keeps the victim subservient (Coker, Smith, McKeown, & King, 2000). Psychological battering differs from psychological abuse in that it centers on the threat of actual physical or sexual abuse to control the behavior of another, whereas emotional abuse involves repeated verbal assaults on the victim's sense of self or self-worth.

Based on 2003 dollars, the estimated annual costs for medical and mental health care and lost productivity due to IPV is $8.3 billion. Severe IPV results in the loss of nearly 8 million days of work productivity for employed women and 5.6 million days of lost household productivity (NCIPC, 2006b).

Intimate partner violence occurs throughout the world in all nations and in all social, economic, religious, and cultural groups. IPV is often referred to as *gender-based violence* because in many cultures it arises in part from women's subordinate social status

FOCUS ON DIVERSITY AND CULTURE Genital Mutilation

Female genital mutilation (FGM) refers to a variety of procedures that damage female genitalia for nonmedical reasons. One such procedure is the clitoridectomy—removal of the clitoris. FGM is a common practice in a number of African, Middle Eastern, and Asian countries. Some immigrant populations in Europe and North America practice it as well. The reasons for FGM involve a combination of cultural, religious, and social factors. Traditionally FGM was practiced by certain members of the community, but there is an alarming trend in that health care providers in some areas have begun to practice it. FGM is typically practiced on girls while they are still in puberty.

Female genital mutilation is a violation of human rights against girls and women. Short-term consequences include severe bleeding and difficulty urinating. Long-term effects include potential complications during childbirth, infertility, and complications requiring further surgery.

The World Health Organization is gravely concerned with the involvement of health care providers in this human rights violation and counsels health care providers not to participate in female genital mutilation (WHO, 2009).

(Ahmed, van Ginneken, Razzaque, & Alam, 2004). Like child abuse, several different forms of IPV occur, including physical and sexual abuse, threats of physical or sexual violence, stalking, and emotional or psychological abuse. Other measures by which intimate partners exert coercive control include threats to children and control of financial assets.

Although most people think of IPV as occurring in heterosexual relationships, there is evidence to suggest that IPV also occurs in same-sex relationships and that IPV "occurs with the same or greater frequency in gay and lesbian communities" as in the general public (Freedberg, 2006, p. 15). For example, in one study of homosexual men in four U.S. cities, 34% of respondents reported psychological or "symbolic" battering by their partners in the prior 5 years, 22% reported physical abuse, and 5% reported sexual abuse (Greenwood et al., 2002). As many as 50,000–100,000 lesbians and 500,000 gay men may be subjected to IPV each year. However, reporting may be inhibited by perceptions of IPV as occurring in "mutual combat" and fear of one's same-sex orientation being "outed" by the sexual partner in retaliation for reporting abuse (Freedberg, 2006).

Intimate partner violence and child abuse tend to co-occur in families. Even when children are not themselves abused, witnessing family violence has profound psychological and social consequences. It is estimated that as many as 10 million children may witness family violence each year (Gomby, 2000).

Intimate partner violence also occurs outside the family constellation. In 2004, the prevalence rate for date rape was 1 per 1,000 population (BJS, 2005b). In the 2005 Youth Risk Behavior Surveillance (YRBS) survey, 9.2% of high school students reported experiencing dating violence and 7.5% were forced to have sexual intercourse (Eaton et al., 2006). In another study of 14-year-old to college-aged women, 32% reported experiencing dating violence. Lifetime risk of dating violence is estimated at 15%, with a 9% risk of rape. In one study, women assaulted by dating partners in high school were found to be at higher risk for revictimization in college (Smith, White, & Holland, 2003).

ABUSE OF PREGNANT WOMEN Pregnancy is a time of increased risk for abuse. There are more incidents of violence during pregnancy than of hypertension, gestational diabetes, or placenta previa, all of which are screened for regularly. Indeed, 16–25% of women report abuse during pregnancy. Pregnant teens have a higher rate of abuse than pregnant adults. It is not unusual for the violence to continue into the postpartum period. A history of abuse is one of the strongest predictors of abuse during pregnancy. Nonpregnant women are usually beaten in the face and chest. Pregnant women tend to be beaten in the abdomen, which can lead to miscarriage, placenta abruption, fetal loss, premature labor, fetal fractures, pelvic fractures, rupture of the uterus, and hemorrhage. Battering during pregnancy is associated with severity of abuse. The man who beats his pregnant partner is an extremely violent and dangerous man. Battering during pregnancy is a risk factor for eventual homicide of the female partner (Kearney, Haggerty, Munro, & Hawkins, 2003; Tan & Gregor, 2006).

The timing of the first prenatal visit is often related to abuse status. Abused women are twice as likely to delay prenatal care until the third trimester. Many abused women report that the abuser forced them to avoid prenatal care by denying them access to transportation.

Physical abuse during pregnancy may be related to ambivalent feelings about the pregnancy, competition for attention with the developing fetus, increased vulnerability of the woman, increased economic pressures, and decreased sexual availability. Unfortunately, abuse of pregnant women is often overlooked by health care professionals, even when the victim appears in the emergency department with bruises, cuts, broken bones, and abdominal injuries.

ETIOLOGY AND RISK FACTORS

Etiology

Interpersonal violence is easy to describe but difficult to explain. There is no single cause of this type of violence. It results from an interaction of biology, personality, relationship, and societal factors that have an impact on individuals and families.

NEUROBIOLOGY Researchers believe that genes and neurotransmitters may contribute to violent behavior. Although a genetic predisposition may make certain behaviors more likely, it does not make them inevitable. Serotonin (5-HT) plays an important role in mood and aggressive behavior: 5-HT calms us through inhibitory control over aggression. Abnormally low levels of 5-HT result in a lack of control, loss of temper, and explosive rage.

Childhood abuse and neglect lead to permanent alterations in the parts of the central nervous system known to be stress responsive. Corticotropin-releasing factor (CRF) is a major regulator of the endocrine, autonomic, immune, and behavioral stress responses. It is thought that stress early in life results in sensitization of the brain to even mild stressors in adulthood, thus contributing to mood and anxiety disorders long after the abuse or neglect has stopped (Griffin, Resick, & Yehuda, 2005).

INTRAPERSONAL THEORY Intrapersonal theory suggests that the cause of violence lies in the personality of the abuser. It is thought that people who are violent choose not to control their expressions of anger and hostility. This lack of self-regulation leads them to overrespond to stress. Poor problem-solving skills and the belief that aggression is a legitimate response to conflict intensify the violence (Close, 2005).

SOCIAL LEARNING THEORY Social learning theory proposes that violence is a learned behavior and that violent people are conditioned to respond aggressively and violently. Young boys are encouraged to demonstrate strength and dominance rather than empathetic and caring attributes. Children learn about violence from observation, from being a victim, and from behaving violently. If the use of violence is rewarded by a gain in power or a reduction in anxiety, the behavior is reinforced. If there is immediate negative reinforcement within the family, a decrease in violent behavior will result. Although learning may have occurred and opportunity is present, the potentially abusive person makes a conscious choice to abuse. The abuser is always solely responsible for the abuse (Tremblay & Nagin, 2005).

In addition to family models, the media expose children to many models of violence. Some movies and television shows demonstrate that "good" people use force to achieve "good" ends. Many of the stories make no attempt to justify the use of force for "good" ends; they simply present endless, senseless acts of cruelty by one human being upon another. With these types of family and media examples, children develop values that tolerate, and even accept as normal, everyday violence between people.

GENDER-BIAS FACTORS In some settings, the structure of the family and society can influence, condone, and even promote interpersonal violence. Some cultures and communities value the subordination of women through power and privilege. In these settings, men abuse because they believe they have a right to do so and because they can get away with it. Violence is a power issue. Unfortunately, victims can learn to become codependent, becoming so confused and desperate that they will accept negative attention as better than no attention. Women may be further marginalized when they are viewed or treated as sexual objects, restricted from decision making processes in their communities and countries, dehumanized with labels, controlled over the rights to their own bodies, and demeaned in value (Downs & Miller, 2002).

Women may be forced to choose between poverty and abuse. It can be difficult for women to find advocates and solutions, especially those who have been stay-at-home mothers who suddenly find themselves needing legal and medical support when they have no source of income or benefits. Some may choose to stay with abusive partners who provide financially for them and their children rather than risk facing poverty.

Risk Factors

Risk factors for abuse include age, gender, psychological factors, a history of abuse in the family, environment, culture, financial dependency, and substance abuse. Risk factors for child abuse and neglect are outlined in Table 31–6.

RISK FACTORS RELATED TO AGE AND PHYSIOLOGIC STATUS Age and physiologic status tend to interact in terms of their influence on family violence. For example, children with disabilities are nearly twice as likely to be abused as those without disabilities (Massey-Stokes & Lanning, 2004). Mental retardation in the child also increases the risk of maltreatment (NCIPC, 2006a). When physical difficulties in the child are combined with immaturity on the part of the parent (e.g., adolescent parents), the potential for abuse is even greater. Older clients made vulnerable by poor health and other forms of dependence, such as dementia, are also at greater risk of abuse than those who are more independent and in better health.

Younger children are more likely than older ones to experience serious injury or death as a result of maltreatment. For example, 38% of juvenile homicide victims are under age 5. Approximately 1,200–1,600 infants experience shaken baby syndrome each year, and death occurs in 25–30% of victims. **Shaken baby syndrome** is a constellation of signs and symptoms that result from violent shaking in an infant or child. Other effects include visual, motor, and cognitive impairment (NCIPC, 2006a).

PRACTICE ALERT

Any infant who arrives in the emergency department with seizures, failure to thrive, vomiting, lethargy, respiratory irregularities, or coma should be evaluated for child abuse, particularly shaken baby syndrome or shaken impact syndrome. Infants have relatively large heads with relatively weak neck muscles. A frustrated adult can shake an infant and cause inertial injuries (acceleration and deceleration) to the head that tear nerve fibers as the brain moves back and forth in the skull. Throwing the infant down onto a solid surface further increases the forces with which the brain hits the back of the skull (Nakagawa & Conway, 2004).

RISK FACTORS RELATED TO GENDER Generally speaking, child maltreatment occurs at similar levels for boys and girls, although young girls are four times more likely to be sexually abused than boys (Stokes-Massey & Lanning, 2004). For example, high school girls are nearly twice as likely as boys to report sexual assault (NCIPC, 2006d). Boys, however, are more likely than girls to die as a result of abuse, accounting for 64% of abuse-related fatalities (Snyder, 2004).

Among adults, women are more likely to experience victimization at the hands of a friend, acquaintance, or intimate partner, while men are more likely to be victimized by strangers (BJS, 2005a). Women experience more domestic violence and men are more often subjected to street violence, which occurs in public places (Steen & Hunskaar, 2004).

TABLE 31–6 **Risk Factors for Child Abuse and Neglect**

FACTORS INCREASING RISK FOR PHYSICAL ABUSE	FACTORS INCREASING RISK FOR SEXUAL ABUSE
Poverty	Absence of natural father or having a stepfather
Violence in the family	Being female
Prematurity or low birth weight	Mother's employment outside the home
Unrelated male primary caretaker	Poor relationship with parent
Parents who were abused as children	Parental relationship characterized by conflict
Age less than 3 years	Parental substance abuse or social isolation
Child disability or condition that requires a great deal of care (e.g., mental retardation, attention deficit/hyperactivity disorder)	
Parental substance abuse or social isolation	

PSYCHOLOGICAL RISK FACTORS Psychological factors serve as both contributors to and consequences of violence. For example, caregiver resentment, fatigue, family conflict, and personality traits have been found to contribute to elder abuse. Similarly, grief at the loss of a loved one may also contribute to abuse. The presence of psychiatric disorders also increases the potential for all forms of violence.

Psychological factors that may contribute to family violence include poor coping skills, the emotional climate in the family, personality traits of the abuser or the victim, and the presence of psychopathology. The abuser's level of emotional intelligence has also been suggested as a factor influencing domestic violence. In one study, perpetrators of IPV scored significantly lower on several components of emotional intelligence than the general population. Specifically, abusers had difficulties with emotional self-awareness, self-regard, assertiveness, independence, problem solving, flexibility, and impulsivity (Winters et al., 2004).

Families with poor coping skills have difficulty dealing with situational stressors; as a result, tension within the family increases, and this tension may result in violence. Constant family crises or upheavals indicative of poor coping abilities are frequently characteristic of abusive families. Types of coping used by victims of abuse may also influence the frequency and severity of violence. For example, some research has found that women who engage in avoidance coping mechanisms are subjected to more violence than women who use more active coping strategies. In addition, women subjected to severe abuse may encounter avoidance behaviors on the part of family and friends, further diminishing their sources of support (Waldrop & Resick, 2004).

The emotional climate in the family can also contribute to abuse. Families that exhibit increased emotional tension and anxiety, with little display of visible affection or emotional support, are considered emotionally impoverished and are at risk for violence. Similarly, family communication patterns that are not nurturing, are destructive, or are ambiguous may also indicate risk for family violence. Couples that experience intimate partner violence have been found to have poorer communication skills and less satisfying relationships than other couples and often engage in mutual exchange of negative communication (McClellan & Killeen, 2000). These couples may also be characterized by poor conflict negotiation skills, poor problem-solving skills, and defensiveness on the part of both members (Lloyd, 2000; Tilley & Brackley, 2005).

The distribution of power within the family is another element of the emotional climate that may lead to abuse. Abusive families are often characterized by autocratic decision making and power struggles between members. Abusers tend to abuse the power they have over other family members when they feel their power is threatened. The importance of power distribution to the risk for abuse of the older adult should not be overlooked. Partners who previously stood up for their rights may become more vulnerable if dementia or a medical illness that results in physical frailty occurs.

Child abusers may exhibit unrealistic expectations of children, particularly as sources of warmth and love. When they are disappointed in these expectations, abuse may occur. For example, children who are irritable, who cry often, or who do not care to be cuddled may be perceived as rejecting the parent. For parents with low self-esteem, this perceived rejection can set the stage for abuse.

RISK FACTORS RELATED TO CULTURE As discussed previously, women are at greater risk of interpersonal violence in cultures that grant men financial and physical control of women. Personal belief in strict gender roles is a risk factor for perpetration of IPV. For example, intimate partner violence in China has been found to be strongly associated with male patriarchal values. Even though Chinese culture has little value for the concept of privacy, IPV is considered a private family affair, and as many as 43% of Chinese women in one study reported IPV victimization at some time in their lives (Xu et al., 2005). Similarly, immigrant South Asian women have been found to be at higher risk than other women for IPV, perhaps in part due to the stresses of immigration and consequent social isolation (Raj & Silverman, 2003). Immigrant women may also be less likely to report IPV because of language barriers or fear of deportation (Dienemann, Glass, & Hyman, 2005). The risk for IPV may be particularly high when couples have differing cultural conceptions of the role of women in society. Cultural accommodations may need to be made by both parties, and this may be difficult if they do not recognize the influence of culture in their expectations (Locsin & Purnell, 2002).

Cultural attitudes that foster abuse of women are not confined to ethnic minority populations. Men from any race or culture may be brought up in an environment which justifies the control and discipline of women. Consistent with the concept of male control over women, U.S. women with higher educational levels than their partners have been found in some studies to be at greater risk for IPV than those with equal or lower education levels because they challenge male superiority (NCIPC, 2006b). It has been suggested that changing these cultural attitudes should be a major focus in the primary prevention of IPV and that interventions should be undertaken particularly with school-aged children to change their perceptions of gender-appropriate roles and behaviors (Gundersen, 2002).

SOCIOECONOMIC RISK FACTORS Women's risk of IPV is increased by financial dependence on their partners, partners' relationships with other women, inability to negotiate condom use, lower levels of education and household income, and cohabitation or short-term relationships with multiple partners (Maman et al., 2002). Childlessness is also a risk for IPV against women in societies where childbearing is considered women's primary function (Koenig, Stephenson, Ahmed, Jejeebhoy, & Campbell, 2006). Cohabitation has also been associated with greater risk for child maltreatment and fatality (Giorgianni, 2003).

IPV is five times more common in households with annual incomes under $15,000 than in those with incomes over $50,000 (Division of Violence Prevention, 2000a). Victims of IPV may also stay in abusive relationships because of limited resource availability and social isolation. Lack of social resources, both tangible social support and emotional support provided by friends and family, has also been linked to child abuse (NCIPC, 2006a). Economic factors and the cultural factor of ageism may contribute to abuse of elderly individuals.

SUBSTANCE ABUSE AND INTERPERSONAL VIOLENCE Alcohol abuse by a male partner was found to be the strongest correlate of intimate partner violence (Coker et al., 2000). Similarly, alcohol and drug abuse by family members are risk factors for child maltreatment (NCIPC, 2006a). Some research suggests, however, that the association between substance use or misuse and violence is mediated by beliefs about substance use. For example, in one study, attitudes approving of marital aggression, perceptions of alcohol use as an excuse for abusive behavior, and expectations of aggressive behavior by someone who has been drinking were linked to IPV among people who drink. Drinkers without these attitudes were less likely to engage in IPV, suggesting that it was not alcohol use *per se* that contributed to IPV, but perceptions of alcohol use and its effects (Field, Caetano, & Nelson, 2004).

Significant numbers of women in treatment for drug abuse have a history of IPV. In fact, data suggest that 25–57% of women in treatment programs experienced IPV in the prior year, compared to 1.5–16% of women in the general population. Research indicates that the relationship between substance abuse and IPV is bidirectional, with substance abuse increasing risk for abuse and also resulting as a means of coping with abuse (El-Bassel, Gilbert, Wu, Go, & Hill, 2005).

OTHER RISK FACTORS Family relationships and dynamics may increase the risk for child maltreatment or serve as protective factors. Family risk factors include social isolation, parental lack of understanding of child development, family disorganization, and lack of family cohesion. Negative parent–child interactions and parental stress levels may also contribute to family violence. Protective factors within families include supportive family relationships, nurturing parenting skills, stable family relationships, household rules, and adequate role models outside the family. Employment and adequate housing also influence interpersonal family violence (NCIPC, 2006a).

For youth, association with delinquent peers, gang involvement, and social rejection by peers may contribute to increased violence. At the community level, social disorganization, diminished economic opportunities, increased transience, and low levels of community participation have been linked to violence among youth. Conversely, religiosity, intolerant attitudes to deviance, family connectedness, high parental performance expectations, and parental supervision have been linked to decreased risk of youth violence, as have commitment to school and involvement in social activities (NCIPC, 2006f).

Family violence frequently occurs in the context of divorce and child custody battles. Granting custody of children to men who have a history of IPV and/or child abuse and granting visitation rights to abusive parents or partners have been regular occurrences in U.S. courts that are viewed as violations of international human rights. Additional court-perpetrated violations of rights include cases in which courts have refused to include evidence of interpersonal violence (Silverman et al., 2004). Sometimes evidence of abuse is scanty or inconclusive, and courts are put in the difficult position of deciding when to restrict custody by or visitation with an abusive partner or parent. Some courts elect to require supervised visitation, in which the noncustodial parent must be supervised either by a social worker or a family friend agreed upon by both parents. In either case, time is limited and scheduling is difficult, further limiting the visitation process. This can be particularly devastating to the parent–child relationship when the parent is not an abuser, but has been falsely accused. On the other hand, visitation or shared custody by an abusive parent can place a child at further risk of abuse. It is not uncommon for courts to require abusive parents to participate in parenting, anger management, and therapy programs.

The availability of lethal weapons, particularly guns, is another social factor that influences violence. In one study, firearms were more likely to be found in homes of women subjected to IPV than in other households, and in two thirds of these homes, intimate partners had either threatened to shoot the women or had actually shot them (Sorenson & Weibe, 2004).

CLINICAL MANIFESTATIONS

Violence results in a variety of physiological and psychological effects for people of all age groups. Violence against women leads to twice as many health care visits and an 800% increase in mental health visits as well as increased risk of hospitalization compared to women who are not abused (Murdaugh, Hunt, Sowell, & Santana, 2004). Approximately 42% of physically abused women and 20% of men require medical care for injuries received. In addition, victims of IPV may experience chronic headaches, back pain, pelvic pain, sexually transmitted diseases, gastrointestinal disorders, and heart conditions. IPV directed at women may also result in injuries to children. For example, children of abused mothers have been found to be 57 times more likely to suffer maltreatment than children whose mothers were not abused (NCIPC, 2006b).

Psychological consequences of abuse are many and varied and may arise both from the experience of being abused and from witnessing abuse. Psychological consequences of IPV for women appear to be mediated by perceptions of their ability to control violence, but the direction of effects is somewhat unusual. For example, in one study women who believed they should be able to control current violence were at greater risk for depression and low self-esteem than those who did not perceive themselves as able to control the abuse. Expectations of abilities to control future abuse, however, were linked to decreased risk for dysphoria and hopelessness and increased self-esteem (Clements, Sabourin, & Spiby, 2004).

Manifestations of Child Abuse

Clinical manifestations of child abuse and sexual abuse in children and adolescents are listed on pages 1954–1955. Behaviors inconsistent with developmental stage may be apparent. For example, the toddler or preschooler may be indiscriminately friendly with unfamiliar adults, including health care providers, rather than demonstrating shyness or anxiety.

CLINICAL MANIFESTATIONS AND THERAPIES Abuse

TYPE OF ABUSE	CLINICAL MANIFESTATIONS	CLINICAL THERAPIES
Child Abuse	■ Bruises or welts in unusual places or in several stages of healing; distinctive shapes ■ Wary of physical contact with adults ■ Behavioral extremes of withdrawal or aggression ■ Burns (especially cigarette burns; immersion burns of hands, feet, or buttocks; rope burns; or distinctively shaped burns) ■ Apprehensive when other children cry ■ Inappropriate response to pain ■ Fractures (multiple or in various stages of healing, inconsistent with explanations of injury) ■ Joint swelling or limited mobility ■ Long-bone deformities ■ Lacerations and abrasions to the mouth, lip, gums, eye, genitalia ■ Human bite marks ■ Signs of intracranial trauma ■ Deformed or displaced nasal septum ■ Bleeding or fluid drainage from the ears or ruptured eardrums ■ Broken, loose, or missing teeth ■ Difficulty in respirations, tenderness or crepitus over ribs ■ Abdominal pain or tenderness ■ Recurrent urinary tract infection ■ Emotional and/or behavioral problems	■ Treatment for physical injuries ■ Therapy may be behavioral, cognitive, group, or play therapy depending on developmental stage ■ Behavioral therapy for perpetrators
Elder Abuse	■ Constant hunger or malnutrition ■ Listlessness ■ Poor hygiene ■ Social isolation ■ Inappropriate dress for the weather ■ Chronic fatigue ■ Unattended medical needs ■ Poor skin integrity or decubiti ■ Contractures ■ Urine burns/excoriation ■ Dehydration ■ Fecal impaction ■ Bruises and welts ■ Withdrawal ■ Burns ■ Confusion ■ Fractures ■ Fear or suspicion of caretaker, family members, health care providers ■ Sprains or dislocations ■ Lacerations or abrasions ■ Evidence of oversedation ■ Inappropriate clothing ■ Failure to meet financial obligations ■ Unmet medical needs	■ Treat physical injuries ■ Treat psychological effect such as depression with medication or therapy ■ Respite services ■ Adult day care ■ Referral to treatment or therapy for perpetrators ■ Transfer of legal authority

CLINICAL MANIFESTATIONS AND THERAPIES **Abuse (continued)**

TYPE OF ABUSE	CLINICAL MANIFESTATIONS	CLINICAL THERAPIES
Intimate Partner Violence	■ Chronic fatigue ■ Casual response to a serious pains ■ Vague complaints, aches, and injury or excessively emotional response to a relatively minor injury ■ Frequent injuries ■ Recurrent sexually transmitted diseases ■ Frequent ambulatory or emergency room visits ■ Muscle tension ■ Nightmares ■ Facial lacerations ■ Depression ■ Injuries to chest, breasts, back, abdomen, or genitalia ■ Anorexia or other eating disorder ■ Bilateral injuries of arms or legs ■ Anxiety ■ Symmetric injuries ■ Drug or alcohol abuse ■ Obvious patterns of belt buckles, bite marks, fist or hand marks ■ Suicide attempts ■ Poor self-esteem ■ Burns of hands, feet, buttocks, or with distinctive patterns ■ Headaches ■ Gastrointestinal or stress ulcers	■ Treat physical injuries and physiologic conditions ■ Treat psychological effects such as depression with medication or therapy ■ Substance abuse counseling for perpetrator and victim, as needed
Sexual Abuse	■ Torn, stained, or bloody underwear ■ Pain or itching in genital areas ■ Engages in fantasy behavior or infantile behavior ■ Bruises or bleeding from external genitalia, vagina, rectum ■ Poor peer relationships ■ Withdrawal ■ Sexually transmitted disease ■ Unwilling to participate in physical activities ■ Swollen or red cervix, vulva, or perineum ■ Wears long sleeves and several layers of clothing even in hot weather ■ Semen around the mouth or genitalia or on clothing ■ Pregnancy ■ Delinquency or running away ■ Inappropriate sexual behavior or mannerisms ■ Regressive behaviors	■ Treatment for physical injuries ■ Therapy may be behavioral, cognitive, group, or play therapy depending on developmental stage ■ Behavioral therapy for perpetrators

For the infant or young child with shaken baby syndrome or shaken child syndrome, the symptoms are those of CNS injury from repeated coup and contrecoup injury. The high water and gelatinous content of the infant's brain makes it highly vulnerable to injury during shaking. Symptoms include vomiting, irritability, fatigue, poor feeding, bradycardia, apnea, enlarged fontanel, and seizures. Bruises are usually not present, but computed tomography (CT) is often definitive for the diagnosis, with radiographs and MRIs used for a thorough diagnostic profile (Carbaugh, 2004: Hymel & Hall, 2005).

Box 31–3 Clinical Manifestations of Child Abuse

- Multiple bruises in various stages of healing
- Scald burns with clear lines of demarcation and in a glove or stocking distribution (see Figure 30–20 in Exemplar 30.1, Burns)
- Rope, belt, or cord marks, usually seen on the mouth, buttocks, back, legs, and arms (see Figure 31–1)
- Burn scars in various stages of healing (see Figure 31–2)
- Multiple fractures in various stages of healing; spiral fractures not explained by accident
- Shortness of breath and distress upon being moved, indicating chest contusions and possible rib fractures
- Sedation from overmedication
- Cranial injuries
- Abdominal injury
- Change in behavior or school performance
- Fear and avoidance of certain people or situations
- Anger and violent play
- Exacerbation of chronic illness (such as diabetes or asthma) because of withholding of medication

Manifestations of physical neglect include undernourishment (evidenced by constantly feeling hungry, hoarding or stealing food, and being underweight), unclean clothes and body, poor dental health (extensive cavities or generally poor condition of teeth), and inappropriate clothing for the season (Box 31–3).

Manifestations of emotional abuse, verbal abuse, emotional neglect, and witnessing domestic violence include fear, poor physical growth, and failure to meet appropriate developmental milestones. The child may have difficulty relating to adults, impaired communication skills, and developmental delays. Behavioral manifestations include anxiety, fear, shame, aggression, delinquency, and depression.

Children who have been sexually abused may exhibit a variety of physical and behavioral signs and symptoms (Box 31–4). Bruising, bleeding, and laceration of the genital area are obvious signs of trauma (Johnson, 2006). However, sexual abuse does not always result in apparent injury. Among the many long-term consequences of child sexual abuse are ongoing feelings of shame, guilt, anger, and hostility; decreased self-esteem, which leads to increased self-destructive behavior and risk of suicide; recurrence of victimization experiences; substance abuse; posttraumatic stress disorder; and eating disorders. Children who have been abused are more likely to abuse others in the future. Factors associated with greater psychological harm to the child include (1) a long period of abuse, (2) use of violent force or threat of violence, (3) abuse involving penetration (intercourse or oral–genital sex), and (4) abuse involving family members, especially the father or stepfather.

Cultural Considerations

It is important to differentiate true child abuse from cultural variations that might inaccurately be assumed to indicate abuse (Figure 31–3A ■ and B). For example, traditional treatment practices are sometimes mistaken for signs of physical abuse. The Chinese practice of cupping, which involves heating a bamboo cup and placing it on the skin, is a traditional treatment for headaches or abdominal pain. The Vietnamese practice of *caogio* (rubbing out the wind), in which a coin or the fingers are forcefully rubbed on the chest, back, or neck, is used to treat minor ailments. Ask about marks on the skin, how they occurred, and what health practices the family uses.

Manifestations of Elder Abuse

The physical symptoms of elder mistreatment are often difficult for clinicians to discern because older adults may suffer from chronic and acute illnesses that mask the presence of mistreatment (Collins, 2006). Cognitively impaired older adults provide an additional challenge. Their subjective reporting may be questioned for accuracy or they may be unable to express the mistreatment situation due to amnesia, *aphasia* (total or partial loss of ability to speak or understand language), *agnosia* (inability to recognize common persons and things), and *apraxia* (inability to perform simple tasks), which commonly occur with dementia. It is often difficult to determine whether the older adult's worsening physical condition is a result of the natural progression of illness or mistreatment on the part of a caregiver. Because some frail older

Box 31–4 Clinical Manifestations of Sexual Abuse in Children and Adolescents

- Vaginal discharge
- Blood-stained underpants or diaper
- Genital redness, pain, itching, or bruising
- Difficulty walking or sitting
- Urinary tract infection
- Sexually transmitted disease
- Somatic complaints, such as headaches or stomachaches
- Sleeping problems, such as nightmares or night terrors
- Bedwetting
- Unwillingness to go to babysitter, family member, neighbor, or other person
- Fear of strangers
- New or excessive sexual curiosity or play
- Constant masturbation
- Curling into fetal position
- Phobias about particular places, people, or things
- Abrupt changes in school performance and attendance
- Changes in eating habits
- Abrupt changes in behavior (especially withdrawal)
- Child or adolescent female acts like a wife or mother
- Precocious or excessively seductive behavior
- Child or adolescent works as a prostitute

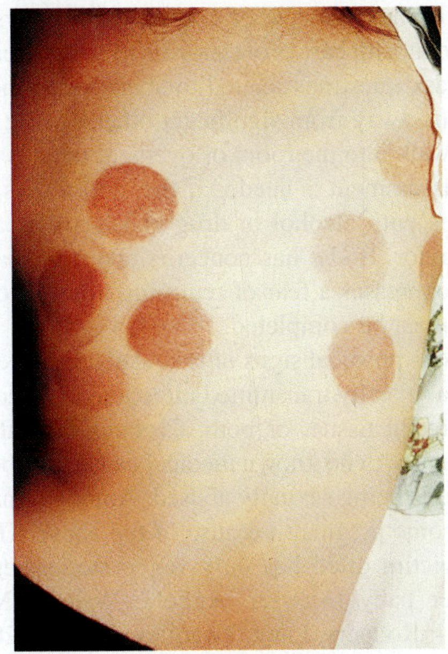

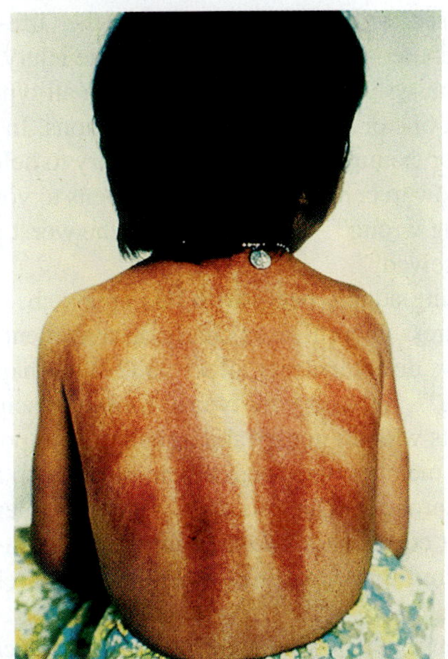

Figure 31–3 ■ It is important to differentiate cultural practices such as *A*, cupping, and *B*, coining, from signs of child abuse.

Source: Used with permission of the American Academy of Pediatrics, Visual Diagnosis of Child Physical Abuse Slide Kit. Photographs copyright © AAP/Kempe.

individuals are prone to underlying conditions that give rise to trauma, such as instability of gait and poor vision resulting in falls, it may be difficult for clinicians to differentiate accidental from willful injuries. The presence of both fresh and healing injuries may suggest ongoing episodes of trauma and represent the need for further investigation to determine whether abuse or neglect may be a contributing factor. Examples include fractures, bruising, and burns (Lachs & Pillemer, 1995).

COLLABORATION

Usually, the best way to treat violent families is a multidisciplinary approach involving nurses, physicians, social workers and protective services personnel, law enforcement and, often, lawyers. Most families are more open to accepting help during a time of crisis than at other times. They most likely will be willing to develop new behavior patterns for a short time following a crisis, but changing behaviors over time requires much difficult work and support. It is not uncommon for family members to return to previous, unhealthy behavior patterns, including those that condone or promote interpersonal violence.

Domestic Violence Shelters

Today's domestic violence shelters offer a broad array of services. In addition to offering immediate shelter for women and their children, they also provide referrals to a number of agencies that provide services as well as group therapy for women and children, advocacy, and parent training. Many have a list of attorneys and other professionals who make their services available at sliding scale fees. Nurses working with women and children should have available the contact information for the domestic violence shelters in their community.

Working With Children

The nurse plays an important role in the multidisiciplinary team providing treatment to the child who is the victim of abuse. The nurse should ensure that the team creates a safe and predictable environment in which the child feels supported, at home, at school, and in whatever therapeutic environment the team chooses for the child.

As part of the team, the nurse should plan interventions that will encourage affective release in a supportive environment. Child victims must be able to experience a range of emotions. Play therapy helps these children play out traumatic themes, fears, and distorted beliefs. It is a nonthreatening way to process thoughts and feelings associated with the abuse, both symbolically and directly. Art therapy provides an opportunity to express feelings for which there are no words. Therapeutic stories present the traumatic issues of abuse, link victims' feelings and behavior, and describe new coping methods. Journal writing can help children over age 10 cope with intrusive thoughts and feelings. They often choose to bring their journal into the one-on-one sessions with their therapist.

NURSING PROCESS

Nurses must be involved in the prevention, detection, and treatment of all forms of abuse. Developing the knowledge base and the ability to identify factors that contribute to abuse help the nurse detect and accurately diagnose the problem and provide appropriate interventions.

Assessment

Given the incidence of abuse, it is logical to assume that every nurse will encounter victims in a variety of clinical settings. Women are often treated for the immediate injury or complaint and dismissed without assessing for the life-threatening condition—abuse—that caused the immediate injury.

During the assessment of every client, in all types of health settings, ask one or two introductory questions. In assessing a child, say, for example, "Moms and Dads try to help their children learn how to behave well. What happens to you when you do something wrong?" Or ask, "What is the worst punishment you ever received?"

In assessing adults, begin with this approach: "One of the sources of stress in our lives is family disagreement. Could you describe how disagreements affect you? What happens when you disagree?" "What is your typical form of discipline?"

For clients who do not speak English, it is important to use a nonfamily member who speaks their language to assist in the assessment process. The use of a nonfamily member helps ensure client confidentiality and safety. Immigrants may need to be reassured that reporting of abuse will not change their immigrant status.

Nurses must be able to recognize clues that indicate the possibility of interpersonal violence. One behavior to look for is the man speaking for the female client in response to questions about the injury. She may seek his approval before answering questions. He may criticize or correct her answers. Often, he may not want health care professionals to talk to her alone. The nurse must ask questions related to abuse when the woman is by herself and away from significant others. Make certain that no one can walk into the room or overhear what is said.

Further assessment is needed if the victim says her partner has problems with alcohol or drug abuse or has a history of violent behavior. If she has concerns about the safety of her children or expresses a fear of returning home, more in-depth assessment must be completed.

The obvious physical signs of sexual abuse in a child are the presence of a sexually transmitted infection, irritated or swollen genitals or rectal tissue, or both. Chronic vaginal or urinary tract infections with no known medical cause may be indicators that the child is being sexually abused. Among female victims, 12–24% become pregnant because of the abuse. The pregnant adolescent victim often has only vague stories regarding the father of her baby (Kawsar, Anfield, Walters, McCabe, & Forster, 2004; Rodgers, Lang, Twamley, & Stein, 2003).

Some children will, consciously or unconsciously, attempt to abuse their bodies either to prevent or to stop the sexual abuse. The child may gain a great deal of weight, hoping to

Assessment Interview Victims of Family Violence

In order to successfully interview suspected victims of abuse it is essential that the victim be separated from the potential abuser. Victims often lie to protect their abuser because of fear of retribution or an unwillingness to prosecute their abuser out of misplaced loyalty. Establishing a trusting relationship, providing support for the client, and taking a professional caring approach can help to overcome the victim's reluctance, but it is not always effective.

BEHAVIORAL ASSESSMENT

- Tell me about how people communicate within your family.
- What types of things cause conflict within your family?
- How is conflict managed or resolved?
- Who in your family loses control of themselves when angry?
- Have you received verbal threats of harm?
- Have you ever been threatened with a knife or gun?
- What happens to you when a family member has violent outbursts? Are you slapped? Hit? Punched? Thrown? Shoved? Kicked? Burned? Beaten up?
- Who in your family has needed emergency medical treatment?
- In what ways have you attempted to stop the violence?
- Have you attempted to leave the situation in the past?
- What happened when you attempted to leave?
- Describe the use of alcohol in your family.
- Describe the use of drugs in your family.

AFFECTIVE ASSESSMENT

- Who do you think is responsible for the use of physical force within your family?
- In what way is this person(s) responsible?
- How much guilt are you experiencing at this time?
- Tell me about your fears. Lack of security? Financial problems? Child care problems? Living apart from spouse? Further physical injury?
- What factors contribute to your feeling of helplessness to leave or stop the abuse?
- How hopeless do you feel about your situation?
- How would you describe your level of depression?

COGNITIVE ASSESSMENT

- Describe your strengths and abilities as a person.
- If you were describing yourself to a stranger, what would you say?
- What are your beliefs about keeping your family together?
- Tell me about your reasons for remaining in this situation. Promises of reform? Material rewards?
- Do you believe or hope the violence will not recur?
- What are your expectations of how children should behave?
- What rights do parents have with their children?
- What rights do spouses have with each other?
- What are the rules about physical force within your family?

SOCIOCULTURAL ASSESSMENT

- How did your parents relate to each other?
- Who enforced discipline when you were a child?
- What type of discipline was used when you were a child?
- What was/is your relationship like with your mother?
- What was/is your relationship like with your father?
- How did you get along with your siblings?
- In your present family, who is the head of the household?
- How are decisions made in your family?
- How are household jobs assigned in your family?
- Describe recent and current stresses on your family. Unemployment? Financial problems? Illness? New family members? Deaths or separations? Child-rearing problems? Change in job status? Increase in conflict? Change in residence?
- To whom can you turn for support in times of stress?
- Describe your social life.
- What types of contact have you had with the legal system? Phoned police? Obtained an order of protection? Obtained a lawyer? Court cases? Protective services?

become so unattractive that the abuser will leave the child alone. If an older child is being abused, a younger sister may become anorexic in an attempt not to mature and experience the same abuse. This lack of care for the body may continue into adult life in an unconscious attempt to maintain distance and avoid intimate relationships.

Questioning families suspected of abuse requires great delicacy and sensitivity. It is suggested that the inexperienced nurse observe the more experienced nurse before attempting to approach a family member. When in doubt, it is always best to defer to a more experienced team member.

Assessing the Older Adult

A multidisciplinary team's comprehensive geriatric assessment of the older adult's cognitive and psychosocial function is essential in identifying elder mistreatment, and the nurse's role is of utmost importance (Baker & Heitkemper, 2005; VanderWeerd, Paveza, & Fulmer, 2006). The nursing history should entail asking older adult clients about the presence of violence in their lives. Research has demonstrated that nurses can accurately identify elder mistreatment cases in busy emergency department settings (Fulmer, Paveza, Abraham, & Fairchild, 2000).

The Hartford Institute for Geriatric Nursing (2007) recommends the Elder Assessment Instrument (EAI) for use in the clinical setting. Screening can facilitate accurate assessment, risk categorization, referral for services, and ultimately protection of the older person who is being mistreated or abused.

Various screening instruments have been developed that aid nurses and other clinicians in undertaking a thorough mistreatment assessment. The EAI (Fulmer & Cahill, 1984; Fulmer, Street, & Carr, 1984) assesses signs and symptoms of elder mistreatment. The nurse should first assess general appearance. An older adult appearing disheveled with poor hygiene warrants further investigation. Common signs of abuse include bruising, malnutrition, burns, excoriations, and fractures. Common clinical manifestations of neglect include dehydration, malnutrition, decubitus ulcers, and contractures. Other signs and symptoms of elder mistreatment include delays between the injury or illness and the seeking of medical treatment, frequent visits to the emergency department, and diagnostic testing results inconsistent with the history given (Lachs & Pillemer, 1995; National Research Council, 2003).

Ideally, the client and the suspected abuser should be interviewed separately, which may reveal inconsistencies. Maintaining a nonjudgmental attitude will enable the nurse to obtain more accurate data. A caregiver's refusal to allow for separate interviews should increase suspicion of elder mistreatment (Fulmer et al., 2005; Nadien, 2006).

Assessing caregiver stress and burden allows for a more complete assessment. Various caregiver assessment questionnaires are available (Friss-Feinberg, 2002).

Diagnosis

There are a number of nursing diagnoses for victims and perpetrators of interpersonal violence (North American Nursing Diagnosis Association, 2007). Priority must be given to critical and serious physical injuries. The severity and potential fatality of the situation must be considered, as well as the needs of dependent children and legal issues surrounding the case. Some appropriate diagnoses include the following:

- Interrupted Family Process related to an inability to manage conflict without violence
- Risk for Other-Directed Violence related to a history of physical force with family or intimate friends
- Impaired Parenting related to abuse or neglect of children with ineffective parenting skills
- Powerlessness related to feelings of being dependent on the abuser
- Chronic Low Self-Esteem related to feeling responsible and guilty for being a victim of interpersonal violence
- Social Isolation related to control by perpetrator and shame regarding family violence
- Ineffective Individual Coping related to being a victim of sexual abuse
- Post-Trauma Syndrome related to being a victim of sexual abuse.

Plan

Based on the assessment data and in collaboration with the client, select goals appropriate to the nursing diagnoses. Two broad goals are:

- Victims remain safe.
- Abusive behavior ends.

Other goals appropriate to victims or perpetrators include the following:

- Victims remain safe and free from harm.
- Victims develop an escape plan.
- Clients manage conflict appropriately.
- Victims verbalize an internal locus of control.
- Clients implement appropriate and safe parenting techniques.
- Clients use community resources.

Once the nursing diagnoses and goals have been identified, the nurse develops the plan of care to assist clients toward a safer and more predictable level of life functioning.

Implementation

The priority of care for victims of abuse is to ensure their safety. It is especially important that children feel personally safe and also that they are kept safe from further emotional damage in interactions with others.

Client at Risk for Other Directed Violence

In the initial contact with family members, ensure their physical safety as much as possible. It is critical to assess the level of danger for the victim; homicide may be a real possibility if previous threats have been made. If an adult is being abused, it is likely that children are being abused. Even if the children are not being physically abused, witnessing violence can be devastating. It is also important to assess the level of danger for the abuser. The severity and duration of the violence are the factors that contribute the most directly to victims killing their abusers in self-defense. If the level of danger is high, follow agency protocol for reporting the abuse to protective services or the police in order to initiate emergency custody placement or removal to a shelter.

Help clients develop a "safe plan" or "escape plan" to use when their safety is threatened. The goal is to escape before violence occurs. Exact and careful preplanning will aid escape during a time when anxiety and fear are at a high level. Items to consider include the following:

- Decide on a quick, safe exit from the home.
- Determine a safe place to go and teach it to the children.
- Put important documents in a secure location (birth certificates, orders of protection, money, medications, list of important phone numbers, few days clothing).
- Have an extra set of car keys.

Client at Risk for Decisional Conflict

Communication among family members is often key to making decisions related to an action plan to stop abuse and maintain safety. Families experiencing violence often have poor communication skills. Nursing interventions can be designed to improve the family members' communication. Improved communication skills will enable family members to resolve issues before they escalate to the point of violence. Using a minor, nonemotional family problem, have family members solve the problem in a democratic manner. Once the process is learned, family members can transfer this knowledge and ability to solve other problems.

Client at Risk for Hopelessness

One of the primary goals of therapy is empowering victims. The process of violence removes all power and control from a person, resulting in low self-esteem, anxiety, depression, and somatic problems. Nurses can change that through a variety of interventions.

Help the client identify past dependency relationships. Identifying patterns will help the client focus on how he or she maintains his or her own feelings of powerlessness.

- Help the client formulate a list of ways he or she is dependent on abuser (e.g., emotional and economic areas of dependency). High levels of dependency make it difficult for victim to leave abuser without intense support.
- Help the client identify intrapersonal and interpersonal strengths. Recognition of strengths will decrease feelings of helplessness.
- Help the client identify aspect(s) of life under his or her control. Provide assertiveness training; caution client that if he or she is still in an abusive situation, assertive behavior may escalate the violence.
- Avoid trying to convince adult victims to leave their abuser. Be willing to support clients in their pain, rather than telling them what to do about their problems. Support and affirm positive choices and decisions they make. For the most adaptive outcome, adult victims must be their own rescuers and take charge of their own safety and protection plan. If they need help with this process they must be taught to ask for that help directly.

Risk for Caregiver Role Strain: Caregiver of an Older Adult

- Support the older adult and caretakers in identifying and expanding social support networks that may decrease the level of stress within the household. Supportive professionals, paraprofessionals, and even friends may be able to help with activities of daily living (ADLs), transportation, financial advice, and assistance with personal problems.
- Assist caregivers in exploring their feelings about the older person in their care. Unexplored and unresolved negative feelings contribute to the potential for violence. Help caregivers identify situations that are disturbing to them. These situations may contribute to neglect or abuse.
- Determine the caretakers' ability to meet their loved one's needs and provide appropriate teaching. Encourage family to formulate alternatives for coping with elderly person in the home.
- Ensure safety of the older adult.

Working with Victims of Abuse

Interventions for victims of abuse include those that are supportive as well as those that help clients begin to build skills necessary for empowerment and recovery.

- Design interventions to increase self-esteem. Both adult and child abuse victims have a continuous internal monologue of negative statements such as "You're weak, stupid, incompetent, unlovable, and unattractive." Negative statements become self-administered abuse and keep the survivor weak and powerless. Help clients become aware of the frequency and intensity of these negative thoughts. Teach them to consciously replace negative thoughts with positive ones. While this is often difficult at first, it becomes easier with practice.
- Because abuse survivors are often anxious, interventions to reduce anxiety are also necessary. Clients who learn progressive relaxation and controlled breathing are often able to avoid full-blown panic attacks. Teach the process, and talk clients through the stages of relaxation until they are able to reduce anxiety by themselves. When they are relaxed, instruct them to imagine a scene in which they feel safe and comfortable. Anytime they need to, they can return to this safe scene where they are in total control.

Treating the Abuser

Most abusers do not seek treatment unless it is court ordered or there are custody issues involved. It is frustrating to intervene with abusers who deny the reality of or responsibility for the violence. Group therapy for abusers is sometimes helpful. The group setting is more effective than individual therapy because interactions with a number of people more successfully address the anger and control problems. The responsibility for aggression is always placed on the aggressor. Issues regarding the patriarchal and power views of relationships are discussed in great depth. Participants are asked to specify their abusive behaviors, identify the intentions behind those behaviors, and examine the effects of the abuse on their victims. Abusers learn that anger can be controlled and that violence is always a *choice*.

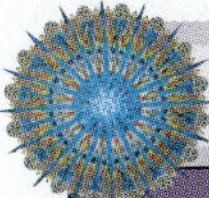

NURSING CARE PLAN An Older Adult With Self-Neglect

ASSESSMENT

Mrs. Baker is brought to the emergency department by ambulance attendants. Her mail carrier noticed that her mail had not been collected for 2 days and called 911. She is in a diabetic coma.

Mrs. Baker's past medical history is significant for heart failure, hypertension, diabetes, peripheral vascular disease, and depression.

A review of her social history reveals that Mrs. Baker is a 70-year-old widow whose only living relatives are her 95-year-old mother who lives in a nursing home 500 miles away and a daughter who lives 70 miles away. She lives alone in a lower-middle-class neighborhood in a modest but run-down home. She has a protective services caseworker who has tried to arrange help, but Mrs. Baker refuses. Her usual routine consists of eating an occasional meal (soup, a sandwich, or cereal), smoking two packs of cigarettes a day, drinking a pint of alcohol every 2 days, and lying on the sofa watching television. She rarely sees her neighbors and does not respond to her physician's request to see him. On occasion, she may answer her telephone or the doorbell. Last year she was the victim of fraud by two men claiming to protect her home from termites and water damage. She realizes she cannot fully maintain her home or herself on her own, but she refuses in-home assistance and is determined to stay in her home, manage her own money and affairs, and die there.

Mrs. Baker remains in the emergency department, receives her insulin, and is stabilized for admission. The nurse is unable to get an accurate history of her medications and cannot tell what she is taking. She refuses to answer any questions about a caregiver. She says she is completely independent and refuses to discuss her financial support. She denies being left alone for long periods of time and says she has all the contact she wants. She says she is able to express her needs and have them met.

Mrs. Baker's vital signs are as follows:

- Temperature: 98°F, oral
- Pulse: 70, regular
- Respiratory rate: 20
- Blood pressure: 210/100

DIAGNOSES

- Coping
- Ineffective Individual Protection
- Ineffective Self-Care Deficits
- Situational Low Self-Esteem
- Social Isolation
- Impaired Risk for Poisoning: Alcohol or Tobacco Abuse

PLANNING

The expected outcomes for the plan of care specify that Mrs. Baker will do the following:

- Become aware of the harmful effects of alcohol and tobacco on overall health status.
- Identify family and community supports that might allow her to return home and achieve her goal of spending the rest of her life there.
- Develop a more trusting and open relationship with her physician regarding her health status.
- Agree to establish a therapeutic relationship with the nurse and develop a mutually acceptable plan to work toward these outcomes.

IMPLEMENTATION

Establish a therapeutic relationship.

- Avoid being judgmental or using scare tactics.
- Encourage a family meeting with the daughter present to talk about health issues in general with Mrs. Baker's permission.
- Begin a mental status and mood assessment to establish the underlying cause of Mrs. Baker's self-neglect.
- Begin a values clarification to establish long-term goals and facilitate end-of-life planning.

EVALUATION

The nurse hopes to work with Mrs. Baker over time and realizes the sensitive nature of self-neglect in older people. The nurse will consider the plan a success based on the following criteria:

- During hospitalization, Mrs. Baker's condition will become stable and physical indicators of health status will improve (dehydration, nutrition, skin integrity, etc.).
- A family meeting will be held to discuss Mrs. Baker's overall health and values.
- She will accept counseling and discuss beginning to decrease her alcohol and tobacco consumption.
- Ongoing assessment of Mrs. Baker's cognitive status, mood, and resources will be conducted as her condition stabilizes.
- Appropriate discharge planning will take place, and safe living arrangements will be identified and used at the time of hospital discharge.

(continued)

NURSING CARE PLAN An Older Adult With Self-Neglect *continued*

CRITICAL THINKING

1. What is your emotional response to the thought of caring for an older person who has been mistreated?
2. Can you identify some unique reasons for elder mistreatment in your community?
3. Have you ever witnessed elder mistreatment during your clinical experiences as a student nurse?
4. Identify actions that can help relieve stress in family caregivers.

When the client is the aggressor, the nurse may take a number of steps to help the client learn how to change his or her behavior. Suggest appropriate expressions of anger such as talking out anger as it occurs; physical exercise; and striking safe, inanimate object (pillow, couch, punching bag). When people can use alternative expression of anger, the use of violence will decrease. Help the client establish limits and definite consequences if violence recurs. Setting and enforcement of limits may lead to the extinction of violence.

Evaluation

The nursing plan of care and client response to treatment may be based on the following outcomes, depending on nursing diagnoses selected:

- Victim remains safe.
- Abusive behavior ends.
- Victim develops an escape plan.
- Client manages conflict appropriately.
- Client verbalizes an internal locus of control.
- Client verbalizes an understanding of normal growth and development of children.
- Client implements appropriate and safe parenting techniques.
- Client utilizes community resources.

HEALTH CARE

Legal Issues

Every state in America has mechanisms for reporting elder mistreatment, and adult protective services (APS) programs exist in each state. Amendments to the Older Americans Act in 1987 included federal definitions of elder abuse. State to state variations do exist (Capezuti, Brush, & Lawson, 1997; Daly & Jogerst, 2006). Standards of care for nursing homes are based on policy stipulated in the Nursing Home Reform Act of 1987 (Omnibus Budget Reconciliation Act, 1987). This law was set forth to prevent substandard care and mistreatment of older adults. Many states currently have mandatory reporting laws for elder mistreatment, in which nurses and other health care practitioners are required by law to report suspected cases. In some states, failure by clinicians to report suspected incidents of mistreatment is a misdemeanor, punishable by fine or penalty (Capezuti et al., 1997). A national study of domestic elder abuse reports made in 1999 for all 50 states and Washington, DC (Jogerst et al., 2003) found that higher investigation rates were associated with a state-mandated reporting requirement and statutes specifying penalties for failure to report elder abuse. Therefore, the findings suggest that when systems are in place to address and resolve reports of mistreatment, health care professionals respond accordingly.

REVIEW Abuse

RELATE: LINK THE CONCEPTS

Linking the exemplar of Abuse with the concept of Development:

1. What protective factors would indicate a child who hasn't experienced abuse? At age 3? At age 15?
2. What factors would put them at risk?

Linking the exemplar of Abuse with the concept of Mood and Affect:

3. What mood and affect would you anticipate an abuse victim might display?
4. What nursing assessment regarding mood and affect would be a priority when admitting a client who was abused by a family member?

READY: GO TO COMPANION SKILLS MANUAL

- Evaluating client safety
- Maintaining nurses' safety
- Assessing home for safe environment
- Assessing for elder abuse

REFER: GO TO MYNURSINGKIT

REFLECT: CASE STUDY

Lucy Barnes, a 30-year-old woman who is 25 weeks pregnant, comes to the emergency department of Parkfield Community Hospital. She says she fell and hit her head at home and is having headaches. During the assessment the nurse notices multiple bruises in various stages of healing over her body and asks Lucy how she got them. Lucy says that she is just clumsy and falls a lot. While the nurse is assessing Lucy, another nurse enters the room to tell Lucy that her boyfriend is there to take her back home. At that point, Lucy becomes frightened and tells the nurse that her boyfriend has hit her many times before and had knocked her down today. She says he has threatened to kill her if she tells anyone and she does not want to leave with him.

1. Identify questions that the nurse could use in continuing her assessment and in documenting the discussion with Lucy.
2. What other people should be involved in Lucy's care in the Emergency Department?
3. Who should make the decision about where Lucy should go?

31.2 ASSAULT AND HOMICIDE

KEY TERMS

Aggravated assault, *1964*
Antisocial behavior, *1964*
Assault, *1963*
Intermittent explosive disorder (IED), *1963*

BASIS FOR SELECTION OF EXEMPLAR

National Center for Health Statistics
Centers for Disease Control and Prevention
Healthy People 2010

LEARNING OUTCOMES

After reading about this exemplar, you will be able to:

1. Describe the psychopathology, etiology, and clinical manifestations of assault and homicide.
2. Identify risk factors associated with assault and homicide.
3. Illustrate the nursing process in providing culturally competent care across the life span for victims of assault and individuals at risk for assault and homicide.
4. Formulate priority nursing diagnoses appropriate for an individual who has been assaulted and individuals at risk for assault and homicide.
5. Create a plan of care for individuals who have been assaulted and those at risk for assault and homicide and their family members.
6. Assess expected outcomes for an individual who has been assaulted or is at risk for assault or homicide.
7. Discuss therapies used in the collaborative care of an individual who has been assaulted or who is at risk for assault and homicide.
8. Employ evidence-based caring interventions for an individual who has been assaulted or is at risk for assault and homicide.

OVERVIEW

Multiple forms of physical assault take place each day in the United States. **Assault** is an "injury from an act of violence where physical force by one or more persons is used with the intent of causing harm, injury, or death to another person; or an intentional poisoning by another person" (CDC, 2007). This definition excludes unintentional acts of violence, such as accidental shootings or drug overdoses; assault involves intent. In 2006, 1.8 million people in the United States were treated for assault-related injuries in emergency departments (CDC, 2006).

PATHOPHYSIOLOGY AND ETIOLOGY

Violence may be a consequence of poor frustration tolerance, ineffective individual coping, impulsivity, and real or imagined threats to the person's territory, body space, or life. Aggressive behavior is a complex phenomenon that may occur in clients with substance use disorders, schizophrenia, mood disorders, borderline personality disorder, and conduct disorder. Aggression may be related to a lower level of activity in the cingulate gyrus and the frontal cortex, resulting in an underactive executive system. The result is a lack of inhibition messages and an inability to moderate aggressive thoughts and behaviors. Reduced activity of serotonin (5-HT), either genetically (50% of the cases) or because of early brain injury (prenatal alcohol exposure), is a risk factor in aggression but is not enough by itself. When low 5-HT is combined with other genetic factors and environmental stressors, impulsiveness and aggression may be triggered. With the onset of environmental stressors, there is a rapid release of norepinepherine (NE), resulting in increased arousal and attention. This may also contribute to an increase in aggressive behavior. Some people taking antidepressant medication that increases NE may experience agitation and irritability as a side effect (Frankle et al., 2005; Perusse & Gendreau, 2005; Pihl & Benkelfat, 2005).

When an individual learns that acting on aggressive impulses brings a kind of relief, that person can rely on aggression as a way to solve problems and relieve frustrations. This makes it very difficult to control angry outbursts. Other factors related to societal violence include personal pressures such as lack of social support, employment difficulties, or financial problems; an easy access to weapons; and the tendency in U.S. culture to condone violence as a solution to problems (Woodside & McClum, 2006).

Explosive behavior may be the result of organic disease, such as temporal lobe epilepsy, dementia, delirium, hypoxia, or hypoglycemia. Explosive behavior may also be related to substance use, substance withdrawal, and antisocial personality disorder. In these situations, the diagnosis of intermittent explosive disorder is not appropriate.

Intermittent explosive disorder (IED) is a *DSM-IV-TR* diagnosis. The affected person has episodes of aggressive impulses that result in serious assaultive acts or destruction of property. The degree of aggressiveness is grossly out of proportion with the associated stress. Clients may experience rage and increased energy during the episode, and depressed mood, fatigue, and remorse after the acts. This disorder results in severe psychosocial and legal consequences. It may begin as early as childhood or as late as the 20s. Among young people, IED is on the increase, and it may set the stage for the onset of other mental disorders. Two things generally set these people off: perceived threats and frustrating situations. For some people it is a temporary condition, while for others it has a long-term course (American Psychiatric Association, 2000; Kessler et al., 2006).

Sociocultural factors play a considerable part in the occurrence of societal violence. Social disorganization theories of homicide, for example, suggest that the inability of communities to realize the common values of their members and maintain social controls on behavior contribute to homicide. In other theoretical perspectives, homicide is an instrumental act designed to obtain money or property denied one because of economic hardship or lack of opportunity. A third perspective posits that homicide arises out of a subculture of violence in which violence is perceived as a legitimate means of conflict resolution (Cubbin et al., 2000).

Etiology

The most extreme form of assault results in homicide; 18,573 homicides occurred in 2006 in the United States. However, homicide rates have declined significantly in recent years, from 10.2 per 100,000 population in 1980 to 6.2 per 100,000 in 2003 (BJS, 2005b; CDC, 2006). These figures are somewhat misleading in that part of the decline in homicide-related fatalities lies in better medical care for those who have been assaulted. Some authors believe a more accurate indicator of societal violence is the rate of aggravated assault. An **aggravated assault** is one in which a weapon is used or in which serious injury is inflicted (U.S. Census Bureau, 2006).

Frequently, societal violence involves the use of weapons, which are readily available among the general public. Evidence of this is seen in the fact that nearly one fifth of California adolescents reported having access to firearms at home (Sorenson & Vittes, 2004). Similarly, 18.5% of high school students in the 2005 Youth Risk Behavior Surveillance (YRBS) survey admitted carrying a weapon in the last 30 days and 6.5% of students carried a weapon to school. In addition, nearly 8% of the students indicated that they had been threatened or injured with a weapon at school. Overall, more than 35% of the students reported being involved in a physical fight in the prior year and 3% reported being injured in a fight (Eaton et al., 2006).

Risk Factors

Risk factors for assault include age, culture, socioeconomic status, and occupational factors. While anyone can be assaulted, it is most often perpetrated on a known associate and is often the result of interfamily conflict.

AGE In the Unites States, homicide is the 4th leading cause of death in children aged 1–9 years, the 3rd leading cause of death in those 10–14 years of age, and the 2nd leading cause among those 15–24 years of age (CDC, 2006). Overall, homicide causes 15% of deaths in the 10- to 24-year-old age group (Grunbaum et al., 2004), with higher rates of occurrence among African American, Hispanic, American Indian/Alaska Native, and Asian/Pacific Islander youth than among White youth (NCIPC, 2006f). Homicide is also the 15th leading cause of death in infants, with the greatest risk of death occurring on the day of birth and 9% of deaths occurring in the first week of life (Division of Violence Prevention, 2002c). Among homicides that occur during the first week of life, 89% of perpetrators are female, usually the mother. Mothers who kill their infants are more likely to be adolescents and have a history of mental illness.

In addition to being victims of violence, youth also perpetrate societal violence. In 2002, juveniles accounted for 12% of all violent crime in the United States, including 5% of murders, 12% of rapes, and 12% of aggravated assaults (Snyder, 2004). Firearms were even more likely to be used by youth for homicide than suicide (73% vs. 62%) (Snyder & Swahn, 2004).

CULTURE Similarly, homicide is the sixth leading cause of death among all African Americans, but fifth among African American men and sixth among American Indian/Alaska Native and Hispanic men. Among women, neither homicide nor suicide ranks in the top 10 causes of death for any racial or ethnic group (National Center for Health Statistics [NCHS], 2005).

Urban settings have higher rates of firearm homicides than rural areas, perhaps due to greater ease of access to firearms (Branas, Nance, Elliott, Richmond, & Schwab, 2004). Similarly, workplaces and other settings with limited visibility, such as poorly lit streets and parking lots, increase the potential for violent victimization.

For youth, association with delinquent peers, gang involvement, and social rejection by peers may contribute to increased violence. At the community level, social disorganization, diminished economic opportunities, increased transience, and low levels of community participation have been linked to violence among youth. Conversely, religiosity, intolerant attitudes to deviance, family connectedness, high parental performance expectations, and parental supervision have been linked to decreased risk of youth violence, as have commitment to school and involvement in social activities (NCIPC, 2006f).

SOCIOECONOMIC FACTORS Community violence is associated with economic inequality. Extremes of poverty and racism contribute to the trauma of children and become breeding grounds for violence, as evidenced by a higher incidence of violence in poor communities. In the United States, 1 in 10 adults and 1 in 5 children live in poverty. Poverty is not an equal-opportunity condition: African American and Latino children, as well as children from mother-only families, are disproportionately poor. Families who are struggling to just put food on the table may have minimal time to supervise the children, who are then more likely to act out.

Poverty also affects the child's chance for school success. Poor academic performance, expulsion, and dropout rates are common indicators of unsuccessful youth functioning. The more children and adolescents are turned off by, and turned away from, the school system, the more they tend to associate with and seek approval from antisocial peers. In addition to poverty, experiencing racism is also a factor. Those who are subjected to racism experience humiliation, powerlessness, and rage and may act out in retaliatory violence. Racism and poverty create chaotic environments, making children vulnerable to violence as victims, witnesses, and perpetrators (Shelton, 2000).

Research has shown that youths who engage in high levels of **antisocial behavior** (behavior that deviates significantly from established norms) are much more likely than other youths to have a biological parent who also engages in antisocial behavior. This association is thought to reflect the genetic transmission of predisposing temperament, the modeling of aggression, and the lack of control over expression of negative emotions. It is also believed that ineffective and inconsistent discipline and poor supervision contribute to antisocial behavior in children (Herrenkohl, Hill, Hawkins, Chung, & Nagin, 2006).

Childhood abuse and neglect place children at increased risk for violent criminal behavior. Child abuse and neglect often occur in chronically dysfunctional families, and it may be difficult to disentangle the effect of abuse and neglect from the effect of other stressors. Children living in abusive and neglectful families may also experience parental separations, poor physical and emotional health of their caretakers, and the need to cope with financial and social problems.

All children tend to make friends with peers who are similar to themselves. This becomes socially significant when antisocial children form groups and reinforce one another's antisocial behavior. By adolescence, violence can be the membership card for entry into some adolescent peer groups. Most studies that compare the relative effects of parental supervision and peer deviance find that peer deviance is a stronger predictor of delinquency than the family.

Another social factor that influences societal violence is media attention. Some authors contend that unbalanced media attention to some types of homicide (e.g., of children or by children) provides the public with an inaccurate view of the problem that hampers their ability to engage in effective problem solving. Others suggest that exposure to media violence is a causal factor in homicide and suicide. The media no longer presents extensive coverage of youth suicides, for example, because of the known effect seen in cluster suicides. The contention is made that similar coverage of adolescent homicide creates inappropriate role models for vulnerable youth. In some counties, in fact, reporting of the names and images of juvenile criminals is prohibited in efforts to prevent "copycat" violence (Grossman, 2000).

The availability of lethal weapons, particularly guns, is another social factor that influences violence. Firearm-associated homicides in the United States exceed those of 25 other developed nations (Hahn et al., 2003b). Firearms are used in approximately 67% of homicides and in 49% of suicides (Office of Statistics and Programming, 2003; U.S. Census Bureau, 2006). In one study, firearms were more likely to be found in homes of women subjected to IPV than in other households, and in two thirds of these homes, intimate partners had either threatened to shoot the women or had actually shot them (Sorenson & Weibe, 2004). Findings of another study indicated that the risk of IPV ending in homicide increased with perpetrator access to a gun and previous threats with a weapon (Campbell et al., 2003). At the community level, areas where household firearm ownership rates are high also have high rates of homicide (Miller, Azrael, & Hemenway, 2002). In the 2005 YRBS, 18.5% of high school students reported carrying a weapon, and more than 5% carried a gun (Eaton et al., 2006), attesting to the easy availability of weapons to U.S. youth.

Although schools are often perceived as safe places for children, violence occurs in schools on a regular basis. From 1994 to 1996, for example, 126 school-related fatalities occurred as a result of homicide and suicide (Division of Violence Prevention, 2003a), and several events included both homicide and suicide (Division of Violence Prevention, 2003b). Frequently, societal violence involves the use of weapons, which are readily available among the general public.

OCCUPATION Occupation is another social factor to be addressed in assessing contributions to societal violence. Assault, homicide, suicide, and intimate partner violence all occur in work settings. The National Institute for Occupational Safety and Health (NIOSH) has defined workplace violence as "violent acts, including physical assaults and threats of assault directed toward individuals at work or on duty" (as quoted in Anderson, 2004, p. 24). Each year more than 1 million workers are assaulted in the work setting, and workplace violence accounts for 15% of all violence affecting the U.S. population 12 years of age and over. Workplace violence results in 1.75 million work days lost each year at a cost of $55 million in lost wages. These figures exclude days lost as annual leave or sick days (Anderson, 2004).

Workplace homicides are the second leading cause of job-related deaths. The workers at greatest risk are those who exchange money with the public, make deliveries, carry passengers in vehicles, work alone or in small groups during late night or early morning hours, or work in community settings in high crime areas. Robbery is the primary motive of job-related homicide; together with disputes among coworkers and with customers or clients they accounted for the most fatalities (OSHA, 2002).

In the United States, health care professionals are at greater risk for violence than other service workers, and nurses are the health care professionals at greatest risk. The U.S. Occupational Safety and Health Administration (OSHA) published Guidelines for Preventing Workplace Violence for Health Care and Social Service Workers in 2002. These guidelines consist of four main components: (1) management commitment and employee involvement, (2) worksite analysis, (3) hazard prevention and control, and (4) safety and health training. The training for employees should include recognizing potential violence, defusing violence, and dealing with the aftermath of violence. Topics suggested for the training programs are as follows:

- The institution's workplace violence prevention policy
- Early recognition of escalating behavior
- Ways of defusing volatile situations, managing anger, and appropriately using medications.

CLINICAL MANIFESTATIONS

It is much better to prevent aggressive behavior than to manage it. In some instances, no matter what preventive actions are undertaken, aggression will erupt. The goal is to decrease the likelihood of this happening; nurses are in the position to identify the potential for aggressive behaviors before outbursts occur.

Several studies have shown that children who witness violence display more internalizing (withdrawn, anxious, depressed) behavior, whereas those who are victims display more externalizing (aggressive, disruptive) behavior. Those children who witness community violence watch from the sidelines, recognizing their own inability to change the situation. This sense of helplessness contributes to internalizing behavior. On the other hand, children who are victimized by

Box 31–5 Warning Signs of Violent Behavior in Children

- Truancy, suspension, and expulsion from school
- Little or no parental or adult supervision
- Is a loner and has few or no friends
- Mistreats animals
- Is a victim of neglect, abuse, or both
- Has been bullied
- History of aggressive and violent behavior
- Has made serious threats of violence
- Psychosis
- Romantic obsessions or erotomanic delusions
- Chemical dependency
- Depression and suicidality
- Pathological blaming, feelings of persecution
- Impaired neurological functioning
- Personality disorder
- Interest in firearms, bombs
- Affiliation with gangs

community violence are more likely to learn aggressive, externalizing behavior as a means of self-protection or a way of relating to others, growing into violent adults.

Thinking drives behavior, and violent individuals think of violent solutions to perceived offenses against them. They may live in an inner fantasy world with frequent thoughts of anger, revenge, and justifiable rage. Crime-prone persons are more likely to display cognitive deficits and distortions and have a tendency to process information incorrectly when making decisions. Crime is a convenient way to satisfy their individual needs, which take precedence over societal responsibilities (Ward & Stewart, 2003).

Aggressive behavior can range from slaps, pushes, or shoves in play to serious attempts to hurt another person. The best predictor of future violence in a client is a *history of violent behavior*. Early warning signs are just that—indicators that a person may need help. Nurses must assess the situation and get help for the client before problems escalate. It is important, however, to avoid inappropriately labeling or stigmatizing because individuals appear to fit a specific profile. Early warning signs should not be used as a rationale to exclude, isolate, or punish an individual. It is important to be aware of false cues—including race, socioeconomic status, cognitive or academic ability, or physical appearance. People who are at risk for violence typically exhibit multiple warning signs, repeatedly, and with increasing intensity (Box 31–5).

Imminent warning signs indicate that a person is very close to behaving in a way that is potentially dangerous to self or others. These signs require an immediate response. No single sign can predict that a dangerous act will occur. Usually, they are presented as a sequence of serious, hostile threats or behaviors directed at peers, family, staff, or other individuals. Imminent warning signs may include the following:

- Serious physical fighting with family or peers
- Severe destruction of property
- Severe rage for seemingly minor reasons
- Detailed threats of lethal violence
- Possession or use of firearms or other weapons
- Other self-injurious behaviors or threats of suicide.

Medication may be necessary to help clients whose aggression is organic in origin.

COLLABORATION

A multidisciplinary approach is necessary when dealing with the violence of assault and homicide. Preventive activities at the community level involve school nurses and counselors, health department nurses, social workers, protective services personnel, police, and workplace programs. Professionals can identify those at risk for victimization and those at risk of committing violent acts and intervene by offering appropriate training, such as anger management or strategies for school safety.

Multidisciplinary approaches are also necessary when working with victims of homicide and assault and their families. Upon arriving at the hospital, a client with a serious gunshot wound, for example, will require care by the trauma team, which may include a trauma physician, a surgeon, several nurses, an infection specialist, a cardiologist, and a pulmonologist. An assault victim who has broken bones will require orthopedic care. The victim and family members may require counseling and spiritual guidance.

Violence Prevention Programs for Children

One way in which many communities are providing a multidisciplinary approach is to offer violence prevention programs in schools, child care centers, churches, and other community programs where children and adults gather. A number of evidence-based curricula exist, which can be offered by nurses, teachers, social workers, or other professionals. Some of the most effective programs include a home teaching component that gets parents involved. Two such violence prevention programs are offered by the Committee for Children (www.cfchildren.org). *Second Step: A Violence Prevention Program* is designed to teach children of various ages how to solve problems and manage anger, and includes a home teaching component. *Steps to Respect: A Bullying Prevention Program* is designed to teach children why bullying is not appropriate, how it affects others, and how to manage their own anger.

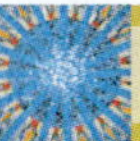

DEVELOPMENTAL CONSIDERATIONS Young Children and Anger Management

As children begin to understand language, we can gradually teach and reinforce some basic principles—not just with words, but also with our actions and example. Here are some concepts to stress and reinforce with young children:

- It's okay to be angry.
- There are "okay" ways and "not okay" ways to show our anger.
- It's not okay to hurt anyone, to break or throw things, or to hurt pets when we are angry.
- It's okay to tell someone that we are angry.
- There are ways to calm ourselves when we are angry.

Source: American Psychological Association. (n.d.). Retrieved September 9, 2009, from http://actagainstviolence.apa.org/materials/publications/act/violenceprevention_childhood.pdf

NURSING PROCESS

The nurse who is caring for a victim of assault needs to document all findings and care in specific detail. The likelihood of the medical record being entered into evidence at the legal proceeding against the person who committed the assault is high, and proper documentation can play a significant role in convicting the criminal. Wounds should be accurately and precisely described, client's emotional state should be described as objectively as possible, and any specimens collected must follow the legal chain of custody procedure.

Assessment

Assessment of risk for violence differs from the assessment of a client who is the victim of violence, except that the nurse's assessment of the client who is a victim should include an assessment of the client's risk for revictimization.

Assessment of Risk in the Community

Assessment related to societal violence may entail identification of risk factors at individual/family or population levels. For example, nurses working with families would assess them for factors that increase their risk for family violence, suicide, or homicide. In addition, nurses would be alert to the signs and symptoms of actual family violence or signs of impending suicide. At the community or population level, nurses would identify risk factors that lend themselves to high incidence and prevalence of societal violence. For example, they would identify unemployment or other causes of social stress (e.g., homelessness, racial/ethnic tension) as risk factors for social violence. Information on risk factors for and the incidence and prevalence of violence would be used to derive nursing diagnoses and to plan strategies to minimize or control societal violence. Because nurses are in a position to intervene with clients at a young age, the focus of this assessment will be the youth at-risk for violent behavior.

Assessment of Victims of Assault or Homicide

Assessment of the victim of assault or homicide will follow the assessment guidelines for trauma that are detailed in the About section of this concept. Primary consideration should be given to assessment of the airway and assessment of hemorrhaging. Assessment of the client prior to discharge should include assessing the risk for revictimization. Nurses should follow agency policy regarding notifying law enforcement or social services.

Diagnosis

Based on assessment data, the nurse formulates nursing diagnoses for the potential perpetrators of community violence. Some examples of possible nursing diagnoses with this population are (North American Nursing Diagnosis Association, 2007):

- Risk for Loneliness related to excessive feelings of isolation and rejection from peers
- Self-Esteem Disturbance related to beliefs of being bullied by others
- Fear related to being a victim of being teased, bullied, ridiculed, or humiliated
- Impaired Social Interaction related to an intolerance for diversity among peers and prejudicial attitudes
- Risk for Violence to Others related to threats of violence, past violent behavior, uncontrolled anger, and possession of firearms or other weapons.

Diagnoses for a victim of assault or attempted homicide is largely dependent on what injuries are incurred and may include the following:

- Deficient Fluid Volume
- Ineffective Breathing Pattern
- Decreased Cardiac Output
- Impaired Spontaneous Ventilation
- Risk Prone Health Behavior
- Impaired Skin Integrity
- Impaired Tissue Integrity.

Plan

Appropriate goals of care are highly dependent on the type and extent of injury, the client's general condition and age, as well as the unique needs of the individual. Broad goals that may be used include the following:

- The client is comfortable and reports pain level of 3 or less.
- The client's fluid status is returned to homeostasis.
- The client verbalizes feelings related to event.
- The client's wounds heal without infection.
- The client will verbalize an internal locus of control.
- The client will use nonviolent expressions of anger and self calming techniques.
- The client will relate appropriately to several peers.
- The client will accept responsibility for his or her own behavior.
- The client will attend school or work.

- The client will receive treatment for injuries sustained during the assault.
- The client will remain free from harm, verbalize feeling safe, and be appropriately supervised (if necessary).
- The client and family will receive referrals for counseling and social support as necessary.
- The family of a homicide victim will receive referrals for grief counseling.

Implementation

Because of the prevalence of youth violence, some of the interventions in this section related to prevention are directed at prevention efforts that may be used with children and adolescents.

Helping Young Children Learn to Manage Anger

Because violence-prone children often experience explosive outbursts, they need to learn *coping skills* to help them avoid aggression in the future. Giving choices to the child who is acting out is often effective. "There are two quieter places you may go to: your room or the deck. Which one would you like?" Each time a choice is given, the child must pause and consider the options. Each pause decreases the amount of energy behind the anger. Giving choices also helps children feel they have some control in the situation. It is best to intervene before the behavior escalates to out-of-control aggression.

Assist in identifying the source of the anger, and establish the expectation that the child can control the behavior. Direct the child to seek assistance before lashing out with aggressive behavior. If appropriate, provide physical outlets for the expression of anger or tension. Help the child identify the benefits of expressing anger in an adaptive, nonviolent way, as well as identify the consequences of inappropriate expression of anger. Teach the child calming measures, such as deep breathing and self-controlled time-outs, when beginning to feel aggressive.

Setting Limits

When working with children and adolescents who have limited self-control, it is critical to set appropriate limits. Limit setting reinforces the predictability of the environment. Learning about and accepting external limits assists these individuals in developing internal controls. If the child or adolescent is institutionalized, the staff should adopt a *solution focus* rather than a *problem focus*, such as "What can we do to solve this problem?" rather than "What is the cause of this problem?" When unwanted behavior occurs, staff should help children identify clearly what the desirable, positive alternative is, in behavioral terms. The nurse may find it helpful to develop *behavioral contracts* with some children. The contract, which is mutually created, has clear behavioral expectations, states how these are to be achieved, and relates achievement to particular rewards. Consequences for inappropriate behavior must be immediate, logical, and appropriate to the child's age.

Facilitating Self-Responsibility

The goal of the interventions is to help children overcome their defensiveness and their tendency to blame others. Children who are at risk for becoming violent often are unable or unwilling to accept responsibility for their choices and behaviors. The nurse may hear, "She started it," or "I couldn't help it; he made me do it." Even young children can be taught the concept of good choices versus bad choices. The nurse needs to establish reasonable and meaningful consequences for both good and bad decisions. Excuses are not accepted for bad choices and the focus returns to the child's personal decisions regarding behavior. If self-esteem is low or the child does not have good coping skills, a defensive coping stance is often assumed. Nursing intervention should aim to provide positive and honest feedback, help the child develop insight about how others perceive him or her, and assist him or her in connecting behavior to his or her feeling of inadequacy.

Improving Socialization

The inability to develop empathy for others decreases a child's social sensitivity and leads to peer disapproval and conflict. Because they are unable to put themselves in another's place, they demonstrate little or no empathy unless it is to manipulate someone. They often have no concept of how they have hurt another's feelings.

Because some of these children have learned violence from being treated disrespectfully, it is helpful if the nurse role-plays positive interactions. Treat the child with warmth, friendliness, humor, empathy, and unconditional positive regard. Minimize the amount of attention given for negative behavior and maximize the amount of attention given for desirable and positive behavior.

Some violence-prone individuals alienate their peers by interrupting others, intruding in particular situations, invading personal space, and treating others' property as if it were their own. When youths experience conflict with peers or adults, they often refuse to back down, even on little points. It is important that the nurse avoid power struggles, which can be damaging to a child's self-esteem. It is better to act as a role model to teach children how to negotiate differences and how to admit to errors.

Nursing interventions are also directed at helping these children establish and maintain social relationships. Being a role model is an effective way to demonstrate social skills such as giving and receiving compliments, sharing, conflict resolution, and personal boundary issues. Because violence-prone children often use anger to control people, they may become abusive, aggressive, or threatening. Feedback and consequences must be immediate to avoid reinforcing this inappropriate behavior.

The nurse should structure the child's environment to allow for success. It is very important to clearly state the rules and expectations. It is important to provide frequent, immediate, and consistent feedback regarding appropriate and inappropriate social behavior. The nurse may select particular peers to interact with the child. It is best to begin with one-on-one interactions. Suggestions include that the child work with one child at the computer, another child while problem solving, and a different child in free play. As the child's social skills improve, two or more children can be included in each of the groups.

Care of the Client With a Gunshot Wound

Gunshot wounds require a specific and sometimes complex set of interventions. As a result, the entire trauma team is usually activated upon receiving notification by law enforcement or emergency services of the imminent arrival of the victim of a gunshot wound.

Possible injuries from gunshot wounds include, but are not limited to, the following:

- Eye injury, skull fracture, brain injury
- Pneumothorax, hemothorax, pulmonary contusion
- Organ and tissue damage, nerve and vascular damage.

Gunshot wounds may be classified in a variety of ways: by nature (e.g., contact or noncontact wound, entry or exit wound), size, or severity. Clinical priorities for the treatment of gunshot wound are as following:

- Maintain airway and assist ventilation as necessary.
- Control hemorrhage.
- Prevent hypothermia.

Rapid, recurrent assessment of neurologic status is also necessary, as is infection control. Bleeding can result in hypovolemia, leading to inadequate perfusion and oxygenation of tissues.

Family members of gunshot victims typically are very upset and often very angry. An experienced nurse should work closely with these families while the victim is being treated.

Gunshot victims may themselves display dangerous behaviors. If law enforcement has not determined that the victim is free of weapons, such an assessment should be done before treatment is initiated. Violent or angry victims may need to be restrained during treatment for the protection of the trauma team. Law enforcement may assign officers to remain present during treatment.

Because the majority of gunshot wounds require an investigation by law enforcement, nurses working in emergency departments and trauma centers should be familiar with their agency's protocols for maintaining evidence required by law enforcement. Often, law enforcement does not want the victim's hands or the area around the victim's wounds cleansed. Clothes and personal items are often wanted as evidence (Taylor, 2009).

Evaluation

Client response to nursing care is evaluated based on the client's nursing diagnoses and specific needs and may include the following:

- Client obtains pain relief allowing for adequate rest and comfort.
- Client seeks counseling as needed to deal with emotions caused by the assault.
- Family provides support and comfort to client.
- Wound heals appropriately.
- Client is able to return to work or school.
- Client accepts responsibility for own actions.

REVIEW Assault and Homicide

RELATE: LINK THE CONCEPTS

Linking the exemplar of Assault and Homicide with the concept of Addition Behaviors:

1. You are caring for a client with addiction to alcohol who presents to the clinic for treatment of injuries incurred when he became assaultive in the bar where he had been drinking. What teaching is appropriate for this client while he is under the influence of alcohol? What follow-up care will you recommend?
2. How will you intervene with the client who threatens to assault you in the emergency room and is known to be under the influence of cocaine?

Linking the exemplar of Assault and Homicide with the concept of Family:

3. What is your priority nursing diagnosis for the family of a client who was assaulted because the client is homosexual?
4. What communication strategy will you use when talking with the 8-year-old child who is visiting his mother shot during a home robbery?

READY: GO TO COMPANION SKILLS MANUAL

- Administering oxygen by cannula, face mask, or face tent
- Inserting an oropharyngeal airway
- Assisting with endotracheal intubation
- Caring for a client on a mechanical ventilator
- Administering automated external defibrillation
- Performing surgical and antisepsis
- Maintaining nurses' safety

REFER: GO TO MYNURSINGKIT

REFLECT: CASE STUDY

Kevin, a 4th grader, told his classmate Tran that he was going to shoot him with a gun if Tran continued making fun of him at school. Tran's parents contacted the children's teacher, Mr. Salazar, expressing strong concerns about the safety of their son and demanding that the school take action against Kevin. During a faculty meeting, Mr. Salazar shared with the other teachers that Kevin is a shy student who had relocated from another state at the beginning of the school year, does not seem to have any friends, and struggles with his studies. Kevin's parents' divorce is still in progress two years after they officially separated; they are still disputing financial and child custody issues. Two months ago, Kevin was arrested for vandalizing his father's car after an argument, but the charges were dropped. This is the first time Kevin has made such a threat at school. Mr. Salazar is asking for input from his colleagues and the school nurse on how to handle the situation.

1. What actions could the nurse take to support the faculty in understanding this student's potential for violence?
2. List at least four warning signs that teachers should watch for to detect the potential for violent behavior from Kevin.
3. List at least three outcomes that would be included in a comprehensive plan of care to address Kevin's aggressive behavior.
4. List at least three actions you would suggest the teachers can take to effectively communicate with this student and deescalate his aggressive behavior.

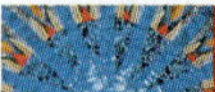

31.3 RAPE-TRAUMA SYNDROME

KEY TERMS

Acquaintance rape, *1970*
Date rape, *1970*
Marital rape, *1970*
Post-traumatic stress disorder (PTSD), *1972*
Rape, *1970*
Rape-trauma syndrome, *1970*

BASIS FOR SELECTION OF EXEMPLAR

Health People 2010

LEARNING OUTCOMES

After reading about this exemplar, you will be able to:

1. Describe the pathophysiology, etiology, and clinical manifestations of rape-trauma syndrome.
2. Identify risk factors associated with rape-trauma syndrome.
3. Illustrate the nursing process in providing culturally competent care across the life span for individuals experiencing rape-trauma syndrome.
4. Formulate priority nursing diagnoses appropriate for an individual experiencing rape-trauma syndrome.
5. Create a plan of care for individuals expereincing rape-trauma syndrome and their family members.
6. Assess expected outcomes for an individual experiencing rape-trauma syndrome.
7. Discuss therapies used in the collaborative care of an individual experiencing rape-trauma syndrome.
8. Employ evidence-based caring interventions for an individual experiencing rape-trauma syndrome.

OVERVIEW

Sexual assault and rape are crimes of violence. The issue is not one of sex but of force, domination, and humiliation. **Rape** refers to any forced sexual activity; the key factor is the absence of consent. The victim's response to this act of violence is referred to as **rape-trauma syndrome**.

There is no typical rape victim. Of reported rapes, however, 90–95% of the victims are female and 90% of the perpetrators are male. Given these percentages, this concept utilizes the male rapist and female victim as the model. Approximately half of rape victims are raped by a spouse, partner, relative, or friend. **Date rape**, also known as **acquaintance rape**, refers to rape by a (usually) new acquaintance with whom the woman has chosen to spend time. Typically, there is less physical violence and more coercion and deception involved in date rapes.

Certain drugs are called "rape drugs" because they can be used to overpower and incapacitate victims to facilitate a sexual assault. Rohypnol is a benzodiazepine drug that is illegal in the United States. Gamma-hydroxybutyrate (GHB) has euphoric and sedative effects. Ketamine is a dissociative general anesthetic used by veterinarians. These drugs are often slipped into a victim's drink without the victim's knowledge or consent. When dissolved, they are colorless, odorless, and often tasteless. All three of these drugs can be fatal when mixed with alcohol.

In 1993, **marital rape** became a crime in all 50 states. Some states, however, still have exemptions from prosecuting husbands for rape. Marital rape is the most prevalent and underreported form of rape; 2 million instances are estimated to occur each year in the United States. Between one third and one half of battered women are raped by their partners. Women who are raped by their husbands or partners are less likely to report the assault or to seek professional help (Rauch & Foa, 2004).

Some men who rape their wives see the rape as punishment for perceived wrongs. Others believe they have a right to sex on demand and that when sex is refused they have a right to take it. For other perpetrators, rape is a way to assert power and control. Some may even try to impregnate their wives to ensure that they will not leave the relationship. Others become angered over pregnancy and increase the level of violence in an attempt to abort the fetus.

The myth of male-on-male rape has been that it occurs only where heterosexual contact is not possible, such as in prisons or in isolated living conditions. As more male rape victims report the crime, however, this myth is being debunked. It is estimated that 5–10% of all sexual assault victims are men. Male victims as a group are more likely to have been beaten and are more reluctant to reveal the sexual component of their assaults. Homosexual victims fear police prejudice, and heterosexual victims feel shame and confusion regarding their own sexuality. Male-on-male rape is not a homosexual attack. Just as in female rape, the issue is one of violence and domination rather than of sex. It should also be noted that men can be raped by women because an erection can be evinced through stimulation, even then the man does not wish to have sex.

PATHOPHYSIOLOGY AND ETIOLOGY

Theorists in many disciplines have studied the crime of rape in an effort to understand the causes and develop preventive measures. Most agree that rape is a crime of violence generated by issues of power and anger rather than by sex drive.

Intrapersonal Factors

Many convicted sex offenders meet the criteria for antisocial, schizoid, paranoid, and narcissistic personality disorders. Rapists are typically young; the average age is 31 years old (U.S. Department of Justice, 2005). Two thirds of sex offenders in prison report being victimized as children (Sexual Abuse Statistics, n.d.).

The causes of rape are many, but the dynamics of the act are that perpetrators abuse their own and others' sexuality as a method of discharging anger and frustration.

Interpersonal Factors

Most rapists do not have normal interpersonal involvements. Preoccupied with their own fantasies, they want to control and dominate others rather than engage in mutually satisfying relationships. With this model in mind, a rapist sees no need for consent to sexual activity, particularly from a wife or partner. The husband may view the rape as merely a disagreement over sexual behavior. If the wife has said she does not want to engage in sex and the husband uses force, her control and autonomy have been violated. When sex occurs without consent, it is rape.

Sociocultural Factors

The acceptance of interpersonal violence in a culture contributes to a higher incidence of rape. Societal approval of the use of intimidation, coercion, and force to achieve a goal promotes an excessive level of violence. Violent behavior is an expression of power and strength, and individual rights are disregarded.

Aggression is learned through three primary sources: family and peers, culture/subculture, and the mass media. The modeling effect occurs when potential offenders see rape scenes and other acts of violence against women in real life or in the media, in slasher and horror films, in violent pornography, video games, and degrading music lyrics. These media contribute to the process of desensitization; with repeated exposure, viewers become numb to the pain, fear, and humiliation of sexual aggression (Huesmann, Moise-Titus, Podolski, & Eron, 2003; Martino et al., 2006).

Gender-Bias Factors

From the gender-bias perspective, rape is the result of long and deeply rooted socioeconomic traditions. Worldwide, men dominate most political and economic activities, and women are viewed as subservient and relatively powerless. At the furthest extreme, women are viewed as property. Sexual gratification is not the prime motive in rape; rather, sex is used to establish or maintain control of one person by another. When women are considered inferior to men, tacit approval is given for coercion and force. These stereotypes support the false beliefs that, at times, women deserve to be raped, that they may want or need to be raped, and that rape does not cause them much physical or emotional damage.

Etiology

Police records indicate that a woman is raped every 6 minutes in the United States. Experts believe that 80% of rapes are unreported. It is believed that one of every three or four American women will be raped or sexually assaulted at least once in her lifetime. In addition, 50% of victims are raped by a spouse, partner, relative, or friend (Rauch & Foa, 2004; Stermac, Dunlap, & Bainbridge, 2005).

Of all rapes of women on college campuses, 50% are date rapes. Women very rarely report rapes when they know their attackers, especially if they are or were in a dating relationship with the attacker. The victim is often blamed by herself and others for being naive or provocative.

Risk Factors

Gender is the primary risk factor for rape. However, according to the World Health Organization (2002), other factors include the following:

- Youth
- Alcohol or drug use
- Having been previously raped or sexually abused
- Having many sexual partners
- Being a sex worker (e.g., prostitute, sex slave)
- Becoming more educated and economically empowered
- Poverty.

Risk factors for perpetrators include the following:

- Alcohol and drug use
- Lacking inhibitions to suppress associations between sex and aggression
- Holding attitudes and beliefs supportive of sexual violence, including coercive sexual fantasies
- A pattern of behavior that is impulsive, antisocial, and hostile toward women
- Associating with sexually aggressive peers
- Having been sexually abused as a child
- Growing up in a family environment characterized by physical violence, little emotional support, and few economic resources.

CLINICAL MANIFESTATIONS

Although some rape survivors do not develop major symptoms in response to the trauma, as many as 25% continue to have signs of impairment a year after the assault. A variety of factors contribute to the response, including age or developmental state, history of prior victimization, the relationship to the offender, precrisis coping abilities, and the ability to use support resources. Response factors related to the rape itself include severity of the rape, duration, frequency, number of offenders, and degree of violence. Environmental factors contributing to a rape victim's response are quality and continuity of social supports and community attitudes and values (American Psychiatric Association, 2000).

Victims of rape have immediate and long-lasting emotional trauma. After a period of shock and disbelief, many experience episodes of fear. Fear can result from a stimulus directly associated with the attack, such as a penis, the act of oral sex, or a person who looks like the offender. There are also fears of rape consequences such as pregnancy; sexually transmitted infections, especially HIV; talking to the police; and testifying in court. In addition, there are fears related to potential future attacks, which underlie fears of getting close to men, of being alone, and of being in a strange place. Typically, the level of fear peaks around the third week, but it may take a long time for the level to decrease.

Immediate responses take place during the acute phase, which occurs immediately following the rape and may continue for a number of weeks. As the victim begins to cope with the rape, he or she enters the reorganizational phase. Symptoms of trauma may continue to occur during this time, as the survivor actively seeks ways to resolve these and to regain control over his or her life. If the survivor is unable to find appropriate treatment and resolution, he or she may develop **post-traumatic stress disorder (PTSD)**, an anxiety disorder that can evolve after exposure to a traumatic or overwhelming event in which an individual's physical health was endangered. See Exemplar 28.5 in Concept 28, Stress and Coping, for more information on PTSD. Survivors who are successful during the reorganizational phase eventually enter the recovery phase.

Physical Injuries

Rape usually results in a number of physical injuries as the result of being beaten, stabbed, or shot. Profuse bleeding and trauma to vital organs may be critical problems. Most likely, the vagina or rectum will be painful or swollen. There may be tearing of the vaginal or rectal wall from forceful insertion of the penis or a foreign object. The throat may be traumatized from forced oral sex or pressure on the throat during the attack.

Immediate Response

Some victims respond immediately with agitated and nonpurposeful behavior. They are brought to the emergency department emotionally distraught and unable to respond to questions about what has occurred. Their level of anxiety may be so high that they may not be able to follow simple directions. Some rape victims may shower or bathe before notifying the police or going to the hospital. This cleaning-up behavior is often an attempt to regain control of oneself by "washing away" the "dirtiness" that many victims feel and trying to counteract feelings of helplessness induced by the rape.

Many victims appear in good control of their feelings and behavior immediately after the rape. This appearance of outward calmness usually indicates a state of numbness, disbelief, and emotional shock. They may say such things as, "This whole thing doesn't seem real," "I must be dreaming. This couldn't have happened," and "I just can't believe this has happened to me." Nurses must recognize that underneath the calmness is acute distress. Assuming that calmness implies no distress increases the chance that the nurse will overlook the person's need for emotional support and intervention.

During the rape, some victims use the defense mechanism of depersonalization or dissociation to cope with the attack. They may exhibit a flat affect and mechanical behavior. By perceiving the attack as "not really happening to me," a victim protects

CLINICAL MANIFESTATIONS AND THERAPIES **Rape-Trauma Syndrome**

PHASE	CLINICAL MANIFESTATIONS	CLINICAL THERAPIES
Acute	Expressive styles vary: ■ Open expression of feelings—confusion, fear, crying, sobbing, pacing, hostility, inappropriate laughter ■ Controlled style—numbness, shock, disbelief, withdrawal ■ Compound reaction—reactivated symptoms of previous conditions, for example, psychotic behavior, depression, suicidal behavior, substance abuse ■ Somatic reactions—tension headache, fatigue, increased startle reaction, nausea, gagging ■ Outward appearance of adjustment with an attempt to restore equilibrium ■ Life activities are renewed, but superficially and mechanically ■ Periods of anxiety, fear, nightmares, depression, guilt, shame, vulnerability, helplessness, isolation, sexual dysfunctions	■ Counseling ■ Therapy ■ Follow-up care for emotional and physical trauma ■ Medication
Reorganization Phase	■ Anger at the assailant, at society, and at the judicial system ■ The need to talk to resolve feelings ■ The survivor seeks family and professional support	■ Therapy ■ Support groups
Post-traumatic stress disorder (if unable to recover)	■ Anxiety ■ Flashbacks ■ Depression ■ Nightmares ■ Withdrawal	■ Therapy ■ Support groups ■ Antidepressants

a sense of integrity. Other victims rely on denial to block out the traumatic experience. The use of these defense mechanisms may continue through initial treatment and should be supported until the person is able to face the reality of the attack.

Depression frequently develops within a few weeks of the assault. This posttrauma depression usually lasts about 3 months, and it is not unusual for the survivor to experience suicidal ideation. For some, the depression will develop into a major depressive disorder necessitating medical intervention.

Rape victims feel physically and emotionally violated, and unclean and contaminated. The loss of control over their bodies and their autonomy leads to feelings of helplessness and vulnerability. They may feel alienated from friends and family, particularly if there is not a strong supportive network. Anger is a healthy response to the violation that has occurred, but the energy of anger must be appropriately discharged so the person does not become obsessed with fantasies of revenge.

Long-Term Response

There may be long-term behavioral characteristics of the rape-trauma syndrome. Some survivors are prone to crying spells that they may or may not be able to explain. Some may have difficulty establishing or maintaining personal relationships, especially with people who remind them of the perpetrator. Many develop problems at work or school. Some report nightmares and have difficulty sleeping. Others develop secondary phobic reactions to people, objects, or situations that remind them of the rape. Sexual dysfunction is not unusual. A woman who is a survivor of partner rape suffers additional problems. Often, she must continue to interact with her rapist because she is dependent on him. She may be forced to pretend—to herself and to family members and friends—that the rape never occurred.

As a direct result of the rape, survivors may experience PTSD, or may turn to alcohol or drugs to numb the emotional pain. Rape survivors are more likely to experience major depressive disorders, anxiety disorders, eating disorders, and sexual problems. They are more likely to attempt suicide than are individuals who have not been raped (Faravelli, Giugni, Salvatori, & Ricca, 2004; Ullman, Filipas, Townsend & Starzynski, 2005).

Some victims go through a period when they blame themselves for the rape. This self-blame may be heard in such statements as, "If only I had taken a different way home," "I should have been able to escape because he didn't have a gun," and "If I were a better wife, he wouldn't have raped me." Remember that the victim is never to blame for this violent crime.

Some survivors develop obsessive thoughts about the rape, which may be severe enough to interfere with daily functioning. Some experience flashbacks, some have violent dreams, and others may be preoccupied with thoughts of future danger. Rape profoundly affects a person's beliefs about the environment. If the assault occurred in the home, the normal feeling of safety within the home will most likely be destroyed. Belief in an inability to protect themselves in the future may lead to social withdrawal or phobic avoidance. Young female survivors, especially, may generalize their fear to the point that it applies to all men or all strange men. Women who have been raped by their husbands often state that their ability to trust the husband or any other man has been destroyed.

Sexual problems are one of the longest lasting effects of rape. Nearly all adult rape survivors feel the need to withdraw from sexual activity for a period. For some, a period of celibacy is necessary to reestablish control and autonomy. Others may choose abstinence because they feel unclean or contaminated. Both the survivor and the sex partner must understand that the need for closeness and nondemanding physical contact continues. Expressing caring and affection through nonsexual touching minimizes the partner's feelings of rejection and reduces the survivor's feelings of self-blame and uncleanliness.

COLLABORATION

A multidisciplary approach to rape-trauma symdrome involves nurses, physicians, and law enforcement immediately after the rape, and mental health professionals for ongoing treatment for emotional trauma. Sexual Assault Nursing Examiners often participate in the assessment process (see Box 31–6). Many communities have victims' advocates who are available to guide rape victims through the process of prosecuting their attacker. These are sometimes volunteers trained by local health departments and district attorneys' offices. Some law enforcement agencies or district attorneys' offices employ trained staff to serve as victims advocates, sometimes through grant funding made possible for the Violence Against Women Act and combinations of federal, state, and private funding.

Diagnostic Tests

While not diagnostic in nature, specimens will likely be collected for the purpose of convicting the rapist, if caught. As a result, chain of custody laws must be followed and vary within jurisdictions. Specimens will include the following:

- Vaginal, oral, and anal swabs for DNA material
- Scrapings from under the client's fingernails for skin samples if the client scratched the rapist
- Combing of pubic hair for rapists DNA
- Collect all clothing worn by the victim if they are brought directly to the ED following the rape.

In addition to the specimens collected for legal purposes, the victim will be tested for sexually transmitted infections and potential pregnancy. Baseline testing is performed at the time of the initial examiniation and then follow-up HIV testing is done at 3, 6, and 12 months. Pregnancy testing related to the rape cannot be accurately performed until the woman has missed her first menstrual period.

Pharmacologic Therapies

Female rape victims may request information about emergency contraception if the attacker did not use a condom. Plan B (levonorgestrel) is available over the counter and may be made available to the client at the facility performing the examination following the attack. The use of this medication is considered controversial by some and the nurse's role is to explain the woman's options and respect her decision regarding whether or not she chooses to take the drug.

Group Therapy

Group therapy provides an opportunity for clients to meet with other survivors of rape in a safe, supportive, and egalitarian setting. In this therapeutic environment, clients' feelings are validated as normal reactions to the assault and clients receive confirmation of their survival behaviors. Support groups may help moderate depression by providing an opportunity to speak openly and network with other survivors and supportive people. Clients may be able to redirect the energy that is often spent on anger and pain into compassionate acts of supporting others. The long-term goal of support groups is to help survivors understand their distress and take charge of their own recovery. Recovery is accomplished by counteracting self-blame, sharing grief, and affirming self and life.

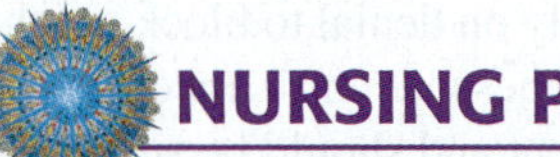

NURSING PROCESS

Priorities of nursing care include treating any acute physical injuries, and supporting the victim throughout the examination. Providing for referrals for follow-up care is essential because the psychological effects of the attack can be pervasive and life changing. Rape support groups are available to meet the client as soon as they present to the emergency department and remain with the client for as long as they are needed.

Assessment

Rape victims must be assessed physically from head to toe for any serious or critical injuries that may have resulted from the assault (Box 31–6). Critical injuries have the highest priority of care.

Rape Victim Assessment

Physical Assessment

Complete a head-to-toe physical assessment with particular attention to the following:

Head and neck

- Evidence of trauma
- Facial bruises
- Facial fractures
- Eyes: swollen, bruised, hemorrhages

Skin

- Bruises
- Genital trauma
- Rectal trauma

Musculoskeletal

- Fractures of the ribs
- Fractures of arms/legs
- Dislocated joints
- Impaired mobility

Abdomen

- Bruises or wounds
- Evidence of internal injuries

Other

- Have physical injuries such as scratches, bruises, and cuts been recorded and photographed?
- Have fingernail scrapings been taken and preserved?
- Has blood typing been done?
- Have smears for sexually transmitted infections been taken of the mouth, throat, vagina, and rectum?
- Have combings of the pubic hair been made and preserved?
- Has genital trauma been recorded and photographed?
- Has rectal trauma been recorded and photographed?
- Have semen specimens been preserved?
- When was the client's last menstrual period?
- Has the clothing been inspected for rips, blood, and stains?
- Has the clothing been preserved?

Behavioral Assessment

- Is the client able to respond verbally to questions?
- Is the client able to follow simple directions?
- Has the client bathed, douched, changed clothes, or done any self-treatment before coming to the hospital?

Affective Assessment

Which of the following emotions is the client experiencing? Describe with objective and subjective data.

- Disbelief
- Shame
- Embarrassment
- Humiliation
- Hopelessness
- Vulnerability
- Anxiety
- Fear
- Guilt
- Anger
- Depression
- Alienation from others

Cognitive Assessment

- Is there evidence of defense mechanisms?
- Is the client confused?
- Has the client been informed of her rights?
- What is the client's attention span like?
- Is the client able to describe what occurred?
- Is the client able to make decisions?
- Whom has the client informed about the rape? Family? Friends? Police?
- Does the client need assistance in telling others?
- Is the client blaming him- or herself for the attack?
- Is the client experiencing flashbacks to the attack?
- What does this event represent to the client?

Sociocultural Assessment

- Who and where are the available support systems for the client? Family? Friends? Advocate? Clergy?
- Is the client in need of temporary shelter?
- Does the client know about available counseling?

Box 31–6 Sexual Assault Nurse Examiner (SANE)

In the 1990s, Sexual Assault Nurse Examiner (SANE) programs were established throughout Canada and the United States to improve the community response to sexual assault victims. The retraumatization of victims in the medical setting in the past included long waits in busy public areas; not being allowed to eat, drink, or urinate to avoid destroying evidence; and being examined by health care professionals untrained in procedures for collection of forensic evidence.

A SANE is a registered nurse who has advanced education and clinical preparation in forensic examination of sexual assault victims. SANEs provide respectful and prompt emergency medical–legal treatment. They offer victims compassionate care for both physical and psychological trauma. SANEs know what forensic evidence to collect and how to document injuries and other legal evidence. SANE programs provide improved medical and legal response to sexual assault victims (Stermac et al., 2005).

Rape usually results in a number of physical injuries. The victim may be beaten, stabbed, or shot. Profuse bleeding and trauma to vital organs may be critical problems. Nongenital physical injuries occur in about 46% of rape cases. Most likely, the vagina or rectum will be sore or swollen. There may be tearing of the vaginal or rectal wall from forceful insertion of the penis or a foreign object. The throat may be traumatized from forced oral sex (Palmer, McNulty, D'Este, & Donovan, 2004).

Before any further medical intervention occurs, clients must be informed of their right to have a rape crisis advocate with them during the assessment process. Victims must also be informed of their rights to

- Have family or friends present during the questioning and examination;
- Have their personal physician notified;
- Privacy during the assessment and treatment process;
- Confidentiality maintained by all members of the staff;
- Gentle and sensitive treatment;
- Detailed explanations of and give consent for all tests and procedures, including photographs; and
- Referrals for follow-up treatment and counseling.

It is important that all health care professionals working with the victim respect the victim's autonomy in order to prevent revictimization. Give the client as much control as possible through every step of the assessment and treatment process. With the victim's permission, perform a vaginal or rectal examination to determine necessary treatment and to provide evidence for legal action. With permission, take photographs of the injuries for legal documentation. The physical assessment process must be carefully documented in writing to assist with possible prosecution of the perpetrator. A complete assessment checklist can be found on page 1974.

Diagnosis

The assessment process provides the data that informs the nursing diagnosis and care plan. The health care team must quickly establish immediate physical and mental status priorities. The team must then give attention to the long-range physical, emotional, social, and legal concerns of the survivor.

Appropriate diagnoses may include the following:

- Rape-Trauma Syndrome
- Acute Confusion
- Impaired Memory
- Risk for Situational Low Self-Esteem.
- Fear.

Plan

It is critical that the client who is the victim of rape have control over the planning process. The client's input regarding both short-term and long-term goals is essential in order to prevent revictimization and to help the client regain control over self and environment. Appropriate short-term goals include the following:

- The client will receive treatment for physical injuries sustained during the rape.
- The client will participate in follow-up care for physical injuries.
- The client will follow a safety plan following release from medical care (e.g., stay with family or friends, change locks on doors, etc.).

It may be more than the client can manage to think beyond the first few days following the rape. The nurse can provide follow-up care to determine when the client is ready to engage further planning. This follow-up care also allows the nurse to reassess how the client is meeting short-term goals. Appropriate long-term goals may include the following:

- The client will gain control over remembering—experiencing decreased flashbacks and nightmares.
- The client will work toward affect tolerance—ability to name feelings, feel them, and endure them without overwhelming arousal or numbing.
- The client will gain mastery over symptoms—anxiety, fear, depression, and sexual problems will decrease or become more tolerable.
- The client will reconnect—increasing his or her ability to trust and attach to others.
- The client will discover or attach some kind of meaning to the event, finding empowerment.

Implementation

Identifying and Prioritizing Concerns

Help clients identify and prioritize immediate concerns. Focusing on immediate problems lessens the client's confusion and the feeling of being overwhelmed. Next, help the

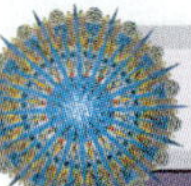

NURSING CARE PLAN **A Client Who Has Been Raped**

ASSESSMENT	DIAGNOSES	PLANNING
Doreen, a graduate student at the local university, is brought to the hospital by the police, who had found her running down the street half-clothed. In the hospital she tells the staff that she had been raped by her date, Mike, another graduate student. She exhibits outward calmness but keeps repeating, "This cannot have happened to me. My friends introduced us and he seemed so nice." She is unable to decide whether or not she wants a physical examination. When asked if she would like the nurse to call one of her friends or her parents, she is unable to decide.	■ Rape-Trauma Syndrome ■ Decisional Conflict ■ Ineffective Coping ■ Ineffective Denial	■ Client will demonstrate abuse recovery as evidenced by verbalizations of details of rape, feeling about rape, and feelings of guilt. ■ Client will demonstrate. coping as evidenced by use of effective coping patterns. ■ Client will use available social support to improve coping. ■ Client will verbalize sense of control.

IMPLEMENTATION

Rape Trauma Treatment
- Refer to rape advocacy program
- Administer medications to prevent STI and pregnancy

Client Teaching
- Support and educate about the physical examination and specimen collection process
- Inform of HIV testing
- Legal procedures available to client

Collect data to include the following:
- Events as client remembers them to have occurred
- Has client showered, bathed or douched since the rape
- Mental and physical state

Collect specimens following chain of custody using Rape Evidence Kits:
- Pubic hair combing over a white paper sealed in an envelope and initialed by nurse
- Fingernail scrapings placed into an envelope that is sealed and initialed by nurse
- Clothing removed and placed in paper bag that is sealed and initialed by nurse
- Oral, rectal, and vaginal samples sealed and taken to laboratory for testing
- All specimens labeled with client's name, medical record number, date, time of collection, and nurse's initials
- Seal all specimens (except for those that go to the lab) in a large bag/folder and initial the seal and attach chain of custody form which must be signed by the person who takes the bag for testing. Attach copy of chain of custody form on the client's medical record

EVALUATION

- Consents to collection of specimen and physical examination to promote conviction of rapist
- Calls her best friend to bring a change of clothing
- Talks with rape counselor
- Relates need for future HIV and pregnancy testing.

CRITICAL THINKING

1. What would you say to Doreen if she refused to have specimens collected or a physical examination at this time?
2. Explain how you would describe emergency contraceptives and their actions.
3. How might this client's emotional state change over the next 24–48 hours?

client use the problem-solving process. Clients need to be empowered to make their own decisions and act on their own behalf. Restoring personal choice is a primary antidote to rape trauma. Informed choices help clients regain control and autonomy, both of which were violated during the rape.

Support Coping Behaviors

Rape is both a personal and family crisis. It is important to support clients and families until they are able to cope with the reality of the assault. Discuss beliefs about postcoital contraception and abortion if appropriate. Pregnancy may result from rape, and clients must have information about available options. The most common medical intervention is a course of hormonal treatment. Elevated doses of oral contraceptive or DES (diethylstilbestrol) may be administered if the woman chooses to prevent conception. Mifepristone (RU-486) is a chemical that greatly diminishes the chance that a fertilized ovum will be implanted or that a placenta will develop. Inform clients about the need for follow-up medical evaluation and treatment for sexually transmitted infections, including a test for HIV.

Help the clients identify immediate concerns and prioritize them. Focusing on immediate problems lessens the client's confusion and feelings of being overwhelmed.

Next, help the client use the problem-solving process. Clients must be empowered to make their own decisions and act on their own behalf. Restoring personal choice is a primary antidote to rape trauma. Informed choices help clients regain control and autonomy, both of which were violated during the rape.

Encourage Calming Techniques

Calming techniques such as muscle relaxation and deep breathing are useful for managing flashbacks. Deep breathing replaces the shallow breathing that occurs in highly anxious states and prevents hyperventilation. The goal is to provide clients with a skillful response so that they can get through the flashback without feeling overwhelmed.

Guided imagery can be used to gain control over remembering the rape, the goal being to reduce the frequency of flashbacks. Instruct clients to assume a comfortable position and close their eyes. Make suggestions that induce relaxation such as describing peaceful images or slow, gentle breathing. Ask clients to imagine surrounding the flashback with a pink bubble. Then have clients let go of the bubble and watch the bubble float off into the universe and disappear. With practice clients will be able to initiate this process at the first sign of an unwanted flashback.

Provide Community Resources

Provide a written list of referrals of community resources before clients are discharged from the emergency department. Sexual assault advocacy programs address a wide range of victim needs, including crisis counseling and emotional support to victims and their families. Crisis intervention counseling can help minimize the long-term emotional and spiritual impact of sexual assault.

Evaluation

Evaluation made within a few days following a rape may reveal new manifestations and require additional planning based on the information elicited through the evaluation process. Additional diagnoses may emerge, such as disturbed body image, ineffective coping, and fear. The role of the nurse at this time is critical, as the nurse is able to provide additional support, client teaching, and referral for which the client may not have been ready earlier.

The long-term goal of intervention is to help rape victims return to their precrisis level or achieve a higher level of functioning. The road to recovery is profoundly personal and uniquely individual. Finally, it is the victim/survivor who determines whether recovery is complete.

Recovery from sexual violence includes clients' ability to demonstrate effective coping strategies, modification of lifestyle and environment as necessary, a decrease in negative feelings, and a decrease in physical symptoms. Spiritual coping is evidenced by their discovery of some tolerable meaning to the trauma and to themselves as trauma survivors.

REVIEW Rape-Trauma Syndrome

RELATE: LINK THE CONCEPTS

Linking the exemplar of Rape-Trauma Syndrome with the concept of Stress and Coping:

1. What teaching would you provide a client with rape-trauma syndrome about managing anxiety?
2. Describe the differences in communication strategy to assess for rape in a 12-year-old child versus a 30-year-old woman.

Linking the exemplar of Rape-Trauma Syndrome with the concept of Self:

3. How will you plan to assist the victim of rape to regain her self-esteem?
4. What interventions can you initiate when collecting specimens for use by the legal system for a client that has been raped to help her maintain a positive self-concept?

READY: GO TO COMPANION SKILLS MANUAL

- Evaluating client safety
- Assessing appearance and mental status

REFER: GO TO MYNURSING KIT

REFLECT: CASE STUDY

Dominique Harris, 23 years old, presented to the emergency department with complaints of difficulty breathing, palpitations, and pressure on her throat. She reports that she has been experiencing those "panic attacks" at least twice a day for the past week. A year ago, she was raped by her boyfriend's brother in the early morning when he offered to drive her home from a fraternity party and attributes the panic attacks to the upcoming rape anniversary. She tells the nurse that she can't stop thinking about what happened to her and feels stupid that she put herself in that situation. The rape resulted in the loss of her relationship with her boyfriend who physically abused her for "seducing his brother." She has missed school and her grades have suffered as a result. She describes her mood as anxious and fearful for the past couple of months and complains that nobody can understand what she went through and how she felt. Dominique reports that she drinks every night to relax but it has not helped much with her ongoing nightmares, her interpersonal relationship difficulties, or the guilt she is feeling about what happened to her. "I should have taken a cab instead of letting him take me home that night."

1. What is the appropriate nursing diagnosis for this client?
2. What interventions would be appropriate?
3. List at least two community resources appropriate for this client.

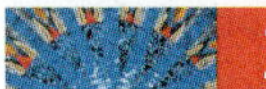

31.4 SUICIDE

KEY TERMS

Chronic self-destructive behavior, *1981*
Lethality, *1982*
Suicidal behavior, *1978*
Suicidal ideation, *1982*
Suicide, *1978*
Suicide attempt, *1982*
Suicide threat, *1982*

BASIS FOR SELECTION FOR EXEMPLAR

Healthy People 2010
National Center for Health Statistics
National Institute of Mental Health
Centers for Disease Control and Prevention

LEARNING OUTCOMES

After reading about this exemplar, you will be able to:

1. Describe the pathophysiology, psychopathology, and clinical manifestations of suicidal ideation and behavior.
2. Identify risk factors associated with suicidal ideation or behaviors.
3. Illustrate the nursing process in providing culturally competent care across the life span for individuals at risk for suicide.
4. Formulate priority nursing diagnoses appropriate for an individual at risk for suicide.
5. Create a plan of care for individuals at risk for suicide and their family members.
6. Assess expected outcomes for an individual at risk for suicide.
7. Discuss therapies used in the collaborative care of an individual at risk for suicide.
8. Employ evidence-based caring interventions for an individual at risk for suicide.

OVERVIEW

Suicide is a worldwide, national, local, and familial problem. Although the definitions of suicidal behavior and suicide overlap, there are slight differences. **Suicidal behavior** can be defined in two ways:

1. The behavior and thoughts leading up to the act of suicide
2. The act of taking one's own life.

The word **suicide** is defined in the following three ways:

1. The act of taking one's own life
2. A person who takes her or his own life
3. The result—survival or death—described as either attempted or completed.

In 2006, suicide was the eleventh leading cause of death in the United States, accounting for 33,300 deaths. The overall rate was 10.9 suicide deaths per 100,000 people (CDC, 2009). An estimated 12–25 attempted suicides occur per every suicide death.

More than 90% of suicide victims have a psychiatric disorder at the time of death. Most psychiatric clients, however, do not commit suicide. People who are severely and persistently mentally ill often commit suicide because of demoralization and depression resulting from years of pain, frustration, and low self-esteem. Spiritually, they may perceive themselves as hopelessly damaged and may lose all sense of purpose and meaning in life.

People attempt and commit suicide for a variety of reasons, including the following:

- Some are driven by delusions or command hallucinations.
- Some see no hope for the future because of depressed feelings related to a chronic or terminal illness.
- Some exhibit faulty thinking processes, believing that there is no other option.
- For some, suicide is a relief from intolerable and inescapable physical or emotional pain.
- Some individuals have experienced so many losses that life is no longer valuable.
- Some have been beset with multiple crises, which have drained their internal and external resources.
- For some, suicide is the ultimate expression of anger toward significant others.

Although an attempt at suicide can be precipitated by many factors, potential suicide victims have a number of characteristics in common that can alert the nurse to the danger of suicide. Previous suicide attempts and a sense of hopelessness or desperation are the most powerful clinical predictors of suicide.

PATHOPHYSIOLOGY AND ETIOLOGY

Suicide is a complex act, and a variety of factors contribute to the behavior. The degree of influence of each factor varies from individual to individual. When risk factors are combined, the likelihood of suicidal behavior is greater, either because internal restraints decrease or excess stress increases suicidal impulses.

Genetics

Adoption studies in the United States and Denmark indicate that there may be a genetic factor in suicidal behavior. Individuals who were adopted at birth and later committed suicide had significantly more biological relatives who had committed suicide than the control group. It is believed that this genetic factor may be an inability to control impulsive behavior, and that either environmental stress or a mental illness may drive the impulsive behavior toward suicide (Mann, Bortinger, Oquendo, Currier, Li, & Brent, 2005).

Neurobiology

Recent research indicates that the primary neurobiological factor in suicide is a disturbance related to serotonin (5-HT) dysfunction. 5-HT is the constraining and anti-impulsive neurotransmitter. Sufficient 5-HT may be related to people's tolerance for adversity, the ability to resist impulsive urges, and the means to find solutions to problems. In people who attempt or commit suicide there is a significant *decrease* in 5-HT, irrespective of the primary psychiatric diagnosis. As levels of 5-HT decrease, people become more impulsive, more aggressive, and lose control more quickly. Interestingly, 5-HT levels increase during pregnancy, and pregnant women are at very low risk for suicide. The fetus produces much of the excess 5-HT, which may be self-protective, by inhibiting self-destructive behaviors by the mother (Joiner, 2005).

Suicide risk is also related to past traumatic brain injury. Aggressive, impulsive children and adults are more likely to sustain a head injury, and head injuries can cause impulsive and aggressive behavior. The final decision to commit suicide may be an impulsive act that is the result of powerful biological processes.

Interpersonal Factors

Suicide may result when people experience social isolation and become alienated from society, family, and friends. Another factor is rapid social change resulting in the loss of previous patterns of social integration. People who have difficulty adapting to the demand of new roles are more likely to view suicide as a solution to their problems.

Loss is closely related to suicide. Certainly, the impact of any loss depends on the significance the person attributes to that loss. Whenever the most important and significant aspects of a person's life are threatened or destroyed, suicide is likely to be considered. Women's motives tend to be interpersonal, that is, related to painful or lost relationships. Men's motives tend to be intrapersonal, that is, related to financial problems or the loss of a job.

Behavioral Theory

Behavioral theorists believe that suicide is often a learned problem-solving behavior. They consider the reinforcements prior to and following attempted suicide. The internal reinforcement is that the behavior itself serves to decrease anxiety. Following the suicidal behavior, the external reinforcement is that the person is removed from the stressful environment and freed from daily pressures. Significant others who were critical may now become supportive. These types of reinforcement are essential in the repetition of suicidal behavior.

Comorbid Disorders

Although most people with mental disorders do not attempt suicide, more than 90% of people who do commit suicide have a diagnosable mental illness at the time of death. Among people with schizophrenia, 20–40% attempt suicide and 10–13% commit suicide; suicide is the leading cause of death in young people with schizophrenia.

For those with mood disorders, the suicide rate is 20%; for those with personality disorder, the rate is 5–10%; and 7% of people with alcohol dependence die by suicide. People with more than one of these disorders may be at very high risk for attempting or completing suicide (Fortune & Hawton, 2005; Simon, 2004).

Remember, people are at risk for suicide throughout the course of treatment for their mental disorder. In some cases, the risk increases as individuals improve. This transient greater risk may be because the person has the energy and the capacity to act on self-destructive plans made earlier in the course of their illness.

People with chronic medical diseases are more likely to commit suicide than those with acute illnesses or without illness. At greatest risk are people with progressive diseases such as cardiovascular disease, chronic obstructive pulmonary disease, seizure disorder, and moderate to severe pain. Moreover, people who take a large number of medications may, as a direct result of the chemical effects on the body, experience a depressive episode that leads to suicide. Substance abuse is a contributing factor for some suicidal people, particularly older men who live alone and have few or no support systems. The use of chemicals may be an attempt to self-medicate to control the symptoms of depression, or it may be a way to overcome inhibitions about the actual act of suicide (Moscicki & Caine, 2004).

Social Factors

More people kill themselves with guns than by all other methods combined, and death by firearms is the fastest growing method of suicide. More than half the teenagers who commit suicide shoot themselves with a gun kept at home. An important social issue is the alarming increase in the number of guns purchased in the United States. Individual Americans now own 200 million guns, which is more than double the number held in 1969. Those who are most vulnerable to impulsive suicide are clearly the most affected by availability of guns. The dramatic increase in suicide in children and adolescents is almost solely due to easy availability of guns (Simon, 2004).

Studies show that people who live in a home in which there is a gun are five times more likely to experience a suicide than people who do not have a gun in the home. Most gun owners state that they keep a gun in their home for "protection" or "self-defense." Only 2% of gun-related deaths in the home are the result of a homeowner shooting an intruder. In contrast, 3% of gun-related deaths are accidental child shootings, 12% are the result of adult partners shooting one another, and 83% are the result of suicide, often by a young person (Simon, 2004).

Etiology

Suicide is a major public health problem in North America and in many countries around the globe. Figure 31–4 ■ depicts U.S. suicide rates by age, gender, and race. The information in Box 31–7 demonstrates that suicide affects all age groups, both genders, and all cultures, religions, and socioeconomic classes. Be aware that any client in a health care, occupational, or community setting may, given the right circumstances, contemplate suicide.

Risk Factors

Risk factors for suicide in the United States include depression or other mental disorders; a family history of abuse, violence, or suicide; substance abuse disorders; exposure to

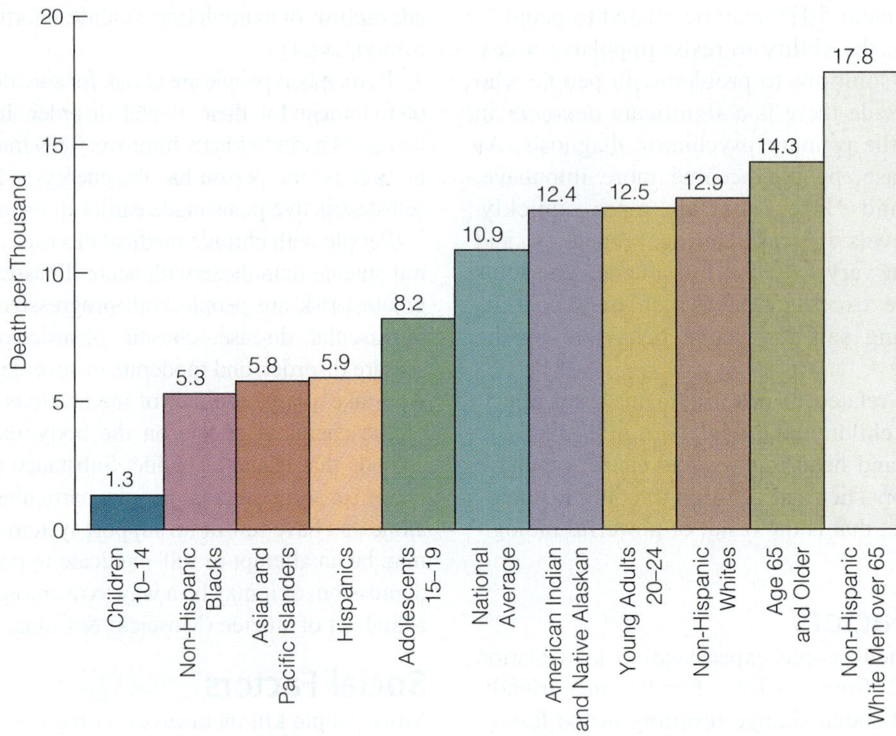

Figure 31–4 ■ Death by suicide according to age, ethnicity, and gender, 2004 (latest available figures). Almost four times as many men as women die by suicide.

Source: Centers for Disease Control and Prevention, National Center for Injury Prevention and Control. Web-based Injury Statistics Query and Reporting System (WISQARS): www.cdc.gov/nclpc.wisqars

suicidal behavior; firearms in the home; or a previous suicide attempt (Box 31–8).

Gender is a risk factor: Almost four times as many males as females die by suicide (CDC, 2006). Male–female differences in rates of completed suicide lie primarily in the lethality of methods most often chosen by men.

Box 31–7 **Suicide Facts, 2007**

- Every 18 minutes, a life is lost to suicide.
- Suicide is now the 11th leading cause of death in the United States across all age groups.
- There are more than 30,000 deaths from suicide in the United States each year.
- More people kill themselves each year than are murdered; for every two people who are murdered, there are three persons who take their own lives.
- In the past 50 years, the number of deaths from suicide in young adults has tripled.
- There are twice as many suicides as deaths due to HIV/AIDS.
- In the month prior to their suicide, 75% of older suicide victims had visited a primary care provider; many had a depressive illness that was not detected.
- More men than women die by suicide; the gender ratio is four males to every one female.
- Over half the deaths from suicide are in adult men ages 25–65.
- Many suicidal people never seek professional care.

Source: National Institute of Mental Health. (2007). *Suicide Facts.*

Age differences are also noted with respect to suicide. Suicide rates are highest among the elderly and increase with age. For example, in 2002, the suicide rate for men 85 years of age and older was 51.1 per 100,000 population, more than twice that for men aged 65–69. Among women, peak suicide rates occurred in the 45–49 age group (8.02 per 100,000 women) (Knox & Caine, 2005). In 2002 and 2003, the suicide rate for people over 65 years of age was 27.23 per 100,000 population for men and 4.43 per 100,000 for women (NCIPC, 2005).

Box 31–8 **Factors Contributing to High Suicidal Risk**

- Euro-American
- Elderly people, especially men, followed by adolescents and college students
- People who are isolated without support systems
- Individuals who are recently unemployed
- Recent loss of a significant relationship
- Separated, divorced, or widowed people
- Social isolation, including rural location
- Presence of a substance use disorder
- Presence of a mental disorder
- Feelings of failure and hopelessness
- Presence of a gun in the home
- Previous suicide attempts
- Positive family history of completed suicide

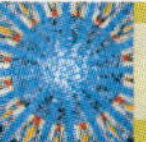

DEVELOPMENTAL CONSIDERATIONS **Suicide**

CHILDREN AND ADOLESCENTS

Suicide was the third leading cause of death for young people ages 15–24 in 2006. Adolescents are more likely to use firearms; young children are more likely to die by suffocation (NIH, 2008).

OLDER ADULTS

People who are 65 and older have the highest suicide rate of all age groups. They comprise only 13% of the population, but they account for 25% of all suicides. In the United States, someone 65 years or older commits suicide every 95 minutes, most frequently with firearms. Suicide rates for men are relatively constant from ages 25–64, but increase significantly after age 65, and men account for 83% of suicides among persons 65 years of age and older (Bruce et al., 2004).

Suicide among older adults may be related to a change in status from autonomy to dependency, accompanied by decreased participation in social activities. Many changes experienced by older adults may contribute to a higher incidence of suicide. Those who experience illness that results in a lower level of functioning may become suicidal. Other factors include loneliness and social isolation, loss of partner and friends, loss of work deemed important by the culture, and outliving resources.

Suicide also occurs at lower, but still alarming, rates among adolescents and young adults, particularly men. For example, suicide is the third leading cause of death among adolescents worldwide (Hindin & Gultiano, 2006), and from 1950 to 2004, the U.S. suicide rate among 10- to 24-year-olds tripled (Aseltine & DeMartino, 2004). In the 2005 Youth Risk Behavior Surveillance (YRBS), nearly 30% of high school students reported being sad or hopeless enough to stop their usual activities, 13.8% had considered suicide, 11.7% had developed a suicide plan, and 8.4% actually attempted suicide, with 2.3% of students requiring medical treatment for a suicide attempt (Eaton et al., 2006). Approximately half of all poisoning incidents among adolescents are due to suicide attempts (NCIPC, 2006c).

Social factors associated with increased suicide potential among adolescents include poor school performance and long absences from school (Thompson, Eggert, Randell, & Pike, 2001), as well as lack of social connectedness and interpersonal conflict (NCIPC, 2006e).

CLINICAL MANIFESTATIONS

Suicide is the most self-destructive behavior. Other typical self-destructive behaviors and self-damaging acts include, but are not limited to, nail biting, hair pulling, self-mutilating behaviors such as scratching or cutting one's wrist or another part of the body, smoking cigarettes, driving recklessly, gambling, drinking alcohol, and using drugs. **Chronic self-destructive behavior** is behavior that harms the self, is habitual, and generally poses a low level of lethality. In general, these behaviors range from relatively innocuous acts at one end of the continuum, such as overeating and gambling, to more lethal ones at the other, such as driving recklessly in a blinding snowstorm. Such self-destructive behaviors can injure one's health and sometimes hasten one's death.

It is important to understand that not all self-destructive individuals (in fact, only about 10% of those who purposefully injure themselves) go on to kill themselves. However, people who are suicidal may manifest several of the behaviors listed in Box 31–9.

Behavior

In addition to exhibiting self-destructive behaviors, people contemplating suicide may exhibit a range of other behaviors. They may make subtle or even overt comments that indicate they feel that suicide is a solution to a problem, a way out. They may mention all the pressure and stress they are experiencing and how helpless they feel. Some may discuss beliefs concerning life after death. Verbal cues are such statements as follows:

- "It won't matter much longer."
- "Will you miss me when I'm gone?"
- "I can't take this much longer."
- "The pain will be over soon."
- "I won't be here when you come back on Monday."
- "You won't have to worry about the money problems much longer."
- "The voices are telling me to hurt myself."

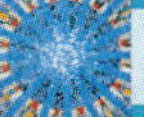

FOCUS ON DIVERSITY AND CULTURE **Suicide Rates**

Euro-Americans have the highest rates of suicide in the United States. The peak age for females is around age 50. For males, the suicide rate continues to increase throughout life; those older than 65 have the highest suicide rate of all groups. Rural men in all age groups have about twice the suicide rate of those men who live in urban areas. Factors may include greater access to firearms and physical and social isolation.

The highest rates of suicide occur among American Indians and Alaska Natives, at 15.1 per 100,000; non-Hispanic whites follow with 13.9 per 100,000 in 2006. The lowest rates of suicide occur among Hispanics, non-Hispanic blacks, and Asian and Pacific Islanders (CDC, 2006).

In general, individuals with strong religious beliefs have a lower rate of suicide. Similarly, cultures with strong religious faith have low suicide rates. Islamic tradition regards suicide as morally wrong and in some Islamic countries, suicide is against the law (Dervic et al., 2004).

Box 31–9 Continuum of Suicidal Behavior

- **Suicidal ideation:** Having thoughts of harming or killing oneself.
- **Suicide threat:** A threat that is more serious than a casual statement of suicidal intent and that is accompanied by other behavior changes. These may include mood swings, temper outbursts, a decline in school or work performance, personality changes, sudden or gradual withdrawal from friends, and other significant changes in attitude.
- **Suicide attempt:** A nonfatal, self-inflicted destructive act with explicit or inferred intent to die. The attempt may be thwarted by another person or by circumstances, it may be planned to avoid serious injury, or it may be one in which the outcome depends on the circumstances and is not under the individual's control. For example, someone who takes a heavy overdose of sleeping pills may or may not be discovered in time.

Certain behaviors may indicate suicidal intentions. Obtaining a weapon such as a gun, a strong rope, or a collection of pills is a strong indicator of impending suicide. Often, people contemplating suicide begin to withdraw from relationships and become more isolated. There may be a change in school or work performance. An increased tendency toward accidents might indicate initial suicidal behavior. Some people may show sudden interest in their life insurance policies, whereas others may make or change in their wills and give personal belongings away. Signs of substance abuse may also be present.

Behavioral characteristics also include choosing a method for suicide. **Lethality** is measured by four factors:

1. The degree of effort it takes to plan the suicide
2. The specificity of the plan
3. The accessibility of the weapon or method
4. The ease by which one may or may not be rescued.

Affect

All the affective characteristics indicative of depression may be associated with people who are suicidal. These include feelings of desolation, guilt, failure, shame, and loss of emotional attachments. A pervading sense of hopelessness has the highest association with suicide. Life is seen as intolerable, with no hope for change or improvement. Some people, when faced with intolerable humiliation, such as scandals or criminal charges, commit what is called a "shame" suicide. In these situations, death is preferable to humiliation.

People have a high degree of ambivalence before making the final decision to commit suicide. An internal conflict exists between the wish to die and the wish to live. If the part that wants to live can be adequately supported during this struggle, the balance may shift in favor of life. Once the decision has been made to commit suicide, conflict and anxiety cease, and the person may appear calm and untroubled. Others may interpret this change in the affective state as an improvement. What appears to be a change for the better in fact may be an indication of the decision to die.

Cognition

Suicidal behavior has a variety of cognitive components. Suicidal people tend to think dichotomously, that is, all-or-none reasoning such as good or bad, right or wrong. This rigid cognitive style makes it difficult for people who are suicidal to problem solve. Recurring thoughts of self-blame, negative self-evaluation, and dire expectations of the future contribute to a hopeless outlook. When people choose to die, they are so distorted by pain—physical, mental, or emotional—that the world is reduced to a solitary alternative. There seems to be only one answer: to die.

Another cognitive component involves fantasies. Unable to see the finality of death, suicidal people sometimes have fantasies about continuing on after death. They may talk about being able to see how people will react to their death or how their children will grow up. Others have expectations about meeting up with departed loved ones after death. Many people eagerly look forward to this reunion with family and friends.

A smaller percentage hopes or believes a suicide attempt will force a solution to interpersonal problems. For some, it is a cry for help. In either case, the suicidal behavior is a form of manipulation. They are so desperate that they can see no other method to resolve problems or get the necessary help.

People with sensory or thought disorders may be potentially suicidal. Command hallucinations are common and may often direct the person to commit suicide. At first, the person may be frightened by the voices, but later the person may become compliant and carry out the command. People with delusions of control or persecution may also be at risk for suicide. If these delusions cannot be managed with treatment, they may believe the only way to escape those who are controlling or persecuting them is to die. It is the ultimate method of getting relief from their extremely painful thoughts.

For those rescued from their suicidal behavior, there is often a change of mind. Either they return to the ambivalent state of thought or they decide they do want to live. Throughout their lives, however, they remain at higher risk for suicide than the general population. It seems that once the decision to die was made in the past, that decision might be easier to make again.

Interpersonal Relationships

People who attempt or commit suicide are often in periods of high stress in their lives. Stressors include under- or unemployment, family disruption, rejection by a significant other, abrupt changes in career responsibilities, and recent catastrophic events. They often have a limited social network, and when their attempts to get support fail, their level of distress increases. When people either have not developed their own coping skills or have exhausted their ability to cope, suicide may be a last, desperate attempt to cope with stress and resolve problems. Parents who have lost a child to a violent death may be so devastated that suicide seems like the only option. This group must be carefully assessed for suicide potential (Murphy, Tapper, Johnson, & Lohan, 2003).

CLINICAL MANIFESTATIONS AND THERAPIES **Suicide**

ETIOLOGY	CLINICAL MANIFESTATIONS	CLINICAL THERAPIES
Suicide	Behavioral ■ Verbal cues ■ Planning	■ Treat underlying condition ■ Behavioral therapy ■ Medication therapy
	Affect ■ Depression ■ Hopelessness	■ Treat underlying condition ■ Behavioral therapy ■ Medication therapy
	Cognition ■ Rigid thinking ■ Fantasies ■ Thought disorders	■ Treat underlying condition ■ Behavioral therapy ■ Medication therapy
	Interpersonal relationships ■ Life stressors ■ Poor support systems ■ Social pressure	■ Behavioral therapy ■ Medication therapy

Social pressures and a lack of resources often result in depression in adolescents who are gay, lesbian, bisexual, or transgendered (GLBT). They are vulnerable to all the stressors of adolescence and the many stressors related to a stigmatized sexual orientation. GLBT youth feel ostracized from the dominant culture because of an absence of role models and distorted media presentations. They may suffer intimidation, ranging from ridicule to threats and physical violence from beatings to rape. For reasons of acceptance and personal safety, GLBT youth hide from their families and the community in which they live. Given this type of social climate, it is no surprise that lesbian and gay youths are six times more likely to commit suicide than heterosexual youths (Huygen, 2006).

When teenage suicides are publicized by the news media or when there are television dramas about suicide, the rate of adolescent suicide increases several weeks after the event. Suicides that are inspired by suicides in this way are called *copycat suicides*. Copycat suicide seems to be an adolescent phenomenon and girls are more susceptible than boys. The potential copycat appears to be a troubled adolescent who empathizes with the pain of the suicidal person and is easily influenced by the media.

COLLABORATION

Collaborative care includes nurses, physicians, and mental health professionals. The treatment team needs to have a realistic approach when planning the care of a suicidal client. It is usually not possible to meet all therapeutic goals in an inpatient setting. Even clients who are suicidal are often discharged well before antidepressant medication is at full therapeutic response. These clients will need intensive monitoring in the community and should be encouraged to maintain contact with a mental health professional in a mental health facility, private office, or suicide and crisis center. The case manager or mental health professional will help the client design a safety plan that will include contact information for support, such as the therapist, a friend or family member, and the suicide hotline and crisis unit telephone numbers.

Pharmacologic Therapies

The suicidal client should be assessed for the presence of comorbid disorders, especially major depressive disorder, bipolar disorder, and post-traumatic stress disorder. Depending on the individual client's manifestations and the presence of comorbid disorders, pharmacologic therapy may be appropriate. The most likely choices of medications for the suicidal client will be antidepressants and mood stabilizers.

ANTIDEPRESSANTS Drugs used to treat depression are categorized as antidepressants. Antidepressants treat major depression by enhancing mood. Antidepressants are also sometimes prescribed to treat anxiety disorders. Recent studies link depression and anxiety to similar neurotransmitter dysfunction, and both seem to respond to treatment with antidepressant medications. Antidepressants are also beneficial in treating psychological and physical signs of pain, especially in clients without major depressive disorder, for example when mood problems are associated with debilitating conditions such as fibromylagia or muscle spasticity. Antidepressants include tricylcic antidepressants (TCAs) and selective serotonin reuptake inhibitors (SSRIs). For more on antidepressants, see the concept of Mood and Affect.

DRUGS FOR BIPOLAR DISORDER Drugs for bipolar disorder are called *mood stabilizers*, because they have the ability to moderate extreme shifts in emotions between mania and depression. Some antiseizure drugs are also used for mood stabilization in bipolar clients. For more on drugs for bipolar disorder, please see Exemplar 20.1, Bipolar Disorders.

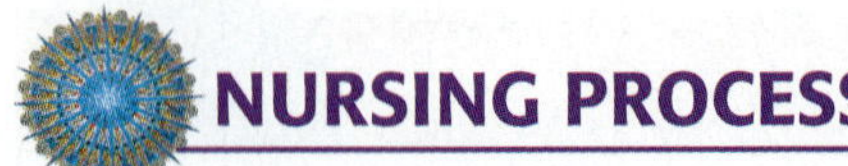

NURSING PROCESS

People who are suicidal are afraid. They fear that no one cares. They may not introduce the topic because they fear being judged or considered weak or "crazy." Suicidal clients may avoid the topic because they do not want to be talked out of suicide. When nurses are confronted with their own fears about discussing suicide, they should remember that no nursing intervention will be effective unless the suicide threat is assessed. If the person is not suicidal, asking the questions will do no damage. But if the person is suicidal and the topic is not discussed, the person has been abandoned while in a dangerously vulnerable position.

Assessment

The nurse may be apprehensive about assessing people who are at risk of attempting or committing suicide. The nurse's reasons may include fear of giving the person the idea of suicide, fear of being incorrect, fear of the person's reaction, and reluctance to discuss a taboo subject. It is important to recognize that *the nurse cannot give the idea of suicide to anyone.* By late childhood or early adolescence, every person knows that suicide is an option for solving problems. Many adults have considered which method they would choose if they were to commit suicide. Thus, even though the topic is taboo under most social conditions, most people have thought about and formed an opinion about suicide.

When assessing people for suicidal potential, use specific words and phrases such as "kill yourself" or "commit suicide." Using a more vague term, such as "want to hurt yourself," may cause some suicidal people to respond negatively. They may not want to cause themselves pain, but they do want to kill themselves. The nurse cannot risk misunderstanding by failing to communicate clearly. Possible ways to introduce the topic of suicide include saying something like, "Often, when people are feeling very upset or depressed, they have thoughts of killing themselves. Have you had any thoughts of wanting to kill yourself?"

It is also important to assess for protective factors (Box 31–10) against suicidal acts. Protective factors include a social support system, problem-solving and coping history, a sense of responsibility to children, pregnancy, hopefulness, fear of suicide, fear of social disapproval, and moral objections to suicide. The more protective factors an individual has, the less likely it is that they will act on suicidal thoughts at vulnerable times.

Box 31–10 Protective Factors

- Intact, positive support systems
- Active religious affiliation or faith
- Presence of dependent young children
- Ongoing supportive relationship with a caregiver
- Absence of a mental disorder or substance abuse
- Living close to medical and mental health resources
- Problem-solving and coping skills

Indications of suicide risk include the following:

- Is there a family history of suicide? Of other forms of violence?
- Do family or cultural views support suicide? Do cultural beliefs lead to stigma and unwillingness to seek help for depression or other problems?
- Does the client hold religious beliefs that would protect against suicide?
- Is there a history of prior suicide attempt(s) by the client or by significant others?
- Is there a history of mental illness? Is the client exhibiting current symptoms of mental illness? Has the client experienced barriers to obtaining mental health services?
- Is there a history of substance abuse by the client or significant others?
- Does the client exhibit impulsive or aggressive behavior?
- Has the client experienced a recent serious loss (particularly in the last 6 months)?
- Does the client have a chronic illness that is severely affecting his or her quality of life?
- Does the client exhibit signs of depression?
- Does the client express feelings of hopelessness or helplessness?
- Does the client talk about wanting to die or express the wish that he or she were dead?
- Does the client express feelings of being a burden to others?
- Does the client express feelings of isolation?
- Does the client display evidence of anxiety, irritability, or panic?
- Does the client fail to refer to future goals or activities?
- Does the client express frequent or persistent thoughts of suicide?
- Has the client developed a carefully thought-out plan for suicide?
- Has the client chosen a lethal method for suicide with reduced likelihood of rescue?
- Does the client have easy access to lethal methods of suicide?
- Is suicide planned for the near future?
- Does the client exhibit behavior designed to "put one's house in order" (e.g., making a will, giving away prized possessions)?
- Does the client engage in behavior that would be likely to result in death (e.g., provoking fights with others, hazardous driving)?
- Has there been extensive media attention to recent suicides?

Diagnosis

Depending on the assessment data, a number of nursing diagnoses may be appropriate. For a person who is suicidal, the most obvious nursing diagnosis is the following:

- Risk for Violence, Self-directed related to active suicidal plan, method available, multiple risk factors, and no protective factors.

If a person has committed suicide, the family may become the client in the short-term, as in the emergency room, or for a longer period, in a community or home setting. Possible nursing diagnoses for family members of suicide victims may be as follows:

- Ineffective Family Coping, Compromised, related to the suicide of a family member
- Spiritual Distress related to questions regarding the death, anger at the deceased, or a struggle with the sense of life's injustices.

Plan

Priorities of care for the client who is suicidal include the following:

- The client will remain safe from self-injury.
- The client will verbalize a decrease in suicidal thoughts and related behaviors.
- The client will develop a no-suicide contract.

Implementation

Suicidal ideation and behaviors are managed within the context of the nurse–client relationship. It is critical to establish rapport and demonstrate empathy with clients who are suicidal. Within the context of the therapeutic alliance, explore and manage thoughts and feelings. Identify the seriousness and extent of client intent, including whether or not the client has a plan for suicide.

Maintain Safety

When clients are severely or extremely suicidal, the first priority of care is client safety. If the client is not in the hospital, someone must remain with the client at all times until he or she can be moved to a safe environment. It is difficult to ensure client safety in the emergency room, on medical-surgical units, and in intensive care units. These facilities hold equipment that can be used to harm oneself and windows that may be opened or broken. Without appropriate supervision, the suicidal client who is not seriously ill may simply walk off the unit and disappear. Most acute care facilities either ask family members to stay with the client at all times or provide a "sitter" to ensure client safety in these nonpsychiatric settings.

Never lecture suicidal clients about the negative consequences of suicide. The goal is to protect clients who are suicidal until they are able to protect themselves. Through active intervention, it is hoped that clients will be able to develop alternative solutions to the difficulties fostering their suicidal intentions.

In a no-harm contract, the client agrees not to act on suicidal impulses. This type of contract may be made verbally or in writing, and is also referred to as a no-suicide contract, or a contract for safety. It is unknown at this time how effective no-harm contracts are in preventing suicide. They are probably only as reliable as the state of the therapeutic alliance that exist between the client and the nurse or health care provider. People who are determined to kill themselves may agree to a contract to avoid detection of their suicidal intent. Rejection of a no-harm contract is generally a more certain indicator of a person's suicide risk status than acceptance of the contract.

Never use a no-harm contract as a substitute for ongoing suicide assessment and maintaining environmental safety. Contracts are adjunct to other safety interventions. No-harm contracts are not appropriate for clients who are agitated, psychotic, or highly impulsive, or for those under the influence of intoxicating substances.

Promote Problem Solving

Suicidal people feel overpowered by life's problems. They may say, "Suicide is the only thing I can do." The nurse's role is one of active participation in problem solving.

Listen carefully and take all suicide talk seriously. Do not try to talk client out of suicidal intentions. Use the problem-solving process regarding the reasons for suicide:

- Have client write out list of reasons to live and reasons to die.
- Have client describe the goal he or she hopes to achieve.
- Remind client that suicide is only one of several possible alternatives.
- Develop a list of alternatives to meet client's goal.
- Discuss potential outcomes of suicide (e.g., "What is the likelihood that you will injure yourself seriously if your attempt is not successful?" and "Will death be the most successful method of meeting your goal?").
- Discuss potential outcomes of other alternatives.

Focus on things that may help the client resist suicidal impulses:

- Discuss death: what it means to client, feelings about death, and what client thinks it will be like.
- Focus on the list of reasons to continue living.

Prevent Future Suicidal Behavior

Discuss with client and family that recurrences of suicidal thoughts and behavior may happen, and encourage client and family to read books about suicide.

Assist client in developing a crisis care card including the following information:

- Names and phone numbers of competent and willing family and friends.
- Numbers of community resources such as hotlines, mental health emergency centers, and local emergency departments.
- Reasonable, nonsuicidal responses to problems.
- A list of activities that have helped in the past.

Support Families of Victims

Suicide has a traumatic effect on the family and friends of the victim. In addition to grief, family and friends must cope with the stigma and cultural taboos associated with suicide. Family and friends are frequently unaware of the danger signs and respond to the suddenness of the death with shock and bewilderment. Some may respond with anger toward the victim and the event. Others may feel betrayed and abandoned. Because society assumes that all survivors must feel guilty and responsible for the suicidal behavior, those who do not experience guilt may wonder why and may feel guilty about not feeling guilty. Some survivors may experience a sense of relief when a suicide ends the physical or mental suffering of a loved one. Other survivors may blame themselves with such thoughts as, "If only I had (not) done X, this would not have happened." Shame and guilt cast family members in the role of murderers, when in truth they, too, are victims. The death of a child, in particular, puts extreme strain on the parents. Because they were unable to protect their child, they may be overwhelmed with feelings of guilt and powerlessness (Simon, 2004).

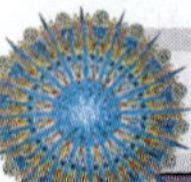

NURSING CARE PLAN A Suicidal Client

ASSESSMENT	DIAGNOSES	PLANNING
Carolyn D., a 19-year-old college student majoring in theater arts, is admitted to the inpatient unit after a heavy night of drinking alcohol that culminated in a suicide attempt. Carolyn's boyfriend has just dropped out of the college they attend—well-known as a "party school"—and returned to his hometown, 1,375 miles away. Three months ago, Carolyn experienced a major injury to her knee. The injury was severe enough to prevent her from achieving her life plan—being a dancer. Her family reports that she became increasingly despondent, saying she had nothing left to live for. They also worry that Carolyn will revert to the drinking problem she had in high school.	■ Hopelessness ■ Ineffective Coping ■ Risk for Suicide	■ Risk for suicide is diminished as demonstrated by mood equilibrium and will to live ■ Demonstrates suicide self-restraint as evidenced by seeking help when feeling self-destructive ■ Verbalizes the desire to live ■ Seeks treatment for substance abuse ■ Client verbalizes a sense of hopefulness about the future

IMPLEMENTATION

- Assist Carolyn to decrease or eliminate self-abusive behaviors.
- Facilitate development of a positive outlook for the future.
- Provide for safety, stabilization, recovery, and maintenance until Carolyn's depression improves.
- Administer antidepressants as ordered.
- Teach visitors about restricted items (razors, scissors, etc).
- Involve family, as client allows, in discharge planning.
- Initiate a multidisciplinary client care conference to develop a plan of care.
- Refer to mental health care provider.
- Initiate suicide precautions.
- Encourage Carolyn to verbalize feelings.
- Contract with the client, as appropriate, for no self-harm for a specific period of time.
- Limit access to windows.
- Consider strategies to decrease isolation and opportunity to act on harmful thoughts.

EVALUATION

Carolyn agrees that she needs help to abstain from alcohol and agrees to be admitted to alcohol rehabilitation facility. She says she would never have harmed herself if she hadn't been drinking, but agrees counseling is required and talks with a psychologist.

CRITICAL THINKING

1. If you are the nurse caring for Carolyn on the medical unit what actions will you take to keep the client safe?
2. Will you notify Carolyn's parents and family of her admission? Explain your answer.
3. What strategies would you promote to Carolyn to reduce hopelessness and have hope for the future?

Many survivors are plagued with real or imagined images of the death scene. Families must also cope with other people seeking details about the death, with others' inability to acknowledge the death, or others even blaming them for the death. Some people develop obsessions about their own suicide. Family survivors enter a higher risk category for suicide; about 20% of them will exhibit suicidal behavior themselves. Having a loved one die is traumatic at any time; having a loved one die as a result of suicide can be overwhelming.

When a client commits suicide, the nurse must quickly intervene to support the family through the crisis. The taboo against suicide makes it difficult for survivors to discuss the situation. Provide the opportunity for family to discuss the death, and allow them to express anger at the victim for abandonment and anger at themselves for not being able to prevent the suicide.

Help family members anticipate future difficulties (e.g., holiday times, anniversary of the death, and suicidal ideation and behavior in other family members). Offer referral to a survivors of suicide support group. If family issues remain unresolved, refer for family therapy.

Combat Desperation and Hopelessness

The nurse is a keeper of hope. It is a privilege to be intimately present with other human souls at some of their darkest moments. Hope is meaningfulness and dignity and a way of relating to oneself and others. Hope is also a way of being with clients. People who are suicidal feel very hopeless. They may need to borrow the nurse's hope until they can regain their own. The nurse sees clients not only as they are at the given moment but also as they can be. They need to hear about their own competence and about their ability to grow and change, especially in times of discouragement and hopelessness.

Evaluation

The outcome in a suicidal crisis is simply to keep the person alive. The outcome for families of suicides is that the family will remain functional as a unit and as individuals. As the client begins to move successfully from a suicidal mindset to a more hopeful, positive mindset, the evaluation process allows for the opportunity to help the client adjust the plan of care and continue moving forward. Expected outcomes will include the following:

- The client will use the problem-solving process.
- The client will discuss his or her personal philosophy of death.
- The client will verbalize a sense of hopefulness regarding the immediate future.
- The client will implement realistic protective factors.
- The client will participate in the plan of care with hope of recovery.

Evaluating One's Own Feelings Following a Client's Suicide

It is necessary for staff members to discuss their feelings and responsibilities in regard to a client's suicide. They will find it helpful to explore concepts of life and death, as well as their moral obligations. If feelings of guilt and failure are not thought about and expressed, individual staff members may project anger and blame onto others or even onto the dead client.

When clients are successful at suicide, nurses can ask themselves several questions to resolve any unnecessary self-blame and guilt:

- Did I take the client's suicidal intentions seriously?
- Did I provide as safe an environment as possible?
- Was the client willing to find alternative solutions?
- Do I have a right to prevent all suicides?
- Does the client have a right to determine her or his own death?
- Am I the only one who is blaming myself?
- What do I need to do to feel less guilty about this death?

REVIEW Suicide

RELATE: LINK THE CONCEPTS

Linking the exemplar of Suicide with the concept of Mood and Affect:

1. Explain the relationship between depression and risk for suicide.
2. What questions will you ask the client you are admitting to the medical/surgical unit who admits to frequent bouts of depression to determine suicide risk?

Linking the exemplar of Suicide with the concept of Comfort:

3. Explain why the client with chronic pain should be assessed for risk of suicide.
4. How will you assess the client living with chronic pain for suicide risk?

READY: GO TO COMPANION SKILLS MANUAL

- Assessing appearance and mental status
- Evaluating client safety
- Assessing home for safe environment

REFER: GO TO MYNURSINGKIT

REFLECT: CASE STUDY

Luis Ramos, a 17-year-old client, presents to the psychiatric facility with his parents. The client is verbally abusive to his parents and staff, stating, "You can't keep me here against my will!" There is blood on his shirt and pants, and his wrists have recently been stitched. His parents say they found him at home in his room with a gun in his hand and his wrists bleeding. He apparently severed a nerve in his wrist, preventing him from being able to pull the trigger of the gun. His mother also says that Luis has been getting progressively worse over the past few months, stating, "After Keisha broke up with him, he lost his job after school, and his grades have been deteriorating. I cannot believe all this over a girl!" When the nurse interviews Luis without his parents, he is visibly upset and preoccupied, and has a hard time concentrating on the questions. He says, "I don't know if I can continue living without her."

1. Based on this initial assessment, what is the most likely cause of Luis's suicide attempt? What types of symptoms is he experiencing? Are there reasons why Luis is experiencing these particular types of symptoms?
2. What should be included in the client/family education and interventions to help Luis cope with his situation?

31.5 UNINTENTIONAL INJURY: MOTOR VEHICLE CRASHES

BASIS OF SELECTION FOR EXEMPLAR

Healthy People 2010

Leading cause of death in North Carolina

LEARNING OUTCOMES

After reading about this exemplar, you will be able to:

1. Describe the pathophysiology resulting from injuries caused by motor vehicle crashes.
2. Identify risk factors associated with motor vehicle crashes.
3. Illustrate the nursing process in providing culturally competent care across the life span for victims of motor vehicle crashes.
4. Formulate priority nursing diagnoses appropriate for an individual who has sustained injury in a motor vehicle crash.
5. Create a plan of caring interventions for individuals who have sustained injury in a motor vehicle crash.
6. Assess expected outcomes for an individual who has sustained injury in a motor vehicle crash.
7. Discuss therapies used in the collaborative care of an individual who has sustained injury in a motor vehicle crash.
8. Employ evidence-based caring interventions for an individual who has sustained injury in a motor vehicle crash.

OVERVIEW

Motor vehicle crashes (MVCs) are a significant cause of injury and death in the U.S. In 2006, 42,600 people were killed in crashes; 75% were vehicle occupants, 11% were on motorcycles, and 14% were pedestrians, cyclists, and others not in vehicles (U.S. National Highway Traffic Safety Administration, 2008). Motor vehicle-related injuries are the leading cause of injury death to people ages 1–34, and the economic toll is in billions of dollars. MVCs are a significant public health concern, and nurses play a key role in prevention.

CAUSES AND RISK FACTORS

According to the National Highway Traffic Safety Administration (NHTSA), alcohol, lack of proper restraints, and speed cause a large percentage of motor vehicle fatalities. Alcohol was responsible for 41% of traffic fatalities in 2006; 33% of the drivers were age 21–24 years old, followed by ages 25–34 (29%) and 35–44 (25%) (NHTSA, 2008). Of the traffic fatalities involving children up to 14 years of age in 2006, 17% involved an alcohol-impaired driver. In 2006, 35% of passenger car occupants in MVC-related fatalities were not restrained, and 39% of the drivers ages 15–20 involved in fatal MVCs were males who were speeding at the time of the crash. The relationship between speeding and alcohol are also implicated; in 2006, 41% of drivers with blood alcohol concentration (BAC) levels of .08 g/dL or higher involved in fatal crashes were speeding. Speed is also a factor in motorcycle fatalities, as is helmet use; 41% of motorcycle drivers and 55% of passengers were not wearing helmets in fatal motorcycle crashes in 2006.

Those at highest risk for motor vehicle-related injury and fatality are males, young children, teen drivers, and older adults (NHTSA, 2008):

- In 2006, males accounted for 70% of traffic fatalities, 69% of pedestrian fatalities, and 88% of cyclist fatalities.
- Child restraint systems are often used incorrectly, and this increases a child's risk of injury in a crash.
- Drivers age 16–19 years old are four times more likely than older drivers to crash; rates are high during the teens' first year of driving, and also increase with the number teen passengers.
- Although older adults tend to drive when conditions are safer and observe posted speed limits, many experience age-related driving problems due to changes to vision and cognition that can affect their driving ability and they are more likely to die from injuries sustained in an MVC.
- It is estimated that drivers over the age of 80 have a crash rate per mile driven equivalent to teenage motorists (Centers for Disease Control, 2007).
- Significant differences in injury rates are observed in various ethnic groups. High rates of motor vehicle death occur in American Indian and Alaska Native youth.

INJURY PREVENTION

Knowledge of the causes and at-risk groups directs prevention efforts. MVC-related injuries and death are preventable, and efforts are proven to work. Injury is the greatest health hazard for adolescents; therefore, injury prevention must be integrated into every health contact with youth.

Many teens learn to drive and have a license by 16 years of age. They often transport friends, get distracted by social interactions in the car, have little experience with actions to take if a car slides or has mechanical problems, may drink and drive, and are often tired when driving.

Several states have instituted graduated driver licensing to help decrease some risks. Graduated driver licensing is an approach used to decrease motor vehicle crashes among novice teen drivers. Common approaches are to increase the period required for a learner's permit, to decrease driving after dark, and to limit passengers in the car. Another method that has been suggested to improve safety records is to involve parents in practice driving times. Parents need support and information as they interact with the teen driver. Video presentations, newsletters, and a parent–teen driving agreement have all been helpful in supporting the family during the first year of a teen's driving experience (Simons-Morton & Ouimet, 2006).

Driving should always be presented as a privilege and a responsibility. Serious consequences such as losing the ability to drive for a time after any infraction can be suggested to parents. Because of the great risk of injury and death from car crashes, ask at each health visit if the teen drives or rides with other teens, what rules parents have established about driving, and whether the teen ever drinks and drives or rides with someone who does. Reinforce the need to wear a lap and shoulder belt at all times and to never drink and drive. Many common injuries are preventable by using protective gear and following safety guidelines. More than 10% of youth rarely or never wear seat belts in automobiles (Centers for Disease Control and Prevention, 2006). Many children ride bicycles, but only about 16–17% are protected by helmet use, contributing to 23,000 bicycle-related head injuries annually. Bike helmets

FOCUS ON DIVERSITY AND CULTURE: Use of Safety Protection

There are marked differences in behaviors that influence unintentional injuries. Although only about 10% of children rarely or never wear a seat belt in the car, almost 18% of black males, 13% of Hispanic males, and 12% of white males do not use seat belts (Centers for Disease Control and Prevention, 2006). Males of all races are therefore more likely to avoid seat belt use than females, but black males are at highest risk. How will you inquire about seat belt use in an open-ended manner during health promotion visits? Consider asking these questions: Where do you usually ride in the car? Who do you usually ride with? Are there seat belts? How often do you use them? Plan strategies to include for all children and families, especially those at high risk of not using seat belts.

could prevent up to 88% of serious brain injuries from bicycle crashes (Centers for Disease Control and Prevention, 2006).

The two leading causes of accidental death in older adults are falls and motor vehicle crashes, respectively. Therefore, it is very important for elderly adults to have their vision and driving ability screened regularly. In the United States, driving is sometimes seen as a right, and many older people are reluctant to relinquish their driver's licenses because they fear loss of independence.

Many older adults restrict their driving to short distances only during the daytime in an effort to compensate for visual impairment. As a result of recent publicity given to older drivers who were involved in fatal pedestrian accidents, many states are struggling to develop systems that would detect older drivers with cognitive and visual impairments on a more timely and accurate basis. Although most states require periodic vision testing for all drivers regardless of age, few require road tests that would simulate actual conditions that an older person may encounter when driving. Such conditions may include driving in the rain and using windshield wipers, encountering oncoming vehicles with headlights on, and driving in bright sunlight with various reflections and solar glare. The debate will continue; however, as young male drivers have the highest accident rates of any age group. Safe driving habits, including avoiding drugs or alcohol, wearing seat belts, obeying the speed limit, and limiting driving in poor weather conditions, are recommended for all drivers regardless of age. Families with concern over an older person's driving safety are urged to observe firsthand the older person's performance behind the wheel. The AARP offers an 8-hour safe driving course in which older people are taught the effects of aging on driving. Many states have medical review boards. In these states, health care providers, law enforcement, family, and even neighbors can refer someone for a medical review of driving privileges. It is not uncommon for family members of older adults or others with diminished capacity to ask the person's physician to make such a referral.

Table 31–7 outlines injury prevention strategies for high-risk groups.

TABLE 31–7 **Strategies for Preventing Motor Vehicle Crashes**

AT-RISK GROUP OR BEHAVIOR	INJURY PREVENTION STRATEGY
Newborn/Infants	■ Choose an infant-only seat or a convertible seat suitable for an infant. ■ Infant rides rear-facing until at least 1 year of age and more than 20 lb. ■ The safest place for all children to ride is in the back seat. Never place a rear-facing car safety seat in the front seat with an active passenger air bag. ■ Use a car safety seat every time the infant is in the car. ■ Read and follow the manufacturer's instructions for the car safety seat and the vehicle owner's manual for installation information. ■ Dress the infant in clothes that allow the straps to go between the legs. Never place blankets under the baby or under the belts. Buckle the baby into the seat, and place blankets over the baby. ■ To make sure the car safety seat is installed correctly and the baby is positioned correctly, go to a car seat inspection station. A certified child passenger safety technician will assist you. Find a list of certified CPS technicians and safety seat inspection stations by state or zip code on the National Highway Traffic Safety Administration website or 1–866-SEAT-CHECK (AAP, 2007c).
Toddlers	Insist on safety seat use for all trips. Use approved safety seat only, such as forward-facing convertible seat. A toddler is not large enough to use car seat belts.
School-Age	■ Verify that the child is belted in properly before starting car. Keep the child in a rear-facing seat until at least 1 year of age and 20 lb, but preferably longer, until achieving the highest weight or height recommended for the seat by the manufacturer. Forward-facing seats and booster seats are used in the backseat. These child restraint systems must be used until the child is 57 inches tall (8–12 years of age) and can safely use regular car safety belts. ■ For children over 40 lb (generally 4–8 years of age), use a belt-positioning, forward-facing booster seat located in the backseat. Always use both lap and shoulder belts. Make sure the lap belt fits low and tight across the lap/upper thigh area and the shoulder belt is snug across the chest and shoulder to avoid abdominal injuries. ■ Children 4'9" and taller can sit in a regular car seat restrained with lap and shoulder belt that are snug and correctly located across the lap and chest. The backseat is preferred for all children and should be the only location used for children 12 years and younger.
Adolescents	■ School-based education programs. ■ Graduated driver's licensing programs. ■ Enforce rules about safe driving. ■ Use seat belts for every trip. ■ Discourage drug and alcohol use. ■ Refer teenagers who are known substance abusers to treatment.

(continued)

TABLE 31–7 Strategies for Preventing Motor Vehicle Crashes (continued)

AT-RISK GROUP OR BEHAVIOR	INJURY PREVENTION STRATEGY
Older adults	■ Regular vision exams ■ Driving ability screenings and community programs ■ Evaluate potential effects of polypharmacy
Alcohol-related	■ Enforcement of minimum drinking age laws ■ Promote transportation alternatives, e.g. designated driver ■ Sobriety checkpoints ■ Treatment for alcohol abusers ■ Conduct community-wide programs
Speeding	■ Observe speed limits ■ Speed limits are enforced
Motorcycle	■ Use helmet ■ Observe speed limits
Pedestrians and Cyclists	Children: Teach young children never to go into the road. A safe, preferably enclosed, play yard is recommended. The child should be supervised at all times. Teach older children safe outside play, especially near streets. Teach biking safety rules and provide safe places for riding. Reinforce use of bike helmet. Adults: Observe bike safety rules; wear helmet.

Collaborative care of the client who has sustained injury in a motor vehicle crash depends on a team approach including health personnel on site, and nurses, physicians, and surgeons at the hospital. Providing trauma care with a team focus helps each team member know his or her role. Prompt delegation of tasks and responsibilities improves the client's chances for survival and decreases the morbidity that may result from traumatic injuries.

Prevention efforts require collaboration as well. Often local fire departments, law enforcement, and health departments will combine to offer awareness campaigns regarding issues related to motor vehicle crashes. Many communities offer programs that provide child car seats free of charge as well as providing training for parents on how to install and use child car seats correctly. Increasingly, states are mandating driver safety training for drivers who receive traffic citations for minor incidents in which no one was injured.

NURSING PROCESS

Nursing care of the client who has been injured begins with a primary assessment and the initiation of collaborative interventions for any life-threatening injuries. Nursing care is directed toward the client's specific responses to trauma.

Assessment

See the About section for a complete assessment of the client experiencing trauma.

For the client who has sustained injury in a motor vehicle crash, primary consideration should be given to the airway: Assess if airway is patent, maintainable, or nonmaintainable. Assess for manifestations of airway obstruction: stridor, tachypnea, bradypnea, cough, cyanosis, dyspnea, decreased or absent breath sounds, changes in oxygen levels, and changes in level of consciousness. Assessing the airway and initiating interventions are the first steps in managing the client with multiple injuries.

Diagnosis

The trauma client has many complex and interrelated actual or potential alterations in health. The nursing care in this section focuses on client and family problems with respirations, infection, immobility, spirituality, and stress. Potential nursing diagnoses include the following:

- Ineffective Airway Clearance
- Risk for Infection
- Impaired Physical Mobility
- Spiritual Distress
- Post-Trauma Syndrome.

Plan

Goals are based on individualized client needs, the type and amount of trauma sustained, and may include the following:

- The client's airway will remain open and free of obstruction.
- The client will retain or regain mobility.

Implementation

As with any traumatic injury, nursing interventions follow the ABCs of trauma. Only after assuring an intact airway, appropriate breathing, and adequate circulation are other issues addressed.

Maintain Airway

The client with multiple injuries is at great risk for developing airway obstruction and apnea. Facial injuries, loose teeth, blood, and vomitus increase the risk for aspiration and obstruction. Neurologic injuries and cerebral edema alter the client's respiratory drive and ability to keep the airway clear.

- Monitor oxygen saturation by applying a pulse oximeter. Adjust oxygen flow to maintain oxygen saturation from

94–100%. Changes in oxygen saturation as measured by the pulse oximeter indicate the effectiveness of the client's airway. Pulse oximetry in clients who have been exposed to carbon monoxide (i.e., house fires) is unreliable since it cannot differentiate carboxyhemoglobin from oxyhemoglobin.

- Monitor level of consciousness. An early sign of an ineffective airway is change in the client's behavior. If the client becomes restless, anxious, combative, or unresponsive, the effectiveness of the airway needs to be immediately evaluated and appropriate interventions initiated.

Prevent Infection

Traumatic injuries are considered dirty wounds. Projectiles enter the body through dirty surfaces and clothing, carrying dirt and debris into the wound. Open fractures provide a portal for the entry of bacteria and dirt. Even with surgical intervention, the wounds often remain contaminated. Risk factors for wound infection include contamination, inadequate wound care, and the condition of the wound at the time of closure. Aseptic techniques used in applying and changing dressings reduce the entry of organisms:

- Use careful hand washing practices. Hand washing remains the single most important factor in preventing the spread of infection.
- Use strict standard precautions and aseptic technique when caring for wounds. Standard precautions are essential to protect the client and the nurse from infection. In addition do the following:
  a. Monitor wounds for odor, redness, heat, swelling, and copious or purulent drainage.
  b. Monitor hidden wounds, such as those under casts, by asking the client whether the pain has increased and observing for increased drainage and heat over the area of the wound.
  c. Ensure that cross-contamination between wounds does not occur. Collect drainage in ostomy bags if it is copious.
- Take and record vital signs, including temperature, every 2–4 hours. Vital signs, particularly an elevated body temperature, indicate the presence of an infection.
- Provide adequate fluids and nutrition. Adequate fluids, calories, and protein are essential to wound healing.
- Assess for manifestations of gas gangrene: fever, pain, and swelling in traumatized tissues; drainage with a foul odor. Gas gangrene is usually caused by the organism *Clostridium perfringens.* This bacterium is found in the soil and can be introduced into the body during a traumatic injury. The organism grows in the tissues, causing necrosis; hydrogen and carbon dioxide are released, with resultant swelling of tissues. If the infection continues, tissues are progressively destroyed, and sepsis and death may result.
- Assess status of tetanus immunization and administer tetanus toxoid or human toxin-antitoxin as prescribed.
- Use strict aseptic technique when inserting catheters, suctioning, administering parenteral medications, or performing any other invasive procedure. Using aseptic technique during invasive procedures reduces the chances of infection.

Ensure Mobility

The client with trauma injuries is often unable to change positions independently and is at risk for complications of the integumentary, cardiovascular, gastrointestinal, respiratory, musculoskeletal, and renal systems. Clients at greatest risk are those who have had multiple injuries, spinal cord injuries, peripheral nerve injuries, and traumatic amputations. Collaborate with the physical therapist and occupational therapist (if available) to determine the most effective types and schedule of exercises and assistive devices:

- If active bleeding or edema is not present, provide active or passive exercises to affected and unaffected extremities at least once every 8 hours. Exercise improves muscle tone, maintains joint mobility, improves circulation, and prevents contractures.
- Help the client turn, cough, and deep breathe, and use the incentive spirometer at least every 2 hours. Changing positions, coughing, deep breathing, and incentive spirometry reduce the risk of integumentary and respiratory complications.
- If the client is unable to be moved and positioned, consider a specialty bed, such as the kinetic continuous rotation bed. The kinetic continuous rotation bed allows continuous turning of the client; the motion decreases pulmonary complications, venous stasis, postural hypotension, urinary stasis, muscle wasting, and bone demineralization.
- Monitor the lower extremities each day for manifestations of deep venous thrombosis: heat, swelling, and pain. Measure and record the circumference of the thigh and calf each day. If antiembolic stockings or intermittent compression stockings are used, remove them for 1 hour during each shift and assess the skin. Venous stasis results when surrounding muscles are unable to contract and help move the blood through the veins. Thrombus (clot) formation in deep veins is a major risk for pulmonary embolism.

Promote Spiritual Comfort

Trauma generally strikes without warning and carries potentially devastating consequences, including severe alterations in the lives of the victim and family, and death. The traumatic death of a loved one may be the most difficult event a family may ever experience. The decision to cease life support systems or to donate organs challenges the family's belief systems and psychological stability. Nursing care of the family (or client) experiencing spiritual distress includes the following:

- Give the family information about the option to donate the client's organs. The decision to donate organs needs to be based on information about the client's condition, prognosis, and criteria by which brain death is determined. It is important to convey to family members that organ donation is only an option and that they should not feel they are obligated to consent or are doing something wrong if they do not consent.
- Encourage the family members to ask questions and express their feelings about the traumatic event and/or organ donation. Allowing families to express their feelings may help prevent long-term consequences such as guilt.

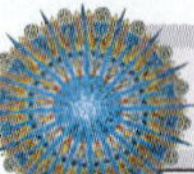

NURSING CARE PLAN **A Client With Multiple Injuries**

Jane Souza is a 25-year-old married woman with two children who provides day care for preschool children in her home. As she is driving the interstate at 65 miles per hour, a car crosses the median and strikes her vehicle head-on. Jane, who is not wearing a seat belt, is thrown forward against the steering wheel. The front of her car is pushed up against her by the car that struck her, entrapping her lower extremities.

After extensive efforts to extricate her from the car, Jane is transported to the local trauma center. She is still conscious, is receiving high-flow oxygen by mask, and has one intravenous line in place. Her vital signs are a palpable systolic blood pressure of 80, a pulse rate of 120, and a respiratory rate of 36. On arrival, she states that she is having difficulty breathing.

ASSESSMENT	DIAGNOSES	PLANNING
■ *Airway:* Maintainable with high-flow oxygen in place. ■ *Breathing:* Respiratory rate of 36, multiple bruising and abrasions on right side of her chest, decreased breath sounds on the right side. ■ *Circulation:* No palpable radial pulses; palpable brachial pulses. Monitor shows sinus tachycardia. No active external bleeding noted. Skin color pale, cool to the touch, and diaphoretic. ■ *Neurologic:* Moved her fingers when asked; complains of difficulty breathing; denies that she is hurt. Pupils 4 mm, equal, and react to light. Has a broken right arm and an open fracture of the left ankle; because of these injuries, extremity movement is limited. Because of Jane's respiratory distress, she is intubated and ventilated with 100% oxygen. Another intravenous line is inserted and O-negative blood administered.	■ Ineffective Breathing Pattern related to multiple bruises and abrasions on the right side of the chest, and respiratory difficulty ■ Deficient Fluid Volume related to acute internal blood loss (presumed because no active bleeding can be found) ■ Risk for Injury related to trauma resuscitation	Client goals are individualized, and may include the following: ■ Maintain adequate oxygenation. ■ Maintain adequate circulating blood volume.

IMPLEMENTATION

- Monitor airway and assist in any needed airway management.
- Explain all procedures.
- Monitor the effects of fluid and blood administration, including any changes in blood pressure and pulse.
- Prepare for transfer to the operating room for emergency surgery.
- Keep family informed about her condition.

EVALUATION

Jane is transferred to the operating room, where it is determined that she has a ruptured spleen and a serious pelvic fracture. Jane's treatment continues in the operating room.

CRITICAL THINKING

1. Is the nursing diagnosis deficient fluid volume appropriate for Jane Souza? Why or why not?
2. The assessment of a client who has experienced trauma is, in order, A = airway, B = breathing, and C = circulation. What is the rationale for this sequence?
3. Following surgery, Jane is moved to the surgical intensive care unit. She is very anxious and restless. What assessments would you make to identify the cause of her restlessness?
4. Infection is a common complication for the trauma client. Describe five risks for infection that are present from the time of injury to the time of hospital discharge.

- Refer the family for follow-up care. Long-term follow-up is important for the family facing the sudden death of a loved one. Grieving is not an overnight process, and providing the family with resources that may be used in the future may help prevent future crises and dysfunction.
- Provide the family of the dying or deceased client a place and time to pray or observe faith rituals together. Provide the family the opportunity to call for the family minister or spiritual leader. Praying or observing faith rituals helps the family begin a healthy process of grieving.
- Be present for the family. The nurse's act of "presencing" provides a level of support and assures the family that they and their loved one are valued and respected. More information about presencing and providing spiritual support can be found in Concept 27, Spirituality.

Provide Support

Post-trauma syndrome is an intense, sustained emotional response to a disastrous event. It is characterized by emotions that range from anger to fear and by flashbacks or psychic numbing. In the initial stage, the client may be calm or may express feelings of anger, disbelief, terror, and shock. In the long-term phase, which begins anywhere from a few days to several months after the event, the client often experiences flashbacks and nightmares of the traumatic event. The client may call on ineffective coping mechanisms, such as alcohol or drugs, and withdraw from relationships. Appropriate interventions may include the following:

- Assess emotional responses while providing physical care. Observe for crying, sleep problems, suspiciousness, and fear during the initial phase of treatment. If the client is unconscious, encourage family members and friends to express their feelings. These assessments provide valuable information about the client's ability to cope with the trauma.
- Be available if the client wishes to talk about the trauma, and encourage expression of feelings. The client may initially deny negative feelings; this denial is a coping mechanism in the initial phase of recovery.
- Teach relaxation techniques, such as deep breathing, progressive muscle relaxation, or imagery. These techniques are often useful in coping when thoughts of the trauma recur.
- Refer the client and family members for counseling, psychotherapy, or support groups as appropriate. Continued therapy may be necessary in assisting the client and family to resolve the acute and long-term effects of trauma.

Facilitate Community-Based Care

Address the following topics to prepare the client and family for home care:

- The type of home environment to which the client will be returning, including any changes that will be required to let the client function in that environment
- Medications, dressings, wound care, equipment, and supplies
- Special diet, if needed
- Rehabilitation plan and its effect on the client's family
- Follow-up appointments with the physician or at the trauma clinic
- Emotional changes that the client may undergo as a result of the trauma
- Helpful resources:
  a. Home health care
  b. Community support groups
  c. National Institute of Neurological Disorders and Stroke.

Evalution

Desired outcome include the following:

- The client's airway will remain free of obstruction.
- The client will remain free from infection.
- The client will retain mobility.
- The client will express relief from fearful emotions.

REVIEW Unintentional Injury: Motor Vehicle Crashes

RELATE: LINK THE CONCEPTS

Linking the exemplar of Unintentional Injury with the concept of Intracranial Regulation:

1. What is the priority of care when your client who experienced a head injury in a car crash has a blood pressure of 90/60 and a heart rate of 51?
2. What caring interventions would you plan with the client who has a head injury from a car crash to prevent the rise of intracranial pressure?

Linking the exemplar of Unintentional Injury with the concept of Perfusion:

3. Describe potential threats to a client's perfusion as a result of a motor vehicle crash? How would this be impacted if the client's mobility was altered due to traction or other immobilizing treatments?
4. How can you promote mobility for a client involved in a motor vehicle crash who has a casted left leg and right arm? How would this plan change if the client was an older adult with diminished mobility prior to the trauma?

READY: GO TO COMPANION SKILLS MANUAL

- Administering oxygen by cannula, face mask, or face tent
- Inserting an oroharyngeal airway
- Assisting with endotracheal intubation
- Caring for the client on a mechanical ventilator
- Clearing an obstructed airway
- Administering automated external defibrillation
- Performing surgical and antisepsis

REFER: GO TO MYNURSINGKIT

REFLECT: CASE STUDY

Laura Mays, age 26, was driving her car and was hit by another car at an intersection. The car that hit her ran a red light. Laura was extracted from her car using the jaws of life and was moaning when initially removed, but was unable to respond verbally. Her pupils were pinpoint and were reactive to light. The paramedics at the scene provided initial emergent care. Her vital signs were T 98, P 110, R 10, and BP 90/50. She had bleeding from facial and scalp lacerations as well as suspected fractured ribs. Since she hit her head and is not conscious, the paramedics also suspect a head injury.

Laura's airway was determined to be patent and she was given oxygen by a bag-mask resuscitator. Her cervical spine was immobilized with a cervical collar and head immobilizer and she was placed on a spine board to prepare for transport to local emergency department. Circulatory status was assessed and an intravenous solution of 0.9% normal saline was begun in the right antecubital area at a rate of 150 ml/hr.

In the emergency room her vital signs were T 98, P 118, R 12, and BP 98/50. IV fluid of normal saline was continued, and a Foley cathether was inserted. Her airway remained patent and oxygen was continued.

1. What are priority nursing diagnosis for Laura?
2. What laboratory and diagnostic tests will the nurse anticipate being ordered?

Adjustment phase Initial phase experienced in response to crisis, characterized by disorganization and unsuccessful attempts to meet the crisis.

Adolescent family A family in which one or more parents are adolescents.

Advance directives Legal documents that allow an individual to plan for health care and/or financial affairs in the event of incapacity.

Aerobic exercise An activity during which the amount of oxygen taken into the body is greater than that used to perform the activity.

Affect The immediate and observable emotional expression of mood, which people communicate verbally and nonverbally; the outward manifestation of what the individual is feeling.

Afterload The force that ventricles must overcome to eject their blood volume.

Ageism A deep and profound prejudice in American society against older adults.

Aggressive behavior Behavior directed toward getting what one wants without considering the feelings of others.

Agnosia The inability to recognize one or more subjects that previously were familiar.

Agnostic A person who doubts the existence of God or a supreme being or believes the existence of God has not been proved.

Agraphia The inability to write properly.

Airborne precautions Used for clients who are known to have or suspected of having serious illnesses transmitted by airborne **droplet nuclei** smaller than 5 microns, such as **tuberculosis.**

Airway resistance The effort or force needed to move oxygen through the trachea to the lungs.

AIDS dementia complex The most common cause of mental status changes for clients with HIV infection. This **dementia** results from a direct effect of the virus on the brain and affects cognitive, motor, and behavioral functioning. Fluctuating memory loss, confusion, difficulty concentrating, lethargy, and diminished motor speed are typical manifestations.

Air trapping Decreased airflow with exhalation caused by edema of the air passages.

Airway remodeling Structural changes of the airway caused by a disease, such as asthma, which in progressive or permanent loss of lung function.

Alcohol withdrawal delirium A medical emergency usually occurring 3 to 5 days following alcohol withdrawal and lasting 2 to 3 days. Characterized by paranoia, disorientation, delusions, visual hallucinations, elevated vital signs, vomiting, diarrhea, and diaphoresis. Also known as **delirium tremens.**

Alcohol withdrawal syndrome Typically begins about 6 to 8 hours after the alcoholic's last drink. Early symptoms include irritability, anxiety, insomnia, tremors, sweating, and a mild tachycardia.

Alcoholic cirrosis A progressive, irreversible liver disorder resulting from excessive consumption of alcohol.

Alcoholism A primary, chronic disease characterized by use or abuse of alcohol; genetic, psychosocial, and environmental factors influence its development and manifestations. Also referred to as **alcohol dependence.**

Alkalosis The condition that results when hydrogen ion concentration falls below normal and the pH level rises above 7.45.

Allergen An environmental or exogenous **antigen** that provokes a hypersensitivity response.

Allergy A hypersensitivity response to environmental or exogenous antigens.

Alogia Limited speech, associated with **catatonic inhibition.**

Allografts Grafts between members of the same species who have different genotypes and HLA antigens. See also *Homograft.*

Allogenic bone marrow transplant A transplant using bone marrow from a matched donor.

Alloimmunization The reaction of the immune system to donated tissue.

Alzheimer's disease The most common kind of **dementia,** Alzheimer's involves progressive dementia, memory loss, and the inability to care for one's self.

Amenorrhea The absence of menstruation.

Amnion A thin protective membrane that contains amniotic fluid.

Amphetamine A powerful stimulant which poses a severe health risk to society due to its devastating physical and neurologic consequences, including amphetamine-induced mental disorders.

Ampulla The outer third of the Fallopian tube, where fertilization usually occurs.

Amniotic fluid The liquid surrounding the fetus in utero. It absorbs shocks, permits fetal movement, and prevents heat loss.

Amyloid plaques Seen in Alzheimer's disease and formed when groups of nerve cells degenerate and clump around the amyloid core in the spaces between the neurons in the brain, they consist primarily of insoluble deposits of beta-amyloid, a protein fragment from a larger protein called amyloid precursor protein (APP), mixed with other neurons and nonnerve cells.

Anaerobic exercise Activity in which the muscles cannot draw out enough oxygen from the bloodstream, and anerobic pathways are used to provide additional energy for storing for a short time.

Anal stimulation The stimulation of the anus with fingers, mouth, or sex toys for sexual pleasure.

Anaphylactic shock Shock resulting from a widespread hypersensitivity reaction (**anaphylaxis**).

Anaphylaxis An acute systemic type I hypersensitivity (allergic) response that may result in shock and death. It occurs in highly sensitive persons following exposure to a specific antigen, usually through injection or ingestion.

Anaplasia The regression of a cell to an immature or undifferentiated cell type.

Anasarca Severe, generalized edema.

Androgen A hormone that stimulates the development and maintenance of male sex characteristics.

Androgyny Flexibility in gender roles.

GLOSSARY

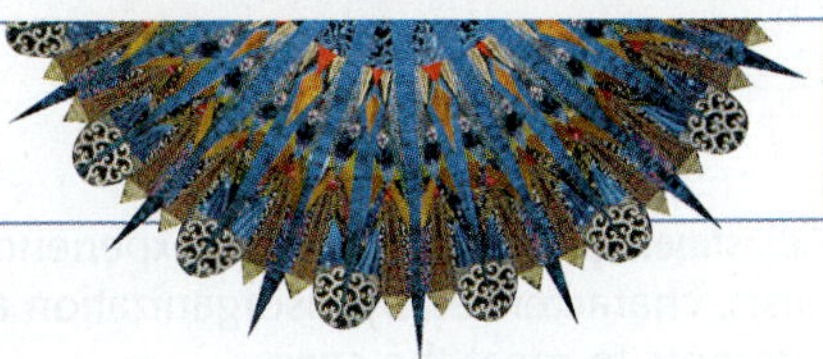

Abortion Loss of pregnancy before the fetus is viable outside the uterus; miscarriage.

Abstinence Voluntarily going without alcohol, drugs, or other pleasurable substances or activities.

Acidosis The condition that results when hydrogen ion concentration increases above normal causing the pH to drop below 7.35.

Acids Substances that releases hydrogen ions in solution.

Accommodation The ability of the eye to adjust to variations in distance; The process of a change whereby cognitive processes mature sufficiently to allow the person to solve problems that were unsolvable before.

Accountability The ability and willingness to assume responsibility for one's actions and to accept the consequences of one's behavior.

Acculturation The process of adapting to the majority culture and accepting it as one's own.

Acquaintance phase The first few days after her child's birth, when the new mother applies herself to the task of getting to know her baby.

Acquired immunity Immunity developed after exposure to a pathogen.

Acquired immunodeficiency disorder (AIDS) An immune system deficit induced by infection by the **human immunodeficiency virus** (HIV), and which is characterized by **opportunistic infections.**

Acromegaly Continued growth of bone from growth hormone hypersecretion.

Actinic keratosis An epidermal skin lesion directly related to chronic sun exposure and photodamage.

Action potential The electrical activity produced by movement of ions across cell membranes that stimulates muscle contraction.

Active immunity Production of antibodies or development of immune lymphocytes against specific antigens with inducing clinical disease.

Active Transport The process by which substances are able to move across cell membranes from a less concentrated solution to a more concentrated one.

Activities of daily living (ADLs) Activities used routinely in daily life, such as grooming, eating, bathing, and dressing.

Activity-exercise pattern A person's routine of exercise, activity, leisure, and recreation, including activities of daily living that require energy expenditure.

Activity tolerance The type and amount of exercise or daily living activities that an individual is able to perform without experiencing adverse effects.

Acute fatigue A sudden onset of physical and mental exhaustion or weariness, particularly after a period of mental or physical stress.

Acute illness An alteration in health or functioning characterized by severe symptoms of relatively short duration.

Acute infection An **infection** that appears suddenly and lasts for a very short time.

Acute lymphocytic leukemia (ALL) The most common type of leukemia in children and young adults, marked by the proliferation of malignant cells that resemble immature lymphocytes.

Acute myeloid leukemia (AML) A disorder characterized by uncontrolled proliferation of myeloblasts and hyperplasia of the bone marrow and spleen.

Acute pain Pain lasting for less than 6 months and has an identifiable cause, such as trauma, surgery, or inflammation. Usually temporary, localized, and of sudden onset.

Acute postinfectious glomerulonephritis (APIGN) Inflammation of the glomerular capillary membrane which is most often seen in children as a response to a group A beta-hemolytic streptococcal infection of the skin or pharynx or as a result of infection by the *Staphylococcus, Pneumococcus,* or *Coxsackie* virus.

Acute renal failure A type of **renal failure** that has an abrupt onset and may be reversed with prompt intervention.

Acute respiratory distress syndrome (ARDS) A disorder with rapid onset characterized by noncardiac pulmonary edema and progressive refractory hypoxemia. ARDS is a life-threatening emergency.

Acute Retroviral Syndrome (ARS) Primary **human immunodeficiency virus** infection.

Acute tubular necrosis (ATN) The destruction of tubular epithelial cells, which causes an abrupt and progressive decline of renal function.

Actual loss A change in or unavailability of something or someone of value that can be recognized by others.

Adaptation Coping behavior; the return to normal functioning, even when homeostasis cannot be regained.

Adaptive functioning The ability of an individual to meet the standards expected for his or her cultural group.

Adaptation phase The phase in crisis in which the individual meets the challenge and uses his or her resources to successfully resolve the crisis.

Adherence Compliance.

Addiction A psychological or physical need for a substance (such as alcohol) or process (such as gambling) to the extent that the individual will risk negative consequences in an attempt to meet the need.

Addictive behaviors Compulsive, problematic patterns of action resulting in psychological and/or physiological dependence.

Adjustment disorder (situational depression) A maladaptive reaction to an identifiable psychosocial stressor or stressors that occurs within 3 months after the onset of the stressor and has persisted for no longer than 6 months.

Adjustment reaction to depressed mood See **postpartum blues.**

Adjustment phase Initial phase experienced in response to crisis, characterized by disorganization and unsuccessful attempts to meet the crisis.

Adolescent family A family in which one or more parents are adolescents.

Advance directives Legal documents that allow an individual to plan for health care and/or financial affairs in the event of incapacity.

Aerobic exercise An activity during which the amount of oxygen taken into the body is greater than that used to perform the activity.

Affect The immediate and observable emotional expression of mood, which people communicate verbally and nonverbally; the outward manifestation of what the individual is feeling.

Afterload The force that ventricles must overcome to eject their blood volume.

Ageism A deep and profound prejudice in American society against older adults.

Aggressive behavior Behavior directed toward getting what one wants without considering the feelings of others.

Agnosia The inability to recognize one or more subjects that previously were familiar.

Agnostic A person who doubts the existence of God or a supreme being or believes the existence of God has not been proved.

Agraphia The inability to write properly.

Airborne precautions Used for clients who are known to have or suspected of having serious illnesses transmitted by airborne **droplet nuclei** smaller than 5 microns, such as **tuberculosis.**

Airway resistance The effort or force needed to move oxygen through the trachea to the lungs.

AIDS dementia complex The most common cause of mental status changes for clients with HIV infection. This **dementia** results from a direct effect of the virus on the brain and affects cognitive, motor, and behavioral functioning. Fluctuating memory loss, confusion, difficulty concentrating, lethargy, and diminished motor speed are typical manifestations.

Air trapping Decreased airflow with exhalation caused by edema of the air passages.

Airway remodeling Structural changes of the airway caused by a disease, such as asthma, which in progressive or permanent loss of lung function.

Alcohol withdrawal delirium A medical emergency usually occurring 3 to 5 days following alcohol withdrawal and lasting 2 to 3 days. Characterized by paranoia, disorientation, delusions, visual hallucinations, elevated vital signs, vomiting, diarrhea, and diaphoresis. Also known as **delirium tremens.**

Alcohol withdrawal syndrome Typically begins about 6 to 8 hours after the alcoholic's last drink. Early symptoms include irritability, anxiety, insomnia, tremors, sweating, and a mild tachycardia.

Alcoholic cirrosis A progressive, irreversible liver disorder resulting from excessive consumption of alcohol.

Alcoholism A primary, chronic disease characterized by use or abuse of alcohol; genetic, psychosocial, and environmental factors influence its development and manifestations. Also referred to as **alcohol dependence.**

Alkalosis The condition that results when hydrogen ion concentration falls below normal and the pH level rises above 7.45.

Allergen An environmental or exogenous **antigen** that provokes a hypersensitivity response.

Allergy A hypersensitivity response to environmental or exogenous antigens.

Alogia Limited speech, associated with **catatonic inhibition.**

Allografts Grafts between members of the same species who have different genotypes and HLA antigens. See also *Homograft.*

Allogenic bone marrow transplant A transplant using bone marrow from a matched donor.

Alloimmunization The reaction of the immune system to donated tissue.

Alzheimer's disease The most common kind of **dementia,** Alzheimer's involves progressive dementia, memory loss, and the inability to care for one's self.

Amenorrhea The absence of menstruation.

Amnion A thin protective membrane that contains amniotic fluid.

Amphetamine A powerful stimulant which poses a severe health risk to society due to its devastating physical and neurologic consequences, including amphetamine-induced mental disorders.

Ampulla The outer third of the Fallopian tube, where fertilization usually occurs.

Amniotic fluid The liquid surrounding the fetus in utero. It absorbs shocks, permits fetal movement, and prevents heat loss.

Amyloid plaques Seen in Alzheimer's disease and formed when groups of nerve cells degenerate and clump around the amyloid core in the spaces between the neurons in the brain, they consist primarily of insoluble deposits of beta-amyloid, a protein fragment from a larger protein called amyloid precursor protein (APP), mixed with other neurons and nonnerve cells.

Anaerobic exercise Activity in which the muscles cannot draw out enough oxygen from the bloodstream, and anerobic pathways are used to provide additional energy for storing for a short time.

Anal stimulation The stimulation of the anus with fingers, mouth, or sex toys for sexual pleasure.

Anaphylactic shock Shock resulting from a widespread hypersensitivity reaction (**anaphylaxis**).

Anaphylaxis An acute systemic type I hypersensitivity (allergic) response that may result in shock and death. It occurs in highly sensitive persons following exposure to a specific antigen, usually through injection or ingestion.

Anaplasia The regression of a cell to an immature or undifferentiated cell type.

Anasarca Severe, generalized edema.

Androgen A hormone that stimulates the development and maintenance of male sex characteristics.

Androgyny Flexibility in gender roles.

Appendixes

Appendix A: NANDA-Approved Nursing Diagnoses
Appendix A can be found in Volume 2.

Appendix B: Diagnostic Studies
Appendix B can be found in Volume 2 and at www.mynursingkit.com.

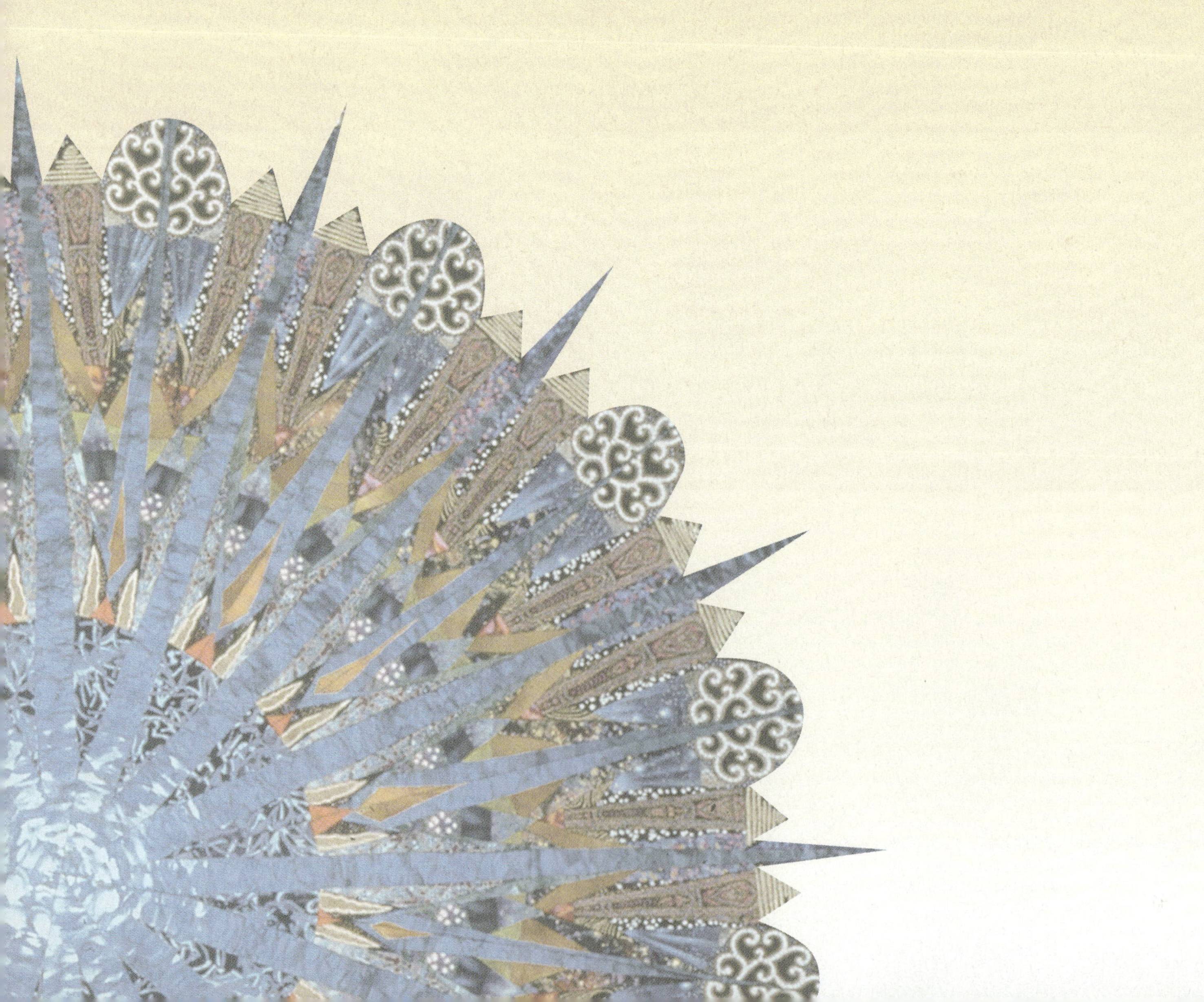

http://publications.nigms.nih.gov/factsheets/trauma_burn_facts.html

National Research Council. (2003). *Elder mistreatment: Abuse, neglect, and exploitation in aging America.* Washington, DC.

Nelson, H., Nygren, P., McInerney, Y., & Klein, J. (2004). Screening women and elderly adults for family and intimate partner violence: A review of the evidence for the U.S. Preventive Services Task Force. *Annals of Internal Medicine, 140*, 387–396.

North American Nursing Diagnosis Association. (2007). *Nursing diagnosis: Definition and classification,* 2007–2008. Philadelphia: Author.

Occupational Safety and Health Administration. (2002). *Workplace violence.* Retrieved from http://www.osha.gov/oshinfo/priorities/ violence.html

Office of Statistics and Programming, National Center for Injury Prevention and Control. (2003). Methods of suicide among persons aged 10–19 years—United states, 1992–2001. *Morbidity and Mortality Weekly Report, 52*, 471–474.

Palmer, C. M., McNulty, A. M., D'Este, C., & Donovan, B. (2004). Genital injuries in women reporting sexual assault. *Sexual Health, 1*(1), 55–59.

Pearsall, C. (2005). Forensic biomarkers of elder abuse. *Journal of Forensic Nursing, 194*, 182–186.

Pihl, R. O., & Benkelfat, C. (2005). Neuromodulators in the development and expression of inhibition and aggression. In R. E. Tremblay, W. W. Hartup, & J. Archer (Eds.), *Developmental origins of aggression* (pp. 261–280). New York: Guilford Press.

Pirkis, J., Goldney, R., & Burgess, P. (2003). Suicidality in the community. In P. Liamputtong & H. Gardner (Eds.), *Health, social change and communities* (pp. 328–339). Oxford: Oxford University Press.

Raj, A., & Silverman, J. G. (2003). Immigrant South Asian women at greater risk for injury from intimate partner violence. *American Journal of Public Health, 93*, 435–437.

Rauch, S. A. M., & Foa, E. B. (2004). Sexual trauma. In B. T. Litz (Ed.), *Early interventions for trauma and traumatic loss* (pp. 216–240). New York: Guilford Press.

Riner, M. E., & Flynn, B. C. (1999). Creating violence-free healthy cities for our youth. *Holistic Nursing Practice, 14*(1), 1–11.

Rodgers, C. S., Lang, A. J., Twamley, E. W., & Stein, M. B. (2003). Sexual trauma and pregnancy. *Journal of Women's Health, 12*(10), 961–970.

Saewyc, E., Skay, C., Richens, K., Reis, E., Poon, C., & Murphy, A. (2006). Sexual orientation, sexual abuse, and HIV-risk behaviors among adolescents in the Pacific Northwest. *American Journal of Public Health, 96*, 1104–1110.

Salter, D., McMillan, D., Richards, M., Talbot, T., Hodges, J., Bentovim, A., et al. (2003). Development of sexually abusive behavior in sexually victimized males. *Lancet, 361*(9356), 471–476.

SAMHSA—Center for Substance Abuse Prevention of the Substance Abuse and Mental Health Services Administration. (2001). *Violence against the elderly.* Rockville, MD: The National Clearinghouse for Alcohol and Drug Information.

Sexual Abuse Statistics. (n.d.). Retrieved October 29, 2009, from http://www.prevent-abuse-now.com/stats.htm

Shelton, D. (2000). Health status of young offenders and their families. *Journal of Nursing Scholarship, 32*(2), 173–178.

Silver, E., Arsenault, L., Langley, J., Caspi, A., & Moffitt, T. E. (2005). Mental disorder and violent victimization in a total birth cohort. *American Journal of Public Health, 95*, 2015–2021.

Silverman, J. G., Mesh, C. M., Cuthbert, C. V., Slote, K., & Bancroft, L. (2004). Child custody determinations in cases involving intimate partner violence: A human rights analysis. *American Journal of Public Health, 94*, 951–957.

Smith, P. H., White, J. W., & Holland, L. J. (2003). A longitudinal perspective on dating violence among adolescent and college-age women. *American Journal of Public Health, 93*, 1104–1109.

Snyder, H. N. (2004). *Juvenile arrests 2002.* Retrieved March 30, 2006, from http://www. ncjrs.gov/html/ojjdp/204608/contents.html

Snyder, H. N., & Swahn, M. H. (2004, March). Juvenile suicides, 1981–1998. *Youth Violence Research Bulletin.* Retrieved March 20, 2004, from http://www.ojp.usdoj.gov/ojjdp

Sorenson, S. B., & Vittes, K. A. (2004). Adolescents and firearms: A California statewide survey. *American Journal of Public Health, 94*, 852–858.

Sorenson, S. B., & Weibe, D. J. (2004). Weapons in the lives of battered women. *American Journal of Public Health, 94*, 1412–1417.

Steen, K., & Hunskaar, S. (2004). Gender and physical violence. *Social Science & Medicine, 59*, 567–571.

Stermac, L., Dunlap, H., & Bainbridge, D. (2005). Sexual assault services delivered by SANES. *Journal of Forensic Nursing, 1*(3), 124–128.

Stinson, C. K., & Robinson, R. (2006). Intimate partner violence: Continuing education for registered nurses. *Journal of Continuing Education in Nursing, 37*(2), 58–62.

Stretesky, P. B., & Lynch, M. J. (2001). The relationship between lead exposure and homicide. *Archives of Pediatrics & Adolescent Medicine, 155*, 579–582.

Swahn, M. H., & Bossarte, R. M. (2006). The associations between victimization, feeling unsafe, and asthma episodes among US high school students. *American Journal of Public Health, 96*, 802–804.

Tam, S., & Neysmith, S. (2006). Disrespect and isolation: Elder abuse in Chinese communities. *Canadian Journal on Aging, 25*(2), 141–151.

Tan, J. C., & Gregor, K. V. (2006). Violence against pregnant women in northwestern Ontario. *Annals of the New York Academy of Sciences, 11*(1087), 320–338.

Taylor, I. (2009). Emergency care of patients with gunshot wounds. *Nursing Standard 23*, 40, 49–56.

Thompson, E. A., Eggert, L. L., Randell, B. P., & Pike, K. C. (2001). Evaluation of indicated suicide risk prevention approaches for potential high school dropouts. *American Journal of Public Health, 91*, 742–752.

Thompson, M. P., Kingree, J. B., & Desai, S. (2004). Gender differences in long-term health consequences of physical abuse of children: Data from a nationally representative survey. *American Journal of Public Health, 94*, 599–604.

Tilley, D. S., & Brackley, M. (2005). Men who batter intimate partners: A grounded theory study of the development of male violence in intimate partner relationships. *Issues in Mental Health Nursing, 26*, 281–297.

Tilley, D. S., & Brackley, M. (2003). Men who batter intimate partners: A grounded theory study of the development of male violence in intimate partner relationships. *Issues in Mental Health Nursing, 26*, 281–297.

Tomita, S. (1999). Exploration of elder mistreatment among the Japanese. In T. Tatara (Ed.), *Understanding elder abuse in minority populations* (pp. 119–139). (CANE File No. N4672-13). New Zealand: MacMillan.

Tremblay, R. E., & Nagin, D. S. (2005). The developmental origins of physical aggression in humans. In R. E. Tremblay, W. W. Hartup, & J. Archer (Eds.), *Developmental origins of aggression* (pp. 83–106). New York: Guilford Press.

United Nations Economic and Social Council. (2002). *Abuse of older persons: Recognizing and responding to abuse of older persons in a global context.* Retrieved June 19, 2006, from http:// www.un.org/ageing/enc52002eng.pdf

U.S. Census Bureau. (2006). *Statistical abstract of the United States, 2006.* Retrieved June 5, 2006, from http://www.census.gov/prod/ 2005pubs/06statab

U.S. Department of Health and Human Services. (2005). *Summary: Child maltreatment 2003.* Retrieved February 20, 2006, from http://www.acf.hhs.gov/programs/cb/pubs/cm03/summary.htm

U.S. Department of Health and Human Services. (2000). *Healthy People 2010: Understanding and improving health* (2nd ed.). Washington, DC: U.S. Government Printing Office.

U.S. Department of Health and Human Services (2006). *Healthy People 2010: Midcourse review.* Washington, DC: U.S. Government Printing Office.

U.S. Department of Justice (2005). Crime and victims statistics. Accessed on February 15, 2008, at www.ojp.usdoj.gov/bjs/cvict.htm

U. S. Department of Justice. (2005). *National Crime Victimizaiton Study.* Retrieved October 19, 2009, from http://www.rainn.org/get-information/statistics/sexual-assault-offenders

Valente, S. M. (2005). Sexual abuse of boys. *Journal of Child and Adolescent Psychiatric Nursing, 18*(1), 10–16.

Waldrop, A. E., & Resick, P. A. (2004). Coping among adult female victims of domestic violence. *Journal of Family Violence, 19*, 291–302.

Walker, L. E. A. (2000). *The battered woman syndrome* (2nd ed.). New York: Springer.

Ward, T., & Stewart, C. (2003). The relationship between human needs and criminogenic needs. *Psychology Crime and Law, 9*, 219–225.

Warne, T., & McAndrew, S. (2005). The shackles of abuse: Unprepared to work at the edges of reason. *Journal of Psychiatric and Mental Health Nursing, 12*(6), 679–686.

Wathen, C. N., & MacMillan, H. L. (2003). Interventions for violence against women: Scientific review. *Journal of the American Medical Association, 289*(5), 589–600.

Winters, J., Clift, R. J., & Dutton, D. G. (2004). An exploratory study of emotional intelligence and domestic abuse. *Journal of Family Violence, 19*, 255–267.

Wood, J. T. (2004). Monsters and victims: Male felons' accounts of intimate partner violence. *Journal of Social and Personal Relationships, 21*, 555–576.

World Health Organization. (2009). Female genital mutilation. Retrieved September 10, 2009, from http://www.who.int/mediacentre/factsheets/fs241/en/

Xu, X., Zhu, F., O'Campo, P., Koenig, M. A., Mock, V., & Campbell, J. (2005). Prevalence of and factors for intimate partner violence in China. *American Journal of Public Health, 95*, 78–85.

Fulmer, T., Paveza, G., Vandeweerd, C., Guadagno, L., Fairchild, S., Norman, R., et al. (2005). Neglect assessment in urban emergency departments and confirmation by an expert clinical team. *Journals of Gerontology: A Biological Sciences and Medical Sciences, 60*(8), 1002–1006.

Fulmer, T., Street, S., & Carr, K. (1984). Abuse of the elderly: Screening and detection. *Journal of Emergency Nursing, 10*(3), 131–140.

Giorgianni, S. J. (Ed.). (2003). *How families matter in health: Challenges of the evolving 21st century family.* New York, NY: Impact Communications.

Gomby, D. S. (2000). Promise and limitations of home visitation. *Journal of the American Medical Association, 284,* 1430–1431.

Goodwin, R. D., Hoven, C. W., Murison, R., & Hotopf, M. (2003). Association between childhood physical abuse and gastrointestinal disorders and migraine in adulthood. *American Journal of Public Health, 94,* 1065–1067.

Greenwood, G. L., Relf, M. V., Huang, B., Pollack, L. M., Canchola, J. A., & Catania, J. A. (2002). Battering victimization among a probability-based sample of men who have sex with men. *American Journal of Public Health, 92,* 1964–1969.

Griffin, M. G., Resick, P. A., & Yehuda, R. (2005). Enhanced cortisol suppression following dexamethasone administration in domestic violence survivors. *American Journal of Psychiatry, 162*(6), 1192–1199.

Grossman, D. (2000). Teaching kids to kill. *National Forum, 80*(4), 10–14.

Grunbaum, J. A., Kann, L., Kinchen, S., Ross, J., Hawkins, J., Lowry, R., et al. (2004). Youth risk behavior surveillance—United States, 2003. *Morbidity and Mortality Weekly Report, 53*(SS-2), 1–96.

Gundersen, L. (2002). Intimate partner violence: The need for primary prevention in the community. *Annals of Internal Medicine, 136,* 637–640.

Hahn, R. A., Biluka, O. O., Crosby, A., Fullilove, M. T., Liberman, A., Moscicki, E. K., et al. (2003b). First reports evaluating the effectiveness of strategies for preventing violence: Firearms laws: Findings from the Task Force on Community Preventive Services. *Morbidity and Mortality Weekly Report, 52*(RR-14), 11–20.

Hartford Institute for Geriatric Nursing. (2007). *Best practices in nursing care to older adults.* New York: New York University Division of Nursing. Try this: Modified Caregiver Strain Index. Retrieved June 16, 2008, from http://www.hartforign.org/publications/trythis/issue14.pdf

Herrenkohl, T. I., Hill, K. G., Hawkins, J. D., Chung, I. J., & Nagin, D. S. (2006). Developmental trajectories of family management and risk for violent behavior in adolescence. *Journal of Adolescent Health, 39*(2), 206–213.

Hindin, M. J., & Gultiano, S. (2006). Associations between witnessing parental domestic violence and experiencing depressive symptoms in Filipino adolescents. *American Journal of Public Health, 96,* 660–663.

Hoffman, K. L., & Edwards, J. N. (2004). An integrated theoretical model of sibling violence and abuse. *Journal of Family Violence, 19,* 185–200.

Hudson, M. F., Armachain, W. D., Beasley, C. M., & Carlson, J. R. (1998). Elder abuse: Two Native American views. *Gerontologist, 38*(5), 538–548.

Hudson, M. F., Beasley, C., Benedict, R. H., Carlson, J. R., Craig, B. F., Herman, C., et al. (2000). Elder abuse: Some Caucasian-American views. *Journal of Elder Abuse and Neglect, 12*(1), 89–114.

Huesmann, L. R., Moise-Titus, J., Podolski, C. L., & Eron, L. D. (2003). Longitudinal relations between children's exposure to TV violence and their aggressive and violent behavior in young adulthood. *Developmental Psychology, 39*(2), 201–221.

Hymel, K. P., & Hall, C. A. (2005). Diagnosing pediatric head trauma. *Pediatric Annals, 34,* 358–370.

Institute of Medicine. (2006). *Improving the quality of health care for mental and substance-use conditions.* Retrieved February 22, 2006, from http://www.nap.edu

Institute of Medicine. (2002). *Confronting chronic neglect: The education and training of health professionals on family violence.* Washington, DC: National Academy Press.

Jech, A. J. (2002). Elder abuse: Mistreatment of older Americans on the rise. *NurseWeek, 15*(23), 22–23.

Johnson, C. F. (2006). Sexual abuse in children. *Pediatrics in Review, 27,* 17–26.

Kaplow, J. B., Dodge, K. A., Amaya-Jackson, L., & Saxe, G. N. (2005). Pathways to PTSD, part II: Sexually abused children. *American Journal of Psychiatry, 162*(7), 1305–1310.

Kawsar, M., Anfield, A., Walters, E., McCabe, S., & Forster, G. E. (2004). Prevalence of sexually transmitted infections and mental health needs of female child and adolescent survivors of rape and sexual assault attending a specialist clinic. *Sexually Transmitted Infections, 80*(2), 138–141.

Kearney, M. H., Haggerty, L. A., Munro, B. H., & Hawkins, J. W. (2003). Birth outcomes and maternal morbidity in abused pregnant women with public versus private health insurance. *Journal of Nursing Scholarship, 35*(4), 345–349.

Kernic, M. A., Wolf, M. E., & Holt, V. L. (2000). Rates and relative risk of hospital admission among women in violent intimate partner relationships. *American Journal of Public Health, 90,* 1416–1420.

Knox, K. L., & Caine, E. D. (2005). Establishing priorities for reducing suicide and its antecedents in the United States. *American Journal of Public Health, 95,* 1898–1903.

Knox, K. L., Conwell, Y., & Caine, E. D. (2004). If suicide is a public health problem, what are we doing to prevent it? *American Journal of Public Health, 94,* 37–45.

Koenig, L. J., Whitaker, D. J., Royce, R. A., Wilson, T. E., Ethier, K., & Fernandez, M. I. (2006). Physical and sexual violence during pregnancy and after delivery: A prospective multistate study of women with or at risk for HIV infection. *American Journal of Public Health, 96,* 1052–1059.

Koenig, M. A., Stephenson, R., Ahmed, S., Jejeebhoy, S. J., & Campbell, J. (2006). Individual and contextual determinants of domestic violence in north India. *American Journal of Public Health, 96,* 132–138.

Kreidler, M. (2005). Group therapy for survivors of childhood sexual abuse who have chronic mental illness. *Archives of Psychiatric Nursing, 19*(4), 176–183.

Lachs, M. S., & Pillemer, K. A. (1995). Abuse and neglect of elderly persons. *New England Journal of Medicine, 332*(7), 437–443.

Lloyd, S. A. (2000). Intimate violence: Paradoxes of romance, conflict, and control. *National Forum, 80*(4), 19–22.

Locsin, R. C., & Purnell, M. J. (2002). Intimate partner violence, culture-centrism, and nursing. *Holistic Nursing Practice, 16*(3), 1–4.

Malecha, A. (2003). Screening for and treating intimate partner violence in the workplace. *AAOHN Journal, 51,* 310–316.

Maman, S., Mbwambo, J. K., Hogan, N. M., Kilonzo, G. P., Campbell, J. C., Weiss, E., et al. (2002). HIV-positive women report more lifetime partner violence: Findings from a voluntary counseling and testing clinic in Dar es Salaam, Tanzania. *American Journal of Public Health, 92,* 1331–1337.

Martino, S. C., Collins, R. L., Elliott, M. N., Strachman, A., Kanouse, D. E., & Berry, S. H. (2006). Exposure to degrading versus nondegrading music lyrics and sexual behavior among youth. *Pediatrics, 118*(2), 430–441.

Marshall, C. E., Benton, D., & Brazier, J. M. (2000). Elder abuse: Using clinical tools to identify clues of mistreatment. *Geriatrics, 55,* 42–53.

Massey-Stokes, M., & Lanning, B. (2004). The role of CSHPs in preventing child abuse and neglect. *Journal of School Health, 74,* 193–194.

McClellan, A. C., & Killeen, M. R. (2000). Attachment theory and violence toward women by male intimate partners. *Journal of Nursing Scholarship, 32,* 353–360.

Miller, M., Azrael, D., & Hemenway, D. (2002). Rates of firearm ownership and homicide across US regions and states, 1988–1997. *American Journal of Public Health, 92,* 1988–1993.

Moon, A., & Benton, D. (2000). Tolerance of elder abuse and attitudes toward third-party intervention among African American, Korean American and White elderly. *Journal of Multicultural Social Work, 8*(3/4), 283–303.

Murdaugh, C., Hunt, S., Sowell, R., & Santana, I. (2004). Domestic violence in Hispanics in the southeastern United States: A survey and needs analysis. *Journal of Family Violence, 19,* 107–115.

Murty, S. A., Peek-Asa, C., Zwerling, C., Stromquist, A. M., Burmeister, L. F., & Merchant, J. A. (2003). Physical and emotional abuse reported by men and women in a rural community. *American Journal of Public Health, 93,* 1073–1075.

Nadien, M. B. (2006). Factors that influence abusive interactions between aging women and their caregivers. *Annals of the New York Academy of Sciences, 1087,* 158–169.

National Center for Health Statistics, National Vital Statistics System. (2008). *Leading Causes of Death by Age Group – United States – 2006.* Retrieved August 23, 2009, from http://www.cdc.gov/injury/Images/LC-Charts/101c%20-%2B

National Center for Health Statistics, National Vital Statistics System. (2007). *Leading causes of injury deaths for children and adolescents by age, external cause, and intent, 2004.* Retrieved February 18, 2009, from http://webapppa.cdc.gov/cgi-bin/broker.exe

National Center for Health Statistics. (2005). *Health United States, 2005 with chartbook on trends in the health of Americans.* Retrieved December 23, 2005, from http://www. cdc.gov/nchs/data/hus/hus05.pdf

National Center for Injury Prevention and Control. (2003). *Costs of intimate partner violence against women in the United States.* Atlanta: Centers for Disease Control and Prevention. Retrieved from http://www.cdc.gov/ncipc

National Center for Injury Prevention and Control. (2004a). *Child maltreatment: Fact sheet.* Atlanta, GA: Centers for Disease Control and Prevention.

National Center for Injury Prevention and Control. (2004b). *Youth violence: Fact sheet.* Atlanta, GA: Centers for Disease Control and Prevention.

National Center for Injury Prevention and Control. (2009a). *Child maltreatment: Fact sheet.* Retrieved June 14, 2006, from http:// www.cdc.gov/ncipc/factsheets/cmfacts.htm

National Center for Injury Prevention and Control. (2006b). *Intimate partner violence: Fact sheet.* Retrieved June 14, 2006, from http://www.cdc.gov/ncipc/factsheets/ipvfacts.htm

National Center for Injury Prevention and Control. (2008d). *Sexual violence: Fact sheet.* Retrieved June 14, 2006, from http://www. cdc.gov/ncipc/factsheets/svfacts.htm

National Center for Injury Prevention and Control. (2008e). *Suicide: Fact sheet.* Retrieved June 14, 2006, from http://www.cdc.gov/ ncipc/factsheets/suifacts.htm

National Center for Injury Prevention and Control. (2009f). *Youth violence: Fact sheet.* Retrieved June 14, 2006, from http://www. cdc.gov/ncipc/factsheets/yvfacts.htm

National Center on Elder Abuse. (2006). Abuse of adults aged 60+: 2004 survey of adult protective services. Retrieved June 16, 2008, from http://www.ncea.aoa.gov/NCEAroot/Main_Site/pdf/2-14-06%2060FACT%20SHEET.pdf

National Center on Elder Abuse. (2000). *What is elder abuse?* http://www.elderabusecenter.org/basic/indes.html

National Center on Elder Abuse. *Trends in elder abuse in domestic settings. Elder abuse information series No. 2.* Washington, DC: National Center on Elder Abuse. Retrieved August 20, 2004, http://www.elderabusecenter.org

National Highway Traffic Safety Administration (NHTSA), Department of Transportation (DOT). (2008) [cited 2008 Oct 22]. Traffic Safety Facts 2006: Alcohol-Impaired Driving. Washington (DC): NHTSA. Retrieved from http://www-nrd.nhtsa.dot.gov/Pubs/810801.PDF

National Highway Traffic Safety Administration (NHTSA), Department of Transportation (DOT). (2006) [cited 2008 March 28].Traffic Safety Facts 2005: Speeding. Washington (DC): NHTSA. Retrieved from http://www-nrd.nhtsa.dot.gov/pdf/nrd-3-/NCSA/TSF2005/SpeedingTSF05.PDF

National Highway Traffic Safety Administration (NHTSA), Department of Transportation (DOT). (2006b) [cited 2008 March 28].Traffic Safety Facts 2005: Young Drivers. Washington (DC): NHTSA. Retrieved from http://www-nrd.nhtsa.dot.govf

National Highway Traffic Safety Administration (NHTSA), Department of Transportation (DOT). (2008). *Traffic Safety Facts: 2006 Data.* Washington (DC): NHTSA's National Center for Statistics and Analysis.

National Highway Traffic Safety Administration (NHTSA), Department of Transportation (DOT). (2008). *Traffic Safety Facts 2006: Older Population.* Washington (DC): 2006.

National Highway Traffic Safety Administration (NHTSA), Department of Transportation (DOT). (2008). *Traffic Safety Facts: 2006 Data.* Washington (DC): NHTSA's National Center for Statistics and Analysis.

National Highway Traffic Safety Administration. (2004). *National standardized child passenger safety training program curriculum.* Washington, DC: Author.

__________. (2004). Retrived October 2, 2006 from http://www.nhtsa.gov

National Institute of General Medical Sciences (NIGMS), National Institutes of Health. (2006). Fact sheet: Trauma, shock, burn and injury: Fact and Figures. Retrieved October 2, 2006, from

express feelings of anger, disbelief, terror, and shock. In the long-term phase, which begins anywhere from a few days to several months after the event, the client often experiences flashbacks and nightmares of the traumatic event. The client may call on ineffective coping mechanisms, such as alcohol or drugs, and withdraw from relationships. Appropriate interventions may include the following:

- Assess emotional responses while providing physical care. Observe for crying, sleep problems, suspiciousness, and fear during the initial phase of treatment. If the client is unconscious, encourage family members and friends to express their feelings. These assessments provide valuable information about the client's ability to cope with the trauma.
- Be available if the client wishes to talk about the trauma, and encourage expression of feelings. The client may initially deny negative feelings; this denial is a coping mechanism in the initial phase of recovery.
- Teach relaxation techniques, such as deep breathing, progressive muscle relaxation, or imagery. These techniques are often useful in coping when thoughts of the trauma recur.
- Refer the client and family members for counseling, psychotherapy, or support groups as appropriate. Continued therapy may be necessary in assisting the client and family to resolve the acute and long-term effects of trauma.

Facilitate Community-Based Care

Address the following topics to prepare the client and family for home care:

- The type of home environment to which the client will be returning, including any changes that will be required to let the client function in that environment
- Medications, dressings, wound care, equipment, and supplies
- Special diet, if needed
- Rehabilitation plan and its effect on the client's family
- Follow-up appointments with the physician or at the trauma clinic
- Emotional changes that the client may undergo as a result of the trauma
- Helpful resources:
  a. Home health care
  b. Community support groups
  c. National Institute of Neurological Disorders and Stroke.

Evalution

Desired outcome include the following:

- The client's airway will remain free of obstruction.
- The client will remain free from infection.
- The client will retain mobility.
- The client will express relief from fearful emotions.

REVIEW Unintentional Injury: Motor Vehicle Crashes

RELATE: LINK THE CONCEPTS

Linking the exemplar of Unintentional Injury with the concept of Intracranial Regulation:

1. What is the priority of care when your client who experienced a head injury in a car crash has a blood pressure of 90/60 and a heart rate of 51?
2. What caring interventions would you plan with the client who has a head injury from a car crash to prevent the rise of intracranial pressure?

Linking the exemplar of Unintentional Injury with the concept of Perfusion:

3. Describe potential threats to a client's perfusion as a result of a motor vehicle crash? How would this be impacted if the client's mobility was altered due to traction or other immobilizing treatments?
4. How can you promote mobility for a client involved in a motor vehicle crash who has a casted left leg and right arm? How would this plan change if the client was an older adult with diminished mobility prior to the trauma?

READY: GO TO COMPANION SKILLS MANUAL

- Administering oxygen by cannula, face mask, or face tent
- Inserting an orohabyngeal airway
- Assisting with endotracheal intubation
- Caring for the client on a mechanical ventilator
- Clearing an obstructed airway
- Administering automated external defibrillation
- Performing surgical and antisepsis

REFER: GO TO MYNURSINGKIT

REFLECT: CASE STUDY

Laura Mays, age 26, was driving her car and was hit by another car at an intersection. The car that hit her ran a red light. Laura was extracted from her car using the jaws of life and was moaning when initially removed, but was unable to respond verbally. Her pupils were pinpoint and were reactive to light. The paramedics at the scene provided initial emergent care. Her vital signs were T 98, P 110, R 10, and BP 90/50. She had bleeding from facial and scalp lacerations as well as suspected fractured ribs. Since she hit her head and is not conscious, the paramedics also suspect a head injury.

Laura's airway was determined to be patent and she was given oxygen by a bag-mask resuscitator. Her cervical spine was immobilized with a cervical collar and head immobilizer and she was placed on a spine board to prepare for transport to local emergency department. Circulatory status was assessed and an intravenous solution of 0.9% normal saline was begun in the right antecubital area at a rate of 150 ml/hr.

In the emergency room her vital signs were T 98, P 118, R 12, and BP 98/50. IV fluid of normal saline was continued, and a Foley cathether was inserted. Her airway remained patent and oxygen was continued.

1. What are priority nursing diagnosis for Laura?
2. What laboratory and diagnostic tests will the nurse anticipate being ordered?

PEARSON
EXPLORE mynursingkit™

MyNursingKit is your one stop for online chapter review materials and resources. Prepare for success with additional NCLEX®-style practice questions, interactive assignments and activities, web links, animations and videos, and more!

Register your access code from the front of your book at **www.mynursingkit.com**.

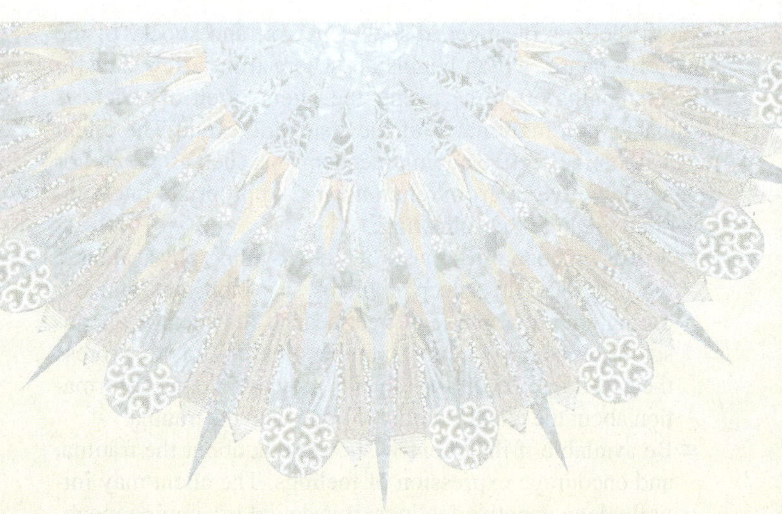

REFERENCES

Abrahams, N., & Jewkes, R. (2005). Effects of South African men's having witnessed abuse of their mothers during childhood on their levels of violence in adulthood. *American Journal of Public Health, 95,* 1811–1816.

Abrams, R. C., Marzuk, P. M., Tardiff, K., & Leon, A. C. (2005). Preference for fall from height as a method of suicide by elderly residents of New York City. *American Journal of Public Health, 95,* 1000–1002.

Ahmed, M. K., van Ginneken, J., Razzaque, A., & Alam, N. (2004). Violent deaths among women of reproductive age in rural Bangladesh. *Social Science & Medicine, 59,* 311–319.

American Psychiatric Association. (2000). *Diagnostic and statistical manual of mental disorders* (4th ed., Text Revision). Washington, DC: Author.

American Psychological Association. (n.d.) Violence prevention in early childhood: how teachers can help. Retrieved September 9, 2009, from http://actagainstviolence.apa.org/materials/publications/act/violenceprevention_childhood.pdf

Anderson, D. G. (2004). Workplace violence in long haul trucking. *AAOHN Journal, 52,* 23–27.

Aseltine, R. H., & DeMartino, R. (2004). An outcome evaluation of the SOS suicide prevention program. *American Journal of Public Health, 94,* 446–451.

Baker, M. W., & Heitkemper M. M. (2005). The roles of nurses on interpersonal teams to combat elder mistreatment. *Nursing Outlook, 53*(5), 253–259.

Branas, C. C., Nance, M. L., Elliott, M. R., Richmond, T. S., & Schwab, C. W. (2004). Urban–rural shifts in intentional firearm death: Different causes, same results. *American Journal of Public Health, 94,* 1750–1755.

Brodowski, M. L., Nolan, C. M., Gaudiosi, J. A., Yuan, Y. Y., Zikratova, L., Oritz, M. J., et al. (2008). Nonfatal maltreatment of infants—United States, October 2005–September 2006. *Morbidity and Mortality Weekly Report, 57,* 336–339.

Bureau of Justice Statistics. (2005a). *Crime characteristics.* Retrieved March 30, 2006, from http://www.ojp.usdoj.gov/bjs/cvict_c.htm

Bureau of Justice Statistics. (2005b). *Criminal victimization.* Retrieved March 30, 2006, from http://www.ojp.usdoj.gov/bjs/cvictgen.htm

Campbell, J. C., Webster, D., Koziol-McLain, J., Block, C., Campbell, D., Curry, M. A., et al. (2003). Risk factors for femicide in abusive relationships: Results from a multisite case control study. *American Journal of Public Health, 93,* 1089–1097.

Canadian Nurses Association. (1992). *Family violence: Clinical guidelines for nurses.* Ottawa: CNA.

Carbaugh, S. F. (2004). Understanding shaken baby syndrome. *Advanced Neonatal Care, 4,* 105–116.

Centers for Disease Control and Prevention, National Center for Injury Prevention and Control. (2009) [cited 2009 June 01]. Web-based Injury Statistics Query and Reporting System (WISQARS) [Online]. Retrieved from www.cdc.gov/injury/wisqars/index.html

Centers for Disease Control and Prevention National Center for Health Statistics. (2008). National Hospital Ambulatory Medical Care Survey: 2006 Emergency Department Summary. Retrieved from http://www.cdc.gov/nchs/data/nhsr/nhsr007.pdf

Centers for Disease Control and Prevention. Web-based Injury Statistics Query and Reporting System (WISQARS) [Online]. (2008) [cited 2008 Jun 16]. National Center for Injury Prevention and Control, Centers for Disease Control and Prevention (producer). Retrieved from www.cdc.gov/ncipc/wisqars

Centers for Disease Control. (2000). *What is domestic violence?* Retrieved from http://www.cdc.gov/ncipc/dvp/fivpt/spotlite/home.htm

Centers for Disease Control and Prevention. (2003a). Domestic violence awareness month, October 2003. *Morbidity and Mortality Weekly Report, 52,* 942.

Centers for Disease Control and Prevention. (2003b). Suicide and attempted suicide. *Morbidity and Mortality Weekly Report, 53,* 471.

Centers for Disease Control and Prevention. (2004). Sexual Assault Awareness Month, April 2004. *Morbidity and Mortality Weekly Report, 53,* 189–190.

Centers for Disease Control and Prevention. (2005a). *Healthy people data.* Retrieved September 5, 2005, from http://wonder.cdc.gov/data2010

Centers for Disease Control and Prevention. (2005b). Sexual assault awareness month—April, 2005. *Morbidity and Mortality Weekly Report, 54,* 311.

Centers for Disease Control and Prevention. (n.d.). *Injury and Violence Prevention.* Retrieved October 20, 2009 from http://www.hhs.gov/opa/pubs/hp2010/hp2010rh_sec2_ivp.pdf

Clements, C. M., Sabourin, C. M., & Spiby, L. (2004). Dysphoria and hopelessness following battering: The role of perceived control, coping, and self-esteem. *Journal of Family Violence, 19,* 25–36.

Close, S. M. (2005). Dating violence prevention in middle school and high school youth. *Journal of Child and Adolescent Psychiatric Nursing, 18*(1), 2–9.

Coker, A. L., Smith, P. H., McKeown, R. E., & King, M. J. (2000). Frequency and correlates of intimate partner violence by type: Physical, sexual, and psychological battering. *American Journal of Public Health, 90,* 553–559.

Collins, K. A. (2006). Elder maltreatment. *Archives of Pathology and Laboratory Medicine, 130,* 1290–1296.

Cubbin, C., Pickle, L. W., & Fingerhut, L. (2000). Social context and geographic patterns of homicide among US black and white males. *American Journal of Public Health, 90,* 579–587.

Dienemann, J., Glass, N., & Hyman, R. (2005). Survivor preferences for response to IPV disclosure. *Clinical Nursing Research, 14,* 215–233.

Dienemann, J. C., & Wiederhorn, N. (2003). A critical pathway for intimate partner violence across the continuum of care. *Journal of Obstetric, Gynecologic, and Neonatal Nursing, 32*(5), 594–603.

Division of Violence Prevention. (2000a). Intimate partner violence among men and women—South Carolina, 1998. *Morbidity and Mortality Weekly Report, 49,* 691–694.

Division of Violence Prevention. (2000b). Use of medical care, police assistance, and restraining orders by women reporting intimate partner violence—Massachusetts, 1996–1997. *Morbidity and Mortality Weekly Report, 49,* 485–488.

Division of Violence Prevention. (2002c). Variation in homicide risk during infancy—United States, 1989–1998. *Morbidity and Mortality Weekly Report, 51,* 187–189.

Division of Violence Prevention. (2003a). School-associated suicides—United States, 1994–1999. *Morbidity and Mortality Weekly Report, 52,* 476–478.

Division of Violence Prevention. (2003b). Suicide attempts and physical fighting among high school students—United States, 2001. *Morbidity and Mortality Weekly Report, 52,* 474–476.

Dong, X., Simon, M. A., Gorbien, M., Percak, J., & Golden, R. (2007). Loneliness in older Chinese adults: A risk factor for elder mistreatment. *Journal of the American Geriatrics Society, 55*(11), 1831–1835.

Downs, W. R., & Miller, B. A. (2002). Treating dual problems of partner abuse and substance abuse. In C. Wekerle & A. Wall (Eds.), *The violence and addiction equation* (pp. 254–274). New York: Brunner-Routledge.

Durose, M. R., Harlow, C. W., Langan, P. A., Motivans, M., Rantala, R. R., & Smith, R. L. (2005). *Family violence statistics: Including statistics on strangers and acquaintances.* Washington, DC: Bureau of Justice Statistics.

Eaton, D. K., Kann, L., Kinchen, S., Ross, J., Hawkins, J., Harris, W. A., et al. (2006). Youth Risk Behavior Surveillance—United States, 2005. *Morbidity and Mortality Weekly Report, 55*(SS-5), 1–108.

El-Bassel, N., Gilbert, L., Wu, E., Go, H., & Hill, J. (2005). Relationship between drug abuse and intimate partner violence: A longitudinal study among women receiving methadone. *American Journal of Public Health, 95,* 465–470.

Federal Bureau of Investigation. (2004). *Work place violence: Issues in response.* Washington, DC: FBI.

Field, C. A., Caetano, R., & Nelson, S. (2004). Alcohol and violence related cognitive risk factors associated with the perpetration of intimate partner violence. *Journal of Family Violence, 19,* 249–253.

Fontes, L. A. (2005). *Child abuse and culture.* New York: Guilford Press.

Foster, E. M., Qaseem, A., & Connor, T. (2004). Can better mental health services reduce the risk of juvenile justice system involvement? *American Journal of Public Health, 94,* 859–865.

Freedberg, P. (2006). Health care barriers and same-sex intimate partner violence: A review of the literature. *Journal of Forensic Nursing, 2*(1), 15–24, 41.

Friss-Feinberg, L. F. (2002). The state of the art: Caregiver assessment in practice settings. *Family Caregiver Alliance.* National Consensus Development Conference Report (Vol. I). San Francisco.

Fulmer, T. (2002). Elder abuse and neglect assessment. *Try this: Best practices in nursing care to older adults.* New York: Hartford Geriatric Institute for Nursing.

Fulmer, T., & Cahill, V. M. (1984). Assessing elder abuse: A study. *Journal of Gerontological Nursing, 10*(12), 16–20.

Fulmer, T., Paveza, G., Abraham, I., & Fairchild, S. (2000). Elder neglect assessment in the emergency department. *Journal of Emergency Nursing, 26*(5), 436–443.

Anemia An abnormally low number of circulating red blood cells (RBCs), low hemoglobin concentration, or both.

Anergic Unable to react to common antigens.

Anergy Fatigue and decreased energy associated with a depressive disorder.

Angle-closure glaucoma A type of **glaucoma** that results from a narrowing of the anterior chamber angle due to corneal flattening or bulging of the iris into the anterior chamber.

Anhedonia The inability to feel pleasure.

Anion Ion that carries a negative charge.

Anorexia Loss of appetite.

Anorexia nervosa A potentially life-threatening disorder characterized by extreme perfectionism, weight fear, significant weight loss, body image disturbances, strenuous exercising, peculiar food-handling patterns, and reductions in heart rate, blood pressure, metabolic rate, and the production of estrogen or testosterone.

Anorgasmia Absence of orgasm.

Antepartum Time between conception and the onset of labor; usually used to describe the period during which a woman is pregnant.

Antibodies Proteins that work against **antigens.**

Antibody-mediated (humoral) immune response Activation of B cells to produce antibodies to respond to antigens such as bacteria, bacterial toxins, and free viruses.

Anticipatory grief Experienced in advance of a loss, such as the wife who grieves before her ailing husband dies.

Anticipatory loss A loss that is experienced before the loss actually occurs. For example, the gradual decline and eventual death of a family member who has Alzheimer's disease.

Antigen Foreign substance that triggers the immune response.

Antigen-antibody complex The complex formed by the binding of an antibody to an antigen.

Antigenic drift Describes small changes that occur continuously as a virus makes copies of itself.

Antiretroviral therapies Pharmacologic therapies that stop or suppress the activity of a retrovirus, preventing further weakening of the immune system and thereby minimizing opportunistic infections.

Antiseptics Agents that inhibit the growth of some microorganisms.

Antisocial personality disorder (ASPD) One of 11 types of **personality disorder** defined by the DSM-IV, ASPD is characterized by a pattern of disregard for and violation of the rights of others.

Anuria The failure of the kidneys to produce urine, resulting in a total lack of urination or output of less than 100 mL per day in an adult.

Aortic stenosis Narrowing of the aortic valve that obstructs blood flow to systemic circulation.

Aphakia Absence of the lens of the eye (e.g., after surgical removal of a cataract).

Aphasia Defective or absent language function.

Aplastic anemia A disorder that results when the bone marrow fails to produce all three types of blood cells.

Apnea Absence of breathing.

Appendectomy Surgical removal of the appendix.

Appendicitis Inflammation of the vermiform appendix.

Apraxia The inability to perform purposeful movements and use objects correctly.

Areflexia The loss of reflex function.

Areola Pigmented ring surrounding the nipple of the breast.

Arterial blood gas (ABG) A laboratory test used to evaluate acid–base balance and gas exchange.

Arteriosclerosis An arterial disorder characterized by thickening, loss of elasticity, and calcification of arterial walls.

Arthroscopy A surgical procedure in which an arthroscope (a thin tube that is lighted and has a camera in one end) is inserted into a joint.

Arthrodesis Joint fusion, a procedure that may be used to stabilize joints such as cervical vertebrae, wrists, and ankles.

Arthroplasty Total joint replacement.

Ascites Excess fluid in the peritoneal cavity.

Asepsis The absence of disease-causing organisms.

Assertive behavior Behavior that consists of expressing one's wishes and opinions, or taking care of oneself, but not at the expense of others.

Assimilation 1. The process of adapting to and integrating characteristics of the dominant culture as one's own. 2. The process by which humans encounter and react to new situations by using the mechanisms they already possess.

Associative play A stage of play in which children play together or share tasks during play.

Astereognosis The inability to identify objects by touch.

Asthma A chronic inflammatory disease of the lungs characterized by recurrent episodes of wheezing, breathlessness, chest tightness, and coughing.

Asystole Cardiac standstill.

Atelectasis Collapse of lung tissue following obstruction of the bronchus or bronchioles.

Atheist An individual who does not believe in God.

Atherosclerosis A form of **arteriosclerosis** in which deposits of fat and fibrin obstruct and harden the arteries.

Atrial gallop A heart sound produced by atrial contraction and ejection of blood into the ventricle during late diastole. Also called the fourth heart sound.

Atrial kick An extra bolus of blood delivered to the ventricles before they contract.

Atrial natriuretic factor (ANF) A peptide-hormone released from cells in the atrium of the heart in response to excess blood volume and stretching of the atrial walls.

Atrial septal defect An opening in the atrial septum that permits left-to-right shunting of blood.

Atrioventricular (AV) canal defect A combination of defects in the atrial and ventricular septa and portions of tricuspid and mitral valves. A complete AV canal defect allows blood to travel freely among all four chambers of the heart.

Atrophy The wasting away or decrease in size of an organ, muscle, or tissue.

Attention deficit disorder (ADD) A variation in central nervous system processing characterized by developmentally inappropriate behaviors involving inattention. When hyperactivity and impulsivity accompany inattention, the disorder is called **attention deficit hyperactivity disorder (ADHD)**.

Attention impairment A condition marked by an inability to process information and respond to such information appropriately; a client with attention impairment will have poor concentration and be easily distracted.

Audiologist A health care professional specializing in identifying, diagnosing, treating and monitoring disorders of the auditory and vestibular portions of the ear.

Aura An olfactory or visual sensory sensation that may provide an early warning sign of a seizure.

Autistim spectrum disorders (ASDs) This term described three of the pervasive developmental disorders that share a number of similarities: autism, Asperger syndrome, and pervasive developmental disorder not otherwise specified (PDD-NOS).

Autoantibodies Antibodies that react to the individual's own tissues.

Autoimmune disorder/disease Failure of immune system to recognize itself, resulting in normal host tissue being targeted by immune defenses.

Autografting A procedure performed in the surgical suite in which part of the client's healthy skin is removed and used to effect permanent skin coverage over the wound area.

Autologous bone marrow transplant Bone marrow transplant using a client's own bone marrow.

Automatism A reaction that occurs automatically, without conscious thought.

Autonomy The state of being independent and self-directed without outside control. **Autonomy** refers to the right to make one's own decisions.

Autonomic dysreflexia An exaggerated sympathetic response that occurs in clients with spinal cord injuries at or above the T6 level. Also called *autonomic hyperreflexia*.

Autosomal chromosomes Genetic material found in the cell nucleus which determines physical characteristics (excluding gender) of the individual.

Autosome A single chromosome from any one of the 22 pairs of chromosomes not involved in sex determination (X or Y); humans have 22 pairs of autosomes.

Avian Influenza Also known as "bird flu," it is a form of influenza that commonly infects birds. This virus has not yet demonstrated the ability to spread between humans; however, concerns are that it will mutate to allow person-to-person spread. This viral strain has a mortality rate of greater than 50% in people who have been infected due to close association with infected birds.

Avoidant personality disorder (APD) One of 11 types of **personality disorders** recognized by the DSM-IV, APD is characterized by a pattern of social withdrawal along with a sense of inadequacy, fear, and hypersensitivity to potential rejection or shame.

Avolition The inability to persist in goal-directed activities.

Awareness The ability to perceive environmental stimuli and body reactions and to respond appropriately through thought and action.

Axial loading The application of vertical force to the spinal column.

Azotemia Increased levels of nitrogenous wastes in the blood.

B Lymphocytes Integral to specific immune response, they are activated and mature into either plasma cells, which secrete antibodies, or memory cells.

Bacilli Rod-shaped bacteria.

Bacteremia The presence of bacteria in the blood.

Bacteria The most common category of infection-causing microorganisms.

Bactericidal agent Destroys bacteria.

Bacteriostatic agent Prevents the growth and reproduction of some bacteria.

Balloon tamponade The inflation of the balloon tip of a multiple-lumen nasogastric tube to control bleeding.

Barotrauma Lung injury caused by alveolar overdistention.

Barrel chest An increase in the anteroposterior chest diameter resulting from air trapping and hyperinflation.

Basal cell carcinoma An epithelial tumor believed to originate either from the basal layer of the epidermis or from cells in the surrounding dermal structures.

Basal metabolic rate The amount of energy expended by the body at rest.

Base excess (BE) A calculated value also known as *buffer base capacity*. The BE measures substances that can accept or combine with hydrogen ions. It reflects the degree of acid–base imbalance by indicating the status of the body's total buffering capacity.

Bases (or **alkalis**) Substances that accept hydrogen ions in solution.

Behavioral therapy A form of therapy in which clients learn techniques to modify or change maladaptive behaviors.

Belief system The way in which a culture explains the mysteries of the universe and life.

Beneficence The act of doing good.

Benign prostatic hypertrophy (BPH) Age-related, nonmalignant enlargement of the prostate gland that decreases the outflow of urine by obstructing the urethra, causing difficult urination.

Bereavement The subjective response experienced by the surviving loved ones after the death of a person with whom they have shared a significant relationship.

Bias A negative belief or preference that is generalized about a group that leads to prejudgment.

Bilevel ventilator (BiPAP) Mechanical ventilation that provides inspiratory positive airway pressure as well as airway support during expiration.

Biliary colic A severe, steady pain in the epigastric region or right upper quadrant of the abdomen.

Binge eating The ingestion of huge amounts of food (about 3,500 kcal) within a short time (about 1 hour).

Binge eating disorder An eating disorder characterized by recurring episodes of **binge eating**, a sense of lack of control and negative feelings about oneself, but without intervening periods of behavior such as self-induced vomiting, purging by laxatives, fasting, or prolonged exercise.

Binge drinking A form of alcoholism in which the addict frequently drinks copious amounts of alcohol in a single session.

Binuclear family A postdivorce family in which the biologic children are members of two nuclear households, both that of the father and that of the mother, and the children alternate between the two homes.

Bioethics The application of ethics to issues of human life or health (e.g., to decisions about abortion or euthanasia).

Biological Rhythm A cyclical event or function that consists of repeated occurrences and repeated, regular intervals between occurrences.

Bipolar disorder A mood disorder characterized by alternating depression and elation, with periods of normal mood in between; also called manic–depressive disorder.

Bisexual An individual who is attracted to members of both sexes.

Bisphosphonates Drugs used to treat osteoporosis that inhibit bone resorption by suppressing osteoclast activity.

Blackouts A form of amnesia about events that occurred during the drinking period, which is seen in the early stages of alcoholism.

Bladder training Gradually increases the bladder capacity by increasing the intervals between voidings and resisting the urge to void.

Blended family A family formed after the death or divorce of a parent, may include stepparents on both sides, stepchildren, half-siblings.

Blepharism Spasms that cause the eye to blink continuously.

Bloodborne pathogens Microorganisms carried in blood and body fluids that are capable of infecting others with serious and difficult to treat viral infections.

Blood flow The volume of blood transported in a vessel, in an organ, or throughout the entire circulation over a given period of time.

Blood pressure The force that blood exerts against the walls of the arteries as it is pumped from the heart.

Blood urea nitrogen (BUN) A measure of blood level of urea, the end product of protein metabolism.

Body image The image of physical self.

Body fluid Any fluid that is essential to homeostasis; water is the primary body fluid.

Body mass index (BMI) A method of comparing weight to height as an indirect measure of body fat.

Body substance isolation (BSI) System that employs generic infection control precautions for all clients, except those with the few airborne diseases.

Body surface area (BSA) The relationship between height and weight measured in square meters.

Bone marrow transplant The treatment of disease by infusing a client with his or her own bone marrow or that of a healthy donor.

Borborygumus Hyperactive, high-pitched, tinkling, rushing, or growling bowel sounds heard in diarrhea or at the onset of bowel obstruction.

Borderline personality disorder (BPD) One of 11 **personality disorders** defined in the DSM-IV, it is marked by unstable interpersonal relationships, self-image, affect, and impulsivness.

Boutonnière deformity A flexion deformity of the PIP joints with extension of the DIP joint.

Boundaries The invisible lines that define the amount and kind of contact allowable among members of the family and between the family and outside systems.

Brachytherapy Radiation treatment given by placing radioactive material directly in or near the target, which is often a tumor.

Bradykinesia Slowed movements due to muscle rigidity.

Bradyphrenia Slowed thinking and a decreased ability to form thoughts, to plan, or to make decisions.

Brain death The cessation and irreversibility of all brain functions, including the brainstem.

Brainstem Contains the midbrain, pons, and medulla oblongata. Located between the cerebrum and spinal cord, the brainstem connects pathways between the higher and lower structures. Ten of the 12 pairs of cranial nerves originate in the brainstem.

Braxton Hicks contractions Intermittent painless uterine contractions that may occur every 10–20 minutes and occur more frequently near the end of pregnancy.

Breakthrough pain A sudden flare or increase in pain despite comfort with or without baseline analgesia.

Breast Mammary gland.

Breast cancer The unregulated growth of abnormal cells in breast tissue.

Brief psychotic disorder Rapid onset of at least one of the following psychotic symptoms: delusions, hallucinations, disorganized speech, or disorganized behavior. The episode lasts at least 1 day but less than 1 month, after which the person returns to the premorbid level of functioning.

Bronchiectasis Chronic dilation of the bronchi and bronchioles.

Bronchiolitis A lower respiratory tract illness that occurs when an infecting agent (virus or bacterium) causes inflammation and obstruction of the small airways.

Bronchogenic carcinomas Tumors of the airway epithelium.

Bruits Blowing sound sometimes heard due to restriction of blood flow through the vessels.

Buffers Substances that prevent major changes in pH by releasing hydrogen ions.

Bulimia nervosa A type of **eating disorder** characterized by cycles of binge eating followed by purging.

Burn An injury resulting from exposure to heat, chemicals, radiation, or electric current.

Burn shock Hypovolemic shock resulting from the shift of a massive amount of fluid from the intracellular and intravascular compartments into the interstitium following burn injury.

Cachexia Physical wasting from weight loss and loss of muscle mass due to the rapid growth and reproduction of cancer cells and their need for increased nutrients.

Caffeine A stimulant that increases the heart rate and acts as a diuretic.

Calcium oxalate A chemical compound from which kidney stones may form.

Calcium phosphate A chemical compound from which kidney stones may form.

Calculi Renal stones.

Cancellous bone The spongy tissue of bone.

Cancer A family of complex diseases with manifestations that vary according to body system and type of tumor cells.

Cancer pain Pain that may result from the direct effects of the disease and its treatment, or it may be unrelated to the disease and its treatment in individuals with cancer.

Cannabis sativa The plant source of marijuana.

Candidiasis A common, opportunistic fungal infection in clients with AIDS.

Carcinogen A substance that causes cancer.

Carcinogenesis The production or origin of cancer.

Cardiac arrest The cessation of heart function.

Cardiac cycle One contraction and relaxation of the heart; a single heartbeat.

Cardiac index The cardiac output adjusted for the client's body size.

Cardiac output The amount of blood pumped by the ventricles into the pulmonary and systemic circulations in 1 minute.

Cardiac reserve The heart's ability to respond to the body's changing need for cardiac output.

Cardinal ligament Major ligament of the uterus containing the uterine artery and vein.

Cardiogenic shock Shock that occurs when the heart's pumping ability is compromised to the point that it cannot maintain cardiac output and adequate tissue perfusion.

Cardiomyopathy Primary abnormality of the heart muscle that affects its structural or functional characteristics.

Cardiopulmonary resuscitation (CPR) A mechanical attempt to maintain tissue perfusion and oxygenation using oral resuscitation and external cardiac compressions.

Carpal spasm Involuntary contraction of the hand and fingers due to decreased calcium levels.

Carrier Human or animal reservoir of a specific infectious agent that usually does not manifest any clinical signs of the disease.

Caseation necrosis A process in which tissue infected with **mycobacterium tuberculosis** dies and forms a cheeselike center in the infectious **bacilli.**

Cast A rigid device applied to immobilize injured bones and promote healing.

Catabolism The breakdown of body proteins.

Cataract An opacification (clouding) of lens of the eye.

Catatonic excitement A positive symptom of **schizophrenia** characterized by hyperactivity and bizarre behavior.

Catatonic inhibition A negative symptom of **schizophrenia** that involves decreased activity level; limited speech; minimal self-care; and, at times, a trancelike state.

Cation An **ion** that carries a positive charge.

Cavitation Formation of a cavity or bubble.

Cell-mediated (cellular) immune response Direct or indirect inactivation of antigen by lymphocytes.

Cellulitis An acute bacterial **infection** of the dermis and underlying connective tissue. Cellulitis is characterized by red or lilac, tender, warm, edematous skin that may have an ill-defined, nonelevated border.

Central nervous system (CNS) One of two principal parts of the neurologic system, the central nervous system consists of the brain and the spinal cord.

Central nervous system depressants Drugs that act to slow brain function, decreasing levels of alertness and awareness. CNS depressants include including barbiturates, benzodiazepines, paraldehyde, meprobamate, and chloral hydrate.

Central pain A type of pain related to a lesion in the brain that may spontaneously produce high-frequency bursts of impulses that are perceived as pain.

Cephalocaudal Growth that proceeds in the direction from head to toe.

Cerebellum Located below the cerebrum and behind the brainstem, it coordinates stimuli from the cerebral cortex to provide precise timing for skeletal muscle coordination and smooth movements.

Cerebral palsy (CP) A group of chronic conditions affecting body movement, coordination, and posture that results from a nonprogressive abnormality of the immature brain.

Cerebrum The largest portion of the brain.

Cerumen Earwax.

Cervical cap A latex cup-shaped device, used with spermicidal cream or jelly, that fits snugly over the cervix and is held in place by suction.

Cervix The narrow neck of the uterus.

Chancre A painless ulceration formed during the first stage of syphilis.

Cheilosis Cracking of lips.

Chemotherapy Cancer treatment involving the use of cytotoxic medications to decrease tumor size, adjunctive to surgery or radiation therapy; or to prevent or treat suspected metastases.

Childless family (also *child-free family*) A family without children.

Chlamydias A group of sexually transmitted infections caused by *Chlamydia trachomatis.*

Chloasma (melasma gravidarum) Brownish pigmentation over the bridge of the nose and the cheeks during pregnancy and in some women who are taking oral contraceptives. Also called *mask of pregnancy.*

Cholangitis Duct inflammation.

Cholecystitis Inflammation of the gallbladder.

Cholelithiasis The formation of stones (*calculi* or *gallstones*) in the gallbladder or biliary duct system.

Chromosomes Tightly coiled strands of DNA within the nucleus that contain genetic information.

Chronic bronchitis A disorder of excessive bronchial mucous secretion.

Chronic fatigue Profound fatigue of long duration that is not improved by rest.

Chronic fatigue syndrome A complex disorder in which the client experiences unrelenting fatigue and associated symptoms that are not alleviated by substantial rest and cannot be otherwise explained for a period of six months or longer.

Chronic illness An alteration in health or function that lasts for an extended period of time, usually six months or longer, and often for the duration of the individual's life.

Chronic infection An **infection** that develops slowly and persists for months or sometimes years.

Chronic intermittent colitis A recurrent form of **ulcerative colitis** characterized by insidious onset, few systemic manifestations, and attacks lasting 1–3 months, which occur at intervals of months to years.

Chronic lymphocytic leukemia (CLL) A disorder characterized by the proliferation and accumulation of small, abnormal, mature lymphocytes in the bone marrow, peripheral blood, and body tissues.

Chronic myeloid leukemia (CML) A disorder characterized by abnormal proliferation of all bone marrow elements.

Chronic obstructive pulmonary disease (COPD) A specific progressive disorder that slowly alters the structures of the respiratory system over time, irreversibly affecting lung function.

Chronic pain Prolonged pain, usually lasting longer than 6 months. It is not always associated with an identifiable cause and is often unresponsive to conventional medical treatment.

Chronic renal failure A type of **renal failure** that progresses slowly with few symptoms until the kidneys are severely damaged and unable to meet the excretory needs of the body.

Chronic venous insufficiency A disorder of inadequate venous return over a prolonged period of time.

Chvostek's sign Facial grimacing caused by repeated contractions of the facial muscle.

Cirrhosis A progressive, irreversible disorder, eventually leading to liver failure; the end stage of chronic liver disease.

Clean A state of **medical asepsis** in which almost all microorganisms are absent.

Clonic phase Typically the second phase in a generalized or tonic-clonic seizure, characterized by alternating muscular contraction and relaxation.

Closed fracture A bone fracture in which the skin remains intact; also known as a simple fracture.

Club drugs Substances popular among adolescents and young adults who frequent dance clubs and "raves," the most common of which is MDMA (methylenedioxymethamphetamine), better known as Ecstasy.

Coarctation of the aorta Narrowing or constriction in the descending aorta, often near the ductus arteriosus or left subclavian artery, which obstructs the systemic blood outflow.

Cocaine A powerful stimulant of natural origin that acts at the nerve terminals to prevent the reuptake of dopamine and norepinephrine, which in turn results in vasoconstriction, tachycardia, and hypertension.

Codependence A cluster of maladaptive behaviors exhibited by significant others of a substance-abusing individual that serves to enable and protect the abuse at the expense of living a full and satisfying life.

Cognition The process by which an individual learns, stores, retrieves, and uses information.

Cognitive development The manner in which people learn to think, reason, and use language.

Cognitive skills Intellectual skills or thought processes that include problem solving, decision making, critical thinking, and creativity.

Coitus interruptus A method of contraception in which the male withdraw from the female's vagina when he feels that ejaculation is impending.

Colectomy Surgical resection and removal of the colon.

Colloids Substances such as large protein molecules that do not readily dissolve into true solutions.

Colloid osmotic pressure A pulling force exerted by colloids that helps maintain the water content of blood by pulling water from the interstitial space into the vascular compartment.

Colon cancer Cancer of the third segment of the large bowel.

Colonization The process by which strains of microorganisms become resident flora, capable of growing and multiplying.

Colorectal cancer Cancer of the colon or rectum.

Colostomy A surgical opening into the colon.

Combined oral contraceptives A combination of estrogen and progestin. Also called birth control pills.

Comfort To ease the grief or trouble of others; to give hope.

Communicable disease An illness that is transmitted directly from one person or animal to another by contact with body fluids, or that is indirectly transmitted by contact with contaminated objects or **vectors**.

Compartment syndrome Condition in which the tissue pressure in a muscle compartment exceeds microvascular pressure, interrupting cellular perfusion.

Compliance The relationship between the volume of the intracranial components and intracranial pressure; the amount of distention or expansion the ventricles can achieve to increase stroke volume.

Complicated grief A form of **grief** in which the individual's strategies to cope with the loss are maladaptive.

Compromised host An individual who is at increased risk of infection.

Comorbidity The presence of one or more additional disease processes.

Concrete thinking A type of thinking characterized by a focus on facts and details and an inability to generalize or think abstractly.

Condom A sheath of synthetic material that covers the penis to prevent conception or disease.

Confabulation Making up information to fill memory gaps; used as defensive mechanism to protect the person's attempt to protect self-esteem when confronted with memory loss.

Confusion An alteration in cognition that makes it difficult to think clearly, focus attention, or make decisions.

Congenital cataracts A type of **cataract** that may appear in a child at birth or in childhood, usually in both eyes.

Congenital heart defect A defect of the heart or great vessels that is present at birth.

Conjugate vera The true conjugate, which extends from the middle of the sacral promontory to the middle of the pubic crest.

Conjunctiva The thin, transparent membrane that covers the anterior surface of the eye and lines the inner surfaces of the eyelids.

Conjunctivitis Inflammation of the **conjunctiva**. The most common eye disease, conjunctivitis is usually caused by a bacterial or viral infection.

Connective tissue Tissue made of fiber that forms the framework for support of the body's tissue and organs.

Consciousness A condition in which the person is aware of self and environment and is able to respond appropriately to stimuli. Full consciousness requires both normal arousal and full cognition.

Consequence-based (teleological) theories Theories that look to the outcomes (consequences) of an action in judging whether that action is right or wrong.

Constipation Fewer than three bowel movements per week or the difficult passage of stools.

Contact precautions Used for clients who are known to have or suspected of having serious illnesses that are easily transmitted by direct contact with the client or by contact with items in the environment, such as *shigella*.

Contingency contracts A reinforcement process. Congingency contracts operate by "if-then" rules. If the client performs a targeted response, such as abstinence from the addictive behavior (gambling, drug use, cutting, etc.), then the client receives desired reinforcers.

Continuous renal replacement therapy (CRRT) A form of **dialysis** in which blood is continuously circulated through a highly porous hemofilter from artery to vein or vein to vein.

Continuous positive airway pressure (CPAP) Mechanical ventilation that applies positive pressure to the airways of a client who is breathing spontaneously. Breathing is client-triggered and pressure controlled. CPAP is used to help maintain open airways and alveoli, decreasing the work of breathing.

Contractility The inherent capability of the cardiac muscle fibers to shorten.

Contracture Permanent shortening of connective tissue.

Contralateral deficit Loss or impairment of sensorimotor functions on the side of the body opposite the side of the brain that is damaged by stroke.

Convergence The medial rotation of the eyeballs so that each is directed toward the viewed object.

Cooperative play The stage of play in which children work together to contribute to a unified whole, such as forming a sports team or dancing in an ensemble.

Corneal abrasion Disruption of the superficial epithelium of the cornea.

Corneal reflex Closure of eyelids (blinking) due to corneal irritation.

Cor pulmonale Right-sided heart failure.

Corpus The upper triangular portion of the uterus, also called the uterine body.

Corpus luteum A small yellow body that develops within a ruptured ovarian follicle.

Coruna The elongated portion of the uterus where the fallopian tubes enter.

Coryza Inflammation of the mucous membranes lining the nose usually associated with nasal discharge.

Couplet Two premature ventricular contractions in a row.

Couvade In some cultures, the male's observance of certain rituals and taboos to signify the transition to fatherhood.

Creatinine clearance A test that uses 24-hour urine and serum creatinine levels to determine the glomerular filtration rate; a sensitive indicator of renal function.

Crepitation A grating sound.

Crohn's disease (also known as regional enteritis) A chronic, relapsing **inflammatory bowel disorder** affecting the GI tract.

Cross-dressing Occurs when an individual of one gender (typically male) dresses in clothing specific to the opposite gender.

Crystalloids Salts that dissolve readily into true solutions.

Cultural deprivation A lack of culturally assistive, supportive, or facilitative acts.

Cultural groups Racial, ethnic, religious, or social groups with specific group behaviors and characteristics that are learned and shared, including language, customs, beliefs, and values.

Cultural values Preferred ways of behaving or thinking that are sustained over time and used to govern a cultural group's actions and decisions.

Culture The patterns of behavior and thinking that people living in social groups learn, develop, and share.

Cultures Laboratory cultivations used to identify probable microorganisms by their characteristics, such as shape, growth patterns, and Gram-staining qualities.

Curling's ulcers Acute ulcerations of the stomach or duodenum that form following a burn injury.

Cyanosis Gray to blue or purple skin color caused by deoxygenated hemoglobin.

Cyclothymic disorder A type of **bipolar disorder** characterized by chronic, fluctuating mood disturbances involving numerous periods of hypomanic symptoms and numerous periods of depressive symptoms.

Cystitis Inflammation of the urinary bladder.

Cytokines Proteins that carry messages for immune system function.

Dawn phenomenon A rise in blood glucose between 4 a.m. and 8 a.m. that is not a response to hypoglycemia.

Dead space Areas of the lung that are ventilated but not perfused.

Death anxiety Worry or fear related to death or dying.

Debridement The process of removing necrotic material, including all loose tissue, wound debris, and eschar (dead tissue), from a wound.

Decibels Units of loudness.

Decompensation Loss of effective compensation.

Declarative memory Memory related to people and facts, is consciously accessible, and can be verbally expressed.

Deep venous thrombosis (DVT) A blood clot that forms along the intimal lining of a large vein.

Defecation The expulsion of feces from the anus and rectum.

Defibrillation An emergency procedure that delivers an electrical shock to stop ventricular fibrillation and return to a rhythm that promotes cardiac output sufficient to sustain life.

Deformation The alteration of the spinal cord and soft tissues caused by abnormal movement.

Dehiscence An unintended separation of wound margins due to incomplete healing.

Dehydration A condition that occurs when a body does not take in as much water as it loses or lacks sufficient reserves to maintain proper function.

Delayed union The prolonged healing of bones beyond the usual time period.

Delirium An acute disorder of cognition that affects functional independence.

Delirium Tremens A medical emergency usually occurring 3–5 days following alcohol withdrawal and lasting 2–3 days. Characterized by paranoia, disorientation, delusions, visual hallucinations, elevated vital signs, vomiting, diarrhea, and diaphoresis. Also known as **alcohol withdrawal delirium**.

Delusion Firm idea or belief not founded in reality.

Denominations Groups of members that adhere to the same practices and beliefs.

Dental caries Cavities.

Dependent personality disorder (DPD) A **personality disorder** marked by a pervasive, excessive, and unrealistic need to be cared for; fear of separation; lack of self-confidence; an inability to make decisions; and an inability to function independently.

Depersonalization A feeling of strangeness or unreality about the self.

Derealization A feeling of disconnection from the environment.

Dermatome An area of skin innervated by the cutaneous branch of one spinal nerve.

Deoxyribonucleic acid (DNA) One of two types of nucleic acid made by cells, DNA contains the genetic instructions for the development and functioning of human beings.

Depolarization The rapid inflow of sodium ions, causing an electrical change in which the inside of a cell becomes positive in relation to the outside; the phase in which the heart contracts as a result of ion channel functions.

Depo-Provera A long-acting progesterone that provides highly effective birth control for 3 months when given as a single injection.

Desaturated blood Blood that is low in oxygen.

Desire phase The first phase of the sexual response cycle; the arousal of sexual interest.

Detrusor muscle The smooth muscle layers of the bladder wall, the detrusor muscle allows the bladder to expand as it fills with urine and contract as it releases urine during voiding.

Development An increase in the complexity and function of skill progression, the individual's capacity and skill to adapt to the environment. Related to **growth**.

Developmental disability Any of a variety of chronic conditions characterized by mental and/or physical impairment.

Developmental stage A level of achievement for a particular segment of a person's life.

Developmental task A skill or behavior pattern learned during stages of development.

Diabetes mellitus Group of chronic disorders of the endocrine pancreas, all categorized under a broad diagnostic label. The condition is characterized by inappropriate hyperglycemia caused by a relative or absolute deficiency of insulin or by a cellular resistance to the action of insulin.

Diabetic ketoacidosis A form of metabolic acidosis induced by stress in a person with type 1 diabetes.

Diabetic nephropathy Disease of the kidneys in clients with diabetes that is characterized by the presence of albumin in the urine, hypertension, edema, and progressive renal insufficiency.

Diabetic neuropathy A disorder of the peripheral nerves and the autonomic nervous system in clients with diabetes, which manifests in one or more of the following: sensory and motor impairment, muscle weakness and pain, cranial nerve disorders, impaired vasomotor function, impaired gastrointestinal function, and impaired genitourinary function.

Diabetic retinopathy The collective name for the changes in the retina that occur in the person with diabetes. The retinal capillary structure undergoes alterations in blood flow, leading to retinal ischemia and a breakdown in the blood retinal barrier.

Diagonal conjugate Distance from the lower posterior border of the symphis pubis to the scaral promontory.

Diaphragm A flexible disk that covers the cervix to prevent conception.

Diaphysis The shaft of the bone.

Dialysate Dialysis solution.

Dialysis A process by which fluids and molecules pass through a semipermeable membrane from an area of higher solute concentration to one of lower solute concentration according to the rules of osmosis.

Diarrhea The passage of liquid feces and an increased frequency of defecation.

Diastole The phase of ventricular relaxation between heartbeats.

Diastolic blood pressure The minimum pressure within the arteries during **diastole**.

Diathermy Treatment with heat generated by high-frequency electrical currents.

Diet recall Client history of intake over a specified period of time.

Differentiation A process occurring over many cell cycles that allows cells to specialize in certain tasks.

Diffusion The continual intermingling of molecules in liquids, gases, or solids brought about by the random movement of the molecules.

Digital rectal examination An examination to detect for abnormalities in the rectum that can be detected through palpation.

Dihydrotestosterone (DHT) Formed in the prostate from testosterone, DHT is the androgen that mediates prostatic growth at all ages.

Dilated cardiomyopathy The most common form of **cardiomyopathy**, in which the heart chambers dilate and ventricular contraction is impaired.

Dirty In **medical asepsis**, a term used to indicate that microorganisms are likely to be present.

Discipline A method of teaching children the rules for how to behave in society and what is expected in different circumstances.

Discrimination The differential treatment of individuals or groups based on categories such as race, age, weight, gender, or social class, that occurs when an individual acts on prejudice and denies other people one or more of their fundamental rights.

Disease A detectable alteration in body function resulting from infection by microorganisms that causes a reduction of capacities or a shortening of the normal life span.

Disease surveillance Monitoring patterns of disease occurrence from cases of infections and communicable diseases reported by health care workers to state officials.

Disenfranchised grief Occurs when a person is unable to acknowledge the loss to other persons.

Disinfectants Agents that destroy pathogens other than spores.

Diskectomy The removal of the nucleus pulposus of an intervertebral disk.

Dissatisfaction problems Issues that arise from unmet sexual needs and expectations.

Disseminated intravascular coagulation (DIC) A complication resulting from prolonged retention of the dead fetus in the mother's womb.

Distributive shock Shock which results from widespread vasodilatation and decreased peripheral resistance. Also called **vasogenic shock.**

Diuresis (polyurea) The production of abnormally large amounts of urine.

Diuretics Pharmacologic agents that increase urine formation and secretion.

Diversity The unique variations among and between individuals, variations that are informed by genetics and cultural background, but that are refined by experience and personal choice.

Diverticula Saclike projections of mucosa through the muscular layer of the colon.

Do-not-resuscitate (DNR or "no-code") order Usually written by the physician for the client who has a terminal illness or is near death, this order is usually based on the wishes of the client and family that no cardiopulmonary resuscitation be performed for respiratory or cardiac arrest.

Do-not-intubate (DNI) order Usually written by the physician for the client who has a terminal illness or is near death, this order is usually based on the wishes of the client and family that no life-saving measures are provided once the client stops breathing.

Dormant Temporarily inactive but not dead.

Double depression A condition in which individuals experience **dysthymic disorder** in combination with **major depressive disorder.**

Down Syndrome A condition associated with mental retardation; Down Syndrome results when an individual is born with an extra chromosome.

Durable power of attorney A document that can delegate the authority to make health, financial, and/or legal decisions on a person's behalf.

Dramatic play The stage of play in which children use props to act out the drama of human life.

Droplet nuclei Residue of evaporated droplets emitted by an infected host; can remain in the air for long periods of time.

Droplet precautions Used for clients who are known to have or suspected of having serious illnesses transmitted by particle droplets larger than 5 microns, such as pertussis or pneumonia.

Duodenal ulcer A **peptic ulcer** occurring in the duodenum.

Dwarfism Excessively short stature, typically resulting from a genetic abnormality.

Dysfunctional uterine bleeding (DUB) Vaginal bleeding that is usually painless but abnormal in amount, duration, or time of occurrence.

Dysmenorrhea Painful menstruation.

Dysparenuria Painful intercourse.

Dysphagia Difficulty swallowing.

Dysplasia A loss of DNA control over differentiation occurring in response to adverse conditions.

Dyspnea Shortness of breath or difficulty breathing.

Dysrhythmias Abnormal heart rate or rhythm.

Dysthymic disorder A chronic disorder in which periods of depressed mood are interspersed with normal mood.

Dystonias Severe muscle spasms, particularly of the back, neck, tongue, and face.

Dysuria Difficult or painful urination.

Eating disorder A set of maladaptive responses to stress or anxiety characterized by obsessions with food and weight, often to the extent that daily functioning is impaired and physical and psychological health are threatened.

Echolalia The compulsive parroting of a word or phrase just spoken by another.

Echopraxia The compulsive imitation of the movements of another.

Eclampsia A major complication of pregnancy characterized by hypertension, albuminuria, oliguria, tonic and clonic convulsions, and coma.

Ecologic theory A theory of development that emphasizes the presence of mutual interactions between the individual and all of life's settings.

Ecomap Visual representation of how the family unit interacts with the external community environment, including schools, religious institutions, occupational duties, and recreational pursuits.

Ectopic beats Impulses originating outside normal conduction pathways of the heart.

Edema Swelling caused by excess fluid trapped in bodily tissue.

Ego The realistic part of the individual, balances the gratification demands of the **id** with the limitations of social and physical circumstances.

Ego-syntonic The perception that one's difficulties in dealing with other people are external.

Ejection fraction The fraction or percent of the diastolic volume that is ejected from the heart during systole.

Elective surgery Performed when surgical intervention is the preferred treatment for a condition that is not imminently life threatening (but may ultimately threaten life or well-being) or to improve the client's life.

Electrocardiogram (ECG) A graphic record of the heart's activity.

Electrocardiography A diagnostic test of cardiac function.

Electroconvulsive therapy (ECT) A treatment procedure during which an electric current is passed through the brain; it is useful to clients with severe depression, acute mania, some psychotic conditions, and those who are acutely suicidal.

Electroencephalogram (EEG) Measures and records the brain's electrical activity.

Electrolyte Charged ion capable of conducting electricity.

Elimination The secretion and excretion of body wastes from the kidneys and intestines.

Embryo The early stage of development of the young of any organism. In humans the embryonic period is from about 2 to 8 weeks' gestation and is characterized by cellular differentiation and predominantly hyperplastic growth.

Embryonic membranes The amnion and chorion.

Embolus Debris that obstructs a blood vessel.

Emergency surgery Surgery that is performed immediately to preserve function or the life of the client.

Emigration The movement of leukocytes through the blood vessel wall into affected tissue spaces in response to illness or injury.

Emotional availability The quality of parent-child interactions, including parental sensitivity, structuring, and degree of intrusiveness and hostility.

Emotions Feeling responses to a wide variety of emotional stimuli.

Emphysema A progressive pulmonary disease characterized by destruction of the walls of the alveoli, with resulting enlargement of abnormal air spaces.

Empyema Accumulation of purulent (infected) exudate in a space, e.g., the pleural cavity or the gallbladder.

Enabling behavior Any action by a person that consciously or unconsciously facilitates substance dependence.

Encapsulated Enclosed.

Encopresis Abnormal elimination pattern characterized by recurrent soling or passage of stool at inappropriate times.

Enculturation The process by which children learn culture from adults.

Endocardial cushions Fetal growth centers for mitral and tricuspid valves and AV septum.

End-of-life The final weeks of life when death is imminent.

End-of-life care The nursing care provided to a client who is dying or who is near death.

Endogenous Developing from within.

Endogenous insulin Insulin that is produced by the body.

Endometrium The innermost mucosal layer of the uterus.

Endotoxins Found in the cell wall of gram-negative bacteria, endotoxins are released only when the cell is disrupted. They act as activators of many human regulatory systems, producing fever, inflammation, and potentially clotting, bleeding, or hypotension when released in large quantities.

End-stage renal disease (ESRD) The final stage of **chronic renal failure**, when the kidneys are unable to excrete metabolic wastes and regulate fluid and electrolyte balance adequately.

Engrossment The characteristic sense of absorption, preoccupation, and interest in the infant demonstrated by fathers during early contact.

Enophthalmos Sunken appearance of the eyes.

Entropion Inversion of the eyelid.

Enuresis Involuntary passing of urine in children after bladder control is achieved.

Eosiniphil A type of leukocyte found in large numbers in the respiratory and gastrointestinal tracts. Eosinophils are thought to be responsible for protecting the body from parasitic worms. They also play a role in hypersensitivity response by inactivating some of the inflammatory chemicals released during the inflammatory response.

Epidemic Widespread outbreak of infectious disease with many infected people.

Epilepsy A chronic disorder characterized by recurrent, unprovoked seizures secondary to a central nervous system (CNS) disorder.

Erectile dysfunction (ED) The inability of the male to attain and maintain an erection sufficient to permit satisfactory sexual intercourse.

Erythema A reddening of the skin.

Eschar Hard, leathery crust that covers a burn wound and harbors necrotic tissue.

Escharotomy Surgical removal of eschar from the torso or extremity to prevent circumferential constriction.

Estrogen The primary hormone responsible for female sex characteristics.

Esotropia Momentary turning inward of the eyes.

Ethnic groups Group of individuals that have common racial characteristics and share a cultural heritage.

Ethics The rules or principles that govern right conduct.

Eustachian tube Connects the middle ear with the nasopharynx to help equalize the pressure in the middle ear with the atmospheric pressure.

Euthanasia From the Greek for painless, easy, gentle, or good death, now commonly used to signify a killing prompted by a humanitarian motive.

Euthyroid A normal thyroid state.

Evisceration Protrusion of body contents through a surgical wound.

Exacerbation A reappearance of symptoms of a chronic illness; sometimes referred to as a *flare.*

Excitement phase The second phase of the sexual response cycle, marked by an increase in the blood flow to various body parts resulting in erection of the penis and clitoris and swelling of the labia, testes, and breasts.

Exercise A type of physical activity defined as a planned, structured, and repetitive bodily movement performed to improve or maintain one or more components of physical fitness.

Exercise intolerance Decreased ability to participate in activities using large skeletal muscles because of fatigue or dyspnea.

Exogenous Developing from outside sources.

Exogenous insulin Insulin from a source outside the body.

Exophthalmos Protruding eyes.

Exotoxins Soluble proteins that microorganisms secrete into surrounding tissue. Exotoxins are highly poisonous, causing cell death and dysfunction.

Expectorate To expel or spit out.

Expressive jargon Using unintelligible words with normal speech intonations as if truly communicating in words.

Expressive speech The ability to speak and be understood by others.

Extended family The relatives of **nuclear** families, such as grandparents, aunts, and uncles.

Extended-kin network family A form of **extended family** in which two nuclear families of primary or unmarried kin live in close proximity to each other and share a social support network, goods, and services.

Extracapsular extraction A surgical treatment for **cataracts** in which the anterior capsule, nucleus, and cortex of the lens are removed, leaving the posterior capsule intact.

Extracapsular fracture A hip fracture involving the trochanteric region.

Extracellular fluid (ECF) Fluid found outside the cells and accounts for about one-third of total body fluid. It is subdivided into compartments. The two main compartments of ECF are intravascular and interstitial.

Extracorporeal shock wave lithotripsy (ESWL) A noninvasive technique for fragmenting kidney stones using shock waves generated outside the body.

Extrapulmonary tuberculosis Results when the disease spreads through the blood and lymph system to other organs.

Extrapyramidal side effects (EPS) A particularly serious set of adverse reactions to antipsychotic drugs. **EPS** include acute dystonia, akathisia, Parkinsonism, and tardive dyskinesia.

Exudate Material, such as fluid and cells, that has escaped from blood vessels during the inflammatory process and is deposited in tissue or on tissue surfaces.

Failure to thrive (FTT) A syndrome in which an infant falls below the fifth percentile for weight and height on a standard growth chart or is falling in percentiles on a growth chart.

Faith To believe in or be committed to something or someone.

Fallopian tubes Tubes that extend from the lateral angle of the uterus and terminate near the ovary. Also called oviducts and uterine tubes.

False pelvis The portion of the pelvis above the linea terminalis, which supports the enlarged pregnant uterus.

Family Individuals who are joined together by marriage, blood, adoption, or residence in the same household.

Family burden The overall level of distress experienced by the family as a result of a family member's mental illness.

Family-centered care Health care that is provided in partnership with the client and family.

Family-centered nursing Nursing that considers the health of the family as a unit in addition to the health of individual family members.

Family cohesion The emotional bonding between family members.

Family communication Includes listening, speaking, self-disclosure, and the abilities of the family as a group.

Family coping mechanisms The behaviors families use to deal with stress or changes imposed from either within or without the family.

Family development The dynamics or changes a family experiences over time, including changes in relationships, communication patterns, roles, and interactions.

Family flexibility The amount of change in a family's leadership, role relationships, relationship rules, and the families ability to respond to stress.

Family recovery Family response to a member's mental illness.

Family support Support from family members as they care for other family members. e.g., one sister relieves another to care for their aging mother over the weekend.

Family therapy A form of therapy in which the family system is treated as a unit and the focus is on family dynamics.

Fasciectomy (fascial excision) Process of excising the wound to the level of fascia.

Fat Embolism Syndrome (FES) Occurs when fat globules lodge in the pulmonary vascular bed or peripheral circulation.

Fatigue A condition characterized by a lack of energy and motivation that may or may not be accompanied by drowsiness.

Febrile seizures Generalized seizures that usually occur in children as the result of rapid temperature rise above 39°C (102°F), usually in association with an acute illness. No evidence of intracranial infection or other defined cause is found.

Fecal impaction A mass or collection of hardened feces in the folds of the rectum.

Fecal incontinence The loss of voluntary ability to control fecal and gaseous discharges through the anal sphincter.

Feces (stool) Body wastes and undigested food eliminated from the bowel.

Feedback The mechanisms by which some of the output of a system is returned to the system as input.

Female orgasmic disorder A sexual arousal cycle that stops before orgasm.

Female reproductive cycle (FRC) The monthly rhythmic changes in sexually mature women; composed of the ovarian cycle, during which ovulation occurs, and the uterine cycle, during which menstruation occurs.

Female sexual arousal disorder Discomfort or pain during sexual intercourse caused by a lack of vaginal lubrication.

Fertility awareness-based methods Contraception based on an understanding of the changes that occur throughout a woman's ovulatory cycle. Also called *natural family planning*.

Fertilization The process by which a sperm fuses with an ovum to form a new diploid cell, or zygote.

Fetal alcohol syndrome A form of mental retardation that results when the developing fetus is exposed to ethyl alcohol.

Fetal demise Intrauterine fetal death (IUFD) occurs after 20 weeks' gestation.

Fetal heart rate (FHR) The number of times the fetal heart beats per minute; normal range is 120 to 160.

Fetal lie Relationship of the cephalocaudal axis (spinal column) of the fetus to the cephalocaudal axis (spinal column) of the woman. The fetus may be in a longitudinal or transverse lie.

Fetal position Relationship of the landmark on the presenting fetal part to the front, sides, or back of the maternal pelvis.

Fetal tachycardia A fetal heart rate of 160 beats per minute or more during a 10-minute period of continuous monitoring.

Fetoscope An adaptation of a stethoscope that facilitates auscultation of the fetal heart rate.

Fetoscopy A technique for directly observing the fetus and obtaining a sample of fetal blood or skin.

Fetus The child in utero from about the seventh to ninth week of gestation until birth.

Fibrin degradation products Potent anticoagulants.

Fibromyalgia A chronic disorder characterized by widespread musculoskeletal pain, fatigue, and multiple **tender points.**

Fidelity A moral principle that obligates the individual to be faithful to agreements and responsibilities one has undertaken.

Filtration A process whereby fluid and solutes move together across a membrane from one compartment to another.

Filtration pressure The pressure in the compartment that results in the movement of the fluid and substances dissolved in fluid out of the compartment.

Fimbria A funnel-like enlargement of the Fallopian tube with many fingerlike projections (fimbriae) reaching out to the ovary.

First heart sound The heart sound produced by the closure of the AV valve, characterized by the syllable "lub."

5 P's of neurovascular assessment Pain, pulse, pallor, paralysis/paresis, paresthesia.

Fixation The immobilization or inability of the individual to proceed to the next developmental stage because of anxiety.

Flaccidity Absence of muscle tone; hypotonia.

Flatulence The presence of excessive amounts of gas in the stomach or intestines.

Flatus Gas or air normally present in the stomach or intestines.

Flight of ideas Rapidly changing, fragmentary thoughts.

Fluid resuscitation The administration of intravenous (IV) fluids to restore the circulating blood volume during the acute period of increasing capillary permeability.

Fluid volume deficit (FVD) (hypovolemia) Loss of both water and electrolytes in similar proportions from the extracellular fluid.

Fluid volume excess (FVE) (hypervolemia) The retention of both water and sodium in similar proportions to normal extracellular fluid (ECF).

Focal seizures (also known as *partial seizures)* Seizures that are caused by abnormal electrical activity in one hemisphere or in a specific area of the cerebral cortex, most often the temporal, frontal, or parietal lobes. The seizure may spread regionally, and the symptoms are related to the region of the cortex that is affected.

Follicle-stimulating hormone (FSH) Hormone produced by the anterior pituitary during the first half of the menstrual cycle, stimulating development of the graafian follicle.

Foramen ovale An opening between the atria of the fetal heart.

Foraminotomy An enlargement of the opening between the disk and the facet joint to remove bony overgrowth.

Forced expiratory volume in 1 second (FEV1) The amount of air that can be exhaled in 1 second as measured by a spirometer.

Foster family A family consisting of one or more adults caring for one or more children from other families when the children can no longer live with their birth parents.

Fourth heart sound A heart sound produced by atrial contraction and ejection of blood into the ventricle during late diastole. Also called **atrial gallop.**

Fracture A break in the continuity of a bone.

Fragile X syndrome A form of mental retardation caused by a single recessive gene abnormality on the X chromosome.

Frank–Starling mechanism An increase in venous return increases ventricular filling and myocardial stretch, which increases the force of contraction.

Friend support Support or assistance from non-family members, such as friends or coworkers, for a family during a time of illness or stress.

Fulguration A procedure that destroys tissue with electrical current.

Fulminant colitis An acute form of **ulcerative colitis** that involves the entire colon; manifestations include severe bloody diarrhea, acute abdominal pain, and fever.

Full-thickness burn A burn that involves all layers of the skin, including the epidermis, the dermis, and the epidermal appendages

Functional assessments Typically a combination of assessments that includes observations of child behavior, responses, and abilities that is used to assess how a child functions on a daily basis in his or her environment and to determine if the child has any developmental delays or special needs.

Functional strength The body's ability to perform work.

Fundus The rounded uppermost portion of the uterus.

Fungi A type of microorganism capable of producing infection. Yeasts and molds are common types of fungi.

Gallstone ileus A large gallstone.

Gamete Female or male germ cell; contains a haploid number of chromosomes.

Gametogenesis The process by which germ cells are produced.

Gastric lavage Irrigation of the stomach with large quantities of normal saline.

Gastric outlet obstruction Obstruction of the pyloric region of the stomach and duodenum that impairs gastric outflow; a potential complication of peptic ulcer disease.

Gastric ulcer A **peptic ulcer** occurring in the stomach.

Gender identity One's self-image as a female or male.

Gender-role behavior The outward expression of a person's sense of maleness or femaleness.

Generalized seizures The result of diffuse electrical activity that often begins in both hemispheres of the brain simultaneously, then spreads throughout the cortex into the brainstem. As a result, movements and spasms displayed by the client are bilateral and symmetric.

Genital herpes A sexually transmitted disease caused by the herpes simplex virus.

Genital intercourse (coitus) Penetration of the vagina by the penis.

Genital warts A sexually transmitted disease caused by the human papillomavirus.

Genogram Visual representation of gender showing lines of birth descent through the generations.

Genotype The pattern of genes on chromosomes.

Gestation Period of intrauterine development from conception through birth; pregnancy.

Gingiva The gum.

Gingivitis Red, swollen gingiva.

Glaucoma A condition characterized by optic neuropathy with gradual loss of peripheral vision and, usually, increased intraocular pressure of the eye.

Global self The collective beliefs and images one holds about oneself.

Global self-esteem How much one likes oneself as a whole.

Glomerular filtration rate (GFR) The rate at which fluid is filtered through the kidneys.

Glomerulonephritis Inflammation of the glomerular capillary membrane.

Glomerulus Found in the nephrons of the kidneys, a tuft of capillaries surrounded by Bowman's capsule.

Glucagon A hormone that stimulates the breakdown of glycogen in the liver, the formation of carbohydrates in the liver, and the breakdown of lipids in both the liver and adipose tissue.

Glucosuria The excretion of glucose in the urine.

Glycogenolysis The breakdown of liver glycogen.

Gluconeogenesis The formation of glucose from fats and proteins.

Goiter An enlarged thyroid gland.

Gonadotropon-releasing hormone (GnRH) A hormone secreted by the hypothalamus that stimulates the anterior pituitary to secrete follicle-stimulating hormone (FSH) and leutenizing hormone (LH).

Goodpasture's syndrome A rare autoimmune disorder of unknown etiology. It is characterized by formation of antibodies to the glomerular basement membrane.

Graafian follicle The ovarian cyst containing the ripe ovum, which secretes estrogens.

Graft-versus-host disease A series of immunologic reactions in response to transplanted cells.

Gram stain A diagnostic test conducted to identify the infecting organisms in urine by shape and characteristic.

Granulation tissue Young connective tissue with new capillaries formed in the healing process.

Grave's disease An autoimmune disorder marked by an enlarged thyroid and the signs of hyperthyroidism.

Grief The total response to the emotional experience related to loss.

Growth Physical change and increase in size.

Glycosuria The excretion of carbohydrates into the urine.

Guillain-Barré syndrome (GBS) An acute inflammatory demyelinating disorder of the peripheral nervous system characterized by an acute onset of motor paralysis (usually ascending).

Gynecomastia Abnormal enlargement of the breast(s) in men.

H_1 Receptors Cellular histamine receptors that are present in the smooth muscle of the vascular system, the bronchial tree, and the digestive tract. Stimulation of these receptors results in itching, pain, edema, bronchoconstriction, and other characteristics symptoms of inflammation and allergy.

H1N1 influenza A form of the influenza virus that consists of avian genes, human genes, and genes from flu viruses typically found in pigs from Asia and Europe. Once mistakenly called "swine flu," it can be spread through human to human transmission.

H_2 Receptors Cellular histamine receptors present primarily in the stomach; their stimulation results in the secretion of large amounts of hydrochloric acid.

Habit training Attempts to keep clients dry by having them void at regular intervals.

Hallucination The perceptions of seeing, hearing, or feeling something that is not there.

Hashimoto's thyroiditis An autoimmune disorder in which antibodies destroy thyroid tissue.

Health A state of complete physical, mental, and social well-being.

Health beliefs Concepts about health that an individual believes are true, regardless of whether or not they are founded in fact.

Health care surrogate An individual selected to make medical decisions when a person is no longer able to make them for himself or herself.

Health literacy The ability to read, understand, and act on health information; includes such tasks as comprehending prescription labels, interpreting appointment slips, completing health insurance forms, and following instructions for diagnostic tests.

Health promotion Any activity undertaken for the purpose of achieving a higher level of health and well-being.

Heart block A block in the normal electrical conduction of the heart.

Heart failure The inability of the heart to pump adequate blood to meet the metabolic demands of the body.

Heart murmur Harsh, blowing sounds caused by disruption of blood flow into the heart, between the chambers of the heart, or from the heart into the pulmonary or aortic systems.

Heaving Lifting of the chest wall during contraction.

Helper T cells Play a vital role in normal immune system function, recognizing foreign antigens and infected cells and activating antibody-producing B cells. They are the primary cells infected by the **human immodeficiency virus.**

HELPP syndrome A cluster of changes including hemolysis, elevated liver enzymes, and low platelet count, sometimes associated with preeclampsia.

Hemanopia The loss of half of the visual field of one or both eyes.

Hematochezia Bright blood in the stool.

Hematocrit A laboratory test that measures the proportion of cells and plasma in blood.

Hematogenous spread Describes the spread of infection or disease through the blood.

Hematopoiesis Blood cell formation.

Hematuria The presence of blood in the urine.

Hemiarthroscopy The surgical replacement of the femoral head with a smooth metal sphere.

Hemiparesis Weakness of the left or right half of the body.

Hemiplegia Paralysis of the left or right half of the body.

Hemodialysis A process by which the client's blood flows through vascular catheters, passes by the **dialysate** in an external machine, and then returns to the client.

Hemodynamics The study of forces involved in blood circulation.

Hemoglobin The oxygen-carrying molecule within red blood cells; a laboratory test to measure the amount of hemoglobin.

Hemoglobinopathy A disorder of hemoglobin.

Hemolytic anemia A disorder that results from the premature destruction of red blood cells.

Hemolysis The destruction of red blood cells; releases hemoglobin into the circulation.

Hemoptysis Bloody sputum.

Hemorrhage Rapid or excessive bleeding.

Hemosiderosis The storage of excessive iron in tissues and organs.

Hemotympanum Bleeding into or behind the tympanic membrane.

Heroin An illicit CNS depressant narcotic that alters perception and produces euphoria.

Hernia A protrusion (such as of the intestine through the inguinal wall or canal).

Herniated intervertebral disk A rupture of the cartilage surrounding the intervertebral disk with protrusion of the nucleus pulposus.

Heterograft (xenograft) Skin used for transplantation that was obtained from an animal, usually a pig.

Heterosexism The view that heterosexuality is the only correct sexual orientation.

Heterosexual An individual who is attracted to members of the opposite sex.

Hip fracture A fracture of the femur at the head, neck, or trochanteric regions.

Histamine A key chemical mediator of inflammation.

Histrionic personality disorder (HPD) One of the 11 types of **personality disorder**, it is characterized by a lifelong tendency for dramatic, egocentric, attention-seeking response patterns.

Holosystolic Term used to describe the sounds heard during the entire phase of systole.

Holy day A day set aside for special religious observance.

Homan's sign Pain in the calf when the foot is dorsiflexed.

Homeostasis The body's tendency to maintain a state of physiologic balance in the presence of constantly changing conditions.

Homophobia The fear, hatred, or mistrust of gays and lesbians often expressed in overt displays of discrimination.

Homograft (allograft) Human skin that has been harvested from cadavers.

Homologous chromosomes The pair of chromosomes that are inherited, one from each parent.

Homosexual An individual who is attracted to members of the same sex.

Hope To expect or desire with confidence.

Hormones Chemical messengers secreted by various glands that exert controlling effects on the cells of the body.

Hormone replacement therapy Administration of hormones, usually estrogen and a progestin, to alleviate the symptoms of menopause.

Hospice care The support and care for persons in the last phase of an incurable disease so that they may live as fully and comfortably as possible.

Human chorionic gonadotropin (hCG) A hormone produced by the chorionic villi which is found in the urine of pregnant women. Also called prolan.

Human Immunodeficiency Virus (HIV) A primary immunodeficiency disorder, which is spread primarily through sexual contact with an infected person. HIV is the virus that causes **acquired immunodeficiency syndrome (AIDS)**.

Humoral immune response Hyperreactive response of B cells characteristic of **systemic lupus erythematosus (SLE)**.

Hyaluronic acid (HA) A lubricating substance in cartilage and joint synovial fluid.

Hydronephrosis Accumulation of urine in the renal pelvis as a result of obstructed outflow.

Hydrostatic pressure The pressure a fluid exerts within a closed system on the walls of its container. The hydrostatic pressure of blood is the force blood exerts against the vascular walls (e.g., the artery walls). The principle involved in hydrostatic pressure is that fluids move from the area of greater pressure to the area of lesser pressure.

Hydroureter Distention of the ureter with urine.

Hyperalgesia Increased response to a pain stimulus because of peripheral sensitization.

Hypercalcemia Elevated blood levels of calcium.

Hypercapnia A condition that results when $PaCO_2$ rises above 45mmHg.

Hyperchloremia Elevated chloride levels in the blood.

Hypercyanotic episode A potentially life-threatening episode of hypoxia.

Hyperemia Increased blood flow to an area.

Hyperextension Forcible backward bending.

Hyperflexion Forcible forward bending.

Hyperglycemia Elevated glucose levels.

Hyperkalemia Elevated potassium levels in the blood.

Hypermagnesemia Elevated magnesium levels in the blood.

Hypernatremia Elevated sodium levels in the blood.

Hyperopia Farsightedness.

Hyperosmolar hyperglycemic state (HHS) A disorder characterized by a plasma osmolarity of 340 mOsm/L or greater, greatly elevated blood glucose levels, and altered levels of consciousness.

Hyperphosphatemia Increased blood levels of phosphate.

Hyperplasia An increase in the number or density of normal cells.

Hypoplastic left heart syndrome One of the most severe congenital heart defects, characterized by absence or stenosis of mitral and aortic valves, an abnormally small left ventricle, a small aorta, and aortic or mitral stenosis or atresia.

Hyperresponsiveness An exaggerated response, as with bronchoconstruction in asthma.

Hypersensitivity An overreaction of the immune system to an antigen or antigens.

Hypersomnia The inability to stay awake during the day, despite obtaining sufficient sleep at night.

Hypertension Excess pressure in the arterial portion of the circulatory system.

Hypertensive emergency A systolic pressure is greater than 180 mmHg and the diastolic pressure higher than 120 mmHg. Also called malignant hypertension.

Hypertensive encephalopathy A syndrome characterized by extremely high blood pressure, altered level of consciousness, increased intracranial pressure, papilledema, and seizures.

Hyperthyroidism A disorder caused by excessive delivery of thyroid hormone to the peripheral tissues. Also called thyrotoxosis.

Hypertonic Refers to solutions that have a higher osmolality than body fluids; 3% sodium chloride is a hypertonic solution.

Hypertonic dehydration (or hypernatremic dehydration). Occurs when sodium loss is proportionately less than water loss.

Hypertrophic cardiomyopathy A disorder characterized by decreased compliance of the left ventricle and hypertrophy of the ventricular muscle mass.

Hypertrophic scar An overgrowth of dermal tissue that remains within the boundaries of the wound.

Hypertrophy Enlargement of glandular cells or muscles.

Hyperventilation Unusually fast respirations, or overbreathing.

Hypervolemia (Fluid volume excess) The retention of both water and sodium in similar proportions to normal extracellular fluid (ECF).

Hypovolemic shock Shock caused by a decrease in intravascular volume.

Hyphema Bleeding into the anterior chamber of the eye.

Hypoactive sexual desire disorder A deficiency in or absence of sexual fantasies and persistently low interest or a total lack of interest in sexual activity.

Hypocalcemia Decreased blood levels of calcium.

Hypocapnia A condition that results when $PaCO_2$ falls below 35 mmHg.

Hypochloremia Decreased blood levels of chloride.

Hypogeusia Diminished sense of taste.

Hypoglycemia Diminished glucose levels.

Hypokalemia Decreased blood levels of potassium.

Hypomagnesemia Decreased blood levels of magnesium.

Hypomania A less extreme form of mania that is not severe enough to markedly impair functioning or require hospitalization.

Hyponatremia Decreased blood levels of sodium.

Hypothyroidism A disorder resulting when the thyroid gland produces an insufficient amount of thyroid hormone.

Hypotonic dehydration (or hyponatremic dehydration) This occurs when fluid loss is characterized by a proportionately greater loss of sodium than water.

Hypoperfusion Decreased blood flow.

Hypophosphatemia Decreased blood levels of phosphate.

Hyposmia Diminished sense of smell.

Hypotonic Refers to solutions that have a lower osmolality than body fluids, such as one-half normal saline (0.45% sodium chloride).

Hypovolemia (Fluid volume deficit) Loss of both water and electrolytes in similar proportions from the extracellular fluid.

Hypoxemia A condition that results when PaO_2 falls below 80 mmHg.

Iatrogenic infection A type of **infection** that results directly from diagnostic or therapeutic procedures.

Id In Freudian terms, the source of instinctive and unconscious psychologic urges.

Ideal self How the individual thinks he/she should be or would prefer to be.

Ileostomy A surgical opening made in the ileum of the small intestine.

Ileus A condition that causes a temporary cessation of the passage of material through the intestines.

Illness A state in which the individual's physical, emotional, intellectual, social, developmental, or spiritual functioning is diminished.

Illness behavior A coping mechanism that includes the ways that an individual describes, monitors, and interprets symptoms, and the individual's ability to take remedial action and use the health care system.

Illusion A distorted perception of actual sensory stimuli.

Immunity The body's natural or induced response to infection and the conditions associated with its response.

Immunization Introduces an **antigen** into the body, allowing **immunity** against a disease to develop naturally.

Immunocompetent Term used to describe clients who have an immune system that identifies antigens and effectively destroys or removes them.

Immunodeficiency A condition that develops when the immune system is incompetent or unable to respond effectively.

Immunoglobulin (Ig) A protein that functions as an antibody.

Immunosuppression Inability of the immune system to respond to an antigen. Occurs in response to disease or medications; may be intentional to prevent rejection of transplants or a side effect of some medications.

Impulsiveness or **Impulsivity** Acting without considering the consequences of one's behavior.

Impulse conduction The transmission of an impulse along the nerve pathways to the spinal cord and directly to the brain.

Incident pain A type of breakthrough pain that is predictable because it is precipitated by an event or activity such as coughing or changing position.

Infection An invasion of the body tissue by microorganisms with the potential to cause illness or disease.

Infectious disease Any communicable disease that is caused by microorganisms that are commonly transmitted from one person to another or from an animal to a person.

Infertility A lack of conception despite unprotected sexual intercourse for at least 12 months.

Inflammation or **Inflammatory response** An adaptive response to what the body sees as harmful, such as an allergen, illness, or injury. Inflammation typically is characterized by pain, heat, redness, and swelling.

Inflammatory bowel disease (IBD) Chronic inflammation of the bowel common to a group of conditions that includes Crohn's disease and ulcerative colitis.

Influenza A highly contagious viral respiratory disease characterized by **coryza** (inflammation of the mucous membranes lining the nose usually associated with nasal discharge), fever, cough, and systemic symptoms such as headache and **malaise** (vague feeling of physical discomfort).

Infundibulopelvic ligament A ligament that suspends and supports the ovaries.

Inhalants Substances inhaled to produce euphoria. Categorized into three types: anesthetics, volatile nitrites, and organic solvents.

Impotence Inability to achieve or maintain an erection.

Input Information, material, or energy that enters a system.

Insensible fluid loss Fluid loss that is not perceptible to the individual.

Insomnia The inability to fall asleep or remain asleep.

Insulin A hormone that facilitates the uptake and use of glucose by cells and prevents an excessive breakdown of glycogen in the liver and muscle.

Insulin reaction Low blood glucose levels, or hypoglycemia. Also called insulin shock.

Intermittent claudication A cramping or aching pain in the calves of the legs, the thighs, and the buttocks that occurs with a predictable level of activity.

Intersex Ambiguous gender.

Interstitial fluid Accounts for approximately 75% of extracellular fluid; intersticial fluid surrounds the cells.

Intimacy A relationship that entails commitment, affective intimacy, cognitive intimacy, physical intimacy, and mutuality.

Intracellular fluid (ICF) Fluid found within the body cells, also called *cellular fluid.*

Intractable seizures Seizures that continue to occur even with optimal medical management.

Intracapsular fracture A hip fracture involving the head or neck of the femur.

Intracranial hypertension A sustained state of **increased intracranial pressure** that is potentially life threatening.

Intracranial regulation The processes that affect intracranial compensation and adaptive neurologic function.

Intradiscal electrothermal therapy (IDET) The use of thermal energy to treat pain from a bulging spinal disk.

Intragenerational family A family in which more than two generations live together.

Intrapartum The time from the onset of true labor until the birth of the infant and expulsion of the placenta.

Intrauterine device (IUD) A small plastic or metal form that is placed in the uterus to prevent implantation of a fertilized ovum.

Intrauterine fetal death (IUFD) Death of a fetus that occurs after 20 weeks gestation; often referred to as **stillbirth** or **fetal demise.**

Intravascular fluid or **plasma** Accounts for approximately 20% of the **extracellular fluid** and is found within the vascular system.

Intravenous pyelography A diagnostic test used to evaluate the structure and excretory function of the kidneys, ureters, and bladder.

In vitro fertilization A process in which a woman's eggs are collected from her ovaries, fertilized in the laboratory, and then placed into her uterus after normal embryo development has begun.

Involuntary admission The detention of a client in a psychiatric or medical facility against the client's will, normally reserved for cases in which the client is a danger to himself or others.

Ion Electrically charged particle.

Iron deficiency anemia A disorder that results when the supply of iron in the body is insufficient for the formation of red blood cells.

Ischemia Insufficient blood supply.

Ischemic Deprived of oxygen.

Ischial spines Prominences that arise near the junction of the ilium and ischium and jut into the pelvic cavity.

Isoelectric line A straight line on an electrocardiograph that indicates the absence of electrical activity.

Isokinetic exercises Resistive exercises that involve muscle contraction or tension against resistance; can be either isotonic or isometric.

Isometric exercises exercises in which muscles contract without moving the joint.

Isotonic A solution that has the same osmolality as body fluids.

Isotonic dehydration (or isonatremic dehydration) A type of fluid imbalance that occurs when fluid loss is not balanced by intake and the losses of water and sodium are in proportion.

Isotonic exercises Exercises in which the muscle shortens to produce muscle contractions and active movement.

Isotonic fluid volume deficit A type of fluid imbalance that occurs when electrolytes are lost along with fluid.

Isotonic imbalance A fluid imbalance that occurs when water and electrolytes are lost or gained in equal proportions, so that the osmolality of body fluids remains constant.

Isthmus That portion of the uterus between the internal cervical os and the endometrial cavity.

Joint arthroplasty The reconstruction or replacement of a joint.

Joint custody Occurs when two parents who are not married have equal responsibility and legal rights for their shared children.

Justice Fairness.

Juvenile Rheumatoid Arthritis (JRA) A chronic inflammatory autoimmune disease diagnosed in children that is characterized by joint inflammation, resulting in decreased mobility, swelling, and pain.

Kaposi's sarcoma (KS) Often the presenting symptom of AIDS, it remains the most common cancer associated with the disease. Kaposi's sarcoma is caused by a virus called the Kaposi sarcoma-associated herpesvirus, also known as human herpesvirus 8.

Karyotype A pictorial analysis of chromosomes.

Keloid A scar that extends beyond the boundaries of the original wound.

Keratotic basal cell carcinoma A type of skin cancer.

Ketonuria The presence of ketones in the urine.

Ketosis An accumulation of ketone bodies produced during oxidation of fatty acids.

Kindling Long-term changes in brain neurotransmission that occur after repeated detoxifications.

Kinesthesia The ability to perceive movement and sense of position.

Kinesthetic A term referring to awareness of the position and movement of body parts.

Korsakoff's psychosis A condition typically seen in alcoholics that is characterized by intact intellectual functioning but an inability to retrieve long-term memory events or retain new information.

Kosher Acceptable or prepared according to Jewish law.

Kussmaul's respirations Deep, rapid respirations associated with compensatory mechanisms.

Labyrinthitis also called **otitis externa** Is inflammation of the inner ear.

Laënnec's cirrhosis A progressive, irreversible liver disorder resulting from excessive alcohol consumption. Also called alcoholic cirrhosis.

Laminectomy The removal of a part of the vertebral lamina.

Laparoscopic cholecystectomy Removal of the gallbladder using an endoscope.

Laxatives Medications that stimulate bowel activity and assist in fecal elimination.

Lead An insulated wire that connects an electrocardiograph to the electrodes attached to the patient.

Learning disabilities Neurological conditions in which the brain cannot receive or process information normally.

Lesbian A woman who prefers relationships with other women.

Leukemia A group of chronic malignant disorders of white blood cells (WBCs) and WBC precursors.

Leukocytes The primary cells involved in both nonspecific and specific immune system responses. Also known as white blood cells (WBCs).

Leukocytosis An increase in the number of leukocytes in the blood (above 10,000/mm^3), in response to infection or inflammation.

Leukopenia A decrease in the number of circulating leukocytes.

Libido The psychic energy that, according to Freud, provides the underlying motivation to human development.

Lifestyle A person's general way of living, including living conditions and individual patterns of behavior that are influenced by sociocultural factors and personal characteristics.

Limit setting Establishing clear and consistent rules or guidelines for child or client behavior.

Lipoatrophy Atrophy of subcutaneous tissues.

Lipodystrophy Excessive growth of subcutaneous tissue.

Lithiasis Stone formation.

Lithotripsy The preferred treatment for urinary calculi, uses sound or shock waves to crush a stone.

Living will A document that provides written directions about life-prolonging procedures to provide instructions when a person can no longer communicate in a life-threatening situation.

Local infection Invasion by a microorganism that is limited to the specific part of the body where the microorganism remains.

Localized responses More common manifestations of type I hypersensitivity, they are typically atopic responses; that is, they have a strong genetic predisposition. Atopic reactions are the result of localized, rather than systemic, IgE-mediated responses to an **allergen**. They are prompted by contact of the allergen with IgE in the bronchial tree, nasal mucosa, and conjunctival tissues.

Locked-in syndrome A state of consciousness in which the client is alert and fully aware of the environment and has intact cognitive abilities but is unable to communicate through speech or movement because of blocked efferent pathways from the brain. Motor paralysis affects all voluntary muscles, although the upper cranial nerves (I through IV) may remain intact, allowing the client to communicate through eye movements and blinking.

Locus of control (LOC) A concept about whether clients believe their health status is under their own or others' control.

Long-term memory The repository for information stored for periods longer than 72 hours and usually weeks and years.

Loose association An indication of disordered thinking characterized by the shifting of verbal ideas from one topic to another, with no apparent relationship between thoughts, and the person speaking being unaware that the topics are unconnected. Commonly seen in **schizophrenia**.

Loss An actual or potential situation in which something that is valued becomes altered or no longer available.

Lower-body obesity Identified by a waist-to-hip ratio of less than 0.8; more commonly seen in women. Also called peripheral obesity.

Lung abscess A local area of necrosis and pus formation within the lung.

Lupus nephritis Inflammation of the kidneys resulting from **systemic lupus erythematosus** (SLE).

Lutenizing hormone (LH) Anterior pituitary hormone responsible for stimulating ovulation and for development of the **corpus luteum**.

Lymphadenopathy The enlargement of lymph nodes (over 1 cm) with or without tenderness. It may be caused by inflammation, infection, or malignancy of the nodes or the regions drained by the nodes.

Lymphangitis **Inflammation** of a lymph vessel.

Lymphocytes Account for 20%–40% of circulating leukocytes. Lymphocytes are the principal effector and regulator cells of specific immune responses to protect the body from microorganisms, foreign tissue, and cell mutations or alterations.

Lyse Disintegrate.

Macrophages Large phagocytes that are important in the body's defense against chronic infections.

Major depressive disorder A mood disorder characterized by loss of interest in life and unresponsiveness, moving from mild to severe, severe lasting at least 2 weeks; also called unipolar disorder.

Major depressive episode Characterized by a change in several aspects of a person's life and emotional state consistently over a period of 14 days or longer.

Malaise Vague feeling of physical discomfort.

Male erectile disorder When a man has erection problems during 25% or more of his sexual interactions.

Male orgasmic disorder Difficulty of a male client to ejaculate.

Malignant Term used to refer to a cell or growth which, if not treated, will recur, continue to grow, and spread to other sites in the body, ending in death.

Malnutrition (also known as **undernutrition)** Health effects due to insufficient nutrient intake or stores.

Mania An abnormal and persistently elevated, expansive, or irritable mood lasting at least one week, significantly impairing social or occupational functioning, and generally requiring hospitalization.

Manipulation Controlling behavior used to exploit others for personal gain.

Margination The accumulation of **leukocytes** along the inner surface of blood vessels. Occurs as part of the inflammatory process.

Massage therapy The scientific manipulation of the soft tissues of the body for the purposes of promoting healing and wellness.

Mast cells Cells that detect foreign agents or injury and respond by releasing histamine, thereby activating the inflammatory process.

Masturbation The self-stimulation of one's genitals for sexual pleasure.

Maternal role attainment The process by which a woman learns mothering behaviors and becomes comfortable with her identity as a mother.

McDonald's sign A probable sign of pregnancy characterized by an ease in flexing the body of the uterus against the cervix.

Mean arterial pressure (MAP) The average pressure in the arterial circulation throughout the cardiac cycle.

Meatus A body passage or opening.

Meconium The first fecal material passed by the newborn, normally up to 24 hours after birth.

Medical asepsis All practices intended to confine a specific microorganism to a specific area, thus limiting the number, growth, and transmission of the microorganism.

Meditation The act of focusing one's thoughts or engaging in self-reflection or contemplation.

Meiosis A reductive division of sex cells, producing ova or sperm with a half set (haploid) of chromosomes.

Melanoma A type of malignant skin cancer.

Melasma gravidarum See chloasma.

Mendelian inheritance Traits that are passed on by a single gene.

Meninges Three connective tissue membranes that cover, protect, and nourish the **central nervous system.**

Menorrhagia Excessive or prolonged menstruation.

Menstruation The periodic shedding of the uterine lining in a woman of childbearing age who is not pregnant.

Menstrual cycle The cyclic phases of **menstruation** that occurs about every 28 days.

Mental retardation Significant limitation in intellectually functioning and adaptive behavior.

Metabolism The process of biochemical reactions occurring in the body's cells that are necessary to sustain life.

Metabolic acidosis (bicarbonate deficit) A disorder characterized by a low pH (< 7.35) and a low bicarbonate (< 22 mEq/L). It may be caused by excess acid in the body or loss of bicarbonate from the body.

Metabolic alkalosis (bicarbonate excess) A disorder characterized by a high pH (> 7.45) and a high bicarbonate (> 26 mEq/L). It may be caused by loss of acid or excess bicarbonate in the body.

Metabolic syndrome A disorder characterized by the presence of three or more of the following: increased waist circumference, hypertension, elevated blood triglycerides and fasting blood glucose, and low HDL cholesterol.

Metaphysic The portion of the bone between the diaphysis and the epiphysis.

Metaplasia A change in the normal pattern of differentiation such that dividing cells differentiate into cell types not normally found at that location in the body.

Metastasis The process by which spreading of malignant neoplasms occurs; the transfer of disease from one organ or part to another.

Metrorrhagia Bleeding between menstrual periods.

Microalbuminuria A low but abnormal level of albumin in the urine.

Microstaging The assessment of the level of invasion of a malignant melanoma and the maximum tumor thickness.

Micturition Releasing urine from the urinary bladder (voiding).

Middle ear effusion Results when negative pressure in the middle ear causes sterile serous fluid to move from the capillaries into the space.

Miliary tuberculosis Results from **hematogenous spread** (through the blood) of the bacilli throughout the body.

Milieu therapy A therapeutic recovery environment that supports behavior changes, teaches new coping skills, and helps the client move from addiction to sobriety.

Milliequivalent The chemical combining power of the ion, or the capacity of cations to combine with anions to form molecules.

Miscarriage The loss of a fetus prior to 20 weeks gestation.

Mitosis The process of cell division.

Modeling Observing the behavior of people who have successfully achieved a goal that one has set for oneself and, through observing, acquiring ideas for behavior and coping strategies.

Monoamine oxidase inhibitor (MAOIs) Drug inhibiting monoamine oxidase, an enzyme that terminates the actions of neurotransmitters such as dopamine, norepinephrine, epinephrine, and serotonin.

Monophasic A term used to describe **rheumatoid arthritis** when it occurs for a limited time and then improves.

Monotheism The belief in the existence of one God.

Mononeuropathies Isolated peripheral neuropathies that affect a single nerve.

Monosomy Absence of a chromosome.

Monro-Kellie hypothesis States that if the volume of any of the three intracranial components (the brain, cerebral spinal fluid, and blood) increases, the volume of the others must decrease to maintain normal pressures in the cranial cavity.

Mood A sustained emotional state and how one feels subjectively.

Mood stabilizers Drugs used for bipolar disorder because they moderate extreme shifts in emotions between mania and depression.

Moral behavior The way in which a person perceives and responds to society's requirements.

Moral development The process of learning to tell the difference between right and wrong and of learning what ought and ought not to be done; the pattern of change in moral behavior that occurs with age.

Moral rules Specific prescriptions for actions.

Morality The requirements necessary for people to live together in society.

Morbid obesity Greater than 200% of ideal body weight.

Morning sickness A term that refers to the nausea and vomiting that a woman may experience in early pregnancy. This lay term is sometimes used because these symptoms frequently occur in the early part of the day and disappear within a few hours.

Morpheaform basal cell carcinoma A type of skin cancer.

Morula Developmental stage of the fertilized ovum in which there is a solid mass of cells.

Mosaicism The expression of two cell lines, each with a different chromosomal number, in an individual.

Mourning The behavioral process through which grief is eventually resolved or altered; it is often influenced by culture, spiritual beliefs, and custom.

Multiculturalism Characterized by many subcultures coexisting within a given society in which no one culture dominates.

Multifocal A term used to describe premature ventricular contractions that arise from different **ectopic** sites.

Multigravida Woman who has been pregnant more than once.

Multipara Woman who has had more than one pregnancy in which the fetus was viable.

Multiple pregnancy More than one fetus in the uterus at the same time.

Multiple sclerosis (MS) A chronic demyelinating neurologic disease of the central nervous system associated with an abnormal immune response to an environmental factor.

Mural thrombi Blood clots in the heart wall.

Mycobacterium tuberculosis The bacteria that causes **tuberculosis**.

Mydriasis Abnormal or excessive dilation of the pupil of the eye, usually caused by a disease or drug.

Myelin sheath The fatty, segmented wrappings that normally protect and insulate nerves.

Myocardial hypertrophy An increase in the size of muscle cells of the myocardium.

Myometrium The middle muscular layer of the uterus.

Myopia Nearsightedness.

Myringotomy An incision of the tympanic membrane.

Myxedema The hypothyroid state, with characteristic accumulation of nonpitting edema in the connective tissues throughout the body.

Myxedema coma A life-threatening complication of long-standing, untreated hypothyroidism, usually triggered by an acute illness or trauma.

Narcissism Self-centered behavior in which the individual feels entitled to special favors due to a mistaken perception being the "center of the universe."

Narcolepsy A disorder characterized by daytime sleep attacks or excessive daytime sleepiness.

Narcissistic personality disorder (NPD) One of the 11 types of **personality disorders**, it is marked by in a pattern of grandiosity, difficulty regulating self-esteem, and the need for admiration and attention from others.

Natural killer cells (NK cells) Large, granular cells found in the spleen, lymph nodes, bone marrow, and blood. They constitute 15% of circulating lymphocytes. NK cells provide immune surveillance and resistance to infection, and they play an important role in the destruction of early malignant cells.

Nature The genetic or hereditary capability of the individual.

Negative feedback Output of a system that returns to the system as input and which inhibits system change.

Negative symptom A loss of normal function normally seen in mentally healthy adults, such as the ability to care for one's self, commonly seen in **schizophrenia**.

Neglect syndrome A disorder of attention that can result from stroke.

Neonatal anemia A disorder caused by blood loss, hemolysis, and impaired red blood cell production related to birth.

Neoplasm A mass of new tissue.

Nephrectomy Removal of a kidney.

Nephritis Inflammation of the kidneys.

Nephrolithiasis The formation of stones in the kidney.

Nephrolithotomy A procedure for removal of a staghorn calculus that invades the calyces and renal parenchyma.

Nephrotoxins Substances which damage nerves or nerve tissue.

Nerve block A chemical interruption of a nerve pathway, affected by injecting a local anesthetic into the nerve.

Neurogenic bladder interference with the normal mechanisms of urine elimination in which the client does not perceive bladder fullness and is unable to control the urinary sphincters; the result of impaired neurologic function.

Neurogenic shock The result of an imbalance between parasympathetic and sympathetic stimulation of vascular smooth muscle.

Neuron The basic cell of the nervous system.

Newborn Infant from birth through the first 28 days of life.

Nicotine A highly addictive chemical that is found in tobacco and enters the body via the lungs (cigarettes, pipes, and cigars) and oral mucous membranes (chewing tobacco as well as smoking).

Nicotine replacement therapy (NRT) A pharmacologic therapy designed to relieve some of the physiologic effects of withdrawal, including cravings, for clients trying to quit smoking or using tobacco. NRT transdermal patches and gums are available over the counter; nicotine inhalers and nasal sprays are available by prescription only.

Nicotinic receptors Found in the hippocampus and involved with new sensory information and memory formation, they are thought to be impaired in clients with **schizophrenia**.

Nidation The cyclical preparation of the uterine lining by steroid hormones for implantation of the embryo.

Neurofibrillary tangles Seen in Alzheimer's clients, they are thick, insoluble clots of protein inside the damaged brain cells or neurons.

Neuropathic pain Experienced by people who have damaged or malfunctioning nerves.

Nociceptors The nerve receptors for pain.

Nocturia Voiding two or more times at night.

Nocturnal emissions Orgasm and emission of semen during sleep.

Nocturnal enuresis Bed-wetting; involuntary urination at night after bladder control is achieved.

Nocturnal frequency The need for older adults to arise during the night to urinate.

Nodular basal cell carcinoma A type of skin cancer.

Noninvasive ventilation (NIV) Ventilator support using a tight-fitting face mask, thus avoiding intubation.

Nonmaleficence The duty to do no harm.

Non-Mendelian inheritance Traits that are passed on by the influence of multiple genes.

Non-small-cell carcinoma Lungs cancers other than small-cell carcinoma.

Nonunion Failure of the ends of the fracture to heal together.

Normal sinus rhythm The normal heart rhythm, in which impulses originate in the SA (sinus) node and travel through all normal conduction pathways without delay.

Nosocomial infections Also known as health care-associated infections (HAIs), infections that are associated with the delivery of health care services in a facility such as a hospital or nursing home.

NREM Sleep Non-rapid-eye-movement sleep; occurs when activity in the **reticular activating system** is inhibited.

Nuclear family A family structure consisting of a husband and wife and their biological children.

Nucleation The formation of a crystal from a liquid.

Nuclectomy The surgical removal of the nucleus pulposus.

Nulligravida A woman who has never been pregnant.

Nullipara A woman who has not given birth to a viable fetus.

Nursing ethics Ethical issues that occur in nursing practice.

Nurture The effects of the environment on an individual's performance.

Nutrients Substances found in food that are used by the body to promote growth, maintenance, and repair.

Nutrition The process by which the body ingests, absorbs, transports, uses, and eliminates nutrients in food.

Nutritional health The physical result of the balance between **nutrient** intake and nutritional requirements.

Nystagmus Involuntary rapid eye movement.

Objective family burden Actual, identifiable family problems associated with the mental illness of a family member.

Obligatory losses Essential fluid losses required to maintain body functioning.

Obesity An excess of adipose tissue.

Obsessive–compulsive personality disorder (OCPD) One of 11 types of **personality disorders,** it is marked by fear and anxiety concerning loss of control over situations, objects, or people.

Obstetric conjugate The distance from the middle of the sacral promontory to an area approximately 1 cm below the pubic crest.

Obstructive shock Shock caused by an obstruction in the heart or great vessels that either impedes venous return or prevents effective cardiac pumping action.

Occult blood Hidden blood.

Occupational exposure Skin, eye, mucous membrane, or parental contact with blood or other potentially infectious materials that may result from the performance of an employee's duties.

Oliguria The production of abnormally small amounts of urine by the kidney.

Oncogenes Genes that promote cell proliferation and are capable of triggering cancerous characteristics.

Oncology The study of cancer.

Oncotic pressure A pulling force exerted by colloids that helps maintain the water content of blood by pulling water from the interstitial space into the vascular compartment.

Oogenesis The process that produces the female gamete, called an ovum (egg).

Open-angle glaucoma The most common form of **glaucoma**, it is a chronic, gradually progressive disease that typically affects both eyes.

Open fracture A fracture in which the skin integrity is disrupted. Also known as a compound fracture.

Open reduction and internal fixation (ORIF) The insertion of nails, screws, plates, or pins to hold fractured bones in place.

Opportunistic infection An invasion of the body tissue by microorganisms appearing in an individual with **immunodeficiency** that would normally not affect an individual with an intact immune system.

Opportunistic pathogen A microorganism that causes disease only in susceptible individuals.

Oral-genital sex Kissing, licking, or sucking of the genitals for sexual pleasure.

Orchiectomy Surgical removal of the testes.

Orgasmic phase The third phase of the sexual response cycle, marked by the involuntary release of sexual tension accompanied by physiological and psychological release.

Orthopnea Difficulty breathing when supine.

Orthopneic position A body position with the head and arms supported on the overbed table to facilitate breathing.

Orthotic devices Orthopedic devices that may include splints or braces applied to reduce strain on a joint.

Osmolality A measure of the concentration of solutes in body fluids. Osmolality is determined by the total solute concentration within a fluid compartment and is measured as parts of solute per kilogram of water.

Osmolar imbalance A fluid imbalance that involves the loss or gain of only water, so that the osmolality of the serum is altered.

Osmosis The movement of water across cell membranes, from the less concentrated solution to the more concentrated solution.

Osmotic pressure The power of a solution to draw water across a semipermeable membrane.

Ossification The development of bone.

Osteoarthritis The most common form of arthritis in older adults. It is caused by chronic degenerative changes in the cartilage and synovial membranes of the joints.

Osteoblasts Cells that form bone.

Osteoclasts Cells that resorb bone.

Osteocytes Cells that maintain bone matrix.

Osteodystrophy A complex bone disease process of chronic kidney disease in which there is increased resorption of bone caused by chronic hyperparathyroidism.

Osteoporosis A metabolic bone disorder characterized by loss of bone mass, increased bone fragility, and increased risk of fractures.

Osteophytes Boney spurs that form when cartilage deteriorates.

Osteotomy An incision into or transection of the bone.

Otitis externa Inflammation of the ear canal. It is often called "swimmer's ear" because it is most frequently found in people who spend significant time in the water.

Otitis interna (also called **labyrinthitis**) An inflammation of the inner ear.

Otitis media Inflammation of the middle ear.

Otoscope A hand-held instrument with a light and a cone-shaped attachment known as the "ear speculum."

Output Energy, material, or information that a system gives out as a result of its processes.

Ovarian cycle The three cyclical phases of oogenesis that occurs about every 28 days.

Ovarian ligaments Ligaments that anchor the lower pole of the ovary to the uterus.

Ovaries Female sex glands in which the ova are formed and in which estrogen and progesterone are produced. Normally, there are two ovaries.

Overnutrition Health effects of excesses in nutrient intake or stores; can be manifested in conditions such as obesity, hypertension, hypercholesterolemia, or toxic levels of stored vitamins or minerals.

Ovulation Normal process of discharging a mature ovum from an ovary approximately 14 days before the onset of menses.

Pacemaker A pulse generator used to provide an electrical stimulus to the heart when the heart fails to generate or conduct its own at a rate that maintains the cardiac output.

Pain An unpleasant sensory and emotional experience associated with actual or potential tissue damage.

$PaCO_2$ A measure of the pressure exerted by dissolved carbon dioxide in the blood and reflects the respiratory component of acid–base regulation and balance because it is regulated by the lungs.

PaO_2 A measure of the pressure exerted by oxygen that is dissolved in the plasma.

Pain threshold The point at which pain is perceived.

Pain tolerance The duration of time or intensity of pain an individual will endure before demonstrating pain responses.

Palliation See **palliative care**.

Palliative care Nursing care that improves the quality of life of clients and their families facing life-threatening illness by preventing, assessing, and treating pain and other physical, psychosocial, and spiritual problems.

Pallidotomy A surgical technique for Parkinson's disease in which the neurosurgeon locates the affected areas of the globus pallidus and destroys the involved tissue in order to improve tremors and mobility.

Pandemic Widespread global outbreak of an infectious disease.

Pannus Granulation tissue.

Para A woman who has borne offspring who reached the age of viability.

Paracentesis Aspiration of fluid from the peritoneal cavity.

Paraplegia Paralysis of the lower portion of the body.

Parallel play A stage of play in which toddlers play side-by-side with similar objects, but do not play together.

Paranoia An extreme suspicion and delusion that one is being followed and that others are trying to harm oneself.

Parasite One of the four categories of microorganisms, parasites live on other organisms.

Parasomnias Behaviors that may interfere with sleep and may occur during sleep.

Parenting The ongoing act of guiding children to learn acceptable behaviors, morals, and rituals of the family and of teaching them to become socially responsible, contributing members of society.

Paresis Weakness.

Parethesia Sensation of prickling, tingling, or numbing.

Perimetrium The outermost layer of the uterus.

Parkinsonism The symptoms of Parkinson's disease; tremors, muscle rigidity, postural instability, and bradykinesia.

Parkinson's disease A degenerative disorder of the central nervous system resulting from the death of neurons that produce the brain neurotransmitter dopamine.

Paroxysmal Abrupt onset and termination.

Paroxysmal nocturnal dyspnea A sudden episode of shortness of breath occurring at night during sleep.

Partial-thickness burns Burns that involve the entire dermis and the papillae of the dermis (superficial partial-thickness burns) or extend into the hair follicles (deep partial-thickness burns).

Passive behavior Behavior that seeks to avoid conflict at any cost, even at the expense of one's own happiness.

Passive immunity Temporary protection—provided by antibodies produced by other people or animals—against disease-producing antigens. Protection is gradually lost when these acquired antibodies are used up either by natural degradation or by combining with the antigen.

Pathogen A microorganism that causes **disease.**

Pathogenicity The ability to produce **disease.**

Pathologic fracture A fracture that results from disease that has weakened the bone.

Patent ductus arteriosis A congenital connection between the great vessels that normally closes after birth, allowing blood from the right and left side of the heart to mix.

Patient-controlled analgesia (PCA) A pump with a control mechanism that allows the client to self-manage pain.

Pauciarticular arthritis A form of **juvenile rheumatoid arthritis** that primarily affects the knees, ankles, and elbows; it occurs more frequently in females.

Pedigree The graphical representation of a family tree.

Pelvic cavity Bony portion of the birth passage; a curved canal with a longer posterior than anterior wall.

Pelvic diaphragm Part of the pelvic floor, composed of deep fascia and the levator ani and the coccygeal muscles.

Pelvic inlet Upper border of the true pelvis.

Pelvic outlet Lower border of the true pelvis.

Penetrating injury A type of eye injury in which the layers of the eye spontaneously reapproximate after entry of a sharp-pointed object or small missile (e.g., a BB) into the globe.

Penumbra A band of minimally perfused cells that surrounds a central core of dead or dying cells.

Peptic ulcers A break in the mucosal lining of the GI tract exposed to acid-pepsin secretions, including the esophagus, stomach, and duodenum.

Peptic ulcer disease (PUD) A break in the mucous lining of the GI tract where it comes in contact with gastric juice.

Perceived loss A **loss** that is experienced by one person but cannot be verified by others.

Perception Awareness and interpretation of stimuli; the ability of the individual to interpret the environment.

Percussion Forceful striking of the skin with cupped hands, sometimes called *clapping.*

Perforating injury A type of eye injury in which the layers of the eye do not spontaneously reapproximate after the entry of a sharp-pointed object or small missile (e.g., a BB) into the globe, which results in rupture of the globe and potential loss of ocular contents.

Perforation Rupture, as in the penetration of ulcer through mucosal wall.

Perinatal loss Death of a fetus or infant that occurs between the time of conception and the end of the newborn period 28 days after birth.

Periodontal disease Gum disease.

Perineal body The wedge-shaped mass of fibromuscular tissue between the lower part of the vagina and the anus.

Perioperative nursing care Nursing care provided during any or all of the three phases of surgery: preoperative, intraoperative, and postoperative.

Peripartum cardiomyopathy A relatively rare but serious dysfunction of the left ventricle that occurs in the last month of pregnancy or the first 5 months postpartum in a woman with no previous history of heart disease.

Peripheral nervous system (PNS) One of two principal parts of the neurologic system, the peripheral nervous system consists of the cranial nerves and the spinal nerves.

Peripheral neuropathy A condition that results when trauma or disease process interferes with innervation of peripheral nerves.

Peripheral vascular disease (PVD) A disorder in which arteriosclerosis and atherosclerosis affects circulation to peripheral tissues, particularly the lower extremities.

Peripheral vascular resistance The opposing forces or impedance to blood flow as the arterial channels become more and more distant from the heart.

Peritoneal dialysis The process by which **dialysate** is instilled into the abdominal cavity through a catheter, allowed to rest there while fluids and molecules exchange, and then removed through the catheter.

Peritonitis Inflammation and bacterial infection of the abdominal area.

Pernicious anemia A disorder that results from a failure to absorb dietary vitamin B12.

Persistent A term used to describe a disease or disorder (such as **rheumatoid arthritis**) that lasts for a period of 3–6 months or longer.

Persistent bacteriuria The reappearance of bacteria in urine due to a persistent source of infection causing repeated infection after the initial cure.

Persistent vegetative state (also called *irreversible coma*) A permanent condition of complete unawareness of self and the environment and loss of all cognitive functions.

Personal identity The conscious sense of individuality and uniqueness that is continually evolving throughout life.

Personality The individual qualities, including habitual behavior patterns, that make a person unique; the outward expression of the inner self.

Personality disorder (PD) is a rigid, stereotyped behavioral pattern that deviates markedly from the norm of an individual's culture and persists throughout the person's life. Personality disorders are characterized by a lifelong maladaptive pattern of perceiving, thinking, and relating that impairs social or occupational functioning.

Personality trait Persistent behavioral pattern.

Pervasive developmental disorders (PDDs) Disorders that begin in early childhood and are characterized by impairments in social interactions and communication. There are five PDDs: autistic spectrum disorder, Asperger syndrome, Rett's disorder, childhood disintegrative disorder, and pervasive developmental disorder not otherwise specified (PDD-NOS).

pH The amount of hydrogen ion concentration of a solution.

Phagocytosis A process by which a foreign agent or target cell is engulfed, destroyed, and digested. Neutrophils and macrophages, known as phagocytes, are the primary cells involved in phagocytosis.

Phantom pain (also **phantom limb syndrome**) A confusing pain syndrome that occurs following surgical or traumatic amputation of a limb. The client experiences pain in the missing body part even though there is complete mental awareness that the limb is gone.

Phase of mutual regulation Time period in which the mother and infant seek to determine the degree of control each partner in their relationship will exert. In this phase of adjustment, a balance is sought between the needs of the mother and the needs of the infant.

Philadelphia chromosome The balanced translocation of chromosome 22 to chromosome 9 associated with chronic myeloid leukemia.

Phimosis Tightness of prepuce that prevents retraction of foreskin.

Phenotype The observable expression of genetic traits.

Photophobia Sensitivity to light.

Physical activity Bodily movement produced by skeletal muscle contraction that increases energy expenditure.

Physiological pain Experienced when an intact, properly functioning nervous system sends signals that tissues are damaged, requiring attention and proper care.

Physiologic anemia of infancy A type of **anemia** that occurs as a result of the normal, gradual drop in hemoglobin for the first 6–12 weeks of life.

Physiologic anemia of pregnancy Apparent anemia that results because during pregnancy the plasma volume increases more than the erythrocytes increase.

Pigmented basal cell carcinoma A type of skin cancer.

Pitting edema Edema that retains indentation caused by pressure.

Placenta A flat, disc-shaped organ that is highly vascular and normally forms in the upper segment of the endometrium of the uterus; exchanges nutrients and gases between the fetus and the mother.

Plaque An invisible soft film that adheres to the enamel surface of teeth; consists of bacteria, saliva molecules, and remnants of epithelial cells and leukocytes.

Plasmapheresis (plasma exchange) Removal of the plasma component from whole blood.

Play therapist A therapist who designs and provides recreational activities to promote emotional and/or physical healing and wellness.

Pleuritic pain Sharp localized chest pain that increases with breathing and coughing.

Pneumatic retinopexy A surgical procedure to correct **retinal detachment** in which air is injected into the vitreous cavity and the client is positioned so that the air bubble pushes the detached portion of the retina into contact with the choroid.

Pneumocystis carinii pneumonia (PCP) An **opportunistic infection** that is not pathogenic in those with intact immune systems.

Pneumomediastinum The presence of air in the mediastinum.

Pneumonia Inflammation of the lung parenchyma (the respiratory bronchioles and alveoli).

Pneumopericardium Air in the pericardial sac.

Pneumothorax A partial lung collapse due to air or gas collecting in the lung or in the pleural space which surrounds the lungs.

Polyarticular arthritis A form of **juvenile rheumatoid arthritis** that involves many joints (five or more), particularly the small joints of the hands and fingers. It may also affect the hips, knees, feet, ankles, and neck.

Polycythemia An increase in the production of red blood cells.

Polycyclic Describes a periodically recurring course of **rheumatoid arthritis.**

Polydipsia Excessive thirst.

Polyp A small vascular growth on the surface of any mucous membrane.

Polyphagia Excessive hunger.

Polysomnography (PSG) A recording of the biophysical changes that a client experiences during sleep.

Polysubstance abuse The simultaneous use of many substances.

Polyneuropathies Bilateral sensory disorders; they are the most common types of neuropathy associated with diabetes.

Polytheism The belief in more than one god.

Polyuria The production of abnormally large amounts of urine.

Positive end-expiratory pressure (PEEP) Mechanical ventilation in which a positive pressure is maintained in the airways during exhalation and between breaths to help keep alveoli open.

Positive feedback Output of a system that returns to the system as input and which promotes system change.

Positive-pressure ventilation A mechanical device that pushes air into the lungs through an invasive device such as endotracheal tube or tracheostomy, rather than drawing air in by negative pressure.

Positive reinforcement Giving rewards such as praise for a learner's achievements.

Positive symptoms Excessive or added behaviors that are not normally seen in healthy adults, such as delusions; commonly seen in **schizophrenia.**

Postcoital contraception A drug taken after intercourse to avoid pregnancy. Also called Plan B or the "morning after pill."

Postconception age periods Period of time in embryonic/fetal development calculated from the time of fertilization of the ovum.

Postictal period Period immediately following seizure activity in which level of consciousness is decreased. The length of the postictal period varies.

Postpartal hemorrhage A loss of blood of greater than 500 mL following birth. The hemorrhage is classified as ***early*** if it occurs within the first 24 hours and ***late*** if it occurs after the first 24 hours.

Postpartum After childbirth.

Postpartum blues A maternal adjustment reaction occurring in the first few postpartal days, characterized by mild depression, tearfulness, anxiety, headache, and irritability.

Postpartum depression A severe form of depression that affects new mothers, often beginning within 3 months of delivery but which may strike at any time during the first year after having a child.

Postpartum psychosis Psychosis occurring within the first 3 months after birth.

Postterm labor Labor that occurs after 42 weeks' gestation.

Postterm newborn Any infant born after 42 weeks' gestation.

Postterm pregnancy Pregnancy that lasts beyond 42 weeks' gestation.

Postural drainage The drainage by gravity of secretions from various lung segments.

PPD Tuberculin skin test.

Prader–Willi syndrome (PWS) A congenital disorder of the 15th chromosome that causes an unrelenting feeling of hunger, but also low muscle tone, short stature, incomplete sexual development, mild to severe mental retardation, and behavioral problems.

Prayer Human communication with divine and spiritual entities.

Preeclampsia Toxemia of pregnancy, characterized by hypertension, albuminuria, and edema.

Prejudice A negative belief or preference that is generalized about a group that leads to prejudgment.

Preload The amount of cardiac muscle fiber tension, or stretch, that exists at the end of diastole.

Premature junctional contractions Beats that occur before the next expected beat of the underlying rhythm.

Premenstrual syndrome (PMS) A complex of manifestations (e.g., mood swings, breast tenderness, fatigue, irritability, food cravings, and depression) that are limited to 3–14 days before menstruation and relieved by the onset of menses.

Prenatal education Programs offered to expectant families, adolescents, women, or partners to provide education regarding the pregnancy, labor, and birth experience.

Presbycusis Age-related loss of the ability to hear high-frequency sounds, may occur because of cochlear hair cell degeneration or loss of auditory neurons in the organ of Corti.

Presbyopia Impaired near vision resulting from a loss of elasticity of the lens related to aging.

Presencing Being present, being there, or just being with a client.

Pretibial myxedema The formation of edematous, erythematous, and sometimes hyperpigmented plaques and nodules that develop bilaterally over the shins and dorsal surface of the feet. A characteristic sign of Grave's disease.

Priapism Persistent, painful erection of the penis.

Primary hypertension A persistently elevated systemic blood pressure, also called *essential hypertension.*

Primigravida A woman who is pregnant for the first time.

Primipara A woman who has given birth to her first child (past the point of viability), whether or not that child is living or was alive at birth.

Principles-based (deontological) theories Theories that involve logical and formal processes and emphasize individual rights, duties, and obligations.

Procedural memory Recall of information that does not require conscious awareness and involves the memory of motor skills and procedures.

Professional support Assistance provided by professionals in the community who exhibit a nonblaming and respectful attitude towards families and clients, and who provide information and help locating community resources.

Progesterone Hormone produced by the corpus luteum, adrenal cortex, and placenta whose function is to stimulate proliferation of the endometrium to facilitate growth of the embryo.

Prone Face-down.

Propioception The body's sense of its position.

Proptosis Forward displacement of the eye.

Prostaglandins (PGs) Complex lipids compounds synthesized by many cells of the body.

Prostate specific antigen (PSA) A protein produced in the cells of the prostate gland.

Prostatectomy Surgical removal of part or all of the prostate gland.

Prostatitis Inflammation of the prostate gland.

Prostatodynia A condition in which the client experiences the symptoms of prostatitis, but shows no evidence of inflammation or infection.

Proteinuria Excess protein in urine.

Protein-calorie malnutrition Problem of clients with long-term deficiencies in caloric intake; characteristics include depressed visceral proteins (e.g., albumin), weight loss, and visible muscle and fat wasting.

Proximodistal Growth that proceeds from the center of the body outward.

Pseudoaddiction A term applied to clients who display drug-seeking behaviors but differ from addicts in that they have true underlying pain for which they are seeking relief. These behaviors will generally stop when adequate pain control is achieved.

Psychiatric (psychosocial) rehabilitation The development of skills and support necessary for successful living, learning, and working in the community.

Psychogenic pain Pain that is experienced in the absence of any diagnosed physiologic cause or event.

Psychomotor retardation A state in which thinking and body movements are noticeably slowed and speech is slowed or absent.

Psychosis (or psychotic disorder) A mental health condition characterized by **delusions** (firm ideas and beliefs not founded in reality), **hallucinations** (perceptions of seeing, hearing, or feeling something that is not there), **illusions** (distorted perceptions of actual sensory stimuli), disorganized behavior, and a difficulty relating to others.

Psychosocial skills Skills which enable a person in crisis to maintain relationships with family and friends throughout and after a crisis period.

Psychostimulants A class of stimulants including cocaine and amphetamines that have a high potential for abuse.

Ptosis Drooping of the eyelid.

Puberty The stage during which an individual reaches sexual maturity.

Pubis Pertaining to the pubes or pubic area.

Puerperium That time immediately following childbirth during which physiologic changes that occurred during pregnancy begin to return to normal.

Pulmonary atresia The absence of communication between the right ventricle and the pulmonary artery.

Pulmonary circulation Consists of the right side of the heart, the pulmonary artery, the pulmonary capillaries, and the pulmonary vein.

Pulmonary edema An abnormal accumulation of fluid in the interstitial tissue and alveoli of the lung.

Pulmonary embolism The obstruction of blood flow in part of the pulmonary vascular system by an **embolus.**

Pulmonary vascular resistance The force or resistance of the blood in the pulmonary circulation.

Pulse pressure The difference between the systolic and diastolic pressure.

Punishment Action taken to enforce rules when a child misbehaves.

Pupillary light reflex Reflex in which the pupil contracts in response to a bright light.

Purging Self-induced vomiting or misuse of laxatives, diuretics, or enemas.

Pursed-lipped breathing Exhaling through a narrow opening between the lips to prolong the expiratory phase in an effort to promote more alveolar emptying while maintaining open alveoli.

Pyelolithotomy An incision into and removal of a stone from the kidney pelvis.

Pyelonephritis Inflammation of the renal pelvis and parenchyma, the functional kidney tissue.

Pyorrhea Advanced **periodontal disease.**

Pyuria Cloudy or pus-filled urine.

Quadriplegia Loss of function of the arms, trunk, legs, and pelvic organs.

Quickening The mother's perception of fetal movement.

Race A term used to described socially defined populations that share genetically transmitted physical characteristics, such as skin color and bone structure.

Radiation cataracts A type of **cataract** that may result from long-term exposure to radiation.

Range of Motion The degree to which a joint can be moved; a measurement of flexon and extension.

Receptive speech The ability to understand the spoken word.

Receptor A nerve cell acts as a receptor by converting the **stimulus** to a nerve impulse. Most receptors are specific, that is, sensitive to only one type of stimulus.

Recovery Return to (or exceed) pre-illness levels of functioning.

Recurrence A later recurrence of a disorder after recovery.

Red blood cell (RBCs, *erythrocytes*) Blood cells shaped like a biconcave disk that contain hemoglobin required for oxygen transport to body tissues; the most common type of blood cell.

Referred pain Pain that is perceived in an area distant from the site of the stimuli.

Reflexes Stimulus–response activities of the body, reflexes are fast, predictable, unlearned, innate, and involuntary reactions to stimuli.

Reflux A backward flow of acidic secretions into the lower esophagus.

Refraction The bending of light rays as they pass from one medium to another medium of different optical density.

Refractory hypoxemia The decrease of particle arterial oxygen despite administration of oxygen at high flow rates.

Refractory period A phase during which myocardial cells resist stimulation.

Refractory septic shock A persistently low mean arterial blood pressure despite vasopressor therapy and adequate fluid resuscitation.

Regeneration The replacement of destroyed tissue cells by cells that are identical or similar in structure and function.

Reinfection The development of a new infection with a different pathogen following successful treatment.

Relapse Return of a disorder soon after recovery.

Relationships-based (caring) theories Theories that stress courage, generosity, commitment, and the need to nurture and maintain relationships.

Relaxation response A healthful physiologic state that can be elicited through deep relaxation breathing with emphasis on a prolonged exhalation phase.

Religion A set of doctrines accepted by a group of people who gather together regularly to worship and that offer a means to relate to God or a higher power; an organized system of beliefs and practices.

REM Sleep Rapid-eye-movement sleep; occurs during sleep about every 90 minutes and lasts 5–30 minutes.

Remission A period during a chronic illness in which the symptoms of the illness disappear; sustained recovery lasting 8 weeks or more.

Renal colic Acute, severe flank pain on the affected side; develops when a stone obstructs the ureter, causing ureteral spasm.

Renal failure A condition in which the kidneys are unable produce urine, resulting in altered fluid, electrolyte, and acid–base balance.

Renal insufficiency Decrease in the kidneys' ability to conserve sodium and concentrate the urine.

Renin-angiotensin-aldosterone system System initiated by specialized receptors in the juxtaglomerular cells of the kidney nephrons that respond to changes in renal perfusion.

Repolarization The process that returns the cell to its resting, polarized state.

Reservoir A source of microorganisms.

Residual urine Urine that remains in the bladder after voiding.

Resilience/resiliency The ability to function with healthy responses, even when experiencing significant stress or adversity.

Resolution phase The fourth and final phase of the sexual response cycle, marked by the return to the unaroused state.

Respiratory acidosis A condition caused by an excess of dissolved carbon dioxide, or carbonic acid. It is characterized by a pH less than 7.35 and a $PaCO_2$ greater than 45 mmHg.

Respiratory alkalosis A condition that results when pH rises above 7.45 and $PaCO_2$ falls below 35 mmHg. It is always caused by **hyperventilation** (unusually fast respiration, or overbreathing), leading to a carbon dioxide deficit.

Respiratory syncytial virus (RSV) A highly contagious respiratory infection that affects almost all children before 2 years of age.

Responsibility The specific accountability or liability associated with the performance of duties of a particular role.

Rest pain Cramping or aching pain in the calves of the legs, the thighs, and the buttocks that occurs while at rest.

Restrictive cardiomyopathy A disorder characterized by rigid ventricular walls that impair diastolic filling.

Retinal detachment Separation of the retina or sensory portion of the eye from the choroid.

Retrograde conduction Cardiac conduction against the normal flow or pattern.

Reward deficiency syndrome The decreased ability to experience pleasure. Reward deficiency syndrome drives the person to seek external forms of gratification through the use of substances, pathological gambling, or other high-risk behaviors.

Rheumatoid arthritis (RA) A chronic systemic autoimmune disease that causes inflammation of connective tissue, primarily in the joints.

Rhinorrhea A runny nose.

Ribonucleic acid (RNA) One of two types of nucleic acid made by cells. Ribonucleic acid is made up of ribose rather than deoxyribose and contains information that has been copied from DNA (the other type of nucleic acid).

Risk Factor A practice, behavior, or environmental factor that has potentially negative affects on individual health.

Role A set of expectations about how the person occupying one position behaves.

Role ambiguity Occurs when expectations are unclear, and when people do not know perform their roles and are unable to predict the reactions of others to their behavior.

Role conflict Emotional conflict arising when competing demands are made on an individual in the fulfillment of his or her multiple social roles.

Role development Socialization into a particular role.

Role mastery Occurs when an individual's behaviors meet social expectations.

Role performance How a person in a particular role behaves related to the behaviors expected of that role.

Role strain The stress or strain experienced by an individual when incompatible behavior, expectations, or obligations are associated with a single social role.

Round ligaments The ligaments that hold the ovaries in place.

Sacral promotory A projection into the pelvic cavity on the anterior upper portion of the sacrum, which serves as a landmark for pelvic measurements.

Saline 0.9% sodium chloride, an isotonic solution.

Satiety The sensation of fullness.

Scheduled toileting Toileting at regular intervals.

Schistocytes Fragmented red blood cells.

Schizoaffective disorder A psychotic disorder with features of both schizophrenia and mood disorders.

Schizoid personality disorder One of 11 types of **personality disorders**, it is characterized by a lifelong pattern of indifference to others and social isolation.

Schizophrenia The most common psychotic disorder, schizophrenia is a combination of disordered thinking, perceptual disturbances, behavioral abnormalities, affective disruptions, and impaired social competency.

Schizophreniform disorder A disorder with rapid onset of psychotic symptoms, very similar to schizophrenia, lasting less than 6 months.

Schizotypal personality disorder One of 11 types of **personality disorders**, it is characterized by a pattern of disturbed interpersonal relationships, thought patterns, appearance, and behavior.

Sciatica Lumbar back pain that radiates down the posterior leg to the ankle.

Scleral buckling A surgical procedure to correct **retinal detachment**.

Seasonal affective disorder (SAD) A mood disorder characterized by depression during fall and winter and normal mood or hypomania during spring and summer.

Second heart sound Produced by closure of the semilunar valves, characterized by the syllable "dub."

Secondary cataracts Can form after surgery to treat another eye disorder, such as glaucoma, or as an effect of medication or another primary disorder.

Secondary hypertension Elevated blood pressure resulting from an identifiable underlying process.

Secondary infertility The inability to conceive after one or more successful pregnancies, or the inability to sustain a pregnancy.

Seizures Periods of abnormal electrical discharges in the brain that cause involuntary movement as well as behavior and sensory alterations.

Selective perception The process of filtering out unnecessary and distracting information in order to focus on what is important at any given moment.

Selective serotonin reuptake inhibitor (SSRI) A drug that selectively inhibits the reuptake of serotonin into nerve terminals; used mostly for depression.

Selectively permeable Refers to membranes separating body fluid compartments across which solutes can move with relative ease.

Self-awareness The relationship between an individual's perception of himself or herself and others' perceptions of him or her.

Self-concept One's mental image of oneself.

Self-esteem One's judgment of one's own worth.

Semen Sperm mixed with seminal fluid, ejaculated during sexual activity.

Sensitization An increased reaction to pain over time, or a reduced threshold for reaction to painful stimuli.

Sensory memory The momentary perception of stimuli from the environment.

Sensory overload An overabundance of sensory stimulation.

Sensory perception The conscious organization and translation of external data or stimuli into meaningful information.

Sensory reception The process of receiving external stimuli or data. External stimuli are **visual** (sight), **auditory** (hearing), **olfactory** (smell), **tactile** (touch), and **gustatory** (taste).

Sepsis 1) The whole body inflammatory process resulting in acute illness; 2) The state of infection.

Septal defect A **congenital heart defect** that connects the right and left side of the heart.

Septicemia A systemic infection caused by **bacteremia**.

Septic shock Altered perfusion resulting from a systemic infection that manifests with hypotension, delayed capillary refill, and inadequate perfusion and oxygenation of vital body tissues.

Seroconversion Antibody response to a disease or vaccine.

Serum bicarbonate (HCO_3^-) reflects the renal regulation of acid–base balance. The normal HCO_3^- value is 22–26 mEq/L.

Serum sickness A systemic type III hypersensitivity response, usually in response to a drug such as penicillin or a sulfonamide.

Sex chromosomes Genetic material found in the cell nucleus that determines the individual's gender.

Sexual aversion disorder A disorder characterized by severe distaste for sexual activity or the thought of sexual activity.

Sexual health The integration of the somatic, emotional, intellectual, and social aspects of sexual being, in ways that are positively enriching and that enhance personality, communication, and love.

Sexual orientation The preference of a person for one sex or the other.

Sexual self-concept How one values oneself as a sexual being.

Shared psychotic disorder A condition that results when a person who is in a close relationship with another person who is delusional comes to share the delusional beliefs.

Shock A clinical syndrome characterized by a systemic imbalance between oxygen supply and demand.

Short-term memory Information held in the brain for immediate use; what one has in mind at a given moment.

Shunt A natural or artificially created tunnel or passage that allows blood to flow through an area.

Sickle cell anemia An inherited chronic anemia marked by defective hemoglobin and the irregular crescent shape of red blood cells.

Sickle cell crisis Severe episodes of fever and intense pain that are the hallmark of sickle cell disease.

Sickle cell disorder A hereditary **hemoglobinopathy**, a type of disorder characterized by replacement of normal hemoglobin with abnormal hemoglobin S (Hgb S) in RBCs.

Sickle cell trait Carrying one copy of the defective sickle cell gene, which can be passed on to children but not usually causing illness.

Single-parent family Family in which only one parent resides in the home and is the primary caretaker and provider for the family.

Situational depression A maladaptive reaction to an identifiable psychosocial stressor or stressors that occurs within 3 months after the onset of the stressor and has persisted for no longer than 6 months.

Sleep An altered state of consciousness in which the individual's perception and reaction to the environment are decreased.

Sleep apnea A disorder characterized by frequent short breathing pauses during sleep.

Sleep architecture The basic organization of normal sleep.

Sleep hygiene Interventions used to promote sleep.

Small cell carcinoma A highly malignant cancer usually associated with the lung.

Sobriety The state of habitual refrain from using alcohol or drugs.

Solitary play A stage of play in which the infant still plays primarily alone, but enjoys the presence of others.

Solutes Substances that dissolve in liquid.

Solvent The component of a solution that can dissolve a **solute**.

Somatic cells Cells that make up the tissue of the body, with a full complement (diploid) of chromsomes, as opposed to sex cells.

Somatic pain Pain arising from nerve receptors originating in the skin or close to the surface of the body.

Somatization The process by which psychological distress is experienced and communicated in the form of somatic symptoms.

Somatostatin A substance (believed to be a neurotransmitter) that inhibits the production of both glucagon and insulin.

Somnology The study of sleep.

Somogyi phenomenon A combination of hypoglycemia during the night with a rebound, morning rise in blood glucose to hyperglycemic levels.

Spasticity Increased muscle tone (hypertonia), usually with some degree of weakness.

Specific defenses Immune system responses directed against identifiable bacteria, viruses, fungi, or other infectious agents.

Specific gravity An indicator of urine concentration that can be performed quickly and easily by nursing personnel.

Specific self-esteem How much one approves of a certain part of oneself.

Spermatogenesis The process by which mature spermatozoa are formed.

Spermicide A cream, jelly, foam, vaginal film, and suppository that is inserted into the vagina before intercourse to destroy sperm and prevent conception.

Spinal cord A continuation of the medulla oblongata, it has the ability to transmit impulses to and from the brain via the ascending and descending pathways.

Spinal cord injury Trauma to the spinal cord that results from excessive force to the spinal column.

Spinal cord stimulation (SCS) A form of therapy used with persistent pain that has not been controlled with less invasive therapies. SCS involves the insertion of an electrode (may be a single channel or multichannel device) adjacent to the spinal cord in the epidural space. The electrode(s) is attached to an impulse-generator (external or implanted) that sends electric impulses to the spinal cord to control pain.

Spinal fusion The insertion of a wedge-shaped piece of bone or bone chips between the vertebrae to stabilize them.

Spinal shock The temporary loss of reflex function due to injury.

Spiritual distress A challenge to the spiritual well-being or to the belief system that provides strength, hope, and meaning to life; a feeling of being separated from interconnectedness with others or with a higher power.

Spiritual skills Skills which help the individual find meaning in and understand the personal significance of an unexpected event.

Spiritual support Assistance to clients and families in providing meaning and sustaining courage during difficult times.

Spiritual well-being A feeling of inner peace and of being generally alive, purposeful, and fulfilled; the feeling is rooted in spiritual values and/or specific religious beliefs.

Spirituality The part of being human that seeks meaningfulness through personal connection, which may include belief in or relationship with some higher power, creative force, driving being, or infinite source of energy.

Splitting The inability to integrate contradictory experiences.

Spontaneous abortion The loss of a fetus prior to 20 weeks gestation; also called **miscarriage**.

Sprain A tearing of ligaments.

Sputum Mucus or mucopurulent matter expectorated from the lungs.

Squamous cell carcinoma A malignant tumor of the squamous epithelium of the skin or mucous membranes.

Staghorn stones See **struvite stones**.

Staging A system of classifying cancer according to the size of the tumor, involvement of lymph nodes, and metastasis to distant sites.

Status asthmaticus A severe, prolonged form of asthma that is difficult to treat.

Status epilepticus A continuous seizure that lasts for more than 30 minutes or a series of seizures during which time consciousness is not regained.

Steatorrhea Excess fat in the feces.

Stem cell transplant The infusion of immature stem cells to replenish a client's blood cell lines, as an alternative to bone marrow transplantation.

Stenosis Narrowing of the valve, valve area, or great artery above the valve.

Step-down therapy A gradual reduction in the dosage and number of drugs used in a therapeutic regimen.

Stepfamily Consists of a biologic parent with children and a new spouse who may or may not have children.

Stereogenesis The ability to perceive and understand an object through touch.

Stereotaxic thalamotomy An x-ray taken during neurosurgery to guide the insertion of a needle into a specific area of the brain.

Stereotyping The act of generalizing that all people in a group are the same.

Stereotypy Rigid and obsessive behavior.

Sterile field An area free of microorganisms.

Sterile technique Practices that keep an area or object free of all microorganisms. Also known as **surgical asepsis**.

Sterilization A process that destroys all microorganisms, including spores and viruses; surgical procedures to permanently prevent pregnancy.

Stigma A collection of negative attitudes and beliefs that lead people to fear, reject, avoid, and discriminate against people with mental illness.

Stillbirth Intrauterine fetal death (IUFD) occurs after 20 weeks' gestation.

Stimulus The agent or act that stimulates a nerve receptor.

Stoma An artificial opening in the abdominal wall; it may be permanent or temporary.

Stress fracture A fracture that results from disease that has weakened the bone.

Striae Whitish-silver stretch marks seen in obesity and during or after pregnancy.

Stroke A condition in which neurologic deficits result from a sudden decrease in blood flow to a localized area of the brain. Also known as cerebrovascular accident.

Stroke volume difference between the end-diastolic volume and the end-systolic volume.

Structural-functional theory Focuses on family structure and function, examining family relationships and how they effect the functions of the family and relationships with other systems.

Struvite stones A type of calculi associated with UTI caused by urease-producing bacteria such as *Proteus.* These stones can grow to become very large, filling the renal pelvis and calyces. They are often called **staghorn stones** because of their shape.

Subculture groups Minority groups characterized by specific norms, beliefs, and values that coexist with a dominant culture.

Subdermal implant Capsules implanted within the skin that slowly release medication, such as for contraception.

Subfertility Occurs when both partners of a couple have reduced fertility.

Subjective family burden The psychological distress of family members in relation to the **objective family burden** of having a family member with a mental illness.

Substance abuse refers to the use of any chemical in a fashion inconsistent with medical or culturally defined social norms despite physical, psychological, or social adverse effects.

Substance dependence A condition in which the client can no longer control use of the substance, continues to use despite adverse effects, and experiences withdrawal symptoms without continued use of the substance.

Subsystem A component of a larger system.

Suctioning Aspirating secretions through a catheter connected to a suction machine or wall suction outlet.

Sudden cardiac death (SCD) Unexpected death occurring within 1 hr of the onset of cardiovascular symptoms.

Sudden infant death syndrome (SIDS) The sudden death of an apparently healthy infant that remains unexplained after other possible causes have been ruled out through autopsy, death scene investigation, and review of the medical history.

Sundowning A behavioral change commonly seen in dementia clients, characterized by increased agitation, time disorientation, and wandering behaviors during afternoon and evening hours; it is accelerated on overcast days.

Superego the conscience of personality, the ego ideal; the source of feelings of guilt, shame, and inhibition.

Superficial basal cell carcinoma A type of skin cancer.

Superficial burn A burn that involves only the epidermal layer of the skin.

Supersaturated urine A condition that results when the concentration of an insoluble salt in the urine is very high.

Supine On the back.

Suprasystem An overarching system to which smaller systems or subsystems belong. For example, the family is the suprasystem of the individual.

Surgical asepsis or **sterile technique** Practices that keep an area or object free of all microorganisms.

Surgical debridement The process of excising a wound to the level of fascia (fascial excision) or sequentially removing thin slices of a burn wound to the level of viable tissue (sequential excision).

Swan-neck deformity Caused by **rheumatoid arthritis**, it is characterized by hyperextension of the proximal interphalangeal (PIP) joints joint with compensatory flexion of the distal interphalangeal (DIP) joints.

Switching A term used in disorders of mood and affect to describe a new illness phase (manic or depressed) without recovery.

Sympathetic tone A state of partial smooth muscle contraction around arteries and veins.

Symphysis pubic Fibrocartilaginous joint between the pelvic bones in the midline.

Synchronized cardioversion Delivery of direct electrical current synchronized with the client's heart rhythm.

Syncope Transient loss of consciousness and muscle tone after exercise or activity.

Synovitis Inflammation of the synovial membrane lining the articular capsule of a joint.

Synovectomy Excision of synovial membrane, this procedure is used as a treatment for **rheumatoid arthritis.**

Syphilis A complex systemic sexually transmitted infection caused by the spirochete *Treponema pallidum*.

System A set of interacting identifiable parts or components.

Systematized delusions A manifestation of **schizophrenia** characterized by an extensively developed central delusional theme from which conclusions are deduced.

Systemic arthritis A form of **juvenile rheumatoid arthritis** that characteristically is manifested by high fever, polyarthritis, and rheumatoid rash. Systemic arthritis also affects internal organs and joints.

Systemic circulation Consists of the left side of the heart, the aorta and its branches, the capillaries that supply the brain and peripheral tissues, the systemic venous system, and the vena cava.

Systemic lupus erythematosus (SLE) A chronic inflammatory connective tissue disease.

Systemic infection Occurs when an invading microorganism spreads and damages different parts of the body.

Systemic Inflammatory Response Syndrome (SIRS) Describes the body's response to a critical illness that can result from an infectious or noninfectious cause precipitating a whole-body inflammatory process.

Systemic vascular resistance The force or resistance of the blood in the body's blood vessels that helps return blood to the heart.

Systems theory The study of how a system operates, including how it interacts with other systems and how its components interact with each other within the system itself.

Systole The phase of ventricular contraction.

Systolic blood pressure The maximum pressure exerted within the arteries when the heart compresses.

T lymphocyte A type of **leukocyte** that matures in the thymus gland and is integral to the specific immune response.

Tachypnea Rapid respirations.

Tangential excision The sequential removal of thin slices of the burn wound to the level of viable tissue.

Tardive dyskinesia A condition characterized by unusual tongue and face movements such as lip smacking and wormlike motions of the tongue.

Tartar A visible, hard deposit of **plaque** and dead bacteria that forms at the gumlines.

Tau A protein found in the neurons.

Teaching A system of activities intended to produce learning.

Temperament The combination of biological and physical characteristics that is specific to each individual and influences personality and behavior.

Tender points refers to tenderness that occurs in precise, localized areas, particularly in the neck, spine, shoulders, and hips.

Tendonitis Inflammation of a tendon.

Teratogen Any chemical that has the potential to harm the fetus, including pesticides, viruses, and medications.

Terminal weaning The gradual withdrawal of mechanical ventilation when survival without assisted ventilation is not expected.

Testosterone The primary male sex hormone produced by the testes.

Tetany Tonic muscle spasms.

Tetraplegia Loss of function of the arms, trunk, legs, and pelvic organs.

Tetralogy of Fallot Consists of four defects—pulmonic stenosis, right ventricular hypertrophy, ventricular-septal defect, and an overriding aorta.

Thalassemia Inherited disorder of hemoglobin synthesis in which either the alpha or beta chains of the hemoglobin molecule are missing or defective.

Therapeutic insemination The deposition of semen at the cervical os or in the uterus by mechanical means.

Third heart sound Sometimes heard after the second heart sound in children, young adults, and pregnant females during the third trimester. Also called a **ventricular gallop.**

Third spacing A shift of fluid from the vascular space into an area where it is not available to support normal physiologic processes.

Thoracentesis Needle insertion into the pleural space to remove fluid accumulation.

Threshold potential The point at which an action potential is capable of being generated.

Thrill A palpable vibration over the precordium or an artery.

Thromboemboli Blood clots.

Throughput The process by which information, energy, or material that enters a system (input) is used by the system.

Thyroidectomy Surgical removal of the thyroid gland.

Thyroiditis Inflammation of the thyroid gland.

Thyroid storm An extreme state of hyperthyroidism, also called thyroid crisis.

Thyrotoxosis A disorder caused by excessive delivery of thyroid hormone to the peripheral tissues.

Tine test A multiple-puncture device is used to introduce tuberculin into the skin.

Tinea pedis Fungal infection of the feet; aka "athlete's foot."

Tinnitus The perception of sound or noise in the ears without stimulus from the environment.

Token economies Formalized programs of contingency contracts.

Tolerance State in which a particular dose elicits a smaller response than it formerly did. With increased tolerance, the individual needs higher and higher doses to obtain the desired response.

Tone The amount of tension or resistance to movement in a muscle.

Tonic phase Initial phase of a generalized seizure, manifested by unconsciousness and continuous muscular contraction.

Tonic-clonic seizures Alternating contraction (tonic phase) and relaxation (clonic phase) of muscles during seizure activity.

Tonicity The osmolality of a solution. Solutions may be termed **isotonic**, **hypertonic**, or **hypotonic**.

Torsades de pointes A type of ventricular tachycardia associated with a prolongation of the QT interval.

Total anomalous pulmonary venous return The pulmonary veins empty into the right atrium, or into veins leading to the right atrium, rather than into the left atrium.

Total lymphoid irradiation A procedure sometimes used in the treatment of **rheumatoid arthritis**; it decreases total lymphocyte levels.

Toxic multinodular goiter A tumor characterized by small, discrete, independently functioning nodules in the thyroid gland tissue that secrete excessive amounts of thyroid hormone.

Toxoplasmosis Space-occupying lesions common in clients with AIDS that may cause headache, altered mental status, and neurologic deficits.

Trachoma A chronic conjunctivitis caused by *Chlamydia trachomatis,* is a significant preventable cause of blindness worldwide.

Traction The application of a straightening or pulling force to return or maintain the fractured bones in normal anatomic position.

Traditional family An autonomous unit in which both parents reside in the home with their children, the mother assuming the nurturing role and the father providing the necessary economic resources.

Transcellular fluid One of the components of **extracellular fluid.** Examples of transcellular fluid are cerebrospinal, pericardial, pancreatic, pleural, intraocular, biliary, peritoneal, and synovial fluids.

Transcendence Person's recognition that there is something other or greater than the self and a seeking and valuing of that greater other, whether it is an ultimate being, force, or value.

Transfusion reaction A type II or cytotoxic hypersensitivity reaction to blood of an incompatible type.

Transgenderism Gradations of human characteristics running from female to male.

Transient ischemic attack (TIA) A brief period of localized cerebral ischemia that causes neurologic deficits lasting for less than 24 hours. Also called a mini-stroke.

Transjugular intrahepatic portosystemic shunt (TIPS) An expandable metal stent inserted through a transcutaneous needle to channel blood from the portal vein into the hepatic vein, bypassing the cirrhotic liver.

Transposition of the great arteries A congenital heart defect in which the pulmonary artery, which is the outflow tract for the left ventricle, and the aorta, which is the outflow tract for the right ventricle, are switched (transposed).

Transplacental immunity **Passive immunity** transferred from mother to infant.

Transsexual An individual who feels his or her sexual anatomy is not consistent with his or her gender identity.

Transverse diameter The largest diameter of the pelvic inlet; helps determine the shape of the inlet.

Traumatic cataracts A type of **cataract** that may result from an injury to the eye.

Tricuspid atresia The absence of the tricuspid valve.

Tricyclic antidepressant (TCA) A class of drugs used in the pharmacotherapy of depression.

Triglycerides Substances formed from dietary fats and carbohydrates in fat cells to store energy.

Triplet Three premature ventricular contractions in a row.

Tripod position A position of sitting and leaning forward.

Trisomy An extra chromosome.

Trousseau's sign Contraction of the hand and fingers in response to occlusion of the blood supply by a blood pressure cuff; caused by decreased blood calcium levels.

True pelvis The portion that lies below the **linea terminalis**, made up of the inlet, cavity and outlet.

Truncus arteriosus A heart defect in which a single large vessel empties both ventricles and provides circulation for the pulmonary, systemic, and coronary circulations.

Tubal ligation A surgical procedure to clip, tie off, band, or plug the fallopian tubes to effect sterilization of a female client.

Tubercle A granulomatous lesion (a sealed-off colony of bacilli) formed from **mycobacterium tuberculosis.**

Tuberculosis (TB) A chronic, recurrent infectious disease caused by **Mycobacterium tuberculosis.** TB usually affects the lungs, but any organ can be affected.

Two-career family A family in which both partners are employed by choice or necessity. A two-career family may or may not have children.

Tympanic membrane A thin, tense membrane which separates the middle ear from the external auditory canal, protecting the middle ear from the external environment.

Ulcer A break in the GI mucosa which develops when the mucosal barrier is unable to protect the mucosa from damage by hydrochloric acid and pepsin, the gastric digestive juices.

Ulcerative colitis A chronic inflammatory bowel disorder that affects the mucosa and submucosa of the colon and rectum.

Ultrafiltration Removal of excess body water using a hydrostatic pressure gradient.

Unconscious mind The part of the individual's mental life of which he or she is unaware.

Undernutrition (also known as **malnutrition**) Health effects due to insufficient nutrient intake or stores.

Unifocal When ventricular impulse arises from one ectopic site.

Unilateral lobar pneumonia A pattern of **pneumonia** in which bacteria tend to be distributed evenly throughout one or more lobes of a single lung.

Universal precautions (UP) Techniques used to decrease the risk of transmitting unidentified pathogens.

Unresolved bacteriuria The presence of bacteria in urine that fails to resolve with treatment.

Upper body obesity Identified by a waist-to-hip ratio of greater than 1 in men or 0.8 in women. Also called central obesity.

Uremia Excessive amounts of urea in the blood.

Ureteral stent A thin catheter inserted into the ureter to provide for urine flow and ureteral support.

Ureterolithotomy An incision in the affected ureter to remove a calculus.

Ureteroplasty The surgical repair of a ureter.

Urgency The sudden, strong desire to **void**.

Uric acid stones Develop when the urine concentration of uric acid is high.

Urinary calculi Stones in the urinary tract.

Urinary drainage system Those organs required to drain urine from the kidneys, including the ureters, urinary bladder, and urethra.

Urinary frequency The need to urinate often.

Urinary hesitancy A delay and difficulty in initiating voiding; often associated with dysuria.

Urinary incontinence Involuntary urination due to the temporary or permanent inability of the external sphincter muscles to control the flow of urine from the bladder.

Urinary reflux Backward flow of urine.

Urinary retention The accumulation of urine in the bladder and inability of the bladder to empty itself, resulting in overdistention of the bladder.

Urinary stasis Stagnation of urinary flow.

Urination Releasing urine from the urinary bladder (voiding).

Uroflowmetry Measures urine flow rate.

Urolithiasis The formation of stones in the urinary tract.

Utilitarianism A form of consequentialist theory that views a good act as one that brings the most good and the least harm for the greatest number of people. This is called the principle of **utility**.

Utility See **utilitarianism**.

Uterosacral ligaments Ligaments that provide support for the uterus and cervix at the level of the ischial spines.

Uterus The hollow muscular organ in which the fertilized ovum is implanted and in which the developing fetus is nourished until birth.

Uveitis Inflammation of the middle layer of the eye called the uvea.

Vaccine Suspensions of whole or fractionated bacteria or viruses that have been treated to make them nonpathogenic; introduced by **immunization** to provoke **active immunity**.

Vagina The muscular and membranous tube that connects the external genitals with the uterus.

Vaginismus The involuntary spasm of the outer one-third of the vaginal muscles, making penetration of the vagina painful and sometimes impossible.

Valsalva maneuver Forced exhalation against a closed glottis.

Vasectomy A procedure to surgically sever the vas deferens on both sides of the scrotum to permanently prevent pregnancy.

Vasogenic shock Shock that results from widespread vasodilatation and decreased peripheral resistance. Also called distributive shock.

Venous stasis The collection and stagnation of blood in the lower extremities.

Venous thrombectomy Surgical removal of a blood clot.

Venous thrombosis A condition in which a blood clot (thrombus) forms on the wall of a vein, accompanied by inflammation of the vein wall and some degree of obstructed venous blood flow.

Ventilation the exchange of oxygen and carbon dioxide.

Ventricular bigeminy A premature ventricular contraction following each normal beat.

Ventricular gallop Sometimes heard after the second heart sound in children, young adults and pregnant females during the third trimester. Also called the **third heart sound**.

Ventricular septal defect An opening in the ventricular septum causes increased pulmonary blood flow.

Ventricular trigeminy A premature ventricular contraction every third beat.

Veracity A moral principle that holds that one should tell the truth and not lie.

Vertical transmission Perinatal transmission of an infection, such as the **human immunodeficiency virus**, from mother to infant.

Very-low-calorie diets A program providing a protein-sparing modified fast (400–800 kcal/day or less) under close medical supervision.

Vesicoureteral reflux A condition in which urine moves from the bladder back toward the kidney; a common risk factor in children who develop **pyelonephritis** that may also be seen in adults whose bladder outflow is obstructed.

Vestibulitis Pain of the outer portion of the vagina upon touch or attempted penetration.

Vibration A series of vigorous quiverings produced by hands that are placed flat against the client's chest wall.

Virchow's triad Three factors associated with thrombophlebitis; stasis of blood, vessel damage, and increased blood coagulability.

Virions Virus able to grow and reproduce outside a host.

Virulence The ability of a microorganism to produce disease.

Virus A type of microorganism that must enter living cells in order to reproduce.

Visceral Of or relating to any large organ in the body.

Visceral pain Pain arising from body organs. It is dull and poorly localized because of the low number of nociceptors.

Viscosupplementation A treatment for osteoarthritis of the knee, involving injecting lubricating substances directly into the knee.

Voiding Releasing urine from the urinary bladder (urinating).

Volatile acid Acids eliminated from the body as a gas.

Volksmann's contracture The impaired mobility of the arm and inability to extend the arm completely, which is a common complication of elbow fractures.

Vulnerable populations Social groups with inadequate access to health care because they lack resources and are exposed to more risk factors.

Vulva The female external genitals.

Vulvodynia Constant, unremitting burning that is localized to the vulva with an acute onset.

Voluntary admission The detention of a client in a psychiatric or medical facility at the client's request.

Weaning The process of removing ventilator support and reestablishing spontaneous, independent respirations; the process of discontinuing breastfeeding and accustoming an infant to another feeding method.

Well-being A subjective perception of feeling well that can be described objectively and measured.

Wellness A state of well-being that encompasses self responsibility, dynamic growth, nutrition, physical fitness, emotional health, preventive health care, and the whole being of the individual.

Wellness diagnosis A term that describes human responses to levels of wellness in an individual, family, or community that have a readiness for enhancement. For example, Readiness for Enhanced Coping.

Wernicke's encephalopathy A condition typically seen in alcoholics which is characterized by ataxia (lack of coordination), abnormal eye movements, and confusion.

World view The way in which people in a culture perceive ideas and attitudes about the world, other people, and life in general.

Xenophobia The fear or dislike of people different from one's self.

Xerostomia Dry mouth.

Zollinger-Ellison syndrome A form of **peptic ulcer disease** caused by a gastrinoma, or gastrin-secreting tumor of the pancreas, stomach, or intestines.

Zygote A fertilized egg.

INDEX

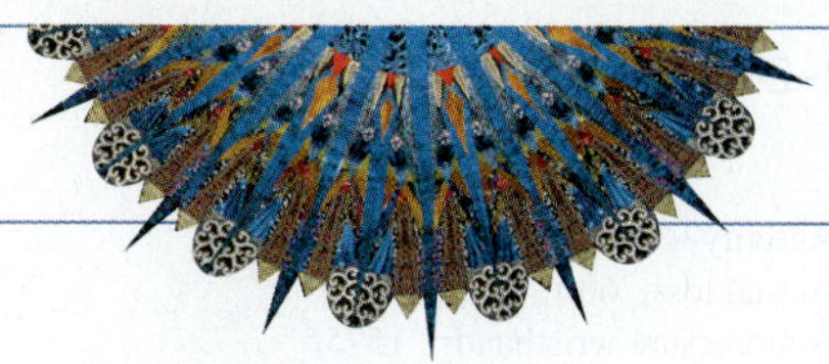

A

Virchow's triad Three factors associated with thrombophlebitis; stasis of blood, vessel damage, and increased blood coagulability.

Virions Virus able to grow and reproduce outside a host.

Virulence The ability of a microorganism to produce disease.

Virus A type of microorganism that must enter living cells in order to reproduce.

Visceral Of or relating to any large organ in the body.

Visceral pain Pain arising from body organs. It is dull and poorly localized because of the low number of nociceptors.

Viscosupplementation A treatment for osteoarthritis of the knee, involving injecting lubricating substances directly into the knee.

Voiding Releasing urine from the urinary bladder (urinating).

Volatile acid Acids eliminated from the body as a gas.

Volksmann's contracture The impaired mobility of the arm and inability to extend the arm completely, which is a common complication of elbow fractures.

Vulnerable populations Social groups with inadequate access to health care because they lack resources and are exposed to more risk factors.

Vulva The female external genitals.

Vulvodynia Constant, unremitting burning that is localized to the vulva with an acute onset.

Voluntary admission The detention of a client in a psychiatric or medical facility at the client's request.

Weaning The process of removing ventilator support and reestablishing spontaneous, independent respirations; the process of discontinuing breastfeeding and accustoming an infant to another feeding method.

Well-being A subjective perception of feeling well that can be described objectively and measured.

Wellness A state of well-being that encompasses self responsibility, dynamic growth, nutrition, physical fitness, emotional health, preventive health care, and the whole being of the individual.

Wellness diagnosis A term that describes human responses to levels of wellness in an individual, family, or community that have a readiness for enhancement. For example, Readiness for Enhanced Coping.

Wernicke's encephalopathy A condition typically seen in alcoholics which is characterized by ataxia (lack of coordination), abnormal eye movements, and confusion.

World view The way in which people in a culture perceive ideas and attitudes about the world, other people, and life in general.

Xenophobia The fear or dislike of people different from one's self.

Xerostomia Dry mouth.

Zollinger-Ellison syndrome A form of **peptic ulcer disease** caused by a gastrinoma, or gastrin-secreting tumor of the pancreas, stomach, or intestines.

Zygote A fertilized egg.

C

F

G

H

I

J

K

L

O

P

Q

R

S

T

U

V